The American Psychiatric Publishing

TEXTBOOK OF

Psychopharmacology

FOURTH EDITION

The American Psychiatric Publishing

TEXTBOOK OF

Psychopharmacology

FOURTH EDITION

Edited by

Alan F. Schatzberg, M.D.
Charles B. Nemeroff, M.D., Ph.D.

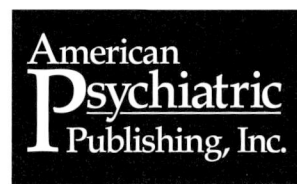

Washington, D.C.
London, England

Note: The authors have worked to ensure that all information in this book is accurate at the time of publication and consistent with general psychiatric and medical standards, and that information concerning drug dosages, schedules, and routes of administration is accurate at the time of publication and consistent with standards set by the U.S. Food and Drug Administration and the general medical community. As medical research and practice continue to advance, however, therapeutic standards may change. Moreover, specific situations may require a specific therapeutic response not included in this book. For these reasons and because human and mechanical errors sometimes occur, we recommend that readers follow the advice of physicians directly involved in their care or the care of a member of their family.

Books published by American Psychiatric Publishing, Inc., represent the views and opinions of the individual authors and do not necessarily represent the policies and opinions of APPI or the American Psychiatric Association.

Diagnostic criteria included in this textbook are reprinted, with permission, from *Diagnostic and Statistical Manual of Mental Disorders*, 4th Edition, Text Revision. Copyright © 2000, American Psychiatric Association.

Copyright © 2009 American Psychiatric Publishing, Inc.
ALL RIGHTS RESERVED
Manufactured in the United States of America on acid-free paper
14 13 12 11 10 09   6 5 4 3 2 1
Fourth Edition

Typeset in Adobe's Goudy and Goudy Sans.

American Psychiatric Publishing, Inc.
1000 Wilson Boulevard
Arlington, VA 22209-3901
www.appi.org

Library of Congress Cataloging-in-Publication Data
The American Psychiatric Publishing textbook of psychopharmacology / edited by Alan F. Schatzberg, Charles B. Nemeroff. — 4th ed.
      p. ; cm.
   Includes bibliographical references and index.
   ISBN 978-1-58562-309-9 (alk. paper)
1. Mental illness—Chemotherapy. 2. Psychotropic drugs. 3. Psychopharmacology. I. Schatzberg, Alan F. II. Nemeroff, Charles B. III. Title: Textbook of psychopharmacology. IV. Title: Textbook of psychopharmacology.
   [DNLM: 1. Psychotropic Drugs—pharmacology. 2. Psychotropic Drugs—therapeutic use. 3. Mental Disorders—drug therapy. 4. Psychopharmacology. QV 77.2 A512 2009]
   RM315.A555 2009
   615′.78—dc22

2008053103

British Library Cataloguing in Publication Data
A CIP record is available from the British Library.

To our lovely and supportive wives,

Nancy S. Schatzberg and Gayle A. Nemeroff,

who encouraged us to spend the many hours dedicated to this project

Contents

PART I

Principles of Psychopharmacology

Robert C. Malenka, M.D., Ph.D., Section Editor

PART II

Classes of Psychiatric Treatments:
Animal and Human Pharmacology

K. Ranga Rama Krishnan, M.D., and Dennis S. Charney, M.D., Section Editors

Antidepressants and Anxiolytics

Antipsychotics

Drugs for Treatment of Bipolar Disorder

PART III

Clinical Psychobiology and Psychiatric Syndromes

David J. Kupfer, M.D., Section Editor

P A R T I V

Psychopharmacological Treatment

David L. Dunner, M.D., Section Editor

PART V

Ethical Issues

Contributors

Elias Aboujaoude, M.D.
Assistant Clinical Professor, Department of Psychiatry and Behavioral Sciences, Stanford University School of Medicine, Stanford, California

W. Stewart Agras, M.D.
Professor of Psychiatry, Department of Psychiatry and Behavioral Sciences, Stanford University School of Medicine, Stanford, California

Jonathan M. Amiel, M.D.
Resident in Psychiatry, Columbia University College of Physicians and Surgeons and the New York State Psychiatric Institute, New York, New York

Josephine Astrid Archer, B.Sc.
Research Student, Centre for Psychiatry, Queen Mary University of London, Barts and The London School of Medicine and Dentistry, London, United Kingdom

Steven E. Arnold, M.D.
Professor and Director, Cellular and Molecular Neuropathology Program, Geriatric Psychiatry Section, Department of Psychiatry, Penn Memory Center, University of Pennsylvania, Philadelphia, Pennsylvania

Christos A. Ballas, M.D.
Assistant Professor of Clinical Psychiatry, Department of Psychiatry, University of Pennsylvania School of Medicine, Philadelphia, Pennsylvania

Jacob S. Ballon, M.D.
Chief Resident, Department of Psychiatry and Behavioral Science, Stanford University, Stanford, California

Matthew J. Bair, M.D., M.S.
Assistant Professor of Medicine, Division of General Internal Medicine and Geriatrics, Department of Medicine, Indiana University School of Medicine; Research Scientist, Regenstrief Institute, Inc.; and Center for Implementing Evidence-Based Practice, Richard Roudebush VA Medical Center, Indianapolis, Indiana

Gregory S. Berns, M.D., Ph.D.
Professor, Department of Psychiatry and Behavioral Sciences, Emory University School of Medicine, Atlanta, Georgia

Elisabeth B. Binder, M.D., Ph.D.
Assistant Professor, Department of Psychiatry and Behavioral Sciences and Department of Human Genetics, Emory University School of Medicine, Atlanta, Georgia; Head, RG Molecular Genetics of Depression, Max Planck Institute of Psychiatry, Munich, Germany

Pierre Blier, M.D., Ph.D.
Professor, Departments of Psychiatry and Cellular/Molecular Medicine, University of Ottawa; Research Director, Mood Disorders Research Unit, University of Ottawa Institute of Mental Health Research, Ottawa, Ontario, Canada

David R. Block, M.D.
Staff Psychiatrist, Student Health Services, San Francisco State University, San Francisco, California

Charles L. Bowden, M.D.
Clinical Professor of Psychiatry and Psychopharmacology, Department of Psychiatry, University of Texas Health Science Center at San Antonio, San Antonio, Texas

Catherine Bresee, M.S.
Senior Research Associate, Department of Psychiatry and Behavioral Neurosciences, Cedars-Sinai Medical Center, Los Angeles, California

Frank W. Brown, M.D.
Associate Professor of Psychiatry and Behavioral Sciences, Emory University School of Medicine, and Chief Medical Officer, Wesley Woods Geriatric Hospital, Emory Health-Care, Atlanta, Georgia

Mary F. Brunette, M.D.
Associate Professor of Psychiatry, Department of Psychiatry, Dartmouth Psychiatric Research Center, Dartmouth Medical School, Hanover, New Hampshire

Peter F. Buckley, M.D.
Professor and Chairman, Department of Psychiatry, and Associate Dean for Leadership Development, Medical College of Georgia, Augusta, Georgia

Joseph R. Calabrese, M.D.
Director, Center for Bipolar Disorder at Case Western Reserve University and University Hospitals Case Medical Center; Professor of Psychiatry, Case Western Reserve University School of Medicine, Cleveland, Ohio

Carla M. Canuso, M.D.
Senior Director, Clinical Development, Ortho-McNeil Janssen Scientific Affairs, LLC, Titusville, New Jersey

Linda L. Carpenter, M.D.
Associate Professor, Department of Psychiatry and Human Behavior, Warren Alpert Medical School of Brown University, Providence, Rhode Island

Dennis S. Charney, M.D.
Dean and Executive Vice President of Academic Affairs, Mount Sinai School of Medicine, New York, New York

Anita H. Clayton, M.D.
David C. Wilson Professor, Department of Psychiatry and Neurobehavioral Sciences, University of Virginia School of Medicine, Charlottesville, Virginia

Emil F. Coccaro, M.D.
Professor and Chair of Psychiatry, Department of Psychiatry, University of Chicago, Chicago, Illinois

Kathryn M. Connor, M.D., M.H.S.
Associate Director of Clinical Research, Clinical Neuroscience and Ophthalmology, Merck & Co, Inc., North Wales, Pennsylvania (formerly Associate Professor, Department of Psychiatry and Behavioral Sciences, Duke University Medical Center, Durham, North Carolina)

Monica Kelly Cowles, M.D., M.S.
Assistant Professor, Department of Psychiatry and Behavioral Sciences, Winship Cancer Institute (WCI), Emory School of Medicine, Atlanta, Georgia

Joseph F. Cubells, M.D., Ph.D.
Associate Professor, Department of Psychiatry and Behavioral Sciences and Department of Human Genetics, Emory University School of Medicine, Atlanta, Georgia

Charles A. Dackis, M.D.
Associate Professor, Department of Psychiatry, and Medical Director of Clinical Services, Presbyterian Medical Center, University of Pennsylvania, Philadelphia, Pennsylvania

Jonathan R. T. Davidson, M.D.
Professor, Department of Psychiatry and Behavioral Sciences, Duke University Medical Center, Durham, North Carolina

Albert A. Davis, B.S.
Department of Neurology, Emory University School of Medicine, Atlanta, Georgia

Karon Dawkins, M.D.
Associate Professor of Psychiatry and Director of General Psychiatry Residency Training, School of Medicine, University of North Carolina at Chapel Hill, Chapel Hill, North Carolina

William C. Dement, M.D., Ph.D.
Lowell W. and Josephine Q. Berry Professor, Department of Psychiatry and Behavioral Sciences, Stanford University School of Medicine, Stanford, California; Director, Stanford Sleep Disorders Center, Palo Alto, California

D. P. Devanand, M.D.
Professor of Clinical Psychiatry and Neurology, College of Physicians and Surgeons, Columbia University; Co-Director, Memory Disorders Center, New York State Psychiatric Institute, New York, New York

C. Lindsay DeVane, Pharm.D.
Professor of Psychiatry and Behavioral Sciences and Director, Laboratory of Drug Disposition and Pharmacogenetics, Department of Psychiatry, Medical University of South Carolina, Charleston, South Carolina

David F. Dinges, Ph.D.
Professor of Psychology in Psychiatry, Chief, Division of Sleep and Chronobiology, Director, Unit for Experimental Psychiatry, Department of Psychiatry, University of Pennsylvania School of Medicine, Philadelphia, Pennsylvania

Barbara D'Orio, M.D., M.P.A.
Associate Professor, Department of Psychiatry and Behavioral Sciences, Emory University School of Medicine, Atlanta, Georgia

David L. Dunner, M.D.
Professor, Department of Psychiatry and Behavioral Sciences, and Director, Center for Anxiety and Depression, University of Washington, Seattle, Washington

Clifford J. Ehmke, M.D.
Department of Psychiatry and Behavioral Sciences, Emory University School of Medicine, Atlanta, Georgia

Dwight L. Evans, M.D.
Ruth Meltzer Professor and Chairman, Professor of Psychiatry, Medicine, and Neuroscience, Department of Psychiatry, University of Pennsylvania School of Medicine, Philadelphia, Pennsylvania

Elise M. Fallucco, M.D.
Clinical Fellow—Child and Adolescent Psychiatry, Washington University School of Medicine, St. Louis, Missouri

Susana V. Fernandez, B.A.
Research Interviewer, Department of Psychiatry, Emory University School of Medicine, Atlanta, Georgia

Adriana E. Foster, M.D.
Assistant Professor, Department of Psychiatry and Health Behavior, Medical College of Georgia, Augusta, Georgia

Marlene P. Freeman, M.D.
Center for Women's Mental Health, Perinatal and Reproductive Psychiatry Clinical Research Program, Massachusetts General Hospital, Boston, Massachusetts; Harvard Medical School

Mark A. Frye, M.D.
Consultant, Department of Psychiatry and Psychology, Director, Mayo Mood Clinic and Research Program, Mayo Clinic, Rochester, Minnesota

Keming Gao, M.D., Ph.D.
Director, Mood and Anxiety Clinic, Assistant Professor of Psychiatry, University Hospitals Case Medical Center, Case Western Reserve University School of Medicine, Cleveland, Ohio

Amir Garakani, M.D.
Visiting Associate, Mount Sinai School of Medicine, New York, New York

Steven J. Garlow, M.D., Ph.D.
Director of Adult Mental Health Services and Emergency Psychiatry, Emory University Hospital; Assistant Professor, Department of Psychiatry and Behavioral Sciences, Emory University School of Medicine, Atlanta Georgia

Steven J. Garlow, M.D., Ph.D.
Assistant Professor, Department of Psychiatry and Behavioral Sciences, Emory University School of Medicine, Atlanta, Georgia

Alan J. Gelenberg, M.D.
President and CEO, Healthcare Technology Systems Inc., Madison, Wisconsin; Clinical Professor of Psychiatry, University of Wisconsin, Madison, Wisconsin; Professor Emeritus of Psychiatry, University of Arizona College of Medicine, Tucson, Arizona

Charles F. Gillespie, M.D., Ph.D.
Assistant Professor, Department of Psychiatry and Behavioral Sciences, Emory University School of Medicine, Atlanta, Georgia

Elizabeth H. Gillespie, D.O.
Child and Adolescent Psychiatry Fellow, Department of Psychiatry and Neurobehavioral Sciences, University of Virginia, Charlottesville, Virginia

Donald C. Goff, M.D.
Director, Schizophrenia Program, Massachusetts General Hospital; Associate Professor of Psychiatry, Harvard Medical School, Boston, Massachusetts

Robert N. Golden, M.D.
Professor of Psychiatry and Dean, School of Medicine and Public Health, University of Wisconsin–Madison, Madison, Wisconsin

Jennifer Gotto, M.D.
Chief, Department of Psychiatry, Division of Supportive Care Medicine, City of Hope Cancer Center, Duarte, California

Todd D. Gould, M.D.
Assistant Professor, Department of Psychiatry, School of Medicine, University of Maryland, Baltimore, Maryland

Anthony A. Grace, Ph.D.
Professor of Neuroscience, Psychiatry, and Psychology, Department of Neuroscience, University of Pittsburgh School of Medicine, Pittsburgh, Pennsylvania

Alan I. Green, M.D.
Raymond Sobel Professor of Psychiatry and Chairman, Department of Psychiatry, Dartmouth Medical School, Hanover, New Hampshire

Raquel E. Gur, M.D., Ph.D.
Professor and Director, Schizophrenia Research Center, Neuropsychiatry Section, Department of Psychiatry, University of Pennsylvania, Philadelphia, Pennsylvania

Ebrahim Haroon, M.D.
Assistant Professor, Department of Psychiatry and Behavioral Sciences, Emory University School of Medicine, Atlanta, Georgia

Christine M. Heim, Ph.D.
Assistant Professor, Department of Psychiatry and Behavioral Sciences, Emory University School of Medicine, Atlanta, Georgia

Eric Hollander, M.D.
Professor of Psychiatry and Director of Clinical Psychopharmacology, Department of Psychiatry, Mount Sinai School of Medicine, New York, New York

Florian Holsboer, M.D., Ph.D.
Director and Professor, Max Planck Institute of Psychiatry, Munich, Germany

Jinger G. Hoop, M.D., M.F.A.
Assistant Professor, Department of Psychiatry and Behavioral Medicine, Medical College of Wisconsin, Milwaukee, Wisconsin

Sandra Juric, B.A.
Research Interviewer, Department of Psychiatry, Emory University School of Medicine, Atlanta, Georgia

Ned H. Kalin, M.D.
Hedberg Professor and Chair, Department of Psychiatry; and Director, HealthEmotions Research Institute, University of Wisconsin School of Medicine and Public Health, Madison, Wisconsin

Walter H. Kaye, M.D.
Professor of Psychiatry and Director of the Eating Disorder Program, Department of Psychiatry, University of California at San Diego, La Jolla, California

Paul E. Keck Jr., M.D.
President–CEO, Lindner Center of HOPE, Mason, Ohio; Lindner Professor of Psychiatry and Neuroscience and Executive Vice Chair, University of Cincinnati College of Medicine, Cincinnati, Ohio

David E. Kemp, M.D.
Director, Mood and Metabolic Clinic, Assistant Professor of Psychiatry, University Hospitals Case Medical Center, Case Western Reserve University School of Medicine, Cleveland, Ohio

Ashley P. Kennedy, B.S.
Department of Psychiatry and Behavioral Sciences, Emory University School of Medicine, Atlanta, Georgia

Terence A. Ketter, M.D.
Professor of Psychiatry and Behavioral Sciences and Chief, Bipolar Disorders Clinic, Stanford University School of Medicine, Stanford, California

Clinton D. Kilts, Ph.D.
Paul Janssen Professor and Vice Chair for Research, Department of Psychiatry and Behavioral Sciences, Emory University School of Medicine, Atlanta, Georgia

Lorrin M. Koran, M.D.
Professor, Department of Psychiatry and Behavioral Sciences, Stanford University School of Medicine, Stanford, California

Ania Korszun, Ph.D., M.D., M.R.C.Psych.
Professor of Psychiatry, Centre for Psychiatry, Queen Mary University of London, Barts and The London School of Medicine and Dentistry, London, United Kingdom

Helena C. Kraemer, Ph.D.
Professor of Biostatistics in Psychiatry, Emerita, Department of Psychiatry and Behavioral Sciences, Stanford University School of Medicine, Stanford, California

Erin E. Krebs, M.D., M.P.H.
Assistant Professor of Medicine, Division of General Internal Medicine and Geriatrics, Department of Medicine, Indiana University School of Medicine; Research Scientist, Regenstrief Institute, Inc.; and Center for Implementing Evidence-Based Practice, Richard Roudebush VA Medical Center, Indianapolis, Indiana

K. Ranga Rama Krishnan, M.D.
Professor and Chairman, Department of Psychiatry and Behavioral Sciences, Duke University Medical Center, Durham, North Carolina; Dean, Duke–NUS Graduate Medical School Singapore

Kurt Kroenke, M.D.
Professor of Medicine, Division of General Internal Medicine and Geriatrics, Department of Medicine, Indiana University School of Medicine; Research Scientist, Regenstrief Institute, Inc.; and Center for Implementing Evidence-Based Practice, Richard Roudebush VA Medical Center, Indianapolis, Indiana

David J. Kupfer, M.D.
Thomas Detre Professor and Chair, Department of Psychiatry, and Professor of Neuroscience, University of Pittsburgh School of Medicine, Pittsburgh, Pennsylvania

James J. Lah, M.D., Ph.D.
Associate Professor, Department of Neurology, Emory University School of Medicine, Atlanta, Georgia

Joseph B. Layde, M.D., J.D.
Professor, Department of Psychiatry and Behavioral Medicine, Medical College of Wisconsin, Milwaukee, Wisconsin

Royce Lee, M.D.
Assistant Professor of Psychiatry, Department of Psychiatry, University of Chicago, Chicago, Illinois

Allan I. Levey, M.D., Ph.D.
Professor and Chair, Department of Neurology, Emory University School of Medicine, Atlanta, Georgia

David A. Lewis, M.D.
UPMC Professor, Translational Neuroscience Program, Departments of Psychiatry and Neuroscience; Director, Center for the Neuroscience of Mental Disorders; and Associate Director for Basic Research, Western Psychiatric Institute and Clinic, University of Pittsburgh School of Medicine, Pittsburgh, Pennsylvania

Jeffrey A. Lieberman, M.D.
Chairman, Department of Psychiatry, College of Physicians and Surgeons, Columbia University; Director, New York State Psychiatric Institute; Director, Lieber Center for Schizophrenia Research; Psychiatrist-in-Chief, New York Presbyterian Hospital and Columbia University Medical Center, New York, New York

David M. Lyons, Ph.D.
Associate Professor, Department of Psychiatry and Behavioral Sciences, Stanford University School of Medicine, Stanford, California

Robert C. Malenka, M.D., Ph.D.
Pritzker Professor of Psychiatry and Behavioral Sciences, Stanford Brain Research Institute, Stanford University School of Medicine, Stanford, California

Husseini K. Manji, M.D., F.R.C.P.C.
Vice President, CNS and Pain, Johnson & Johnson Pharmaceutical Research & Development, Titusville, New Jersey

Stephen R. Marder, M.D.
Professor and Director, Section on Psychosis, Semel Institute of Neuroscience and Human Behavior, University of California at Los Angeles; Director, Desert Pacific Mental Illness Research, Education, and Clinical Center, West Los Angeles Veterans Administration Medical Center, Los Angeles, California

Sanjay J. Mathew, M.D.
Director, Mood and Anxiety Disorders Program, and Associate Professor of Psychiatry, Mount Sinai School of Medicine, New York, New York

Helen S. Mayberg, M.D.
Professor, Department of Psychiatry and Behavioral Sciences, and Professor, Department of Neurology, Emory University School of Medicine, Atlanta, Georgia

W. Vaughn McCall, M.D., M.S.
Professor and Chair, Department of Psychiatry and Behavioral Medicine, Wake Forest University School of Medicine; Medical Director, Sleep Center, Wake Forest University Baptist Medical Center, Winston-Salem, North Carolina

William M. McDonald, M.D.
Professor of Psychiatry and J.B. Fuqua Chair for Late-Life Depression, Emory University School of Medicine; Chief, Division of Geriatric Psychiatry, Director, Fuqua Center for Late-Life Depression, Atlanta, Georgia

Susan L. McElroy, M.D.
Chief Research Officer, Lindner Center of HOPE, Mason, Ohio; Professor of Psychiatry and Neuroscience, University of Cincinnati College of Medicine, Cincinnati, Ohio

Thomas W. Meeks, M.D.
Assistant Professor of Psychiatry, Division of Geriatric Psychiatry, University of California–San Diego, VA San Diego Healthcare System, San Diego, California

Darlene S. Melchitzky, M.S.
Research Principal, Department of Psychiatry, University of Pittsburgh School of Medicine, Pittsburgh, Pennsylvania; Laboratory Director, Department of Biology, Mercyhurst College, Erie, Pennsylvania

Emmanuel Mignot, M.D., Ph.D.
Howard Hughes Medical Institute Investigator; Professor of Psychiatry and Behavioral Sciences, Stanford University School of Medicine, Stanford, California; Director, Center for Narcolepsy, Stanford Sleep Research Center, Palo Alto, California

Andrew H. Miller, M.D.
Professor, Department of Psychiatry and Behavioral Sciences, Winship Cancer Institute (WCI), Emory School of Medicine, Atlanta, Georgia

Kazuo Mishima, M.D., Ph.D.
Director, National Institute of Mental Health, National Center of Neurology and Psychiatry, Kodaira, Tokyo, Japan

Katherine Marshall Moore, M.D.
Consultant, Department of Psychiatry and Psychology, Director, Mayo Clinic Anxiety Disorders Clinic, Mayo Clinic, Rochester, Minnesota

David J. Muzina, M.D.
Director, Center for Mood Disorders Treatment and Research, Associate Professor of Medicine, Cleveland Clinic Neurological Institute, Cleveland, Ohio

Henry A. Nasrallah, M.D.
Professor of Psychiatry and Neuroscience, Department of Psychiatry, University of Cincinnati College of Medicine, Cincinnati, Ohio

J. Craig Nelson, M.D.
Professor of Psychiatry, Leon J. Epstein, M.D., Chair in Geriatric Psychiatry, Director of Geriatric Psychiatry, University of California–San Francisco

Charles B. Nemeroff, M.D., Ph.D.
Reunette W. Harris Professor, Department of Psychiatry and Behavioral Sciences, Emory University, Atlanta, Georgia

Alexander Neumeister, M.D.
Associate Professor of Psychiatry and Director of the Molecular Imaging Program of the Clinical Neurosciences Division, Yale University School of Medicine, West Haven, Connecticut

John W. Newcomer, M.D.
Gregory B. Couch Professor of Psychiatry, Psychology and Medicine and Medical Director, Center for Clinical Studies, Washington University School of Medicine, St. Louis, Missouri

D. Jeffrey Newport, M.D.
Associate Professor, Department of Psychiatry, Emory University School of Medicine, Atlanta, Georgia

Linda Nicholas, M.D.
Professor of Psychiatry, School of Medicine, University of North Carolina at Chapel Hill, Chapel Hill, North Carolina

Seiji Nishino, M.D., Ph.D.
Professor of Psychiatry and Behavioral Sciences, Stanford University School of Medicine, Stanford, California; Director, Sleep and Circadian Neurobiology Laboratory, Stanford Sleep Research Center, Palo Alto, California

Sandhaya Norris, M.D.
Physician, Mood Disorders Research Unit, University of Ottawa Institute of Mental Health Research, Ottawa, Ontario, Canada

Charles P. O'Brien, M.D., Ph.D.
Kenneth Appel Professor, Department of Psychiatry, University of Pennsylvania, Philadelphia, Pennsylvania

Giuseppe Pagnoni, Ph.D.
Dip. Scienze Biomediche, Sezione Fisiologia, Università di Modena e Reggio Emilia, Modeno, Italy

Daniel S. Pine, M.D.
Chief of Developmental Studies, Mood and Anxiety Disorders Program, National Institute of Mental Health, Bethesda, Maryland

Steven R. Pliszka, M.D.
Professor and Vice Chair, Chief, Division of Child and Adolescent Psychiatry, Department of Psychiatry, The University of Texas Health Science Center at San Antonio

Bruce G. Pollock, M.D., Ph.D.
Professor and Head, Division of Geriatric Psychiatry, University of Toronto Faculty of Medicine; Sandra A. Rotman Chair in Neuropsychiatry, Rotman Research Institute, Baycrest; Vice President of Research, Centre for Addiction and Mental Health, Toronto, Ontario, Canada

Robert M. Post, M.D.
Clinical Professor of Psychiatry, George Washington University, Washington, DC, and Penn State College of Medicine, Hershey, Pennsylvania; Head, Bipolar Collaborative Network, Bethesda, Maryland

David C. Purselle, M.D., M.S.
Assistant Professor, Department of Psychiatry and Behavioral Sciences, Emory University School of Medicine; Director of Acute Mental Health Services, Veterans Affairs Medical Center, Atlanta, Georgia

Charles L. Raison, M.D.
Assistant Professor, Department of Psychiatry and Behavioral Sciences, Winship Cancer Institute (WCI), Emory School of Medicine, Atlanta, Georgia

B. Ashok Raj, M.D.
Physician Researcher, University of South Florida College of Medicine, Tampa, Florida

Mark Hyman Rapaport, M.D.
Chairman, Department of Psychiatry and Neurosciences, Cedars-Sinai Medical Center; Professor of Psychiatry and Biobehaviorial Sciences and Polier Family Endowed Chair for Schizophrenia and Related Disorders, David Geffen School of Medicine, University of California–Los Angeles

Mark M. Rasenick, Ph.D.
Professor of Physiology and Biophysics and Psychiatry, Departments of Physiology and Biophysics and Psychiatry, University of Illinois at Chicago, Chicago, Illinois

Martin Reite, M.D.
Diplomate, American Board of Sleep Medicine; Diplomate, American Board of Psychiatry and Neurology; Clinical Professor, Department of Psychiatry and Medical Director, Neuromagnetic Imaging Lab, University of Colorado School of Medicine, Denver, Colorado

Karl Rickels, M.D.
Stuart and Emily B.H. Mudd Professor of Behavior and Reproduction in Psychiatry, Department of Psychiatry, University of Pennsylvania, Philadelphia, Pennsylvania

Laura Weiss Roberts, M.D., M.A.
Charles E. Kubly Professor and Chairman, Department of Psychiatry and Behavioral Medicine, Medical College of Wisconsin, Milwaukee, Wisconsin

Donald S. Robinson, M.D.
Consultant, Worldwide Drug Development, Shelburne, Vermont

Steven P. Roose, M.D.
Professor of Clinical Psychiatry, College of Physicians and Surgeons, Columbia University; Co-Director, Neuropsychiatric Research Clinic, New York State Psychiatric Institute, New York, New York

Patrick H. Roseboom, Ph.D.
Associate Scientist in Psychiatry and Lecturer in Pharmacology, University of Wisconsin School of Medicine and Public Health, Madison, Wisconsin

Jerrold F. Rosenbaum, M.D.
Chief of Psychiatry, Massachusetts General Hospital; Stanley Cobb Professor of Psychiatry, Harvard Medical School, Boston, Massachusetts

J. Amiel Rosenkranz, Ph.D.
Assistant Professor, Department of Cellular and Molecular Pharmacology, Rosalind Franklin University of Medicine and Science, North Chicago, Illinois

Carl Salzman, M.D.
Professor of Psychiatry, Harvard Medical School, Beth Israel Deaconess Medical Center, Boston, Massachusetts

Alan F. Schatzberg, M.D.
Kenneth T. Norris Jr. Professor and Chair, Department of Psychiatry and Behavioral Sciences, Stanford University School of Medicine, Stanford, California

S. Charles Schulz, M.D.
Professor and Head, Department of Psychiatry, University of Minnesota School of Medicine, Riverside, Minneapolis

Zafar A. Sharif, M.D.
Associate Clinical Professor of Psychiatry, Department of Psychiatry, College of Physicians and Surgeons, Columbia University, New York, New York

David V. Sheehan, M.D., M.B.A.
Distinguished University Health Professor, University of South Florida College of Medicine, Tampa, Florida

Daphne Simeon, M.D.
Associate Professor, Department of Psychiatry, Mount Sinai School of Medicine, New York, New York

George M. Simpson, M.D.
Interim Chair and Professor of Research Psychiatry, Department of Psychiatry and the Behavioral Sciences, USC Keck School of Medicine, Los Angeles, California

Diane M. Sloan, Pharm.D.
Senior Medical Director, Advogent, Wayne, New Jersey

Joseph K. Stanilla, M.D.
Assistant Professor of Psychiatry, Jefferson Medical College of Thomas Jefferson University, Philadelphia, Pennsylvania

Zachary N. Stowe, M.D.
Professor, Department of Psychiatry and Department of Gynecology/Obstetrics, Emory University School of Medicine, Atlanta, Georgia

Michael A. Strober, Ph.D.
Franklin Mint Chair in Eating Disorders and Professor of Psychiatry, Semel Institute for Neuroscience and Human Behavior and Stewart and Lynda Resnick Neuropsychiatric Hospital, David Geffen School of Medicine, University of California at Los Angeles, Los Angeles, California

Steven T. Szabo, Ph.D.
Mood and Anxiety Disorders Program, Laboratory of Molecular Pathophysiology, National Institute of Mental Health, National Institutes of Health, Bethesda, Maryland

Rajiv Tandon, M.D.
Chief of Psychiatry, State of Florida Program of Mental Health, Department of Children and Families, Tallahassee, Florida

Pierre N. Tariot, M.D.
Director, Memory Disorders Center, Banner Alzheimer's Institute; and Research Professor of Psychiatry, University of Arizona College of Medicine, Phoenix, Arizona

Michael E. Thase, M.D.
Professor, Department of Psychiatry, University of Pennsylvania School of Medicine, Philadelphia Veterans Affairs Medical Center, Philadelphia, Pennsylvania; and Adjunct Professor, University of Pittsburgh Medical Center, Pittsburgh, Pennsylvania

Gary D. Tollefson, M.D., Ph.D.
CEO/President, Orexigen Therapeutics, La Jolla, California

Karen Dineen Wagner, M.D., Ph.D.
Marie B. Gale Centennial Professor and Vice-Chair, Department of Psychiatry and Behavioral Sciences; Director, Division of Child and Adolescent Psychiatry, The University of Texas Medical Branch, Galveston, Texas

Po W. Wang, M.D.
Clinical Associate Professor, Department of Psychiatry and Behavioral Sciences, Stanford University School of Medicine, Stanford, California

Margaret B. Weigel, M.D.
Assistant Professor, Department of Psychiatry and Behavioral Sciences, Emory University School of Medicine; Staff Physician, Veterans Affairs Medical Center, Atlanta, Georgia

Anthony R. West, Ph.D.
Associate Professor, Department of Neuroscience, The Chicago Medical School of Rosalind Franklin University of Medicine and Science, North Chicago, Illinois

Christopher B. Wiegand, M.D.
Clinical Assistant Professor of Psychiatry, Department of Psychiatry, University of Arizona College of Medicine, Tucson, Arizona

Donna A. Wirshing, M.D.
Associate Professor, Semel Institute of Neuroscience and Human Behavior, David Geffen School of Medicine, University of California at Los Angeles; West Los Angeles Veterans Administration Medical Center, Los Angeles, California

Joanne D. Wojcik, P.M.H.C.N.S.-B.C.
Instructor in Psychiatry and Associate Director, Commonwealth Research Center and the Massachusetts Mental Health Center, Department of Psychiatry, Harvard Medical School, Boston, Massachusetts

Tsung-Ung W. Woo, M.D., Ph.D.
Assistant Professor of Psychiatry, Beth Israel Deaconess Medical Center and McLean Hospital, Department of Psychiatry, Harvard Medical School, Boston, Massachusetts

Frank D. Yocca, Ph.D.
Vice President and Head, CNS and Pain Discovery, AstraZeneca Pharmaceuticals Co., Wilmington, Delaware

Kimberly A. Yonkers, M.D.
Associate Professor, Departments of Psychiatry, Obstetrics, Gynecology and Reproductive Sciences, Yale School of Medicine, New Haven, Connecticut

Elizabeth Ann Young, M.D.
Professor of Psychiatry, Department of Psychiatry, University of Michigan, Ann Arbor, Michigan

Jiang-Zhou Yu, M.D., Ph.D.
Research Assistant Professor, Departments of Physiology and Biophysics and Psychiatry, University of Illinois at Chicago, Chicago, Illinois

Janos Zahajszky, M.D.
Medical Director of Outpatient Mental Health, California Pacific Medical Center, San Francisco, California

Wei Zhang, M.D., Ph.D.
Director, Anxiety and Traumatic Stress Program, Department of Psychiatry and Behavioral Sciences, Duke University Medical Center, Durham, North Carolina

Charles F. Zorumski, M.D.
Samuel B. Guze Professor of Psychiatry, Department of Psychiatry, Washington University School of Medicine, St. Louis, Missouri

Disclosure of Interests

The following contributors to this textbook have indicated a financial interest in or other affiliation with a commercial supporter, manufacturer of a commercial product, and/or provider of a commercial service as listed below:

Elias Aboujaoude, M.D.   *Research Support:* Eli Lilly and Forest Laboratories (as co-investigator in clinical trials).

Matthew J. Bair, M.D., M.S.   *Advisory Board:* Abbott, and Ortho-McNeil-PriCare Division.

Christos A. Ballas, M.D.   *Speakers Bureau:* AstraZeneca, Cephalon, and Pfizer; *Consultant:* AstraZeneca, GlaxoSmithKline, Pfizer, and Wyeth.

Pierre Blier, M.D., Ph.D.   *Grant/Grant/Research Support:* Eli Lilly, Forest Laboratories, Lundbeck, Sepracor, and Wyeth-Ayerst; *Consultant/Advisory Board:* Eli Lilly, Forest Laboratories, Lundbeck, Sepracor, and Wyeth-Ayerst; *Speakers Bureau:* Eli Lilly, Forest Laboratories, Lundbeck, Sepracor, and Wyeth-Ayerst.

Elisabeth B. Binder, M.D., Ph.D.   *Grant/Research Support:* Doris Duke Foundation, GlaxoSmithKline, NARSAD, National Institutes of Health, and Pfizer; *Speaker's Honorarium:* AstraZeneca.

Charles L. Bowden, M.D.   *Grant/Research Support:* Abbott Laboratories, Bristol-Myers Squibb, Elan Pharmaceuticals, GlaxoSmithKline, Janssen, Lilly Research, National Institute of Mental Health, Parke Davis, R. W. Johnson Pharmaceutical Institute, SmithKlineBeecham, and Stanley Medical Research Foundation, *Consultant:* Abbott Laboratories, GlaxoSmithKline, Janssen, Lilly Research, Sanofi-Synthelabo, and UCB Pharma; *Speakers Bureau:* Abbott Laboratories, AstraZeneca, GlaxoSmithKline, Janssen, Lilly Research, and Pfizer.

Peter F. Buckley, M.D.   *Grant/Research Support:* Astra Zeneca, National Institute of Mental Health, Janssen Pharmaceutica, Pfizer, Solvay, and Wyeth; *Consultant (Honorarium/Expenses):* Janssen Pharmaceutica and National Institute of Mental Health.

Joseph R. Calabrese, M.D.   *Grant/Research Support:* Abbott, AstraZeneca, Cleveland Foundation, GlaxoSmithKline, Janssen, Lilly, NARSAD, Repligen, and Stanley Medical Research Institute; *Federal Funding:* Department of Defense, Health Resources Services Administration, and National Institute of Mental Health; *Advisory Board:* Abbott, AstraZeneca, Bristol-Myers Squibb, France Foundation, GlaxoSmithKline, Janssen, Johnson & Johnson Pharmaceutical Research & Development, and Solvay/Wyeth; *CME Activities:* AstraZeneca, Bristol-Myers Squibb, France Foundation, GlaxoSmithKline, Janssen, Johnson & Johnson, and Solvay/Wyeth.

Carla M. Canuso, M.D.   *Employed by:* Ortho-McNeil Janssen Scientific Affairs; *Stock:* Johnson & Johnson.

Linda L. Carpenter, M.D.   *Grant/Research Support:* NARSAD, National Institute of Mental Health, Pfizer, Sepracor, and UCB Pharma; *Consultant/Advisory Board:* Abbott, Bristol-Myers Squibb, Cyberonics, Medtronic, Novartis, Pfizer, Sepracor, and Wyeth; *Honoraria for CME:* APA, Cyberonics, and Wyeth; *Speakers Bureau:* AstraZeneca, Cyberonics, and Pfizer; *Travel Support:* Neuronetics.

Anita H. Clayton, M.D.   *Grant/Research Support:* BioSame Pharmaceuticals, Boehringer-Ingelheim, Bristol-Myers Squibb, Eli Lilly, Forest Pharmaceuticals, GlaxoSmithKline, Neuronetics, Pfizer, Sanofi-Aventis, and Wyeth; *Consultant/Advisory Board:* Boehringer-Ingelheim, Bristol-Myers Squibb, Eli Lilly, Fabre-Kramer Pharmaceuticals, GlaxoSmithKline, Novartis Pharmaceuticals, Pfizer, Vela Pharmaceuticals, and Wyeth; *Speakers Bureau/Honoraria:* Eli Lilly, GlaxoSmithKline, Pfizer, and Wyeth.

Emil F. Coccaro, M.D.   *Consultant:* Azevan Pharmaceuticals.

Kathryn M. Connor, M.D., M.H.S.   *Employed by:* Merck & Co, Inc.

Joseph F. Cubells, M.D., Ph.D.   *Grant/Research Support:* NARSAD, National Institute on Drug Abuse, National Institute of Mental Health, and The Robert W. Woodruff Fund of Emory University.

D. P. Devanand, M.D.   *Research Support:* Eli Lilly, Forest Labs, and GlaxoSmithKline, and Wyeth.

C. Lindsay DeVane, Pharm.D.   *Grant/Research Support:* National Institute on Drug Abuse and National Institute of Mental Health; *Consultant:* Bristol-Myers Squibb, CME, Eli Lilly, GlaxoSmithKline, Janssen Pharmaceuticals, Medscape, Novadel Pharma, Primedia Healthcare, and Theracos.

David F. Dinges, Ph.D.   *Grant/Research Support:* Cephalon, and Merck; *Consultant/Scientific Advisor:* Arena Pharmaceuticals, Cephalon, GlaxoSmithKline, ILSI North America, Mars Masterfoods, Merck, Neurogen, Novartis, Pfizer, Procter & Gamble, and Takeda;

Barbara D'Orio, M.D., M.P.A.   *Grant/Research Support:* American Foundation for Suicide Prevention, Emory Medical Care Foundation, and National Institute of Mental Health.

David L. Dunner, M.D.   *Grant/Research Support:* Bristol-Myers Squibb, Cyberonics, Eli Lilly, Forest, GlaxoSmithKline, Janssen, Pfizer, and Wyeth; *Consultant/Advisory Board:* Bristol-Myers Squibb, Cypress, Corcept, Eli Lilly, Forest, GlaxoSmithKline, Janssen, Novartis, Otsuka, Pfizer, Roche Diagnostics, Shire, Somerset, and Wyeth; *Speakers Bureau:* Bristol-Myers Squibb, Eli Lilly, Forest, GlaxoSmithKline, Organon, Pfizer, and Wyeth.

Susana V. Fernandez, B.A.   *Research Support:* National Institutes of Health.

Marlene P. Freeman, M.D.   *Research Support:* Forest, Institute for Mental Health Research (Arizona), Lilly, National Institute of Mental Health, Pronova Biocare (research materials), Reliant (for investigator-initiated trials), and U.S. Food and Drug Administration.

Mark A. Frye, M.D.   *Research Support:* Abbott Laboratories, Cephalon, GlaxoSmithKline, Janssen Pharmaceutica, and Pfizer; *Consultant:* Abbott Laboratories, Bristol-Myers Squibb, Eli Lilly, GlaxoSmithKline, Janssen Pharmaceutica, Organon, and Otsuka Pharmaceuticals; *CME Supported Activities:* AstraZeneca, Bristol-Myers Squibb, Eli Lilly, GlaxoSmithKline, Organon, and Otsuka Pharmaceuticals; *Travel Support:* Bristol-Myers Squibb, Cephalon, Organon, and Otsuka Pharmaceuticals.

Keming Gao, M.D., Ph.D.   *Grant/Research Support:* Abbott, AstraZeneca, GlaxoSmithKline, and NARSAD; *Speakers Bureau:* AstraZeneca.

Steven J. Garlow, M.D., Ph.D.   *Grant/Research Support:* Janssen Pharmaceutical, NARSAD, and National Institute of Mental Health; *Consultant:* Eli Lilly, and Solvay Pharmaceuticals; *Scientific Advisor/Grant Review:* American Foundation for Suicide Prevention, Constella Group, and Oak Ridge Associated Universities; *Honoraria:* CME; *Speakers Bureau:* Eli Lilly, and Pfizer.

Alan J. Gelenberg, M.D.   *Research Support:* Novartis Pharmaceuticals; *Consultant:* AstraZeneca, Best Practice, Cyberonics, Eli Lilly, Forest, GlaxoSmithKline, Novartis, Pfizer, and Wyeth; *Stock Options:* Vela Pharmaceuticals.

Charles F. Gillespie, M.D., Ph.D.   *Grant/Research Support:* APIRE/Wyeth, National Institute on Drug Abuse, and NARSAD; *Review Board:* CME outfitters.

Donald C. Goff, M.D.   *Research Support:* Bristol-Myers Squibb, Cephalon, Dainippon Sumitomo, Eli Lilly, Janssen Pharmaceuticals, Letters and Science, Organon, Pfizer, Primedia, Proteus, SG Cowen, Solvay/Wyeth, Vanda Pharmaceuticals, Verusmed, Vista Research, Xenoport, and Xytis.

Anthony A. Grace, Ph.D.   *Grant/Research Support:* Lundbeck Pharmaceuticals; *Consultant:* Johnson & Johnson, and Taisho Pharmaceuticals.

Alan I. Green, M.D.   *Research Support:* AstraZeneca, Bristol-Myers, Cyberonics, Forest, Janssen, Lilly, and Novartis; *Consultant/Advisory Board:* AstraZeneca, Cyberonics, Janssen, and Lilly; *Stock:* Johnson & Johnson, and Meylau.

Raquel E. Gur, M.D., Ph.D.   *Investigator:* AstraZeneca.

Eric Hollander, M.D.   *Research Support:* Abbott, FDA (Oprah products), National Institute on Drug Abuse, National Institute of Mental Health, National Institute of Neurological Disorders and Stroke, Ortho-McNeil, and Pfizer; *Consultant:* Abbott, and Neuropharm.

Florian Holsboer, M.D., Ph.D.   *Shareholder:* Amectis Pharmaceuticals, Corcept, and Neurocrine.

Ned H. Kalin, M.D.   *Research Support/Consultant/Speakers Bureau:* Amgen, AstraZeneca, Bristol-Myers Squibb, Corcept, CeNeRx Biopharma, Cypress Biosciences, Cyberonics, Forest Laboratories, GlaxoSmithKline, Janssen Pharmaceutica, Johnson & Johnson, Lilly, National Institute of Mental Health, Neurocrine Bio, Neuronetics, Pfizer Pharmaceuticals, Sanofi-Synthelabo, Stanley Foundation, and Wyeth-Ayerst; *Editor: Nature* and *Psychoneuroendocrinology* (Elsevier); *Field Editor: Neuropsychopharmacology; Stock/Equity Holdings:* Corcept, CeNeRx, and Neurocrine Biosciences; *Owner:* Promoter Neurosciences; *Patents:* U.S. Patent No. 7,071,323—Kalin NH, Landry CF, Nanda SA, Roseboom PH: Promoter sequences for corticotropin-releasing factor CRF2alpha and method of identifying agents that alter the activity of the promoter sequences; U.S. Patent No. 7,087,385—Kalin NH, Nanda SA, Roseboom PH: Promoter sequences for urocortin 2 and the use thereof; U.S. Patent No. 7,122,650—Kalin NH, Nanda SA, and Roseboom PH: Promoter sequences for corticotropin-releasing factor binding protein and use thereof; U.S. Patent Application No. 10/896544—Bakshi VP, Kalin NH, Nanda SA, Roseboom PH: Method of reducing CRF receptor mRNA.

Paul E. Keck Jr., M.D.   *Research Support:* Abbott Laboratories, AstraZeneca, Bristol-Myers Squibb, GlaxoSmithKline, Eli Lilly, Janssen Pharmaceutica, National Institute of Mental Health, National Institute on Drug Abuse, Pfizer, and UCB Pharma; *Consultant:* Bristol-Myers Squibb, Eli Lilly, Forest Laboratories, Organon, and Pfizer; *Patents:* U.S. Patent No. 6,387,956—Shapira NA, Goldsmith TD, Keck PE Jr. (University of Cincinnati): Methods of treating obsessive-compulsive spectrum disorder comprises the step of administering an effective amount of tramadol to an individual. Filed March 25, 1999; approved May 14, 2002.

David E. Kemp, M.D.   *Consultant:* Abbott, Bristol-Myers Squibb, and Wyeth.

Terence A. Ketter, M.D.   *Grant/Research Support:* Abbott Laboratories, AstraZeneca, Bristol-Myers Squibb, Eisai, Elan Pharmaceuticals, Eli Lilly, GlaxoSmithKline, Janssen Pharmaceutica Products, Novartis Pharmaceuticals Group, Repligen, Shire Pharmaceuticals, Solvay Pharmaceuticals, and Wyeth Pharmaceuticals; *Consultant:* Abbott Laboratories, AstraZeneca Pharmaceuticals, Bristol-Myers Squibb, Cephalon, Corcept Therapeutics, Elan Pharmaceuticals, Eli Lilly, Forest Laboratories, GlaxoSmithKline, Janssen Pharmaceutica Products, Jazz Pharmaceuticals, Merck, Novartis Pharmaceuticals, Pfizer, Repligen, Shire Pharmaceuticals Group, Solvay Pharmaceuticals, UCB Pharmaceuticals, and Wyeth Pharmaceuticals; *Lecture Honoraria:* Abbott Laboratories, AstraZeneca Pharmaceuticals, Bristol-Myers Squibb, Eli Lilly, GlaxoSmithKline, Janssen Pharmaceutica Products, Novartis Pharmaceuticals, Pfizer, and Shire Pharmaceuticals Group.

Clinton Kilts, Ph.D.   *Grant/Research Support:* National Institutes of Health; *Consultant/Advisory Board:* Forest Laboratories, H. Lundbeck A/S, and Solvay Pharmaceuticals; *Patents:* U.S. Serial No. 6,375990 B1, Method and Devices for Transdermal Delivery of Lithium, Co-holder with C.B. Nemeroff, M.D., Ph.D.; *Endowed Chair:* Paul Janssen Endowed Chair of Neuropsychopharmacology, Emory University.

Lorrin M. Koran, M.D.   *Grant Support:* Eli Lilly; *Consultant:* Jazz Pharmaceuticals.

K. Ranga Rama Krishnan, M.D.   *Consultant:* Amgen, Bristol-Myers Squibb, CeNeRx, Corcept, GlaxoSmithKline, Johnson & Johnson, Lundbeck, Merck, Organon, Pfizer, Sepracor, Somerset, and Wyeth.

Kurt Kroenke, M.D.   *Research Support:* Eli Lilly, and Pfizer; *Honoraria:* Eli Lilly, and Forest.

David J. Kupfer, M.D.   *Consultant:* Servier Amerique.

Allan I. Levey, M.D., Ph.D.   *Grant:* Acadia Pharmaceuticals.

David A. Lewis, M.D.   *Research Support:* Merck, and Pfizer; *Consultant:* BMS, Pfizer, Sepracor, and Wyeth.

Jeffrey A. Lieberman, M.D.   *Research Support:* Acadia, Bristol-Myers Squibb, GlaxoSmithKline, Janssen, Merck, Organon, and Pfizer; *Consultant:* Eli Lilly, and Pfizer; *Advisory Board:* AstraZeneca, Eli Lilly, GlaxoSmithKline, Lundbeck, Organon, and Pfizer; *Patent:* Repligen.

David M. Lyons, Ph.D. *Grant/Research Support:* Public Health Service Grants DA16902, MH77884, and MH47573, Pritzker Neuropsychiatric Disorders Research Consortium which is supported by the Pritzker Neuropsychiatric Disorders Research Fund. A shared intellectual property agreement exists between the Pritzker Neuropsychiatric Disorders Research Fund and the University of Michigan, the University of California, and Stanford University to encourage the development of appropriate findings for research and clinical applications.

Husseini K. Manji, M.D., F.R.C.P.C. The work presented in Chapter 1 was undertaken under the auspices of the National Institute of Mental Health Intramural Program. Dr. Manji is now at Johnson & Johnson Pharmaceutical Research & Development.

Stephen R. Marder, M.D. *Research Support:* Allon, Epix, Merck, and Novartis; *Consultant/Advisory Board:* Abbott, Acadia, Bristol-Myers Squibb, GlaxoSmithKline, Lundbeck, Memory, Otsuka, Pfizer, and Wyeth.

Sanjay Mathew, M.D. *Grant/Research Support:* Alexza Pharmaceuticals, General Clinical Research Center at Mount Sinai School of Medicine, National Alliance for Research in Schizophrenia and Depression, National Institute of Mental Health Career Development Award K23MH0 69656, U19-MH-069056, and Novartis; *Compensation:* AstraZeneca, Jazz Pharmaceuticals, and Pfizer; *Patent:* Inventor on a use patent of ketamine for the treatment of depression. If ketamine were shown to be effective in the treatment of depression and received approval from the U.S. Food and Drug Administration (FDA) for this indication, Dr. Mathew could benefit financially.

Helen S. Mayberg, M.D. *Consultant:* Advanced Neuromodel Systems (ANS); *Licensing of IP:* ANS.

W. Vaughn McCall, M.D., M.S. *Research Support:* GlaxoSmithKline, MECTA, Mini Mitter, Neurocrine, Sanofi, Sepracor, Somaxon, and Wyeth; *Speakers Bureau:* GlaxoSmithKline, Sanofi, and Sepracor.

William M. McDonald, M.D. *Grant/Research Support:* Boehringer Ingelheim, Fuqua Foundation, Janssen, National Institute of Mental Health, National Institute of Neurological Disorders and Stroke, and NeuroNetics; *Consultant:* Bristol-Myers Squibb, Forest, Janssen, and NeuroNetics; *Speakers Bureau:* Bristol-Myers Squibb, Forest, Janssen, and Solvay.

Susan L. McElroy, M.D. *Research Support:* Abbott Laboratories, AstraZeneca, Bristol-Myers Squibb, Eisai, Eli Lilly, Forest Labs, GlaxoSmithKline, Janssen Pharmaceutica, Jazz Pharmaceuticals, National Institute of Mental Health, OREXIGEN Therapeutics, Ortho-McNeil Pharmaceutical, Pfizer, Sanofi-Synthelabo, Somaxon Pharmaceuticals, Stanley Medical Research Institute, and Takeda Pharmaceutical (serves as principal or co-investigator); *Consultant/Advisory Board:* Abbott Laboratories, AstraZeneca, Eli Lilly, GlaxoSmithKline, Janssen Pharmaceutica, Ortho-McNeil Pharmaceutical, and Wyeth-Ayerst; *Patents:* U.S. Patent No. 6,323,236B2, Use of Sulfamate Derivatives for Treating Impulse Control Disorders, and along with the patent's assignee, University of Cincinnati, Cincinnati, OH, receives payments from Johnson & Johnson Pharmaceutical Research & Development, L.L.C., which has exclusive rights under the patent.

Andrew H. Miller, M.D. *Research Support:* Centers for Disease Control and Prevention, GlaxoSmithKline, Janssen/Johnson & Johnson, National Institutes of Health, and Schering-Plough; *Consultant/Advisory Board:* Centocor, and Schering-Plough.

David J. Muzina, M.D. *Grant/Research Support:* Abbott Labs, Bristol-Myers Squibb, Eli Lilly, GlaxoSmithKline, Novartis, Repligen, and Wyeth Pharmaceuticals; *Speaking/Advisory Honoraria:* AstraZeneca, GlaxoSmithKline, and Pfizer.

Henry A. Nasrallah, M.D. *Grant/Research Support:* AstraZeneca, GlaxoSmithKline, Janssen, Lilly, National Institute of Mental Health, Pfizer, and Sanofi-Aventis; *Consultant:* Abbott, AstraZeneca, Janssen, and Pfizer; *Advisory Board:* Abbott, AstraZeneca, Janssen, and Pfizer, *Speakers Bureau:* Abbott, AstraZeneca, Janssen, and Pfizer.

J. Craig Nelson, M.D. *Advisory Board:* Biovail, Bristol-Myers Squibb, Corcept, Eli Lilly, Forest, GlaxoSmithKline, Novartis, Orexigen, Organon, and Pfizer; *Consultant:* Bristol-Myers Squibb, Corcept, Forest, Merck, and Orexigen.

Charles B. Nemeroff, M.D., Ph.D. *Research Support/Board of Directors/Equity Holdings:* American Foundations for Suicide Prevention (AFSP), CeNeRx, Corcept, George West Mental Health Foundation, Mt. Cook, National Alliance for Research on Schizophrenia and Depression (NARSAD), National Institute of Mental Health, NovaDel Pharmaceuticals, and Reevax; *Scientific Advisory Board:* AstraZeneca, Forest Laboratories, Johnson & Johnson, NARSAD, PharmaNeuroboost, and Quintiles.

D. Jeffrey Newport, M.D., M.Div. *Research Support:* Eli Lilly, GlaxoSmithKline, Janssen, NARSAD, National Institutes of Health, and Wyeth; *Speaker's Honoraria:* AstraZeneca, Eli Lilly, GlaxoSmithKline, and Pfizer.

Linda Nicholas, M.D. *Speakers Bureau:* AstraZeneca.

Seiji Nishino, M.D., Ph.D. *Research Support:* Johnson & Johnson (The Effects of H3 Antagonists on Sleep in Narcoleptic Mice), Jazz Pharmaceuticals (A Retrospective Chart Study of the Pediatric Management of Narcolepsy, Narcolepsy in African Americans, and Narcolepsy in African American Patients-Hypocretin deficiency without cataplexy).

Charles P. O'Brien, M.D., Ph.D. *Consultant/Advisory Board:* Alkermes, Cephalon, Forest, and McNeil.

Steven R. Pliszka, M.D. *Research Support:* AstraZeneca, Eli Lilly, and McNeil Pediatrics; *Consultant:* Ortho-McNeil Scientific, and Shire; *Speakers Bureau:* McNeil Pediatrics, and Shire.

Bruce G. Pollock, M.D., Ph.D. *Grant/Research Support:* National Institutes of Health, and Janssen Pharmaceuticals; *Advisory Board:* Forest Laboratories; *Consultant:* Lundbeck, and Takeda; *Speakers Bureau:* Forest, and Lundbeck; *Faculty:* Lundbeck Institute.

Robert M. Post, M.D. *Consultant/Speakers Bureau:* Abbott, AstraZeneca, BMS, and GlaxoSmithKline.

David C. Purselle, M.D., M.S. *Speakers Bureau:* Pfizer; *Faculty:* Lilly.

Charles L. Raison, M.D. *Consultant/Advisory Board:* Centocor, Lilly, Schering, and Wyeth; *Speakers Bureau:* Lilly, and Wyeth.

Mark Hyman Rapaport, M.D.   *Grant/Research Support:* Astra-Zeneca, National Center for Complementary and Alternative Medicine, National Institute of Mental Health, and Solvay; *Consultant:* Cyberonics, Janssen Pharmaceutica, NCCR, National Institute of Mental Health, Pfizer, Solvay, and Wyeth; *Speakers Bureau:* Forest Labs, and Wyeth.

Karl Rickels, M.D.   *Grant/Research Support:* AstraZeneca, Bristol-Myers Squibb, Forest Laboratories, Cephalon, Epix Pharmaceuticals, Genaissance Pharmaceuticals, Kramer-Fabre, Merck, National Institute of Mental Health, Pamlab, Pfizer, Somerset Pharmaceuticals, and Wyeth Lab; *Honoraria/Consultant/Advisory Board:* Cephalon, DOV Pharmaceuticals, Eli Lilly, Medicinova, Novartis Pharmaceuticals, Pfizer, PreDix Pharmaceuticals, and Sanofi-Synthelabo Research.

Donald S. Robinson, M.D.   *Employed by:* Worldwide Drug Development.

Patrick H. Roseboom, Ph.D.   *Co-Owner:* Promoter Neurosciences; *Patents:* U.S. Patent No. 7,071,323—Kalin NH, Landry CF, Nanda SA, Roseboom PH: Promoter sequences for corticotropin-releasing factor CRF2alpha and method of identifying agents that alter the activity of the promoter sequences; U.S. Patent No. 7,087,385—Kalin NH, Nanda SA, Roseboom PH: Promoter sequences for urocortin 2 and the use thereof; U.S. Patent No. 7,122,650—Kalin NH, Nanda SA, and Roseboom PH: Promoter sequences for corticotropin-releasing factor binding protein and use thereof; U.S. Patent Application No. 10/896544—Bakshi VP, Kalin NH, Nanda SA, Roseboom PH: Method of reducing CRF receptor mRNA.

Jerrold F. Rosenbaum, M.D.   *Consultant:* Neuronetics, Organon, Somaxon Pharm, and Supernus; *Advisory Board:* Forest, Lilly, MedAvante, Novartis Pharm, Sanofi Pharm, and Wyeth Pharm; *Speakers Bureau:* Boehringer Ingelheim Italia, and Primedia Health Care (Educational Content Development); *Equity Holdings:* Compellis, MedAvante, and Somaxon.

Alan F. Schatzberg, M.D.   *Consultant:* Abbott, BrainCells, CeNeRx, Corcept (co-founder), Eli Lilly, Forest Labs, Merck, Neuronetics, Novartis, Pathways Diagnostics, PharmaNeuroBoost, Quintiles, Synosis, and Wyeth; *Speakers Bureau:* GlaxoSmithKline; *Equity Holdings:* Corcept, Forest, Merck, Neurocrine, and Pfizer; *Patents:* Named inventor on pharmacogenetic use patents on prediction of antidepressant response.

S. Charles Schulz, M.D.   *Grant/Research Support:* Abbott, AstraZeneca, Eli Lilly, and MIND Institute; *Consultant:* AstraZeneca, Eli Lilly, and Vanda; *Honoraria:* AstraZeneca, and Eli Lilly; *Speakers Bureau:* AstraZeneca, BMS, and Eli Lilly.

Zafar A. Sharif, M.D.   *Advisory Board:* Bristol-Myers Squibb, and Janssen Pharmaceutica; *Speakers Bureau:* Bristol-Myers Squibb, and Janssen Pharmaceutica.

David V. Sheehan, M.D., M.B.A.   *Grant/Research Support:* Abbott Laboratories, Andote Foundation, AstraZeneca, Avera Pharmaceuticals, Bristol-Myers Squibb, Burroughs Wellcome, Eisai, Eli Lilly, Forest Laboratories, GlaxoSmithKline, Glaxo-Wellcome, International Clinical Research (ICR), Janssen Pharmaceutica, Jazz Pharmaceuticals, Kali-Duphar, Mead Johnson, MediciNova, Merck Sharp & Dohme, National Institute on Drug Abuse, National Institutes of Health, Novartis Pharmaceuticals Corp., Parke-Davis, Pfizer, Quintiles, Sandoz Pharmaceuticals, Sanofi-Aventis, Sanofi-Synthelabo Recherche, SmithKlineBeecham, TAP Pharmaceuticals, United Bioscience, The Upjohn Company, Warner Chilcott, Wyeth-Ayerst, and Zeneca Pharmaceuticals; *Consultant:* Abbott Laboratories, Alexa, Alza Pharmaceuticals, Applied Health Outcomes/XCENDA, AstraZeneca, Avera Pharmaceuticals, Bristol-Myers Squibb, Cephalon, Cortex Pharmaceutical, Cypress Bioscience, Eisai, Eli Lilly, Forest Laboratories, GlaxoSmithKline, INC Research, Janssen Pharmaceutica, Jazz Pharmaceuticals, Labopharm, Layton Bioscience, Lilly Research Laboratories, Lundbeck, Denmark, MediciNova, National Anxiety Awareness Program, National Anxiety Foundation, National Depressive & Manic Depressive Association, Organon, Orion Pharma, Parexel International Corporation, Pfizer, Pharmacia, Pharmacia & Upjohn, Pierre Fabre, France, Roche, Sanofi-Aventis, Sanofi-Synthelabo Recherche, Sepracor, Shire Laboratories, Inc., SmithKlineBeecham, Solvay Pharmaceuticals, Takeda Pharmaceuticals, Targacept, The Upjohn Company, Tikvah Therapeutics, Titan Pharmaceuticals, Wyeth-Ayerst, and ZARS; *Speakers Bureau:* Abbott Laboratories, AstraZeneca, Boehringer Ingelheim, Boots Pharmaceuticals, Bristol-Myers Squibb, Burroughs Wellcome, Charter Hospitals, Ciba Geigy, Dista Products Company, Eli Lilly, Excerpta Medica Asia, Glaxo Pharmaceuticals, GlaxoSmithKline, Hospital Corporation of America, Humana, ICI, Janssen Pharmaceutica, Kali-Duphar, Marion Merrill Dow, McNeil Pharmaceuticals, Mead Johnson, Merck Sharp & Dohme, Novo Nordisk, Organon, Parke-Davis, Pfizer, Pharmacia & Upjohn, Rhone Laboratories, Rhone-Poulenc Rorer Pharmaceuticals, Roerig, Sandoz Pharmaceuticals, Sanofi-Aventis, Schering Corporation, SmithKlineBeecham, Solvay Pharmaceuticals, TAP Pharmaceuticals, The Upjohn Company, Warner Chilcott, and Wyeth-Ayerst; *Stock:* Medical Outcome Systems.

George M. Simpson, M.D.   *Grant Support:* AstraZeneca, Janssen, and Pfizer; *Consultant:* Janssen, Merck, and Pfizer.

Diane M. Sloan, Pharm.D.   *Employed by:* Advogent (a medical communications agency that does work with Wyeth Pharmaceuticals).

Zachary N. Stowe, M.D.   *Grant/Research Support:* GlaxoSmithKline, National Institutes of Health, and Wyeth; *Advisory Board:* BMS, GlaxoSmithKline, and Wyeth; *Speaker's Honoraria:* Eli Lilly, GlaxoSmithKline, Pfizer, and Wyeth.

Pierre N. Tariot, M.D. *Grant/Research Support:* Abbott Laboratories, AstraZeneca, Alzheimer's Association, Arizona Department of Health Services, Bristol-Myers Squibb, Eisai, Elan, Eli Lilly, Forest Laboratories, GlaxoSmithKline, Institute for Mental Health Research, Janssen Pharmaceutica, Merck, Mitsubishi Pharma Corporation, Myriad Pharmaceuticals, NIA, National Institute of Mental Health, Neurochem, Ono Pharmaceuticals, Pfizer, Sanofi-Synthelabo, Schwabe, Takeda Pharmaceuticals North America, and Wyeth Laboratories; *Consultant:* Abbott Laboratories, AstraZeneca, Bristol-Myers Squibb, Eisai, Eli Lilly, Forest Laboratories, GlaxoSmithKline, Janssen Pharmaceutica, Memory Pharmaceuticals, Merck, Myriad Pharmaceuticals, Novartis AG, Pfizer, Sanofi-Synthelabo, Schwabe, and Takeda Pharmaceuticals North America; *Speakers Bureau:* AstraZeneca, Eisai, Forest Pharmaceuticals, and Pfizer; *Educational Fees:* AstraZeneca, Eisai, Forest Laboratories, Lundbeck, and Pfizer; *Patents:* Biomarkers of Alzheimer's Disease.

Michael E. Thase, M.D. *Consultant/Advisory Board:* AstraZeneca, Bristol-Myers Squibb, Cephalon, Cyberonics, Eli Lilly, Forest Pharmaceuticals, GlaxoSmithKline, Janssen Pharmaceutica, MedAvante, Neuronetics, Novartis, Organon, Sepracor, Shire, Supernus Pharmaceuticals, and Wyeth-Ayerst Laboratories; *Speakers Bureau:* AstraZeneca, Bristol-Myers Squibb, Cyberonics, Eli Lilly, GlaxoSmithKline, Organon, Sanofi Aventis, and Wyeth-Ayerst Laboratories; *Royalty/Patent/Other Income:* American Psychiatric Publishing, Guilford Publications, Herald House, and W.W. Norton; *Equity Holdings:* MedAvante; *Expert Testimony:* Jones Day and Phillips Lyttle, and Pepper Hamilton.

Gary D. Tollefson, M.D., Ph.D. *Employed by:* Orexigen Therapeutics.

Karen D. Wagner, M.D., Ph.D. *Research Support:* National Institute of Mental Health; *Consultant/Advisory Board:* Abbott Laboratories, AstraZeneca, Bristol-Myers Squibb, Eli Lilly, Forest Laboratories, Janssen, Novartis, Otsuka, Pfizer, Sanofi Aventis, and Solvay.

Margaret B. Weigel, M.D. *Grant/Stipend Support:* Novartis Pharmaceuticals, and Ono.

Donna A. Wirshing, M.D. *Speakers Bureau:* Bristol-Myers Squibb, and Pfizer.

Frank D. Yocca, Ph.D. *Employed by:* AstraZeneca Pharmaceuticals Co.

Kimberly A. Yonkers, M.D. *Grant Support:* Lilly, National Institute of Mental Health, Pfizer, and Wyeth.

Jiang-Zhou Yu, M.D., Ph.D. *Grant Support:* Bristol-Myers Squibb, and ONO Pharmaceuticals.

The following contributors stated that they had no competing interests during the year preceding manuscript submission:

W. Stewart Agras, M.D.; Jonathan M. Amiel, M.D.; Josephine Astrid Archer, B.Sc.; Gregory S. Berns, M.D., Ph.D.; David R. Block, M.D.; Catherine Bresee, M.S.; Frank W. Brown, M.D.; Mary F. Brunette, M.D.; Monica Kelly Cowles, M.D., M.S.; Charles A. Dackis, M.D.; Albert A. Davis, B.S.; Karon Dawkins, M.D.; Clifford J. Ehmke, M.D.; Dwight L. Evans, M.D.; Amir Garakani, M.D.; Elizabeth H. Gillespie, D.O.; Robert N. Golden, M.D.; Todd D. Gould, M.D.; Ebrahim Haroon, M.D.; Christine Heim, Ph.D.; Jinger G. Hoop, M.D., M.F.A.; Walter H. Kaye, M.D.; Ashley P. Kennedy, B.S.; Ania Korszun, Ph.D., M.D., M.R.C.Psych.; Helena C. Kraemer, Ph.D.; Erin E. Krebs, M.D., M.P.H.; Joseph B. Layde, M.D., J.D.; Thomas W. Meeks, M.D.; Darlene S. Melchitzky, M.S.; Emmanuel Mignot, M.D., Ph.D.; Kazuo Mishima, M.D., Ph.D.; Katherine Marshall Moore, M.D.; Alexander Neumeister, M.D.; Sandhaya Norris, M.D.; Giuseppe Pagnoni, Ph.D.; Daniel S. Pine, M.D.; B. Ashok Raj, M.D.; Mark M. Rasenick, Ph.D.; Martin Reite, M.D.; Laura Weiss Roberts, M.D., M.A.; J. Amiel Rosenkranz, Ph.D.; Carl Salzman, M.D.; Daphne Simeon, M.D.; Joseph K. Stanilla, M.D.; Michael A. Strober, Ph.D.; Steven T. Szabo, Ph.D.; Rajiv Tandon, M.D.; Anthony R. West, Ph.D.; Po W. Wang, M.D.; Joanne D. Wojcik, P.M.H.C.N.S.–B.C.; Tsung-Ung W. Woo, M.D.; Janos Zahajszlay, M.D.; Charles F. Zorumski, M.D.

Introduction

Psychopharmacology has developed as a medical discipline over approximately the past five decades. The discoveries of the earlier effective antidepressants, antipsychotics, and mood stabilizers were invariably based on serendipitous observations. The repeated demonstration of efficacy of these agents then served as an impetus for considerable research into the neurobiological bases of their therapeutic effects and of emotion and cognition themselves, as well as the biological basis of the major psychiatric disorders. Moreover, the emergence of an entire new multidisciplinary field, neuropsychopharmacology, which has led to newer specific agents to alter maladaptive central nervous system processes or activity, was another by-product of these early endeavors. The remarkable proliferation of information in this area—coupled with the absence of any comparable, currently available text—led us to edit the first edition of *The American Psychiatric Press Textbook of Psychopharmacology*, published in 1995. The response to that edition was overwhelmingly positive. In the second edition, published in 1998, we expanded considerably on the first edition, covering a number of areas in much greater detail, adding several new chapters, and updating all of the previous material. Again, the response was positive. We then presented a third edition in 2004 with virtually all new material, and now this fourth edition has updated the previous material and added several chapters on important (often emerging) areas not previously covered.

In order for the reader to appreciate and integrate the rich amount of information about pharmacological agents, we have attempted in all editions to provide sufficient background material to understand more easily how drugs work and why, when, and in whom they should be used. For this fourth edition, we have updated all the material, often adding new contributors as well as adding several new chapters, and thus expanding the scope and length of the text. The textbook consists of five major parts. The first section, "Principles of Psychopharmacology," was edited by Robert Malenka and provides a theoretical background for the ensuing parts. It includes chapters on neurotransmitters; signal transduction and second messengers; molecular biology; chemical neuroanatomy; electrophysiology; animal models of psychiatric disorders; psychoneuroendocrinology, pharmacokinetics; and pharmacodynamics; psychoneuroimmunology; brain imaging in psychopharmacology; and statistics/clinical trial design.

The second part, "Classes of Psychiatric Treatments: Animal and Human Pharmacology," presents information by classes of drugs and is coedited by K. Ranga Rama Krishnan and Dennis Charney. For each drug within a class, data are reviewed on preclinical and clinical pharmacology, pharmacokinetics, indications, dosages, and cognate issues. This section is pharmacopoeia-like. Individual chapters are now generally dedicated to individual agents (e.g., paroxetine, venlafaxine). We include data not only on currently available drugs in the United States but also on medications that will in all likelihood become available in the near future. We have not only updated all the material but invited new authors on many chapters to provide fresh insights.

The third part, "Clinical Psychobiology and Psychiatric Syndromes," edited by David Kupfer, reviews data on the biological underpinnings of specific disorders—for example, major depression, bipolar disorder, and panic disorder. The chapter authors in this section comprehensively review the biological alterations described for each of the major psychiatric disorders, allowing the reader to better understand current psychopharmacological approaches as well as to anticipate future developments.

The fourth part, "Psychopharmacological Treatment," edited by David Dunner, reviews state-of-the-art therapeutic approaches to patients with major psychiatric disorders as well as to those in specific age groups or circumstances: childhood disorders, emergency psychiatry, pregnancy and postpartum, and so forth. Here, too, new contributors provide fresh looks at important clinical topics. This section provides the reader with specific information about drug selection and prescription. We have added a new chapter on chronic pain syndromes.

Last, we have added a new chapter on ethical considerations in psychopharmacological treatment and research, providing the reader with a thoughtful overview of this important area.

This textbook would not have been possible without the superb editorial work of the section editors—as well as, of course, the authors of the chapters, who so generously gave of their time. In addition, we wish to thank Editorial Director John McDuffie of American Psychiatric Publishing and his staff for their editorial efforts. In particular, we appreciate the major efforts of Bessie Jones, Acquisitions Coordinator; Greg Kuny, Managing Editor; Tammy J. Cordova, Graphic Design Manager; Susan Westrate, Prepress Coordinator; Judy Castagna, Manufacturing Manager; Melissa Coates, Assistant Editor; and Rebecca Richters, Senior Editor. Finally, we extend our thanks to Tina Coltri-Marshall at the University of California–Davis, Rebecca Wyse at Stanford University, and Janice Dell at Emory University for their invaluable editorial assistance.

Alan F. Schatzberg, M.D.
Charles B. Nemeroff, M.D., Ph.D.

PART I

Principles of
Psychopharmacology

Robert C. Malenka, M.D., Ph.D., Section Editor

Neurotransmitters, Receptors, Signal Transduction, and Second Messengers in Psychiatric Disorders

Steven T. Szabo, Ph.D.

Todd D. Gould, M.D.

Husseini K. Manji, M.D., F.R.C.P.C.

This chapter serves as a primer on the recent advances in our understanding of neural function both in health and in disease. It is beyond the scope of this chapter to cover these important areas in extensive detail, and readers are referred to outstanding textbooks that are entirely devoted to the topic (Cooper et al. 2001; Kandel et al. 2000; Nestler et al. 2001; Squire et al. 2003). Here, we focus on the principles of neurotransmission and second-messenger generation that we believe are critical for an understanding of the biological bases of major psychiatric disorders, as well as the mechanisms by which effective treatments may exert their beneficial effects. In particular, it is our goal to lay the groundwork for the subsequent chapters, which focus on individual disorders and their treatments.

Although this chapter is intended to provide a general overview on neurotransmitter and second-messenger function, whenever possible we emphasize the neuropsychiatric relevance of specific observations. In the chapter proper, we outline principles that are of utmost importance to the study and practice of psychopharmacology; in the figure legends, we provide additional details for the interested reader.

What Are Neurotransmitters?

Several criteria have been established for a neurotransmitter, including 1) it is synthesized and released from neurons; 2) it is released from nerve terminals in a chemically or pharmacologically identifiable form; 3) it interacts with postsynaptic receptors and brings about the same effects as are seen with stimulation of the presynaptic neuron; 4) its interaction with the postsynaptic receptor displays a specific pharmacology; and 5) its actions are terminated by active processes (Kandel et al. 2000; Nestler et al. 2001). However, our growing appreciation of the complexity of the central nervous system (CNS) and of the existence of numerous molecules that exert *neuro-*

The work presented in this chapter was undertaken under the auspices of the National Institute of Mental Health Intramural Program. Dr. Manji is now at Johnson & Johnson Pharmaceutical Research & Development.

The authors thank Ioline Henter for assistance in the preparation of this chapter.

modulatory and *neurohormonal* effects has blurred the classical definition of neurotransmitters somewhat, and even well-known neurotransmitters do not meet all these criteria under certain situations (Cooper et al. 2001).

Most neuroactive compounds are small polar molecules that are synthesized in the CNS via local machinery or are able to permeate the blood–brain barrier. To date, more than 50 endogenous substances have been found to be present in the brain that appear to be capable of functioning as neurotransmitters. There are many plausible explanations for why the brain would need so many transmitters and receptor subtypes to transmit messages. Perhaps the simplest explanation is that the sheer complexity of the CNS results in many afferent nerve terminals impinging on a single neuron. This requires a neuron to be able to distinguish the multiple information conveying inputs. Although this can be accomplished partially by spatial segregation, it is accomplished in large part by chemical coding of the inputs—that is, different chemicals convey different information. Moreover, as we discuss in detail later, the evolution of multiple receptors for a single neurotransmitter means that the same chemical can convey different messages depending on the receptor subtypes it acts on. Additionally, the firing pattern of neurons is also a means of conveying information; thus, the firing activities of neurons in the brain differ widely, and a single neuron firing at different frequencies can even release different neuroactive compounds depending on the firing rate (e.g., the release of peptides often occurs at higher firing rates than that which is required to release monoamines). These multiple mechanisms to enhance the diversity of responses—chemical coding, spatial coding, frequency coding—are undoubtedly critical in endowing the CNS with its complex repertoire of physiological and behavioral responses (Kandel et al. 2000; Nestler et al. 2001). Finally, the existence of multiple neuroactive compounds also provides built-in safeguards to ensure that vital brain circuits are able to partially compensate for loss of function of particular neurotransmitters.

Receptors

An essential property of any living cell is its ability to recognize and respond to external stimuli. Cell surface receptors have two major functions: recognition of specific molecules (neurotransmitters, hormones, growth factors, and even sensory signals) and activation of "effectors." Binding of the appropriate agonist (i.e., neurotransmitter or hormone) externally to the receptor alters the confor-

mation (shape) of the protein. Cell surface receptors use a variety of membrane-transducing mechanisms to transform an agonist's message into cellular responses. In neuronal systems, the most typical responses ultimately (in some cases rapidly, in others more slowly) involve changes in transmembrane voltage and hence neuronal changes in excitability. Collectively, the processes are referred to as *transmembrane signaling* or *signal transduction mechanisms*. These processes are not restricted to neurons. For example, astrocytes, which were once thought to be unrelated to neurotransmission, have recently been demonstrated to possess voltage-regulated anion channels (VRAC), which not only transport Cl^- but also allow efflux of amino acids such as taurine, glutamate, and aspartate (Mulligan and MacVicar 2006).

Interestingly, although increasing numbers of potential neuroactive compounds and receptors continue to be identified, it has become clear that translation of the extracellular signals (into a form that can be interpreted by the complex intracellular enzymatic machinery) is achieved through a relatively small number of cellular mechanisms. Generally speaking, these transmembrane signaling systems, and the receptors that utilize them, can be divided into four major groups (Figure 1–1):

- Those that are relatively self-contained in structure and whose message takes the form of transmembrane ion fluxes (**ionotropic**)
- Those that are multicomponent in nature and generate intracellular second messengers (**G protein–coupled**)
- Those that contain intrinsic enzymatic activity (**receptor tyrosine kinases and phosphatases**)
- Those that are cytoplasmic and translocate to the nucleus to directly regulate transcription (gene expression) after they are activated by lipophilic molecules (often hormones) that enter the cell (**nuclear receptors**)

Ionotropic Receptors

The first class of receptors contains in their molecular complex an intrinsic *ion channel*. Receptors of this class include those for a number of amino acids, including glutamate (e.g., the NMDA [N-methyl-D-aspartate] receptor) and GABA (γ-aminobutyric acid via the $GABA_A$ receptor), as well as the nicotinic acetylcholine (ACh) receptor and the serotonin$_3$ (5-HT_3) receptor. Ion channels are integral membrane proteins that are directly responsible for the electrical activity of the nervous system by virtue of their regulation of the movement of ions across membranes. Receptors containing intrinsic ion channels have been called *ionotropic* and are generally composed of four or five subunits that open transiently when neurotransmitter binds, allowing ions to flow into (e.g., Na^+, Ca^{2+}, Cl^-) or out of (e.g., K^+) the neuron, thereby generating synaptic potential (see Figure 1–1).

Often, the ionotropic receptors can be composed of different compositions of the different subunits, thereby providing the system with considerable flexibility. For example, there is extensive research into the potential development of an anxiolytic that is devoid of sedative effects by targeting $GABA_A$ receptor subunits present in selected brain regions. In general, neurotransmission that is mediated by ionotropic receptors is very fast, with ion channels opening and closing within milliseconds, and regulates much of the tonic excitatory (e.g., glutamate-mediated) and inhibitory (e.g., GABA-mediated) activity in the CNS; as we discuss below, many of the classical neurotransmitters (e.g., monoamines) exert their effects on a slower time scale and are therefore often considered to be modulatory in their effects.

G Protein–Coupled Receptors

Most receptors in the CNS do not have intrinsic ionic conductance channels within their structure but instead regulate cellular activity by the generation of various "second messengers." Receptors of this class do not generally interact directly with the various second-messenger-generating enzymes but instead transmit information to the appropriate "effector" by the activation of interposed coupling proteins. These are the G protein–coupled receptor families. The G *protein–coupled receptors* (GPCRs, which constitute more than 80% of all known receptors in the body, and number about 300) all span the plasma membrane seven times (see Figure 1–1). GPCRs have been the focus of extensive research in psychiatry in recent years (Catapano and Manji 2007). The amino terminus is on the outside of the cell and plays a critical role in recognition of the ligand; the carboxy terminus and third intracellular loop are inside the cell and regulate not only coupling to different G proteins but also "cross talk" between receptors and desensitization (see Figure 1–1).

G proteins are so named because of their ability to bind the guanine nucleotides guanosine triphosphate (GTP) and guanosine diphosphate (GDP). Receptors coupled to G proteins include those for catecholamines, serotonin, ACh, various peptides, and even sensory signals such as light and odorants (Table 1–1). As we discuss

later in the chapter, multiple subtypes of G proteins are known to exist, and they play critical roles in amplifying and integrating signals.

Autoreceptors and Heteroreceptors

Autoreceptors are receptors located on neurons that produce the endogenous ligand for that particular receptor (e.g., a serotonergic receptor on a serotonergic neuron). By contrast, *heteroreceptors* are receptor subtypes that are present on neurons that do not contain an endogenous ligand for that particular receptor subtype (e.g., a serotonergic receptor located on a dopaminergic neuron).

Two major classes of autoreceptors play very important roles in fine-tuning neuronal activity. *Somatodendritic autoreceptors* are present on cell bodies and dendrites and exert critical roles in regulating *the firing rate of neurons*. In general, activation of somatodendritic autoreceptors (e.g., α_2-adrenergic receptors for noradrenergic neurons, serotonin1A [5-HT_{1A}] receptors for serotonergic neurons, dopamine2 [D_2] receptors for dopaminergic neurons) inhibits the firing rate of the neurons by opening K^+ channels and by reducing cyclic adenosine monophosphate (cAMP) levels, both of which may be important in psychiatric disease. For example, TREK-1 is a background K^+ channel regulator protein important in 5-HT transmission and potentially in mood-like behavior regulation in mice (Heurteaux et al. 2006). Fundamental mechanisms of neuronal transmission—such as K^+ channels, which regulate membrane potentials—may relate to global alterations in brain functioning relevant to psychiatry.

The second major class of autoreceptors, *nerve terminal autoreceptors*, play an important role in regulating *the amount of neurotransmitter released per nerve impulse*, generally by closing nerve terminal Ca^{2+} channels. Both of these types of autoreceptors are *typically* members of the G protein–coupled receptor family. Neurotransmitter release is known to be triggered by influx and alterations of intracellular calcium, with the functioning of three types of SNARE (soluble *N*-ethylmaleimide–sensitive factor attachment protein [SNAP] receptor) proteins exerting critical roles. Recent advances in our understanding of the distinct kinetics of neurotransmitter release modulators, such as botulinum and tetanus neurotoxins, suggest that these induce prominent alterations in synaptobrevin and syntaxin, leading to calcium-independent mechanisms of neurotransmitter regulation (Sakaba et al. 2005). Most synapses are dependent on influx of Ca^{2+} through voltage-gated calcium channels for presynaptic neurotransmitter release; in the retina, however, this influx of

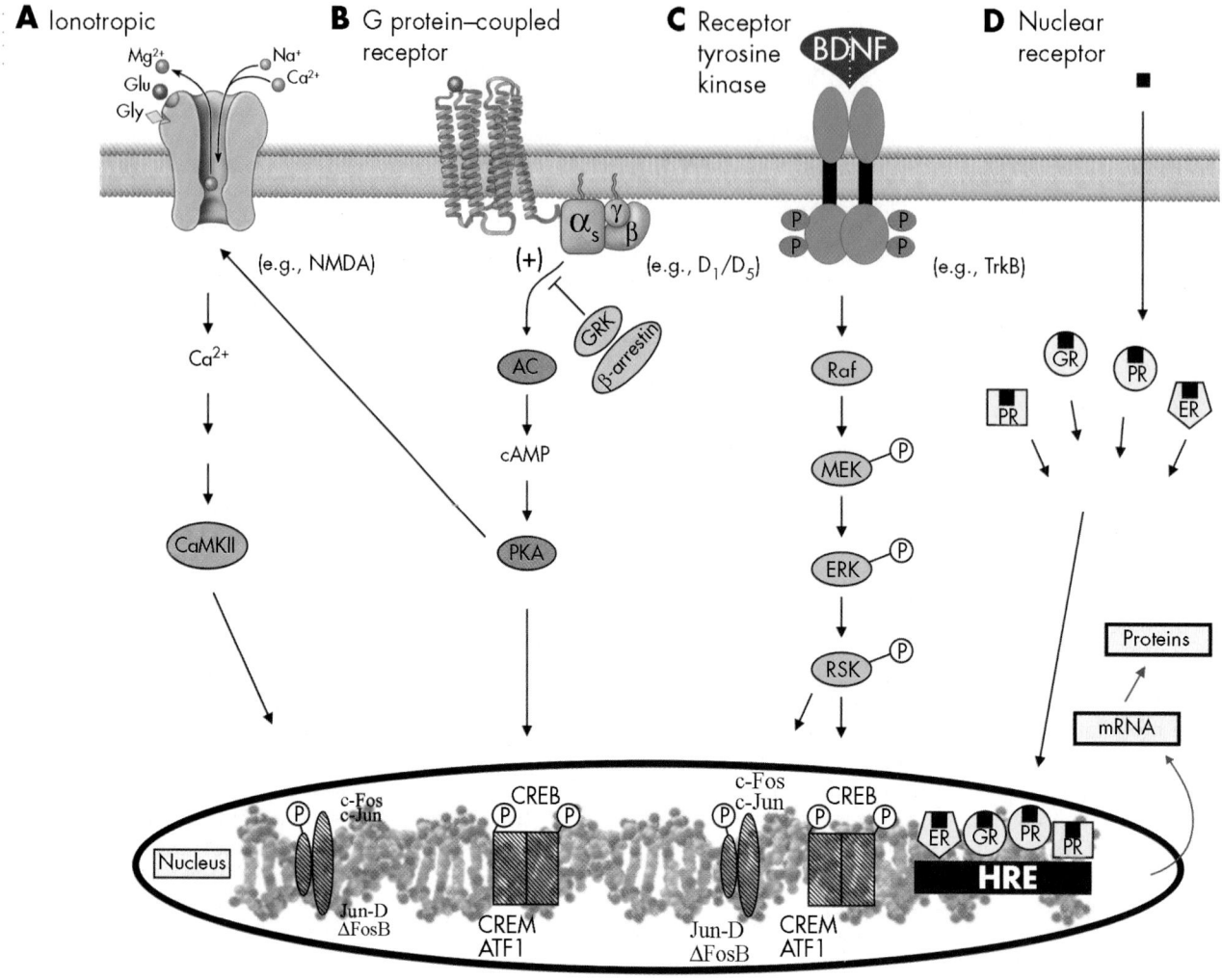

calcium occurs via glutamatergic AMPA receptors (Chavez et al. 2006). Beyond the receptor level, presynaptic SAD, an intracellular serine threonine kinase, is associated with the active zone cytomatrix that regulates neurotransmitter release (Inoue et al. 2006). These recent data further exemplify the dynamic nature and ongoing advancement of our knowledge pertaining to basic processes involved in neurotransmitter regulation that may possibly aid in advancing treatment of psychopathology.

G Protein–Coupled Receptor Regulation and Trafficking

The mechanism by which GPCRs translate extracellular signals into cellular changes was once envisioned as a simple linear model. It is now known, however, that the activity of GPCRs is subject to at least three additional principal modes of regulation: desensitization, downregulation, and trafficking (Carman and Benovic 1998) (Figure 1–2).

Desensitization, the process by which cells rapidly adapt to stimulation by agonists, is generally believed to occur by two major mechanisms: homologous and heterologous.

Homologous desensitization is receptor specific; that is, only the receptor actively being stimulated becomes desensitized. This form of desensitization occurs via a family of kinases known as G protein–coupled kinases (GRKs). When a receptor activates a G protein and causes dissociation of the α subunit from the βγ subunits (discussed in detail later), the βγ subunits are able to provide an "anchoring surface" for the GRKs to allow them to come into the proximity of the activated receptor and phosphorylate it. This phorphorylation then recruits another family of proteins known as *arrestins*, which physically interfere with the coupling of the phosphorylated receptor and the G protein, thereby dampening the signal. This form of desensitization is very rapid and usually transient (i.e., the receptors get dephosphorylated and return to the baseline state). However, if the stimulation of the receptor is ex-

---

FIGURE I–I.   Major receptor subtypes in the central nervous system (*opposite page*).

This figure depicts the four major classes of receptors in the CNS. **(A)** *Ionotropic receptors.* These receptors comprise multiple protein subunits that are combined in such a way as to create a central membrane pore through this complex, allowing the flow of ions. This type of receptor has a very rapid response time (milliseconds). The consequences of receptor stimulation (i.e., excitatory or inhibitory) depend on the types of ions that the receptor specifically allows to enter the cell. Thus, for example, Na^+ entry through the NMDA (*N*-methyl-D-aspartate) receptor depolarizes the neuron and brings about an excitatory response, whereas Cl^- efflux through the γ-aminobutyric acid type A ($GABA_A$) receptor hyperpolarizes the neuron and brings about an inhibitory response. Illustrated here is the NMDA receptor regulating a channel permeable to Ca^{2+}, Na^+, and K^+ ions. The NMDA receptors also have binding sites for glycine, Zn^{2+}, phencyclidine (PCP), MK801/ketamine, and Mg^{2+}; these molecules are able to regulate the function of this receptor. **(B)** *G protein–coupled receptors* (GPCRs). The majority of neurotransmitters, hormones, and even sensory signals mediate their effects via seven transmembrane domain–spanning receptors that are G protein–coupled. The amino terminus of the G protein is on the outside of the cell and plays an important role in the recognition of specific ligands; the third intracellular loop and carboxy terminus of the receptor play an important role in coupling to G proteins and are sites of regulation of receptor function (e.g., by phosphorylation). All G proteins are heterotrimers (consisting of α, β, and γ subunits). The G proteins are attached to the membrane by isoprenoid moieties (fatty acid) via their γ subunits. Compared with the ionotropic receptors, GPCRs mediate a slower response (on the order of seconds). Detailed depiction of the activation of G protein–coupled receptors is given in Figure 1–2. Here we depict a receptor coupled to the G protein G_s (the *s* stands for stimulatory to the enzyme adenylyl cyclase [AC]). Activation of such a receptor produces activation of AC and increases in cAMP levels. G protein–coupled pathways exhibit major amplification properties, and, for example, in model systems researchers have demonstrated a 10,000-fold amplification of the original signal. The effects of cAMP are mediated largely by activation of protein kinase A (PKA). One major downstream target of PKA is CREB (cAMP response element–binding protein), which may be important to the mechanism of action of antidepressants. **(C)** *Receptor tyrosine kinases.* These receptors are activated by neurotrophic factors and are able to bring about acute changes in synaptic function, as well as long-term effects on neuronal growth and survival. These receptors contain intrinsic tyrosine kinase activity. Binding of the ligand triggers receptor dimerization and transphosphorylation of tyrosine residues in its cytoplasmic domain, which then recruits cytoplasmic signaling and scaffolding proteins. The recruitment of effector molecules generally occurs via interaction of proteins with modular binding domains SH2 and SH3 (named after homology to the src oncogenes–src homology domains); SH2 domains are a stretch of about 100 amino acids that allows high-affinity interactions with certain phosphotyrosine motifs. The ability of multiple effectors to interact with phosphotyrosines is undoubtedly one of the keys to the pleiotropic effects that neurotrophins can exert. Shown here is a tyrosine kinase receptor type B (TrkB), which upon activation produces effects on the Raf, MEK (mitogen-activated protein kinase/ERK), extracellular response kinase (ERK), and ribosomal S6 kinase (RSK) signaling pathway. Some major downstream effects of RSK are CREB and stimulation of factors that bind to the AP-1 site (c-Fos and c-Jun). **(D)** *Nuclear receptors.* These receptors are transcription factors that regulate the expression of target genes in response to steroid hormones and other ligands. Many hormones (including glucocorticoids, gonadal steroids, and thyroid hormones) are able to rapidly penetrate into the lipid bilayer membrane, because of their lipophilic composition, and thereby directly interact with these cytoplasmic receptors inside the cell. Upon activation by a hormone, the nuclear receptor–ligand complex translocates to the nucleus, where it binds to specific DNA sequences, referred to as *hormone responsive elements* (HREs), and regulates gene transcription. Nuclear receptors often interact with a variety of coregulators that promote transcriptional activation when recruited (coactivators) and those that attenuate promoter activity (corepressors). However, nongenomic effects of neuroactive steroids have also been documented, with the majority of evidence suggesting modulation of ionotropic receptors. This figure illustrates both the genomic and the nongenomic effects. ATF1 = activation transcription factor 1; BDNF = brain-derived neurotrophic factor; CaMKII = Ca^{2+}/calmodulin–dependent protein kinase II; CREM = cyclic adenosine 5′-monophosphate response element modulator; D_1 = dopamine$_1$ receptor; D_5 = dopamine$_5$ receptor; ER = estrogen receptor; GR = glucocorticoid receptor; GRK = G protein–coupled receptor kinase; P = phosphorylation; PR = progesterone receptor.

---

cessive and prolonged, it leads to an internalization of the receptor, and often its degradation, a process referred to as *downregulation*.

Heterologous desensitization is not receptor specific and is mediated by second-messenger kinases such as protein kinase A (PKA) and protein kinase C (PKC). Thus, when a receptor activates PKA, the activated PKA is capable of phosphorylating (and thereby desensitizing) not only that particular receptor but also other receptors that are present in proximity and have the correct phosphorylation motif, thereby producing heterologous desensitization.

Upon prolonged or repeated activation of receptors by agonist ligands, the process of receptor *downregulation* is observed. Downregulation is associated with a reduced number of receptors detected in cells or tissues, thereby leading to attenuation of cellular responses (Carman and

Benovic 1998). The process of GPCR sequestration is mediated by a well-characterized endocytic pathway involving the concentration of receptors in clathrin-coated pits and subsequent internalization and recycling back to the plasma membrane (Tsao and von Zastrow 2000). Endocytosis can thus clearly serve as a primary mechanism to attenuate signaling by rapidly and reversibly removing receptors from the cell surface. However, emerging evidence suggests additional functions of endocytosis and receptor trafficking in mediating GPCR signaling by way of certain effector pathways, most notably mitogen-activated protein (MAP) kinase cascades (discussed in greater detail later). There is also evidence that endocytosis of GPCRs may be required for certain signal transduction pathways leading to the nucleus (Tsao and von Zastrow 2000). These diverse functions of GPCR endocytosis and traf-

TABLE 1–1.　Key features of G protein subunits

G PROTEIN CLASS	MEMBERS	EFFECTOR(S)/FUNCTIONS	EXAMPLES OF RECEPTORS
α_i	$G\alpha_{i1-3}$, $G\alpha_o$	AC (+)	α_2, D_2, A_1, μ, M_2, 5-HT$_{1A}$
		Ligand-type Ca^{2+} channels (+)	Olfactory signals
	$G\alpha_z$, $G\alpha_{t1-2}$	K$^+$ channels (+)	
		Ca^{2+} channels (−)^a	GABA$_B$
		Cyclic GMP	Retinal rods, cones (rhodopsins)
		Phosphodiesterase (+) ($G\alpha_{t1-2}$)	
α_q	$G\alpha_q$, $G\alpha_{11}$, $G\alpha_{14}$, $G\alpha_{15}$, $G\alpha_{16}$	PLC-β (+)	TxA$_2$, 5-HT$_{2C}$, M_1, M_3, M_5, α_1
α_{12}	$G\alpha_{12}$, $G\alpha_{13}$	RGS domain–containing rho exchange factors	TxA$_2$, thrombin
β^b	β (×5)	AC type I (−); AC types II, IV (potentiation)	
		PLC (+)	
		Receptor kinases (+)	
		Inactivates α_s	
γ	γ (×12)	$\beta\gamma$ required for interaction of α subunit with receptor	

Note.　AC=adenylyl cyclase; A_1, A_2=adenosine receptor subtypes; β_1, α_1, α_2=adrenergic receptor subtypes; C=cholera toxin; D_1, D_2=dopamine receptor subtypes; $G\alpha_t$=olfactory, but also found in limbic areas; $G\alpha_s$=stimulatory; $G\alpha_t$=transducin; GABA$_B$=γ-aminobutyric acid receptor subtype; 5-HT$_{1A}$, 5-HT$_{2C}$=serotonin receptor subtypes; M_1, M_2, M_3, M_5=muscarinic receptor subtypes; μ=opioid μ receptor; P=pertussis toxin; PLC=phospholipase C; RGS=regulators of G protein signaling; TxA$_2$=thromboxane A_2 receptor.
^{a}Although regulation of Na$^+$/H$^+$ exchange and Ca^{2+} channels by $G\alpha_{1-2}$ and $G\alpha_{1-3}$ has been demonstrated in artificial systems in vitro, these findings await definitive confirmation.
^{b}Effectors are regulated by $\beta\gamma$ subunits as a dimer.

ficking are leading to unexpected insights into the biochemical and functional properties of endocytic vesicles. Indeed, there is considerable excitement about our growing understanding of the diverse molecular mechanisms for signaling specificity and receptor trafficking, and the possibility that this knowledge could lead to highly selective therapeutics.

Receptor Tyrosine Kinases

The receptor tyrosine kinases, as their name implies, contain intrinsic tyrosine kinase activity and are generally utilized by growth factors, such as neurotrophic factors, and cytokines. Binding of an agonist initiates receptor dimerization and transphosphorylation of tyrosine residues in its cytoplasmic domain (Patapoutian and Reichardt 2001) (see Figure 1–1). The phosphotyrosine residues of the receptor function as binding sites for recruiting specific cytoplasmic signaling and scaffolding proteins. The ability of multiple effectors to interact with phosphotyrosines is undoubtedly one of the keys to the

pleiotropic effects that neurotrophins can exert. These pleiotropic and yet distinct effects of growth factors are mediated by varying degrees of activation of three major signaling pathways: the MAP kinase pathway, the phosphoinositide-3 (PI$_3$) kinase pathway, and the phospholipase C (PLC)–γ1 pathway (see Figure 1–9 later in this chapter).

Nuclear Receptors

Nuclear receptors are transcription factors that regulate the expression of target genes in response to steroid hormones and other ligands. Many hormones (including glucocorticoids, gonadal steroids, and thyroid hormones) are able to rapidly penetrate into the lipid bilayer membrane, because of their lipophilic composition, and thereby directly interact with these cytoplasmic receptors inside the cell (see Figure 1–1). Upon activation by a hormone, the nuclear receptor–ligand complex translocates to the nucleus, where it binds to specific DNA sequences referred to as *hormone-responsive elements* (HREs), and subse-

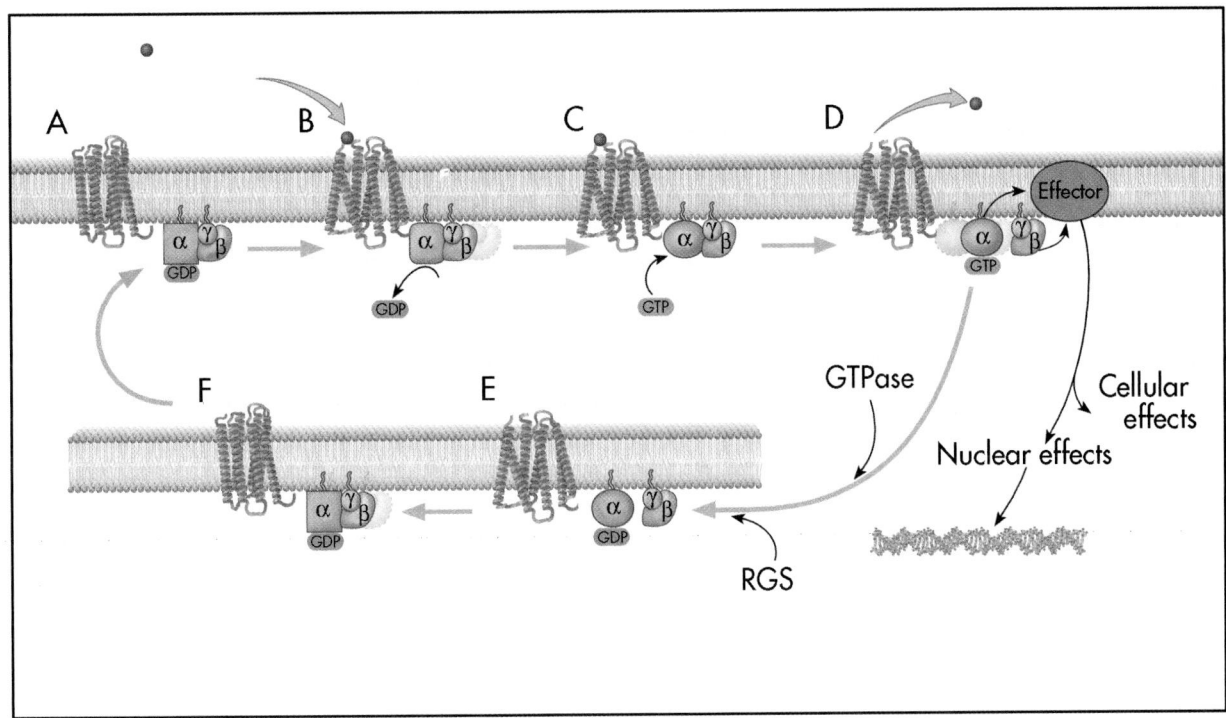

FIGURE 1–2.   G protein–coupled receptors and G protein activation.

All G proteins are heterotrimers consisting of α, β, and γ subunits. The receptor shuttles between a low-affinity form that is not coupled to a G protein and a high-affinity form that is coupled to a G protein. **(A)** At rest, G proteins are largely in their inactive state, namely, as αβγ heterotrimers, which have GDP (guanosine diphosphate) bound to the α subunit. **(B)** When a receptor is activated by a neurotransmitter, it undergoes a conformational (shape) change, forming a transient state referred to as a *high-affinity ternary complex,* comprising the agonist, receptor in a high-affinity state, and G protein. A consequence of the receptor interaction with the G protein is that the GDP comes off the G protein α subunit, leaving a very transient empty guanine nucleotide binding domain. **(C)** Guanine nucleotides (generally GTP) quickly bind to this nucleotide binding domain; thus, one of the major consequences of active receptor–G protein interaction is to facilitate guanine nucleotide exchange—this is basically the "on switch" for the G protein cycle. **(D)** A family of GTPase-activating proteins for G protein–coupled receptors has been identified, and they are called regulators of G protein signaling (RGS) proteins. Since activating GTPase activity facilitates the "turn off" reaction, these RGS proteins are involved in dampening the signal. Binding of GTP to the α subunit of G proteins results in subunit dissociation, whereby the α-GTP dissociates from the βγ subunits. Although not covalently bound, the β and γ subunits remain tightly associated and generally function as dimers. The α-GTP and βγ subunits are now able to activate multiple diverse effectors, thereby propagating the signal. While they are in their active states, the G protein subunits can activate multiple effector molecules in a "hit and run" manner; this results in major signal amplification (i.e., one active G protein subunit can activate multiple effector molecules; see Figure 1–11). The activated G protein subunits also dissociate from the receptor, converting the receptor to a low-affinity conformation and facilitating the dissociation of the agonist from the receptor. The agonist can now activate another receptor, and this also results in signal amplification. Together, these processes have been estimated to produce a 10,000-fold amplification of the signal in certain models. **(E)** Interestingly, the α subunit has intrinsic GTPase activity, which cleaves the third phosphate group from GTP (G-P-P-P) to GDP (G-P-P). Since α-GDP is an inactive state, the GTPase activity serves as a built-in timing mechanism, and this is the "turn off" reaction. **(F)** The reassociation of α-GDP with βγ is thermodynamically favored, and the reformation of the inactive heterotrimer (αβγ) completes the G protein cycle.

quently regulates gene transcription (Mangelsdorf et al. 1995; Truss and Beato 1993). Nuclear receptors often interact with a variety of coregulators that promote transcriptional activation when recruited (*coactivators*) and those that attenuate promoter activity (*corepressors*).

With this overview of neurotransmitters and receptor subtypes, we now turn to a discussion of selected individual neurotransmitters and neuropeptides before discussing the intricacies of cellular signal transduction systems.

Neurotransmitter and Neuropeptide Systems

Serotonergic System

Largely on the basis of the observation that most current effective antidepressants and antipsychotics target these systems, the monoaminergic systems (e.g., serotonin, norepinephrine, dopamine) have been extensively studied. Serotonin (5-HT) was given that name because of its activity as an endogenous vasoconstrictor in blood serum (Rapport et al. 1947). It was later acknowledged as being the same molecule (secretin) found in the intestinal mucosa and that is "secreted" by chromaffin cells (Brodie 1900). Following these findings, 5-HT soon became characterized as being a neurotransmitter in the CNS (Bogdansky et al. 1956).

5-HT-producing cell bodies in the brain are localized in the central gray, in the surrounding reticular formation, and in cell clusters located in the center, and thus the name *raphe* (from Latin, meaning midline) was adopted (Figure 1–3A) (discussed more extensively in Chapter 4, "Chemical Neuroanatomy of the Primate Brain"). The dorsal raphe (DR), the largest brain stem 5-HT nucleus, contains approximately 50% of the total 5-HT neurons in the mammalian CNS; in contrast, the medial raphe (MR) comprises 5% (Descarries et al. 1982; Wiklund and Bjorklund 1980). Serotonergic neurons project widely throughout the CNS rather than to discrete anatomical locations (as the dopaminergic neurons appear to do; see Figure 1–4A later in this chapter), leading to the suggestion that 5-HT exerts a major *modulatory* role throughout the CNS (Reader 1980). Interestingly, evidence suggests that infralimbic and prelimbic regions of the ventral medial prefrontal cortex (mPFCv) in rats are responsible for detecting whether a stressor is under the organism's control. When a stressor is controllable, stress-induced activation of the dorsal raphe nucleus is inhibited by the mPFCv, and the behavioral sequelae of the uncontrollable stress response are blocked (Amat et al. 2005). The organism's ability to regulate 5-HT neuron activity and function has been a major ongoing focus of psychiatric disorder research and treatments.

The precursor for 5-HT synthesis is L-tryptophan, an amino acid that comes primarily from the diet and crosses the blood–brain barrier through a carrier for large neutral amino acids. Tryptophan hydroxylase (TrpH) is the rate-limiting enzyme in serotonin biosynthesis (Figure 1–3B), and polymorphisms in this enzyme have been extensively investigated in psychiatric disorders, with equivocal results to date. A more fruitful research strategy in humans has been tryptophan depletion via dietary restriction to study the role of serotonin in the pathophysiology and treatment of psychiatric disorders (Bell et al. 2001). These studies have indicated that tryptophan depletion produces a rapid depressive relapse in patients treated with selective serotonin reuptake inhibitors (SSRIs) but not in those treated with norepinephrine reuptake inhibitors; the data suggesting induction of depressive symp-

toms in remitted patients or individuals with family histories of mood disorders are more equivocal (Bell et al. 2001).

Serotonin Transporters

As is the case for many classical neurotransmitters, termination of the effects of 5-HT in the synaptic cleft is brought about in large part by an active reuptake process mediated by the 5-HT transporter (5-HTT). 5-HT is taken up into the presynaptic terminals, where it is metabolized by the enzyme monoamine oxidase (MAO) or sequestered into secretory vesicles by the vesicle monoamine transporter (see Figure 1–3B). This presumably underlies the mechanism by which MAO inhibitors initiate their therapeutic effects; that is, the blockade of monoamine breakdown results in increasing the available pool for release when an action potential invades the nerve terminal. It is now well established that many tricyclic antidepressants and SSRIs exert their initial primary pharmacological effects by binding to the 5-HTT and blocking 5-HT reuptake, thereby increasing the intrasynaptic levels of 5-HT, which initiates a cascade of downstream effects (see Figure 1–3B for details). It has been hypothesized that the first step in 5-HT transport involves the binding of 5-HT to the 5-HTT and then a co-transport with Na^+, while the second step involves the translocation of K^+ across the membrane to the outside of the cell. SSRIs bind to the same site on the transporter as 5-HT itself. Recently, elegant biochemical and mutagenesis experiments have elucidated a leucine transporter from bacterial species, providing information that may aid in unraveling the complex process by which mammalian transporters couple ions and substrates to mediate neurotransmitter clearance (Henry et al. 2006).

In the brain, 5-HTTs have been radiolabeled with [3H]-imipramine (Hrdina et al. 1985; Langer et al. 1980) and with SSRIs such as [3H]cyanoimipramine (Wolf and Bobik 1988), [3H]paroxetine (Habert et al. 1985), and [3H]citalopram (D'Amato et al. 1987). The regional distribution of 5-HTT corresponds to discrete regions of rat brain known to contain cell bodies of 5-HT neurons and synaptic axon terminals, most notably the cerebral cortex, neostriatum, thalamus, and limbic areas (Cooper et al. 2001; Hrdina et al. 1990; Madden 2002). The specific cellular localization of 5-HTT in the CNS has also been accomplished by using site-specific antibodies (Lawrence et al. 1995a). Immunohistochemical studies utilizing antibodies against the 5-HT carrier have revealed both neuronal and glial staining in areas of the rat brain containing 5-HT somata and terminals (i.e., DR and hippoc-ampus) (Lawrence et al. 1995b). Experimental alter-ations of 5-HTT in young mice for a brief period during early development indicate abnormal emotional behav-ior in the same mice later in life, similar to the phenotype in mice where 5-HTT is deficient throughout life (An-sorge et al. 2004). This suggests the necessity of 5-HT early in emotional development and provides a possible mechanism by which genetic changes in the 5-HTT sys-tem may lead to susceptibility to developing psychiatric diseases such as depression (Caspi et al. 2003). Further-more, 5-HT uptake ability has been documented in pri-mary astrocyte cultures (Kimelberg and Katz 1985) and has been postulated to account for considerable 5-HT up-take in the frontal cortex and periventricular region (Ravid et al. 1992). Since 5-HTT is transcribed from a single copy gene, abnormalities in platelet 5-HTT have been postulated to reflect CNS abnormalities (Owens and Nemeroff 1998). A number of studies on platelet 5-HTT density have been undertaken using [3H]imip-ramine binding or [3H]paroxetine binding in mood disor-ders. Although the results of these studies are not entirely consistent, in toto the results suggest that the B_{max} value for platelet 5-HT density is significantly lower in de-pressed subjects compared with healthy control subjects (Owens and Nemeroff 1998).

Serotonin Receptors

In 1957, the existence of two separate 5-HT receptors was first proposed primarily because of the opposing phenom-enon this neurotransmitter produces in reference to cho-linergic mediation of smooth muscle contraction (Gad-dum and Picarelli 1957). Today, through the use of more precise molecular cloning and pharmacological and bio-chemical studies, seven distinct 5-HT receptor families have been identified (5-HT$_{1-7}$), many of which contain several subtypes. With the exception of the 5-HT$_3$ recep-tor, which is an excitatory ionotropic receptor, all of the other 5-HT receptors are GPCRs. The 5-HT$_{1A,B,D,E,F}$ receptor subtypes are negatively coupled to adenylyl cyclase, the 5-HT$_{2A,B,C}$ subtypes are positively coupled to PLC, and the 5-HT$_{4,5,6,7}$ subtypes are positively coupled to adenylyl cyclase (see Figure 1–3B) (Humphrey et al. 1993).

5-HT$_1$ receptors.   5-HT$_{1A}$ receptors are found in par-ticularly high density in several limbic structures, includ-ing the hippocampus, septum, amygdala, and entorhinal cortex, as well as on serotonergic neuron cell bodies,

where they serve as autoreceptors regulating 5-HT neu-ronal firing rates (Blier et al. 1998; Cooper et al. 2001; Pa-zos and Palacios 1985). The highest density of labeling is found in the DR, with lower densities observed in the re-maining raphe nuclei (Pazos and Palacios 1985). The density and mRNA expression of 5-HT$_{1A}$ receptors ap-pear insensitive to reductions in 5-HT transmission asso-ciated with lesioning the raphe or administering the sero-tonin-depleting agent *p*-chlorophenylalanine (PCPA). Similarly, elevation of 5-HT transmission resulting from chronic administration of an SSRI or monoamine oxidase inhibitor (MAOI) does not consistently alter 5-HT$_{1A}$ re-ceptor density or mRNA in the cortex, hippocampus, amygdala, or hypothalamus. In contrast to the insensitiv-ity to 5-HT, 5-HT$_{1A}$ receptor density is downregulated by adrenal steroids. Postsynaptic 5-HT$_{1A}$ receptor gene ex-pression is under tonic inhibition by adrenal steroids in the hippocampus and some other regions. Thus, in ro-dents, hippocampal 5-HT$_{1A}$ receptor mRNA expression is increased by adrenalectomy and decreased by cortico-sterone administration or chronic stress. The stress-induced downregulation of 5-HT$_{1A}$ receptor expression is prevented by adrenalectomy. Mineralocorticoid receptor stimulation has the most potent effect on downregulating 5-HT$_{1A}$ receptors, although glucocorticoid receptor stim-ulation also contributes to this effect.

In addition to being expressed on neurons, postsynap-tic 5-HT$_{1A}$ receptors are also abundantly expressed by as-trocytes and some other glia (Whitaker-Azmitia et al. 1990) (see Figure 1–7 later in this chapter). Stimulation of astrocyte-based 5-HT$_{1A}$ sites causes astrocytes to acquire a more mature morphology and to release the trophic factor S-100β, which promotes growth and arborization of sero-tonergic axons. Administration of 5-HT$_{1A}$ receptor an-tagonists, antibodies to S-100β, or agents that deplete 5-HT produces similar losses of dendrites, spines, and/or synapses in adult and developing animals—effects that are blocked by administration of 5-HT$_{1A}$ receptor ago-nists or SSRIs. These observations have led to the hy-pothesis that a reduction of 5-HT$_{1A}$ receptor function may play an important role in mood disorders that are known to be associated with glial reductions (Manji et al. 2001). The use of conditional knockouts of the 5-HT$_{1A}$ receptor, in which gene expression is altered only in par-ticular anatomical regions and/or during particular times, has illustrated the caution necessary in attributing com-plex behaviors to simple "too much" or "too little" neuro-transmitter/receptor hypotheses. Using a knockout/res-cue approach with regional and temporal specificity, Gross et al. (2002) demonstrated that the anxiety-related

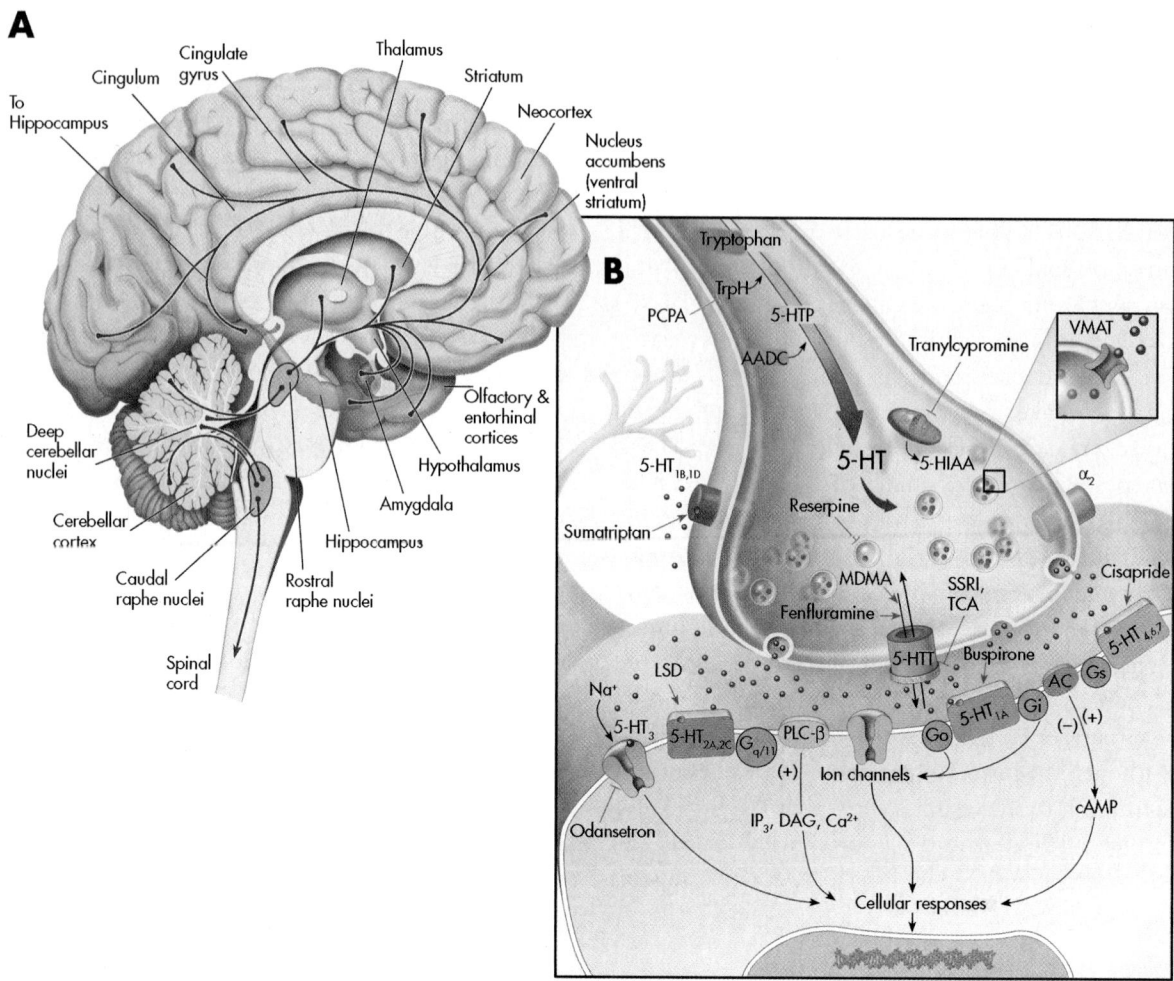

effect of the 5-HT$_{1A}$ receptor knockout was actually developmental. Specifically, expression limited to the hippocampus and cortex during early postnatal development was sufficient to counteract the anxious phenotype of the mutant, even though the receptor was still absent in adulthood (Gross et al. 2002). As is discussed in the chapters on antidepressants and anxiolytics (see Chapters 12–26), there is growing interest in the observation that antidepressants enhance hippocampal neurogenesis (Duman 2002; Malberg et al. 2000). It is noteworthy that preliminary data suggest that 5-HT$_{1A}$ receptor activation is required for SSRI-induced hippocampal neurogenesis in mice (Jacobs et al. 2000). Altering 5-HT levels with the SSRI fluoxetine does not affect division of stem cells in the dentate gyrus, but rather increases symmetric divisions of an early progenitor cell class that exists after stem cell division (Encinas et al. 2006).

5-HT$_{1A}$ receptors are now known to utilize a variety of signaling mechanisms to bring about their effects in distinct brain areas. Thus, somatodendritic 5-HT$_{1A}$ re-

ceptors appear to inhibit the firing of serotonergic neurons by opening a K$^+$ channel through a pertussis toxin–sensitive G protein (likely G$_o$, discussed later in the section on G proteins) (Andrade et al. 1986), as well as by reducing cAMP levels. Postsynaptic 5-HT$_{1A}$ receptors appear to exert many of their effects by inhibiting adenylyl cyclase via G$_i$ (De Vivo and Maayani 1990) but have also been demonstrated to potentiate the activity of certain adenylyl cyclases (Bourne and Nicoll 1993) and to stimulate inositol-1,4,5-triphosphate (IP$_3$) production and activate PKC (Y.F. Liu and Albert 1991).

5-HT$_{1D}$ receptors are virtually absent in the rodent but have been detected in guinea pig and man (Bruinvels et al. 1993). On the basis of an approximately 74% sequence homology, it has been proposed that 5-HT$_{1B}$ receptors are the rodent homolog of 5-HT$_{1D}$ receptors (see Saxena et al. 1998). Furthermore, the distribution of the 5-HT$_{1D}$ receptors in guinea pig and man is roughly equivalent to that of the 5-HT$_{1B}$ receptors in the rat (Bruinvels et al. 1993). Both 5-HT$_{1B}$ and 5-HT$_{1D}$ receptors have

FIGURE 1-3. The serotonergic system *(opposite page)*.

This figure depicts the location of the major serotonin (5-HT)–producing cells (raphe nuclei) innervating brain structures **(A),** and various cellular regulatory processes involved in serotonergic neurotransmission **(B).** 5-HT neurons project widely throughout the CNS and innervate virtually every part of the neuroaxis. L-Tryptophan, an amino acid actively transported into presynaptic 5-HT-containing terminals, is the precursor for 5-HT. It is converted to 5-hydroxytryptophan (5-HTP) by the rate-limiting enzyme tryptophan hydroxylase (TrpH). This enzyme is effectively inhibited by the drug *p*-chlorophenylalanine (PCPA). Aromatic amino acid decarboxylase (AADC) converts 5-HTP to 5-HT. Once released from the presynaptic terminal, 5-HT can interact with a variety (15 different types) of presynaptic and postsynaptic receptors. Presynaptic regulation of 5-HT neuron firing activity and release occurs through somatodendritic 5-HT_{1A} (not shown) and $5\text{-HT}_{1B,1D}$ autoreceptors, respectively, located on nerve terminals. Sumatriptan is a $5\text{-HT}_{1B,1D}$ receptor agonist. (The antimigraine effects of this agent are likely mediated by local activation of this receptor subtype on blood vessels, which results in their constriction.) Buspirone is a partial 5-HT_{1A} agonist that activates both pre- and postsynaptic receptors. Cisapride is a preferential 5-HT_4 receptor agonist that is used to treat irritable bowel syndrome as well as nausea associated with antidepressants. The binding of 5-HT to G protein receptors (G_o, G_i, etc.) that are coupled to adenylyl cyclase (AC) and phospholipase C–β (PLC-β) will result in the production of a cascade of second-messenger and cellular effects. Lysergic acid diethylamide (LSD) likely interacts with numerous 5-HT receptors to mediate its effects. Pharmacologically this ligand is often used as a 5-HT_2 receptor agonist in receptor binding experiments. Ondansetron is a 5-HT_3 receptor antagonist that is marketed as an antiemetic agent for chemotherapy patients but is also given to counteract side effects produced by antidepressants in some patients. 5-HT has its action terminated in the synapse by rapidly being taken back into the presynaptic neuron through 5-HT transporters (5-HTT). Once inside the neuron, it can either be repackaged into vesicles for reuse or undergo enzymatic catabolism. The selective 5-HT reuptake inhibitors (SSRIs) and older-generation tricyclic antidepressants (TCAs) are able to interfere/block the reuptake of 5-HT. 5-HT is then metabolized to 5-hydroxyindoleacetic acid (5-HIAA) by monoamine oxidase (MAO), located on the outer membrane of mitochondria or sequestered and stored in secretory vesicles by vesicle monoamine transporters (VMATs). Reserpine causes a depletion of 5-HT in vesicles by interfering with uptake and storage mechanisms (depressive-like symptoms have been reported with this agent). Tranylcypromine is an MAO inhibitor (MAOI) and an effective antidepressant. Fenfluramine (an anorectic agent) and MDMA ("Ecstasy") are able to facilitate 5-HT release by altering 5-HTT function. DAG=diacylglycerol; 5-HTT=serotonin transporter; IP_3=inositol-1,4,5-triphosphate.
Source. Adapted from Cooper JR, Bloom FE, Roth RH: *The Biochemical Basis of Neuropharmacology*, 7th Edition. New York, Oxford University Press, 2001. Copyright 1970, 1974, 1978, 1982, 1986, 1991, 1996, 2001 by Oxford University Press, Inc. Used by permission of Oxford University Press, Inc. Modified from Nestler et al. 2001.

been proposed to represent the major nerve terminal autoreceptors regulating the amount of 5-HT released per nerve impulse (Pineyro and Blier 1999) (see Figure 1–3B). Like 5-HT_{1A} receptors, 5-HT_{1B} and 5-HT_{1D} receptors inhibit cAMP formation and stimulate IP_3 production and activate PKC (Schoeffter and Bobirnac 1995). As we discuss later, this appears to be the case for many receptors coupled to G_i and G_o (see Table 1–1). The α subunits of the G protein (α_i and α_o) inhibit adenylyl cyclase and regulate ion channels, respectively, whereas the βγ subunits activate PLC isozymes to stimulate IP_3 production and activate PKC.

Finally, it should be noted that the 5-HT_{1C} receptor classification has been revoked, as these receptors have structural and transductional similarities to the 5-HT_2 receptor class (Hoyer et al. 1986; Saxena et al. 1998).

5-HT_2 receptors.   There are three subtypes of 5-HT_2 receptors: 5-HT_{2A}, 5-HT_{2B}, and 5-HT_{2C}. The highest level of 5-HT_{2A} binding sites and mRNA for these receptors exists in the cortex, and these receptors have been implicated in the psychotomimetic effects of agents like lysergic acid diethylamide (LSD) (for a review, see Aghajanian and Marek 1999). In addition, lesioning of 5-HT neurons with 5,7-DHT does not reduce the 5-HT_2 receptor density reported in brain regions (Hoyer et al. 1986),

indicating that these receptors are primarily (if not exclusively) postsynaptic. Autoradiography performed with the potent and selective radioligand [^{3}H]MDL 100,907 has localized 5-HT_{2A} receptors to many similar brain regions in the rat and primate brain (Lopez-Gimenez et al. 1997). Recent experiments show that mice expressing 5-HT_{2A} receptors only in the frontal cortex have conserved receptor signaling and behavioral responses to hallucinogenic drugs similar to those of wild-type littermates, suggestive of cortical importance (Gonzalez-Maeso et al. 2007). Competition studies with other radioligands (Westphal and Sanders-Bush 1994) and their mRNA distribution indicate that 5-HT_{2C} receptors are considerably widespread throughout the CNS, with the highest density in the choroid plexus (Hoffman and Mezey 1989). 5-HT_{2B} receptors are detected sparingly in the brain and are more prominently located in the fundus, gut, kidney, lungs, and heart (Hoyer et al. 1986).

Several antidepressants (e.g., mianserin, mirtazapine) and antipsychotics (e.g., clozapine) bind to 5-HT_2 receptors, raising the possibility that blockade of 5-HT_2 receptors may play an important role in the therapeutic efficacy of these agents. Indeed, a leading hypothesis concerning the mechanism of action of atypical antipsychotic agents suggests that the ratio of D_2/5-HT_2 blockade confers "atypicality" properties on many currently available antipsychotic agents (Meltzer 2002). Evidence from animal experiments in which cortical 5-HT$_{2A}$ receptors are disrupted indicates a specific role of these receptors in modulation of conflict anxiety without affecting fear conditioning and depression-like behaviors (Weisstaub et al. 2006). Furthermore, chronic administration of many antidepressants downregulates 5-HT$_2$ receptors, suggesting that this effect may be important for their efficacy (J. A. Scott and Crews 1986); however, chronic electroconvulsive shock (ECS) appears to upregulate 5-HT$_2$ expression, precluding a simple mechanism for antidepressant efficacy. The obesity seen in 5-HT$_{2C}$ knockout animals suggests that in addition to histamine receptor blockade, 5-HT$_{2C}$ blockade may play a role in the weight gain observed with certain psychotropic agents; this is an area of considerable current research. In keeping, recent evidence suggests that the weight gain "orexigenic" properties of atypical antipsychotics are likely due to potent activation of hypothalamic AMP-kinase through histamine$_1$ (H$_1$) receptors (Kim et al. 2007). The regulation of 5-HT$_2$ receptors is intriguing, as not only is it important in psychiatric disorders and therapeutic benefit, but both agonists and antagonists appear to cause an internalization of the receptor. Moreover, emerging data suggest that mRNA editing may play an important role in regulating the levels and activity of this receptor subtype (Niswender et al. 1998). All of the 5-HT$_2$ receptor subtypes are linked to the phosphoinositide signaling system, and their activation produces IP$_3$ and diacylglycerol (DAG), via PLC activation (Conn and Sanders-Bush 1987) (see Figure 1–3B).

An exciting recent pharmacogenetic investigation searched for genetic predictors of treatment outcome in 1,953 patients with major depressive disorder who were treated with the antidepressant citalopram in the Sequenced Treatment Alternatives to Relieve Depression (STAR*D) study and prospectively assessed (McMahon et al. 2006). In a split-sample design, a selection of 68 candidate genes was genotyped, with 768 single-nucleotide-polymorphism markers chosen to detect common genetic variation. A significant and reproducible association was detected between treatment outcome and a marker in HTR2A ($P = 1 \times 10^{-6}$ to 3.7×10^{-5} in the total sample). The "A" allele (associated with better outcome) was six times more frequent in white than in black participants, for whom treatment was also less effective in this sample (McMahon et al. 2006). The "A" allele may thus contribute to racial differences in outcomes of antidepressant treatment. Taken together with prior neurobiological findings, these new genetic data make a compelling

case for a key role of HTR2A in the mechanism of antidepressant action.

5-HT$_{3–7}$ receptors.   Unlike the other 5-HT receptors, 5-HT$_3$ receptors are ligand-gated ion channels capable of mediating fast synaptic responses (see Figure 1–3B). The cis-trans isomerization and molecular rearrangement at proline 8 is the structural mechanism that opens the 5-HT$_3$ receptor protein pore (Lummis et al. 2005). 5-HT$_3$ receptors are present in multiple brain areas, including the hippocampus, dorsal motor nucleus of the solitary tract, and area postrema (Laporte et al. 1992). The 5-HT$_3$ receptor is effectively modulated by a variety of compounds, such as alcohols and anesthetics, and antagonists against this receptor are used as effective antiemetics in patients who are undergoing chemotherapy (e.g., ondansetron). 5-HT$_4$, 5-HT$_6$, and 5-HT$_7$ are GPCRs that are preferentially coupled to Gs and activate adenylyl cyclases (see Figure 1–3B). 5-HT$_4$ receptors are able to modulate the release of monoamines and GABA in the brain. 5-HT$_5$ receptors are located in the hypothalamus, hippocampus, corpus callosum, cerebral ventricles, and glia (Hoyer et al. 2002). The 5-HT$_{5A}$ receptor is negatively coupled to adenylyl cyclase, whereas the 5-HT$_{5B}$ receptor does not involve cAMP accumulation or phosphoinositide turnover. 5-HT$_6$ receptors are located in the striatum, amygdala, nucleus accumbens, hippocampus, cortex, and olfactory tubercle (Hoyer et al. 2002). Of interest, many antipsychotic agents and antidepressants have high affinity for 5-HT$_6$ receptors and act as antagonists at this receptor. 5-HT$_7$ receptors have been localized to the cerebral cortex, medial thalamic nuclei, substantia nigra, central gray, and dorsal raphe nucleus (Hoyer et al. 2002). It appears that chronic treatment with antidepressants is able to downregulate this receptor, whereas acute stress has been reported to alter 5-HT$_7$ expression (Sleight et al. 1995; Yau et al. 2001).

Dopaminergic System

Dopamine (DA) was originally thought to simply be a precursor of norepinephrine (NE) and epinephrine synthesis, but the demonstration that its distribution in the brain was quite distinct to that of NE led to extensive research demonstrating its role as a unique critical neurotransmitter. DA synthesis requires transport of the amino acid L-tyrosine across the blood–brain barrier and into the cell. Once tyrosine enters the neuron, the rate-limiting step for DA synthesis is conversion of L-tyrosine to L-dihydroxyphenylalanine (L-dopa) by the enzyme tyrosine hydroxylase (TH); L-dopa is readily converted to dopamine and, hence, is used as a precursor strategy to correct a dopamine deficiency in the treatment of Parkinson's disease (Figure 1–4B). The activity of TH can be regulated by many factors, including the activity of catecholamine neurons; furthermore, catecholamines function as end-product inhibitors of TH by competing with a tetrahydrobiopterin cofactor (Cooper et al. 2001).

In contrast to the widespread 5-HT and NE projections, DA neurons form more discrete circuits, with the nigrostriatal, mesolimbic, tuberoinfundibular, and tuberohypophysial pathways comprising the major CNS dopaminergic circuits (Figure 1–4A). The nigrostriatal circuit is composed of DA neurons from the mesencephalic reticular formation (region A8) and the pars compacta region of the substantia nigra (region A9) of the mesencephalon. These neurons give rise to axons that travel via the medial forebrain bundle to innervate the caudate nucleus and putamen (see Anden et al. 1964; Ungerstedt 1971). The DA neurons that make up the nigrostriatal circuit have been assumed to be critical for maintaining normal motor control, since destruction of these neurons is associated with Parkinson's disease; however, it is now clear that these projections subserve a variety of additional functions. For example, recent evidence from human brain imaging studies indicates that a subject's ability to choose rewarding actions during instrumental learning tasks can be modulated by administration of drugs that enhance or reduce striatal DA receptor activation. This further implies that the DA reward pathway in the brain is likely convergent on many discrete brain circuits and neurotransmitter alterations, and it shows that striatal activity can also account for how the human brain proceeds toward making future decisions based on reward prediction (Pessiglione et al. 2006).

The mesolimbic DA circuit consists of DA neurons located in the midbrain just medial to the A9 cells in an area termed the ventral tegmental area (VTA) (Cooper et al. 2001; Nestler et al. 2001; Squire et al. 2003). This circuit shares some similarities to the nigrostriatal circuit in that it is a parallel circuit consisting of axons that make up the medial forebrain bundle. However, these axons ascend through the lateral hypothalamus and project to the nucleus accumbens, olfactory tubercle, bed nucleus of the stria terminalis, lateral septum, and frontal, cingulate, and entorhinal regions of the cerebral cortex (Cooper et al. 2001). This circuit innervates many limbic structures known to play critical roles in motivational, motor, and reward pathways and has therefore been implicated in a va-

riety of clinical conditions, including psychosis and drug abuse (Cooper et al. 2001). Data also suggest a potential role for dopamine—and, in particular, mesolimbic pathways—in the pathophysiology of bipolar mania as well as bipolar and unipolar depression (Beaulieu et al. 2004; Dunlop and Nemeroff 2007; Goodwin and Jamison 2007; Roybal et al. 2007). It is perhaps surprising that the role of the dopaminergic system in the pathophysiology of mood disorders has not received greater study, since it represents a prime candidate on a number of theoretical grounds. The motoric changes in bipolar disorder are perhaps the most defining characteristics of the illness, ranging from the near-catatonic immobility of depressive states to the profound hyperactivity of manic states. Similarly, loss of motivation is one of the central features of depression, whereas anhedonia and "hyperhedonic states" are among the most defining characteristics of bipolar depression and mania, respectively. In this context, it is noteworthy that the midbrain dopaminergic system is known to play a critical role in regulating not only motoric activity but also motivational and reward circuits. It is clear that motivation and motor function are closely linked and that motivational variables can influence motor output both qualitatively and quantitatively. Furthermore, there is considerable evidence that the mesolimbic dopaminergic pathway plays a crucial role in the selection and orchestration of goal-directed behaviors, particularly those elicited by incentive stimuli (Goodwin and Jamison 2007).

The firing pattern of mesolimbic DA neurons appears to be an important regulatory mechanism; thus, in rats, electrical or glutamatergic stimulation of medial prefrontal cortex elicits a burst firing pattern of dopaminergic cells in the VTA and increases DA release in the nucleus accumbens (Murase et al. 1993; Taber and Fibiger 1993). The burst firing of DA cell activity elicits more terminal DA release per action potential than the nonbursting pacemaker firing pattern (Roth et al. 1987). The phasic burst firing of DA neurons and accompanying rise in DA release normally occur in response to primary rewards (until they become fully predicted) and reward-predicting stimuli. Such a role has also been postulated to provide a neural mechanism by which prefrontal cortex dysfunction could alter hedonic perceptions and motivated behavior in mood disorders (Drevets et al. 2002). Recent studies indicate that the amygdala is important in learning new cocaine drug-seeking responses as well as the habit-forming properties of cocaine (Lee et al. 2005), expanding our knowledge of drug addiction circuits in the brain.

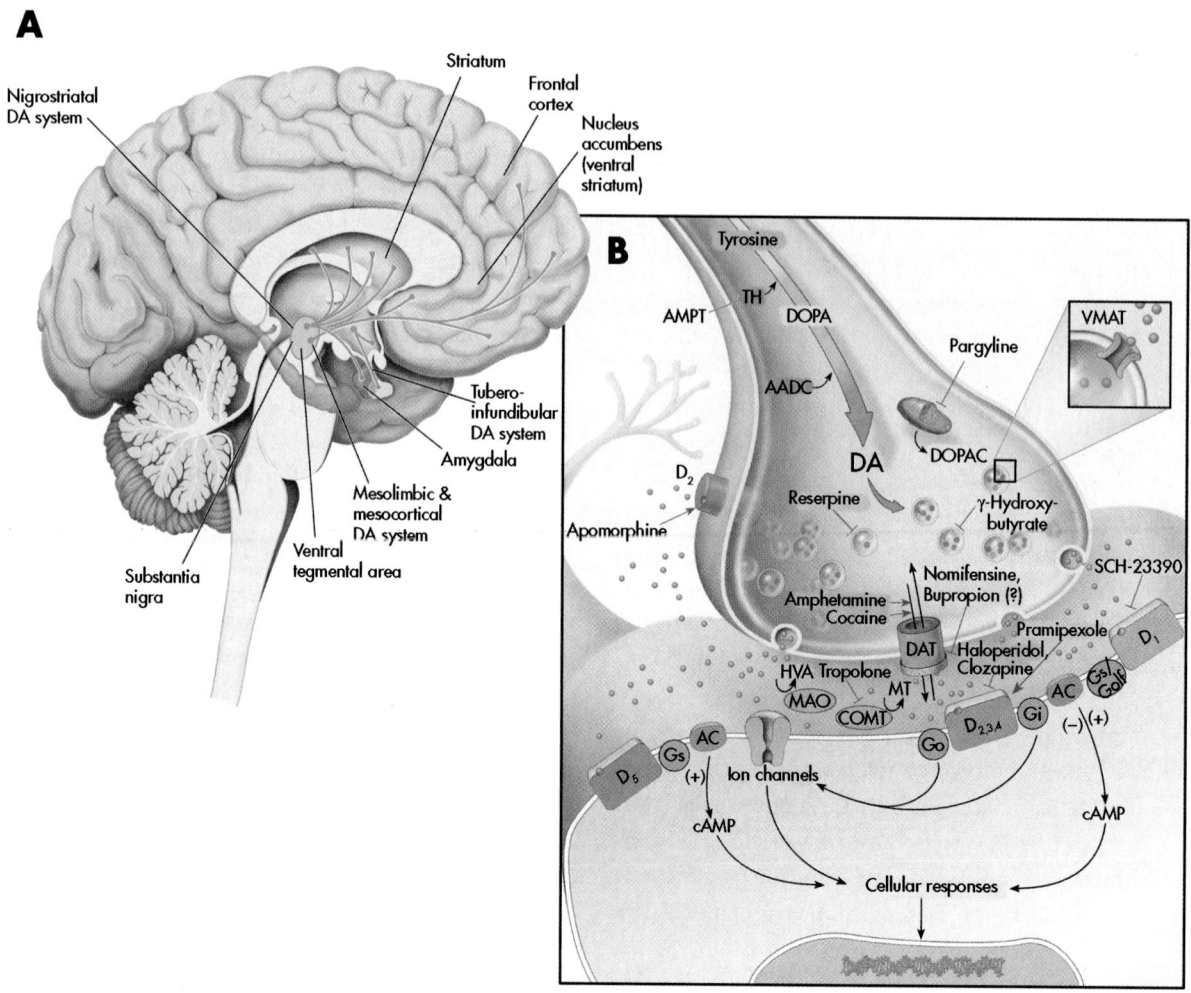

Dopamine Transporters

As with serotonin, the DA signal in the synaptic cleft is terminated primarily by reuptake into the presynaptic terminal. The dopamine transporter (DAT) comprises 12 putative transmembrane domains and is located somatodendritically as well as on DA nerve terminals (see Figure 1–4B). Like other monoamine transporters, the DAT functions as a Na^+/K^+ pump to clear DA from the synaptic cleft upon its release. However, data suggest that many drugs of abuse are capable of altering the function of these transporters. Thus, the amphetamines are thought to mediate their effects, in part, by reversing the direction of the transporter so that it *releases* DA. Cocaine is capable of blocking the reuptake of DAT, leading to an increase in DA in the synaptic cleft. Of interest, altered neuronal long-term potentiation in the VTA in response to chronic cocaine exposure has been recently linked to drug-associated memory and likely contributes to the powerful addictive potential of this drug of abuse (Q.S.

Liu et al. 2005). DA in the medial frontal cortex is taken up predominantly by the NE transporter. Although the precise functional significance of this finding is not currently known, it goes against the dogma of transporters being able to selectively take up only their respective neurotransmitter. Furthermore, this provides a mechanism by which NE reuptake–inhibiting antidepressants may also increase synaptic levels of DA in the frontal cortex, effects that may be therapeutically very important.

Dopaminergic Receptors

The existence of two subtypes of DA receptors, dopamine$_1$ (D_1) and dopamine$_2$ (D_2), was initially established using classic pharmacological techniques in the 1970s (Stoof and Kebabian 1984). Subsequent molecular biological studies have shown that the D_1 family contains both the D_1 and dopamine$_5$ (D_5) receptors, whereas the D_2 family contains the D_2, dopamine$_3$ (D_3), and dopamine$_4$ (D_4) receptors (Cooper et al. 2001). D_1 receptor family members

FIGURE 1–4. The dopaminergic system *(opposite page)*.

This figure depicts the dopaminergic projections throughout the brain **(A)** and various regulatory processes involved in dopaminergic neurotransmission **(B)**. The amino acid l-tyrosine is actively transported into presynaptic dopamine (DA) nerve terminals, where it is ultimately converted into DA. The rate-limiting step is conversion of L-tyrosine to L-dihydroxyphenylalanine (L-dopa) by the enzyme tyrosine hydroxylase (TH). α-Methyl-*p*-tyrosine (AMPT) is a competitive inhibitor of tyrosine hydroxylase and has been used to assess the impact of reduced catecholaminergic function in clinical studies. The production of DA requires that L-aromatic amino acid decarboxylase (AADC) act on L-dopa. Thus, the administration of L-dopa to patients with Parkinson's disease bypasses the rate-limiting step and is able to produce DA quite readily. DA has its action terminated in the synapse by rapidly being taken back into the presynaptic neuron through DA transporters (DATs). DA is then metabolized to dihydroxyphenyla-lanine (DOPAC) by intraneuronal monoamine oxidase (MAO; preferentially by the MAO-B subtype) located on the outer membrane of mito-chondria, or is sequestered and stored in secretory vesicles by vesicle monoamine transporters (VMATs). Reserpine causes a depletion of DA in vesicles by interfering and irreversibly damaging uptake and storage mechanisms. γ-Hydroxybutyrate inhibits the release of DA by blocking impulse propagation in DA neurons. Pargyline inhibits MAO and may have efficacy in treating parkinsonian symptoms by augmenting DA levels through inhibition of DA catabolism. Other clinically used inhibitors of MAO are nonselective and thus likely elevate the levels of DA, norepinephrine, and serotonin. Once released from the presynaptic terminal (because of an action potential and calcium influx), DA can interact with five different G protein–coupled receptors (D_1–D_5), which belong to either the D_1 or D_2 receptor family. Presynaptic regulation of DA neuron firing activity and release occurs through somatodendritic (not shown) and nerve terminal D_2 autoreceptors, respectively. Pramipexole is a D_2/D_3 receptor agonist and has been documented to have efficacy as an augmentation strategy in cases of treatment-resistant depression and in the management of Parkinson's disease. The binding of DA to G protein receptors (G_o, G_i, etc.) positively or negatively coupled to adenylyl cyclase (AC) results in the activation or inhibition of this enzyme, respectively, and the production of a cascade of second-messenger and cellular effects (see diagram). Apomorphine is a D_1/D_2 receptor agonist that has been used clinically to aid in the treatment of Parkinson's disease. (SKF-82958 is a pharmacologically selective D_1 receptor agonist.) SCH-23390 is a D_1/D_5 receptor antagonist. There are likely physiological differences between D_1 and D_5 receptors, but the current unavailability of selective pharmacological agents has precluded an adequate differentiation thus far. Haloperidol is a D_2 receptor antagonist, and clozapine is a nonspecific D_2/D_4 receptor antagonist (both are effective antipsychotic agents). Once inside the neuron, DA can either be repackaged into vesicles for reuse or undergo enzymatic catabolism. Nomifensine is able to interfere/block the reuptake of DA. The antidepressant bupropion has affinity for the dopaminergic system, but it is not known whether this agent mediates its effects through DA or possibly by augmenting other monoamines. DA can be degraded to homovanillic acid (HVA) through the sequential action of catechol-O-methyltransferase (COMT) and MAO. Tropolone is an inhibitor of COMT. Evidence suggests that the COMT gene may be linked to schizophrenia (Akil et al. 2003).

Source.   Adapted from Cooper JR, Bloom FE, Roth RH: *The Biochemical Basis of Neuropharmacology,* 7th Edition. New York, Oxford University Press, 2001. Copyright 1970, 1974, 1978, 1982, 1986, 1991, 1996, 2001 by Oxford University Press, Inc. Used by permission of Oxford University Press, Inc.

were originally defined solely on the ability to stimulate adenylyl cyclase (AC), while the D_2 family inhibited the enzyme. Interestingly, DA receptors complexed with subunits from other subclasses of DA receptors within a receptor family are able to form distinct hetero-oligomeric receptors (also termed "kissing cousin receptors"). Notably, hetero-oligomeric D_1–D_2 receptor complexes in the brain require binding to active sites of both receptor subtypes to induce activation of the hetero-oligomeric receptor complex. These receptors have been demonstrated to use traditional D_1 receptor intracellular signaling components of $G_{q/11}$ and Ca^{2+}/calmodulin–dependent protein kinase II (CaMKII) second-messenger activation as demonstrated in the nucleus accumbens (Rashid et al. 2007). This work suggests possible avenues through which the brain might use different receptor subunit proportions to further fine-tune brain neurophysiology.

D_1 and D_5 receptors.   The D_1 and D_5 receptors stimulate adenylyl cyclase activity via the activation of G_s or G_{olf} (a G protein originally thought to be present exclusively in olfactory tissue but now known to be abundantly present in limbic areas) (see Figure 1–4B). Other second-

messenger pathways have also been reported to be activated by D_1 receptors, effects that may play a role in the reported D_1–D_2 cross-talk (Clark and White 1987). The frontal cortex contains almost exclusively D_1 receptors (Clark and White 1987), suggesting that this receptor may play an important role in higher cognitive function and perhaps in the actions of medications like methylphenidate. The D_5 receptor is a neuron-specific receptor that is located primarily in limbic areas of the brain.

D_2 receptors.   Four types of D_2 receptors have been identified. The two subtypes of D_2 receptors (the short and long forms, D_{2S} and D_{2L}, respectively) are derived from alternative splicing of the D_2 gene. Although a seemingly identical pharmacological profile for these receptors exists, there are undoubtedly (yet to be discovered) physiological differences between the two subtypes. D_2 receptors mediate their cellular effects via the G_i/G_o proteins and thereby several effectors (see Figure 1–4B). In addition to the well-characterized inhibition of adenylyl cyclase, D_2 receptors in different brain areas also regulate PLC, bring changes in K^+ and Ca^{2+} currents, and possibly regulate phospholipase A_2. D_2 receptors are located on cell bodies and nerve terminals of DA neurons and function as autoreceptors. Thus, activation of somatodendritic D_2 receptors reduces DA neuron firing activity, likely via opening of K^+ channels, whereas activation of nerve-terminal D_2 autoreceptors reduces the amount of DA released per nerve impulse, in large part by closing voltage-gated Ca^{2+} channels. As discussed extensively in Chapters 27 and 46, D_2 receptors have long been implicated in the pathophysiology and treatment of schizophrenia. Recently, transgenic mice overexpressing D_2 receptors in the striatum have been found to display many phenotypic hallmarks of schizophrenia (Kellendonk et al. 2006).

D_3 receptors. D_3 receptors possess a different anatomical distribution than do D_2 receptors and, because of their preferential limbic expression, have been postulated to represent an important target for antipsychotic drugs. Numerous studies have investigated the position association of a polymorphism in the coding sequence of the D_3 receptor with schizophrenia, with equivocal results. It has been suggested that brain-derived neurotrophic factor (BDNF) may regulate behavioral sensitization via its effects on D_3 receptor expression (Guillin et al. 2001).

D_4 receptors.   The D_4 receptor has received much interest in psychopharmacological research in recent years because of the fact that clozapine has a high affinity for this receptor. Studies are currently under way that are investigating more selective D_4 antagonists as adjunctive agents in the treatment of schizophrenia. Furthermore, considerable attention has focused on the possibility that genetic D_4 variants may be associated with thrill-seeking behavior (Zuckerman 1985), attention-deficit/hyperactivity disorder (Roman et al. 2001), and responsiveness to clozapine (Van Tol et al. 1992).

Noradrenergic System

Named *sympathine* because it was initially encountered as being released by sympathetic nerve terminals, the molecule was later given the name *norepinephrine* after meeting the criteria for a neurotransmitter in the CNS (see Cooper et al. 2001). NE is produced from the amino acid precursor L-tyrosine found in neurons in the brain, chromaffin cells, sympathetic nerves, and ganglia. The enzyme dopamine β-hydroxylase (DBH) converts DA to NE, and as is the case for DA synthesis, tyrosine hydroxylase is the rate-limiting enzyme for NE synthesis (Figure 1–5B). The dietary depletion of tyrosine and α-methyl-*p*-tyrosine (a TH inhibitor) has played an important part in efforts

aimed at delineating the role of catecholamines in the pathophysiology and treatment of mood and anxiety disorders (Coupland et al. 2001; McCann et al. 1995).

There are seven NE cell groups in the mammalian CNS, designated A1 through A7. In the brain stem, these are the lateral tegmental neurons (A5 and A7) and the locus coeruleus (A6) (Dahlstrom 1971) (see Figure 1–5B). In general, the projections from A5 and A7 are more restricted to brain stem areas and do not interact with those of A6. The term *locus coeruleus* (LC) was derived from the Greek because of its saddle shape and its "bluish color" (*caeruleum*). The LC is the most widely projecting CNS nucleus known (Foote et al. 1983), responsible for approximately 90% of the NE innervation of the forebrain and 70% of the total NE in the brain (Figure 1–5A). Indeed, the LC NE neurons, although small in number, constitute a diffuse system of projections to widespread brain areas via highly branched axons. The extensive efferent innervation suggests that the LC plays a modulatory and integrative role, rather than a role in specific sensory or motor processing (Foote et al. 1983).

A number of physiological roles have been ascribed to the LC, notably in the control of vigilance and the initiation of adaptive behavioral responses (Foote et al. 1983). Considerable data support the hypothesis that NE neurons in the LC constitute a CNS response or defense system, since the neurons are activated by "challenges" in both the behavioral/environmental and the physiological domains (Jacobs et al. 1991). Thus, while a variety of sensory stimuli are capable of increasing LC activity, noxious or stressful stimuli are particularly potent in this regard. Moreover, considerable evidence also supports a role for LC NE neurons in the learning of aversively motivated tasks and in the conditioned response to stressful stimuli (Rasmussen et al. 1986a, 1986b), with obvious implications for a variety of psychiatric conditions (see Gould et al. 2003; Szabo and Blier 2001). Indeed, tonic activation of the LC appears to occur preferentially in the response to stressful stimuli, in contrast to stimuli limited to simply evoking activation or arousal (Rasmussen et al. 1986a, 1986b).

Norepinephrine Transporter

The norepinephrine transporter (NET), the first of the monoamine transporters to be cloned in humans, transports NE from the synaptic cleft back into the neuron (Pacholczyk et al. 1991). Like other monoamine transporters, NET comprises 12 putative transmembrane domains, and autoradiography with various NE reuptake inhibitors has

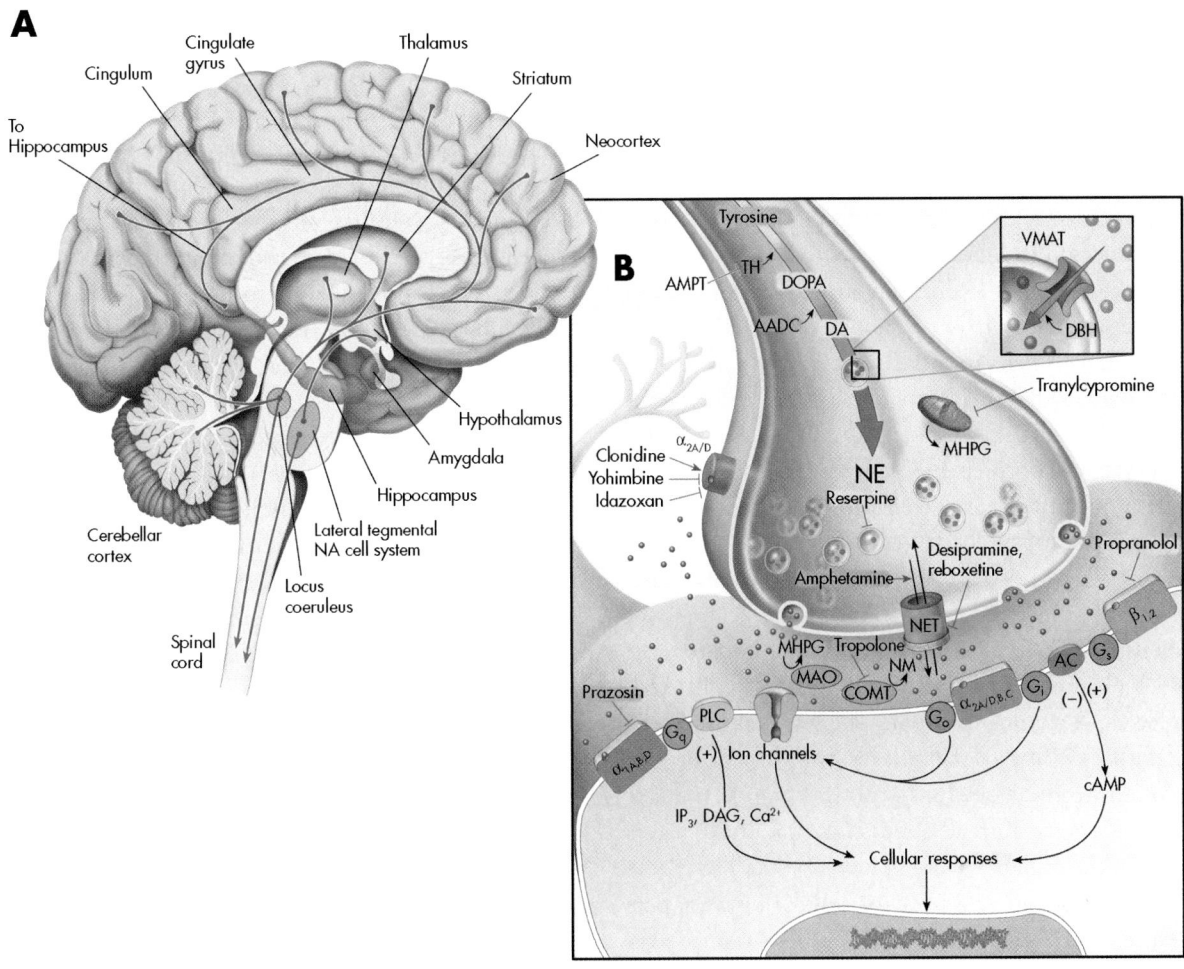

FIGURE 1–5. The noradrenergic system.

This figure depicts the noradrenergic projections throughout the brain **(A)** and the various regulatory processes involved in norepinephrine (NE) neurotransmission **(B)**. NE neurons innervate nearly all parts of the neuroaxis, with neurons in the locus coeruleus being responsible for most of the NE in the brain (90% of NE in the forebrain and 70% of total NE in the brain). The amino acid L-tyrosine is actively transported into presynaptic NE nerve terminals, where it is ultimately converted into NE. The rate-limiting step is conversion of L-tyrosine to L-dihydroxyphenylalanine (L-dopa) by the enzyme tyrosine hydroxylase (TH). α-Methyl-*p*-tyrosine (AMPT) is a competitive inhibitor of tyrosine hydroxylase and has been used to assess the impact of reduced catecholaminergic function in clinical studies. Aromatic amino acid decarboxylase (AADC) converts L-dopa to dopamine (DA). L-dopa then becomes decarboxylated by decarboxylase to form dopamine (DA). DA is then taken up from the cytoplasm into vesicles, by vesicle monoamine transporters (VMATs), and hydroxylated by dopamine β-hydroxylase (DBH) in the presence of O₂ and ascorbate to form NE. Normetanephrine (NM), which is formed by the action of COMT (catechol-O-methyltransferase) on NE, can be further metabolized by monoamine oxidase (MAO) and aldehyde reductase to 3-methoxy-4-hydroxyphenylglycol (MHPG). Reserpine causes a depletion of NE in vesicles by interfering with uptake and storage mechanisms (depressive-like symptoms have been reported with this hypertension). Once released from the presynaptic terminal, NE can interact with a variety of presynaptic and postsynaptic receptors. Presynaptic regulation of NE neuron firing activity and release occurs through somatodendritic (not shown) and nerve-terminal α₂ adrenoreceptors, respectively. Yohimbine potentiates NE neuronal firing and NE release by blocking these α₂ adrenoreceptors, thereby disinhibiting these neurons from a negative feedback influence. Conversely, clonidine attenuates NE neuron firing and release by activating these receptors. Idazoxan is a relatively selective α₂ adrenoreceptor antagonist primarily used for pharmacological purposes. The binding of NE to G protein receptors (Gₒ, Gᵢ, etc.) that are coupled to adenylyl cyclase (AC) and phospholipase C–β (PLC-b) produces a cascade of second-messenger and cellular effects (see diagram and later sections of the text). NE has its action terminated in the synapse by rapidly being taken back into the presynaptic neuron via NE transporters (NETs). Once inside the neuron, it can either be repackaged into vesicles for reuse or undergo enzymatic degradation. The selective NE reuptake inhibitor and antidepressant reboxetine and older-generation tricyclic antidepressant desipramine are able to interfere/block the reuptake of NE. On the other hand, amphetamine is able to facilitate NE release by altering NET function. Green spheres represent DA neurotransmitters; blue spheres represent NE neurotransmitters. DAG=diacylglycerol; IP₃=inositol-1,4,5-triphosphate.

Source. Adapted from Cooper JR, Bloom FE, Roth RH: *The Biochemical Basis of Neuropharmacology,* 7th Edition. New York, Oxford University Press, 2001. Copyright 1970, 1974, 1978, 1982, 1986, 1991, 1996, 2001 by Oxford University Press, Inc. Used by permission of Oxford University Press, Inc. Modified from Nestler et al. 2001.

been used to determine the brain distribution of NET. A high level of NET is found in the LC, with moderate to high levels found in the dentate gyrus, raphe nuclei, and hippocampus (Tejani-Butt and Ordway 1992; Tejani-Butt et al. 1990). This pattern of expression is consistent with the NE innervation to these structures. The NET is expressed mainly on NE terminals, as demonstrated by a drastic reduction in labeling following NE destruction with the neurotoxin 6-hydroxydopamine or DSP-4 (Tejani-Butt and Ordway 1992; Tejani-Butt et al. 1990).

The NET is dependent on extracellular Na^+ to mediate NE reuptake and the effectiveness of NE reuptake inhibitors in inhibiting NE reuptake (Bruss et al. 1997, 1999; Harder and Bonisch 1985). The uptake of NE is Cl^- dependent, meaning that the electrogenic process of NE transport is Na^+ and Cl^- driven (Harder and Bonisch 1985). In addition to the electrogenic process, the NET demonstrates properties of a channel-like pore, in that it can transport NE showing an infinite stoichiometry that can be blocked by cocaine and desipramine (Galli et al. 1995, 1996). A number of studies suggest that NET can be regulated by diverse stimuli, neuronal activity, and peptide hormones, as well as protein kinases. Indeed, studies have shown that all monoaminergic transporters (5-HTT, DAT, and NET) are rapidly regulated by direct or receptor-mediated activation of cellular kinases, particularly PKC (Bauman et al. 2000). PKC activation results in an activity-dependent transporter phosphorylation and sequestration. Protein phosphatase–1/2A (PP-1/PP-2A) inhibitors, such as okadaic acid and calyculin A, also promote monoaminergic transporter phosphorylation and functional downregulation (Bauman et al. 2000). These phenomena that occur beyond the receptor level may well be important in the long-term actions of psychotropic drugs known to regulate protein kinases (G. Chen et al. 1999; Manji and Lenox 1999).

Adrenergic Receptors

The α and β catecholamine receptors were first discovered more than 50 years ago (Alhquist 1948) and later subdivided further into α_1, α_2, and β_1, β_2, and β_3 adrenoreceptors—all of which are GPCRs—on the basis of molecular cloning and pharmacological and biochemical studies (see Figure 1–5B).

α **receptors.** There are three subtypes of α_1 receptors, denoted 1A, 1B, and 1D; they are all positively coupled to PLC and possibly phospholipase A_2 (see Figure 1–5B). The α_2 family comprises the 2A/D, 2B, and 2C subtypes, which couple negatively to adenylyl cyclase and regulate

K^+ and Ca^{2+} channels (see Figure 1–5B). The 2A, 2B, and 2C adrenoceptors correspond to the human genes α_2-C10, α_2-C2, and α_2-C4, respectively (see Bylund et al. 1994). The bovine, guinea pig, rat, and mouse a_{2D} adrenoreceptor is thought to be a species homolog or variant of the human α_{2A} adrenoreceptor (Bylund et al. 1994) and is often referred to as $\alpha_{2A/D}$. The α_2 receptors represent autoreceptors for NE neurons, and blockade of these autoreceptors results in increased NE release—a biochemical effect that has been postulated to play a role in the mechanisms of action of selected antidepressants (e.g., mianserin, mirtazapine) and antipsychotics (e.g., clozapine). In the LC, α_2-adrenergic receptors converge onto similar K^+ channels as μ opioid receptors, and this convergence has been postulated to represent a mechanism for the efficacy of clonidine (an α_2 agonist) in attenuating some of the physical symptoms of opioid withdrawal. The α_2 antagonist yohimbine, which robustly increases NE neuron firing and NE release, has been used as a provocative challenge in clinical studies of anxiety disorders and as an antidepressant-potentiating agent. Given that NE neurons colocalize and release orexins, it is of interest that this neuropeptide has been implicated in sleep disorders and hypoglycemia through its glucose-sensing tandem-pore K^+ (K^{2P}) effects in coordinating arousal (M.M. Scott et al. 2006).

β **receptors.** The β receptor family comprises β_1, β_2, and β_3 adrenoreceptors, which are all positively coupled to adenylyl cyclase (Bylund et al. 1994) (see Figure 1–5B). As is discussed in greater detail in the chapters on antidepressants and anxiolytics (see Chapters 12–26), most effective antidepressants produce a downregulation/desensitization of β_1 receptors in rat forebrain, leading to the suggestion that these effects may play a role in their therapeutic efficacy. Interestingly, β receptors have also been shown to play a role in regulating emotional memories, leading to the proposal that β antagonists may have utility in the treatment of posttraumatic stress disorder (PTSD) (Cahill et al. 1994; Przybyslawski et al. 1999). β_3 receptors are not believed to be present in the CNS but are abundantly expressed on brown fat, where they exert lipolytic and thermogenic effects. Not surprisingly, there is active research attempting to develop selective β_3 agonists for the treatment of obesity.

Cholinergic System

ACh is the only major low-molecular-weight neurotransmitter substance that is not derived from an amino acid (Kandel et al. 2000). ACh is synthesized from acetyl coenzyme A and choline in nerve terminals via the enzyme choline acetyltransferase (ChAT). Choline is transported into the brain by uptake from the bloodstream and enters the neuron via both high-affinity and low-affinity transport processes (Cooper et al. 2001). In addition to the "standard" ChAT pathway, there are several additional possible mechanisms by which ACh can be synthesized; the precise roles of these additional pathways and their physiological relevance in the CNS remain to be fully elucidated (Cooper et al. 2001). The highest activity of ChAT is observed in the interpeduncular nucleus, caudate nucleus, corneal epithelium, retina, and central spinal roots. In contrast to the other transmitters discussed thus far (which are most dependent on reuptake mechanisms), ACh has its signal terminated primarily by the enzyme acetylcholinesterase, which degrades ACh (Figure 1–6B). Not surprisingly, therapeutic strategies to increase synaptic ACh levels (e.g., for the treatment of Alzheimer's disease) have focused on inhibiting the activity of cholinesterases.

Several cholinergic pathways have been proposed, but until recently the circuits had not been worked out in the brain because of the lack of appropriate techniques. The development of tract tracing and histochemical techniques has provided a clearer picture of the cholinergic pathways. In brief, cholinergic neurons can act as local circuit neurons (interneurons) and are found in the caudate putamen, nucleus accumbens, olfactory tubercle, and islands of Calleja complex (Cooper et al. 2001). They do, however, also serve to function as projection neurons that connect different brain regions; one fairly well-characterized pathway runs from the septum to the hippocampus (Figure 1–6A). The basal forebrain cholinergic complex is composed of cholinergic neurons originating from the medial septal nucleus, diagonal band nuclei, substantia innominata, magnocellular preoptic field, and nucleus basalis. These nuclei project cholinergic neurons to the entire nonstriatal telencephalon, pontomesencephalotegmental cholinergic complex, thalamus, and other diencephalic loci (see Figure 1–6A). Descending cholinergic projections from these nuclei also innervate pontine and medullary reticular formations, deep cerebellar and vestibular nuclei, and cranial nerve nuclei (Cooper et al. 2001).

Cholinergic Receptors

There are two major distinct classes of cholinergic receptors, the *muscarinic* and *nicotinic* receptors. Five muscarinic receptors (M_1 through M_5) have been cloned (Kandel et al. 2000). These receptors are G protein–coupled and act

either by regulating ion channels (in particular, K^+ or Ca^{2+}) or through being linked to second-messenger systems. Generally speaking, M_1, M_3, and M_5 are coupled to phosphoinositol hydrolysis, whereas M_2 and M_4 are coupled to inhibition of adenylyl cyclase and regulation of K^+ and Ca^{2+} channels (Cooper et al. 2001) (see Figure 1–6B).

By contrast, the nicotinic receptors are ionotropic receptors, and at least seven different functional receptors (based on different subunit composition) have been identified. Biochemical and biophysical data indicate that the nicotinic receptors in the muscle are formed from five protein subunits, with the stoichiometry of $\alpha_2\beta\gamma\delta$ (Kandel et al. 2000). The binding of ACh molecules on the α subunit is necessary for channel activation. By contrast, neuronal nicotinic receptors contain only two types of subunits (α and β), with the α occurring in at least seven different forms and the β in three (Cooper et al. 2001). Nicotinic receptors may be the targets of considerable cross-talk, as a variety of kinases (including PKA, PKC, and tyrosine kinases) are able to regulate the sensitivity of this receptor. A number of regulatory mechanisms exist. For example, the mammalian prototoxin lynx1 acts as an allosteric modulator of nicotinic acetylcholine receptors (Miwa et al. 2006).

From a clinical standpoint, Freedman et al. (1997) demonstrated that in a cohort of patients with schizophrenia, abnormal P50 auditory evoked potentials were linked to a susceptibility locus for this disease on chromosome 15. Notably, this is where a nicotinic receptor subunit is found, providing indirect support for the longstanding contention that the high rates of cigarette smoking in patients with schizophrenia may represent (at least in part) an attempt to correct an underlying nicotinic receptor defect.

Glutamatergic System

Glutamate and aspartate are the two major excitatory amino acids in the CNS and are present in high concentrations (Nestler et al. 2001; Squire et al. 2003). As the principal mediators of excitatory synaptic transmission in the mammalian brain, they participate in wide-ranging aspects of both normal and abnormal CNS function. Physiologically, glutamate appears to play a prominent role in synaptic plasticity, learning, and memory. However, glutamate can also be a potent neuronal excitotoxin under a variety of experimental conditions, triggering either rapid or delayed neuronal death. Unlike the monoamines, which require transport of amino acids through the blood–brain barrier, glutamate and aspartate cannot adequately

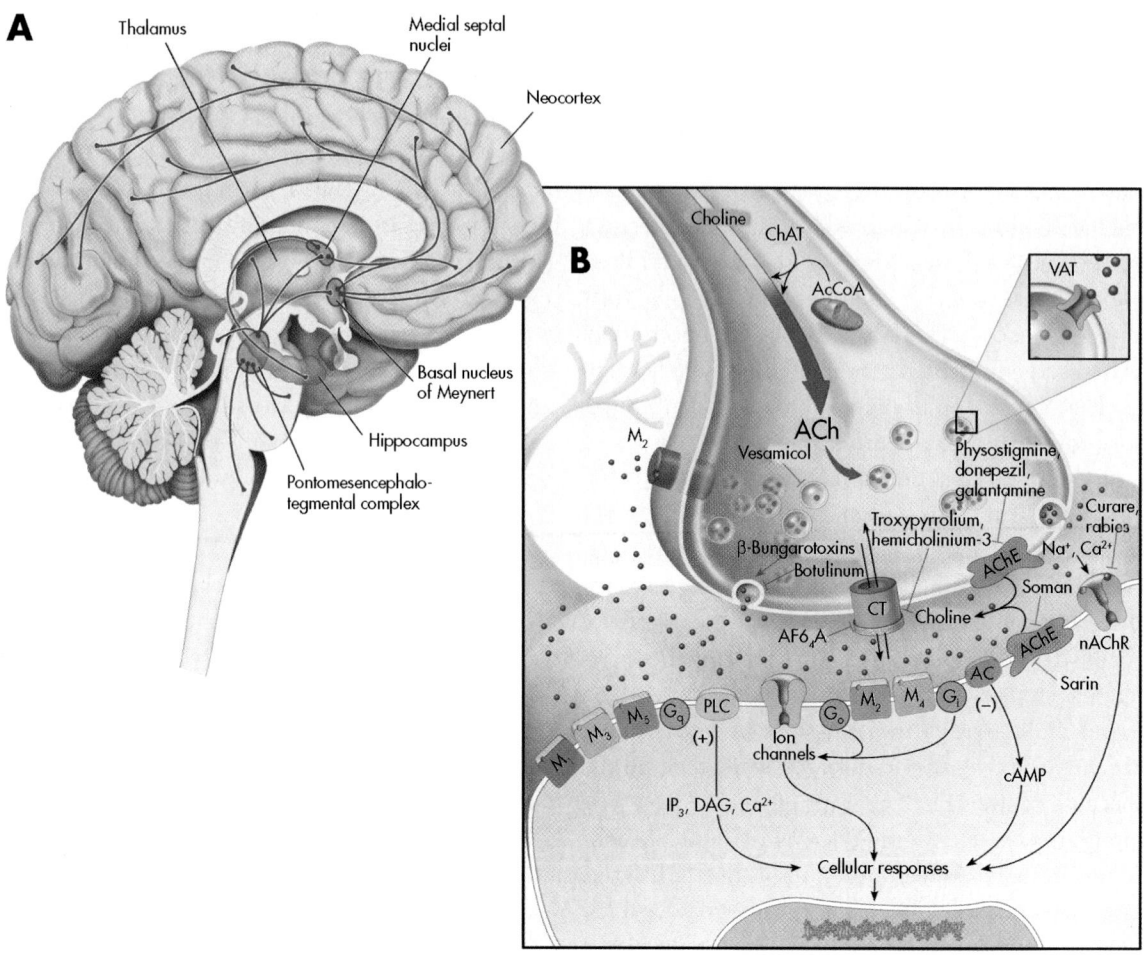

FIGURE 1–6. The cholinergic system.

This figure depicts the cholinergic pathways in the brain **(A)** and various regulatory processes involved in cholinergic neurotransmission **(B).** Choline crosses the blood–brain barrier to enter the brain and is actively transported into cholinergic presynaptic terminals by an active uptake mechanism (requiring ATP). This neurotransmitter is produced by a single enzymatic reaction in which acetyl coenzyme A (AcCoA) donates its acetyl group to choline by means of the enzyme choline acetyltransferase (ChAT). AcCoA is primarily synthesized in the mitochondria of neurons. Upon its formation, acetylcholine (ACh) is sequestered into secretory vesicles by vesicle ACh transporters (VATs), where it is stored. Vesamicol effectively blocks the transport of ACh into vesicles. An agent such as β-bungarotoxin or AF_64A is capable of increasing synaptic concentration of ACh by acting as a releaser and a noncompetitive reuptake inhibitor, respectively. In turn, agents such as botulinum toxin are able to attenuate ACh release from nerve terminals. Once released from the presynaptic terminals, ACh can interact with a variety of presynaptic and postsynaptic receptors. In contrast to many other monoaminergic neurotransmitters, the ACh signal is terminated primarily by degradation by the enzyme acetylcholinesterase (AChE) rather than by reuptake. Interestingly, AChE is present on both presynaptic and postsynaptic membranes and can be inhibited by physostigmine (reversible) and soman (irreversible). Currently, AChE inhibitors such as donepezil and galantamine are the only classes of agents that are FDA approved for the treatment of Alzheimer's disease. ACh receptors are of two types: muscarinic (G protein–coupled) and nicotinic (ionotropic). Presynaptic regulation of ACh neuron firing activity and release occurs through somatodendritic (not shown) and nerve terminal M2 autoreceptors, respectively. The binding of ACh to G protein–coupled muscarinic receptors that are negatively coupled to adenylyl cyclase (AC) or coupled to phosphoinositol hydrolysis produces a cascade of second-messenger and cellular effects (see diagram). ACh also activates ionotropic nicotinic receptors (nAChRs). ACh has it action terminated in the synapse through rapid degradation by AChE, which liberates free choline to be taken back into the presynaptic neuron through choline transporters (CTs). Once inside the neuron, it can be reused for the synthesis of ACh, can be repackaged into vesicles for reuse, or undergoes enzymatic degradation. There are some relatively new agents that selectively antagonize the muscarinic receptors, such as CI-1017 for M_1, methoctramine for M_2, 4-DAMP for M_3, PD-102807 for M_4, and scopolamine (hardly a new agent) for M_5 (although it also has affinity for M3 receptor). nAChR or nicotine receptors are activated by nicotine and the specific alpha(4)beta(2*) agonist metanicotine. Mecamylamine is an AChR antagonist. DAG=diacylglycerol; IP_3=inositol-1,4,5-triphosphate.

Source.   Adapted from Cooper JR, Bloom FE, Roth RH: *The Biochemical Basis of Neuropharmacology,* 7th Edition. New York, Oxford University Press, 2001. Copyright 1970, 1974, 1978, 1982, 1986, 1991, 1996, 2001 by Oxford University Press, Inc. Used by permission of Oxford University Press, Inc. Modified from Nestler et al. 2001.

penetrate into the brain from the periphery and are produced locally by specialized brain machinery. The metabolic and synthetic enzymes responsible for the formation of these nonessential amino acids are located in glial cells as well as neurons (Squire et al. 2003).

The major metabolic pathway in the production of glutamate is derived from glucose and the transamination of α-ketoglutarate; however, a small proportion of glutamate is formed directly from glutamine. The latter is actually synthesized in glia, via an active process (requiring adenosine triphosphate [ATP]), and is then transported to neurons where glutaminase is able to convert this precursor to glutamate (Figure 1–7). Following release, the concentration of glutamate in the extracellular space is highly regulated and controlled, primarily by a Na$^+$-dependent reuptake mechanism involving several transporter proteins.

The major glutamate transporter proteins found in the CNS include the excitatory amino acid transporters (EAATs) EAAT1 (or GLAST-1), EAAT2 (or GLT-1), and EAAT3 (or EAAC1), with EAAT2 being the most predominantly expressed form in the forebrain. Additionally, these transporters are differentially expressed in specific cell types, with EAAT1 and EAAT2 being found primarily in glial cells and EAAT3 being localized in neurons. EAAT4 is mainly localized in cerebellum. The physiological events regulating the activity of the glutamate transporters are not well understood, although there is evidence that phosphorylation of the transporters by protein kinases may differentially regulate glutamate transporters and therefore glutamate reuptake (Casado et al. 1993; Conradt and Stoffel 1997; Pisano et al. 1996). Glutamate concentrations have been shown to rise to excitotoxic levels within minutes following traumatic or ischemic injury, and there is evidence that the function of the glutamate transporters becomes impaired under these excitotoxic conditions (Faden et al. 1989). It is surprising that the glutamatergic system has only recently undergone extensive investigation with regard to its possible involvement in the pathophysiology of mood disorders, since it is the major excitatory neurotransmitter in the CNS and known to play a role in regulating the threshold for excitation of most other neurotransmitter systems. Although direct evidence for glutamatergic excitotoxicity in bipolar disorder is lacking and the precise mechanisms underlying the cell atrophy and death that occur in recurrent mood disorders are unknown, considerable data have shown that impairments of the glutamatergic system play a major role in the morphometric changes observed with severe stresses (McEwen 1999; Sapolsky 2000).

It is now clear that modification of the levels of synaptic AMPA-type glutamate receptors—in particular by receptor subunit trafficking, insertion, and internalization—is a critically important mechanism for regulating various forms of synaptic plasticity and behavior. Recent studies have identified region-specific alterations in expression levels of AMPA and NMDA glutamate receptor subunits in subjects with mood disorders (Beneyto et al. 2007). Supporting the suggestion that abnormalities in glutamate signaling may be involved in mood pathophysiology, AMPA receptors have been shown to regulate affective-like behaviors in rodents. AMPA antagonists have been demonstrated to attenuate amphetamine- and cocaine-induced hyperactivity and psychostimulant-induced sensitization and hedonic behavior (Goodwin and Jamison 2007).

Glutamatergic Receptors

The many subtypes of glutamatergic receptors in the CNS can be classified into two major subtypes: ionotropic and metabotropic receptors (see Figure 1–7).

Ionotropic glutamate receptors. The ionotropic glutamate receptor ion channels are assemblies of homo- or hetero-oligomeric subunits integrated into the neuron's membrane. Every channel is assembled of (most likely) four subunits associated into a dimer of dimers as has been observed in crystallographic studies (Ayalon and Stern-Bach 2001; Madden 2002). Every subunit consists of an extracellular amino-terminal and ligand binding domain, three transmembrane domains, a reentrant pore loop (located between the first and second transmembrane domains), and an intracellular carboxyl-terminal domain (Hollmann et al. 1994). The subunits associate through interactions between their amino-terminal domains, forming a dimer that undergoes a second dimerization mediated by interactions between the ligand binding domains and/or between transmembrane domains (Ayalon and Stern-Bach 2001; Madden 2002). Three different subgroups of glutamatergic ion channels have been identified on the basis of their pharmacological ability to bind different synthetic ligands, each of which is composed of a different set of subunits. The three subgroups are the NMDA receptors, the AMPA (α-amino-3-hydroxy-5-methyl-4-isoxazole propionic acid) receptors, and the kainate receptor. The latter two groups are often referred to together as the "non-NMDA" receptors, but they undoubtedly subserve unique functions (see Figure 1–7). In the adult mammalian brain, NMDA and AMPA glutamatergic receptors are collocated in approximately 70% of the synapses (Bek-

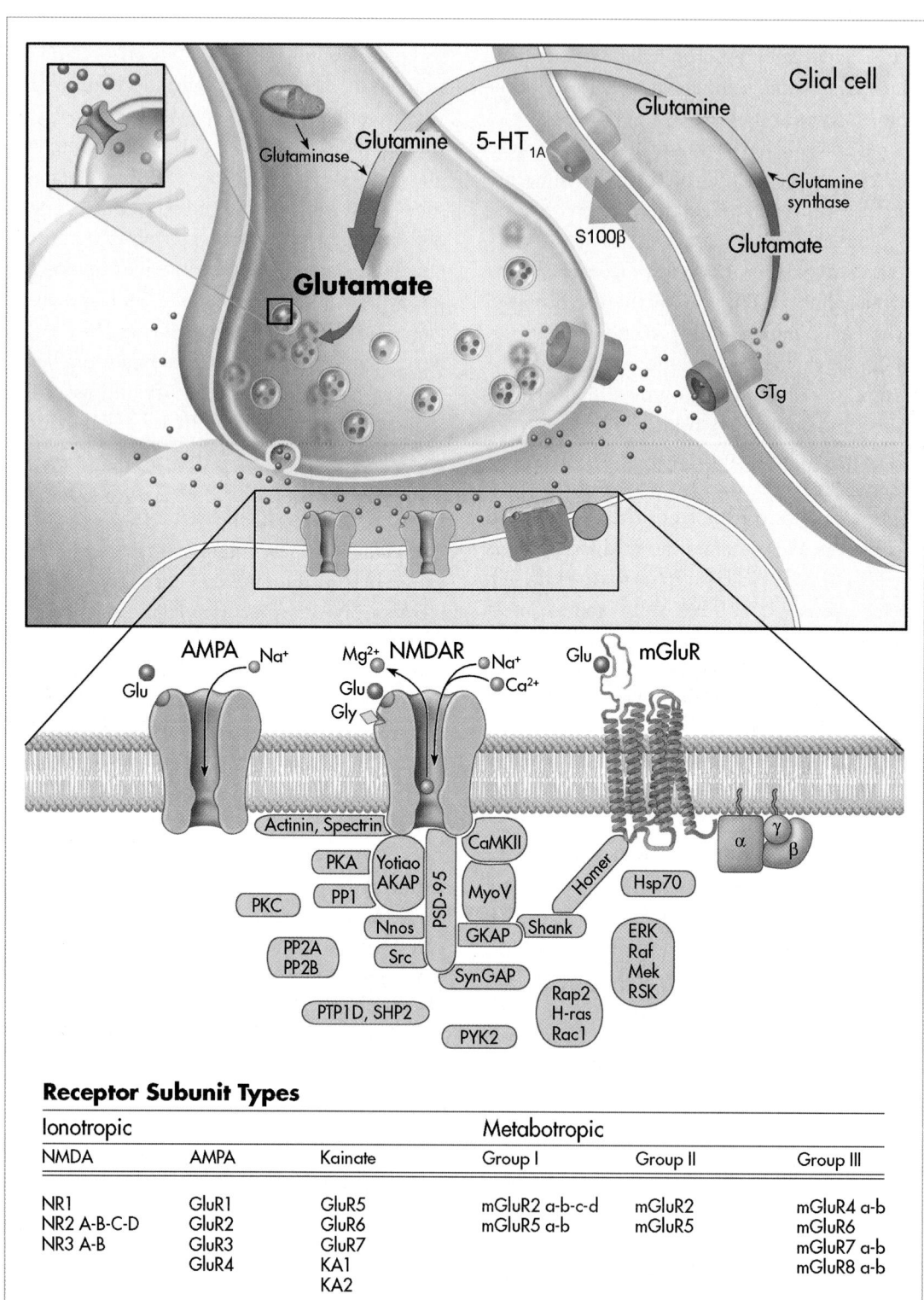

Receptor Subunit Types

Ionotropic			Metabotropic		
NMDA	AMPA	Kainate	Group I	Group II	Group III
NR1	GluR1	GluR5	mGluR2 a-b-c-d	mGluR2	mGluR4 a-b
NR2 A-B-C-D	GluR2	GluR6	mGluR5 a-b	mGluR5	mGluR6
NR3 A-B	GluR3	GluR7			mGluR7 a-b
	GluR4	KA1			mGluR8 a-b
		KA2			

FIGURE 1-7. The glutamatergic system (*opposite page*).

This figure depicts the various regulatory processes involved in glutamatergic neurotransmission. The biosynthetic pathway for glutamate involves synthesis from glucose and the transamination of α-ketoglutarate; however, a small proportion of glutamate is formed more directly from glutamine by glutamine synthetase. The latter is actually synthesized in glia and, via an active process (requiring ATP), is transported to neurons, where in the mitochondria glutaminase is able to convert this precursor to glutamate. Furthermore, in astrocytes glutamine can undergo oxidation to yield α-keto-glutarate, which can also be transported to neurons and participate in glutamate synthesis. Glutamate is either metabolized or sequestered and stored in secretory vesicles by vesicle glutamate transporters (VGluTs). Glutamate can then be released by a calcium-dependent excitotoxic process. Once released from the presynaptic terminal, glutamate is able to bind to numerous excitatory amino acid (EAA) receptors, including both ionotropic (e.g., NMDA [*N*-methyl-D-aspartate]) and metabotropic (mGluR) receptors. Presynaptic regulation of glutamate release occurs through metabo-tropic glutamate receptors (mGluR2 and mGluR3), which subserve the function of autoreceptors; however, these receptors are also located on the postsynaptic element. Glutamate has its action terminated in the synapse by reuptake mechanisms utilizing distinct glutamate transporters (labeled VGT in figure) that exist on not only presynaptic nerve terminals but also astrocytes; indeed, current data suggest that astrocytic glutamate uptake may be more important for clearing excess glutamate, raising the possibility that astrocytic loss (as has been documented in mood disorders) may contribute to deleterious glutamate signaling, but more so by astrocytes. It is now known that a number of important intracellular proteins are able to alter the function of glutamate receptors (see diagram). Also, growth factors such as glial-derived neurotrophic factor (GDNF) and S100β secreted from glia have been demonstrated to exert a tremendous influence on glutamatergic neurons and synapse formation. Of note, serotonin$_{1A}$ (5-HT$_{1A}$) receptors have been documented to be regulated by antidepressant agents; this receptor is also able to modulate the release of S100β. AKAP = A kinase anchoring protein; CaMKII = Ca2+/calmodulin–dependent protein kinase II; ERK = extracellular response kinase; GKAP = guanylate kinase–associated protein; Glu = glutamate; Gly = glycine; GTg = glutamate transporter glial; GTn = glutamate transporter neuronal; Hsp70 = heat shock protein 70; MEK = mitogen-activated protein kinase/ERK; mGluR = metabotropic glutamate receptor; MyoV = myosin V; NMDAR = NMDA receptor; nNOS = neuronal nitric oxide synthase; PKA = phosphokinase A; PKC = phosphokinase C; PP-1, PP-2A, PP-2B = protein phosphatases; RSK = ribosomal S6 kinase; SHP2 = src homology 2 domain–containing tyrosine phosphatase.

Source. Adapted from Cooper JR, Bloom FE, Roth RH: *The Biochemical Basis of Neuropharmacology,* 7th Edition. New York, Oxford University Press, 2001. Copyright 1970, 1974, 1978, 1982, 1986, 1991, 1996, 2001 by Oxford University Press, Inc. Used by permission of Oxford University Press, Inc. Modified from Nicholls 1994.

kers and Stevens 1989). By contrast, at early stages of development, synapses are more likely to contain only NMDA receptors. Radioligand binding studies have shown that NMDA and AMPA receptors are found in high density in the cerebral cortex, hippocampus, striatum, septum, and amygdala.

NMDA receptors. The NMDA receptor is activated by glutamate and requires the presence of a co-agonist, namely glycine or D-serine, to be activated, a process that likely varies in importance according to brain region (Panatier et al. 2006). However, the binding of both glutamate and glycine is still not sufficient for the NMDA receptor channel to open, since at resting membrane potential, the NMDA ion channel is blocked by Mg^{2+} ions. Only when the membrane is depolarized (e.g., by the activation of AMPA or kainate receptors on the same postsynaptic neuron) is the Mg^{2+} blockade relieved. Under these conditions, the NMDA receptor channel will open and permit the entry of both Na^+ and Ca^{2+} (see Figure 1–7).

The NMDA receptor channel is composed of a combination of NR1, NR2A, NR2B, NR2C, NR2D, NR3A, and NR3B subunits (see Figure 1–7). The binding site for glutamate has been localized to the NR2 subunit, and the site for the co-agonist glycine has been localized to the NR1 subunit, which is required for receptor function.

Two molecules of glutamate and two of glycine are thought to be necessary to activate the ion channel. Within the ion channel, two other sites have been identified—the sigma (σ) site and the phencyclidine (PCP) site. The hallucinogenic drug PCP, ketamine, and the experimental drug dizocilpine (MK-801) all bind at the latter site and are considered noncompetitive receptor antagonists that inhibit NMDA receptor channel function.

In clinical psychiatric studies, ketamine has been shown to transiently induce psychotic symptoms in schizophrenic patients and to produce antidepressant effects in some depressed patients (Krystal et al. 2002). Building on these preclinical and preliminary clinical data, recent clinical trials have investigated the clinical effects of glutamatergic agents in subjects with mood disorders. Recent clinical studies have demonstrated effective and rapid antidepressant action of glutamatergic agents, including ketamine, an NMDA receptor antagonist, and riluzole, a glutamate release inhibitor (Sanacora et al. 2007; Zarate et al. 2006a). These and other data have led to the hypothesis that alterations in neural plasticity in critical limbic and reward circuits, mediated by increasing the postsynaptic AMPA-to-NMDA throughput, may represent a convergent mechanism for antidepressant action (Zarate et al. 2006b). This line of research holds considerable promise for developing new treatments for depression and bipolar disorder. The NMDA receptor agonists glycine, D-serine, and D-cycloserine have been shown to improve cognition and decrease negative symptoms in patients with schizophrenia who are receiving antipsychotics (Coyle et al. 2002). NMDA receptors in the amygdala may also be of critical importance in the process of transforming a fixed and consolidated fear memory to a labile state (Ben Mamou et al. 2006).

NMDA receptors play a critical role in regulating synaptic plasticity (Malenka and Nicoll 1999). The best-studied forms of synaptic plasticity in the CNS are *long-term potentiation* (LTP) and *long-term depression* (LTD) of excitatory synaptic transmission. The molecular mechanisms of LTP and LTD have been extensively characterized and have been proposed to represent cellular models of learning and memory (Malenka and Nicoll 1999). Induction of LTP and LTD in the CA1 region of the hippocampus and in many regions of the brain has now clearly been demonstrated to be dependent on NMDA receptor activation. During NMDA receptor–dependent synaptic plasticity, Ca^{2+} influx through NMDA receptors can activate a wide variety of kinases and/or phosphatases that in turn modulate synaptic strength. An important development was the finding that two of the primary molecules involved—CaMKII and the NMDA subtype of glutamate receptor—form a tight complex with each other at the synapse (Lisman and McIntyre 2001). Interestingly, this binding appears to enhance both the autophosphorylation of the kinase and the ability of the entire holoenzyme, which has 12 subunits, to become hyperphosphorylated (Lisman and McIntyre 2001). This hyperphosphorylated state has been postulated to represent a "memory switch" that can lead to long-term strengthening of the synapse by multiple mechanisms. One important mechanism involves direct phosphorylation of the glutamate-activated AMPA receptors, which increases their conductance. Furthermore, CaMKII, once bound to the NMDA receptor, may organize additional anchoring sites for AMPA receptors at the synapse. Switching of synaptic NMDA receptor subunits, which bind CaMKII, for other NMDA receptor subunits having no affinity for this enzyme dramatically reduces LTP, demonstrating that glutamate and calcium signaling interactions are critical for learning and memory (Barria and Malinow 2005).

While the NMDA receptor clearly plays important roles in plasticity, abundant evidence has shown that excessive glutamatergic signaling is also involved in neuronal toxicity. With anoxia or hypoglycemia, the highly energy-dependent uptake mechanisms that keep glutamate compartmentalized in presynaptic terminals fail. Within minutes, glutamate is massively released into the synaptic space, resulting in activation of excitatory amino acid receptors. This leads to depolarization of target neurons via AMPA and kainate receptors and then to inappropriate and excessive activation of NMDA receptors. Considerable data suggest that the large excess of Ca^{2+} entering cells via the NMDA receptor channel may represent an important step in the rapid cell death that occurs via excitotoxicity.

AMPA receptors. The AMPA receptor is stimulated by the presence of glutamate and characteristically produces a fast excitatory synaptic signal that is responsible for the initial reaction to glutamate in the synapse. In fact, as discussed above, it is generally believed that it is the activation of the AMPA receptor that results in neuronal depolarization sufficient to liberate the Mg^{2+} cation from the NMDA receptor, thereby permitting its activation. The AMPA receptor channel is composed of the combination of the GluR1, GluR2, GluR3, and GluR4 subunits and requires two molecules of glutamate to be activated (see Figure 1–7). AMPA receptors have a lower affinity for glutamate than does the NMDA receptor, thereby allowing for more rapid dissociation of glutamate and, therefore, a rapid deactivation of the AMPA receptor (for a review, see Dingledine et al. 1999).

Studies have indicated that AMPA receptor subunits are direct substrates of protein kinases and phosphatases. Phosphorylation of the receptor subunits regulates not only the intrinsic channel properties of the receptor but also the interaction of the receptor with associated proteins that modulate the membrane trafficking and synaptic targeting of the receptors (discussed in Malinow and Malenka 2002). Additionally, protein phosphorylation of other synaptic proteins has been proposed to indirectly modulate AMPA receptor function by affecting the macromolecular complexes that are important for the presence of AMPA receptors at the synaptic plasma membrane (Malinow and Malenka 2002; Nestler et al. 2001). Studies have been elucidating the cellular mechanisms by which AMPA receptor subunit insertion and trafficking occur and have revealed two major mechanisms (Malinow and Malenka 2002; Nestler et al. 2001). The first mechanism is used for GluR1-containing AMPA receptor insertion and is regulated by activity. The second mechanism is governed by constitutive receptor recycling, mainly through GluR2/3 heteromers in response to activity-dependent signals. Data suggest that AMPA receptor subunit trafficking may play an important role in neuropsychiatric disorders. Thus, Nestler and associates have shown that the ability of drugs of abuse to elevate levels of the GluR1 subunit of AMPA glutamate receptors in the VTA of the midbrain is crucial for the development of sensitization (Carlezon and Nestler 2002). They have demonstrated that even transient increases in GluR1 levels within VTA neurons can trigger complex cascades of other molecular adaptations in these neurons and, within larger neural circuits, can cause enduring changes in the responses of the brain to drugs of abuse. Chronic lithium and valproate have been shown to reduce GluR1 expression in hippocampal synaptosomes, effects that may play a role in the delayed therapeutic effects of these agents (Du et al. 2003; Szabo et al. 2002).

Recent studies have sought to test the hypothesis that "antidepressant anticonvulsants," like traditional antidepressants, can enhance surface AMPA receptors (Du et al. 2007). It was found that the predominantly antidepressant anticonvulsants lamotrigine and riluzole significantly enhanced the surface expression of GluR1 and GluR2 in a time- and dose-dependent manner in cultured hippocampal neurons. By contrast, the predominantly antimanic anticonvulsant valproate significantly reduced surface expression of GluR1 and GluR2. Concomitant with the GluR1 and GluR2 changes, the peak value of depolarized membrane potential evoked by AMPA was significantly higher in lamotrigine- and riluzole-treated neurons, supporting the surface receptor changes. In addition, lamotrigine and riluzole, as well as the traditional antidepressant imipramine, increased GluR1 phosphorylation at GluR1 (S845) in the hippocampus after chronic in vivo treatment.

Recent clinical research has demonstrated a robust and rapid antidepressant effect of ketamine; studies were therefore undertaken to test the hypothesis that ketamine brings about its rapid antidepressant effect by enhancing AMPA relative to NMDA throughput (Maeng et al. 2008). Although the AMPA antagonist NBQX was without behavioral effects alone, it blocked the antidepressant-like effects of ketamine. AMPA antagonists also blocked ketamine-induced changes in hippocampal GluR1 AMPA receptor phosphorylation. Together, these results suggest that regulating AMPA relative to NMDA throughput in critical neuronal circuits may play an important role in antidepressant action.

Kainate receptors. The kainate receptor has pre- and postsynaptic roles, sharing some properties with AMPA receptors. It is composed of the combination of the GluR5, GluR6, GluR7, KA1, and KA2 subunits (see Figure 1–7). The precise role of kainate receptors in the ma-

ture CNS remains to be fully elucidated, although the activity of the receptors clearly plays a role in synaptic function in many brain areas. Increasing data suggest the involvement of aberrant synaptic plasticity in the pathophysiology of bipolar disorder. Kainate receptors contribute to synaptic plasticity in different brain regions involved in mood regulation, including the prefrontal cortex, hippocampus, and amygdala. GluR6 (GRIK2) is a subtype of kainate receptor whose chromosomal loci of 6q16.3–q21 have been identified as potentially harboring genetic polymorphism(s) contributing to an increased risk of mood disorders. The role of GluR6 in modulating animal behaviors correlated with mood symptoms was investigated using GluR6 knockout and wild-type mice (Shaltiel et al. 2008). GluR6 knockout mice appeared to attain normal growth and showed no neurological abnormalities. GluR6 mice showed increased basal- or amphetamine-induced activity, were extremely aggressive, took more risks, and consumed more saccharin (a measure of hedonic drive). Notably, most of these aberrant behaviors responded to chronic lithium administration. These results suggest that abnormalities in kainate receptor throughput generated by GluR6 gene disruption may lead to the concurrent appearance of a constellation of behaviors related to manic symptoms, including persistent hyperactivity; escalated irritability, aggression, and risk taking; and hyperhedonia.

Metabotropic glutamate receptors. The metabotropic glutamate receptors (mGluRs) are G protein–coupled receptors. The eight types of receptors that currently have been cloned can be organized into three different subgroups (groups I, II, and III) based largely on the signaling transduction pathways that they activate (see Figure 1–7). These receptors have a large extracellular N-terminal consisting of two lobes forming a "venus flytrap" binding pocket involved in glutamate recognition and a cysteine-rich extracellular domain that connects with seven transmembrane domains separated by short intra- and extracellular loops (see Figure 1–7). The intracellular loop plays an important role in the coupling with and selectivity of the G protein. The cytoplasmic carboxyl-terminal domain is variable in length and is involved with G protein activation and coupling efficacy (Bruno et al. 2001; Conn and Pin 1997).

The mGluR group I includes the mGluR1 (a, b, c, d), and mGluR5 (a, b) receptors (see Figure 1–7). They preferentially interact with the $G\alpha_{q/11}$ subunit of G proteins, leading to activation of the IP_3/calcium and DAG/PKC cascades. The receptors are located on both pre- and postsynaptic neurons. Group II metabotropic receptors include mGluR2 and mGluR3, which have been best characterized as inhibiting adenylyl cyclase but, like many receptors coupled to G_i/G_o, may also regulate ion channels. Group III receptors, which include mGluR4 (a, b), mGluR6, mGluR7 (a, b), and mGluR8 (a, b), are reported to produce inhibition of adenylyl cyclase as well, but also to interact with the phosphodiesterase enzyme regulating guanosine monophosphate (cGMP) levels (Cooper et al. 2001; Squire et al. 2003). The group II and III receptors are located in the presynaptic membrane and, because of their coupling with G_i/G_o proteins, appear to negatively modulate glutamate and GABA neurotransmission output when activated (i.e., they serve as inhibitory auto- and heteroreceptors). Preclinical studies suggest that mGlu group II and III receptors are "extrasynaptic" in their localization; that is, they are located some distance from the synaptic cleft and are thus activated only under conditions of excessive (pathological?) glutamate release, when there is sufficient glutamate to diffuse out of the synapse to these receptors (Schoepp 2001). In preclinical studies, mGluR2/3 agonists have been demonstrated to exert anxiolytic, antipsychotic, and neuroprotective properties (Schoepp 2001).

Glycine

Glycine is a nonessential amino acid that also functions as a neurotransmitter in the CNS. Although the exact metabolic pathway for glycine production has yet to be fully elucidated, evidence suggests that glycine may be produced in the CNS by two distinct pathways. First, glycine is produced from serine by the enzyme serine-*trans*-hydroxymethylase in a reversible folate-dependent reaction (Cooper et al. 2001; Squire et al. 2003). Additionally, glycine may be produced from glyoxylate by the enzyme D-glycerate dehydrogenase. This amino acid is found in higher concentrations in the spinal cord than in the rest of the CNS. Glycine acts as an inhibitory neurotransmitter predominantly in the brain stem and spinal cord (Nestler et al. 2001). As discussed earlier, a very important role that glycine also plays is to augment the NMDA-mediated frequency of NMDA receptor channel opening. This effect is strychnine-insensitive and pharmacologically suggests that the actions of glycine on NMDA receptor function are different from its effect on the spinal cord, where glycine's inhibitory effect is blocked by strychnine (Cooper et al. 2001). The allosteric modulation of NMDA receptors via a glycine-insensitive site is further underscored by receptor binding

experiments yielding an anatomic distribution similar to that of NMDA receptors. Functionally, it has been postulated that glycine is able to augment the NMDA-mediated responses by speeding up the recovery process of the receptor (Cooper et al. 2001). Given the ability of glycine to alter NMDA function, glycine may be beneficial in the treatment of schizophrenia (Coyle et al. 2002).

GABAergic System

γ-Aminobutyric acid—the major inhibitory neurotransmitter system in the CNS—is one of the most abundant neurotransmitters, and GABA-containing neurons are located in virtually every area of the brain. Unlike the monoamines, GABA occurs in the brain in high concentrations in the order of micromoles per milligrams (about 1,000-fold higher than concentrations of monoamines) (Cooper et al. 2001; Nestler et al. 2001; Squire et al. 2003). GABA is produced when glucose is converted to α-ketoglutarate, which is then transaminated to glutamate by GABA α-oxoglutarate transaminase (GABA-T). Glutamic acid is decarboxylated by glutamic acid decarboxylase, which leads to the formation of GABA (Figure 1–8). Indeed, the neurotransmitter and the rate-limiting enzyme are localized together in the brain and at approximately the same concentration. Catabolism of GABA occurs via GABA-T, which is also important in the synthesis of this transmitter.

The function of this dual-role enzyme becomes apparent when placed in the context of its role in the metabolic process. GABA-T converts GABA to succinic acid, and subsequent removal of the amino group yields α-ketoglutarate. Thus, α-ketoglutarate is able to be used by GABA-T in GABA biosynthesis as mentioned above (Cooper et al. 2001). This process, called the GABA *shunt*, maintains a steady GABA supply in the brain. As with the monoamines, the major mechanism by which the effects of GABA are terminated in the synaptic cleft is by reuptake through GABA transporters. The GABA transporters have a high affinity for GABA and mediate their reuptake via a Na^+ and Cl^- gradient (Squire et al. 2003).

Detailed studies from the Rajkowska laboratory (Grazyna Rajkowska, The University of Mississippi Medical Center, Jackson, MS) have measured the density and size of calbindin-immunoreactive neurons (presumed to be GABAergic) in layers II and III of the dorsolateral prefrontal cortex, revealing a 43% reduction in the density of these neurons in patients with major depressive disorder compared with controls (discussed in Goodwin and Jamison 2007). Of particular note, in the rostral orbitofrontal cortex, there was a trend toward a negative correlation between the duration of depression and the size of neuronal cell bodies, suggesting changes associated with disease progression. Valproate has also been shown to have neurogenic effects in at least one study. In cultured embryonic rat cortical cells and striatal primordial stem cells, valproate markedly increased the number and percentage of primarily GABAergic neurons and promoted neurite outgrowth (Laeng et al. 2004).

GABA Receptors

There are two major types of well-characterized GABA receptors, $GABA_A$ and $GABA_B$, and most neurons in the CNS possess at least one of these types. The $GABA_A$ receptor is the more prevalent of the two in the mammalian CNS and as a result has been extensively studied and characterized. $GABA_A$ contains an integral transmembrane chloride channel, which is opened upon receptor activation, generally resulting in hyperpolarization of the neuron (i.e., suppressing excitability). The GABA receptor is a heteropentameric glycoprotein of approximately 275 kDa composed of a combination of multiple polypeptide subunits. $GABA_A$ displays enormous heterogeneity, being composed of a combination of five classes of polypeptide subunits (α, β, γ, δ, ϵ), of which there are at least 18 total subtypes. The various receptors display variation in functional pharmacology, hinting at the multiple finely tuned roles that inhibitory neurotransmission plays in brain function.

It is now well established that benzodiazepines (BZDs) function by binding to a potentiator site on the $GABA_A$ receptor, increasing the amplitude and duration of inhibitory postsynaptic currents in response to GABA binding. Coexpression of additional γ subunits is believed to be necessary for the potentiation of GABA-mediated responses by BZDs. In addition to BZDs, barbiturates and ethanol are also believed to exert many of their effects by potentiating the opening of the $GABA_A$ receptor chloride channel (see Figure 1–8). As noted earlier, $GABA_A$ receptors have a widespread distribution in the brain, and the majority of these receptors in the brain are targets of the currently available BZDs. For this reason, there has been considerable interest in determining if the desirable and undesirable effects of BZDs can be differentiated on the basis of the presence of different subunit composition. Much of the work has used gene knockout technology; thus, mutation of the BZD-binding site of the α_1 subunit

in mice blocks the sedative, anticonvulsive, and amnesic, but not the anxiolytic, effects of diazepam (see Gould et al. 2003; Mohler et al. 2002). In contrast, the α_2 subunit (expressed highly in the cortex and hippocampus) is necessary for diazepam anxiolysis and myorelaxation. Thus, there is now optimism that an α_2-selective ligand will soon provide effective acute treatment of anxiety disorders without the unfavorable side-effect profile of current BZDs. A compound with this preferential affinity has already been demonstrated to exert fewer sedative/depressant effects than diazepam in rat behavioral studies (see Gould et al. 2003; Mohler et al. 2002).

The phosphorylation of $GABA_A$ receptors is another mechanism by which this receptor complex can be regulated in function and expression. In this context, it is noteworthy that studies have reported that knockout mice deficient in PKC ϵ isoforms show reduced anxiety and alcohol consumption and an enhanced response to the effects of BZDs (discussed in Gould et al. 2003). Furthermore, different $GABA_A$ receptor subunit partnerships, such as α_1/δ, mediate tonic inhibitory currents in the hippocampus and are highly sensitive to low concentrations of ethanol (Glykys et al. 2007).

The $GABA_B$ receptors are coupled to G_i and G_o and thereby regulate adenylyl cyclase activity (generally inhibit), K^+ channels (open), and Ca^{2+} channels (close). $GABA_B$ receptors can function as an autoreceptor but are also found abundantly postsynaptically on non-GABAergic neurons. Of interest, there is mounting evidence that receptor dimerization may be required for the activation of $GABA_B$ and possibly other G protein–coupled receptors; although receptor dimerization has long been known to occur for growth factor and JAK (Janus tyrosine kinase)/STAT (signal transducers and activators of transcription) receptors (discussed later in this chapter), this was not expected for GPCRs. However, studies have reported that coexpression of two $GABA_B$ receptor subunits—subunit 1 ($GABA_B R1$) and subunit 2 ($GABA_B R2$)—is necessary for the formation of a functional $GABA_B$ receptor (Bouvier 2001). Some data suggest that $GABA_B R2$ may be necessary for proper protein folding of $GABA_B R1$ (acting as a molecular chaperone) in the endoplasmic reticulum, but this remains to be definitively established. Support for the physiological relevance of this dimerization comes from studies showing that the $GABA_B$ R1 and R2 subunits can be co-immunoprecipitated in rat cortical membrane preparations (Kaupmann et al. 1997); thus, the dimerization is not simply an in vitro phenomenon.

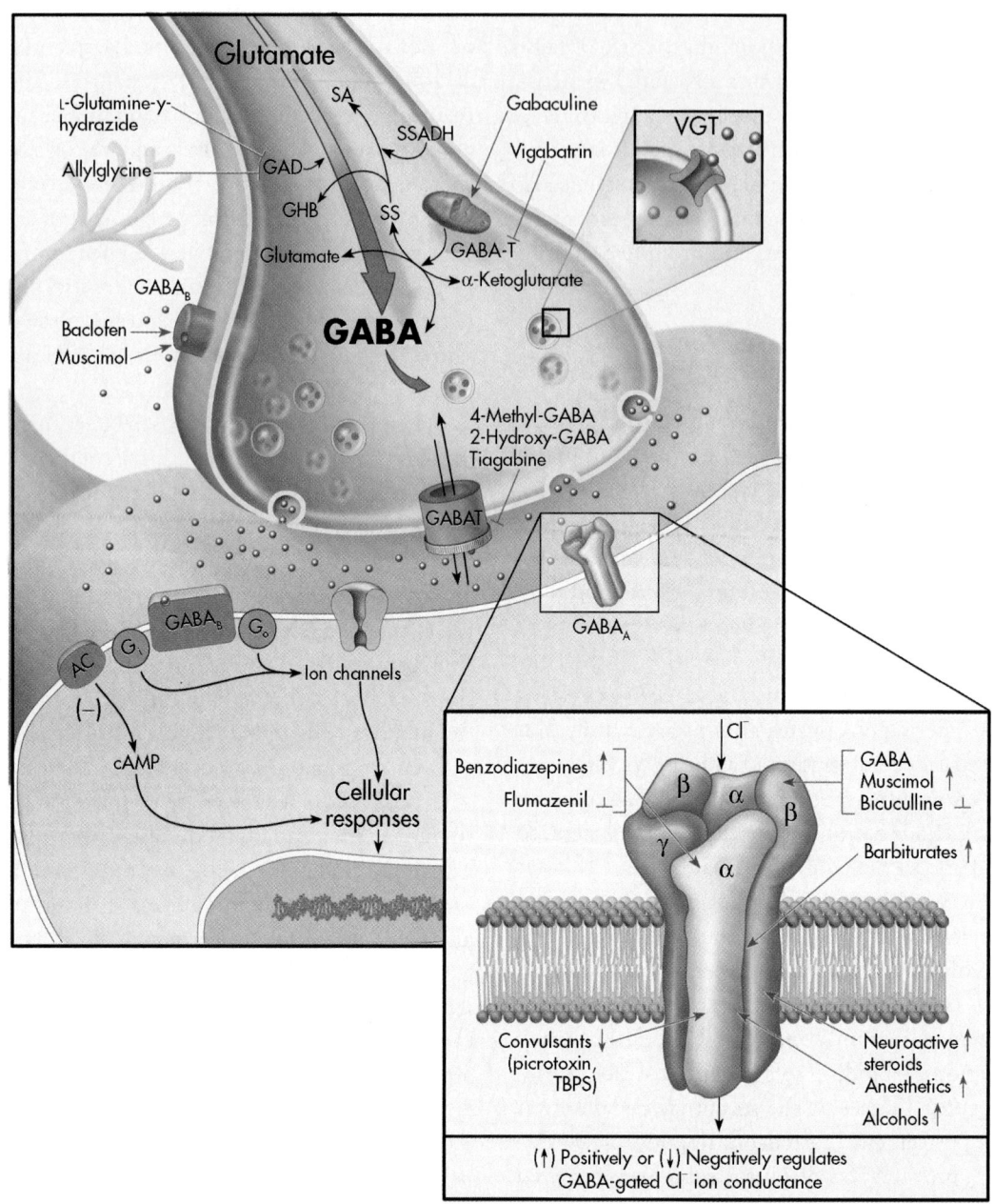

Purinergic Neurotransmission: Focus on Adenosine

It has been known for quite some time that ATP is capable of exerting profound effects on the nervous system (Drury and Szent-Györgyi 1929). However, adenosine and adenosine nucleotides have gained acceptance as neuroactive substances in the CNS only relatively recently (Cooper et al. 2001). Adenosine is released from neurons and glia, but many of the neurotransmitter criteria outlined in the beginning of this chapter are not met.

Nonetheless, adenosine is able to activate many cellular functions that are able to produce changes in neuronal and behavioral states. For example, adenosine is able to stimulate cAMP in vitro in brain slices, and caffeine (which in addition to being a phosphodiesterase inhibitor is a well-known adenosine receptor antagonist) is able to block this response.

Four adenosine receptors have been cloned (A_1, A_{2A}, A_{2B}, and A_3), each of which exhibits unique tissue distribution, ligand binding affinity (nanomolar range), and signal transduction mechanisms (Cooper et al. 2001).

FIGURE 1–8. The GABAergic system (*opposite page*).

This figure depicts the various regulatory processes involved in GABAergic neurotransmission. The amino acid (and neurotransmitter) glutamate serves as the precursor for the biosynthesis of γ-aminobutyric acid (GABA). The rate-limiting enzyme for the process is glutamic acid decarboxylase (GAD), which utilizes pyridoxal phosphate as an important cofactor. Furthermore, agents such as L-glutamine-γ-hydrazide and allylglycine inhibit this enzyme and, thus, the production of GABA. Once released from the presynaptic terminal, GABA can interact with a variety of presynaptic and postsynaptic receptors. Presynaptic regulation of GABA neuron firing activity and release occurs through somatodendritic (not shown) and nerve-terminal $GABA_B$ receptors, respectively. Baclofen is a $GABA_B$ receptor agonist. The binding of GABA to ionotropic $GABA_A$ receptors and metabotropic $GABA_B$ receptors mediates the effects of this receptor. The $GABA_B$ receptors are thought to mediate their actions by being coupled to Ca^{2+} or K^+ channels via second-messenger systems. Many agents are able to modulate $GABA_A$ receptor function. Benzodiazepines, such as diazepam, increase Cl^- permeability, and there are numerous available antagonists directed against this site. There is also a distinctive barbiturate binding site on $GABA_A$ receptors, and many psychotropic agents are capable of influencing the function of this receptor (see blown-up diagram). GABA is taken back into presynaptic nerve endings by a high-affinity GABA uptake transporter (GABAT) similar to that of the monoamines. Once inside the neuron, GABA can be broken down by GABA transaminase (GABA-T), which is localized in the mitochondria; GABA that is not degraded is sequestered and stored into secretory vesicles by vesicle GABA transporters (VGTs), which differ from VMATs in their bioenergetic dependence. The metabolic pathway that produces GABA, mostly from glucose, is referred to as the *GABA shunt*. The conversion of α-ketoglutarate into glutamate by the action of GABA-T and GAD catalyzes the decarboxylation of glutamic acid to produce GABA. GABA can undergo numerous transformations, of which the simplest is the reduction of succinic semialdehyde (SS) to γ-hydroxybutyrate (GHB). On the other hand, when SS is oxidized by succinic semialdehyde dehydrogenase (SSADH), the production of succinic acid (SA) occurs. GHB has received attention because it regulates narcoleptic episodes and may produce amnestic effects. The mood stabilizer and antiepileptic drug valproic acid is reported to inhibit SSADH and GABA-T. TBPS = *t*-butylbicyclophosphorothionate.

Source. Adapted from Cooper JR, Bloom FE, Roth RH: *The Biochemical Basis of Neuropharmacology,* 7th Edition. New York, Oxford University Press, 2001. Copyright 1970, 1974, 1978, 1982, 1986, 1991, 1996, 2001 by Oxford University Press, Inc. Used by permission of Oxford University Press, Inc.

Currently available data suggest that the high-affinity adenosine receptors (A_1 and A_{2A}) may be activated under normal physiological conditions, whereas in pathological states such as hypoxia and inflammation (in which high adenosine concentrations [micromolar range] are present), low-affinity A_{2B} and A_3 receptors are also activated. A_{2B} receptors are expressed in low levels in the brain but are ubiquitous in the rest of the body, whereas A_{2A} receptors are found in high concentrations in areas of the brain that receive dopaminergic projections (i.e., striatum, nucleus accumbens, and olfactory tubercle) (Nestler et al. 2001). Given this receptor's distribution and the inverse relationship between DA and adenosine, it has been postulated that A_{2A} antagonists may have some utility in the treatment of Parkinson's disease (Nestler et al. 2001). The mood stabilizer and antiepileptic drug carbamazepine acts as an antagonist of the A1 subtype and also decreases protein levels of the receptor (for a review, see Gould et al. 2002).

Adenosine is widely regarded as important in the homeostasis of blood flow and metabolic demands in peripheral tissue physiology. Adenosine is also able to alter the function (both pre- and postsynaptically) of numerous neurotransmitters and their receptors, including NMDA, metabotropic glutamate receptors, ionotropic nicotinic receptors, NE, 5-HT, DA, GABA, and various peptidergic receptors. Recent evidence implicates adenosine as a fatigue factor in the decrease of cholinergic activity–arousal via presynaptic inhibition of glutamate release

(Brambilla et al. 2005). In addition, P2X (ligand-gated ion channels) and P2Y (G protein–coupled receptors) are purine receptors that can be activated by ATP. It has been demonstrated that ATP is released from astrocytes (through an unknown mechanism) and that the release is accompanied by glutamate release (Ca^{2+}-dependent) (Innocenti et al. 2000). However, more data suggest that it may be adenosine (that is derived from ATP) that serves as the true ligand for these purinergic receptors (Fields and Stevens-Graham 2002). The ATP/adenosine is then able to activate purine receptors (P_{2Y} receptors) on neighboring astrocytes, and this stimulates Ca^{2+} influx and subsequent release of glutamate and ATP to then impact other astrocytes and neurons. This may be a critical component in the communication process between glial cells, as well as representing a signaling molecule from glia to neurons (Fields and Stevens-Graham 2002).

Peptidergic Neurotransmission

Neuropeptides have garnered increasing attention as critical modulators of CNS function. In general, peptide transmitters are released from neurons when they are stimulated at higher frequencies from those required to facilitate release of traditional neurotransmitters, but they can also be collocated and coreleased together with other neurotransmitters (Cooper et al. 2001; Nestler et al. 2001). Modulation of the firing rate pattern of neurons and subsequent release of neurotransmitters and peptides in a circumscribed fashion are likely important in the basal functioning of the brain as well as response to specific stimuli. For instance, cannabinoids, an example of a neuropeptide neurotransmitter, do not alter the firing rates of hippocampal neurons but instead change the temporal coordination of those neurons, an effect that correlates with memory deficits in individuals (Soltesz and Staley 2006). Virtually every known mammalian bioactive peptide is synthesized first as a precursor protein in which product peptides are flanked by cleavage sites. Neuropeptides are generally found in large dense-core vesicles, whereas other neurotransmitters, such as the monoamines, are packaged in small synaptic vesicles (approximately 50 nm) and are usually half the size of their peptidergic counterparts (Kandel et al. 2000; Squire et al. 2003).

Space limitations preclude an extensive discussion of the diverse array of neuropeptides known to exist in the mammalian brain. Table 1–2 highlights some of the major neuropeptides that may be of particular psychiatric relevance. In the remainder of this section, the basic aspects of peptidergic transmission are highlighted vis-à-vis an overview of opioidergic neurotransmission.

Opioids are a family of peptides that occur endogenously in the brain (endorphins), as botanicals, or as drugs. Pro-opiomelanocortin (POMC), proenkephalin-derived peptides, and prodynorphin-derived peptides yield opioid peptides upon cleavage. Three opioid peptide families currently exist: enkephalins, endorphins, and dynorphins. There are also three types of opioid receptors—namely, μ, δ, and κ—each of which is further subclassified. POMC gene expression occurs in various areas of the brain as well as other tissues. POMC has tissue- and cell-specific regulatory factors at every step from gene transcription to its posttranslational processing. Opioid peptides are stored in large dense-core vesicles and are coreleased from neurons that usually contain a classical neurotransmitter agent (e.g., glutamate and norepinephrine). Opioids activate a variety of signal transduction processes, and different mechanisms in their regulation are in place for different cell types. The opioid receptors are G protein–coupled receptors and exert their cellular effects by inhibiting adenylyl cyclase and regulating K^+ and Ca^{2+} channels, via activation of G_i/G_o. Recently opiorphin, an endogenously derived enkephalin that inactivates zinc ectopeptidase, has been described as equal to morphine in the suppression of pain (Wisner et al. 2006). Although opiates are widely associated with and used therapeutically in pain modulation, recent evidence indicates that dynorphin can actually activate bradykinin receptors and contribute to neuropathic pain (Altier and

Zamponi 2006). The continued study of the opioid system and the second-messenger changes brought about by the chronic administration of opioids has greatly facilitated our understanding of the molecular and cellular effects of drugs of abuse and the potential to develop novel therapeutics (Nestler et al. 2001).

Neurotrophins

Neurotrophins are a family of regulatory factors that mediate the differentiation and survival of neurons, as well as the modulation of synaptic transmission and synaptic plasticity (Patapoutian and Reichardt 2001; Poo 2001). The neurotrophin family now includes, among others, nerve growth factor (NGF), brain-derived neurotrophic factor (BDNF), neurotrophin-3 (NT_3), neurotrophin-4/5 ($NT_{4/5}$), and neurotrophin-6 (NT_6) (Patapoutian and Reichardt 2001). These various proteins are closely related in terms of sequence homology and receptor specificity. They bind to and activate specific tyrosine receptor kinases belonging to the Trk family of receptors, including TrkA, TrkB, and TrkC, and a pan-neurotrophin receptor p75 (Patapoutian and Reichardt 2001; Poo 2001). Additionally, there are two isoforms of TrkB receptors: the full-length TrkB and the truncated form of TrkB, which does not contain the intracellular tyrosine kinase domain (Fryer et al. 1996). The truncated form of TrkB can thus function as a dominant-negative inhibitor for the TrkB receptor tyrosine kinase, thereby providing another mechanism to regulate BDNF signaling in the CNS (Eide and Virshup 2001; Gonzalez et al. 1999).

Neurotrophins can be secreted constitutively or transiently, and often in an activity-dependent manner. Observations support a model in which neurotrophins are generally secreted from the dendrite and act retrogradely at presynaptic terminals, where they act to induce long-lasting modifications (Poo 2001). Within the neurotrophin family, BDNF is a potent physiological survival factor that has also been implicated in a variety of pathophysiological conditions, such as Parkinson's disease, Alzheimer's disease, diabetic peripheral neuropathy, and psychiatric disorders (Malberg et al. 2000; Nagatsu et al. 2000; Pierce and Bari 2001; Salehi et al. 1998). In particular, a genetic variant of BDNF (Val66Met) has been associated with risk for development of mood disorders in humans, as well as with mood- and anxiety-related behaviors and response to antidepressant medications in animal models (Z.Y. Chen et al. 2006; Neves-Pereira et al. 2002; Sklar et al. 2002). Recent data also support a role for this polymorphism in human brain development and

TABLE 1–2. Selected peptides and their presumed relevance to psychiatric disorders and treatment

GROUP	POTENTIAL CLINICAL REFERENCE
Opioid and related peptides	
Endorphin	All of these peptides may be involved in opiate dependence/drug abuse; possible antidepressant activity; chronic pain
Enkephalin	
Dynorphin	
Nociceptin	
Gut-derived peptides	
VIP	Sexual behavior
CCK	Anxiety/panic
Gastrin	
Secretin	Autism?
Somatostatin	Mood disorders and treatment
Tachykinin peptides	
Substance P	NK$_1$ receptor antagonists may alleviate depression/anxiety
Substance K	Regulated by antipsychotics
Neuromedin N	Regulated by lithium
Pituitary peptides	
Oxytocin	Affiliative behavior
Vasopressin	Potential novel anxiolytics?
ACTH	Dysregulated in mood disorders
MSH	
Hypothalamic releasing factors	
CRF	Strongly implicated in depressive and anxiety symptoms; potential target for novel treatments
TRF	Potential antidepressant effects
GHRF	
LHRF	
Others	
Calcitonin gene–related peptide	Regulated by ECT and lithium
Angiotensin	Mood disorders, bipolar disorder
Neurotensin	Regulated by antipsychotics and stimulants
Leptin	Satiety signal; involved in diagnosis and in treatment-induced appetite/weight changes?
CART	Drug addiction, eating disorders
Galanin	Potentially relevant for Alzheimer's diagnosis and other cognitive disorders
Neuropeptide Y	Potential endogenous anxiolytic; regulated by antidepressants/lithium; reduced by early maternal separation
Orexin/hypocretin	Narcolepsy; sleep abnormalities in other disorders?

Note.   This table summarizes selected peptides and their presumed relevance for psychiatric disorders and their treatment; it is not meant to be an exhaustive listing of findings. It should also be noted that in some cases—for example, CRF (mood/anxiety), NPY and neurotensin (regulation by medications), oxytocin (affiliative behavior), and orexin (narcolepsy)—the data are quite convincing. In many of the other examples noted, the evidence must be considered preliminary but is, in our opinion, quite noteworthy and warrants further investigation. ACTH = adrenocorticotropic hormone; CART = cocaine- and amphetamine-related transcript; CCK = cholecystokinin; CRF = corticotropin-releasing factor; ECT = electroconvulsive therapy; GHRF = growth hormone–releasing factor; LHRF = luteinizing hormone–releasing factor; MSH = melanocyte-stimulating hormone; NPY = neuropeptide Y; TRF = thyrotropin-releasing factor; VIP = vasoactive intestinal peptide.

function (Frodl et al. 2007; Kleim et al. 2006). The cellular actions of BDNF are mediated through two types of receptors: a high-affinity tyrosine receptor kinase (TrkB) and a low-affinity pan-neurotrophin receptor (p75) (see Figure 1–1 for details). TrkB is preferentially activated by BDNF and NT4/5 and appears to mediate most of the cellular responses to these neurotrophins (Du et al. 2003; Poo 2001).

Binding of BDNF initiates TrkB dimerization and transphosphorylation of tyrosine residues in its cytoplasmic domain (Patapoutian and Reichardt 2001), a process that involves cAMP activation (Ji et al. 2005). Binding of cytoplasmic src homology 2 (SH2) domain–containing scaffolding proteins—including Shc and Grb-2, which recognize specific phosphotyrosine residues on the receptor—can thus result in the recruitment of a variety of effector molecules. This recruitment of effector molecules generally occurs via interaction of proteins with modular binding domains SH2 and SH3 (named after homology to the src oncogenes—src homology domains). The ability of multiple effectors to interact with phosphotyrosines is undoubtedly one of the keys to the pleiotropic effects that neurotrophins can exert. The physiological effects of neurotrophins are mediated by varying degrees of activation of three major signaling pathways—the Ras/MAP kinase pathway, the phosphoinositide-3 kinase (PI$_3$K) pathway, and the phospholipase C–γ1 (PLC-γ1) pathway (Figure 1–9). Among these pathways, the effects of the PI$_3$K pathway and the MAP kinase pathway have traditionally been linked to the cell survival effects of neurotrophins (Patapoutian and Reichardt 2001) (see Figure 1–9). A series of studies by Duman (2002) have shown that BDNF and TrkB are upregulated by antidepressant treatment. The "neurotrophin hypothesis of depression" has enjoyed heuristic value in reconceptualizing mood disorders as arising from abnormalities in neural plasticity cascades. The demonstration that decreases in hippocampal BDNF levels are correlated with stress-induced depressive behaviors and that antidepressant treatment enhances BDNF expression has generated considerable interest. It is now accepted that the main function of BDNF in the adult brain is regulating synaptic plasticity rather than mediating neuronal survival. Exciting results show that BDNF is first synthesized as a precursor proBDNF, which is then proteolytically cleaved to mature BDNF (mBDNF). ProBDNF and mBDNF facilitate LTD and LTP, respectively, suggesting opposing cellular functions. Finally, BDNF plays different and perhaps opposing roles in the brain stress versus reward system (discussed in Martinowich et al. 2007).

Retrograde Transportation of Neurotrophin Receptors as Signal to the Cell Body

Unlike most other internalized receptors, which are usually degraded after internalization, neurotrophin–Trk complexes in endocytotic vesicles function as signal transducers and provide a mechanism for long-range signaling in the neuronal cytoplasm. Several studies have provided support for the retrograde transportation model of neurotrophin–Trk complexes; these studies indicate that endocytotic vesicles containing neurotrophin–Trk complexes may be functionally active and should be viewed as activated signaling complexes that spread the cytosolic signaling of neurotrophin–Trk complexes to distant parts of the neuron via active transport mechanisms. Intriguingly, as has been shown with another tyrosine kinase (ErbB4 receptor tyrosine kinase), other hitherto unappreciated mechanisms, such as cleavage of receptor fragments, may also be operative in trafficking signals from extracellular receptors to intracellular and nuclear targets (Ni et al. 2001). Whether such novel signaling mechanisms are also utilized by neurotrophin receptors will undoubtedly be the focus of considerable future research.

Regulation of Neurotrophin Signaling by Neuronal Activity

The neurotrophic functions of neurotrophins depend in large part on a cytoplasmic signal-transduction cascade, whose efficacy may be influenced by the presence of electrical activity in the neuron. Seizure activity, as well as nonseizure activity of a frequency or intensity capable of inducing LTP, has been shown to elevate BDNF mRNA levels and to facilitate the release of BDNF from hippocampal and cortical neurons (Poo 2001). Although BDNF was originally considered to be transported only retrogradely, evidence indicates that BDNF can also act anterogradely to modulate synaptic plasticity (Poo 2001). High-frequency neuronal activity and synaptic transmission have also been shown to elevate the number of TrkB receptors on the surface of cultured hippocampal neurons through activation of the CaMKII pathway and may therefore facilitate the synaptic action of BDNF (Du et al. 2000). Thus, electrically active nerve terminals may be more susceptible to synaptic potentiation by secreted neurotrophins than are inactive terminals. Neuronal or synaptic activity is also known to promote the effects of neurotrophins on the survival of cultured retinal ganglion cells; here, neuronal or synaptic activity elevates cAMP levels to enhance the responsiveness of the neuron to

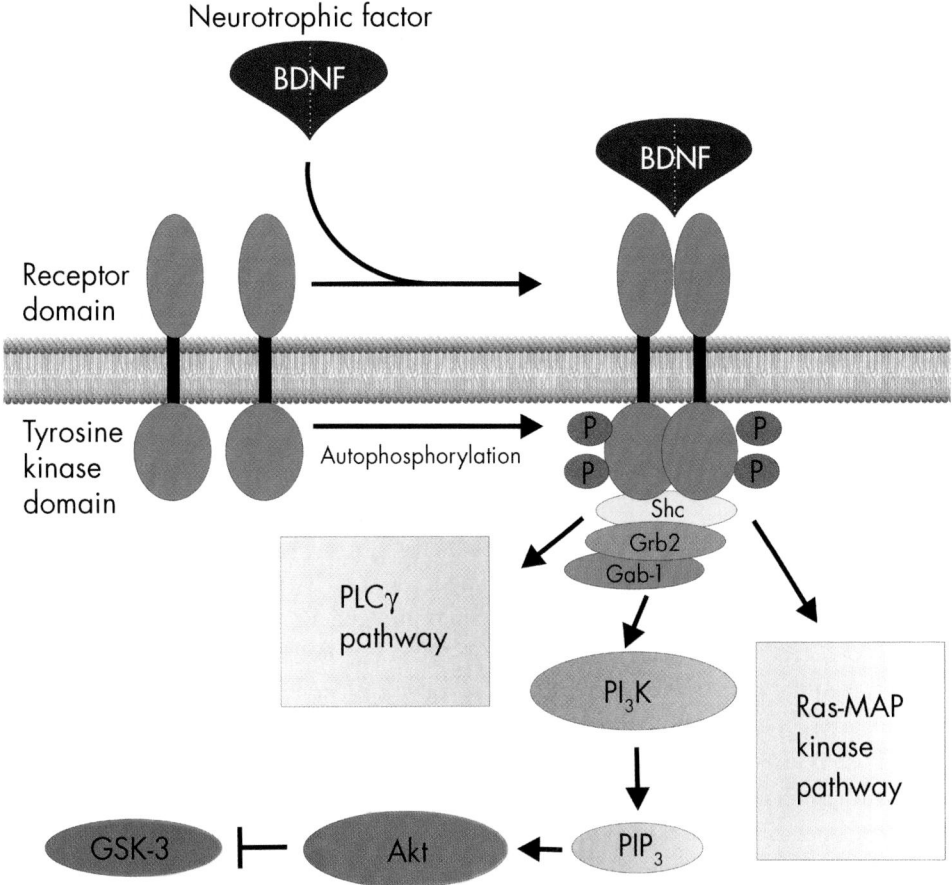

FIGURE 1–9. Neurotrophic cascades.

Cell survival is dependent on neurotrophic factors, such as brain-derived neurotrophic factor (BDNF) and nerve growth factor, and the expression of these factors can be induced by synaptic activity. Phosphorylation of tyrosine receptor kinase (Trk) receptors activates a critical signaling pathway, the Ras/MAP kinase pathway (see Figure 1–15). Phosphorylated Trk receptors also recruit the phosphoinositide-3 kinase (PI$_3$K) pathway through at least two distinct pathways, the relative importance of which differs between neuronal subpopulations. In many neurons, Ras-dependent activation of PI$_3$K is the most important pathway through which neurotrophins promote cell survival (not shown; see text). In some cells, as shown in the figure, PI$_3$K can also be directly activated through adaptor proteins (Shc, Grb-2, and Gab-1). PI$_3$K directly regulates certain cytoplasmic apoptotic pathways. Akt phosphorylates the pro-apoptotic Bcl-2 family member BAD (Bcl-xl/Bcl-2–associated death promoter), thereby inhibiting BAD's pro-apoptotic functions (Datta et al. 1997). Akt may also promote survival in an indirect fashion by regulating another major signaling enzyme: glycogen synthase kinase–3 (GSK-3) (Woodgett 2001). Interestingly, lithium is an inhibitor of GSK-3. Phosphorylated Trk receptors also recruit phospholipase C–γ1 (PLC-γ1). The Trk kinase then phosphorylates and activates PLC-γ1, which acts to hydrolyze phosphatidylinositides to generate diacylglycerol (DAG) and inositol-1,4,5-triphosphate (IP$_3$). Antidepressant medication and mood stabilizers increase levels of BDNF and other neurotrophic factors, suggesting a therapeutic relevance.

neurotrophins, apparently by recruiting extra TrkB receptors to the plasma membrane (Meyer-Franke et al. 1998). Moreover, the internalization of BDNF receptor TrkB is also upregulated by activity as a retrograde signal to the cell body in cultured hippocampal neurons (this regulation is discussed in some detail in Du et al. 2003). The activity-dependent regulation of BDNF signaling on BDNF synthesis and release, TrkB insertion onto neuronal surfaces, and activated TrkB tyrosine kinase internalization are crucial for its influence on synaptic plasticity and neuronal survival.

Cytokines and JAK/ STAT–Coupled Receptors

There is mounting evidence that many psychiatric disorders may be associated with altered immune function. Even more convincing is the evidence that numerous medical disorders and treatments that regulate immune function are associated with psychiatric symptomatology (Evans et al. 2001). Thus, the mechanism by which the immune system is able to mediate its effects through specified signaling pathways in the CNS will undoubtedly be of increasing importance in our understanding of these complex disorders.

Numerous cytokines and growth factors are able to activate the JAK/STAT pathway; here we focus on interferons as a prototype. *Interferons* are cytokines that subserve important antiviral, antigrowth, and immunomodulatory activities (Larner and Keightley 2000). The interferon/cytokine receptor family is a group of receptors that, on binding to an extracellular site, produce dimerization or higher-order clustering. Unlike the tyrosine kinase type receptors (Trk), these receptors associate intrinsically in a noncovalent constitutive manner with proteins of the JAK (Janus tyrosine kinase) family to mediate their effects. Signal transducers and activators of transcription (STATs), which are SH2 domain–containing transcription factors, are required for the actions of many other cytokines and growth factors.

There are two types of receptors for which interferons, on binding to the extracellular part of the receptor, are able to rapidly induce corresponding genes: interferon-α/β (IFN-α/β), or type I receptors; and IFN-γ, or type II receptors. The interferon-stimulated gene factors, which are more commonly known as STATs, bind to enhancers in the promoter regions of type I and type II receptor genes to mediate transcription (Larner and Keightley 2000). It should be mentioned that in addition to interferon, interleukin-6 and prolactin are other cytokines whose effects have been documented to be mediated by STATs. STATs are modified through tyrosine kinases and are necessary for activation of early response genes on interferon binding to the receptor. Thus, the Janus tyrosine kinases (JAK1–3 and TYK2) are important in the regulation of interferon-mediated cellular effects.

Evidence suggests that IFN-α/β cluster in receptor complexes, and upon ligand binding, these proteins are able to mediate some of the receptor–effector responses of interferons. Type I interferon receptors consist of two subunits (IFNAR1 and IFNAR2), of which the IFNAR2 subunit has three isoforms (IFNAR2a, IFNAR2b, and IFNAR2c). Upon binding of interferon to IFN-α, the IFNAR2c subunit is necessary for the activation of the JAK/STAT pathway. Initially, interferons bind to two sites—IFNAR1 and IFNAR2—which heterodimerize, and then the activation of TYK2 and JAK ensues to phosphorylate the receptor (Larner and Keightley 2000). Other phosphatases and kinases are also able to interact with type I interferon receptors to produce a cascade of intercellular effects.

Nuclear Hormones: Focus on Steroids

In contrast to the other neuroactive compounds we have discussed thus far, many hormones (including cortisol, gonadal steroids, and thyroid hormones) are able to rapidly penetrate into the lipid bilayer membrane because of their lipophilic composition (Kandel et al. 2000). Retinoic acid (vitamin A) has recently been shown to be involved in sleep, as well as learning and memory formation (Drager 2006). Nuclear receptors are transcription factors that regulate the expression of target genes in response to steroid hormones and other ligands. Approximately 50 nuclear receptors are known to exist, and their structure is defined by a number of signature functional domains. Generally, nuclear receptors comprise an amino-terminal activation function, the DNA-binding domain, a hinge region, and a carboxy-terminal ligand-binding domain containing a second activation function (Kandel et al. 2000). Upon activation by a hormone, the steroid receptor–ligand complex translocates to the nucleus, where it binds to specific DNA sequences referred to as *hormone responsive elements* (HREs), which subsequently regulate gene transcription (Mangelsdorf et al. 1995; Truss and Beato 1993) (see Figure 1–1). It is now known that nuclear receptors are markedly regulated by additional "accessory proteins." *Nuclear receptor coregulators* are cellular factors that complement nuclear receptors' function as mediators of the cellular response to endocrine signals. They are generally divisible into coregulators that promote transcriptional activation when recruited (coactivators) and those that attenuate promoter activity (corepressors).

In addition to the traditional view of steroid hormone action, it is now clear, however, that steroid hormones also have so-called nongenomic effects that include changes in neurotransmitter receptors, other membrane receptors, and second-messenger systems. These effects are less well characterized, but evidence for their existence includes modulation of neural activity in brain areas where there are few, if any, gonadal steroid receptors; there is also evidence showing that estrogen directly and rapidly inhibits calcium channels in neurons (McEwen 1999; Mermelstein et al. 1996). A growing body of data is also demonstrating bidirectional cross-talk between nuclear receptors and GPCRs. Thus, for example, gonadal steroids have long been known to modulate the activity of monoaminergic neurons and receptors. More recently, it has been shown that β-adrenergic and dopamine D_1 receptors are capable of transactivating glucocorticoid and progesterone receptors, respectively. *Neuroactive steroid* is the term used for a steroid that is able not only to bind to its respective intracellular receptor and become rapidly translocated to the nucleus but also to alter neuronal excitability via interactions with certain neurotransmitter receptors (Rupprecht 2003) (see Figure 1–1). Many of the above-mentioned neuroactive steroids are capable of altering neuronal excitability by interacting with $GABA_A$ receptors. Studies using chimeras of $GABA_A$/glycine receptors suggest an allosteric action of neuroactive steroids at the *N*-terminal side of the middle of the second transmembrane domain of the GABA receptor β_1 and/or α_2 subunits (Rick et al. 1998). However, no direct binding of the steroid to the receptor has been demonstrated. In addition to $GABA_A$ receptors, other members of the ligand-gated ion channel family (including $5\text{-}HT_3$, glycine, nicotinic, ACh, and glutamate receptors) have been postulated to represent targets for neuroactive steroids (Rupprecht 2003).

In view of the $GABA_A$-enhancing potential of 3α-reduced neuroactive steroids, these steroids have been suggested to possess sleep-modulating or -promoting (Mendels and Chernik 1973), anticonvulsant (Frye and Scalise 2000), anxiolytic (Crawley et al. 1986), and neuroprotective (Rupprecht 2003) properties. Finally, it has been postulated that neuroactive steroids may also contribute to psychiatric symptoms sometimes observed during pregnancy and in the postpartum period (Pearson Murphy et al. 2001).

Unconventional Transmitters: Focus on Gases

Many of the unconventional transmitters do not fit the well-accepted neurotransmitter criteria mentioned at the beginning of this chapter. A handful of unconventional transmitters have been characterized and may ultimately prove to have relevance for neuropsychiatric disorders; here, we limit ourselves to a discussion of the gases nitric oxide (NO) and carbon monoxide (CO), which have been demonstrated to exhibit neurotransmitter-like properties in the brain (Dawson and Snyder 1994). The gases, as a result of being small and uncharged, are able to permeate the lipid bilayer and enter the neuron and directly affect certain second-messenger generating systems directly.

Synthesis of NO is derived from arginine via an enzymatic reaction involving NO synthase, flavin adenine dinucleotide, and flavin mononucleotide enzyme (Cooper et al. 2001). Currently, there are three different variations of NO synthase, which arise from different genes that share approximately 50% sequence homology. The neuronal NO synthase is activated by Ca^{2+} and calmodulin and is also regulated by phosphorylation, which decreases its function. NO is released from both neurons and glia and can activate the enzyme guanylate cyclase to augment cGMP concentrations, thereby regulating a variety of neurotransmitter systems (Cooper et al. 2001) (Figure 1–10). These effects likely occur via the activation of protein kinase G (termed G because it is activated by cGMP), but this remains to be definitely established. Notably, endocannabinoids, a class of fatty acid derivatives that bind to cannabinoid receptors, exert prominent effects on NO signaling (Alger 2005).

CO appears to be formed in neurons exclusively by heme oxygenase–2 (HO-2), which cleaves the heme ring, releasing biliverdin, expelling iron from the heme ring, and releasing a one-carbon fragment as CO. HO-2 activity occurs in neuronal populations in numerous parts of the brain and is dynamically regulated by neuronal impulses through a kinase cascade in which PKC activates casein kinase–2, which in turn phosphorylates and activates HO-2. HO-2 activity generates low micromolar concentrations of CO in the brain.

Similar to NO, CO augments cGMP levels to produce its effects in the brain. Additionally, protein carboxyl methylation and phospholipid methylation involve *S*-adenosylmethionine acting as the methyl donor. Protein carboxyl methylation and phospholipid methylation are able to impact certain aspects of brain function (i.e., calmodulin-linked enzymes), and indeed both NO and CO have been implicated in long-term neural alterations such as learning and memory. Thus, it has been presumed that these gases could influence events in the nucleus, such as transcription. When released from postsynaptic neurons, these gases have feedback potential that impacts neurotransmitter release, states of neuronal activity, and notably learning and memory.

Signal Transduction Pathways

Signal transduction refers to the processes by which extracellular stimuli are transferred to—and propagated as—intracellular signals (Figure 1–11). Multicomponent cellular-signaling pathways interact at various levels, thereby forming complex networks that allow the cell to receive, process, and respond to information (Bhalla and Iyengar 1999; Bourne and Nicoll 1993). These networks facilitate

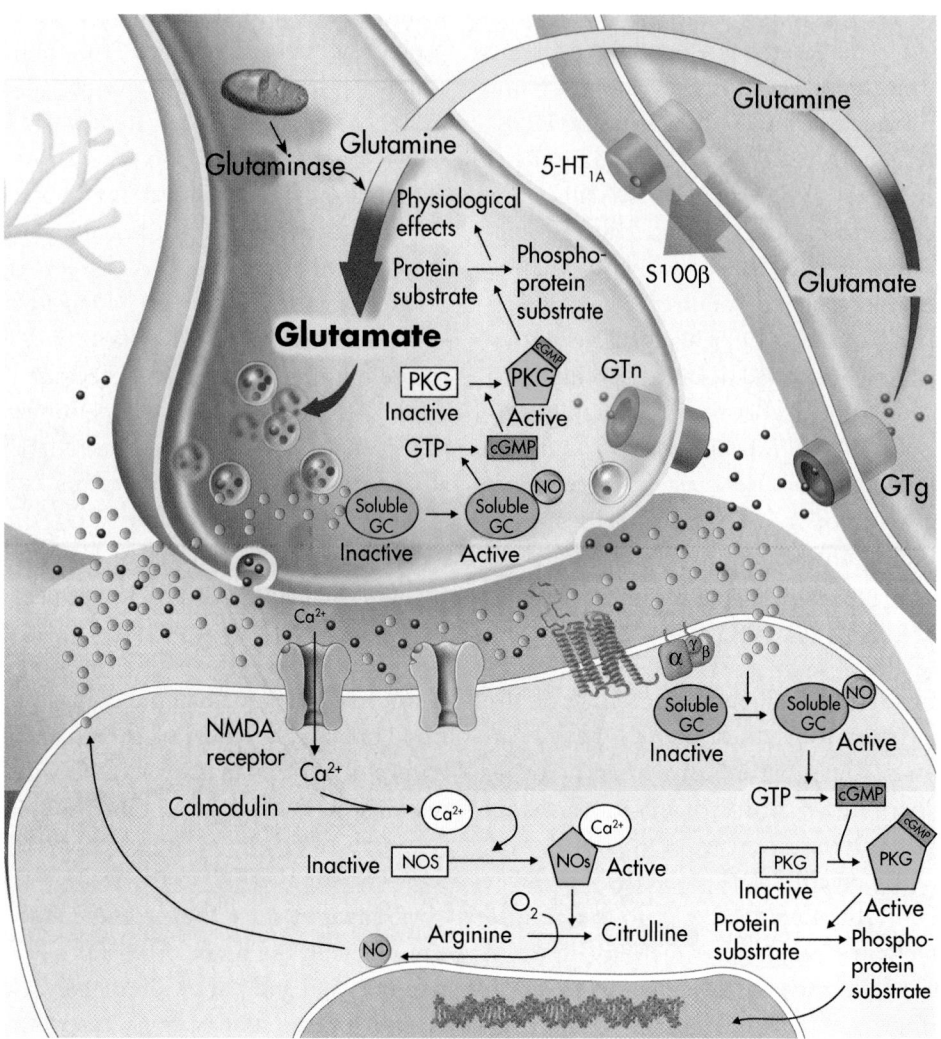

FIGURE 1–10. Nitric oxide as a signaling molecule.

This figure depicts the various regulatory processes involved in nitric oxide (NO) signaling. Reactive oxygen species, in particular several gases, represent yet another means by which the brain is able to transmit messages. NO is formed via NO synthase (NOS), an enzyme that is generally activated by Ca^{2+}-calmodulin. As such, Ca^{2+} entry into cells via NMDA (*N*-methyl-D-aspartate) receptor activation is an important means of activating NOS. NOS yields NO by converting arginine to citrulline using O_2. NO then converts GTP to cGMP, which then is able to target soluble guanylyl cyclases (GCs) (enzymes that are similar to adenylyl cyclases but are activated by cGMP rather than cAMP). cGMP then activates the protein kinase (PKG) and, through the conversion of ATP to ADP, phosphorylates many proteins to bring about the physiological effects of NO. Once produced, NO is then able to diffuse out of the neuron and act on other cells as a signaling molecule. Interestingly, NO is able to also diffuse back to the presynaptic terminal, acting as a *retrograde transmitter*, and is thought to be important in reshaping synaptic connections (i.e., it has been linked to long-term potentiation). NO is labeled in yellow; glutamate is labeled in purple. GTg=glial transporter for glutamate; GTn=neuronal transporter for glutamate; 5-HT$_{1A}$=serotonin$_{1A}$ receptor; S100β=calcium-binding protein expressed primarily by astrocytes.

Source. Adapted from Girault J-A, Greengard P: "Principles of Signal Transduction," in *Neurobiology of Mental Illness.* Edited by Charney DS, Nestler EJ, Bunney BS. New York, Oxford University Press, 1999. Copyright 1999, Oxford University Press. Used with permission.

the integration of signals across multiple time scales, the generation of distinct outputs that depend on input strength and duration, and the regulation of intricate feed-forward and feedback loops (Bhalla and Iyengar 1999). These properties of signaling networks suggest that they play critical roles in cellular memory; thus, cells with different histories, and therefore expressing different repertoires of signaling molecules, interacting at different levels, may respond quite differently to the same signal over time. Given their widespread and crucial role in the integration, regulation, amplification, and fine-tuning of physiological processes, it is not surprising that abnormalities in signaling pathways have now been identified in a variety of human diseases (Simonds 2003; Spiegel 1998).

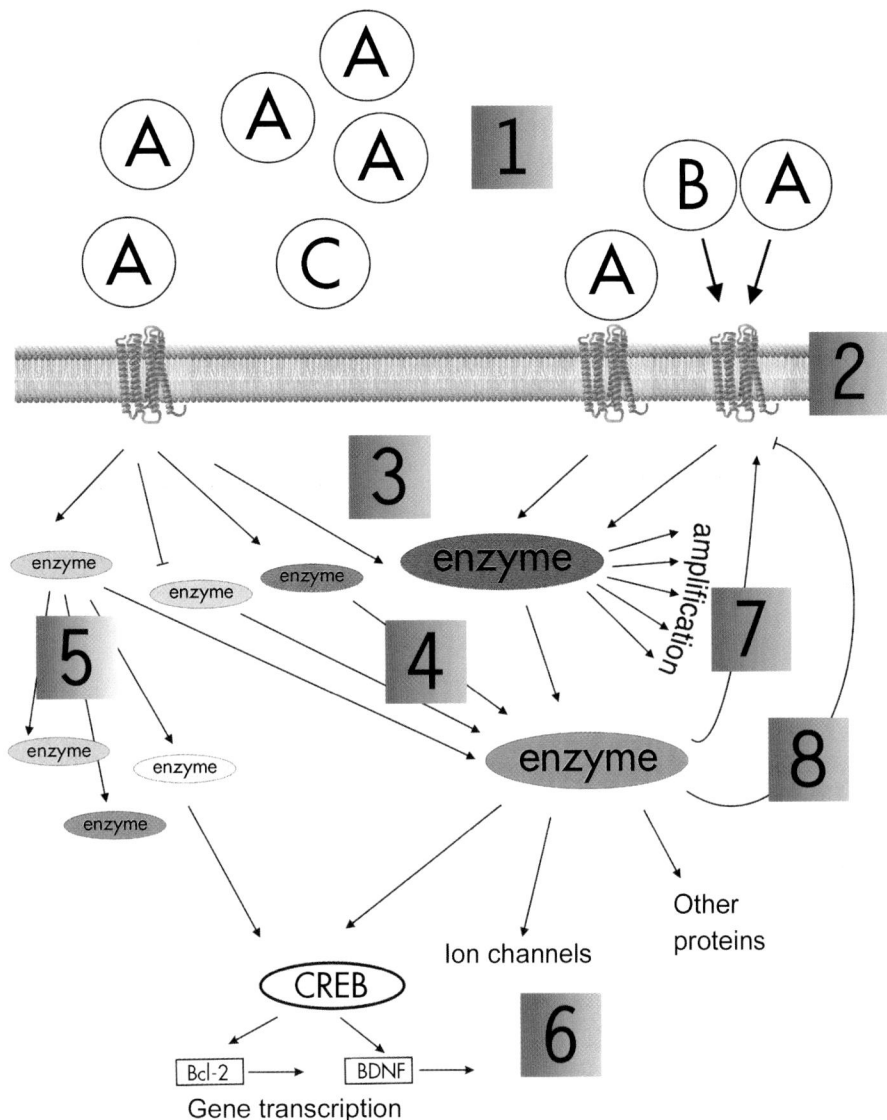

FIGURE 1–11. Principles of signal transduction.

As described in the text, neurons regulate signaling pathways through multiple mechanisms and at multiple levels. Neuronal circuits possess a large number of extracellular neuroactive molecules (**1**; labeled **A, B,** and **C**) that can interact with multiple receptors (**2**). Binding of neuroactive molecules to receptors can result in stimulation and/or attenuation of multiple cellular signaling pathways (**3**), depending on the type of receptor, location in the central nervous system, and activity of other signaling pathways within the cell. Thus, the potential is there to greatly amplify the signals. This signaling can then converge on one signaling pathway (**4**) or diverge into many signaling pathways (**5**). Activation of signaling pathways alters gene transcription and activity of proteins such as ion channels and other signaling molecules (**6**). Additionally, activation of signaling pathways can both positively (**7**) and negatively (**8**) regulate the function of extracellular receptors. Bcl-2 = an anti-apoptotic protein; BDNF = brain-derived neurotrophic factor; CREB = cAMP response element–binding protein.

Pertinent to the present discussion is the observation that a variety of diseases manifest a relatively circumscribed symptomatology, despite the widespread, often ubiquitous expression of the affected signaling proteins.

Although complex signaling networks are likely present in all eukaryotic cells and control various metabolic, humoral, and developmental functions, they may be especially important in the CNS, where they serve the critical roles of first amplifying and "weighting" numerous extracellularly generated neuronal signals and then transmitting these integrated signals to effectors, thereby forming the basis for a complex information-processing network (Bourne and Nicoll 1993; Manji 1992). The high degree of complexity generated by these signaling networks may be one mechanism by which neurons acquire the flexibility for generating the wide range of responses observed in the nervous system. These pathways are thus undoubtedly involved in regulating such diverse vegetative functions as mood, appetite, and wakefulness and are therefore likely to be involved in the pathophysiology of a variety of psychiatric disorders and their treatments.

G Proteins

As mentioned already, G proteins were originally named because of their ability to bind the guanine nucleotides guanosine triphosphate and guanosine diphosphate. Receptors coupled to G proteins include those that respond to catecholamines, serotonin, ACh, various peptides, and even sensory signals such as light and odorants. G_s and G_i were among the first G proteins identified and received their names because of their ability to stimulate or inhibit adenylyl cyclase. Since that time, a multitude of G protein subunits have been identified by a combination of biochemical and molecular cloning techniques. Indeed, genes for 16 $G\alpha$ subunits are known and give rise via alternative splicing to at least 20 mature $G\alpha$ subunits with differential tissue expression (Simonds 2003) (see Table 1–1). There are four homology-based subfamilies of $G\alpha$ subunits: the G_s subfamily, whose members stimulate adenylyl cyclase; the G_i subfamily, which includes G_{i1-3} and G_z, which inhibit adenylyl cyclase; the G_q subfamily, whose members activate PLC-β; and the G_{12} subfamily, whose members interact with regulators of G protein signaling (RGS) domain–containing Rho exchange factors (see Table 1–1 and Figure 1–2) (Simonds 2003). Genes encoding 5 $G\beta$ isoforms and 12 different $G\gamma$ subunits are known in humans; effectors of $G\beta\gamma$ complexes include ion channels, isoforms of adenylyl cyclase, isoforms of PLC-β, and MAP kinase pathways (Simonds 2003) (see Table 1–1).

G Protein Function

G proteins function in the context of two interrelated cycles: a cycle of subunit association and dissociation and a cycle of GTP binding and hydrolysis (discussed in detail in the legend to Figure 1–2). G protein heterotrimers consist of $G\alpha$, $G\beta$, and $G\gamma$ subunits at a 1:1:1 stoichiometry and are named according to decreasing mass, with the α subunits having an apparent mass of 40–52 kDa, β subunits having an apparent mass of 35–36 kDa, and γ subunits having an apparent mass of 5–20 kDa. The different types of G protein have been named on the basis of the distinct α subunits they possess (i.e., G_s represents G proteins containing $G\alpha_s$). This classification system arose from the erroneous assumption that it was only the α sub-

units that were responsible for the proteins' specific functional activity; it is now known that the β and γ subunits exert a number of functional effects on their own (see Table 1–1) and are not simply "anchoring proteins" for α subunits. Although the β and γ subunits are not covalently bound, they are tightly linked by noncovalent coiled-coil interactions; thus, they are generally assumed to function as $\beta\gamma$ dimers. It is very likely that different $\beta\gamma$ subunits exert different effects on α subunits and effectors (e.g., $\beta_2\gamma_2$ behaves differently from $\beta_2\gamma_3$), but the delineation of the differential effects of the different subunit compositions is still in its infancy.

Mediation of neurotransmitter–neurotransmitter and receptor–receptor interactions. The CNS is remarkably complex, both anatomically and chemically, with a remarkable convergence of different receptors in common cortical layers and considerable convergence of neurotransmitter action. A single neuron in the brain receives thousands of synaptic inputs on the cell body and dendrites, and neuronal response is also modulated by a variety of hormonal and neurohormonal substances that are not dependent on synaptic organization (Kandel et al. 2000). The neuron needs to integrate all the synaptic and nonsynaptic inputs impinging on it; this integration of a multitude of signals determines the ultimate excitability, firing pattern, and response characteristics of the neuron, which are then conveyed to succeeding targets via synaptic transmission. How does the single neuron decipher and integrate the multitude of signals it receives and, additionally, generate unique responses to each of these signals or combinations of signals?

Not only do G proteins amplify signals, but they also appear to form the basis of a complex information-processing network in the plasma membrane (Bhalla and Iyengar 1999; Manji 1992). Thus, the ability of G proteins to interact with multiple receptors provides an elegant mechanism to organize the signals from these multiple receptors and to transmit them to a relatively much smaller number of effectors. Signals from a variety of receptors can be "weighted" according to their intrinsic ability to activate a given G protein and integrated to stimulate a single second-messenger pathway (see Figure 1–11). Similarly, the dual (positive and negative) regulation of adenylyl cyclase by G proteins allows for stimulatory and inhibitory signals for these pathways to be "balanced" at the G protein level, yielding an integrated output. Thus, G proteins provide the first opportunity for signals from different receptors to be integrated. This complex web of interactions linking receptors, G proteins, and their effectors with signals con-

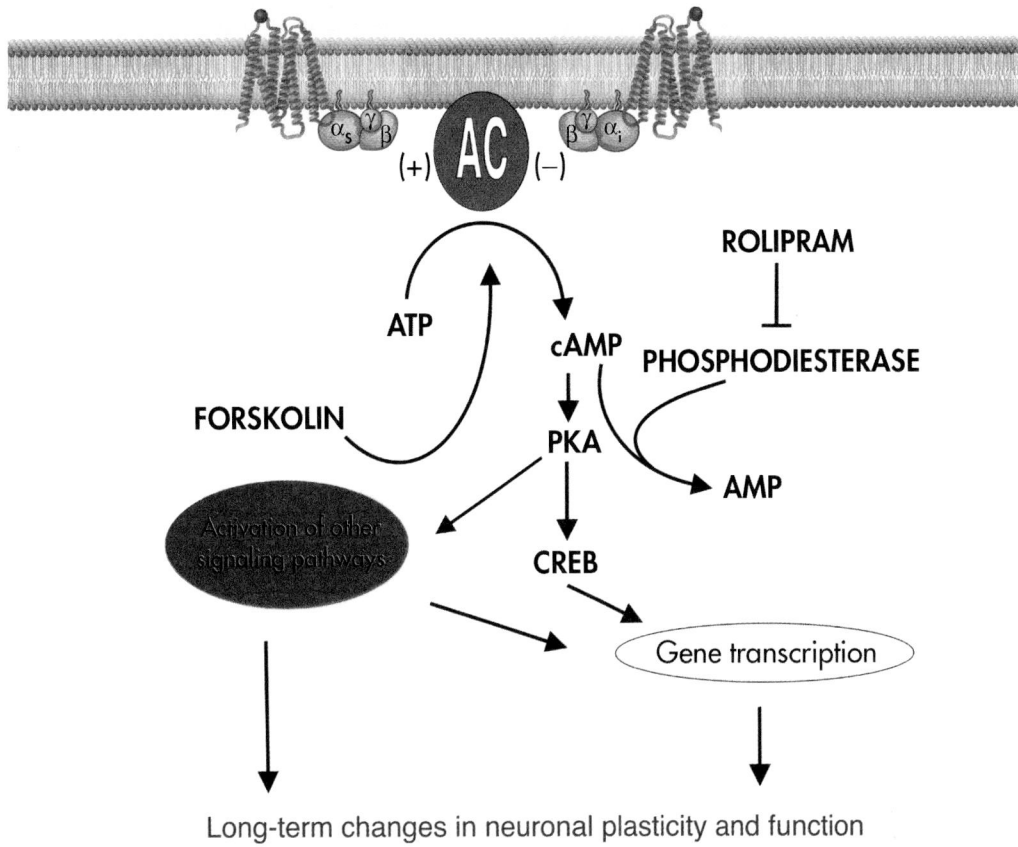

FIGURE 1–12. cAMP signaling pathway.

Receptors can be positively (e.g., β-adrenergic, D₁) or negatively (e.g., 5-HT₁A, D₂) coupled to adenylyl cyclase (AC) to regulate cAMP levels. The effects of cAMP are mediated largely by activation of protein kinase A (PKA). One major downstream target of PKA is CREB (cAMP response element–binding protein). After activation, the phosphorylated CREB binds to the cAMP response element (CRE), a gene sequence found in the promoter of certain genes; data suggest that antidepressants may activate CREB, thereby bringing about increased expression of a major target gene, BDNF. Phosphodiesterase is an enzyme that breaks down cAMP to AMP. Some antidepressant treatments have been found to upregulate phosphodiesterase. Drugs like rolipram, which inhibit phosphodiesterase, may be useful as adjunct treatments for depression. Forskolin is an agent used in preclinical research to stimulate adenylyl cyclase.

verging to shared detectors appears to be crucial for the integrative functions performed by the CNS.

Abnormalities in a variety of human diseases have now been clearly shown to arise from primary abnormalities in G protein signaling cascades and in the G protein subunits themselves (for an excellent discussion, see Simonds 2003; Spiegel 1998). To date, the direct evidence for the involvement of G proteins in psychiatric disorders is more limited. Thus, although elevations in the levels of Gα_s have been found in postmortem brain and peripheral tissue in bipolar disorder, a mutation in the Gα_s gene has not yet been identified (discussed in Manji and Lenox 1999). There is, however, convincing evidence that chronic lithium administration attenuates the functioning of both G_s and G_i, resulting in an elevation of basal cAMP levels but dampened receptor-mediated effects. The allosteric modulation of G proteins has been pro-

posed to play a role in lithium's long-term prophylactic efficacy in protecting susceptible individuals from cyclic affective episodes induced spontaneously or by stress or drugs (e.g., antidepressant, stimulant) (G. Chen et al. 1999; Gould and Manji 2002).

The cAMP signaling cascade. G proteins control intracellular cAMP levels by mediating the ability of neurotransmitters to activate or inhibit adenylyl cyclase (Figure 1–12; see also Figure 1–2). The mechanism by which neurotransmitters stimulate adenylyl cyclase is well established. Activation of those neurotransmitter receptors that couple to G_s results in the generation of free Gα_s subunits that bind to and directly activate adenylyl cyclase. A similar mechanism appears to be the case for Gα_olf, a type of G protein (structurally related to Gα_s) that is enriched in olfactory epithelium and dopamine-rich areas of the brain and mediates the ability of odorant receptors and D_1 receptors to stimulate adenylyl cyclase. The mechanism by which neurotransmitters inhibit adenylyl cyclase and decrease neuronal levels of cAMP is somewhat less clear, and more than one mechanism may be operative. By analogy with the action of G_s, it was originally proposed that activation of neurotransmitter receptors that couple to Gi results in the generation of free $G\alpha_i$ subunits, which could bind to, and thereby directly inhibit, adenylyl cyclase. While this mechanism may be operative, there are also data to suggest that $\beta\gamma$ subunit complexes, generated by the release of $G\alpha_i$, might directly inhibit certain forms of adenylyl cyclase or might bind and "tie up" free $G\alpha_s$ subunits in the membrane.

It is now clear that there are several forms of adenylyl cyclase that make up a distinct enzyme family; these various forms are differentially regulated and display distinct distributions in nervous and nonnervous tissues. For example, type I is found predominantly in brain, whereas types II and IV, although abundantly expressed in the brain, have a more widespread distribution. The topographical structure of the adenylyl cyclase proteins resembles that of membrane transporters and ion channels. However, there is currently no convincing evidence of a transporter or channel function for mammalian adenylyl cyclases.

As would be predicted, the different forms of adenylyl cyclase are regulated by distinct mechanisms. Type I through IV enzymes differ in their ability to be regulated by Ca^{2+} and calmodulin. Types I and III are stimulated by Ca^{2+}-calmodulin complexes, whereas types II and IV are insensitive. Perhaps the most intriguing regulation is that by the G protein β and γ subunits. Thus, it is now clear that when type II adenylyl cyclase is concurrently stimulated by a stimulatory receptor (e.g., β-adrenergic receptor), the $\beta\gamma$ subunits released from an "inhibitory receptor" (e.g., 5-HT_{1A}, α_2, $GABA_B$) can, in fact, *robustly potentiate* the cAMP response (Bourne and Nicoll 1993). Type II adenylyl cyclase thus serves as a "coincidence detector" in the CNS, capable of temporally and spatially integrating signals to bring about dramatically different effects. An additional important mechanism by which adenylyl cyclase can be regulated is by cross-talk with protein kinase C, thereby linking receptors linked to stimulation of adenylyl cyclase and those linked to the turnover of membrane phosphoinositides. The physiological effects of cAMP are mediated primarily by activation of protein kinase A, an enzyme that phosphorylates and regulates many proteins, including ion channels, cytoskeletal elements, transcription factors, and other enzymes. Indeed, one major CNS target for the actions of PKA is the

transcription factor CREB (cAMP response element–binding protein), which plays a major role in long-term neuroplasticity and is an indirect target of antidepressants (Duman 2002) (see Figure 1–12). As we discuss in greater detail below, phosphorylation and dephosphorylation reactions play a major role in regulating a variety of long-term neuroplastic events in the CNS.

Phosphoinositide/Protein Kinase C

Phosphoinositide

Although inositol phospholipids are relatively minor components of cell membranes, they play a major role in receptor-mediated signal transduction pathways. They are involved in a diverse range of responses, such as cell division, secretion, and neuronal excitability and responsiveness. In many cases, $G_{q/11}$ is involved, and it is believed that $G\alpha_{q/11}$ directly binds to and activates phospholipase C (Figure 1–13). In other cases, however, it is the $\beta\gamma$ subunits released upon activation of receptors coupled to G_i/G_o that bring about activation of the enzyme PLC to produce the intracellular second messengers sn-1,2-diacylglycerol (DAG; an endogenous activator of PKC) and inositol-1,4,5-triphosphate (IP_3). IP_3 binds to the IP_3 receptor and facilitates the release of calcium from intracellular stores, in particular the endoplasmic reticulum (see Figure 1–13). The released calcium then interacts with various proteins in the cell, including the important family of calmodulins (Ca^{2+}-receptor protein calmodulin, or CaM) (discussed later in this chapter; Figure 1–14). Calmodulins then activate calmodulin-dependent protein kinases (CaMKs), which affect the activity of diverse proteins, including ion channels, signaling molecules, proteins that regulate apoptosis, scaffolding proteins, and transcription factors (Miller 1991; Soderling 2000).

IP_3 can be metabolized both by dephosphorylation to form inositol-1,4-P_2 and by phosphorylation to form inositol-1,3,4,5-P_4 (IP_4), which has been proposed to be involved in the entry of Ca^{2+} into cells from extracellular sources. Recycling of IP_3 is important for continuation of phosphoinositide hydrolysis in response to extracellular signals. This is achieved by the enzyme inositol monophosphatase (IMPase), which is the rate-limiting enzyme that converts IP_3 back to phosphoinositide-4,5-bisphosphate (PIP_2). Without this enzyme, PIP_2 cannot be recycled adequately, potentially leading to low levels of PIP_2 and inhibition of the signaling cascades involving DAG and IP_3. Lithium, at therapeutically relevant concentrations, is a noncompetitive inhibitor of IMPase (for a review, see Gould et al. 2003). This has led to the "inositol

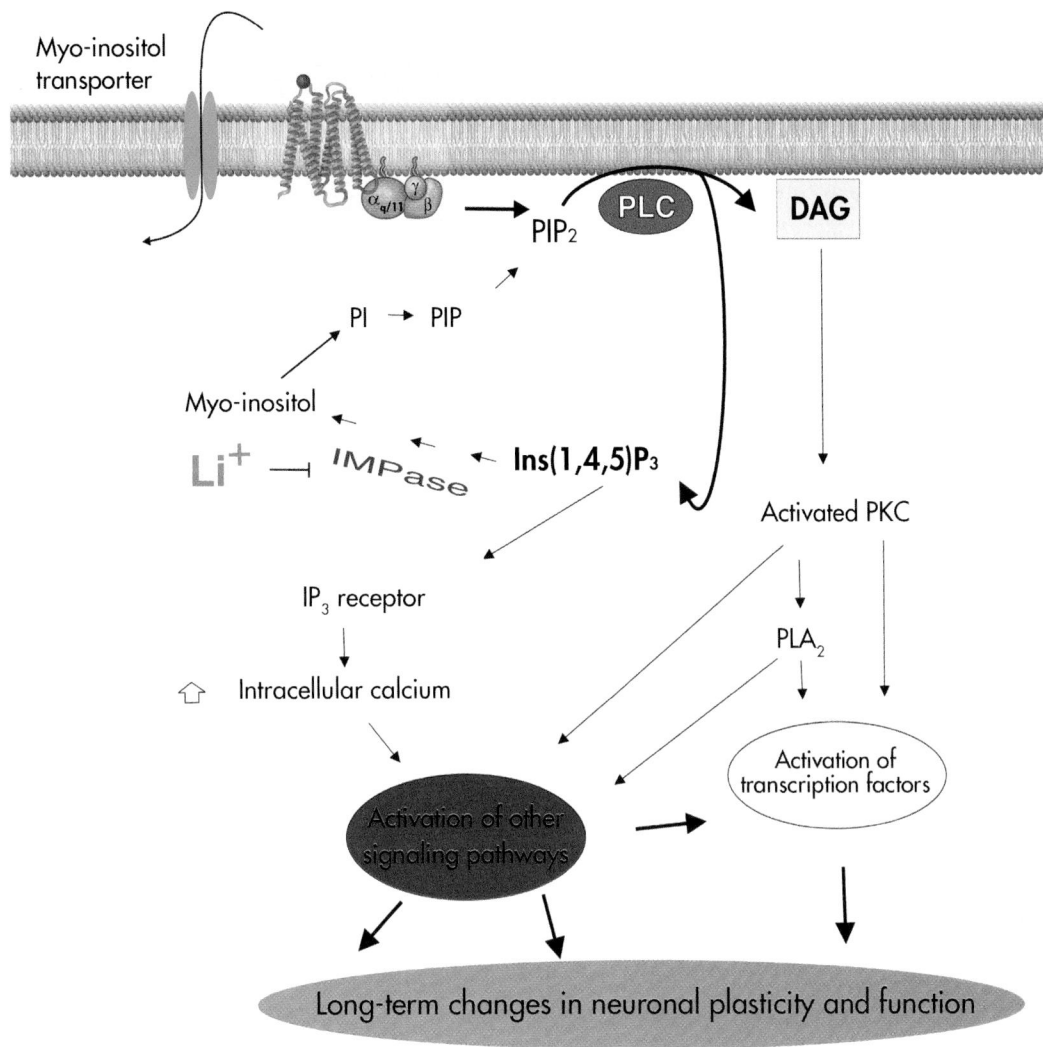

FIGURE 1–13. Phosphoinositide (PI) signaling pathway.

A number of receptors in the CNS (including M_1, M_3, M_5, 5-HT$_{2C}$) are coupled, via $G\alpha_{q/11}$, to activation of PI hydrolysis. Activation of these receptors induces phospholipase C (PLC) hydrolysis of phosphoinositide-4,5-bisphosphate (PIP$_2$) to sn-1,2-diacylglycerol (DAG) and inositol-1,4,5-triphosphate (IP$_3$). DAG activates protein kinase C (PKC), an enzyme that has many effects, including the activation of phospholipase A$_2$ (PLA$_2$), an activator of arachidonic acid signaling pathways. IP$_3$ binds to the IP$_3$ receptor, which results in the release of intracellular calcium from intracellular stores, most notably the endoplasmic reticulum. Calcium is an important signaling molecule and initiates a number of downstream effects such as activation of calmodulins and calmodulin-dependent protein kinases (see Figure 1–15). IP$_3$ is recycled back to PIP$_2$ by the enzymes inositol monophosphatase (IMPase) and inositol polyphosphatase (IPPase; not shown), both of which are targets of lithium. Thus, lithium may initiate many of its therapeutic effects by inhibiting these enzymes, thereby bringing about a cascade of downstream effects involving PKC and gene expression changes.

Source. Adapted from Gould TD, Chen G, Manji HK: "Mood Stabilizer Pharmacology." *Clinical Neuroscience Research* 2:193–212, 2003. Copyright 2003, Elsevier. Used with permission.

depletion hypothesis," which posits that lithium brings about a reduction in the levels of inositol by inhibiting the activity of this "recycling enzyme." Although lithium does reduce inositol levels in the areas of the brain in bipolar patients (Moore et al. 1999), this likely represents an upstream "initiating event," which brings about downstream changes in PKC and regulates gene expression, which may be ultimately responsible for some of its ther-

apeutic effects (see Figure 1–13) (Brandish et al. 2005; Gould et al. 2003; Manji and Lenox 1999).

Protein Kinase C

Ca^{2+}-activated, phospholipid-dependent protein kinase (protein kinase C, or PKC) is a ubiquitous enzyme, highly enriched in brain, where it plays a major role in regulating both pre- and postsynaptic aspects of neurotransmission (Nishizuka 1992; Stabel and Parker 1991). PKC is one of the major intracellular mediators of signals generated upon external stimulation of cells via a variety of neurotransmitter receptors (including muscarinic [M_1, M_3, M_5], noradrenergic [α_1], and serotonergic [5-HT$_2$] receptors) that induce the hydrolysis of various membrane phospholipids.

Activation of PKC by DAG appears to involve the binding of the lipid to a specific regulatory site on the enzyme, resulting in an increase in the Ca^{2+} affinity, and thus its stimulation at physiological ionic concentrations. Ca^{2+} is also believed to contribute to PKC activation by facilitating the interaction of the enzyme with the lipid bilayer and hence with acidic phospholipids and DAG. PKC is now known to exist as a family of closely related subspecies, has a heterogeneous distribution in brain (with particularly high levels in presynaptic nerve terminals), and, together with other kinases, appears to play a crucial role in the regulation of synaptic plasticity and various forms of learning and memory. The multiple closely related PKC isoforms are all activated by phospholipids and DAG, albeit with slightly different kinetics. The isoforms can be subclassified according to Ca^{2+} dependence: the "conventional" PKCs (α, βI, βII, γ) are dependent on Ca^{2+} for activity, whereas several others, termed "novel" (δ, ε, η, θ) and "atypical" (ι, λ, ζ), are calcium independent (Nishizuka 1992). The conventional, novel, and atypical isozymes all share activation by phospholipids or DAG and an autoinhibitory pseudosubstrate region, which maintains the enzyme in an inactive state until activated. However, the subgroups are activated by different activators. The conventional PKCs require calcium, acidic phospholipids, and DAG for activation; the novel PKCs do not require calcium, and the atypical PKCs do not require calcium or DAG. PKC isozymes that do not share the pseudosubstrate region (μ/PKD and υ) have been described, which suggests a possible different mode of action.

The differential tissue distribution of PKC isozymes, as well as the fact that several isoforms are expressed within a single cell type, suggests that each isozyme may exert distinct cellular functions. At present, it is unclear whether such putative functional specificity arises from differential in vivo activation, differential substrate specificity, or a combination thereof. PKC has many growth-regulating properties in immature cells and has additional cell-specific responses in individual mature cells (Kanashiro and Khalil 1998). One protein whose activity is modulated by PKC is myristoylated alanine-rich C kinase

substrate (MARCKS). This protein functions as a regulated crossbridge between actin and the plasma membrane, contributing to the cytoskeleton of the cell and subsequently to neuronal plasticity (Aderem 1992) (see Figure 1–13). PKC is also an important activator of phospholipase A_2, thus linking the phosphoinositide cycle with arachidonic acid pathways (see Figure 1–13). Arachidonic acid functions as an important mediator of second-messenger pathways within the brain and is regulated by chronic lithium (Axelrod et al. 1988; Rapoport 2001). The activation of phospholipase A_2 by PKC (and other pathways) results in arachidonic acid release from membrane phospholipids (Axelrod 1995). This release of arachidonic acid from cellular membrane allows for the subsequent formation of a number of eicosanoid metabolites such as prostaglandins and thromboxanes. These metabolites mediate numerous subsequent intracellular responses and, because of their lipid permeable nature, transsynaptic responses.

PKC also has been demonstrated to be active in many other cellular processes, including stimulation of transmembrane glucose transport, secretion, exocytosis, smooth muscle contraction, gene expression, modulation of ion conductance, cell proliferation, and desensitization of extracellular receptors (Nishizuka 1992). One of the best-characterized effects of PKC activation in the CNS is the facilitation of neurotransmitter release. Studies have suggested that PKC activation may facilitate neurotransmitter release via a variety of mechanisms, including modulating several ionic conductances regulating Ca^{2+} influx, upstream steps regulating release of Ca^{2+} from intracellular stores, recruitment of vesicles to at least two distinct vesicle pools, and the Ca^{2+} sensitivity of the release process itself (discussed in Bown et al. 2002). Abundant data also suggest that the PKC signaling pathway may play an important role in the pathophysiology and treatment of bipolar disorder (Manji and Lenox 1999). Thus, elevations in PKC isozymes have been reported in postmortem brain and platelets in bipolar patients; more importantly, in animal and cell-based models, lithium and valproate exert strikingly similar effects on PKC isozymes and substrates in a time frame mimicking their therapeutic actions.

A recent whole-genome association study of bipolar disorder has further implicated this pathway. Of the risk genes identified, the one demonstrating by far the strongest association with bipolar disorder was diacylglycerol kinase, an immediate regulator of PKC (Baum et al. 2008). In animal models of mania, several studies have demonstrated that both acute and chronic amphetamine exposure produces an alteration in PKC activity and its relative cytosol-to-membrane distribution, as well as the phosphorylation of a major PKC substrate, GAP-43, which has been implicated in long-term alterations of neurotransmitter release. Increased hedonistic drive and increased tendency to abuse drugs are well-known facets of manic behavior; notably, PKC inhibitors attenuate these important aspects of the manic-like syndrome in rodents (Einat and Manji 2006; Einat et al. 2007). Recent preclinical studies have specifically investigated the antimanic effects of tamoxifen (since this is the only CNS-penetrant PKC inhibitor available for humans). These studies showed that tamoxifen significantly reduced amphetamine-induced hyperactivity and risk-taking behavior (Einat et al. 2007). Finally, with respect to cognitive dysfunction associated with mania, Birnbaum et al. (2004) demonstrated that excessive activation of PKC dramatically impaired the cognitive functions of the prefrontal cortex and that inhibition of PKC protected cognitive function. In summary, preclinical biochemical and behavioral data support the notion that PKC activation may result in manic-like behaviors, whereas PKC inhibition may be antimanic. These preclinical data, along with animal studies discussed above, have prompted clinical studies of PKC inhibitors and mood dysregulation. A number of small studies have found that tamoxifen, a nonsteroidal antiestrogen and a PKC inhibitor at high concentrations, possesses antimanic efficacy (Bebchuk et al. 2000; Kulkarni et al. 2006). Most recently, a double-blind, placebo-controlled trial of tamoxifen in the treatment of acute mania was undertaken (Zarate et al. 2007). Subjects showed significant improvement in mania on tamoxifen compared with placebo as early as 5 days, and the effect size for the drug difference was very large after 3 weeks.

Calcium

Calcium is a very common signaling element and plays a critical role in the CNS by regulating the activity of diverse enzymes and facilitating neurotransmitter release (see Figure 1–14). Importantly, excessively high levels of calcium are also a critical mediator of cell death cascades within neurons, necessitating diverse homeostatic mechanisms to regulate intracellular calcium levels very precisely. Thus, although the external level of Ca2+ is approximately 2 mM, the resting intracellular Ca2+ concentrations (Ca^{2+}_i) are in the range of 100 nM (that is, 2×10^4 *lower*) (Rasmussen 1989). Neuronal stimulation by depolarization or receptor activation activates phosphoinositol turnover and increases Ca^{2+}_i by one to two orders of magnitude as a result of release of Ca^{2+} from intracellular stores and/or influx of Ca^{2+} through ion channels (Rink 1988). Acting via intracellular proteins such as calmodulin and enzymes such as PKC, calcium ions influence synthesis and release of neurotransmitters (Parnas and Segel 1989), receptor signaling (Rasmussen 1986), and neuronal periodicity (Matthews 1986).

Many proteins bind Ca^{2+}; these are classified as either "buffering" or "triggering" and include calcium pumps, calbindin, calsequestrin, calmodulin, PKC, phospholipase A_2, and calcineurin (see Figure 1–14). Once stability of intracellular calcium is accomplished, transient low-magnitude changes can serve an important signaling function. Importantly, calcium action is locally mediated; that is, because of the high concentration of calcium-binding proteins, it is estimated that the free Ca^{2+} ion diffuses only approximately 0.5 µM and is free for around 50 µsec before encountering a Ca^{2+}-binding protein. Ca^{2+} is sequestered in the endoplasmic reticulum (which serves as a vast web and framework for Ca^{2+}-binding proteins to capture and sequester Ca^{2+}). Ca^{2+} buffering/triggering proteins are nonuniformly distributed, and thus there is considerable subcellular variation of Ca^{2+} concentrations (e.g., near a Ca^{2+} channel).

Calcium is generally mobilized in one of two ways in the cell, either by mobilization from intracellular stores or by selective diffusion across plasma membrane ion channels (see Figure 1–14). Ca^{2+} ions pass the membrane through more or less specific channels regulated by changes of membrane potential or transmitter binding. This Ca^{2+} influx lasts until Ca^{2+} levels reach a critical level in the submembranal compartment; a potassium current is then activated that repolarizes the membrane. This Ca^{2+}-dependent potassium current represents a strong inhibitory mechanism of the single neuron itself without synaptic input. Its attractiveness for psychiatry lies in its sensitivity to modulatory influences: many amines, peptides, or drugs with relevance in the etiology and/or treatment of these disorders (e.g., norepinephrine, dopamine, corticotrophin-releasing factor [CRF], caffeine, neuroleptics) modify (i.e., increase or decrease) this potassium current. When activation of the potassium pump is decreased, the capacity for negative feedback after excitation becomes impaired and the neuron switches to a state of higher activation, coincidentally with increased calcium influx. Such an overdrive in calcium currents and discharge activity could be a functional prerequisite for states of pathological activity, possibly underlying neuropsychiatric symptoms such as epilepsy, mania, or depression.

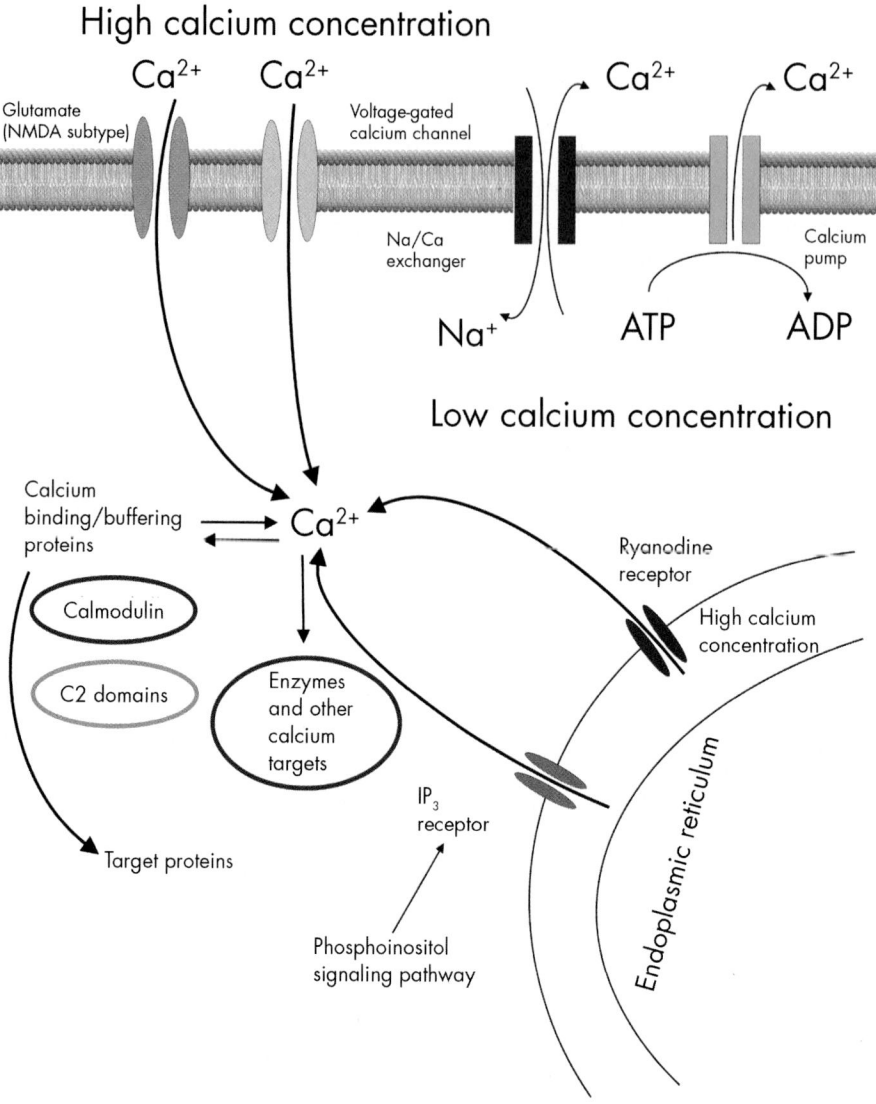

FIGURE 1–14.   Calcium-mediated signaling.

In neurons, Ca^{2+}-dependent processes represent an intrinsic nonsynaptic feedback system that provides competence for adaptation to different functional tasks. Ca^{2+} is generally mobilized in one of two ways in the cells: either by mobilization from intracellular stores (e.g., from the endoplasmic reticulum) or from outside of the cell via plasma membrane ion channels and certain receptors (e.g., NMDA [N-methyl-D-aspartate]). The external concentration of Ca^{2+} is approximately 2 mM, yet resting intracellular Ca^{2+} concentrations are in the range of 100 nM (2×10^4 *lower*). Local high levels of calcium result in activation of enzymes, signaling cascades, and, at extremes, cell death. Release of intracellular stores of calcium is primarily regulated by inositol-1,4,5-triphosphate (IP_3) receptors that are activated upon generation of IP_3 by phospholipase C (PLC) activity, and the ryanodine receptor that is activated by the drug ryanodine. Many proteins bind Ca2+ and are classified as either "buffering" or "triggering." These include calcium pumps, calbindin, calsequestrin, calmodulin, PKC, phospholipase A_2, and calcineurin. Once stability of intracellular calcium is accomplished, transient low-magnitude changes can serve an important signaling function. Calcium action is *local*. Because of the high concentration of calcium-binding proteins, it is estimated that the free Ca^{2+} ion diffuses only approximately 0.5 µM and is free for about 50 µsec before encountering a Ca^{2+}-binding protein. Ca^{2+} is sequestered in the endoplasmic reticulum (which serves as a vast web and framework for Ca2+-binding proteins to capture and sequester Ca^{2+}). Ca^{2+} buffering/triggering proteins are nonuniformly distributed, so there is considerable subcellular variation of Ca^{2+} concentrations (e.g., near a Ca^{2+} channel). The primary mechanism for Ca^{2+} calcium exit from the cell is either via sodium-calcium exchange or by means of a calcium pump.

Ca^{2+} released intracellularly is regulated both positively and negatively, resulting in the generation of dynamic Ca^{2+} waves. Once intracellular Ca^{2+} levels are increased, this triggers/activates a number of proteins (e.g., adenylyl cyclase type I, CaMKs, PKC, calpain [a protease], calcineurin [a protein phosphatase]). In neurons, Ca^{2+}-dependent processes represent an intrinsic nonsynaptic feedback system that provides the competence for adaptation to different functional tasks (see Figure 1–14). Regulation of intracellular Ca^{2+} could be of particular relevance to the study of psychiatric disorders, because the same elevation of intracellular Ca^{2+} may facilitate or inhibit a given function, depending on the target enzyme, the phase of the cell cycle, the intracellular effector protein, and the Ca^{2+}-dependent process. In addition, higher or more sustained increases of intracellular Ca^{2+} may inhibit the same function that smaller elevations facilitate (Wolff et al. 1977), so that elevated intracellular Ca^{2+} can produce excessive activation of some systems and inhibition of others. A polymorphism in PPP3CC, a component of the calcium-dependent protein phosphatase calcineurin, has been associated with risk of developing schizophrenia in at least two patient populations (Gerber et al. 2003; Y.L. Liu et al. 2007).

Signaling Cascades Generally Utilized by Neurotrophic Receptors in the CNS

The pleiotropic and often profound effects (e.g., neuronal growth, differentiation, survival) of neurotrophins and growth factors in the CNS are generally mediated by varying degrees of activation of three major signaling pathways: MAP kinase (extracellular response kinase [ERK]) pathway, the phosphoinositol-3 kinase pathway, and the phospholipase C–γ1 pathway (see Figure 1–9). Among these pathways, the effects of the PI3K pathway and the MAP kinase pathway have been most directly linked to the cell survival effects of neurotrophins (Patapoutian and Reichardt 2001).

MAP Kinase Cascade

MAP kinases are abundantly present in brain and have been postulated to play a major role in a variety of long-term CNS functions, in both the developing and the mature CNS (Fukunaga and Miyamoto 1998; Kornhauser and Greenberg 1997; Matsubara et al. 1996; Robinson et al. 1998). With respect to their actions in the mature CNS, MAP kinases have been implicated in mediating neurochemical processes associated with long-term facilitation (Martin et al. 1997), long-term potentiation (English and Sweatt 1996, 1997), associative learning (Atkins

et al. 1998), one-trial and multitrial classical conditioning (Crow et al. 1998), long-term spatial memory (Blum et al. 1999), and modulation of the addictive effects of abused drugs (Lu et al. 2005). They have also been postulated to integrate information from multiple infrequent bursts of synaptic activity (Murphy et al. 1994). Importantly for the present discussion, MAP kinase pathways have been demonstrated to regulate the responses to environmental stimuli and stressors in rodents (Xu et al. 1997) and to couple PKA and PKC to CREB protein phosphorylation in area CA1 of the hippocampus (Roberson et al. 1996, 1999). These studies suggest the possibility of a broad role for the MAP kinase cascade in regulating gene expression in long-term forms of synaptic plasticity (Roberson et al. 1999). For example, it has recently been shown that CREB modulates excitability of neurons of the nucleus accumbens, which helps to limit behavioral sensitivity to cocaine in rodent models (Dong et al. 2006). Thus, overall, the data suggest that MAP kinases play important physiological roles in the mature CNS and, furthermore, may be important targets for the actions of CNS-active agents (Nestler 1998).

Growth factors acting through specific receptors (e.g., BDNF acting on TrkB) activate the Ras/MAP kinase signaling cascade (Figure 1–15). Among the targets of the MAP kinase pathway is ribosomal S6 kinase (RSK). RSK phosphorylates CREB and other transcription factors. Studies have demonstrated that the activation of the MAP kinase pathway can inhibit apoptosis by inducing the phosphorylation and inactivation of the pro-apoptotic protein BAD (Bcl-xl/Bcl-2–associated death promoter) and increasing the expression of the anti-apoptotic protein Bcl-2 (the latter effect likely involves CREB) (Bonni et al. 1999; Riccio et al. 1997). Phosphorylation of BAD occurs via activation of RSK. RSK phosphorylates BAD and thereby promotes its inactivation. Activation of RSK also mediates the actions of the MAP kinase cascade and neurotrophic factors on the expression of Bcl-2. RSK can phosphorylate CREB, leading to the expression of genes with neurotrophic functions, such as Bcl-2 and BDNF (see Figure 1–15). Treatment with mood-stabilizing drugs activates the ERK (extracellular signal–regulated kinase) pathway in brain regions involved in mood regulation (reviewed in G. Chen and Manji 2006). Earlier work showed that lithium and valproate induce AP-1 and CREB transcription factors and enhance expression of the bcl-2 gene. Later, it was found that chronic lithium or valproate treatment promotes neurogenesis in the hippocampus, an effect mediated at least in part by activation of the ERK pathway (see G. Chen and Manji 2006).

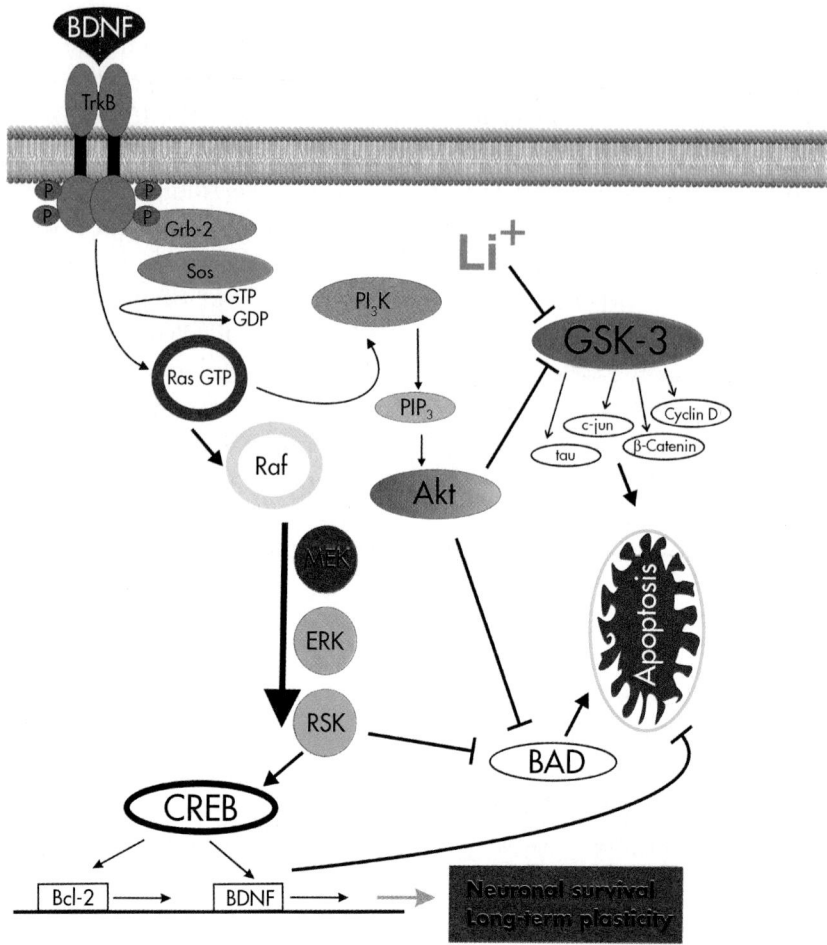

FIGURE 1–15. MAP (mitogen-activated protein) kinase signaling pathway.

The influence of neurotrophic factors on cell survival is mediated by activation of the MAP kinase cascade and other neurotrophic cascades. Activation of neurotrophic factor receptors referred to as tyrosine receptor kinases (Trks) results in activation of the MAP kinase cascade via several intermediate steps, including phosphorylation of the adaptor protein Shc and recruitment of the guanine nucleotide exchange factor Sos. This results in activation of the small guanosine triphosphate–binding protein Ras, which leads to activation of a cascade of serine/threonine kinases. This includes Raf, MAP kinase kinase (MEK), and MAP kinase (also referred to as extracellular response kinase, or ERK). One target of the MAP kinase cascade is the ribosomal S6 kinases, known as RSK, which influences cell survival in at least two ways. RSK phosphorylates and inactivates the pro-apoptotic factor BAD (Bcl-xl/Bcl-2–associated death promoter). RSK also phosphorylates cAMP response element–binding protein (CREB) and thereby increases the expression of the anti-apoptotic factor Bcl-2 and brain-derived neurotrophic factor (BDNF). Ras also activates the phosphoinositol–3 kinase (PI₃K) pathway, a primary target of which is the enzyme glycogen synthase kinase (GSK-3). Activation of the PI₃ kinase pathway deactivates GSK-3. GSK-3 has multiple targets in cells, including transcription factors (β-catenin and c-Jun) and cytoskeletal elements such as tau. Many of the targets of GSK-3 are pro-apoptotic when activated. Thus, deactivation of GSK-3 via activation of the PI₃K pathway results in neurotrophic effects. Lithium inhibits GSK-3, an effect that may be, at least in part, responsible for lithium's therapeutic effects. These mechanisms underlie many of the long-term effects of neurotrophins, including neurite outgrowth, cytoskeletal remodeling, and cell survival.
Source. Adapted from Gould TD, Chen G, Manji HK: "Mood Stabilizer Psychopharmacology." *Clinical Neuroscience Research* 2:193–212, 2002. Copyright 2002, Elsevier. Used with permission.

Inactivation of the ERK pathway in the CNS induces animal behavioral alterations reminiscent of manic symptoms, which are likely to depend on ERK's effect on distinct brain regions and the presence of interacting molecules (Shaltiel et al. 2007). Moreover, ERK knockout mice display behavioral abnormalities related to manic symptoms. These data support a clinical role for the ERK pathway in therapeutic action of mood stabilizers. Never-

theless, the possible role of this pathway in the pathophysiology of bipolar disorder has yet to be elucidated.

PI₃ Kinase–Akt Pathway

The PI₃K–Akt pathway is also particularly important for mediating neuronal survival in a wide variety of circumstances. Trk receptors can activate PI₃K through at least two distinct pathways, the relative importance of which differs between neuronal subpopulations. In many neurons, Ras-dependent activation of PI_3K is the most important pathway through which neurotrophins promote cell survival (see Figure 1–15). In some cells, however, PI_3K can also be activated through three adaptor proteins: Shc, Grb-2, and Gab-1. Binding to phosphorylated tyrosine 490 of Shc results in recruitment of Grb-2 (see Figure 1–9). Phosphorylated Grb-2 provides a docking site for Gab-1, which in turn is bound by PI_3K (Brunet et al. 2001). PI_3K directly regulates certain cytoplasmic apoptotic pathways. Akt has been proposed to act both prior to the release of cytochrome c by pro-apoptotic Bcl-2 family members and subsequent to the release of cytochrome c by regulating components of the apoptosome. Akt phosphorylates the pro-apoptotic Bcl-2 family member BAD, thereby inhibiting BAD's pro-apoptotic functions (see Figure 1–15) (Datta et al. 1997).

Another important target of Akt is the enzyme glycogen synthase kinase–3 (GSK-3) (see Figures 1–11 and 1–15). GSK-3 is a serine/threonine kinase that is, in general, constitutively active in cells. It is found in two forms—α and β—and currently appears to be the only kinase significantly *directly* inhibited by lithium (Davies et al. 2000; Klein and Melton 1996; Stambolic et al. 1996). It may thus represent a target of the development of novel medications for the treatment of bipolar disorder (Gould and Manji 2005). While most research has focused on the β isoform, available evidence suggests that the two forms may have very similar—though not absolutely identical—biological properties (Ali et al. 2001; Plyte et al. 1992). GSK-3 was named on the basis of its originally described function as a kinase that inactivates glycogen synthase. Following insulin receptor stimulation, PI_3K and Akt are activated, and this results in the phosphorylation and concomitant inactivation of GSK-3. Inactivated GSK-3 no longer phosphorylates glycogen synthase, allowing the formation of glycogen from glucose (Cohen and Frame 2001; Woodgett 2001).

In addition to regulation by Akt, other kinases, including p70 S6 kinase, RSK, and cAMP-dependent protein kinase (PKA), appear to deactivate GSK-3 by phosphorylation (Cohen and Frame 2001; Grimes and Jope 2001). The effect of GSK-3 on transcription factors such as c-Jun, heat shock factor–1 (HSF-1), nuclear factor of activated T-cells (NFAT), and β-catenin (see below) has drawn considerable interest and is particularly noteworthy (Frame and Cohen 2001; Grimes and Jope 2001) (see Figure 1–15). Generally, GSK-3 activity results in suppression of the activity of transcription. Conversely, inac-

tivation of GSK-3 appears to activate these transcription factors (Grimes and Jope 2001). Thus, GSK-3 is well positioned to receive signals from multiple diverse signal pathways, a function that is undoubtedly critical in the CNS.

GSK-3 is also a critical regulator of the Wnt pathway. Wnt is a family of secreted glycoproteins that are well known to have important roles in development. Signaling through Wnt glycoproteins results in inactivation of GSK-3 and a subsequent increase in the transcription factor β-catenin. Furthermore, some studies suggest a role for β-catenin (and Wnt) in synaptic plasticity (Salinas 1999; Salinas and Hall 1999). Additional studies have suggested that β-catenin itself may play an important role for this protein in the function of the brain. Indeed, upregulation of this protein is sufficient to cause the formation of gyri and sulci in the mouse brain, a finding observed only in higher mammals, and is suggestive of an important role in higher mammalian cognitive functions (Chenn and Walsh 2002).

PLC-γ1 Pathway

Phosphorylated Trk receptors also recruit PLC-γ1 (see Figure 1–9). The Trk kinase then phosphorylates and activates PLC-γ1, which acts to hydrolyze phosphatidylinositides to generate DAG and IP_3. IP_3 induces the release of Ca^{2+} stores, increasing levels of cytoplasmic Ca^{2+} and thereby activating many pathways controlled by Ca^{2+}. It has been shown that neurotrophins activate protein kinase C δ, which is required for activation of the ERK cascade and for neurite outgrowth (Patapoutian and Reichardt 2001). As discussed previously, emerging data suggest that the regulation of hippocampal LTP by TrkB receptors is mediated primarily through the PLC-γ cascade (for details, see Minichiello et al. 2002).

Phosphorylation/Dephosphorylation

For many proteins, a change in charge and conformation due to the addition or removal of phosphate groups results in alterations in their intrinsic functional activity. Although proteins are covalently modified in many other ways—for example, by ADP ribosylation, acylation (acetylation, myristoylation), carboxymethylation, and glycosylation—none of these mechanisms appear to be as widespread and readily subject to regulation by physiological stimuli as phosphorylation. Indeed, protein phosphorylation/dephosphorylation represents a pathway of fundamental importance in the chemistry of biological regulation (see Nestler et al. 2001). Virtually all types of extracellular signals are known to produce many of their diverse physiological effects by regulating the state of phosphorylation of specific proteins in the cells that they target.

The phosphate group provides an unwieldy negative charge that often interacts with the catalytic and other regions of enzymes. The addition of a phosphate often results in conformational changes in proteins. In the case of enzymes, this change may increase (more commonly) or decrease the affinity of an enzyme for its substrate. Thus, phosphorylation may result in a change in kinase activity, a change in phosphatase activity, or the marking of a protein for cleavage by proteases. The catalytic activity of an enzyme can be switched on or off, or an ion channel can be opened or closed. For many other proteins, phosphorylation-induced changes in charge and conformation result in alterations in the affinity of the proteins for other molecules. For example, phosphorylation alters the affinity of numerous enzymes for their cofactors and end-product inhibitors, phosphorylation of receptors can alter their affinity for G proteins, and phosphorylation of some nuclear transcription factors alters their DNA-binding properties. Therefore, phosphorylation can produce varied effects on cellular physiology and ultimately can have major behavioral manifestations.

Protein kinases are classified by the residues that they phosphorylate, with the two major classes being serine/threonine kinases and tyrosine kinases. Most phosphorylation (>95%) of proteins occurs on serine residues, a small amount (about 3%–4%) on threonine residues, and very little (0.1%) on tyrosine residues (but, as discussed earlier, the tyrosine kinases can be very important for neurotrophic signaling). In all cases, the kinases catalyze the transfer of the terminal (γ) phosphate group of ATP to the hydroxyl moiety in the respective amino acid residue, a process that requires Mg^{2+}. Within cells, protein kinases often form sequential pathways, whereby one kinase phosphorylates/activates another, which phosphorylates/activates another kinase, and so forth. In this manner, signals can be propagated within cells, allowing ample opportunity (see below) for the signal to be altered by other intracellular signals, often in a cell type–specific manner, allowing for considerable "fine-tuning."

Although clearly playing critical roles in modulating the function of proteins by catalyzing the cleavage of the phosphoester bond, *protein phosphatases* have not been as extensively studied as kinases. In the CNS, phosphatases often function as a molecular "off switch," thereby decreasing the activity of enzymes and the intracellular signaling pathways they control. However, it is clear that

protein phosphatases are much more than simple off switches. Thus, in an elegant series of studies, Greengard and associates demonstrated that a major CNS phosphoprotein, known by the acronym DARPP-32 (dopamine and cAMP-regulated phosphoprotein, 32 kDa), brings about many of its long-term neuroplastic effects by regulating the activity of a protein phosphatase (protein phosphatase–1; PP-1) (for a review, see Greengard 2001a). Thus, they demonstrated that the DARPP-32/PP-1 pathway integrates information from a variety of neurotransmitters and produces a coordinated response involving numerous downstream physiological effectors. DARPP-32 phosphorylation by PKA is regulated by the actions of various neurotransmitters, principally dopamine acting at D_1 receptors but also a variety of other neurotransmitters (Greengard 2001b; Nestler et al. 2001). Phospho-DARPP-32, by inhibiting the activity of PP-1, acts in a synergistic manner with different protein kinases (primarily PKA and PKC) to increase the level of phosphorylation of various downstream effector proteins and thereby long-term neuronal adaptations that have also been implicated in the actions of drugs of abuse and antidepressants (Greengard 2001b; Nestler et al. 2001).

While propagation of signals may be very immediate, even short-term phosphorylation of many types of proteins can have long-term effects, resulting in "molecular and cellular memory." Indeed, various forms of learning and memory are known to be regulated, in large part, by phosphorylation events. Short-term memory may involve the phosphorylation of presynaptic or postsynaptic proteins in response to synaptic activity, a process that results in transient facilitation or inhibition of synaptic transmission. Long-term memory may involve phosphorylation of proteins that play a role in the regulation of gene expression, which would result in more permanent modifications of synaptic transmission, potentially via structural brain changes (Malenka and Nicoll 1999). As discussed, long-term potentiation, one of the most extensively studied models of learning and memory, is believed to be initiated through short-term changes in Ca^{2+}-dependent protein phosphorylation and maintained by long-term changes in gene expression. There is also growing appreciation that protein phosphatases play a critical role in the *extinction* of memory. Thus, abundant data now suggest that rather than representing a passive process, "forgetting" is more an *active process of memory erasure* (discussed in Genoux et al. 2002). In an elegant series of behavioral studies using transgenic mice, Genoux et al. (2002) provided strong evidence that PP-1 is involved in forgetting rather than in preventing the encoding of memory. Although the precise mechanisms by which PP-1 brings about these effects remain to be fully elucidated, these investigators postulate that CaMKII and the GluR1 subunit of the AMPA receptor play important roles. These findings may have major implications for the ultimate development of agents that could be used to facilitate the erasure of traumatic memories—for example, in PTSD.

Conclusion

In this chapter, we have attempted to provide an overview of some fundamental aspects of neurotransmitters, signal transduction pathways, and second messengers. For most psychiatrists, molecular and cellular biology have not traditionally played a major role in day-to-day clinical practice. However, new insights into the molecular and cellular basis of disease and drug action are being generated at an ever-increasing rate and will ultimately result in a transformation of our understanding and management of diseases. Indeed, the last decade of the twentieth century was truly a remarkable one for biomedical research. The "molecular medicine revolution" has utilized the power of sophisticated cellular and molecular biological methodologies to tackle many of society's most devastating illnesses. The rate of progress has been exciting indeed, and hundreds of G protein–coupled receptors and dozens of G proteins and effectors have now been identified and characterized at the molecular and cellular levels. These efforts have allowed the study of a variety of human diseases that are caused by abnormalities in cell-to-cell communication; studies of such diseases are offering unique insights into the physiological and pathophysiological functioning of many cellular transmembrane signaling pathways.

Psychiatry, like much of the rest of medicine, has entered a new and exciting age demarcated by the rapid advances and the promise of molecular and cellular biology and neuroimaging. There is a growing appreciation that severe psychiatric disorders arise from abnormalities in cellular plasticity cascades, leading to aberrant information processing in synapses and circuits mediating affective, cognitive, motoric, and neurovegetative functions. Thus, these illnesses can be best conceptualized as genetically influenced disorders of synapses and circuits rather than simply as deficits or excesses in individual neurotransmitters (Carlson et al. 2006). Furthermore, many of these pathways play critical roles not only in synaptic (and therefore behavioral) plasticity but also in long-term atrophic processes. Targeting these cascades in treatment

may stabilize the underlying disease process by reducing the frequency and severity of the profound mood cycling that contributes to morbidity and mortality. The role of cellular signaling cascades offers much explanatory power for understanding the complex neurobiology of bipolar illness (Goodwin and Jamison 2007). Signaling cascades regulate the multiple neurotransmitter and neuropeptide systems implicated in psychiatric disorders and are targets for the most effective treatments. The highly integrated monoamine and prominent neuropeptide pathways are known to originate in and project heavily to limbic-related regions, such as the hippocampus, hypothalamus, and brain stem, which are likely associated with neurovegetative symptoms. Abnormalities in cellular signaling cascades that regulate diverse physiological functions likely explain the tremendous medical comorbidity associated with psychiatric disorders.

References

Aderem A: The MARCKS brothers: a family of protein kinase C substrates. Cell 71:713–716, 1992

Aghajanian GK, Marek GJ: Serotonin and hallucinogens. Neuropsychopharmacology 21 (2, suppl):16S–23S, 1999

Akil M, Kolachana BS, Rothmond DA, et al: Catechol-O-methyltransferase genotype and dopamine regulation in the human brain. J Neurosci 23:2008–2013, 2003

Alger BE: Endocannabinoid identification in the brain: studies of breakdown lead to breakthrough, and there may be NO hope. Sci STKE 2005(309):pe51, 2005

Alhquist R: A study of adrenergic receptors. Am J Physiol 153:586–590, 1948

Altier C, Zamponi GW: Opioid, cheating on its receptors, exacerbates pain. Nat Neurosci 9:1534–1540, 2006

Ali A, Hoeflich KP, Woodgett JR: Glycogen synthase kinase–3: properties, functions, and regulation. Chem Rev 101:2527–2540, 2001

Amat J, Baratta MV, Paul E, et al: Medial prefrontal cortex determines how stressor controllability affects behavior and dorsal raphe nucleus. Nat Neurosci 8:365–371, 2005

Anden NE, Magnusson T, Rosengren E: On the presence of dihydroxyphenylalanine decarboxylase in nerves. Experientia 20:328–329, 1964

Andrade R, Malenka RC, Nicoll RA: A G protein couples serotonin and GABAB receptors to the same channels in hippocampus. Science 234:1261–1265, 1986

Ansorge MS, Zhou M, Lira A, et al: Early life blockade of the 5-HT transporter alters emotional behavior in adult mice. Science 306:879–881, 2004

Atkins CM, Selcher JC, Petraitis JJ, et al: The MAPK cascade is required for mammalian associative learning. Nat Neurosci 1:602–609, 1998

Axelrod J: Phospholipase A2 and G proteins. Trends Neurosci 18:64–65, 1995

Axelrod J, Burch RM, Jelsema CL: Receptor-mediated activation of phospholipase A2 via GTP-binding proteins: arachidonic acid and its metabolites as second messengers. Trends Neurosci 11:117–123, 1988

Ayalon G, Stern-Bach Y: Functional assembly of AMPA and kainate receptors is mediated by several discrete protein-protein interactions. Neuron 31:103–113, 2001

Barria A, Malinow R: NMDA receptor subunit composition controls synaptic plasticity by regulating binding to CaMKII. Neuron 48:289–301, 2005

Baum AE, Akula N, Cabanero M, et al: A genome-wide association study implicates diacylglycerol kinase eta (DGKH) and several other genes in the etiology of bipolar disorder. Mol Psychiatry 13:197–207, 2008

Bauman AL, Apparsundaram S, Ramamoorthy S, et al: Cocaine and antidepressant-sensitive biogenic amine transporters exist in regulated complexes with protein phosphatase 2A. J Neurosci 20:7571–7578, 2000

Bekkers JM, Stevens CF: NMDA and non-NMDA receptors are co-localized at individual excitatory synapses in cultured rat hippocampus. Nature 341:230–233, 1989

Bell C, Abrams J, Nutt D: Tryptophan depletion and its implications for psychiatry. Br J Psychiatry 178:399–405, 2001

Beaulieu JM, Sotnikova TD, Yao WD, et al: Lithium antagonizes dopamine-dependent behaviors mediated by an AKT/glycogen synthase kinase 3 signaling cascade. Proc Natl Acad Sci U S A 101:5099–5104, 2004

Bebchuk JM, Arfken CL, Dolan-Manji S, et al: A preliminary investigation of a protein kinase C inhibitor in the treatment of acute mania. Arch Gen Psychiatry 57:95–97, 2000

Beneyto M, Kristiansen LV, Oni-Orisan A, et al: Abnormal glutamate receptor expression in the medial temporal lobe in schizophrenia and mood disorders. Neuropsychopharmacology 32:1888–1902, 2007

Ben Mamou C, Gamache K, Nader K: NMDA receptors are critical for unleashing consolidated auditory fear memories. Nat Neurosci 9:1237–1239, 2006

Bhalla US, Iyengar R: Emergent properties of networks of biological signaling pathways. Science 283:381–387, 1999

Birnbaum SG, Yuan PX, Wang M, et al: Protein kinase C overactivity impairs prefrontal cortical regulation of working memory. Science 306:882–884, 2004

Blier P, Pineyro G, el Mansari M, et al: Role of somatodendritic 5-HT autoreceptors in modulating 5-HT neurotransmission. Ann N Y Acad Sci 861:204–216, 1998

Blum S, Moore AN, Adams F, et al: A mitogen-activated protein kinase cascade in the CA1/CA2 subfield of the dorsal hippocampus is essential for long-term spatial memory. J Neurosci 19:3535–3544, 1999

Bogdansky D, Pletscher A, Brodie B, et al: Identification and assay of serotonin in brain. J Pharmacol Exp Ther 117:88–98, 1956

Bonni A, Brunet A, West AE, et al: Cell survival promoted by the Ras-MAPK signaling pathway by transcription-dependent and -independent mechanisms. Science 286:1358–1362, 1999

Bourne HR, Nicoll R: Molecular machines integrate coincident synaptic signals. Cell 72 (suppl):65–75, 1993

Bouvier M: Oligomerization of G-protein–coupled transmitter receptors. Nat Rev Neurosci 2:274–286, 2001

Bown CD, Wang JF, Chen B, et al: Regulation of ER stress proteins by valproate: therapeutic implications. Bipolar Disord 4:145–151, 2002

Brambilla D, Chapman D, Greene R: Adenosine mediation of presynaptic feedback inhibition of glutamate release. Neuron 46:275–283, 2005

Brandish PE, Su M, Holder DJ: Regulation of gene expression by lithium and depletion of inositol in slices of adult rat cortex. Neuron 45:861–872, 2005

Brodie B: The immediate action of an intravenous injection of blood serum. J Physiol (Lond) 26:48–71, 1900

Bruinvels AT, Palacios JM, Hoyer D: 5-Hydroxytryptamine1 recognition sites in rat brain: heterogeneity of non-5-hydroxytryptamine1A/1C binding sites revealed by quantitative receptor autoradiography. Neuroscience 53:465–473, 1993

Brunet A, Datta SR, Greenberg ME: Transcription-dependent and -independent control of neuronal survival by the PI3K-Akt signaling pathway. Curr Opin Neurobiol 11:297–305, 2001

Bruno V, Battaglia G, Copani A, et al: An activity-dependent switch from facilitation to inhibition in the control of excitotoxicity by group I metabotropic glutamate receptors. Eur J Neurosci 13:1469–1478, 2001

Bruss M, Porzgen P, Bryan-Lluka LJ, et al: The rat norepinephrine transporter: molecular cloning from PC12 cells and functional expression. Brain Res Mol Brain Res 52:257–262, 1997

Bruss M, Bonisch H, Buhlen M, et al: Modified ligand binding to the naturally occurring Cys-124 variant of the human serotonin 5-HT1B receptor. Pharmacogenetics 9:95–102, 1999

Bylund DB, Eikenberg DC, Hieble JP, et al: International Union of Pharmacology nomenclature of adrenoceptors. Pharmacol Rev 46:121–136, 1994

Cahill L, Prins B, Weber M, et al: Beta-adrenergic activation and memory for emotional events. Nature 371:702–704, 1994

Carlezon WA Jr, Nestler EJ: Elevated levels of GluR1 in the midbrain: a trigger for sensitization to drugs of abuse? Trends Neurosci 25:610–615, 2002

Carlson PJ, Singh JB, Zarate CA Jr, et al: Neural circuitry and neuroplasticity in mood disorders: insights for novel therapeutic targets. NeuroRx 3:22–41, 2006

Carman CV, Benovic JL: G-protein–coupled receptors: turn-ons and turn-offs. Curr Opin Neurobiol 8:335–344, 1998

Casado M, Bendahan A, Zafra F, et al: Phosphorylation and modulation of brain glutamate transporters by protein kinase C. J Biol Chem 268:27313–27317, 1993

Caspi A, Sugden K, Moffitt TE, et al: Influence of life stress on depression: moderation by a polymorphism in the 5-HTT gene. Science 301:386–389, 2003

Catapano L, Manji HK: G protein–coupled receptors in major psychiatric disorders. Biochim Biophys Acta 1768:976–993, 2007

Chavez AE, Singer JH, Diamond JS: Fast neurotransmitter release triggered by Ca influx through AMPA-type glutamate receptors. Nature 443:705–708, 2006

Chen G, Manji HK: The extracellular signal-regulated kinase pathway: an emerging promising target for mood stabilizers. Curr Opin Psychiatry 19:313–323, 2006

Chen G, Hasanat KA, Bebchuk JM, et al: Regulation of signal transduction pathways and gene expression by mood stabilizers and antidepressants. Psychosom Med 61:599–617, 1999

Chen ZY, Jing D, Bath KG, et al: Genetic variant BDNF (Val66Met) polymorphism alters anxiety-related behavior. Science 314:140–143, 2006

Chenn A, Walsh CA: Regulation of cerebral cortical size by control of cell cycle exit in neural precursors. Science 297:365–369, 2002

Clark D, White FJ: D1 dopamine receptor—the search for a function: a critical evaluation of the D1/D2 dopamine receptor classification and its functional implications. Synapse 1:347–388, 1987

Cohen P, Frame S: The renaissance of GSK3. Nat Rev Mol Cell Biol 2:769–776, 2001

Conn PJ, Pin JP: Pharmacology and functions of metabotropic glutamate receptors. Annu Rev Pharmacol Toxicol 37:205–237, 1997

Conn PJ, Sanders-Bush E: Central serotonin receptors: effector systems, physiological roles and regulation. Psychopharmacology (Berl) 92:267–277, 1987

Conradt M, Stoffel W: Inhibition of the high-affinity brain glutamate transporter GLAST-1 via direct phosphorylation. J Neurochem 68:1244–1251, 1997

Cooper JR, Bloom FE, Roth RH: The Biochemical Basis of Neuropharmacology, 7th Edition. New York, Oxford University Press, 2001

Coupland N, Zedkova L, Sanghera G, et al: Response to pentagastrin after acute phenylalanine and tyrosine depletion in healthy men: a pilot study. J Psychiatry Neurosci 26:247–251, 2001

Coyle JT, Tsai G, Goff DC: Ionotropic glutamate receptors as therapeutic targets in schizophrenia. Curr Drug Targets CNS Neurol Disord 1(2):183–189, 2002

Crawley JN, Glowa JR, Majewska MD, et al: Anxiolytic activity of an endogenous adrenal steroid. Brain Res 398:382–385, 1986

Crow T, Xue-Bian JJ, Siddiqi V, et al: Phosphorylation of mitogen-activated protein kinase by one-trial and multi-trial classical conditioning. J Neurosci 18:3480–3487, 1998

Dahlstrom A: Regional distribution of brain catecholamines and serotonin. Neurosci Res Program Bull 9:197–205, 1971

D'Amato RJ, Largent BL, Snowman AM, et al: Selective labeling of serotonin uptake sites in rat brain by [3H]citalopram contrasted to labeling of multiple sites by [3H]imipramine. J Pharmacol Exp Ther 242:364–371, 1987

Datta SR, Dudek H, Tao X, et al: Akt phosphorylation of BAD couples survival signals to the cell-intrinsic death machinery. Cell 91:231–241, 1997

Davies SP, Reddy H, Caivano M, et al: Specificity and mechanism of action of some commonly used protein kinase inhibitors. Biochem J 351(pt 1):95–105, 2000

Dawson TM, Snyder SH: Gases as biological messengers: nitric oxide and carbon monoxide in the brain. J Neurosci 14:5147–5159, 1994

Descarries L, Watkins KC, Garcia S, et al: The serotonin neurons in nucleus raphe dorsalis of adult rat: a light and electron microscope radioautographic study. J Comp Neurol 207:239–254, 1982

De Vivo M, Maayani S: Stimulation and inhibition of adenylyl cyclase by distinct 5-hydroxytryptamine receptors. Biochem Pharmacol 40:1551–1558, 1990

Dingledine R, Borges K, Bowie D, et al: The glutamate receptor ion channels. Pharmacol Rev 51:7–61, 1999

Dong Y, Green T, Saal D, et al: CREB modulates excitability of nucleus accumbens neurons. Nat Neurosci 9:475–477, 2006

Drager UC: Retinoic acid signaling in the functioning brain. Sci STKE (324):pe10, 2006

Drevets WC, Bogers W, Raichle ME: Functional anatomical correlates of antidepressant drug treatment assessed using PET measures of regional glucose metabolism. Eur Neuropsychopharmacol 12:527–544, 2002

Drury AN, Szent-Györgyi A: The physiological activity of adenine compounds with especial reference to their action upon the mammalian heart. J Physiol 68:213–237, 1929

Du J, Feng L, Yang F, et al: Activity- and Ca(2+)-dependent modulation of surface expression of brain-derived neurotrophic factor receptors in hippocampal neurons. J Cell Biol 150:1423–1434, 2000

Du J, Gould TD, Manji HK: Neurotrophic signaling in mood disorders, in Signal Transduction and Human Disease. Edited by Finkel T, Gutkind JS. New York, Wiley, 2003, pp 411–445

Du J, Wei Y, Chen Z, et al: The anticonvulsants lamotrigine, riluzole and valproate differentially regulate AMPA receptor trafficking: relationship to clinical effects in mood disorders. Neuropsychopharmacology 32:793–802, 2007

Duman RS: Synaptic plasticity and mood disorders. Mol Psychiatry 7 (suppl 1):S29–S34, 2002

Dunlop BW, Nemeroff CB: The role of dopamine in the pathophysiology of depression. Arch Gen Psychiatry 64:327–337, 2007

Eide EJ, Virshup DM: Casein kinase I: another cog in the circadian clockworks. Chronobiol Int 18:389–398, 2001

Einat H, Manji HK: Cellular plasticity cascades: genes-to-behavior pathways in animal models of bipolar disorder. Biol Psychiatry 59:1160–1171, 2006

Einat H, Yuan P, Szabo ST, et al: Protein kinase C inhibition by tamoxifen antagonizes manic-like behavior in rats: implications for the development of novel therapeutics for bipolar disorder. Neuropsychobiology 55:123–131, 2007

Encinas JM, Vaahtokari A, Enikolopov G: Fluoxetine targets early progenitor cells in the adult brain. Proc Natl Acad Sci U S A 103:8233–8238, 2006

English JD, Sweatt JD: Activation of p42 mitogen-activated protein kinase in hippocampal long term potentiation. J Biol Chem 271:24329–24332, 1996

English JD, Sweatt JD: A requirement for the mitogen-activated protein kinase cascade in hippocampal long term potentiation. J Biol Chem 272:19103–19106, 1997

Evans DL, Leary JH 3rd, Jaso-Friedmann L: Nonspecific cytotoxic cells and innate immunity: regulation by programmed cell death. Dev Comp Immunol 25:791–805, 2001

Faden AI, Demediuk P, Panter SS, et al: The role of excitatory amino acids and NMDA receptors in traumatic brain injury. Science 244:798–800, 1989

Fields RD, Stevens-Graham B: New insights into neuron-glia communication. Science 298:556–562, 2002

Foote SL, Bloom FE, Aston-Jones G: Nucleus locus ceruleus: new evidence of anatomical and physiological specificity. Physiol Rev 63:844–914, 1983

Frame S, Cohen P: GSK3 takes centre stage more than 20 years after its discovery. Biochem J 359 (pt 1):1–16, 2001

Freedman R, Coon H, Myles-Worsley M, et al: Linkage of a neurophysiological deficit in schizophrenia to a chromosome 15 locus. Proc Natl Acad Sci U S A 94:587–592, 1997

Frodl T, Schule C, Schmitt G, et al: Association of the brain-derived neurotrophic factor Val66Met polymorphism with reduced hippocampal volumes in major depression. Arch Gen Psychiatry 64:410–416, 2007

Frye CA, Scalise TJ: Anti-seizure effects of progesterone and 3α,5α-THP in kainic acid and perforant pathway models of epilepsy. Psychoneuroendocrinology 25:407–420, 2000

Fryer RH, Kaplan DR, Feinstein SC, et al: Developmental and mature expression of full-length and truncated TrkB receptors in the rat forebrain. J Comp Neurol 374:21–40, 1996

Fukunaga K, Miyamoto E: Role of MAP kinase in neurons. Mol Neurobiol 16:79–95, 1998

Gaddum JH, Picarelli ZP: Two kinds of tryptamine receptor. Br J Pharmacol 12:323–328, 1957

Galli A, DeFelice LJ, Duke BJ, et al: Sodium-dependent norepinephrine-induced currents in norepinephrine-transporter–transfected HEK-293 cells blocked by cocaine and antidepressants. J Exp Biol 198(pt 10):2197–2212, 1995

Galli A, Blakely RD, DeFelice LJ: Norepinephrine transporters have channel modes of conduction. Proc Natl Acad Sci U S A 93:8671–866, 1996

Genoux D, Haditsch U, Knobloch M, et al: Protein phosphatase 1 is a molecular constraint on learning and memory. Nature 418:970–975, 2002

Gerber DJ, Hall D, Miyakawa T, et al: Evidence for association of schizophrenia with genetic variation in the 8p21.3 gene, PPP3CC, encoding the calcineurin gamma subunit. Proc Natl Acad Sci U S A 100:8993–8998, 2003

Glykys J, Peng Z, Chandra D, et al: A new naturally occurring GABA(A) receptor subunit partnership with high sensitivity to ethanol. Nat Neurosci 10:40–48, 2007

Gonzalez M, Ruggiero FP, Chang Q, et al: Disruption of Trkb-mediated signaling induces disassembly of postsynaptic receptor clusters at neuromuscular junctions. Neuron 24:567–583, 1999

Gonzalez-Maeso J, Weisstaub NV, Zhou M, et al: Hallucinogens recruit specific cortical 5-HT(2A) receptor-mediated signaling pathways to affect behavior. Neuron 53:439–452, 2007

Goodwin FK, Jamison KR: Manic-Depressive Illness: Bipolar Disorders and Recurrent Depression. New York, Oxford University Press, 2007

Gould T, Manji H: Signaling pathways in the pathophysiology of mood disorders. J Psychosom Res 53:687–697, 2002

Gould T, Manji HK: Glycogen synthase kinase-3: a putative molecular target for lithium mimetic drugs. Neuropsychopharmacology 30:1223–1237, 2005

Gould T, Chen G, Manji HK: Mood stabilizer psychopharmacology. Clinical Neuroscience Research 2:193–212, 2002

Gould T, Gray NA, Manji HK: The cellular neurobiology of severe mood and anxiety disorders: implications for the development of novel therapeutics, in Molecular Neurobiology for the Clinician (Review of Psychiatry Series, Vol 22, No 3; Oldham JM, Riba MB, series eds). Edited by Charney DS. Washington, DC, American Psychiatric Publishing, 2003, pp 123–227

Greengard P: The neurobiology of dopamine signaling. Biosci Rep 21:247–269, 2001a

Greengard P: The neurobiology of slow synaptic transmission. Science 294:1024–1030, 2001b

Grimes CA, Jope RS: The multifaceted roles of glycogen synthase kinase 3β in cellular signaling. Prog Neurobiol 65:391–426, 2001

Gross C, Zhuang X, Stark K, et al: Serotonin1A receptor acts during development to establish normal anxiety-like behaviour in the adult. Nature 416:396–400, 2002

Guillin O, Diaz J, Carroll P, et al: BDNF controls dopamine D3 receptor expression and triggers behavioural sensitization. Nature 411:86–89, 2001

Habert E, Graham D, Tahraoui L, et al: Characterization of [3H]paroxetine binding to rat cortical membranes. Eur J Pharmacol 118:107–114, 1985

Harder R, Bonisch H: Effects of monovalent ions on the transport of noradrenaline across the plasma membrane of neuronal cells (PC-12 cells). J Neurochem 45:1154–1162, 1985

Heurteaux C, Lucas G, Guy N, et al: Deletion of the background potassium channel TREK-1 results in a depression-resistant phenotype. Nat Neurosci 9:1134–1141, 2006

Henry LK, Defelice LJ, Blakely RD: Getting the message across: a recent transporter structure shows the way. Neuron 49:791–796, 2006

Hoffman BJ, Mezey E: Distribution of serotonin 5-HT1C receptor mRNA in adult rat brain. FEBS Lett 247:453–462, 1989

Hollmann M, Maron C, Heinemann S: N-Glycosylation site tagging suggests a three transmembrane domain topology for the glutamate receptor GluR1. Neuron 13:1331–1343, 1994

Hoyer D, Pazos A, Probst A, et al: Serotonin receptors in the human brain, II: characterization and autoradiographic localization of 5-HT1C and 5-HT2 recognition sites. Brain Res 376:97–107, 1986

Hoyer D, Hannon JP, Martin GR: Molecular, pharmacological and functional diversity of 5-HT receptors. Pharmacol Biochem Behav 71:533–554, 2002

Hrdina PD, Pappas BA, Roberts DC, et al: Relationship between levels and uptake of serotonin and high affinity [3H]imipramine recognition sites in the rat brain. Can J Physiol Pharmacol 63:1239–1244, 1985

Hrdina PD, Foy B, Hepner A, et al: Antidepressant binding sites in brain: autoradiographic comparison of [3H]paroxetine and [3H]imipramine localization and relationship to serotonin transporter. J Pharmacol Exp Ther 252:410–418, 1990

Humphrey PP, Hartig P, Hoyer D: A proposed new nomenclature for 5-HT receptors. Trends Pharmacol Sci 14:233–236, 1993

Innocenti B, Parpura V, Haydon PG: Imaging extracellular waves of glutamate during calcium signaling in cultured astrocytes. J Neurosci 20:1800–1808, 2000

Inoue E, Mochida S, Takagi H, et al: SAD: a presynaptic kinase associated with synaptic vesicles and the active zone cytomatrix that regulates neurotransmitter release. Neuron 50:261–275, 2006

Jacobs BL, Abercrombie ED, Fornal CA, et al: Single-unit and physiological analyses of brain norepinephrine function in behaving animals. Prog Brain Res 88:159–165, 1991

Jacobs BL, Praag H, Gage FH: Adult brain neurogenesis and psychiatry: a novel theory of depression. Mol Psychiatry 5:262–269, 2000

Ji Y, Pang PT, Feng L, et al: Cyclic AMP controls BDNF-induced TrkB phosphorylation and dendritic spine formation in mature hippocampal neurons. Nat Neurosci 8:164–172, 2005

Kanashiro CA, Khalil RA: Signal transduction by protein kinase C in mammalian cells. Clin Exp Pharmacol Physiol 25:974–985, 1998

Kandel ER, Schwartz JH, Jessell TM: Principles of Neural Science. New York, McGraw-Hill, 2000

Kaupmann K, Huggel K, Heid J, et al: Expression cloning of GABA(B) receptors uncovers similarity to metabotropic glutamate receptors. Nature 386:239–246, 1997

Kellendonk C, Simpson EH, Polan HJ, et al: Transient and selective overexpression of dopamine D2 receptors in the striatum causes persistent abnormalities in prefrontal cortex functioning. Neuron 49:603–615, 2006

Kim SF, Huang AS, Snowman AM, et al: From the Cover: Antipsychotic drug-induced weight gain mediated by histamine H1 receptor-linked activation of hypothalamic AMP-kinase. Proc Natl Acad Sci U S A 104:3456–3459, 2007

Kimelberg HK, Katz DM: High-affinity uptake of serotonin into immunocytochemically identified astrocytes. Science 228:889–891, 1985

Kleim JA, Chan S, Pringle E, et al: BDNF val66met polymorphism is associated with modified experience-dependent plasticity in human motor cortex. Nat Neurosci 9:735–737, 2006

Klein PS, Melton DA: A molecular mechanism for the effect of lithium on development. Proc Natl Acad Sci U S A 93:8455–8459, 1996

Kornhauser JM, Greenberg ME: A kinase to remember: dual roles for MAP kinase in long-term memory. Neuron 18:839–842, 1997

Krystal JH, Anand A, Moghaddam B: Effects of NMDA receptor antagonists: implications for the pathophysiology of schizophrenia. Arch Gen Psychiatry 59:663–664, 2002

Kulkarni J, Garland KA, Scaffidi A, et al: A pilot study of hormone modulation as a new treatment for mania in women with bipolar affective disorder. Psychoneuroendocrinology 31:543–547, 2006

Laeng P, Pitts RL, Lemire AL, et al: The mood stabilizer valproic acid stimulates GABA neurogenesis from rat forebrain stem cells. J Neurochem 91:238–251, 2004

Langer SZ, Moret C, Raisman R, et al: High-affinity [3H]imipramine binding in rat hypothalamus: association with uptake of serotonin but not of norepinephrine. Science 210:1133–1135, 1980

Laporte AM, Koscielniak T, Ponchant M, et al: Quantitative autoradiographic mapping of 5-HT3 receptors in the rat CNS using [125I]iodo-zacopride and [3H]zacopride as radioligands. Synapse 10:271–281, 1992

Larner AC, Keightley A: The Jak/Stat signaling cascade: its role in the biological effects of interferons, in Signaling Networks and Cell Cycle Control: The Molecular Basis of Cancer and Other Diseases. Edited by Gutkind JS. Totowa, NJ, Humana Press, 2000, pp 393–409

Lawrence JA, Charters AR, Butcher SP, et al: 5-HT transporter antibodies as a tool in serotonergic synaptosomal isolation. Biochem Soc Trans 23 (1, suppl):115S, 1995a

Lawrence JA, Charters AR, Butcher SP, et al: Recognition of 5-HT transporter by antipeptide antibodies. Biochem Soc Trans 23 (3, suppl):473S, 1995b

Lee JL, Di Ciano P, Thomas KL: Disrupting reconsolidation of drug memories reduces cocaine-seeking behavior. Neuron 47:795–801, 2005

Lisman JE, McIntyre CC: Synaptic plasticity: a molecular memory switch. Curr Biol 11(19):R788–R791, 2001

Liu QS, Pu L, Poo MM: Repeated cocaine exposure in vivo facilitates LTP induction in midbrain dopamine neurons. Nature 437:1027–1031, 2005

Liu YF, Albert PR: Cell-specific signaling of the 5-HT1A receptor: modulation by protein kinases C and A. J Biol Chem 266:23689–23697, 1991

Liu YL, Fann CS, Liu CM, et al: More evidence supports the association of PPP3CC with schizophrenia. Mol Psychiatry 12:966–974, 2007

Lopez-Gimenez JF, Mengod G, Palacios JM, et al: Selective visualization of rat brain 5-HT2A receptors by autoradiography with [3H]MDL 100,907. Naunyn Schmiedebergs Arch Pharmacol 356:446–454, 1997

Lu L, Hope BT, Dempsey J, et al: Central amygdala ERK signaling pathway is critical to incubation of cocaine craving. Nat Neurosci 8:212–219, 2005

Lummis SC, Beene DL, Lee LW: Cis-trans isomerization at a proline opens the pore of a neurotransmitter-gated ion channel. Nature 438:248–252, 2005

Madden DR: The structure and function of glutamate receptor ion channels. Nat Rev Neurosci 3:91–101, 2002

Maeng S, Zarate CA, Du J, et al: Cellular mechanisms underlying the antidepressant effects of ketamine: role of alpha-amino-3-hydroxy-5-methylisoxazole-4-propionic acid receptors. Biol Psychiatry 63:349–352, 2008

Malberg JE, Eisch AJ, Nestler EJ, et al: Chronic antidepressant treatment increases neurogenesis in adult rat hippocampus. J Neurosci 20:9104–9110, 2000

Malenka RC, Nicoll RA: Long-term potentiation—a decade of progress? Science 285:1870–1874, 1999

Malinow R, Malenka RC: AMPA receptor trafficking and synaptic plasticity. Annu Rev Neurosci 25:103–126, 2002

Mangelsdorf D, Thummel C, Beato M, et al: The nuclear receptor superfamily: the second decade. Cell 83:835–839, 1995

Manji HK: G proteins: implications for psychiatry. Am J Psychiatry 149:746–760, 1992

Manji HK, Lenox RH: Ziskind-Somerfeld Research Award. Protein kinase C signaling in the brain: molecular transduction of mood stabilization in the treatment of manic-depressive illness. Biol Psychiatry 46:1328–1351, 1999

Manji HK, Drevets WC, Charney DS: The cellular neurobiology of depression. Nat Med 7:541–547, 2001

Martin KC, Michael D, Rose J, et al: MAP kinase translocates into the nucleus of the presynaptic cell and is required for long-term facilitation in Aplysia. Neuron 18:899–912, 1997

Martinowich K, Manji HK, Lu B: New insights into BDNF function in depression and anxiety. Nat Neurosci 10:1089–1093, 2007

Matsubara M, Kusubata M, Ishiguro K, et al: Site-specific phosphorylation of synapsin I by mitogen-activated protein kinase and Cdk5 and its effects on physiological functions. J Biol Chem 271:21108–21113, 1996

Matthews EK: Calcium and membrane permeability. Br Med Bull 42:391–397, 1986

McCann UD, Thorne D, Hall M, et al: The effects of l-dihydroxyphenylalanine on alertness and mood in alpha-methyl-para-tyrosine-treated healthy humans: further evidence for the role of catecholamines in arousal and anxiety. Neuropsychopharmacology 13:41–52, 1995

McEwen BS: Stress and hippocampal plasticity. Annu Rev Neurosci 22:105–122, 1999

McMahon FJ, Burnevich S, Charney DS, et al: Variation in the gene encoding the serotonin 2A receptor is associated with outcome of antidepressant treatment. Am J Hum Genet 78:804–814, 2006

Meltzer HY: Action of atypical antipsychotics. Am J Psychiatry 159:153–154; discussion 154–155, 2002

Mendels J, Chernik DA: The effect of lithium carbonate on the sleep of depressed patients. Int Pharmacopsychiatry 8:184–192, 1973

Mermelstein PG, Becker JB, Surmeier DJ: Estradiol reduces calcium currents in rat neostriatal neurons via a membrane receptor. J Neurosci 16:595–604, 1996

Meyer-Franke A, Wilkinson GA, Kruttgen A, et al: Depolarization and cAMP elevation rapidly recruit TrkB to the plasma membrane of CNS neurons. Neuron 21:681–693, 1998

Miller RJ: The control of neuronal Ca2+ homeostasis. Prog Neurobiol 37:255–285, 1991

Minichiello L, Calella AM, Medina DL, et al: Mechanism of TrkB-mediated hippocampal long-term potentiation. Neuron 36:121–137, 2002

Miwa JM, Stevens TR, King SL, et al: The prototoxin lynx1 acts on nicotinic acetylcholine receptors to balance neuronal activity and survival in vivo. Neuron 51:587–600, 2006

Mohler H, Fritschy JM, Rudolph U: A new benzodiazepine pharmacology. J Pharmacol Exp Ther 300:2–8, 2002

Moore GJ, Bebchuk JM, Parrish JK, et al: Temporal dissociation between lithium-induced changes in frontal lobe myo-inositol and clinical response in manic-depressive illness. Am J Psychiatry 156:1902–1908, 1999

Mulligan SJ, MacVicar BA: VRACs CARVe a path for novel mechanisms of communication in the CNS. Sci STKE (357):pe42, 2006

Murase S, Mathe JM, Grenhoff J, et al: Effects of dizocilpine (MK-801) on rat midbrain dopamine cell activity: differential actions on firing pattern related to anatomical localization. J Neural Transm Gen Sect 91:13–25, 1993

Murphy TH, Blatter LA, Bhat RV, et al: Differential regulation of calcium/calmodulin-dependent protein kinase II and p42 MAP kinase activity by synaptic transmission. J Neurosci 14(3, pt 1):1320–1331, 1994

Nagatsu T, Mogi M, Ichinose H, et al: Changes in cytokines and neurotrophins in Parkinson's disease. J Neural Transm Suppl 60:277–290, 2000

Nestler EJ: Antidepressant treatments in the 21st century. Biol Psychiatry 44:526–533, 1998

Nestler EJ, Hyman SE, Malenka RC: Molecular Neuropharmacology: A Foundation for Clinical Neuroscience. New York, McGraw-Hill, 2001

Neves-Pereira M, Mundo E, Muglia P, et al: The brain-derived neurotrophic factor gene confers susceptibility to bipolar disorder: evidence from a family based association study. Am J Hum Genet 71:651–655, 2002

Ni C, Murphy P, Golde TE, et al: γ-Secretase cleavage and nuclear localization of ErbB-4 receptor tyrosine kinase. Science 294:2179–2181, 2001

Nicholls DG: Proteins, Transmitters and Synapses. Cambridge, MA, Blackwell Science, 1994

Nishizuka Y: Intracellular signaling by hydrolysis of phospholipids and activation of protein kinase C. Science 258:607–614, 1992

Niswender CM, Sanders-Bush E, Emeson RB: Identification and characterization of RNA editing events within the 5-HT2C receptor. Ann N Y Acad Sci 861:38–48, 1998

Owens MJ, Nemeroff CB: The serotonin transporter and depression. Depress Anxiety 8 (suppl 1):5–12, 1998

Pacholczyk T, Blakely RD, Amara SG: Expression cloning of a cocaine- and antidepressant-sensitive human noradrenaline transporter. Nature 350:350–354, 1991

Panatier A, Theodosis DT, Mothet JP, et al: Glia-derived D-serine controls NMDA receptor activity and synaptic memory. Cell 125:775–784, 2006

Parnas H, Segel LA: Facilitation as a tool to study the entry of calcium and the mechanism of neurotransmitter release. Prog Neurobiol 32:1–9, 1989

Patapoutian A, Reichardt LF: Trk receptors: mediators of neurotrophin action. Curr Opin Neurobiol 11:272–280, 2001

Pazos A, Palacios JM: Quantitative autoradiographic mapping of serotonin receptors in the rat brain, I: serotonin-1 receptors. Brain Res 346:205–230, 1985

Pearson Murphy BE, Steinberg SI, Hu FY, et al: Neuroactive ring A–reduced metabolites of progesterone in human plasma during pregnancy: elevated levels of 5α-dihydroprogesterone in depressed patients during the latter half of pregnancy. J Clin Endocrinol Metab 86:5981–5987, 2001

Pessiglione M, Seymour B, Flandin G, et al: Dopamine-dependent prediction errors underpin reward-seeking behaviour in humans. Nature 442:1042–1045, 2006

Pierce RC, Bari AA: The role of neurotrophic factors in psychostimulant-induced behavioral and neuronal plasticity. Rev Neurosci 12:95–110, 2001

Pineyro G, Blier P: Autoregulation of serotonin neurons: role in antidepressant drug action. Pharmacol Rev 51:533–591, 1999

Pisano P, Samuel D, Nieoullon A, et al: Activation of the adenylate cyclase–dependent protein kinase pathway increases high affinity glutamate uptake into rat striatal synaptosomes. Neuropharmacology 35:541–547, 1996

Plyte SE, Hughes K, Nikolakaki E, et al: Glycogen synthase kinase-3: functions in oncogenesis and development. Biochim Biophys Acta 1114:147–162, 1992

Poo MM: Neurotrophins as synaptic modulators. Nat Rev Neurosci 2:24–32, 2001

Przybyslawski J, Roullet P, Sara SJ: Attenuation of emotional and nonemotional memories after their reactivation: role of beta adrenergic receptors. J Neurosci 19:6623–6628, 1999

Rajkowska G: Cell pathology in mood disorders. Semin Clin Neuropsychiatry 7:281–292, 2002

Rapoport SI: In vivo fatty acid incorporation into brain phospholipids in relation to plasma availability, signal transduction and membrane remodeling. J Mol Neurosci 16:243–261; discussion 279–284, 2001

Rapport M, Green AR, Page I: Serum vasoconstrictor (serotonin): isolation and characterization. J Biol Chem 176:1248–1251, 1947

Rashid AJ, So CH, Kong MM, et al: D1-D2 dopamine receptor heterooligomers with unique pharmacology are coupled to rapid activation of Gq/11 in the striatum. Proc Natl Acad Sci U S A 104:654–659, 2007

Rasmussen H: The calcium messenger system (I). N Engl J Med 314:1094–1101, 1986

Rasmussen H: The cycling of calcium as an intracellular messenger. Sci Am 261:66–73, 1989

Rasmussen K, Morilak DA, Jacobs BL: Single unit activity of locus coeruleus neurons in the freely moving cat, I: during naturalistic behaviors and in response to simple and complex stimuli. Brain Res 371:324–334, 1986a

Rasmussen K, Strecker RE, Jacobs BL: Single unit response of noradrenergic, serotonergic and dopaminergic neurons in freely moving cats to simple sensory stimuli. Brain Res 369:336–340, 1986b

Ravid R, Van Zwieten EJ, Swaab DF: Brain banking and the human hypothalamus—factors to match for, pitfalls and potentials. Prog Brain Res 93:83–95, 1992

Reader TA: Microiontophoresis of biogenic amines on cortical neurons: amounts of NA, DA and 5-HT ejected, compared with tissue content. Acta Physiol Lat Am 30:291–304, 1980

Riccio A, Pierchala BA, Ciarallo CL, et al: An NGF-TrkA-mediated retrograde signal to transcription factor CREB in sympathetic neurons. Science 277:1097–1100, 1997

Rick CE, Ye Q, Finn SE, et al: Neurosteroids act on the GABA(A) receptor at sites on the N-terminal side of the middle of TM2. Neuroreport 9:379–383, 1998

Rink TJ: A real receptor-operated calcium channel? Nature 334:649–650, 1988

Roberson ED, English JD, Sweatt JD: A biochemist's view of long-term potentiation. Learn Mem 3:1–24, 1996

Roberson ED, English JD, Adams JP, et al: The mitogen-activated protein kinase cascade couples PKA and PKC to cAMP response element binding protein phosphorylation in area CA1 of hippocampus. J Neurosci 19:4337–4348, 1999

Robinson MJ, Stippec SA, Goldsmith E, et al: A constitutively active and nuclear form of the MAP kinase ERK2 is sufficient for neurite outgrowth and cell transformation. Curr Biol 8:1141–1150, 1998

Roman T, Schmitz M, Polanczyk G, et al: Attention-deficit hyperactivity disorder: a study of association with both the dopamine transporter gene and the dopamine D4 receptor gene. Am J Med Genet 105:471–478, 2001

Roth BL, McLean S, Zhu XZ, et al: Characterization of two [3H]ketanserin recognition sites in rat striatum. J Neurochem 49:1833–1838, 1987

Roybal K, Theobold D, Graham A, et al: Mania-like behavior induced by disruption of CLOCK. Proc Natl Acad Sci U S A 104:6406–11, 2007

Rupprecht R: Neuroactive steroids: mechanisms of action and neuropsychopharmacological properties. Psychoneuroendocrinology 28:139–168, 2003

Sakaba T, Stein A, Jahn R: Distinct kinetic changes in neurotransmitter release after SNARE protein cleavage. Science 309:491–494, 2005

Salehi A, Verhaagen J, Swaab DF: Neurotrophin receptors in Alzheimer's disease. Prog Brain Res 117:71–89, 1998

Salinas PC: Wnt factors in axonal remodelling and synaptogenesis. Biochem Soc Symp 65:101–109, 1999

Salinas PC, Hall AC: Lithium and synaptic plasticity. Bipolar Disord 1:87–90, 1999

Sanacora G, Kendell SF, Levin Y, et al: Preliminary evidence of riluzole efficacy in antidepressant-treated patients with residual depressive symptoms. Biol Psychiatry 61:822–825, 2007

Sapolsky RM: The possibility of neurotoxicity in the hippocampus in major depression: a primer on neuron death. Biol Psychiatry 48:755–765, 2000

Saxena PR, De Vries P, Villalon CM: 5-HT1-like receptors: a time to bid goodbye. Trends Pharmacol Sci 19:311–316, 1998

Schoeffter P, Bobirnac I: 5-Hydroxytryptamine 5-HT1D receptors mediating inhibition of cyclic AMP accumulation in Madin-Darby canine kidney (MDCK) cells. Naunyn Schmiedebergs Arch Pharmacol 352:256–262, 1995

Schoepp DD: Unveiling the functions of presynaptic metabotropic glutamate receptors in the central nervous system. J Pharmacol Exp Ther 299:12–20, 2001

Scott JA, Crews FT: Down-regulation of serotonin2, but not of β-adrenergic receptors during chronic treatment with amitriptyline is independent of stimulation of serotonin2 and β-adrenergic receptors. Neuropharmacology 25:1301–1306, 1986

Scott MM, Marcus JN, Elmquist JK: Orexin neurons and the TASK of glucosensing. Neuron 50:665–667, 2006

Shaltiel G, Chen G, Manji HK: Neurotrophic signaling cascades in the pathophysiology and treatment of bipolar disorder. Curr Opin Pharmacol 7:22–26, 2007

Shaltiel G, Maeng S, Malkesman O, et al: Evidence for the involvement of the kainate receptor subunit GluR6 (GRIK2) in mediating behavioral displays related to behavioral symptoms of mania. Mol Psychiatry 13:858–872, 2008

Simonds WF: Dysfunction of G protein–regulated pathways and endocrine diseases, in Signal Transduction and Human Disease. Edited by Finkel T, Gutkind JS. New York, Wiley, 2003, pp 201–231

Sklar P, Gabriel SB, McInnis MG, et al: Family-based association study of 76 candidate genes in bipolar disorder: BDNF is a potential risk locus. Brain-derived neurotrophic factor. Mol Psychiatry 7:579–593, 2002

Sleight AJ, Carolo C, Petit N, et al: Identification of 5-hydroxytryptamine7 receptor binding sites in rat hypothalamus: sensitivity to chronic antidepressant treatment. Mol Pharmacol 47:99–103, 1995

Soderling TR: CaM-kinases: modulators of synaptic plasticity. Curr Opin Neurobiol 10:375–380, 2000

Soltesz I, Staley K: High times for memory: cannabis disrupts temporal coordination among hippocampal neurons. Nat Neurosci 9:1526–1533, 2006

Spiegel AM: G Proteins, Receptors, and Disease. Totowa, NJ, Humana Press, 1998

Squire LR, Bloom FE, McConnell SK, et al: Fundamental Neuroscience. New York, Academic Press, 2003

Stabel S, Parker PJ: Protein kinase C. Pharmacol Ther 51:71–95, 1991

Stambolic V, Ruel L, Woodgett JR: Lithium inhibits glycogen synthase kinase–3 activity and mimics wingless signalling in intact cells. Curr Biol 6:1664–1668, 1996

Stoof JC, Kebabian JW: Two dopamine receptors: biochemistry, physiology and pharmacology. Life Sci 35:2281–2296, 1984

Szabo ST, Blier P: Response of the norepinephrine system to antidepressant drugs. CNS Spectr 6:679–684, 2001

Szabo ST, Du J, Gray N, et al: Mood stabilizer lithium regulates the synaptic and total protein expression of AMPA glutamate receptors in vitro and in vivo. Annual IRP Scientific Retreat, 2002

Taber MT, Fibiger HC: Electrical stimulation of the medial prefrontal cortex increases dopamine release in the striatum. Neuropsychopharmacology 9:271–275, 1993

Tejani-Butt SM, Ordway GA: Effect of age on [3H]nisoxetine binding to uptake sites for norepinephrine in the locus coeruleus of humans. Brain Res 583:312–315, 1992

Tejani-Butt SM, Brunswick DJ, Frazer A: [3H]Nisoxetine: a new radioligand for norepinephrine uptake sites in brain. Eur J Pharmacol 191:239–243, 1990

Truss M, Beato M: Steroid hormone receptors: interaction with deoxyribonucleic acid and transcription factors. Endocr Rev 14:459–479, 1993

Tsao P, von Zastrow M: Downregulation of G protein–coupled receptors. Curr Opin Neurobiol 10:365–369, 2000

Ungerstedt U: Stereotaxic mapping of the monoamine pathways in the rat brain. Acta Physiol Scand Suppl 367:1–48, 1971

Van Tol HH, Wu CM, Guan HC, et al: Multiple dopamine D4 receptor variants in the human population. Nature 358:149–152, 1992

Weisstaub NV, Zhou M, Lira A, et al: Cortical 5-HT2A receptor signaling modulates anxiety-like behaviors in mice. Science 313:536–540, 2006

Westphal RS, Sanders-Bush E: Reciprocal binding properties of 5-hydroxytryptamine type 2C receptor agonists and inverse agonists. Mol Pharmacol 46:937–942, 1994

Whitaker-Azmitia PM, Shemer AV, Caruso J, et al: Role of high affinity serotonin receptors in neuronal growth. Ann N Y Acad Sci 600:315–330, 1990

Wiklund L, Bjorklund A: Mechanisms of regrowth in the bulbospinal serotonin system following 5,6-dihydroxytryptamine induced axotomy, II: fluorescence histochemical observations. Brain Res 191:109–127, 1980

Wisner A, Dufour E, Messaoudi M, et al: Human opiorphin, a natural antinociceptive modulator of opioid-dependent pathways. Proc Natl Acad Sci U S A 103:17979–17984, 2006

Wolf WA, Bobik A: Effects of 5,6-dihydroxytryptamine on the release, synthesis, and storage of serotonin: studies using rat brain synaptosomes. J Neurochem 50:534–542, 1988

Wolff DJ, Poirier PG, Brostrom CO, et al: Divalent cation binding properties of bovine brain Ca2+-dependent regulator protein. J Biol Chem 252:4108–4117, 1977

Woodgett JR: Judging a protein by more than its name: gsk-3. Sci STKE (100):RE12, 2001

Xu Q, Fawcett TW, Gorospe M, et al: Induction of mitogen-activated protein kinase phosphatase–1 during acute hypertension. Hypertension 30(1, pt 1):106–111, 1997

Yau JL, Noble J, Seckl JR: Acute restraint stress increases 5-HT7 receptor mRNA expression in the rat hippocampus. Neurosci Lett 309:141–144, 2001

Zarate CA Jr, Singh J, Carlson PJ, et al: A randomized trial of an N-methyl-D-aspartate antagonist in treatment-resistant major depression. Arch Gen Psychiatry 63:856–864, 2006a

Zarate CA Jr, Singh J, Manji HK: Cellular plasticity cascades: targets for the development of novel therapeutics for bipolar disorder. Biol Psychiatry 59:1006–1020, 2006b

Zarate CA Jr, Singh J, Carlson PJ, et al: Efficacy of a protein kinase c inhibitor (tamoxifen) in the treatment of acute mania: a pilot study. Bipolar Disord 9:561–570, 2007; erratum in: Bipolar Disord 9:932, 2007

Zuckerman M: Sensation seeking, mania, and monoamines. Neuropsychobiology 13:121–128, 1985

CHAPTER 2

Basic Principles of Molecular Biology and Genomics

Jiang-Zhou Yu, M.D., Ph.D.

Mark M. Rasenick, Ph. D.

In June 2000, it was announced that both a corporate effort and a government consortium had succeeded in sequencing all of the human genome. This was followed by the publication of that sequence in February 2001 (Lander et al. 2001; Venter et al. 2001). For anyone involved in biology or medicine, these events represented a revolution in the technical and conceptual approach to both research and therapy.

It seems that humans are far less complex than most scientists had previously thought. Rather than having 100,000–150,000 genes, as was once the belief, humans may have only about 30,000 genes. At this point, not all of those genes have an identified function, and it is becoming clear that many gene products have more than one function. Perhaps more importantly, genes that have been identified in a single cell type may have an entirely different function in other cell types. Some other genes may enjoy a brief and transient expression during the process of embryonic development only to play an entirely different role in the adult. Truly understanding those genes and gene products will revolutionize all of science, and this may be especially true for psychiatry.

Consider that prior to identification of the genome, psychiatric genomics has been limited to studies of chromosomal linkage wherein a putative gene for a disorder could be roughly localized to a given region of a chromosome. The burgeoning understanding of the human genome now occurring has led to a rudimentary understanding of genetic variation among humans. In many humans, a single base or single nucleotide is modified, and it is a combination of knowing the entire genetic code and determining aberrations in individuals with disease that will allow the pinpointing of specific genes associated with psychiatric diseases.

New advances and technology are also furthering our understanding of the genome. Microarrays, which permit one to put several genes on a chip, show the ability of a given cell or tissue to activate given genes. Sometimes, during a disease process, inappropriate genes are activated or inactivated. Identification of these genes also helps to shed light on the disease process and on possible therapy. At the same time that rapid advances are being made in understanding the genome, rapid advances in molecular biology are allowing the manipulation of genes and proteins in individual nerve cells. The development of molecular and cellular models for neuropsychiatric disease has also permitted tremendous advancement in our understanding of both biochemical defects and possible new approaches toward ameliorating those defects.

In this chapter, we present information about genetics, genomics, and the genome and explain modern molecular biology and the investigative methods used in that field. We also discuss pathophysiology, as related to neuropsychiatry and molecular strategy, and introduce findings from studies on the cell biology of the neuron that help us to understand both psychopharmacology and the biology of the brain and mind.

Cell Biology of the Neuron

To appreciate the molecular biology presented in this chapter, it is necessary to describe the components of the neuron that process signals that directly or indirectly modify the aspects of the genome described below. Neurons—specialized cells that function to transmit signals to other neurons, muscles, and secretory cells—contain four basic domains (Figure 2–1), and these domains serve to receive signals, process and integrate signals, conduct impulses, and release transmitter.

The nucleus resides in the cell body (the signal processing domain) and contains the DNA that codes for the genes expressed by neurons. Activation of a given gene results in the generation of a messenger RNA (mRNA), which is then translated into a protein (see below). Although such events are common to all cells, neural cells are unique in some aspects of molecular signaling. Of importance, the variety of gene expression is far greater in the brain than in any other organ or tissue. Some estimates are that in aggregate, the brain expresses as much as 10 times the number of genes expressed in any other tissue. This does not mean that individual neurons undergo a much greater gene expression. Rather, it suggests an extraordinary heterogeneity among neurons and glia, which allows for a rich regulation when those neurons and glia assemble into the elaborate network of the human brain.

mRNA molecules exported from the nucleus are translated into proteins by ribosomes in the endoplasmic reticulum. Note that most of the protein production occurs in the cell body, although there is also some mRNA in the dendrites (Steward and Wallace 1995). This means that newly made proteins must be transported from that cell body to the axon terminal, a distance as great as 1 m. These proteins are often packaged in vesicles, and specialized "motor" molecules transport packaged proteins down microtubule "tracks" at the cost of adenosine triphosphate (ATP) hydrolysis (Setou et al. 2000).

Essential Principles of Gene Expression

Genes and DNA

The DNA double helix transmits genetic information from generation to generation and is the repository of information required to guide an organism's development and interaction with the environment. The role of DNA in storing and transferring hereditary information depends on the innate properties of its four constituent bases. There are two purine bases, adenine (A) and guanine (G), and two pyrimidine bases, cytosine (C) and thymine (T). Within the DNA double helix, A is complementary to T, and G is complementary to C. Each block of DNA that codes for a single RNA or protein is called a *gene*, and the entire set of genes in a cell, organelle, or virus forms its *genome*. Cells and organelles may contain more than one copy of their genome. There are 46 chromosomes in a typical human cell; when "unraveled," the total DNA of a single cell is approximately 1 m in length. The 46 human chromosomes consist of 22 pairs of autosomes and 2 sex chromosomes, either XX for females or XY for males. Such a large amount of genetic material is effectively packaged into a cell nucleus, which is also the site of DNA replication and transcription. Only a small percentage of chromosomal DNA in the human genome is responsible for encoding the genes that act as a template for RNA strands; there are approximately 20,000–25,000 genes total, of which about 10,000–15,000 genes are expressed in any individual cell.

Among RNA strands, only ribosomal RNA (rRNA), transfer RNA (tRNA), and small nuclear RNA (snRNA) have independent cellular functions. Most cellular RNA, mRNA, serves as a template for protein synthesis. RNA, like DNA, is also composed of four nucleotide building blocks. However, in RNA, the nucleotide uracil (U) takes the place of thymine (T), and RNA is a flexible single strand that is free to fold into a variety of conformations. Thus, the functional versatility of RNA greatly exceeds that of DNA.

Chromosomal DNA contains both genes and more extensive intergenic regions. Some regions of DNA in genes act as the template for RNA, but some regions are responsible for regulatory functions. The distribution of genes on chromosomes is not uniform: some chromosomal regions, and indeed whole chromosomes, are richly endowed with genes, whereas other regions are more amply supplied with noncoding DNA. Regulation of gene expression conferred by the nucleotide sequence of a DNA molecule is referred to as *cis*-regulation, because the regulatory and transcribed regions occur on the same DNA molecule. *cis*-Regulatory elements that determine the transcription start site of a gene are called *basal* (or *core*) *promoters*; other *cis*-regulatory elements are responsible for tethering different activators and repressor proteins to DNA. There are specific regions of DNA that bind to regulatory proteins. These regulatory proteins may be encoded at any regions in the genome, and because they are not coded by the stretch of DNA to which

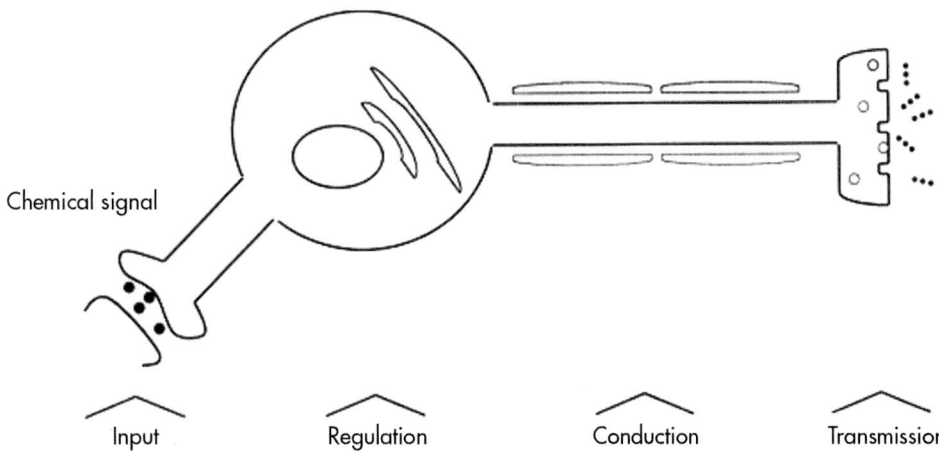

Chemical signal

Input Regulation Conduction Transmission

FIGURE 2–1. Diagram of a typical neuron.

As described in the text, this neuron is divided into zones for the reception of signals (input=dendrites), integration of signals (regulation=nucleus and soma), conduction of signals (axon), and transmission of signals (axon terminal).

they bind, they are sometimes called *trans*-acting factors. *Trans*-acting factors that regulate the transcription of DNA are also called *transcription factors*.

DNA Replication

Chromosomal DNA must be replicated to coordinate with cell division. Replication begins at a sequence called the *origin of replication*. It involves the separation of the double helix DNA strands over a short length and the binding of enzymes, including DNA and RNA polymerases. During DNA replication, each existing strand of DNA serves as a template for the synthesis of a new double helix that contains one old strand and one strand that is newly synthesized but complementary. This process is known as *semiconservative replication*. In the process of cell division, each of the 46 double helices is replicated and folded into chromosomes.

Transcription

Only a fraction of all the genes in a genome are expressed in a given cell or at a given time. These genes undergo the process of *transcription*, in which an RNA molecule complementary to one of the gene's DNA strands is synthesized in a 5′ to 3′ direction, using nucleotide triphosphates. Transcription can be classified into three discrete steps: initiation, mRNA chain elongation, and chain termination. Transcriptional regulation may occur at any step in the process; however, initiation appears to be the primary control point because, in a sense, it is the rate-limiting step. Localization of the transcription start site and regulation of the rate of transcription are essential to

initiation. The *cis-* and *trans*-acting factors described above all regulate the initiation of transcription.

Translation

Each mRNA in a cell can code for the primary amino acid sequence of a protein, using a triplet of nucleotides (codon) to represent each of the amino acids. Some amino acids are represented by more than one codon, because there are more triplet codons than there are amino acids. The codons in mRNA do not interact directly with the amino acids they specify. The translation of the individual codons of mRNA into protein depends on the presence of another RNA molecule, tRNA, which has a cloverleaf structure. On the top leaf of the tRNA structure, three nucleotides form a complementary codon (an anticodon) to each mRNA nucleotide triplet. Thus, each mRNA nucleotide triplet can code for a specific amino acid. Each tRNA carries an amino acid corresponding to its anticodon, and when thus "charged," the complex is termed *aminoacyl-tRNA*. Anticodons of aminoacyl-tRNA bind with mRNA codons in ribosomes. Ribosomes, a complex of rRNA and enzymes needed for translation, provide the structure on which tRNA can bind with the codons of mRNA in sequential order.

Initiation of protein synthesis involves the assembly of the components of the translation system. These components include the two ribosomal subunits, the mRNA to be translated, the aminoacyl-tRNA specified by the first codon in the message, guanosine triphosphate (GTP), and initiation factors that facilitate the assembly of this initiation complex. In eukaryotes, there are at least 12 distinct translation initiation factors (Roll-Mecak et al. 2000). After the ribosome recognizes the specific start site on the mRNA sequence, which is always the codon AUG coding for methionine, it slides along the mRNA molecule strand and translates the nucleotide sequence one codon at a time, adding amino acids to the growing end of the polypeptide chain (the elongation process). During elongation, the ribosome moves from the 5'-end to the 3'-end of the mRNA that is being translated. The binding of GTP to the elongation factor tu (EFtu) promotes the binding of aminoacyl-tRNA to the ribosome (Wieden et al. 2002). When the ribosome finds a stop codon (UAA, UGA, or UAG) in the message RNA, the mRNA, the tRNA, and the newly synthesized protein are released from the ribosomes, with the help of release factors that also bind GTP. The translation process is stopped, and a nascent protein exists.

It is noteworthy that initiation, elongation, and release factors undergo a conformational change upon the binding of GTP. In this regard, they are similar to the G proteins (both heterotrimeric G proteins and small "ras-like" G proteins) involved in cellular signaling (Halliday et al. 1984; Kaziro et al. 1991).

Regulation of Gene Expression

Chromatin and DNA Methylation

Biophysics and molecular biology have revealed that chromatin consists of a repetitive nucleoprotein complex, the nucleosome. This particle consists of a histone octamer, with two copies of each of the histones (H2A, H2B, H3, and H4), wrapped by 147 base pairs of DNA. In the octamer, histones H3 and H4 are assembled in a tetramer, which is flanked by two H2A–H2B dimers. A variable length of DNA completes the second turn around the histone octamer and interacts with a fifth histone, H1. H2A, H2B, H3, and H4 are variously modified at their amino- and carboxyl-terminal tails to influence the dynamics of chromatin structure and function (Ballestar and Esteller 2002; Keshet et al. 1986; Kornberg and Lorch 1999; Strahl and Allis 2000). Although chromatin provides structure to chromosomes, it also plays a critical role in transcriptional regulation in eukaryotes because it can repress gene expression by inhibiting the ability of transcription factors to access DNA. In fact, chromatin ensures that genes are inactive until their expression is commanded. In the activation process, cells must attenuate nucleosome-mediated repression of an appropriate subset of genes by means of activator proteins that modify chromatin structure. An activator protein displaces nucleosomes, which permits a complex of proteins (general transcription factors) to bind DNA at a promoter and to recruit RNA polymerase.

Cytosine methylation at CpG dinucleotides is the most common modification of the eukaryotic genome. In vertebrates, methylation occurs globally throughout the genome, with the exception of CpG islands. These are CG-rich regions of DNA that stretch for an average of ~1 kilobase (kb), coincident with the promoters of 60% of human RNA polymerase II–transcribed genes. Methylation of cytosines at CpG represses transcription (Ballestar and Esteller 2002). *Genetic imprinting,* a process by which particular paternal or maternal genes are inactivated throughout a species, is at least partly controlled by DNA methylation. Specific proteins binding to methylated DNA may establish a bridge between chromatin and DNA methylation. They recruit histone deacetylases (HDACs) to activate a methylated promoter, which in turn deacetylates histones, leading to a repressed state (Ballestar and Esteller 2002; Keshet et al. 1986).

RNA Polymerases

There are three distinct classes of RNA polymerase—RNA polymerase I, RNA polymerase II, and RNA polymerase III—in the nucleus of eukaryotic cells, and they are designed to carry out transcription. RNA polymerase I synthesizes large rRNA molecules. RNA polymerase II is mainly used to yield mRNA and, subsequently, proteins. RNA polymerase III produces snRNA, small rRNA, and tRNA molecules. Each class of RNA polymerase recognizes particular types of genes. However, RNA polymerases do not bind to DNA directly. Rather, they are recruited to DNA by other proteins that bind to promoters (Figure 2–2).

mRNA is transcribed from DNA by RNA polymerase II with heterogeneous nuclear RNA (hnRNA), an intermediate product. The core promoter recognized by RNA polymerase II is the TATA box (Hogness box), a sequence rich in nucleotides A and T, which is usually located 25–30 bases upstream of the transcription start site. The TATA box determines the start site of transcription and orients the basal transcription complex that binds to DNA and recruits RNA polymerase II to the TATA box; thus, it establishes the 5' to 3' direction in which RNA polymerase II synthesizes RNA. The formation of the basal transcription complex is promoted by a *TATA binding protein* (TBP) that binds to a core promoter, together

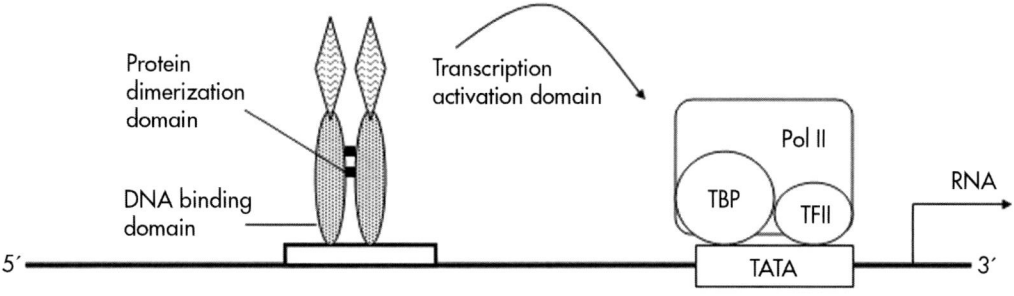

FIGURE 2–2. Transcription factors and RNA polymerase II complex.

Typical transcription factors contain DNA-binding domains, protein dimerization domains, and transcription activation domains. Some transcription factors (e.g., cAMP response element–binding protein [CREB]) may be modified by phosphorylation. The transcription activation domain interacts with an RNA polymerase II (Pol II) complex to induce transcription. TATA binding protein (TBP) binds to the TATA box element and associates with general transcription factors (TFII). This gene transcription apparatus recruits Pol II to the appropriate gene.

with multiple TBP-associated factors and other general transcription factors. *Enhancers* are DNA sequences that increase the rate of initiation of transcription by RNA polymerase II through its interaction with transcription factors, which can be located "upstream" or "downstream" of the transcription start site. Enhancer elements are important to cell-specific and stimulus-dependent expression of hnRNA. Some RNA polymerase II species, including those for many genes that are expressed in neurons, lack a TATA box and possess instead an *initiator*, a poorly conserved genetic promoter element.

Transcription Factors

Transcription factors act as the key regulators of gene expression. Sequence-specific transcription factors typically contain physically distinct functional domains (see Figure 2–2). Numerous transcription factors have been found. Some of them translocate to the nucleus to bind their *cis*-regulatory elements in response to activation reaction, such as nuclear factor κB (NF-κB). However, some transcription factors are already bound to their cognate *cis*-regulatory elements in the nucleus under basal conditions and are converted into transcriptional activators by phosphorylation. cAMP (cyclic 3′-5′-adenosine monophosphate) response element–binding protein (CREB), for example, is bound to regions of DNA, called *cAMP response elements* (CREs), before cell stimulation. CREB can promote transcription when it is phosphorylated on a serine residue (ser133), because phosphorylated CREB can interact with a coactivator, CREB-binding protein, which in turn contacts and activates the basal transcription complex. Of interest, CREB-binding protein possesses intrinsic histone acetyltransferase

(HAT) activity. The activity of most transcription factors is regulated through second-messenger pathways. CREB can be activated via phosphorylation at ser133 by second messengers, such as cAMP, Ca++, and growth factors (Figure 2–3).

CREB is a molecule that is widely implicated in learning and memory in many species. Mice expressing mutant CREB isoforms show impaired memory, but this is dependent on the genetic background of the mice (Graves et al. 2002). CREB-binding protein (CBP) is a transcriptional coactivator with CREB. A partial-knockout mouse model, in which CBP activity is lost, exhibits learning deficiencies (Oike et al. 1999). Further, Rubinstein-Taybi syndrome (RTS) is an autosomal-dominant dysmorphic syndrome that results in severe impairment of learning and memory. The RTS gene has been mapped to chromosome 16 and identified as CBP. The loss of function of CBP is likely one important contributing factor to the learning and memory defects seen in RTS (Murata et al. 2001; Oike et al. 1999; Petrij et al. 1995).

Posttranscriptional Modification of RNA

The mRNA of prokaryotes can be used without any modification to direct protein synthesis, but posttranscription processing of mRNA is needed in eukaryotes. The DNA sequences that code for mRNA (exons) are frequently interrupted by intervening DNA sequences (introns). When a protein-coding gene is first transcribed, the hnRNA contains both exons and introns. Before the transcript exits the nucleus, its introns are removed and its exons are spliced to form mature mRNA (Figure 2–4). The hnRNA that is synthesized by RNA polymerase has a 7-methyl-guanosine "cap" added at the 5′ end. The cap

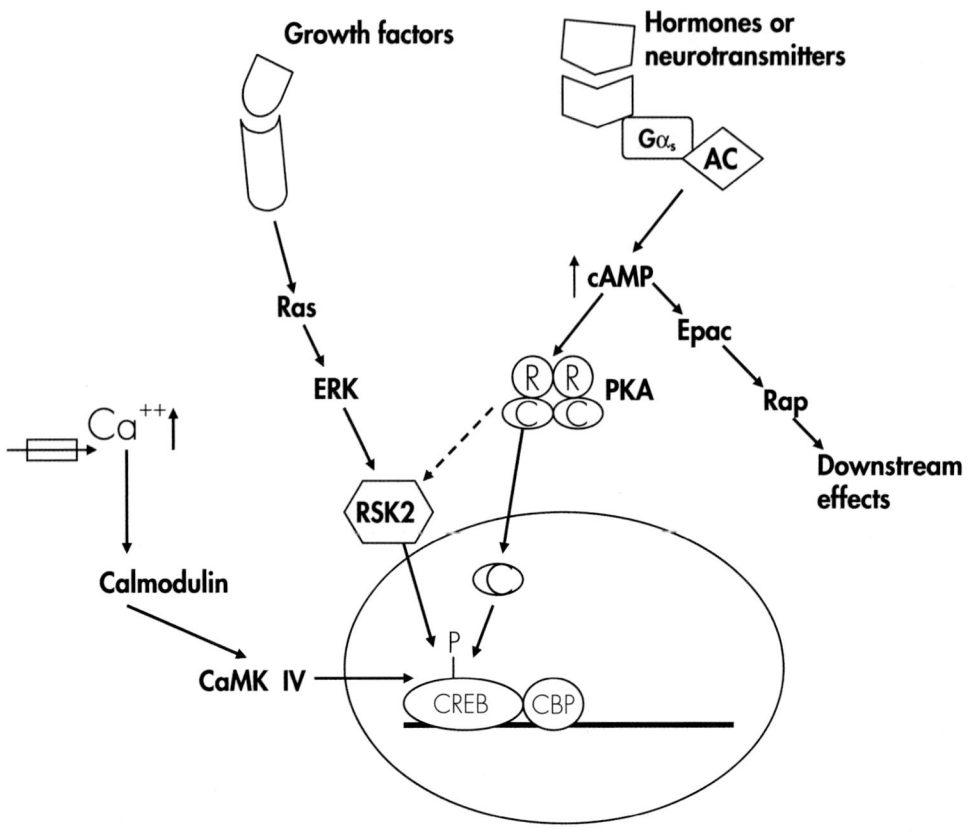

FIGURE 2–3. Activation of cAMP response element–binding protein (CREB) via different signal transduction pathways.

Signal cascades are activated by external stimuli, such as hormones or neurotransmitters and growth factors. *Arrows* indicate the interaction between pathways. AC=adenylyl cyclase; C=catalytic subunits of PKA; Ca^{++}=calcium; CaMK IV=calmodulin-dependent kinase IV; cAMP=cyclic 3'-5'-adenosine monophosphate; CBP=CREB-binding protein; Epac=exchange protein activated by cAMP; ERK=extracellular-regulated kinase; $G\alpha_s$=α subunit of the stimulatory G protein; P=phosphorylation; PKA=cAMP–dependent protein kinase; R=regulatory subunits of PKA; Rap and Ras = small GTPases (small proteins that bind to guanosine triphosphate [GTP]); RSK2=ribosomal S6 kinase 2.

appears to facilitate the initiation of translation and to help stabilize the mRNA. In addition, most eukaryotic mRNA has a chain of 40–200 adenine nucleotides attached to the 3′ end of the mRNA. The poly (A) tail is not transcribed from DNA; rather, it is added after transcription by the nuclear enzyme poly (A) polymerase. The poly (A) tail may help stabilize the mRNA and facilitate mRNA exit from the nucleus. After the mRNA enters the cytoplasm, the poly (A) tail is gradually shortened.

RNA Editing

RNA editing has been detected in eukaryotes ranging from single-celled protozoa to mammals and plants and is now recognized as a type of RNA process (posttranscriptional modification of RNA) that differs from the established processes of RNA splicing, 5′ end formation, and 3′

endonucleolytic cleavage and polyadenylation (DeCerbo and Carmichael 2005; Kable et al. 1997). The conversion of adenosine to inosine was observed first in yeast tRNA (Grosjean et al. 1996) but has since been detected in viral RNA transcripts and mammalian cellular RNA (Bass 1997; Simpson and Emeson 1996). The inosine residues generated from adenosines can alter the coding information of the transcripts, as inosine is synonymous for guanosine during transcript translation. For example, upon A-to-I editing, the CAC codon for histamine is transformed to CIC, coding for arginine. RNA editing can have dramatic consequences for the expression of genetic information, and in a number of cases it has been shown to lead to the expression of proteins not only with altered amino acid sequences from those predicted from the DNA sequence but also with altered biological functions (Bass 2002; Burns et al. 1997).

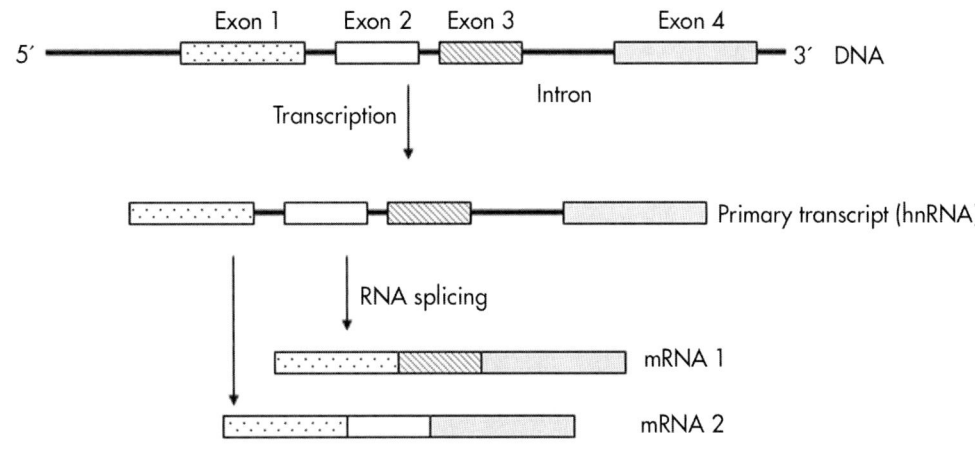

FIGURE 2–4. Transcription and RNA splicing.

The horizontal black line between exons indicates an intron. The region before the first exon is the 5′ regulatory region of the gene, such as a TATA box. There also are *cis*-regulatory elements in introns and downstream of the last exon. The heterogeneous nuclear RNA (hnRNA), containing both exons and introns, is spliced to form mRNA. mRNAs are then exported from the nucleus to the cytoplasm, where they will direct the synthesis of distinct proteins.

The enzymes for RNA editing are referred to as *adenosine deaminases that act on RNA* (ADARs). ADARs target RNA that is double-stranded and convert adenosines to inosines by catalyzing a hydrolytic deamination at the adenine base (Bass 2002). Mammals have several ADARs, of which two (ADAR1 andADAR2) are expressed in most tissues of the body (Seeburg and Hartner 2003). RNA editing may also catalyze the conversion of one or a few adenosines in a transcript to inosines (Maas et al. 1997; Stuart and Panigrahi 2002). On the other hand, RNA editing can convert numerous adenosines to inosines in RNA. This type of editing is thought to be the result of aberrant production of dsRNA (DeCerbo and Carmichael 2005) and has been suggested to lead to RNA degradation (Scadden and Smith 2001), nuclear retention (Zhang and Carmichael 2001), or even gene silencing (Wang et al. 2005).

The 5-HT$_{2C}$ receptor is a G protein–coupled receptor that is well known to have variants generated by A-to-I editing (Burns et al. 1997). 5-HT$_{2C}$ receptor transcripts can be edited at up to five sites, potentially generating 24 different receptor versions, and hence a diverse receptor population. The RNA-edited 5-HT$_{2C}$ receptor affects ligand affinity and the efficacy of G protein coupling (Berg et al. 2001; Wang et al. 2000; Yang et al. 2004). The unedited form of the 5-HT$_{2C}$ receptor has the highest affinity to serotonin and exhibits constitutive activity independent of serotonin levels. When RNA is edited, the basal activity of the 5-HT$_{2C}$ receptor is suppressed, and agonist potency and efficacy are modified.

Modification of the Nascent Polypeptide Chain

The posttranslational modifications described above occur after translation is initiated. They may include removal of part of the translated sequence or the covalent addition of one or more chemical groups that are required for protein activity. Some of these modifications, such as glycosylation or prenylation, represent an obligatory step in the synthesis of the "finished" protein product. In addition, many proteins may be activated or inactivated by the covalent attachment of a variety of chemical groups. Phosphorylation, glycosylation, hydroxylation, and prenylation are common types of covalent alterations in posttranslational modifications. A number of different enzymes coordinate these processes, and they represent a major portion of the events of cellular signaling.

Approaches to Determining and Manipulating Gene Expression

Changes in gene expression within the central nervous system (CNS) have profound effects on all other aspects of the organism. Changes in gene expression are causally associated not only with the development of the CNS but also with the complex phenomena of brain function, such as memory formation, learning, cognition, and affective state. Changes in gene expression likely underlie the pathogenesis of many sporadic or inherited CNS-related disorders, such as Alzheimer's disease, Huntington's disease, depression, and schizophrenia. Thus, insight into and characterization of gene expression profiles are necessary steps for understanding how the brain functions at the molecular level and how malfunction will result in disease. Molecular biological and genomic technologies such as gene mapping and cloning, DNA libraries, gene transfection and expression, and gene knockout and gene targeting have provided numerous benefits to neuropsychopharmacology. Genomic methods applied to pedigree and population samples of patients with psychiatric disorders may soon make it possible to identify genes contributing to the etiology and pathogenesis of these diseases and to provide a potential basis for new therapies.

Cloning of DNA

The cloning of DNA confers the ability to replicate and amplify individual pieces of genes. Cloning can be performed with genomic DNA or complementary DNA (cDNA). cDNA is synthesized artificially from mRNA in

vitro with the aid of *reverse transcriptase*. Cloned genomic DNA may contain any stretch of DNA, either introns or exons, whereas cloned cDNA consists only of exons. For cloning (see Figure 2–5 for outline of the process), the desired pieces of DNA (often called "inserts") are connected with the DNA of genetically engineered vectors or plasmids, and the vectors are introduced into hosts, such as bacteria or mammalian cells. A DNA library is a collection of cloned restriction fragments of the DNA of an organism that consists of random pieces of genomic DNA (i.e., genomic library) or cDNA (i.e., cDNA library). Complete cDNA libraries contain all of the mRNA molecules expressed in a certain tissue. Sometimes cDNA libraries can be made from a specific tissue in a distinct circumstance. For example, a cDNA library could be made from cerebral cortex in rats undergoing transient forebrain ischemia (Abe et al. 1993).

The cloning of disease-related genes is an important step toward insight into the pathogenesis of diseases and development of new drugs against these diseases. If a pro-

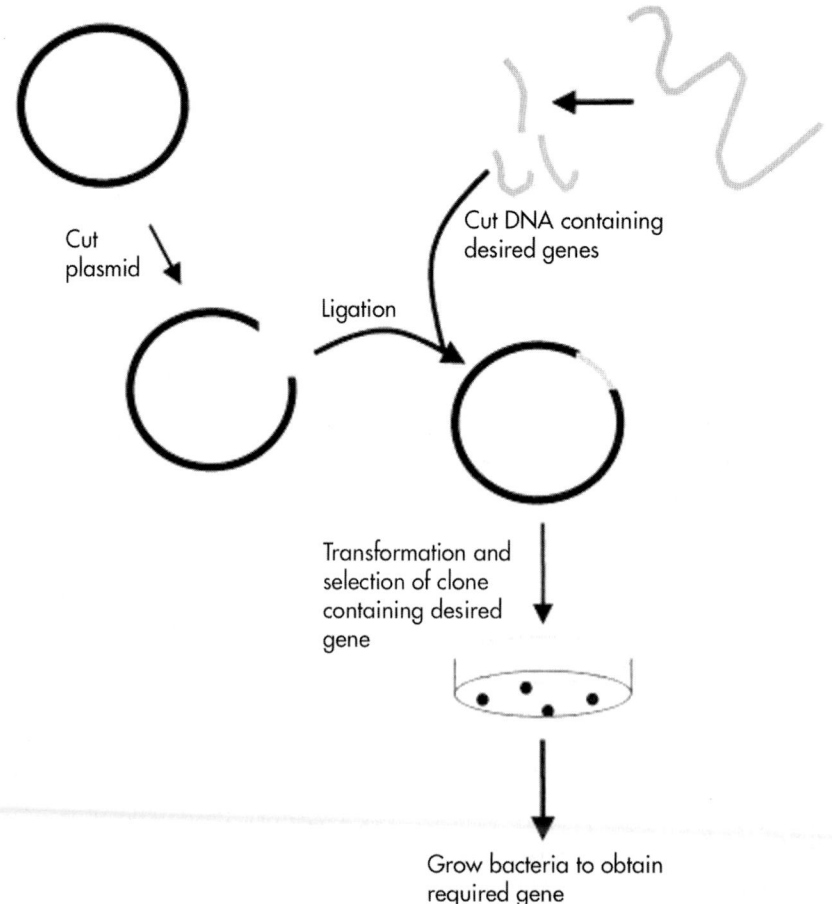

FIGURE 2–5.   Outline of gene cloning.

See text for details.

tein is suspected of involvement in pathogenesis, a nucleic acid sequence can be deduced from the partial amino acid sequence. cDNA libraries are screened with the partial sequence in order to fish out a complete clone of interest. The isolated cDNA molecules are used to infect bacteria, which amplify the cloned cDNA. Bacteria expressing these cDNA molecules will often make the protein of interest, which can be detected with antibody. A variation on the above technique uses antibodies against the purified proteins to screen a DNA library transfected into bacteriophages. The bacteriophages containing the "right" cDNA can be retrieved, and the sequence of cDNA can be analyzed.

Polymerase Chain Reaction

Polymerase chain reaction (PCR) is a rapid procedure for in vitro enzymatic amplification of specific segments of DNA. Amplification of the genes of interest occurs by selecting and synthesizing "primers"—stretches of DNA that span the region of interest to be "filled in"—and by heating DNA to make it single stranded, allowing polymerase and primers to bind. The polymerase then reads the "blank" stretch of DNA between the primers and synthesizes DNA corresponding to the region of interest. This is usually done in "thermal cyclers" that heat the DNA at regular intervals and allow "cycles" of PCR to amplify the genes repetitively. To avoid continual addition of polymerase, the DNA polymerase used is often from bacteria that inhabit hot springs or hot ocean vents. This polymerase is not denatured by heating and can therefore support several cycles of PCR.

A variation on PCR is reverse transcriptase PCR (or RT-PCR), in which the RNA is the template. Reverse transcriptase (the "RT" of RT-PCR) is employed to synthesize cDNA from the RNA. Enzymatic amplification of this cDNA is then accomplished with PCR.

Real-time PCR is based on the method of RT-PCR, following the reverse transcription of RNA into cDNA. Real-time PCR requires suitable detection chemistries to report the presence of PCR products, as well as an instrument to monitor the amplification in real time through recording of the change in fluorescence (Wittwer et al. 1997). Generally, chemistries in PCR consist of fluorescent probes. Several probes exist, including DNA-binding dyes like EtBr or SYBR green I, hydrolysis probes (5′-nuclease probes), and hybridization probes (Valasek and Repa 2005). Each type of probe has its own unique characteristics, but the strategy for each is to link a change in fluorescence to amplification of DNA (Kubista et al. 2006; Lind

et al. 2006). The instrumentation to detect the production of PCR must be able to input energy for excitation of fluorescent chemistries at the desired wavelength and simultaneously detect a particular emission wavelength. Many instrument platforms are available for real-time PCR. The major differences among them are the excitation and emission wavelengths that are available, speed, and the number of reactions that can be run in parallel (Kubista 2004).

Positional Cloning

Disease genes can sometimes be isolated with the aid of *positional cloning,* a process also known as *reverse genetics* (Collins 1995). Positional cloning is the process used to identify a disease gene, based only on knowledge of its chromosomal location, without any knowledge of the biological function of the gene. Positional cloning requires a genetic map of unique DNA segments or genes (genetic markers), with known chromosomal location, that exist in several alternative forms (alleles). These allelic variations (polymorphisms) allow comparisons of the wild type as the "diseased" genotype.

Linkage analysis is a method of localizing one or more genes influencing a trait to specific chromosomal regions. This is performed by examining the cosegregation of the phenotype of interest with genetic markers. Relatives who are phenotypically alike will share common alleles at markers surrounding the genes influencing the phenotype, whereas other relatives (i.e., those who are phenotypically dissimilar) will not carry these alleles. To carry out linkage analyses, investigators need, minimally, a set of families in which phenotyped individuals have known relationships to one another and the genotypes of these individuals, including one or more genetic markers.

Once the chromosomal location of the disease gene has been ascertained, the area of chromosomal DNA can be cloned. Until recently, the process of positional cloning involved laborious efforts to build a physical map and to sequence the region. (The sequencing of the human genome has obviated this step.) Physical maps can be produced by isolating and linking together yeast and/or bacterial artificial chromosomes containing segments of human DNA from the region. These fragments are then sequenced and ordered, and from these data, the genomic DNA sequence for the region of the candidate gene region is determined.

Differential Display

The technique of differential display is designed to determine the complement of genes being expressed (mRNAs) by a tissue or an organ at a given point in time. The establishment of differential display is dependent on the random amplification and subsequent size separation of cDNA molecules (Liang et al. 1992). With RT-PCR amplification with specific oligo-T primers (one- or two-base anchored oligo-dT primers, such as oligo-T-XC, oligo-T-XG, oligo-T-XT, and oligo-T-XA; X = G/A/C), four separate cDNA synthesis reactions are performed. These cDNA synthesis reactions form the four pools of cDNA for one original mRNA population. The resulting cDNA molecules from each RT-PCR reaction are amplified, using the same primer of the reverse transcription step plus randomly chosen primers. Because the randomly chosen primers will anneal at various locations upstream of the oligo-T site, many individual cDNA fragments of different sizes are amplified in each PCR reaction. cDNA fragments derived from different original mRNA populations are sized and then separated on parallel gels to analyze the presence of unique bands. The differentially expressed cDNA fragments can be excised from gels, cloned, and further characterized by a variety of technologies based on different purposes, such as in situ hybridization, sequences, and Northern blot analysis.

Differential display is a useful tool in identifying region-specific mRNA transcripts in brain. The molecular markers for these regions can be found by screening for gene expression in specific brain regions or nuclei (Mizushima et al. 2000; Tochitani et al. 2001). In addition, under different stimulation or behavioral conditions, the changes in gene expression can be explored by differential display (Hong et al. 2002; Q.R. Liu et al. 2002; Mello et al. 1997; Tsai et al. 2002). This technique has even been adapted to indicate the RNA expression profile of an individual neuron (Eberwine et al. 1992). Many genes related to ischemia or Alzheimer's disease in the CNS were also isolated by means of differential display (Doyu et al. 2001; Imaizumi et al. 1997; Tanaka et al. 2002). Genes that are activated in response to chronic drug treatment (e.g., opiates or antidepressants) can also be identified this way. Furthermore, as described later in this chapter (see "Microarray Technology"), streamlined technologies (gene arrays) are now available for this purpose.

Gene Delivery Into Mammalian Cells

The introduction of recombinant DNA (including desired genes) into cells is becoming an increasingly important strategy for understanding certain gene functions in neurons or glia. These advances in gene function studies have benefited the diagnosis of, and therapy for, a variety of disorders that affect the CNS. The delivery of desired genes into cells may also provide the technological base for insight into molecular mechanisms of brain function and, ultimately, for gene therapy in the CNS.

Vectors and Delivery

For gene transfer, it is necessary to incorporate the desired cDNA into various vectors, such as appropriate plasmids or replication-deficient viruses. Vectors used for transfection generally possess two essentially independent functions: 1) carrying genes to the target cell and 2) expressing the genes properly in the target cell. There are currently many commercial vectors with different features from which to choose, and the choice is dependent on the purpose of the experiments and on the characterizations of exogenous desired genes. In one form of transfection, *stable transfection,* cells expressing the gene of interest can be actively selected by a marker (e.g., neomycin resistance genes, *Neo*), and the cDNA or other type of foreign DNA is stably integrated into the DNA of a chromosome. In *transient transfection,* however, cells express the gene of interest for a few days. Cells for hosting the foreign DNA can be either established cell lines or primary cultured neuronal cells. The desired cDNA delivered into cells may be native genes, fragments of the genes, mutant genes, or chimeric genes.

The main barrier to the delivery of DNA into cells is getting the foreign DNA through the cellular membrane. Over the past decades, various methods have been developed to convey the foreign DNA molecules into mammalian cells. These include chemical or physical techniques, such as calcium phosphate coprecipitation of DNA, liposome fusion, electroporation, microinjection, ballistic injection, and viral infection. At present, methods dependent on incorporation of DNA into cationic liposomes (e.g., lipofectin) are used most widely. These methods of transfection are accessible to both cell lines and cultured primary neuronal cells. The ratio of DNA to liposomal suspension, cell density, and time duration of exposure to the DNA–liposomal complex must be optimized for each cell type in culture.

Viral Vectors

Over the past few years, several viral vectors with low toxicity, high infection rate, and persistent expression have extended the methodology of delivery of genes to mammalian cells. These viruses include DNA viruses, such as adenoviruses and adeno-associated viruses, herpes simplex viruses, and RNA retroviruses. Recently, as a result of advances in genetic manipulation, adenoviruses and adeno-associated viruses have been more widely applied to gene transfer. The advantages of adenoviruses are 1) the ability to carry large sequences of foreign DNA, 2) the ability to infect a broad range of cell types, and 3) an almost 100% expression of the foreign gene in cells.

Human adenovirus is a large DNA virus (36 kb of DNA) composed of early genes (from *E1* to *E4*) and later genes (*L1* to *L5*). Wild-type adenovirus cannot be applied to gene transfer, because it causes a lytic infection. Thus, recombinant adenoviruses with defects of some essential viral genes are used for gene delivery. These recently developed adenoviral expression systems are safe; such systems have the capacity for large DNA inserts and allow for relatively simple adenoviral production (Harding et al. 1997; He et al. 1998).

The process of gene transfer into cells (cell lines and primary cells) via recombinant adenoviruses is simple, but the optimal viral titer, the time of exposure to virus, and the multiplicity of infection should be optimized for each cell type. Cell lines and a variety of primary neuronal cells have been infected by adenoviruses (Barkats et al. 1996; Chen and Lambert 2000; Hughes et al. 2002; Koshimizu et al. 2002; Slack et al. 1996). In addition, recombinant adenoviruses containing the desired genes can be delivered to neurons in vivo via intracerebral injection into particular brain areas (Bemelmans et al. 1999; Benraiss et al. 2001; Berry et al. 2001; Neve 1993).

Identification of Ectopic Gene Expression

After delivery of the desired genes into cells, identification of their proper expression is necessary. The general strategies for identification (Chalfie et al. 1994; Kohara et al. 2001; Yu and Rasenick 2002; Yu et al. 2002b) include

1. The measurement of some functional changes elicited by gene expression in targeted cells. If an enzyme is expressed, this would involve measuring the activity of that enzyme.
2. The detection of the proteins coded by the desired genes by techniques relying on antibodies, such as western blot, immunoprecipitation, and immunocytochemistry. Expression of the desired genes tagged with some epitopes, such as HA, GST, and His-tag, can also be determined with antibodies directed against these epitopes.
3. The use of green fluorescent protein (GFP) as an indicator. GFP, a protein from the jellyfish *Aequorea victoria*, can be either cotransfected with the desired

genes or fused with the desired genes before incorporation into cells. The fluorescence from GFP is easy to detect using fluorescent microscopy, and this allows the monitoring of gene expression in living cells. Furthermore, if GFP is fused with the gene of interest, its fluorescence provides a useful tool for studying the function and cellular localization of proteins coded by the genes of interest.

At this point, several different "colors" have been developed through mutation of the initial GFP gene (Shaner et al. 2005). Depending on the wavelengths of excitation, they can be used to localize multiple protein species, or fluorescence resonance energy transfer (FRET) can be used to demonstrate that two target proteins are in close (<10 nm) proximity. FRET uses two fluors with little spectral overlap and depends on the emission of one of the fluors exciting the other.

Inhibition of Cellular Gene Expression

RNA Interference

The previous edition of this textbook (2004) mentioned RNA interference as a new technique with great potential for simple manipulation of gene expression. In September 2006, Andrew Z. Fire and Craig C. Mello were awarded a Nobel Prize for this versatile discovery. RNA interference (RNAi) is believed to be a biologically conserved function in a wide range of eukaryotic species. It may play a role in protection against double-stranded RNA viruses (Sijen et al. 2001) and genome-invading transposable elements (Provost et al. 2002; Volpe et al. 2002). Triggered by dsRNA, RNAi identifies and destroys the mRNA that shares homology with the dsRNA. Thus, the expression of a particular gene can be suppressed by introducing dsRNA whose antisense strand sequence matches the mRNA sequence. Fire et al. (1998) first described RNAi in the nematode *Caenorhabditis elegans* as sequence-specific gene silencing in response to double-stranded RNA. The mechanism of RNAi is partly understood, and key proteins involved in the pathway have been identified. In brief, the basic process of RNAi involves the following steps. In a first initiation step, Dicer, an enzyme of the RNase III family, initiates ATP-dependent fragmentation of long dsRNA into 21- to 25-nucleotide double-stranded fragments, termed *small interfering RNAs* (siRNAs). These siRNAs are specifically characterized by overhanging 3′ ends of two nucleotides and phosphorylated 5′ ends. The siRNA duplexes bind with Dicer, which facilitates the formation of an siRNA/multiprotein complex called *RISC loading complex* (RLC). The siRNA duplex in RLC then unwinds (which requires the protein Ago2) to form an active *RNA-induced silencing complex* (RISC) that contains a single-stranded RNA (called the *guide strand*). The RISC recognizes the target RNA through Watson–Crick base pairing with the guide strand and cleaves the target RNA. Finally, the RISC releases its cleaved product and goes on to catalyze a new cycle of target recognition and cleavage (Figure 2–6) (Tomari and Zamore 2005; Xia et al. 2005).

RNAi Knockdown of Gene Expression

Knockdown of gene expression is accomplished by designing siRNA sequences that target the coding and noncoding regions of the candidate mRNAs with perfect complementarity. In mammalian cells, administration of siRNAs is effective in short-term investigations. Introduction of siRNA into cells is accomplished by transfection or electroporation of either the specific siRNA itself or small hairpin RNA (shRNA) in which the hair loop is rapidly cleaved to produce siRNA. Most of the proposed applications of RNAi incorporate 21-nt siRNA duplexes with 2-nt 3′ overhangs, which after chemical synthesis allow large-scale and uniform production of siRNA molecules that are also amenable to stabilizing chemical modifications. Several commercial entities involved in the manufacturing of siRNAs provide effective design algorithms online, which are based on a combination of mRNA target sequence and secondary structures. In some siRNA–target combinations, the use of longer dsRNAs can increase the potency of RNAi (Kim et al. 2005; Siolas et al. 2005).

For stable longer-term suppression, a gene construct coding for the shRNA with a Pol III or a Pol II promoter can be applied (Brummelkamp et al. 2002; Y. Shi 2003; Yu et al. 2002a). RNA Pol II and III promoters are used to drive expression of shRNA constructs (Amarzguioui et al.

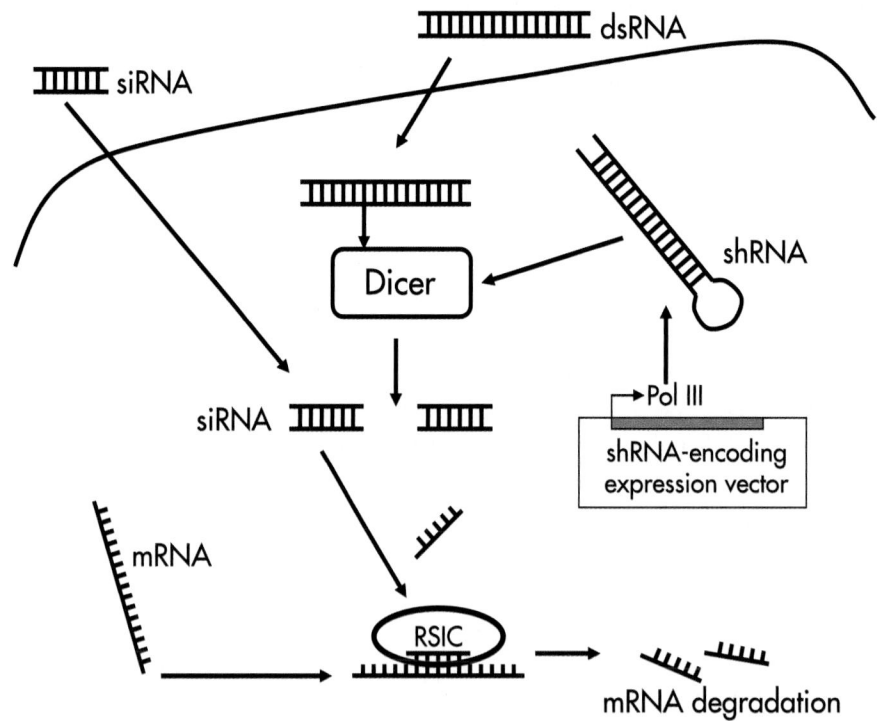

FIGURE 2–6. Schematic of the mechanism of RNA interference (RNAi) posttranscriptional knockdown of a gene product.

The procedure starts with introduction (transfection, electroporation, or injection) of double-stranded RNA (dsRNA) or small interfering RNA (siRNA) into cells, or expression of small hairpin RNA (shRNA) in cells with vectors encoding shRNAs. The cellular ribonuclease (RNase) Dicer recognizes the long dsRNA molecules and shRNA. Subsequently the dsRNA is cleaved, resulting in 21-nt RNA duplexes, the siRNAs. These siRNA molecules are then incorporated into the RNA-induced silencing complex (RISC) multiprotein complex, where they are unwound by an adenosine triphosphate (ATP)–dependent process, transforming the complex into an active state. Activated RISC uses one strand of the RNA as a bait to bind homologous RNA molecules. The target RNA is cleaved and degraded, resulting in gene silencing.

2005), depending on the type of expression required. Pol III promoters drive high levels of constitutive shRNA expression, and their transcription initiation points and termination signals are well defined. Pol II promoter–driven shRNAs can be expressed tissue-specifically (Zeng et al. 2002). Expressed shRNAs are efficiently incorporated into RISC, leading to a more potent inhibition of target gene expression. Generally, viral vectors such as adenovirus, lentivirus, or adeno-associated virus can carry the inhibitory construct into cells to achieve adequate expression for knockdown (Kim and Rossi 2007).

RNAi Applications

RNAi is a straightforward method for inducing sequence-specific silencing of one or more genes of interest with the introduction of siRNAs. It has been a powerful tool to investigate gene function. Studies using RNAi have been performed in neuronal cells to examine the functional roles of individual genes in developing growth cones and neurite outgrowth (Eriksson et al. 2007; Hengst et al. 2006; J. Liu et al. 2007; Schmitz et al. 2007; Yanaka et al. 2007), ion channels (Geng et al. 2004; Lauver et al. 2006; Tahiliani et al. 2007), apoptosis (Yano et al. 2007; Zhang et al. 2007), and a variety of signaling pathways (Meuer et al. 2007; Sanada and Tsai 2005; G.X. Shi et al. 2006; Yamada et al. 2005). Furthermore, RNAi is now being used for the knockdown of gene expression in animals. It appears to apply in virtually all mammalian species, as exemplified by its capability for silencing genes in mice, rats, and goats (Peng et al. 2006; Zhou et al. 2007). Inducible RNAi based on the Cre-loxP system has also been developed in transgenic mice, enabling the investigator to control gene silencing spatially and temporally (Chang et al. 2004; Coumoul et al. 2005; Xia et al. 2006). Thus, it is possible to rapidly establish human genetic diseases as a whole-animal model without the difficulty and expense of embryonic stem cell and gene targeting.

RNAi can knock down specific genes, making it evident that RNAi may be used to disrupt the expression of disease-associated genes for therapeutic purposes. Recent findings have highlighted the possibility of RNAi as a potential therapeutic approach to many human diseases, although a number of challenges need to be addressed, such as the safety concerns and effective delivery of RNAi therapy. RNAi-based therapies for age-related macular degeneration (AMD) and respiratory syncytial virus (RSV) have already reached clinical trials. Moreover, therapies based on RNAi are also in preclinical development for other viral diseases (Rossi 2006), neurodegenerative disorders (Raoul et al. 2006; Xia et al. 2005), and cancers (Pai et al. 2006).

RNAi has become a frequently used tool in a wide range of biomedical research. It has provided a convenient method to study gene function via application of RNAi to cell lines, cultures, and embryonic stem cells. It is anticipated that new uses for this tool will continue to proliferate.

Antisense Oligonucleotides

Antisense oligonucleotides (AOs) are short sequences of nucleotide with about 20 bases that are complementary to some regions of the specific mRNA sequence of interest. When cells take up the short DNA molecules, synthesis of the protein from the specific mRNA is inhibited. The mechanism by which AO blocks the specific protein production remains unclear. Interfering with the selected mRNA stability or its translation may be one potential mechanism (Phillips et al. 1996). Because of specificity, effectiveness, and reversibility, cell-based antisense experiments have proven useful in studying gene and protein function.

Proteomic Techniques for Altering Cellular Function

Not all manipulations of gene products are made at the gene level. It is possible to modify cell function by interfering directly with gene products (i.e., the proteomic strategy). One mechanism for such manipulation involves adding peptides that correspond to the active regions of proteins. These peptides bind to the molecular targets of those proteins within the cell and block the downstream effects. Sometimes these peptides can mimic the effect of the larger peptide. For example, a peptide corresponding to the carboxyl-terminal region of a G protein (which interacts with G protein–coupled receptors) was used to block the interaction between receptors and G proteins while "mimicking" the G protein to shift the receptor into a "high affinity" agonist-binding state (Rasenick et al. 1994). Although this strategy usually involves adding peptides to cells made permeable with a detergent or with electric current, it is also possible to incorporate DNA plasmids encoding peptides into cells (Gilchrist et al. 1999).

Another proteomic strategy for manipulating cellular processes involves expression of "dominant-negative" proteins that are generated in sufficient amount to block the activity of the native protein in the cell. Usually this strategy involves the construction of a mutant protein that is similar to the protein of interest but deficient at some active site. This inactive mutant protein, expressed in considerable excess over the native protein, competes with the native protein for target sites and inhibits its activity (Osawa and Johnson 1991).

Proteomics and Beyond

Shotgun proteomics takes its name from shotgun DNA sequencing, in which long DNA sequences are disassembled into shorter, easily readable components and reassembled. Shotgun proteomics works in much the same way as the proteome of a cell is digested, subjected to analysis on mass spectrometry, and "reassembled" into proteins identified through a sophisticated bioinformatic analysis of the protein "fingerprint." At first glance, such an approach might seem problematic, as a tripeptide would have the same mass regardless of the order of the amino acids; however, ionization of the peptide reveals the order of the amino acids. It is the computational algorithms that allow this identification. A recent review explains this in language that any biologist (or psychiatrist) can understand (Marcotte 2007).

Analysis of the proteome has the potential to yield much more information than simply the identity of the proteins being expressed in a given cell at a given time. Drugs that mimic, antagonize, or alter metabolism of neurotransmitters and neuromodulators comprise the vast majority of the current psychiatric armamentarium. These drugs, often used chronically, have been shown to have long-term effects, altering second-messenger systems. These second messengers (e.g., cAMP, inositol-1,4,5-triphosphate [IP_3], cyclic guanosine monophosphate [cGMP]) activate or inhibit enzymes that modify proteins covalently. Phosphorylation, prenylation, and glycosylation are examples of these modifications, all of which can be determined in mass spectroscopic proteomic analysis.

In addition to—and, in part, due to—the modifications discussed above, molecules involved in neurotransmitter response and responsiveness move among cellular compartments in response to neurotransmitters, neuromodulators, and drugs that affect these. A simple example might be the agonist-induced depalmitoylation of the α subunit of the stimulatory G protein ($G_s\alpha$) that results in its translocation from the plasma membrane (Wedegaertner and Bourne 1994; Yu and Rasenick 2002). We have demonstrated that this translocation is due to collection of G proteins in lipid rafts structures that either amplify or attenuate signaling (Allen et al. 2005, 2007). A catalog of these protein shifts during disease or response to drug can be easily assembled.

As noted above, G protein–coupled receptors comprise targets for a major component of drugs used in psychiatry. Curiously, many of these drugs were thought to have a single site of action until a screening/informatics approach was applied to them. Receptoromics allows screening of compounds for their agonist or antagonist effects on receptors measured through batteries of cells selectively expressing a single species of G protein–coupled receptor (or other receptor or transporter). Results from these studies have been both informative and surprising (Strachan et al. 2006). For example, atypical antipsychotics have been selected for their antagonist properties at the 5-HT_{2A} receptor. Some of these drugs, such as olanzapine, have been associated with excessive weight gain, and this appears to be due to interaction with H_1 receptors—not related to the therapeutic profile of the drug. Other effective antipsychotic drugs may owe their efficacy to actions at a panel of receptors that, when combined, contribute to a therapeutic whole. The ability to screen libraries of compounds against a large number of receptor targets makes design and identification of new drugs an exciting possibility.

Transgenic and Gene-Targeting Techniques

Over the past two decades, progress in the development of molecular genetic methods has enabled the manipulation of genes in intact organisms, such as mice. The technologies have provided a powerful and useful tool that allows the study of gene function and promotes understanding of the molecular mechanisms of disorders of the brain and mind. The mouse genome is by far the most accessible mammalian genome for manipulation. Many successful procedures for introducing new genes, expressing elevated levels of genes, and eliminating or altering the function of identified target genes have been reported. Many mouse models produced by manipulating genes may be used in a variety of fields relevant to neuroscience. It is noteworthy, however, that behavioral studies in mice lag far behind those in rats. For this reason, genetically induced behavioral alterations in mice must be interpreted with caution (Lucki et al. 2001).

Generally, transgenic mice are those expressing exogenous DNA because of the insertion of a gene into the mouse genome. Usually that gene is randomly located within the mouse genome, often as several copies. The use of transgenic mice has represented a major strategy for the investigation of genetic questions since the feasibility and reproducibility of stably introducing DNA by micro-injection into individual male mouse embryos were established (Markert 1983). In DNA constructs used for the generation of transgenic mice, the gene of interest is located 3′ to promoter sequences to produce a desired distribution of gene expression. The selection of the promoter is the most important consideration in generating transgenic mice. Some promoters, such as platelet-derived growth factor (PDGF), thy1 (a cell surface glyco-sylphosphatidylinositol-linked glycoprotein), prin (PrP), neuron-specific enolase (NSE), and glial fibrillary acidic protein (GFAP), have demonstrated the ability to direct high-level expression of exogenous genes in brain and/or in the neurons of mice (Hsiao et al. 1996; Kan et al. 2004; Nolte et al. 2001; Sturchler-Pierrat et al. 1997). This level of expression can be modified by incorporation of a "tet-on" or "tet-off" vector into the desired inserted gene. Depending on the nature of the switch (on or off), the mouse will express the gene of interest when ingesting (or taken off) doxycycline.

"Gene targeting" refers to the homologous recombination that occurs between a specifically designed targeting construct and the chromosomal target of interest, in which recombination at the target locus leads to replacement of the native target sequence with construct sequence. The method enables the precise introduction of a mutant into one of many murine genes and has proven invaluable in examining the roles of gene functions in complex biological processes. Most of the target constructs are used to disrupt a target and to eliminate gene function (conventional "knockout"). Generally, a gene-targeting construct that contains positive–negative selection markers is prepared such that the target gene is interrupted by the gene for neomycin resistance, which also serves as a positive selection marker, and a thymidine kinase (TK; Gusella et al. 1983) gene is adjacent to either one or both ends of the homologous genomic sequence for negative selection. The positive–negative deletion scheme is employed to enrich for homologous recombination.

The targeting construct is often introduced into mouse embryonic stem (ES) cells by electroporation. Cells that fail to integrate the targeting construct into the genome are killed by application of neomycin in the culture medium (positive selection). The majority of the remaining cells, in which the entire construct (including the TK gene) inserts randomly, will die as a result of the incorporation of ganciclovir or fialuridine (inactive thymidine analogs), which block DNA synthesis. Homologous recombinant clones that do not contain the TK gene are used to prepare chimeric mice. Cells from these clones are microinjected into the fluid-filled cavity of 3.5-day-old embryos at the blastocyst stage. The injected embryos are then surgically transferred into the uterus of pseudopregnant females. These animals will give birth to chimeric mice. Breeding can be used to generate mice that are heterozygous and homozygous for the mutation. Homozygous mutants may express the gene of interest in any cell of the body (Figure 2–7).

Use of Mutant Mice in Studies of Brain Disease

Transgenic mice produced by this method are generally gain-of-function mutants, because the transgene is designed either to express a novel gene product or to disrupt a normal gene product by expressing a "dominant-negative" alternative. It is also possible to put a DNA fragment in an opposite direction and hence to produce transgenic mice expressing antisense RNA, which will reduce gene function (Jouvenceau et al. 1999; Katsuki et al. 1988). Expression of mutant amyloid precursor protein (APP) or presenilin 1 (PS1) in mice has generated many animal models that may be related to Alzheimer's disease. These transgenic mice have facilitated studies of the pathogenesis, molecular mechanisms, and behavioral abnormalities of Alzheimer's disease (Bornemann and Staufenbiel 2000; Janus et al. 2001). Nevertheless, because the transgene integrates into the mouse genome randomly and often exists as several copies, the interpretation of studies with transgenic mice is difficult.

Experiments with knockout mice have provided novel insights into the functional roles of neuronal genes and, in some cases, animal models relevant to brain disorders. The targeted mutants in a gene of interest, however, can sometime lead to embryonic lethality in mice, thus obscuring the particular role of that gene in a target tissue or in the adult. Furthermore, in some instances, genes related to the gene that was eliminated undergo increased expression in the knockout mice. In this case, the related gene compensates for the gene of interest and yields a phenotype that resembles the "normal" animal. This has been seen for the knockouts of the axonal microtubule-associated protein tau (Takei et al. 2000). Here, we take Huntington's disease to exemplify the use of transgenic mice in the study of neurological and psychiatric disease.

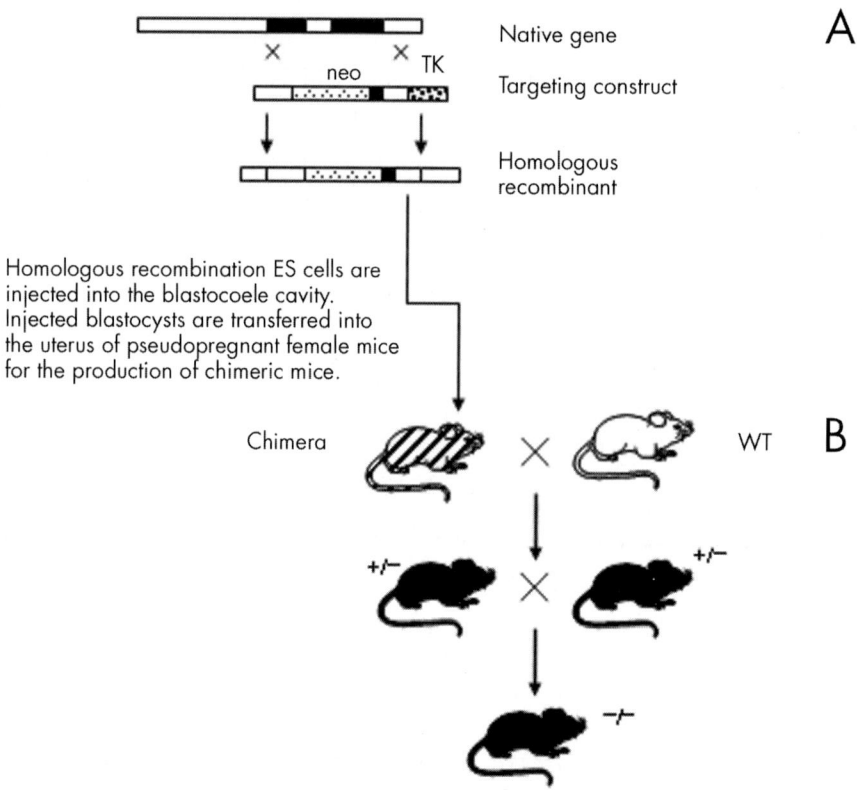

FIGURE 2–7.   Conventional gene disruption ("knockout").

(A) Producing chimeric mice. First, a mutant allele is produced by replacing the coding exons of the desired gene with a neomycin (neo) cassette and transferring it into embryonic stem (ES) cells. Second, genetically altered ES cells are reintroduced into a developing blastocyst, where they contribute to the developing embryo. **(B) Breeding chimeric mice.** When the germ cells of the resulting chimeric mouse (chimera) are ES cell–derived (germ-line mutation), the heterozygotes (+/–) can be produced by breeding. One-half of the offspring will be heterozygous. The heterozygous animals may be bred to produce homozygous mice (–/–). TK = thymidine kinase; WT = wild type.

Huntington's disease (HD) is a genetic neurological disorder that is inherited in an autosomal dominant manner. The gradual atrophy of the striatum is its pathological hallmark. It has a prevalence of 3–10 affected subjects per 100,000 individuals in Western Europe and North America (Gil and Rego 2008). The first symptoms generally appear in middle age, and the disease is progressive and invariably fatal 15–20 years after its onset (Ho et al. 2001). HD is caused by an expansion of cytosine-adenine-guanine (CAG) repeats in exon 1 of the *HD* gene. The *HD* gene is located on the short arm of chromosome 4 (4p63) and encodes the protein huntingtin, composed of more than 3,100 amino acids with a polyglutamine tail, which is widely expressed throughout the body in both neuronal and nonneuronal cells.

The function of huntingtin has been revealed with different research approaches, especially those with transgenic mice. Engineered knockout mice that disrupt exon 4 (Duyao et al. 1995), exon 5 (Nasir et al. 1995), or the promoter (Zeitlin et al. 1995) of mouse gene homology,

hdh, showed embryonic lethality. A subsequent study using mutant human huntingtin to compensate for the absence of endogenous huntingtin rescued the embryonic lethality of mice homozygous for a targeted disruption of the hdh gene (Leavitt et al. 2001). These suggest its essential role for normal embryonic development. Moreover, condition knockout mice indicated that huntingtin is also required throughout life, because adult mice are sterile, develop a progressive motor phenotype, and with short life span after inactivating hdh gene during adulthood (Dragatsis et al. 2000). Furthermore, overexpression of wild-type huntingtin, bearing 12 glutamine residues, in transgenic mice brought significant protection against apoptosis triggered by NMDA (Leavitt et al. 2006), suggesting that huntingtin may play a role in cellular apoptosis.

As mentioned above, HD is a neurodegenerative disorder caused by uninterrupted CGA trinucleotide repeats that located near the 5′-end in exon 1. Consequently, mutant huntingtin bears a string of consecutive glutamine residues in the NH2-terminal, 17 amino acids downstream of the initiator (Gil and Rego 2008). The length of glutamine residues in NH2-terminal of mutant huntingtin is the primary and predominant determinant for severity of HD. To elucidate the mechanism of neurodegeneration in HD, multiple mouse models of HD have been established. These models vary in terms of the site of transgene incorporation, promoter used, gene expression levels, CAG repeat length, and background mouse strain used. These transgenic models have facilitated investigations into potential pathogenic mechanisms of HD. At present, there are three categories of mouse model:

1. *Mice expressing exon-1 fragments of human huntingtin gene (HD) containing polyglutamine mutations (R6/1, R6/2, and R6/5).* This transgenic mouse carries exon 1 of the *HD* gene with 115–155 CAG repeats. The transgene protein contains the first 69 amino acids of huntingtin in addition to the number of residues encoded by the CAG repeats. Extensive neuropathological analysis has been performed on the brains is R6/2 mice. The mice display subtle motor and learning deficits at approximately 1 month and overt symptoms appear by 2 months, and they usually die at 3 or 4 months (Carter et al. 1999; Lione et al. 1999; Murphy et al. 2000). It is worthy to note that the characteristic nuclear inclusions were first detected with antibodies against the *N*-terminal portion of huntingtin in R6/2 mice. R6/2 mice show measurable deficits in motor behavior that increase progressively until death. R6/2 mice are a model of *HD* to aim at studying the severity of motor symptoms or the course of the disease. In R6/2 mice, many neurotransmitter receptors, such as NMDA, AMPA, mGluR2, DA, and GABA, display abnormal response to their ligands (Ali and Levine 2006; Cepeda et al. 2004; Cha et al. 1998; Dunah et al. 2002; Starling et al. 2005).

2. *Mice expressing the full-length human HD gene.* Yeast artificial chromosomes (YACs) were used to create a YAC transgenic mouse model of HD that expresses the full-length human HD gene. The transgenic mice express human transgenic huntingtin with 18, 46, 72, or 128 polyglutamine repeats. The YAC mice with 72 CGA repeats develop a progressive motor phenotype, neuronal dysfunction, and selective striatal neurodegeneration similar to that seen in HD by a 12-month timeline. YAC mice with 128 CAG repeats (YAC128 mice) exhibit initial hyperactivity, followed by the onset of motor deficits and finally hypokinesis, which show phenotypic uniformity with low interanimal variability present. The motor deficit in the YAC128 mice is highly correlated with striatal neuronal loss, providing a structural correlate for the behavioral changes (Hodgson et al. 1999; Slow et al. 2003). These lines of transgenic mice may be extremely useful for preclinical experimental therapeutics.

3. *Knock-in HD transgenic mice.* In knock-in mice, a mutated DNA sequence is exchanged for the endogenous sequence without any other disruption of the gene. To establish the line of knock-in HD mice, CGA repeats in the murine *hdh* gene were replaced with human mutant CAG repeats. These mice are characterized by a biphasic progression in behavioral anomalies, and the nuclear inclusions appear late and are preceded by nuclear staining for huntingtin, followed by the presence of microaggregates of the mutant protein in the nucleus and the neuropil (Menalled et al. 2002, 2003, 2005). These knock-in mice are considered to be an ideal genetic model of HD to evaluate the effectiveness of new therapies and to study the mechanisms involved in the neuropathology of HD.

The above examples illustrate both the potential and the current promise of manipulation of the mouse genome for the study of human neuropsychiatric disease.

Microarray Technology

Since the mid-1990s, a new and advanced microarray technology was developed that allows the study of gene expression. This technology is proving to be a powerful research tool for gaining insight into the study of gene expression and gene structure. The main large-scale application of the microarray is *comparative expression analysis*. However, studies of DNA variation are also possible with microarray techniques, as are pharmacogenetics applications.

For DNA microarrays, DNA sequences, DNA inserts of a library from PCR amplifications, cDNA clones, or synthetic oligonucleotides can be immobilized on an impermeable rigid support (e.g., glass) in matrix spots. These microarrays can be hybridized to labeled cDNA probes prepared from the mRNA extracted from the cell and tissue of interest. The hybridization of the probe to each array component is measured to provide a quantitative measure of the abundance of each array component in the probe. Currently, oligonucleotide-based DNA chips are generated by the in situ synthesis of short (20- to 30-nucleotide) DNA fragments by either photolithography on a chip (developed by Affymetrix, Santa Clara, CA) or ink-jet technology (developed by Rosetta Inpharmatics, Kirkland, WA). The latter offers more speed in producing an array and increases the number of elements that can be arrayed on a single chip. Hybridization to short oligonucleotides on a chip has a lower threshold of specificity than the older hybridization techniques, but it is a more comprehensive and extremely rapid screening mechanism. The application of DNA microarray technology has been used recently for characterizing gene expression profiles in human diseases, such as multiple sclerosis (Whitney et al. 1999), cancers (Perou et al. 1999), and various neurodegenerative diseases (Ginsberg et al. 2000).

In principle, any type of ligand-binding assay that relies on the product formation of an immobilized capture molecule and a "binder" present in the surrounding solution can be miniaturized, parallelized, and performed in a microarray format (Templin et al. 2002). Many microarray-based assays have emerged; these include studies of DNA–protein interaction in a microarray format (Bulyk et al. 1999), enzyme–substrate arrays (Zhu et al. 2000), and protein–protein binding assays (Zhu et al. 2001). Microarray-based technology is likely to accelerate basic research in the area of molecular interactions and has the potential to change the diagnostic methods used for a variety of human diseases.

Conclusion

Rapid advances in the identification of the human genome and in the methodology for genetic manipulation have combined to open a window into the brain. We are accumulating knowledge of human gene mutations and their connection to neurological and psychiatric diseases at a rapid pace. As genes are being identified, the proteins for which they code are also becoming known. With this knowledge, the pathogenic mechanism of some diseases is becoming apparent. Understanding these maladies at the molecular level is likely to lead to new methods of diagnosis and novel approaches to therapy.

References

Abe K, Sato S, Kawagoe J, et al: Isolation and expression of an ischaemia-induced gene from gerbil cerebral cortex by subtractive hybridization. Neurol Res 15:23–28, 1993

Allen JA, Yu JZ, Donati RJ, et al: Beta-adrenergic receptor stimulation promotes G alpha s internalization through lipid rafts: a study in living cells. Mol Pharmacol 67:1493–1504, 2005

Allen JA, Halverson-Tamboli RA, Rasenick MM: Lipid raft microdomains and neurotransmitter signalling. Nat Rev Neurosci 8:128–140, 2007

Ali NJ, Levine MS: Changes in expression of N-methyl-D-aspartate receptor subunits occur early in the R6/2 mouse model of Huntington's disease. Dev Neurosci 28:230–238, 2006

Amarzguioui M, Rossi JJ, Kim D: Approaches for chemically synthesized siRNA and vector-mediated RNAi. FEBS Lett 579:5974–5981, 2005

Ballestar E, Esteller M: The impact of chromatin in human cancer: linking DNA methylation to gene silencing. Carcinogenesis 23:1103–1109, 2002

Barkats M, Bemelmans AP, Geoffroy MC, et al: An adenovirus encoding CuZnSOD protects cultured striatal neurones against glutamate toxicity. Neuroreport 7:497–501, 1996

Bass BL: RNA editing and hypermutation by adenosine deamination. Trends Biochem Sci 22:157–162, 1997

Bass BL: RNA editing by adenosine deaminases that act on RNA. Annu Rev Biochem 71:817–846, 2002

Bemelmans AP, Horellou P, Pradier L, et al: Brain-derived neurotrophic factor-mediated protection of striatal neurons in an excitotoxic rat model of Huntington's disease, as demonstrated by adenoviral gene transfer. Hum Gene Ther 10:2987–2997, 1999

Benraiss A, Chmielnicki E, Lerner K, et al: Adenoviral brain-derived neurotrophic factor induces both neostriatal and olfactory neuronal recruitment from endogenous progenitor cells in the adult forebrain. J Neurosci 21:6718–6731, 2001

Berg KA, Cropper JD, Niswender CM, et al: RNA-editing of the 5-HT(2C) receptor alters agonist-receptor-effector coupling specificity. Br J Pharmacol 134:386–392, 2001

Berry M, Barrett L, Seymour L, et al: Gene therapy for central nervous system repair. Curr Opin Mol Ther 3:338–349, 2001

Bornemann KD, Staufenbiel M: Transgenic mouse models of Alzheimer's disease. Ann N Y Acad Sci 908:260–266, 2000

Brummelkamp TR, Bernards R, Agami R: A system for stable expression of short interfering RNAs in mammalian cells. Science 296:550–553, 2002

Bulyk ML, Gentalen E, Lockhart DJ, et al: Quantifying DNA-protein interactions by double-stranded DNA arrays. Nat Biotechnol 17:573–577, 1999

Burns CM, Chu H, Rueter SM, et al: Regulation of serotonin-2C receptor G-protein coupling by RNA editing. Nature 387:303–308, 1997

Carter RJ, Lione LA, Humby T, et al: Characterization of progressive motor deficits in mice transgenic for the human Huntington's disease mutation. J Neurosci 19:3248–3257, 1999

Cepeda C, Starling AJ, Wu N, et al: Increased GABAergic function in mouse models of Huntington's disease: reversal by BDNF. J Neurosci Res 78:855–867, 2004

Cha JH, Kosinski CM, Kerner JA, et al: Altered brain neurotransmitter receptors in transgenic mice expressing a portion of an abnormal human huntington disease gene. Proc Natl Acad Sci U S A 95:6480–6485, 1998

Chalfie M, Tu Y, Euskirchen G, et al: Green fluorescent protein as a marker for gene expression. Science 263:802–805, 1994

Chang HS, Lin CH, Chen YC, et al: Using siRNA technique to generate transgenic animals with spatiotemporal and conditional gene knockdown. Am J Pathol 165:1535–1541, 2004

Chen H, Lambert NA: Endogenous regulators of G protein signaling proteins regulate presynaptic inhibition at rat hippocampal synapses. Proc Natl Acad Sci U S A 97:12810–12815, 2000

Collins FS: Positional cloning moves from perditional to traditional. Nat Genet 9:347–350, 1995

Coumoul X, Shukla V, Li C, et al: Conditional knockdown of Fgfr2 in mice using Cre-LoxP induced RNA interference. Nucleic Acids Res 33:e102, 2005

DeCerbo J, Carmichael GG: SINEs point to abundant editing in the human genome. Genome Biol 6:216, 2005

Doyu M, Sawada K, Mitsuma N, et al: Gene expression profile in Alzheimer's brain screened by molecular indexing. Brain Res Mol Brain Res 87:1–11, 2001

Dragatsis I, Levine MS, Zeitlin S: Inactivation of Hdh in the brain and testis results in progressive neurodegeneration and sterility in mice. Nature genetics 26:300–306, 2000

Dunah AW, Jeong H, Griffin A, et al: Sp1 and TAFII130 transcriptional activity disrupted in early Huntington's disease. Science 296:2238–2243, 2002

Duyao MP, Auerbach AB, Ryan A, et al: Inactivation of the mouse Huntington's disease gene homolog Hdh. Science 269:407–410, 1995

Eberwine J, Yeh H, Miyashiro K, et al: Analysis of gene expression in single live neurons. Proc Natl Acad Sci U S A 89:3010–3014, 1992

Eriksson M, Taskinen M, Leppa S: Mitogen activated protein kinase-dependent activation of c-Jun and c-Fos is required for neuronal differentiation but not for growth and stress response in PC12 cells. J Cell Physiol 210:538–548, 2007

Fire A, Xu S, Montgomery MK, et al: Potent and specific genetic interference by double-stranded RNA in Caenorhabditis elegans. Nature 391:806–811, 1998

Geng C, Pellegrino A, Bowman J, et al: Complete RNAi rescue of neuronal degeneration in a constitutively active Drosophila TRP channel mutant. Biochim Biophys Acta 1674:91–97, 2004

Gil JM, Rego AC: Mechanisms of neurodegeneration in Huntington's disease. Eur J Neurosci 27:2803–2820, 2008

Gilchrist A, Bunemann M, Li A, et al: A dominant-negative strategy for studying roles of G proteins in vivo. J Biol Chem 274:6610–6616, 1999

Ginsberg SD, Hemby SE, Lee VM, et al: Expression profile of transcripts in Alzheimer's disease tangle-bearing CA1 neurons. Ann Neurol 48:77–87, 2000

Graves L, Dalvi A, Lucki I, et al: Behavioral analysis of CREB alpha-delta mutation on a B6/129 F1 hybrid background. Hippocampus 12:18–26, 2002

Grosjean H, Auxilien S, Constantinesco F, et al: Enzymatic conversion of adenosine to inosine and to N1-methylinosine in transfer RNAs: a review. Biochimie 78:488–501, 1996

Gusella JF, Wexler NS, Conneally PM, et al: A polymorphic DNA marker genetically linked to Huntington's disease. Nature 306:234–238, 1983

Halliday KR, Stein PJ, Chernoff N, et al: Limited trypsin proteolysis of photoreceptor GTP-binding protein: light- and GTP-induced conformational changes. J Biol Chem 259:516–525, 1984

Harding TC, Geddes BJ, Noel JD, et al: Tetracycline-regulated transgene expression in hippocampal neurones following transfection with adenoviral vectors. J Neurochem 69:2620–2623, 1997

He TC, Zhou S, da Costa LT, et al: A simplified system for generating recombinant adenoviruses. Proc Natl Acad Sci U S A 95:2509–2514, 1998

Hengst U, Cox LJ, Macosko EZ, et al: Functional and selective RNA interference in developing axons and growth cones. J Neurosci 26:5727–5732, 2006

Ho LW, Brown R, Maxwell M, et al: Wild type huntingtin reduces the cellular toxicity of mutant huntingtin in mammalian cell models of Huntington's disease. J Med Genet 38:450–452, 2001

Hodgson JG, Agopyan N, Gutekunst CA, et al: A YAC mouse model for Huntington's disease with full-length mutant huntingtin, cytoplasmic toxicity, and selective striatal neurodegeneration. Neuron 23:181–192, 1999

Hong J, Yoshida K, Rosner MR: Characterization of a cysteine proteinase inhibitor induced during neuronal cell differentiation. J Neurochem 81:922–934, 2002

Hsiao K, Chapman P, Nilsen S, et al: Correlative memory deficits, Abeta elevation, and amyloid plaques in transgenic mice. Science 274:99–102, 1996

Hughes SM, Moussavi-Harami F, Sauter SL, et al: Viral-mediated gene transfer to mouse primary neural progenitor cells. Mol Ther 5:16–24, 2002

Imaizumi K, Tsuda M, Imai Y, et al: Molecular cloning of a novel polypeptide, DP5, induced during programmed neuronal death. J Biol Chem 272:18842–18848, 1997

Janus C, Phinney AL, Chishti MA, et al: New developments in animal models of Alzheimer's disease. Curr Neurol Neurosci Rep 1:451–457, 2001

Jouvenceau A, Potier B, Battini R, et al: Glutamatergic synaptic responses and long-term potentiation are impaired in the CA1 hippocampal area of calbindin D(28k)-deficient mice. Synapse 33:172–180, 1999

Kable ML, Heidmann S, Stuart KD: RNA editing: getting U into RNA. Trends Biochem Sci 22:162–166, 1997

Kan L, Hu M, Gomes WA, Kessler JA: Transgenic mice overexpressing BMP4 develop a fibrodysplasia ossificans progressiva (FOP)-like phenotype. Am J Pathol 165:1107–1115, 2004

Katsuki M, Sato M, Kimura M, et al: Conversion of normal behavior to shiverer by myelin basic protein antisense cDNA in transgenic mice. Science 241:593–595, 1988

Kaziro Y, Itoh H, Kozasa T, et al: Structure and function of signal-transducing GTP-binding proteins. Annu Rev Biochem 60:349–400, 1991

Keshet I, Lieman-Hurwitz J, Cedar H: DNA methylation affects the formation of active chromatin. Cell 44:535–543, 1986

Kim DH, Rossi JJ: Strategies for silencing human disease using RNA interference. Nat Rev Genet 8:173–184, 2007

Kim DH, Behlke MA, Rose SD, et al: Synthetic dsRNA Dicer substrates enhance RNAi potency and efficacy. Nat Biotechnol 23:222–226, 2005

Kohara K, Kitamura A, Morishima M, et al: Activity-dependent transfer of brain-derived neurotrophic factor to postsynaptic neurons. Science 291:2419–2423, 2001

Kornberg RD, Lorch Y: Twenty-five years of the nucleosome, fundamental particle of the eukaryote chromosome. Cell 98:285–294, 1999

Koshimizu H, Araki T, Takai S, et al: Expression of CD47/integrin-associated protein induces death of cultured cerebral cortical neurons. J Neurochem 82:249–257, 2002

Kubista M: Nucleic acid-based technologies: application amplified. Pharmacogenomics 5:767–773, 2004

Kubista M, Andrade JM, Bengtsson M, et al: The real-time polymerase chain reaction. Mol Aspects Med 27:95–125, 2006

Lander ES, Linton LM, Birren B, et al: Initial sequencing and analysis of the human genome. Nature 409:860–921, 2001

Lauver A, Yuan LL, Jeromin A, et al: Manipulating Kv4.2 identifies a specific component of hippocampal pyramidal neuron A-current that depends upon Kv4.2 expression. J Neurochem 99:1207–1223, 2006

Leavitt BR, Guttman JA, Hodgson JG, et al: Wild-type huntingtin reduces the cellular toxicity of mutant huntingtin in vivo. Am J Hum Genet 68:313–324, 2001

Leavitt BR, van Raamsdonk JM, Shehadeh J, et al: Wild-type huntingtin protects neurons from excitotoxicity. J Neurochem 96:1121–1129, 2006

Liang P, Averboukh L, Keyomarsi K, et al: Differential display and cloning of messenger RNAs from human breast cancer versus mammary epithelial cells. Cancer Res 52:6966–6968, 1992

Lind K, Stahlberg A, Zoric N, et al: Combining sequence-specific probes and DNA binding dyes in real-time PCR for specific nucleic acid quantification and melting curve analysis. Biotechniques 40:315–319, 2006

Lione LA, Carter RJ, Hunt MJ, et al: Selective discrimination learning impairments in mice expressing the human Huntington's disease mutation. J Neurosci 19:10428–10437, 1999

Liu J, Lamb D, Chou MM, et al: Nerve growth factor-mediated neurite outgrowth via regulation of Rab5. Mol Biol Cell 18:1375–1384, 2007

Liu QR, Zhang PW, Zhen Q, et al: KEPI, a PKC-dependent protein phosphatase 1 inhibitor regulated by morphine. J Biol Chem 277:13312–13320, 2002

Lucki I, Dalvi A, Mayorga AJ: Sensitivity to the effects of pharmacologically selective antidepressants in different strains of mice. Psychopharmacology (Berl) 155:315–322, 2001

Maas S, Melcher T, Seeburg PH: Mammalian RNA-dependent deaminases and edited mRNAs. Curr Opin Cell Biol 9:343–349, 1997

Mangiarini L, Sathasivam K, Seller M, et al: Exon 1 of the HD gene with an expanded CAG repeat is sufficient to cause a progressive neurological phenotype in transgenic mice. Cell 87:493–506, 1996

Marcotte EM: How do shotgun proteomics algorithms identify proteins? Nat Biotechnol 25:755–757, 2007

Markert CL: Fertilization of mammalian eggs by sperm injection. J Exp Zool 228:195–201, 1983

Mello CV, Jarvis ED, Denisenko N, et al: Isolation of song-regulated genes in the brain of songbirds. Methods Mol Biol 85:205–217, 1997

Menalled LB: Knock-in mouse models of Huntington's disease. NeuroRx 2:465–470, 2005

Menalled LB, Sison JD, Wu Y, et al: Early motor dysfunction and striosomal distribution of huntingtin microaggregates in Huntington's disease knock-in mice. J Neurosci 22:8266–8276, 2002

Menalled LB, Sison JD, Dragatsis I, et al: Time course of early motor and neuropathological anomalies in a knock-in mouse model of Huntington's disease with 140 CAG repeats. J Comp Neurol 465:11–26, 2003

Meuer K, Suppanz IE, Lingor P, et al: Cyclin-dependent kinase 5 is an upstream regulator of mitochondrial fission during neuronal apoptosis. Cell Death Differ 14:651–661, 2007

Mizushima K, Miyamoto Y, Tsukahara F, et al: A novel G-protein-coupled receptor gene expressed in striatum. Genomics 69:314–321, 2000

Murata T, Kurokawa R, Krones A, et al: Defect of histone acetyltransferase activity of the nuclear transcriptional coactivator CBP in Rubinstein-Taybi syndrome. Hum Mol Genet 10:1071–1076, 2001

Murphy KP, Carter RJ, Lione LA, et al: Abnormal synaptic plasticity and impaired spatial cognition in mice transgenic for exon 1 of the human Huntington's disease mutation. J Neurosci 20:5115–5123, 2000

Nasir J, Floresco SB, O'Kusky JR, et al: Targeted disruption of the Huntington's disease gene results in embryonic lethality and behavioral and morphological changes in heterozygotes. Cell 81:811–823, 1995

Neve RL: Adenovirus vectors enter the brain. Trends Neurosci 16:251–253, 1993

Nolte C, Matyash M, Pivneva T, et al: GFAP promoter-controlled EGFP-expressing transgenic mice: a tool to visualize astrocytes and astrogliosis in living brain tissue. Glia 33:72–86, 2001

Oike Y, Hata A, Mamiya T, et al: Truncated CBP protein leads to classical Rubinstein-Taybi syndrome phenotypes in mice: implications for a dominant-negative mechanism. Hum Mol Genet 8:387–396, 1999

Osawa S, Johnson GL: A dominant negative G alpha s mutant is rescued by secondary mutation of the alpha chain amino terminus. J Biol Chem 266:4673–4676, 1991

Pai SI, Lin YY, Macaes B, et al: Prospects of RNA interference therapy for cancer. Gene Ther 13:464–477, 2006

Peng S, York JP, Zhang P: A transgenic approach for RNA interference-based genetic screening in mice. Proc Natl Acad Sci U S A 103:2252–2256, 2006

Perou CM, Jeffrey SS, van de Rijn M, et al: Distinctive gene expression patterns in human mammary epithelial cells and breast cancers. Proc Natl Acad Sci U S A 96:9212–9217, 1999

Petrij F, Giles RH, Dauwerse HG, et al: Rubinstein-Taybi syndrome caused by mutations in the transcriptional co-activator CBP. Nature 376:348–351, 1995

Phillips MI, Ambuhl P, Gyurko R: Antisense oligonucleotides for in vivo studies of angiotensin receptors. Adv Exp Med Biol 396:79–92, 1996

Provost P, Silverstein RA, Dishart D, et al: Dicer is required for chromosome segregation and gene silencing in fission yeast cells. Proc Natl Acad Sci U S A 99:16648–16653, 2002

Raoul C, Barker SD, Aebischer P: Viral-based modelling and correction of neurodegenerative diseases by RNA interference. Gene Ther 13:487–495, 2006

Rasenick MM, Watanabe M, Lazarevic MB, et al: Synthetic peptides as probes for G protein function. Carboxyl-terminal G alpha s peptides mimic Gs and evoke high affinity agonist binding to beta-adrenergic receptors. J Biol Chem 269:21519–21525, 1994

Roll-Mecak A, Cao C, Dever TE, et al: X-Ray structures of the universal translation initiation factor IF2/eIF5B: conformational changes on GDP and GTP binding. Cell 103:781–792, 2000

Rossi JJ: RNAi as a treatment for HIV-1 infection. Biotechniques Suppl:25–29, 2006

Sanada K, Tsai LH: G protein betagamma subunits and AGS3 control spindle orientation and asymmetric cell fate of cerebral cortical progenitors. Cell 122:119–131, 2005

Scadden AD, Smith CW: Specific cleavage of hyper-edited dsRNAs. Embo J 20:4243–4252, 2001

Schmitz C, Kinge P, Hutter H: Axon guidance genes identified in a large-scale RNAi screen using the RNAi-hypersensitive Caenorhabditis elegans strain nre-1(hd20) lin-15b(hd126). Proc Natl Acad Sci U S A 104:834–839, 2007

Seeburg PH, Hartner J: Regulation of ion channel/neurotransmitter receptor function by RNA editing. Curr Opin Neurobiol 13:279–283, 2003

Setou M, Nakagawa T, Seog DH, et al: Kinesin superfamily motor protein KIF17 and mLin-10 in NMDA receptor-containing vesicle transport. Science 288:1796–1802, 2000

Shaner NC, Campbell RE, Steinbach PA, et al: Improved monomeric red, orange and yellow fluorescent proteins derived from Discosoma sp. red fluorescent protein. Nat Biotechnol 22:1567–1572, 2004

Shaner NC, Steinbach PA, Tsien RY: A guide to choosing fluorescent proteins. Nat Methods 2:905–909, 2005

Shi GX, Rehmann H, Andres DA: A novel cyclic AMP-dependent Epac-Rit signaling pathway contributes to PACAP38-mediated neuronal differentiation. Mol Cell Biol 26:9136–9147, 2006

Shi Y: Mammalian RNAi for the masses. Trends Genet 19:9–12, 2003

Sijen T, Fleenor J, Simmer F, et al: On the role of RNA amplification in dsRNA-triggered gene silencing. Cell 107:465–476, 2001

Simpson L, Emeson RB: RNA editing. Annu Rev Neurosci 19:27–52, 1996

Siolas D, Lerner C, Burchard J, et al: Synthetic shRNAs as potent RNAi triggers. Nat Biotechnol 23:227–231, 2005

Slack RS, Belliveau DJ, Rosenberg M, et al: Adenovirus-mediated gene transfer of the tumor suppressor, p53, induces apoptosis in postmitotic neurons. J Cell Biol 135:1085–1096, 1996

Slow EJ, van Raamsdonk J, Rogers D, et al: Selective striatal neuronal loss in a YAC128 mouse model of Huntington disease. Hum Mol Genet 12:1555–1567, 2003

Starling AJ, Andre VM, Cepeda C, et al: Alterations in N-methyl-D-aspartate receptor sensitivity and magnesium blockade occur early in development in the R6/2 mouse model of Huntington's disease. J Neurosci Res 82:377–386, 2005

Steward O, Wallace CS: mRNA distribution within dendrites: relationship to afferent innervation. J Neurobiol 26:447–449, 1995

Strachan RT, Ferrara G, Roth BL: Screening the receptorome: an efficient approach for drug discovery and target validation. Drug Discov Today 11:708–716, 2006

Strahl BD, Allis CD: The language of covalent histone modifications. Nature 403:41–45, 2000

Stuart K, Panigrahi AK: RNA editing: complexity and complications. Mol Microbiol 45:591–596, 2002

Sturchler-Pierrat C, Abramowski D, Duke M, et al: Two amyloid precursor protein transgenic mouse models with Alzheimer disease-like pathology. Proc Natl Acad Sci U S A 94:13287–13292, 1997

Tahiliani M, Mei P, Fang R, et al: The histone H3K4 demethylase SMCX links REST target genes to X-linked mental retardation. Nature 447:601–605, 2007

Takei Y, Teng J, Harada A, et al: Defects in axonal elongation and neuronal migration in mice with disrupted tau and map 1b genes. J Cell Biol 150:989–1000, 2000

Tanaka S, Kitagawa K, Ohtsuki T, et al: Synergistic induction of HSP40 and HSC70 in the mouse hippocampal neurons after cerebral ischemia and ischemic tolerance in gerbil hippocampus. J Neurosci Res 67:37–47, 2002

Templin MF, Stoll D, Schrenk M, et al: Protein microarray technology. Trends Biotechnol 20:160–166, 2002

Tochitani S, Liang F, Watakabe A, et al: The occ1 gene is preferentially expressed in the primary visual cortex in an activity-dependent manner: a pattern of gene expression related to the cytoarchitectonic area in adult macaque neocortex. Eur J Neurosci 13:297–307, 2001

Tomari Y, Zamore PD: Perspective: machines for RNAi. Genes Dev 19:517–529, 2005

Tsai K, Chen S, Ma Y, et al: sgk, a primary glucocorticoid-induced gene, facilitates memory consolidation of spatial learning in rats. Proc Natl Acad Sci U S A 99:3990–3995, 2002

Valasek MA, Repa JJ: The power of real-time PCR. Adv Physiol Educ 29:151–159, 2005

Venter JC, Adams MD, Yan C, et al: The sequence of the human genome. Science 291:1304–1351, 2001

Volpe TA, Kidner C, Hall IM, et al: Regulation of heterochromatic silencing and histone H3 lysine-9 methylation by RNAi. Science 297:1833–1837, 2002

Wang Q, O'Brien PJ, Chen CX, et al: Altered G protein-coupling functions of RNA editing isoform and splicing variant serotonin2C receptors. J Neurochem 74:1290–1300, 2000

Wang Q, Zhang Z, Blackwell K, et al: Vigilins bind to promiscuously A-to-I-edited RNAs and are involved in the formation of heterochromatin. Curr Biol 15:384–391, 2005

Wedegaertner PB, Bourne HR: Activation and depalmitoylation of Gs alpha. Cell 77:1063–1070, 1994

Whitney LW, Becker KG, Tresser NJ, et al: Analysis of gene expression in multiple sclerosis lesions using cDNA microarrays. Ann Neurol 46:425–428, 1999

Wieden HJ, Gromadski K, Rodnin D, et al: Mechanism of elongation factor (EF)-Ts-catalyzed nucleotide exchange in EF-Tu: contribution of contacts at the guanine base. J Biol Chem 277:6032–6036, 2002

Wittwer CT, Herrmann MG, Moss AA, et al: Continuous fluorescence monitoring of rapid cycle DNA amplification. Biotechniques 22:130–131, 134–138, 1997

Xia XG, Zhou H, Xu Z: Promises and challenges in developing RNAi as a research tool and therapy for neurodegenerative diseases. Neurodegener Dis 2:220–231, 2005

Xia X, Zhou H, Huang Y, et al: Allele-specific RNAi selectively silences mutant SOD1 and achieves significant therapeutic benefit in vivo. Neurobiol Dis 23:578–586, 2006

Yamada T, Sakisaka T, Hisata S, et al: RA-RhoGAP, Rap-activated Rho GTPase-activating protein implicated in neurite outgrowth through Rho. J Biol Chem 280:33026–33034, 2005

Yanaka N, Nogusa Y, Fujioka Y, et al: Involvement of membrane protein GDE2 in retinoic acid-induced neurite formation in Neuro2A cells. FEBS Lett 581:712–718, 2007

Yang W, Wang Q, Kanes SJ, et al: Altered RNA editing of serotonin 5-HT2C receptor induced by interferon: implications for depression associated with cytokine therapy. Brain Res Mol Brain Res 124:70–78, 2004

Yano M, Nakamuta S, Shiota M, et al: Gatekeeper role of 14-3-3tau protein in HIV-1 gp120-mediated apoptosis of human endothelial cells by inactivation of Bad. AIDS 21:911–920, 2007

Yu JZ, Rasenick MM: Real-time visualization of a fluorescent G(alpha)(s): dissociation of the activated G protein from plasma membrane. Mol Pharmacol 61:352–359, 2002

Yu JZ, DeRuiter SL, Turner DL: RNA interference by expression of short-interfering RNAs and hairpin RNAs in mammalian cells. Proc Natl Acad Sci U S A 99:6047–6052, 2002a

Yu JZ, Kuret J, Rasenick MM: Transient expression of fluorescent tau proteins promotes process formation in PC12 cells: contributions of the tau C-terminus to this process. J Neurosci Res 67:625–633, 2002b

Zeitlin S, Liu JP, Chapman DL, et al: Increased apoptosis and early embryonic lethality in mice nullizygous for the Huntington's disease gene homologue. Nat Genet 11:155–163, 1995

Zeng Y, Wagner EJ, Cullen BR: Both natural and designed micro RNAs can inhibit the expression of cognate mRNAs when expressed in human cells. Mol Cell 9:1327–1333, 2002

Zhang Z, Carmichael GG: The fate of dsRNA in the nucleus: a p54(nrb)-containing complex mediates the nuclear retention of promiscuously A-to-I edited RNAs. Cell 106:465–475, 2001

Zhang Z, Yang X, Zhang S, et al: BNIP3 upregulation and EndoG translocation in delayed neuronal death in stroke and in hypoxia. Stroke 38:1606–1613, 2007

Zhou H, Falkenburger BH, Schulz JB, et al: Silencing of the Pink1 gene expression by conditional RNAi does not induce dopaminergic neuron death in mice. Int J Biol Sci 3:242–250, 2007

Zhu H, Klemic JF, Chang S, et al: Analysis of yeast protein kinases using protein chips. Nat Genet 26:283–289, 2000

Zhu H, Bilgin M, Bangham R, et al: Global analysis of protein activities using proteome chips. Science 293:2101–2105, 2001

CHAPTER 3

Genetics and Genomics

Elisabeth B. Binder, M.D., Ph.D.

Joseph F. Cubells, M.D., Ph.D.

Genetics and genomics have become among the most important tools in modern psychiatric research. Spurred by the completion of the human genome sequence in February 2001, the number of psychiatric genetic studies has increased dramatically in the past two decades (Lander et al. 2001; Venter et al. 2001). The following chapter will attempt to cover the basic methodologies and concepts, and define key terms, currently used in psychiatric genetics and genomics. Our goal is to facilitate interpretation by working physicians and scientists in the field of psychopharmacology of the avalanche of genetic and genomic data that are accumulating in the human neuroscience literature. Throughout this chapter, terms in common use in the genetics and genomics literature will be italicized upon their first use and definition.

Epidemiological Basis for Genetic Contributions to Neurobehavioral Disorders

Insights From Adoption and Twin Studies

Genetic epidemiological studies have established that most psychiatric disorders, as well as many nonpathological human behavioral traits, have a substantial genetic component. Investigations in genetic epidemiology therefore provide the scientific foundation for molecular genetic and genomic studies of human behavior and behavioral disorders (Kendler 1993, 2001; Plomin and Kosslyn 2001). Genetic epidemiology uses family, twin, and adoption studies to assess the contribution of familial, environmental, and genetic factors to a trait of interest. Family studies can establish that a given disorder "runs in families" but cannot easily distinguish whether such familiality is due to genetic or environmental factors. An everyday example of the distinction between *genetic* and *familial* (but environmental) traits is the difference between the ability to acquire language (a *genetic* trait that distinguishes humans from other species) and the native language spoken by a given person, which is *familial*, but entirely environmentally determined.

Adoption and twin studies distinguish between genetic and environmental influences on traits by accounting for each separately. Adoption studies investigate whether an individual's risk for a psychiatric disease depends on the mental health status of the biological or adoptive parents to disentangle genetic (i.e., similarity to biological parents, who have had little or no interaction with the adoptee) from environmental (i.e., similarity to adoptive parents, who have provided the adoptee with his or her family/social environment) influence (Cadoret 1986; Tienari and Wynne 1994; Tienari et al. 2004). Practical, ethical, and legal obstacles make large-scale adoption studies very difficult to conduct. Twin studies, while also quite challenging, are more tractable, and large twin registries are now available across the world (Busjahn 2002). These studies have provided the bulk of strong evidence supporting genetic contributions to psychiatric disorders and human behavioral traits.

In twin studies one determines what the probability of one twin being affected with a given trait or disorder,

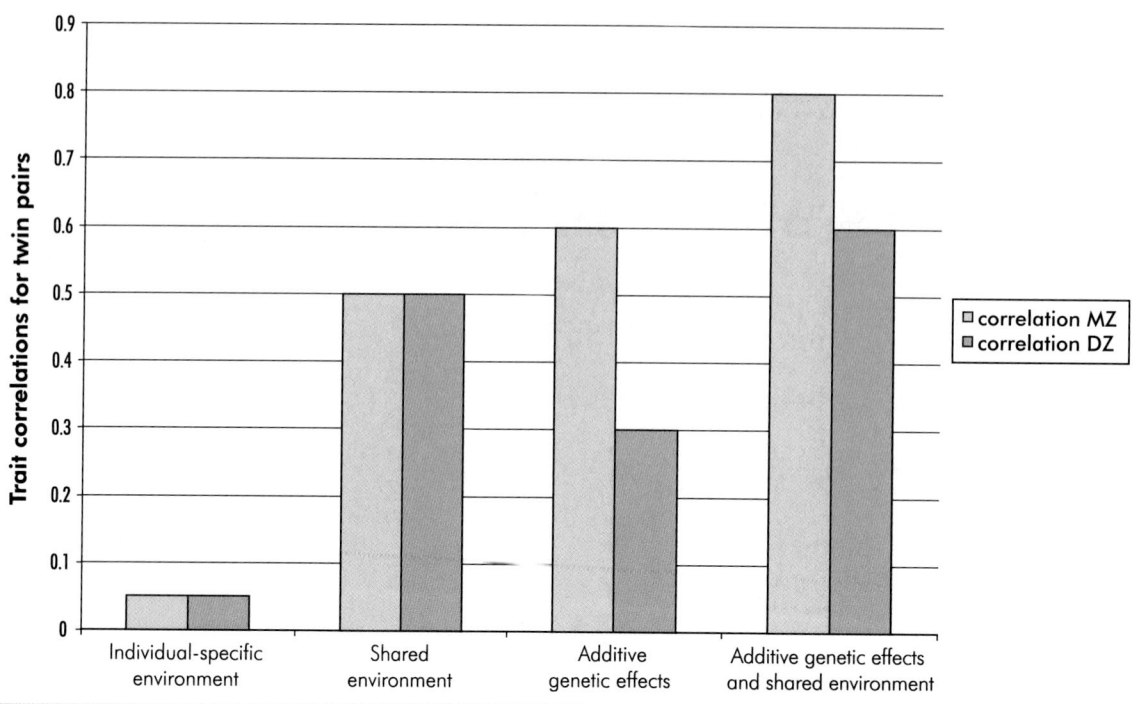

FIGURE 3–1.   Patterns of intrapair correlations and source of variance implied.

Intrapair correlations around zero imply effects of individual-specific environment. Equal intrapair correlations greater than zero that are equal for monozygotic (MZ) and dizygotic (DZ) twins imply effects of shared environment. Correlations for MZ twins that are twice as great as those for DZ twins imply additive genetic effects. Correlations for MZ twins that are greater than—but not twice as great as—those for DZ twins imply additive genetic effects and shared environment effects. The correlations of less than 1.0 in the last three examples are likely mediated by individual-specific environment effects.

given the affectation status of the co-twin. This degree of correlation between twins for the investigated trait is then compared between monozygotic (MZ) and dizygotic (DZ) twins to gain information on the degree of genetic and environmental influence on a certain trait. MZ twins result from a separation of the zygote to yield two genetically identical embryos. DZ twins result from the separate fertilization of two eggs in the same pregnancy. DZ twins thus only share on average 50% of their genes, similar to siblings born in separate pregnancies. While neither the pre- or postnatal environments of twins are perfectly identical, to a first approximation MZ and DZ twins are equally correlated for relevant environmental exposures (Kendler and Gardner 1998). The trait correlation between MZ and DZ twins therefore allows estimation of the degree to which additive genetic, shared, or individual-specific environment contributes to the likelihood of a given trait. Figure 3–1 summarizes relative contributions of each factor, estimated from patterns of correlation between MZ and DZ twins (for a methodological review of this topic, see Bulik et al. 2000).

Twin studies have firmly established important genetic contributions for all psychiatric disorders, with *her-*

itability estimates (i.e., the proportion of risk for a disorder attributable to the additive effects of genes) ranging from 30% from 80% for most common psychiatric disorders (see Table 3–1). Interestingly, the importance of shared environment seems to be of significant relevance mostly in schizophrenia, whereas in most other disorders, including anxiety and mood disorders, individual-specific but not shared environment is the major environmental contributor to susceptibility.

Genetic epidemiology can also contribute to the exploration of more complex questions, such as whether genetic risk factors are shared among different psychiatric disorders and gender and whether they can moderate the effects of environmental risk factors (Kendler 2001) and can thus lead the design of follow-up molecular genetic studies. For example, a twin study has suggested that genetic risk factors for major depression could in part act by increasing vulnerability to stressful life events (Kendler 1995). This finding has been corroborated in recent years by the now well-replicated interaction of functional alleles of the locus encoding the serotonin transporter protein with stressful life events to predict depression (Caspi et al. 2003; Kaufman et al. 2004; Kendler et al. 2005;

TABLE 3–1. Heritability scores for major psychiatric illnesses, with focus on results of recent meta-analyses

DISORDER	HERITABILITY	N IN META-ANALYSIS	REFERENCES
Autism	>0.8		Bailey et al. 1995; Rutter 2000
Schizophrenia	0.81 (0.73–0.9)	12 studies (Sweden, US, England, Norway, Denmark, Finland, Germany)	Sullivan et al. 2003 (meta-analysis)
Bipolar disorder	0.79–0.85		Kendler et al. 1995b; McGuffin et al. 2003
Major depression	0.37 (0.31–0.42)	5 studies (UK, Sweden, US), N>21,000	Sullivan et al. 2000 (meta-analysis)
Panic disorder	0.43 (0.32–0.53)	3 studies, N>9,000	Hettema et al. 2001 (meta-analysis)
Generalized anxiety disorder	0.32 (0.24–0.39)	2 studies, N>12,000	Hettema et al. 2001 (meta-analysis)
Specific phobias	0.25–0.35		Kendler et al. 1992, 2001b
Social phobias	0.20–0.30		Kendler et al. 1992, 2001b
Agoraphobia	0.37–0.39		Kendler et al. 1992, 2001b
Obsessive-compulsive disorder	0.45–0.65 (children) 0.27–0.47 (adults)		van Grootheest et al. 2005 (review)
Anorexia nervosa	0.56 (0.00–0.86)	Swedish twin registry, N>30,000	Bulik et al. 2006
Bulimia nervosa	0.28–0.83		Bulik et al. 2000 (review)
Alcohol dependence	0.48–0.73 (men) 0.51–0.65 (women)		Tyndale 2003 (review)
Nicotine addiction	0.4–0.7		Li 2003; Tyndale 2003 (reviews)
Antisocial personality disorder	0.32	51 studies	Rhee and Waldman 2002 (meta-analysis)

Sjoberg et al. 2006; Surtees et al. 2006; Wilhelm et al. 2006). Genetic epidemiological and more specifically twin studies have therefore been an important foundation of psychiatric genetics and are likely to continue to contribute more elaborate disease models for future molecular genetic analysis. The major limitation of these studies, however, is that the estimated heritability using twin studies is only an estimate of the aggregate genetic effect. Heritability does not give information on the contributions of specific genes to risk for a disorder. These questions, the answers to which ultimately will shed light on the underlying developmental neurobiology underlying psychiatric illness, require molecular genetic methods.

Psychiatric Disorders Are Complex Genetic Disorders

Genetic epidemiological studies have also established that psychiatric disorders are likely not single-gene disorders inherited in a *Mendelian* fashion (i.e., in a clear recessive, dominant, or X-linked fashion), although rare fami-

lies in which psychiatric phenotypes are inherited this way have been reported (Brunner et al. 1993). A genetic disorder can be complex for several reasons:

- *Incomplete penetrance*. Not everybody carrying the disease allele(s) becomes ill.
- *Phenocopy*. Individuals, even within the same families, can exhibit similar or identical traits because of environmental factors.
- *Locus heterogeneity*. Variants in different genes can lead to similar or identical disease phenotypes.
- *Allelic heterogeneity*. Different patterns of variation within the same gene or genes can lead to similar or identical disease phenotypes.
- *Polygenic inheritance*. Additive or interactive effects of variation at multiple genes (i.e., *epistatic effects*) are necessary for an illness to manifest.
- *Gene–environment interaction*. A disorder manifests in response to environmental factors only in the context of predisposing genetic variants. An extreme example of such interaction is phenylketonuria, where exposure

to dietary phenylalanine causes severe neurobehavioral impairment in individuals carrying two mutant copies of the locus encoding phenylalanine hydroxylase; limitation of dietary phenylalanine prevents the neurobehavioral disorder.

- *High frequency of the disorder and the predisposing alleles.* It appears increasingly likely that common disorders such as schizophrenia, diabetes mellitus, stroke, or hypertension represent final common outcomes to a variety of combinations of environmental and genetic predisposing factors. Thus, two individuals, even within the same family, might manifest clinically indistinguishable disorders for different reasons.
- *Other genetic mechanisms of inheritance.* Alternative genetic mechanisms—for example, mitochondrial inheritance or alteration of the genome across generations, such as occurs in trinucleotide-repeat-expansion disorders (e.g., Huntington's disease, fragile X syndrome) or in epigenetic disorders—may be operable in producing a disorder. *Epigenetic disorders* result from alterations in the genetic material that do not involve changes in the base pair sequence of DNA. Examples of epigenetic disease include the imprinted disorders Angelman syndrome and Prader-Willi syndrome, in which parent-of-origin–dependent chemical modification of DNA produces different phenotypic outcomes from the same chromosomal deletion. Newton and Duman recently reviewed possible roles of epigenetic mechanisms in the action of psychotropic drugs (Newton and Duman 2006) and in neuronal plasticity (Duman and Newton 2007).

From the cumulative evidence of psychiatric genetic studies so far, one can conclude that psychiatric disorders best fit a polygenic mode of inheritance, with two or more polymorphic loci contributing to these disorders, including unipolar depression (Johansson et al. 2001; Kendler et al. 2006), bipolar disorder (Blackwood and Muir 2001), schizophrenia (Sobell et al. 2002), and autism (Folstein and Rosen-Sheidley 2001). However, it is still relatively unclear how many loci contribute to each disorder. The inheritance of schizophrenia, for example, fits models including only a few loci as well as very large numbers of loci (Risch 1990a, 1990b; Sullivan et al. 2003). Data from gene-mapping studies suggest that different loci are indeed likely to contribute to schizophrenia and bipolar disorder in different individuals or families (meta-analyses [Levinson et al. 2003; Lewis et al. 2003; Segurado et al. 2003]), strongly supporting the hypothesis that locus heterogeneity is an important factor in schizophrenia. Thus,

Bleuler (1951) appears to have been correct when he referred to dementia praecox as "the group of schizophrenias."

As already noted, susceptibility genes are likely to interact with environment, gender, and other genes, making the search for genes for psychiatric disorders even more complex (Kendler and Greenspan 2006). Twin studies have produced evidence of genetic interactions with stressful life events predicting major depression (Kendler et al. 1995a) and with early rearing environment to predict schizophrenia, conduct disorder, and drug abuse (Cadoret et al. 1995a, 1995b; Tienari et al. 2004). These gene–environment interactions have now been substantiated by several molecular genetic studies (e.g., Binder et al. 2008; Bradley et al. 2008; Caspi et al. 2002, 2003, 2005), suggesting that future genetic and genomic studies will need to include analysis of both sets of factors. Furthermore, it is likely that there are gender-specific predisposing genes for psychiatric disorders. Data from twin studies suggest that the combined genetic factors predisposing to major depression, phobias, and alcoholism may differ in some respects for men and women (Kendler and Prescott 1999; Kendler and Walsh 1995; Kendler et al. 2001a, 2002, 2006; Prescott and Kendler 2000; Prescott et al. 2000), and this has been supported in molecular genetic studies by the identification of gender-specific loci for major depression (e.g., Abkevich et al. 2003; Zubenko et al. 2002). Finally, gene–gene interactions may be relevant for these disorders (Risch 1990b).

Response to Drug Treatment

In contrast to disease susceptibility, genetic epidemiological studies on responses to psychotropic drugs are rare. There is some evidence from family studies that suggests an important contribution of genetic factors in antidepressant response. Already in the early 1960s, studies on the effects of tricyclic antidepressants (TCAs) in relatives suggested that response to these drugs was similar among family members (Angst 1961; Pare et al. 1962). O'Reilly et al. (1994) reported a familial aggregation of response to tranylcypromine, a monoamine oxidase inhibitor, in a large family with major depression. These initial reports were followed by only a few systematic studies. Franchini et al. (1998) indicated a possible genetic basis of response to the selective serotonin reuptake inhibitor (SSRI) fluvoxamine in 45 pairs of relatives. In light of these data, some groups have used or proposed to use response to certain antidepressant drugs or mood stabilizers as an additional phenotype in classical linkage analyses for mood disorders in the hope of identifying genetically more homogeneous families (Serretti et al. 1998; Turecki et al. 2001).

Nonetheless, family studies supporting a genetic basis of response to psychotropic drugs are sparse, certainly reflecting the extreme difficulties inherent in conducting well-controlled family studies of therapeutic responses to medications. It has been proposed that genetic modifiers for response to treatment to psychotropic drugs may be easier to detect than associations with disease susceptibility, as the genetic contribution to these traits may be less complex (Weinshilboum 2003). So far, the data are insufficient to support or refute that contention.

Human Genetic Variation

As mentioned above, genetic epidemiological studies can only indicate the presence of an aggregate genetic effect but not which type and how many variations contribute to the effect. This next section will give an overview of the types of variation that occur in the human genome and will provide examples for implications of each of them for psychiatric disorders (see also Figure 3–2).

Variation on a Chromosomal Scale

Variation in Chromosomal Number

The human genome has approximately 3 billion bases that are distributed over 23 chromosome pairs, with 22 pairs of autosomes and 1 pair of sex chromosomes, X and Y. The most obvious genetic variations can be observed at the light microscope level in the karyotype. This approach visualizes metaphase chromosomes using histological procedures, allowing identification of each specific pair of chromosomes and variations in the total number of chromosomes, such as unisomies and trisomies. Several of the known variations of total chromosome number have an associated psychiatric phenotype. For example, Down syndrome is a complex neurodevelopmental disorder that results in variable levels of mental retardation, and in old age, dementia strikingly similar to Alzheimer's disease (Visootsak and Sherman 2007). Down syndrome results from *trisomy 21* (i.e., inheritance of three copies of chromosome 21, due to meiotic nondysjunction during oogenesis). Turner syndrome, in which there is only a single X chromosome (i.e., an XO karyotype), is associated with nonverbal learning disabilities, particularly in arithmetic, select visuospatial skills, and processing speed (Sybert and McCauley 2004).

Translocations

Karyotypic examination and other cytogenetic techniques such as fluorescent in situ hybridization (FISH) can reveal additional large-scale chromosomal abnormalities, such as translocations, deletions, or duplications of large regions of chromosomes. In a large Scottish pedigree, a balanced translocation between chromosomes 1 and 11 appears causally linked to a series of major psychiatric disorders, including schizophrenia, bipolar disorder, recurrent major depression, and conduct disorder (St. Clair et al. 1990). This *balanced translocation* (which exchanged parts of chromosome 1 with parts of chromosome 11 to produce two abnormal chromosomes, but no net loss of chromosomal material) disrupts two genes at the translocation breakpoint on chromosome 1, termed "disrupted in schizophrenia" (DISC) 1 and 2 (Millar et al. 2000, 2001). Subsequent molecular analysis has provided strong evidence that variation in *DISC1* can alter the risk for schizophrenia; the locus is presently considered by most a "confirmed" schizophrenia locus (Porteous et al. 2006).

Deletions

Microdeletions occurring on the long arm of chromosome 22 have received considerable attention as cytogenetic risk factors for the development of schizophrenia (Karayiorgou and Gogos 2004). The 22q11 deletion syndrome (DS), in which 1.5–3 million base pairs of DNA are missing on one copy of 22q, includes a spectrum of disorders affecting structures associated with development of the fourth branchial arch and migration of neural crest cells (e.g., the great vessels of the heart, the oropharynx, facial midline, and thymus and parathyroid glands). Originally described as distinct disease syndromes prior to the elucidation of their common molecular etiology, 22q11DS includes velocardiofacial syndrome (VCFS), DiGeorge syndrome, and conotruncal anomaly face syndrome. Following an initial report of early-onset psychosis in patients with VCFS (Shprintzen et al. 1992), Pulver and colleagues examined psychiatric symptoms in adults with VCFS (Pulver et al. 1994) and in a cohort of patients ascertained for schizophrenia (Karayiorgou et al. 1995). The latter study identified two previously undiagnosed cases in 200 patients, verified by fluorescent in situ hybridization to carry 22q11 deletions. These findings, together with earlier reports of suggestive linkage of 22q11–22q12 (Gill et al. 1996; Pulver et al. 2000), strongly suggested that a gene or genes in the 22q11DS region could contribute to risk for schizophrenia.

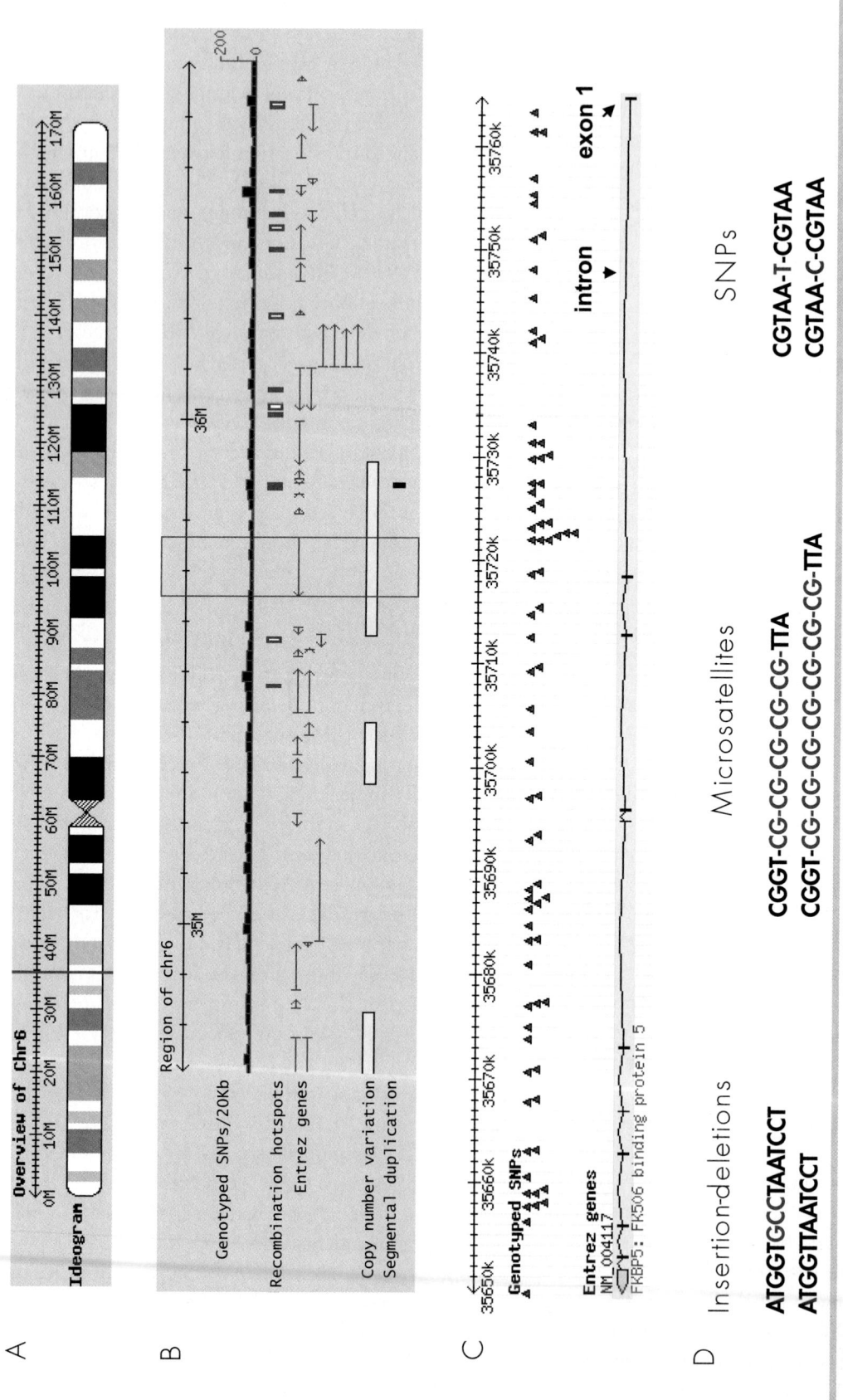

FIGURE 3–2.   Chromosomes, genes, and genetic variation.

Panel A shows a representation of chromosome 6 (Chr6), which spans 170 megabases of DNA. **Panel B** shows a zoomed-in representation of the area highlighted in red in panel A. This region contains 31 genes within 2 megabases. In the region shown, three copy number variants (CNVs) have been identified. All three span several genes. The *arrows* indicate the direction of transcription and translation of the respective genes. In the region shown, three copy number variants (CNVs) have been identified. All three span several genes. **Panel C** shows a zoomed-in representation of the gene for FK506 binding protein 5 (*FKBP5*) highlighted with a red frame in panel B. The gene spans 115 kilobases and is composed of 11 exons (translated into protein). The intervening introns are transcribed into RNA but are spliced out to form the mature mRNA that serves as the template for translation. The transcription start is at exon 1. In this gene, more than 60 SNPs have been genotyped within the HapMap Project. Their positions are indicated by the *triangles*. **Panel D** shows sequence examples for three common polymorphisms.

Source.   Representations from www.hapmap.org.

Duplications

Duplications of the long arm of chromosome 15 (15q11–13) are the most frequent cytogenetic anomalies in autism spectrum disorders, occurring in approximately 1%–2% of cases (Cook 2001). This duplication syndrome cannot be clinically differentiated from idiopathic autism spectrum disorders (Veenstra-VanderWeele and Cook 2004), indicating that a complete workup of autism should include testing for this cytogenetic abnormality, as well as for several others (Martin and Ledbetter 2007). Interestingly, deletion of this same region of 15q is associated with Angelman syndrome when the deletion occurs on the maternal copy of chromosome 15, and with Prader-Willi syndrome when the deletion occurs on the paternal chromosome (or more rarely, when two maternal copies of chromosome 15 are present, and the paternal chromosome is missing entirely, a condition known as *maternal disomy*). Both syndromes manifest as quite distinct but dramatic neurobehavioral disorders (Nicholls and Knepper 2001; Vogels and Fryns 2002).

Molecular Variation in the Genome

The majority of genetic and genomic studies in neuropsychiatry conducted to date have examined variation at the molecular level, which would be undetectable with methods appropriate for the kinds of variation described above. To introduce this section, we provide basic definitions of terms.

Definition of Alleles, Genotypes, Haplotypes

The definition of alleles, genotypes, and haplotypes is common to all the types of polymorphisms discussed below. An *allele* is a variation in DNA sequence that occurs at a particular *polymorphic* site on one chromosome. Every individual with a normal set of chromosomes has two alleles for each polymorphism on the *autosomes* (nonsex chromosomes, numbers 1–22). On the sex chromosomes, men have only one allele each for all polymorphisms located on the X and Y chromosomes, whereas women carry two copies of each X-linked allele. A *genotype* is the combined description for the variation at a particular corresponding point on homologous chromosomes and is expressed as two alleles. When the alleles on both chromosomes are the same, it is a *homozygous* genotype. When the alleles differ, it is a *heterozygous* genotype. A *haplotype*, a term derived from abbreviation of "haploid genotype," is the sequence of alleles along an adjacent series of polymorphic sites on a single chromosome. When

genotypic data are available from three generations, haplotypes in the third generation can be unambiguously deduced. In the absence of sufficient family-based data (e.g., in case–control studies of unrelated individuals), some haplotypes are ambiguous because the combination of genotypes at the polymorphic sites under study can be explained by more than one set of possible chromosomal arrangements of the component alleles. In such cases, methods such as estimation maximization (EM) can be used to infer the most likely haplotype (Hawley and Kidd 1995; Long et al. 1995).

Copy Number Variation

Genome-scale investigations enabled by the sequencing of the human genome and the advent of microarray-based comparative genomic hybridization have recently revealed a previously unappreciated form of polymorphic variation in the human genome: chromosomal regions containing one or more genes can sometimes be deleted or, alternatively, occur in multiple copies, with the number of copies differing among individuals (Nadeau and Lee 2006; Sebat et al. 2004). Such *copy number variants* (CNVs) occur normally in human populations, and a preliminary map of such variants is now available (Redon et al. 2006). They have recently been associated with marked differences in gene expression (Stranger et al. 2007). CNVs can also be associated with predisposition to disease, including neurobehavioral disorders such as autism and schizophrenia (International Schizophrenia Consortium 2008; Sebat et al. 2007; Stefansson et al. 2008). Research in this exciting new area is in its infancy but has already contributed importantly to the genetics of psychiatric disorders (Cook and Scherer 2008).

Copy number variation of the cytochrome P450 gene *CYP2D6*, which is important for the metabolism of many antidepressants, neuroleptics, and mood stabilizers (Kirchheiner et al. 2004), provides a prominent example of the importance of CNVs to pharmacogenetics. The presence in the genome of copy-number variation at this locus was inferred through biochemical–genetic studies predating the molecular era and was subsequently confirmed by molecular studies. The reported range of copy numbers of *CYP2D6* is from 0 to 13. The number of functional *CYP2D6* gene copies directly correlates with plasma levels of metabolized drugs, such as the TCA nortriptyline (Bertilsson et al. 2002). Patients with 0 or 1 functional copy of the gene attain therapeutic plasma levels of nortriptyline with very low doses and can easily reach potentially toxic concentrations with typical or high doses. Patients with 2–4 copies, on the other hand, would require high-normal doses to even reach therapeutic plasma levels (Kirchheiner et al. 2001). In the case of the one reported patient with 13 gene copies, even high-normal doses did not produce therapeutic plasma concentrations (Dalen et al. 1998).

Insertion/Deletion Polymorphisms

Microscopic insertions and deletions (much smaller than CNVs—on the order of one to hundreds of base pairs [bp]) are another important type of genetic variation. The most famous insertion/deletion polymorphism in psychiatric genetics is a common functional polymorphism in the promoter region of the serotonin transporter gene *SLC6A4*, referred to as the 5-HT transporter gene–linked polymorphic region (*5-HTTLPR*). It consists of a repetitive region containing 16 imperfect repeat units of 22 bp, located approximately 1,000 bp upstream of the transcriptional start site (Heils et al. 1996; Lesch et al. 1996). The *5-HTTLPR* is polymorphic because of the insertion/deletion of the repeat units 6–8 (of the 16 repeats), which produces a short (S) allele that is 44 bp shorter than the long (L) allele. Although the *5-HTTLPR* was originally described as biallelic, rare (<<5%) very-long and extra-long alleles have been described in Japanese and African Americans (Gelernter et al. 1999). Numerous additional variants within the repetitive region also occur (Nakamura et al. 2000). Thus, although most studies continue to treat this complex region as biallelic, this is an oversimplification that may be hiding additional genetic information. The *5-HTTLPR* has been associated with different basal activity of the transporter, most likely related to differential transcriptional activity (Heils et al. 1996; Lesch et al. 1996). The long variant (L allele) of this polymorphism has been shown to lead to a higher serotonin reuptake by the transporter in vitro. It is also noteworthy that the function of this insertion/deletion polymorphism may be influenced by a single nucleotide polymorphism (SNP) that occurs with the L allele (Hu et al. 2006). However a positron emission tomography study could not identify differences in serotonin transporter binding potential by *5-HTTLPR* genotype, even when including the information of the additional SNP, in healthy control subjects or patients with major depression (Parsey et al. 2006). This polymorphism has shown associations with a multitude of psychiatric disorders and related phenotypes. The best established are an association with response to treatment with SSRI (Serretti et al. 2007) and the moderation of the influence of life events on the development of depression (Caspi et al. 2003; Kaufman et al. 2004; Kendler et al. 2005; Surtees et al. 2006; Wilhelm et al. 2006; Zalsman et al. 2006).

Microsatellites: STRs and VNTRs

A very important class of polymorphisms, upon which molecular linkage studies and some association studies were based until very recently, is *microsatellite* markers, also called *short tandem repeats* (STRs) or *variable number of tandem repeats* (VNTRs). The polymorphisms consist of simple sequences, such as GT or GATA, that are repeated a variable number of times. An individual may thus have 5 GT repeats at a specific locus on one chromosome and 7 such repeats on the other. When these regions are amplified by *polymerase chain reaction* (PCR), a technique for producing many copies of a specific small portion of the genome based on DNA polymerase activity directed by specific DNA sequences, the difference in number of repeats results in differences in the length of the amplified fragments (a difference of 4 bp in the current example), allowing efficient genotyping of these polymorphisms by gel electrophoresis, which separates DNA fragments according to length. About 30,000 of these polymorphisms are now known in the human genome (Kawashima et al. 2006; Tamiya et al. 2005), and they have served as markers for genomewide linkage analysis (see "Linkage Studies" subsection below for more detail). VNTRs, however, not only serve as genetic markers for linkage analysis but also may produce functional variation within genes. An important example of such functional variation is a VNTR in the 3′ untranslated region (UTR) of the dopamine transporter gene (DAT). The repeat element consists of a 40-bp sequence that can occur with 3–11 repeats, with 9 and 10 repeats being the most common (Vandenbergh et al. 1992). Different effects of the 9 or 10 repeats on gene expression and DAT binding using single photon emission computed tomography (SPECT) in humans have been reported, although the direction of these differences is controversial (Greenwood and Kelsoe 2003; Inoue-Murayama et al. 2002; Martinez et al. 2001; Mill et al. 2002, 2005; van Dyck et al. 2005; VanNess et al. 2005), with the 9 or the 10 repeat alleles respectively associated with higher expression of the DAT gene and higher DAT binding in different studies. Another example of a functional VNTR (48-bp repeat) is a polymorphism in the third exon of the *DRD4* locus (the locus encoding the D_4 dopamine receptor), which results in a variable number of glutamine residues in the third intracellular loop of the dopamine D_4 receptor protein

(Van Tol et al. 1992). The allelomorphic proteins differ in their ligand-binding affinities, but all couple to G proteins (Van Tol et al. 1992). Both polymorphisms have been associated with a multitude of psychiatric and behavioral phenotypes (many of which require further investigation before their validity can be established with confidence).

Single Nucleotide Polymorphisms

The polymorphisms that have revolutionized (not only) psychiatric genetics are SNPs (Altshuler et al. 2000; Sachidanandam et al. 2001). SNPs consist of a single-base difference at a particular site in the genome—in two-thirds of cases, a cytosine (C)-to-thymidine (T) exchange. Although theoretically the presence of all four different bases at an SNP is possible, the vast majority of SNPs have only two alleles, although SNPs with three or four different alleles have occasionally been reported. As of June 2008, close to 10 million SNPs have been catalogued in public databases (such as dbSNP [http://www.ncbi.nlm.nih.gov/projects/SNP]). SNPs are so far the most common type of genetic variation and may represent up to 90% of all genetic variations (although this estimate may need revision as knowledge about CNVs accumulates). Besides being very common (SNPs occur, on average, every 300 bases), SNPs are also amenable to high-throughput genotyping methods (Kim and Misra 2007; Kwok 2000). Since SNPs are common (essentially every gene of interest has a number of known SNPs) and cheap to genotype, they have become the markers of choice for psychiatric genetic studies. SNPs are now replacing STRs in genomewide linkage studies, as more genetic information can be gleaned from 5,000–6,000 common SNPs across the genome than from the 300–400 markers typical of STR-based genome scans. SNPs are also the backbone of genetic association analysis.

Besides serving as genetic markers for chromosomal loci in association studies, SNPs can also have functional relevance themselves. SNPs in regulatory regions can alter the transcriptional regulation of a gene, SNPs in regions relevant for mRNA splicing can alter splice sites, and SNPs in protein-coding exons can encode differences in primary amino acid sequence. Interestingly, when one considers the occurrence of SNPs across the genome, one observes that SNPs are most dense in intergenic and intronic regions, while they are scarcer in putative regulatory regions and exons, suggesting selection against putatively functional variants (Altshuler et al. 2000; Sachidanandam et al. 2001). Within exons, SNPs that will not cause an amino acid exchange due to the degenerate code are called *synonymous* SNPs as opposed to *nonsynonymous* SNPs, which lead to amino acid substitution. One nonsynonymous SNP that has repeatedly been associated with psychiatric phenotypes is a valine-to-methionine exchange at amino acid position 108/158 in the soluble (S) or membrane-bound (MB) form of the catechol-O-methyltransferase (COMT) peptide sequence due to a G-to-A exchange at position 472 of exon 4. This amino acid exchange dramatically affects the temperature lability of this enzyme, with the methionine allelomorphic protein having only one-fourth of the enzyme activity at 37°C as the valine allelomorph (Lachman et al. 1996; Lotta et al. 1995). It is presumed that individuals with the Val/Val genotype have a more rapid inactivation of centrally released dopamine than individuals with the other genotypes, following an additive genetic model. This polymorphism seems to impact dopamine transmission, particularly in the frontal cortex, where expression of the dopamine transporter protein is relatively low, and has been associated with differences in executive cognition and functional activity of the prefrontal cortex during working memory tasks (Egan et al. 2001; Goldberg et al. 2003; Joober et al. 2002; Mattay et al. 2003). While it was hypothesized that this polymorphism could also alter the risk for schizophrenia (particularly since COMT resides in the 22q11 region, the deletion of which has been associated with schizophrenia), larger association studies and meta-analyses do not fully support that conclusion (Fan et al. 2005).

Identification of Disease Loci

These next paragraphs will describe specific examples of the different molecular genetic strategies to identify susceptibility genes for psychiatric disorders. We will also discuss potential problems that hinder the identification of such genes.

Cytogenetic Studies

Disruption of chromosomal integrity by rare events such as balanced translocations has facilitated gene discovery in a variety of diseases and has significant promise for similar applications in psychiatric illness (Pickard et al. 2005). Advances in techniques such as chromosome painting, FISH, and, most recently, genomewide analysis of CNVs using microarrays have made it possible to identify disruptions in chromosomal architecture to single-base resolution, thus facilitating identification of specific genes in families cosegregating mental illness and cytogenetic abnormalities. Such data may then be used to generate testable hypotheses about the role of a particular gene in disease pathophysiology. The *DISC1* and *DISC2* genes provide clear examples of specific genes implicated in mental illness following their discovery through careful molecular analysis of a cytogenetic anomaly. Since much more work has been published on *DISC1*, we focus on that locus here.

As noted previously, *DISC1* was initially identified by cytogenetic studies in which a large Scottish family with numerous relatives affected by major psychiatric illness was shown to carry a balanced (1;11) (q42;q14.3) translocation that cosegregates with the presence of psychiatric illness. Linkage analysis using psychiatric diagnosis as a phenotype and the translocation as a genetic marker yielded highly significant evidence supporting linkage of the translocation to psychiatric illness, and particularly to schizophrenia (Blackwood et al. 2001; St. Clair et al. 1990). The translocation was shown to disrupt *DISC1* and *DISC2* on chromosome 1 (Millar et al. 2000, 2001), whereas no known genes were disrupted on chromosome 11. *DISC1* was shown to encode a novel protein, with no known related proteins, that subsequently has been shown to play important roles in several key neuronal functions, including axonal transport and regulation of G protein–mediated intracellular signaling (Porteous et al. 2006).

Linkage Studies

In the 1980s and 1990s, many genes for Mendelian disorders were successfully identified using linkage analysis in large families. Linkage relies on the principle that on average, chromosomes from parents differ from those of offspring by only one meiotic crossover event. During *meiosis*, the cell divisions that produce gametes by reducing the diploid genome (i.e., two chromosomes of each pair per cell) to a haploid genome (one copy of each chromosome per spermatocyte or ooctye), homologous grandparental chromosomes (i.e., paternal and maternal to the parents of the offspring of interest) make physical contact and exchange homologous regions (referred to as *crossing over*) to give rise to a new set of chromosomes in which each gametic chromosome is a mix of grandparental sequences. This crossing-over process produces *recombination* that can then be tracked using molecular markers to delineate the ancestral origin of each chromosomal region in the offspring. Classically, linkage studies use anywhere from several hundred up to a few thousand micro-

satellite markers, evenly spaced across the genome. These markers are then genotyped in large families in which the disease of interest is common. To identify positions in the genome that may be involved in the disease, one tracks whether marker alleles are inherited by affected relatives more often than expected by chance (i.e., linkage tests whether a particular chromosomal region *cosegregates* with the disease). A quantitative measure of the likelihood of a particular pattern of marker–disease cosegregation is the *logarithm of odds (LOD) score*. As the name implies, the LOD score is logarithmic, with LOD = 1 corresponding to 1:10 odds, LOD = 2 to 1:100 odds, and so forth. Because of the high a priori probability that a given region is *not* linked to a given phenotype, a LOD score of 3.3 or greater is usually required before significant linkage is accepted (Lander and Schork 1994). The results of linkage analyses are usually presented as plots of LOD scores at each marker, which are arranged in their known order across individual chromosomes or the entire genome. These plots show a pattern of peaks and valleys. Linkage peaks identify chromosomal regions (i.e., loci) where the LOD score is high, suggesting a high probability that a disease-linked variant resides nearby. Due to the spacing of the markers and their multiallelic properties, the identified regions are usually large, comprising up to tens of mega bases and harboring dozens of genes (which are then referred to as *positional candidates* because they reside under the linkage peak). Linkage peaks need to be followed up with additional *fine mapping* using denser marker maps, including SNPs, to narrow in on the candidate gene(s) of interest.

While classical linkage approaches have been very successful in identifying monogenic diseases that follow clear, simple patterns of inheritance, they have been far less successful in complex psychiatric disease. Parametric linkage analysis requires the specification of an inheritance model (e.g., recessive or dominant), information we do not have for psychiatric disorders as they clearly do not follow Mendelian inheritance. In addition, each family may have a different pattern of inheritance, so that specifying one model for several pedigrees may decrease the power to detect a signal in some of the families. Nonparametric linkage analyses that are mode of inheritance independent have been developed to address this problem. Also, linkage analysis requires that each person in a pedigree be designated as either affected or unaffected, so one must decide, for example, in which category to place individuals with a single major depressive episode in a bipolar pedigree. Linkage analysis studies therefore often run several different models and may also use different definitions of affected status and then report the best LOD score, but here the threshold for significance also has to be adjusted for additional multiple testing, so that even higher LOD scores are required for statistical significance. Linkage analyses in psychiatric disorders are further complicated by the fact that they explore complex psychiatric diseases, with likely multiple (possibly additive or interacting) susceptibility genes and a strong environmental component, all of which cannot be modeled easily in these analyses. It is therefore not surprising that linkage analyses have yielded very inconsistent data in the past. In an effort to overcome these problems by sheer sample size, large meta-analyses have been conducted for linkage scans in schizophrenia and bipolar disorder (Badner and Gershon 2002; Levinson et al. 2003). In schizophrenia, for example, 20 scans with 1,208 pedigrees and 2,945 affected individuals have been used for a combined analysis (Lewis et al. 2003). This study yielded a locus on chromosome 2 segregating with schizophrenia with genomewide significance after correction for multiple testing, and 10 further regions have been identified as strong schizophrenia candidates. A similar meta-analysis was also conducted for bipolar disorder (Segurado et al. 2003), with 948 affected when bipolar I and schizoaffective disorder, bipolar type, were included as diagnoses and 1,733 when bipolar II disorder was also included. In this analysis, none of the linkage peaks reached genomewide significance. These findings suggest that in bipolar disorder the effects of individual genes may be small, thus requiring even greater sample sizes, or that heterogeneity across families is substantial.

Association Studies

Association studies are usually performed in case–control studies of unrelated individuals. In such studies, allele frequencies of markers are compared between a case and a control population. Association has been shown to have more power than linkage studies to detect susceptibility genes that exert only a small effect on disease risk (Risch and Merikangas 1996). Considering the strong evidence supporting complex inheritance for most psychiatric disorders, it appears that association studies are the optimal study design to identify and/or test candidate genes for these disorders. Nonetheless, association studies have been fraught with failures to replicate initially reported associations. For example, several meta-analyses of association studies of the *DRD3* locus, encoding the dopamine D_3 receptor, yielded conflicting results on whether a true association exists between an SNP in exon 2, which

encodes either serine or glycine at amino acid position 9 (ser9gly), and risk for schizophrenia (Dubertret et al. 1998; Jonsson et al. 2003, 2004; Williams et al. 1998). Critical evaluation of such controversies requires an understanding of several key concepts, which are important for the design and interpretation of association studies.

Linkage Disequilibrium

Association studies rely on the principle that even unrelated individuals share very small stretches of chromosomal DNA derived from a distant common ancestor. In the case of a disease-predisposing mutation, some proportion of ill individuals will share that mutation arising from an original common ancestor. As the variant is passed down from generation to generation, meiotic recombination events will shrink the size of the initial piece of ancestral chromosome that is inherited together with the disease mutation. On these small ancestral stretches of chromosome (perhaps several thousand to several hundred thousand bp in length), nonfunctional "marker" polymorphisms close to the disease mutation will "ride" through generations together with the disease variant. Such markers (SNPs, for example) can thus serve as surrogate "tags" for the disease mutation. Note, however, that as generations pass and individuals become ever more distant relatives (to a point where social/cultural "memory" of genetic relationship is usually lost), different families will produce recombination events at different points near the disease mutation. Therefore, at a population level, unrelated individuals carrying the disease marker will carry variable lengths of DNA on which markers linked to the disease variant ride. Stated another way, unrelated individuals carrying the disease variant will carry *haplotypes* that become more similar to each other as the boundaries of the haplotypes are moved closer to the disease variant. Thus, the closer a marker is to the disease variant, the more likely it is to be originally linked to the variant. When a marker is close enough to a disease marker that the number of recombination events in the population has not yet completely randomized, and the chance is that it is on the same ancestral stretch of DNA (haplotype) as the disease variant, the marker and the disease variant are correlated and are said to be in *linkage disequilibrium* (LD). Knowing the allele of a marker variant in LD with a disease variant can therefore predict the allele of the disease variant (i.e., the marker and the disease variant are not statistically independent).

Several factors influence the length of DNA over which LD occurs. The most important are the geographic origins of the population from which an individual is drawn and the history of that population. For example, sub-Saharan African populations are ancient and reflect the greatest proportions of the total human pool of variation, because most of the human species' history predates migration of humans out of Africa. Therefore, on average, sub-Saharan African populations have undergone the greatest number of recombination events since a given pair of unrelated individuals shared a common ancestor. Those individuals thus share only short stretches of ancestral chromosomes (which are said to be *identical by descent*, or IBD). Non-African populations all derive from a relatively small number of migrants who left Africa within approximately the last 100,000 years. Thus, Europeans, or Eastern Asians, or Native Americans share longer stretches of DNA IBD within their respective continental groups than do sub-Saharan Africans (Daly et al. 2001; Gabriel et al. 2002; Patil et al. 2001; Reich et al. 2001). On the other extreme, individuals from reproductively isolated populations, in which a small recent founder population has expanded with little admixture (i.e., introduction of outside individuals into the mating pool), share longer blocks of ancestral chromosomes IBD (Shifman and Darvasi 2001). An example of such an isolate is the Icelandic population, which derives almost exclusively from a small number of migrants who arrived on the island only several hundred years ago (Helgason et al. 2003).

Another factor contributing to the complexity of patterns of LD is the fact that recombination events do not occur with the same likelihood across all parts of the genome (Phillips et al. 2003; Reich et al. 2002). In addition to a general pattern in which more telomeric regions of chromosomes are more likely to recombine than centromeric regions, specific "hot spots" of recombination have been identified that are spaced unevenly along chromosomes. This variation across the genome in the likelihood of recombination results in the observation that there are stretches in the genome (sometimes referred to as *blocks*) that have undergone relatively little recombination over the generations and therefore exhibit strong LD among SNPs in the region. Such regions of high LD can span millions of bases, whereas other regions in the same population have recombined more frequently, resulting in very short blocks of LD (e.g., <5,000 bp). It is important to note that the observed haplotypes formed by the SNPs within a given stretch of chromosome usually represent only a small proportion of all possible haplotypes (for SNPs, the number of possible haplotypes = 2^n, where n = the number of SNPs defining the haplotype). For this reason, such regions of high LD are also called *haplotype*

blocks (Daly et al. 2001; Gabriel et al. 2002; Patil et al. 2001; Reich et al. 2001).

The HapMap Project.   The HapMap Project is cataloguing LD structure (International HapMap Consortium 2003). This international consortium has set out to identify all ancestral or haplotype blocks in four different populations: Caucasian Utah Mormons, Sub-Saharan African Yorubans, Han Chinese, and Japanese. Currently, phase 2 of the project, with genotype data on SNPs with an average density of 1 SNP/1,000 bp, is available online (www.hapmap.org). These publicly available data allow identification of the number of SNPs necessary to tag all ancestral blocks for a given gene, region of interest, or even the whole genome (Cardon and Abecasis 2003; Need and Goldstein 2006). While the data generated in this project have been invaluable for the field, one has to evaluate carefully whether the LD structure of the populations characterized in HapMap is representative for the selected study population. HapMap tag SNPs seem to perform reasonably well in most populations, the only caveat being that tag SNPs from Yorubans are not optimal for other African populations, especially African Americans, as they are an admixed population in which the African ancestors of the population came from a larger geographical area (predominantly along the western coast of Sub-Saharan Africa) than did the Yoruban population (Conrad et al. 2006; de Bakker et al. 2006).

Linkage disequilibrium and replication of association studies.   As already noted, the literature contains myriad reported genetic associations to psychiatric disorders that have not replicated in subsequent studies. The most important reason for such nonreplication is that until recently, the vast majority of association studies have been grossly underpowered and have examined only one or a few SNPs. Given the huge a priori odds against a true genetic association at a given locus, even for candidate genes that "make biological sense," many reported associations are likely to be due to chance.

However, even when a disorder-predisposing variant does occur within a candidate gene (i.e., when a true genetic association exists), several factors can lead to nonreplication of association results. Differences in LD patterns between the population of the initial and the replication study can be one reason for such nonreplication. If a marker polymorphism is in strong or complete LD with a true disease-predisposing variant at a given locus, then typing the marker in a sufficiently large case–control study will detect an association to the disease, because the allelic variation at the marker accurately "tags" the true disease-predisposing variant. If an association is detected, then replication is imperative. However, if an independent sample of cases and controls derives from a population with a different ancestry, and hence a different pattern of LD between the marker and the true disease variant, the power of the originally "positive" marker to detect the association can be greatly reduced if the marker does not tag the disease-predisposing variant as well (i.e., power is reduced to the degree that LD between the marker and the disease-predisposing variant is lower). One implication of the foregoing scenario is that adequate evaluation of a given candidate gene requires examination of a number of SNPs across that gene sufficient to represent most of the common sequence variation in the gene: from this principle derives the concept of "tagging SNPs" (International HapMap Consortium 2003; Johnson et al. 2001). Useful software is now publicly available that enables investigators to search the SNP databases and select SNPs that meet a desired criterion of correlation (LD) with each other. Selecting "tagging SNPs" in this way accomplishes two important goals. First, as just discussed, such selection allows the researcher to capture most of the common variation at a candidate gene. Second, selecting tagging SNPs allows the researcher to avoid the unnecessary cost and effort of genotyping redundant SNPs. Among the most useful and widely used software for selecting tagging SNPs is Haploview, developed by Daly and colleagues (Barrett et al. 2005).

One attractive strategy for increasing the likelihood that a given candidate polymorphism is relevant to disease is to focus on variants that clearly alter the structure or regulation of gene products. While it certainly makes sense that polymorphisms that definitely alter protein structure or gene expression (the most obvious type being nonsynonymous SNPs) might be expected to alter more complex phenotypes, it is also quite possible that a presumed functional variant may in fact only be in LD with the real causal mutation. For example, some evidence suggests that the *COMT* Val/Met polymorphism discussed above is merely a marker for an upstream schizophrenia-associated variant (Bray et al. 2003; Shifman et al. 2002). As already discussed, variable LD of the Val/Met variant with some other true schizophrenia-predisposing variant could explain the inconsistent results of the numerous association studies of this polymorphism in schizophrenia.

Stringent testing of the functionality of a specific human polymorphism is currently difficult. Almost invariably, tests of presumed functional variants also examine

other known or unknown polymorphisms due to LD with those other variants. Even if correlations with functional readouts are observed, such as changes in expression or function in lymphoblastoid cell lines or differences in imaging parameters, one cannot definitely conclude that the specific polymorphism typed is necessarily the functional one. To test this, one would need to hold all other genetic parameters in the experiment constant and just manipulate the variant of interest on the same ancestral chromosome. So far these very stringent criteria for establishing functionality are rarely met, including for the most commonly genotyped "functional" variants in psychiatric genetics.

One should also note that recent data from the Encyclopedia of DNA Elements (ENCODE) project suggest that the regulation of transcription is much more complicated and widespread than previously assumed (ENCODE Project Consortium 2007). SNPs in *genomic deserts* (no genes close by) may be as important for gene transcription regulation as SNPs located in classical promoter elements.

Population Stratification

Frequencies of specific alleles can vary to a great degree among different populations. The approximate frequency of the S allele of the *5-HTTLPR*, for example, is 40%–50% in European, 70%–80% in East Asians, and 25% in African populations (Gelernter et al. 1999). Spurious associations can thus be found if subjects for a genetic association study are sampled from genetically different subpopulations (with different marker allele frequencies) in different proportions in cases and controls, for example. This could occur if an outcome is more prevalent in one subpopulation, perhaps because of different environmental exposure, so that individuals from this subpopulation will be represented more frequently in the case as opposed to the control group. Differences in allele frequencies between comparison groups can thus result from differences in the population structure of the sample alone, without any causal relationship to the outcome of interest. This problem is called *population stratification* and is exemplified by the hypothetical example of the "chopsticks gene" (Hamer and Sirota 2000).

Several methods have been developed to address population stratification in genetic association studies. Family-based approaches to genetic association studies, such as the transmission disequilibrium test (TDT; Spielman et al. 1993) and the haplotype relative risk (HRR) method (Knapp et al. 1993), are robust to population stratification. In the TDT, rather than compare allele frequencies between cases and controls, genotypes are determined in probands and their parents. To be informative, at least one parent must be heterozygous at the marker of interest (this is one of the disadvantages of the method in its original form: in some cases, not all families can be used). The allele transmitted to the proband from each parent is recorded, as well as the nontransmitted allele. Under the null hypothesis of no linkage or association, the expected chance of each allele's transmission is 50%. Significant deviations from that chance provide evidence for association (and linkage) between the trait and the marker. The HRR method is similar, except that the frequency of the nontransmitted alleles is compared to that of the transmitted alleles over a large number of families. Each family thus provides its own control—since the proband is always matched for the population background of the parents, population stratification cannot arise.

Recently, methods based on the TDT have been developed to allow transmission disequilibrium testing in larger family groups. Such family-based association tests offer the advantage of using more of the available genetic information from each family (Horvath et al. 2001). The major disadvantage of the family-based methods is that it is often impractical to gather families, especially in disorders such as schizophrenia or substance dependence, which are often associated with familial estrangement, or age-related disorders such as Alzheimer's disease, where surviving relatives (especially parents) may not be available. An additional problem with family-based association studies is they generally have less statistical power than case–control studies (Risch and Merikangas 1996).

To control for population stratification in case–control studies, two sets of methods have been developed, both of which estimate, and then correct for, the degree of stratification between comparison groups by typing a series of unlinked markers across the genome (Devlin and Roeder 1999; Pritchard et al. 2000). Using these methods, called *structured association* (Rosenberg et al. 2002) and *genomic control* (Devlin and Roeder 1999), one can only determine stratification of the level of the whole sample. A refinement of these methods employs ancestry informative markers (AIMs), which can estimate the proportional genetic heritage from predefined ethnicities for each individual (Montana and Pritchard 2004; Parra et al. 2001). As opposed to the first approaches, AIMs are not randomly selected unlinked markers, but markers are chosen to exhibit large differences in allele frequencies between specified populations (Northern Europeans vs. sub-Saharan Africans, for example). Using such markers,

one can demonstrate that some populations, such as self-identified African Americans and European Americans, may show substantial admixture of European, African, and (to a lesser degree) Native American chromosomal ancestry (Parra et al. 1998, 2001). Each individual's proportion of predefined chromosomal ancestry can be estimated and then used as a covariate to correct for stratification in association analysis (Frudakis et al. 2003).

Correction for Multiple Testing

The ease and cost-effectiveness with which SNPs or other markers can now be genotyped have led to the advent of whole-genome association studies, in which 100,000–1,000,000 SNPs are typed in large case–control comparisons. This approach, while creating the exciting opportunity to scan the genome in a non-hypothesis-driven manner for genetic associations, suffers from the difficult problem that the number of statistical tests in each association study is enormous, and thus the likelihood of false-positive associations is high. In a simple example, when one performs 100 statistical tests, one would expect that 5 of them would show a P value of <0.05 just by chance. To decrease the likelihood of reporting and following false-positive associations, methods to correct for multiple testing have been developed. The simplest and most common is the Bonferroni correction, in which the alpha level required for statistical significance overall is divided by the number of statistical tests and thus, in this case, the number of tested SNPs. However, because not all SNPs are independent (see "Linkage Disequilibrium" subsection above), Bonferroni correction is often overly conservative. Newer methods of correcting for multiple testing take into account the LD among the tested SNPs (e.g., Nyholt 2004). An alternative is permutation-based methods, in which the outcome status (e.g., case or control status) is randomly assigned and the genotypes remain fixed. The association statistic is recalculated for every permutation, and all P values are noted. This allows estimation of the number of P values that are as small as or smaller than the P value based on the correct assignment of outcome status (Churchill and Doerge 1994). The corrected empirical P value then is the number of P values smaller than the empirical one/number of total iterations. Because permutation-based correction can be computationally intensive, newer, faster methods have been developed (Dudbridge and Koeleman 2004; Seaman and Muller-Myshok 2005). Another method to control for multiple tests is the false discovery rate (Benjamini and Hochberg 1995). In this method one controls the expected proportion of false positives in a list of potential positive associations. It is a less conservative comparison procedure with greater power than the methods mentioned above but at a cost of increasing the likelihood of obtaining type I errors.

While stringent correction for multiple testing reduces the likelihood of reporting false-positive associations, true association may be dismissed as false positives because, while nominally significant, the association does not reach the set threshold for correction for multiple testing. Some researchers thus advocate a two-step design for association studies, in which a first sample is used as an exploratory sample, in which the alpha levels are more liberal, and then nominally associated SNPs are tested in a second replication sample. Only associations that show significance in both samples are considered as potential true positives. This approach has, for example, been used in the pharmacogenetic association study of the Sequenced Treatment Alternatives to Relieve Depression (STAR*D) sample (McMahon et al. 2006).

Genomewide Association Studies

New Possibilities Due to the Human Genome Project

Despite 30–40 years of intense research on a series of promising markers, none has thus far been validated as diagnostic tools or predictors of treatment response. In addition, most of the past approaches were hypothesis driven, relying on our limited knowledge of the pathophysiology of psychiatric disorders. With the sequence of the human genome having being publicly available since February 2001 (Lander et al. 2001; Venter et al. 2001), an array of novel research tools has become available that may yield unbiased, hypothesis-free insight into the pathophysiological underpinnings of certain psychiatric disorders. These novel tools combine knowledge of the sequence of the human genome with miniaturized assays amenable to high-throughput processing for a parallel analysis of the whole genome. Using these, one can investigate the whole genome at the level of the DNA (genomics), all expressed mRNA (expressomics—or, more commonly, expression array or microarray analysis), and all proteins (proteomics) in a single experiment. These three approaches have to deal with increasing levels of complexity, because the approximately 25,000 predicted human genes are expected to give rise to at least 10 times as many protein isoforms with a multitude of posttranslational modifications, such as phosphorylation and glyco-

sylation. Using these unbiased whole genome–based approaches, novel pathways and molecules involved in the pathogenesis of psychiatric disorders may be identified. This chapter will mostly focus on genomewide SNP association studies and their impact on psychiatric genetics; we recommend several reviews on the impact of microarray analysis and proteomics on pathophysiological concepts in psychiatry (Freeman and Hemby 2004; Ginsberg et al. 2004; Mirnics et al. 2006; Tannu and Hemby 2006) for additional information in these areas.

Genomewide SNP Arrays

How many SNPs? The presence of linkage disequilibrium in the human genome allows the investigator to evaluate a large extent of the common genetic variation with selected markers. Estimates of the number of SNPs necessary to account for most of the common sequence variation across the genome (e.g., to account for SNPs with minor allele frequencies of 1% or greater) have varied over time, with estimates ranging from as few as 10,000–100,000 to over a million SNPs. Thanks to the HapMap and the ENCODE resequencing projects (International HapMap Consortium 2003 and www.hapmap.org), we are starting to have a better idea of how efficiently we have and can cover the genetic information using SNP assays. These massive genotyping and resequencing projects have confirmed the segments of long LD in the genome and thus the possibility of using tag SNPs (see discussion above) for each of these segments. Using the data from several hundred thousand SNPs should be sufficient to cover most common variants in Caucasians; more SNPs will be necessary in African populations with shorter LD distances (for a review, see Hirschhorn and Daly 2005). Based on the information in the HapMap and ENCODE databases, Barrett and Cardon (2006) estimated the coverage of commercially available whole-genome SNP panels from Illumina (www.Illumina.com) and Affymetrix (www.affymetrix.com). The Illumina 300k chip offered coverage of 75% in Caucasians and the Affymetrix 500K 65%. These values dropped dramatically for Yorubans, to 28% and 41%, respectively. While these whole-genome arrays with 300,000 to 500,000 SNP assays offered relatively good coverage of more common variants, rare SNPs are not well covered. While these earlier arrays still had relatively substantial holes in the genomewide coverage, especially in African populations, the development in this area is exponential. For example, Affymetrix now offers a 1.8 million SNP array, and Illumina a 1 million SNP chip. Incomplete coverage should soon become a problem of the past (Schuster 2008).

A major drawback of whole-genome LD-based approaches to association testing, such as those just outlined, is that the majority of sequence variation in the genome is *rare*, with minor allele frequencies too small to be detected with any power by even very dense maps of SNPs. Thus, to the degree that the genetic underpinnings of complex diseases deviate from the "common disease, common variant" hypothesis, whole-genome SNP scans will be inadequate to detect associated genes (Zwick et al. 2000). This concern is not merely theoretical. Thus, it is abundantly clear that in Mendelian diseases, such as cystic fibrosis, where variation at only one *locus* accounts for the disease, a multitude of very rare *sequence variants* are causal in different families. Rare variation also clearly contributes to complex diseases. For example, in familial autism, a subgroup of families who exhibit linkage to markers on chromosome 17q (Sutcliffe et al. 2005) has demonstrated that a series of rare functional variants at *SLC6A4*, the serotonin transporter locus, accounts for much of the observed linkage in these families. Common variation at the locus (e.g., the *5-HTTLPR* discussed above) did not contribute to linkage to the disorder in these families. In all likelihood, complex disorders will represent a mixture of contributions from rare and common variants, so that methods appropriate for both types of variation will need to be developed and implemented. In regard to rare variation, the advent of whole-genome resequencing may contribute importantly to identifying such variants.

How many individuals?   Genomewide associations require massive correction for multiple testing so that P values below 10^{-7} or smaller have to be achieved for genomewide significance. These necessary low alpha levels, together with the expected low odds ratios (ORs) associated with identified susceptibility variants, require large sample sizes for adequate power. For example, to detect the effect of a susceptibility allele that has a frequency of 20% and an OR of 1.3 with a power of at least 80% and an even more liberal alpha level of 10^{-6}, more than 2,500 cases are necessary. If the allele is rarer (e.g., 10% carriers), at least 6,000 cases would be required (W.Y. Wang et al. 2005). Given that epidemiological studies suggest small effect sizes of multiple genes for psychiatric disorders, these calculations would apply to this field as well.

How to reduce false-positive findings?   Because whole-genome association studies use a large number of tests, very

strict levels of significance have been proposed (7.2×10^{-8}; Dudbridge and Gusnanto 2008). While this strategy may avoid a large number of false positives (at least 25,000 SNPs are expected to show association with a P value of 0.05 or smaller in a set of 500,000 SNPs), true positives may also be missed. This is especially relevant given that most studies in psychiatric genetics will likely be underpowered to detect relevant effect sizes of 1.3 or smaller with rarer alleles. One possibility to reduce false negatives due to overly stringent correction for multiple testing would be to genotype all SNPs in a smaller fraction of the sample (discovery sample) and use a liberal P value to select SNPs that are then genotyped in a second larger sample (confirmation sample). Only SNPs passing this second stage would then be selected for replication in an independent sample (Hirschhorn and Daly 2005; H. Wang et al. 2006). Recently, guidelines for replicating genotype–phenotype associations, with focus on whole-genome associations, have been put forward (Chanock et al. 2007).

Another strategy is to use convergent evidence from other genomewide approaches, such as linkage analyses, expression microarrays, and proteomics. While such studies have not yet been published for whole-genome SNP association studies, this strategy has been successful with microarray and linkage data. John Kelsoe and his colleagues used an approach that combined microarray analysis of animal models of mania and linkage analysis in families with bipolar disorder to identify G protein–coupled receptor kinase 3 (*GRK3*) as a promising candidate gene. This gene is involved in the homologous desensitization of G protein–coupled receptors. The group had initially identified a linkage peak for bipolar disorder on chromosome 22q (Kelsoe et al. 2001; Lachman et al. 1997). That linked region, however, spanned 32 cM, making it a challenging task to identify the causal gene by fine-mapping strategies. The group then used microarray analysis of different brain regions in methamphetamine-treated rats and identified several genes that were regulated by this treatment that also mapped to previous linkage peaks with bipolar disorder (Niculescu et al. 2000). One of these was *GRK3*, which maps to 22q. In addition to being regulated in the animal model, protein levels for this gene were also found to be decreased in a subset of patient lymphoblastoid cell lines, and the magnitude of the decrease correlated with disease severity. By using resequencing and SNP genotyping strategies, the group confirmed the association of 5'UTR and promoter variants of this gene with bipolar disorder (Barrett et al. 2003).

Current Results From Genomewide SNP Association Studies

In a landmark paper, Risch and Merikangas (1996) suggested that genomewide association studies will have more power to detect disease genes for complex diseases than family-based studies. This bold suggestion was postulated 5 years before the sequence of the human genome was available and SNPs emerged as potential tools for this type of study. Now, more than 10 years later, genomewide association studies with hundreds of thousands of SNPs in thousands of affected individuals and controls are identifying novel hypothesis-free candidate genes for complex disorders. In the past few years, a number of large multicenter studies have identified novel candidate genes for diabetes type 1 and type 2, metabolic diseases, several types of cancer, age-related macular degeneration, and a series of autoimmune disorders using this approach (Altshuler et al. 2008). A series of genomewide association studies have now been published for addiction, bipolar disorder, unipolar depression, schizophrenia, autism, and attention-deficit hyperactivity disorder (Psychiatric GWAS Consortium Steering Committee 2009). By early 2009, genomewide association studies in 47 samples from these disorders will be completed, with well over 50,000 independent individuals in these studies. Whole-genome SNP association studies have been successful in bipolar disorder, and polymorphisms in the genes encoding ankyrin G (*ANK3*) and the alpha 1C subunit of the L-type voltage-gated calcium channel (*CACNA1C*) have emerged as new candidates for this disorder from data combining several large samples (Ferreira et al. 2008; Schulze et al. 2008). The latter gene family may also be of relevance in schizophrenia (Moskvina et al. 2008). Interestingly, the independent samples (Baum et al. 2008a, 2008b; Craddock et al. 2008; Sklar et al. 2008; Wellcome Trust Case Control Consortium 2007) mostly yielded no genomewide significant associations or could not be replicated in single association studies, showing the importance of large sample sizes for these studies. The single genomewide association study on unipolar depression published by the end of 2008, starting with data from the Genetic Association Information Network (GAIN) initiative of the National Institutes of Health, did not show replication of the strongest, but not genomewide significant hit in five other samples with a total of more than 7,000 cases and controls (Sullivan et al. 2008a). Whole-genome SNP association studies for schizophrenia have also been less convincing than for bipolar disorder (Kirov et al. 2008; Lencz et al. 2007; Shifman et al. 2008; Sullivan

et al. 2008b). The largest replication attempt of genomewide association studies in schizophrenia, with more than 16,000 individuals, points to a locus around zinc finger protein 804A (*ZNF804A*) that reaches genomewide significance when patients with bipolar disorder are included in the meta-analysis (O'Donovan et al. 2008). Genomewide genetics studies in schizophrenia seem to point to the importance of a combination of rare and common variants in this disorder, possibly explaining the relative lack of genomewide significant hits in genomewide association studies. A whole-genome association study in schizophrenic patients revealed a colony-stimulating factor receptor (*CSF2RA*) and an interleukin receptor (*IL3RA*) as potential novel candidate genes for this disorder (Lencz et al. 2007). From this study in two independent samples, the authors could identify an association with disease of common haplotypes in these two genes and also discovered an excess of rare nonsynonymous mutations in these genes, thus supporting a model in which both common and rare mutations can contribute to disease susceptibility (Lewis et al. 2003). The importance of rare variants and specifically structural variants in schizophrenia has been underlined by two large international genomewide studies identifying a series of CNVs associated with the disorder, confirming previous hits in neurodevelopmental genes from earlier linkage and candidate gene association studies (International Schizophrenia Consortium 2008; Stefansson et al. 2008).

The first sets of genomewide association data in psychiatric genetics provide new insights into these disorders. Although promising, these new data raise several important issues:

1. *Multiple genes of small effects contribute to psychiatric disease.* To identify these effects with sufficient power, large sample sizes of several thousand cases will be required, and international collaborations are essential.

2. *Comparison with other complex diseases.* The Wellcome Trust Case Control Consortium (2007) has published whole-genome association data for 14,000 cases of seven disorders and 3,000 common controls. In this study, 2,000 cases of bipolar disorder were examined next to cases of coronary artery disease, Crohn's disease, hypertension, rheumatoid arthritis, and diabetes type 1 and type 2. The direct comparison of this association study for bipolar disorder with association in the other tested disorders is very interesting. In bipolar disorder, no really strong clusters of association could be determined. For diabetes type 1, with a similar heritability (around 80%), on the other hand, at least five

very strong clusters of association could be identified, and even coronary artery disease and diabetes type 2, disorders with a prominent environmental component and lower heritabilities, showed several clusters of very strong association. Psychiatric disorders may thus be even more complex than other complex disorders. The fact that bipolar disorder, the most heritable affective disorder, did not perform well in the Wellcome Trust Case Control Consortium analysis in comparison with diabetes and coronary artery disease, for example, shows that psychiatric genetics needs to invest in the identification of reliable biological phenotypes that better cluster genetically homogeneous patient groups.

3. *Importance of a mix of common and rare variants, with rare variants likely predominating in autism and schizophrenia.* Linkage and association studies will need to be combined with resequencing studies to identify these rare variants.

4. *Importance of structural variations in psychiatric genetics.* In schizophrenia and autism, investigation of structural variation has proven to be a very powerful tool to dissect the genetics of these disorders (Cook and Scherer 2008; Marshall et al. 2008; Sebat et al. 2007; St. Clair 2009; Szatmari et al. 2007; Weiss et al. 2008). We are awaiting similar studies in other psychiatric disorders.

Gene–Environment Interactions

To date, most genetic association studies have searched for simple associations between sequence variants and psychiatric disorders. This approach ignores the clear reality that environmental factors contribute importantly to psychiatric illness. While many such factors remain unknown, several clearly are known. For example, it is becoming increasingly clear that early childhood traumatic experiences substantially increase the risk of major depression and other mood disorders. In their landmark paper, now replicated by several groups, Caspi et al. (2003) showed that genotype at the *5-HTTLPR* interacts with exposure to early trauma to increase the risk of depression differentially in carriers of the S allele. From a theoretical perspective, searching for such gene–environment interactions makes sense. Thus, any statistical interaction is bound at the upper end of its effect size by the magnitude of the main effects being considered. When environmental factors such as early trauma, which have large effect sizes, are examined together with genetic factors, which are expected generally to have small effect sizes, the result

can be greater power to detect gene–environment interactions than main effects of the gene. Thus, an argument can be made (which by no means is accepted by all) that future genetic studies of psychiatric disorders and other complex disorders should be based on models that incorporate both genetic and environmental factors.

Conclusion

Taken together, epidemiological, cytogenetic, linkage, and association studies in psychiatric genetics to date paint a picture of highly complex genetic influences on psychiatric disorders. As Kendler (2005) pointed out, the phrase "a gene for…" will very likely *not* apply to psychiatric genetics. And, as Kendler went on to note, "The impact of individual genes on risk for psychiatric illness is small, often nonspecific, and embedded in a complex causal pathway" (Kendler 2005, p. 1243). The field may need to adopt strategies that are better adapted to the most likely disease models. In the following we will mention some of the proposed strategies to address this issue.

First, we may need to reconsider the way we define cases or the phenotype of interest. Our current classification schemes are not likely directly reflective of the underlying biology—and thus the genetic determinants—of psychiatric disease. The currently used diagnostic algorithms (DSM-IV-TR [American Psychiatric Association 2000] and ICD-10 [World Health Organization 1992]) group diagnoses by symptoms and clinical course, characteristics that may reflect not a common biology but rather a final common pathway of several different pathophysiological disturbances. That recognition has led some to propose the use of intermediate phenotypes—including neurophysiological, biochemical, cognitive, and endocrine measures (Gottesman and Gould 2003; Hasler et al. 2004)—in psychiatric genetic studies in order to create biologically more homogeneous subgroups of patients and thus to increase the power to detect case–control associations. Another important consideration is that a number of symptoms are common to several different DSM-IV-TR diagnoses, and the genetic susceptibility to develop these symptoms may be common across disorders. In fact, there is evidence that the major psychiatric disorders may share susceptibility genes. A series of linkage peaks and candidate gene associations overlaps between bipolar disorder and schizophrenia, for example (Craddock et al. 2006), and the cytogenetic disruption of *DISC1* leads to a variety of severe psychiatric disorders, ranging from recurrent unipolar disorder to schizophrenia (St. Clair et al. 1990).

Second, environmental measures should be included more consistently in genetic studies, including whole-genome association studies. Epidemiological (Kendler 1995) as well as molecular genetic studies have now repeatedly demonstrated the importance of gene–environment interactions in psychiatric disease (Caspi and Moffitt 2006). Genetic effects may be obscured by unmeasured environmental effects, so that different environmental exposures in replication samples may be one source of non-replication of genetic association.

Finally, one should not forget that SNPs are just the most common and convenient type of genetic variant. Other types of variation, such as CNVs, may be equally important (Redon et al. 2006; Sebat et al. 2004). Newer versions of whole-genome arrays now try to cover most copy number variations known to date, and association with these may lead to surprising findings.

References

Abkevich V, Camp NJ, Hensel CH, et al: Predisposition locus for major depression at chromosome 12q22–12q23.2. Am J Hum Genet 73:1271–1281, 2003

Altshuler D, Pollara VJ, Cowles CR, et al: An SNP map of the human genome generated by reduced representation shotgun sequencing. Nature 407:513–516, 2000

Altshuler D, Daly MJ, Lander ES: Genetic mapping in human disease. Science 322:881–888, 2008

American Psychiatric Association: Diagnostic and Statistical Manual of Mental Disorders, 4th Edition, Text Revision. Washington, DC, American Psychiatric Association, 2000

Angst J: A clinical analysis of the effects of Tofranil in depression: longitudinal and follow-up studies. Treatment of blood relations. Psychopharmacologia 2:381–407, 1961

Badner JA, Gershon ES: Meta-analysis of whole-genome linkage scans of bipolar disorder and schizophrenia. Mol Psychiatry 7:405–411, 2002

Bailey A, Le Couteur A, Gottesman I, et al: Autism as a strongly genetic disorder: evidence from a British twin study. Psychol Med 25:63–77, 1995

Barrett JC, Cardon LR: Evaluating coverage of genome-wide association studies. Nat Genet 38:659–662, 2006

Barrett JC, Fry B, Maller J, et al: Haploview: analysis and visualization of LD and haplotype maps. Bioinformatics 21:263–265, 2005

Barrett TB, Hauger RL, Kennedy JL, et al: Evidence that a single nucleotide polymorphism in the promoter of the G protein receptor kinase 3 gene is associated with bipolar disorder. Mol Psychiatry 8:546–557, 2003

Baum AE, Akula N, Cabanero M, et al: A genome-wide association study implicates diacylglycerol kinase eta (DGKH) and several other genes in the etiology of bipolar disorder. Mol Psychiatry 13:197–207, 2008a

Baum AE, Hamshere M, Green E, et al: Meta-analysis of two genome-wide association studies of bipolar disorder reveals important points of agreement. Mol Psychiatry 13:466–467, 2008b

Benjamini Y, Hochberg Y: Controlling the false discovery rate: a practical and powerful approach to multiple testing. Journal of the Royal Statistical Society, Series B (Methodological) 57:289–300, 1995

Bertilsson L, Dahl ML, Dalen P, et al: Molecular genetics of CYP2D6: clinical relevance with focus on psychotropic drugs. Br J Clin Pharmacol 53:111–122, 2002

Binder EB, Bradley RG, Liu W, et al: Association of FKBP5 polymorphisms and childhood abuse with risk of posttraumatic stress disorder symptoms in adults. JAMA 299:1–15, 2008

Blackwood D, Muir W: Molecular genetics and the epidemiology of bipolar disorder. Ann Med 33:242–247, 2001

Blackwood DH, Fordyce A, Walker MT, et al: Schizophrenia and affective disorders—cosegregation with a translocation at chromosome 1q42 that directly disrupts brain-expressed genes: clinical and P300 findings in a family. Am J Hum Genet 69:428–433, 2001

Bleuler M: Psychiatry of cerebral diseases. BMJ 2:1233–1238, 1951

Bradley RG, Binder EB, Epstein MP, et al: Influence of child abuse on adult depression: moderation by the corticotropin-releasing hormone receptor gene. Arch Gen Psychiatry 65:190–200, 2008

Bray NJ, Buckland PR, Williams NM, et al: A haplotype implicated in schizophrenia susceptibility is associated with reduced COMT expression in human brain. Am J Hum Genet 73:152–161, 2003

Brunner HG, Nelen M, Breakefield XO, et al: Abnormal behavior associated with a point mutation in the structural gene for monoamine oxidase A. Science 262:578–580, 1993

Bulik CM, Sullivan PF, Wade TD, et al: Twin studies of eating disorders: a review. Int J Eat Disord 27:1–20, 2000

Bulik CM, Sullivan PF, Tozzi F, et al: Prevalence, heritability, and prospective risk factors for anorexia nervosa. Arch Gen Psychiatry 63:305–312, 2006

Busjahn A: Twin registers across the globe: what's out there in 2002? Twin Res 5:v–vi, 2002

Cadoret RJ: Adoption studies: historical and methodological critique. Psychiatr Dev 4:45–64, 1986

Cadoret RJ, Yates WR, Troughton E, et al: Adoption study demonstrating two genetic pathways to drug abuse. Arch Gen Psychiatry 52:42–52, 1995a

Cadoret RJ, Yates WR, Troughton E, et al: Genetic-environmental interaction in the genesis of aggressivity and conduct disorders. Arch Gen Psychiatry 52:916–924, 1995b

Cardon LR, Abecasis GR: Using haplotype blocks to map human complex trait loci. Trends Genet 19:135–140, 2003

Caspi A, Moffitt TE: Gene-environment interactions in psychiatry: joining forces with neuroscience. Nat Rev Neurosci 7:583–590, 2006

Caspi A, McClay J, Moffitt TE, et al: Role of genotype in the cycle of violence in maltreated children. Science 297:851–854, 2002

Caspi A, Sugden K, Moffitt TE, et al: Influence of life stress on depression: moderation by a polymorphism in the 5-HTT gene. Science 301:386–389, 2003

Caspi A, Moffitt TE, Cannon M, et al: Moderation of the effect of adolescent-onset cannabis use on adult psychosis by a functional polymorphism in the catechol-O-methyltransferase gene: longitudinal evidence of a gene x environment interaction. Biol Psychiatry 57:1117–1127, 2005

Chanock SJ, Manolio T, Boehnke M, et al: Replicating genotype-phenotype associations. Nature 447:655–660, 2007

Churchill GA, Doerge RW: Empirical threshold values for quantitative trait mapping. Genetics 138:963–971, 1994

Conrad DF, Jakobsson M, Coop G, et al: A worldwide survey of haplotype variation and linkage disequilibrium in the human genome. Nat Genet 38:1251–1260, 2006

Cook EH Jr: Genetics of autism. Child Adolesc Psychiatr Clin N Am 10:333–350, 2001

Cook EH Jr, Scherer SW: Copy-number variations associated with neuropsychiatric conditions. Nature 455:919–923, 2008

Craddock N, O'Donovan MC, Owen MJ: Genes for schizophrenia and bipolar disorder? Implications for psychiatric nosology. Schizophr Bull 32:9–16, 2006

Craddock N, Jones L, Jones IR, et al: Strong genetic evidence for a selective influence of GABA(A) receptors on a component of the bipolar disorder phenotype. Mol Psychiatry 2008 Jul 1 [Epub ahead of print]

Dalen P, Dahl ML, Ruiz ML, et al: 10-Hydroxylation of nortriptyline in white persons with 0, 1, 2, 3, and 13 functional CYP2D6 genes. Clin Pharmacol Ther 63:444–452, 1998

Daly MJ, Rioux JD, Schaffner SF, et al: High-resolution haplotype structure in the human genome. Nat Genet 29:229–232, 2001

de Bakker PI, Burtt NP, Graham RR, et al: Transferability of tag SNPs in genetic association studies in multiple populations. Nat Genet 38:1298–1303, 2006

Devlin B, Roeder K: Genomic control for association studies. Biometrics 55:997–1004, 1999

Dubertret C, Gorwood P, Ades J, et al: Meta-analysis of DRD3 gene and schizophrenia: ethnic heterogeneity and significant association in Caucasians. Am J Med Genet 81:318–322, 1998

Dudbridge F, Gusnanto A: Estimation of significance thresholds for genomewide association scans. Genet Epidemiol 32:227–234, 2008

Dudbridge F, Koeleman BP: Efficient computation of significance levels for multiple associations in large studies of correlated data, including genomewide association studies. Am J Hum Genet 75:424–435, 2004

Duman RS, Newton SS: Epigenetic marking and neuronal plasticity. Biol Psychiatry 62:1–3, 2007

Egan MF, Goldberg TE, Kolachana BS, et al: Effect of COMT Val108/158 Met genotype on frontal lobe function and risk for schizophrenia. Proc Natl Acad Sci U S A 98:6917–6922, 2001

ENCODE Project Consortium: Identification and analysis of functional elements in 1% of the human genome by the ENCODE pilot project. Nature 447:799–816, 2007

Fan JB, Zhang CS, Gu NF, et al: Catechol-O-methyltransferase gene Val/Met functional polymorphism and risk of schizophrenia: a large-scale association study plus meta-analysis. Biol Psychiatry 57:139–144, 2005

Ferreira MA, O'Donovan MC, Meng YA, et al: Collaborative genome-wide association analysis supports a role for ANK3 and CACNA1C in bipolar disorder. Nat Genet 2008 Aug 17 [Epub ahead of print]

Folstein SE, Rosen-Sheidley B: Genetics of autism: complex aetiology for a heterogeneous disorder. Nat Rev Genet 2:943–955, 2001

Franchini L, Serretti A, Gasperini M, et al: Familial concordance of fluvoxamine response as a tool for differentiating mood disorder pedigrees. J Psychiatr Res 32:255–259, 1998

Freeman WM, Hemby SE: Proteomics for protein expression profiling in neuroscience. Neurochem Res 29:1065–1081, 2004

Frudakis T, Thomas M, Gaskin Z, et al: Sequences associated with human iris pigmentation. Genetics 165:2071–2083, 2003

Gabriel SB, Schaffner SF, Nguyen H, et al: The structure of haplotype blocks in the human genome. Science 296:2225–2229, 2002

Gelernter J, Cubells JF, Kidd JR, et al: Population studies of polymorphisms of the serotonin transporter protein gene. Am J Med Genet 88:61–66, 1999

Gill M, Vallada H, Collier D, et al: A combined analysis of D22S278 marker alleles in affected sib-pairs: support for a susceptibility locus for schizophrenia at chromosome 22q12. Schizophrenia Collaborative Linkage Group (Chromosome 22). Am J Med Genet 67:40–45, 1996

Ginsberg SD, Elarova I, Ruben M, et al: Single-cell gene expression analysis: implications for neurodegenerative and neuropsychiatric disorders. Neurochem Res 29:1053–1064, 2004

Goldberg TE, Egan MF, Gscheidle T, et al: Executive subprocesses in working memory: relationship to catechol-O-methyltransferase Val158Met genotype and schizophrenia. Arch Gen Psychiatry 60:889–896, 2003

Gottesman II, Gould TD: The endophenotype concept in psychiatry: etymology and strategic intentions. Am J Psychiatry 160:636–645, 2003

Greenwood TA, Kelsoe JR: Promoter and intronic variants affect the transcriptional regulation of the human dopamine transporter gene. Genomics 82:511–520, 2003

Hamer D, Sirota L: Beware the chopsticks gene. Mol Psychiatry 5:11–13, 2000

Hasler G, Drevets WC, Manji HK, et al: Discovering endophenotypes for major depression. Neuropsychopharmacology 29:1765–1781, 2004

Hawley ME, Kidd KK: HAPLO: a program using the EM algorithm to estimate the frequencies of multi-site haplotypes. J Hered 86:409–411, 1995

Heils A, Teufel A, Petri S, et al: Allelic variation of human serotonin transporter gene expression. J Neurochem 66:2621–2624, 1996

Helgason A, Nicholson G, Stefansson K, et al: A reassessment of genetic diversity in Icelanders: strong evidence from multiple loci for relative homogeneity caused by genetic drift. Ann Hum Genet 67:281–297, 2003

Hettema JM, Neale MC, Kendler KS: A review and meta-analysis of the genetic epidemiology of anxiety disorders. Am J Psychiatry 158:1568–1578, 2001

Hirschhorn JN, Daly MJ: Genome-wide association studies for common diseases and complex traits. Nat Rev Genet 6:95–108, 2005

Horvath S, Xu X, Laird NM: The family based association test method: strategies for studying general genotype–phenotype associations. Eur J Hum Genet 9:301–306, 2001

Hu XZ, Lipsky RH, Zhu G, et al: Serotonin transporter promoter gain-of-function genotypes are linked to obsessive-compulsive disorder. Am J Hum Genet 78:815–826, 2006

Inoue-Murayama M, Adachi S, Mishima N, et al: Variation of variable number of tandem repeat sequences in the 3′-untranslated region of primate dopamine transporter genes that affects reporter gene expression. Neurosci Lett 334:206–210, 2002

International HapMap Consortium: The International HapMap Project. Nature 426:789–796, 2003

International Schizophrenia Consortium: Rare chromosomal deletions and duplications increase risk of schizophrenia. Nature 455:237–241, 2008

Johansson C, Jansson M, Linner L, et al: Genetics of affective disorders. Eur Neuropsychopharmacol 11:385–394, 2001

Johnson GC, Esposito L, Barratt BJ, et al: Haplotype tagging for the identification of common disease genes. Nat Genet 29:233–237, 2001

Jonsson EG, Flyckt L, Burgert E, et al: Dopamine D3 receptor gene Ser9Gly variant and schizophrenia: association study and meta-analysis. Psychiatr Genet 13:1–12, 2003

Jonsson EG, Kaiser R, Brockmoller J, et al: Meta-analysis of the dopamine D3 receptor gene (DRD3) Ser9Gly variant and schizophrenia. Psychiatr Genet 14:9–12, 2004

Joober R, Gauthier J, Lal S, et al: Catechol-O-methyltransferase Val-108/158-Met gene variants associated with performance on the Wisconsin Card Sorting Test. Arch Gen Psychiatry 59:662–663, 2002

Karayiorgou M, Gogos JA: The molecular genetics of the 22q11-associated schizophrenia. Brain Res Mol Brain Res 132:95–104, 2004

Karayiorgou M, Morris MA, Morrow B, et al: Schizophrenia susceptibility associated with interstitial deletions of chromosome 22q11. Proc Natl Acad Sci U S A 92:7612–7616, 1995

Kaufman J, Yang BZ, Douglas-Palumberi H, et al: Social supports and serotonin transporter gene moderate depression in maltreated children. Proc Natl Acad Sci U S A 101:17316–17321, 2004

Kawashima M, Tamiya G, Oka A, et al: Genomewide association analysis of human narcolepsy and a new resistance gene. Am J Hum Genet 79:252–263, 2006

Kelsoe JR, Spence MA, Loetscher E, et al: A genome survey indicates a possible susceptibility locus for bipolar disorder on chromosome 22. Proc Natl Acad Sci U S A 98:585–590, 2001

Kendler KS: Twin studies of psychiatric illness. Current status and future directions. Arch Gen Psychiatry 50:905–915, 1993

Kendler KS: Genetic epidemiology in psychiatry. Taking both genes and environment seriously. Arch Gen Psychiatry 52:895–899, 1995

Kendler KS: Twin studies of psychiatric illness: an update. Arch Gen Psychiatry 58:1005–1014, 2001

Kendler KS: "A gene for...": the nature of gene action in psychiatric disorders. Am J Psychiatry 162:1243–1252, 2005

Kendler KS, Gardner CO Jr: Twin studies of adult psychiatric and substance dependence disorders: are they biased by differences in the environmental experiences of monozygotic and dizygotic twins in childhood and adolescence? Psychol Med 28:625–633, 1998

Kendler KS, Greenspan RJ: The nature of genetic influences on behavior: lessons from "simpler" organisms. Am J Psychiatry 163:1683–1694, 2006

Kendler KS, Prescott CA: A population-based twin study of lifetime major depression in men and women. Arch Gen Psychiatry 56:39–44, 1999

Kendler KS, Walsh D: Gender and schizophrenia. Results of an epidemiologically based family study. Br J Psychiatry 167:184–192, 1995

Kendler KS, Neale MC, Kessler RC, et al: The genetic epidemiology of phobias in women. The interrelationship of agoraphobia, social phobia, situational phobia, and simple phobia. Arch Gen Psychiatry 49:273–281, 1992

Kendler KS, Kessler RC, Walters EE, et al: Stressful life events, genetic liability, and onset of an episode of major depression in women. Am J Psychiatry 152:833–842, 1995a

Kendler KS, Pedersen NL, Neale MC, et al: A pilot Swedish twin study of affective illness including hospital- and population-ascertained subsamples: results of model fitting. Behav Genet 25:217–232, 1995b

Kendler KS, Gardner CO, Neale MC, et al: Genetic risk factors for major depression in men and women: similar or different heritabilities and same or partly distinct genes? Psychol Med 31:605–616, 2001a

Kendler KS, Myers J, Prescott CA, et al: The genetic epidemiology of irrational fears and phobias in men. Arch Gen Psychiatry 58:257–265, 2001b

Kendler KS, Jacobson KC, Myers J, et al: Sex differences in genetic and environmental risk factors for irrational fears and phobias. Psychol Med 32:209–217, 2002

Kendler KS, Kuhn JW, Vittum J, et al: The interaction of stressful life events and a serotonin transporter polymorphism in the prediction of episodes of major depression: a replication. Arch Gen Psychiatry 62:529–535, 2005

Kendler KS, Gatz M, Gardner CO, et al: A Swedish national twin study of lifetime major depression. Am J Psychiatry 163:109–114, 2006

Kim S, Misra A: SNP genotyping: technologies and biomedical applications. Annu Rev Biomed Eng 9:289–320, 2007

Kirchheiner J, Brosen K, Dahl ML, et al: CYP2D6 and CYP2C19 genotype-based dose recommendations for antidepressants: a first step towards subpopulation-specific dosages. Acta Psychiatr Scand 104:173–192, 2001

Kirchheiner J, Nickchen K, Bauer M, et al: Pharmacogenetics of antidepressants and antipsychotics: the contribution of allelic variations to the phenotype of drug response. Mol Psychiatry 9:442–473, 2004

Kirov G, Zaharieva I, Georgieva L, et al: A genome-wide association study in 574 schizophrenia trios using DNA pooling. Mol Psychiatry 2008 Mar 11 [Epub ahead of print]

Knapp M, Seuchter SA, Baur MP: The haplotype-relative-risk (HRR) method for analysis of association in nuclear families. Am J Hum Genet 52:1085–1093, 1993

Kwok PY: High-throughput genotyping assay approaches. Pharmacogenomics 1:95–100, 2000

Lachman HM, Papolos DF, Saito T, et al: Human catechol-O-methyltransferase pharmacogenetics: description of a functional polymorphism and its potential application to neuropsychiatric disorders. Pharmacogenetics 6:243–250, 1996

Lachman HM, Kelsoe JR, Remick RA, et al: Linkage studies suggest a possible locus for bipolar disorder near the velo-cardio-facial syndrome region on chromosome 22. Am J Med Genet 74:121–128, 1997

Lander ES, Schork NJ: Genetic dissection of complex traits. Science 265:2037–2048, 1994

Lander ES, Linton LM, Birren B, et al: Initial sequencing and analysis of the human genome. Nature 409:860–921, 2001

Lencz T, Morgan TV, Athanasiou M, et al: Converging evidence for a pseudoautosomal cytokine receptor gene locus in schizophrenia. Mol Psychiatry 12:572–580, 2007

Lesch KP, Bengel D, Heils A, et al: Association of anxiety-related traits with a polymorphism in the serotonin transporter gene regulatory region. Science 274:1527–1531, 1996

Levinson DF, Levinson MD, Segurado R, et al: Genome scan meta-analysis of schizophrenia and bipolar disorder, part I: methods and power analysis. Am J Hum Genet 73:17–33, 2003

Lewis CM, Levinson DF, Wise LH, et al: Genome scan meta-analysis of schizophrenia and bipolar disorder, part II: schizophrenia. Am J Hum Genet 73:34–48, 2003

Li MD: The genetics of smoking related behavior: a brief review. Am J Med Sci 326:168–173, 2003

Long JC, Williams RC, Urbanek M: An E-M algorithm and testing strategy for multiple-locus haplotypes. Am J Hum Genet 56:799–810, 1995

Lotta T, Vidgren J, Tilgmann C, et al: Kinetics of human soluble and membrane-bound catechol-O-methyltransferase: a revised mechanism and description of the thermolabile variant of the enzyme. Biochemistry 34:4202–4210, 1995

Marshall CR, Noor A, Vincent JB, et al: Structural variation of chromosomes in autism spectrum disorder. Am J Hum Genet 82:477–488, 2008

Martin CL, Ledbetter DH: Autism and cytogenetic abnormalities: solving autism one chromosome at a time. Curr Psychiatry Rep 9:141–147, 2007

Martinez D, Gelernter J, Abi-Dargham A, et al: The variable number of tandem repeats polymorphism of the dopamine transporter gene is not associated with significant change in dopamine transporter phenotype in humans. Neuropsychopharmacology 24:553–560, 2001

Mattay VS, Goldberg TE, Fera F, et al: Catechol O-methyltransferase val158-met genotype and individual variation in the brain response to amphetamine. Proc Natl Acad Sci U S A 100:6186–6191, 2003

McGuffin P, Rijsdijk F, Andrew M, et al: The heritability of bipolar affective disorder and the genetic relationship to unipolar depression. Arch Gen Psychiatry 60:497–502, 2003

McMahon FJ, Buervenich S, Charney D, et al: Variation in the gene encoding the serotonin 2A receptor is associated with outcome of antidepressant treatment. Am J Hum Genet 78:804–814, 2006

Mill J, Asherson P, Browes C, et al: Expression of the dopamine transporter gene is regulated by the 3′ UTR VNTR: evidence from brain and lymphocytes using quantitative RT-PCR. Am J Med Genet 114:975–979, 2002

Mill J, Asherson P, Craig I, et al: Transient expression analysis of allelic variants of a VNTR in the dopamine transporter gene (DAT1). BMC Genet 6:3, 2005

Millar JK, Wilson-Annan JC, Anderson S, et al: Disruption of two novel genes by a translocation co-segregating with schizophrenia. Hum Mol Genet 9:1415–1423, 2000

Millar JK, Christie S, Anderson S, et al: Genomic structure and localisation within a linkage hotspot of Disrupted In Schizophrenia 1, a gene disrupted by a translocation segregating with schizophrenia. Mol Psychiatry 6:173–178, 2001

Mirnics K, Levitt P, Lewis DA: Critical appraisal of DNA microarrays in psychiatric genomics. Biol Psychiatry 60:163–176, 2006

Montana G, Pritchard JK: Statistical tests for admixture mapping with case-control and cases-only data. Am J Hum Genet 75:771–789, 2004

Moskvina V, Craddock N, Holmans P, et al: Gene-wide analyses of genome-wide association data sets: evidence for multiple common risk alleles for schizophrenia and bipolar disorder and for overlap in genetic risk. Mol Psychiatry 2008 Dec 9 [Epub ahead of print]

Nadeau JH, Lee C: Genetics: copies count. Nature 439:798–799, 2006

Nakamura M, Ueno S, Sano A, et al: The human serotonin transporter gene linked polymorphism (5-HTTLPR) shows ten novel allelic variants. Mol Psychiatry 5:32–38, 2000

Need AC, Goldstein DB: Genome-wide tagging for everyone. Nat Genet 38:1227–1228, 2006

Newton SS, Duman RS: Chromatin remodeling: a novel mechanism of psychotropic drug action. Mol Pharmacol 70:440–443, 2006

Nicholls RD, Knepper JL: Genome organization, function, and imprinting in Prader-Willi and Angelman syndromes. Annu Rev Genomics Hum Genet 2:153–175, 2001

Niculescu AB 3rd, Segal DS, Kuczenski R, et al: Identifying a series of candidate genes for mania and psychosis: a convergent functional genomics approach. Physiol Genomics 4:83–91, 2000

Nyholt DR: A simple correction for multiple testing for single-nucleotide polymorphisms in linkage disequilibrium with each other. Am J Hum Genet 74:765–769, 2004

O'Donovan MC, Craddock N, Norton N, et al: Identification of loci associated with schizophrenia by genome-wide association and follow-up. Nat Genet 2008 Jul 30 [Epub ahead of print]

O'Reilly RL, Bogue L, Singh SM: Pharmacogenetic response to antidepressants in a multicase family with affective disorder. Biol Psychiatry 36:467–471, 1994

Pare CM, Rees L, Sainsbury MJ: Differentiation of two genetically specific types of depression by the response to anti-depressants. Lancet 2(7270):1340–1343, 1962

Parra EJ, Marcini A, Akey J, et al: Estimating African American admixture proportions by use of population-specific alleles. Am J Hum Genet 63:1839–1851, 1998

Parra EJ, Kittles RA, Argyropoulos G, et al: Ancestral proportions and admixture dynamics in geographically defined African Americans living in South Carolina. Am J Phys Anthropol 114:18–29, 2001

Parsey RV, Hastings RS, Oquendo MA, et al: Effect of a triallelic functional polymorphism of the serotonin-transporter-linked promoter region on expression of serotonin transporter in the human brain. Am J Psychiatry 163:48–51, 2006

Patil N, Berno AJ, Hinds DA, et al: Blocks of limited haplotype diversity revealed by high-resolution scanning of human chromosome 21. Science 294:1719–1723, 2001

Phillips MS, Lawrence R, Sachidanandam R, et al: Chromosome-wide distribution of haplotype blocks and the role of recombination hot spots. Nat Genet 33:382–387, 2003

Pickard BS, Millar JK, Porteous DJ, et al: Cytogenetics and gene discovery in psychiatric disorders. Pharmacogenomics J 5:81–88, 2005

Plomin R, Kosslyn SM: Genes, brain and cognition. Nat Neurosci 4:1153–1154, 2001

Porteous DJ, Thomson P, Brandon NJ, et al: The genetics and biology of DISC1—an emerging role in psychosis and cognition. Biol Psychiatry 60:123–131, 2006

Prescott CA, Kendler KS: Influence of ascertainment strategy on finding sex differences in genetic estimates from twin studies of alcoholism. Am J Med Genet 96:754–761, 2000

Prescott CA, Aggen SH, Kendler KS: Sex-specific genetic influences on the comorbidity of alcoholism and major depression in a population-based sample of US twins. Arch Gen Psychiatry 57:803–811, 2000

Pritchard JK, Stephens M, Donnelly P: Inference of population structure using multilocus genotype data. Genetics 155:945–959, 2000

Psychiatric GWAS Consortium Steering Committee: A framework for interpreting genome-wide association studies of psychiatric disorders. Mol Psychiatry 14:10–17, 2009

Pulver AE, Nestadt G, Goldberg R, et al: Psychotic illness in patients diagnosed with velo-cardio-facial syndrome and their relatives. J Nerv Ment Dis 182:476–478, 1994

Pulver AE, Mulle J, Nestadt G, et al: Genetic heterogeneity in schizophrenia: stratification of genome scan data using cosegregating related phenotypes. Mol Psychiatry 5:650–653, 2000

Redon R, Ishikawa S, Fitch KR, et al: Global variation in copy number in the human genome. Nature 444:444–454, 2006

Reich DE, Cargill M, Bolk S, et al: Linkage disequilibrium in the human genome. Nature 411:199–204, 2001

Reich DE, Schaffner SF, Daly MJ, et al: Human genome sequence variation and the influence of gene history, mutation and recombination. Nat Genet 32:135–142, 2002

Rhee SH, Waldman ID: Genetic and environmental influences on antisocial behavior: a meta-analysis of twin and adoption studies. Psychol Bull 128:490–529, 2002

Risch N: Genetic linkage and complex diseases, with special reference to psychiatric disorders. Genet Epidemiol 7:3–16; discussion 17–45, 1990a

Risch N: Linkage strategies for genetically complex traits, I: multilocus models. Am J Hum Genet 46:222–228, 1990b

Risch N, Merikangas K: The future of genetic studies of complex human diseases. Science 273:1516–1517, 1996

Rosenberg NA, Pritchard JK, Weber JL, et al: Genetic structure of human populations. Science 298:2381–2385, 2002

Rutter M: Genetic studies of autism: from the 1970s into the millennium. J Abnorm Child Psychol 28:3–14, 2000

Sachidanandam R, Weissman D, Schmidt SC, et al: A map of human genome sequence variation containing 1.42 million single nucleotide polymorphisms. Nature 409:928–933, 2001

Schulze TG, Detera-Wadleigh SD, Akula N, et al: Two variants in Ankyrin 3 (ANK3) are independent genetic risk factors for bipolar disorder. Mol Psychiatry 2008 Dec 16 [Epub ahead of print]

Schuster SC: Next-generation sequencing transforms today's biology. Nat Methods 5(1):16–18, 2008

Seaman SR, Muller-Myshok B: Rapid simulation of P values for product methods and multiple-testing adjustments in association studies. Am J Hum Genet 76:399–408, 2005

Sebat J, Lakshmi B, Troge J, et al: Large-scale copy number polymorphism in the human genome. Science 305:525–528, 2004

Sebat J, Lakshmi B, Malhotra D, et al: Strong association of de novo copy number mutations with autism. Science 316:445–449, 2007

Segurado R, Detera-Wadleigh SD, Levinson DF, et al: Genome scan meta-analysis of schizophrenia and bipolar disorder, part III: bipolar disorder. Am J Hum Genet 73:49–62, 2003

Serretti A, Franchini L, Gasperini M, et al: Mode of inheritance in mood disorder families according to fluvoxamine response. Acta Psychiatr Scand 98:443–450, 1998

Serretti A, Kato M, De Ronchi D, et al: Meta-analysis of serotonin transporter gene promoter polymorphism (5-HTTLPR) association with selective serotonin reuptake inhibitor efficacy in depressed patients. Mol Psychiatry 12:247–257, 2007

Shifman S, Darvasi A: The value of isolated populations. Nat Genet 28:309–310, 2001

Shifman S, Bronstein M, Sternfeld M, et al: A highly significant association between a COMT haplotype and schizophrenia. Am J Hum Genet 71:1296–1302, 2002

Shifman S, Johannesson M, Bronstein M, et al: Genome-wide association identifies a common variant in the reelin gene that increases the risk of schizophrenia only in women. PLoS Genet 4(2):e28, 2008

Shprintzen RJ, Goldberg R, Golding-Kushner KJ, et al: Late-onset psychosis in the velo-cardio-facial syndrome. Am J Med Genet 42:141–142, 1992

Sjoberg RL, Nilsson KW, Nordquist N, et al: Development of depression: sex and the interaction between environment and a promoter polymorphism of the serotonin transporter gene. Int J Neuropsychopharmacol 9:443–449, 2006

Sklar P, Smoller JW, Fan J, et al: Whole-genome association study of bipolar disorder. Mol Psychiatry 13:558–569, 2008

Sobell JL, Mikesell MJ, McMurray CT: Genetics and etiopathophysiology of schizophrenia. Mayo Clin Proc 77:1068–1082, 2002

Spielman RS, McGinnis RE, Ewens WJ: Transmission test for linkage disequilibrium: the insulin gene region and insulin-dependent diabetes mellitus (IDDM). Am J Hum Genet 52:506–516, 1993

St. Clair D: Copy number variation and schizophrenia. Schizophr Bull 35:9–12, 2009

St. Clair D, Blackwood D, Muir W, et al: Association within a family of a balanced autosomal translocation with major mental illness. Lancet 336:13–16, 1990

Stefansson H, Rujescu D, Cichon S, et al: Large recurrent microdeletions associated with schizophrenia. Nature 455:232–236, 2008

Stranger BE, Forrest MS, Dunning M, et al: Relative impact of nucleotide and copy number variation on gene expression phenotypes. Science 315:848–853, 2007

Sullivan PF, Neale MC, Kendler KS: Genetic epidemiology of major depression: review and meta-analysis. Am J Psychiatry 157:1552–1562, 2000

Sullivan PF, Kendler KS, Neale MC: Schizophrenia as a complex trait: evidence from a meta-analysis of twin studies. Arch Gen Psychiatry 60:1187–1192, 2003

Sullivan PF, de Geus EJ, Willemsen G, et al: Genome-wide association for major depressive disorder: a possible role for the presynaptic protein piccolo. Mol Psychiatry 2008a Dec 9 [Epub ahead of print]

Sullivan PF, Lin D, Tzeng JY, et al: Genomewide association for schizophrenia in the CATIE study: results of stage 1. Mol Psychiatry 13:570–584, 2008b

Surtees PG, Wainwright NW, Willis-Owen SA, et al: Social adversity, the serotonin transporter (5-HTTLPR) polymorphism and major depressive disorder. Biol Psychiatry 59:224–229, 2006

Sutcliffe JS, Delahanty RJ, Prasad HC, et al: Allelic heterogeneity at the serotonin transporter locus (SLC6A4) confers susceptibility to autism and rigid-compulsive behaviors. Am J Hum Genet 77:265–279, 2005

Sybert VP, McCauley E: Turner's syndrome. N Engl J Med 351:1227–1238, 2004

Szatmari P, Paterson AD, Zwaigenbaum L, et al: Mapping autism risk loci using genetic linkage and chromosomal rearrangements. Autism Genome Project Consortium. Nat Genet 39:319–328, 2007

Tamiya G, Shinya M, Imanishi T, et al: Whole genome association study of rheumatoid arthritis using 27 039 microsatellites. Hum Mol Genet 14:2305–2321, 2005

Tannu NS, Hemby SE: Methods for proteomics in neuroscience. Prog Brain Res 158:41–82, 2006

Tienari PJ, Wynne LC: Adoption studies of schizophrenia. Ann Med 26:233–237, 1994

Tienari P, Wynne LC, Sorri A, et al: Genotype-environment interaction in schizophrenia-spectrum disorder: long-term follow-up study of Finnish adoptees. Br J Psychiatry 184:216–222, 2004

Turecki G, Grof P, Grof E, et al: Mapping susceptibility genes for bipolar disorder: a pharmacogenetic approach based on excellent response to lithium. Mol Psychiatry 6:570–578, 2001

Tyndale RF: Genetics of alcohol and tobacco use in humans. Ann Med 35:94–121, 2003

van Dyck CH, Malison RT, Jacobsen LK, et al: Increased dopamine transporter availability associated with the 9-repeat allele of the SLC6A3 gene. J Nucl Med 46:745–751, 2005

van Grootheest DS, Cath DC, Beekman AT, et al: Twin studies on obsessive-compulsive disorder: a review. Twin Res Hum Genet 8:450–458, 2005

Van Tol HH, Wu CM, Guan HC, et al: Multiple dopamine D4 receptor variants in the human population. Nature 358:149–152, 1992

Vandenbergh DJ, Persico AM, Hawkins AL, et al: Human dopamine transporter gene (DAT1) maps to chromosome 5p15.3 and displays a VNTR. Genomics 14:1104–1106, 1992

VanNess SH, Owens MJ, Kilts CD: The variable number of tandem repeats element in DAT1 regulates in vitro dopamine transporter density. BMC Genet 6:55, 2005

Veenstra-VanderWeele J, Cook EH Jr: Molecular genetics of autism spectrum disorder. Mol Psychiatry 9:819–832, 2004

Venter JC, Adams MD, Myers EW, et al: The sequence of the human genome. Science 291:1304–1351, 2001

Visootsak J, Sherman S: Neuropsychiatric and behavioral aspects of trisomy 21. Curr Psychiatry Rep 9:135–140, 2007

Vogels A, Fryns JP: The Prader-Willi syndrome and the Angelman syndrome. Genet Couns 13:385–396, 2002

Wang H, Thomas DC, Pe'er I, et al: Optimal two-stage genotyping designs for genome-wide association scans. Genet Epidemiol 30:356–368, 2006

Wang WY, Barratt BJ, Clayton DG, et al: Genome-wide association studies: theoretical and practical concerns. Nat Rev Genet 6:109–118, 2005

Weinshilboum R: Inheritance and drug response. N Engl J Med 348:529–537, 2003

Weiss LA, Shen Y, Korn JM, et al: Association between microdeletion and microduplication at 16p11.2 and autism. N Engl J Med 358:667–675, 2008

Wellcome Trust Case Control Consortium: Genome-wide association study of 14,000 cases of seven common diseases and 3,000 shared controls. Nature 447:661–678, 2007

Wilhelm K, Mitchell PB, Niven H, et al: Life events, first depression onset and the serotonin transporter gene. Br J Psychiatry 188:210–215, 2006

Williams J, Spurlock G, Holmans P, et al: A meta-analysis and transmission disequilibrium study of association between the dopamine D3 receptor gene and schizophrenia. Mol Psychiatry 3:141–149, 1998

World Health Organization: The ICD-10 Classification of Mental and Behavioural Disorders: Clinical Descriptions and Diagnostic Guidelines. Geneva, World Health Organization, 1992

Zalsman G, Huang YY, Oquendo MA, et al: Association of a triallelic serotonin transporter gene promoter region (5-HTTLPR) polymorphism with stressful life events and severity of depression. Am J Psychiatry 163:1588–1593, 2006

Zubenko GS, Hughes HB 3rd, Maher BS, et al: Genetic linkage of region containing the CREB1 gene to depressive disorders in women from families with recurrent, early onset, major depression. Am J Med Genet 114:980–987, 2002

Zwick ME, Cutler DJ, Chakravarti A: Patterns of genetic variation in Mendelian and complex traits. Annu Rev Genomics Hum Genet 1:387–407, 2000

CHAPTER 4

Chemical Neuroanatomy of the Primate Brain

Darlene S. Melchitzky, M.S.

David A. Lewis, M.D.

Other chapters in this textbook address the questions of how psychotropic medications affect the brain to reduce the severity of the clinical features and symptoms of psychiatric disorders and to produce the side effects that frequently accompany their administration. Appropriately, much attention has been directed toward the neurotransmitter systems that are the targets of these medications. A potential consequence of this emphasis is the idea, in its simplest form, that an excess or deficit in the functional activity of a given neurotransmitter is the pathophysiological basis for the clinical features of interest. Although variants of this view have been very useful in motivating investigations of the molecular underpinnings and biochemical features of neurotransmitter systems and in spurring the development of novel psychopharmacological agents that influence these systems, in the extreme case this perspective tends to consider a given psychiatric disorder as the consequence *solely* of the postulated disturbance in a neurotransmitter system.

In addition to this limited conceptual perspective, neurotransmitter-based views of psychiatric disorders sometimes seem to attribute behavioral, emotional, or cognitive functions to neurotransmitters instead of explicitly recognizing that neurotransmitters have defined actions on receptors, whereas behaviors, emotions, and cognitive abilities represent emergent properties of the integrated activity of large networks of neurons. This view of psychiatric disorders was influenced, at least in part, by extrapolations from earlier successes in the study of Parkinson's disease, which was then viewed as a single-neurotransmitter (i.e., dopamine) disease resulting from a localized neuropathology (e.g., cell death in the substantia nigra).

In recent years, however, greater attention has been given to neural circuitry–based views of psychiatric disorders that reflect a fuller appreciation of the fact that neurotransmitters act in an anatomically constrained fashion to produce specific biochemical effects at the cellular level and that the localization of function(s) is a consequence of the flow of information processing through the neural circuits formed by neurotransmitter systems (Lewis 2002). Consequently, the goal of this chapter is to provide a brief overview of the major neurotransmitter systems of the primate brain, with reference to the rodent brain where appropriate, and to consider these systems within the context of the anatomical pathways in which they participate.

Neuroanatomy of the Dopamine System

The precursor for dopamine (DA), and all catecholamines, is the amino acid tyrosine. The rate-limiting step in DA synthesis is the conversion of tyrosine to L-dihydroxyphenylalanine (L-dopa) by the enzyme tyrosine hydroxylase. DA is then formed by decarboxylation of L-dopa via the enzyme L-aromatic amino acid decarboxylase. DA neurotransmission is terminated through the actions of the dopamine transporter (DAT) (Jaber et al. 1997), although in some areas where the amount of DAT is low, metabolism also plays a role. The DAT accomplishes this task by transporting DA back into the nerve terminal. DA, and all catecholamines, can also be deactivated by degradation via the enzymes monoamine oxidase (MAO) and catechol-O-methyltransferase (COMT) (Cooper et al. 1996). MAO metabolizes DA into its aldehyde metabolite, and COMT breaks down DA to 3-methoxytyramine. The role of COMT in regulating DA levels appears to depend on brain region (see subsection below titled "Projection Sites") as well as on the presence of two isoforms of the enzyme created by a valine-for-methionine substitution at codon 108/105 in the COMT gene (Chen et al. 2004).

Antibodies against DA, tyrosine hydroxylase, and DAT have all been used to map the locations of DA cell bodies, dendrites, and axons (Akil and Lewis 1993; Gaspar et al. 1989; Lewis et al. 1988a, 2001; Williams and Goldman-Rakic 1993). A detailed description of the DA system in the primate brain can be found in Lewis and Sesack (1997).

Cell Locations

The majority of DA cells, which synthesize approximately three-quarters of all the DA in the brain, are located in the anterior midbrain or mesencephalon (Figure 4–1). Although the mesencephalic DA neurons of the primate brain have been parcellated into distinct nuclei, most of these cell groups are interconnected by regions that contain a mixture of cell bodies with different morphological characteristics. These features make it difficult to draw precise boundaries between nuclei, and most investigators agree that DA neurons form a continuum (Moore and Bloom 1978) that extends caudally from the mammillary bodies to the pedunculopontine nucleus.

The substantia nigra contains the majority of DA neurons in the primate brain and is subdivided into two main regions, the substantia nigra pars compacta and the substantia nigra pars reticulata (Figure 4–2) (Arsenault et al. 1988; Felten and Sladek 1983). The DA neurons in the substantia nigra pars compacta form a dense zone located in the dorsal region of the substantia nigra. Some DA neurons are located along the dorsal portion of the substantia nigra pars compacta in an area referred to as the pars dorsalis (Poirier et al. 1983). The neurons of the monkey sub-

stantia nigra pars compacta are considered to correspond to the A9 region in the rodent (Dahlström and Fuxe 1964). The caudal substantia nigra pars compacta has distinct columns of cells that extend deeply into the ventrally located substantia nigra pars reticulata (Haber and Fudge 1997). Most neurons within the substantia nigra pars reticulata do not contain DA and use γ-aminobutyric acid (GABA) as a neurotransmitter (Smith et al. 1987).

The neurons within these subdivisions of the substantia nigra differ in their expression of the messenger RNAs (mRNAs) for both tyrosine hydroxylase and DAT. For example, the substantia nigra pars compacta neurons have higher levels of both tyrosine hydroxylase and DAT mRNAs than do cells in the substantia nigra pars dorsalis (Haber et al. 1995). This difference is of interest, given that the neurons in the substantia nigra pars compacta and substantia nigra dorsalis project to different brain regions (see subsection below titled "Projection Sites"). Interestingly, tyrosine hydroxylase mRNA levels in the substantia nigra pars dorsalis and ventral cell columns are associated with the COMT genotype. Specifically, individuals with the val/val genotype express higher levels of tyrosine hydroxylase mRNA than do individuals with the val/met genotype (Akil et al. 2003).

The ventral tegmental area, which is located immediately medial to the substantia nigra, contains DA neurons that are smaller and less densely packed than those in the substantia nigra pars compacta (Arsenault et al. 1988). This group of neurons corresponds to the A10 group of Dahlström and Fuxe (1964), but the boundaries of this region are less well developed in primates than in rodents. As in the substantia nigra dorsalis, DA neurons in the ventral tegmental area contain lower levels of both tyrosine hydroxylase and DAT mRNA than do cells in the substantia nigra pars compacta (Haber et al. 1995).

A third group of DA neurons, the retrorubral area, resides in the caudal midbrain at the level of the medial lemniscus (Arsenault et al. 1988). This group of neurons corresponds to the A8 group of Dahlström and Fuxe (1964). The DA neurons in the retrorubral area are smaller and more dispersed than those located in the substantia nigra (Arsenault et al. 1988).

Several hypothalamic nuclei, including the arcuate, periventricular, paraventricular, and supraoptic nuclei, also contain DA neurons (Arsenault et al. 1988). These DA cell groups correspond to the A11–A15 groups of Dahlström and Fuxe (1964). The DA neurons located within the hypothalamus differ from those located in the mesencephalon in at least two ways. First, the projections of hypothalamic DA neurons are much shorter, extending

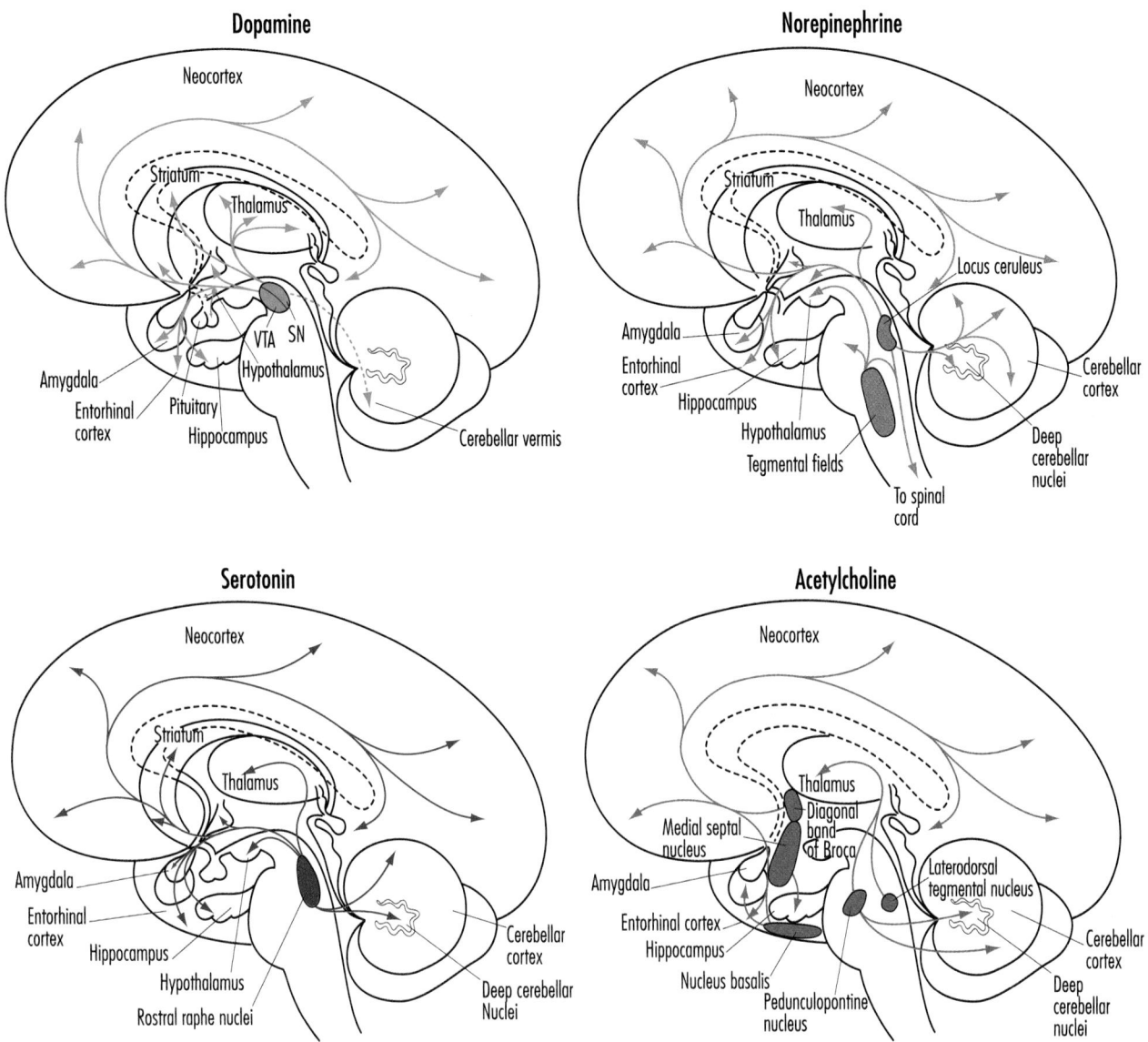

FIGURE 4–1. Projections of dopamine-, norepinephrine-, serotonin-, and acetylcholine-containing neurons in the human brain.

SN = substantia nigra; VTA = ventral tegmental area.
Source. Adapted from Heimer 1995.

only to the intermediate lobe of the pituitary and the median eminence. Second, unlike the DA neurons in the substantia nigra, ventral tegmental area, and retrorubral area, most of the DA neurons in the hypothalamus do not express the DAT protein (Ciliax et al. 1995, 1999).

Interestingly, recent studies using large-scale gene expression profiling techniques have revealed differences in gene expression across the various groups of DA neurons (Greene 2006). For example, genes involved in energy metabolism and mitochondria are more highly expressed in neurons of the substantia nigra than in neurons of the

ventral tegmental area (Chung et al. 2005). This suggests that DA neurons in the substantia nigra may rely more on oxidative energy metabolism, are under greater metabolic stress, and thus may be more vulnerable to degeneration, such as in Parkinson's disease (Greene et al. 2005).

Projection Sites

The striatum, including the caudate, putamen, and nucleus accumbens, is a major projection target of the DA neurons in the substantia nigra (see Figure 4–2). Indeed,

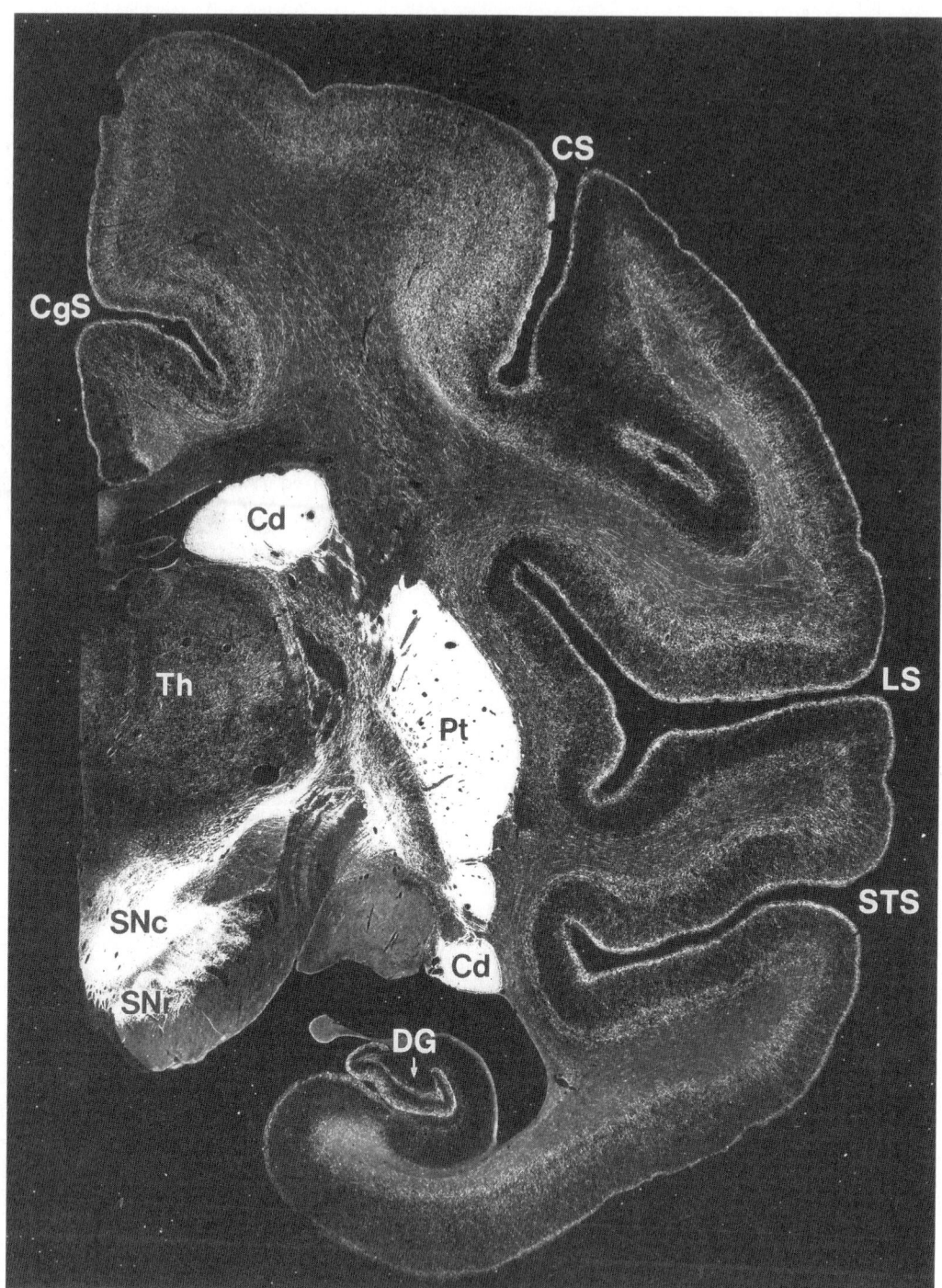

FIGURE 4–2. Low-power darkfield photomicrograph of a coronal section through macaque monkey brain processed for dopamine transporter (DAT) immunoreactivity.

Consistent with its localization to dopaminergic structures, intense DAT immunoreactivity (DAT-IR) is evident in the substantia nigra pars compacta (SNc) and pars reticulata (SNr), as well as in the nigrostriatal projection to the caudate (Cd) and putamen (Pt) nuclei. Also note the marked differences in density of DAT-IR axons across the cortical regions on this section. DAT-IR axons are also present in areas not traditionally thought to contain DA axons, such as the dentate gyrus (DG) and the thalamus (Th). Scale bar = 2.0 mm. CgS = cingulate sulcus; CS = central sulcus; LS = lateral sulcus; STS = superior temporal sulcus.

Source.   Reprinted from Lewis DA, Melchitzky DS, Sesack SR, et al: "Dopamine Transporter Immunoreactivity in Monkey Cerebral Cortex: Regional, Laminar and Ultrastructural Localization." *Journal of Comparative Neurology* 432:119–138, 2001. Copyright 2001, Wiley. Used with permission.

this nigrostriatal projection is the largest DA system projection in the brain. Specifically, DA neurons in the substantia nigra pars compacta provide the majority of this projection, with cells in the substantia nigra dorsalis, ventral tegmental area, and retrorubral area furnishing minor projections to the striatum (Haber and Fudge 1997).

The cerebral cortex is another major projection site of DA neurons, and this projection arises from cells within the substantia nigra dorsalis, ventral tegmental area, and retrorubral area (Lewis et al. 1988b; Williams and Goldman-Rakic 1998). Although early studies suggested that DA projections to the neocortex in the primate were restricted to frontal and temporal regions, it has since been demonstrated that essentially all cortical regions in the primate are innervated by DA axons, although the density of innervation differs substantially across regions (Gaspar et al. 1989; Lewis et al. 1987, 2001; Williams and Goldman-Rakic 1993). In both nonhuman primate and human brains, the motor and premotor cortices, as well as certain areas of the prefrontal (Figure 4–3) and posterior parietal cortices, contain a high density of DA axons. In these areas, DA axons are present in all cortical layers. In the prefrontal cortex, areas 9 and 24 contain the greatest density of DA axons; areas 11, 12, 13, and 25 have an intermediate density; and areas 10 and 46 have the lowest density of DA axons (Figure 4–4). The presence of dense DA innervation in some areas of prefrontal cortex and the well-documented deficits in prefrontal cortical activity in schizophrenia suggest that there may be an abnormality in the DA axons in the prefrontal cortex of patients with schizophrenia. Indeed, postmortem studies indicate that the total lengths of tyrosine hydroxylase- and DAT-containing axons are significantly reduced in the dorsolateral prefrontal cortex of patients with schizophrenia (Akil et al. 1999). These findings suggest that the cortical DA signal might be diminished in schizophrenia as a result of reduced content of tyrosine hydroxylase per axon, reduced density of DA axons, or both. Other cortical regions, such as association areas in the temporal cortex within the lateral sulcus (see Figure 4–2), contain intermediate levels of DA axons, whereas primary sensory cortices (e.g., visual cortex) generally have low densities of DA axons (Lewis et al. 1987, 2001). Furthermore, DA axons are present only in layers 1 and 6 in the sparsely innervated sensory regions and in layers 1–3 and 5–6 in the regions that have a moderate density of DA axons.

The regional and laminar distributions of DA axons in the primate cerebral cortex differ from those present in the rodent. For example, DA innervation of the rodent cortex is principally restricted to the medial prefrontal and anterior cingulate regions (Berger et al. 1991), in contrast to the widespread DA innervation of the primate cerebral cortex (Lewis et al. 1987, 2001). This expansion of cortical DA innervation in the primate correlates with an increased number of neurons in the ventral mesencephalon (Bjorklund and Dunnett 2007). At the laminar level, DA axons are denser in layers 1–3 in the primate (see Figure 4–3), whereas DA axons in the rodent are confined to layers 5–6. The expansion of DA innervation in primates to additional areas, such as sensory and motor cortices, suggests that DA has additional functions, such as the processing of sensorimotor information, in the human brain, which may be important in movement disorders like Parkinson's disease (Berger et al. 1991).

Ultrastructural investigations of DA-containing axon terminals in the primate cortex have revealed that many do not form conventional synaptic specializations (Beaudet and Descarries 1984; Smiley and Goldman-Rakic 1993). In addition, DA receptors have been identified on spines that are not in direct contact with DA-containing axon terminals (Smiley et al. 1994), and the DA transporter has been localized at a distance from synaptic sites (Lewis et al. 2001; Sesack et al. 1998). For example, in rodent and primate prefrontal cortex, the DA transporter is localized in preterminal axons as opposed to axon terminals (where it is heavily localized in the striatum), limiting the ability of the transporter to regulate extracellular DA levels. In association with this difference, COMT appears to have a more significant role in regulating DA levels in the prefrontal cortex than in subcortical structures (Tunbridge et al. 2004). Polymorphisms in the *COMT* gene lead to protein products with marked differences in enzymatic activity (Chen et al. 2004). Thus, the COMT genotype determines DA levels in the prefrontal cortex and may be important in functions in which the level of DA activity at D_1 receptors plays a role (e.g., working memory). Indeed, individuals with the *COMT* Val allele (high enzyme activity, low DA levels) perform poorly on working memory tasks compared with individuals with the *COMT* Met allele (low enzyme activity, high DA levels) (Egan et al. 2001), and it has been suggested that the COMT genotype is important in the etiology and pathogenesis of schizophrenia (Lewandowski 2007).

Besides the striatum, other subcortical structures, such as the amygdala and the hippocampus, receive projections from DA neurons. In the amygdala, DA axons originating from the ventral tegmental area and substantia nigra dorsalis are predominantly found in the central, basal, and lateral nuclei (Ciliax et al. 1999). In rodents, a projection from the ventral tegmental area and substantia

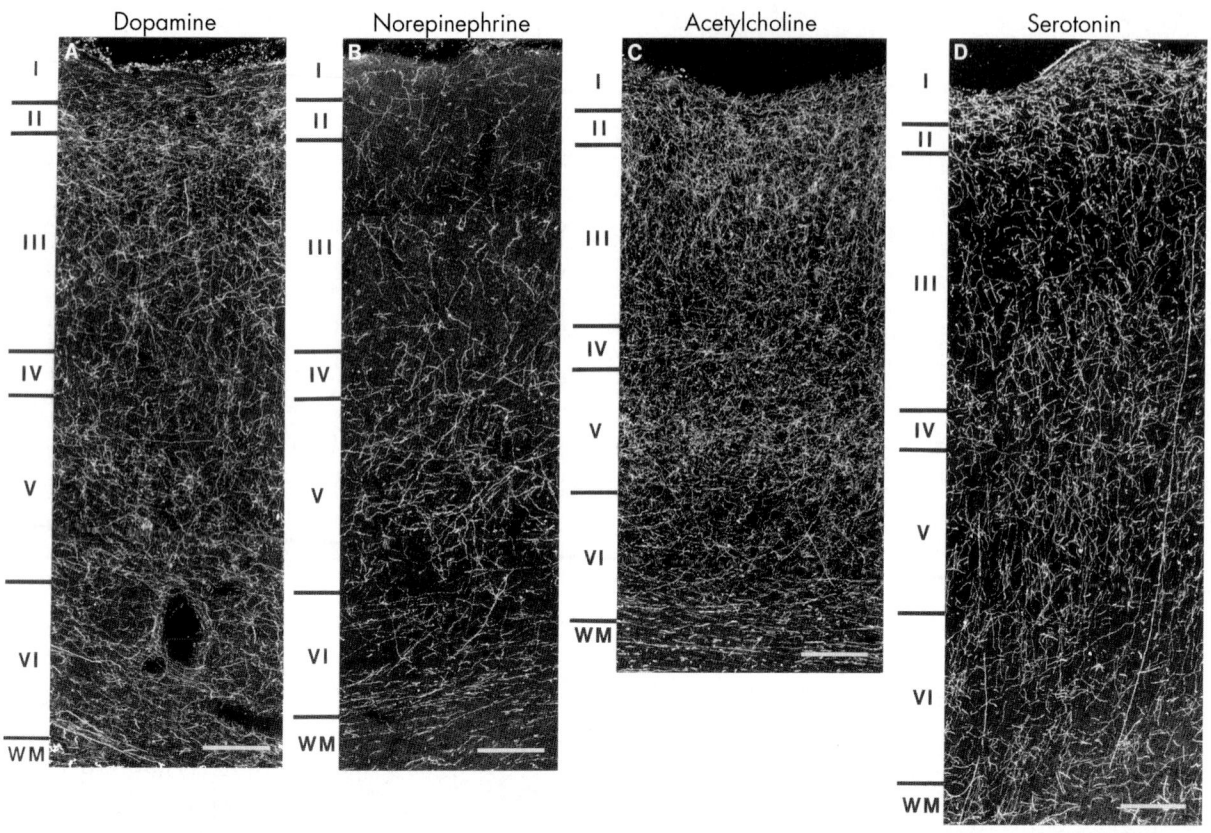

FIGURE 4–3.   Darkfield photomicrographs of (A) tyrosine hydroxylase–, (B) dopamine β-hydroxylase–, (C) choline acetyltransferase–, and (D) serotonin-immunoreactive axons in area 9 of macaque monkey prefrontal cortex.

Note the differences in relative density and the distinctive laminar distribution of each afferent system. Scale bar = 200 μm. WM = white matter.

Source.   Adapted from Lewis et al. 1992.

nigra pars compacta to the hippocampus has been demonstrated. A similar projection has not been reported in primates. However, tyrosine hydroxylase- and DAT-immunoreactive axons have been localized only to the dentate gyrus of the hippocampus in the macaque monkey (Lewis et al. 2001; Samson et al. 1990). DA axons have also been identified in the primate thalamus (Melchitzky and Lewis 2001; Sanchez-Gonzalez et al. 2005) and cerebellum (Melchitzky and Lewis 2000), two brain regions traditionally thought not to receive DA innervation (Moore and Bloom 1978; Steriade et al. 1997). In the thalamus, the mediodorsal, midline, lateral posterior, and ventral lateral nuclei contain the greatest density of DA axons (Melchitzky and Lewis 2001; Sanchez-Gonzalez et al. 2005). Within the mediodorsal nucleus, the ventrolateral portion, which includes both the densocellular and the parvocellular subdivisions, has the highest density of DAT-immunoreactive axons (Figure 4–5). The DA projections to the thalamus arise from DA neurons in the

substantia nigra pars dorsalis, ventral tegmental area, and retrorubral area (Melchitzky et al. 2006; Sanchez-Gonzalez et al. 2005) as well as from hypothalamic DA neurons (Sanchez-Gonzalez et al. 2005). The widespread origins of the thalamic DA projections have led to the proposal of a novel dopaminergic system (Sanchez-Gonzalez et al. 2005); however, other evidence indicates that the thalamic projections share anatomical features with the mesocortical DA system (Melchitzky et al. 2006). In the cerebellum, DAT-immunoreactive axons have been localized only to the granule cell layer of the vermis, with lobules VIIIB and IX showing the greatest density of labeled axons (Figure 4–6). Given that both the mediodorsal nucleus of the thalamus and the posterior vermis of the cerebellum are areas reported to be dysfunctional in schizophrenia (Andreasen et al. 1996; Popken et al. 2000; Tran et al. 1998; Young et al. 2000), the identification of DA axons in these brain regions may be of importance to the pathophysiology and treatment of this disease.

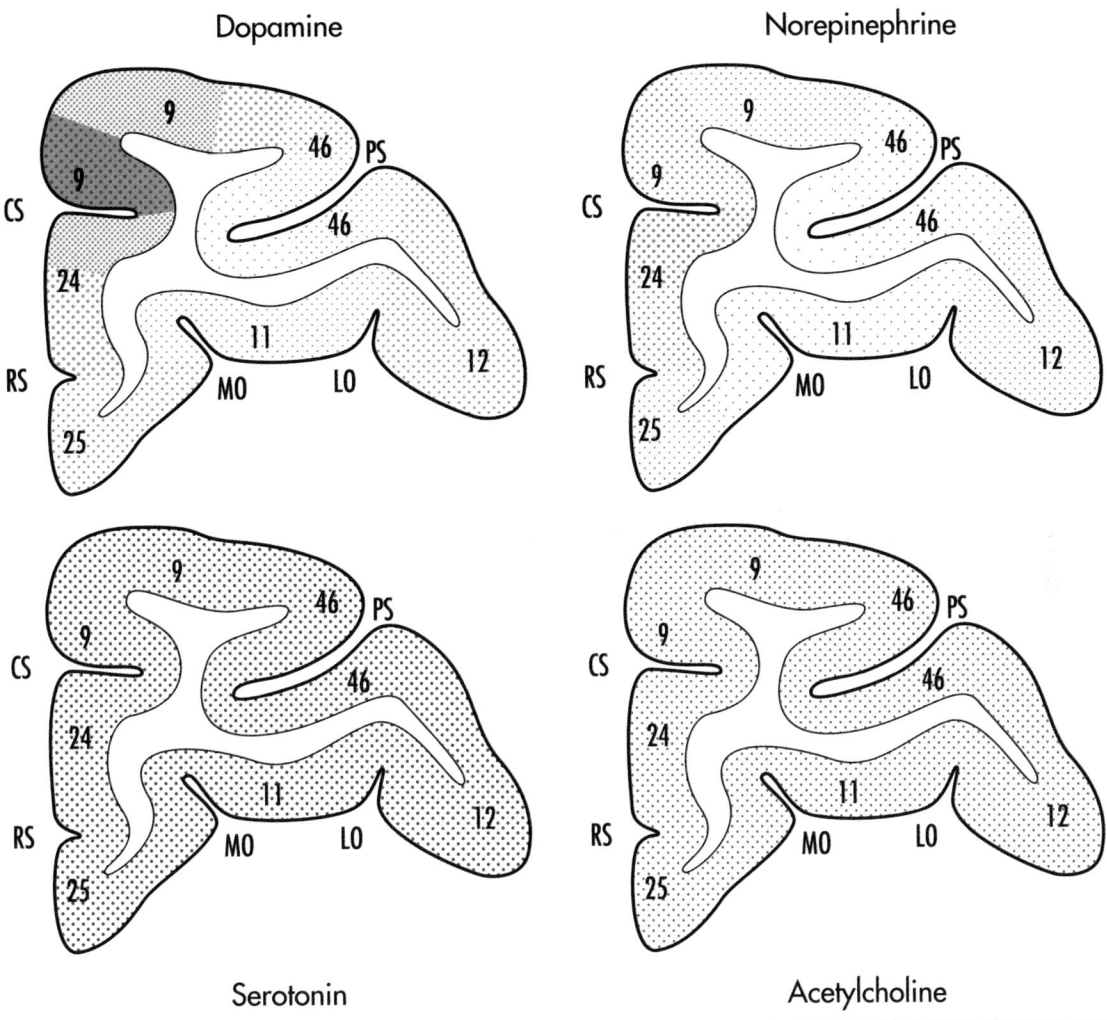

Dopamine

Norepinephrine

Serotonin

Acetylcholine

FIGURE 4–4. Schematic representation of coronal sections from macaque monkey prefrontal cortex illustrating the relative densities of dopamine, norepinephrine, serotonin, and acetylcholine axons.

Numbers refer to the cortical areas described by Walker (1940). CS = cingulate sulcus; LO = lateral orbital sulcus; MO = medial orbital sulcus; PS = principal sulcus; RS = rostral sulcus.
Source. Adapted from Lewis 1992.

Receptors

Five genes encoding five unique DA receptors have been identified. All of these receptors belong to the superfamily of seven-transmembrane-domain G protein–coupled receptors. As implied by the name, the receptor protein spans the plasma membrane seven times, and these receptors are linked to specific G proteins, through which activation of these receptors affects intracellular mechanisms in the postsynaptic cell. Pharmacologically, these receptors can be grouped into two general classes, the D_1 and D_2 subtypes. The D_1 receptor subtype includes the D_1 and D_5 receptors, and the D_2 receptor subtype consists of the D_2, D_3, and D_4 receptors. Interestingly, the D_5 receptor has a 10-fold higher affinity for DA than the D_1 recep-

tor, although the D_1 receptor is more prevalent (described in detail later in this section) (Meador-Woodruff 1994). The D_2 subtype receptors are targeted by many antipsychotic medications.

The mRNAs encoding the different DA receptors have distinct anatomical distributions. The following description of the localization of DA receptor mRNA is based mostly on data from rodents, but data from studies in primates are included when available. In addition, data from autoradiographic and/or immunocytochemical investigations of receptor and protein localization, respectively, are discussed where appropriate. D_1 receptor mRNA is present at high levels in the caudate, putamen, nucleus accumbens, and amygdala and at lower levels in

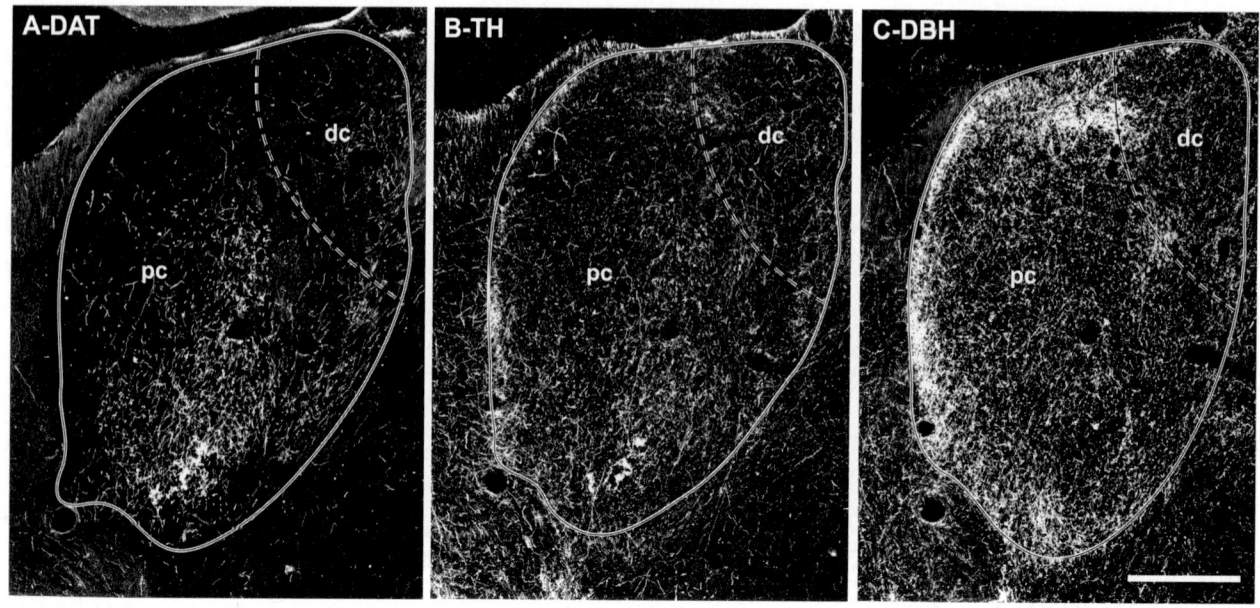

FIGURE 4–5.   Darkfield photomicrographs of adjacent sections through the caudal part of the mediodorsal thalamic nucleus in macaque monkey labeled for (A) dopamine transporter (DAT), (B) tyrosine hydroxylase (TH), and (C) dopamine β-hydroxylase (DBH).

Note that the DAT- and TH-immunoreactive axons are primarily located in the ventral portion of the mediodorsal thalamic nucleus. In contrast, DBH-immunoreactive axons are present throughout the mediodorsal thalamic nucleus. Scale bar = 700 μm. dc = densocellular; pc = parvocellular.

Source.   Reprinted from Melchitzky DS, Lewis DA: "Dopamine Transporter–Immunoreactive Axons in the Mediodorsal Thalamic Nucleus of the Macaque Monkey." *Neuroscience* 103:1033–1042, 2001. Copyright 2001, Elsevier. Used with permission.

the septal region, hippocampus, thalamus, cerebellum, and cerebral cortex (Hurd et al. 2001; Jaber et al. 1996; Meador-Woodruff et al. 1996). In the cerebellum, D_1 receptor mRNA is expressed in the anterior lobules within the granular cell layer (Mengod et al. 1991). D_1 receptor mRNA is found in all layers of the cerebral cortex, but cortical regions exhibit different laminar patterns (Meador-Woodruff et al. 1991). Brain regions that do not contain D_1 receptor mRNA include the substantia nigra pars compacta and the ventral tegmental area (Meador-Woodruff 1994). In addition, the D_1 receptor has been localized, using a type-specific antibody and immunocytochemistry, in the primate prefrontal and premotor cortices and in the hippocampus (Bergson et al. 1995). In these regions, the D_1 receptor is predominantly located postsynaptically in dendritic spines. The D_1 receptor protein has also been localized to the medium-sized GABA neurons in the caudate nucleus (Bergson et al. 1995). A positron emission tomography study revealed an increase in the binding of NNC112, a D_1 receptor ligand, in drug-free and drug-naive schizophrenia patients, consistent with a compensatory D_1 receptor upregulation in response to reduced DA levels (Abi-Dargham et al. 2002).

Thus, both postmortem anatomical and neuroimaging studies indicate decreased DA in the prefrontal cortex of subjects with schizophrenia. Brain regions that do not contain D_1 receptor mRNA include the substantia nigra pars compacta and the ventral tegmental area (Hurd et al. 2001; Meador-Woodruff 1994).

Regions of the brain that contain high levels of D_2 receptor mRNA include the caudate, putamen, nucleus accumbens, ventral tegmental area, and substantia nigra (Hurd et al. 2001; Jaber et al. 1996; Meador-Woodruff et al. 1996). Within the latter two areas, D_2 receptors are predominantly located presynaptically and where they regulate dopamine synthesis and release. The D_2 receptor mRNA is present at lower levels in the septal region, amygdala, hippocampus, thalamus, cerebellum, and cerebral cortex (Jaber et al. 1996; Meador-Woodruff 1994). In the cerebellum, lobules IX and X, which contain DA axons (Melchitzky and Lewis 2000), have the greatest concentrations of D_2 receptor mRNA (Mengod et al. 1992) and also express the D_2 receptor protein (Khan et al. 1998). Limbic regions of the brain, such as the nucleus accumbens, have the highest density of D_3 receptor mRNA in the brain (Jaber et al. 1996; Meador-Woodruff 1994).

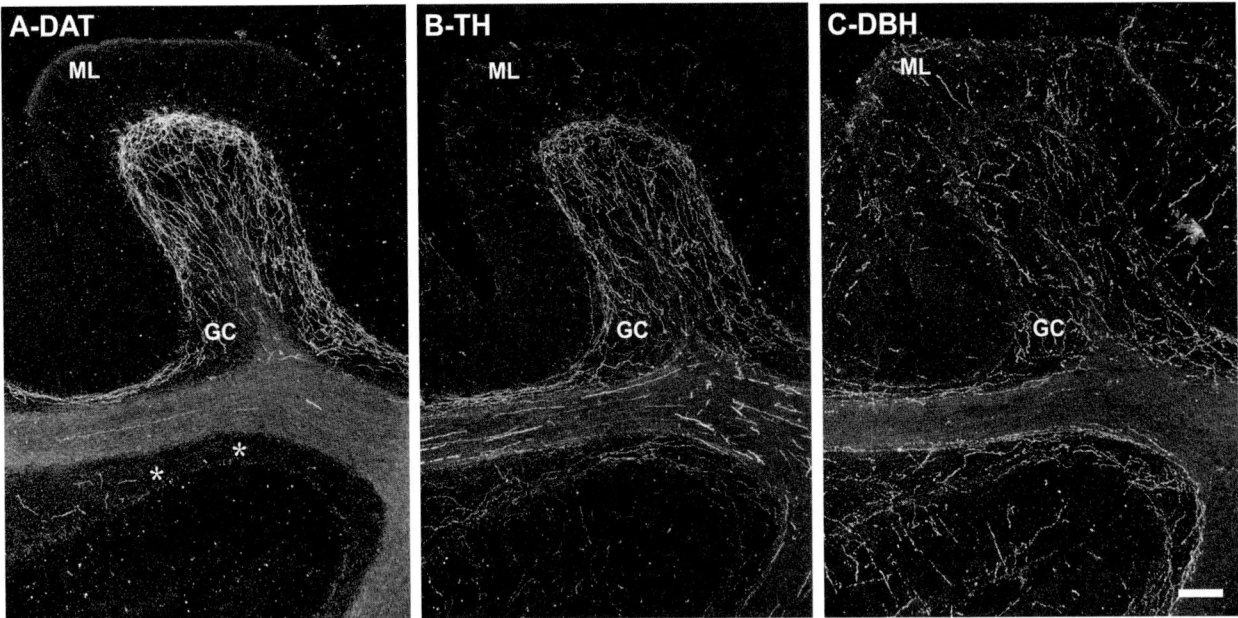

FIGURE 4–6.   Darkfield photomicrographs of (A) dopamine transporter (DAT)–, (B) tyrosine hydroxylase (TH)–, and (C) dopamine β-hydroxylase (DBH)–immunoreactive axons in adjacent sections through vermal lobule VIIIB of macaque monkey cerebellum.

Note that both the TH- and DAT-immunoreactive axons are primarily restricted to the granule cell layer (GC), with some clusters of axons extending into the Purkinje cell layer. TH-immunoreactive axons are also present in the molecular layer (ML), but no DAT-immunoreactive axons are detectable in this layer. In contrast, DBH-immunoreactive axons are distributed across all layers. In addition, the restricted lobular distribution of DAT-immunoreactive axons is illustrated by the marked paucity of these axons in the GC (*asterisks in B*) of the folium across the white matter, whereas the density of DBH-immunoreactive axons does not seem to differ across lobules. Scale bar = 150 μm.
Source.   Reprinted from Melchitzky DS, Lewis DA: "Tyrosine Hydroxylase- and Dopamine Transporter–Immunoreactive Axons in the Primate Cerebellum: Evidence for a Lobular- and Laminar-Specific Dopamine Innervation." *Neuropsychopharmacology* 22:466–472, 2000. Copyright 2000, Elsevier. Used with permission.

The substantia nigra, ventral tegmental area, septal region, thalamus, cerebellum, and cerebral cortex contain moderate to low levels of the mRNA for this receptor. In addition, lobules 9 and 10 of the cerebellar vermis express the D_3, as well as the D_2, receptor mRNA (Diaz et al. 1995; Mengod et al. 1992).

The D_4 and D_5 receptor mRNAs are not as highly expressed in the brain as are the mRNAs for the D_1–D_3 receptors (Jaber et al. 1996; Meador-Woodruff 1994). Low levels of D_4 receptor mRNA have been localized to the substantia nigra, nucleus accumbens, ventral tegmental area, hippocampus, amygdala, and cerebral cortex. In addition, the D_4 receptor protein is found in the cerebral cortex and hippocampus, where it is localized to both pyramidal and GABA-containing cells (Mrzljak et al. 1996). The D_5 receptor is the least widely distributed DA receptor, with low levels of mRNA present in the hippocampus, cerebellum, and thalamus (Jaber et al. 1996; Meador-Woodruff 1994). However, visualization of D_5 receptors with a type-specific antibody and immunocytochemistry has revealed that in the primate brain, the D_5 receptor is located in prefrontal, premotor, and mesolimbic cortices, as well as in the hippocampus (Bergson et al. 1995).

Neuroanatomy of the Norepinephrine System

The initial steps in the biosynthesis of norepinephrine (NE) are identical to those for DA. The rate-limiting step is the conversion of the amino acid tyrosine into L-dihydroxyphenylalanine, or L-dopa, via the enzyme tyrosine hydroxylase. NE is then formed from dopamine by the enzyme dopamine-β-hydroxylase. As for the other monoamines, NE neurotransmission is terminated through the actions of the NE transporter protein. A detailed description of the primate NE system can be found in Foote (1997).

Cell Locations

NE-containing neurons in the central nervous system are located predominantly in the medulla and pons (see Figure 4–1). The principal noradrenergic cell group is the locus coeruleus, the largest group of NE-containing neurons in the mammalian brain. In addition, it is the source of most of the ascending noradrenergic projections. The locus coeruleus is composed of a compact collection of neurons located in the dorsal pons, medial to the mesencephalic tract of the trigeminal nerve. In primate species, NE-containing neurons of the locus coeruleus, like the DA neurons of the substantia nigra, are heavily pigmented with neuromelanin, particularly in mature individuals (Manaye et al. 1995). Consistent with the role of NE in mood disorders, decreases in the neuronal density of locus coeruleus neurons have been reported in postmortem studies of patients with depression (Ressler and Nemeroff 2000).

NE-containing cells are also present in the caudal medulla, including the intermediate reticular zone and the lateral paragigantocellularis nucleus, as well as in the nucleus ambiguus. Collectively, these groups are known as the *lateral ventral tegmental fields* (Cooper et al. 1996).

Projection Sites

The cerebral cortex is a major recipient of noradrenergic projections, specifically those coming from the locus coeruleus (Gatter and Powell 1977; Porrino and Goldman-Rakic 1982). All areas of the cerebral cortex receive these projections; however, certain areas have higher densities of NE axons than other areas. For example, primary somatosensory and visual cortices have a very high density of NE axons, whereas prefrontal cortical areas (see Figure 4–3) are less densely innervated (Lewis and Morrison 1989; Morrison et al. 1982). Within the prefrontal cortex, the distribution of NE axons is similar to that of DA axons, with areas 9 and 24 having the highest density of NE axons; areas 11, 12, 13, and 25 having an intermediate density of NE axons; and areas 10 and 46 having the lowest density of NE axons (see Figure 4–4). These innervation patterns exhibit interesting comparisons and contrasts with those of DA axons. For example, the primary motor cortex contains high densities of both DA and NE axons, whereas the adjacent primary somatosensory cortex contains a very high density of NE axons but a low density of DA axons (Lewis and Morrison 1989; Morrison et al. 1982).

Other brain regions innervated by the locus coeruleus include the thalamus, cerebellar cortex, hypothalamus, and amygdala. Within the thalamus, the different nuclei display varied densities of NE axons. For example, in the primate, the mediodorsal thalamic nucleus contains a high density of NE axons (see Figure 4–5) (Melchitzky and Lewis 2001), whereas the lateral geniculate nucleus is sparsely innervated (Morrison and Foote 1986). By contrast, the different regions of the cerebellar cortex (i.e., the vermis, intermediate zones, and hemispheres) are all moderately innervated by noradrenergic axons (see Figure 4–6) (Melchitzky and Lewis 2000). In addition, unlike the distribution of DA axons, NE axons are found in both the granule cell and molecular layers. Within the hypothalamus and amygdala, the paraventricular and basolateral nuclei, respectively, contain the highest density of NE axons in these structures (Ginsberg et al. 1993; Li et al. 2001).

The noradrenergic nuclei in lateral tegmental fields appear to project exclusively to the brain stem and spinal cord in primates. By contrast, in rodents, these nuclei have been shown to also project to subcortical structures, such as the amygdala and septum (Delfs et al. 2000; Zardetto-Smith and Gray 1995).

Receptors

The receptors that recognize NE, the α and β adrenoceptors, belong to the G protein superfamily of receptors. Thus, similar to DA, NE elicits responses in the postsynaptic cell via G protein–mediated second-messenger systems. Both α and β adrenoceptors have two subtypes, namely the α_1 and α_2 adrenoceptors and the β_1 and β_2 adrenoceptors (Cooper et al. 1996). All of these receptors are widely distributed across the cerebral cortex, although their regional and laminar patterns differ. For example, in primate prefrontal cortex, autoradiography using appropriate ligands demonstrated that the α_1 and α_2 adrenoceptors are prominent in layers 1–superficial 3, whereas the highest density of β_1 and β_2 adrenoceptors is in layers deep 3–4 (Goldman-Rakic et al. 1990). Furthermore, in the human brain, α_1 adrenoceptors are also present in high density in the cortex, as well as in regions of the thalamus, hypothalamus, and hippocampus (Palacios et al. 1987). Stimulation of α_2 adrenoceptors in the frontal cortex appears to improve attention, raising the possibility of adrenergic system–targeted therapies for attention-deficit disorders and disorders associated with cognitive deficits, such as Alzheimer's disease and schizophrenia (Stahl 1998).

In the rodent, the mRNA for the β_1 adrenoreceptor is localized to many areas, including cerebral cortex, reticular nucleus of the thalamus, deep cerebellar nuclei, brain stem nuclei, and spinal cord, while the mRNA for the β_2 adrenoreceptor has a more restricted distribution to the olfactory bulb, hippocampus, cerebellar cortex, and intralaminar thalamic nuclei (Nicholas et al. 1993). Autoradiographic studies have also revealed high densities of the β adrenoreceptors in the striatum, the hippocampus and the cerebral cortex in human brain (Pazos et al. 1985). Lower densities of β adrenoreceptors have been found in the thalamus, hypothalamus, and amygdala and the molecular and granule cell layers of the cerebellar cortex (Pazos et al. 1985). Dysregulation of noradrenergic transmission via β adrenoreceptors has been implicated in the pathophysiology of depression. For example, postmortem studies have revealed increased binding of β adrenoreceptors in the frontal cortex of suicide victims (Mann et al. 1986).

Neuroanatomy of the Serotonin System

Only 2% of the serotonin (5-hydroxytryptamine [5-HT]) in the body is found in the brain. The neurons within the brain synthesize 5-HT, starting with the amino acid tryptophan, which is then hydroxylated via the enzyme tryptophan hydroxylase to form 5-hydroxytryptophan. 5-HT is then formed by decarboxylation of 5-hydroxytryptophan. Similar to DA, reuptake via the serotonin transporter (SERT) is the principal mechanism for terminating serotonergic neurotransmission. SERT also regulates the availability—and hence the signaling potential—of released 5-HT. Consequently, the strength of 5-HT activity at 5-HT receptors is inversely proportional to the number of functional SERT molecules present at the presynaptic membrane. Selective serotonin reuptake inhibitors (SSRIs) and related antidepressant drugs exploit this relationship by blocking the reuptake of 5-HT by SERT, thus increasing the levels of 5-HT in the synaptic cleft. In humans, the gene encoding for SERT exists in both long and short forms, with the short form resulting in lower levels of SERT expression. Azmitia and Gannon (1986) have provided a detailed description of the primate 5-HT system.

Cell Locations

The highest concentration of 5-HT–containing neurons in the mammalian brain is found in the raphe nuclei of the brain stem (see Figure 4–1). The cellular morphology and anatomical distribution of 5-HT neurons indicate that the raphe nuclei can be divided into rostral and cau-

dal brain stem groups in the monkey and human brain stem (Hornung 2003). The principal subdivisions of the rostral raphe nuclei consist of the median raphe, dorsal raphe, and caudal linear nuclei located in the pons and midbrain. The caudal raphe nuclei consist of the raphe pallidus, raphe obscurus, and raphe magnus located in the caudal pons and medulla. The rostral raphe nuclei provide the bulk of the ascending axonal projections to the cerebral cortex and other subcortical structures, whereas the caudal raphe nuclei give rise to descending projections to the lower brain stem and spinal cord (Hornung 2003). Because of the functional and clinical importance of the 5-HT input to the cerebral cortex and limbic forebrain provided by the rostral nuclei, the following anatomical description of the 5-HT system will focus on the rostral raphe nuclei and their axonal projections.

The most rostral 5-HT neurons are located in the interpeduncular nucleus of the ventral mesencephalon (Hornung 2003). The caudal linear nucleus, located dorsal and caudal to the interpeduncular nucleus, lies between the red nuclei and contains both 5-HT and DA neurons. The most diverse of the raphe nuclei is the dorsal raphe nucleus (Baker et al. 1990). It is located in the central gray matter ventral to the cerebral aqueduct and fourth ventricle. On the basis of the topography and density of neurons in the primate, the dorsal raphe can be subdivided into five distinct subnuclei. Of these subnuclei, the ventrolateral subnucleus exhibits the highest density of 5-HT neurons in the entire brain stem (Baker et al. 1990). Postmortem studies have revealed abnormalities such as increased mRNA and protein levels of tryptophan hydroxylase, the rate-limiting enzyme in the synthesis of 5-HT, in the dorsal raphe nucleus of suicide victims (Bach-Mizrachi et al. 2006). The median raphe extends from the caudal midbrain into the rostral pons (Tork and Hornung 1990). Serotonin neurons in the rostral level of the median raphe are densely packed along the midline, whereas at caudal levels, the nucleus expands laterally to form its characteristic barrel-shaped appearance. The barrel-like appearance is formed by the development of the paramedian raphe nuclei, which straddle the midline and contain both 5-HT neurons and 5-HT axons that arise from more caudal levels.

Projection Sites

The cerebral cortex is a major recipient of 5-HT axons arising from the mesencephalon. The heaviest projections to the frontal cortex, including prefrontal (see Figure 4–3) and motor cortices, arise from the dorsal raphe

(M.A. Wilson and Molliver 1991). The median raphe and supralemniscal group project equally to the parietal, occipital, and frontal cortices. Unlike DA axons in the DA system, 5-HT axons are homogeneously distributed across different cortical areas, with the greatest density of axons usually present in the middle cortical layers (Morrison and Foote 1986). Furthermore, within cortical areas such as the prefrontal cortex, the density of 5-HT axons across regions is homogeneous (see Figure 4–4).

Although this area has been less well studied in primates, investigations in rodents suggest that the median raphe and dorsal raphe projections to the cerebral cortex are distinct in a number of respects (Mamounas and Molliver 1991). The cortical 5-HT axons originating from the median raphe are characterized by the presence of large spherical varicosities with thin intervaricose segments that give these axons a beaded appearance. In contrast, cortical axons originating from the dorsal raphe are fine and tortuous, with irregularly spaced small varicosities. Most cortical regions contain both types of 5-HT axons; however, the intracortical distribution of 5-HT axons is not uniform. For example, in the primate prefrontal cortex, the fine axons are present in all layers but are more abundant in layers 3–6, whereas the beaded axons predominate in layers 1–2 (Smiley and Goldman-Rakic 1996). These distinct morphological features of 5-HT axons, together with the unique topographical distributions, suggest that different functional roles for the two 5-HT fiber systems may exist. For example, in both rodents and primates, administration of amphetamine derivatives, such as methylenedioxyamphetamine and p-chloroamphetamine, causes selective degeneration of fine 5-HT-containing axons, whereas the beaded axons are spared (Mamounas and Molliver 1991; Molliver et al. 1990).

Interestingly, the effects of SSRIs differ based on the brain region and cellular localization of SERT. For example, blocking SERT in 5-HT projection fields (e.g., in the cerebral cortex) increases 5-HT levels and signaling at all available 5-HT receptors. By contrast, blocking SERT at the 5-HT cell body level (e.g., in the raphe nuclei) leads to increased activation of 5-HT_1 autoreceptors (see subsection below titled "Receptors"), ultimately resulting in reduction of overall 5-HT function. Eventually, 5-HT output is increased through desensitization of 5-HT_1 autoreceptors by SSRIs.

With regard to 5-HT synapses in primate cortex, the presence of 5-HT-labeled varicosities does not necessarily correspond to 5-HT synaptic specializations. In fact, it has been reported that more than three-quarters of 5-HT varicosities in the primate cortex do not form identifiable

synaptic specializations, even though many had synaptic vesicles and accumulated 5-HT immunoreactivity (Smiley and Goldman-Rakic 1996). These observations suggest that 5-HT release, like that of DA, may occur at sites other than identified synapses and support the concept that nonsynaptic mechanisms of 5-HT neurotransmission are present in the primate cortex.

The raphe nuclei also project to a number of subcortical structures. The rostral group, including the caudal linear and dorsal raphe nuclei, project to the caudate, putamen, substantia nigra, and thalamus. In the primate, the 5-HT innervation of the thalamus is heterogeneous and widespread. The midline, rostral intralaminar, and reticular nuclei are the most densely innervated, whereas the ventral anterior and habenula are sparsely innervated (Lavoie and Parent 1991). The median raphe and the interfascicular subnucleus of the dorsal raphe project to limbic structures such as the hippocampus, amygdala, and septum. Serotonin neurons in both the median raphe and dorsal raphe contain highly collocated axons that innervate multiple terminal fields. This axonal organization pattern suggests that functionally related nuclei can be innervated by the same group of 5-HT neurons or even the same individual neuron.

Receptors

Physiological and biochemical studies have revealed that multiple receptors exist for 5-HT and that many of these receptors have subtypes. To date, 14 5-HT receptors have been identified. The current classification of 5-HT receptors is based on structural characteristics and the second-messenger systems that are utilized. All but one of the 5-HT receptors belong to the G protein receptor superfamily. The exception is the 5-HT_3 receptor, which belongs to the ligand-gated ion channel family (Peroutka 1997).

As with the other monoamine systems, the distribution of 5-HT receptors has been studied mostly in rodents by localization of receptor mRNAs. However, studies conducted in human subjects reveal receptor mRNA distributions similar to those in rodents. The 5-HT_1 receptor has six subtypes, 5-HT_{1A-F} (Peroutka 1997). Several of the 5-HT_1 subtypes—5-HT_{1A}, 5-HT_{1B}, and 5-HT_{1D}—appear to also function presynaptically, because the mRNA for these subtypes has been localized to 5-HT-containing neurons in both the dorsal and median raphe. Thus, these receptors also function as autoreceptors, regulating the firing of raphe neurons. In addition, 5-HT_{1A} and 5-HT_{1B} receptors, as revealed by immunocytochemistry and autoradiography, are present in the cerebral cortex as well as other projection sites of the dorsal raphe and median raphe (DeFelipe et al. 2001; Goldman-Rakic et al. 1990; Jakab and Goldman-Rakic 2000; Mengod et al. 1996).

The 5-HT$_2$ receptor has three subtypes, 5-HT$_{2A-C}$ (Peroutka 1997). The most widely studied of these is the 5-HT$_{2A}$ subtype, the mRNA of which is most abundant in the cerebral cortex. In most cortical areas, layers 1 and 3–4 have a higher density of 5-HT$_{2A}$ mRNA levels than layers 2 and 5–6 (Lopez-Gimenez et al. 2001b). In monkey prefrontal cortex, the 5-HT$_{2A}$ receptor appears to be expressed by pyramidal cells as well as in the parvalbumin-containing subclass of nonpyramidal neurons (Jakab and Goldman-Rakic 2000), which provide potent inhibitory input to pyramidal cells. Subcortical structures, including the caudate, putamen, substantia nigra, and inferior olive, also express 5-HT$_{2A}$ mRNA (Lopez-Gimenez et al. 2001b). The anatomical localization of the 5-HT$_{2B}$ receptor has not been extensively studied, but the cerebral cortex has been shown to contain the mRNA for this receptor (Mengod et al. 1996). The 5-HT$_{2B}$ receptor mRNA is also localized to the cerebral cortex, whereas the 5-HT$_{2C}$ receptor mRNA has been identified in the hypothalamus and medulla (Mengod et al. 1996). The mRNA for the 5-HT$_{2C}$ receptor has been localized to layer 5 of cerebral cortex, nucleus accumbens, caudate, putamen, septal nuclei, diagonal band, ventral striatum, and extended amygdala (Lopez-Gimenez et al. 2001a). Increased binding of both 5-HT$_{1A}$ and 5-HT$_{2A}$ receptors has been found in the prefrontal cortex of suicide victims (Mann et al. 1986), possibly representing an upregulation of receptors due to decreased serotonergic transmission.

The 5-HT$_3$ receptor mRNA has been identified in rodent cerebral cortex, where it was found to be collocated with GABA-containing neurons (Tecott et al. 1993). In addition, in monkey prefrontal cortex, the 5-HT$_3$ receptor has been localized to small GABA-containing neurons that also express substance P and the calcium-binding protein calbindin (Jakab and Goldman-Rakic 2000).

The anatomical distribution of the 5-HT$_4$ receptor has been examined by autoradiography in human brain, and areas with the highest levels of receptors are in the basal ganglia nuclei (caudate, putamen, nucleus accumbens, globus pallidus, and substantia nigra) and the hippocampus, specifically area CA1 and subiculum (Varnas et al. 2003). In neocortex, the superficial layers have higher levels of 5-HT$_4$ receptor than the deeper cortical layers.

In rodent brain, the 5-HT$_7$ receptor protein is found in the cerebral cortex, hippocampus, thalamus, and hypothalamus, with a somatodendritic localization in these areas (Neumaier et al. 2001). In human brain, 5-HT$_7$ receptors, visualized via autoradiography, are also found in the cerebral cortex, hippocampus, and thalamus, as well as in the caudate and putamen (Martin-Cora and Pazos 2004).

The anatomical localization of the remaining 5-HT receptors (i.e., 5-HT$_{5A-B}$, 5-HT$_6$) has not been as well studied. However, mRNA for these receptor subtypes appears to be predominantly localized to subcortical structures, such as the caudate, nucleus accumbens, hippocampus, thalamus, and amygdala.

Neuroanatomy of the Acetylcholine System

Acetylcholine (ACh) is phylogenetically a very old molecule that is widely distributed in eukaryotic as well as prokaryotic cells. Furthermore, ACh is found in many non-neuronal tissues, in which it appears to modulate basic cellular actions. ACh is formed by the synthesis of acetyl coenzyme A and choline via the enzyme choline acetyltransferase. Acetyl coenzyme A is available from mitochondria, and choline is obtained through the diet. ACh is rapidly inactivated in the synaptic cleft by the enzyme acetylcholinesterase. The activity of both choline acetyltransferase and acetylcholinesterase is reduced in the frontal and temporal cortices of patients with Alzheimer's disease, and the decrease in choline acetyltransferase activity is associated with the presence of the apolipoprotein epsilon 4 (*ApoE*-ε4) allele (Lai et al. 2006).

The presence of ACh-containing cell bodies and axons has been demonstrated by the use of histochemical procedures to visualize the acetylcholinesterase molecule, as well as by the use of specific antibodies directed against choline acetyltransferase. Immunocytochemical identification of ACh-containing axons using choline acetyltransferase antibodies is the preferred method, because acetylcholinesterase may not be a specific marker of cholinergic structures. A detailed review of the primate cholinergic system can be found in De Lacalle and Saper (1997).

Cell Locations

ACh-containing neurons are located in two main groups in the brain (see Figure 4–1). The basal forebrain cholinergic complex is located near the inferior surface of the telencephalon, between the hypothalamus and orbital cortex. This complex includes the medial septal nucleus, the diagonal band of Broca, the nucleus basalis (also known as the basal nucleus of Meynert), the magnocellular preoptic area, and the substantia innominata. All of these regions are characterized by the presence of large ACh-containing multipolar neurons (Semba and Fibiger 1989).

The pontomesencephalotegmental cholinergic complex consists of the pedunculopontine nucleus, which is located along the dorsolateral aspect of the superior cerebellar peduncle, and the laterodorsal tegmental nucleus in the ventral part of the periaqueductal gray. Similar to the cells in the basal forebrain complex, the pontomesencephalotegmental complex is also characterized by the presence of large ACh-containing cells (Semba and Fibiger 1989).

In addition to these cell groups, ACh-containing neurons are also present in all nuclei of the striatum (i.e., the caudate, putamen, and nucleus accumbens). However, these cholinergic cells are interneurons and thus do not project out of the striatum (Cooper et al. 1996).

Projection Sites

The cerebral cortex is a major recipient of cholinergic projections, which originate predominantly from the basal forebrain complex. The organization of these projections in the primate is similar to that in the rodent. In general, these projections are topographically organized, with a distinct population of neurons projecting to a particular location in the cortex.

The distribution of ACh-containing axons in the cerebral cortex is heterogeneous, with paralimbic areas having the greatest density of ACh-containing axons. The sensory and association regions of neocortex are less densely innervated by cholinergic axons than are the paralimbic areas. For example, in human brain, the density of cholinergic axons is lowest in the primary visual cortex; moderate in association areas, including parts of the prefrontal (see Figure 4–3) and parietal cortices; and highest in the paralimbic entorhinal and cingulate cortices (Mesulam et al. 1992). The density of cholinergic axons also differs within a cortical region. In monkey prefrontal cortex, there is a rostral to caudal increase in the density of ACh-containing axons, so that area 10 at the frontal pole has a lower density of cholinergic axons than does area 9, which is less densely innervated than the more caudal area 8B. Furthermore, the more caudal premotor (area 6) and motor (area 4) cortices have the highest density of ACh-containing axons in the frontal lobe (Lewis 1991). However, cholinergic axons are distributed homogeneously across prefrontal areas at the same rostrocaudal level (see Figure 4–4).

The distribution of ACh-containing axons across the cortical layers is also heterogeneous. In general, layers 1–2 and 5 have the highest density of cholinergic axons, whereas layer 4 has the lowest density of ACh-containing axons (Lewis 1991; Mesulam et al. 1992).

The hippocampus is also densely innervated by cholinergic axons. These projections arise from the medial septal and diagonal band of Broca nuclei of the basal forebrain complex (Kitt et al. 1987). The molecular layer of the dentate gyrus and the CA2, CA3, and CA4 subsectors of the hippocampus contain the highest densities of ACh-containing axons (Mesulam et al. 1992). Although the densities of ACh-containing fibers in the CA1 subsector and subiculum are lower than those in the other portions of the hippocampus, they are still more densely innervated than most cortical areas (Mesulam et al. 1992).

The amygdala also receives projections from the basal forebrain cholinergic complex. Within the amygdala, all nuclei are densely innervated by ACh-containing axons, with the basolateral nucleus having the highest density (Mesulam et al. 1992). Retrograde tracing has demonstrated that this projection principally arises from the nucleus basalis (Kitt et al. 1987).

In the rodent, the reticular nucleus of the thalamus and the interpeduncular nucleus are densely innervated by cholinergic axons originating from the nucleus of the diagonal band of Broca and the nucleus basalis, respectively. These projections have not been investigated in the primate (Semba and Fibiger 1989).

The thalamus is densely innervated by cholinergic axons, which originate from the pedunculopontine and laterodorsal tegmental nuclei (Semba and Fibiger 1989). In addition, acetylcholinesterase activity and immunoreactivity for choline acetyltransferase have revealed a heterogeneous distribution of cholinergic axons within the thalamus. For example, in the primate, the midline, intralaminar, anterodorsal, lateral mediodorsal, and medial pulvinar nuclei contain very high levels of cholinergic axons (Barbas et al. 1991; Cavada et al. 1995). A similar pattern of cholinergic axons is found in the rodent (Levey et al. 1987).

The pedunculopontine and laterodorsal tegmental nuclei project to other subcortical structures, including the lateral hypothalamus, the superior colliculus, and the lateral preoptic area. However, these projections have only been investigated in rodents (Semba and Fibiger 1989).

Receptors

ACh receptors have been divided into two main classes, the muscarinic and nicotinic receptors. There are five (M_1–M_5) subtypes of the muscarinic receptor, all of which are coupled to G proteins and linked to a variety of second-messenger systems. Neuronal nicotinic receptors are formed from five membrane-spanning subunits situated around a central pore. The neuronal nicotinic receptor has two subunits, α and β; the α subunit has seven different forms, and the subunits that form $\alpha\beta$ combinations include α_2–α_6 and β_2–β_4 (Dani and Bertrand 2007). Homomeric and heteromeric nicotinic receptors can be formed from the α_7–α_{10} subunits. The nicotinic receptors are ionotropic, acting directly on sodium channels.

Most of the studies investigating the localization of ACh receptors in the brain have employed autoradiography, utilizing tritiated nicotine or receptor subtype-specific ligands. For example, the M_1 and M_2 receptor subtypes have been shown to be present in many regions of the cerebral cortex, including the frontal, parietal, and occipital cortices (Flynn and Mash 1993). Specifically, the overall densities of the M_1 and M_2 receptor subtypes are similar, but the laminar distributions vary across the cortex (Lidow et al. 1989). In parietal, occipital, and motor cortices, both receptor subtypes are concentrated in the superficial layers. In contrast, the M_1 and M_2 subtypes are evenly distributed across the cortical layers in the prefrontal cortex. Subcortical structures show a varied distribution of muscarinic receptors. The striatum has a high density of M_1, M_2, and M_3 receptors, with M_3 receptors localized to the anterior and dorsal caudate nucleus and M_1 receptors more prevalent in the ventromedial caudate and medial globus pallidus (Flynn and Mash 1993). Low levels of M_1 and M_3 receptors are found in the thalamus, hypothalamus, and brain stem. In Alzheimer's disease, M_1 and M_2 receptors, as measured by autoradiography, are reduced in the frontal cortex and hippocampus, respectively, whereas M_3 and M_4 receptors appear to be unaffected (Rodriguez-Puertas et al. 1997).

The distribution of tritiated nicotine binding sites is similar in both rat and monkey brains. For example, in both species, dense labeling occurs in sensory- and motor-related thalamic nuclei, the dentate gyrus of the hippocampus, and layer 3 of the cerebral cortex (Clarke 1989). Furthermore, the anatomical distributions of mRNA for the nicotinic ACh receptor subunits have been investigated in the monkey brain. The α_4 and β_2 receptor subunits are the most widely distributed, with highest densities in the dorsal thalamus and the DA-containing nuclei of the mesencephalon (Han et al. 2000). Consistent with the well-known involvement of the cholinergic system in Alzheimer's disease, the densities of α_4 and β_2 nicotinic receptors are reduced in the temporal and frontal cortices of patients with this disease (Lai et al. 2006).

Several lines of evidence support a role for the α_7 receptor subunit in the pathophysiology of sensory gating deficits in schizophrenia. For example, a postmortem study has shown that binding of α-bungarotoxin, which most likely corresponds to nicotinic receptors containing the α_7 subunit (Leonard et al. 2000), is reduced in the hippocampus of patients with schizophrenia (Freedman et al. 1995). In addition, sensory gating deficits are improved by nicotine in subjects with schizophrenia as well as in their unaffected family members (Adler et al. 1998). Interestingly, unlike control subjects, who show an upregulation of nicotinic receptors in association with smoking, individuals with schizophrenia exhibit lower binding of nicotinic receptors at every level of smoking history (Breese et al. 2000).

Endocannabinoid System

The endocannabinoid system is an endogenous signaling system composed of endocannabinoids, their receptors, and the proteins involved in their synthesis and degradation (Pazos et al. 2005). Anandamide and 2-arachidonoylglycerol, the two principal endocannabinoids in the brain, bind to and activate the G protein–coupled cannabinoid receptors, CB_1 and CB_2. The CB_1 receptor, the predominant endocannabinoid receptor in the brain, mediates most of the behavioral effects of endogenous and exogenous cannabinoids (Zimmer et al. 1999). The CB_2 receptor is principally expressed in non-neural tissues, such as immune system organs (e.g., spleen). CB_1 receptors are located primarily on presynaptic axon terminals and mediate the retrograde signaling of endocannabinoids in synaptic plasticity processes, such as depolarization-induced suppression of inhibition (Alger 2002).

Distribution of the CB_1 receptor is widespread, with many areas of the brain expressing high levels (Figure 4–7). Specifically, the neocortex, hippocampus, amygdala, globus pallidus, and cerebellum all exhibit high densities of the CB_1 receptor (Biegon and Kerman 2001; Eggan and Lewis 2007; Herkenham et al. 1991). Within the primate cerebral cortex, association regions, such as the prefrontal cortex, contain the highest levels of CB_1-immunoreactive axons, whereas primary sensory regions, particularly primary visual cortex, have the lowest densities (Eggan and Lewis 2007). Within the prefrontal cortex, dorsolateral area 46 contains the highest densities of CB_1-immunoreactive axons. The density of CB_1-labeled axons in the hippocampus is similar to that in the prefrontal cortex. Interestingly, within the amygdala, the corti-

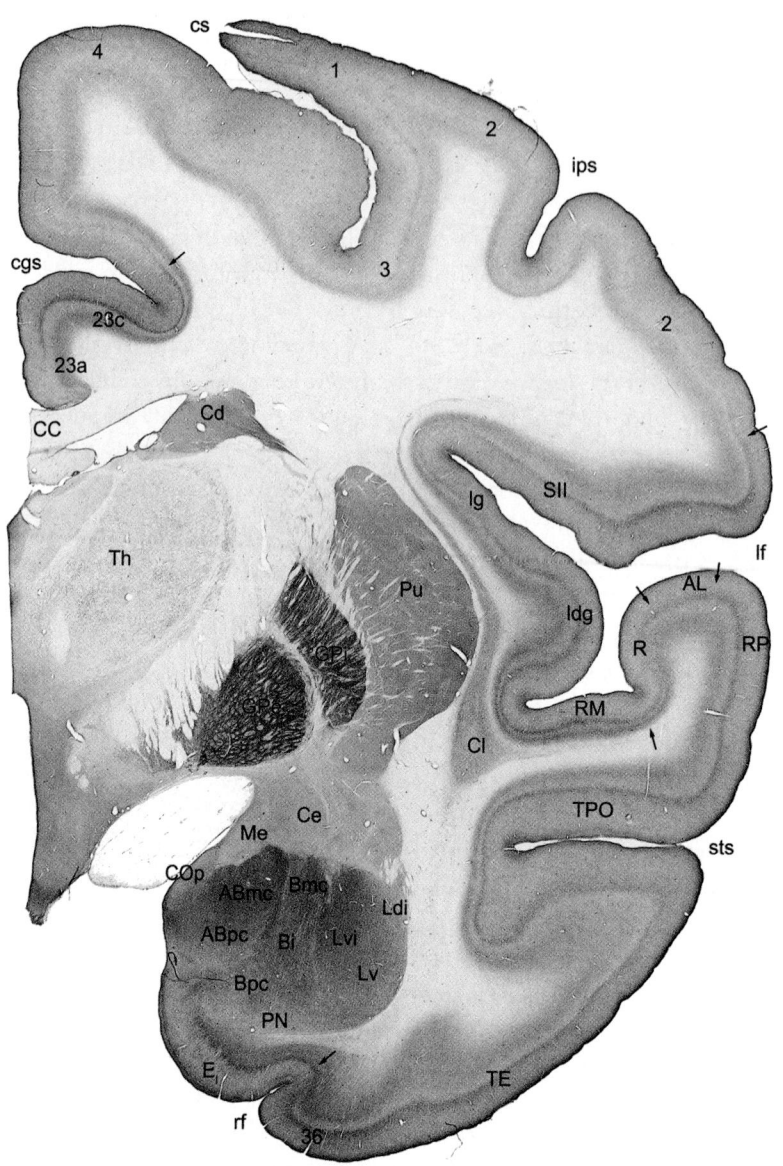

FIGURE 4–7.   Brightfield photomicrograph of a coronal section through macaque monkey brain illustrating the distribution of cannabinoid CB$_1$ receptor–immunoreactive axons.

Association areas such as the cingulate cortex (area 32), insula (Ig, Idg), auditory association cortex (RP), and entorhinal cortex (E$_I$) have an overall higher density of CB$_1$-immunoreactive axons than do primary somatosensory areas (areas 3, 1, 2) and primary motor cortex (area 4). Note the distinct differences in laminar distribution of labeled processes at the boundaries of some cytoarchitectonic regions (*arrows*). In subcortical structures, the intensity of CB$_1$ immunoreactivity is high in the claustrum (Cl), the basal and lateral nuclei of the amygdala, and both segments of the globus pallidus (GP); intermediate to low in the caudate (Cd) and putamen (Pu) and the central and medial nuclei of the amygdala; and not detectable in the thalamus (Th). Scale bar = 2 mm. ABmc = accessory basal nucleus, magnocellular division; ABpc = accessory basal nucleus, parvicellular division; Bi = basal nucleus, intermediate division; Bmc = basal nucleus, magnocellular division; Bpc = basal nucleus, parvicellular division; CC = corpus callosum; Cd = caudate; Ce = central amygdaloid nucleus; Cgs = cingulate sulcus; Cl = claustrum; COp = posterior cortical nucleus; cs = central sulcus; E$_I$ = entorhinal cortex, intermediate field; GPe = globus pallidus, external; GPi = globus pallidus, internal; Idg = insula, dysgranular; Ig = insula, granular; ips = intraparietal sulcus; Ldi = lateral nucleus, dorsal intermediate division; lf = lateral fissure; Lv = lateral nucleus, ventral division; Lvi = lateral nucleus, ventral intermediate division; Me = medial amygdaloid nucleus; PN = paralaminar nucleus; Pu = putamen; R = rostral auditory area (core primary auditory); rf = rhinal fissure; RM = rostromedial auditory belt; RP = rostral auditory parabelt; SII = second somatosensory cortex; sts = superior temporal sulcus; TE = inferotemporal cortex; Th = thalamus; TPO = temporal parieto-occipital associated area in sts.

Source.   Reprinted from Eggan SM, Lewis DA: "Immunocytochemical Distribution of the Cannabinoid CB$_1$ Receptor in the Primate Neocortex: A Regional and Laminar Analysis." *Cerebral Cortex* 17:175–191, 2007. Copyright 2007, Oxford. Used with permission.

cal-like basolateral complex has a higher density of CB_1 axons than does the striatal-like central and medial nuclei (Figure 4–7). Of the basal ganglia nuclei, the globus pallidus has the highest and the striatum the lowest levels of CB_1 immunoreactivity. As is evident in Figure 4–7, the thalamus is completely devoid of CB_1 axons.

In the neocortex, the CB_1 receptor is highly expressed in the subpopulation of GABA-containing inhibitory interneurons (Marsicano and Lutz 1999) that also synthesize the neuropeptide cholecystokinin (Bodor et al. 2005). In addition, in rodent hippocampus (Katona et al. 1999) and monkey prefrontal cortex (Melchitzky et al. 2007), CB_1-immunoreactive axons have been shown to be collocated with cholecystokinin. This association of CB_1 with GABA neurons in the prefrontal cortex suggests that the endocannabinoid system may be involved in cognitive processing as well as in disorders characterized by impaired cognition, such as schizophrenia. Indeed, cannabis use impairs cognitive processes such as working memory (D'Souza et al. 2004) and has been associated with an increased risk for schizophrenia (Smit et al. 2004). In addition, a reduction in CB_1 mRNA levels in the prefrontal cortex of subjects with schizophrenia (Eggan et al. 2008) provides further evidence for a role of the endocannabinoid system in the pathophysiology of schizophrenia.

Excitatory and Inhibitory Amino Acid Neurotransmitters in the Context of Neural Circuitry

The amino acid neurotransmitters are the most abundant and widely used neurotransmitters in the brain. The excitatory neurotransmitter glutamate and the inhibitory neurotransmitter GABA are the predominant transmitters in both the local and long-range circuits that form distributed neural networks. In the brain, L-glutamate is synthesized in axon terminals from glucose (via the Krebs cycle) or from glutamine that is converted into glutamate by the enzyme glutaminase. The synaptic action of glutamate is terminated by the glutamate transporter, which is located on the presynaptic axon terminal. GABA is synthesized in the brain by the decarboxylation of L-glutamic acid, which is catalyzed by the enzyme glutamic acid decarboxylase. As in other neurotransmitter systems, the synaptic action of GABA is terminated by the GABA transporter. In the following section, we focus on the cell types and projections utilizing these two neurotransmitters in the neocortex, basal ganglia, and thala-

mus, given that these brain regions have been implicated in the pathophysiology of a number of psychiatric disorders.

Cerebral Cortex

Pyramidal cells, the predominant projection neurons of the cerebral cortex, utilize glutamate as their neurotransmitter. Most pyramidal neurons are characteristically shaped and possess a single apical dendrite that extends toward the pial surface. In addition, several basilar dendrites extend from the base of the cell body in a radial fashion. Dendritic spines, short extensions of the dendritic shafts, coat both apical and basilar dendrites. Pyramidal neurons have principal axons that enter the white matter and project to other cortical regions, as well as axon collaterals that travel either horizontally or vertically within the gray matter. In all cortical areas, pyramidal cells are located in layers 2–6, and the laminar location of a pyramidal cell often indicates its projection target. For example, cortically projecting pyramidal neurons are predominantly located in layer 3, whereas striatal- and thalamic-projecting cells reside in layers 5 and 6, respectively (DeFelipe and Farinas 1992).

Nonpyramidal neurons are the other major class of cortical neuron, and the majority (90%) of these neurons utilize GABA as their neurotransmitter. Also known as interneurons, the axons of cortical GABA cells arborize within the gray matter and thus do not project out of the cortical region in which they reside. As many as 12 different subtypes of GABA neurons can be found in the cortex, and these can be distinguished biochemically, electrophysiologically, and morphologically (Figure 4–8) (Fairen et al. 1984; Krimer et al. 2005; Lund and Lewis 1993). For example, subpopulations of GABA cells can be distinguished by the presence of certain neuropeptides or calcium-binding proteins (Condé et al. 1994; Gabbott and Bacon 1996). In addition, the organization of the axonal arbor and synaptic targets of the axon terminals differ greatly across these different subtypes (Lund and Lewis 1993). As depicted in Figure 4–8, the chandelier class of GABA cell expresses the calcium-binding protein parvalbumin (DeFelipe et al. 1989; Lund and Lewis 1993) and has axon terminals that are arrayed as distinct vertical structures, termed *cartridges* (Fairen and Valverde 1980; Goldman-Rakic and Brown 1982). These axon terminals form inhibitory or symmetric synapses exclusively with the axon initial segments of pyramidal cells (DeFelipe et al. 1985). Parvalbumin-containing basket neurons form symmetric synapses with the cell bodies and dendrites of pyramidal neurons (Melchitzky et al. 1999; Williams et al. 1992). Parvalbumin-containing neurons are predominantly located in layers 3 and 4. Martinotti cells contain somatostatin and form symmetric synapses with the tuft dendrites of pyramidal neurons (Kawaguchi and Kubota 1997; Wang et al. 2004) and, to a lesser extent, with the dendrites of GABA neurons (Melchitzky and Lewis 2008). Double bouquet neurons have radially oriented axonal arbors and contain either somatostatin and the calcium-binding protein calbindin (DeFelipe 1993) or the calcium-binding protein calretinin (Condé et al. 1994). The somatostatin- and calbindin-containing double bouquet cells form symmetric synapses with the distal dendritic shafts and spines of pyramidal neurons. By contrast, the calretinin-containing double bouquet cells form symmetric synapses predominantly with the dendritic shafts of other GABA neurons (Gonchar and Burkhalter 1999; Meskenaite 1997), although they also target distal dendritic shafts and spines of pyramidal neurons to a lesser extent (Melchitzky et al. 2005). Calretinin-containing Cajal-Retzius cells reside solely in layer 1 and target the tuft dendrites of pyramidal neurons. These subpopulations of GABA neurons have differing laminar patterns of distribution (see Figure 4–8). For example, in the prefrontal cortex, layers deep 3 and 4 have the majority of parvalbumin-containing neurons (Condé et al. 1994; Gabbott and Bacon 1996); layers 2, superficial 3, and 5 have the greatest density of somatostatin-containing neurons (Lewis et al. 1986); and layer 2 has the highest density of calretinin-containing cells (Condé et al. 1994; Gabbott and Bacon 1996).

Multiple lines of evidence show that GABA neurons in monkey prefrontal cortex are involved in working memory tasks. For example, fast-spiking neurons are active during the delay period of working memory tasks (Wilson et al. 1994), and injection of GABA antagonists into the prefrontal cortex disrupts working memory (Sawaguchi et al. 1989). Patients with schizophrenia perform poorly on working memory tasks (Weinberger et al. 1986), and postmortem studies have demonstrated alterations in markers of GABA neurotransmission in the prefrontal cortex of schizophrenic subjects. For example, reduced mRNA for the 67 kiloDalton isoform of glutamic acid decarboxylase, the principal determinant of GABA synthesis, is one of the most consistent findings in postmortem studies of individuals with schizophrenia (Akbarian and Huang 2006). In addition, mRNA levels of parvalbumin and somatostatin, but not of calretinin, are reduced in the prefrontal cortex of subjects with schizophrenia (Hashimoto et al. 2003, 2008).

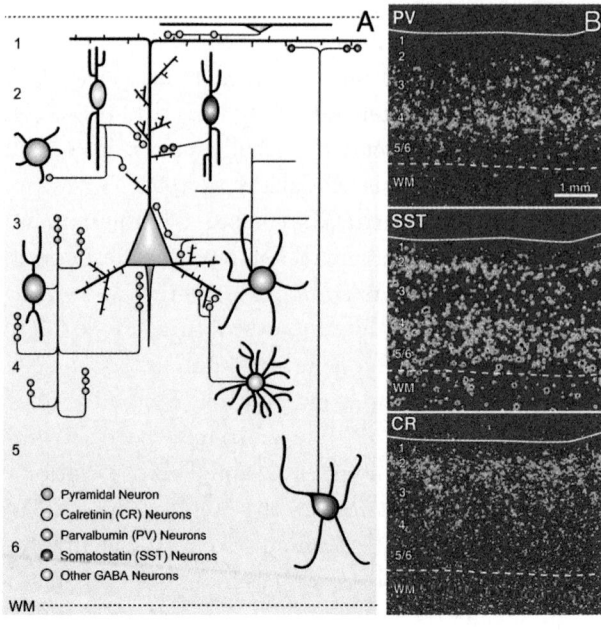

FIGURE 4–8.   (A) Schematic illustration of synaptic contacts between different subpopulations of GABA neurons and a layer 3 pyramidal neuron in monkey prefrontal cortex.

(A) The indicated synaptic connections of each subpopulation of GABA neuron are based on previous studies (see text for details).

(B) Film autoradiograms showing signals for parvalbumin (PV), somatostatin (SST), and calretinin (CR) mRNAs in human prefrontal cortex.

(B) Note the different laminar distribution of these three subclasses of GABA neurons. GABA = γ-aminobutyric acid; WM = white matter.

Source.   Adapted from Gonzalez-Burgos G, Hashimoto T, Lewis DA: "Inhibition and Timing in Cortical Neural Circuits" (Images in Neuroscience). *American Journal of Psychiatry* 164:12, 2007. Copyright 2007, American Psychiatric Association. Used with permission.

Thalamus

The dorsal thalamus is a heterogeneous structure composed of numerous nuclei that are distinguished on the basis of their location, cytoarchitecture, and connections with other brain regions. The projection or relay neurons within these nuclei use glutamate as their neurotransmitter and thus provide excitatory input to their target regions. For example, the axon terminals that project from the thalamus to primary sensory cortices contain glutamate immunoreactivity and form Gray's type I synapses (Kharazia and Weinberg 1994).

There are two groups of GABA-containing neurons in the primate thalamus: the interneurons, whose axons and actions are confined within the various dorsal thalamic nuclei, and the neurons of the reticular nucleus. All of the neurons in the reticular nucleus are GABAergic, and they provide extensive projections to the nuclei of the dorsal thalamus, the principal and possibly sole target of the reticular nucleus (Steriade et al. 1997). Thus, as in the cortex, the activity of the long-range excitatory projections from the thalamus is regulated by inhibitory inputs from nearby GABA neurons.

Basal Ganglia

The basal ganglia consist of the striatum (comprising the caudate nucleus, putamen, and nucleus accumbens), the globus pallidus (internal and external segments), and the substantia nigra pars reticulata. The internal segment of the globus pallidus and the substantia nigra pars reticulata are often grouped together and are referred to as the output nuclei of the basal ganglia. In contrast to the cortex and thalamus, the projection neurons of the basal ganglia utilize GABA as a neurotransmitter. For example, the GABA-containing medium spiny neurons of the striatum, which are the principal target of the excitatory projections from cortical pyramidal cells (Alexander and Crutcher 1990), project to the output nuclei of the basal ganglia (Figure 4–9). These medium spiny striatal neurons express substance P and dynorphin as well as GABA (Gerfen and Young 1988). The GABA projection neurons of the output nuclei of the basal ganglia project to the thalamus, where they form inhibitory contacts with thalamic projection neurons. This pathway from the striatum through the output nuclei of the basal ganglia to the thalamus is known as the "direct" pathway through the basal ganglia, and it results in disinhibition of the thalamus, which in turn sends a glutamatergic projection back to the cerebral cortex (Alexander and Crutcher 1990). In the "indirect" pathway (see Figure 4–9), GABA- and enkephalin-containing neurons in the striatum project to the external segment of the globus pallidus (Gerfen and Young 1988), where they target GABA projection neurons. The axons of these pallidal projection neurons target glutamate-containing cells in the subthalamic nucleus, which then project to GABA neurons of the output nuclei of the basal ganglia. Similar to the direct pathway, the output nuclei of the basal ganglia send GABAergic projections to the thalamus. In both the direct and indirect pathways, the cerebral cortex sends glutamatergic projections to the striatum and receives glutamatergic input from the thalamus, thus forming a corticostriatal circuit (see Figure 4–9). DA released from

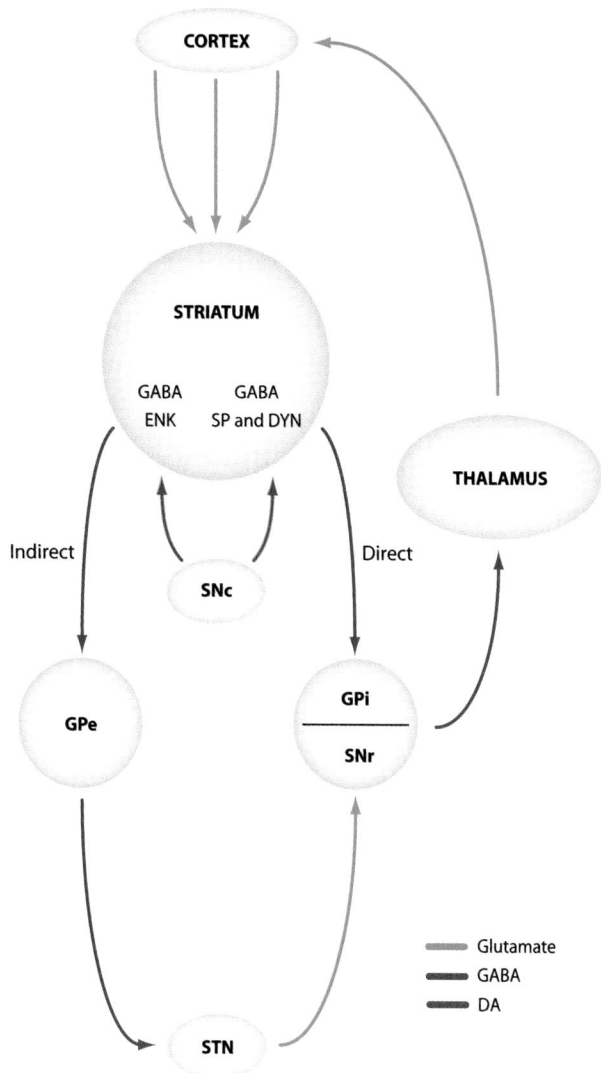

FIGURE 4–9. Schematic diagram of basal ganglia circuitry, illustrating the direct and indirect pathways.

See text for details. DA = dopamine; DYN = dynorphin; ENK = enkephalin; GABA = γ-aminobutyric acid; GPe = external globus pallidus; GPi = internal globus pallidus; SNc = substantia nigra pars compacta; SNr = substantia nigra pars reticulata; SP = substance P; STN = subthalamic nucleus.

Source. Adapted from Parent A, Sato F, Wu Y, et al: "Organization of the Basal Ganglia: The Importance of Axonal Collateralization." *Trends in Neurosciences* 23:S20–S27, 2000. Copyright 2000, Elsevier. Used with permission.

neurons in the substantia nigra pars compacta appears to facilitate transmission through the direct pathway, via D_1 receptors on the substance P/dynorphin cells, and to inhibit transmission through the indirect pathway, via D_2 receptors on the enkephalin cells (Albin et al. 1989; Gerfen et al. 1990).

The nigrostriatal projection constitutes one of the major inputs to the basal ganglia. The striatum reciprocates and sends projections back to the midbrain DA neurons (Figure 4–10), forming a striatonigrostriatal circuit. The midbrain DA neurons can be divided into two tiers: the dorsal tier (which includes neurons of the dorsal substantia nigra pars compacta, the ventral tegmental area, and the retrorubral group) and the ventral tier (composed of the densocellular and cell column neurons of the substantia nigra pars compacta) (Haber and Fudge 1997). As illustrated in Figure 4–10, there is an inverse dorsal–ventral topographical organization to the projection from the dorsal and ventral DA neurons to the striatum (Haber 2003). For example, dorsally and medially located DA neurons project to the ventral and medial parts of the striatum (red and yellow pathways in Figure 4–10), whereas ventrally and laterally located DA neurons project to the dorsal and lateral parts of the striatum (green and blue pathways in Figure 4–10). Another prominent input to the striatum derives from the cerebral cortex, and this projection has a topographic organization related to that of the striatonigrostriatal pathway (see Figure 4–10). The orbital and medial prefrontal cortices project to the ventral striatum, the dorsolateral prefrontal cortex projects to the central striatum, and the premotor and motor cortices project to the dorsolateral striatum. These topographies create limbic, associative, and motor pathways (red/orange, yellow, and green/blue, respectively, in Figure 4–10) within the corticostriatalcortical and striatonigrostriatal projections.

Neuropeptides

Neuropeptides are generally thought to modulate the effects of classical neurotransmitters and are often collocated with neurotransmitters within neurons. This section focuses on six neuropeptides that have been implicated in the pathophysiology of psychiatric disorders.

Corticotropin-Releasing Factor

Corticotropin-releasing factor (CRF) is best known as a hormone that is secreted by the hypothalamus and that stimulates adrenocorticotropic hormone (ACTH) release from the pituitary, which results in the production of cortisol by the adrenal glands. Specifically, CRF is localized to neurons of the paraventricular nucleus in the hypothalamus, which send axons to the median eminence. CRF-containing cells are also localized to other hypothalamic nuclei, such as the medial preoptic area and the

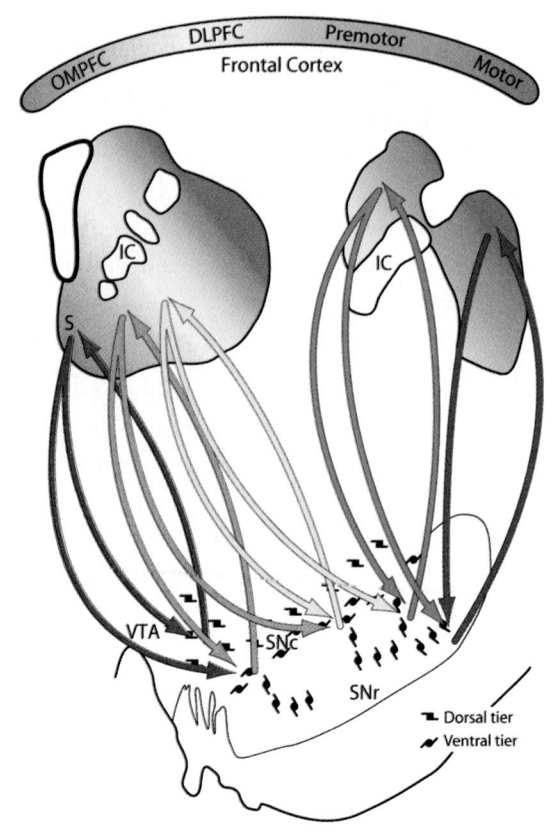

FIGURE 4–10. Organization of striatonigralstriatal projections.

The organization of functional corticostriatal inputs (red = limbic, green = associative, blue = motor) is illustrated (see text for details). DL-PFC = dorsolateral prefrontal cortex; IC = internal capsule; OMPFC = orbital and medial prefrontal cortex; SNc = substantia nigra pars compacta; SNr = substantia nigra pars reticulata. VTA = ventral tegmental area.

Source. Adapted from Haber SN, Fudge JH, McFarland NR: "Striatonigrostriatal Pathways in Primates Form an Ascending Spiral From the Shell to the Dorsolateral Striatum." *Journal of Neuroscience* 20:2369–2382, 2000. Copyright 2000, Society for Neuroscience. Used with permission.

dorsomedial, arcuate, and mammillary nuclei (DeSouza and Grigoriadis 2002), as well as to the amygdala and bed nucleus of the stria terminalis (Keller et al. 2006). Besides the median eminence, CRF axons are present in the cerebral cortex, brain stem (including the locus coeruleus), and spinal cord. To date, two CRF receptors have been identified, CRF$_1$ and CRF$_2$. CRF$_1$ receptors are expressed in the pituitary, cerebral cortex, hippocampus, amygdala, and medial septum, and CRF$_2$ receptors are localized to the hypothalamic nuclei, lateral septum, and bed nucleus of the stria terminalis (Keller et al. 2006).

It has been hypothesized that hyperactivity of hypothalamic CRF might underlie the hypercortisolemia and contribute to the symptomatology seen in major depression (Aborelius et al. 1999). Furthermore, given that both NE and DA have been shown to be involved with stress as well as with depression, the presence of CRF-containing axons in NE- and DA-containing nuclei provides another mechanism by which CRF can affect stress responses (Austin et al. 1997).

CRF also appears to have effects on cognitive processing. Of interest, CRF is found in GABA-containing cells in the cerebral cortex, with the highest densities of these cells found in prefrontal, insular, and cingulate cortices (DeSouza and Grigoriadis 2002). In addition, cortical CRF has also been implicated in major depression and in Alzheimer's disease. For example, a decrease in CRF binding sites in the frontal cortex of suicide victims compared with normal controls has been demonstrated (Mitchell 1998). Furthermore, in postmortem tissue from individuals with Alzheimer's disease, CRF-containing axons are associated with amyloid deposits in the cerebral cortex (Powers et al. 1987); reduced CRF levels in frontal, temporal, and parietal cortices are correlated with the severity of dementia (Davis et al. 1999).

Neuropeptide Y

Neuropeptide Y (NPY) is a 36–amino acid peptide that, along with its receptors, is widely distributed within the central nervous system (Wettstein et al. 1995). The regions of the human brain that contain high densities of NPY-containing neurons include the striatum and amygdala, with the hypothalamus, cerebral cortex, hippocampus, periaqueductal gray, and basal forebrain having moderate levels of NPY-containing cells (Schwartzberg et al. 1990). Five G protein–coupled NPY receptor subtypes, termed Y_1–Y_5, have been identified and cloned (Redrobe et al. 2002). The NPY receptors Y_1 and Y_2 are the most abundant and are found in the cerebral cortex, thalamus, brain stem, and hypothalamus (Redrobe et al. 2002). In addition to its role in regulating eating behavior, NPY has been implicated in affective disorders. For example, in a rodent model of depression, chronic antidepressant treatment increased NPY and Y_1 mRNA levels (Caberlotto et al. 1998). In humans, cerebrospinal fluid and plasma levels of NPY are lower in depressed patients than in controls (Nilsson et al. 1996; Westrin et al. 1999), and these levels increase after electroconvulsive therapy (Mathé et al. 1996). In addition, NPY mRNA is reduced in the prefrontal cortex of subjects with bipolar disorder (Caberlotto and Hurd 2001) and subjects with schizophrenia (Hashimoto et al. 2008).

Substance P

Substance P is a member of the family of neuropeptides known as the tachykinins, which also includes neurokinin A and B. The actions of these neuropeptides are mediated through the specific G protein–coupled receptors NK_1, NK_2, and NK_3, and substance P is the preferred agonist for the NK_1 receptor (Hökfelt et al. 2001). Substance P is found throughout the nervous system. In particular, substance P is expressed in brain regions that appear to be involved in emotion, such as the amygdala, periaqueductal gray, and hypothalamus (Pioro et al. 1990). In addition, substance P is collocated with serotonin in approximately 50% of the dorsal raphe neurons in the human brain (Baker et al. 1991; Sergeyev et al. 1999), and a large number of serotonin-containing dorsal raphe neurons express the NK_1 receptor (Lacoste et al. 2006).

Studies in animals have suggested that substance P, besides having a role in pain and inflammation, may also be involved in anxiety and in neurochemical responses to stress. For example, injection of substance P into periaqueductal gray matter produced anxiety-like behavior in rats (Aguiar and Brandao 1996). Furthermore, in guinea pigs subjected to maternal separation, the number of neurons with NK_1 receptor internalization increased in the basolateral amygdala (Kramer et al. 1998).

Substance P also appears to be involved in depression. For example, elevated concentrations of substance P have been reported in the cerebrospinal fluid of depressed patients (Rimon et al. 2002).

Neurotensin

Neurotensin is a tridecapeptide found throughout the brain, with high tissue concentrations in the amygdala, lateral septum, bed nucleus of the stria terminalis, substantia nigra, and ventral tegmental area (Caceda et al. 2006). Similarly, neurotensin-immunoreactive neurons are found in the amygdala, bed nucleus of the stria terminalis, lateral septum, and preoptic and lateral hypothalamus (Geisler et al. 2006). Three types of neurotensin receptors have been cloned, NTS_1–NTS_3, with NTS_1 and NTS_2 being G protein–coupled receptors and NTS_3 belonging to the vacuolar sorting receptor family (Caceda et al. 2006). High levels of mRNA for all three of these receptor types are found in the substantia nigra and amygdala.

Neurotensin has a strong association with the dopaminergic system, as evidenced by the heavy neurotensin innervation of nuclei that have high densities of DA cells or axons, such as the ventral tegmental area and the amygdala, respectively (Geisler et al. 2006). In addition, the majority of DA neurons in the ventral tegmental area express NTS$_1$ (Fassio et al. 2000), and neurotensin axons in this area arise from the preoptic and lateral hypothalamus (Zahm et al. 2001). Because of the role of DA in neuropsychiatric disorders such as schizophrenia, the localization and function of neurotensin in the brain have been widely studied. One of the most consistent findings is reduced cerebrospinal fluid concentrations of neurotensin in neuroleptic-naive people diagnosed with schizophrenia (Sharma et al. 1997). In addition, clinically effective antipsychotic drug treatment may increase cerebrospinal fluid neurotensin levels in schizophrenia (Sharma et al. 1997). Neurotensin has also been implicated in Parkinson's disease, which involves the progressive loss of DA neurons in the striatum. For example, decreases in neurotensin receptor binding as well as in NTS$_1$ receptor mRNA have been found in the substantia nigra and striatum of patients with Parkinson's disease (Yamada et al. 1995).

Somatostatin

The neuropeptide somatostatin was first identified in the hypothalamus as a tetradecapeptide (Brazeau et al. 1973). Other peptides of the somatostatin family, all of which are derived from the prosomatostatin protein, include somatostatin-28 and somatostatin-28$_{1-12}$ (Benoit et al. 1982). The hypothalamus and limbic regions such as the amygdala and hippocampus have large numbers of somatostatin-containing neurons. A small number of somatostatin neurons are localized to the cerebral cortex and are particularly abundant in layers 2–3 and layers 5–6 (Epelbaum et al. 1994). Somatostatin-containing neurons in the cerebral cortex have a nonpyramidal morphology and contain GABA (Hendry et al. 1984). The principal somatostatinergic tract projects from the anterior periventricular nucleus of the hypothalamus to the median eminence (Patel 1999). This projection inhibits secretion of growth hormone, thyroid-stimulating hormone, and prolactin from the adenohypophysis (Epelbaum et al. 1994). The actions of somatostatin are mediated by five distinct subtypes of G protein–coupled receptors, SST$_1$–SST$_5$. The SST$_2$ receptor undergoes alternative splicing that results in two forms, SST$_{2A}$ and SST$_{2B}$ (Epelbaum et al. 1994). Although all somatostatin receptors appear to be present in the brain (Patel 1999), the SST$_2$ receptor is the most widely studied. In rodent brain, the SST$_{2A}$ receptor protein has been localized to the cerebral cortex, basal ganglia, and hippocampus (Dournaud et al. 1996; Hervieu and Emson 1998).

The widespread distribution of somatostatin cells and receptors reflects the varied physiological actions that somatostatin release has in the nervous system, ranging from thermoregulation to cognitive functions such as learning and memory (Epelbaum et al. 1994). Deficits in the somatostatin system in Alzheimer's disease are some of the most consistent findings in this neurodegenerative disease. Decreases in cerebrospinal fluid somatostatin levels, selective degeneration of cortical somatostatin neurons, and reduction in cortical somatostatin receptors have all been found in Alzheimer's disease (Bissette 1997).

Somatostatin has also been implicated in the pathophysiology of schizophrenia. For example, studies have revealed decreased expression of somatostatin mRNA in the prefrontal cortex of individuals with schizophrenia (Hashimoto et al. 2008), specifically in layers 2–6 (Morris et al. 2008).

Orexins

The orexin neuropeptides, orexin A and orexin B (also known as hypocretin A and hypocretin B), were identified in the late 1990s as endogenous ligands for two orphan G protein–coupled receptors (de Lecea et al. 1998; Sakurai et al. 1998). Orexin A and orexin B are derived from a single precursor gene, prepro-orexin. Because neurons in the lateral hypothalamic area, a region with an established role in feeding behavior, produce these neuropeptides, Sakurai et al. (1998) named them orexins, based on the Greek word for appetite, *orexis*. Neurons producing orexin are also located in posterior and perifornical hypothalamus. Estimates of the number of orexin neurons range from 3,000 in rat brain (Nambu et al. 1999) to 7,000 in human brain (Peyron et al. 1998). Orexin neurons project throughout the brain, with the exception of the cerebellum (Figure 4–11). Interestingly, orexin neurons project to most of the monoaminergic (substantia nigra, locus coeruleus, dorsal raphe) and cholinergic (medial septum, pedunculopontine, laterodorsal tegmental) nuclei (Sakurai 2007). Orexin neurons also have widespread projections throughout the cerebral cortex. Areas containing high densities of orexin axons include the paraventricular thalamic nucleus, the arcuate nucleus of the hypothalamus, the locus coeruleus, and the dorsal raphe nucleus (Nambu et al. 1999).

The multiple actions of orexin are mediated by two types of G protein–coupled receptors, orexin 1 and orexin 2, which display high homology. In concert with the widespread projections of orexin neurons, the orexin receptors are located throughout the brain (Marcus et al.

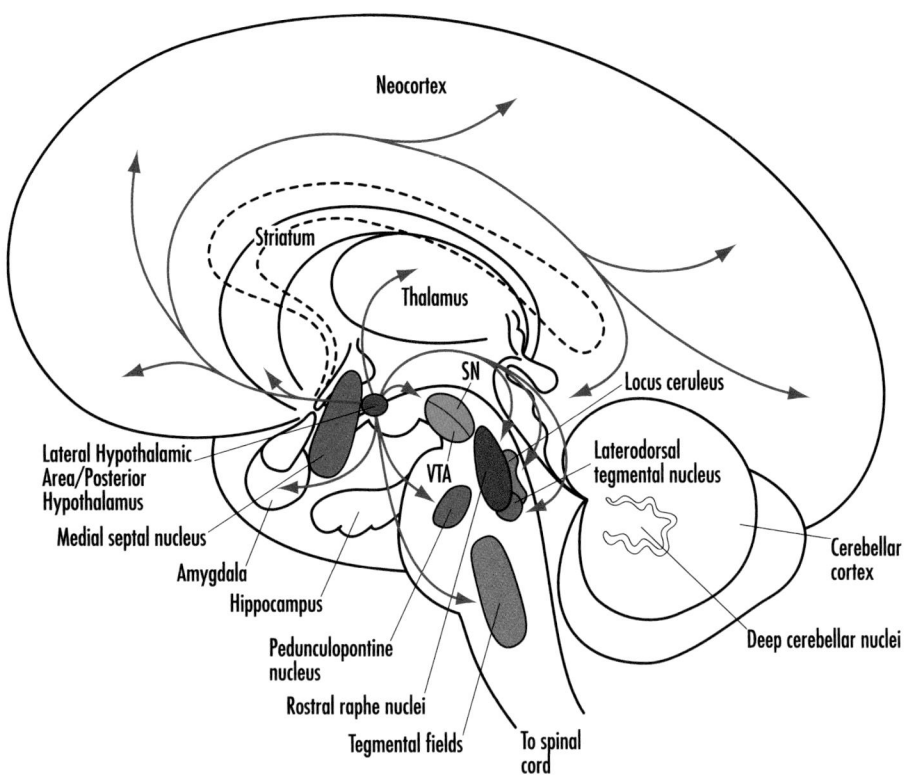

FIGURE 4–11. Projections of orexin-containing neurons in the human brain.

SN = substantia nigra; VTA = ventral tegmental area.

Source. Adapted from Heimer 1995.

2001). For example, the mRNA for orexin 1 is found in the prefrontal cortex, the CA2 field of the hippocampus, the paraventricular thalamic nucleus, the ventromedial hypothalamic nucleus, and the locus coeruleus. The distribution of the mRNA for orexin 2 is somewhat complementary to that of orexin 1 in that it is found in the piriform cortex, CA3 field of the hippocampus, rhomboid thalamic nucleus, dorsomedial hypothalamic nucleus, and tuberomammillary nucleus (Marcus et al. 2001). Some regions of the brain, such as the raphe nuclei, ventral tegmental area, and substantia nigra, express both orexin receptors.

The location of orexin-containing neurons in the feeding center of the brain (lateral hypothalamic area) and the projections of orexin neurons to neuronal systems involved in sleep and wakefulness (locus coeruleus, raphe nuclei, and laterodorsal/pedunculopontine tegmental nuclei) and reward (ventral tegmental area) illustrate the variety of functions in which orexin neurons participate (Harris and Aston-Jones 2006). Supporting orexin's involvement in feeding behavior, administration of an anti-orexin antibody or an orexin 1 receptor antagonist to rats reduces food intake (Haynes et al. 2002; Yamada et al.

2000). Numerous studies in both animals and humans show that orexin deficiency is the main cause of narcolepsy. For example, mice that lack the orexin gene exhibit physiological symptoms similar to those of human narcolepsy (Chemelli et al. 1999). More direct evidence of orexin's role in narcolepsy is that postmortem examination of the brains of narcolepsy patients revealed an 85%–95% reduction in the number of orexin-immunoreactive neurons (Thannickal et al. 2000). A recent study of an orexin receptor antagonist demonstrated the usefulness of this drug in inducing sleep without cataplexy (Brisbare-Roch et al. 2007), providing hope to people who suffer from sleeping disorders like narcolepsy. Current treatments for narcolepsy include addictive amphetamine-like drugs, but patients taking these drugs rarely become addicted (Harris and Aston-Jones 2006). This finding has led to speculation that orexins may also be involved in reward processing and addiction. For example, orexin neurons activate ventral tegmental DA neurons, which, through their projections to the nucleus accumbens, form the "reward" pathway. In addition, in rodents, administration of orexin directly into the ventral tegmental area reinstates an extinguished drug preference (Harris et al. 2005).

Conclusion

This chapter reviews the basic framework of the anatomical distribution of the major neurochemical systems in the primate brain, including the anatomical determinants of where neurotransmitters are released and where they produce their effects. These organizational schema provide important constraints on the actions of the neurotransmitters and neuromodulators. In addition, the consequences of the cellular actions and of pharmacological manipulations of their synthesis, release, reuptake, and receptor binding depend on the rich and diverse interplay across these neurochemical systems. Clearly, a major challenge for the future involves the elucidation of these interactions and the characterization of how these interactions are disturbed in psychiatric disorders. Such information is critical for identification and validation of potential molecular targets for the rational development of new pharmacotherapies for psychiatric illnesses.

References

Abi-Dargham A, Mawlawi O, Lombardo I, et al: Prefrontal dopamine D1 receptors and working memory in schizophrenia. J Neurosci 22:3708–3719, 2002

Aborelius L, Owens MJ, Plotsky PM, et al: The role of corticotropin-releasing factor in depression and anxiety disorders. J Endocrinol 160:1–12, 1999

Adler LE, Olincy A, Waldo MC, et al: Schizophrenia, sensory gating, and nicotinic receptors. Schizophr Bull 24:189–202, 1998

Aguiar MS, Brandao ML: Effects of microinjections of the neuropeptide substance P in the dorsal periaqueductal gray on the behaviour of rats in the plus-maze test. Physiol Behav 60:1183–1186, 1996

Akbarian S, Huang HS: Molecular and cellular mechanisms of altered GAD1/GAD67 expression in schizophrenia and related disorders. Brain Res Brain Res Rev 52:293–304, 2006

Akil M, Lewis DA: The dopaminergic innervation of monkey entorhinal cortex. Cerebral Cortex 3:533–550, 1993

Akil M, Kolachana BS, Rothmond DA, et al: Catechol-O-methyltransferase genotype and dopamine regulation in the human brain. J Neurosci 23:2008–2013, 2003

Akil M, Pierri JN, Whitehead RE, et al: Lamina-specific alterations in the dopamine innervation of the prefrontal cortex in schizophrenic subjects. Am J Psychiatry 156:1580–1589, 1999

Albin RL, Young AB, Penney JB. The functional anatomy of basal ganglia disorders. Trends Neurosci 12:366–375, 1989

Alexander GE, Crutcher MD: Functional architecture of the basal ganglia circuits: neural substrates of parallel processing. Trends Neurosci 13:266, 1990

Alger BE: Retrograde signaling in the regulation of synaptic transmission: focus on endocannabinoids. Prog Neurobiol 68:247–286, 2002

Andreasen NC, O'Leary DS, Cizaldo T, et al: Schizophrenia and cognitive dysmetria: a positron-emission tomography study of dysfunctional prefrontal-thalamic-cerebellar circuitry. Proc Natl Acad Sci U S A 93:9985–9990, 1996

Arsenault MY, Parent A, Seguela P, et al: Distribution and morphological characteristics of dopamine-immunoreactive neurons in the midbrain of the squirrel monkey (Saimiri sciureus). J Comp Neurol 267:489–506, 1988

Austin MC, Rhodes JL, Lewis DA: Differential distribution of corticotropin-releasing hormone immunoreactive axons in monoaminergic nuclei of the human brainstem. Neuropsychopharmacology 17:326–341, 1997

Azmitia EC, Gannon PJ: The primate serotonergic system: a review of human and animal studies and a report on Macaca fascicularis. Adv Neurol 43:407–468, 1986

Bach-Mizrachi H, Underwood MD, Kassir SA, et al: Neuronal tryptophan hydroxylase mRNA expression in the human dorsal and median raphe nuclei: major depression and suicide. Neuropsychopharmacology 31:814–824, 2006

Baker KG, Halliday GM, Tork I: Cytoarchitecture of the human dorsal raphe nucleus. J Comp Neurol 301:147–161, 1990

Baker KG, Halliday GM, Hornung JP, et al: Distribution, morphology and number of monoamine-synthesizing and substance P–containing neurons in the human dorsal raphe nucleus. Neuroscience 42:757–775, 1991

Barbas H, Henion TH, Dermon CR: Diverse thalamic projections to the prefrontal cortex in the rhesus monkey. J Comp Neurol 313:65–94, 1991

Beaudet A, Descarries L: Fine structure of monoamine axon terminals in cerebral cortex, in Monoamine Innervation of Cerebral Cortex. Edited by Descarries L, Reader TR, Jasper HH. New York, Alan R Liss, 1984, pp 77–93

Benoit R, Ling N, Alford B, et al: Seven peptides derived from prosomatostatin in rat brain. Biochem Biophys Res Commun 107:944–950, 1982

Berger B, Gaspar P, Verney C: Dopaminergic innervation of the cerebral cortex: unexpected differences between rodents and primates. Trends Neurosci 14:21–27, 1991

Bergson C, Mrzljak L, Smiley JF, et al: Regional, cellular, and subcellular variations in the distribution of D1 and D5 dopamine receptors in primate brain. J Neurosci 15:7821–7836, 1995

Biegon A, Kerman IA: Autoradiographic study of pre- and postnatal distribution of cannabinoid receptors in human brain. Neuroimage 14:1463–1468, 2001

Bissette G: Neuropeptides and Alzheimer's disease pathology. Ann N Y Acad Sci 814:17–29, 1997

Bjorklund A, Dunnett SB: Dopamine neuron systems in the brain: an update. Trends Neurosci 30:194–202, 2007

Bodor AL, Katona I, Nyiri G, et al: Endocannabinoid signaling in rat somatosensory cortex: laminar differences and involvement of specific interneuron types. J Neurosci 25:6845–6856, 2005

Brazeau P, Vale W, Burgus R, et al: Hypothalamic polypeptide that inhibits the secretion of immunoreactive pituitary growth hormone. Science 179:77–79, 1973

Breese CR, Lee MJ, Adams CE, et al: Abnormal regulation of high affinity nicotinic receptors in subjects with schizophrenia. Neuropsychopharmacology 23:351–364, 2000

Brisbare-Roch C, Dingemanse J, Koberstein R, et al: Promotion of sleep by targeting the orexin system in rats, dogs and humans. Nat Med 13:150–155, 2007

Caberlotto L, Fuxe K, Overstreet DH, et al: Alterations in neuropeptide Y and Y1 receptor mRNA expression in brains from an animal model of depression: region specific adaptation after fluoxetine treatment. Brain Res Mol Brain Res 59:58–65, 1998

Caberlotto L, Hurd YL: Neuropeptide Y Y(1) and Y(2) receptor mRNA expression in the prefrontal cortex of psychiatric subjects. Relationship of Y(2) subtype to suicidal behavior. Neuropsychopharmacology 25:91–97, 2001

Caceda R, Kinkead B, Nemeroff CB: Neurotensin: role in psychiatric and neurological diseases. Peptides 27:2385–2404, 2006

Cavada C, Compañy T, Hernández-González A, et al: Acetylcholinesterase histochemistry in the macaque thalamus reveals territories selectively connected to frontal, parietal and temporal association cortices. J Chem Neuroanat 8:245–257, 1995

Chemelli RM, Willie JT, Sinton CM, et al: Narcolepsy in orexin knockout mice: molecular genetics of sleep regulation. Cell 98:437–451, 1999

Chen J, Lipska BK, Halim N, et al: Functional analysis of genetic variation in catechol-O-methyltransferase (COMT): effects on mRNA, protein, and enzyme activity in postmortem human brain. Am J Hum Genet 75:807–821, 2004

Chung CY, Seo H, Sonntag KC, et al: Cell type-specific gene expression of midbrain dopaminergic neurons reveals molecules involved in their vulnerability and protection. Hum Mol Genet 14:1709–1725, 2005

Ciliax BJ, Heilman C, Demchyshyn LL, et al: The dopamine transporter: immunochemical characterization and localization in brain. J Neurosci 15:1714–1723, 1995

Ciliax BJ, Drash GW, Staley JK, et al: Immunocytochemical localization of the dopamine transporter in human brain. J Comp Neurol 409:38–56, 1999

Clarke PB: Mapping of brain nicotinic receptors by autoradiographic techniques and the effect of experimental lesions. Prog Brain Res 79:65–71, 1989

Condé F, Lund JS, Jacobowitz DM, et al: Local circuit neurons immunoreactive for calretinin, calbindin D-28k, or parvalbumin in monkey prefrontal cortex: distribution and morphology. J Comp Neurol 341:95–116, 1994

Cooper JR, Bloom FE, Roth RH: The Biochemical Basis of Neuropharmacology. New York, Oxford University Press, 1996

D'Souza DC, Perry E, MacDougall L, et al: The psychotomimetic effects of intravenous delta-9-tetrahydrocannabinol in healthy individuals: implications for psychosis. Neuropsychopharmacology 29:1558–1572, 2004

Dahlström A, Fuxe K: Evidence for the existence of monoamine neurons in the central nervous system, I: demonstration of monoamines in the cell bodies of brain stem neurons. Acta Physiol Scand Suppl 232:1–55, 1964

Dani JA, Bertrand D: Nicotinic acetylcholine receptors and nicotinic cholinergic mechanisms of the central nervous system. Annu Rev Pharmacol Toxicol 47:699–729, 2007

Davis KL, Mohs RC, Marin DB, et al: Neuropeptide abnormalities in patients with early Alzheimer disease. Arch Gen Psychiatry 56:981–987, 1999

De Lacalle S, Saper CB: The cholinergic system in the primate brain: basal forebrain and pontine-tegmental cell groups, in Handbook of Chemical Neuroanatomy: The Primate Nervous System, Vol 13. Edited by Bloom FE, Björklund A, Hökfelt T. Amsterdam, The Netherlands, Elsevier Science, 1997, pp 217–262

de Lecea L, Kilduff TS, Peyron C, et al: The hypocretins: hypothalamus-specific peptides with neuroexcitatory activity. Proc Natl Acad Sci U S A 95:322–327, 1998

DeFelipe J: Neocortical neuronal diversity: chemical heterogeneity revealed by colocalization studies of classic neurotransmitters, neuropeptides, calcium-binding proteins, and cell surface molecules. Cereb Cortex 3:273–289, 1993

DeFelipe J, Farinas I: The pyramidal neuron of the cerebral cortex: morphological and chemical characteristics of the synaptic inputs. Prog Neurobiol 39:563–607, 1992

DeFelipe J, Hendry SHC, Jones EG, et al: Variability in the terminations of GABAergic chandelier cell axons on initial segments of pyramidal cell axons in the monkey sensory-motor cortex. J Comp Neurol 231:364–384, 1985

DeFelipe J, Hendry SHC, Jones EG: Visualization of chandelier cell axons by parvalbumin immunoreactivity in monkey cerebral cortex. Proc Natl Acad Sci U S A 86:2093–2097, 1989

DeFelipe J, Arellano JI, Gómez A, et al: Pyramidal cell axons show a local specialization for GABA and 5-HT inputs in monkey and human cerebral cortex. J Comp Neurol 433:148–155, 2001

Delfs JM, Zhu Y, Druhan JP, et al: Noradrenaline in the ventral forebrain is critical for opiate withdrawal-induced aversion. Nature 403:430–434, 2000

DeSouza EB, Grigoriadis DE: Corticotropin-releasing factor: physiology, pharmacology, and role in central nervous system disorders, in Neuropsychopharmacology: The Fifth Generation of Progress. Edited by Davis KL, Charney DS, Coyle JT, et al. New York, Lippincott Williams & Wilkins, 2002, pp 91–107

Diaz J, Lévesque D, Lammers CH, et al: Phenotypical characterization of neurons expressing the dopamine D3 receptor in the rat brain. Neuroscience 65:731–745, 1995

Dournaud P, Gu YZ, Schonbrunn A, et al: Localization of the somatostatin receptor SST2A in rat brain using a specific anti-peptide antibody. J Neurosci 16:4468–4478, 1996

Egan MF, Goldberg TE, Kolachana BS, et al: Effect of COMT Val 108/158 Met genotype on frontal lobe function and risk for schizophrenia. Proc Natl Acad Sci U S A 98:6917–6922, 2001

Eggan SM, Lewis DA: Immunocytochemical distribution of the cannabinoid CB1 receptor in the primate neocortex: a regional and laminar analysis. Cereb Cortex 17:175–191, 2007

Eggan SM, Hashimoto T, Lewis DA: Reduced cortical cannabinoid 1 receptor messenger RNA and protein expression in schizophrenia. Arch Gen Psychiatry 65:1–13, 2008

Epelbaum J, Dournaud P, Fodor M, et al: The neurobiology of somatostatin. Crit Rev Neurobiol 8:25–44, 1994

Fairen A, Valverde F: A specialized type of neuron in the visual cortex of cat: a Golgi and electron microscope study of chandelier cells. J Comp Neurol 194:761–779, 1980

Fairen A, DeFelipe J, Regidon J: Nonpyramidal neurons, general account. Cereb Cortex 1:201–245, 1984

Fassio A, Evans G, Grisshammer R, et al: Distribution of the neurotensin receptor NTS1 in the rat CNS studied using an amino-terminal directed antibody. Neuropharmacology 39:1430–1442, 2000

Felten DL, Sladek JR: Monoamine distribution in primate brain, V: monoaminergic nuclei: anatomy, pathways and local organization. Brain Res Bull 10:171–284, 1983

Flynn DD, Mash DC: Distinct kinetic binding properties of N-[3H]-methylscopolamine afford differential labeling and localization of M1, M2, and M3 muscarinic receptor subtypes in primate brain. Synapse 14:283–296, 1993

Foote SL: The primate locus coeruleus: the chemical neuroanatomy of the nucleus, its efferent projections, and its target receptors, in Handbook of Chemical Neuroanatomy: The Primate Nervous System, Part I. Edited by Bloom FE, Björklund A, Hökfelt T. New York, Elsevier Sciences, 1997, pp 187–215

Freedman R, Hall M, Adler LE, et al: Evidence in postmortem brain tissue for decreased numbers of hippocampal nicotinic receptors in schizophrenia. Biol Psychiatry 38:22–33, 1995

Gabbott PLA, Bacon SJ: Local circuit neurons in the medial prefrontal cortex (areas 24a,b,c, 25 and 32) in the monkey, I: cell morphology and morphometrics. J Comp Neurol 364:567–608, 1996

Gaspar P, Berger B, Fabvret A, et al: Catecholamine innervation of the human cerebral cortex as revealed by comparative immunohistochemistry of tyrosine hydroxylase and dopamine-beta-hydroxylase. J Comp Neurol 279:249–271, 1989

Gatter KC, Powell TPS: The projection of the locus coeruleus upon the neocortex in the macaque monkey. Neuroscience 2:441–445, 1977

Geisler S, Berod A, Zahm DS, et al: Brain neurotensin, psychostimulants, and stress—emphasis on neuroanatomical substrates. Peptides 27:2364–2384, 2006

Gerfen CR, Young WS III: Distribution of striatonigral and striatopallidal peptidergic neurons in both patch and matrix compartments: an in situ hybridization histochemistry and fluorescent retrograde tracing study. Brain Res 460:161–167, 1988

Gerfen CR, Engver TM, Mahan LC, et al: D1 and D2 dopamine receptor-regulated gene expression of striatonigral and striatopallidal neurons. Science 250:1429–1432, 1990

Ginsberg SD, Hof PR, Young WG, et al: Noradrenergic innervation of the hypothalamus of rhesus monkeys: distribution of dopamine-beta-hydroxylase immunoreactive fibers and quantitative analysis of varicosities in the paraventricular nucleus. J Comp Neurol 327:597–611, 1993

Goldman-Rakic PS, Brown RM: Postnatal development of monoamine content and synthesis in the cerebral cortex of rhesus monkeys. Dev Brain Res 4:339–349, 1982

Goldman-Rakic PS, Lidow MS, Gallagher DW: Overlap of dopaminergic, adrenergic, and serotonergic receptors and complementarity of their subtypes in primate prefrontal cortex. J Neurosci 10:2125–2138, 1990

Gonchar Y, Burkhalter A: Connectivity of GABAergic calretinin-immunoreactive neurons in rat primary visual cortex. Cereb Cortex 9:683–696, 1999

Greene JG: Gene expression profiles of brain dopamine neurons and relevance to neuropsychiatric disease. J Physiol 575:411–416, 2006

Greene JG, Dingledine R, Greenamyre JT: Gene expression profiling of rat midbrain dopamine neurons: implications for selective vulnerability in parkinsonism. Neurobiol Dis 18:19–31, 2005

Haber SN: The primate basal ganglia: parallel and integrative networks. J Chem Neuroanat 26:317–330, 2003

Haber SN, Fudge JL: The primate substantia nigra and VTA: integrative circuitry and function. Crit Rev Neurobiol 11:323–342, 1997

Haber SN, Ryoo H, Cox C, et al: Subsets of midbrain dopaminergic neurons in monkeys are distinguished by different levels of mRNA for the dopamine transporter: comparison with the mRNA for the D2 receptor, tyrosine hydroxylase and calbindin immunoreactivity. J Comp Neurol 362:400–410, 1995

Han Z-Y, Le Novere N, Zoli M, et al: Localization of nAChR subunit mRNAs in the brain of Macaca mulatta. Eur J Neurosci 12:3664–3674, 2000

Harris GC, Aston-Jones G: Arousal and reward: a dichotomy in orexin function. Trends Neurosci 29:571–577, 2006

Harris GC, Wimmer M, Aston-Jones G: A role for lateral hypothalamic orexin neurons in reward seeking. Nature 437:556–559, 2005

Hashimoto T, Volk DW, Eggan SM, et al: Gene expression deficits in a subclass of GABA neurons in the prefrontal cortex of subjects with schizophrenia. J Neurosci 23:6315–6326, 2003

Hashimoto T, Arion D, Volk DW, et al: Alterations in GABA-related transcriptome in the dorsolateral prefrontal cortex of subjects with schizophrenia. Mol Psychiatry 13:147–161, 2008

Haynes AC, Chapman H, Taylor C, et al: Anorectic, thermogenic and anti-obesity activity of a selective orexin-1 receptor antagonist in ob/ob mice. Regul Pept 104:153–159, 2002

Heimer L: The Human Brain and Spinal Cord: Functional Neuroanatomy and Dissection Guide, 2nd Edition. New York, Springer-Verlag, 1995

Hendry SHC, Jones EG, Emson PC. Morphology, distribution, and synaptic relations of somatostatin- and neuropeptide Y-immunoreactive neurons in rat and monkey neocortex. J Neurosci 4:2497–2517, 1984

Herkenham M, Lynn AB, Johnson MR, et al: Characterization and localization of cannabinoid receptors in rat brain: a quantitative in vitro autoradiographic study. J Neurosci 11:563–583, 1991

Hervieu G, Emson PC: Visualisation of non-glycosylated somatostatin receptor two (ngsst2) immunoreactivity in the rat central nervous system. Brain Res Mol Brain Res 58:138–155, 1998

Hökfelt T, Pernow B, Wahren J: Substance P: a pioneer amongst neuropeptides. J Intern Med 249:27–40, 2001

Hornung JP: The human raphe nuclei and the serotonergic system. J Chem Neuroanat 26:331–343, 2003

Hurd YL, Suzuki M, Sedvall GC: D1 and D2 dopamine receptor mRNA expression in whole hemisphere sections of the human brain. J Chem Neuroanat 22:127–137, 2001

Jaber M, Robinson SW, Missale C, et al: Dopamine receptors and brain function. Neuropharmacology 35:1503–1519, 1996

Jaber M, Jones S, Giros B, et al: The dopamine transporter: a crucial component regulating dopamine transmission. Mov Disord 12:629–633, 1997

Jakab RL, Goldman-Rakic PS: Segregation of serotonin 5-HT2A and 5-HT3 receptors in inhibitory circuits of the primate cerebral cortex. J Comp Neurol 417:337–348, 2000

Katona I, Sperlagh B, Sik A, et al: Presynaptically located CB1 cannabinoid receptors regulate GABA release from axon terminals of specific hippocampal interneurons. J Neurosci 19:4544–4558, 1999

Kawaguchi Y, Kubota Y: GABAergic cell subtypes and their synaptic connections in rat frontal cortex. Cereb Cortex 7:476–486, 1997

Keller PA, McCluskey A, Morgan J, et al: The role of the HPA axis in psychiatric disorders and CRF antagonists as potential treatments. Arch Pharm (Weinheim) 339:346–355, 2006

Khan ZU, Gutiérrez A, Martín R, et al: Differential regional and cellular distribution of dopamine D2-like receptors: an immunocytochemical study of subtype-specific antibodies in rat and human brain. J Comp Neurol 402:353–371, 1998

Kharazia VN, Weinberg RJ: Glutamate in thalamic fibers terminating in layer IV of primary sensory cortex. J Neurosci 14:6021–6032, 1994

Kitt CA, Mitchell SJ, DeLong MR, et al: Fiber pathways of basal forebrain cholinergic neurons in monkeys. Brain Res 406:192–206, 1987

Kramer MS, Cutler N, Feighner J, et al: Distinct mechanism for antidepressant activity by blockade of central substance P receptors. Science 281:640, 1998

Krimer LS, Zaitsev AV, Czanner G, et al: Cluster analysis-based physiological classification and morphological properties of inhibitory neurons in layers 2–3 of monkey dorsolateral prefrontal cortex. J Neurophysiol 94:3009–3022, 2005

Lacoste B, Riad M, Descarries L: Immunocytochemical evidence for the existence of substance P receptor (NK1) in serotonin neurons of rat and mouse dorsal raphe nucleus. Eur J Neurosci 23:2947–2958, 2006

Lai MK, Tsang SW, Garcia-Alloza M, et al: Selective effects of the APOE epsilon4 allele on presynaptic cholinergic markers in the neocortex of Alzheimer's disease. Neurobiol Dis 22:555–561, 2006

Lavoie B, Parent A: Serotonergic innervation of the thalamus in the primate: an immunohistochemical study. J Comp Neurol 312:1–18, 1991

Leonard S, Breese C, Adams C, et al: Smoking and schizophrenia: abnormal nicotinic receptor expression. Eur J Pharmacol 393:237–242, 2000

Levey AI, Hallanger AE, Wainer BH: Choline acetyltransferase immunoreactivity in the rat thalamus. J Comp Neurol 257:317–332, 1987

Lewandowski KE: Relationship of catechol-O-methyltransferase to schizophrenia and its correlates: evidence for associations and complex interactions. Harv Rev Psychiatry 15:233–244, 2007

Lewis DA: Distribution of choline acetyltransferase immunoreactive axons in monkey frontal cortex. Neuroscience 40:363–374, 1991

Lewis DA: The catecholaminergic innervation of primate prefrontal cortex. J Neural Transm Suppl 36:179–200, 1992

Lewis DA: Neural circuitry approaches to understanding the pathophysiology of schizophrenia, in Neuropsychopharmacology: The Fifth Generation of Progress. Edited by Davis KL, Charney DS, Coyle JT, et al. Philadelphia, PA, Lippincott Williams & Wilkins, 2002, pp 729–743

Lewis DA, Morrison JH: The noradrenergic innervation of monkey prefrontal cortex: a dopamine-beta-hydroxylase immunohistochemical study. J Comp Neurol 282:317–330, 1989

Lewis DA, Sesack SR: Dopamine systems in the primate brain, in Handbook of Chemical Neuroanatomy. Edited by Bloom FE, Björklund A, Hökfelt T. Amsterdam, The Netherlands, Elsevier Science, 1997, pp 261–373

Lewis DA, Campbell MJ, Morrison JH: An immunohistochemical characterization of somatostatin-28 and somatostatin-28 (1–12) in monkey prefrontal cortex. J Comp Neurol 248:1–18, 1986

Lewis DA, Campbell MJ, Foote SL, et al: The distribution of tyrosine hydroxylase–immunoreactive fibers in primate neocortex is widespread but regionally specific. J Neurosci 7:279–290, 1987

Lewis DA, Foote SL, Goldstein M, et al: The dopaminergic innervation of monkey prefrontal cortex: a tyrosine hydroxylase immunohistochemical study. Brain Res 449:225–243, 1988a

Lewis DA, Morrison JH, Goldstein M. Brainstem dopaminergic neurons project to monkey parietal cortex. Neurosci Lett 86:11–16, 1988b

Lewis DA, Hayes TL, Lund JS, et al: Dopamine and the neural circuitry of primate prefrontal cortex: implications for schizophrenia research. Neuropsychopharmacology 6:127–134, 1992

Lewis DA, Melchitzky DS, Sesack SR, et al: Dopamine transporter immunoreactivity in monkey cerebral cortex: regional, laminar and ultrastructural localization. J Comp Neurol 432:119–138, 2001

Li R, Nishijo H, Wang Q, et al: Light and electron microscopic study of cholinergic and noradrenergic elements in the basolateral nucleus of the rat amygdala: evidence for interactions between the two systems. J Comp Neurol 439:411–425, 2001

Lidow MS, Gallagher DW, Rakic P, et al: Regional differences in the distribution of muscarinic cholinergic receptors in macaque cerebral cortex. J Comp Neurol 289:247–259, 1989

Lopez-Gimenez JF, Mengod G, Palacios JM, et al: Regional distribution and cellular localization of 5-HT2C receptor mRNA in monkey brain: comparison with [3H]mesulergine binding sites and choline acetyltransferase mRNA. Synapse 42:12–26, 2001a

Lopez-Gimenez JF, Vilaró MT, Palacios JM, et al: Mapping of 5-HT2A receptors and their mRNA in monkey brain: [3H]MDL100,907 autoradiography and in situ hybridization studies. J Comp Neurol 429:571–589, 2001b

Lund JS, Lewis DA: Local circuit neurons of developing and mature macaque prefrontal cortex: Golgi and immunocytochemical characteristics. J Comp Neurol 328:282–312, 1993

Mamounas LA, Molliver ME: Evidence for dual serotonergic projections to neocortex: axons from the dorsal and median raphe nuclei are differentially vulnerable to the neurotoxin p-chloroamphetamine (PCA). Exp Neurol 102:23–36, 1991

Manaye KF, McIntire DD, Mann DM, et al: Locus coeruleus cell loss in the aging human brain: a non-random process. J Comp Neurol 358:79–87, 1995

Mann JJ, Stanley M, McBride PA, et al: Increased serotonin2 and beta-adrenergic receptor binding in the frontal cortices of suicide victims. Arch Gen Psychiatry 43:954–959, 1986

Marcus JN, Aschkenasi CJ, Lee CE, et al: Differential expression of orexin receptors 1 and 2 in the rat brain. J Comp Neurol 435:6–25, 2001

Marsicano G, Lutz B: Expression of the cannabinoid receptor CB1 in distinct neuronal subpopulations in the adult mouse forebrain. Eur J Neurosci 11:4213–4225, 1999

Martin-Cora FJ, Pazos A: Autoradiographic distribution of 5-HT7 receptors in the human brain using [3H]mesulergine: comparison to other mammalian species. Br J Pharmacol 141:92–104, 2004

Mathé AA, Rudorfer WV, Stenfors C, et al: Effects of electroconvulsive treatment on somatostatin, neuropeptide Y, endothelin, and neurokinin A concentrations in cerebrospinal fluid of depressed patients. Depression 3:250–256, 1996

Meador-Woodruff JH: Update on dopamine receptors. Ann Clin Psychiatry 6:79, 1994

Meador-Woodruff JH, Mansour A, Civelli O, et al: Distribution of D2 dopamine receptor mRNA in the primate brain. Prog Neuropsychopharmacol Biol Psychiatry 15:885–893, 1991

Meador-Woodruff JH, Damask SP, Wang J, et al: Dopamine receptor mRNA expression in the human striatum and neocortex. Neuropsychopharmacology 15:17–29, 1996

Melchitzky DS, Lewis DA: Tyrosine hydroxylase- and dopamine transporter-immunoreactive axons in the primate cerebellum: evidence for a lobular- and laminar-specific dopamine innervation. Neuropsychopharmacology 22:466–472, 2000

Melchitzky DS, Lewis DA: Dopamine transporter-immunoreactive axons in the mediodorsal thalamic nucleus of the macaque monkey. Neuroscience 103/4:1035–1044, 2001

Melchitzky DS, Lewis DA: Dendrite-targeting GABA neurons in monkey prefrontal cortex: Comparison of somatostatin- and calretinin-immunoreactive axon terminals. Synapse 62:456–465, 2008

Melchitzky DS, Sesack SR, Lewis DA: Parvalbumin-immunoreactive axon terminals in macaque monkey and human prefrontal cortex: laminar, regional and target specificity of type I and type II synapses. J Comp Neurol 408:11–22, 1999

Melchitzky DS, Eggan SM, Lewis DA: Synaptic targets of calretinin-containing axon terminals in macaque monkey prefrontal cortex. Neuroscience 130:185–195, 2005

Melchitzky DS, Erickson SL, Lewis DA: Dopamine innervation of the monkey mediodorsal thalamus: location of projection neurons and ultrastructural characteristics of axon terminals. Neuroscience 143:1021–1030, 2006

Melchitzky DS, Eggan SM, Mackie K, et al: Localization of cannabinoid CB1 receptor and cholecystokinin immunoreactivity in monkey prefrontal cortex. Soc Neurosci Abstracts 190:6, 2007

Mengod G, Vilaró MT, Niznik HB, et al: Visualization of a dopamine D1 receptor mRNA in human and rat brain. Mol Brain Res 10:185–191, 1991

Mengod G, Vilaró MT, Landwehrmeyer GB, et al: Visualization of dopamine D1, D2 and D3 receptor mRNAs in human and rat brain. Neurochem Int 20 (suppl):S33–S43, 1992

Mengod G, Vilaró MT, Raurich A, et al: 5-HT receptors in mammalian brain: receptor autoradiography and in situ hybridization studies of new ligands and newly identified receptors. Histochem J 28:747–758, 1996

Meskenaite V: Calretinin-immunoreactive local circuit neurons in area 17 of the cynomolgus monkey, Macaca fascicularis. J Comp Neurol 379:113–132, 1997

Mesulam M-M, Hersh LB, Mash DC, et al: Differential cholinergic innervation within functional subdivisions of the human cerebral cortex: a choline acetyltransferase study. J Comp Neurol 318:316–328, 1992

Mitchell AJ: The role of corticotropin releasing factor in depressive illness: a critical review. Neurosci Biobehav Rev 22:635–651, 1998

Molliver ME, Berger UV, Mamounas LA, et al: Neurotoxicity of MDMA and related compounds: anatomic studies. Ann N Y Acad Sci 600:649–661, 1990

Moore RY, Bloom FE: Central catecholamine neuron systems: anatomy and physiology of the dopamine systems. Annu Rev Neurosci 1:129–169, 1978

Morris HM, Hashimoto T, Lewis DA: Alterations in somatostatin mRNA expression in the dorsolateral prefrontal cortex of subjects with schizophrenia or schizoaffective disorder. Cerebral Cortex 18:1575–1587, 2008

Morrison JH, Foote SL: Noradrenergic and serotonergic innervation of cortical, thalamic, and tectal visual structures in Old and New World monkeys. J Comp Neurol 243:117–138, 1986

Morrison JH, Foote SL, O'Connor D, et al: Laminar, tangential and regional organization of the noradrenergic innervation of monkey cortex: dopamine-beta-hydroxylase immunohistochemistry. Brain Res Bull 9:309–319, 1982

Mrzljak L, Bergson C, Pappy M, et al: Localization of dopamine D4 receptors in GABAergic neurons of the primate brain. Nature 381:245–248, 1996

Nambu T, Sakurai T, Mizukami K, et al: Distribution of orexin neurons in the adult rat brain. Brain Res 827:243–260, 1999

Neumaier JF, Sexton TJ, Yracheta J, et al: Localization of 5-HT(7) receptors in rat brain by immunocytochemistry, in situ hybridization, and agonist stimulated cFos expression. J Chem Neuroanat 21:63–73, 2001

Nicholas AP, Pieribone VA, Hökfelt T: Cellular localization of messenger RNA for beta-1 and beta-2 adrenergic receptors in rat brain: an in situ hybridization study. Neuroscience 56:1023–1039, 1993

Nilsson C, Karlsson G, Blennow K, et al: Differences in neuropeptide Y-like immunoreactivity of the plasma and platelets of human volunteers and depressed patients. Peptides 17:359–362, 1996

Palacios JM, Hoyer D, Cortes R: Alpha1-adrenoceptors in the mammalian brain: similar pharmacology but different distribution in rodents and primates. Brain Res 419:65–75, 1987

Patel YC: Somatostatin and its receptor family. Front Neuroendocrinol 20:157–198, 1999

Pazos A, Probst A, Palacios JM: Beta-adrenoceptor subtypes in the human brain: autoradiographic localization. Brain Res 358:324–328, 1985

Pazos MR, Nunez E, Benito C, et al: Functional neuroanatomy of the endocannabinoid system. Pharmacol Biochem Behav 81:239–247, 2005

Peroutka SJ: 5-Hydroxytryptamine receptor subtypes, in Serotonin Receptors and Their Ligands. Edited by Oliver B, van Wijngaarden I, Soudijn W. Amsterdam, The Netherlands, Elsevier Science, 1997, pp 3–13

Peyron C, Tighe DK, van den Pol AN, et al: Neurons containing hypocretin (orexin) project to multiple neuronal systems. J Neurosci 18:9996–10015, 1998

Pioro EP, Mai JM, Cuello AC: Distribution of substance-P- and enkephalin-immunoreactive neurons and fibers, in The Human Nervous System. Edited by Paxinos G. New York, Academic Press, 1990, pp 1051–1094

Poirier LJ, Giguère M, Marchand R: Comparative morphology of the substantia nigra and ventral tegmental area in the monkey, cat and rat. Brain Res Bull 11:371–397, 1983

Popken GJ, Bunney WE Jr, Potkin SG, et al: Subnucleus-specific loss of neurons in medial thalamus of schizophrenics. Proc Natl Acad Sci U S A 97:9276–9280, 2000

Porrino LJ, Goldman-Rakic PS: Brainstem innervation of prefrontal and anterior cingulate cortex in the rhesus monkey revealed by retrograde transport of HRP. J Comp Neurol 205:63–76, 1982

Powers RE, Walker LC, DeSouza EB, et al: Immunohistochemical study of neurons containing corticotropin-releasing factor in Alzheimer's disease. Synapse 1:405–410, 1987

Redrobe JP, Dumont Y, Quirion R: Neuropeptide Y (NPY) and depression: from animal studies to the human condition. Life Sci 71:2921–2937, 2002

Ressler KJ, Nemeroff CB: Role of serotonergic and noradrenergic systems in the pathophysiology of depression and anxiety disorders. Depress Anxiety 12 (suppl 1):2–19, 2000

Rimon R, Le Greves P, Nyberg F, et al: Elevation of substance P-like peptides in the CSF of psychiatric patients. Biol Psychiatry 19:509–516, 2002

Rodriguez-Puertas R, Pascual J, Vilaro T, et al: Autoradiographic distribution of M1, M2, M3, and M4 muscarinic receptor subtypes in Alzheimer's disease. Synapse 26:341–350, 1997

Sakurai T: The neural circuit of orexin (hypocretin): maintaining sleep and wakefulness. Nat Rev Neurosci 8:171–181, 2007

Sakurai T, Amemiya A, Ishii M, et al: Orexins and orexin receptors: a family of hypothalamic neuropeptides and G protein-coupled receptors that regulate feeding behavior. Cell 92:573–585, 1998

Samson Y, Wu JJ, Friedman AH, et al: Catecholaminergic innervation of the hippocampus in the cynomolgus monkey. J Comp Neurol 298:250–263, 1990

Sanchez-Gonzalez MA, Garcia-Cabezas MA, Rico B, et al: The primate thalamus is a key target for brain dopamine. J Neurosci 25:6076–6083, 2005

Sawaguchi T, Matsumura M, Kubota K: Delayed response deficits produced by local injection of bicuculline into the dorsolateral prefrontal cortex in Japanese macaque monkeys. Exp Brain Res 75:457–469, 1989

Schwartzberg M, Unger J, Weindl A, et al: Distribution of neuropeptide Y in the prosencephalon of man and cotton-head tamarin (Saguinus oedipus): colocalization with somatostatin in neurons of striatum and amygdala. Anat Embryol (Berl) 181:157–166, 1990

Semba K, Fibiger HC: Organization of the central cholinergic systems. Prog Brain Res 79:37–63, 1989

Sergeyev V, Hökfelt T, Hurd Y: Serotonin and substance P co-exist in dorsal raphe neurons of the human brain. Neuroreport 10:3967–3970, 1999

Sesack SR, Hawrylak VA, Matus CV, et al: Dopamine axon varicosities in the prelimbic division of the rat prefrontal cortex exhibit sparse immunoreactivity for the dopamine transporter. J Neurosci 18:2697–2708, 1998

Sharma RP, Janicak PG, Bissette G, et al: CSF neurotensin concentrations and antipsychotic treatment in schizophrenia and schizoaffective disorder. Am J Psychiatry 154:1019–1021, 1997

Smiley JF, Goldman-Rakic PS: Heterogeneous targets of dopamine synapses in monkey prefrontal cortex demonstrated by serial section electron microscopy: a laminar analysis using the silver-enhanced diaminobenzidine sulfide (SEDS) immunolabeling technique. Cereb Cortex 3:223–238, 1993

Smiley JF, Goldman-Rakic PS: Serotonergic axons in monkey prefrontal cerebral cortex synapse predominantly on interneurons as demonstrated by serial section electron microscopy. J Comp Neurol 367:431–443, 1996

Smiley JF, Levey AI, Ciliax BJ, et al: D1 dopamine receptor immunoreactivity in human and monkey cerebral cortex: predominant and extrasynaptic localization in dendritic spines. Proc Natl Acad Sci U S A 91:5720–5724, 1994

Smit F, Bolier L, Cuijpers P: Cannabis use and the risk of later schizophrenia: a review. Addiction 99:425–430, 2004

Smith Y, Parent A, Seguela P, et al: Distribution of GABA-immunoreactive neurons in the basal ganglia of the squirrel monkey (Saimiri sciureus). J Comp Neurol 259:50–64, 1987

Stahl SM: Basic psychopharmacology of antidepressants, part 1: antidepressants have seven distinct mechanisms of action. J Clin Psychiatry 59 (suppl 4):5–14, 1998

Steriade M, Jones EG, McCormick DA: Thalamus: Organisation and Function. Amsterdam, The Netherlands, Elsevier Science, 1997

Tecott LH, Maricq AV, Julius D: Nervous system distribution of the serotonin 5-HT3 receptor mRNA. Proc Natl Acad Sci U S A 90:1430–1434, 1993

Thannickal TC, Moore RY, Nienhuis R, et al: Reduced number of hypocretin neurons in human narcolepsy. Neuron 27:469–474, 2000

Tork I, Hornung JP: Raphe nuclei and the serotonergic system, in The Human Nervous System. Edited by Paxinos G. New York, Academic Press, 1990, pp 1001–1022

Tran KD, Smutzer GS, Doty RL, et al: Reduced Purkinje cell size in the cerebellar vermis of elderly patients with schizophrenia. Am J Psychiatry 155:1288–1290, 1998

Tunbridge EM, Bannerman DM, Sharp T, et al: Catechol-O-methyltransferase inhibition improves set-shifting performance and elevates stimulated dopamine release in the rat prefrontal cortex. J Neurosci 24:5331–5335, 2004

Varnas K, Halldin C, Pike VW, et al: Distribution of 5-HT4 receptors in the postmortem human brain—an autoradiographic study using [125I]SB 207710. Eur Neuropsychopharmacol 13:228–234, 2003

Walker AE: A cytoarchitectural study of the prefrontal area of the macaque monkey. J Comp Neurol 73:59–86, 1940

Wang Y, Toledo-Rodriguez M, Gupta A, et al: Anatomical, physiological and molecular properties of Martinotti cells in the somatosensory cortex of the juvenile rat. J Physiol 561:65–90, 2004

Weinberger DR, Berman KF, Zec RF: Physiologic dysfunction of dorsolateral prefrontal cortex in schizophrenia, I: regional cerebral blood flow evidence. Arch Gen Psychiatry 43:114–124, 1986

Westrin Å, Ekman R, Träskman-Bendz L: Alterations of corticotropin releasing hormone (CRH) and neuropeptide Y (NPY) plasma levels in mood disorder patients with a recent suicide attempt. Eur Neuropsychopharmacol 9:205–211, 1999

Wettstein JG, Earley B, Junien JL: Central nervous system pharmacology of neuropeptide Y. Pharmacol Ther 65:397–414, 1995

Williams SM, Goldman-Rakic PS: Characterization of the dopaminergic innervation of the primate frontal cortex using a dopamine-specific antibody. Cereb Cortex 3:199–222, 1993

Williams SM, Goldman-Rakic PS: Widespread origin of the primate mesofrontal dopamine system. Cereb Cortex 8:321–345, 1998

Williams SM, Goldman-Rakic PS, Leranth C: The synaptology of parvalbumin-immunoreactive neurons in primate prefrontal cortex. J Comp Neurol 320:353–369, 1992

Wilson FA, O'Scalaidhe SP, Goldman-Rakic PS: Functional synergism between putative gamma-aminobutyrate-containing neurons and pyramidal neurons in prefrontal cortex. Proc Natl Acad Sci U S A 91:4009–4013, 1994

Wilson MA, Molliver ME: The organization of serotonergic projections to cerebral cortex in primates: retrograde transport studies. Neuroscience 44:555–570, 1991

Yamada H, Okumura T, Motomura W, et al: Inhibition of food intake by central injection of anti-orexin antibody in fasted rats. Biochem Biophys Res Commun 267:527–531, 2000

Yamada M, Yamada M, Richelson E: Heterogeneity of melanized neurons expressing neurotensin receptor messenger RNA in the substantia nigra and the nucleus paranigralis of control and Parkinson's disease brain. Neuroscience 64:405–417, 1995

Young KA, Manaye KF, Liang C-L, et al: Reduced number of mediodorsal and anterior thalamic neurons in schizophrenia. Biol Psychiatry 47:944–953, 2000

Zahm DS, Grosu S, Williams EA, et al: Neurons of origin of the neurotensinergic plexus enmeshing the ventral tegmental area in rat: retrograde labeling and in situ hybridization combined. Neuroscience 104:841–851, 2001

Zardetto-Smith AM, Gray TS: Catecholamine and NPY efferents from the ventrolateral medula to the amygdala in the rat. Brain Res Bull 38:253–260, 1995

Zimmer A, Zimmer AM, Hohmann AG, et al: Increased mortality, hypoactivity, and hypoalgesia in cannabinoid CB1 receptor knockout mice. Proc Natl Acad Sci U S A 96:5780–5785, 1999

Electrophysiology

Anthony A. Grace, Ph.D.

J. Amiel Rosenkranz, Ph.D.

Anthony R. West, Ph.D.

Several approaches can be used to analyze the structure and function of the nervous system in health and disease. Many of these techniques—for example, the biochemical analysis of neurotransmitter and metabolite levels, anatomical studies of axonal projection sites or neurotransmitter enzymes, and molecular biological studies of messenger levels and turnover—examine the nervous system at the level of groups or populations of neurons. In contrast, by its very nature, electrophysiology is oriented toward the physiological analysis of individual neurons. In this chapter, we describe preparations and techniques that are in a general sense applicable to many systems, with specific examples from the dopaminergic system to draw on our field of expertise.

The use of electrophysiological techniques for the analysis of neuronal physiology depends on the unique properties of the neuronal membrane. Like many other cell types, the neuron possesses an electrochemical gradient across its membrane. The electrochemical gradient itself is a product of two forces: 1) an electrical potential force derived from the voltage difference between the inside and the outside of the cell and 2) a chemical potential force resulting from the unequal distribution of ions across the membrane. Cells set up and maintain this electrochemical gradient because of the selective permeability of their membranes to particular ionic species. Thus, the membrane has a rather high degree of permeability to ions such as potassium but is relatively impermeable to ions such as sodium and calcium.

In the resting state, cells have a very low internal concentration of sodium and calcium. To achieve this state, the cell must expend energy (in the form of adenosine triphosphate [ATP] hydrolysis) to extrude sodium from the intracellular space in exchange for potassium ions. The extrusion of sodium sets up both a chemical gradient (because sodium attempts to exist in equal concentrations across the membrane) and an electrical gradient (because sodium is positively charged and is not freely permeable across the membrane; thus, net positive charges are being removed from inside the cell). To partially counter this electrical gradient, potassium—which is more permeable—flows down the electrical gradient to become concentrated inside the cell. However, during this process, the cell is also setting up an opposing chemical gradient, because potassium is achieving higher concentrations within the cell in comparison with the extracellular environment. When the electrical force drawing potassium into the cell balances the chemical force of the concentration gradient forcing potassium out of the cell, the membrane is at equilibrium—with high extracellular sodium concentrations, relatively high intracellular potassium concentrations, and a transmembrane potential causing the inside of the cell to be negatively charged with respect to its environment.

A typical resting membrane potential for a neuron is rather small, being on the order of -70 mV with respect to the extracellular fluid. In actuality, potassium itself is not freely permeable. A small electrochemical gradient exists in most neurons that attempts to force potassium out of the cell and draw the membrane potential to more negative values. Although the scenario is somewhat more complicated than this (e.g., involving charged proteins and other ionic species with selective permeabilities), this description approximates how a cell gains an electrochemical gradient via the energy-dependent extrusion of sodium.

Note that neurons are not the only cells that have transmembrane potentials. In fact, all living cells have an electrochemical gradient across their membranes that they use for transporting glucose and other essential materials and accumulating them against a concentration gradient. Such energy-dependent processes are usually coupled to other gradients from which they derive this energy. For example, a compound may be taken up and concentrated by linking its transport to sodium, which itself has a large electrochemical gradient in the opposite direction. What makes the neuron unique is its ability to rapidly change the permeability of its membrane to one or more ion species in a regenerative manner. This process underlies the generation of an action potential, sets up active propagation of an action potential down an axon, and triggers the procedure that ultimately results in neurotransmitter release. It also provides the electrophysiologist with a measure of neuronal activity that can be assayed by recording the electrical activity generated by the neuron.

The *action potential* is an active regenerative phenomenon, which means that the events that initiate the action potential also serve as the force that drives this event to completion. Normally, a given neuron receives information in the form of synaptic potentials. For example, an axon terminal synapsing on the neuron releases a neurotransmitter, which binds to the neuron and selectively alters the permeability of its membrane by opening ion channels linked to its binding site. An ion channel that opens in response to a neurotransmitter is referred to as a *ligand-gated channel*. If the neurotransmitter activates a channel that increases the permeability of the membrane to a negatively charged ion present in high concentrations in the extracellular fluid (e.g., chloride), the influx of chloride down its electrochemical gradient causes a negative shift in the membrane potential of the cell, thereby increasing the potential difference across the membrane, or a hyperpolarization of the cell. If activation of this channel causes a positively charged ion such as sodium to flow down its electrochemical gradient and into the cell, it will cause a brief decrease in the membrane potential (i.e., a depolarization) of the neuron.

Because a change in the membrane potential alters the electrochemical gradient of potassium across the membrane, potassium ions will flow through their respective channels to restore the membrane to its resting level. Thus, a neurotransmitter that depolarizes the membrane causes an efflux of potassium ions and a return of the membrane potential to resting levels. However, if the depolarization is large enough, another type of channel is activated—the *voltage-gated* or *voltage-dependent sodium channel*. In response to a given level of depolarization, this channel increases its permeability to sodium to allow more of this ion to enter the cell. The result is a further depolarization of the membrane and consequently an increased activation of this voltage-dependent channel. Because of the positive-feedback nature of this event, it is referred to as *regenerative*, because the depolarization augments the very factor that causes the cell to be depolarized. The membrane potential at which this regenerative process is initiated is thus the threshold potential for action potential generation, with a hyperpolarization of the cell causing a decrease in its excitability and a depolarization increasing the likelihood that it will generate an action potential.

The regenerative depolarization of the membrane has limits, however. One limit is the equilibrium potential for sodium. The *equilibrium potential* is the membrane potential at which the electrochemical gradient for a particular ion is zero, with no net flux of the ion across a membrane. This would occur when the membrane potential is sufficiently positive to oppose the further influx of the positively charged sodium ion across its concentration gradient. Although this potential is usually about +40 mV in many cells, the action potential does not actually reach this value. Instead, another voltage-activated channel that is selectively permeable to potassium is activated. The resultant massive increase in potassium permeability starts to return the membrane potential to its original state, thereby inactivating the regenerative sodium conductance. The increased potassium permeability is sufficient to drive the membrane potential negative to the resting potential and toward the equilibrium potential for potassium (i.e., approximately −80 to −90 mV) before the subsequent decrease in voltage-dependent potassium conductance returns the membrane to its original resting state.

The equilibrium potential of an ion determines the net effect that opening its associated ion channels will have on the neuron. The equilibrium potential occurs when the membrane is depolarized or hyperpolarized sufficiently to offset exactly the effects of the concentration gradient on the ion; as a result, no net flux of this ion crosses the membrane. For example, because of the very high concentration of sodium outside the neuron compared with inside the cell, the large concentration gradient for sodium across the membrane attempts to force sodium into the neuron. Therefore, to oppose this concentration gradient, the membrane potential of the neuron would have to be highly positive to provide an electrical gradient of equivalent force. This occurs at approximately +40 mV for sodium. However, potassium's equilibrium potential is about 10–20 mV more negative than its resting potential, which is partly the result of ATP hydrolysis that exchanges extruded sodium for potassium. As a result, increasing potassium permeability causes a hyperpolarization of the neuron because of an efflux of potassium down its concentration gradient.

Chloride is another common ionic species. This ion is negatively charged and therefore has an electrical gradient that would act against its entering the cell. However, the concentration of chloride is so much higher in the extracellular fluid that the chemical gradient predominates. As a result, opening chloride ion channels causes chloride to flow into the cell, hyperpolarizing the membrane (Figure 5–1). In fact, the opening of chloride ion channels is the mechanism through which the primary inhibitory neurotransmitter in the brain (i.e., γ-aminobutyric acid [GABA]) decreases neuronal activity.

Neurons within the vertebrate nervous system have additional conductances that provide them with unique functions. One of these conductances is the voltage-gated calcium conductance. Like sodium, calcium exists in higher concentrations outside the neuron compared with inside the cell. However, the gradient is even more extreme than it is for sodium. Even though much less calcium than sodium is present in the extracellular fluid, the equilibrium potential for calcium is almost +240 mV because of the extremely low intracellular concentration of this ion. The neuron maintains this low intracellular concentration so as to use this ion for specialized purposes. Thus, calcium influx causes neurotransmitter release, activates calcium-gated ion channels, and triggers second-messenger systems (e.g., calcium-regulated protein kinase). Calcium channels, like their sodium counterparts, are also voltage gated and cause calcium influx into the neuron during the action potential. Furthermore, calcium can influence the excitability of the cell by activating the calcium-activated potassium current, which then causes a large membrane hyperpolarization after the spike, known as an *afterhyperpolarization*, that delays the occurrence of a subsequent spike in that neuron. After entering the neuron, calcium is rapidly sequestered into intracellular organelles to terminate its action and reset the neuron before the next event. Therefore, calcium can alter the physiological activity and the biochemical properties of the neuron it affects (Llinás 1988).

In addition to the role of ion channels in setting the resting membrane potential, generating the action potential, and repolarizing the membrane potential, they can have a more subtle effect on aspects of electrophysiological function. For example, by regulating properties of the neuronal membrane, such as the amplitude and speed of the neuronal voltage response to inputs, ion channels can regulate neuronal responses to synaptic inputs. By modulation of these parameters, ion channels influence the integration of multiple synapses (temporal and spatial integration) and ultimately regulate the ability of synaptic inputs to depolarize membrane potentials and drive the generation of action potentials. Furthermore, neurotransmitters such as acetylcholine and monoamines can influence these same parameters through modulation of ion channels.

Electrophysiological Techniques

Through use of a broad range of electrophysiological techniques to assess information about a neuron, such as those described earlier in this chapter, experiments can be designed to investigate differences in the physiological properties of neurons of interest, the interaction between neurotransmitter systems involved in behavioral or pathological conditions, and the mode of action of pathomimetic or psychotherapeutic agents. In attempting to gain such information, it is important to note that there is no "best" technique. Each approach has its relative strengths and weaknesses, and only through integrating information gained at these various levels will a more complete comprehension of neuronal function be achieved.

Numerous parameters of neuronal activity can be assessed electrophysiologically. These parameters can be selectively assessed depending on the method of recording used. Six recording methods are reviewed here: electroencephalographic (EEG) recordings, field potential recordings, single-unit extracellular recordings, intracellular recordings, patch clamp recordings, and whole-cell recordings. Which parameter is measured is essentially a function of the type of electrode used.

Electroencephalographic Recordings

In recording EEGs, the desired signal is very small in amplitude; thus, a large electrode that sums activity over large regions of the brain surface is used. Although this technique is less invasive than others, the information it yields is comparatively narrow, in that a large array of

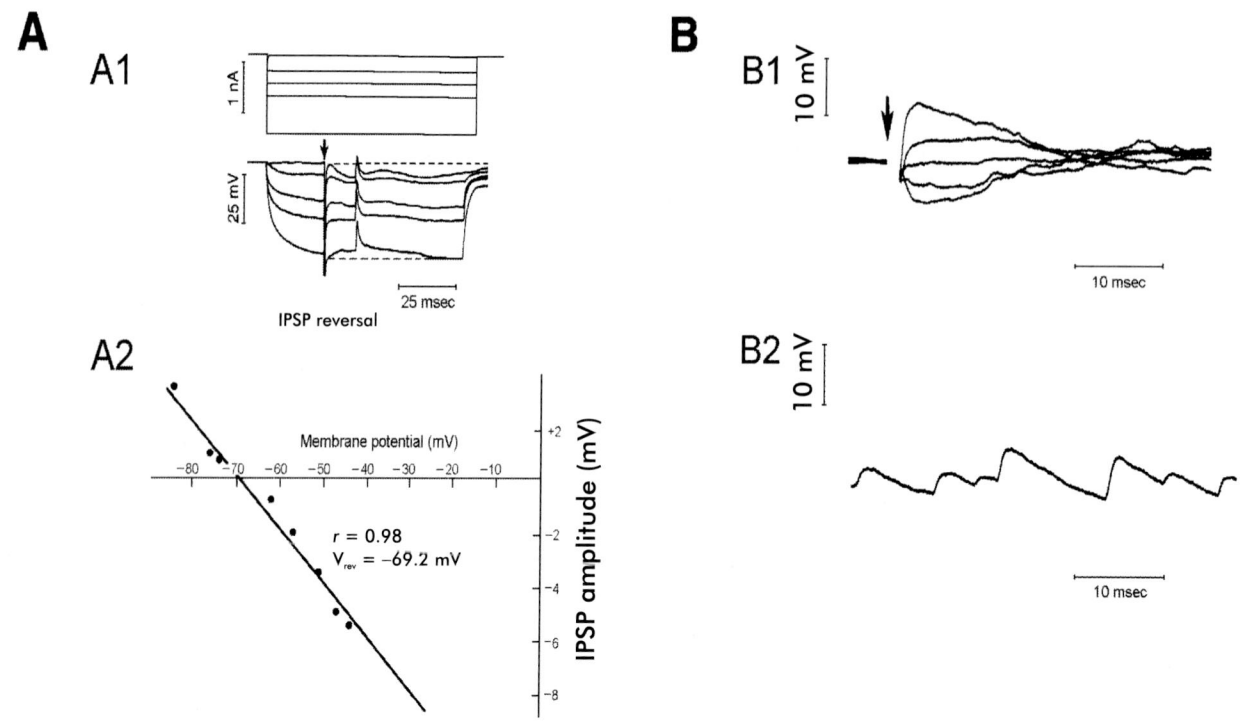

FIGURE 5–1. Determining the ionic nature of a synaptic event.

At least three techniques can be used to determine the ionic species that mediates a synaptic response: determining the reversal potential of the ion, reversing the membrane potential deflection produced by changing the concentration gradient of the ion across the membrane, and determining the reversal potential (or blocking the synaptic response) after applying a specific ion channel blocker. In this figure, three techniques are used to illustrate the involvement of a chloride ion conductance increase evoked in dopamine-containing neurons by stimulation of the striatonigral γ-aminobutyric acid (GABA)ergic projection. **(A)** The reversal potential of a response may be determined by examining the amplitude of the response as the membrane potential of the neuron is varied. In this example, we superimposed several responses of the neuron evoked at increasingly hyperpolarized membrane potentials *(top traces)*, with the membrane potential altered by injecting current through the electrode and into the neuron *(bottom traces=current injection)*. **(A1)** A synaptic response in the form of an inhibitory postsynaptic potential (IPSP) is evoked in a dopamine neuron by stimulating the GABAergic striatonigral pathway *(arrow)*. When increasing amplitudes of hyperpolarizing current *(lower traces)* are injected into the neuron through the electrode, a progressive hyperpolarization of the membrane occurs *(top traces)*. As the membrane is made more negative, the IPSP diminishes in amplitude, eventually being replaced by a depolarizing response. **(A2)** Plotting the amplitude of the evoked response *(y-axis)* against the membrane potential at which it was evoked *(x-axis)* illustrates how the synaptic response changes with membrane potential. The membrane voltage at which the synaptic response is equal to zero (i.e., ~69.2 mV in this case) is the reversal potential of the ion mediating the synaptic response (i.e., the potential at which the electrochemical forces working on the ion are zero). Therefore, there is no net flux of ions that cross the membrane. At more negative membrane potentials, the flow of the ion is reversed, causing the chloride ion (in this case) to exit the cell and result in a depolarization of the membrane. **(B)** The flow of an ion across a membrane may also be altered by changing the concentration gradient of the ion across the membrane. Normally, chloride ions flow from the outside of the neuron (where they are present at a higher concentration) to the inside of the neuron (where their concentration is lower), causing the membrane potential to become more negative. In this case, the concentration of chloride ions across the membrane of the dopamine neuron is reversed by using potassium chloride as the electrolyte in the intracellular recording electrode. **(B1)** Soon after the neuron is impaled with the potassium chloride–containing electrode, stimulation of the striatonigral pathway *(arrow)* evokes an IPSP *(bottom trace)*. However, as the recording is maintained, chloride is diffusing from the electrode into the neuron, causing the electrochemical gradient to decrease progressively over time. As a result, each subsequent stimulation pulse evokes a smaller IPSP, eventually causing the IPSP to reverse to a depolarization *(top trace)*. The depolarization is caused by an efflux of chloride ions out of the neuron and down its new electrochemical gradient. This has caused the reversal potential of the chloride-mediated response to change from a potential that was negative to the resting potential to one that is now positive to the resting potential. **(B2)** After injecting chloride ions into the neuron, spontaneously occurring IPSPs that were not readily observed in the control case are now readily seen as reversed IPSPs (i.e., depolarizations) occurring in this dopamine neuron recorded in vivo.

neurons must be simultaneously activated for the potentials to be recorded at the scalp. As a result, stimulus presentation and EEG averaging are typically required to separate the signal desired from the background noise.

Field Potential Recordings

The next level of analysis is the recording of field potentials. This method uses a recording electrode with a smaller tip and a higher resistance than that for EEG elec-

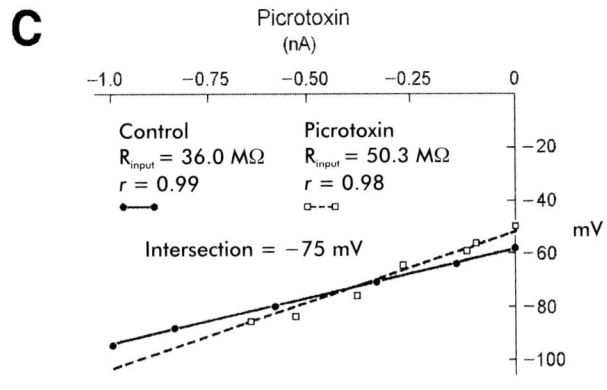

FIGURE 5–1.   Determining the ionic nature of a synaptic event (*continued*).

(C) Another means for determining the ionic conductance involved in a response is by using a specific ion channel blocker. This can be done in two ways: by using the drug to block an evoked response or (as shown in this example) by examining the effects of administering the drug on the neuron to determine whether the cell is receiving synaptic events that alter the conductance of the membrane to this ion. To do this, the current–voltage relationship of the cell is first established. This is done by injecting hyperpolarizing current pulses into the neuron (*x-axis*) and recording the membrane potential that is present during the current injection (*y-axis*). These values are then plotted on the graph (*filled circles*), with the resting membrane potential being the membrane potential at which no current is being injected into the neuron (*y-intercept*). The slope of the resultant regression line (*solid line*) is equal to the input resistance of the neuron (Rinput = 36 megohms). After administration of the chloride ion channel blocker picrotoxin (*open boxes*), a new current–voltage relationship is established in a similar manner. Picrotoxin caused a depolarization of the membrane (y-intercept of dashed line is more positive) and an increase in the neuron input resistance (the slope of the dashed line is larger). The intersection of the membrane current–voltage plots obtained before and after picrotoxin administration is then calculated. By definition, this point of intersection (i.e., ~75 mV) is the reversal potential of the response to picrotoxin, because a neuron at this membrane potential would show no net change in membrane potential on drug administration.
Source.   Adapted from Grace AA, Bunney BS: "Opposing Effects of Striatonigral Feedback Pathways on Midbrain Dopamine Cell Activity." *Brain Research* 333:271–284, 1985. Copyright 1985, Elsevier. Used with permission.

trodes, and the electrophysiological measures are confined to a small population of neurons surrounding the electrode tip. This technique still depends on the simultaneous activation of a number of cells; however, because the electrode is inserted into the brain, the cells do not have to be at the surface of the skull as in the EEG recordings. Furthermore, the activation can consist of stimulation of an afferent pathway. Nonetheless, the array of neurons sampled must have a common orientation for the massed activity to be measurable. Therefore, such measures are typically restricted to cortical structures such as

the neocortex and hippocampus. With this method, the current resulting from the parallel activation of excitatory and inhibitory afferents can be measured as well as the electrophysiological response of a population of neurons to such stimulation.

On the other hand, even in structures without a parallel orientation of neurons, field recordings have been useful in evaluating changes in afferent synaptic strength. For example, field recordings have been particularly effective in examining phenomena manifesting synaptic plasticity, such as long-term potentiation. By measuring the fields generated by stimulating afferent inputs, one can evaluate how effective synaptic pathways are in driving a region and how this effectiveness can be modified by experience. Therefore, learning paradigms, behavioral conditioning, and drug sensitization have all been shown to alter evoked field potentials within functional pathways in the brain (e.g., Goto and Grace 2005b).

Single-Unit Extracellular Recordings

The next level of recording involves examining the electrophysiology of individual neurons with extracellular single-unit recording techniques. This technique requires that an electrode be placed in close proximity to a single neuron to record its spike discharge. An electrode with a smaller tip and a higher resistance than those used for recording field potentials results in the sampling of a smaller volume of tissue (i.e., the somata of individual neurons). Because the region sampled by the electrode is small, the signal is larger in amplitude and the background noise is less. This allows easy recording of the spontaneous spike discharge of a single neuron within the brain of a living (but typically anesthetized) animal. The cells examined are located through use of an atlas and a stereotaxic apparatus. The stereotaxic apparatus holds the head of the animal in a precise orientation so that a brain atlas may be used to place the recording electrodes accurately within the region of the brain desired. Furthermore, if a dye is dissolved in the electrolyte within the recording pipette, the dye may be ejected into the recording site for subsequent histological verification of the region recorded.

Because the recording electrode is placed near the outside surface of the neuron, there is less of a concern that the activity recorded is a result of damage to the neuron itself, as may be the case with intracellular recording techniques. Furthermore, many neurons may be sampled in a given animal. However, as a consequence, the amount of information that can be obtained from a neuron is limited. Typically, the research is relegated to recording infor-

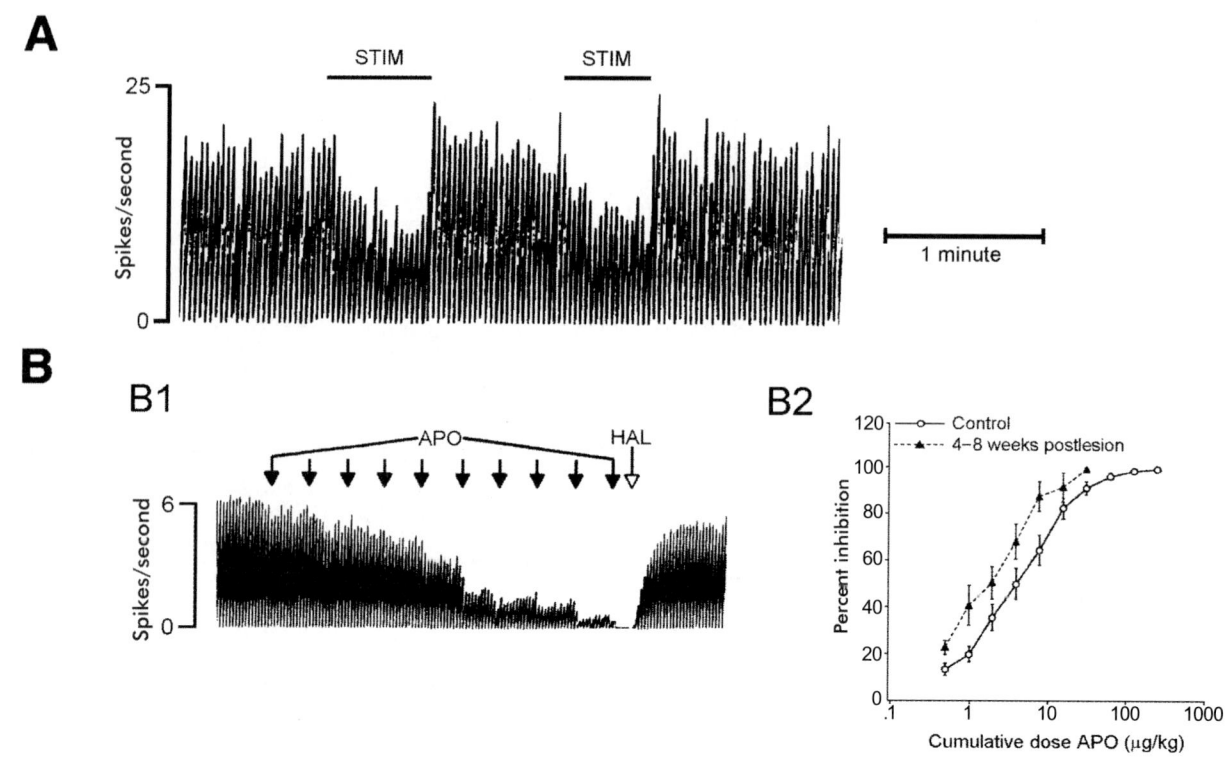

FIGURE 5–2. Detection of changes in firing rates and pattern of spike discharge by extracellular recording measurements.

Extracellular recording techniques are an effective means of assessing the effects of afferent pathway stimulation or drug administration on neuron activity. On the other hand, the measurements that can be made are typically restricted to changes in firing rates or in the pattern of spike discharge. **(A)** This firing rate histogram illustrates the response of a substantia nigra–zona reticulata neuron to stimulation of the γ-aminobutyric acid (GABA)ergic striatonigral pathway. A common method for illustrating how a manipulation affects the firing rate of a neuron is by constructing a firing rate histogram. This is typically done by using some type of electronic discriminator and counter to count the number of spikes that a cell fires in a given time. In this example, the counter counts spikes over a 10-second interval and converts this number to a voltage, which is then plotted on a chart recorder. The counter then resets to zero and begins counting spikes over the next 10-second interval. Therefore, in this firing rate histogram, the height of each vertical line is proportional to the number of spikes that the cell fires during each 10-second interval, with the calibration bar on the left showing the equivalent firing frequency in spikes per second. During the period at which the striatonigral pathway is stimulated (*horizontal bars above trace marked "STIM"*), the cell is inhibited, as reflected by the decrease in the height of the vertical lines. When the stimulation is terminated, a rebound activation of cell firing is observed. **(B)** In this figure, a similar histogram is used to illustrate the effects of a drug on the firing of a neuron. **(B1)** This figure shows the well-known inhibition of dopamine neuron firing rate on administration of the dopamine agonist apomorphine (APO). Each of the filled arrows represents the intravenous administration of a dose of APO. After the cell is completely inhibited, the specificity of the response is tested by examining the ability of the dopamine antagonist haloperidol (HAL *[open arrow]*) to reverse this response. Typically, drug sensitivity is determined by administering the drug in a dose–response fashion. This is done by giving an initial drug dose that is subthreshold for altering the firing rate of the cell. The first dose is then repeated, with each subsequent dose given being twice that of the previous dose. This is continued until a plateau response is achieved (in this case, a complete inhibition of cell discharge). **(B2)** The drug is administered in a dose–response manner to facilitate the plotting of a cumulative dose–response curve, with drug doses plotted on a logarithmic scale (i.e., a log dose–response curve). To compare the potency of two drugs or the sensitivity of two cells to the same drug, a point on the curve is chosen during which the fastest rate of change of the response is obtained. The point usually chosen is that at which the drug dose administered causes 50% of the maximal change obtained (i.e., the ED_{50}). As is shown in this example, the dopamine neurons recorded after a partial dopamine depletion (*dashed line*) are substantially more sensitive to inhibition by APO than the dopamine neurons recorded in control (*solid line*) rats.

mation related to action potential firing (e.g., the firing rate of the neuron, its pattern of spike discharge, and how these states of activity may be affected by stimulation of an afferent pathway or administration of a drug [Figure 5–2]). Nonetheless, when combined with the appropriate pharmacological techniques, extracellular recording has yielded a substantial amount of valuable information related to drug action or neuronal interconnections of physiologically important neuronal types. For example, by using a series of coordinated pharmacological and physiological techniques, we were able to define a unique extracellular waveform as that associated with the discharge of

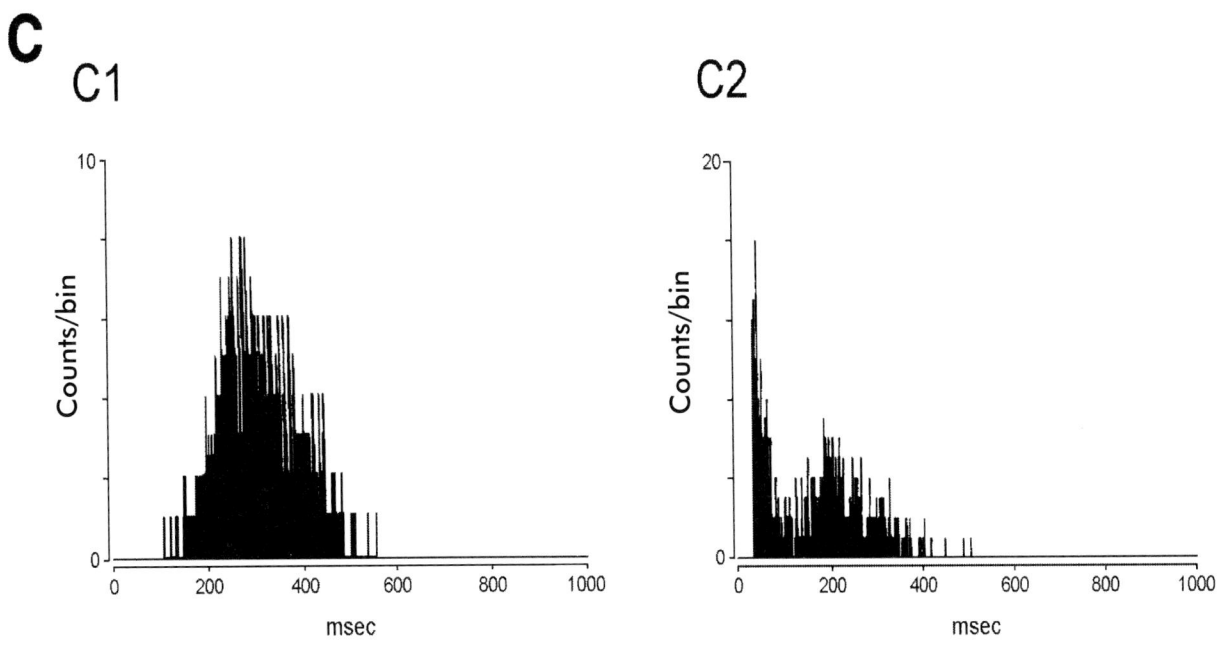

C

C1

C2

FIGURE 5–2. Detection of changes in firing rates and pattern of spike discharge by extracellular recording measurements (*continued*).

(C) In addition to determining the firing rate of a neuron, extracellular recording techniques may be used to assess the effects of drugs on the pattern of spike discharge. This is typically done by plotting an interspike interval histogram. In this paradigm, a computer is connected to a spike discriminator, and a train of about 500 spikes is analyzed. The computer is used to time the delay between subsequent spikes in the train (i.e., the time interval between spikes) and plots this in the form of a histogram, in which the x-axis represents time between subsequent spikes and the y-axis shows the number of interspike intervals that had a specific delay (bin=range of time; e.g., for 1-msec bins, all intervals between 200.0 and 200.99 msec). **(C1)** The cell is firing irregularly (as shown by the primarily normal distribution of intervals around 200 msec), with some spikes occurring after longer-than-average delays (i.e., bins greater than 400 msec, probably caused by spontaneous inhibitory postsynaptic potentials [IPSPs] delaying spike occurrence). **(C2)** In contrast, this cell is firing in bursts, which consist of a series of 3–10 spikes with comparatively short interspike intervals (i.e., approximately 70 msec) separated by long delays between bursts (i.e., events occurring at greater than 150-msec intervals). The computer determined that in this case, the cell was discharging 79% of its spikes in bursts, compared with 0% in *(C1)*.

Source. (A) Adapted from Grace AA, Bunney BS: "Opposing Effects of Striatonigral Feedback Pathways on Midbrain Dopamine Cell Activity." *Brain Research* 333:271–284, 1985. Copyright 1985, Elsevier. Used with permission. (B) Adapted from Pucak ML, Grace AA: "Partial Dopamine Depletions Result in an Enhanced Sensitivity of Residual Dopamine Neurons to Apomorphine." *Synapse* 9:144–155, 1991. Copyright 1991, Wiley. Used with permission. (C) Adapted from Grace AA, Bunney BS: "The Control of Firing Pattern in Nigral Dopamine Neurons: Single Spike Firing." *Journal of Neuroscience* 4:2866–2876, 1984a. Copyright 1984, Society for Neuroscience. Used with permission.

a dopamine-containing neuron (Bunney et al. 1973; Grace and Bunney 1983). This provided the basis for studies that yielded information defining the mode of action of antipsychotic drugs (Bunney and Grace 1978; Grace 1992).

Extracellular recordings from neurons measure the current flow generated around a neuron as it generates spikes. For this reason, extracellular action potentials generally are composed of two components: a positive-going component followed by a negative-going component. The positive-going component is a reflection of the ion flux across the neuronal membrane surrounding the electrode that occurs during the depolarizing phase of the action potential, with the negative phase reflecting the

repolarization. Because the extracellular recording electrode is measuring current across the membrane occurring in concert with changes in intracellular membrane potential and because current is defined in terms of the first derivative (i.e., rate of change) of voltage, the extracellularly recorded action potential (or spike) waveform is typically a first derivative of the action potential voltage with respect to time (Terzuolo and Araki 1961). This phenomenon underlies the biphasic nature of the extracellularly recorded event (Figure 5–3). Furthermore, the recorded spike is largest when the recording electrode is placed near the active site of spike generation because the current density is greatest (and thus the voltage drop induced across the electrode largest) at this site.

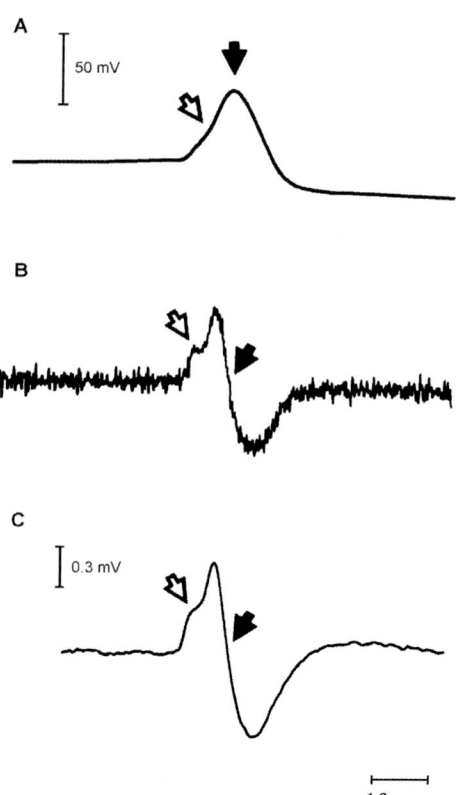

FIGURE 5–3.   Relationship between action potentials recorded intracellularly and those recorded extracellularly from dopamine-containing neurons.

(A) During intracellular recordings, an action potential is initiated from a negative resting membrane potential (e.g., ~55 mV), reaches a peak membrane potential *(solid arrow)*, and is followed by a repolarization of the membrane and usually an afterhyperpolarization. An inflection in the rising phase of the spike *(open arrow)* is often observed. This reflects the delay between the initial segment spike that initiates the action potential (occurring prior to the open arrow) and the somatodendritic action potential that it triggers (occurring after the open arrow). **(B)** A computer was used to differentiate the membrane voltage deflection occurring in the action potential in *(A)* with respect to time, resulting in a pattern that shows the rate of change of membrane voltage. Note that the inflection is exaggerated *(open arrow)*, and the peak of the action potential crosses zero *(solid arrow)*, because at the peak of a spike, the rate of change reaches zero before reversing to a negative direction. **(C)** A trace showing a typical action potential in a dopamine neuron recorded extracellularly. The extracellular action potential resembles the differentiated intracellular action potential in *(B)*. This is because the extracellular electrode is actually measuring the current crossing the membrane during the action potential and is therefore, by definition, equivalent to the absolute value of the first derivative of the voltage trace in *(A)*. The amplitude of the extracellular spike is indicated in volts, because the parameter measured is actually the voltage drop produced across the electrode tip by the current flux and is therefore much smaller than the actual membrane voltage change that occurs in *(A)*.

Source.   Adapted from Grace AA, Bunney BS: "Intracellular and Extracellular Electrophysiology of Nigral Dopaminergic Neurons, I: Identification and Characterization." *Neuroscience* 10:301–315, 1983. Copyright 1983, International Brain Research Organization. Used with permission.

Intracellular Recordings

With intracellular recording, an electrode with a much smaller tip and a much higher electrical resistance than that used with extracellular recording is inserted into the membrane of the neuron. Although the tip of the electrode is smaller, the signal measured is much larger than that with extracellular recording, because it measures the potential difference across the membrane directly rather than relying on transmembrane current density changes outside the neuron. As a result, one can measure electrical activity occurring within the neuron that would be nearly impossible to measure extracellularly, such as spontaneously occurring or evoked (via afferent pathway stimulation) electrical potentials generated by neurotransmitter release (or postsynaptic potentials). Furthermore, because the membrane potential of the neuron may be altered by injecting depolarizing or hyperpolarizing current into the cell through the electrode, the equilibrium potential (also known as the reversal potential) of the response may be determined. In addition, the overall conductance of the membrane may be measured by injecting known levels of current and measuring the membrane voltage deflection produced. By applying this information using Ohm's law, the input resistance of the cell can be determined. This could be important in assessing drug effects. A drug could increase the input resistance of the membrane, making it more responsive to current generated by afferent synapses, without changing the membrane potential of the neuron. Indeed, such a condition has been proposed to underlie the mechanism through which norepinephrine exerts a "modulatory" action—that is, increasing the amplitude of the response of a neuron to a stimulus without affecting its basal firing rate (which has also been described as increasing its "signal-to-noise" ratio; Freedman et al. 1977; Woodward et al. 1979).

The intracellular recording electrode can also be used to inject specific substances into the neuron. For example, second messengers or calcium chelators can be introduced into the neuron to examine how they regulate the excitability and modulate the baseline activity of the neuron or how they affect the neuron's response to drugs (Figure 5–4). Furthermore, by injecting the neuron with a fluorescent dye or enzymatic marker, the morphology of the specific cell impaled may be recovered and examined (Figure 5–5). This technique can be combined with immunocytochemistry to examine the neurotransmitter synthesized by the cell under study (e.g., Grace and Onn 1989).

Inserting an electrode into the membrane of a cell to measure transmembrane voltage and manipulating its

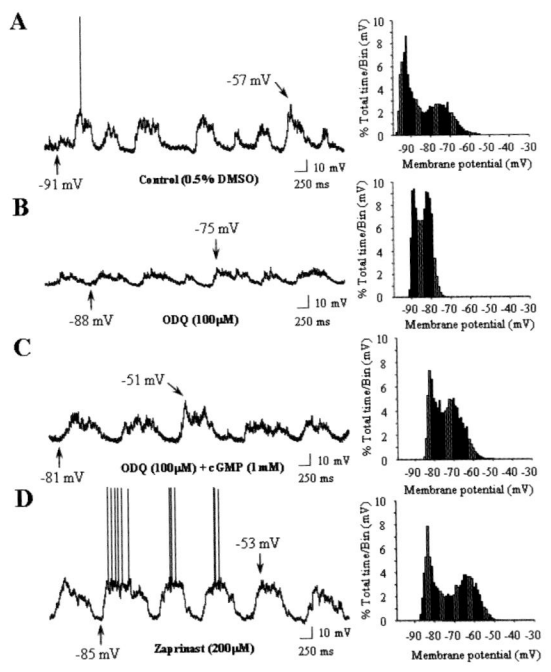

FIGURE 5-4. *(continued)*

solution of dimethylsulfoxide (DMSO); B) the drug 1*H*-[1,2,4]oxadiazole[4,3-a]quinoxalin-1-one (ODQ), which blocks cGMP synthesis by inhibiting the synthetic enzyme guanylyl cyclase; C) ODQ plus cGMP; or D) the drug zaprinast, which inhibits phosphodiesterase enzymes responsible for degrading cGMP. **(A)** *Left:* After vehicle injection, striatal neurons exhibited typical rapid spontaneous shifts in steady-state membrane potential and irregular spontaneous spike discharge. *Right:* Time interval plots of membrane potential activity recorded from control neurons demonstrated bimodal membrane potential distributions indicative of bistable membrane activity. **(B)** *Left:* Striatal neurons recorded after ODQ injection exhibited significantly lower-amplitude depolarizing events compared with vehicle-injected controls and rarely fired action potentials. *Right:* The depolarized portion of the membrane potential distribution of neurons recorded after ODQ injection was typically shifted leftward (i.e., hyperpolarized) compared with controls. **(C)** *Left:* Striatal neurons recorded after ODQ and cGMP coinjection rarely fired action potentials but exhibited high-amplitude depolarizing events with extraordinarily long durations. *Right:* The membrane potential distribution of neurons recorded after ODQ and cGMP coinjection was similar to that of controls, indicating that cGMP partially reversed some of the effects of ODQ. **(D)** *Left:* Striatal neurons recorded after intracellular injection of zaprinast exhibited high-amplitude depolarizing events with extraordinarily long durations. Additionally, all of the cells fired action potentials at relatively high rates (0.4–2.2 Hz). *Right:* The membrane potential distribution of these neurons was typically shifted rightward (i.e., depolarized) compared with controls. Because zaprinast blocks the degradation of endogenous cGMP, we can conclude that basal levels of cGMP depolarize the membrane potential of striatal neurons and facilitate spontaneous postsynaptic potentials. *Arrows* indicate the membrane potential at its maximal depolarized and hyperpolarized levels.

Source. Adapted from West AR, Grace AA: "The Nitric Oxide–Guanylyl Cyclase Signaling Pathway Modulates Membrane Activity States and Electrophysiological Properties of Striatal Medium Spiny Neurons Recorded In Vivo." *Journal of Neuroscience* 24:1924–1935, 2004. Copyright 2004, Society for Neuroscience. Used with permission.

FIGURE 5-4. Effects of intracellular manipulations of cGMP levels on basal activity of striatal medium spiny neurons.

Intracellular application of selective pharmacological agents enables the investigator to examine the direct effects of these agents on the membrane activity of single neurons as well as to manipulate intracellular second-messenger systems. This figure demonstrates that manipulation of intracellular cyclic guanosine monophosphate (cGMP) levels potently and specifically modulates the membrane activity of striatal medium spiny neurons in a manner that cannot be achieved by extracellular application of drugs. Striatal neurons were recorded after intracellular application (~5 minutes) of either A) vehicle (control), a 0.5%

membrane by injecting current are commonly known as *current clamp*, because the amount and direction of ionic current crossing the membrane of the cell can be controlled by the experimenter, such as when determining the reversal potential of a response. Another technique that is effective in neurophysiological research is the use of *voltage clamping*. With voltage clamping, the membrane potential of the neuron is maintained at a set voltage level by injecting current into the cell. This is achieved by rapid feedback electronics that adjusts the current injected to accurately offset any factors that may act to change this potential. Thus, when the neuron is exposed to a drug that opens ion channels, the effect of the ionic influx is precisely counterbalanced by altering the current injected into the neuron by the voltage clamp device. The amount of additional current that must be injected into the neuron to maintain the membrane potential at its set point is therefore the inverse of the transmembrane

current generated in response to the drug. By using specific ion channel blockers or by altering the extracellular ionic environment of the neuron, the precise ionic mechanism and conductance changes induced in a neuron by a drug or neurotransmitter may be determined.

Patch Clamp Recordings

A final level of analysis to be discussed is one directed at assessing the response of individual ionic channels in the membrane of a neuron. Actually, this technique may be described more as a type of high-resolution extracellular recording. In this method, a glass pipette with a comparatively large tip is drawn, and the tip is fire-polished until it is very smooth. The electrode tip is then placed against the membrane surface of a neuron under visual control. Typically, the neuronal membrane is first cleaned of debris with a jet of fluid to permit a tight seal between the

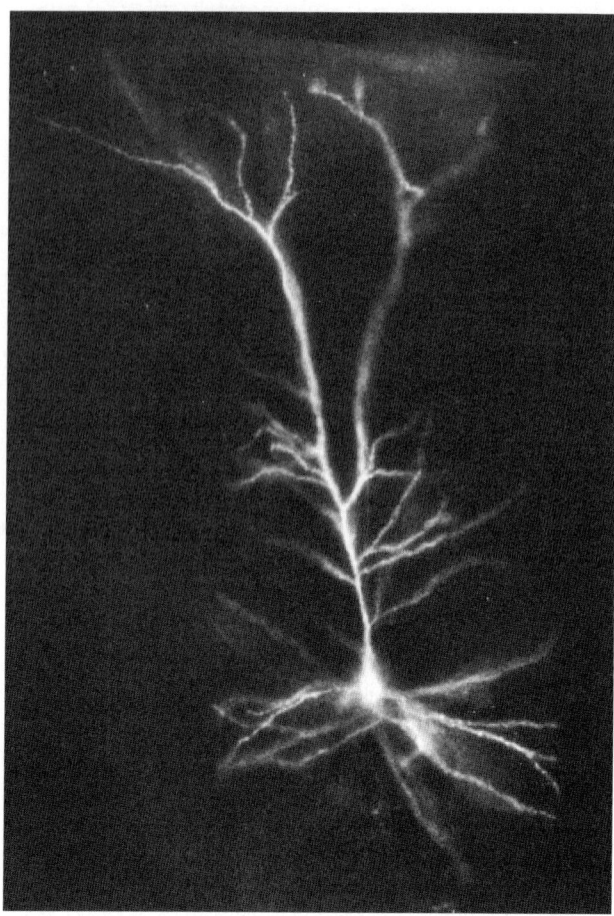

FIGURE 5–5.   Intracellular staining of neuron recorded intracellularly.

During intracellular recordings, the recording pipette is filled with an electrolyte to enable the transmission of membrane voltage deflections to the preamplifier. The electrode may also be filled with substances, such as a morphological stain, for injection into the impaled neuron. In this example, the electrode was filled with the highly fluorescent dye Lucifer yellow. Because this dye has a negative charge at neutral pH, it may be ejected from the electrode by applying a negative current across the electrode, with the result that the Lucifer yellow carries the negative current flow from the electrode and into the neuron. Because this dye diffuses rapidly in water, it quickly fills the entire neuron impaled. The tissue is then fixed in a formaldehyde compound, the lipids clarified by dehydration-defatting or by using dimethylsulfoxide (Grace and Llinás 1985), and the tissue examined under a fluorescence microscope. In this case, a brightly fluorescing pyramidal neuron in layer 3 of the neocortex of a guinea pig is recovered.

electrode and the membrane. A small suction is then applied to the pipette to tighten its seal with the membrane. Because such an attachment provides a high-resistance junction with the membrane, the minute transmembrane currents that are generated as a result of the opening and closing of individual ionic channels may be monitored. The biophysical characteristics (e.g., open time, inactiva-

tion rate) of specific ion channels and how they may be modified by drugs applied via the pipette lumen or to other regions of the neuron being studied can be determined.

Whole-Cell Recordings

A technology widely used in neuropharmacology research is whole-cell recordings. This technique is a modification of the patch clamp technique. The membrane patch underlying the electrode is ruptured, typically by applying a small suction through the pipette, which results in the interior of the electrode becoming continuous with the intracellular fluid. The combination of a tight giga-ohm seal around the electrode–cell membrane junction and the very low resistance of the electrode–intracellular patch has several major advantages: the recordings are very low noise, and the low resistance of the electrodes can minimize errors that may arise during voltage clamp recordings or distort the recorded voltage response to a current input.

When combined with infrared video microscopy techniques, which allow both the large electrode tip and the cell to which it is to be attached to be visualized (Figure 5–6), recordings can be made from specific cell types or from cells labeled with a retrogradely transported fluorescent dye. Although such a preparation has many unique and powerful advantages, this low-resistance junction is also subject to the introduction of artifacts. This is particularly true in cases in which the response to be measured is mediated by diffusible second messengers: the large bore of the attached electrode has been reported to dialyze intracellular constituents from the cell into the electrode. When this process happens, the experimenter often observes a rundown of the response, in which the current gradually decreases with time as a result of loss of the intracellular milieu. To test for this possibility, investigators often rely on a "perforated patch" technique, in which the patch pipette is filled with the ionophore nystatin, gramicidin, or others. When a patch pipette of this type is attached to the cell surface, these channel ionophores are incorporated into the membrane section adjacent to the bore of the electrode. As a result, a low-resistance access to the intracellular space is obtained without the need for rupturing the membrane.

When penetrating at the level of the soma, the somatic current clamp and voltage clamp recordings are capable of measuring the voltage and conductance changes that occur at the soma or proximal dendrites. As a result,

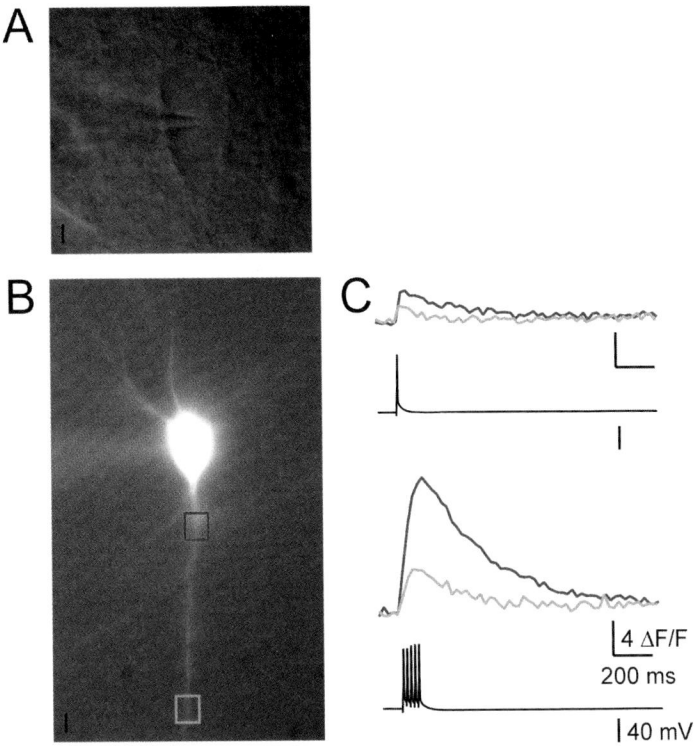

FIGURE 5–6. Patch clamp electrophysiology and calcium imaging.

By combining patch clamping with injection of selective dyes, the dynamics of calcium can be imaged in real time within isolated neurons. **(A)** Using infrared differential interference contrast (IR-DIC) microscopy, the image of a patch pipette can be observed attached to a neuron during a whole-cell electrophysiology experiment. Note the relatively large size of the pipette tip *(coming from the left side of the image)*. Calibration bar = 2 μm. **(B)** After filling the neuron with a calcium-sensitive dye, bis-Fura 2, the live neuron can be imaged with a fluorescence microscope. The dye takes about 10 minutes to fill the neuron after rupturing the patch membrane. Calibration bar = 10 μm. **(C)** A unique property of the dye bis-Fura 2 is that it changes its fluorescence properties as it binds calcium. This can be observed by the changes in the fluorescence signal in response to a single *(top)* or five *(bottom)* action potentials. The fluorescence traces correspond to two regions, one close to the cell body *(red box* and *red trace)* and one farther out in the apical dendrite *(orange box, orange trace)*. In this way, one can observe changes in calcium dynamics and how they correspond to activity states within single neurons.

the complex membrane dynamics and synaptic events that occur along the dendritic tree cannot be resolved by somatic penetration in neurons with a complex morphology. One powerful application of patch recording techniques is targeted recordings of dendrites and presynaptic terminals, structures previously not accessible to direct electrophysiological measurement. Recordings at dendritic sites have demonstrated dendritic membrane properties that often are quite distinct from properties determined from somatic recordings. From these findings, it can be inferred that dendrites are not just extensions of the soma but also play an active role in the propagation of postsynaptic potentials from the synapse to the soma.

However, many structures, such as finer dendrites and smaller axonals, are still resistant to direct electrophysiological measurement with patch electrodes. Another technique that allows for examination of minute struc-

tures is the use of fluorescent dyes. Two basic classes of dyes are commonly used: 1) dyes sensitive to changes in ion concentration, which indirectly reflect the membrane potential, and 2) dyes sensitive to voltage changes, with fluorescence directly responsive to changes of membrane potential. Because these dyes readily diffuse throughout the neuron, real-time imaging of changes in dye fluorescence can be performed in live cells (see Figure 5–6). Although the temporal resolutions and signal-to-noise ratios of imaging technologies do not rival those achievable with direct electrical recordings, imaging allows examination of minute structures and wide spatial regions. Major drawbacks of this technique include the toxicity of some dyes and the phototoxicity induced by light sources used to excite the dyes. More recently, this technique has been applied in vivo, providing new avenues for study of neuronal function.

Preparations Used in Electrophysiological Research

As with the various types of recordings that can be done, several preparations also can be used in this analysis. No single preparation is "best"; instead, each has specific advantages and shortcomings. A more complete picture of the functioning of a system can be gained by taking advantage of the unique perspective provided by each preparation and designing the experiments accordingly. Except for the first category listed below, all preparations pertain to the mammalian vertebrate.

Simpler Nervous Systems—Invertebrates and Lower Vertebrate Preparations

We include a reference to simpler nervous systems for completeness; more comprehensive reviews of the use of nonmammalian model systems can be found elsewhere (Kandel 1978). However, depending on the application, use of these preparations may yield varying degrees of relevance. With respect to the use of phylogenetically lower species as models for psychopharmacological studies in humans, much of the data related to anatomy, cellular physiology, and behavior would be of limited value. The nervous system of these organisms is substantially different from those of vertebrates and humans, even at the single neuronal level. As a result, information derived from these systems is likely to be substantially less applicable to behavioral control in the mammalian class. Nonetheless, several unique advantages are associated with the study of the nervous systems of these organisms: the nervous system is more accessible, the small number of neurons allows for simple and replicable identification of specific neurons, the large neuronal size enables more stable impalement and more complex procedures, and so on. Furthermore, information about the study of some second-messenger systems or receptor transduction mechanisms appears to be more directly transferable to the vertebrate. Thus, it appears that nature is more likely to conserve the most basic functional units of neurotransmitter actions throughout phylogeny, with decreasing levels of homology as the functional units are assembled into more complex systems of neurons and networks.

In Vivo Electrophysiological Recordings

Protocols that use the in vivo preparation focus on the living, intact, anesthetized animal as the subject of the study. Recording the activity of neurons in the intact animal has numerous advantages over studies of isolated tissues. For example, the health of the tissue or neuron under study is more easily maintained and monitored. Furthermore, the neuron can be examined in its normal ionic and cellular microenvironment, with its normal complement of afferent connections intact. In addition, neurons recorded in vivo are more likely to be spontaneously active, facilitating the use of extracellular recordings and investigations into the actions of inhibitory neurotransmitters.

With respect to psychopharmacological research, the in vivo preparation provides the most direct link between neurophysiology and behavior. A drug that elicits a characteristic behavioral response can be administered systemically to examine how the drug affects neurons that are likely to participate in the behavioral response. For similar reasons, this preparation is also the most effective for investigating the mode of action of psychoactive drugs on specific neuronal systems. Although the precise locus of action through which the systemically administered drugs achieve these effects may be difficult to determine directly, whether a given drug ultimately influences the activity of a neuronal system of interest can be determined.

Experimental parameters present difficulties that, although not insurmountable, add complexity to the experimental paradigm. For example, the researcher cannot visually identify the nucleus or the cell to be recorded and must often rely on indirect techniques for cell identification. However, methods are available to enhance the ability to identify cell types. Thus, unlike the in vitro preparations, cells may be identified with respect to the projection sites of their axons by employing antidromic activation—that is, stimulation of the axon terminal region to evoke an action potential that is conducted back down the axon and subsequently recorded at the soma. Furthermore, by using in vivo intracellular recording, the neuron in question may be stained with dye and its location, morphology, and neurotransmitter content identified post hoc by various histochemical and immunocytochemical techniques (e.g., Grace and Bunney 1983; Onn et al. 1994). In addition, although the precise locus of action of systemically administered drugs cannot be determined, the drug effects obtained can be compared with those produced by directly applying the drug to the neuron through microiontophoresis (Figure 5–7) (Bloom 1974). With microiontophoresis, the drug is applied locally to the recording site, affecting the soma and proximal dendrites of the neuron recorded. However, this may be a shortcoming when the afferents to be examined synapse distally on the dendritic tree of the neuron.

A

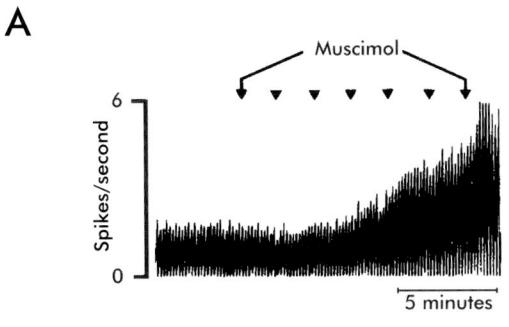

B

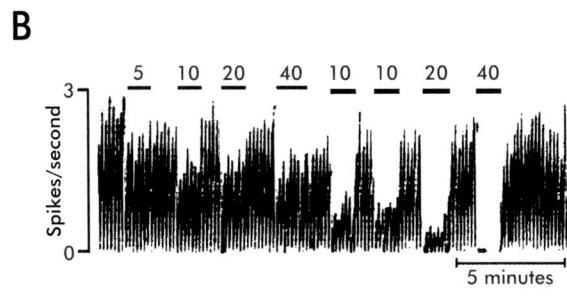

FIGURE 5–7. Determining the effects of systemic and direct drug administration on neuronal activity.

There are several means of applying drugs to a neuron to examine their actions. During in vivo recording, drugs may be administered systemically (i.e., intravenously, intraperitoneally, subcutaneously, intraventricularly, intramuscularly) or directly to the neuron by microiontophoresis or pressure ejection. **(A)** Systemic administration of a drug is useful for determining how a drug affects neurons in the intact organism, regardless of whether the action is direct or indirect. In this case, intravenous administration of the γ-aminobutyric acid (GABA) agonist muscimol (*solid arrows*) causes a dose-dependent increase in the firing rate of this dopamine-containing neuron. **(B)** In contrast, direct administration of a drug to a neuron will provide information about the site of action of the drug, at least as it concerns the discharge of the neuron under study. In this case, GABA is administered directly to a dopamine neuron by microiontophoresis. In this technique, several drug-containing pipettes are attached to the recording electrode. The pH of the drug solutions is adjusted to ensure that the drug molecules are in a charged state (e.g., GABA is used at pH = 4.0 to give it a positive charge), and the drug is ejected from the pipette tip by applying very small currents to the drug-containing pipette. Because the total diameter of the microiontophoretic pipette tip is only about 5 μm, the drugs ejected typically affect only the cell being recorded. In this case, GABA is applied to a dopamine neuron by microiontophoresis; the horizontal bars show the time during which the current is applied to the drug-containing pipette, and the amplitude of the current (indicated in nA) is listed above each bar. Note that, unlike the excitatory effects produced by a systemically administered GABA agonist in (A), direct application of GABA will inhibit dopamine neurons. This has been shown to be caused by inhibition of a much more GABA-sensitive inhibitory interneuron by the systemically administered drug and illustrates the need to compare systemic drug administration with direct drug administration to ascertain the site of action of the drug of interest.

Source. Adapted from Grace AA, Bunney BS: "Opposing Effects of Striatonigral Feedback Pathways on Midbrain Dopamine Cell Activity." *Brain Research* 333:271–284, 1985. Copyright 1985, Elsevier. Used with permission.

A technique that overcomes this shortcoming is the use of combined microdialysis and intracellular recording. In this approach, a microdialysis probe is used for *delivering* a drug to the region surrounding the neuron (Figure 5–8). To preserve the tissue surrounding the probe, the probe is lowered at a rate of 3–6 microns per second using a micromanipulator (West et al. 2002b). The microdialysis probe is then allowed to equilibrate for approximately 2–3 hours, and sharp-electrode intracellular recordings are conducted within 500 micrometers of the active surface of the probe. Provided that the probe has been inserted with care, the passive membrane properties, spontaneous spike activity, and spike characteristics of striatal and cortical neurons recorded during perfusion of artificial cerebrospinal fluid are found to be similar to those of neurons recorded in animals without microdialysis. The viability of neurons recorded proximal to the microdialysis probe is further evidenced by the increase in membrane excitability and spontaneous activity occurring within minutes after introduction of excitatory amino acid agonists (glutamate, N-methyl-D-aspartate [NMDA]) or the GABA$_A$ receptor antagonist bicuculline into the perfusate. Conversely, local reverse dialysis of tetrodotoxin eliminates

action potentials and the spontaneous plateau depolarizations in prefrontal cortex neurons, indicating that these properties are dependent on synaptic inputs to these neurons. Given these findings, it is clear that this combination method has unique properties in comparison with local application via microiontophoresis. Thus, the site of application will span several hundred micrometers and thereby affect a microcircuit, including the distal dendrites and neighboring neurons of the neuron impaled. Moreover, by applying a neurotransmitter antagonist, one can ascertain the baseline effect of spontaneous neurotransmitter action on a neuron being recorded (West and Grace 2002). This approach has recently been applied to single-unit extracellular recordings (West et al. 2002a) and field potential recordings (Lavin et al. 2005; Goto and Grace 2005a, 2005b).

On the other hand, the properties that confer distinct advantages on the in vivo preparation with respect to examining how drugs act in the intact organism also limit the type of data that may be collected. Regarding drug administration, some drugs are not easily applied via microdialysis or do not readily cross the blood–brain barrier, or they may actually produce their direct actions outside of

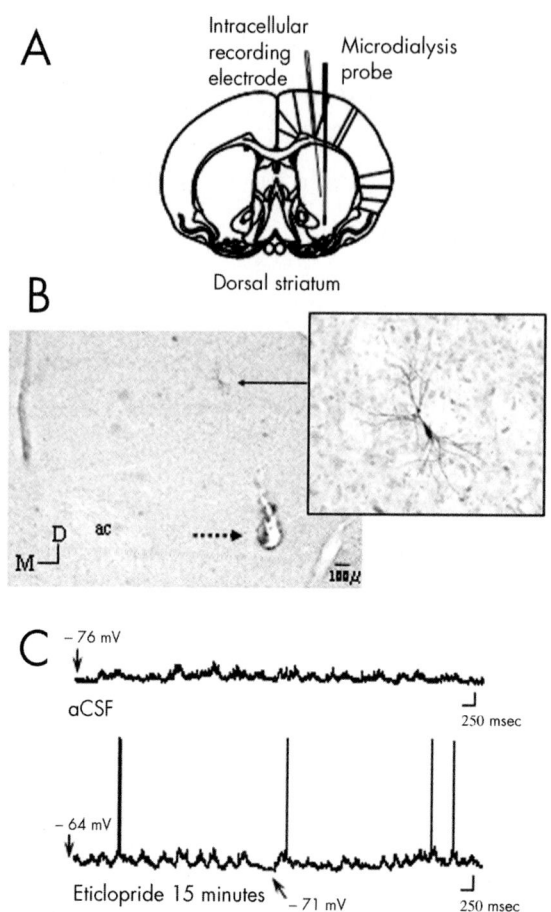

FIGURE 5–8.   Use of a microdialysis probe for delivering drugs locally during in vivo recordings to affect local circuits.

(A) In this schematic diagram, the relationship between the microdialysis probe and the intracellular recording electrode is depicted. In this case, the neuron recorded is in the striatum. The active surface of the microdialysis probe is shown in gray; this is the area through which the compound is delivered. The probe is implanted very slowly so as not to disrupt the tissue (i.e., 3–6 μm per second) and is perfused with artificial cerebrospinal fluid for 2–4 hours to allow equilibration and settling of the tissue prior to recording. The intracellular recording electrode is then advanced, and a neuron is impaled. After recording baseline activity for 10 minutes, the perfusate is changed to a drug-containing solution to examine the effects on the neuron. **(B)** The histology taken after the recording shows the track of the microdialysis probe; the termination site of the probe tip is indicated by a *dashed arrow*. To confirm that the neuron recorded was near the probe, the neuron is filled with a stain (in this case, biocytin) so as to allow visualization of the neuron. In this case, the neuron was confirmed to be a medium spiny striatal neuron (*magnified in insert*). ac = anterior commissure. **(C)** Recordings taken from the neuron labeled in B. The *top trace* shows the activity of the neuron while the microdialysis probe is being perfused with artificial cerebrospinal fluid. The neuron demonstrates a healthy resting membrane potential, and spontaneously occurring postsynaptic potentials are evident. The *lower trace* shows the same neuron 15 minutes after switching to a perfusate containing the dopamine D_2 antagonist eticlopride. The neuron shows a strong depolarization of the resting potential (by 12 mV) as well as increased postsynaptic potential activity and spontaneous spike firing. Since the eticlopride is blocking the effects of dopamine that is being released spontaneously from dopamine terminals in this region, we can conclude that basal levels of dopamine D_2 receptor stimulation cause a tonic hyperpolarization of the neuronal membrane and suppress spontaneous excitatory postsynaptic potentials.

Source.   Adapted from West AR, Grace AA "Opposite Influences of Endogenous Dopamine D_1 and D_2 Receptor Activation on Activity States and Electrophysiological Properties of Striatal Neurons: Studies Combining In Vivo Intracellular Recordings and Reverse Microdialysis." *Journal of Neuroscience* 22:294–304, 2002. Copyright 2002, Society for Neuroscience. Used with permission.

the brain via an effect on peripheral organs. Thus, although dopamine cells can be excited by microiontophoretic administration of cholecystokinin (Skirboll et al. 1981), the excitation produced by systemic administration of this peptide is mediated peripherally and affects

the brain via the vagus (Hommer et al. 1985). In addition, the inability to control the microenvironment of the neuron restricts the analysis of the ionic mechanisms underlying cell firing or drug action because the researcher cannot readily control the precise drug concentration or the ionic composition of the fluid surrounding the neuron. There is also difficulty in segregating local actions of drugs versus those imposed on afferent neurons or their local axon terminals. Therefore, whereas the in vivo preparation affords many advantages with respect to examining how behaviorally or therapeutically effective drugs may exert their actions through defined neuronal systems, examination of the site of action or the membrane mechanisms underlying these responses is more readily accessible with in vitro systems.

In Vitro Electrophysiological Recordings From Brain Slices

Recordings of neurons maintained in vitro have led to significant advances in understanding the ionic mechanisms underlying neurotransmitter and drug actions. This preparation consists of slices 300–400 μm thick cut from the brain of an animal soon after decapitation. If this procedure is done carefully and the brain slices are rapidly placed into oxygenated physiological saline, the neurons within the slices will remain alive and healthy, often for 10 hours or more. Because the neurons are recorded in a chamber with oxygenated media superfused over the slice, several advantages may be realized:

1. Both intracellular and extracellular recordings are more stable because blood and breathing pulsations are absent.
2. Visual control over electrode placement is achieved.
3. The ionic composition of the microenvironment may be controlled precisely.
4. Little interference from the activity of long-loop afferents occurs, and the near-absence of spontaneous spike discharge limits the contribution of local circuit neurons to the responses.

Furthermore, in contrast to microiontophoresis, the concentration of drug in the solution can be controlled precisely. This preparation is also the most complex that can be used for patch clamp recordings because debris may be removed and the patch pipette placed on selected neurons under visual control with a high-resolution optics system (Edwards et al. 1989).

Nonetheless, because of the isolated nature of this system, the results obtained may not precisely reflect the physiology of the intact system. For example, dopamine neurons recorded in vivo have been characterized by their burst-firing discharge pattern (Grace and Bunney 1984a), which appears to be important in regulating neurotrans-

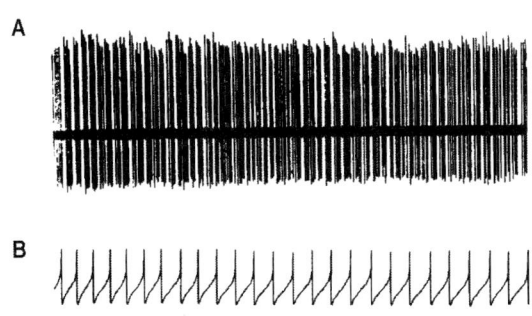

FIGURE 5–9. Variation (sometimes substantial) in patterns of activity of a neuron type, depending on the preparation in which it is recorded.

(A) Extracellular recordings of a dopamine neuron in an intact anesthetized rat (i.e., in vivo) illustrate the typical irregular firing pattern of the cell, with single spikes occurring intermixed with bursts of action potentials. (B) In contrast, intracellular recordings of a dopamine neuron in an isolated brain slice preparation (i.e., in vitro) illustrate the pacemaker pattern that occurs exclusively in identified dopamine neurons in this preparation. For dopamine neurons, a pacemaker firing pattern is rarely observed in vivo, and burst firing has never been observed in the in vitro preparation. However, although the activity recorded in vitro is obviously an abstraction compared with the firing pattern of this neuron in vivo, a comparative study in each preparation does provide the opportunity to examine factors that may underlie the modulation of firing pattern in this neuronal type.

Source. Adapted from Grace AA: "The Regulation of Dopamine Neuron Activity as Determined by In Vivo and In Vitro Intracellular Recordings," in *The Neurophysiology of Dopamine Systems.* Edited by Chiodo LA, Freeman AS. Detroit, MI, Lake Shore Publications, 1987, pp. 1–67 (Copyright 1987, Lake Shore Publications. Used with permission); and Grace AA, Bunney BS: "Intracellular and Extracellular Electrophysiology of Nigral Dopaminergic Neurons, I: Identification and Characterization." *Neuroscience* 10:301–315, 1983. Copyright 1983, International Brain Research Organization. Used with permission.

mitter release (Gonon 1988). However, dopamine neurons recorded in vitro do not fire in bursting patterns (Grace and Onn 1989) (Figure 5–9). On the other hand, this distinction provides what may be an ideal system for examining the factors that cause in vivo burst firing. Therefore, the most complete model of the functioning of a system or of its response to drug application can be derived by comparing the results obtained in vitro with those in the intact organism.

Recordings From Dissociated Neurons and Neuronal Cell Cultures

Recordings from isolated neurons are actually a subset of in vitro recording methods, with many of the same advantages in terms of accessibility and stability. Furthermore, because the neurons can be completely visualized, advanced techniques such as patch clamping are more easily done. A unique advantage of this system can be obtained by coculturing different neuronal populations. For example, defining the effects of a noradrenergic synapse on a hippocampal pyramidal neuron more precisely may be possible by coculturing these cell types and allowing them to make synapses. In this way, the researcher has visual control over impaling neurons that constitute a presynaptic and postsynaptic pairing. On the other hand, the synapses formed are not necessarily limited to those that occur naturally in the intact organism, in terms of both the location of the synapse on the neuron and the classes of neurons that are interconnected. Furthermore, the altered neuronal morphology present in these preparations may modify the response of the neurons to drugs. Nonetheless, when the analysis is limited to well-defined responses, such as second-messenger actions or ion channel measures, this system affords an unparalleled level of accessibility.

Relationship Between Biochemical and Electrophysiological Measures of Neuronal Activity

The methods outlined here are directed at analyzing the activity of individual neurons as a means of assessing their role in pharmacological responses or behavioral actions. This is based on the premise that the discharge of a neuron in some manner reflects its release of a transmitter onto a postsynaptically located target neuron. As such, biochemical measures of neurotransmitter levels would be predicted to correspond to the activity changes occurring during electrophysiological recordings from neurons (Roth 1987). In several cases, such approaches have helped to define the physiological relevance of recorded neuron activity. One case in which this has proven valuable is in the analysis of firing pattern. For example, dopamine neurons, like many other cell types in the central nervous system, are capable of discharging trains of action potentials in two patterns of activity: single spiking and burst firing. However, their range of firing rates is comparatively restricted, with most cells firing only between 2 and 8 Hz. Nonetheless, information on the temporal relationship between spikes and bursts (Grace and Bunney 1984a) has been used in in vivo voltammetry studies to measure dopamine levels. Dopamine cells firing in bursts will release two to three times more neurotransmitter per spike from their terminals than those discharging at sim-

ilar frequencies but in a steady firing pattern (Gonon 1988). Therefore, in this case, knowledge of the physiological firing pattern provided information to the electrochemist that resulted in the elucidation of the physiological consequence of burst firing in this system.

However, the extrapolation between biochemical and electrophysiological measures may not always be valid. Thus, recordings from single neurons may not necessarily reflect the activity across the population of neurons of interest. Therefore, a drug that exerts an action via activation of the nonfiring population of neurons may be overlooked if its actions are assessed on single spontaneously discharging neurons (Bunney and Grace 1978; Grace and Bunney 1984b). Furthermore, the response may be confined to a topographically defined subset of neurons mediating a particular response (e.g., a change in the activity of neurons regulating movement of the leg would not be predicted if the response involves a reaching movement of the arm). With respect to biochemical measurements, actions of transmitters at presynaptic terminals could dramatically alter the amount of neurotransmitter they release independent of neuronal discharge (e.g., Grace 1991). On the other hand, electrophysiological measurements enable researchers to examine responses that occur very rapidly. Indeed, a massive but transient activation of spike discharge in a neuronal system may evoke a substantial behavioral response, whereas biochemical measurements of neurotransmitter release performed over a long time course may dilute the impact of the transient event. Therefore, although the results obtained from each measure may not be directly comparable, the electrophysiological measurements are better optimized for detecting transient events.

Summary

In this chapter, we reviewed several electrophysiological techniques and preparations used in the analysis of nervous system function. Each approach is characterized by a set of unique advantages and potential shortcomings inherent in the method. Nonetheless, it should be apparent that no single technique has an overwhelming advantage in psychopharmacological research. Instead, by matching the preparation to the question at hand, and through the judicious comparison of data obtained from intact versus isolated preparations, the various limitations may be systematically overcome to yield a more broadly applicable model of psychopharmacological action.

References

Bloom FE: To spritz or not to spritz: the doubtful value of aimless iontophoresis. Life Sci 14:1819–1834, 1974

Bunney BS, Grace AA: Acute and chronic haloperidol treatment: comparison of effects on nigral dopaminergic cell activity. Life Sci 23:1715–1728, 1978

Bunney BS, Walters JR, Roth RH, et al: Dopaminergic neurons: effect of antipsychotic drugs and amphetamine on single cell activity. J Pharmacol Exp Ther 185:560–571, 1973

Edwards FA, Konnerth A, Sakmann B, et al: A thin slice preparation for patch clamp recordings from neurons of the mammalian central nervous system. Pflugers Arch 414:600–612, 1989

Freedman R, Hoffer BJ, Woodward DJ, et al: Interaction of norepinephrine with cerebellar activity evoked by mossy and climbing fibers. Exp Neurol 55:269–288, 1977

Gonon FG: Nonlinear relationship between impulse flow and dopamine released by rat midbrain dopaminergic neurons as studied by in vivo electrochemistry. Neuroscience 24:19–28, 1988

Goto Y, Grace AA: Dopaminergic modulation of limbic and cortical drive of nucleus accumbens in goal-directed behavior. Nat Neurosci 8:805–812, 2005a

Goto Y, Grace AA: Dopamine-dependent interactions between limbic and prefrontal cortical plasticity in the nucleus accumbens: disruption by cocaine sensitization. Neuron 47:255–266, 2005b

Grace AA: Phasic versus tonic dopamine release and the modulation of dopamine system responsivity: a hypothesis for the etiology of schizophrenia. Neuroscience 41:1–24, 1991

Grace AA: The depolarization block hypothesis of neuroleptic action: implications for the etiology and treatment of schizophrenia. J Neural Transm 36 (suppl):91–131, 1992

Grace AA, Bunney BS: Intracellular and extracellular electrophysiology of nigral dopaminergic neurons, I: identification and characterization. Neuroscience 10:301–315, 1983

Grace AA, Bunney BS: The control of firing pattern in nigral dopamine neurons: burst firing. J Neurosci 4:2877–2890, 1984a

Grace AA, Bunney BS: The control of firing pattern in nigral dopamine neurons: single spike firing. J Neurosci 4:2866–2876, 1984b

Grace AA, Bunney BS: Opposing effects of striatonigral feedback pathways on midbrain dopamine cell activity. Brain Res 333:271–284, 1985

Grace AA, Llinás R: Dehydration-induced morphological artifacts in intracellularly stained neurons: circumvention using rapid DMSO clearing. Neuroscience 16:461–475, 1985

Grace AA, Onn SP: Morphology and electrophysiological properties of immunocytochemically identified rat dopamine neurons recorded in vitro. J Neurosci 9:3463–3481, 1989

Hommer DW, Palkovits M, Crawley JN, et al: Cholecystokinin-induced excitation in the substantia nigra: evidence for peripheral and central components. J Neurosci 5:1387–1392, 1985

Kandel ER: A Cell-Biological Approach to Learning (Grass Lecture Monograph 1). Bethesda, MD, Society for Neuroscience, 1978, pp 1–90

Lavin A, Nogueira L, Lapish CC, et al: Mesocortical dopamine neurons operate in distinct temporal domains using multimodal signals. J Neurosci 25:5013–5023, 2005

Llinás RR: The intrinsic electrophysiological properties of mammalian neurons: a new insight into CNS function. Science 242:1654–1664, 1988

Onn SP, Berger TW, Grace AA: Identification and characterization of striatal cell subtypes using in vivo intracellular recording and dye-labelling in rats, III: morphological correlates and compartmental localization. Synapse 16:231–254, 1994

Roth RH: Biochemical correlates of the electrophysiological activity of dopaminergic neurons: reflections on two decades of collaboration with electrophysiologists, in Neurophysiology of Dopaminergic Systems—Current Status and Clinical Perspectives. Edited by Chiodo LA, Freeman AS. Detroit, MI, Lake Shore Publications, 1987, pp 187–203

Skirboll LR, Grace AA, Hommer DW, et al: Peptide-monoamine coexistence: studies of the actions of a cholecystokinin-like peptide on the electrical activity of midbrain dopamine neurons. Neuroscience 6:2111–2124, 1981

Terzuolo CA, Araki T: An analysis of intra- versus extracellular potential changes associated with activity of single spinal motoneurons. Ann N Y Acad Sci 94:547–558, 1961

West AR, Grace AA: Opposite influences of endogenous dopamine D1 and D2 receptor activation on activity states and electrophysiological properties of striatal neurons: studies combining in vivo intracellular recordings and reverse microdialysis. J Neurosci 22:294–304, 2002

West AR, Galloway, MP, Grace AA: Regulation of striatal dopamine neurotransmission by nitric oxide: effector pathways and signaling mechanisms. Synapse 44:227–245, 2002a

West AR, Moore H, Grace AA: Direct examination of local regulation of membrane activity in striatal and prefrontal cortical neurons in vivo using simultaneous intracellular recording and microdialysis. J Pharmacol Exp Ther 301:867–877, 2002b

Woodward DJ, Moises HC, Waterhouse BD, et al: Modulatory actions of norepinephrine in the central nervous system. Fed Proc 38:2109–2116, 1979

CHAPTER 6

Animal Models

David M. Lyons, Ph.D.

Practical limitations and ethical concerns restrict opportunities for randomized, controlled trials of potentially new drug treatments for human psychiatric disorders. Prospects for discovering the neural mechanisms of action of established therapeutic drugs are also less prevalent in psychiatry than other fields of medicine, because biopsies of diseased brain tissue in humans are seldom performed. Animal models are therefore essential for screening new drugs and for understanding how drug therapies in humans restore the neural basis of mental health. This chapter addresses the validity, utility, and limitations of animal models in psychopharmacological research.

Model Types and Validity

Two principal types of animal models are prevalent in psychopharmacology. *Assay models* are used to screen drugs with unknown therapeutic potential and need not resemble anything seen in a psychiatric disorder. The validity of assay models is determined by their ability to predict that a drug reliably belongs to a therapeutic class. In rats, for example, passive avoidance deficits induced by olfactory bulbectomies are reversed by antidepressants but not by psychostimulants, neuroleptics, or anticholinergics (Song and Leonard 2005). New drugs with unknown therapeutic potential that reverse bulbectomy-induced deficits in rats are therefore considered to be possible antidepressants. Assay models also satisfy additional criteria, including ease of use, high throughput capacity, reproducibility, and economic concerns.

The second principal type of animal model simulates an aspect of interest in a psychiatric disorder. *Simulation*

models are used to investigate the biology of psychiatric disorders or the mechanisms of action of psychotherapeutic drugs. In addition to the criterion of *predictive validity* described above for assay models, simulation models are often evaluated for two other aspects of validity.

Face validity refers to phenomenological similarities between the animal model and the human psychiatric condition. As originally proposed by McKinney and Bunney (1969), animal models of human mental illness have a high degree of face validity when the following criteria are met: the model is produced by etiological factors known to produce the human disorder, the model resembles the behavioral manifestations and symptoms of the human disorder, the model has an underlying physiology similar to the human disorder, and the model responds to therapeutic treatments known to be effective in human psychiatric patients. How these criteria are evaluated and established has been described in detail elsewhere (McKinney 2001; Weiss and Kilts 1998).

Construct validity refers to the theoretical rationale for linking a psychiatric disorder to an endpoint measured in the animal model. To establish construct validity, a theory for understanding a disorder is mapped or shown to be equivalent to an endpoint in the animal model (Sarter and Bruno 2002). Disease heterogeneity and related concerns that no single animal model can capture the complexities of an entire disorder have shifted attention away from modeling disorders as a whole (McKinney 2001; Insel 2007) to focus on psychiatric endophenotypes (Gould and Gottesman 2006). The endophenotype strategy presupposes that each disorder comprises behavioral, physiological, neuroanatomical, cellular, and molecular components that are more proximal to causal risk factors than are the actual disorders defined in DSM-IV-TR (American Psychiatric Association 2000; Arguello and Gogos 2006). Psychiatric endophenotypes are conceptualized as mediating the link between genetic or environmental risk factors and the resulting disorder (Figure 6–1). Precise delineation of endophenotypes also serves to highlight the fact that certain features of psychiatric disorders—for example, diminished verbal recall, self-conscious emotions, delusions of control, impaired theory of mind, and suicidal ideation— are likely unique to humans. Many other endophenotypes are, however, amenable to modeling in animal research, as will be described in the following sections of this chapter.

Features that confer a high degree of validity for simulation models are often poorly suited for animal assay models used in drug screening research. An example is the typical delay in response onset for conventional antidepressants. On the other hand, simulation models that achieve all three aspects of validity may be better suited to identify substantively new drugs that differ from those used to establish an assay model. Excessive reliance on assay models may increase the tendency to perpetuate the same side effects as those produced by known medications. The following sections selectively illustrate how animal models have advanced our understanding of the psychopharmacology and biology of depressive disorders.

Learned Helplessness

One of the earliest and most studied models of depression emerged from now classic studies of learned helplessness (Overmier and Seligman 1967; Seligman and Maier 1967) and uncontrollable stress (Weiss 1968). Animals exposed to uncontrollable stress, but not those exposed to controllable stress, exhibit diminished reactivity to rewarding stimulation, altered sleep patterns, social impairments, and deficits in learning appropriate avoidance–escape behavior (Maier 2001; Vollmayr et al. 2004; Weiss and Kilts 1998). Exposure to uncontrollable stress also induces significant changes in noradrenergic (Weiss 1991), serotonergic (Maier and Watkins 2005), and GABAergic (Minor and Hunter 2002) brain systems hypothesized to mediate the behavioral endpoints measured in learned helplessness models. Avoidance–escape deficits in rats are reversed by subchronic treatment with known antidepressants, including tricyclic antidepressants (TCAs), monoamine oxidase inhibitors (MAOIs), selective serotonin reuptake inhibitors (SSRIs), and atypical antidepressants. Stimulants, neuroleptics, sedatives, and anxiolytics do not reverse learned helplessness effects (Weiss and Kilts 1998).

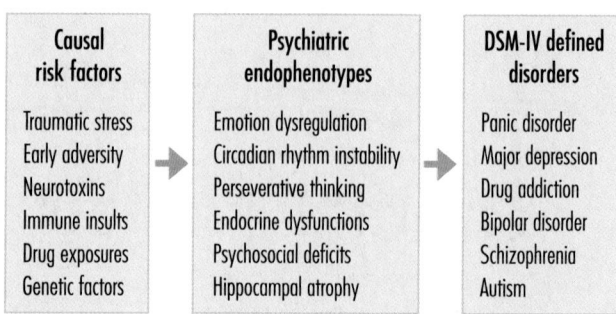

FIGURE 6–1. Psychiatric endophenotypes mediate the link between causal risk factors and the resulting psychiatric disorders defined in DSM-IV-TR. Representative examples and nonexhaustive lists of risk factors, endophenotypes, and disorders are provided to illustrate this theoretical framework for psychiatry neuroscience and psychopharmacological research.

These and related findings demonstrate that learned helplessness models have a high degree of validity in terms of etiology (uncontrollable stress), behavioral symptoms (anhedonia, passivity, disrupted sleep), pathophysiology (sensitization of serotonergic neurons), and response to conventional antidepressants. In rats, however, learned helplessness persists only for several days, whereas depression in humans may last for months. A possible explanation for this discrepancy is that rats do not spontaneously generate perseverative memories or ruminations about their experiences beyond the context in which the experiences occurred. By reminding rats of a stressful experience through repeated exposure to contextual cues, Maier (2001) discovered that learned helplessness manifestations in rats can be prolonged. These findings lend support to the view that stressful perseverative thinking plays a prominent role in the maintenance of human depressive disorders (Brosschot et al. 2006; Nolen-Hoeksema 2000).

Chronic Stress

Chronic stress models in rodents prevent acclimatization by presenting a variety of stressors in an unpredictable sequence over several weeks. Rats exposed to immobilization, immersion in cold water, and other stressors fail to show the typical increase in open-field activity observed in rats not exposed to chronic stress (Katz et al. 1981). A variety of antidepressants restore normal open-field activity in rats exposed to chronic stress, whereas nonantidepressants do not reproduce this effect (Willner 1990). A modified version of the chronic stress model employs milder manipulations, such as exposure to flashing lights, intermittent white noise, and short-term deprivation of food or water. After several weeks of chronic mild stress, rats exhibit decreased consumption of a palatable sucrose solution (Willner 1997). This measure of anhedonia is restored to normal in rats who receive concurrent treatment with an antidepressant during exposure to stress (three different TCAs and two atypical antidepressants were effective in restoring normal consumption behavior). Evidence that antidepressants reverse the anhedonic effects of chronic stress by potentiating dopamine neurotransmission comes from studies in which the therapeutic response to TCAs was reversed by administration of dopamine receptor antagonists (Willner 1997). These findings concur with numerous studies linking dopamine neurotransmission with stress (Pani et al. 2000), reward processing (Martin-Soelch et al. 2001), and the neural mechanisms of action for antidepressants (Willner et al. 2005).

In the original chronic stress model, it was reported that sustained elevations in glucocorticoid levels were restored to normal by antidepressants (Katz and Sibel 1982; Katz et al. 1981). These findings are of interest because patients with major depression often present with increased levels of the glucocorticoid stress hormone cortisol (see Chapter 45, "Neurobiology of Mood Disorders"). In rodents, however, chronically elevated glucocorticoid levels are difficult to maintain (Rivier and Vale 1987; E.A. Young and Akil 1985), and rodent models often rely on manipulations that differ from the stressors that induce or exacerbate depression in humans. An intriguing exception is the visible burrow model, which enables small groups of rats to produce natural stress-engendering social interactions well suited for behavioral, neural, and hormonal investigations of stress pathophysiology (Blanchard et al. 1995).

Social Loss

Life events that signify loss or departure from the social network are risk factors for the development of hypercortisolism and depression in humans (Biondi and Picardi 1996; Kendler et al. 2002). A model of social loss–induced hypercortisolism based on species-typical patterns of social organization has been developed in squirrel monkeys (Parker et al. 2003). In their natural environment, squirrel monkeys live in sexually segregated groups. Adult males and females within a group spend most of their time with same-sex companions, and social interactions between the sexes are limited to mating activities (Lyons et al. 1992). When adults are separated from same-sex companions, they respond with increased cortisol levels that frequently persist for several weeks (Lyons and Levine 1994; Lyons et al. 1999). Hypercortisolism occurs not only when monkeys are separated and temporarily housed alone but also when males and females are housed without same-sex companions in male–female pairs and when males are housed without male companions in multifemale groups (Mendoza et al. 1991).

Hypercortisolism in this animal model is initially driven by hypersecretion of adrenocorticotropic hormone (ACTH). This finding concurs with the widely held view that stress induces hypothalamic release of corticotropin-releasing factor (CRF), which stimulates pituitary secretion of ACTH and thereby triggers secretion of cortisol from the adrenal cortex (see Chapter 7, "Psychoneuroendocrinology"). In socially separated monkeys, however, cortisol levels remain elevated while significant reductions occur in plasma levels of ACTH (Lyons and Levine 1994). Low ACTH levels also occur in the context of hypercortisolism in humans with major depression (Murphy 1991). Despite reductions in ACTH, hypercortisolism is maintained because of enhanced adrenal responsiveness to ACTH in socially separated monkeys (Lyons et al. 1995) and in humans with major depression (Plotsky et al. 1998). The low ACTH levels seen in major depression are also observed in response to administration of CRF (Gold et al. 1986). Metyrapone blockade of cortisol biosynthesis abolishes the attenuated ACTH response to exogenous CRF (von Bardeleben et al. 1988), and metyrapone alone increases baseline ACTH levels in humans with major depression (E.A. Young et al. 1997) and monkeys subjected to social separation (Lyons et al. 1999). These results together suggest that hypercortisolism inhibits the response to excessive CRF at the level of pituitary corticotrophs. Evidence that hypercortisolism and excessive CRF are also involved in behavioral and not just neuroendocrine aspects of depression in humans comes from animal models described in the next section.

Physiological Manipulations

Direct administration of naturally occurring neuropeptides, hormones, and cytokines has been used in animal models to identify physiological factors that induce behavioral symptoms of depression in humans. For example, chronic stress levels of cortisol systemically administered to squirrel monkeys impair prefrontal-dependent cognitive control of impulsive behavior (Lyons et al. 2000).

Cortisol administered to healthy humans induces prefrontal-dependent cognitive impairments that resemble those that are caused in humans by prefrontal lesions (Lupien et al. 1999; A.H. Young et al. 1999). Humans with psychotic major depression consistently present with endogenous hypercortisolism (Nelson and Davis 1997), and patients with psychotic major depression are impaired on standardized tests of prefrontal cognitive functions (Schatzberg et al. 2000). Based on these findings, drugs that block cortisol at the receptor level are now being tested as novel treatments for psychotic major depression (DeBattista and Belanoff 2006) and bipolar disorder (A.H. Young 2006).

In various animals, administration of CRF in the brain increases heart rate, arterial blood pressure, limbic brain glucose metabolism, and depressive- and anxiety-like behavior (Heinrichs and Koob 2004; Lowry and Moore 2006; Strome et al. 2002). Conversely, mice genetically engineered to be deficient in the CRF type 1 receptor (CRF-R1) demonstrate diminished depressive- and anxiety-like behavior in response to CRF administration (Muller et al. 2003). These findings from animal models support clinical studies of depression in humans (Nemeroff and Vale 2005) and suggest that drugs that dampen CRF signaling may be therapeutic for patients with depressive disorders. Receptors for CRF, and particularly CRF-R1, are therefore targets of interest in contemporary drug development (Chen 2006).

In rodents and monkeys, peripheral administration of proinflammatory cytokines (i.e., interleukin-1) mimics the effects of stress as a cause of so-called sickness behavior (Hennessy et al. 2001). Sickness behavior in animals is characterized by anhedonia, reduced activity, diminished social and sexual interests, increased sleep, and behaviors reminiscent of depression in humans. Administration of interferon, a potent inducer of proinflammatory mediators, triggers depression in a subset of humans receiving interferon treatment for cancer or hepatitis C (Asnis and De La Garza 2006). These findings suggest that drugs that block proinflammatory mediators may be novel antidepressants. Recent support for this possibility comes from a guinea pig model of stress-induced sickness behavior (Hennessy et al. 2007).

Early Life Stress

Early exposure to parental neglect, child abuse, and severe forms of stress is a risk factor for the development of mood and anxiety disorders. Rhesus macaque monkeys raised without mothers tend to exhibit depression-like behavior (Kraemer 1997), fragmented sleep patterns (Kaemingk and Reite 1987), and excessive consumption of alcohol (Fahlke et al. 2000). Ecologically informed studies of maternal availability have identified similar effects in primate psychosocial development. Bonnet macaque monkeys raised by mothers in stressful variable-demand foraging conditions are impaired on tests of psychosocial and emotional functions (Rosenblum and Andrews 1994). These same monkeys in early adulthood exhibit elevated cerebrospinal fluid levels of monoamines, somatostatin, and CRF (Coplan et al. 2006). Prenatal stress decreases hippocampal volume and inhibits neurogenesis in the dentate gyrus of adolescent rhesus monkey offspring (Coe et al. 2003). Conversely, all known antidepressants increase neurogenesis in the dentate gyrus, as modeled in adult monkeys (Perera et al. 2007), tree shrews (Czeh et al. 2001), and rodents (Drew and Hen 2007).

Hippocampal volumes are smaller in humans with major depression compared with healthy control subjects (Videbech and Ravnkilde 2004), and preliminary evidence in humans suggests that prior exposure to early life stress causes hippocampal volume loss (Vythilingam et al. 2002). To test this hypothesis, we recently examined early life stress and hippocampal volume variation in squirrel monkeys (Lyons et al. 2007). Paternal half-siblings raised apart from one another by different mothers in the absence of fathers were randomized to intermittent postnatal stress or no-stress conditions from 10 to 21 weeks of age. After weaning, at 9 months of age, all monkeys were socially housed in identical conditions. Sexual maturity occurs at 2–3 years of age, and the average maximum squirrel monkey life span is 21 years (Brady 2000). In early adulthood, at 5 years of age, hippocampal volumes were determined in vivo from T1-weighted brain images acquired by magnetic resonance imaging (MRI).

Hippocampal volumes did not differ with respect to prior postnatal stress versus no-stress conditions in squirrel monkeys (Lyons et al. 2001). Rhesus monkeys raised in social isolation do not show hippocampal atrophy despite striking changes in other brain systems and associated behavior (Sanchez et al. 1998). In keeping with studies of humans (Sullivan et al. 2001; van Erp et al. 2004), however, significant heritabilities were discerned by paternal half-sibling analysis of squirrel monkey hippocampal volumes (Lyons et al. 2001). These and related findings suggest that the morphology of specific brain regions is determined in part by genes (Lyons 2002). Moreover, we found that small hippocampal volumes predicted increased stress levels of ACTH after pretreatment with saline or hydrocortisone (Lyons et al. 2007). Small hippocampal volumes may be a risk factor for, and not just an effect of, impaired regulation of the hypothalamic-pituitary-adrenal (HPA) axis response to stress. Similar studies in humans are needed to determine whether small hippocampi are a marker for HPA axis dysregulation in major depression.

Genetic Manipulations

Major depression is a heritable disorder that likely involves multiple genes, each with small effects (Wong and Licinio 2001). Targeted gene deletions and gene transfers in animal models are beginning to elucidate the functional significance of potentially relevant genes (Insel 2007). Consider, for example, dysregulation of the HPA axis evinced in depression by an increase in cortisol levels (see Chapter 45, "Neurobiology of Mood Disorders"). Receptors for cortisol are densely expressed in the prefrontal cortex (Webster et al. 2002), where they function as transcription factors that regulate gene expression (Chrousos and Kino 2005). Hundreds of genes in prefrontal cortex appear to be differentially expressed in humans with a history of major depression based on postmortem analysis of whole-genome microarray data (Choudary et al. 2005; Evans et al. 2004; Iwamoto et al. 2004; Sequeira et al. 2006). Genetic manipulations of receptors for cortisol are not yet feasible in human patients but have recently been studied in various animal models (Boyle et al. 2005; Kaufer et al. 2004; Ridder et al. 2005; Wei et al. 2004). These studies suggest that high-throughput technologies designed to identify candidate genes regulated by receptors for cortisol may yield novel targets for the development of new antidepressants.

Another promising genetic approach involves selective breeding of rodents and subsequent genomewide scans to identify predisposing candidate genes. An intriguing example is the swim-test-susceptible rat, which is bred for extreme passivity in response to uncontrollable stress (Weiss and Kilts 1998). In the swim-test-susceptible rat, eight different antidepressants restore normal swim-test activity after exposure to uncontrollable stress. Four drugs that produce false-positive results in swim tests administered to normal rats (Porsolt et al. 1991) all fail to restore normal swim-test activity in swim-test-susceptible rats. None of the eight tested antidepressants have any effect on a selectively bred line of swim-test-resistant rats, indicating that the detection of antidepressants is best achieved with genetically susceptible rats (Weiss and Kilts 1998). This

model is well suited to identify genes involved in a common mechanism of action of diverse antidepressants.

A related strategy combining genetic and developmental approaches to investigate gene–environment interactions is exemplified by studies of BALB/cByJ mice, which typically are more reactive to stress than C57BL/6ByJ mice (Anisman et al. 1998). When stress-susceptible BALB/cByJ mouse pups are raised by stress-resistant C57BL/6ByJ dams, the development of excessive reactivity to stress is diminished in the cross-fostered pups. However, when stress-resistant C57BL/6ByJ pups are raised by stress-susceptible BALB/cByJ dams, the development of subsequent stress reactivity is not affected in the cross-fostered pups. This model demonstrates that genetic factors affect mother–infant interactive styles, which in turn influence the subsequent development of stress susceptibility in mice.

A complementary approach involves targeted disruptions of gene expression in specific brain regions only during critical periods of postnatal brain development. An example is provided by mice engineered to lack the serotonin$_{1A}$ receptor (5-HT1AR) protein. These mice exhibit increased anxiety-like behavior on a variety of tests. Selective expression of 5-HT1AR in the hippocampus and cortex, but not the raphe nuclei, restores to normal the behavior of 5-HT1AR knockout mice (Gross et al. 2002). Additional evidence suggests that tissue-specific 5-HT1AR expression during postnatal development, but not in adulthood, is necessary to achieve the behavioral rescue effect. This model indicates that developmental changes in 5-HT1AR gene expression within specific brain regions are involved in the emergence of anxiety-like behavior in adulthood.

Utility and Limitations

Most animal models used to study aspects of depression in humans have utilized males, but the prevalence of depression in humans is nearly two times higher in women than in men (Shively et al. 2005). Another limitation of animal models is the tendency to focus on single factors as the cause of depression in humans (Willner 1990). In certain cases, one causal factor may be identified, but more often than not, depression evolves from a nexus of causal risk factors that accumulate over the life span (Kendler et al. 2002). Attempts to model aspects of depression in animals based on one causal factor may be impractical if no single factor is sufficiently potent to trigger the development of depression in humans.

Prefrontal cortical enlargement in humans and associated cognitive complexities raise additional concerns for animal models of psychiatric disorders (Keverne 2004). The difficulty stems from problems in identifying homologous brain regions in humans and animals (Porrino and Lyons 2000; Preuss 1995; Sasaki et al. 2004), especially for the rodents now widely used in neuroscience research. Transgenic mouse models likewise require homologous genes, and the resulting mouse phenotypes are not necessarily isomorphic with the human condition, because genes expressed on different backgrounds can produce different phenotypes (Yoshiki and Moriwaki 2006).

Despite these concerns, many important aspects of human psychiatric disorders are amenable to modeling in animal research. Because the life span of most animals is shorter than that of humans, longitudinal studies of development are facilitated by animal models. Randomized, controlled experiments can be conducted in animals without the common confounds that characterize clinical studies, such as comorbidity, polydrug abuse, and medication effects. Animal models also provide brain tissue of the highest possible quality for cellular and molecular research. Discoveries first made in clinical settings and subsequently tested in animals form the foundation of psychiatric neuroscience and will continue to play a key role in psychopharmacological research.

References

American Psychiatric Association: Diagnostic and Statistical Manual of Mental Disorders, 4th Edition, Text Revision. Washington, DC, American Psychiatric Association, 2000

Anisman H, Zaharia MD, Meaney MJ, et al: Do early life events permanently alter behavioral and hormonal responses to stressors? Int J Dev Neurosci 16:149–164, 1998

Arguello PA, Gogos JA: Modeling madness in mice: one piece at a time. Neuron 52:179–196, 2006

Asnis GM, De La Garza R 2nd: Interferon-induced depression in chronic hepatitis C: a review of its prevalence, risk factors, biology, and treatment approaches. J Clin Gastroenterol 40:322–335, 2006

Biondi M, Picardi A: Clinical and biological aspects of bereavement and loss-induced depression: a reappraisal. Psychother Psychosom 65:229–245, 1996

Blanchard DC, Spencer RL, Weiss SM, et al: Visible burrow system as a model of chronic social stress: behavioral and neuroendocrine correlates. Psychoneuroendocrinology 20:117–134, 1995

Boyle MP, Brewer JA, Funatsu M, et al: Acquired deficit of forebrain glucocorticoid receptor produces depression-like changes in adrenal axis regulation and behavior. Proc Natl Acad Sci U S A 102:473–478, 2005

Brady AG: Research techniques for the squirrel monkey (Saimiri). ILAR J 41:10–18, 2000

Brosschot JF, Gerin W, Thayer JF: The perseverative cognition hypothesis: a review of worry, prolonged stress-related physiological activation, and health. J Psychosom Res 60:113–124, 2006

Chen C: Recent advances in small molecule antagonists of the corticotropin-releasing factor type-1 receptor-focus on pharmacology and pharmacokinetics. Curr Med Chem 13:1261–1282, 2006

Choudary PV, Molnar M, Evans SJ, et al: Altered cortical glutamatergic and GABAergic signal transmission with glial involvement in depression. Proc Natl Acad Sci U S A 102:15653–15658, 2005

Chrousos GP, Kino T: Intracellular glucocorticoid signaling: a formerly simple system turns stochastic. Sci STKE (304):pe48, 2005

Coe CL, Kramer M, Czeh B, et al: Prenatal stress diminishes neurogenesis in the dentate gyrus of juvenile rhesus monkeys. Biol Psychiatry 54:1025–1034, 2003

Coplan JD, Smith EL, Altemus M, et al: Maternal-infant response to variable foraging demand in nonhuman primates: effects of timing of stressor on cerebrospinal fluid corticotropin-releasing factor and circulating glucocorticoid concentrations. Ann N Y Acad Sci 1071:525–533, 2006

Czeh B, Michaelis T, Watanabe T, et al: Stress-induced changes in cerebral metabolites, hippocampal volume, and cell proliferation are prevented by antidepressant treatment with tianeptine. Proc Natl Acad Sci U S A 98:12796–12801, 2001

DeBattista C, Belanoff J: The use of mifepristone in the treatment of neuropsychiatric disorders. Trends Endocrinol Metab 17:117–121, 2006

Drew MR, Hen R: Adult hippocampal neurogenesis as target for the treatment of depression. CNS Neurol Disord Drug Targets 6:205–218, 2007

Evans SJ, Choudary PV, Neal CR, et al: Dysregulation of the fibroblast growth factor system in major depression. Proc Natl Acad Sci U S A 101:15506–15511, 2004

Fahlke C, Lorenz JG, Long J, et al: Rearing experiences and stress-induced plasma cortisol as early risk factors for excessive alcohol consumption in nonhuman primates. Alcohol Clin Exp Res 24:644–650, 2000

Gold PW, Loriaux DL, Roy A, et al: Responses to corticotropin-releasing hormone in the hypercortisolism of depression and Cushing's disease. Pathophysiological and diagnostic implications. N Engl J Med 314:1329–1335, 1986

Gould TD, Gottesman II: Psychiatric endophenotypes and the development of valid animal models. Genes Brain Behav 5:113–119, 2006

Gross C, Zhuang X, Stark K, et al: Serotonin1A receptor acts during development to establish normal anxiety-like behaviour in the adult. Nature 416:396–400, 2002

Heinrichs SC, Koob GF: Corticotropin-releasing factor in brain: a role in activation, arousal, and affect regulation. J Pharmacol Exp Ther 311:427–440, 2004

Hennessy MB, Deak T, Schiml-Webb PA: Stress-induced sickness behaviors: an alternative hypothesis for responses during maternal separation. Dev Psychobiol 39:76–83, 2001

Hennessy MB, Schiml-Webb PA, Miller EE, et al: Anti-inflammatory agents attenuate the passive responses of guinea pig pups: evidence for stress-induced sickness behavior during maternal separation. Psychoneuroendocrinology 32:508–515, 2007

Insel TR: From animal models to model animals. Biol Psychiatry 62:1337–1339, 2007

Iwamoto K, Kakiuchi C, Bundo M, et al: Molecular characterization of bipolar disorder by comparing gene expression profiles of postmortem brains of major mental disorders. Mol Psychiatry 9:406–416, 2004

Kaemingk K, Reite M: Social environment and nocturnal sleep: studies in peer-reared monkeys. Sleep 10:542–550, 1987

Katz RJ, Sibel M: Animal model of depression: tests of three structurally and pharmacologically novel antidepressant compounds. Pharmacol Biochem Behav 16:973–977, 1982

Katz RJ, Roth KA, Carroll BJ: Acute and chronic stress effects on open field activity in the rat: implications for a model of depression. Neurosci Biobehav Rev 5:247–251, 1981

Kaufer D, Ogle WO, Pincus ZS, et al: Restructuring the neuronal stress response with anti-glucocorticoid gene delivery. Nat Neurosci 7:947–953, 2004

Kendler KS, Gardner CO, Prescott CA: Toward a comprehensive developmental model for major depression in women. Am J Psychiatry 159:1133–1145, 2002

Keverne EB: Understanding well-being in the evolutionary context of brain development. Philos Trans R Soc Lond B Biol Sci 359:1349–1358, 2004

Kraemer GW: Psychobiology of early social attachment in rhesus monkeys. Clinical implications. Ann N Y Acad Sci 807:401–418, 1997

Lowry CA, Moore FL: Regulation of behavioral responses by corticotropin-releasing factor. Gen Comp Endocrinol 146:19–27, 2006

Lupien SJ, Gillin CJ, Hauger RL: Working memory is more sensitive than declarative memory to the acute effects of corticosteroids: a dose-response study in humans. Behav Neurosci 113:420–430, 1999

Lyons DM: Stress, depression, and inherited variation in primate hippocampal and prefrontal brain development. Psychopharmacol Bull 36:27–43, 2002

Lyons DM, Levine S: Socioregulatory effects on squirrel monkey pituitary-adrenal activity: a longitudinal analysis of cortisol and ACTH. Psychoneuroendocrinology 19:283–291, 1994

Lyons DM, Mendoza SP, Mason WA: Sexual segregation in squirrel monkeys (Saimiri sciureus): a transactional analysis of adult social dynamics. J Comp Psychol 106:323–330, 1992

Lyons DM, Ha CM, Levine S: Social effects and circadian rhythms in squirrel monkey pituitary-adrenal activity. Horm Behav 29:177–190, 1995

Lyons DM, Wang OJ, Lindley SE, et al: Separation induced changes in squirrel monkey hypothalamic-pituitary-adrenal physiology resemble aspects of hypercortisolism in humans. Psychoneuroendocrinology 24:131–142, 1999

Lyons DM, Lopez JM, Yang C, et al: Stress-level cortisol treatment impairs inhibitory control of behavior in monkeys. J Neurosci 20:7816–7821, 2000

Lyons DM, Yang C, Sawyer-Glover AM, et al: Early life stress and inherited variation in monkey hippocampal volumes. Arch Gen Psychiatry 58:1145–1151, 2001

Lyons DM, Parker KJ, Zeitzer JM, et al: Preliminary evidence that hippocampal volumes in monkeys predict stress levels of adrenocorticotropic hormone. Biol Psychiatry 62:1171–1174, 2007

Maier SF: Exposure to the stressor environment prevents the temporal dissipation of behavioral depression/learned helplessness. Biol Psychiatry 49:763–773, 2001

Maier SF, Watkins LR: Stressor controllability and learned helplessness: the roles of the dorsal raphe nucleus, serotonin, and corticotropin-releasing factor. Neurosci Biobehav Rev 29:829–841, 2005

Martin-Soelch C, Leenders KL, Chevalley AF, et al: Reward mechanisms in the brain and their role in dependence: evidence from neurophysiological and neuroimaging studies. Brain Res Brain Res Rev 36:139–149, 2001

McKinney WT: Overview of the past contributions of animal models and their changing place in psychiatry. Semin Clin Neuropsychiatry 6:68–78, 2001

McKinney WT Jr, Bunney WE Jr: Animal model of depression, I: review of evidence: implications for research. Arch Gen Psychiatry 21:240–248, 1969

Mendoza SP, Lyons DM, Saltzman W: Sociophysiology of squirrel monkeys. Am J Primatol 23:37–54, 1991

Minor TR, Hunter AM: Stressor controllability and learned helplessness research in the United States: sensitization and fatigue processes. Integr Physiol Behav Sci 37:44–58, 2002

Muller MB, Zimmermann S, Sillaber I, et al: Limbic corticotropin-releasing hormone receptor 1 mediates anxiety-related behavior and hormonal adaptation to stress. Nat Neurosci 6:1100–1107, 2003

Murphy BE: Steroids and depression. J Steroid Biochem Mol Biol 38:537–559, 1991

Nelson JC, Davis JM: DST studies in psychotic depression: a meta-analysis. Am J Psychiatry 154:1497–1503, 1997

Nemeroff CB, Vale WW: The neurobiology of depression: inroads to treatment and new drug discovery. J Clin Psychiatry 66 (suppl 7):5–13, 2005

Nolen-Hoeksema S: The role of rumination in depressive disorders and mixed anxiety/depressive symptoms. J Abnorm Psychol 109:504–511, 2000

Overmier JB, Seligman ME: Effects of inescapable shock upon subsequent escape and avoidance responding. J Comp Physiol Psychol 63:28–33, 1967

Pani L, Porcella A, Gessa GL: The role of stress in the pathophysiology of the dopaminergic system. Mol Psychiatry 5:14–21, 2000

Parker KJ, Schatzberg AF, Lyons DM: Neuroendocrine aspects of hypercortisolism in major depression. Horm Behav 43:60–66, 2003

Perera TD, Coplan JD, Lisanby SH, et al: Antidepressant-induced neurogenesis in the hippocampus of adult nonhuman primates. J Neurosci 27:4894–4901, 2007

Plotsky PM, Owens MJ, Nemeroff CB: Psychoneuroendocrinology of depression. Hypothalamic-pituitary-adrenal axis. Psychiatr Clin North Am 21:293–307, 1998

Porrino LJ, Lyons D: Orbital and medial prefrontal cortex and psychostimulant abuse: studies in animal models. Cereb Cortex 10:326–333, 2000

Porsolt RD, Lenegre A, McArthur RA: Pharmacological models of depression, in Animal Models in Psychopharmacology. Edited by Olivier B, Mos J, Slangen JL. Basel, Switzerland, Birkhauser Verlag, 1991, pp 137–159

Preuss TM: Do rats have prefrontal cortex? The Rose-Woolsey-Akert program reconsidered. J Cogn Neurosci 7:1–24, 1995

Ridder S, Chourbaji S, Hellweg R, et al: Mice with genetically altered glucocorticoid receptor expression show altered sensitivity for stress-induced depressive reactions. J Neurosci 25:6243–6250, 2005

Rivier C, Vale W: Diminished responsiveness of the hypothalamic-pituitary-adrenal axis of the rat during exposure to prolonged stress: a pituitary-mediated mechanism. Endocrinology 121:1320–1328, 1987

Rosenblum LA, Andrews MW: Influences of environmental demand on maternal behavior and infant development. Acta Paediatr Suppl 397:57–63, 1994

Sanchez MM, Hearn EF, Do D, et al: Differential rearing affects corpus callosum size and cognitive function of rhesus monkeys. Brain Res 812:38–49, 1998

Sarter M, Bruno JP: Animal models in biological psychiatry, in Biological Psychiatry. Edited by D'haenen H, den Boer JA, Willner P. New York, Wiley, 2002, pp 1–8

Sasaki M, Tohyama K, Matsunaga S, et al: MRI identification of dorsal hippocampus homologue in human brain. Neuroreport 15:2173–2176, 2004

Schatzberg AF, Posener JA, DeBattista C, et al: Neuropsychological deficits in psychotic versus nonpsychotic major depression and no mental illness. Am J Psychiatry 157:1095–1100, 2000

Seligman ME, Maier SF: Failure to escape traumatic shock. J Exp Psychol 74:1–9, 1967

Sequeira A, Gwadry FG, Ffrench-Mullen JM, et al: Implication of SSAT by gene expression and genetic variation in suicide and major depression. Arch Gen Psychiatry 63:35–48, 2006

Shively CA, Register TC, Friedman DP, et al: Social stress-associated depression in adult female cynomolgus monkeys (Macaca fascicularis). Biol Psychol 69:67–84, 2005

Song C, Leonard BE: The olfactory bulbectomised rat as a model of depression. Neurosci Biobehav Rev 29:627–647, 2005

Strome EM, Wheler GH, Higley JD, et al: Intracerebroventricular corticotropin-releasing factor increases limbic glucose metabolism and has social context-dependent behavioral effects in nonhuman primates. Proc Natl Acad Sci U S A 99:15749–15754, 2002

Sullivan EV, Pfefferbaum A, Swan GE, et al: Heritability of hippocampal size in elderly twin men: equivalent influence from genes and environment. Hippocampus 11:754–762, 2001

van Erp TG, Saleh PA, Huttunen M, et al: Hippocampal volumes in schizophrenic twins. Arch Gen Psychiatry 61:346–353, 2004

Videbech P, Ravnkilde B: Hippocampal volume and depression: a meta-analysis of MRI studies. Am J Psychiatry 161:1957–1966, 2004

Vollmayr B, Bachteler D, Vengeliene V, et al: Rats with congenital learned helplessness respond less to sucrose but show no deficits in activity or learning. Behav Brain Res 150:217–221, 2004

von Bardeleben U, Stalla GK, Muller OA, et al: Blunting of ACTH response to human CRH in depressed patients is avoided by metyrapone pretreatment. Biol Psychiatry 24:782–786, 1988

Vythilingam M, Heim C, Newport J, et al: Childhood trauma associated with smaller hippocampal volume in women with major depression. Am J Psychiatry 159:2072–2080, 2002

Webster MJ, Knable MB, O'Grady J, et al: Regional specificity of brain glucocorticoid receptor mRNA alterations in subjects with schizophrenia and mood disorders. Mol Psychiatry 7:985–994, 924, 2002

Wei Q, Lu XY, Liu L, et al: Glucocorticoid receptor overexpression in forebrain: a mouse model of increased emotional lability. Proc Natl Acad Sci U S A 101:11851–11856, 2004

Weiss JM: Effects of coping responses on stress. J Comp Physiol Psychol 65:251–260, 1968

Weiss JM: Stress-induced depression: critical neurochemical and electrophysiologial changes, in Neurobiology of Learning, Emotion and Affect. Edited by Madden J. New York, Raven, 1991, pp 123–154

Weiss JM, Kilts CD: Animal models of depression and schizophrenia, in The American Psychiatric Press Textbook of Psychopharmacology, 2nd Edition. Edited by Schatzberg AF, Nemeroff CB. Washington, DC, American Psychiatric Press, 1998, pp 89–131

Willner P: Animal models of depression: an overview. Pharmacol Ther 45:425–455, 1990

Willner P: Validity, reliability and utility of the chronic mild stress model of depression: a 10-year review and evaluation. Psychopharmacology (Berl) 134:319–329, 1997

Willner P, Hale AS, Argyropoulos S: Dopaminergic mechanism of antidepressant action in depressed patients. J Affect Disord 86:37–45, 2005

Wong ML, Licinio J: Research and treatment approaches to depression. Nat Rev Neurosci 2:343–351, 2001

Yoshiki A, Moriwaki K: Mouse phenome research: implications of genetic background. ILAR J 47:94–102, 2006

Young AH: Antiglucocorticoid treatments for depression. Aust N Z J Psychiatry 40:402–405, 2006

Young AH, Sahakian BJ, Robbins TW, et al: The effects of chronic administration of hydrocortisone on cognitive function in normal male volunteers. Psychopharmacology (Berl) 145:260–266, 1999

Young EA, Akil H: Corticotropin-releasing factor stimulation of adrenocorticotropin and beta-endorphin release: effects of acute and chronic stress. Endocrinology 117:23–30, 1985

Young EA, Lopez JF, Murphy-Weinberg V, et al: Normal pituitary response to metyrapone in the morning in depressed patients: implications for circadian regulation of corticotropin- releasing hormone secretion. Biol Psychiatry 41:1149–1155, 1997

CHAPTER 7

Psychoneuroendocrinology

Ania Korszun, Ph.D., M.D., M.R.C.Psych.

Josephine Astrid Archer, B.Sc.

Elizabeth Ann Young, M.D.

An association between hormones and psychiatric disorders has been long recognized, but it is only in the past few decades that we have reached an understanding of the mechanisms underlying this association. A full account of the myriad ways in which the various endocrine systems influence neurobehavioral function would be beyond the scope of a single chapter. We will therefore focus on examples of promising research directions in this area: namely, how the stress and reproductive hormone axes contribute to the pathoetiology of psychiatric conditions, in particular mood and anxiety disorders.

Major depression is considered to be a maladaptive, exaggerated response to stress, and although it is accompanied by abnormalities in multiple endocrine systems, it is the hypothalamic-pituitary-adrenal (HPA) axis that is the main component of the physiological stress response that plays the key role. Stressful life events, particularly those related to loss, have a strong causal relationship with depressive episodes. However, not all people who experience such events develop depression, and an individual's vulnerability to depression depends on the interaction of genetic, developmental, and environmental factors. In addition to the role of the HPA axis in depression, there is growing evidence of HPA axis abnormalities in anxiety disorders and posttraumatic stress disorder (PTSD).

Hypothalamic-Pituitary-Adrenal Axis

The HPA axis transforms stressful stimuli into hormonal messages that enable the organism to adapt to environ-

mental change and to maintain the body's homeostasis. Corticotropin-releasing hormone (CRH) is synthesized in the hypothalamus and is stimulated by stressors, which can be either "physical" (e.g., exercise, starvation) or "psychological" (e.g., perceived danger, stressful life events). The HPA axis is closely linked to the autonomic nervous system, and brain stem catecholamine systems can also "activate" CRH release (Herman et al. 1990; Plotsky 1987; Plotsky et al. 1989). CRH stimulates secretion of pituitary adrenocorticotropic hormone (ACTH), resulting in the secretion of glucocorticoids by the adrenal cortex in a feedforward cascade. Cortisol is the main glucocorticoid, and its secretion is tightly controlled by negative feedback effects of glucocorticoids at both pituitary and brain sites. These comprise very rapid real-time inhibition of the stress response that prevents oversecretion of glucocorticoids (Keller-Wood and Dallman 1984) and results in a slower effect on messenger ribonucleic acid (mRNA) and subsequent protein stores for both CRH and the ACTH precursor, pro-opiomelanocortin (Roberts et al. 1979) (Figure 7–1).

Stressful stimuli activate all levels of the HPA axis, causing increases in CRH, ACTH, and cortisol secretion. However, these increases are superimposed on an intrinsic circadian pattern of HPA activity driven by the suprachiasmatic nucleus (SCN) (Krieger 1979). HPA axis hormone secretion is pulsatile in nature, with the trough of integrated secretion occurring in the evening and early night and the peak of secretion occurring just before awakening; active secretion continues throughout the morning

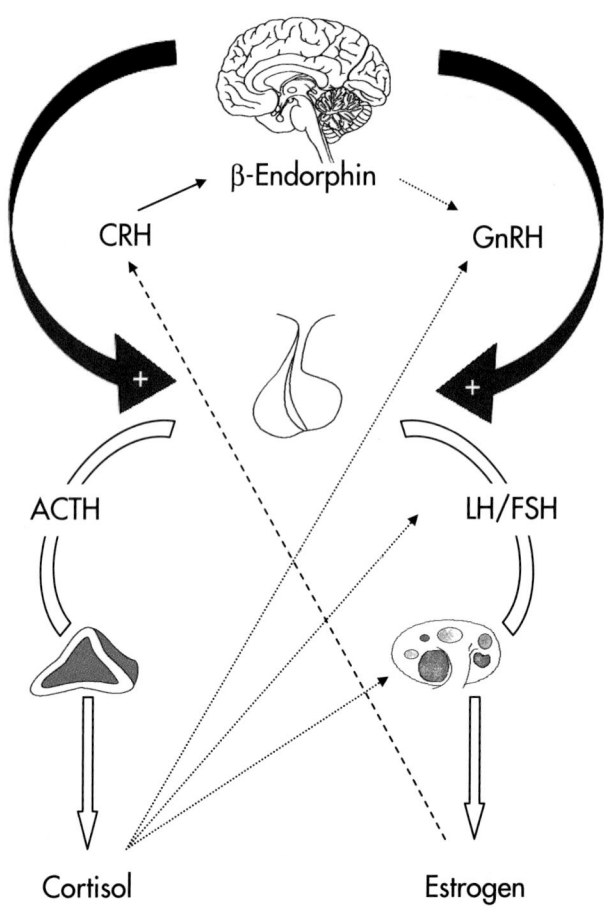

FIGURE 7–1. The hypothalamic-pituitary-adrenal axis.

ACTH = adrenocorticotropic hormone; CRH = corticotropin-releasing hormone; FSH = follicle-stimulating hormone; GnRH = gonadotropin-releasing hormone; LH = luteinizing hormone.

and early afternoon. This rhythm persists even in the absence of corticosteroid feedback (e.g., adrenalectomy [Jacobson et al. 1989]), and there is evidence that there are intrinsic neural elements responsible for both initiation and inhibition of the CRH/ACTH/cortisol circadian rhythm and that glucocorticoids merely act to dampen the overall amount of secretion (Kwak et al. 1993).

HPA Axis in Depression and Anxiety Disorders

Depression

Overactivity of the HPA axis as manifested by an increase in cortisol secretion is now a well-established phenomenon in depression (Carroll et al. 1976; Sachar et al. 1973). The first studies (Sachar et al. 1973) showed that up to 50% of depressed patients have higher mean plasma cor-

tisol concentrations and an increased number and duration of cortisol secretory episodes, suggesting increased cortisol secretory activity. Numerous studies have subsequently validated these findings (Carroll et al. 1976; Halbreich et al. 1985; Krishnan et al. 1990a; Pfohl et al. 1985; Rubin et al. 1987). As many as two-thirds of endogenously depressed patients fail to suppress cortisol, or show an early escape of cortisol, following overnight administration of 1 mg of dexamethasone (using a cortisol cutoff of 5 μg/dL to define "escape") (Carroll et al. 1981). While nonsuppression of cortisol in response to dexamethasone is strongly associated with endogenous depression, this finding is less robust in outpatients with depression. Although both hypercortisolemia and feedback abnormalities in response to dexamethasone are present in depressed patients, they do not necessarily occur in the same individuals (Carroll et al. 1981; Halbreich et al. 1985). Other abnormalities, such as reduced glucocorticoid fast feedback (Young et al. 1991) and a blunted ACTH response to exogenous CRH, have also been reported in depressed patients (Gold et al. 1986; Holsboer et al. 1984; Young et al. 1990).

The blunted response to CRH appears to be dependent on increased baseline cortisol, since blockade of cortisol production with metyrapone normalizes the ACTH response (Von Bardeleben et al. 1988; Young et al. 1995). It was expected that the increased cortisol would be accompanied by an increased level of ACTH in plasma, but this has been difficult to validate, although several studies (Linkowski et al. 1985; Pfohl et al. 1985; Young et al. 2001) have demonstrated small differences in mean 24-hour plasma ACTH levels between healthy control subjects and depressed subjects. The demonstration of enhanced sensitivity to ACTH 1–24 in depressed patients suggests that increased ACTH secretion is not necessarily the cause of increased cortisol secretion (Amsterdam et al. 1983). However, other studies using very low "threshold" doses of ACTH 1–24 have not been able to demonstrate increased sensitivity to ACTH in depressed patients (Krishnan et al. 1990b), which suggests that increased cortisol secretion is secondary to increased ACTH secretion. Our 24-hour studies of ACTH and cortisol secretion demonstrated that subjects with increased mean cortisol also demonstrated increased mean ACTH, supporting a central origin of the HPA axis overactivity (Young et al. 2001). Further studies with metyrapone in major depression also support the presence of increased central nervous system (CNS) drive, at least in the evening (Young et al. 1994, 1997). It appears likely that there is increased CRH/ACTH secretion, which is then probably amplified by the adrenal, leading to increased cortisol secretion.

These changes in cortisol secretion are commonly considered to be "state" changes that resolve when the depression resolves. However, almost all studies examining the HPA axis in major depression in euthymic subjects have examined patients on tricyclic antidepressants, which exert direct effects on the HPA axis. Three of our recent studies in epidemiological samples and a recent British study (Bhagwagar et al. 2003) found that salivary cortisol is increased in subjects with *lifetime* major depression, most of whom had no current mood symptoms (Bhagwagar et al. 2003; Young et al. 2000a). The overall picture suggests that depression generally shows both an increase in activity of circadian activational elements of the system and reduced feedback inhibition.

Anxiety Disorders

The HPA axis has also been studied in patients with anxiety disorders, particularly panic disorder, with and without comorbid major depression. Both the cortisol response to dexamethasone and the response to CRH have been examined in pure panic disorder without comorbid depression. The earliest study with dexamethasone demonstrated a 15% nonsuppression rate in panic disorder (Curtis et al. 1982). A number of other studies have since been conducted, and the overall incidence of cortisol nonsuppression is 17% in panic disorder (13 studies), while the incidence for major depression is 50% (Heninger 1990). Grunhaus et al. (1987) compared patients with major depression to those with major depression with panic disorder and found a similar rate of cortisol nonsuppression following dexamethasone administration (approximately 50%) in the two populations, suggesting that the presence of comorbid panic disorder had little impact beyond that of depression on dexamethasone nonsuppression. In CRH challenge tests, panic disorder patients have demonstrated a decreased integrated ACTH response relative to control subjects in some studies (Holsboer et al. 1987; Roy-Byrne et al. 1986) but a normal response in others (Brambilla et al. 1992). Similar to findings in depression, "baseline" plasma cortisol was increased in panic patients who showed blunted CRH responses. A study of CRH challenge in panic disorder patients (Curtis et al. 1997) demonstrated a normal response to CRH challenge.

Studies of the HPA axis in social phobia have not found evidence of baseline hyperactivity by urinary free cortisol (Uhde et al. 1994), although few challenges other than a social speaking task have been used. Public speaking challenges in anxiety disorders do not support an exaggerated ACTH or cortisol response to this stressor (Gerra et al. 2000; Levin et al. 1993; Martel et al. 1999). A few studies in children with anxiety disorders have also examined the HPA axis. Children with anxiety disorders coming in for a CO_2 challenge demonstrated elevated "basal" cortisol in those who panicked in response to CO_2, suggesting that increased reactivity to a threatening situation (i.e., anticipation of a procedure that would cause discomfort) was linked to activation of the HPA axis (Coplan et al. 2002). This interpretation is further supported by an extremely large study of basal 24-hour cortisol in normal children and children with either anxiety disorders or major depression, which found lower nighttime cortisol and a sluggish morning rise in cortisol in children with an anxiety disorder. This suggests that anxiety disorders lead to stress hyperreactivity (in the case of anxious children, in the context of a threatening experimental procedure of CO_2) with compensatory decreased basal cortisol secretion (24-hour study) (Feder et al. 2004).

Overall, the studies to date do not suggest HPA axis hyperactivity in anxiety disorders to the same extent as shown in depression (Abelson and Curtis 1996). Feedback elements are generally normal, and the abnormalities that do exist may reflect "extrinsic" factors that contribute to heightened reactivity within activational elements of the system. The question of whether stress-activated HPA axis elements are abnormal in comorbid major depression and anxiety has not yet been well studied.

Posttraumatic Stress Disorder

Given the stress-related etiology of PTSD, it was expected that PTSD patients would show HPA axis abnormalities similar to those seen in depressed patients or chronically stressed animals, but this has not always been the case. An initial study (Mason et al. 1986) found that urinary free cortisol (UFC) excretion was *lower* in PTSD than in major depression. However, another study (Pitman and Orr 1990) found *increased* UFC excretion in outpatient PTSD veterans compared with combat-exposed control subjects without PTSD. Since then, there have been various findings, but the most comprehensive studies of PTSD, those by Yehuda and colleagues (for a review, see Yehuda 2002), continue to show low cortisol and enhanced cortisol suppression in response to dexamethasone in combat veterans with PTSD. Interestingly, the presence of comorbid major depression does not change the neuroendocrine picture. The main criticism of this body of work is that the sample comprised only male combat veterans and therefore is not representative, given that in the community, it is women who are most likely to experience PTSD (Breslau et al. 1991, 1995; Kessler et al. 1995). Furthermore, significant confounds with current and past alcohol and substance abuse occur in the veteran population.

Several studies have sought to address this problem, with the majority examining women with a history of childhood sexual abuse. While some studies have demonstrated increased UFC in women with PTSD or a history of abuse compared with control subjects (Lemieux and Coe 1995), others have demonstrated similar plasma cortisol (Rasmusson et al. 2001), and still others have found lower cortisol and enhanced cortisol suppression in response to dexamethasone (Stein et al. 1997). Yehuda (2002) examined Holocaust survivors, who were also predominantly exposed early in life, and observed lower UFC and enhanced cortisol suppression following dexamethasone administration in this population. The issue of comorbid depression in the PTSD population has not been well addressed, with most studies including comorbid individuals and few analyzing the data by the presence or absence of comorbid depression. The exception is the studies of Heim et al. (2001), which focused on childhood abuse and major depression and examined multiple HPA axis challenges in the same subjects. These studies found an effect of early abuse (with comorbid PTSD in 11 of 13 subjects) and major depression on stress reactivity, with both increased ACTH and cortisol response to the stressor compared with either healthy control subjects or depressed patients without childhood abuse. In this same cohort, there was a blunted response to CRH challenge in patients who had major depression with or without childhood abuse, but an increased response to CRH in those with early abuse but without major depression. The abused subjects also showed a blunted cortisol response to ACTH 1–24. Thus, childhood abuse produced an increased pituitary response with adaptive adrenal compensation, a change compatible with low or normal basal cortisol. Furthermore, lower cortisol and enhanced feedback to low-dose dexamethasone were found in the same subjects (Newport et al. 2004) regardless of the presence or absence of PTSD as the primary diagnosis, thus indicating enhanced feedback.

Epidemiologically based samples in adults have focused on natural disasters and have generally examined exposure with high and low PTSD symptoms (Anisman et al. 2001; Davidson and Baum 1986; Fukuda et al. 2000) but without diagnostic information. However, one study

(Maes et al. 1998) that examined PTSD subjects recruited from community disasters demonstrated increased UFC in PTSD. In general, community-based studies suggest that exposure to disaster increases plasma (Fukuda et al. 2000) and saliva cortisol (Anisman et al. 2001) and UFC (Davidson and Baum 1986). Studies examining motor vehicle accident survivors (Hawk et al. 2000) found no difference in cortisol between those with and without PTSD 6 months later. Studies of male and female adults with exposure to mixed traumas have found either no effect of PTSD on basal cortisol (Kellner et al. 2002, 2003) or elevated basal cortisol (Atmaca et al. 2002; Lindley et al. 2004). Our analysis of recent trauma exposure in two community samples (Young and Breslau 2004a, 2004b; Young et al. 2004) found increased cortisol in those with past-year exposure to trauma, but no effect of greater than 1 year past trauma exposure and no effect of childhood abuse on basal saliva cortisol or UFC. To add further complexity, the majority of studies of trauma and PTSD included subjects with comorbid depression, and in most studies, the majority of subjects had both PTSD and major depression. The PTSD studies generally report comorbid depression in their subjects; however, studies of depression often fail to measure and report trauma histories. As a result, documented depression confounds much of the PTSD HPA axis literature, and undocumented trauma and abuse may confound some of the depression HPA axis literature.

In addition to the issue of exposure to trauma, the persistence of the neuroendocrine changes following recovery from PTSD is unclear. In an early study, Yehuda et al. (1995) reported that Holocaust survivors with past but not current PTSD demonstrated normal UFC, while later studies of offspring of Holocaust survivors (Yehuda et al. 2002) suggested that changes in cortisol may persist beyond the duration of the symptoms and thus may represent a marker of underlying vulnerability to PTSD. The large analysis by Boscarino (1996) of cortisol data from several thousand combat veterans showed a very small effect of PTSD on basal cortisol, but a very clear effect of combat exposure, with increasing levels of severity of combat exposure associated with increasingly lower cortisol.

Our recent studies of cortisol in PTSD from two epidemiological samples (Young and Breslau 2004a, 2004b; Young et al. 2004) demonstrated normal UFC and saliva cortisol in community-based individuals with "pure" and comorbid PTSD. The studies also demonstrated a clear effect of lifetime comorbid major depression on cortisol, showing increased HPA axis activation in the late afternoon/evening in patients with both major depression and PTSD. Furthermore, the elevated HPA drive demonstrated by increased evening cortisol levels was greater in the comorbid group than the elevation already documented in pure major depression.

Studies examining the response to low-dose dexamethasone in PTSD veterans found enhanced feedback to dexamethasone in veterans who met criteria for PTSD, regardless of the presence of comorbid major depression (Yehuda et al. 2002). Similar enhanced cortisol suppression in response to dexamethasone administration has been found in Holocaust survivors with PTSD and their offspring. In the studies of Yehuda (2002) as well as the report by Stein et al. (1997), the enhanced suppression was also paired with low baseline cortisol, although other studies did not replicate this finding (Kellner et al. 2004a, 2004b).

In a CRH challenge study in combat-related PTSD, there was a normal to increased plasma cortisol at the time of challenge (Smith et al. 1989) and a decreased ACTH response in subjects with high baseline cortisol. Another study of women with PTSD and a history of childhood abuse (Rasmusson et al. 2001) showed enhanced cortisol response to CRH and to exogenous ACTH infusion, as well as a trend toward higher 24-hour UFC. Interestingly, all the women with PTSD had either past or current major depression, so comorbidity was the rule. In the study by Heim et al. (2001) examining response to CRH in women with major depression with and without childhood abuse, 14 of 15 major depressive disorder patients with childhood abuse also met criteria for PTSD. This group with comorbid major depression and PTSD demonstrated a blunted ACTH response to CRH challenge similar to that observed in major depression without PTSD. The abused groups also demonstrated lower baseline and stimulated cortisol both in response to CRH challenge and following ACTH infusion. These same groups of women showed a significantly *greater* HPA response to the Trier Stress Test, despite *smaller* responses to CRH challenge (Heim et al. 2000).

Several additional studies have evaluated response to stressors. Our early study (Liberzon et al. 1999) using combat noise versus white noise in male veterans with PTSD showed elevated basal and postprovocation cortisol compared with combat controls but no real evidence of a difference between the combat and white-noise days. A study by Bremner et al. (2003) of PTSD subjects of both sexes used a stressful cognitive challenge and found elevated basal saliva cortisol and continued higher cortisol

for 60 minutes postchallenge. Eventually the saliva cortisol of the PTSD group returned to the same level as that of controls, raising the issue of whether the "basal" samples were truly basal or were influenced by the anticipatory challenge. Similar data were found in a study (Elzinga et al. 2003), using trauma scripts, in women with childhood abuse and PTSD compared with abused women with no PTSD. In that study, salivary cortisol was again significantly elevated at baseline, increased in response to the challenge (whereas controls showed no response), and then greatly decreased following the stressor, compatible with "basal" levels already reflecting exaggerated stress sensitivity in this group. Using a 1-minute cold pressor test, a recent study (Santa Ana et al. 2006) compared the ACTH and cortisol response in PTSD subjects with either childhood trauma or adult trauma with that of control subjects and found lower basal cortisol in the childhood abuse group. However, their data do not support an actual change in ACTH or cortisol in response to the stressor in any group, so it is difficult to interpret their findings as reflecting differences in stress response. In addition, sampling was very infrequent and therefore inadequate to characterize the time course to a very *brief* stressor. Overall, the existing stress data suggest an exaggerated stress response in PTSD.

Furthermore, the challenge studies certainly suggest that the picture is complicated in PTSD with comorbid depression; the findings of some studies look like depression while others look quite different—for example, showing a smaller response to ACTH infusion whereas patients with major depression show an augmented response. Age of trauma exposure may be one reason for contradictory data. Finally, one study by Yehuda (2002) of combat veterans with PTSD demonstrated greater rebound ACTH secretion compared with controls following administration of metyrapone in the morning, indicating that increased CRH drive is present in the morning but is normally restrained by cortisol feedback. The other two studies examining metyrapone challenge in PTSD found a normal ACTH response to afternoon or overnight metyrapone as well as a normal response to cortisol infusion in PTSD subjects and panic disorder subjects (Kanter et al. 2001; Kellner et al. 2004a, 2004b). In summary, these data suggest that there may be no simple relationship between diagnostic categories and specific HPA axis abnormalities. Timing of trauma or of onset of depression or anxiety disorders may differentially affect the HPA axis profile, although definitive studies have not been done.

Depression and Reproductive Hormone Changes

In women with a previous episode of depression, times of rapidly changing gonadal steroid concentrations, such as those occurring premenstrually or postpartum, mark particularly vulnerable times for the occurrence of depressive symptoms. Several studies have shown that in women, a history of depression increases the risk of both postpartum "blues" and postpartum major depression (O'Hara 1986; O'Hara et al. 1991; Reich and Winokur 1970) and that hormonal changes occurring premenstrually may affect mood (Halbreich et al. 1984, 1986). When they were euthymic, 62% of women with a history of major depressive episodes reported the occurrence of premenstrual mood changes and biological symptoms typical of major depressive disorder. Other studies found a relationship between the rise in estrogen and testosterone levels and the rising incidence of depression in girls during adolescence (Angold et al. 1999). More recently in two epidemiological cohorts (Cohen et al. 2006; Freeman et al. 2006), there was an increased incidence of depressive symptoms and major depression during the menopausal transition. Both high and low estrogen were associated with depression (Freeman et al. 2004, 2006), and the variability in estrogen levels may drive depression—that is, those women who show rapid changes from high to low estrogen and vice versa are those who develop depressive symptoms during the perimenopause transition. This suggests that examining the reproductive axis in depression may be a fruitful area of psychoneuroendocrine research.

Hypothalamic-Pituitary-Gonadal Axis

The secretion of the principal gonadal steroids, estrogen and progesterone, is governed by cyclic changes in ovarian follicular and corpus luteum development over the course of the menstrual cycle. Critical to the proper functioning and timing of the monthly hormonal cycle is the pulsatile secretion of gonadotropin-releasing hormone (GnRH). GnRH secretion from the hypothalamus drives the secretion of luteinizing hormone (LH) and follicle-stimulating hormone (FSH) from pituitary gonadotropes (Midgley and Jaffe 1971). During the early follicular phase, FSH plays the major role in maturing the follicle (diZerega and Hodgen 1981), and the developing follicle secretes increasing amounts of estradiol as it matures. Maturation-induced increases in estradiol exert a nega-

tive feedback on FSH secretion and both negative and delayed positive feedback effects on LH secretion (Karsch et al. 1983). The change in estradiol feedback from negative to positive late in the follicular phase is complemented by rising progesterone and results in the midcycle surge in LH necessary for ovulation. Following ovulation, progesterone levels continue to rise as a result of active secretion from the corpus luteum. LH secretion is necessary for the maintenance of the corpus luteum and subsequent estrogen and progesterone secretion and also facilitates estradiol production by the follicle and controls the secretion of hormones by the corpus luteum but is inhibited by progesterone (Chabbert et al. 1998). In the absence of fertilization, regression of the corpus luteum occurs, with the subsequent fall in estrogen and progesterone leading to the onset of menses.

The pulsatile secretion of GnRH is driven by a pulse generator in the arcuate nucleus of the hypothalamus (Knobil 1990). This pulsatile pattern of GnRH secretion is critical for the control of serum LH, FSH, and ovulation. Indeed, continuous administration of the GnRH agonist leuprolide in a nonpulsatile pattern suppresses ovulation as effectively as does inadequate secretion of GnRH. Studies in primates with arcuate lesions have demonstrated that administration of GnRH pulses in frequencies that are too fast or too slow results in low serum concentrations of LH (Belchetz et al. 1978).

LH secretory pulses in the peripheral circulation are used as the marker of GnRH secretory pulses. In humans, the follicular phase of the menstrual cycle is characterized by reasonably constant amplitude LH pulses every 1–2 hours (Reame et al. 1984). During the luteal phase, pulse amplitude becomes much more variable and pulse frequency decreases. The slowing of the LH pulses during the luteal phase is due to the actions of progesterone on the GnRH pulse generator (Goodman and Karsch 1980; Soules et al. 1984; Steele and Judd 1986). Gonadal steroids exert negative feedback effects on the amplitude and frequency of GnRH pulses and through this mechanism (in addition to direct actions on the pituitary) inhibit the secretion of LH and FSH. Likewise, central opioids, particularly β-endorphin, exert a tonic inhibition on GnRH secretion (Ferin and Vande 1984). Circadian changes in LH secretion are not as prominent as those of the HPA axis (Jaffe et al. 1990). During puberty and following recovery from anorexia- or exercise-induced amenorrhea, nighttime secretion of LH becomes particularly prominent. Furthermore, nighttime slowing of LH pulses during the early follicular phase also occurs in normal women (Soules et al. 1985).

Effect of HPA Axis on the Reproductive Axis

Stress has long been known to inhibit the reproductive axis, and the work of Christian (1971) demonstrating infertility secondary to high population density is often cited as a seminal report. Shortly after the isolation and sequencing of CRH, it was demonstrated in rats that CRH inhibited LH secretion (Rivier and Vale 1984) and GnRH secretion (Petraglia et al. 1987), and further primate studies showed inhibition of LH secretion by injection of CRH (Olster and Ferin 1987).

While early studies used peripheral administration of high doses of CRH, subsequent studies demonstrated that intracerebrovascular administration of CRH demonstrated much greater potency and confirmed a central site of action of the inhibition, pointing to direct inhibition of GnRH by CRH (Gambacciani et al. 1986; Nikolarakis et al. 1986a, 1986b; Olster and Ferin 1987; Petraglia et al. 1987). However, the peripheral administration of CRH also demonstrated an opioid-mediated inhibition by CRH that could be abolished by dexamethasone pretreatment, suggesting a role for pituitary-derived opioids, most probably β-endorphin from anterior pituitary corticotropes. Anatomical studies demonstrate that CRH neurons synapse with GnRH neurons (MacLusky et al. 1988); in vitro studies demonstrate that CRH can function as a secretagogue for β-endorphin secretion from the arcuate β-endorphin system (Nikolarakis et al. 1986a). Studies in primates by the Knobil laboratory (Williams et al. 1990) recording multiunit activity from the arcuate nucleus (i.e., the GnRH pulse generator) demonstrated that CRH administration induced inhibition of the rhythmic firing of the arcuate nucleus accompanying LH secretory pulses, as well as abolishing LH pulses. Studies with a CRH antagonist, α-helical CRH$_{9-41}$, demonstrated the antagonist's ability to reverse stress-induced LH suppression in rats, confirming a central CRH-based mechanism by which stress inhibits LH secretion (Rivier et al. 1986). While the primate and rat studies have clearly pointed to CRH as the primary mechanism by which stress inhibits GnRH release, this is not true in all species (e.g., central CRH has no effect on GnRH or LH secretion in sheep [Tilbrook et al. 1999]), and some stressors act through cortisol (Debus et al. 2002). The demonstration of a central CRH effect on GnRH release does not preclude an effect of cortisol in both rats and primates, including humans.

So is there evidence that cortisol may also be involved in the inhibition of reproductive function? Several studies have demonstrated that ACTH administration reduces the increase in serum LH concentrations following ovariectomy or orchidectomy in rats (Mann et al. 1982; Schwartz and Justo 1977). This effect is dependent on the presence of the adrenal but could also involve adrenal production of gonadal steroids, which is regulated by ACTH (Putnam et al. 1991). Glucocorticoids also exert inhibitory effects on GnRH secretion or LH responsiveness to GnRH, including direct effects of cortisol on the gonadotrope (Suter and Schwartz 1985). Radovick et al. (1990) demonstrated a glucocorticoid-responsive element (GRE) on the *GnRH* gene, providing the potential for glucocorticoids to modulate *GnRH* gene expression. Diminished LH response to GnRH following long-term prednisolone treatment has been found in women (Sakakura et al. 1975). Patients with Cushing's disease, in which cortisol is increased but central CRH is likely to be low because of excessive glucocorticoid feedback on paraventricular nucleus of the hypothalamus CRH, show inhibition of LH secretion. Recent studies in ewes have found that 1) LH secretory amplitude is clearly inhibited by stress; 2) the effects of stress or endotoxin are reversed by metyrapone inhibition of cortisol synthesis; and 3) infusion of stress levels of cortisol can produce inhibition of LH pulse amplitude but not frequency, which is blocked by RU486, a glucocorticoid receptor antagonist (Breen et al. 2004; Debus et al. 2002). Finally, a recent study of exercise-induced reproductive abnormalities in adolescent girls concluded that "in active adolescents, increased cortisol concentration may…precede gonadotropin changes seen with higher levels of fitness" (Kasa-Vubu et al. 2004, p. 1). These data suggest that cortisol, in addition to central CRH, may also play a role in LH disruption.

Other studies in humans have linked hypothalamic-pituitary-gonadal (HPG) axis abnormalities to HPA axis activation. These include exercise-induced amenorrhea, anorexia nervosa, and hypothalamic amenorrhea. In all three syndromes, hypercortisolemia has been observed, indicating overactivity of the HPA axis (Berga et al. 1989; Casanueva et al. 1987; Hohtari et al. 1988; Loucks et al. 1989; Suh et al. 1988; Villanueva et al. 1986). In all three syndromes, CRH has been used as a challenge to evaluate pituitary and adrenal function. The response to exogenous CRH challenge demonstrates diminished ACTH or cortisol responses, suggesting that high baseline cortisol exerts negative-feedback effects on the hormonal responses to CRH (Berger et al. 1983; Biller et al. 1990; Gold et al. 1986; Hohtari et al. 1991). In anorexia nervosa, the hormonal abnormalities in both HPA and HPG axes are secondary to weight loss. Weight restriction and low body weight are also observed in exercise-induced amenorrhea, and low body weight has been reported in hypothalamic amenorrhea. Even relatively mild degrees of weight loss in normal-weight or obese subjects can lead to disturbances in both axes, as manifested by resistance to dexamethasone and by disturbances in menstrual regularity or amenorrhea (Berger et al. 1983; Edelstein et al. 1983; Pirke et al. 1985). Consequently, these three syndromes present with evidence of increased HPA axis activation and disrupted HPG functioning and amenorrhea. The disturbances in LH secretion in anorexia nervosa and hypothalamic amenorrhea have been evaluated primarily by examining the characteristics of LH pulsatile activity. In anorexia nervosa, LH secretory patterns may revert to prepubertal levels of low nonpulsatile secretion or to a pubertal pattern of entrainment of LH secretion to the sleep cycle. Studies by Reame et al. (1985) in women with hypothalamic amenorrhea demonstrated that LH secretion in the follicular phase is slowed to the rate normally observed during the luteal phase. In these individuals, LH and FSH responses to GnRH appear normal, indicating that the reduced pulse frequency is not secondary to pituitary changes but presumably due to changes in the GnRH pulse generator. Figure 7–2 summarizes the various levels at which hormones of the HPA axis may impinge on the reproductive axis. Despite suggestions that reproductive hormones may play a role in mood disorders, the HPG axis has received little examination in depression.

Reproductive Abnormalities in Depression

In depression, response to GnRH has been assessed by several groups. Some studies have reported a normal LH and FSH response to GnRH in pre- and postmenopausal women (Unden et al. 1988; Winokur et al. 1982). However, given the major differences in LH pulse amplitude and mean LH levels between follicular and luteal phases, it would be extremely difficult to observe a difference in basal LH secretion between major depression and control women without strict control of menstrual cycle phase. However, Brambilla et al. (1990) noted a decreased LH response to GnRH in both premenopausal and postmenopausal women, with lower baseline LH concentrations in postmenopausal depressed women. It may be that the increased secretion of LH following removal of the negative feedback of gonadal steroids in postmenopausal women unmasks a decrease in LH secretion that is not as easily observed in women with intact estrogen and progesterone feedback. Other studies examining depressed patients of both sexes, which were not analyzed separately, observed

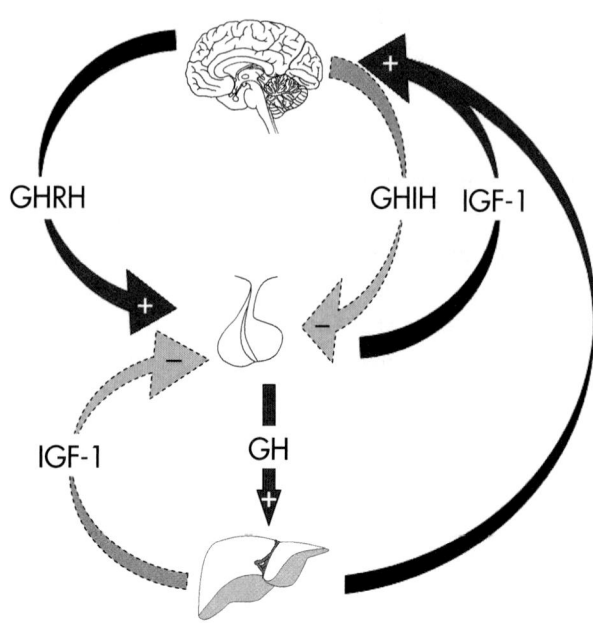

FIGURE 7–2. Effects of the hypothalamic-pituitary-adrenal axis on the hypothalamic-pituitary-gonadal axis.

GH = growth hormone; GHIH = growth hormone–inhibiting hormone; GHRH = growth hormone–releasing hormone; IGF-1 = insulin-like growth factor 1.

no change in baseline or GnRH-stimulated LH and FSH secretion (Unden et al. 1988).

Only recently have studies begun to focus on the pulsatile rhythm of LH secretion in women with major depression. Thus far, there have been only four published studies examining pulsatile LH secretion in depressed women: two by Meller et al. (1997, 2001), a third by us (Young et al. 2000b), and a fourth looking at the data from both Meller and Young with spectral analysis (Grambsch et al. 2004). The data from the Meller studies showed slower LH frequency in the follicular phase. Our data revealed significantly lower estradiol in the follicular phase in a small sample of depressed women. Since our publication in December 2000, a large-scale epidemiological study by Harlow et al. (2003) has found that earlier menopause is accompanied by lower estradiol in perimenopausal depressed women. Thus, three recent carefully done studies using modern techniques with sophisticated analyses have found evidence of reproductive axis abnormalities in depressed women. One study of the reproductive axis in men with major depression (Schweiger et al. 1999) also revealed decreased testosterone and a trend for slower LH pulses, suggesting that abnormalities in the reproductive axis are also found in men. Consequently, further studies on the reproductive axis in depression are indicated.

Estrogen and Depression

Because of increased incidence of depression at critical hormonal transition phases such as postpartum and perimenopause, much speculation has taken place about estrogen's role as a precipitant. Recent studies have found increased incidence of depressive symptoms and major depression during the menopause transition (Cohen et al. 2006; Freeman et al. 2006). The initial findings of Freeman et al. (2004) in regard to estrogen were that both high and low estrogen levels were associated with depression. More recently, the data suggest that variability in estrogen levels may drive depression. A model of differential sensitivity to estrogen has been proposed for premenstrual dysphoric disorder (PMDD) and also by Cohen et al. (2006) to explain the findings of increased depression during the menopause transition. Increased FSH, suggesting ovarian aging, and overall low or variable estrogen were also found to be strongly associated with depression (Freeman et al. 2006). And in the Freeman et al. study, PMDD was associated with depression during the menopause transition. Furthermore, the central effects of estrogen are intriguing and lend credence to a possible role of estrogen in modulating critical neuronal systems involved in depression. Studies in nonhuman primates have confirmed that estrogen increases tryptophan hydroxylase, the rate-limiting step in serotonin synthesis (Bethea et al. 2002). Estrogen also decreases serotonin$_{1A}$ (5-HT$_{1A}$) autoreceptor binding, which would serve to increase serotonin levels at the synapse (Bethea et al. 2002). Estrogen modulates the serotonin transporter, leading to decreases in the transporter mRNA but increases in the transporter expression in the hypothalamus (Bethea et al. 2002). Estrogen also decreases monoamine oxidase A activity, which would potentiate actions of norepinephrine in the synapse, and increases tyrosine hydroxylase, the critical first enzyme for synthesis of norepinephrine (Bethea et al. 2002). However, use of estrogen as a treatment has produced mixed results, perhaps because not all studies have targeted women with changing estrogen levels. Early studies found an effect of high-dose estrogen augmentation on response to antidepressants (Klaiber et al. 1979; Shapira et al. 1985). In situations of recent-onset estrogen deficiency such as postpartum and perimenopause, estrogen has been demonstrated to be an effective treatment for depression in randomized, controlled trials (Gregoire et al. 1996; Schmidt et al. 2000; Soares et al.

2001). However, randomized, controlled trials examining the effects of estrogen on mood in postmenopausal women have been negative (Hlatky et al. 2002; Morrison et al. 2004), suggesting a loss of beneficial mood response to estrogen following prolonged periods without estrogen. Finally, if data on estrogen's role in *inhibiting* the HPA axis in normal women are correct, then lower estradiol in depressed women would result in exacerbation of the HPA axis abnormalities seen in major depression, and these may need to be corrected along with changing the ovarian hormone milieu.

Premenstrual Dysphoric Disorder

One of the most well-studied mood disorders, with respect to the influence of ovarian steroids on mood, is PMDD. In any studies of this disorder, it is necessary to define carefully the study population and limit both endocrine investigations and treatment to women with clear luteal phase depressive symptoms who are well during the follicular phase; many more women report significant variations in mood premenstrually in retrospective reports than are found to have symptoms with prospective studies. In a study that used optimal sampling frequency to investigate LH and FSH, pulse frequency, and amplitude in follicular, midluteal, and late luteal phases of the menstrual cycle and examined estradiol and progesterone levels at these three time points, there was no difference between estradiol and progesterone at any time point between women with PMDD and control women (Reame et al. 1992). LH pulse frequency was also similar in both groups, with parallel changes across the menstrual cycle. Thus, these and earlier data (Rubinow et al. 1988) do not suggest an alteration in GnRH secretion or ovarian steroids in women with PMDD. Nevertheless, several studies have suggested that hormone manipulations can improve the symptoms.

One of the best-documented effective treatments is elimination of menstrual cycling with leuprolide, a GnRH agonist that improves mood. A number of studies found that leuprolide was highly effective in reducing symptom severity and cyclicity in PMDD patients (Mortola et al. 1991; Rosenbaum et al. 1996; Schmidt et al. 1998), although an increased rate of depressive-like symptoms has also been reported during leuprolide treatment (Steingold et al. 1987; Zorn et al. 1990). Leuprolide also leads to hypoestrogenism, which affects both bone density and cardiovascular disease; thus, it is necessary to add both steroid hormones. In the study by Mortola et al. (1991), just the addition of a placebo, with the suggestion that it might make mood symptoms worse, caused a significant worsening in mood symptoms. However, addition of conjugated equine estrogen with or without medroxyprogesterone acetate (MPA) while patients were still on leuprolide did not lead to a relapse in depressive symptoms. Not all studies have agreed that progesterone can be added back without significant worsening of symptoms. Schmidt and colleagues studied a group of women with PMDD whose symptoms were significantly improved by leuprolide, as well as a group of control women with no previous mood symptoms who were also taking leuprolide. They demonstrated a return of symptoms following administration of estradiol or progesterone but not with placebo. In the control women, none of the hormone replacements altered mood (Rubinow and Schmidt 2006). Finally, progesterone itself has been used for the treatment of PMDD despite its documented lack of effectiveness. The results of a recent Cochrane Database review of 17 randomized, placebo-controlled trials were equivocal, and the authors were unable to determine whether progesterone was useful or ineffective in the treatment of PMDD. They concluded that there was not enough evidence to say whether progesterone was helpful or ineffective (Ford et al. 2006).

Since it is generally believed that the symptoms of PMDD are related to delayed effects of progesterone on mood, several studies have investigated the effects of RU486, a progesterone antagonist, on mood symptoms. In the studies of Schmidt et al. (1991), creation of an artificial follicular phase during the second half of the menstrual cycle by the use of RU486 plus human chorionic gonadotropin did not result in a reduction of mood symptoms. Likewise, blockade of progesterone's action led to early menses, with depressive symptoms still occurring. The study by Chan et al. (1994), using a randomized, double-blind, placebo-controlled crossover design for 6 months, showed no effectiveness of RU486 on mood symptoms. Thus, although it is generally believed that PMDD is related to changes in CNS neurotransmitter systems caused by progesterone, the data do not support the conclusion that progesterone blockade affects these mood symptoms. Rubinow and Schmidt (2006) have proposed that PMDD represents an abnormal response to normal hormone changes or levels that occurs in a small proportion of genetically susceptible women and is most likely associated with gene polymorphisms involved in the gonadal steroid signaling pathway.

Another period of increased vulnerability to depression in women is the postpartum period. Although it is known that this period is accompanied by a sudden drop in progesterone and estradiol levels, there is limited information available on how this relates to the onset of depression. Postpartum depression is associated with a history of depression (O'Hara 1986; O'Hara et al. 1991), marital disharmony, and a higher number of stressful life events in the previous year (Cox et al. 1982). Gregoire et al. (1996) reported that transdermal estrogen is an effective treatment for depression. However, the group of women studied was small, heterogeneous, and ill-defined, and no information was available on whether these women had a new onset of depression or a prior psychiatric history. Furthermore, some of the patients were being concurrently treated with antidepressants.

Growth Hormone and the Hypothalamic-Pituitary-Somatotrophic Axis

Growth hormone (GH) or somatotropin is another stress-sensitive neuroendocrine system. GH is synthesized by the anterior pituitary, and although it can be used as an endpoint in itself for neuroendocrine research in psychiatry, its predominant use is as a marker of the integrity of the noradrenergic system following challenge. The hypothalamic-pituitary-somatotrophic (HPS) axis is under complex regulatory control that is not yet fully understood since cross-species variations in GH regulation make it difficult to extrapolate to humans from animal studies. It is well established, however, that the final common pathways for control of GH release from the pituitary are hypothalamic growth hormone–releasing hormone (GHRH) (stimulation) and somatostatin (inhibition). The wide variety of metabolic, endocrine, and neural influences that alter GH secretion do so primarily through effects on GHRH and/or somatostatin. Neural influences may be mediated by noradrenergic, cholinergic, dopaminergic, γ-aminobutyric acid (GABA)–ergic, and serotonergic neurotransmission. Clear physiological regulatory roles, however, have only been well documented in humans for noradrenergic and cholinergic inputs. Dopamine, serotonin, and GABAergic drugs can alter GH release but do so in contradictory ways, depending on the experimental paradigm, leaving their roles as GH regulatory agents uncertain at present (Devesa et al. 1992; Muller 1987). In humans, GH is released by acute stress, but is suppressed by chronic stress. Chronic psychosocial stress in children can result in growth arrest and even short stature and delayed puberty. A variety of other endocrine, metabolic, and physiological factors can influence GH release, although the mechanisms by which they do so are not clear. Factors that can inhibit GH release include free fatty acids (Penalva et al. 1990) and, most importantly for this review, CRH (Corsello et al. 1992) and glucocorticoids (del Balzo et al. 1990; Giustina and Wehrenberg 1992). Studies by Wiedemann et al. (1991) examined GH secretion in healthy control subjects given hourly pulses of ACTH (1 µg) or h-CRH (10 µg) between 9 A.M. and 6 P.M. to induce hypercortisolemia. They found an increase in the number of GH pulses and amount of GH secreted during the daytime but did not find an increase in the total 8 A.M. to 3 A.M. GH secretion because of blunted nighttime secretion. This pattern is similar to that seen in depressed patients (Mendlewicz et al. 1985) who have increased daytime GH secretion and reduced sleep-related GH secretion, suggesting a similar mechanism may occur in depressed patients. However, our own studies of 26 premenopausal women with major depression and 26 age- and menstrual-cycle-day-matched control women examining 10-minute secretion of GH for 24 hours found no changes in GH secretion (Amsterdam et al. 1989).

Current evidence suggests that the normal episodic GH secretory pattern is shaped by an alternating rhythm of GHRH and somatostatin release (Plotsky and Vale 1985), which has been called the hypothalamic-somatotroph rhythm (HSR) (Devesa et al. 1992). This is not a regular alternation but consists rather of four to eight short pulses of GH secretion distributed irregularly over a 24-hour period, the largest one occurring shortly after the onset of sleep. The significant role of somatostatin in shaping the HSR is evidenced by its persistence in the face of a constant GHRH infusion (Hulse et al. 1986; Vance et al. 1985). The intrinsic HSR, in turn, appears to shape the response to exogenous GHRH (Devesa et al. 1989, 1990, 1991a, 1992; Tannenbaum and Ling 1984). The response is greatest if GHRH is given while plasma GH is rising or near the peak of a pulse, presumably indicating that somatostatin is suppressed. The GH response is minimal if GHRH is given while plasma GH is low and stable, presumably indicating predominance of the somatostatin effect. Currently available human data therefore suggest that clonidine exerts a major effect on GH release via suppression of somatostatin-mediated inhibition.

It appears that cholinergically mediated suppression of somatostatin plays a significant role in regulating nocturnal GH release (Ghigo et al. 1990; Mendelson et al. 1978; Peters et al. 1986). Factors that can enhance GH release include estrogen (Devesa et al. 1991b; Ho et al. 1987), thyroid-releasing hormone, vasoactive intestinal

peptide, hypoglycemia, sleep, exercise, and stress (Devesa et al. 1992; Muller 1987; Uhde et al. 1992). Finally, GH exerts a negative feedback inhibition of its own secretion (Devesa et al. 1992; Muller 1987). It appears to act at the level of the hypothalamus and/or median eminence to stimulate somatostatin release (Devesa et al. 1992). It may also inhibit GHRH release (Devesa et al. 1992). GH also stimulates the production of somatomedin-C/insulin-like growth factor 1 (IGF-1) in peripheral tissues, including liver. Somatomedin-C in turn has a dual inhibitory feedback effect. It directly suppresses GH secretion at the pituitary level and stimulates somatostatin release at the hypothalamic level (Devesa et al. 1992). Levels of somatomedin-C correlate positively with, and can be used to infer, systemic GH levels during the past 8–12 hours (Copeland et al. 1980; Ross et al. 1987; Vance et al. 1985). Measurement of somatomedin-C levels thus can provide another means of evaluating the overall functional status of the HPS axis.

Growth Hormone Studies in Psychiatric Disorders

Adrenergic input to the HPS axis is mediated primarily by the α_2-adrenergic receptor. α_2-Adrenergic agonism is a potent stimulus for GH secretion, the effect being blocked by corresponding antagonists (Devesa et al. 1992; Muller 1987). α-Adrenergic stimulation of GH release may also be antagonized by β-adrenergic agonism (Devesa et al. 1992), but the β-adrenergic-receptor-mediated influences are less well researched. In humans, the evidence suggests that the GH-releasing effect of α_2-adrenergic agonism may be due primarily to inhibition of somatostatin release, with perhaps a secondary stimulation of GHRH. This is based on two main types of evidence. First, for at least 2 hours after a supramaximal dose of GHRH (200 µg), the pituitary is refractory to a repeated dose of GHRH, but the α_2-adrenergic agonist clonidine (Valcavi et al. 1988) or insulin-induced hypoglycemia (Shibasaki et al. 1985) will still evoke a vigorous GH response. Presumably, if the GH-releasing cells are unresponsive to GHRH, clonidine must stimulate GH release through a non-GHRH mechanism, the most likely alternative being inhibition of somatostatin release. Similarly, insulin-induced hypoglycemia is thought to stimulate noradrenergic outflow, which then suppresses somatostatin secretion (Shibasaki et al. 1985). Whereas the GH response to GHRH depends on the point in the HSR rhythm at which the GHRH is given, the response to clonidine does not (Devesa et al. 1990, 1991a, 1992), again suggesting that clonidine acts through a non-GHRH mechanism, again presumably somatostatin.

Downregulation of GH release in response to clonidine presumably occurs in response to chronic, excessive noradrenergic outflow from the locus coeruleus, which is thought to play a role in anxiety states (Uhde et al. 1992). The blunted GH response to clonidine in panic disorder has been replicated in 8 of 10 studies from 6 of 7 different clinical research groups (Abelson et al. 1991, 1992; Amsterdam et al. 1989; Charney and Heninger 1986; Coplan et al. 1993; Nutt 1989; Schittecatte et al. 1988, 1992; Uhde et al. 1986, 1991). Both failures to replicate (Schittecatte et al. 1988, 1992) were by the same group. One of those studies (Schittecatte et al. 1988) involved only seven subjects, and blunting was absent only in the female subjects, in whom birth control pills or menstrual cycle phase can obscure blunting. Blunted GH response to clonidine is seen in generalized anxiety disorder (Abelson et al. 1991) and social anxiety disorder (Uhde et al. 1991) but not in obsessive-compulsive disorder (OCD) (Hollander et al. 1991; Lee et al. 1990). It has also recently been reported in patients with PTSD (Morris et al. 2004). It is unlikely that the GH blunting seen in anxiety disorders is an artifact of tricyclic exposure, given that in our own work, 10 of 12 anxiety patients with blunted responses had no significant prior exposure to tricyclic antidepressants (Abelson et al. 1992) and our recent findings demonstrate a blunted response in subjects with anxiety (predominantly social phobia) with no tricyclic exposure (Cameron et al. 2004). The nonspecificity of the GH response to clonidine suggests that it could be a secondary response to the presence of a psychiatric disorder. However, the absence of blunting in patients with OCD (Lee et al. 1990), schizophrenia (Lal et al. 1983), or heroin abuse (Facchinetti et al. 1985) argues against this interpretation. Although the replicability of the blunted GH response to clonidine in panic disorder is well established, the mechanism remains less certain. It has been thought to reflect subsensitivity (downregulation) of postsynaptic α_2-adrenergic receptors (Siever et al. 1982). Our own data support the presence of blunted GH response to clonidine in social anxiety disorder, suggesting that excessive noradrenergic tone is also present in this form of anxiety (Cameron et al. 2004). These data are consistent with the hypothesis that excessive noradrenergic outflow from the locus coeruleus plays a pivotal role in anxiety states (Charney and Heninger 1986).

Numerous studies have also demonstrated reduced GH responses to clonidine in patients with major and melancholic depression (Amsterdam and Maislin 1990; Amsterdam et al. 1989; Charney et al. 1982; Checkley et al. 1981; Corn et al. 1984; Lesch et al. 1988; Siever and Uhde 1984), but not all studies have replicated these findings (Gann et al. 1995; Katona et al. 1993; Mitchell et al. 1991; Schittecatte et al. 1989, 1994). In particular, more recent studies have not found a blunted GH response to clonidine. It is unclear whether diagnostic changes and subject selection have affected these failures to replicate, given that several investigators found differences between endogenous and nonendogenous depression, with more severe blunting in the endogenous groups (Amsterdam et al. 1989; Checkley et al. 1984; Matussek and Laakmann 1981; Matussek et al. 1980). Furthermore, most of the studies in depression were done before it was realized that menstrual status (i.e., pre- vs. postmenopausal), menstrual cycle phase, and prior tricyclic exposure affected the GH response to clonidine. In particular, patients with endogenous depression are more likely to have been older and postmenopausal, both factors that decrease the GH response. The altered GH response to clonidine is thought to result from α_2-noradrenergic receptor downregulation, since studies using either GHRH, which acts directly at the pituitary, or apomorphine, which acts via dopamine input to the GH system, demonstrate normal GH response in depressed patients (Amsterdam and Maislin 1990; Corn et al. 1984; Krishnan et al. 1988; Lesch et al. 1988; Thomas et al. 1959). Again, this is consistent with increased central noradrenergic activation in depression, similar to that hypothesized in panic disorder. Our own recent studies (Cameron et al. 2004) found a normal GH response to clonidine in patients with "pure" depression (i.e., patients who did not meet criteria for any anxiety disorders). All of our patients had been off any psychotropic drugs for at least 6 months. Furthermore, there was no relationship between dimensional measures of anxiety or dimensional measures of depression and GH response. Patients with melancholic depression did not differ from nonmelancholic patients or control subjects. Subjects with a high Hamilton Anxiety Scale (Ham-A) score (≥ 20, $n=13$) did not differ from their matched controls. Thus, our data suggest that blunted GH response to clonidine challenge is specific to anxiety disorders and is not seen with less severe forms of anxiety or with depression in the absence of an anxiety disorder.

Conclusion

In this chapter we have reviewed ways in which hormonal systems may be altered in psychiatric disorders that may be linked to the pathoetiology of the disorders. The evidence is strongest for the HPA system, which has been implicated in at least two disorders, depression and PTSD, both disorders clearly linked to stress-based etiologies. The evidence for abnormalities in reproductive hormones is still small, but this is a subject of continued investigation. Most notably, abnormalities of reproductive hormones have not been found in PMDD, the disorder most responsive to changing reproductive hormone milieu. Finally, hormones can be used as markers of the functioning of CNS neurotransmitters or receptors, as is the case for GH. As neuroimaging ligands are developed to directly measure these receptors, the latter role of neuroendocrinology may be useful. Many of the critical hormones, like cortisol and estradiol, regulate many other critical neurotransmitter systems, such as serotonin, as well as regulating gene transcription. The area of psychoneuroendocrinology continues to expand, and in combination with the major advances occurring throughout the field of psychiatry, it will become possible to identify the genetic and molecular mechanisms involved in psychiatric disorders, thereby leading to the development of better treatments.

References

Abelson JL, Curtis GC: Hypothalamic-pituitary-adrenal axis activity in panic disorder: 24-hour secretion of corticotropin and cortisol. Arch Gen Psychiatry 53:323–331, 1996

Abelson JL, Glitz D, Cameron OG, et al: Blunted growth hormone response to clonidine in patients with generalized anxiety disorder. Arch Gen Psychiatry 48:157–162, 1991

Abelson JL, Glitz D, Cameron OG, et al: Endocrine, cardiovascular, and behavioral responses to clonidine in patients with panic disorder. Biol Psychiatry 32:18–25, 1992

Amsterdam JD, Maislin G: Comparison of growth hormone response after clonidine and insulin hypoglycemia in affective illness. Biol Psychiatry 28:308–314, 1990

Amsterdam JD, Winokur A, Abelman E, et al: Cosyntropin (ACTH alpha 1–24) stimulation test in depressed patients and healthy subjects. Am J Psychiatry 140:907–909, 1983

Amsterdam JD, Maislin G, Skolnick B, et al: Multiple hormone responses to clonidine administration in depressed patients and healthy volunteers. Biol Psychiatry 26:265–278, 1989

Angold A, Costello EJ, Erkanli A, et al: Pubertal changes in hormone levels and depression in girls. Psychol Med 29:1043–1053, 1999

Anisman H, Griffiths J, Matheson K, et al: Posttraumatic stress symptoms and salivary cortisol levels. Am J Psychiatry 158:1509–1511, 2001

Atmaca M, Kuloglu M, Tezcan E, et al: Neopterin levels and dexamethasone suppression test in posttraumatic stress disorder. Eur Arch Psychiatry Clin Neurosci 252:161–165, 2002

Belchetz PE, Plant TM, Nakai Y, et al: Hypophysial responses to continuous and intermittent delivery of hypothalamic gonadotropin-releasing hormone. Science 202:631–633, 1978

Berga SL, Mortola JF, Girton L, et al: Neuroendocrine aberrations in women with functional hypothalamic amenorrhea. J Clin Endocrinol Metab 68:301–308, 1989

Berger M, Pirke KM, Doerr P, et al: Influence of weight loss on the dexamethasone suppression test. Arch Gen Psychiatry 40:585–586, 1983

Bethea CL, Lu NZ, Gundlah C, et al: Diverse actions of ovarian steroids in the serotonin neural system. Front Neuroendocrinol 23:41–100, 2002

Bhagwagar Z, Hafizi S, Cowen PJ: Increase in concentration of waking salivary cortisol in recovered patients with depression. Am J Psychiatry 160:1890–1891, 2003

Biller BM, Federoff HJ, Koenig JI, et al: Abnormal cortisol secretion and responses to corticotropin-releasing hormone in women with hypothalamic amenorrhea. J Clin Endocrinol Metab 70:311–317, 1990

Boscarino JA: Posttraumatic stress disorder, exposure to combat, and lower plasma cortisol among Vietnam veterans: findings and clinical implications. J Consult Clin Psychol 64:191–201, 1996

Brambilla F, Maggioni M, Ferrari E, et al: Tonic and dynamic gonadotropin secretion in depressive and normothymic phases of affective disorders. Psychiatry Res 32:229–239, 1990

Brambilla F, Bellodi L, Perna G, et al: Psychoimmunoendocrine aspects of panic disorder. Neuropsychobiology 26:12–22, 1992

Breen KM, Stackpole CA, Clarke IJ, et al: Does the type II glucocorticoid receptor mediate cortisol-induced suppression in pituitary responsiveness to gonadotropin-releasing hormone? Endocrinology 145:2739–2746, 2004

Bremner JD, Vythilingam M, Vermetten E, et al: Cortisol response to a cognitive stress challenge in posttraumatic stress disorder (PTSD) related to childhood abuse. Psychoneuroendocrinology 28:733–750, 2003

Breslau N, Davis GC, Andreski P, et al: Traumatic events and posttraumatic stress disorder in an urban population of young adults. Arch Gen Psychiatry 48:216–222, 1991

Breslau N, Davis GC, Andreski P: Risk factors for PTSD-related traumatic events: a prospective analysis. Am J Psychiatry 152:529–535, 1995

Cameron OG, Abelson JL, Young EA: Anxious and depressive disorders and their comorbidity: effect on central nervous system noradrenergic function. Biol Psychiatry 56:875–883, 2004

Carroll BJ, Curtis GC, Mendels J: Neuroendocrine regulation in depression, I: limbic system-adrenocortical dysfunction. Arch Gen Psychiatry 33:1039–1044, 1976

Carroll BJ, Feinberg M, Greden JF, et al: A specific laboratory test for the diagnosis of melancholia: standardization, validation, and clinical utility. Arch Gen Psychiatry 38:15–22, 1981

Casanueva FF, Borras CG, Burguera B, et al: Steroids and neuroendocrine function in anorexia nervosa. J Steroid Biochem 27:635–640, 1987

Chabbert BN, Djakoure C, Maitre SC, et al: Regulation of the human menstrual cycle. Front Neuroendocrinol 19:151–186, 1998

Chan AF, Mortola JF, Wood SH, et al: Persistence of premenstrual syndrome during low-dose administration of the progesterone antagonist RU 486. Obstet Gynecol 84:1001–1005, 1994

Charney DS, Heninger GR: Abnormal regulation of noradrenergic function in panic disorders. Effects of clonidine in healthy subjects and patients with agoraphobia and panic disorder. Arch Gen Psychiatry 43:1042–1054, 1986

Charney DS, Heninger GR, Sternberg DE, et al: Adrenergic receptor sensitivity in depression: effects of clonidine in depressed patients and healthy subjects. Arch Gen Psychiatry 39:290–294, 1982

Checkley SA, Slade AP, Shur E: Growth hormone and other responses to clonidine in patients with endogenous depression. Br J Psychiatry 138:51–55, 1981

Checkley SA, Glass IB, Thompson C, et al: The GH response to clonidine in endogenous as compared with reactive depression. Psychol Med 14:773–777, 1984

Christian JJ: Population density and reproductive efficiency. Biol Reprod 4:248–294, 1971

Cohen LS, Soares CN, Vitonis AF, et al: Risk for new onset of depression during the menopausal transition: the Harvard study of moods and cycles. Arch Gen Psychiatry 63:385–390, 2006

Copeland KC, Underwood LE, Van Wyk JJ: Induction of immunoreactive somatomedin C human serum by growth hormone: dose-response relationships and effect on chromatographic profiles. J Clin Endocrinol Metab 50:690–697, 1980

Coplan JD, Rosenblum L, Friedman S, et al: Noradrenergic/serotonergic interaction in panic disorder. Presented at the 13th National Conference of the Anxiety Disorders Association of America, Charleston, SC, March 19–21, 1993

Coplan JD, Moreau D, Chaput F, et al: Salivary cortisol concentrations before and after carbon-dioxide inhalations in children. Biol Psychiatry 51:326–333, 2002

Corn TH, Hale AS, Thompson C, et al: A comparison of the growth hormone responses to clonidine and apomorphine in the same patients with endogenous depression. Br J Psychiatry 144:636–639, 1984

Corsello SM, Tofani A, Della CS, et al: Activation of cholinergic tone by pyridostigmine reverses the inhibitory effect of corticotropin-releasing hormone on the growth hormone-releasing hormone-induced growth hormone secretion. Acta Endocrinol (Copenh) 126:113–116, 1992

Cox JL, Connor Y, Kendell RE: Prospective study of the psychiatric disorders of childbirth. Br J Psychiatry 140:111–117, 1982

Curtis GC, Cameron OG, Nesse RM: The dexamethasone suppression test in panic disorder and agoraphobia. Am J Psychiatry 139:1043–1046, 1982

Curtis GC, Abelson JL, Gold PW: Adrenocorticotropic hormone and cortisol responses to corticotropin-releasing hormone: changes in panic disorder and effects of alprazolam treatment. Biol Psychiatry 41:76–85, 1997

Davidson LM, Baum A: Chronic stress and posttraumatic stress disorders. J Consult Clin Psychol 54:303–308, 1986

Debus N, Breen KM, Barrell GK, et al: Does cortisol mediate endotoxin-induced inhibition of pulsatile luteinizing hormone and gonadotropin-releasing hormone secretion? Endocrinology 143:3748–3758, 2002

del Balzo P, Salvatori R, Cappa M, et al: Pyridostigmine does not reverse dexamethasone-induced growth hormone inhibition. Clin Endocrinol (Oxf) 33:605–612, 1990

Devesa J, Lima L, Lois N, et al: Reasons for the variability in growth hormone (GH) responses to GHRH challenge: the endogenous hypothalamic-somatotroph rhythm (HSR). Clin Endocrinol (Oxf) 30:367–377, 1989

Devesa J, Arce V, Lois N, et al: Alpha 2-adrenergic agonism enhances the growth hormone (GH) response to GH-releasing hormone through an inhibition of hypothalamic somatostatin release in normal men. J Clin Endocrinol Metab 71:1581–1588, 1990

Devesa J, Diaz MJ, Tresguerres JA, et al: Evidence that alpha 2-adrenergic pathways play a major role in growth hormone (GH) neuroregulation: alpha 2-adrenergic agonism counteracts the inhibitory effect of muscarinic cholinergic receptor blockade on the GH response to GH-releasing hormone, while alpha 2-adrenergic blockade diminishes the potentiating effect of increased cholinergic tone on such stimulation in normal men. J Clin Endocrinol Metab 73:251–256, 1991a

Devesa J, Lois N, Arce V, et al: The role of sexual steroids in the modulation of growth hormone (GH) secretion in humans. J Steroid Biochem Mol Biol 40:165–173, 1991b

Devesa J, Lima L, Tresguerres JA: Neuroendocrine control of growth-hormone secretion in humans. Trends Endocrinol Metab 3:175–183, 1992

diZerega GS, Hodgen GD: Folliculogenesis in the primate ovarian cycle. Endocr Rev 2:27–49, 1981

Edelstein CK, Roy-Byrne P, Fawzy FI, et al: Effects of weight loss on the dexamethasone suppression test. Am J Psychiatry 140:338–341, 1983

Elzinga BM, Schmahl CG, Vermetten E, et al: Higher cortisol levels following exposure to traumatic reminders in abuse-related PTSD. Neuropsychopharmacology 28:1656–1665, 2003

Facchinetti F, Volpe A, Nappi G, et al: Impairment of adrenergic-induced proopiomelanocortin-related peptide release in heroin addicts. Acta Endocrinol (Copenh) 108:1–5, 1985

Feder A, Coplan JD, Goetz RR, et al: Twenty-four-hour cortisol secretion patterns in prepubertal children with anxiety or depressive disorders. Biol Psychiatry 56:198–204, 2004

Ferin M, Vande WR: Endogenous opioid peptides and the control of the menstrual cycle. Eur J Obstet Gynecol Reprod Biol 18:365–373, 1984

Ford O, Lethaby A, Mol B, et al: Progesterone for premenstrual syndrome. Cochrane Database Syst Rev (4):CD003415, 2006

Freeman EW, Sammel MD, Liu L, et al: Hormones and menopausal status as predictors of depression in women in transition to menopause. Arch Gen Psychiatry 61:62–70, 2004

Freeman EW, Sammel MD, Lin H, et al: Associations of hormones and menopausal status with depressed mood in women with no history of depression. Arch Gen Psychiatry 63:375–382, 2006

Fukuda S, Morimoto K, Mure K, et al: Effect of the Hanshin-Awaji earthquake on posttraumatic stress, lifestyle changes, and cortisol levels of victims. Arch Environ Health 55:121–125, 2000

Gambacciani M, Yen SS, Rasmussen DD: GnRH release from the mediobasal hypothalamus: in vitro inhibition by corticotropin-releasing factor. Neuroendocrinology 43:533–536, 1986

Gann H, Riemann D, Stoll S, Berger, M, et al: Growth hormone response to growth hormone-releasing hormone and clonidine in depression. Biol Psychiatry 38:325–329, 1995

Gerra G, Zaimovic A, Zambelli U, et al: Neuroendocrine responses to psychological stress in adolescents with anxiety disorder. Neuropsychobiology 42:82–92, 2000

Ghigo E, Arvat E, Mazza E, et al: Failure of pyridostigmine to increase both basal and GHRH-induced GH secretion in the night. Acta Endocrinol (Copenh) 122:37–40, 1990

Giustina A, Wehrenberg WB: The role of glucocorticoids in the regulation of growth-hormone secretion—mechanisms and clinical significance. Trends Endocrinol Metab 3:306–311, 1992

Gold PW, Loriaux DL, Roy A, et al: Responses to corticotropin-releasing hormone in the hypercortisolism of depression and Cushing's disease: pathophysiologic and diagnostic implications. N Engl J Med 314:1329–1335, 1986

Goodman RL, Karsch FJ: Pulsatile secretion of luteinizing hormone: differential suppression by ovarian steroids. Endocrinology 107:1286–1290, 1980

Grambsch P, Young EA, Meller WH: Pulsatile luteinizing hormone disruption in depression. Psychoneuroendocrinology 29:825–829, 2004

Gregoire AJ, Kumar R, Everitt B, et al: Transdermal oestrogen for treatment of severe postnatal depression. Lancet 347:930–933, 1996

Grunhaus L, Flegel P, Haskett RF, et al: Serial dexamethasone suppression tests in simultaneous panic and depressive disorders. Biol Psychiatry 22:332–338, 1987

Halbreich U, Vital-Herne J, Goldstein S, et al: Sex differences in biological factors putatively related to depression. J Affect Disord 7:223–233, 1984

Halbreich U, Asnis GM, Shindledecker R, et al: Cortisol secretion in endogenous depression, I: basal plasma levels. Arch Gen Psychiatry 42:904–908, 1985

Halbreich U, Endicott J, Goldstein S, et al: Premenstrual changes and changes in gonadal hormones. Acta Psychiatr Scand 74:576–586, 1986

Harlow BL, Wise LA, Otto MW, et al: Depression and its influence on reproductive endocrine and menstrual cycle markers associated with perimenopause: the Harvard Study of Moods and Cycles. Arch Gen Psychiatry 60:29–36, 2003

Hawk LW, Dougall AL, Ursano RJ, et al: Urinary catecholamines and cortisol in recent-onset posttraumatic stress disorder after motor vehicle accidents. Psychosom Med 62:423–434, 2000

Heim C, Newport DJ, Heit S, et al: Pituitary-adrenal and autonomic responses to stress in women after sexual and physical abuse in childhood. JAMA 284:592–597, 2000

Heim C, Newport DJ, Bonsall R, et al: Altered pituitary-adrenal axis responses to provocative challenge tests in adult survivors of childhood abuse. Am J Psychiatry 158:575–581, 2001

Heninger GR: A biological perspective on comorbidity of major depressive disorder and panic disorder, in Comorbidity of Mood and Anxiety Disorders. Edited by Maser JD, Cloninger CR. Washington, DC, American Psychiatric Press, 1990, pp 381–401

Herman JP, Wiegand SJ, Watson SJ: Regulation of basal corticotropin-releasing hormone and arginine vasopressin messenger ribonucleic acid expression in the paraventricular nucleus: effects of selective hypothalamic deafferentations. Endocrinology 127:2408–2417, 1990

Hlatky MA, Boothroyd D, Vittinghoff E, et al: Quality-of-life and depressive symptoms in postmenopausal women after receiving hormone therapy: results from the Heart and Estrogen/Progestin Replacement Study (HERS) trial. JAMA 287:591–597, 2002

Ho KY, Evans WS, Blizzard RM, et al: Effects of sex and age on the 24-hour profile of growth hormone secretion in man: importance of endogenous estradiol concentrations. J Clin Endocrinol Metab 64:51–58, 1987

Hohtari H, Elovainio R, Salminen K, et al: Plasma corticotropin-releasing hormone, corticotropin, and endorphins at rest and during exercise in eumenorrheic and amenorrheic athletes. Fertil Steril 50:233–238, 1988

Hohtari H, Salminen-Lappalainen K, Laatikainen T: Response of plasma endorphins, corticotropin, cortisol, and luteinizing hormone in the corticotropin-releasing hormone stimulation test in eumenorrheic and amenorrheic athletes. Fertil Steril 55:276–280, 1991

Hollander E, DeCaria C, Nitescu A, et al: Noradrenergic function in obsessive-compulsive disorder: behavioral and neuroendocrine responses to clonidine and comparison to healthy controls. Psychiatry Res 37:161–177, 1991

Holsboer F, Von Bardeleben U, Gerken A, et al: Blunted corticotropin and normal cortisol response to human corticotropin-releasing factor in depression. N Engl J Med 311:1127, 1984

Holsboer F, Von Bardeleben U, Buller R, et al: Stimulation response to corticotropin-releasing hormone (CRH) in patients with depression, alcoholism and panic disorder. Horm Metab Res Suppl 16:80–88, 1987

Hulse JA, Rosenthal SM, Cuttler L, et al: The effect of pulsatile administration, continuous infusion, and diurnal variation on the growth hormone (GH) response to GH-releasing hormone in normal men. J Clin Endocrinol Metab 63:872–878, 1986

Jacobson L, Akana SF, Cascio CS, et al: The adrenocortical system responds slowly to removal of corticosterone in the absence of concurrent stress. Endocrinology 124:2144–2152, 1989

Jaffe RB, Plosker S, Marshall L, et al: Neuromodulatory regulation of gonadotropin-releasing hormone pulsatile discharge in women. Am J Obstet Gynecol 163(5 pt 2):1727–1731, 1990

Kanter ED, Wilkinson CW, Radant AD, et al: Glucocorticoid feedback sensitivity and adrenocortical responsiveness in posttraumatic stress disorder. Biol Psychiatry 50:238–245, 2001

Karsch FJ, Foster DL, Bittman EL, et al: A role for estradiol in enhancing luteinizing hormone pulse frequency during the follicular phase of the estrous cycle of sheep. Endocrinology 113:1333–1339, 1983

Kasa-Vubu JZ, Sowers M, Ye W, et al: Differences in endocrine function with varying fitness capacity in postpubertal females across the weight spectrum. Arch Pediatr Adolesc Med 158:333–340, 2004

Katona CL, Healy D, Paykel ES, et al: Growth hormone and physiological responses to clonidine in depression. Psychol Med 23:57–63, 1993

Keller-Wood ME, Dallman MF: Corticosteroid inhibition of ACTH secretion. Endocr Rev 5:1–24, 1984

Kellner M, Baker DG, Yassouridis A, et al: Mineralocorticoid receptor function in patients with posttraumatic stress disorder. Am J Psychiatry 159:1938–1940, 2002

Kellner M, Yassouridis A, Hubner R, et al: Endocrine and cardiovascular responses to corticotropin-releasing hormone in patients with posttraumatic stress disorder: a role for atrial natriuretic peptide? Neuropsychobiology 47:102–108, 2003

Kellner M, Otte C, Yassouridis A, et al: Overnight metyrapone and combined dexamethasone/metyrapone tests in post-traumatic stress disorder: preliminary findings. Eur Neuropsychopharmacol 14:337–339, 2004a

Kellner M, Schick M, Yassouridis A, et al: Metyrapone tests in patients with panic disorder. Biol Psychiatry 56:898–900, 2004b

Kendell RE: Emotional and physical factors in the genesis of puerperal mental disorders. J Psychosom Res 29:3–11, 1985

Kessler RC, Sonnega A, Bromet E, et al: Posttraumatic stress disorder in the National Comorbidity Survey. Arch Gen Psychiatry 52:1048–1060, 1995

Klaiber EL, Broverman DM, Vogel W, et al: Estrogen therapy for severe persistent depressions in women. Arch Gen Psychiatry 36:550–554, 1979

Knobil E: The GnRH pulse generator. Am J Obstet Gynecol 163(5 pt 2):1721–1727, 1990

Krieger DT: Rhythms in CRH, ACTH and corticosteroids. Endocr Rev 1:123, 1979

Krishnan KR, Manepalli AN, Ritchie JC, et al: Growth hormone-releasing factor stimulation test in depression. Am J Psychiatry 145:90–92, 1988

Krishnan KR, Ritchie JC, Saunders W, et al: Nocturnal and early morning secretion of ACTH and cortisol in humans. Biol Psychiatry 28:47–57, 1990a

Krishnan KR, Ritchie JC, Saunders WB, et al: Adrenocortical sensitivity to low-dose ACTH administration in depressed patients. Biol Psychiatry 27:930–933, 1990b

Kwak SP, Morano MI, Young EA, et al: Diurnal CRH mRNA rhythm in the hypothalamus: decreased expression in the evening is not dependent on endogenous glucocorticoids. Neuroendocrinology 57:96–105, 1993

Lal S, Nair NP, Thavundayil JX, et al: Clonidine-induced growth hormone secretion in chronic schizophrenia. Acta Psychiatr Scand 68:82–88, 1983

Lee MA, Cameron OG, Gurguis GN, et al: Alpha 2-adrenoreceptor status in obsessive-compulsive disorder. Biol Psychiatry 27:1083–1093, 1990

Lemieux AM, Coe CL: Abuse-related posttraumatic stress disorder: evidence for chronic neuroendocrine activation in women. Psychosom Med 57:105–115, 1995

Lesch KP, Laux G, Erb A, et al: Growth hormone (GH) responses to GH-releasing hormone in depression: correlation with GH release following clonidine. Psychiatry Res 25:301–310, 1988

Levin AP, Saoud JB, Strauman T, et al: Responses of generalized and discrete social phobics during public speaking. J Anxiety Disord 7:207–221, 1993

Liberzon I, Abelson JL, Flagel SB, et al: Neuroendocrine and psychophysiologic responses in PTSD: a symptom provocation study. Neuropsychopharmacology 21:40–50, 1999

Lindley SE, Carlson EB, Benoit M: Basal and dexamethasone suppressed salivary cortisol concentrations in a community sample of patients with posttraumatic stress disorder. Biol Psychiatry 55:940–945, 2004

Linkowski P, Mendlewicz J, Leclercq R, et al: The 24-hour profile of adrenocorticotropin and cortisol in major depressive illness. J Clin Endocrinol Metab 61:429–438, 1985

Loucks AB, Mortola JF, Girton L, et al: Alterations in the hypothalamic-pituitary-ovarian and the hypothalamic-pituitary-adrenal axes in athletic women. J Clin Endocrinol Metab 68:402–411, 1989

MacLusky NJ, Naftolin F, Leranth C: Immunocytochemical evidence for direct synaptic connections between corticotropin-releasing factor (CRF) and gonadotrophin-releasing hormone (GnRH)-containing neurons in the preoptic area of the rat. Brain Res 439:391–395, 1988

Maes M, Lin A, Bonaccorso S, et al: Increased 24-hour urinary cortisol excretion in patients with post-traumatic stress disorder and patients with major depression, but not in patients with fibromyalgia. Acta Psychiatr Scand 98:328–335, 1998

Mann DR, Jackson GG, Blank MS: Influence of adrenocorticotropin and adrenalectomy on gonadotropin secretion in immature rats. Neuroendocrinology 34:20–26, 1982

Martel FL, Hayward C, Lyons DM, et al: Salivary cortisol levels in socially phobic adolescent girls. Depress Anxiety 10:25–27, 1999

Mason JW, Giller EL, Kosten TR, et al: Urinary free-cortisol levels in posttraumatic stress disorder patients. J Nerv Ment Dis 174:145–149, 1986

Matussek N, Laakmann G: Growth hormone response in patients with depression. Acta Psychiatr Scand Suppl 290:122–126, 1981

Matussek N, Ackenheil M, Hippius H, et al: Effect of clonidine on growth hormone release in psychiatric patients and controls. Psychiatry Res 2:25–36, 1980

Meller WH, Zander KM, Crosby RD, et al: Luteinizing hormone pulse characteristics in depressed women. Am J Psychiatry 154:1454–1455, 1997

Meller WH, Grambsch PL, Bingham C, et al: Hypothalamic pituitary gonadal axis dysregulation in depressed women. Psychoneuroendocrinology 26:253–259, 2001

Mendelson WB, Sitaram N, Wyatt RJ, et al: Methoscopolamine inhibition of sleep-related growth hormone secretion. Evidence for a cholinergic secretory mechanism. J Clin Invest 61:1683–1690, 1978

Mendlewicz J, Linkowski P, Kerkhofs M, et al: Diurnal hypersecretion of growth hormone in depression. J Clin Endocrinol Metab 60:505–512, 1985

Midgley AR Jr, Jaffe RB: Regulation of human gonadotropins, X: episodic fluctuation of LH during the menstrual cycle. J Clin Endocrinol Metab 33:962–969, 1971

Mitchell P, Smythe G, Parker G, et al: Growth hormone and other hormonal responses to clonidine in melancholic and nonmelancholic depressed subjects and controls. Psychiatry Res 37:179–193, 1991

Morris P, Hopwood M, Maguire K, et al: Blunted growth hormone response to clonidine in post-traumatic stress disorder. Psychoneuroendocrinology 29:269–278, 2004

Morrison MF, Kallan MJ, Ten HT, et al: Lack of efficacy of estradiol for depression in postmenopausal women: a randomized, controlled trial. Biol Psychiatry 55:406–412, 2004

Mortola JF, Girton L, Fischer U: Successful treatment of severe premenstrual syndrome by combined use of gonadotropin-releasing hormone agonist and estrogen/progestin. J Clin Endocrinol Metab 72:252A–252F, 1991

Muller EE: Neural control of somatotropic function. Physiol Rev 67:962–1053, 1987

Newport DJ, Heim C, Bonsall R, et al: Pituitary-adrenal responses to standard and low-dose dexamethasone suppression tests in adult survivors of child abuse. Biol Psychiatry 55:10–20, 2004

Nikolarakis KE, Almeida OF, Herz A: Corticotropin-releasing factor (CRF) inhibits gonadotropin-releasing hormone (GnRH) release from superfused rat hypothalami in vitro. Brain Res 377:388–390, 1986a

Nikolarakis KE, Almeida OF, Herz A: Inhibition of LH release by CRF may be partially mediated through hypothalamic beta-endorphin release. NIDA Res Monogr 75:403–405, 1986b

Nutt DJ: Altered central alpha 2-adrenoceptor sensitivity in panic disorder. Arch Gen Psychiatry 46:165–169, 1989

O'Hara MW: Social support, life events, and depression during pregnancy and the puerperium. Arch Gen Psychiatry 43:569–573, 1986

O'Hara MW, Schlechte JA, Lewis DA, et al: Prospective study of postpartum blues: biologic and psychosocial factors. Arch Gen Psychiatry 48:801–806, 1991

Olster DH, Ferin M: Corticotropin-releasing hormone inhibits gonadotropin secretion in the ovariectomized rhesus monkey. J Clin Endocrinol Metab 65:262–267, 1987

Penalva A, Gaztambide S, Vazquez JA, et al: Role of cholinergic muscarinic pathways on the free fatty acid inhibition of GH responses to GHRH in normal men. Clin Endocrinol (Oxf) 33:171–176, 1990

Peters JR, Evans PJ, Page MD, et al: Cholinergic muscarinic receptor blockade with pirenzepine abolishes slow wave sleep-related growth hormone release in normal adult males. Clin Endocrinol (Oxf) 25:213–217, 1986

Petraglia F, Sutton S, Vale W, et al: Corticotropin-releasing factor decreases plasma luteinizing hormone levels in female rats by inhibiting gonadotropin-releasing hormone release into hypophysial-portal circulation. Endocrinology 120:1083–1088, 1987

Pfohl B, Sherman B, Schlechte J, et al: Pituitary-adrenal axis rhythm disturbances in psychiatric depression. Arch Gen Psychiatry 42:897–903, 1985

Pirke KM, Schweiger U, Lemmel W, et al: The influence of dieting on the menstrual cycle of healthy young women. J Clin Endocrinol Metab 60:1174–1179, 1985

Pitman RK, Orr SP: Twenty-four-hour urinary cortisol and catecholamine excretion in combat-related posttraumatic stress disorder. Biol Psychiatry 27:245–247, 1990

Plotsky PM: Facilitation of immunoreactive corticotropin-releasing factor secretion into the hypophysial-portal circulation after activation of catecholaminergic pathways or central norepinephrine injection. Endocrinology 121:924–930, 1987

Plotsky PM, Vale W: Patterns of growth hormone-releasing factor and somatostatin secretion into the hypophysial-portal circulation of the rat. Science 230:461–463, 1985

Plotsky PM, Cunningham ET Jr, Widmaier EP: Catecholaminergic modulation of corticotropin-releasing factor and adrenocorticotropin secretion. Endocr Rev 10:437–458, 1989

Putnam CD, Brann DW, Mahesh VB: Acute activation of the adrenocorticotropin-adrenal axis: effect on gonadotropin and prolactin secretion in the female rat. Endocrinology 128:2558–2566, 1991

Radovick S, Wondisford FE, Nakayama, Y, et al: Isolation and characterization of the human gonadotropin-releasing hormone gene in the hypothalamus and placenta. Mol Endocrinol 4:476–480, 1990

Rasmusson AM, Lipschitz DS, Wang S, et al: Increased pituitary and adrenal reactivity in premenopausal women with posttraumatic stress disorder. Biol Psychiatry 50:965–977, 2001

Reame N, Sauder SE, Kelch RP, et al: Pulsatile gonadotropin secretion during the human menstrual cycle: evidence for altered frequency of gonadotropin-releasing hormone secretion. J Clin Endocrinol Metab 59:328–337, 1984

Reame NE, Sauder SE, Case GD, et al: Pulsatile gonadotropin secretion in women with hypothalamic amenorrhea: evidence that reduced frequency of gonadotropin-releasing hormone secretion is the mechanism of persistent anovulation. J Clin Endocrinol Metab 61:851–858, 1985

Reame NE, Marshall JC, Kelch RP: Pulsatile LH secretion in women with premenstrual syndrome (PMS): evidence for normal neuroregulation of the menstrual cycle. Psychoneuroendocrinology 17:205–213, 1992

Reich T, Winokur G: Postpartum psychoses in patients with manic depressive disease. J Nerv Ment Dis 151:60–68, 1970

Rivier C, Vale W: Influence of corticotropin-releasing factor on reproductive functions in the rat. Endocrinology 114:914–921, 1984

Rivier C, Rivier J, Vale W: Stress-induced inhibition of reproductive functions: role of endogenous corticotropin-releasing factor. Science 231:607–609, 1986

Roberts JL, Budarf ML, Baxter JD, et al: Selective reduction of proadrenocorticotropin/endorphin proteins and messenger ribonucleic acid activity in mouse pituitary tumor cells by glucocorticoids. Biochemistry 18:4907–4915, 1979

Rosenbaum AH, Ginsberg K, Rosenberg R, et al: Treatment for major depression and manic-depressive illness with gonadotropin-releasing hormone agonist therapy (abstract). International Society of Psychoneuroendocrinology XXVIIth Congress, Cascais, Portugal, August 1996

Ross RJ, Tsagarakis S, Grossman A, et al: GH feedback occurs through modulation of hypothalamic somatostatin under cholinergic control: studies with pyridostigmine and GHRH. Clin Endocrinol (Oxf) 27:727–733, 1987

Roy-Byrne PP, Uhde TW, Post RM, et al: The corticotropin-releasing hormone stimulation test in patients with panic disorder. Am J Psychiatry 143:896–899, 1986

Rubin RT, Poland RE, Lesser IM, et al: Neuroendocrine aspects of primary endogenous depression, I: cortisol secretory dynamics in patients and matched controls. Arch Gen Psychiatry 44:328–336, 1987

Rubinow DR, Schmidt PJ: Gonadal steroid regulation of mood: the lessons of premenstrual syndrome. Front Neuroendocrinol 27:210–216, 2006

Rubinow DR, Hoban MC, Grover GN, et al: Changes in plasma hormones across the menstrual-cycle in patients with menstrually related mood disorder and in control subjects. Am J Obstet Gynecol 158:5–11, 1988

Sachar EJ, Hellman L, Roffwarg HP, et al: Disrupted 24-hour patterns of cortisol secretion in psychotic depression. Arch Gen Psychiatry 28:19–24, 1973

Sakakura M, Takebe K, Nakagawa S: Inhibition of luteinizing hormone secretion induced by synthetic LRH by long-term treatment with glucocorticoids in human subjects. J Clin Endocrinol Metab 40:774–779, 1975

Santa Ana EJ, Saladin ME, Back SE, et al: PTSD and the HPA axis: differences in response to the cold pressor task among individuals with child vs. adult trauma. Psychoneuroendocrinology 31:501–509, 2006

Schittecatte M, Charles G, Depauw Y, et al: Growth hormone response to clonidine in panic disorder patients. Psychiatry Res 23:147–151, 1988

Schittecatte M, Charles G, Machowski R, et al: Growth hormone response to clonidine in untreated depressed patients. Psychiatry Res 29:199–206, 1989

Schittecatte M, Ansseau M, Charles G, et al: Growth hormone response to clonidine in male patients with panic disorder untreated by antidepressants. Psychol Med 22:1059–1062, 1992

Schittecatte M, Charles G, Machowski R, et al: Effects of gender and diagnosis on growth hormone response to clonidine for major depression: a large-scale multicenter study. Am J Psychiatry 151:216–220, 1994

Schmidt PJ, Nieman LK, Grover GN, et al: Lack of effect of induced menses on symptoms in women with premenstrual syndrome. N Engl J Med 324:1174–1179, 1991

Schmidt PJ, Nieman LK, Danaceau MA, et al: Differential behavioral effects of gonadal steroids in women with and in those without premenstrual syndrome. N Engl J Med 338:209–216, 1998

Schmidt PJ, Nieman L, Danaceau MA, et al: Estrogen replacement in perimenopause-related depression: a preliminary report. Am J Obstet Gynecol 183:414–420, 2000

Schwartz NB, Justo SN: Acute changes in serum gonadotrophins and steroids following orchidectomy in the rat: role of the adrenal gland. Endocrinology 100:1550–1556, 1977

Schweiger U, Deuschle M, Weber B, et al: Testosterone, gonadotropin, and cortisol secretion in male patients with major depression. Psychosom Med 61:292–296, 1999

Shapira B, Oppenheim G, Zohar J, et al: Lack of efficacy of estrogen supplementation to imipramine in resistant female depressives. Biol Psychiatry 20:576–579, 1985

Shibasaki T, Hotta M, Masuda A, et al: Plasma GH responses to GHRH and insulin-induced hypoglycemia in man. J Clin Endocrinol Metab 60:1265–1267, 1985

Siever LJ, Uhde TW: New studies and perspectives on the noradrenergic receptor system in depression: effects of the alpha 2-adrenergic agonist clonidine. Biol Psychiatry 19:131–156, 1984

Siever LJ, Uhde TW, Silberman EK, et al: Growth hormone response to clonidine as a probe of noradrenergic receptor responsiveness in affective disorder patients and controls. Psychiatry Res 6:171–183, 1982

Smith MA, Davidson J, Ritchie JC, et al: The corticotropin-releasing hormone test in patients with posttraumatic stress disorder. Biol Psychiatry 26:349–355, 1989

Soares CN, Almeida OP, Joffe H, et al: Efficacy of estradiol for the treatment of depressive disorders in perimenopausal women: a double-blind, randomized, placebo-controlled trial. Arch Gen Psychiatry 58:529–534, 2001

Soules MR, Steiner RA, Clifton DK, et al: Progesterone modulation of pulsatile luteinizing hormone secretion in normal women. J Clin Endocrinol Metab 58:378–383, 1984

Soules MR, Steiner RA, Cohen NL, et al: Nocturnal slowing of pulsatile luteinizing hormone secretion in women during the follicular phase of the menstrual cycle. J Clin Endocrinol Metab 61:43–49, 1985

Steele PA, Judd SJ: Role of endogenous opioids in reducing the frequency of pulsatile luteinizing hormone secretion induced by progesterone in normal women. Clin Endocrinol (Oxf) 25:669–674, 1986

Stein MB, Yehuda R, Koverola C, et al: Enhanced dexamethasone suppression of plasma cortisol in adult women traumatized by childhood sexual abuse. Biol Psychiatry 42:680–686, 1997

Steingold KA, Cedars M, Lu JK, et al: Treatment of endometriosis with a long-acting gonadotropin-releasing hormone agonist. Obstet Gynecol 69(3 pt 1):403–411, 1987

Suh BY, Liu JH, Berga SL, et al: Hypercortisolism in patients with functional hypothalamic-amenorrhea. J Clin Endocrinol Metab 66:733–739, 1988

Suter DE, Schwartz NB: Effects of glucocorticoids on secretion of luteinizing hormone and follicle-stimulating hormone by female rat pituitary cells in vitro. Endocrinology 117:849–854, 1985

Tannenbaum GS, Ling N: The interrelationship of growth hormone (GH)-releasing factor and somatostatin in generation of the ultradian rhythm of GH secretion. Endocrinology 115:1952–1957, 1984

Thomas GJ, Moore RY, Harvey JA, et al: Relations between the behavioral syndrome produced by lesions in the septal region of the forebrain and maze learning of the rat. J Comp Physiol Psychol 52:527–532, 1959

Tilbrook AJ, Canny BJ, Stewart BJ, et al: Central administration of corticotrophin releasing hormone but not arginine vasopressin stimulates the secretion of luteinizing hormone in rams in the presence and absence of testosterone. J Endocrinol 162:301–311, 1999

Uhde TW, Vittone BJ, Siever LJ, et al: Blunted growth hormone response to clonidine in panic disorder patients. Biol Psychiatry 21:1081–1085, 1986

Uhde TW, Tancer ME, Black B, et al: Phenomenology and neurobiology of social phobia: comparison with panic disorder. J Clin Psychiatry 52 (suppl):31–40, 1991

Uhde TW, Tancer ME, Rubinow DR, et al: Evidence for hypothalamo-growth hormone dysfunction in panic disorder: profile of growth hormone (GH) responses to clonidine, yohimbine, caffeine, glucose, GRF and TRH in panic disorder patients versus healthy volunteers. Neuropsychopharmacology 6:101–118, 1992

Uhde TW, Tancer ME, Gelernter CS, et al: Normal urinary free cortisol and postdexamethasone cortisol in social phobia: comparison to normal volunteers. J Affect Disord 30:155–161, 1994

Unden F, Ljunggren JG, Beck-Friis J, et al: Hypothalamic-pituitary-gonadal axis in major depressive disorders. Acta Psychiatr Scand 78:138–146, 1988

Valcavi R, Dieguez C, Page MD, et al: Alpha-2-adrenergic pathways release growth hormone via a non-GRF-dependent mechanism in normal human subjects. Clin Endocrinol (Oxf) 29:309–316, 1988

Vance ML, Kaiser DL, Evans WS, et al: Evidence for a limited growth hormone (GH)-releasing hormone (GHRH)-releasable quantity of GH: effects of 6-hour infusions of GHRH on GH secretion in normal man. J Clin Endocrinol Metab 60:370–375, 1985

Villanueva AL, Schlosser C, Hopper B, et al: Increased cortisol production in women runners. J Clin Endocrinol Metab 63:133–136, 1986

Von Bardeleben U, Stalla GK, Muller OA, et al: Blunting of ACTH response to human CRH in depressed patients is avoided by metyrapone pretreatment. Biol Psychiatry 24:782–786, 1988

Wiedemann K, Von Bardeleben U, Holsboer F: Influence of human corticotropin-releasing hormone and adrenocorticotropin upon spontaneous growth hormone secretion. Neuroendocrinology 54:462–468, 1991

Williams CL, Nishihara M, Thalabard JC, et al: Corticotropin-releasing factor and gonadotropin-releasing hormone pulse generator activity in the rhesus monkey: electrophysiological studies. Neuroendocrinology 52:133–137, 1990

Winokur A, Amsterdam J, Caroff S, et al: Variability of hormonal responses to a series of neuroendocrine challenges in depressed patients. Am J Psychiatry 139:39–44, 1982

Yehuda R: Current status of cortisol findings in post-traumatic stress disorder. Psychiatr Clin North Am 25:341–368, 2002

Yehuda R, Kahana B, Schmeidler J, et al: Impact of cumulative lifetime trauma and recent stress on current posttraumatic stress disorder symptoms in holocaust survivors. Am J Psychiatry 152:1815–1818, 1995

Yehuda R, Halligan SL, Grossman R, et al: The cortisol and glucocorticoid receptor response to low dose dexamethasone administration in aging combat veterans and holocaust survivors with and without posttraumatic stress disorder. Biol Psychiatry 52:393–403, 2002

Young EA, Breslau N: Cortisol and catecholamines in posttraumatic stress disorder: an epidemiologic community study. Arch Gen Psychiatry 61:394–401, 2004a

Young EA, Breslau N: Saliva cortisol in posttraumatic stress disorder: a community epidemiologic study. Biol Psychiatry 56:205–209, 2004b

Young EA, Watson SJ, Kotun J, et al: Beta-lipotropin-beta-endorphin response to low-dose ovine corticotropin releasing factor in endogenous depression. Preliminary studies. Arch Gen Psychiatry 47:449–457, 1990

Young EA, Haskett RF, Murphy-Weinberg V, et al: Loss of glucocorticoid fast feedback in depression. Arch Gen Psychiatry 48:693–699, 1991

Young EA, Haskett RF, Grunhaus L, et al: Increased evening activation of the hypothalamic-pituitary-adrenal axis in depressed patients. Arch Gen Psychiatry 51:701–707, 1994

Young EA, Akil H, Haskett RF, et al: Evidence against changes in corticotroph CRF receptors in depressed patients. Biol Psychiatry 37:355–363, 1995

Young EA, Lopez JF, Murphy-Weinberg V, et al: Normal pituitary response to metyrapone in the morning in depressed patients: implications for circadian regulation of corticotropin-releasing hormone secretion. Biol Psychiatry 41:1149–1155, 1997

Young EA, Aggen SH, Prescott CA, et al: Similarity in saliva cortisol measures in monozygotic twins and the influence of past major depression. Biol Psychiatry 48:70–74, 2000a

Young EA, Midgley AR, Carlson NE, et al: Alteration in the hypothalamic-pituitary-ovarian axis in depressed women. Arch Gen Psychiatry 57:1157–1162, 2000b

Young EA, Carlson NE, Brown MB: Twenty-four-hour ACTH and cortisol pulsatility in depressed women. Neuropsychopharmacology 25:267–276, 2001

Young EA, Tolman R, Witkowski K, et al: Salivary cortisol and posttraumatic stress disorder in a low-income community sample of women. Biol Psychiatry 55:621–626, 2004

Zorn JR, Mathieson J, Risquez F, et al: Treatment of endometriosis with a delayed release preparation of the agonist D-Trp6-luteinizing hormone-releasing hormone: long-term follow-up in a series of 50 patients. Fertil Steril 53:401–406, 1990

CHAPTER 8

Principles of Pharmacokinetics and Pharmacodynamics

C. Lindsay DeVane, Pharm.D.

Pharmacokinetics is defined as the study of the time course of drugs and their metabolites through the body. *Pharmacodynamics* is defined as the study of the time course and intensity of pharmacological effects of drugs. A convenient lay description of these terms is that pharmacokinetics describes what the body's physiology does to a drug, and pharmacodynamics describes what a drug does to the body. Although clinicians are more interested in drug effects than drug concentrations, these disciplines are closely connected. Pharmacokinetic and pharmacodynamic variability is a major determinant of the dose–effect relationship in patients (Figure 8–1). There is increasing recognition that genetic variability—in the form of polymorphic genes controlling the transcription of proteins involved in drug-metabolizing enzymes, drug transporters, and drug targets—is a substantial determinant of pharmacokinetic and pharmacodynamic variability. An integrated knowledge of these areas is essential in the drug development process and can be instrumental in individualizing dosage regimens for specific patients.

The dose and the frequency of dosing necessary to produce the desired pharmacological response from psychoactive drugs differ widely among patients. This variability in the drug dose–effect relationship is not surprising, given the large differences in patients' physiology, ages, range of severity of illness, activity of drug metabolizing enzymes and transporters, renal function, and other variables. Thus, a rational approach to drug dosage regimens, based on scientific principles, is needed to reach therapeutic objectives without either underdosing (and

obtaining an unsatisfactory response) or overdosing (and risking intolerability or toxicity).

The interface between pharmacokinetics and pharmacodynamics, where drugs interact with molecular targets at an effect site (see Figure 8–1), is increasingly becoming the focus of research. The ability to link drug concentrations with pharmacodynamic effects using mathematical models has improved greatly in recent years with the availability of new computer software. Population pharmacokinetic/pharmacodynamic modeling enables definition of the relationship between drug concentration and effect in individuals from vulnerable populations such as children, pregnant women, and the elderly where only sparse data may be available (Bies et al. 2004). Covariants such as age, gender, genotype of drug-metabolizing enzymes, and concomitant treatment with other drugs can be easily incorporated into these models and tested for their significance in influencing drug concentration and effects (DeVane et al. 2006). Measurements of plasma drug concentration are easily performed with sensitive analytical methods including gas and liquid chromatography and mass spectrometry.

In recent years, our understanding of the role of drug transporters and of gene expression of intestinal and hepatic enzymes in influencing drug movement within the body has increased considerably. Extensive contributions to our understanding of the sources of variability in pharmacokinetic/pharmacodynamic response have come from the field of pharmacogenetics. Genetic polymorphisms in drug-metabolizing enzymes enhance or diminish the

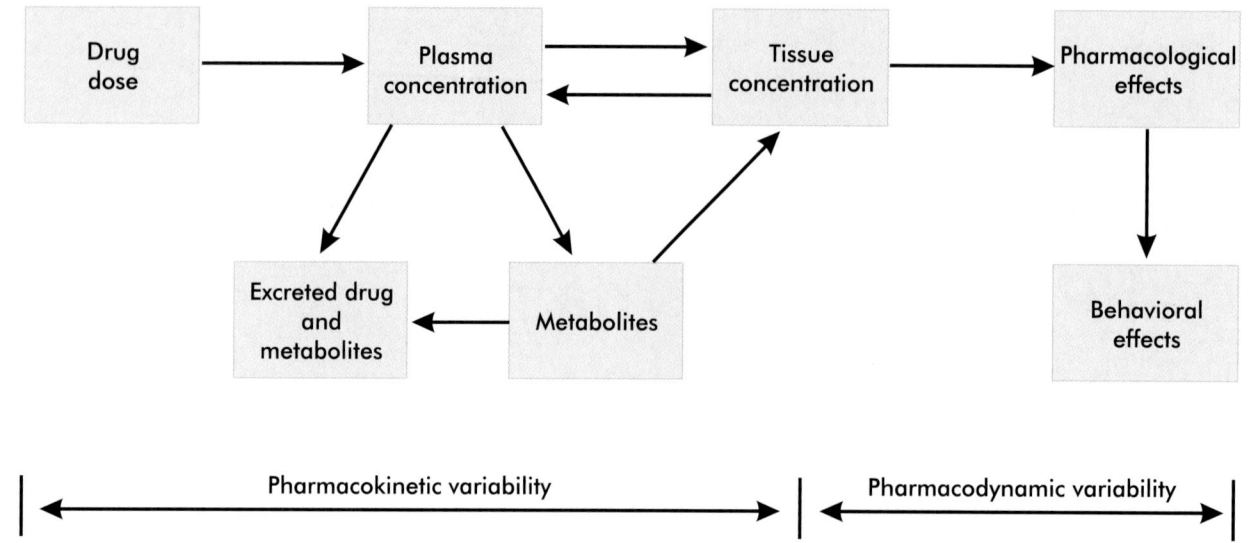

FIGURE 8–1.   Pharmacokinetic and pharmacodynamic variability as determinants of the dose–effect relationship.

body's ability to biotransform a variety of substrate drugs. A large number of defective alleles have been discovered, some of which have functional significance. On the pharmacodynamic side of the dose–effect relationship, the significance of polymorphisms in drug targets is an intense area of investigation. One of the most studied polymorphisms is in the promoter region of the gene encoding the serotonin transporter (5-HTT) and consists of the insertion or deletion of a 44–base pair sequence, giving rise to two variants: long (L) and short (S). A meta-analysis of 15 studies representing 1,435 patients concluded that patients with the SS genotype are less likely to reach remission during selective serotonin reuptake inhibitor (SSRI) therapy and require a longer treatment period for 50% symptom improvement (Serretti et al. 2007).

Although the discipline of pharmacokinetics relies heavily on mathematical description and prediction of the time course of drugs in the body, the purpose of this chapter is to explain basic principles of pharmacokinetics and how they interface with pharmacodynamics to provide insight into observed dose–effect relationships that can aid in developing drug dosage regimens. The fundamental concepts of pharmacokinetics have not changed since the initial publication of this chapter. These principles are reviewed here, and the interface of pharmacokinetics with the discipline of pharmacogenetics—the study of the genetic basis for differences in drug effects—is discussed as a essential component of variability in drug dose–effect relationships in psychopharmacology (see Figure 8–1).

Pharmacokinetics

A human pharmacokinetic study typically results in a mathematical description of drug concentration changes in plasma over time. The value of these data and of their use varies according to patient circumstances. During drug development, this knowledge is essential to develop guidelines for ensuring safe and effective dosage regimens in clinical trials. In clinical practice, plasma concentration measurements are useful to guide dosage adjustments to reach targeted steady-state concentrations of lithium, some anticonvulsant mood stabilizers, and clozapine. In the United States, the low utilization of tricyclic antidepressants and conventional antipsychotics has narrowed the scope of plasma drug concentration monitoring in psychiatry. However, a resurgence of interest is occurring as the search for biomarkers of drug efficacy and tolerability is increasing in drug development (Sunderland et al. 2005). Even without patient-specific drug concentration data, some knowledge of population pharmacokinetic parameters is clinically useful. Population estimates of drug and metabolite half-life can predict the time required for washout from the body once drug dosing is discontinued. This is useful for predicting the overlap of drug in the body when switching among antidepressants or antipsychotics, the presence of drug in the body during anesthesia for surgical procedures, and the probability of a drug–drug interaction when initiating new pharmacotherapy. Such information is useful when prescribing fluoxetine, for example, which produces an active metabolite, norfluoxetine, with an elimination half-life estimated between 4 and 16 days. Thus, an interval as long as 1 month may be necessary after discontinuing fluoxetine before initiating treatment with a monoamine oxidase (MAO) inhibitor to minimize the possibility of developing a serotonin syndrome. The use of slow-release microspheres for injection of risperidone results in an extended drug half-life that predicts continual accumulation to a steady state over four injections given every 2 weeks and sustained drug concentration in plasma for 4–6 weeks after the last injection (Gefvert et al. 2005). The fundamental description of drug disposition begins with studies of single drug doses.

Single-Dose Drug Disposition

Absorption

The route of administration is a major determinant of the onset and duration of a drug's pharmacological effects. Intravenous injection ensures that all of the administered drug is available to the circulation. The rate of drug injection or infusion can be used to control completely the rate of drug availability. However, few psychopharmacological drugs are administered intravenously. Intramuscular administration is commonly thought to produce a rapid onset of effect, but exceptions have been documented. For example, drug absorption by this route was slow and erratic with chlordiazepoxide (Greenblatt et al. 1974). The recent availability of intramuscular forms of some atypical antipsychotics will be advantageous for treating psychotic states when rapid tranquilization is desired and oral administration is impractical. For drugs that are equally well absorbed by the intramuscular and oral routes of administration, the total systemic exposure (as reflected in the area under the plasma concentration–time curve [AUC]) from the two routes should be similar, as should the elimination half-life. A major difference is that the rate of absorption from the intramuscular route may be more rapid. Intramuscular administration of olanzapine 5 mg produced a maximum plasma concentration five times higher than the maximum plasma concentration produced by a 5-mg oral dose with a similar AUC from both routes of administrations (Bergstrom et al. 1999). Most psychoactive drugs are highly lipophilic compounds, which are well absorbed when taken orally. More than 60% of the drugs available on the market are for oral use because of the ease of administration and efficiency of absorption, together with greater patient compliance.

Drug absorption is usually a passive process occurring in the small intestine. The efficiency of oral absorption is influenced by the physiological state of the patient, by

formulation factors, and by the timing of administration around meals. Most drugs are best absorbed on an empty stomach. The presence of food or antacids in the stomach usually decreases the rate of drug absorption. Exceptions are sometimes noted. Coadministration of sertraline with food increased peak plasma concentration by approximately 25% and decreased time to peak concentration from 8 hours to 5 hours, with a negligible effect on the AUC (Ronfeld et al. 1997). A partial explanation for this finding is that a food-induced increase in hepatic blood flow could allow more unabsorbed drug to escape first-pass hepatic uptake and metabolism. The significance of this food–drug interaction is doubtful, given that sertraline's therapeutic benefits are reported in association with chronic daily administration. The rate of drug absorption is important when a rapid onset of effect is needed. Normally, the presence of food can be expected to reduce the peak drug concentration achieved in blood or plasma and prolong the time following an oral dose to reach the maximum plasma concentration. The absolute amount of drug absorbed may or may not be affected. Acute drug effects are facilitated by administration apart from meals. Sedative-hypnotic drugs are examples of drugs for which the rate of absorption is clinically meaningful (Greenblatt et al. 1978).

Formulation factors are especially meaningful when a drug effect is associated with achieving a minimal effective concentration (MEC) in plasma. Figure 8–2 shows the predicted plasma concentration–time curves of a drug following a rapid intravenous injection (I), an oral formulation that is completely absorbed with no presystemic elimination (II), an incompletely absorbed oral formulation (III), and an extended-release formulation that results in slow absorption of drug (IV). A formulation with poor bioavailability (III) may not result in a plasma concentration above the MEC, whereas a drug whose absorption is delayed (IV) may retard the onset of effect but maintain an effective concentration for a period similar to the more rapidly available formulations (I, II). The principle of an MEC may apply in antipsychotic therapy, where minimal occupancy of dopamine D_2 receptors during a dosage interval may be needed for optimal therapeutic benefit.

Recent research in pharmaceutical science has resulted in a variety of systems for controlling the release of oral drugs. These include coated systems, with a core of active drug surrounded by a slow-releasing film; matrix systems, with active drug distributed in erodible gel matrices, and other hydrophilic, swellable, or erodible polymers to slowly dissolve and release drug at predictable rates to produce one or more peak concentrations during a dosage in-

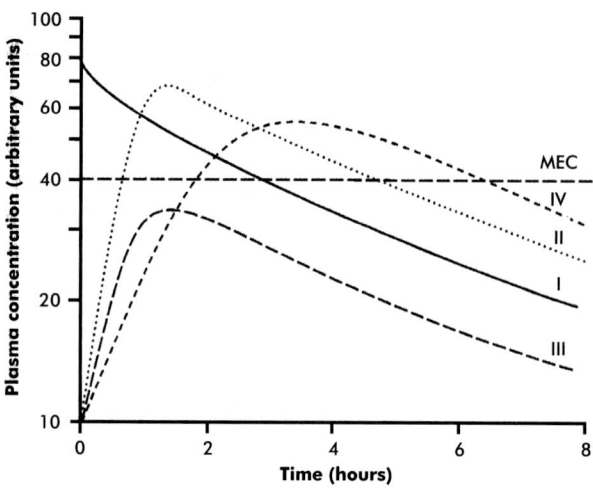

FIGURE 8–2. Predicted plasma concentration curves following single doses of a drug by rapid intravenous injection (I), a dosage form with complete bioavailability (II), a dosage form with reduced bioavailability (III), and an extended-release dosage form that reduces the rate but not the completeness of absorption (IV).

MEC = minimal effective concentration.

terval. Bupropion, paroxetine, venlafaxine, and the psychostimulants used to treat attention-deficit/hyperactivity disorder (ADHD) are examples of drugs whose clinical utility has been improved by reformulation as sustained- or extended-release dosage forms. Among the immediate-release dosage formulations, a general rank order of products providing the most rapid to the slowest rate of drug release for oral absorption is solutions, suspensions, tablets, enteric- or film-coated tablets, and capsules. Regardless of the dosage formulation selected, the last several hours of declining drug concentration in plasma occur in parallel, because drug elimination rate is unaffected by its rate or extent of absorption (see Figure 8–2). The time at which a terminal elimination phase is clearly observable following a single dose may be delayed, but the terminal elimination half-life is unchanged. Formulation into sustained- or slow-release tablets or capsules may allow drugs with short elimination half-lives, which must be given multiple times per day to maintain an effective concentration, to be effective when administered once or twice daily.

Presystemic Elimination

Many drugs undergo extensive metabolism as they move from the gastrointestinal tract to the systemic circulation (i.e., as they pass through the gastrointestinal membranes

and hepatic circulation during absorption). This process is known as the *first-pass effect* or *presystemic elimination* and is an important determinant of drug bioavailability after oral administration. Several factors are potentially important in influencing the degree of first-pass effect. A first-pass effect is usually indicated by either a decreased amount of parent drug reaching the systemic circulation or an increased quantity of metabolites after oral administration compared with parenteral dosing. This process is important in the formation of active metabolites for psychoactive drugs and is a major source of pharmacokinetic variability (George et al. 1982).

Presystemic metabolism of drugs is extensively accomplished by cytochrome P450 (CYP) enzymes in the luminal epithelium of the small intestine (Kolars et al. 1992). CYP3A4 represents approximately 70% of total cytochrome P450 in the human intestine. Many useful psychopharmacological drugs are CYP3A4 substrates. Examples of these drugs are listed in Table 8–1 along with substrates, inhibitors, and inducers of other major human CYP isoforms. The liver contains about two- to fivefold greater amounts of CYP3A protein (nmol/mg protein) compared with the intestine (de Waziers et al. 1990). Nevertheless, intestinal CYP3A4 has a profound effect on presystemic drug metabolism. Up to 43% of orally administered midazolam, for example, is metabolized as it passes through the intestinal mucosa (Paine et al. 1996). The exposure of drugs to gut CYP3A4 is not limited by binding to plasma proteins, as can occur with hepatic metabolism. Slower blood flow may also contribute to intestinal metabolism, thereby compensating for the lower quantity of CYP3A4 in the gut compared with the liver.

Certain foods, such as grapefruit juice, can substantially alter the bioavailability of some drugs. Components in grapefruit juice—which contains a variety of suspect candidates, including naringin, other flavonoids, bergamottin, and other furanocoumarins—inhibit intestinal CYP3A4-mediated first-pass metabolism (Paine et al. 2005). The maximal effect can occur within 30 minutes of ingestion of juice. Grapefruit juice may also inhibit the efflux transport of drugs by P-glycoprotein (P-gp) and multidrug resistance protein 2 (MRP2), which are efflux transporters expressed in the human small intestine. The more completely studied of these drug transporters is the transmembrane pump P-gp (also known as the multidrug resistance protein), which causes the adenosine triphosphate (ATP)–dependent efflux of a diverse range of drugs from cells. The distribution of P-gp includes the epithelial cells lining the luminal surface of enterocytes in the small intestine and kidney, making P-gp a critical determinant

TABLE 8–1. Substrates, inhibitors, and inducers of the major human liver cytochrome P450 (CYP) enzymes involved in drug metabolism

CYP ENZYME	SUBSTRATES	INHIBITORS[a]	INDUCERS
CYP1A2	Caffeine,[b] clozapine, duloxetine, haloperidol,[b] imipramine,[b] phenacetin, tacrine, theophylline,[b] verapamil,[b] warfarin[b]	Cimetidine, fluoro-quinolones (cipro-floxacin, norfloxacin), fluvoxamine	Charcoal-broiled beef, cigarette smoke, cruciferous vegetables, marijuana smoke, omeprazole
CYP2A6	Coumarin, nicotine	Tranylcypromine	Barbiturates
CYP2B6	Bupropion, cyclophosphamide, diazepam,[b] nicotine, tamoxifen		Phenobarbital, cyclo-phosphamide (in vitro)
CYP2C9	Amitriptyline,[b] diclofenac, metoclopramide, phenytoin, propranolol,[b] tetrahydrocannabinol,[b] tolbutamide, warfarin[b]	Disulfiram, fluconazole, fluvoxamine, d-propoxyphene, sulfaphenazole	Rifampin, phenytoin, secobarbital
CYP2C19	Amitriptyline,[b] clomipramine,[b] desmethyldiazepam,[b] diazepam,[b] ibuprofen, imipramine,[b] S-mephenytoin, moclobemide, naproxen, omeprazole,[b] piroxicam, tenoxicam	Omeprazole	Rifampin
CYP2D6	Amitriptyline,[b] codeine,[b] debrisoquine, desipramine, dextromethorphan, duloxetine, haloperidol,[b] imipramine,[b] metoclopramide, metoprolol, mexiletine, nortriptyline, ondansetron,[b] orphenadrine, paroxetine, pindolol, propafenone, propranolol,[b] risperidone, sparteine, thioridazine, timolol, venlafaxine[b]	Cimetidine, fluoxetine, paroxetine, quinidine, sertraline	None documented in vivo
CYP2E1	Caffeine,[b] dapsone,[b] ethanol	Disulfiram	Ethanol
CYP3A4	Alprazolam, amiodarone, amitriptyline,[b] astemizole, bupropion, caffeine,[b] carbamazepine, cisapride, clarithromycin, clonazepam, codeine,[b] cortisol, cyclosporin, dapsone,[b] desmethyldiazepam,[b] diazepam,[b] diltiazem, erythromycin, estradiol, ethinylestradiol, fluoxetine, haloperidol,[b] imipramine,[b] lidocaine, loratadine, lovastatin, midazolam, nefazodone, nicardipine, nifedipine, omeprazole,[b] ondansetron, orphenadrine, progesterone, quinidine, rifampin, sertraline, tamoxifen, terfenadine, testosterone, trazodone, triazolam, venlafaxine,[b] verapamil,[b] zolpidem	Cimetidine, erythromycin, fluoxetine, fluvoxamine, indinavir, ketoconazole, naringenin, nefazodone, ritonavir, saquinavir, sertraline (weak)	Barbiturates, carbamazepine, dexamethasone, phenytoin, rifampin, St. John's wort

[a]Inhibitory potency varies greatly (see text).
[b]More than one CYP enzyme is known to be involved in the metabolism of these drugs.
Source. Ketter et al. 1995; Nemeroff et al. 1996; Schmider et al. 1996.

of oral drug bioavailability and biliary and renal excretion for many drugs (Benet et al. 1999; Silverman 1999). P-gp is also expressed on the luminal surface of the endothelial cells making up the blood–brain barrier and other critical organs. In the gut, P-gp works in concert with CYP3A4 to limit the intestinal absorption of drugs that are common substrates for both proteins.

Changing the route of administration to avoid presystemic metabolism can have a therapeutic advantage. When given orally, selegiline, an irreversible inhibitor of MAO, is substantially converted to several metabolites through extensive first-pass metabolism. Transdermal dosing with drug contained in a removable patch adhering to the skin results in higher systemic exposure to selegiline and lower exposure to metabolites. This allows greater central nervous system (CNS) exposure to selegiline from a given dose to inhibit MAO relative to the required dose from oral administration (Azzaro et al. 2007). Buccal or sublingual administration can also avoid some presystemic drug elimination (Markowitz et al. 2006).

In summary, an important pharmacokinetic principle is that the choice of drug formulation and the route of administration can determine the rate at which the drug and metabolites appear in the systemic circulation. This rate may be manipulated to retard the magnitude of the peak plasma drug concentration when a high peak concentration is related to the occurrence of adverse effects. For example, slow-release formulations of lithium and paroxetine reduce gastrointestinal side effects (DeVane 2003). Alternatively, rapid absorption may be desirable to achieve immediate pharmacological effects.

Distribution

Drug distribution to tissues begins almost simultaneously with absorption into the systemic circulation. The rate at which distribution occurs will partially influence the onset of pharmacological response. Access to effect sites depends on membrane permeability, the patient's state of hydration, regional blood flow, and other physiological variables. There is increasing evidence that drug transporters in the blood–brain barrier influence drug passage to and accumulation in the brain. Sadeque et al. (2000) demonstrated that loperamide, a potent opiate used to reduce gut motility and not normally distributed to the CNS, produced typical opiate depressant effects on respiratory drive when coadministered with quinidine, a P-gp inhibitor. Physicochemical properties influencing the rate of drug distribution to effect sites include lipid solubility, ionizability, and affinity for plasma proteins and tissue components. Diazepam is highly lipophilic, and its onset of effect is rapid as a result of its entry into the brain within minutes after oral administration (Greenblatt et al. 1980). The concentration of diazepam at its effect site may fall so precipitously as a result of redistribution that its duration of action after an initial dose is shorter than would be expected based on its elimination half-life.

Frequently, the intensity and duration of the pharmacological effect of a second drug dose, taken immediately after cessation of the effect of the first dose, are greater and longer, respectively, than the intensity and duration of the effect of the first dose. This is known as the *second-dose effect* in pharmacokinetics (DeVane and Liston 2001). When dosing is repeated before the previous dose has been eliminated from the body, the second and subsequent doses produce a greater effect than the initial dose, but the relative intensity of subsequent doses diminishes. This second-dose effect occurs, regardless of the half-life of the drug, when dosing is repeated in response to the observed effect. Common examples of this phenomenon include the self-administration of caffeine and the administration of certain anesthetics.

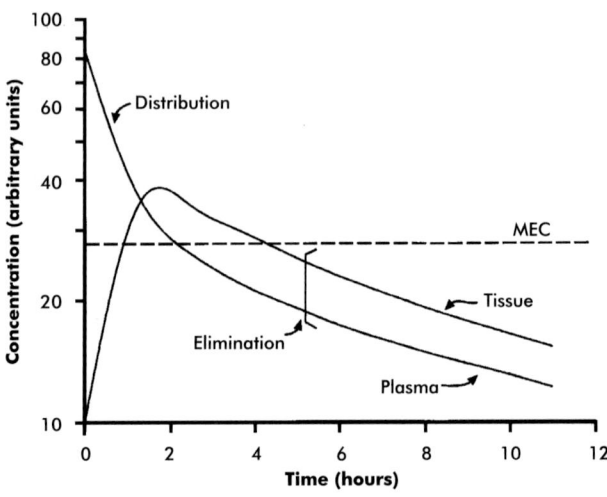

FIGURE 8–3. Predicted concentration of a drug in plasma and tissue following a rapid intravenous injection.

MEC=minimal effective concentration.

The predicted time course of drug concentration in plasma and in tissue following a single intravenous drug injection is shown in Figure 8–3. Drug concentration in plasma rapidly declines in a manner consistent with the extensive distribution of the compound out of the systemic circulation. Drug concentration in tissue rapidly increases during this time. Pharmacological effects may not occur immediately but may be delayed until the tissue concentration at the effect site rises above an MEC. An equilibrium eventually occurs between drug in plasma and in tissue. Concentrations from this time forth decline in parallel during a terminal elimination phase.

The observed time course of drug concentration changes in plasma has frequently been considered in the pharmacokinetic literature to confer the characteristics on the body of a two-compartment mathematical model (Gibaldi and Perrier 1975). Many drugs appear to be absorbed into a central compartment composed of the circulation and rapidly equilibrating tissues and then distributed to less accessible tissues, which collectively form a peripheral compartment. This compartmentalization of drug concentration greatly aids mathematical analysis of pharmacokinetic data but is clearly an oversimplification, because drug concentrations determined in animal studies can vary over orders of magnitude among different tissues (DeVane and Simpkins 1985).

Even though the drug concentration can vary widely among tissues, equilibrium eventually occurs between drug concentration in plasma and in tissue (see Figure 8–

| Plasma | Tissue |

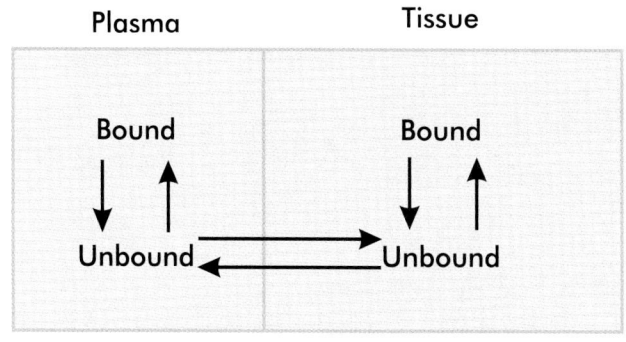

FIGURE 8–4. Effect of protein binding on distribution of drug between plasma and tissue.

3). The concentration of drug in brain tissue may be substantially different—higher or lower—from that in plasma, but renal and hepatic elimination of drug from the central compartment reducing the plasma drug concentration should be mirrored by a proportional reduction of drug concentration from the brain or other tissues. For this reason, an MEC determined from plasma data may reflect an MEC at the effect site. The distribution of a drug in the body largely depends on the drug's relative binding affinity to plasma proteins and tissue components and the capacity of tissues for drug binding. This pharmacokinetic principle is illustrated in Figure 8–4. Only unbound drug is capable of distributing between plasma and tissues. Different degrees of plasma protein binding among antidepressants, for example, cannot be used to draw valid conclusions about the availability of drug to exert pharmacological effects at the site of action (DeVane 1994). The nonspecific binding of drugs to tissue components complicates the interpretation of the significance of plasma protein–binding differences among drugs. Drug binding in tissues cannot be measured directly in vivo and must be inferred using mathematical models and/or in vitro methods.

Most drugs circulate in the blood bound to plasma proteins, principally albumin or alpha-1-acid glycoprotein. Many psychotropic drugs are highly protein bound, frequently to a degree greater than 90%. Displacement of drug from plasma protein–binding sites may result from drug–drug interactions. This situation should lead to more unbound drug being available for distribution to peripheral tissues and interaction with receptor sites (see Figure 8–4). As a result, potentially greater pharmacological effects, either beneficial or detrimental, may be expected. However, there are few documented examples in which the above events occurred with psychoactive drugs

and led to significant clinical consequences. Compensatory changes occur in the body to buffer the impact of drug-binding interactions (DeVane 2002). When plasma protein binding is restrictive regarding the drug's hepatic and/or renal elimination, the increased free drug concentration in plasma will be a transient effect as more free (non-protein-bound) drug becomes available to routes of elimination. Total (bound plus free) drug concentration in plasma will eventually return to a predisplacement value. The conclusion of several authoritative reviews is that plasma protein–binding displacement interactions are rarely a major source of variability in psychopharmacology (DeVane 2002; Greenblatt et al. 1982; Rolan 1994; Sellers 1979).

Elimination

Drugs are eliminated or cleared from the body through renal excretion in an unchanged or conjugated form; through biotransformation, primarily in the liver, to polar metabolites; or through both of these mechanisms (see Figure 8–1). *Clearance* is defined as the volume of blood or other fluid from which drug is irreversibly removed per unit of time. Thus, clearance units are volume per time. Drug clearance is analogous to creatinine clearance by the kidney. From the blood that delivers drug to the liver, or any other eliminating organ, an extraction occurs as blood travels through the organ. Because drug extraction by the liver and other organs is rarely 100%, the portion that escapes presystemic elimination reaches the systemic circulation intact. Plasma protein binding, as mentioned above, can restrict the organ extraction process, depending on the specific drug. If a drug were to be completely extracted, then clearance would equal the blood flow to the organ. An average hepatic blood flow is 1,500 mL/minute. When drug is eliminated by additional organs, the total clearance is an additive function of all the individual organ clearances. Clearance values reported in excess of 1,500 mL/minute for many psychopharmacological drugs are reflective of presystemic elimination (DeVane 1994). When the drug dose and bioavailability are constant, then clearance is the pharmacokinetic parameter that determines the extent of drug accumulation in the body to a steady state. In contrast, elimination half-life is useful to reflect the rate, but not the extent, of drug accumulation.

Elimination half-life is defined as the time required for the amount of drug in the body, or drug concentration, to decline by 50%. This parameter is commonly determined after a single-dose pharmacokinetic study or after drug discontinuation in a multiple-dose study. In either situation, drug concentration decline in plasma can be followed by multiple blood sampling. Half-life is easily determined by graphical means or by inspection, as long as data are used from the terminal log-linear portion of the elimination curve (see Figures 8–2 and 8–3). Knowledge of a drug's elimination half-life is particularly useful for designing multiple-dosing regimens.

Multiple Dosing to Steady State

Multiple drug doses usually are required in the pharmacotherapy of mental illness. During a multiple-dosing regimen, second and subsequent drug doses are usually administered before sufficient time has elapsed for the initial dose to be completely eliminated from the body. This process results in drug accumulation, as illustrated in Figure 8–5. When drug elimination follows a linear or first-order process, the amount of drug eliminated over time is proportional to the amount of drug available for elimination (Gibaldi and Perrier 1975). Accumulation does not occur indefinitely; rather, it reaches a steady state. A *steady state* exists when the amount of drug entering the body is equal to the amount leaving the body. From a practical standpoint, this definition means that after a period of continuous dosing, the body retains a pool of drug molecules from several doses, and the drug eliminated each day is replaced by an equivalent amount of newly administered drug. The time required from the first administered dose to the point at which an approximate steady state occurs is equivalent to the total of four to five elimination half-lives. The same amount of time is required for a new steady state to be achieved after an increase or decrease in the daily dosing rate or for a drug to wash out of the body after dosing is discontinued (see Figure 8–5).

The term *steady state* is a misnomer in that a true drug steady state occurs only with a constant-rate intravenous infusion. Because of the concurrent processes of drug absorption, distribution, and elimination, drug concentration is constantly changing in plasma and tissues during an oral dosing regimen. A peak and a trough concentration occur within each dosage interval. The average steady-state concentration occurs somewhere between these extremes and is determined by the daily dose and the drug's total body clearance for that individual.

On reaching a steady-state concentration, the average concentration and the magnitude of the peaks and troughs may be manipulated according to established pharmacokinetic principles. Figure 8–6 shows the predicted plasma concentration changes based on drug doses given every

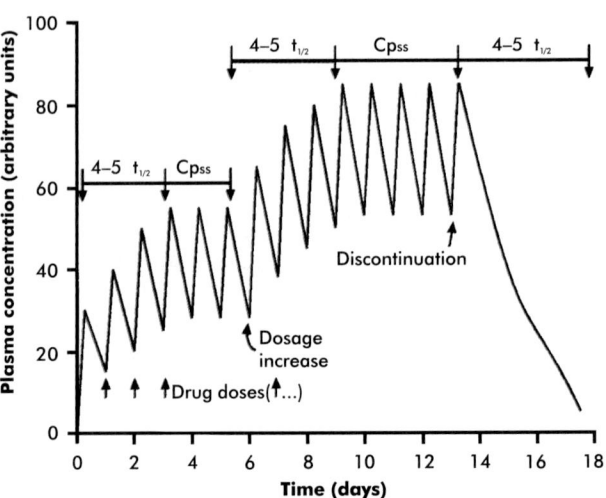

FIGURE 8–5. Accumulation of drug during multiple dosing.

It takes four to five half-lives (4–5 $t_{1/2}$) to achieve initial steady state (Cp_{ss}) on a constant dosage regimen, to achieve a new steady state after an increase in dosage, or to wash out drug from the body after discontinuation. The average steady-state concentration lies somewhere between the peaks and troughs of drug concentration during a dosage interval.

24 hours. The selected dose does not produce a high enough average steady-state concentration to reach the desired concentration range between an MEC and a concentration threshold associated with an increased risk of toxicity. By doubling the dose and keeping the dosage interval constant, the average steady-state concentration increases, but the magnitude of the peak and trough concentration difference also increases. These changes are consistent with the pharmacokinetic principles of superposition and linearity (Gibaldi and Perrier 1975).

Linearity refers to maintaining a stable clearance across the usual dosage range. Within the linear dose range, the magnitude of a dosage increase results in a proportional change in steady-state concentration (see Figure 8–6). The magnitude of the dose change theoretically superimposes on the new peak and trough concentration. In Figure 8–6, doubling the daily dose results in an adequate average steady-state concentration, but the new peak and trough concentration values cause both an increased risk of toxicity and an inadequate concentration declining below the MEC for a portion of each dosage interval. An alternative is to increase the total daily dose and divide it into more frequent administrations. This is accomplished by administering the original dose every 12 hours instead of every 24 hours. The new average steady-state concentration remains within the desired range, and

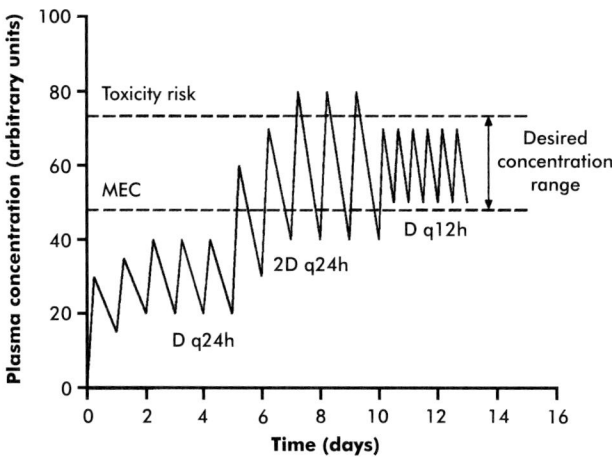

FIGURE 8-6. Predicted plasma concentration changes from administering either a selected dose (D) every 24 hours (D q24h), twice the dose every 24 hours (2D q24h), or the original dose every 12 hours (D q12h).

MEC = minimal effective concentration.

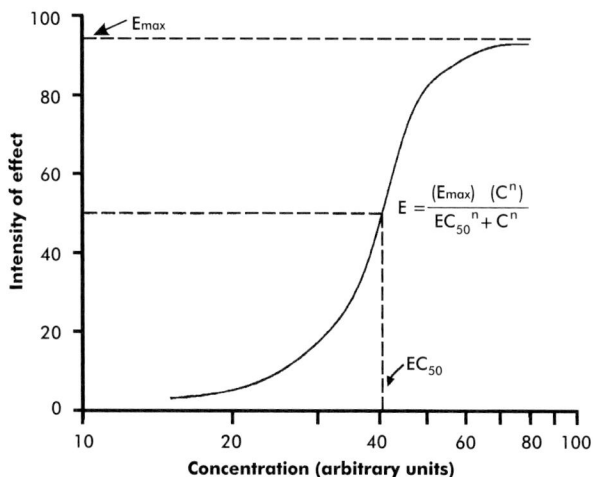

FIGURE 8-7. The sigmoid maximum effect (E_{max}) pharmacodynamic model relates concentration (C) to intensity of effect (E).

EC_{50} is the concentration that produces half of the E_{max}, and n is an exponent that relates to the shape of the curve.

the differences between the peak and trough concentrations are reduced to an acceptable fluctuation.

Selection of a proper drug dosage regimen must consider both the amount of drug administered and the frequency of administration. Some drugs with half-lives long enough to be administered once daily may not be suitable for administration every 24 hours because toxicity may be precipitated by an excessive peak concentration in a single dose. Examples include lithium and clozapine. Once-daily dosing with lithium may produce gastrointestinal intolerance, and clozapine is dosed two or more times each day to avoid peak concentrations that might predispose to seizure activity. Bupropion was initially formulated to be dosed multiple times a day to avoid high peak concentrations in plasma for this same reason but reformulation into an extended-release tablet allows once-daily administration. When high peak concentration is tolerable, then the dosage interval can theoretically be extended beyond 1 day by giving larger amounts of drug in single doses less frequently. This principle applies to fluoxetine, which is available as a 90-mg capsule for once-weekly administration.

Pharmacodynamics

Pharmacodynamic variability may exceed pharmacokinetic variability (see Figure 8–1). The drug dose or concentration that produces a pharmacological effect differs widely among patients. Similarly, pharmacological effects can vary widely among patients with a comparable plasma concentration of drug.

The principles of dosage regimen design discussed above rely heavily on the existence of a functional relationship between the concentration at an effect site and the intensity of the response produced. Many observed processes in nature behave according to the sigmoid relationship shown in Figure 8–7. At a low dose or concentration, only a marginal effect is produced. As drug dose or concentration increases, the intensity of effect (E) increases until a maximum effect (E_{max}) is achieved. This response is observed as a plateau in the sigmoid dose–effect curve (see Figure 8–7). Further dosage increases do not produce a greater effect.

The sigmoid dose–effect relationship in Figure 8–7 has practical applications to psychopharmacology. The increase in drug response that results from an increase in dosage depends on the shape and steepness of the theoretical dose–response curve for each patient and the starting point on the curve when a dosage is changed. At low doses or concentrations, a substantial dose increase may be necessary to achieve an effect. In a linear part of the relationship, dosage increases should result in proportional increases in effect. In the higher dose or concentration range, a further increase will not produce a significant increase in effect because of diminishing returns. This phenomenon is likely caused by the saturation of enzyme-binding sites or receptors by drug molecules above a critical concentration.

The general equation shown in Figure 8–7 describes the sigmoid relationship between concentration and response (i.e., intensity of effect). The response is usually measured as a percentage change or the difference from the baseline effect. C is the drug concentration, and EC_{50} is the effective concentration that produces half of the E_{max}. Theoretically, n is an integer reflecting the number of molecules that bind to a specific drug receptor. Practically, it is a parameter that determines the sigmoid shape of the concentration–effect relationship. Pharmacokinetic–pharmacodynamic models have found wide application in psychopharmacology—for example, relating concentration to electroencephalogram parameters, psychomotor reaction times, and subjective effects from drugs of abuse (Dingemanse et al. 1988).

Drugs rarely have a single pharmacological effect or interact with only a single receptor population or molecular target. Drugs generally have affinity for multiple receptors; therefore, several theoretical concentration–effect relationships can exist for a given drug. Dose–response curves are shown in Figure 8–8 for a drug that produces a therapeutic effect and mild and severe toxicity. The greater the separation between the curves for therapeutic and toxic effects, the more safely the drug can be administered in increasing doses to achieve therapeutic goals. Estimates of these interrelationships are made in preclinical animal studies and Phase I human studies for drugs in development. In clinical practice, the degree of separation between these curves and their steepness will show both inter- and intraindividual variability. Concurrent medical illness may predispose patients to side effects by effectively causing a shift to the left in one or both of the concentration–toxicity curves. This narrows the range over which doses can be safely administered without incurring adverse effects. The EC_{50} in Figure 8–8 produces negligible toxicity. Increasing the concentration with a dosage increase to gain an increased response can only be accomplished at the expense of mild toxicity. As the dosage and concentration increase, therapeutic effects approach a plateau, and small increments in concentration result in a disproportionate change in toxicity.

The pharmacodynamic relationships considered above are most reproducible when pharmacological effects are direct and closely related to plasma concentration. In Figure 8–9, the concentration–effect relationship is shown as a function of drug concentration changes over time. In Figure 8–9A, the changes in effect are almost superimposable with the increase and decrease in concen-

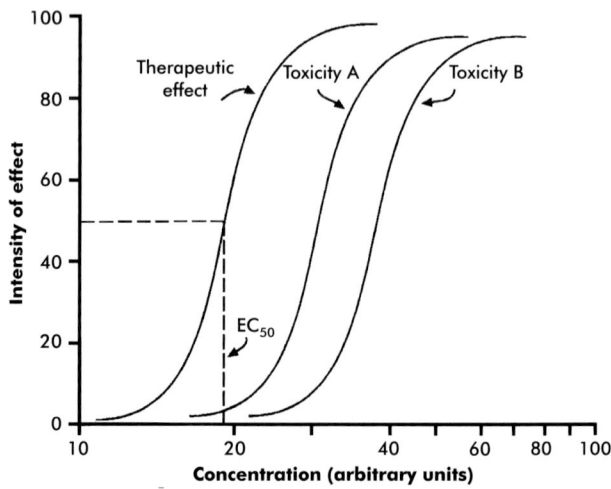

FIGURE 8–8. Concentration–effect curves for a drug that produces a therapeutic effect and mild (A) and severe (B) toxicity.

The concentration is shown for a therapeutic effect that produces 50% of the maximum effect (EC_{50}).

tration. This type of relationship often reflects a direct action of the drug with a single receptor. This straightforward relationship is generally not observed in psychopharmacology.

In Figure 8–9B, the response has begun to diminish with time before concentration begins to decline. This type of plot is known as a *clockwise hysteresis curve*. The observed effect may be explained by the development of tolerance. The time course of tolerance to psychoactive drug effects varies from minutes to weeks. Acute tolerance to some euphoric effects of cocaine can occur following a single dose (Foltin and Fischman 1991). Tolerance to the sedative effects of various drugs may take weeks. The mechanisms operative in the development of tolerance include acute depletion of a neurotransmitter or cofactor, homeostatic changes in receptor sensitivity from blockade of various transporters, or receptor agonist or antagonist effects. Ultimately, cellular responses to chronic treatment with drugs can alter gene transcription factors as mediators of physical and psychological aspects of tolerance (Nestler 1993).

A time delay in response occurs when effects are increasing and are maintained despite decreasing plasma drug concentration (see Figure 8–9C). This results in a *counterclockwise hysteresis curve*. A pharmacokinetic explanation of this lag in response may involve a delay in reaching the critical drug MEC at the effect site until the plasma concentration has already begun to decline. Alternatively, response may depend on multiple "downstream"

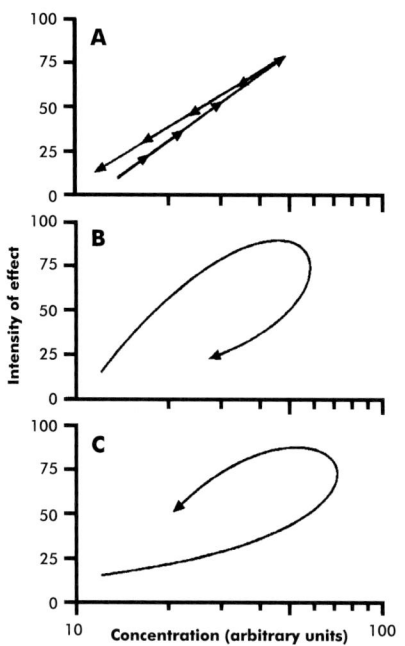

FIGURE 8–9. Theoretical relationships of drug concentration versus intensity of effect.

Drug concentration changes occur in the direction of the arrow. Effects superimposable on concentration changes (**A**) suggest a direct and reversible interaction between drug and receptor, a clockwise hysteresis curve (**B**) suggests the development of tolerance, and a counterclockwise curve (**C**) suggests an indirect effect or the presence of an active metabolite.

receptor effects. This theory likely accounts for the counterclockwise hysteresis curve observed between plasma drug concentration and growth hormone response in plasma after an intravenous alprazolam challenge (Osman et al. 1991). Response may increase despite a decreasing drug concentration when a metabolite contributes to the observed effects. To overcome these complications, kinetic dynamic models can incorporate an "effect" compartment (see Figure 8–1). The effect site equilibrates with plasma after a finite time, which can be assigned a half-life. Models can also incorporate the presence of metabolites (Dingemanse et al. 1988).

Variability in the Dose–Effect Relationship

A major challenge of treating mental illness with drugs is that both pharmacokinetic and pharmacodynamic variability complicate the dose–effect relationship. The presence of active metabolites, the influence of pharmacogenetics, and the effects of combining two or more drugs

contribute to variability. Noncompliance with the prescribed treatment plan on the part of the patient can seriously undermine reliability in the expected effects from pharmacotherapy. Physiological differences between patients are another source of variability. The effects of age, weight, and hepatic and other disease states are major factors in pharmacokinetics and pharmacodynamics that indicate the need for individualization of therapy.

Active Metabolites

With the exceptions of lithium and gabapentin, which are renally excreted, drugs used in clinical psychopharmacology are cleared partially or completely by metabolism, primarily in the liver. Many psychoactive drugs produce pharmacologically active metabolites that distribute to the effect sites (see Figure 8–1) to produce pharmacological effects. Like their precursors, metabolites may have multiple pharmacological effects that may be similar to or different from those of the parent drug. Sertraline's metabolite, desmethylsertraline, has about 10% of the activity of sertraline in inhibiting the serotonin (5-HT) transporter, but the metabolite is equipotent with sertraline in its affinity for the hepatic isoenzyme CYP2D6 (Fuller et al. 1995). The major metabolite of risperidone, 9-hydroxyrisperidone, has pharmacological effects similar to its precursor as a dopamine type 2 (D_2) and serotonin type 2 (5-HT_2) antagonist but differs in its affinity for and inhibition of the drug transporter P-gp (Zhu et al. 2007).

When switching therapy from one drug or drug class to another, the presence of any active metabolites should be considered (Garattini 1985). Norfluoxetine, for example, has an average half-life of 8–9 days, much longer than the average of 2–3 days for fluoxetine, its parent drug (DeVane 1994), and is an equipotent serotonin reuptake inhibitor. It may take several weeks for this metabolite to clear the body after discontinuation of fluoxetine (Pato et al. 1991). A similar situation applies to aripiprazole and its active metabolite, dehydro-aripiprazole, which have elimination half-lives of 75 hours and 94 hours, respectively.

Metabolites will accumulate to a steady state in the body in relation to their elimination half-lives and not those of their parent drugs. For a drug that is nearly completely metabolized in the liver, a characteristic of numerous psychoactive drugs, the produced metabolites will always have an elimination half-life that is equal to or longer than the half-life of the parent drug. This is a logical conclusion of considering that a metabolite cannot be eliminated faster than it is formed. Of course, administration of the metabolite as a separate molecular entity apart from the parent drug would produce a drug concentration–time curve independent of any influence of the metabolite being formed from a precursor in vivo. For some drugs, the full expression of direct pharmacological effects may not be expected until both the drug and any important active metabolites have all attained their steady-state concentration. For drugs producing indirect effects when the response depends on second messengers or a cascade of receptor actions, the waiting period for fully expressed effects may be even longer.

Stereochemistry

Stereochemistry or chirality of drug molecules is an increasingly important consideration in pharmacokinetics. Many psychoactive drugs exist as two or more stereoisomers or enantiomers with distinctly different biological properties and are marketed as the racemic (i.e., 50:50) mixtures of both isomers. Although enantiomers have identical physicochemical properties, they are often recognized as distinct entities by biological systems and may bind to transport proteins, drug-metabolizing enzymes, and pharmacological effect sites with different affinities. As a result, one enantiomer may possess a significant pharmacological effect, while the other stereoisomer may lack similar effects or produce different effects. Enantiomers may also differ in their absorption, metabolism, protein binding, and excretion, leading to substantial differences in pharmacokinetic properties (DeVane and Boulton 2002). Furthermore, one isomer may modify the effects of the other.

The development of single-isomer drugs may offer advantages over use of the racemic mixture. Potential advantages include a less complex and more selective pharmacological profile, a potential for an improved therapeutic index, a more simplified pharmacokinetic profile, a reduced potential for complex drug interactions, and a more definable relationship between plasma drug concentration and effect. Examples of racemic mixtures in current use include methadone, methylphenidate, bupropion, venlafaxine, fluoxetine, and citalopram. Clearly, each drug needs to be considered individually with regard to its development as a single stereoisomer formulation. Recent examples of successful switches to single isomers are escitalopram and dexmethylphenidate.

Pharmacogenetics

Inheritance accounts for a large part of the variations observed in the ability to eliminate drugs (see Figure 8–1) among individuals. This forms the basis of *pharmacogenet-*

ics, which is defined as the study of the genetic contribution to the variability in drug response (Kalow et al. 1986; Price Evans 1993). This term was originally applied to the effect on pharmacokinetics, while pharmacogenomics dealt specifically with genes mediating drug response. More recently, the terms have been used interchangeably. Numerous association studies have been performed of genetic polymorphisms of molecular targets as predictors of disease susceptibility, specific drug response, and tolerability. This topic is covered in the chapter addressing pharmacogenomics (see Chapter 3, "Genetics and Genomics"). The genetic differences in pharmacokinetics that have been detected apply mostly to drug metabolism. The renal clearance of drugs appears to be similar in age- and weight-matched healthy subjects with no defined genetic polymorphisms. Genetic polymorphisms have been identified and defined for some drug transporters, primarily P-gp, and several hepatic enzymes important for the cellular transport and metabolism of many drugs used in psychopharmacology. These genetic polymorphisms are summarized in Table 8–2.

P-gp, as the most thoroughly studied drug transporter, appears to be significantly involved in the disposition of a variety of psychoactive drugs (Mahar Doan et al. 2002) (see Table 8–2). More than 70 polymorphisms have been reported in the *ABCB1* gene that encodes for P-gp, and three single-nucleotide polymorphisms (SNPs) of P-gp have been associated with functional changes in P-gp activity. The majority of SNP-related reports focus on the silent C3435T SNP of exon 26. It has been associated with changes in expression resulting in increased serum concentrations of digoxin and fexofenadine (Hoffmeyer et al. 2000; Kurata et al. 2002). There is emerging evidence that haplotypes of P-gp SNPs may influence drug-resistant epilepsy (Siddiqui et al. 2003), access of drugs to the brain (Brunner et al. 2005), and placental transfer of psychoactive drugs (Rahi et al. 2007). Theoretically, P-gp substrates may act as competitive inhibitors of P-gp, so that drug–drug interactions may also involve P-gp (Wang et al. 2006).

Genetic polymorphism in a drug-metabolizing enzyme can result in subpopulations of people who may deviate substantially from the population mean in their ability to metabolize substrates of the affected enzyme. People who are poor metabolizers constitute at least 1% of the population, but the majority of people are normal or rapid metabolizers, and some are identified as ultrarapid metabolizers due to duplicate or multiple genes. The genetic polymorphisms in listed Table 8–2 were identified mostly as a result of adverse drug reactions to typical drug

TABLE 8–2. Some genetically determined variations influencing drug pharmacokinetics

PROTEIN (MAJOR POLYMORPHISMS)	FREQUENCY OF POOR METABOLIZERS OR DYSFUNCTIONAL PHENOTYPES	CLINICAL CONSEQUENCES	EXAMPLE SUBSTRATES
P-glycoprotein (T1236C, G2677T, C3435T)	Unknown	Increased drug bioavailability	Digoxin, fexofenadine, methadone, olanzapine, aripiprazole, risperidone, paliperidone, citalopram, sertraline, amitriptyline, buspirone, clozapine, fluvoxamine, haloperidol, nortriptyline, venlafaxine
CYP2D6	5%–10% Caucasians 3% Blacks 1% Asians 1% Arabs	High drug concentrations; possible toxicity	Desipramine, nortriptyline, codeine, dextromethorphan
CYP2C9	10% Caucasians 1%–3% Blacks 0%–2% Asians	Reduced substrate clearance	Tolbutamide, S-warfarin, phenytoin
CYP2C19	3%–5% Caucasians 15%–20% Asians	High drug concentrations; increased sedation and possible toxicity	Diazepam, S-mephenytoin
NAT-2	40%–60% Caucasians 10%–20% Asians and Eskimos	Greater toxicity; peripheral neuritis; skin eruptions	Procainamide, hydralazine
Plasma cholinesterase	<1%; many atypical cholinesterase forms	Prolonged apnea	Succinylcholine

Note. CYP=cytochrome P450; NAT-2=*N*-acetyltransferase 2.

Source. Kalow and Genest 1957; Lockridge 1990; Meyer et al. 1990; Price Evans 1993; Relling et al. 1991.

doses. Subsequent studies have used debrisoquine, sparteine, and dextromethorphan as probe drugs to calculate a metabolic ratio (MR) as an index of the relative ability of an individual to metabolize CYP2D6 substrates, thereby providing a phenotype identity. The MR is equal to the concentration of parent drug divided by the concentration of the major metabolite determined in the urine excreted during a timed interval following an oral dose. Similar methodology has been applied to study the metabolism of prototype substrates for a variety of hepatic enzymes (Price Evans 1993).

The results of many pharmacogenetic studies appear similar to the frequency distribution histograms in Figure 8–10. The frequency in Figure 8–10A is expected when enzyme activity is distributed normally within a population without genetic polymorphisms. The range of values for the MR may be broad, which reflects a large variability in oxidation reaction capacity in the study population. Thus, vastly different dosages are required for many patients. The bimodal distribution in Figure 8–10B is a typical finding for an enzyme that has a genetic polymorphism. Values above the antimode for the reference (or "probe") drug define poor metabolizers, who are clearly differentiated from normal or extensive metabolizers. The probe drug need not be metabolized by only one enzyme, which characterizes the use of caffeine for phenotyping the enzyme activity of *N*-acetyltransferase and CYP1A2, but the overlap of other enzymes should be minimal to produce the specific metabolite of interest (Denaro et al. 1996). Comparison of MRs between many patients of different ethnic origins has yielded measures of variability in enzyme activity in the population (Lin et al. 1996). The widespread availability of a commercial microarray chip for genotyping limited CYP enzymes has eliminated the need to perform phenotyping procedures in most circumstances. While a genotypical extensive metabolizer may be phenotypically a poor metabolizer, the opposite situation does not occur.

The potential clinical consequences of being a poor metabolizer will vary according to the activity of the administered drug and any active metabolites. When the

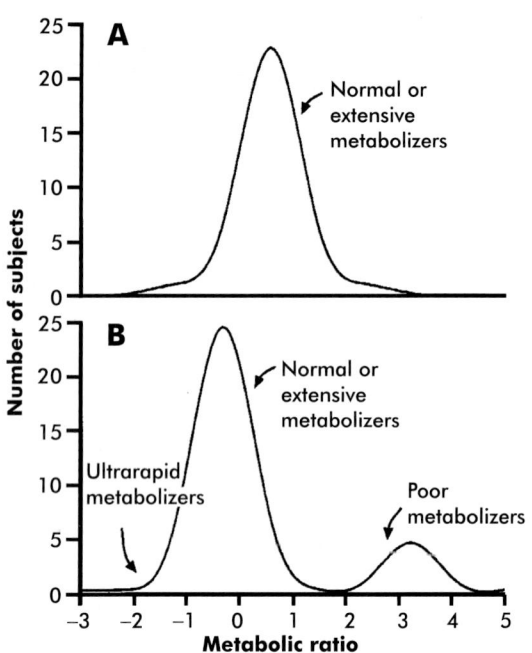

FIGURE 8–10. Theoretical frequency histograms of the distribution of the metabolic ratio of a model substrate showing a unimodal distribution among a population of normal or extensive metabolizers (A) and a bimodal distribution among a population including poor metabolizers and ultrarapid metabolizers (B).

drug is active and a pathway is affected (a situation that usually produces an inactive metabolite), higher drug concentrations can be expected. This result can lead to an exaggerated response and potential toxicity. The most serious consequences would be expected from drugs with a narrow therapeutic window (see Table 8–1). For example, when perphenazine (a drug with a narrow therapeutic window) was given to elderly patients who were poor metabolizers of CYP2D6, extrapyramidal side effects were exaggerated (Pollock et al. 1995). If the therapeutic effects depend on the formation of an active metabolite, diminished response can be expected from a lower concentration of metabolite in poor metabolizers. For example, normal doses of codeine, which is partially metabolized to the more potent morphine, may provide an inadequate analgesic effect.

For CYP2D6, the poor-metabolizer status is inherited as an autosomal recessive trait. At least 70 different alleles have been defined for the *CYP2D6* gene, and many types of null mutations result in impaired CYP2D6 activity (Gonzalez and Idle 1994). Methods based on polymerase chain reaction (PCR) have a high sensitivity for detecting the mutant alleles and can establish a genotype. This procedure can be beneficial in drug development to test compounds that are CYP2D6 substrates and in some forensic circumstances to help establish the cause of excessive drug concentrations. Genetic phenotyping is potentially more clinically useful than genotyping and can be done when patients are drug free to characterize their relative ability to metabolize CYP2D6 substrates. About 1% of Caucasians are ultrarapid metabolizers because of an amplification of the functional *CYP2D6* gene (Johansson et al. 1993). These patients have the lowest MR when phenotyped with a CYP2D6 substrate with a high urinary concentration of metabolite and a low parent drug concentration (see Figure 8–10B). The implication is that these individuals will often require very high drug doses. Research is needed to support phenotyping and genotyping as an aid in the initial selection of drugs and drug doses for individualizing medicine.

Of the human cytochrome P450 enzymes, three families (CYP1, CYP2, and CYP3) are involved in drug metabolism (Guengerich 1992; Wrighton and Stevens 1992). The enzymes most relevant to psychopharmacology were listed in Table 8–1. Interindividual differences in the expression and catalytic activities of cytochrome P450 result in a large variation in the in vivo metabolism of drugs. The average immunoquantified levels of the various specific P450 enzymes in 60 human liver microsomal samples were reported by Shimada et al. (1994). Benet et al. (1996) and Wrighton and Stevens (1992) estimated the participation of the liver cytochrome P450 enzymes in drug metabolism based on known substrates and pathways (see Table 8–1). These values are compared in Table 8–3. CYP3A has the highest level of P450 in the liver and participates in the metabolism of the largest number of drugs. Together, CYP3A and CYP2D6 participate in the metabolism of an estimated 80% of currently used drugs.

In 2004, the U.S. Food and Drug Administration approved the AmpliChip CYP450 Test (Roche Diagnostics Corporation, Indianapolis, IN) as a regulated pharmacogenetic test. This device uses a DNA microarray platform to assess the presence of the polymorphic form of the *CYP2D6* and *CYP2C19* genes. As these enzymes metabolize a substantial number of psychoactive drugs, use of this device should facilitate individualized medicine in psychiatry. Unfortunately, research demonstrating a clinical benefit from use of this technology is lacking.

In summary, recent pharmacogenetic investigations have yielded fruitful data relating to the causes of pharmacokinetic variability in the dose–effect relationship. The polymorphism of molecular drug targets in the brain

TABLE 8–3. Comparison of average immunoquantified levels of the various cytochrome P450 (CYP) enzymes in liver microsomes, with their estimated participation in drug metabolism

CYP ENZYME	AVERAGE IMMUNOQUANTIFIED LEVEL IN HUMAN LIVER MICROSOMAL SAMPLES (%)[a]	ESTIMATED PARTICIPATION IN DRUG METABOLISM (%)[b]
1A2	13	<10
2A6	4	<10
2B6	0.2	(Marginal)
2E1	7	<10
2C	18	10
2D6	1.5	30
3A	29	50
Unidentified	27.3	
Total	100	

[a]Shimada et al. 1994.
[b]Benet et al. 1996; Wrighton and Stevens 1992.

is a source of pharmacodynamic variability. This topic is covered in the chapter addressing pharmacogenomics (see Chapter 3, "Genetics and Genomics"). Pharmacogenetic studies have extensively used metabolic phenotyping with model substrates for specific enzymes to characterize several genetic polymorphisms (see Table 8–2). The practical implications of metabolic phenotyping are most meaningful when the metabolic pathways of therapeutically administered drugs are known and when drug concentration has been correlated to either therapeutic or toxic effects (Gonzalez and Idle 1994). In this situation, knowledge of enzyme activity will serve as a guide to initial dosing and also allow a prediction of the significance of potential drug–drug interactions.

Drug Interactions

Drugs are frequently coadministered to achieve therapeutic effects from the combined actions at effect sites or to treat the adverse effects caused by one drug with another. Drug combinations routinely used include hypnotics with antidepressants, anticholinergic–antiparkinsonian drugs with antipsychotics, benzodiazepines with SSRIs, and mood stabilizers with antipsychotics. The use of more than one antidepressant or antipsychotic in combination for specific patients is increasingly encountered in clinical practice (Papakostas et al. 2007). When more than one drug is administered concurrently to a patient, the drugs may interact either in a positive manner or in a negative or undesired way because of either pharmacodynamic or pharmacokinetic mechanisms.

Pharmacodynamic interactions are likely to occur when the combination of an MAO inhibitor and an SSRI produces a serotonin syndrome and when the combination of ethanol and a benzodiazepine leads to psychomotor impairment. Two drugs may have affinity for the same receptor sites in the brain and produce additive or synergistic effects, or their actions may oppose each other through antagonistic interactions at receptor sites. Most often, pharmacodynamic mechanisms are not such obvious causes of drug interactions and are usually less easily determined and investigated than pharmacokinetic interactions.

The kinetics of drug interactions has been extensively described and is a routine focus of clinical investigations as part of drug development (Brosen 1996; Rowland and Matin 1973). Two major mechanisms of drug interactions involve an alteration of metabolism through either induction or inhibition of hepatic cytochrome P450 enzymes. Major differences exist in the pharmacokinetic consequences of these interactions. The expected changes are illustrated in Figures 8–11 and 8–12. In Figure 8–11, the steady-state plasma concentration of drug A following continuous intermittent dosing is altered by the addition of an enzyme inducer. After the inducer is started, the effects on the steady-state concentration of drug A do not occur for several days while additional enzyme that metabolizes drug A is synthesized. Ultimately, an increase in the metabolic clearance of drug A accompanied by a decrease in its steady-state plasma concentration occurs. The degree to which clearance is increased will depend on the relative importance of the particular induced enzymes

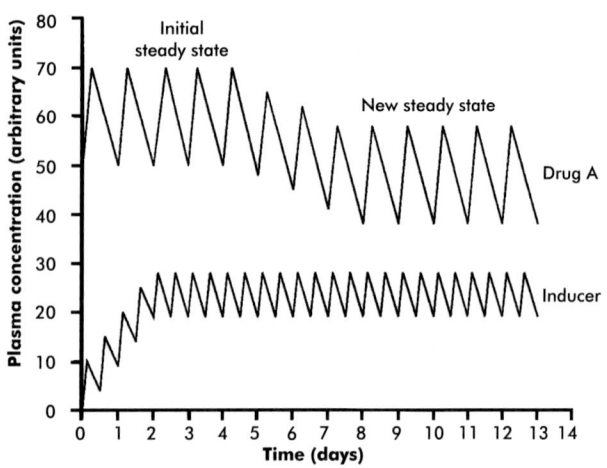

FIGURE 8-11. Predicted plasma concentration changes from the coadministration of an inducer of the metabolism of drug A.

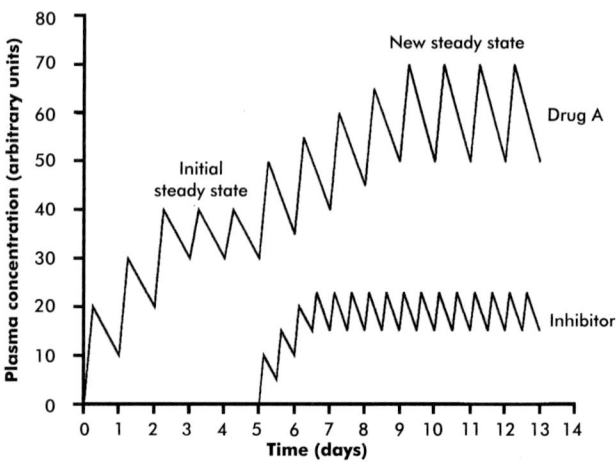

FIGURE 8-12. Predicted plasma concentration changes from the coadministration of an inhibitor of the metabolism of drug A.

in the overall elimination of drug A and the dose and potency of the inducer. A clinically significant example of this type of interaction is the loss of oral contraceptive effect by carbamazepine induction of CYP3A4. The time required for a new steady state of drug A to occur following enzyme induction and the extent to which plasma concentrations decrease will depend on how marked a change in clearance occurs and the resulting change in drug half-life.

In contrast to the delayed effects of an inducer on drug A, the addition of an inhibitor causes an immediate increase in the plasma concentration of drug A (see Figure 8–12). This increase occurs as a result of a competitive inhibition of the relevant hepatic enzyme. Drug A's plasma concentration rises to a new steady state consistent with a change in its clearance. The time required to achieve the new steady state is greater than the time to achieve the initial steady state, because the half-life is now prolonged relative to its original value. The full effect of an inhibitory interaction may not be realized until the inhibitor also reaches a steady state, because the degree of inhibition will also depend on the concentration of the inhibitor (Houston 1994; von Moltke et al. 1994, 1995).

Drug interactions are graded phenomena. The degree of interaction depends on the concentration of interacting drugs and, therefore, on the dose and timing of administration. Drug interactions are most likely to be detected when therapy with an interacting drug is initiated or discontinued. The clinical significance will depend on the particular drugs involved, the physiological state of the patient, the presence of concurrent illness, and other fac-

tors. Drugs with a narrow concentration range over which therapeutic effects are present without incurring toxicity are more likely to be involved in clinically significant drug interactions. These drugs include theophylline, some antiepileptic drugs, and antiarrhythmics (see Table 8–1).

When selecting a specific drug from a class of drugs to treat mental illness, its efficacy, safety, cost, and history of response are pertinent considerations. The introduction of the SSRIs has emphasized the critical importance of also considering potential drug interactions (Brosen 1996). Some of these antidepressants have been shown in vitro and in vivo to be potent inhibitors of specific cytochrome P450 isoenzymes (Crewe et al. 1992; Nemeroff et al. 1996; von Moltke et al. 1994, 1995). The most thoroughly studied reaction is the competitive inhibition of CYP2D6. Pharmacokinetic studies in healthy volunteers have provided a rank order of the potency for increasing the plasma concentration of model substrates. Case reports in patients have confirmed the existence of some interactions, and many others remain theoretical possibilities. Table 8–4 provides an overall ranking of the cytochrome P450 inhibitory potential of the antidepressants based on both in vitro and in vivo data. The rational selection of an antidepressant should include consideration of its potential enzyme inhibition when therapy is to be combined with substrates listed in Table 8–1, which may be inhibited by the specific antidepressant. Reviews (Harvey and Preskorn 1996; Nemeroff et al. 1996) describe the specific in vivo reports in more detail. While numerous interactions are possible, their clinical significance is a topic that continues to be debated (DeVane 2006; Pres-

TABLE 8–4. Newer antidepressants and cytochrome P450 (CYP) enzyme inhibitory potential

DRUG	CYP1A2	CYP2C9/19	CYP2D6	CYP3A4
Bupropion	0	0	+++	0
Citalopram	0	0	+	0
Duloxetine	0	0	++	0
Escitalopram	0	0	0	0
Fluoxetine (metabolite)	0	++	++++ (++++)	++ (+++)
Fluvoxamine	++++	+++	0	+++
Mirtazapine	0	0	0	0
Nefazodone	0	0	0	++++
Paroxetine	0	0	++++	0
Sertraline (metabolite)	0	+ (+)	+ (++)	++ (++)
Venlafaxine (metabolite)	0	0	0 (+)	0

Note. 0=unknown or insignificant; +=mild and usually insignificant; ++=moderate and possibly significant; +++=moderate and usually significant; ++++=potent.

Source. In vivo and in vitro results: Crewe et al. 1992; Nemeroff et al. 1996; von Moltke et al. 1994, 1995.

korn and Werder 2006). Compensatory mechanisms and patterns of practice that minimize the expression of significant interactions include parallel pathways of drug elimination, dose dependence of inhibition and induction, initiating dosage at lower starting doses, and careful attention to patient response (DeVane 2006). Although some interactions have an unequivocal high likelihood for adverse events (e.g., drug combinations that can result in a serotonin syndrome), severe adverse interactions appear to be rare events.

The selection of a drug based on its cytochrome P450 inhibitory potential should not be limited to the newer antidepressants (see Table 8–4). Combining any two drugs that are substrates for the same enzyme increases the likelihood of competitive enzyme inhibition. All of the substrates listed in Table 8–1 are potential inhibitors. For example, nortriptyline, desipramine, and thioridazine are potent inhibitors of CYP2D6. In vitro methods using microsomal incubations to predict in vivo interactions have appeared and are based on accepted pharmacokinetic principles (Gillette 1971; Houston 1994; von Moltke et al. 1994, 1995). These screening techniques are now used extensively in the pharmaceutical industry in drug development. The knowledge of isoenzyme-specific metabolism of new and established drugs is expanding rapidly and holds promise for further enabling the selection of combined pharmacotherapy based on pharmacokinetic principles.

The increasingly recognized role of drug transporters in the disposition of psychoactive drugs has led to the proposition that inhibition or induction of transporter activity may be involved as a mechanism of drug interactions. Risperidone and its metabolite paliperidone, along with some antidepressants, have been shown in vitro to be inhibitors of P-gp (Doran et al. 2005; Zhu et al. 2007). Reports of clinically significant interactions related to these effects have yet to emerge.

Conclusion

The use of drugs in psychopharmacology can be problematic as a result of pharmacokinetic and pharmacodynamic variability in the dose–effect relationship. Some sources of variability can be controlled through application of pharmacokinetic principles in dosage regimen design and therapeutic drug monitoring. Understanding of pharmacodynamic principles contributes to individualization of dosage regimens. The database on the genetic contribution to drug response and the interactions between drugs is rapidly expanding. Future application of this knowledge will further enhance pharmacotherapy for mentally ill patients.

References

Azzaro AJ, Ziemniak J, Kemper E, et al: Selegiline transdermal system: an examination of the potential for CYP450-dependent pharmacokinetic interactions with 3 psychotropic medications. J Clin Pharmacol 47:146–158, 2007

Benet LZ, Kroetz DL, Sheiner LB: Pharmacokinetics: the dynamics of drug absorption, distribution, and elimination, in Goodman and Gilman's The Pharmacological Basis of Therapeutics, 9th Edition. Edited by Hardman JG, Limbird LE. New York, McGraw-Hill, 1996, pp 3–27

Benet LZ, Izumi T, Zhang Y, et al: Intestinal MDR transport proteins and P-450 enzymes as barriers to oral drug delivery. J Control Release 62:25–31, 1999

Bergstrom R, Mitchell M, Jewell H, et al: Examination of the safety, tolerance, and pharmacokinetics of intramuscular (IM) olanzapine compared to oral olanzapine in healthy subjects. Schizophr Res 36:305–306, 1999

Bies RR, Feng Y, Lotrich FE, et al: Utility of sparse concentration sampling for citalopram in elderly clinical trial subjects. J Clin Pharmacol 44:1352–1359, 2004

Brosen K: Are pharmacokinetic drug interactions with the SSRIs an issue? Int Clin Psychopharmacol 11 (suppl 1):23–27, 1996

Brunner M, Langer O, Sunder-Plassmann R, et al: Influence of functional haplotypes in the drug transporter gene ABCB1 on central nervous system drug distribution in humans. Clin Pharmacol Ther 78:182–190, 2005

Crewe HK, Lennard MS, Tucker GT, et al: The effect of selective serotonin re-uptake inhibitors on cytochrome P4502D6 (CYP2D6) activity in human liver microsomes. Br J Clin Pharmacol 34:262–265, 1992

Denaro CP, Wilson M, Jacob P 3rd, et al: Validation of urine caffeine metabolite ratios with use of stable isotope-labeled caffeine clearance. Clin Pharmacol Ther 59:284–296, 1996

DeVane CL: Pharmacokinetics of the newer antidepressants: clinical relevance. Am J Med 97 (suppl 6A):13–23, 1994

DeVane CL: Clinical significance of drug plasma protein binding and binding displacement drug interactions. Psychopharmacol Bull 36:5–21, 2002

DeVane CL: Immediate-release versus controlled-release formulations: pharmacokinetics of newer antidepressants in relation to nausea. J Clin Psychiatry 64 (suppl 18):14–19, 2003

DeVane CL: Antidepressant-drug interactions are potentially but rarely clinically significant. Neuropsychopharmacology 31:1594–1604, 2006

DeVane CL, Boulton DW: Great expectations in stereochemistry: focus on antidepressants. CNS Spectr 7 (4 suppl 1):28–33, 2002

DeVane CL, Liston HL: An explanation of the second-dose effect in pharmacokinetics and its meaning for clinical psychopharmacology. Psychopharmacol Bull 35:42–52, 2001

DeVane CL, Simpkins JM: Pharmacokinetics of imipramine and its major metabolites in pregnant rats and their fetuses treated with a single dose. Drug Metab Dispos 13:438–442, 1985

DeVane CL, Stowe ZN, Donovan JL, et al: Therapeutic drug monitoring of psychoactive drugs during pregnancy in the genomic era: challenges and opportunities. J Psychopharmacol 20 (4 suppl):54–59, 2006

de Waziers I, Cugnenc PH, Yang CS, et al: Cytochrome P450 isoenzymes, epoxide hydrolase and glutathione transferases in rat and human hepatic and extrahepatic tissues. J Pharmacol Exp Ther 253:287–294, 1990

Dingemanse J, Danhof M, Briemer DD: Pharmacokinetic-pharmacodynamic modeling of CNS drug effects: an overview. Pharmacol Ther 38:1–52, 1988

Doran A, Obach RS, Smith BJ, et al: The impact of P-glycoprotein on the disposition of drugs targeted for indications of the central nervous system: evaluation using the mdr1a/b knockout mouse model. Drug Metab Dispos 33:165–174, 2005

Foltin RW, Fischman MW: Smoked and intravenous cocaine in humans: acute tolerance, cardiovascular and subjective effects. J Pharmacol Exp Ther 257:247–261, 1991

Fuller RW, Hemrick-Luecke SK, Litterfield ES, et al: Comparison of desmethylsertraline with sertraline as a monoamine uptake inhibitor in vivo. Life Sci 19:135–149, 1995

Garattini S: Active drug metabolites: an overview of their relevance in clinical pharmacokinetics. Clin Pharmacokinet 19:216–227, 1985

Gefvert O, Eriksson B, Persson P, et al: Pharmacokinetics and D2 receptor occupancy of long-acting injectable risperidone (Risperdal Consta) in patients with schizophrenia. Int J Neuropsychopharmacol 8:27–36, 2005

George CF, Shand DG, Renwick AG (eds): Presystemic Drug Elimination. London, Butterworth Scientific, 1982

Gibaldi M, Perrier D: Pharmacokinetics. New York, Marcel Dekker, 1975

Gillette JR: Techniques for studying drug metabolism in vitro, in Fundamentals of Drug Metabolism. Edited by La Du BN, Mandel HG, Way EL. Baltimore, MD, Williams & Wilkins, 1971, pp 400–418

Gonzalez FJ, Idle JR: Pharmacogenetic phenotyping and genotyping: present status and future potential. Clin Pharmacokinet 26:59–70, 1994

Greenblatt DJ, Shader RI, Koch-Wiser J, et al: Slow absorption of intramuscular chlordiazepoxide. N Engl J Med 291:1116–1118, 1974

Greenblatt DJ, Allen MD, MacLaughlin DS, et al: Diazepam absorption: effect of antacids and food. Clin Pharmacol Ther 24:600–609, 1978

Greenblatt DJ, Allen MD, Harmatz JS, et al: Diazepam disposition determinants. Clin Pharmacol Ther 27:301–312, 1980

Greenblatt DJ, Sellers EM, Doch-Weser J: Importance of protein binding for the interpretation of serum or plasma drug concentrations. J Clin Pharmacol 22:259–263, 1982

Guengerich FP: Human cytochrome P-450 enzymes. Life Sci 50:1471–1478, 1992

Harvey AT, Preskorn SH: Cytochrome P450 enzymes: interpretation of their interactions with selective serotonin reuptake inhibitors, part I. J Clin Psychopharmacol 16:273–285, 1996

Hoffmeyer S, Burk O, von Rischter O, et al: Functional polymorphisms of the human multidrug-resistance gene: multiple sequence variations and correlation of one allele with P-glycoprotein expression and activity in vivo. Proc Natl Acad Sci U S A 97:3473–3478, 2000

Houston JB: Utility of in vitro drug metabolism data in predicting in vivo metabolic clearance. Biochem Pharmacol 47:1469–1479, 1994

Johansson I, Lundqvist E, Bertilsson L, et al: Inherited amplification of an active gene in the cytochrome P450 CYP2D locus as a cause of ultrarapid metabolism of debrisoquin. Proc Natl Acad Sci U S A 90:11825–11829, 1993

Kalow W, Genest K: A method for the detection of atypical forms of human serum cholinesterase. Can J Biochem Physiol 35:339–346, 1957

Kalow W, Goedde WH, Agarwal DP: Ethnic Differences in Reactions to Drugs and Xenobiotics. New York, Alan R Liss, 1986

Ketter TA, Flockhart DA, Post RM, et al: The emerging role of cytochrome P450 3A in psychopharmacology. J Clin Psychopharmacol 15:387–398, 1995

Kolars JC, Schmiedlin-Ren P, Schuetz JD, et al: Identification of rifampin-inducible P450IIIA4 (CYP3A4) in human small bowel enterocytes. J Clin Invest 90:1871–1878, 1992

Kurata Y, Ieri I, Kimura M, et al: Role of human MDR1 gene polymorphism in bioavailability and interaction of digoxin, a substrate of P-glycoprotein. Clin Pharmacol Ther 72:209–219, 2002

Lin K-M, Poland RE, Wan Y-JY, et al: The evolving science of pharmacogenetics: clinical ethnic perspectives. Psychopharmacol Bull 32:205–217, 1996

Lockridge O: Genetic variants of human serum cholinesterase influence metabolism of the muscle relaxant succinylcholine. Pharmacol Ther 47:35–60, 1990

Mahar Doan KM, Humphreys JE, Webster LO, et al: Passive permeability and P-glycoprotein-mediated efflux differentiate central nervous system and non-CNS marketed drugs. J Pharmacol Exp Ther 303:1029–1037, 2002

Markowitz JS, DeVane CL, Malcolm RJ, et al: Pharmacokinetics of olanzapine after single-dose oral administration of standard tablet versus normal and sublingual administration of an orally disintegrating tablet in normal volunteers. J Clin Pharmacol 46:164–171, 2006

Meyer UA, Zanger UM, Grant D, et al: Genetic polymorphisms of drug metabolism. Adv Drug Res 19:197–241, 1990

Nemeroff CB, DeVane CL, Pollock BG: Newer antidepressants and the cytochrome P450 system. Am J Psychiatry 153:311–320, 1996

Nestler EJ: Cellular responses to chronic treatment with drugs of abuse. Crit Rev Neurobiol 7:23–39, 1993

Osman OT, DeVane CL, Greenblatt DJ, et al: Pharmacokinetic and dynamic correlates of intravenous alprazolam challenge. Clin Pharmacol Ther 50:656–662, 1991

Paine MF, Shen DD, Kunze KL, et al: First-pass metabolism of midazolam by the human intestine. Clin Pharmacol Ther 60:14–24, 1996

Paine MF, Criss AB, Watkins PB: Two major grapefruit juice components differ in time to onset of intestinal CYP3A4 inhibition. J Pharmacol Exp Ther 312:1151–1160, 2005

Papakostas GI, Shelton RC, Smith J, et al: Augmentation of antidepressants with atypical antipsychotic medications for treatment-resistant major depressive disorder: a meta-analysis. J Clin Psychiatry 68:826–831, 2007

Pato M, Murphy DL, DeVane CL: Sustained plasma concentrations of fluoxetine and/or norfluoxetine four and eight weeks after fluoxetine discontinuation. J Clin Psychopharmacol 11:224–225, 1991

Pollock BG, Mulsant BH, Sweet RA, et al: Prospective cytochrome P450 phenotyping for neuroleptic treatment in dementia. Psychopharmacol Bull 31:327–331, 1995

Preskorn S, Werder S: Detrimental antidepressant drug-drug interactions: are they clinically relevant? Neuropsychopharmacology 31:1605–1612, 2006

Price Evans DA: Genetic Factors in Drug Therapy. Cambridge, MA, Cambridge University Press, 1993

Rahi M, Heikkinen T, Hartter S, et al: Placental transfer of quetiapine in relation to P-glycoprotein activity. J Psychopharmacol 21:751–756, 2007

Relling MV, Cherrie J, Schell MJ, et al: Lower prevalence of the debrisoquin oxidative poor metabolizer phenotype in American black versus white subjects. Clin Pharmacol Ther 50:308–313, 1991

Rolan PE: Plasma protein binding displacement interactions—why are they still regarded as clinically important? Br J Clin Pharmacol 37:125–128, 1994

Ronfeld RA, Wilner KD, Baris BA: Sertraline. Chronopharmacokinetics and the effect of coadministration with food. Clin Pharmacokinet 32 (suppl 1):50–55, 1997

Rowland M, Matin SB: Kinetics of drug-drug interactions. J Pharmacokinet Biopharm 1:553–567, 1973

Sadeque AJM, Wandel C, He H, et al: Increased drug delivery to the brain by P-glycoprotein inhibition. Clin Pharmacol Ther 68:231–237, 2000

Schmider J, Greenblatt DJ, von Moltke LL, et al: Relationship of in vitro data on drug metabolism to in vivo pharmacokinetics and drug interactions: implications for diazepam disposition in humans. J Clin Psychopharmacol 16:267–272, 1996

Sellers EM: Plasma protein displacement interactions are rarely of clinical significance. Pharmacology 18:225–227, 1979

Serretti A, Kato M, De Ronchi D, et al: Meta-analysis of serotonin transporter gene promoter polymorphism (5-HTTLPR) association with selective serotonin reuptake inhibitor efficacy in depressed patients. Mol Psychiatr 12:247–257, 2007

Shimada T, Yamazaki H, Mimura M, et al: Interindividual variations in human liver cytochrome P-450 enzymes involved in the oxidation of drugs, carcinogens and toxic chemicals: studies with liver microsomes of 30 Japanese and 30 Caucasians. J Pharmacol Exp Ther 270:414–423, 1994

Siddiqui A, Reinhold K, Weale ME, et al: Association of multidrug resistance in epilepsy with a polymorphism in the drug-transporter gene ABCB1. N Engl J Med 348:1442–1448, 2003

Silverman JA: Multidrug-resistance transporters. Pharm Biotechnol 12:353–86, 1999

Sunderland T, Gur RE, Arnold SE: The use of biomarkers in the elderly: current and future challenges. Biol Psychiatry 58:272–276, 2005

von Moltke LL, Greenblatt DJ, Cotreau-Bibbo MM, et al: Inhibition of desipramine hydroxylation in vitro by serotonin-reuptake-inhibitor antidepressants, and by quinidine and ketoconazole: a model system to predict drug interactions in vivo. J Pharmacol Exp Ther 268:1278–1283, 1994

von Moltke LL, Greenblatt DJ, Court MH, et al: Inhibition of alprazolam and desipramine hydroxylation in vitro by paroxetine and fluvoxamine: comparison with other selective serotonin reuptake inhibitor antidepressants. J Clin Psychopharmacol 15:125–131, 1995

Wang JS, DeVane CL, Gibson BB, et al: Population pharmacokinetic analysis of drug-drug interactions among risperidone, bupropion, and sertraline in CF1 mice. Psychopharmacology (Berl) 183:490–499, 2006

Wrighton SA, Stevens JC: The human hepatic cytochromes P450 involved in drug metabolism. Crit Rev Toxicol 22:1–21, 1992

Zhu H-J, Wang J-S, Markowitz JS, et al: Risperidone and paliperidone inhibit P-glycoprotein activity in vitro. Neuropsychopharmacology 32:757–764, 2007

Brain–Immune System Interactions

Relevance to the Pathophysiology and Treatment of Neuropsychiatric Disorders

Charles L. Raison, M.D.

Monica Kelly Cowles, M.D., M.S.

Andrew H. Miller, M.D.

Although once considered heresy, the notion that meaningful interactions occur between the brain and the immune system has become scientific dogma. This change in scientific orthodoxy results from more than 30 years of research demonstrating that brain-mediated events, such as psychological stress and depression, can alter peripheral immune system functioning and, conversely, that changes in peripheral immune functioning, such as those that occur during illness, can profoundly affect the brain, leading to clinically meaningful changes in mood, anxiety, and cognition. In this chapter, we provide an overview of brain–immune system interactions that are of potential relevance to the field of psychiatry.

This effort needs to be understood within the far wider context of psychoneuroimmunology, which is the interdisciplinary field that focuses on brain–mind–immune system interactions. When Robert Ader first coined the term *psychoneuroimmunology* as a title for his textbook on brain–immune system interactions in 1981, the resulting text filled a single slim volume (Ader 1981). In contrast, the most recent edition fills two volumes, each running more than 1,000 pages, and covers topics as diverse as gene–ribonucleic acid interactions within the cellular nucleus and the effects of spirituality on the immune system (Ader 2007).

The Immune System: An Overview

When considered in the broadest sense as the process whereby organisms maintain functional and organizational integrity against foreign encroachment, immunity is clearly a prerequisite to life itself. Given this, it is not surprising that even the simplest of organisms demonstrate immune functioning, which is consistent with the notion that immunity arose early in the evolution of life on earth (Maier and Watkins 1998). In vertebrates, the immune system has evolved a wide array of separate, but cooperative, mechanisms that serve to attack invading pathogens, destroy tumor cells, and remove and repair damaged tissue. From an evolutionary perspective, the high rate of autoimmune disorders, such as multiple sclerosis and rheumatoid arthritis, suggests that the adaptive advantages of robust immune system functioning outweigh the frequently disastrous consequences engendered when the immune system overreacts and begins attacking the self (Nesse and Williams 1994). The immune system review that follows is necessarily simplified. More extensive discussions of the immune system can be found elsewhere (Abbas and Lichtman 2005; Rabin 1999; Roitt et al. 1998).

Innate Versus Acquired Immunity

A primary distinction within the immune system is between innate immunity (also known as natural or nonspecific immunity) and acquired (or specific) immunity. Innate immunity provides a first line of defense by attacking foreign substances rapidly in a nonspecific manner, without requiring that a specific antigen (or antibody-generating molecule) be recognized (Table 9–1). Although this lack of antigenic specificity precludes the development of an immunological memory to speed the response should a pathogen be encountered again in the future, the nonselectivity of the innate immune system allows for a rapid response to a wide variety of environmental assaults. The immediate response sets in motion a complicated series of processes that contribute to activation of the acquired immune system, which responds more slowly, but far more selectively, to the particular invading entity. An acquired immune response requires specific recognition of a foreign substance and allows for the establishment of memory cells that react far more quickly when the same substance is again encountered. Finally, both innate and acquired immune systems contain mechanisms to control and extinguish activation; therefore, immune activity, with its attendant metabolic costs and danger of self-attack, does not become self-perpetuating.

Innate immunity begins with the skin and other mucosal surfaces lining the gastrointestinal and respiratory tracts, which provide a physiochemical barrier to invasion by foreign pathogens. When these surfaces are breached, phagocytic cells, such as macrophages, microglia (in the brain), and certain dendritic cells, recognize invading pathogens through relatively crude pattern-recognition molecules referred to as toll-like receptors and, depending on the cell type, ultimately engulf and destroy these foreign agents. Upon activation, these cells and other participants in the early innate immune response (e.g., natural killer [NK] cells) release soluble, proteinaceous, immune mediators known as cytokines. Cytokines that mediate innate immunity include the type I interferons, which have direct antiviral effects, and proinflammatory cytokines. Of these, interleukin-1 (IL-1), interleukin-6 (IL-6), and tumor necrosis factor–α (TNF-α) are important in inducing inflammation at the site of pathogen invasion or tissue damage. IL-6 also plays a central role in stimulating the liver to produce a host of acute-phase reactants, such as C-reactive protein; α_1-acid glycoprotein; complement C3; haptoglobin; α_2-macroglobulin; α_1-antitrypsin; ceruloplasmin; and α-, β-, and γ-fibrinogen (Baumann and Gauldie 1994). These proteins, which make up the acute-phase response, serve to both facilitate destruction of foreign substances and limit tissue damage from immune activation. In addition to the release of cytokines and acute-phase proteins, other molecules are induced, including chemokines and adhesion molecules, which assist in the recruitment of multiple cell types to the site of infection and/or tissue damage and destruction. Depending on the magnitude of the innate immune response, relevant cytokines can enter the peripheral blood or activate local afferent nerve fibers and have potent effects on the neuroendocrine system, especially the hypothalamic-pituitary-adrenal (HPA) axis and the central nervous system (CNS), where they mediate many symptoms of illness, including fever, loss of appetite, social withdrawal, and sleep changes (Maier et al. 1998). These behavioral changes are believed to subserve the metabolic demands inherent in the task of fighting infection and maintaining an elevated body temperature.

Acquired immunity relies on hematopoietically derived lymphocytes, which have the ability to specifically recognize an astoundingly wide array of foreign substances. These lymphocytes fall into two general categories. T lymphocytes mature in the thymus and mediate cellular immunity, which is essential for protection against intracellular pathogens, such as viruses and mycobacteria. B lymphocytes mature in the bone marrow and produce antibodies that are especially effective in neutralizing bloodborne and extracellular pathogens, such as parasites, viruses in replication phase, and many species of bacteria. A further key function of the acquired immune system is to screen out lymphocytes that might react against self-molecules. When this essential function fails, autoimmune conditions can result.

Like innate immunity, acquired immunity utilizes soluble cytokine mediators. It is generally recognized that an acquired immune response develops along one of two lines, Th1 or Th2, on the basis of the cytokine profiles induced by T-helper CD4 cells (Elenkov and Chrousos 1999). A Th1 response is characterized by cytokines that promote cell-mediated inflammatory reactions, such as delayed-type hypersensitivity (DTH). These cytokines include interleukin-2 (IL-2), interleukin-12 (IL-12), tumor necrosis factor–β (TNF-β), and interferon-γ (IFN-γ). Cytokines generated by T-helper cells during a Th2 immune response include interleukin-4 (IL-4), interleukin-9 (IL-9), and interleukin-10 (IL-10). IL-6 is also produced by CD4 cells during a Th2-type acquired immune response. The development of a Th2 response favors antibody production, may provide protection against parasites, and is associated with allergic and hypersensitivity reactions.

TABLE 9–1. Major divisions of the immune response

| | | ACQUIRED IMMUNE RESPONSE | |
	INNATE IMMUNE RESPONSE	CELLULAR RESPONSE	HUMORAL RESPONSE
Effector cells	Phagocytes (macrophages, neutrophils), NK cells	Th1 lymphocytes, cytolytic T lymphocytes	Th2 lymphocytes, B lymphocytes
Soluble mediators	Complement, acute-phase reactants		Antibodies
Representative cytokines	TNF-α, IL-1 α and β, IL-6	IL-2, IL-12, IFN-γ	IL-4, IL-10

Note. IFN = interferon; IL = interleukin; NK = natural killer; Th1 = T-helper 1; Th2 = T-helper 2; TNF = tumor necrosis factor.

An acquired immune system response consists of three phases: an induction phase, in which the system detects the presence of antigen; an activation phase, in which the presence of antigen triggers the expansion of antigen-specific T and B cells; and an effector phase, in which the foreign substance is cleared from the body (Miller et al. 2000). In this process, the acquired immune system utilizes and empowers many innate immune elements. For example, the coating of bacteria by B cell–produced antibodies enhances the ability of innate immune system phagocytes to destroy pathogens. Like other complicated physiological response systems, the immune response has built-in negative feedback elements that have evolved to limit immune reactivity once the pathogenic challenge has been met. Other bodily systems, including the HPA axis, perform important extrinsic immunomodulatory roles, and when functioning optimally, these systems limit inflammation and immune system proliferation. A final feature of the acquired immune system, which is central to its functioning, is the formation of long-lived B and T lymphocytes that serve as memory cells for recognizing an antigen should it be encountered in the future. This mechanism accounts for the ability of acquired immunity to mount far more rapid and effective responses to previously seen antigens. It also provides the physiological basis for the effectiveness of vaccines, which activate acquired immunity toward a specific pathogen without inducing illness.

Brain to Body: Central Nervous System Effects on the Immune System

Despite the fact that a general belief in the ability of psychological states to affect health has been apparent since antiquity, scientific formulations, until recently, have tended to view the CNS and the immune system as separate and noninteracting entities. Indeed, the immune system has historically been conceptualized as autonomous and self-contained, with a purpose that begins and ends with the tasks of protection against infection and malignancy and the repair of damaged tissue. Such a view tends to preclude any physiological mechanism by which mental events might directly affect immune functioning. However, in the 1970s, researchers made the startling discovery that the immune system was amenable to classical Pavlovian conditioning (Ader and Cohen 1975). Numerous studies have confirmed and extended this initial insight and established beyond argument the ability of brain states to significantly modulate immune system functioning. The majority of these studies have focused on the effects of stress on the immune response. Virtually every type of stressor, ranging from laboratory stressors (e.g., public speaking, mental arithmetic) to more naturalistic stressors (e.g., bereavement, loneliness, and academic examinations), has demonstrated a measurable effect on the immune response, including effects on various aspects of both innate and acquired immunity (Raison et al. 2002). Although the relationship between stress and immunity is quite complex, more acute and/or mild stressors, in general, tend to be associated with activation of immune responses, whereas more chronic and intense stressors tend to be associated with activated innate immune system elements and impaired acquired immune system responses. The health relevance of these stress-related immune changes has been demonstrated in studies that have shown an association between chronic stress and increased susceptibility to the common cold, reduced antibody responses to vaccination, and delayed wound healing (Cohen et al. 1991; Glaser et al. 1992; Kiecolt-Glaser et al. 1995). In addition, stress, as well as depression, has been linked to increased morbidity and mortality in infectious diseases (e.g., HIV infection), neoplastic diseases (including breast cancer and malignant melanoma), diabetes, and cardiovascular disease (Evans et al. 2005; Fenton and Stover 2006; Leserman et al. 1999; Raison and Miller 2003a).

Effects of Depression and Stress on Acquired Immune (Lymphocyte) Responses

In psychiatry, the practical import of connections between brain outflow pathways and the immune system has been best documented in the effects of stress-related disorders, especially major depression, on immune functioning. Despite a significant degree of heterogeneity across individual studies, significant evidence suggests that patients with major depression demonstrate a number of immune changes similar to those seen in individuals undergoing chronic and/or severe stress (Herbert and Cohen 1993; Zorrilla et al. 2001). This is hardly surprising, given the many indices of stress system hyperactivity that are apparent in patients with major depression, including increased corticotropin-releasing hormone (CRH) and cortisol production (Pariante et al. 1995) and augmented sympathetic nervous system (SNS) activity as manifested in part by increased peripheral blood catecholamines (Veith et al. 1994; Wong et al. 2000). Enumerative immune changes shared by major depression and chronic/severe stress include a decrease in lymphocytes, B cells, and T cells and an increase in the ratio of CD4 to CD8 T cell subsets (Herbert and Cohen 1993). Shared functional changes include a decrease in NK cell activity and lymphocyte proliferation in response to nonspecific mitogens (Herbert and Cohen 1993; Zorrilla et al. 2001).

In a meta-analysis examining the issue, major depression was found to have a larger effect than stress on these immune variables (Zorrilla et al. 2001) (Table 9–2). It is important to note, however, that major depression is a heterogeneous condition and that immune changes are not uniform across all patients. Indeed, inhibited lymphocyte responses tend to be most striking in patients who are older, are hospitalized, or have more severe and/or melancholic types of depression (Miller 1998; Schleifer et al. 1989). In addition, the sleep changes common in depression are known to alter lymphocyte responses, especially NK cell activity (NKCA), even in the absence of other depressive symptoms (Irwin et al. 1996). Nonetheless, it does not appear that these factors completely account for the association between major depression and alterations in measures of the number and function of lymphocyte subsets (Herbert and Cohen 1993).

TABLE 9–2.   Immune alterations in major depression

Increased white blood cells

Increased neutrophil percentage

Decreased lymphocyte percentage

Increased CD4-to-CD8 ratio

Decreased natural killer cell activity

Decreased mitogen-induced lymphocyte proliferation

Increased interleukin-6

Increased haptoglobin

Increased prostaglandin E_2

Compared with chronic/severe stress, major depression has been less well characterized in terms of effects on in vivo functional immunity; however, the little evidence that is available suggests that depression, like chronic/severe stress, may impair T-cell function in ways that are relevant to disease vulnerability. For example, although it is not known whether major depression is associated with an increase in antibody titers to latent viruses, one study reports that patients with major depression have a marked decrease in the ability to generate lymphocytes that respond to the herpes zoster virus (Irwin et al. 1998). Also consistent with impaired T-cell function in depression is the observation that depressed patients, especially those with melancholia, demonstrate impaired DTH (Hickie et al. 1993).

Effects of Depression and Stress on Innate Immune Inflammatory Responses

Although stress and depression have been most often seen as suppressing lymphocyte function, emerging data suggest that such a conclusion oversimplifies the complexities of the mammalian immune response to environmental perturbation and that stress indeed may also activate certain aspects of the immune system (Raison and Miller 2001; Raison et al. 2006). For example, stress exposure in animals and humans has been shown to increase the expression of innate immune cytokines (Goebel et al. 2000; Maier and Watkins 1998; Paik et al. 2000), activate microglia (Frank et al. 2007), and sensitize subsequent immune responses to inflammatory immune challenge (Johnson et al. 2004). Peripheral production of either IL-1β or its soluble receptor antagonist (sIL-1ra), as well as IL-6, has been reported to be increased in the context of several acutely stressful situations, including exercise, academic examinations, and laboratory stressors (Ackerman et al.1998; Goebel et al. 2000; Maes et al. 1998; Pace et al. 2006; Paik et al. 2000; Steptoe et al. 2001). While the mechanism by which stress induces cytokine production has yet to be fully elucidated, it has been shown that catecholamines may play an important role. In particular, β- but not α-adrenoreceptors are critical for central production of inflammatory cytokines, whereas both α- and β-adrenoreceptors contribute to the induction of plasma cytokines following stress (Johnson et al. 2005). These effects of stress appear to be mediated in part by activation of inflammatory signaling pathways including nuclear factor kappa B (NF-κB), which is a linchpin in the initiation of the inflammatory response following the stimulation of toll-like receptors as well as relevant cytokine receptors (Bierhaus et al. 2003).

A growing database suggests that depression (in addition to stress) in both medically healthy and medically ill patients is associated with innate immune system activation (Andrei et al. 2007; Kim et al. 2007; Lesperance et al. 2004; Maes 1999; Musselman et al. 2001b; Raison et al. 2006). Findings consistent with inflammatory activation in depression include increased plasma and cerebrospinal fluid (CSF) concentrations of inflammatory cytokines, increased in vitro production of proinflammatory cytokines from stimulated peripheral blood mononuclear cells, increased acute-phase proteins (and decreased negative acute-phase proteins), increased chemokines and adhesion molecules, and increased production of prostaglandins (Kim et al. 2007; Maes 1999; Raison et al. 2006). Based on meta-analyses, increases in peripheral blood IL-6 and C-reactive protein are two of the most reliable inflammatory biomarkers associated with depression (Zorrilla et al. 2001). Indeed, careful studies examining IL-6 across the circadian cycle have shown a reverse circadian pattern of IL-6 in depressed patients, with markedly elevated levels of this cytokine compared with control subjects during the morning hours (Alesci et al. 2005). Interestingly, given the role of IL-6 and C-reactive protein in predicting disease outcome in both cardiovascular disorders and diabetes (Ridker et al. 2000a, 2000b), as well as data indicating that inflammation may play a role in cancer (Aggarwal et al. 2006), the relationship between depression and activation of the innate immune inflammatory response may provide a mechanism that explains the negative impact of depression on a number of illnesses (Evans et al. 2005). Moreover, immune activation in major depression may be involved in several of the pathophysiological changes that are common in the context of depression, including bone loss, insulin resistance, cachexia, increased body temperature, and hippocampal

volume loss (Raison et al. 2006). Interestingly, activation of innate immune responses following stress and depression may also contribute to stress- and depression-induced decreases in acquired immune (lymphocyte) responses. For example, administration of IL-1ra prior to stressor exposure has been found to reduce the inhibitory impact of stress on antibody production (Moraska et al. 2002).

There are a number of potential factors that may contribute to increased innate immune responses in depressed patients. One factor that has received special attention is body mass index (BMI). BMI has been reliably correlated with peripheral markers of inflammation including IL-6, in part related to the capacity of adipocytes to produce inflammatory cytokines (Schaffler et al. 2007). Relevant in this regard, an analysis of data from the Third National Health and Nutrition Examination Survey revealed that after adjustment for a multitude of variables, including BMI, there was a strong association between major depression and elevated levels of C-reactive protein in men but not women (Ford and Erlinger 2004). Early life stress is another factor that may be involved. For example, males with current major depression and increased early life stress exhibited significantly greater increases in IL-6 and NF-κB DNA binding following a psychosocial stressor compared with control subjects (Pace et al. 2006).

Given the anti-inflammatory properties of glucocorticoids (Rhen and Cidlowski 2005) (see below for further discussion of the immunological effects of glucocorticoids), it might be expected that patients with depression who have decreased glucocorticoid sensitivity, as manifested by nonsuppression of cortisol on the dexamethasone suppression test (DST), would be especially prone to showing evidence of immune activation. Some evidence suggests that this is indeed the case. Compared with patients with depression who have normal in vivo glucocorticoid sensitivity, patients who are DST nonsuppressors demonstrate increased plasma concentrations of the acute-phase reactant α_1-glycoprotein, as well as increased in vitro mitogen-stimulated IL-6 production (Sluzewska 1999). Glucocorticoid resistance, as assessed by the DST, has been associated with a poor response to antidepressant treatment (Holsboer 2000). Of interest, in light of the relationship between DST nonsuppression and increased inflammatory activity, findings suggest that patients with depression who are treatment resistant are more likely than patients who are treatment responders to show evidence of increased inflammatory activity, including increased plasma concentrations of acute-phase proteins, IL-6, and the soluble receptor for IL-6 (sIL-6r), which synergistically enhances IL-6 activity (Raison et al. 2006; Sluzewska 1999). Moreover, depressed patients who exhibit a decrease in unstimulated TNF-α during antidepressant treatment are more likely to respond than those whose TNF-α remains elevated (Lanquillon et al. 2000).

Other Psychiatric Disorders and the Immune Response

Some evidence suggests that other stress-related neuropsychiatric conditions may be associated with immune activation, although these conditions are less well characterized than major depression. These disorders include posttraumatic stress disorder (PTSD), chronic fatigue syndrome (CFS), seasonal affective disorder (SAD), and fibromyalgia. Patients with combat-related PTSD have been reported to demonstrate increased plasma concentrations of IL-1 and increased CSF concentrations of IL-6 (Baker et al. 2001; Spivak et al. 1997). PTSD following civilian disasters appears to be associated with elevated plasma concentrations of IL-6 and its soluble receptor (Maes et al. 1999c). Although not found consistently (Maes et al. 1999c), both severity of symptoms and duration of illness have been reported to correlate positively with indices of immune activation in PTSD (Miller et al. 2001; Spivak et al. 1997).

A growing body of literature suggests that patients exposed to early life trauma may be especially vulnerable to the development of psychophysical disorders (e.g., CFS, fibromyalgia) that are characterized by complaints of chronic pain, fatigue, and cognitive difficulties of unknown etiology (Heim et al. 1997). Consistent with this, these disorders have also been associated with evidence of increased inflammatory activity. For example, it has been reported that both CFS and fibromyalgia are accompanied by an increase in acute-phase reactants and increased plasma concentrations and/or peripheral blood mononuclear cell production of proinflammatory cytokines, including IL-1, IL-6, and TNF-α (Borish et al. 1998; Cannon et al. 1999; Gupta et al. 1997; Maes et al. 1999b). Of note, one report indicates that SAD, a condition with significant symptom overlap with CFS and fibromyalgia, may be characterized by increased plasma concentrations of IL-6 (Leu et al. 2001).

Finally, although the picture is far less clear, there has been speculation that immune system activation may contribute to the pathophysiology of psychotic disorders, including schizophrenia, possibly related to an autoimmune diathesis (Pearce 2001; Rothermundt et al.

2001). Elevated levels of cytokines and their receptors, including IL-2, sIL-2, and IL-6, have been reported in the blood and CSF of patients with schizophrenia, and a high level of CSF IL-2 has been found to predict subsequent schizophrenic relapse (Rothermundt et al. 2001). In a related fashion, consideration has been given to the role of viral infection early in development (Pearce 2001), based on seasonal birth patterns that have been reliably replicated in large epidemiological studies of patients with schizophrenia. These findings are consistent with in utero infections of relevant brain structures, including the hippocampus, during critical periods of development (especially during the second trimester) (Pearce 2001). Moreover, cross-reactivity between brain antigens and antigens of infectious agents may contribute not only to schizophrenia but also to the neurological and psychiatric complications associated with streptococcal infection (i.e., pediatric autoimmune neuropsychiatric disorders associated with streptococcal infections [PANDAS]) (Snider and Swedo 2000).

Mediating Pathways

Underlying the ability of the CNS to affect the immune system is a host of connections between autonomic and neuroendocrine pathways and immune system elements. Immune cells are able to directly respond to brain outflow pathways via receptors for small-molecule neurotransmitters, adrenal and gonadal steroids, hypothalamic-releasing factors, and other neuropeptides (Raison et al. 2002). Specific receptor densities vary among immune cell types, and these variations correlate with cell sensitivity to a given ligand.

Autonomic Nervous System

It is well known that sympathetic and parasympathetic pathways within the autonomic nervous system (ANS) interact to maintain homeostasis in a variety of physiological states, including regulation of the immune response. In addition to expressing receptors for autonomic and neuroendocrine signaling molecules, immune cells and tissues are innervated by fibers derived from the ANS, together comprising a neural pathway which can reflexively regulate the immune response (Czura et al. 2007; Downing and Miyan 2000; Miller 1998; Raison et al. 2002; Sanders and Kavelaars 2007; Tracey 2002). For example, the sympathetic branch of the ANS sends fibers into immune tissues in association with the vascular supply. Within tissue parenchyma, these fibers are associated with vascular smooth muscle cells, where they regulate vascular tone. In addition, sympathetic nerve terminals have been observed by electron microscopy to exist in close approximation with lymphocytes and macrophages. Thus, the sympathetic branch of the ANS appears able to influence the immune system either by changing the vascular tone and blood flow into lymphoid organs or by directly influencing immune cell function via locally released neurotransmitters, especially norepinephrine and neuropeptides such as neuropeptide Y, substance P, vasoactive intestinal peptide, calcitonin gene–related peptide, and CRH, which, in turn, interact with specific receptors on nearby immune cells (Bellinger et al. 1997; Czura et al. 2007).

Initial conceptualizations of the effect of the SNS on immune functioning tended to view the system as being primarily immunosuppressive. Catecholamines are well known to diminish NKCA and nonspecific mitogen-stimulated lymphocyte proliferation and appear to be the primary mediators of rapid immune changes in humans in response to acute stress paradigms (Raison and Miller 2001). Many of the immunosuppressive effects of catecholamines result from β-adrenergic receptor activation: blocking the β receptor obviates many of the stress-related immune alterations, especially those that occur in solid immune tissues, such as the spleen (Benschop et al. 1994; Cunnick et al. 1990; Rabin 1999; Sanders et al. 2007).

However, in recent years, it has become evident that the immune system effects of both norepinephrine and epinephrine cannot be adequately subsumed under a single rubric of immunosuppression. Indeed, as noted above, it has become apparent that catecholamines also have immune-activating effects, given data that catecholamines can stimulate the production of proinflammatory cytokines, especially IL-6, both in the periphery and in the CNS and activate inflammatory signaling cascades (Bierhaus et al. 2003; Johnson et al. 2005; Norris and Benveniste 1993; Papanicolaou et al. 1998). The ability of catecholamines to induce inflammation may be related in part to a "switch" that occurs whereby protein kinase A activation leads to β-adrenergic receptor phosphorylation, which in turn switches β-receptor signaling from G_s to G_i. G_i has been associated with activation of the ras inflammatory signaling cascade (Daaka et al. 1997). Of note, catecholamines also appear to favor the development of Th1 cellular immune responses and promote the production of the Th1 cytokine IFN-γ (Kohm and Sanders 2000). Consistent with this, β-adrenergic receptors are found on Th1 CD4 T cells, but not on Th2 cells (Kohm and Sanders 2000).

In addition to immune regulation by the sympathetic branch, the parasympathetic branch of the ANS has been shown to contribute to the regulation of innate immune responses via an efferent neural signaling pathway referred to as the *cholinergic anti-inflammatory pathway* (Tracey 2002). The existence of this pathway was initially identified in studies showing that stimulation of the vagus nerve attenuates immune system activation and the physiological signs of septic shock in response to lipopolysaccharide, a key component of gram-negative bacterial cell walls (Borovikova et al. 2000). Follow-up studies have determined that vagal release of acetylcholine, which in turn interacts with the α7 subunit of the nicotinic AChR (α7 nAChR) on relevant immune cells, is capable of suppressing production of cytokines, including TNF-α, via inhibitory effects on nuclear translocation of NF-κB (Altavilla et al. 2006; Guarini et al. 2003) and activation of Janus kinase (JAK) 2 signal transducers and activators of transcriptions (STAT) 3 (de Jonge et al. 2005; Pavlov and Tracey 2005). Subsequent studies have established that cytokine production is inhibited by efferent vagal pathways in the context of a variety of inflammatory processes, including myocardial ischemia, hemorrhagic shock, ischemia/reperfusion, and pancreatitis (Altavilla et al. 2006; Guarini et al. 2003; Mioni et al. 2005; van Westerloo et al. 2006; H. Wang et al. 2004). It also has been shown that both vagus nerve stimulation and α7nAChR agonists inhibit production of a number of proinflammatory cytokines, including TNF, IL-1, IL-6, IL-8, and high-mobility group box 1 (HMGB1) (H. Wang et al. 2004). Of note, a specific αnAChR-dependent vagus nerve pathway to the spleen has been identified that inhibits proinflammatory cytokine production during endotoxemia and polymicrobial sepsis. Furthermore, both splenectomy and vagotomy interrupt the cholinergic anti-inflammatory response (Huston et al. 2006). Taken together, these findings suggest that in addition to effects on cellular signaling, there are anatomical and hard-wired components of the cholinergic anti-inflammatory pathway.

Hypothalamic-Pituitary-Adrenal Axis

In concert with the ANS, the HPA axis serves as a central component of the mammalian stress response system. Although glucocorticoids, which represent the final product of HPA axis activation, have long been viewed as immunosuppressive because of their well-documented ability to suppress inflammation (largely through protein–protein interactions between the glucocorticoid receptor and

NF-κB) (Rhen et al. 2005), it is increasingly recognized that HPA axis effects on immunity are complex (Dhabhar et al. 1995). This complexity arises from the fact that HPA axis effects on the immune system depend on numerous factors, including the immune compartment that is assessed, the element of the HPA axis being evaluated (i.e., CRH vs. cortisol), and the duration and timing relative to the immune response and stressor application. Thus, for example, glucocorticoids are known to acutely diminish CD4 cell counts in the blood; however, at the same time, glucocorticoids enhance CD4-mediated DTH reactions in the skin, through their effects on lymphocyte trafficking (Dhabhar 1998). Moreover, different HPA axis elements demonstrate divergent immune system effects. For example, the end result of CRH-induced HPA axis activation is proinflammatory cytokine suppression, and yet studies demonstrate that the direct effect of CRH on proinflammatory cytokine production may be stimulatory (Labeur et al. 1995; Paez Pereda et al. 1995).

Finally, the effect of glucocorticoids on naturalistic measures of immunity, such as DTH, depends on both the concentration and the duration of glucocorticoids within the immune compartment under consideration. Thus, low doses of glucocorticoids applied for brief periods have been shown in rodents to stimulate DTH, whereas higher (or more protracted) glucocorticoid exposure suppresses DTH (Dhabhar and McEwen 1999).

CRH applied within the CNS suppresses several measures of immunity, including splenic NKCA, mitogen-stimulated lymphocyte proliferation, and in vivo and in vitro antibody formation, as well as T-cell responses to T-cell receptor antibody (Caroleo et al. 1993; Irwin et al. 1988; Labeur et al. 1995; Rassnick et al. 1994). CRH-overproducing mice demonstrate a profound decrease in the number of B cells and severely diminished primary and memory antibody responses (Stenzel-Poore et al. 1994). These immunosuppressive effects appear to be mediated by stress response outflow pathways activated by CRH, given that blockade of the SNS abolishes CRH effects on NKCA and adrenalectomy obviates CRH effects on lymphocyte proliferation (Irwin et al. 1988; Labeur et al. 1995). In addition, the B-cell decreases in CRH-overproducing mice are consistent with the marked reduction in rodent B cells observed after chronic glucocorticoid exposure (Miller et al. 1994).

In contradistinction to its immunosuppressive properties, CRH has also been shown to enhance proinflammatory cytokine production in animals and humans when administered peripherally or within the CNS. Chronic intracerebroventricular administration of CRH to rats leads to induction of IL-1β messenger RNA (mRNA) in splenocytes, and acute intravenous administration in humans has been reported to cause a fourfold increase in the induction of IL-1α (Labeur et al. 1995; Schulte et al. 1994). Similarly, the addition of CRH to in vitro mononuclear cell preparations induces the release of IL-1 and IL-6 (Leu and Singh 1992; Paez Pereda et al. 1995). Both chronic and acute CRH infusion have also been reported to increase production of the immunoregulatory cytokine IL-2 in humans and animals (Labeur et al. 1995; Schulte et al. 1994). In addition to potential proinflammatory activities of CRH within the CNS, peripheral production of CRH has been demonstrated in inflammatory diseases, such as ulcerative colitis and arthritis, in which it appears to act as a local proinflammatory agent (Karalis et al. 1997; Nishioka et al. 1996).

Of all neurotransmitters or hormones known to modulate immune functioning, the actions of glucocorticoids, although complicated, are probably best understood (Raison et al. 2002). Identified effects of glucocorticoids on the immune (and inflammatory) system include

- Modulation of immune cell trafficking throughout the body (Dhabhar et al. 1995)
- Modulation of cell death pathways (i.e., apoptosis) (McEwen et al. 1997)
- Inhibition of arachidonic acid pathway products (e.g., prostaglandins) that mediate inflammation and sickness symptoms (e.g., fever) (Goldstein et al. 1992)
- Modulation of Th1/Th2 cellular immune response patterns in a manner that inhibits Th1 (cell-mediated) responses and promotes Th2 (antibody) responses (Elenkov and Chrousos 1999)
- Inhibition of T-cell– and NK-cell–mediated cytotoxicity (Raison et al. 2002)
- Inhibition of cytokine production and function through interaction of glucocorticoid receptors with transcription factors (NF-κB, in particular), which, in turn, regulate cytokine gene expression and/or the expression of cytokine-inducible genes (McKay and Cidlowski 1999)

Although, as discussed below, glucocorticoids may actually enhance certain aspects of naturalistic immune functioning when produced for brief periods at low to moderate doses in the context of acute and/or mild stress, glucocorticoids, in general, play a primary role in restraining excessive or prolonged inflammatory activation (Munck 1989). This property has long been exploited by modern medicine for the treatment of autoimmune and other chronic inflammatory conditions, with the result that glucocorticoids remain a cornerstone of our anti-inflammatory armamentarium. Consistent with their pharmacological uses, glucocorticoids have been shown to be essential for inflammatory regulation in response to immune system activation. For example, neutralization of endogenous glucocorticoid function results in enhanced pathology and mortality in animals exposed to lipopolysaccharide, as well as other inflammatory stimulators, such as streptococcal cell wall antigen or myelin basic protein (Bertini et al. 1988; Sternberg et al. 1989). Similarly, rodents that have been rendered glucocorticoid deficient by adrenalectomy have markedly increased death rates following infection with murine cytomegalovirus, an effect that arises from unrestrained activity of the proinflammatory cytokine TNF-α (Ruzek et al. 1999).

Body to Brain: Immune System Effects on Central Nervous System Functioning

Immune System to Brain Signaling Pathways

The field of psychoneuroimmunology is based on the existence of bidirectional communication pathways between the brain and the immune system. This implies that just as the CNS is capable of modulating immunity, the immune system can alter functioning within the CNS. Although researchers historically were first interested in pathways by which the brain affects immunity, the past 10–15 years have seen a groundswell of interest in the ways in which the immune system contributes to the development of psychopathology.

Underpinning this growing interest is an increasing appreciation for the multiple ways in which proinflammatory cytokines are able to signal the brain and change CNS function (Table 9–3). Although the brain was historically considered an "immune privileged" organ, protected from immune system activity by the blood–brain barrier, it is now clear that cytokines released in the periphery rapidly affect CNS functioning via at least four pathways that are not mutually exclusive (Raison et al. 2002). Proinflammatory cytokines injected into the abdominal cavity (intraperitoneal) have been shown to activate the vagus nerve, resulting in the independent production of proinflammatory cytokines within the CNS, especially in the hypothalamus and hippocampus, which are regions of central importance for the regulation of the

TABLE 9–3. Evidence that cytokines can alter central nervous system function

1. Cytokines released peripherally have access to the brain.

   Passage through leaky regions in the blood–brain barrier (e.g., circumventricular organs)

   Active transport

   Activation of intermediary cell types (e.g., endothelial cells) that produce relevant second messengers (e.g., prostaglandins, nitric oxide)

   Transmission of cytokine signals through afferent nerve fibers (e.g., vagus)

2. A cytokine network exists within the brain.

   Glia (especially microglia) and neurons express/produce cytokines and express cytokine receptors

3. Cytokines have effects on neurotransmitter turnover, neuroendocrine function, synaptic plasticity, and behavior (sickness behavior).

ANS and emotion (Maier et al. 1998). Recent studies suggest that in addition to activating the vagus nerve, proinflammatory cytokines in the blood are able to signal the CNS by entering through "leaky" regions lacking a fully formed blood–brain barrier, such as the circumventricular organs, and, from there, to circulate in CSF to other brain regions (Rivest et al. 2000). Bloodborne proinflammatory cytokines can also communicate with the brain through intermediaries, without themselves entering the CNS parenchyma, for example, by acting on cells of the brain endothelium or choroid plexus and inducing the release of secondary messengers, such as prostaglandins and nitric oxide (Rivest et al. 2000). Finally, active transport across the blood–brain barrier provides another mechanism by which small quantities of proinflammatory cytokines may gain access to the CNS (Banks 2006; Banks et al. 1995; Plotkin et al. 1996).

Once proinflammatory cytokines have gained access to the CNS through any of the routes outlined above, the inflammatory signal appears to be amplified by a cytokine network within the brain itself (Quan et al. 1999). It has already been noted that cytokines produced in the periphery stimulate the production of proinflammatory cytokines, such as IL-1, IL-6, and TNF-α, in a number of brain regions (Dantzer and Kelley 2007; Gatti and Bartfai 1993; Laye et al. 1994; Quan et al. 1999). Receptors for proinflammatory cytokines are found in the brain, especially in areas that are of central importance to homeostatic and emotional regulation, such as the hypothalamus and hippocampus (Benveniste 1998). Among neural cells, activated microglia are capable of producing significant amounts of proinflammatory cytokines, which, in turn, are potent activators of glial cells (Schobitz et al. 1994). Of interest, growing evidence suggests that non-immunological stressors can induce cytokine expression in the brain, likely due in part to stress-induced activation of microglia (Frank et al. 2007). These data suggest that CNS cytokine pathways may participate in the response of an organism to a wide variety of environmental perturbations. Consistent with this finding, proinflammatory cytokines have been implicated in the modulation of circadian functioning, especially the sleep–wake cycle (Hohagen et al. 1993; Opp 2005).

Sickness Behavior and the Development of Depression in the Medically Ill

It has long been known that rates of major depression, as well as milder forms of mood disturbance, are many times more common in people with medical illnesses than in the general population (Evans et al. 1999). Although this has been typically ascribed to the overwhelming psychological stress frequently engendered by being seriously ill, more recent attention has been paid to the idea that immune system activation, which typically accompanies medical illness, may itself biologically predispose patients to depression (Raison and Nemeroff 2000). Evidence for this comes from the observation that rates of depression are significantly elevated in a wide variety of medical conditions including inflammatory and autoimmune disorders such as multiple sclerosis and rheumatoid arthritis, as well as illnesses such as cardiovascular disease, diabetes, and cancer, which are increasingly being recognized as having an important inflammatory component (Aggarwal et al. 2006; Blake and Ridker 2002; Evans et al. 2005). Moreover, prospective studies of conditions that are characterized by episodic immune dysregulation, such as multiple sclerosis or herpes infection, typically find that depression immediately precedes, rather than follows, episodes of disease exacerbation, suggesting that depressive symptoms associated with these conditions may result from underlying immune system activity rather than arising from a psychological reaction to exacerbation of the illness (Foley et al. 1992; Hickie and Lloyd 1995). Finally, as noted above, numerous groups have shown that when compared with similar patients without a current mood disorder, plasma concentrations of proinflammatory cytokines are significantly higher in medically ill patients with major depression versus those without (Raison et al. 2006). For example, IL-6 is elevated in depressed patients with cancer (Musselman et al. 2001b), and C-reac-

tive protein is elevated in depressed patients with both acute coronary syndromes and chronic heart failure (Andrei et al. 2007; Lesperance et al. 2004).

More direct evidence that inflammatory processes may contribute to psychopathology, especially in the context of medical illness, comes from many studies in humans and animals demonstrating that the administration of proinflammatory cytokines reliably induces changes in mood, cognition, and behavior similar to those commonly observed in patients with mood and anxiety disorders, as well as in psychophysical conditions such as CFS and fibromyalgia (Dantzer and Kelley 2007; Raison et al. 2006). This constellation of immune-induced changes, alternately referred to as "sickness syndrome" or "sickness behavior," consists of dysphoria, anhedonia, fatigue, social withdrawal, hyperalgesia, and cognitive and sleep disturbances, as well as decreases in appetite and libido (Kent et al. 1992). Although seen in response to infection, the full syndrome can be reproduced in animals and humans by administration of innate immune cytokines, such as IFN-α, IL-1, TNF-α, and IL-6, as well as IL-2, even in the absence of infection (Raison et al. 2002).

Results from studies utilizing positron emission tomography (PET) and functional magnetic resonance imaging (fMRI) provide further evidence that peripheral cytokine activity can induce centrally mediated behavioral changes. These and other imaging modalities provide a means by which various behavioral alterations can be associated with specific brain regions. For example, during an fMRI task of visuospatial attention, in comparison with control subjects, patients administered IFN-α exhibited significantly greater activation of the dorsal anterior cingulate cortex (dACC) that highly correlated with the number of task-related errors (Capuron et al. 2005). Interestingly, increased dACC activity during cognitive tasks has also been demonstrated in patients vulnerable to mood disorders, such as those with high trait anxiety, neuroticism, or obsessive-compulsive disorder (Capuron et al. 2005). IFN-α has also been shown to lead to changes in basal ganglia metabolic activity as measured by PET that resemble those seen in Parkinson's disease. These changes also correlate with IFN-α–induced fatigue-related symptoms and may be a function of IFN-α effects on dopamine metabolism (Capuron et al. 2007).

Blocking cytokine activity with an IL-1 receptor antagonist, α-melanocyte-stimulating hormone, or IL-10 diminishes or prevents the development of sickness behavior in laboratory animals, even when such behavior develops as a result of psychological stress (Milligan et al. 1998). Similarly, etanercept, a novel agent that blocks

TNF-α activity, has been reported to improve energy and overall emotional functioning in patients with rheumatoid arthritis, a condition characterized by increased proinflammatory cytokine activity (Mathias et al. 2000). TNF antagonists have recently been shown to reduce depressive symptoms in patients with several autoimmune conditions (Persoons et al. 2005; Tyring et al. 2006). Further evidence that cytokine-induced behavioral toxicity is related to major depression comes from studies showing that in humans and animals, antidepressants are able to abolish or attenuate the development of sickness behavior in response to cytokine administration (Musselman et al. 2001a; Yirmiya et al. 2001).

Pathways by Which Inflammatory Cytokines Produce Neuropsychiatric Disturbance

In keeping with the observation that antidepressants mitigate emotional and behavioral symptoms resulting from immune system activation, significant evidence demonstrates that inflammatory cytokines affect neurotransmitters and neuroendocrine pathways that are regulated by currently available antidepressants and that have been implicated in the pathophysiology of depression and other stress-related neuropsychiatric disorders. It is increasingly recognized that these effects on the CNS and its outflow pathways may provide a physiological basis for the observation that immune activation frequently produces neuropsychiatric disturbance (Table 9–4).

Effects on Monoamine Neurotransmitters

In laboratory animals, the acute intracerebral administration of IL-1 produces a rapid and significant increase in norepinephrine and serotonin (5-HT) turnover in several brain regions (Linthorst et al. 1995a, 1995b). Far less is known about the effect of chronic proinflammatory cytokine exposure on functioning of monoamine systems in either animals or humans; however, cytokines, including IFN-α, have been shown to diminish 5-HT availability as a result of a cytokine-mediated enhancement in the activity of indoleamine 2,3-dioxygenase (IDO), an enzyme that shunts tryptophan metabolism away from 5-HT toward kynurenine and quinolinic acid, which is known to have neurotoxic properties (Dantzer et al. 2007; Raison et al. 2006). Tryptophan is the primary precursor of 5-HT, and depletion of tryptophan has been associated with the precipitation of mood disturbances in vulnerable patients (Moore et al. 2000). Moreover, significant evidence suggests that serotonergic neurotransmission is decreased in

TABLE 9–4. Potential mechanisms by which cytokines may influence behavior

Activation of corticotropin-releasing hormone pathways

Alteration of monoamine metabolism

Induction of the euthyroid sick syndrome

Disruption of glucocorticoid receptor signaling

Alteration of regional brain activity

Inhibition of relevant growth factors

many patients with depression (Owens and Nemeroff 1998). It has also been shown that proinflammatory cytokines, via p38 mitogen-activated protein kinase (MAPK)–linked pathways, can increase the expression and function of synaptic reuptake pumps for serotonin (and norepinephrine), potentially further contributing to reduced synaptic availability of mood-relevant monoamines (Zhu et al. 2005, 2006). Of interest, the development of major depression in the context of chronic IFN-α treatment has been shown to correlate closely with decreased plasma concentrations of tryptophan, possibly as a result of increased IDO activity, consistent with the idea that cytokine-induced decrements in 5-HT availability may contribute to the development of depression (Capuron et al. 2002b). Furthermore, treatment with paroxetine attenuates the behavioral consequences of IFN-α–mediated tryptophan depletion (Capuron et al. 2003a). In addition to the effects of chronic cytokine exposure on serotonergic transmission, both IL-2 and IFN-α, when they are administered chronically, have been reported to alter dopamine metabolism, and as noted above, IFN-α has been shown to lead to altered metabolic activity in brain regions high in dopaminergic neurocircuits including the basal ganglia (Capuron et al. 2007; Lacosta et al. 2000; Shuto et al. 1997).

Effects on the Thyroid Axis

Medical illness is often associated with a state of functional thyroid deficiency known as euthyroid sick syndrome (ESS) (Papanicolaou 2000). In its early stages, ESS is characterized by normal thyroid-stimulating hormone (TSH) and thyroxine (T_4) levels, but by reduced levels of triiodothyronine (T_3), which is the more biologically active form of thyroid hormone. In later stages of ESS, T_4 levels are also decreased. Evidence suggests that proinflammatory cytokines promote this condition via direct effects on the thyroid gland, as well as by inhibition of enzymes responsible for peripheral conversion of T_4 to T_3, especially in the liver (Papanicolaou 2000). It is well known that decreased thyroid functioning is associated with the development of symptoms of depression, and functional abnormalities of the thyroid axis are observed in many patients with major depression who do not have clinically obvious thyroid disease (Musselman and Nemeroff 1996).

Effects on the Hypothalamic-Pituitary-Adrenal Axis

Inflammatory cytokines have well-described effects on the HPA axis that are consistent with changes frequently seen in patients with major depression, including increased production of CRH and cortisol and decreased tissue sensitivity to glucocorticoid hormones (Capuron et al. 2003a; Hasler et al. 2004; Pace et al. 2007; Silverman et al. 2005). Although cytokines have been shown to be capable of activating the HPA axis at multiple levels, with a resultant increase in glucocorticoid release, significant evidence suggests that a major final common pathway for cytokine activation involves stimulation of CRH production in the paraventricular nucleus (PVN) of the hypothalamus (Besedovsky and del Rey 1996). Several lines of evidence suggest that this increase in CRH activity may contribute to cytokine-induced depression/sickness behavior. CRH has behavioral effects in animals that are similar to those seen in patients with depression and/or sickness syndrome, including alterations in appetite, activity, and sleep (Owens and Nemeroff 1991). Patients with major depression frequently demonstrate increased CRH production, as assessed by increased CRH in CSF, increased messenger RNA in the PVN, downregulated frontal CRH receptors, and a blunted adrenocorticotropic hormone (ACTH) response to CRH challenge (likely reflecting downregulation of pituitary CRH receptors) (Owens and Nemeroff 1993). Agents that block the CRH type I receptor have been shown to have antidepressant and anxiolytic effects in humans (Zobel et al. 2000). In animals, blocking CRH reverses some of the behavioral sequelae of proinflammatory cytokine administration (Dantzer 2001). Indirect evidence for a role of CRH in cytokine-induced depression in humans comes from a study in which individuals who developed depression during IFN-α administration exhibited significantly higher ACTH and cortisol responses to the first injection of IFN-α compared with control subjects (Capuron et al. 2003b). These findings suggest that sensitized CRH pathways may serve as a vulnerability factor for cytokine-induced behavioral changes.

In addition to direct stimulatory effects on CRH within the CNS, in vivo and in vitro studies suggest that inflammation may induce resistance to circulating glu-

cocorticoids in nervous, endocrine, and immune system tissues (Pariante and Miller 2001; Raison and Miller 2003b). This is of great potential relevance, given the high rates of relative glucocorticoid resistance in HPA axis tissues (as assessed in vivo by the DST or the dexamethasone–CRH stimulation test) and the immune system (as measured in vitro) seen in patients with major depression and in animals and humans exposed to chronic and/or severe stressors (Holsboer 2000). Supporting a role for cytokines in the induction of glucocorticoid resistance is the observation that many chronic inflammatory conditions, including steroid-resistant asthma, rheumatoid arthritis, multiple sclerosis, and HIV infection, are characterized by a decrease in sensitivity to glucocorticoids (Raison et al. 2002). In HIV infection, glucocorticoid resistance has been shown to correlate with increased IFN-α plasma levels (Norbiato et al. 1998).

There are several mechanisms by which proinflammatory cytokines can disrupt glucocorticoid receptor (GR) function and contribute to glucocorticoid resistance. In addition to downregulating the expression of GR protein, proinflammatory cytokines have been found to increase the expression of the inert β isoform of the GR (Oakley et al. 1996). Exposure of cells that constitutively express both GR-α (the active isoform) and GR-β to either TNF-α or IL-1β in vitro results in a marked increase in GR-β production, which is associated with the development of glucocorticoid resistance, as evidenced by a significant reduction in dexamethasone-stimulated activity of a GR-sensitive reporter gene in cytokine-treated cells (Webster et al. 2001). That overproduction of the negative GR-β isoform has a clinically relevant effect on glucocorticoid sensitivity is suggested by several recent studies documenting that patients with a variety of inflammatory and immune system disorders, including asthma, ulcerative colitis, and chronic lymphocytic leukemia, whose conditions are resistant to steroid treatment demonstrate a significantly increased GR-β to GR-α ratio (Honda et al. 2000; Leung 1997; Shahidi et al. 1999; Sousa et al. 2000).

Another mechanism by which inflammatory cytokines may attenuate GR signal transduction and, hence, cause glucocorticoid resistance is through induction of inflammatory signaling pathways that directly influence GR function (Pace et al. 2007). For example, adding IL-1α to an in vitro preparation of mouse fibroblast cells has been shown to suppress the ability of dexamethasone to induce translocation of the GR from the cytoplasm to its site of action in the nucleus (Pariante et al. 1999). This IL-1α–mediated blockade of GR translocation from the cytoplasm to the cellular nucleus inhibits GR activity, as indicated by a decrease in the ability of dexamethasone to activate a glucocorticoid-sensitive reporter gene construct. The signaling pathways involved in this effect include p38 MAPK, which has been shown to phosphorylate the GR (X. Wang et al. 2004). Other inflammatory signaling pathways have also been shown to alter GR function, including NF-κB, Jun N-terminal kinase (JNK), and STAT5 (Pace et al. 2007).

Psychopharmacological Implications of Brain–Immune System Interactions

Antidepressants and Immune System Activation

The term *antidepressant* has been depicted, more than once, as a misnomer, given the wide spectrum of activity evinced by these pharmacological agents. Adding to this activity spectrum are findings that antidepressants have clear immunomodulatory effects in animals and humans. In general, antidepressants have been found to decrease immune responsiveness (Kenis and Maes 2002). Because of this, these agents may be of benefit for a wide range of symptoms that arise in the context of immune activation. Of special interest, given the ability of inflammatory cytokines to induce sickness behavior and/or major depression, a number of antidepressants have been reported to attenuate proinflammatory cytokine production, not just from peripheral immune cells (Maes 1999) but also from within the CNS, where desipramine has been reported to diminish TNF-α release within the locus coeruleus (Ignatowski and Spengler 1994). Interestingly in this regard, the antidepressant efficacy of desipramine during the forced-swim test has been shown to be dependent on reductions in neuronal production of TNF-α and can be reversed by exogenous TNF-α coadministered with the antidepressant (Reynolds et al. 2004). Desipramine has also been shown to lower peripheral TNF-α production in response to lipopolysaccharide (LPS) administration—an effect that was associated with abrogation of the depressive-like behavioral effects of LPS (Shen et al. 1999). The heterocyclic antidepressant bupropion has been similarly noted to markedly diminish TNF-α production following LPS administration in animals (Brustolim et al. 2006). Of note, concomitant with attenuating proinflammatory cytokine production, antidepressants enhance production of the anti-inflammatory cytokine IL-10 (Maes et al. 1999d).

In addition to potential direct effects on cytokine production, antidepressants impact neuroendocrine and neurotransmitter systems in ways known to diminish inflammatory activity. For example, all antidepressants appear to downregulate the overproduction of CRH and cortisol that frequently occurs in the context of major depression. Much evidence suggests that this downregulation results from the ability of antidepressants to enhance glucocorticoid signaling via increased glucocorticoid receptor functioning, which, in turn, leads to a restoration of glucocorticoid-mediated inhibitory control on the HPA axis (Pariante and Miller 2001). Because CRH has been shown to directly stimulate proinflammatory cytokine production, antidepressants may modulate inflammatory activity in part by diminishing CRH production. Glucocorticoid receptors, in addition to inhibiting CRH release in the hypothalamus, also mediate the well-characterized anti-inflammatory properties of glucocorticoids. It is likely that antidepressants decrease inflammatory activity in part via their ability to potentiate glucocorticoid receptor functioning (Pariante and Miller 2001). Antidepressants also normalize the hyperactivity of the locus coeruleus and SNS frequently seen in major depression (Ressler and Nemeroff 1999). Because catecholamines have been shown to enhance proinflammatory activity, the ability of antidepressants to normalize catecholaminergic functioning would be expected to diminish inflammatory activity. Finally, antidepressants are known to enhance functioning in intracellular second-messenger systems (such as the cyclic adenosine monophosphate [cAMP] cascade) known to suppress the activation of genes that encode for the production of proinflammatory cytokines (Duman et al. 2001).

Whatever the mechanism, it is clear from studies in animals and humans that antidepressants effectively diminish many physical, emotional, cognitive, and behavioral symptoms that arise in the context of immune system activation (Capuron et al. 2002a). In animals, pretreatment with a number of antidepressants has been shown to prevent or diminish the development of sickness syndrome in response to either pathogen or cytokine exposure (Yirmiya et al. 2001). In humans, pretreatment with an antidepressant has been shown in a double-blind, placebo-controlled trial to significantly reduce the development of major depression in patients receiving high doses of the proinflammatory cytokine IFN-α for the treatment of malignant melanoma (Musselman et al. 2001a). In this study, 45% of patients receiving placebo had developed major depression within 3 months of starting IFN-α, compared with only 11% receiving the selective serotonin reuptake inhibitor paroxetine. Of interest, however, paroxetine was not equally efficacious for all the symptoms associated with sickness syndrome. Specifically, the antidepressant significantly reduced the symptoms of depressed mood, anxiety, and poor cognitive functioning but was no more effective than placebo in the treatment of somatic or neurovegetative symptoms, such as fatigue and anorexia, suggesting that these symptom domains may have nonoverlapping etiologies (Capuron et al. 2002a). Consistent with this finding, neurovegetative symptoms tended to develop early (and to persist) in the course of IFN-α treatment in a majority of patients, whereas symptoms of depressed mood, anxiety, and cognitive disturbance tended to develop insidiously over weeks or months of treatment in a smaller percentage of patients (Trask et al. 2000). The success of pretreatment strategies in preventing the development of neuropsychiatric disorders in medically ill patients at high risk for mood disorders is intriguing and suggests that prophylactic antidepressants may be considered in other medical contexts, such as for patients about to undergo treatment with radiation and/or chemotherapy, as well as for patients about to undergo major surgery.

There are also data to suggest that antipsychotics, although not as well studied as antidepressants, may have immunological effects relevant to their mechanism of action. Intriguing in this regard is a study demonstrating increased antipsychotic efficacy in patients with schizophrenia treated with the combination of the cyclooxygenase-2 inhibitor celecoxib, an anti-inflammatory drug, and risperidone versus risperidone plus placebo (Müller et al. 2002).

Immune System Interventions for Behavioral Symptoms

Given that proinflammatory cytokines induce depressive syndromes, and given that many medically healthy patients with depression appear to demonstrate increased inflammatory activity, it is logical to inquire as to whether agents that directly target inflammatory mediators, such as anti-inflammatory agents and drugs that disrupt cytokines and their cytokine signaling pathways (e.g., NF-κB, p38 MAPK), might be of benefit in the treatment of both stress- and immune-related neurobehavioral disorders. Indeed, in a recent double-blind, randomized, placebo-controlled study, patients with major depressive disorder who took celecoxib as an adjunct to reboxetine experienced a significantly greater therapeutic benefit than those taking reboxetine alone (Müller et al. 2006). In ani-

mal models, endogenous inhibitors of proinflammatory cytokines, such as the soluble receptor antagonist for IL-1 (sIL-1ra), have been reported to attenuate or abolish sickness symptoms following endotoxin or cytokine administration (Maier and Watkins 1998). Of interest, in addition to direct anti-inflammatory activities, sIL-1ra also blocks many of the sequelae of psychological stress in rodents. For example, direct injection of sIL-1ra blunts HPA axis responses to psychological stressors, such as restraint, and prevents stress from causing learned helplessness (a frequent animal model for depression) (Maier and Watkins 1998). Administration of IL-ra has also been shown to reverse the inhibitory effects of stress on the expression of brain-derived neurotrophic factor in the dentate gyrus of the rat hippocampus (Barrientos et al. 2003). Of note, mice whose TNF-α receptor genes have been knocked out exhibit an antidepressant phenotype and are resistant to anxiety-conditioning paradigms and virus-induced anxiety behaviors (Silverman et al. 2004, 2007; Simen et al. 2006). Of further relevance to the behavioral effects of targeting cytokines such as TNF-α are data demonstrating improvements in behavioral symptoms in patients with inflammatory and autoimmune disorders who are receiving therapies that block TNF-α activity (e.g., etanercept, infliximab). For example, significant improvement in emotional well-being has been observed in patients treated with these agents for psoriasis, rheumatoid arthritis, and ankylosing spondylitis (Braun et al. 2007; Katugampola et al. 2007; Mathias et al. 2000). Most relevant, however, was a recent double-blind, placebo-controlled trial of etanercept for the treatment of psoriasis, in which patients who received active drug exhibited significantly greater improvement in depressive symptoms compared with placebo-treated patients, independent of the effect of the drug on disease activity (Tyring et al. 2006). Although the risk of side effects with cytokine antagonists is relatively low, when adverse events do occur, they can be serious, including life-threatening infections, reactivation of tuberculosis, congestive heart failure, lymphoma, induction of autoantibodies, and a lupus-like reaction.

Treatment of chronic pain, with or without the presence of mood symptoms, is another burgeoning area of translational drug discovery. Data from animal models suggest that proinflammatory cytokines, specifically IL-1 and TNF, play a pivotal role in the creation and maintenance of neuropathic pain (Marchand et al. 2005; Moalem and Tracey 2006). These findings led to the hypothesis that IL-10, an anti-inflammatory cytokine, may prove to be a promising therapeutic option via attenuation of IL-1 and TNF activity. Indeed, it has been shown in animal studies that IL-10, via intrathecal IL-10 gene therapy, is effective in the control of both acute and chronic pain (Ledeboer et al. 2007; Milligan et al. 2006).

It has been suggested that the increased prevalence of major depression observed in the Western world over the past half-century may be caused, at least in part, by a decrease in the consumption of omega-3 fatty acids (Maes et al. 1999a), which are well known to have anti-inflammatory effects via the inhibition of prostaglandins and proinflammatory cytokines. Consistent with this, populations that consume diets high in omega-3 fatty acids (found especially in fish) appear to have diminished rates of major depression (Tanskanen et al. 2001). Conversely, patients with major depression have been reported to have decreased serum concentrations of omega-3 fatty acids (Maes et al. 1999a; Tiemeier et al. 2003). These observations suggest that the administration of omega-3 fatty acids might be beneficial to patients with mood disorders. Preliminary studies have indeed shown that adjunctive administration of omega-3 fatty acids under double-blind, placebo-controlled conditions significantly improves persistent mood symptoms in patients with depression (Peet and Horrobin 2002) and decreases disease relapse in patients with bipolar disorder (Stoll et al. 1999). Low omega-3 fatty acid levels may also contribute to the increased rates of depression in the medically ill, in particular in patients with cardiovascular disease. In a study evaluating patients 2 months after an acute coronary event (myocardial infarction or unstable angina), patients with comorbid major depression had significantly lower levels of omega-3 fatty acids (Frasure-Smith et al. 2004) than their nondepressed counterparts. Given that low omega-3 fatty acid levels are associated with mood disorders (Parker et al. 2006), in addition to increased levels of inflammation (Simopoulos 2002), an increased risk for coronary artery disease (Kris-Etherton et al. 2003), and fatal arrhythmias (Leaf et al. 2003), further studies evaluating the effects of omega-3 supplements in at-risk populations are warranted.

References

Abbas AK, Lichtman AH: Basic Immunology: Functions and Disorders of the Immune System, 2nd Edition. Philadelphia, PA, WB Saunders, 2004

Ackerman KD, Martino M, Heyman R, et al: Stressor-induced alteration of cytokine production in multiple sclerosis patients and controls. Psychosom Med 60:484–491, 1998

Ader R: Psychoneuroimmunology. New York, Academic Press, 1981

Ader R: Psychoneuroimmunology, 4th Edition. Burlington, MA, Elsevier Academic Press, 2007

Ader R, Cohen N: Behaviorally conditioned immunosuppression. Psychosom Med 37:333–340, 1975

Aggarwal BB, Shishodia S, Sandur SK, et al: Inflammation and cancer: how hot is the link? Biochem Pharmacol 72:1605–1621, 2006

Alesci S, Martinez PE, Kelkar S, et al: Major depression is associated with significant diurnal elevations in plasma interleukin-6 levels, a shift of its circadian rhythm, and loss of physiological complexity in its secretion: clinical implications. J Clin Endocrinol Metab 90:2522–2530, 2005

Altavilla D, Guarini S, Bitto A, et al: Activation of the cholinergic anti-inflammatory pathway reduces NF-kappab activation, blunts TNF-alpha production, and protects against splanchic artery occlusion shock. Shock 25:500–506, 2006

Andrei AM, Fraguas R Jr, Telles RM, et al: Major depressive disorder and inflammatory markers in elderly patients with heart failure. Psychosomatics 48:319–324, 2007

Baker DG, Ekhator NN, Kasckow JW, et al: Plasma and cerebrospinal fluid interleukin-6 concentrations in posttraumatic stress disorder. Neuroimmunomodulation 9:209–217, 2001

Banks WA: The blood-brain barrier in psychoneuroimmunology. Neurol Clin 24:413–419, 2006

Banks WA, Kastin AJ, Broadwell RD: Passage of cytokines across the blood-brain barrier. Neuroimmunomodulation 2:241–248, 1995

Barrientos RM, Sprunger DB, Campeau S, et al: Brain-derived neurotrophic factor mRNA downregulation produced by social isolation is blocked by intrahippocampal interleukin-1 receptor antagonist. Neuroscience 121:847–853, 2003

Baumann H, Gauldie J: The acute phase response (comments). Immunol Today 15:74–80, 1994

Bellinger D, Felten SY, Lorton D, et al: Innervation of the lymphoid organs and neurotransmitter–lymphocyte interactions, in Immunology of the Nervous System. Edited by Keane RW, Hickey WF. New York, Oxford University Press, 1997, pp 226–332

Benschop RJ, Nieuwenhuis EE, Tromp EA, et al: Effects of beta-adrenergic blockade on immunologic and cardiovascular changes induced by mental stress. Circulation 89:762–769, 1994

Benveniste EN: Cytokine actions in the central nervous system. Cytokine Growth Factor Rev 9:259–275, 1998

Bertini R, Bianchi M, Ghezzi P: Adrenalectomy sensitizes mice to the lethal effects of interleukin 1 and tumor necrosis factor. J Exp Med 167:1708–1712, 1988

Besedovsky HO, del Rey A: Immune-neuro-endocrine interactions: facts and hypotheses. Endocrinol Rev 17:64–102, 1996

Bierhaus A, Wolf J, Andrassy M, et al: A mechanism converting psychosocial stress into mononuclear cell activation. Proc Natl Acad Sci U S A 100:1920–1925, 2003

Blake GJ, Ridker PM: Tumour necrosis factor-alpha, inflammatory biomarkers, and atherogenesis. Eur Heart J 23:345–347, 2002

Borish L, Schmaling K, DiClementi JD, et al: Chronic fatigue syndrome: identification of distinct subgroups on the basis of allergy and psychologic variables. J Allergy Clin Immunol 102:222–230, 1998

Borovikova LV, Ivanova S, Zhang M, et al: Vagus nerve stimulation attenuates the systemic inflammatory response to endotoxin. Nature 405:458–462, 2000

Braun J, McHugh N, Singh A, et al: Improvement in patient-reported outcomes for patients with ankylosing spondylitis treated with etanercept 50 mg once-weekly and 25 mg twice-weekly. Rheumatol (Oxf) 46:999–1004, 2007

Brustolim D, Ribeiro-dos-Santos R, Kast RE, et al: A new chapter opens in anti-inflammatory treatments: the antidepressant bupropion lowers production of tumor necrosis factor-alpha and interferon-gamma in mice. Int Immunopharmacol 6:903–907, 2006

Cannon JG, Angel JB, Ball RW, et al: Acute phase responses and cytokine secretion in chronic fatigue syndrome. J Clin Immunol 19:414–421, 1999

Capuron L, Gumnick JF, Musselman DL, et al: Neurobehavioral effects of interferon-alpha in cancer patients: phenomenology and paroxetine responsiveness of symptom dimensions. Neuropsychopharmacology 26:643–652, 2002a

Capuron L, Ravaud A, Neveu PJ, et al: Association between decreased serum tryptophan concentrations and depressive symptoms in cancer patients undergoing cytokine therapy. Mol Psychiatry 7:468–473, 2002b

Capuron L, Neurauter G, Musselman DL, et al: Interferon-alpha-induced changes in tryptophan metabolism: relationship to depression and paroxetine treatment. Biol Psychiatry 54:906–914, 2003a

Capuron L, Raison CL, Musselman DL, et al: Association of exaggerated HPA axis response to the initial injection of interferon-alpha with development of depression during interferon-alpha therapy. Am J Psychiatry 160:1342–1345, 2003b

Capuron L, Pagnoni G, Demetrashvili M, et al: Anterior cingulate activation and error processing during interferon-alpha treatment. Biol Psychiatry 58:190–196, 2005

Capuron L, Pagnoni G, Demetrashvili MF, et al: Basal ganglia hypermetabolism and symptoms of fatigue during interferon-alpha therapy. Neuropsychopharmacology 32:2384–2392, 2007

Caroleo MC, Pulvirenti L, Arbitrio M, et al: Evidence that CRH microinfused into the locus coeruleus decreases cell-mediated immune response in rats. Funct Neurol 8:271–277, 1993

Cohen S, Tyrrell DA, Smith AP: Psychological stress and susceptibility to the common cold (comments). N Engl J Med 325:606–612, 1991

Cunnick JE, Lysle DT, Kucinski BJ, et al: Evidence that shock-induced immune suppression is mediated by adrenal hormones and peripheral beta-adrenergic receptors. Pharmacol Biochem Behav 36:645–651, 1990

Czura CJ, Rosas-Ballina M, Tracey KJ: Cholinergic regulation of inflammation, in Psychoneuroimmunology, 4th Edition. Edited by Ader R. Burlington, MA, Elsevier Academic Press, 2007, pp 85–96

Daaka Y, Luttrell LM, Lefkowitz RJ: Switching of the coupling of the beta2-adrenergic receptor to different G proteins by protein kinase A. Nature 390:88–91, 1997

Dantzer R: Cytokine-induced sickness behavior: where do we stand? Brain Behav Immun 15:7–24, 2001

Dantzer R, Kelley KW: Twenty years of research on cytokine-induced sickness behavior. Brain Behav Immun 21:153–160, 2007

de Jonge WJ, van der Zanden EP, The FO, et al: Stimulation of the vagus nerve attenuates macrophage activation by activating the Jak2-STAT3 signaling pathway. Nat Immunol 6:844–851, 2005

Dhabhar FS: Stress-induced enhancement of cell-mediated immunity. Ann N Y Acad Sci 840:359–372, 1998

Dhabhar FS, McEwen BS: Enhancing versus suppressive effects of stress hormones on skin immune function. Proc Natl Acad Sci U S A 96:1059–1064, 1999

Dhabhar FS, Miller AH, McEwen BS, et al: Effects of stress on immune cell distribution. Dynamics and hormonal mechanisms. J Immunol 154:5511–5527, 1995

Downing JE, Miyan JA: Neural immunoregulation: emerging roles for nerves in immune homeostasis and disease. Immunol Today 21:281–289, 2000

Duman RS, Nakagawa S, Malberg J: Regulation of adult neurogenesis by antidepressant treatment. Neuropsychopharmacology 25:836–844, 2001

Elenkov IJ, Chrousos G: Stress hormones, Th1/Th2 patterns, pro/anti-inflammatory cytokines and susceptibility to disease. Trends Endocrinol Metab 10:359–368, 1999

Evans DL, Staab JP, Petitto JM, et al: Depression in the medical setting: biopsychological interactions and treatment considerations. J Clin Psychiatry 60 (suppl 4):40–55; discussion 56, 1999

Evans DL, Charney DS, Lewis L, et al: Mood disorders in the medically ill: scientific review and recommendations. Biol Psychiatry 58:175–189, 2005

Fenton WS, Stover ES: Mood disorders: cardiovascular and diabetes comorbidity. Curr Opin Psychiatry 19:421–427, 2006

Foley FW, Traugott U, LaRocca NG, et al: A prospective study of depression and immune dysregulation in multiple sclerosis. Arch Neurol 49:238–244, 1992

Ford DE, Erlinger TP: Depression and C-reactive protein in US adults: data from the Third National Health and Nutrition Examination Survey. Arch Intern Med 164:1010–1014, 2004

Frank MG, Baratta MV, Sprunger DB, et al: Microglia serve as a neuroimmune substrate for stress-induced potentiation of CNS pro-inflammatory cytokine responses. Brain Behav Immun 21:47–59, 2007

Frasure-Smith N, Lesperance F, Julien P: Major depression is associated with lower omega-3 fatty acid levels in patients with recent acute coronary syndromes. Biol Psychiatry 55:891–896, 2004

Gatti S, Bartfai T: Induction of tumor necrosis factor-alpha mRNA in the brain after peripheral endotoxin treatment: comparison with interleukin-1 family and interleukin-6. Brain Res 624:291–294, 1993

Glaser R, Kiecolt-Glaser JK, Bonneau RH, et al: Stress-induced modulation of the immune response to recombinant hepatitis B vaccine. Psychosom Med 54:22–29, 1992

Goebel MU, Mills PJ, Irwin MR, et al: Interleukin-6 and tumor necrosis factor-alpha production after acute psychological stress, exercise, and infused isoproterenol: differential effects and pathways. Psychosom Med 62:591–598, 2000

Goldstein R, Bowen DL, Fauci AS: Adrenal corticosteroids, in Inflammation: Basic Principles and Clinical Correlates. Edited by Gallin JI, Goldstein IM, Snyderman R. New York, Raven, 1992, pp 1061–1082

Guarini S, Altavilla D, Cainazzo MM, et al: Efferent vagal fibre stimulation blunts nuclear factor-kappaB activation and protects against hypovolemic hemorrhagic shock. Circulation 107:1189–1194, 2003

Gupta S, Aggarwal S, See D, et al: Cytokine production by adherent and non-adherent mononuclear cells in chronic fatigue syndrome. J Psychiatr Res 31:149–156, 1997

Hasler G, Drevets WC, Manji HK, et al: Discovering endophenotypes for major depression. Neuropsychopharmacology 29:1765–1781, 2004

Heim C, Owens MJ, Plotsky PM, et al: The role of early adverse life events in the etiology of depression and posttraumatic stress disorder. Focus on corticotropin-releasing factor. Ann N Y Acad Sci 821:194–207, 1997

Herbert TB, Cohen S: Depression and immunity: a meta-analytic review. Psychol Bull 113:472–486, 1993

Hickie I, Lloyd A: Are cytokines associated with neuropsychiatric syndromes in humans? Int J Immunopharmacol 17: 677–683, 1995

Hickie I, Hickie C, Lloyd A, et al: Impaired in vivo immune responses in patients with melancholia. Br J Psychiatry 162:651–657, 1993

Hohagen F, Timmer J, Weyerbrock A, et al: Cytokine production during sleep and wakefulness and its relationship to cortisol in healthy humans. Neuropsychobiology 28:9–16, 1993

Holsboer F: The corticosteroid hypothesis of depression. Neuropsychopharmacology 23:477–501, 2000

Honda M, Orii F, Ayabe T, et al: Expression of glucocorticoid receptor beta in lymphocytes of patients with glucocorticoid-resistant ulcerative colitis. Gastroenterology 118:859–866, 2000

Huston JM, Ochani M, Rosas-Ballina M, et al: Splenectomy inactivates the cholinergic antiinflammatory pathway during lethal endotoxemia and polymicrobial sepsis. J Exp Med 203:1623–1628, 2006

Ignatowski TA, Spengler RN: Tumor necrosis factor-alpha: presynaptic sensitivity is modified after antidepressant drug administration. Brain Res 665:293–299, 1994

Irwin M, Hauger RL, Brown M, et al: CRF activates autonomic nervous system and reduces natural killer cytotoxicity. Am J Physiol 255 (5 pt 2):R744–R747, 1988

Irwin M, McClintick J, Costlow C, et al: Partial night sleep deprivation reduces natural killer and cellular immune responses in humans. FASEB J 10:643–653, 1996

Irwin M, Costlow C, Williams H, et al: Cellular immunity to varicella-zoster virus in patients with major depression. J Infect Dis 178 (suppl 1):S104–S108, 1998

Johnson JD, O'Connor KA, Watkins LR, et al: The role of IL-1beta in stress-induced sensitization of proinflammatory cytokine and corticosterone responses. Neuroscience 127:569–577, 2004

Johnson JD, Campisi J, Sharkey CM, et al: Catecholamines mediate stress-induced increases in peripheral and central inflammatory cytokines. Neuroscience 135:1295–1307, 2005

Karalis K, Muglia LJ, Bae D, et al: CRH and the immune system. J Neuroimmunol 72:131–136, 1997

Katugampola RP, Lewis VJ, Finlay AY: The Dermatology Life Quality Index: assessing the efficacy of biological therapies for psoriasis. Br J Dermatol 156:945–950, 2007

Kenis G, Maes M: Effects of antidepressants on the production of cytokines. Int J Neuropsychopharmacol 5:401–412, 2002

Kent S, Bluthe RM, Kelley KW, et al: Sickness behavior as a new target for drug development. Trends Pharmacol Sci 13:24–28, 1992

Kiecolt-Glaser JK, Marucha PT, Malarkey WB, et al: Slowing of wound healing by psychological stress (comments). Lancet 346:1194–1196, 1995

Kim YK, Na KS, Shin KH, et al: Cytokine imbalance in the pathophysiology of major depressive disorder. Prog Neuropsychopharmacol Biol Psychiatry 31:1044–1053, 2007

Kohm AP, Sanders VM: Norepinephrine: a messenger from the brain to the immune system. Immunol Today 21:539–542, 2000

Kris-Etherton PM, Harris WS, Appel LJ: Fish consumption, fish oil, omega-3 fatty acids, and cardiovascular disease. Arterioscler Thromb Vasc Biol 23:e20–e30, 2003

Labeur MS, Arzt E, Wiegers GJ, et al: Long-term intracerebroventricular corticotropin-releasing hormone administration induces distinct changes in rat splenocyte activation and cytokine expression. Endocrinology 136:2678–2688, 1995

Lacosta S, Merali Z, Anisman H: Central monoamine activity following acute and repeated systemic interleukin-2 administration. Neuroimmunomodulation 8:83–90, 2000

Lanquillon S, Krieg JC, Bening-Abu-Shach U, et al: Cytokine production and treatment response in major depressive disorder. Neuropsychopharmacology 22:370–379, 2000

Laye S, Parnet P, Goujon E, et al: Peripheral administration of lipopolysaccharide induces the expression of cytokine transcripts in the brain and pituitary of mice. Brain Res Mol Brain Res 27:157–162, 1994

Leaf A, Kang JX, Xiao YF, et al: Clinical prevention of sudden cardiac death by n-3 polyunsaturated fatty acids and mechanism of prevention of arrhythmias by n-3 fish oils. Circulation 107:2646–2652, 2003

Ledeboer A, Jekich BM, Sloane EM, et al: Intrathecal interleukin-10 gene therapy attenuates paclitaxel-induced mechanical allodynia and proinflammatory cytokine expression in dorsal root ganglia in rats. Brain Behav Immun 21:686–698, 2007

Leserman J, Jackson ED, Petitto JM, et al: Progression to AIDS: the effects of stress, depressive symptoms, and social support. Psychosom Med 61:397–406, 1999

Lesperance F, Frasure-Smith N, Theroux P, et al: The association between major depression and levels of soluble intercellular adhesion molecule 1, interleukin-6, and C-reactive protein in patients with recent acute coronary syndromes. Am J Psychiatry 161:271–277, 2004

Leu SJ, Singh VK: Stimulation of interleukin-6 production by corticotropin-releasing factor. Cell Immunol 143:220–227, 1992

Leu SJ, Shiah IS, Yatham LN, et al: Immune-inflammatory markers in patients with seasonal affective disorder: effects of light therapy. J Affect Disord 63:27–34, 2001

Leung DY: Atopic dermatitis: immunobiology and treatment with immune modulators. Clin Exp Immunol 107 (suppl 1):25–30, 1997

Linthorst AC, Flachskamm C, Holsboer F, et al: Intraperitoneal administration of bacterial endotoxin enhances noradrenergic neurotransmission in the rat preoptic area: relationship with body temperature and hypothalamic-pituitary-adrenocortical axis activity. Eur J Neurosci 7:2418–2430, 1995a

Linthorst AC, Flachskamm C, Muller-Preuss P, et al: Effect of bacterial endotoxin and interleukin-1 beta on hippocampal serotonergic neurotransmission, behavioral activity, and free corticosterone levels: an in vivo microdialysis study. J Neurosci 15:2920–2934, 1995b

Maes M: Major depression and activation of the inflammatory response system. Adv Exp Med Biol 461:25–46, 1999

Maes M, Song C, Lin A, et al: The effects of psychological stress on humans: increased production of pro-inflammatory cytokines and a Th1-like response in stress-induced anxiety. Cytokine 10:313–318, 1998

Maes M, Christophe A, Delanghe J, et al: Lowered omega 3 poly-unsaturated fatty acids in serum phospholipids and cholesteryl esters of depressed patients. Psychiatry Res 85:275–291, 1999a

Maes M, Libbrecht I, Van Hunsel F, et al: The immune-inflammatory pathophysiology of fibromyalgia: increased serum soluble gp130, the common signal transducer protein of various neurotrophic cytokines. Psychoneuroendocrinology 24:371–383, 1999b

Maes M, Lin AH, Delmeire L, et al: Elevated serum interleukin-6 (IL-6) and IL-6 receptor concentrations in posttraumatic stress disorder following accidental man-made traumatic events. Biol Psychiatry 45:833–839, 1999c

Maes M, Song C, Lin AH, et al: Negative immunoregulatory effects of antidepressants: inhibition of interferon-gamma and stimulation of interleukin-10 secretion. Neuropsychopharmacology 20:370–379, 1999d

Maier SF, Watkins LR: Cytokines for psychologists: implications of bidirectional immune-to-brain communication for understanding behavior, mood, and cognition. Psychol Rev 105:83–107, 1998

Maier SF, Goehler LE, Fleshner M, et al: The role of the vagus nerve in cytokine-to-brain communication. Ann N Y Acad Sci 840:289–300, 1998

Marchand F, Perretti M, McMahon SB: Role of the immune system in chronic pain. Nature Reviews Neuroscience 6:521–532, 2005

Mathias SD, Colwell HH, Miller DP, et al: Health-related quality of life and functional status of patients with rheumatoid arthritis randomly assigned to receive etanercept or placebo. Clin Ther 22:128–139, 2000

McEwen BS, Biron CA, Brunson KW, et al: The role of adrenocorticoids as modulators of immune function in health and disease: neural, endocrine and immune interactions. Brain Res Brain Res Rev 23:79–133, 1997

McKay LI, Cidlowski JA: Molecular control of immune/inflammatory responses: interactions between nuclear factor-kappa B and steroid receptor-signaling pathways. Endocrinol Rev 20:435–459, 1999

Miller AH: Neuroendocrine and immune system interactions in stress and depression. Psychiatr Clin North Am 21:443–463, 1998

Miller AH, Spencer RL, Hassett J, et al: Effects of selective type I and II adrenal steroid agonists on immune cell distribution. Endocrinology 135:1934–1944, 1994

Miller AH, Pearce B, Pariante C: Immune system and central nervous system interactions, in Kaplan and Sadock's Comprehensive Textbook of Psychiatry, Vol 1. Philadelphia, PA, Lippincott Williams & Wilkins, 2000, pp 113–133

Miller RJ, Sutherland AG, Hutchison JD, et al: C-reactive protein and interleukin 6 receptor in post-traumatic stress disorder: a pilot study. Cytokine 13:253–255, 2001

Milligan ED, Nguyen KT, Deak T, et al: The long term acute phase-like responses that follow acute stressor exposure are blocked by alpha-melanocyte stimulating hormone. Brain Res 810:48–58, 1998

Milligan ED, Sloane EM, Langer SJ, et al: Repeated intrathecal injections of plasmid DNA encoding interleukin-10 produce prolonged reversal of neuropathic pain. Pain 126:294–308, 2006

Mioni C, Bazzani C, Giuliani D, et al: Activation of an efferent cholinergic pathway produces strong protection against myo-cardial ischemia/reperfusion injury in rats. Crit Care Med 33:2621–2628, 2005

Moalem G, Tracey DJ: Immune and inflammatory mechanisms in neuropathic pain. Brain Res Rev 51:240–264, 2006

Moore P, Landolt HP, Seifritz E, et al: Clinical and physiological consequences of rapid tryptophan depletion (comment). Neuropsychopharmacology 23:601–622, 2000

Moraska A, Campisi J, Nguyen KT, et al: Elevated IL-1beta contributes to antibody suppression produced by stress. J Appl Physiol 93:207–215, 2002

Müller N, Riedel M, Scheppach C, et al: Beneficial antipsychotic effects of celecoxib add-on therapy compared to risperidone alone in schizophrenia. Am J Psychiatry 159:1029–1034, 2002

Müller N, Schwarz MJ, Dehning S, et al: The cyclooxygenase-2 inhibitor celecoxib has therapeutic effects in major depression: results of a double-blind, randomized, placebo controlled, add-on pilot study to reboxetine. Mol Psychiatry 11:680–684, 2006

Munck A: Glucocorticoid physiology and homeostasis in relation to anti-inflammatory actions, in Anti-Inflammatory Steroid Action: Basic and Clinical Aspects. New York, Academic Press, 1989, pp 30–47

Musselman DL, Nemeroff CB: Depression and endocrine disorders: focus on the thyroid and adrenal system. Br J Psychiatry 30 (suppl):123–128, 1996

Musselman DL, Lawson DH, Gumnick JF, et al: Paroxetine for the prevention of depression induced by high-dose interferon alfa (comments). N Engl J Med 344:961–966, 2001a

Musselman DL, Miller AH, Porter MR, et al: Higher than normal plasma interleukin-6 concentrations in cancer patients with depression: preliminary findings. Am J Psychiatry 158:1252–1257, 2001b

Nesse RM, Williams GC: Why We Get Sick. New York, Times Books, 1994

Nishioka T, Kurokawa H, Takao T, et al: Differential changes of corticotropin releasing hormone (CRH) concentrations in plasma and synovial fluids of patients with rheumatoid arthritis (RA). Endocr J 43:241–247, 1996

Norbiato G, Bevilacqua M, Vago T, et al: Glucocorticoid resistance and the immune function in the immunodeficiency syndrome. Ann N Y Acad Sci 840:835–847, 1998

Norris JG, Benveniste EN: Interleukin-6 production by astrocytes: induction by the neurotransmitter norepinephrine. J Neuroimmunol 45:137–145, 1993

Oakley RH, Sar M, Cidlowski JA: The human glucocorticoid receptor beta isoform. Expression, biochemical properties, and putative function. J Biol Chem 271:9550–9559, 1996

Opp MR: Cytokines and sleep. Sleep Med Rev 9:355–364, 2005

Owens MJ, Nemeroff CB: Physiology and pharmacology of corticotropin-releasing factor. Pharmacol Rev 43:425–473, 1991

Owens MJ, Nemeroff CB: The role of corticotropin-releasing factor in the pathophysiology of affective and anxiety disorders: laboratory and clinical studies. Ciba Found Symp 172:296–308; discussion 308–216, 1993

Owens MJ, Nemeroff CB: The serotonin transporter and depression. Depress Anxiety 8 (suppl 1):5–12, 1998

Pace TW, Mletzko TC, Alagbe O, et al: Increased stress-induced inflammatory responses in male patients with major depression and increased early life stress. Am J Psychiatry 163:1630–1633, 2006

Pace TW, Hu F, Miller AH: Cytokine-effects on glucocorticoid receptor function: relevance to glucocorticoid resistance and the pathophysiology and treatment of major depression. Brain Behav Immun 21:9–19, 2007

Paez Pereda M, Sauer J, Perez Castro C, et al: Corticotropin-releasing hormone differentially modulates the interleukin-1 system according to the level of monocyte activation by endotoxin. Endocrinology 136:5504–5510, 1995

Paik IH, Toh KY, Lee C, et al: Psychological stress may induce increased humoral and decreased cellular immunity. Behav Med 26:139–141, 2000

Papanicolaou DA: Euthyroid sick syndrome and the role of cytokines. Rev Endocr Metab Disord 1:43–48, 2000

Papanicolaou DA, Wilder RL, Manolagas SC, et al: The pathophysiologic roles of interleukin-6 in human disease. Ann Intern Med 128:127–137, 1998

Pariante CM, Miller AH: Glucocorticoid receptors in major depression: relevance to pathophysiology and treatment. Biol Psychiatry 49:391–404, 2001

Pariante CM, Nemeroff CB, Miller AH: Glucocorticoid receptors in depression. Isr J Med Sci 31:705–712, 1995

Pariante CM, Pearce BD, Pisell TL, et al: The proinflammatory cytokine, interleukin-1alpha, reduces glucocorticoid receptor translocation and function. Endocrinology 140:4359–4366, 1999

Parker G, Gibson NA, Brotchie H, et al: Omega-3 fatty acids and mood disorders. Am J Psychiatry 163:969–978, 2006

Pavlov VA, Tracey KJ: The cholinergic anti-inflammatory pathway. Brain Behav Immun 19:493–499, 2005

Pearce BD: Schizophrenia and viral infection during neurodevelopment: a focus on mechanisms. Mol Psychiatry 6:634–646, 2001

Peet M, Horrobin DF: A dose-ranging study of the effects of ethyl-eicosapentaenoate in patients with ongoing depression despite apparently adequate treatment with standard drugs. Arch Gen Psychiatry 59:913–919, 2002

Persoons P, Vermeire S, Demyttenaere K, et al: The impact of major depressive disorder on the short- and long-term outcome of Crohn's disease treatment with infliximab. Aliment Pharmacol Ther 22:101–110, 2005

Plotkin SR, Banks WA, Kastin AJ: Comparison of saturable transport and extracellular pathways in the passage of interleukin-1 alpha across the blood-brain barrier. J Neuroimmunol 67:41–47, 1996

Quan N, Stern EL, Whiteside MB, et al: Induction of pro-inflammatory cytokine mRNAs in the brain after peripheral injection of subseptic doses of lipopolysaccharide in the rat. J Neuroimmunol 93:72–80, 1999

Rabin BS: Stress, Immune Function, and Health: The Connection. New York, Wiley, 1999

Raison CL, Miller AH: The neuroimmunology of stress and depression. Semin Clin Neuropsychiatry 6:277–294, 2001

Raison CL, Miller AH: Depression in cancer: new developments regarding diagnosis and treatment. Biol Psychiatry 54:283–294, 2003a

Raison CL, Miller AH: When not enough is too much: the role of insufficient glucocorticoid signaling in the pathophysiology of stress-related disorders. Am J Psychiatry 160:1554–1565, 2003b

Raison CL, Nemeroff CB: Cancer and depression: prevalence, diagnosis, and treatment. Home Health Care Consultant 7:34–41, 2000

Raison CL, Gumnick JF, Miller AH: Neuroendocrine-immune interactions: implications for health and behavior, in Hormones, Brain and Behavior, Vol 5. San Diego, CA, Academic Press, 2002, pp 209–261

Raison CL, Capuron L, Miller AH: Cytokines sing the blues: inflammation and the pathogenesis of depression. Trends Immunol 27:24–31, 2006

Rassnick S, Sved AF, Rabin BS: Locus coeruleus stimulation by corticotropin-releasing hormone suppresses in vitro cellular immune responses. J Neurosci 14:6033–6040, 1994

Ressler KJ, Nemeroff CB: Role of norepinephrine in the pathophysiology and treatment of mood disorders. Biol Psychiatry 46:1219–1233, 1999

Reynolds JL, Ignatowski TA, Sud R, et al: Brain-derived tumor necrosis factor-alpha and its involvement in noradrenergic neuron functioning involved in the mechanism of action of an antidepressant. J Pharmacol Exp Ther 310:1216–1225, 2004

Rhen T, Cidlowski JA: Antiinflammatory action of glucocorticoids—new mechanisms for old drugs. N Engl J Med 353:1711–1723, 2005

Ridker PM, Hennekens CH, Buring JE, et al: C-reactive protein and other markers of inflammation in the prediction of cardiovascular disease in women. N Engl J Med 342:836–843, 2000a

Ridker PM, Rifai N, Stampfer MJ, et al: Plasma concentration of interleukin-6 and the risk of future myocardial infarction among apparently healthy men. Circulation 101:1767–1772, 2000b

Rivest S, Lacroix S, Vallieres L, et al: How the blood talks to the brain parenchyma and the paraventricular nucleus of the hypothalamus during systemic inflammatory and infectious stimuli. Proc Soc Exp Biol Med 223:22–38, 2000

Roitt I, Bostoff J, Male D: Immunology. New York, CV Mosby, 1998

Rothermundt M, Arolt V, Bayer TA: Review of immunological and immunopathological findings in schizophrenia. Brain Behav Immun 15:319–339, 2001

Ruzek MC, Pearce BD, Miller AH, et al: Endogenous glucocorticoids protect against cytokine-mediated lethality during viral infection. J Immunol 162:3527–3533, 1999

Sanders V, Kavelaars A: Adrenergic regulation of immunity, in Psychoneuroimmunology, 4th Edition. Edited by Ader R. Burlington, MA, Elsevier Academic Press, 2007, pp 63–84

Schaffler A, Scholmerich J, Salzberger B: Adipose tissue as an immunological organ: toll-like receptors, C1q/TNFs and CTRPs. Trends Immunol 28:393–399, 2007

Schleifer SJ, Keller SE, Bond RN, et al: Major depressive disorder and immunity. Role of age, sex, severity, and hospitalization. Arch Gen Psychiatry 46:81–87, 1989

Schobitz B, De Kloet ER, Holsboer F: Gene expression and function of interleukin 1, interleukin 6 and tumor necrosis factor in the brain. Prog Neurobiol 44:397–432, 1994

Schulte HM, Bamberger CM, Elsen H, et al: Systemic interleukin-1 alpha and interleukin-2 secretion in response to acute stress and to corticotropin-releasing hormone in humans. Eur J Clin Invest 24:773–777, 1994

Shahidi H, Vottero A, Stratakis CA, et al: Imbalanced expression of the glucocorticoid receptor isoforms in cultured lymphocytes from a patient with systemic glucocorticoid resistance and chronic lymphocytic leukemia. Biochem Biophys Res Commun 254:559–565, 1999

Shen Y, Connor TJ, Nolan Y, et al: Differential effect of chronic antidepressant treatments on lipopolysaccharide-induced depressive-like behavioural symptoms in the rat. Life Sci 65:1773–1786, 1999

Shuto H, Kataoka Y, Horikawa T, et al: Repeated interferon-alpha administration inhibits dopaminergic neural activity in the mouse brain. Brain Res 747:348–351, 1997

Silverman MN, Miller AH, Biron CA, et al: Characterization of an interleukin-6- and adrenocorticotropin-dependent, immune-to-adrenal pathway during viral infection [see comment]. Endocrinology 145:3580–3589, 2004

Silverman MN, Pearce BD, Biron CA, et al: Immune modulation of the hypothalamic-pituitary-adrenal (HPA) axis during viral infection. Vir Immunol 18:41–78, 2005

Silverman MN, Macdougall MG, Hu F, et al: Endogenous glucocorticoids protect against TNF-alpha-induced increases in anxiety-like behavior in virally infected mice. Mol Psychiatry 12:408–417, 2007

Simen BB, Duman CH, Simen AA, et al: TNFalpha signaling in depression and anxiety: behavioral consequences of individual receptor targeting. Biol Psychiatry 59:775–785, 2006

Simopoulos AP: Omega-3 fatty acids in inflammation and autoimmune diseases. J Am Coll Nutr 21:495–505, 2002

Sluzewska A: Indicators of immune activation in depressed patients. Adv Exp Med Biol 461:59–73, 1999

Snider LA, Swedo SE: Pediatric obsessive-compulsive disorder. JAMA 284:3104–3106, 2000

Sousa AR, Lane SJ, Cidlowski JA, et al: Glucocorticoid resistance in asthma is associated with elevated in vivo expression of the glucocorticoid receptor beta-isoform. J Allergy Clin Immunol 105:943–950, 2000

Spivak B, Shohat B, Mester R, et al: Elevated levels of serum interleukin-1 beta in combat-related posttraumatic stress disorder. Biol Psychiatry 42:345–348, 1997

Stenzel-Poore MP, Heinrichs SC, Rivest S, et al: Overproduction of corticotropin-releasing factor in transgenic mice: a genetic model of anxiogenic behavior. J Neurosci 14(5, pt 1):2579–2584, 1994

Steptoe A, Willemsen G, Owen N, et al: Acute mental stress elicits delayed increases in circulating inflammatory cytokine levels (comments). Clin Sci 101:185–192, 2001

Sternberg EM, Hill JM, Chrousos GP, et al: Inflammatory mediator-induced hypothalamic-pituitary-adrenal axis activation is defective in streptococcal cell wall arthritis-susceptible Lewis rats. Proc Natl Acad Sci U S A 86:2374–2378, 1989

Stoll AL, Severus WE, Freeman MP, et al: Omega 3 fatty acids in bipolar disorder: a preliminary double-blind, placebo-controlled trial (comments). Arch Gen Psychiatry 56:407–412, 1999

Tanskanen A, Hibbeln JR, Tuomilehto J, et al: Fish consumption and depressive symptoms in the general population in Finland. Psychiatr Serv 52:529–531, 2001

Tiemeier H, van Tuijl HR, Hofman A, et al: Plasma fatty acid composition and depression are associated in the elderly: the Rotterdam Study. Am J Clin Nutr 78:40–46, 2003

Tracey KJ: The inflammatory reflex. Nature 420:853–859, 2002

Trask P, Esper P, Riba M, et al: Psychiatric side effects of interferon therapy: prevalence, proposed mechanisms, and future directions. J Clin Oncol 18:2316–2326, 2000

Tyring S, Gottlieb A, Papp K, et al: Etanercept and clinical outcomes, fatigue, and depression in psoriasis: double-blind placebo-controlled randomised phase III trial [see comment]. Lancet 367:29–35, 2006

van Westerloo DJ, Giebelen IA, Florquin S, et al: The vagus nerve and nicotinic receptors modulate experimental pancreatitis severity in mice. Gastroenterology 130:1822–1830, 2006

Veith RC, Lewis N, Linares OA, et al: Sympathetic nervous system activity in major depression. Basal and desipramine-induced alterations in plasma norepinephrine kinetics. Arch Gen Psychiatry 51:411–422, 1994

Wang H, Liao H, Ochani M, et al: Cholinergic agonists inhibit HMGB1 release and improve survival in experimental sepsis. Nat Med 10:1216–1221, 2004

Wang X, Wu H, Miller AH: Interleukin 1alpha (IL-1alpha) induced activation of p38 mitogen-activated kinase inhibits glucocorticoid receptor function. Mol Psychiatry 9:65–75, 2004

Webster JC, Oakley RH, Jewell CM, et al: Proinflammatory cytokines regulate human glucocorticoid receptor gene expression and lead to the accumulation of the dominant negative beta isoform: a mechanism for the generation of glucocorticoid resistance. Proc Natl Acad Sci U S A 98:6865–6870, 2001

Wong ML, Kling MA, Munson PJ, et al: Pronounced and sustained central hypernoradrenergic function in major depression with melancholic features: relation to hypercortisolism and corticotropin-releasing hormone. Proc Natl Acad Sci U S A 97:325–330, 2000

Yirmiya R, Pollak Y, Barak O, et al: Effects of antidepressant drugs on the behavioral and physiological responses to lipopolysaccharide (LPS) in rodents. Neuropsychopharmacology 24:531–544, 2001

Zhu CB, Carneiro AM, Dostmann WR, et al: p38 MAPK activation elevates serotonin transport activity via a trafficking-independent, protein phosphatase 2A-dependent process. J Biol Chem 280:15649–15658, 2005

Zhu CB, Blakely RD, Hewlett WA: The proinflammatory cytokines interleukin-1beta and tumor necrosis factor-alpha activate serotonin transporters. Neuropsychopharmacology 31:2121–2131, 2006

Zobel AW, Nickel T, Kunzel HE, et al: Effects of the high-affinity corticotropin-releasing hormone receptor 1 antagonist R121919 in major depression: the first 20 patients treated. J Psychiatr Res 34:171–181, 2000

Zorrilla E, Luborsky L, McKay JR, et al: The relationship of depression and stressors to immunological assays: a meta-analytic review. Brain Behav Immun 15:199–226, 2001

CHAPTER 10

Brain Imaging in Psychopharmacology

Ebrahim Haroon, M.D.

Giuseppe Pagnoni, Ph.D.

Christine M. Heim, Ph.D.

Gregory S. Berns, M.D., Ph.D.

Helen S. Mayberg, M.D.

Functional brain imaging refers to a class of techniques that noninvasively measure correlates of neural activity. Positron emission tomography (PET) and functional magnetic resonance imaging (fMRI) are the two technologies most commonly used today to study the human brain "in action." The explosion of information about human brain function occurring in the past decade has resulted in large part from these two techniques. As will be described in this chapter, PET imaging has made considerable contributions to our understanding of the mechanisms of drug action, mostly through application of radiopharmaceutical labeling of neurotransmitter receptors. fMRI, on the other hand, has gained rapid acceptance because of the widespread availability of magnetic resonance imaging (MRI) scanners, the lack of radioactive exposure, and the better image resolution offered.

The advent of neuroimaging techniques for probing in vivo human brain function undoubtedly represents a major milestone in the scientific endeavor of understanding the relationship between mental disorders and the brain. The development of the specific tools employed in brain mapping, although fairly recent, has already produced an impressive amount of experimental data, whose potential informational content is most likely being underexploited at the present time (Van Horn and Gazzaniga 2002). The neuroimaging approach offers the unique possibility of noninvasively investigating the neurophysiological, neuroanatomical, and neurochemical correlates of the living, performing human individual. As a complement to classical neuropsychology, this approach represents an unprecedented break from the necessity of lesion studies for the inference of structure–function relationships in the human brain. Furthermore, a neuroimaging assay can typically acquire data simultaneously from the entire cerebral system, thereby allowing the study of the distributed processing properties of the brain (Friston 2002). Those properties represent a fundamental and distinctive feature of massively parallel processing systems

Portions of this chapter are reprinted from Berns GS: "Functional Neuroimaging." *Life Sciences* 65:2531–2540 1999. Copyright 1999, Elsevier Science. Used with permission.

but are not easily penetrated with the standard neurophysiological methods employed in the animal, such as intracortical electrode recording, which can probe only a limited number of sites simultaneously.

Neuroimaging Techniques

Neuroimaging is a generic term for a number of techniques and methods aimed at detecting meaningful information through the acquisition of brain images of different kinds. The presentation of different classification criteria may help the reader to get a sense of this rich but often confounding landscape. A first classification may be technology based:

- MRI
- PET
- Single photon emission computed tomography (SPECT)
- Electroencephalography (EEG)
- Magnetoencephalography (MEG)

Each of the above technologies requires different hardware, and each measures different physical quantities. It should be noted that whereas PET and SPECT employ radioactive tracers that limit their repeated use on the same subject, the other techniques are noninvasive and therefore allow more latitude in regard to experimental design and the subsequent statistical treatment of the data. MRI and PET/SPECT scanners are able to implement different imaging protocols, according to the specific acquisition modality employed (MRI) or the nature of the injected radioisotope (PET/SPECT). More recently, the availability of combined PET–computed tomography (PET–CT) and PET–MRI scanners has yielded an added dimension to our capacity to understand human brain in action (Blodgett et al. 2007).

The neurally related variable that is actually imaged may provide an alternative classification framework:

- *Vascular (or hemodynamic) effects engendered by neural activity:* PET ($H_2^{15}O$), fMRI (blood oxygenation level–dependent [BOLD] contrast, perfusion imaging), SPECT
- *Metabolic demand:* PET (^{18}fluorodeoxyglucose)
- *Receptor density:* PET/SPECT (radioligands)
- *Neurochemistry:* Magnetic resonance spectroscopy (MRS)
- *Connectivity pathways:* MRI (diffusion tensor imaging), fMRI-based functional connectivity analysis

- *Surface electromagnetic effects of brain activity:* EEG/MEG
- *Morphometry of brain structures:* MRI

We begin this chapter with current thoughts on the physiological basis of functional imaging and the phenomenon of neural activation it attempts to study (referred to as "neurovascular coupling") and then proceed to examine the two major functional imaging modalities of relevance to psychiatry—PET and fMRI. The section on fMRI will also incorporate basic principles of MRI. We end the chapter with a brief review of magnetic resonance (MR)–based structural imaging modalities and how they might confer newer insights into the understanding of mental illness and development of newer treatments. The focus is intended to be on how these imaging methods are used to better understand psychopharmacology. More details on individual disorders will be available in their respective sections.

Functional Imaging and Correlates of Neural Activity

It has been known for more than 100 years that blood flow to the brain increases in a regionally specific manner, according to mental activity. The father of modern psychology, William James, was aware of observations relating regional brain pulsation to mental activity (James 1890). Paul Broca, known primarily for his observations on the effects of left frontal lesions on language, performed several experiments relating regional brain temperature to cognitive function (Broca 1879). But it was not until the 1950s, when Seymour Kety and Louis Sokoloff developed the autoradiographic technique for quantitatively measuring regional blood flow, that specific cognitive functions could be directly mapped in the living brain (Kety 1965).

Both PET and fMRI rely on the fact that blood flow increases in areas where neuronal activity increases, and most studies implicitly assume the validity of this relationship. It is easy to see the link in terms of an increased metabolic demand. The activation of a neural circuit is a complex network of electrochemical processes that requires energy. The most demanding processes, in terms of energy expenditure, are those related to synaptic activity, which results in breakdown of energy stores in the neuron in the form of adenosine triphosphate (ATP) molecules. To replace the ATP energy stores degraded by the increased metabolic demand, a surge in the concentration of glucose and oxygen is necessary, which results in increased blood flow to the activated region. It is this vascular or *hemodynamic* response to neural activity—that is, the variation in regional cerebral blood flow (rCBF)—that is the quantity actually measured in the majority of brain activation studies with fMRI and PET/SPECT (Arthurs and Boniface 2002; Jueptner and Weiller 1995). Thus, the hemodynamic response represents an *indirect* assay of neural activity (Villringer and Dirnagl 1995). It is important to note that the hemodynamic response *lags behind* the actual neural activity by a few seconds. The hemodynamic response is also blurred in the spatial domain compared with the underlying neural activity. This imposes limits on the spatiotemporal resolution of blood flow methods, independently of technology improvement.

A special caveat should be noted concerning the interpretation of rCBF results. The measurement of task-related variations of rCBF does not provide any clear indication about the nature of the underlying neural activity (i.e., whether it is excitatory or inhibitory), although hypotheses have been proposed for and argued against a bias favoring excitatory contributions (Heeger et al. 1999; Tagamets and Horwitz 2001; Waldvogel et al. 2000). The construction of specific inferences about the actual state of activity—actively excited or actively inhibited—of brain regions showing an increase in rCBF during an experimental task would require the integration of information from many different sources (e.g., electrophysiology, neurochemistry, cytoarchitectonics).

In summary, despite the fact that the physiological and biochemical processes linking the neural activity and the hemodynamic response have not been clarified yet, the empirical relationship between these parameters appears to be both reliable and reproducible in a variety of contexts. The validity of fMRI measurements of signal change as an assay of neural activity has been documented using electrophysiological techniques such as neuronal field potentials (Logothetis et al. 2001).

Positron Emission Tomography

PET was developed from in vivo autoradiographic techniques. In an autoradiographic procedure, an animal is typically injected with a biologically interesting compound synthesized with a radioisotope (e.g., ^{3}H). When the animal is sacrificed, the local tissue radioactivity is easily quantified. Although autoradiography yields exquisitely detailed pictures of brain activity, it can only be applied in animals, and the animals must be sacrificed to obtain the brain tissue. Although these techniques were in use in the 1950s and 1960s, the development of an in vivo method applicable to humans awaited technological advancements from the "silicon revolution"—namely, the availability of high-quality inexpensive crystal detectors and the huge advancements in computing power realized in the late 1970s.

PET requires three basic technologies: the production of positron-emitting compounds, the ability to detect simultaneously emitted gamma rays, and the computational power to reconstruct the sources of emission. Positrons, or positively charged electrons (antimatter), have a particular advantage over other radioactive compounds. When a positron encounters an electron, the two annihilate each other, and their collective energy is transformed into two high-energy photons that are emitted in exactly opposite directions. Because the photons travel 180° apart, it is easy to arrange a ring of detectors to determine where the annihilation occurred. When two detectors are activated simultaneously, then one knows that the emission occurred somewhere along the line connecting the two detectors. By collecting the counts over a period of time, say 60 seconds, and over a full sphere surrounding the subject's head, it becomes possible to reconstruct the geometry of the source.

Positrons are produced indirectly, through the radioactive decay of particular isotopes. The most commonly used isotopes (carbon-11 [^{11}C], oxygen-15 [^{15}O], fluorine-18 [^{18}F], nitrogen-13 [^{13}N]) are produced in a cyclotron by the bombardment of targets with high-energy protons. This results in a gas (e.g., ^{15}O$_2$), which can then be used in any chemical reaction (e.g., oxidation–reduction reaction with product H$_2$^{15}O). After appropriate purification procedures, these compounds can then be injected intravenously into a human subject, and they flow to the brain in about 20 seconds. The isotope undergoes radioactive decay by positron emission, and the half-life depends on the particular isotope (e.g., 2 minutes for ^{15}O).

Because the photons emitted during positron decay are fairly high in energy (511-keV gamma rays), they tend to pass through matter with relative ease. A specialized detector, called a scintillation detector, is required to accurately count the decays in a directional fashion. PET scanners consist of rings of these detectors arranged in parallel planes. An individual detector would be constructed from a scintillating crystal, either bismuth germanate (BGO) or lutetium oxyorthosilicate (LSO), and amplification electronics. When a gamma ray enters the crystal, it loses its energy through either the photoelectric or Compton effect, which results in the production of electrons. These electrons further interact with the crystal, resulting in the production of visible wavelength photons. These photons are then detected and amplified by a photomultiplier tube and converted into an electrical pulse. A "coincidence circuit" allows for the identification of the detector that picks up the 180°-emitted gamma ray.

Depending on the injected molecule, a particular regional distribution will occur. In the case of $H_2^{15}O$, it will follow the rCBF. Other compounds will cross the blood–brain barrier and bind to specific receptors, in which case the distribution of radioactivity will reflect receptor concentration. Fluorodeoxyglucose-18 (^{18}FDG), a commonly used tracer, is metabolized by hexokinase during glycolysis, like glucose. Unlike glucose-6 phosphate, ^{18}FDG is not metabolized further and thus accumulates intracellularly, yielding a measurement of local metabolic activity (Kennedy et al. 1976; Reivich et al. 1979).

Types of PET Studies

Most PET neuroimaging studies can be grouped into one of three categories: metabolic, blood flow, or receptor studies.

Metabolic PET Studies

Metabolic studies use ^{18}FDG to measure regional glucose metabolism. ^{18}FDG, like all ^{18}F compounds, has the advantage of a relatively long half-life (110 minutes). This allows the synthesis to be performed in one location, the subject injection in another location, and the scanning in yet another location. In fact, one can have a subject doing a particular task in a location remote from the PET scanner and inject ^{18}FDG, which will be trapped in brain regions according to the local metabolic rate. This has an obvious advantage in situations in which placing the subject in the scanner would alter the conditions of the task. For example, ^{18}FDG is used commonly in sleep studies. The main disadvantage is that the long half-life results in effectively no temporal resolution. This offers a time-averaged snapshot of a particular brain state, and the state is averaged over 20–60 minutes. Figure 10–1 shows functional localization of an epileptic focus in the right temporal lobe during presurgical workup.

Most of the FDG uptake studies are based on the assumption that the glucose uptake and neural activity at the synaptic level might be coupled. A caveat must be borne in mind when evaluating studies using FDG-PET. Glutamate is the main excitatory neurotransmitter in the brain, and it is removed from the synapse through a process of uptake by astroglial tissues, thus terminating neural activation (Magistretti and Pellerin 1999). But recent studies have shown that uptake of glutamate by astroglia can by itself stimulate glucose (and FDG) uptake (Magistretti 2006). In fact, deactivation might actually be coupled with increased glucose uptake in a variety of conditions (Magistretti 2006). Thus, the same problems that accompany studies of fMRI—i.e., whether the signal is actively excitatory versus actively inhibitory—are present in FDG-PET studies as well.

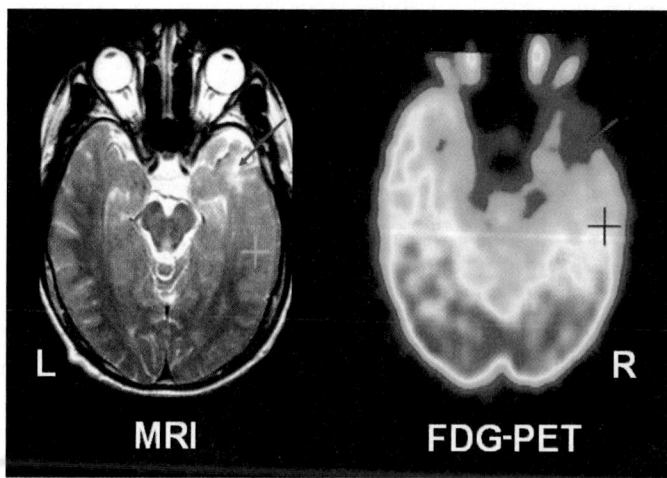

FIGURE 10–1.   Functional localization of an epileptic focus in the right temporal lobe during presurgical workup using magnetic resonance imaging (MRI) and fluorodeoxyglucose positron emission tomography (FDG-PET).

Source.   Image courtesy of Carolyn C. Meltzer, M.D.

Blood Flow PET Studies

Blood flow studies use $H_2{}^{15}O$ to measure changes in local brain blood flow (Herscovitch et al. 1983; Mintun et al. 1984). As noted earlier, blood flow is an indirect measure of local synaptic activity. Because ^{15}O has a short half-life (2 minutes), several administrations can be performed in one session. A typical $H_2{}^{15}O$ study would have 8–16 injections and scans for each subject. The experimental design would manipulate the task that the subject performs during each scan. Each scan lasts about 1 minute, with 8–10 minutes between scans (5 half-lives). $H_2{}^{15}O$ studies not only allow for multiple conditions to be studied, but they also allow for the repetition of conditions, increasing statistical power. The main disadvantage is that because of the short half-life, the $H_2{}^{15}O$ must be produced reliably and in close proximity to the scanner.

Receptor-Mapping PET Studies

Receptor studies use radioligands—chemicals incorporating a positron-emitting isotope into a molecule whose pharmacokinetics are already known. Ideally, these ligands bind specifically to one receptor type. Most of these studies are of the mapping type, which shows the distribution of a particular receptor in the brain (e.g., dopamine type 2 [D_2] receptor). Here, the measured radioactivity reflects both the local concentration of receptors (B_{max}) and the affinity of the ligand for the receptor (measured by K_D, the equilibrium dissociation constant). If the ligand acts as a competitive antagonist, then the *apparent* affinity is also affected by the concentration of the endogenous neurotransmitter. The analysis can be simplified by considering the ratio of B_{max} to K_D, termed the *binding potential* (BP). Ligands undergo both specific and nonspecific binding. Typically, one is interested only in the specific binding (i.e., to the receptor of interest). Use of a reference tissue that is known to have a low receptor concentration allows one to subtract out the nonspecific binding (e.g., the cerebellum has a low concentration of D_2 receptors). In this case, the difference in distribution for the two tissues is directly proportional to the BP. Ligands require a more involved synthesis than either water or ^{18}FDG, and their use is a race against the clock as the isotope decays. The end product must meet several requirements: high specific activity (amount of radioactivity per mole), high radiochemical purity, and sterility. ^{18}F ligands are easier to synthesize because of their long half-life, but ^{11}C ligands (20-minute half-life) have a higher potential for biological relevance. These will be discussed in the next section, which addresses psychopharmacological applications of PET tracers and ligands.

Clinical Applications of PET and SPECT in Psychopharmacology

PET-based receptor imaging has provided us with a window to view the complex functioning of brain systems involved in mediating treatment response to psychopharmacological agents. A snapshot of available radionuclide-binding modalities is provided in Table 10–1. Using PET-based radioligands, it has been possible to visualize density, distribution, and occupancy of neural receptors and transporters before, during, and after drug therapy (Talbot and Laruelle 2002). Details about use of neuroimaging methods in individual psychiatric disorders will be described in detail in later chapters pertaining to these disorders. In the following sections, specific examples will be provided to illustrate the use of imaging methods to answer pertinent questions of relevance to psychopharmacology.

Neurotransmitter Synthesizing Systems

Appropriate availability of neurotransmitters and neuromodulators is essential to normal neurological and psychological function. Dysfunction or degeneration of neurons that synthesize these substances can lead to various disorders. For example, Parkinson's disease is caused by selective degeneration of the dopamine-synthesizing neurons of the nigrostriatal system. Uptake of [^{18}F] DOPA, which selectively labels aromatic L-amino acid decarboxylase (AADC), a critical enzyme in the synthesis of dopamine, has been used to estimate both the number of surviving cells and AADC activity among nigral neurons, thus providing a tool to understand the connection between dopamine dysfunction and clinical symptom evolution (Cropley et al. 2006; Ravina et al. 2005). PET scanning using [^{11}C] methyl-L-tryptophan, which is a marker of serotonin (5-HT) synthesis, is being used in identifying overactive serotonin-synthesizing systems in differentiating epileptogenic from nonepileptogenic lesions in tuberous sclerosis (Luat et al. 2007) prior to neurosurgery. In a similar vein, recent functional imaging techniques have combined with neurosurgical treatments such as deep brain stimulation to study brain imaging biomarkers of treatment response (Carbon and Eidelberg 2002).

Neurotransmitter Binding Sites

PET imaging has been used to identify binding sites of neurotransmitters of relevance to psychiatric disorders, in order to characterize patients and inform treatment decisions based on mechanisms of drug action. For instance, studies with ligands that bind to D_2 receptors have in-

TABLE 10–1.   Pharmacoimaging in psychiatry

IMAGING MODALITY	LABELING AGENT	BINDING SITE	CLINICAL FOCUS AND TYPE OF PHARMACOLOGICAL PROBE
Dopamine			
PET	[^{18}F] DOPA	Aromatic L-amino acid decarboxylase	Viability of dopamine-synthesizing neurons Probe type: enzyme labeling ligand
PET	[^{11}C] methylphenidate, [^{11}C] cocaine, [^{123}I] β-CIT, [^{11}C] WIN 35428	Dopamine uptake receptor	Synaptic dopamine availability and correlation with cognition Probe type: reuptake transporter ligand
PET	[^{11}C] raclopride, [^{11}C] FLB 457, [^{18}F] fallipiride, [^{11}C] NPA	D_2 receptor	Binding and affinity and occupancy of D_2 receptors by antipsychotics Probe type: postsynaptic (PS) receptor ligand
PET	[^{11}C] NNC-112, [^{11}C] SCH 23390	D_1 receptor	Role of dopamine in cognition Probe type: PS receptor ligand
SPECT	[^{123}I] iodobenzamide	D_2 receptor	Hyperresponse of dopamine secretion in schizophrenia Probe type: PS receptor ligand
Serotonin			
PET	[^{11}C] methyl-L-tryptophan	5-HT synthesis	A marker of 5-HT biosynthesis Probe type: precursor ligand
PET	[^{18}F] setoperone, [^{18}F] ketanserin, [^{18}F] altanserin	5-HT_{2A} receptor	Serotonin turnover among suicidal and depressed patients Probe type: PS receptor ligand
PET	[^{11}C] WAY-100685	5-HT_{1A} receptor	Antidepressant efficacy studies Type: autoreceptor ligand
PET	[^{11}C] McN-5652, [^{11}C] DASB	SERT	Antidepressant binding efficacy Probe type: reuptake site ligand
SPECT	[^{123}I] β-CIT, [^{123}I] ADAM	SERT; type: same as above	Antidepressant binding efficacy Probe type: reuptake site ligand
SPECT	[^{123}I] 5-I-R91150	5-HT_{2A} receptor	Serotonin turnover Probe type: PS receptor ligand
Amino acid transmitters: GABA/glutamate			
SPECT	[^{123}I] iomazenil	Benzodiazepine receptor	GABA levels in anxiety states Probe type: PS receptor ligand
Magnetic resonance spectroscopy	None	None	Concentrations of GABA, glutamate Probe type: metabolomic approach
Beta-amyloid imaging			
PET	[^{18}F] FDDNP, [^{11}C] PIB, [^{11}C] SB	Beta-amyloid plaque	Progression of senile plaques in Alzheimer's disease Probe type: ligand of pathological deposit

Note.   5-HT = serotonin (5-hydroxytryptamine); GABA = γ-aminobutyric acid; PET = positron emission tomography; SERT = serotonin transporter; SPECT = single photon emission computed tomography.

formed us that lower binding affinity, faster dissociation, and optimal occupancy at usually prescribed doses of D_2 receptor antagonists might form the basis of atypical antipsychotic drug action (Kapur and Remington 2001). Studies reporting increased binding of serotonin type 2A (5-HT_{2A}) receptors using agents such as ^{18}F-altanserin in frontal cortex (Brodmann area [BA] 9) and their association with increased pessimism and self-injurious and suicidal behavior have added to our understanding of depression (Meyer et al. 2003). Alterations in the function of γ-aminobutyric acid (GABA) systems in posttraumatic stress disorder (PTSD) and panic disorder have been reported based on decreased binding of (^{123}I)iomazenil to benzodiazepine receptors in the BA 9 region of these patients (Bremner et al. 2000).

Neurotransmitter Reuptake Site Binding Studies

Drugs that bind to and inhibit the serotonin reuptake transporter (SERT) have been shown to be associated with symptomatic recovery from depression in a large number of patients (Nemeroff 2007). Radioligands that show high specificity for binding to SERT, such as [^{11}C] 3-amino-4-(2-dimethylaminomethyl-phenylsulfanyl)-benzonitrile (^{11}C DASB), have been used to study the site occupancy levels of selective serotonin reuptake inhibitors (SSRIs) and how these values correlate with clinical efficacy (Meyer 2007). These methods have led to reformulation of clinical algorithms in the management of depressive disorders. Suicide remains a serious risk among all psychiatric patients, and the role of SERT in the expression of suicide has been studied using PET ligands (Purselle and Nemeroff 2003). Dopamine transporter (DAT) ligands have also been used to study cognitive and motor dysfunction in Parkinson's disease (Cropley et al. 2006; Ravina et al. 2005), and the same methods are currently being applied to investigate conditions such as attention-deficit/hyperactivity disorder (ADHD).

Neurotransmitter Autoreceptor Binding Methods

Synaptic turnover of serotonin secretion is regulated by two processes—by SERT-mediated reuptake and by negative feedback mediated through serotonin type 1A (5-HT$_{1A}$) autoreceptors. Downregulation of 5-HT$_{1A}$ receptors may be associated with antidepressant efficacy and might also explain the delay in the onset of clinical response after being started on SSRIs (Blier and Ward 2003). Radioligands such as [^{11}C] WAY-100865 have been used to study the dynamics of 5-HT$_1$ receptors (Fisher et al. 2006). This methodology has also made contributions to better understanding how serotonergic system imbalances disrupt mood-regulating neural circuitry, resulting in depressive disorders (Fisher et al. 2006).

Pathological Cerebral Deposits

Degenerative disorders such as Alzheimer's disease have acquired critical relevance, given the larger proportion of aging population in the modern society. Since the pathological changes associated with neurodegeneration (such as beta-amyloid deposits, neurofibrillary tangles, and decreased metabolic activity) often precede clinical disease by several decades, early identification of these changes is of paramount importance. Three different ligands have been reported recently, all of them with the ability to detect intracerebral beta-amyloid deposition with high accuracy using PET radiotracer technology: [^{18}F] FDDNP (Small et al. 2006), [^{11}C] PIB (Pittsburgh Compound–B) (Klunk et al. 2004), and [^{11}C] SB (Ono et al. 2003). Such compounds have potential clinical applications in that they may help identify patients with mild cognitive impairment (MCI) who are at increased risk of converting to dementia (Mathis et al. 2005).

PET Tracers of Cerebral Metabolism and Blood Flow

PET has been used to assess functional activity of brain regions, both in the resting state and in response to various stimuli. The methods used include use of FDG-PET and radioactive [^{15}O] H$_2$O-PET to study metabolic activity and blood flow, respectively. Figure 10–2A shows a picture of increased cerebral blood flow to paralimbic regions during a sad mood induction task (to be described later) using H$_2$O-PET. In contrast, Figure 10–2B shows metabolic activity differences among depressed versus healthy patients using FDG-PET. These modalities have been effectively used to study a variety of mental phenomena and have been of considerable benefit in enhancing our understanding of psychiatric disorders. Of particular interest have been studies using PET to understand the biological basis of schizophrenia (Fujimoto et al. 2007; Lange et al. 2005), bipolar disorder (Post et al. 2003), depression (Mayberg 2003b; Neumeister et al. 2004), substance abuse and craving (Kilts et al. 2004), PTSD (Bremner 2007), ADHD (Schweitzer et al. 2003), and Alzheimer's disease (Small 1996). Most of the studies of psychiatric disorders have shown generally similar patterns of resting blood flow and metabolic abnormalities in using PET. That said, such identified patterns have not yet proven adequately consistent to warrant use of PET as a diagnostic procedure in an individual patient. Notably, only resting-state FDG-PET scanning has undergone repeated sensitivity and specificity testing to be considered useful and reliable for the diagnosis of Alzheimer's disease in patients with progressive cognitive disturbance and presumed dementia (Silverman et al. 2002). Nonetheless, research studies using these methods have provided considerable new in-

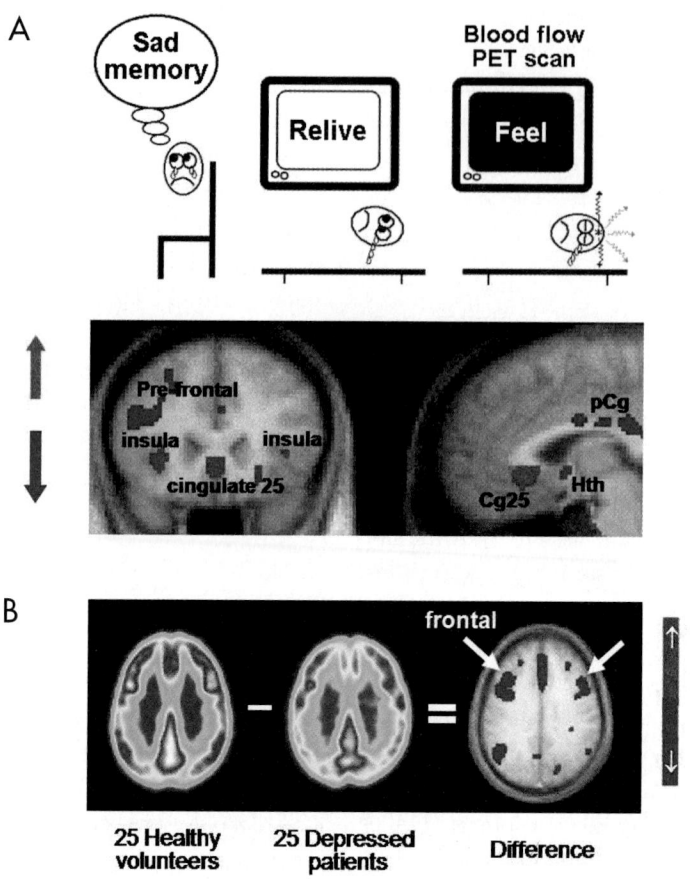

FIGURE 10–2.   (A) Task-induced increased cerebral blood flow using H₂O-PET. (B) FDG-PET resting-state contrasts among depressed patients versus healthy control subjects.

FDG = fluorodeoxyglucose; PET = positron emission tomography; Cg25 = subgenual cingulate; pCg = posterior cingulate; Hth = hypothalamus.

Source.   (A) Adapted from Mayberg HS, Liotti M, Brannan SK, et al.: "Reciprocal Limbic-Cortical Function and Negative Mood: Converging PET Findings in Depression and Normal Sadness." *American Journal of Psychiatry* 156:675–682, 1999. Copyright 1999, American Psychiatric Association. Used with permission. (B) Image courtesy of Helen Mayberg, M.D.

sights into disease pathophysiology as well as mechanisms mediating treatment response (Erritzoe et al. 2003; Evans et al. 2006; Mayberg 2003a; Roffman et al. 2005).

Magnetic Resonance Imaging

The basis of MRI technology rests on the magnetic properties of the hydrogen atom, which, as a component of water, is found ubiquitously in organic tissues (water constitutes roughly 80% of brain weight). The nucleus of a hydrogen atom, a single proton, is characterized by an intrinsic magnetic moment, called *spin*. The protons in tissue are normally oriented in random directions, but if an external magnetic field is applied, they will tend to align with the field. Quantum mechanics and statistical physics dictate that spins can orient either in the direction of the

applied field (*parallel*) or in the direction opposite to it (*anti-parallel*), but on average the parallel orientation will gain a weak majority. This situation will result in a net magnetic moment induced by the external field in the tissue; in other words, the tissue will become slightly magnetized. The external (or *main*) field in an MR environment is provided by a powerful electromagnet whose intensity is typically 1.5 tesla for clinical scanners (for comparison, the electromagnets used in car demolition lots have a similar strength), and up to 7 tesla for human research scanners. The intensity of the induced magnetization is dependent on the proton distribution (i.e., on the local molecular characteristic of the tissue). Although this induced magnetization could, in principle, provide a contrast signal resolving different types of tissues (e.g., gray matter, white matter, cerebrospinal fluid) into an image of anatomical detail, the magnitude of this effect is in practice so small that it does not lend itself to direct measurement.

The way in which MRI actually recovers its signal is by first perturbing the examined system. This instrumental perturbation is performed by applying short radiofrequency (RF) pulses that, when appropriately tuned, are able to transiently tip the orientation of the spins away from the applied magnetic field. However, the tendency of the spins is to return to the orientation coherent with the applied magnetic field, given that the latter state is characterized by a lower energy. The relaxation process occurs through the emission of an RF wave that is detected by the same RF hardware that emits the excitation pulses. In MR terminology, this is referred to as the RF coil, which has the form of a small cylindrical cage that surrounds the subject's head in the scanner. The emitted RF wave—or, more precisely, the temporal signature of its decay as the excited spins relax—constitutes the actual MR signal and depends on the molecular characteristics of the local tissue, as well on the particular sequence of excitation pulses employed. The details of the physics that specify how appropriate pulse sequences can be engineered to acquire images of the brain system with different physiological meaning are beyond the scope of this discussion, and the interested reader is directed elsewhere (e.g., Buxton 2002).

The spin relaxation measured with MRI can be decomposed into longitudinal and transverse components, which are only partially related. The measurement of the relaxation time of the longitudinal component, called *T1*, provides images in which the contrast between different types of tissue (notably, gray matter, white matter, and cerebrospinal fluid) is maximized. Such *T1-weighted images* are capable of defining the anatomy of the living brain with great precision and are therefore used as an anatomical reference for most of the neuroimaging studies. An image of the entire brain, with a resolution, or voxel size, of 1 mm^3 (*voxel* stands for "volume pixel," the unitary element of a three-dimensional image), can be acquired on a 1.5-tesla clinical scanner in less than 6 minutes.

The measurement of the relaxation time of the transverse component, which can be further split between the T2 and the T2* characteristic times, provides images that are influenced by the local inhomogeneity of the magnetic field, which in turn is increased by the local blood perfusion. In particular, T2*-weighted images are characterized by a contrast that highlights changes in vascular dynamics that accompany neural activity and are thus employed in functional mapping studies. The advent of a very fast technique for the acquisition of T2*-weighted images, called *echoplanar imaging* (EPI), allows the collection of an entire brain volume in 3–4 seconds and has been instrumental in the rapid development of functional MRI. The ultrarapid acquisition of EPI images and the nature of the detected T2* signal, which tends to become negligible when integrated over very small voxels, limit the resolution of standard EPI images, which typically have a voxel size of 3–4 mm per side. The use of particular technical and experimental arrangements has allowed, in special cases, the achievement of submillimetric precision, such as that required for the imaging of the columnar organization of visual cortex (Menon and Goodyear 1999). Table 10–2 includes the multiple applications of MR-based technologies in psychopharmacology.

Functional MRI

Functional magnetic resonance imaging, or fMRI, refers to a variant of MRI that is sensitive to local changes in deoxyhemoglobin concentration. The increase in regional blood flow, as engendered by neural activation, overshoots the oxygen consumption. This results in an apparent *decrease* in deoxyhemoglobin. In the 1930s, Linus Pauling had observed that the amount of oxygen carried by hemoglobin is inversely proportional to the degree to which it perturbed a magnetic field. This property of differential paramagnetism was finally demonstrated in vivo in the late 1980s, and fMRI was born (Ogawa et al. 1992; Thulborn et al. 1982).

The BOLD Signal in Functional MRI

Functional MRI exploits the fact that deoxyhemoglobin has paramagnetic properties and oxyhemoglobin does not. Deoxyhemoglobin disturbs the local magnetic environment, causing the surrounding protons to dephase even faster than they would otherwise (Figure 10–3).

Because neuronal activity leads to an overactive increase in blood flow, this actually decreases the amount of deoxyhemoglobin relative to oxyhemoglobin. Because less deoxyhemoglobin means less rapid spin dephasing, this increase in blood flow appears as an increase in MR signal. This is called the blood oxygenation level–dependent (BOLD) signal. In response to a regionally specific neuronal activation, the BOLD signal will usually increase by an amount on the order of 1% on a standard 1.5-tesla clinical scanner. The intensity of the signal is proportional to the strength of the main magnetic field—for example, it will double in the case of a 3-tesla scanner.

The temporal resolution of fMRI is determined both by the hemodynamic response and the physical con-

TABLE 10–2.   Use of magnetic resonance imaging (MRI) in psychopharmacology research

TYPE OF IMAGING	TECHNIQUE	METHOD OF ANALYSIS	USED TO MEASURE
Structural MRI (sMRI)	Voxel-based morphometry (VBM)	Automated	Volume of brain regions in brain disorders and ischemic lesions
sMRI	Region of interest (ROI) analysis	Manual	Same as above to measure volumes and ischemic brain lesions (hyperintensities)
Functional MRI (fMRI)	BOLD technique (described in text)	Computerized algorithm	Area of activation in response to cognitive/affective challenge
Functional connectivity analysis	Resting-state activity, independent component analysis (ICA), structural equation modeling	Computerized algorithms, statistical models	Connectivity between different components of neural network during various mental states
Diffusion-based MRI	Diffusion-weighted, perfusion-weighted, diffusion tensor imaging (DTI)	Computerized algorithms	Tissue integrity by imaging water diffusion in restricted and free space, used in diagnosis of stroke and neurodegeneration
Diffusion tensor tractography	DTI-based imaging and fiber tracking	Computerized algorithms	Anatomical white matter tract connectivity between brain locations
Magnetic resonance spectroscopy	Detect concentration of specific metabolites in cerebral regions	Automated and voxel based (manual)	Neuronal/glial metabolic abnormalities in localized in single or multiple voxels
Innovative in vivo magnetic resonance approaches			
Neuroimaging genomics	fMRI activations to challenges in various genotypes	Computerized genotyping	Identification of candidate disease-associated genes among genetically distinct populations (COMT, BDNF, 5-HTTLPR polymorphisms)
sMRI + fMRI	Data fusion using joint independent component analysis (jICA) of simultaneously recorded structural and functional data	Computerized algorithms	Structural and functional disconnection in mental disorders
Virtual reality (VR)–fMRI	VR-based cognitive challenges	Computerized	Cerebral activation in real-life scenarios (spatial recognition memory)
Hyperscanning	Online linkage of two fMRI scanners in different locations	Web based	Cerebral activation changes during social interactions (social neuroscience technique)

Note.   5-HTTLPR = serotonin transporter–linked polymorphic region; BDNF = brain-derived neurotrophic factor; BOLD = blood oxygenation level–dependent; COMT = catechol-O-methyltransferase.

straints of the scanner magnetic fields. The hemodynamic response generally lags the neural activity by 3–5 seconds and may extend upward to 10–15 seconds (Figure 10–4). The rate at which the scanner can acquire images is influenced by the desired resolution. Generally, the more slices and the finer the resolution within each slice, the longer a whole-brain acquisition takes. While an individual slice can be acquired in as little as 60 milliseconds, whole-brain imaging usually requires about 2–3 seconds.

Whereas fMRI measurements are easy to perform, there are specific limitations with BOLD imaging.

1. The BOLD effect originates from venous vessels (capillaries, venules, and veins), so the signal is not exactly collocated either with the locus of neural activity or with the arterial supply. This spatial error may, however, be negligible for brain-mapping studies employing a standard spatial resolution (voxel size ~50 mm^3).

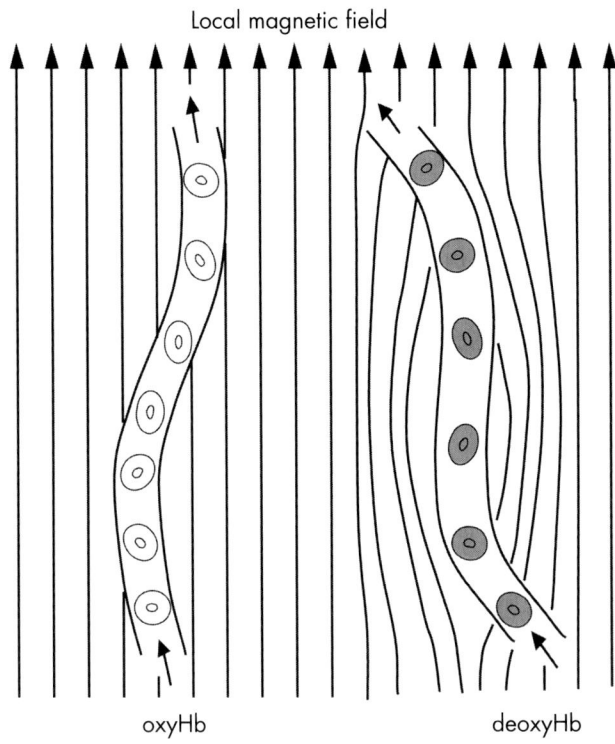

Local magnetic field

oxyHb   deoxyHb

FIGURE 10–3. Schematic diagram of the effect of hemoglobin (Hb) on the local magnetic field of brain tissue.

Only deoxyhemoglobin (deoxyHb) has paramagnetic properties and locally distorts the field, leading to faster spin dephasing.

Source. Reprinted from Pagnoni G, Berns GS: "Brain Imaging in Psychopharmacology," in *The American Psychiatric Publishing Textbook of Psychopharmacology,* 3rd Edition. Edited by Schatzberg AF, Nemeroff CB. Washington, DC, 2003, pp. 163–172. Copyright 2003, American Psychiatric Publishing, Inc. Used with permission.

2. Bulk head motion and physiological pulsation (heart pulse, respiration) artifacts. For the motion, head movement should be restrained while maintaining a comfortable situation for the subject.

3. Susceptibility artifacts. The fact that BOLD detects local changes in magnetic susceptibility (due to the variation in deoxyhemoglobin concentration) renders it vulnerable to the large discontinuity that exists at the interfaces between bone/air and bone/liquid. In these regions, the steep variations in tissue density cause a distortion of the local magnetic field, resulting in both a spatial distortion of the image and a drop in the BOLD signal. This makes it difficult to detect the small changes associated with deoxyhemoglobin variations. The problematic regions are notably the orbitofrontal cortex and the inferior part of the temporal lobes, which unfortunately are the locus of many interesting neuropsychological processes.

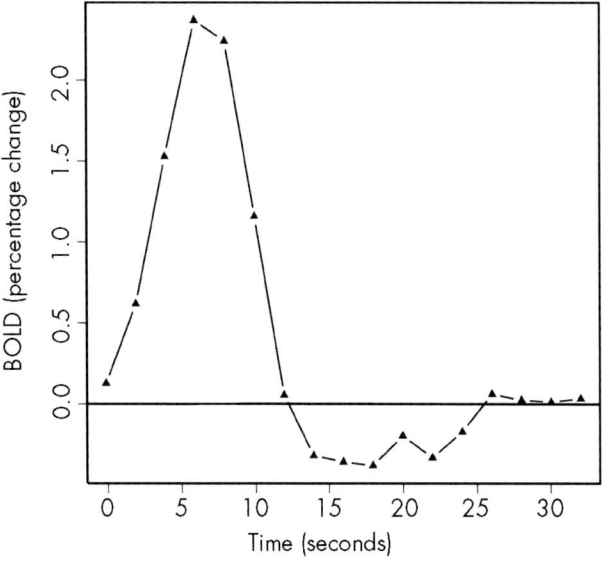

FIGURE 10–4. Relative blood oxygenation level–dependent (BOLD) response to 1-second visual stimulation.

These functional magnetic resonance imaging (fMRI) data are from the occipital cortex and were obtained in a healthy volunteer in a 3-tesla scanner. The amplitude of the signal is about 2%, with the peak 5–8 seconds after the stimulus.

Source. Reprinted from Pagnoni G, Berns GS: "Brain Imaging in Psychopharmacology," in *The American Psychiatric Publishing Textbook of Psychopharmacology,* 3rd Edition. Edited by Schatzberg AF, Nemeroff CB. Washington, DC, 2003, pp. 163–172. Copyright 2003, American Psychiatric Publishing, Inc. Used with permission.

Functional MRI Experimental Designs

The particular characteristics of fMRI (i.e., its noninvasiveness and its spatiotemporal resolution) allow for its use in a variety of experimental designs. Two commonly employed schemas are block design and event-related design.

In a *block design* experiment, the experimental conditions alternate in blocks of some tens of seconds, each consisting of multiple repetitions of the same condition. In the subsequent statistical analysis, the scans acquired during the same block are pooled together to give an average effect. In an *event-related design*, each single experimental event/stimulus is modeled separately, which usually allows more latitude both in terms of the analysis (one can, for instance, separate the scan corresponding to a correct behavioral response from the scans corresponding to the subject's errors) and of the experiment itself (for instance, one can alternate between events of different types to avoid effects related to habituation). The analysis of such studies relies on the assumption of linearity in the BOLD response: if events of the same type are presented not too closely one to the other (the "linearity" seems to break down with an interstimulus interval of 1–2 seconds), then the resulting BOLD signal is simply the sum of the BOLD responses for the individual events.

Comparison of PET and Functional MRI

The advantages and disadvantages of PET versus fMRI are summarized in Table 10–3.

Applications of Functional MRI in Psychopharmacological Research

At the time of writing this chapter, most of the applications of fMRI methods have been experimental—for example, helping investigators map areas of functional activation in response to cognitive and affective tasks. Similarly, several novel and innovative uses of imaging methods are seen in the literature, and the field has evolved considerably since the previous edition of this textbook. A few of these advances will be reviewed in this section and are also included in Table 10–2.

Neural activation in response to tasks. Measurement of neural activation patterns in response to specific tasks, using fMRI, has been particularly useful in elucidating the neural mechanisms contributing to the development of psychiatric disorders. Thus, specific tasks can be constructed that target specific emotional or cognitive behaviors that are altered in a given disorder. This research strategy allows delineation of neural pathways involved in the generation of specific symptoms and behaviors. A few examples of commonly used paradigms are discussed below.

Mood/self-referential paradigms. As an example, a core feature of depression involves negative bias and anhedonia, suggesting specific alterations in neural pathways mediating salience, self-reference, and reward. Accordingly, several fMRI studies reported failed activation of dorsomedial prefrontal cortex (BA 10) in depressed patients in response to positive words or pictures (Le Bastard et al. 2003; Mitterschiffthaler et al. 2003). Interestingly, activation of this region is also seen in tasks requiring self-referencing in healthy subjects (Craik et al. 1999; Fossati et al. 2003). A depression-specific pattern has been described using an emotional "Go/No-Go task" that identified blunted responses in reward circuits in response to neutral words but exaggerated responses in self-referential areas of the rostral cingulate and medial frontal cortex in

response to sad words (Elliott et al. 2002). Such sensitive tasks can plausibly be used as outcome measures in the evaluation of the efficacy of antidepressant treatments.

Facial expression–processing paradigms. Another task frequently used across a range of disorders involves the presentation of faces with different emotional expressions, such as angry, sad, fearful, happy, and neutral. Such faces can be either overtly presented or may be hidden behind a mask, depending on the study hypothesis. With overt presentation, subjects typically perform a behavioral task related to classifying some aspect of the faces. Application of such tasks in fMRI studies has produced a large amount of data regarding the neural basis of emotional processing in healthy subjects, reporting robust activation of the amygdala in response to emotional faces (Whalen et al. 1998). Of note, patients with depression, anxiety disorders, and PTSD exhibit increased amygdala responses to the presentation of fearful or angry faces (Rauch et al. 2000; Shin et al. 2005; Whalen et al. 2002). The paradigm has also proven useful to evaluate treatment effects of antidepressant drugs (Sheline et al. 2001), as well as temperamental or genetic contributions to emotional processing (Hariri et al. 2002; Stein et al. 2007). Similar strategies have identified antidepressant-induced changes with other tasks (Fu et al. 2007).

Cognitive "working memory" paradigms. Another common task used to identify neurocognitive changes is the so-called n-back task. The n-back task is a working memory task that reflects prefrontal cortical function. The n-back task has been used in fMRI studies to identify altered neural circuits in a variety of disorders, including schizophrenia and depression (Harvey et al. 2005; Meyer-Lindenberg and Weinberger 2006). The "n-back" working memory test (Owen et al. 2005) involves visual presentation of letter stimuli at previously chosen intervals and epochs (e.g., 2-second interval for 30-second epochs). The baseline (control) condition is usually a 0-back condition in which subjects are required to press a button with the right index finger when the stimulus (e.g., the letter "x") appears. In the experimental condition (1-, 2-, or 3-back), subjects are required to press a button if the presented stimulus is the same as a stimulus presented n trials previously ($n=1$, $n=2$, or $n=3$). The level of task difficulty and the condition are varied in a previously specified order throughout the scan time. Subject performance during scanning in regard to accuracy (number of target stimuli correctly identified) and response time (RT) is usually recorded. Interestingly, findings vary

TABLE 10-3. Advantages and disadvantages of positron emission tomography (PET) versus functional magnetic resonance imaging (fMRI)

Advantages of PET versus fMRI

Quiet (good for acoustic stimulation); fMRI may have noise >90 dB

Less sensitive to movement artifact

Allows metabolic and receptor mapping

Allows imaging of brain regions that are typically difficult to image with fMRI because of the presence of a susceptibility artifact (orbitofrontal cortex, inferior temporal lobe) that causes both distortion and loss of signal

Allows the use of standard measurement devices (physiological, behavioral) inside the scanner (i.e., avoids the complication for the need of specially designed MRI-compatible hardware)
(In the MRI environment, the presence of a very strong static magnetic field commands the use of diamagnetic components; moreover, every electric device in the scanner room needs to be carefully shielded to prevent interference problems to and from the scanner. Scanning is not used in patients who have pacemakers or ferromagnetic metal parts in their bodies.)

Disadvantages of PET versus fMRI

Injection of a radioactive isotope precludes the use of PET for longitudinal studies in which the same subjects are scanned repeatedly over an extended period of time.

PET provides an integral measure (over time) of brain activity (for activation techniques), with a temporal resolution on the order of minutes because of the lifetime of the isotope. By comparison, fMRI has a temporal resolution on the order of seconds. This prevents the use of sophisticated, event-related designs with PET. Also, the number of images typically collected with PET on a single subject rarely exceeds a dozen, thereby limiting the statistical treatment in the analysis of the data.

Spatial resolution is more limited with PET than with fMRI.

Cyclotron must be located nearby.

PET is more expensive than fMRI (utilization costs per hour: fMRI, ~$500; PET, ~$2,000).

The acquisition procedure is time-consuming and requires more resources. (One scan typically lasts ~3 hours [fMRI typically lasts <1 hour]. In comparison, the MRI experimental setup is easier to perform and can be operated by just one person.)

across disorders, suggesting differing impacts of underlying pathophysiology on networks mediating these behaviors. For example, increased prefrontal activity is seen in depressed patients relative to control subjects performing this task, an effect amplified by task difficulty (Harvey et al. 2005). On the other hand, several studies have reported that schizophrenic patients demonstrate deficits in activation of the prefrontal cortex during this task, thought to reflect alterations in dopamine functioning. Normalization of neural activation patterns by antipsychotic drugs is associated with response to treatment. The *n*-back task has also been useful in identifying genetic contributions to schizophrenia risk (Meyer-Lindenberg and Weinberger 2006). Bookheimer et al. (2000) used a verbal memory paradigm, in which patients memorized unrelated pairs of words during scanning, to study hippocampal activation in patients at risk of developing Alzheimer's disease. Not only did the carriers of the apolipoprotein epsilon 4 (*ApoE*-ε4)++ allele (higher risk of dementia) show greater hippocampal activation, but this baseline activation pattern predicted longitudinal cognitive decline.

Reward-processing paradigms. Reward-processing paradigms are commonly used in studying substance use and craving, but also in studying anhedonia in both depression and schizophrenia. In addiction studies, typically the patient, while lying in a scanner, is presented with multiple contexts associated with drug abuse, and activation of reward-processing circuitry is studied. Zink et al. (2006) used fMRI to study activation of the basal ganglia (a key component of reward circuitry) of healthy volunteers in response to salient stimuli with high motivational relevance. Figure 10–5 illustrates differential activation patterns in the ventral striatum in response to wins versus monetary losses during a gambling task, as measured with fMRI. The concept of "intertemporal discounting" is often used to describe choosing between discounted immediate reward to delayed reward at a rate that is much higher in value. Patients with impulse-control disorders such as pathological gambling show considerable variation in their tendency to use intertemporal discounting (Dixon et al. 2006). A recent study using fMRI reported that increased activation of paralimbic cortex was associated when choosing smaller/earlier rewards while fronto/parietal activation

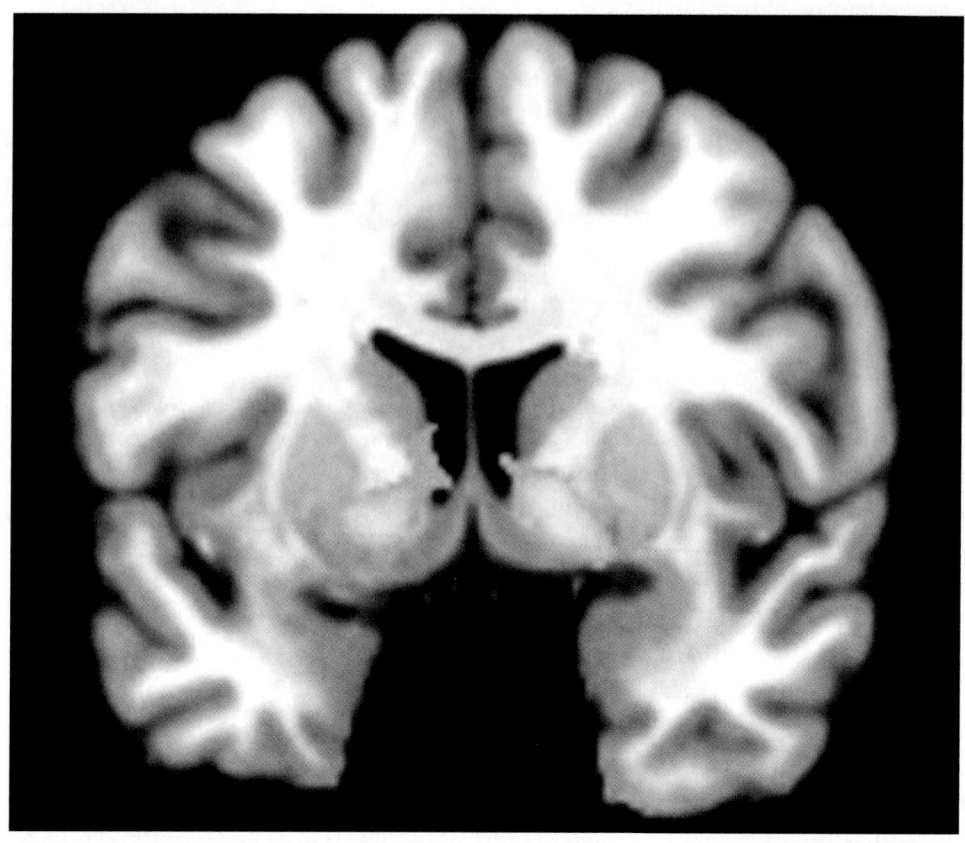

FIGURE 10–5.   Ventral striatum activation for wins versus monetary losses during a gambling task, as visualized with functional magnetic resonance imaging (fMRI).

Source.   Image courtesy of Giuseppe Pagnoni, Ph.D.

was seen when making the larger/later (opposite) type of choice (McClure et al. 2004). Studies such as these might help us develop brain activation–based biomarkers of complex disorders such as pathological gambling and substance abuse. A recent innovation in this field has been the development of "hyperscanning"—a method by which a person in an fMRI scanner at one location can interact with another person in another scanner using World Wide Web–based connectivity (Montague et al. 2002). Thus, the brain structures that are activated during social interactions could be studied using this technology.

Summary of neural activation paradigms.   In conclusion, these examples illustrate the potential of fMRI activation studies in probing brain–behavior relationships in psychiatric disorders, owing to the flexibility of fMRI paradigm design as well as the large variety of standardized tasks and possibility to develop novel tasks.

Neuroimaging genomics.   Despite the substantial advances in the pharmacotherapy of psychiatric disorders, re-

sponse rates of patients remain unsatisfactory. For example, only 40%–70% of depressed patients adequately respond to 6 weeks of treatment with a single antidepressant drug. The factors that determine whether or not a patient will favorably respond to a specific drug are poorly understood, and there are no established strategies for clinicians to decide whether a patient might benefit from psychotherapy rather than pharmacotherapy (Binder and Holsboer 2006). Similarly, there is considerable individual variability in the response to antipsychotic drugs in patients with schizophrenia, which remains unexplained, and some but not other patients experience debilitating side effects (Reynolds et al. 2006). In concert with the rapid advances in the field of molecular genetics, there has been increasing recognition that genes influence individual differences in treatment response, as studied in the field of pharmacogenetics (see Chapter 3, "Genetics and Genomics"). Neuroimaging techniques have substantial potential to further the field of pharmacogenetics. There has been a surge of studies in recent years using neuroimaging to describe genetically determined differences in brain structure and function. Research strategies include neuroimaging studies in twin populations, unaffected individuals with high familial risk for a specific disorder (i.e., healthy siblings of patients), and groups of individuals with different variants of functional polymorphisms in genes involved in brain development or behavior (Hariri et al. 2006; Meyer-Lindenberg and Weinberger 2006; Peper et al. 2007). Such studies not only advance our understanding of individual differences in cognitive and emotional behaviors, and the mechanisms involved in mental disorders, but also elucidate genetically determined variations in neural systems that are targeted by specific treatments. For example, one recent study found that the functional Val66Met polymorphism in the brain-derived neurotrophic factor (BDNF) gene moderates the association between depression and hippocampal volume loss. Carriers of the Met allele had smaller hippocampal volumes than subjects who were homozygous for the Val allele (Frodl et al. 2007). These findings suggest that the Met allele conveys increased risk for smaller hippocampi and susceptibility to depression. Because antidepressants stimulate neurogenesis in the hippocampus, carriers of the Met allele may be particularly responsive to antidepressant drugs.

In the area of schizophrenia research, it has been shown that a genetic variation (Val[108/158]Met) of catechol-O-methyltransferase (COMT), an important enzyme that degrades cortical dopamine at the synapse, is associated with deficits in working memory and prefrontal cortical activation in response to a working memory task. Specifically, carriers of the Val allele exhibit more deficits and less prefrontal cortical activation compared with subjects homozygous for the Met allele, likely reflecting low synaptic dopamine availability due to greater COMT activity, potentially increasing risk of developing schizophrenia (Meyer-Lindenberg and Weinberger 2006). Interestingly, the same polymorphism predicts effects of antipsychotic treatment on prefrontal cortical function in schizophrenic patients, as measured by fMRI, contributing to individual differences in treatment response (Bertolino et al. 2004). Based on such findings, COMT inhibitors are being investigated in the treatment of cognitive symptoms in schizophrenia.

Of course, in studying the effects of genes on neural responses to drugs, factors that interact with genes in shaping brain structure and function—for example, environmental factors across development—must be considered as well. In another example, it has been found that a functional polymorphism in the promoter region of the serotonin transporter gene—5-HTTLPR polymorphism (SCL6A4)—moderates the relationship between stress,

including child maltreatment, and depression (Caspi et al. 2003; Kaufman et al. 2004; Kendler et al. 2005). Carriers of the short (S) allele had increased depression risk in relation to stress, whereas subjects homozygous for the long (L) allele were resilient even in the context of severe stress. Remarkably, S allele carriers demonstrate increased amygdala activation as well as decreased functional connectivity between amygdala and inhibitory prefrontal cortical regions in response to emotional stimuli, compared with L/L allele carriers (Hariri et al. 2002; Heinz et al. 2005; Pezawas et al. 2005). Of note, both the SCL6A4 polymorphism and developmental stress have been associated with treatment response to serotonergic drugs (Nemeroff et al. 2003; Reimold et al. 2007). Accordingly, neuroimaging is evolving as a valuable tool to evaluate gene–environment–drug interactions at the neural level. Such studies, taken together, have the potential to yield diagnostic markers to guide treatment decisions and identify targets for the prevention of manifest disorders in subjects at risk.

Default or resting-state functional imaging. Most studies reviewed so far have used challenges or probes that elicit neural activation and blood flow responses that could be captured by fMRI or PET scanners. Several authors have consistently found evidence for the existence of a "default" neural network that preferentially shows greater activity during restful or passive cognitive states (Buckner and Vincent 2007; Gusnard et al. 2001). High activity of these regions (posterior cingulate; inferior parietal and medial frontal cortices) during periods of wakeful rest and passive self-reflection have led some to hypothesize that this activity may "consolidate the past, stabilize brain ensembles, and prepare us for the future" (Buckner and Vincent 2007, p. 1066). Abnormalities in the functional connectivity of this network in psychiatric disorders such as schizophrenia (Bluhm et al. 2007), depression (Greicius et al. 2007), dementia (Rombouts et al. 2005), autism (Cherkassky et al. 2006), and multiple sclerosis (Lowe et al. 2002) have been reported. It is possible that further research into these default networks might yield key diagnostic or pathological information about various psychiatric disorders.

Application of virtual reality–based techniques to functional imaging. Most of the recently available challenge tasks used in functional imaging are based on tasks or tests standardized for clinical testing. A major criticism of this approach has been that it might not be reflective of real-life situations. Consequently, some authors use virtual reality (VR)–based techniques to overcome this criticism. Ability to remember places and navigate through a VR-based city (similar to spatial memory testing in rodents) has been used in an fMRI environment to study activity of parietal and temporal cortices (Spiers and Maguire 2006).

Statistical modeling methods.   A complex array of data is now available using functional and structural imaging methods in multiple states of activation within subjects and between groups, necessitating the use of elegant multivariate and multifactorial models (such as independent component analysis). A detailed description of these techniques is beyond the scope of this chapter and has been undertaken elsewhere (Pearlson and Calhoun 2007). Thus, using the related approach of structural equation modeling, it has been possible to compare functional activation changes across multiple scans and states: depressed subjects versus control subjects, treatment responders versus nonresponders, medication responders versus cognitive-behavioral therapy responders, and so forth (Chen et al. 2007). Use of such models has provided Chen and colleagues with the opportunity to identify and classify depression phenotypes at the level of neural systems, with future implications for evidence-based treatment selection.

Structural MRI: Overview and Use in Psychopharmacological Research

As indicated in Table 10–2, MR technology has also provided important information on structural abnormalities in various psychiatric disorders. Use of these methods in the understanding of psychiatric disorders and their treatment will be addressed in the chapters on individual disorders. Only a general introduction will be provided here.

Volumetric Methods

Magnetic resonance–based volumetric methods involve estimating volumes of cerebral structures using MR images. They may be divided into two different types—automated (voxel-based morphometry [VBM]) and manual (region of interest [ROI]) methods. A detailed review of these methods is provided elsewhere (Pearlson and Calhoun 2007). Using volumetric studies of hippocampus in depression, Sheline et al. (2002) described a subtype of depression associated with hippocampal volume loss, memory impairment, and hippocampal loss of 5-HT$_{2A}$ receptors. The alteration of cerebral structure by medications has been reported as well. G.J. Moore et al. (2000) reported that lithium administration led to a 3% increase in

the volume of gray matter within a period of about 4 weeks. Psychiatric disorders are clinically heterogeneous entities and such structural MRI–based studies have helped us to characterize more specific pathological subtypes of depression. T2-weighted MRI studies have also been used to identify and rate subcortical hyperintensities, the increase of which is believed to result in late-life cerebrovascular disease and late-life depression (Alexopoulos et al. 1997; Kumar et al. 2002; Parsey and Krishnan 1997).

Diffusion Tensor Imaging and Tractography

Most of the previously described volumetric methods focus on gray matter structures as opposed to diffusion tensor imaging (DTI) and associated techniques that image white matter. DTI technologies image water diffusion to study the directionality and integrity of white matter connections between different locations of the brain (Kubicki et al. 2007). These studies advance the hypothesis that psychiatric disorders are characterized by altered connectivity ("disconnection syndromes"). These studies are beginning to help us understand the basis of cerebral organization and connectivity and how it might be affected in psychiatric disorders such as autism (Alexander et al. 2007), late-life depression (Taylor et al. 2007), and schizophrenia (Nestor et al. 2007).

Magnetic Resonance Spectroscopy

MRS technology is based on the fact that MR acquisition involves receiving echoed RF waves of multiple cellular chemical constituents. The individual chemical and metabolite constituents could be measured by suppressing the resonance frequency of water molecules. A detailed exposition of the various types of MRS techniques is beyond the scope of this chapter, and the reader is referred to excellent reviews on the topic (Mason and Krystal 2006; C.M. Moore et al. 1999). Among the markers currently being researched are N-acetylaspartate (NAA), glutamate/glutamine (glx), myoinositol (mI), choline (Cho), glutathione, creatine, GABA, phosphomonoester (PME), and phosphodiester (PDE) (Lyoo and Renshaw 2002). An example of an MRS spectrum from a healthy control subject is provided in Figure 10–6. Using this approach, Frye et al. (2007)were able not only to demonstrate elevated glutamate/glutamine (glx) in anterior cingulate/medial prefrontal areas of patients with bipolar depression but also to document the reduction of glutamine among patients who showed clinical response to treatment with lamotrigine. Using proton MRS, C.M. Moore et al. (2007) measured multiple metabolites in the

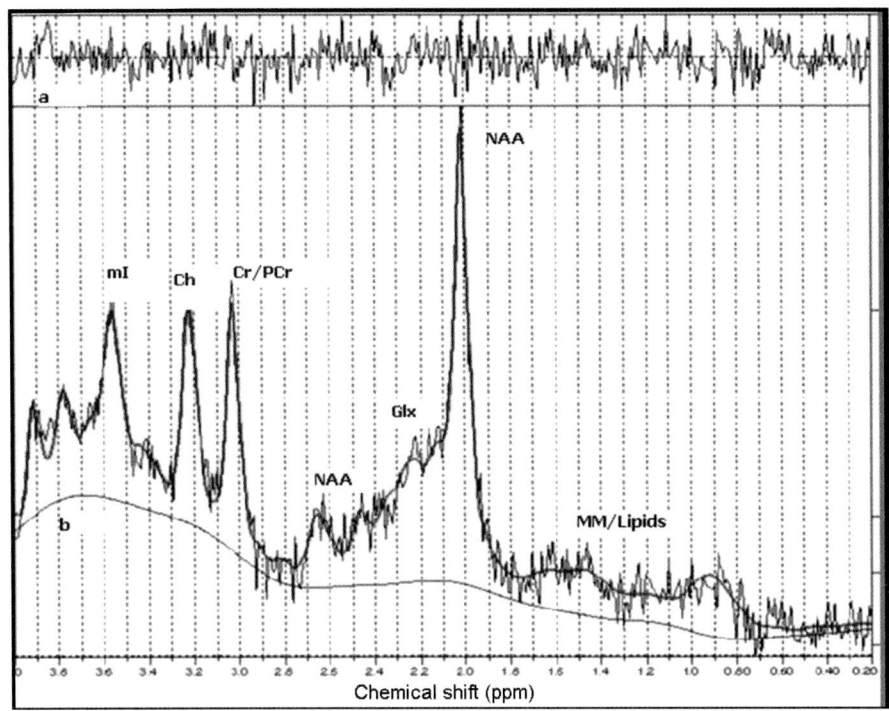

FIGURE 10–6. Proton magnetic resonance spectroscopy (MRS) spectrum from right dorsolateral prefrontal cortex voxel of a healthy individual.

MM = macromolecules; NAA = *N*-acetylaspartate; Glx = glutamate/glutamine; Cr/PCr = creatine/phosphocreatine; Ch = choline; mI = myoinositol.

Source. Reprinted from Haroon E, Watari K, Thomas MA, et al.: "Prefrontal Myo-Inositol Concentration and Visuospatial Functioning Among Diabetic Depressed Patients." *Psychiatry Research: Neuroimaging* 171:10–19, 2009. Copyright 2009, Elsevier Ltd. Used with permission.

anterior cingulate cortex (ACC) of children with bipolar disorder and reported decreased glutamine concentrations in the presence of normal glutamate levels. Using another sample of adult patients, these same authors reported that anterior cingulate cortex glutamine levels were elevated rapidly following administration of the anticonvulsant topiramate (C.M. Moore et al. 2006). Using MRS technology, Sanacora et al. (2003) reported that cortical GABA concentrations increased following a course of electroconvulsive therapy and used this information to hypothesize that this increase in GABA might be associated with clinical recovery. Thus, MRS might provide very useful biomarkers of neural functioning and disease states among patients with psychiatric disorders.

Electromagnetic Measures of Brain Activity

The recording of the group electrical activity of neuronal assemblies is possible in human subjects with the techniques of EEG and MEG. In these techniques, electrical activity is recorded extracranially from the scalp of the individual in a noninvasive way (Bearden 2007). The appeal of these techniques is the extremely high temporal resolution (~msec), which allows one to follow the measurement of global patterns of neural activity in real time. Also, the electrical signal is directly related to the neural activity (in contrast to methods such as PET and fMRI, which rely on indirect assessment of neural activity through vascular effects), although the recorded electrical signals still represent an average over extended regions of the brain. This high temporal resolution makes them ideal candidates for studying synchrony phenomena (Tononi and Edelman 1998; Varela et al. 2001). Although considerable limitations and constraints exist in regard to spatial localization of activity across brain regions, these have mostly been overcome through technical and mathematical means. In spite of this, the spatial resolution, which depends also on the number of electrodes at one's disposal, remains quite poor in comparison with that achievable with fMRI and is on the order of 1 centimeter. Also, the signals are quite weak, so the task has to be repeated a large number of times (tens or even hundreds).

The electromagnetic techniques record the scalp distribution of the field produced by the sum of mainly postsynaptic potentials of the neurons, each of which can be conceptualized as an electric dipole. EEG detects the electrical potential of the field, and MEG detects the magnetic component. The two techniques have very different technical requirements. EEG uses relatively simple equipment, basically a multielectrode helmet, an amplifying and filtering device, and a computer (Ebner et al. 1999). MEG, by contrast, employs cutting-edge technology (Ioannides 2006), because the detection of a magnetic field intensity as weak as the one produced by the brain (~20,000 billion times weaker than the intensity of the Earth's magnetic field) requires the use of superconducting coil units based on superconducting quantum interference device (SQUID) technology. These units need to be specially cooled to a temperature near absolute zero. To avoid the intrusion of electromagnetic interference from the environment, the recording takes place in a room that has been appropriately shielded.

A minimum of 32 scalp electrodes is needed to localize the sources of the recorded potential EEG, but high-density arrays of 128 or 256 electrodes are now common. MEG commonly employs arrays of 100–300 detectors. The intensity of the EEG or MEG response is typically very low, and it takes generally a large number of repetitions (~100) of the task/stimulus presentation (*trial*) to achieve a sufficient power. The time series from each of the recording units is then segmented according to the stimulus delivery sequence, and these temporally realigned segments are averaged together to obtain a waveform that represents the mean time course of the response to the trial for that recording location (*evoked potentials*). By combining these waveforms from all of the detectors, one can obtain a map of the surface field distribution at each time interval inside the trial window. Both EEG and MEG are essentially surface techniques: because the intensity of the electromagnetic field decreases rapidly with distance, the detection of neural signals is restricted to the sources closest to the detectors—that is, the neocortex. The activity of subcortical regions is very difficult to detect.

Use of Electroencephalography and Magnetoencephalography in Psychopharmacology

While these techniques carry considerable potential, their use in psychopharmacology remains elusive. The use of EEG and related technology of evoked potentials has helped contribute considerably to our understanding of

the pathophysiology of schizophrenia (Ford and Mathalon 2005; Turetsky et al. 1998). Tucker et al. (2003) used dense-array EEG to study frontolimbic responsiveness in patients with moderate depression. A potential for the use of EEG technology used in conjunction with fMRI in study of analgesia and pain management has been recommended by some authors (Wise and Tracey 2006). Pizzagalli et al. (2003) combined PET and EEG technologies using a source localization technique to identify disruption of frontocingulate connectivity among patients with depression. Studies such as these provide critical information that can complement and enhance our understanding of functional imaging approaches.

Conclusion

Contemporary brain imaging methods provide a variety of strategies to probe structural, functional, and chemical abnormalities in specific neural circuits relevant to psychiatric disease. Such studies are having a considerable impact on our conceptualization of these disorders, with potential impacts on diagnosis (Mayberg 2003a), clinical management (monitoring occupancy, or PIB changes with treatment [Klunk et al. 2004]), and novel treatment development (Mayberg et al. 2005). Brain imaging in psychopharmacology can be categorized both by the scanning technology (e.g., MRI, PET, or EEG) and by its purpose (e.g., activation, resting state, behavioral, biochemical, or receptor mapping). Receptor-mapping studies have clearly added to our ability to understand mechanisms of action of psychopharmacological agents and their side-effect profiles. Activation studies, which indirectly measure neuronal activity vis-à-vis changes in cerebral blood flow, have become widely used with fMRI technology, providing new insights into behaviorally specific subcircuits. Structural MRI studies have also begun to yield considerable data enabling a better understanding of how the disease processes are regionally localized, where to target for functional imaging, and where to obtain specimens for postmortem histopathological analysis. Multimodal imaging through the combination of fMRI, PET, structural MRI, MRS, and electromagnetic measurements (EEG, MEG) offers the promise of identifying both neuronal and chemical changes related to brain function.

References

Alexander AL, Lee JE, Lazar M, et al: Diffusion tensor imaging of the corpus callosum in autism. Neuroimage 34:61–73, 2007

Alexopoulos GS, Meyers BS, Young RC, et al: "Vascular depression" hypothesis. Arch Gen Psychiatry 54:915–922, 1997

Arthurs OJ, Boniface S: How well do we understand the neural origins of the fMRI BOLD signal? Trends Neurosci 25:27–31, 2002

Bearden S: EEG reviewing/recording strategy. Am J Electroneurodiagnostic Technol 47:1–19, 2007

Bertolino A, Caforio G, Blasi G, et al: Interaction of COMT (Val(108/158)Met) genotype and olanzapine treatment on prefrontal cortical function in patients with schizophrenia. Am J Psychiatry 161:1798–1805, 2004

Binder EB, Holsboer F: Pharmacogenomics and antidepressant drugs. Ann Med 38:82–94, 2006

Blier P, Ward NM: Is there a role for 5-HT1A agonists in the treatment of depression? Biol Psychiatry 53:193–203, 2003

Blodgett TM, Meltzer CC, Townsend DW: PET/CT: form and function. Radiology 242:360–385, 2007

Bluhm RL, Miller J, Lanius RA, et al: Spontaneous low-frequency fluctuations in the BOLD signal in schizophrenic patients: anomalies in the default network. Schizophr Bull 33:1004–1012, 2007

Bookheimer SY, Strojwas MH, Cohen MS, et al: Patterns of brain activation in people at risk for Alzheimer's disease. N Engl J Med 343:450–456, 2000

Bremner JD: Functional neuroimaging in post-traumatic stress disorder. Expert Rev Neurother 7:393–405, 2007

Bremner JD, Innis RB, White T, et al: SPECT [I-123]iomazenil measurement of the benzodiazepine receptor in panic disorder. Biol Psychiatry 47:96–106, 2000

Broca P: Sur les températures morbides locales. Bulletin de l'Académie de. Medecine 8:1331–1347, 1879

Buckner RL, Vincent JL: Unrest at rest: default activity and spontaneous network correlations. Neuroimage 37:1091–1096, 2007

Buxton RB: Introduction to Functional Magnetic Resonance Imaging: Principles and Techniques. Cambridge, UK, Cambridge University Press, 2002

Carbon M, Eidelberg D: Modulation of regional brain function by deep brain stimulation: studies with positron emission tomography. Curr Opin Neurol 15:451–455, 2002

Caspi A, Sugden K, Moffitt TE, et al: Influence of life stress on depression: moderation by a polymorphism in the 5-HTT gene. Science 301:386–389, 2003

Chen CH, Ridler K, Suckling J, et al: Brain imaging correlates of depressive symptom severity and predictors of symptom improvement after antidepressant treatment. Biol Psychiatry 62:407–414, 2007

Cherkassky VL, Kana RK, Keller TA, et al: Functional connectivity in a baseline resting-state network in autism. Neuroreport 17:1687–90, 2006

Craik FIM, Moroz TM, Moscovitch M, et al: In search of the self: a positron emission tomography investigation. Psychological Science 10:26–34, 1999

Cropley VL, Fujita M, Innis RB, et al: Molecular imaging of the dopaminergic system and its association with human cognitive function. Biol Psychiatry 59:898–907, 2006

Dixon MR, Jacobs EA, Sanders S: Contextual control of delay discounting by pathological gamblers. J Appl Behav Anal 39:413–422, 2006

Ebner A, Sciarretta G, Epstein CM, et al: EEG instrumentation. The International Federation of Clinical Neurophysiology. Electroencephalogr Clin Neurophysiol Suppl 52:7–10, 1999

Elliott R, Rubinsztein JS, Sahakian BJ, et al: The neural basis of mood-congruent processing biases in depression. Arch Gen Psychiatry 59:597–604, 2002

Erritzoe D, Talbot P, Frankle WG, et al: Positron emission tomography and single photon emission CT molecular imaging in schizophrenia. Neuroimaging Clin N Am 13:817–832, 2003

Evans KC, Dougherty DD, Pollack MH, et al: Using neuroimaging to predict treatment response in mood and anxiety disorders. Annu Clin Psychiatry 18:33–42, 2006

Fisher PM, Meltzer CC, Ziolko SK, et al: Capacity for 5-HT1A-mediated autoregulation predicts amygdala reactivity. Nat Neurosci 9:1362–1363, 2006

Ford JM, Mathalon DH: Corollary discharge dysfunction in schizophrenia: can it explain auditory hallucinations? Int J Psychophysiol 58:179–189, 2005

Fossati P, Hevenor SJ, Graham SJ, et al: In search of the emotional self: an FMRI study using positive and negative emotional words. Am J Psychiatry 160:1938–1945, 2003

Friston K: Beyond phrenology: what can neuroimaging tell us about distributed circuitry? Annu Rev Neurosci 25:221–250, 2002

Frodl T, Schule C, Schmitt G, et al: Association of the brain-derived neurotrophic factor Val66Met polymorphism with reduced hippocampal volumes in major depression. Arch Gen Psychiatry 64:410–416, 2007

Frye MA, Watzl J, Banakar S, et al: Increased anterior cingulate/medial prefrontal cortical glutamate and creatine in bipolar depression. Neuropsychopharmacology 32:2490–2499, 2007

Fu CH, Williams SC, Brammer MJ, et al: Neural responses to happy facial expressions in major depression following antidepressant treatment. Am J Psychiatry 164:599–607, 2007

Fujimoto T, Takeuch K, Matsumoto T, et al: Abnormal glucose metabolism in the anterior cingulate cortex in patients with schizophrenia. Psychiatry Res 154:49–58, 2007

Greicius MD, Flores BH, Menon V, et al: Resting-state functional connectivity in major depression: abnormally increased contributions from subgenual cingulate cortex and thalamus. Biol Psychiatry 62:429–437, 2007

Gusnard DA, Raichle ME, Raichle ME: Searching for a baseline: functional imaging and the resting human brain. Nat Rev Neurosci 2:685–694, 2001

Hariri AR, Mattay VS, Tessitore A, et al: Serotonin transporter genetic variation and the response of the human amygdala. Science 297:400–403, 2002

Hariri AR, Drabant EM, Weinberger DR: Imaging genetics: perspectives from studies of genetically driven variation in serotonin function and corticolimbic affective processing. Biol Psychiatry 59:888–897, 2006

Harvey PO, Fossati P, Pochon JB, et al: Cognitive control and brain resources in major depression: an fMRI study using the n-back task. Neuroimage 26:860–869, 2005

Heeger DJ, Boynton GM, Demb JB, et al: Motion opponency in visual cortex. J Neurosci 19:7162–7174, 1999

Heinz A, Braus DF, Smolka MN, et al: Amygdala-prefrontal coupling depends on a genetic variation of the serotonin transporter. Nat Neurosci 8:20–21, 2005

Herscovitch P, Markham J, Raichle ME: Brain blood flow measured with H2(15)O, I: theory and error analysis. J Nucl Med 24:782–789, 1983

Ioannides AA: Magnetoencephalography as a research tool in neuroscience: state of the art. Neuroscientist 12:524–544, 2006

James W: The Principles of Psychology. New York, Henry Holt, 1890

Jueptner M, Weiller C: Does measurement of regional cerebral blood flow reflect synaptic activity? Implications for PET and fMRI. Neuroimage 2:148–156, 1995

Kapur S, Remington G: Dopamine D(2) receptors and their role in atypical antipsychotic action: still necessary and may even be sufficient. Biol Psychiatry 50:873–883, 2001

Kaufman J, Yang BZ, Douglas-Palumberi H, et al: Social supports and serotonin transporter gene moderate depression in maltreated children. Proc Natl Acad Sci U S A 101:17316–17321, 2004

Kendler KS, Kuhn JW, Vittum J, et al: The interaction of stressful life events and a serotonin transporter polymorphism in the prediction of episodes of major depression: a replication. Arch Gen Psychiatry 62:529–535, 2005

Kennedy C, Des Rosiers MH, Sakurada O, et al: Metabolic mapping of the primary visual system of the monkey by means of the autoradiographic [14C]deoxyglucose technique. Proc Natl Acad Sci U S A 73:4230–4234, 1976

Kety SS: Biochemistry and mental function. Nature 208:1252–1257, 1965

Kilts CD, Gross RE, Ely TD, et al: The neural correlates of cue-induced craving in cocaine-dependent women. Am J Psychiatry 161:233–241, 2004

Klunk WE, Engler H, Nordberg A, et al: Imaging brain amyloid in Alzheimer's disease with Pittsburgh Compound-B. Ann Neurol 55:306–319, 2004

Kubicki M, McCarley R, Westin CF, et al: A review of diffusion tensor imaging studies in schizophrenia. J Psychiatr Res 41:15–30, 2007

Kumar A, Mintz J, Bilker W, et al: Autonomous neurobiological pathways to late-life major depressive disorder: clinical and pathophysiological implications. Neuropsychopharmacology 26:229–236, 2002

Lange C, Kracht L, Herholz K, et al: Reduced glucose metabolism in temporo-parietal cortices of women with borderline personality disorder. Psychiatry Res 139:115–126, 2005

Le Bastard G, Fossati P, Pochon JB, et al: Self-referential processing and emotional bias in depression: a fMRI study (poster #49). Presented at: Ninth International Conference of Functional Mapping of the Human Brain. New York City, NY, June 2003

Logothetis NK, Pauls J, Augath M, et al: Neurophysiological investigation of the basis of the fMRI signal. Nature 412:150–157, 2001

Lowe MJ, Phillips MD, Lurito JT, et al: Multiple sclerosis: low-frequency temporal blood oxygen level-dependent fluctuations indicate reduced functional connectivity initial results. Radiology 224:184–192, 2002

Luat AF, Makki M, Chugani HT: Neuroimaging in tuberous sclerosis complex. Curr Opin Neurol 20:142–150, 2007

Lyoo IK, Renshaw PF: Magnetic resonance spectroscopy: current and future applications in psychiatric research. Biol Psychiatry 51:195–207, 2002

Magistretti PJ: Neuron-glia metabolic coupling and plasticity. J Exp Biol 209:2304–2311, 2006

Magistretti PJ, Pellerin L: Cellular mechanisms of brain energy metabolism and their relevance to functional brain imaging. Philos Trans R Soc Lond B Biol Sci 354:1155–1163, 1999

Mason GF, Krystal JH: MR spectroscopy: its potential role for drug development for the treatment of psychiatric diseases. NMR Biomed 19:690–701, 2006

Mathis CA, Klunk WE, Price JC, et al: Imaging technology for neurodegenerative diseases: progress toward detection of specific pathologies. Arch Neurol 62:196–200, 2005

Mayberg HS: Modulating dysfunctional limbic-cortical circuits in depression: towards development of brain-based algorithms for diagnosis and optimised treatment. Br Med Bull 65:193–207, 2003a

Mayberg HS: Positron emission tomography imaging in depression: a neural systems perspective. Neuroimaging Clin N Am 13:805–815, 2003b

Mayberg HS, Lozano AM, Voon V, et al: Deep brain stimulation for treatment-resistant depression. Neuron 45:651–660, 2005

McClure SM, Laibson DI, Loewenstein G, et al: Separate neural systems value immediate and delayed monetary rewards. Science 306:503–507, 2004

Menon RS, Goodyear BG: Submillimeter functional localization in human striate cortex using BOLD contrast at 4 Tesla: implications for the vascular point-spread function. Magn Reson Med 41:230–235, 1999

Meyer-Lindenberg A, Weinberger DR: Intermediate phenotypes and genetic mechanisms of psychiatric disorders. Nat Rev Neurosci 7:818–827, 2006

Meyer JH: Imaging the serotonin transporter during major depressive disorder and antidepressant treatment. J Psychiatry Neurosci 32:86–102, 2007

Meyer JH, McMain S, Kennedy SH, et al: Dysfunctional attitudes and 5-HT2 receptors during depression and self-harm. Am J Psychiatry 160:90–99, 2003

Mintun MA, Raichle ME, Kilbourn MR, et al: A quantitative model for the in vivo assessment of drug binding sites with positron emission tomography. Ann Neurol 15:217–227, 1984

Mitterschiffthaler MT, Kumari V, Malhi GS, et al: Neural response to pleasant stimuli in anhedonia: an fMRI study. Neuroreport 14:177–182, 2003

Montague PR, Berns GS, Cohen JD, et al: Hyperscanning: simultaneous fMRI during linked social interactions. Neuroimage 16:1159–1164, 2002

Moore CM, Frederick BB, Renshaw PF: Brain biochemistry using magnetic resonance spectroscopy: relevance to psychiatric illness in the elderly. J Geriatr Psychiatry Neurol 12:107–117, 1999

Moore CM, Wardrop M, deB Frederick B, et al: Topiramate raises anterior cingulate cortex glutamine levels in healthy men: a 4.0 T magnetic resonance spectroscopy study. Psychopharmacology (Berl) 188:236–243, 2006

Moore CM, Frazier JA, Glod CA, et al: Glutamine and glutamate levels in children and adolescents with bipolar disorder: a 4.0-T proton magnetic resonance spectroscopy study of the anterior cingulate cortex. J Am Acad Child Adolesc Psychiatry 46:524–534, 2007

Moore GJ, Bebchuk JM, Wilds IB, et al: Lithium-induced increase in human brain gray matter. Lancet 356:1241–1242, 2000

Nemeroff CB: Prevalence and management of treatment-resistant depression. J Clin Psychiatry 68 (suppl 8):17–25, 2007

Nemeroff CB, Heim CM, Thase ME, et al: Differential responses to psychotherapy versus pharmacotherapy in patients with chronic forms of major depression and childhood trauma. Proc Natl Acad Sci U S A 100:14293–14296, 2003

Nestor PG, Kubicki M, Spencer KM, et al: Attentional networks and cingulum bundle in chronic schizophrenia. Schizophr Res 90:308–315, 2007

Neumeister A, Nugent AC, Waldeck T, et al: Neural and behavioral responses to tryptophan depletion in unmedicated patients with remitted major depressive disorder and controls. Arch Gen Psychiatry 61:765–773, 2004

Ogawa S, Tank DW, Menon R, et al: Intrinsic signal changes accompanying sensory stimulation: functional brain mapping with magnetic resonance imaging. Proc Natl Acad Sci U S A 89:5951–5955, 1992

Ono M, Wilson A, Nobrega J, et al: 11C-labeled stilbene derivatives as Abeta-aggregate-specific PET imaging agents for Alzheimer's disease. Nucl Med Biol 30:565–571, 2003

Owen AM, McMillan KM, Laird AR, et al: N-back working memory paradigm: a meta-analysis of normative functional neuroimaging studies. Hum Brain Mapp 25:46–59, 2005

Parsey RV, Krishnan KR: A new MRI ratio method for in-vivo estimation of signal hypointensity in aging and Alzheimer's disease. Prog Neuropsychopharmacol Biol Psychiatry 21:1257–1267, 1997

Pearlson GD, Calhoun V: Structural and functional magnetic resonance imaging in psychiatric disorders. Can J Psychiatry 52:158–166, 2007

Peper JS, Brouwer RM, Boomsma DI, et al: Genetic influences on human brain structure: a review of brain imaging studies in twins. Hum Brain Mapp 28:464–473, 2007

Pezawas L, Meyer-Lindenberg A, Drabant EM, et al: 5-HTTLPR polymorphism impacts human cingulate-amygdala interactions: a genetic susceptibility mechanism for depression. Nat Neurosci 8:828–834, 2005

Pizzagalli DA, Oakes TR, Davidson RJ: Coupling of theta activity and glucose metabolism in the human rostral anterior cingulate cortex: an EEG/PET study of normal and depressed subjects. Psychophysiology 40:939–949, 2003

Post RM, Speer AM, Hough CJ, et al: Neurobiology of bipolar illness: implications for future study and therapeutics. Ann Clin Psychiatry 15:85–94, 2003

Purselle DC, Nemeroff CB: Serotonin transporter: a potential substrate in the biology of suicide. Neuropsychopharmacology 28:613–619, 2003

Rauch SL, Whalen PJ, Shin LM, et al: Exaggerated amygdala response to masked facial stimuli in posttraumatic stress disorder: a functional MRI study. Biol Psychiatry 47:769–776, 2000

Ravina B, Eidelberg D, Ahlskog JE, et al: The role of radiotracer imaging in Parkinson disease. Neurology 64:208–215, 2005

Reimold M, Smolka MN, Schumann G, et al: Midbrain serotonin transporter binding potential measured with [(11)C]DASB is affected by serotonin transporter genotype. J Neural Transm 114:635–639, 2007

Reivich M, Kuhl D, Wolf A, et al: The [18F]fluorodeoxyglucose method for the measurement of local cerebral glucose utilization in man. Circulation Research 44:127–137, 1979

Reynolds GP, Templeman LA, Godlewska BR: Pharmacogenetics of schizophrenia. Expert Opin Pharmacother 7:1429–1440, 2006

Roffman JL, Marci CD, Glick DM, et al: Neuroimaging and the functional neuroanatomy of psychotherapy. Psychol Med 35:1385–1398, 2005

Rombouts SA, Barkhof F, Goekoop R, et al: Altered resting state networks in mild cognitive impairment and mild Alzheimer's disease: an fMRI study. Hum Brain Mapp 26:231–239, 2005

Sanacora G, Mason GF, Rothman DL, et al: Increased cortical GABA concentrations in depressed patients receiving ECT. Am J Psychiatry 160:577–579, 2003

Schweitzer JB, Lee DO, Hanford RB, et al: A positron emission tomography study of methylphenidate in adults with ADHD: alterations in resting blood flow and predicting treatment response. Neuropsychopharmacology 28:967–973, 2003

Sheline YI, Barch DM, Donnelly JM, et al: Increased amygdala response to masked emotional faces in depressed subjects resolves with antidepressant treatment: an fMRI study. Biol Psychiatry 50:651–658, 2001

Sheline YI, Mittler BL, Mintun MA: The hippocampus and depression. Eur Psychiatry 17 (suppl 3):300–305, 2002

Shin LM, Wright CI, Cannistraro PA, et al: A functional magnetic resonance imaging study of amygdala and medial prefrontal cortex responses to overtly presented fearful faces in posttraumatic stress disorder. Arch Gen Psychiatry 62:273–281, 2005

Silverman DH, Cummings JL, Small GW, et al: Added clinical benefit of incorporating 2-deoxy-2-[18F]fluoro-D-glucose with positron emission tomography into the clinical evaluation of patients with cognitive impairment. Mol Imaging Biol 4:283–293, 2002

Small GW: Neuroimaging and genetic assessment for early diagnosis of Alzheimer's disease. J Clin Psychiatry 57 (suppl 14):9–13, 1996

Small GW, Kepe V, Ercoli LM, et al: PET of brain amyloid and tau in mild cognitive impairment. N Engl J Med 355:2652–2663, 2006

Spiers HJ, Maguire EA: Spontaneous mentalizing during an interactive real world task: an fMRI study. Neuropsychologia 44:1674–1682, 2006

Stein MB, Simmons AN, Feinstein JS, et al: Increased amygdala and insula activation during emotion processing in anxiety-prone subjects. Am J Psychiatry 164:318–327, 2007

Tagamets M-A, Horwitz B: Interpreting PET and fMRI measures of functional neural activity: the effects of synaptic inhibition on cortical activation in human imaging studies. Brain Res Bull 54:267–273, 2001

Talbot PS, Laruelle M: The role of in vivo molecular imaging with PET and SPECT in the elucidation of psychiatric drug action and new drug development. Eur Neuropsychopharmacol 12:503–511, 2002

Taylor WD, Bae JN, MacFall JR, et al: Widespread effects of hyperintense lesions on cerebral white matter structure. AJR Am J Roentgenol 188:1695–1704, 2007

Thulborn KR, Waterton JC, Matthews PM, et al: Oxygenation dependence of the transverse relaxation time of water protons in whole blood at high field. Biochimugia Biophysica Acta 714:265–270, 1982

Tononi G, Edelman GM: Consciousness and complexity. Science 282:1846–1851, 1998

Tucker DM, Luu P, Frishkoff G, et al: Frontolimbic response to negative feedback in clinical depression. J Abnorm Psychol 112:667–678, 2003

Turetsky BI, Colbath EA, Gur RE: P300 subcomponent abnormalities in schizophrenia, I: physiological evidence for gender and subtype specific differences in regional pathology. Biol Psychiatry 43:84–96, 1998

Van Horn JD, Gazzaniga MS: Databasing fMRI studies towards a "discovery science" of brain function. Nat Rev Neurosci 3:314–318, 2002

Varela F, Lachaux JP, Rodriguez E, et al: The brainweb: phase synchronization and large-scale integration. Nature Reviews Neuroscience 2:229–239, 2001

Villringer A, Dirnagl U: Coupling of brain activity and cerebral blood flow: basis of functional neuroimaging. Cerebrovasc Brain Metab Rev 7:240–276, 1995

Waldvogel D, van Gelderen P, Muellbacher W, et al: The relative metabolic demand of inhibition and excitation. Nature 406:995–998, 2000

Whalen PJ, Rauch SL, Etcoff NL, et al: Masked presentations of emotional facial expressions modulate amygdala activity without explicit knowledge. J Neurosci 18:411–418, 1998

Whalen PJ, Shin LM, Somerville LH, et al: Functional neuroimaging studies of the amygdala in depression. Semin Clin Neuropsychiatry 7:234–242, 2002

Wise RG, Tracey I: The role of fMRI in drug discovery. J Magn Reson Imaging 23:862–876, 2006

Zink CF, Pagnoni G, Chappelow J, et al: Human striatal activation reflects degree of stimulus saliency. Neuroimage 29:977–983, 2006

CHAPTER 11

Statistics, Placebo Response, and Clinical Trial Design in Psychopharmacology

Helena C. Kraemer, Ph.D.

Alan F. Schatzberg, M.D.

D rug development is a highly complex process that involves multiple steps of preclinical and clinical pharmacological refinement and testing. Preclinical studies include assessing drug bioavailability, metabolism, and toxicity; effects on known biological targets (e.g., receptor binding); and performance in various animal models of pathology. After sufficient data are obtained in animal studies, drug testing in humans can begin. In the United States, human clinical trials are divided into four phases. Phase I involves testing multiple doses of a drug for bioavailability, pharmacokinetics, and side effects. Phase II studies are dose-finding studies in patients with a given disorder. They can be open-label or double-blind trials. Phase III generally includes pivotal double-blind trials for demonstrating efficacy and safety/tolerability. Phase IV trials, which take place after a drug has received U.S. Food and Drug Administration (FDA) approval and is on the market, are conducted to help clarify potential uses of the drug.

Generally, efficacy is established via a randomized, controlled trial (RCT) in which a test drug is compared with a so-called placebo and/or an active compound. An RCT is an experiment designed to establish the efficacy of a treatment by comparing the responses in two or more groups of patients sampled from a relevant clinical population, with one group randomly assigned to receive the treatment of interest and a second group randomly as-

signed to receive a control treatment, in which all subjects are enrolled, treated, and uniformly followed over the same time period (Meinert 1986). In contrast, experiments that are performed under any of the following circumstances are not RCTs:

1. Using human tissues or animals
2. For purposes other than establishing efficacy of a treatment
3. Comparing groups of patients who were selected rather than randomly assigned to receive a given treatment (observational, or *quasi-randomized*, clinical trials)
4. Assessing response to a treatment in absence of a control group (e.g., pre–post study designs)
5. Comparing a group of patients given a treatment versus another group given another treatment observed at different times or places (e.g., historical control subjects)

Although the basic premise underlying the RCT has remained the same over the past half century, RCTs today differ from RCTs of the 1950s. Advances have occurred not only in statistical methodology but also in research methods; studies are now better designed to promote the replicability of the results and thus to protect the validity of inferences drawn from RCTs and applied to patient populations. The basic premise underlying the RCT defines the "causal effect of treatment (T) on an individual patient" as a comparison between a patient's response to T with what the outcome in that same patient would have been if that patient had not been given T (Rubin 1974, 2004). The condition proposed to represent what would have happened if that patient had not been given T is generally called the *control* or *comparison* group (hereafter referred to as C).

Unfortunately, there is no way to assess response to any treatment for an individual patient under two conditions, T and C, simultaneously. If a treatment were given to the same patient at different times, the condition of the patient might change between the first and second time (*secular trends*), or the response to treatment the first time may influence the response to treatment the second time (*carryover effects*). Consequently, how much of any difference seen between the two responses is attributable to T per se and how much is attributable to other, extraneous influences cannot be ascertained. Thus, the causal effect of T in an individual patient cannot be assessed. However, what cannot be done with an individual patient can be done with a clinical population. Patients in a representative sample from the clinical population of interest can be randomly assigned to receive either T or C. Under optimal conditions in a rigorously controlled study, the average responses in the two groups are estimates of what the average responses to receiving T and to not receiving T would be within the entire population, and the comparison between them is an estimate of the average causal effect of T on the population sampled.

In designing an optimal RCT the following issues need to be considered, all of which we address at least briefly in this chapter:

- Specific indications and populations to be studied
- Drug formulation and doses to be used
- Route and time of administration
- Instruments to be used as outcome measures
- What the comparison groups should be
- Power analysis and statistical analysis tools

The question of what the comparison groups should be is especially important. The issue of whether to compare the treatment with a placebo or an active control has become a contentious social and ethical issue as well as a scientific issue, particularly regarding psychiatric patients with severe disorders such as schizophrenia, and we focus strongly on that issue in this chapter.

Indications

An indication for a drug is really an administrative approval by a regulatory authority (in the United States, the FDA) for a company to market and sell a product for a specific clinical need. To establish efficacy in treating psychiatric illness, the FDA has generally required statistically significant results in trials. Generally the requirement has been for more than one statistically significant study outcome, although there have been exceptions to this rule. Historically, indications have revolved around syndromes (e.g., treatment of major depression or schizophrenia). More recently, the FDA has shown greater flexibility with approvals for drugs to treat symptom dimensions—e.g., agitation—that transcend underlying syndromes.

The population to be sampled is a matter of some importance because one cannot generalize the result beyond the population the sample actually represents. Thus, for example, a study that samples alcoholic patients but excludes those with comorbidities will generate a sample that represents a small fraction of the population with that disorder (Humphreys and Weisner 2000; Humphreys et al. 2005). Whether or not some advantage is found for T over C in such a nonrepresentative subpopulation gives little insight as to whether that same advantage pertains in the majority of people with the disorder.

The choice of population to be sampled is also crucial to differentiating efficacy from effectiveness. *Efficacy* refers to the extent to which T produces a beneficial result under ideal conditions; *effectiveness* refers to the extent to which T produces a beneficial result when used as it would be in actual clinical practice (Hoagwood et al. 1995). Both issues are best addressed with RCTs. One crucial difference between RCTs geared toward establishing efficacy and those geared toward establishing effectiveness is the population that the RCT researchers choose to sample. RCTs directed more toward establishing efficacy usually set very narrow inclusion/exclusion criteria, focusing on the subpopulation of patients with the disorder who are most likely to comply and to respond well. In contrast, RCTs directed more toward effectiveness try to use patients who are representative of all those with the disorder who might benefit from that treatment for their disorder. The primary reason for exclusion from effectiveness RCTs is usually that there is some reason to believe that either T or C is contraindicated (e.g., pregnancy excludes women in many drug studies) or the patient is unwilling to sign an informed consent form. Because the sample in an efficacy study is chosen to be more compliant and responsive, and is typically more homogeneous than that in an effectiveness study, sample sizes are likely to be much smaller than those in an effectiveness study, and effect sizes much larger.

The earliest studies of a particular drug are likely to be efficacy studies in order to establish that the drug works at least under optimal conditions. For pivotal studies, hypotheses are stated a priori. Generally, these take the form that a tested treatment will be superior to a comparator in reducing a given set of symptoms over a specific duration of treatment. A statistical analysis plan is developed to test the a priori hypothesis. The most influential studies on clinical practice, however, are likely to be effectiveness studies, for they inform clinicians about which treatments might benefit the patients they are likely to see.

Clinical development of psychiatric agents is such that approval for indications are usually for adults (i.e., over the age of 18 years) and for both sexes. Specific additional approvals can be sought for children and the elderly. Obviously, in disorders that occur primarily in childhood (e.g., attention-deficit/hyperactivity disorder), studies may begin with youths.

Establishing Diagnoses

Establishing an accurate diagnosis is generally done according to criteria from an established classification system—for example, the *Diagnostic and Statistical Manual of Mental Disorders*, 4th Edition, Text Revision (DSM-IV-TR; American Psychiatric Association 2000). Criteria can be checked off using an unstructured clinical interview or by using a structured instrument—the Scheduled Clinical Interview for DSM-IV (SCID). The latter is more time-consuming but can offer greater information on diagnoses, particularly in cases of psychiatric comorbidity. Obviously, the use of the SCID requires training and assessment for interrater reliability, as well as monitoring over the course of the trial to prevent "slippage" of diagnostic standards.

Rating Instruments

Because in psychiatry we do not yet have reliable biological measures (e.g., a serum lipid panel) to assess efficacy, we rely on objective rating instruments applied by an observer or on self-reporting. Before being used in a study on drug efficacy, the instruments need to be assessed for both validity and clinical relevancy, and reliability and consistency must be established in the population to be sampled and in the hands of the RCT research staff. This is particularly true in multisite RCTs, where special efforts are

necessary to ensure that the primary outcome measure is the same across the sites. Lack of reliability, lack of consistency between raters, or lack of consistency across sites in a multisite RCT is likely to lead to a failed RCT, one unable to establish statistically significant differences between T and C.

An RCT should have only one primary outcome being measured—or very few—and all the decisions in study design, measurement, and analysis are directed toward generating valid and powerful tests for that primary outcome. Other outcomes can be assessed in the study, as long as they do not compromise assessment of the primary outcome and do not impose undue burden on patients and research staff that would lead to dropouts and diminished reliability of measures. Outcome assessments that amplify or elucidate the primary outcome results are generally listed as secondary outcomes. Finally, it is necessary at baseline to collect enough information to well characterize the sample, both sociodemographically and clinically, to check the adequacy of randomization in producing two groups assigned to T and C that are comparable at baseline.

Such baseline data also are valuable in post hoc exploratory analyses to assess the possibility of moderators of treatment response (identification of subpopulations that have different effect sizes) (Kraemer 2008; Kraemer et al. 2006, 2008).

During treatment, there may be repeated assessments of the primary and secondary outcomes, which can be used in analysis of results using methods such as hierarchical modeling that generally deal much more effectively with dropouts and missing data; such methods usually increase the power to detect T versus C effects without requiring an increase in the sample size. Events or changes that happen during the treatment may also be used in post hoc analysis to identify mediators (possible mechanisms) that indicate how and why T works better than C (or does not), which can then lead to improved treatments for evaluation in future studies.

Such descriptive statistics or the results of post hoc analyses lead not to conclusions but rather to hypotheses that would be tested in future RCTs, but they are essential to the advancement of treatments.

In seeking approval for an indication, observer-rated instruments are generally preferred over self-reports. However, some studies employ self-report measures to test secondary hypotheses. Over time, a commonly used measure may be supplanted by another that is believed to more accurately reflect specific symptoms to be studied. Some of these scales are quite different from each other.

For example, the Montgomery-Åsberg Depression Rating Scale (MADRS) has been used in antidepressant trials as an alternative to the Hamilton Rating Scale for Depression (Ham-D) because the former focuses less on anxiety symptoms and more on core depression. Other scales may be expansions on existing ones, adding items to focus on specific symptoms in a particular disorder. An example is the use of the Positive and Negative Syndrome Scale (PANSS) for schizophrenia. The scale is an expansion of the classic Brief Psychiatric Rating Scale (BPRS). Detailed descriptions of rating scales can be found in a source textbook edited by Rush et al. (2008).

Application of a validated and reliable instrument still requires that raters be trained and that a high degree of agreement (interrater reliability) be found among raters, both cross-sectionally and over time. This generally requires formally training raters and then testing multiple raters on patient vignettes to establish interrater reliability. In many cases, patient interviews might be videotaped and randomly selected videotapes submitted to independent experts to assess the reliability and consistency of ratings. Again, this is particularly important with multisite RCTs.

Symptom Severity Criteria

Historically, minimal levels of symptom severity on rating scales have been incorporated into study inclusion criteria. These criteria are aimed at ensuring that patients have at least a minimum level of symptom severity at baseline to allow for assessing relative effects of a therapy. Issues arise in implementing these inclusion criteria, particularly a possible inflation of rating scale scores to ensure inclusion. This can become an important issue in studies with relatively few patients. To counter possible severity rating inflation, several tactics have been employed, including audio- or videotaping of entry interviews with subsequent quality review; use of self-reporting or an interview rating done outside the study for inclusion; not specifying minimal entry symptom severity criteria to the investigator; and ensuring that there is funding to cover the costs of screening failures.

Whenever entry criteria specify a threshold inclusion, there is the risk of regression to the mean in both the T and C groups. Although regression to the mean (Campbell and Kenny 1999) in an RCT does not bias the comparison of T versus C effects, the use of an entry criterion may focus attention on the very subgroup in which T is least, rather than most, effective, which might lead to a failed RCT. The alternative is to include all those in

whom clinicians might use T rather than C (effectiveness criteria) and then use post hoc moderator analyses to determine whether those within a certain range of baseline severity are likely to have the greatest effect sizes.

Trial Duration, Drug Dosage, and Route of Administration

Protocol development requires specifying the duration of the trial a priori. The optimal duration varies across disorders. For example, for acute treatment of major depression, commonly 6–8 weeks of active treatment are employed; for mania, 3 weeks' duration is common. The shorter trial length for acute mania is used for convenience to allow sufficient time to assess a novel therapy without an unduly long duration of placebo treatment that would discourage enrollment.

Route of administration and specific dosage regimens are determined for each agent and vary according to the agent's physical properties (e.g., half-life, absorption) as well as the indication. (These are frequently determined in Phase II trials.) Drugs that can be prescribed once per day are obviously more convenient to administer than are agents that require multiple daily dosing, so manufacturers strive for once-daily dosing.

Statistical Issues in Planning

Sampling, Randomization, and Blinding

The basics strategies of the RCT methodology are simple: appropriate patient sampling, choice of control group, randomization, and blinded assessment. However, each basic requirement can be satisfied in a myriad of ways, only some of which are valid in a particular RCT. What is ideal in one RCT may be either precluded or the worst choice in another. However, if all is done appropriately in the particular context of the RCT, nonrandom differences in response between the T and C groups reported as a *statistically significant* effect of T versus C are attributable to the treatment (thus the effect of T) rather than to biases in sampling, group assignment, measurement, or analysis.

Given that randomization is done to generate two random samples from the same population, any postrandomization removal of patients from the sample has the potential of biasing those samples relative to each other, and relative to the parent population. Consequently, RCT methodology also requires analysis of results *by intention to treat*. Every patient randomly assigned to a group (i.e., with the intention to treat) must be considered in the analysis comparing responses in the T and the C groups. In absence of an intention-to-treat analysis, when there is any postrandomization removal of patients from the randomized sample, the trial is no longer an RCT, because it is not based on comparison with randomized treatment and control groups. It is in this context that repeated measures of the primary outcome over the duration of treatment are particularly useful, for partial response data can be used to impute values for missing data or postdropout data, thus minimizing the associated loss of power.

To ensure that response is measured exactly the same in T and C groups, either objective outcome measures should be used or the assessor should be unaware of the treatment group to which a subject was assigned (i.e., "blinded").

Statistical Significance and Clinical Significance (Effect Sizes)

It must be emphasized that a *statistically significant* effect of T, with $P<0.05$, merely means that the data satisfy minimal requirements to show a nonrandom difference between T and C. If $P<0.01$ or $P<0.001$, etc., the data satisfy more than minimal requirements, but the conclusion remains only that there is a nonrandom difference between T and C. Thus, a statistically significant effect of T may or may not be large, important, or of any clinical significance.

To show that a statistically significant effect of T is of clinical significance as well, descriptive statistics and an effect size should be reported (as required by the Consolidated Standards of Reporting Trials [CONSORT] guidelines) (Altman et al. 2001; Rennie 1996). For example, how likely is a patient given T to have a response that is clinically preferable to the response of a patient given C (an effect size called *area under the curve* [AUC]) (Acion et al. 2006; Grissom 1994; Kraemer and Kupfer 2006)? Or how many patients would have to be given T to have one more "success" than if they had all been given C (another effect size, called *number needed to treat*) (Altman et al. 2001; Grissom and Kim 2005; Kraemer and Kupfer 2006; Wen et al. 2005)?

By the time there is rationale and justification to propose an RCT to compare T versus C, it is very unlikely that the null hypothesis of randomness is exactly true (Jones and Tukey 2000; Meehl 1967). In any case, with the best possible RCT, there is still a 5% chance of a false-positive result even if the null hypothesis of randomness is

exactly true. Thus, given a large enough sample size, and/or given enough RCTs comparing T versus C, every T could eventually be declared statistically significantly better than any C. Accordingly, in recent years the costs of exclusive emphasis on statistical significance have been recognized. There is now growing emphasis on reporting effect sizes that are clinically interpretable (Altman et al. 2001; Grissom and Kim 2005; Kraemer and Kupfer 2006).

Choice of Control Group

Among all the myriad sampling, design, and analysis questions that need to be addressed in proposing an RCT, the most contentious continues to be: What is C?; that is, what is the appropriate control group (or set of groups) in a particular RCT? More specifically, when is a placebo control group the appropriate choice? If not a placebo control group, then what? These are the questions to which we here turn our attention, questions that continue to be the focus of much disagreement and argument, even among experts in RCT methodology or application, ranging from many who propose that a placebo control group *always* be included in an RCT to some others who propose that it *never* be included.

In what follows we consider a variety of options for a control group, beginning with a few options that are, by strict definition, not RCTs. It is important to realize why these options are considered unacceptable, for those are the same considerations that apply when considering other possible choices for control groups, particularly that of a placebo control group. Then we discuss the choice of the placebo control group in some detail, ending with consideration of the *treatment-as-usual* (TAU) control group and the *standard-of-treatment* control group, the most common alternatives to the placebo control group.

Each Patient as His or Her Own Control (Pre–Post Study Design)

The very simplest, but unacceptable, proposal is to compare patients' conditions prior to and after treatment with T, with no control group and no randomization (hence not an RCT). Any change in condition beyond that consistent with random variation is taken to indicate a treatment effect. Researchers unable to detect a statistically significant difference between T and C groups in an RCT often report such pre–post comparisons as indicating an equally beneficial "effect" in the groups, a misinterpretation of statistical significance.

With any treatment, even a completely inert placebo, it is very unusual, given a large enough sample size, to *not* see a statistically significant change in patients' conditions pre- and posttreatment. Such a change is attributable not to the effect of that treatment but rather to artifacts of various kinds that a control group is meant to "control" for, as discussed below:

1. The first artifact is statistical regression to the mean (Blomqvist 1986; Campbell and Kenny 1999; Davis 1976; Senn 1997; Stigler 1997). Patients are selected for participation because they have symptoms of a disorder severe enough to require treatment (especially if there is an explicit cutoff point on severity required for inclusion), and frequently the outcome measures evaluate severity of the same symptoms. However, assessment of symptom severity at entry is never completely reliable. With error of measurement due to day-to-day inconsistencies in patients' conditions, coupled with assessor bias and random error, patients with a false-positive assessment at entry are included in the study, but patients in the population with a false-negative assessment at entry are excluded. In the absence of any effect of treatment on their clinical condition, those patients with a false-positive assessment at study entry are likely to later have their symptoms be assessed as closer to their true level, creating the false appearance of overall improvement.

2. Second are expectation effects. Both patients and assessors hope and expect to see improvement after onset of treatment. As Yogi Berra is reported to have said: "If I hadn't believed it, I wouldn't have seen it!" The power of suggestion is very strong, particularly in the process of recruitment into an RCT. The informed consent process, as well as patients' awareness of physicians' sworn obligation to do no harm, combined with the patients' pain, needs, and hopes, tends to bolster expectation effects.

3. Third are possible secular trends both in the condition of the patients and in the measurements of response. In some cases, patients with a disorder, receiving only the close and caring attention given in both T and C groups, spontaneously improve. At the same time, how assessors view a patient's response can change over time. With blinding, these effects are the same for patients in the T and C groups.

The cumulative effect of these and other artifactual influences constitutes the *placebo response*, which is experienced by those in *both* the T and C groups, whatever C

might be, but which is expressed in its pure form in a placebo control group. With randomization to the T and C groups and blinded assessment, the effect attributable to T is the differential response of the T and C groups, not the responses to T or to C separately. Thus, pre–post comparisons within a single treatment group may be of some clinical interest, and worth reporting, but are not adequate to establish the efficacy or effectiveness of any treatment.

Historical Control Groups

The pre–post treatment comparison as an indicator of treatment effect does away with the RCT requirements of a control group, of randomization, and of evaluator blinding. Another unacceptable alternative acknowledges the necessity of a control group but tries to do away with randomization and blinding: the *historical control group*. Here, as in pre–post studies, all patients recruited into the study receive T. However, information is obtained from clinical records and from past RCTs and other research studies on what happened to patients who received C—a historical rather than a concurrent control group. The treatment effect is then inferred from comparisons of the T group with the historical control group.

It has long been known that when one recruits patients from different sources (e.g., different sites, different recruitment pools, or at different times), what is seen, even in response to the same treatment in samples satisfying the same inclusion/exclusion criteria, is different. It is usually hoped that the effects of T versus C within each source are much the same (generalizability) in patients recruited from different sources, but the responses within the individual T and C groups are expected to differ sharply in patients recruited from one source versus another. With a historical control group, any difference seen may be due wholly or in part to site/time/context effects rather than being due to the effect of T versus C, and the effect size that is estimated and tested is not valid for establishing the efficacy or effectiveness of a treatment.

Withhold Treatment: Waiting List Control Groups

Yet another proposal, one consistent with RCT methodology but still questionable, is to randomly assign patients either to the T group or to a *waiting list control group*. Those in the waiting list control group are asked to refrain from seeking treatment for their disorder for the duration of the RCT, at the end of which they are given T if they then wish to receive it.

There is an ethical problem here. Patients being recruited into an RCT suffer from some disorder for which they seek help. It is difficult in many cases for clinical researchers to maintain *clinical equipoise*—defined as "a state of genuine uncertainty on the part of the clinical investigator regarding the comparative therapeutic merits of each arm in a trial" (Freedman 1987)—when the choices are between using a treatment that has a rationale, and for which there is justification for a belief that it might be helpful, and denying treatment for the duration of the study. Clinical equipoise is not solely an issue related to ethics. Lack of clinical equipoise often has repercussions for the scientific validity of the RCT, because when researchers are sure that T is better than the selected C, it is difficult to ensure the scientific objectivity necessary to the design, conduct, and analysis of the trial in order to produce a balanced and fair comparison of T versus C.

Clearly, if the disorder that the patients have is not serious, disabling, or painful; if it is unlikely to worsen with a delay in treatment; and particularly if no treatments are available for the condition outside the RCT that the patients would have had access to had they not been in the RCT, there is no convincing ethical argument for withholding treatment. However, it is not the ethical considerations but rather practical considerations that make the choice of withholding treatment untenable.

When patients seeking help for a disorder are able to obtain treatment from clinicians in their community, patients are less likely to volunteer for an RCT in which they take a chance of having such help withheld. Thus, the sample that is recruited into an RCT with a waiting list control group is likely to be nonrepresentative of the population with the disorder, often missing adequate representation of those most seriously affected by the disorder and those most anxious to be relieved of the effects of the disorder.

Moreover, after randomization, patients in the control group are more likely to drop out to seek outside help, introducing bias to the RCT and loss of power. Indeed, in many cases, clinicians observing patients in the waiting list control group often relent and transfer patients from the control group to treatment group prior to the end of the RCT, because of clinical ethical concerns.

Technically, this is a valid RCT proposal, because there is a C (in this case, temporary withholding of treatment) and randomization to T and C groups. However, in waiting list–controlled RCTs, it is very difficult to blind assessment of the outcomes. Patients are often very aware that they are receiving no treatment for their disorder and such awareness can color all measures of response. Consequently, the problems of sample bias, measurement bias, missing data, dropouts, loss of power, and bias in resulting effect sizes militate against choosing a waiting list control group in most cases.

Placebo Control Groups

A *placebo* is defined as an inert medication or procedure, one that is selected specifically because it cannot affect the underlying process of the disorder: a saline injection, a sugar pill. When a patient given placebo appears to respond, such a response is often mistakenly labeled a *placebo effect*. However, since this response cannot be attributed to the placebo, the more appropriate label is *placebo response*. As noted above, the placebo response is experienced both by those receiving T and those receiving C, but it is experienced in its pure form only by those in a placebo control group (see "Each Patient as His or Her Own Control [Pre–Post Study Design]").

Because of the artifacts associated with pre–post study designs (regression to the mean, expectation effects, secular trends in the clinical condition of the patient or in the measurement process, etc.), it is very common for patients randomly assigned to placebo treatment to appear to respond favorably. In fact, it is reasonable to expect that given a large enough sample size, one will always find a statistically significant placebo response.

There has long been discussion of how one might 1) understand the placebo response and 2) reduce the placebo response in RCTs to make it easier to detect the efficacy or effectiveness of treatment versus placebo. That portion of placebo response related to artifacts, however, is already well understood. They are controlled in well-designed RCTs to the extent that is possible, by use of reliable measures and consistent application of measurement protocols over the course of the RCT.

Clinically, the most interesting aspect of placebo response is the expectation effect in both patients and assessors of response. Why would we want to reduce such expectation effects? Such expectations have a great deal to do with compliance and cooperation of patients during RCTs, as well as with their potential response to treatment. It would certainly be worthwhile to understand on whom one might expect strong expectation effects, how and why they exist, and exactly how they influence clinical response to treatment. But the goal would be to consider how to *increase* expectation effects to maximize the efficacy or effectiveness of any treatment, rather than to *reduce* them.

Like the waiting list control group, the placebo control group amounts to a withholding of treatment for the duration of the study. However, having a placebo control group repairs many, though not all, of the technical problems associated with a waiting list control group. One clear advantage is that use of a placebo control group facilitates blinding of outcome measurement. Thus, the problem of measurement bias expected in waiting list–controlled RCTs can be obviated in a placebo-controlled trial.

In the past, many patients did not actually understand what a placebo was, and when U.S. drug studies are conducted in Third World countries, this problem is still of concern. With the growing sophistication of medical consumers and medical advocates, however, and with the increasing scrutiny of how the placebo group is described in informed consent forms, this is less of a problem today. As is the case for use of waiting list control groups, patients with the greatest impairment from their disorder—who are most anxious to get relief, most in need of effective treatment, and most likely to cooperate and comply with treatment—are less likely to be willing to agree to randomization in a placebo-controlled trial. Moreover, their primary care physicians often have the same reaction and are reluctant to recommend participation in an RCT for those most in need of treatment. Thus, placebo-controlled trials run a strong risk of having a nonrepresentative sample from the relevant clinical population. Accordingly, the CONSORT guidelines for reporting the results of an RCT (Altman et al. 2001) ask that researchers provide a patient flowchart that includes how many patients were eligible for the RCT and how many refused participation. This information sheds light on the possible sample bias in any RCT but particularly in a placebo-controlled one.

Moreover, the problems that waiting list–controlled RCTs have with dropouts can be exacerbated (Kemmler et al. 2005) by substituting a placebo control group. Now patients in *both* the active treatment and placebo control groups are equally aware that they might be receiving a placebo. Patients in either group who do not experience the relief from their disorder that they hope for are likely to suspect that they are in the placebo control group, and thus are likely to drop out of the RCT. Again, their physicians, observing no amelioration of symptoms, may add to the problem by recommending dropping out and initiation of what they would consider effective treatment. Once again, such concerns are reflected in the CONSORT guidelines (Altman et al. 2001) with the requirement that researchers report the number of patients randomly assigned to each group (the intention-to-treat

samples) and the number that drop out in each group, with reasons for such dropouts. This information is intended to help assess the possible biases that might result from such dropouts.

The RCT requirement that all randomly assigned patients be considered in assessing the treatment effect (an intention-to-treat analysis) in the face of any appreciable dropout is difficult to comply with. Although imputation methods, both simple and complex, are often used, there is no imputation procedure that completely corrects for the impact of dropouts or missing data on an RCT that are directly related to the experiences of patients with the treatment that they were assigned to receive. The fact that a placebo control often increases the risk for dropouts and missing data is thus an important consideration.

Although missing data and dropouts remain major issues in considering the use of placebo control groups, the major source of contention arises not from the theory of RCTs, or from the implementation problems of RCTs, but rather from the ethics of proposing a placebo-controlled RCT in the first place and from the clinical value of the results of a placebo-controlled RCT. To understand these arguments, let us consider a few specific contexts in which placebo control groups might be considered.

When Is Use of a Placebo Control Group Unarguable?

When usual treatment is no treatment.   Little or no argument about the choice of placebo as the control group in an RCT occurs when the usual treatment by clinicians in the community is no treatment at all. Then, using a placebo in the control group mimics clinicians' recommendations exactly in providing no treatment that can influence the disorder.

In such cases, patients may be better off volunteering for participation in an RCT, where they have at least a chance of being assigned to receive an effective treatment. Patients might actually respond better to a placebo in an RCT than to absence of treatment in the community because of one of the artifactual responses that the control group controls for. For example, the attention, care, and scrutiny provided to patients in an RCT are usually far beyond those provided in usual clinical practice, and that may benefit patients. For all these reasons, when usual care in the community is no treatment, patients have strong inducement to volunteer to participate in a placebo-controlled RCT.

Moreover, in this situation patients have little inducement to drop out of the RCT, for nothing is available as an alternative in the community that can be better than what is offered in the placebo control group, and what is offered in the T group may improve their condition. Thus, when usual treatment in the community is no treatment, placebo control groups are the only choice, and an excellent choice at that.

In seeking FDA approval.   Even when there are treatments thought to be effective in the community for a disorder (often other drug companies' products), drug companies generally prefer placebo control groups in studies directed to the FDA for drug approval.

The FDA requires that the drug company provide "proof that a drug has a therapeutic effect in at least some patients," and "no requirements are imposed regarding the 'representativeness'" of a study sample vis-à-vis the population of patients from which it is drawn" (Leber and Davis 1998, p. 179).

Moreover, the FDA does not set any criteria for a *clinically* significant effect, although it generally—as noted above in the "Indications" section—requires demonstration in more than one RCT of a *statistically* significant effect. Thus, drug companies prefer to use a control group in which response is minimized to that associated with unavoidable artifacts of participating in an RCT, because having such a control group maximizes the chance of finding a statistically significant effect. Given that the sample size necessary to demonstrate a statistically significant effect is smallest when the effect size is largest, the easiest way to achieve drug approval is to use very stringent inclusion/exclusion criteria that favor recruitment into the RCT of only those most likely to respond well to the drug (an efficacy trial) and a placebo control group that minimizes the benefit in the control group. Pharmaceutical companies are then doing exactly what they need to do to satisfy FDA requirements to market their drugs.

What the FDA requires or accepts depends on how it interprets the mandate from the U.S. Congress, under which it operates, and what drug companies do is determined by what the FDA requires and accepts. For these reasons, issues related to the use of placebo control groups in RCTs that are performed to establish the efficacy or effectiveness of treatments in clinical populations might well be considered separately from issues related to FDA requirements for drug approval and drug companies' efforts to satisfy those requirements.

However, as described above, the results of studies funded by drug companies to gain FDA approval of an agent may not generalize to the type of patients clinicians are treating. Even within the limited populations actually studied in some such studies, the clinical benefits of the drug may well be statistically significantly better, but not clinically significantly better, than the effects of withholding treatment (i.e., as in placebo control groups), or the drug's effects may be both statistically and clinically worse than the effects of whatever treatments clinicians are already using for their patients.

Such considerations relate closely to present-day concerns about conflict-of-interest issues when academic researchers are associated with studies funded by drug companies and explain the requirements of many research journals and professional organizations that such conflicts of interests be reported when presenting results of such studies.

In medical experiments.   Another situation is a medical experiment that is not a clinical trial. Basic researchers in pharmacology, for example, might be interested in the pharmacokinetics of a particular drug in human subjects, not in the efficacy or effectiveness of that drug in any patient population. To test their hypotheses, a control group, randomization, and blinding may also be necessary. However, in many cases, the individuals recruited into such a study are not patients with a disorder but simply volunteers, and the outcomes are focused not on the clinical benefits or harm to patients but rather on aspects of the drug, such as rates of drug absorption and elimination. In many such situations, a placebo control group is the only scientifically valid choice to test hypotheses. Because the focus here is not on establishing the efficacy or effectiveness of a treatment, this is a *medical experiment* but is not that specific type of medical experiment called the *clinical trial.* Such medical experiments are fundamental to progress in basic science and translational research.

The issues about the use of human subjects in medical experiments, including that of using placebo control subjects, are specific to the particular research question being addressed in a study and are generally different from those in an RCT. These are issues that institutional review boards must assess for each individual research project. Informed consent forms for such studies should not describe the study as an RCT and should spell out clearly that the focus of the study is to further biochemical or pharmacological knowledge about the drug, not (at least not in the near future) to improve treatment for any patients with a disorder.

In testing a supplemental treatment. In many cases, an RCT is performed to test whether a new treatment that is used as a supplement to an established treatment is more effective or efficacious than the standard treatment alone. This is a case in which there are few, if any, reservations to the use of a placebo to control the artifactual effects of offering two treatments rather than one. All patients would receive the standard treatment and then be randomly assigned to supplementation with either the new treatment or a placebo. If researchers find a statistically and clinically significant difference between the two groups, it would represent not an effect of the new treatment but rather an additive or interactive effect of the old and new treatments together. Here few people would have ethical or scientific concerns about the use of a placebo control group.

Placebo Control Groups: Arguments Pro and Con

As we have seen, the arguments against the use of placebo control groups are seldom absolute. Few would argue against using placebo control groups when the usual treatment is no treatment. Few would argue against using placebo control groups when a new treatment is tested as a supplement to an old treatment. The general argument against the use of placebo control groups can be summarized as: There are often better alternatives for a control group than placebo control subjects, alternatives that are better clinically and ethically, and often the scientific quality and clinical impact of RCTs using alternative control groups are preferable.

On the other hand, Leber (2000, p. 699), for example, has argued that "in the evaluation of drugs intended for the management of psychiatric illness, placebo control groups are indispensable, a fact that has been recognized for almost half a century by literally generations of investigators working in the fields of clinical pharmacology and psychopharmacology." Yet A. Bradford Hill (1963), often recognized as the father of RCTs, stated the following: "Is it ethical to use a placebo? The answer to this question will depend, I suggest, upon whether there is already available an orthodox treatment of proved or accepted use." The arguments about placebo control groups among those most knowledgeable about RCTs have been around as long as RCTs have been around (Rothman and Michels 1994).

Arguments for the necessity of placebo control groups are often made on philosophical grounds (Leber 2000) or in terms of convenience to researchers because placebo-controlled RCTs take less time and effort and require less funding (with their smaller sample sizes). However, RCTs are *clinical* trials proposed to address *clinical* issues, not philosophical or logistical ones. To benefit clinical decision making, hence medical consumers and clinicians, the crucial question is this: Is T clinically preferable to C in the population studied? If physicians in the community are using a range of treatments that they believe to be effective, there is little value in demonstrating that a new treatment is better than withholding treatment altogether (as in a placebo control group).

Others argue, not for the necessity of placebo control groups but for their acceptability, that placebos do no *lasting* or *irrevocable* harm. For example, numerous studies have demonstrated that the suicide risk among psychiatric patients receiving a placebo is not such as to preclude the ethical use of placebos in that context (Khan et al. 2000, 2001, 2006; Storosum et al. 2005). However, the Hippocratic oath's requirement to "do no harm" is not restricted to lasting or irrevocable harm. It is not the prerogative of the medical researcher to stipulate how much potential harm to a patient is acceptable. Rather, it is the duty of the medical researcher to assure patients that, to the best of current medical knowledge, the harm that may occur if they participate in the RCT would not be greater than if they chose not to participate in the RCT, and may well be less.

Alternative Control Groups

Treatment-as-Usual Control Groups

For a variety of reasons, from the perspective of a patient or a clinician, the most attractive choice for a comparison group is one that uses what clinicians are currently using: the TAU (treatment-as-usual) control group. Here patients are recruited into the study and randomly assigned either to T, the new treatment under study, or to the treatment they would have received if they had not entered the RCT. The responses in both groups are monitored using the same protocol, with evaluators blinded to group membership. The research question is whether it can be shown, beyond reasonable doubt, that T produces better results than what community clinicians generally achieve.

Because patients who enter such an RCT receive at least the treatment that they would have received had they not entered the RCT (TAU), or perhaps receive a treatment for which there is a rationale and justification for a belief that it might be better (T), such a control group is an inducement to participation. Moreover, since dropping out of the study generally means getting what is now the control treatment, there is little inducement to drop out. Clearly, patients and treatment providers cannot be blinded to the treatment choice, although assessors of treatment response can be.

Objections to this choice of control group generally come from researchers, who correctly point out that community clinicians do not all use the same treatment, and many use treatments that are known to be far from optimal (or use optimal treatment in a less-than-optimal fashion). Far greater variability in response is likely in a TAU control group than there would be if one particular treatment were specified for a control group, or if placebo were used, and greater variability than in the T group. Consequently, the sample size has to be larger to achieve adequate power than with a specific choice of comparator treatment or with a placebo as the control intervention.

Clearly, with TAU as the control condition, greater detail is needed in reporting results. It is important to report which treatments were being used by community clinicians and to explore whether some of those treatments were likely to be better or worse than T (hypotheses to perhaps be tested in future RCTs). However, all in all, TAU is a viable choice for a control condition in an RCT to document whether T is a better choice in general than what is already available in the community.

Standard-of-Treatment Control Groups

Another viable option is that of selecting and delivering what, on the basis of past, independently replicated RCTs, appears to be the most effective of the treatments in use in the community. This allays many of the problems with TAU control groups, because now the one control treatment can be optimally delivered by research staff, decreasing the heterogeneity within the control group. Also, blinding can now be more complete and effective. Moreover, patients can be assured that current medical knowledge indicates that the treatment in the control group is as good as or better than what they would receive if they were not in the study, which again is an inducement both to participate in the RCT and to not drop out. If there is persuasive evidence that the new treatment T is indeed superior (or at least equivalent) to others currently available, significant findings in such a study might well convince clinicians to use T rather than whatever treatment they had been using.

Equivalence and Noninferiority RCTs

The RCT methodology was originally established to establish the efficacy or effectiveness of a treatment, to establish whether T is better than C. In recent years, attention has also been paid to issues of clinical significance, as well as to *noninferiority* and *equivalence*. Misconceptions concerning statistical significance, clinical significance, equivalence, and noninferiority have unnecessarily confused the issue of the placebo control.

The basic requirements of an RCT still apply to equivalence and noninferiority trials: the necessity of an appropriate control group, randomization to T versus C groups, blinded assessment of response, and analysis by intention to treat. In the study population, there is an unknown effect size, delta (δ), that is zero when there is absolutely no differential response between T and C, is positive when T tends to be better than C, and is negative when C tends to be better than T. One way of stating the purpose of an RCT is that it is meant to estimate that unknown effect size (Borenstein 1994, 1997, 1998).

The usual two-tailed null hypothesis significance test seeks to prove beyond reasonable doubt that δ is not zero. In designing such a study, a value of δ, the threshold of clinical significance, is designated—say, δ^*. The test is then structured so that when $\delta = 0$, the probability of a significant result is less than, say, 5% (the significance level). When the magnitude of δ is greater than δ^*, the probability of a significant result is greater than, say, 80% (adequate power). Given the fact that when there is sufficient rationale and justification for proposing an RCT there is almost no realistic chance that the effect size is exactly zero, achieving statistical significance in an RCT is generally a matter of having a large enough sample size in a well-designed study with reliable outcome measures. To indicate the possible clinical significance of a statistically significant finding, the effect size and its confidence interval should be reported (as per CONSORT guidelines).

Another way of saying the same thing: with the study design described above, there is a better than 80% probability that a two-tailed 95% confidence interval for the unknown true effect size δ will not include $\delta = 0$, whenever the true effect size is greater than the critical value δ^*.

In contrast, to show that T is clinically superior to C, one needs to show that the entire confidence interval for that effect size is greater than δ^*. To show that T and C are clinically equivalent, one needs to show that the confidence interval lies completely between $-\delta^*$ and δ^*. To show the noninferiority of T to C, one needs to show that the entire confidence interval is less than $-\delta^*$.

One can always demonstrate either noninferiority or equivalence, simply by using unreliable outcome measures, allowing deviations from treatment and measurement protocols, etc. That is, a badly conducted trial will result in an attenuated effect size between any two drugs, an effect size closer to zero, that can almost always be labeled as a noninferior or equivalent result.

This issue is highly relevant to the valid interpretation of study results because of a common confusion between a result being *non–statistically significant* and two drugs showing *equivalence*. To report a non–statistically significant result is only to admit that the sample size was not large enough, the design not powerful enough, or the measures not reliable enough to demonstrate beyond reasonable doubt that $\delta \neq 0$. That is nowhere near the same thing as reporting a demonstration beyond reasonable doubt that $-\delta^* < \delta < \delta^*$ (i.e., equivalence). As the old saying goes: "Absence of proof is not proof of absence."

In particular, if one randomly assigned subjects in an RCT to one of two treatment groups (T1 or T2) or to a placebo control group (C) and found no statistically significant difference between T1 and T2 but found statistically significant differences both between T1 and C and between T2 and C, that tells nothing about the possible clinical equivalence of T1 and T2. All one would know is that both T1 and T2 were shown to be better than (not necessarily even clinically superior to) placebo; the sample was not large enough to detect whatever difference there might be between T1 and T2. Any conclusion comparing T1 and T2 would be exactly the same whether or not the placebo control group were included in the design. Yet many arguments for the use of a placebo control group inappropriately reflect an effort to use the placebo control as a decoy to interpret results comparing T1 and T2.

But finally, why would it be important to establish beyond reasonable doubt the clinical equivalence of two treatments, particularly when such a result can be obtained through poor study design (e.g., choice of measurement) and execution of the RCT? Often when this question is asked, whether of a drug company representative or of an academic researcher, a complete answer often contains an implicit reinterpretation of equivalence as superiority. For example: Two treatments might have equivalent effects in reducing symptoms, but one might have a better side-effect profile. Or the two treatments might have equivalent effects in terms of both symptom reduction and side effects, but one may be far less costly or have greater ease of use than the other. In all such cases, the goal of the RCT should be to establish the clinical preference for one treatment or the other over the control condition by using an outcome measure sensitive to the specific ways one drug might be clinically preferable to another. But that would then be not an equivalence study but rather the usual type of RCT, with a primary outcome reflecting the particular way in which T is hypothesized to be superior to C.

Statistical Analysis and Power

Threaded through all the above issues are implicit considerations of statistical analysis and power. Every single decision about research design has some impact on the appropriate choice of analysis and on the power to detect clinically significant effects. In fact, the major difference between well-designed and well-executed present-day RCTs and those done 50 years ago stems from advances in methods of statistical analysis of results and better understanding of the concept and application of power in designing RCTs.

With the simplest possible design, randomly assigning a representative sample of patients to a treatment (T) or control (C) condition, with a binary primary outcome—"success" versus "failure"—the analytic method would be a 2×2 (treatment $\times$ outcome) χ^2 test. This is the least powerful design (Cohen 1983; Kraemer 1991; Kraemer and Thiemann 1987, 1989; MacCallum et al. 2002), and the study thus requires perhaps twice, perhaps 10 times, as many patients for adequate power compared with studies with other designs. A valid choice? Yes. A wise choice? No.

Suppose we merely substituted that binary primary outcome with a dimensional one—for example, symptom level at the end of treatment—and proposed to use the most common RCT analysis method: the two-sample t test. Immediately, there would be an increase of power (thus requiring a smaller sample size for adequate power). If the goal is to detect a moderate effect (number needed to treat [NNT] ~4), for a 5% two-tailed test one would require 63 patients per group or a total of 126 patients. Detecting a small effect (NNT ~9) would require 389 patients per group, and detecting a large effect (NNT ~2) would require only 26 patients per group.

The two-sample t test is valid when the outcomes being measured are approximately normally distributed with equal variances in the two groups, but many clinically meaningful outcomes have asymmetrical distributions, have long tails, or occur with unequal variances in the two groups. Then one might use instead the nonparametric Wilcoxon rank sum test (Mann-Whitney test). When the t test gives valid results, the Mann-Whitney test is also valid and has quite similar power. However, the nonparametric test is valid in many circumstances when the t test is not. This illustrates two general principles: the choice of the outcome measure must be in accordance with the choice of the analytic procedure, and better selection of the outcome measure has a major impact on the study's power and thus the necessary sample size.

If one uses any of the above for an RCT of depressed patients, most of the sample would be female; for an RCT of schizophrenic patients, most of the sample would be male. In many cases, it is proposed to stratify such sample populations in order to equalize the representation of males and females. Is this wise?

If it is decided that stratification is warranted, to be valid the analytic procedure must acknowledge that stratification. For a binary outcome, one might use a logistic regression analysis and for a dimensional outcome, a linear regression analysis, with treatment group, stratum (here, gender), and their interaction as independent variables in each case.

One common analytic error is to assume that the interaction does not exist and to use analysis of covariance with gender as the covariate. If that interaction does exist in the study population and is ignored in the analysis, it often compromises the significance level, and thus the validity of the test, and almost inevitably reduces the power. But if the interaction is included in the analysis, care must be taken to properly center all the independent variables to produce clinically interpretable results (Kraemer and Blasey 2004).

If this is done correctly, the interaction test assesses whether the treatment effect in women is different from the effect in men, and the main effect of treatment assesses whether the average treatment effect across men and women is nonrandom. When there is an interaction effect in the study population, the main effect of treatment in this analysis is not the same as the effect of treatment assessed in an unstratified sample. The crucial issue then is which treatment effect is of interest—the effect in the total population or the average effect across the subpopulations defined by the strata.

If the decision is that the sample should be stratified, the sample size needed for adequate power is likely to increase, and the logistical difficulty of accumulating a stratified sample is likely to be much greater. If, for example, 80% of those with the disorder of interest are women, but it is decided that 50% of the sample in the RCT should be women, one will have to work much harder to recruit that oversampling of men into the study. Thus, careful thought should be given to whether the rationale and justification for stratification are strong enough to necessitate larger samples, more complex analyses, and a shift in the hypothesis being tested.

The difficulty of such decisions is exacerbated when researchers (or reviewers) seek to control for multiple covariates (e.g., gender, age, ethnicity, initial severity of the disorder). To truly control the study for the effects of such

variables, one stratifies the sample. However, with gender (two possibilities), age (say, five age groups), ethnicity (say, five ethnic groups), and initial severity (say, three levels), one has $2\times5\times5\times3=150$ strata, and one would have to recruit adequate numbers into each stratum (for optimal power, an equal number into each stratum). If even a minimal number of patients per stratum were specified, say, 10 per stratum (5 randomized to T and 5 to C), the minimal sample size would be 1,500!

If these stratification variables are not very strongly associated with treatment effect, the result is a study with less power than would be achieved with a simple design. If there are collinearities among these variables (say, women and older patients tend to have high higher initial disease severity), the power to detect treatment effects might also be reduced. One of the least wise decisions in RCT design is to try to control for the effects of too many variables, and many experienced biostatisticians argue against any stratification of the sample unless the primary hypotheses concern moderators of treatment outcome.

Researchers and review committees, however, often propose another tactic: Instead of controlling for the effects of these baseline variables through stratification, adjust for them in a mathematical model. Now the sample would continue to be 80% women, but the analysis would include consideration of both treatment and gender. What then often happens in analysis is exclusion of all interactions. Without adjustment, the two-sample t test has $N-2$ degrees of freedom (the larger the number of degrees of freedom, other things being equal, the greater the power), but with a single covariate, that becomes $N-4$ ($N-2^2$), and with four covariates, it becomes $N-32$ ($N-2^5$). As noted above, if such interactions exist in the study population and are excluded in the model, the significance level may be compromised and power is almost inevitably lost. Thus, if covariates are to be included, their interactions must be as well. Unless inclusion of those variables has a major strengthening effect on effect size, this inevitably means a loss of power. Finally and perhaps most important, collinearity effects resulting from associations between the variables included cost even more power. Again, most experienced biostatisticians argue against adjusting for the effects of baseline variables in the absence of a strong rationale and empirical justification for doing so.

On the other hand, in a multisite RCT, stratification by site is built into the design and must be included in the analysis, and even then, many researchers and reviewers choose to ignore it. Multisite RCTs often show that site differences are a major source of variance in the outcome measurements (MTA Cooperative Group 1999). The most convincing demonstration of the almost-ubiquitous nature of site differences is not from an RCT but from a study of inbred strains of mice in a genetics study (Crabbe et al. 1999) under controlled laboratory conditions. Even then, site differences occurred. In an RCT, if samples are drawn from different sites, or in different time spans, or at the same site at the same time but using different recruitment strategies (e.g., referrals from doctors versus responses to advertisement), one should always expect that these differences will affect the primary outcome. Thus, randomization must be done within each such stratum, and comparison of T versus C must be a pooled comparison of the within-stratum comparisons of T versus C (Kraemer and Robinson 2005).

Thus far we have focused on assessing a single primary outcome at the end of treatment, whether a binary success/failure or a dimensional outcome, and have recommended against using a binary outcome. But, some would argue, some outcomes are by their nature binary: either the patient dies or not, the patient recovers or not, the disease remits or not. Are we not then obliged to use a binary outcome, and "take the hit" by increasing the sample size manyfold?

Outcomes such as these occur over the course of time, and at different times for different patients. By simply reorienting the analysis to examination of the time to the event, one moves from a binary outcome to a dimensional one. This is the situation in which survival analyses become the analytic procedure of choice: Kaplan-Meier estimation-of-survival curves within each group (Kaplan and Meier 1958), comparison of these survival curves in the T versus C groups, and use of the Cox proportional model (Andersen et al. 1985), for example, when there are strata or covariates to be considered. Although the sample sizes for adequate power will be somewhat greater than with other dimensional outcomes (because some patients will be censored, i.e., they will not have had the outcome occur before the end of study), the sample size here will be much smaller than when using a binary outcome, and more useful clinical information will be obtained.

Also, with dimensional outcome measurement, modern analytic tools can lead to increased power without increasing sample size. For example, instead of assessing the outcome using only the endpoint of treatment, one could assess that outcome measure at baseline and at fixed times during the treatment period. Random regression models (also known as hierarchical models, or growth curves; Berger 1986; deLeeuw and Kreft 1986; Ware 1985) basically model the trajectory of response within each patient

and then test whether the trajectories of response in the T group are clinically preferable to those in the C group. Because multiple measures per patient are used to characterize each patient's response, reliability is increased, and thus power is increased. Moreover, in the case of missing data or dropouts, partial data on the trajectory per patient enable stronger imputation methods to facilitate intention-to-treat analyses. Quite aside from the multiple statistical advantages of designing studies with repeated measures of outcomes over time, such information is often clinically informative in guiding clinicians to recognize early those patients who are unlikely to ever respond to a given treatment.

This discussion barely scratches the surface of analytic methods available, but illustrates two general principles:

1. For adequate power and to best inform clinical decision making, characterize the response of each individual patient as precisely and concisely as possible (using reliable measures, preferably dimensional, with repeated measures over time). That might sometimes complicate the analysis, but analytic methods are generally available to take advantage of such precision.
2. Design the study to answer the primary research question, not to answer all possible questions that might arise. Leave those to secondary or exploratory post hoc analyses. Do not stratify the study population unless the design requires multiple sites or recruitment sources or the primary research question is about the strata. Do not try to control or adjust for all possible influences on treatment effect; instead, focus on controlling those factors empirically shown to strongly influence treatment effect.

Summary

The sine qua non of an RCT is that there be a control or comparison group, with an appropriate sample of patients randomly assigned to the treatment and control groups, with blinded assessment of outcome, and with analysis by intention to treat. A reasonable analogy of conducting an RCT is that it is like juggling many balls, trying to keep them all in the air at the same time: choice of control group, randomization, blinding, sampling, treatment protocol, measurement protocol, and fidelity to the protocols during the study, analysis, and interpretation of results, etc. The more research questions that are to be addressed in a particular RCT, and the more complex each research question is, the more balls are being juggled and the more slippery they are. Moreover, as soon as one ball drops, the others are likely also to follow. Any mistake in sampling, for example, is likely to have repercussions in analysis and interpretation of results. Poor measurement (e.g., use of a binary primary outcome) will have an effect on design (sample size). Improved design (e.g., repeated measures of the primary outcome) will have an effect on analysis and interpretation of results. For this reason, the best studies result when there is a focus on the primary research question, when all research decisions are made to protect the integrity of and amplify the answers to that primary research question. When the effort is made to answer as many questions as possible in one study, e.g., addressing multiple outcomes, or controlling or adjusting for multiple variables, RCTs tend not to answer any research questions well at all.

The choice of an appropriate control group is context specific but should take into consideration ethical and clinical as well as scientific issues. On the issue of using placebo control groups, we distinguished RCTs to establish the efficacy or effectiveness of a drug from studies done for the purpose of gaining FDA approval of a drug versus randomized medical experiments to explicate basic science questions, which are often performed with subjects who are not patients and for purposes that have little or nothing to do with efficacy or effectiveness of treatments.

We have discussed in detail when it is best and least controversial to use a placebo control group (i.e., when there is no better alternative to placebo) and when it may be more appropriate to use a TAU control group or a standard-of-care control group, particularly in cases where withholding treatment, as would be done with placebo control subjects, raises ethical questions as well as logistical questions.

Using placebo control groups as a foil to understand differences not seen between two active treatments is often based on a misinterpretation of statistical significance. Moreover, use of placebo control groups as an aid in establishing equivalence or noninferiority is questionable, because what may appear to be equivalence is often related to poor study execution rather than to actual equivalence between treatments. Also, it is not clear why equivalence is important to clinical decision making.

In short, in some circumstances using a placebo control group is the only choice, and in others using a placebo control group is the best choice. There are also circumstances in which ethical, clinical, and scientific interests are best served by using other types of control groups. Finally, there have been circumstances in which inclusion of placebo control groups has misled thinking about the effects of other drugs.

References

Acion L, Peterson JJ, Temple S, et al: Probabilistic index: an intuitive non-parametric approach to measuring the size of treatment effects. Stat Med 25:591–602, 2006

Altman DG, Schulz KF, Hoher D, et al: The revised CONSORT statement for reporting randomized trials: explanation and elaboration. CONSORT Group (Consolidated Standards of Reporting Trials). Ann Intern Med 134:663–694, 2001

American Psychiatric Association: Diagnostic and Statistical Manual of Mental Disorders, 4th Edition, Text Revision. Washington, DC, American Psychiatric Association, 2000

Andersen PK, Borch-Johnsen K, Deckert T, et al: A Cox regression model for the relative mortality and its application to diabetes mellitus survival data. Biometrics 41:921–932, 1985

Berger MPF: A comparison of efficiencies of longitudinal, mixed longitudinal, and cross-sectional designs. Journal of Educational Statistics 11:171–181, 1986

Blomqvist N: On the bias caused by regression toward the mean in studying the relation between change and the initial value. J Clin Periodontol 13:34–37, 1986

Borenstein M: The case for confidence intervals in controlled clinical trials. Control Clin Trials 15:411–428, 1994

Borenstein M: Hypothesis testing and effect size estimation in clinical trials. Ann Allergy Asthma Immunol 78:5–16, 1997

Borenstein M: The shift from significance testing to effect size estimation, in Comprehensive Clinical Psychology (Bellak AS, Hersen M, editors-in-chief), Vol 3: Research Methods (Schooler NR, volume editor). Burlington, MA, Elsevier Science, 1998, pp 319–349

Campbell DT, Kenny DA: A Primer on Regression Artifacts. New York, Guilford, 1999

Cohen J: The cost of dichotomization. Applied Psychological Measurement 7:249–253, 1983

Crabbe JC, Wahlsten D, Dudek BC: Genetics of mouse behavior: interactions with laboratory environment. Science 284:1670–1672, 1999

Davis CE: The effect of regression to the mean in epidemiologic and clinical studies. Am J Epidemiol 104:493–498, 1976

deLeeuw J, Kreft I: Random coefficient models for multilevel analysis. Journal of Educational Statistics 11:57–85, 1986

Freedman B: Equipoise and the ethics of clinical research. N Engl J Med 317:141–145, 1987

Grissom RJ: Probability of the superior outcome of one treatment over another. J Appl Psychol 79:314–316, 1994

Grissom RJ, Kim JJ: Effect Sizes for Research: A Broad Practical Approach. Mahwah, NJ, Lawrence Erlbaum, 2005

Hoagwood K, Hibbs E, Brent D, et al: Introduction to the special section: efficacy and effectiveness in studies of child and adolescent psychotherapy. J Consult Clin Psychol 63:683–687, 1995

Hill AB: Medical ethics and controlled trials. BMJ 1(5337):1043–1049, 1963

Humphreys K, Weisner C: Use of exclusion criteria in selecting research patients and its effect on the generalizability of alcohol treatment outcome studies. Am J Psychiatry 157:588–594, 2000

Humphreys K, Weingardt KR, Horst D, et al: Prevalence and predictors of research participant eligibility criteria in alcohol treatment outcome studies, 1970–98. Addiction 100:1249–1257, 2005

Jones LV, Tukey JW: A sensible formulation of the significance test. Psychol Methods 5:411–414, 2000

Kaplan EL, Meier P: Nonparametric estimation from incomplete observations. J Am Stat Assoc 53:457–481, 562–563, 1958

Kemmler G, Hummer M, Widschwendter C, et al: Dropout rates in placebo-controlled and active-control clinical trials of antipsychotic drugs. Arch Gen Psychiatry 62:1305–1312, 2005

Khan A, Warner HA, Brown WA: Symptom reduction and suicide risk in patients treated with placebo in antidepressant clinical trials: an analysis of the Food and Drug Administration database. Arch Gen Psychiatry 57:311–317, 2000

Khan A, Khan SR, Leventhal RM, et al: Symptom reduction and suicide risk among patients treated with placebo in antipsychotic clinical trials: an analysis of the Food and Drug Administration database. Am J Psychiatry 158:1449–1454, 2001

Khan A, Kolts RL, Brodhead AE, et al: Suicide risk analysis among patients assigned to psychotropics and placebo. Psychopharmacol Bull 39:6–14, 2006

Kraemer HC: To increase power in randomized clinical trials without increasing sample size. Psychopharmacol Bull 27:217–224, 1991

Kraemer HC: Toward non-parametric and clinically meaningful moderators and mediators. Stat Med 27:1679–1692, 2008

Kraemer HC, Blasey C: Centring in regression analysis: a strategy to prevent errors in statistical inference. Int J Methods Psychiatr Res 13:141–151, 2004

Kraemer HC, Kupfer DJ: Size of treatment effects and their importance to clinical research and practice. Biol Psychiatry 59:990–996, 2006

Kraemer HC, Robinson TN: Are certain multicenter randomized clinical trial structures misleading clinical and policy decisions? Contemp Clin Trials 26:518–529, 2005

Kraemer HC, Thiemann S: How Many Patients? Statistical Power Analysis in Research. Newbury Park, CA, Sage, 1987

Kraemer HC, Thiemann SA: A strategy to use "soft" data effectively in randomized clinical trials. J Consult Clin Psychol 57:148–154, 1989

Kraemer HC, Frank E, Kupfer DJ: Moderators of treatment outcomes: clinical, research, and policy importance. JAMA 296:1286–1289, 2006

Kraemer HC, Kiernan M, Essex MJ, et al: How and why criteria defining moderators and mediators differ between the Baron and Kenny and MacArthur approaches. Health Psychol 27:S101–S108, 2008

Leber P: The use of placebo control groups in the assessment of psychiatric drugs: an historical context. Biol Psychiatry 47:699–706, 2000

Leber PD, Davis CS: Threats to the validity of clinical trials employing enrichment strategies for sample selection. Control Clin Trials 19:178–187, 1998

MacCallum RC, Zhang S, Preacher KJ, et al: On the practice of dichotomization of quantitative variables. Psychol Methods 7:19–40, 2002

Meehl PE: Theory testing in psychology and physics: a methodological paradox. Philos Sci 34:103–115, 1967

Meinert CL: Clinical Trials: Design, Conduct, and Analysis. New York, Oxford University Press, 1986

MTA Cooperative Group: A 14-month randomized clinical trial of treatment strategies for attention-deficit/hyperactivity disorder. Arch Gen Psychiatry 56:1073–1086, 1999

Rennie D: How to report randomized controlled trials: the CONSORT Statement. JAMA 276.649, 1996

Rothman KJ, Michels KB: The continuing unethical use of placebo controls. N Engl J Med 331:394–398, 1994

Rubin DB: Estimating causal effects of treatments in randomized and nonrandomized studies. J Educ Psychol 66:688–701, 1974

Rubin DB: Teaching statistical inference for causal effects in experiments and observational studies. Journal of Educational and Behavioral Statistics 29:343–367, 2004

Rush AJ Jr, First MB, Blacker D (eds): Handbook of Psychiatric Measures, 2nd Edition. Washington, DC, American Psychiatric Publishing, 2008

Senn S: Regression to the mean. Stat Methods Med Res 6:99–102, 1997

Stigler SM: Regression towards the mean, historically considered. Stat Methods Med Res 6:103–114, 1997

Storosum JG, Wohlfarth T, Gispen-de Wied CC, et al: Suicide risk in placebo-controlled trials of treatment for acute manic episode and prevention of manic-depressive episode. Am J Psychiatry 162:799–802, 2005 (Comment in: Am J Psychiatry 163:329, 2006)

Ware JH: Linear models for the analysis of longitudinal studies. Am Stat 39:95–101, 1985

Wen L, Badgett R, Cornell J: Number needed to treat: a descriptor for weighing therapeutic options. Am J Health Syst Pharm 62:2031–2036, 2005

PART II

Classes of Psychiatric Treatments:
Animal and Human Pharmacology

K. Ranga Rama Krishnan, M.D., and Dennis S. Charney, M.D.,
Section Editors

Antidepressants and Anxiolytics

CHAPTER 12

Tricyclic and Tetracyclic Drugs

J. Craig Nelson, M.D.

The tricyclic antidepressant agents hold an important place in the history of treatments for depression. They were the first class of antidepressant compounds to be widely used in depression and remained the first-line treatment for more than 30 years. The observation of their activity led to theories of drug action involving norepinephrine and serotonin. Indeed, this "psychopharmacological bridge" suggested that alterations of these neurotransmitters might cause depression (Bunney and Davis 1965; Prange 1965; Schildkraut 1965). The tricyclics were extensively studied, and through this study the field developed several principles for the management of depressive illness. For example, in addition to understanding the need for adequate dose and duration during acute treatment, the importance of continuation treatment was described. The adverse events associated with these agents required that psychiatrists become familiar with a variety of syndromes, such as anticholinergic delirium, delayed cardiac conduction, precipitation of acute glaucoma, and orthostatic hypotension. The observation that tricyclic plasma concentrations varied widely stimulated interest in understanding the metabolism of tricyclic drugs. The field was introduced to the concepts of polymorphisms in the mephenytoin and debrisoquine pathways (later relabeled the cytochrome P450 [CYP] 2C19 and 2D6 pathways), which in part explained the widely varying blood levels. Knowledge of the widely varying drug concentrations raised questions about the relationships of clinical activity and drug concentrations. Although effects of antipsychotics and a few other drugs on tricyclic plasma levels had been described in the 1970s, it was the observation of the effect of fluoxetine on desipramine coupled with the aggressive marketing of the

selective serotonin reuptake inhibitors (SSRIs) that greatly expanded our awareness of and knowledge about drug interactions. Finally, our knowledge of how these drugs worked became the basis for the discovery of new drugs such as the SSRIs.

History and Discovery

Although iminodibenzyl had been synthesized in 1889 (Byck 1975), it was not until after 1948 that derivatives of this compound were investigated for their potential usefulness in human subjects. Ironically, the properties that were of interest—the antihistaminic and sedative actions—would later be viewed as the "side effects" of these compounds. In the 1950s, investigation of one of these compounds led to the serendipitous observation that chlorpromazine had "antipsychotic" effects (Delay and Deniker 1952). The tricyclic compound imipramine was closely related to chlorpromazine, differing only in the substitution of an ethylene linkage for sulfur. In 1957, Roland Kuhn, a Swiss psychiatrist, investigated the clinical effects of imipramine in human subjects in part to determine if its sedative properties would be useful (Kuhn 1958, 1970). He found that imipramine was not useful for calming agitated patients; however, he observed that it did appear to ameliorate symptoms in depressed patients. As with lithium and chlorpromazine earlier, the discovery of the psychotropic effects of the tricyclics was a chance observation.

After imipramine was introduced, several other antidepressant compounds were developed and marketed. These compounds had a basic tricyclic structure and also shared many of the secondary effects for which the tricyclics came to be known. Later, other heterocyclic compounds, such as maprotiline, were also marketed. These agents had somewhat similar structures and secondary effects.

Structure–Activity Relations

Tricyclic and tetracyclic compounds are categorized on the basis of their chemical structure (Figure 12–1). The tricyclics have a central three-ring structure, hence the name. The tertiary-amine tricyclics, such as amitriptyline and imipramine, have two methyl groups at the end of the side chain. These compounds can be demethylated to secondary amines, such as desipramine and nortriptyline. The tetracyclic compound maprotiline (Ludiomil) has a four-ring central structure. Five tertiary amines have been marketed in the United States—amitriptyline (Elavil), clomipramine (Anafranil), doxepin (Sinequan), imipramine (Tofranil), and trimipramine (Surmontil). The three secondary-amine compounds are desipramine (Norpramin, Pertofrane), nortriptyline (Aventyl, Pamelor), and protriptyline (Vivactil). All of these compounds, in addition to amoxapine (Asendin) and maprotiline (Ludiomil), have been approved for use in major depression with the exception of clomipramine (Anafranil), which in the United States is approved for use only in obsessive-compulsive disorder (OCD).

Although the tricyclics are named for their central three-ring structure, the nature of the side chain appears more important for their function. The tertiary tricyclic agents—amitriptyline, imipramine, and clomipramine—are more potent in blocking the serotonin transporter. The secondary tricyclics are much more potent in blocking the norepinephrine transporter (Table 12–1) (Bolden-Watson and Richelson 1993; Tatsumi et al. 1997).

The nature of the central three-ring structure produces other differences. For example, amitriptyline and nortriptyline share a similar dibenzocycloheptadiene structure, although their side chains are identical to those of imipramine and desipramine, respectively. Similar to the imipramine–desipramine pair, amitriptyline and nortriptyline have similar differences in potency in blocking the serotonin and norepinephrine transporters; however, compared with imipramine, amitriptyline is more anticholinergic and antihistaminic, has greater α_1-adrenergic receptor blockade, and is somewhat more potent in blocking the serotonin transporter (see Table 12–1) (Cusack et al. 1994; Richelson and Nelson 1984; Tatsumi et al. 1997).

Of the tricyclics, clomipramine is the most potent in blocking the serotonin transporter, although its metabo-

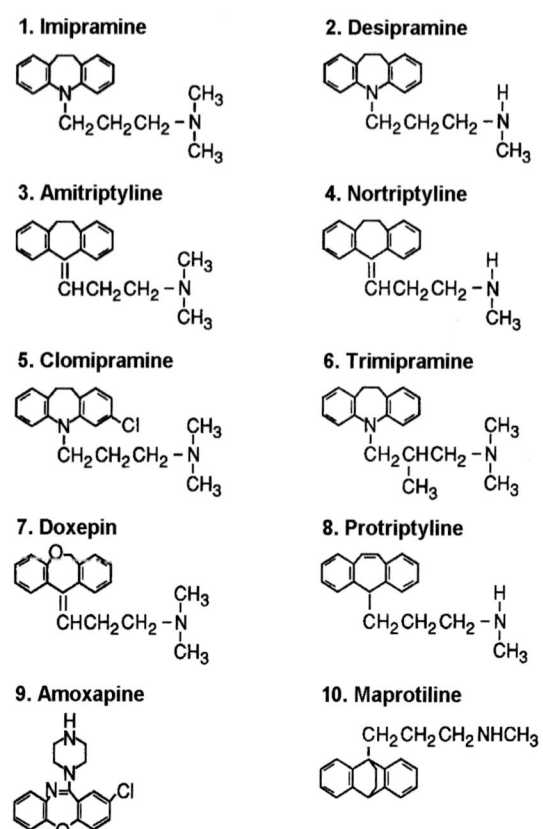

FIGURE 12–1. Drugs marketed in the United States as tricyclics (1–9) and a tetracyclic (10).

Source. Reprinted from Potter WZ, Manji HK, Rudorfer MV: "Tricyclics and Tetracyclics," in *The American Psychiatric Press Textbook of Psychopharmacology,* Second Edition. Edited by Schatzberg AF, Nemeroff CB. Washington, DC, American Psychiatric Press, 1998, p. 200. Copyright 1998, American Psychiatric Press, Inc. Used with permission.

lite desmethylclomipramine is a potent norepinephrine reuptake inhibitor (Hall and Ogren 1981). Doxepin is structurally most similar to amitriptyline but is more similar in functional potency to imipramine (Pinder et al. 1977). Doxepin is the most antihistaminic of these compounds. Protriptyline is structurally most similar to nortriptyline but is more slowly cleared (has a longer elimination half-life) and is given in doses about one-third those of nortriptyline (Moody et al. 1977).

The structure of amoxapine differs from the structures of the other tricyclics. With a central three-ring structure and a side chain that differ from those of the tricyclics, amoxapine is structurally more similar to the neuroleptic loxapine, from which it is derived. Similar to the secondary tricyclics, it is a potent norepinephrine reuptake inhibitor. Unlike all of the other compounds in this group, amoxapine, and particularly its metabolite 7-hydroxy-

TABLE 12–1. Affinity of tricyclics and tetracyclics for the neurotransmitter transporters and specific receptors (expressed as equilibrium dissociation constants)

	POTENCY UPTAKE BLOCKADE			RECEPTOR BINDING AFFINITY					
DRUG	5-HT	NE	DA	α_1	α_2	H_1	M_1	5-HT$_{1A}$	5-HT$_2$
Amitriptyline	4.3	35	3,250	27	940	1.1	18	450	18
Amoxapine	58.0	16	4,310	50	2,600	25	1,000	220	1.0
Clomipramine	0.28	38	2,190	38	3,200	31	37	7,000	27
Desipramine	17.6	0.83	3,190	130	7,200	110	198	6,400	350
Doxepin	68.0	29.5	12,100	24	1,100	0.24	80	276	27
Imipramine	1.4	37	8,500	90	3,200	11	90	5,800	150
Maprotiline	5,800.0	11.1	1,000	90	9,400	2	570	12,000	120
Nortriptyline	18.0	4.37	1,140	60	2,500	10	150	294	41
Protriptyline	19.6	1.41	2,100	130	6,600	25	25	3,800	67
Trimipramine	149.0	2,450	3,780	24	680	0.27	58	8,400	32
Reference									
Pentolamine				15					
Yohimbine					1.6				
D-Chlorpheniramine						15			
Atropine							2.4		
Serotonin								0.72	
Ketanserin									2.5

Note. Affinity and potency=equilibrium dissociation constants in molarity. α_1=α_1-adrenergic; α_2=α_2-adrenergic; DA=dopamine; 5-HT=serotonin; 5-HT$_{1A}$=serotonin$_{1A}$; 5-HT$_2$=serotonin$_2$; H$_1$=histamine$_1$; M$_1$=muscarinic$_1$; NE=norepinephrine.
Source. Uptake potency data adapted from Tatsumi et al. 1997. Receptor affinity data adapted from Richelson and Nelson 1984.

amoxapine, blocks postsynaptic dopamine receptors (Coupet et al. 1979). As a result, it is the only compound in the group that has antipsychotic activity in addition to antidepressant effects.

Maprotiline also differs from the others in this group. Although maprotiline is referred to as a heterocyclic or tetracyclic, these terms do not explain its inclusion in the group. The side chain, however, is identical to that in desipramine, nortriptyline, and protriptyline. As would be predicted from this similarity, maprotiline is most potent in blocking the norepinephrine transporter (Randrup and Braestrup 1977).

As discussed below, it is important to remember that in humans, the tertiary tricyclic compounds are demethylated to secondary tricyclic compounds, all of which are potent norepinephrine reuptake inhibitors. As a result, when these tertiary compounds are administered to humans subjects, the effects of both the metabolite and the parent have to be taken into account.

Pharmacological Profile

Reuptake Blockade

Early in the history of the tricyclic and tetracyclic antidepressants, the ability of these compounds to block the transporter site for norepinephrine was described (Axelrod et al. 1961) (see Table 12–1). The tertiary amines have greater affinity for the serotonin transporter, whereas the secondary amines are relatively more potent at the norepinephrine transporter. During the administration of amitriptyline, imipramine, or clomipramine, these tertiary amines are demethylated to secondary amines; thus, both serotonergic and noradrenergic effects occur. In addition, because dopamine is inactivated by norepinephrine transporters in the frontal cortex (Bymaster et al. 2002), norepinephrine reuptake inhibitors would be expected to increase dopamine concentrations in that region.

Receptor Sensitivity Changes

The initial reuptake blockade described above is followed by a sequence of events (Blier et al. 1987; Charney et al. 1991; Tremblay and Blier 2006). The tertiary tricyclic compounds inhibit the uptake of serotonin, and serotonin levels rise. As the result of inhibitory feedback from the presynaptic somatodendritic serotonin$_{1A}$ (5-HT$_{1A}$) autoreceptor, the firing rate of the presynaptic serotonin neuron falls, and concentrations of 5-hydroxyindoleacetic acid (5-HIAA), the major metabolite of serotonin, decline rapidly. During a 10- to 14-day period, the presynaptic autoreceptor is desensitized, and at this point, the tonic firing rate returns to its pretreatment rate. With both a normal firing rate and reuptake blockade, serotonin transmission is enhanced.

The tricyclic agents also sensitize or upregulate postsynaptic 5-HT$_{1A}$ receptors (de Montigny and Aghajanian 1978). These changes further enhance the effects of serotonin. The changes in pre- and postsynaptic receptor sensitivity occur over a 2-week period. Consequently, the timing of these changes is more consistent with the onset of early antidepressant response than with the initial uptake blockade (Charney et al. 1991).

The tricyclics also have actions at the 5-HT$_2$ receptor. Depression is associated with an increase in postsynaptic 5-HT$_2$ receptor density (Arora and Meltzer 1989; Cheetham et al. 1988; Stanley and Mann 1983; Yates et al. 1990). A variety of antidepressants, including the tricyclics, downregulate the 5-HT$_2$ receptors (Goodwin et al. 1984; Peroutka and Snyder 1980). The 5-HT$_2$ receptors mediate excitatory effects, whereas the 5HT$_{1A}$ receptors generally have inhibitory effects; thus, these two systems act in opposition. In preclinical experiments, when the 5-HT$_2$ receptor was blocked by an antagonist, the effects of serotonin were enhanced (Lakoski and Aghajanian 1985; Marek et al. 2003). Some of the tricyclics—particularly doxepin, amitriptyline, and amoxapine—have 5-HT$_2$ antagonist properties relatively comparable to their reuptake potency (see Table 12–1) (Tatsumi et al. 1997). These properties should enhance their serotonergic effects.

The sequence of events with chronic dosing in the noradrenergic system is more complicated (Tremblay and Blier 2006). As in the serotonergic system, reuptake inhibition results in a rapid decline in norepinephrine turnover, as reflected by a fall in concentrations of 3-methoxy-4-hydroxyphenylglycol (MHPG), a metabolite of norepinephrine, and attenuation of the firing rate of the noradrenergic neuron. This effect appears to be mediated by the presynaptic somatodendritic α_2-adrenergic autoreceptor, which provides inhibitory feedback to the presynaptic neuron. In contrast to the serotonergic system, the firing rate of noradrenergic neurons remains inhibited with chronic treatment (Szabo and Blier 2001), suggesting that somatodendritic α_2 receptors do not desensitize. Norepinephrine concentrations do increase at postsynaptic sites such as the hippocampus and frontal cortex. This may indicate desensitization of terminal α_2 autoreceptors.

With chronic treatment, the postsynaptic β-adrenergic receptor is downregulated or decreased in density. In fact, downregulation of the β-adrenergic receptor was once proposed as a mechanism of tricyclic action (Sulser et al. 1978; Vetulani and Sulser 1975). Current evidence suggests that β-adrenergic receptor downregulation is more likely a compensatory change. Overall, chronic administration of a noradrenergic reuptake inhibitor appears to override the downregulation of the postsynaptic β-receptor, resulting in enhanced noradrenergic transmission. This effect is manifested as enhanced formation of the second messenger cyclic adenosine monophosphate (cAMP) (Duman et al. 1997) and is reflected clinically by a persistent increase in heart rate (Roose et al. 1998; Rosenstein and Nelson 1991).

Alternatively, some of the actions of noradrenergic reuptake inhibitors may be mediated by postsynaptic α_1 and α_2 receptors, which do not appear to be downregulated during chronic treatment. The net effect of norepinephrine reuptake inhibitors on noradrenergic transmission during chronic treatment is further complicated by regional differences in the adrenergic receptors. Nevertheless, the antidepressant effects of norepinephrine reuptake inhibitors do appear to be mediated by norepinephrine, because inhibition of catecholamine synthesis with α-methyl-p-tyrosine (AMPT) results in relapse of depressive symptoms (H.L. Miller et al. 1996).

Secondary Effects

The tricyclic and tetracyclic compounds also have a variety of other actions mediated by other receptors (Cusack et al. 1994; Richelson and Nelson 1984) (see Table 12–1). For example, these compounds block muscarinic receptors, producing anticholinergic effects. Although these anticholinergic effects have generally been thought to mediate adverse effects, a recent double-blind, randomized crossover study in 19 subjects with major depression found that the anticholinergic drug scopolamine had a beneficial effect on depressive and anxious symptoms (Furey and Drevets 2006). The tricyclics also block histamine$_1$ (H$_1$) receptors and α_1- and α_2-adrenergic receptors, resulting in a variety of other effects (as discussed in the next section). Tricyclics act on fast sodium channels, which explains their adverse cardiac effects. Although the actions of tricyclics on sodium channels have traditionally been considered problematic for patients with depression, these same actions may contribute to the beneficial effects of tricyclics on pain (Priest and Kaczorowski 2007). The potency of secondary effects of the tricyclics and tetracyclics varies considerably. Amitriptyline is the most anticholinergic not only of the agents in this group but also of all antidepressants. Desipramine is the least anticholinergic among the tricyclics. Doxepin is the most potent H_1 antagonist in this group, although another antidepressant, mirtazapine, is even more potent. The consequences of these secondary effects are discussed below.

Pharmacokinetics and Disposition

Absorption

Absorption of the tricyclic and tetracyclic drugs occurs in the small intestine and is rapid and reasonably complete. Peak levels are reached within 2–8 hours following ingestion. Exceptions include protriptyline (peak levels reached between 6 and 12 hours after ingestion) and maprotiline (peak levels not reached until 8 hours or longer). Although peak levels may have implications for side effects, which can occur quickly, the timing of peak levels is relatively unimportant with respect to efficacy because the antidepressant action of these drugs occurs over several weeks.

Volume of Distribution

The tricyclic and tetracyclic compounds are basic lipophilic amines and are concentrated in a variety of tissues throughout the body. As a result, they have a high volume of distribution. For example, concentrations of these drugs in cardiac tissue exceed concentrations in plasma.

Plasma Protein Binding

The tricyclic and tetracyclic compounds are extensively bound to plasma proteins (e.g., 90% or greater) because of their lipid solubility. Exceptions are the hydroxy metabolites, which have lower plasma protein binding than the parent compounds.

First-Pass Metabolism

Following absorption, the tricyclics are taken up in the circulation but pass first through the liver, and metabo-

lism of the drug begins—the so-called first-pass effect. As a result, the amount of the compound that enters the systemic circulation is reduced.

Hepatic Metabolism

Hepatic metabolism is the principal method of clearance for the tricyclic and tetracyclic compounds. Only a small portion of drug is eliminated by the kidney. Rates of hepatic metabolism vary widely from person to person, resulting in dramatic differences in steady-state plasma concentrations. Elimination half-lives for most of the tricyclic and tetracyclic compounds average about 24 hours or longer; thus, the drugs can be given once a day (Table 12–2). Amoxapine has a shorter half-life than the other tricyclics and is an exception.

Hepatic metabolism of the tricyclics and tetracyclics occurs along two principal metabolic pathways. *Demethylation of the side chain* converts the tertiary amines to secondary amines—for example, amitriptyline is converted to nortriptyline—and the characteristics of the compound are altered. The tertiary amines are relatively more serotonergic, whereas the demethylated amines are relatively more noradrenergic. The other pathway in hepatic metabolism is *hydroxylation of the ring structure*. Hydroxylation results in the formation of hydroxy metabolites. In some cases, the levels of the metabolite are substantial. The concentration of 10-hydroxynortriptyline usually exceeds that of the parent compound (Bertilsson et al. 1979). Usually 2-hydroxydesipramine is present at levels approximately 40%–50% of those present in the parent compound, but these ratios are quite variable, depending on the rate of hydroxylation (Bock et al. 1983; Potter et al. 1979). Thus, in extensive metabolizers, the ratio of hydroxy metabolite to parent compound can be quite high, but total drug levels are low. Hydroxyimipramine and hydroxyamitriptyline are present at very low concentrations and are clinically unimportant. The hydroxy metabolites are then conjugated and excreted. The conjugated metabolites are not active.

Hydroxynortriptyline and hydroxydesipramine both block the norepinephrine transporter (Bertilsson et al. 1979; Potter et al. 1979). Both have been shown to have antidepressant activity (Nelson et al. 1988b; Nordin et al. 1987). The potency of hydroxydesipramine is comparable to that of the parent compound in terms of norepinephrine reuptake blockade. There are two isomers of hydroxynortriptyline, *E*- and *Z*-10-hydroxynortriptyline. *E*-10-hydroxynortriptyline is present at levels four times higher than those of the *Z* isomer and is about 50% as potent as

TABLE 12–2.   Dosage, clearance, and apparent therapeutic plasma concentrations of tricyclics and tetracyclics

	PLASMA		THERAPEUTIC	
DRUG	HALF-LIFE (HOURS)	CLEARANCE (L/HOUR)	DOSAGE RANGE (MG/DAY)	PLASMA LEVEL (NG/ML)
Tertiary tricyclics				
Amitriptyline	5–45	20–70	150–300	
Clomipramine	15–60	20–120	150–300	>150[a]
Doxepin	10–25	40–60	150–300	
Imipramine	5–30	30–100	150–300	>200[a]
Trimipramine	15–40	40–105		
Secondary tricyclics				
Desipramine	10–30	80–170	75–300	>125
Nortriptyline	20–55	15–80	50–150	50–150
Protriptyline	55–200	5–25	15–60	
Tetracyclics				
Amoxapine	5–10	225–275	150–300	
Maprotiline	25–50	15–35	100–225	

[a]Total concentration of the parent compound and the desmethyl metabolite.

Source.   Adapted from Nelson JC: "Tricyclic and Tetracyclic Drugs," in *Comprehensive Textbook of Psychiatry/VII*, 7th Edition. Edited by Kaplan HI, Sadock BJ. Baltimore, MD, Lippincott Williams & Wilkins, 2000, p. 2494. Copyright 2000, Lippincott Williams & Wilkins. Used with permission.

nortriptyline in blocking norepinephrine uptake. The clinical significance of high levels of less potent hydroxynortriptyline is not entirely clear. In particular, it is not clear whether high levels of less potent hydroxynortriptyline might interfere with the action of nortriptyline—a question of interest because such an effect might explain the therapeutic window described for this drug. Both hydroxynortriptyline and hydroxydesipramine are less anticholinergic than their parent compounds. The hydroxy metabolites may have other effects. Early studies suggested that hydroxynortriptyline concentrations were disproportionately associated with cardiac conduction abnormalities (Schneider et al. 1988; Young et al. 1985), but later studies indicated that the E enantiomer of 10-hydroxynortriptyline was less cardiotoxic (Pollock et al. 1992).

The principal metabolic pathway for amoxapine is hydroxylation, during which 7-hydroxyamoxapine and 8-hydroxyamoxapine are produced (Coupet et al. 1979). These compounds differ: 7-hydroxyamoxapine has high-potency neuroleptic properties but a short half-life; 8-hydroxyamoxapine is metabolized more slowly and appears to contribute to the drug's antidepressant action.

In recent years, identification of the specific isoenzyme pathways involved in the metabolism of a variety of drugs, including the tricyclics, has been the focus of intensive study. The CYP2D6 pathway appears responsible for hydroxylation of desipramine and nortriptyline (Brosen et al. 1991). In fact, desipramine has been considered the prototypic substrate for CYP2D6 because it has no other major metabolic pathways. Demethylation of the tertiary-amine compounds appears to involve a number of CYP isoenzymes, including 1A2, 3A4, and 2C19. These hepatic isoenzymes are under the control of specific genes, and the gene loci have been identified for several of these isoenzymes, including CYP2D6. Approximately 5%–10% of Caucasians are homozygous for the recessive autosomal 2D6 trait, resulting in deficient hydroxylation of desipramine and nortriptyline (Brosen et al. 1985; Evans et al. 1980). These individuals are termed *poor metabolizers*, while those with adequate 2D6 enzyme are referred to as *extensive metabolizers*. Approximately 20% of individuals of Asian descent have a genetic polymorphism resulting in deficient CYP2C19 metabolism. This pathway is involved in the metabolism of the tertiary tricyclic compounds.

The variability in plasma concentrations that results from these metabolic differences is substantial. For example, in a sample of 83 inpatients who were given a fixed dose of 2.5 mg/kg of desipramine, we observed steady-state plasma concentrations ranging from 20 ng/mL to 934 ng/mL (Nelson 1984). Even among extensive metabolizers, there can be variability in the rates of metabolism, resulting in the term *ultrarapid metabolizers*. Various methods have been used to phenotype the individuals who are slow or fast metabolizers. For example, formation of the debrisoquine metabolite in the urine has been used to characterize the metabolic rate of CYP2D6 (Brosen et al. 1991; Evans et al. 1980). Recent work in this area has shifted to genotyping the involved isoenzymes. In clinical practice, blood levels of the compounds themselves are more often used as a crude index of the rate of metabolism.

As noted above, desipramine has often been used as a substrate for 2D6 because 2D6 is the only major metabolic pathway for this compound. While desipramine may be useful for examination of 2D6 inhibition, it may overestimate the magnitude of drug interactive effects for those agents that have multiple pathways.

Steady-State Concentrations

Steady state is an important pharmacological concept for clinicians to understand if drug monitoring is employed. Steady state is that point, on a fixed dose, at which plasma concentrations of the drug reach a plateau. Steady state is achieved after five half-lives. At this point, the concentration of the drug should be 97% of the maximal concentration achieved for that dose. In fact, after three half-lives, the drug will have achieved about 87% of the steady-state concentration. If blood level monitoring is employed, a sample is drawn before the next dose is given, usually in the morning after the patient's level has reached a steady state. Steady-state drug concentrations should remain relatively stable as long as the dose is constant, the patient is compliant, and no interactive drugs are added.

The day-to-day biological variability of drug concentrations at steady state is not frequently described. In inpatients at steady state, the coefficient of variation (SD/mean) of desipramine is approximately 10%–15% (J.C. Nelson, unpublished data, 1985). In outpatients, this variability may increase. This means that if the average plasma concentration is 150 ng/mL, two-thirds of samples obtained will be ±10%, or between 135 ng/mL and 165 ng/mL. Research studies of drug concentrations usually employ an average of two or three plasma samples to reduce the effect of this variability. If only one sample is drawn, the clinician needs to remember that even if the laboratory error is low, there will be moderate biological variability. Single blood levels are better viewed as estimates than as precise measures.

When the drug concentration is measured, the total of both the free and bound drug is reported. Few laboratories are prepared to measure free levels, yet drug concentrations in the cerebrospinal fluid are proportional to the free levels. The *free concentration* is dependent on dose and hepatic clearance but is not affected by plasma protein binding (Greenblatt et al. 1998). The latter is often misunderstood. Factors that affect plasma proteins—malnutrition, inflammation—may lead to changes in the bound fraction, but the absolute free concentration is unaffected. If another drug affects binding, the absolute free concentration remains unaffected. In these instances, the *free fraction* may change because the bound portion declines, not because there is a change in the free concentration.

Linear Kinetics

Most of the tricyclics have linear kinetics; that is, concentration increases in proportion to dose within the therapeutic range. There are exceptions. Desipramine, for example, appears to have nonlinear kinetics in the usual dose range (Nelson and Jatlow 1987). Rapid metabolizers of desipramine are most likely to display nonlinear changes during the time when the dose is increasing. In these patients, a disproportionate rise in the drug concentration occurs when the dose is increased. In cases of overdose, nonlinear changes are more likely to occur, and the clinician cannot assume that usual rates of drug elimination will be maintained.

Effects of Aging

Many changes in the pharmacodynamics and pharmacokinetics of drug treatment occur with aging, yet some may be relatively unimportant (Greenblatt et al. 1998). The ratio of fat to lean body mass increases, and cardiac output and hepatic blood flow decrease. There may be further changes associated with medical illness. But the clinical importance of these changes is usually relatively minor because of the dramatic variability of hepatic metabolism. Age-related changes in metabolism vary with the isoenzymes involved. The activity of the CYP3A4 pathway does slow with age (von Moltke et al. 1995). Most studies of the tertiary amines, such as imipramine, suggest that concentrations of these drugs are increased somewhat in older individuals (Abernathy et al. 1985; Benetello et al.

1990; Furlanut and Benetello 1990). Alternatively, most studies of nortriptyline (Bertilsson 1979; Katz et al. 1989; Smith et al. 1980; Young et al. 1984; Ziegler and Biggs 1977) and desipramine (Abernathy et al. 1985; Nelson et al. 1985, 1995) indicate that ratios of blood level to dosage of these drugs are relatively unaffected by aging, suggesting that the 2D6 isoenzyme is not similarly affected. In addition, the relationship of nortriptyline and desipramine plasma concentrations to therapeutic effects appears to be relatively similar in younger and older adults (Katz et al. 1989; Nelson et al. 1985, 1995; Young et al. 1988). Renal clearance of the hydroxy metabolites does decrease with age (Nelson et al. 1988a; Young et al. 1984). As a result, concentrations of hydroxynortriptyline may be substantially elevated in older patients.

In children, the clearance of tricyclic compounds is increased. Half-lives of imipramine are shorter and ratios of desmethylimipramine to imipramine are higher, consistent with more rapid metabolism (Geller 1991; Rapoport and Potter 1981). Alternatively, a study of desipramine in children found that the clearance of both desipramine and hydroxydesipramine was increased so that hydroxy metabolite–parent compound ratios were not elevated (Wilens et al. 1992).

Relationship of Plasma Concentration to Clinical Action

Plasma Concentration and Response

Marked interindividual variability of tricyclic plasma concentrations was described by Hammer and Sjöqvist in 1967. This finding suggested that drug level monitoring might ensure that therapeutic blood levels are achieved and might help to avoid toxic levels. In carefully selected inpatients with endogenous or melancholic major depression, treatment with adequate levels of imipramine or desipramine resulted in robust response rates of about 85% (Glassman et al. 1977; Nelson et al. 1982). For several years, the relationship of tricyclic blood levels to response and the utility of monitoring blood levels were the focus of considerable attention and debate.

A task force of the American Psychiatric Association (1985) that reviewed these studies concluded that relationships between plasma level and response had been demonstrated for imipramine, desipramine, and nortriptyline (see Table 12–2). For imipramine, drug levels above 200 ng/mL were more effective than lower levels (Glassman et al. 1977; Reisby et al. 1977). For desipramine, levels above 125 ng/mL were more effective (Nel-

son et al. 1982). For both desipramine and imipramine, blood levels in excess of 300 ng/mL were more likely to be associated with serious side effects. Effective plasma concentrations were also established for nortriptyline, but the relationship appeared to be curvilinear. For this drug, plasma levels between 50 ng/mL and 150 ng/mL were more effective than lower or higher levels (Åsberg et al. 1971; Kragh-Sørenson et al. 1973, 1976).

For amitriptyline, it has been more difficult to establish a therapeutic relationship between plasma levels and response (American Psychiatric Association 1985). In part, this difficulty may be related to the fact that during amitriptyline administration, three active compounds are present (amitriptyline, nortriptyline, and hydroxynortriptyline), and it is unclear if their effects are additive or if there is a more complicated relationship (Breyer-Pfaff et al. 1982). During amitriptyline administration, responders usually have total amitriptyline and nortriptyline levels in the neighborhood of 150–250 ng/mL (Kupfer et al. 1977), but there is not good agreement between studies. For clomipramine, blood levels of 150–300 ng/mL (total of clomipramine and desmethylclomipramine) have been suggested for antidepressant effectiveness. Higher levels are usually employed in the treatment of OCD. The data relating blood levels and response are limited for the other tricyclic and tetracyclic compounds.

The therapeutic utility of blood level monitoring has been the subject of controversy. Blood level–response relationships have been demonstrated in melancholic inpatients. But similar relationships have proven difficult to demonstrate in depressed outpatients. In outpatients, drug–placebo differences are often small, and the effect of drug treatment is harder to detect. Depressed outpatients may be more heterogeneous and include individuals who are not responsive to any drug treatment. Finally, many studies are not designed to detect blood level–response relationships. Fixed dosing is required, and the plasma concentrations achieved must fall above and below the suspected threshold. If all patients achieve adequate drug concentrations, no relationship with response will be found. It is logical to conclude that blood level relationships determined in severely depressed inpatients might be used as a guide for treatment of outpatients, but this assumption has not been empirically validated.

Plasma Concentration and Toxicity

The alternative question is whether blood level monitoring might help to avoid toxicity. A variety of data support this view. The risk of delirium is substantially increased at amitriptyline plasma concentrations above 450 ng/mL and is moderately increased at concentrations above 300 ng/mL (Livingston et al. 1983; Preskorn and Simpson 1982). But amitriptyline is the most anticholinergic tricyclic and is most likely to produce delirium. The risk of first-degree atrioventricular block is also increased with plasma concentrations of imipramine greater than 350 ng/mL (Preskorn and Irwin 1982). The risk of seizures also increases at higher doses and, presumably, higher blood levels, although a clear plasma-level threshold for seizures has not been demonstrated. Following overdose, tricyclic blood levels greater than 1,000 ng/mL can be achieved, and the risks of delirium, stupor, cardiac abnormalities, and seizures are all substantially increased (Preskorn and Irwin 1982; Rudorfer and Young 1980; Spiker et al. 1975).

The value of blood level monitoring to avoid serious adverse effects has been hard to demonstrate because rates of serious toxicity are low so that large samples are required to demonstrate any increase in risk at higher blood levels. For some adverse reactions (e.g., delirium), early warning signs may prompt dose reduction. Alternatively, there may be no warning for seizures or cardiac arrhythmia, and blood level monitoring might be most useful for reducing the risk of those adverse events.

If blood level monitoring is undertaken, the clinician needs to remember that the patient needs to be at steady state, the blood sample should be drawn before the next dose (a trough level), and the sample should be sent to the laboratory promptly. For a quantitative estimate the laboratory will usually employ high-performance liquid chromatography (HPLC). In a competent laboratory, the coefficient of variation for an HPLC assay is usually less than 10%. This assay is relatively specific; however, other drugs can interfere. Because there are many modifications of the HPLC technique, the interfering drugs will vary by site. Under the best of circumstances, there will still be biological variability of the compound (discussed earlier in subsection "Steady-State Concentrations"). Add to this occasional missed doses or laboratory problems, and there will be considerable sample-to-sample variability. For these reasons, the clinician should not view the concentration reported as a precise measure. Yet, because concentrations vary across such a wide range, it may be very helpful to know if the level is low (e.g., 25–75 ng/mL), moderate (e.g., 100–300 ng/mL), or high (e.g., 300–1,000 ng/mL).

Prospective Dosing Techniques

Conventional dosing requires administration of a given dose for a long enough period of time to determine whether that dose is effective. Sometimes two or three trials are needed to determine the effective dose. The possibility of rapid dosage adjustment using plasma levels was suggested when several investigators demonstrated a relationship between an initial timed blood sample and the final steady-state level (Alexanderson 1972; Brunswick et al. 1979; Cooper and Simpson 1978; Potter et al. 1980). This method appeared most applicable for nortriptyline, which has linear kinetics, but was also useful for desipramine, because the targeted level was within a broad range. Clinical studies using blood levels to adjust dose were reported for amitriptyline (Dawling et al. 1984; Madakasira and Khazanie 1985), but sedation and anticholinergic side effects limited the rate at which the dose could be adjusted. Alternatively, a clinical study using rapid dosing of desipramine found that treatment could be initiated at full dose once the dose needed to reach a therapeutic level was determined from a 24-hour blood level following a test dose (Nelson et al. 1987). Sixteen of the 18 patients who completed treatment had plasma levels within the targeted range, and side effects appeared to be no greater than those experienced with more gradual dosing.

The practical application of these methods was limited by laboratory issues. The laboratory performing the assay had to be prepared to determine drug concentrations accurately at very low levels (below the therapeutic range) and had to be able to report results quickly. Most labs were not prepared to do either. A more practical and clinically feasible method is to start the drug at a low or moderate fixed dose, obtain a blood sample after 5–7 days on that dose, and then make further adjustments based on that level.

There are exceptions. Elderly depressed patients often require gradual dosing in order to assess tolerance. In panic patients, lower starting doses are employed to avoid exacerbation of panic attacks.

Mechanism of Action

Early biochemical theories of depression were in large part based on the knowledge of drug action. The observation that the tricyclic agents increased the availability of norepinephrine and serotonin suggested that depression resulted from a deficit in these neurotransmitters (Bunney and Davis 1965; Prange 1965; Schildkraut 1965). This work stimulated interest in the role of these neurotransmitters in the etiology of depression, and several abnormalities were identified. Yet, it remains unclear which, if any, of these abnormalities play a central role in causing depression or are responsible for the vulnerability to becoming depressed.

Recent challenge studies in depressed patients do confirm that the actions of antidepressant drugs are mediated by serotonin and norepinephrine. For example, administration of a tryptophan-free diet rapidly depletes serotonin and, in depressed patients who have been successfully treated, causes relapse (Delgado et al. 1990). In addition, tryptophan depletion caused relapse in patients who were treated with serotonergic agents, whereas those who were treated with norepinephrine reuptake inhibitors were relatively unaffected. Alternatively, administration of AMPT, which interrupts the synthesis of catecholamines, caused relapse in patients who were being successfully treated with noradrenergic agents but not those receiving serotonergic drugs (Delgado et al. 1993). Tryptophan depletion in untreated depressed patients, however, had no effect on the patients' depression. These studies provide supporting evidence that serotonin and norepinephrine mediate antidepressant effects, but they do not necessarily imply that alterations in these neurotransmitter systems are central to the pathophysiology of depression.

The synaptic effects of tricyclic and tetracyclic agents on norepinephrine and serotonin transporters and receptors were described in detail earlier (see section "Pharmacological Profile" earlier in this chapter).

The early theories of depression that focused on depletion of norepinephrine or serotonin suggested that it might be possible to identify "serotonergic" and "noradrenergic" depressions and that such identification would help the clinician select the appropriate type of antidepressant (Beckmann and Goodwin 1975; Maas et al. 1972). A number of studies investigated the predictive value of urinary MHPG, a metabolite of norepinephrine, but a definite predictive link with a noradrenergic antidepressant was not established. Some of these studies were, in part, hampered by the use of agents such as amitriptyline and imipramine, which are not very selective. However, even those studies that examined the ability of MHPG to predict response to more selective agents, such as zimelidine, fluoxetine, and desipramine, failed to demonstrate clear predictive utility (Bowden et al. 1993; Potter 1984). The data, taken together, suggest that urinary MHPG is not a clinically useful predictor. Nevertheless, these studies do not rule out the possibility that there are depressions in which serotonin or norepinephrine plays a relatively more prominent role.

More recently, research into the mechanism of action of the tricyclics and other antidepressant drugs has shifted

to include consideration of factors affecting postsynaptic signal transduction (Manji et al. 1995). These factors include coupling of G proteins to the adrenergic receptor or to adenylyl cyclase and the activity of membrane phospholipases and protein kinases. Other novel targets, including glucocorticoid receptors (Barden 1996), neurotrophic factors (Duman et al. 1997), and gene expression (Lesch and Manji 1992; Nibuya et al. 1996; Schwaninger et al. 1995), have been explored.

Indications and Efficacy

Major Depression

The efficacy of the tricyclic and tetracyclic compounds in major depression is well established. The evidence for their effectiveness has been reviewed previously (Agency for Health Care Policy and Research 1993; Davis and Glassman 1989). Imipramine is the most extensively studied tricyclic antidepressant, in part because for many years it was the standard agent against which other new drugs were compared. In 30 of 44 placebo-controlled studies, imipramine was more effective than placebo. If data from these studies are combined, 65% of 1,334 patients *completing* treatment with imipramine were substantially improved, whereas 30% of those on placebo improved. *Intention-to-treat* response rates for placebo-controlled studies of imipramine in outpatients were 51% for imipramine and 30% for placebo (Agency for Health Care Policy and Research 1993). In most comparison studies, the other tricyclic and tetracyclic antidepressants have been found to be comparable to imipramine in efficacy.

The tricyclic compounds are also effective when used for maintenance treatment. Early studies demonstrated that maintenance treatment with a tricyclic would reduce the relapse rate associated with placebo by about 50% (Davis 1976). These studies, however, usually employed low doses. Subsequently, the Pittsburgh group found that imipramine, at full dose, effectively maintained nearly 80% of the depressed patients for a 3-year period compared with 10% of those on placebo (Frank et al. 1990). In this study, maintenance psychotherapy had an intermediate effect, with about 30% of the patients remaining well. Although this seminal study demonstrated the impressive value of maintenance treatment with full-dose imipramine, the magnitude of the findings may reflect characteristics of the sample treated. The sample comprised patients with recurrent depression who might have been expected to do poorly on placebo. In addition, the patients selected for the study had a history of symptom-free periods between prior episodes, suggesting that these patients might be more likely (than patients with a history of residual symptoms) to have a complete response to treatment. In practice, clinicians may encounter patients with chronic depression, patients with residual symptoms, or patients with comorbid medical and psychiatric disorders. For such patients, drug treatment may be more effective than placebo, but the actual number of patients whose depression remains in remission may be lower.

The U.S. Food and Drug Administration (FDA) has approved all of the tricyclic and tetracyclic compounds discussed in this chapter for the treatment of depression with the exception of clomipramine. In Europe, clomipramine is also used for depression; in fact, it is regarded by many as the most potent antidepressant.

Melancholia or Severe Depression

The efficacy of the tricyclic compounds appears to vary in different subtypes of depression. Four decades ago, when Kuhn studied imipramine, the prevailing view was that it was essential to establish efficacy of an antidepressant in patients with endogenous depression or at least in those with severe depression (Kuhn 1970). The early studies of imipramine and the other tricyclic compounds were frequently conducted in hospitalized patients with severe or endogenous depression, and in these patients the tricyclics were found to be effective. In fact, these agents may be especially effective in this group. Two studies of imipramine and desipramine found rates of response of about 85% in severely depressed hospitalized patients who did not have a refractory history, did not have prominent personality disorder, received an adequate plasma concentration of the drug, and completed treatment (Glassman et al. 1977; Nelson et al. 1982).

When the SSRIs were introduced, it was suggested that they might be less effective than the tricyclic antidepressants in treating severe or melancholic depression. In a large meta-analysis of more than 100 studies comparing tricyclic antidepressants and SSRIs, Anderson (2000) found that in general, these agents had comparable efficacy. When individual agents and patient characteristics were considered, the only tricyclic agent that appeared to be more effective than the SSRIs was amitriptyline, and the only patient characteristic was inpatient status. In a separate meta-analysis of 25 inpatient studies (Anderson 1998), the advantage of the tricyclics appeared limited to those with dual action, namely amitriptyline and clomipramine. Two of the most frequently cited studies in this regard were the two Danish University Antidepressant Group (1986, 1990) studies that found clomipramine to be more effective than paroxetine or citalopram in severely depressed inpatients. Recent clinical trials of antidepressants were usually conducted in outpatients with depression of moderate severity. In outpatients, the designation of melancholia does not appear to predict an advantage for tricyclic antidepressants versus SSRIs (Anderson and Tomenson 1994; Montgomery 1989). Although the question of the best treatment for severely melancholic inpatients lingers, the expense of these studies, and the shift in practice to treatment of depression in outpatient settings, has substantially decreased interest in this question.

Anxious Depression

Anxious depression is not recognized in DSM-IV-TR (American Psychiatric Association 2000) as a subtype of depression; nevertheless, it has been frequently studied. Three of the tricyclic and tetracyclic compounds—doxepin, amoxapine, and maprotiline—have received FDA approval for use in patients with depression and symptoms of anxiety. For many years, clinical lore suggested that amitriptyline was most effective for anxious depression. Direct comparison studies, however, have found little indication that one of these compounds is better than another for treatment of anxious depression. Depressed patients who are anxious may respond less well than less anxious patients. This has been observed with amitriptyline (Kupfer and Spiker 1981), imipramine (Roose et al. 1986), and desipramine (Nelson et al. 1994). Yet these drugs are still more effective than placebo in anxious depressed patients, and it is not established that other classes of antidepressants are more effective in these patients.

Atypical Depression

A series of studies by the Columbia University Group examined the efficacy of imipramine in depressed patients with atypical features (Liebowitz et al. 1984, 1988). These depressed patients had reactive mood and reversed vegetative symptoms, severe fatigue, or rejection sensitivity. Imipramine was more effective than placebo but significantly less effective than the monoamine oxidase inhibitor (MAOI) phenelzine. Other investigators have reported the value of switching from a tricyclic to an MAOI in tricyclic-refractory depressed patients, especially those with atypical features (McGrath et al. 1987; Thase et al. 1992). In fact, the validity and utility of the atypical subtype of depression were in large part supported by this observed difference. However, this subtype has not been shown to be preferentially responsive to SSRIs (Fava et al. 1997), nor has any second-generation antidepressant been shown to be superior to any other in treating atypical depression.

Psychotic Depression

In 1975, Glassman et al. observed that imipramine was less effective in patients with major depression who had delusions. Later, Chan et al. (1987), in reviewing several studies addressing this question and involving more than 1,000 patients, found that antidepressants—usually tricyclics—given alone were effective in approximately two-thirds of the nonpsychotic patients but only about one-third of those with psychotic features. Although the definition of psychosis has undergone several changes, currently it is defined in DSM-IV-TR as major depression with delusions or hallucinations. Several open studies reviewed elsewhere (Nelson 1987) and one prospective study (Spiker et al. 1985) found that the tricyclics, when combined with an antipsychotic, are effective in psychotic depression.

Anton and Burch (1990) suggested that because of its antipsychotic effects, amoxapine might be effective for psychotic depression. In a double-blind study, these researchers demonstrated that amoxapine was comparable in efficacy to the combination of perphenazine and amitriptyline in treating psychotic depression (Anton and Burch 1990).

Bipolar Depression

Thirty years ago, it was suggested that the MAOI antidepressants might be more effective than the tricyclics in treating bipolar depression (Himmelhoch et al. 1972). Later, Himmelhoch et al. (1991) demonstrated in a double-blind study that tranylcypromine was more effective than imipramine for bipolar depression. In addition, tricyclics are more likely than other agents to induce mania (Weir and Goodwin 1987). As a result, the tricyclics are not recommended for monotherapy of bipolar depression.

Chronic Major Depression and Dysthymia

Imipramine appears to be effective in treating chronic depression and dysthymia and to be relatively comparable to sertraline in efficacy (Keller et al. 1998; Kocsis et al. 1988; Thase et al. 1996). Imipramine and desipramine have both been studied in controlled trials and have been found to be more effective than placebo both for acute treatment and for maintenance treatment (N.L. Miller et al. 2001).

Late-Life Depression

Gerson et al. (1988) reviewed the studies of tricyclic antidepressants reported prior to 1986. They found 13 placebo-controlled trials but noted several problems, such as lack of diagnostic criteria, inclusion of younger patients, and dosing issues. Although tricyclics were effective, overall drug and placebo response rates in these older patients appeared to be lower than rates in nonelderly patients (Agency for Health Care Policy and Research 1993). Katz et al. (1990) performed one of the first placebo-controlled trials of nortriptyline in the treatment of patients older than 80 years living in a residential care facility. Nortriptyline was more effective than placebo. The doses employed and levels achieved were similar to those in younger subjects. This study remains the only study to date showing an advantage for an antidepressant over placebo in depressed patients older than 75 years.

Depression in Children

In children and adolescents, the tricyclic antidepressants have not demonstrated superiority over placebo (Ryan 1992).

Obsessive-Compulsive Disorder

Unlike depression, which responds to a variety of antidepressant agents, OCD appears to require treatment with a serotonergic agent. Clomipramine, the most serotonergic of the tricyclics, is approved by the FDA for use in OCD, and its efficacy in this disorder is well established (Greist et al. 1995). Studies comparing its effectiveness with noradrenergic agents such as desipramine found that clomipramine was substantially superior (Leonard et al. 1989). Although the SSRIs are effective in treating OCD, there is a suggestion that clomipramine may be superior (Greist et al. 1995). Whether this putative superiority is due to the dual mechanism of clomipramine or to other factors is unclear.

Panic Disorder

None of the tricyclic or tetracyclic drugs is approved for use in panic disorder. Yet imipramine was the first drug described for use in this disorder (Klein 1964). In fact, observation of the effects of imipramine helped to establish the diagnostic utility of panic disorder. The efficacy of both tertiary and secondary tricyclics has been demonstrated in controlled trials (Jobson et al. 1978; Munjack et al. 1988; Zitrin et al. 1980). In treating this disorder, the drug is initiated at a low dose to avoid exacerbation of panic symptoms.

Attention-Deficit/Hyperactivity Disorder

The efficacy of the stimulant drugs in treating attention-deficit/hyperactivity disorder (ADHD) is well established. The tricyclics, especially desipramine, also appear to be of value. In one study, desipramine, given at doses greater than 4 mg/kg for 3–4 weeks, was effective in two-thirds of the children, whereas placebo was effective in only 10% (Biederman et al. 1989). Desipramine was also found to be more effective than placebo in adults with ADHD (Wilens et al. 1996). One of the advantages of desipramine is its low potential for abuse. Unfortunately, five cases of sudden death were reported in the early 1990s in children being treated with desipramine (Riddle et al. 1991, 1993). All were under the age of 12 years. As a result, desipramine is now contraindicated in children younger than 12 years (discussed in greater detail below; see section "Side Effects and Toxicology"). Given that tricyclics as a group share the same adverse cardiac effects, there is reason to be concerned that other tricyclics might also have safety issues in young children.

Pain Syndromes

The tricyclics and maprotiline have been widely used in various chronic pain syndromes. In a review of the literature, O'Malley et al. (1999) identified 56 controlled studies involving tricyclic antidepressant therapy for various pain syndromes, including headache (21 studies), fibromyalgia (18 studies), functional gastrointestinal syndromes (11 studies), idiopathic pain (8 studies), and tinnitus (2 studies), and Salerno et al. (2002) identified 7 more placebo-controlled trials of tricyclics or maprotiline used for chronic back pain. These agents were quite effective; in fact, the mean effect size (0.87) and the drug–placebo difference in response rates (32%) observed in pain syndromes are more robust than those usually observed in placebo-controlled studies in depression. In studies in which depression was also assessed, improvement in pain appeared to be independent of improvement in depression. Thus, the analgesic effects of these compounds were not simply the result of their antidepressant effects.

The mechanism of these agents' analgesic effects appears to differ from that of their antidepressant effects. The antinociceptive actions of the antidepressants result from actions on descending norepinephrine and serotonin pathways in the spinal cord (Yoshimura and Furue 2006). In animals, norepinephrine reuptake inhibitors and combined norepinephrine–serotonin reuptake inhibitors appear to be more potent than SSRIs (Mochizucki 2004). In humans, there is some evidence that the combined-action agents amitriptyline and clomipramine are more effective than the SSRI fluoxetine (Max et al. 1992) or the norepinephrine-selective agents maprotiline (Eberhard et al. 1988) and nortriptyline (Panerai et al. 1990). In humans, antidepressant dosing and timing of effects for pain differ from those observed in depression. For example, usual dosages of amitriptyline required for pain management (≤75 mg/day) are lower than those required to treat depression (15–300 mg/day), and response occurs more quickly, usually within the first 1 or 2 weeks.

Other Indications

Imipramine has been used for treatment of nocturnal enuresis in children with FDA approval, and controlled trials indicate that it is clearly effective (Rapoport et al. 1980). The dose of imipramine is usually 25–50 mg at bedtime. Amitriptyline and nortriptyline also appear to be useful, although they are not approved for use in this disorder. The mechanism of action is unclear but may in part be anticholinergic. It is not clear, however, that the risk of cardiac problems would be substantially less with tricyclics other than desipramine in children younger than 12 years, although the low doses required may reduce this risk.

Tricyclic antidepressant drugs have been extensively studied in patients with schizophrenia. However, in the absence of a major depressive syndrome, these agents appear to be of limited value (Siris et al. 1978).

Side Effects and Toxicology

The delineation of side effects during the treatment of depressed patients is complicated because depression itself is accompanied by a variety of somatic symptoms. For example, headache, constipation, and drowsiness—symptoms usually considered as "side effects"—have been observed in more than 50% of untreated inpatients with major depression if these symptoms were each directly assessed (Nelson et al. 1984). During treatment, patients may be quick to label these somatic symptoms as side effects even if the symptoms were preexisting. Another manifestation of this issue is the rate of spontaneously reported "side effects" on placebo in clinical trials. One of the best examples is headache. Clinical trial data for recently marketed antidepressants indicate that the rate of headaches on placebo in depressed outpatients ranges from 17% to 24% (Physicians' Desk Reference 2002). For fluoxetine, sertraline, paroxetine, and bupropion, the rate for drug was only 1%–2% higher than that for placebo. For venlafaxine XR and citalopram, the rate of headaches was higher for placebo than for drug. A strong argument can be made that headache is usually a symptom of depression. Of course, these mean values conceal the possibility that a symptom may worsen or emerge during treatment in some patients and improve with treatment in others. In groups of patients, however, the strongest predictor of overall somatic symptom severity is the severity of the depression at the time of assessment (Nelson et al. 1984), and the best intervention may be more aggressive treatment.

Another general factor contributing to side effects is the patient's vulnerability. For example, one of the best predictors of orthostatic hypotension during treatment is the presence of orthostatic hypotension prior to treatment (Glassman et al. 1979). Seizures are most likely in a patient with a history of seizures (Rosenstein et al. 1993). Cardiac conduction problems are most likely to occur in patients with preexisting conduction delay (Roose et al. 1987a).

The final manifestation of somatic symptoms during treatment is the net result of the interaction of direct effects of the medication on specific organs, the indirect effects of the medication on depression and its associated somatic symptoms, and the patient's vulnerability to certain symptoms. The attribution of cause—that is, whether a physical symptom is a "side effect" of a drug or a symptom of depression—involves a judgment about whether the symptom is new or has worsened during drug treatment.

Antidepressant drugs do, of course, have direct effects on a variety of organs and can produce adverse effects. The in vitro potency or affinity of antidepressant compounds for various receptor sites (see Table 12–1) is one method for comparing the likelihood that various agents will produce specific side effects. A related issue is how the in vitro potency of a secondary effect relates to the potency of the primary action of the drug. If the secondary effect is more potent, it will occur at concentrations below the therapeutic level of the drug. An example for the tricyclics is orthostatic hypotension, which often manifests at plasma concentrations below the usual antidepressant threshold. Alternatively, in patients without preexisting medical illness, the proarrhythmic and proconvulsant effects of the tricyclic antidepressants are uncommon at therapeutic concentrations but become more frequent at levels encountered in overdose.

Central Nervous System Effects

The principal action of the tricyclic and tetracyclic agents in the central nervous system is to alleviate depression. In particular, they reduce the symptoms of depres-

sion rather than simply elevating mood. Nondepressed subjects given imipramine may feel sleepy, quieter, lightheaded, clumsy, and tired. These effects are generally unpleasant (DiMascio et al. 1964).

The anticholinergic and antihistaminic effects of the tricyclics and tetracyclics can produce confusion or delirium. The incidence of delirium is dose-dependent and increases at blood levels above 300 ng/mL. One study reported that 67% of patients with blood levels above 450 ng/mL developed delirium when receiving the tertiary amines, particularly amitriptyline (Livingston et al. 1983; Preskorn and Simpson 1982). The clinician should be alert to the possibility of delirium in a patient whose depression is worsening during treatment. This can be especially problematic in patients with psychotic depression. Patients with concurrent dementia are particularly vulnerable to the development of delirium, and the more anticholinergic tricyclics should be avoided in these patients. Intramuscular or intravenous physostigmine can be used to reverse or reduce the symptoms of delirium. Although physostigmine may represent a useful diagnostic test, its short duration of action makes the continued use of this agent difficult.

Seizures can occur with all of the tricyclic and tetracyclic agents and are dosage- and blood level–related (Rosenstein et al. 1993). For clomipramine, the risk for seizures is reported to be 0.5% at dosages up to 250 mg/day. At dosages above 250 mg/day, the seizure risk increases to 1.67% (new drug application data on file with the FDA). For maprotiline, the overall risk of seizures is reported to be 0.4%, but, again, this risk increases at dosages above the maximum recommended dose of 225 mg/day (Dessain et al. 1986). The seizure risk for some of the older compounds was not as well established at the time of marketing. A retrospective meta-analysis of imipramine found an estimated seizure rate of 1 per 1,000 patients receiving less than 200 mg/day (Peck et al. 1983). At dosages above 200 mg/day, the rate was 0.6%. Another large review (Jick et al. 1983) found similar dose-dependent rates for amitriptyline and doxepin. Rates of 1%–4% have been reported at doses between 250 mg/day and 450 mg/day, but the samples in these studies were often small, and the confidence intervals for these rates were large. Consistent with a dose-dependent effect, the risk of seizures is substantially increased following overdose (Spiker et al. 1975). Seizure rates for the secondary amines have not been well described. Because the risk of convulsions is clearly increased in patients with predisposing factors such as a prior history of seizures, brain injury, or presence of neuroleptics; because the rates are low (e.g., 1/100); and because sample size in drug trials is often on the order of 200 patients, inclusion of a few patients who have a significant vulnerability to seizures can have a marked effect on the rate of seizures reported. The mechanism by which tricyclics produce seizures is not well understood. It has been suggested that antidepressant drugs induce convulsions by acting at the γ-aminobutyric acid (GABA) receptor chloride–ionophore complex, where they inhibit chloride conductance (Escorihuela et al. 1989; Malatynska et al. 1988).

A fine, rapid tremor can occur with use of tricyclic agents. Because this tremor is dose dependent, tends to occur at higher levels, and is not a typical depressive symptom, development of a tremor may be a clinical indicator of an elevated blood level (Nelson et al. 1984). Dose reduction will often lead to improvement in the tremor.

Because the 7-hydroxy metabolite of amoxapine has neuroleptic properties, administration of amoxapine carries the potential risk of neuroleptic malignant syndrome, which has been reported (Lesaca 1987; Madakasira 1989; Taylor and Schwartz 1988; Washington et al. 1989), and tardive dyskinesia. The occurrence of these adverse events is rare; however, the seriousness of the risk and the availability of many alternatives suggest that use of amoxapine should be reserved for patients whose clinical condition warrants the use of an agent with antipsychotic properties.

Anticholinergic Effects

The tricyclics block muscarinic receptors and can cause a variety of anticholinergic side effects, such as dry mouth, constipation, blurred vision, and urinary hesitancy. These effects can precipitate an ocular crisis in patients with narrow-angle glaucoma. The tricyclic and tetracyclic compounds vary substantially in their muscarinic potency (see Table 12–1). Amitriptyline is the most potent, followed by clomipramine. Of the tricyclics, desipramine is the least anticholinergic. Amoxapine and maprotiline also have minimal anticholinergic effects. Anticholinergic effects can contribute to tachycardia, but tachycardia also occurs as a result of stimulation of β-adrenergic receptors in the heart. Thus, tachycardia regularly occurs in patients receiving desipramine, which is minimally anticholinergic (Rosenstein and Nelson 1991).

Although anticholinergic effects may be annoying, they are usually not serious. They can, however, become severe. An ocular crisis in patients with narrow-angle glaucoma is an acute condition associated with severe pain. Urinary retention can be associated with stretch injuries to the bladder. Constipation can progress to severe

obstipation. (Paralytic ileus has been described but is rare.) In these conditions, medication must be discontinued and appropriate supportive measures instituted. Elderly patients are at greatest risk for severe adverse consequences. The frequency of severe anticholinergic adverse reactions is increased by concomitant neuroleptic administration. Use of nortriptyline or desipramine, either of which is less anticholinergic, can help to reduce the likelihood of these problems.

Anticholinergic effects may benefit from other interventions. Bethanechol (Urecholine) at a dosage of 25 mg three or four times a day may be helpful in patients with urinary hesitancy. The regular use of stool softeners helps to manage constipation. Patients with narrow-angle glaucoma who are receiving pilocarpine eyedrops regularly can be treated with a tricyclic, as can those who have had an iridectomy. Tricyclic agents do not affect patients with chronic open-angle glaucoma.

Antihistaminic Effects

Several of the tricyclic compounds and maprotiline have clinically significant antihistaminic effects. Doxepin is the most potent H_1 receptor blocker in this group. It is more potent than the commonly administered antihistamine diphenhydramine. More recently, however, it has been surpassed by mirtazapine and olanzapine, which are even more potent antihistamines. Central H_1 receptor blockade can contribute to sedation and delirium and also appears to be related to the increased appetite and associated weight gain that patients may develop with chronic treatment. Because of their sedating effects, the tricyclic antidepressants, especially amitriptyline, have been used as hypnotics. Given their cardiac effects and the frequency of lethal overdose, this practice should be discouraged.

Cardiovascular Effects

Orthostatic hypotension is one of the most common reasons for discontinuation of tricyclic antidepressant treatment (Glassman et al. 1979). It can occur with all of the tricyclics but appears to be less pronounced with nortriptyline (Roose et al. 1981; Thayssen et al. 1981). The α_1-adrenergic blockade associated with the tricyclics contributes to orthostatic hypotension; however, it is the postural reflex that is primarily affected. Resting supine blood pressure may be unaffected or can even be elevated (Walsh et al. 1992). Orthostatic hypotension is most likely to occur or is most severe in patients who have preexisting orthostatic hypotension (Glassman et al. 1979).

It is also aggravated by concurrent antihypertensive medications, especially volume-depleting diuretic agents. The elderly are more likely to have preexisting hypotension and are also more vulnerable to the consequences of orthostatic hypotension, such as falls and hip fractures.

Often, orthostatic hypotension occurs at low blood levels, so that dosage reduction is not a helpful management strategy. Gradual dose adjustment may allow accommodation to the subjective experience of light-headedness, but the actual orthostatic blood pressure changes do not accommodate within a reasonable period of time (e.g., 4 weeks) (Roose et al. 1998). Thus, unless the plasma level is elevated and the dose can be reduced, patients who experience serious symptomatic orthostatic hypotension may not be treatable with a tricyclic antidepressant. Fludrocortisone (Florinef) has been used to raise blood pressure, but in this author's experience it is not very effective. If patients are receiving antihypertensives, it may be possible and helpful to reduce the dose of these agents.

Desipramine has been reported to raise supine blood pressure in younger patients, although it is not clear this effect is limited to that age group (Walsh et al. 1992). This effect may be similar to that reported for venlafaxine.

Tachycardia occurs with all the tricyclics, not just the more anticholinergic agents. Both supine and postural pulse changes can occur, and the standing pulse can be markedly elevated. A relatively recent study of nortriptyline, dosed to a therapeutic plasma concentration, found a mean pulse rise of 11% (8 beats per minute) (Roose et al. 1998). Patients do not accommodate to the pulse rise, which can persist for months. Tachycardia is more prominent in younger patients, who appear more sensitive to sympathomimetic effects, and is one of the most common reasons for drug discontinuation in adolescents. A persistent pulse rise in older patients, however, increases cardiac work and may be clinically significant in patients with ischemic heart disease.

The effect of tricyclic antidepressants on cardiac conduction has been a subject of great interest. Cardiac arrhythmia is the principal cause of death following overdose (Biggs et al. 1977; Pimentel and Trommer 1994; Spiker et al. 1975). As a result of this observation, for many years there was great concern about the use of tricyclic antidepressants in patients with and without heart disease. The effect of these agents has now been well described. Apparently, through inhibition of Na^+/K^+-ATPase, the tricyclics stabilize electrically excitable membranes and delay conduction, particularly His ventricular conduction. Consequently, the tricyclics have type I antiarrhythmic qualities or quinidine-like effects.

At therapeutic blood levels, the tricyclics can have beneficial effects on ventricular excitability. In patients with preexisting conduction delay, however, the tricyclic antidepressants can further delay conduction and cause heart block (Glassman and Bigger 1981; Roose et al. 1987b). A pretreatment QTc interval of 450 milliseconds or greater indicates that conduction is already delayed, that a tricyclic may aggravate this condition, and that the patient is not a candidate for tricyclic antidepressant treatment. High drug plasma levels further increase the risk of cardiac toxicity. For example, first-degree atrioventricular heart block is increased with imipramine plasma concentrations above 350 ng/mL (Preskorn and Irwin 1982).

The tricyclic antidepressants do not reduce cardiac contractility or cardiac output (Hartling et al. 1987; Roose et al. 1987a). Studies using radionuclide angiography indicate no adverse effect of imipramine or doxepin on cardiac output, even in patients with diminished left ventricular ejection fractions. But orthostatic hypotension was common in these studies and could be severe in these patients.

Glassman et al. (1993), noting that the type I antiarrhythmic drugs given following myocardial infarction actually increased the risk of sudden death, suggested that the tricyclics may pose similar risks. The risk of sudden death is also increased when heart rate variability is reduced, and the tricyclics reduce heart rate variability (Roose et al. 1998).

As mentioned earlier (see subsection "Attention-Deficit/Hyperactivity Disorder"), sudden death has been reported in five children under the age of 12 years who were receiving desipramine (Riddle et al. 1991, 1993). It was suggested that the immature conduction system in some children might render them more vulnerable to the cardiac effects of desipramine. Subsequently, a study was conducted in 71 children with 24-hour cardiac monitoring (Biederman et al. 1993). No cardiac abnormalities were observed. Wilens et al. (1992) examined the possibility that hydroxydesipramine might reach unusually high levels in children and adolescents, but such levels were not found. A study of electrocardiographic parameters in that sample failed to show a relationship between those parameters and concentrations of desipramine or hydroxydesipramine (Wilens et al. 1993). Although these studies failed to reveal a mechanism for the sudden deaths reported, they do suggest that these events are not predictable, that they are not dose-dependent cardiac effects, and that usual blood level or electrocardiogram monitoring is not likely to identify those at risk.

To summarize the clinical implications of these cardiac effects, the clinician may wish to consider the following. In adults without cardiac disease, orthostatic hypotension may occur with tricyclic use, but conduction problems are not likely. In patients with preexisting conduction delay, the tricyclics may cause heart block. In patients with ischemic heart disease, continued use of tricyclics will increase cardiac work and reduce heart rate variability, possibly increasing the risk of sudden death. Children younger than 12 years also appear vulnerable to the risk of sudden death during tricyclic administration, possibly because of cardiac conduction effects or reduced heart rate variability. Cardiac arrhythmia is the most common cause of death with tricyclic overdose. These cardiac safety issues, coupled with the recently reported safety of the SSRI sertraline when administered for depression following myocardial infarction (Glassman et al. 2002), indicate that the tricyclics are relatively contraindicated in patients with ischemic heart disease and that their use should be reserved for patients whose illnesses are refractory to other treatments.

Hepatic Effects

Acute hepatitis has been associated with administration of imipramine (Horst et al. 1980; Moskovitz et al. 1982; Weaver et al. 1977) and desipramine (Powell et al. 1968; Price and Nelson 1983). Mild increases of liver enzymes (less than three times normal) are not uncommon and usually can be monitored safely over a period of days or weeks without apparent harmful consequences. These changes in liver enzymes do not appear to be related to drug concentrations (Price et al. 1984). Acute hepatitis is relatively uncommon but can occur. The etiology is not well established but in some cases appears to be a hypersensitivity reaction. It is characterized by very high enzyme levels (e.g., aspartate aminotransferase [AST] levels >800), which develop within days. The enzyme pattern can be either hepatocellular or cholestatic. Enzyme changes may precede clinical symptoms, especially in the hepatocellular form. If a random blood test indicates mildly elevated liver enzymes, enzyme levels can be followed for a few days. Because of the rapid rise in liver enzyme levels in acute hepatitis, that condition will become evident quickly and will be easily distinguished from mild, persistent enzyme level elevations.

Acute hepatitis is a dangerous and potentially fatal condition. The antidepressant must be discontinued and should not be introduced again because the next reaction may be more severe. Unfortunately, it is not uncommon for the patient to be receiving several medications, so that the offending agent may be hard to identify. The risk of severe drug-induced hepatitis is not well established. This author has observed four cases associated with desipramine in the course of treating approximately 500 patients.

Other Side Effects

Increased sweating can occur with the tricyclic compounds and occasionally can be marked. The mechanism for this symptom is unclear but may be associated with noradrenergic effects. Another side effect for which the mechanism is unclear is carbohydrate craving. This effect, when coupled with antihistaminic effects, can lead to significant weight gain. One report of outpatients treated with amitriptyline found an average gain of 7 kg during a 6-month period (Berken et al. 1984). Weight gain appears to be greater with the tertiary compounds (Fernstrom et al. 1986) and is less common with nortriptyline, desipramine, and protriptyline. Sexual dysfunction has been described with the tricyclics but generally is less common with this group than during treatment with the SSRIs. This side effect appears to be associated with the more serotonergic compounds and does occur with clomipramine. Tricyclic antidepressants can cause allergic skin rashes, which are sometimes associated with photosensitivity reactions. Various blood dyscrasias also have been reported; fortunately, these are very rare.

Overdose

Because antidepressants are used for depressed patients who are at risk for overdose, the lethality of antidepressant drugs in overdose is of great concern. A tricyclic overdose of 10 times the total daily dose can be fatal (Gram 1990; Rudorfer and Robins 1982). Death most commonly occurs as a result of cardiac arrhythmia. However, seizures and central nervous system depression can occur. Although the use of tricyclics for the treatment of depression has declined, amitriptyline remains widely used for other disorders, such as pain.

The total number of deaths associated with amitriptyline is comparable to that for all other tricyclics and tetracyclics combined. Overdoses often include multiple drugs. In 2006, the American Association of Poison Control Centers (Bronstein et al. 2007) began reporting deaths based on single substance ingestions, which gives a more accurate estimate of lethality. There were 2,730 ingestions of amitriptyline, with 6 deaths, and 1,938 ingestions of all other tricyclic and tetracyclic antidepressants, with 6 deaths. By comparison, there were 19,598 ingestions of various SSRIs, with 3 deaths. The mortality rate for the cyclic antidepressants was 257 per 100,000, while the rate for the SSRIs was 15.3 per 100,000, a 17-fold difference. All of the tricyclic and tetracyclic compounds are dangerous in overdose. Desipramine appears to have a particularly high fatality rate. Amoxapine has been reported to produce high rates of seizure in overdose. But the differences among these drugs are relatively minor in comparison with the improved safety of the second-generation antidepressant agents.

Teratogenicity

Although it would be ideal to discontinue all drugs during pregnancy, the patient and physician are faced with a dilemma. The risk of relapse is a serious concern in patients with recurrent depression because the risk may be increased during pregnancy or the postpartum period. This risk is particularly high for patients with a prior history of depression during or following pregnancy. The long history of tricyclic use without observation of birth defects argues for the safety of these agents. Of course, the patient must be informed of the possible risks and benefits of taking the drug and of discontinuing treatment before making a decision.

If tricyclics are continued during pregnancy, dosage adjustment may be required because of metabolic changes related to the pregnancy (Altshuler and Hendrick 1996). Drug withdrawal following delivery can occur in the infant and is characterized by tachypnea, cyanosis, irritability, and poor sucking reflex. The drugs in this class should be discontinued 1 week prior to delivery if possible. The tricyclics are excreted in breast milk at concentrations similar to those in plasma. The actual quantity delivered, however, is very small, so that drug levels in the infant are usually undetectable (Rudorfer and Potter 1997).

Drug–Drug Interactions

Pharmacodynamic Interactions

Pharmacodynamic interactions are those in which the action of one drug affects the action of the other. More commonly, the effects of the two drugs are additive and result in an adverse event. Perhaps the best example is the interaction of the tricyclics with MAOI drugs. The most dangerous sequence is to give a large dose of a tricyclic to a patient who is already taking an MAOI. This can result in a sudden increase in catecholamines and a potentially

fatal hypertensive reaction. These two compounds have been used together to treat patients with refractory depression (Goldberg and Thornton 1978; Schuckit et al. 1971). Treatment is begun with lower doses, and either the two compounds are started together or the tricyclic is started first. Once begun, coadministration may actually reduce the risk of tyramine reactions (Pare et al. 1985); however, because the protective effect is variable and unpredictable, the usual MAOI diet is maintained.

Perhaps the most common pharmacodynamic interaction is when two psychotropic drugs are added together, resulting in increased sedation. This interaction might occur when tricyclics are combined with antipsychotic agents or with benzodiazepines. Other pharmacodynamic interactions can occur. By blocking the transporters, the tricyclics block the uptake and thus interfere with the action of guanethidine. Desipramine and the other tricyclics reduce the effect of clonidine.

Quinidine is an example of a drug with a potential dynamic and kinetic interaction with tricyclics. Because the tricyclics have quinidine-like effects, the effects of tricyclics and quinidine on cardiac conduction are potentially additive. In addition, quinidine is a potent CYP2D6 isoenzyme inhibitor that can raise tricyclic levels, further adding to the problem.

Pharmacokinetic Interactions

Recently, pharmacokinetic interactions have received considerable attention. One type of pharmacokinetic interaction is enzyme inhibition. A number of drugs can block the metabolic pathways of the tricyclics, resulting in higher and potentially toxic levels. Desipramine has been of particular interest because its metabolism is fairly simple, occurring via the CYP2D6 isoenzyme. Because there are no major alternative pathways, inhibition of CYP2D6 can result in very high desipramine plasma levels, and toxicity can occur (Preskorn et al. 1990). A number of drugs inhibit 2D6. Quinidine, mentioned above, is a very potent 2D6 inhibitor. Other drugs commonly used in psychiatry that inhibit CYP2D6 include the SSRIs fluoxetine and paroxetine, duloxetine, bupropion, and some antipsychotics. Fluoxetine and paroxetine at usual doses raise desipramine levels, on average, three- to fourfold in extensive metabolizers (Preskorn et al. 1994). In slow metabolizers, enzyme inhibitors have less of an effect, because the patients are already deficient in the enzyme and the drug level is already high. In ultrarapid metabolizers, fluoxetine and paroxetine may cause a greater increase in desipramine levels, but these patients are likely to have very low initial desipramine levels. Sertraline 50 mg/day increases desipramine levels, on average, about 30%–40%, which is not a clinically meaningful difference (Preskorn et al. 1994). At higher doses, there is proportionally greater inhibition, but the increase is still substantially less than the 300%–400% increase that occurs with fluoxetine or paroxetine. The magnitude of the effect of bupropion on CYP2D6 has not been reported but appears to be clinically significant. Venlafaxine, nefazodone, mirtazapine, and citalopram appear to have minimal effects on 2D6. 2D6 inhibitors would be expected to block nortriptyline metabolism, but the magnitude of this interaction has not been well studied.

Antipsychotic agents such as chlorpromazine and perphenazine also inhibit 2D6 (Gram et al. 1974; Nelson and Jatlow 1980). At usual doses, perphenazine raises desipramine levels, on average, twofold, but this effect varies with dose and with the neuroleptic employed. Haloperidol can also inhibit the CYP2D6 pathway, but in this author's experience, this effect is not likely to be clinically meaningful at low dosages (e.g., <10 mg/day).

Because the tertiary tricyclics are metabolized by several pathways (CYP1A2, 3A4, 2C19), a selective inhibitor of one pathway would be likely to have less of an effect on these compounds. Drug interactions with the tertiary amines do occur but appear to be less robust. Methylphenidate appears to inhibit demethylation of imipramine to desipramine. At this point, numerous drug interactions have been described, although many are of doubtful clinical significance (for comprehensive reviews, see Nemeroff et al. 1996; Pollock 1997).

The other type of pharmacokinetic drug interaction is enzyme induction. The result of this interaction may render the drug acted upon ineffective. Unlike enzyme inhibition, which occurs quickly, enzyme induction requires synthesis of new enzyme. As a result, the full effect of an enzyme inducer may take 2–3 weeks to develop. If the inducer is discontinued, the effect takes 2–3 weeks to dissipate. Barbiturates and carbamazepine are potent inducers of CYP3A4. Phenytoin also can induce this enzyme, but its effects on the tricyclics appear to be less dramatic. Although CYP2D6 is a noninducible isoenzyme, phenobarbital reduces the availability of desipramine substantially. Apparently when CYP3A4 is induced, it becomes an important metabolic pathway for desipramine and the other tricyclics. In this author's experience, it can be difficult to attain an effective blood level of desipramine in the presence of a barbiturate.

Nicotine induces the CYP1A2 pathway and may lower concentrations of the tertiary tricyclics, but the secondary tricyclics (e.g., desipramine, nortriptyline) appear to be less affected.

Alcohol has a complicated interaction with the tricyclics. Acute ingestion of alcohol can reduce first-pass metabolism, resulting in higher tricyclic levels. Because tricyclic overdose is often associated with alcohol ingestion, this is an important interaction, resulting in higher tricyclic levels. Alternatively, chronic use of alcohol appears to induce hepatic isoenzymes and may lower tricyclic levels (Shoaf and Linnoila 1991).

The tricyclics themselves produce some enzyme inhibition, but few clinically significant interactions have been described. The tertiary tricyclics compete with warfarin for some metabolic enzymes (e.g., CYP1A2) and may raise warfarin levels.

Conclusion

The tricyclic drugs were the mainstay of treatment for depression for three decades. Although the second-generation antidepressants appear to be better tolerated, no new agent has been shown to be more effective than the tricyclics, and if anything, there has been concern that the new agents may be less effective. The tricyclics were "dirty" drugs; that is, they had multiple actions. Although their side effects have been emphasized, these multiple actions may have contributed to their efficacy. Not only does amitriptyline block uptake of 5-HT, but its metabolite blocks uptake of norepinephrine, and in addition, amitriptyline is a 5-HT$_2$ antagonist. The principal drawback of this class of agents is the risk of serious cardiac adverse effects. They can aggravate arrhythmia in patients with preexisting conduction delay. They also may increase the risk of sudden death in children and in patients with ischemic heart disease. Moreover, a week's supply of medication taken in overdose could be fatal. As noted, even though the use of the tricyclics has diminished, amitriptyline remains a common cause of death by overdose in the United States. Because of these adverse effects, it is unlikely that there will be a resurgence of interest in the tricyclics. Nevertheless, the efficacy of these agents across a range of disorders, including pain, suggests the possible advantage of antidepressant drugs with multiple actions.

References

Abernathy DR, Greenblatt DJ, Shader RI: Imipramine and desipramine disposition in the elderly. J Pharmacol Exp Ther 232:183–188, 1985

Agency for Health Care Policy and Research: Clinical Practice Guideline: Depression in Primary Care: Treatment of Major Depression, Vol 2. Rockville, MD, U.S. Government Printing Office, 1993

Alexanderson B: Pharmacokinetics of nortriptyline in man after single and multiple oral doses: the predictability of steady-state plasma concentrations from single-dose plasma-level data. Eur J Clin Pharmacol 4:82–91, 1972

Altshuler LL, Hendrick VC: Pregnancy and psychotropic medication: changes in blood levels. J Clin Psychopharmacol 16:78–80, 1996

American Psychiatric Association: Diagnostic and Statistical Manual of Mental Disorders, 4th Edition, Text Revision. Washington, DC, American Psychiatric Association, 2000

American Psychiatric Association Task Force: Tricyclic antidepressants—blood level measurements and clinical outcome: an APA Task Force report. Task Force on the Use of Laboratory Tests in Psychiatry. Am J Psychiatry 142:155–162, 1985

Anderson I: SSRIs versus tricyclics antidepressants in depressed inpatients: a meta-analysis of efficacy and tolerability. Depress Anxiety 7 (suppl 1):11–17, 1998

Anderson I: Selective serotonin reuptake inhibitors versus tricyclics antidepressant: a meta-analysis of efficacy and tolerability. J Affect Disord 58:19–36, 2000

Anderson I, Tomenson B: A meta-analysis of the efficacy of selective serotonin reuptake inhibitors compared to tricyclic antidepressants in depression (abstract). Neuropsychopharmacology 10 (suppl):106, 1994

Anton RF, Burch EA: Amoxapine versus amitriptyline combined with perphenazine in the treatment of psychotic depression. Am J Psychiatry 147:1203–1208, 1990

Arora RC, Meltzer HY: Serotonergic measures in the brains of suicide victims: 5-HT2 binding sites in frontal cortex of suicide victims and control subjects. Am J Psychiatry 146:730–736, 1989

Åsberg M, Cronholm B, Sjöqvist F, et al: Relationship between plasma level and therapeutic effect of nortriptyline. BMJ 3:331–334, 1971

Axelrod J, Whitby LG, Herting G: Effect of psychotropic drugs on the uptake of H3-norepinephrine by tissues. Science 133:383–384, 1961

Barden N: Modulation of glucocorticoid receptor gene expression by antidepressant drugs. Pharmacopsychiatry 29:12–22, 1996

Beckmann H, Goodwin FK: Antidepressant response to tricyclics and urinary MHPG in unipolar patients. Arch Gen Psychiatry 32:17–22, 1975

Benetello P, Furlanut M, Zara G, et al: Imipramine pharmacokinetics in depressed geriatric patients. Int J Clin Pharmacol Res 10:191–195, 1990

Berken GN, Weinstein DO, Stern WC: Weight gain: a side effect of tricyclic antidepressants. J Affect Disord 7:133–138, 1984

Bertilsson L, Mellstrom B, Sjöqvist P: Pronounced inhibition of noradrenaline uptake by 10-hydroxy metabolites of nortriptyline. Life Sci 25:1285–1292, 1979

Biederman J, Baldessarini RJ, Wright V, et al: A double-blind placebo-controlled study of desipramine in the treatment of ADD, I: efficacy. J Am Acad Child Adolesc Psychiatry 32:805–813, 1989

Biederman J, Baldessarini RJ, Goldblatt A, et al: A naturalistic study of 24-hour electrocardiographic recording and echocardiographic findings in children and adolescents treated with desipramine. J Am Acad Child Adolesc Psychiatry 32:805–813, 1993

Biggs JT, Spiker DG, Petit JM, et al: Tricyclic antidepressant overdose. JAMA 238:135–138, 1977

Blier P, de Montigny C, Chaput Y: Modification of the serotonin system by antidepressant treatments: implications for the therapeutic response in major depression. J Clin Psychopharmacol 7:24S–35S, 1987

Bock J, Nelson JC, Gray S, et al: Desipramine hydroxylation: Variability and effect of antipsychotic drugs. Clin Pharmacol Ther 33:190–197, 1983

Bolden-Watson C, Richelson E: Blockade of newly developed antidepressants of biogenic amine uptake into rat brain synaptosomes. Life Sci 52:1023–1029, 1993

Bowden CL, Schatzberg AF, Rosenbaum A, et al: Fluoxetine and desipramine in major depressive disorder. J Clin Psychopharmacol 13:305–310, 1993

Breyer-Pfaff U, Gaertner HJ, Kreuter F, et al: Antidepressive effect and pharmacokinetics of amitriptyline with consideration of unbound drug and 10-hydroxynortriptyline plasma levels. Psychopharmacology (Berl) 76:240–244, 1982

Bronstein AC, Spyker DA, Cantilena LR, et al: 2006 Annual Report of the American Association of Poison Control Centers' National Poison Data System (NPDS). Clin Toxicol 45:815–917, 2007

Brosen K, Otton SV, Gram LF: Sparteine oxidation polymorphism in Denmark. Acta Pharmacol Toxicol 57:357–360, 1985

Brosen K, Zeugin T, Myer UA: Role of P450IID6, the target of the sparteine/debrisoquin oxidation polymorphism, in the metabolism of imipramine. Clin Pharmacol Ther 49:609–617, 1991

Brunswick DJ, Amsterdam JD, Mendels J, et al: Prediction of steady-state imipramine and desmethylimipramine plasma concentrations from single dose data. Clin Pharmacol Ther 25:605–610, 1979

Bunney WE, Davis JM: Norepinephrine in depressive reactions: a review. Arch Gen Psychiatry 13:483–494, 1965

Byck R: Drugs and the treatment of psychiatric disorders, in The Pharmacological Basis of Therapeutics, 5th Edition. Edited by Gilman AG, Goodman IS. New York, Macmillan, 1975, pp 152–200

Bymaster FP, Katner JS, Nelson DL, et al: Atomoxetine increases extracellular levels of norepinephrine and dopamine in prefrontal cortex of rat: a potential mechanism for efficacy in attention deficit/hyperactivity disorder. Neuropsychopharmacology 27:699–711, 2002

Chan CH, Janicak PG, Davis JM: Response of psychotic and nonpsychotic depressed patients to tricyclic antidepressants. J Clin Psychiatry 48:197–200, 1987

Charney DS, Delgado PL, Price LH, et al: The receptor sensitivity hypothesis of antidepressant action: a review of antidepressant effects on serotonin function, in The Role of Serotonin in Psychiatric Disorders. Edited by Brown SL, van Praag HM. New York, Brunner/Mazel, 1991, pp 29–56

Cheetham SC, Crompton MR, Katona CLE, et al: Brain 5-HT2 receptor binding in suicide victims. Brain Res 443:272–280, 1988

Cooper TB, Simpson GM: Prediction of individual dosage of nortriptyline. Am J Psychiatry 135:333–335, 1978

Coupet I, Rauh CE, Szucs-Myers VA, et al: 2-Chloro-11(pipera-zinyl)[b,f][1,4]oxazepine (amoxapine), an antidepressant with antipsychotics properties—a possible role for 7-hydroxyamoxapine. Biochem Pharmacol 28:2514–2515, 1979

Cusack B, Nelson A, Richelson E: Binding of antidepressants to human brain receptors: focus on newer generation compounds. Psychopharmacology 114:559–565, 1994

Danish University Antidepressant Group: Citalopram: clinical effect profile in comparison with clomipramine. A controlled multicenter study. Psychopharmacology (Berl) 90:131–138, 1986

Danish University Antidepressant Group: Paroxetine: a selective serotonin reuptake inhibitor showing better tolerance, but weaker antidepressant effect than clomipramine in a controlled multicenter study. J Affect Disord 18:289–299, 1990

Davis JM: Overview: maintenance therapy in psychiatry, II: affective disorders. Am J Psychiatry 133:1–13, 1976

Davis JM, Glassman AH: Antidepressant drugs, in Comprehensive Textbook of Psychiatry. Edited by Kaplan HI, Sadock BJ. Baltimore, MD, Williams & Wilkins, 1989, pp 1627–1655

Dawling S, Ford S, Rangedara DC, et al: Amitriptyline dosage prediction in elderly patients from plasma concentration at 24 hours after a single 100 mg dose. Clin Pharmacokinet 9:261–266, 1984

Delay J, Deniker P: Trente-huit cas de psychoses traitees par la cure prolongee et continue de 4560 RP. Le Congres des Al. et Neurol. de Langue Fr. in Compte rendu du Congres. Masson et Cie, Paris, 1952

Delgado PL, Charney DS, Price LH, et al: Serotonin function and the mechanism of antidepressant action. Reversal of antidepressant-induced remission by rapid depletion of plasma tryptophan. Arch Gen Psychiatry 47:411–418, 1990

Delgado PL, Miller HL, Salomon RM, et al: Monoamines and the mechanism of antidepressant action: effects of catecholamine depletion on mood of patients treated with antidepressants. Psychopharmacol Bull 29:389–396, 1993

de Montigny C, Aghajanian GK: Tricyclic antidepressants: long-term treatment increases responsivity of rat forebrain neurons to serotonin. Science 202:1303–1306, 1978

Dessain EC, Schatzberg AF, Woods BT, et al: Maprotiline treatment in depression: a perspective on seizures. Arch Gen Psychiatry 43:86–90, 1986

DiMascio A, Heninger G, Klerman GL: Psychopharmacology of imipramine and desipramine: a comparative study of their effects in normal males. Psychopharmacologia 5:361–371, 1964

Duman RS, Heninger GR, Nestler EJ: A molecular and cellular theory of depression. Arch Gen Psychiatry 54:597–606, 1997

Eberhard G, von Knorring L, Nilsson HL, et al: A double-blind randomized study of clomipramine versus maprotiline in patients with idiopathic pain syndromes. Neuropsychobiology 19:25–34, 1988

Escorihuela RM, Boix F, Corda MG, et al: Chronic but not acute antidepressant treatment increases pentetrazol-induced convulsions in mice. J Pharm Pharmacol 41:143–144, 1989

Evans DAP, Mahgoub A, Sloan TP, et al: A family and population study of the genetic polymorphism of debrisoquin oxidation in a white British population. J Med Genet 17:102–105, 1980

Fava M, Uebelacker LA, Alpert JE, et al: Major depression subtypes and treatment response. Biol Psychiatry 42:568–576, 1997

Fernstrom MD, Krowinski RL, Kupfer DJ: Chronic imipramine treatment and weight gain. Psychiatr Res 17:269–273, 1986

Frank E, Kupfer DJ, Perel JM, et al: Three-year outcomes for maintenance therapies in recurrent depression. Arch Gen Psychiatry 47:1093–1099, 1990

Furey ML, Drevets WC: Antidepressant efficacy of the antimuscarinic drug scopolamine: a randomized, placebo-controlled clinical trial. Arch Gen Psychiatry 63:1121–1129, 2006

Furlanut M, Benetello P: The pharmacokinetics of tricyclic antidepressant drugs in the elderly. Pharmacol Res 22:15–25, 1990

Geller B: Psychopharmacology of children and adolescents: pharmacokinetics and relationships of plasma/serum levels to response. Psychopharmacol Bull 27:401–409, 1991

Gerson SC, Plotkin DA, Jarvik LF: Antidepressant drug studies, 1964 to 1986: empirical evidence for aging patients. J Clin Psychopharmacol 8:311–322, 1988

Glassman AH, Bigger JT: Cardiovascular effects of therapeutic doses of tricyclic antidepressants. Arch Gen Psychiatry 38:815–820, 1981

Glassman AH, Kantor S, Shostak M: Depression, delusions, and drug response. Am J Psychiatry 132:716–719, 1975

Glassman AH, Perel JM, Shostak M, et al: Clinical implications of imipramine plasma levels for depressive illness. Arch Gen Psychiatry 34:197–204, 1977

Glassman AH, Bigger JT Jr, Giardina EV, et al: Clinical characteristics of imipramine induced orthostatic hypotension. Lancet 1(8114):468–472, 1979

Glassman AH, Roose SP, Bigger JT Jr: The safety of tricyclic antidepressants in cardiac patients: risk/benefit reconsidered. JAMA 269:2673–2675, 1993

Glassman AH, O'Connor CM, Califf RM, et al: Sertraline treatment of major depression in patients with acute MI or unstable angina. JAMA 288:701–709, 2002

Goldberg RS, Thornton WE: Combined tricyclic-MAOI therapy for refractory depression: a review, with guidelines for appropriate usage. J Clin Pharmacol 18:143–147, 1978

Goodwin GM, Green AR, Johnson P: 5-HT2 receptor characteristics in frontal cortex and 5-HT2 receptor mediated head-twitch behavior following antidepressant treatment to mice. Br J Pharmacol 83:235–242, 1984

Gram LF: Inadequate dosing and Pharmacokinetic variability as confounding factors in assessment of efficacy of antidepressants. Clin Neuropharmacol 13 (suppl):S35–S44, 1990

Gram LF, Overo KF, Kirk L: Influence of neuroleptics and benzodiazepines on metabolism of tricyclic antidepressants in man. Am J Psychiatry 131:863–866, 1974

Greenblatt DJ, Moltke LL, Shader RI: Pharmacokinetics of psychotropic drugs, in Geriatric Psychopharmacology. Edited by Nelson JC. New York, Marcel Dekker, 1998, pp 27–41

Greist JH, Jefferson JW, Kobak KA, et al: Efficacy and tolerability of serotonin transport inhibitors in obsessive-compulsive disorder: a meta-analysis. Arch Gen Psychiatry 52:53–60, 1995

Hall H, Ogren SO: Effects of antidepressant drugs on different receptors in the brain. Eur Pharmacol 70:393–407, 1981

Hammer W, Sjöqvist F: Plasma levels of monomethylated tricyclic antidepressants during treatment with imipramine-like compounds. Life Sci 6:1895–1903, 1967

Hartling OJ, Marving J, Knudsen P, et al: The effect of the tricyclic antidepressant drug, nortriptyline on left ventricular ejection fraction and left ventricular volumes. Psychopharmacology 91:381–383, 1987

Himmelhoch JM, Detre T, Kupfer DJ, et al: Treatment of previously intractable depressions with tranylcypromine and lithium. J Nerv Ment Dis 155:216–220, 1972

Himmelhoch JM, Thase ME, Mallinger AG, et al: Tranylcypromine versus imipramine in anergic bipolar depression. Am J Psychiatry 148:910–916, 1991

Horst DA, Grace ND, Le Compte PM: Prolonged cholestasis and progressive hepatic fibrosis following imipramine therapy. Gastroenterology 79:550–554, 1980

Jick H, Dinan BJ, Hunter JR, et al: Tricyclic antidepressants and convulsions. J Clin Psychopharmacol 3:182–185, 1983

Jobson K, Linnoila M, Gillam J, et al: Successful treatment of severe anxiety attacks with tricyclic antidepressants: a possible mechanism of action. Am J Psychiatry 135:863–864,1978

Katz IR, Simpson GM, Jethanandani V, et al: Steady state pharmacokinetics of nortriptyline in the frail elderly. Neuropsychopharmacology 2:229–236, 1989

Katz IR, Simpson GM, Curlik SM, et al: Pharmacologic treatment of major depression for elderly patients in residential care settings. J Clin Psychiatry 51 (7, suppl):41–47, 1990

Keller MB, Gelenberg AJ, Hirschfeld RMA, et al: The treatment of chronic depression: a double-blind, randomized trial of sertraline and imipramine. J Clin Psychiatry 59(pt 2):598–607, 1998

Klein DF: Delineation of two drug responsive anxiety syndromes. Psychopharmacologia 5:397–408, 1964

Kocsis JH, Frances AJ, Voss CB, et al: Imipramine treatment for chronic depression. Arch Gen Psychiatry 45:253–257, 1988

Kragh-Sørenson P, Åsberg M, Eggert-Hansen C: Plasma nortriptyline levels in endogenous depression. Lancet 1(7795):113–115, 1973

Kragh-Sørenson P, Hansen CE, Baastrup PC, et al: Self-inhibiting action of nortriptyline antidepressant effect at high plasma levels: a randomized double-blind study controlled by plasma concentrations in patients with endogenous depression. Psychopharmacologia 45:305–312, 1976

Kuhn R: The treatment of depressive states with G22355 (imipramine hydrochloride). Am J Psychiatry 115:459–464, 1958

Kuhn R: The imipramine story, in Discoveries in Biological Psychiatry. Edited by Ayd FJ, Blackwell B. Philadelphia, PA, JB Lippincott, 1970, pp 205–217

Kupfer D, Hanin I, Spiker DG, et al: Amitriptyline plasma levels and clinical response in primary depression. Clin Pharmacol Ther 22:904–911, 1977

Kupfer DJ, Spiker DG: Refractory depression: prediction of nonresponse by clinical indicators. J Clin Psychiatry 42:307–312, 1981

Lakoski JM, Aghajanian GK: Effects of ketanserin on neuronal responses to serotonin in the prefrontal cortex, lateral geniculate and dorsal raphe nucleus. Neuropharmacology 24:265–273, 1985

Leonard HL, Swedo S, Rapoport JL, et al: Treatment of obsessive compulsive disorder in children and adolescents with clomipramine and desipramine: a double-blind crossover comparison. Arch Gen Psychiatry 46:1088–1092, 1989

Lesaca T: Amoxapine and neuroleptic malignant syndrome. Am J Psychiatry 144:1514, 1987

Lesch KP, Manji HK: Signal-transducing G proteins and antidepressant drugs: evidence for modulation of alpha subunit gene expression in rat brain. Biol Psychiatry 32:549–579, 1992

Liebowitz MR, Quitkin FM, Stewart JW, et al: Phenelzine vs imipramine in atypical depression. Arch Gen Psychiatry 41:669–677, 1984

Liebowitz MR, Quitkin FM, Stewart JW, et al: Antidepressant specificity in atypical depression. Arch Gen Psychiatry 45:129–137, 1988

Livingston RL, Zucker DK, Isenberg K, et al: Tricyclic antidepressants and delirium. J Clin Psychiatry 44:173–176, 1983

Maas JW, Fawcett JA, Dekirmenjian H: Catecholamine metabolism, depressive illness, and drug response. Arch Gen Psychiatry 26:353–363, 1972

Madakasira S: Amoxapine-induced neuroleptic malignant syndrome. DICP 23:50–55, 1989

Madakasira S, Khazanie PG: Reliability of Amitriptyline dose prediction based on single-dose plasma levels. Clin Pharmacol Ther 37:145–149, 1985

Malatynska E, Knapp RJ, Ikeda M, et al: Antidepressants and seizure-interactions at the GABA-receptor chloride-ionophore complex. Life Sci 43:303–307,1988

Manji HK, Potter WZ, Lenox RH: Signal transduction pathways: molecular targets for lithium's actions. Arch Gen Psychiatry 52:531–543, 1995

Marek GJ, Carpenter LL, McDougle CJ, et al: Synergistic action of 5-HT2A antagonists and selective serotonin reuptake inhibitors in neuropsychiatric disorders Neuropsychopharmacology 28:402–412, 2003

Max MB, Lynch SA, Muir J, et al: Effects of desipramine, amitriptyline, and fluoxetine on pain in diabetic neuropathy. N Engl J Med 326:1250–1256, 1992

McGrath PJ, Stewart JW, Harrison W, et al: Treatment of tricyclic refractory depression with a monoamine oxidase inhibitor antidepressant. Psychopharmacol Bull 23:169–172, 1987

Miller HL, Delgado PL, Salomon RM, et al: Clinical and biochemical effects of catecholamine depletion on antidepressant-induced remission of depression. Arch Gen Psychiatry 53:117–128, 1996

Miller NL, Kocsis JH, Leon AC, et al: Maintenance desipramine for dysthymia: a placebo-controlled study. J Affect Disord 64:231–237, 2001

Mochizucki D: Serotonin and noradrenaline reuptake inhibitors in animal models of pain. Hum Psychopharmacol 19 (suppl 1): S15–S19, 2004

Montgomery SA: The efficacy of fluoxetine as an antidepressant in the short and long term. Int Clin Psychopharmacol 4 (suppl):113–119, 1989

Moody JP, Whyte SF, MacDonald AJ, et al: Pharmacokinetic aspects of protriptyline plasma levels. Eur J Clin Pharmacol 11:51–56, 1977

Moskovitz R, DeVane CL, Harris R, et al: Toxic hepatitis and single daily dosage imipramine therapy. J Clin Psychiatry 43:165–166, 1982

Munjack DJ, Usigli R, Zulueta A, et al: Nortriptyline in the treatment of panic disorder and agoraphobia with panic attacks. J Clin Psychopharmacol 8:204–207, 1988

Nelson JC: Use of desipramine in depressed inpatients. J Clin Psychiatry 45:10–15, 1984

Nelson JC: The use of antipsychotic drugs in the treatment of depression, in Treating Resistant Depression. Edited by Zohar J, Belmaker RH. New York, PMA Publishing, 1987, pp 131–146

Nelson JC, Jatlow P: Neuroleptic effect on desipramine steady state plasma concentrations. Am J Psychiatry 137:1232–1234, 1980

Nelson JC, Jatlow PI: Nonlinear desipramine kinetics: prevalence and importance. Clin Pharmacol Ther 41:666–670, 1987

Nelson JC, Jatlow P, Quinlan DM, et al: Desipramine plasma concentrations and antidepressant response. Arch Gen Psychiatry 39:1419–1422, 1982

Nelson JC, Jatlow PI, Quinlan DM: Subjective complaints during desipramine treatment: relative importance of plasma drug concentrations and the severity of depression. Arch Gen Psychiatry 41:55–59, 1984

Nelson JC, Jatlow P, Mazure C: Desipramine plasma levels and response in elderly melancholics. J Clin Psychopharmacol 5:217–220, 1985

Nelson JC, Jatlow PI, Mazure C: Rapid desipramine dose adjustment using 24-hour levels. J Clin Psychopharmacol 7:72–77, 1987

Nelson JC, Mazure C, Attilasoy E, et al: Hydroxy-desipramine in the elderly. J Clin Psychopharmacol 8:428–433, 1988a

Nelson JC, Mazure C, Jatlow PI: Antidepressant activity of 2-hydroxy-desipramine. Clin Pharmacol Ther 44:283–288, 1988b

Nelson JC, Mazure CM, Jatlow PI: Characteristics of desipramine refractory depression. J Clin Psychiatry 55:12–19, 1994

Nelson JC, Mazure CM, Jatlow PI: Desipramine treatment of major depression in patients over 75 years of age. J Clin Psychopharmacol 15:99–105, 1995

Nemeroff CB, DeVane CL, Pollock BG: Newer antidepressants and the cytochrome P450 system. Am J Psychiatry 153:311–320, 1996

Nibuya M, Nestler EJ, Duman RS: Chronic antidepressant administration increases the expression of cAMP response element-binding protein (CREB) in rat hippocampus. J Neurosci 16:2365–2372, 1996

Nordin C, Bertilsson L, Siwers B: Clinical and biochemical effects during treatment of depression with nortriptyline—the role of 10-hydroxynortriptyline. Clin Pharmacol Ther 42:10–19, 1987

O'Malley PG, Jackson JL, Santoro J, et al: Antidepressant therapy for unexplained symptoms and symptom syndromes. J Fam Pract 48:980–990, 1999

Panerai AE, Monza G, Movilia P, et al: A randomized, within-patient, cross-over, placebo-controlled trial on the efficacy and tolerability of the tricyclic antidepressants chlorimipramine and nortriptyline in central pain. Acta Neurol Scand 82:34–38, 1990

Pare CMB, Mousawi MA, Sandler M, et al: Attempts to attenuate the "cheese effect": combined drug therapy in depressive illness. J Affect Disord 9:137–141, 1985

Peck AW, Stern WC, Watkinson C: Incidence of seizures during treatment with tricyclic antidepressant drugs and bupropion. J Clin Psychiatry 44 (5, pt 2):197–201, 1983

Peroutka SJ, Snyder SH: Long term antidepressant treatment decreases spiroperidol-labeled serotonin receptor binding. Science 210:88–90, 1980

Physicians' Desk Reference. Montvale, NJ, Medical Economics Company, 2002

Pimentel L, Trommer L: Cyclic antidepressant overdoses: a review. Emerg Med Clin North Am 12:533, 1994

Pinder RM, Brogden RN, Speight TM, et al: Doxepin up-to-date: a review of its pharmacological properties and therapeutic efficacy with particular reference to depression. Drugs 13:161–218, 1977

Pollock BG: Drug interactions, in Geriatric Psychopharmacology. Edited by Nelson JC. New York, Marcel Dekker, 1997, pp 43–60

Pollock BG, Everett G, Perel JM: Comparative cardiotoxicty of nortriptyline and its isomeric 10-hydroxymetabolites. Neuropsychopharmacology 6:1–10, 1992

Potter WZ: Psychotherapeutic drugs and biogenic amines: current concepts and therapeutic indications. Drugs 28:127–143, 1984

Potter WZ, Calil NM, Manian AA, et al: Hydroxylated metabolites of tricyclic antidepressants: preclinical assessment of activity. Biol Psychiatry 14:601–613, 1979

Potter WZ, Zavadil AP, Kopin IJ, et al: Single-dose kinetics predict steady-state concentrations of imipramine and desipramine. Arch Gen Psychiatry 36:314–320, 1980

Powell WJ, Koch-Weser J, Williams RA: Lethal hepatic necrosis after therapy with imipramine and desipramine. JAMA 206:1791–1792, 1968

Prange AI: The pharmacology and biochemistry of depression. Dis Nerv Syst 25:217–221, 1965

Preskorn SH, Irwin HA: Toxicity of tricyclic antidepressants: kinetics, mechanism, intervention: a review. J Clin Psychiatry 43:151–156, 1982

Preskorn SH, Simpson S: Tricyclic antidepressant–induced delirium and plasma drug concentration. Am J Psychiatry 139:822–823, 1982

Preskorn SH, Beber JH, Faul JC, et al: Serious adverse effects of combining fluoxetine and tricyclic antidepressants. Am J Psychiatry 147:532, 1990

Preskorn SH, Alderman J, Chung M, et al: Pharmacokinetics of desipramine co-administered with sertraline or fluoxetine. J Clin Psychopharmacol 14:90–98, 1994

Price LH, Nelson JC: Desipramine associated hepatitis. J Clin Psychopharmacology 3:243–246, 1983

Price LH, Nelson JC, Jatlow P: Effects of desipramine on clinical liver function tests. Am J Psychiatry 414:798–800, 1984

Priest BT, Kaczorowski GJ: Blocking sodium channels to treat neuropathic pain. Expert Opin Ther Targets 11:291–306, 2007

Randrup A, Braestrup C: Uptake inhibition of biogenic amines by newer antidepressant drugs: relevance to the dopamine hypothesis of depression. Psychopharmacology (Berl) 53:309–314, 1977

Rapoport J, Potter WZ: Tricyclic antidepressants: use in pediatric psychopharmacology, in Pharmacokinetics: Youth and Age. Edited by Raskin A, Robinson D. Amsterdam, The Netherlands, Elsevier, 1981, pp 105–123

Rapoport JL, Mikkelson EJ, Zavadil AP, et al: Childhood enuresis, II: psychopathology, tricyclic concentrations in plasma and anti-enuretic effect. Arch Gen Psychiatry 37:1146–1152, 1980

Reisby N, Gram LF, Bech P, et al: Imipramine: clinical effects and pharmacokinetic variability. Psychopharmacology 54:263–272, 1977

Richelson E, Nelson A: Antagonism by antidepressants of neurotransmitter receptors of normal human brain in vitro. J Pharmacol Exp Ther 230:94–102, 1984

Riddle MA, Nelson JC, Kleinman CS, et al: Sudden death in children receiving Norpramin: a review of three reported cases and commentary. J Am Acad Child Adolesc Psychiatry 30:104–108, 1991

Riddle MA, Geller B, Ryan N: Another sudden death in a child treated with desipramine. J Am Acad Child Adolesc Psychiatry 32:792–797, 1993

Roose SP, Glassman AH, Siris SG, et al: Comparison of imipramine and nortriptyline-induced orthostatic hypotension: a meaningful difference. J Clin Psychopharmacol 1:316–319, 1981

Roose SP, Glassman AH, Walsh BT, et al: Tricyclic nonresponders, phenomenology and treatment. Am J Psychiatry 143:345–348, 1986

Roose SP, Glassman AH, Giardina EG, et al: Cardiovascular effects of imipramine and bupropion in depressed patients with congestive heart failure. J Clin Psychopharmacol 7:247–251, 1987a

Roose SP, Glassman AH, Giardina EG, et al: Tricyclic antidepressants in depressed patients with cardiac conduction disease. Arch Gen Psychiatry 44:273–275, 1987b

Roose S, Laghrissi-Thode F, Kennedy JS, et al: A comparison of paroxetine and nortriptyline in depressed patients with ischemic heart disease. JAMA 279:287–291, 1998

Rosenstein DL, Nelson JC, Jacobs JC: Seizures associated with antidepressants: a review. J Clin Psychiatry 54:289–299, 1993

Rosenstein DL, Nelson JC: Heart rate during desipramine treatment as an indicator of beta1-adrenergic function. Society of Biological Psychiatry Scientific Program. Biol Psychiatry 29:132A, 1991

Rudorfer MV, Potter WZ: The role of metabolites of antidepressant in the treatment of depression. CNS Drugs 7:273–312, 1997

Rudorfer MV, Robins E: Amitriptyline overdose: clinical effects of tricyclic antidepressant plasma levels. J Clin Psychiatry 43:457–460, 1982

Rudorfer MV, Young RC: Desipramine: cardiovascular effects and plasma levels. Am J Psychiatry 137:984–986, 1980

Ryan ND: The pharmacologic treatment of child and adolescent depression. Psychiatric Clin North Am 15:29–40, 1992

Salerno SM, Browning R, Jackson JL: The effect of antidepressant treatment on chronic back pain. Arch Intern Med 162:19–24, 2002

Schildkraut JJ: The catecholamine hypothesis of affective disorders: a review of supporting evidence. Am J Psychiatry 122:509–522, 1965

Schneider LS, Cooper TB, Severson JA, et al: Electrocardiographic changes with nortriptyline and 10-hydroxynortriptyline in elderly depressed outpatients. J Clin Psychopharmacol 8:402–408, 1988

Schuckit M, Robins E, Feighner J: Tricyclic antidepressants and monoamine oxidase inhibitors: combination therapy in the treatment of depression. Arch Gen Psychiatry 24:509–514, 1971

Schwaninger M, Schofl C, Blume R, et al: Inhibition by antidepressant drugs of cyclic AMP response element-binding protein/cyclic AMP response element-directed gene transcription. Mol Pharmacol 47:1112–1118, 1995

Shoaf SE, Linnoila M: Interaction of ethanol and smoking on the pharmacokinetics and pharmacodynamics of psychotropic medications. Psychopharmacol Bull 27: 577–594, 1991

Siris SG, van Kammen DP, Docherty JP: Use of antidepressant drugs in schizophrenia. Arch Gen Psychiatry 35:1368–1377, 1978

Smith RC, Reed K, Leelavathi DE, et al: Pharmacokinetics and the effects of nortriptyline in geriatric depressed patients. Psychopharmacol Bull 16:54–57, 1980

Spiker DG, Weiss JC, Chang S, et al: Tricyclic antidepressant overdose: clinical presentation and plasma levels. Clin Pharmacol Ther 18:539–546, 1975

Spiker DG, Weiss JC, Dealy RS, et al: The pharmacologic treatment of delusional depression. Am J Psychiatry 142:430–436, 1985

Stanley M, Mann JJ: Increased serotonin-2 binding sites in frontal cortex of suicide victims. Lancet 1(8318):214–216, 1983

Sulser F, Vetulani J, Mobley PL: Mode of action of antidepressant drugs. Biochem Pharmacol 27:257–261, 1978

Szabo ST, Blier P: Effect of the selective noradrenergic reuptake inhibitor reboxetine on the firing activity of noradrenaline and serotonin neurons. Eur J Neurosci 13:2077–2087, 2001

Tatsumi M, Groshan K, Blakely RD, et al: Pharmacological profile of antidepressants and related compounds at human monoamine transporters. Eur J Pharmacol 340:249, 1997

Taylor NE, Schwartz HI: Neuroleptic malignant syndrome following amoxapine overdose. J Nerv Ment Dis 176:249–251, 1988

Thase ME, Malinger AG, McKnight D, et al: Treatment of imipramine-resistant recurrent depression, IV: a double-blind crossover study of tranylcypromine for anergic bipolar depression. Am J Psychiatry 149:195–198, 1992

Thase ME, Fava M, Halbreich U, et al: A placebo-controlled, randomized clinical trial comparing sertraline and imipramine for the treatment of dysthymia. Arch Gen Psychiatry 53:777, 1996

Thayssen P, Bjerre M, Kragh-Sorenson P, et al: Cardiovascular effects of imipramine and nortriptyline in elderly patients. Psychopharmacology 74:360–364, 1981

Tremblay P, Blier P: Catecholaminergic strategies for the treatment of major depression. Curr Drug Targets 7:149–158, 2006

Vetulani J, Sulser F: Action of various antidepressant treatments reduces reactivity of noradrenergic cyclic AMP generating systems in limbic forebrain. Nature 257:395–496, 1975

von Moltke LL, Greenblatt DJ, Harmatz JS, et al: Psychotropic drug metabolism in old age: principles and problems of assessment, in Psychopharmacology: The Fourth Generation of Progress. Edited by Bloom FE, Kupfer DJ. New York, Raven, 1995, pp 1461–1469

Walsh T, Hadigan CM, Wong LM: Increased pulse and blood pressure associated with desipramine treatment of bulimia nervosa. J Clin Psychopharmacol 12:163–168, 1992

Washington C, Haines KA, Tam CW: Amoxapine-induced neuroleptic malignant syndrome. DICP 23:713, 1989

Weaver GA, Pavinoc D, Davis JS: Hepatic sensitivity to imipramine. Dig Dis 22:551–553, 1977

Weir TA, Goodwin FK: Can antidepressants cause mania and worsen the course of affective illness? Am J Psychiatry 144:1403–1411, 1987

Wilens TE, Biederman J, Baldessarini RJ, et al: Developmental changes in serum concentrations of desipramine and 2-hydroxydesipramine during treatment with desipramine. J Am Acad Child Adolesc Psychiatry 31:691–698, 1992

Wilens TE, Biederman J, Baldessarini RJ, et al: Electrocardiographic effects of desipramine and 2-hydroxydesipramine in children, adolescents, and adults treated with desipramine. J Am Acad Child Adolesc Psychiatry 32:789–804, 1993

Wilens TE, Biederman J, Prince J, et al: Six week, double-blind, placebo-controlled study of desipramine for adult attention deficit hyperactivity disorder. Am J Psychiatry 153:1147–1153, 1996

Yates M, Leake A, Candy JM, et al: 5-HT2 receptor changes in major depression. Biol Psychiatry 27:489–496, 1990

Yoshimura M, Furue H: Mechanisms for the anti-nociceptive actions of the descending noradrenergic and serotonergic systems in the spinal cord. J Pharmacol Sci 101:107–117, 2006

Young RC, Alexopoulos GS, Shamoian CA, et al: Plasma 10-hydroxy-nortriptyline in elderly depressed patients. Clin Pharmacol Ther 35:540–544, 1984

Young RC, Alexopoulos GS, Shamoian CA, et al: Plasma 10-hydroxynortriptyline and ECG changes in elderly depressed patients. Am J Psychiatry 142:866–868, 1985

Young RC, Alexopoulos GS, Shindledecker R, et al: Plasma 10-hydroxynortriptyline and therapeutic response in geriatric depression. Neuropsychopharmacology 1:213–215, 1988

Ziegler VE, Biggs JT: Tricyclic plasma levels: effect of age, race, sex, and smoking. JAMA 238:2167–2169, 1977

Zitrin CM, Klein DF, Woerner MG: Treatment of agoraphobia with group exposure in vivo and imipramine. Arch Gen Psychiatry 37:63–72, 1980

CHAPTER 13

Fluoxetine

Janos Zahajszky, M.D.

Jerrold F. Rosenbaum, M.D.

Gary D. Tollefson, M.D., Ph.D.

The introduction of fluoxetine as the first selective serotonin reuptake inhibitor (SSRI) approved in the United States, initially for the treatment of depression, represents an important advance in psychopharmacology and has been the catalyst for much subsequent basic and clinical research. Considerable evidence has demonstrated that fluoxetine, like other SSRIs, has a broad spectrum of clinical indications. There is a consensus, however, that the commercial success of fluoxetine (and subsequently marketed SSRIs) derived from its advantageous safety profile, which propelled SSRIs to dominance in the antidepressant drug market. Fluoxetine, under the brand name Prozac, became a cultural icon—a symbol of the growth in antidepressant prescribing and depression recognition. Consequently, it also became a focus of controversies about rare events attributed to side effects, such as violent acts and suicide, and a symbol of the medicalization of mental health concerns. Fluoxetine was also the first of the SSRI blockbuster drugs to become available in generic form; ironically, with decreased cost has come decreased market share, likely reflecting the reduction in marketing and availability of office samples. Although SSRIs, as a class, share several common features, individual agents, such as fluoxetine, also have unique characteristics.

History and Discovery

Serotonin (5-HT) is an indoleamine with wide distribution in plants, animals, and humans. Pioneering histochemistry by Falck et al. (1962) found that 5-HT was localized within specific neuronal pathways and cell bodies. These originate principally from two discrete nuclei, the medial and dorsal raphe. Across animal species, 5-HT innervation is widespread. Although regional variations exist, several limbic structures manifest especially high levels of 5-HT (A.H. Amin et al. 1954).

However, 5-HT levels in the central nervous system (CNS) represent only a small fraction of 5-HT found in the body (Bradley 1989). Because 5-HT does not cross the blood–brain barrier, it must be synthesized locally. 5-HT is released into the synapse from the cytoplasmic and vesicular reservoirs (Elks et al. 1979). Following release, 5-HT is principally inactivated by reuptake into nerve terminals through a sodium/potassium (Na^+/K^+) adenosine triphosphatase (ATPase)–dependent carrier (Shaskan and Snyder 1970). The transmitter is subsequently subject to either degradation by monoamine oxidase (MAO) or vesicular restorage. Abnormalities in central 5-HT function have been hypothesized to underlie disturbances in mood, anxiety, satiety, cognition, aggression, and sexual drives, to highlight a few. As described by Fuller (1985), there are several loci at which therapeutic drugs might alter 5-HT neurotransmission (Figure 13–1). The explosion of knowledge regarding the serotonergic

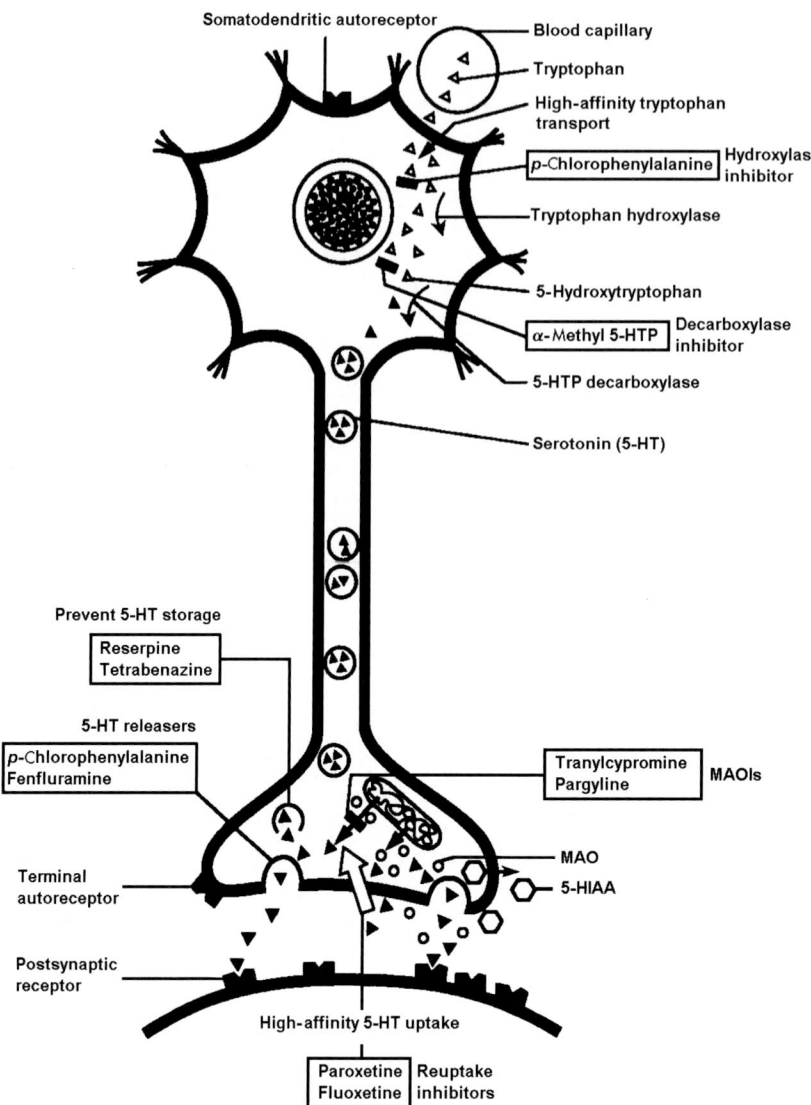

FIGURE 13-1. Serotonin (5-HT) neuron showing the main steps in the life cycle of 5-HT and the sites at which drugs act.

For clarity, drugs acting at 5-HT receptors have been omitted. 5-HIAA = 5-hydroxyindoleacetic acid; 5-HTP = 5-hydroxytryptophan; MAO = monoamine oxidase; MAOI = monoamine oxidase inhibitor.

Source. Reprinted from Marsden CA: "The Neuropharmacology of Serotonin in the Central Nervous System," in *Selective Serotonin Re-Uptake Inhibitors*. Edited by Feighner JP, Boyer WF. Chichester, England, Wiley, 1991, pp. 11–35. Copyright 1991, John Wiley and Sons Limited. Reproduced with permission.

system can largely be traced to the development of compounds, such as fluoxetine, that block the reuptake of this neurotransmitter.

Structure–Activity Relations

Drugs that inhibit 5-HT reuptake vary in their selectivity (Table 13–1). Despite the tendency to lump the contemporary SSRIs into the same class designation, significant structural and activity differences exist. Their chemical structures help illustrate this diversity (Figures 13–2 and 13–3). In contrast to paroxetine and sertraline, which exist as single isomers, fluoxetine, like citalopram, is a racemate. The family of SSRIs manifests diverse structural and activity relations. Such data are in vitro and thus subject to methodological variability (Thomas et al. 1987). Fluoxetine is less potent than paroxetine in vitro and less selective for 5-HT reuptake inhibition, relative to norepinephrine (NE), than citalopram. However, note that in

TABLE 13–1. Inhibition of [³H]monoamine uptake into rat brain synaptosomes in vitro

	K_i (NM)		
COMPOUND	[³H]-5-HT	[³H]-NE	[³H]-DA
Paroxetine	1.1	350	2,000
Citalopram	1.8	8,800	>10,000
Fluvoxamine	6.2	1,100	>10,000
Sertraline	7.3	1,400	230
Clomipramine	7.4	96	9,100
Fluoxetine	25	500	4,200
Amitriptyline	87	79	4,300

Note. DA=dopamine; 5-HT=serotonin; NE=norepinephrine.
Source. Relative values from a series of related trials from Boyer and Feighner 1991.

vitro potency does not necessarily equate with in vivo dosing experience, clinical efficacy, or adverse-event profile.

Although the tricyclic antidepressants (TCAs), like the SSRIs, antagonize 5-HT receptors (Dempsey et al. 2005; Eisensamer et al. 2003), they also exhibit inhibitory activity at other receptor targets mediating their adverse-event profile (Hall and Ogren 1981; Snyder and Yamamura 1977; U'Prichard et al. 1978). These include histaminergic, α_1-adrenergic, and muscarinic receptors. For

fluoxetine, the median inhibitory concentration (IC_{50}) at histaminergic and adrenergic sites is in the micromolar range and thus unlikely to be of clinical significance. Activity at the muscarinic receptor is negligible for fluoxetine. Stauderman et al. (1992) reported that fluoxetine and paroxetine inhibit the binding of ³H-nitrendipine to L-type calcium channels; however, this was at concentrations that were probably in excess of those achieved during in vivo treatment of depression.

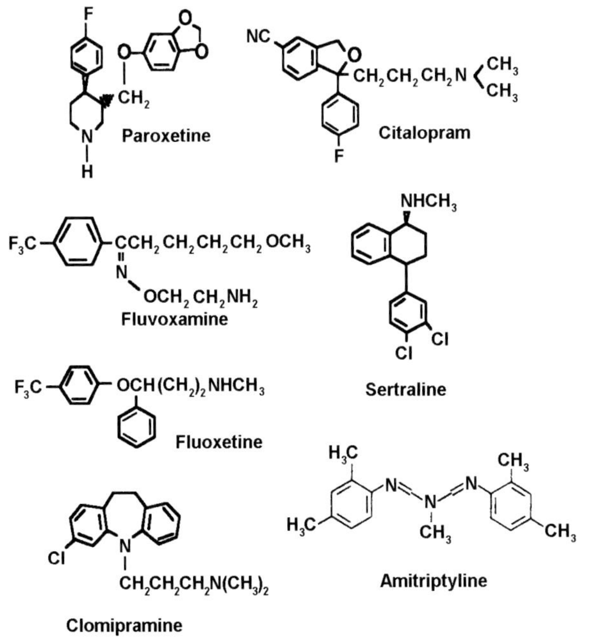

In summary, in vitro radioligand-binding techniques showed that fluoxetine had a lower probability of many of the troublesome side effects associated with TCAs and was relatively selective in its 5-HT reuptake inhibition. (For a general review of the synaptic effects of several SSRIs, compared with other antidepressants, see Richelson 1996.)

Pharmacological Profile

Serotonin

The action of any SSRI extends beyond the inhibition of 5-HT reuptake. At least 14 different 5-HT receptor subtypes reside at pre- and postsynaptic locations (Fuller 1996). Serotonin$_{1A}$ (5-HT$_{1A}$) binding sites include both somatodendritic and presynaptic autoreceptors (which inhibit 5-HT firing) and postsynaptic receptors. The lat-

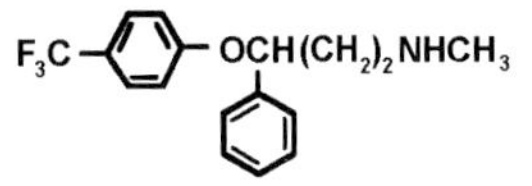

FIGURE 13–2. Chemical structures of selective serotonin reuptake inhibitors and some tricyclic antidepressants.

FIGURE 13–3. Chemical structure of fluoxetine.

ter are predominantly hippocampal, and their sensitivity is increased after chronic antidepressant exposure (Aghajanian et al. 1988; Elena Castro et al. 2003).

After chronic administration, many antidepressants downregulate or reduce the density of serotonin$_2$ (5-HT$_2$) binding sites in rat frontal cortex (Peroutka and Snyder 1980). Some, but not all, SSRIs have been associated with this effect (Fraser et al. 1988), and fluoxetine has been demonstrated to normalize 5-HT$_{1A}$ density in rats (Sodero et al. 2006). SSRIs, as a drug class, have been reported to normalize both 5-HT$_{1A}$ and 5-HT$_2$ receptor density among patients with depression (Leonard 1992).

The mechanisms by which fluoxetine and other SSRIs interact with the human serotonin transporter (SERT) are not yet fully understood. Some evidence suggests that fluoxetine's effect on SERT is partially based on SERT promoter polymorphism; it can lead to increased or decreased SERT expression, depending on an individual's genotype (Little et al. 2006). Further studies have shown that SERT may also be inhibited at the posttranslational stage, likely through multiple binding sites on the SERT molecule itself (Henry et al. 2006; Iceta et al. 2007).

Fluoxetine transiently inhibits dorsal raphe firing, decreases terminal autoreceptor function, and ultimately increases net 5-HT synaptic transmission within CA3 pyramidal cells in the hippocampus (Blier et al. 1988). Electrophysiological studies indicate that most antidepressants enhance net 5-HT transmission after chronic administration (Blier et al. 1990), albeit at different loci: the TCAs via enhanced sensitivity of postsynaptic 5-HT$_{1A}$ receptors, and the SSRIs (and MAO inhibitors [MAOIs]) via reduced sensitivity of somatodendritic (5-HT$_{1A}$) and terminal (serotonin$_{1D}$ [5-HT$_{1D}$]) autoreceptors. SSRIs and TCAs also exert an inhibitory effect on 5-HT$_3$ receptors in a noncompetitive fashion (Eisensamer et al. 2003). These observations of different mechanisms may help to explain why certain depressive symptoms that do not respond to one class of antidepressant will respond to another class and may also explain the enhanced response reported when combinations of antidepressant agents are used.

Norepinephrine

Chronic administration of most somatic treatments for depression downregulates or reduces the density of β-adrenergic binding sites in the brain (Bergstrom and Kellar 1979). These treatments include traditional NE-specific and mixed uptake inhibitors (Charney et al. 1981). However, results with the SSRIs have been less

consistent (Johnson 1991). Despite its in vitro 5-HT selectivity, fluoxetine has been observed, with autoradiography, to induce β-adrenergic receptor downregulation. It has also been shown in at least one study to increase extracellular NE concentrations in rat prefrontal cortex after acute systemic administration; this effect was not observed with other SSRIs tested (Bymaster et al. 2002). Fluoxetine has also been demonstrated to potentiate the noradrenergic effects of bupropion (Li et al. 2002).

Most studies with SSRIs have not shown a consistent change in β-adrenergic binding or β-adrenergic-stimulated cyclic adenosine monophosphate (cAMP) production. However, Baron et al. (1988) reported that fluoxetine, when it was coadministered with desipramine, augmented the reduction in cortical β-adrenergic receptors expected with desipramine alone. In contrast, investigations with fluvoxamine, paroxetine, and citalopram have not yielded consistent results. In general, the greater the 5-HT selectivity of a compound, the less in vitro evidence for β-adrenergic downregulation has been seen. Thus, β-adrenergic downregulation may not be essential for clinical efficacy.

Current data do not support a significant effect on α-adrenergic receptor affinity or density by the SSRIs. Studies using radiolabeling to investigate fluoxetine (Wong et al. 1985) have shown relative inactivity at this site. Fluoxetine has been reported to reduce desipramine-induced release of growth hormone after 4 weeks of treatment (O'Flynn et al. 1991). This effect suggests a possible indirect activity at the α$_2$-adrenergic receptor.

In summary, although relative differences in adrenoreceptor affinity exist across the SSRI class, and fluoxetine may have more adrenergic activity than some of the other SSRIs, the clinical significance of these differences appears to be negligible.

Dopamine

Animal studies provide evidence that the serotonergic system may exert tonic inhibition on the central dopaminergic system. Serotonin has also been shown to decrease the generation of dopaminergic cells from mesencephalic precursors in rats, an effect mediated by 5-HT$_4$ and 5-HT$_7$ receptors found on glial cells (Parga et al. 2007). Thus, fluoxetine might diminish dopaminergic transmission consistent with anecdotes of extrapyramidal side effects (EPS) during fluoxetine therapy (Bouchard et al. 1989). 5-HT agonists, however, also exert a facilitatory influence on dopamine (DA) release (Benloucif and Galloway 1991), which can be antagonized by the 5-HT$_1$

blocker pindolol, and evidence suggests that SSRIs may actually sensitize mesolimbic DA receptors (Arnt et al. 1984a, 1984b). Furthermore, repeated administration of fluoxetine, citalopram, or paroxetine to rats increased spontaneous dopaminergic neuronal activity (Sekine et al. 2007), and chronic fluoxetine treatment also increased brain-derived neurotrophic factor (BDNF) expression within rat dopaminergic regions (Molteni et al. 2006).

Many structurally diverse antidepressants are associated with a net enhancement of mesolimbic DA (see Klimek and Maj 1990). The benefits of antidepressants in an animal model of depression can be antagonized by a dopamine$_1$ (D$_1$) (SCH-23390) or dopamine$_2$ (D$_2$) blocker (sulpiride) (Sampson et al. 1991). Repeated administration of several SSRIs was found to increase the hypermotility response to several dopaminergic agents, including amphetamine, methylphenidate (Arnt et al. 1984b), quinpirole (Maj et al. 1984), and apomorphine (Plaznik and Kostowski 1987).

The induction of catalepsy or the inhibition of apomorphine-induced catalepsy is not a property of the SSRIs. Both citalopram and fluoxetine have been inactive in displacing D$_2$ blockers (Peroutka and Snyder 1980). Baldessarini et al. (1992) reported that fluoxetine "even at high doses or with repeated treatment" demonstrated "no significant inhibition of the DA metabolism—increasing actions of haloperidol" (p. 191).

In summary, fluoxetine enhances central 5-HT transmission through increased output and/or increased postsynaptic receptor sensitivity (Blier et al. 1987). Fluoxetine's overall effects on the noradrenergic and dopaminergic systems are less straightforward and are also less likely to play a role in the drug's antidepressant effects. However, such changes alone, in any of the neurotransmitter systems, do not guarantee a clinically meaningful response (Charney et al. 1984). A change in baseline 5-HT function or a "permissive" set of interactions with other collocated neurotransmitter receptors is likely involved in the highly individualized responses in patients with depression.

Pharmacokinetics and Disposition

As demonstrated in Table 13–2, considerable pharmacokinetic variability exists within the SSRI class (Leonard 1992). Of particular note, discussion of drug half-life must also include consideration of the presence or absence of active metabolites. Fluoxetine is extensively metabolized by the liver's cytochrome P450 (CYP) system to its active

metabolite, norfluoxetine. Fluoxetine is a potent CYP2D6 inhibitor, and norfluoxetine has a moderate inhibitory effect on CYP3A4 (Hemeryck and Belpaire 2002). The elimination half-life of norfluoxetine (4–16 days) is significantly longer than that of fluoxetine (4–6 days); in fact, norfluoxetine's half-life is the longest of any of the SSRIs or their active metabolites (see Table 13–2). Half-life is not significantly affected by hemodialysis or renal impairment (Aronoff et al. 1984).

The relatively long half-life of fluoxetine confers greater protection from the discontinuation syndrome that is associated with abrupt discontinuation or noncompliance related to interruption of treatment than more rapidly cleared SSRIs. Conversely, more prolonged vigilance for drug–drug interactions following discontinuation is required for fluoxetine; for example, a 5-week washout from fluoxetine is recommended before initiating an MAOI (Ciraulo and Shader 1990; Lane and Baldwin 1997). Variability in drug half-life is associated with a range in time to steady-state plasma concentrations, which does not clearly predict or correlate with onset of antidepressant activity.

Mechanism of Action

In the absence of pharmacological manipulation, the reuptake of 5-HT into the presynaptic nerve terminal typically leads to its inactivation. Fluoxetine, through blockade of the reuptake process, acutely enhances serotonergic neurotransmission by permitting 5-HT to act for an extended period of time at synaptic binding sites. A net result is an acute increase in synaptic 5-HT. One difference separating SSRIs from direct-acting agonists is that SSRIs are dependent on neuronal release of 5-HT for their action—that is, SSRIs can be considered augmenters of basal physiological signals, but they are not direct stimulators of postsynaptic receptor function and they are dependent on presynaptic neuronal integrity. These pharmacodynamic features might explain SSRI nonresponse. If the release of 5-HT from presynaptic neuronal storage sites is substantially compromised, and in turn, if net synaptic 5-HT concentration is negligible, a clinically meaningful response to an SSRI would not be expected.

Serotonin receptors also include a family of presynaptic autoreceptors that suppress the further release of 5-HT, thus limiting the degree of postsynaptic receptor stimulation that can be achieved. de Montigny et al. (1989) investigated the mechanism of action of several SSRIs and suggested that the enhanced efficacy of serotonergic syn-

TABLE 13–2.   A comparison of several selective serotonin reuptake inhibitors

	FLUOXETINE	PAROXETINE	SERTRALINE	CITALOPRAM	FLUVOXAMINE	ESCITALOPRAM
Volume of distribution (L/kg)	3–40	17	20	12–16	>5	12–16
Percentage protein bound	94	95	99	80	77	56
Peak plasma level (hours)	6–8	2–8	6–8	1–6	2–8	5
Parent half-life (hours)	24–72	20	24–26	33	15	27–32
Major metabolite half-life	4–16 days	NA	66 hours	NA	NA	NA
Standard dose range (mg)	20–80	10–50	50–200	10–40	50–300	10–20
Absorption altered by fast or fed status	No	No	Yes	No	No	No
Altered half-life in geriatric patient	No	Yes	Yes	Yes	No	Yes
Reduced clearance in renal patients[a]	±	+	±	±	±	±

Note.   NA = not applicable.
[a]+=yes; ±=somewhat/mixed.

aptic transmission is not the result of increased postsynaptic sensitivity. Rather, longer-term SSRI treatment induced a desensitization of somatodendritic and terminal 5-HT autoreceptors. This desensitization would permit 5-HT neurons to reestablish a normal rate of firing, despite sustained reuptake blockade. These neurons could then release a greater amount of 5-HT (per impulse) into the synaptic cleft. This modification reportedly occurs over a time course that is compatible with the antidepressant response.

Indications and Efficacy

The U.S. Food and Drug Administration (FDA)–labeled indications for fluoxetine are major depressive disorder, obsessive-compulsive disorder (OCD), panic disorder, bulimia nervosa, and premenstrual dysphoric disorder (PMDD). We will review these as well as some other disorders for which fluoxetine is commonly used.

Major Depressive Disorder

Placebo-controlled, double-blind trials have established the superiority of fluoxetine over placebo (Kasper et al. 1992). Statistically significant reductions from baseline in the Hamilton Rating Scale for Depression (Ham-D; Hamilton 1960) score have been seen as early as the second week of treatment; however, the rate and quality of response to any SSRI are highly individualized (range, 10–42 days). Overall, the efficacy of fluoxetine has been

found to be comparable to or slightly better than that of conventional TCAs (Cipriani et al. 2005; Wernicke et al. 1987) and comparable to that of venlafaxine (Nemeroff et al. 2007; Schatzberg and Roose 2006). Notwithstanding, in a survey of 439 clinicians, about one-quarter indicated that they believed SSRIs to be the most efficacious antidepressant class, despite a lack of clear empirical evidence (Petersen et al. 2002). Within the class of SSRIs, there is no clear and consistent evidence for superior effectiveness of one agent over another in primary care settings (Kroenke et al. 2001).

In general, the range for dose titration with most SSRIs is relatively narrow (see Table 13–2), and higher dosages are more often associated with increased adverse events (Altamura et al. 1988; M. Amin et al. 1989). Schweizer et al. (1990) reported that in a study of 108 subjects treated with 20 mg of fluoxetine for 3 weeks and then randomly assigned to either 20 mg or 60 mg for another 5 weeks, both groups did equally well after 8 weeks.

However, early implementation of high-dose therapy may be appropriate in some circumstances. Conversion of nonresponders by prescribing at the higher end of the dose range has been described with fluoxetine (Fava et al. 1992). Unfortunately, plasma-level studies have contributed little toward the understanding of the dose–response relationship. Most studies have failed to confirm any relationship between clinical response and plasma concentration with fluoxetine (Kelly et al. 1989). This suggests that synaptic concentrations and/or pharmacodynamic effects are not accurately reflected by plasma levels.

Continued efficacy of fluoxetine during maintenance therapy has been established in several trials (Danion 1989; Dufour 1987; Ferrey et al. 1989; Montgomery et al. 1988; Reimherr et al. 1998). One trial reported a recurrence in 54 of 94 placebo subjects (57%) versus 23 of 88 fluoxetine-maintained subjects (26%) (*P*<0.0001) who had at least 4.5 months of recovery before randomization (Montgomery et al. 1988). Study participants were required to have had at least two previous episodes.

Although fluoxetine is perceived as "activating," considerable evidence supports its utility in depression with anxious features. Montgomery (1989a) conducted a meta-analysis of several fluoxetine trials that indicated efficacy in depression featuring anxiety and psychomotor agitation. Similar findings have been reported by Jouvent et al. (1989) and Beasley et al. (1991).

In an attempt to improve compliance with long-term antidepressant treatment, a once-weekly formulation of fluoxetine was developed and approved. Although the concept appears reasonable and the preparation, a once-weekly enteric-coated 90-mg tablet, is safe and efficacious for continuation treatment (Schmidt et al. 2000), this formulation has not attracted widespread use, which suggests that a once-daily formulation may be convenient enough for most patients.

Obsessive-Compulsive Disorder

Clomipramine, a potent inhibitor of both 5-HT and NE reuptake, was observed more than 30 years ago to reduce obsessive-compulsive symptoms (Renynghe de Voxurie 1968). The superior benefit of this potent serotonergic TCA over desipramine represents a cornerstone in the 5-HT hypothesis of OCD (Benkelfat et al. 1989). Fluoxetine has been shown to be effective in OCD independent of a patient's comorbid mood status (Jenike et al. 1989). Patients who have OCD may require higher doses of medication and longer treatment periods than do patients with depression to determine response. Currently, clomipramine and the SSRIs are considered to be the first-line agents for treatment of OCD (Kaplan and Hollander 2003).

A precise explanation of this selective 5-HT advantage in OCD is unknown. A heightened level of metabolic activity in the orbital region and caudate dysfunction have been reported by Baxter et al. (1992) and may be normalized by either somatic (fluoxetine 60–80 mg) or behavioral interventions. Hypersensitivity of the serotonergic system has been theorized. Receptor downregulation associated with long-term SSRI therapy has been

offered as a potential explanation of clinical response (Zohar et al. 1988). This hypothetical neuroadaptation is supported by a positive correlation between symptomatic improvement from baseline and cerebrospinal fluid (CSF) 5-hydroxyindoleacetic acid (5-HIAA) (Thorén et al. 1980) or platelet 5-HT concentration (Flament et al. 1985). Chronic administration of fluoxetine attenuates ipsapirone-induced hypothermia and adrenocorticotropic hormone (ACTH) and cortisol release among patients with primary OCD. Although these data support a model of drug-induced 5-HT$_{1A}$ subsensitivity and/or dampened postreceptor signal, the magnitude of change fails to correlate with the degree of clinical improvement (Lesch et al. 1991). An SSRI-mediated decrease in 5-HT responsivity is consistent with the observed latency in symptomatic improvement.

Because OCD is a chronic disorder, prolonged fluoxetine therapy may be necessary. In patients whose symptoms have been minimally or only moderately reduced with SSRI treatment, numerous augmentation strategies have been proposed, including tryptophan, fenfluramine, lithium, buspirone, trazodone, or a neuroleptic (see Goodman et al. 1992). In addition, fluoxetine has shown efficacy in children and adolescents with OCD (Geller et al. 2001). In so-called OCD spectrum disorders, such as skin picking (Bloch et al. 2001) and body dysmorphic disorder (Phillips et al. 2002), controlled trials also indicate efficacy for fluoxetine.

Panic Disorder

SSRIs are the drugs of choice in the prevention of panic attacks and in the treatment of panic disorder. Positive results from double-blind, placebo-controlled trials in patients with panic disorder are available for fluoxetine (Michelson et al. 2001). In general, patients with panic disorder need a low initial dose of fluoxetine (e.g., 10 mg); however, often usual antidepressant dosing for optimal response (e.g., 20–80 mg) is required. The initial low dose serves to minimize early side effects in anxious patients who are particularly sensitive to somatic symptoms of anxiety, and it sets the stage for long-term compliance. The recurrent and chronic nature of panic disorder requires individual medication regimens that may include multiple agents as well as variable dosages.

Eating Disorders

Manipulation of central 5-HT results in significantly altered feeding behaviors (e.g., an increased satiety response) (Carruba et al. 1986). Blundell (1986) reported that pharmacological enhancement of 5-HT reduced meal size, rate of eating, and body weight. The predominant locus of this 5-HT effect is likely within the hypothalamus and may be mediated through gene expression of neuropeptide Y (NPY) and pro-opiomelanocortin (POMC) (Myung et al. 2005). In general, the ability of an antidepressant to diminish appetite and, in turn, to reduce weight is related to its ability to block 5-HT uptake (Angel et al. 1988). One exception may be paroxetine, a highly potent 5-HT uptake inhibitor that, compared with conventional TCAs, was associated with a similar proportion of subjects in clinical trial experience reporting weight gain (Dechant and Clissold 1991). Paroxetine, compared with fluoxetine and sertraline over time in patients with depression, was associated with more significant weight gain (Fava et al. 2000). Selective 5-HT$_{1A}$ activation in some patients may influence weight gain (Dourish et al. 1986).

Bulimia Nervosa

5-HT involvement in bulimia nervosa has been based on several observations (Jimerson et al. 1989; Kaye et al. 1988). Kaye et al. (1988) hypothesized that variations in the ratio of tryptophan to other amino acids, consequent to recurrent bingeing and vomiting, mediated both satiety and mood. Some patients with bulimia nervosa, independent of mood status, manifest a blunted prolactin response to m-chlorophenylpiperazine (m-CPP). This has been interpreted as evidence of postsynaptic 5-HT hypersensitivity within select hypothalamic pathways (Brewerton et al. 1990).

Goldbloom et al. (1988) reported that the V$_{max}$ (maximum velocity)—the maximum amount of substrate per unit of time that an enzyme can break down or synthesize at saturation (i.e., when all of the enzyme's active sites are filled)—of platelet 5-HT uptake was increased among bulimic patients without depression. Jimerson et al. (1989) observed a significant inverse association between CSF 5-HIAA and symptom severity. However, much of the support for a 5-HT role in bulimia nervosa comes from pharmacotherapeutic experience. Agents with at least some degree of 5-HT uptake inhibition have been useful in bulimia nervosa (see Brewerton et al. 1990).

Clinical trials with fluoxetine have found a positive treatment effect on binge eating and purging behaviors (Goldstein et al. 1995). In a large placebo-controlled trial, Enas et al. (1989) studied dosing of 20 mg versus 60 mg of fluoxetine in 382 female outpatients with bu-

limia. A clinical benefit was observed in binge frequency, purging, mood, and carbohydrate craving. In a smaller study of 91 female patients in a primary care setting, women assigned to fluoxetine kept more physician appointments, exhibited greater reductions in binge eating and vomiting, and had a greater improvement in psychological symptoms than those assigned to placebo (Walsh et al. 2004). Continued treatment with fluoxetine is associated with improvement and decreased risk of relapse (Romano et al. 2002).

Anorexia Nervosa

A 5-HT disturbance in anorexia nervosa was postulated by Fanelli et al. (1986). Coppen et al. (1976) reported a reduction in plasma L-tryptophan among patients with anorexia. Others have observed that platelet imipramine binding is decreased (Weizman et al. 1986); however, these findings have not been uniformly replicated. Brewerton et al. (1990) suggested that hypothalamic 5-HT responsivity at or beyond postsynaptic sites is abnormal in subjects with anorexia nervosa.

Pharmacological trials with SSRIs in patients with anorexia nervosa have been relatively sparse. Kaye et al. (1991) suggested that fluoxetine may help maintain body weight in patients with anorexia nervosa who have gained weight. This group also completed a similar study with fluoxetine under controlled conditions, suggesting some benefit for fluoxetine in improving outcome and preventing relapse (Kaye et al. 2001). On the other hand, Walsh et al. (2006) found no benefit for continued treatment with fluoxetine after weight restoration in a randomized, double-blind, placebo-controlled trial of 93 patients. Efficacy of SSRIs has been linked to the food obsessions of many patients with eating disorders.

Premenstrual Dysphoric Disorder

Several randomized, blinded, placebo-controlled trials that used various diagnostic criteria and outcome measures have established the efficacy and tolerability of fluoxetine in the treatment of PMDD (Menkes et al. 1993; Pearlstein et al. 1997; Steiner et al. 1995; Su et al. 1993, 1997; Wood et al. 1992). In the largest study, 313 women with DSM-III-R–defined late luteal phase dysphoric disorder (American Psychiatric Association 1987) received 20 mg of fluoxetine, 60 mg of fluoxetine, or placebo daily for six menstrual cycles after a two-cycle placebo washout period (Steiner et al. 1995). One hundred eighty women completed the study. Both doses of fluoxetine were superior to placebo, beginning at the first menstrual cycle and continuing throughout the six cycles. More patients treated with 60 mg of fluoxetine discontinued because of adverse events than did patients treated with 20 mg of fluoxetine or placebo. More patients treated with placebo discontinued because of lack of response than did patients treated with either fluoxetine dose. In a subsequent study of 34 women, fluoxetine was significantly superior to bupropion and placebo in treating PMDD (Pearlstein et al. 1997).

Anger and Aggression

Diminished serotonergic activity has been implicated in the personality features of impulsivity, anger, hostility, and aggression (Coccaro et al. 1989). These clinical attributes best associate with DSM-IV (American Psychiatric Association 1994) Cluster B personality disorders. Fluoxetine reduced impulsivity in small groups of patients with borderline personality disorder (Cornelius et al. 1991; Norden 1989). Fluoxetine significantly reduced anger attacks in patients with and without depression (Fava et al. 1991, 1993, 1996; Rubey et al. 1996; Salzman et al. 1995).

Posttraumatic Stress Disorder

Fluoxetine significantly reduced symptoms of posttraumatic stress disorder (PTSD), compared with placebo, in 64 patients (veterans and nonveterans), as measured by the Clinician-Administered PTSD Scale (CAPS) (Van der Kolk et al. 1994). It also showed efficacy by week 6 in a large double-blind, placebo-controlled trial (Martenyi et al. 2002).

Premature Ejaculation

SSRIs, including fluoxetine, are effective in the treatment of premature ejaculation, although increased latency to ejaculation is highest with paroxetine (Waldinger et al. 1998). In a 1-year follow-up study, patients treated with fluoxetine (20 mg/day or less) in combination with sexual behavior therapy reported significant improvement in ejaculation latency (Graziottin et al. 1996). Another study demonstrated efficacy from a weekly fluoxetine dose of 90 mg (Manasia et al. 2003). Clear-cut dosing recommendations have not been clarified, however, and titration (upward or downward) may be necessary.

Pain Syndromes

Fluoxetine has shown efficacy in reducing pain associated with diabetic neuropathy (Max et al. 1992). Fluoxetine (20 mg/day) improved scores on measures of pain and dis-

comfort in subjects with fibromyalgia, compared with subjects on placebo (Arnold et al. 2002; Goldenberg et al. 1996). The effect of fluoxetine combined with amitriptyline was superior to the effect of either agent used alone. Fluoxetine reduced the number of attacks in patients with migraine headaches (Saper et al. 1994). More recent work has demonstrated that antidepressants that also affect the NE system (i.e., serotonin–norepinephrine reuptake inhibitors [SNRIs]) are more effective than the SSRIs in treating neuropathic pain (Mochizucki 2004; L.H. Pedersen et al. 2005). In fact, the SNRI duloxetine has received FDA approval for the treatment of neuropathic pain.

Alcohol Abuse and Dependence

A substantial amount of evidence supports a 5-HT dysfunction in alcohol abuse and dependence. Animal studies have shown that increased 5-HT levels reduce alcohol consumption (Farren 1995). For example, Murphy et al. (1988) reported beneficial effects with fluoxetine and fluvoxamine in reducing alcohol intake in a rat model.

Although results are not consistent, some clinical trials with SSRIs have reported reduced alcohol consumption in patients with and without depression, in contrast to patients treated with TCAs, which have less robust efficacy (Cornelius et al. 1997; Lejoyeux 1996). A precise mechanism for the role of SSRIs in the treatment of alcohol dependence is not understood. To date, the beneficial effect, if any, appears to be independent of antidepressant activity (Naranjo et al. 1986, 1990). More work is needed to determine the specific patient subpopulations that might benefit most from SSRIs (see Gorelick 1989).

From a risk–benefit assessment, it is reassuring that fluoxetine does not appear to potentiate the effects of ethanol (Lemberger et al. 1985) and does not carry a high risk of fatal poisoning when taken in combination with alcohol (Koski et al. 2005). SSRIs may help selected patients with alcohol dependence in recovery when these drugs are used as part of a multifaceted treatment program.

Obesity

SSRIs have been extensively investigated for an effect on food consumption. This interest stems from evidence that perturbation of 5-HT receptors modifies animal feeding behavior (Garattini et al. 1986). This modification appears to be independent of a local gastrointestinal effect (e.g., the perception of nausea). 5-HT innervation to the hypothalamus influences satiety and may selectively affect carbohydrate consumption (Wurtman et al. 1981). In one large trial, 458 patients were treated for 52 weeks with fluoxetine (60 mg/day) or placebo (Goldstein et al. 1994). Weight loss was significantly greater in the fluoxetine-treated group at 28 weeks, but not at 52 weeks. Long-term benefits may be better sustained when fluoxetine is combined with behavior modification (Marcus et al. 1990).

The broad involvement of the serotonergic system in modulating behavior and cognition supports the wide potential utility of SSRIs.

Other Medical Conditions

Fluoxetine has been evaluated and observed to be efficacious in a variety of medical conditions, including post-stroke depression, fibromyalgia, chronic pain, and depression in cancer patients. It has also proved useful in some patients with chronic fatigue syndrome.

Side Effects and Toxicology

Safety and a favorable side-effect profile, as well as the lack of multiple receptor affinity that mediates adverse events associated with TCAs, distinguish fluoxetine and other SSRIs from TCAs. Medications in the SSRI class generally have similar side-effect profiles.

For most patients, SSRIs are better tolerated than TCAs, based on the number of early trial discontinuations attributable to an adverse event (see Boyer and Feighner 1991). In general, for three-arm trials, the incidence of early discontinuation due to an adverse event was 5%–10% for placebo, 10%–20% for SSRIs, and 30%–35% for TCAs. The SSRIs, presumably by enhancement of 5-HT within the CNS, may induce agitation, anxiety, sleep disturbance, tremor, sexual dysfunction (primarily anorgasmia), or headache. Baseline clinical features do not appear to predispose patients to these adverse events (Montgomery 1989b). Although CNS adverse events may occur with SSRIs, Kerr et al. (1991) suggested that these drugs have a more favorable profile of behavioral toxicity overall than do conventional TCAs.

Because the enteric nervous system is richly innervated by 5-HT, adverse events may include altered gastrointestinal motility and nausea. Certain autonomic adverse events, including dry mouth, sweating, and weight change, also occur.

Fluoxetine decreases rapid eye movement (REM) and increases non–rapid eye movement (NREM) sleep at dose ranges of 5–40 mg/kg in rodent models (Gao et al.

1992). This is a common property of many antidepressant medications. Of interest, fluoxetine induces higher rates of sedation as dosages are increased.

As was discussed earlier in this chapter, fluoxetine is unlikely to alter DA function; nonetheless, some side effects, such as hyperprolactinemia, extrapyramidal symptoms, sexual and cognitive dysfunction, galactorrhea, mammary hypertrophy, and gynecomastia, have been attributed to SSRI effects on the dopaminergic system (Damsa et al. 2004). Anecdotal reports of EPS (Meltzer et al. 1979) associated with SSRIs are not more frequent than those reported historically with TCAs (Fann et al. 1976; Zubenko et al. 1987), MAOIs (Teusink et al. 1984), or trazodone (Papini et al. 1982). Very rare events, including arthralgia, lymphadenopathy, syndrome of inappropriate antidiuretic hormone (SIADH) secretion, agranulocytosis, and hypoglycemia, have been reported during clinical trials or postmarketing surveillance; however, causality typically is uncertain.

One additional rare and life-threatening event associated with all SSRIs (and, more prominently, their interaction with MAOIs or other 5-HT enhancers) is the central 5-HT syndrome. This phenomenon appears to represent an overactivation of central 5-HT receptors and may manifest with features such as abdominal pain, diarrhea, sweating, fever, tachycardia, elevated blood pressure, altered mental state (e.g., delirium), myoclonus, increased motor activity, irritability, hostility, and mood change. Severe manifestations of this syndrome can induce hyperpyrexia, cardiovascular shock, or death. There are insufficient data to rate one MAOI or SSRI as more or less likely to be associated with 5-HT syndrome. The risk of 5-HT syndrome seems to be increased when an SSRI is administered temporally with a second 5-HT–enhancing agent (e.g., an MAOI) (Marley and Wozniak 1984a, 1984b). When switching from an SSRI to an MAOI, drug half-life (and that of any active metabolite, where applicable) should serve as a guide to the length of the washout period. A standard recommendation is to wait at least five times the half-life of the SSRI or its metabolite, whichever is longer, before administering the next serotonergic agent (for a review, see Lane and Baldwin 1997). For fluoxetine, this means a minimum 5-week washout period.

Although some variability in adverse-event frequency has been reported among the SSRIs, all of the SSRIs are characterized by the above-mentioned features. Tolerance to an adverse event may change with dose and/or length of exposure; higher doses are typically associated with higher rates of adverse events (Bressa et al. 1989). Many events, such as activation, are transient, usually beginning early in the course of therapy and then remitting (Beasley et al. 1991). Comparisons between A.M. and P.M. administration did not identify differences in efficacy (Usher et al. 1991). Individual patient differences suggest the need for some flexibility in dosing schedules. TCAs behave like type IA antiarrhythmics; therefore, in a dose-dependent fashion, they may retard His-Purkinje conduction. SSRIs are essentially devoid of this property. In clinical trials, the incidence of increased heart rate or conduction disturbance has been very low with fluoxetine (Fisch 1985). For a review of the relative side-effect profiles of TCAs and SSRIs, see Brambilla et al. (2005).

Specific Issues

Suicidality

Evidence implicating 5-HT in suicide or violence is compelling. Reduced CSF 5-HIAA concentrations correlate highly with completed suicides in patients with depression (Edman et al. 1986; Ninan et al. 1984). In vitro binding assays have shown an increased density (B_{max}) of 5-HT_2 receptors in individuals with depression and suicidal tendencies (Pandey et al. 1990). Both observations are consistent with a relative state of 5-HT depletion among subjects with suicidal tendencies. The American College of Neuropsychopharmacology (1992) reviewed evidence showing that antidepressants result in substantial improvement or remission of suicidal ideation and impulses in the vast majority of patients. SSRIs were thought to potentially "carry a lower risk for suicide than older tricyclic antidepressants" (p. 181) when taken in overdose. Furthermore, the task force stated that no evidence indicated that SSRIs triggered emergent suicidal ideation above base rates associated with depression. In addition, Warshaw and Keller (1996) determined that fluoxetine use did not increase the rate of suicide in a group of 654 patients with anxiety disorders. In a large retrospective review of patients receiving one or more of 10 antidepressants (including fluoxetine), Jick et al. (1995) concluded that the risk for suicide was similar among all agents.

Concern about suicidality surged in 2003 after the industry alerted the FDA that there might be an increased risk of suicide-related adverse events in children being treated with paroxetine. The FDA's review of available data found that approximately 4% of children taking SSRI medications reported or exhibited suicidal thinking or behavior (including suicide attempts), twice the rate of those taking placebo. No completed suicides occurred among nearly 2,200 children treated with SSRIs, however.

The FDA's review was followed by a number of other studies examining this issue, including a meta-analysis of 24 pediatric trials of nine antidepressant drugs by Hammad et al. (2006). These authors found a modestly increased risk of suicidality (risk ratio=1.66) for SSRIs in depression trials (95% confidence interval=1.02–2.68). This risk must be balanced against the benefit—in the form of general improvement in mood and overall functioning—experienced by most depressed patients when they are placed on antidepressant therapy. In most cases, the therapeutic benefit of SSRIs will outweigh the risk of increased suicidal thoughts or behaviors (Bridge et al. 2007).

Black Box Warning

On March 22, 2004, the FDA issued a public health advisory warning of the risk of worsened depression and suicidality in children and adolescents being treated with antidepressant medications. This was followed by placement of a black box warning on the packaging of all antidepressant medications, revised in 2006 to include adults through age 25 years (for the full text of the 2007 revision, see http://www.fda.gov/cder/drug/antidepressants/antidepressants_label_change_2007.pdf).

Pregnancy and Lactation

Given the widespread use of SSRIs and the high prevalence of mood disorders during the childbearing years, it is likely that these agents are being used during pregnancy and breast feeding. Published information about the use and safety of SSRIs in this special population is greatest for fluoxetine. Goldstein et al. (1997) evaluated the outcomes of 796 prospectively identified pregnancies with confirmed first-trimester exposure to fluoxetine. Historical reports of newborn surveys were used for comparison. Abnormalities were observed in 5% of the fluoxetine-exposed newborns, which was consistent with historical controls.

Pregnancy outcomes and follow-up cognitive and behavioral assessments of 135 children exposed in utero to a TCA or fluoxetine (55 infants) were compared with those in a control group of infant–mother pairs (Nulman et al. 1997). The incidence of major malformations and perinatal complications was similar among the three groups. No statistically significant differences in mean global intelligence quotient (IQ) scores or language development were found in the children of mothers who received a TCA or fluoxetine or control mothers. There were also no differences among the groups on several behavioral assessments. The results of children exposed during the first trimester were not different from those of children exposed throughout the pregnancy. Prospectively derived data are not available for paroxetine, sertraline, fluvoxamine, or citalopram.

Fluoxetine is secreted into breast milk (Hendrick et al. 2001). The implications of this minimal exposure are unclear, but one naturalistic study (Taddio et al. 1996) and two case reports (Burch and Wells 1992; Isenberg 1990), with a total of 13 infants, noted no adverse effects in these infants during the short-term study periods. One case report did describe adverse events in a breast-fed infant whose mother was taking fluoxetine (Lester et al. 1993).

Fractures

Several studies have found a 1.5- to twofold increase in the risk of bone fractures in elderly patients taking TCAs or SSRIs. In a cohort study of more than 8,000 community-dwelling older women followed for almost 5 years, the risk of nonspinal fractures increased by a factor of 1.7 for those taking TCAs or SSRIs (Ensrud et al. 2003). More recently, a randomized cohort of 5,008 community-dwelling adults older than 50 years followed for a 5-year period found a 2.1-fold increase in the rate of fractures for those taking SSRIs (Richards et al. 2007). In this study, SSRI use was also associated with increased risk of falls, lower bone mineral density at the hip, and a trend toward lower bone mineral density at the spine in a dose- dependent fashion.

Animal models have so far failed to consistently demonstrate significant changes in bone architecture as a result of SSRI exposure, and the exact mechanism by which SSRIs may lead to fractures in humans is still unclear. There does appear to be, however, a functional serotonin 5-HT system in osteoclasts and osteoblasts involving both receptor activation and 5-HT reuptake (Battaglino et al. 2007).

SSRI Discontinuation Syndrome

Discontinuation symptoms have been described with several classes of antidepressants, including TCAs and MAOIs. SSRI discontinuation symptoms have been reported most frequently with paroxetine (short elimination half-life and no active metabolite) and least frequently with fluoxetine (long elimination half-lives of parent compound and active metabolite) (Haddad 1997; Stahl et al. 1997). SSRIs are not drugs of abuse; when these agents are discontinued, patients show neither the characteristic abstinence syndrome of CNS-depressant withdrawal nor drug-seeking behavior. The most com-

mon physical symptoms are dizziness, nausea and vomiting, fatigue, lethargy, flulike symptoms (e.g., aches and chills), and sensory and sleep disturbances. The psychological symptoms most commonly reported are anxiety, irritability, and crying spells. For most patients, the discontinuation symptoms are different from the adverse effects that they may have experienced while taking an SSRI. Discontinuation symptoms most often emerge within 1–3 days (Schatzberg et al. 1997).

Until recently, most information about SSRI discontinuation syndrome came from case reports or retrospective analyses. Rosenbaum et al. (1998) compared the effects of a 5- to 8-day abrupt discontinuation period from fluoxetine, paroxetine, or sertraline in three groups of patients with depression receiving maintenance therapy. Patients from the paroxetine and sertraline groups had a significant increase in adverse events, whereas patients in the fluoxetine group experienced no increase in adverse events.

In a more extended evaluation, the effects of abrupt discontinuation of fluoxetine were studied in 195 patients with depression (Zajecka et al. 1998). Patients whose depression remitted while taking fluoxetine were randomly assigned to continue fluoxetine (20 mg/day) or to discontinue abruptly to placebo, and they were monitored for 6 weeks. Reports of adverse events were similar for both groups.

In summary, SSRIs with short half-lives (paroxetine and fluvoxamine) and related drugs, such as venlafaxine, should be tapered. Fluoxetine does not require tapering because of its extended half-life.

Overdose

A major advantage of SSRIs, relative to other antidepressants, has been their superior therapeutic index (Cooper 1988; O.L. Pedersen et al. 1982). The number of deaths per 1 million prescriptions, across several SSRIs (0–6), is substantially lower than that for conventional TCAs (8–53) or MAOIs (0–61) (Leonard 1992).

Borys et al. (1992) reported on 234 cases of fluoxetine overdose (serum level = 232–1,390 ng/mL) obtained in a prospective multicenter study. Fluoxetine was the sole ingestant in 87 cases; in the remaining 147 cases, it was taken in combination with alcohol and/or other drugs. Common symptoms included tachycardia, sedation, tremor, nausea, and emesis. The authors concluded that the emergent symptoms were minor and of short duration; thus, aggressive supportive care "is the only intervention necessary" (p. 115).

Drug–Drug Interactions

Although the potential for significant interactions exists, SSRIs are unlikely to be associated with many of the conventional problems seen with the earlier antidepressants. These problems include the cumulative CNS-depressant effects with alcohol, anticholinergic agents, or antihistaminic compounds. The structural differences among SSRIs (see Figure 13–2) offer a basis for some intraclass differences. Lithium concentrations are generally unaffected.

One potential for clinically relevant antidepressant pharmacokinetic interactions is based on the drug effect on the cytochrome P450 family of enzymes (Brosen and Gram 1989). For example, SSRIs are both substrates for and inhibitors of oxidation via cytochrome P450 2D6. Crewe et al. (1992) ranked the potency of 2D6 inhibition for serotonergic antidepressants, revealing the most clinically relevant effects on 2D6 for paroxetine and fluoxetine and less relevant effects for sertraline, fluvoxamine, citalopram, clomipramine, and amitriptyline.

Through inhibition of 2D6, fluoxetine may elevate the concentration of concomitantly administered drugs that rely on this enzyme for metabolism. This has particular clinical relevance when the second agent has a narrow therapeutic index. Examples of such agents include flecainide, quinidine, carbamazepine, propafenone, TCAs, and several antipsychotics (Rudorfer and Potter 1989). The clinical consequence of such an interaction may either enhance or impair efficacy and/or heighten the adverse-event profile.

The data with respect to fluoxetine's inhibition of other cytochrome P450 enzymes, such as 3A3/4, 2C9, and 2C19, are less consistent, but the potential for interaction exists.

Conclusion

Fluoxetine has been shown to be a safe and effective drug that has proved to be better tolerated than TCAs and to have a superior safety profile in overdose for patients with comorbid medical illness. Evidence suggests a broad utilitarian role for fluoxetine across a spectrum of psychopathology.

References

Aghajanian JK, Sprouse JS, Rasmussen K: Electrophysiology of central serotonin receptor subtypes, in The Serotonin Receptors. Edited by Sanders-Bush E. Clifton, NJ, Humana Press, 1988, pp 225–252

Altamura AC, Montgomery SA, Wernicke JF: The evidence for 20 mg a day of fluoxetine as the optimal dose in the treatment of depression. Br J Psychiatry 153:109–112, 1988

American College of Neuropsychopharmacology: Suicidal behavior and psychotropic medication (consensus statement). Neuropsychopharmacology 8:177–183, 1992

American Psychiatric Association: Diagnostic and Statistical Manual of Mental Disorders, 3rd Edition, Revised. Washington, DC, American Psychiatric Association, 1987

American Psychiatric Association: Diagnostic and Statistical Manual of Mental Disorders, 4th Edition. Washington, DC, American Psychiatric Association, 1994

Amin AH, Crawford TBB, Gaddum JH: The distribution of substance P and 5-hydroxytryptamine in the central nervous system of the dog. J Physiol (Lond) 126:596–618, 1954

Amin M, Lehmann H, Mirmiran J: A double blind, placebo-controlled, dose-finding study with sertraline. Psychopharmacol Bull 25:164–167, 1989

Angel I, Taranger MA, Claustrey Y, et al: Anorectic activities of serotonin uptake inhibitors: correlation with their potencies at inhibiting serotonin uptake in vivo and with 3H-mazindol binding in vitro. Life Sci 43:651–658, 1988

Arnold LM, Hess EV, Hudson JI, et al: A randomized, placebo-controlled, double-blind, flexible-dose study of fluoxetine in the treatment of women with fibromyalgia. Am J Med 112:191–197, 2002

Arnt J, Hyttel J, Overo FK: Prolonged treatment with the specific 5-HT uptake inhibitor citalopram: effect on dopaminergic and serotonergic functions. Pol J Pharmacol Pharm 36:221–230, 1984a

Arnt J, Overo KF, Hyttel J, et al: Changes in rat dopamine and serotonin function in vivo after prolonged administration of the specific 5-HT uptake inhibitor citalopram. Psychopharmacology (Berl) 84:457–465, 1984b

Aronoff GR, Bergstrom RF, Pottratz ST, et al: Fluoxetine kinetics and protein binding in normal and impaired renal function. Clin Pharmacol Ther 36:138–144, 1984

Baldessarini RJ, Marsh ER, Kula NS: Interactions of fluoxetine with metabolism of dopamine and serotonin in rat brain regions. Brain Res 579:152–156, 1992

Baron BM, Ogden AM, Siegel BW, et al: Rapid down-regulation of β-adrenoceptors by co-administration of desipramine and fluoxetine. Eur J Pharmacol 154:125–134, 1988

Battaglino R, Vokes M, Schulze-Spate U, et al: Fluoxetine treatment increases trabecular bone formation in mice. J Cell Biochem 100:1387–1394, 2007

Baxter LR, Schwartz JM, Bergman KS, et al: Caudate glucose metabolic rate changes with both drug and behavior therapy for obsessive-compulsive disorder. Arch Gen Psychiatry 49:681–689, 1992

Beasley CM, Sayler ME, Bosomworth JC, et al: High-dose fluoxetine: efficacy and activating-sedating effects in agitated and retarded depression. J Clin Psychopharmacol 11:166–174, 1991

Benkelfat C, Murphy DL, Zohar J, et al: Clomipramine in obsessive-compulsive disorder: further evidence for a serotonergic mechanism of action. Arch Gen Psychiatry 46:23–28, 1989

Benloucif S, Galloway MP: Facilitation of dopamine release in vivo by serotonin agonists: studied with microdialysis. Eur J Pharmacol 200:1–8, 1991

Bergstrom DA, Kellar JK: Adrenergic and serotonergic receptor binding in rat brain after chronic desmethyl imipramine treatment. J Pharmacol Exp Ther 209:256–261, 1979

Blier P, de Montigny C, Chaput Y: Modifications of the serotonin system by antidepressant treatments: implications for the therapeutic response in major depression. J Clin Psychopharmacol 7 (suppl):24S–35S, 1987

Blier P, Chaput Y, de Montigny C: Long-term 5-HT reuptake blockade, but not monoamine oxidase inhibition, decreases the function of terminal 5-HT autoreceptors: an electrophysiological study in the rat brain. Naunyn Schmiedebergs Arch Pharmacol 337:246–254, 1988

Blier P, de Montigny C, Chaput Y: A role for the serotonin system in the mechanism of action of antidepressants. J Clin Psychiatry 51 (suppl 4):14–20, 1990

Bloch MR, Elliott M, Thompson H, et al: Fluoxetine in pathologic skin-picking: open-label and double-blind results. Psychosomatics 42:314–319, 2001

Blundell JE: Serotonin manipulations and the structure of feeding behaviour. Appetite 7 (suppl):39–56, 1986

Borys DJ, Setzer SC, Ling LJ, et al: Acute fluoxetine overdose: a report of 234 cases. Am J Emerg Med 10:115–120, 1992

Bouchard RH, Pourcher E, Vincent P: Fluoxetine and extrapyramidal side effects. Am J Psychiatry 146:1352–1353, 1989

Boyer WF, Feighner JP: The efficacy of selective serotonin uptake inhibitors in depression, in Selective Serotonin Uptake Inhibitors. Edited by Feighner JP, Boyer WF. Chichester, England, Wiley, 1991, pp 89–108

Bradley PB: Introduction to Neuropharmacology. Boston, MA, Wright, 1989

Brambilla P, Cipriani A, Hotopf M, et al: Side-effect profile of fluoxetine in comparison with other SSRIs, tricyclic and newer antidepressants: a meta-analysis of clinical trial data. Pharmacopsychiatry 38:69–77, 2005

Bressa GM, Brugnoli R, Pancheri P: A double-blind study of fluoxetine and imipramine in major depression. Int Clin Psychopharmacol 4 (suppl 1):69–73, 1989

Brewerton TD, Brandt HA, Lessem MD, et al: Serotonin in eating disorders, in Serotonin in Major Psychiatric Disorders. Edited by Coccaro EF, Murphy DL. Washington, DC, American Psychiatric Press, 1990, pp 153–184

Bridge JA, Iyengar S, Salary CB, et al: Clinical response and risk for reported suicidal ideation and suicide attempts in pediatric antidepressant treatment: a meta-analysis of randomized controlled trials. JAMA 297:1683–1696, 2007

Brosen K, Gram LF: Clinical significance of the sparteine/debrisoquine oxidation polymorphism. Eur J Clin Pharmacol 36:537–547, 1989

Burch KJ, Wells BG: Fluoxetine/norfluoxetine concentrations in human milk. Pediatrics 89:676–677, 1992

Bymaster FP, Zhang W, Carter PA, et al: Fluoxetine, but not other selective serotonin uptake inhibitors, increases norepinephrine and dopamine extracellular levels in prefrontal cortex. Psychopharmacology (Berl) 160:353–361, 2002

Carruba MO, Mantegazza P, Memo M, et al: Peripheral and central mechanisms of action of serotoninergic anorectic drugs. Appetite 7 (suppl):105–113, 1986

Charney DS, Menkes DB, Heninger GR: Receptor sensitivity and the mechanism of action of antidepressant treatment. Arch Gen Psychiatry 38:1160–1180, 1981

Charney DS, Heninger GR, Sternberg DE: Serotonin function and mechanism of action of antidepressant treatment. Arch Gen Psychiatry 41:359–365, 1984

Cipriani A, Brambilla P, Furukawa T, et al: Fluoxetine versus other types of pharmacotherapy for depression. Cochrane Database Syst Rev (4):CD004185, 2005

Ciraulo DA, Shader RI: Fluoxetine drug-drug interactions, I: antidepressants and antipsychotics. J Clin Psychopharmacol 10:48–50, 1990

Coccaro EF, Siever LJ, Klar HM, et al: Serotonergic studies in patients with affective and personality disorders: correlates with suicidal and impulsive aggressive behavior. Arch Gen Psychiatry 46:587–599, 1989

Cooper GL: The safety of fluoxetine—an update. Br J Psychiatry 153:77–86, 1988

Coppen AJ, Gupta RK, Eccleston EG, et al: Plasma tryptophan in anorexia nervosa (letter). Lancet 1(7966):961, 1976

Cornelius JR, Soloff PH, Perel JM, et al: A preliminary trial of fluoxetine in refractory borderline patients. J Clin Psychopharmacol 11:116–120, 1991

Cornelius JR, Salloum IM, Ehler JG, et al: Fluoxetine in depressed alcoholics: a double-blind, placebo-controlled trial. Arch Gen Psychiatry 54:700–705, 1997

Crewe HK, Lennard MS, Tucker GT, et al: The effect of selective serotonin reuptake inhibitors on the cytochrome P4502D6 (CYP2D6) activity in human liver microsomes. Br J Clin Pharmacol 34:262–265, 1992

Damsa C, Bumb A, Bianchi-Demicheli F, et al: "Dopamine-dependent" side effects of selective serotonin reuptake inhibitors: a clinical review. J Clin Psychiatry 65:1064–1068, 2004

Danion JM: The effectiveness of fluoxetine in acute studies and long-term treatment, in Psychiatry Today: VIII World Congress of Psychiatry Abstracts. Edited by Stefanis CN, Soldatos CR, Rabavilas AD. New York, Elsevier, 1989, p 334

de Montigny C, Chaput Y, Blier P: Long-term tricyclic and electroconvulsive treatment increases responsiveness of dorsal hippocampus 5-HT1A receptors: an electrophysiological study. Soc Neurosci Abstracts 15:854, 1989

Dechant KL, Clissold SP: Paroxetine. Drugs 41:225–253, 1991

Dempsey CM, Mackenzie SM, Gargus A, et al: Serotonin (5-HT), fluoxetine, imipramine and dopamine target distinct 5-HT receptor signaling to modulate Caenorhabditis elegans egg-laying behavior. Genetics 169:1425–1436, 2005

Dourish CT, Hutson PH, Kennett GA, et al: 8-OH-DPAT-induced hyperphagia: its neural basis and possible therapeutic relevance. Appetite 7 (suppl):127–140, 1986

Dufour H: Fluoxetine: long-term treatment and prophylaxis in depression. Paper presented at the International Fluoxetine Symposium, Tyrol, Austria, October 13–17, 1987

Edman G, Åsberg M, Levander S, et al: Skin conductance habituation and cerebrospinal fluid 5-hydroxyindoleacetic acid in suicidal patients. Arch Gen Psychiatry 43:586–592, 1986

Eisensamer B, Rammes G, Gimpl G, et al: Antidepressants are functional antagonists at the serotonin type 3 (5-HT3) receptor. Mol Psychiatry 8:994–1007, 2003

Elena Castro M, Diaz A, del Olmo E, et al: Chronic fluoxetine induces opposite changes in G protein coupling at pre and postsynaptic 5-HT1A receptors in rat brain. Neuropharmacology 44:93–101, 2003

Elks ML, Youngblood WW, Kizer JS: Serotonin synthesis and release in brain slices, independence of tryptophan. Brain Res 172:471–486, 1979

Enas GG, Pope HJ, Levine LR: Fluoxetine and bulimia nervosa: double-blind study, in 1989 New Research Program and Abstracts, American Psychiatric Association 142nd Annual Meeting, San Francisco, CA, May 6–11, 1989. Washington, DC, American Psychiatric Association, 1989, p 204

Ensrud KE, Blackwell T, Mangione CM, et al: Central nervous system active medications and risk for fractures in older women. Arch Intern Med 163:949–957, 2003

Falck B, Hillarp N-A, Thieme G, et al: Fluorescence of catecholamines and related compounds condensed with formaldehyde. J Histochem Cytochem 10:348–354, 1962

Fanelli FR, Cangiano C, Cecil F, et al: Plasma tryptophan and anorexia in human cancer. Eur J Cancer Clin Oncol 22:89–95, 1986

Fann WE, Sullivan JL, Richman BW: Dyskinesias associated with tricyclic antidepressants. Br J Psychiatry 128:490–493, 1976

Farren CK: Serotonin and alcoholism: clinical and experimental research. Journal of Serotonin Research 2:9–26, 1995

Fava M, Rosenbaum JF, McCarthy M, et al: Anger attacks in depressed outpatients and their response to fluoxetine. Psychopharmacol Bull 27:275–280, 1991

Fava M, Rosenbaum JF, Cohen L, et al: High dose fluoxetine in the treatment of depressed patients not responsive to a standard dose of fluoxetine. J Affect Disord 25:229–234, 1992

Fava M, Rosenbaum JF, Pava JA, et al: Anger attacks in unipolar depression, I: clinical correlates and response to fluoxetine treatment. Am J Psychiatry 150:1158–1163, 1993

Fava M, Alpert J, Nierenberg AA, et al: Fluoxetine treatment of anger attacks: a replication study. Ann Clin Psychiatry 8:7–10, 1996

Fava M, Judge R, Hoog SL, et al: Fluoxetine versus sertraline and paroxetine in major depressive disorder: changes in weight with long-term treatment. J Clin Psychiatry 61:863–867, 2000

Ferrey G, Gailledrau J, Beuzen JN: The interest of fluoxetine in prevention of depressive recurrences, in Psychiatry Today: VIII World Congress of Psychiatry Abstracts. Edited by Stefanis CN, Soldatos CR, Rabavilas AD. New York, Elsevier, 1989, p 99

Fisch C: Effect of fluoxetine on the electrocardiogram. J Clin Psychiatry 46:42–44, 1985

Flament MF, Rapoport JL, Berg CJ, et al: Clomipramine treatment of childhood obsessive-compulsive disorder: a double-blind, controlled study. Arch Gen Psychiatry 42:977–983, 1985

Fraser A, Offord SJ, Lucki I: Regulation of serotonin receptors and responsiveness in the brain, in The Serotonin Receptors. Edited by Sanders-Bush E. Clifton, NJ, Humana Press, 1988, pp 319–362

Fuller RW: Drugs altering serotonin synthesis and metabolism, in Neuropharmacology of Serotonin. Edited by Green AR. New York, Oxford University Press, 1985, pp 1–20

Fuller RW: Mechanisms and functions of serotonin neuronal systems: opportunities for neuropeptide interactions. Ann N Y Acad Sci 780:176–184, 1996

Gao B, Duncan WC Jr, Wehr ATA: Fluoxetine decreases brain temperature and REM sleep in Syrian hamsters. Psychopharmacology (Berl) 106:321–329, 1992

Garattini S, Mennini T, Bendotti C, et al: Neurochemical mechanism of action of drugs which modify feeding via the serotonergic system. Appetite 7 (suppl):15–38, 1986

Geller DA, Hoog SL, Heiligenstein JH, et al: Fluoxetine treatment for obsessive-compulsive disorder in children and adolescents: a placebo-controlled clinical trial. J Am Acad Child Adolesc Psychiatry 40:773–779, 2001

Goldbloom DS, Hicks LK, Garfinkel PE: Platelet serotonin uptake in bulimia nervosa, in 1988 New Research Program and Abstracts, American Psychiatric Association 141st Annual Meeting, Montreal, Quebec, Canada, May 7–12, 1988. Washington, DC, American Psychiatric Association, 1988, p 137

Goldenberg D, Mayskiy M, Mossey C, et al: A randomized, double-blind crossover trial of fluoxetine and amitriptyline in the treatment of fibromyalgia. Arthritis Rheum 39:1852–1859, 1996

Goldstein DJ, Rampey AH, Enas GG, et al: Fluoxetine: a randomized clinical trial in the treatment of obesity. Int J Obes Relat Metab Disord 18:129–135, 1994

Goldstein DJ, Wilson MG, Thompson VL, et al: Long-term fluoxetine treatment of bulimia nervosa. Br J Psychiatry 166:660–666, 1995

Goldstein DJ, Corbin LA, Sundell KL: Effects of first-trimester fluoxetine exposure on the newborn. Obstet Gen 89 (5, pt 1):713–718, 1997

Goodman WK, McDougle CJ, Price LH: Pharmacotherapy of obsessive-compulsive disorder. J Clin Psychiatry 53 (suppl 4):29–37, 1992

Gorelick DA: Serotonin uptake blockers and the treatment of alcoholism. Recent Dev Alcohol 7:267–281, 1989

Graziottin A, Montorsi F, Guazzoni G, et al: Combined fluoxetine and sexual behavioral therapy for premature ejaculation: one-year follow-up analysis of results, complications and success predictors (abstract). J Urol 155 (5, suppl):497A, 1996

Haddad P: Newer antidepressants and the discontinuation syndrome. J Clin Psychiatry 58 (suppl 7):17–21, 1997

Hall H, Ogren SO: Effects of antidepressant drugs on different receptors in rat brain. Eur J Pharmacol 70:393–407, 1981

Hamilton M: A rating scale for depression. J Neurol Neurosurg Psychiatry 23:56–62, 1960

Hammad TA, Laughren T, Racoosin J: Suicidality in pediatric patients treated with antidepressant drugs. Arch Gen Psychiatry 63:332–339, 2006

Hemeryck A, Belpaire FM: Selective serotonin reuptake inhibitors and cytochrome P-450 mediated drug-drug interactions: an update. Curr Drug Metab 3:13–37, 2002

Hendrick V, Stowe ZN, Altshuler LL et al: Fluoxetine and norfluoxetine concentrations in nursing infants and breast milk. Biol Psychiatry 50:775–782, 2001

Henry LK, Field JR, Adkins EM, et al: Tyr-95 and Ile-172 in transmembrane segments 1 and 3 of human serotonin transporters interact to establish high affinity recognition of antidepressants. J Biol Chem 281:2012–2023, 2006

Iceta R, Mesonero JE, Alcalde AI: Effect of long-term fluoxetine treatment on the human serotonin transporter in Caco-2 cells. Life Sci 80:1517–1524, 2007

Isenberg KE: Excretion of fluoxetine in human breast milk (letter). J Clin Psychiatry 51:169, 1990

Jenike MA, Buttolph L, Baer L, et al: Open trial of fluoxetine in obsessive-compulsive disorder. Am J Psychiatry 146:909–911, 1989

Jick SS, Dean AD, Jick H: Antidepressants and suicide. BMJ 310:215–218, 1995

Jimerson DC, Lesem MD, Kaye WH, et al: Serotonin and symptom severity in eating disorders (abstract). Biol Psychiatry 25 (suppl 7A):141A, 1989

Johnson AM: The comparative pharmacological properties of selective serotonin reuptake inhibitors in animals, in Selective Serotonin Uptake Inhibitors. Edited by Feighner JP, Boyer WF. Chichester, England, Wiley, 1991, pp 37–70

Jouvent R, Baruch P, Ammar S, et al: Fluoxetine efficacy in depressives with impulsivity vs blunted affect, in Psychiatry Today: VIII World Congress of Psychiatry Abstracts. Edited by Stefanis CN, Soldatos CR, Rabavilas AD. New York, Elsevier, 1989, p 398

Kaplan A, Hollander E: A review of pharmacologic treatments for obsessive-compulsive disorder. Psychiatr Serv 54:1111–1118, 2003

Kasper S, Fuger J, Moller H-J: Comparative efficacy of antidepressants. Drugs 43 (suppl 2):11–23, 1992

Kaye WH, Gwirtsman HE, Brewerton TD, et al: Bingeing behavior and plasma amino acids: a possible involvement of brain serotonin in bulimia nervosa. Psychiatry Res 23:31–43, 1988

Kaye WH, Weltzin TE, Hsu LK, et al: An open trial of fluoxetine in patients with anorexia nervosa. J Clin Psychiatry 52:464–471, 1991

Kaye WH, Nagat T, Weltzin TE, et al: Double-blind, placebo controlled administration of fluoxetine in restricting- and restricting-purging-type anorexia nervosa. Biol Psychiatry 49:644–652, 2001

Kelly MW, Perry J, Holstad SG, et al: Serum fluoxetine and norfluoxetine concentrations and antidepressant response. Ther Drug Monit 11:165–170, 1989

Kerr JS, Sherwood N, Hindmarch I: The comparative psychopharmacology of 5-HT reuptake inhibitors. Hum Psychopharmacol 6:313–317, 1991

Klimek V, Maj J: Repeated administration of antidepressant drugs enhanced agonist affinity for mesolimbic D-2 receptors. J Pharm Pharmacol 41:555–558, 1990

Koski A, Vuori E, Ojanpera I: Newer antidepressants: evaluation of fatal toxicity index and interaction with alcohol based on Finnish postmortem data. Int J Legal Med 119:344–348, 2005

Kroenke K, West SL, Swindle R, et al: Similar effectiveness of paroetine, fluoxetine, and sertraline in primary care: a randomized trial. JAMA 286:2947–2955, 2001

Lane R, Baldwin D: Selective serotonin reuptake inhibitor-induced serotonin syndrome: review. J Clin Psychopharmacol 17:208–221, 1997

Lejoyeux M: Use of serotonin (5-hydroxytryptamine) reuptake inhibitors in the treatment of alcoholism. Alcohol 31 (suppl 1):69–75, 1996

Lemberger L, Rowe H, Bergstrom RF, et al: Effect of fluoxetine on psychomotor performance, physiologic response and kinetics of ethanol. Clin Pharmacol Ther 37:658–664, 1985

Leonard BE: Pharmacological differences of serotonin reuptake inhibitors and possible clinical relevance. Drugs 43 (suppl 2):3–10, 1992

Lesch KP, Hoh A, Schulte HM, et al: Obsessive-compulsive disorder. Psychopharmacology 105:415–420, 1991

Lester BM, Cucca J, Andreozzi BA, et al: Possible association between fluoxetine hydrochloride and colic in an infant. J Am Acad Child Adolesc Psychiatry 32:1253–1255, 1993

Li SX, Perry KW, Wong DT: Influence of fluoxetine on the ability of bupropion to modulate extracellular dopamine and norepinephrine concentrations in three mesocorticolimbic areas of rats. Neuropharmacology 42:181–190, 2002

Little KY, Zhang L, Cook E: Fluoxetine-induced alterations in human platelet serotonin transporter expression: serotonin transporter polymorphism effects. J Psychiatry Neurosci 31:333–339, 2006

Maj J, Rogoz Z, Skuza G, et al: Repeated treatment with antidepressant drugs potentiates the locomotor response to (+)-amphetamine. J Pharm Pharmacol 36:127–130, 1984

Manasia P, Pomerol J, Ribe N, et al: Comparison of the efficacy and safety of 90 mg versus 20 mg fluoxetine in the treatment of premature ejaculation. J Urol 170:164–165, 2003

Marcus MD, Wing RR, Ewing L, et al: Double-blind, placebo-controlled trial of fluoxetine plus behavior modification in the treatment of obese binge eaters and non-binge eaters. Am J Psychiatry 147:876–881, 1990

Marley E, Wozniak KM: Interactions of a non-selective monoamine oxidase inhibitor, phenelzine, with inhibitors of 5-hydroxytryptamine, dopamine or noradrenaline re-uptake. J Psychiatr Res 18:173–189, 1984a

Marley E, Wozniak KM: Interactions of non-selective monoamine oxidase inhibitors, tranylcypromine and nialamide, with inhibitors of 5-hydroxytryptamine, dopamine or noradrenaline re-uptake. J Psychiatr Res 18:191–203, 1984b

Martenyi F, Brown EB, Zhang H, et al: Fluoxetine versus placebo in posttraumatic stress disorder. J Clin Psychiatry 63:199–206, 2002

Max MB, Lynch SA, Muir J, et al: Effects of desipramine, amitriptyline, and fluoxetine on pain in diabetic neuropathy. N Engl J Med 326:1250–1256, 1992

Meltzer HY, Young M, Metz J, et al: Extrapyramidal side effects and increased serum prolactin following fluoxetine, a new antidepressant. J Neural Transm 45:165–175, 1979

Menkes DB, Taghavi E, Mason PA, et al: Fluoxetine's spectrum of action in premenstrual syndrome. Int Clin Psychopharmacol 8:95–102, 1993

Michelson D, Allgulander C, Dantendorfer K, et al: Efficacy of usual antidepressant dosing regimens of fluoxetine in panic disorder: randomized placebo-controlled trial. Br J Psychiatry 179:514–518, 2001

Mochizucki D: Serotonin and noradrenaline reuptake inhibitors in animal models of pain. Hum Psychopharmacol 19 (suppl 1):S15–S19, 2004

Molteni R, Calabrese F, Bedogni F, et al: Chronic treatment with fluoxetine upregulates cellular BDNF mRNA expression in rat dopaminergic regions. Int J Neuropsychopharmacol 9:307–317, 2006

Montgomery SA, Dufour H, Brion S, et al: The prophylactic efficacy of fluoxetine in unipolar depression. Br J Psychiatry 153:69–76, 1988

Montgomery SA: Fluoxetine in the treatment of anxiety, agitation and suicidal thoughts, in Psychiatry Today: VIII World Congress of Psychiatry Abstracts. Edited by Stefanis CN, Soldatos CR, Rabavilas AD. New York, Elsevier, 1989a, p 335

Montgomery SA: New antidepressants and 5-HT uptake inhibitors. Acta Psychiatr Scand 80 (suppl 350):107–116, 1989b

Murphy JM, Waller MB, Gatto GJ, et al: Effects of fluoxetine on the intragastric self-administration of ethanol in the alcohol preferring P line of rats. Alcohol 5:283–286, 1988

Myung CS, Kim BT, Choi SH, et al: Role of neuropeptide Y and proopiomelanocortin in fluoxetine-induced anorexia. Arch Pharm Res 28:716–721, 2005

Naranjo CA, Kadlec KE, Sanhueza P, et al: Fluoxetine differentially alters alcohol intake and other consummatory behaviors in problem drinkers. Clin Pharmacol Ther 47:490–498, 1990

Naranjo CA, Sellers EM, Lawrin MO: Modulation of ethanol intake by serotonin uptake inhibitors. J Clin Psychiatry 47 (suppl 4):16–22, 1986

Nemeroff CB, Thase ME; EPIC 014 Study Group: A double-blind, placebo-controlled comparison of venlafaxine and fluoxetine treatment in depressed outpatients. J Psychiatr Res 41:351–359, 2007

Ninan PT, van-Kammen DP, Scheinin M, et al: CSF 5-hydroxyindoleactic acid levels in suicidal schizophrenic patients. Am J Psychiatry 141:566–569, 1984

Norden MJ: Fluoxetine in borderline personality disorder. Prog Neuropsychopharmacol Biol Psychiatry 13:885–893, 1989

Nulman I, Rovet J, Stewart DE, et al: Neurodevelopment of children exposed in utero to antidepressant drugs. N Engl J Med 336:258–262, 1997

O'Flynn K, O'Keane V, Lucey JV, et al: Effect of fluoxetine on noradrenergic mediated growth hormone release: a double-blind, placebo-controlled study. Biol Psychiatry 30:377–382, 1991

Pandey GN, Pandey SC, Janicak PG, et al: Platelet serotonin-2 receptor binding sites in depression and suicide. Biol Psychiatry 28:215–222, 1990

Papini M, Martinetti MJ, Pasquinelli A: Trazodone symptomatic extrapyramidal disorders of infancy and childhood. Ital J Neurol Sci 3:161–162, 1982

Parga J, Rodriguez-Pallares J, Munoz A, et al: Serotonin decreases generation of dopaminergic neurons from mesencephalic precursors via serotonin type 7 and type 4 receptors. Dev Neurobiol 67:10–22, 2007

Pearlstein TB, Stone AB, Lund SA, et al: Comparison of fluoxetine, bupropion, and placebo in the treatment of premenstrual dysphoric disorder. J Clin Psychopharmacol 17:261–266, 1997

Pedersen LH, Nielsen AN, Blackburn-Munro G: Anti-nociception is selectively enhanced by parallel inhibition of multiple subtypes of monoamine transporters in rat models of persistent and neuropathic pain. Psychopharmacology (Berl) 182:551–561, 2005

Pedersen OL, Kragh-Sorenson P, Bjerre M, et al: Citalopram, a selective serotonin reuptake inhibitor: clinical antidepressive and long-term effect—a phase II study. Psychopharmacology (Berl) 77:199–204, 1982

Peroutka SJ, Snyder SH: Long-term antidepressant treatment decreases spiroperidol-labelled serotonin receptor binding. Science 210:88–90, 1980

Petersen T, Dording C, Neault NB, et al: A survey of prescribing practices in the treatment of depression. Prog Neuropsychopharmacol Biol Psychiatry 26:177–187, 2002

Phillips KA, Albertini RS, Rasmussen SA: A randomized placebo-controlled trial of fluoxetine in body dysmorphic disorder. Arch Gen Psychiatry 59:381–388, 2002

Plaznik A, Kostowski W: The effects of antidepressants and electroconvulsive shocks on the functioning of the mesolimbic dopaminergic system: a behavioural study. Eur J Pharmacol 135:389–396, 1987

Reimherr FW, Amsterdam JD, Quitkin FM, et al: Optimal length of continuation therapy in depression: a prospective assessment during long-term fluoxetine treatment. Am J Psychiatry 155:1247–1253, 1998

Renynghe de Voxurie GE: Anafranil (G34586) in obsessive neurosis. Acta Neurol Belg 68:787–792, 1968

Richards JB, Papaioannou A, Adachi JD, et al: Effect of selective serotonin reuptake inhibitors on the risk of fracture. Arch Intern Med 167:188–194, 2007

Richelson E: Synaptic effects of antidepressants. J Clin Psychopharmacol 16 (suppl 2):1S–9S, 1996

Romano SJ, Halmi KA, Sarkar NP, et al: A placebo-controlled study of fluoxetine in continued treatment of bulimia nervosa after successful acute fluoxetine treatment. Am J Psychiatry 159:96–102, 2002

Rosenbaum JF, Fava M, Hoog SL, et al: Selective serotonin reuptake inhibitor discontinuation syndrome: a randomized clinical trial. Biol Psychiatry 44:77–87, 1998

Rubey RN, Johnson MR, Emmanuel N, et al: Fluoxetine in the treatment of anger: an open clinical trial. J Clin Psychiatry 57:398–401, 1996

Rudorfer MV, Potter WZ: Combined fluoxetine and tricyclic antidepressants. Am J Psychiatry 146:562–564, 1989

Salzman C, Wolfson AN, Schatzberg A, et al: Effect of fluoxetine on anger in symptomatic volunteers with borderline personality disorder. J Clin Psychopharmacol 15:23–29, 1995

Sampson D, Willner P, Muscat R: Reversal of antidepressant action by dopamine antagonists in an animal model of depression. Psychopharmacology (Berl) 104:491–495, 1991

Saper JR, Silberstein SD, Lake AE 3rd, et al: Double-blind trial of fluoxetine: chronic daily headache and migraine. Headache 34:497–502, 1994

Schatzberg A, Roose S: A double-blind, placebo-controlled study of venlafaxine and fluoxetine in geriatric outpatients with major depression. Am J Geriatr Psychiatry 14:361–370, 2006

Schatzberg AF, Haddad P, Kaplan EM, et al: Serotonin reuptake discontinuation syndrome: a hypothetical definition (discontinuation consensus panel). J Clin Psychiatry 58 (suppl 7):5–10, 1997

Schmidt ME, Fava M, Robinson JM, et al: The efficacy and safety of a new enteric-coated formulation of fluoxetine given once weekly during the continuation treatment of major depressive disorder. J Clin Psychiatry 61:851–857, 2000

Schweizer E, Rickels K, Amsterdam JD, et al: What constitutes an adequate antidepressant trial for fluoxetine? J Clin Psychiatry 51:8–11, 1990

Sekine Y, Suzuki K, Ramachandran PV, et al: Acute and repeated administration of fluoxetine, citalopram, and paroxetine significantly alters the activity of midbrain dopamine neurons in rats: an in vivo electrophysiological study. Synapse 61:72–77, 2007

Shaskan EG, Snyder SH: Kinetics of serotonin accumulation into slices from rat brain: relationship to catecholamine uptake. J Pharmacol Exp Ther 175:404–418, 1970

Snyder SH, Yamamura HI: Antidepressants and the muscarinic acetylcholine receptor. Arch Gen Psychiatry 34:236–239, 1977

Sodero AO, Orsingher OA, Ramirez OA: Altered serotonergic function of dorsal raphe nucleus in perinatally protein-deprived rats: effects of fluoxetine administration. Eur J Pharmacol 532:230–235, 2006

Stahl MMS, Lindquist M, Pettersson M, et al: Withdrawal reactions with selective serotonin reuptake inhibitors as reported to the WHO system. Eur J Clin Pharmacol 53:163–169, 1997

Stauderman KA, Gandhi DC, Jones DJ: Fluoxetine-induced inhibition of synaptosomal [3H] 5-HT release: possible calcium-channel inhibition. Life Sci 50:2125–2138, 1992

Steiner M, Steinberg S, Stewart D, et al: Fluoxetine in the treatment of premenstrual dysphoria. N Engl J Med 332:1529–1534, 1995

Su T-P, Danaceau M, Schmidt PJ, et al: Fluoxetine in the treatment of patients with premenstrual syndrome. Biol Psychiatry 33:159A–160A, 1993

Su T-P, Schmidt PJ, Danaceau MA, et al: Fluoxetine in the treatment of premenstrual dysphoria. Neuropsychopharmacology 16:346–356, 1997

Taddio A, Ito S, Koren G: Excretion of fluoxetine and its metabolite, norfluoxetine, in human breast milk. J Clin Pharmacol 36:42–47, 1996

Teusink JP, Alexopoulos GS, Shamoian CA: Parkinsonian side effects induced by a monoamine oxidase inhibitor. Am J Psychiatry 141:118–119, 1984

Thomas DR, Nelson DR, Johnson AM: Biochemical effects of the antidepressant paroxetine, a specific 5-hydroxytryptamine uptake inhibitor. Psychopharmacology (Berl) 93:193–200, 1987

Thorén P, Asberg M, Bertilsson L, et al: Clomipramine treatment of obsessive-compulsive disorder, II: biochemical aspects. Arch Gen Psychiatry 37:1289–1294, 1980

U'Prichard DC, Greenberg DA, Sheehan PB, et al: Tricyclic antidepressants: therapeutic properties and affinity for a-noradrenergic receptor binding sites in the brain. Science 199:197–198, 1978

Usher RW, Beasley CM, Bosomworth JC: Efficacy and safety of morning versus evening fluoxetine administration. J Clin Psychiatry 52:134–136, 1991

Van der Kolk BA, Dreyfuss D, Michaels M, et al: Fluoxetine in posttraumatic stress disorder. J Clin Psychiatry 55:517–522, 1994

Waldinger MD, Hengeveld MW, Zwinderman AH, et al: Effect of SSRI antidepressants on ejaculation: a double-blind, randomized, placebo-controlled study with fluoxetine, fluvoxamine, paroxetine and sertraline. J Clin Psychopharmacology 18:274–281, 1998

Walsh BT, Fairburn CG, Mickley D, et al: Treatment of bulimia nervosa in a primary care setting. Am J Psychiatry 161:556–561, 2004

Walsh BT, Kaplan AS, Attia E, et al: Fluoxetine after weight restoration in anorexia nervosa: a randomized controlled trial. JAMA 295:2605–2612, 2006

Warshaw MG, Keller MB: The relationship between fluoxetine use and suicidal behavior in 654 subjects with anxiety disorders. J Clin Psychiatry 57:158–166, 1996

Weizman R, Carmi M, Tyano S, et al: High affinity [3H] imipramine binding and serotonin uptake to platelets of adolescent females suffering from anorexia nervosa. Life Sci 38:1235–1242, 1986

Wernicke JF, Bremner JD, Bosomworth J, et al: The efficacy and safety of fluoxetine in the long-term treatment of depression. Paper presented at the International Fluoxetine Symposium, Tyrol, Austria, October 13–17, 1987

Wong DT, Reid LR, Bymaster FP, et al: Chronic effects of fluoxetine, a selective inhibitor of serotonin uptake, on neurotransmitter receptors. J Neural Transm 64:251–269, 1985

Wood SH, Mortola JF, Chan Y-F, et al: Treatment of premenstrual syndrome with fluoxetine: a double-blind placebo-controlled crossover study. Obstet Gen 80:339–344, 1992

Wurtman JJ, Wurtman RJ, Growdon JH, et al: Carbohydrate craving in obese people: suppression by treatments affecting serotonergic transmission. Int J Eat Disord 1:2–15, 1981

Zajecka J, Fawcett J, Amsterdam J, et al: Safety of abrupt discontinuation of fluoxetine: a randomized, placebo-controlled study. J Clin Psychiatry 18:193–197, 1998

Zohar J, Insel TR, Zohar-Kadouch RC, et al: Serotonergic responsivity in obsessive-compulsive disorder: effects of chronic clomipramine treatment. Arch Gen Psychiatry 45:167–172, 1988

Zubenko GS, Cohen BM, Lipinski JF: Antidepressant-related akathisia. J Clin Psychopharmacol 7:254–257, 1987

CHAPTER 14

Sertraline

David R. Block, M.D.

Kimberly A. Yonkers, M.D.

Linda L. Carpenter, M.D.

History and Discovery

Research has implicated dysregulation of serotonin (5-HT) in mood and anxiety disorders. Despite the effectiveness of the monoamine oxidase inhibitors (MAOIs) and tricyclic antidepressants (TCAs), which exert their effects by inhibiting the enzymatic degradation and reuptake of monoamines, respectively, side effects and potential serious adverse events limited their utility. Researchers thus identified compounds that are selective in blocking neurotransmitter reuptake and yet have little agonist and antagonist activity at receptors thought to be associated with adverse effects. Sertraline [(+)-cis-(1S,4S)-4-(3,4-dichlorophenyl)-1,2,3,4-tetrahydro-N-methyl-1-naphthylamine], a naphthylamino compound that is structurally different from MAOIs and TCAs (Figure 14–1), is one of this class of drugs (Guthrie 1991; Heym and Koe 1988).

For the 12 months ending June 2006, it has been estimated that sales of sertraline (under the brand name Zoloft) in the United States exceeded $3 billion (Rancourt 2006). In August 2006, a generic formulation of ser-

traline became available in the United States, and within the first 2 weeks of its availability, the substitution rate exceeded 77% (Block 2006).

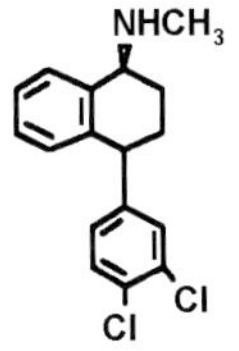

Structure–Activity Relations

Sertraline hydrochloride specifically blocks the reuptake of 5-HT in the soma and terminal regions of serotonergic neurons. The ability of sertraline to inhibit 5-HT reuptake is approximately 20-fold higher than its capacity to inhibit uptake of either norepinephrine or dopamine (DA) (Heym and Koe 1988). However, sertraline is more potent at blocking DA receptor uptake than are other selective serotonin reuptake inhibitors (SSRIs) and TCAs (Hiemke and Härtter 2000; Richelson 1994).

Serotonin neurons in the midbrain raphe nuclei have inhibitory autoreceptors in both the soma (serotonin$_{1A}$ [5-HT$_{1A}$] receptors) and terminal area (serotonin$_{1B}$ [5-HT$_{1B}$] receptors) that are stimulated by the acute increase in 5-HT. Thus, the immediate effect of serotonin transporter (5-HTT) blockade is to increase the amount of 5-HT in axosomatic synapses and to decrease neuronal firing (Blier 2001; Blier et al. 1990; Heym and Koe 1988). Over several weeks, these autoreceptors are desensitized and firing rates increase.

Unlike the older TCAs, sertraline has little appreciable antagonistic effect on histamine$_1$ (H$_1$), muscarinic, or dopamine$_2$ (D$_2$) receptors and thus is associated with few difficulties with severe constipation, drowsiness, and dry

FIGURE 14–1. Chemical structure of sertraline.

mouth (Hiemke and Härtter 2000; Richelson 1994). The antagonism of α_1-adrenoreceptors by sertraline is at least 10-fold more than that of other SSRIs (Hiemke and Härtter 2000), although this antagonism does not translate into clinically meaningful hypotension or reflex tachycardia. However, there is a report suggesting that sertraline decreases sympathetic nervous system activity, a property consistent with α receptor blockade (Shores et al. 2001). It is also possible that the decrease in sympathetic response is related to stimulation of the 5-HT$_{1A}$ receptors noted above. Given that sertraline and other medications in its class exhibit anxiolytic effects, it is possible that the decrease in sympathetic activity is related to these effects.

Sertraline is metabolized to desmethylsertraline (see section "Pharmacokinetics and Distribution" below). This compound is approximately one-tenth as active in blocking the reuptake of 5-HT; it also lacks antidepressant activity in animal models (Heym and Koe 1988).

Pharmacological Profile

Among the various antidepressant agents that block the 5-HTT, sertraline is second only to paroxetine in potency for 5-HT reuptake blockade, as demonstrated in animal models (Hiemke and Härtter 2000; Owens et al. 2001; Richelson 1994). The selectivity of sertraline over norepinephrine follows that of escitalopram (Hiemke and Härtter 2000; Owens et al. 2001), although other work suggests greater selectivity for fluvoxamine than for sertraline (Richelson 1994). The relative selectivity for the 5-HTT, compared with the dopamine transporter (DAT), is lowest for sertraline (Owens et al. 2001).

Sertraline exhibits inhibitory activity on several cytochrome P450 (CYP) enzymes. The ability of the compound to slightly elevate dextromethorphan and desipramine supports modest inhibition of CYP2D6 (Hiemke and Härtter 2000; Ozdemir et al. 1998; Preskorn 1996). It has little appreciable inhibition of CYP1A2, even when used at higher doses (Ozdemir et al. 1998). A very mild elevation of CYP2C9/10 substrates has been found in several studies (Preskorn 1996). Sertraline has complex effects on the CYP3A3/4 enzyme system: it initially shows slight inhibition, but it also induces this system, albeit modestly, over time (Preskorn 1996).

Pharmacokinetics and Distribution

Sertraline is absorbed slowly via the gastrointestinal tract, with peak plasma levels occurring between 6 and 8 hours

after ingestion (Warrington 1991). The delay in achieving peak levels may be the result of enterohepatic circulation (Hiemke and Härtter 2000; van Harten 1993). When sertraline is taken with food, the peak level decreases to about 5.5 hours ("Zoloft" 2001). The medication is more than 95% protein bound; however, because it binds weakly to α_1-glycoproteins, it does not cause substantial displacement of other protein-bound drugs (Preskorn 1996).

The volume of distribution (V_d) of sertraline is large in that it exceeds 20 L/kg. The distribution is larger in young females than in young males (Warrington 1991). In animal models, the concentration of sertraline is 40 times higher in brain than in plasma (Hiemke and Härtter 2000).

The elimination half-life of sertraline is 26–32 hours, and steady-state levels are achieved after 7 days. Sertraline shows linear pharmacokinetics within a range of 50–200 mg/day (Warrington 1991) and does not appear to inhibit or induce its own metabolism. Peak plasma levels are somewhat lower in young males, compared with females and older males (Ronfeld et al. 1997; Warrington 1991; "Zoloft" 2001), and the elimination rate constant is higher in young males than in females or older males (0.031/hour in young males; 0.022/hour in young females and 0.019/hour in older males and females).

In children between the ages of 6 and 17 years, weight-corrected metabolism is more rapid. The maximum concentration and area under the curve (AUC) are 22% lower than in adults. Despite the greater efficiency, the smaller body mass found in children suggests that lower dosages should be used ("Zoloft" 2001).

Sertraline is metabolized in the liver via oxidative metabolism; the concentration of the primary metabolite, desmethylsertraline, is up to threefold higher than that of the parent compound (Hiemke et al. 1991; Ronfeld et al. 1997; Warrington 1991). Desmethylsertraline levels are also lower in young males than in females and elderly males. The peak concentration (t_{max}) of desmethylsertraline is attained more quickly in young females than in young males (6 hours in young females vs. 9 hours in young males, 8 hours in older females, and 14 hours in older males) (Warrington 1991). The half-life of desmethylsertraline is 1.6–2.0 times that of the parent compound (Warrington 1991).

As mentioned above, desmethylsertraline is the major metabolite of sertraline; minor metabolites include a ketone and an alcohol compound (Warrington 1991). Less than 0.2% of an oral dose of sertraline is excreted unchanged in urine, whereas approximately 50% is found in feces. The enzymes involved in metabolism of sertraline to desmethylsertraline remain unclear (Greenblatt et al. 1999). Although six different CYP enzymes have the capacity to catalyze this reaction, none accounts for more than 25% of sertraline's clearance. The contribution of each CYP enzyme is dependent on not only the protein's activity on the substrate, as evidenced through in vitro models, but also the abundance of the enzyme. Given these properties, one computer model found that the greatest contribution to the demethylation of sertraline is from 2C9 (~23%), with 3A4 and 2C19 each contributing about 15%, 2D6 adding 5%, and 2B6 contributing 2% to the process (Greenblatt et al. 1999; Lee et al. 1999). The percentages could vary in a particular individual, depending on the amount of enzyme available or enzyme inhibition that occurs. However, given that multiple CYP enzymes are involved in this metabolic process, concurrent medications with specific CYP inhibition are not likely to impair metabolism of sertraline (Greenblatt et al. 1999).

Patients with liver disease experience decreased sertraline metabolism (Hiemke and Härtter 2000). For individuals with mild liver impairment, the half-life of drug may be increased threefold ("Zoloft" 2001). It is likely to be greater in patients with severe impairment, such as in those with cirrhosis. On the other hand, renal impairment does not appreciably influence the metabolism of sertraline (Hiemke and Härtter 2000).

Mechanism of Action

The means by which antidepressants exert their therapeutic action is still unknown, although some of the properties noted above have been related to hypothetical mechanisms (Blier 2001; Blier et al. 1990). As previously noted, the immediate effect of sertraline is to decrease neuronal firing rates. This is followed by normalization and an increase in firing rates, as autoreceptors are desensitized. Normalization in firing coincides with the time course of patient improvement in depressive symptoms and has been theoretically linked to the mechanism of action. It has been suggested that the downregulation of autoreceptors is important in correcting the depressive disorder (Blier 2001; Blier et al. 1990). However, the activity of noradrenergic neurons is also affected. As activity in the presynaptic neuron increases, noradrenergic neurons are stimulated by postsynaptic 5-HT receptors located on noradrenergic nerve terminals. This leads to eventual downregulation of β-adrenergic receptors, a property caused by many, but not all, antidepressant agents (Frazer and Scott 1994; Guthrie 1991).

Not inconsistent with the above are more recent results suggesting that SSRI treatment decreases production of 5-HT$_{1B}$ messenger RNA (mRNA), the message for a regulatory autoreceptor on dorsal raphe neurons that controls the amount of 5-HT released with each impulse (Anthony et al. 2000). Again, the decrease in mRNA production coincides temporally with the time frame for SSRI therapeutic effects.

Indications and Efficacy

Sertraline is currently approved by the U.S. Food and Drug Administration (FDA) for the treatment of major depressive disorder (MDD), obsessive-compulsive disorder (OCD) and pediatric OCD, posttraumatic stress disorder (PTSD), panic disorder, premenstrual dysphoric disorder (PMDD), and, most recently, social anxiety disorder. Some of the pivotal studies using this compound for these indications are reviewed below.

Major Depressive Disorder

The efficacy of sertraline in the treatment of MDD was established by a number of placebo-controlled trials for acute-phase therapy (Fabre et al. 1995; Opie et al. 1997; Reimherr et al. 1990). In a multicenter trial, 369 patients were randomly assigned to a fixed dose of sertraline (50 mg, 100 mg, or 200 mg daily) or placebo for 6 weeks (Fabre et al. 1995). Patients at all doses of sertraline showed approximately equivalent improvement, which was greater than placebo for most measures, including the total Hamilton Rating Scale for Depression (Ham-D) score, Beck subscale of the Ham-D, and the Clinical Global Impressions (CGI) Scale score. The combined effect size for sertraline, compared with placebo, was 0.31 (Davidson et al. 2002).

Sertraline was compared with amitriptyline and placebo in a multicenter trial of 448 patients (Reimherr et al. 1990). Sertraline was dosed flexibly up to 200 mg daily, and amitriptyline was administered at dosages as high as 150 mg/day. Both active treatments were superior to placebo, as indicated by Ham-D and CGI scores; similarly, response rates (rates at which patients attained a 50% decrease in the Ham-D or a CGI score of 1 or 2) were higher with the active treatment compared with placebo. Comparisons of sertraline and amitriptyline showed superiority on the Ham-D for amitriptyline until about week 3, after which both treatments were equivalent; response rates were nonsignificantly higher in the amitriptyline group. The effect size for sertraline, compared with placebo, in this study was 0.45 (Davidson et al. 2002).

A recent study sponsored by the National Institute of Mental Health (NIMH) that compared the acute-phase efficacy of *Hypericum perforatum* (St. John's wort), sertraline, and placebo in the acute-phase treatment of MDD had more equivocal results (Davidson et al. 2002). The study enrolled 340 patients with MDD for 8 weeks of treatment. Average patient age ranged from 40 to 43 years, and 37%–40% were male. The dosage of sertraline was flexibly titrated to 50–150 mg daily, although patients were at the highest dose for no more than 2 weeks. At study endpoint, there were no statistically significant differences in full response, defined as a CGI Scale score of ≤2 and a Ham-D score of ≤8. However, more patients had a partial response (CGI ≤2, 50% improvement on the Ham-D, but not full response) in the sertraline group (26%), compared with the placebo (13%) and *Hypericum* (16%) groups. Sertraline was also statistically superior to both placebo and *Hypericum* when the CGI Scale was used as a continuous measure. The effect size for sertraline, compared with placebo, was 0.24 with the Ham-D and 0.41 with the CGI Scale (Davidson et al. 2002). The difference between sertraline and placebo may have failed to achieve significance in some tests because the sample size may have been inadequate given the effect size.

In a multicenter study of 235 men and 400 women with either chronic MDD (enduring at least 2 years) or MDD superimposed on dysthymic disorder, probands were randomly assigned to 12 weeks of either sertraline or imipramine in a 2:1 ratio (Kornstein et al. 2000). Treatment was double-blind, and participants had their medication titrated to a maximum total daily dose of 200 mg of sertraline or 300 mg of imipramine. Full remission was defined as a CGI–Improvement (CGI-I) score of ≤2 and a 24-item Ham-D (Ham-D_{24}) score of <7; criteria for satisfactory response were a decrease in the Ham-D_{24} to 50% of baseline, an absolute score of ≤15, a CGI–Severity of Illness (CGI-S) score of ≤3, and a CGI-I score of ≤2, but no full remission. Remission occurred in 36% and 40% of the sertraline and the imipramine groups, respectively. Satisfactory response rates were 22% and 21% for the sertraline and the imipramine groups, respectively.

An interesting finding from this study is that men and women had differential response rates to sertraline and imipramine (Kornstein et al. 2000). The remission and satisfactory response groups were combined for this analysis. When these criteria and an intent-to-treat group were used, it was found that 57% of women, but only 46% of men, responded to sertraline. Response was somewhat better for imipramine, compared with sertraline, among men (62% for imipramine and 45% for sertraline). Response rates were more rapid for men assigned to imipramine and for women given sertraline and did not differ if only completers were used in the analysis. Premenopausal women were more likely to respond to sertraline, while postmenopausal women were equally likely to respond to either agent.

Sertraline has been shown to be effective for maintenance-phase treatment, generally in patients with MDD (Doogan and Caillard 1992) and in patients with chronic MDD (defined as MDD enduring at least 2 years or co-occurring with dysthymic disorder) (Keller et al. 1999). The Doogan and Caillard (1992) study included more than 450 patients with MDD (17-item Ham-D [Ham-D_{17}]>17) who entered 8 weeks of acute-phase treatment with sertraline, dosed flexibly between 50 and 200 mg daily; 68% of those patients responded, and 300 patients entered double-blind, placebo-controlled maintenance therapy. After 44 weeks of maintenance treatment, 13% of sertraline-treated patients, compared with 46% of placebo-treated patients, experienced a relapse.

The utility of sertraline in preventing illness recurrence has been explored using data from the chronic depression maintenance trial discussed above (Keller et al. 1999). Fifty-five percent of the acute-phase responders (378 of the total 426 patients who received sertraline) began continuation-phase treatment, and 169 patients continued to meet the criteria for remission (CGI-I score of 1 or 2 and a Ham-D score of <8); 161 patients entered maintenance treatment and were randomly assigned to 52 weeks of treatment with either placebo or a flexible dose of sertraline (maximum 200 mg daily). More than 60% of those entering maintenance treatment were female and had a current episode of depression that exceeded 8 years in duration. Sertraline significantly outperformed placebo for all outcome measures, which included the Ham-D, CGI Scale, Beck Depression Inventory (BDI), Cornell Dysthymia Scale, and Montgomery-Åsberg Depression Rating Scale; 20% of sertraline-treated patients and 50% of placebo-treated patients experienced illness recurrence.

In addition to the above trials, several studies found sertraline to be at least as effective as TCAs in treating younger adults (Cohn et al. 1990; Lydiard et al. 1997; Moller et al. 1998) and elderly patients (Bondareff et al. 2000; Finkel et al. 1999; Forlenza et al. 2001) with MDD. Sertraline has been shown to be as beneficial as nortriptyline in women with postpartum major depression (Wisner et al. 2006). Furthermore, sertraline may also confer a prophylactic advantage in women at high risk for developing postpartum depression (Wisner et al. 2004). Other trials show roughly equivalent response between sertraline and other SSRIs (Aguglia et al. 1993; Franchini et al. 1997; Nemeroff et al. 1996; Newhouse et al. 2000; Stahl 2000). A recent study suggests that the combination of liothyronine and sertraline enhances the antidepressant effect of the latter and leads to higher remission rates (Cooper-Kazaz et al. 2007).

Obsessive-Compulsive Disorder

Several multicenter trials find benefit of sertraline over placebo in the acute- and maintenance-phase treatment of OCD in adults. One earlier, smaller study failed to show superiority of sertraline over placebo, perhaps because of the limited sample size ($n = 19$) or the treatment-resistant characteristics of the cohort (Jenike et al. 1990). Larger-scale studies with diverse patients had differing results. In a 12-week flexible-dose study (Kronig et al. 1999), 167 patients were randomly assigned to placebo or sertraline. Between 53% and 57% of the subjects were male, and the average age was 37–38 years. The mean daily dose of sertraline at endpoint was 165 mg (SD = 55 mg). By week 3, significant differences between drug and placebo emerged. Forty-one percent of patients receiving sertraline and 23% of patients receiving placebo achieved a CGI-I score of 1 or 2 at endpoint.

A fixed-dose study (Greist et al. 1995) also found superior results with three different doses of sertraline, compared with placebo, over 1 year. Three hundred twenty-five subjects with OCD from 11 sites were randomly assigned to 12 weeks of double-blind treatment with one of three fixed doses of sertraline (50, 100, or 200 mg) or placebo after a 1-week washout period. At the end of this period, all treatment responders were offered enrollment in an additional 40 weeks of treatment. Forty percent of sertraline responders versus 26% of placebo responders entered the second phase of the study, a significant difference ($P = 0.025$). In fact, over the full 52 weeks of the study, subjects treated with sertraline demonstrated significantly greater improvement than subjects given placebo, based on efficacy measures that included the Children's Yale-Brown Obsessive Compulsive Scale (CY-BOCS) ($F_{1,289} = 7.06$, $P = 0.001$), the NIMH–Global Obsessive-Compulsive Scale (NIMH-GOCS) ($F_{1,311} = 11.22$, $P = 0.0009$), the CGI Scale ($F_{1,311} = 8.09$, $P = 0.005$), and the CGI-I ($F_{1,311} = 7.18$, $P = 0.0007$).

Some evidence suggests that higher amounts of sertraline may be helpful for patients who fail to respond at standard dosages. In one study, 66 patients with OCD who failed to respond to sertraline therapy at doses of 200 mg/daily after 16 weeks of treatment were randomly assigned to continue on the same dose for an additional 12 weeks or to increase their dose to 250–400 mg/daily (Ninan et al. 2006). At the end of the trial, those receiving higher doses had greater improvement in Y-BOCS scores, though responder rates (at least a 25% decrease in Y-BOCS scores and a CGI-I rating ≤3) between the two groups were similar.

Other studies supporting the utility of sertraline in OCD include head-to-head comparison studies with other antidepressants (Bergeron et al. 2002; Bisserbe et al. 1995; Hoehn-Saric et al. 2000). In a comparison of lower-dose sertraline with cognitive-behavioral group therapy, both treatments were shown to be efficacious, though OCD patients treated with group therapy had greater reduction in symptoms (Sousa and Isolan 2006).

Pediatric Obsessive-Compulsive Disorder

Sertraline is approved for use in children for the treatment of OCD. In a 12-week double-blind, placebo-controlled, parallel-group, multicenter study, March et al. (1998) found that children and adolescents treated with sertraline showed significant improvement on several efficacy measures, compared with placebo. One hundred eighty-seven subjects (107 children, ages 6–12 years, and 80 adolescents, ages 13–17 years) were randomly assigned to receive either sertraline (92 subjects) or placebo (95 subjects). The mean dosage at endpoint was 167 mg/day for sertraline and 180 mg/day for placebo. Subjects who were treated with sertraline showed significantly greater improvement than placebo on the Y-BOCS (−6.8 and −3.4, respectively; $P = 0.005$), NIMH-GOCS (−2.2 and −1.3, respectively; $P = 0.02$), and CGI-I (2.7 and 3.3, respectively; $P = 0.002$). The authors reported a small number of dropouts because of adverse events and overall found sertraline to be a safe, well-tolerated treatment for this age group. In children and adolescents treated with sertraline over 12 months (at doses between 50–200 mg/daily over 52 weeks), evidence suggests that acute response can convert to full or partial remission of symptoms with longer-term treatment (Wagner et al. 2003).

Posttraumatic Stress Disorder

The efficacy of sertraline for the treatment of PTSD is supported by two large multicenter, acute-phase, double-blind, placebo-controlled studies (Brady et al. 2000; Davidson et al. 2001), a long-term treatment study (Londborg et al. 2001), and a relapse prevention trial (Davidson et al. 2001). In one acute-phase trial (Davidson et al.

2001), 208 civilian patients were randomly assigned to either sertraline or placebo for 12 weeks of treatment. The symptom reductions with active treatment were about 50% for reexperiencing/intrusion, just under 50% for avoidance/numbing, and 40% for arousal. The probability of response, defined as a CGI Scale score of 1 or 2 and a minimal 30% decrease in the Clinician-Administered PTSD Scale—Part 2 (CAPS-2), was 0.65 in sertraline-treated patients and 0.38 in placebo-treated patients at 12 weeks. Approximately 40% of each group had comorbid MDD, and baseline 21-item Ham-D scores were around 21. Of interest, there were no significant differences among groups in this depression measure at 12 weeks, suggesting that depression in the context of PTSD may be more treatment refractory. An acute-phase study by Brady et al. (2000) had similar results. Although both studies concluded that sertraline was a well-tolerated and effective treatment for PTSD, findings from a recent Department of Veterans Affairs (VA) medical center study failed to show that sertraline was more efficacious than placebo in patients with predominantly combat-related PTSD (Friedman et al. 2007). It has been proposed that patients in VA settings may constitute a special population with particularly treatment-refractory PTSD.

The acute-phase efficacy of sertraline in treating PTSD in the studies reviewed above (Brady et al. 2000; Davidson et al. 2001) was significant for women; however, it failed to achieve significance, compared with placebo, for men. Some research suggests treatment efficacy may vary between men and women and the type of traumas experienced. Other research has shown no significant gender differences in patients with combat-related PTSD in response to sertraline (Friedman et al. 2007). The overall sex difference in response is not attributable to inclusion of studies with "treatment-resistant" male VA patients, because the lack of difference occurred with civilian males. Reasons for the sex difference in efficacy findings are not clear. One possible explanation is that women are more likely to experience sexual or physical trauma and childhood abuse than men, and perhaps the nature of the trauma itself may alter response to medication (Stein et al. 2006). However, it is intriguing that, compared with men, women appeared to have a superior response to sertraline in the chronic depression study reviewed above.

The long-term benefit of sertraline in the treatment of PTSD has also been shown in a study by Londborg et al. (2001). Subjects who had completed 12 weeks of double-blind, placebo-controlled acute-phase treatment for PTSD with sertraline (Brady et al. 2000) were eligible for enrollment in a 24-week open-label continuation study (Londborg et al. 2001). This study, which included 252 patients, found that 92% of those who responded to acute-phase treatment with sertraline sustained their response over 36 weeks. Furthermore, 54% of patients with minimal acute-phase response went on to respond during the subsequent continuation of treatment. Londborg et al. (2001) found that about 20%–25% of the total improvement in PTSD symptoms seen over the full 36 weeks of treatment occurred during the continuation phase (weeks 12–36). The greatest improvement over time was among patients who were originally considered "nonresponders" in the acute phase. On the basis of these data, the authors concluded that as many as one-third of PTSD patients may require longer treatment to achieve a clinically significant response.

Davidson et al. (2001) furthered the aforementioned work by examining the efficacy of sertraline in maintaining improvement in PTSD symptoms, as well as in preventing the relapse of these symptoms, in a 28-week double-blind continuation study. Ninety-six patients were randomly assigned to receive either sertraline or placebo. At the end of the study, sertraline was found to be significantly superior to placebo in preventing relapse of PTSD, as defined by three primary outcome measures: relapse (sertraline vs. placebo, 5.3% and 26.1%, respectively; $P<0.02$), relapse or discontinuation due to clinical deterioration (sertraline vs. placebo, 15.8% and 45.7%, respectively; $P=0.005$), and acute exacerbation (sertraline vs. placebo, 15.8% and 52.2%, respectively; $P<0.001$). Relative risk of relapse (RR) after discontinuing sertraline was 6.35. Other outcomes were relapse or discontinuation due to clinical deterioration (RR=4.48 for patients switched to placebo, compared with those maintained on sertraline) and acute exacerbation of symptoms (RR=5.82 of placebo over sertraline). On measures of symptom severity, patients who were treated with sertraline demonstrated changes on their scores on the Davidson Trauma Scale ($P=0.008$), Impact of Event Scale ($P<0.03$), and CGI-S ($P=0.002$), compared with placebo subjects.

Panic Disorder

Sertraline has also proven effective in the treatment of panic disorder, as demonstrated by a number of studies. In a 12-week randomized, placebo-controlled, flexible-dose multicenter study of outpatients with panic disorder (with and without agoraphobia) but without depression (Pohl et al. 1998), sertraline was superior to placebo on a number of efficacy measures. One hundred sixty-eight patients meeting DSM-III-R (American Psychiatric Association 1987) criteria for panic disorder without depression were randomly assigned to receive sertraline (80 patients) or placebo (88 patients) after a 2-week single-blind lead-in. Mean dosage at endpoint for sertraline-treated patients was 126 mg/day (SD = 62 mg/day), and the reduction in frequency of panic attacks was significantly greater for those treated with sertraline compared with those on placebo (77% vs. 51%, respectively). The mean number of limited-symptom attacks for the sertraline group also decreased significantly more than for those given placebo (5.9 [SD = 8.8] and 2.4 [SD = 7.0], respectively). Other outcomes that reached statistical significance included scores on the CGI-S ($F_{1,145} = 13.35$, $P<0.001$) and CGI-I ($F_{1,146} = 15.83$, $P<0.001$) Scales, as well as ratings on the Quality of Life Enjoyment and Satisfaction Questionnaire ($F_{1,125} = 7.94$, $P = 0.006$). Similar results were reported by Pollack et al. (1998), who randomly assigned 178 patients to sertraline or placebo.

A fixed-dose study employed 50 mg, 100 mg, or 200 mg of sertraline or placebo for 12 weeks (Londborg et al. 1998). Outcomes, including number of panic attacks and limited-symptom attacks, severity of anticipatory anxiety, dimensional anxiety measures, and global measures of improvement, showed that sertraline, at all doses, was significantly superior to placebo. Pooled sertraline data indicated a 65% reduction in the number of panic attacks, compared with a 39% decrease in the placebo group. Effect sizes, or the magnitude of difference between the two treatments, for the three doses were 0.58 (50 mg), 0.41 (100 mg), and 0.60 (200 mg). Response rates did not differ significantly between fixed-dose groups. In the above panic studies, the authors reported a low incidence of attrition secondary to sertraline adverse events, concluding that sertraline is a safe, as well as effective, treatment for patients with panic disorder.

Premenstrual Dysphoric Disorder

In one of the first multicenter trials to test the efficacy of an antidepressant agent for PMDD, sertraline was compared with placebo (Yonkers et al. 1997). Either placebo or sertraline, administered flexibly and daily, was given to 243 women. After three menstrual cycles of treatment, total daily rating scores had decreased by 32% and 11% in the sertraline- and placebo-treated groups, respectively. Both emotional and physical symptom clusters had improved by 32% with sertraline treatment, a reduction that was about threefold higher than the change seen with placebo. At the endpoint, CGI-I scores of 1 or 2 were

achieved by 62% and 34% of those assigned to sertraline and placebo, respectively.

In a second multicenter trial, it was shown that sertraline treatment could be commenced halfway through the menstrual cycle (i.e., at ovulation) and still be more effective than placebo (Halbreich et al. 2002). In this three-cycle flexible-dose study, 281 women were randomly assigned to receive total daily doses of 50–100 mg of sertraline or placebo. The responder rates in this study, after three cycles of luteal-phase treatment, were 50% and 26% for sertraline and placebo, respectively. As with the daily treatment study, improvement in functional impairment paralleled symptomatic improvement. Only 8% of the women taking sertraline and 1% of the women receiving placebo discontinued the study because of side effects. The efficacy of this platform of drug administration for women with PMDD potentially revolutionizes treatment approaches because many women with PMDD prefer to avoid taking medication during nonsymptomatic periods.

Social Anxiety Disorder

Several studies have established the efficacy of sertraline in the treatment of social anxiety disorder (also known as social phobia). In one of the earliest studies, sertraline treatment (at flexible doses of 50–100 mg/day) showed a statistically significant improvement compared with placebo, as measured by the Liebowitz Social Anxiety Scale (LSAS) (Katzelnick et al. 1995). A large double-blind, placebo-controlled study followed more than 200 Canadian outpatients with generalized social phobia for 20 weeks, measuring response on CGI-I scores and mean reductions on the social phobia subscale of the Marks Fear Questionnaire and the Brief Social Phobia scale (Van Ameringen et al. 2001). Fifty-three percent of patients treated with sertraline, compared with only 29% of patients receiving placebo, were either much or very much improved by the study's end, as measured by CGI-I scores. Statistically significant changes favoring sertraline were seen on the other two study measures as well. When subjects who responded to sertraline were randomly assigned to continue sertraline or switch to placebo for an additional 24 weeks, the relative risk of relapse for those who were randomized to placebo was greater than 10 (Walker et al. 2000).

Liebowitz et al. (2003) demonstrated that sertraline caused a significant reduction in LSAS scores and produced a greater proportion of responders after 12 weeks of treatment (at doses up to 200 mg/daily) compared to placebo. In a placebo-controlled study comparing sertraline, exposure therapy, or combined treatment involving over 380 Norwegian patients with generalized social phobia in general practices, sertraline alone or in combination with exposure therapy yielded statistically significant improvements in CGI social phobia scores, whereas exposure therapy alone did not (Blomhoff et al. 2001). Additional studies have commented on the efficacy of sertraline in the treatment of social phobia in adults (Czepowicz et al. 1995; Munjack et al. 1995; Roberts et al. 1995). While not FDA approved in the pediatric population, sertraline has been well tolerated and has shown efficacy in childhood social anxiety disorder (Compton et al. 2001).

Off-Label Use

Sertraline has also been studied for off-label use in the treatment of a variety of disorders. Sertraline has been used in a number of studies for treatment of a wide range of neurological conditions, including Alzheimer's dementia (Lyketsos et al. 2000; Magai et al. 2000; Volicer et al. 1994), depression associated with Parkinson's disease (Antonini et al. 2006; Hauser and Zesiewicz 1997; Meara and Hobson 1998), and depression-linked fatigue in multiple sclerosis (Mohr et al. 2003).

Sertraline has also demonstrated success in the treatment of depression in patients with schizophrenia (Addington et al. 2002; Kirli and Caliskan 1998; Mulholland et al. 2003). Several studies have established the benefit of sertraline in generalized anxiety disorder (GAD). Two randomized trials showed the superiority of sertraline over placebo (Allgulander et al. 2004; Brawman-Mintzer et al. 2006) and similar efficacy as paroxetine (Ball et al. 2005) in GAD. Sertraline has been studied for use in a number of impulse-control disorders, with mixed results. In combination with habit reversal training, sertraline has been utilized in the treatment of trichotillomania, with good outcomes (Dougherty et al. 2006). However, a trial of sertraline in patients with pathological gambling did not show any superiority in control of gambling behaviors compared with placebo (Saiz-Ruiz et al. 2005). Some studies suggest a role for sertraline in the treatment of several types of eating disorders, including anorexia nervosa (Santonastaso et al. 2001), bulimia nervosa (Milano et al. 2004), binge-eating disorder (Leombruni et al. 2006; McElroy el al. 2000), and night-eating syndrome (O'Reardon et al. 2006).

There have been a limited number of studies examining the potential for sertraline in substance use disorders. Trials of sertraline in alcohol (Kranzler et al. 2006), methamphetamine (Shoptaw et al. 2006), and cocaine dependence (Winhusen et al. 2005) do not suggest any benefit in helping curb substance abuse.

In a placebo-controlled trial (Rynn et al. 2001), sertraline was both effective and safe in children with GAD. Sertraline has also been used successfully in the treatment of children and adolescents with major depression and dysthymic disorder (Ambrosini et al. 1999; Nixon et al. 2001). Pervasive developmental disorder has been successfully treated with sertraline, according to at least two studies (Hellings et al. 1996; McDougle et al. 1998).

Sertraline is one of the few antidepressants that has been shown to be safe and effective for the treatment of depression in patients with cardiovascular disease. In a well-publicized study by the Sertraline Antidepressant Heart Attack Randomized Trial (SADHART) Group, 369 patients with a recent myocardial infarction or hospitalization for unstable angina who also met criteria for a current major depressive episode were randomly assigned to sertraline (at flexible dosages of 50–200 mg/daily) or placebo for 24 weeks (Glassman et al. 2002). The main outcome measure was change from baseline left ventricular ejection fraction (LVEF) and secondary measures included scores on the Ham-D and CGI-I Scale. Not only was there no statistical difference in LVEF between the two patient groups, but patients treated with sertraline had fewer severe cardiovascular events (though this did not reach statistical significance). Sertraline was also superior to placebo in improving CGI scores, though no significant difference was seen in Ham-D scores. In a separate analysis of the SADHART data, patients treated with sertraline experienced fewer psychiatric or cardiovascular hospitalizations during the treatment period (O'Connor et al. 2005).

While the mechanism of cardiovascular benefit is not entirely clear, sertraline may decrease platelet adherence, thus decreasing the likelihood of recurrent myocardial events (McFarlane et al. 2001; Shapiro et al. 1999). Sertraline has also been shown to improve quality-of-life measurements in depressed patients with acute coronary syndrome (Swenson et al. 2003) and stroke (Murray et al. 2005).

Sertraline has been studied in patients with cancer who do not have MDD, but have some symptoms of the disorder. In a double-blind, controlled trial of almost 200 patients with advanced disease, Stockler et al. (2007) showed that sertraline had no benefit over placebo in ameliorating depression, anxiety, fatigue, or sense of well-being after 8 weeks of treatment.

TCAs have long been used for their analgesic properties, though side effects can sometimes impair efficacy. A

10-week study of sertraline in 50 patients with chronic tension headaches showed a decline in analgesic medication use, suggesting sertraline may be a good alternative for patients who cannot tolerate the adverse events associated with TCAs (Singh and Misra 2002).

Several studies have used sertraline to treat the side effect of premature ejaculation (Arafa and Shamloul 2006; Balbay et al. 1998; Biri et al. 1998; McMahon 1998; Mendels et al. 1995). The side effect of sexual dysfunction associated with the medication may underlie the success found by these investigators.

A number of studies have highlighted the effective use of sertraline in treating aggressive behaviors (Buck 1995; Feder 1999), specifically in patients with personality disorders (Kavoussi et al. 1994) and Huntington's disease (Ranen et al. 1996).

Sertraline has been used to improve pathological crying and pseudobulbar-type affects (Benedek and Peterson 1995; Mukand et al. 1996; Okun et al. 2001; Peterson et al. 1996).

In at least two studies, sertraline has been shown to be effective in preventing dialysis-induced hypotension, a condition that can be exacerbated by other antidepressive agents (Dheenan et al. 1998). Sertraline has also been used to treat pruritus associated with cholestatic liver disease (Mayo et al. 2007) and severe, refractory tinnitus (Zoger at al. 2006).

Another proposed off-label use for sertraline is the alleviation of hot flashes associated with menopause (Gordon et al. 2006; Grady et al. 2007; Plouffe et al. 1997) and tamoxifen treatment for breast cancer (Kimmick et al. 2006) in women and in men following medical castration for advanced prostate cancer (Roth and Scher 1998), suggesting that 5-HT may play a role in vasomotor instability associated with hormonal changes. One study suggested that response to sertraline in hot flashes is related to activity level, education, and menopausal status (Kerwin et al. 2007).

Side Effects and Toxicology

Sertraline has been demonstrated to have a low incidence of anticholinergic, sedative, or cardiovascular effects because of its low affinity for adrenergic, cholinergic, histaminergic, or benzodiazepine receptors. However, sertraline was associated with a number of adverse effects in premarketing evaluation, the most common of which included gastrointestinal disturbance (nausea, 27%; diarrhea/loose stools, 21%), sleep disturbance (insomnia,

22%; somnolence, 14%), headache (26%), dry mouth (15%), and sexual dysfunction (ejaculation failure, 14%; decreased libido, 6%). Other side effects reported by subjects, described as frequent (i.e., they occurred in at least 1 of 100 subjects) in premarketing pooled data from clinical trials, include impotence, palpitations, chest pain, hypertonia, hypoesthesia, increased appetite, back pain, asthenia, malaise, weight gain, myalgia, yawning, rhinitis, and tinnitus ("Zoloft" 2001).

Since sertraline has been approved for use, there have been a number of reports of different adverse events associated with its use. Sertraline and other SSRIs have been associated with instances of hyponatremia, as well as with the syndrome of inappropriate antidiuretic hormone (SIADH) secretion (see Bouman et al. 1997; Bradley et al. 1996; Catalano et al. 1996; Goldstein et al. 1996; Kessler and Samuels 1996). Bradley et al. (1996), in a review of the literature, noted that the average age of patients experiencing SIADH is over 70 years, suggesting that the elderly may be more vulnerable to age-related changes in water balance, which may make them more susceptible to developing SIADH with an SSRI. Furthermore, the authors suggested that sertraline may have some effect on vasopressin secretion, although they stated that there have been no controlled studies to confirm this link.

Extrapyramidal side effects (EPS), including dyskinesias, dystonias, and akathisia, have also been seen with sertraline use, although they are infrequent (Altshuler and Szuba 1994; Lambert et al. 1998; Madhusoodanan and Brenner 1997; Opler 1994). Hamilton and Opler (1992) suggested that the underlying mechanism of SSRI-induced akathisia is serotonergic inhibition of the nigrostriatal DA pathway, which can be associated with parkinsonism (Leo et al. 1995; Pina Latorre et al. 2001). Madhusoodanan and Brenner (1997), in a case report of choreiform dyskinesia and EPS associated with sertraline therapy, proposed that 5-HT-driven antagonism of dopaminergic transmission in the nigrostriatal pathway, as well as in the ventral tegmental area (VTA), may be responsible for the development of EPS.

Sexual side effects are a well-known side effect of SSRIs, including sertraline. A recent Cochrane Database review noted that while there is currently limited evidence available, some trials suggest that the addition of sildenafil or bupropion can reduce antidepressant-induced erectile dysfunction in men (Rudkin et al. 2004).

Other adverse events associated with sertraline are rare and include seizures (Raju et al. 2000; Saraf and Schrader 1999), stuttering (Brewerton et al. 1996; Christensen et al. 1996; McCall 1994), altered platelet function and bleeding time (Calhoun and Calhoun 1996; Mendelson 2001), and galactorrhea (Bronzo and Stahl 1993; Lesaca 1996). A recent study of children and adolescents with epilepsy and depression demonstrated sertraline's efficacy in treating depressive symptoms while maintaining good seizure control (Thome-Souza et al. 2007). Urinary hesitancy and retention have been reported in a few cases in women (Lowenstein et al. 2007).

As with all other antidepressants, sertraline carries an FDA black box warning regarding increased risk of suicidality in children and adolescents. Interestingly, one study of suicidal thinking and behavior in more than 700 seniors with late-life depression showed no increase in suicidality in those treated with sertraline versus placebo (Nelson et al. 2007).

Sertraline has also been associated with a discontinuation syndrome. Leiter et al. (1995) described two cases in which patients experienced a constellation of symptoms, including alterations in mood, cognition, energy, gait, and equilibrium, in addition to gastrointestinal symptoms, headaches, and paresthesias. Elsewhere there have been reports of insomnia, impaired short-term memory, myalgias, dyspnea, and chills without fevers (Louie et al. 1994). On the other hand, in a systematic 28-week study involving panic disorder patients (Rapaport et al. 2001), abrupt discontinuation of sertraline was primarily associated only with insomnia (15.7% of patients randomly assigned to placebo vs. 4.3% continuing on sertraline) and dizziness (4.3% of patients continuing to take sertraline and 16.4% switched to placebo). There was no statistically significant deterioration in headache or in general malaise.

Drug–Drug Interactions

Sertraline has a number of drug–drug interactions of which clinicians need to be aware. Because the drug is tightly bound to plasma proteins, caution should be employed when sertraline is used in combination with pharmaceuticals possessing similar characteristics, such as warfarin, and prothrombin time should be monitored when sertraline and warfarin are used concurrently ("Zoloft" 2001). The potential for serotonin syndrome may be increased when sertraline is combined with other SSRIs, serotonin–norepinephrine reuptake inhibitors, or triptans used for the acute treatment of migraines. The administration of sertraline and MAOIs is contraindicated because of the significant risk of serotonin syndrome with this combination.

As discussed earlier, sertraline inhibits a number of enzymes in the cytochrome P450 system, most significantly CYP2D6. However, the degree of inhibition is relatively minor in comparison with other SSRIs, such as fluoxetine and paroxetine (Preskorn et al. 2007). Because TCAs are substrates of CYP2D6, drug levels and dosages need to be closely monitored when TCAs are used in combination with sertraline.

Conclusion

Controlled clinical trials support the efficacy of sertraline in the treatment of a variety of disorders, including mood disorders, such as MDD and PMDD, and anxiety disorders, such as OCD, PTSD, and social phobia. It may be that response is somewhat more favorable in younger women with mood disorders, perhaps because women are more likely to have anxious symptoms. Uncontrolled studies suggest an expanded role for sertraline in a variety of other conditions that require further evaluation. The safety profile is superior to that of the older antidepressant agents, thus increasing the potential target population of patients with mood and anxiety disorders.

References

Addington DD, Azorin JM, Falloon IR, et al: Clinical issues related to depression in schizophrenia: an international survey of psychiatrists. Acta Psychiatr Scand 105:189–195, 2002

Aguglia E, Casacchia M, Cassano G, et al: Double-blind study of the efficacy and safety of sertraline versus fluoxetine in major depression. Int Clin Psychopharmacol 8:197–202, 1993

Allgulander C, Dahl AA, Austin C, et al: Efficacy of sertraline in a 12-week trial for generalized anxiety disorder. Am J Psychiatry 161:1642–1649, 2004

Altshuler LL, Szuba MP: Course of psychiatric disorders in pregnancy. Dilemmas in pharmacologic management. Neurol Clin 12:613–635, 1994

Ambrosini P, Wagner K, Biederman J, et al: Multicenter open-label sertraline study in adolescent outpatients with major depression. J Am Acad Child Adolesc Psychiatry 38:566–572, 1999

American Psychiatric Association: Diagnostic and Statistical Manual of Mental Disorders, 3rd Edition, Revised. Washington, DC, American Psychiatric Association, 1987

Anthony J, Sexton T, Neumaier J: Antidepressant-induced regulation of 5-HT 1B mRNA in rat dorsal raphe nucleus reverses rapidly after drug discontinuation. J Neurosci Res 61:82–87, 2000

Antonini A, Tesei S, Zecchinelli A, et al: Randomized study of sertraline and low-dose amitriptyline in patients with Parkinson's disease and depression: effect on quality of life. Mov Disord 21:1119–1122, 2006

Arafa M, Shamloul R: Efficacy of sertraline hydrochloride in treatment of premature ejaculation: a placebo-controlled study using a validated questionnaire. Int J Impot Res 18:534–538, 2006

Balbay M, Yildiz M, Salvarci A, et al: Treatment of premature ejaculation with sertraline. Int Urol Nephrol 30:81–83, 1998

Ball SG, Kuhn A, Wall D, et al: Selective serotonin reuptake inhibitor treatment for generalized anxiety disorder: a double-blind, prospective comparison between paroxetine and sertraline. J Clin Psychiatry 66:94–99, 2005

Benedek D, Peterson K: Sertraline for treatment of pathological crying. Am J Psychiatry 152:953–954, 1995

Bergeron R, Ravindran A, Chaput Y, et al: Sertraline and fluoxetine treatment of obsessive-compulsive disorder: results of a double-blind, 6-month treatment study. J Clin Psychopharmacol 22:148–154, 2002

Biri H, Isen K, Sinik Z, et al: Sertraline in the treatment of premature ejaculation: a double-blind placebo controlled study. Int Urol Nephrol 30:611–615, 1998

Bisserbe J, Lane R, Flament M: A double-blind comparison of sertraline and clomipramine in outpatients with obsessive-compulsive disorder. Eur Psychiatry 12:82–93, 1995

Blier P: Pharmacology of rapid-onset antidepressant treatment strategies. J Clin Psychiatry 62:12–17, 2001

Blier P, de Montigny C, Chaput Y: A role for the serotonin system in the mechanism of action of antidepressant treatments: preclinical evidence. J Clin Psychiatry 51 (4, suppl):14–20, 1990

Block J: Zoloft erosion outpaces recent generic launches. "The Pink Sheet" Daily. September 5, 2006. Available at: www.thepinksheetdaily.com. Accessed November 2007.

Blomhoff S, Haug TT, Hellstrom K, et al: Randomised controlled general practice trial of sertraline, exposure therapy and combined treatment in generalized social phobia. Br J Psychiatry 179:23–30, 2001

Bondareff W, Alpert M, Friedhoff A, et al: Comparison of sertraline and nortriptyline in the treatment of major depressive disorder in late life. Am J Psychiatry 157:729–736, 2000

Bouman W, Johnson H, Trescoli-Serrano C, et al: Recurrent hyponatremia associated with sertraline and lofepramine. Am J Psychiatry 154:580, 1997

Bradley M, Foote E, Lee E, et al: Sertraline-associated syndrome of inappropriate antidiuretic hormone: case report and review of the literature. Pharmacotherapy 16:680–683, 1996

Brady K, Pearlstein T, Asnis G, et al: Efficacy and safety of sertraline treatment of posttraumatic stress disorder. JAMA 283:1837–1844, 2000

Brawman-Mintzer O, Knapp RG, Rynn M, et al: Sertraline treatment for generalized anxiety disorder: a randomized, double-blind, placebo-controlled study. J Clin Psychiatry 67:874–881, 2006

Brewerton T, Markowitz J, Keller S, et al: Stuttering with sertraline. J Clin Psychiatry 57:90–91, 1996

Bronzo M, Stahl S: Galactorrhea induced by sertraline. Am J Psychiatry 150:1269, 1993

Buck O: Sertraline for reduction of violent behavior. Am J Psychiatry 152:953, 1995

Calhoun J, Calhoun D: Prolonged bleeding time in a patient treated with sertraline. Am J Psychiatry 153:443, 1996

Catalano G, Kanfer S, Catalano M, et al: The role of sertraline in a patient with recurrent hyponatremia. Gen Hosp Psychiatry 18:278–283, 1996

Christensen R, Byerly M, McElroy R: A case of sertraline-induced stuttering. J Clin Psychopharmacol 16:92–93, 1996

Cohn CK, Shrivastava R, Mendels J, et al: Double-blind, multicenter comparison of sertraline and amitriptyline in elderly depressed patients. J Clin Psychiatry 51 (12, suppl B):28–33, 1990

Compton S, Grant P, Chrisman A, et al: Sertraline in children and adolescents with social anxiety disorder: an open trial. J Am Acad Child Adolesc Psychiatry 40:564–571, 2001

Cooper-Kazaz R, Apter JT, et al: Combined treatment with sertraline and liothyronine in major depression: a randomized, double-blind, placebo-controlled trial. Arch Gen Psychiatry 64:679–688, 2007

Czepowicz V, Johnson M, Lydiard R, et al: Sertraline in social phobia. J Clin Psychopharmacol 15:372–373, 1995

Davidson J, Rothbaum B, van der Kolk B, et al: Multicenter, double-blind comparison of sertraline and placebo in the treatment of posttraumatic stress disorder. Arch Gen Psychiatry 58:485–492, 2001

Davidson J, Tharwani H, Connor K: Davidson Trauma Scale (DTS): normative scores in the general population and effect sizes in placebo-controlled SSRI trials. Depress Anxiety 15:75–78, 2002

Dheenan S, Venkatesan J, Grubb B, et al: Effect of sertraline hydrochloride on dialysis hypotension. Am J Kidney Dis 31:624–630, 1998

Doogan DP, Caillard V: Sertraline in the prevention of depression. Br J Psychiatry 160:217–222, 1992

Dougherty DD, Loh R, Jenike MA, et al: Single modality versus dual modality treatment for trichotillomania: sertraline, behavioral therapy, or both? J Clin Psychiatry 67:1086–1092, 2006

Fabre L, Abuzzahab F, Amin M, et al: Sertraline safety and efficacy in major depression: a double-blind fixed dose comparison with placebo. Biol Psychiatry 38:592–602, 1995

Feder R: Treatment of intermittent explosive disorder with sertraline in 3 patients. J Clin Psychiatry 60:195–196, 1999

Finkel S, Richter E, Clary C, et al: Comparative efficacy of sertraline vs. fluoxetine in patients age 70 or over with major depression. Am J Geriatr Psychiatry 7:221–227, 1999

Forlenza O, Almeida O, Stoppe A, et al: Antidepressant efficacy and safety of low-dose sertraline and standard-dose imipramine for the treatment of depression in older adults: results from a double-blind, randomized, controlled clinical trial. Int Psychogeriatr 13:75–84, 2001

Franchini L, Gasperini M, Perez J, et al: A double-blind study of long-term treatment with sertraline or fluvoxamine for prevention of highly recurrent unipolar depression. J Clin Psychiatry 58:104–107, 1997

Frazer A, Scott PA: Onset of action of antidepressant treatments: neuropharmacological aspects. Int Acad Biomed Drug Res 9:1–7, 1994

Friedman MJ, Marmar CR, Baker DG, et al: Randomized, double-blind comparison of sertraline and placebo for posttraumatic stress disorder in a Department of Veterans Affairs setting. J Clin Psychiatry 68:711–720, 2007

Glassman A, O'Connor C, Califf R, et al: Sertraline treatment of major depression in patients with acute MI or unstable angina. JAMA 6:701–709, 2002

Goldstein L, Barker M, Segall F, et al: Seizure and transient SIADH associated with sertraline. Am J Psychiatry 153:732, 1996

Gordon PR, Kerwin JP, Boesen KG, et al: Sertraline to treat hot flashes: a randomized controlled, double-blind, crossover trial in a general population. Menopause 13:568–575, 2006

Grady D, Cohen B, Tice J, et al: Ineffectiveness of sertraline for treatment of menopausal hot flashes: a randomized controlled trial. Obstet Gynecol 109:823–840, 2007

Greenblatt D, von Moltke L, Harmatz J, et al: Human cytochromes mediating sertraline biotransformation: seeking attribution. J Clin Psychopharmacol 19:489–493, 1999

Greist J, Jefferson J, Kobak K, et al: A 1 year double-blind placebo-controlled fixed dose study of sertraline in the treatment of obsessive-compulsive disorder. Int Clin Psychopharmacol 10:57–65, 1995

Guthrie S: Sertraline: a new specific serotonin reuptake blocker. DICP 25:952–961, 1991

Halbreich U, Bergeron R, Yonkers K, et al: Efficacy of intermittent, luteal phase sertraline treatment of premenstrual dysphoric disorder. Obstet Gynecol 100:1219–1229, 2002

Hamilton M, Opler L: Akathisia, suicidality, and fluoxetine. J Clin Psychiatry 53:401–406, 1992

Hauser R, Zesiewicz T: Sertraline for the treatment of depression in Parkinson's disease. Mov Disord 12:756–759, 1997

Hellings J, Kelley L, Gabrielli W, et al: Sertraline response in adults with mental retardation and autistic disorder. J Clin Psychiatry 57:333–336, 1996

Heym J, Koe BK: Pharmacology of sertraline: a review. J Clin Psychiatry 49:40–45, 1988

Hiemke C, Härtter S: Pharmacokinetics of selective serotonin reuptake inhibitors. Pharmacol Ther 85:11–28, 2000

Hiemke C, Jussofie A, Juptner M: Evidence that 3-alpha-hydroxy-5-alpha-pregnan-20-one is a physiologically relevant modulator of GABA-ergic neurotransmission. Psychoneuroendocrinology 16:517–523, 1991

Hoehn-Saric R, Ninan P, Black D, et al: Multicenter double-blind comparison of sertraline and desipramine for concurrent obsessive-compulsive and major depressive disorders. Arch Gen Psychiatry 57:76–82, 2000

Jenike M, Baer L, Summergrad P, et al: Sertraline in obsessive-compulsive disorder: a double-blind comparison with placebo. Am J Psychiatry 147:923–928, 1990

Katzelnick DJ, Kobak KA, Greist JH, et al: Sertraline for social phobia: a double-blind, placebo-controlled crossover study. Am J Psychiatry 152:1368–1371, 1995

Kavoussi R, Liu J, Coccaro E: An open trial of sertraline in personality disordered patients with impulsive aggression. J Clin Psychiatry 55:137–141, 1994

Keller M, Kocsis J, Thase M, et al: Maintenance phase efficacy of sertraline for chronic depression: a randomized controlled trial. JAMA 280:1665–1672, 1999

Kerwin JP, Gordon PR, Senf JH: The variable response of women with menopausal hot flashes when treated with sertraline. Menopause 14:841–845, 2007

Kessler J, Samuels S: Sertraline and hyponatremia. N Engl J Med 335:524, 1996

Kimmick GG, Lovato J, McQuellon R, et al: Randomized, double-blind, placebo-controlled, crossover study of sertraline (Zoloft) for the treatment of hot flashes in women with early stage breast cancer taking tamoxifen. Breast J 12:114–122, 2006

Kirli S, Caliskan M: A comparative study of sertraline versus imipramine in postpsychotic depressive disorder of schizophrenia. Schizophr Res 33:103–111, 1998

Kornstein S, Schatzberg A, Thase M, et al: Gender differences in treatment response to sertraline versus imipramine in chronic depression. Am J Psychiatry 157:1445–1452, 2000

Kranzler HR, Mueller T, Cornelius J, et al: Sertraline treatment of co-occurring alcohol dependence and major depression. J Clin Psychopharmacol 26:13–20, 2006

Kronig M, Apter J, Asnis G, et al: Placebo-controlled, multicenter study of sertraline treatment for obsessive-compulsive disorder. J Clin Psychopharmacol 19:172–176, 1999

Lambert M, Trutia C, Petty F, et al: Extrapyramidal adverse effects associated with sertraline. Prog Neuropsychopharmacol Biol Psychiatry 22:741–748, 1998

Lee A, Chan W, Harralson A, et al: The effects of grapefruit juice on sertraline metabolism: an in vitro and in vivo study. Clin Ther 21:1890–1899, 1999

Leiter F, Nierenberg A, Sanders K, et al: Discontinuation reactions following sertraline. Biol Psychiatry 38:694–695, 1995

Leo R, Lichter D, Hershey L: Parkinsonism associated with fluoxetine and cimetidine: a case report. J Geriatr Psychiatry Neurol 8:231–233, 1995

Leombruni P, Piero A, Brustolin A, et al: A 12 to 24 weeks pilot study of sertraline treatment in obese women binge eaters. Hum Psychopharmacol 21:181–188, 2006

Lesaca T: Sertraline and galactorrhea. J Clin Psychopharmacol 16:333–334, 1996

Liebowitz MR, DeMartinis NA, Weihs K, et al: Efficacy of sertraline in severe generalized social anxiety disorder: results of a double-blind, placebo-controlled study. J Clin Psychiatry 64:785–792, 2003

Londborg P, Wolkow R, Smith W, et al: Sertraline in the treatment of panic disorder. Br J Psychiatry 173:54–60, 1998

Londborg P, Hegel M, Goldstein S, et al: Sertraline treatment of posttraumatic stress disorder: results of 24 weeks of open-label continuation treatment. J Clin Psychiatry 62: 325–331, 2001

Louie AK, Lannon RA, Ajari LJ: Withdrawal reaction after sertraline discontinuation. Am J Psychiatry 151:450–451, 1994

Lowenstein L, Mueller ER, Sharma S, et al: Urinary hesitancy and retention during treatment with sertraline. Int Urogynecol J Pelvic Floor Dysfunct 18:827–829, 2007

Lydiard RB, Stahl S, Hertzman M, et al: A double-blind, placebo-controlled study comparing the effects of sertraline versus amitriptyline in the treatment of major depression. J Clin Psychiatry 58:484–491, 1997

Lyketsos C, Sheppard J, Steele C, et al: Randomized, placebo-controlled, double-blind clinical trial of sertraline in the treatment of depression complicating Alzheimer's disease: initial results from the Depression in Alzheimer's Disease study. Am J Psychiatry 157:1686–1689, 2000

Madhusoodanan S, Brenner R: Reversible choreiform dyskinesia and extrapyramidal symptoms associated with sertraline therapy. J Clin Psychopharmacol 17:138–139, 1997

Magai C, Kennedy G, Cohen C, et al: A controlled clinical trial of sertraline in the treatment of depression in nursing home patients with late-stage Alzheimer's disease. Am J Geriatr Psychiatry 8:66–74, 2000

March J, Biederman J, Wolkow R, et al: Sertraline in children and adolescents with obsessive-compulsive disorder: a multicenter randomized controlled trial. JAMA 280:1752–1756, 1998

Mayo MJ, Handem I, Saldana S, et al: Sertraline as a first-line treatment for cholestatic pruritus. Hepatology 45:666–674, 2007

McCall W: Sertraline induced stuttering. J Clin Psychiatry 55:316, 1994

McDougle C, Brodkin E, Naylor S, et al: Sertraline in adults with pervasive developmental disorders: a prospective open-label investigation. J Clin Psychopharmacol 18:62–66, 1998

McElroy S, Casuto L, Nelson E, et al: Placebo-controlled trial of sertraline in the treatment of binge eating disorder. Am J Psychiatry 157:1004–1006, 2000

McFarlane A, Kamath M, Fallen E, et al: Effect of sertraline on the recovery rate of cardiac autonomic function in depressed patients after acute myocardial infarction. Am Heart J 142:617–623, 2001

McMahon C: Treatment of premature ejaculation with sertraline hydrochloride. Int J Impot Res 10:181–184, 1998

Meara J, Hobson P: Depression, anxiety and hallucinations in Parkinson's disease. Elder Care 10 (suppl 4–5), 1998

Mendels J, Camera A, Sikes C: Sertraline treatment for premature ejaculation. J Clin Psychopharmacol 15:341–346, 1995

Mendelson S: Platelet function and sertraline. Am J Psychiatry 158:823–824, 2001

Milano W, Petrella C, Sabatino C, et al: Treatment of bulimia nervosa with sertraline: a randomized control trial. Adv Ther 21:232–237, 2004

Mohr DC, Hart SL, Goldberg A: Effects of treatment for depression on fatigue in multiple sclerosis. Psychosom Med 65:542–547, 2003

Moller J, Gallinat J, Hegerl U, et al: Double-blind, multicenter comparative study of sertraline and amitriptyline in hospitalized patients with major depression. Pharmacopsychiatry 31:170–177, 1998

Mukand J, Kaplan M, Senno R, et al: Pathological crying and laughing: treatment with sertraline. Arch Phys Med Rehabil 77:1309–1311, 1996

Mulholland C, Lynch G, King DJ, et al: A double-blind, placebo-controlled trial of sertraline for depressive symptoms in patients with stable, chronic schizophrenia. J Psychopharmacol 17:107–112, 2003

Munjack D, Flowers C, Eagan T: Sertraline in social phobia. Anxiety 1:196–198, 1995

Murray V, von Arbin M, Bartfai A, et al: Double-blind comparison of sertraline and placebo in stroke patients with minor depression and less severe major depression. J Clin Psychiatry 66:708–716, 2005

Nelson JC, Delucchi K, Schneider L: Suicidal thinking and behavior during treatment with sertraline in late-life depression. Am J Geriatr Psychiatry 15:573–580, 2007

Nemeroff CB, DeVane CL, Pollock BJ: Newer antidepressants and the cytochrome P450 system. Am J Psychiatry 153:311–320, 1996

Newhouse P, Krishnan K, Doraiswamy P, et al: A double-blind comparison of sertraline and fluoxetine in depressed elderly outpatients. J Clin Psychiatry 61:559–568, 2000

Ninan PT, Koran LM, Kiev A, et al: High-dose sertraline strategy for non-responders to acute treatment for obsessive-compulsive disorder: a multicenter double-blind trial. J Clin Psychiatry 67:15–22, 2006

Nixon M, Milin R, Simeon J, et al: Sertraline effects in adolescent major depression and dysthymia: a six month open trial. J Child Adolesc Psychopharmacol 11:131–142, 2001

Okun M, Riestra A, Nadeau S: Treatment of ballism and pseudobulbar affect with sertraline. Arch Neurol 58:1682–1684, 2001

Opie J, Gunn K, Katz E: A double-blind placebo-controlled multicenter study of sertraline in the acute and continuation treatment of major depression. Psychiatry 12:34–41, 1997

Opler L: Sertraline and akathisia. Am J Psychiatry 151:620–621, 1994

O'Connor CM, Glassman AH, Harrison DJ: Pharmacoeconomic analysis of sertraline treatment of depression in patients with unstable angina or a recent myocardial infarction. J Clin Psychiatry 66:346–352, 2005

O'Reardon JP, Allison KC, Martino NS, et al: A randomized, placebo-controlled trial of sertraline in the treatment of night eating syndrome. Am J Psychiatry 163:893–898, 2006

Owens MJ, Knight DL, Nemeroff CB: Second-generation SSRIs: human monoamine transporter binding profile of escitalopram and R-fluoxetine. Soc Biol Psychiatry 50:345–350, 2001

Ozdemir V, Naranjo C, Herrmann N, et al: The extent and determinants of changes in CYP2D6 and CYP1A2 activities with therapeutic doses of sertraline. J Clin Psychopharmacol 18:55–61, 1998

Peterson K, Armstrong S, Moseley J: Pathologic crying responsive to treatment with sertraline. J Clin Psychopharmacol 16:333, 1996

Pina Latorre M, Modrego P, Rodilla F, et al: Parkinsonism and Parkinson's disease associated with long-term administration of sertraline. J Clin Pharm Ther 26:111–112, 2001

Plouffe L, Trott E, Largoza M, et al: An open trial of sertraline for menopausal hot flashes: potential involvement of serotonin in vasomotor instability. Delaware Med J 69:481–482, 1997

Pohl R, Wolkow R, Clary C: Sertraline in the treatment of panic disorder: a double-blind multicenter trial. Am J Psychiatry 155:1189–1195, 1998

Pollack M, Otto M, Worthington J, et al: Sertraline in the treatment of panic disorder: a flexible-dose multicenter trial. Arch Gen Psychiatry 55:1010–1016, 1998

Preskorn S: Effects of antidepressants on the cytochrome P450 system. Am J Psychiatry 153:1655–1670, 1996

Preskorn SH, Shah R, Neff M, et al: The potential for clinically significant drug-drug interactions involving the CYP 2D6 system: effects with fluoxetine and paroxetine versus sertraline. J Psychiatr Pract 13:5–12, 2007

Raju G, Kumar T, Khanna S: Seizures associated with sertraline. Can J Psychiatry 45:491, 2000

Rancourt J: Teva Launches First Generic Zoloft. "The Pink Sheet" Daily. August 14, 2006. Available at: www.thepinksheet-daily.com. Accessed November 2007.

Ranen N, Lipsey J, Treisman G, et al: Sertraline in the treatment of severe aggressiveness in Huntington's disease. J Neuropsychiatry Clin Neurosci 8:338–340, 1996

Rapaport M, Wolkow R, Rubin A, et al: Sertraline treatment of panic disorder: results of a long-term study. Acta Psychiatr Scand 104:289–298, 2001

Reimherr FW, Chouinard G, Cohn CK, et al: Antidepressant efficacy of sertraline: a double-blind, placebo- and amitriptyline-controlled multicenter comparison study in outpatients with major depression. J Clin Psychiatry 51 (12, suppl B):18–27, 1990

Richelson E: Pharmacology of antidepressants—characteristics of the ideal drug. Mayo Clin Proc 69:1069–1081, 1994

Roberts J, Wohlreich G, Santos A: Sertraline in the treatment of social phobia. Am J Psychiatry 152:810–811, 1995

Ronfeld RA, Tremaine LM, Wilner KD: Pharmacokinetics of sertraline and its N-demethyl metabolite in elderly and young male and female volunteers. Clin Pharmacokinet 32 (suppl 1):22–30, 1997

Roth A, Scher H: Sertraline relieves hot flashes secondary to medical castration as treatment of advanced prostate cancer. Psychooncology 7:129–132, 1998

Rudkin L, Taylor MJ, Hawton K: Strategies for managing sexual dysfunction induced by antidepressant medication. Cochrane Database Syst Rev (4):CD003382, 2004

Rynn M, Siqueland L, Rickels K: Placebo-controlled trial of sertraline in the treatment of children with generalized anxiety disorder. Am J Psychiatry 158:2008–2014, 2001

Saiz-Ruiz J, Blanco C, Ibáñez A, et al: Sertraline treatment of pathological gambling: a pilot study. J Clin Psychiatry 66:28–33, 2005

Santonastaso P, Friederici S, Favaro A: Sertraline in the treatment of restricting anorexia nervosa: an open controlled trial. J Child Adolesc Psychopharmacol 11:143–150, 2001

Saraf M, Schrader G: Seizure associated with sertraline. Aust N Z J Psychiatry 33:944–945, 1999

Shapiro P, Lesperance F, Frasure-Smith N, et al: An open-label preliminary trial of sertraline for treatment of major depression after acute myocardial infarction (the SADHAT Trial). Am Heart J 137:1100–1106, 1999

Shoptaw S, Huber A, Peck J, et al: Randomized, placebo-controlled trial of sertraline and contingency management for the treatment of methamphetamine dependence. Drug Alcohol Depend 85:12–18, 2006

Shores M, Pascualy M, Lewis N, et al: Short-term sertraline treatment suppresses sympathetic nervous system activity in healthy human subjects. Psychoneuroendocrinology 26:433–439, 2001

Singh NN, Misra S: Sertraline in chronic tension-type headache. J Assoc Physicians India 50:873–878, 2002

Sousa MB, Isolan LR: A randomized clinical trial of cognitive-behavioral group therapy and sertraline in the treatment of obsessive-compulsive disorder. J Clin Psychiatry 67:1133–1139, 2006

Stahl S: Placebo-controlled comparison of the selective serotonin reuptake inhibitors citalopram and sertraline. Biol Psychiatry 48:894–901, 2000

Stein DJ, van der Kolk BA, Austin C, et al: Efficacy of sertraline in posttraumatic stress disorder secondary to interpersonal trauma or childhood abuse. Ann Clin Psychiatry 18:243–249, 2006

Stockler MR, O'Connell R, Nowak AK, et al: Effect of sertraline on symptoms and survival in patients with advanced cancer, but without major depression: a placebo-controlled double-blind randomized trial. Lancet Oncol 8:603–612, 2007

Swenson JR, O'Connor CM, Barton D, et al: Influence of depression and effect of treatment with sertraline on quality of life after hospitalization for acute coronary syndrome. Am J Cardiol 92:1271–1276, 2003

Thome-Souza MS, Kuczynski E, Valente KD: Sertraline and fluoxetine: safe treatments for children and adolescents with epilepsy and depression. Epilepsy Behav 10:417–425, 2007

Van Ameringen M, Lane R, Walker J, et al: Sertraline treatment of generalized social phobia: a 20 week, double-blind, placebo-controlled study. Am J Psychiatry 158:275–281, 2001

van Harten J: Clinical pharmacokinetics of selective serotonin reuptake inhibitors. Clin Pharmacokinet 24:203–220, 1993

Volicer L, Rheaume Y, Cyr D: Treatment of depression in advanced Alzheimer's disease using sertraline. J Geriatr Psychiatry Neurol 7:227–229, 1994

Wagner KD, Cook EH, Chung H, et al: Remission status after long-term sertraline treatment of pediatric obsessive-compulsive disorder. J Child Adolesc Psychopharmacol 13 (suppl 1):S53–S60, 2003

Walker JR, Van Ameringen MA, Swinson R, et al: Prevention of relapse in generalized social phobia: results of a 24-week study in responders to 20 weeks of sertraline treatment. J Clin Psychopharmacol 20:636–644, 2000

Warrington SJ: Clinical implications of the pharmacology of sertraline. Int Clin Psychopharmacol 6:11–21, 1991

Winhusen TM, Somoza EC, Harrer JM, et al: A placebo-controlled screening trial of tiagabine, sertraline and donepezil as cocaine dependence treatments. Addiction 100 (suppl 1):68–77, 2005

Wisner KL, Perel JM, Peindl KS, et al: Prevention of postpartum depression: a pilot randomized clinical trial. Am J Psychiatry 161:1290–1292, 2004

Wisner KL, Hanusa BH, Perel JM, et al: Postpartum depression: a randomized trial of sertraline versus nortriptyline. J Clin Psychopharmacol 26:353–360, 2006

Yonkers KA, Halbriech U, Freeman E, et al: Symptomatic improvement of premenstrual dysphoric disorder with sertraline treatment. JAMA 278:983–988, 1997

Zoger S, Svedlund J, Holgers KM: The effects of sertraline on severe tinnitus suffering—a randomized, double-blind, placebo-controlled study. J Clin Psychopharmacol 26:32–39, 2006

Zoloft (sertraline hydrochloride) tablets and oral concentrate (package insert). New York, Pfizer, 2001

CHAPTER 15

Paroxetine

Clifford J. Ehmke, M.D.
Charles B. Nemeroff, M.D., Ph.D.

Paroxetine (Paxil) is classified as one of the serotonin reuptake inhibitors (SRIs) because of its potent inhibition of presynaptic serotonin (5-HT) uptake. It is also a relatively potent norepinephrine (NE) reuptake inhibitor, particularly at higher doses, leading some to argue for its inclusion in the growing class of acknowledged dual serotonin–norepinephrine reuptake inhibitors (SNRIs). Since its approval for the treatment of depression, paroxetine has been demonstrated to be effective and has been approved for a broad spectrum of anxiety disorders, including panic disorder, obsessive-compulsive disorder (OCD), social anxiety disorder, generalized anxiety disorder (GAD), and posttraumatic stress disorder (PTSD). Moreover, studies have demonstrated the efficacy of paroxetine in premenstrual dysphoric disorder (PMDD), postmenopausal hot flashes, and child and adolescent OCD and social anxiety disorder. Paroxetine is still one of the most prescribed antidepressant medications in the United States because of its proven efficacy, as demonstrated in randomized, double-blind clinical trials, and its much improved tolerability compared with tricyclic antidepressants (TCAs) and monoamine oxidase inhibitors (MAOIs). Although paroxetine shares many characteristics with other members of the SRI class, its unique pharmacological characteristics and clinical database are reviewed, with particular attention to the clinical setting.

History and Discovery

The synthesis of the first SRI, fluoxetine, in 1972 marked the inception of an exciting new era of scientific and clin-

ical innovation in the field of psychiatry (Wong et al. 1995). Prior to this discovery, psychiatrists had only a few classes of pharmacological treatments for managing depression and anxiety. These medications, including TCAs, MAOIs, and benzodiazepines, were indeed efficacious; however, they were poorly tolerated and, therefore, quite limited in usefulness.

Shortly after the introduction of fluoxetine into the U.S. market in 1988, a marked increase in research led to the development of other SRIs, which ultimately proved effective in a wide array of psychiatric disorders. In 1992, paroxetine became the third SRI to be approved by the U.S. Food and Drug Administration (FDA) for the treatment of depression. Since then, it has also obtained FDA approval for the treatment of all five DSM-IV-TR (American Psychiatric Association 2000) anxiety disorders: panic disorder, OCD, PTSD, social anxiety disorder, and GAD. Paroxetine is available in 10-, 20-, 30-, and 40-mg tablets and in suspension form. A controlled-release (CR) formulation is available in 12.5-, 25-, and 37.5-mg tablets. It exhibits equal or better efficacy than the paroxetine immediate-release (IR) formulation, as well as clear advantages in tolerability (Golden et al. 2002).

Structure–Activity Relations and Pharmacological Profile

Paroxetine is a phenylpiperidine derivative chemically unrelated to any other antidepressant (Bourin et al. 2001) (Figure 15–1). As noted above, it has been traditionally codified with the SRI class of drugs and is indeed the most

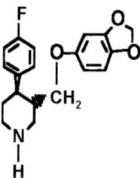

FIGURE 15–1.   Chemical structure of paroxetine.

potent inhibitor of the serotonin transporter (5-HTT) within this group of compounds (Frazer 2001). By comparison, sertraline has about one-half and fluoxetine has only one-tenth the affinity of paroxetine for the human 5-HTT (Owens et al. 1997). Positron emission tomography (PET) reveals that 85%–100% of 5-HTT binding sites are occupied in the amygdala and midbrain following 20- to 40-mg daily doses of paroxetine in human subjects (Kent et al. 2002; Meyer et al. 2001). Paroxetine-induced antagonism of the 5-HTT is prolonged following single-dose administration, and transporter binding is maintained for up to 14 days after 4 weeks of treatment in rodents, suggesting that it dissociates slowly from the 5-HTT binding site (Magnussen et al. 1982; Thomas et al. 1987).

Data from both humans and rodents, using the transfected human norepinephrine transporter (NET), have revealed that paroxetine is the most potent inhibitor of the NET among drugs classified as SRIs. Despite its relatively high affinity for the NET, paroxetine has a higher affinity for the 5-HTT (Finley 1994). Ex vivo experiments in rats demonstrated a 21% and 34% inhibition of the NET within the central nervous system (CNS) at serum concentrations of 100–500 ng/mL and >500 ng/mL, respectively (Owens et al. 2000). Results from an ex vivo study of patients with depression demonstrated substantial NET antagonism at serum concentrations attained with paroxetine IR dosages of 40 mg/day and higher (Gilmor et al. 2002) (Figure 15–2). These results have recently been replicated in depressed patients in a high-dose, forced-titration protocol comparing paroxetine CR dosages of 12.5 and 75 mg/day with venlafaxine XR dosages of 75–375 mg/day. Both medications produced dose-dependent inhibition of the 5-HTT and NET. Maximal 5-HTT inhibition for paroxetine and venlafaxine was 90% and 85%, respectively, whereas maximal NET inhibition for the two drugs was 33% and 61% (Owens et al. 2008). Such data reflect the inhibitory activity of both medications at the NET and 5-HTT within the CNS. The utility of ex vivo studies is best understood with respect to bioavailability. Paroxetine, which is highly pro-

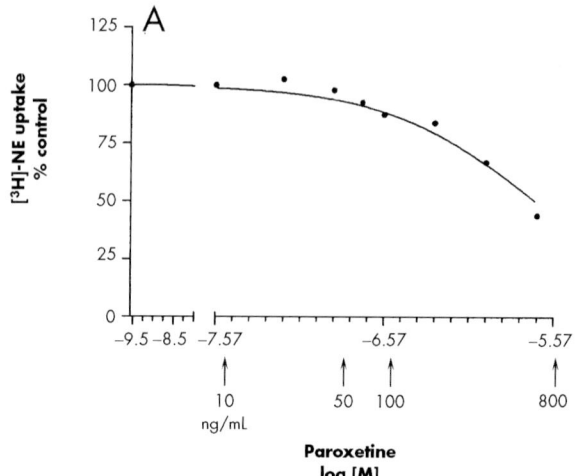

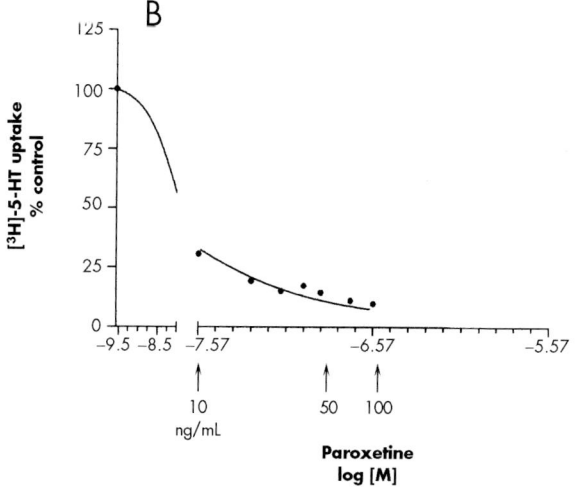

FIGURE 15–2.   Norepinephrine and serotonin uptake inhibition versus serum paroxetine concentration.

Standard curves for paroxetine inhibition of NE (**A**) and 5-HT (**B**) resulting from NET and 5-HTT antagonism, respectively. Note that at 100 ng/mL of paroxetine, which represents a typical therapeutic dose, there is a 15% decrease in NE uptake and a 90% decrease in 5-HT uptake. Transporter inhibition occurs in a dose-dependent manner. 5-HT = serotonin; 5-HTT = serotonin transporter; NE = norepinephrine; NET = norepinephrine transporter. *Source.*   Gilmor et al. 2002.

tein bound, must pass through the blood–brain barrier in order to interact with the NET and thereby contribute to the antidepressant effect of the drug (Frazer 2001). Because the ex vivo studies utilize transfected cells in tissue culture exposed to patient sera, only free drug that is not protein bound is available to interact in the NE uptake assay. These results can therefore be extrapolated to pharmacological effects in the CNS. Whether the NET antagonism observed in these ex vivo studies has clinical significance in terms of additional efficacy in comparison with drugs that solely block 5-HT reuptake will need to be further studied.

Paroxetine's role as a norepinephrine reuptake inhibitor (NRI) has implications for interpreting the results of head-to-head comparisons with other antidepressants. The minimal NET activity observed at more conventional doses of paroxetine necessitates that clinical trials comparing it with established SNRIs (Goldstein et al. 2004; Shelton et al. 2005) would have to employ doses much higher than 20 mg in order to be considered a valid comparison. It currently remains somewhat controversial whether the combination of 5-HTT and NET inhibition is associated with greater antidepressant efficacy (J.C. Nelson 1998; J.C. Nelson et al. 1991, 2004; Seth et al. 1992; Thase et al. 2001). Additionally, it remains to be discovered what magnitude of NE reuptake inhibition would result in increased efficacy and/or decreased latency of antidepressant effect.

Paroxetine has no appreciable affinity for the dopamine transporter (DAT) or for dopamine$_1$ (D$_1$), dopamine$_2$ (D$_2$), serotonin$_{1A}$ (5-HT$_{1A}$), serotonin$_{2A}$ (5-HT$_{2A}$), α_1- and α_2-adrenergic, and histamine$_1$ (H$_1$) receptors, indicating that it is a relatively "clean" drug, particularly when compared with the older generation of antidepressants, such as TCAs and MAOIs (Hyttel 1994; Owens et al. 1997). It is distinguished from sertraline by its high affinity for the NET and low affinity for the DAT. Sertraline, in contrast, has a very high affinity for the DAT but no affinity for the NET (Tulloch and Johnson 1992). The affinity of paroxetine for the muscarinic cholinergic receptor is approximately 22 nmol, which is similar to that of desipramine, though paroxetine is used in lower doses than desipramine and is therefore less anticholinergic than this TCA. However, this property may account for its mild anticholinergic side effects, including dry mouth, blurry vision, and constipation (Owens et al. 1997). However, compared with nortriptyline, paroxetine has virtually no measurable anticholinergic activity in geriatric patients treated for depression (Pollock et al. 1998). Table 15–1 shows a comparison of paroxetine and other available antidepressants in terms of their affinity for various neurotransmitter receptors and monoamine transporters.

Pharmacokinetics and Disposition

Paroxetine is well absorbed from the alimentary tract, and absorption is not affected by the presence or absence of food (Kaye et al. 1989). Being a highly lipophilic compound, paroxetine is readily distributed into peripheral tissues and exhibits a high volume of distribution, ranging from 3.1 to 28 L/kg (Kaye et al. 1989). Once absorbed, paroxetine is reportedly 95% bound to serum proteins (Kaye et al. 1989), though we have observed protein binding of 85% in our studies (M.J. Owens and C.B. Nemeroff, unpublished observations, June 1997). Oral bioavailability is affected by extensive first-pass metabolism, which is carried out by a high-affinity, low-capacity hepatic enzyme system (Lane 1996). With serial dosing, bioavailability increases as this metabolic system becomes saturated and a larger proportion of parent compound en-

TABLE 15–1. Inhibition constants (K$_i$, nmol/L) of various antidepressants for various transporters and receptors in human and animal cells

COMPOUND	5-HTT[a]	NET[a]	H$_1$[b]	α_1[a]	α_2[a]	MUSCARINIC[c]
Paroxetine	0.07	85	>10,000	1,000	4,000	42
Sertraline	0.15	800	5,000	36	470	230
Fluoxetine	1	800	1,000	1,300	3,000	500
Venlafaxine	7.5	2,300	>10,000	>10,000	>100,000	>10,000
Desipramine	22	0.63	30	23	1,400	37
Nefazodone	450	600	30	6	85	4,500
Citalopram	16.2	>10,000	300	>10,000	>10,000	>10,000
Escitalopram	6.6	>10,000	1,500	>10,000	>10,000	>10,000

Note.   5-HTT = serotonin transporter; NET = norepinephrine transporter.
[a]Human cortex.
[b]Guinea pig brain.
[c]Rat cortex.

ters the systemic circulation (Kaye et al. 1989). Steady-state concentrations of paroxetine, following oral dosing, exhibit wide intersubject variability (Sindrup et al. 1992a). Following 30 days of daily administration of 30 mg of paroxetine, steady-state plasma concentrations ranged from 8.6 to 105 ng/mL (Kaye et al. 1989). Such variability has been considered inconsequential because a consistent relationship between paroxetine levels and clinical response or adverse outcome has not been found (see Tasker et al. 1989). However, higher plasma concentrations are associated with a greater magnitude of both 5-HTT and NET inhibition (Gilmor et al. 2002).

Strong in vivo and in vitro evidence points to the hepatic cytochrome P450 (CYP) 2D6 enzyme system as the rate-limiting mechanism in the metabolism of paroxetine (Crewe et al. 1992; Sindrup et al. 1992a). Genetic studies have demonstrated up to 40 polymorphisms of the 2D6 enzyme, which likely explain, at least in part, the wide-ranging differences in pharmacokinetic parameters observed among individuals (Lane 1996). Phenotypically, individual probands can be categorized as poor, extensive, or ultrarapid metabolizers and will have very high, low, or very low serum paroxetine concentrations, respectively (Charlier et al. 2003). Patients with negligible or diminished 2D6 activity are poor metabolizers of paroxetine and other 2D6-dependent substrates and are thought to use alternative enzyme systems (Gunasekara et al. 1998; Lane 1996). The 2D6 enzyme system is believed to be primarily responsible for the initial step in the metabolism of paroxetine in extensive and ultrarapid metabolizers, carrying out oxidation of the methylenedioxy bridge. The resulting unstable catechol intermediate is methylated and subsequently conjugated into polar compounds by the addition of a glucuronide or sulfate moiety and is then excreted into urine and feces (Haddock et al. 1989). These conjugated entities are the major circulating metabolites of paroxetine; however, unlike the metabolites of other SRIs, such as fluoxetine or sertraline, they exhibit minimal in vitro monoamine uptake inhibition and likely do not contribute any therapeutic activity (DeVane 1992; Haddock et al. 1989).

Paroxetine is the most potent inhibitor of the 2D6 enzyme system of all of the SRIs ($K_i = 0.15 \mu M$) (Crewe et al. 1992; Nemeroff et al. 1996). Studies in healthy volunteers show that the drug continues to cause meaningful inhibition of 2D6 up to 5 days postdiscontinuation (Liston et al. 2002). As both a substrate for and an inhibitor of its own metabolism, paroxetine has a nonlinear pharmacokinetic profile, such that higher doses produce disproportionately greater plasma drug concentrations as the enzyme be-

comes saturated and, therefore, less available for metabolic activity (Preskorn 1993). Peak plasma concentration is attained in approximately 5 hours, and plasma steady-state concentration is achieved within 4–14 days, following oral administration of paroxetine IR (Kaye et al. 1989). The terminal half-life ($t_{1/2}$) of the parent compound is approximately 1 day and increases at higher doses, consequent to autoinhibition of 2D6 (Preskorn 1993). The pharmacokinetic properties of paroxetine appear to be affected by age. Bayer et al. (1989) reported a threefold increase in maximum plasma concentration in elderly subjects, compared with younger subjects, following a single dose of paroxetine. Furthermore, $t_{1/2}$ in the elderly subgroup was extended by nearly 100%. Although there was significant overlap in both pharmacokinetic parameters between the age groups studied, the clinical principle of "start low and go slow" regarding medication treatment in older patients applies to paroxetine.

Patients with renal and hepatic insufficiency are often subject to alterations in metabolism and clearance of drugs, compared with healthy subjects. In individuals with renal impairment, both half-life and maximum plasma levels of paroxetine have been shown to increase relative to the extent of renal disease (Doyle et al. 1989). In a single-dose study, no significant difference was observed in pharmacokinetic outcomes in patients with cirrhosis of the liver, compared with healthy volunteers (Krastev et al. 1989); however, subsequent data revealed considerable elevations in steady-state concentration and $t_{1/2}$ of paroxetine following 14 days of administration of paroxetine in individuals with severe liver disease (Dalhoff et al. 1991). Accordingly, patients with substantial renal or hepatic dysfunction should initially be treated with a lower dose of paroxetine than is generally recommended to avoid potential side effects associated with unusually high plasma paroxetine levels.

Paroxetine CR was designed to slow absorption and delay the release of paroxetine until after the tablet has passed the stomach. The dissolution rate of paroxetine CR after single dosing is about 4–5 hours. It is completely absorbed and otherwise exhibits the same pharmacokinetic parameters with regard to $t_{1/2}$ and nonlinearity as the IR formulation. Following absorption, paroxetine CR is extensively distributed and highly protein bound. Paroxetine CR causes increased plasma concentrations of paroxetine in patients with renal and hepatic dysfunction, and lower doses are therefore recommended for these patients (Paxil CR 2002).

Paroxetine mesylate is a generic formulation of the compound in which a methanesulfonic acid moiety is attached to the compound during the salification process instead of the hydrochloric acid used in paroxetine hydrochloride. It is currently available in some European countries including Holland and Denmark. Although currently there are no studies available comparing its efficacy or bioequivalence to paroxetine hydrochloride, there are several published case reports indicating problems of efficacy and tolerability in patients switched from paroxetine hydrochloride to paroxetine mesylate (Borgherini 2003) and this warrants further investigation.

Pharmacogenomics

The subject of pharmacogenomics has been of increasing interest to researchers and clinicians in all branches of contemporary medicine, including psychiatry. Inquiries into this field have been undertaken to gain a better understanding of the mechanisms by which variation between individuals occurs in clinical response to psychopharmacological treatment. Although pharmacogenetic principles are covered more thoroughly elsewhere in this text (see Chapter 3, "Genetics and Genomics"), here we will briefly focus on some of the recent work as applied to paroxetine. Specific attention will be paid to aspects of drug–gene interactions that affect tolerance and efficacy.

As previously described in this chapter, paroxetine's primary mode of action is likely mediated by its binding to the serotonin transporter (5-HTT). A well-known polymorphism (5-HT transporter gene–linked polymorphic region [5-HTTLPR]) has been located in the promoter region of the gene (SLC6A4) that encodes 5-HTT, resulting in two alleles referred to as "long" and "short." It has been proposed that this polymorphism might be a pharmacogenetic marker for antidepressant efficacy with some evidence that the short form, or S allele, results in reduced efficacy to SRI medications, including paroxetine (Zanardi et al. 2000). This finding was replicated in a study that included severity of drug-induced adverse events, dosing compliance indices, and discontinuations due to adverse events as main outcome measures in elderly depressed patients treated with paroxetine. The data revealed that subjects carrying the S allele experienced more severe adverse events, achieved lower final daily doses, and had more discontinuations during the course of the study. When, however, these subjects reached doses comparable with those of the homozygous L/L sample, efficacy measures were quite similar, albeit slower to exert maximal benefit, indicating that the main effect of the S allele was on the tolerability of paroxetine rather than

its efficacy (G.M. Murphy et al. 2004). In the only known head-to-head comparison of paroxetine and another SRI, in regard to the 5-HTTLPR polymorphism, a sample of 81 depressed Japanese patients were treated with either paroxetine or fluvoxamine. The results showed that although both drugs had similar efficacy in L-carrying probands, S/S homozygotes responded significantly better to paroxetine (Kato et al. 2005).

Another intriguing locus that has been studied as a possible genetic marker for antidepressant efficacy is the 102 T/C single-nucleotide polymorphism (SNP) in the serotonin$_{2A}$ (5-HT$_{2A}$) gene (*5HTR2A*). A second study, using the same patient sample and the same outcome measures as those of G.M. Murphy et al. (2004), was used to evaluate the role of the 102 T/C SNP in medication intolerance. Survival analysis showed a more or less linear relationship between the number of C alleles and the odds of patients discontinuing paroxetine therapy due to untoward effects (G.M. Murphy et al. 2003). Of note, when these investigators similarly studied the effect of genetic polymorphisms at the hepatic CYP2D6 gene, of which there are 40 known alleles, no signal could be detected with regard to tolerance or efficacy of paroxetine. The authors conclude that pharmacodynamic differences among patients, particularly at the *5HTR2A* site, appear to have a greater impact on paroxetine tolerability than pharmacokinetic variables.

Mechanism of Action

Despite almost four decades of intensive investigation directed at understanding the pathogenesis and pathophysiology of depression and related psychiatric disorders and the precise mechanism(s) of the therapeutic action of antidepressants, the answers to these questions remain elusive.

Early theorists suggested a causal association between an aberration in synaptic monoamine neurotransmitter concentrations and depression, based largely on the precipitation of depressive symptoms in a significant number of individuals treated with the antihypertensive agent reserpine, a monoamine-depleting drug (Goodwin and Bunney 1971). The once-celebrated "monoamine hypothesis of depression" provided the theoretical framework for the development and investigation of successive generations of antidepressants. This hypothesis, although seminal, has since been challenged as being too simplistic to explain either the pathophysiological underpinnings of depression or the mechanisms of action of antidepressants

(Duman et al. 1997; Ressler and Nemeroff 2000). Antidepressants that effectively increase monoamine neurotransmitter concentrations in the synapse, such as MAOIs, TCAs, SRIs, and SNRIs, clearly implicate the serotonergic and noradrenergic neuronal systems as targets of action of these drugs; however, drug binding to a specific receptor or transporter and consequent manipulation of its affiliated neural circuitry do not necessarily equate to the ultimate mechanism of action of a pharmacological agent (Dubovsky 1994). Although our understanding of antidepressant pharmacology and the biology of depression has grown exponentially, the relationship between the evident pharmacodynamic actions of antidepressants and their well-documented therapeutic effects remains relatively obscure.

Paroxetine and all of the other SRIs cause immediate elevations in extracellular fluid 5-HT concentrations in serotonergic synapses, resulting from the decreased 5-HT clearance associated with 5-HTT inhibition (Wagstaff et al. 2002). Blier et al. (1990) demonstrated that administration of paroxetine initially causes a paradoxical *decrease* in 5-HT neurotransmission, likely caused by activation of a negative feedback system mediated by increased 5-HT binding to the 5-HT_{1A} autoreceptor and subsequent diminution in serotonergic neural activity. After 2 weeks of paroxetine treatment, a desensitization of the 5-HT_{1A} autoreceptors occurs and is associated with an increase in serotonergic neurotransmission (Chaput et al. 1991). The delayed changes in 5-HT_{1A} receptor sensitivity and 5-HT neurotransmission seen after long-term paroxetine administration are temporally associated with clinical improvement, hinting at a possible mechanistic link.

These and related findings led to the study of pindolol, a nonselective β-adrenergic receptor antagonist/5-HT_{1A} antagonist, as a novel approach to accelerate the therapeutic response to SRIs, as well as to convert SRI nonresponders to responders. Preclinical studies revealed greater and more persistent increases in extracellular 5-HT concentrations after treatment with pindolol and an SRI than after treatment with an SRI alone (Dreshfield et al. 1996; Hjorth 1993; Sharp et al. 1997). This observation, coupled with the hypothesis that blockade of the presynaptic 5-HT_{1A} autoreceptor might serve to avert the initial reduction in serotonergic transmission induced by SRI treatment, suggested that the combination of pindolol and paroxetine might produce a more rapid and more robust clinical response (Perez et al. 1999).

Results from open studies supported both hypotheses (Artigas et al. 1994; Blier and Bergeron 1995). Double-blind, placebo-controlled trials also indicated that the addition of pindolol (2.5–5 mg three times a day) to paroxetine in the early phase of treatment for major depression might decrease latency to clinical improvement. However, the augmentation of clinical efficacy with pindolol was not compelling, especially in individuals refractory to monotherapy with paroxetine (Bordet et al. 1998; Perez et al. 1999; Tome et al. 1997; Zanardi et al. 1997). Currently, the available data do not support the use of pindolol to accelerate or augment the efficacy of paroxetine or other SRIs. To be fair, at the doses of pindolol used, PET imaging revealed that only a relatively low percentage of 5-HT_{1A} binding sites were occupied; therefore, the studies should be repeated with adequate doses of pindolol or another 5-HT_{1A} autoreceptor antagonist (Martinez et al. 2000).

Consistent with the potency of paroxetine in blocking NE reuptake are reports that it increases NE concentrations in extracellular fluid, as demonstrated by microdialysis techniques (Hajos-Korcsok et al. 2000). Although not studied extensively, chronic treatment with paroxetine, unlike TCAs such as desipramine, does not produce downregulation of postsynaptic β-adrenergic receptor binding sites in cerebral cortex and hippocampus (Duman et al. 1997).

While 5-HT and β-adrenergic receptor adaptation remains an attractive area of research, attention has increasingly been focused on postreceptor intracellular signal transduction changes observed after long-term antidepressant treatment. Chronic administration of antidepressants has been shown to activate second-messenger systems, such as cyclic adenosine monophosphate (cAMP) and tyrosine kinase B, associated with hippocampal neurons (Duman 1998). Data derived from postmortem human brain tissue studies suggest increased levels of brain-derived neurotrophic factor (BDNF) within the hippocampus of subjects with depression who had been treated with antidepressants, compared with control subjects with depression who had been nonmedicated (Chen et al. 2001). It has been suggested that neuronal injury mediated by stress-related illnesses, such as depression and anxiety, may be reversed by antidepressant-induced increases in BDNF expression in the CNS posited to contribute to clinical response (Duman 1998). Antidepressants from diverse classes, including SRIs, have all been shown to increase the rate of neurogenesis in the hippocampus of adult animals (Duman et al. 2001).

A recent boon to the study of antidepressant effect has been the development and fine-tuning of techniques in the field of functional brain imaging. One study compared the modulation of cortical-limbic systems in depressed patients who were treated with either paroxetine or cognitive-behavioral therapy (CBT) (Mayberg et al. 2004). PET was used to obtain images serially during the course of treatment and revealed interesting distinctions in brain activity in response to the two treatment modalities. Paroxetine responders experienced significant increases in prefrontal cortical activity in the setting of decreases in hippocampal and subgenual cingulate processing. This is in marked contrast to treatment-emergent changes seen in the CBT group in which patients developed increases in hippocampal and dorsal cingulate metabolism subsequent to subtle decreases in dorsal, ventral, and medial frontal cortical processing. The implication is that antidepressant therapy seems to entail a "bottom up" approach distinguishable from the "top down" effect seen with CBT. These results may help explain why combination treatment with antidepressants and various psychotherapies consistently outperforms monotherapy, particularly in moderate to severe depression.

Another major advance in the study of antidepressant action has been the link between paroxetine and the corticotropin-releasing factor (CRF)/hypothalamic-pituitary-adrenal (HPA) axis. It is well established that a sizeable percentage of patients with depression exhibit HPA axis hyperactivity and hypersecretion of CRF from hypothalamic and extrahypothalamic circuits (Heim and Nemeroff 1999). Early life stress, as exemplified by maternal separation, is associated with profound hyperactivity of the HPA axis and increased CRF messenger RNA (mRNA) expression (Nemeroff 1996; Newport et al. 2002). In adult animals, these effects are reversed by chronic, but not acute, paroxetine treatment. Thus, paroxetine exerts multiple effects on neurotransmitter systems implicated in the pathophysiology of mood and anxiety disorders, including 5-HT, NE, and CRF.

Indications and Efficacy

Depression

Comparison With Other Agents

Tricyclic and tetracyclic antidepressants.   The efficacy of paroxetine in major depression has been established in several randomized, placebo-controlled studies, as well as in studies comparing the effects of paroxetine with those of active comparators, including fluoxetine, TCAs, and other agents. The preponderance of early data with paroxetine in establishing efficacy in depression was

in comparison trials with TCAs, particularly imipramine and amitriptyline, and placebo. The earliest placebo-controlled trials used 10–50 mg of paroxetine and were 6 weeks in duration. Outcome variables typically used were the Hamilton Rating Scale for Depression (Ham-D), the Montgomery-Åsberg Depression Rating Scale (MADRS), and the Clinical Global Impressions (CGI) Scale. These trials demonstrated the clear superiority of paroxetine over placebo in the treatment of major depression (Claghorn et al. 1992; Kiev 1992; Rickels et al. 1989; Smith and Glaudin 1992).

A meta-analysis by Montgomery (2001) compared the efficacy and tolerability of paroxetine with those of TCAs, including amitriptyline, imipramine, clomipramine, doxepin, and nortriptyline, and the tetracyclic antidepressants mianserin and maprotiline. Studies included in the meta-analysis were randomized, double-blind, and parallel-group in design; were 6 weeks or less in duration; and employed the Ham-D as the primary outcome measure. Results from the pooled data of 3,758 hospitalized and ambulatory patients from 39 studies showed no overall significant difference in antidepressant response rates between paroxetine and TCAs or tetracyclics, based on a ≥50% reduction in the Ham-D total score or in remission rates, defined as an endpoint Ham-D score of ≤8. Clearly, paroxetine is better tolerated than the TCAs and related heterocyclic antidepressants in terms of lower rates of discontinuation attributed to adverse events. In addition, paroxetine had a greater effect on concomitant anxiety associated with depression, compared with all other studied medications, except clomipramine, which was equally efficacious with regard to anxiolysis.

Despite the overwhelming evidence supporting the equivalent antidepressant efficacy of paroxetine and TCAs, one notable exception exists. The Danish University Antidepressant Group (1990) conducted a multicenter double-blind, placebo-controlled, fixed-dose investigation comparing the efficacy and tolerability of paroxetine (30 mg/day) with clomipramine (150 mg/day) and found nonresponder rates to be significantly greater in the paroxetine group. Whereas most of the data supporting the clinical superiority of paroxetine are derived from outpatient studies, the Danish University Antidepressant Group (1990) study comprised only inpatients. These data appear to argue for relative greater efficacy of clomipramine in severe depression; however, two notable confounds exist here. First, higher dosages of paroxetine (e.g., 50–60 mg/day) might well show equivalent efficacy with clomipramine, especially in view of the NET findings described above. Second, Ham-D scores reported in this study were no more severe than those in the outpatient trials, making it difficult to draw any conclusions regarding relative superiority of clomipramine based on severity of depression. All other published studies comparing paroxetine with clomipramine have shown no difference in efficacy in outpatients with depression; paroxetine is, of course, uniformly better tolerated (Guillibert et al. 1989; Pelicier and Schaeffer 1993; Ravindran et al. 1997).

Other SRIs.   Because the SRIs, as a class, have become the first-line pharmacological agents in the treatment of depression and a number of anxiety disorders, the results of a large number of studies, mostly sponsored by the pharmaceutical industry, are available. To date, fluoxetine, fluvoxamine, and sertraline have been compared with paroxetine in the treatment of major depression. In addition, given the favorable response of SRIs in several anxiety disorders, clinical trials have compared the clinical ameliorative effects of paroxetine with those of other SRIs on anxiety symptoms associated with depression.

De Wilde et al. (1993) found, at various time points during the trial, statistically significant advantages of paroxetine (20–40 mg/day) over fluoxetine (20–60 mg/day) in total Ham-D score and anxiety subscore. However, by the end of the 6-week study, there was no difference noted in any outcome variable. Geretsegger et al. (1994) studied a group of geriatric patients with severe depression (n = 106) and found a significantly greater proportion of patients treated with paroxetine (20–40 mg/day) than fluoxetine (20–60 mg/day) to have a ≥50% reduction in total Ham-D and MADRS scores by the end of the study; however, no difference was observed in terms of response based on the CGI Scale or between-group differences in MADRS or Ham-D at the termination of the study. Other studies have found paroxetine and fluoxetine to be equally effective in the treatment of major depression and associated anxiety (Chouinard et al. 1999; Fava et al. 1998, 2000; Tignol 1993).

Similar results have been observed in trials comparing paroxetine and sertraline. Zanardi et al. (1996) studied a small group (n = 46) of hospitalized patients with psychotic depression and found rates of response to both medications among study completers to be comparable. The intent-to-treat analysis in this trial revealed sertraline (150 mg/day) to be more effective than paroxetine (50 mg/day). The authors suggested that the difference might be attributable to the disproportionately high dropout rate (41%) in the paroxetine group, likely caused by the rapid paroxetine dose titration, compared with the dropout rate in the sertraline group. In the only published study comparing paroxetine and sertraline in a 6-month trial, the two medications had similar antidepressant efficacy and similar ratings on quality-of-life measures (Aberg-Wistedt et al. 2000).

Kiev and Feiger (1997) reported that paroxetine (20–50 mg/day) and fluvoxamine (50–150 mg/day) had equivalent efficacy in the treatment of depression.

Other agents.   Paroxetine has also been compared with nefazodone, mirtazapine, bupropion, moclobemide, duloxetine, venlafaxine, and investigational agents such as substance P (neurokinin 1 [NK_1]) antagonists in the treatment of depression. Nefazodone (200–600 mg/day) and paroxetine (20–40 mg/day) were shown to possess similar efficacy and tolerability in an 8-week randomized, double-blind trial of 206 outpatients with moderate to severe depression (Baldwin et al. 1996). In this study, 42.3% of patients in the paroxetine-treated group and 39.7% of patients in the nefazodone-treated group achieved ≥50% reduction in the Ham-D intent-to-treat analysis. Furthermore, both groups had similar significant reductions in associated anxiety. In a study comparing paroxetine (20–40 mg/day) and mirtazapine (15–45 mg/day) in 275 outpatients with major depression, both medications fared equally well in terms of efficacy and tolerability (Benkert et al. 2000). There was evidence of a slightly faster onset of action with mirtazapine, as determined by significant reductions in the 17-item Ham-D and Hamilton Anxiety Scale (Ham-A) scores by week 1 of the study, compared with paroxetine.

A recent randomized open trial was conducted in Italy comparing paroxetine with moclobemide, a reversible MAOI widely prescribed in Europe for the treatment of depression (Pini et al. 2003). The results suggested greater efficacy for paroxetine in the treatment of major depressive disorder with comorbid panic disorder; however, these data are limited by lack of double-blinding.

The SNRI venlafaxine was compared with paroxetine in a population of hospitalized and ambulatory patients with treatment resistance to two or more antidepressants (Poirier and Boyer 1999). Venlafaxine (200–300 mg/day) was superior to paroxetine (30–40 mg/day) in bringing treatment-refractory patients into remission, defined as total Ham-D score of ≤10 at study end (37% vs. 18%, respectively). It should be noted that this definition of remission departs from the customary criterion of Ham-D total score ≤7 and that the study period was rather short (4 weeks), limiting comparison with data from longer-term parallel-group studies with a more standard definition of remission. In the meta-analysis of the venlafaxine worldwide database, in which venlafaxine showed a slight statistically significant advantage in efficacy over SRIs as a class, there was no such difference demonstrated between venlafaxine and paroxetine (Nemeroff et al. 2003). A more recent comparison between venlafaxine XR and paroxetine demonstrated higher rates of remission with venlafaxine in the maintenance treatment of depression (Shelton et al. 2005). An important caveat in interpreting these results is that the doses of paroxetine used never exceeded 20 mg/day and are therefore indicative of only minimal NE reuptake antagonism. Similarly, a study comparing paroxetine with the SNRI duloxetine (40–80 mg/day) revealed higher probability of remission with duloxetine 80 mg/day than with paroxetine (57% and 34%, respectively) (Goldstein et al. 2004). Again, paroxetine was administered to test subjects at the "selective" serotonergic dose of 20 mg/day, too low to exhibit true SNRI activity.

Paroxetine has also been compared with investigational agents such as substance P (NK_1) receptor antagonists. In the Merck-sponsored NK_1 receptor antagonist trials in major depression, paroxetine 20 mg/day was superior to both placebo and the putative novel agent (Cutler et al. 2000).

Depression in the Elderly

Geriatric depression deserves special attention because it is a particularly common, debilitating, and potentially life-threatening disorder (see Weihs et al. 2000). A large number of studies have been conducted with a variety of medications, particularly TCAs and SRIs, in geriatric patients with depression. SRIs are currently the treatment of choice in this population because of their demonstrated efficacy and their relative safety over TCAs and MAOIs. Paroxetine has been shown to be effective in treating individuals with late-life depression in a number of parallel-group trials. Hutchinson et al. (1992) reported that paroxetine (20–30 mg/day) and amitriptyline (50–100 mg/day) were equally effective in a 6-week trial, as determined by similar rates of response and a somewhat faster onset of action for paroxetine. Another study comparing paroxetine (20–30 mg/day) and amitriptyline (50–150 mg/day) yielded similar results, although the time to response was identical between the two agents (Geretsegger et al. 1995). Clomipramine (75 mg/day) and paroxetine (30 mg/day) were equally effective in patients (ages ≥60 years) with depression, as determined by a change in Ham-D and Widlocher Scale scores (Guillibert et al.

1989). Although dropout rates secondary to adverse events were similar, CNS and anticholinergic side effects, not surprisingly, were more frequent in the clomipramine group (41% vs. 18%). Mulsant et al. (1999) reported similar response rates for nortriptyline (mean dosage = 51.4 mg/day) and paroxetine (mean dosage = 23 mg/day) in 80 geriatric patients with depression. The two drug groups had comparable dropout rates.

In view of evidence that elderly patients with depression are more likely to experience earlier relapses than nonelderly depressed patients following successful treatment (Zis et al. 1980), Bump et al. (2001) conducted a study, funded by the National Institute of Mental Health (NIMH), that compared paroxetine (10–40 mg/day) and nortriptyline (20–125 mg/day) in an 18-month, open-label continuation and maintenance trial. No significant differences in rates of relapse (15% for paroxetine and 9.5% for nortriptyline) or time to relapse (60.3 weeks for paroxetine and 58.8 weeks for nortriptyline) were noted. Maintenance efficacy was likewise investigated by Reynolds et al. (2006) using monthly interpersonal psychotherapy (IPT) as a comparator. Patients 70 years or older with major depression who responded to combined treatment with paroxetine and IPT were significantly less likely to have recurrent depression if they received 2 years of maintenance paroxetine compared with placebo. Conversely, maintenance psychotherapy in the absence of drug was ineffective in preventing recurrence. The researchers concluded that the number needed to treat with paroxetine to prevent 1 recurrence was 4 (95% confidence interval [CI] = 2.3–10.9).

In a study by Schöne and Ludwig (1993), paroxetine (20–40 mg/day) was superior in efficacy to fluoxetine (20–60 mg/day) in elderly patients using response rates (≥50% reduction in Ham-D score) as the measure of improvement. Improvements in cognitive function, as measured by the Sandoz Clinical Assessment Geriatric (SCAG) Scale, were similar in both groups at the end of 6 weeks; however, there appeared to be a more rapid response with paroxetine (Gunasekara et al. 1998). A subsequent trial also found paroxetine to be more effective in improving cognitive function at early time points and by study end (Geretsegger et al. 1994). In both studies, paroxetine and fluoxetine were shown to be well tolerated. Weihs et al. (2000) compared paroxetine (10–40 mg/day) and bupropion sustained-release (SR) (100–300 mg/day) in 100 elderly patients with major depression and found similar improvements in all outcomes and comparably low discontinuation rates secondary to adverse events by study end.

One element of concern in treating the frail elderly with paroxetine is the fear of possible anticholinergic side effects. This population is, of course, susceptible to cognitive decline caused by muscarinic antagonist drugs, which can, in some cases, lead to frank delirium. This concern was formally tested in a study of paroxetine effects on mood and cognition in depressed elderly patients without dementia using fluoxetine as a comparator because of the latter drug's minimal anticholinergic activity (Cassano et al. 2002). The results revealed that paroxetine did not cause cognitive decline but rather produced marked improvement on neuropsychological test scores in depressed elderly patients.

Long-Term Treatment

It is now well recognized that because unipolar depression is often a chronic and recurrent disorder, the prevention of recurrence should be a primary aim. Although there are considerable data supporting the efficacy of paroxetine in short-term trials, only a handful of studies have evaluated its effectiveness in maintaining remission following an acute episode of depression over an extended period.

In a large multicenter open-label trial, Duboff (1993) treated 433 patients with paroxetine (mean dose = 32.9 mg) for 54 weeks. Subjects had moderate to severe depression (mean 17-item Ham-D baseline score = 27.9), and most subjects (81%) had a history of depressive episodes. Approximately two-thirds of the subjects were judged responders (Ham-D score ≤8) at 54 weeks. Nineteen percent of the subjects suffered a relapse (Ham-D score ≥18 at some time point), and 30% withdrew from the study because of adverse events. A 3-year extension study of 110 patients demonstrated the continued antidepressant effects of paroxetine.

Montgomery and Dunbar (1993) studied 172 patients with major depression who had had two or more previous depressive episodes in an 8-week open-label trial with paroxetine (20–40 mg/day), followed by a double-blind, placebo-controlled 1-year extension phase for the acute-treatment responders. The authors reported significantly higher rates of relapse in placebo recipients (43%), compared with paroxetine-treated patients (16%).

Claghorn and Feighner (1993) compared paroxetine (10–50 mg/day), imipramine (65–275 mg/day), and placebo in 717 patients with major depression. Similar rates of response among all three groups were noted after 1 year, following a blinded 6-week acute course of therapy. However, more placebo-treated patients withdrew from the long-term trial because of lack of efficacy (22%) than did

those treated with paroxetine (12%) or imipramine (4%). Moreover, 25% of the placebo group relapsed, compared with 15% of the paroxetine group and 4% of the imipramine group. A substantially greater percentage of patients in the imipramine group (35%) withdrew from the study because of adverse events than in the group receiving paroxetine (15%) or placebo (9%).

In all three studies cited above, the paroxetine doses used in the long-term phases were those typically used in the acute studies (20–40 mg). Thus, for maintenance therapy for depression, the recommended dose of paroxetine is the dose that was effective during the acute phase.

In most patients with an acute major depressive episode, an initial daily dose of 20 mg is usually sufficient for the duration of the illness episode, at least using response as an endpoint (Dunner and Dunbar 1992). However, to improve the likelihood of remission, we recommend increasing the dosage in 10-mg increments per week—up to 50 mg/day or more of the IR form and up to 75 mg/day of the CR form (Nemeroff 1993). Elderly patients and those with renal and hepatic dysfunction should be initiated at a lower dose, with gradual dose titration to therapeutic effect, while monitoring for side effects.

Bipolar Depression

Patients with bipolar disorder present significant clinical challenges, not the least of which are episodes of bipolar depression; nearly 50% of such patients are unresponsive to the antidepressant effects of lithium alone (Sachs 1996). This is a particularly difficult clinical problem because antidepressants may precipitate manic episodes in patients with bipolar disorder.

Two paroxetine studies have demonstrated the efficacy and safety of this SRI in treating patients with this often treatment-refractory disorder. In one study with lithium-treated patients, Bauer et al. (1999) found paroxetine (20–40 mg/day) to be superior to amitriptyline (75–150 mg/day), on the basis of the Ham-D and CGI–Severity of Illness (CGI-S) scores, although relatively low doses of amitriptyline were used in the 6-week study. In a multicenter double-blind, placebo-controlled comparison trial, Nemeroff et al. (2001) found no difference in response rates among paroxetine (20–50 mg/day), imipramine (150–300 mg/day), and placebo in patients stabilized on a regimen of lithium in a 10-week trial; however, both antidepressants were superior to placebo in treating patients with bipolar disorder with serum lithium concentrations ≤0.8 mEq/L. A study of 27 patients with bipolar I and II disorders receiving a mood stabilizer (lithium or divalproex) at the time of the study evaluated the addition of a second mood stabilizer or paroxetine for the treatment of depression (Young et al. 2000). Both treatment conditions were found to be effective, although patients in the mood stabilizer plus paroxetine group experienced fewer side effects and were more likely to complete the study. Sachs et al. (2007) did not find any difference between paroxetine (10–40 mg/day), bupropion SR (150–375 mg/day), and placebo in a 26-week placebo-controlled study of antidepressant augmentation of mood stabilizer therapy in 366 patients with bipolar depression. Paroxetine was not associated with an increased rate of switch into mania or hypomania in any of these studies.

Depression Associated With Medical Illness

It has been increasingly recognized that depression frequently occurs as a "co-traveler" with a number of medical conditions, and paroxetine has been studied and found to be efficacious in several of these disorders, including rheumatoid arthritis, irritable bowel syndrome, and, most recently, interferon-α-induced depression in malignant melanoma patients (Bird and Broggini 2000; Masand et al. 2001; Musselman et al. 2001). The Musselman et al. (2001) study is a true landmark in the field, because it demonstrated, for the first time, the prevention of an induced depression by pretreatment with paroxetine (Figure 15–3). The association between ischemic heart disease (IHD) and depression has also been extensively studied. Individuals with IHD have a greater risk than the general population for developing depression, and patients with depression are more likely to develop IHD and cerebrovascular disease than are individuals without depression (Anda et al. 1993; Frasure-Smith et al. 1993; J.M. Murphy et al. 1987; Musselman et al. 2007; Simonsick et al. 1995).

Increased platelet reactivity has been observed in individuals with depression, which may explain the increased vulnerability to IHD in this population (Musselman et al. 1996). One study demonstrated normalization of platelet activity in patients with depression, following 6 weeks of treatment with paroxetine 20 mg/day (Musselman et al. 2000). It is unclear whether the antidepressant action of paroxetine or a direct pharmacological effect of the drug on platelet activity resulted in the observed outcome, but the preponderance of evidence with other SRIs supports the latter hypothesis (Serebruany et al. 2003).

Although the physiological association between depression and IHD is still obscure, there is ample evidence

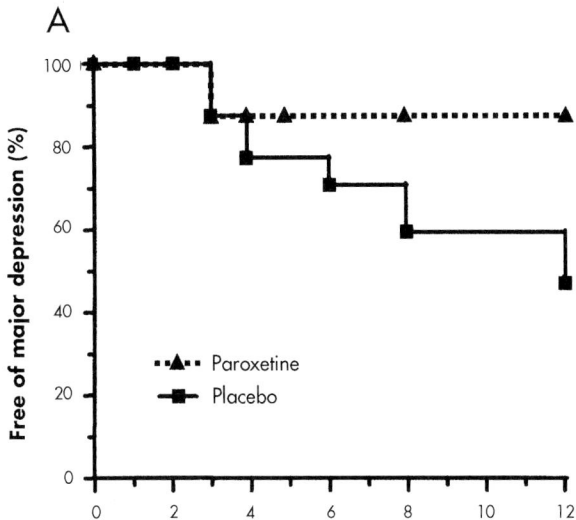

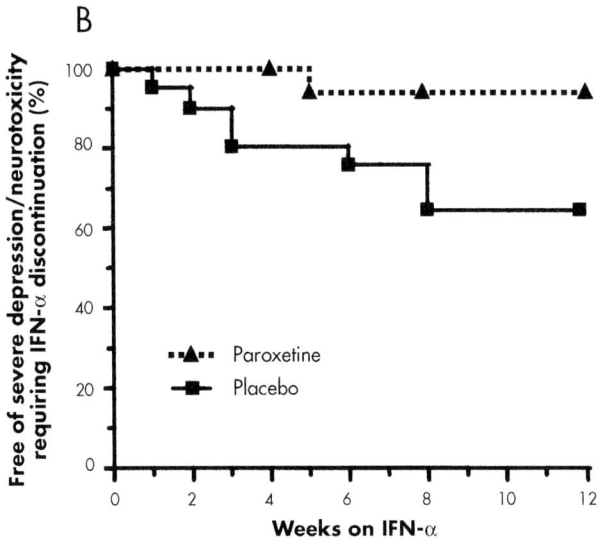

FIGURE 15–3. Paroxetine effect on interferon-α (IFN-α)–induced depression.

Kaplan-Meier analysis of the percentage of patients in the placebo and paroxetine groups who were free of major depression (**A**) and of severe depression, requiring the discontinuation of IFN-α (**B**). *Source.* Musselman et al. 2000.

that the treatment of depression and comorbid IHD with SRIs is safe and effective and that it reduces the risk of adverse cardiac events (Roose and Spatz 1999). In a landmark study, Roose et al. (1998) reported that paroxetine and nortriptyline were both effective in treating depression in elderly patients with severe heart disease but that paroxetine had a superior safety and tolerability profile. It is currently unknown whether early recognition and treatment of depression will reduce the risk of future cardiac disease.

Childhood and Adolescent Depression

The subject of the role of paroxetine in the treatment of depression in children and adolescents has been one of great controversy and media attention. On June 19, 2003, the FDA released a statement regarding a possible increased risk of suicidal thinking and suicide attempts in children and adolescents 18 years of age and younger treated with paroxetine for major depressive disorder (U.S. Food and Drug Administration 2003). The statement was based on data from three well-controlled unpublished studies, each showing no benefit for paroxetine above placebo in the treatment of pediatric depression. In addition to the lack of demonstrable efficacy for paroxetine, the data were troubling in that they revealed a two- to threefold increase in suicidal ideation and suicide attempts for paroxetine compared with placebo (3.4% and 1.2%, respectively).

These data contrasted with those of an earlier study supporting the efficacy of paroxetine in the treatment of depression in this population. Keller et al. (2001) conducted a randomized, double-blind study of adolescents (ages 12–18 years) that compared paroxetine with placebo. Paroxetine demonstrated a significant advantage over placebo in most, but not all, outcome variables. It is, however, notable that they reported a rate of suicidal behavior/ideation in the paroxetine group of 5.4%; the rate of the placebo arm was not contained in the report.

More recently, Emslie et al. (2006) reported that paroxetine was no more efficacious than placebo in the treatment of pediatric depression. Using the Children's Depression Rating Scale—Revised, they found that at week 8 of treatment, the total adjusted mean changes in score from baseline for patients receiving paroxetine and placebo were –22.58 and 23.38 points, respectively. In this trial, rates of suicidal ideation and behavior were comparable between the paroxetine (1.92%) and placebo (0.98%) groups. An important distinction between the above-mentioned studies was that Emslie et al. (2006) used lower doses of paroxetine than did Keller et al. (2001); mean dosages were 20.4 and 28 mg/day, respectively. This difference is highly relevant, given that paroxetine has been shown to exhibit marked nonlinear kinetics in children. Findling et al. (1999) showed that an increase in dosage from 10 to 20 mg results in a sixfold increase in child serum paroxetine levels.

The FDA's black box warning concerning antidepressant use and suicidality risk in children and adolescents has already had a major adverse impact on SRI prescribing in the under-18 age group (Nemeroff et al. 2007). For the first time in a decade, an increase in teenage suicide rates has been noted, perhaps due to the decrease in antidepressant prescribing.

Obsessive-Compulsive Disorder

Prior to the introduction of SRIs, the most effective pharmacological treatment for OCD was clomipramine. Early studies showed that patients with both OCD and depressive symptoms fared better on clomipramine than patients treated with other available TCAs (Pigott and Seay 1999). Later work revealed that clomipramine was effective in treating OCD, independent of the presence or severity of comorbid depressive symptoms (Fineberg et al. 1992).

The notable efficacy of clomipramine in OCD was attributed to its remarkable potency as a 5-HT reuptake inhibitor (Benfield et al. 1980). The 5-HTT-specific action of clomipramine, coupled with its specificity in targeting obsessive-compulsive symptoms, led to the formulation of the "serotonin hypothesis of OCD," which posited disturbed 5-HT neurotransmission in OCD (see D.L. Murphy et al. 1989; Zohar and Insel 1987). Consequently, researchers focused their efforts on identifying and developing other agents that were effective in treating OCD, without the unfavorable side effects of TCAs, including their anticholinergic, antihistaminergic, and antiadrenergic properties.

Currently, among the SRIs, fluvoxamine, fluoxetine, sertraline, citalopram, and paroxetine have been shown to be effective, in comparisons with placebo, in the treatment of OCD in randomized, double-blind trials (Greist et al. 1995; Montgomery et al. 2001). Although two meta-analyses assessing the efficacy and tolerability of clomipramine and SRIs in OCD seemed to favor clomipramine in terms of overall effectiveness (Greist et al. 1995; Piccinelli et al. 1995), the only placebo-controlled multicenter study to compare clomipramine (50–250 mg/day) directly with an SRI, paroxetine (20–60 mg/day), revealed equal efficacy (Zohar and Judge 1996). Moreover, significantly more patients receiving clomipramine dropped out of the study because of side effects compared with patients receiving either paroxetine or placebo. These results suggest that paroxetine is a safe and effective treatment for OCD and is preferable to clomipramine as a first-line agent.

More recent work in the field of functional brain imaging has elucidated paroxetine's effect on neural processing in patients suffering from OCD. Saxena et al. (2002) demonstrated that paroxetine treatment led to significant decreases in metabolic activity in the right caudate, bilat-

regimen was not tested against standard fixed-dosing schedules. It is likewise unknown whether such "drug holidays" lead to better adherence or outcomes.

Menopausal Vasomotor Symptoms

In addition to its proven efficacy in PMDD, paroxetine (20 mg/day) was shown to be effective in the treatment of postmenopausal hot flashes in breast cancer survivors with chemotherapy-induced ovarian failure in two open trials (Stearns et al. 2000; Weitzner et al. 2002; for a review, see Bordeleau et al. 2007) and in a double-blind study (Stearns et al. 2005). Paroxetine CR (25 mg/day) was subsequently found to be efficacious in treating perimenopausal hot flashes in a placebo-controlled trial (Stearns et al. 2003). The drug's usefulness in this setting is underscored by recent concerns about the safety of hormone replacement therapy (HRT), hitherto the treatment of choice (H.D. Nelson et al. 2002). For clinicians and patients concerned about the long-term consequences of estrogen replacement in treating hot flashes, paroxetine provides a reasonable alternative.

Side Effects and Toxicology

The popularity of SRIs, as a class, in the treatment of psychiatric disorders is owed not to their superiority in efficacy over their predecessors but rather to their overall tolerability and safety. In general, SRIs share a common profile in terms of severity and frequency of side effects. The side-effect profile of paroxetine has been studied extensively in comparison studies with other psychotropic medications and placebo. The most commonly cited adverse experiences in patients treated with paroxetine are, in order of frequency, nausea, headache, somnolence, dry mouth, asthenia, sweating, constipation, dizziness, and tremor (Boyer and Blumhardt 1992).

According to the worldwide preregistration clinical trial database, anticholinergic side effects, tremor, dizziness, postural hypotension, and somnolence were more common in comparison drugs—generally TCAs—in mostly short-term studies (Jenner 1992). Nausea and abnormal ejaculation were more frequently reported with paroxetine than with active controls. In these early trials, a greater proportion of patients in the antidepressant comparison and placebo groups withdrew because of adverse events than did patients in the paroxetine group. According to preregistration data, 13% of patients taking paroxetine dropped out prior to study's end because of side effects, compared with 19% for other agents and 5% for placebo. The most common side effect associated with early termination for paroxetine was nausea. Clinical experience demonstrates that this significant complaint can be mitigated with a conservative starting dose and administration with food, as well as with the use of the CR form of the compound. Furthermore, patients reported that nausea diminishes markedly with prolonged administration, a phenomenon also noted in long-term trials (Jenner 1992).

According to the limited data available comparing paroxetine directly with other newer-generation antidepressants, notably venlafaxine, sertraline, and fluoxetine, tolerability was similar and early termination rates were also comparable (Aberg-Wistedt et al. 2000; Ballus et al. 2000; Poirier and Boyer 1999; Schöne and Ludwig 1993; Tignol 1993). A possible exception to this might be mirtazapine. As described earlier in this chapter (see "Pharmacogenomics" section), the presence of the S allele in the 5-HTT gene and the C allele in the 5-HT$_{2A}$ receptor gene both confer lower tolerability and earlier discontinuation in patients taking paroxetine. Neither of these polymorphisms had any effect on tolerability of mirtazapine, which demonstrated lower rates of adverse events and discontinuation in comparison with paroxetine (G.M. Murphy et al. 2003, 2004). As noted earlier, elderly patients do not appear to be more susceptible to the side effects of paroxetine, and cognitive function remains intact or improves during treatment (Cassano et al. 2002; Nebes et al. 1999).

The paroxetine CR formulation has been compared with paroxetine IR in a placebo-controlled, randomized trial (Golden et al. 2002). Although the frequency of reported side effects was similar between the two active agents, paroxetine CR was significantly less likely to induce nausea (14%), compared with paroxetine IR (23%), in the first week of treatment. A later comparison that used time to discontinuation and economic costs as primary outcome measures found that patients on the CR formulation remained on therapy longer, resulting in better outcomes and lower health care costs (Sheehan et al. 2004). Because nausea is the most frequently reported side effect associated with paroxetine treatment and because it often results in medication discontinuation, paroxetine CR may offer a clinical advantage over the IR formulation in terms of improved treatment compliance and overall clinical effectiveness.

Sexual Side Effects

Sexual dysfunction is a liability associated with many psychotropic medications, and the full scope of this problem is only recently gaining its deserved recognition. When assessing emergence of side effects, most clinical studies rely on spontaneous reporting of adverse experiences. Because most patients do not feel comfortable reporting sexual side effects, it is not surprising that treatment-emergent sexual dysfunction is often underreported in these trials. In one prospective study, specific inquiry about sexual dysfunction with treatment of fluoxetine, paroxetine, sertraline, or fluvoxamine resulted in nearly a threefold increase in reporting of sexual problems, compared with only spontaneous communication (Montejo-Gonzalez et al. 1997).

Typically, data derived from clinical studies estimate sexual disability attributed to SRIs to be less than 20%, whereas in clinical practice the incidence appears to be significantly higher, perhaps as high as 40%. This side effect clearly has an adverse effect on medication adherence, partly because discussion of sexual issues is difficult for patients and clinicians alike. Although all SRIs and venlafaxine have been associated with male and female sexual dysfunction, there is a prevailing view among clinicians that this side effect might be more problematic with paroxetine, although few controlled data are available to address this issue. In a comparison study of 200 subjects treated with paroxetine, fluoxetine, fluvoxamine, or sertraline, paroxetine treatment was associated with higher rates of anorgasmia or difficulty with ejaculation and impotence in both men and women (Montejo-Gonzalez et al. 1997). Significant differences among the four drugs were not noted with respect to decrease in libido, delay in orgasm, or patient attitude toward treatment-induced sexual disability. In a large cross-sectional observational study ($N=6,297$) conducted by Clayton et al. (2002), paroxetine was associated with the highest prevalence of overall sexual dysfunction, compared with a wide range of novel antidepressants, including mirtazapine, venlafaxine, sertraline, citalopram, fluoxetine, nefazodone, and bupropion. However, a significant difference between paroxetine and the other agents was observed with only fluoxetine, bupropion, and nefazodone. Waldinger et al. (1998) studied 51 men without depression who had premature ejaculation and noted greater delay in time to ejaculation during paroxetine treatment, compared with treatment with fluoxetine, fluvoxamine, and sertraline.

The above findings have led to the use of paroxetine and other SRIs in the treatment of premature ejaculation (PE) in men (Balon 1996). Head-to-head comparisons between paroxetine and other antidepressants in the treatment of PE currently exist only for dapoxetine and mirtazapine. Safarinejad (2006) used a measure called the Intravaginal Ejaculatory Latency Time (IELT) to test paroxetine's effectiveness in slowing down male climax versus dapoxetine, a short-acting SRI that is currently awaiting FDA approval for the treatment of PE. Male patients taking paroxetine in a randomized, double-blind fashion showed IELT increases from a mean of 31 seconds at baseline to 370 seconds with treatment, whereas subjects taking dapoxetine (38 seconds to 179 seconds) or placebo (34 seconds to 55 seconds) did not fare as well. Ejaculatory latency was likewise compared, using the IELT measure, between paroxetine and mirtazapine. In a 6-week double-blind study, treatment with paroxetine (20 mg/day), but not mirtazapine (30 mg/day), resulted in significant delays in orgasm and ejaculation in men with PE (Waldinger et al. 2003).

Sexual side effects emerge in a dose-dependent fashion and do not appear to diminish with prolonged administration. Strategies to lessen the impact of psychotropic medications on sexual function include using dosage reduction, changing to a different antidepressant with lesser sexual side-effect liability, and adding an agent, such as sildenafil, yohimbine, buspirone, cyproheptadine, amantadine, methylphenidate, or bupropion, to reverse the sexual side effects (Rosen et al. 1999). Controlled studies demonstrating the efficacy of these agents are largely lacking, with one exception. Ephedrine, an α- and β-adrenergic agonist previously shown to enhance genital blood flow in women, was evaluated in 19 women experiencing SRI-induced sexual dysfunction from paroxetine, sertraline, or fluoxetine (Meston 2004). Although ephedrine (50 mg taken within 1 hour of sexual activity onset) significantly improved self-reported scores of desire and orgasm intensity compared with baseline, these measures, in addition to sexual arousal and satisfaction, were also similarly enhanced by placebo.

Suicidality

Apprehension surrounding the alleged relationship between SRIs and suicide first gained media attention in the late 1980s, largely due to incidental reports of supposed SRI-induced suicide and homicide circulated in the lay press. The issue once again gained international attention in October 2004, when the FDA ordered drug companies to place a black box warning on all antidepressants, stating that suicidal behavior might increase in children and adolescents taking these drugs. The FDA based this decision on a pooled analysis of 24 antidepressant trials involving more than 4,400 children and adolescents. Paroxetine was not singled out in this analysis, and, indeed, the warning applies to all antidepressants. Data on paroxetine and suicidal behavior in pediatric depression are covered more specifically in the "Childhood and Adolescent Depression" subsection earlier in this chapter.

Concerns about a link between antidepressant usage and suicidal ideation led FDA regulators to request that antidepressant manufacturers examine their databases for a similar link in adult patients. GlaxoSmithKline (Paxil/Seroxat) responded by supporting a meta-analysis of its clinical data comparing suicidality between paroxetine and placebo. The researchers found that 0.32% (11 of 3,455) of people taking paroxetine for depression attempted suicide, compared with 0.05% (1 of 1,978) of depressed patients taking placebo, an odds ratio of 6.7 (see GlaxoSmithKline 2006). Incidences of completed suicide in both samples were exceedingly rare, with one reported in the paroxetine sample versus none reported with placebo. Such data need to be considered cautiously for several reasons. First, it should be noted that neither suicidal ideation nor self-harming behaviors were among the main outcome measures in any of the pooled studies. Procedures to assess suicidality are not standardized and are based largely on unsolicited and unstructured reports and observations. Second, transient suicidal thinking must be viewed in the context of the overall risk–benefit analysis of paroxetine in the treatment of adults with major depressive disorder, an illness for which there is robust evidence supporting its efficacy.

In late 2006, an FDA advisory panel used the above data, along with findings from a total of 372 randomized, placebo-controlled antidepressant trials (involving close to 100,000 adult patients), in their decision to recommend that the black box warning be extended to cover young adults up to their mid-20s (U.S. Food and Drug Administration 2007). They reported that in patients 18–24 years of age, antidepressant use was associated with four cases of suicidal ideation per 1,000 patients treated, whereas drug therapy for patients older than 30 years was unequivocally protective against suicidality. The decision to extend the warning was made despite evidence that the initial warning might have had dangerous, unintended consequences for children and adolescents suffering from depression in the United States. Nemeroff et al. (2007) analyzed prescription data and physician surveys detailing prescription practices to identify trends in antidepressant use among children and adolescents. They found that from April 2002 to February 2004, antidepressant prescriptions among children and teens increased by an average of 0.79% a month. Between February 2004 and July 2004, prescriptions declined by an average of 4% a month.

The latter period corresponds with the time that the initial FDA advisory committee was holding highly publicized hearings regarding a link between antidepressant treatment and suicide attempts in depressed children. The Centers for Disease Control and Prevention (2007) recently reported that suicide rates in American children and adolescents increased by a staggering 18% in 2004 after 10 straight years of steady decline.

Suicide and attempted suicide were the main outcome measures in a recently published highly powered cohort study in which 15,390 patients, representing all subjects hospitalized in Finland for a confirmed suicide attempt between January 1997 and December 2003, were followed prospectively to ascertain whether active antidepressant treatment was associated with change in risk compared with patients taking no medication (Tiihonen et al. 2006). The investigators concluded that current SRI treatment across age groups was associated with a substantial decrease in overall mortality (relative risk of 0.59). Paroxetine was noted to confer increased risk of death in the population of patients between the ages of 10 and 19 years (relative risk: 5.44) compared with subjects who were not taking an antidepressant during the follow-up period. This was a naturalistic study, and it should be emphasized that patients are most likely to opt for antidepressant treatment when they are most depressed and that severe depression is a risk factor for suicide attempts. Still, it should also be noted that patients 10–19 years of age had higher risks of suicidal ideation with paroxetine than with other SRIs studied in the trial.

Theories attempting to explain the possible association between antidepressants and the onset of suicidality have been a part of psychiatric folklore since these medicines became available decades ago. Paroxetine in particular has several characteristics that may explain its implication in suicidal adverse events in children and adolescents with major depressive disorder. As previously noted, it has nonlinear kinetics, such that small dosage increases produce dramatic increases in child serum levels. Such high levels could lead to activation, akathisia, or disinhibition, any of which might explain suicidal thoughts or acts (Brent 2004). This effect is even more dramatic in those children who are slow metabolizers of the CYP2D6 isoenzyme (roughly 10% of the Caucasian population) (Riddle 2004). Additionally, paroxetine has a relatively short half-life (11 hours vs. 5 days with fluoxetine), and limited dosing adherence, not uncommon in children and teens, could lead to SRI discontinuation syndrome and dysphoria (Brent 2004). Another possibility is that paroxetine, along with venlafaxine and other NE-acting antidepressants that have similar links to suicidal risk in depressed children, might lead to manic or mixed-episode switching in children or adolescents who have undiagnosed bipolar disorder (Rihmer and Akiskal 2006). These possibilities require further study to elucidate.

Regardless of whether the association between antidepressants and transient suicidal activation in young people is causal, clinicians should inform their patients about the possible risks and should monitor depressed patients closely once paroxetine or any other antidepressants are prescribed, particularly during the early phase of treatment. The FDA advisory committee has made it clear that the black box warning should not dissuade physicians from prescribing antidepressants to patients in need (U.S. Food and Drug Administration 2007).

Medical Safety

Paroxetine treatment in clinical trials has not been associated with any significant abnormalities in standard laboratory tests, including hematological indices and chemistry panels, electroencephalogram (EEG), or electrocardiogram (ECG). One possible concern regarding paroxetine had been the potential for decreased heart rate variability (HRV), because depressed patients have been shown to exhibit lower HRV than nondepressed persons and this decrease represents a significant risk factor for myocardial infarction (Gorman and Sloan 2000). Moreover, NE reuptake–inhibiting antidepressant drugs have been shown to cause further decreases in this electrophysiological variable (Rechlin 1994). Decreases in HRV have been implicated in increased cardiovascular mortality (Carney et al. 2005), and depression itself has been conclusively shown to be a risk factor in the development of heart disease (Musselman et al. 1998). Davidson et al. (2005) demonstrated that paroxetine (doses up to 40 mg/day) resulted in lower NET occupancy compared with venlafaxine XR (doses up to 225 mg/day). In contrast to venlafaxine, paroxetine had no effect on HRV, as measured by changes in R-R interval during forced 10-second breaths and respiratory sinus arrhythmia (RSA) during paced breathing. Further comparisons of the effects of antidepressant medications on HRV are warranted.

Paroxetine and other SRIs have been implicated in precipitation of the syndrome of inappropriate antidiuretic hormone (SIADH), particularly in elderly individuals, which resolves on discontinuation of the medication (Strachan and Shepherd 1998). The potential for paroxetine-induced hyponatremia was prospectively evaluated in a 12-week open trial involving depressed male and fe-

male subjects between the ages of 63 and 90 years (Fabian et al. 2004). Hyponatremia, defined as plasma sodium levels lower than 135 mEq per liter, developed in 9 of the 75 total subjects (12%), in most cases within 10 days of initiation. Risk factors for developing hyponatremia were low body mass index (BMI) and low starting plasma sodium levels. These results underscore the importance of monitoring electrolytes closely in geriatric patients treated with paroxetine and other antidepressants.

Discontinuation Syndrome

Following closely on the heels of the widespread use of SRIs came the realization that abrupt discontinuation of these drugs often precipitates the emergence of unpleasant symptoms. This constellation of psychological and physical symptoms, which may appear upon treatment interruption, is referred to as the "SRI discontinuation syndrome." Postmarketing data gathered in the United Kingdom reported the occurrence of withdrawal-related events to be greater in paroxetine-treated patients (5.1% of total adverse drug events) than in patients treated with sertraline (0.9%), fluvoxamine (0.4%), or fluoxetine (0.2%), with a mean duration of 10.2 days (Price et al. 1996). Rosenbaum et al. (1998) compared paroxetine with fluoxetine and sertraline, following, on average, nearly 12 months of open-label treatment in 242 patients with major depression to assess the emergence of withdrawal symptoms in a double-blind, placebo-substitution fashion. The authors found paroxetine to be associated with a significantly greater mean score on the discontinuation-emergent signs and symptoms (DESS) checklist than both sertraline and fluoxetine. Both paroxetine and sertraline were associated with significant deterioration in depressive symptoms, as rated by the 28-item Ham-D and MADRS, during the 5- to 7-day placebo substitution. The most common symptoms attributed to paroxetine discontinuation were nausea, dizziness, insomnia, headache, and nervousness. Withdrawal in all groups was resolved upon subsequent reintroduction of medication.

These findings were confirmed in another blinded, placebo-substitution study, which reported a significantly greater total number of adverse events in paroxetine-treated patients with depression versus either fluoxetine or sertraline, as early as day 2 of active drug withdrawal (see Michelson et al. 2000). Similar liability was associated with paroxetine in terms of the 21-item Ham-D and State Anxiety Inventory scores, as well as changes in standing and orthostatic heart rate. Discontinuation was more recently compared between paroxetine and agomelatine, a mixed melatonergic and serotonergic agonist currently under FDA evaluation for the treatment of depression. In a double-blind, placebo-controlled discontinuation study, 192 depressed patients who had experienced sustained remission on either drug were randomly assigned to continue active treatment or to receive placebo for a 2-week follow-up period (Montgomery et al. 2004). During the first week postrandomization, placebo substitution resulted in considerable discontinuation symptoms in the paroxetine group (active dosage = 20 mg/day) but none in patients taking agomelatine (active dosage = 25 mg/day). These effects were not observed into the second week of discontinuation for either drug.

The studies noted above tested treatment discontinuation effects over a minimum of 5–8 days. Newer trials have evaluated the effects of shorter-term interruptions (3–5 days) similar to what a patient would experience if he or she were to inadvertently miss just a few doses. Following brief treatment interruption with placebo, Judge et al. (2002) found that paroxetine cessation led to significant discontinuation-emergent events, whereas fluoxetine-treated patients were not symptomatic. It was surmised that fluoxetine's long half-life conferred a protective effect during interruption. Paroxetine fared better during brief discontinuation in comparison with escitalopram. Measurements on the DESS checklist indicated that there were no significant differences between the two drugs when randomly replaced with placebo for 3- to 5-day periods (Baldwin et al. 2006), as both medications showed similar degrees of SRI withdrawal. The researchers did note that paroxetine (mean dosage = 26.3 mg/day) was significantly more likely to cause discontinuation side effects in comparison with escitalopram (mean dosage = 13.9 mg/day) during a taper period at the end of the trial in which higher-dosed subjects in either group were switched to lower doses for a week and lower-dosed subjects were switched to alternate-day dosing for a week prior to complete cessation.

Results from these studies suggest that the abrupt cessation of paroxetine is associated with the SRI discontinuation syndrome in approximately one-third of patients. This syndrome has been attributed to the short half-life of paroxetine, relative to that of other SRIs, as well as to the lack of any active metabolites (Michelson et al. 2000). Symptoms occur as early as the second day after a missed dose and may persist for several days. To mitigate the emergence of withdrawal symptoms, practitioners are advised to gradually taper the dose of paroxetine when discontinuing this medication in their patients. Despite the potential for "withdrawal" reactions after abrupt discontinuation of paroxetine, venlafaxine, duloxetine, and other antidepressants, there is no clinical evidence for dose escalation, craving, or drug-seeking behavior associated with dependence liability or "addiction" (Inman et al. 1993; Johnson et al. 1998; Sharma et al. 2000).

Overdoses with paroxetine are rarely associated with morbidity or mortality, which stands in stark contrast to the situation with the TCAs, with their low therapeutic index, or venlafaxine (Buckley et al. 2003; Cheeta et al. 2004). In the clinical trials program prior to FDA registration of paroxetine, 16 patients had ingested an overdose (doses of up to 850 mg of paroxetine); all patients recovered uneventfully (Jenner 1992). A review examining the American Association of Poison Control Centers (AAPCC) and FDA adverse events databases, as well as a MEDLINE literature search, revealed a total of 28 fatalities involving paroxetine overdoses; however, in nearly all cases, either coingestants were involved or causality could not be ascertained (Barbey and Roose 1998). In the overwhelming majority of intentional overdoses of paroxetine, individuals recovered without incident. Consequently, paroxetine can be safely prescribed in patients in whom impulsivity and suicidality are present.

Pregnancy and Lactation

One of the most challenging questions faced by patients and health care practitioners in family planning is whether to initiate or continue antidepressant therapy during conception, pregnancy, and the postpartum period. In exploring the risk–benefit analysis, one needs to consider the potential teratogenic risk of exposure of the antidepressant to the infants against the risks to the unborn children of women with untreated depression during pregnancy.

Newborns of women with depression have been shown to have a disproportionately higher risk of lower birth weight, preterm delivery, and small size for gestational age (Steer et al. 1992). Additionally, women with depression have higher rates of smoking and alcohol consumption, which represent further risks to pregnancy outcome (Zuckerman et al. 1989). Laboratory animal studies have demonstrated no significant effects of paroxetine in offspring of exposed pregnant mice in terms of early developmental tasks, locomotor and exploratory behavior, or cognition (Christensen et al. 2000; Coleman et al. 1999). In human studies, placental passage of paroxetine from mothers to developing infants was assessed by comparing maternal serum SRI concentrations with those found in cord blood at the time of delivery (Hendrick et al. 2003b). Paroxetine and sertraline had lower ratios of umbilical cord–maternal serum drug concentrations compared with citalopram and fluoxetine. Furthermore, unlike fluoxetine and sertraline, paroxetine cord blood concentrations did not correlate with maternal dosing, suggesting that an increase in maternal medication dose during pregnancy will not necessarily be accompanied by a comparable increase in fetal paroxetine exposure.

Clinical studies of paroxetine in the setting of pregnancy suggest that gestational exposure might have transient negative effects on newborn infants, particularly if the mother is treated during the third trimester. A prospective cohort study compared perinatal outcomes of 55 pregnant mothers treated with paroxetine, at various doses, during the third trimester with those of 27 mothers treated with paroxetine during one or both of the first two trimesters. A third sample was a control group of 27 expectant females treated with other medications classified as nonteratogenic. In this trial, Costei et al. (2002) found that third-trimester paroxetine exposure was associated with significant increases in neonatal distress (odds ratio = 9.53) compared with the other two groups. The most commonly observed forms of distress were characterized as respiratory distress and hypoglycemia. Results like these have stirred debate among neonatologists as to whether newborn distress attributed to SRIs is a manifestation of toxicity or of withdrawal (Stiskal 2005). Numerous case reports and case series have described transient neonatal symptoms following in utero exposure to SRI antidepressants, and these include (but are not limited to) tremor, hypertonicity, irritability, and poor feeding (Knoppert et al. 2006). Large trials correlating neonatal distress symptoms with infant serum drug levels, however, have not been performed thus far with paroxetine. Reduced or absent CYP2D6 isoenzyme activity associated with high paroxetine concentrations and hyperserotonergic states has been suggested as a putative mechanism for infant distress in many cases (Laine et al. 2004). Conversely, it has also been argued that in view of paroxetine's short half-life, neonatal distress is more likely to be caused by an SRI discontinuation effect (Stiskal 2006). The question is somewhat muddied by the fact that both hyper- and hyposerotonergic states can result in similar symptoms in newborns, such as restlessness and rigidity (Einarson and Koren 2006). The differential diagnosis between SRI neonatal withdrawal and serotonergic symptoms has important ramifications, given that withdrawal would be optimally treated with an SRI. In contrast, such treatment may endanger babies exhibiting serotonin toxicity.

Another significant clinical question is whether paroxetine is associated with teratogenicity. The results of an unpublished study conducted by GlaxoSmithKline (Paxil) led the FDA to warn that paroxetine may increase the risk of major congenital malformations. In a retrospective analysis of data from two U.S. managed-care insurance databases, pregnancy outcomes from a sample of 3,581 gravid mothers (ages 12–49 years) who were taking antidepressants were studied (see GlaxoSmithKline 2005). Of the 18 total medications compared, including other SRIs, SNRIs, TCAs, and newer drugs, only paroxetine had an increased risk of malformations that was significantly greater than that of other antidepressants (odds ratio = 2.20). Several organ systems, including the gastrointestinal, genitourinary, and central nervous systems, were affected in similar proportions. The most common cardiovascular anomalies were ventricular septal defects. The study did not include pregnant women without antidepressant exposure; however, the accepted prevalence of major congenital malformations for all births in the United States is roughly 3%, while the absolute rate observed among first-trimester paroxetine-exposed infants in this study was 4%. A 1% increase in absolute risk over baseline translates to a need for 100 pregnant women to take paroxetine during the first trimester before additional harm would come to 1 infant. Limitations of this study include its retrospective design, lack of controls, lack of clinical details about individual cases, and the fact that it represents a post hoc secondary analysis.

These data are contradicted by several other trials that might be considered more scientifically valid, given their prospective nature. In a cohort study, Kulin et al. (1998) compared rates of major congenital malformations in 237 pregnant women treated with paroxetine, fluvoxamine, or sertraline and found no significant differences among the medication groups compared with control groups. More recently, Hendrick et al. (2003a) followed a total of 138 pregnant females treated with paroxetine, fluoxetine, or sertraline and found that rates of neonatal complications and congenital malformations were lower (1.4%) than rates in the general population. There were no significant differences among individual antidepressants when compared with each other. In a postmarketing surveillance report, 137 pregnancies involving maternal exposure to paroxetine were cited, with no infant abnormalities noted (Inman et al. 1993). In spite of these more reassuring data, the American College of Obstetricians and Gynecologists Committee on Obstetric Practice (2006) has recommended that paroxetine be avoided in women who are pregnant or planning to become pregnant.

Whether a woman decides to begin or continue paroxetine for the treatment of depression during pregnancy, the clinician is advised to monitor for relapse because one study demonstrated that higher doses are often needed, especially in the early third trimester, to effect or maintain disease remission (Hostetter et al. 2000). Another time of increased risk is the postpartum period, when women are at a threefold higher relative risk for depression compared with non-child-bearing women (Cox et al. 1993). It is estimated that 13% of women develop depression following childbirth (O'Hara and Swain 1996). Furthermore, children of women with postpartum depression suffer from a number of social and intellectual impairments thought to be associated with compromised mother–infant bonding (A. Stein et al. 1991). Consequently, postpartum depression represents a significant health risk to both mother and child, and treatment with antidepressants during this period is often necessary.

Balanced against the established hazards associated with postpartum depression is the potential risk of exposure to antidepressants by the nursing infant. Breast feeding has long been advocated by health care providers for improved mother–child interaction and for infant health. In women with postpartum depression, the decision to breast feed, therefore, presents a dilemma. The emerging data appear to allay the concern of the exposure of SRIs, including paroxetine, to infants through breast milk. Like other antidepressants, paroxetine is secreted into breast milk, with greater concentrations found in hindmilk than foremilk (Ohman et al. 1999; Stowe et al. 2000). In a prospective study involving 16 women with postpartum depression treated with paroxetine, the sera of nursing infants were analyzed for the presence of paroxetine at several time points following maternal administration of paroxetine. Paroxetine was undetectable in all infants (Stowe et al. 2000). The authors cautioned against interpreting the findings to suggest that there is no infant exposure to paroxetine through breast milk because it is indeed found in breast milk, albeit in very low concentrations. Nevertheless, in view of the undetectable concentrations in infant blood, the exposure appears to be minimal. Furthermore, no obvious alterations in infant behavior or temperament have been observed in the breast-fed children of women treated with paroxetine in the short term. These data suggest that the benefits of breast-feeding can be maintained in women treated with paroxetine with minimal apparent risk of exposure to the infant. This issue is described in considerable detail elsewhere in this textbook (see Chapter 64, "Psychopharmacology During Pregnancy and Lactation").

Drug–Drug Interactions

Many medications rely on common metabolic processes for biotransformation into an active agent or inactive metabolite. As such, the likelihood that pharmacokinetic interactions among prescription and over-the-counter medications may lead to adverse outcomes becomes greater as medications with shared metabolic pathways are administered concurrently. As noted previously, paroxetine is primarily dependent on the CYP2D6 enzyme for conversion into its inactive metabolites (Hiemke and Härtter 2000). Paroxetine is not only a substrate for this system but also an inhibitor; therefore, other drugs that use this hepatic enzyme are potentially subject to decreased clearance and subsequent increased plasma concentrations (Sindrup et al. 1992b). Concern is greatest for potential drug–drug interactions when the affected medication has a low therapeutic index.

Medications that are CYP2D6 dependent include many antipsychotics, TCAs, type IC antiarrhythmics, β-adrenergic agents, trazodone, and dextromethorphan (Nemeroff et al. 1996). Most reports of interactions between these medications and paroxetine are published as case reports from which firm conclusions regarding causality cannot be drawn (Lane 1996). In regard to the TCAs, Brøsen et al. (1993) and Alderman et al. (1997) demonstrated, in prospective studies, that desipramine concentrations increased by 364% and 358%, respectively, when coadministered with paroxetine. Imipramine levels are also increased with the coadministration of paroxetine (Albers et al. 1996).

Antipsychotics are often prescribed with paroxetine in the treatment of psychotic depression and in the treatment of negative symptoms in schizophrenia or as augmentation therapy in patients with primary mood disorders. Paroxetine does not appear to potentiate the sedative effects of haloperidol (Cooper et al. 1989). Dystonia resulting from the combination of paroxetine and haloperidol has been reported (Budman et al. 1995). In one prospective study, clozapine levels increased by an average of 40% over controls when coadministered with SRIs, including paroxetine, at a mean dose of 31.2 mg (Centorrino et al. 1996). In another study using a lower dose of paroxetine (20 mg), no significant increases in clozapine concentrations were noted (Wetzel et al. 1998). These findings indicate that caution should be exercised when paroxetine and clozapine are prescribed together, particularly at higher doses of paroxetine. Case reports have demonstrated possible exaggerated extrapyramidal side effects when paroxetine was administered with per-phenazine, molindone, and pimozide (Horrigan and Barnhill 1994; Malek-Ahmadi and Allen 1995; Ozdemir et al. 1997).

A number of medications that are bound to plasma proteins are capable of displacing or being displaced by highly protein-bound drugs, such as paroxetine, resulting in a potentially significant increase in the free concentration of the drug, although this mechanism rarely, if ever, is clinically meaningful (Preskorn 1993). In a prospective study with 27 patients, 5 patients developed mild bleeding when paroxetine was added to ongoing treatment with warfarin, although concentrations of warfarin and paroxetine, as well as prothrombin time, did not change significantly (Bannister et al. 1989). Although an explanation for an increased propensity for bleeding is unclear, it is recommended that anticoagulation parameters be carefully monitored when warfarin and paroxetine are co-prescribed. Digoxin levels are unaffected by paroxetine treatment (Bannister et al. 1989), and lithium concentrations are also unchanged by paroxetine administration (Haenen et al. 1995).

In prospective studies involving the antiepileptic/mood stabilizers valproate and carbamazepine, as well as the anticonvulsant phenytoin, coadministration with paroxetine did not cause any significant changes in plasma levels of these drugs (Andersen et al. 1991; Kaye et al. 1989). In contrast, both phenytoin and carbamazepine have been shown to decrease plasma paroxetine concentrations by 28% (Kaye et al. 1989) and 55% (Hiemke and Härtter 2000), respectively. Valproate may increase plasma paroxetine concentrations (Andersen et al. 1991). Cimetidine, which is a potent inhibitor of the CYP2D6 isoenzyme, has been shown to result in a 50% elevation of paroxetine concentrations (Bannister et al. 1989). The clinical significance of the overall deviations in serum paroxetine concentration at steady state caused by these agents is minor because of wide interindividual pharmacokinetic variability, high therapeutic index, and lack of a concentration–efficacy relationship with paroxetine (Gunasekara et al. 1998).

Sedation is a possible side effect associated with barbiturates, benzodiazepines, and ethanol. Paroxetine does not potentiate the psychomotor effects of amobarbital, oxazepam, or alcohol (Cooper et al. 1989). No clinical or pharmacokinetic interaction was noted when paroxetine and diazepam were coadministered in a prospective study (Bannister et al. 1989).

Combination of medications that enhance serotonergic activity may result in the so-called serotonin syn-

drome, which may manifest as agitation, myoclonus, hyperreflexia, diarrhea, sweating, delirium, fever, elevated blood pressure, and possibly death (Weiner et al. 1997). Following case reports describing the emergence of this syndrome with the combination use of fluoxetine and MAOIs, the concomitant use of MAOIs with any of the SRIs is absolutely contraindicated, and a washout period of 14 days is recommended when switching from one agent to another (Gunasekara et al. 1998; Weiner et al. 1997). Evidence for the serotonin syndrome with paroxetine, in combination with other drugs, has been documented in case reports for moclobemide (Hawley et al. 1996), nefazodone (John et al. 1997), dextromethorphan (Skop et al. 1994), imipramine (Weiner et al. 1997), trazodone (Reeves and Bullen 1995), and others. The combination of SRIs and sumatriptan, a serotonin$_{1D}$ (5-HT$_{1D}$) receptor agonist used in the treatment of migraine, was previously discouraged because of the theoretical risk of precipitation of the serotonin syndrome; however, a series of six cases, one involving paroxetine, of concurrent sumatriptan and SRI administration demonstrated no adverse events (Leung and Ong 1995). This lack of interaction has been confirmed in a prospective trial (Franklin et al. 1996).

Overall, paroxetine may be safely administered with other medications, as clinically indicated. Coadministration with an MAOI is absolutely contraindicated, and careful monitoring is advised when TCAs, warfarin, and clozapine are used in conjunction with paroxetine. As with any medication, clinicians are advised to minimize polypharmacy and remain vigilant to the possibility of drug–drug interactions (see Table 15–2 for the important drug–drug interactions with paroxetine).

TABLE 15–2. Potential drug–drug interactions involving paroxetine

Monoamine oxidase inhibitors	Clinically significant
Tricyclic antidepressants	Clinically significant
Type IC antiarrhythmics	Probably significant
β-Adrenergic antagonists	Probably significant
Antiepileptic agents	Probably significant
Cimetidine	Probably significant
Typical antipsychotics	Possibly significant
Warfarin	Possibly significant
Clozapine	Inconclusive
Lithium	Not clinically significant
Digoxin	Not clinically significant

Conclusion

Paroxetine has been demonstrated to be an effective treatment for several psychiatric disorders, including major depression and virtually all of the anxiety disorders. It is well tolerated with convenient once-daily dosing and is available in both IR and CR formulations. Most patients can expect symptomatic relief within 4 weeks, and some patients as early as 2 weeks. Concern for pharmacokinetic interactions with other drugs is minimal, although concomitant MAOI use is contraindicated. Overdosage rarely results in significant toxicity, rendering paroxetine a judicious choice among available psychotropics for the impulsive or suicidal patient. Paroxetine should be used cautiously in the treatment of pediatric anxiety disorders and sparingly in child and adolescent patients with depression. Its use in pregnancy remains controversial and requires more data to resolve safety concerns. In the postpartum setting, however, nursing very likely poses a negligible exposure risk to infants of mothers receiving treatment with paroxetine.

Paroxetine, with its wide application and favorable safety profile, represents an important member of the SRI class of drugs, although it appears to behave as an SNRI at higher doses. It continues to be evaluated for efficacy in the treatment of other psychiatric and nonpsychiatric disorders.

References

Aberg-Wistedt A, Agren H, Ekselius L, et al: Sertraline versus paroxetine in major depression: clinical outcome after six months of continuous therapy. J Clin Psychopharmacol 20:645–652, 2000

Albers LJ, Reist C, Helmeste D: Paroxetine shifts imipramine metabolism. Psychiatry Res 59:186–196, 1996

Alderman J, Preskorn SH, Greenblatt DJ, et al: Desipramine pharmacokinetics when coadministered with paroxetine or sertraline in extensive metabolizers. J Clin Psychopharmacol 17:284–291, 1997

American College of Obstetricians and Gynecologists (ACOG) Committee on Obstetric Practice: ACOG Committee Opinion No. 354: Treatment with selective serotonin reuptake inhibitors during pregnancy. Obstet Gynecol 108:1601–1603, 2006

American Psychiatric Association: Diagnostic and Statistical Manual of Mental Disorders, 3rd Edition. Washington, DC, American Psychiatric Association, 1980

American Psychiatric Association: Diagnostic and Statistical Manual of Mental Disorders, 4th Edition, Text Revision. Washington, DC, American Psychiatric Association, 2000

Anda R, Williamson D, Jones D, et al: Depressed affect, hopelessness, and the risk of ischemic heart disease in a cohort of US adults. Epidemiology 4:285–294, 1993

Andersen BB, Mikkelsen M, Vesterager A, et al: No influence of the antidepressant paroxetine on carbamazepine, valproate and phenytoin. Epilepsy Res 10:201–204, 1991

Artigas F, Perez V, Alvarez E: Pindolol induces a rapid improvement of depressed patients treated with serotonin reuptake inhibitors. Arch Gen Psychiatry 51:248–251, 1994

Bakker A, van Dyck R, Spinhoven P, et al: Paroxetine, clomipramine, and cognitive therapy in the treatment of panic disorder. J Clin Psychiatry 60:831–838, 1999

Baldwin DS: Clinical experience with paroxetine in social anxiety disorder. Int Clin Psychopharmacol 15 (suppl 1):19–24, 2000

Baldwin DS, Hawley CJ, Abed RT, et al: A multicenter double-blind comparison of nefazodone and paroxetine in the treatment of outpatients with moderate-to-severe depression. J Clin Psychiatry 57 (suppl 2):46–52, 1996

Baldwin DS, Bobes J, Stein DJ, et al: Paroxetine in social phobia/social anxiety disorder. Br J Psychiatry 175:120–126, 1999

Baldwin DS, Cooper JA, Huusom AK, et al: A double-blind, randomized, parallel-group, flexible-dose study to evaluate the tolerability, efficacy and effects of treatment discontinuation with escitalopram and paroxetine in patients with major depressive disorder. Int Clin Psychopharmacol 21:159–169, 2006

Ballenger JC, Wheadon DE, Steiner M, et al: Double-blind, fixed dose, placebo-controlled study of paroxetine in the treatment of panic disorder. Am J Psychiatry 155:36–42, 1998

Ballus C, Quiros G, de Flores T, et al: The efficacy and tolerability of venlafaxine and paroxetine in outpatients with depressive disorder or dysthymia. Int Clin Psychopharmacol 15:43–48, 2000

Balon R: Antidepressants in the treatment of premature ejaculation. J Sex Marital Ther 22:85–96, 1996

Bannister SJ, Houser VP, Hulse JD, et al: Evaluation of the potential for interaction of paroxetine with diazepam, cimetidine, warfarin, and digoxin. Acta Psychiatr Scand Suppl 350:102–106, 1989

Barbey JT, Roose SP: SSRI safety in overdose. J Clin Psychiatry 59 (suppl 15):42–48, 1998

Bauer M, Zaninelli R, Müller-Oerhlinghausen B, et al: Paroxetine and amitriptyline augmentation of lithium in the treatment of major depression: a double-blind study. J Clin Psychopharmacol 19:164–171, 1999

Bayer AJ, Roberts NA, Allen EA, et al: The pharmacokinetics of paroxetine in the elderly. Acta Psychiatr Scand Suppl 350:152–155, 1989

Benfield D, Harris C, Luscombe D: Some psychopharmacological aspects of desmethylclomipramine. Postgrad Med 56:13–18, 1980

Benkert O, Szegedi A, Kohnen R: Mirtazapine compared with paroxetine in major depression. J Clin Psychiatry 61:656–663, 2000

Bielski RJ, Bose A, Chang CC: A double-blind comparison of escitalopram and paroxetine in the long-term treatment of generalized anxiety. Ann Clin Psychiatry 17:65–69, 2005

Bird H, Broggini M: Paroxetine versus amitriptyline for the treatment of depression associated with rheumatoid arthritis: a randomized, double blind, parallel group study. J Rheumatol 27:2791–2797, 2000

Blier P, Bergeron R: Effectiveness of pindolol with selected antidepressant drugs in the treatment of major depression. J Clin Psychopharmacol 15:217–222, 1995

Blier P, de Montigny C, Chaput Y: A role for the serotonin system in the mechanism of action of antidepressant treatments: preclinical evidence. J Clin Psychiatry 51 (suppl 4):14–20, 1990

Bordeleau L, Pritchard K, Loprinzi C, et al: Therapeutic options for the management of hot flashes in breast cancer survivors: an evidence-based review. Clin Ther 29:230–241, 2007

Bordet R, Thomas P, Dupuis B: Effect of pindolol on onset of action of paroxetine in the treatment of major depression: intermediate analysis of a double-blind, placebo-controlled trial. Reseau de Recherche et d'Experimentation Psychopharmacologique. Am J Psychiatry 155:1346–1351, 1998

Borgherini G: The Bioequivalence and Therapeutic Efficacy of Generic Versus Brand-Name Psychoactive Drugs. Clin Therapeutics 25:1578–1593, 2003

Bourin M, Chue P, Guillon Y: Paroxetine: a review. CNS Drug Rev 7:22–47, 2001

Boyer WF, Blumhardt CL: The safety profile of paroxetine. J Clin Psychiatry 53 (suppl 2):61–66, 1992

Brady K, Pearlstein T, Asnis GM, et al: Efficacy and safety of sertraline treatment of posttraumatic stress disorder: a randomized controlled trial. JAMA 283:1837–1844, 2000

Bremner JD, Vermetten E, Charney DS et al: Long-term treatment with paroxetine increases verbal declarative memory and hippocampal volume in post traumatic stress disorder. Biol Psychiatry 54:693–702, 2003

Brent DA: Paroxetine and the FDA [comment]. J Am Acad Child Adolesc Psychiatry 43:127–128, 2004

Brøsen K, Hansen JG, Nielsen KK, et al: Inhibition of paroxetine of desipramine metabolism in extensive but not in poor metabolizers of sparteine. Eur J Clin Pharmacol 44:349–355, 1993

Buckley NA, Whyte IM, Dawson AH: Relative toxicity of venlafaxine and selective serotonin reuptake inhibitors in overdose compared to tricyclic antidepressants. Q J Med 96:369–374, 2003

Budman CL, Sherling M, Bruun RD: Combined pharmacotherapy risk. J Am Acad Child Adolesc Psychiatry 34:263–264, 1995

Bump GM, Mulsant BH, Pollock BG, et al: Paroxetine versus nortriptyline in the continuation and maintenance treatment of depression in the elderly. Depress Anxiety 13:38–44, 2001

Carney RM, Blumenthal JA, Freedland KE, et al: Low heart rate variability partially explains the effect on post-MI mortality. Arch Intern Med 165:1486–1491, 2005

Cassano GB, Puca F, Scapicchio PL, et al: Paroxetine and fluoxetine effects on mood and cognitive functions in depressed nondemented elderly patients. J Clin Psychopharmacol 63:396–402, 2002

Centers for Disease Control and Prevention: Suicide trends among youths and young adults aged 10–24—United States, 1990–2004. MMWR Morb Mortal Wkly Rep 56:905–908, 2007

Centorrino F, Baldessarini RJ, Frankenburg FR, et al: Serum levels of clozapine and norclozapine in patients treated with selected serotonin reuptake inhibitors. Am J Psychiatry 153:820–822, 1996

Chaput Y, de Montigny C, Blier P, et al: Presynaptic and postsynaptic modifications of the serotonin system by long-term administration of antidepressant treatments. Neuropsychopharmacology 5:219–229, 1991

Charlier C, Broly F, Plomteux G, et al: Polymorphisms in the CYP 2D6 gene: association with plasma concentrations of fluoxetine and paroxetine. Ther Drug Monit 25:738–742, 2003

Cheeta S, Schifano F, Oyefeso A, et al: Antidepressant-related deaths and antidepressant prescriptions in England and Wales, 1998–2000. Br J Psychiatry 184:41–47, 2004

Chen B, Dowlatshahi D, MacQueen GM, et al: Increased hippocampal BDNF immunoreactivity in subjects treated with antidepressant medication. Biol Psychiatry 50:260–265, 2001

Chouinard G, Saxena B, Belanger MC, et al: A Canadian multicenter, double-blind study of paroxetine and fluoxetine in major depressive disorder. J Affect Disord 54:39–48, 1999

Christensen HD, Rayburn WF, Gonzalez CL: Chronic prenatal exposure to paroxetine (Paxil) and cognitive development of mice offspring. Neurotoxicol Teratol 22:733–739, 2000

Claghorn JL, Feighner JP: A double-blind comparison of paroxetine with imipramine in the long-term treatment of depression. J Clin Psychopharmacol 13 (suppl 2):23–27, 1993

Claghorn JL, Kiev A, Rickels K: Paroxetine versus placebo: a double-blind comparison in depressed patients. J Clin Psychiatry 53:434–438, 1992

Clayton AH, Pradko JF, Croft HA, et al: Prevalence of sexual dysfunction among newer antidepressants. J Clin Psychiatry 63:357–366, 2002

Cohen LS, Soares CN, Steiner M, et al: Paroxetine controlled release for premenstrual dysphoric disorder: a double-blind, placebo-controlled trial. Psychosom Med 66:707–713, 2004

Coleman FH, Dix C, Gonzalez CL, et al: Behavioral changes in developing mice after prenatal exposure to paroxetine (Paxil). Am J Obstet Gynecol 181:1166–1171, 1999

Condon JT: The premenstrual syndrome: a twin study. Br J Psychiatry 162:481–486, 1993

Cooper SM, Jackson D, Loudon JM, et al: The psychomotor effects of paroxetine alone and in combination with haloperidol, amylobarbitone, oxazepam or alcohol. Acta Psychiatr Scand Suppl 350:53–55, 1989

Costei AM, Kozer E, Koren G, et al: Perinatal outcome following third trimester exposure to paroxetine. Arch Pediatric Adolesc Med 156:1129–1132, 2002

Cox JL, Murray D, Chapman G: A controlled study on the onset, duration and prevalence of postnatal depression. Br J Psychiatry 163:27–31, 1993

Crewe HK, Lennard MS, Tucker GT, et al: The effect of selective serotonin re-uptake inhibitors on cytochrome P450 2D6 (CYP2D6) activity in human liver microsomes. Br J Clin Pharmacol 34:262–265, 1992

Cutler NR, Kramer MS, Reines SA, et al: Single site results from a multicenter study of efficacy and safety of MK-869, an NK-1 antagonist, in patients with major depressive disorder (abstract S.05.4). Int J Neuropsychopharmacol 3 (suppl 1):S7, 2000

Czepowicz VD, Johnson MR, Lydiard RB, et al: Sertraline in social phobia. J Clin Psychopharmacol 15:372–373, 1995

Dalhoff K, Almadi TP, Bjerrum K, et al: Pharmacokinetics of paroxetine in patients with cirrhosis. Eur J Clin Pharmacol 41:351–354, 1991

Danish University Antidepressant Group: Paroxetine: a selective reuptake inhibitor showing better tolerance, but weaker antidepressant effect than clomipramine in a controlled multicenter study. J Affect Disord 18:289–299, 1990

Davidson J, Watkins L, Nemeroff CB, et al: Effects of paroxetine and venlafaxine XR on heart rate variability in depression. J Clin Psychopharmacol 25:480–484, 2005

DeVane CL: Pharmacokinetics of the selective serotonin reuptake inhibitors. J Clin Psychiatry 53 (suppl 2):13–20, 1992

De Wilde J, Spiers R, Mertens C, et al: A double-blind, comparative, multicentre study comparing paroxetine with fluoxetine in depressed patients. Acta Psychiatr Scand 87:141–145, 1993

Dimmock PW, Wyatt KM, Jones PW, et al: Efficacy of selective serotonin-reuptake inhibitors in premenstrual syndrome: a systematic review. Lancet 356:1131–1136, 2000

Doyle GD, Laher M, Kelly JG, et al: The pharmacokinetics of paroxetine in renal impairment. Acta Psychiatr Scand Suppl 350:89–90, 1989

Dreshfield LJ, Wong DT, Perry KW, et al: Enhancement of fluoxetine-dependent serotonin (5HT) levels by (-) pindolol, an antagonist at 5HT1A receptors. Neurochem Res 21:557–562, 1996

Duboff EA: Long-term treatment of major depressive disorder with paroxetine. J Clin Psychopharmacol 13 (suppl 2):28–33, 1993

Dubovsky SL: Beyond the serotonin reuptake inhibitors: rationales for the development of new serotonergic agents. J Clin Psychiatry 55 (suppl 2):34–44, 1994

Duman RS: Novel therapeutic approaches beyond the serotonin receptor. Biol Psychiatry 44:324–335, 1998

Duman RS, Heninger GR, Nestler EJ: A molecular and cellular theory of depression. Arch Gen Psychiatry 54:597–606, 1997

Duman RS, Nakagawa S, Malberg J: Regulation of adult neurogenesis by antidepressant treatment. Neuropsychopharmacology 25:836–844, 2001

Dunner DL, Dunbar GC: Optimal dose regimen for paroxetine. J Clin Psychiatry 53 (suppl 2):21–26, 1992

Einarson A, Koren G: Defective alleles may not have contributed to adverse effects. Ther Drug Monit 28:142–143, 2006

Emslie GJ, Wagner KD, Wilkinson C, et al: Paroxetine treatment in children and adolescents with major depressive disorder: a randomized, multicenter, double-blind, placebo-controlled trial. J Am Acad Child Adolesc Psychiatry 45:709–719, 2006

Eriksson E, Hedberg HA, Andersch B, et al: The serotonin reuptake inhibitor paroxetine is superior to the noradrenaline reuptake inhibitor maprotiline in the treatment of premenstrual syndrome. Neuropsychopharmacology 12:167–176, 1995

Fabian TJ, Amico JA, Pollock BG, et al: Paroxetine-induced hyponatremia in older adults: a 12-week prospective study. Arch Intern Med 164:327–332, 2004

Fava M, Amsterdam JD, Deltito JA, et al: A double-blind study of paroxetine, fluoxetine, and placebo in outpatients with major depression. Ann Clin Psychiatry 10:145–150, 1998

Fava M, Rosenbaum JF, Hoog SL, et al: Fluoxetine versus sertraline and paroxetine in major depression: tolerability and efficacy in anxious depression. J Affect Disord 59:119–126, 2000

Findling RL, Reed MD, Myers C, et al: Paroxetine pharmacokinetics in depressed children and adolescents. J Am Acad Child Adolesc Psychiatry 38:952–959, 1999

Fineberg NA, Bullock T, Montgomery DB: Serotonin reuptake inhibitors are the treatment of choice in obsessive compulsive disorder. Int Clin Psychopharmacol 7 (suppl 1):43–47, 1992

Finley PR: Selective serotonergic reuptake inhibitors: pharmacologic profiles and potential therapeutic distinctions. Ann Pharmacother 28:1359–1369, 1994

Franklin M, Odintiadis EM, Clement PJ, et al: Sumatriptan in plasma by HPLC with coulometric detection: effect of paroxetine treatment on plasma sumatriptan concentrations (abstract). Eur Neuropsychopharmacol 6 (suppl 3):40, 1996

Frasure-Smith N, Lesperance F, Talajic M: Depression following myocardial infarction: impact on 6-month survival. JAMA 270:1819–1825, 1993

Frazer A: Serotonergic and noradrenergic reuptake inhibitors: prediction of clinical effects from in vitro potencies. J Clin Psychiatry 62 (suppl 12):16–23, 2001

Geller DA, Wagner KD, Gardiner C, et al: Paroxetine treatment in children and adolescents with obsessive-compulsive disorder: a randomized, multicenter, double-blind, placebo-controlled trial. J Am Acad Child Adolesc Psychiatry 43:1387–1396, 2004

Geretsegger C, Böhmer F, Ludwig M: Paroxetine in the elderly depressed patient: randomized comparison with fluoxetine of efficacy, cognitive and behavioural effects. Int Clin Psychopharmacol 9:25–29, 1994

Geretsegger C, Stuppaeck CH, Mair M, et al: Multicenter double blind study of paroxetine and amitriptyline in elderly depressed inpatients. Psychopharmacology 199:277–281, 1995

Gilmor ML, Owens MJ, Nemeroff CB: Inhibition of norepinephrine uptake in patients with major depression treated with paroxetine. Am J Psychiatry 159:1702–1710, 2002

GlaxoSmithKline: Paroxetine Adult Suicidality Analysis: Major Depressive Disorder and Non-Major Depressive Disorder. Briefing Document. Update April 5, 2006. Available at: http://www.gsk.com/media/paroxetine/briefing_doc.pdf.

GlaxoSmithKline: Important Prescribing Information. December 2005. Available at: http://www.gsk.com/media/paroxetine/paxil_letter_e3.pdf.

Golden RN, Nemeroff CB, McSorley P, et al: Efficacy and tolerability of controlled-release and immediate-release paroxetine in the treatment of depression. J Clin Psychiatry 63:577–584, 2002

Goldstein DJ, Lu Y, Demitrack MA, et al: Duloxetine in the treatment of depression: a double-blind placebo-controlled comparison with paroxetine. J Clin Psychopharmacol 24:389–399, 2004

Goodwin FK, Bunney WF: Depressions following reserpine: a reevaluation. Semin Psychiatry 3:435–448, 1971

Gorman JM, Sloan RP: Heart rate variability in depression and anxiety disorders. Am Heart J 140:77–83, 2000

Grados MA, Riddle MA, Nestadt G, et al: The familial phenotype of obsessive-compulsive disorder in relation to tic disorders: the Hopkins OCD family study. Biol Psychiatry 50:55–65, 2001

Greist JH, Jefferson JW, Kobak KA, et al: Efficacy and tolerability of serotonin transport inhibitors in obsessive-compulsive disorder. Arch Gen Psychiatry 52:53–60, 1995

Guillibert E, Pelicier Y, Archambault JC, et al: A double-blind, multicentre study of paroxetine versus clomipramine in depressed elderly patients. Acta Psychiatr Scand Suppl 350:132–134, 1989

Gunasekara NS, Noble S, Benfield P: Paroxetine: an update of its pharmacology and therapeutic use in depression and a review of its use in other disorders. Drugs 55:85–120, 1998

Haddock RE, Johnson AM, Langley PF, et al: Metabolic pathway of paroxetine in animals and man and the comparative pharmacological properties of its metabolites. Acta Psychiatr Scand Suppl 350:24–26, 1989

Haenen J, DeBleeker E, Mertens C, et al: An interaction study of paroxetine on lithium levels in depressed patients on lithium therapy. Eur J Clin Res 7:161–167, 1995

Hajos-Korcsok E, McTavish SF, Sharp T: Effect of a selective 5-hydroxytryptamine reuptake inhibitor on brain extracellular noradrenaline: microdialysis studies using paroxetine. Eur J Pharmacol 407:101–107, 2000

Hawley CJ, Quick SJ, Ratnam S, et al: Safety and tolerability of combined treatment with moclobemide and SSRIs: a systemic study of 50 patients. Int Clin Psychopharmacol 11:187–191, 1996

Heim C, Nemeroff CB: The impact of early adverse experiences on brain systems involved in the pathophysiology of anxiety and affective disorders. Biol Psychiatry 46:1509–1522, 1999

Hendrick V, Smith LM, Altshuler L, et al: Birth outcomes after prenatal exposure to antidepressant medication. Am J Obstet Gynecol 188:812–815, 2003a

Hendrick V, Stowe ZN, Haynes D, et al: Placental passage of antidepressant medications. Am J Psychiatry 160:993–996, 2003b

Hiemke C, Härtter S: Pharmacokinetics of selective serotonin reuptake inhibitors. Pharmacol Ther 85:11–28, 2000

Hirschfeld RMA: Panic disorder: diagnosis, epidemiology, and clinical course. J Clin Psychiatry 57 (suppl 10):3–8, 1996

Hjorth S: Serotonin 5HT1A autoreceptor blockade potentiates the ability of the 5-HT reuptake inhibitor citalopram to increase nerve terminal output of 5-HT in vivo: a microdialysis study. J Neurochem 60:776–779, 1993

Horrigan JP, Barnhill LJ: Paroxetine-pimozide drug interaction. J Am Acad Child Adolesc Psychiatry 33:1060–1061, 1994

Hostetter A, Stowe ZN, Strader JR, et al: Dose of selective serotonin uptake inhibitors across pregnancy: clinical implications. Depress Anxiety 11:51–57, 2000

Hutchinson DR, Tong S, Moon CA, et al: Paroxetine in the treatment of elderly depressed patients in general practice: a double-blind comparison with amitriptyline. Int Clin Psychopharmacol 6 (suppl 4):43–51, 1992

Hyttel J: Pharmacological characterization of selective serotonin reuptake inhibitors (SSRIs). Int Clin Psychopharmacol 9 (suppl 1):19–26, 1994

Inman W, Kubota K, Pearce G, et al: PEM report number 6: paroxetine. Pharmacoepidemiol Drug Saf 2:393–422, 1993

Jenner PN: Paroxetine: an overview of dosage, tolerability, and safety. Int Clin Psychiatry 6 (suppl 4):69–80, 1992

John L, Perreault M, Tao T: Serotonin syndrome associated with nefazodone and paroxetine. Ann Emerg Med 29:287, 1997

Johnson H, Bouman WP, Lawton J: Withdrawal reaction associated with venlafaxine. BMJ 317:787, 1998

Judd LL, Kessler RC, Paulus MP, et al: Comorbidity as a fundamental feature of generalized anxiety disorder: results from the National Comorbidity Study (NCS). Acta Psychiatr Scand Suppl 393:6–11, 1998

Judge R, Parry MG, Quail D, Jacobson JG: Discontinuation symptoms: comparison of brief interruption in fluoxetine and paroxetine treatment. Int Clin Psychopharmacol 17:217–225, 2002

Kato M, Ikenaga Y, Kinoshita T, et al: Controlled clinical comparison of paroxetine and fluvoxamine considering the serotonin transporter promoter polymorphism. Int Clin Psychopharmacol 20:151–156, 2005

Katzelnick DJ, Kobak KA: Sertraline for social phobia: a double-blind, placebo-controlled crossover study. Am J Psychiatry 152:1368–1371, 1995

Kaye CM, Haddock RE, Langley PF, et al: A review of the metabolism and pharmacokinetics of paroxetine in man. Acta Psychiatr Scand Suppl 350:60–75, 1989

Keller MB, Ryan ND, Strober M, et al: Efficacy of paroxetine in the treatment of adolescent major depression: a randomized, controlled trial. J Am Acad Child Adolesc Psychiatry 40:762–772, 2001

Kent JM, Coplan JD, Lombardo I, et al: Occupancy of brain serotonin transporters during treatment with paroxetine in patients with social phobia: a positron emission tomography study with [11C] McN 5652. Psychopharmacology (Berl) 164:341–348, 2002

Kessler RC, McGonagle KA, Zhao S, et al: Lifetime and 12-month prevalence of DSM-III-R psychiatric disorders in the United States: results from the National Comorbidity Study. Arch Gen Psychiatry 51:8–19, 1994

Kessler RC, Sonnega A, Bromet E, et al: Posttraumatic stress disorder in the National Comorbidity Survey. Arch Gen Psychiatry 52:1048–1060, 1995

Kiev A: A double-blind, placebo-controlled study of paroxetine in depressed outpatients. J Clin Psychiatry 53 (2, suppl):27–29, 1992

Kiev A, Feiger A: A double-blind comparison of fluvoxamine and paroxetine in the treatment of depressed outpatients. J Clin Psychiatry 58:146–152, 1997

Knoppert DC, Nimkar R, Principi T, et al: Paroxetine toxicity in a newborn after in utero exposure: clinical symptoms correlate with serum levels. Ther Drug Monit 28:5–7, 2006

Krastev Z, Terziivanov D, Vlahov V, et al: The pharmacokinetics of paroxetine in patients with liver cirrhosis. Acta Psychiatr Scand Suppl 350:91–92, 1989

Kulin NA, Pastuszak A, Sage SR, et al: Pregnancy outcome following maternal use of the new selective serotonin reuptake inhibitors. JAMA 279:609–610, 1998

Laine K, Kytola J, Bertilsson L: Severe adverse effects in a newborn with two defective CYP2D6 alleles after exposure to paroxetine during late pregnancy. Ther Drug Monit 26:685–687, 2004

Lane RM: Pharmacokinetic drug interaction potential of selective serotonin reuptake inhibitors. Int Clin Psychopharmacol 11 (suppl 5):31–61, 1996

Lecrubier Y, Judge R: Long-term evaluation of paroxetine, clomipramine and placebo in panic disorder. Collaborative Paroxetine Panic Study Investigators. Acta Psychiatr Scand 95:153–160, 1997

Lecrubier Y, Bakker A, Dunbar G, et al: A comparison of paroxetine, clomipramine and placebo in the treatment of panic disorder. Acta Psychiatr Scand 95:145–152, 1997

Leung M, Ong M: Lack of an interaction between sumatriptan and selective serotonin reuptake inhibitors. Headache 35:488–489, 1995

Liebowitz MR, Gelenberg AJ, Munjack D: Venlafaxine extended release vs placebo and paroxetine in social anxiety disorder. Arch Gen Psychiatry 62:190–198, 2005

Liston HL, DeVane CL, Goldman J, et al: Differential time course of cytochrome P450 2D6 enzyme inhibition by fluoxetine, sertraline, and paroxetine in healthy volunteers. J Clin Psychopharmacol 22:169–173, 2002

Lydiard RB, Bobes J: Therapeutic advances: paroxetine for the treatment of social anxiety disorder. Depress Anxiety 11:99–104, 2000

Magnussen I, Tønder K, Engbaek F: Paroxetine, a potent selective long-acting inhibitor of synaptosomal 5-HT uptake in mice. J Neural Transm 55:217–226, 1982

Malek-Ahmadi P, Allen SA: Paroxetine-molindone interaction. J Clin Psychiatry 56:82–83, 1995

Mancini C, van Amerigen M: Paroxetine in social phobia. J Clin Psychiatry 57:519–522, 1996

Marshall RD, Schneier FR, Fallow BA, et al: An open trial of paroxetine in patients with noncombat-related, chronic posttraumatic stress disorder. J Clin Psychiatry 18:10–18, 1998

Marshall RD, Beebe KL, Oldham M, et al: Efficacy and safety of paroxetine treatment for chronic PTSD: a fixed dose, placebo-controlled study. Am J Psychiatry 158:1982–1988, 2001

Martinez D, Broft A, Laruelle M: Pindolol augmentation of antidepressant treatment: recent contributions from brain imaging studies. Biol Psychiatry 48:844–853, 2000

Masand PS, Gupta S, Schwartz T, et al: Paroxetine in patients with irritable bowel syndrome (IBS): a pilot open-label study. Paper presented at the New Clinical Drug Evaluation Unit (NCDEU), Phoenix, AZ, May 2001

Mayberg H, Bieling P, Kennedy S, et al: Modulation of cortical-limbic pathways in major depression: treatment-specific effects of cognitive behavioral therapy. Arch Gen Psychiatry 61:34–41, 2004

Meston CM: A randomized, placebo-controlled, crossover study of ephedrine for SSRI-induced female sexual dysfunction. J Sex Marital Ther 30:57–68, 2004

Meyer JH, Wilson AA, Ginovart N, et al: Occupancy of serotonin transporters by paroxetine and citalopram during treatment of depression: a [11C]DASB PET imaging study. Am J Psychiatry 158:1843–1849, 2001

Michelson D, Fava M, Amsterdam J, et al: Interruption of selective serotonin reuptake inhibitor treatment. Br J Psychiatry 176:363–368, 2000

Montejo-Gonzalez AL, Llorca G, Izquierdo JA, et al: SSRI-induced sexual dysfunction: fluoxetine, paroxetine, sertraline, and fluvoxamine in a prospective, multicenter, and descriptive clinical study of 344 patients. J Sex Marital Ther 23:176–194, 1997

Montgomery SA: A meta-analysis of the efficacy and tolerability of paroxetine versus tricyclic antidepressants in the treatment of major depression. Int Clin Psychopharmacol 16:169–178, 2001

Montgomery SA, Dunbar G: Paroxetine is better than placebo in relapse prevention and the prophylaxis of recurrent depression. Int Clin Psychopharmacol 8:189–195, 1993

Montgomery SA, Kasper S, Lemming OM, et al: Citalopram 20 mg, 40 mg and 60 mg are all effective and well tolerated compared to placebo in obsessive-compulsive disorder. Int Clin Psychopharmacol 16:75–86, 2001

Montgomery SA, Kennedy SH, Burrows GD, et al: Absence of discontinuation symptoms with agomelatine and occurrence of discontinuation symptoms with paroxetine: a randomized, double-blind, placebo-controlled discontinuation study. Int Clin Psychopharmacol 19:271–280, 2004

Mulsant BH, Pollock BG, Nebes RD, et al: A double-blind randomized comparison of nortriptyline and paroxetine in the treatment of late-life depression: 6-week outcome. J Clin Psychiatry 60 (suppl 20):16–20, 1999

Murphy DL, Zohar J, Benkelfat M, et al: Obsessive-compulsive disorder as a 5-HT subsystem-related behavioural disorder. Br J Psychiatry 155 (suppl 8):15–24, 1989

Murphy GM Jr, Kremer C, Rodrigues HE, et al: Pharmacogenetics of antidepressant medication intolerance. Am J Psychiatry 160:1830–1835, 2003

Murphy GM Jr, Hollander SB, Schatzberg AF, et al: Effects of the serotonin transporter gene promoter polymorphism on mirtazapine and paroxetine efficacy and adverse events in geriatric major depression. Arch Gen Psychiatry 61:1163–1169, 2004

Murphy JM, Monson RR, Olivier DC, et al: Affective disorders and mortality: a general population study. Arch Gen Psychiatry 44:473–480, 1987

Musselman DL, Tomer A, Manatunga AK, et al: Exaggerated platelet reactivity in major depression. Am J Psychiatry 153:1313–1317, 1996

Musselman DL, Evans DL, Nemeroff CB: The relationship of depression to cardiovascular disease: epidemiology, biology and treatment. Arch Gen Psychiatry 55:580–592, 1998

Musselman DL, Marzec UM, Manatunga A, et al: Platelet reactivity in depressed patients treated with paroxetine: preliminary findings. Arch Gen Psychiatry 57:875–882, 2000

Musselman DL, Lawson DH, Gumnick JF, et al: Paroxetine for the prevention of depression induced by high-dose interferon alpha. N Engl J Med 344:961–966, 2001

Musselman DL, Cowles MC, McDonald WM, et al: Effects of mood and anxiety disorders on the cardiovascular system (chapter 95), in Hurst's The Heart, 12th Edition. Edited by Fuster V, O'Rourke R, Walsh R, Poole-Wilson P. New York, McGraw-Hill Professional, 2007, pp 2189–2210

Nebes RD, Pollock BG, Mulsant BH, et al: Cognitive effects of paroxetine in older depressed patients. J Clin Psychiatry 60 (suppl 20):26–29, 1999

Nelson HD, Humphrey LL, Nygren P, et al: Postmenopausal hormone replacement therapy: scientific review. JAMA 288:872–881, 2002

Nelson JC: Synergistic benefits of serotonin and noradrenaline reuptake inhibition. Depress Anxiety 7 (suppl 1):5–6, 1998

Nelson JC, Mazure CM, Bowers MB Jr, et al: A preliminary, open study of the combination of fluoxetine and desipramine for rapid treatment of major depression. Arch Gen Psychiatry 48:303–307, 1991

Nelson JC, Mazure CM, Jatlow PI, et al: Combining norepinephrine and serotonin reuptake inhibition mechanisms for treatment of depression: a double-blind, randomized study. Biol Psychiatry 55:296–300, 2004

Nemeroff CB: Paroxetine: an overview of the efficacy and safety of a new selective serotonin reuptake inhibitor in the treatment of depression. J Clin Psychopharmacol 13 (suppl 2):10–17, 1993

Nemeroff CB: The corticotropin-releasing factor (CRF) hypothesis of depression. Mol Psychiatry 1:336–342, 1996

Nemeroff CB, DeVane CL, Pollock BG: Newer antidepressants and the cytochrome P450 system. Am J Psychiatry 153:311–320, 1996

Nemeroff CB, Evans DL, Laszlo G, et al: Double-blind, placebo-controlled comparison of imipramine and paroxetine in the treatment of bipolar depression. Am J Psychiatry 158:906–912, 2001

Nemeroff CB, Etsuah AR, Willard LB, et al: Venlafaxine and SSRIs: pooled remission analysis (New Research Abstract NR263). Program and abstracts of the American Psychiatric Association 156th Annual Meeting, San Francisco, CA, May 17–22, 2003

Nemeroff CB, Kalali A, Schatzberg A, et al: Impact of publicity concerning pediatric suicidality data on physician practice patterns in the United States. Arch Gen Psychiatry 64:466–472, 2007

Newport J, Stowe ZN, Nemeroff CB: Parental depression: animal models of an adverse life event. Am J Psychiatry 158:1265–1283, 2002

Oehrberg S, Christiansen PE, Behnke K, et al: Paroxetine in the treatment of panic disorder. Br J Psychiatry 167:374–379, 1995

O'Hara MW, Swain AM: Rates and risk of postpartum depression: a meta-analysis. Int Rev Psychiatry 8:37–54, 1996

Ohman R, Hägg S, Carleborg L, et al: Excretion of paroxetine into breast milk. J Clin Psychiatry 60:519–523, 1999

Owens MJ, Morgan WN, Plott SJ, et al: Neurotransmitter receptor and transporter binding profiles of antidepressants and their metabolites. J Pharmacol Exp Ther 283:1305–1322, 1997

Owens MJ, Knight DJ, Nemeroff CB: Paroxetine binding to the rat norepinephrine transporter in vivo. Biol Psychiatry 47:842–845, 2000

Owens MJ, Krulewicz S, Simon JS, et al: Estimates of serotonin and norepinephrine transporter inhibition in depressed patients treated with paroxetine or venlafaxine. Neuropsychopharmacology 33:3201–3212, 2008

Ozdemir V, Naranjo CA, Herrmann N, et al: Paroxetine potentiates central nervous system side effects of perphenazine: contribution of cytochrome P4502D6 inhibition in vivo. Clin Pharmacol Ther 62:334–347, 1997

Paxil (package insert). Research Triangle Park, NC, GlaxoSmithKline, 2001

Paxil CR (package insert). Research Triangle Park, NC, GlaxoSmithKline, 2002

Pelicier Y, Schaeffer P: Multicenter double-blind study comparing the efficacy and tolerance of paroxetine and clomipramine in reactive depression in the elderly patient. Encephale 19:257–261, 1993

Perez V, Soler J, Puigdemont D, et al: A double-blind, placebo-controlled trial of pindolol augmentation in depressive patients resistant to serotonin reuptake inhibitors. Arch Gen Psychiatry 56:375–379, 1999

Piccinelli M, Pini S, Bellantuono C, et al: Efficacy of drug treatment in OCD: a meta-analysis review. Br J Psychiatry 166:424–443, 1995

Pigott TA, Seay SM: A review of selective serotonin reuptake inhibitors in obsessive-compulsive disorder. J Clin Psychiatry 60:101–106, 1999

Pini S, Amador XF, Cassano GB, et al: Treatment of depression with comorbid anxiety disorders: differential efficacy of paroxetine versus moclobemide. Int Clin Psychopharmacol 18:15–21, 2003

Poirier MF, Boyer P: Venlafaxine and paroxetine in treatment-resistant depression. Br J Psychiatry 175:12–16, 1999

Pollack MH, Rocco Z, Goddard A, et al: Paroxetine in the treatment of generalized anxiety disorder: results of a placebo-controlled, flexible-dosage trial. J Clin Psychiatry 62:350–357, 2001

Pollock GB, Mulsant BH, Nebes R, et al: Serum anticholinergicity in elderly depressed patients treated with paroxetine or nortriptyline. Am J Psychiatry 155:1110–1112, 1998

Preskorn SH: Pharmacokinetics of antidepressants: why and how they are relevant to treatment. J Clin Psychiatry 54 (suppl 9):14–34, 1993

Price JS, Waller PC, Wood SM, et al: A comparison of the postmarketing safety of four selective serotonin re-uptake inhibitors including the investigation of symptoms occurring on withdrawal. Br J Clin Psychopharmacol 42:757–763, 1996

Rasmussen SA, Eisen JL, Pato MT: Current issues in the pharmacologic management of obsessive compulsive disorder. J Clin Psychiatry 54 (suppl 6):4–9, 1993

Ravindran AV, Judge R, Hunter BN, et al: A double-blind, multicenter study in primary care comparing paroxetine and clomipramine in patients with depression and associated anxiety. J Clin Psychiatry 58:112–118, 1997

Rechlin T: The effect of amitriptyline, doxepin, fluvoxamine and paroxetine treatment on heart rate variability. J Clin Psychopharmacol 14:392–395, 1994

Reeves R, Bullen J: Serotonin syndrome produced by paroxetine and low-dose trazodone. Psychosomatics 36:159–160, 1995

Ressler KJ, Nemeroff CB: Role of serotonergic and noradrenergic systems in the pathophysiology of depression and anxiety disorders. Depress Anxiety 12 (suppl 1):2–19, 2000

Reynolds CF 3rd, Dew MA, Kupfer DJ, et al: Maintenance treatment of major depression in old age. N Engl J Med 354:1130–1138, 2006

Rickels K, Amsterdam J, Clary C, et al: A placebo-controlled, double-blind, clinical trial of paroxetine in depressed outpatients. Acta Psychiatr Scand Suppl 350:117–123, 1989

Rickels K, Zaninelli R, Sheehan D, et al: Paroxetine treatment of generalized anxiety disorder: a double-blind, placebo-controlled study. Am J Psychiatry 160:749–756, 2003

Riddle MA: Paroxetine and the FDA [comment]. J Am Acad Child Adolesc Psychiatry 43:128–130, 2004

Rihmer Z, Akiskal H: Do antidepressants threaten depressives? Towards a clinically judicious formulation of the antidepressant-suicidality FDA advisory in light of declining national suicide statistics from many countries. J Affect Disord 94:3–13, 2006

Rocca P, Fonzo V, Scotta M, et al: Paroxetine efficacy in the treatment of generalized anxiety disorder. Acta Psychiatr Scand 95:444–450, 1997

Roose SP, Spatz E: Treatment of depression in patients with heart disease. J Clin Psychiatry 60 (suppl 20):34–37, 1999

Roose SP, Laghrissi-Thode F, Kennedy JS, et al: Comparison of paroxetine and nortriptyline in depressed patients with ischemic heart disease. JAMA 279:287–291, 1998

Rosen RC, Lane RM, Menza M: Effects of SSRIs on sexual function: a critical review. J Clin Psychiatry 19:67–85, 1999

Rosenbaum JF, Fava M, Hoog SL, et al: Selective serotonin reuptake inhibitor discontinuation syndrome: a randomized clinical trial. Biol Psychiatry 44:77–87, 1998

Roy-Byrne PP: Generalized anxiety and mixed anxiety-depression: association with disability and health care utilization. J Clin Psychiatry 57 (suppl 7):86–91, 1996

Sachs GS: Treatment-resistant bipolar depression. Psychiatr Clin North Am 19:215–236, 1996

Sachs GS, Nierenberg MD, Thase ME, et al: Effectiveness of adjunctive antidepressant treatment for bipolar depression. N Engl J Med 356:1711–1722, 2007

Safarinejad MR: Comparison of dapoxetine versus paroxetine in patients with premature ejaculation: a double-blind, placebo-controlled, fixed-dose, randomized study. Clin Neuropharmacol 29:243–252, 2006

Saxena S, Brody AL, Ho ML, et al: Differential cerebral metabolic changes with paroxetine treatment of obsessive-compulsive disorder vs major depression. Arch Gen Psychiatry 59:250–261, 2002

Saxena S, Brody AL, Ho ML, et al: Differential brain metabolic predictors of response to paroxetine in obsessive-compulsive disorder versus major depression. Am J Psychiatry 160:522–532, 2003

Schöne W, Ludwig M: A double-blind study of paroxetine compared with fluoxetine in geriatric patients with major depression. J Clin Psychopharmacol 13 (6 suppl 2):34S–39S, 1993

Serebruany VL, Glassman AH, O'Connor CM: Platelet/endothelial biomarkers in depressed patients treated with the selective serotonin reuptake inhibitor sertraline after acute coronary events. Circulation 108:939, 2003

Seth R, Jennings AL, Bindman J, et al: Combination treatment with noradrenaline and serotonin reuptake inhibitors in resistant depression. Br J Psychiatry 161:562–565, 1992

Sharma A, Goldberg MJ, Cerimele BJ: Pharmacokinetics and safety of duloxetine, a dual-serotonin and norepinephrine reuptake inhibitor. J Clin Pharmacol 40:161–167, 2000

Sharp T, Umbers V, Gartside SE: Effect of a selective 5-HT reuptake inhibitor in combination with 5-HT1A and 5-HT1B receptor antagonists on extracellular 5-HT in rat frontal cortex in vivo. Br J Pharmacol 121:941–946, 1997

Sheehan DV, Eaddy M, Regan T, et al: Evaluating the economic consequences of early antidepressant treatment discontinuation: a comparison between controlled-release and immediate-release paroxetine. J Clin Psychopharmacol 24:544–548, 2004

Shelton C, Entsuah R, Padmanabhan SK, et al: Venlafaxine XR demonstrates higher rates of sustained remission compared to fluoxetine, paroxetine or placebo. Int Clin Psychopharmacol 20:233–238, 2005

Simonsick EM, Wallace RB, Blazer DG, et al: Depressive symptomatology and hypertension-associated morbidity and mortality in older adults. Psychosom Med 57:427–435, 1995

Sindrup SH, Brøsen K, Gram LF: Pharmacokinetics of the selective serotonin reuptake inhibitor paroxetine: nonlinearity and relation to the sparteine oxidation polymorphism. Clin Pharmacol Ther 51:288–295, 1992a

Sindrup SH, Brøsen K, Gram LF, et al: The relationship between paroxetine and sparteine oxidation polymorphism. Clin Pharmacol Ther 51:278–287, 1992b

Skop BP, Finkelstein JA, Mareth TR: The serotonin syndrome associated with paroxetine, an over-the-counter cold remedy, and vascular disease. Am J Emerg Med 12:642–644, 1994

Smith WT, Glaudin V: A placebo-controlled trial of paroxetine in the treatment of major depression. J Clin Psychiatry 53 (suppl):36–39, 1992

Stearns V, Isaacs C, Rowland J, et al: A pilot trial assessing the efficacy of paroxetine hydrochloride (Paxil) in controlling hot flashes in breast cancer survivors. Ann Oncol 11:17–22, 2000

Stearns V, Beebe KL, Iyengar M, et al: Paroxetine controlled release in the treatment of menopausal hot flashes: a randomized controlled trial. JAMA 289:2827–2834, 2003

Stearns V, Slack R, Isaacs C, et al: Paroxetine is an effective treatment for hot flashes: results from a prospective randomized clinical trial. J Clin Oncol 23:6919–6930, 2005

Steer RA, Scholl TO, Hediger ML, et al: Self-reported depression and negative pregnancy outcomes. J Clin Epidemiol 45:1093–1099, 1992

Stein A, Gath DH, Bucher J, et al: The relationship between postnatal depression and mother/child interaction. Br J Psychiatry 158:46–52, 1991

Stein DJ, Versiani M, Hair T, et al: Efficacy of paroxetine for relapse prevention in social anxiety disorder: a 24-week study. Arch Gen Psychiatry 59:1111–1118, 2002

Stein MB, Chartier MJ, Hazen AL, et al: Paroxetine in the treatment of generalized social phobia: open-label treatment and double-blind, placebo-controlled discontinuation. J Clin Psychopharmacol 16:218–222, 1996

Stein MB, Liebowitz MR, Lydiard RB, et al: Paroxetine treatment of generalized social phobia (social anxiety disorder): a randomized controlled trial. JAMA 280:708–713, 1998

Steiner M, Born L: Diagnosis and treatment of premenstrual dysphoric disorder: an update. Int Clin Psychopharmacol 15 (suppl 3):5–17, 2000

Steiner M, Pearlstein T: Premenstrual dysphoria and the serotonin system: pathophysiology and treatment. J Clin Psychiatry 61 (suppl 12):17–21, 2000

Steiner M, Hirschberg AL, Van Erp E, et al: Luteal phase dosing with paroxetine controlled release (CR) in the treatment of premenstrual dysphoric disorder. Am J Obstet Gynecol 193:352–360, 2005

Stiskal JA: Defective alleles may not have contributed to adverse effects. Ther Drug Monit 27:683, 2005

Stiskal JA: Defective alleles may not have contributed to adverse effects [comment]. Ther Drug Monit 28:142, 2006

Stocchi F, Nordera G, Jokinen RH, et al: Efficacy and tolerability of paroxetine for the long-term treatment of generalized anxiety disorder. Paroxetine Generalized Anxiety Disorder Study Team. J Clin Psychiatry 64:250–258, 2003

Stowe ZN, Cohen L, Hostetter A, et al: Paroxetine in human breast milk and nursing infants. Am J Psychiatry 157:185–189, 2000

Strachan J, Shepherd J: Hyponatremia associated with the use of selective serotonin re-uptake inhibitors. Aust N Z J Psychiatry 32:295–298, 1998

Sunblad C, Wikander I, Andersch B, et al: A naturalistic study of paroxetine in premenstrual syndrome: efficacy and side-effects during ten cycles of treatment. Eur Neuropsychopharmacol 7:201–206, 1997

Tasker TCG, Kaye CM, Zussman BD, et al: Paroxetine plasma levels: lack of correlation with efficacy or adverse events. Acta Psychiatr Scand Suppl 350:152–155, 1989

Thase ME, Entsuah AR, Rudolph RL: Remission rates during treatment with venlafaxine or selective serotonin reuptake inhibitors. Br J Psychiatry 178:234–241, 2001

Thomas DR, Nelson DR, Johnson AM: Biochemical effects of the antidepressant paroxetine, a specific 5-hydroxytryptamine uptake inhibitor. Psychopharmacology (Berl) 93:193–200, 1987

Tignol J: A double-blind, randomized, fluoxetine-controlled, multicenter study of paroxetine in the treatment of depression. J Clin Psychopharmacol 13 (suppl 2):18–22, 1993

Tiihonen J, Lonnqvist J, Haukka J, et al: Antidepressants and the risk of suicide, attempted suicide, and overall mortality in a nationwide cohort. Arch Gen Psychiatry 63:1358–1367, 2006

Tome MB, Isaac MT, Harte R, et al: Paroxetine and pindolol: a randomized trial of serotonergic receptor blockade in the reduction of antidepressant latency. Int Clin Psychopharmacol 12:81–89, 1997

Tucker P, Zaninelli R, Yehuda R, et al: Paroxetine in the treatment of chronic posttraumatic stress disorder: results of a placebo-controlled, flexible dosage trial. J Clin Psychiatry 62:860–868, 2001

Tucker P, Beebe KL, Nawar O, et al: Paroxetine treatment of depression with posttraumatic stress disorder: effects on autonomic reactivity and cortisol secretion. J Clin Psychopharmacol 24:131–140, 2004

Tulloch IF, Johnson AM: The pharmacologic profile of paroxetine, a new selective serotonin reuptake inhibitor. J Clin Psychiatry 53 (suppl):7–12, 1992

U.S. Food and Drug Administration: FDA Statement Regarding the Antidepressant Paxil for Pediatric Population. June 19, 2003. Available at: http://www.fda.gov/bbs/topics/AN-SWERS/2003/ANS01230.html. Accessed September 2008.

U.S. Food and Drug Administration: New Warnings Proposed for Antidepressants. May 3, 2007. (FDA Consumer Health Information, Consumer Updates archive) Available at: http://www.fda.gov/consumer/updates/antidepressants050307.html. Accessed September 2008.

van Amerigen M, Mancini C, Streiner DL: Fluoxetine efficiency in social phobia. J Clin Psychiatry 54:27–32, 1993

van der Kolk BA, Dreyfuss D, Michaels M, et al: Fluoxetine in posttraumatic stress disorder. J Clin Psychiatry 55:517–522, 1994

van Vliet IM, den Boer JA, Westenberg HG: Psychopharmacologic treatment of social phobia: a double blind placebo controlled study with fluvoxamine. Psychopharmacology 115:128–134, 1994

Wagner KD, Berard R, Machin A, et al: A multicenter, randomized, double-blind, placebo-controlled trial of paroxetine in children and adolescents with social anxiety disorder. Arch Gen Psychiatry 61:1153–1162, 2004

Wagstaff AJ, Cheer SM, Matheson AJ, et al: Paroxetine: an update of its use in psychiatric disorders in adults. Drugs 62:655–703, 2002

Waldinger MD, Hengeveld MW, Zwinderman AH, et al: Effect of SSRI antidepressants on ejaculation: a double-blind, randomized, placebo-controlled study with fluoxetine, fluvoxamine, paroxetine, and sertraline. J Clin Psychopharmacol 18:274–281, 1998

Waldinger MD, Zwinderman AH, Olivier B: Antidepressants and ejaculation: a double-blind, randomized, fixed-dose study with mirtazapine and paroxetine. J Clin Psychopharmacol 23:467–470, 2003

Weihs KL, Settle EC, Batey SR, et al: Bupropion sustained-release versus paroxetine for the treatment of depression in the elderly. J Clin Psychiatry 61:196–202, 2000

Weiner AL, Tilden FF, McKay CA: Serotonin syndrome: case report and review of the literature. Conn Med 61:717–721, 1997

Weissman MM, Klerman GL, Markowitz JS, et al: Suicidal ideation and suicide attempts in panic disorder and attacks. N Engl J Med 321:1209–1214, 1989

Weitzner MA, Moncello J, Jacobsen PB, et al: A pilot trial of paroxetine in the treatment of hot flashes and associated symptoms associated with breast cancer. J Pain Symptom Manage 23:337–345, 2002

Wetzel H, Anghelescu I, Szegedi A, et al: Pharmacokinetic interactions of clozapine with selective serotonin reuptake inhibitors: differential effects of fluvoxamine and paroxetine in a prospective study. J Clin Psychopharmacol 18:2–9, 1998

Wittchen HU, Zhao S, Kessler RC, et al: DSM-III-R generalized anxiety disorder in the National Comorbidity Study. Arch Gen Psychiatry 51:355–364, 1994

Wong DT, Bymaster FP, Engleman EA: Prozac (fluoxetine, Lilly 110140), the first selective serotonin uptake inhibitor and an antidepressant drug: twenty years since its first publication. Life Sci 57:411–441, 1995

Yonkers KA, Gullion C, Williams BA, et al: Paroxetine as a treatment for premenstrual dysphoric disorder. J Clin Psychopharmacol 16:3–8, 1996

Young LT, Joffe RT, Robb JC, et al: Double-blind comparison of a second mood stabilizer versus an antidepressant to an initial mood stabilizer for the treatment of patients with bipolar depression. Am J Psychiatry 157:124–126, 2000

Zanardi R, Franchini L, Gasperini M, et al: Double-blind controlled trial of sertraline versus paroxetine in the treatment of delusional depression. Am J Psychiatry 153:1631–1633, 1996

Zanardi R, Artigas F, Franchini L, et al: How long should pindolol be associated with paroxetine to improve the antidepressant response? J Clin Psychopharmacol 17:446–450, 1997

Zanardi R, Benedetti F, Smeraldi E, et al: Efficacy of paroxetine in depression is influenced by a functional polymorphism within the promoter of the serotonin transporter gene. J Clin Psychopharmacol 20:105–107, 2000

Zis AP, Grof P, Webster M, et al: Prediction of relapse in recurrent affective disorder. Psychopharmacol Bull 16:47–49, 1980

Zohar J, Insel TR: Obsessive-compulsive disorder: psychobiological approaches to diagnosis, treatment, and pathophysiology. Biol Psychiatry 22:667–687, 1987

Zohar J, Judge R: Paroxetine versus clomipramine in the treatment of obsessive-compulsive disorder. Br J Psychiatry 169:468–474, 1996

Zuckerman B, Amaro H, Bauchner H, et al: Depressive symptoms during pregnancy: relationship to poor health behaviors. Am J Obstet Gynecol 160:1107–1111, 1989

CHAPTER 16

Fluvoxamine

Elias Aboujaoude, M.D.

Lorrin M. Koran, M.D.

Fluvoxamine is a member of the selective serotonin re-uptake inhibitor (SSRI) family of drugs. Initially manufactured by Duphar Laboratories in the United Kingdom in 1971, fluvoxamine was registered as an antidepressant in Switzerland in 1983, becoming the first drug in the now hugely popular SSRI class to reach the market (Freeman 1991). Since its introduction, fluvoxamine has undergone a wide range of trials to assess its therapeutic potential in depression and across several anxiety disorders, including obsessive-compulsive disorder (OCD). Fluvoxamine has been available in the United States since 1994, when it received U.S. Food and Drug Administration (FDA) approval for the treatment of OCD (Ware 1997). More than 28 million people worldwide have been treated with fluvoxamine (Buchberger and Wagner 2002).

Structure–Activity Relations

Fluvoxamine belongs to the 2-aminoethyl oxime ethers of the aralkyl ketones, a unique chemical series unrelated to tricyclic antidepressants or other SSRIs. Fluvoxamine maleate is chemically identified as 5-methoxy-4′-(trifluoromethyl) valerophenone-(E)-O-(2-aminoethyl) oxime maleate (1:1). Its empirical formula is $C_{15}H_{21}O_2N_2F_3 \cdot C_4H_4O_4$, and its molecular weight is 434.4. Unlike the other SSRIs, fluvoxamine does not have an asymmetric carbon and hence does not have a chiral center or exist in stereoisomers. It is a whitish, odorless crystalline powder that is only sparingly soluble in water. It possesses local irritant properties that preclude its parenteral use ("Fluvoxamine" 2002). Figure 16–1 shows the molecular structure of fluvoxamine.

Mechanism of Action

Like other SSRIs, fluvoxamine binds to the presynaptic serotonin transporter (SERT) and prevents it from absorbing serotonin back into the presynaptic terminals, where it is metabolized by monoamine oxidases or stored in secretory vesicles. This has the net effect of increasing serotonin in the synaptic cleft. How these actions translate into efficacy for depression or anxiety remains the subject of investigation, especially because clinical improvement typically takes several weeks, whereas the drug's effect in enhancing monoamine neurotransmission is almost immediate. As a result, downstream mechanisms have been hypothesized to explain the therapeutic effects of SSRIs. These mechanisms include 5-HT_{1A} autoreceptor desensitization (Stahl 1998), increased sensitivity of the D_2-like receptors in the nucleus accumbens (Gershon et al. 2007), enhanced neurogenesis in the hippocampus (Dranovsky and Hen 2006), cyclic adenosine monophosphate (cAMP)–mediated activation of the pathway for cAMP response element–binding protein brain-derived neurotrophic factor (CREB-BDNF) (Gershon et al. 2007), and individual pharmacogenomic factors that de-

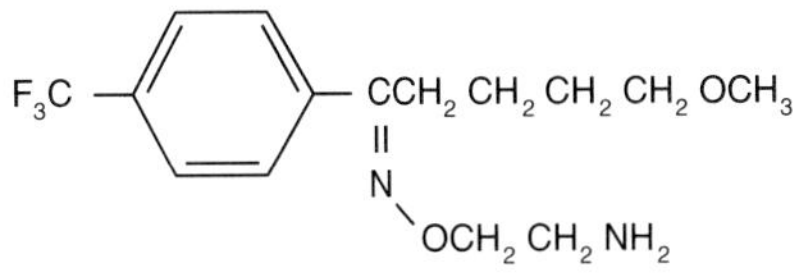

FIGURE 16–1. Chemical structure of fluvoxamine.

termine how SSRIs interact with specific gene variants of the serotonin transporter (Mancama and Kerwin 2003).

Recent research has examined the putative role of the sigma-1 receptor in the mechanism of action of SSRIs and the pathophysiology of various psychiatric illnesses, including major depression. Sigma-1 receptors are thought to exert potent modulatory effects on several neurotransmitter systems, including the serotonergic, glutamatergic, noradrenergic, and dopaminergic pathways. Studies using positron emission tomography have demonstrated that fluvoxamine's affinity for the sigma-1 receptor in the human brain is higher than that of any of the other SSRIs (Ishikawa et al. 2007).

Pharmacological Profile

Although the data are somewhat inconsistent, in vitro and in vivo studies suggest that fluvoxamine is a more potent inhibitor of serotonin reuptake than the tricyclic antidepressants, including clomipramine, but less potent than the other SSRIs. Fluvoxamine also is very selective for the human serotonin transporter ($K_i = 2.3$ nmol/L) and has only minimal affinity for the human norepinephrine and dopamine transporters ($K_i = 1,427$ and $16,790$ nmol/L, respectively) (Owens et al. 2001). Fluvoxamine also has minimal affinity for the muscarinic, α_1-adrenergic, histaminic, and 5-HT$_{2C}$ receptors and possesses no monoamine oxidase–inhibiting properties (Lapierre et al. 1983; Owens et al. 2001; Palmer and Benfield 1994; Ware 1997; Westenberg and Sadner 2006).

Pharmacokinetics and Disposition

After oral administration, fluvoxamine is almost entirely absorbed from the gastrointestinal tract, regardless of the presence of food (Van Harten 1995). However, despite complete absorption, oral bioavailability (i.e., the amount available in systemic circulation in intact form) is only 53% (DeVane 2003; DeVane and Gill 1997) due to first-pass hepatic metabolism. Following single-dose administration, peak plasma concentrations are reached within 2–8 hours, and steady-state concentration is achieved within 10 days (Van Harten 1995). At steady state, fluvoxamine appears to display nonlinear pharmacokinetics over its therapeutic dosage range, with disproportionately higher plasma concentrations at higher dosages. Plasma concentration, however, shows no consistent correlation with efficacy or severity of side effects, suggesting that plasma concentration monitoring is of limited value.

The mean half-life of fluvoxamine is 15 hours (range: 8–28 hours). This relatively short half-life makes twice-daily dosing preferable. Although psychoactive medications with relatively short half-lives are more likely to cause discontinuation syndromes if stopped abruptly, this effect appears to be rare with fluvoxamine (Buchberger and Wagner 2002), especially in comparison with paroxetine, an SSRI with a somewhat longer half-life but worse discontinuation problems (Pae and Patkar 2007). A possible explanation for this difference is provided from fluorine-19 magnetic resonance spectroscopy (^{19}F MRS) data showing that fluvoxamine is more slowly eliminated from the brain than from plasma (mean ratio of brain elimination half-life to plasma half-life = 2.4) (Strauss et al. 1998).

Because of its lipophilicity, fluvoxamine is widely distributed and is found in higher concentrations in the brain and other major organs than in plasma (Benfield and Ward 1986). For this reason, it is unnecessary to give replacement doses of fluvoxamine to patients receiving hemodialysis for severe renal dysfunction: re-equilibration should occur, with drug being recruited from tissues to plasma (DeVane and Gill 1997).

Compared with other SSRIs, fluvoxamine's rate of protein binding is relatively low, at 77% (DeVane and Gill 1997). Only escitalopram has a lower protein-binding rate (56%) (Rao 2007). Low protein binding can be advantageous, because interactions through drug displacement are less likely to occur when multiple medications that are bound to the same proteins are coadministered. Protein binding is also important in determining the hemodialyzability of drugs.

At least 11 products of fluvoxamine hepatic metabolism have been identified, but none are thought to be pharmacologically active (DeVane and Gill 1997; Palmer and Benfield 1994; Ruijten et al. 1984). Metabolism is thought to occur primarily through oxidative demethylation, although the exact enzyme systems involved in fluvoxamine breakdown have not been fully elucidated. Only minimal amounts of fluvoxamine (3%) are excreted unchanged by the kidneys, suggesting that renal impairment should not significantly alter fluvoxamine's pharmacokinetics (Van Harten 1995).

Because hepatic clearance is decreased in patients with liver disease and in elderly patients, dosage adjustments are sometimes necessary in these populations (DeVane and Gill 1997; Van Harten et al. 1993). No gender-based differences in fluvoxamine concentration seem to exist in adults, although most pharmacokinetic data were obtained from male subjects (DeVane and Gill 1997).

Studies examining the pharmacokinetics of fluvoxamine among children and adolescents have found a higher area under the curve (AUC) in children compared with adolescents, with the difference being more pronounced among female children, suggesting that lower drug dosages may be sufficient in this group. No appreciable pharmacokinetic differences were observed between the adolescent and adult groups ("Fluvoxamine" 2002).

Indications and Efficacy

Depression

The first trial to assess the role of fluvoxamine in the treatment of depression dates back to 1976. We identified 38 randomized, single- or double-blind studies conducted since then to test the antidepressant efficacy of fluvoxamine against placebo, SSRIs (sertraline, fluoxetine, citalopram, and paroxetine), serotonin–norepinephrine reuptake inhibitors (SNRIs; venlafaxine and milnacipran), tricyclic antidepressants (clomipramine, imipramine, desipramine, amitriptyline, and nortriptyline), tetracyclic antidepressants (mianserin and maprotiline), and a reversible inhibitor of monoamine oxidase (moclobemide). These trials varied widely in design, including the diagnostic and inclusion criteria utilized, the requirement for a washout period before initiation of study drug, and the way treatment response was defined. However, taken together, these studies support the efficacy and safety of fluvoxamine in the treatment of mild, moderate, and severe depression—including psychotic depression—across all age groups and in both inpatient and outpatient settings (Fukuchi and Kanemoto 2002; Haffmans et al. 1996; Kiev and Feiger 1997; Otsubo et al. 2005; Rapaport et al. 1996; Rossini et al. 2005; Ware 1997; Zanardi et al. 2000; Zohar et al. 2003). Among all studies, none showed fluvoxamine to be inferior in efficacy to another active comparator when a priori response criteria were applied. Study durations ranged from 4 to 7 weeks, and dosages ranged from 50 to 300 mg/day. Furthermore, the benefits from fluvoxamine seem to be sustained over the long term. In a double-blind, placebo-controlled study assessing the efficacy of fluvoxamine continuation treatment, fluvoxamine at 100 mg/day was significantly superior to placebo in preventing symptom recurrence over the 1-year maintenance period (Terra and Montgomery 1998).

Obsessive-Compulsive Disorder in Adults

Clomipramine is the only tricyclic antidepressant with established efficacy in OCD. Given that clomipramine is also the most serotonergic drug in its class, its efficacy supported the hypothesis that serotonin pathways are implicated in the pathophysiology of OCD. When fluvoxamine, a drug that is more potent and selective for the serotonin transporter than clomipramine, became available in the early 1980s, researchers quickly became interested in exploring its potential efficacy in the treatment of OCD. The first formal testing took place in 1987: a positive single-blind trial of 10 subjects with OCD (Price et al. 1987). Since then, multiple randomized studies have established fluvoxamine's efficacy and safety in the treatment of OCD, regardless of the presence or severity of comorbid depression. These trials have compared fluvoxamine with placebo, clomipramine, and other SSRIs.

In randomized, double-blind comparisons with placebo, subjects were given fluvoxamine 100–300 mg/day for 6–10 weeks. Significant improvements in scores on the Yale-Brown Obsessive Compulsive Scale (Y-BOCS) and other primary and secondary outcome measures were observed after a 3- to 4-week delay. Overall, response rates ranged from 38% to 52% (vs. 0% to 18% for placebo) (Figgitt and McClellan 2000).

We identified five published double-blind comparisons of fluvoxamine and clomipramine, both dosed at ≤300 mg/day, involving a total of 531 subjects and lasting 9–10 weeks (Figgitt and McClellan 2000; Freeman et al. 1994; Koran et al. 1996; Milanfranchi et al. 1997; Mundo et al. 2000, 2001). All of these studies demonstrated equal efficacy for the two agents (range of response rates: 56%–85% for fluvoxamine and 53%–83% for clomipramine). In the largest of these comparisons, 227 subjects meeting DSM-III-R (American Psychiatric Association 1987) criteria for OCD were randomly assigned to either fluvoxamine or clomipramine (both at 150–300 mg/day) for 10 weeks. At study end, rates of response (defined as ≤35% improvement in Y-BOCS score) were similar for the two drugs (62% for fluvoxamine vs. 65% for clomipramine, P=NS). However, fluvoxamine was better tolerated than clomipramine, as evidenced by its much lower rate of premature withdrawal due to side effects (8% for fluvoxamine vs. 16% for clomipramine) (Mundo et al. 2001). Only one published study has compared fluvoxamine with other SSRIs. This small 10-week single-blind study of 30 subjects randomly assigned to fluvoxamine, paroxetine, or citalopram suggested similar efficacy among the three agents (Mundo et al. 1997).

Data also suggest that long-term maintenance treatment with fluvoxamine following acute response is protective against OCD relapse. A 2-year open-label follow-up study in 130 subjects who had responded to a 6-month course of fluvoxamine 300 mg/day, clomipramine 150 mg/day, or fluoxetine 40 mg/day showed that for all three agents, maintenance treatment at full or half dosages was significantly superior to treatment discontinuation in preventing OCD relapse (Ravizza et al. 1996).

Use of fluvoxamine in the short term has been reported to enhance the efficacy of behavioral therapy in patients with OCD. In a 9-week study that compared 58 evaluable subjects who received exposure therapy in combination with fluvoxamine (≤300 mg/day) or placebo, the response rate (≥35% reduction in Y-BOCS score) was higher in the fluvoxamine group than in the placebo group (87.5% vs. 60%, $P \leq 0.05$) (Hohagen et al. 1998). In another study in 60 subjects with OCD, fluvoxamine (≤300 mg/day) combined with either antiexposure or exposure therapy significantly reduced daily rituals, compared with placebo combined with exposure therapy ($P = 0.02$), in the first 2 months of treatment, although this superior response did not persist at subsequent follow-up points (Cottraux et al. 1993).

The long-term benefit of fluvoxamine relative to behavioral treatment was explored in a study of 102 subjects recruited 5 years after completing two 16-week studies that tested the effectiveness of cognitive therapy alone, exposure response prevention alone, or cognitive-behavioral therapy in combination with fluvoxamine (Van Oppen et al. 2005). The original sample included 122 subjects. At the 5-year follow-up point, the clinical benefits to patients who had received cognitive therapy alone, exposure response prevention alone, or cognitive-behavioral therapy with fluvoxamine were maintained. Significantly more subjects who were still on antidepressants had received fluvoxamine in the controlled trials, suggesting that subjects who were randomized to the fluvoxamine group in the original trials tended to stay on the drug. However, more than 63% of subjects had received some form of additional psychological or pharmacological treatment in the intervening 5 years, making the results difficult to interpret. More than half (53.5%) of subjects no longer met DSM-III-R criteria for OCD at follow-up, and only 5% showed signs of deterioration.

Obsessive-Compulsive Disorder in Children and Adolescents

OCD often manifests in childhood or adolescence. Early intervention could potentially alter what is often a chronic waxing and waning course, but few pharmacological options for OCD have been adequately studied in this patient population. The safety and efficacy of fluvoxamine 50–200 mg/day were assessed in a 10-week double-blind, placebo-controlled multisite study involving 120 subjects ages 8–17 years with DSM-III-R–defined OCD. Response was defined as a reduction of at least 25% in the Children's Yale-Brown Obsessive Compulsive Scale (CY-BOCS) score. Mean CY-BOCS scores were significantly lower in the fluvoxamine group than in the placebo group as early as week 1 and remained lower at weeks 2, 3, 4, 6, and 10 ($P<0.05$). End-of-study response rates were 42% for the fluvoxamine group and 26% for the placebo group ($P=0.065$). The most common side effects (>10% rate than placebo) were insomnia and asthenia (Riddle et al. 2001).

Panic Disorder

SSRIs are considered a first-line treatment for panic disorder. Several small randomized, double-blind, placebo-controlled studies lasting 6–8 weeks were conducted in the 1990s to assess the efficacy of fluvoxamine 50–300 mg/day in the treatment of subjects with DSM-III-R–defined panic disorder. These studies generally showed favorable results compared with placebo, reporting reductions of 54%–100% in the weekly rate of panic attacks (Figgitt and McClellan 2000). More recently, a large multisite study was conducted in 188 subjects who met DSM-III-R criteria for panic disorder with or without agoraphobia, recruited from four centers in the United States. Subjects were randomly assigned to receive 8 weeks of fluvoxamine 100–300 mg/day or placebo. At study end, significantly more subjects in the fluvoxamine group were free from panic attacks (69% vs. 46%, $P=0.002$). An early onset of action was also seen: between-group differences in the proportion of subjects free from panic attacks at week 1 were significant in favor of fluvoxamine ($P<0.05$) (Asnis et al. 2001).

Limited comparative data suggest equal efficacy between fluvoxamine and the tricyclic antidepressant imipramine (both at dosages ≤300 mg/day) in the treatment of panic disorder, as well as a possible potentiating effect of fluvoxamine when combined with cognitive or exposure therapy (Figgitt and McClellan 2000).

Social Anxiety Disorder

Selective serotonin reuptake inhibitors are considered the first-line treatment for social anxiety disorder (social phobia). The largest double-blind, placebo-controlled study to assess the effectiveness of fluvoxamine in the treatment of social anxiety disorder recruited 92 subjects meeting DSM-IV (American Psychiatric Association 1994) criteria for social phobia from four centers in the United States (M. B. Stein et al. 1999). Subjects were randomly assigned to receive fluvoxamine (50–300 mg/day) or placebo. The primary outcome measure was the proportion of subjects at study end with a rating of much or very much improved on the global improvement item of the Clinical Global Impressions Scale. Secondary outcome measures included the Liebowitz Social Anxiety Scale (LSAS). Using last-observation-carried-forward analysis to interpret results from 86 evaluable subjects, the investigators determined that significantly more patients receiving fluvoxamine than receiving placebo had responded (43% vs. 23%, $P = 0.04$). The decrease in Liebowitz Social Anxiety Scale score was 22 for the fluvoxamine group versus 8 for placebo group (M. B. Stein et al. 1999). More recently, a controlled-release (CR) formulation of fluvoxamine showed similarly good results in two randomized, double-blind studies (Davidson et al. 2004; Westenberg et al. 2004). In February 2008, this formulation was approved by the FDA for the treatment of social anxiety disorder and OCD.

Posttraumatic Stress Disorder

Small open-label studies suggest a role for fluvoxamine in the treatment of posttraumatic stress disorder (PTSD) (Davidson et al. 1998; Figgitt and McClellan 2000; Marmar et al. 1996; Tucker et al. 2000). Twenty-four Dutch World War II veterans with chronic PTSD showed significant improvement on a PTSD self-rating scale after a 12-week course of fluvoxamine at ≤300 mg/day ($P = 0.04$). Improvement was seen across several key PTSD symptoms, including reductions in nightmares, flashbacks, insomnia, and survival guilt (De Boer et al. 1992). More recently, a 14-week open-label trial of fluvoxamine (100–300 mg/day) in the treatment of 15 U.S. veterans with combat-related PTSD reported a statistically significant decrease at study end in the Clinician-Administered PTSD Scale (CAPS) total score ($P < 0.001$), as well as in the intrusion and avoidance subscales (both $P < 0.001$) (Escalona et al. 2002).

Obsessive-Compulsive Spectrum Disorders

Because of their established role in the treatment of OCD, SSRIs (including fluvoxamine) have been tested in other disorders considered to be part of the obsessive-compulsive spectrum, including trichotillomania, compulsive buying disorder, pathological gambling, and body dysmorphic disorder. These conditions share with OCD features such as intrusive, anxiety-laden thoughts and a drive to perform a pathological behavior that can help relieve anxiety. However, like other SSRIs, fluvoxamine has produced inconsistent results when tested in these disorders.

For instance, in an open-label study of fluvoxamine in subjects with compulsive buying disorder, 9 of 10 participants improved (Black et al. 1997). However, two double-blind, placebo-controlled studies failed to show benefit for fluvoxamine over placebo (Black et al. 2000; Ninan et al. 2000).

Similarly, one double-blind study with placebo crossover and one single-blind study ($N = 15$ and 10, respectively) in subjects with pathological gambling suggested that fluvoxamine might be beneficial (Hollander et al. 1998, 2000). However, a larger 6-month double-blind, placebo-controlled study in 32 subjects with pathological gambling failed to show a separation between fluvoxamine 200 mg/day and placebo (Blanco et al. 2002).

Body dysmorphic disorder (or delusional disorder, somatic type) has also been conceptualized to be part of the obsessive-compulsive spectrum of conditions. Three prospective open-label trials of fluvoxamine (≤300 mg/day for 10–16 weeks) involving a total of 75 subjects reported response rates of 63%–67% (Perugi et al. 1996; Phillips et al. 1998, 2001). These findings, however, have not been confirmed in double-blind studies.

Finally, a 12-week open-label study of fluvoxamine 300 mg/day in 21 subjects with trichotillomania found only minor differences on some measures of improvement between pre- and posttreatment (Stanley et al. 1997).

Eating Disorders

Bulimia nervosa is characterized by binge-eating episodes that are accompanied by pathological compensatory measures, including self-induced vomiting, laxative abuse, fasting, and excessive exercising. Seventy-two subjects with bulimia nervosa treated successfully with psychotherapy were randomly assigned to receive fluvoxamine (100–300 mg/day) or placebo and were followed for 12 weeks. Fluvoxamine was significantly superior to placebo in protecting against relapse to bulimic behavior during the study period (*P*<0.05) (Fichter et al. 1996). A small 12-week double-blind, placebo-controlled study in 12 subjects with DSM-IV–defined bulimia nervosa suggested that fluvoxamine 200 mg/day was superior to placebo for acute treatment of bulimia nervosa (Milano et al. 2005).

The hallmark of binge-eating disorder is recurrent binge-eating episodes without accompanying purging. A 9-week double-blind, placebo-controlled study in 85 subjects with DSM-IV–defined binge-eating disorder found that fluvoxamine (50–300 mg/day) was significantly more effective than placebo in reducing binge-eating frequency (*P*<0.05) (Hudson et al. 1998).

Side Effects and Toxicology

The SSRIs, including fluvoxamine, represent an improvement in tolerability over the tricyclic antidepressants, including less likelihood of anticholinergic, cardiotoxic, and epileptogenic side effects, as well as relative safety in overdose. With the goal of assessing safety, data from 34,587 patients enrolled in 66 postmarketing fluvoxamine clinical studies were combined in a global database. The majority of these studies were conducted in patients with depression. Some studies lacked a placebo arm or relied on voluntary reporting of side effects by subjects, which likely led to underestimation of side effects. Fluvoxamine dosages employed in these studies ranged from 50 to 300 mg/day taken over 4–52 weeks. Both "adverse events" and "serious adverse events" were analyzed (Wagner et al. 1994). Of subjects enrolled in the analysis of the postmarketing trials, 14% discontinued prematurely because of side-effect rates. The most frequent reasons for early discontinuation due to adverse events were nausea and vomiting (4.6% and 1.7%, respectively). In the sample overall, the adverse events reported at greater than 5% incidence were nausea, somnolence, and asthenia (15.7%, 6.4%, and 5.1%, respectively). The rate of weight gain was only 1%. Sexual side effects were not mentioned in the analysis, suggesting that fewer than 1% of subjects in these studies reported such effects (only side effects with >1% incidence were listed), although a separate prospective open-label study specifically designed to assess the incidence of SSRI-induced sexual dysfunction in men (*n*=152) and women (*n*=192) showed statistically similar rates for fluvoxamine, fluoxetine, sertraline, and paroxetine (range: 54.4%–64.7%) (Montejo-Gonzales et al. 1997). "Serious adverse events" were defined, according to FDA guidelines, as events that are fatal, life-threatening, permanently disabling, necessitate hospitalization, or lead to cancer, overdose, or congenital anomaly. Approximately 2% of the fluvoxamine-exposed population reported at least one serious adverse event. The most commonly reported adverse event was hospitalization (1.6%), followed by emergence of suicidality (0.66%—which includes suicide attempts in 0.3%). The rate of completed suicide was 0.03%. The incidence of seizures was only 0.005% (Wagner et al. 1994).

Other studies have assessed changes in laboratory values or vital signs in fluvoxamine-exposed subjects. One database of standard metabolic lab results and complete blood counts was compiled from 1,630 subjects enrolled in 17 studies. Another database assessed vital signs in 9,689 subjects enrolled in 37 studies. No consistent treatment-related changes were seen in either study (Wagner et al. 1994).

Postmarketing surveillance usually relies on spontaneous self-reports from patients, health care providers, and health authorities. Because it covers millions of exposed patients in varied clinical settings, such surveillance can reveal a drug's rare side effects, although it also tends to underestimate common, expected side effects that often go unreported. A review covering 17 years of postmarketing surveillance of patients exposed to fluvoxamine (Buchberger and Wagner 2002) analyzed 6,658 individual reports, including 16,110 adverse drug reactions. The frequency of death while taking fluvoxamine was calculated at 0.9 death per 100,000 patients. Suicide, mostly by overdose, was the cause of death in nearly half of these cases, but only 1.2% of overdoses involved fluvoxamine alone. The rate of suicidality (ideation, attempts, and completed suicides) was estimated at 2.81 events per 100,000 patients. Drug interactions were reported at a rate of 0.85 case per 100,000 patients; the most commonly reported interaction was with clozapine. Switch to mania and discontinuation syndrome were also rare, occurring at rates of 0.47 and 0.38 events per 100,000 patients, respectively. Serotonin syndrome was even less frequent (Buchberger and Wagner 2002).

Drug–Drug Interactions

Fluvoxamine's inhibitory effect on some cytochrome P450 (CYP) enzymes has been well documented. Fluvoxamine is a potent inhibitor of CYP1A2. Drugs partially metabolized by CYP1A2 whose levels may rise as a result of fluvoxamine's inhibition of this isozyme include tizanidine, tertiary-amine tricyclic antidepressants (imipramine, amitriptyline, clomipramine), clozapine, tacrine, theophylline, propranolol, and caffeine. For this reason, it has been recommended that doses of theophylline and clozapine be reduced when either of these agents is coadministered with fluvoxamine (DeVane and Gill 1997).

Fluvoxamine also inhibits CYP2C19 and CYP3A4 (DeVane and Gill 1997). CYP2C19 metabolizes warfarin, and elevations in warfarin concentration have been reported in patients taking fluvoxamine. As a result, closer monitoring of anticoagulation status is indicated in these patients. Alprazolam and diazepam are metabolized in part through CYP3A4, and fluvoxamine has been shown to prolong their elimination (DeVane and Gill 1997). Carbamazepine is partially metabolized through CYP3A4, and elevated carbamazepine levels have been documented in patients concomitantly taking fluvoxamine (Palmer and Benfield 1994). Other drugs metabolized in part through CYP3A4 that may be affected by fluvoxamine include pimozide, methadone, and thioridazine. Also, because of the serious QT interval prolongation that can occur when terfenadine or astemizole is combined with the potent CYP3A4 inhibitor ketoconazole, it is recommended that fluvoxamine be avoided in patients who require these antihistamines (DeVane and Gill 1997). Fluvoxamine is contraindicated for use with thioridazine, tizanidine, pimozide, alosetron, ramelteon, and MAOIs (Fluvoxamine CR 2008).

No appreciable drug interactions exist between fluvoxamine and lithium, digoxin, or alcohol ("Fluvoxamine" 2002).

Pregnancy and Lactation

Pregnancy and the postpartum are considered to be relatively high-risk periods for depressive episodes. The decision to administer antidepressant treatment to a pregnant or breast-feeding woman can be difficult and should involve careful evaluation of the severity of the symptoms, the patient's psychiatric history (including her history during and following previous pregnancies), self-care while pregnant, the effects of depression on mother–infant bonding, and the availability of other treatments and support. The FDA lists fluvoxamine under Pregnancy Category C, meaning that risk to the fetus cannot be ruled out, and only limited fluvoxamine-specific data exist to help guide clinicians and patients. One study tried to assess teratogenic or perinatal effects relating to fluvoxamine exposure in utero in 92 pregnant women, 37 of whom were taking concomitant medications. No signifi-

cant difference in adverse events was seen compared with the control group (Gentile 2005).

Very limited case reports, covering only 8 infants exposed to fluvoxamine through lactation, have been published. No adverse events were reported in any of the infants. Fluvoxamine was not detected in 4 exposed infants in one case report, and another suggested normal development 2–3 years following lactation in 2 infants (Gentile 2005).

Conclusion

In 1983, fluvoxamine became the first member of the hugely popular SSRI family to be available on the market. Since then, more than 28 million adults and children have been prescribed fluvoxamine for a variety of psychiatric conditions including major depression, OCD, panic disorder, social anxiety disorder, impulse-control disorders, and eating disorders. Considering the number and size of double-blind, placebo-controlled clinical trials conducted, major depression and OCD have received the most attention, and hence have the strongest database supporting the use of fluvoxamine in their treatment. Looking at these studies in their totality and at the available postmarketing surveillance data, one can conclude that at the commonly used doses of 50–300 mg/day, fluvoxamine is well tolerated and shares the superior side-effect and safety profile of the SSRIs as compared with tricyclic antidepressants. However, fluvoxamine's pharmacodynamic and pharmacokinetic properties, including its inhibitory effects on some CYP enzymes, help differentiate it from other SSRIs.

Compared with other SSRIs, fluvoxamine is relatively selective for the serotonin transporter, and it is less protein-bound than fluoxetine, paroxetine, or sertraline. Adverse events from drug–drug interactions with fluvoxamine are rare, but caution should be exercised when combining fluvoxamine, a potent inhibitor of CYP1A2, with substrates of this isozyme, including theophylline, clozapine, and (to a lesser degree) carbamazepine. Through inhibition of CYP2C19 and CYP3A4, fluvoxamine could also interact with substrates of these isozymes, including coumadin, terfenadine, astemizole, alprazolam, and diazepam.

Fluvoxamine's relatively short half-life makes twice-daily dosing preferable but does not seem to lead to a significant discontinuation syndrome on abrupt discontinuation. A controlled-release formulation that can be dosed once daily has been investigated in OCD and social anxiety clinical trials, with positive efficacy and tolerability reported (Davidson et al. 2004; Hollander et al. 2003; D.J. Stein et al. 2003; Westenberg et al. 2004). This formulation became available in the United States in 2008.

References

American Psychiatric Association: Diagnostic and Statistical Manual of Mental Disorders, 3rd Edition, Revised. Washington, DC, American Psychiatric Association, 1987

American Psychiatric Association: Diagnostic and Statistical Manual of Mental Disorders, 4th Edition. Washington, DC, American Psychiatric Association, 1994

Asnis GM, Hameedi FA, Goddard AW, et al: Fluvoxamine in the treatment of panic disorder: a multicenter double-blind, placebo-controlled study in outpatients. Psychiatry Res 103:1–14, 2001

Benfield P, Ward A: Fluvoxamine: a review of its pharmacodynamic and pharmacokinetic properties, and therapeutic efficacy in depressive illness. Drugs 32:313–334, 1986

Black DW, Monahan P, Gabel J: Fluvoxamine in the treatment of compulsive buying. J Clin Psychiatry 58:159–163, 1997

Black DW, Gabel J, Hansen J, et al: A double-blind comparison of fluvoxamine versus placebo in the treatment of compulsive buying disorder. Ann Clin Psychiatry 12:205–211, 2000

Blanco C, Petkova E, Ibanez A, et al: A pilot placebo-controlled study of fluvoxamine for pathological gambling. Ann Clin Psychiatry 14:9–15, 2002

Buchberger R, Wagner W: Fluvoxamine: safety profile in extensive post-marketing surveillance. Pharmacopsychiatry 35:101–108, 2002

Cottraux J, Mollard E, Bouvard M, et al: Exposure therapy, fluvoxamine, or combination treatment in obsessive-compulsive disorder: one-year follow up. Psychiatry Res 49:63–75, 1993

Davidson JR, Weisler RH, Malik M, et al: Fluvoxamine in civilians with posttraumatic stress disorder. J Clin Psychopharmacol 18:93–95, 1998

Davidson J, Yaryura-Tobias J, DuPont R, et al: Fluvoxamine controlled-release formulation for the treatment of generalized social anxiety disorder. J Clin Psychopharmacol 24:118–125, 2004

De Boer M, Op den Velde W, Falger PJ, et al: Fluvoxamine treatment for chronic PTSD: a pilot study. Psychother Psychosom 57:158–163, 1992

DeVane CL: Pharmacokinetics, drug interactions and tolerability of paroxetine and paroxetine CR. Psychopharmacol Bull 37 (suppl 1):29–41, 2003

DeVane CL, Gill HS: Clinical pharmacokinetics of fluvoxamine: applications to dosage regimen design. J Clin Psychiatry 58 (suppl 5):7–14, 1997

Dranovsky A, Hen R: Hippocampal neurogenesis: regulation by stress and antidepressants. Biol Psychiatry 59:1136–1143, 2006

Escalona R, Canive JM, Calais LA, et al: Fluvoxamine treatment in veterans with combat-related post-traumatic stress disorder. Depress Anxiety 15:29–33, 2002

Fichter MM, Kruger R, Rief W, et al: Fluvoxamine in prevention of relapse in bulimia nervosa: effects on eating-specific psychopathology. J Clin Psychopharmacol 16:9–18, 1996

Figgitt DP, McClellan KJ: Fluvoxamine: an updated review of its use in the management of adults with anxiety disorders. Drugs 60:925–954, 2000

Fluvoxamine, in Physicians' Desk Reference, 56th Edition. Montvale, NJ, Medical Economics Company, 2002

Fluvoxamine CR (package insert). Palo Alto, CA, Jazz Pharmaceuticals Inc, February 2008. Available at: http://www.luvoxcr.com/LUVOX-CR-PI.pdf. Accessed December 2008.

Freeman CP, Trimble MR, Deakin JF, et al: Fluvoxamine versus clomipramine in the treatment of obsessive compulsive disorder: a multicenter, randomized, double-blind, parallel group comparison. J Clin Psychiatry 55:301–305, 1994

Freeman CP: Fluvoxamine: clinical trials and clinical use. J Psychiatry Neurosci 16 (2 suppl 1):19–25, 1991

Fukuchi T, Kanemoto K: Differential effects of milnacipran and fluvoxamine, especially in patients with severe depression and agitated depression: a case-control study. Int Clin Psychopharmacol 17:53–58, 2002

Gentile S: The safety of newer antidepressants in pregnancy and breastfeeding. Drug Saf 28:137–152, 2005

Gershon AA, Vishne T, Grunhaus L: Dopamine D2-like receptors and the antidepressant response. Biol Psychiatry 61:145–153, 2007

Haffmans PM, Timmerman L, Hoogduin CA: Efficacy and tolerability of citalopram in comparison with fluvoxamine in depressed outpatients: a double-blind, multicentre study. The LUCIFER Group. Int Clin Psychopharmacol 11:157–164, 1996

Hohagen F, Winkelmann G, Rasche-Ruchle H, et al: Combination of behaviour therapy with fluvoxamine in comparison with behaviour therapy and placebo: results of a multicentre study. Br J Psychiatry Suppl (35):71–78, 1998

Hollander E, DeCaria CM, Mari E, et al: Short-term single-blind fluvoxamine treatment of pathological gambling. Am J Psychiatry 155:1781–1783, 1998

Hollander E, DeCaria CM, Finkell JN, et al: A randomized double-blind fluvoxamine/placebo crossover trial in pathologic gambling. Biol Psychiatry 47:813–817, 2000

Hollander E, Koran LM, Goodman WK, et al: A double-blind, placebo-controlled study of the efficacy and safety of controlled-release fluvoxamine in patients with obsessive-compulsive disorder. J Clin Psychiatry 64:640–647, 2003

Hudson JI, McElroy SL, Raymond NC, et al: Fluvoxamine in the treatment of binge-eating disorder: a multicenter placebo-controlled, double-blind trial. Am J Psychiatry 155:1756–1762, 1998

Ishikawa M, Ishiwata K, Ishii K, et al: High occupancy of sigma-1 receptors in the human brain after single oral administration of fluvoxamine: a positron emission tomography study using [(11)C]SA4503. Biol Psychiatry 62:878–883, 2007

Kiev A, Feiger A: A double-blind comparison of fluvoxamine and paroxetine in the treatment of depressed outpatients. J Clin Psychiatry 58:146–152, 1997

Koran LM, McElroy SL, Davidson JR, et al: Fluvoxamine versus clomipramine for obsessive-compulsive disorder: a double-blind comparison. J Clin Psychopharmacol 16:121–129, 1996

Lapierre YD, Rastogi RB, Singhal RL: Fluvoxamine influences serotonergic system in the brain: neurochemical evidence. Neuropsychobiology 10:213–216, 1983

Mancama D, Kerwin RW: Role of pharmacogenomics in individualizing treatment with SSRIs. CNS Drugs 17:143–151, 2003

Marmar CR, Schoenfeld F, Weiss DS, et al: Open trial of fluvoxamine treatment for combat-related posttraumatic stress disorder. J Clin Psychiatry 57 (suppl 8):66–70, 1996

Milanfranchi A, Ravagli S, Lensi P, et al: A double-blind study of fluvoxamine and clomipramine in the treatment of obsessive-compulsive disorder. Int Clin Psychopharmacol 12:131–136, 1997

Milano W, Siano C, Putrella C, et al: Treatment of bulimia nervosa with fluvoxamine: a randomized controlled trial. Adv Ther 22:278–283, 2005

Montejo-Gonzalez AL, Llorca G, Izquierdo JA, et al: SSRI-induced sexual dysfunction: fluoxetine, paroxetine, sertraline, and fluvoxamine in a prospective, multicenter, and descriptive clinical study of 344 patients. J Sex Marital Ther 23:176–194, 1997

Mundo E, Bianchi L, Bellodi L: Efficacy of fluvoxamine, paroxetine, and citalopram in the treatment of obsessive-compulsive disorder: a single-blind study. J Clin Psychopharmacol 17:267–271, 1997

Mundo E, Maina G, Uslenghi C: Multicenter, double-blind comparison of fluvoxamine and clomipramine in the treatment of obsessive-compulsive disorder. Int Clin Psychopharmacol 15:69–76, 2000

Mundo E, Rouillon F, Figuera ML, et al: Fluvoxamine in obsessive-compulsive disorder: similar efficacy but superior tolerability in comparison with clomipramine. Hum Psychopharmacol 16:461–468, 2001

Ninan PT, McElroy SL, Kane CP, et al: Placebo-controlled study of fluvoxamine in the treatment of patients with compulsive buying. J Clin Psychopharmacol 20:362–366, 2000

Otsubo T, Akimoto Y, Yamada H, et al: A comparative study of the efficacy and safety profiles between fluvoxamine and nortriptyline in Japanese patients with major depression. Pharmacopsychiatry 38:30–35, 2005

Owens JM, Knight DL, Nemeroff CB: Second generation SSRIs: human monoamine transporter binding profile of escitalopram and R-fluoxetine. Biol Psychiatry 50:345–350, 2001

Pae CU, Patkar AA: Paroxetine: current status in psychiatry. Expert Rev Neurother 7:107–120, 2007

Palmer KJ, Benfield P: Fluvoxamine: an overview of its pharmacological properties and review of its therapeutic potential in nondepressive disorders. CNS Drugs 1:57–87, 1994

Perugi G, Giannotti D, Di Vaio S, et al: Fluvoxamine in the treatment of body dysmorphic disorder (dysmorphophobia). Int Clin Psychopharmacol 11:247–254, 1996

Phillips KA, Dwight MM, McElroy SL: Efficacy and safety of fluvoxamine in body dysmorphic disorder. J Clin Psychiatry 59:165–171, 1998

Phillips KA, McElroy SL, Dwight MM, et al: Delusionality and response to open-label fluvoxamine in body dysmorphic disorder. J Clin Psychiatry 62:87–91, 2001

Price LH, Goodman WK, Charney DS, et al: Treatment of severe obsessive-compulsive disorder with fluvoxamine. Am J Psychiatry 144:1059–1061, 1987

Rao N: The clinical pharmacokinetics of escitalopram. Clin Pharmacokinet 46:281–290, 2007

Rapaport M, Coccaro E, Sheline Y, et al: A comparison of fluvoxamine and fluoxetine in the treatment of major depression. J Clin Psychopharmacol 16:373–378, 1996

Ravizza L, Barzega G, Bellino S, et al: Drug treatment of obsessive-compulsive disorder (OCD): long-term trial with clomipramine and selective serotonin reuptake inhibitors (SSRIs). Psychopharmacol Bull 32:167–173, 1996

Riddle MA, Reeve EA, Yaryura-Tobias JA, et al: Fluvoxamine for children and adolescents with obsessive compulsive disorder: a randomized, controlled, multicenter trial. J Am Acad Child Adolesc Psychiatry 40:222–229, 2001

Rossini D, Serretti A, Franchini L, et al: Sertraline versus fluvoxamine in the treatment of elderly patients with major depression: a double-blind, randomized trial. J Clin Psychopharmacol 25:471–475, 2005

Ruijten HM, de Bree H, Borst AJ, et al: Fluvoxamine: metabolic fate in animals. Drug Metab Dispos 12:82–92, 1984

Stahl SM: Mechanism of action of selective serotonin reuptake inhibitors: serotonin receptors and pathways mediate therapeutic effects and side effects. J Affect Disord 51:215–235, 1998

Stanley MA, Breckenridge JK, Swann AC, et al: Fluvoxamine treatment of trichotillomania. J Clin Psychopharmacol 17:278–283, 1997

Stein DJ, Westenberg HG, Yang H et al: Fluvoxamine CR in the long-term treatment of social anxiety disorder: the 12- to 24-week extension phase of a multicentre, randomized, placebo-controlled trial. Int J Neuropsychopharmacol 6:317–323, 2003

Stein MB, Fyer AJ, Davidson JR, et al: Fluvoxamine treatment of social phobia (social anxiety disorder): a double-blind, placebo-controlled study. Am J Psychiatry 156:756–760, 1999

Strauss WL, Layton ME, Dager SR: Brain elimination half-life of fluvoxamine measured by 19F magnetic resonance spectroscopy. Am J Psychiatry 155:380–384, 1998

Terra JL, Montgomery SA: Fluvoxamine prevents recurrence of depression: results of a long-term, double-blind, placebo-controlled study. Int Clin Psychopharmacol 13:55–62, 1998

Tucker P, Smith KL, Marx B, et al: Fluvoxamine reduces physiologic reactivity to trauma scripts in posttraumatic stress disorder. J Clin Psychopharmacol 20:367–372, 2000

Van Harten J: Overview of the pharmacokinetics of fluvoxamine. Clin Pharmacokinet 29 (suppl 1):1–9, 1995

Van Harten J, Duchier J, Devissaguet JP, et al: Pharmacokinetics of fluvoxamine maleate in patients with liver cirrhosis after single-dose oral administration. Clin Pharmacokinet 24:177–182, 1993

Van Oppen P, Van Balkom AJ, de Haan E, et al: Cognitive therapy and exposure in vivo alone and in combination with fluvoxamine in obsessive-compulsive disorder: a 5-year follow-up. J Clin Psychiatry 66:1415–1422, 2005

Wagner W, Zaborny BA, Gray TE: Fluvoxamine: a review of its safety in world-wide studies. Int Clin Psychopharmacol 9:223–227, 1994

Ware MR: Fluvoxamine: a review of the controlled trials in depression. J Clin Psychiatry 58 (suppl 5):15–23, 1997

Westenberg HG, Sadner C: Tolerability and safety of fluvoxamine and other antidepressants. Int J Clin Pract 60:482–491, 2006

Westenberg HG, Stein DJ, Yang H, et al: A double-blind placebo-controlled study of controlled release fluvoxamine for the treatment of generalized social anxiety disorder. J Clin Psychopharmacol 24:49–55, 2004

Zanardi R, Franchini L, Serretti A, et al: Venlafaxine versus fluvoxamine in the treatment of delusional depression: a pilot double-blind controlled study. J Clin Psychiatry 61:26–29, 2000

Zohar J, Keegstra H, Barrelet L: Fluvoxamine as effective as clomipramine against symptoms of severe depression: results from a multicentre, double-blind study. Hum Psychopharmacol 18:113–119, 2003

CHAPTER 17

Citalopram and *S*-Citalopram

Patrick H. Roseboom, Ph.D.

Ned H. Kalin, M.D.

Citalopram (Celexa) and its pharmacologically active enantiomer, S-citalopram (Lexapro), are among the most selective serotonin (5-HT) reuptake inhibitors available. Both drugs are widely prescribed and have been shown in large-scale controlled trials to be effective in the treatment of depression; S-citalopram has also been shown in large-scale controlled trials to be effective in the treatment of anxiety disorders. In addition, both drugs are well tolerated in patients and show a low potential for pharmacokinetic drug interactions. Citalopram and S-citalopram have similar efficacy in the treatment of depression, with some studies suggesting a modest superiority of S-citalopram over citalopram in some measures of efficacy, including a possibly faster onset of therapeutic effect for S-citalopram. Antagonism of the effects of S-citalopram by R-citalopram has been invoked to explain the purported therapeutic differences between the two drugs. In addition, the affinity of citalopram for histamine receptors appears to reside in the R-enantiomer, suggesting that S-citalopram has a decreased potential for antihistaminergic side effects. Whether the postulated superiority of S-citalopram over citalopram is clinically meaningful in psychiatric practice requires further study.

History and Discovery

Citalopram (Lu 10-171), 1-(3-[dimethylamino]propyl)-1-(p-fluorophenyl)-5-phthalancarbonitrile, is a bicyclic phthalane derivative (molecular weight = 405.35 Da) with a chemical structure that is distinct from other antidepressants. The pharmacology of citalopram was first described in 1977 (Christensen et al. 1977; Hyttel 1977b). Citalopram was discovered in a series of ring system substitutions of phthalane derivatives and was shown to be a very potent inhibitor of 5-HT reuptake in both in vitro and in vivo models (Hyttel 1977b, 1978). In contrast, it was not active in models of norepinephrine (NE) reuptake, and it inhibited dopamine (DA) reuptake only at extremely high concentrations. In addition, it did not affect the activity of monoamine oxidase (MAO) (Hyttel 1977b). It was subsequently discovered that all of the inhibitory activity of citalopram on 5-HT reuptake resides in the S-(+)-enantiomer (S-citalopram) (Hyttel et al. 1992). Originally introduced in Denmark in 1989, citalopram was approved by the U.S. Food and Drug Administration (FDA) for the treatment of depression in July 1998. S-citalopram received FDA approval for the treatment of major depressive disorder in August 2002 and for the treatment of generalized anxiety disorder (GAD) in December 2003.

Structure–Activity Relations

Citalopram has a single chiral center (Figure 17–1). A chiral center is an atom surrounded by an asymmetrical arrangement of atoms such that the three-dimensional configuration is not superimposable on its mirror image. At this chiral center, there are two possible stereoisomers. Often, drugs are produced as a mixture of both stereoisomers; this is referred to as the racemate. However, pharmacological activity or unwanted toxicity may reside in only one of the stereoisomers. Therefore, producing a formulation that contains only one stereoisomer has the po-

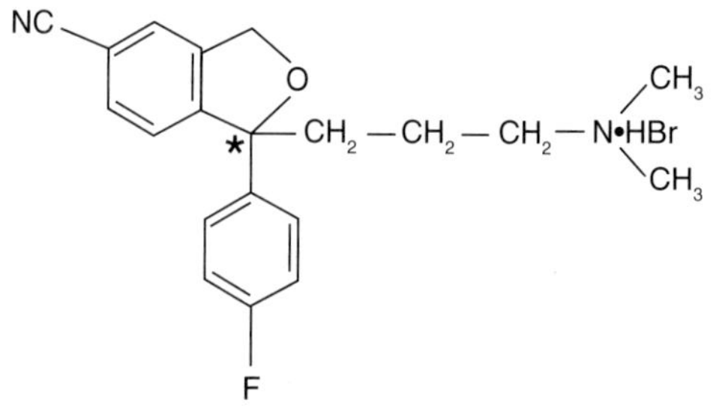

FIGURE 17–1.   Chemical structure of citalopram.
Asterisk (*) indicates chiral center.

tential to improve efficacy and limit toxicity while also extending the period of patent protection for the compound. Increasingly, drug companies are performing "chiral switches" and converting the formulation of a drug from the racemate to one pure enantiomer (Agranat et al. 2002). This is the case with citalopram, which was originally characterized and marketed as the racemate, but subsequently the single stereoisomer of citalopram, S-citalopram, has been developed for the treatment of depression and other psychiatric disorders.

Preclinical studies indicate that inhibition of 5-HT transporter activity resides in the S-enantiomer (Hyttel et al. 1992), with S-citalopram being 30-fold more potent than R-citalopram at inhibiting 5-HT transport (Owens et al. 2001). Molecular modeling has suggested that the lower potency of R-citalopram may be due to steric hindrance associated with the interaction of R-citalopram with the primary binding site on the 5-HT transporter (Ravna et al. 2003). S-citalopram also appears to be more selective than R-citalopram both in terms of inhibition of monoamine reuptake and in terms of neurotransmitter receptor interactions (Owens et al. 2001). Additionally, there is some in vitro evidence that S-citalopram has a slightly lower potential to interact with the liver cytochrome P450 (CYP) system compared with R-citalopram, thus decreasing the likelihood of drug–drug interactions at the level of drug metabolism (von Moltke et al. 2001).

A possible explanation for the postulated modest superiority of S-citalopram over citalopram in some measures of antidepressant efficacy is provided by the evidence that the R-enantiomer of citalopram may interfere with the activity of the S-enantiomer (Sanchez 2006). The ability of R-citalopram to antagonize the effects of S-citalopram has been obtained from a variety of behavioral (Fish et al. 2004; Sanchez and Kreilgaard 2004; Sanchez et al. 2003b, 2003c) and physiological (El Mansari et al. 2005, 2007; Mork et al. 2003) assays. This antagonism has

been hypothesized to result from a kinetic interaction at the level of the 5-HT transporter (Storustovu et al. 2004).

Pharmacological Profile

Citalopram

Citalopram is one of the most selective of the selective 5-HT reuptake inhibitors (SSRIs) approved to date, with a 524-fold lower potency for inhibiting the human NE transporter and a >10,000-fold lower potency for inhibiting the human DA transporter (Owens et al. 2001). In addition, citalopram has low affinity for a wide variety of neurotransmitter receptors, including dopamine$_1$ (D$_1$) and dopamine$_2$ (D$_2$); serotonin$_{1A}$ (5-HT$_{1A}$), serotonin$_{2A}$ (5-HT$_{2A}$), and serotonin$_{2C}$ (5-HT$_{2C}$); α$_1$-, α$_2$-, and β-adrenergic; muscarinic cholinergic (Hall et al. 1984; Hyttel 1982, 1994; Hyttel and Larsen 1985; Richelson and Nelson 1984); and γ-aminobutyric acid (GABA) and opiate receptors (Hyttel et al. 1995). Citalopram has been reported to have submicromolar affinity for the histamine$_1$ (H$_1$) receptor (Hyttel 1994; Richelson and Nelson 1984), but recent evidence indicates that this is true only for the R-enantiomer (Owens et al. 2001). Citalopram does not show significant inhibition of MAO (Hyttel 1977b).

Behavioral studies have shown citalopram to be a potent and selective inhibitor of 5-HT reuptake. In mice, citalopram is potent at potentiating the L-5-hydroxytryptophan (L-5-HTP) or tryptophan-induced 5-HT syndrome (Christensen et al. 1977; Hyttel 1994). In rats, citalopram decreases spontaneous tail flicks that are induced by p-chloroamphetamine, which acts by entering 5-HT neurons through the 5-HT transporter. In contrast, citalopram is ineffective in models that reflect in vivo inhibition of DA and NE reuptake (Hyttel 1994).

Citalopram is active in various behavioral models related to antidepressant activity. For example, in rats citalopram reverses helpless behavior in the learned helplessness paradigm (Martin et al. 1990), and it reverses the effects of chronic mild stress-induced decreases in sucrose consumption (Papp et al. 2002; Przegalinski et al. 1995). In mice, citalopram reverses the immobility induced by forced swimming in a confined space (Sanchez and Meier 1997). Citalopram also has antiaggressive activity in animal models, as shown by a decrease in isolation-induced aggressive behavior in male mice that have been pretreated with the 5-HT precursor L-5-HTP (Sanchez and Hyttel 1994). Citalopram is also active in various behavioral models designed to predict anxiolytic activity. For example, in rats, citalopram antagonizes freezing behavior produced by conditioned fear (Inoue 1993), and in both rats and mice, citalopram increases exploratory behavior in a black-and-white approach–avoidance test box (Sanchez 1995).

Similar to other SSRIs, citalopram potentiates the effects of some pharmacological agents. For example, the anticonvulsant activity of diphenylhydantoin administered prior to electroshock-induced convulsions in mice (Hyttel et al. 1995) and the antinociceptive effects of opiates administered prior to the hot plate test in rats are potentiated (Larsen and Hyttel 1985; Sugrue 1979).

S-Citalopram

S-citalopram is also a highly potent inhibitor of 5-HT reuptake, with a K_i for binding to the human 5-HT transporter of 1.1 nM compared with a K_i of 1.9 nM for citalopram and 36 nM for *R*-citalopram (Owens et al. 2001). S-citalopram is the most selective SSRI approved for clinical use, with a 2,600-fold lower potency for inhibiting the human NE transporter and a >45,000-fold lower potency for inhibiting the human DA transporter. S-citalopram also has no appreciable binding affinity for a large number of other neurotransmitter receptors, including all those mentioned above in relation to the selectivity of citalopram (Owens et al. 2001; Sanchez et al. 2003a). S-citalopram displays a weak affinity ($K_i = 100$ nM) for binding to the σ_1 receptor, with both citalopram and *R*-citalopram displaying a similar affinity. Finally, there is a low level of binding affinity ($K_i = 181$ nM) displayed by *R*-citalopram for the histamine H_1 receptor (Owens et al. 2001), which could explain any antihistaminergic side effects that may be associated with citalopram.

S-citalopram also has potent activity in various in vivo paradigms (for a review, see Sanchez et al. 2003a). For example, in an in vivo model of 5-HT reuptake inhibition, S-citalopram potentiates the L-5-HTP-induced 5-HT syndrome. S-citalopram is also active in behavioral models of antidepressant, antiaggressive, and anxiolytic activity. In mice, S-citalopram reverses the immobility induced by forced swimming. S-citalopram is also potent at inhibiting aggressive behavior in male mice following pretreatment with L-5-HTP. Finally, S-citalopram has anxiolytic-like activity, as shown in mice by an increase in exploratory activity in the black-and-white approach–avoidance test box and in rats by inhibition of ultrasonic vocalization induced by foot shock. In these in vivo paradigms, the potency of S-citalopram ranges from similar to citalopram to approximately twofold greater than citalopram. In contrast, in the majority of these paradigms *R*-citalopram is severalfold less potent than either S-citalopram or citalopram.

Pharmacokinetics and Disposition

Citalopram

Citalopram is well absorbed after oral administration, with an absolute bioavailability for citalopram tablets of 80% compared with intravenous administration (Joffe et al. 1998). The peak plasma concentration is normally observed 2–4 hours following an oral dose (Kragh-Sorensen et al. 1981). The bioavailability of citalopram is not affected by food (Baumann and Larsen 1995), and it is subject to very little first-pass metabolism (Kragh-Sorensen et al. 1981). The apparent volume of distribution is 12–16 L/kg (Kragh-Sorensen et al. 1981; Overo 1982), which indicates that the drug distributes widely. There is a linear relationship between steady-state plasma concentration and dose (Bjerkenstedt et al. 1985), and plasma protein binding is approximately 80% (Baumann and Larsen 1995). Because citalopram is less strongly protein bound than many other compounds, it is less susceptible to drug–drug interactions at the level of protein binding. Systemic clearance of citalopram was determined to be 0.3–0.4 L/minute in a study of healthy volunteers given a single intravenous dose. This value indicates a low hepatic extraction ratio (Baumann and Larsen 1995). In a separate study, the renal clearance of citalopram was determined to be approximately 0.05–0.08 L/minute (Sindrup et al. 1993).

Racemic citalopram undergoes *N*-demethylation by the hepatic P450 system to the major metabolite, monodesmethylcitalopram (DCT). In vitro studies using human liver microsomes and heterologously expressed individual human cytochromes indicate that CYP2C19, CYP3A4, and CYP2D6 all contribute approximately equally to the formation of DCT (Kobayashi et al. 1997; Rochat et al. 1997; von Moltke et al. 1999). DCT also undergoes N-demethylation to the minor metabolite didesmethylcitalopram (DDCT) by the actions of CYP2D6 (Sindrup et al. 1993; von Moltke et al. 2001). Compared with citalopram, DCT is 4 times less potent than an SSRI and 11 times more potent than an NE reuptake inhibitor (Hyttel 1982). Because DCT only weakly crosses the blood–brain barrier and usually is present at significantly lower concentrations than citalopram, the contribution of DCT to the antidepressant efficacy of citalopram is likely negligible (van Harten 1993). Clinical studies indicate that the half-lives for citalopram, DCT, and DDCT are approximately 36 hours, 50 hours, and 100 hours, respectively (Dalgaard and Larsen 1999; Kragh-Sorensen et al. 1981; Overo 1982). In a study in which a single radioactive dose of citalopram was administered to volunteers,

75% of the radioactivity was recovered in the urine and 10% in the feces. The radioactivity in the urine corresponded to citalopram (26%), DCT (19%), and DDCT (9%) (Dalgaard and Larsen 1999). The remainder was composed of the N-oxide derivative of citalopram (7%) and the glucuronide conjugates of citalopram (14%), DDCT (6%), and citalopram acid (12%).

The potential for drug–drug interactions at the level of inhibition of liver metabolism is low for both citalopram and S-citalopram (see below). In vitro studies show that citalopram only weakly inhibits CYP1A2 and CYP2C19 and does not significantly inhibit CYP2C9, CYP2E1, and CYP3A (von Moltke et al. 1999). Citalopram is a relatively weak inhibitor of CYP2D6.

Because citalopram is metabolized by human cytochromes that display genetic polymorphisms, it is possible that metabolism of citalopram may display genetic variability. In a study of 69 depressed patients who were phenotyped as extensive and poor metabolizers of the CYP2C19 pathway (mephenytoin), poor metabolizers had significantly higher ratios of citalopram to DCT compared with extensive metabolizers, indicating that the metabolism of citalopram is impaired in poor metabolizers (Baumann et al. 1996). Similar results were seen in two separate studies involving 24 healthy male volunteers and 77 healthy Chinese volunteers in which steady-state plasma concentrations of citalopram were elevated in poor metabolizers of the CYP2C19 pathway (Sindrup et al. 1993; Yu et al. 2003). Additionally, both of these studies showed that the further metabolism of DCT to DDCT was impaired in poor metabolizers of the CYP2D6 pathway (Baumann et al. 1996; Sindrup et al. 1993). Taken together, these data provide evidence for the roles of CYP2C19 and CYP2D6 in the metabolism of citalopram.

The effects of age and physiological status on the metabolism of citalopram have also been studied. In elderly patients (Overo et al. 1985; Uehlinger et al. 1995) and patients with liver disease (Joffe et al. 1998), the clearance of citalopram is decreased, and a decrease in dosage may be necessary for these patients. In a study of seven patients, renal insufficiency did not have a significant effect on the plasma concentration of citalopram (Joffe et al. 1998). Therefore, reduced renal function does not have a major impact on the kinetics of citalopram, and dosage adjustment may not be necessary. It should be noted that the data for the effects of renal insufficiency were following a single dose. No published studies have yet reported the effects of impaired kidney function in chronic treatment of patients with citalopram.

S-Citalopram

The clinical pharmacokinetic characteristics of S-citalopram have recently been reviewed and are similar to those described for citalopram (N. Rao 2007). The pharmacokinetic characteristics of S-citalopram are essentially the same regardless of whether patients are given a single oral dose of 20 mg of S-citalopram or 40 mg of racemic citalopram (which contains 20 mg of S-citalopram). This indicates that there is no pharmacokinetic interaction or interconversion between R-citalopram and S-citalopram (N. Rao 2007; Sogaard et al. 2005). The human cytochromes involved in the metabolism of S-citalopram and its metabolite S-DCT are the same as those reported for racemic citalopram (von Moltke et al. 2001). The average half-lives of the two enantiomers differ. In one study of five hospitalized depressed patients, the half-life of S-citalopram (42 ± 13 h) was shorter than that of the R-enantiomer (R-citalopram; 66 ± 11 h). Likewise, the half-life of the major metabolite S-DCT (93 ± 35 h) was significantly shorter than that of R-DCT (228 ± 148 h) (Voirol et al. 1999). The shorter reported half-life for S-citalopram is consistent with the trend toward lower steady-state plasma concentrations of S-citalopram and S-DCT compared with R-citalopram and R-DCT in patients (Bondolfi et al. 1996; Foglia et al. 1997; Sidhu et al. 1997).

Both S-citalopram and R-citalopram and their metabolites show weak or negligible inhibition in vitro of the various liver P450 enzymes (von Moltke et al. 2001). In a clinical study, S-citalopram did show some inhibition of CYP2D6, measured as a change in the pharmacokinetics of the CYP2D6 substrate metoprolol, but to a significantly lesser extent compared with paroxetine or fluoxetine (Preskorn et al. 2007). It should be noted that both R-DDCT and S-DDCT show moderate potency for inhibiting CYP2C19, but this is unlikely to be clinically relevant since the median inhibitory concentration (IC_{50}) values for CYP2C19 are more than two orders of magnitude above the low plasma concentrations achieved for these two metabolites (Baumann and Larsen 1995). The only substantial inhibition of CYP2D6 that has been noted in vitro results from R-DCT ($IC_{50}=25.5$ μM), which is still an order of magnitude less potent than paroxetine ($IC_{50}=2.6$ μM) (von Moltke et al. 2001). However, this inhibitory activity of the metabolite of R-citalopram suggests a lower potential for S-citalopram to inhibit liver P450 enzymes compared with racemic citalopram.

Mechanism of Action

The majority of studies on mechanism of action have focused on citalopram, with a relatively limited number of studies using S-citalopram. Because the antidepressant activity of citalopram results from S-citalopram, the majority of the conclusions from these studies pertain to both citalopram and S-citalopram. Studies that specifically utilized S-citalopram are reviewed in the S-citalopram section that immediately follows.

Citalopram

Citalopram is a potent and selective inhibitor of 5-HT reuptake and acts by binding directly to the 5-HT transporter. In vitro studies demonstrate that citalopram blocks 5-HT reuptake by rabbit thrombocytes (Hyttel 1977b), rat brain synaptosomes (Hyttel 1978, 1982; Richelson and Pfenning 1984; Vaatstra et al. 1981; Waldmeier et al. 1979), rat brain slices (Classen et al. 1984; Dyck 1984; Galzin et al. 1985), and rat lung slices (Drew and Siddik 1980). Blockade of 5-HT reuptake is of the competitive type, as shown in thrombocytes and synaptosomes, and the accumulation of 5-HT is not due to citalopram-induced 5-HT release (Hyttel 1977b, 1978). This is consistent with experiments demonstrating that citalopram does not alter spontaneous release of endogenous or preloaded 5-HT from rat cortical slices, but it does increase the electrically induced release of 5-HT (Baumann and Waldmeier 1981). The IC_{50} values for 5-HT reuptake in rat brain synaptosomes are 3.9 nM (citalopram), 2.1 nM (S-citalopram), and 275 nM (R-citalopram) (Sanchez and Brennum 2000).

Citalopram is one of the most selective inhibitors of radioligand binding to the 5-HT transporter versus the NE transporter. The K_i for inhibiting [^{3}H]citalopram binding to rat cortical membranes was 0.75 nM, compared with 3,042 nM for inhibiting [^{3}H]nisoxetine binding. A similar selectivity was found for inhibiting the binding of the same radioligands to the cloned human 5-HT and NE transporters expressed in transfected cells. In addition, the K_is for inhibiting [^{3}H]5-HT and [^{3}H]NE reuptake into these transfected cells were 8.9 nM and 30,285 nM, respectively (Owens et al. 1997). Citalopram appears to bind at or near the site that 5-HT occupies during transport (Barker et al. 1998).

Citalopram, at doses that profoundly affect 5-HT reuptake, does not alter the endogenous levels of 5-HT, NE, or DA in the rat brain (Hyttel 1977b). Inhibition of 5-HT reuptake should result in an increase in synaptic levels of 5-HT, resulting in decreased 5-HT neuronal firing via feedback inhibition. This inhibition should decrease 5-HT synthesis and turnover, and this effect has been observed following administration of citalopram to rats (Hyttel 1977a).

As with other SSRIs, acute administration of citalopram to rats increases extracellular 5-HT in the raphe nucleus (Invernizzi et al. 1992). Acute citalopram also potently inhibits the firing of 5-HT neurons in the dorsal raphe nucleus (DRN), presumably through activation of 5-HT$_{1A}$ autoreceptors (Arborelius et al. 1995; Chaput et al. 1986). The inhibition of 5-HT neurons in the raphe nucleus is thought to limit the ability of a single administration of SSRIs to increase extracellular 5-HT in frontal brain regions that receive projections from the raphe nucleus. As expected, coadministration of 5-HT autoreceptor antagonists blocks the ability of acute citalopram to inhibit firing of DRN neurons (Arborelius et al. 1995) and increases the ability of citalopram to elevate extracellular 5-HT levels in various forebrain regions (Hjorth 1993; Hjorth et al. 1996; Invernizzi et al. 1997). This acute effect of citalopram on 5-HT neurons in the DRN is also seen in mice, but not in knockout mice, where the target for the actions of citalopram, the 5-HT transporter, has been eliminated (la Cour et al. 2001).

Some studies of the interaction between antidepressants and the 5-HT transporter indicate that in addition to the primary high-affinity binding site, there is also a second low-affinity allosteric site. The high-affinity site is responsible for inhibition of 5-HT transport, whereas the allosteric site modulates the dissociation rate of ligand binding at the high-affinity site (Neubauer et al. 2006; Plenge et al. 1991). When citalopram binds to the allosteric site, it is thought to inhibit the dissociation of citalopram from the primary binding site, thereby enhancing the inhibition of 5-HT transport (Plenge and Mellerup 1997). Interestingly, both enantiomers of citalopram bind to this site to inhibit dissociation of citalopram with S-citalopram being three to five times more potent than R-citalopram at binding to this allosteric site (Chen et al. 2005).

Because antidepressants usually require weeks of administration to be therapeutically beneficial, several studies have described how repeated dosing alters the effects of citalopram on serotonergic neuronal function. Much as with other SSRIs, the ability of citalopram to inhibit the firing of 5-HT neurons in the DRN is greatly reduced after 14 days of repeated administration (Chaput et al. 1986). This is associated with an increase in the ability of citalopram to elevate the extracellular levels of 5-HT in the cortex (Invernizzi et al. 1994). These two effects appear to result from a desensitization of 5-HT$_{1A}$ autoreceptors because repeated citalopram administration decreases the effectiveness of 5-HT$_{1A}$ agonists to inhibit firing of 5-HT neurons in the DRN (Chaput et al. 1986) and to decrease extracellular 5-HT levels in the rat forebrain (Cremers et al. 2000; Invernizzi et al. 1994). It should be noted, however, that one study failed to demonstrate a chronic citalopram-induced desensitization of 5-HT$_{1A}$ autoreceptors (Hjorth and Auerbach 1994). This adaptive change of 5-HT$_{1A}$ receptors following repeated administration of citalopram, as well as other SSRIs, has been postulated to underlie the slow onset of antidepressant efficacy that is observed clinically (Blier and de Montigny 1994).

Evidence suggests that a variety of antidepressants, including those that block monoamine reuptake or metabolism, produce their therapeutic response in part by overcoming depression-associated decreases in neurogenesis and synaptogenesis. Brain-derived neurotrophic factor (BDNF), which supports neuroplasticity, has been implicated in both the pathophysiology of depression and the therapeutic response to antidepressants. Citalopram has been shown to affect BDNF expression and signaling through the primary BDNF receptor, TrkB. In terms of BDNF expression, citalopram increases the levels of BDNF mRNA in various subregions of the ventral hippocampus either alone or in combination with exercise (wheel running) in rats (Russo-Neustadt et al. 2004). Citalopram, like several other antidepressants, also induces signaling through TrkB. Acute injection of citalopram into rats results in a significant increase in the autophosphorylation of TrkB within the rat anterior cingulate and dentate gyrus within 60 minutes (Rantamaki et al. 2007). Acute citalopram treatment was also associated with activation of TrkB-associated phospholipase Cγ1 and an increase in the phosphorylation of the transcription factor cAMP response element–binding protein (CREB). The relevance of these findings is shown by the abolishment of the effects of citalopram in the forced-swim test in transgenic mice lacking functional TrkB receptors (Rantamaki et al. 2007). Finally, there are preliminary clinical data suggesting that a polymorphism within the coding region for BDNF (Val66Met) is associated with the therapeutic response to citalopram. In Korean patients with major depressive disorder, responders to 8 weeks of citalopram treatment were more likely to have the Met allele (Val/Met or Met/Met) (78.9%) compared with nonresponders (46.2%) (Choi et al. 2006).

A number of studies have implicated the 5-HT$_{2A}$ receptor in a variety of neuropsychiatric disorders (Norton and Owen 2005), and there is evidence implicating the 5-HT$_{2A}$ receptor in the mechanism of action of antidepressants. For example, preclinical studies show that a number of antidepressant treatments, including citalopram administration, downregulate brain 5-HT$_{2A}$ receptors in a time frame that corresponds to the onset of therapeutic effect in humans (Chen and Lawrence 2003; Peremans et al. 2005; Strome et al. 2005). In addition, antagonism of rodent 5-HT$_{2A}$ receptors blocks the stress-induced reduction in BDNF mRNA (Vaidya et al. 1997). In a large-scale clinical study involving 1,953 patients who participated in the STAR*D trial, a survey of 768 single-nucleotide polymorphisms (SNPs) contained in 68 candidate genes identified a significant association between a polymorphism contained in the second intron of the gene for the 5-HT$_{2A}$ receptor (rs7997012) and treatment response to citalopram. This was observed in the initial discovery sample ($n = 859$), which consisted of two-thirds of the total number of subjects in the study, and was confirmed in a replication sample ($n = 438$) consisting of the remaining one-third of the subjects (McMahon et al. 2006). Specifically, those patients who were homozygous for the A allele had an 18% lower risk of treatment failure compared with patients who were homozygous for the G allele. Importantly, this allele was six times more frequent in white compared with black patients, and this was associated with a poorer response to citalopram therapy in the black patient population. While perhaps relevant to clinical work, the functional significance of this intronic polymorphism on the 5-HT$_{2A}$ receptor has yet to be determined.

S-Citalopram

Like citalopram, S-citalopram is a potent and highly selective inhibitor of 5-HT reuptake that acts by binding directly to the 5-HT transporter. Acute treatment with S-citalopram inhibits the firing of 5-HT neurons in the DRN presumably through 5-HT-dependent activation of 5-HT$_{1A}$ autoreceptors (Sanchez et al. 2003a). Additionally, the adaptive changes in the sensitivity of 5-HT$_{1A}$ autoreceptors that are postulated to underlie the onset of antidepressant efficacy have also been shown to occur following S-citalopram treatment. Specifically, desensitization of 5-HT$_{1A}$ autoreceptors in the rat prefrontal cortex was reported following chronic treatment with S-citalopram (Ceglia et al. 2004). Antidepressants have also been postulated to work through changes in neuronal plasticity. S-citalopram has been shown to affect cytogenesis within the brain. Cytogenesis refers to the proliferation of new cells that may subsequently differentiate into neurons (neurogenesis). For example, S-citalopram treatment for 4 weeks reverses the decrease in cytogenesis that occurs in the subgranular zone of the dentate gyrus in the ventral hippocampus as a result of 2 weeks of chronic mild stress exposure. Importantly, this effect was only seen in a subgroup of rats for which S-citalopram reversed chronic mild stress-induced anhedonia; those rats that did not have this behavioral effect did not show the change in cytogenesis (Jayatissa et al. 2006). Because the majority of newly formed cells within the subgranular zone will divide and, if they survive, differentiate into neurons, the authors speculate that the changes in cytogenesis will ultimately affect the number of new neurons that are formed within the granular cell layer of the dentate gyrus.

Indications and Efficacy

Depression

Citalopram

The efficacy of citalopram in the treatment of depression has been shown in at least 11 placebo-controlled clinical trials (for a review, see Keller 2000). In addition to the independently published reports described below, meta-analyses of multiple placebo-controlled studies reported similar findings (Bech and Cialdella 1992; Montgomery et al. 1994). In the United States, three large multicenter clinical trials were conducted. In a 4-week trial, a variable dosage paradigm ranging from 20 mg to 80 mg per day was utilized among 180 patients with depression or melancholia. At the end of the study, patients on citalopram showed a significant improvement on the Hamilton Rating Scale for Depression (Ham-D), the Clinical Global Impressions (CGI) Scale, and the Zung Self-Rating Depression Scale compared with placebo. The improvement in the Ham-D score was seen as early as 1 week (Mendels et al. 1999).

In a second trial, patients ($n = 650$) with moderate to severe depression were assigned a fixed dosage of 10, 20, 40, or 60 mg of citalopram or placebo for 6 weeks (Feighner and Overo 1999). Citalopram was significantly more efficacious than placebo ($P<0.05$) based on reductions in the Ham-D and Montgomery-Åsberg Depression Rating Scale (MADRS) scores, and the CGI–Improvement (CGI-I) and CGI–Severity of Illness (CGI-S) ratings. All four doses of citalopram significantly improved the Ham-D score ($P<0.01$), and the response rate with all four doses was significantly greater than with placebo.

A third placebo-controlled study compared the efficacy of citalopram (20–60 mg/day) with that of another SSRI, sertraline (50–150 mg/day), in 323 patients with DSM-IV (American Psychiatric Association 1994)–defined major depression. Both treatments produced significantly greater improvement than placebo in the Ham-D score ($P<0.05$), the MADRS score ($P<0.01$), the CGI-S rating ($P<0.05$), and the CGI-I rating ($P<0.05$) (Stahl 2000).

Sequenced Treatment Alternatives to Relieve Depression (STAR*D) trial. The effectiveness of citalopram has also been demonstrated in a study designed to simulate real-world conditions for the treatment of depression. Treatment with citalopram was used in the first phase of the Sequenced Treatment Alternatives to Relieve Depression (STAR*D) trial. This large-scale multicenter study enrolled 4,041 patients with nonpsychotic major depression from 23 psychiatric and 18 primary care settings across the United States in a test of various antidepressant therapies (Rush et al. 2004). The first phase of the study consisted of 12 weeks of treatment with a flexible dosage of citalopram initiated at 20 mg/day and gradually increased on an individualized basis to 60 mg/day, and the primary outcome measure was depression remission defined as a score of ≤7 on the 17-item Ham-D (Ham-D$_{17}$) or a score of ≤5 on the 16-item Quick Inventory of Depressive Symptomatology, Self-Report (QIDS-SR). Response rates were defined as ≥50% reduction in the QIDS-SR score. Approximately 80% of the 2,876 patients who were included in an analysis of the first phase of the study had chronic or recurrent major depression, with most of these patients having a variety of other comorbid general medical and psychiatric conditions. The mean daily dose of citalopram at study exit was 41.8 mg, the remission rates were 28% (Ham-D) and 33% (QIDS-SR), and the response rate was 47% (QIDS-SR) (Trivedi et al. 2006). These response and remission rates are comparable to those found in controlled 8-week clinical trials examining the efficacy of acute antidepressant treatment.

Long-term treatment with citalopram. Early discontinuation of antidepressant treatment is associated with depression relapse. To prevent relapse, it is recommended that antidepressant treatment should be continued for at least 4–6 months (Montgomery 1996). Two placebo-controlled studies indicate that for patients with an acute therapeutic response to citalopram, continuation of citalopram therapy at the same dose (20, 40, or 60 mg/day) for 24 additional weeks significantly decreases the relapse rate compared with placebo (Montgomery et al. 1993; P. Robert and Montgomery 1995). These studies suggest that citalopram may be effective in continuation therapy to prevent depression relapse. Depression also tends to be a recurrent illness, and many patients experience multiple episodes within a lifetime. Two studies have shown that long-term (at least 48 weeks) administration of citalopram at the same fixed dose at which patients initially showed therapeutic response (20–60 mg/day) can significantly increase the time before depression recurs in adult patients (18–65 years) and in the elderly (≥65 years) (Hochstrasser et al. 2001; Klysner et al. 2002). These studies suggest that long-term administration of citalopram may be beneficial in patients who have a history of recurrent depression.

S-Citalopram

A number of placebo-controlled clinical trials and retrospective analyses have demonstrated the efficacy of S-citalopram in the treatment of major depression. In addition, several clinical studies have directly compared S-citalopram to citalopram and a variety of other antidepressants. In general, S-citalopram was at least as effective as other widely used antidepressants, and in some clinical trials it has been suggested to be superior to other antidepressants based on modestly greater changes in various depression rating scales, especially in severely depressed patients. In addition, also based on depression rating scales, S-citalopram has been suggested in a few clinical trials to possibly have a faster onset of therapeutic effect occurring as early as 1 week. The details of these studies are reviewed below. Whether the modest differences between S-citalopram and other antidepressants in controlled clinical trials translate into a therapeutically meaningful difference in the treatment of depression in psychiatric practice remains to be demonstrated.

Three placebo-controlled clinical trials have demonstrated the efficacy of S-citalopram in treatment of depression. Results of a double-blind, placebo-controlled, fixed-dose multicenter clinical trial ($n = 491$) revealed that S-citalopram produced significant improvement compared with placebo at both doses tested (10 mg/day or 20 mg/day) (Burke et al. 2002). Significant improvement was seen within 1 week, and S-citalopram at 10 mg/day was at least as effective as citalopram at 40 mg/day in improving depressive symptomatology by the end of the 8-week study. Similar results were seen in another study in which patients receiving 10 mg/day of S-citalopram ($n = 191$) showed significant improvement compared with placebo ($n = 189$) by the end of the 8-week study (Wade et al. 2002).

In a separate double-blind study, citalopram (20–40 mg/day; $n = 160$) and S-citalopram (10–20 mg/day; $n = 155$) were compared with placebo ($n = 154$) in the treatment of primary care patients with major depression (MADRS scores ≥22 and ≤40) (Lepola et al. 2003; Montgomery et al. 2001b). Treatment with S-citalopram resulted in significantly greater improvement compared with placebo after 1 week. This difference was maintained through week 8, and the adjusted mean change in MADRS score was 2.9 points ($P = 0.002$). Treatment with S-citalopram also produced a significantly greater improvement compared with placebo on the CGI-I and CGI-S subscales from week 1 onward. In contrast, treatment with citalopram demonstrated superiority to placebo only at week 8 and only on the CGI-I scale. At the end of the study, significantly more patients had responded (defined as ≥50% decrease in MADRS total score) to S-citalopram (63.7%) than to either citalopram (52.6%; $P = 0.021$) or placebo (48.2%; $P = 0.009$).

Comparison of S-citalopram with citalopram. Two clinical trials that did not include a placebo control have compared S-citalopram to citalopram. In a 24-week double-blind, fixed-dosage study, S-citalopram at 10 mg/day ($n = 195$) was compared with citalopram at 20 mg/day ($n = 182$) in a primary care setting (Colonna et al. 2005). In this study, S-citalopram was as effective as citalopram as assessed by a decrease in the total MADRS score using a repeated-measures analysis of covariance (ANCOVA) to assess treatment response at all time points. Based on the mean change from baseline in the CGI-S score, S-citalopram was superior to citalopram by week 24. Interestingly, exploratory analysis revealed a statistically significant greater response to S-citalopram over citalopram in moderately depressed subjects (MADRS score ≥22 and <30) in the change in MADRS score and CGI-S score from baseline at both 8 and 24 weeks. Finally, the effectiveness of long-term treatment was evidenced by the observation that more than half of the patients (55% and 51% for S-citalopram and citalopram, respectively) who had not responded by week 8 were in remission by week 24. In a second study, S-citalopram at 20 mg/day ($N = 138$) was compared with citalopram at 40 mg/day ($n = 142$) in the outpatient treatment of major depressive disorder (Moore et al. 2005). The mean change in total MADRS score was greater in the S-citalopram group (-22.4 ± 12.9) than in the citalopram group (-20.3 ± 12.7; $P < 0.05$). In addition, there were more treatment responders (defined as a decrease from initial MADRS score of ≥50%) in the S-citalopram group (76.1%) than in the citalopram group (56.1%; *P*<0.01).

Finally, three pooled analyses suggest that S-citalopram has a faster onset of clinical effect when compared with citalopram (Gorman et al. 2002; Kasper et al. 2006; Lepola et al. 2004). In these studies, a significantly greater therapeutic response compared with placebo was achieved within 1 week for S-citalopram (10–20 mg/day), whereas citalopram (20–40 mg/day) required approximately 4 weeks of treatment. Whether this study observation results in a clinically meaningful faster onset of therapeutic effect requires further analysis.

Comparison of *S*-citalopram with other antidepressants.   The antidepressant efficacy of S-citalopram has been compared with that of several other commonly used SSRIs. Two published long-term randomized, double-blind studies directly compared S-citalopram with paroxetine. In a flexible-dosage study, S-citalopram at 10–20 mg/day was compared with paroxetine at 20–40 mg/day, and in a fixed dosage study S-citalopram at 20 mg/day was compared with paroxetine at 40 mg/day (Baldwin et al. 2006a; Boulenger et al. 2006). S-citalopram was found to be at least as effective as—and, in some measures, possibly modestly superior to—paroxetine in the treatment of severe depression (baseline MADRS total score ≥30). Specifically, in the severely depressed, treatment with 20 mg/day S-citalopram (*n*=228) produced greater improvement than treatment with 40 mg/day paroxetine (*n*=223). The mean change in total MADRS score at the end of 24 weeks of treatment was –25.2 points with S-citalopram and –23.1 points with paroxetine (*P*<0.05), and the percentage of remitters (MADRS≤12) was 75% with S-citalopram and 67% with paroxetine (*P*<0.05) (Boulenger et al. 2006). In addition, S-citalopram (10–20 mg/day) compared with paroxetine (20–40 mg/day) had fewer adverse events associated with treatment discontinuation (Baldwin et al. 2006a). When compared with sertraline in a randomized, double-blind trial, S-citalopram (10 mg/day) was as effective as sertraline (50–200 mg/day) in treating depression, and the two drugs had similar tolerability (Ventura et al. 2007). Finally, in a randomized, double-blind trial, S-citalopram (10 mg/day; *n*=173) was compared with fluoxetine (20 mg/day; *n*=164) and placebo (*n*=180) in the treatment of depression in the elderly (ages 65–93 years) (Kasper et al. 2005a). At the conclusion of the 8-week study, S-citalopram was numerically superior to fluoxetine in reducing mean total MADRS score from baseline, although neither drug was statistically superior to placebo.

There are also a large number of retrospective pooled analyses that have compared S-citalopram with other SSRIs. In general, these trials provide evidence that S-citalopram has a slightly superior efficacy compared with other SSRIs (fluoxetine, sertraline, and paroxetine) based on improvement in ratings on depression scales or percentage of depressed patients experiencing a therapeutic response or remission (Einarson 2004; Kennedy et al. 2006; Llorca et al. 2005).

Several clinical trials have compared S-citalopram with the serotonin–norepinephrine reuptake inhibitors (SNRIs) venlafaxine and duloxetine. In two randomized, double-blind trials (Bielski et al. 2004; Montgomery et al. 2004), S-citalopram was shown to be as effective as venlafaxine extended-release (XR) in the treatment of major depressive disorder, and S-citalopram had significantly better tolerability. One trial was a fixed-dosage study where S-citalopram at 20 mg/day was compared with venlafaxine XR at 225 mg/day, and the other was a flexible-dosage study in which S-citalopram at 10–20 mg/day was compared with venlafaxine XR at 75–150 mg/day. A retrospective analysis of these two clinical trials (Montgomery and Andersen 2006) suggested that treatment with S-citalopram was superior to treatment with venlafaxine XR for patients who were severely depressed (MADRS score ≥30). S-citalopram was compared with duloxetine in two randomized, double-blind clinical trials (Nierenberg et al. 2007; Wade et al. 2007). In these two studies, S-citalopram had either similar or slightly superior efficacy compared with duloxetine in terms of improvement of depressive symptoms, with S-citalopram having a better tolerability profile. Both of these were fixed-dosage studies, with S-citalopram at 10 mg/day compared with duloxetine at 60 mg/day in one study (Nierenberg et al. 2007) and S-citalopram at 20 mg/day compared with duloxetine at 60 mg/day in the other study (Wade et al. 2007).

Finally, in a retrospective analysis of two randomized, double-blind, placebo-controlled studies (Clayton et al. 2006), S-citalopram had a similar antidepressant efficacy compared with bupropion extended-release, while S-citalopram interfered with sexual functioning in a significantly greater proportion of patients. In both of these similarly designed flexible-dosage studies, S-citalopram at 10–20 mg/day was compared with both bupropion at 300–450 mg/day and placebo.

Long-term treatment with *S*-citalopram.   The effectiveness of S-citalopram in the prevention of relapse following resolution of a depressive episode was demonstrated in a placebo-controlled clinical trial (Rapaport et al. 2004) in which patients who responded to 8 weeks of open-label treatment with S-citalopram (10–20 mg/day) were randomly assigned to receive placebo (n=93) or S-citalopram (10–20 mg/day; n=181) for 36 additional weeks. The time to relapse was significantly longer in the S-citalopram group compared with the placebo group (P=0.013), and a significantly smaller percentage of patients relapsed in the S-citalopram group (26%) compared with the placebo group (40%; P=0.01). The effectiveness of long-term S-citalopram therapy in the prevention of recurrence of depression was tested in a group of patients who had been diagnosed with recurrent major depressive disorder (Kornstein et al. 2006). Patients who responded to 16 weeks of open-label treatment with a flexible dosage of S-citalopram (10–20 mg/day) were randomly assigned to receive either placebo (n=66) or a fixed dose of S-citalopram (10 or 20 mg/day; n=73) for an additional 52 weeks. Time to recurrence was significantly longer in the S-citalopram group compared with the placebo group (P<0.001).

S-citalopram treatment of depression with comorbid anxiety disorders. Major depressive disorder with comorbid anxiety has been associated with a poorer prognosis. To assess the effectiveness of S-citalopram in depressed patients with high levels of anxiety, a pooled analysis was performed on three clinical trials that focused on a subpopulation of depressed patients who had baseline inner tension scores (MADRS item 3) of ≥4 (Bandelow et al. 2007). S-citalopram (10–20 mg/day; n=131) produced a significantly greater mean change from baseline in the MADRS total score compared with placebo (n=128) at weeks 1, 4, 6, and 8, whereas citalopram (20–40 mg/day; n=132) was not superior to placebo until weeks 6 and 8. In addition, the response to S-citalopram exceeded that of citalopram in weeks 1, 6, and 8. Similarly, a prospective open-label trial completed by 649 depressed patients demonstrated that 12 weeks of treatment with S-citalopram (10–20 mg/day) was effective in relieving the symptoms of depression regardless of whether the patients had a comorbid anxiety disorder (Olie et al. 2007). These studies indicate that S-citalopram is effective in relieving depression in those patients who also experience high levels of anxiety.

Depression in Children and Adolescents

Citalopram

Fluoxetine is currently the only FDA-approved medication for the treatment of depression in children 8 years and older. In addition, the FDA has mandated the place-ment of black box warnings on product labels to indicate that there is a potential for increased suicidality associated with the use of SSRIs in patients younger than 25 years. Nevertheless, a recent meta-analysis of pediatric trials conducted between 1988 and 2006 indicated that the benefits of antidepressant treatment of the young outweigh the risks (Bridge et al. 2007). Only a limited number of clinical studies have examined the effectiveness of citalopram and S-citalopram in the treatment of depression in the young, and the efficacy of these two drugs in this patient group requires further study. Citalopram showed a modest superiority over placebo in the treatment of depression in a double-blind trial involving 174 children and adolescent (ages 7–17 years). The response rate (defined as a score of ≤28 on the Children's Depression Rating Scale–Revised) at week 8 was 36% in patients receiving 20 mg/day citalopram compared with 24% in patients receiving placebo (Wagner et al. 2004). Conversely, citalopram (10–40 mg/day) was not superior to placebo in a clinical trial involving 244 adolescents (ages 13–18 years) receiving treatment for 12 weeks. The percentage of responders and remitters based on the MADRS and the Schedule for Affective Disorders and Schizophrenia for School-Aged Children–Present Episode (Kiddie-SADS-P) scores did not significantly differ between the two groups. Interestingly, there was a significantly better response to citalopram compared with placebo in those patients (approximately one-third of total patients) who were not receiving psychotherapy during the trial (von Knorring et al. 2006). Finally, in an open-label trial conducted in Iran of citalopram (10–40 mg/day) in children and adolescents (ages 8–17 years) with major depressive disorder, 22 out of 24 subjects had a ≥50% decrease in their Ham-D score at the end of 6 weeks of treatment (Shirazi and Alaghband-Rad 2005). While citalopram was effective in this patient sample, the authors noted that 5 of the patients switched to mania during the study. Clearly, additional clinical trials are required to establish the efficacy and safety of citalopram in the treatment of childhood depression.

S-Citalopram

One published clinical trial has examined the effectiveness of S-citalopram in the treatment of depression in children and adolescents (Wagner et al. 2006). In this randomized, double-blind trial in adolescents (ages 6–17 years) with major depression, treatment with 10–20 mg/day S-citalopram (n=131) was not significantly better than treatment with placebo (n=133).

Posttraumatic Stress Disorder

Citalopram

No large-scale double-blind, placebo-controlled trials have evaluated the effectiveness of citalopram in the treatment of PTSD. However, a number of small-scale open-label trials with citalopram suggest that it may be effective in the treatment of PTSD in adults (English et al. 2006; Tucker et al. 2004) and adolescents (Seedat et al. 2002).

S-Citalopram

Only one published open-label trial (n = 24) has examined the effectiveness of S-citalopram in the treatment of combat veterans with PTSD (S. Robert et al. 2006). At the end of this 12-week study, S-citalopram (starting at 10 mg/day and increased to 20 mg/day at week 4) improved symptoms based on a variety of PTSD and depression rating scales, suggesting that it may be an effective treatment for PTSD.

Bipolar Disorder

Citalopram

One pilot study has addressed the effectiveness of citalopram as an adjunctive treatment in bipolar disorder (Schaffer et al. 2006). In this 12-week double-blind trial, 20 patients who were currently being treated with first-line mood stabilizers were randomly assigned to receive flexible dosing of either citalopram (10–50 mg/day) or an additional mood stabilizer, lamotrigine (12.5–200 mg/day). At the end of the study, treatment with either citalopram or lamotrigine produced a similar and statistically significant improvement in depression based on the magnitude of the mean decrease in total MADRS score. In this study, one patient in each of the two treatment groups switched to hypomania, which is consistent with the known risk of antidepressant-induced mood elevation in association with treatment of bipolar disorder (Henry et al. 2001). A large-scale placebo-controlled study is necessary to demonstrate the efficacy of using citalopram for acute treatment of depression in bipolar disorder.

S-Citalopram

To date, no published randomized, controlled trials have examined the effectiveness of S-citalopram as an adjuvant therapy for the treatment of bipolar depression. In the only published clinical trial, the effectiveness of S-citalopram was examined in a 12-week open-label study of 20 patients with type I or type II bipolar depression (Fonseca et al. 2006). In these patients, the addition of 20 mg/day S-citalopram to their mood stabilizer therapy significantly improved their depression as measured by a decrease in the Ham-D total score. It should be noted that 1 patient switched to mania and 2 patients displayed mild symptoms of hypomania. Additional large-scale placebo-controlled trials are necessary to fully evaluate the utility of S-citalopram in the treatment of bipolar depression.

Obsessive-Compulsive Disorder

Citalopram

To date, a limited number of clinical studies have evaluated the effectiveness of citalopram in the treatment of obsessive-compulsive disorder (OCD). In the only published large-scale double-blind, placebo-controlled study of citalopram in treatment of OCD (Montgomery et al. 2001a), 401 patients were randomly assigned to receive placebo or a fixed dose of citalopram at 20, 40, or 60 mg/day for 12 weeks. The study was conducted at 53 centers in 12 different countries. All three doses of citalopram were significantly more effective than placebo, as measured on the Yale-Brown Obsessive Compulsive Scale (Y-BOCS) change score. There was no significant difference between the individual doses of citalopram; however, the highest response rate, as determined by a 25% improvement in Y-BOCS score, was 65% for the 60 mg/day group, as compared with 52% and 57.4% for the 40 mg/day and 20 mg/day groups, respectively. The drug was well tolerated, with only 4–6 patients withdrawing from the study in each group due to adverse events. Citalopram appears to be effective in treating both obsessions and compulsions based on similar results from the Y-BOCS obsessional and compulsive subscores. For both of these subscores, there was a trend for a more rapid onset of effect with higher doses of citalopram. The authors of the study concluded that treatment with citalopram is an effective therapy for OCD and that the higher dose of 60 mg/day may possibly give a better therapeutic response with a more rapid onset. Further analysis of this study was done to identify factors that may predict response to citalopram therapy of OCD. The authors concluded that subjects with a longer history of OCD, more severe OCD symptoms, or previous exposure to SSRIs were less likely to be responders in the citalopram trial (D.J. Stein et al. 2001). This conclusion is similar to that reported for other drugs used in the treatment of OCD.

Three small clinical trials, all lacking placebo control groups, have been published. A 24-week open-label pilot study of 29 patients with OCD showed that 76% of patients receiving 40–60 mg/day of citalopram had decreased symptoms as evaluated by various self- and observer-rated scales such as the Y-BOCS (Koponen et al. 1997). A single blind study (raters were blind, but not patients) with 30 patients compared the efficacy of citalopram (20–60 mg/day; n=11) to fluvoxamine (150–300 mg/day; n=10) and paroxetine (20–60 mg/day; n=9) in a 10-week trial (Mundo et al. 1997). All three groups showed significant improvement, and there was no significant difference in the response for the three groups. The other published study examined the effects of citalopram in children. Twenty-three children (ages 9–18 years) were enrolled in a 10-week open-label design. Citalopram (10–40 mg/day) was beneficial, with 75% of participants showing at least moderate improvement with greater than 20% change in children's Y-BOCS. Only limited conclusions can be drawn from this study due to the possible presence of comorbid illness, the lack of a placebo control, and the fact that all participants received cognitive and behavioral treatment along with the medication (Thomsen 1997). A long-term follow-up to this study revealed that the clinical effectiveness of citalopram (20–70 mg/day) in the long-term therapy of OCD was comparable to that of other SSRIs in children and adolescents and that further improvement can be achieved by extending the treatment period up to 1 year (Thomsen et al. 2001).

S-Citalopram

The effectiveness of S-citalopram in the treatment of OCD has been demonstrated in a 24-week multicenter double-blind, placebo-controlled clinical trial (D.J. Stein et al. 2007). In this study patients were randomly assigned to receive placebo (n=115), S-citalopram at either 10 mg/day (n=116) or 20 mg/day (n=116), or paroxetine at 40 mg/day (n=119). Based on the primary efficacy measure of a change in Y-BOCS total score from baseline to week 12, S-citalopram at 20 mg/day and paroxetine at 40 mg/day produced a significant improvement compared with placebo, and by week 24 all treatments were superior to placebo. The effectiveness of both the 20 mg/day S-citalopram and the 40 mg/day paroxetine was evident by week 6. In some of the secondary measures, S-citalopram at 20 mg/day was superior to placebo at an earlier time point compared with the reference treatment of paroxetine at 40 mg/day, leading the authors to suggest that S-citalopram should be considered a treatment of choice for OCD.

One large-scale study has examined the ability of long-term treatment with S-citalopram to prevent relapse of OCD in patients who respond to initial treatment (Fineberg et al. 2007). In the first part of the study, 468 patients enrolled in a 16-week open-label treatment phase with either 10 or 20 mg/day S-citalopram. At the end of this phase, 320 patients were defined as responders (Y-BOCS total score decrease by ≥25%) and were entered into the 24-week double-blind relapse prevention phase. Patients were randomly assigned to receive either placebo (n=157) or S-citalopram (10 or 20 mg/day; n=163) at the dosage they received during the treatment phase. S-citalopram showed superiority over placebo in the primary analysis (time to relapse; P<0.001). A statistically significant greater percentage of patients relapsed in the placebo group (52%) compared with the S-citalopram group (23%), as defined by a Y-BOCS total score increase of ≥5 or a lack of efficacy as determined by the investigator.

Generalized Anxiety Disorder

Citalopram

There are no published large-scale randomized, double-blind clinical trials examining the effectiveness of citalopram in the treatment of GAD. As described in the next section, all large-scale trials have focused on the development of S-citalopram for the treatment of GAD. One pilot study examined open-label treatment with citalopram in 13 patients suffering from GAD. In this study citalopram treatment (10–60 mg/day) for 12 weeks produced a significant reduction in GAD symptoms and a marked improvement in social and occupational functioning (Varia and Rauscher 2002).

S-Citalopram

The efficacy of S-citalopram in the treatment of GAD has been established is several randomized, controlled clinical trials (Baldwin and Nair 2005). The effectiveness of acute treatment (up to 12 weeks) of GAD has been examined in four clinical trials. Three of these studies had a flexible-dosage, randomized, double-blind, placebo-controlled design and were subjected to pooled analysis (Davidson et al. 2004; Goodman et al. 2005; D.J. Stein et al. 2005). The intent-to-treat population of the pooled study consisted of 840, patients with 421 receiving S-citalopram (10–20 mg/day) and 419 receiving placebo. S-citalopram was superior to placebo in all three studies based on the change in Hamilton Anxiety Scale (Ham-A) total score from baseline to week 8. A significantly greater fraction of patients receiving S-citalopram were responders (47.5%) versus placebo (28.6%), with response defined as a reduction in total Ham-A score of 50% or more. By-visit analyses revealed a significantly greater response for S-citalopram compared with placebo by weeks 1 or 2 for all secondary efficacy measures (Goodman et al. 2005). Finally, S-citalopram was effective in patients with above-median severity of depressive symptoms at baseline (Ham-D$_{17}$>12) (D.J. Stein et al. 2005). The fourth study used a fixed-dosage, double-blind design and compared three doses of S-citalopram—5 mg/day (n=134), 10 mg/day (n=136), and 20 mg/day (n=133)—with paroxetine 20 mg/day (n=139) and with placebo (n=139) (Baldwin et al. 2006b). The primary outcome measure was the adjusted mean change in the Ham-A total score from baseline to week 12. By this measure, both 10 and 20 mg/day S-citalopram were superior to placebo, whereas 5 mg/day S-citalopram and 20 mg/day paroxetine were not. The last observation carried forward (LOCF) analysis revealed that S-citalopram at 10 mg/day was also superior to 20 mg/day paroxetine at week 12. In terms of the time course of the therapeutic response, the separation of active drug from placebo was evident by week 4 onward for 10 and 20 mg/day S-citalopram, whereas 20 mg/day paroxetine was superior to placebo only at week 10.

The efficacy of S-citalopram in the long-term treatment of GAD has been demonstrated in two controlled clinical trials. In one study, subjects who completed one of the three short-term (8-week) clinical trials described in the preceding paragraph were given the option of entering a 24-week flexible-dosage, open-label study (Davidson et al. 2005). The patients were placed on a dose of 10 mg/day S-citalopram, and those patients who had not responded by the end of 4 weeks were given the option of increasing the dosage to 20 mg/day. Of the 526 patients who entered the extension study, 299 (56.8%) completed the 24-week study. Of these, 92% were responders (CGI-I score ≤2) at the end of the study. The average Ham-A score decreased from 13.1 at baseline to 6.9 at the conclusion of the study. In a separate randomized, double-blind, flexible-dosage study, the long-term efficacy of S-citalopram (10–20 mg/day; n=61) was compared with paroxetine (20–50 mg/day; n=62) over 24 weeks (Bielski et al. 2005). The proportions of patients receiving S-citalopram and paroxetine that met the criteria for a satisfactory response (CGI-I≤2) were 65.0% and 55.7% at week 8 and 78.3% and 62.3% at week 24, respectively. Although a greater percentage of patients re-

sponded to S-citalopram, the difference was not statistically significant.

The efficacy of long-term therapy with S-citalopram in the prevention of relapse of GAD was evaluated in patients who had initially responded to acute treatment (Allgulander et al. 2006). The initial phase of the study was a 12-week open-label trial of patients with a primary diagnosis of GAD (Ham-A total score ≥20) and used a fixed dose of 20 mg/day S-citalopram. Of the 491 patients who participated in this phase, 375 had a satisfactory response (Ham-A total score ≤10) and were randomly assigned to the double-blind relapse prevention phase of the study, in which treatment was continued with either placebo (n=188) or S-citalopram (20 mg/day; n=187) for an additional 24–76 weeks. A statistically significant smaller proportion of patients relapsed (increase in Ham-A total score of ≥15 or a lack of efficacy as judged by the investigator) in the S-citalopram group (19%) compared with the placebo group (56%). S-citalopram was well tolerated, with 8% of patients withdrawing due to adverse events compared with 7% of placebo-treated patients.

Panic Disorder

Citalopram

Few well-controlled studies have evaluated the effectiveness of citalopram in the treatment of panic disorder. In a 1-year placebo-controlled, double-blind study, 475 patients were assigned to either placebo or one of three fixed dosage ranges of citalopram (10 or 15 mg/day, 20 or 30 mg/day, or 40 or 60 mg/day) or one dosage range of clomipramine (60 or 90 mg/day). After an 8-week acute treatment period, 279 patients agreed to continue their double-blind treatment at the assigned dose. Patients receiving clomipramine or the two highest dosage ranges of citalopram showed significant improvement compared with placebo in a variety of anxiety rating scales including the Clinical Anxiety Scale (CAS) panic attack item. The authors concluded that citalopram in the dosage range of 20–60 mg/day was an effective long-term therapy for the management of panic disorder (Lepola et al. 1998).

In a single-blind variable-dosage study (Perna et al. 2001), 58 patients were randomly assigned to groups for treatment with either citalopram or paroxetine (both at doses of 20–50 mg/day). By day 60, 86% of patients receiving citalopram and 84% of patients receiving paroxetine responded well to treatment as determined by a 50% reduction from baseline of both the Panic Associated Symptoms Scale (PASS) and the Sheehan Disability

Scale (SDS) global scores (Perna et al. 2001). There was no significant difference found between the two drugs. While both drugs were well tolerated, sexual side effects and weight gain were frequent. By day 60 of the study, 41% of patients on citalopram and 48% of patients on paroxetine reported sexual dysfunctions, and 37% of patients on citalopram and 40% of patients on paroxetine reported weight gain. An additional small-scale study (Rampello et al. 2006) demonstrated that citalopram and S-citalopram had similar effectiveness in the management of panic attacks, with a suggestion that S-citalopram had a faster onset of action. This study is described in more detail in the S-citalopram section below. While these studies have a limited number of subjects and lack a placebo control group, they do provide a preliminary indication that citalopram may be effective in the treatment of panic disorder. To conclusively demonstrate the effectiveness of citalopram, additional large placebo-controlled studies are necessary.

S-Citalopram

S-citalopram has been evaluated for effectiveness in the treatment of panic disorder in two clinical trials. In a 10-week randomized, double-blind, placebo-controlled, flexible-dosage study S-citalopram (5–10 mg/day) was compared with citalopram (10–20 mg/day) and placebo in patients with a diagnosis of panic disorder with or without agoraphobia (Stahl et al. 2003). The primary measure of efficacy was the number of panic attacks at week 10 relative to baseline as assessed by the Modified Sheehan Panic and Anticipatory Anxiety Scale (PAAS). The relative panic attack frequency was significantly lower in the S-citalopram group ($n=125$) compared with the placebo group ($n=114$; $P=0.04$), and at the end of the study there was a greater proportion of patients with zero panic attacks in the S-citalopram group (50%) compared with the placebo group (38%) that was marginally significant ($P=0.051$). There was no significant difference with the citalopram treatment group ($n=112$) in these two measures. Both S-citalopram and citalopram significantly improved panic disorder symptoms and severity relative to placebo at the end of the study, as measured by several different assessment scales.

The second clinical study was a smaller-scale 8-week open-label community-based comparison trial that examined the effectiveness of S-citalopram (10 mg/day; $n=20$) and citalopram (20 mg/day; $n=20$) in the treatment of panic attacks in the elderly (Rampello et al. 2006). Both drugs produced a similar decrease in the weekly rate of

panic attacks and decreases in both Ham-A and Cooper Disability Scores, with no significant difference between drugs at the end of the study. However, a significant improvement from baseline was evident for S-citalopram as early as 2 weeks ($P<0.001$), whereas the effectiveness of citalopram was not evident until 4 weeks ($P<0.01$), suggesting a faster onset of clinical effect with S-citalopram.

Social Anxiety Disorder

Citalopram

A large-scale double-blind, placebo-controlled study demonstrated that paroxetine is effective in the treatment of social anxiety disorder, suggesting that other SSRIs may be effective in the treatment of this disorder (M.B. Stein et al. 1998). While there are no such published large-scale, placebo-controlled studies with citalopram, case reports indicate that citalopram may have efficacy in the treatment of social anxiety disorder (Bouwer and Stein 1998; Lepola et al. 1994, 1996; Simon et al. 2001). In addition, one 12-week, small-scale ($N=21$) flexible-dose, open-label study demonstrated the effectiveness of citalopram (20–60 mg/day) in relieving the symptoms of social anxiety disorder in patients who suffered from comorbid depression (Schneier et al. 2003).

S-Citalopram

Two large-scale multinational, multicenter clinical trials have demonstrated the effectiveness of S-citalopram in the treatment of social anxiety disorder. In a 24-week fixed-dosage trial (Lader et al. 2004), patients with a diagnosis of social anxiety disorder were randomly assigned to double-blind treatment with placebo ($n=166$), 5 mg/day S-citalopram ($n=167$), 10 mg/day S-citalopram ($n=167$), 20 mg/day S-citalopram ($n=170$), or 20 mg/day paroxetine ($n=169$). Based on the mean change from baseline in the Liebowitz Social Anxiety Scale (LSAS) total score, there was a statistically superior therapeutic effect compared with placebo by week 12 using observed cases analysis for all doses of S-citalopram and the 20 mg/day paroxetine. Further improvement was seen by week 24 for all doses of S-citalopram and paroxetine, and the 20 mg/day S-citalopram was superior to the 20 mg/day paroxetine. The mean reduction in LSAS score from baseline was significant for 5 mg/day and 20 mg/day S-citalopram by week 2 and for 10 mg/day S-citalopram by week 4. Finally, treatment with 20mg/day S-citalopram showed superiority over 20 mg/day paroxetine by week 16. In a second study of 12 weeks (Kasper et al. 2005b), patients were randomly assigned to double-blind treatment with either placebo ($n = 177$) or 10–20 mg/day S-citalopram ($n = 181$). Based on the mean change from baseline in the LSAS score, S-citalopram produced a superior therapeutic response compared with placebo ($P = 0.005$). A greater percentage of patients responded to treatment (defined as a CGI-I score of 1 or 2) from the S-citalopram group (54%) compared with the placebo group (39%; $P < 0.001$). This improvement was associated with a lessening of symptoms as measured with work and social components of the SDS.

Because social anxiety disorder is a chronic illness, pharmacological treatment should be effective over extended periods of time to prevent illness relapse. One study has examined the ability of S-citalopram treatment for up to 24 weeks to prevent relapse of social anxiety disorder following successful short-term therapy (Montgomery et al. 2005). In the first phase of this trial, patients took part in a 12-week open-label, flexible-dosage (10–20 mg/day S-citalopram) study. Of the 517 patients who enrolled in the study, 371 responded to treatment. The responders were then entered into a 24-week double-blind trial, receiving either a fixed-dosage of S-citalopram (10 or 20 mg/day; $n = 190$) or placebo ($n = 181$). Significantly fewer patients relapsed at both doses of S-citalopram (22%) compared with placebo (50%), with relapse being 2.8 times more likely with placebo treatment than with S-citalopram treatment ($P < 0.001$).

Anxiety Associated With Major Depression

Citalopram

A retrospective study of 2,000 depressed patients enrolled in eight different double-blind, placebo-controlled clinical trials revealed that citalopram was effective in relieving the symptoms of anxiety in depressed patients based on a greater decrease from baseline in the anxiety factor of the Ham-D compared with placebo (Flicker and Hakkarainen 1998). The incidence of activating side effects (i.e., insomnia, nervousness, anxiety, agitation, and tremor) was similar to that for placebo. The authors concluded that citalopram was effective in the treatment of anxious depression, with a low potential for producing activating side effects. Another double-blind, placebo-controlled study involving 323 patients diagnosed with DSM-IV-defined major depression revealed a significant antianxiety effect of citalopram (20–60 mg/day) compared with placebo based on decreases in the Ham-A score (Stahl 2000). In the same study, sertraline (50–150 mg/day) did not show significant antianxiety activity.

S-Citalopram

The effectiveness of S-citalopram in the treatment of anxiety symptoms associated with major depressive disorder has been evaluated in a pooled analysis of five clinical trials (Bandelow et al. 2007). These placebo-controlled trials were originally designed to examine the effectiveness of S-citalopram in treating major depression, and three of them included a comparison to citalopram. In the pooled analysis, S-citalopram (10–20 mg/day) was consistently superior to placebo in relieving the anxious symptoms associated with the depression as revealed in several different assessments of anxiousness. For example, when pooling data from all five trials and using the change from baseline in inner tension score (item 3 from MADRS), S-citalopram ($n = 850$) was superior to placebo ($n = 737$) from week 1 through week 8. Citalopram also showed superiority to placebo in the majority of the anxiety measures in the three clinical trials in which it was included. The analyses presented in this pooled study indicate that S-citalopram is effective in relieving anxiety symptoms in depressed patients.

Eating Disorders

Citalopram

SSRIs are often used in the treatment of eating disorders such as bulimia, anorexia, and binge-eating disorder (Carter et al. 2003). However, the effectiveness of citalopram in the treatment of eating disorders has not been tested in any published large-scale trials. A small-scale ($n = 18$) open-label trial indicated that citalopram (20 mg/day) may be effective in the treatment of bulimia and anorexia (Calandra et al. 1999), although another report questioned the effectiveness of citalopram in the treatment of anorexia (Bergh et al. 1996). More recently, a small-scale, double-blind clinical trial was performed in which patients diagnosed with binge-eating disorder were randomly assigned to receive citalopram (20–60 mg/day; $n = 19$) or placebo ($n = 19$) (McElroy et al. 2003). Compared with patients on placebo, patients receiving citalopram for 6 weeks significantly improved based on a variety of measures including frequency of binge eating ($P = 0.003$), frequency of binge days ($P < 0.001$), body mass index ($P < 0.001$), and weight ($P < 0.001$). In the treatment of bulimia nervosa there is one published single-blind trial that compared citalopram (20–40 mg/day; $n = 19$) with fluoxetine (20–60 mg/day; $n = 18$) and demonstrated a similar efficacy between these two drugs in the relief of eating psychopathology (Leombruni et al. 2006). These studies are preliminary, and a clear demonstration of the effectiveness of citalopram in the treatment of eating disorders requires further study.

S-Citalopram

One small-scale study has examined the effectiveness of high-dose S-citalopram therapy in the treatment of binge-eating disorder associated with obesity (Guerdjikova et al. 2008). In this 12-week double-blind study treatment with a flexible dosage of S-citalopram (10–30 mg/day; $n=21$) was compared with placebo ($n=23$). S-citalopram treatment was associated with significant reductions in weight, body mass index, and global severity of illness scores; however, due to limitations in statistical power, the authors could not make conclusions about the ability of S-citalopram to reduce the frequency of binge eating. Clearly, additional larger clinical trials are necessary to assess the effectiveness of S-citalopram in the treatment of eating disorders.

Poststroke Depression

Citalopram

Depression is a common complication that occurs in approximately 20% of stroke victims (Robinson 2003). Citalopram has demonstrated efficacy in the treatment of poststroke depression in a controlled clinical trial. A 6-week double-blind, placebo-controlled study demonstrated that citalopram (10–40 mg/day) was significantly better than placebo in treating poststroke depression (Andersen et al. 1994). Significant improvement was seen with the Ham-D and MADRS scores compared with placebo. This significant effect was seen only in patients who became depressed 7 weeks or more after the stroke. For patients who became depressed 2–6 weeks after the stroke, recovery from depression occurred within 1 month, independent of the treatment, indicating a high level of spontaneous recovery. Additionally, in a randomized, double-blind study in which citalopram (20 mg/day) was compared only with reboxetine (4 mg/day), 16 weeks of citalopram treatment was particularly effective in poststroke patients suffering from anxious depression (Rampello et al. 2004). In the treatment of poststroke crying, a small ($n=16$) double-blind, placebo-controlled study demonstrated that citalopram (10–20 mg/day) was effective in relieving poststroke pathological crying compared with placebo (Andersen et al. 1993). In a variable-dose study involving 32 patients receiving either citalopram or paroxetine, citalopram (10–40 mg/day) was comparable to paroxetine (10–40 mg/day) in relieving the symptoms of pathological crying or laughing following brain injury (Muller et al. 1999).

S-Citalopram

The effectiveness of S-citalopram in the treatment of poststroke depression has been tested in one double-blind, placebo-controlled clinical trial (Robinson et al. 2008). This 12-month trial, conducted with nondepressed patients within 3 months of an acute stroke, contained a double-blinded comparison between a placebo treatment group ($n=58$) and an S-citalopram treatment group (5–10 mg/day; $n=59$) and a nonblinded comparison with a problem-solving therapy group ($n=59$). Using a conservative intention-to-treat method of analyzing the data, the study showed that the likelihood of developing depression was greater in the placebo group (34.5%) compared with the S-citalopram group (23.1%; $P<0.01$). While the problem-solving therapy group had a lower incidence of depression (30.5%) compared with the placebo group, the difference did not reach statistical significance. This study provides a preliminary indication that S-citalopram therapy may afford some protection against the development of poststroke depression, but additional studies are necessary to conclusively demonstrate this.

Dementia

Citalopram

The effectiveness of citalopram in relieving various emotional disturbances associated with dementia was compared with placebo in a double-blind multicenter clinical trial. Of the 89 patients included in the efficacy analyses, 65 had senile dementia of the Alzheimer type (SDAT)/Alzheimer's disease (AD) and 24 had vascular dementia; the average age of the patients was 77.6 years. In the patients with SDAT/AD, treatment with citalopram (10–30 mg/day) significantly improved emotional bluntness, confusion, irritability, anxiety, fear/panic, depressed mood, and restlessness compared with placebo (Nyth and Gottfries 1990). This improvement was not seen in patients suffering from vascular dementia. A separate 6-week placebo-controlled study examined the effects of citalopram in elderly depressed patients ($n=149$) with and without dementia. In this study, depressed patients with and without dementia receiving either 20 mg/day or 30 mg/day of citalopram showed significantly greater improvement in depressive symptoms compared with those receiving placebo. It is noteworthy that there was also improvement on several measures on the Gottfries-Brane-Steen scale of cognitive function in the subgroup of depressed patients with dementia (Nyth et al. 1992). In another randomized, double-blind trial involving 336 elderly depressed patients with and without dementia, 12 weeks of treatment with either citalopram (20–40 mg/day) or mianserin (30–60 mg/day) was effective in relieving the symptoms of depression, although it should be noted that the magnitude of response was lower in the patients with dementia (Karlsson et al. 2000). Finally, a randomized, double-blind, placebo-controlled trial involving 85 nondepressed elderly inpatients with dementia compared the effectiveness of citalopram and perphenazine in the treatment of behavioral disturbances. In this study, citalopram (20 mg/day) was more effective than perphenazine (0.1 mg/kg/day) in the acute relief of both psychotic symptoms and emotional disturbances associated with dementia (Pollock et al. 2002). Taken together, these studies provide a preliminary indication that citalopram may be effective in the management of the emotional disturbances, including depression, associated with dementia in the elderly.

S-Citalopram

There are no published large-scale clinical trials evaluating the effectiveness of S-citalopram in treating mood disturbances associated with dementia in elderly patients. In an 8-week open-label treatment study involving 12 patients diagnosed with depression of AD (for definition, see Olin et al. 2002), S-citalopram (10–20 mg/day) was effective in relieving the symptoms of depression but showed no improvement in cognition (V. Rao et al. 2006).

Side Effects and Toxicology

Citalopram

In a meta-analysis of 746 depressed patients who participated in several short-term clinical trials, the most common adverse events associated with citalopram were nausea and vomiting (20%), increased sweating (18%), and dry mouth and headache (17%) (Baldwin and Johnson 1995). Analysis of an integrated safety database, which includes data from 3,107 patients enrolled in 24 clinical trials, indicated that in placebo-controlled trials, nausea, dry mouth, somnolence, increased sweating, tremor, diarrhea, and ejaculatory failure of mild to moderate severity occurred with significantly greater frequency with citalopram compared with placebo (Muldoon 1996). The inci-

dences of these adverse events were less than 10% above those seen with placebo and were comparable to those seen with other SSRIs. Citalopram had a tolerability that was superior to that of the TCAs, with the exception that nausea and ejaculatory failure occurred with a 5% greater frequency with citalopram (Keller 2000).

It is well known that administration of SSRIs can produce sexual side effects such as anorgasmia and ejaculatory failure. Some reports have suggested that citalopram may be associated with a lower incidence of sexual side effects (Waldinger et al. 2001). However, other reports indicate that the rate of sexual side effects seen with citalopram is similar to that seen with other SSRIs (Ekselius and von Knorring 2001). For example, using the Changes in Sexual Functioning Questionnaire (CSFQ), the percentage of patients receiving citalopram that rated as experiencing sexual dysfunction was approximately 40% in the overall patient group and approximately 30% in the subpopulation of patients free of other probable causes of sexual dysfunction. These two rates were similar to those reported for all other SSRIs used in the study (Clayton et al. 2002).

At therapeutic doses, citalopram does not have significant cardiovascular effects. Analysis of ECG data from prospective studies in healthy volunteers and patients as well as retrospective ECG data from all clinical trials conducted from 1978 to 1996 (a total of 40 trials) concluded that citalopram was without significant effect on cardiac conduction and repolarization (Rasmussen et al. 1999). The only significant cardiovascular effect was a small reduction in heart rate (≤8 beats/minute). There are some reports of citalopram producing cardiovascular abnormalities in association with overdose (Catalano et al. 2001). Citalopram has been associated with ECG abnormalities and seizure at doses over 600 mg/day.

S-Citalopram

In general, the side effects associated with S-citalopram are similar to those observed with citalopram. In the three placebo-controlled clinical trials that have been performed with S-citalopram, a dosage of 10 mg/day produced rates of discontinuation due to adverse events that did not differ from those in the placebo group (Burke et al. 2002; Montgomery et al. 2001b; Wade et al. 2002). In the one trial that included an S-citalopram dosage of 20 mg/day, the rate of discontinuation was 10.4%, which was greater than the placebo rate of 2.5% (Burke et al. 2002). In addition, the rate of adverse events overall in the 20 mg/day S-citalopram group (85.6%) was significantly greater than that in the placebo group (70.5%). Regardless of dose, the adverse events that have been reported to occur more frequently with S-citalopram compared with placebo are nausea, diarrhea, insomnia, dry mouth, and ejaculatory disorder, with nausea being reported most frequently, at a rate of 15% (McRae 2002). No published studies have reported clinically significant findings in laboratory test values, vital signs, weight gain or loss, or electrocardiogram values.

Specific Effects and Syndromes

Hyponatremia

The use of SSRIs as a class has been associated with hyponatremia (Guay 2000) that is defined as a serum sodium concentration below 130 mEq/L and is characterized initially by nausea and malaise and subsequently by headache, lethargy, muscle cramps, disorientation, and restlessness. If serum sodium concentrations fall below 120 mEq/L, this can lead to seizures, coma, and respiratory arrest. The reported frequency of hyponatremia associated with SSRI use varies considerably, from 0.5% to 32%, with a greater incidence associated with older patients. The mechanism for SSRI-induced hyponatremia is unclear but may result from the syndrome of inappropriate secretion of antidiuretic hormone (SIADH). Citalopram and S-citalopram have been shown to produce hyponatremia in case reports involving the elderly (Covyeou and Jackson 2007; Fisher et al. 2002), and this information was recently reviewed (Jacob and Spinler 2006). In addition to advanced age, other factors that may increase the likelihood of hyponatremia include female gender, concurrent diuretic use, low body weight, and recent pneumonia. Treatment of SSRI-induced hyponatremia usually involves fluid restriction and/or administration of a loop diuretic such as furosemide and may include discontinuation of the SSRI.

Discontinuation Syndrome

The abrupt cessation of antidepressant therapy can result in a "discontinuation syndrome" characterized by dizziness, nausea and vomiting, lethargy, and flu-like symptoms. Other effects include dysphoric mood, irritability, agitation, paresthesias (such as electric shock sensations), anxiety, confusion, headache, emotional lability, insomnia, and hypomania. This syndrome is more common with short-half-life SSRIs such as paroxetine and less common with long-half-life SSRIs such as fluoxetine. The data obtained from clinical trials suggest that the ad-

verse events associated with discontinuation of citalopram tend to be mild and transient (Markowitz et al. 2000; Montgomery et al. 1993). In terms of S-citalopram, a meta-analysis of five clinical studies on treatment of major depressive disorder, GAD, and social anxiety disorder that ranged in duration from 8 weeks to 27 weeks showed that S-citalopram (5–20 mg/day; n = 1,051) had significantly fewer discontinuation symptoms compared with paroxetine (20–40 mg/day; n = 336) and venlafaxine (75–150 mg/day; n = 124), two short-half-life antidepressants commonly associated with treatment discontinuation syndrome (Baldwin et al. 2007). However, S-citalopram did show significantly more discontinuation symptoms compared with placebo (n = 239), with some of the more common symptoms being dizziness, irritability, nervousness, and sweating. The incidence of these symptoms tended to increase with the dose of S-citalopram that was being administered prior to discontinuation. Dose tapering is recommended for patients discontinuing treatment with citalopram or S-citalopram.

Treatment-Emergent Suicidal Ideation and Suicide

Considerable attention has been focused in recent years on the possibility that antidepressant drugs, especially SSRIs, may lead to an increase in suicidal ideation in some patients, particularly at the onset of therapy (Jick et al. 2004). This issue is of great concern in young patients and was described earlier in the chapter (see section "Depression in Children and Adolescents"). In studies involving adults, several meta-analyses of large-scale clinical trial data obtained with a variety of antidepressants have demonstrated no increase in the relative risk of suicide compared with placebo (Beasley et al. 1991; Khan et al. 2003; Storosum et al. 2001). In the case of citalopram, analyses of data obtained from 17 controlled clinical trials involving 5,000 patients indicate that the group of patients receiving citalopram had the lowest rate of suicide compared with the groups receiving placebo, tricyclic antidepressants, or other SSRIs (Nemeroff 2003). The risk of suicide associated with S-citalopram was evaluated based on data contained in the Summary Basis of Approval reports obtained from the FDA (Khan and Schwartz 2007). This study did not detect a significantly greater rate of suicide in the S-citalopram group compared with either the citalopram or the placebo group. There was also no indication that S-citalopram increased suicidal behavior in major depressive disorder and anxiety disorders in a meta-analysis of the S-citalopram clinical trials database consisting of

2,277 S-citalopram-treated patients and 1,814 placebo-treated patients (Pedersen 2005).

While the data do not indicate a significantly greater risk of suicide in patients receiving either citalopram or S-citalopram compared with placebo, most antidepressant studies do show that a limited number of patients will exhibit increased suicidal ideation upon initiation of therapy. Family and twin studies provide some evidence of a genetic influence on suicidal behavior, and it has been postulated that treatment-emergent suicidal ideation may also be genetically linked. Interestingly, a recent study involving patients participating in the STAR*D trial demonstrated a significant association between citalopram treatment-emergent suicidal ideation in men and polymorphisms near the gene for the transcription factor CREB (Perlis et al. 2007). This protein is of great interest because it mediates the effects of second messengers on new gene transcription and has been implicated in antidepressant action and suicide (Dowlatshahi et al. 1998; Dwivedi et al. 2003).

Drug–Drug Interactions

Because multiple P450 enzymes (CYP2C19, CYP3A4, and CYP2D6) contribute equally to the metabolism of citalopram and S-citalopram, inhibition of any one of these enzymes by another drug is unlikely to significantly impact the overall metabolism of citalopram or S-citalopram. Consistent with this, there are relatively few reports in the literature of drug–drug interactions involving citalopram or S-citalopram.

Antipsychotics

While citalopram has not been shown to increase the levels of concomitantly administered antipsychotics (Syvalahti et al. 1997), there are studies showing that the administration of antipsychotics, including levomepromazine and alimemazine, increases the levels of citalopram and its major metabolite DCT (Gram et al. 1993; Oyehaug et al. 1984). Additionally, a study involving 169 psychiatric patients demonstrated that concomitant administration of a neuroleptic, a benzodiazepine, or a TCA resulted in small but significant elevations of citalopram concentrations (Leinonen et al. 1996).

Antidepressants

The administration of relatively high doses of citalopram (40–60 mg/day) did not affect the plasma concentrations of amitriptyline, clomipramine, or maprotiline in five case studies (Baettig et al. 1993). In contrast, citalopram was shown to increase the level of the metabolite of imipramine, desipramine, by 50% without changing the concentration of the parent compound (Gram et al. 1993). This latter finding may result from competition between DCT, the major metabolite of citalopram, and desipramine for metabolism by CYP2D6. In terms of SSRIs, coadministration of citalopram with fluoxetine or fluvoxamine significantly increased the plasma concentration of the S-citalopram enantiomer. The elevated S-citalopram levels most likely result from the known inhibitory activity of fluvoxamine and fluoxetine on the activity of CYP2C19 and CYP2D6 (Bondolfi et al. 1996, 2000).

Benzodiazepines and Mood Stabilizers

There is little evidence of clinically significant pharmacokinetic interactions between citalopram and either benzodiazepines or mood stabilizers, including lithium (Baumann et al. 1996; Gram et al. 1993; Sproule et al. 1997).

Monoamine Oxidase Inhibitors

Because of the possibility of a potentially fatal phamacodynamic interaction resulting in the serotonin syndrome, neither citalopram nor S-citalopram should be administered with an MAO inhibitor or within 14 days of discontinuing an MAO inhibitor.

Conclusion

Citalopram and S-citalopram are highly selective 5-HT reuptake inhibitors that are well tolerated and effective in the treatment of depression, with S-citalopram also having proven efficacy in large-scale clinical trials in the treatment of GAD. While the use of citalopram and S-citalopram in the treatment of other psychiatric conditions has not been as thoroughly studied, the few well-controlled trials that have been completed suggest that both drugs may have a significant role in treating a wide range of psychiatric illnesses, including panic disorder, social anxiety disorder, anxiety associated with depression, and OCD. An advantage of citalopram and S-citalopram compared with some other common SSRIs is a relatively weak inhibition of liver cytochrome P450 enzymes, which reduces the potential for adverse pharmacokinetic drug–drug interactions. In addition, because S-citalopram does not share with citalopram a modest affinity for the histamine H_1 receptor, it may have a lower potential for anti-histaminergic side effects compared with citalopram, a difference that has yet to be demonstrated in a clinical trial. There are a number of clinical trials comparing S-citalopram with a variety of other antidepressants, including citalopram and venlafaxine, that suggest that S-citalopram may have a faster onset of antidepressant efficacy and modest superiority in the treatment of the severely depressed. More extensive experience with S-citalopram is necessary to conclusively determine whether its statistically significant superiority to citalopram and other SSRIs in clinical studies translates into the "real world" of psychiatric practice.

References

Agranat I, Caner H, Caldwell J: Putting chirality to work: the strategy of chiral switches. Nat Rev Drug Discov 1:753–768, 2002

Allgulander C, Florea I, Huusom AK: Prevention of relapse in generalized anxiety disorder by escitalopram treatment. Int J Neuropsychopharmacol 9:495–505, 2006

American Psychiatric Association: Diagnostic and Statistical Manual of Mental Disorders, 4th Edition. Washington, DC, American Psychiatric Association, 1994

Andersen G, Vestergaard K, Riis JO: Citalopram for post-stroke pathological crying. Lancet 342:837–839, 1993

Andersen G, Vestergaard K, Lauritzen L: Effective treatment of poststroke depression with the selective serotonin reuptake inhibitor citalopram. Stroke 25:1099–1104, 1994

Arborelius L, Nomikos GG, Grillner P, et al: 5-HT1A receptor antagonists increase the activity of serotonergic cells in the dorsal raphe nucleus in rats treated acutely or chronically with citalopram. Naunyn Schmiedebergs Arch Pharmacol 352:157–165, 1995

Baettig D, Bondolfi G, Montaldi S, et al: Tricyclic antidepressant plasma levels after augmentation with citalopram: a case study. Eur J Clin Pharmacol 44:403–405, 1993

Baldwin D, Johnson FN: Tolerability and safety of citalopram. Rev Contemp Pharmacother 6:315–325, 1995

Baldwin DS, Nair RV: Escitalopram in the treatment of generalized anxiety disorder. Expert Rev Neurother 5:443–449, 2005

Baldwin DS, Cooper JA, Huusom AK, et al: A double-blind, randomized, parallel-group, flexible-dose study to evaluate the tolerability, efficacy and effects of treatment discontinuation with escitalopram and paroxetine in patients with major depressive disorder. Int Clin Psychopharmacol 21:159–169, 2006a

Baldwin DS, Huusom AK, Maehlum E: Escitalopram and paroxetine in the treatment of generalised anxiety disorder: randomised, placebo-controlled, double-blind study. Br J Psychiatry 189:264–272, 2006b

Baldwin DS, Montgomery SA, Nil R, et al: Discontinuation symptoms in depression and anxiety disorders. Int J Neuropsychopharmacol 10:73–84, 2007

Bandelow B, Andersen HF, Dolberg OT: Escitalopram in the treatment of anxiety symptoms associated with depression. Depress Anxiety 24:53–61, 2007

Barker EL, Perlman MA, Adkins EM, et al: High affinity recognition of serotonin transporter antagonists defined by species-scanning mutagenesis. An aromatic residue in transmembrane domain I dictates species-selective recognition of citalopram and mazindol. J Biol Chem 273:19459–19468, 1998

Baumann P, Larsen F: The pharmacokinetics of citalopram. Rev Contemp Pharmacother 6:287–295, 1995

Baumann PA, Waldmeier PC: Further evidence for negative feedback control of serotonin release in the central nervous system. Naunyn Schmiedebergs Arch Pharmacol 317:36–43, 1981

Baumann P, Nil R, Souche A, et al: A double-blind, placebo-controlled study of citalopram with and without lithium in the treatment of therapy-resistant depressive patients: a clinical, pharmacokinetic, and pharmacogenetic investigation. J Clin Psychopharmacol 16:307–314, 1996

Beasley CM Jr, Dornseif BE, Bosomworth JC, et al: Fluoxetine and suicide: a meta-analysis of controlled trials of treatment for depression. BMJ 303:685–692, 1991

Bech P, Cialdella P: Citalopram in depression—meta-analysis of intended and unintended effects. Int Clin Psychopharmacol 6 (suppl 5):45–54, 1992

Bergh C, Eriksson M, Lindberg G, et al: Selective serotonin reuptake inhibitors in anorexia. Lancet 348:1459–1460, 1996

Bielski RJ, Ventura D, Chang CC: A double-blind comparison of escitalopram and venlafaxine extended release in the treatment of major depressive disorder. J Clin Psychiatry 65:1190–1196, 2004

Bielski RJ, Bose A, Chang CC: A double-blind comparison of escitalopram and paroxetine in the long-term treatment of generalized anxiety disorder. Ann Clin Psychiatry 17:65–69, 2005

Bjerkenstedt L, Flyckt L, Overo KF, et al: Relationship between clinical effects, serum drug concentration and serotonin uptake inhibition in depressed patients treated with citalopram. A double-blind comparison of three dose levels. Eur J Clin Pharmacol 28:553–557, 1985

Blier P, de Montigny C: Current advances and trends in the treatment of depression. Trends Pharmacol Sci 15:220–226, 1994

Bondolfi G, Chautems C, Rochat B, et al: Nonresponse to citalopram in depressive patients: pharmacokinetic and clinical consequences of a fluvoxamine augmentation. Psychopharmacology (Berl) 128:421–425, 1996

Bondolfi G, Lissner C, Kosel M, et al: Fluoxetine augmentation in citalopram nonresponders: pharmacokinetic and clinical consequences. Int J Neuropsychopharmacol 3:55–60, 2000

Boulenger JP, Huusom AK, Florea I, et al: A comparative study of the efficacy of long-term treatment with escitalopram and paroxetine in severely depressed patients. Curr Med Res Opin 22:1331–1341, 2006

Bouwer C, Stein DJ: Use of the selective serotonin reuptake inhibitor citalopram in the treatment of generalized social phobia. J Affect Disord 49:79–82, 1998

Bridge JA, Iyengar S, Salary CB, et al: Clinical response and risk for reported suicidal ideation and suicide attempts in pediatric antidepressant treatment: a meta-analysis of randomized controlled trials. JAMA 297:1683–1696, 2007

Burke WJ, Gergel I, Bose A: Fixed-dose trial of the single isomer SSRI escitalopram in depressed outpatients. J Clin Psychiatry 63:331–336, 2002

Calandra C, Gulino V, Inserra L, et al: The use of citalopram in an integrated approach to the treatment of eating disorders: an open study. Eat Weight Disord 4:207–210, 1999

Carter WP, Hudson JI, Lalonde JK, et al: Pharmacologic treatment of binge eating disorder. Int J Eat Disord 34 Suppl:S74–S88, 2003

Catalano G, Catalano MC, Epstein MA, et al: QTc interval prolongation associated with citalopram overdose: a case report and literature review. Clin Neuropharmacol 24:158–162, 2001

Ceglia I, Acconcia S, Fracasso C, et al: Effects of chronic treatment with escitalopram or citalopram on extracellular 5-HT in the prefrontal cortex of rats: role of 5-HT1A receptors. Br J Pharmacol 142:469–478, 2004

Chaput Y, de Montigny C, Blier P: Effects of a selective 5-HT reuptake blocker, citalopram, on the sensitivity of 5-HT autoreceptors: electrophysiological studies in the rat brain. Naunyn Schmiedebergs Arch Pharmacol 333:342–348, 1986

Chen F, Lawrence AJ: The effects of antidepressant treatment on serotonergic and dopaminergic systems in Fawn-Hooded rats: a quantitative autoradiography study. Brain Res 976:22–29, 2003

Chen F, Larsen MB, Neubauer HA, et al: Characterization of an allosteric citalopram-binding site at the serotonin transporter. J Neurochem 92:21–28, 2005

Choi MJ, Kang RH, Lim SW, et al: Brain-derived neurotrophic factor gene polymorphism (Val66Met) and citalopram response in major depressive disorder. Brain Res 1118:176–182, 2006

Christensen AV, Fjalland B, Pedersen V, et al: Pharmacology of a new phthalane (Lu 10-171), with specific 5-HT uptake inhibiting properties. Eur J Pharmacol 41:153–162, 1977

Classen K, Gothert M, Schlicker E: Effects of DU 24565 (6-nitroquipazine) on serotonergic and noradrenergic neurones of the rat brain and comparison with the effects of quipazine. Naunyn Schmiedebergs Arch Pharmacol 326:198–202, 1984

Clayton AH, Pradko JF, Croft HA, et al: Prevalence of sexual dysfunction among newer antidepressants. J Clin Psychiatry 63:357–366, 2002

Clayton AH, Croft HA, Horrigan JP, et al: Bupropion extended release compared with escitalopram: effects on sexual functioning and antidepressant efficacy in 2 randomized, double-blind, placebo-controlled studies. J Clin Psychiatry 67:736–746, 2006

Colonna L, Andersen HF, Reines EH: A randomized, double-blind, 24-week study of escitalopram (10 mg/day) versus citalopram (20 mg/day) in primary care patients with major depressive disorder. Curr Med Res Opin 21:1659–1668, 2005

Covyeou JA, Jackson CW: Hyponatremia associated with escitalopram. N Engl J Med 356:94–95, 2007

Cremers TI, Spoelstra EN, de Boer P, et al: Desensitisation of 5-HT autoreceptors upon pharmacokinetically monitored chronic treatment with citalopram. Eur J Pharmacol 397:351–357, 2000

Dalgaard L, Larsen C: Metabolism and excretion of citalopram in man: identification of O-acyl- and N-glucronides. Xenobiotica 29:1033–1041, 1999

Davidson JR, Bose A, Korotzer A, et al: Escitalopram in the treatment of generalized anxiety disorder: double-blind, placebo controlled, flexible-dose study. Depress Anxiety 19:234–240, 2004

Davidson JR, Bose A, Wang Q: Safety and efficacy of escitalopram in the long-term treatment of generalized anxiety disorder. J Clin Psychiatry 66:1441–1446, 2005

Dowlatshahi D, MacQueen GM, Wang JF, et al: Increased temporal cortex CREB concentrations and antidepressant treatment in major depression. Lancet 352:1754–1755, 1998

Drew R, Siddik ZH: Effect of a specific 5-HT uptake inhibitor (citalopram) on drug accumulation by rat lung slices. Pharmacology 20:27–31, 1980

Dwivedi Y, Rao JS, Rizavi HS, et al: Abnormal expression and functional characteristics of cyclic adenosine monophosphate response element binding protein in postmortem brain of suicide subjects. Arch Gen Psychiatry 60:273–282, 2003

Dyck LE: Tryptamine transport in rat brain slices: a comparison with 5- hydroxytryptamine. Neurochem Res 9:617–628, 1984

Einarson TR: Evidence based review of escitalopram in treating major depressive disorder in primary care. Int Clin Psychopharmacol 19:305–310, 2004

Ekselius L, von Knorring L: Effect on sexual function of long-term treatment with selective serotonin reuptake inhibitors in depressed patients treated in primary care. J Clin Psychopharmacol 21:154–160, 2001

El Mansari M, Sanchez C, Chouvet G, et al: Effects of acute and long-term administration of escitalopram and citalopram on serotonin neurotransmission: an in vivo electrophysiological study in rat brain. Neuropsychopharmacology 30:1269–1277, 2005

El Mansari ME, Wiborg O, Mnie-Filali O, et al: Allosteric modulation of the effect of escitalopram, paroxetine and fluoxetine: in-vitro and in-vivo studies. Int J Neuropsychopharmacol 10:31–40, 2007

English BA, Jewell M, Jewell G, et al: Treatment of chronic posttraumatic stress disorder in combat veterans with citalopram: an open trial. J Clin Psychopharmacol 26:84–88, 2006

Feighner JP, Overo K: Multicenter, placebo-controlled, fixed-dose study of citalopram in moderate-to-severe depression. J Clin Psychiatry 60:824–830, 1999

Fineberg NA, Tonnoir B, Lemming O, et al: Escitalopram prevents relapse of obsessive-compulsive disorder. Eur Neuropsychopharmacol 17:430–439, 2007

Fish EW, Faccidomo S, Gupta S, et al: Anxiolytic-like effects of escitalopram, citalopram, and R-citalopram in maternally separated mouse pups. J Pharmacol Exp Ther 308:474–480, 2004

Fisher A, Davis M, Croft-Baker J, et al: Citalopram-induced severe hyponatraemia with coma and seizure. Case report with literature and spontaneous reports review. Adverse Drug React Toxicol Rev 21:179–187, 2002

Flicker C, Hakkarainen H: Citalopram in anxious depression: anxiolytic effects and lack of activation. Biol Psychiatry 43:1S–133S, 1998

Foglia JP, Pollock BG, Kirshner MA, et al: Plasma levels of citalopram enantiomers and metabolites in elderly patients. Psychopharmacol Bull 33:109–112, 1997

Fonseca M, Soares JC, Hatch JP, et al: An open trial of adjunctive escitalopram in bipolar depression. J Clin Psychiatry 67:81–86, 2006

Galzin AM, Moret C, Verzier B, et al: Interaction between tricyclic and nontricyclic 5-hydroxytryptamine uptake inhibitors and the presynaptic 5-hydroxytryptamine inhibitory autoreceptors in the rat hypothalamus. J Pharmacol Exp Ther 235:200–211, 1985

Goodman WK, Bose A, Wang Q: Treatment of generalized anxiety disorder with escitalopram: pooled results from double-blind, placebo-controlled trials. J Affect Disord 87:161–167, 2005

Gorman JM, Korotzer A, Su G: Efficacy comparison of escitalopram and citalopram in the treatment of major depressive disorder: pooled analysis of placebo-controlled trials. CNS Spectr 7:40–44, 2002

Gram LF, Hansen MG, Sindrup SH, et al: Citalopram: interaction studies with levomepromazine, imipramine, and lithium. Ther Drug Monit 15:18–24, 1993

Guay DR: Hyponatremia associated with selective serotonin reuptake inhibitors: clinical review. Consult Pharm 15:160–177, 2000

Guerdjikova AI, McElroy SL, Kotwal R, et al: High-dose escitalopram in the treatment of binge-eating disorder with obesity: a placebo-controlled monotherapy trial. Hum Psychopharmacol 23:1–11, 2008

Hall H, Sallemark M, Wedel I: Acute effects of atypical antidepressants on various receptors in the rat brain. Acta Pharmacol Toxicol (Copenh) 54:379–384, 1984

Henry C, Sorbara F, Lacoste J, et al: Antidepressant-induced mania in bipolar patients: identification of risk factors. J Clin Psychiatry 62:249–255, 2001

Hjorth S: Serotonin 5-HT1A autoreceptor blockade potentiates the ability of the 5-HT reuptake inhibitor citalopram to increase nerve terminal output of 5-HT in vivo: a microdialysis study. J Neurochem 60:776–779, 1993

Hjorth S, Auerbach SB: Lack of 5-HT1A autoreceptor desensitization following chronic citalopram treatment, as determined by in vivo microdialysis. Neuropharmacology 33:331–334, 1994

Hjorth S, Bengtsson HJ, Milano S: Raphe 5-HT1A autoreceptors, but not postsynaptic 5-HT1A receptors or beta-adrenoceptors, restrain the citalopram-induced increase in extracellular 5-hydroxytryptamine in vivo. Eur J Pharmacol 316:43–47, 1996

Hochstrasser B, Isaksen PM, Koponen H, et al: Prophylactic effect of citalopram in unipolar, recurrent depression: placebo-controlled study of maintenance therapy. Br J Psychiatry 178:304–310, 2001

Hyttel J: Effect of a selective 5-HT uptake inhibitor—Lu 10-171—on rat brain 5-HT turnover. Acta Pharmacol Toxicol (Copenh) 40:439–446, 1977a

Hyttel J: Neurochemical characterization of a new potent and selective serotonin uptake inhibitor: Lu 10-171. Psychopharmacology (Berl) 51:225–233, 1977b

Hyttel J: Effect of a specific 5-HT uptake inhibitor, citalopram (Lu 10-171), on 3H-5-HT uptake in rat brain synaptosomes in vitro. Psychopharmacology (Berl) 60:13–18, 1978

Hyttel J: Citalopram—pharmacological profile of a specific serotonin uptake inhibitor with antidepressant activity. Prog Neuropsychopharmacol Biol Psychiatry 6:277–295, 1982

Hyttel J: Pharmacological characterization of selective serotonin reuptake inhibitors (SSRIs). Int Clin Psychopharmacol 9 (suppl 1):19–26, 1994

Hyttel J, Larsen JJ: Serotonin-selective antidepressants. Acta Pharmacol Toxicol (Copenh) 56:146–153, 1985

Hyttel J, Bogeso KP, Perregaard J, et al: The pharmacological effect of citalopram resides in the (S)-(+)-enantiomer. J Neural Transm Gen Sect 88:157–160, 1992

Hyttel J, Arnt J, Sanchez C: The pharmacology of citalopram. Rev Contemp Pharmacother 6:271–285, 1995

Inoue T: Effects of conditioned fear stress on monoaminergic systems in the rat brain. Hokkaido Igaku Zasshi 68:377–390, 1993

Invernizzi R, Belli S, Samanin R: Citalopram's ability to increase the extracellular concentrations of serotonin in the dorsal raphe prevents the drug's effect in the frontal cortex. Brain Res 584:322–324, 1992

Invernizzi R, Bramante M, Samanin R: Chronic treatment with citalopram facilitates the effect of a challenge dose on cortical serotonin output: role of presynaptic 5-HT1A receptors. Eur J Pharmacol 260:243–246, 1994

Invernizzi R, Velasco C, Bramante M, et al: Effect of 5-HT1A receptor antagonists on citalopram-induced increase in extracellular serotonin in the frontal cortex, striatum and dorsal hippocampus. Neuropharmacology 36:467–473, 1997

Jacob S, Spinler SA: Hyponatremia associated with selective serotonin-reuptake inhibitors in older adults. Ann Pharmacother 40:1618–1622, 2006

Jayatissa MN, Bisgaard C, Tingstrom A, et al: Hippocampal cytogenesis correlates to escitalopram-mediated recovery in a chronic mild stress rat model of depression. Neuropsychopharmacology 31:2395–2404, 2006

Jick H, Kaye JA, Jick SS: Antidepressants and the risk of suicidal behaviors. JAMA 292:338–343, 2004

Joffe P, Larsen FS, Pedersen V, et al: Single-dose pharmacokinetics of citalopram in patients with moderate renal insufficiency or hepatic cirrhosis compared with healthy subjects. Eur J Clin Pharmacol 54:237–242, 1998

Karlsson I, Godderis J, Augusto De Mendonca Lima C, et al: A randomised, double-blind comparison of the efficacy and safety of citalopram compared to mianserin in elderly, depressed patients with or without mild to moderate dementia. Int J Geriatr Psychiatry 15:295–305, 2000

Kasper S, de Swart H, Friis Andersen H: Escitalopram in the treatment of depressed elderly patients. Am J Geriatr Psychiatry 13:884–891, 2005a

Kasper S, Stein DJ, Loft H, et al: Escitalopram in the treatment of social anxiety disorder: randomised, placebo-controlled, flexible-dosage study. Br J Psychiatry 186:222–226, 2005b

Kasper S, Spadone C, Verpillat P, et al: Onset of action of escitalopram compared with other antidepressants: results of a pooled analysis. Int Clin Psychopharmacol 21:105–110, 2006

Keller MB: Citalopram therapy for depression: a review of 10 years of European experience and data from US clinical trials. J Clin Psychiatry 61:896–908, 2000

Kennedy SH, Andersen HF, Lam RW: Efficacy of escitalopram in the treatment of major depressive disorder compared with conventional selective serotonin reuptake inhibitors and venlafaxine XR: a meta-analysis. J Psychiatry Neurosci 31:122–131, 2006

Khan A, Schwartz K: Suicide risk and symptom reduction in patients assigned to placebo in duloxetine and escitalopram clinical trials: analysis of the FDA Summary Basis of Approval reports. Ann Clin Psychiatry 19:31–36, 2007

Khan A, Khan S, Kolts R, et al: Suicide rates in clinical trials of SSRIs, other antidepressants, and placebo: analysis of FDA reports. Am J Psychiatry 160:790–792, 2003

Klysner R, Bent-Hansen J, Hansen HL, et al: Efficacy of citalopram in the prevention of recurrent depression in elderly patients: placebo-controlled study of maintenance therapy. Br J Psychiatry 181:29–35, 2002

Kobayashi K, Chiba K, Yagi T, et al: Identification of cytochrome P450 isoforms involved in citalopram N-demethylation by human liver microsomes. J Pharmacol Exp Ther 280:927–933, 1997

Koponen H, Lepola U, Leinonen E, et al: Citalopram in the treatment of obsessive-compulsive disorder: an open pilot study. Acta Psychiatr Scand 96:343–346, 1997

Kornstein SG, Bose A, Li D, et al: Escitalopram maintenance treatment for prevention of recurrent depression: a randomized, placebo-controlled trial. J Clin Psychiatry 67:1767–1775, 2006

Kragh-Sorensen P, Overo KF, Petersen OL, et al: The kinetics of citalopram: single and multiple dose studies in man. Acta Pharmacol Toxicol (Copenh) 48:53–60, 1981

la Cour CM, Boni C, Hanoun N, et al: Functional consequences of 5-HT transporter gene disruption on 5-HT(1a) receptor-mediated regulation of dorsal raphe and hippocampal cell activity. J Neurosci 21:2178–2185, 2001

Lader M, Stender K, Burger V, et al: Efficacy and tolerability of escitalopram in 12- and 24-week treatment of social anxiety disorder: randomised, double-blind, placebo-controlled, fixed-dose study. Depress Anxiety 19:241–248, 2004

Larsen JJ, Hyttel J: 5-HT-uptake inhibition potentiates antinociception induced by morphine, pethidine, methadone and ketobemidone in rats. Acta Pharmacol Toxicol (Copenh) 57:214–218, 1985

Leinonen E, Lepola U, Koponen H, et al: The effect of age and concomitant treatment with other psychoactive drugs on serum concentrations of citalopram measured with a nonenantioselective method. Ther Drug Monit 18:111–117, 1996

Leombruni P, Amianto F, Delsedime N, et al: Citalopram versus fluoxetine for the treatment of patients with bulimia nervosa: a single-blind randomized controlled trial. Adv Ther 23:481–494, 2006

Lepola U, Koponen H, Leinonen E: Citalopram in the treatment of social phobia: a report of three cases. Pharmacopsychiatry 27:186–188, 1994

Lepola U, Leinonen E, Koponen H: Citalopram in the treatment of early onset panic disorder and school phobia. Pharmacopsychiatry 29:30–32, 1996

Lepola UM, Wade AG, Leinonen EV, et al: A controlled, prospective, 1-year trial of citalopram in the treatment of panic disorder. J Clin Psychiatry 59:528–534, 1998

Lepola UM, Loft H, Reines EH: Escitalopram (10–20 mg/day) is effective and well tolerated in a placebo-controlled study in depression in primary care. Int Clin Psychopharmacol 18:211–217, 2003

Lepola U, Wade A, Andersen HF: Do equivalent doses of escitalopram and citalopram have similar efficacy? A pooled analysis of two positive placebo-controlled studies in major depressive disorder. Int Clin Psychopharmacol 19:149–155, 2004

Llorca PM, Azorin JM, Despiegel N, et al: Efficacy of escitalopram in patients with severe depression: a pooled analysis. Int J Clin Pract 59:268–275, 2005

Markowitz JS, DeVane CL, Liston HL, et al: An assessment of selective serotonin reuptake inhibitor discontinuation symptoms with citalopram. Int Clin Psychopharmacol 15:329–333, 2000

Martin P, Soubrie P, Puech AJ: Reversal of helpless behavior by serotonin uptake blockers in rats. Psychopharmacology (Berl) 101:403–407, 1990

McElroy SL, Hudson JI, Malhotra S, et al: Citalopram in the treatment of binge-eating disorder: a placebo-controlled trial. J Clin Psychiatry 64:807–813, 2003

McMahon FJ, Buervenich S, Charney D, et al: Variation in the gene encoding the serotonin 2A receptor is associated with outcome of antidepressant treatment. Am J Hum Genet 78:804–814, 2006

McRae AL: Escitalopram. Curr Opin Investig Drugs 3:1225–1229, 2002

Mendels J, Kiev A, Fabre LF: Double-blind comparison of citalopram and placebo in depressed outpatients with melancholia. Depress Anxiety 9:54–60, 1999

Montgomery SA: Efficacy in long-term treatment of depression. J Clin Psychiatry 57:24–30, 1996

Montgomery SA, Andersen HF: Escitalopram versus venlafaxine XR in the treatment of depression. Int Clin Psychopharmacol 21:297–309, 2006

Montgomery SA, Rasmussen JG, Tanghoj P: A 24-week study of 20 mg citalopram, 40 mg citalopram, and placebo in the prevention of relapse of major depression. Int Clin Psychopharmacol 8:181–188, 1993

Montgomery SA, Pedersen V, Tanghoj P, et al: The optimal dosing regimen for citalopram—a meta-analysis of nine placebo-controlled studies. Int Clin Psychopharmacol 9 (suppl 1):35–40, 1994

Montgomery SA, Kasper S, Stein DJ, et al: Citalopram 20 mg, 40 mg and 60 mg are all effective and well tolerated compared with placebo in obsessive-compulsive disorder. Int Clin Psychopharmacol 16:75–86, 2001a

Montgomery SA, Loft H, Sanchez C, et al: Escitalopram (S-enantiomer of citalopram): clinical efficacy and onset of action predicted from a rat model. Pharmacol Toxicol 88:282–286, 2001b

Montgomery SA, Huusom AK, Bothmer J: A randomised study comparing escitalopram with venlafaxine XR in primary care patients with major depressive disorder. Neuropsychobiology 50:57–64, 2004

Montgomery SA, Nil R, Durr-Pal N, et al: A 24-week randomized, double-blind, placebo-controlled study of escitalopram for the prevention of generalized social anxiety disorder. J Clin Psychiatry 66:1270–1278, 2005

Moore N, Verdoux H, Fantino B: Prospective, multicentre, randomized, double-blind study of the efficacy of escitalopram versus citalopram in outpatient treatment of major depressive disorder. Int Clin Psychopharmacol 20:131–137, 2005

Mork A, Kreilgaard M, Sanchez C: The R-enantiomer of citalopram counteracts escitalopram-induced increase in extracellular 5-HT in the frontal cortex of freely moving rats. Neuropharmacology 45:167–173, 2003

Muldoon C: The safety and tolerability of citalopram. Int Clin Psychopharmacol 11 (suppl 1):35–40, 1996

Muller U, Murai T, Bauer-Wittmund T, et al: Paroxetine versus citalopram treatment of pathological crying after brain injury. Brain Inj 13:805–811, 1999

Mundo E, Bianchi L, Bellodi L: Efficacy of fluvoxamine, paroxetine, and citalopram in the treatment of obsessive-compulsive disorder: a single-blind study. J Clin Psychopharmacol 17:267–271, 1997

Nemeroff CB: Overview of the safety of citalopram. Psychopharmacol Bull 37:96–121, 2003

Neubauer HA, Hansen CG, Wiborg O: Dissection of an allosteric mechanism on the serotonin transporter: a cross-species study. Mol Pharmacol 69:1242–1250, 2006

Nierenberg AA, Greist JH, Mallinckrodt CH, et al: Duloxetine versus escitalopram and placebo in the treatment of patients with major depressive disorder: onset of antidepressant action, a non-inferiority study. Curr Med Res Opin 23:401–416, 2007

Norton N, Owen MJ: HTR2A: association and expression studies in neuropsychiatric genetics. Ann Med 37:121–129, 2005

Nyth AL, Gottfries CG: The clinical efficacy of citalopram in treatment of emotional disturbances in dementia disorders. A Nordic multicentre study. Br J Psychiatry 157:894–901, 1990

Nyth AL, Gottfries CG, Lyby K, et al: A controlled multicenter clinical study of citalopram and placebo in elderly depressed patients with and without concomitant dementia. Acta Psychiatr Scand 86:138–145, 1992

Olie JP, Tonnoir B, Menard F, et al: A prospective study of escitalopram in the treatment of major depressive episodes in the presence or absence of anxiety. Depress Anxiety 24:318–324, 2007

Olin JT, Katz IR, Meyers BS, et al: Provisional diagnostic criteria for depression of Alzheimer disease: rationale and background. Am J Geriatr Psychiatry 10:129–141, 2002

Overo KF: Kinetics of citalopram in man: plasma levels in patients. Prog Neuropsychopharmacol Biol Psychiatry 6:311–318, 1982

Overo KF, Toft B, Christophersen L, et al: Kinetics of citalopram in elderly patients. Psychopharmacology 86:253–257, 1985

Owens MJ, Morgan WN, Plott SJ, et al: Neurotransmitter receptor and transporter binding profile of antidepressants and their metabolites. J Pharmacol Exp Ther 283:1305–1322, 1997

Owens MJ, Knight DL, Nemeroff CB: Second-generation SSRIs: human monoamine transporter binding profile of escitalopram and R-fluoxetine. Biol Psychiatry 50:345–350, 2001

Oyehaug E, Eide G, Salvesen B: Effect of phenothiazines on citalopram steady-state kinetics in psychiatric patients. Nord Pharma Acta 46:37–46, 1984

Papp M, Nalepa I, Antkiewicz-Michaluk L, et al: Behavioural and biochemical studies of citalopram and WAY 100635 in rat chronic mild stress model. Pharmacol Biochem Behav 72:465–474, 2002

Pedersen AG: Escitalopram and suicidality in adult depression and anxiety. Int Clin Psychopharmacol 20:139–143, 2005

Peremans K, Audenaert K, Hoybergs Y, et al: The effect of citalopram hydrobromide on 5-HT2A receptors in the impulsive-aggressive dog, as measured with 123I-5-I-R91150 SPECT. Eur J Nucl Med Mol Imaging 32:708–716, 2005

Perlis RH, Purcell S, Fava M, et al: Association between treatment-emergent suicidal ideation with citalopram and polymorphisms near cyclic adenosine monophosphate response element binding protein in the STAR*D study. Arch Gen Psychiatry 64:689–697, 2007

Perna G, Bertani A, Caldirola D, et al: A comparison of citalopram and paroxetine in the treatment of panic disorder: a randomized, single-blind study. Pharmacopsychiatry 34:85–90, 2001

Plenge P, Mellerup ET: An affinity-modulating site on neuronal monoamine transport proteins. Pharmacol Toxicol 80:197–201, 1997

Plenge P, Mellerup ET, Laursen H: Affinity modulation of [3H]imipramine, [3H]paroxetine and [3H]citalopram binding to the 5-HT transporter from brain and platelets. Eur J Pharmacol 206:243–250, 1991

Pollock BG, Mulsant BH, Rosen J, et al: Comparison of citalopram, perphenazine, and placebo for the acute treatment of psycho-sis and behavioral disturbances in hospitalized, demented patients. Am J Psychiatry 159:460–465, 2002

Preskorn SH, Greenblatt DJ, Flockhart D, et al: Comparison of duloxetine, escitalopram, and sertraline effects on cytochrome P450 2D6 function in healthy volunteers. J Clin Psychopharmacol 27:28–34, 2007

Przegalinski E, Moryl E, Papp M: The effect of 5-HT1A receptor ligands in a chronic mild stress model of depression. Neuropharmacology 34:1305–1310, 1995

Rampello L, Chiechio S, Nicoletti G, et al: Prediction of the response to citalopram and reboxetine in post-stroke depressed patients. Psychopharmacology (Berl) 173:73–78, 2004

Rampello L, Alvano A, Raffaele R, et al: New possibilities of treatment for panic attacks in elderly patients: escitalopram versus citalopram. J Clin Psychopharmacol 26:67–70, 2006

Rantamaki T, Hendolin P, Kankaanpaa A, et al: Pharmacologically diverse antidepressants rapidly activate brain-derived neurotrophic factor receptor TrkB and induce phospholipase-C gamma signaling pathways in mouse brain. Neuropsychopharmacology 32:2152–2162, 2007

Rao N: The clinical pharmacokinetics of escitalopram. Clin Pharmacokinet 46:281–290, 2007

Rao V, Spiro JR, Rosenberg PB, et al: An open-label study of escitalopram (Lexapro) for the treatment of "depression of Alzheimer's disease" (dAD). Int J Geriatr Psychiatry 21:273–274, 2006

Rapaport MH, Bose A, Zheng H: Escitalopram continuation treatment prevents relapse of depressive episodes. J Clin Psychiatry 65:44–49, 2004

Rasmussen SL, Overo KF, Tanghoj P: Cardiac safety of citalopram: prospective trials and retrospective analyses. J Clin Psychopharmacol 19:407–415, 1999

Ravna AW, Sylte I, Dahl SG: Molecular mechanism of citalopram and cocaine interactions with neurotransmitter transporters. J Pharmacol Exp Ther 307:34–41, 2003

Richelson E, Nelson A: Antagonism by antidepressants of neurotransmitter receptors of normal human brain in vitro. J Pharmacol Exp Ther 230:94–102, 1984

Richelson E, Pfenning M: Blockade by antidepressants and related compounds of biogenic amine uptake into rat brain synaptosomes: most antidepressants selectively block norepinephrine uptake. Eur J Pharmacol 104:277–286, 1984

Robert P, Montgomery SA: Citalopram in doses of 20–60 mg is effective in depression relapse prevention: a placebo-controlled 6 month study. Int Clin Psychopharmacol 10 (suppl 1):29–35, 1995

Robert S, Hamner MB, Ulmer HG, et al: Open-label trial of escitalopram in the treatment of posttraumatic stress disorder. J Clin Psychiatry 67:1522–1526, 2006

Robinson RG: Poststroke depression: prevalence, diagnosis, treatment, and disease progression. Biol Psychiatry 54:376–387, 2003

Robinson RG, Jorge RE, Moser DJ, et al: Escitalopram and problem-solving therapy for prevention of poststroke depression: a randomized controlled trial. JAMA 299:2391–2400, 2008

Rochat B, Amey M, Gillet M, et al: Identification of three cytochrome P450 isozymes involved in N-demethylation of citalopram enantiomers in human liver microsomes. Pharmacogenetics 7:1–10, 1997

Rush AJ, Fava M, Wisniewski SR, et al: Sequenced treatment alternatives to relieve depression (STAR*D): rationale and design. Control Clin Trials 25:119–142, 2004

Russo-Neustadt AA, Alejandre H, Garcia C, et al: Hippocampal brain-derived neurotrophic factor expression following treatment with reboxetine, citalopram, and physical exercise. Neuropsychopharmacology 29:2189–2199, 2004

Sanchez C: Serotonergic mechanisms involved in the exploratory behaviour of mice in a fully automated two-compartment black and white text box. Pharmacol Toxicol 77:71–78, 1995

Sanchez C: The pharmacology of citalopram enantiomers: the antagonism by R-citalopram on the effect of S-citalopram. Basic Clin Pharmacol Toxicol 99:91–95, 2006

Sanchez C, Brennum LT: The S-enantiomer of citalopram (Lu 26-054) is a highly selective and potent serotonin reuptake inhibitor. Biol Psychiatry 47:88S, 2000

Sanchez C, Hyttel J: Isolation-induced aggression in mice: effects of 5-hydroxytryptamine uptake inhibitors and involvement of postsynaptic 5-HT1A receptors. Eur J Pharmacol 264:241–247, 1994

Sanchez C, Kreilgaard M: R-citalopram inhibits functional and 5-HTP-evoked behavioural responses to the SSRI, escitalopram. Pharmacol Biochem Behav 77:391–398, 2004

Sanchez C, Meier E: Behavioral profiles of SSRIs in animal models of depression, anxiety and aggression: are they all alike? Psychopharmacology (Berl) 129:197–205, 1997

Sanchez C, Bergqvist PB, Brennum LT, et al: Escitalopram, the S-(+)-enantiomer of citalopram, is a selective serotonin reuptake inhibitor with potent effects in animal models predictive of antidepressant and anxiolytic activities. Psychopharmacology (Berl) 167:353–362, 2003a

Sanchez C, Gruca P, Bien E, et al: R-citalopram counteracts the effect of escitalopram in a rat conditioned fear stress model of anxiety. Pharmacol Biochem Behav 75:903–907, 2003b

Sanchez C, Gruca P, Papp M: R-citalopram counteracts the antidepressant-like effect of escitalopram in a rat chronic mild stress model. Behav Pharmacol 14:465–470, 2003c

Schaffer A, Zuker P, Levitt A: Randomized, double-blind pilot trial comparing lamotrigine versus citalopram for the treatment of bipolar depression. J Affect Disord 96:95–99, 2006

Schneier FR, Blanco C, Campeas R, et al: Citalopram treatment of social anxiety disorder with comorbid major depression. Depress Anxiety 17:191–196, 2003

Seedat S, Stein DJ, Ziervogel C, et al: Comparison of response to a selective serotonin reuptake inhibitor in children, adolescents, and adults with posttraumatic stress disorder. J Child Adolesc Psychopharmacol 12:37–46, 2002

Shirazi E, Alaghband-Rad J: An open trial of citalopram in children and adolescents with depression. J Child Adolesc Psychopharmacol 15:233–239, 2005

Sidhu J, Priskorn M, Poulsen M, et al: Steady-state pharmacokinetics of the enantiomers of citalopram and its metabolites in humans. Chirality 9:686–692, 1997

Simon NM, Sharma SG, Worthington JJ, et al: Citalopram for social phobia: a clinical case series. Prog Neuropsychopharmacol Biol Psychiatry 25:1469–1474, 2001

Sindrup SH, Brosen K, Hansen MG, et al: Pharmacokinetics of citalopram in relation to the sparteine and the mephenytoin oxidation polymorphisms. Ther Drug Monit 15:11–17, 1993

Sogaard B, Mengel H, Rao N, et al: The pharmacokinetics of escitalopram after oral and intravenous administration of single and multiple doses to healthy subjects. J Clin Pharmacol 45:1400–1406, 2005

Sproule BA, Naranjo CA, Brenner KE, et al: Selective serotonin reuptake inhibitors and CNS drug interactions: a critical review of the evidence. Clin Pharmacokinet 33:454–471, 1997

Stahl SM: Placebo-controlled comparison of the selective serotonin reuptake inhibitors citalopram and sertraline. Biol Psychiatry 48:894–901, 2000

Stahl SM, Gergel I, Li D: Escitalopram in the treatment of panic disorder: a randomized, double-blind, placebo-controlled trial. J Clin Psychiatry 64:1322–1327, 2003

Stein DJ, Montgomery SA, Kasper S, et al: Predictors of response to pharmacotherapy with citalopram in obsessive-compulsive disorder. Int Clin Psychopharmacol 16:357–361, 2001

Stein DJ, Andersen HF, Goodman WK: Escitalopram for the treatment of GAD: efficacy across different subgroups and outcomes. Ann Clin Psychiatry 17:71–75, 2005

Stein DJ, Andersen EW, Tonnoir B, et al: Escitalopram in obsessive-compulsive disorder: a randomized, placebo-controlled, paroxetine-referenced, fixed-dose, 24-week study. Curr Med Res Opin 23:701–711, 2007

Stein MB, Liebowitz MR, Lydiard RB, et al: Paroxetine treatment of generalized social phobia (social anxiety disorder): a randomized controlled trial. JAMA 280:708–713, 1998

Storosum JG, van Zwieten BJ, van den Brink W, et al: Suicide risk in placebo-controlled studies of major depression. Am J Psychiatry 158:1271–1275, 2001

Storustovu S, Sanchez C, Porzgen P, et al: R-citalopram functionally antagonises escitalopram in vivo and in vitro: evidence for kinetic interaction at the serotonin transporter. Br J Pharmacol 142:172–180, 2004

Strome EM, Clark CM, Zis AP, et al: Electroconvulsive shock decreases binding to 5-HT2 receptors in nonhuman primates: an in vivo positron emission tomography study with [18F]setoperone. Biol Psychiatry 57:1004–1010, 2005

Sugrue MF: On the role of 5-hydroxytryptamine in drug-induced antinociception. Br J Pharmacol 65:677–681, 1979

Syvalahti EK, Taiminen T, Saarijarvi S, et al: Citalopram causes no significant alterations in plasma neuroleptic levels in schizophrenic patients. J Int Med Res 25:24–32, 1997

Thomsen PH: Child and adolescent obsessive-compulsive disorder treated with citalopram: findings from an open trial of 23 cases. J Child Adolesc Psychopharmacol 7:157–166, 1997

Thomsen PH, Ebbesen C, Persson C: Long-term experience with citalopram in the treatment of adolescent OCD. J Am Acad Child Adolesc Psychiatry 40:895–902, 2001

Trivedi MH, Rush AJ, Wisniewski SR, et al: Evaluation of outcomes with citalopram for depression using measurement-based care in STAR*D: implications for clinical practice. Am J Psychiatry 163:28–40, 2006

Tucker P, Ruwe WD, Masters B, et al: Neuroimmune and cortisol changes in selective serotonin reuptake inhibitor and placebo treatment of chronic posttraumatic stress disorder. Biol Psychiatry 56:121–128, 2004

Uehlinger C, Nil R, Amey M, et al: Citalopram-lithium combination treatment of elderly depressed patients: a pilot study. Int J Geriatr Psychiatry 10:281–287, 1995

Vaatstra WJ, Deiman-Van Aalst WM, Eigeman L: Du 24565, a quipazine derivative, a potent selective serotonin uptake inhibitor. Eur J Pharmacol 70:195–202, 1981

Vaidya VA, Marek GJ, Aghajanian GK, et al: 5-HT2A receptor-mediated regulation of brain-derived neurotrophic factor mRNA in the hippocampus and the neocortex. J Neurosci 17:2785–2795, 1997

van Harten J: Clinical pharmacokinetics of selective serotonin reuptake inhibitors. Clin Pharmacokinet 24:203–220, 1993

Varia I, Rauscher F: Treatment of generalized anxiety disorder with citalopram. Int Clin Psychopharmacol 17:103–107, 2002

Ventura D, Armstrong EP, Skrepnek GH, et al: Escitalopram versus sertraline in the treatment of major depressive disorder: a randomized clinical trial. Curr Med Res Opin 23:245–250, 2007

Voirol P, Rubin C, Bryois C, et al: Pharmacokinetic consequences of a citalopram treatment discontinuation. Ther Drug Monit 21:263–266, 1999

von Knorring AL, Olsson GI, Thomsen PH, et al: A randomized, double-blind, placebo-controlled study of citalopram in adolescents with major depressive disorder. J Clin Psychopharmacol 26:311–315, 2006

von Moltke LL, Greenblatt DJ, Grassi JM, et al: Citalopram and desmethylcitalopram in vitro: human cytochromes mediating transformation, and cytochrome inhibitory effects. Biol Psychiatry 46:839–849, 1999

von Moltke LL, Greenblatt DJ, Giancarlo GM, et al: Escitalopram (S-citalopram) and its metabolites in vitro: cytochromes mediating biotransformation, inhibitory effects, and comparison to R-citalopram. Drug Metab Dispos 29:1102–1109, 2001

Wade A, Michael Lemming O, Bang Hedegaard K: Escitalopram 10 mg/day is effective and well tolerated in a placebo-controlled study in depression in primary care. Int Clin Psychopharmacol 17:95–102, 2002

Wade A, Gembert K, Florea I: A comparative study of the efficacy of acute and continuation treatment with escitalopram versus duloxetine in patients with major depressive disorder. Curr Med Res Opin 23:1605–1614, 2007

Wagner KD, Robb AS, Findling RL, et al: A randomized, placebo-controlled trial of citalopram for the treatment of major depression in children and adolescents. Am J Psychiatry 161:1079–1083, 2004

Wagner KD, Jonas J, Findling RL, et al: A double-blind, randomized, placebo-controlled trial of escitalopram in the treatment of pediatric depression. J Am Acad Child Adolesc Psychiatry 45:280–288, 2006

Waldinger MD, Zwinderman AH, Olivier B: SSRIs and ejaculation: a double-blind, randomized, fixed-dose study with paroxetine and citalopram. J Clin Psychopharmacol 21:556–560, 2001

Waldmeier PC, Baumann PA, Maitre L: CGP 6085 A, a new, specific, inhibitor of serotonin uptake: neurochemical characterization and comparison with other serotonin uptake blockers. J Pharmacol Exp Ther 211:42–49, 1979

Yu BN, Chen GL, He N, et al: Pharmacokinetics of citalopram in relation to genetic polymorphism of CYP2C19. Drug Metab Dispos 31:1255–1259, 2003

Monoamine Oxidase Inhibitors

K. Ranga Rama Krishnan, M.D.

History and Discovery

Monoamine oxidase inhibitors (MAOIs) were first identified as effective antidepressants in the late 1950s. An early report suggested that iproniazid, an antitubercular agent, had mood-elevating properties in patients who had been treated for tuberculosis (Bloch et al. 1954). Following these observations, two studies confirmed that iproniazid did indeed have antidepressant properties (Crane 1957; Kline 1958). Zeller (1963) reported that iproniazid caused potent inhibition of monoamine oxidase (MAO) enzymes both in vivo and in vitro in the brain. He also reported that the medication reversed some of the actions of reserpine. Because reserpine produced significant depression as a side effect, it was suggested that iproniazid might have mood-elevating properties.

The use of iproniazid soon fell into disfavor because of its significant hepatotoxicity. Other MAOIs, both hydrazine derivatives (e.g., isocarboxazid and phenylhydrazine) and nonhydrazine derivatives (e.g., tranylcypromine), were introduced. These MAOIs were not specific for any subtype of MAO enzyme, and they were irreversible inhibitors of MAO (see next section, "Monoamine Oxidase"). Their use has been rather limited because hypertensive crisis by the MAOIs may occur in some patients from potentiation of the pressor effects of amines (such as tyramine) in food (Blackwell et al. 1967).

In the past few years, there has been a resurgence of interest in the development of new monoamine oxidase inhibitors—that is, in those MAOIs that are more selective for specific subtypes of MAO enzyme and in those that are reversible in nature. Newer MAOIs, such as L-deprenyl (selegiline hydrochloride), a monoamine oxi-

dase B (MAO-B) inhibitor, have been introduced (Table 18–1). Reversible monoamine oxidase A (MAO-A) inhibitors, such as moclobemide, have been introduced in Europe but are not yet available in the United States.

Monoamine Oxidase

A and B Isoenzymes

MAO is widely distributed in mammals. Two isoenzymes, MAO-A and MAO-B, are of special interest in psychiatry (Cesura and Pletscher 1992). Both are present in the central nervous system (CNS) and in some peripheral organs. Both MAO-A and MAO-B are present in discrete cell populations within the CNS. MAO-A is present in both dopamine (DA) and norepinephrine (NE) neurons, whereas MAO-B is present to a greater extent in serotonin (5-HT)–containing neurons. They are also present in nonaminergic neurons in various subcortical regions of the brain. Glial cells also express MAO-A and MAO-B (Cesura and Pletscher 1992).

The physiological functions of these two isoenzymes have not been fully elucidated. The main substrates for MAO-A are epinephrine, NE, and 5-HT. The main substrates for MAO-B are phenylethylamine, phenylethanolamine, tyramine, and benzylamine. DA and tryptamine are metabolized by both isoenzymes. The localization of the MAO subtypes does not fully correspond to the neurons containing the substrates. The reason for this discrepancy is unknown. The occurrence of the MAO-B form in 5-HT neurons may actually protect these neurons from amines (other than 5-HT) that could be toxic to them (Cesura and Pletscher 1992).

TABLE 18–1.   Classification of monoamine oxidase inhibitor (MAOI) drugs by structure, selectivity, and reversibility

DRUG	HYDRAZINE	SELECTIVE	REVERSIBLE
Phenelzine	Yes	No	No
Isocarboxazid	Yes	No	No
Tranylcypromine	No	No	No
Selegiline	No	Yes[a,b]	No
Moclobemide	No	Yes[c]	Yes
Brofaromine	No	Yes[c]	Yes

[a]Selective for MAO-B at lower doses.
[b]Becomes nonselective at higher doses.
[c]Selective for MAO-A.

The primary structures of MAO-A and MAO-B have been fully described. MAO-A has 527 amino acids, and MAO-B has 520 amino acids. About 70% of the amino acid sequence of the two forms is homologous. The genes for both isoenzymes are located on the short arm of the human X chromosome. MAO-A and MAO-B are linked and have been located in the XP11.23–P11 and XP22.1 regions, respectively. The genes are about 70 kilobases and consist of about 15 exons and 14 introns. MAO-A has two messenger RNA (mRNA) transcripts of 2.1 and 5.0 kilobytes in length. MAO-B has a 3-kb mRNA single transcript (Cesura and Pletscher 1992). A rare inherited disorder, Norrie's disease, is characterized by deletion of both genes; patients with this disorder have very severe mental retardation and blindness.

The subunit composition of MAO is unknown. The enzyme is primarily found in the outer mitochondrial membrane; flavin adenine dinucleotide (FAD) is a cofactor for both MAO-A and MAO-B.

Because the cofactor domain is the same for both of the MAO isoenzymes, the structural differences responsible for substrate specificity are believed to lie in regions of the protein that bind to the hydrophobic moiety of the substrate. Although DA is considered to be a mixed substrate for both MAO-A and MAO-B, the breakdown of DA in the striatal regions of the brain is preferentially by MAO-B. In other regions, MAO-A may be more important. There may be regional differences as to which isoenzyme is responsible for the metabolism of other biogenic amines that are substrates for both forms of MAO (Cesura and Pletscher 1992).

Enzyme Kinetics

The enzyme kinetics of MAO-A have not been well studied. The enzyme kinetics for MAO-B, for which more in-

formation is available, depend on the nature of the substrate. Some substrates (e.g., tyramine) go through ping-pong mechanisms characterized by first oxidation of the amine to the imine form that is subsequently released from the reduced enzyme before reoxidation of the latter occurs. Other substrates (e.g., benzylamine) involve formation of a tertiary complex with the enzyme and oxygen (Husain et al. 1982; Pearce and Roth 1985; Ramsay and Singer 1991).

Mechanism of Action

The target function of MAOIs is regulation of the monoamine content within the nervous system. Because MAO is bound to the outer surface of the plasma membrane of the mitochondria, in neurons MAO is unable to deaminate amines that are present inside stored vesicles and can metabolize only amines that are present in the cytoplasm. As a result, MAO maintains a low cytoplasmic concentration of amines within the cells. Inhibition of neuronal MAO produces an increase in the amine content in the cytoplasm. Initially, it was believed that the therapeutic action of MAOIs was a result of this amine accumulation (Finberg and Youdim 1984; Murphy et al. 1984, 1987). More recently, it has been suggested that secondary adaptive mechanisms may be important for the antidepressant action of these agents.

After several weeks of treatment, MAOIs produce effects, such as a reduction in the number of β-adrenoreceptors, α_1- and α_2-adrenoreceptors, and serotonin$_1$ (5-HT$_1$) and serotonin$_2$ (5-HT$_2$) receptors. These changes are similar to those produced by the chronic use of tricyclic antidepressants (TCAs) and other antidepressant treatment (DaPrada et al. 1984, 1989).

MAOIs can be subdivided on the basis of not only the particular type of enzyme inhibition but also the type of inhibition they produce (reversible or irreversible). The reversible MAOIs are basically chemically inert substrate analogs. MAOIs are recognized as substrates by the enzyme and are converted into intermediates by the normal mechanism. These converted compounds react to the inactive site of the enzyme and form a stable bound enzyme. This effect occurs gradually, and there is usually a correlation between the plasma concentration of the reversible inhibitors and pharmacological action.

Pharmacological Profile

The classic MAOIs inhibit both forms of the enzyme and are divided into two main subtypes: hydrazine and nonhydrazine derivatives. The hydrazine derivatives, two of which (phenelzine and isocarboxazid) are currently available, are related to iproniazid. The nonhydrazine irreversible MAOI is tranylcypromine, which is chemically similar to amphetamine. Clorgyline is an example of an irreversible inhibitor of MAO-A, whereas selegiline is an irreversible inhibitor of MAO-B. The only reversible inhibitor of MAO-A available anywhere is moclobemide.

Three classic MAOIs (i.e., tranylcypromine, phenelzine, and isocarboxazid) are of clinical interest. Clinicians must recognize that these drugs not only inhibit MAO but also exert other actions that may be clinically relevant. Thus, these compounds can block MAO uptake—tranylcypromine more than isocarboxazid or phenelzine. In addition, because tranylcypromine is structurally similar to amphetamine, it is believed to exert stimulant-like actions in the brain. Many issues are common to all three of these MAOIs.

Indications and Efficacy

Major and Atypical Depression

Many studies have examined the efficacy of MAOIs in the treatment of different types of depression. MAOIs have been effective in the treatment of major depression or atypical depression (Davidson et al. 1987a; Himmelhoch et al. 1982, 1991; Johnstone 1975; Johnstone and Marsh 1973; McGrath et al. 1986; Paykel et al. 1982; Quitkin et al. 1979, 1990, 1991; Rowan et al. 1981; Thase et al. 1992; Vallejo et al. 1987; White et al. 1984; Zisook et al. 1985). Although early studies of relatively low-dose regimens suggested that the efficacy of MAOIs was lower than that of TCAs, more recent studies have documented that their efficacy is comparable (Table 18–2).

TABLE 18–2. Indications for use of monoamine oxidase inhibitors (MAOIs)

DEFINITELY EFFECTIVE	OTHER POSSIBLE USES
Atypical depression	OCD
Major depression	Narcolepsy
Dysthymia	Headache
Melancholia	Chronic pain syndrome
Panic disorder	GAD
Bulimia	
Atypical facial pain	
Anergic depression	
Treatment-resistant depression	
Parkinson's disease[a]	

Note. GAD=generalized anxiety disorder; OCD=obsessive-compulsive disorder.
[a]Selegiline is the only MAOI that is useful in the treatment of Parkinson's disease.

Quitkin et al. (1979, 1991) reviewed both phenelzine and tranylcypromine studies in patients with either atypical neurotic depression or melancholic depression. The authors reported that phenelzine appeared to be effective for the treatment of atypical depression.

Relatively few studies of endogenous depression in patients have been done. From the limited number of initial patient studies, it is difficult to conclude that phenelzine is effective in the treatment of these patients. In addition, very few well-controlled studies of tranylcypromine, compared with placebo, have been done. Three of the four studies that compared tranylcypromine with placebo showed that tranylcypromine was more effective. In one study, a nonsignificant trend was found favoring tranylcypromine. More recently, studies have documented the efficacy of tranylcypromine in treating anergic depression and, at high doses, treatment-resistant depression (Himmelhoch et al. 1982, 1991; Thase et al. 1992; White et al. 1984). In the Sequenced Treatment Alternatives to Relieve Depression (STAR*D) study, patients who had failed to respond to at least three treatment options were randomly assigned to tranylcypromine or a combination of venlafaxine and mirtazapine. Remission rates were modest for both the tranylcypromine group and the extended-release venlafaxine plus mirtazapine group, and the rates were not statistically different between groups (McGrath et al. 2006).

The heterogeneity of acetylation rate may account for some of the variance in response to phenelzine (Johnstone 1975; Johnstone and Marsh 1973; Paykel et al. 1982; Rowan et al. 1981). One-half of the patients in a given population are often slow acetylators. An initial study by Johnstone and Marsh (1973) suggested that slow acetylators improve more with phenelzine than do fast acetylators. Other groups have been unable to confirm the relation between acetylation, acetylator type, and response to MAOIs.

MAOIs are used in a wide range of psychiatric disorders. Early studies suggested that MAOIs are particularly effective in patients who have atypical depression, originally defined as depression with anxiety or chronic pain, reversed vegetative symptoms, and rejection sensitivity (Quitkin et al. 1990).

The concept of atypical depression remains controversial and has not been completely validated. In general, patients with atypical depression have an earlier age at onset than do patients with melancholic depression, and the prevalence of dysthymia, alcohol abuse, sociopathy, and atypical depression is increased in the relatives of patients with atypical depression. The best differentiating criterion appears to be that phenelzine and other irreversible MAOIs are more effective than TCAs in treating these patients (Cesura and Pletscher 1992; Quitkin et al. 1990; Zisook et al. 1985).

Some studies have also suggested that MAOIs are effective in treating typical major depression and melancholic depression (Davidson et al. 1987a; McGrath et al. 1986; Vallejo et al. 1987).

Panic Disorder

Both single- and double-blind studies have found that phenelzine and iproniazid are effective in treating panic disorder (Lydiard et al. 1989; Quitkin et al. 1990; Tyrer et al. 1973). About 50%–60% of patients with panic disorder respond to MAOIs. In the early stages of treatment, patients may have a worsening of symptoms. This is reduced in clinical practice by combining the MAOI with a benzodiazepine for the initial phase of the study. It has been suggested that in addition to its antipanic effect, phenelzine has an antiphobic action (Kelly et al. 1971). The time course of effect and the dose used are similar to those for major depression.

Social Phobia

Liebowitz et al. (1992) reported that phenelzine is effective in treating social phobia. In an open-label study, Versiani et al. (1988) suggested that tranylcypromine is effec-

tive. Versiani et al. (1992) also demonstrated the efficacy of moclobemide in a double-blind study. In clinical experience, about 50% of patients respond to MAOIs, and the onset of response is gradual (usually about 2–3 weeks).

Obsessive-Compulsive Disorder

Although initial case reports suggested that MAOIs may be effective in obsessive-compulsive disorder (Jenike 1981), no double-blind studies have indicated efficacy.

Posttraumatic Stress Disorder

The classic MAOI phenelzine has been proven effective for the treatment of posttraumatic stress disorder (PTSD) in single-blind trials (Davidson et al. 1987b) and a double-blind crossover trial (Kosten et al. 1991).

Generalized Anxiety Disorder

MAOIs are not usually used to treat generalized anxiety disorder (GAD) because the risk–benefit ratio favors the use of selective serotonin reuptake inhibitors (SSRIs), azaspirones, or benzodiazepines. When they are used, MAOIs are used primarily for treating treatment-resistant GAD.

Bulimia Nervosa

Both phenelzine and isocarboxazid have been shown to be effective in treating some symptoms of bulimia nervosa (Kennedy et al. 1988; McElroy et al. 1989; Walsh et al. 1985, 1987).

Premenstrual Dysphoria

Preliminary studies and clinical experience suggest that MAOIs may be effective in the treatment of premenstrual dysphoria (Glick et al. 1991).

Chronic Pain

MAOIs are believed to be effective in the treatment of atypical facial pain and other chronic pain syndromes. However, only limited data on these conditions are available.

Neurological Diseases

The classic MAOIs have not been found to be effective for treating neurological disorders such as Parkinson's disease and Alzheimer's dementia. However, the MAO-B inhibitor selegiline has been shown to be effective in slowing the progression of Parkinson's disease (Cesura and Pletscher 1992), but the mechanism underlying this effect is unknown.

Side Effects and Toxicology

The side effects of MAOIs are generally more severe or frequent than those of other antidepressants (Zisook 1984). The most frequent side effects include dizziness, headache, dry mouth, insomnia, constipation, blurred vision, nausea, peripheral edema, forgetfulness, fainting spells, trauma, hesitancy of urination, weakness, and myoclonic jerks. Loss of weight and appetite may occur with isocarboxazid use (Davidson and Turnbull 1982). Hepatotoxicity is more rare with the currently available MAOIs, compared with iproniazid. However, liver enzymes, such as aspartate transaminase (AST) and alanine transaminase (ALT), are elevated in 3%–5% of patients. Liver function tests must be done only when patients have symptoms like malaise, jaundice, and excessive fatigue.

Some side effects first emerge during maintenance treatment (Evans et al. 1982). These side effects include weight gain (which occurs in almost one-half of patients), edema, muscle cramps, carbohydrate craving, sexual dysfunction (usually anorgasmia), pyridoxine deficiency (see Goodheart et al. 1991), hypoglycemia, hypomania, urinary retention, and disorientation. Peripheral neuropathy (Goodheart et al. 1991) and speech blockage (Goldstein and Goldberg 1986) are rare side effects of MAOIs. Weight gain is more of a problem with hydrazine compounds, such as phenelzine, than with tranylcypromine. Therefore, weight gain that is caused by hydrazine derivatives is an indication to switch to tranylcypromine. Edema is also more common with phenelzine than with tranylcypromine.

The management of some of these side effects can be problematic. Orthostatic hypotension is common with MAOIs. Addition of salt and salt-retaining steroids, such as fluorohydrocortisone, is sometimes effective in treating orthostatic hypotension. Elastic support stockings are also helpful. Small amounts of coffee or tea taken during the day also keep the blood pressure elevated. The dose of fluorohydrocortisol should be adjusted carefully because in elderly patients it could provoke cardiac failure resulting from fluid retention.

Sexual dysfunction that occurs with these compounds is also difficult to treat. Common problems include anorgasmia, decreased libido, impotence, and delayed ejaculation (Harrison et al. 1985; Jacobson 1987). Cyprohepta-

dine is sometimes effective in treating sexual dysfunction like anorgasmia. Bethanechol may also be effective in some patients.

Insomnia occasionally occurs as an intermediate or late side effect of these compounds. Changing the time of administration does not seem to help much, although dosage reduction may be helpful. Adding trazodone at bedtime is effective, but this should be done with caution. Myoclonic jerks, peripheral neuropathy, and paresthesia, when present, are also difficult to treat. When a patient has paresthesia, the clinician should evaluate for peripheral neuropathy and pyridoxine deficiency. In general, patients taking MAOIs should also take concomitant pyridoxine therapy. When myoclonic jerks occur, patients can be treated with cyproheptadine.

MAOIs also have the potential to suppress anginal pain; therefore, coronary artery disease could be overlooked or underestimated.

Patients with hyperthyroidism are more sensitive to MAOIs because of their overall sensitivity to pressor amines. MAOIs can also worsen hypoglycemia in patients taking hypoglycemic agents like insulin.

Dietary Interactions

After the introduction of MAOIs, several reports of severe headaches in patients who were taking these compounds were published ("Cheese and Tranylcypromine" 1970; Cronin 1965; Hedberg et al. 1966; Simpson and Gratz 1992). These headaches were caused by a drug–food interaction. The risk of such an interaction is highest for tranylcypromine and lower for phenelzine, provided that the dose of the latter remains low. The interaction of MAOIs with food has been attributed to increased tyramine levels. Tyramine, which has a pressor action, is present in a number of foodstuffs. It is normally broken down by the MAO enzymes and has both direct and indirect sympathomimetic actions. The classic explanation of this side effect may not be entirely accurate; in fact, it has been suggested that the potentiation of tyramine by an MAOI may be secondary to increased release of NE rather than to the MAOI. Adrenaline would increase the indirect sympathetic activity of tyramine. The spontaneous occurrence of hypertensive crises in a few patients lends support to this hypothesis (O'Brien et al. 1992; Zajecka and Fawcett 1991).

The tyramine effect of food is potentiated by MAOIs 10- to 20-fold. A mild tyramine interaction occurs with about 6 mg of tyramine; 10 mg can produce a moderate episode, and 25 mg can produce a severe episode that is characterized by hypertension, occipital headache, palpitations, nausea, vomiting, apprehension, occasional chills, sweating, and restlessness. On examination, neck stiffness, pallor, mild pyrexia, dilated pupils, and motor agitation may be seen. The reaction usually develops within 20–60 minutes after ingestion of food. Occasionally, the reaction can be very severe and may lead to alteration of consciousness, hyperpyrexia, cerebral hemorrhage, and death. Death is exceedingly rare and has been calculated to be about 0.01%–0.02% for all patients taking tranylcypromine.

The classic treatment of the hypertensive reaction is phentolamine (5 mg) administered intravenously (Youdim et al. 1987; Zisook 1984). More recently, nifedipine, a calcium channel blocker, has been shown to be effective. Nifedipine has an onset of action of about 5 minutes, and it lasts approximately 3–5 hours; in fact, some clinicians have suggested that patients should carry nifedipine with them for immediate use in the event of a hypertensive crisis.

Because of the drug interaction of the classic MAOIs with food, clinicians usually make several dietary recommendations (Table 18–3). These recommendations are quite varied.

All of the MAOI diets recommend restriction of cheese (with the exception of cream cheese and cottage cheese), red wine, sherry, liqueurs, pickled fish, overripe (aged) fruit, brewer's yeast, fava beans, beef and chicken liver, and fermented products. Other diets also recommend restriction of all alcoholic beverages, coffee, chocolate, colas, tea, yogurt, soy sauce, avocados, and bananas. The more restrictive the diet, the greater the risk of patient noncompliance. Furthermore, many of the compounds—for example, avocados and bananas—rarely cause hypertensive crisis. For example, an interaction may occur only if overripe fruit is eaten or, in the case of bananas, if the skin is eaten (which is an uncommon practice in the United States). Similarly, unless a person ingests large amounts of caffeine, the interaction is usually not clinically significant.

In evaluating patients who have had a drug–food reaction, it is also important to evaluate the hypertensive reaction and differentiate it from histamine headache, which can occur with an MAOI. Histamine headaches are usually accompanied by hypotension, colic, loose stools, salivation, and lacrimation (Cooper 1967). The clinician should provide oral instructions, as well as printed cards, outlining these instructions to patients who are taking classic MAOIs.

In addition to the food interaction, drug interactions are extremely important (see next section, "Drug–Drug

TABLE 18–3. Food restrictions for monoamine oxidase inhibitors (MAOIs)

TO BE AVOIDED	TO BE USED IN MODERATION
Cheese (except for cream cheese)	Coffee
Overripe (aged) fruit (e.g., banana peel)	Chocolate
Fava beans	Colas
Sausage, salami	Tea
Sherry, liqueurs	Soy sauce
Sauerkraut	Beer, other wines
Monosodium glutamate	
Pickled fish	
Brewer's yeast	
Beef and chicken liver	
Fermented products	
Red wine	

Interactions"). Each patient should be given a card indicating that he or she is taking an MAOI and instructions that the card should be carried at all times. A medical bracelet indicating that the wearer takes an MAOI is also a good idea.

Drug–Drug Interactions

The extensive inhibition of MAO enzymes by MAOIs raises the potential for a number of drug interactions (Table 18–4). Of particular importance, many over-the-counter medications can interact with MAOIs. These medications include cough syrups containing sympathomimetic agents, which in the presence of an MAOI can precipitate a hypertensive crisis.

Another area of caution is the use of MAOIs in patients who need surgery. In this situation, interactions include those with narcotic drugs, especially meperidine. Meperidine administered with MAOIs can produce a syndrome characterized by coma, hyperpyrexia, and hypertension. This syndrome has been reported primarily with phenelzine; however, it has also been reported with tranylcypromine (Mendelson 1979; Stack et al. 1988). Stack et al. (1988) noted that this syndrome is most likely to occur with meperidine and that it may be related to that drug's serotonergic properties. Similar reactions have not been reported to any significant extent with other narcotic analgesics such as morphine and codeine. In fact, many patients probably receive these medications with-

TABLE 18–4. Drug interactions with monoamine oxidase inhibitors (MAOIs)

DRUG	INTERACTION	COMMENT
Other MAOIs (e.g., furazolidone, pargyline, procarbazine)	Potentiation of side effects; convulsions possible	Allow at least 1 week before changing MAOI
Tricyclic antidepressants (TCAs) (e.g., maprotiline, bupropion)	Severe side effects, such as hypertension and convulsions, possible	Allow at least 2 weeks before changing MAOI; combinations have been used occasionally for refractory depression
Carbamazepine	Low possibility of interaction; similar to TCAs	Same as for TCAs
Cyclobenzaprine	Low possibility of interaction; similar to TCAs	Same as for TCAs
Selective serotonin reuptake inhibitors (SSRIs)	Serotonin syndrome	Avoid combinations; allow at least 2 weeks before changing MAOI and 5 weeks if switching from fluoxetine to MAOI
Stimulants (e.g., methylphenidate, dextroamphetamine)	Potential for increased blood pressure (hypertension)	Avoid combination
Buspirone	Potential for increased blood pressure (hypertension)	Avoid use; if used, monitor blood pressure
Meperidine	Severe, potentially fatal interaction possible (see text)	Avoid combination
Dextromethorphan	Reports of brief psychosis	Avoid high doses
Direct sympathomimetics (e.g., L-dopa)	Increased blood pressure	Avoid use, if possible; if they need to be used, use with caution
Indirect sympathomimetics	Hypertensive crisis possible	Avoid use
Oral hypoglycemics (e.g., insulin)	Worsening of hypoglycemia possible	Monitor blood sugar levels and adjust medications
Fenfluramine	Serotonin syndrome possible	Avoid use
L-Tryptophan	Serotonin syndrome possible	Avoid use

out problems. Only a small fraction of patients may have this interaction, and it could reflect an idiosyncratic effect. In general, current opinion favors the use of morphine or fentanyl when intra- or postoperative narcotics are needed in patients taking MAOIs.

The issue of whether directly acting sympathomimetic amines interact with MAOIs is more controversial. Intravenous administration of sympathomimetic amines to patients receiving MAOIs does not provoke hypertension. When a bolus infusion of catecholamines is given to healthy volunteer subjects who have been taking phenelzine or tranylcypromine for 1 week, a potentiation of the pressor effect of phenylephrine occurs, but no clinically significant potentiation of cardiovascular effects of NE, epinephrine, or isoproterenol occurs (Wells 1989).

In general, direct sympathomimetic amine–MAOI interactions do not appear to produce significant cardiovascular problems. However, there is a low incidence of hypertensive episodes in the presence of indirect sympathomimetics. Ideally, these compounds should not be used in those patients who are receiving MAOIs. A direct-acting compound is preferable to an indirect-acting compound.

Caution should be exercised when using MAOIs in patients with pheochromocytoma and cardiovascular, cerebrovascular, and hepatic disease. Because phenelzine tablets contain gluten, they should not be given to patients with celiac disease.

Specific Monoamine Oxidase Inhibitors

Phenelzine

Phenelzine, a hydrazine derivative, is a potent MAOI and the best studied among the MAOIs.

Pharmacokinetics

Phenelzine is a substrate as well as an inhibitor of MAO, and major identified metabolites of phenelzine include phenylacetic acid and p-hydroxyphenylacetic acid. Phenelzine undergoes acetylation, and therefore drug levels are lower in fast acetylators than in slow acetylators. However, because phenelzine is an irreversible inhibitor, plasma concentrations are not relevant. The antidepressant effect, the degree of inhibition of MAO, and the amount of free phenelzine excreted in the urine are all significantly greater in slow acetylators than in fast acetylators (Baker et al. 1999).

Efficacy

Phenelzine is useful in the treatment of major depression, atypical depression, panic disorder, social phobia, and atypical facial pain (see section "Indications and Efficacy" presented earlier in this chapter).

Side Effects

The primary side effects of phenelzine are similar to those of other MAOIs. Hepatitis secondary to phenelzine may occur. This effect is quite rare (<1 in 30,000). The most difficult side effect, often leading to discontinuation, is postural hypotension.

Contraindications

The contraindications to phenelzine include known sensitivity to the drug, pheochromocytoma, congestive heart failure, and history of liver disease. (In addition, see sections "Dietary Interactions" and "Drug–Drug Interactions" presented earlier in this chapter.)

Isocarboxazid

Isocarboxazid is a hydrazine type of MAOI.

Pharmacokinetics

Isocarboxazid is rapidly absorbed from the gastrointestinal tract and is metabolized in the liver. It is primarily excreted as hippuric acid. Its half-life is of little interest because it is an irreversible MAOI. Chemically, isocarboxazid is 5-methyl-3-isoxazolecarboxylic acid 2-benzylhydrazide. Isocarboxazid is a colorless crystalline substance with very little taste.

Efficacy

Isocarboxazid is the least studied of the MAOIs. Its indications are similar to those of the other MAOIs.

Side Effects

The side effects of isocarboxazid are similar to those of phenelzine. Postural hypotension is the most common problem.

Contraindications

The contraindications to isocarboxazid are similar to those of phenelzine.

Tranylcypromine

Tranylcypromine, a nonhydrazine reversible MAOI, increases the concentration of NE, epinephrine, and 5-HT in the CNS. When tranylcypromine is discontinued, about 5 days are needed for recovery of MAO function. Tranylcypromine has a mild stimulant effect.

Pharmacokinetics

Limited data exist on pharmacokinetics. Tranylcypromine is excreted within 24 hours. The dynamic effect lasts for up to 5 days after withdrawal. There is considerable debate about whether it is metabolized to amphetamine; most studies in the literature indicate that this does not occur.

Efficacy

Tranylcypromine's indications are similar to those of other MAOIs (see section "Indications and Efficacy" presented earlier in this chapter).

Side Effects

The side effects of tranylcypromine are similar to those of other MAOIs. In addition, problems with physical dependence on tranylcypromine have been reported. Thus, withdrawal symptoms, such as anxiety, restlessness, depression, and headache, may occur. Syndrome of inappropriate antidiuretic hormone (SIADH) has been reported with tranylcypromine. Rare cases of toxic hepatitis have been reported. Tranylcypromine can lead to increased agitation, insomnia, and restlessness, compared with phenelzine.

Contraindications

The contraindications to tranylcypromine are the same as those for phenelzine. In addition, in view of the greater potential for hypertensive episodes, tranylcypromine should be used with particular caution in patients with cerebrovascular or cardiovascular disease.

Moclobemide

Moclobemide, a reversible inhibitor of MAO-A enzyme (Amrein et al. 1989), has a higher potency in vivo than in vitro. Therefore, it has been suggested that moclobemide is a prodrug and that it is metabolized to a form with higher affinity for MAO-A than the parent compound. After single- or repeated-dose moclobemide administration, the recovery of MAO-A activity is much shorter than that seen with other MAOIs, including clorgyline, an irreversible inhibitor of MAO-A. One of the metabolites of moclobemide does inhibit MAO-B; however, this action is minimally significant in humans. When administered to rats, moclobemide increases the concentration of 5-HT, NE, epinephrine, and DA in rat brain (see Haefely et al. 1992). These effects are short-lasting, and they parallel the time course of MAO-A inhibition. In addition, unlike irreversible inhibitors, repeated administration does not increase the inhibition.

In animals, moclobemide only partially potentiates the blood pressor effect of oral tyramine. This is because it is a reversible inhibitor with a low affinity for the MAO isoenzymes and is easily displaced by the pressor amines ingested in food. On the basis of these studies, moclobemide is thought to be safer than irreversible MAOIs.

Pharmacokinetics

After oral administration of moclobemide, peak plasma concentrations are reached within 1 hour. The drug is about 50% bound to plasma proteins and is extensively metabolized; only 1% of the compound is excreted (unchanged) in the urine. The half-life of the compound is approximately 12 hours. Moclobemide is extensively metabolized; 95% of the administered dose is excreted in the urine. The metabolites are pharmacologically inactive. The presence of food reduces the rate (but not the extent) of moclobemide absorption.

Efficacy

Moclobemide has been studied in all types of depressive disorders (Gabelic and Kuhn 1990; Larsen et al. 1991; Rossel and Moll 1990). Controlled trials have found that it is superior to placebo. In addition, moclobemide has been found to be as effective as imipramine, desipramine, clomipramine, and amitriptyline in the treatment of depression. The dosage required is 300–600 mg/day.

Unlike the classic MAOIs, moclobemide has been found to be effective in treating both endogenous and nonendogenous depression. In addition, in combination with antipsychotics, the drug seems to be effective in treating psychotic depression (Amrein et al. 1989). Moclobemide has also been effective in treating bipolar endogenous depression.

Versiani et al. (1992) compared phenelzine, moclobemide, and placebo and reported that both phenelzine and moclobemide were superior to placebo in treating patients with social phobia. Given the efficacy of classic MAOIs in the treatment of other psychiatric disorders, such as bulimia, panic disorder, and PTSD, it is likely that patients with such disorders would respond to the reversible MAOIs. Additional trials of moclobemide are required to confirm its utility in other psychiatric disorders.

Side Effects

Nausea was the only side effect noted to be greater in patients taking moclobemide than in patients taking placebo. Thus, the profile of moclobemide seems to be ideal in that it causes few or no major side effects. Case reports have shown no toxicity after overdoses of up to 20 g (Amrein et al. 1989).

Dietary Interactions

Intravenous tyramine pressor tests indicate that a single dose of moclobemide increases tyramine sensitivity (Cusson et al. 1991). However, this increase is marginal, compared with the increase associated with other MAOIs. Under most conditions, there appears to be limited drug–food interaction. However, to minimize even mild tyramine pressor effects, it would be preferable to administer moclobemide after a meal rather than before it. In a study in which tyramine was administered in doses of up to 100 mg, inpatients pretreated with moclobemide had no significant changes in blood pressure. The drug also has minimal effect on cognitive performance and no effect on body weight or hematological parameters (Wesnes et al. 1989; Youdim et al. 1987).

Drug–Drug Interactions

Several studies have examined potential drug–drug interactions with moclobemide (Amrein et al. 1992). No drug interaction with lithium or in combination with TCAs has been reported. Moclobemide has also been combined with fluoxetine and other SSRIs with no significant interaction. No interactions with benzodiazepines or neuroleptics have been reported (Amrein et al. 1992). Parallel data suggest that moclobemide can potentiate the effects of meperidine; therefore, the narcotic–MAOI interaction may occur. Until proven otherwise, it would be prudent to avoid the combination of moclobemide with opiates like meperidine. A pharmacokinetic interaction has been observed with cimetidine that requires the reduction of the moclobemide dose because cimetidine reduces the clearance of moclobemide.

Selegiline Hydrochloride

Selegiline hydrochloride is an irreversible MAO-B inhibitor (Cesura and Pletscher 1992). Its primary use is in the treatment of Parkinson's disease, as an adjunct to L-dopa and carbidopa. The average dosage for Parkinson's disease is 5–10 mg/day. The exact mechanism of action of MAO-B in Parkinson's disease is unknown (Gerlach et al. 1996; Hagan et al. 1997; Lyytinen et al. 1997).

Pharmacokinetics

Selegiline is metabolized to levoamphetamine, methamphetamine, and N-desmethylselegiline. Selegiline hydrochloride undergoes significant first-pass metabolism following oral administration. Transdermal delivery avoids the first-pass effect and provides greater levels of unchanged drug and reduced levels of metabolites compared with the oral regimen. The time to reach the peak is less than 1 hour. The elimination half-life of selegiline is about 1.5 hours. There is at least a threefold increase in the area under the curve (AUC) of selegiline with food (Mahmood 1997).

Efficacy

The efficacy of selegiline in treating depression has not been well studied. The few studies that have examined its utility have been equivocal. The dose required for treating depression may be much higher than that required to treat Parkinson's disease. Clinical experience suggests that dosages of 20–40 mg/day are needed. At these dosages, dietary interactions could occur. Early studies have reported that selegiline is of modest benefit in patients with Alzheimer's disease (Lawlor et al. 1997). Quitkin et al. (1984) showed that L-deprenyl was superior to 6 weeks of placebo administered to patients with depression in a separate double-blind study. Dosages of more than 10–20 mg/day were needed.

Side Effects

Selegiline has been found to have no adverse effects when combined with other antidepressants during treatment of depression in patients with Parkinson's disease. The few side effects that have been noted with selegiline include nausea, dizziness, and light-headedness. When the drug is abruptly discontinued, nausea, hallucinations, and confusion have been reported.

Dietary Interactions

Because MAO-B is not involved in the intestinal tyramine interaction, dietary interaction with selegiline (at low dosages, i.e., 5–10 mg/day) would probably be minimal; therefore, no drug interactions have been reported. An interaction between selegiline and narcotics has been reported and should be kept in mind.

Selegiline Transdermal System

The selegiline transdermal system (STS) was developed to overcome limitations of orally administered MAOIs, particularly dietary tyramine restrictions. The system does not overcome drug–drug interactions. It bypasses the gut, thereby reducing drug–food interactions. The pharmacokinetic and pharmacodynamic properties promote the inhibition of MAO-A and MAO-B in the CNS while avoiding significant inhibition of intestinal and liver MAO-A enzymes. Three different strengths of Emsam patch are currently marketed: 20 mg/20 cm^2, 30 mg/30 cm^2, and 40 mg/40 cm^2. The three patch sizes deliver 24-hour doses of selegiline averaging 6 mg, 9 mg, and 12 mg, respectively. Use of the lowest-dosage Emsam 6-mg/24-hour patch does not call for dietary modification. A restricted "MAOI diet" is advised for the higher-dosage Emsam 9-mg/24-hour patch and the 12-mg/24-hour patch to avoid any risk of hypertensive crisis. Patients are strongly advised to follow these restrictions.

Pharmacokinetics

Following dermal application of the selegiline patch, 25%–30% of the selegiline content on average is delivered systemically over 24 hours. Consequently, the degree of drug absorption is one-third higher than the average amounts of 6–12 mg/24 hours. In comparison with oral dosing, transdermal dosing results in substantially higher exposure to selegiline and lower exposure to metabolites.

Efficacy

The efficacy of STS as a treatment for major depressive disorder was established in two placebo-controlled studies of 6 and 8 weeks' duration in adult outpatients with major depressive disorder. In both studies, patients were randomly assigned to double-blind treatment with drug patch or placebo. The 6-week trial showed that 6 mg/24 hours was significantly more effective than placebo, as assessed by scores on the 17-item Hamilton Rating Scale for Depression (Ham-D) (Amsterdam 2003). In an 8-week dosage titration trial, depressed patients receiving the drug patch (starting dose was 6 mg/24 hours, with possible increases to 9 mg/24 hours or 12 mg/24 hours based on clinical response) showed significant improvement compared with those receiving placebo on the primary outcome measure, the 28-item Ham-D total score (Feiger et al. 2006). In another trial, 322 patients meeting DSM-IV-TR (American Psychiatric Association 2000) criteria for major depressive disorder who had responded during an initial 10-week open-label treatment phase were randomly assigned either to continuation at the same dose or to placebo under double-blind conditions for observation of relapse. In this double-blind phase, patients receiving continued selegiline transdermal experienced a significantly longer time to relapse (Amsterdam and Bodkin 2006).

Drug–Drug Interactions

Potential drug interactions for STS are the same as for other MAOIs.

Conclusion

Various MAOIs have been shown to be effective in treating a wide variety of psychiatric disorders, including depression, panic disorder, social phobia, and PTSD. The classic MAOIs are currently used only rarely as first-line medication because of potential dietary interactions and other long-term side effects. The reversible inhibitors of MAO-A enzyme, such as moclobemide, which have fewer side effects and no dietary restrictions compared with classic MAOIs, are unlikely to be introduced in the United States. In fact, the risk–benefit ratio for these compounds is highly favorable, compared with other antidepressants. The MAO-B inhibitor selegiline is used to reduce the progression of Parkinson's disease. Its utility in treating other degenerative disorders is currently being assessed. The selegiline transdermal system reduces dietary interactions when used at low doses and is now approved for the treatment of major depression. New applications and a wider use of these compounds may be found in the near future.

References

American Psychiatric Association: Diagnostic and Statistical Manual of Mental Disorders, 4th Edition, Text Revision. Washington, DC, American Psychiatric Association, 2000

Amrein R, Allen SR, Guentert TW, et al: Pharmacology of reversible MAOIs. Br J Psychiatry 144:66–71, 1989

Amrein R, Guntert TW, Dingemanse J, et al: Interactions of moclobemide with concomitantly administered medication: evidence from pharmacological and clinical studies. Psychopharmacology (Berl) 106 (suppl):S24–S31, 1992

Amsterdam JD: A double-blind, placebo-controlled trial of the safety and efficacy of selegiline transdermal system without dietary restrictions in patients with major depressive disorder. J Clin Psychiatry 64:208–214, 2003

Amsterdam JD, Bodkin JA: Selegiline transdermal system in the prevention of relapse of major depressive disorder: a 52-week, double-blind, placebo-substitution, parallel-group clinical trial. J Clin Psychopharmacol 26:579–586, 2006

Baker GB, Urichuk LJ, McKenna KF, et al: Metabolism of monoamine oxidase inhibitors. Cell Mol Neurobiol 19:411–426, 1999

Blackwell B, Marley E, Price J, et al: Hypertensive interactions between monoamine oxidase inhibitors and food stuffs. Br J Psychiatry 113:349–365, 1967

Bloch RG, Doonief AS, Buchberg AS, et al: The clinical effect of isoniazid and iproniazid in the treatment of pulmonary tuberculosis. Ann Intern Med 40:881–900, 1954

Cesura AM, Pletscher A: The new generation of monoamine oxidase inhibitors. Prog Drug Res 38:171–297, 1992

Cheese and tranylcypromine (letter). BMJ 3(5718):354, 1970

Cooper AJ: MAO inhibitors and headache (letter). BMJ 2:420, 1967

Crane GE: Iproniazid (Marsilid) phosphate, a therapeutic agent for mental disorders and debilitating disease. Psychiatry Research Reports 8:142–152, 1957

Cronin D: Monoamine-oxidase inhibitors and cheese (letter). BMJ 5469:1065, 1965

Cusson JR, Goldenberg E, Larochelle P: Effect of a novel monoamine oxidase inhibitor, moclobemide, on the sensitivity to intravenous tyramine and norepinephrine in humans. J Clin Pharmacol 31:462–467, 1991

DaPrada M, Kettler R, Burkard W, et al: Moclobemide, an antidepressant with short-lasting MAO-A inhibition: brain catecholamines/tyramine pressor effects in rats, in Monoamine Oxidase and Disease. Edited by Tipton K, Dostert P, Strolin Benedetti M. New York, Academic Press, 1984, pp 137–154

DaPrada M, Kettler R, Keller HH, et al: Neurochemical profile of moclobemide, a short-acting and reversible inhibitor of monoamine oxidase type A. J Pharmacol Exp Ther 248:400–414, 1989

Davidson J, Turnbull C: Loss of appetite and weight associated with the monoamine oxidase inhibitor isocarboxazid. J Clin Psychopharmacol 2:263–266, 1982

Davidson J, Raft D, Pelton S: An outpatient evaluation of phenelzine and imipramine. J Clin Psychiatry 48:143–146, 1987a

Davidson J, Walker JI, Kilts C: A pilot study of phenelzine in the treatment of post-traumatic stress disorder. Br J Psychiatry 150:252–255, 1987b

Evans DL, Davidson J, Raft D: Early and late side effects of phenelzine. J Clin Psychopharmacol 2:208–210, 1982

Feiger AD, Rickels K, Rynn MA, et al: Selegiline transdermal system for the treatment of major depressive disorder: an 8-week, double-blind, placebo-controlled, flexible-dose titration trial. J Clin Psychiatry 67:1354–1361, 2006

Finberg JPM, Youdim MBH: Reversible monoamine oxidase inhibitors and the cheese effect, in Monoamine Oxidase and Disease: Prospects for Therapy With Reversible Inhibitors. Edited by Tipton KF, Dostert P, Strolin Benedetti M. New York, Academic Press, 1984, pp 479–485

Gabelic I, Kuhn B: Moclobemide (Ro 11–1163) versus tranylcypromine in the treatment of endogenous depression (abstract). Acta Psychiatr Scand Suppl 360:63, 1990

Gerlach M, Youdim MB, Riederer P: Pharmacology of selegiline. Neurology 47 (6, suppl 3):S137–S145, 1996

Glick R, Harrison W, Endicott J, et al: Treatment of premenstrual dysphoric symptoms in depressed women. J Am Med Womens Assoc 46:182–185, 1991

Goldstein DM, Goldberg RL: Monoamine oxidase inhibitor-induced speech blockage (case report). J Clin Psychiatry 47:604, 1986

Goodheart RS, Dunne JW, Edis RH: Phenelzine associated peripheral neuropathy: clinical and electrophysiologic findings. Aust N Z J Med 21:339–340, 1991

Haefely W, Burkard WP, Cesura AM, et al: Biochemistry and pharmacology of moclobemide: a prototype RIMA. Psychopharmacology (Berl) 106 (suppl):S6–S15, 1992

Hagan JJ, Middlemiss DN, Sharpe PC, et al: Parkinson's disease: prospects for improved drug therapy. Trends Pharmacol Sci 18:156–163, 1997

Harrison WM, Stewart J, Ehrhardt AA, et al: A controlled study of the effects of antidepressants on sexual function. Psychopharmacol Bull 21:85–88, 1985

Hedberg DL, Gordon MW, Glueck BC Jr: Six cases of hypertensive crisis in patients on tranylcypromine after eating chicken livers. Am J Psychiatry 122:933–937, 1966

Himmelhoch JM, Fuchs CZ, Symons BJ: A double-blind study of tranylcypromine treatment of major anergic depression. J Nerv Ment Dis 170:628–634, 1982

Himmelhoch JM, Thase ME, Mallinger AG, et al: Tranylcypromine versus imipramine in anergic bipolar depression. Am J Psychiatry 148:910–916, 1991

Husain M, Edmondson DE, Singer TP: Kinetic studies on the catalytic mechanism of liver monoamine oxidase. Biochemistry 21:595–600, 1982

Jacobson JN: Anorgasmia caused by an MAOI (letter). Am J Psychiatry 144:527, 1987

Jenike MA: Rapid response of severe obsessive-compulsive disorder to tranylcypromine. Am J Psychiatry 138:1249–1250, 1981

Johnstone EC: Relationship between acetylator status and response to phenelzine. Mod Probl Pharmacopsychiatry 10:30–37, 1975

Johnstone EC, Marsh W: The relationship between response to phenelzine and acetylator status in depressed patients. Proc R Soc Lond B Biol Sci 66:947–949, 1973

Kelly D, Mitchell-Heggs N, Sherman D: Anxiety and the effects of sodium lactate assessed clinically and physiologically. Br J Psychiatry 119:129–141, 1971

Kennedy SH, Warsh JJ, Mainprize E, et al: A trial of isocarboxazid in the treatment of bulimia. J Clin Psychopharmacol 8:391–396, 1988

Kline NS: Clinical experience with iproniazid (Marsilid). J Clin Exp Psychopathol 19 (suppl 1):72–78, 1958

Kosten TR, Frank JB, Dan E, et al: Pharmacotherapy for posttraumatic stress disorder using phenelzine or imipramine. J Nerv Ment Dis 179:366–370, 1991

Larsen JK, Gjerris A, Holm P, et al: Moclobemide in depression: a randomized, multicentre trial against isocarboxazide and clomipramine emphasizing atypical depression. Acta Psychiatr Scand 84:564–570, 1991

Lawlor BA, Aisen PS, Green C, et al: Selegiline in the treatment of behavioural disturbance in Alzheimer's disease. Int J Geriatr Psychiatry 12:319–322, 1997

Liebowitz MR, Schneier F, Campeas R, et al: Phenelzine vs atenolol in social phobia: a placebo-controlled comparison. Arch Gen Psychiatry 49:290–300, 1992

Lydiard RB, Laraia MT, Howell EF, et al: Phenelzine treatment of panic disorder: lack of effect on pyridoxal phosphate levels. J Clin Psychopharmacol 9:428–431, 1989

Lyytinen J, Kaakkola S, Ahtila S, et al: Simultaneous MAO-B and COMT inhibition in L-dopa-treated patients with Parkinson's disease. Mov Disord 12:497–505, 1997

Mahmood I: Clinical pharmacokinetics and pharmacodynamics of selegiline. An update. Clin Pharmacokinet 33:91–102, 1997

McElroy SL, Keck PE Jr, Pope HG Jr, et al: Pharmacological treatment of kleptomania and bulimia nervosa. J Clin Psychopharmacol 9:358–360, 1989

McGrath PJ, Stewart JW, Harrison W, et al: Phenelzine treatment of melancholia. J Clin Psychiatry 47:420–422, 1986

McGrath PJ, Stewart JW, Fava M, et al: Tranylcypromine versus venlafaxine plus mirtazapine following three failed antidepressant medication trials for depression: a STAR*D report. Am J Psychiatry 163:1531–1541, 2006

Mendelson G: Narcotics and monoamine oxidase-inhibitors (letter). Med J Aust 1:400, 1979

Murphy DL, Garrick NA, Aulakh CS, et al: New contribution from basic science of understanding the effects of monoamine oxidase inhibiting antidepressants. J Clin Psychiatry 45:37–43, 1984

Murphy DL, Sunderland T, Garrick NA, et al: Selective amine oxidase inhibitors: basic to clinical studies and back, in Clinical Pharmacology in Psychiatry. Edited by Dahl SG, Gram A, Potter W. Berlin, Springer Verlag, 1987, pp 135–146

O'Brien S, McKeon P, O'Regan M, et al: Blood pressure effects of tranylcypromine when prescribed singly and in combination with amitriptyline. J Clin Psychopharmacol 12:104–109, 1992

Paykel ES, West PS, Rowan PR, et al: Influence of acetylator phenotype on antidepressant effects of phenelzine. Br J Psychiatry 141:243–248, 1982

Pearce LB, Roth JA: Human brain monoamine oxidase type B: mechanism of deamination as probed by steady-state methods. Biochemistry 24:1821–1826, 1985

Quitkin F, Rifkin A, Klein DF: Monoamine oxidase inhibitors: a review of antidepressant effectiveness. Arch Gen Psychiatry 36:749–760, 1979

Quitkin FM, Liebowitz MR, Stewart JW, et al: l-Deprenyl in atypical depressives. Arch Gen Psychiatry 41:777–781, 1984

Quitkin FM, McGrath PJ, Stewart JW, et al: Atypical depression, panic attacks, and response to imipramine and phenelzine: a replication. Arch Gen Psychiatry 47:935–941, 1990

Quitkin FM, Harrison W, Stewart JW, et al: Response to phenelzine and imipramine in placebo nonresponders with atypical depression: a new application of the crossover design. Arch Gen Psychiatry 48:319–323, 1991

Ramsay RR, Singer TP: The kinetic mechanisms of monoamine oxidases A and B. Biochem Soc Trans 19:219–223, 1991

Rossel L, Moll E: Moclobemide versus tranylcypromine in the treatment of depression. Acta Psychiatr Scand Suppl 360:61–62, 1990

Rowan PR, Paykel ES, West PS, et al: Effects of phenelzine and acetylator phenotype. Neuropharmacology 20(12B):1353–1354, 1981

Simpson GM, Gratz SS: Comparison of the pressor effect of tyramine after treatment with phenelzine and moclobemide in healthy male volunteers. Clin Pharmacol Ther 52:286–291, 1992

Stack CG, Rogers P, Linter SPK: Monoamine oxidase inhibitors and anaesthesia: a review. Br J Anaesth 60:222–227, 1988

Thase ME, Mallinger AG, McKnight D, et al: Treatment of imipramine-resistant recurrent depression, IV: a double-blind crossover study of tranylcypromine for anergic bipolar depression. Am J Psychiatry 149:195–198, 1992

Tyrer PJ, Candy J, Kelly D: A study of the clinical effects of phenelzine and placebo in the treatment of phobic anxiety. Psychopharmacologia 32:237–254, 1973

Vallejo J, Gasto C, Catalan R, et al: Double-blind study of imipramine versus phenelzine in melancholias and dysthymic disorders. Br J Psychiatry 151:639–642, 1987

Versiani M, Mundim FD, Nardi AE, et al: Tranylcypromine in social phobia. J Clin Psychopharmacol 8:279–283, 1988

Versiani M, Nardi AE, Mundim FD, et al: Pharmacotherapy of social phobia: a controlled study with moclobemide and phenelzine. Br J Psychiatry 161:353–360, 1992

Walsh BT, Stewart JW, Roose SP, et al: A double-blind trial of phenelzine in bulimia. J Psychiatr Res 19:485–489, 1985

Walsh BT, Gladis M, Roose SP, et al: A controlled trial of phenelzine in bulimia. Psychopharmacol Bull 23:49–51, 1987

Wells DG: MAOI revisited. Can J Anaesth 36:64–74, 1989

Wesnes KA, Simpson PM, Christmas L, et al: Acute cognitive effects of moclobemide and trazodone, alone and in combination with alcohol, in the elderly. Br J Clin Pharmacol 27:647P–648P, 1989

White K, Razani J, Cadow B, et al: Tranylcypromine vs nortriptyline vs placebo in depressed outpatients: a controlled trial. Psychopharmacology (Berl) 82:258–262, 1984

Youdim MBH, DaPrada M, Amrein R (eds): The cheese effect and new reversible MAO-A inhibitors. Proceedings of the Round Table of the International Conference on New Directions in Affective Disorders, Jerusalem, Israel, April 5–9, 1987

Zajecka J, Fawcett J: Susceptibility to spontaneous MAOI hypertensive episodes (letter). J Clin Psychiatry 52:513–514, 1991

Zeller EA: Diamine oxidase, in The Enzymes, 2nd Edition, Vol 8. Edited by Boyer PD, Lardy H, Myrback K. London, Academic Press, 1963, pp 313–335

Zisook S: Side effects of isocarboxazid. J Clin Psychiatry 45 (7, part 2):53–58, 1984

Zisook S, Braff DL, Click MA: Monoamine oxidase inhibitors in the treatment of atypical depression. J Clin Psychopharmacol 5:131–137, 1985

CHAPTER 19

Trazodone and Nefazodone

Robert N. Golden, M.D.

Karon Dawkins, M.D.

Linda Nicholas, M.D.

Trazodone was among the earliest "second generation" antidepressants to become available for clinical use in the United States in the early 1980s. Its side-effect profile and potential toxicity were considerably different from and, in many instances preferable to, those of the original antidepressants (i.e., the monoamine oxidase inhibitors [MAOIs] and tricyclic antidepressants [TCAs]). Several years later, its pharmacological "cousin," nefazodone, joined the growing armamentarium of effective antidepressant medications.

Trazodone

History and Discovery

Trazodone was first synthesized in Italy about three decades ago, and clinical studies began in the United States in 1978. Trazodone was different from the conventional antidepressants that were available at that time in several ways. It was the first triazolopyridine derivative to be developed as an antidepressant. In addition, it was developed as an outgrowth of a specific hypothesis (i.e., that depression is caused by an imbalance in the brain mechanisms responsible for the emotional integration of adverse unpleasant experiences). For this reason, new animal models that measured the response to noxious stimuli or situations were used as screening tests for developing the drug. In fact, trazodone is inactive in classic antidepressant screening tests, such as the reserpine model, the potentiation of

yohimbine toxicity, and the behavioral despair/forced swim paradigm, yet it inhibits painful and conditioned emotional responses (Silvestrini 1980). Trazodone shares with the phenothiazines the ability to suppress self-stimulation behavior and amphetamine effects, and it produces substantial blockade of α-adrenergic receptors. In sharp contrast to most other antidepressants available at the time of its development, trazodone showed minimal effects on muscarinic cholinergic receptors.

In 1982, trazodone was introduced for clinical use in the United States under the brand name Desyrel. It quickly became a widely prescribed medication, capturing up to one-third of the American market. More recently, the availability of the extremely popular selective serotonin reuptake inhibitors (SSRIs) has led to a decline in trazodone use. The medication is now available in generic formulation.

Structure–Activity Relations

Trazodone is chemically unrelated to other antidepressant drugs, although it does resemble some of the side-chain components of TCAs and the phenothiazines. Its structure (Figure 19–1) includes a triazole moiety that may be linked to its antidepressant activity.

Pharmacological Profile

The effects of trazodone on serotonergic systems are complex. Trazodone is a relatively weak SSRI, compared with

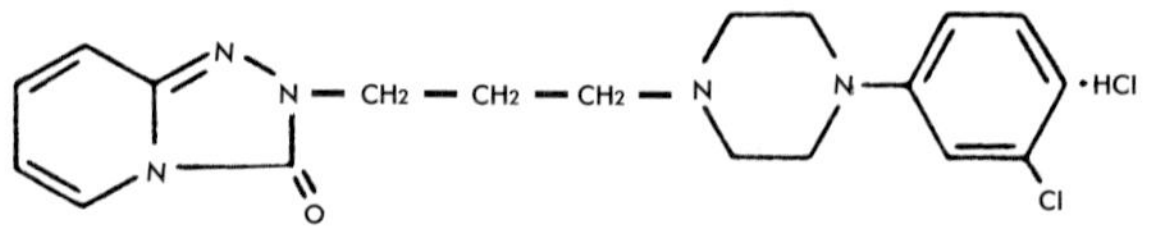

FIGURE 19-1.   Chemical structure of trazodone.

the more potent SSRIs such as fluoxetine or paroxetine. However, it is relatively *specific* for serotonin (5-HT) uptake inhibition, with minimal effects on norepinephrine (NE) or dopamine reuptake (Hyttel 1982). In the rat, systemic administration of trazodone leads to fivefold increases in extracellular 5-HT concentrations in the frontal cortex, which can be blocked by pretreatment with fluoxetine. Direct administration into the frontal cortex via reverse dialysis also elicits increases in extracellular 5-HT levels that are reduced by local perfusion of ketanserin. Thus, trazodone appears to increase extracellular 5-HT concentrations through a combination of mechanisms involving the 5-HT transporter (5-HTT) and the serotonin$_{2A/2C}$ (5-HT$_{2A/2C}$) receptors (Pazzagli et al. 1999). In addition, trazodone has some 5-HT receptor antagonist activity, particularly at serotonin$_{1A}$ (5-HT$_{1A}$), serotonin$_{1C}$ (5-HT$_{1C}$), and serotonin$_2$ (5-HT$_2$) receptor subtypes (Haria et al. 1994). Furthermore, its active metabolite, *m*-chlorophenylpiperazine (m-CPP), is a potent direct 5-HT agonist. Thus, trazodone can be viewed as a mixed serotonergic agonist–antagonist, with the relative amount of m-CPP accumulation affecting the relative degree of the predominant agonist activity.

In vivo, trazodone is virtually devoid of anticholinergic activity, and in clinical studies, the incidence of anticholinergic side effects is similar to that seen with placebo. Trazodone is a relatively weak blocker of presynaptic α$_2$-adrenergic receptors and a relatively potent antagonist of postsynaptic α$_1$-adrenergic receptors. The latter property probably accounts for its propensity to cause orthostatic hypotension. Trazodone has moderate antihistaminergic (histamine$_1$ [H$_1$] receptor) activity.

Pharmacokinetics and Disposition

Trazodone is well absorbed after oral administration, with peak blood levels occurring about 1 hour after dosing when the drug is taken on an empty stomach and about 2 hours after dosing when the drug is taken with food. Trazodone is 89%–95% bound to plasma protein. Elimination appears to be biphasic, consisting of an initial alpha phase followed by a slower beta phase, with half-lives of 3–6 and 5–9 hours, respectively. Bioavailability is not influenced by age or by food intake. Gender differences are inconsistent.

Trazodone undergoes extensive hepatic metabolism, including hydroxylation, splitting at the pyridine ring, oxidation, and *N*-oxidation. Less than 1% of the drug is excreted unchanged in feces and urine. The active metabolite m-CPP is cleared more slowly than the parent compound (4- to 14-hour half-life) and reaches higher concentrations in the brain than in plasma (Caccia et al. 1981). The cytochrome P450 (CYP) 2D6 and 3A microsomal enzyme systems also appear to play a role in trazodone metabolism. CYP3A inhibitors (e.g., ketoconazole, ritonavir, indinavir) inhibit trazodone clearance (see Zalma et al. 2000), and ketoconazole inhibits m-CPP formation (Rotzinger et al. 1998).

The relation between steady-state blood levels and clinical response to trazodone is unclear. In a study involving geriatric patients, plasma concentrations of trazodone were lower in responders compared with nonresponders (Spar 1987). However, this study was limited by the lack of a fixed-dose design (increasing the chances that patients who were destined to be nonresponders would have continued dose increases, yielding relatively higher plasma levels) and a small sample size. Another study of geriatric patients found a positive relation between steady-state trazodone plasma concentrations and clinical response in a sample of 11 subjects (Monteleone and Gnocchi 1990).

Mechanism of Action

The ultimate mechanism of action of trazodone remains unclear. Although the drug is often referred to as a 5-HT reuptake inhibitor, such labeling overlooks the complexity of its effects on this neurotransmitter system. Binding studies confirm that trazodone has relative selectivity for 5-HT reuptake sites (Hyttel 1982); however, in vivo, it blocks the head twitch response induced by classic 5-HT agonists in animals. The potent 5-HT agonist properties of trazodone's major metabolite, m-CPP, may play a role in the mechanism of action of the parent compound. Trazodone, unlike the vast majority of antidepressants, does not produce downregulation of β-adrenergic receptors in rat cortex (Sulser 1983).

Indications and Efficacy

The primary indication for trazodone is the treatment of major depression. In a review of the double-blind studies published after the release of trazodone in this country, Schatzberg (1987) found the therapeutic efficacy of trazodone to be similar to that of TCAs in patients with either endogenous or nonendogenous depression. A review of the European literature by Lader (1987) yielded similar findings: data from open and double-blind trials suggest that the antidepressant efficacy of trazodone is comparable to that of amitriptyline, doxepin, and mianserin. Also, trazodone showed anxiolytic properties, low cardiotoxicity, and relatively mild side effects in the European studies.

Questions have been raised about the effectiveness of trazodone in treating severely ill patients, especially those with prominent psychomotor retardation (Klein and Muller 1985). Shopsin et al. (1981) pointed out that in several unpublished double-blind, controlled studies, the rates of clinical response to trazodone were low (i.e., 10%–20%). Lader (1987) acknowledged that the numbers of patients with psychomotor retardation in the reported studies are too small to resolve the controversy regarding the efficacy of trazodone in this population.

The performance of trazodone, in direct comparisons with other second-generation antidepressants, has been mixed. In a double-blind, placebo-controlled comparison with venlafaxine, the final response rates were 55% for placebo, 60% for trazodone, and 72% for venlafaxine. Trazodone was more effective than venlafaxine in ameliorating sleep disturbances and was associated with the most dizziness and somnolence (Cunningham et al. 1994). In a double-blind comparison, response rates for trazodone and bupropion were 46% and 58%, respectively (see Weisler et al. 1994). In a double-blind study of 200 hospitalized patients with moderate to severe major depressive episode, mirtazapine yielded greater reductions in depression ratings than did trazodone (van Moffaert et al. 1995).

Because trazodone has minimal anticholinergic activity, it was especially welcomed as a treatment for geriatric patients with depression when it first became available. Three double-blind studies reported that trazodone has antidepressant efficacy similar to that of other antidepressants in geriatric patients (Gerner 1987). However, a side effect of trazodone, orthostatic hypotension, which may cause dizziness and increase the risk of falls, can have devastating consequences in elderly patients; thus, this side effect, along with sedation, often makes trazodone less acceptable in this population, compared with newer compounds that share its lack of anticholinergic activity but not the rest of its side-effect profile. Still, trazodone is often helpful for geriatric patients with depression who have severe agitation and insomnia. A recent survey of British geropsychiatrists identified trazodone as one of their most popular adjuncts or alternatives to atypical antipsychotics in the management of behavioral symptoms in the elderly (Condren and Cooney 2001). A randomized, controlled trial found that trazodone, haloperidol, behavioral management techniques, and placebo each produced comparable modest reductions in agitation associated with Alzheimer's disease (Teri et al. 2001). Another double-blind study reported comparable therapeutic effects for trazodone and haloperidol in the treatment of dementia-associated agitated behaviors, with more common adverse effects in the latter group (Sultzer et al. 1997). A recent Cochrane Database review found insufficient evidence to support trazodone as a treatment for the behavioral and psychological symptoms of dementia, although the review could not conclude that trazodone was ineffective, given the limited number of eligible studies (Martinon-Torres et al. 2004).

Trazodone has also been reported to have antianxiety properties. In a randomized, double-blind, placebo-controlled trial, the anxiolytic efficacy of trazodone was comparable to that of diazepam in weeks 3–8 of treatment for generalized anxiety disorder, although patients treated with diazepam had greater improvement during the first 2 weeks of treatment (Rickels et al. 1993). Early case reports had indicated that trazodone is associated with improvement in obsessive-compulsive disorder, but a double-blind, placebo-controlled study found that trazodone lacked antiobsessional effects (Pigott et al. 1992).

Many clinicians use low-dose trazodone as an alternative to benzodiazepines for the treatment of insomnia. Two recent reviews found that trazodone is the second most prescribed agent for insomnia, even though there is minimal evidence to support its use for this indication (Mendelson 2005; Rosenberg 2006). Mendelson (2005) noted that there are few data to support trazodone's use in primary insomnia, because most studies have been limited to patients with depression. In addition, the available literature is characterized by small sample sizes, limited control groups, and weak statistical analyses. Rosenberg (2006) arrived at very similar conclusions. Controlled trials have confirmed trazodone's efficacy (at doses of 50–100 mg) in treating insomnia that occurs as a side effect of some antidepressants (Nierenberg et al. 1994). A retrospective analysis at a Department of Veterans Affairs (VA) medical center found that approximately 24% of patients receiving trazodone were taking other primary antidepressants (Clark and Alexander 2000). Another VA study of patients with posttraumatic stress disorder (PTSD) found that of those patients who were able to tolerate trazodone (60 of 72 patients), 92% reported that it improved sleep onset and 78% reported that it improved sleep maintenance (Warner et al. 2001).

Trazodone has been investigated as a treatment for adjustment disorders in medically ill populations. A randomized, double-blind study found a trend toward greater efficacy in trazodone, compared with clorazepate, in the management of adjustment disorders in patients with breast cancer (Razavi et al. 1999). A similar trend was noted in a study of adjustment disorders in patients who tested positive for HIV (DeWit et al. 1999).

A handful of reports have described the use of trazodone in the treatment of bulimia nervosa, including a well-designed placebo-controlled trial that found trazodone to be superior to placebo in reducing the frequency of episodes of binge eating and vomiting (Hudson et al. 1989). In addition, trazodone has been found to be effective in the treatment of erectile dysfunction in some (e.g., Lance et al. 1995), but not all (e.g., Costabile and Spevak 1999), studies.

Whether prescribed as an antidepressant or a hypnotic, trazodone should always be initiated at a low dose and increased gradually, based on clinical response and tolerance to side effects. For the treatment of a major depressive episode, the suggested initial dosage is 150 mg/day, with increases of 50-mg increments every 3–4 days. Doses may be divided, although many patients prefer bedtime dosing because of the sedating effects. The maximum dosage recommended for outpatients is 400 mg/day, although for inpatients with more severe depression, dosages up to 600 mg/day have been used. When trazodone is prescribed as a hypnotic agent, the usual dose is 50 mg at bedtime, although some patients may require as little as 25 mg or as much as 200–300 mg.

Side Effects and Toxicology

Because of its lack of anticholinergic side effects, trazodone is especially useful in situations in which antimuscarinic effects are particularly problematic (e.g., in patients with prostatic hypertrophy, closed-angle glaucoma, or severe constipation). Trazodone's propensity to cause sedation is a dual-edged sword. For many patients, the relief from agitation, anxiety, and insomnia can be rapid; for other patients, including those individuals with considerable psychomotor retardation and feelings of low energy, therapeutic doses of trazodone may not be tolerable because of sedation.

Trazodone elicits orthostatic hypotension in some patients, probably as a consequence of α_1-adrenergic receptor blockade. Trazodone-related syncope in the elderly has been described in the literature (Nambudiri et al.

1989). A study of nursing home residents, however, found no increased rate of falls during the initiation of trazodone therapy, compared with tricyclic or SSRI therapy (Thapa et al. 1998). By contrast, trazodone was found to be among the top three medications associated with orthostatic hypotension in patients attending a VA geriatric clinic (Poon and Braun 2005). Case reports have noted cardiac arrhythmias emerging in relation to trazodone treatment, both in patients with preexisting mitral valve prolapse and in patients with negative personal and family histories of cardiac disease (see Janowsky et al. 1983; Lippman et al. 1983; Winkler et al. 2006).

A relatively rare, but dramatic, side effect associated with trazodone is priapism. More than 200 cases have been reported (Thompson et al. 1990), and the manufacturer estimates that the incidence of any abnormal erectile function is approximately 1 in 6,000 male patients treated with trazodone. The risk for this side effect appears to be greatest during the first month of treatment at low dosages (i.e., <150 mg/day). Early recognition of any abnormal erectile function, including prolonged or inappropriate erections, is important and should prompt discontinuation of trazodone treatment. Clinical reports have also described trazodone-associated psychosexual side effects in women, including increased libido (Gatrell 1986), priapism of the clitoris (Pescatori et al. 1993), and spontaneous orgasms (Purcell and Ghurye 1995).

Mania has been observed in association with trazodone treatment (as with nearly all antidepressants), including in patients with bipolar disorder as well as in patients with previous diagnoses of unipolar depression. Terao (1993) found that the switch process occurs more rapidly in trazodone-treated patients than in fluoxetine-treated patients.

Trazodone appears to be *relatively* safer than TCAs, MAOIs, and a few of the other second-generation antidepressants in overdose situations, especially when it is the only agent taken. Fatalities are rare, and uneventful recoveries have been reported after ingestion of doses as high as 6,000–9,200 mg (Ayd 1984). In one report, 9 of 294 cases of overdose were fatal, and all 9 patients had also taken other central nervous system (CNS) depressants (Gamble and Peterson 1986). When trazodone overdoses occur, clinicians should carefully monitor for hypotension, a potentially serious toxic effect. In a report of a fatal trazodone overdose, torsades de pointes and complete atrioventricular block developed, along with subsequent multiple organ failure, with a trazodone plasma concentration of 25.4 μg/mL on admission (de Meester et al. 2001).

Drug–Drug Interactions

Trazodone can potentiate the effects of other CNS depressants. Patients should be warned about increased drowsiness and sedation when trazodone is combined with other CNS depressants, including alcohol.

The combination of trazodone with an MAOI, as with other antidepressants, should be handled with great caution, although there are case reports of the successful combination of trazodone with an MAOI (Zimmer et al. 1984). Development of the serotonin syndrome has been associated with the combination of trazodone with other proserotonergic agents, including an MAOI (plus methylphenidate) (Bodner et al. 1995), buspirone (Goldberg and Huk 1992), paroxetine (Reeves and Bullen 1995), nefazodone (Margolese and Chouinard 2000), and lithium plus amitriptyline (Nisijima et al. 1996). The addition of fluoxetine to trazodone treatment led to increases in plasma concentrations of both trazodone and m-CPP (Maes et al. 1997).

Trazodone inhibits the antihypertensive effects of clonidine (Georgotas et al. 1982). On the other hand, trazodone itself can cause hypotension, especially orthostatic hypotension, and the manufacturer states in the package insert for Desyrel that concomitant administration of trazodone with antihypertensive therapy may require a reduction in the dose of the antihypertensive agent.

Drug–drug interactions with anticoagulants are of great concern, given the potentially serious consequences of too much or too little anticoagulant effect. Three clinically significant cases of suspected trazodone–warfarin interactions were described in a retrospective chart review (Small and Giamonna 2000). The initiation of trazodone treatment was associated with a subsequent decrease in prothrombin time (PT) and international normalized ratio (INR) that could not be explained by other factors. Conversely, in a patient who stopped trazodone, PT and INR increased.

Recently, combined administration of the antibiotic linezolid and trazodone has been associated with emergence of serotonin syndrome (Bergeron et al. 2005).

Nefazodone

History and Discovery

Trazodone's sedative properties and association with orthostatic hypotension eventually inspired an effort to discover a modified molecule, utilizing receptor-binding techniques, which would possess a more desirable pharmacological profile. This led to the development of nefazodone (Taylor et al. 1986), which became available for clinical use in the United States in 1994. Nefazodone can be considered a member of the trazodone family because they share a common active metabolite.

Structure–Activity Relations

Nefazodone is a phenylpiperazine compound. Its chemical structure, shown in Figure 19–2, is similar to that of trazodone.

Pharmacological Profile

Nefazodone is a 5-HT_2 receptor antagonist and a weak inhibitor of 5-HT and NE reuptake. It has little affinity for α_2-adrenergic, β-adrenergic, or 5-HT_{1A} receptors, and its affinity for the α_1-adrenergic receptor is less than that of trazodone (Eison et al. 1990). Nefazodone is inactive at most other receptor-binding sites, including H_1, muscarinic, dopamine, benzodiazepine, γ-aminobutyric acid (GABA), μ opiate, and calcium channel receptors (Taylor et al. 1986).

Nefazodone demonstrates several of the classic preclinical characteristics of antidepressants. It prevents reserpine-induced ptosis in mice and reverses learned helplessness in rats. The effects of nefazodone on electrophysiological measures of serotonergic systems are similar to those of many other effective antidepressants (Blier et al. 1990). In humans, nefazodone does not suppress rapid eye movement (REM) sleep, in contrast to most other antidepressants (Sharpley et al. 1996).

Pharmacokinetics and Disposition

Nefazodone is rapidly and completely absorbed and is then extensively metabolized, resulting in a low (about 20%) and variable absolute bioavailability. The plasma half-life is only 2–4 hours. Nefazodone has three active metabolites: desethyl hydroxynefazodone (triazole dione), hydroxynefazodone, and m-CPP. Triazole dione is a specific 5-HT_2 antagonist with weaker affinity for that re-

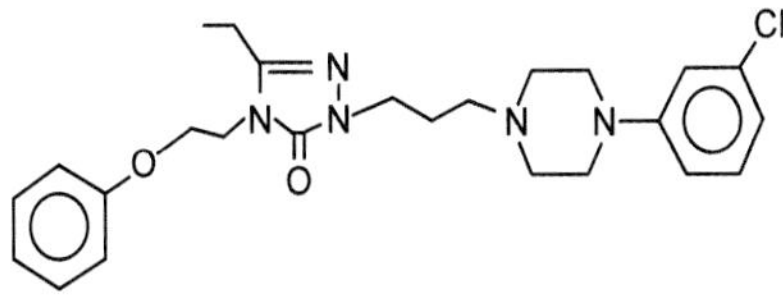

FIGURE 19–2. Chemical structure of nefazodone.

ceptor than the parent compound and no appreciable effects on 5-HT reuptake. With a plasma half-life of 18 hours, triazole dione predominates in the plasma, occurring at concentrations approaching four times that of the parent compound. Hydroxynefazodone has similar affinities for the 5-HT$_2$ receptor and 5-HT reuptake site as the parent compound. Its plasma half-life is between 1.5 and 4 hours, and at steady state, plasma concentrations are approximately 40% of the parent compound. m-CPP is a direct agonist at the 5-HT$_1$, 5-HT$_2$, and serotonin$_3$ (5-HT$_3$) receptors, with one order of magnitude higher affinity for 5-HT$_{2C}$ receptors. m-CPP has a plasma half-life of 4–8 hours, and its plasma concentrations are only 7% of those seen with the parent compound (DeVane et al. 2002; Eison et al. 1990; Mayol et al. 1994).

In rodent studies, there are striking differences in the brain-to-blood partition of nefazodone and its metabolites. The ratios of m-CPP to nefazodone concentrations in the brain are 47:1 and 10:1 in the mouse and rat, respectively. Brain concentrations of hydroxynefazodone in the rat are less than 10% of those in plasma, suggesting very poor blood–brain barrier penetration. Thus, despite its relatively lower plasma concentrations, m-CPP has substantial presence in the brain, whereas the in vivo activity of hydroxynefazodone may be mostly the result of its biotransformation to m-CPP (Nacca et al. 1998).

Nefazodone has nonlinear kinetics, which result in greater than proportional mean plasma concentrations with higher doses. Similar kinetics for nefazodone and hydroxynefazodone are seen in poor and extensive metabolizers, whereas m-CPP is eliminated more slowly by poor metabolizers. Nefazodone is extensively (99%) but loosely protein bound. It does not displace chlorpromazine, desipramine, diazepam, diphenylhydantoin, lidocaine, prazosin, propranolol, verapamil, or warfarin (Bristol-Myers Squibb Pharmaceutical Research Institute, data on file, June 1994). In patients with hepatic cirrhosis, single-dose nefazodone and hydroxynefazodone levels are about twice as high as in healthy volunteers, but the difference decreases to approximately 25% at steady state. Exposure to m-CPP is about two- to threefold greater in patients with cirrhosis, and exposure to triazole dione is similar after a single dose and at steady state (Barbhaiya et al. 1995).

Mechanism of Action

The mechanism of action of nefazodone is poorly understood. The manufacturer indicates that nefazodone antagonizes 5-HT$_2$ receptors and also inhibits neuronal up-

take of both 5-HT and NE (Serzone [package insert] 2002). Several reviews refer to nefazodone as a "dual acting" antidepressant, suggesting that it enhances both serotonergic and noradrenergic neurotransmission via uptake blockade. Although it is accurate to characterize nefazodone as having similar effects on the 5-HTT and NE transporter, such a description is potentially misleading. Nefazodone's inhibition of NE reuptake is weaker than that of the SSRI fluoxetine, and approximately three orders of magnitude weaker than what is seen with conventional NE reuptake inhibitors, such as desipramine. Furthermore, nefazodone's inhibition of 5-HT reuptake is nearly identical to that of desipramine and more than 100-fold less than that of fluoxetine (Bolden-Watson and Richelson 1993). Thus, the "dual action" of nefazodone refers to minimal, albeit equal, effects on 5-HT and NE reuptake inhibition.

In a study examining the clinical psychobiological effects of nefazodone and SSRIs in patients with depression, the latter treatment yielded decreases from mean baseline platelet 5-HT content that were significantly greater than the effects of nefazodone, suggesting that therapeutic doses of nefazodone do not cause sustained 5-HT uptake inhibition at the platelet 5-HTT (Narayan et al. 1998). The active metabolite m-CCP, which appears to predominate in the brain because of greater penetration of the blood–brain barrier (for details, see Nacca et al. 1998), may play an important role in the mechanism of action.

Indications and Efficacy

In three of four Phase III imipramine- and placebo-controlled studies, nefazodone was found to be an effective antidepressant with similar efficacy to imipramine; in one of these studies, neither active drug had significantly greater efficacy than did placebo. The incidence of premature treatment discontinuation and side effects was higher for the imipramine group than for the nefazodone treatment group (Rickels et al. 1995). In a double-blind study without a placebo control group, there was no significant difference in the clinical responses to nefazodone and sertraline in outpatients with depression, and sertraline had negative effects on sexual function and satisfaction (Feiger et al. 1996). A similar study in outpatients with moderate to severe depression found no difference between nefazodone and paroxetine in treatment outcome or discontinuation because of adverse events (Baldwin et al. 1996). Hospitalized patients with severe major depression achieved higher response rates to nefazodone, compared with placebo (Feighner et al. 1998). In contrast, a European study of patients with moderate to severe major depression reported that the efficacy of amitriptyline (50–200 mg/day) was clearly superior to that of nefazodone (100–400 mg/day) (Ansseau et al. 1994). In one of the first studies to include psychotherapy, Keller et al. (2000) compared nefazodone, cognitive-behavioral therapy (CBT), and a combination of these two treatments in a double-blind study of patients with chronic major depressive disorder. Each monotherapy yielded a response rate of 48%, whereas the combined treatment had a greater efficacy (73%). When patients who failed to respond to 12 weeks of treatment with either nefazodone or cognitive-behavioral analysis system psychotherapy are then switched to the other treatment, significant symptom improvement is achieved (Schatzberg et al. 2005). Nefazodone has also been shown to be effective in the continuation phase of treatment in double-blind studies with and without placebo controls (Anton et al. 1994; Baldwin et al. 2001; Feiger et al. 1999).

The usual starting dosage of nefazodone, as recommended by the manufacturer, is 200 mg/day in two divided doses. The suggested dosage range is 300–600 mg/day. Increases should be in increments of 100–200 mg/day at weekly intervals. The manufacturer points out that the starting dosage in elderly or debilitated patients should be lowered to 100 mg/day, again taken in two divided doses, and the rate of titration in these patient populations should be adjusted accordingly (Serzone [package insert] 2002). In a recent review expanding on this guideline, Zajecka et al. (2002) reported that in studies comparing low-dosage (50–250 mg/day) and high-dosage (100–500 mg/day) nefazodone, better clinical response was obtained in the latter group, and the mean effective dosage ranged from 375 to 460 mg/day. A lower starting dose should be considered when switching to nefazodone from an SSRI if a full washout has not been completed. The authors also cite data suggesting that once-daily bedtime dosing is safe, well tolerated, and effective (Zajecka et al. 2002).

Nefazodone has also been studied in other specific patient populations, including patients with substance abuse disorders. In a double-blind, placebo-controlled study, nefazodone was found to be safe and effective in the treatment of depression in patients with alcohol dependence, although it did not add any advantage over psychoeducational group intervention in terms of drinking outcomes (Roy-Byrne et al. 2000). A double-blind, controlled study found that nefazodone was not efficacious for the treatment of alcohol dependence (Kranzler et al. 2000). A recent randomized, placebo-controlled, double-blind multicenter study compared nefazodone versus placebo and CBT versus nondirective group counseling (GC) for relapse prevention in alcohol dependence. Two hundred forty-two male patients with alcohol dependence received either nefazodone plus GC or CBT or placebo plus GC or CBT. There were no differences between the four groups in cumulative days of abstinence or amount of alcohol consumed during specified time periods during the initial 12-week study phase. After 1 year, the only significant difference between the groups was higher alcohol consumption in the nefazodone plus GC group, raising concerns that nefazodone may potentially increase the risk of relapse (Wetzel et al. 2004). A 10-week randomized, double-blind, placebo-controlled trial found no difference between nefazodone and placebo in the treatment of inhaled cocaine dependence (Passos et al. 2005). An 8-week double-blind, placebo-controlled trial of nefazodone in patients with cocaine dependence and comorbid depressive symptoms found equivalent improvements in self-reported cocaine use, psychosocial functioning, and mood in the nefazodone and placebo treatment groups (Ciraulo et al. 2005).

A 1998 open-label study found nefazodone to be effective in the treatment of social phobia (Worthington et al. 1998), but a more recent randomized, double-blind trial in 105 patients with generalized social phobia found no difference between nefazodone and placebo on the primary outcome measures (van Ameringen et al. 2007). Open-label studies with relatively small sample sizes have described the efficacy of nefazodone in the treatment of PTSD (Hidalgo et al. 1999), panic disorder (Bystritsky et al. 1999), generalized anxiety disorder (Hedges et al. 1996), chronic fatigue syndrome (Goodnick and Jorge 1999), chronic daily headache prophylaxis (Saper et al. 2001), depression in HIV-seropositive outpatients (Elliot et al. 1999), and seasonal affective disorder in women (Shen et al. 2005). A few open-label reports described the efficacy of nefazodone in the treatment of late luteal phase dysphoric disorder; however, a double-blind, controlled study reported no significant difference compared with placebo (Landen et al. 2001).

Side Effects and Toxicology

Nefazodone has been found to be safe and well tolerated in clinical trials that included approximately 2,250 patients. Side effects that occur more frequently in patients who receive nefazodone, compared with placebo, include dizziness, asthenia, dry mouth, nausea, and constipation. There was no evidence of cardiac dysfunction or cardiotoxicity in a careful review of more than 2,000 patients. Nefazodone modestly reduced resting pulse rate and supine blood pressure, but orthostatic hypotension was rare (Fontaine 1993).

Preskorn (1995) found that the total cumulative incidence of treatment-emergent adverse effects for nefazodone was lower than that of imipramine or fluoxetine. The most common placebo-adjusted adverse effects associated with nefazodone were dry mouth (7.5%), somnolence (5.8%), dizziness (5.6%), nausea (5.5%), constipation (3.3%), blurred vision (3.2%), and postural hypotension (2.6%). In the premarketing clinical trials, based on experience with approximately 3,500 patients, the rate of discontinuation due to adverse events for nefazodone was lower than that for imipramine and was comparable to that of fluoxetine (Robinson et al. 1996).

There are several reported cases of nefazodone-induced liver failure, including some in which there was irreversible damage (Aranda-Michel et al. 1999; Lucena et al. 1999; Schirren and Baretton 2000). The manufacturer issued a black box warning in the package insert, which describes a reported rate of life-threatening liver failure in this country of 1 per 250,000–300,000 patient-years of nefazodone treatment. Recommendations include avoiding the initiation of nefazodone treatment in patients with active liver disease or elevated baseline serum transaminases (because preexisting abnormalities can complicate patient monitoring); advising patients to be alert for signs and symptoms of liver dysfunction and to report any such occurrences to their doctor immediately; and discontinuing treatment if clinical signs or symptoms suggest liver failure. Any patient who develops evidence of liver damage, such as serum aspartate aminotransferase (AST) or alanine aminotransferase (ALT) levels that are three times greater than the upper limit of normal, while taking nefazodone should have the medication withdrawn and should never be reexposed.

Nefazodone appears to have advantages over SSRIs in terms of treatment-associated sexual dysfunction. An open-label multicenter prospective study of 1,022 patients with previously normal sexual function found substantially higher rates of treatment-associated sexual dysfunction with SSRIs (ranging from 58% to 73%), compared with nefazodone (8%) (Montejo et al. 2001). In a study of 105 patients with depression who had developed adverse sexual side effects attributable to sertraline, random double-blind assignment to either nefazodone or sertraline found significantly lower rates of reemergent sexual dysfunction with nefazodone (26%), compared with sertraline (76%), and the former group was more satisfied with sexual functioning than the latter group (Ferguson et al.

2001). In a recent cross-sectional study of more than 6,000 outpatients, nefazodone and bupropion were found to be associated with lower risk for sexual dysfunction, compared with SSRIs, mirtazapine, and venlafaxine (Clayton et al. 2002).

In a recent review of 1,338 humans with exposure to nefazodone poisoning, there were no reported deaths, and in the 45 cases for which estimated doses were available, no dose–response relationship emerged. The most common findings were drowsiness, nausea, and dizziness. The most common serious clinical effect was hypotension, reported in 1.6% of cases. No patients required intubation, mechanical ventilation, or vasopressors, and this analysis suggests that nefazodone appears to have low toxicity in overdose situations (Benson et al. 2000).

Other rare nefazodone side effects have been described. An unusual visual side effect, akinetopsia (characterized by the inability to perceive motion in a normal, smooth fashion), as well as persistent strobelike images and visual trails behind moving objects, has been reported (Horton and Trobe 1999). A case report of nefazodone-induced mania supports the popular clinical opinion that probably all effective antidepressants can stimulate the switch process (Jeffries and Al-Jeshi 1995). There is a single case report of nefazodone-induced clitoral priapism lasting 3 days (Brodie-Meijer et al. 1999).

Drug–Drug Interactions

The manufacturer of triazolam warns that its concurrent use with nefazodone is contraindicated because of nefazodone's significant inhibition of oxidative metabolism mediated by CYP3A. Increases in the plasma concentration of digoxin occur with concurrent nefazodone administration, and although the increases are relatively modest, the combined administration of these two drugs should be avoided, in light of the narrow therapeutic index for digoxin. Nefazodone increases the plasma concentrations of terfenadine and loratadine (with associated QTc prolongation), carbamazepine (Abernethy et al. 2001; Laroudie et al. 2000), and cyclosporin (Wright et al. 1999). No significant pharmacokinetic or pharmacodynamic interactions have been noted between nefazodone and lorazepam, lithium, alcohol, cimetidine, propranolol, warfarin, or theophylline (Greene and Barbhaiya 1997).

Conclusion

Trazodone, one of the first second-generation antidepressants, and its pharmacological "cousin," nefazodone, do not readily fit within the conventional classifications of antidepressants. Do any common themes link these two "miscellaneous" medications?

In a way, trazodone and nefazodone (as well as bupropion and the tertiary-amine TCAs) remind us of the potential importance of metabolites in the clinical profile of pharmacological agents. m-CPP, the shared active metabolite of trazodone and nefazodone, may play a role in their mechanisms of action. Future research should clarify the specific role of this metabolite and its potential utility in therapeutic blood level monitoring.

Another theme is the important advantage for clinicians in understanding the basic pharmacology of a drug. Many side effects can be understood, or even predicted, on the basis of the pharmacological profiles of a medication. Thus, the propensity of trazodone to evoke orthostatic hypotension makes sense in light of its effects on α-adrenergic receptors.

A review of trazodone also points out that "side effects" can potentially be exploited in the service of helping patients with conditions that are outside the realm of a drug's initial indication. The sedative properties of trazodone have led to its use in treating both primary and secondary insomnia (even in the absence of a strong evidence base to support this indication). The relatively rare side effect of priapism sparked several clinical studies in patients with erectile dysfunction, although the results to date are mixed. Thus, when thinking about side effects, one should consider the adage "One man's ceiling is another man's floor"; a clinical effect of a medication that is troubling to certain patients might potentially find use in treating targeted symptoms of other conditions.

Finally, each novel antidepressant adds to our available tools for the treatment of depression. Although we do not have a "perfect" antidepressant therapy that is safe and effective for all patients, novel compounds provide clinicians with additional options and flexibility in selecting the best available approach for each individual patient.

References

Abernethy DR, Barbey JT, Franc J, et al: Loratadine and terfenadine interaction with nefazodone: both antihistamines are associated with QTc prolongation. Clin Pharmacol Ther 69:96–103, 2001

Ansseau M, Darimont P, Lecoq A, et al: Controlled comparison of nefazodone and amitriptyline in major depressive inpatients. Psychopharmacology (Berl) 115:254–260, 1994

Anton SF, Robinson DS, Roberts DL, et al: Long-term treatment of depression with nefazodone. Psychopharmacol Bull 30:165–169, 1994

Aranda-Michel J, Koehler A, Bejarano PA, et al: Nefazodone-induced liver failure: report of three cases. Ann Intern Med 130:285–288, 1999

Ayd FJ Jr: Pharmacology update: which antidepressant to choose, II: the overdose factor. Psychiatric Annals 14:212–214, 1984

Baldwin DS, Hawley CJ, Abed RT, et al: A multicenter double-blind comparison of nefazodone and paroxetine in the treatment of outpatients with moderate-to-severe depression. J Clin Psychiatry 57 (suppl 2):46–52, 1996

Baldwin DS, Hawley CJ, Mellors K, et al: A randomized, double-blind controlled comparison of nefazodone and paroxetine in the treatment of depression: safety, tolerability and efficacy in continuation phase treatment. J Psychopharmacol 15:161–165, 2001

Barbhaiya RJ, Sukla UA, Matarakam CS, et al: Single- and multiple-dose pharmacokinetics of nefazodone in patients with hepatic cirrhosis. Clin Pharmacol Ther 58:390–398, 1995

Bergeron L, Boule M, Perreault S: Serotonin toxicity associated with concomitant use of linezolid. Ann Pharmacother 39:956–961, 2005

Benson BE, Mathiason M, Dahl B, et al: Toxicities and outcomes associated with nefazodone poisoning: an analysis of 1,338 exposures. Am J Emerg Med 18:587–592, 2000

Blier P, de Montigny C, Chaput Y: A role for the serotonin system in the mechanism of action of antidepressant treatments: preclinical evidence. J Clin Psychiatry 51 (suppl 4):14–20, 1990

Bodner RA, Lynch T, Lewis L, et al: Serotonin syndrome. Neurology 45:219–223, 1995

Bolden-Watson C, Richelson E: Blockade by newly developed antidepressants of biogenic amine uptake into rat brain synaptosomes. Life Sci 52:1023–1029, 1993

Brodie-Meijer CC, Diemont WL, Buijs PJ: Nefazodone-induced clitoral priapism. Int Clin Psychopharmacol 14:257–258, 1999

Bystritsky A, Rosen R, Suri R, et al: Pilot open-label study of nefazodone in panic disorder. Depress Anxiety 10:137–139, 1999

Caccia S, Ballabio M, Fanelli R, et al: Determination of plasma and brain concentrations of trazodone and its metabolite, 1-m-chlorophenylpiperazine, by gas-liquid chromatography. J Chromatogr 210:311–318, 1981

Ciraulo DA, Knapp C, Rotrosen J, et al: Nefazodone treatment of cocaine dependence with comorbid depressive symptoms. Addiction 100 (suppl 1):23–31, 2005

Clark NA, Alexander B: Increased rate of trazodone prescribing with bupropion and selective serotonin reuptake inhibitors versus tricyclic antidepressants. Ann Pharmacother 34:1007–1012, 2000

Clayton AH, Pradko JF, Croft HA, et al: Prevalence of sexual dysfunction among newer antidepressants. J Clin Psychiatry 63:357–366, 2002

Condren CM, Cooney C: Use of drugs by old age psychiatrists in the treatment of psychotic and behavioural symptoms in patients with dementia. Aging Ment Health 5:235–241, 2001

Costabile RA, Spevak M: Oral trazodone is not effective therapy for erectile dysfunction: a double-blind, placebo-controlled trial. J Urol 161:1819–1822, 1999

Cunningham LA, Borison RL, Carman JS, et al: A comparison of venlafaxine, trazodone, and placebo in major depression. J Clin Psychopharmacol 14:99–106, 1994

de Meester A, Carbutti G, Gabriel L, et al: Fatal overdose with trazodone: case report and literature review. Acta Clin Belg 56:258–261, 2001

DeVane CL, Grothe DR, Smith SL: Pharmacology of antidepressants: focus on nefazodone. J Clin Psychiatry 63 (suppl 1):10–17, 2002

DeWit S, Cremers L, Hirsch D, et al: Efficacy and safety of trazodone versus clorazepate in the treatment of HIV-positive subjects with adjustment disorders: a pilot study. J Int Med Res 27:223–232, 1999

Eison AS, Eison MS, Torrente JR, et al: Nefazodone: preclinical pharmacology of a new antidepressant. Psychopharmacol Bull 26:311–315, 1990

Elliot AJ, Russo J, Bergam K, et al: Antidepressant efficacy in HIV-seropositive outpatients with depressive disorder: an open trial of nefazodone. J Clin Psychiatry 60:226–231, 1999

Feiger A, Kiev A, Shriastava RK, et al: Nefazodone versus sertraline in outpatients with major depression: focus on efficacy, tolerability, and effects on sexual function and satisfaction. J Clin Psychiatry 57 (suppl 2):53–62, 1996

Feiger AD, Bielski RJ, Bremner J, et al: Double-blind, placebo substitution study of nefazodone in the prevention of relapse during continuation treatment of outpatients with major depression. Int Clin Psychopharmacol 14:19–28, 1999

Feighner J, Targum SD, Bennett ME, et al: A double-blind, placebo-controlled trial of nefazodone in the treatment of patients hospitalized for major depression. J Clin Psychiatry 59:246–253, 1998

Ferguson JM, Shrivastava RK, Stahl SM, et al: Reemergence of sexual dysfunction in patients with major depressive disorder: double-blind comparison of nefazodone and sertraline. J Clin Psychiatry 62:24–29, 2001

Fontaine R: Novel serotonergic mechanisms and clinical experience with nefazodone. Clin Neuropharmacol 16 (suppl 3): S45–S50, 1993

Gamble DE, Peterson LG: Trazodone overdose: four years of experience from voluntary reports. J Clin Psychiatry 47:544–546, 1986

Gatrell N: Increased libido in women receiving trazodone. Am J Psychiatry 143:781–782, 1986

Georgotas A, Forsell TL, Mann JJ, et al: Trazodone hydrochloride: a wide spectrum antidepressant with a unique pharmacological profile. Pharmacotherapy 2:255–265, 1982

Gerner RH: Geriatric depression and treatment with trazodone. Psychopathology 20:82–91, 1987

Goldberg RJ, Huk M: Serotonin syndrome from trazodone and buspirone (letter). Psychosomatics 33:235–236, 1992

Goodnick PJ, Jorge CM: Treatment of chronic fatigue syndrome with nefazodone. Am J Psychiatry 156:797–798, 1999

Greene DS, Barbhaiya RH: Clinical pharmacokinetics of nefazodone. Clin Pharmacokinet 33:260–275, 1997

Haria M, Fitton A, McTavish D: Trazodone: a review of its pharmacology, therapeutic use in depression and therapeutic potential in other disorders. Drugs Aging 4:331–335, 1994

Hedges DW, Reimherr FW, Strong RE, et al: An open trial of nefazodone in adult patients with generalized anxiety disorder. Psychopharmacol Bull 32:671–676, 1996

Hidalgo R, Hertzberg MA, Mellman T, et al: Nefazodone in posttraumatic stress disorder: results from six open-label trials. Int Clin Psychopharmacol 14:61–68, 1999

Horton JC, Trobe JD: Akinetopsia from nefazodone toxicity. Am J Ophthalmol 28:530–531, 1999

Hudson JI, Pope HG Jr, Keck PE Jr, et al: Treatment of bulimia nervosa with trazodone: short-term response and long-term follow-up. Clin Neuropharmacol 12 (suppl 1):38–46, 1989

Hyttel J: Citalopram—pharmacologic profile of a specific serotonin uptake inhibitor with antidepressant activity. Prog Neuropsychopharmacol Biol Psychiatry 6:277–295, 1982

Janowsky D, Curtis G, Zisook S, et al: Ventricular arrhythmias possibly aggravated by trazodone. Am J Psychiatry 140:796–797, 1983

Jeffries JJ, Al-Jeshi A: Nefazodone-induced mania. Can J Psychiatry 40:218, 1995

Keller MB, McCullough JP, Klein DN, et al: A comparison of nefazodone, the cognitive behavioral-analysis system of psychotherapy, and their combination for the treatment of chronic depression. N Engl J Med 342:1462–1470, 2000

Klein HE, Muller N: Trazodone in endogenous depressed patients: a negative report and a critical evaluation of the pertaining literature. Prog Neuropsychopharmacol Biol Psychiatry 9:173–186, 1985

Kranzler HR, Modesto-Lowe V, Van Kirk J: Naltrexone vs nefazodone for treatment of alcohol dependence: a placebo controlled trial. Neuropsychopharmacology 22:493–503, 2000

Lader M: Recent experience with trazodone. Psychopathology 20 (suppl 1):39–47, 1987

Lance R, Albo M, Costabile RA, et al: Oral trazodone as empirical therapy for erectile dysfunction: a retrospective review. Urology 46:117–120, 1995

Landen M, Ericksson O, Sundblad C, et al: Compounds with affinity for serotonergic receptors in the treatment of premenstrual dysphoria: a comparison of buspirone, nefazodone and placebo. Psychopharmacology (Berl) 155:292–298, 2001

Laroudie C, Salazar DE, Cosson JP, et al: Carbamazepine–nefazodone interaction in healthy subjects. J Clin Psychopharmacol 20:46–53, 2000

Lippman S, Bedford P, Manshadi M, et al: Trazodone cardiotoxicity (letter). Am J Psychiatry 140:1383, 1983

Lucena MI, Andrade RJ, Gomez-Outes A, et al: Acute liver failure after treatment with nefazodone. Dig Dis Sci 44:2577–2579, 1999

Maes M, Westenberg H, Vandoolaeghe E, et al: Effects of trazodone and fluoxetine in the treatment of major depression: therapeutic pharmacokinetic and pharmacodynamic interactions through formation of meta-chlorophenylpiperazine. J Clin Psychopharmacol 17:358–364, 1997

Margolese HC, Chouinard G: Serotonin syndrome from the addition of low-dose trazodone to nefazodone. Am J Psychiatry 157:1022, 2000

Martinon-Torres G, Fioravanti M, Grimley EJ: Trazodone for agitation in dementia. Cochrane Database Syst Rev (4):CD004990, 2004

Mayol RF, Cole CA, Luke GM, et al: Characterization of the metabolites of the antidepressant drug nefazodone in human urine and plasma. Drug Metab Dispos 22:304–311, 1994

Mendelson WB: A review of the evidence for the efficacy and safety of trazodone in insomnia. J Clin Psychiatry 66:469–476, 2005

Montejo AL, Llorca G, Izquierdo JA, et al: Incidence of sexual dysfunction associated with antidepressant agents: a prospective multicenter study of 1022 outpatients. J Clin Psychiatry 62 (suppl 3):10–21, 2001

Monteleone P, Gnocchi G: Evidence for a linear relationship between plasma trazodone levels and clinical response in depression in the elderly. Clin Neuropharmacol 13 (suppl 1):84–89, 1990

Nacca A, Guiso G, Fracasso C, et al: Brain-to-blood partition and in vivo inhibition of 5-hydroxytryptamine reuptake and quipazine-mediated behaviour of nefazodone and its main active metabolites in rodents. Br J Pharmacol 125:1617–1623, 1998

Nambudiri DE, Mirchandani IC, Young RC: Two more cases of trazodone-related syncope in the elderly. J Geriatr Psychiatry Neurol 2:225, 1989

Narayan M, Anderson G, Cellar J, et al: Serotonin transporter-blocking properties of nefazodone assessed by measurement of platelet serotonin. J Clin Psychopharmacol 18:67–71, 1998

Nierenberg A, Adler LA, Peselow E, et al: Trazodone for antidepressant-associated insomnia. Am J Psychiatry 151:1069–1072, 1994

Nisijima K, Shimizu M, Abe T, et al: A case of serotonin syndrome induced by concomitant treatment with low-dose trazodone and amitriptyline and lithium. Int Clin Psychopharmacol 11:289–290, 1996

Passos SR, Camacho LA, Lopes CS, et al: Nefazodone in outpatient treatment of inhaled cocaine dependence: a randomized double-blind placebo-controlled trial. Addiction 100:489–494, 2005

Pazzagli M, Giovannini MG, Pepeu G: Trazodone increases extracellular serotonin levels in the frontal cortex of rats. Eur J Pharmacol 383:249–257, 1999

Pescatori ES, Engelman JC, Davis G, et al: Priapism of the clitoris: a case report following trazodone use. J Urol 149:1557–1559, 1993

Pigott TA, Leheureux F, Rubenstein CS, et al: A double-blind, placebo-controlled study of trazodone in patients with obsessive-compulsive disorder. J Clin Psychopharmacol 12:156–162, 1992

Poon IO, Braun U: High prevalence of orthostatic hypotension and its correlation with potentially causative medications among elderly veterans. J Clin Ther 30:173–178, 2005

Preskorn SH: Comparison of the tolerability of bupropion, fluoxetine, imipramine, nefazodone, paroxetine, sertraline, and venlafaxine. J Clin Psychiatry 56 (suppl):12–21, 1995

Purcell P, Ghurye R: Trazodone and spontaneous orgasms in an elderly postmenopausal woman: a case report. J Clin Psychopharmacol 15:293–295, 1995

Razavi D, Kormoss N, Collard A, et al: Comparative study of the efficacy and safety of trazodone versus clorazepate in the treatment of adjustment disorders in cancer patients: a pilot study. J Int Med Res 27:264–272, 1999

Reeves RR, Bullen JA: Serotonin syndrome produced by paroxetine and low-dose trazodone. Psychosomatics 36:159–160, 1995

Rickels K, Downing R, Schweizer E, et al: Antidepressants for the treatment of generalized anxiety disorder: a placebo-controlled comparison of imipramine, trazodone, and diazepam. Arch Gen Psychiatry 50:884–895, 1993

Rickels K, Robinson DS, Schweizer E, et al: Nefazodone: aspects of efficacy. J Clin Psychiatry 56 (suppl 6):43–46, 1995

Robinson DS, Roberts DL, Smith JM, et al: The safety profile of nefazodone. J Clin Psychiatry 57 (suppl 2):31–38, 1996

Rosenberg RP: Sleep maintenance insomnia: strengths and weaknesses of current pharmacologic therapies. Ann Clin Psychiatry 18:49–56, 2006

Rotzinger S, Fang J, Baker GB: Trazodone is metabolized to m-chlorophenylpiperazine by CYP3A4 from human sources. Drug Metab Dispos 26:572–575, 1998

Roy-Byrne PP, Pages KP, Russo JE, et al: Nefazodone treatment of major depression in alcohol-dependent patients: a double-blind, placebo-controlled trial. J Clin Psychopharmacol 20:129–136, 2000

Saper JR, Lake AE, Tepper SJ: Nefazodone for chronic daily headache prophylaxis: an open-label study. Headache 41:465–474, 2001

Schatzberg AF: Trazodone: a 5-year review of antidepressant efficacy. Psychopathology 20 (suppl 1):48–56, 1987

Schatzberg AF, Rush AJ, Arnow BA, et al: Chronic depression: medication (nefazodone) or psychotherapy (CBASP) is effective when the other is not. Arch Gen Psychiatry 62:513–520, 2005

Schirren CA, Baretton G: Nefazodone-induced acute liver failure. Am J Gastroenterol 95:1596–1597, 2000

Serzone (package insert). Princeton, NJ, Bristol-Myers Squibb, February 2002

Sharpley AL, Williamson DJ, Attenburrow ME, et al: The effects of paroxetine and nefazodone on sleep: a placebo controlled trial. Psychopharmacology (Berl) 126:50–54, 1996

Shen J, Kennedy SH, Levitan RD, et al: The effects of nefazodone on women with seasonal affective disorder: clinical and polysomnographic analyses. J Psychiatry Neurosci 30:11–16, 2005

Shopsin B, Cassano GB, Conti L: An overview of new "second generation" antidepressant compounds: research and treatment implications, in Antidepressants: Neurochemical, Behavioral and Clinical Perspectives. Edited by Enna SJ, Molick J, Richelson E. New York, Raven, 1981, pp 219–251

Silvestrini G: Introductory remarks on trazodone and its position in treatment of psychiatric diseases, in Trazodone: A New Broad-Spectrum Antidepressant (Proceedings of the Symposium of the 11th Congress of the Collegium Internationale Neuro-Psychopharmacologicum, Vienna 1978). Edited by Gershon ES, Rickels K, Silvestrini G. Amsterdam, Excerpta Medica, 1980, pp 34–38

Small NL, Giamonna KA: Interaction between warfarin and trazodone. Ann Pharmacother 34:734–736, 2000

Spar JE: Plasma trazodone concentrations in elderly depressed inpatients: cardiac effects and short-term efficacy. J Clin Psychopharmacol 7:406–409, 1987

Sulser F: Mode of action of antidepressant drugs. J Clin Psychiatry 44 (5 pt 2):14–20, 1983

Sultzer DL, Gray KF, Gunay I, et al: A double-blind comparison of trazodone and haloperidol for treatment of agitation in patients with dementia. Am J Geriatr Psychiatry 5:60–69, 1997

Taylor DP, Smith DW, Hyslop DK, et al: Receptor binding and atypical antidepressant drug discovery, in Receptor Binding in Drug Research. Edited by O'Brien RA. New York, Marcel Dekker, 1986, pp 151–165

Terao T: Comparison of manic switch onset during fluoxetine and trazodone treatment. Biol Psychiatry 33:477–478, 1993

Teri L, Logsdon RG, Peskind E, et al: Treatment of agitation in AD: a randomized, placebo-controlled clinical trial. Neurology 55:1271–1278, 2001

Thapa PB, Gideon P, Cost TW, et al: Antidepressants and the risk of falls among nursing home residents. N Engl J Med 339:875–882, 1998

Thompson JW Jr, Ware MR, Blashfield RK: Psychotropic medication and priapism: a comprehensive review. J Clin Psychiatry 51:430–433, 1990 van Ameringen M, Mancini C, Oakman J, et al: Nefazodone in the treatment of generalized social phobia: a randomized, placebo-controlled trial. J Clin Psychiatry 68:288–295, 2007

van Moffaert M, de Wilde J, Vereecken A, et al: Mirtazapine is more effective than trazodone: a double-blind controlled study in hospitalized patients with major depression. Int Clin Psychopharmacol 10:3–9, 1995

Warner MD, Dorn MR, Peabody CA: Survey on the usefulness of trazodone in patients with PTSD with insomnia or nightmares. Pharmacopsychiatry 34:128–131, 2001

Weisler RH, Johnston JA, Lineberry CG, et al: Comparison of bupropion and trazodone for the treatment of major depression. J Clin Psychopharmacol 14:170–179, 1994

Wetzel H, Szegedi A, Scheurich A, et al: Combination treatment with nefazodone and cognitive-behavioral therapy for relapse prevention in alcohol-dependent men: a randomized controlled study. J Clin psychiatry 65:1406–1413, 2004

Winkler D, Ortner R, Pjrek E, et al: Trazodone-induced cardiac arrhythmias: a report of two cases. Hum Psychopharm Clin Exp 21:61–62, 2006

Worthington JJ 3rd, Zucker BG, Fones CS, et al: Nefazodone for social phobia: a clinical case series. Depress Anxiety 8:131–133, 1998

Wright DH, Lake KD, Bruhn PH, et al: Nefazodone and cyclosporine drug-drug interaction. J Heart Lung Transplant 18:913–915, 1999

Zajecka J, McEnany GW, Lusk KM: Antidepressant dosing and switching guidelines: focus on nefazodone. J Clin Psychiatry 63:42–47, 2002

Zalma A, von Moltke LL, Granda BW, et al: In vitro metabolism of trazodone by CYP3A: inhibition by ketoconazole and human immunodeficiency viral protease inhibitors. Biol Psychiatry 47:655–661, 2000

Zimmer B, Daly F, Benjamin L: More on combination antidepressant therapy. Arch Gen Psychiatry 41:527–528, 1984

CHAPTER 20

Bupropion

Anita H. Clayton, M.D.

Elizabeth H. Gillespie, D.O.

History and Discovery

Bupropion was discovered more than 40 years ago when investigators were searching for an antidepressant with a novel mechanism of action and safer side-effect profile. Synthesized in 1966, this unique compound, different from tricyclic antidepressants (TCAs) and monoamine oxidase inhibitors (MAOIs), was found to have antidepressant activity in animal models that are predictive of antidepressant activity in humans (Soroko and Maxwell 1983). Bupropion was discovered to have minimal sympathomimetic and anticholinergic side effects and a safer pharmacological and biochemical profile in comparison with other antidepressants. Although both bupropion and selective serotonin reuptake inhibitors (SSRIs) were developed with similar goals in mind, their mechanisms of action are unique (Hudziak and Rettew 2004; Soroko and Maxwell 1983). Bupropion is classified as an aminoketone antidepressant (Mehta 1983). Its mechanism of action is thought to be via dual inhibition of norepinephrine and dopamine reuptake (NDRI) without clinically significant serotonin reuptake inhibition (Horst and Preskorn 1998; Stahl et al. 2004). Both bupropion and SSRIs appear to be equally efficacious in the treatment of major depression (Feighner et al. 1991). The sustained-release (bupropion SR) formulation, approved in 1996, has also proved to be significantly better than placebo in preventing depression relapse (Weihs et al. 2002). Bupropion's tolerability is superior to that of SSRIs, with minimal effects on weight, less sedation, minimal withdrawal symptoms upon discontinuation, and fewer or no sexual side effects (Thase et al. 2005).

Besides treatment of major depression, bupropion has proven effective across a wide range of depressive conditions, subtypes, and comorbidities (Clayton 2007). These include major depression with concomitant anxiety, depression in the elderly, smoking cessation, attention-deficit/hyperactivity disorder (ADHD), obesity, hypoactive sexual desire disorder, and seasonal affective disorder (SAD). It has also been effective in bipolar depression and as an augmentation agent in patients with partial response to SSRIs. Overall, bupropion is a unique antidepressant with a broad therapeutic spectrum and a superior tolerability profile.

Bupropion first received U.S. Food and Drug Administration (FDA) approval in 1985. It was on the brink of release when a study by Horne et al. (1988) reported that 4 of 55 subjects with bulimia experienced seizures during treatment with the medication. Bupropion was withdrawn from the market pending additional investigation of its effects on seizure thresholds. Further research revealed that the risk of seizures increased from 0.3% to 0.4% at dosages of 450 mg/day to almost 2% at dosages of 600 mg/day. Bupropion was reintroduced in 1989 with a maximum recommended dosage of 450 mg/day (Davidson 1989). The original immediate-release (IR) formulation of bupropion was dosed three times daily. In an effort to improve tolerability and safety, a sustained-release (SR) formulation of bupropion, dosed twice daily, was subsequently introduced, and a once-daily extended-release (XL) formulation became available in 2003. Bupropion XL is now the most commonly prescribed formulation, as once-daily dosing is thought to optimize tolerability and adherence (McLaughlin et al. 2007).

Among its many uses stated above, this medication was also FDA approved for the indication of smoking cessation under the name Zyban in 1997, and bupropion XL was FDA approved for prophylaxis of seasonal depression in 2006. Over time, investigators continue to discover more uses and indications for this multifaceted medication.

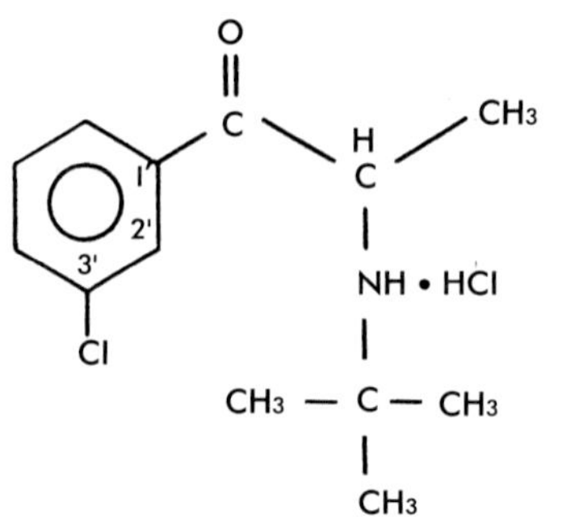

Structure–Activity Relations

Bupropion, 2-(tert-butylamino)-1-(3'-chlorophenyl)propan-1-one, is a monocyclic antidepressant and member of the aminoketone group (Figure 20–1). It was designed as a simple chemical structure that would, in vivo, result in relatively innocuous metabolites (Mehta 1983). Bupropion works as an organic base with a high degree of both water and lipid solubility, resulting in good systemic absorption. Its benign side-effect profile in comparison with that of tricyclic and tetracyclic antidepressants is due to the absence of heterocyclic rings as well as other common functional groups (Mehta 1983). Bupropion has little potential for abuse (Griffith et al. 1983). Mehta (1983) discussed the many significant differences between the chemical structures of bupropion and psychostimulants and accounted for the varying pharmacological and clinical effects (Hudziak and Rettew 2004).

Pharmacological Profile

Although similar to classical antidepressants such as TCAs and SSRIs in therapeutic efficacy, bupropion is considered to be an atypical antidepressant with a mixed neuropharmacological profile. Bupropion inhibits the reuptake of dopamine (DA) and norepinephrine (NE) by acting as a nonselective inhibitor of the dopamine transporter (DAT) and the norepinephrine transporter (NET). Studies show that bupropion also acts as an antagonist to nicotinic acetylcholine (nACh) receptors. Alternatively, bupropion does not act as an inhibitor of monoamine oxidase A or B, nor are the effects of bupropion mediated by serotonin (Ascher et al. 1995).

Dwoskin et al. (2006) reported that bupropion inhibits DA reuptake into rat striatal synaptosomes, NE reuptake into rat hypothalamic synaptosomes, and, less potently, serotonergic reuptake into rat hypothalamic synaptosomes (Ascher et al. 1995; Dwoskin et al. 2006;

FIGURE 20–1.   Chemical structure of bupropion.

Ferris and Beaman 1983; Ferris et al. 1982; Workman and Short 1993). In fact, Ferris et al. (1983) reported that bupropion is six times more potent than imipramine in blocking DA reuptake.

Recent studies demonstrate that bupropion also raises DA concentrations by causing a rapid and reversible increase in vesicular DA reuptake via cellular redistribution of the vesicular monoamine transporter (VMAT2) protein. By increasing the presynaptic pool of DA available for release, the concentration of DA in the extracellular space is further augmented, adding to the therapeutic efficacy of this compound (Dwoskin et al. 2006; Rau et al. 2005).

Although more is known about the dopaminergic effects of bupropion, interaction with the noradrenergic system also plays an important role in the drug's antidepressant activity. Bupropion is a weak competitive inhibitor of NE; in comparison with imipramine, it is 65-fold less potent (Ferris and Beaman 1983).

Along with inhibiting DA reuptake and NE function, bupropion has also been found to act as an nACh receptor antagonist. Research with various cellular expression systems has elucidated the ability of bupropion to interact with specific nACh receptors. Bupropion has been shown to work by noncompetitive inhibition of nACh receptors (Dwoskin et al. 2006). This action may partially contribute to the efficacy of bupropion not only as an antidepressant but also as an agent for tobacco cessation.

It has been noted that bupropion shares some structural and neurochemical properties with sympathomimetics and has a phenylethylamine skeleton similar to that of amphetamine. Although it resembles amphetamine in certain structural aspects, bupropion does not increase the spontaneous release of catacholamines in rat striatum and hypothalamus. A study by Griffith et al. (1983) examining the effect of bupropion and amphetamine in previous amphetamine abusers concluded that bupropion had little abuse potential in humans.

Although a great deal remains to be learned about the complete pharmacological profile of bupropion, what we do know is significant. In summary, bupropion is known to be an atypical antidepressant with a mixed pharmacological profile. It exerts its effect by blocking DA and NE reuptake as well as by antagonizing nACh receptors. It does not work through inhibition of monoamine oxidase and does not block serotonin reuptake. As Dwoskin et al. (2006) emphasized, in the future it will be important to elucidate which specific mechanism, or combination of mechanisms, is responsible for the clinical efficacy of bupropion.

Pharmacokinetics and Disposition

Bupropion is rapidly absorbed in the gastrointestinal tract after oral administration (Findlay et al. 1981; Jefferson et al. 2005). Absorption has been found to be close to 100% (Schroeder 1983). After first-pass metabolism, systemic bioavailability of the drug is decreased (Jefferson et al. 2005; Schroeder 1983). Peak plasma levels occur within 2 hours for the IR preparation. As expected, absorption is prolonged for the SR and XL formulations, for which peak plasma concentrations occur at 3 and 5 hours, respectively (Jefferson et al. 2005). Although absorption times differ, the three forms are considered to be bioequivalent (Fava et al. 2005; Jefferson et al. 2005; Physicians' Desk Reference 2005). Food does not impair absorption, and protein binding ranges from 82% to 88%. Jefferson et al. (2005) noted that this level of protein binding is not high and is not likely to be of clinical importance. The elimination half-life for bupropion is 21(±9) hours, and the half-life for hydroxybupropion, the major metabolite of bupropion, is close to 20 (±5) hours (Clayton 2007; Jefferson et al. 2005). Steady state occurs in 7–10 days. Finally, excretion in the urine occurs with 0.5% of the drug unchanged (Findlay et al. 1981).

Bupropion is extensively metabolized by the liver. The major metabolite, hydroxybupropion, is formed by cytochrome P450 (CYP) 2B6 (Hesse et al. 2000; Kirchheiner et al. 2003). The peak plasma concentration of hydroxybupropion at steady state is four- to sevenfold higher than that of bupropion. Although CYP2B6 is the primary isoenzyme involved in bupropion's metabolism, other isoforms, including 1A2, 2A6, 2CP, 2D6, 2E1, and 3A4, play a small role (Hesse et al. 2000; Kirchheiner et al. 2003). Bupropion inhibits CYP2B6 and therefore may interfere with drugs that are metabolized by this enzyme, such as desipramine and nortriptyline (Hesse et al. 2000; Jefferson et al. 2005).

Besides hydroxybupropion, other active metabolites of bupropion are threohydrobupropion and erythrohydrobupropion. These two pharmacologically active metabolites have the capacity to accumulate at levels nearly five times greater than the parent compound and can have half-lives up to 43 hours (Golden et al. 1988; Jefferson et al. 2005; Posner et al. 1985; Preskorn et al. 1990).

In examining the pharmacokinetics of bupropion in regard to gender, age, and smoking status, no significant effect has been found and definitive results have been inconclusive (Daviss et al. 2006; Hsyu et al. 1997; Jefferson et al. 2005; Stewart et al. 2001; Sweet et al. 1995). Nevertheless, it is important to monitor elderly patients more closely as they often have greater clinical issues with tolerability. One study with the elderly found evidence for an extended half-life of bupropion and for accumulation of metabolites (Sweet et al. 1995). For patients with impaired renal function, dosing should be initiated at lower levels. Worrall et al. (2004) showed that accumulation of two of the metabolites of bupropion—hydroxybupropion and threohydrobupropion—was significantly elevated in patients with end-stage renal disease compared with historical controls. Moreover, the metabolism of bupropion is also negatively affected in hepatic disease. Two studies have found increased levels of both bupropion and hydroxybupropion or of bupropion alone in patients with hepatic dysfunction (DeVane et al. 1990; Jefferson et al. 2005; Physicians' Desk Reference 2005). These results prompted the manufacturer to recommend that bupropion be used with caution in patients with mild to moderate liver disease and with extreme caution in patients with severe liver disease (Physicians' Desk Reference 2005).

Mechanism of Action

Despite considerable time and energy spent in elucidating bupropion's mechanism of action, what we know is limited. Preclinical data indicate that bupropion does not work by binding to postsynaptic histamine, α- or β-adrenergic, or serotonin receptors, nor does it inhibit monoamine oxidase (Ascher et al. 1995; Baldessarini 2001; Fava et al. 2005; Stahl et al. 2004). Thus, it is the only newer antidepressant without substantial serotonergic activity (Ascher et al. 1995; Richelson 1996; Stahl et al. 2004). Most researchers believe, and there is strong evidence to support, that the neurochemical mechanisms mediating the antidepressant effects of bupropion are from DA and NE reuptake inhibition. As discussed earlier, evidence shows that bupropion is a nonselective inhibitor of the

DAT and the NET and is also an antagonist at neuronal nACh receptors (Dwoskin et al. 2006).

Bupropion's three major metabolites—hydroxybupropion, threohydrobupropion, and erythrohydrobupropion—play a crucial role in its antidepressant activity (Physicians' Desk Reference 2005). Together, bupropion and its active metabolites have been shown to decrease the reuptake of NE and DA into rat striatal and rat hypothalamic synaptosomes (Ascher et al. 1995; Ferris and Beaman 1983; Ferris et al. 1983; Miller et al. 2002). Moreover, in vitro studies have demonstrated that bupropion and its active metabolites inhibit both the NE and the DA human transporters (described in Fava et al. 2005).

Although other antidepressants often produce their effects by downregulation of the postsynaptic noradrenergic receptors, bupropion differs in how it interacts with noradrenergic systems in that it decreases the firing rate of neurons in the locus coeruleus in a dose-dependent manner (B.R. Cooper et al. 1994; T.B. Cooper et al. 1984). Acute administration of bupropion not only decreases firing of brain stem NE and DA neurons but also increases extracellular NE and DA concentrations in the nucleus accumbens (Fava et al. 2005). Furthermore, the efficacy of bupropion and hydroxybupropion has been shown to decrease in animal models when NE- or DA-blocking drugs are administered (B.R. Cooper et al. 1980).

Indications and Efficacy

Primary Indications

Depression

The efficacy of bupropion for the treatment of major depressive disorder is supported by many clinical trials. All three forms have proven to be equally useful in the treatment of depression. In 1983, Fabre et al. published results of a multicenter trial showing that bupropion IR at dosages of 300–600 mg/day was significantly better than placebo in reducing symptoms of depression. This was followed by a 6-week double-blind, placebo-controlled five-center trial by Lineberry et al. (1990), which supported the conclusion that bupropion IR 300 mg/day was more efficacious than placebo in treating major depressive disorder. In evaluations against TCAs such as doxepin, amitriptyline, and imipramine in several clinical trials, bupropion was demonstrated to be equally efficacious (Branconnier et al. 1983; Feighner et al. 1986; Mendels et al. 1983). These studies also noted the more benign side-effect profile and improved tolerability of bupropion IR in comparison with

TCAs. In 1991, Feighner et al. examined the efficacy of bupropion and fluoxetine in treating depressed outpatients and found it to be comparable. In addition, similar effectiveness in treating depression was also found between trazodone and bupropion IR (Weisler et al. 1994).

After the development of bupropion SR, many studies followed comparing bupropion SR with SSRIs, including fluoxetine, sertraline, and paroxetine. In most studies, the effective daily dosage of bupropion SR was between 300 mg and 400 mg. All studies demonstrated that bupropion's effectiveness in treating symptoms of depression was equal to that of SSRIs (Coleman et al. 1999, 2001; Croft et al. 1999; Kavoussi et al. 1997; Weihs et al. 2000). In 2005, a meta-analysis of remission rates using all existing bupropion SR versus SSRI comparative trials was conducted by Thase et al. (2005). This analysis also found that remission rates with these two types of antidepressants were essentially the same. Although bupropion SR and SSRIs both were generally well tolerated, bupropion SR treatment was associated with less sexual dysfunction (Thase et al. 2005). Bupropion SR has also been shown to prevent relapse of depressive symptoms when given up to 1 year (Weihs et al. 2002).

Like bupropion IR and bupropion SR, the third and most recently released formulation of this NDRI, bupropion XL, has also been studied in regard to its effectiveness in treating depressive symptoms. In two 8-week placebo-controlled comparative trials with bupropion XL and escitalopram, pooled analysis confirmed equivalent efficacy of the two agents based on mean change in Hamilton Rating Scale for Depression (Ham-D; Hamilton 1960) score. Both antidepressants produced remission rates greater than the rate with placebo alone (Clayton et al. 2006). Other studies comparing bupropion XL with the serotonin and norepinephrine reuptake inhibitor (SNRI) venlafaxine XR demonstrated clinical equivalence for the two drugs in the treatment of depression. However, a study that used higher dosages of bupropion XL (300–450 mg/day) found statistically significantly higher remission rates for bupropion XL relative to venlafaxine XR (Thase et al. 2006).

It is also important to note that for patients who are unable to tolerate or fail to respond to SSRIs, bupropion may be added. Studies have shown bupropion to be efficacious for treatment of major depressive disorder not only as monotherapy but also as an augmenting agent with SSRIs or SNRIs (Bodkin et al. 1997; DeBattista et al. 2003; Fava et al. 2003; Ferguson et al. 1994; Lam et al. 2004; Rush et al. 2006; Spier 1998; Stern et al. 1983; Trivedi et al. 2006).

Depression in the elderly.   Depression in the elderly is often underdiagnosed and may go untreated. Elderly patients with depression frequently report less specific symptoms, such as insomnia, anorexia, and low energy, instead of admitting to depressed mood (Birrer and Vemuri 2004). Bupropion has been found to be an effective antidepressant in elderly patients (Birrer and Vemuri 2004; Branconnier et al. 1983; Weihs et al. 2000). An early study concluded that bupropion had therapeutic advantages over TCAs because it alleviated depressive symptoms without producing sedation or anticholinergic side effects, such as dry mouth, constipation, or confusion (Branconnier et al. 1983). A later study comparing bupropion SR and paroxetine noted that although both agents were effective in treating depression, bupropion SR had a more favorable side-effect profile (Weihs et al. 2000). Like bupropion SR, bupropion XL has proven efficacious for treatment of depression in the elderly (Clayton 2007). A recent study examining gender- and age-related differences in treatment of depressive symptoms, anxious and somatic symptoms, and insomnia found SSRIs and bupropion to be equally effective (Papakostas et al. 2007).

Depression with decreased energy, interest, and pleasure.   Bupropion XL has been studied specifically in patients with a retarded–anergic profile. Jefferson et al. (2006) showed that bupropion XL was more effective than placebo in treatment of patients with decreased energy, pleasure, and interest. This is the first study to look at those parameters exclusively. The unique NDRI mechanism of action of bupropion may play a role in its effectiveness in treating these symptoms (Jefferson et al. 2006).

Anxiety symptoms in depression.   Studies have demonstrated the effectiveness of bupropion dosages of 300–400 mg/day in reducing symptoms of anxiety (Fabre et al. 1983). Moreover, bupropion and SSRIs appear to be equally effective in this realm (Feighner et al. 1991; Weihs et al. 2000). In 2001, Trivedi et al. published results of a study examining the effects of bupropion SR versus sertraline on anxiety in depressed patients. This was a retrospective, pooled analysis of two 8-week double-blind, placebo-controlled trials that used the Hamilton Anxiety Scale (Ham-A) and the 21-item Hamilton Rating Scale for Depression (Ham-D-21) to measure symptoms. Results revealed that both bupropion SR and sertraline were superior to placebo in allaying depressive symptoms; however, treatment of anxious symptoms did not significantly differ from placebo for either active medication. The study concluded that bupropion and SSRIs were comparable in

their antidepressant and anxiolytic effects in patients with major depressive disorder. Neither was favored for more specific management of anxiety (Trivedi et al. 2001). A more recent meta-analysis comparing efficacy of bupropion and selective serotonin reuptake inhibitors for treatment of anxious symptoms in major depressive disorder came to a similar conclusion. The study found that both classes of medication led to a similar degree of improvement in anxiety symptoms, with no significant difference in the severity of residual anxiety symptoms (Papakostas et al. 2008).

Bipolar depression.   A small number of studies have demonstrated the advantages of bupropion in the treatment of depression in bipolar disorder (Haykal and Akiskal 1990; Shopsin 1983; Wright et al. 1985). Although these investigations yielded positive results, they were limited by small numbers of subjects and were uncontrolled. A study by Sachs et al. (1994) comparing bupropion and desipramine in the treatment of bipolar depression suggested that bupropion may have a lower rate of precipitation of mania. Another study comparing the effect of bupropion SR versus topiramate, as an add-on agent for bipolar depression in patients already taking lithium or valproate, demonstrated no difference in response. Regarding change from baseline, a significant reduction in depressive symptoms occurred with both medications. This study reported no cases of affective switching in either arm (McIntyre et al. 2002).

Seasonal Affective Disorder

Bupropion XL is the first, and currently the only, medication to have a labeled indication for the preventive treatment of SAD. A study published in 1992 initially suggested bupropion's efficacy as treatment for SAD (Dilsaver et al. 1992). In 2005, Modell et al. published results of three prospective randomized, placebo-controlled prevention trials involving 1,042 outpatients with a diagnosis of SAD. Patients received 150–300 mg/day of bupropion XL or placebo in autumn while they were still well. Bupropion XL reduced the frequency of emergence of SAD by 44% and protected against the recurrence of seasonal major depressive episodes. Furthermore, there was no noticeable increase in major depressive episodes following discontinuation of bupropion in the springtime (Modell et al. 2005).

Smoking Cessation

The smoking cessation activity of bupropion was first noted after researchers observed unplanned suspension of smoking in depressed subjects who were being treated with bupropion (Hudziak and Rettew 2004). In 1997, Hurt et al. published the results of a double-blind, placebo-controlled trial of bupropion SR therapy for smoking cessation. Six hundred and fifteen subjects received bupropion SR at dosages of 100, 150, or 300 mg/day for 7 weeks, with a target quit date of 1 week after beginning treatment. Brief counseling was also provided. Rates of smoking cessation at the end of 7 weeks were 29% for the 100-mg group, 39% for the 150-mg group, and 44% for the 300-mg group, versus 10% for placebo. At 1 year, rates for the three bupropion dosage groups were 20%, 23%, and 23%, respectively, compared with 12% for the placebo group. Cessation rates for the two higher dosages were significantly better than the rate for placebo. This trial concluded that bupropion SR is an effective agent for smoking cessation (Hurt et al. 1997).

A later placebo-controlled study compared bupropion SR alone, nicotine patch alone, bupropion SR plus nicotine patch, and placebo. At 1 year, rates of smoking cessation were significantly higher in both the bupropion monotherapy group and the bupropion plus nicotine patch group than in the placebo group or the nicotine patch monotherapy group (Jorenby et al. 1999). In 2004, Killen et al. published results of the first study in adolescent smokers. In that study, 211 adolescent smokers (ages 15–18 years) were randomly assigned to two groups. One group received the nicotine patch plus placebo, and the other received the nicotine patch plus bupropion SR 150 mg/day. Both groups also received relapse prevention skills training. Results did not show a significant treatment effect but did reveal an overall reduction in cigarette consumption per day and maintenance of this reduction over time (Killen et al. 2004).

Clinical trials have demonstrated that bupropion SR is effective in improving initial and long-term abstinence rates and may be helpful in preventing relapse. Hays et al. (2001) showed that subjects who had successfully stopped smoking for 7 weeks with bupropion treatment had a significant delay in smoking relapse with continued bupropion SR therapy compared with placebo. More recently, however, a trial looking specifically at extended treatment with bupropion SR for smoking cessation reported that bupropion SR did not surpass placebo (Killen et al. 2006). In the first study arm, 362 adult smokers received 11 weeks of open-label treatment consisting of bupropion SR, nicotine patch, and relapse prevention training. In the second arm of the study, subjects were randomly assigned to placebo or bupropion SR for 14 weeks of extended treatment. Whereas higher abstinence rates with

bupropion SR than with placebo were found at week 25 (42% vs. 38%), abstinence rates were about the same at week 52 (33% vs. 34%). Another interesting finding this study uncovered was that men were more likely than women to abstain from smoking.

Although more work needs to be done in areas of relapse prevention and long-term abstinence, it is clear that bupropion SR is helpful in smoking cessation. Many of theses studies were instrumental in the approval of bupropion SR for smoking cessation. Recommended dosages are 150 mg/day for 3 days, with an increase to 150 mg two times a day for 7–12 weeks. The patient should set a quit date of 1–2 weeks after treatment has been initiated. In 2003, Ferry and Johnston published a 5-year review of efficacy and safety data for bupropion SR in smoking cessation since its approval in 1997 for that indication. A risk–benefit analysis assuming a 30% 1-year quit rate found that 19 lives were saved out of 10,000 subjects and that 86 of the cases of smoking-attributed morbidity were avoided compared with a 0.22% chance of experiencing an adverse effect from bupropion SR (Ferry and Johnston 2003).

Other Uses

Attention-Deficit/Hyperactivity Disorder

Currently there is no FDA indication for this use, but studies have demonstrated that bupropion may also be helpful is treating symptoms of ADHD in both children and adults. Clinical trials in children with ADHD have shown bupropion to be a safe and effective alternative for treatment of this disorder (Conners et al. 1996; Simeon et al. 1986). A comparison trial of bupropion and methylphenidate demonstrated that both drugs were effective in the treatment of ADHD and had similar efficacy (Barrickman et al. 1995). Bupropion has also been studied in adults with ADHD and has demonstrated statistically significant symptom improvement in this population (Wilens et al. 2001). In a meta-analysis by Peterson et al. (2008), long-acting forms of bupropion appeared to exhibit similar clinical effectiveness compared with long-acting stimulants in adults. An open trial by Riggs et al. (1998) suggested that bupropion may also be useful for treatment of ADHD in adolescents with both conduct disorder and substance abuse (Riggs et al. 1998).

Currently, bupropion is thought of as a useful second-line agent in the treatment of ADHD and may be more favorable with comorbid conduct disorder or substance abuse (Riggs et al. 1998; Wilens et al. 2001). More studies are needed to further establish the efficacy of bupropion for use in this realm.

Obesity

One of the well-known characteristics of bupropion is that it is usually not associated with weight gain as are many other classes of antidepressants. Alternatively, mild weight loss has been noted in many clinical trials. To further investigate this observation, Gadde et al. (2001) conducted a randomized, placebo-controlled trial investigating the tolerability and efficacy of bupropion for weight loss in 50 obese women using bupropion (100–400 mg/day) versus placebo. All subjects kept a food journal and were placed on a 1,600 kcal/day diet. Results revealed bupropion to be more effective than placebo in achieving weight loss at 8 weeks. At 24 weeks, responders to bupropion had lost an average of 13% of their baseline body weight (Gadde et al. 2001). Following this initial study for bupropion and weight loss, two larger studies confirmed these results (Anderson et al. 2002; Jain et al. 2002). A more recent randomized, open-label study found that combination treatment with zonisamide and bupropion resulted in more weight loss than treatment with zonisamide alone. Eighteen obese women were randomly assigned to receive either combination therapy or zonisamide monotherapy. For those who completed the study, women in the combination group lost an average of 8.1 kg, versus an average of 3.0 kg for women in the monotherapy group (Gadde et al. 2007). Although bupropion is not FDA approved for weight reduction, it may mitigate weight gain in patients being treated for depression.

Sexual Dysfunction

Studies by Segraves et al. (2001) demonstrated that bupropion may be helpful in treatment of hypoactive sexual desire disorder (HSDD). More recently, a double-blind, placebo-controlled trial supported this finding and also revealed increases in sexual arousal, orgasm completion, and sexual satisfaction in women with HSDD receiving bupropion (Segraves et al. 2004). Another study of bupropion SR treatment of patients with SSRI-induced sexual dysfunction found that bupropion improved desire to engage in sexual activity and increased frequency of engaging in sexual activity (Clayton et al. 2004). Further studies have also demonstrated that bupropion may be helpful for treatment of sexual disorders in both men and women (Modell et al. 2000).

Side Effects and Toxicology

Thousands of clinical trials and millions of patient exposures reveal bupropion to be a safe and generally well tolerated medication across populations. Because of its unique mechanism of action and structure, its reported side effects are somewhat different than with other antidepressants.

In a series of large randomized, placebo-controlled multicenter trials evaluating the safety of bupropion SR in the treatment of depressed outpatients, Settle et al. (1999) found that the most commonly reported adverse events (occurring in >5% of subjects) were headache, dry mouth, nausea, insomnia, constipation, and dizziness. Only three of these—dry mouth, nausea, and insomnia—occurred at higher rates in patients taking bupropion SR than in those receiving placebo. The rate of discontinuation due to adverse events was low: 7% for bupropion SR, compared with 4% for placebo. Rash, nausea, agitation, and migraine were the most common adverse effects leading to discontinuation (Settle et al. 1999). Similarly favorable safety and tolerability findings were reported for continuation-phase bupropion SR treatment in a longer-term (up to 44 weeks) relapse prevention trial (Weihs et al. 2002).

Adverse events associated with bupropion XL are presented in Table 20–1. This table is based on combined results from four different studies previously discussed: the two escitalopram studies (Clayton et al. 2006); the venlafaxine XR study (Thase et al. 2006); and the reduced energy, pleasure, and interest study (Jefferson et al. 2006). These data indicate that the most common side effects of bupropion XL are similar to those of other formulations. Fatigue and somnolence were associated more with escitalopram, whereas bupropion XL caused more dry mouth. Compared with bupropion XL, venlafaxine XR was found to be associated with more dry mouth, nausea, diarrhea, somnolence, sedation, and yawning. These data indicate that bupropion XL does not appear to cause somnolence (Clayton et al. 2006).

A review by Fava et al. (2005) presented similar conclusions, supporting the evidence that bupropion causes much less somnolence than SSRIs. Moreover, insomnia, a known adverse effect of bupropion, occurs at rates similar to those seen with SSRIs (Fava et al. 2005).

Other important adverse events that have been reported with bupropion may include seizure, allergic reaction, or vital sign changes. These are less common but could possibly be more harmful. Allergic reactions, in-

TABLE 20–1.   Frequency of adverse events: comparison studies of bupropion XL versus escitalopram, venlafaxine XR, and placebo in patients with MDD

| | Bupropion XL | | Comparison Agent | | | | | |
| | | | Escitalopram | | Venlafaxine XR | | Placebo | |
Adverse event	N	N (%)	N	N (%)	N	N (%)	N	N (%)
Dry mouth	579	120 (21)	281	37 (13)	174	51 (29)	412	38 (9)
Dizziness	135	14 (10)	—	—	—	—	139	3 (2)
Nausea	303	39 (13)	—	—	174	45 (26)	139	7 (5)
Insomnia	411	49 (12)	281	28 (10)	—	—	412	23 (6)
Anxiety	135	8 (6)	—	—	—	—	139	1 (<1)
Dyspepsia	135	8 (6)	—	—	—	—	139	0 (0)
Sinusitis	135	7 (5)	—	—	—	—	139	3 (2)
Tremor	135	7 (5)	—	—	—	—	139	0 (0)
Fatigue	276	12 (4)	281	39 (14)	—	—	273	16 (6)
Constipation	276	26 (9)	281	9 (3)	—	—	273	16 (6)
Irritability	276	14 (5)	281	3 (1)	—	—	273	10 (4)
Somnolence	444	10 (2)	281	22 (8)	174	12 (7)	273	14 (5)
Decreased appetite	444	19 (4)	281	16 (6)	174	12 (7)	273	10 (4)
Nasopharyngitis	444	31 (7)	281	14 (5)	174	9 (5)	273	8 (3)
Diarrhea	168	9 (5)	—	—	174	17 (10)	—	—
Sedation	168	2 (1)	—	—	174	10 (6)	—	—
Yawning	444	2 (<1)	281	15 (5)	174	12 (7)	273	3 (1)

Note.   Data combined from Clayton et al. 2006; Jefferson et al. 2006; Thase et al. 2006. Reporting frequencies and percentages varied across these three studies. MDD = major depressive disorder; XL/XR = extended release.

Source.   Reprinted from Clayton AH: "Extended-Release Bupropion: An Antidepressant With a Broad Spectrum of Therapeutic Activity." *Expert Opinion on Pharmacotherapy* 8:457–466, 2007. Copyright 2007, Informa Healthcare, Informa UK Ltd. Used with permission.

cluding rash, arthralgias, fever, and serum sickness–like reactions, have all been reported (Kanani et al: 2000; McCollom et al. 2000). In light of these data, it is important to fully evaluate any reports of hypersensitivity when administering bupropion.

Screening for a history of seizure disorder or other organic brain disease should be performed before commencing a trial of bupropion. Seizure has been reported at a rate of 0.1% at dosages up to 300 mg/day with bupropion SR, with a dose-related effect (Dunner et al. 1998). This rate is similar to that of other newer antidepressants, such as SSRIs and mirtazapine, but lower than the rate associated with therapeutic doses of TCAs (Montgomery 2005).

Although cases of spontaneous hypertension with bupropion therapy have been reported, clinical trials have also shown minimal changes in heart rate and blood pressure (Settle et al. 1999). In a smoking cessation study, patients receiving combination treatment with both bupropion SR and a nicotine patch had a higher incidence of new or worsening hypertension compared with patients receiving either treatment alone or placebo (Jorenby et al. 1999). Thase et al. (2008) conducted a dose–response study to evaluate the potential of bupropion to elevate blood pressure. Bupropion SR dosages of 150–400 mg/day were administered to 296 nondepressed volunteers with mild hypertension. Results revealed that bupropion SR did not separate from placebo on blood pressure changes. However, clinicians should be aware that elevated blood pressure is a possibility with bupropion therapy and should monitor patients accordingly.

Many agents used to treat depression have been associated with weight gain. This effect is thought to be due to an affinity for the H_1 histamine receptor, which is not a factor with bupropion. In fact, mild weight loss over time, instead of weight gain, has been reported with bupropion treatment (Harto-Truax et al. 1983). Studies have shown bupropion XL to be associated with a loss of 0.1–1.1 kg in the short term, compared with placebo, which was linked with a small gain of 0.1–0.8 kg (Jefferson et al. 2006; Modell et al. 2005; Thase et al. 2006). In a longer-term depression relapse prevention study, Croft et al. (2002) observed that patients with a higher body mass index at baseline experienced greater weight loss with bupropion XL.

Another difference in bupropion's tolerability compared with other antidepressants is the lower incidence of sexual dysfunction. A comparative meta-analysis of bupropion SR and SSRIs concluded that bupropion SR therapy resulted in lower rates of sexual dysfunction than did SSRI therapy (Thase et al. 2005). Orgasmic dysfunction, sexual arousal disorder, and sexual desire disorder

were all less frequent with bupropion SR. Notably, the risk of sexual dysfunction with bupropion SR in this study was comparable to that with placebo. Data from two comparative studies also confirm lower rates of sexual dysfunction with bupropion SR than with the SSRI escitalopram (Clayton et al. 2006). Furthermore, a large study published in 2002 examining the prevalence of sexual dysfunction among outpatients on monotherapy with newer antidepressants found that the odds of developing sexual dysfunction were four to six times greater with SSRIs or venlafaxine XR than with bupropion SR (Clayton et al. 2002). As a result of these data, studies have examined bupropion as an antidote for SSRI-induced sexual dysfunction. A placebo-controlled comparative trial of bupropion SR treatment in 42 patients with SSRI-induced sexual dysfunction concluded that bupropion SR improved both desire to engage in sexual activity and frequency of engaging in sexual activity relative to placebo (Clayton et al. 2004). Use of bupropion for the treatment of SSRI-induced sexual dysfunction has not yet been approved by the FDA. Further investigation is needed.

Overall, at approved dosages, bupropion is a safe medication for depression in most populations and has an excellent tolerability profile. Although safe in general, bupropion can be fatal with high blood levels. Serious medical consequences such as hypertension, acidosis, sinus tachycardia, seizures, cardiotoxicity with QRS widening, and even death have all been reported with overdoses of bupropion (Bhattacharjee et al. 2001; Curry et al. 2005; Shrier et al. 2000).

On initiation of bupropion therapy, it is usually not necessary to obtain routine laboratory evaluations, although cases of elevated serum transaminase (Oslin and Duffy 1993) and rare cases of hepatitis (Hu et al. 2000) have been reported. Other unexpected changes in laboratory values have also occurred with bupropion therapy and include false-positive urine amphetamine screening results (Weintraub and Linder 2000).

Unfortunately, there is little evidence about the safety of bupropion in pregnancy. In a recent study by Cole et al. (2007), bupropion exposure in the first trimester was not associated with teratogenic effects.

Drug–Drug Interactions

As discussed earlier, the major pathway for metabolism of bupropion to its primary metabolite, hydroxybupropion, occurs through the cytochrome P450 system in the liver. The main enzyme responsible for this metabolism is CYP2B6. Competitive inhibition of metabolism could occur with other drugs processed by this enzyme, such as paroxetine, sertraline, diazepam, clonazepam, clopidogrel, ritonavir, and efavirenz (Hesse et al. 2000; Jefferson et al. 2005). A study examining the effects of concurrent use of lopinavir/ritonavir on bupropion pharmacokinetics in 12 healthy subjects found that maximum plasma concentrations of bupropion and hydroxybupropion decreased by 57% and 31%, respectively (Hogeland et al. 2007).

Bupropion and hydroxybupropion are also inhibitors of CYP2D6, an essential enzyme that plays a role in the metabolism of several classes of medications, including antidepressants, β-blockers, and antiarrhythmic agents (Wilkinson 2005). Studies of the effects of bupropion on CYP2D6 activity are limited (Jefferson et al. 2005). Coadministration of bupropion SR with desipramine, a drug extensively metabolized by CYP2D6, results in decreased clearance of desipramine and increased maximum plasma concentrations and area under the curve of desipramine (Jefferson et al. 2005). Similarly, in an 8-week open-label study of bupropion SR coadministered with venlafaxine, paroxetine, or fluoxetine, venlafaxine metabolism was inhibited and higher concentrations of venlafaxine were found. No significant interaction effects were seen for paroxetine or fluoxetine (Kennedy et al. 2002). Other agents known to induce various metabolic pathways have also been shown to affect the metabolism of bupropion. Carbamazepine, which induces CYP2B6, 3A4, and 1A2 activity, has been shown to decrease bupropion concentrations but increase hydroxybupropion concentrations.

Bupropion should also be used with caution if coadministered with other agents that can lower the seizure threshold, such as tramadol, other antidepressants, or antipychotics (Delanty et al. 1998; Gardner et al. 2000). It should also be used with caution in patients who abuse alcohol, as this population may have increased risk for seizures (Dunner et al. 1998). In addition, because bupropion increases DA reuptake, additive effects with other dopaminergic agents (e.g., levodopa) have been observed (Goetz et al. 1984).

Conclusion

Bupropion is unique in that it works as a DA and NE reuptake inhibitor and acts as an antagonist of nACh receptors. Unlike other newer agents, it has very little serotonergic activity and therefore produces a different side-effect profile. Bupropion may be the antidepressant of choice for patients who cannot tolerate or do not respond to SSRIs. While currently indicated for major depressive disorder, for tobacco dependence, and for prevention of SAD, bupropion has also proven useful in many other circumstances, such as child and adult ADHD, obesity, and sexual disorders. For more specific treatment of depression with decreased energy and interest, for depression with concomitant anxiety, and for bipolar depression, bupropion may be beneficial. Bupropion may also be used to augment other antidepressants in the treatment of major depressive disorder and to reverse SSRI-induced side effects. Greater tolerability, including low risk of weight gain, less sedation, and fewer sexual side effects, adds to its value as an effective antidepressant.

References

Anderson JW, Greenway FL, Fujioka K, et al: Bupropion SR enhances weight loss: a 48-week double-blind, placebo-controlled trial. Obes Res 10:633–641, 2002
Ascher JA, Cole JO, Colin JN, et al: Bupropion: a review of its mechanism of antidepressant activity. J Clin Psychiatry 56:395–401, 1995
Baldessarini RJ: Drugs and the treatment of psychiatric disorders: depression and anxiety disorders, in Goodman and Gilman's The Pharmacological Basis of Therapeutics. New York, McGraw-Hill, 2001, pp 447–483
Barrickman LL, Perry PJ, Allen AJ, et al: Bupropion versus methylphenidate in the treatment of attention-deficit hyperactivity disorder. J Am Acad Child Adolesc Psychiatry 34:649–657, 1995
Bhattacharjee C, Smith M, Todd F, et al: Bupropion overdose: a potential problem with the new "miracle" anti-smoking drug. Int J Clin Pract 55:221–222, 2001
Birrer RB, Vemuri SP: Depression in later life: a diagnostic and therapeutic challenge. Am Fam Physician 69:2375–2382, 2004
Bodkin JA, Lasser RA, Wines JD Jr, et al: Combining serotonin reuptake inhibitors and bupropion in partial responders to antidepressant monotherapy. J Clin Psychiatry 58:137–145, 1997
Branconnier RJ, Cole JO, Ghazvinian S, et al: Clinical pharmacology of bupropion and imipramine in elderly depressives. J Clin Psychiatry 44:130–133, 1983
Clayton AH: Extended-release bupropion: an antidepressant with a broad spectrum of therapeutic activity? Expert Opin Pharmacother 8:457–466, 2007
Clayton AH, Pradko JF, Croft HA, et al: Prevalence of sexual dysfunction among newer antidepressants. J Clin Psychiatry 63:357–366, 2002
Clayton AH, Warnock JK, Kornstein SG, et al: A placebo-controlled trial of bupropion SR as an antidote for selective serotonin reuptake inhibitor–induced sexual dysfunction. J Clin Psychiatry 65:62–67, 2004
Clayton AH, Croft HA, Horrigan JP, et al: Bupropion extended release compared with escitalopram: effects on sexual functioning and antidepressant efficacy in 2 randomized, double-blind, placebo-controlled studies. J Clin Psychiatry 67:736–746, 2006
Cole JA, Modell JG, Haight BR, et al: Bupropion in pregnancy and the prevalence of congenital malformations. Pharmacoepidemiol Drug Saf 16:474–484, 2007

Coleman CC, Cunningham LA, Foster VJ, et al: Sexual dysfunction associated with the treatment of depression: a placebo-controlled comparison of bupropion sustained release and sertraline treatment. Ann Clin Psychiatry 11:205–215, 1999

Coleman CC, King BR, Bolden-Watson C, et al: A placebo-controlled comparison of the effects on sexual functioning of bupropion sustained release and fluoxetine. Clin Ther 23:1040–1058, 2001

Conners CK, Casat CD, Gualtieri CT, et al: Bupropion hydrochloride in attention deficit disorder with hyperactivity. J Am Acad Child Adolesc Psychiatry 35:1314–1321, 1996

Cooper BR, Hester TJ, Maxwell RA: Behavioral and biochemical effects of the antidepressant bupropion (Wellbutrin): evidence for selective blockade of dopamine uptake in vivo. J Pharmacol Exp Ther 215:127–134, 1980

Cooper BR, Wang CM, Cox RF, et al: Evidence that the acute behavioral and electrophysiological effects of bupropion (Wellbutrin) are mediated by a noradrenergic mechanism. Neuropsychopharmacology 11:133–141, 1994

Cooper TB, Suckow RF, Glassman A: Determination of bupropion and its major basic metabolites in plasma by liquid chromatography with dual-wavelength ultraviolet detection. J Pharm Sci 73:1104–1107, 1984

Croft H, Settle E Jr, Houser T, et al: A placebo-controlled comparison of the antidepressant efficacy and effects on sexual functioning of sustained-release bupropion and sertraline. Clin Ther 21:643–658, 1999

Croft H, Houser TL, Jamerson BD, et al: Effect on body weight of bupropion sustained-release in patients with major depression treated for 52 weeks. Clin Ther 24:662–672, 2002

Curry SC, Kashani JS, LoVecchio F, et al: Intraventricular conduction delay after bupropion overdose. J Emerg Med 29:299–305, 2005

Davidson J: Seizures and bupropion: a review. J Clin Psychiatry 50:256–261, 1989

Daviss WB, Perel JM, Birmaher B, et al: Steady-state clinical pharmacokinetics of bupropion extended-release in youths. J Am Acad Child Adolesc Psychiatry 45:1503–1509, 2006

DeBattista C, Solvason HB, Poirier J, et al: A prospective trial of bupropion SR augmentation of partial and non-responders to serotonergic antidepressants. J Clin Psychopharmacol 23:27–30, 2003

Delanty N, Vaughan CJ, French JA: Medical causes of seizures. Lancet 352:383–390, 1998

DeVane CL, Laizure SC, Stewart JT, et al: Disposition of bupropion in healthy volunteers and subjects with alcoholic liver disease. J Clin Psychopharmacol 10:328–332, 1990

Dilsaver SC, Qamar AB, Del Medico VJ: The efficacy of bupropion in winter depression: results of an open trial. J Clin Psychiatry 53:252–255, 1992

Dunner DL, Zisook S, Billow AA, et al: A prospective safety surveillance study for bupropion sustained-release in the treatment of depression. J Clin Psychiatry 59:366–373, 1998

Dwoskin LP, Rauhut AS, King-Pospisil KA, et al: Review of the pharmacology and clinical profile of bupropion, an antidepressant and tobacco use cessation agent. CNS Drug Rev 12:178–207, 2006

Fabre LF, Brodie HK, Garver D, et al: A multicenter evaluation of bupropion versus placebo in hospitalized depressed patients. J Clin Psychiatry 44:88–94, 1983

Fava M, Papakostas GI, Petersen T, et al: Switching to bupropion in fluoxetine-resistant major depressive disorder. Ann Clin Psychiatry 15:17–22, 2003

Fava M, Rush AJ, Thase ME, et al: 15 years of clinical experience with bupropion HCl: from bupropion to bupropion SR to bupropion XL. Prim Care Companion J Clin Psychiatry 7:106–113, 2005

Feighner J, Hendrickson G, Miller L, et al: Double-blind comparison of doxepin versus bupropion in outpatients with a major depressive disorder. J Clin Psychopharmacol 6:27–32, 1986

Feighner JP, Gardner EA, Johnston JA, et al: Double-blind comparison of bupropion and fluoxetine in depressed outpatients. J Clin Psychiatry 52:329–335, 1991

Ferguson J, Cunningham L, Merideth C, et al: Bupropion in tricyclic antidepressant nonresponders with unipolar major depressive disorder. Ann Clin Psychiatry 6:153–160, 1994

Ferris RM, Beaman OJ: Bupropion: a new antidepressant drug, the mechanism of action of which is not associated with down-regulation of postsynaptic beta-adrenergic, serotonergic (5-HT2), alpha 2-adrenergic, imipramine and dopaminergic receptors in brain. Neuropharmacology 22:1257–1267, 1983

Ferris RM, Maxwell RA, Cooper BR, et al: Neurochemical and neuropharmacological investigations into the mechanisms of action of bupropion HCl—a new atypical antidepressant agent. Adv Biochem Psychopharmacol 31:277–286, 1982

Ferris RM, Cooper BR, Maxwell RA: Studies of bupropion's mechanism of antidepressant activity. J Clin Psychiatry 44:74–78, 1983

Ferry L, Johnston JA: Efficacy and safety of bupropion SR for smoking cessation: data from clinical trials and five years of postmarketing experience. Int J Clin Pract 57:224–230, 2003

Findlay JW, Van Wyck Fleet J, Smith PG, et al: Pharmacokinetics of bupropion, a novel antidepressant agent, following oral administration to healthy subjects. Eur J Clin Pharmacol 21:127–135, 1981

Gadde KM, Parker CB, Maner LG, et al: Bupropion for weight loss: an investigation of efficacy and tolerability in overweight and obese women. Obes Res 9:544–551, 2001

Gadde KM, Yonish GM, Foust MS, et al: Combination therapy of zonisamide and bupropion for weight reduction in obese women: a preliminary, randomized, open-label study. J Clin Psychiatry 68:1226–1229, 2007

Gardner JS, Blough D, Drinkard CR, et al: Tramadol and seizures: a surveillance study in a managed care population. Pharmacotherapy 20:1423–1431, 2000

Goetz CG, Tanner CM, Klawans HL: Bupropion in Parkinson's disease. Neurology 34:1092–1094, 1984

Golden RN, De Vane CL, Laizure SC, et al: Bupropion in depression. The role of metabolites in clinical outcome. Arch Gen Psychiatry 45:145–149, 1988

Griffith JD, Carranza J, Griffith C, et al: Bupropion: clinical assay for amphetamine-like abuse potential. J Clin Psychiatry 44:206–208, 1983

Hamilton M: A rating scale for depression. J Neurol Neurosurg Psychiatry 23:56–62, 1960

Harto-Truax N, Stern WC, Miller LL, et al: Effects of bupropion on body weight. J Clin Psychiatry 44:183–186, 1983

Haykal RF, Akiskal HS: Bupropion as a promising approach to rapid cycling bipolar II patients. J Clin Psychiatry 51:450–455, 1990

Hays JT, Hurt RD, Rigotti NA, et al: Sustained-release bupropion for pharmacologic relapse prevention after smoking cessation: a randomized, controlled trial. Ann Intern Med 135:423–433, 2001

Hesse LM, Venkatakrishnan K, Court MH, et al: CYP2B6 mediates the in vitro hydroxylation of bupropion: potential drug interactions with other antidepressants. Drug Metab Dispos 28:1176–1184, 2000

Hogeland GW, Swindells S, McNabb JC, et al: Lopinavir/ritonavir reduces bupropion plasma concentrations in healthy subjects. Clin Pharmacol Ther 81:69–75, 2007

Horne RL, Ferguson JM, Pope HG Jr, et al: Treatment of bulimia with bupropion: a multicenter controlled trial. J Clin Psychiatry 49:262–266, 1988

Horst WD, Preskorn SH: Mechanisms of action and clinical characteristics of three atypical antidepressants: venlafaxine, nefazodone, bupropion. J Affect Disord 51:237–254, 1998

Hsyu PH, Singh A, Giargiari TD, et al: Pharmacokinetics of bupropion and its metabolites in cigarette smokers versus nonsmokers. J Clin Pharmacol 37:737–743, 1997

Hu KQ, Tiyyagura L, Kanel G, et al: Acute hepatitis induced by bupropion. Dig Dis Sci 45:1872–1873, 2000

Hudziak JJ, Rettew DC: Bupropion, in The American Psychiatric Publishing Textbook of Psychopharmacology, 3rd Edition. Edited by Schatzberg AF, Nemeroff CB. Washington, DC, American Psychiatric Publishing, 2004, pp 327–339

Hurt RD, Sachs DP, Glover ED, et al: A comparison of sustained-release bupropion and placebo for smoking cessation. N Engl J Med 337:1195–1202, 1997

Jain AK, Kaplan RA, Gadde KM, et al: Bupropion SR vs placebo for weight loss in obese patients with depressive symptoms. Obes Res 10:1049–1056, 2002

Jefferson JW, Pradko JF, Muir KT: Bupropion for major depressive disorder: pharmacokinetic and formulation considerations. Clin Ther 27:1685–1695, 2005

Jefferson JW, Rush AJ, Nelson JC, et al: Extended-release bupropion for patients with major depressive disorder presenting with symptoms of reduced energy, pleasure, and interest: findings from a randomized, double-blind, placebo-controlled study. J Clin Psychiatry 67:865–873, 2006

Jorenby DE, Leischow SJ, Nides MA, et al: A controlled trial of sustained-release bupropion, a nicotine patch, or both for smoking cessation. N Engl J Med 340:685–691, 1999

Kanani AS, Kalicinsky C, Warrington RJ, et al: Serum sickness–like reaction with bupropion sustained release. Can J Allergy Clin Immunol 5:27–29, 2000

Kavoussi RJ, Segraves RT, Hughes AR, et al: Double-blind comparison of bupropion sustained release and sertraline in depressed outpatients. J Clin Psychiatry 58:532–537, 1997

Kennedy SH, McCann SM, Masellis M, et al: Combining bupropion SR with venlafaxine, paroxetine, or fluoxetine: a preliminary report on pharmacokinetic, therapeutic, and sexual dysfunction effects. J Clin Psychiatry 63:181–186, 2002

Killen JD, Robinson TN, Ammerman S, et al: Randomized clinical trial of the efficacy of bupropion combined with nicotine patch in the treatment of adolescent smokers. J Consult Clin Psychol 72:729–735, 2004

Killen JD, Fortmann SP, Murphy GG, et al: Extended treatment with bupropion SR for cigarette smoking cessation. J Consult Clin Psychol 74:286–294, 2006

Kirchheiner J, Klein C, Meineke I, et al: Bupropion and 4-OH-bupropion pharmacokinetics in relation to genetic polymorphisms in CYP2B6. Pharmacogenetics 13:619–626, 2003

Lam RW, Hossie H, Solomons K, et al: Citalopram and bupropion-SR: combining versus switching in patients with treatment-resistant depression. J Clin Psychiatry 65:337–340, 2004

Lineberry CG, Johnston JA, Raymond RN, et al: A fixed-dose (300 mg) efficacy study of bupropion and placebo in depressed outpatients. J Clin Psychiatry 51:194–199, 1990

McCollom RA, Elbe DH, Ritchie AH: Bupropion-induced serum sickness–like reaction. Ann Pharmacother 34:471–473, 2000

McIntyre RS, Mancini DA, McCann S, et al: Topiramate versus bupropion SR when added to mood stabilizer therapy for the depressive phase of bipolar disorder: a preliminary single-blind study. Bipolar Disord 4:207–213, 2002

McLaughlin T, Hogue SL, Stang PE: Once-daily bupropion associated with improved patient adherence compared with twice-daily bupropion in treatment of depression. Am J Ther 14:221–225, 2007

Mehta NB: The chemistry of bupropion. J Clin Psychiatry 44:56–59, 1983

Mendels J, Amin MM, Chouinard G, et al: A comparative study of bupropion and amitriptyline in depressed outpatients. J Clin Psychiatry 44:118–120, 1983

Miller DK, Sumithran SP, Dwoskin LP: Bupropion inhibits nicotine-evoked [(3)H]overflow from rat striatal slices preloaded with [(3)H]dopamine and from rat hippocampal slices preloaded with [(3)H]norepinephrine. J Pharmacol Exp Ther 302:1113–1122, 2002

Modell JG, May RS, Katholi CR: Effect of bupropion SR on orgasmic dysfunction in nondepressed subjects: a pilot study. J Sex Marital Ther 26:231–240, 2000

Modell JG, Rosenthal NE, Harriett AE, et al: Seasonal affective disorder and its prevention by anticipatory treatment with bupropion XL. Biol Psychiatry 58:658–667, 2005

Montgomery SA: Antidepressants and seizures: emphasis on newer agents and clinical implications. Int J Clin Pract 59:1435–1440, 2005

Oslin DW, Duffy K: The rise of serum aminotransferases in a patient treated with bupropion. J Clin Psychopharmacol 13:364–365, 1993

Papakostas GI, Kornstein SG, Clayton AH, et al: Relative antidepressant efficacy of bupropion and the selective serotonin reuptake inhibitors in major depressive disorder: gender-age interactions. Int Clin Psychopharmacol 22:226–229, 2007

Papakostas GI, Trivedi MH, Alpert JE, et al: Efficacy of bupropion and the selective serotonin reuptake inhibitors in the treatment of anxiety symptoms in major depressive disorder: a meta-analysis of individual patient data from 10 double-blind, randomized clinical trials. J Psychiatr Res 42:134–140, 2008

Peterson K, McDonagh MS, Fu R: Comparative benefits and harms of competing medications for adults with attention-deficit hyperactivity disorder: a systematic review and indirect comparison meta-analysis. Psychopharmacology 197:1–11, 2008

Physicians' Desk Reference: Wellbutrin (bupropion) tablets, Wellbutrin SR (bupropion) and Wellbutrin XL (bupropion), in Physicians' Desk Reference. Montvale, NJ, Thomson PDR, 2005, pp 1655–1659, 1659–1663, 1663–1668

Posner J, Bye A, Dean K, et al: The disposition of bupropion and its metabolites in healthy male volunteers after single and multiple doses. Eur J Clin Pharmacol 29:97–103, 1985

Preskorn SH, Fleck RJ, Schroeder DH: Therapeutic drug monitoring of bupropion. Am J Psychiatry 147:1690–1691, 1990

Rau KS, Birdsall E, Hanson JE, et al: Bupropion increases striatal vesicular monoamine transport. Neuropharmacology 49:820–830, 2005

Richelson E: Synaptic effects of antidepressants. J Clin Psychopharmacol 16:1S–7S; discussion 7S–9S, 1996

Riggs PD, Leon SL, Mikulich SK, et al: An open trial of bupropion for ADHD in adolescents with substance use disorders and conduct disorder. J Am Acad Child Adolesc Psychiatry 37:1271–1278, 1998

Rush AJ, Trivedi MH, Wisniewski SR, et al: Bupropion-SR, sertraline, or venlafaxine-XR after failure of SSRIs for depression. N Engl J Med 354:1231–1242, 2006

Sachs GS, Lafer B, Stoll AL, et al: A double-blind trial of bupropion versus desipramine for bipolar depression. J Clin Psychiatry 55:391–393, 1994

Schroeder DH: Metabolism and kinetics of bupropion. J Clin Psychiatry 44:79–81, 1983

Segraves RT, Croft H, Kavoussi R, et al: Bupropion sustained release (SR) for the treatment of hypoactive sexual desire disorder (HSDD) in nondepressed women. J Sex Marital Ther 27:303–316, 2001

Segraves RT, Clayton AH, Croft H, et al: Bupropion sustained release for the treatment of hypoactive sexual desire disorder in premenopausal women. J Clin Psychopharmacol 24:339–342, 2004

Settle EC, Stahl SM, Batey SR, et al: Safety profile of sustained-release bupropion in depression: results of three clinical trials. Clin Ther 21:454–463, 1999

Shopsin B: Bupropion's prophylactic efficacy in bipolar affective illness. J Clin Psychiatry 44:163–169, 1983

Shrier M, Diaz JE, Tsarouhas N: Cardiotoxicity associated with bupropion overdose. Ann Emerg Med 35:100, 2000

Simeon JG, Ferguson HB, Van Wyck Fleet J: Bupropion effects in attention deficit and conduct disorders. Can J Psychiatry 31:581–585, 1986

Soroko FE, Maxwell RA: The pharmacologic basis for therapeutic interest in bupropion. J Clin Psychiatry 44:67–73, 1983

Spier SA: Use of bupropion with SRIs and venlafaxine. Depress Anxiety 7:73–75, 1998

Stahl SM, Pradko JF, Haight BR, et al: A review of the neuropharmacology of bupropion, a dual norepinephrine and dopamine reuptake inhibitor. Prim Care Companion J Clin Psychiatry 6:159–166, 2004

Stern WC, Harto-Truax N, Bauer N: Efficacy of bupropion in tricyclic-resistant or intolerant patients. J Clin Psychiatry 44:148–152, 1983

Stewart JJ, Berkel HJ, Parish RC, et al: Single-dose pharmacokinetics of bupropion in adolescents: effects of smoking status and gender. J Clin Pharmacol 41:770–778, 2001

Sweet RA, Pollock BG, Kirshner M, et al: Pharmacokinetics of single- and multiple-dose bupropion in elderly patients with depression. J Clin Pharmacol 35:876–884, 1995

Thase ME, Haight BR, Richard N, et al: Remission rates following antidepressant therapy with bupropion or selective serotonin reuptake inhibitors: a meta-analysis of original data from 7 randomized controlled trials. J Clin Psychiatry 66:974–981, 2005

Thase ME, Clayton AH, Haight BR, et al: A double-blind comparison between bupropion XL and venlafaxine XR: sexual functioning, antidepressant efficacy, and tolerability. J Clin Psychopharmacol 26:482–488, 2006

Thase ME, Haight BR, Johnson MC, et al: A randomized, double-blind, placebo-controlled study of the effect of sustained-release bupropion on blood pressure in individuals with mild untreated hypertension. J Clin Psychopharmacol 28:302–307, 2008

Trivedi MH, Rush AJ, Carmody TJ, et al: Do bupropion SR and sertraline differ in their effects on anxiety in depressed patients? J Clin Psychiatry 62:776–781, 2001

Trivedi MH, Fava M, Wisniewski SR, et al: Medication augmentation after the failure of SSRIs for depression. N Engl J Med 354:1243–1252, 2006

Weihs KL, Settle EC Jr, Batey SR, et al: Bupropion sustained release versus paroxetine for the treatment of depression in the elderly. J Clin Psychiatry 61:196–202, 2000

Weihs KL, Houser TL, Batey SR, et al: Continuation phase treatment with bupropion SR effectively decreases the risk for relapse of depression. Biol Psychiatry 51:753–761, 2002

Weintraub D, Linder MW: Amphetamine positive toxicology screen secondary to bupropion. Depress Anxiety 12:53–54, 2000

Weisler RH, Johnston JA, Lineberry CG, et al: Comparison of bupropion and trazodone for the treatment of major depression. J Clin Psychopharmacol 14:170–179, 1994

Wilens TE, Spencer TJ, Biederman J, et al: A controlled clinical trial of bupropion for attention deficit hyperactivity disorder in adults. Am J Psychiatry 158:282–288, 2001

Wilkinson GR: Drug metabolism and variability among patients in drug response. N Engl J Med 352:2211–2221, 2005

Workman EA, Short DD: Atypical antidepressants versus imipramine in the treatment of major depression: a meta-analysis. J Clin Psychiatry 54:5–12, 1993

Worrall SP, Almond MK, Dhillon S: Pharmacokinetics of bupropion and its metabolites in hemodialysis patients who smoke:a single dose study. Nephron Clin Pract 97:c83–c89, 2004

Wright G, Galloway L, Kim J, et al: Bupropion in the long-term treatment of cyclic mood disorders: mood stabilizing effects. J Clin Psychiatry 46:22–25, 1985

CHAPTER 21

Mirtazapine

Alan F. Schatzberg, M.D.

History and Discovery

Mirtazapine, originally known as ORG 3770, was first synthesized by the Department of Medicinal Chemistry of NV Organon in the Netherlands (Kaspersen et al. 1989). First approved for use in major depression in the Netherlands in 1994, mirtazapine was introduced in the United States in 1996. The new drug application consisted of 47 Phase II/III clinical trials involving 2,796 mirtazapine-treated patients, 605 placebo-treated patients, and 1,161 active-control patients (Fawcett and Barkin 1998b).

Structure–Activity Relations

Mirtazapine is a member of the piperazinoazepines, a class of chemical compounds that is unrelated to any other class used in the treatment of psychiatric conditions (Maris et al. 1999) (Figure 21–1). Mirtazapine is also known by its chemical name, 1,2,3,4,10,14b-hexahydro-2-methyl-pyrazino[2,1-a]pyridol[2,3-c]benzazepine (Dahl et al. 1997; Dodd et al. 2000).

Pharmacological Profile

Mirtazapine is described as a noradrenergic and specific serotonergic antidepressant (NaSSA) (Holm and Markham 1999; Kent 2000; Nutt 1998). It is a potent serotonin$_2$ (5-HT$_2$), serotonin$_3$ (5-HT$_3$), and central α_2-adrenergic receptor antagonist (De Boer 1996; De Boer et al. 1995; Kooyman et al. 1994). Antagonism of 5-HT$_2$ and 5-HT$_3$ receptors results in an increase in serotonin$_{1A}$ (5-HT$_{1A}$) receptor–mediated transmission and, thus, a more specific effect on serotonergic transmission, relative to the selective serotonin reuptake inhibitor (SSRI) class of antidepressants (Bengtsson et al. 2000; Berendsen and Broekkamp 1997; Kent 2000). In addition, because α_2-adrenergic receptors normally act to inhibit transmission at serotonergic and noradrenergic axon terminals, mirtazapine acts to increase the release of both serotonin (5-HT) and norepinephrine (NE) via blockade of central α_2 receptors (Numazawa et al. 1995).

Mirtazapine has no significant affinity for dopamine (DA) receptors, low affinity for muscarinic cholinergic receptors (De Boer 1996), and high affinity for histamine$_1$ (H$_1$) receptors (De Boer 1996). Mirtazapine appears to have no effect on 5-HT and DA reuptake and only a minimal effect on NE reuptake (De Boer 1996; Kent 2000). The drug appears to significantly reduce cortisol levels (Laakmann et al. 2004; Schmid et al. 2006).

Pharmacokinetics and Disposition

Absorption

Mirtazapine is well absorbed from the gastrointestinal tract, and bioavailability does not appear to be affected by

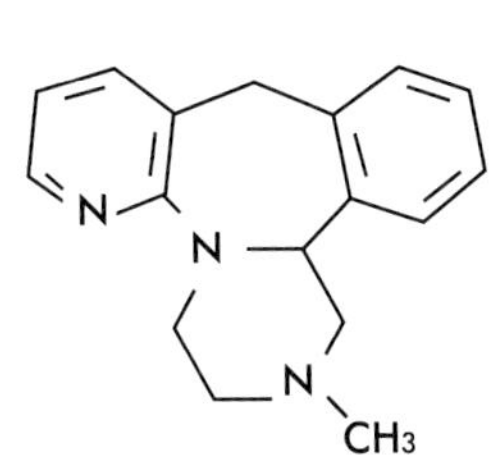

FIGURE 21–1. Chemical structure of mirtazapine.

the presence of food in the stomach (Fawcett and Barkin 1998b). An oral rapidly disintegrating tablet has been well studied and available for several years (Benkert et al. 2006).

Distribution

Mirtazapine appears to be 85% bound to plasma proteins (Fawcett and Barkin 1998b).

Metabolism

Mirtazapine is primarily metabolized by the liver via demethylation and hydroxylation, followed by glucuronide conjugation (Fawcett and Barkin 1998b; Remeron package insert 2002). Its major metabolite, desmethylmirtazapine, is weakly active but present in lower serum concentrations than is the parent compound (Fawcett and Barkin 1998b; Kent 2000). Mirtazapine lacks both autoinduction and autoinhibition of hepatic cytochrome P450 (CYP) enzymes (Fawcett and Barkin 1998b). Although in vitro studies do not demonstrate inhibitory effect, mirtazapine is a substrate for CYP1A2, 2D6, and 3A4 (Fawcett and Barkin 1998b; Remeron package insert 2002). Mirtazapine is a mild competitive inhibitor of CYP2D6 (Barkin et al. 2000; Fawcett and Barkin 1998b).

Elimination

Mirtazapine and its metabolites are eliminated primarily in the urine (up to 75%) and feces (up to 15%) (Fawcett and Barkin 1998b). The elimination half-life of mirtazapine is 20–40 hours (Fawcett and Barkin 1998b; Remeron package insert 2002; Stimmel et al. 1997). Of note, the clearance of mirtazapine may be affected by hepatic or renal impairment (Fawcett and Barkin 1998b). The elimination half-life may increase by 30%–40% in patients with hepatic impairment (Fawcett and Barkin 1998b; Kent 2000). In patients with moderate to severe renal impairment, the clearance of mirtazapine may be decreased by 30%–50% (Fawcett and Barkin 1998b; Kent 2000; Remeron package insert 2002).

Indications and Efficacy

Major Depression

Pooled data from the 6-week U.S. clinical trials that were part of the new drug application showed that approximately 50% of mirtazapine-treated patients and 20% of placebo-controlled patients achieved at least a 50% improvement in scores on the Hamilton Rating Scale for Depression (Ham-D) (Fawcett and Barkin 1998b).

In a randomized, double-blind, placebo-controlled study of 90 patients with major depression, mirtazapine treatment resulted in clinically significant reductions in Ham-D scores by study endpoint at 6 weeks, although improvement was noted as early as the first week (Claghorn and Lesem 1995).

A meta-analysis of four randomized, double-blind 6-week studies demonstrated mirtazapine to be as effective as amitriptyline in the treatment of major depression, but with significantly fewer anticholinergic, serotonergic, and cardiovascular adverse effects (Stahl et al. 1997).

In a multicenter randomized, double-blind study comparing mirtazapine and fluoxetine, both medications were found to be well tolerated in the treatment of major depression, although the former was noted to demonstrate a significantly greater improvement in Ham-D scores, beginning in the third week of treatment (Wheatley et al. 1998).

When mirtazapine was compared with paroxetine in a randomized, double-blind study of 275 patients with major depression, the two drugs were found to be, overall, equally well tolerated and efficacious, but mirtazapine was noted to result in significantly lower Ham-D and Hamilton Anxiety Scale (Ham-A) scores at week 1 (Benkert et al. 2000).

Similarly, when compared with citalopram in a multicenter randomized, double-blind, 8-week study of 270 patients with major depression, mirtazapine was equally well tolerated and efficacious at study endpoint, but significantly more effective on Ham-A, Montgomery-Åsberg Depression Rating Scale (MADRS), and Clinical Global Impression (CGI) Scale scores by week 2 (Leinonen et al. 1999).

Of interest, in a multicenter randomized, double-blind 8-week study comparing two antidepressants with both serotonergic and noradrenergic activity, mirtazapine was found to be equal in efficacy to venlafaxine in the treatment of major depression with melancholic features, although it demonstrated a trend, which was not statistically significant, toward a higher percentage of responders and remitters (Guelfi et al. 2001).

The sleep effects of mirtazapine in major depression were recently reported by Steiger's group (Schmid et al. 2006). Mirtazapine improved sleep continuity by day 2 of therapy, and the effect was sustained for at least 4 weeks. At day 28, significant increases in slow-wave and low-delta sleep were also observed.

Treatment Failure With a Selective Serotonin Reuptake Inhibitor

In an 8-week open-label study of 103 outpatients with DSM-IV (American Psychiatric Association 1994) major depressive disorder complicated by failure to respond to (or intolerance of) treatment with fluoxetine, paroxetine, or sertraline, approximately one-half of the outpatients demonstrated a 50% reduction in the 17-item Ham-D (Ham-D-17) score when switched to treatment with mirtazapine (Fava et al. 2001).

In a 4-week study of patients with persistent major depression, despite adequate antidepressant monotherapy, augmentation with mirtazapine resulted in a 45% remission rate, compared with a 13% remission rate among patients receiving placebo augmentation (Carpenter et al. 2002). Of note, in this latter study, there were no significant differences in terms of side effects between patients treated with mirtazapine augmentation and patients receiving placebo augmentation (Carpenter et al. 2002).

In level 3 of the Sequenced Treatment Alternatives to Relieve Depression (STAR*D) trial, mirtazapine was compared with nortriptyline in patients who had failed to respond to two previous consecutive trials with antidepressants (Fava et al. 2006). Level 1 of STAR*D employed citalopram; level 2 employed a switch to another drug or augmentation. Nortriptyline produced higher remission rates than did mirtazapine (19.8% vs. 12.3%); however, the difference was not statistically significant.

Patients With Depression and Sexual Dysfunction

In an open-label study of 103 patients with depression treated with mirtazapine, 54% of patients who had reported poor or very poor sexual functioning during prior treatment with an SSRI described an improvement in sexual functioning by study endpoint (Fava et al. 2001).

Similarly, Gelenberg et al. (2000) reported 58% of patients with prior SSRI-induced sexual dysfunction had a return of normal sexual functioning when they switched to treatment with mirtazapine.

In contrast, augmentation with mirtazapine was no more effective than placebo augmentation in reversing SSRI-associated sexual side effects in patients with fluoxetine-associated sexual dysfunction (Michelson et al. 2002).

Depression in Elderly Patients

In a study of 150 outpatients (ages between 55 and 80 years) with moderate to severe depression, mirtazapine was found to be effective, safe, and well tolerated (Halikas 1995). In this 6-week trial, 50% of the mirtazapine-treated patients and 35% of the placebo-treated patients demonstrated at least a 50% reduction in Ham-D score (Halikas 1995). In another blinded study, mirtazapine was significantly more effective than paroxetine at weeks 1, 2, 3, and 6, but not at week 8, in subjects older than 65 years (Schatzberg et al. 2002). Differences were observed primarily on measures of anxiety and sleep. Apolipoprotein epsilon 4 (*ApoE*-ε4) carrier status predicted a positive response to mirtazapine (Murphy et al. 2003).

An oral disintegrating tablet has been studied in the elderly and appears to be well tolerated (Nelson et al. 2007; Varia et al. 2007).

Patients With Comorbid and Primary Symptoms of Anxiety

Meta-analyses of placebo-controlled studies of patients with depression and associated symptoms of anxiety have demonstrated that mirtazapine-treated patients exhibit significantly greater improvement in symptoms of anxiety (Fawcett and Barkin 1998a; Nutt 1998), beginning as early as the first week of treatment (Fawcett and Barkin 1998a).

In an 8-week open-label study of 10 patients with major depressive disorder and comorbid generalized anxiety disorder, mirtazapine treatment resulted in significant decreases in Ham-D and Ham-A scores, with improvement beginning as early as the first week of treatment (Goodnick et al. 1999).

Dysthymia

In a 10-week open-label trial of the use of mirtazapine in 15 patients with dysthymic disorder, 8 patients demonstrated at least a 40% reduction in Ham-D scores, and 4 of these 8 patients exhibited a remission of symptoms by study endpoint (Dunner et al. 1999).

Posttraumatic Stress Disorder

In an 8-week open-label study of six patients with severe chronic posttraumatic stress disorder (PTSD), mirtazapine treatment resulted in one-half of the patients demonstrating at least a 50% reduction in CGI score and significant reductions on scales of PTSD severity (Connor et al. 1999).

In a 6-week double-blind comparison study, mirtazapine was compared with sertraline in Korean veterans with PTSD (Chung et al. 2004). At study endpoint, mirtazapine was statistically significantly superior to sertraline on several measures (e.g., Clinician-Administered PTSD Scale—Part 2 [CAPS-2]). Efficacy was apparently maintained to 24 weeks (Kim et al. 2005).

Social Phobia

Mirtazapine was compared with placebo in a 10-week double-blind comparison study in 66 women with social phobia. Mirtazapine appeared to separate from placebo on several primary measures of social phobia symptoms (Muehlbacher et al. 2005).

Generalized Anxiety Disorder

In an open-label trial of mirtazapine treatment in 44 adult patients with generalized anxiety disorder, response criteria were achieved in 80% of patients (Gambi et al. 2005). Controlled trial data are not available.

Obsessive-Compulsive Disorder

Koran et al. (2005) reported on a two-phase study (a 12-week open-label phase followed by an 8-week double-blind discontinuation phase) of mirtazapine (maximum dosage = 60 mg/day) in 30 patients with obsessive-compulsive disorder (OCD). In the 8-week discontinuation phase, mirtazapine was significantly more effective than placebo in preventing symptom recurrence.

Mirtazapine augmentation of citalopram was assessed in 49 nondepressed OCD patients (Pallanti et al. 2004). Subjects were treated with citalopram plus placebo or citalopram plus mirtazapine under single-blind conditions. Mirtazapine appeared to speed the response to citalopram but not to improve overall response.

Sleep Disorders

Because of its sedating properties in depression, mirtazapine has recently been studied in patients with primary sleep disorders. In a double-blind crossover study in 7 patients with obstructive sleep apnea, mirtazapine dosages of 4.5 and 15 mg/day produced significantly greater reductions (on the order of 46%–52%) in apnea–hypopnea index (AHI) scores in comparison with placebo (Carley et al. 2007). However, the authors' concerns regarding weight gain and sedation led them to not recommend it at this time as a primary therapy.

Chronic or Recurrent Pain

A number of case reports indicate mirtazapine could be beneficial in chronic recurrent pain. A 56-year-old man with an 11-year history of treatment-refractory cluster headaches who was treated for 6 weeks with mirtazapine (30 mg/day) experienced rapid reduction in frequency and intensity of cluster attacks, with a concomitant decreased need for interventions, such as oxygen therapy and sumatriptan (Nutt 1999). A 47-year-old man with chronic pain symptoms resulting from a severe fall injury and major depression was treated unsuccessfully with amitriptyline, fluoxetine, and bupropion; however, the patient demonstrated significant improvement in symptoms of depression and pain, beginning 1 month after initiating mirtazapine (Brannon and Stone 1999). Another case report described a patient who was successfully treated with mirtazapine for major depression. The patient was also able to successfully abort migraine headaches with an extra dose of 7.5 mg of mirtazapine (Brannon et al. 2000). Finally, a report on four patients with phantom limb pain noted improvement in all cases (Kuiken et al. 2005).

A large series of 600 patients with comorbid pain and depression treated with mirtazapine has been reported in Germany (Freynhagen et al. 2006). The drug appeared to reduce pain effectively in this sample, with a relatively low-order risk of side effects (7%) at a mean dosage of 35 mg/day.

The drug at 15–30 mg/day has also been reported to be effective in a double-blind crossover study in 24 nondepressed patients with chronic tension headaches (Bendtsen and Jensen 2004). Area under the curve (intensity times duration) for headache was significantly lower for drug than placebo.

Oncology

Theobold (2000) described a case of a 59-year-old patient with B-cell lymphoma recurrence treated with mirtazapine with a resolution of symptoms of depression, combined with a significant improvement in prior symptoms of anorexia and weight loss, by the end of 6 weeks of treatment.

A case series of 20 breast cancer and gynecological patients treated with mirtazapine demonstrated a significant reduction in symptoms of depression, anxiety, nausea, anorexia, and insomnia in 19 of the patients, as well as a lack of adverse drug interactions when combined with the usual treatment regimen, including chemotherapy (Thompson 2000).

A 7-week open-label, crossover trial of mirtazapine in 20 patients with cancer revealed significant improvements in mood, anxiety, insomnia, appetite, weight, and pain symptoms by the study endpoint (Theobold et al. 2002).

It has been suggested that mirtazapine could prove to be a safe and effective adjunct to cancer chemotherapy because of its ability to treat nausea via a 5-HT$_3$ receptor antagonism effect; insomnia, anorexia, and weight loss via H$_1$ receptor antagonism; symptoms of depression via enhanced 5-HT and noradrenergic transmission by way of α_2, 5-HT$_2$, and 5-HT$_3$ receptor blockade; and symptoms of anxiety via 5-HT$_2$ and 5-HT$_3$ receptor antagonism (Kast 2001).

Obstetrics/Gynecology

A review of seven cases of pregnant patients with treatment-refractory hyperemesis gravidarum and symptoms of depression and anxiety revealed that treatment with mirtazapine resulted in resolution of symptoms without adverse impact on the newborns (Saks 2001).

Waldinger et al. (2000) described four cases in which women (ages between 39 and 60 years) experienced a near-complete resolution of symptoms of hot flushes and perspiration within the first week of treatment with mirtazapine.

An 8-week open-label trial of mirtazapine in 22 menopausal patients receiving estrogen replacement therapy who had major depression demonstrated an almost 90% remission rate among the study completers (Joffe et al. 2001).

Pediatric Depression and Anxiety

Mirtazapine has been assessed in several trials involving children or adolescents with major depression or anxiety disorders. In one trial of 24 adolescents with major depression, patients responded well to the drug, with no dropouts due to side effects (Haapasalo-Pesu et al. 2004). In another small open-label trial in 18 patients with social phobia, mirtazapine also demonstrated efficacy (Mrakotsky et al. 2008). Although there was a very high dropout rate, most of the discontinuations were not due to side effects.

Pervasive Developmental Disorders

In an open-label study on the use of mirtazapine in 26 patients with pervasive developmental disorders, 35% of subjects demonstrated significant improvement on CGI scores with respect to symptoms of aggression, self-injury, irritability, hyperactivity, anxiety, depression, and insomnia (Posey et al. 2001).

Depression in Alzheimer's Disease

Raji and Brady (2001) described three cases of patients with comorbid Alzheimer's dementia (Mini-Mental State Exam [MMSE] scores of 21/30, 11/30, and 18/30) and depressive symptomatology who were treated safely with mirtazapine. The patients demonstrated significant improvement in appetite, weight loss, sleep disturbances, anxiety, mood, anhedonia, and energy level.

Schizophrenia

The utility of mirtazapine in the treatment of the negative symptoms of schizophrenia has been examined. In a 6-week double-blind, randomized, placebo-controlled trial, addition of mirtazapine to haloperidol in the treatment of schizophrenia demonstrated a statistically significant reduction in Positive and Negative Syndrome Scale (PANSS) scores, as well as in CGI–Severity and CGI–Improvement scores (Berk et al. 2001). In addition, PANSS negative symptom scores in this study were found to be reduced by 42% in the group of patients who received adjunctive mirtazapine, compared with the group who received placebo (Berk et al. 2001). Furthermore, the latter finding was not correlated with Ham-D scores at study endpoint, which suggests that the effect of mirtazapine on diminution of negative symptoms in schizophrenia is not a result of improvement in mood symptoms (Berk et al. 2001).

Akathisia

Poyurovsky et al. (2003, 2006) conducted two double-blind, placebo-controlled studies of mirtazapine treatment of antipsychotic-induced akathisia in patients with schizophrenia. In the first study (Poyurovsky et al. 2003), mirtazapine 15 mg/day was compared with placebo in 26 patients. The drug was significantly superior to placebo. In the second study (Poyurovsky et al. 2003), mirtazapine at the same dose was compared with propranolol 80 mg/day or placebo in 90 patients. Both drugs separated from placebo, but propranolol was associated with significantly greater bradycardia and hypotension.

Side Effects and Toxicology

In an open-label study of 103 outpatients with DSM-IV major depressive disorder, the most commonly reported side effects with mirtazapine were somnolence (49.5%), increased appetite (29.7%), and weight gain (22.8%) (Fava et al. 2001).

In a double-blind, placebo-controlled study of outpatients with depression, somnolence, increased appetite, and weight gain were the most commonly reported side effects associated with mirtazapine treatment (Claghorn and Lesem 1995).

In a review of data from the clinical development program for mirtazapine, the only adverse effects that occurred at a higher incidence with mirtazapine versus placebo were excessive sedation, increased appetite, weight gain, and dry mouth (Montgomery 1995). Also reported in this review was the observation that these side effects were typically mild and transient in nature and that they decreased with time and often diminished with increased dose (Montgomery 1995).

Side effects typical of SSRIs, such as nausea, diarrhea, and sexual dysfunction, appear to occur less frequently in patients treated with mirtazapine (Boyarsky et al. 1999; Farah 1998; Montgomery 1995; Stimmel et al. 1997).

Mirtazapine also appears to be well tolerated in elderly patients. The most common side effects reported, including somnolence, increased appetite, weight gain, and dry mouth, are of the same type as those reported in younger adults (Fawcett and Barkin 1998b; Halikas 1995).

Mirtazapine appears to have a very low incidence of causing clinically relevant laboratory abnormalities, such as transient rise in liver enzymes (2%) and severe neutropenia (0.1%) (Claghorn and Lesem 1995; Fawcett and Barkin 1998b; Kent 2000; Montgomery 1995).

Mirtazapine appears to have no clinically significant effects on seizure threshold or on the cardiovascular system (Claghorn and Lesem 1995; Fawcett and Barkin 1998b; Kent 2000; Montgomery 1995).

Of note, the noradrenergic effects of mirtazapine appear to be dose dependent and increase significantly at dosages >15 mg/day. As such, sedation associated with the affinity for H_1 receptors and typically experienced at dosages of ≤15 mg/day may be counteracted by an increasing noradrenergic neurotransmission at dosages ≥30 mg/day (Claghorn and Lesem 1995; Kent 2000). Likewise, it is also hypothesized that the risk of weight gain with mirtazapine is diminished at dosages ≥30 mg/day (Barkin et al. 2000; Fawcett and Barkin 1998b).

Use During Pregnancy and Lactation

A recent study conducted across six countries (Djulus et al. 2006) assessed the risk associated with exposure to mirtazapine during pregnancy. Birth outcomes were examined for three groups: pregnant women taking mirtazapine, disease-matched pregnant women taking other antidepressants, and pregnant women exposed to nonteratogens. There were approximately 100 patients per group. The rate of spontaneous abortions in the mirtazapine group (19%) was similar to that in the other antidepressant group (17%) and in the nonteratogen control group (11%). The rate of prematurity was significantly higher in the mirtazapine group (10%) versus the nonteratogen group (2%). The prematurity rate in the group taking other antidepressants was 7%. The rate of major malformations was not elevated in the mirtazapine group.

In a study of 8 women taking mirtazapine while breast feeding, concentrations of mirtazapine or desmethylmirtazapine were measured in milk and plasma (Kristensen 2007). Low infant doses were observed, leading the authors to conclude that the drug is safe for lactating women who breast feed.

Overdose

Mirtazapine appears to be safe in overdose. In one report (Holzbach et al. 1998), the cases of two patients who had overdosed with 30–50 times the average daily dose of mirtazapine were presented. In each case, the patient recovered fully and without any complications. The first patient was a 44-year-old woman with a diagnosis of major depression who attempted suicide with 900 mg of mirtazapine, combined with an unknown quantity of amitriptyline and 0.5 L of wine. On admission to the hospital, the patient was somnolent and depressed but with normal vital signs, electrocardiogram, and neurological examination.

The second patient reported by Holzbach et al. (1998) was a 51-year-old woman with a diagnosis of major depression who attempted suicide with 1,500 mg of mirtazapine and 1 L of wine. Somnolence, minor sinus tachycardia, and mild leukocytosis were noted in this patient on admission to the hospital.

Overall, symptoms reported in cases of mirtazapine overdose include disorientation, drowsiness, impaired memory, and tachycardia (Fawcett and Barkin 1998b; Kent 2000; Montgomery 1995; Stimmel et al. 1997).

A review of 117 mirtazapine overdoses (average ingestion: 450 mg) in Scotland revealed the adverse consequences to be relatively mild (Waring et al. 2007). Decreased consciousness was seen in 27% of subjects; 30% demonstrated tachycardia.

Drug–Drug Interactions

In vitro data suggest that mirtazapine is unlikely to have clinically significant effects on the metabolism of drugs by cytochrome P450 enzymes (Barkin et al. 2000; Fawcett and Barkin 1998b; Kent 2000). Analysis of data from the clinical development program for mirtazapine and postmarketing surveillance reveal no clinically relevant drug–drug interactions occurring with the concomitant use of medications, such as opiates, anticonvulsants, analgesics, antihypertensives, diuretics, or nonsteroidal anti-inflammatory drugs (NSAIDs) (Barkin et al. 2000; Fawcett and Barkin 1998b). However, few formal drug interaction studies involving mirtazapine have been performed (Barkin et al. 2000; Fawcett and Barkin 1998b; Holm and Markham 1999). Of note, a recent study of elderly patients with depression allowed for patients to be on drugs that are CYP2D6 substrates (Schatzberg et al. 2002). In this latter study, no increase in side effects was observed in these patients, compared with patients who were not taking CYP2D6 substrate agents (Schatzberg et al. 2002).

Conclusion

In conclusion, mirtazapine is derived from the piperazinoazepine class of compounds and, as such, is structurally unrelated to any other psychotropic medication. Mirtazapine is also unique as an antidepressant because of its 5-HT$_2$, 5-HT$_3$, and α_2 receptor antagonist pharmacodynamic profile, which results in enhancement of noradrenergic and serotonergic transmission. It is an antidepressant that has been shown to be efficacious and well tolerated in the treatment of depression, and there are suggestions that it may be effective in a number of other medical and psychiatric conditions. Mirtazapine has also been suggested as a treatment intervention that may offer a more rapid amelioration of symptoms of depression and anxiety, compared with other antidepressants. The most common side effects reported with mirtazapine include somnolence, increased appetite, weight gain, and dry mouth. It otherwise appears to be a medication that is free of many of the adverse effects typical of the SSRIs, especially sexual dysfunction.

Furthermore, mirtazapine appears to be well tolerated and equally effective in the treatment of geriatric depression. In addition, mirtazapine appears to be safe in overdose, with case reports documenting complete and uncomplicated recovery following ingestion of up to 50 times the average daily dose. Finally, mirtazapine appears devoid of clinically significant drug–drug interactions, although larger formal clinical trials are still needed to verify this.

References

American Psychiatric Association: Diagnostic and Statistical Manual of Mental Disorders, 4th Edition. Washington, DC, American Psychiatric Association, 1994

Barkin RL, Schwer W, Barkin SJ: Recognition and management of depression in primary care: a focus on the elderly. A pharmacotherapeutic overview of the selection process among the traditional and new antidepressants. Am J Ther 7:205–226, 2000

Bendtsen L, Jensen R: Mirtazapine is effective in the prophylactic treatment of chronic tension-type headache. Neurology 62:1706–1711, 2004

Bengtsson HJ, Kele J, Johansson J, et al: Interaction of the antidepressant mirtazapine with α_2 adrenoceptors modulating the release of 5-HT in different rat brain regions in vivo. Naunyn Schmiedebergs Arch Pharmacol 362:406–412, 2000

Benkert O, Szegedi A, Kohnen R: Mirtazapine compared with paroxetine in major depression. J Clin Psychiatry 61:656–663, 2000

Benkert O, Szegedi A, Philipp M, et al: Mirtazapine orally disintegrating tables versus venlafaxine extended release: a double-blind, randomized multicenter trial comparing the onset of antidepressant response in patients with major depressive disorder. J Clin Psychopharmacol 26:75–78, 2006

Berendsen HHG, Broekkamp CLE: Indirect in vivo 5-HT1A-agonistic effects of the new antidepressant mirtazapine. Psychopharmacology (Berl) 133:275–282, 1997

Berk M, Ichim C, Brook S: Efficacy of mirtazapine add on therapy to haloperidol in the treatment of the negative symptoms of schizophrenia: a double-blind randomized placebo-controlled study. Int Clin Psychopharmacol 16:87–92, 2001

Boyarsky BK, Haque W, Rouleau MR, et al: Sexual functioning in depressed outpatients taking mirtazapine. Depress Anxiety 9:175–179, 1999

Brannon GE, Stone KD: The use of mirtazapine in a patient with chronic pain. J Pain Symptom Manage 18:382–385, 1999

Brannon GE, Rolland PD, Gary JM: Use of mirtazapine as prophylactic treatment for migraine headache. Psychosomatics 41:153–154, 2000

Carley DW, Olopade C, Ruigt GS, et al: Efficacy of mirtazapine in obstructive sleep apnea syndrome. Sleep 30:35–41, 2007

Carpenter LL, Yasmin S, Price L: A double-blind, placebo-controlled study of antidepressant augmentation with mirtazapine. Biol Psychiatry 51:183–188, 2002

Chung MY, Min KH, Jun YJ, et al: Efficacy and tolerability of mirtazapine and sertraline in Korean veterans with posttraumatic stress disorder: a randomized open label trial. Hum Psychopharmacol 19:489–494, 2004

Claghorn JL, Lesem MD: A double-blind placebo-controlled study of Org 3770 in depressed outpatients. J Affect Disord 34:165–171, 1995

Connor KM, Davidson JRT, Weisler RH, et al: A pilot study of mirtazapine in post-traumatic stress disorder. Int Clin Psychopharmacol 14:29–31, 1999

Dahl ML, Voortman G, Alm C, et al: In vitro and in vivo studies on the disposition of mirtazapine in humans. Clin Drug Invest 13:37–46, 1997

De Boer T: The pharmacologic profile of mirtazapine. J Clin Psychiatry 57 (suppl 4):19–25, 1996

De Boer T, Ruigt GCF, Berendsen HHG: The α-2 adrenoceptor antagonist Org 3770 (mirtazapine, Remeron®) enhances noradrenergic and serotonergic transmission. Hum Psychopharmacol Clin Exp 10 (suppl):S107–S118, 1995

Djulus J, Koren G, Einarson TR, et al: Exposure to mirtazapine during pregnancy: a prospective, comparative study of birth outcomes. J Clin Psychiatry 67:1280–1284, 2006

Dodd S, Burrows GD, Norman TR: Chiral determination of mirtazapine in human blood plasma by high-performance liquid chromatography. J Chromatogr B Biomed Sci Appl 748:439–443, 2000

Dunner DL, Hendrickson HE, Bea C, et al: Dysthymic disorder: treatment with mirtazapine. Depress Anxiety 10:68–72, 1999

Farah A: Lack of sexual adverse effects with mirtazapine. Am Health Syst Pharm 55:2195–2196, 1998

Fava M, Dunner DL, Greist JH, et al: Efficacy and safety of mirtazapine in major depressive disorder patients after SSRI treatment failure: an open-label trial. J Clin Psychiatry 62:413–420, 2001

Fava M, Rush AJ, Wisniewski SR, et al: A comparison of mirtazapine and nortriptyline following two consecutive failed medication treatments for depressed outpatients: a STAR*D report. Am J Psychiatry 163:1161–1172, 2006

Fawcett J, Barkin RL: A meta-analysis of eight randomized, double-blind controlled clinical trials of mirtazapine for the treatment of patients with major depression and symptoms of anxiety. J Clin Psychiatry 59:123–127, 1998a

Fawcett J, Barkin RL: Review of the results from clinical studies on the efficacy, safety and tolerability of mirtazapine for the treatment of patients with major depression. J Affect Disord 51:267–285, 1998b

Freynhagen R, Muth-Selbach U, Lipfert P, et al: The effect of mirtazapine in patients with chronic pain and concomitant depression. Curr Med Res Opin 22:257–264, 2006

Gambi F, De Berardis D, Campanello D, et al: Mirtazapine treatment of generalized anxiety disorder: a fixed dose, open label study. J Psychopharmacol 19:483–487, 2005

Gelenberg AJ, Laukes C, McGauhey C, et al: Mirtazapine substitution in SSRI-induced sexual dysfunction. J Clin Psychiatry 61:356–360, 2000

Goodnick PJ, Puig A, DeVane CL, et al: Mirtazapine in major depression with comorbid generalized anxiety disorder. J Clin Psychiatry 60:446–448, 1999

Guelfi JD, Ansseau M, Timmerman L, et al: Mirtazapine versus venlafaxine in hospitalized severely depressed patients with melancholic features. J Clin Psychopharmacol 21:425–431, 2001

Haapasalo-Pesu KM, Vuola T, Lahelma L, et al: Mirtazapine in the treatment of adolescents with major depression: an open-label, multicenter pilot study. J Child Adolesc Psychopharmacol 14:175–184, 2004

Halikas JA: Org 3770 (mirtazapine) versus trazodone: a placebo controlled trial in depressed elderly patients. Hum Psychopharmacol 10:125–133, 1995

Holm KJ, Markham A: Mirtazapine: a review of its use in major depression. Drugs 57:607–631, 1999

Holzbach R, Jahn H, Pajonk FG, et al: Suicide attempts with mirtazapine overdose without complications. Biol Psychiatry 44:925–926, 1998

Joffe H, Groninger H, Soares C, et al: An open trial of mirtazapine in menopausal women with depression unresponsive to estrogen replacement therapy. J Womens Health Gend Based Med 10:999–1004, 2001

Kaspersen FM, van Rooij FAM, Sperling EMG: The synthesis of Org 3770 labeled with 3-H, 13-C and 14-C. J Labelled Comp Radiopharma 27:1055–1068, 1989

Kast RE: Mirtazapine may be useful in treating nausea and insomnia of cancer chemotherapy. Support Care Cancer 9:469–470, 2001

Kent JM: SNaRIs, NaSSAs, and NaRIs: new agents for the treatment of depression. Lancet 355:911–918, 2000

Kim W, Pae CU, Chae JH, et al: The effectiveness of mirtazapine in the treatment of post-traumatic stress disorder: a 24-week continuation therapy. Psychiatry Clin Neurosci 59:743–747, 2005

Kooyman AR, Zwart R, Vanderheijden PM, et al: Interaction between enantiomers of mianserin and Org 3770 at 5-HT3 receptors in cultured mouse neuroblastoma cells. Neuropsychopharmacology 33:501–510, 1994

Koran LM, Gamel NN, Choung HW, et al: Mirtazapine for obsessive-compulsive disorder: an open trial followed by double-blind discontinuation. J Clin Psychiatry 66:515–520, 2005

Kristensen JH, Ilett KF, Rampono J, et al: Transfer of the antidepressant mirtazapine into breast milk. Br J Clin Pharmacol 63:322–327, 2007

Kuiken TA, Schechtman L, Harden RN: Phantom limb pain treatment with mirtazapine: a case series. Pain Pract 5:356–360, 2005

Laakmann G, Hennig J, Baghai T, et al: Mirtazapine acutely inhibits salivary cortisol concentrations in depressed patients. Ann N Y Acad Sci 1032:279–282, 2004

Leinonen E, Skarstein J, Behnke K, et al: Efficacy and tolerability of mirtazapine versus citalopram: a double-blind, randomized study in patients with major depressive disorder. Int Clin Psychopharmacol 14:329–337, 1999

Maris FA, Dingler E, Niehues S: High-performance liquid chromatographic assay with fluorescence detection for the routine monitoring of the antidepressant mirtazapine and its desmethyl metabolite in human plasma. J Chromatogr B Biomed Sci Appl 721:309–316, 1999

Michelson D, Kociban K, Tamura R, et al: Mirtazapine, yohimbine or olanzapine augmentation therapy for serotonin reuptake-associated female sexual dysfunction: a randomized, placebo controlled trial. J Psychiatr Res 36:147–152, 2002

Montgomery SA: Safety of mirtazapine: a review. Int Clin Psychopharmacol 10 (suppl 4):37–45, 1995

Mrakotsky C, Masek B, Biederman J, et al: Prospective open-label pilot trial of mirtazapine in children and adolescents with social phobia. J Anxiety Disord 22:88–97, 2008

Muehlbacher M, Nickel MK, Nickel C, et al: Mirtazapine treatment of social phobia in women: a randomized, double-blind, placebo-controlled study. J Clin Psychopharmacol 25:580–582, 2005

Murphy GM, Kremer C, Rodrigues H, et al: The apolipoprotein E epsilon4 allele and antidepressant efficacy in cognitively intact elderly depressed patients. Biol Psychiatry 54:665–673, 2003

Nelson JC, Holden K, Roose S, et al: Are there predictors of outcome in depressed elderly nursing home residents during treatment with mirtazapine orally disintegrating tablets? Int J Geriatr Psychiatry 22:999–1003, 2007

Numazawa R, Yoshioka M, Matsumoto M, et al: Pharmacological characterization of α-2 adrenoceptor regulated serotonin release in the rat hippocampus. Neurosci Lett 192:161–164, 1995

Nutt DJ: Efficacy of mirtazapine in clinically relevant subgroups of depressed patients. Depress Anxiety 7 (suppl 1):7–10, 1998

Nutt D: Treatment of cluster headache with mirtazapine. Headache 39:586–587, 1999

Pallanti S, Quercioli L, Bruscoli M: Response acceleration with mirtazapine augmentation of citalopram in obsessive-compulsive disorder patients without comorbid depression: a pilot study. J Clin Psychiatry 65:1394–1399, 2004

Posey DJ, Guenin KD, Kohn AE, et al: A naturalistic open-label study of mirtazapine in autistic and other pervasive developmental disorders. J Child Adolesc Psychopharmacol 11:267–277, 2001

Poyurovsky M, Epshtein S, Fuchs C, et al: Efficacy of low-dose mirtazapine in neuroleptic-induced akathisia: a double-blind randomized placebo-controlled pilot study. J Clin Psychopharmacol 23:305–308, 2003

Poyurovsky M, Pashinian A, Weizman R, et al: Low-dose mirtazapine: a new option in the treatment of antipsychotic-induced akathisia. A randomized, double-blind, placebo- and propranolol-controlled trial. Biol Psychiatry 59:1071–1077, 2006

Raji MA, Brady SR: Mirtazapine for treatment of depression and comorbidities in Alzheimer's disease. Ann Pharmacother 35:1024–1027, 2001

Remeron (package insert). Physicians' Desk Reference, 56th Edition. Montvale, NJ, Medical Economics Company, 2002

Saks BR: Mirtazapine: treatment of depression, anxiety, and hyperemesis gravidarum in the pregnant patient: a report of 7 cases. Arch Women Ment Health 3:165–170, 2001

Schatzberg AF, Kremer C, Rodrigues HE, et al: Double-blind randomized comparison of mirtazapine and paroxetine in elderly depressed patients. Am J Geriatr Psychiatry 10:541–550, 2002

Schmid DA, Wichniak A, Uhr M, et al: Changes of sleep architecture, spectral composition of sleep EEG, the nocturnal secretion of cortisol, ACTH, GH, prolactin, melatonin, ghrelin, and leptin, and the DEX-CRH test in depressed patients during treatment with mirtazapine. Neuropsychopharmacology 31:832–844, 2006

Stahl S, Zivkov M, Reimitz PE, et al: Meta-analysis of randomized, double-blind, placebo-controlled, efficacy and safety studies of mirtazapine versus amitriptyline in major depression. Acta Psychiatr Scand Suppl 391:22–30, 1997

Stimmel GL, Dopheide JA, Stahl SM: Mirtazapine: an antidepressant with noradrenergic and specific serotonergic effects. Pharmacotherapy 17:10–21, 1997

Theobold DE: A patient with B-cell lymphoma and major depression treated with mirtazapine. Primary Care and Cancer 20:61–63, 2000

Theobold DE, Kirsh KE, Holtszclaw E, et al: An open-label, crossover trial of mirtazapine (15 and 30 mg) in cancer patients with pain and other distressing symptoms. J Pain Symptom Manage 23:442–447, 2002

Thompson DS: Mirtazapine for the treatment of depression and nausea in breast and gynecological oncology. Psychosomatics 41:356–359, 2000

Varia I, Venkataraman S, Hellegers C, et al: Effect of mirtazapine orally disintegrating tablets on health-related quality of life in elderly depressed patients with comorbid medical disorders: a pilot study. Psychopharmacol Bull 40:47–56, 2007

Waldinger MD, Berendsen HHG, Schweitzer DH: Treatment of hot flushes with mirtazapine: four case reports. Maturitas 36:165–168, 2000

Waring WS, Good AM, Bateman DN: Lack of significant toxicity after mirtazapine overdose: a five-year review of cases admitted to a regional toxicology unit. Clin Toxicol (Phila) 45:45–50, 2007

Wheatley DP, Van Moffaert M, Timmerman L, et al: Mirtazapine: efficacy and tolerability in comparison with fluoxetine in patients with moderate to severe major depressive disorder. J Clin Psychiatry 59:306–312, 1998

Venlafaxine and Desvenlafaxine

Michael E. Thase, M.D.

Diane M. Sloan, Pharm.D.

History and Discovery

The drug known as venlafaxine was first synthesized in the early 1980s and was found to block the uptake of serotonin (5-HT) and, with lower potency, norepinephrine (NE), in rat brain synaptosomal preparations (Muth et al. 1986). Subsequently, it was shown to have in vivo activity in animal models of depression and to have little affinity for muscarinic or histaminergic postsynaptic receptors (Bolden-Watson and Richelson 1993; Muth et al. 1986). As such, venlafaxine was predicted to have a better tolerability profile than the tricyclic antidepressants (TCAs). Several early randomized, controlled trials (RCTs) confirmed that venlafaxine had antidepressant effects comparable to those of TCAs, with fewer side effects attributable to anticholinergic and antihistaminergic activity (see, for example, T.R. Einarson et al. 1999). The initial formulation of venlafaxine—now known as venlafaxine immediate-release (IR)—was approved by the U.S. Food and Drug Administration (FDA) for treatment of depression in 1994. An extended-release (XR) formulation was introduced a little more than 3 years later. Generic formulations of venlafaxine IR began to be introduced in 2007.

O-desmethylvenlafaxine (ODV), or simply desvenlafaxine, the primary active metabolite of venlafaxine, was introduced in 2008 as desvenlafaxine succinate, a sustained-release formulation for treatment of depression. Like venlafaxine, desvenlafaxine is classified as a serotonin–norepinephrine reuptake inhibitor (SNRI) and has minimal effects on other neurotransmitter receptors. Desvenlafaxine was developed in the hope of improving on the strengths of the parent drug. In vitro studies indicate that desvenlafaxine is somewhat more potent for blockade of norepinephrine transporters than the parent drug; the succinate salt was chosen to enhance bioavailability (Deecher et al. 2006). To date, desvenlafaxine's efficacy has been established in a series of placebo-controlled RCTs of major depressive disorder (MDD).

Structure–Activity Relations

Venlafaxine and desvenlafaxine are bicyclic phenylethylamine compounds and are structurally and chemically unrelated to all other available antidepressants and anxiolytics, including other antidepressants classified as SNRIs (Figure 22–1).

Pharmacological Profile

As noted above, venlafaxine and desvenlafaxine inhibit the neuronal reuptake of 5-HT and NE in in vitro and ex vivo experimental paradigms (Bolden-Watson and Richelson 1993; Muth et al. 1986; Owens et al. 1997). Venlafaxine and desvenlafaxine do not inhibit the enzyme monoamine oxidase and have little or no in vitro affinity for muscarinic, cholinergic, histaminergic H_1, and α-adrenergic receptors (Bolden-Watson and Richelson 1993; Muth et al. 1986).

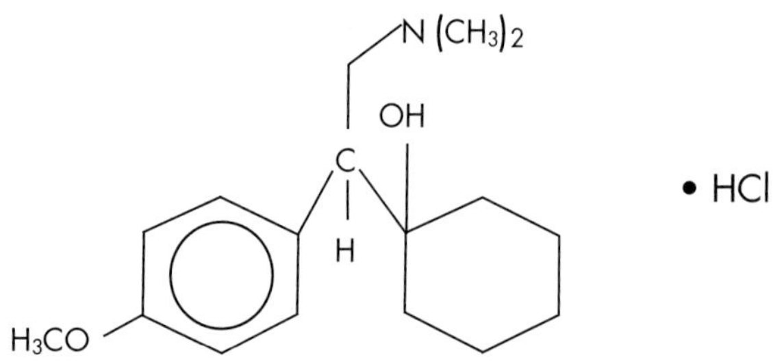

FIGURE 22–1. Chemical structure of venlafaxine hydrochloride.

Pharmacokinetics and Disposition

After oral administration, venlafaxine and desvenlafaxine are well absorbed from the gastrointestinal tract and undergo extensive first-pass metabolism in the liver. Given that ODV is the only major metabolite of venlafaxine with relevant activity, desvenlafaxine has no active metabolites. Coadministration with food decreases the rate but not the extent of absorption (Troy et al. 1997b). Peak plasma concentrations are achieved within 2 hours for venlafaxine and within 3 hours for ODV following ingestion of the IR formulation (Troy et al. 1995b). Venlafaxine XR is absorbed more slowly than the IR formulation (peak plasma concentrations are achieved within 5.5 hours for venlafaxine and within 9 hours for ODV), resulting in lower peak and higher trough plasma concentrations. The extent of absorption and bioavailability of the two formulations of venlafaxine is comparable (Troy et al. 1997a). Steady-state plasma concentrations of both the parent drug and ODV are reached within 3–4 days of therapy.

Venlafaxine exhibits linear kinetics over a dosage range of 75–450 mg/day (Klamerus et al. 1992). The same is true for ODV across a range of 50–400 mg/day. Renal elimination is the primary route of excretion for both venlafaxine and ODV (S.R. Howell et al. 1993). Clearance of ODV (half-life = 10 hours) is slower than that of venlafaxine (half-life = 4 hours); therefore, most patients treated with venlafaxine have higher steady-state plasma concentrations of ODV than of the parent drug (Klamerus et al. 1992). Both venlafaxine and ODV are minimally bound to plasma albumin at therapeutic concentrations (27% and 30%, respectively).

The recommended starting dosage of venlafaxine is 75 mg/day (either divided into two or three doses of the IR or once-daily dosing of the XR formulation) for most therapeutic indications; a lower starting dosage may be used when treating the elderly or patients with a history of tol-

erability problems. The IR formulation is available in 25-, 37.5-, 50-, 75-, 100-, and 150-mg tablets. The XR formulation is available in 37.5-, 75-, and 150-mg capsules; attempts to develop a greater dosage strength failed because some people found a capsule of that size too large to easily swallow. Once-daily dosing with the XR formulation achieves bioavailability (i.e., >90%) nearly equivalent to that of twice-daily dosing with the IR formulation (Troy et al. 1997a). The XR formulation may be taken in either the morning or evening, and bioavailability is not affected by coadministration with food (Troy et al. 1997a).

The recommended starting dose of desvenlafaxine is 50 mg/day. A larger (100-mg) capsule is also available.

The results of fixed-dose studies of venlafaxine suggest dose-dependent efficacy in MDD (Kelsey 1996; Khan et al. 1998; Rudolph et al. 1998c; Thase et al. 2006b). Perhaps most importantly, a large amount of data from RCTs suggests that patients who do not respond to lower dosages often benefit from dosage increases (Costa e Silva 1998; Diaz-Martinez et al. 1998; Dierick et al. 1996; Mehtonen et al. 2000; Thase et al. 2006b). As reviewed elsewhere (Thase 2006), there is relatively little evidence of a dose–response relationship in treatment of anxiety disorders. Whereas the original form of venlafaxine was approved for treatment at doses of up to 375 mg/day (divided bid or tid), the manufacturer "capped" the recommended maximum daily dosage of XR at 225 mg because of a lack of data on the safety and tolerability of once-daily therapy at higher doses. Although some clinicians disregard this arbitrary restriction, it is true that the incidence of elevated blood pressure during venlafaxine therapy is heavily dose dependent (Thase 1998), and if only for this reason, vigilance is warranted when higher-dose therapy is indicated.

Less is known about the dose–response characteristics of desvenlafaxine. Early experiences with the compound in RCTs of MDD suggested that dosages above 200 mg/day may convey no additional efficacy and have a significantly higher incidence of side effects (DeMartinis et al. 2007; Septien-Velez et al. 2007). Although the full therapy development program has not yet been published, the minimum therapeutic dosage is 50 mg/day, and dosages above 100 mg/day are not recommended by the manufacturer. Whether patients who do not respond to 50 mg/day will benefit from upward titration to higher dosages has not yet been demonstrated.

Clearance of venlafaxine and desvenlafaxine is reduced among patients with cirrhosis or severe renal disease (Troy et al. 1994); therefore, dosing should be adjusted downward accordingly. In the absence of formal studies to inform such decisions, a 50% reduction in dosage and slower titration (i.e., at least 7–10 days between adjustments) of both the parent drug and desvenlafaxine are generally recommended. In otherwise healthy elders, adjustments in dosing of venlafaxine do not appear to be necessary (Klamerus et al. 1996). However, initiation of treatment with a lower starting dose, and slower subsequent titration, is a sensible approach when treating frail elders or medically complicated patients. Specific studies of desvenlafaxine in older, medically complex patients have not yet been undertaken.

Mechanism of Action

The mechanism of action of both venlafaxine and desvenlafaxine is believed to be inhibition of 5-HT and NE reuptake. From the beginning, comparisons with the first medication to be considered a "dual reuptake inhibitor," the TCA clomipramine, have been inevitable. Venlafaxine is also a weak inhibitor of dopamine reuptake in vitro (Muth et al. 1986), although this effect probably is not clinically significant at routine therapeutic doses. Consistent with this view are the results of one recent in vivo study of healthy volunteers, which found essentially no blockade of the dopamine transporter with venlafaxine dosages of 75 and 150 mg/day (Shang et al. 2007).

There is good evidence that venlafaxine and desvenlafaxine are more potent inhibitors of 5-HT reuptake than of NE reuptake (Bolden-Watson and Richelson 1993; Deecher et al. 2006; Vaishnavi et al. 2004). It has long been suggested that this relationship underpins the ascending dose–response relationship of venlafaxine (Kelsey 1996; Thase 1996). Moreover, some argue that venlafaxine is essentially an SSRI at the lowest therapeutic dosage (i.e., 75 mg/day) and that the noradrenergic effect is progressively recruited as the dose is increased (Kelsey 1996). There are both experimental (Harvey et al. 2000) and clinical (Davidson et al. 2005; R. Entsuah and Gao 2002; Rudolph et al. 1998a; Thase 1998; Thase et al. 2006b) data that are consistent with such a relationship. Nevertheless, significant effects on autonomic measures of noradrenergic function are evident at 37.5- and 75-mg/day dosages (Bitsios et al. 1999; Siepmann et al. 2007). Until it is possible to directly image NE transporter occupancy in vivo, this question cannot be definitively answered.

Indications and Efficacy

Venlafaxine XR is approved by the FDA for the treatment of MDD, generalized anxiety disorder (GAD), social anx-

iety disorder, and panic disorder. Venlafaxine IR and desvenlafaxine are approved only for the treatment of MDD.

Although venlafaxine has not been formally approved for treatment of other psychiatric disorders, there is evidence that it also has efficacy in other disorders that are responsive to SSRIs, including obsessive-compulsive disorder (OCD), posttraumatic stress disorder (PTSD), and premenstrual dysphoric disorder (PMDD). Given that desvenlafaxine is the active metabolite of venlafaxine, it is likely to be effective in every disorder that is responsive to the parent drug.

Major Depressive Disorder

The antidepressant efficacy of venlafaxine has been established in a large number of placebo-controlled, randomized trials (Cunningham 1997; Guelfi et al. 1995; Khan et al. 1991; Mendels et al. 1993; Rudolph et al. 1998c; Schweizer et al. 1991; Shrivastava et al. 1994; Thase 1997), including studies focusing on depressed patients with associated symptoms of anxiety (Feighner et al. 1998; Khan et al. 1998; Rudolph et al. 1998b). In published studies employing SSRIs as active comparators, venlafaxine therapy has been found to be comparable or superior to therapy with fluoxetine (Alves et al. 1999; Clerc et al. 1994; Costa e Silva 1998; De Nayer et al. 2002; Dierick et al. 1996; Keller et al. 2007a; Nemeroff and Thase 2007; Rudolph and Feiger 1999; Rudolph et al. 1998a; Schatzberg and Roose 2006; Silverstone and Ravindran 1999; Tylee et al. 1997; Tzanakaki et al. 2000), sertraline (Mehtonen et al. 2000; Rush et al. 2006; Shelton et al. 2006; Sir et al. 2005), paroxetine (Ballus et al. 2000; McPartlin et al. 1998; Poirier and Boyer 1999), and citalopram (Allard et al. 2004). Results of two studies comparing venlafaxine and escitalopram have yielded somewhat conflicting results (Bielski et al. 2004; Montgomery et al. 2004b), with comparability in the latter study and trends favoring the SSRI in the former study, which employed rapid titration to maximum FDA-approved doses (Bielski et al. 2004). A pooled analysis of these two trials also found a significant advantage for escitalopram among the subset of patients with higher pretreatment depression severity (Montgomery and Andersen 2006). Comparative studies of desvenlafaxine and SSRIs are under way, but results are not yet available.

Results from meta-analyses of early published and unpublished studies comparing venlafaxine and SSRIs provided some evidence that venlafaxine may produce a significantly greater antidepressant response than fluoxetine and perhaps than SSRIs as a class (T.R. Einarson et al. 1999; Smith et al. 2002; Stahl et al. 2002; Thase et al.

2001). In the meta-analysis by Thase et al. (2001), for example, the magnitude of this effect was a 10% higher rate of remission (as defined by a total score of 7 or less on the 17-item Hamilton Rating Scale for Depression), which was comparable to the magnitude of the effect favoring the SSRIs over placebo. The advantage versus fluoxetine was subsequently confirmed by an independent meta-analysis conducted by the Cochrane group (Cipriani et al. 2006), although this was not observed in the largest prospective head-to-head RCT (Keller et al. 2007a), which examined the outcomes of 1,096 patients with recurrent MDD across 10 weeks of double-blind therapy.

Results of the most comprehensive meta-analysis of RCTs comparing venlafaxine and SSRIs undertaken to date are consistent with the hypothesis that venlafaxine therapy has significantly greater efficacy than fluoxetine alone and than the SSRIs as a class (Nemeroff et al. 2008). Working with individual patient data from all of the manufacturer-sponsored double-blind RCTs conducted worldwide ($N=34$ studies), the antidepressant efficacy of venlafaxine, various SSRIs (fluoxetine, paroxetine, sertraline, citalopram, or fluvoxamine), and placebo (9 studies) across up to 8 weeks of therapy were compared in more than 8,500 adults with MDD. The absolute difference in remission rates was found to be 6%, favoring the SNRI (95% confidence interval = 3.8%–8.1%) (Figure 22–2). The difference was again statistically significant for the more numerous studies using fluoxetine as a comparator but not for the comparisons of the other SSRIs individually. A secondary analysis utilizing the funnel plot method, which also included results of all other known comparative studies of venlafaxine and SSRIs, yielded confirmatory results (Nemeroff et al. 2008). Although statistical significance was observed, the modest magnitude of the difference across studies falls below the standard for clinical significance suggested by the Cochrane group (e.g., Cipriani et al. 2006).

With respect to other newer antidepressants, two studies comparing venlafaxine and mirtazapine therapies (Benkert et al. 2006; Guelfi et al. 2001) found trends favoring the latter compound early in the course of treatment but comparable efficacy at study endpoint. Mirtazapine, which is a potent blocker of histamine and 5-HT$_2$ receptors, also had a significant advantage in relief of insomnia in both of these studies. One relatively large outpatient study contrasting bupropion, a norepinephrine-dopamine reuptake inhibitor (NDRI), and venlafaxine XR found a comparable overall pattern of efficacy, with the NDRI having a significant advantage in terms of a lower incidence of sexual side effects and a higher propor-

tion of patients achieving remission at study endpoint (Thase et al. 2006a). The latter finding, which was discrepant from levels of symptom reduction and response rates, may be attributable to the special nature of the study population (i.e., relatively younger, sexually active patients). A pair of studies contrasting venlafaxine and the other widely available SNRI, duloxetine, found no differences in efficacy at either the primary or secondary study endpoints (Perahia et al. 2008). In the pooled data set of those two studies, several tolerability indices favored venlafaxine early in the course of therapy, whereas there were fewer discontinuation symptoms in the duloxetine group following cessation of study therapy.

Several studies have evaluated the utility of venlafaxine therapy in bipolar depression. In the first, a double-blind, placebo-controlled study, the efficacy and safety of venlafaxine treatment were compared in 17 patients with bipolar II disorder and 31 patients with unipolar depression (Amsterdam 1998). Patients were randomly assigned to 6 weeks of double-blind treatment with once- versus twice-daily venlafaxine IR (up to 225 mg/day). Overall, similar efficacy was observed in unipolar and bipolar patients, although a more rapid reduction of symptoms was observed by week 2 of treatment among bipolar patients who completed the entire trial. No episodes of drug-induced hypomania or rapid cycling were observed.

Vieta et al. (2002) compared therapy with venlafaxine or paroxetine in a double-blind study of 60 bipolar I patients taking concomitant mood stabilizers. Results suggested comparable efficacy and tolerability, although the patients treated with venlafaxine had a higher rate of treatment-induced mania (13%) than the group treated with paroxetine (3%).

Venlafaxine was contrasted with bupropion and sertraline in 174 bipolar I and II patients taking concomitant mood stabilizers (Post et al. 2006). Again, there was no difference in efficacy, but the rate of treatment-emergent affective switches was significantly higher for the patients randomly assigned to the SNRI compared with those assigned to the other two antidepressants.

Venlafaxine is one of the preferred choices for patients who have not responded to other first-line antidepressants (Thase et al. 2000). Two recent RCTs compared venlafaxine with other treatment options after nonresponse to an initial course of SSRI therapy (Baldomero et al. 2005; Rush et al. 2006). Despite a number of differences in design, these studies yielded almost identical results, with a modest numeric advantage in remission rates for the SNRI versus a second trial within the SSRI class. Results were statistically significant in a larger study (Baldomero et al.

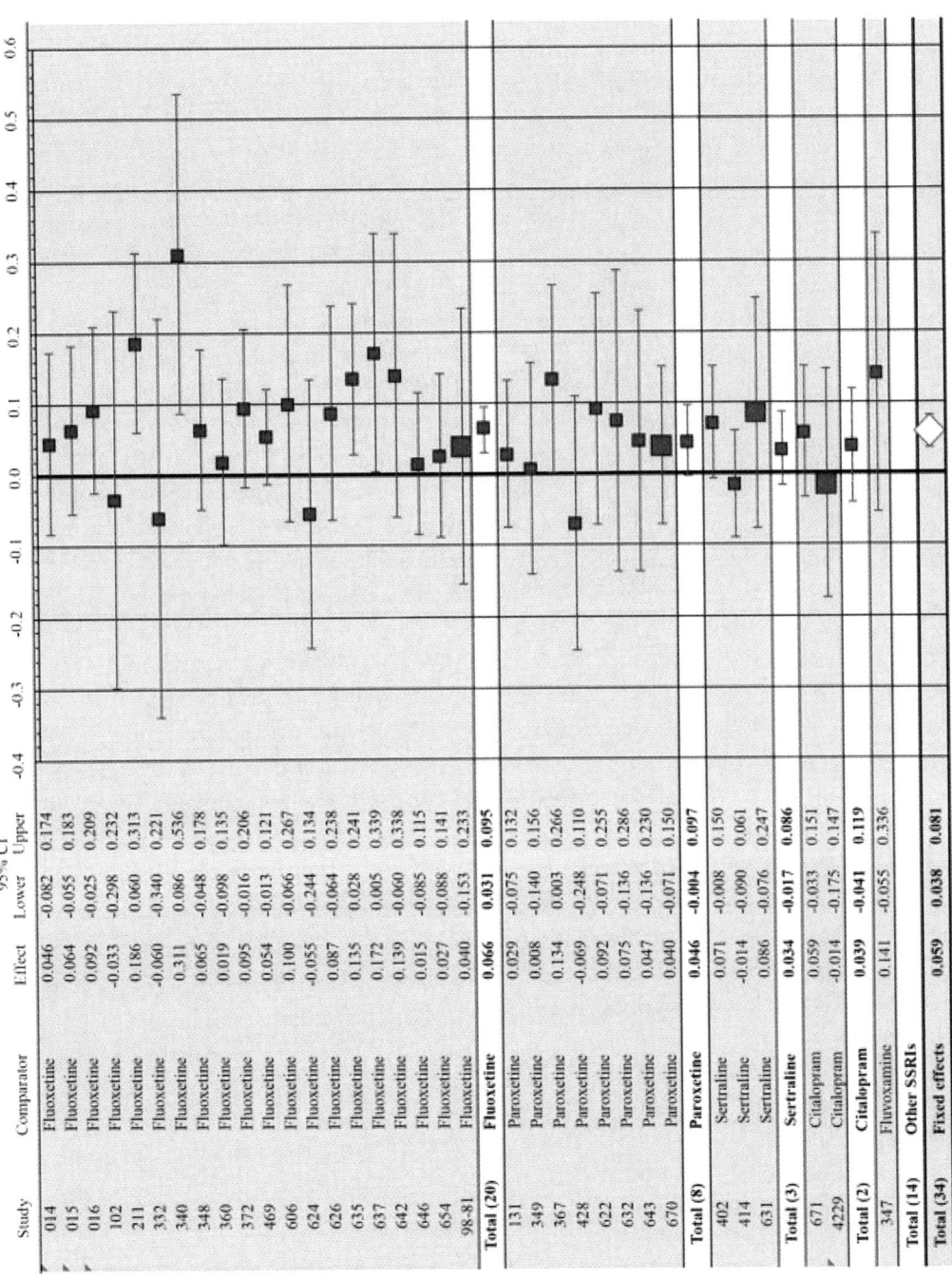

FIGURE 22–2. Rate differences for remission and 95% confidence intervals for venlafaxine versus selective serotonin reuptake inhibitors (SSRIs).

Remission is defined as a 17-item Hamilton Rating Scale for Depression (Ham-D-17) score of 7 or less for 33 of the 34 studies. One study (4229; Allard et al. 2004) did not use the Ham-D, and remission was defined as a Montgomery-Åsberg Depression Rating Scale score of 10 or less. Remission rate differences for the individual studies ranged from –7% to 31%; differences numerically favored venlafaxine in 28 studies (although only 5 reached statistical significance), with 6 studies numerically favoring the SSRIs.

Source. Reprinted from Nemeroff CB, Entsuah R, Benattia I, et al.: "Comprehensive Analysis of Remission (COMPARE) With Venlafaxine Versus SSRIs." *Biological Psychiatry* 63:424–434, 2008. Copyright 2008, Elsevier. Used with permission.

2005), which was conducted in Spain, but did not reach significance in the smaller study, which was conducted in the United States as part of the Sequenced Treatment Alternatives to Relieve Depression (STAR*D) project (Rush et al. 2006). Another study within the STAR*D program contrasted the combination of venlafaxine and mirtazapine (n=51) versus the monoamine oxidase inhibitor (MAOI) tranylcypromine (n=58) among MDD patients who had not responded to three consecutive prospective medication trials (McGrath et al. 2006). Although the two strategies did not differ with respect to the primary outcome variable (remission rates were only 14% and 7% for the combination and MAOI strategies, respectively), patients treated with the combination strategy had significantly greater symptom reduction and a higher study completion rate than patients treated with the MAOI.

Venlafaxine has not been studied in combination with antipsychotic medication for patients with psychotic depression. One study did, however, compare double-blind therapy with either venlafaxine IR (300 mg/day) or fluvoxamine (300 mg/day) as monotherapies in 28 psychotically depressed patients (Zanardi et al. 2000). Findings strongly favored the group receiving fluvoxamine (response rates: 79% vs. 50%), although such an apparently large difference was not statistically significant in this small study. Regardless, venlafaxine should not be thought of as a stand-alone therapy for patients with psychotic depression.

Earlier longer-term open-label trials suggested that venlafaxine had sustained efficacy across 12 months of continued therapy (Magni and Hackett 1992; Tiller et al. 1992). Results of a pooled analysis of the extension phases of four randomized, double-blind, controlled studies in outpatients with major depression demonstrated that the rate of relapse at 6 months and 1 year was significantly lower in the venlafaxine-treated group than in the placebo-treated group (A.R. Entsuah et al. 1996). Double-blind, placebo-controlled studies subsequently confirmed the efficacy of venlafaxine treatment for prevention of relapse during 6 months of continuation treatment (Simon et al. 2004) and for prevention of recurrence during 12 months (Kocsis et al. 2007; Montgomery et al. 2004a) and 24 months (Keller et al. 2007b) of maintenance-phase therapy.

Generalized Anxiety Disorder

Venlafaxine XR was approved by the FDA for treatment of GAD on the basis of a series of placebo-controlled RCTs (Allgulander et al. 2001; Davidson et al. 1999; Gelenberg et al. 2000; Nimatoudis et al. 2004; Rickels et al. 2000), including two trials that evaluated efficacy across

6 months of therapy (Allgulander et al. 2001; Gelenberg et al. 2000). Across studies, the efficacy of doses ranging from 75 mg/day to 225 mg/day was established versus placebo, with little evidence of dose–response relationships for both efficacy and tolerability.

To date, there have been no studies of higher-dose venlafaxine therapy for GAD. Only a handful of studies have been completed comparing venlafaxine XR with other medications with established efficacy in GAD. Superiority to buspirone was found on some (but not all) measures in the one study that was undertaken (Davidson et al. 1999). In the single study that compared venlafaxine XR with the benzodiazepine diazepam (Hackett et al. 2003), the two treatments were comparably effective, although neither active therapy was statistically more effective than placebo.

Two comparative studies have contrasted venlafaxine XR with SSRIs in GAD. In the first, a randomized but open-label trial comparing venlafaxine XR and paroxetine in 60 outpatients, Kim et al. (2006) reported comparable efficacy and tolerability. In the second study (Bose et al. 2008), a relatively large (N=392) RCT, venlafaxine XR and escitalopram were contrasted. Overall, there were no significant differences between the two therapies. However, venlafaxine XR was statistically significantly more effective than placebo on the primary outcome measure (whereas escitalopram was not), and attrition due to side effects was significantly greater in the venlafaxine arm than in the placebo arm (whereas the difference in attrition between the escitalopram and placebo arms was not statistically significant).

Social Anxiety Disorder

Venlafaxine XR was approved for treatment of social anxiety disorder on the basis of a series of RCTs that confirmed its efficacy and safety relative to placebo across up to 6 months of double-blind therapy (Allgulander et al. 2004; Liebowitz et al. 2005a, 2005b; Rickels et al. 2004; Stein et al. 2005). As was the case in GAD, effective doses ranged from 75 mg/day to 225 mg/day, with little evidence of an ascending dose–response relationship. In the two studies that included paroxetine as an active comparator, venlafaxine therapy was at least as effective and as well tolerated as the SSRI (Allgulander et al. 2004; Liebowitz et al. 2005a).

Panic Disorder

Although promising results in panic disorder were apparent in an early placebo-controlled study utilizing the IR formulation (Pollack et al. 1996), the research that ultimately led to a formal FDA indication was largely delayed until after studies of the XR formulation were completed in MDD, GAD, and social anxiety disorder. Antipanic efficacy was demonstrated in three placebo-controlled studies of acute-phase therapy, including one 10-week flexible-dose study (Bradwejn et al. 2005) and two 12-week fixed-dose studies investigating 75 mg/day and 150 mg/day (Pollack et al. 2007a) or 75 mg/day and 225 mg/day (Pollack et al. 2007b). These studies, which incorporated a 37.5-mg starting dose to minimize early side effects, established an effective dosage range of 75–225 mg/day. Two of the placebo-controlled studies also included paroxetine (40 mg/day) as an active comparator (Pollack et al. 2007a, 2007b). Overall, two fixed doses of venlafaxine XR (75 mg/day and 150 mg/day) were comparable to paroxetine in both efficacy and tolerability. In the single RCT that included a fixed-dose 225-mg/day arm, the higher dose of venlafaxine therapy was significantly more effective than paroxetine on several secondary outcome measures, including the proportion of patients who experienced complete relief from full symptom panic attacks (70% vs. 58%) (Pollack et al. 2007b). Sustained efficacy was demonstrated in one longer-term study using a classic relapse prevention design, in which patients who responded to 12 weeks of open-label therapy with venlafaxine XR (75–225 mg/day) were randomly allocated to 6 additional months of double-blind therapy with either the active drug or placebo (Ferguson et al. 2007).

Other Anxiety Disorders

Early studies of venlafaxine therapy of PTSD have been reviewed by Pae et al. (2007). Results of two large RCTs demonstrated the efficacy of venlafaxine XR versus placebo (Davidson et al. 2006a, 2006b). The first trial, which enrolled 573 adults scoring at least 60 on the Clinician-Administered PTSD Scale (CAPS-SX17), compared venlafaxine XR (range=37.5–300 mg/day; mean dosage=225 mg/day), sertraline (range=25–200 mg/day; mean dosage=151 mg/day), and matching placebo across 12 weeks of double-blind treatment. Venlafaxine XR therapy was significantly more effective than placebo, as measured by change in CAPS-SX17 scores and remission rates at study endpoint, whereas sertraline was not. There were, however, no significant differences in efficacy between the two active therapies. Final remission rates were 30%, 24%, and 20% for the SNRI, SSRI, and placebo groups, respectively. In the second study, which enrolled 329 adults meeting the same entry criteria, venlafaxine XR (mean dosage=222 mg/day) was compared with placebo across up to 6 months of double-blind therapy. The efficacy of the SNRI was documented by significant effects on all primary and secondary outcome measures, with final remission rates of 51% and 38% for the venlafaxine XR and placebo groups, respectively.

The results of an initial open-label case series (Rauch et al. 1996) suggested that venlafaxine would also be a useful treatment of OCD. Indeed, results of a 12-week single-blind study indicated that venlafaxine might be at least as effective as clomipramine and significantly better tolerated (Albert et al. 2002). However, the manufacturer did not pursue a large-scale registration program for this indication, and the smaller-scale studies that have been performed do not reveal particular advantages as compared to approved SSRIs such as paroxetine (see the review by Thase 2006).

Premenstrual Dysphoric Disorder

A randomized, double-blind, placebo-controlled study evaluated the efficacy of venlafaxine IR for the treatment of PMDD in 157 women treated across four menstrual cycles (Freeman et al. 2001). Dosages ranged from 50 mg/day to 200 mg/day, with adjustments for adverse events or lack of efficacy early in each cycle. Analysis of daily symptom rating scores revealed significantly greater improvement in the venlafaxine group compared with the placebo group at endpoint in the primary factors of emotion, function, physical symptoms, and pain. In a second small pilot study of intermittent (premenstrual) dosing, Cohen et al. (2004) treated 11 women with PMDD who had not responded to a single-blind placebo lead-in. Nine of the 11 responded to the two 14-day courses of venlafaxine XR 75–112.5 mg/day. The medication was well tolerated, and intermittent dosing was not associated with significant discontinuation symptoms. Further studies are needed to ascertain the longer-term efficacy of venlafaxine treatment for PMDD.

Treatment of Children and Adolescents

Venlafaxine XR was being evaluated for treatment of MDD, GAD, and social anxiety disorder in pediatric populations at the time that concerns about the potential for antidepressants to induce suicidal ideation and behaviors in children began to surface in 2003–2004. Although the manufacturer chose not to pursue further formal indications in any pediatric disorder, results of the five completed studies have been published and include a pair of studies in MDD (Emslie et al. 2007), two RCTs in GAD (Rynn et al. 2007), and one study in social anxiety disorder (March et al. 2007). Results in the depression studies (pooled $N = 334$) were mixed: venlafaxine XR was significantly more effective than placebo among participants ages 12–17 years but not among children ages 7–11 years. In the pooled data set, venlafaxine XR therapy was associated with an increased risk of treatment-emergent suicidal and aggressive behaviors compared with placebo (Emslie et al. 2007). In the pair of GAD studies (pooled $N = 330$), venlafaxine XR was significantly more effective than placebo in the pooled data set; one study was unequivocally positive, but the second study failed to separate between drug and placebo on the primary dependent measure (Rynn et al. 2007). In the social anxiety disorder study ($N = 293$), venlafaxine XR also was significantly more effective than placebo on both primary and secondary outcome measures (March et al. 2007).

Side Effects and Toxicology

The side-effect profile of the IR formulation of venlafaxine was superior to the TCAs, although not quite as favorable as the SSRIs (Preskorn 1995). In the meta-analysis of Nemeroff et al. (2008), for example, 11% of the venlafaxine-treated patients withdrew from therapy because of adverse events, compared with 9% of patients treated with SSRIs. As an SNRI, the tolerability profile of venlafaxine includes all of the characteristic side effects associated with 5-HT uptake inhibition (i.e., nausea, insomnia, tremor, and sexual dysfunction) as well as side effects attributable to NE reuptake inhibition (i.e., sweating and dry mouth). The major advantage of the XR formulation, aside from permitting once-daily dosing, is a somewhat lower incidence of nausea during the first weeks of therapy (Cunningham 1997). To date, no comparative study of venlafaxine and an SSRI has included a detailed assessment of sexual dysfunction. The results of studies focused on detection of sexual dysfunction during antidepressant treatment suggest that venlafaxine and the SSRI are associated with similar risks (Clayton et al. 2002; Kennedy et al. 2000; Montejo et al. 2001).

Like the SSRIs, venlafaxine does not affect cardiac conduction and does not lower the seizure threshold (at least at therapeutic doses). Unlike the SSRIs, however, venlafaxine is associated with a small increase in pulse rate and a dose-dependent increased risk of elevated blood pressure (Thase 1998). Experience with the IR formulation in studies of MDD indicated that the risk of sustained high blood pressure increased from 3% to 7% at dosages of 100–225 mg/day and to 13% at dosages above 300 mg/day (Thase 1998). In the studies of the XR formu-

lation, which limited the maximum dosage to 225 mg/day, the increased risk was only 3% in patients with MDD and 0.5% in patients with GAD. Nevertheless, the manufacturer continues to recommend that all patients receiving venlafaxine have regular monitoring of blood pressure. In practice, it is prudent to record blood pressure prior to initiating venlafaxine therapy and to monitor serially if dosages above 225 mg/day are prescribed. More careful monitoring is warranted for patients with preexisting high blood pressure and for the elderly.

Similar to most other antidepressants, venlafaxine is classified as pregnancy Category C, indicating that there are no adequate and well-controlled studies in pregnant women and that the drug should be used during pregnancy only if it is clearly needed. Results of a multicenter case–control study evaluating pregnancy outcome following gestational exposure to venlafaxine ($n = 150$), SSRIs ($n = 150$), or other drugs ($n = 150$) revealed no evidence that venlafaxine therapy increases the risk of major fetal malformations (A. Einarson et al. 2001).

As with other psychotropic medications, venlafaxine and its metabolites are excreted in human breast milk. Reports by Ilett et al. (1998, 2002) of the distribution of venlafaxine in human milk and its effects in breast-fed infants demonstrated that the mean infant dose exposure was approximately 6%–7% of the maternal dose, which is below the 10% notional level of concern. No adverse effects were noted in any of the infants (Ilett et al. 2002). Although these data support the use of venlafaxine in pregnant or breast-feeding women, the findings are preliminary, and the available safety data remain limited. The decision to use venlafaxine in pregnancy or lactation should be made on the basis of an individual risk–benefit assessment.

Precipitous withdrawal of venlafaxine can result in a characteristic "discontinuation" profile, including dizziness, dry mouth, insomnia, nausea, nervousness, sweating, anorexia, diarrhea, somnolence, and sensory disturbances (Haddad 2001). Venlafaxine therapy therefore should not be discontinued abruptly, and whenever possible, a taper schedule of no more than 75 mg/day/week is strongly recommended. It is important to note that the discontinuation schedule used in clinical trials was based on only 6- to 12-week durations of treatment. In practice, longer tapering schedules may be required, depending on the dose, the duration of therapy, and the individual patient. Clinicians should counsel patients about the possibility of adverse effects following abrupt discontinuation of treatment.

In the 13-plus years since its initial introduction, there has been extensive experience with venlafaxine overdose. A number of fatal overdoses have been reported, primarily involving combinations of venlafaxine and other drugs and/or alcohol (Banham 1998; Kunsman et al. 2000; Long et al. 1997; Parsons et al. 1996). In nonfatal overdoses, electrocardiogram changes (e.g., prolongation of QT interval, bundle branch block, QRS prolongation), sinus and ventricular tachycardia, bradycardia, hypotension, altered level of consciousness (ranging from somnolence to coma), serotonin syndrome, and seizures have been reported (C. Howell et al. 2007; Whyte et al. 2003). In an analysis of fatal poisoning with antidepressants in the United Kingdom, Buckley and McManus (2002) used a statistic known as the fatal toxicity index (FTI), which was defined by the number of overdose deaths per million prescriptions, to compare the relative risks of different antidepressants. They found that venlafaxine had a significantly higher FTI than the SSRIs (13.2 vs. 0.7–3.0). The authors suggested that these data could mean that venlafaxine should not be used as a first-line treatment for patients with suicidal ideation. However, many nonpharmacological factors can contribute to the likelihood of a fatal overdose, particularly patient risk factors. In this regard, two studies have documented that the patients who are selected for treatment with venlafaxine are at greater inherent suicide risk than are patients selected for treatment with SSRIs (Mines et al. 2005; Rubino et al. 2007). Adjustment for these risk factors greatly reduced the difference in FTI between venlafaxine and the SSRIs (Rubino et al. 2007). Although the potential for lethality in overdose certainly warrants ongoing study, the current state of the evidence does not indicate that venlafaxine therapy should be avoided in patients at risk for suicidal behavior.

Drug–Drug Interactions

Venlafaxine undergoes extensive metabolism in the liver by the cytochrome P450 (CYP) enzyme system, particularly by the CYP2D6 isoenzyme. Patients who are "poor CYP2D6 metabolizers," whether genetically or by taking drugs that inhibit this enzyme, thus have increased concentrations of the parent drug relative to ODV. Although it could be argued that this should not affect response, given that the parent drug and ODV are nearly pharmacologically equipotent, poor metabolizers of CYP2D6 may be at greater risk for side effects (McAlpine et al. 2007; Shams et al. 2006). Such patients thus could potentially be better candidates for therapy with desvenlafaxine than the parent drug.

Despite being a substrate for CYP2D6, venlafaxine and ODV are among the weakest of inhibitors of this isoenzyme (Alfaro et al. 2000; Amchin et al. 2001; Ball et al. 1997). In vitro and in vivo studies have shown that venlafaxine and ODV cause little or no inhibition of other CYP isoenzymes, including 1A2, 2C9, 2C19, and 3A4 (Ball et al. 1997; Owen and Nemeroff 1998). Although it does not appear to have significant affinity for CYP3A4, venlafaxine has been shown to decrease blood levels of the protease inhibitor indinavir, a substrate of CYP3A4 (Levin et al. 2001). Neither the mechanism nor the clinical significance of this interaction is known, but it is of concern given the critical nature of treatment with protease inhibitors.

As SNRIs, both venlafaxine and desvenlafaxine are contraindicated in patients taking MAOIs, because of the risk of serotonin syndrome. This is as true for the newer transdermally delivered formulation of selegiline as it is with the older agents. As with cyclic antidepressants and SSRIs, venlafaxine or desvenlafaxine treatment should not be initiated until 2 weeks after discontinuation of an MAOI, and MAOI therapy should not be initiated until at least 7 days after discontinuation of venlafaxine or desvenlafaxine.

Venlafaxine and desvenlafaxine appear to have no clinically significant interactions with lithium (Troy et al. 1996), diazepam (Troy et al. 1995a), or alcohol (Troy et al. 1997c).

Conclusion

Venlafaxine, the first widely used member of the SNRI class, appears to be at least as effective as other first-line antidepressants and has an overall safety profile that is closer to the SSRIs than the TCA. There is evidence of a modest efficacy advantage compared with fluoxetine and perhaps to the SSRIs as a class, although to date a significant efficacy advantage has not been demonstrated against other specific members of the class, most particularly escitalopram. Venlafaxine also has established efficacy for treatment of GAD, social anxiety disorder, and panic disorder. Generic formulations of venlafaxine IR are now available, although the more heavily prescribed XR formulation, which is patent-protected for several more years, offers the advantages of once-daily dosing and a lower incidence of nausea during the first few weeks of therapy. ODV, the primary active metabolite of venlafaxine, was introduced as antidepressant (desvenlafaxine succinate) in 2008. Desvenlafaxine offers several advantages over venlafaxine XR in terms of simpler dosing (e.g., lower starting dose, lower minimum therapeutic dose, no active metabolite, and possibly less need for upward dosage titration); beyond this, however, the relative merits of the two drugs have not yet been assessed. Both drugs have a low potential for cytochrome P450–mediated drug–drug interactions and are associated with dose-dependent increases in blood pressure.

References

Albert U, Aguglia E, Maina G, et al: Venlafaxine versus clomipramine in the treatment of obsessive-compulsive disorder: a preliminary single-blind, 12-week, controlled study. J Clin Psychiatry 63:1004–1009, 2002

Alfaro CL, Lam YW, Simpson J, et al: CYP2D6 inhibition by fluoxetine, paroxetine, sertraline, and venlafaxine in a crossover study: intraindividual variability and plasma concentration correlations. J Clin Pharmacol 40:58–66, 2000

Allard P, Gram L, Timdahl K, et al: Efficacy and tolerability of venlafaxine in geriatric outpatients with major depression: a double-blind, randomised 6-month comparative trial with citalopram. Int J Geriatr Psychiatry 19:1123–1130, 2004

Allgulander C, Hackett D, Salinas E: Venlafaxine extended release (ER) in the treatment of generalised anxiety disorder: twenty-four-week placebo-controlled dose-ranging study. Br J Psychiatry 179:15–22, 2001

Allgulander C, Mangano R, Zhang J, et al: Efficacy of venlafaxine ER in patients with social anxiety disorder: a double-blind, placebo-controlled, parallel-group comparison with paroxetine. SAD 388 Study Group. Hum Psychopharmacol 19:387–396, 2004

Alves C, Cachola I, Brandao J: Efficacy and tolerability of venlafaxine and fluoxetine in outpatients with major depression. Prim Care Psychiatry 5:57–63, 1999

Amchin J, Ereshefsky L, Zarycranski W, et al: Effect of venlafaxine versus fluoxetine on metabolism of dextromethorphan, a CYP2D6 probe. J Clin Pharmacol 41:443–451, 2001

Amsterdam J: Efficacy and safety of venlafaxine in the treatment of bipolar II major depressive episode. J Clin Psychopharmacol 18:414–417, 1998

Baldomero EB, Ubago JG, Cercós CL, et al: Venlafaxine extended release versus conventional antidepressants in the remission of depressive disorders after previous antidepressant failure: ARGOS study. Depress Anxiety 22:68–76, 2005

Ball SE, Ahern D, Scatina J, et al: Venlafaxine: in vitro inhibition of CYP2D6 dependent imipramine and desipramine metabolism: comparative studies with selected SSRIs, and effects on human hepatic CYP3A4, CYP2C9 and CYP1A2. Br J Clin Pharmacol 43:619–626, 1997

Ballus C, Quiros G, De Flores T, et al: The efficacy and tolerability of venlafaxine and paroxetine in outpatients with depressive disorders or dysthymia. Int Clin Psychopharmacol 15:43–48, 2000

Banham ND: Fatal venlafaxine overdose. Med J Aust 169:445–448, 1998

Benkert O, Szegedi A, Philipp M, et al: Mirtazapine orally disintegrating tablets versus venlafaxine extended release: a double-blind, randomized multicenter trial comparing the onset of antidepressant response in patients with major depressive disorder. J Clin Psychopharmacol 26:75–78, 2006

Bielski RJ, Ventura D, Chang CC: A double-blind comparison of escitalopram and venlafaxine extended release in the treatment of major depressive disorder. J Clin Psychiatry 65:1190–1196, 2004

Bitsios P, Szabadi E, Bradshaw CM: Comparison of the effects of venlafaxine, paroxetine and desipramine on the pupillary light reflex in man. Psychopharmacology (Berl) 143:286–292, 1999

Bolden-Watson C, Richelson E: Blockade by newly developed antidepressants of biogenic amine uptake into rat brain synaptosomes. Life Sci 52:1023–1029, 1993

Bose A, Korotzer A, Gommoll C, et al: Randomized placebo-controlled trial of escitalopram and venlafaxine XR in the treatment of generalized anxiety disorder. Depress Anxiety 25:854–861, 2008

Bradwejn J, Ahokas A, Stein DJ, et al: Venlafaxine extended-release capsules in panic disorder: flexible-dose, double-blind, placebo-controlled study. Br J Psychiatry 187:352–359, 2005

Buckley NA, McManus PR: Fatal toxicity of serotoninergic and other antidepressant drugs: analysis of United Kingdom mortality data. BMJ 325:1332–1333, 2002

Cipriani A, Barbui C, Brambilla P, et al: Are all antidepressants really the same? The case of fluoxetine: a systematic review. J Clin Psychiatry 67:850–864, 2006

Clayton AH, Pradko JF, Croft HA, et al. Prevalence of sexual dysfunction among newer antidepressants. J Clin Psychiatry 63:357–366, 2002

Clerc GE, Ruimy P, Verdeau-Palles J: A double-blind comparison of venlafaxine and fluoxetine in patients hospitalized for major depression and melancholia. The Venlafaxine French Inpatient Study Group. Int Clin Psychopharmacol 9:139–143, 1994

Cohen LS, Soares CN, Lyster A, et al: Efficacy and tolerability of premenstrual use of venlafaxine (flexible dose) in the treatment of premenstrual dysphoric disorder. J Clin Psychopharmacol 24:540–543, 2004

Costa e Silva J: Randomized, double-blind comparison of venlafaxine and fluoxetine in outpatients with major depression. J Clin Psychiatry 59:352–357, 1998

Cunningham LA: Once-daily venlafaxine extended release (XR) and venlafaxine immediate release (IR) in outpatients with major depression. Venlafaxine XR 208 Study Group. Ann Clin Psychiatry 9:157–164, 1997

Davidson JR, DuPont RL, Hedges D, et al: Efficacy, safety, and tolerability of venlafaxine extended release and buspirone in outpatients with generalized anxiety disorder. J Clin Psychiatry 60:528–535, 1999

Davidson J, Watkins L, Owens M, et al: Effects of paroxetine and venlafaxine XR on heart rate variability in depression. J Clin Psychopharmacol 25:480–484, 2005

Davidson J, Baldwin D, Stein DJ, et al: Treatment of posttraumatic stress disorder with venlafaxine extended release: a 6-month randomized controlled trial. Arch Gen Psychiatry 63:1158–1165, 2006a

Davidson J, Rothbaum BO, Tucker P, et al: Venlafaxine extended release in posttraumatic stress disorder: a sertraline- and placebo-controlled study. J Clin Psychopharmacol 26:259–267, 2006b

Deecher DC, Beyer CE, Johnston G, et al: Desvenlafaxine succinate: a new serotonin and norepinephrine reuptake inhibitor. J Pharmacol Exp Ther 318:657–665, 2006

DeMartinis NA, Yeung PP, Entsuah R, et al: A double-blind, placebo-controlled study of the efficacy and safety of desvenlafaxine succinate in the treatment of major depressive disorder. J Clin Psychiatry 68:677–688, 2007

De Nayer A, Geerts S, Ruelens L, et al: Venlafaxine compared with fluoxetine in outpatients with depression and concomitant anxiety. Int J Neuropsychopharmacol 5:115–120, 2002

Diaz-Martinez A, Benassinni O, Ontiveros A, et al: A randomized, open-label comparison of venlafaxine and fluoxetine in depressed outpatients. Clin Ther 20:467–476, 1998

Dierick M, Ravizza L, Realini R, et al: A double-blind comparison of venlafaxine and fluoxetine for treatment of major depression in outpatients. Prog Neuropsychopharmacol Biol Psychiatry 20:57–71, 1996

Einarson A, Fatoye B, Sarkar M, et al: Pregnancy outcome following gestational exposure to venlafaxine: a multicenter prospective controlled study. Am J Psychiatry 158:1728–1730, 2001

Einarson TR, Arikian SR, Casciano J, et al: Comparison of extended-release venlafaxine, selective serotonin reuptake inhibitors, and tricyclic antidepressants in the treatment of depression: a meta-analysis of randomized controlled trials. Clin Ther 21:296–308, 1999

Emslie GJ, Findling RL, Yeung PP, et al: Venlafaxine ER for the treatment of pediatric subjects with depression: results of two placebo-controlled trials. J Am Acad Child Adolesc Psychiatry 46:479–488, 2007

Entsuah AR, Rudolph RL, Hackett D, et al: Efficacy of venlafaxine and placebo during long-term treatment of depression: a pooled analysis of relapse rates. Int Clin Psychopharmacol 11:137–145, 1996

Entsuah R, Gao B: Global benefit-risk evaluation of antidepressant action: comparison of pooled data for venlafaxine, SSRIs, and placebo. CNS Spectr 7:882–888, 2002

Feighner JP, Entsuah A, McPherson MK: Efficacy of once-daily venlafaxine extended release (XR) for symptoms of anxiety in depressed outpatients. J Affect Disord 47:55–62, 1998

Ferguson JM, Khan A, Mangano R, et al: Relapse prevention of panic disorder in adult outpatient responders to treatment with venlafaxine extended release. J Clin Psychiatry 68:58–68, 2007

Freeman EW, Rickels K, Yonkers KA, et al: Venlafaxine in the treatment of premenstrual dysphoric disorder. Obstet Gynecol 98:737–744, 2001

Gelenberg AJ, Lydiard RB, Rudolph RL, et al: Efficacy of venlafaxine extended-release capsules in nondepressed outpatients with generalized anxiety disorder: a 6-month randomized controlled trial. JAMA 283:3082–3088, 2000

Guelfi JD, White C, Hackett D, et al: Effectiveness of venlafaxine in patients hospitalized for major depression and melancholia. J Clin Psychiatry 56:450–458, 1995

Guelfi JD, Ansseau M, Timmerman L, et al: Mirtazapine versus venlafaxine in hospitalized severely depressed patients with melancholic features. J Clin Psychopharmacol 21:425–431, 2001

Hackett D, Haudiquet V, Salinas E: A method for controlling for a high placebo response rate in a comparison of venlafaxine XR and diazepam in the short-term treatment of patients with generalised anxiety disorder. Eur Psychiatry 18:182–187, 2003

Haddad PM: Antidepressant discontinuation syndromes. Drug Saf 24:183–197, 2001

Harvey AT, Rudolph RL, Preskorn SH: Evidence of the dual mechanisms of action of venlafaxine. Arch Gen Psychiatry 57:503–509, 2000

Howell C, Wilson AD, Waring WS: Cardiovascular toxicity due to venlafaxine poisoning in adults: a review of 235 consecutive cases. Br J Clin Pharmacol 64:192–197, 2007

Howell SR, Husbands GE, Scatina JA, et al: Metabolic disposition of 14C-venlafaxine in mouse, rat, dog, rhesus monkey and man. Xenobiotica 23:349–359, 1993

Ilett KF, Hackett LP, Dusci LJ, et al: Distribution and excretion of venlafaxine and O-desmethylvenlafaxine in human milk. Br J Clin Pharmacol 45:459–462, 1998

Ilett KF, Kristensen JH, Hackett LP, et al: Distribution of venlafaxine and its O-desmethyl metabolite in human milk and their effects in breastfed infants. Br J Clin Pharmacol 53:17–22, 2002

Keller MB, Trivedi MH, Thase ME, et al: The Prevention of Recurrent Episodes of Depression with Venlafaxine for Two Years (PREVENT) study: outcomes from the acute and continuation phases. Biol Psychiatry 62:1371–1379, 2007a

Keller MB, Trivedi MH, Thase ME, et al: The Prevention of Recurrent Episodes of Depression with Venlafaxine for Two Years (PREVENT) Study: outcomes from the 2-year and combined maintenance phases. J Clin Psychiatry 68:1246–1256, 2007b

Kelsey JE: Dose-response relationship with venlafaxine. J Clin Psychopharmacol 16:21S–26S, 1996

Kennedy SH, Eisfeld BS, Dickens SE, et al: Antidepressant-induced sexual dysfunction during treatment with moclobemide, paroxetine, sertraline, and venlafaxine. J Clin Psychiatry 61:276–281, 2000

Khan A, Fabre LF, Rudolph R: Venlafaxine in depressed outpatients. Psychopharmacol Bull 27:141–144, 1991

Khan A, Upton GV, Rudolph RL, et al: The use of venlafaxine in the treatment of major depression and major depression associated with anxiety: a dose-response study. J Clin Psychopharmacol 18:19–25, 1998

Kim TS, Pae CU, Yoon SJ, et al: Comparison of venlafaxine extended release versus paroxetine for treatment of patients with generalized anxiety disorder. Psychiatry Clin Neurosci 60:347–351, 2006

Klamerus KJ, Maloney K, Rudolph RL, et al: Introduction of a composite parameter to the pharmacokinetics of venlafaxine and its active O-desmethyl metabolite. J Clin Pharmacol 32:716–724, 1992

Klamerus KJ, Parker VD, Rudolph RL, et al: Effects of age and gender on venlafaxine and O-desmethylvenlafaxine pharmacokinetics. Pharmacotherapy 16:915–923, 1996

Kocsis JH, Thase ME, Trivedi MH, et al: Prevention of recurrent episodes of depression with venlafaxine ER in a 1-year maintenance phase from the PREVENT Study. J Clin Psychiatry 68:1014–1023, 2007

Kunsman GW, Kunsman CM, Presses CL, et al: A mixed-drug intoxication involving venlafaxine and verapamil. J Forensic Sci 45:926–928, 2000

Levin GM, Nelson LA, DeVane CL, et al: A pharmacokinetic drug-drug interaction study of venlafaxine and indinavir. Psychopharmacol Bull 35:62–71, 2001

Liebowitz MR, Gelenberg AJ, Munjack D: Venlafaxine extended release vs placebo and paroxetine in social anxiety disorder. Arch Gen Psychiatry 62:190–198, 2005a

Liebowitz MR, Mangano RM, Bradwejn J, et al: A randomized controlled trial of venlafaxine extended release in generalized social anxiety disorder. SAD Study Group. J Clin Psychiatry 66:238–247, 2005b

Long C, Crifasi J, Maginn D, et al: Comparison of analytical methods in the determination of two venlafaxine fatalities. J Anal Toxicol 21:166–169, 1997

Magni G, Hackett D: An open label evaluation of the long-term safety and clinical acceptability of venlafaxine in depressed patients. Clin Neuropharmacol 15 (suppl 1):323B, 1992

March JS, Entusah AR, Rynn M, et al: A randomized controlled trial of venlafaxine ER versus placebo in pediatric social anxiety disorder. Biol Psychiatry 62:1149–1154, 2007

McAlpine DE, O'Kane DJ, Black JL, et al: Cytochrome P450 2D6 genotype variation and venlafaxine dosage. Mayo Clin Proc 82:1065–1068, 2007

McGrath PJ, Stewart JW, Fava M, et al: Tranylcypromine versus venlafaxine plus mirtazapine following three failed antidepressant medication trials for depression: a STAR*D report. Am J Psychiatry 163:1531–1541, 2006

McPartlin GM, Reynolds A, Anderson C, et al: A comparison of once-daily venlafaxine XR and paroxetine in depressed outpatients treated in general practice. Prim Care Psychiatry 4:127–132, 1998

Mehtonen OP, Sogaard J, Roponen P, et al: Randomized, double-blind comparison of venlafaxine and sertraline in outpatients with major depressive disorder. Venlafaxine 631 Study Group. J Clin Psychiatry 61:95–100, 2000

Mendels J, Johnston R, Mattes J, et al: Efficacy and safety of bid doses of venlafaxine in a dose-response study. Psychopharmacol Bull 29:169–174, 1993

Mines D, Hill D, Yu H, Novelli L: Prevalence of risk factors for suicide in patients prescribed venlafaxine, fluoxetine, and citalopram. Pharmacoepidemiol Drug Saf 14:367–372, 2005

Montejo AL, Llorca G, Izquierdo JA, et al: Incidence of sexual dysfunction associated with antidepressant agents: a prospective multicenter study of 1022 outpatients. J Clin Psychiatry 62:10–21, 2001

Montgomery SA, Andersen HF: Escitalopram versus venlafaxine XR in the treatment of depression. Int Clin Psychopharmacol 21:297–309, 2006

Montgomery SA, Entsuah R, Hackett D, et al: Venlafaxine versus placebo in the preventive treatment of recurrent major depression. Venlafaxine 335 Study Group. J Clin Psychiatry 65:328–36, 2004a

Montgomery SA, Huusom AK, Bothmer J: A randomised study comparing escitalopram with venlafaxine XR in primary care patients with major depressive disorder. Neuropsychobiology 50:57–64, 2004b

Muth EA, Haskins JT, Moyer JA, et al: Antidepressant biochemical profile of the novel bicyclic compound Wy-45,030, an ethyl cyclohexanol derivative. Biochem Pharmacol 35:4493–4497, 1986

Nemeroff CB, Thase ME, EPIC 014 Study Group: A double-blind, placebo-controlled comparison of venlafaxine and fluoxetine treatment in depressed outpatients. J Psychiatr Res 41:351–359, 2007

Nemeroff CB, Entsuah R, Benattia I, et al: Comprehensive Analysis of Remission (COMPARE) with venlafaxine versus SSRIs. Biol Psychiatry 63:424–434, 2008

Nimatoudis I, Zissis NP, Kogeorgos J, et al: Remission rates with venlafaxine extended release in Greek outpatients with generalized anxiety disorder: a double-blind, randomized, placebo controlled study. Int Clin Psychopharmacol 19:331–336, 2004

Owen JR, Nemeroff CB: New antidepressants and the cytochrome P450 system: focus on venlafaxine, nefazodone, and mirtazapine. Depress Anxiety 7 (suppl 1):24–32, 1998

Owens MJ, Morgan WN, Plott SJ, Nemeroff CB: Neurotransmitter receptor and transporter binding profile of antidepressants and their metabolites. J Pharmacol Exp Ther 283:1305–1322, 1997

Pae CU, Lim HK, Ajwani N, et al: Extended-release formulation of venlafaxine in the treatment of post-traumatic stress disorder. Expert Rev Neurother 7:603–615, 2007

Parsons AT, Anthony RM, Meeker JE: Two fatal cases of venlafaxine poisoning. J Anal Toxicol 20:266–268, 1996

Perahia DG, Pritchett YL, Kajdasz DK, et al: A randomized, double-blind comparison of duloxetine and venlafaxine in the treatment of patients with major depressive disorder. J Psychiatr Res 42:22–34, 2008

Poirier M-F, Boyer P: Venlafaxine and paroxetine in treatment-resistant depression: double-blind, randomised comparison. Br J Psychiatry 175:12–16, 1999

Pollack MH, Worthington JJ 3rd, Otto MW, et al: Venlafaxine for panic disorder: results from a double-blind, placebo-controlled study. Psychopharmacol Bull 32:667–670, 1996

Pollack MH, Lepola U, Koponen H, et al: A double-blind study of the efficacy of venlafaxine extended-release, paroxetine, and placebo in the treatment of panic disorder. Depress Anxiety 24:1–14, 2007a

Pollack M, Mangano R, Entsuah R, et al: A randomized controlled trial of venlafaxine ER and paroxetine in the treatment of outpatients with panic disorder. Psychopharmacology (Berl) 194:233–342, 2007b

Post RM, Altshuler LL, Leverich GS, et al: Mood switch in bipolar depression: comparison of adjunctive venlafaxine, bupropion and sertraline. Br J Psychiatry 189:124–131, 2006

Preskorn SH: Comparison of the tolerability of bupropion, fluoxetine, imipramine, nefazodone, paroxetine, sertraline, and venlafaxine. J Clin Psychiatry 56:12–21, 1995

Rauch SL, O'Sullivan RL, Jenike MA: Open treatment of obsessive-compulsive disorder with venlafaxine: a series of ten cases. J Clin Psychopharmacol 16:81–84, 1996

Rickels K, Pollack MH, Sheehan DV, et al: Efficacy of extended-release venlafaxine in nondepressed outpatients with generalized anxiety disorder. Am J Psychiatry 157:968–974, 2000

Rickels K, Mangano R, Khan A: A double-blind, placebo-controlled study of a flexible dose of venlafaxine ER in adult outpatients with generalized social anxiety disorder. J Clin Psychopharmacol 24:488–496, 2004

Rubino A, Roskell N, Tennis P, et al: Risk of suicide during treatment with venlafaxine, citalopram, fluoxetine, and dothiepin: retrospective cohort study. BMJ 334:242, 2007

Rudolph RL, Feiger AD: A double-blind, randomized, placebo-controlled trial of once-daily venlafaxine extended release (XR) and fluoxetine for the treatment of depression. J Affect Disord 56:171–181, 1999

Rudolph RL, Entsuah R, Aguiar L, et al: Early onset of antidepressant activity of venlafaxine compared with placebo and fluoxetine in outpatients in a double-blind study (abstract). Eur Neuropsychopharmacol 8:S142, 1998a

Rudolph RL, Entsuah R, Chitra R: A meta-analysis of the effects of venlafaxine on anxiety associated with depression. J Clin Psychopharmacol 18:136–44, 1998b

Rudolph RL, Fabre LF, Feighner JP, et al: A randomized, placebo-controlled, dose-response trial of venlafaxine hydrochloride in the treatment of major depression. J Clin Psychiatry 59:116–122, 1998c

Rush AJ, Trivedi MH, Wisniewski SR, et al: Bupropion-SR, sertraline, or venlafaxine-XR after failure of SSRIs for depression. STAR*D Study Team. N Engl J Med 354:1231–1242, 2006

Rynn MA, Riddle MA, Yeung PP, et al: Efficacy and safety of extended-release venlafaxine in the treatment of generalized anxiety disorder in children and adolescents: two placebo-controlled trials. Am J Psychiatry 164:290–300, 2007

Schatzberg A, Roose S: A double-blind, placebo-controlled study of venlafaxine and fluoxetine in geriatric outpatients with major depression. Am J Geriatr Psychiatry 14:361–370, 2006

Schweizer E, Weise C, Clary C, et al: Placebo-controlled trial of venlafaxine for the treatment of major depression. J Clin Psychopharmacol 11:233–236, 1991

Septien-Velez L, Pitrosky B, Padmanabhan SK, et al: A randomized, double-blind, placebo-controlled trial of desvenlafaxine succinate in the treatment of major depressive disorder. Int Clin Psychopharmacol 22:338–347, 2007

Shams ME, Arneth B, Hiemke C, et al: CYP2D6 polymorphism and clinical effect of the antidepressant venlafaxine. J Clin Pharmacol Ther 31:493–502, 2006

Shang Y, Gibbs MA, Marek GJ, et al: Displacement of serotonin and dopamine transporters by venlafaxine extended release capsule at steady state: a [123I]2beta-carbomethoxy-3beta-(4-iodophenyl)-tropane single photon emission computed tomography imaging study. J Clin Psychopharmacol 27:71–75, 2007

Shelton RC, Haman KL, Rapaport MH, et al: A randomized, double-blind, active-control study of sertraline versus venlafaxine XR in major depressive disorder. J Clin Psychiatry 67:1674–1681, 2006

Shrivastava RK, Cohn C, Crowder J, et al: Long-term safety and clinical acceptability of venlafaxine and imipramine in outpatients with major depression. J Clin Psychopharmacol 14:322–329, 1994

Siepmann T, Ziemssen T, Mueck-Weymann M, et al: The effects of venlafaxine on autonomic functions in healthy volunteers. J Clin Psychopharmacol 27:687–691, 2007

Silverstone PH, Ravindran A: Once-daily venlafaxine extended-release (XR) compared with fluoxetine in outpatients with depression and anxiety. J Clin Psychiatry 60:22–28, 1999

Simon JS, Aguiar LM, Kunz NR, et al: Extended-release venlafaxine in relapse prevention for patients with major depressive disorder. J Psychiatr Res 38:249–257, 2004

Sir A, D'Souza RF, Uguz S, et al: Randomized trial of sertraline versus venlafaxine XR in major depression: efficacy and discontinuation symptoms. J Clin Psychiatry 66:1312–1320, 2005

Smith D, Dempster C, Glanville J, et al: Efficacy and tolerability of venlafaxine compared with selective serotonin reuptake inhibitors and other antidepressants: a meta-analysis. Br J Psychiatry 180:396–404, 2002

Stahl SM, Entsuah R, Rudolph RL: Comparative efficacy between venlafaxine and SSRIs: a pooled analysis of patients with depression. Biol Psychiatry 52:1166–1174, 2002

Stein MB, Pollack MH, Bystritsky A, et al: Efficacy of low and higher dose extended-release venlafaxine in generalized social anxiety disorder: a 6-month randomized controlled trial. Psychopharmacology (Berl) 177:280–288, 2005

Thase ME: Antidepressant options: venlafaxine in perspective. J Clin Psychopharmacol 16:10S–18S, 1996

Thase ME: Efficacy and tolerability of once-daily venlafaxine extended release (XR) in outpatients with major depression. The Venlafaxine XR 209 Study Group. J Clin Psychiatry 58:393–398, 1997

Thase ME: Effects of venlafaxine on blood pressure: a meta-analysis of original data from 3744 depressed patients. J Clin Psychiatry 59:502–508, 1998

Thase ME: Treatment of anxiety disorders with venlafaxine XR. Expert Rev Neurother 6:269–282, 2006

Thase ME, Friedman ES, Howland RH: Venlafaxine and treatment-resistant depression. Depress Anxiety 12:55–62, 2000

Thase ME, Entsuah AR, Rudolph RL: Remission rates during treatment with venlafaxine or selective serotonin reuptake inhibitors. Br J Psychiatry 178:234–221, 2001

Thase ME, Clayton AH, Haight BR, et al: A double-blind comparison between bupropion XL and venlafaxine XR: sexual functioning, antidepressant efficacy, and tolerability. J Clin Psychopharmacol 26:482–488, 2006a

Thase ME, Shelton RC, Khan A: Treatment with venlafaxine extended release after SSRI nonresponse or intolerance: a randomized comparison of standard- and higher-dosing strategies. J Clin Psychopharmacol 26:250–258, 2006b

Tiller J, Johnson G, O'Sullivan B, et al: Venlafaxine: a long-term study (abstract). Clin Neuropharmacol 14:342B, 1992

Troy SM, Schultz RW, Parker VD, et al: The effect of renal disease on the disposition of venlafaxine. Clin Pharmacol Ther 56:14–21, 1994

Troy SM, Lucki I, Peirgies AA, et al: Pharmacokinetic and pharmacodynamic evaluation of the potential drug interaction between venlafaxine and diazepam. J Clin Pharmacol 35:410–419, 1995a

Troy SM, Parker VD, Fruncillo RJ, et al: The pharmacokinetics of venlafaxine when given in a twice-daily regimen. J Clin Pharmacol 35:404–409, 1995b

Troy SM, Parker VD, Hicks DR, et al: Pharmacokinetic interaction between multiple-dose venlafaxine and single-dose lithium. J Clin Pharmacol 36:175–181, 1996

Troy SM, DiLea C, Martin PT, et al: Pharmacokinetics of once-daily venlafaxine extended release (XR) in healthy volunteers. Curr Ther Res 58:504–514, 1997a

Troy SM, Parker VP, Hicks DR, et al: Pharmacokinetics and effect of food on the bioavailability of orally administered venlafaxine. J Clin Pharmacol 37:954–61, 1997b

Troy SM, Turner MB, Unruh M, et al: Pharmacokinetic and pharmacodynamic evaluation of the potential drug interaction between venlafaxine and ethanol. J Clin Pharmacol 37:1073–1081, 1997c

Tylee A, Beaumont G, Bowden MW, et al: A double-blind, randomized, 12-week comparison of the safety and efficacy of venlafaxine and fluoxetine in moderate to severe major depression in general practice. Prim Care Psychiatry 3:51–58, 1997

Tzanakaki M, Guazzelli M, Nimatoudis I, et al: Increased remission rates with venlafaxine compared with fluoxetine in hospitalized patients with major depression and melancholia. Int Clin Psychopharmacol 15:29–34, 2000

Vaishnavi SN, Nemeroff CB, Plott SJ, et al: Milnacipran: a comparative analysis of human monoamine uptake and transporter binding affinity. Biol Psychiatry 55:320–322, 2004

Vieta E, Martinez-Aran A, Goikolea JM, et al: A randomized trial comparing paroxetine and venlafaxine in the treatment of bipolar depressed patients taking mood stabilizers. J Clin Psychiatry 63:508–512, 2002

Whyte IM, Dawson AH, Buckley NA: Relative toxicity of venlafaxine and selective serotonin reuptake inhibitors in overdose compared to tricyclic antidepressants. QJM 96:369–374, 2003

Zanardi R, Franchini L, Serretti A, et al: Venlafaxine versus fluvoxamine in the treatment of delusional depression: a pilot double-blind controlled study. J Clin Psychiatry 61:26–29, 2000

CHAPTER 23

Duloxetine and Milnacipran

Sandhaya Norris, M.D.

Pierre Blier, M.D., Ph.D.

Duloxetine was first synthesized in the 1980s and subsequently patented in 1991. The U.S. Food and Drug Administration (FDA) did not approve this drug for the treatment of major depressive disorder and diabetic neuropathy, however, until the third quarter of 2004. This long delay occurred because the drug was initially tested in depressed patients at low dosages of 5–20 mg/day, which were not efficacious. Duloxetine has received approval in most countries worldwide since then but became available in Canada only in 2008. It is also approved in the United States for generalized anxiety disorder and fibromyalgia. Milnacipran was approved in France for the treatment of depression in 1996 but only recently was approved for use in North America for patients with fibromyalgia.

Structure–Activity Relations

Duloxetine and milnacipran (Figure 23–1), along with venlafaxine, are antidepressant medications that can act as serotonin (5-hydroxytryptamine; 5-HT) and norepinephrine reuptake inhibitors. Whereas selective serotonin reuptake inhibitors (SSRIs) target only the 5-HT transporter (5-HTT), the dual-acting medications have the potential to inhibit both the 5-HTT and the norepinephrine transporter (NET). Collectively, these three medications are referred to as serotonin–norepinephrine reuptake inhibitors (SNRIs). Several lines of evidence have to be considered, however, to determine at which concentrations SNRIs are indeed effective dual reuptake inhibitors. This is of crucial importance in estimating their potency in clinical settings.

Pharmacological Profiles

In Vitro Assessments

The first data to consider in determining the biochemical profile of reuptake inhibitors are their affinity values for membranal carriers. These values can be calculated by determining the concentration of a medication necessary to displace 50% of the specific binding of a standard ligand for a given transporter subtype in a lyzed cell preparation (K_i). This technique generally provides rough estimates of the potential for drugs to inhibit reuptake. A somewhat more indicative approach consists of determining the concentrations of drugs necessary to inhibit the uptake of transmitters in intact cells from either animal brains or human cell lines. These physiological results are more reliable than mere binding data because of the integrity of the tissue. Indeed, recent data indicate that the binding of some norepinephrine reuptake blockers varies markedly when they are tested in membrane preparations versus intact cells, whereas with other agents, such as the tricyclic antidepressants (TCAs), it does not (Mason et al. 2007). As can be seen in Table 23–1, not only do the absolute potencies vary between the two preparations, their ratios vary as well.

In Vivo Assessments

Ideally, the potency of reuptake inhibitors in animal experiments should be assessed in vivo with the medications administered systemically. One common technique is to conduct microdialysis studies whereby extracellular levels

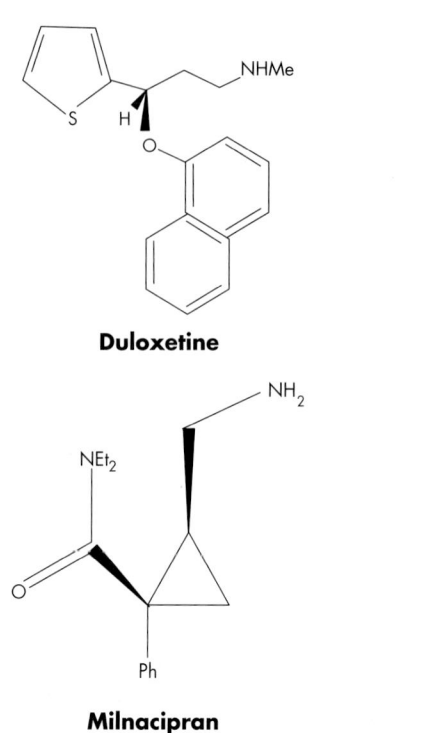

Duloxetine

Milnacipran

FIGURE 23–1. Chemical structures of duloxetine and milnacipran.

of neurotransmitters are estimated from the perfusion of an artificial cerebrospinal fluid. Data generated with duloxetine in rats indicate that it first enhances brain levels of 5-HT, and that with increasing doses it increases norepinephrine levels (Koch et al. 2003). In the case of milnacipran, the levels of 5-HT and norepinephrine are generally enhanced to the same extent (in guinea pigs; Moret and Briley 1997), although pronounced regional differences have been observed. For instance, milnacipran is six times more potent in the rat hypothalamus than in the midbrain raphe nuclei and the frontal cortex (Bel and Artigas 1999). These results suggest that milnacipran may not readily penetrate the blood–brain barrier.

Potency can also be assessed in vivo using electrophysiological approaches. For instance, by determining the capacity of reuptake inhibitors to suppress the firing of 5-HT and norepinephrine neurons, reliable potency estimates can be obtained. As reuptake transporters are dose-dependently inhibited from their systemic injection, 5-HT and norepinephrine accumulate at the cell body level of such neurons that will activate their respective autoreceptors, thereby decreasing firing activity. Using this approach, duloxetine suppresses the firing rate of 5-HT neurons by 50% with an intravenous dose of 0.1 mg/kg and suppresses the firing rate of norepinephrine neurons to

the same level with a dose of 0.5 mg/kg (Kasamo et al. 1996). This in vivo ratio of 1:5 is quite different from the in vitro affinity ratio of 1:12 (Vaishnavi et al. 2004; see Table 23–1). In contrast, using the same in vivo technique, the dose of milnacipran necessary to inhibit the firing rate of 5-HT neurons by 50% is 5.7 mg/kg (Mongeau et al. 1998). The latter results therefore suggest that milnacipran is much less potent in inhibiting 5-HT reuptake than duloxetine.

Assessments of 5-HT and Norepinephrine Reuptake in Humans

Reuptake of neurotransmitters in humans cannot be assessed as directly as it can in the brains of laboratory animals. Several approaches can, however, provide useful estimates. For instance, 5-HT reuptake inhibition can be estimated using blood platelet uptake of radioactive 5-HT because platelets do not synthesize 5-HT and they have a 5-HTT that is nearly identical to the one present on 5-HT neurons in the brain. And because more than 90% of the 5-HT in blood is in platelets, whole blood can be used to measure 5-HT depletion by a reuptake inhibitor, making assessment simpler. Using this peripheral assay, duloxetine produces a dose-dependent depletion of the 5-HT level that reaches only about 60% with a 60-mg dose, an effect that is significantly inferior to that seen with the TCA clomipramine at a dose of 100 mg (Turcotte et al. 2001). Likewise, milnacipran produces a 64% inhibition of 5-HT uptake with the usual recommended dose of 100 mg (Puozzo et al. 1985). Using a similar assay, SSRIs produce a greater than 80% inhibition with clinically effective doses (Gilmor et al. 2002).

Occupancy of the 5-HTT in the human brain is possible to assess directly using carbon 11 (^{11}C)–labeled ligands of these transporters and positron emission tomography (PET). The minimal effective doses of the SSRIs and venlafaxine for treating depression all result in at least 80% occupancy of the 5-HTT (Meyer et al. 2004). A daily dose of 60 mg, but not 40 mg, of duloxetine produces sustained 80% occupancy (Takano et al. 2006). To our knowledge, milnacipran has not been tested using this approach.

Occupancy of the NET in the human brain is currently not possible because a PET ligand, validated with standard norepinephrine reuptake inhibitors (NRIs), is still lacking. A variety of peripheral measures can, however, be used. In particular, the intravenous tyramine pressor test has produced consistent results. Tyramine penetrates into peripheral norepinephrine terminals through

TABLE 23–1. In vitro affinity and inhibition values for milnacipran and duloxetine for human reuptake transporters

	SEROTONIN TRANSPORTER	NOREPINEPHRINE TRANSPORTER	DOPAMINE TRANSPORTER
Affinity values, K_i (nM)			
Milnacipran	8.4	22	ND
Duloxetine	0.1	1.2	230
Inhibition values, K_i (nM)			
Milnacipran	151	68	ND
Duloxetine	3.7	20	439

Note. ND=Not detectable; values for duloxetine for the dopamine transporter are not physiologically significant.
Source. Adapted from Vaishnavi et al. 2004.

the NET and releases norepinephrine in a calcium-independent manner, thereby transiently elevating the systolic blood pressure. Any drug effectively blocking the NET attenuates this pressor response in a dose-dependent manner. The SSRIs paroxetine and sertraline do not affect this response, whereas the TCAs desipramine, nortriptyline, and clomipramine attenuate it, as is also the case with the selective NRIs maprotiline, reboxetine, and atomoxetine (Blier et al. 2007; Gobbi et al. 2003; Harvey et al. 2000; Slater et al. 2000; Turcotte et al. 2001). Venlafaxine significantly attenuates the tyramine response only at dosages in the 225–375 mg/day range in depressed patients (Aldosary et al. 2007; Debonnel et al. 2007). Duloxetine exerts a clear effect only at 120 mg/day (Vincent et al. 2004), whereas milnacipran, to our knowledge, has not been tested using this model. A variety of other peripheral measures suggest that duloxetine may begin to inhibit norepinephrine reuptake at 60 mg/day (Chalon et al. 2003; Turcotte et al. 2001; Vincent et al. 2004).

Taken together, these results obtained in humans indicate that duloxetine is a potent 5-HT reuptake inhibitor at a dosage of 60 mg/day. The exact degree of norepinephrine reuptake inhibition occurring in humans at 60 mg/day remains uncertain, but at 120 mg/day it reaches a physiologically relevant level without any doubt. A definite answer to the degree of norepinephrine reuptake inhibition produced by duloxetine in the human brain awaits both the availability of a PET ligand for the NET and a comparison with clinically effective doses of selective NRIs such as desipramine. Such experiments will also serve to determine the NET reserve beyond which the overall function of the norepinephrine system is altered, as was determined for the 5-HTT (i.e., 80%; Meyer et al. 2004).

With regard to milnacipran, it appears that it acts preferentially on the norepinephrine reuptake process because it has been easy to find evidence of this action in the brain of laboratory animals even with low doses, whereas 5-HT reuptake inhibition can only be documented with high doses. Robust 5-HT reuptake inhibition (>80%) in humans appears to be achieved only with supratherapeutic doses (i.e., 300–400 mg; Palmier et al. 1989).

Mechanism of Action

Administration of SNRIs results in a rapid inhibition of reuptake transporters in the brain. However, their therapeutic effect on depression is delayed at least 2 weeks. Extensive electrophysiological and microdialysis studies in laboratory animals have provided consistent results showing a similar delay before SNRIs produce a net enhancement of 5-HT and/or norepinephrine transmission, thereby explaining their therapeutic lag in treating depression (see Blier 2006 for a review). In brief, SNRIs that are potent 5-HT reuptake inhibitors initially suppress the firing of 5-HT neurons through the activation of 5-HT_{1A} autoreceptors on their cell bodies, as a result of 5-HTT inhibition. After 2–3 weeks of sustained administration, the firing rate returns to normal in the presence of sustained reuptake inhibition, due to 5-HT_{1A} autoreceptor desensitization. At this time, there is a net enhancement of 5-HT transmission in the forebrain (Bel and Artigas 1993; Blier and de Montigny 1983; Rueter et al. 1998a, 1998b).

Regarding SNRI inhibition of the NET, the firing rate of norepinephrine neurons is promptly diminished as a result of the activation of the α_2-adrenergic autoreceptors on their cell bodies. After 2–3 weeks of sustained administration, the firing rate remains attenuated because the cell body α_2-adrenergic autoreceptors do not become desensitized. In contrast, α_2-adrenergic autoreceptors on norepinephrine terminals generally do become desensitized, leading to a net enhancement of norepinephrine transmission in the forebrain in the presence of sustained norepinephrine reuptake inhibition (Invernizzi and Garattini 2004; Rueter et al. 1998a, 1998b; Szabo and Blier 2001).

Pharmacokinetics and Disposition

Absorption and Distribution

Duloxetine is available in an enteric formulation. It is rapidly absorbed after oral administration, and its absorption is not altered by food. Plasma levels are proportional to doses, up to the maximum recommended dose of 60 mg twice daily. It is highly bound to plasma proteins, to an extent of about 90%. Its plasma elimination half-life is approximately 12 hours (Sharma et al. 2000). With repeated administration, duloxetine levels therefore reach a steady-state level after about 3 days.

Milnacipran has low (13%) and nonsaturable plasma protein binding. It is rapidly absorbed after oral administration and has high bioavailability, and its absorption is not affected by food intake. It has no active metabolite, and its elimination half-life is 8 hours. Steady-state levels are thus achieved within 3 days, with no drug accumulation occurring during prolonged dosing, and the drug is cleared from the body within 3 days of treatment cessation. It is eliminated by the kidneys as essentially the parent compound and glucuronide, the inactive glucuronic acid conjugate (Puozzo and Leonard 1996).

Metabolism and Elimination

Duloxetine is extensively metabolized through various pathways (Skinner et al. 2003). Numerous metabolites are found in circulation, none of which is believed to contribute to its therapeutic activity. Duloxetine is metabolized mainly by cytochrome P450 1A2 and 2D6 isoenzymes.

The cytochrome P450 system is not involved in the metabolism of milnacipran (Briley 1998). Its metabolism is mediated mainly through phase II conjugation. Approximately 50%–60% of the drug is recovered in the urine as the parent compound and 20% as its glucuronic acid conjugate, the remainder being excreted mainly as an N-dealkyl metabolite and its glucuronic acid conju-

gate, and in negligible amounts as an N-didealkyl metabolite and a hydroxy metabolite (Puozzo et al. 2002).

Indications and Efficacy

Duloxetine has been approved by the FDA for use in treating major depressive disorder, diabetic peripheral neuropathic pain, fibromyalgia, and generalized anxiety disorder; it is also approved in Europe for treating stress urinary incontinence. Additional common off-label uses include other neuropathic pain/chronic pain disorders.

Milnacipran is used to treat major depressive disorder in various countries, although it has not yet received FDA approval for that indication. It was recently approved in the United States for the treatment of fibromyalgia.

Depression

Duloxetine

To date, 12 placebo-controlled studies have evaluated the antidepressant efficacy of duloxetine at dosages of 40–120 mg/day. Many of these had an active drug comparator group. Efficacy was measured by remission, the optimal outcome measure, or by response. Remission can be operationally defined as a score of less than or equal to 7 on the 17-item Hamilton Rating Scale for Depression (Ham-D) or a score of less than or equal to 10 on the Montgomery-Åsberg Depression Rating Scale (MADRS). Response is often defined as a 50% reduction in the MADRS or Ham-D score from baseline to endpoint. These studies and non-placebo-controlled duloxetine trials are summarized in Tables 23–2 and 23–3.

Head-to-head comparisons with SSRIs have yielded mixed results, which appear to be heavily influenced by dosing regimens (see Tables 23–2 and 23–3). In a recent 8-week, placebo-controlled comparison of duloxetine 60 mg/day and escitalopram 10 mg/day, the two drugs produced similar statistically significant improvement versus placebo on the primary efficacy measure of onset of efficacy and similar response and remission rates at endpoint (Nierenberg et al. 2007).

In a recent meta-analysis of six Phase II/III studies that compared duloxetine with two SSRIs (fluoxetine or paroxetine) in outpatients with major depressive disorder, duloxetine 40–120 mg/day was reported to be an effective antidepressant, with an overall efficacy profile equal to that of fluoxetine and paroxetine at 20 mg/day (Thase et al. 2007). For patients stratified as having moderate to severe symptoms, the remission rates with duloxetine

TABLE 23–2. Duloxetine versus placebo and/or active SSRI or SNRI comparator in acute studies (≤12 weeks) of depression

Study	Duration (weeks)	Sample size	Duloxetine Dosage (mg/day)	Comparator Used	Comparator Dosage (mg/day)	Placebo?	Results
Goldstein et al. 2002	8	173	120	Fluoxetine	20	Yes	Duloxetine>placebo No difference with fluoxetine
Nemeroff et al. 2002[a]	8	194	120	Fluoxetine	20	Yes	No difference in remission rates at endpoint
Nemeroff et al. 2002[a]	8	354	40, 80	Paroxetine	20	Yes	No difference in remission rates at endpoint
Detke et al. 2002b	9	245	60	None	—	Yes	Duloxetine>placebo
Detke et al. 2002a	9	267	60	None	—	Yes	Duloxetine>placebo
Goldstein et al. 2004	8	353	40, 80	Paroxetine	20	Yes	Duloxetine 80 (but not 40)>placebo No difference between duloxetine 80 and paroxetine
Detke et al. 2004	8	354	80, 120	Paroxetine	20	Yes	Duloxetine (80 and 120)>placebo Paroxetine=placebo
Perahia et al. 2006b	8	392	80, 120	Paroxetine	20	Yes	Duloxetine (80 and 120)>placebo Paroxetine=placebo
Raskin et al. 2007	8	311	60	None	—	Yes	Duloxetine>placebo
Nierenberg et al. 2007	8	684	60	Escitalopram	10	Yes	No difference between any groups at endpoint
Khan et al. 2007	8	278	60	Escitalopram	10–20	No	Escitalopram>duloxetine
Brecht et al. 2007	8	327	60	None	—	Yes	Duloxetine>placebo
P. Lee et al. 2007	8	478	60	Paroxetine	20	No	Duloxetine=paroxetine
Perahia et al. 2008	12	667	120	Venlafaxine	225	No	Duloxetine=venlafaxine

Note. SNRI=serotonin–norepinephrine reuptake inhibitor; SSRI=selective serotonin reuptake inhibitor. ">" denotes significantly greater effect; "=" denotes no difference.
[a]These failed studies were reported in this review but were not conducted by Dr. Nemeroff.

TABLE 23–3. Duloxetine versus placebo and/or active SSRI comparator in continuation studies (>12 weeks) of depression

Study	Duration (weeks)	Sample size	Duloxetine Dosage (mg/day)	Comparator Used	Comparator Dosage (mg/day)	Placebo?	Results
Pigott et al. 2007	32	684	60–120	Escitalopram	10–20	Yes	Duloxetine=escitalopram; placebo group underpowered due to length of trial
Wade et al. 2007	24	295	60	Escitalopram	20	No	Duloxetine=escitalopram

Note. SSRI=selective serotonin reuptake inhibitor. "=" denotes no difference.

were statistically superior to those with the SSRIs (see Table 23–3). Another recent meta-analysis of nine randomized, controlled trials (RCTs) evaluating high doses of duloxetine in patients with severe depression concluded that duloxetine 120 mg/day produced significantly greater baseline-to-endpoint improvement than placebo on several of the 17 Ham-D items (Shelton et al. 2007).

Milnacipran

A meta-analysis of three short-term (4- to 8-week), double-blind, acute efficacy multicenter trials in inpatients and outpatients with moderate to severe depression found that milnacipran exerts a superior antidepressant effect compared with placebo at dosages of 50 and 100 mg twice daily but not at a dosage of 25 mg twice a day (Lecrubier et al. 1996; Macher et al. 1989).

Several studies have compared milnacipran with SSRIs or TCAs in the treatment of depression (Table 23–4). In comparison with the TCA imipramine, milnacipran has been noted to have equal efficacy, but superior tolerability (Puech et al. 1997). A recent meta-analysis concluded that there is insufficient evidence to suggest a difference in response rates between milnacipran and any SSRI: Pooling response rates of the agents revealed an overall response rate of 62.1% for milnacipran and 57.5% for the SSRIs (Papakostas and Fava 2007). To date, no continuation studies (>12 weeks' duration) have been published comparing the efficacy of milnacipran to that of any SSRI. There is no maximal recommended dose of milnacipran, but it is important to mention that the highest daily dose tested so far, 300 mg, was tested in only 41 patients and for only 2 weeks (Ansseau et al. 1991).

Generalized Anxiety Disorder

Three placebo-controlled studies have had positive results showing a therapeutic action with duloxetine in patients with generalized anxiety disorder (Allgulander et al. 2007). Dosing strategies are similar to those used in major depression.

Neuropathic Pain/Chronic Pain

TCAs and SNRIs clearly produce significant relief of physical symptoms such as pain in depression and in a variety of pain syndromes (Stahl et al. 2005). Potentiation of the activity of 5-HT and norepinephrine is believed to result in central pain inhibition through descending modulatory pathways (Sussman 2003).

Duloxetine

Duloxetine exerts a prompt and substantial analgesic effect beyond its antidepressant action (Perahia et al. 2006a). Duloxetine has shown efficacy in the treatment of diabetic peripheral neuropathy in randomized, placebo-controlled trials (Fishbain et al. 2006; Wernicke et al. 2006). Response tends to occur early in therapy and has been associated with significant improvement in functional outcomes (Armstrong et al. 2007; Pritchett et al. 2007b).

In a recent 8-week study of patients with major depressive disorder and at least moderate pain of unknown etiology, a fixed dosage of duloxetine (60 mg/day) significantly reduced pain measures at endpoint from baseline compared with placebo (Brecht et al. 2007). The mean average pain score at 8 weeks was close to 3 on the Brief Pain Inventory—Short Form, which can be considered a mild level of pain compared with the moderate or higher levels of pain indicated by baseline scores (Brecht et al. 2007). Similarly, elderly patients with depression treated with duloxetine (60 mg/day) for 8 weeks reported significantly greater improvement in back pain scores and amount of time in pain compared with placebo recipients (Raskin et al. 2007).

An RCT of duloxetine 60 mg/day demonstrated greater efficacy than placebo in reducing overall shoulder pain and back pain in depressed patients, as well as time spent with pain (Detke et al. 2002b). Overall pain severity and back pain improved the most. Improvements were assessed with the visual analog scales of pain severity, measuring overall pain, back pain, headaches, shoulder pain, interference with daily activities, and time in pain.

Milnacipran

The capacity of milnacipran to relieve chronic pain has been reported in open trials, but no RCTs have been published to date.

Fibromyalgia

A 12-week RCT of duloxetine 120 mg/day versus placebo in patients with fibromyalgia, some of whom were also diagnosed with depression, found significant improvement in pain scores in duloxetine recipients and greater improvement in tender points compared with placebo recipients (Arnold et al. 2005). Duloxetine 120 mg/day improved fibromyalgia symptoms and pain severity regardless of the extent of the accompanying depressive disorder. The drug has received FDA approval for this indication.

TABLE 23–4. Milnacipran versus placebo and/or active SSRI comparator in acute studies (≤12 weeks) of depression

Study	Duration (weeks)	Sample size	Milnacipran Dosage (mg/day)	Comparator used	Comparator Dosage (mg/day)	Placebo?	Results
Macher et al. 1989	4	58	100	None	—	Yes	Milnacipran>placebo
Ansseau et al. 1991	4	127	150–300	Fluvoxamine	200	No	Milnacipran=fluvoxamine
Ansseau et al. 1994	6	190	100[a]	Fluoxetine	20	No	Fluoxetine>milnacipran
Lecrubier et al. 1996[b]	6–8	644	50, 100, 200	None	—	Yes	Milnacipran 100 and 200 (but not 50)>placebo
Guelfi et al. 1998	12	289	100–200	Fluoxetine	20	No	Milnacipran=fluoxetine
Clerc 2001	6	113	100	Fluvoxamine	200	No	Milnacipran>fluvoxamine
Sechter et al. 2004	6	302	100	Paroxetine	20	No	Milnacipran=paroxetine
M.S. Lee et al. 2005	6	70	100	Fluoxetine	20	No	Milnacipran=fluoxetine

Note. SSRI=selective serotonin reuptake inhibitor. ">" denotes significantly greater effect; "=" denotes no difference.
[a]Milnacipran was given once daily; this was in contrast to the other studies, in which it was administered on a twice-daily basis.
[b]This is a composite of two positive controlled studies.

A placebo-controlled study of milnacipran in fibromyalgia patients showed that 37% of the patients treated with 100 mg of milnacipran twice daily experienced a significant reduction in pain intensity of 50% or more compared with 14% of placebo recipients (Vitton et al. 2004). Here, too, milnacipran recently received FDA approval for this indication.

Stress Urinary Incontinence

Duloxetine has been investigated in the treatment of stress urinary incontinence, with 40 mg twice daily being the recommended dosage (Norton et al. 2002). Serotonin and norepinephrine increase excitatory glutamate transmission in the Onuf nucleus in the sacral spinal cord, which facilitates urethral sphincter contraction (Thor 2003). This is presumably the mechanism for the beneficial effect of duloxetine in the treatment of this problem.

The capacity of milnacipran to treat stress urinary incontinence has not been reported to date.

Side Effects and Toxicology

Duloxetine

In clinical trials to date, the safety and tolerability of duloxetine in the dosage range of 40–120 mg/day have been assessed. In an 8-month study, the most common treatment-emergent adverse events included nausea, dry mouth, vomiting, yawning, and night sweats (Pigott et al. 2007). Most of these emerged early, within the first 8 weeks. Other studies have reported insomnia, somnolence, headaches, ejaculation disorders, diarrhea, constipation, and dizziness as common adverse events with duloxetine (Detke et al. 2002a, 2002b; Khan et al. 2007; Nierenberg et al. 2007).

The rates of nausea with duloxetine appear to be comparable to those found with other SNRIs and with SSRIs. Nausea is transient and usually present at treatment initiation. A starting dosage of 60 mg/day appears to provide the best combination of clinical response and tolerability (Bech et al. 2006; Pritchett et al. 2007a). Clinicians may, however, consider starting at a lower dosage, 30 mg/day, for patients for whom tolerance is a concern. Duloxetine 30 mg/day offers the advantage of a lower rate of nausea as a treatment-emergent adverse event (in one study, 16% vs. 33% with duloxetine 60 mg/day; Dunner et al. 2005). A recent study indicates that the tolerability of duloxetine at an initial dosage of 60 mg/day can be improved if the drug is taken with food, to the point of being compa-

rable to the tolerability at an initial dosage of 30 mg/day (Whitmyer et al. 2007).

Duloxetine has not been associated with weight gain, and in one study it was in fact noted to be associated with a mean 1-kg weight loss (Nierenberg et al. 2007). This decrease was a statistically significant difference compared with the lack of effect that placebo and escitalopram had on weight. Changes in blood pressure and heart rate do not appear to be clinically significant. Pooled data on 735 patients treated with duloxetine 40–120 mg/day showed that 0.7% had a 10-mm Hg increase in systolic or diastolic blood pressure compared with 0.4% of patients receiving placebo. Heart rate was increased by less than 1 beat per minute (Schatzberg 2003).

Rates of sexual dysfunction, including anorgasmia, erectile dysfunction, delayed ejaculation, and decreased libido, appear to be low with duloxetine. Researchers found that after 8 months, categorical outcomes shown on a questionnaire about changes in sexual functioning did not differ significantly between duloxetine and escitalopram groups (Pigott et al. 2007). In clinical practice, however, sexual dysfunction with any drug that potentially inhibits 5-HT reuptake does create some problems in a significant proportion of patients.

Rates of discontinuation due to adverse events have not differed significantly in placebo and active comparator groups in acute or longer-term studies. However, it appears that study subjects who discontinue duloxetine due to adverse events often do so during the early study visits (Nierenberg et al. 2007; Perahia et al. 2008; Pigott et al. 2007), which may suggest poorer initial tolerability.

Milnacipran

Analysis of a database of more than 3,300 patients concluded that the adverse-event profile of milnacipran is comparable to that of the SSRIs, except that with the SSRIs a higher frequency of nausea and anxiety is seen, whereas milnacipran is associated with a higher incidence of dysuria (Puech et al. 1997). Weight gain is uncommon, and sedation may be reported. Data on the occurrence of sexual dysfunction with milnacipran have not been reported, but its prevalence is estimated to be low compared with the prevalence of sexual dysfunction seen with venlafaxine and much lower than that seen with SSRIs (Stahl et al. 2005). The lower incidence of nausea and sexual dysfunction with milnacipran versus SSRIs may be taken as indirect evidence of its lower 5-HT reuptake inhibition potential, these two treatment-emergent adverse events being classically induced by potent 5-HT reuptake inhibitors.

Blood pressure increases with milnacipran are minimal. A 12-week randomized, double-blind study comparing milnacipran dosages of 100 mg/day and 200 mg/day versus fluoxetine 20 mg/day in 289 depressed inpatients found no significant changes in blood pressure in any of the group (Guelfi et al. 1998). Tachycardia, a heart rate of greater than 100 beats per minute, was seen in 0% of patients receiving fluoxetine, 3% of patients receiving milnacipran 100 mg/day, and 6% of patients receiving milnacipran 200 mg/day. A review of more than 4,000 patients treated with milnacipran showed that the mean increase in blood pressure was less than 1 mm Hg and the mean increase in heart rate was 3.6 beats per minute (Puech et al. 1997). Given that an increase of heart rate is a thumbprint of potent norepinephrine reuptake inhibition, this increase is consistent with the capacity of milnacipran to effectively block norepinephrine reuptake. No cardiotoxicity has been reported with overdoses of up to 2.8 g/day, which is 28 times the recommended daily dose (Montgomery et al. 1996).

Analysis of the long-term safety of milnacipran (in 715 patients receiving milnacipran for >6 months, 189 for >12 months, as reported by Puech et al. 1997) has shown that most adverse events appear within the first 3 months of treatment and that the incidence decreases steadily thereafter. More important, no treatment-emergent adverse events developed during long-term treatment.

Drug–Drug Interactions

Inhibitors of cytochrome P450 1A2, such as ciprofloxacin, increase plasma levels of duloxetine, and their use may require that duloxetine dosages be reduced or that duloxetine use be avoided. When duloxetine is coadministered with a cytochrome P450 2D6 inhibitor of moderate potency, such as bupropion or diphenhydramine, duloxetine levels may increase. Generally, however, such alterations of duloxetine levels are not clinically significant.

Duloxetine does not inhibit or induce the activity of cytochrome P450 1A2, 2C9, or 3A4 systems. It does, however, moderately inhibit the activity of the 2D6 isoenzyme. If duloxetine is prescribed with an agent metabolized by 2D6, clinicians should use doses that are approximately half those usually recommended for the concomitant medication. Duloxetine does not potentiate the psychotropic effects of ethanol or benzodiazepines.

Because milnacipran is not metabolized by the cytochrome P450 pathways, it does not produce pharmacokinetic drug–drug interactions. However, both milnacipran and duloxetine can have a serious, potentially lethal pharmacodynamic interaction if given concomitantly with a monoamine oxidase inhibitor (MAOI) due to the risk of serotonin syndrome. To avoid this catastrophic outcome, an MAOI must never be administered until at least 5 days after duloxetine or milnacipran has been discontinued. A longer washout period must be respected when switching from an MAOI to an SNRI. A washout period of at least 14 days should elapse before starting any SNRI.

Conclusion

At their minimal effective dosages, duloxetine (60 mg/day) and milnacipran (100 mg/day) potently block the reuptake of 5-HT and norepinephrine, respectively. In the case of duloxetine, it is difficult to imagine that increasing the subtherapeutic dosage of 40 mg/day, at which it does not perform as an SSRI, to 60 mg/day would produce marked norepinephrine reuptake inhibition when the in vivo 5-HT–norepinephrine reuptake potency ratio is 1:5. In the case of milnacipran, a 100-mg dose produces suboptimal platelet 5-HT reuptake inhibition. Duloxetine at its maximal recommended dosage (120 mg/day) and milnacipran in its upper therapeutic range (200 mg/day) are dual reuptake inhibitors, but none of the three SNRIs currently available can be considered a balanced serotonin–norepinephrine reuptake inhibitor.

Duloxetine and milnacipran have demonstrated efficacy for the treatment of depression and pain syndromes, with emerging evidence also suggesting a potential role for duloxetine in the treatment of stress urinary incontinence and some anxiety disorders. These medications are generally well tolerated, with most adverse events occurring early in treatment, being mild to moderate in severity, and having a tendency to decrease or disappear with continued treatment.

Either of these two drugs may be used as a first-line treatment for depression because they are not toxic in overdosage and they can be used at therapeutic dosages from treatment initiation onward with minimal side effects. Furthermore, data suggest that treatment with a dual reuptake inhibitor is superior to treatment with an antidepressant with only one mechanism of action, such as an SSRI (Nemeroff et al. 2008; Poirier and Boyer 1999; Thase et al. 2007). Consequently, duloxetine and milnacipran may be useful in patients whose conditions have been resistant to treatment with SSRIs or NRIs, provided that they are used at dosages in the upper end of the therapeutic range.

References

Aldosary F, Tremblay P, Hébert, C, et al: Venlafaxine and atomoxetine, but not paroxetine, dose-dependently inhibit the in vivo function of the norepinephrine reuptake transport system in depressed patients. Paper presented at the annual meeting of the American College of Neuropsychopharmacology, Boca Raton, FL, December 2007

Allgulander C, Hartford J, Russell J, et al: Pharmacotherapy of generalized anxiety disorder: results of duloxetine treatment from a pooled analysis of three clinical trials. Curr Med Res Opin 23:1245–1252, 2007

Ansseau M, von Frenckell R, Gérard MA, et al: Interest of a loading dose of milnacipran in endogenous depressive inpatients. Comparison with the standard regimen and with fluvoxamine. Eur Neuropsychopharmacol 1:113–121, 1991

Ansseau M, Pampart P, Troisfontaines B, et al: Controlled comparison of milnacipran and fluoxetine in major depression. Psychopharmacology (Berl) 114:131–137, 1994

Armstrong DG, Chappell AS, Le TK, et al: Duloxetine for the management of diabetic peripheral neuropathic pain: evaluation of functional outcomes. Pain Med 8:410–418, 2007; erratum in: Pain Med 8:690, 2007

Arnold LM, Rosen A, Pritchett YL, et al: A randomized, double-blind, placebo-controlled trial of duloxetine in the treatment of women with fibromyalgia with or without major depressive disorder. Pain 119:5–15, 2005

Bech P, Kajdasz DK, Porsdal V: Dose-response relationship of duloxetine in placebo-controlled clinical trials in patients with major depressive disorder. Psychopharmacology (Berl) 188:273–280, 2006

Bel N, Artigas F: Chronic treatment with fluvoxamine increases extracellular serotonin in frontal cortex but not in raphe nuclei. Synapse 15:243–245, 1993

Bel N, Artigas F: Modulation of the extracellular 5-hydroxytryptamine brain concentrations by the serotonin and noradrenaline reuptake inhibitor, milnacipran: microdialysis studies in rats. Neuropsychopharmacology 21:745–754, 1999

Blier P: Dual serotonin and norepinephrine reuptake inhibitors: focus on their differences. International Journal of Psychiatry in Clinical Practice 10 (suppl 2):22–32, 2006

Blier P, de Montigny C: Electrophysiological investigations on the effect of repeated zimelidine administration on serotonergic neurotransmission in the rat. J Neurosci 3:1270–1278, 1983

Blier P, Saint-André E, Hébert C, et al: Effects of different doses of venlafaxine on serotonin and norepinephrine reuptake in healthy volunteers. Int J Neuropsychopharmacol 10:41–50, 2007

Brecht S, Courtecuisse C, Debieuvre C, et al: Efficacy and safety of duloxetine 60 mg once daily in the treatment of pain in patients with major depressive disorder and at least moderate pain of unknown etiology: a randomized controlled trial. J Clin Psychiatry 68:1707–1716, 2007

Briley M: Milnacipran, a well tolerated specific serotonin and norepinephrine reuptake inhibiting antidepressant. CNS Drug Rev 4:137–148, 1998

Chalon SA, Granier LA, Vandenhende FR, et al: Duloxetine increases serotonin and norepinephrine availability in healthy subjects: a double-blind, controlled study. Neuropsychopharmacology 28:1685–1693, 2003

Clerc G; Milnacipran/Fluvoxamine Study Group: Antidepressant efficacy and tolerability of milnacipran: a dual serotonin and noradrenaline reuptake inhibitor; a comparison with fluvoxamine. Int Clin Psychopharmacol 16:145–151, 2001

Debonnel G, Saint-André E, Hébert C, et al: Differential physiological effects of a low dose and high doses of venlafaxine in major depression. Int J Neuropsychopharmacol 10:51–61, 2007

Detke MJ, Lu Y, Goldstein DJ, et al: Duloxetine 60 mg once daily dosing versus placebo in the acute treatment of major depression. J Psychiatr Res 36:383–390, 2002a

Detke MJ, Lu Y, Goldstein DJ, et al: Duloxetine, 60 mg once daily, for major depressive disorder: a randomized double-blind placebo-controlled trial. J Clin Psychiatry 63:308–315, 2002b

Detke MJ, Wiltse CG, Mallinckrodt CH, et al: Duloxetine in the acute and long-term treatment of major depressive disorder: a placebo- and paroxetine-controlled trial. Eur Neuropsychopharmacol 14:457–470, 2004

Dunner DL, Wohlreich MM, Mallinckrodt CH, et al: Clinical consequences of initial duloxetine dosing strategies: comparison of 30 and 60 mg QD starting doses. Current Therapeutic Research 66:522–540, 2005

Fishbain D, Berman K, Kajdasz DK: Duloxetine for neuropathic pain based on recent clinical trials. Curr Pain Headache Rep 10:199–204, 2006

Gilmor ML, Owens MJ, Nemeroff CB: Inhibition of norepinephrine uptake in patients with major depression treated with paroxetine. Am J Psychiatry 159:1702–1710, 2002

Gobbi G, Slater S, Boucher N, et al: Neurochemical and psychotropic effects of bupropion in healthy male subjects. J Clin Psychopharmacol 23:233–239, 2003

Goldstein DJ, Mallinckrodt CH, Lu Y, et al: Duloxetine in the treatment of major depressive disorder: a double-blind clinical trial. J Clin Psychiatry 63:225–231, 2002

Goldstein DJ, Lu Y, Detke MJ, et al: Duloxetine in the treatment of depression: a double-blind placebo-controlled comparison with paroxetine. J Clin Psychopharmacol 24:389–399, 2004

Guelfi JD, Ansseau M, Corruble E, et al: A double-blind comparison of the efficacy and safety of milnacipran and fluoxetine in depressed inpatients. Int Clin Psychopharmacol 13:121–128, 1998

Harvey AT, Rudolph RL, Preskorn SH: Evidence of the dual mechanisms of action of venlafaxine. Arch Gen Psychiatry 57:503–509, 2000

Invernizzi RW, Garattini S: Role of presynaptic alpha2-adrenoceptors in antidepressant action: recent findings from microdialysis studies. Prog Neuropsychopharmacol Biol Psychiatry 28:819–827, 2004

Kasamo K, Blier P, de Montigny C: Blockade of the serotonin and norepinephrine uptake processes by duloxetine: in vitro and in vivo studies in the rat brain. J Pharmacol Exp Ther 277:278–286, 1996

Khan A, Bose A, Alexopoulos GS, et al: Double-blind comparison of escitalopram and duloxetine in the acute treatment of major depressive disorder. Clin Drug Investig 27:481–492, 2007

Koch S, Hemrick-Luecke SK, Thompson LK, et al: Comparison of effects of dual transporter inhibitors on monoamine transporters and extracellular levels in rats. Neuropharmacology 45:935–944, 2003

Lecrubier Y, Pletan Y, Solles A, et al: Clinical efficacy of milnacipran: placebo-controlled trials. Int Clin Psychopharmacol 11 (suppl 4):29–33, 1996

Lee MS, Ham BJ, Kee BS, et al: Comparison of efficacy and safety of milnacipran and fluoxetine in Korean patients with major depression. Curr Med Res Opin 21:1369–1375, 2005

Lee P, Shu L, Xu X, et al: Once-daily duloxetine 60 mg in the treatment of major depressive disorder: multicenter, double-blind, randomized, paroxetine-controlled, non-inferiority trial in China, Korea, Taiwan and Brazil. Psychiatry Clin Neurosci 61:295–307, 2007

Macher JP, Sichel JP, Serre C, et al: Double-blind placebo-controlled study of milnacipran in hospitalized patients with major depressive disorders. Neuropsychobiology 22:77–82, 1989

Mason JN, Deecher DC, Richmond RL, et al: Desvenlafaxine succinate identifies novel antagonist binding determinants in the human norepinephrine transporter. J Pharmacol Exp Ther 323:720–729, 2007

Meyer JH, Wilson AA, Sagrati S, et al: Serotonin transporter occupancy of five selective serotonin reuptake inhibitors at different doses: an [11C]DASB positron emission tomography study. Am J Psychiatry 161:826–835, 2004

Mongeau R, Weiss M, de Montigny C, et al: Effect of acute, short- and long-term milnacipran administration on rat locus coeruleus noradrenergic and dorsal raphe serotonergic neurons. Neuropharmacology 37:905–918, 1998

Montgomery SA, Prost JF, Solles A, et al: Efficacy and tolerability of milnacipran: an overview. Int Clin Psychopharmacol 11 (suppl 4):47–51, 1996

Moret C, Briley M: Effects of milnacipran and pindolol on extracellular noradrenaline and serotonin levels in guinea pig hypothalamus. J Neurochem 69:815–822, 1997

Nemeroff CB, Schatzberg AF, Goldstein DJ, et al: Duloxetine for the treatment of major depressive disorder. Psychopharmacol Bull 36:106–132, 2002

Nemeroff CB, Entsuah R, Benattia I, et al: Comprehensive analysis of remission (COMPARE) with venlafaxine versus SSRIs. Biol Psychiatry 63:424–434, 2008

Nierenberg AA, Greist JH, Mallinckrodt CH, et al: Duloxetine versus escitalopram and placebo in the treatment of patients with major depressive disorder: onset of antidepressant action, a non-inferiority study. Curr Med Res Opin 23:401–416, 2007

Norton PA, Zinner NR, Yalcin I, et al: Duloxetine versus placebo in the treatment of urinary stress incontinence. Am J Obstet Gynecol 187:40–48, 2002

Palmier C, Puozzo C, Lenehan T, et al: Monoamine uptake inhibition by plasma from healthy volunteers after single oral doses of the antidepressant milnacipran. Eur J Clin Pharmacol 37:235–238, 1989

Papakostas GI, Fava M: A meta-analysis of clinical trials comparing milnacipran, a serotonin-norepinephrine reuptake inhibitor, with a selective serotonin reuptake inhibitor for the treatment of major depressive disorder. Eur Neuropsychopharmacol 17:32–36, 2007

Perahia DG, Gilaberte I, Wang F, et al: Duloxetine in the prevention of relapse of major depressive disorder: double-blind placebo-controlled study. Br J Psychiatry 188:346–353, 2006a

Perahia DG, Wang F, Mallinckrodt CH, et al: Duloxetine in the treatment of major depressive disorder: a placebo- and paroxetine-controlled trial. Eur Psychiatry 21:367–378, 2006b

Perahia DG, Pritchett YL, Kajdasz DK, et al: A randomized, double-blind comparison of duloxetine and venlafaxine in the treatment of patients with major depressive disorder. J Psychiatr Res 42:22–34, 2008

Pigott TA, Prakash A, Arnold LM, et al: Duloxetine versus escitalopram and placebo: an 8 month, double-blind trial in patients with major depressive disorder. Curr Med Res Opin 23:1303–1318, 2007

Poirier MF, Boyer P: Venlafaxine and paroxetine in treatment-resistant depression: double-blind, randomised comparison. Br J Psychiatry 175:12–16, 1999

Pritchett YL, Marciniak MD, Corey-Lisle PK, et al: Use of effect size to determine optimal dose of duloxetine in major depressive disorder. J Psychiatr Res 41:311–318, 2007a

Pritchett YL, McCarberg BH, Watkin JG, et al: Duloxetine for the management of diabetic peripheral neuropathic pain: response profile. Pain Med 8:397–409, 2007b

Puech A, Montgomery SA, Prost JF, et al: Milnacipran, a new serotonin and noradrenaline reuptake inhibitor: an overview of its antidepressant activity and clinical tolerability. Int Clin Psychopharmacol 12:99–108, 1997

Puozzo C, Lambe R, Briley M: Inhibition of tritiated 5-hydroxytryptamine uptake in platelets by plasma from volunteers after a single oral dose of F2207, midalcipran, a novel antidepressant. Br J Clin Pharmacol 20:293P, 1985

Puozzo C, Leonard BE: Pharmacokinetics of milnacipran in comparison with other antidepressants. Int Clin Psychopharmacol 2 (suppl 4):15–27, 1996

Puozzo C, Panconi E, Deprez D: Pharmacology and pharmacokinetics of milnacipran. Int Clin Psychopharmacol 17 (suppl 1): S25–S35, 2002

Raskin J, Wiltse CG, Siegal A, et al: Efficacy of duloxetine on cognition, depression, and pain in elderly patients with major depressive disorder: an 8-week, double-blind, placebo-controlled trial. Am J Psychiatry 164:900–909, 2007

Rueter LE, de Montigny C, Blier P: Electrophysiological characterization of the effect of long-term duloxetine administration on the rat serotonergic and noradrenergic systems. J Pharmacol Exp Ther 285:404–412, 1998a

Rueter LE, Kasamo K, de Montigny C, et al: Effect of long-term administration of duloxetine on the function of serotonin and noradrenaline terminals in the rat brain. Naunyn-Schmiedebergs Arch Pharmacol 357:600–610, 1998b

Schatzberg AF: Efficacy and tolerability of duloxetine, a novel dual reuptake inhibitor, in the treatment of major depressive disorder. J Clin Psychiatry 64 (suppl 13):30–37, 2003

Sechter D, Vandel P, Weiller E, et al: A comparative study of milnacipran and paroxetine in outpatients with major depression. J Affect Disord 83:233–236, 2004

Sharma A, Goldberg MJ, Cerimele BJ: Pharmacokinetics and safety of duloxetine, a dual-serotonin and norepinephrine reuptake inhibitor. J Clin Pharmacol 40:161–167, 2000

Shelton RC, Prakash A, Mallinckrodt CH, et al: Patterns of depressive symptom response in duloxetine-treated outpatients with mild, moderate or more severe depression. Int J Clin Pract 61:1337–1348, 2007

Skinner MH, Kuan HY, Pan A, et al: Duloxetine is both an inhibitor and a substrate of cytochrome P450 2D6 in healthy volunteers. Clin Pharmacol Ther 73:170–177, 2003

Slater S, Gobbi G, Boucher N, et al: Effect of reboxetine on the norepinephrine reuptake processes in healthy male subjects (abstract). New Clinical Drug Evaluation Unit 40:208, 2000

Stahl S, Grady M, Moret C, et al: SNRIs: their pharmacology, clinical efficacy, and tolerability in comparison with other classes of antidepressants. CNS Spectr 10:732–747, 2005

Sussman N: SNRIs versus SSRIs: mechanism of action in treating depression and painful physical symptoms. Prim Care Companion J Clin Psychiatry 5 (suppl 7):19–26, 2003

Szabo ST, Blier P: Effect of the selective noradrenergic reuptake inhibitor reboxetine on the firing activity of noradrenaline and serotonin neurons. Eur J Neurosci 13:2077–2087, 2001

Takano A, Suzuki K, Kosaka J, et al: A dose-finding study of duloxetine based on serotonin transporter occupancy. Psychopharmacology (Berl) 185:395–399, 2006

Thase ME, Pritchett YL, Ossanna MJ, et al: Efficacy of duloxetine and selective serotonin reuptake inhibitors: comparisons as assessed by remission rates in patients with major depressive disorder. J Clin Psychopharmacol 27:672–676, 2007

Thor KB: Serotonin and norepinephrine involvement in efferent pathways to the urethral rhabdosphincter: implications for treating stress urinary incontinence. Urology 62 (suppl 1):3–9, 2003

Turcotte JE, Debonnel G, de Montigny C, et al: Assessment of the serotonin and norepinephrine reuptake blocking properties of duloxetine in healthy subjects. Neuropsychopharmacology 24:511–521, 2001

Vaishnavi SN, Nemeroff CB, Plott SJ, et al: Milnacipran: a comparative analysis of human monoamine uptake and transporter binding affinity. Biol Psychiatry 55:320–322, 2004

Vincent S, Bieck PR, Garland EM, et al: Clinical assessment of norepinephrine transporter blockade through biochemical and pharmacological profiles. Circulation 109:3202–3207, 2004

Vitton O, Gendreau M, Gendreau J, et al: A double-blind placebo-controlled trial of milnacipran in the treatment of fibromyalgia. Hum Psychopharmacol 19 (suppl 1):S27–S35, 2004

Wade A, Gembert K, Florea I: A comparative study of the efficacy of acute and continuation treatment with escitalopram versus duloxetine in patients with major depressive disorder. Curr Med Res Opin 23:1605–1614, 2007

Wernicke JF, Pritchett YL, D'Souza DN, et al: A randomized controlled trial of duloxetine in diabetic peripheral neuropathic pain. Neurology 67:1411–1420, 2006

Whitmyer VG, Dunner DL, Kornstein SG, et al: A comparison of initial duloxetine dosing strategies in patients with major depressive disorder. J Clin Psychiatry 68:1921–1930, 2007

CHAPTER 24

Benzodiazepines

David V. Sheehan, M.D., M.B.A.

B. Ashok Raj, M.D.

History and Discovery

In spite of adverse publicity and a problematic public image, the most widely prescribed psychiatric medication in the United States over the past several years is not an antidepressant, an atypical antipsychotic, or a mood stabilizer but the benzodiazepine alprazolam, with 31 million prescriptions issued in 2001 (see Stahl 2002).

The first benzodiazepine, chlordiazepoxide (Librium), was patented in 1959. Diazepam was introduced in 1963, and numerous derivatives of this drug have since been introduced into the market. The triazolobenzodiazepine alprazolam was introduced in 1981 and revolutionized the treatment of anxiety disorders when it was shown to be effective in the treatment of panic disorder (Chouinard et al. 1983; D. V. Sheehan et al. 1982). It was the first benzodiazepine to be approved by the U.S. Food and Drug Administration (FDA) for the treatment of panic disorder. Since then, clonazepam, another high-potency benzodiazepine, has also received approval from the FDA for the treatment of panic disorder.

Benzodiazepines were widely prescribed in the 1960s, 1970s, and 1980s for pathological anxiety by psychiatrists, family practitioners, and internists who knew they were effective and relatively safe when compared with prior anxiolytic medications such as the barbiturates and meprobamate. However, since the 1990s, benzodiazepines have increasingly been displaced by the selective serotonin reuptake inhibitors (SSRIs) as the clinician's first choice for the treatment of anxiety disorders (Kramer 1993). The SSRIs are safer and better tolerated than the tricyclic antidepressants and have been shown to be efficacious in a number of different anxiety disorders. In addition, they do not have the dependence, withdrawal, alcohol interaction, and abuse liability of the benzodiazepines. In the United States, benzodiazepine use between 1979 and 1990 decreased from 11.1% to 8.3%. At this time, 35 benzodiazepine products are available worldwide; of these, only 15 are marketed in the United States. Under the Controlled Substances Act (1970), benzodiazepines fall under Schedule IV and are classified as depressants.

Despite these drawbacks, benzodiazepines are often used as an adjunctive treatment with an SSRI or as the primary treatment for the patient with no response or only a partial response to the SSRI. The net result is only a small decline in the recommendation for a benzodiazepine (Uhlenhuth et al. 1999). One user in four uses the benzodiazepine for a year or longer. Among those using it as a hypnotic, 14% reported long-term use (Balter 1991). Rates of use increase with age. Persons older than 65 years account for 27% of all benzodiazepine prescriptions and 38% of all benzodiazepine hypnotics (IMS America 1991). In recent years, there has been a shift to the use of short-half-life benzodiazepines. The use of benzodiazepine hypnotics has remained stable (Woods et al. 1992).

Structure–Activity Relations

Currently marketed benzodiazepines are similar in that they have the 1,4-benzodiazepine ring system (see, e.g., Figure 24–1). Modification of this ring system results in benzodiazepines with somewhat different properties. In-

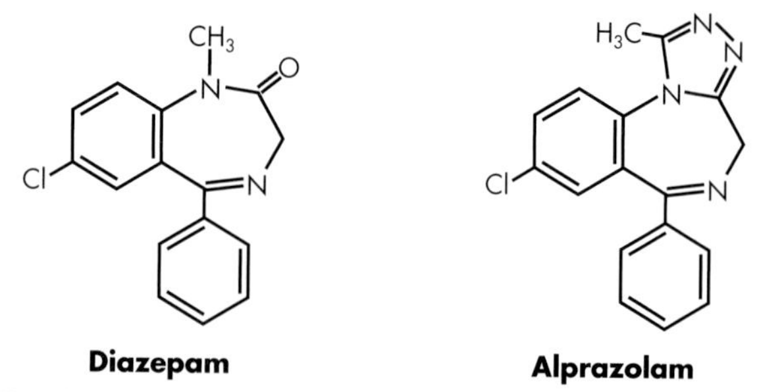

FIGURE 24–1. Chemical structures of diazepam and alprazolam.

creasing the electron-attracting ability of the attachment at the R1 position increases its potency. Alprazolam, a triazolobenzodiazepine, is formed by the addition of a heterocyclic ring that joins the benzodiazepine ring at its 1 and 2 positions (see Figure 24–1) (Sternbach 1982).

Pharmacokinetics and Disposition

Knowledge of benzodiazepine pharmacokinetics helps the clinician choose the most appropriate benzodiazepine for the patient and also guides in its correct use. Benzodiazepines differ in their pharmacokinetic properties, such as absorption, distribution, and elimination (Table 24–1). On the other hand, all benzodiazepines are similar in that to some degree they all exhibit anxiolytic, muscle-relaxant, sedative-hypnotic, and anticonvulsant properties. The belief that one benzodiazepine is primarily anxiolytic while another is primarily hypnotic is not based on scientific evidence (Greenblatt et al. 1983a, 1983b). The preferential selection of a benzodiazepine for one market over another is usually dictated by its pharmacokinetic properties. This, however, is not true for the nonbenzodiazepine hypnotics zolpidem and zaleplon, as they are selective for the benzodiazepine$_1$ (ω_1) receptor only.

Rate of Absorption

Benzodiazepines that are rapidly absorbed from the gastrointestinal tract enter and peak in the circulation quickly and have a quicker onset of action than those that are absorbed more slowly. Diazepam and clorazepate are rapidly absorbed and act quickly, chlordiazepoxide and lorazepam have intermediate rates of absorption and onset of action, while prazepam is slowly absorbed and has a slower onset of action.

Gastrointestinal absorption of benzodiazepines is dictated by intrinsic physiochemical properties of the drug

and characteristics of the formulation such as particle size (Greenblatt et al. 1983a, 1983b). Benzodiazepine absorption when given intramuscularly is dictated by other factors. For example, chlordiazepoxide and lorazepam when given orally are absorbed at similar rates in the gastrointestinal tract. When given intramuscularly, lorazepam is more reliably, rapidly, and completely absorbed than chlordiazepoxide (Greenblatt et al. 1979, 1982b, 1983a, 1983b).

Lipophilicity

The lipid solubility (lipophilicity) of a benzodiazepine at physiological pH influences the rate at which it crosses the blood–brain barrier by passive diffusion from the circulation, and this, in turn, determines the rapidity of onset of action and intensity of effect (Greenblatt et al. 1983a, 1983b). Highly lipophilic drugs cross the blood–brain barrier rapidly, and although all benzodiazepines are highly lipophilic, they differ in their degree of lipophilicity. As diazepam is more lipophilic than lorazepam or chlordiazepoxide, patients are more likely to experience rapid anxiety reduction and onset of side effects with the former.

Duration of Action

With benzodiazepines, the duration of therapeutic action is determined mainly by the rate and extent of drug distribution rather than by the rate of elimination. Benzodiazepine distribution is largely determined by its lipophilicity. Diazepam, which has a longer half-life than lorazepam, has a shorter duration of clinical action after a single dose. The reason for this is that diazepam, because of its greater lipid solubility, is more extensively distributed to peripheral sites, particularly to fat tissue. Consequently, it is more rapidly moved out of the blood and brain into inactive storage sites and its central nervous system (CNS) effects are more rapidly ended. Conversely, less lipophilic benzodiazepines maintain their effective brain concentrations longer because they are less extensively distributed to the periphery (Greenblatt et al. 1983a, 1983b).

Rate of Elimination

The rate of elimination (elimination half-life) influences the speed and extent of accumulation and the time to reach a steady state. It also influences the time for drug washout after termination of multiple doses. Accumulation is slow and extensive when the half-life is long. When the rate of metabolic removal equals the rate of ingestion,

TABLE 24–1. Pharmacokinetics of benzodiazepines

GROUP	MEDICATION	METABOLISM	CYP ENZYME(S)	$T_{1/2}$, HOURS	K_i
Desmethyldiazepam	Diazepam	Oxidation	2C19, 3A4	26–50	9.6
	Bromazepam	Oxidation	3A4	1–5	NA
	Prazepam	Oxidation		>21	NA
	Chlordiazepoxide	Oxidation	3A4	>21	NA
Desalkylflurazepam	Flurazepam	Oxidation		40–120	NA
	Clonazepam	Oxidation		24–56	0.5
Triazolobenzodiazepine	Triazolam	Oxidation	3A4	2–4	0.4
	Alprazolam	Oxidation	3A4	10–15	4.8
Imidazobenzodiazepine	Midazolam	Oxidation	3A4	1–3	0.4
Thienodiazepine	Brotizolam	Oxidation	3A4	4–8	0.9
	Nitrazepam	Reduction	3A4, 2D6	20–50	11.5
	Flunitrazepam	Reduction		10–25	3.8
Oxazolobenzodiazepine	Oxazepam	Glucuronidation		5–15	17.2
	Lorazepam	Glucuronidation		10–20	3.8
	Temazepam	Glucuronidation		6–16	23.0

Note. CYP = cytochrome P450; K_i = kinetic inhibition constant value (nM); NA = not available.

the drug is said to have reached steady state. A useful rule of thumb is that when treatment has been in progress for at least four to five times as long as the elimination half-life, then the accumulation process is more than 90% complete (Greenblatt et al. 1983a, 1983b). When drugs with long elimination half-lives are stopped, they are washed out slowly, and the symptoms recur gradually over a period of days, with less intense or sudden rebound phenomena (Greenblatt et al. 1981, 1982a; Kales et al. 1982). Side effects from long-term treatment with long-half-life benzodiazepines last longer than with short-half-life benzodiazepines. Because of greater drug accumulation with long-half-life benzodiazepines, frequent drowsiness and sedation are a theoretical concern (Greenblatt et al. 1981). Tolerance to sedation occurs with long-term use, even though the plasma drug level remains the same. However, as a matter of caution, it is prudent to choose a benzodiazepine with a shorter or intermediate half-life for the elderly (Greenblatt et al. 1982c), individuals operating equipment, and those engaged in high-level intellectual tasks.

Biotransformation Pathway

Benzodiazepines are metabolized in the liver by microsomal oxidation or by glucuronide conjugation. The oxidation pathway is influenced by hepatic disease, age, several medical illnesses, and a number of drugs that impair oxidizing capacity, such as cimetidine, estrogens, and the hydrazine monoamine oxidase inhibitors (MAOIs). These factors usually magnify the side effects of the benzodiazepine. Consequently, in the elderly and in individuals with liver disease, benzodiazepines that are conjugated (e.g., temazepam, oxazepam, and lorazepam) are safer than benzodiazepines that are metabolized by oxidation (e.g., diazepam and alprazolam). This is the reason why a patient who is taking alprazolam at a stable dose will report that sedation is potentiated more by the addition of a hydrazine MAOI than by a tricyclic antidepressant.

Dosing: Sustained-Release Formulations

Dosing schedules of benzodiazepines should be dictated by knowledge about the rate of distribution rather than by information about elimination half-life. Patients who require several daily doses often feel as if they are on a roller coaster. They experience peaks of mild sedation followed by troughs of mild anxiety. This can lead to "clock watching" (Herman et al. 1987). Sustained-release formulations of several benzodiazepines have been introduced to correct this problem and are promoted as providing 24 hours of anxiolysis. In our experience, the sustained-release forms of alprazolam, clorazepate, diazepam, and adinazolam have a duration of therapeutic action of approximately 12 hours.

Sustained-release alprazolam has recently been approved by the FDA for use in panic disorder and has been available in 51 countries for some time. The medication in sustained-release alprazolam is enmeshed in a hydroxypropyl–methylcellulose matrix that releases the compound slowly and consistently over several hours so that the patient receives a constant dose of medication for a more extended period than in the immediate-release formulation and a therapeutic benefit lasting 11±4 hours (D. V. Sheehan 1993; D. V. Sheehan et al. 1996).

A number of clinical trials, with a total of 893 patients, have investigated the efficacy and safety of sustained-release alprazolam in the treatment of panic disorder (Alexander 1993; Pecknold et al. 1993, 1994; Schweizer 1993; Stahl 1993). The results of these studies suggest that sustained-release alprazolam, administered once in the morning, is superior to placebo and is equal to comparable doses of alprazolam in its compressed or immediate-release tablet form administered in four divided doses. When given in fixed doses twice daily, sustained-release alprazolam was found to be superior to placebo and also appeared to cause fewer CNS side effects than with single-dose administration. Given in a single dose at bedtime, it was not more effective than placebo.

These studies do not answer practical clinical questions such as how to adjust dosing during a switch from the compressed-tablet to the extended-release formulation of a benzodiazepine. A methodology for switching patients from a stable maintenance dose of the compressed-tablet formulation of alprazolam to the extended-release formulation was described by D. V. Sheehan et al. (1996). This methodology, developed in connection with a 9-week open-label crossover study, relies on the use of a patient diary in which the patient records hourly anxiolytic benefit on a 0–10 scale as well as any side effects. During the first week, while patients were still taking the compressed-tablet formulation, they were instructed to keep hourly recordings of the degree of anxiolytic effect and any side effects they experienced after the first morning dose. They were further instructed to wait until they saw a dip in efficacy (evidence of a loss of therapeutic action documented in their diary records) before taking a second dose. This made it possible to establish the average time it took for the first dose to lose therapeutic effect, which was labeled as the endpoint of duration of therapeutic action (DOA). Once the DOA of an effective dose was established, efforts were directed to adjusting the distribution of doses to provide optimal control. At the end of 3 weeks, all patients were switched to an equivalent dose of sustained-release

alprazolam in 0.5- or 1.0-mg tablets. At the switch, the total number of milligrams of the compressed-tablet formulation of alprazolam taken before 5:00 P.M. was converted into the morning dose of sustained-release alprazolam, and the total number of milligrams of the compressed-tablet formulation taken after 5:00 P.M. was converted into the evening dose of sustained-release alprazolam.

With this methodology, equivalent efficacy for the compressed-tablet and sustained-release formulations was found on weekly ratings of anxiety. At the end of the study (week 9), diary records provided evidence of the considerably longer mean duration of therapeutic action of the sustained-release formulation compared with the compressed-tablet formulation: 11.3±4.2 hours (range=3–24 hours) versus 5.1±1.7 hours (range=3–11 hours). The major advantage of the sustained-release form is the convenience of less frequent dosing. Since most (81%) of the patients in the described study (D. V. Sheehan et al. 1996) required only once- or twice-daily dosing, compliance is likely to be higher.

When doses were adjusted with patient input to achieve a smooth therapeutic effect over 24 hours (as reflected in symptom scale scores), the majority reported the best effects with two-thirds of the total daily dose in the morning (8:00 A.M.) and one-third of the total daily dose in the evening (7:00 P.M.) (D. V. Sheehan et al. 1996, 2007). While this may seem odd, there are several explanations for this phenomenon. One explanation is "the second-dose effect in pharmacokinetics" (DeVane and Liston 2001). The effect of a second dose of a medication is always more intense and lasts longer than the effect of the first dose. However, this relative increase in effect diminishes with subsequent doses. When dosing is repeated in response to the observed effect, the second-dose effect occurs regardless of the half-life of the drug. Another explanation is that the individual sleeps during much of the time when the second dose of the day (taken in the evening) is active. During sleep, the individual is less aware of feedback indicating a need for full anxiolytic effect. Yet another explanation is that the anxious patient reports more anxiety in the morning. To better control this early-day anxiety, the patient feels a need for a slightly higher dose at that time. The study by D. V. Sheehan et al. (1996) reaffirms that the half-life of a benzodiazepine does not predict its duration of action. It also provides the clinician with a methodology for switching patients on a regular compressed-tablet formulation of a benzodiazepine to the extended-release formulation of that benzodiazepine (D. V. Sheehan et al. 1996, 2007).

Mechanism of Action

Benzodiazepines produce anxiolysis by their effect on the γ-aminobutyric acid (GABA)–benzodiazepine receptor complex. GABA is synthesized from glutamic acid, which is also the most abundant free amino acid in the CNS. Like serotonin, norepinephrine, and dopamine neurons, the presynaptic GABA neuron has a reuptake pump that transports GABA from the synapse for storage or destruction by GABA transaminase. GABA has two target receptors, $GABA_A$ and $GABA_B$. The chloride ion channel is controlled by $GABA_A$. A number of nearby receptors have the ability to allosterically modulate the $GABA_A$ receptor. These include receptors for benzodiazepines, for nonbenzodiazepine sedatives like zolpidem and zaleplon, for barbiturates, for alcohol, for neuroactive steroids, and for the proconvulsant picrotoxin. The $GABA_B$ receptor has two dissimilar subunits that comprise the functional receptor ($GABA_{B1}$ and $GABA_{B2}$). Six $GABA_{B1}$ isoforms (1a through 1f) have been reported (Dawson et al. 2005). The $GABA_B$ receptor is not allosterically modulated by benzodiazepines but is known to bind to the muscle relaxant baclofen.

Four distinct pharmacological properties have been described for the benzodiazepine receptor: anxiolytic, hypnotic, anticonvulsant, and muscle relaxation effects. Anxiolytic and sedative-hypnotic actions are mainly mediated by the ω_1 receptor and muscle relaxation through the benzodiazepine$_2$ (ω_2) receptor. Most benzodiazepines interact with both these receptor subtypes. The benzodiazepine$_3$ (ω_3) receptor is found mostly outside the CNS, and its role is unclear at this time. Typically, when GABA occupies the $GABA_A$ receptor site, the chloride channel is opened up a little, and this effect is inhibitory. If at the same time a benzodiazepine binds to the nearby benzodiazepine receptor, the $GABA_A$ receptor is allosterically modulated, and GABA exerts a greater effect on the chloride channel and conductance. Although GABA works alone at the GABA receptor, it works better in the presence of a benzodiazepine. The benzodiazepine, on the other hand, in the absence of GABA cannot influence the chloride channel by itself.

The $GABA_A$ receptor–chloride ion channel complex has a transmembrane pentameric structure. There are five subunits selected from eight polypeptide classes: α, β, γ, δ, ε, π, ρ, and τ. Several of these classes have subunits that have been characterized (6 α, 3 β, 3 γ, and 2 δ variants). As a consequence, there is the potential for the existence of a large number of receptor isoforms. The coassembly of an α, a β, and a γ subunit produces a high-affinity benzodiazepine binding site. Benzodiazepines also potentiate combinations of α and γ, or β and γ, subunits. On the other hand, benzodiazepines do not potentiate combinations of α and β subunits even though they are functional $GABA_A$ receptors. The α subunit seems to dictate the pharmacology of the benzodiazepine receptor site. Combinations with α_1 have different pharmacology compared with combinations with α_2 or other alpha variants. Sedation and anticonvulsant activity are mediated by the α_1 subunit and anxiolysis by the α_2 subunit (Low et al. 2000; Mohler et al. 2002). It has been suggested that benzodiazepine-induced hyperphagia is mediated by the α_2 and α_3 subtypes (Cooper 2005).

Therapeutic Uses

Because of their multiple pharmacological actions, benzodiazepines have been found useful in many areas of medical practice, such as induction of anesthesia, use as a muscle relaxant, and control of seizures. It is beyond the scope of this chapter to elaborate on these uses.

In psychiatry, benzodiazepines are used to control anxiety, to treat insomnia, and to acutely manage agitation and withdrawal syndromes. Surprisingly, in the treatment of anxiety disorders, benzodiazepines have a greater impact in some disorders than others. In panic disorder, they have a significant impact on all dimensions of the illness, with the exception of depression. Alprazolam, for example, has been shown to be effective in panic disorder at a mean dosage of 5.7 mg/day (range=1–10 mg/day) (Ballenger et al. 1988; Chouinard et al. 1982; Cross National Collaborative Panic Study 1992; D.V. Sheehan et al. 1982, 1984, 1993). Rapid improvement can be observed within the first week in terms of decreased panic attacks, phobic fears and avoidance, anticipatory anxiety, and disability. These benefits have been shown to persist during a follow-up period of 8 months (Schweizer et al. 1993). Efficacy has also been shown for lorazepam (Rickels and Schweizer 1986) and clonazepam (Pollack et al. 1993; Tesar et al. 1991). In the latter study, clonazepam 2.5 mg/day was as effective and well tolerated as alprazolam 5.3 mg/day.

Despite the well-documented efficacy of benzodiazepines in panic disorder, they have been displaced in clinical practice by the SSRIs. However, it is common practice to initiate treatment with both classes of drug simultaneously and then withdraw the benzodiazepine after 6 weeks. The benefits and practicality of this approach to treating panic disorder have been reinforced by the findings from a 12-week study (Goddard et al. 2001) in which patients with panic disorder were treated with open-label sertraline and double-blind clonazepam or placebo. After 4 weeks of combination treatment, the adjunct medication (clonazepam or placebo) was tapered over 3 weeks and then discontinued. All patients received sertraline monotherapy for the last 4 weeks of the study. The group randomized to sertraline and clonazepam had fewer dropouts (25% vs. 38%) and separated as early as week 1 from the sertraline–placebo group on the Panic Disorder Severity Scale (PDSS). These findings have been further reaffirmed by a recent double-blind, placebo-controlled study (Goddard et al. 2008) in which patients were randomly assigned to flexible-dose treatment with either sertraline plus placebo or sertraline plus extended-release alprazolam for 4 weeks, followed by a 4-week taper from the benzodiazepine, followed by 4 weeks on sertraline alone. Onset of benefit was faster in the initial weeks on the SSRI–benzodiazepine combination, and the dropout rate was lower in this group, but withdrawal symptoms were significantly higher in the benzodiazepine–SSRI group. At the end of 12 weeks, there was no difference in efficacy between the two groups (Goddard et al. 2008). The American Psychiatric Association (1998) guidelines for the treatment of panic disorder recommending SSRI monotherapy as the treatment of first choice has failed to achieve traction, since more than two-thirds of the SSRI prescriptions were accompanied by a concomitant benzodiazepine. The above studies by Goddard et al. (2008) lend justification to the rationale for using the combination treatment more frequently and blessing it as a reasonable alternative first-line treatment for many patients with panic disorder.

Three double-blind studies have shown efficacy for benzodiazepines in the treatment of social phobia. In the first study (Gelernter et al. 1991), alprazolam demonstrated only limited efficacy relative to other treatments. At week 12 (end of study), 69% of phenelzine-, 38% of alprazolam-, 24% of cognitive-behavioral-, and 20% of placebo-treated patients had responded. In the second study (Davidson et al. 1993), at the end of 10 weeks of treatment, 78% of social phobia patients treated with clonazepam, compared with only 20% of those treated with placebo, responded. The mean dosage of clonazepam at endpoint was 2.4 mg/day. Bromazepam, a benzodiazepine not available in the United States, was found to be effective in a 12-week double-blind, placebo-controlled study of social phobia at a mean dosage of 21 mg/day, but it took 8 weeks for bromazepam to separate from placebo (Versiani et al. 1997).

In two parallel and concurrent studies (D. V. Sheehan et al. 1990a, 1990b), we demonstrated that the sustained-release formulation of the benzodiazepine adinazolam was effective in panic disorder and generalized anxiety disorder (GAD). However, the dose of adinazolam needed to treat GAD effectively was higher than the dose needed to treat panic disorder. Endpoint scores on the Hamilton Anxiety Scale (Ham-A) were lower (better) in the patients with panic disorder, even though the mean effective dose of adinazolam was lower than in the GAD patients. This suggests that, contrary to prior assumptions, benzodiazepines in general, and adinazolam in particular, are less effective in GAD than in panic disorder. This has some support from findings in a double-blind, placebo-controlled study (Rickels et al. 1993) showing that the tricyclic antidepressant imipramine was better than diazepam in the treatment of nondepressed GAD patients over 8 weeks. Imipramine showed a trend to be significantly better on the primary outcome measure scale (Ham-A) and was statistically superior to diazepam on the Psychic Anxiety factor of the Ham-A. Psychic anxiety includes the items of worry, anxious mood, tension, fears, and concentration problems. Diazepam and imipramine had identical endpoint Ham-A Somatic Anxiety factor scores, suggesting that they are equally effective against the somatic anxiety symptoms in GAD. This suggests that imipramine is a better "anti-worry" medication than the benzodiazepine. Patients treated with diazepam had an earlier response than those taking imipramine.

Generally, benzodiazepines are thought to be ineffective in the treatment of obsessive-compulsive disorder (OCD). In a small crossover study, clonazepam was reported as effective in treating OCD (Hewlett et al. 1992).

The strongest evidence for effective pharmacotherapy in posttraumatic stress disorder (PTSD) is with SSRIs. A meta-analysis of six studies showed a correlation between greater serotonergic activity and higher effect size (Penava et al. 1996–1997). Another meta-analysis of medications in treating PTSD found effect sizes of 0.49 and 1.38 for benzodiazepines and SSRIs, respectively (Van Etten and Taylor 1998). In a study of 13 trauma survivors treated prophylactically within 2–18 days of their trauma with lorazepam or clonazepam for 6 months, the subjects did not do any better than a matched untreated group in terms of PTSD symptoms at the 6-month evaluation (Gelpin et al. 1996).

Benzodiazepines have potential for benefit in the acute management of mania, as they can rapidly induce sleep with earlier resolution of the mania and allow for lower doses of antipsychotics in the acute phase (Nowlin-

Finch et al. 1994). Antimanic effects have been described for clonazepam. In a double-blind, crossover study, clonazepam was more efficacious than lithium and also had a faster onset of action (Chouinard et al. 1983). It has been reported that clonazepam is more effective in acute mania than lorazepam (Bradwejn et al. 1990).

Intramuscular clonazepam has been compared with intramuscular haloperidol in the management of acute psychotic agitation. Clonazepam use reduced agitation, but haloperidol use had a more rapid onset (Chouinard et al. 1993). Individuals with schizophrenia have high levels of anxiety and frequently experience panic attacks. High-potency benzodiazepines as adjunctive therapy have been shown to benefit schizophrenic patients, with or without panic attacks, in the short term. But long-term use is problematic given this population's poor adherence to therapeutic regimens, their propensity to substance abuse and dependence, and the dangers of benzodiazepine dependence and withdrawal syndromes with chronic use (Wolkowitz and Pickar 1991). Overall, it appears that benzodiazepines have a role in the acute management of agitation, and their use can reduce the need for or the dose of antipsychotics used.

Side Effects and Toxicology

Benzodiazepines are among the safest of drugs, but unwanted effects do occur. The first 1,4-benzodiazepines, such as diazepam and flurazepam, had slow rates of elimination and low receptor-binding affinities. Their main side effect was excessive daytime sleepiness. The late 1970s saw the introduction of the 1,4-benzodiazepines flunitrazepam and lorazepam, which had shorter half-lives and were more potent. These drugs were associated with enhanced efficacy but also with more rapid development of tolerance and significant withdrawal problems. The triazolobenzodiazepines were introduced in the 1980s and were even more potent and had even shorter half-lives. They have also been found to be associated with amnesia, daytime anxiety, early-morning insomnia, and withdrawal problems such as rebound insomnia, anxiety, and seizures (Noyes et al. 1986).

Sedation and drowsiness are common, occurring in 4%–9% of patients taking benzodiazepines. Ataxia occurs in up to 2%. The drowsiness tends to disappear with time or a reduction in dose (Greenblatt et al. 1982b; R.R. Miller 1973; Svenson and Hamilton 1966). Several lines of investigation suggest that benzodiazepines may impair psychomotor performance. Most benzodiazepines, shortly after administration, at their peak concentration cause anterograde amnesia (Lister et al. 1988). These effects are dependent on potency and route of administration. For example, with a low-potency drug such as diazepam, the risk of amnesia is highest with intravenous, less with intramuscular, and rare with oral administration (Bixler et al. 1979). It has been shown that when given orally, lorazepam and flunitrazepam cause more amnesia than diazepam and flurazepam (Magbagbeola 1974). Triazolam, a very potent triazolobenzodiazepine, is reported to cause significantly more memory impairment than other hypnotics such as flurazepam and temazepam (Greenblatt et al. 1989; Ogura et al. 1980; Roth et al. 1980; Scharf et al. 1988). Overall, this memory impairment does appear to be independent of the degree of sedation produced by the drug (Scharf et al. 1988). Also of great significance is that benzodiazepine-treated subjects are often unaware or underestimate the extent of their memory impairment (Roach and Griffiths 1985, 1987).

Hyperexcitability phenomena such as early-morning awakening and rebound anxiety and nervousness are more likely with the short-half-life, high-potency benzodiazepines such as triazolam, alprazolam, lorazepam, and brotizolam (Kales et al. 1983, 1986, 1987; Vela-Bueno et al. 1983). Treatment-emergent hostility (Rosenbaum et al. 1984) may be seen in up to 10% of patients being treated with benzodiazepines. This is most likely to happen early in treatment, is unrelated to pretreatment impulsivity, and has been reported with all benzodiazepines with the exception of oxazepam. Treatment-emergent mania has been reported with alprazolam (Goodman and Charney 1987; Pecknold and Fleury 1986; Strahan et al. 1985). Depression may also emerge with treatment (Pollack et al. 1986). We have seen increased dreaming in some patients, and there are case reports of reversible hepatitis (Judd et al. 1986), ejaculatory inhibition (Munjack and Crocker 1986), and inhibition of female orgasm (Sangal 1985).

Since the 1960s, benzodiazepines have been known to produce anterograde amnesia. Initially, it was believed that this effect happened only with intravenous use. But now the effect is well documented, even with oral dosing (Lister 1985). It is likely that the amnestic effects are produced by interference with the transfer of information from very-short-term memory to long-term memory storage areas. The deficit is therefore one of disrupted consolidation and not impairment of memory retrieval. The degree of amnesia can range from minimal inability to retain isolated pieces of information to total inability to recall any activities that occurred during a specific period.

Whether some benzodiazepines are more likely than others to produce amnesia remains an unresolved question.

Triazolam 0.5 mg has been compared with 30 mg of temazepam in immediate and delayed recall. In tests of delayed recall, triazolam consistently caused anterograde amnesia. No effects were found in immediate recall in both drugs (Scharf et al. 1988). Retrograde facilitation was better with triazolam than with temazepam. Triazolam, lorazepam, and alprazolam are the compounds that show the most amnestic potential. Compared with temazepam and clorazepate, they also tend to be those with the greater benzodiazepine receptor affinities, lower volumes of distribution, and less lipophilicity (Nutt et al. 1989). It is not clear if chronic dosing with benzodiazepines aggravates the problem. One study comparing lorazepam and alprazolam suggested that memory impairment dissipates beyond the single-dose administration period (Kumar et al. 1987). Another area of concern is that the long-term use of benzodiazepines may lead to cognitive and other impairments that persist long after the drug has been discontinued. Abnormal computed tomography (CT) scans were reported in long-term users of benzodiazepines in one study (Lader et al. 1984) but not in others (Poser et al. 1983; Rickels 1985). Busto et al. (2000) found no difference in the CT brain scans of patients taking benzodiazepines compared with control subjects. Paulus et al. (2005) reported a dose-dependent decreased activation in bilateral amygdala and insula by lorazepam during emotion processing. No other positron emission tomography or functional magnetic resonance imaging studies that might inform this question are yet available. Long-term benzodiazepine users have been compared with control subjects and found to have cognitive impairments that reversed on reexamination after taper (Golombok et al. 1988; Lucki et al. 1986; Rickels et al. 1999; Sakol and Power 1988). Another study found that after long-term use, if the benzodiazepine is stopped, there was only partial recovery even after 6 months (Tata et al. 1994).

Drug–Drug Interactions

Antacids slow benzodiazepine absorption, as aluminum delays gastric emptying (Greenblatt et al. 1983a, 1983b). An acid medium is needed for conversion of clorazepate to desmethyldiazepam, the active metabolite, which is then absorbed (Shader et al. 1978).

In the liver, benzodiazepines are metabolized by oxidation, reduction, or conjugation. Alprazolam, diazepam, clorazepate, prazepam, chlordiazepoxide, bromazepam, and halazepam are metabolized by oxidation; nitrazepam by reduction; and lorazepam, oxazepam, and temazepam by conjugation. Inhibitors of the oxidase system prolong the half-life of benzodiazepines that are metabolized by this system. This accentuates the side effects, notably the sedation, ataxia, slurred speech, and imbalance. A decrease in dosage may solve this problem, or a switch to a benzodiazepine that is metabolized by conjugation may be needed. MAOIs, cimetidine (Greenblatt et al. 1984), and oral contraceptives inhibit the oxidative system. There is a decline in this system with age or liver disease. In the elderly, there is a 50% decrease in clearance, with a four- to ninefold increase in half-life and a two- to fourfold increase in the volume of distribution (Peppers 1996). Due to the decreased clearance of lorazepam, lower doses of the benzodiazepine are recommended in patients taking valproate or probenecid. Phenytoin and barbiturates (Scott et al. 1983) cause hepatic enzyme induction and reduce benzodiazepine half-life. Heparinized patients (Routledge et al. 1980) should have partial thromboplastin time (PTT) monitored more closely, as PTT is prolonged by benzodiazepines. Benzodiazepines increase digoxin levels (Castillo-Ferrando et al. 1980; Tollefson et al. 1984), increasing the chance of digoxin toxicity. As antidepressants like fluoxetine or nefazodone and protease inhibitors like indinavir sulfate inhibit the cytochrome P450 enzyme 3A4, they inhibit the metabolism of triazolobenzodiazepines such as midazolam, alprazolam, and triazolam. Inhibition of the gag reflex can occur with benzodiazepine administration (Nutt et al. 1989), increasing the risk for aspiration in patients with nausea and vomiting.

Clinical Issues

Despite decades of research, the optimal extent and duration of appropriate benzodiazepine use in the treatment of anxiety and related disorders remain unresolved. This is primarily because of concerns expressed by prescribers, regulators, and the public about issues such as tolerance, dependence, and abuse liability of this class of medication.

Tolerance

In a study of persistent users of alprazolam and lorazepam, Romach et al. (1995) found that most were not abusing these benzodiazepines, nor were they addicted to them; rather, they were using them appropriately for a chronic disorder and at a constant or a decreasing dose. Soumerai et al. (2003) found a lack of relationship between long-term use of benzodiazepines and escalation to high doses in 2,440 long-term (at least 2 years) users of benzodiazepines and that escalation to a high dose was very rare. Superior results with benzodiazepines are only achieved long term by careful attention to dose adjustment guidelines. The benefits are usually apparent within 2–3 weeks of starting the drug. At this stage, patients often report that the medication is no longer working as well as it did initially. Concurrently, the side effects have also subsided, because of tolerance. If the dose is adjusted up to the next level, the patient again usually gets benefit and continues to do well for another 4–6 weeks. At this stage, tolerance may yet again develop, with the patient losing some benefit and side effects. At this point, adjustment of the dose upward results in benefit again. Physicians may be concerned that there will be no end to this upward adjustment of the dose. However, with effective benzodiazepine therapy, there is a limit to the number of such plateaus that patients go through before reaching their final effective dose. Typically, this dose is reached by the second or third plateau, usually around week 10 or 12. Failure to identify and take appropriate action during these early troughs of partial tolerance in the initial weeks of treatment is common. Sometimes, patients will unilaterally increase the dosage to achieve benefit. The clinician should not take this to be evidence of addictive behavior. Benzodiazepines differ with regard to the degree and timeline for the development of tolerance. As a general rule, long-half-life benzodiazepines such as flurazepam, quazepam, diazepam, and clonazepam tend to be effective for a month or longer before tolerance is exhibited. On the other hand, short-half-life benzodiazepines such as triazolam, alprazolam, temazepam, and lorazepam lose some of their initial efficacy sooner, sometimes in just over a week (Bayer et al. 1986; Bixler et al. 1978; Kales et al. 1986, 1987).

One milligram of alprazolam is approximately equivalent to 0.7 milligrams of clonazepam, to 10 milligrams of diazepam, and to 1 milligram of lorazepam. The cross-tolerance between the benzodiazepines, although good, is not perfect, and it is preferable not to switch patients abruptly from one benzodiazepine to another.

Withdrawal

A withdrawal syndrome is defined as a predictable constellation of signs and symptoms involving altered CNS activity (e.g., tremor, convulsions, or delirium) after the abrupt discontinuation of, or rapid decrease in, dosing of the drug (Rinaldi et al. 1988). Typically, a withdrawal syndrome from short-half-life benzodiazepines will intensify by the second day, will usually have peaked by day 5, and will begin to decrease and taper off by day 10. After 2 weeks, withdrawal symptoms have usually become minimal or absent. Drug factors associated with withdrawal symptoms include length of use, dose, potency, and rate of discontinuation. Psychic, physical, and perceptual symptoms can be observed during withdrawal. The most common are anxiety, restlessness, irritability, insomnia, agitation, muscle tension, weakness, aches and pains, blurred vision, and racing heart, in that order (O'Brien 2005). Nausea, sweating, runny nose, hypersensitivity to stimuli, and tremor are less frequent. Severe withdrawal symptoms, such as psychosis, seizures, hallucinations, paranoid delusions, and persistent tinnitus, are relatively rare and are more likely to occur in abrupt withdrawal from high doses of high-potency benzodiazepines and in the elderly (American Psychiatric Association 1990; Lader 1990; Petturson and Lader 1991).

The minimum duration of use after which clinically significant withdrawal symptoms can be expected has not been definitively determined. At the end of any course of treatment with therapeutic doses and of duration greater than 3–6 weeks, withdrawal of the benzodiazepine should be done as a slow taper. This reduces the risk of unpleasant withdrawal symptoms and the danger of withdrawal seizures and minimizes rebound reactivation of the underlying anxiety disorder (Fontaine et al. 1984; Pecknold et al. 1988; Power et al. 1985).

We recommend that alprazolam or clonazepam not be withdrawn at a rate faster than 0.5 mg every 2–3 weeks. If the drug is tapered at this rate, it is very unlikely that you will see a withdrawal seizure. In a patient taking either drug at a dosage of 6 mg/day, it may take a few months to complete taper on such a slow withdrawal schedule. However, there are no clinical reasons to taper more rapidly. All pharmaceutical companies manufacturing benzodiazepines and the FDA should encourage physicians to withdraw patients from all benzodiazepines at much slower rates than those currently recommended in order to prevent these complications. The recommended rate of withdrawal from alprazolam, for example, is not faster than 0.5 mg every 3 days. In our opinion this rate is too fast. All patients should be advised about the dangers of abruptly stopping the medication, and this should be documented. A systematic review of the literature on this topic in the Cochrane Database recommended slow withdrawal over 10 weeks (Denis et al. 2006).

A number of factors are thought to influence the severity of the withdrawal syndrome. Withdrawal is more difficult with the use of short-half-life drugs, higher doses, long duration of use, rapid tapering, a diagnosis of panic disorder, and certain personality traits (Rickels et al. 1988, 1990; Schweizer et al. 1990). Eighteen percent of patients taking diazepam for 14–22 weeks had withdrawal symptoms, and 43% had withdrawal symptoms after 8 months of use (Rickels et al. 1983). Thirty-five percent of patients taking alprazolam (2–10 mg/day) for 8 weeks had withdrawal symptoms (Pecknold 1993; Pecknold et al. 1993). The first 50% of taper can be done fairly quickly over a 2- to 4-week period. It may be helpful to stay at this dose for several weeks or even a few months before proceeding with the remaining 50% taper at a very slow rate. Early dropouts from taper were found to score higher on the Dependence factor of the Minnesota Multiphasic Personality Inventory compared with late-taper dropouts and those who tapered successfully (Schweizer et al. 1998). In a 3-year follow-up of patients who had participated in a benzodiazepine taper program, it was found that of those who tapered successfully, 73% remained benzodiazepine free. Among those who were able to reduce intake by 50%, only 39% were benzodiazepine free at the end of 3 years. In the group that could not tolerate taper at all, only 14% were benzodiazepine free (Rickels et al. 1991).

A variety of medications have been tried as adjuncts to facilitate taper. Propranolol (Tyrer et al. 1981), progesterone (Schweizer et al. 1995), and dothiepin (Tyrer et al. 1996) were not better than placebo. Buspirone (Lader and Olajide 1987; Rickels 1988; Schweizer and Rickels 1986) was ineffective in patients who had used benzodiazepines for a year or longer but was of some benefit in those who had used lorazepam for a period of 3 months or less (Pancheri et al. 1995). Some benefit for carbamazepine at dosages of 200 to 600 mg/day has been reported (Klein et al. 1986; Neppe and Sindorf 1991; Schweizer et al. 1991; Swantek et al. 1991).

Addiction Potential

In our zeal to heal an anxiety disorder, are we creating a population of addicts? There is much misinformation and concern generated because terms like *addiction* are used without precise definition and pejoratively. Terms such as *addiction, physical dependency,* and *withdrawal syndrome* are often used interchangeably. There is a presumption that a medicine's being associated with a withdrawal syndrome is evidence that the medicine is addicting. Some clinicians believe that benzodiazepines that require frequent dosing during the day are more addicting than those that require

less frequent dosing. In fact, frequency of dosing is a function of the duration of therapeutic action of the drug rather than of any innate addiction potential of the drug.

DSM-IV-TR (American Psychiatric Association 2000) defines *substance (drug) dependence* as a maladaptive pattern of substance use leading to clinically significant impairment or distress, as manifested by three (or more) of the criteria shown in Table 24–2 occurring at any time in the same 12-month period. *Addiction*, in contrast, is defined as a chronic disorder associated with compulsive use of a drug, resulting in physical, psychological, or social harm to the user and continued use despite that harm (Rinaldi et al. 1988). Addiction involves both intense drug-seeking behavior and difficulty in stopping the drug use. If these criteria are used, benzodiazepines are not addictive drugs. *Physical dependence* is different from addiction and is defined as a physiological state of adaptation to a drug, with the development of tolerance to the drug's effects and the emergence of a withdrawal syndrome during prolonged abstinence. During withdrawal after chronic use, biochemical, physiological, or behavioral problems may be triggered. When used on a regular schedule, benzodiazepines are associated with physical dependence, as opposed to drug dependence or DSM-IV-TR "substance dependence," and have a withdrawal syndrome. In *psychological dependence* (Rinaldi et al. 1988), there is a state of emotional craving either to experience the drug's positive effect or to avoid the negative effects associated with its absence. This can lead to compulsive drug-seeking behavior.

Abuse

Studies of abuse use four criteria for benzodiazepine abuse. A benzodiazepine is being abused if it is taken 1) to get high, 2) to promote psychological regression, 3) at doses higher than prescribed, and 4) after the medical indication has passed (Dietch 1983). On the basis of this definition, the data suggest that the incidence of benzodiazepine abuse in clinical practice is low.

A U.S. national health survey in 1979 found that 1.6% of subjects studied used benzodiazepines regularly for at least 1 year (Mellinger et al. 1984). In another study of anxiolytic medication users in the United States, 15% used these drugs daily for more than 1 year (Balter et al. 1984). In a London general practice, 1.6% used benzodiazepines for more than 1 year (Salinsky and Dore 1987). In an Australian general practice study, 10% of first-time benzodiazepine users were still using them with no dose increase after 6 months (Mant et al. 1988). The incidence

TABLE 24–2.   DSM-IV-TR criteria for substance dependence

A maladaptive pattern of substance use, leading to clinically significant impairment or distress, as manifested by three (or more) of the following, occurring at any time in the same 12-month period:

    (1) tolerance, as defined by either of the following:

        (a) a need for markedly increased amounts of the substance to achieve intoxication or desired effect

        (b) markedly diminished effect with continued use of the same amount of the substance

    (2) withdrawal, as manifested by either of the following:

        (a) the characteristic withdrawal syndrome for the substance (refer to criteria A and B of the criteria sets for withdrawal from the specific substances)

        (b) the same (or a closely related) substance is taken to relieve or avoid withdrawal symptoms

    (3) the substance is often taken in larger amounts or over a longer period than was intended

    (4) there is a persistent desire or unsuccessful efforts to cut down or control substance use

    (5) a great deal of time is spent in activities necessary to obtain the substance (e.g., visiting multiple doctors or driving long distances), use the substance (e.g., chain-smoking), or recover from its effects

    (6) important social, occupational, or recreational activities are given up or reduced because of substance use

    (7) the substance use is continued despite knowledge of having a persistent or recurrent physical or psychological problem that is likely to have been caused or exacerbated by the substance (e.g., current cocaine use despite recognition of cocaine-induced depression, or continued drinking despite recognition that an ulcer was made worse by alcohol consumption)

Source.   Reprinted from American Psychiatric Association: Diagnostic and Statistical Manual of Mental Disorders, 4th Edition, Text Revision. Washington, DC, American Psychiatric Association, 2000. Copyright 2000, American Psychiatric Association. Used with permission.

of benzodiazepine dependence in the therapeutic setting (among those for whom the drug is medically correctly prescribed) was estimated to be 1 case in 50 million patient-months (Marks 1978). Of these cases, 92% were associated with alcohol or other drugs of abuse. This estimate is probably on the low side since it is based on the number of published cases of dependence from 1961 to 1977. There is a positive correlation between benzodiazepine use and psychiatric morbidity (Fichter et al. 1989; Pakesch et al. 1989; Salinsky and Dore 1987; Schwartz and Blank 1991). "Benzodiazepine dependence" was diagnosed in only 150 cases (0.5%) of 33,000 consecutive admissions between 1974 and 1983 at a German psychiatric hospital. In contrast, 18.5% of admissions in 1984 ("quarterly incidence") were found to involve long-term users of benzodiazepines (Laux and Konig 1987).

In Basel, Switzerland, with a catchment area of 300,000 people, physicians were surveyed on the prevalence of benzodiazepine abuse in their patients. Only 31 patients were identified—a prevalence of 0.01%, or 1 in 10,000. An additional 88 polysubstance abusers were identified (Ladewig and Grossenbacher 1988). In a small prospective study involving 71 outpatients treated with benzodiazepines for a diagnosis of major depression or an anxiety disorder, no evidence of benzodiazepine abuse was found. Five patients (7%) with a diagnosis of major

depression misused benzodiazepines (Garvey and Tollefson 1986). Another study prospectively followed 99 anxiety disorder patients with a history of alcohol abuse and dependence and 244 without such a history. Over the 12 months of the study, only minor differences in the use of benzodiazepines were noted for the groups. The authors concluded that in patients with an anxiety disorder, the presence or absence of a history of alcohol use disorder was not a strong predictor of future abuse (Mueller et al. 1996). In a random sample of all psychiatric hospitalizations over 15 years (1967–1983) in Sweden (n = 32,679), Allgulander (1989) found only 38 admissions for substance dependence on sedative hypnotics. Twenty-one of the 38 had polysubstance abuse, and 17 had sedative-hypnotic abuse. In another study of all medical and psychiatric hospitalizations (n = 1.6 million) in Stockholm County, Allgulander (1996) found that 0.04% of "prescribed medication" users (including benzodiazepines) were ever admitted for medical problems relating to their drug use. In a study of 5,426 physicians randomly selected from the U.S. physicians American Medical Association database, Hughes et al. (1992) found that although 11.9% had used benzodiazepines in the past year, only 0.6% met DSM-III-R (American Psychiatric Association 1987) criteria for benzodiazepine abuse and 0.5% met criteria for benzodiazepine dependence. In 1990, the American Psychiatric Association task force concluded that benzodiazepines were not normally drugs of abuse, but noted that people who abused alcohol, cocaine, and opiates were at increased risk for benzodiazepine abuse (Salzman 1991).

Although some patients undergoing chronic therapy increase their benzodiazepine dose over time—39% in one study (Khan et al. 1981) and 50% in another (Maletzky and Klotter 1976)—the mean increase is only a small one. A number of studies have noted no increase in dosage with chronic therapy of duration from 1 to 2.5 years, even though many of the patients had residual symptoms that would have benefited from a dose increase or more intensive or additional treatment strategies (Pollack et al. 1986; D.V. Sheehan 1987). It has been reported that nonanxious subjects and those with low anxiety levels find benzodiazepines dysphoric (Reed et al. 1965), prefer placebo to diazepam (Johanson and Uhlenhuth 1978, 1980), or rate their mood as less happy and pleasant after they were given 10 mg of diazepam (Svenson et al. 1980).

Although the data suggest that the prevalence of benzodiazepine abuse or dependence is generally low, this is not true among those who abuse alcohol and other drugs. In a study of chronic alcoholic individuals who were high consumers of benzodiazepines, 17% got their benzodiazepines from nonmedical sources (Busto et al. 1983). In a study of 1,000 admissions to an alcohol treatment unit, 35% of patients used benzodiazepines, but only 10% of the total sample were considered abusers or misusers (Ashley et al. 1978). A study of 427 patients seeking treatment in Toronto who met DSM-III (American Psychiatric Association 1980) criteria for alcohol abuse or dependence found that 40% were recent users and 20% had a lifetime history of benzodiazepine abuse or dependence. Women, unemployed individuals, and those with personality disorder were at higher risk for dependence. The current benzodiazepine users were more likely to endorse psychological distress and depression and have a lifetime history of an anxiety disorder (H.E. Ross 1993). On the other hand, only 5% of 108 alcoholic patients treated for a year with benzodiazepines for anxiety and tension showed evidence of abuse, and 94% felt it helped them function and remain out of hospital (Rothstein et al. 1976). Benzodiazepine abuse liability has been shown for abstinent alcoholic men (Ciraulo et al. 1988) and in the sons and daughters of alcoholic individuals (Ciraulo et al. 1989, 1996). Enhanced sensitivity to the effects of benzodiazepines on frontal electroencephalographic activity was found to correlate with euphoric subjective responses in abstinent alcoholic individuals (Ciraulo et al. 1997).

Benzodiazepines were the primary drug of abuse in one-third of polydrug abusers (Busto et al. 1986), in 29% of 113 drug abusers admitting to the street purchase of diazepam in the previous month (Woody et al. 1975), and in 40% of patients at a methadone maintenance clinic (Woody et al. 1973). The principal reasons for benzodiazepine use among drug addicts are self-treatment of withdrawal symptoms, relief from rebound dysphoria, or potentiation of alcohol or street drug effects (Petera et al. 1987). In one study at an addictions treatment center, 100% of urine samples tested were positive for benzodiazepines and 44% were positive for multiple benzodiazepines, nonprescribed (Igochi et al. 1993). A survey of patients at three different methadone maintenance clinics found that 78%–94% admitted to a lifetime use of benzodiazepines and 44%–66% admitted to use in the prior 6 months. They also expressed a preference for diazepam, lorazepam, and alprazolam over chlordiazepoxide and oxazepam (Darke et al. 1995). Intravenous benzodiazepine use is more likely in polydrug users. In Australia, 48% of heroin users sampled injected benzodiazepines, with diazepam and temazepam being the most frequent. In the United Kingdom, the preference was for temazepam (Lader 1994; J. Ross et al. 1997). Snorting of benzodiazepines by cocaine addicts has been reported (M.F. Sheehan et al. 1991), primarily as a means of blunting the anxiogenic effect of cocaine and allowing for a more pleasant and "less edgy" high from that drug. There is minimal evidence that sustained-release formulations may have less potential for abuse than do immediate-release formulations (Mumford et al. 1995). Flunitrazepam (Rohypnol), a benzodiazepine that is not legally available in the United States, has been popular as a party drug and is sold as "rophies," "roofies," and "roach." When mixed with alcohol, it has very strong sedating and amnestic properties and has been used as a "date rape" drug. Overall, the existing evidence suggests that the prevalence of benzodiazepine abuse is uncommon, except among those individuals who abuse alcohol and or other drugs.

Despite extensive data and discussion on this topic, the issue remains and will continue to be controversial, with strong opinions held by opposing camps. Klerman characterized these camps as "pharmacological Calvinism" and "psychotropic hedonism," respectively (Klerman 1972; Rosenbaum 2005). The pharmacological Puritans or Stoics consider anxiety to be a lesser evil than the damage that may result from psychomotor impairment (including falls in the elderly) and the risks of abuse and dependence, especially in view of the fact that alternative treatments (antidepressants and cognitive-behavior therapy) are available (Geppert 2007). The psychotropic hedonists or the Epicureans consider anxiety disorder to be more hazardous than the aforementioned risks; they believe that an anxious patient has a right to seek a life free from anxiety and fear, and they trust the patient's ability to manage this controlled substance without abuse (Geppert 2007). The middle ground suggests that we should not hesitate to prescribe benzodiazepines when it is reasonable, but that we should exercise restraint in using them when we see any evidence of abuse (Pomeranz 2007). Attempts to restrict benzodiazepine prescription have had mixed results (Schwartz 1992; Schwartz and Blank 1991). For example, the triplicate prescription program instituted in 1989 by New York State with the intent to restrict benzodiazepine prescriptions resulted in increased use of older, more dangerous sedative-hypnotics such as barbiturates and meprobamate and an increase in prescriptions for benzodiazepines in the neighboring state of New Jersey (Hemmelgarn et al. 1997; Schwartz 1992; Schwartz and Blank 1991).

Medicolegal Issues

In addition to issues of dependence and withdrawal described in the previous section, there are a number of potential medicolegal pitfalls in using benzodiazepines. These include issues of teratogenicity, injury, and interaction with substances.

Benzodiazepines and Pregnancy

Since anxiety disorders have their highest incidence in women during their childbearing years, the clinician may have to advise patients who are planning a pregnancy or who become pregnant while taking a benzodiazepine.

First and Second Trimesters

An important concern in the first and second trimesters is the possibility of teratogenic effects. Diazepam and desmethyldiazepam cross the placental barrier easily, and concentrations are higher in fetal blood than in maternal blood (Idanpaan-Heikkila et al. 1971). Early concern over benzodiazepine exposure in pregnancy arose because benzodiazepines act on GABA receptors and GABA is involved in palate shelf reorientation (Wee and Zimmermann 1983; Zimmermann and Wee 1984). Benzodiazepine receptors have been found in fetuses of 12–15 weeks

(Aaltonen et al. 1983). The teratogenic effects of benzodiazepines, however, are a matter of controversy. Exposure to benzodiazepines has been associated with teratogenic effects, including facial clefts and skeletal anomalies in the newborn in some animal studies (R.P. Miller and Becker 1975; Walker and Patterson 1974; Wee and Zimmermann 1983; Zimmermann 1984; Zimmermann and Wee 1984) but not in others (Beall 1972; Chesley et al. 1991). Early studies in humans, including retrospective and case–control studies, reported an increased risk of oral clefts associated with diazepam (Aarskog 1975; Livezey et al. 1986; Safra and Oakley 1975; Saxen 1975; Saxen and Lahti 1974). These results, however, have been criticized on methodological grounds and are contradicted by more recent prospective studies, case–control studies, and meta-analyses that show no increased risk of oral clefts related to benzodiazepine use in pregnancy (Altshuler et al. 1996; Bracken 1986; Czeizel 1988; Dolovich et al. 1998; Ornoy et al. 1998; Pastuszak et al. 1996; Rosenberg et al. 1983; Shiono and Mills 1984).

Other anomalies, including inguinal hernia, pyloric stenosis, and congenital heart defects, have been reported with first-trimester use (Bracken and Holfred 1981); hemangiomas and cardiovascular defects have been associated with second-trimester use (Bracken and Holfred 1981). Isolated cases of skeletal defects such as spina bifida, absence of left forearm, syndactyly, and absence of both thumbs have also been reported following benzodiazepine use in pregnancy (Briggs et al. 1998; Istvan 1970; New Zealand Committee on Adverse Drug Reactions 1969; Ringrose 1972), and other malformations, including dysmorphic features, growth aberrations, and abnormalities of the CNS, have been attributed to benzodiazepines (Hartz et al. 1975; Laegreid et al. 1989; Milkovich and van den Berg 1974). Pooled data from seven cohort studies, however, do not support an association between fetal exposure to benzodiazepines and major malformations (Dolovich et al. 1998).

Third Trimester and Labor

Two concerns associated with benzodiazepine use in the last trimester and through delivery are the possibilities of CNS depression and a withdrawal syndrome. Signs of CNS depression may include hypotonia, lethargy, sucking difficulties, decreased fetal movements, loss of cardiac beat-to-beat variability, respiratory depression, and thermogenesis. These symptoms in the neonate are more likely with higher doses and longer duration of benzodiazepine use by the mother. There have been numerous reports of "floppy infant syndrome" in babies born to women taking diazepam long term during pregnancy (Gillberg 1977; Haram 1977; Rowlatt 1978; Spreight 1977). Neonatal withdrawal symptoms may include hyperactivity and irritability. The occurrence of neonatal withdrawal symptoms is well documented (Barry and St. Clair 1987; Briggs et al. 1998; Cree et al. 1973; Fisher et al. 1985; Gillberg 1977; Haram 1977). Symptoms may be present at birth or appear weeks later and may continue for a period of time (Besunder and Blumer, in Schardein 1993). Elimination of benzodiazepines in the infant is slow, and it is believed that increased blood concentrations, together with an immature blood–brain barrier, contribute to newborns being more sensitive to these medications than are adults (Pastuszak et al. 1996).

Diazepam in isolated doses is safe during labor (Briggs et al. 1998). There are conflicting reports on the effect of benzodiazepines on Apgar scores. Lowered Apgar scores have been reported with benzodiazepine use in some studies (Berdowitz et al. 1981; McElhatton 1994). One study found that diazepam reduced Apgar scores only when doses greater than 30 mg were administered during labor (Cree et al. 1973). Benzodiazepines do not appear to significantly affect fetal pH (Haram 1977). Diazepam contains a buffer, sodium benzoate, that displaces bilirubin from albumin in vitro (Haram 1977). Perhaps for this reason, parenteral diazepam given during labor has been associated with a dose-dependent elevation of neonatal serum bilirubin concentration secondary to delayed bilirubin metabolism (Haram 1977).

Evaluation of the Evidence on Benzodiazepine Teratogenicity

Approximately 3% of all pregnancies end with the delivery of an abnormal live-born infant; only about 3% of these are associated with known teratogenic exposure (Coustan and Carpenter 1985). In the Collaborative Perinatal Project, the overall infant malformation rate was 6.5% (Heinonen et al. 1977).

Several sources of bias must be considered in evaluating the data on benzodiazepine teratogenicity (Dolovich et al. 1998). Retrospective studies have been criticized for "recall bias" as well as confounding and ascertainment bias. Patients using benzodiazepines tend to be a little older, and their anxiety disorder may lead to increased use of cigarettes, alcohol, caffeine, or analgesics, all of which have been associated with complications in pregnancy. Because of their well-known muscle-relaxant and catecholamine-reducing properties, it is conceivable, but not

established, that benzodiazepines might prevent spontaneous abortions of an already malformed fetus. It is also possible that the underlying anxiety disorder itself may be associated with fetal complications (Cohen et al. 1989; Crandon 1979; Istvan 1986). Large population studies are needed in order to control for these confounding factors. In the meantime, the direction of the evidence would suggest that caution and conservative advice are prudent.

Advice to Patients Planning a Pregnancy

If a patient taking a benzodiazepine plans a pregnancy, it is best to advise her to be off the medicine during her pregnancy. Benzodiazepines should always be discontinued very slowly. Some patients are unable to complete taper or tolerate the recurrence of their anxiety disorder and the consequent disability in work, social life, and family life. It is best in all cases to make an attempt to discontinue the benzodiazepine in the hope that the patient will manage without it before conceiving. Patients who are unable or unwilling to stop their benzodiazepine should be encouraged to use the lowest dose possible, preferably on an as-needed schedule. All patients are encouraged to have discontinued their benzodiazepine before the last 2 months of pregnancy. Withdrawal from benzodiazepines in a premature infant could tip the balance against healthy survival. It is common for panic disorder patients to experience a significant worsening of their panic disorder during the postpartum period. The benzodiazepine can be restarted immediately postpartum if they agree not to breast feed.

Management During an Unplanned Pregnancy

It is estimated that almost half of all pregnancies in the United States are unplanned (Skrabanek 1992). It is not unusual for a patient who has been taking a benzodiazepine for months or years to come to a regular office visit and announce that she is pregnant. She now wonders whether she should abruptly stop the benzodiazepine or have a therapeutic abortion. The first recommendation is to ensure that the patient does not abruptly stop the benzodiazepine. Abrupt withdrawal could precipitate a withdrawal seizure and even a miscarriage. Typically, by the time she realizes that she is pregnant, the period for organogenesis (8–9 weeks) is past. The first step is to spend time discussing these issues with the pregnant patient and her family and then enter a detailed record of this discussion into the medical record. Consulting with a colleague on this issue for a second opinion may be helpful. The patient can be told that there is no compelling data to support the view that discontinuing the benzodiazepine will decrease the earlier-mentioned expected 3% risk of having a fetal complication (Coustan and Carpenter 1985). However, physicians prefer their pregnant patients to not be taking any medication, as the patients in these 3% of cases might blame the complication on the benzodiazepine, even if there is no association, and sue them. The next step is to plan carefully with her a very slow withdrawal of the benzodiazepine over weeks rather than over days. A therapeutic abortion is not indicated after routine use of a benzodiazepine in the first or second trimester, as the associated abnormalities are rarely life-threatening.

Breast Feeding

Early on, neonates were found to have only limited capacity to metabolize diazepam (Morselli et al. 1973). Benzodiazepines are excreted in breast milk (Llewellyn and Stowe 1998). Because of the neonate's limited capacity to metabolize these drugs, they can potentially accumulate and cause sedation, lethargy, and loss of weight in the nursing infant. Although the extent to which benzodiazepines actually accumulate in the serum of breast-feeding infants is a matter of debate (Birnbaum et al. 1999), and three decades of studies support a low incidence of toxicity and adverse effects (Birnbaum et al. 1999; Llewellyn and Stowe 1998), caution taking benzodiazepines while breast-feeding is advised. Individualized risk–benefit assessments are recommended with the goal of minimizing, if not avoiding, infant exposure to benzodiazepines in breast milk.

Psychomotor Impairment

Another area of risk of benzodiazepine use relates to issues of psychomotor impairment resulting in injury. Examination of the medical records of a group of benzodiazepine users and nonusers who were part of a health maintenance organization found that the benzodiazepine users were more likely to experience at least one episode of accident-related health care and a greater number of accident-related inpatient days and also utilized significantly more non-accident-related health care services than did nonusers. Accident-related utilization of health care was more likely in the first month after the drug was prescribed (Oster et al. 1987). In the elderly, the issue of benzodiazepine use increasing the risk for falls and fractures is of great concern because hip fractures are associated with increased morbidity and mortality. A number of studies (Boston Collaborative Drug Surveillance Program 1973; Cummings et al. 1995; Greenblatt et al. 1977; Hemmel-

garn et al. 1997; Ray et al. 1992; Roth et al. 1980) have found a greater risk for falls with the use of long-half-life benzodiazepines, and others (Cumming and Klineberg 1993; Herings et al. 1995; Leipzig et al. 1999) have found the risk to be greater with short-half-life drugs. A more recent study (Wang et al. 2001) found the risk for hip fracture in the elderly to be the same with the use of short- or long-half-life benzodiazepines. They did find that the risk increased when benzodiazepine dosages were >3 mg/day in diazepam equivalents. They also found the greatest risk to be shortly after initiation of therapy and after 1 month of continuous use. A 5-year prospective cohort study followed a large group of elderly people newly exposed to benzodiazepines (Tamblyn et al. 2005). The risk of injury varied by benzodiazepine, was independent of its half-life, and was highest for oxazepam, flurazepam, and chlordiazepoxide. The elderly using benzodiazepines are at greater risk of a motor vehicle accident (Hemmelgarn et al. 1997). On the other hand, a study of the effect of New York State requiring triplicate forms for prescribing benzodiazepines showed that despite a 50% drop in the number of prescriptions written, there was no significant change in age-adjusted risk for hip fractures (Wagner et al. 2007).

Patients receiving benzodiazepines are nearly five times more likely than nonusers to experience a serious motor vehicle accident (Skegg et al. 1979). In the first 2 weeks of benzodiazepine use, there is a severalfold excess risk for hospitalization related to accidental injury compared with persons using antidepressants or antipsychotics (Neutel 1995).

In a review of minor tranquilizers and psychomotor performance, the data overall support impairment by the few compounds studied—diazepam, lorazepam, and alprazolam. Generally, behavioral tolerance does not develop with chronic dosing (Smiley 1987). The problem with the psychomotor (driving) studies is that it is not clear how well these mirror real-life situations. In terms of utilization of medical services due to accidents, it is not yet resolved how much is due to the drug and how much is due to the illness itself, as there are no placebo-controlled studies. However, it is good practice to warn patients about the potential for sedation and psychomotor impairment with benzodiazepine use. They should be advised to be cautious when performing skilled tasks, driving, or working with machinery.

Patients should be advised to avoid the use of alcohol or sedating antihistamines when taking benzodiazepines, as there are potentially serious additive effects (Van Steveninck et al. 1996). Ethanol has effects on the GABA–

benzodiazepine receptor complex. Brain benzodiazepine levels are influenced by alcohol ingestion. Alcohol decreases triazolam levels, increases diazepam levels, and does not change chlordiazepoxide levels (Castaneda et al. 1996).

The best protection is a discussion of these issues with the patient prior to prescribing a benzodiazepine. This discussion, including cautionary statements about driving or using dangerous appliances, should be documented in the chart at the start of therapy. The patient should be educated about potentiation by alcohol or other sedating drugs. He or she should be strongly advised never to abruptly discontinue the medicine because of a risk of seizures (Noyes et al. 1986), and this should be documented. Prescribing benzodiazepines for patients with a current or lifetime history of substance abuse or dependence should be done infrequently and only after documenting a risk–benefit discussion in the chart. It is good practice to routinely screen for substance abuse before prescribing a benzodiazepine and to document that this was done. In one outpatient clinic, there was no information about alcohol use recorded in the charts of 57% of patients prescribed benzodiazepines (Graham et al. 1992).

Conclusion

Benzodiazepines, if given in adequate doses, are effective in the treatment of anxiety. They have a lower mortality and morbidity per million prescriptions than some of the alternatives (Girdwood 1972). They are quicker in onset of action, easier for the clinician to use, associated with better compliance, and less subjectively disruptive for the patient than any of the other medication alternatives. Until they are replaced by another class of medicine that is safer, better tolerated, and as rapidly effective, it is likely that they will continue to be prescribed to a significant proportion of patients. It is also likely that we will see a shift toward the use of sustained-release formulations of benzodiazepines, since these formulations may have less abuse liability (Mumford et al. 1995) and blunt the peaks of toxicity and the troughs of symptom recurrence that are often problematic in the chronic management of such patients.

References

Aaltonen L, Erkkola R, Kanto J: Benzodiazepine receptors in the human fetus (letter). Biology of the Neonate 44:54, 1983

Aarskog D: Associations between maternal intake of diazepam and oral clefts (letter). Lancet 2(7941):921, 1975

Alexander PE: Alprazolam-XR in the treatment of panic disorder: results of a randomized, double-blind, fixed-dose, placebo-controlled, multicenter study. Psychiatric Annals 23 (suppl 10):14–19, 1993

Allgulander C: Psychoactive drug use in a general population sample, Sweden: correlates with perceived health, psychiatric diagnoses, and mortality in an automated record-linkage study. Am J Public Health 79:1006–1010, 1989

Allgulander C: Addiction in sedative-hypnotics. Hum Psychopharmacol 119:S49–S54, 1996

Altshuler LL, Cohen L, Szuba MP, et al: Pharmacologic management of psychiatric illness during pregnancy: dilemmas and guidelines. Am J Psychiatry 153:592–606, 1996

American Psychiatric Association: Diagnostic and Statistical Manual of Mental Disorders, 3rd Edition. Washington, DC, American Psychiatric Association, 1980

American Psychiatric Association: Diagnostic and Statistical Manual of Mental Disorders, 3rd Edition, Revised. Washington, DC, American Psychiatric Association, 1987

American Psychiatric Association: Benzodiazepine Dependence, Toxicity, and Abuse: A Task Force Report of the American Psychiatric Association. Washington, DC, American Psychiatric Association, 1990

American Psychiatric Association: Practice guideline for the treatment of patients with panic disorder. Am J Psychiatry 155 (suppl 5):1–34, 1998

American Psychiatric Association: Diagnostic and Statistical Manual of Mental Disorders, 4th Edition, Text Revision. Washington, DC, American Psychiatric Association, 2000

Ashley MJ, LeRiche WH, Olin GS, et al: "Mixed" (drug abusing) and "pure" alcoholics: a socio-medical comparison. Br J Addict 73:19–34, 1978

Ballenger JC, Burrows G, Dupont RL, et al: Alprazolam in panic disorder and agoraphobia: results from a multicenter study. Arch Gen Psychiatry 45:413–422, 1988

Balter MB: Prevalence of medical use of prescription drugs. Presentation at Evaluation of the Impact of Prescription Drug Diversion Control Systems on Medical Practice and Patient Care: Possible Implications for Future Research (NIDA Technical Review), Bethesda, MD, 1991

Balter MB, Manheimer DI, Mellinger GD, et al: A cross national comparison of anti-anxiety/sedative drug use. Current Medical Research Opinion 8 (suppl 4):5P20, 1984

Barry WS, St. Clair SM: Exposure to benzodiazepines in utero. Lancet 1(8547):1436–1437, 1987

Bayer AJ, Bayer EM, Pathy MSJ, et al: A double blind controlled study of chlormethiazole and triazolam and hypnotics in the elderly. Acta Psychiatr Scand 73:104–111, 1986

Beall JR: Study of the teratogenic potential of oral diazepam and SCH 12041. Can Med Assoc J 106:1061, 1972

Berdowitz RL, Coustan DR, Mochizuke T (eds): Handbook for Prescribing Medications During Pregnancy. Boston, MA, Little, Brown, 1981

Birnbaum CS, Cohen LS, Bailey JW, et al: Serum concentrations of antidepressants and benzodiazepines in nursing infants: a case series. Pediatrics 104(1):e11, 1999

Bixler EO, Kales A, Soldatos CR, et al: Effectiveness of temazepam with short, intermediate and long term use: sleep laboratory evaluation. J Clin Pharmacol 18:110–118, 1978

Bixler EO, Scharf MB, Soldatos CR, et al: Effects of hypnotic drugs on memory. Life Sci 25:1379–1388, 1979

Boston Collaborative Drug Surveillance Program: Clinical depression of the central nervous system due to diazepam and chlordiazepoxide in relation to cigarette smoking and age. N Engl J Med 288:277–280, 1973

Bracken MB: Drug use in pregnancy and congenital heart disease in offspring (letter). N Engl J Med 314:1120, 1986

Bracken MB, Holfred TR: Exposure to prescribed drugs in pregnancy and association with congenital malformations. Obstet Gynecol 58:336–344, 1981

Bradwejn J, Shriqui C, Koszycki D, et al: Double-blind comparison of the effects of clonazepam and lorazepam in acute mania. J Clin Psychopharmacol 10:403–408, 1990

Briggs GG, Yaffe SJ, Freeman RK: Drugs in Pregnancy and Lactation: A Reference Guide to Fetal and Neonatal Risk, 5th Edition. Baltimore, MD, Williams & Wilkins, 1998

Busto U, Simpkins J, Sellers EM, et al: Objective determination of benzodiazepine use and abuse in alcoholics. Br J Addict 78:429–435, 1983

Busto U, Sellers EM, Naranjo CA, et al: Patterns of benzodiazepine abuse and dependence. Br J Addict 81:87–94, 1986

Busto UE, Bremner KE, Knight K, et al: Long-term benzodiazepine therapy does not result in brain abnormalities. J Clin Psychopharmacol 20:2–6, 2000

Castaneda R, Sussman N, Westreich L, et al: A review of the effects of moderate alcohol intake on the treatment of anxiety and mood disorders. J Clin Psychiatry 57:207–212, 1996

Castillo-Ferrando JR, Garcia M, Carmona J, et al: Digoxin levels and diazepam. Lancet 2(8190):368, 1980

Chesley S, Lumpkin M, Schatzki A, et al: Prenatal exposure to benzodiazepine, I: prenatal exposure to lorazepam in mice alters open-field activity and GABA receptor function. Neuropharmacology 30:53–58, 1991

Chouinard G, Annable L, Fontaine R, et al: Alprazolam and the treatment of generalized anxiety and panic disorders: a double-blind placebo controlled study. Psychopharmacology (Berl) 77:229–233, 1982

Chouinard G, Young SN, Annable L: Antimanic effect of clonazepam. Biol Psychiatry 18:451–466, 1983

Chouinard G, Annable L, Turnier L, et al: Double blind randomized clinical trial of rapid tranquilization with IM clonazepam and IM haloperidol in agitated psychotic patients with manic symptoms. Can J Psychiatry 38 (suppl 4):S114–S120, 1993

Ciraulo DA, Barnhill JG, Greenblatt DJ, et al: Abuse liability and clinical pharmacokinetics in alcoholic men. J Clin Psychiatry 49:333–337, 1988

Ciraulo DA, Ban JG, Ciraulo AM, et al: Parental alcoholism as a risk factor in benzodiazepine abuse: a pilot study. Am J Psychiatry 146:1333–1335, 1989

Ciraulo DA, Sarid-Segal O, Knapp C, et al: Liability to alprazolam abuse in daughters of alcoholics. Am J Psychiatry 153:956–958, 1996

Ciraulo DA, Barbell JG, Ciraulo AM, et al: Alterations in pharmacodynamics of anxiolytics in abstinent alcoholic men: subjective responses, abuse liability and electroencephalographic effects of alprazolam, diazepam, and buspirone. J Clin Pharmacol 37:64–73, 1997

Cohen LS, Rosenbaum JF, Heller VL: Panic attack–associated placental abruption: a case report. J Clin Psychiatry 50:266–267, 1989

Controlled Substances Act: Title II of the Comprehensive Drug Abuse Prevention and Control Act of 1970 (Pub. L. 91–513, 84 Stat. 1236, enacted 1970-10-27, codified at 21 U.S.C. § 801 et. seq.)

Cooper SJ: Palatability-dependent appetite and benzodiazepines: new directions from the pharmacology of GABA(A) receptor subtypes. Appetite 44:133–150, 2005

Coustan DR, Carpenter MW: The use of medication and pregnancy. Resid Staff Physician 31:64, 1985

Crandon AJ: Maternal anxiety and neonatal well-being. J Psychosom Res 23:113–115, 1979

Cree JE, Meyer J, Hailey DM: Diazepam in labor: its metabolism and effect on the clinical condition of thermogenesis of the newborn. BMJ 4:251–255, 1973

Cross National Collaborative Panic Study, Second Phase Investigators: Drug treatment of panic disorder: comparative efficacy of alprazolam, imipramine, and placebo. Br J Psychiatry 160:191–201, 1992

Cumming RG, Klineberg RJ: Psychotropics, thiazide diuretics and hip fracture in the elderly. Med J Aust 158:414–417, 1993

Cummings SR, Nevitt MC, Browner WS, et al: Risk factors for hip fracture in white women. N Engl J Med 332:767–773, 1995

Czeizel A: Lack of evidence of teratogenicity of benzodiazepine drugs in Hungary. Reprod Toxicol 1(3):183–188, 1988

Darke SG, Ross JE, Hall WD: Benzodiazepine use among injecting heroin users. Med J Aust 162:645–647, 1995

Davidson JRT, Potts NLS, Richichi E, et al: Treatment of social phobia with clonazepam and placebo. J Clin Psychopharmacol 13:423–428, 1993

Dawson GR, Collinson N, Atack JR: Development of subtype selective GABAa modulators. CNS Spectr 10:21–27, 2005

Denis C, Fatseas M, Lavie E, et al: Pharmacological interventions' for benzodiazepine monodependence management in outpatient settings. Cochrane Database Syst Rev (3):CD005194, 2006

DeVane CL, Liston HL: An explanation of the second-dose effect in pharmacokinetics and its meaning for clinical psychopharmacology. Psychopharmacol Bull 35:42–52, 2001

Dietch J: The nature and extent of benzodiazepine abuse: an overview of recent literature. Hosp Community Psychiatry 34:1139–1145, 1983

Dolovich LR, Addis A, Vaillancourt JM, et al: Benzodiazepine use in pregnancy and major malformations or oral cleft: meta-analysis of cohort and case-control studies. BMJ 317:839–843, 1998

Fichter MM, Witzke W, Leibl K, et al: Psychotropic drug use in representative community sample: the Upper Bavarian West German Study. Acta Psychiatr Scand 80:68–77, 1989

Fisher JB, Edgren BE, Mammel MC, et al: Neonatal apnea associated with maternal clonazepam therapy: a case report. Obstet Gynecol 66 (suppl):34–35, 1985

Fontaine RG, Chouinard G, Annable L: Rebound anxiety in anxious patients after abrupt withdrawal of benzodiazepine treatment. Am J Psychiatry 141:848–852, 1984

Garvey MJ, Tollefson GD: Prevalence of misuse of prescribed benzodiazepines in patients with primary anxiety disorder or major depression. Am J Psychiatry 143:1601–1603, 1986

Gelernter CS, Uhde TW, Cimbolic P, et al: Cognitive-behavioral and pharmacologic treatment of social phobia: a controlled study. Arch Gen Psychiatry 48:938–945, 1991

Gelpin E, Bonne O, Peri T, et al: Treatment of recent trauma survivors with benzodiazepines: a prospective study. J Clin Psychiatry 57:390–394, 1996

Geppert CMA: The religion of benzodiazepines. Psychiatric Times 17–18, April 2007

Gillberg C: "Floppy infant syndrome" and maternal diazepam (letter). Lancet 2(8031):244, 1977

Girdwood RH: Death after taking medicaments. Br J Psychiatry 1(906):501, 1972

Goddard AW, Brouette T, Almai A, et al: Early coadministration of clonazepam with sertraline for panic disorder. Arch Gen Psychiatry 58:681–686, 2001

Goddard AW, Sheehan DV, Rickels K: A Double blind placebo controlled study comparing sertraline plus placebo and sertraline plus alprazolam XR in the treatment of panic disorder. Presented at Anxiety Disorders Association of America annual meeting, Savannah, GA, March 2008

Golombok S, Moodley P, Lader M: Cognitive impairment in long-term benzodiazepine users. Psychol Med 18:365–374, 1988

Goodman WK, Charney DS: A case of alprazolam but not lorazepam inducing manic symptoms. J Clin Psychiatry 48:117–118, 1987

Graham AV, Parran TV, Jaen CR: Physician failure to record alcohol use history when prescribing benzodiazepines. J Subst Abuse 4:179–185, 1992

Greenblatt DJ, Allen MD, Shader RI: Toxicity of high dose flurazepam in the elderly. Clin Pharmacol Ther 21:355–361, 1977

Greenblatt DJ, Shader RI, Franke K, et al: Pharmacokinetics and bioavailability of intravenous, intramuscular, and oral lorazepam in humans. J Pharm Sci 68:57–63, 1979

Greenblatt DJ, Divoll M, Harmatz JS, et al: Kinetics and clinical effects of flurazepam in young and elderly noninsomniacs. Clin Pharmacol Ther 30:475–486, 1981

Greenblatt DJ, Divoll M, Abernethy DR, et al: Benzodiazepine hypnotics: kinetic and therapeutic options. Sleep 5 (suppl 1): S18–S27, 1982a

Greenblatt DJ, Divoll M, Harmatz JS, et al: Pharmacokinetic comparison of sublingual lorazepam with intravenous, intramuscular, and oral lorazepam. J Pharm Sci 71:248–252, 1982b

Greenblatt DJ, Sellers EM, Shader RI: Drug therapy: drug distribution in old age. N Engl J Med 306:1081–1088, 1982c

Greenblatt DJ, Shader RI, Abernethy DR: Drug therapy: current status of benzodiazepines, part 1. N Engl J Med 309:354–358, 1983a

Greenblatt DJ, Shader RI, Abernethy DR: Drug therapy: current status of benzodiazepines, part 2. N Engl J Med 309:410–416, 1983b

Greenblatt DJ, Abernethy DR, Morse DS, et al: Clinical importance of the interaction of diazepam and cimetidine. N Engl J Med 310:1639–1643, 1984

Greenblatt DJ, Harmatz JS, Engelhardt N, et al: Pharmacokinetic determinants of dynamic differences among three benzodiazepine hypnotics: flurazepam, temazepam, and triazolam. Arch Gen Psychiatry 46:326–332, 1989

Haram K: Floppy infant syndrome and maternal diazepam. Lancet 2(8038):612–613, 1977

Hartz SC, Heinonen OP, Shapiro S, et al: Antenatal exposure to meprobamate and chlordiazepoxide in relation to malformations, mental development, and childhood mortality. N Engl J Med 292:726–728, 1975

Heinonen OP, Stone D, Shapiro S: Birth Defects and Drugs in Pregnancy. Littleton, MA, PSG, 1977

Hemmelgarn B, Suissa S, Huang A, et al: Benzodiazepine use and the risk of motor vehicle crash in the elderly. JAMA 278:27–31, 1997

Herings RM, Stricker BH, de Boer A, et al: Benzodiazepines and the risk of falling leading to femur fractures: dosage more important than elimination half-life. Arch Intern Med 155:1801–1807, 1995

Herman JB, Brotman AW, Rosenbaum JF: Rebound anxiety in panic disorder patients treated with shorter acting benzodiazepines. J Clin Psychiatry 48 (suppl):22–28, 1987

Hewlett WA, Vinogradov S, Agras WS: Clomipramine, clonazepam and clonidine treatment of obsessive compulsive disorder. J Clin Psychopharmacol 12:420–430, 1992

Hughes PH, Brandenburg N, Baldwin DC, et al: Prevalence of substance use among US physicians. JAMA 267:2333–2339, 1992

Idanpaan-Heikkila JE, Jouppila PI, Puolakka JO, et al: Placental transfer in fetal metabolism of diazepam in early human pregnancy. Am J Obstet Gynecol 109:1011–1016, 1971

Igochi MY, Handelsman L, Bickel WK, et al: Benzodiazepine and sedative use/abuse by methadone maintenance clients. Drug Alcohol Depend 32:257–266, 1993

IMS America: National Disease and Therapeutic Index (NDTI). Plymouth Meeting, PA, IMS America, 1991

Istvan EJ: Drug associated congenital abnormalities (letter). Can Med Assoc J 103:1394, 1970

Istvan J: Stress, anxiety and birth outcomes: a critical review of the evidence. Psychol Bull 100:331–348, 1986

Johanson CE, Uhlenhuth EH: Drug self-administration in humans. NIDA Res Monogr July(20):68–85, 1978

Johanson CE, Uhlenhuth EH: Drug preference and mood in humans: diazepam. Psychopharmacology (Berl) 71:269–273, 1980

Judd FK, Norman TR, Marriott PF, et al: A case of alprazolam-related hepatitis (letter). Am J Psychiatry 143:388–389, 1986

Kales A, Bixler EO, Soldatos CR, et al: Quazepam and flurazepam: long-term use and extended withdrawal. Clin Pharmacol Ther 32:781–788, 1982

Kales A, Soldatos CR, Bixler EO, et al: Early morning insomnia with rapidly eliminated benzodiazepines. Science 220:95–97, 1983

Kales A, Bixler EO, Soldatos CR, et al: Lorazepam: effects on sleep and withdrawal phenomena. Pharmacology 32:121–130, 1986

Kales A, Bixler EO, Vela-Bueno A, et al: Alprazolam: effects on sleep and withdrawal phenomena. J Clin Pharmacol 27:508–515, 1987

Khan A, Hornblow AR, Walshe JWB: Benzodiazepine dependence: a general practice survey. N Z Med J 93:19–21, 1981

Klein E, Uhde TW, Post RM: Preliminary evidence for the utility of carbamazepine in alprazolam withdrawal. Am J Psychiatry 143:235–236, 1986

Klerman GL: Psychotropic hedonism vs. pharmacological Calvinism. Hastings Cent Rep 2:1–3, 1972

Kramer PD: Listening to Prozac. New York, Penguin Books, 1993

Kumar R, Mac DS, Gabrielli WF Jr, et al: Anxiolytics and memory: a comparison of lorazepam and alprazolam. J Clin Psychiatry 48:158–160, 1987

Lader M: Benzodiazepine withdrawal, in Handbook of Anxiety, Vol 4. Edited by Noyer R, Roth M, Burrows GD. Amsterdam, Elsevier, 1990, pp 57–71

Lader M: Anxiolytic drugs: dependence, addiction and abuse. Eur Neuropsychopharmacol 4:85–91, 1994

Lader M, Olajide D: A comparison of buspirone and placebo in relieving benzodiazepine withdrawal symptoms. J Clin Psychopharmacol 7:11–15, 1987

Lader MH, Ron M, Petursson H: Computed axial brain tomography in long term benzodiazepine users. Psychol Med 14:203–206, 1984

Ladewig D, Grossenbacher H: Benzodiazepine abuse in patients of doctors in domiciliary practice in the Basle area. Pharmacopsychiatry 21:104–108, 1988

Laegreid L, Olegard R, Walstrom J, et al: Teratogenic effects of benzodiazepine use during pregnancy. J Pediatr 114:126–131, 1989

Laux G, Konig W: Long term use of benzodiazepines in psychiatric inpatients. Acta Psychiatr Scand 76:64–70, 1987

Leipzig RM, Cumming RG, Tinetti ME: Drugs and falls in older people: a systematic review and meta-analysis, I: psychotropic drugs. J Am Geriatr Soc 47:30–39, 1999

Lister RG: The amnestic action of benzodiazepines in man. Neuroscience Behavior Research 9:87–94, 1985

Lister RG, Weingartner H, Eckhardt MJ, et al: Clinical relevance of effects of benzodiazepines on learning and memory. Psychopharmacol Ser 6:117–127, 1988

Livezey GT, Marczynski TJ, McGrew A, et al: Prenatal exposure to diazepam: late postnasal teratogenic effect. Neurotoxicology Teratology 8:433–440, 1986

Llewellyn A, Stowe ZN: Psychotropic medications in lactation. J Clin Psychiatry 59 (suppl 2):41–52, 1998

Low K, Crestani F, Keist R et al: Molecular and neuronal substrate for the selective attenuation of anxiety. Science 290:131–134, 2000

Lucki I, Rickels K, Geller AM: Chronic use of benzodiazepines and psychomotor and cognitive test performance. Psychopharmacology (Berl) 88:426–433, 1986

Magbagbeola JAO: A comparison of lorazepam and diazepam as oral premedicants for surgery under regional anaesthesia. Br J Anaesth 46:449–451, 1974

Maletzky BM, Klotter J: Addiction to diazepam. Int J Addict 11:95–115, 1976

Mant A, Duncan-Jones P, Saltman D, et al: Development of long term use of psychotropic drugs by general practice patients. BMJ 296:251–254, 1988

Marks J: The Benzodiazepines. Lancaster, England, MTP Press, 1978

McElhatton PR: The effects of benzodiazepine use during pregnancy and lactation. Reprod Toxicol 8:461–475, 1994

Mellinger GD, Balter MB, Uhlenhuth EH: Prevalence and correlates of the long-term regular use of anxiolytics. JAMA 251:375–379, 1984

Milkovich L, van den Berg BJ: Effects of prenatal meprobamate and chlordiazepoxide hydrochloride on human embryonic and fetal development. N Engl J Med 291:1268–1271, 1974

Miller RP, Becker BA: Teratogenicity of oral diazepam and diphenylhydantoin in mice. Toxicol Appl Pharmacol 32:53–61, 1975

Miller RR: Drug surveillance utilizing epidemiologic methods: a report from the Boston Collaborative Drug Surveillance Program. Am J Hosp Pharm 30:584–592, 1973

Mohler H, Fritschy JM, Rudolph U: A new benzodiazepine pharmacology. J Pharmacol Exp Ther 300:2–8, 2002

Morselli PL, Principi N, Tognoni G, et al: Diazepam elimination and premature and full-term infants and children. J Perinat Med 1(2):133–141, 1973

Mueller TI, Goldenberg IM, Gordon AL, et al: Benzodiazepine use in anxiety disordered patients with and without a history of alcoholism. J Clin Psychiatry 57:83–89, 1996

Mumford GK, Evans SM, Fleishaker JC, et al: Alprazolam absorption kinetics affects abuse liability. Clin Pharmacol Ther 57:356–365, 1995

Munjack DJ, Crocker B: Alprazolam induced ejaculatory inhibition (letter). J Clin Psychopharmacol 6:57–58, 1986

Neppe VM, Sindorf J: Carbamazepine for high dose diazepam withdrawal in opiate users. J Nerv Ment Disord 179:234–235, 1991

Neutel CI: Risk of traffic accident injury after a prescription for a benzodiazepine. Ann Epidemiol 5:239–244, 1995

New Zealand Committee on Adverse Drug Reactions: Fourth Annual Report. N Z Med J 70:118–122, 1969

Nowlin-Finch NL, Altshuler LL, Szuba MP, et al: Rapid resolution of first episodes of mania: sleep related? J Clin Psychiatry 55:26–29, 1994

Noyes R Jr, Perry PJ, Crowe RR, et al: Seizures following the withdrawal of alprazolam. J Nerv Ment Dis 174:50–52, 1986

Nutt D, Adinoff B, Linnoila M: Benzodiazepines in the treatment of alcoholism, in Recent Developments in Alcoholism, Vol 8. Edited by Galanter M. New York, American Society of Addiction Medicine and Research Society of Alcoholism/Plenum Press, 1989, pp 283–313

O'Brien CP: Benzodiazepine use, abuse, and dependence. J Clin Psychiatry 66 (suppl 2):28–33, 2005

Ogura C, Nakazawa K, Majima K, et al: Residual effects of hypnotics: triazolam, flurazepam, and nitrazepam. Psychopharmacology (Berl) 68:61–65, 1980

Ornoy A, Arnon J, Shechtman S, et al: Is benzodiazepine use during pregnancy really teratogenic? Reprod Toxicol 12:511–515, 1998

Oster G, Russell MW, Huse DM, et al: Accident- and injury-related health-care utilization among benzodiazepine users and nonusers. J Clin Psychiatry 48 (12, suppl):17–21, 1987

Pakesch G, Loimer N, Rasinger E, et al: The prevalence of psychoactive drug intake in a metropolitan population. Pharmacopsychiatry 2:61–65, 1989

Pancheri P, Casacchia M, Stratta P, et al: Assessment of the efficacy of buspirone in patients affected by generalized anxiety disorder, shifting to buspirone from prior treatment with lorazepam. J Clin Psychopharmacol 15:12–19, 1995

Pastuszak A, Milich V, Chan S, et al: Prospective assessment of pregnancy outcome following first trimester exposure to benzodiazepines. Can J Clin Pharmacol 3:167–171, 1996

Paulus MP, Feinstein JS, Castillo G, et al: Dose-dependent decease of activation in bilateral amygdale and insula by lorazepam during motion processing. Arch Gen Psychiatry 62:282–288, 2005

Pecknold JC: Discontinuation reactions to alprazolam in panic disorder. J Psychiatry Res 27 (suppl 1):155–170, 1993

Pecknold JC, Fleury D: Alprazolam-induced manic episode in two patients with panic disorder. Am J Psychiatry 143:652–653, 1986

Pecknold JC, Swinson RP, Kuch K, et al: Alprazolam in panic disorder and agoraphobia: results from a multicenter trial, III: discontinuation effects. Arch Gen Psychiatry 45:429–436, 1988

Pecknold J, Alexander PE, Munjack D: Alprazolam-XR in the management of anxiety: discontinuation. Psychiatric Annals 23 (10, suppl):38–44, 1993

Pecknold J, Lorenz L, Munjack D, et al: A double-blind, placebo-controlled study with alprazolam and extended-release alprazolam in the treatment of panic disorder. J Clin Psychopharmacol 14:314–321, 1994

Penava SJ, Otto MW, Pollack MH, et al: Current status of pharmacotherapy for PTSD: an effect size analysis of controlled studies. Depress Anxiety 4:240–242, 1996–1997

Peppers MP: Benzodiazepines for alcohol withdrawal in the elderly and in patients with liver disease. Pharmacotherapy 16:49–58, 1996

Petera KMH, Tulley M, Jenner FA: The use of benzodiazepines among street drug addicts. Br J Addict 82:511, 1987

Petturson H, Lader MH: Withdrawal from long term benzodiazepine treatment. BMJ 283:643–645, 1991

Pollack MH, Tesar GE, Rosenbaum JF, et al: Clonazepam in the treatment of panic disorder and agoraphobia: a one-year follow-up. J Clin Psychopharmacol 6:302–304, 1986

Pollack MH, Otto MW, Tesar GE, et al: Long-term outcome after acute treatment with alprazolam or clonazepam for panic disorder. J Clin Psychopharmacol 13:257–263, 1993

Pomeranz JM: Risk versus benefit of benzodiazepines Psychiatric Times 22–26, August 2007

Poser W, Poser S, Roscher D, et al: Do benzodiazepines cause cerebral atrophy (letter)? Lancet 1(8326 Pt 1):715, 1983

Power KG, Jerrom DWA, Simpson RJ, et al: Controlled study of withdrawal symptoms and rebound anxiety after a six week course of diazepam for generalized anxiety disorder. BMJ 290:1246–1248, 1985

Ray WA, Fought RL, Decker MD: Psychoactive drugs and the risk of injurious motor vehicle crashes in elderly drivers. Am J Epidemiol 136:873–883, 1992

Reed CF, Witt PN, Peakall DB: Freehand copying of a geometric pattern as a test for sensory-motor disturbance. Percept Mot Skills 20:941, 1965

Rickels K: Clinical management of benzodiazepine dependence (letter). BMJ 291:1649, 1985

Rickels K: Long-term treatment of anxiety and risk of withdrawal: prospective comparison of clorazepate and buspirone. Arch Gen Psychiatry 45:444–450, 1988

Rickels K, Schweizer EE: Benzodiazepines for treatment of panic attacks: a new look. Psychopharmacol Bull 23:93–99, 1986

Rickels K, Case WG, Downing RW, et al: Long-term diazepam, therapy and clinical outcome. JAMA 250:767–771, 1983

Rickels K, Schweizer E, Case WG, et al: Benzodiazepine dependence, withdrawal severity, and clinical outcome: effects of personality. Psychopharmacol Bull 24:415–420, 1988

Rickels K, Schweizer E, Case WG, et al: Long-term therapeutic use of benzodiazepines, I: effects of abrupt discontinuation. Arch Gen Psychiatry 47:899–907, 1990

Rickels K, Case WG, Schweizer E, et al: Long-term benzodiazepine users 3 years after participation in a discontinuation program. Am J Psychiatry 148:757–761, 1991

Rickels K, Downing R, Schweizer E, et al: Antidepressants for the treatment of generalized anxiety disorder: a placebo-controlled comparison of imipramine, trazodone, and diazepam. Arch Gen Psychiatry 50:884–895, 1993

Rickels K, Lucki I, Schweizer E, et al: Psychomotor performance of long term benzodiazepine users, before, during and after benzodiazepine discontinuation. J Clin Psychopharmacol 19:107–113, 1999

Rinaldi RD, Steindler EM, Wilford BB, et al: Clarification and standardization of substance abuse terminology. JAMA 259:555–557, 1988

Ringrose CAD: The hazard of neurotrophic drugs in the fertile years. Can Med Assoc J 106:1058, 1972

Roach JD, Griffiths RR: Comparison of triazolam and pentobarbital: performance impairment, subjective effects and abuse liability. J Pharmacol Exp Ther 234:120–133, 1985

Roach JD, Griffiths RR: Lorazepam and meprobamate dose effects in humans: behavioral effects and abuse liability. J Pharmacol Exp Ther 243:978–988, 1987

Romach M, Busto U, Somer MA, et al: Clinical aspects of the chronic use of alprazolam and lorazepam. Am J Psychiatry 152:1161–1167, 1995

Rosenbaum JF: Attitudes towards benzodiazepines over the years. J Clin Psychiatry 66 (suppl 2):4–8, 2005

Rosenbaum JF, Woods SW, Groves JE, et al: Emergence of hostility during alprazolam treatment. Am J Psychiatry 141:792–793, 1984

Rosenberg L, Mitchell AA, Parsells JL, et al: Lack of relation of oral clefts to diazepam use during pregnancy. N Engl J Med 309:1282–1285, 1983

Ross HE: Benzodiazepine use and anxiolytics abuse and dependence in treated alcoholics. Addiction 88:209–218, 1993

Ross J, Darke S, Hall W: Transitions between routes of benzodiazepine administration among heroin users in Sydney. Addiction 92:697–705, 1997

Roth T, Hartse KM, Saab PG, et al: The effects of flurazepam, lorazepam and triazolam on sleep and memory. Psychopharmacology (Berl) 70:231–237, 1980

Rothstein E, Cobble JC, Sampson N: Chlordiazepoxide: long-term use in alcoholism. Ann N Y Acad Sci 273:381–384, 1976

Routledge PA, Kitchell BB, Bjornson TD, et al: Diazepam and N-desmethyldiazepam redistribution after heparin. Clin Pharmacol Ther 27:528–532, 1980

Rowlatt RJ: Effective maternal diazepam on the newborn (letter). BMJ 1(6118):985, 1978

Safra MJ, Oakley GP: Association between cleft lip with or without cleft palate and prenatal exposure to diazepam. Lancet 2(7933):478–480, 1975

Sakol MS, Power KG: The effects of long term benzodiazepine treatment and graded withdrawal on psychomotor performance. Psychopharmacology (Berl) 95:135–138, 1988

Salinsky JV, Dore CJ: Characteristics of long term benzodiazepine users in general practice. J R Coll Gen Pract 37:202–204, 1987

Salzman C: APA Task Force report on benzodiazepine dependence, toxicity, and abuse. Am J Psychiatry 148:151–152, 1991

Sangal R: Inhibited female orgasm as a side effect of alprazolam (letter). Am J Psychiatry 142:1223–1224, 1985

Saxen I: Associations between oral clefts and drugs taken during pregnancy. Int J Epidemiol 4:37–44, 1975

Saxen I, Lahti A: Cleft lip and palate in Finland: incidence, secular, seasonal, and geographical variations. Teratology 9:217–224, 1974

Schardein JL (ed): Chemically Induced Birth Defects, 2nd Edition. New York, Marcel Dekker, 1993

Scharf MB, Fletcher K, Graham JP: Comparative amnesic effects of benzodiazepine hypnotic agents. J Clin Psychiatry 49:134–137, 1988

Schwartz HI: An empirical review of the impact of triplicate prescription of benzodiazepines. Hosp Community Psychiatry 43:382–385, 1992

Schwartz HI, Blank K: Regulation of benzodiazepine prescribing practices: clinical implications. Gen Hosp Psychiatry 13:219–224, 1991

Schweizer E: Once daily control of panic disorder: evidence from a placebo controlled study of alprazolam-XR. Psychiatric Annals 23 (10, suppl):32–37, 1993

Schweizer E, Rickels K: Failure of buspirone and placebo in relieving benzodiazepine withdrawal symptoms. Am J Psychiatry 143:1590–1592, 1986

Schweizer E, Rickels K, Case WG, et al; Long-term therapeutic uses of benzodiazepines, II: effects of gradual taper. Arch Gen Psychiatry 47:908–915, 1990

Schweizer E, Rickels K, Case WG, et al: Carbamazepine treatment in patients discontinuing long term benzodiazepine therapy: effects on withdrawal severity and outcome. Arch Gen Psychiatry 48:448–452, 1991

Schweizer E, Rickels K, Weiss S, et al: Maintenance drug treatment of panic disorder, I: results of a prospective, placebo controlled comparison of alprazolam and imipramine. Arch Gen Psychiatry 50:51–60, 1993

Schweizer E, Case WG, Garcia-Espana F, et al: Progesterone co-administration in patients discontinuing benzodiazepine therapy: effects on withdrawal severity and taper outcome. Psychopharmacology (Berl) 117:424–429, 1995

Schweizer E, Rickels K, DeMartinis N, et al: The effect of personality on withdrawal severity and taper outcome in benzodiazepine patients. Psychol Med 28:713–720, 1998

Scott AK, Kher AS, Steele WH, et al: Oxazepam pharmacokinetics in patients with epilepsy treated long term with phenytoin alone or in combination with phenobarbitone. Br J Clin Pharmacol 16:441–444, 1983

Shader RI, Georgotas A, Greenblatt DJ, et al: Impaired absorption of desmethyldiazepam from clorazepate by magnesium aluminum hydroxide. Clin Pharmacol Ther 24:308–315, 1978

Sheehan DV: Benzodiazepines in panic disorder and agoraphobia. J Affect Disord 13:169–181, 1987

Sheehan DV: Why sustained release formulations? Practical considerations in the management of patients with anxiety. Psychiatric Annals October 23 (suppl 10):3–7, 1993

Sheehan DV, Uzogara E, Coleman JH, et al: The treatment of panic attacks with agoraphobia with alprazolam and ibuprofen: a controlled study. Presentation at the annual meeting of the American Psychiatric Association, Toronto, Canada, May 1982

Sheehan DV, Coleman JH, Greenblatt DJ, et al: Some biochemical correlates of panic attacks with agoraphobia and their response to a new treatment. J Clin Psychopharmacol 4:66–75, 1984

Sheehan DV, Raj BA, Harnett-Sheehan K, et al: Adinazolam sustained release formulation in the treatment of generalized anxiety disorder. J Anxiety Disord 4:239–246, 1990a

Sheehan DV, Raj BA, Harnett-Sheehan K, et al: Adinazolam sustained release formulation in the treatment of panic disorder. Irish J Psychol Med 7:124–128, 1990b

Sheehan DV, Raj BA, Harnett-Sheehan K, et al: The relative efficacy of high dose buspirone and alprazolam in the treatment of panic disorder: a double blind placebo controlled study. Acta Psychiatr Scand 88:1–11, 1993

Sheehan DV, Raj BA, Dorotheo J, et al: Method for assessing the duration of therapeutic action and milligram equivalence of anxiolytics. Anxiety 2:40–46, 1996

Sheehan DV, Harnett-Sheehan K, Raj BA: The speed of onset of action of alprazolam-XR compared to alprazolam-CT in panic disorder. Psychopharmacol Bull 40:63–81, 2007

Sheehan MF, Sheehan DV, Torres A, et al: Snorting benzodiazepines. Am J Drug Alcohol Abuse 17:457–468, 1991

Shiono PH, Mills JL: Oral clefts and diazepam use during pregnancy. N Engl J Med 311:919–920, 1984

Skegg DCG, Richards SM, Doll R: Minor tranquilizers and road accidents. BMJ 1(6168):917–919, 1979

Skrabanek P: Smoking and statistical overkill. Lancet 340:1208–1209, 1992

Smiley A: Effects of minor tranquilizers and antidepressants on psychomotor performance. J Clin Psychiatry 48 (12, suppl): 22–28, 1987

Soumerai AB, Simoni-Wastila L, Singer C, et al: Lack of relationship between long-term use of benzodiazepines and escalation to high dosages. Psychiatr Serv 54:1006–1011, 2003

Spreight AN: Floppy-infant syndrome and maternal diazepam and/or nitrazepam (letter). Lancet 2(8043):878, 1977

Stahl SM: Alprazolam-XR: dosage considerations. Psychiatric Annals 23 (10, suppl):27–31, 1993

Stahl SM: Don't ask, don't tell, but benzodiazepines are still the leading treatments for anxiety disorder. J Clin Psychiatry 63:756–757, 2002

Sternbach LH: The discovery of CNS active 1,4-benzodiazepines (chemistry), in Pharmacology of Benzodiazepines. Edited by Usdin E, Skolnick P, Tallman JR, et al. London, Macmillan, 1982, pp 7–14

Strahan A, Rosenthal J, Kaswan M, et al: Three case reports of acute paroxysmal excitement associated with alprazolam treatment. Am J Psychiatry 142:859–861, 1985

Svenson EM, Persson L, Sjoberg L: Mood effects of diazepam and caffeine. Psychopharmacology (Berl) 62:73, 1980

Svenson SE, Hamilton RG: A critique of over emphasis on side effects with the psychotropic drugs: an analysis of 18,000 chlordiazepoxide treated cases. Current Therapeutic Research 8:455–464, 1966

Swantek SS, Grossberg GT, Neppe VM, et al: The use of carbamazepine to treat benzodiazepine withdrawal in a geriatric population. J Geriatr Psychiatry Neurol 4:106–115, 1991

Tamblyn R, Abrahamowicz M, du Berger R, et al: A 5-year prospective assessment of the risk associated with individual benzodiazepines and doses in new elderly users. J Am Geriatr Soc 53:233–241, 2005

Tata PR, Rollings J, Collins M, et al: Lack of cognitive recovery following withdrawal from benzodiazepine use. Psychol Med 24:203–213, 1994

Tesar GE, Rosenbaum JF, Pollack MH, et al: Double-blind, placebo-controlled comparison of clonazepam and alprazolam for panic disorder. J Clin Psychiatry 52:69–76, 1991

Tollefson G, Lesar T, Groble D, et al: Alprazolam-related digitoxin toxicity. Am J Psychiatry 141:1612–1613, 1984

Tyrer P, Rutherford D, Huggett T: Benzodiazepine withdrawal symptoms and propranolol. Lancet 1(8219):520–522, 1981

Tyrer P, Ferguson B, Hallstrom C, et al: A controlled trial of dothiepin and placebo in treating benzodiazepine withdrawal symptoms. Br J Psychiatry 168:457–461, 1996

Uhlenhuth EH, Balter MB, Ban TA, et al: International study of expert judgment on therapeutic use of benzodiazepines and other psychotherapeutic medications, VI: trends in recommendations for the pharmacotherapy of anxiety disorders, 1992–1997. Depress Anxiety 9:107–116, 1999

Van Etten ML, Taylor S: Comparative efficacy of treatments for posttraumatic stress disorder: a meta-analysis. Clin Psychol Psychother 5:126–144, 1998

Van Steveninck AL, Gieschke R, Shoemaker RC, et al: Pharmacokinetic and pharmacodynamic interactions of bretazenil and diazepam with alcohol. Br J Clin Pharmacol 41:565–573, 1996

Vela-Bueno A, Oliveros JC, Dobladez-Blanco B, et al: Brotizolam: a sleep laboratory evaluation. Eur J Clin Pharmacol 25: 53–56, 1983

Versiani M, Nardi AE, Figueira I, et al: Double blind placebo controlled trial with bromazepam in social phobia. Serie psicofarmacologia J Bras Psiquiatr 46:167–171, 1997

Wagner AK, Ross-Degnan D, Gurwitz JH, et al: Effect of New York State regulatory action on benzodiazepine prescribing and hip fracture rates. Ann Intern Med 146:96–103, 2007

Walker BE, Patterson A: Induction of cleft palate in mice by tranquillizers and barbiturates. Teratology 10:159–163, 1974

Wang PS, Bohn RL, Glynn RJ, et al: Hazardous benzodiazepine regimens in the elderly: effects of half-life, dosage, and duration on risk of hip fracture. Am J Psychiatry 158:892–898, 2001

Wee EL, Zimmermann EF: Involvement of GABA in palate morphogenesis and its relation to diazepam teratogenesis in two mouse strains. Teratology 28:15–22, 1983

Wolkowitz OM, Pickar D. Benzodiazepines in the treatment of schizophrenia: a review and reappraisal. Am J Psychiatry 148:714–726, 1991

Woods JH, Katz JL, Winger G: Benzodiazepines: use, abuse, and consequences. Pharmacol Rev 44:151–347, 1992

Woody GE, Mintz G, Ottare K, et al: Diazepam use by patients in a methadone program: how serious a problem? J Psychedelic Drugs 7:373, 1973

Woody GE, O'Brien CP, Greenstein R: Misuse and abuse of diazepam: an increasingly common medical problem. Int J Addict 10:843–848, 1975

Zimmermann EF: Neuropharmacologic teratogenesis and neurotransmitter regulation of palate development. American Journal of Mental Deficits 88:548–558, 1984

Zimmermann EF, Wee EL: Role of neurotransmitters in palate development. Current Topics in Developmental Biology 19:37–63, 1984

CHAPTER 25

Buspirone and Gepirone

Donald S. Robinson, M.D.

Karl Rickels, M.D.

Frank D. Yocca, Ph.D.

Evidence of altered central serotonergic function exists for several of the psychiatric disorders, especially the mood and anxiety disorders. Discovery of the serotonin$_{1A}$ (5-HT$_{1A}$) receptor was instrumental in linking modulation of serotonin neurotransmission to anxiety symptoms. Similarly, the tricyclic antidepressants (TCAs) and the selective serotonin reuptake inhibitors (SSRIs) implicated serotonin in the pathophysiology and treatment of depression.

The notion that serotonin (5-HT) plays a role in the treatment of anxiety initially arose from the discovery that both acute and chronic administration of benzodiazepines reduced turnover of 5-HT in rat brain and that administration of para-chlorophenylalanine (pCPA), an inhibitor of serotonin synthesis, mimics the effects of benzodiazepines in behavioral models of anxiety utilizing a conflict paradigm (Wise et al. 1972). Subsequent characterization of subtypes of 5-HT receptor, especially the 5-HT$_{1A}$ and 5-HT$_2$ receptors, and discovery of the 5-HT$_{1A}$ receptor partial agonist buspirone inferred that serotonin plays a key role in anxiolysis (Eison and Eison 1994). Because both the benzodiazepines and buspirone were found to pharmacologically reduce 5-HT impulse flow, albeit by different mechanisms, it was hypothesized that enhanced serotonergic tone might be an underlying factor in the etiology of anxiety disorders.

The 5-HT$_{1A}$ Receptor

The development of specific pharmacological ligands in combination with molecular cloning and subsequent expression in heterologous systems has led to the unequivocal identification of 14 different 5-HT receptor subtypes (Hoyer et al. 2002). Except for the 5-HT$_3$ receptor, all 5-HT receptor subtypes are members of the large family of seven transmembrane domain G protein–coupled receptors (Pierce et al. 2002). The 5-HT$_{1A}$ receptor is one of the most important receptors in this class and of the subfamily that couples negatively to adenylyl cyclase (De Vivo and Maayani 1986). It has been the most extensively studied 5-HT receptor because 1) identification of the selective agonists, including 8-OH-DPAT (Hamon et al. 1984) and the azapirones, and specific receptor antagonists (WAY-100635; Fletcher et al. 1996) have allowed for strict pharmacological classification; 2) it is the first 5-HT receptor to be cloned and sequenced (Fargin et al. 1988; Kobilka et al. 1987); 3) polyclonal antibodies have been generated for subcellular distribution studies in brain (Azmetia et al. 1996; El Mestikawy et al. 1990); and 4) human, rat, and mouse receptors have been cloned and sequenced (Albert et al. 1998; Charest et al. 1993; Fargin et al. 1988) in support of the translational studies. Furthermore, several studies have determined that the 5-HT$_{1A}$ receptor may play a role in neural development (del Olmo et al. 1998; Gross et al. 2002). Taken together with the recent implications of a salutary effect of chronic SSRI treatment on neurogenesis (Duman et al. 2001) and the fact that 5-HT$_{1A}$ agonists exhibit positive treatment effects in both anxiety and depressive states (Robinson et al. 1989a), the body of evidence suggests that this receptor plays a central role in neuropsychiatric disorders.

Distribution and Function

The regional distribution of the 5-HT$_{1A}$ receptors was established using both selective agonist and antagonist ligands with antibodies that were raised against unique peptide sequences within the receptor protein as well as mRNA densities. Studies utilizing the full agonist [^{3}H]8-OH-DPAT (8-hydroxy-2-[N-dipropylamino]-tetralin) and the putative 5-HT$_{1A}$ receptor antagonist ligand [^{3}H]WAY-100635 reveal high levels of specific binding in hippocampus, raphe nuclei, amygdala, hypothalamus, and cortex (Burnet et al. 1997; Palacios et al. 1990). The results with autoradiography were mirrored by the finding of localization of messenger RNA (mRNA) densities in these regions as well (Burnet et al. 1995; Chalmers and Watson 1991). At the subcellular level, the receptor was found to be localized on cell bodies and dendrites of 5-HT–containing neurons projecting to limbic brain regions. In limbic regions receiving input from 5-HT–containing neurons, particularly hippocampus and cortex, 5-HT$_{1A}$ receptors are located predominantly postsynaptically (Palacios et al. 1990; Riad et al. 2000).

Pharmacological and Clinical Implications

The high regional density of 5-HT$_{1A}$ receptors in midbrain, hippocampus, and limbic areas of the brain is consistent with the notion that 5-HT neurotransmission modulates mood and anxiety. These brain regions of high density of 5-HT$_{1A}$ receptors play key roles in regulating diverse vital processes, including thermoregulation, endocrine function, appetite, aggressive and sexual behavior, and mood. Mice lacking the 5-HT$_{1A}$ receptor gene exhibit various manifestations of anxious behavior with stress (Parks et al. 1998) and exhibit increased autonomic hyperactivity when exposed to foot shock (Pattij et al. 2002).

5-HT$_{1A}$ receptors located on 5-HT–containing neurons in midbrain raphe regions modulate release of 5-HT at synapses in forebrain. These somatodendritic autoreceptors control impulse flow (Yocca 1990), synthesis (Yocca 1990), and release (Sharp et al. 1989) of neurotransmitter from ascending 5-HT–containing neurons. Postmortem study of suicide victims reveals enhanced ra-

dioligand binding of [^{3}H]8-OH-DPAT to the inhibitory 5-HT$_{1A}$ autoreceptors located in the dorsal raphe, providing pharmacological evidence in support of the hypothesis that depressed suicide victims may have diminished activity of 5-HT neurons (Stockmeier et al. 1998). Blunted 5-HT$_{1A}$ receptor–mediated response of corticosteroids has been reported in patients with major depressive disorder (MDD), suggesting that there is desensitization of these receptors in patients with anxiety and depression (Lesch 1992; Rausch et al. 1990; Stahl 1992). In regions postsynaptic to ascending raphe neurons such as prefrontal cortex, altered levels of 5-HT$_{1A}$ receptor binding have been found in the prefrontal cortex of depressed suicide victims (Matsubara et al. 1991), although conflicting evidence exists (Arranz et al. 1994; Cheetham et al. 1990).

The 5-HT$_{1A}$ Receptor and Partial Agonists

Given the large body of work implicating 5-HT in the etiology and treatment of affective disorders, and the role of the 5-HT$_{1A}$ receptor in the control of central 5-HT neurotransmission, it is not surprising to find that drugs targeting this receptor would have an impact in the treatment of mood disorders. It would seem logical to implicate this receptor because 5-HT–acting drugs, such as TCAs and monoamine oxidase inhibitors (MAOIs), increase synaptic concentrations of the neurotransmitter. Furthermore, there is a region-dependent difference in responses to 5-HT$_{1A}$ agonists at pre- and postsynaptic 5-HT$_{1A}$ receptors. This may be attributable to a difference in regional receptor reserve (Meller et al. 1990; Yocca et al. 1992). Therefore, the proper degree of agonism at both pre- and postsynaptic 5-HT$_{1A}$ receptors may be critical to achieving an optimal level of efficacy/tolerability using this pharmacological approach.

Drugs acting as partial agonists represent an attractive strategy for discovery of new psychiatric agents, potentially offering therapeutic advantages (Yocca and Altar 2006). It is postulated that this emerging class of successful central nervous system drugs acts in part by signal attenuation at one or multiple target receptors. Partial agonist compounds, such as buspirone and aripiprazole, produce a desired therapeutic response, with excellent safety and tolerability. Interestingly, among the first drugs in this category were selective partial agonists of 5-HT$_{1A}$ receptors. These agents have undergone extensive clinical development for treatment of both generalized anxiety disorder (GAD) and MDD. As yet, only buspirone has received marketing approval. Gepirone, a 5-HT$_{1A}$ agonist with greater intrinsic activity postsynaptically, has been extensively investigated as an anxiolytic and as an antidepressant agent. A new drug application (NDA) for gepirone extended-release (ER) for treatment of MDD recently failed to obtain U.S. Food and Drug Administration (FDA) approval. An NDA for GAD and hyposexual desire disorder by the drug sponsor is under consideration. Several other selective 5-HT$_{1A}$ agonists (ipsapirone, flesinoxan, tandospirone) have been unsuccessful in clinical development for a target clinical indication of either GAD or MDD.

Buspirone

History and Development

Buspirone hydrochloride, an azaspirodecanedione derivative (Figure 25–1), was synthesized in 1968 in the laboratories of Mead Johnson by Wu et al. (1969). Based on positive findings in conditioned-avoidance testing in rats, buspirone was originally studied clinically as a putative antipsychotic agent. It was projected to be largely devoid of the typical side effects of the antipsychotic class of drugs, but clinical trials failed to demonstrate usefulness in the treatment of schizophrenia (Sathananthan et al. 1975). Further study revealed that a single dose of buspirone had a marked taming effect in aggressive monkeys (Tompkins et al. 1980). In various behavioral models of anxiety in rodents, buspirone inhibited foot shock–induced fighting and prevented shock-induced suppression of drinking behavior, both screening tests predictive of anxiolytic effects (Riblet et al. 1982). At that time, minimal data were available on the molecular pharmacology of buspirone. However, Riblet et al. (1982) reported that buspirone displaced [^{3}H]spiperone from dopamine D$_2$ receptors in rat striatal membranes with an IC$_{50}$ of 260 nM and demonstrated a right shift in binding activity in the presence of guanosine triphosphate (GTP), suggesting that it was a D$_2$ agonist. Until the subsequent finding of high affinity binding to the newly discovered 5-HT$_{1A}$ receptor some 4 years later, the basis for the anxiolytic activity of buspirone was thought to be dopaminergic in origin.

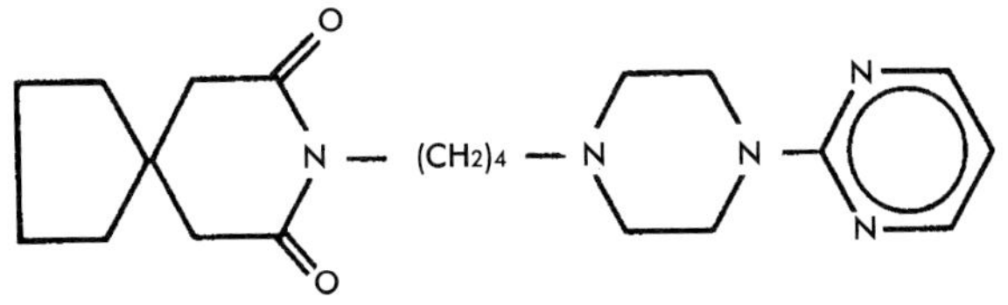

A Phase II proof-of-concept study in patients with DSM-II (American Psychiatric Association 1968) anxiety disorder demonstrated significant anxiolytic treatment effects of buspirone compared with placebo (Goldberg and Finnerty 1979), leading to a full-scale clinical development as an antianxiety agent (Robinson 1991).

Pharmacological Profile

Buspirone is relatively inactive in receptor binding studies in vitro at noradrenergic, cholinergic, and histaminergic sites. It does not displace [^{3}H]diazepam or [^{3}H]nitrazepam from the benzodiazepine receptor complex or affect γ-aminobutyric acid (GABA) modulation of the benzodiazepine binding site (Riblet et al. 1982). Although buspirone does displace [^{3}H]spiperone from rat striatal membranes at relatively high concentrations (Mennini et al. 1986, 1987), dopamine receptor binding is believed to play no role in either the therapeutic or side effects of buspirone (Eison et al. 1991).

The discovery that nanomolar quantities of buspirone displaced [^{3}H]5-HT from hippocampal membranes (Glaser and Traber 1983) led to elucidation of interactions of buspirone with specific central 5-HT receptors. Buspirone was found to inhibit [^{3}H]5-HT binding to cortical and hippocampal membranes (Skolnick et al. 1985). Later, it was determined that buspirone selectively displaced [^{3}H]8-OH-DPAT from 5-HT$_{1A}$ receptor binding sites in rat hippocampal membranes with high affinity (24 nM) (Yocca 1990).

The antianxiety properties of buspirone appear to be exerted through its actions at both pre- and postsynaptic 5-HT$_{1A}$ receptors (Eison and Eison 1994; Yocca 1990). At presynaptic 5-HT$_{1A}$ receptors located in the dorsal raphe, buspirone acts as a full agonist, inhibiting neuronal 5-HT synthesis and firing, whereas at postsynaptic receptors in hippocampus and cortex, it functions as a partial agonist. It is postulated that the anxiolytic effect of buspirone is dependent on its serotonergic actions in the presence of a preexisting deficiency of this neurotransmitter.

Buspirone does differ from benzodiazepines because of its lack of inhibition of spontaneous motor activity, effects on motor coordination, and induction of the serotonin syndrome in rats (Eison et al. 1991). Buspirone lacks abuse potential and does not impair psychomotor performance either alone or in combination with ethanol, unlike the benzodiazepines (Smiley 1987; Sussman and Chow 1988). The behavioral effects of buspirone and benzodiazepines differ in a number of animal models of anxiety (Barrett and Witkin 1991). Unlike benzodiaz-

FIGURE 25–1. Chemical structure of buspirone.

epines, buspirone does not uniformly increase punished or conflict responding in rats and monkeys, and when increased responding is observed, the magnitude of response tends to be less than that of a benzodiazepine.

By contrast, in pigeons buspirone enhances punished response with a magnitude equivalent to benzodiazepines. This finding is characteristic of the 5-HT_{1A} receptor agonists, including 8-OH-DPAT, gepirone, and agents of this class. Other classes of psychotropic drugs—for example, TCAs, SSRIs, opioids, antipsychotics, and psychomotor stimulants—do not increase responding in this behavioral model. Buspirone also enhances exploratory and social interaction behaviors in rodents, similar to the benzodiazepines.

Of interest, 5-HT_{1A} agonists also demonstrate activity in an animal model of depression. Similar to imipramine, desipramine, and fluoxetine, 5-HT_{1A} agonists such as 8-OH-DPAT and the azapirones buspirone, gepirone, ipsapirone, and tandospirone produce antidepressant-like behavior in the forced-swim test in rats (Wieland and Lucki 1990). This occurs in the absence of changes in locomotor activity and is not diminished by pretreatment with the 5-HT synthesis inhibitor pCPA, suggesting that 5-HT_{1A} agonists produce an antidepressant response through postsynaptic effects on 5-HT_{1A} receptors. The major azapirone metabolite, 1-(2-pyrimidinyl) piperazine (1-PP), is devoid of behavioral activity in this test. The finding of activity in a preclinical model of depression comports with clinical studies of both buspirone and gepirone, which are indicative of antidepressant effects.

Pharmacokinetics and Disposition

With oral administration, buspirone is subject to extensive first-pass metabolism, with an elimination half-life of 3 to 4 hours (mean) in normal subjects (Gammans and Johnston 1991). In the liver, buspirone undergoes extensive metabolic transformation by cytochrome P450 3A4 enzymes. Ingestion of food prolongs the elimination half-life of buspirone, as is also the case with significant hepatic and renal impairment. The pharmacokinetics of buspirone in elderly patients do not differ importantly from those in young adults (Gammans et al. 1989).

It was known that buspirone had three major metabolites of varying pharmacological activities: 5-hydroxybuspirone (5-OH-Bu), 8-hydroxybuspirone (8-OH-Bu), and 1-PP. Because buspirone blocks α_2-adrenergic receptors, it is postulated that unwanted noradrenergic effects of 1-PP might be deleterious in patients experiencing benzodiazepine withdrawal or panic attacks. The poten-

tial therapeutic advantage, if any, of 5-HT_{1A} partial agonists lacking the 1-PP metabolite is presently unknown.

Identification of 6-Hydroxybuspirone as a Major Active Metabolite

More recently, conversion of buspirone to the metabolite 6-hydroxybuspirone (6-OH-Bu) by means of biotransformation in human liver microsomes was identified as the predominant metabolic pathway involved in the hepatic clearance of buspirone (Zhu et al. 2005). Plasma levels of 6-OH-Bu were found to be 40-fold greater than those of buspirone following oral administration in humans (Dockens et al. 2006). In vitro, 6-OH-Bu demonstrates high affinity (25 nM) and partial agonist activity for the 5-HT_{1A} receptor, whereas 6-OH-Bu in vivo exhibits anxiolytic activity in the fear-induced ultrasonic vocalization paradigm (F. D. Yocca, unpublished observations, June 1998). The plasma clearance, volume of distribution, and elimination half-life of 6-OH-Bu are similar to those of buspirone, but the bioavailability of 6-OH-Bu is significantly greater (19% vs. 1.4%; Wong et al. 2007). As with buspirone, 6-OH-Bu demonstrates in vivo occupancy of 5-HT_{1A} receptors after intravenous administration in rats, with a fourfold greater potency exhibited in dorsal raphe than in the hippocampus (Wong et al. 2007). Taken together, these findings suggest that 6-OH-Bu contributes significantly to the therapeutic effect of buspirone.

Switching From Benzodiazepine Therapy to Buspirone

A major pharmacodynamic interaction occurs in patients previously treated with benzodiazepines on switching to buspirone. Both tolerability and the therapeutic response to buspirone differ significantly in anxious patients naive to benzodiazepine treatment compared with patients previously treated with a benzodiazepine (DeMartinis et al. 2000; Schweizer and Rickels 1986). Meta-analysis of placebo-controlled efficacy trials of buspirone revealed that GAD patients with either no prior benzodiazepine treatment or temporally remote benzodiazepine treatment (>6 months previously) improved more with buspirone therapy than patients recently treated with a benzodiazepine. The mechanism of this pharmacodynamic interaction is not established, but it may reflect a subtle underlying benzodiazepine withdrawal syndrome (possibly exacerbated by 1-PP). It is also possible that previously treated patients might be preconditioned by benzodiazepine therapy and hold expectations involving the mildly euphoriant, sedating properties of a benzodiazepine. One wonders if successful past treatment with a benzodiazepine influences future attempts to treat anxiety with a nonbenzodiazepine such as buspirone. In the placebo-controlled trials, patients who had received recent prior benzodiazepine therapy and were randomly assigned to the benzodiazepine treatment group may have benefited from reinstitution of benzodiazepine treatment, with resultant amelioration of an unrecognized (subclinical) withdrawal syndrome.

Mechanism of Action

While it has been clearly established that the anxiolytic effects of buspirone are mediated by its actions on 5-HT receptors in the limbic system (Eison and Eison 1994; Yocca 1990), buspirone also has unrelated neuroendocrine effects reflective of a complex pharmacology. Preclinical studies have shown buspirone possesses characteristics of both a D_2 agonist and antagonist in addition to being a 5-HT$_{1A}$ agonist. These pharmacological attributes are important in understanding the neuroendocrine actions of buspirone, because it is well established that prolactin is regulated by the neurotransmitter dopamine acting via D_2 receptors in the anterior pituitary gland. Furthermore, the evidence indicates that 5-HT$_{1A}$ receptors regulate neuroendocrine hormones, such as growth hormone, adrenocorticotropic hormone (ACTH) release, and corticosterone (Gilbert et al. 1988; Pan and Gilbert 1992; Van de Kar et al. 1985). This notion was further substantiated in a study by Vicentic et al. (1998) in which increases in plasma levels of oxytocin, ACTH, and corticosterone induced by the selective 5-HT$_{1A}$ agonist 8-OH-DPAT were blocked by administration of the selective 5-HT$_{1A}$ antagonist WAY-100635.

Meltzer and Fleming (1982) showed that buspirone produces a dose-dependent increase in rat plasma prolactin levels. Furthermore, buspirone has been shown to antagonize the inhibitory effects of dopamine on prolactin release from the rat pituitary gland in vitro, illustrative of its partial agonist activity at D_2 receptors (Meltzer et al. 1991). Buspirone enhances secretion of corticosterone in rats, whereas in patients it increases prolactin, growth hormone, and corticosterone levels when administered orally (Meltzer et al. 1991). In healthy volunteers, buspirone, ipsapirone, and gepirone have been shown to increase plasma cortisol, prolactin, and growth hormone and to decrease body temperature (Cowen et al. 1990). Buspirone stimulation of prolactin and corticosterone secretion in the rat is enhanced by pretreatment with pCPA, whereas spiperone inhibits buspirone-induced increases in rat corticosterone secretion (Meltzer et al.

1991). Pindolol, a 5-HT$_{1A}$ antagonist, does not block the buspirone-induced increase in prolactin (Meltzer et al. 1991). Taken together, these results suggest that the neuroendocrine effects of buspirone in rat and man are complex, exhibiting pharmacological properties of both a dopamine antagonist and a 5-HT$_{1A}$ agonist.

Indications and Efficacy

Generalized Anxiety Disorder

The efficacy of buspirone was established in a series of well-controlled trials conducted in the 1970s and 1980s in a patient population with the DSM-II diagnosis of anxiety disorder (Robinson 1991). The clinical development program of buspirone as an anxiolytic agent was undertaken after positive findings in a placebo-controlled proof-of-concept study in anxious patients (Goldberg and Finnerty 1979). It is of interest that the study investigators commented on the possibility that buspirone possesses antidepressant as well as anxiolytic properties. In a series of Phase III placebo-controlled clinical trials comparing buspirone and diazepam, the efficacy of these two anxiolytics was comparable in patients fulfilling diagnostic criteria for DSM-II anxiety neurosis (Boehm et al. 1990a; Goldberg and Finnerty 1982; Rickels et al. 1982). In these double-blind dosage titration studies, buspirone and diazepam were prescribed on a thrice-daily schedule in dosages (mean) ranging from 20 to 25 mg/day during 4 weeks of treatment.

By the time the FDA granted marketing approval of buspirone in 1986, the newest DSM classification system, DSM-III (American Psychiatric Association 1980), had replaced anxiety neurosis with the diagnostic category of GAD. As a result of this change, retrospective statistical analyses of the placebo-controlled efficacy trials were carried out. Analyses of Hamilton Anxiety Scale (Ham-A; Hamilton 1959) and other symptom ratings were found to be consistent with a diagnosis of DSM-III GAD, so buspirone received FDA-approved labeling for this clinical indication.

In the controlled trials, buspirone was noted to have a slightly slower onset of therapeutic effect than the benzodiazepines (Enkelmann 1991; Pecknold et al. 1989; Rickels 1990). This perceived slower onset of effect was attributable to differences between buspirone and benzodiazepines in early relief of somatic anxiety symptoms but was not due to a difference in relief of psychic anxiety symptoms. It was postulated that absence of sedation with buspirone contributed to a perception of more gradual onset of anxiolytic effect, because relief of somatic anxiety, particularly insomnia, was only manifest with buspirone treatment after psychic anxiety symptoms had abated, whereas the immediate sedating properties of benzodiazepines accounted for a perception of faster onset of therapeutic benefit. A similar slower onset of effectiveness in anxiety disorders occurs with imipramine (Rickels et al. 1993) and SSRI treatment (Rickels et al. 2003).

A longer-term 6-month double-blind comparative trial of buspirone and benzodiazepines found a similar slow onset of anxiolytic effect with buspirone compared with clorazepate during the first 4 weeks of treatment (Rickels et al. 1988). However, with ongoing treatment the therapeutic response to the two drugs was thereafter similar. On double-blind termination of treatment after 6 months, patients who stopped clorazepate abruptly relapsed during a 4-week observation period, whereas the buspirone group experienced no symptom changes. These findings confirmed the observation of others (Fontaine et al. 1984; Noyes et al. 1988) that rapid return of symptoms on discontinuation of clorazepate is attributable to a benzodiazepine withdrawal syndrome and not to recrudescence of symptoms of the underlying anxiety disorder, because this did not occur with abrupt discontinuation of buspirone.

Possible clinical benefit of buspirone therapy on the benzodiazepine withdrawal syndrome was assessed in 15 chronic anxiety patients representing 146 cumulative years of tranquilizer exposure who had previously failed in attempts at both abrupt and gradual withdrawal of benzodiazepine treatment (Schweizer and Rickels 1986). In this study, addition of buspirone overlapping with tapering of benzodiazepine dosage failed to ameliorate benzodiazepine withdrawal symptoms, and none of the patients could be maintained on buspirone alone after complete withdrawal of benzodiazepine treatment. In several other studies, buspirone appears to have only modest beneficial effect on the benzodiazepine withdrawal syndrome (DeMartinis et al. 2000; Shiaie et al. 1995; Udelman and Udelman 1990).

Since the approval and availability of buspirone for clinical use, a limited number of well-controlled efficacy trials in GAD were conducted. One reason for this was its relatively short product life cycle and the fact that the drug sponsor was developing a successor to buspirone, the azapirone analog gepirone. After buspirone's approval, several placebo-controlled efficacy studies in anxiety disorders were conducted, and they reported that it had significant anxiolytic properties (Enkelmann 1991; Laakman et al. 1998; Lader and Scotto 1998; Murphy et al.

1989; Pecknold et al. 1989; Scheibe 1996). In a family practice setting, Boehm et al. (1990a) studied 60 patients with anxiety disorder in a placebo-controlled trial comparing the benzodiazepine clobazam and buspirone. In this 3-week treatment trial, treatment with clobazam and buspirone was equally effective and superior to placebo in relieving anxiety, as measured by the Ham-A and the Clinical Global Impressions–Improvement (CGI-I) scale.

In a large placebo-controlled, fixed-dose multicenter study comparing buspirone and venlafaxine extended-release (XR) in GAD, neither venlafaxine XR nor buspirone differed significantly from placebo on the primary efficacy outcome measure, Ham-A total score (Davidson et al. 1999). On several secondary outcome measures, buspirone treatment appeared less effective than venlafaxine XR but did result in significant improvement in CGI-I scores compared with placebo treatment. One limitation of this trial was utilization of a fixed-dose study design, which underestimates treatment effects as compared with a flexible-dose study design in depression efficacy trials (Robinson and Khan 2004).

Acute treatment of chronically anxious patients is often best managed initially with a benzodiazepine; however, longer-term use of a benzodiazepine can lead to physical dependence and symptom chronicity. For this reason, some patient populations are inappropriate for benzodiazepine therapy due to history of substance abuse or potential risk of cognitive impairment. When initiating therapy with buspirone, one should inform the patient that it is less sedating, with a more gradual onset of action, than benzodiazepine treatment. Patients can be reassured that if they require long-term drug therapy, buspirone will not lead to physical dependence or withdrawal symptoms on discontinuation. Patients also should be informed that acute or long-term treatment with buspirone does not impair cognition or ability to acquire new coping skills (Rickels and Schweizer 1990).

Long-term follow-up at 40 months of patients who previously completed a prior 6-month controlled trial comparing buspirone and clorazepate revealed that none of the buspirone-treated patients was taking either a regular or as-needed anxiolytic medication, whereas 30% of patients originally treated with clorazepate still required daily benzodiazepine therapy, and an additional 24% took benzodiazepines intermittently. Thus, more than 50% of patients treated for 6 months with clorazepate, but none of the buspirone-treated patients, were taking ongoing anxiolytic medication after 3 years (Rickels and Schweizer 1990). Scheibe (1996) reported similar observations in long-term follow-up of an acute efficacy controlled trial of patients with anxiety disorders. In this latter study, at 40 months 38% of buspirone-treated patients still required buspirone therapy, whereas 64% of patients treated with lorazepam required benzodiazepine medication.

The therapeutic advantages of buspirone treatment in elderly anxious patients include the fact the drug both is nonsedating and spares cognitive and memory functions. Buspirone has been studied in elderly patients with anxiety symptoms in a double-blind, placebo-controlled trial and shown to be safe and effective (Boehm et al. 1990b). Meta-analyses of several multicenter trials of buspirone in elderly patients also indicated that the drug is very safe and well tolerated by older patients (Ritchie and Cox 1993; Robinson et al. 1988).

Panic Disorder

Buspirone treatment has been evaluated in patients with panic disorder in placebo-controlled trials (Pohl et al. 1989; Sheehan et al. 1990). These trials did not find that buspirone diminished the number of panic attacks significantly. However, meta-analysis of the double-blind, three-arm multicenter trials comparing buspirone, imipramine, and placebo treatment found that both imipramine and buspirone had significant anxiolytic effects in panic disorder (Robinson et al. 1989b). Absence of buspirone effect on number of panic attacks is not surprising, given the findings of preclinical testing showing that buspirone causes increased firing rates of the locus coeruleus (Eison and Temple 1986) and noradrenergic hyperactivity (Charney and Heninger 1985), both manifestations of panic disorder.

Mixed Anxiety–Depression and Major Depressive Disorder

It was observed in early trials of patients with anxiety disorder and subsyndromal depression that depressive symptoms also improved significantly during buspirone treatment (Feighner et al. 1982; Goldberg and Finnerty 1979). This generated interest in the potential antidepressant properties of buspirone because of the high comorbidity of GAD and MDD (T.A. Brown and Barlow 1992). It has been suggested that GAD and MDD may exhibit differing clinical manifestations of a single underlying diathesis. Genetic studies in patients with MDD and GAD suggest that the genetic vulnerability for both disorders is largely shared (Kendler et al. 1992). Wray et al. (2007) recently described a likely genetic association between variants of the gene *PlexinA2* and anxiety disorders, providing potential evidence for the adult neurogenesis theory of depression.

Several placebo-controlled trials of buspirone have been conducted in patients with MDD and significant associated anxiety symptoms (Rickels et al. 1991; Robinson et al. 1990). For inclusion, patients with MDD were eligible if their Hamilton Rating Scale for Depression (Ham-D; Hamilton 1960) and Ham-A scores were 18 or greater and 15 or greater, respectively. Following a starting dosage of 5 mg thrice daily for 3 days, the daily dosage in these dosage titration studies ranged up to a maximum of buspirone 90 mg/day (mean, ~50 mg/day). Buspirone treatment was found to be superior to placebo treatment, with a global response rate based on CGI-I score of 70% for buspirone and 35% for placebo (Rickels et al. 1991). In a subsequent placebo-controlled study involving 177 geriatric depressed outpatients, Schweizer et al. (1998) compared buspirone and imipramine treatment for 8 weeks. There was a statistically significant treatment effect for both buspirone (mean daily dose, ~50 mg) and imipramine (mean daily dose, ~90 mg) compared with placebo treatment. Global improvement (CGI-I) with buspirone and imipramine was 80% and 86%, respectively, compared with 49% with placebo treatment.

Open-label augmentation of SSRI treatment of partially responding depressed patients leads to further improvement (Dimitriou and Dimitriou 1998; Gonul et al. 1999; Jacobsen 1991; Landren et al. 1998). These findings were recently confirmed in a report of the Sequenced Treatment Alternatives to Relieve Depression (STAR*D) program. Patients who initially failed an adequate therapeutic trial with an SSRI responded when their medication was augmented with either buspirone or bupropion (Trivedi et al. 2006).

We speculate that had the sponsor pursued an antidepressant clinical indication rather than a GAD indication, buspirone might well have become the first 5-HT$_{1A}$ partial antagonist to be developed as an antidepressant drug. Presently, buspirone lives in the shadows of the antidepressant drugs with high clinical exposure and promotion. The fact that the product life cycle of buspirone was relatively short (as mentioned earlier) while all of the SSRIs pursued a clinical indication for GAD served to limit clinical investigation of buspirone's full therapeutic profile.

Nonapproved Clinical Indications

Potential clinical indications for buspirone treatment unapproved by the FDA were recently reviewed by Rickels et al. (2003). Only a few of these buspirone studies and potential clinical indications are mentioned here. Two small double-blind clinical trials indicated modest efficacy of buspirone over placebo in the symptomatic treatment of postmenopausal syndrome (C.S. Brown et al. 1990; Rickels et al. 1989). Several placebo-controlled trials showed that smoking cessation is facilitated by buspirone therapy (Hilleman et al. 1992; West et al. 1991); its main effect, however, is in smokers who are also highly anxious (Cinciripini et al. 1995). Buspirone has been assessed in a few double-blind, placebo-controlled trials involving anxious outpatients with coexisting alcohol use disorders and found to be efficacious (Rickels et al. 2003). Because buspirone lacks abuse potential and has negligible additive effects on psychomotor and cognitive functions when coadministered with alcohol (Mattila et al. 1982), it has therapeutic benefit in the management of alcohol abuse and dependence. In a recent placebo-controlled trial, buspirone was found to be efficacious in ameliorating symptoms of opioid withdrawal (Buydens-Branchey et al. 2005).

Recently, Lee et al. (2005) reported a placebo-controlled study showing beneficial effects of buspirone in migraine patients with anxiety symptoms. Buspirone has also been evaluated under double-blind conditions in patients with aggressive behavior and agitation. In a study of 26 patients Cantillon et al. (1996) demonstrated significantly greater decrease in tension with buspirone compared with haloperidol in patients with Alzheimer's disease.

Dosage and Administration

The recommended dosage of buspirone for the treatment of GAD is 15–20 mg/day initially, prescribed in divided doses, with dosage increases to 30 mg/day if indicated. The maximal daily dosage recommended is 45 mg in the United Kingdom and 60 mg in the United States. It should be mentioned, however, that in the double-blind MDD trials (described earlier), the maximal dosage allowed was 90 mg/day. Thus, higher dosages of buspirone than those prescribed for anxiety disorders may be required in the treatment of MDD, either as monotherapy or as augmentation of an SSRI.

Side Effects and Toxicology

Newton et al. (1986), summarizing data from 17 clinical trials, reported the incidence of frequently reported adverse events during buspirone treatment: dizziness (12%), drowsiness (10%), nausea (8%), headache (6%), nervousness (5%), fatigue (4%), insomnia (3%), light-headedness (3%), dry mouth (3%), and excitement (2%). No deaths by overdose of buspirone occurred during preap-

proval clinical development. Interestingly, patients given buspirone had similar incidences of drowsiness, insomnia, fatigue, and dry mouth as with placebo treatment, and no treatment-emergent sexual dysfunction was observed.

Extensive preclinical and clinical testing indicates that buspirone lacks abuse potential, unlike alcohol and benzodiazepines (Balster 1991). A large number of psychomotor function studies, including evaluation of complex motor driving skills and memory tasks, have documented absence of impairment with buspirone administration, unlike alcohol and the benzodiazepines (Boulenger et al. 1989; Greenblatt et al. 1994; Lucki et al. 1987; Smiley and Moskowitz 1986). Since buspirone's general availability in clinical practice, no deaths attributable to buspirone overdose alone have occurred to our knowledge. Buspirone remains an unusually safe and well-tolerated medication with no abuse liability and few drug–drug interactions except for those associated with concurrent use with MAOIs.

Drug–Drug Interactions

Buspirone does not inhibit P450 enzymes, although it causes modest elevations of haloperidol and cyclosporin A levels. Buspirone has relatively few pharmacodynamic interactions with other psychotropic drugs. Because coadministration of buspirone with MAOIs carries the potential risk of serotonin syndrome, it is contraindicated in the buspirone labeling; however, cautious use of this combination has been regarded as being safe if clinically indicated (Ciraulo and Shader 1990).

Gepirone

History and Development

Gepirone, an azapirone analog of buspirone, is a substituted imide synthesized in 1986 by Bristol-Myers Squibb (refer to Figure 25–2 for chemical structure). The structural alteration (gem-dimethyl substitution) between buspirone and gepirone produces a major pharmacological difference—that is, negligible D_2 receptor affinity. Gepirone exhibits a 30- to 50-fold reduction in affinity for D_2 receptors (New 1990). The fact that gepirone has high affinity and greater intrinsic activity for postsynaptic 5-HT_{1A} receptors yet lacks appreciable affinity for D_2 receptors and has activity in a variety of preclinical anxiolytic and antidepressant models supports the notion that the antidepressant properties of azapirones reside in the agonist interaction at 5-HT_{1A} receptors. Like buspirone,

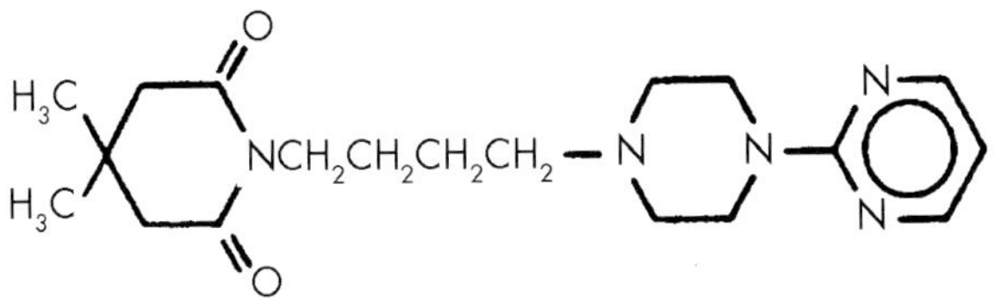

FIGURE 25–2. Chemical structure of gepirone.

gepirone is chemically unrelated to the benzodiazepines and lacks sedative-hypnotic, anticonvulsant, and muscle-relaxant properties.

Given its preclinical pharmacological profile of selective action on serotonergic neurotransmission and its more complete agonist profile at postsynaptic 5-HT$_{1A}$ receptors, gepirone was initially developed as a dual anti-anxiety and antidepressant agent utilizing an immediate-release formulation. Because of its short elimination half-life and suboptimal tolerability, an extended-release formulation was deemed desirable, and clinical development was switched to gepirone ER. In 1993, gepirone was out-licensed to Fabre-Kramer, and in partnership with Organon, the clinical development of gepirone ER for MDD continued. The decision by Bristol-Myers Squibb to out-license gepirone was based on competing depression programs within the company at that time. Organon submitted an NDA for treatment of MDD in October 1999. In its review of the application, the FDA cited insufficient evidence of efficacy due to lack of the requisite two positive well-controlled (pivotal) efficacy trials. Fabre-Kramer reassumed responsibility for gepirone and undertook additional clinical development for treatment of depression. An NDA submitted in 2007 did not receive FDA approval. Further studies with gepirone ER in depression are planned, and clinical indications for GAD and hyposexual desire disorder are being considered by the drug sponsor.

Mechanism of Action

A number of important in vitro and in vivo pharmacological studies have been undertaken with gepirone. At both pre- and postsynaptic 5-HT$_{1A}$ receptors in native tissue, gepirone displaces [^{3}H]8-OH-DPAT from bovine dorsal raphe rat hippocampal membranes with similar affinity, which is approximately fourfold less potent than buspirone (Yocca 1990). Presynaptically, gepirone exhibits potent agonist properties. This is evident in studies measuring markers of presynaptic 5-HT$_{1A}$ receptor stimulation (reduced accumulation of 5-HT [Yocca 1990]), reduction

in hippocampal 5-HT levels measured through microdialysis (Sharp et al. 1989), and reduction in firing of 5-HT–containing dorsal raphe neurons (Blier and de Montigny 1987). At postsynaptic 5-HT$_{1A}$ receptors, gepirone displays partial agonist properties, albeit with less potency but greater intrinsic activity than buspirone (Yocca 1990). The partial agonist nature of gepirone was demonstrated in an elegant study by Andrade and Nicoll (1987). Microiontophoretic administration of gepirone, similar to 5-HT, hyperpolarizes rat hippocampal pyramidal neurons through an interaction with 5-HT$_{1A}$ receptors, only to a lesser degree. When gepirone and 5-HT are microiontophoretically applied simultaneously, gepirone antagonizes the full agonist effect of 5-HT. This study demonstrates the pharmacological versatility of a compound with partial agonist properties, which can function as either a receptor agonist or antagonist depending on ambient conditions. Gepirone lacks appreciable affinity for other monoamine or benzodiazepine receptors and does not bind to neurotransmitter transporter sites.

Chronic treatment with gepirone produces downregulation of 5-HT$_2$ receptors, a characteristic shared by mechanistically distinct agents with antidepressant properties (Yocca et al. 1991). Furthermore, similar to SSRIs, continuous treatment with gepirone desensitizes dorsal raphe 5-HT$_{1A}$ receptors, favoring enhanced serotonergic neuronal signaling (Blier and de Montigny 1987).

Gepirone is similar to buspirone in demonstrating activity in a variety of animal models that predict clinical effect for anxiety and depression. In preclinical anxiety models, gepirone was active in the rat Vogel conflict and open-field test (Stefanski et al. 1992), the rat social stress test (Tomatzky and Miczek 1995), the rat ultrasonic vocalization test (Cullen and Rowan 1994), and the rat fear-potentiated startle paradigm (Kehne et al. 1988). In depression models, gepirone has activity in several behavioral models, including learned helplessness (Giral et al. 1988; Martin et al. 1990) and the forced-swim test (Detke et al. 1995) in rats.

In a series of neuroendocrine studies in rodents and man (Anderson et al. 1990; Cowen et al. 1990), gepirone was observed to be similar to buspirone in that it significantly increases plasma levels of ACTH, β-endorphin, cortisol, prolactin, and growth hormone, accompanied by decreases in body temperature. The fact that prolactin levels are increased by gepirone, which lacks appreciable affinity for dopamine D$_2$ receptors, indicates that this prolactin effect of buspirone may result from multiple receptor interactions.

Pharmacokinetics and Disposition

Gepirone is well absorbed orally, with time to peak plasma concentration (T_{max}) approximately 1 hour. The T_{max} of gepirone is significantly delayed by food ingestion. Gepirone is subject to extensive first-pass metabolism (15% bioavailability), undergoing rapid biotransformation with a short plasma elimination half-life. Gepirone ER formulations have been developed, yielding significantly lower maximum plasma concentrations (C_{max}) and longer T_{max} than gepirone (Timmer and Sitsen 2003). Gepirone ER once daily has a similar area under the curve (AUC) as the gepirone immediate-release preparation administered twice daily. C_{max} of the 1-PP metabolite of gepirone is significantly lower with gepirone ER administration, and the T_{max} is longer. Fluctuations in plasma gepirone concentrations are considerably less with gepirone ER than with the immediate-release formulation.

1-PP, one of two major metabolites of gepirone, possesses activity as a presynaptic α_2-adrenoreceptor antagonist but is thought to lack intrinsic antidepressant effects. Plasma concentrations of 1-PP exceed gepirone plasma levels (Tay et al. 1993) with extended-release formulations, although 1-PP levels are lower than with the immediate-release formulations.

The in vivo physiological effects exerted by gepirone may in part reside in 3-hydroxygepirone, which is an active metabolite of gepirone and has lower plasma concentrations with the ER preparation compared with the immediate-release formulation. It exhibits affinity and full agonist activity at the 5-HT$_{1A}$ receptor ($K_i = 58$ nM) and antidepressant activity in preclinical models (Ward et al. 2000). Furthermore, and like gepirone, 3-hydroxygepirone inhibits the firing of dorsal raphe neurons and produces a desensitization of rat somatodendritic 5-HT$_{1A}$ receptors after chronic exposure (Blier et al. 2000).

Indications and Efficacy

The immediate-release formulation of gepirone was extensively studied for a clinical indication in both the anxiety and depressive disorders. In a placebo-controlled trial comparing gepirone with diazepam in GAD, Rickels et al. (1997) found gepirone somewhat less effective than diazepam, with inferior tolerability and excessive dropouts. These results were consistent with those of other trials with the gepirone immediate-release formulation. Studies in depressive disorders with immediate-release gepirone indicated that it possessed antidepressant properties (Jenkins et al. 1990; McGrath et al. 1994; Robinson et al. 1989a).

Because of tolerability concerns with short-acting immediate-release formulations of gepirone, clinical development was switched to gepirone ER, with a major focus on treatment of MDD. Preliminary placebo-controlled studies provided evidence of the efficacy of gepirone ER in MDD (Feiger 1996; Wilcox et al. 1996). Feiger (1996) compared gepirone ER, imipramine, and placebo in an 8-week trial involving patients with DSM-III-R (American Psychiatric Association 1987) major depression. At dosages ranging from 10 to 60 mg/day, gepirone ER was significantly more effective than placebo treatment as measured by both the 17-item and 28-item versions of the Ham-D, with comparable efficacy to imipramine (150–300 mg/day). Gepirone ER was generally better tolerated than imipramine, with fewer anticholinergic and sexual side effects and with an adverse effect pattern typical of other azapirone agents, predominantly dizziness, lightheadedness, and nausea.

A well-controlled efficacy trial comparing gepirone ER and placebo in MDD has been reported that demonstrates gepirone's therapeutic benefit in the treatment of major depression (Feiger et al. 2003). In this 8-week trial involving 204 patients (gepirone $n = 101$, placebo $n = 103$), treatment with gepirone ER was initiated at a dosage of 20 mg/day and increased to 40 mg/day after 3 days; further dosage increase to 60 mg/day at week 2 was permitted if clinically indicated. Remission rates at week 8 were 24.8% for gepirone ER and 14.9% for placebo treatment ($P < 0.05$). The CGI responder rates were 43.6% and 35.6%, respectively. With gepirone ER, 82% of patients experienced a treatment-emergent adverse event, whereas for placebo patients 56% experienced an adverse event. Ten patients (9.8%) and 3 patients (2.8%) on gepirone and placebo, respectively, terminated treatment prematurely due to adverse events. Based on results on the Derogatis Interview for Sexual Functioning—Self Report questionnaire (Derogatis 1997), there was no evidence that gepirone caused treatment-related sexual dysfunction. A second placebo-controlled trial of gepirone ER for the treatment of MDD has been conducted, providing evidence for antidepressant effectiveness of gepirone (Bielski et al. 2008).

In a 1-year relapse prevention study of the efficacy and tolerability for continuation treatment of major depression, gepirone ER was associated with a significantly lower relapse rate (23.0% vs. 34.7%) than placebo treatment (Keller et al. 2005). In a retrospective subgroup analysis of patients with significant anxiety symptoms associated with MDD, Alpert et al. (2004) reported gepirone ER to be superior to placebo treatment based on outcomes of several efficacy measures, including improvement in total scores on the Ham-D and global response rates.

Side Effects and Toxicology

Gepirone has a safety profile similar to that of buspirone, with dizziness, nausea, light-headedness, and insomnia the most commonly reported adverse events (Fitton and Benfield 1994). Treatment with gepirone ER, which has a lower incidence of side effects than the immediate-release formulation at therapeutic doses, is not associated with weight gain, sexual dysfunction, or sedation (Feiger et al. 2003).

Conclusion

Discovery of the 5-HT_{1A} receptor was instrumental in linking modulation of 5-HT neurotransmission to anxiety symptoms. Buspirone, a partial agonist of the 5-HT_{1A} receptor, is the first of a new class of antianxiety agents approved for treatment of GAD and anxiety with associated depressive symptoms. An ER formulation of gepirone, a more complete 5-TH_{1A} receptor agonist, has been shown to have antidepressant efficacy in several placebo-controlled trials. Clinical development of gepirone ER for indications in treatment of depression and anxiety disorders is ongoing.

References

Albert PR, Morris SJ, Ghahremani MH, et al: A putative α-helical Gβγ–coupling domain in the second intracellular loop of the 5-HT1A receptor. Ann N Y Acad Sci 861:146–161, 1998

Alpert JE, Franznick DA, Hollander SB, et al: Gepirone extended-release treatment of anxious depression: evidence from a retrospective subgroup analysis of inpatients with major depressive disorder. J Clin Psychiatry 65:1069–1025, 2004

American Psychiatric Association: Diagnostic and Statistical Manual of Mental Disorders, 2nd Edition. Washington, DC, American Psychiatric Association, 1968

American Psychiatric Association: Diagnostic and Statistical Manual of Mental Disorders, 3rd Edition. Washington, DC, American Psychiatric Association, 1980

American Psychiatric Association: Diagnostic and Statistical Manual of Mental Disorders, 3rd Edition, Revised. Washington, DC, American Psychiatric Association, 1987

Anderson IM, Cowen PJ, Grahame-Smith DG: The effects of gepirone on neuroendocrine function and temperature in humans. Psychopharmacology 100:498–503, 1990

Andrade R, Nicoll RA: Novel anxiolytics discriminate between postsynaptic serotonin receptors mediating different physiological responses on single neurons of the rat hippocampus. Naunyn Schmiedebergs Arch Pharmacol 336:5–10, 1987

Arranz B, Eriksson A, Mellerup P, et al: Brain 5-HT1A and 5-HT1D and 5-HT2 receptors in suicide victims. Biol Psychiatry 35:457–463, 1994

Azmetia EC, Gannon PJ, Kheck NM, et al: Cellular localization of the 5-HT1A receptor in primate brain neurons and glial cells. Neuropsychopharmacology 14:35–46, 1996

Balster RL: Preclinical studies of the abuse potential of buspirone, in Buspirone: Mechanisms and Clinical Aspects. Edited by Tunnicliff G, Eison AS, Taylor DP. New York, Academic Press, 1991, pp 97–107

Barrett JE, Witkin JM: Buspirone in animal models of anxiety, in Buspirone: Mechanisms and Clinical Aspects. Edited by Tunnicliff G, Eison AS, Taylor DP. New York, Academic Press, 1991, pp 37–79

Bielski RJ, Cunningham L, Harrigan JP, et al: Gepirone extended release in treatment of adult outpatients with major depressive disorder: a double-blind, randomized, placebo-controlled, parallel group study. J Clin Psychiatry 69:571–577, 2008

Blier P, de Montigny C: Modification of the 5HT neuron properties by sustained administration of the 5-HT1A agonist gepirone: electrophysiological studies in rat brain. Synapse 1:470–480, 1987

Blier P, Haddjeri N, Dong J: Effect of 5-HT1A receptor agonist ORG 33062 (gepirone) and its metabolite ORG 25907 (3-OH-gepirone) on the 5-HT system in the rat brain (abstract). J Am Coll Neuropsychopharmacol Abs 140:306, 2000

Boehm C, Placchi M, Stallone R, et al: A double-blind comparison of buspirone, clobazam, and placebo in patients with anxiety treated in a general practice setting. J Clin Psychopharmacol 10:385–425, 1990a

Boehm C, Robinson DS, Gammans RE, et al: Buspirone therapy in anxious elderly patients: a controlled clinical trial. J Clin Psychopharmacology 10 (suppl):47–51, 1990b

Boulenger JP, Gram LF, Jolicouer FB, et al: Repeated administration of buspirone: absence of pharmacodynamic or pharmacokinetic interaction with triazolam. Hum Psychopharmacol 8:117–124, 1989

Brown CS, Ling FW, Farmer RG, et al: Buspirone in the treatment of premenstrual syndrome. Drug Ther Bull 8 (suppl):112–116, 1990

Brown TA, Barlow D: Comorbidity among anxiety disorders: implications for treatment and DSM-IV. J Consult Clin Psychol 60:835–844, 1992

Burnet PW, Eastwood SL, Lacey K, et al: The distribution of 5-HT1A and 5-HT2A receptor mRNA in human brain. Brain Res 676:157–168, 1995

Burnet PW, Eastwood SL, Harrison PJ: [3H]WAY-100635 for 5-HT1A receptor autoradiography in human brain: a comparison with [3H]8-OH-DPAT and demonstration of increased binding in the frontal cortex in schizophrenia. Neurochem Int 30:565–574, 1997

Buydens-Branchey L, Branchey M, Reel-Brander C: Efficacy of buspirone in the treatment of opioid withdrawal. J Clin Psychopharmacol 25:230–236, 2005

Cantillon M, Brunswick R, Molina D, et al: Buspirone versus haloperidol: a double-blind trial for agitation in a nursing home population with Alzheimer's disease. Am J Geriatr Psychiatry 4:236–267, 1996

Chalmers DT, Watson SJ: Comparative anatomical distribution of 5-HT1A receptor mRNA and 5-HT1A binding in rat brain:

a combined in situ hybridization/in vitro receptor autoradiographic study. Brain Res 561:51–60, 1991

Charest A, Wainer BH, Albert PR: Cloning and differentiation-induced expression of a murine serotonin1A receptor in a septal cell line. J Neurosci 13:5164–5171, 1993

Charney DS, Heninger GR: Noradrenergic function and the mechanism of action of antianxiety treatment, I: the effect of long-term alprazolam treatment. Arch Gen Psychiatry 42:458–467, 1985

Cheetham SC, Crompton MR, Katona CL, et al: Brain 5-HT-1 binding sites in depressed suicides. Psychopharmacol 102:544–548, 1990

Cinciripini PM, Lapitsky L, Seay S, et al: A placebo-controlled evaluation of the effects of buspirone on smoking cessation: differences between high- and low-anxiety smokers. J Clin Psychopharmacol 15:182–191, 1995

Ciraulo DA, Shader RL: Question the experts: safety of buspirone with an MAOI. J Clin Psychopharmacol 10:306, 1990

Cowen PJ, Anderson IM, Grahame-Smith DG: Neuroendocrine effects of azapirones. J Clin Psychopharmacol 10 (suppl):21S–25S, 1990

Cullen WK, Rowan MJ: Gepirone and 1-(2-pyrimidinyl)-piperazine-induced reduction of aversively evoked ultrasonic vocalization in the rat. Pharmacol Biochem Behav 48:301–306, 1994

Davidson JRT, DuPont RL, Hedges D, et al: Efficacy, safety, and tolerability of venlafaxine extended release and buspirone in outpatients with generalized anxiety disorder. J Clin Psychiatry 60:528–535, 1999

De Vivo M, Maayani S: Characterization of the 5-hydroxytryptamine1A receptor-mediated inhibition of forskolin-stimulated adenylate cyclase activity in guinea pig and rat hippocampal membranes. J Pharmacol Exp Ther 238:248–253, 1986

del Olmo E, Lopez-Gimenez JF, Vilaro MT, et al: Early localization of mRNA coding for 5-HT1A receptors in human brain during development. Mol Brain Res 60:123–126, 1998

DeMartinis N, Rynn M, Rickels K, et al: Prior benzodiazepine use and buspirone response in the treatment of generalized anxiety disorder. J Clin Psychiatry 61:91–94, 2000

Derogatis LR: The Derogatis Interview for Sexual Functioning (DISF/DISF-SR): an introductory report. J Sex Marital Ther 23:291–304, 1997

Detke MJ, Rickels M, Lucki I: Active behaviors in the rat forced swimming test differentially produced by serotonergic and noradrenergic antidepressants. Psychopharmacology 121:66–72, 1995

Dimitriou EC, Dimitriou CE: Buspirone augmentation of antidepressant therapy. J Clin Psychopharmacol 18:465–469, 1998

Dockens RC, Salazar DE, Fulmor E, et al: Pharmacokinetics of a newly identified active metabolite of buspirone after administration of buspirone over its therapeutic range. J Clin Pharmacol 46:1308–1312, 2006

Duman RS, Nakagawa S, Malberg J: Regulation of adult neurogenesis by antidepressant treatment. Neuropsychopharmacology 25:836–844, 2001

Eison AS, Eison MS: Serotonergic mechanisms in anxiety. Prog Neuropsychopharmacol Biol Psychiatry 18:47–62, 1994

Eison AS, Temple DL: Buspirone: review of its pharmacology and current perspectives on its mechanism of action. Am J Med 80:1–9, 1986

Eison AS, Yocca FD, Taylor DP: Mechanism of action of buspirone: current perspectives, in Buspirone: Mechanisms and Clinical Aspects. Edited by Tunnicliff G, Eison AS, Taylor DP. New York, Academic Press, 1991, pp 3–17

El Mestikawy S, Riad M, Laport AM: Production of specific anti-rat 5-HT1A receptor antibodies in rabbits injected with a synthetic peptide. Neurosci Lett 118:189–192, 1990

Enkelmann R: Alprazolam versus buspirone in the treatment of outpatients with generalized anxiety disorder. Psychopharmacology 105:428–432, 1991

Fargin A, Raymond JR, Lohse MJ, et al: The genomic clone G-21 which resembles a β-adrenergic receptor sequence encodes the 5-HT1A receptor. Nature 335:358–360, 1988

Feiger A: A double-blind comparison of gepirone extended release, imipramine, and placebo in the treatment of outpatient major depression. Psychopharmacology Bull 32:659–665, 1996

Feiger AD, Heiser JF, Smith WT, et al: Gepirone extended-release: new evidence for efficacy in the treatment of major depressive disorder. J Clin Psychiatry 64:243–249, 2003

Feighner JP, Merideth CH, Hendrickson GA: A double-blind comparison of buspirone and diazepam in outpatients with generalized anxiety disorder. J Clin Psychiatry 43:103–107, 1982

Fitton A, Benfield P: Gepirone in depression and anxiety disorders. CNS Drugs 1:388–398, 1994

Fletcher A, Forster EA, Bill DJ, et al: Electrophysiology, biochemical, neurohormonal and behavioral studies with WAY-100635, a potent, selective and silent 5-HT1A receptor antagonist. Behav Brain Res 73:337–353, 1996

Fontaine R, Chouinard G, Annable L: Rebound anxiety in anxious patients after abrupt withdrawal of benzodiazepine treatment. Am J Psychiatry 141:848–852, 1984

Gammans RE, Johnston RE: Metabolism, pharmacokinetics, and toxicology of buspirone, in Buspirone: Mechanisms and Clinical Aspects. Edited by Tunnicliff G, Eison AS, Taylor DP. New York, Academic Press, 1991, pp 233–260

Gammans RE, Westrick ML, Shea JP, et al: Pharmacokinetics of buspirone in elderly subjects. J Clin Pharmacol 29:72–78, 1989

Gilbert F, Dourish CT, Brazell C: Relationship of increased food intake and plasma ACTH levels to 5-HT1A receptor activation in rats. Psychoneuroendocrinology 13:471–478, 1988

Giral P, Martin P, Soubrie P, et al: Reversal of helpless behavior in rats by putative 5-HT-1(a) agonists. Biol Psychiatry 23:237–242, 1988

Glaser HL, Traber J: Buspirone: action on serotonergic receptors in calf hippocampus. Eur J Pharmacol 88:137–138, 1983

Goldberg HL, Finnerty R: The comparative efficacy of buspirone and diazepam in the treatment of anxiety. Am J Psychiatry 136:1184–1187, 1979

Goldberg HL, Finnerty R: Comparison of buspirone in two separate studies. J Clin Psychiatry 43:87–91, 1982

Gonul AS, Oguz A, Yabanoglu I, et al: Buspirone and pindolol in augmentation therapy of treatment-resistant depression. Eur J Neuropsychopharmacology 9 (suppl):S215, 1999

Greenblatt DJ, Harmatz JS, Gouthro TA, et al: Distinguishing a benzodiazepine agonist (triazolam) from a nonagonist anxiolytic (buspirone) by electroencephalography: kinetic studies. Clin Pharmacol Ther 56:100–111, 1994

Gross C, Zhuang X, Stark K, et al: Serotonin1A receptor acts during development to establish normal anxiety-like behavior in the adult. Nature 416:396–400, 2002

Hamilton M: The assessment of anxiety states by rating. J Med Psychol 32:50–55, 1959

Hamilton M: A rating scale for depression. J Neurol Neurosurg Psychiatry 23:56–62, 1960

Hamon M, Bourgoin S, Gozlan H, et al: Biochemical evidence for the 5-HT agonist properties of PAT (8-hydroxy-2-(di-n-propylamino)tetralin) in the rat brain. Eur J Pharmacol 100:263–276, 1984

Hilleman DE, Mohiuddin SM, Del Core MG, et al: Effect of buspirone on withdrawal symptoms associated with smoking cessation. Arch Gen Psychiatry 152:73–77, 1992

Hoyer D, Hannon JP, Martin GR: Molecular, pharmacological and functional diversity of 5-HT receptors. Pharmacol Biochem Behav 71:533–554, 2002

Jacobsen FM: Possible augmentation of antidepressant response by buspirone. J Clin Psychiatry 52:217–220, 1991

Jenkins SW, Robinson DS, Fabre LF, et al: Gepirone in the treatment of major depression. J Clin Psychopharmacol 10 (suppl): 77S–85S, 1990

Kehne JH, Cassella JV, Davis M: Anxiolytic effects of buspirone and gepirone in the fear-potentiated startle paradigm. Psychopharmacology 94:8–13, 1988

Keller MB, Ruwe FJJ, Janssens CJJG, et al: Relapse prevention with gepirone ER in outpatients with major depression. J Clin Psychopharmacol 25:79–84, 2005

Kendler KS, Nearle MC, Kessler RC, et al: Major depression and generalized anxiety disorder: same genes, (partly) different environments? Arch Gen Psychiatry 49:716–722, 1992

Kobilka BK, Frielle T, Collins S, et al: An intronless gene encoding a potential member of the family of receptors coupled to guanine nucleotide regulatory proteins. Nature 329:75–79, 1987

Laakman G, Schule C, Lorkowski G, et al: Buspirone and lorazepam in the treatment of generalized anxiety disorder in outpatients. Psychopharmacology 136:357–366, 1998

Lader M, Scotto JC: A multicenter double-blind comparison of hydroxyzine, buspirone and placebo in patients with generalized anxiety disorder. Psychopharmacology 139:402–406, 1998

Landren M, Bjorling G, Agren H, et al: A randomized, double-blind, placebo-controlled trial of buspirone in combination with an SSRI in patients with treatment-refractory depression. J Clin Psychiatry 59:664–668, 1998

Lee ST, Park JH, Kim M: Efficacy of the 5-HT1A agonist, buspirone hydrochloride, in migraineurs with anxiety: a randomized, prospective, parallel group, double-blind, placebo-controlled study. Headache 45:1004–1011, 2005

Lesch KP: The ipsapirone/5-HT1A receptor challenge in anxiety disorders and depression, in Serotonin 1A Receptors in Depression and Anxiety. Edited by Stahl S, Gastpar M, Keppel Hesselink JM, et al. New York, Raven, 1992, pp 387–407

Lucki I, Rickels K, Giesecke A, et al: Differential effects of the anxiolytic drugs, diazepam and buspirone on memory function. Br J Clin Pharmacol 23:207–211, 1987

Martin P, Beninger RJ, Hamon M, et al: Antidepressant-like action of 8-OH-DPAT, a 5-HT1A agonist, in the learned helplessness paradigm: evidence for a postsynaptic mechanism. Behav Brain Res 38:135–144, 1990

Matsubara S, Arora RC, Meltzer HY: Serotonergic measures in suicide brain: 5-HT1A binding sites in the frontal cortex of suicide victims. J Neural Transm 85:181–194, 1991

Mattila MJ, Aranko K, Seppala T: Acute effects of buspirone and alcohol on psychomotor skills. J Clin Psychiatry 43:56–60, 1982

McGrath PJ, Stewart JW, Quitkin FM, et al: Gepirone treatment of atypical depression: preliminary evidence of serotonergic involvement. J Clin Psychopharmacol 14:347–352, 1994

Meller E, Goldstein M, Bohmaker K: Receptor reserve for 5-hydroxtryptamine1A-mediated inhibition of serotonin synthesis: possible relationship to the anxiolytic properties of 5-hydroxytryptamine1A agonists. Mol Pharmacol 37:231–237, 1990

Meltzer HY, Fleming R: Effect of buspirone on prolactin and growth hormone secretion in laboratory rodents and man. J Clin Psychiatry 43:76–80, 1982

Meltzer HY, Gudelsky GA, Lowy MT, et al: Neuroendocrine effects of buspirone: mediation by dopaminergic and serotonergic mechanisms, in Buspirone: Mechanisms and Clinical Aspects. Edited by Tunnicliff G, Eison AS, Taylor DP. New York, Academic Press, 1991, pp 177–192

Mennini T, Gobbi M, Ponzio F, et al: Neurochemical effects of buspirone in rat hippocampus: evidence for selective activation of 5HT neurons. Arch Int Pharmacodyn Ther 279:40–49, 1986

Mennini T, Caccia C, Garattini S: Mechanism of action of anxiolytic drugs. Prog Drug Res 31:315–347, 1987

Murphy SM, Owen R, Tyrer P: Comparative assessment of efficacy and withdrawal symptoms after 6 and 12 weeks' treatment with diazepam or buspirone. Br J Psychiatry 154:529–534, 1989

New JS: The discovery and development of buspirone: a new approach to the treatment of anxiety. Med Res Rev 3:283–326, 1990

Newton RE, Maruncyz JD, Alderdice MT, et al: Review of the side effect profile of buspirone. Am J Med 80 (suppl):17–21, 1986

Noyes R, Garvey MJ, Cooke BL, et al: Benzodiazepine withdrawal: a review of the evidence. J Clin Psychiatry 49:383–389, 1988

Palacios JM, Waeber C, Hoyer D, et al: Distribution of serotonin receptors. Ann N Y Acad Sci 600:36–52, 1990

Pan LH, Gilbert F: Activation of 5-HT1A receptor subtype in the paraventricular nuclei of the hypothalamus induces CRH and ACTH release in the rat. Neuroendocrinology 56:797–802, 1992

Parks CL, Robinson PS, Sibille E, et al: Increased anxiety of mice lacking the serotonin1A receptor. Proc Natl Acad Sci U S A 95:10734–10739, 1998

Pattij T, Groenick L, Hijzen TH, et al: Autonomic changes associated with enhanced anxiety in 5-HT1A receptor knockout mice. Neuropsychopharmacology 27:380–390, 2002

Pecknold JC, Matas M, Howarth BG, et al: Evaluation of buspirone as an antianxiety agent: buspirone and diazepam versus placebo. Am J Psychiatry 34:766–771, 1989

Pierce KL, Premont RT, Lefkowitz RJ: Seven-transmembrane receptors. Nat Rev Mol Cell Biol 3:639–650, 2002

Pohl R, Balon R, Yeragani VK, et al: Serotonergic anxiolytics in the treatment of panic disorders: a controlled study with buspirone. Psychopathology 22 (suppl):60–67, 1989

Rausch JL, Stall SM, Hauger RL: Cortisol and growth hormone responses to the 5-HT1A agonist gepirone in depressed patients. Biol Psychiatry 28:73–78, 1990

Riad M, Garcia S, Watkins KC, et al: Somatodendritic localization of 5-HT1A and pre-terminal axonal localization of 5-HT1B serotonin receptors in adult rat brain. J Comp Neurol 417:181–194, 2000

Riblet LA, Taylor DP, Eison MS, et al: Pharmacology and neurochemistry of buspirone. J Clin Psychiatry 43:81–86, 1982

Rickels K: Buspirone in clinical practice. J Clin Psychiatry 51 (suppl):51–54, 1990

Rickels K, Schweizer E: The clinical course and long-term management of generalized anxiety disorder. J Clin Psychopharmacol 19:101S–105S, 1990

Rickels K, Weisman K, Norstad M, et al: Buspirone and diazepam in anxiety: a controlled study. J Clin Psychiatry 43:81–86, 1982

Rickels K, Schweizer E, Csanalosi I, et al: Long-term treatment of anxiety and risk of withdrawal. Arch Gen Psychiatry 45:444–450, 1988

Rickels K, Freeman E, Sondheimer S: Buspirone in treatment of premenstrual syndrome. Lancet 1(8641):777, 1989

Rickels K, Amsterdam JD, Clary C, et al: Buspirone in major depression: a controlled study. J Clin Psychiatry 52:34–38, 1991

Rickels K, Downing R, Schweizer E, et al: Antidepressants for the treatment of generalized anxiety disorder: a placebo-controlled comparison of imipramine, trazodone, and diazepam. Arch Gen Psychiatry 50:884–895, 1993

Rickels K, Schweizer E, DeMartinis N, et al: Gepirone and diazepam in generalized anxiety disorder: a placebo-controlled trial. J Clin Psychiatry 17:272–277, 1997

Rickels K, Khalid-Kahn S, Rynn M: Buspirone in the treatment of anxiety disorders, in Anxiety Disorders. Edited by Nutt DJ, Ballenger JC. Oxford, England, Blackwell Publishing, 2003, pp 381–397

Ritchie LD, Cox J: A multicenter study of buspirone in the treatment of anxiety disorders in the elderly. Br J Clin Res 4:131–139, 1993

Robinson DS: Buspirone in the treatment of anxiety, in Buspirone: Mechanisms and Clinical Aspects. Edited by Tunnicliff G, Eison AS, Taylor DP. New York, Academic Press, 1991, pp 3–17

Robinson DS, Khan A: Dosing strategies for antidepressant clinical trials: a commentary. J Clin Psychopharmacol 24:1–3, 2004

Robinson DS, Napoliello MJ, Schenk J: The safety and usefulness of buspirone as an anxiolytic drug in elderly versus young patients. Clin Ther 10:740–746, 1988

Robinson DS, Alms DR, Shrotriya RC, et al: Serotonergic anxiolytics and treatment of depression. Psychopathology 22 (suppl):27–36, 1989a

Robinson DS, Shrotriya RC, Alms KR, et al: Treatment of panic disorder: nonbenzodiazepine anxiolytics, including buspirone. Psychopharmacol Bull 25:21–26, 1989b

Robinson DS, Rickels K, Feighner J, et al: Clinical effects of the 5-HT1A partial agonists in depression: a composite analysis of buspirone in the treatment of depression. J Clin Psychopharmacol 10:67S–76S, 1990

Sathananthan GL, Sanghvi I, Phillips N, et al: Correlation between neuroleptic potential and stereotypy. Curr Ther Res 18:701–705, 1975

Scheibe G: Four-year follow-up in 40 outpatients with anxiety disorders: buspirone versus lorazepam. Eur J Psychiatry 10:25–34, 1996

Schweizer E, Rickels K: Failure of buspirone to manage benzodiazepine withdrawal. Am J Psychiatry 143:12, 1986

Schweizer E, Rickels K, Hassman, et al: Buspirone and imipramine for the treatment of major depression in the elderly. J Clin Psychiatry 59:175–183, 1998

Sharp T, Bramwell SR, Grahame-Smith DG: 5-HT1A agonists reduce 5-hydroxytryptamine release in rat hippocampus in vivo as determined by brain microdialysis. Br J Pharmacol 96:283–290, 1989

Sheehan DV, Raj AB, Harnett-Sheehan K, et al: Is buspirone effective in panic disorder? J Clin Psychopharmacol 10:3–11, 1990

Shiaie RD, Pancheri P, Casacchia M, et al: Assessment of the efficacy of buspirone in patients affected by generalized anxiety disorder, shifting to buspirone from prior treatment with lorazepam: a placebo-controlled, double-blind study. J Clin Psychopharmacol 15:12–19, 1995

Skolnick P, Weissman BA, Youdim MBH: Monoaminergic involvement in the pharmacologic actions of buspirone. Br J Pharmacol 86:637–644, 1985

Smiley A: Effects of minor tranquilizers and antidepressants on psychomotor performance. J Clin Psychiatry 49 (suppl):22–28, 1987

Smiley A, Moskowitz H: The effect of chronically administered buspirone and diazepam on driver steering control. Am J Med 80:22–29, 1986

Stahl SM: Serotonin receptors and the mechanism of action of antidepressant drugs: postmortem, platelet, and neuroendocrine studies in depressed patients, in Serotonin 1A Receptors in Depression and Anxiety. Edited by Stahl S, Gastpar M, Keppel Hesselink JM, et al. New York, Raven, 1992, pp 135–162

Stefanski R, Palejko W, Kostowski W: The comparison of benzodiazepine derivatives and serotonergic agonist and antagonists in two animal models of anxiety. Neuropharmacology 31:1251–1258, 1992

Stockmeier CA, Shapiro LA, Dilley GE, et al: Increase in serotonin-1A autoreceptors in the midbrain of suicide victims with major depression: postmortem evidence for decreased serotonin activity. J Neurosci 18:7394–7401, 1998

Sussman N, Chow JCY: Current issues in benzodiazepine use of anxiety disorders. Psychiatr Ann 18:139–145, 1988

Tay LK, Sciacca MA, Sostrin MB, et al: Effect of food on the bioavailability of gepirone in humans. J Clin Pharmacol 33:631–635, 1993

Timmer CJ, Sitsen JMA: Pharmacokinetic evaluation of gepirone immediate-release capsules and gepirone extended-release tablets in healthy volunteers. J Pharmaceutical Sci 92:1773–1778, 2003

Tomatzky W, Miczek KA: Alcohol, anxiolytics and the social stress test. Psychopharmacol 121:66–72, 1995

Tompkins EC, Clemento AJ, Taylor DP, et al: Inhibition of aggressive behavior in rhesus monkeys by buspirone. Res Commun Psychol Psychiatr Res 5:337–352, 1980

Trivedi M, Fava M, Wiesnewski SR, et al: Medication augmentation after failure of SSRIs for depression. N Engl J Med 354:1243–1252, 2006

Udelman HD, Udelman DL: Concurrent use of buspirone in anxious patients during withdrawal from alprazolam therapy. J Clin Psychiatry 51 (suppl):91–96, 1990

Van de Kar LD, Karteszi M, Bethea CL, et al: Serotonergic stimulation of prolactin and corticosterone secretion is mediated by different pathways from the mediobasal hypothalamus. Neuroendocrinology 41:380–384, 1985

Vicentic A, Li Q, Battaglia G, et al: WAY-100635 inhibits 8-OH-DPAT-stimulated oxytocin, ACTH and corticosterone, but not prolactin secretion. Eur J Pharmacol 346:261–266, 1998

Ward NM, Drinkenburg WH, Shahid M: The preclinical antidepressant profile of the 5-HT1A receptor agonist ORG 33062 (gepirone) and its metabolite ORG 25907 (3-OH-gepirone) (abstract). J Am Coll Neuropsychopharmacol Abs 59:264, 2000

West R, Hajek P, McNeill A: Effect of buspirone on cigarette withdrawal symptoms and short-term abstinence rates in a smokers' clinic. Psychopharmacology 104:91–96, 1991

Wieland S, Lucki I: Antidepressant-like activity of 5-HT1A agonists measured with the forced swim test. Psychopharmacology 101:497–504, 1990

Wilcox CS, Ferguson JM, Dale JL, et al: A double-blind trial of low- and high-dose ranges of gepirone-ER compared with placebo in the treatment of depressed outpatients. Psychopharmacol Bull 32:335–342, 1996

Wise CD, Berger BD, Stein L: Benzodiazepines: anxiety reducing activity by reduction of serotonin turnover in the brain. Science 177:180–183, 1972

Wong H, Dockens RA, Pajor L, et al: 6-Hydroxybuspirone is a major active metabolite of buspirone: assessment of pharmacokinetics and 5-hydroxytryptamine1A receptor occupancy in rats. Drug Metab Dispos 35:1387–1392, 2007

Wray NR, James MR, Mah SP, et al: Anxiety and comorbid measures associated with PLXNA2. Arch Gen Psychiatry 64:318–3236, 2007

Wu YH, Smith KR, Rayburn JW, et al: Psychosedative agents: N-(4-phenyl-1-piperazinylalkyl)-substituted cyclic imides. J Med Chem 12:876–881, 1969

Yocca FD: Neurochemistry and neurophysiology of buspirone and gepirone: interactions at presynaptic and postsynaptic 5-HT1A receptors. J Clin Psychiatry 10:6S–12S, 1990

Yocca F, Altar CA: Partial agonism of dopamine, serotonin and opiate receptors in psychiatry. Drug Discovery Today: Therapeutic Strategies 3:429–435, 2006

Yocca FD, Eison AS, Hyslop DK, et al: Unique modulation of central 5-HT-2 binding sites and 5-HT-2 receptor mediated behavior by continuous gepirone treatment. Life Sci 49:1777–1785, 1991

Yocca FD, Iben L, Meller E: Lack of apparent receptor reserve at postsynaptic 5-HT1A receptors negatively coupled to adenylyl cyclase activity in rat hippocampal membranes. Mol Pharmacol 41:1066–1072, 1992

Zhu M, Zhao W, Jimenez H, et al: Cytochrome P450 3A-mediated metabolism of buspirone in human liver microsomes. Drug Metab Dispos 33:500–507, 2005

CHAPTER 26

Putative New-Generation Antidepressants

Florian Holsboer, M.D., Ph.D.

For the past half-century, antidepressant development has been dominated by drugs that interfere with monoamine neurotransmitters. Some progress regarding safety and adverse effects is undeniable, and the increasing specificity of most current antidepressants targeting exclusively monoamines accounts for this improvement. Nevertheless, existing antidepressants exhibit limited efficacy and protracted onset of action, and we still do not know whether the pharmacological actions delineated thus far are those that account for the clinical benefits of these drugs in 60%–70% of patients with depression. Severe depression poses a particularly difficult problem, because failure to achieve clinical remission yields the risks of extended illness duration and chronicity (Nemeroff 2007). Elucidation of crucial steps in the mechanism of action of current antidepressants could yield an array of new drug candidates. The alternative route to developing better antidepressants relies on the increasing knowledge of the pathophysiology of depression emerging from clinical research and well-founded hypotheses derived from animal models. Despite huge research efforts by both academic and pharmaceutical industry investigators, none of the many discoveries of mechanisms involved in depression-related behavior has yet been translated into clinical application.

This chapter highlights some of the progress made, discusses the impediments to discovery of promising new drug candidates, and offers proposals for how an integration of systemic approaches and hypothesis-driven research may ultimately help us to identify and develop better antidepressants.

Targeting the Stress Hormone System

In response to any kind of stress, the pituitary gland secretes adrenocorticotropic hormone (ACTH), which at the level of the adrenal cortex leads to increased synthesis and release of cortisol (corticosterone in rodents). Many research reports agreed that the key neuropeptides accounting for peripheral increase of stress hormones are corticotropin-releasing hormone (CRH; also known as corticotropin-releasing factor [CRF]) and vasopressin, both synthesized in specialized neurons in the hypothalamus (paraventricular nuclei), from which they reach the anterior pituitary via portal vessels. These neuroendocrine activities are closely associated with a large number of other neural projections resulting in neuropeptide release in many brain areas that were implicated in the neuroanatomy of depression and anxiety (de Kloet et al. 2005). Those extrahypothalamic structures include the central nucleus of the amygdala, the hippocampus, the locus coeruleus, and cortical structures such as the prefrontal cortex.

Also several vasopressinergic subsystems exist. One is particularly well characterized, as it consists of magnocellular neurons of the supraoptic and paraventricular nuclei from where axons project to the posterior pituitary eliciting secretion of vasopressin into the systemic circulation. Upon appropriate stimulation, this mechanism regulates a variety of physiological activities, including renal water absorption and hepatic glycogenolysis. More important in this context is a vasopressin subsystem inducing central release into brain areas that are considered to be involved in the pathogenesis of depression and anxiety. There, vasopressin elevations induce a number of behavioral responses to many stressors. Both neuropeptides, CRH and vasopressin, are involved in the adaptation to stress, as they elicit a number of behavioral responses that are suited to cope optimally with a threat. Over extended periods of time, however, these initially beneficial effects reverse into increased liability for anxiety- and depression-like behavior (Landgraf 2006).

There is good evidence from clinical research that both neuropeptides are elevated in depression. Such evidence includes elevations of CRH and vasopressin in the cerebrospinal fluid (CSF) and increased expression of these neuropeptides in the brains (specifically the hypothalamus and prefrontal cortex) of depressed patients, as well as indirect evidence from neuroendocrine function tests (Scott and Dinan 2002). For example, if a patient with depression is treated with a low dose of dexamethasone, this results in suppression of ACTH, as the precursor of this hormone is negatively controlled by glucocorticoid receptors, to which dexamethasone binds. At the same time, the brain is deprived of the corticosteroid signal, since endogenous cortisol is decreased and cannot be replaced by dexamethasone, because at the low dosages used, this synthetic steroid does not enter the brain. This results in elevation of neuropeptide activation of the hypothalamic-pituitary-adrenal (HPA) axis aimed at reinstatement of appropriate corticosteroid levels. If dexamethasone-pretreated patients with depression receive a test dose of CRH, an excessive release of ACTH and cortisol occurs (Ising et al. 2006). It is assumed that this release is mediated by the induced elevation of vasopressin, which is normally negatively regulated by endogenous corticosteroids. As a result, the endogenously elevated vasopressin and the exogenously administered CRH amplify each other's effects at the level of the anterior pituitary to produce excessive ACTH and cortisol secretions. This finding is one cornerstone of the corticosteroid receptor hypothesis, which postulates that impaired intracellular signaling of steroid-activated hormone receptors (glucocorticoid receptors [GRs] and mineralocorticoid receptors [MRs]) results in inappropriately high and enduring secretions of CRH and vasopressin in the brain and of ACTH and cortisol in the periphery (Holsboer 2000). The stress hormone cortisol easily crosses the blood–brain barrier. Because a host of genes expressed in the brain are activated or suppressed by corticosteroids, mostly via regulatory response elements, it is not surpris-

ing that continuous overexposure of the brain to cortisol also produces behavioral changes (McEwen 2004). Such changes include labile, mostly depressed, mood. Similarly, depression is the most frequent psychopathology among patients with Cushing's syndrome, a disorder characterized by unrestrained hypophyseal–adrenal cortex activity. Another behavioral sequel of hypercortisolism is cognitive deficit, which is well known to be associated with depression. Other clinical features induced by hypercortisolism are suppressed hippocampal neurogenesis (see section "Enhancing Neogenesis of Brain Cells" later in this chapter) and the metabolic syndrome, both of which are frequent concomitants of severe major depression. Some depressed patients also show psychotic features. Since hypercortisolism (whether caused by a hormone-secreting tumor or by corticosteroid medications) also often produces psychotic features, it was hypothesized that the psychotic symptoms are mainly produced by corticosteroid excess (Schatzberg et al. 1985).

As a consequence of these abnormalities induced by various stress hormones, the potential role of stress hormones in the pathogenesis of depression has been hypothesized. Three complementary lines of pharmacological interventions are currently the focus of antidepressant drug discovery and development programs: glucocorticoid receptor antagonists, vasopressin receptor antagonists, and CRH receptor antagonists (Figure 26–1).

Corticotropin-Releasing Hormone Receptor Antagonists

CRH exerts its actions through two different G protein–coupled receptors: CRH_1 and CRH_2. The two receptor subtypes are unequally expressed in the brain, where they bind not only to CRH but also to three other CRH-related peptides: urocortin I (UCN I), stresscopin-related peptide (also called UCN II), and stresscopin (UCN III). UCN I binds with equal affinity to both CRH_1 and CRH_2 receptors, while UCN II and III preferentially bind to CRH_2 receptors and have low affinity for CRH_1 receptors (Grigoriades 2005). The differential expression and function of CRH receptor subtypes in the brain holds particular relevance in regard to the question of whether CRH_1 receptors or CRH_2 receptors are preferred targets for drug interventions (Table 26–1).

CRH_1 Receptor Antagonists

As mentioned, a large number of studies using animal models clearly indicated that CRH accounts for many signs and symptoms of depression, including a host of

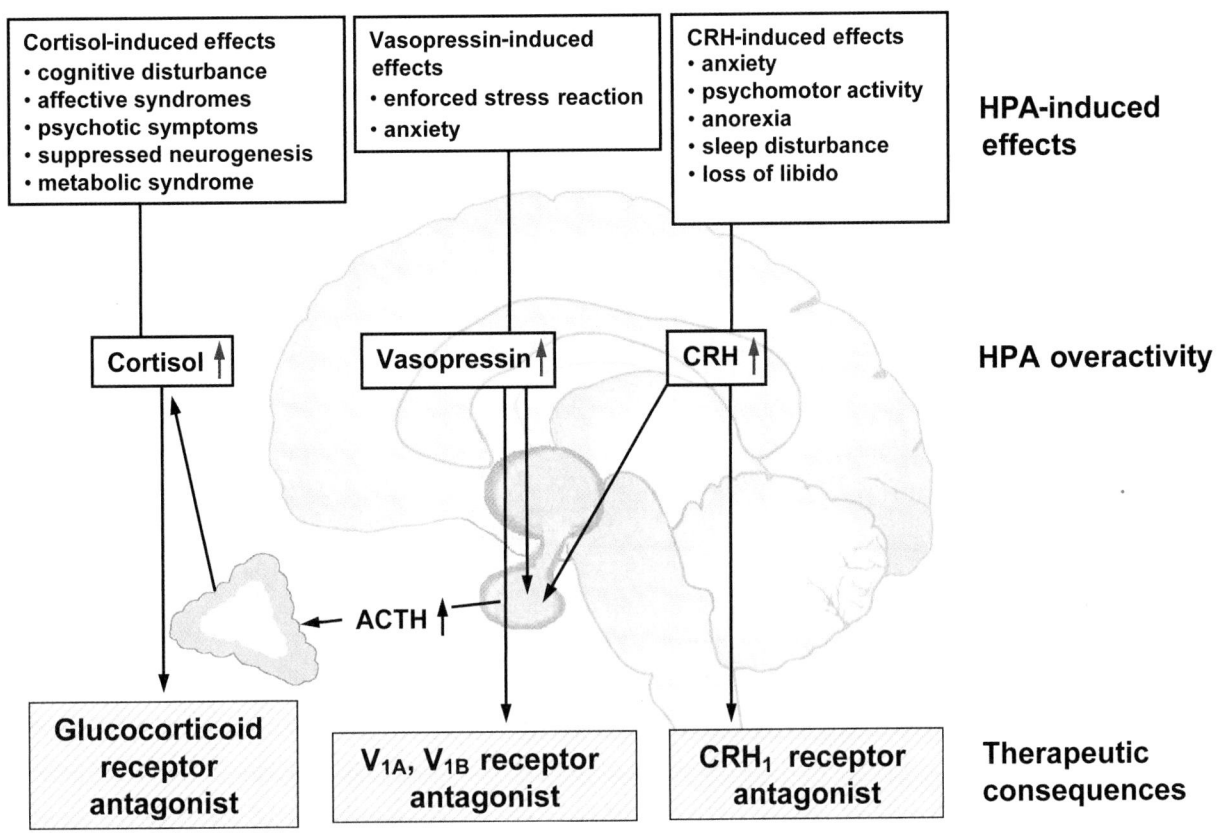

FIGURE 26–1. Targeting stress hormone abnormalities as putative treatment options.

Activation of the hypothalamic-pituitary-adrenal (HPA) system results in elevation of corticotropin-releasing hormone (CRH), vasopressin, and cortisol, which produce several signs and symptoms of depression and anxiety. Blocking the actions of these neuropeptides at the receptor level provides a new lead for antidepressant and anxiolytic drug discovery. ↑=increased.

stress-related features such as anxiety, sleeplessness, decreased appetite, decreased sexual interest, psychomotor agitation, and others. All of these findings were derived from studies that either injected CRH into the rodent brain and measured behavioral changes or used mice where CRH was overexpressed in the brain (Heinrichs and Koob 2004). That these behavioral effects of CRH can be targeted by interfering with CRH/CRH_1 receptor signaling was first shown with peptidergic CRH receptor antagonists (α-helical CRH [9–42], D-Phe-CRH [12–41], and astressin), which all were only poorly selective. Another line of evidence emerged from experiments that used antisense probes directed against CRH_1 receptor messenger RNA (mRNA), thus preventing translation into receptor proteins (Liebsch et al. 1999). These studies showed that the specific antisense probes resulted not only in reduced CRH but also in decreased stress-elicited anxiety-like behavior. Questions regarding specificity of effects by central peptide injections or antisense probes prompted the generation of mouse mutants where the

CRH_1 receptor was deleted by genetic engineering, which confirmed the preeminent role of CRH_1 receptors (Smith et al. 1998; Timpl et al. 1998). The most compelling evidence came from a mouse mutant where the CRH_1 receptor was conditionally deleted, resulting in a functional CRH_1 receptor depletion restricted to the limbic system (Mueller et al. 2003). This finding was important, because in mutants where the CRH_1 receptor is also nonfunctional in the periphery (primarily the pituitary), the abnormal stress hormone regulation had to be considered as a potential confounder (Mueller and Holsboer 2006). This mouse model confirmed that CRH_1 receptors in the brain are responsible for anxiety-like behavior and supported that antagonism of CRH_1 receptor activity may provide a novel hypothesis-driven pharmacological strategy for treatment of stress-related disorders such as depression and anxiety.

A number of small nonpeptidergic molecules with good oral bioavailability and rapid penetration across the blood–brain barrier have been developed and tested in

TABLE 26–1. Expression of CRH and CRH receptors in the rodent central nervous system

BRAIN REGION/STRUCTURE	MAIN FUNCTION	CRH	CRH₁ RECEPTOR	CRH₂ RECEPTOR
Telencephalon				
Prefrontal and cingulate cortex	Motivational and emotional aspects of memory and cognition	X	X	
Hippocampal formation	Spatial learning and memory Participation in HPA axis negative feedback Cognitive components in anxiety and depression	X	X	X
Nucleus accumbens	Reward and addictive behavior	X		
Lateral septum	Anxiety Locomotor regulation	X		X
Bed nucleus stria terminalis	Control of HPA and gonadal axes	X	X	
Central nucleus of the amygdala	Autonomic regulation in stressful situations Control of CRH release in PVN	X		
Basolateral amygdala	Conditional aspects of fear memory Motivational aspects of memory Anxiety Reward-related learning		X	
Diencephalon				
Paraventricular nucleus of the hypothalamus	HPA axis control Autonomic control over descending pathways	X		X
Dorsomedial nucleus of the hypothalamus	Autonomic regulation		X	
Brain stem				
Lateral dorsal tegmentum	Arousal and attention processes REM sleep	X	X	
Pedunculopontine nucleus of reticular formation	Arousal Control of voluntary movements REM sleep		X	
Periaqueductal gray	Arousal Pain modulation Continence and micturition Anxiety Defensive behavior Reproductive behavior	X	X	X
Dorsal raphe	Arousal and consciousness Sleep rhythms Main source of serotonergic release in forebrain			X
Locus coeruleus	Arousal and vigilance Decision-making modulation Cognitive and arousal deregulation in depression/anxiety-related behavior Autonomic regulation under stress conditions Modulation of CRH release from PVN Main source of forebrain noradrenergic innervation	X		
Parabraquial nucleus	Control of parasympathetic visceral sensory information sent toward forebrain	X	X	

TABLE 26–1. Expression of CRH and CRH receptors in the rodent central nervous system *(continued)*

		CRH/CRH RECEPTOR EXPRESSION		
BRAIN REGION/STRUCTURE	MAIN FUNCTION	CRH	CRH$_1$ RECEPTOR	CRH$_2$ RECEPTOR
Nucleus of the solitary tract	Visceral special and general sensory information Autonomic regulation			X
Cerebellum	Motor control of movement Postural reflexes	X	X	
Pituitary				
Anterior pituitary	Control of multiple endocrine and metabolic systems		X	

Note. CRH = corticotropin-releasing hormone; HPA = hypothalamic-pituitary-adrenal; PVN = paraventricular nucleus of the hypothalamus; REM = rapid eye movement.

Source. Cummings et al. 1983; van Pett et al. 2000.

preclinical models of depression and anxiety. The inconsistencies of some of the test results can be ascribed to the fact that the animal models used were validated for the discovery of antidepressants acting at monoamine transmitter reuptake transporters (Markou 2005). This is exemplified by the recent observation that mice that overexpress CRH conditionally in the brain display hyperactivity when exposed to the forced-swim test (A. Lu et al. 2008), with enhanced struggling and reduced floating times. When treated with DMP-696, a selective CRH$_1$ receptor antagonist, struggling time decreased while floating increased. This observation is in opposition to the behavioral changes observed in wild-type mice, which when treated with antidepressants exhibit decreases in floating relative to struggling (Markou 2005). In wild-type mice, where depression- or anxiety-like behavior is absent, most CRH$_1$ receptor antagonists produced reduced immobility similar to that observed after administration of monoamine-based antidepressants. The relevance of the affective state at baseline, which is now deemed pertinent for interpretation of drug effects on a stress-related behavior, is demonstrated in rat and mouse lines that have been selectively and bidirectionally bred for extremes in trait anxiety. As a result, rats and mice with high innate anxiety-like behavior as assessed on the elevated plus-maze are now available (Keck et al. 2001; Landgraf et al. 2007; Wigger et al. 2004). As illustrated in Figure 26–2, mice with innate high anxiety respond to the CRH$_1$ receptor antagonist DMP-696 with reduced anxiety-like behavior, again underscoring the importance of baseline behavior in the assessment of a drug's effects.

Although a large number of small-molecule CRH$_1$ receptor antagonists have been discovered over the past 20 years, only a few of these have entered clinical development, and none has yet found its way to the market (Valdez 2006). A number of clinical trials are still under way, but few clinical data have yet been published. The first study reported was an open-label trial designed to assess the safety of R 121919 (also known as NBI-30775). This molecule binds specifically and with high affinity (K$_i$ = 3.5 nmol/L) to cloned human CRH$_1$ receptors, can be orally administered, and crosses the blood–brain barrier easily. The excellent preclinical profile of this compound made it a preferred candidate for clinical development. The clinical evaluation was designed as an open-label trial to study safety and tolerability (Zobel et al. 2000). Additionally, changes in psychopathology scores, laboratory examinations, and sleep performance, including polysomnography, were recorded. The study population was split into equally sized groups that received either 5–40 mg/day (lower dosages) or 40–80 mg/day (higher dosages) over 30 days. As illustrated in Figure 26–3, in both dosage escalation panels, marked reductions in depression and anxiety scores on patient and clinician scales were observed. The patient group receiving higher dosages showed markedly greater improvement. In fact, in the higher-dosage panel, 8 of 10 patients met the criterion of treatment response (i.e., ≤50% reduction in the Hamilton Rating Scale for Depression [Ham-D] baseline score), and 6 of 10 patients were classified as in remission (i.e., a Ham-D score of ≤8 points at study endpoint). In the low-dosage panel, only 5 of 10 patients were responders, and only 3 of 10 achieved remission. Any conclusions based on a small open-label trial are limited. Nevertheless, when the effect size obtained after a treatment period of 29 days was compared with that obtained from a control trial of the selective se-

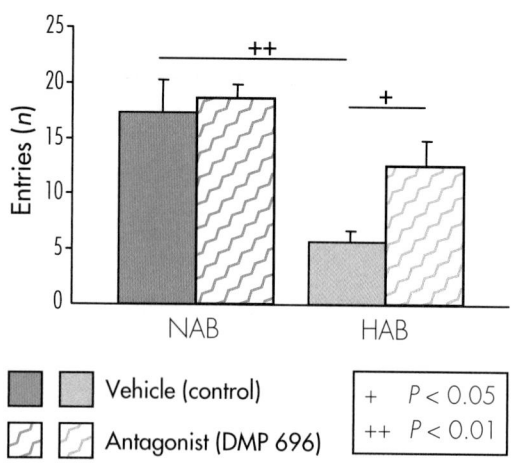

FIGURE 26–2.   Effects of a selective CRH₁ receptor antagonist on number of entries into open arms of elevated plus-maze.

Mice selectively bred for high anxiety-like behavior (HAB) assessed on the elevated plus-maze show increased CRH expression in the PVN (not shown). When HAB mice are treated with a selective CRH₁ receptor antagonist, their behavior normalizes and becomes indistinguishable from that of mice with normal anxiety-like behavior (NAB). *Hatched bars* indicate pretreatment with the CRH₁ receptor antagonist DMP-696. CRH = corticotropin-releasing hormone; CRH₁ = corticotropin-releasing hormone 1 receptor; CRH₂ = corticotropin-releasing hormone 2 receptor; PVN = paraventricular nucleus of the hypothalamus.
Source.   M. Bunck (Max Planck Institute of Psychiatry, Munich), personal communication, August 2006.

rotonin reuptake inhibitor (SSRI) paroxetine conducted over the same observation period under identical study conditions (Nickel et al. 2003), no significant differences between the two drugs were observed, which—within the inherent limitations of such an analysis—suggests that the clinical profiles of R 121919 and paroxetine are similar.

Extensive laboratory examinations, including clinical chemistry and hematology, electroencephalography, and electrocardiography, failed to show any adverse effects of R 121919, regardless of dosage (Künzel et al. 2003). The drug's safety was also confirmed in an in-depth hormonal analysis of all endocrine systems in which it was demonstrated that the pituitary–adrenocortical response to an intravenously administered test dose of 100 µg human CRH was not affected by the drug (Zobel et al. 2000). This finding is of particular importance, because it confirms that even if a dose is administered that effectively blocks central CRH₁ receptors, there are still sufficient CRH₁ receptors available at the anterior pituitary corticotrophs that can be stimulated by CRH. Thus, the stress

hormone system remains responsive to CRH, and treated patients do not develop drug-induced Addison's disease.

Disturbed sleep is a cardinal symptom of depression. Polysomnographic studies have demonstrated that patients with depression have increased rapid eye movement (REM) sleep density and decreased slow-wave sleep. The latter feature is reported to be induced by CRH in both animals and humans (Steiger 2007). A sleep electroencephalogram (EEG) analysis in a random subgroup of patients treated with R 121919 revealed increased slow-wave sleep and decreased REM sleep density (Held et al. 2004). The latter effect was more pronounced among patients receiving the higher dose of R 121919. These studies, as well as EEG studies in transgenic mice centrally overexpressing CRH, raise the possibility that the amount of REM sleep may serve as a biomarker identifying individuals with excessive central CRH secretion (M. Kimura [Max Planck Institute of Psychiatry, Munich], personal communication, July 2008). Despite these very promising early clinical results, further development of R 121919 was discontinued because of suspected liver toxicity at high dosages.

Another CRH₁ receptor antagonist, the nonpeptide tricyclic NBI-34041, was recently clinically investigated. This compound can also be orally administered, passes the blood–brain barrier, and binds to CRH₁ receptors with high affinity ($K_i = 4.0$ nmol/L). A randomized, double-blind, placebo-controlled study administered three different dosages of NBI-34041 (10, 50, and 100 mg/day) to 24 healthy male volunteers. The study was designed to evaluate whether the investigational drug would decrease the stress hormone response to a psychosocial stressor (Ising et al. 2007). For that purpose, the Trier Social Stress Test (TSST) was applied. The TSST is a standardized public-speaking procedure involving a mock job interview and performance of mental arithmetic (Kirschbaum et al. 1993). During and following the test paradigm, plasma ACTH and cortisol concentration–time curves were monitored. All subjects responded to the psychosocial stressor comparably in regard to tension or vigor required for achieving optimal performance (Dickman 2002). However, as illustrated in Figure 26–4, plasma ACTH and cortisol response was attenuated when the study participants were pretreated with NBI-34041. As was observed with R 121919, none of the administered drug dosages prompted a decreased release of plasma ACTH and cortisol in response to an intravenously administered test dose of CRH (Ising et al. 2007). The huge basic science database contrasts with the paucity of clinical reports using

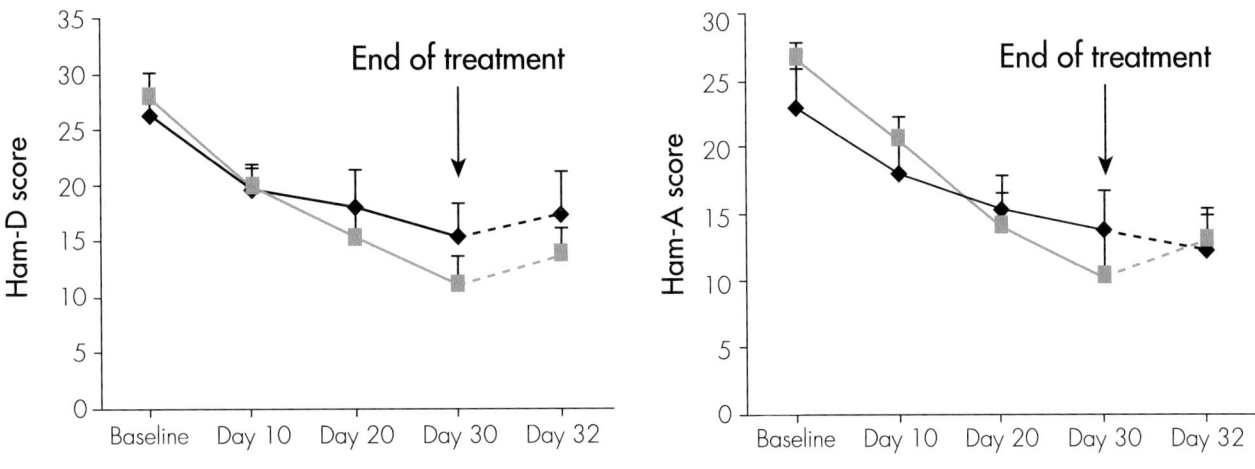

FIGURE 26-3. Results from an open-label proof-of-concept study suggest the potential usefulness of a CRH_1 receptor antagonist in severely depressed patients.

Two patient samples (n=10 each) with severe major depression were treated with R 121919, a selective high-affinity CRH_1 receptor antagonist. Two different dosage escalation panels with weekly increases from 5–20 mg to 40 mg (*black lines*) and from 40–60 mg to 80 mg (*green lines*) were administered, resulting in significantly decreased severity scores on both depression (Hamilton Rating Scale for Depression [Ham-D]) and anxiety (Hamilton Anxiety Scale [Ham-A]) scales. Note that after cessation of active treatment, clinical worsening of depressive and anxiety symptoms was observed. CRH=corticotropin-releasing hormone 1 receptor.
Source.   Adapted from Zobel et al. 2000.

CRH_1 receptor antagonists. In fact, a number of unreported clinical trials were discontinued because of toxic side effects. Importantly, these adversities do not question the pharmacological principle of muting CRH/CRH_1 receptor signaling, as toxicity of investigational CRH_1 receptor antagonists was observed in tissues not carrying CRH_1 receptors.

Even after a CRH_1 receptor antagonist has cleared all of the hurdles required to enter the market, it remains undecided what the ultimate role of these agents in clinical practice will be. To establish a clinical differentiation against current antidepressants or new drugs that act at different pathways, at least two imminent questions must be addressed: 1) Do CRH_1 receptor antagonists act preferentially in patients with documented HPA axis hyperactivity? and 2) Are CRH_1 receptor antagonists best used as treatment alternatives to current antidepressants or as adjuncts to improve time to onset and remission rate?

Regarding the first question, the available data—although limited—suggest that current neuroendocrine HPA tests only poorly predict CRH_1 receptor antagonist treatment outcome (Zobel et al. 2000). In fact, from results both in transgenic mice carrying the CRH_1 receptor gene deletions and in depressed patients undergoing HPA tests, it can be concluded that disturbed central CRH/CRH_1 receptor signaling is not necessarily reflected by peripheral pituitary–adrenocortical measures (Mueller et al.

2003). Ideally, positron emission tomography (PET) quantification of central CRH_1 receptors with PET-active CRH ligands could yield biomarkers to identify patients who might benefit from such a treatment. It would come as no surprise if a number of clinical trials using traditional study designs would fail to demonstrate beneficial effects of CRH_1 receptor antagonists in depression and anxiety disorders. In the absence of biomarkers to identify patients with excessive CRH/CRH_1 receptor signaling, such studies will not be helpful in exploiting the beneficial effects of CRH_1 receptor antagonists, as they would leave unrevealed how many patients in the CRH_1 receptor antagonist group are indeed central CRH hypersecreters. PET studies using appropriate CRH_1 receptor ligands would be needed to identify patients who are potential CRH_1 receptor antagonist responders. As mentioned above, the possibility of using sleep EEG–derived REM sleep measures to identify CRH hypersecretion deserves further study. The possibility that CRH_1 receptor antagonists might be well suited as adjunctive treatments is supported by a large number of studies showing that normalization of initially disturbed HPA axis activity underlies almost all antidepressant treatments, preceding the resolution of depressive symptoms (Ising et al. 2006). It may be worth testing whether the combination of an antidepressant and a CRH_1 receptor antagonist might offer an advantage over treatment with one or the other modality.

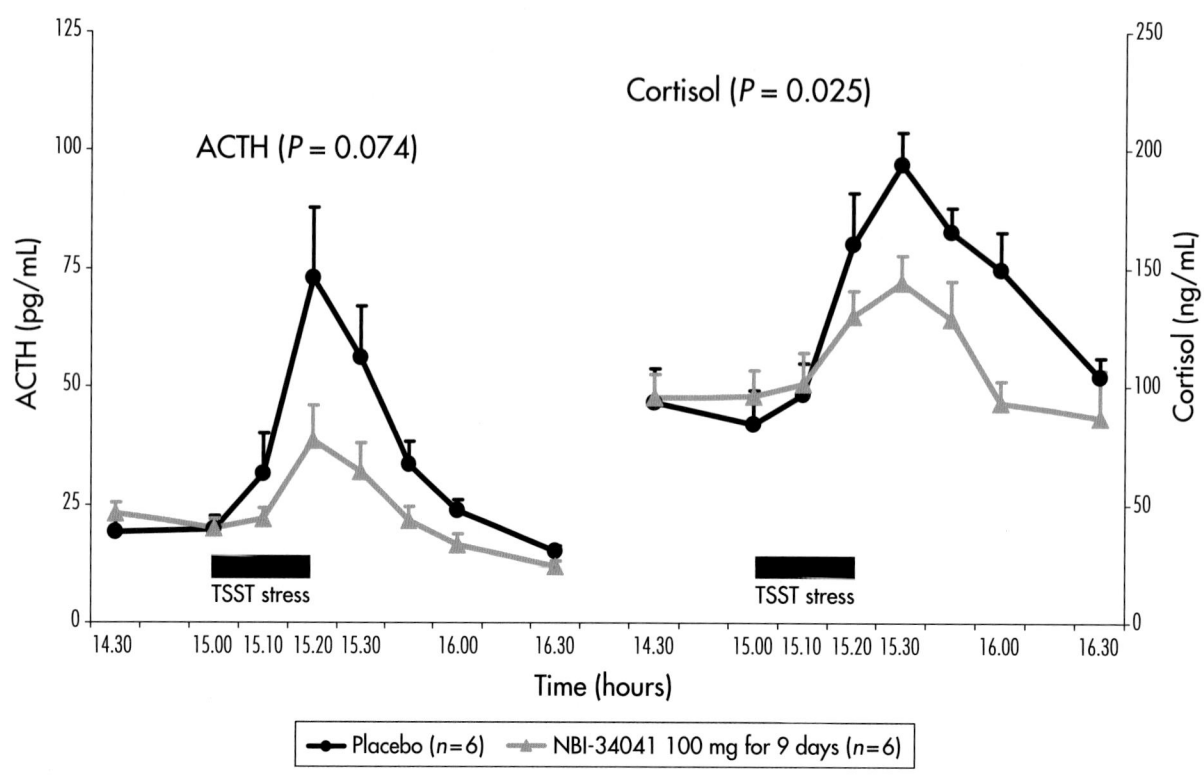

FIGURE 26–4. A CRH$_1$ receptor antagonist attenuates stress-elicited hormone response.

When challenged with a psychosocial stressor, healthy subjects pretreated with the CRH$_1$ receptor antagonist NBI-34041 showed lower secretion of ACTH and cortisol than did untreated subjects. ACTH = adrenocorticotropic hormone; CRH$_1$ = corticotropin-releasing hormone 1 receptor; TSST = Trier Social Stress Test.
Source. Adapted from Ising et al. 2007.

CRH$_2$ Receptor Antagonists

Much less effort has been devoted to evaluating the potential of CRH$_2$ receptor antagonists as drug targets. In fact, the physiological role of CRH/CRH$_2$ receptor signaling is less well elucidated, although several studies have demonstrated that this pathway is involved in stress response, cardiovascular function, and gastric motility. CRH$_2$ receptors seem to have a dual mode of action. In the acute (early) phase of stress, the CRH$_2$ receptor is activated through CRH and stresscopin (UCN III), increasing anxiety-like behavior. The CRH$_2$ receptor is also activated in the recovery phase, but in this phase it contributes to reduced emotionality (Hsu and Hsueh 2001). Three lines of CRH$_2$ receptor–deficient mice have been generated, which also failed to provide a clear picture regarding the behavioral response to blockade of CRH/CRH$_2$ receptor signaling. In two lines of CRH$_2$ receptor knockout mice, increased anxiety-like behavior was found (Bale et al. 2000; Kishimoto et al. 2000), but in the third line, no behavioral changes could be detected (Coste et al. 2000). A mouse line in which both CRH$_1$ and CRH$_2$ receptors were deleted was dominated by the effect of lacking CRH$_1$ receptors (Preil et al. 2001). Because no studies are available that use selective CRH$_2$ receptor antagonists, one can only speculate that such drugs may—through their action at the gastrointestinal tract—alleviate anorexia. Some drug companies are currently studying whether CRH$_2$ receptors are potential drug targets.

Vasopressin Receptor Antagonists

Given the clear indications that pharmacological interference with central vasopressin signaling pathways might be an alternative approach for treatment of stress-related disorders, surprisingly little research efforts aiming at vasopressin receptor antagonists have yet been reported. Three vasopressin receptor subtypes—V$_{1A}$, V$_{1B}$ (often termed V$_3$), and V$_2$—have been cloned. Through V$_{1B}$ receptors, found at the pituitary and central (mainly limbic) structures, vasopressin participates in regulation of the HPA axis by enhancing the release of ACTH and amplifying the action of CRH at corticotrophs (Gillies et al. 1982).

The relevance of this dual action has been demonstrated also in humans, where coadministration of vasopressin and CRH was shown to overcome dexamethasone-induced suppression of ACTH (von Bardeleben et al. 1985). Neither neuropeptide, when given alone, elicited substantial ACTH release (von Bardeleben et al. 1985). In contrast, dexamethasone-pretreated depressed patients show high ACTH release when CRH is administered. This was taken as a conjectural indication of increased limbic vasopressin production and secretion. Also, postmortem studies showed elevated vasopressin in the hypothalamus of depressed subjects (Purba et al. 1996). While V_{1A} receptors are expressed in the brain and are well documented to be involved in many stress-related behaviors (e.g., processing of social stimuli [Bielsky et al. 2005]), current pharmacological efforts are directed toward V_{1B} receptors (Serradeil-Le Gal et al. 2005). One compound, SSR-149415, a selective orally active V_{1B} receptor antagonist, may serve here as an example (Griebel et al. 2002). Recently, a rat strain was generated by selective breeding that shows high innate anxiety (Wigger et al. 2004). These animals overexpress vasopressin in both magnocellular and paraventricular hypothalamic nuclei (Keck et al. 2002). The reason for this overexpression is a polymorphism in the vasopressin gene promoter of these rats, resulting in impaired repression of gene activity (Murgatroyd et al. 2004). When treated with the SSRI paroxetine, the vasopressin gene expression was decreased in parallel with normalization of initially excessive HPA activity (Keck et al. 2003). Apparently existing drugs also interfere with the vasopressin system. From an alternative strategy (i.e., genetically engineered mice), a role for vasopressin V_{1B} signaling was suggested in the finding that V_{1B} receptor–knockout mice presented with reduced aggression and also changes in social recognition (Wersinger et al. 2002). These and other related findings led research at Sanofi to develop SSR-149415 as a selective V_{1B} receptor antagonist (Griebel et al. 2002). This drug was capable of suppressing in a dose-dependent fashion the potentiating effect of vasopressin on CRH-elicited ACTH release. This effect was absent if a selective V_{1B} receptor antagonist was coadministered. Likewise, the stress hormone increases evoked by exposure of mice to the forced-swim test were reduced when the animals were pretreated with SSR-149415. The preclinical behavioral profile of SSR-149415 further indicated that this compound exerts anxiolytic activity in various firmly established test batteries (Serradeil-Le Gal et al. 2002). The results from standard behavioral screens for antidepressant drug candidates showed promising results. Of particular interest here was that the antidepressant-like behavioral changes induced by SSR-149415 were also observed in hypophysectomized rats, underscoring that the effects were not secondary to the neuroendocrine actions of the drug but through brain V_{1B} receptors, which are not linked to the stress hormone control. Because SSR-149415 and related compounds seem to have a favorable preclinical profile, including safety and tolerability in humans (Serradeil-Le Gal et al. 2005), we will soon learn whether V_{1B} receptor antagonists provide an alternative or complementary approach to existing antidepressants.

Glucocorticoid Receptor Antagonists

Rapid activation of the stress hormone system in response to a threat is essential for an individual's health, but equally important is the appropriate curtailment of stress hormone secretion (de Kloet et al. 2005). If this is not achieved and HPA activity remains elevated, a number of changes occur that range from cognitive disturbance, labile mood, and psychotic features to alteration in peripheral metabolism and immune defense. The sustained hyperactivity of the stress hormone system among depressed patients is reflected by hypersecretion of ACTH and cortisol at baseline and altered responses to a number of neuroendocrine function tests. An explanation of disturbed stress hormone regulation and its far-reaching effects on the development and course of depression is provided by the aforementioned corticosteroid receptor hypothesis of depression (Holsboer 2000). According to this hypothesis, signaling via corticosteroid receptors in the brain is impaired in depression. Two corticosteroid receptors are present in the brain—the GR and the MR, which usually form homodimers (GRGR, MRMR). Under certain circumstances, they also form heterodimers (GRMR), provided they are expressed in the same nerve cell, which occurs mainly in the hippocampus (Trapp et al. 1994). The GR is widely expressed in neurons and glial cells in limbic and cortical brain locations and has 10-fold lower affinity for cortisol (humans) and corticosterone (rodents) than the MR (de Kloet et al. 2005). Both receptors have important tasks in adapting to stressful stimuli. MR, which is already substantially occupied by cortisol under resting conditions, sets the thresholds at the onset of the stress response by determining the degree to which the CRH/CRH_1 receptor system gets activated. As a consequence, cortisol secretion is increased, which activates previously unoccupied GRs. On the behavioral side, this facilitates adaptation, promotes memory storage, and prepares coping. These behavioral changes via MR and GR, together with responses elicited from CRH and vasopressin receptors, are essential to adapt to the stressors (de Kloet et al. 2005). When sufficiently activated, GR suppresses further elevation of glucocorticoids via a number of negative feedback actions. At the same time, a huge number of genes in the brain are regulated by ligand-activated corticosteroid receptors. Prominent examples for these repressive effects of ligand-activated GRs are CRH, vasopressin, and brain-derived neurotrophic factor (BDNF). Given their postulated roles in the development and course of depression, it is obvious that impaired corticosteroid receptor function will have consequences not only for HPA activity but also for cognition, mood, and metabolic features, such as development of the metabolic syndrome. Since stress exposure is often a trigger for the onset of depression for patients with a susceptibility to depression, resilience would imply a high threshold for induction of CRH/CRH_1 receptor signaling. This threshold can be increased by increased MR (de Kloet et al. 2005). In this context, it is important to note that a number of studies have shown that the earliest detectable mode of antidepressant action is increased expression of MR, which is followed by increased GR (Herr et al. 2003; Reul et al. 1993). The clinical relevance of these experiments in rats is reflected by a study that administered spironolactone, an MR antagonist, in conjunction with antidepressant treatment and observed worsened clinical outcome (Holsboer 1999).

The opposing effects of GR and MR are further illustrated by studies with GR antagonists such as mifepristone (RU-486), which was reported to ameliorate psychotic symptoms in patients with Cushing's syndrome, a disorder characterized by unrestrained ACTH and cortisol secretion. A number of reports have suggested that mifepristone is also capable of mitigating psychotic symptoms in patients with psychotic depression (deBattista et al. 2006). This clinical condition is almost always associated with elevated plasma cortisol concentrations. Perhaps GR antagonists in combination with an antidepressant would be superior to standard treatment for psychotic depression, which currently combines neuroleptic drugs with antidepressants. This would be in line with a recent study showing that combination therapy with amitriptyline and haloperidol and monotherapy with trimipramine were equally effective in the treatment of psychotic depression (Künzel et al. 2008). Trimipramine is an antidepressant that effectively suppresses HPA activity (Holsboer-Trachsler et al. 1991).

Because mifepristone acts quickly and produces much fewer side effects compared with antipsychotic drugs, it would be desirable if this or another GR antagonist could provide an alternative to antipsychotics in the treatment of psychotic depression. Currently, several large controlled studies are under way, although no conclusive results are yet available. In particular, it will be crucial to ascertain whether positive response to mifepristone in combination with antidepressants is limited to those patients showing hypercortisolism. Indeed, the dopamine hypothesis of psychotic depression formulated by Schatzberg et al. (1985) suggested that this subtype is caused by a pathophysiology that is distinct from other forms of depression. Yet some questions need to be addressed by basic research, because it is not yet firmly established how GR antagonists may exert their beneficial effects on psychopathology. The possibilities range from suppression of stimulant effects of corticosteroids on dopaminergic neurotransmission, as suggested by Piazza et al. (1996), to neuroprotective effects (Crochemore et al. 2005; Mayer et al. 2006). The latter aspect is highlighted by studies that compared the effects of MR and GR on neuronal survival and again showed that MR and GR have opposing effects. In this context, it is of interest that rat hippocampal neurons exposed to amyloid β-protein (a cytotoxic peptide associated with plaque formation in brains of patients with Alzheimer's disease) are protected from cell death when treated with mifepristone (Behl et al. 1997).

Inhibitors of Glucocorticoid Synthesis

A crucial step in the biosynthesis of cortisol is the substitution of a hydroxyl group at the C11 position of ring C. This biosynthetic step is blocked by metyrapone, which inhibits this C11 hydroxylation by blocking the hydroxylating enzyme. Indeed, in small studies, metyrapone produced beneficial effects in depressed patients. In a double-blind, randomized clinical trial, metyrapone supplementation improved both time to onset of action and clinical outcome under two different antidepressants, nefazodone (a mixed serotonin [5-HT] reuptake inhibitor and 5-HT_{2A}/5-HT_{2C} antagonist) and the 5-HT reuptake inhibitor fluvoxamine (Jahn et al. 2004). Regarding the mechanism underlying this interesting observation, glucocorticoid-lowering effects may play a crucial role, but also the biochemical consequences of the enzyme block are to be considered under metyrapone treatment. In the absence of a negative feedback signal via cortisol, corticosteroids that are not hydroxylated at the C11 position are produced at a much higher rate as the adrenal gland becomes continuously overactivated by ACTH. The resulting high levels of 11-deoxycortisol and several other neurosteroids may also have favorable influences on affect and cognition via positive allosteric modulation of γ-aminobutyric acid type A ($GABA_A$) receptors by so-called neuroactive steroids (Rupprecht and Holsboer 1999).

Agomelatine

It has been observed that several chronobiological aspects are impaired among depressed individuals. These circadian fluctuations encompass body temperature, hormone secretory patterns, and sleep–wake cycle during depressive episodes, which normalize once a patient is remitted (Duncan 1996). Based on these longitudinal observations, it was hypothesized that these circadian changes are causally related to depression and that drug-enforced reinstatement may be a promising treatment modality. Melatonin produced in the pineal gland is the prototypical chronobiotic regulator of all these rhythms by acting via two distinct cell membrane–located receptors, MT_1 and MT_2. When these receptors are genetically deleted in transgenic mice, behavioral changes are observed that resemble a depression-like phenotype (Larson et al. 2006; Weil et al. 2006). These and other related findings prompted the development of a drug that mimics the effects of melatonin at both MT receptors, and upon entering the brain, it would resynchronize altered chronobiological rhythms (Hamon and Bourgoin 2006). Agomelatine fulfills these expectations and acts as an agonist at MT_1 and MT_2 receptors. In addition, agomelatine is a 5-HT_{2C} antagonist. Several controlled clinical trials have confirmed the antidepressant efficacy of agomelatine (Kennedy and Emsley 2006). In one of these studies, 106 patients treated with agomelatine were compared with 105 patients receiving placebo, in an intent-to-treat population suffering from a major depressive episode and scoring on the 17-item version of the Ham-D with identical scores. At the end of the 6-week treatment period, agomelatine-treated patients had improvement from a score of 26.5±2.8 to 14.1±7.7, while placebo-treated patients improved from a baseline of 26.7±3.0 to 16.5±7.4 after 6 weeks. This difference of 15% was small but significant and was equivalent to reported drug–placebo differences observed in comparable studies (Thase et al. 2005). Apart from the favorable side-effect profile, two characteristics of agomelatine make this an attractive medication:

1. In depressed patients, agomelatine demonstrated sleep EEG changes consistent with the expectation of a 5-HT_{2C} receptor agonist (e.g., increased slow-wave sleep without affecting REM sleep). In addition, subjective sleep (onset and duration) and daytime alertness were improved as well (Kupfer 2006).

2. Antidepressant-related sexual dysfunction has received increasing attention given the association of SSRIs with diminished libido and difficulties in achieving orgasm (Clayton et al. 2002). In studies of agomelatine's effects on human sexual function, no agomelatine-induced sexual dysfunction was observed (Hamon and Bourgoin 2006). This is unsurprising, as it is known that melatonin exerts a facilitatory influence on sexual behavior.

The slight but significant superiority of agomelatine over placebo and its specific clinical profile, particularly the sleep-improving effects, seem to support the chronobiological diathesis of depression. However, it needs to be kept in mind that agomelatine is also a 5-HT_{2C} receptor antagonist, which may account for these clinical observations. As the anxiolytic actions of agomelatine are not prevented by melatonin receptor antagonists (Millan et al. 2005), it remains to be clarified which pharmacological action—MT receptor agonism or 5-HT_{2C} receptor antagonism—accounts for its psychotropic effects. Whatever the relative contribution of agomelatine's diverse pharmacological properties might be, this novel drug has a novel clinical profile and may provide a further argument that acting on different targets at the same time can be advantageous over highly specific compounds.

Glutamatergic System

From recent investigations, evidence has emerged that glutamate and other amino acid neurotransmitters are involved in the pathophysiology and treatment of depression (Kugaya and Sanacora 2005; Paul and Skolnick 2003). Although not always conclusive, in vivo magnetic resonance imaging (MRI) studies have revealed altered glutamate levels in various brain areas (Auer et al. 2000; Sanacora et al. 2004), as well as in the CSF (Frye et al. 2007), of depressed patients. Also postmortem studies pointed to an abnormal glutamate receptor expression in the locus coeruleus and medial temporal lobe of depressed subjects (Beneyto et al. 2007; Karolewicz et al. 2004). Glial cells are of considerable importance in maintaining proper function of the glutamatergic system. Therefore, it is of interest that studies provided morphometric evidence for glial cell pathology in patients with depression, mainly in prefrontal cortical regions, which confirms glutamatergic abnormality in this clinical condition (Rajkowska et al. 1999). These findings were corroborated by more recent reports, which found decreased levels of glial fibrillary acidic protein (a glial marker) or reduced numbers of glial cells in the anterior cingulate cortex in the brains of subjects with major depressive disorder (Cotter et al. 2001).

Glutamate is the major excitatory neurotransmitter in the brain; it is ubiquitously present at high concentrations (8–10 mmol/kg) in brain tissue. In comparison, brain monoamine concentrations are in the micromolar range. The glutamatergic system plays a role in a wide area of functions, including learning and memory. The effects of glutamate are conveyed by ionotropic and metabotropic receptors located in pre- and postsynaptic neuron membranes as well as on glial cells. The removal of glutamate from the synaptic cleft is achieved by an excitatory amino acid transporter (EAAT) located at neurons and glial cells. Given the relative abundance of glial cells over neurons, most of the glutamate clearance of synaptic clefts is by glial cell uptake. The EAATs are important in maintaining neuronal function, particularly in terminating the postsynaptic action of glutamate and reducing potentially toxic extracellular glutamate concentrations (Shigeri et al. 2004). If glutamate is not efficiently removed from the synaptic cleft, the continuous activation at postsynaptic ionotropic and metabotropic glutamate receptors may result in nerve cell death. In fact, these two glutamate receptor types also mediate glucocorticoid-induced apoptosis in hippocampal cells (J. Lu et al. 2003). Against this background, it is obvious that glial pathology, as observed in brains of depressed patients, may in conjunction with hypercortisolism account for the reported alterations of brain morphology. In fact, a number of studies showed that not only neurogenesis but also development of new glial cells is impaired by stressors, thus precipitating glutamate excess and cell death, ultimately rendering the brain susceptible to the development of mood disorders.

Based on the hypothesis that as a consequence of glial dysfunction, glutamatergic hyperactivity is one mechanism involved in the pathogenesis of depression, several glutamate receptor antagonists have been studied (Alt et al. 2005; Swanson et al. 2005b). Most studies used N-methyl-D-aspartate (NMDA) and α-amino-3-hydroxy-5-methylisoxazole-4-propionic acid (AMPA) receptor antagonists, which had been introduced as neuroprotectants in neurodegenerative diseases. Because some of these compounds also produced antidepressant-like behavioral changes in preclinical animal experiments, clin-

ical trials were initiated to study their possible antidepressant effects. In fact, mood-elevating effects were reported from the NMDA receptor antagonists amantadine and D-cycloserine, which are used for other clinical indications (e.g., tuberculosis). Moreover, the β-lactam antibiotic ceftriaxone, which increases glutamate uptake via enhancement of glutamate transporter function, showed antidepressant-like properties in mice tested in a series of preclinical models predictive for antidepressants (Mineur et al. 2007). Also, the NMDA receptor antagonist ketamine showed antidepressant-like effects in several animal experiments, which is in line with a recently reported anxiolytic and antidepressant-like phenotype of mouse mutants, where NMDA receptor function was decreased by deletion of a crucial receptor subunit (Miyamoto et al. 2002).

In a randomized, double-blind, placebo-controlled study, a single dose of ketamine 0.5 mg/kg intravenously administered to patients with major depression was found to exert a rapid (2 hours postinfusion) and transient (1 week) antidepressant effect (Zarate et al. 2006a). While the clinical use of ketamine is limited because of its potential psychotomimetic effects, this study result will trigger development of other NMDA receptor antagonists and probe their postulated utility. Recently, also memantine, an NMDA receptor antagonist approved for the treatment of Alzheimer's disease, was studied regarding antidepressant effects (Zarate et al. 2006b). In a double-blind, placebo-controlled trial, 32 subjects with major depression were randomly assigned to receive memantine (2–20 mg/day) or placebo. In contrast to the study using ketamine, no treatment effect under memantine was observed. Possibly the low to moderate NMDA receptor affinity of memantine in comparison with ketamine may account for the observed discrepancy.

Also, AMPA receptors are considered a drug target for antidepressants, mainly because 1) positive allosteric modulators of AMPA receptors increase brain levels of BDNF and 2) AMPA receptor potentiators are active in rodent models predictive for antidepressant efficacy. It is not clear how AMPA receptor potentiation may achieve this effect, but it is remarkable that also current antidepressants such as SSRIs positively modulate AMPA receptors, supporting the view that interference with glutamate receptors—specifically, the AMPA receptor subtype—is a general mechanism of antidepressant action (Alt et al. 2005). There is little doubt that glutamate-acting drugs will become more important in future drug discovery and development of antidepressants. Their ultimate role is difficult to predict. It may be speculated that in accordance with the considerations made in the previous paragraphs, targeting only a glutamatergic mechanism is not appropriate for reinstating brain function in depression. Instead, monoaminergic and glutamatergic targets are to be modified in concert to achieve antidepressive effects. A recent study by Sanacora et al. (2007), in which riluzole, a drug that decreases glutamate release and increases glutamate uptake, was added to ongoing antidepressant medication to 10 patients who had not responded to standard treatment, is of particular interest. In this pilot study, riluzole combined with standard antidepressants produced an antidepressant effect, suggesting a role for this drug as a potentiator of monoamine-mediated antidepressant effects.

Several candidate antidepressants and anxiolytics act on glutamate systems. For example, the dual-action serotonin–norepinephrine reuptake inhibitor milnacipran, launched as an antidepressant in Europe and recently approved for the treatment of fibromyalgia in the United States, is an AMPA receptor antagonist. The metabotropic glutamate 2/3 agonist LY544344 is currently in development as an anxiolytic drug (Kellner et al. 2005). All other research programs, mainly targeting AMPA and NMDA receptors, are in early clinical development (Markou 2007).

Neuropeptides

Over the past 20 years, an impressive amount of data has been accumulated that indicates strongly that neuropeptides play a role as brain neurotransmitters. Many studies—ranging from administration of neuropeptides into specific brain areas of animal models to studies using interference RNA directed against mRNA of neuropeptides or their receptors to transgenic mice overexpressing neuropeptides or carrying corresponding null mutations of ligands and receptors—point to neuropeptide receptors as potential drug targets for the treatment of depression and anxiety disorders (Holmes et al. 2003). This approach is not limited to the neuropeptides related to the stress hormone system, as illustrated in a previous paragraph, but includes many other neuropeptides and their receptors. Some of these, considered to be of particular interest, are briefly reviewed here.

Substance P/Neurokinin 1 Receptor

More than 75 years ago, von Euler and Gaddum (1931) discovered an 11–amino acid peptide, called substance P, that proved to be the preferred ligand at the neurokinin 1

(NK$_1$) receptor. NK$_1$ receptors are highly expressed in the spinal cord, brain stem, and limbic system. Substance P was originally thought to be a mediator of pain, and the first NK$_1$ receptor antagonists were evaluated for their potential as analgesics. While these studies failed, a report by Kramer et al. (1998) demonstrated that the NK$_1$ receptor antagonist MK-869 (aprepitant) is indeed an effective antidepressant, superior to placebo and equal in potency to paroxetine. Unfortunately, a number of replication studies (e.g., Keller et al. 2006) produced mixed results, prompting most pharmaceutical companies to discontinue their NK$_1$ receptor antagonist programs. That is disappointing, because a number of clinical and basic studies strongly supported the theory that blockade of the substance P/NK$_1$ receptor signaling cascade may represent a novel antidepressant mechanism. For example, substance P was found to be elevated in patients with depression and to increase in response to stress (Geracioti et al. 2006). This is in agreement with reports of decreased central NK$_1$ receptors in depression (Stockmeier et al. 2002). If substance P is administered centrally to animals, a number of behavioral changes are induced that resemble anxiogenic and depressogenic response patterns, including not only behavioral but also cardiovascular and other vegetative changes (Stout et al. 2001). In agreement with these observations are findings obtained from substance P– and NK$_1$–knockout mice, which showed reduced anxiety- and depression-like behavior (Bilkei-Gorzo and Zimmer 2005). Despite some disillusionment regarding the utility of NK$_1$ receptor antagonists in clinical practice, the chapter does not seem to be closed on these agents, and a recent report on the efficacy and safety of a novel compound, L759274, supports this view (Kramer et al. 2004).

Galanin

Galanin, a 30–amino acid neuropeptide, is widely distributed in the central nervous system, where it exerts its action via three receptor subtypes: Gal$_1$, Gal$_2$, and Gal$_3$. Norepinephrine (NE) neurons in the locus coeruleus as well as 5-HT neurons in the dorsal raphe nucleus can synthesize galanin, and in vivo microdialysis studies suggested that galanin plays an important role as a modulator of NE and 5-HT release (Z.Q. Xu et al. 1998; Yoshitake et al. 2004). A relationship to mood, anxiety, and stress response was derived from studies that injected galanin into the rat brain and observed anxiolytic effects (X. Lu et al. 2005). Also a study that administered galanin to depressed patients and measured psychopathology and recorded the sleep EEG reported antidepressant-like effects (Murck et al. 2004). Further support comes from investigations that administered antidepressants and found that they activated galanin expression in the dorsal raphe nucleus. Studying individual galanin receptors, current antidepressants seem to shift galanin neurotransmission from a predominant galanin/Gal3 receptor pathway toward a galanin/Gal$_{1,2}$ receptor signaling. These observations suggested that the Gal3 receptor is a potential drug target. In fact, several Gal3 receptor antagonists (e.g., SNAP 37889 and SNAP 398299) have been developed and are currently under investigation (Swanson et al. 2005a). Alternatively, stimulating Gal1 or Gal2 receptors is also an option. Accordingly, a potent, highly selective Gal2 receptor agonist, galmic, which is orally available and passes the blood–brain barrier, was synthesized (Ceide et al. 2004). At present it is difficult to predict whether modulators of Gal receptors will play a role in future drug development. If so, they may be used to enhance the effects of the monoamine-based antidepressants.

Orexigenic Peptides

Body weight is regulated by a homeostatic control system in which the brain—in particular, the hypothalamus—senses and integrates incoming signals and coordinates appetite by releasing orexigenic neuropeptides. Among these, at least three -melanin-concentrating hormone (MCH), neuropeptide Y (NPY), and orexin—have been linked to the pathogenesis of depression. Subsequently, their signaling pathways have been investigated to identify potential drug targets.

Melanin-Concentrating Hormone 1 Receptor Antagonists

MCH is a 19–amino acid polypeptide mainly produced in the lateral hypothalamus, where projections to many brain areas originate. The effects of MCH in humans are mediated via two G protein–coupled receptors: MCH1 and MCH2. Because of MCH and MCH1 receptor expression in frontal cortical regions, nucleus accumbens, dorsal raphe nucleus, amygdala, and hippocampus, this system has primarily been studied in the context of depression (Shimazaki et al. 2006). In mice, where the MCH2 receptor does not exist, MCH overexpression is associated not only with increased feeding behavior but also with a depression-like phenotype. In agreement, MCH1 knockout mice showed decreased anxiety-like and depression-like behavior. In line with a depressogenic effect of MCH are

neuropeptide-induced elevations of HPA activity via increased CRH secretion and enhanced anxiety- and depression-like behavior in several behavioral tests. Likewise, an MCH1 receptor antagonist (GW-3430) blocked the neuroendocrine and behavioral effects of MCR only in wild-type mice, but not in mice where the MCH1 receptor was deleted (Smith et al. 2006). These and other complementary studies prompted the development of MCH1 receptor antagonists, and several compounds are currently characterized.

SNAP-7941 is a high-affinity antagonist ligand for the MCH1 receptor and proved to be a centrally active anorectic compound that, according to long-term observations in animals with diet-induced obesity, may serve as an antiobesity drug, since it produced a sustained and consistent decrease in food consumption and body weight. In extension of these studies on food intake, SNAP-7941 was also tested in behavioral paradigms predictive of antidepressant- or anxiolytic-like effects. The results from these experiments provided strong support for the MCH1 receptor as a regulator of mood (Borowsky et al. 2002). It is not yet clear whether these depressogenic and anxiogenic effects are mediated by MCH-induced activation of CRH/CRH1 receptor pathways. Studies in which MCH is administered to CRH1 receptor knockout mice or mice pretreated with a CRH1 receptor antagonist would help to clarify this issue. Currently, several pharmaceutical companies are developing MCH1 receptor antagonists (e.g., ATC0065, ATC0175) that have shown anxiolytic- and antidepressant-like activity in mice and rats (Chaki et al. 2005). Recently, another MCH1 receptor antagonist (SNAP-94847) has been described that has an anxiolytic- and antidepressant-like profile that is clearly distinct from that of current antidepressants (David et al. 2007; Roy et al. 2007). If the antidepressant-like effect in combination with the anorectic effect of MCH1 receptor antagonists could be translated into a clinical medication, it may be particularly useful for those patients whose depression is characterized by reduced activity and weight gain, often termed atypical depression. Also, some psychotropic drugs (e.g., mirtazapine, olanzapine, but also some SSRIs) increase body weight in some patients. These would benefit from coadministration of an MCH1 receptor antagonist.

Neuropeptide Y Receptor Agonists

Neuropeptide Y is a 36–amino acid polypeptide that is abundantly present in many brain areas, including the locus coeruleus (where it is coexpressed with NE), hippocampus, hypothalamus, amygdala, nucleus accumbens, and neocortex. Actions of NPY are mediated in the brain via three different G protein–coupled receptors: Y_1, Y_2, and Y_5. Some clinical data point to decreased activation of NPY/$Y_{1,5}$ signaling in patients with depression (Redrobe et al. 2002), which agrees with findings from animal experiments showing that activation of Y_1 and Y_5 receptors in the amygdala produces anxiolytic-like effects (Kask et al. 2002; Primeaux et al. 2005; Sajdyk et al. 2002). The link between NPY and mood has also been confirmed by studies demonstrating increased anxiety-like behavior in NPY-null mutant mice (Palmiter et al. 1998). In addition, transgenic rats overexpressing NPY in the hippocampus demonstrate a remarkable resilience toward stress exposure (Vezzani et al. 1999). The mechanism underlying the stress-buffering effects of NPY remains to be elucidated. Possibly NPY potentiates the anxiolytic effects of GABA and inhibits glutamate release. Whether the pharmaceutical industry will pursue the development of NPY receptor agonists, specifically Y_1 or Y_5 agonists, is yet not clear.

Orexin Receptor Antagonists

Orexin-A and orexin-B (also named hypocretin 1 and hypocretin 2) are two neuropeptides produced by a cluster of neurons in the posterior lateral hypothalamus. They were originally implicated in the control of food intake (Samson and Resch 2000). The orexin neurons innervate many brain regions that drive arousal and attention, including the locus coeruleus (where noradrenergic projections emerge) and the dorsal raphe nucleus (from which serotonergic projections emerge). These neuroanatomical findings and the corresponding distribution of orexin receptors (OX_1 and OX_2) triggered research efforts investigating other effects than feeding behavior. Most interest has been attracted by findings that orexin/$OX_{1,2}$ signaling is involved in behavioral activity, wakefulness, arousal, and attention (Kilduff and Peyron 2000). The role of orexin as a major component of sleep–wake regulation has been strongly supported by findings in patients with narcolepsy. Patients suffering from this sleep disorder have excessive daytime sleepiness, episodes of muscle weakness (cataplexy) triggered by emotional stimuli, and intrusive REM sleep. These patients have degenerated orexin-producing hypothalamic neurons and decreased orexin in the CSF (Mignot et al. 2002; Nishino et al. 2000; Thanickal et al. 2000).

These findings stimulated the search for drugs that block orexin/$OX_{1,2}$ signaling, and the effects of the first

$OX_{1,2}$ receptor antagonists in rats, dogs, and humans were recently reported (Brisbare-Roch et al. 2007). Administration of ACT-0788573, an orally available tetrahydroisoquinoline derivative that readily passes the blood–brain barrier, was found to decrease alertness, without signs of cataplexy. These behavioral effects were uniform in all three species tested. In the sleep EEG in rats, both REM and non-REM sleep were increased, and in human volunteers, a shortened latency to stage 2 sleep was recorded during a daytime nap opportunity. In the absence of an all-night polysomnography, no conclusion about whether $OX_{1,2}$ antagonists restored physiological sleep patterns can be drawn. When compared with 10 mg zolpidem, a short-acting nonbenzodiazepine $GABA_A$ receptor modulator, the orexin receptor blocker had a longer duration of action. ACT-0788573 produced fewer side effects in comparison with zolpidem. This first report of a single dose administered to healthy volunteers does not allow one to predict whether this new class of drug might also be effective for long-term administration in patients suffering from insomnia. However, given that disturbed sleep is a cardinal symptom among depressed patients, coadministration of an $OX_{1,2}$ receptor antagonist might be a worthwhile strategy. This possibility is particularly compelling because some antidepressants preferentially prescribed to improve sleep (e.g., mirtazapine) also tend to increase body weight. Orexin$_{1,2}$ receptor antagonists are devoid of such adverse effects and, on the contrary, may help maintain body weight.

Targeting Signaling Pathways

Phosphodiesterase Inhibitors

By inhibiting presynaptic monoamine reuptake transporters, antidepressants enhance activation of postsynaptic G protein–coupled receptors to which NE and 5-HT selectively bind. In response to ligand binding, the receptor, when coupled to a stimulatory G protein (G_s), activates the enzyme adenylate cyclase, which results in increased cyclic adenosine monophosphate (cAMP) levels. Most of the effects of cAMP are mediated by activation of protein kinase A (PKA). One of the downstream targets of PKA is CREB (cAMP response element binding protein), which is believed to play a key role in antidepressant-induced mechanisms (Nestler et al. 2002). The activation of CREB via phosphorylation is a mechanism common to nearly all antidepressants, once they were chronically administered. Antidepressants also upregulate expression of CREB, and several studies link CREB expression and activation to antidepressant treatment response, possibly via expression of BDNF, whose gene activity is in part regulated by binding of phosphorylated CREB. In the light of this hypothesized mechanism, elevated levels of cAMP are essential to promote this action.

cAMP is degraded by a phosphodiesterase (PDE) into adenosine monophosphate (Figure 26–5). cAMP is a ubiquitous second messenger, responsible for a multitude of physiological functions, which involve activation of transcription factors by phosphorylation. Not surprisingly, the inactivation of cAMP by PDE is complicated. To date, 11 families of PDEs have been identified, which generate 30 different isoforms that are able to degrade cAMP (Houslay and Adams 2003). The PDE4 family has received particular attention, because over 20 years ago a PDE4 inhibitor, rolipram, had been discovered and developed by Schering Pharmaceuticals (Wachtel 1983). Rolipram was shown to be an inhibitor of cAMP-specific PDE4. Members of this PDE subfamily are encoded by four PDE4 genes, which encode over 16 different isoforms. In animal models as well as in small clinical trials, rolipram was demonstrated to exert antidepressant effects (Fujimaki et al. 2000; Hebenstreit et al. 1989). Its side-effect profile, particularly nausea and vomiting, prompted discontinuation of its clinical development.

The interest in PDE4 inhibitors, however, is still alive, and a growing body of research focused on neurobiology of depression and antidepressant mechanisms may ultimately result in an upsurge of novel PDE4 inhibitors. One possible way of using this unique mechanism would be elucidation of the brain area–specific expression of the four PDE4 subtypes (PDE4A–D), for which, as mentioned before, multiple isoforms exist. Based on the hypothesis that activation of CREB by phosphorylation in the hippocampus is an important common pathway of almost all antidepressants, it would be useful to know whether a specific PDE4 subtype exists in this brain area that is different from the PDE4 subtypes in areas that mediate nausea and vomiting. Recently a transgenic mouse model for emesis was studied, where either PDE4B or PDE4D genes were deficient (Robichaud et al. 2002). This study concluded that inhibition of the PDE4D subtype mediates the emetic side effects observed under rolipram. Interestingly, the PDE4D subtype is predominantly expressed in the area postrema, known to be involved in emesis.

The new possibilities available in pharmaceutical industry to develop assays for very specific potential targets, that allow screening of huge compound libraries, will

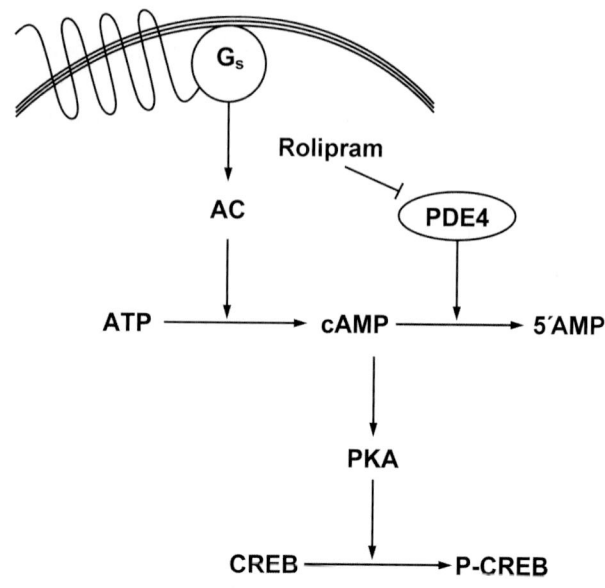

FIGURE 26–5.   Mode of action of rolipram.

Rolipram inhibits phosphodiesterase inhibitor 4 (PDE4), thus preventing degradation of cAMP into systems of 5′AMP and enhancing phosphorylation of transcriptional factors (e.g., CREB via protein kinase A [PKA]). 5′AMP=adenosine-5′-monophosphate; AC=adenylate cyclase; cAMP=cyclic adenosine monophosphate; CREB=cAMP response element binding protein; G_s=stimulatory G protein.

hopefully result in new lead compounds selectively inhibiting those PDE4 subtypes that are directly involved in the antidepressant effects of this class of drugs (Zhang et al. 2002). Such discovery programs can possibly capitalize on the recent disclosure of the crystal structure of PDE4B complexed with rolipram (R.X. Xu et al. 2004).

Glycogen Synthase Kinase–3 Inhibitors

The search for targets of mood-stabilizing lithium salts led to glycogen synthase kinase–3 (GSK-3), and more recently, preclinical evidence implicates modulation of GSK-3 in the mechanism of action of mood stabilizers (Gould and Manji 2005) and current antidepressant medications (Eldar-Finkelman 2002). GSK-3 is found as two isoforms, GSK-3α and GSK-3β, that have a 97% sequence homology and also have similar biological effects. GSK-3 is a kinase that is ubiquitously expressed in the brain and is involved in many signaling pathways. The best elaborated pathways comprise Wnt signaling, insulin signaling, and neurotrophic signaling (Gould et al. 2006). Lithium was found to decrease GSK-3 at therapeutic dosages, and the effect of GSK-3 inhibition was shown in vivo by increase of β-catenin, which acts as a cellular transcription factor and is inactivated by GSK-3. After

Antipsychotics

CHAPTER 27

Classic Antipsychotic Medications

Henry A. Nasrallah, M.D.

Rajiv Tandon, M.D.

History and Discovery

Prior to the introduction of classic antipsychotic medications in the 1950s, treatment for psychotic disorders primarily consisted of humane containment and supportive care. A variety of remedies without empirical support were popular in different cultures for brief periods of time but went out of vogue because they were ineffective. One approach to the treatment of psychosis that survived through the ages was the use of reserpine as a folk medicine in India. In the Ayurveda (the traditional Indian medical system originating 5,000 years ago), Sarpagundha (*Rauwolfia serpentina*, or Indian snakeroot, from which reserpine is derived) was recommended as the treatment for "unmada" (psychosis). In the early 1950s, reserpine was found to improve psychosis and reduce violent behavior in clinical trials among aggressive mentally ill patients in state hospitals in New York and California, and this led to its introduction as an antipsychotic in 1954 (2 years after chlorpromazine). However, reserpine's popularity declined after 1957 because of its high level of side effects and low safety index. Although the use of reserpine has been completely discontinued in some countries (e.g., the United Kingdom) because of its significant drug interactions and adverse effects, it is available in the United States, where it is still used, albeit very infrequently, as an alternative or augmentation treatment in patients with schizophrenia refractory to other antipsychotic treatment.

Chlorpromazine, the first of the "classic" antipsychotics, heralded a pharmacological revolution in psychiatry with its introduction in 1952. The discovery of chlorpromazine was serendipitous and owes much to the need of Allied forces during World War II to find a synthetic antimalarial treatment, given that access to many quinine-producing areas of the world had been blocked by Japanese forces. Paul Ehrlich had noted in 1891 that methylene blue, a phenothiazine derivative, effectively treated symptoms of malaria (Travis 1991). A new group of compounds was synthesized by substituting chains on the central nitrogen atom of the phenothiazine ring. Although these phenothiazine derivatives were found to be inactive as antimalarial drugs, they were noted to have potent antihistaminic properties.

Scientists at Rhône-Poulenc in France found that one of the aminoalkyl phenothiazines, promethazine, had more pronounced sedative properties than other antihistamines. This effect was noted in 1949 by Henri Laborit, an anesthesiologist and surgeon in the French navy who had researched various synthetic antihistamines as a way of "potentiating" anesthetics for use in surgical patients to decrease the morbidity and mortality from surgically induced shock. Promethazine was one of the agents he tested. His observation that administration of a "lytic cocktail" (a mixture of a narcotic, sedating, and hypnotic drug) to induce an "artificial hibernation" was successful in decreasing patient anxiety led to a further search by the Rhône-Poulenc scientists for other phenothiazine derivatives with similar effects. Paul Charpentier, a company chemist and phenothiazine specialist, had synthesized a new phenothiazine, chlorpromazine, which was first tested by S. Couvoisier in rodents and dogs in 1950. It was found to prolong barbiturate-induced sleep, to prevent apomorphine-induced emesis, and to inhibit conditioned avoidance–escape responses. When Laborit used this drug on his surgical patients, he noted that some of them, without losing consciousness, became very relaxed and appeared indifferent to what was occurring around them. He later referred to this effect as a "chemical lobotomy."

On the basis of these observations, Laborit recommended the drug to his psychiatric colleagues at the Val-de-Grace military hospital in Paris. Their success in treating a young male patient with mania at the Sainte-Anne mental hospital in Paris was noted by two French psychiatrists, Jean Delay and Pierre Deniker. In March 1952, they began the treatment of a small group of hospitalized psychotic patients with chlorpromazine alone. Delay and Deniker reported the drug's amazing treatment successes at the June 1952 meeting of the Medical Psychological Society. The use of chlorpromazine quickly spread to Canada, where Heinz Lehmann at the Verdun Hospital in Montreal treated a large cohort of acute schizophrenic patients with the drug. After 4–5 weeks of treatment, many of the patients were practically symptom-free.

In the United States, chlorpromazine was first used by psychiatrist William Long, medical director of McLean Hospital in Boston. Subsequently, the results of a successful open-label trial in September 1953 by a psychiatrist, Willis Bower, also at McLean, were published in the *New England Journal of Medicine* in October 1954. The definitive evidence of chlorpromazine's efficacy was established following completion of a large controlled study by the U.S. Veterans Administration Collaborative Study Group in 1960.

After the successes of chlorpromazine, numerous other phenothiazines were synthesized and tested. Many other drugs, which were slightly different in structure from the phenothiazines but nonetheless effective as antipsychotics, were also produced. These included drugs such as haloperidol and thiothixene. The last of these drugs approved by the U.S. Food and Drug Administration (FDA) was molindone, introduced in 1975. Of the 51 classic antipsychotics (representing 8 different chemical classes) available in the world (Table 27–1), 12 are currently available in the United States.

The ability of chlorpromazine and other conventional antipsychotics to suppress psychotic symptoms (delusions, hallucinations, and bizarre behavior) had a profound impact on chronically hospitalized psychiatric populations worldwide. Massive numbers of psychiatric patients were discharged from state hospitals to the community. This period of deinstitutionalization led to a de-

TABLE 27–1. First-generation antipsychotics (n=51)

I. Phenothiazines
   A. Aliphatic side chain (low/medium-potency agents)
      Chlorproethazine, chlorpromazine, cyamemazine, levomepromazine, promazine, triflupromazine
   B. Piperidine side chain (low/medium-potency agents)
      Mesoridazine, pericyazine, piperacetazine, pipotiazine, propericiazine, sulforidazine, thioridazine
   C. Piperazine side chain (medium/high-potency agents)
      Acetophenazine, butaperazine, dixyrazine, fluphenazine, perazine, perphenazine, prochlorperazine, thiopropazate, thioproperazine, trifluoperazine
II. Butyrophenones (high-potency agents)
    Benperidol, bromperidol, droperidol, fluanisone, haloperidol, melperone, moperone, pipamperone, timiperone, trifluperidol
III. Thioxanthenes (low/medium-potency agents)
     Chlorprothixene, clopenthixol, flupenthixol, thiothixene, zuclopenthixol
IV. Dihydroindolones (low/medium-potency agents)
    Molindone, oxypertine
V. Dibenzepines (low/medium-potency agents)
   Clotiapine, loxapine
VI. Diphenylbutylpiperidines (high-potency agents)
    Fluspirilene, penfluridol, pimozide
VII. Benzamides (low-potency agents)
     Nemonapride, sulpiride, sultopride, tiapride
VIII. Iminodibenzyl (medium-potency agents)
      Clocapramine, mosapramine

crease in the number of patients in state and county mental hospitals in the United States from 559,000 in 1955 to 338,000 in 1970 to 107,000 in 1988, an 80% decrease over 30 years. Initially, this led to enthusiasm about the possibility that patients with schizophrenia and other psychoses would be able to function well in the community. However, it soon became apparent that improvement with antipsychotic treatment was incomplete, and common lack of compliance, with subsequent relapses, led to frequent rehospitalization (i.e., the "revolving door phenomenon"). Many patients stopped their medications shortly after hospital discharge, preferring life with psychosis to intolerable movement disorders. Depot preparations introduced in the 1970s helped reduce the rate of relapse due to noncompliance. However, only a minority of patients received depot antipsychotics, and the search for a safer class of drugs with better tolerability eventually led to the development of the second-generation (atypical) antipsychotics (SGAs).

Shortly after the widespread use of chlorpromazine, psychiatrists began observing that treated patients frequently manifested signs and symptoms of parkinsonism. Along with other side effects such as dystonia and akathisia, these are collectively referred to as *extrapyramidal side effects* (EPS) because they involve involuntary muscle movements. In a 1961 report, the prevalence of antipsychotic-induced EPS was estimated at 40%. Because of the high rate of movement disorders associated with antipsychotic treatment, many psychiatrists believed EPS to be an unavoidable accompaniment of antipsychotic action; in fact, the onset of some EPS was considered to indicate achievement of a necessary dose (*neuroleptic threshold*). The first report of persistent orobuccal movements (later labeled *tardive dyskinesia*) came from France in 1959. The pervasiveness and significant adverse consequences of short-term and long-term motor side effects associated with classic antipsychotic drugs led to a search for antipsychotic drugs that would be as efficacious but without the risk of EPS.

Clozapine, a dibenzodiazepine synthesized in 1959, was the first antipsychotic drug without EPS (i.e., atypical). It was first marketed in 1972 in Europe but was withdrawn in some countries in 1975 after several reports of fatalities secondary to agranulocytosis. Clozapine was not introduced in the United States until 1989, after convincing studies demonstrated its efficacy in neuroleptic-refractory patients, but with the requirement for mandatory weekly leukocyte counts. Several other atypical agents have been launched in the past 15 years and are reported to be associated with far lower levels of EPS and a broader spectrum of efficacy (see Chapters 28–33 in this textbook). Since then, use of the classic antipsychotics (also referred to as traditional, conventional, or first-generation antipsychotics [FGAs]) has steadily declined, especially in the United States—they currently aggregate less than 10% of all antipsychotic prescriptions in the country.

SGAs have increasingly replaced FGAs around the world and have almost completely supplanted FGAs in the United States because of their presumed greater efficacy and better safety/tolerability profiles. However, results of recent government-sponsored studies in the United States (Clinical Antipsychotic Trials of Intervention Effectiveness [CATIE]) and the United Kingdom (Cost Utility of the Latest Antipsychotic Drugs in Schizophrenia Study [CUtLASS]) have challenged the current worldview of the greater effectiveness of SGAs over FGAs and are reinvigorating interest in the utility and clinical applicability of classic antipsychotics.

Structure–Activity Relations

Phenothiazines

Members of the phenothiazine class of classic antipsychotics share the same basic phenothiazine ring but differ in substitutions at both their R1 and R2 positions (Figure 27–1). Based on the side chain attached to the nitrogen atom in the middle ring (R1), the phenothiazines are further subdivided into three subtypes: aliphatic, piperidine, and piperazine phenothiazines. There is much more variety in the substitutions at the second carbon atom; generally more negatively charged (electrophilic) groups tend to result in stronger binding to dopamine receptors. These electrophilic groups weaken the aromatic bonds within the phenothiazine ring by partially drawing bonding electrons into their orbit.

Aliphatic Phenothiazines

The aliphatic phenothiazines share a dimethylamide substitution at their tenth carbon. Chlorpromazine (Thorazine or Largactil) is the prototypical member of this class and remains the aliphatic phenothiazine most widely used throughout the world. With a chlorine atom attached to its second carbon, chlorpromazine is heavily sedating because of its high level of anticholinergic, anti-α-adrenergic, and antihistaminergic actions.

Piperidine Phenothiazines

Piperidine phenothiazines are named for the presence of a piperidine ring at their tenth carbon. Although members of this group have similar efficacy and side effects compared with aliphatic phenothiazines, they are notable for having a less potent effect on nigrostriatal dopamine$_2$ (D$_2$) receptors and a higher level of anticholinergic activity; consequently they are associated with a lower frequency of EPS. Thioridazine (Mellaril) and its metabolite, mesoridazine (Serentil), are the only piperidines available within the United States. The use of these agents has been virtually extinguished by a black box warning about significant QTc prolongation that was added to their product label in 2000.

Piperazine Phenothiazines

With a substitution of a piperazine group at the tenth carbon of a phenothiazine, the piperazines have greatly increased D$_2$ blockade and a lower affinity to muscarinic, α-adrenergic, and histaminergic receptors. Some of the most potent conventional antipsychotics available in the

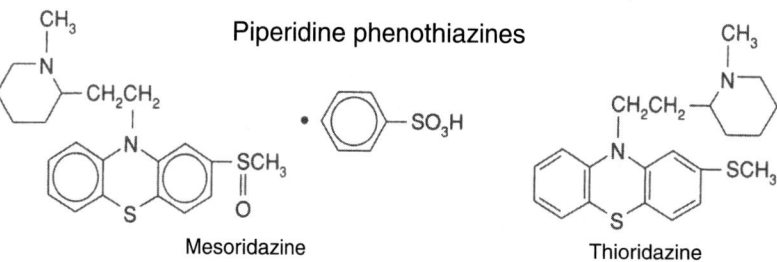

FIGURE 27–1.   Chemical structures of various classic antipsychotics.

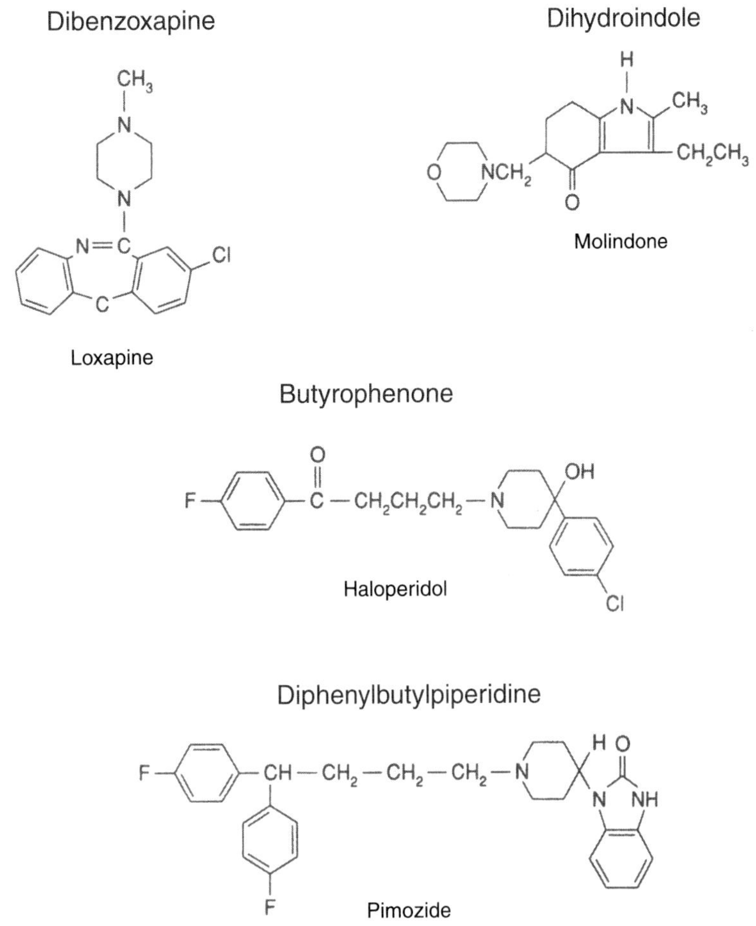

Dibenzoxapine

Dihydroindole

Molindone

Loxapine

Butyrophenone

Haloperidol

Diphenylbutylpiperidine

Pimozide

FIGURE 27–1. Chemical structures of various classic antipsychotics (*continued*).

United States, including fluphenazine (Prolixin), perphenazine (Trilafon), and trifluoperazine (Stelazine), belong to this class. The well-known antiemetic prochlorperazine (Compazine) is also part of this class; although approved for the treatment of psychosis, it is rarely utilized as an antipsychotic.

Thioxanthenes

Structurally and pharmacologically similar to the phenothiazines, the thioxanthenes also differ widely in their pharmacological profiles based on similar side-chain substitutions (see Figure 27–1). For instance, chlorprothixene shares the same dimethylamide and chloride substitution as chlorpromazine, with which it also shares its pharmacological profile. Thiothixene (Navane) has both a piperazine side chain and a strongly electrophilic substitution [$SO_2N(CH_3)CH_3$], thus sharing the pharmacological profile of the piperazines. Of further interest, the thioxanthene ring, which differs from the phenothiazine ring by having a carbon atom at its tenth position, has two

optically active isomers, or enantiomers. Of the two isomers of the ring, the *cis* isomer exerts greater dopaminergic receptor blockade than the *trans* isomer.

Butyrophenones

The butyrophenone class has a piperidine ring with a three-carbon chain ending in a carbonyl-substituted p-fluorobenzene ring. Butyrophenones differ on the basis of the substitutions present within their piperidine rings (see Figure 27–1). Haloperidol, arguably the best-known classic antipsychotic, is the most widely used member of this class. Sharing a similar pharmacological profile but having a lower level of activity within the nigrostriatal pathway, another phenothiazine, droperidol, is available only in an intramuscular form for the indication of nausea. Both haloperidol and droperidol are strong dopamine receptor antagonists and show little antimuscarinic, antihistaminergic, and antiadrenergic activity. Although widely used in the past as an antipsychotic, droperidol is approved by the FDA only for use as an antiemetic, and its use has recently declined due to its QTc-prolonging effects.

Spiperone, one of the most potent dopamine antagonists in existence, is utilized as a D_2, dopamine$_3$ (D_3), and dopamine$_4$ (D_4) receptor radiolabel for research purposes exclusively.

Dibenzoxazepines

Loxapine, the only FDA-approved agent within the dibenzoxazepine class, is composed of a tricyclic ring structure with a seven-member central ring. It has a piperazine side chain and chlorine at position R2 (see Figure 27–1). It exhibits an intermediate level of D_2 blockade, as well as some serotonin$_2$ (5-HT$_2$) antagonism. Its side-effect profile is characterized by intermediate sedation and autonomic effects. Loxapine has the distinction of being the most "atypical" of the classic antipsychotics because it is structurally similar to the dibenzodiazepine clozapine. Another notable feature of loxapine is that one of its metabolites, amoxapine, is marketed as an antidepressant with antipsychotic effects.

Dihydroindoles

Molindone is the only member of the dihydroindoles available in the United States. Sharing a similar structure with the indoleamines (see Figure 27–1), such as serotonin, molindone has the distinction of being the only classic antipsychotic not associated with any weight gain or a lowering of the seizure threshold.

Diphenylbutylpiperidines

Pimozide, the only agent within the diphenylbutylpiperidine class available in the United States, is approved only for the treatment of Tourette's syndrome and has the distinction of possessing the highest selectivity and potency for dopamine D_2 receptors among the conventional antipsychotics. It significantly prolongs the QTc interval, and this has limited its utilization. Derived from benperidol, pimozide shares many characteristics of the butyrophenones (see Figure 27–1).

Benzamides and Iminodibenzyl Agents

Sulpiride, the prototypical substituted benzamide, is a relatively selective dopamine D_2 antagonist and lacks significant activity on cholinergic, histaminergic, or noradrenergic receptors. Because of this relative selectivity and a lower propensity to cause EPS, sulpiride is one of the more common classic antipsychotics utilized in Europe (e.g., it was utilized in about half the patients assigned to receive an FGA in the CUtLASS study). Structurally related to metoclopramide, sulpiride has also been used for the treatment of peptic ulcer and vertigo. No classic antipsychotic agent from either the benzamide or the iminodibenzyl classes is available in the United States.

Pharmacological Profile

The classic conventional antipsychotic drugs have a multitude of effects on various physiological variables through their antagonistic actions on different neurotransmitter systems. The antipsychotic effects of these agents are believed to occur primarily through antagonism of D_2-type dopaminergic receptors. Historically, blockade of D_2 receptors was believed to be indispensable for the treatment of psychosis, although the efficacy of weak D_2 blockers such as clozapine called this theory into question at one time. The major therapeutic, as well as adverse, effects of D_2 antagonism have been conceptualized in the context of the major dopaminergic tracts present in the brain, which include the mesocortical, mesolimbic (A10), tuberoinfundibular (A12), and nigrostriatal (A8 and A9) tracts (Figure 27–2).

Although the effects of D_2 blockade on the mesocortical and mesolimbic dopaminergic systems are believed to represent the putative mechanism of action of conventional antipsychotics, excessive blockade of these tracts is also believed to result in a number of adverse cognitive and behavioral side effects. Such side effects are frequently observed in both animals and human subjects. One such side effect is *ataraxia*, a state of relative indifference to the environment leading to behavioral inhibition and diminished emotional responsiveness. Inhibition of conditioned avoidance and other learned behaviors is observed in rodent models. Although operant-conditioned reward-seeking behaviors are diminished in rat models, one notable exception is the relative increase in cocaine self-administration. One might argue that this correlates with reported anhedonia in human subjects, as well as an increase in cocaine abuse often present within the human population treated with conventional antipsychotics. D_2 receptor antagonism in the mesocortical dopaminergic pathway leads to a blunting of cognition (bradyphrenia) and avolition–apathy—sometimes referred to as the *neuroleptic-induced deficit syndrome*—that can be difficult to differentiate from the primary negative symptoms of schizophrenic illness itself. Although conventional antipsychotics exhibit a ro-

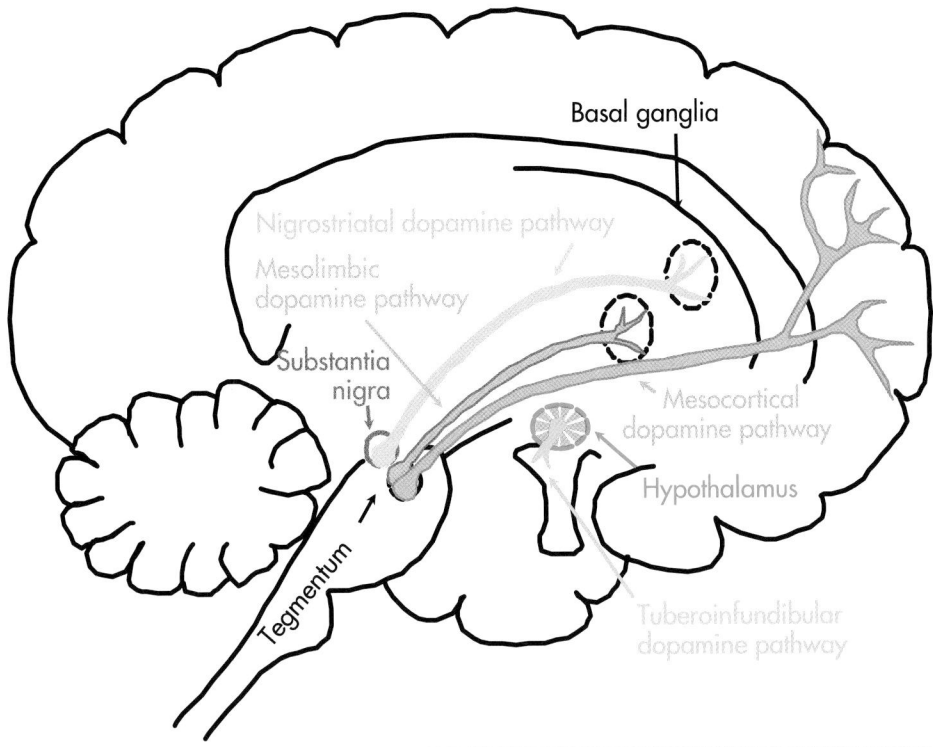

FIGURE 27–2. Dopaminergic pathways of the brain.

bust "tranquilizing" action, they do not induce a state of coma or anesthesia even at very high doses.

Blockade of the tuberoinfundibular tract projecting to the hypothalamus and pituitary gland results in multiple neuroendocrine side effects processed through the pituitary gland. Although dopamine is involved in enhancing the release of most pituitary hormones, it is actually responsible for the tonic inhibition of prolactin release. With significant dopaminergic blockade of the tuberoinfundibular tract, prolactin release is no longer prevented, and the release of other pituitary hormones is no longer enhanced. High levels of prolactin combined with decreased levels of follicle-stimulating hormone and luteinizing hormone often result in amenorrhea, galactorrhea, gynecomastia, decreased bone density, impaired libido, and erectile dysfunction.

High levels of D_2 dopaminergic blockade within the nigrostriatal system, which projects to the basal ganglia and caudate, produce some of the most undesirable side effects of conventional antipsychotics. Movement disorders and EPS such as akathisia, resting tremor, rigidity, and hypokinesia were once believed to be necessary "evidence" of a therapeutic antipsychotic dosage. However, the advent of the new-generation antipsychotics that are associated with minimal EPS conclusively dispensed with this misconception. At higher levels of D_2 blockade, one may also observe a generalized dystonia, catalepsy, and a rigid, immobile catatonic state that may be accompanied by waxy flexibility.

Classic antipsychotic agents have varying degrees of activity at serotonergic, cholinergic, noradrenergic, histaminergic, and other nondopaminergic receptors. Although it is unclear whether any of these activities contribute to or interfere with their efficacy in the treatment of psychotic symptoms, they clearly result in a variety of adverse effects. Because of differences in the pharmacological activity of different classic antipsychotic agents at these receptors, there are predictable differences in their side-effect profiles.

Pharmacokinetics and Disposition

Generally, the pharmacokinetic profiles of the conventional antipsychotics remain poorly understood. Many hundreds of potential metabolites remain undiscovered, even for some of the extensively studied agents. The physiological activity of several metabolites has also not been precisely defined. However, several general statements can be made concerning the classic antipsychotics as a group.

Administration and Absorption

Many of the conventional antipsychotics are available in both oral and intramuscular formulations. Although relatively common in the past, intravenous usage of the parenteral forms of haloperidol, chlorpromazine, and other antipsychotics is not FDA approved. Oral administration of the conventional antipsychotics results in adequate but variable absorption. Calcium-containing food or antacids, coffee, and heavy nicotine use may decrease absorption from the gastrointestinal tract. Peak plasma levels with oral preparations are generally reached in 1–4 hours, with these levels being reached slightly more rapidly with liquid concentrates. All of the agents are highly lipophilic, leading to increased distribution in brain tissue relative to plasma. Oral preparations are extensively metabolized in the liver during their first pass through portal circulation by undergoing any number of transformations, including glucuronidation, oxidation, reduction, and methylation. Steady-state levels are reached in a period of four to five times the half-life of the drug in question.

Intramuscular administration results in faster, more predictable absorption, with peak plasma levels in 30–60 minutes and clinical efficacy as rapidly as 15 minutes. With intramuscular or intravenous administration, plasma levels may be as high as four times those of the oral route because of circumvention of the hepatic first-pass metabolism.

Although 10 classic antipsychotics are available in a long-acting (depot) formulation around the world, haloperidol and fluphenazine are the only antipsychotics currently available in such a formulation in the United States. Although fluphenazine was the first antipsychotic to be released in a long-acting form as an enanthate ester, the longer-lasting decanoate forms of both haloperidol and fluphenazine later became more popular secondary to a lower frequency of side effects. In a decanoate preparation, the antipsychotic drug is esterified to a lipid side chain and suspended in sesame oil. The injection is administered into a major muscle, and the drug is slowly released to the bloodstream through the oil over time. As the esterified version of the drug diffuses into other tissues, the ester chain is hydrolyzed, resulting in the smooth release of the drug in question. This results in the smooth and progressive release of these long-acting agents between scheduled injections. Fluphenazine decanoate can be given every 2–3 weeks on the basis of its half-life of 7–10 days, while haloperidol decanoate may be given every 3–4 weeks because of its longer half-life. These preparations require from 3 to 6 months (four to five times the half-life) to

reach steady-state levels and are eliminated slowly from the body, with plasma concentrations detectable for many months after discontinuation of the drug. Their bioavailability relative to oral administration is twofold greater.

Distribution

Most of the conventional antipsychotics are highly protein-bound (85%–90%). This feature is of importance when other highly protein-bound medications are used concomitantly because of the risk of increasing levels of free or unbound drugs into the toxic range. The antipsychotic drugs are highly lipophilic, which allows unbound portions of the drug to readily cross the blood–brain barrier with concentrations twofold higher in the brain than in the peripheral circulation. The drugs also readily cross the placenta to the fetus in pregnancy. The lipophilic properties of these drugs also allow for large amounts of the drugs to be stored in bodily tissues (i.e., fat, lungs, liver, kidneys, and spleen), leading to high apparent volumes of distribution, generally in the 10- to 40-L/kg range. This property prevents them from being removed from the body effectively via dialysis in cases of overdose.

Metabolism

The conventional antipsychotics are metabolized in the liver by hydroxylation and demethylation to forms that are more soluble and readily excreted by the kidneys and in the feces. Many of these compounds undergo further glucuronidation and remain active as dopamine receptor antagonists. Because of the many active metabolites of the antipsychotic agents, it has not been possible to obtain meaningful correlations between plasma levels and clinical response. Factors such as age, genetic variability among individuals, and coadministration of other drugs cause plasma levels to diverge widely (10- to 20-fold) among individuals.

The majority of conventional antipsychotics are metabolized by the cytochrome P450 (CYP) enzyme subfamilies. Since 2D6 is important for the metabolism of many of these antipsychotics, genetic variation in the rate of 2D6 metabolism should be considered, especially since most conventional antipsychotics inhibit 2D6 as well. It is estimated that 5%–10% of Caucasians poorly metabolize medications through the CYP2D6 pathway, and a higher proportion among African Americans as well. Ultrarapid 2D6 metabolizers have been described in other populations. CYP1A2 and 3A4 subfamily enzymes are also involved in the metabolism of some classic antipsychotics, and this may be relevant to understanding drug–drug interactions of those agents.

Excretion

The major routes of excretion of the classic antipsychotics are through urine and feces by way of bile. These drugs are also excreted in sweat, saliva, tears, and breast milk. Elimination half-life varies from 18 to 40 hours for these drugs. Lower doses of antipsychotics are generally needed in elderly patients because of decreased renal clearance. Because of the long elimination half-lives of these agents, once-a-day dosing is possible for each of these agents following stabilization.

Mechanism of Action

Initial hypotheses centered on the role of dopamine as the major factor in the pathophysiology of psychosis. Carlsson and Lindqvist (1963) first demonstrated an increase in dopamine metabolites following antipsychotic administration. This increase was shown to be a result of dopaminergic blockade, resulting in an increased rate of turnover. Reserpine reduces dopaminergic activity by blocking the uptake and storage of dopamine into synaptic vesicles by inhibiting the vesicular monoamine transporters (VMATs). Amphetamine intoxication served as a drug-induced model of the positive symptoms of schizophrenia. Drugs that blocked dopaminergic receptors, specifically the D_2 receptor, were noted to have greater efficacy and potency as antipsychotics. Since dopaminergic agonists exacerbate psychosis and dopaminergic blockade treats it, dopamine has held central importance in our conceptualization of the neuropharmacology of schizophrenia. Initially, dopamine turnover appears to be increased, as measured by an increase in central nervous system (CNS) metabolites such as homovanillic acid. It is thought that ultimate efficacy may result when this trend is reversed by subsequent receptor supersensitization and ultimate decreases in dopaminergic turnover. The time course of the antipsychotic effect of these agents suggests that both the initial and persistent dopamine D_2 receptor blockade and the more gradually developing depolarization blockade are relevant to antipsychotic action.

The contrast between the efficacies of promazine and chlorpromazine lies in chlorpromazine's tighter affinity to the D_2 receptor. Although structurally related to chlorpromazine, promazine, with its weak binding to the D_2 receptor, resulted in poor antipsychotic efficacy beyond mere sedation. However, although chlorpromazine is more potent than promazine, it remains one of the least potent D_2 receptor antagonists. A 100-mg dose of chlorpromazine is roughly equivalent to 5 mg of trifluoperazine and 2 mg of haloperidol. The potency of a classic antipsychotic is determined by its affinity for the D_2 receptor. High-potency agents with the greatest D_2 affinity are utilized in single-digit total daily doses, whereas low-potency agents are utilized in triple-digit total daily doses.

As additional antipsychotic drugs were developed, the goal of minimizing the sedative, anticholinergic, and autonomic side-effect profiles common among lower-potency antipsychotics was met by the development of drugs that more potently block D_2 receptors, such as the butyrophenones. EPS were considered a sign of therapeutic antipsychotic dosage by early clinicians, who failed to realize the serious impact on the patients of long-term EPS associated with excessive D_2 blockade. Decades later, positron emission tomography (PET) data revealed that a D_2 receptor occupancy of 65%–70% correlates with maximal antipsychotic efficacy, with prolactin elevation appearing beyond 72% D_2 occupancy and EPS appearing beyond 78% D_2 occupancy without any increase in benefits at higher rates of occupancy. Despite the fact that classic antipsychotic agents have been utilized in the treatment of schizophrenia and other psychotic disorders for over half a century, it is still unclear if this 65%–70% occupancy has to be continuously maintained or intermittently achieved (tight versus loose D_2 receptor binding). The importance of 5-HT_{2A} blockade in possible amelioration of EPS was later incorporated into the design of the SGAs discussed elsewhere in this text (see Chapters 28–33).

Indications and Efficacy

Schizophrenia and Schizoaffective Disorder

Conventional antipsychotics are best known for the treatment and maintenance of the psychotic (also known as positive) symptoms of schizophrenia. The major putative mechanism of action is via D_2 blockade of the mesolimbic and mesocortical tracts. In many individuals, this blockade results in a measurable decrease in the positive symptoms of schizophrenia, including hallucinations, delusions, and behavioral disorganization. However, negative and cognitive symptoms of schizophrenia respond less robustly. In fact, they may be worsened by blockade of mesocortical tracts that play roles in cognition and hedonic reinforcement.

TABLE 27–2.   Comparison of CUtLASS band I and CATIE phase I

	COST UTILITY OF THE LATEST ANTIPSYCHOTIC DRUGS IN SCHIZOPHRENIA STUDY (CUtLASS), BAND I	CLINICAL ANTIPSYCHOTIC TRIALS OF INTERVENTION EFFECTIVENESS (CATIE), PHASE I
Subjects		
Diagnosis of schizophrenia	75%	100%
Mental illness duration (chronic illness)	14 years	16 years
First-episode patients (excluded)	Very few (13% of total)	Excluded (0% of total)
Baseline antipsychotic	82% on FGA	15% on FGA
Baseline Positive and Negative Syndrome Scale (PANSS) total score (moderate illness on average)	72.2	75.7
Methods		
When conducted	1999–2003	2001–2004
Study duration	12 months	18 months
Randomized assignment to	FGA or SGA class (50%) (50% FGA on sulpiride)	One of 5 agents (4 SGAs, 1 FGA) (20% FGA)
Antipsychotic switching (both are switching studies)	All patients switched agents 49% switched class 51% stayed in same class	15% continued on same agent 57% actually switched agents 28% antipsychotic-free at baseline and started new agent
Comparison groups	FGA versus SGA arms	Five antipsychotic arms
Primary outcome measure	Quality of life	All-cause antipsychotic discontinuation
Clinical care and primary outcome assessment	Medication blinded to raters but not to patients and physicians	Medication blinded to patients and physicians

Note.   In both studies, patients were at low risk for developing extrapyramidal side effects (EPS) because of inclusion/exclusion criteria and process of study. In both studies, baseline EPS ratings were low despite chronicity and the fact that most patients were receiving antipsychotic treatment. FGA = first-generation antipsychotic; SGA = second-generation antipsychotic.
Source.   Adapted from Tandon et al. 2008.

The failure to improve the negative symptoms of schizophrenia is one of the major drawbacks of the classic antipsychotics. In fact, the EPS induced by the FGAs can worsen negative and cognitive symptoms by inducing bradykinesia and bradyphrenia. Another major limitation is the lack of improvement of positive symptoms (i.e., refractoriness) in about 25% of schizophrenia patients and partial response (i.e., treatment resistance) in another 25%. The discovery that clozapine is more effective than classic antipsychotics in treatment-refractory patients and is devoid of the risk of EPS and tardive dyskinesia led to the introduction of the SGAs. Six additional SGAs (risperidone, olanzapine, quetiapine, ziprasidone, aripiprazole, and paliperidone) have been introduced in the United States, and they have almost completely supplanted FGAs because of their presumed greater efficacy

and better safety/tolerability. However, the greater costs of SGAs, the concern that their benefits were not being realized consistently, and the realization that most of our recent information about these agents derives from industry-sponsored clinical trials (the results of which often contain discrepancies) led to the implementation of two large-scale government-sponsored studies in the United States (CATIE) and the United Kingdom (CUtLASS) between 1999 and 2004. Although findings of both of these studies indicate an absence of any greater effectiveness of SGAs over FGAs on preliminary review, a closer examination of the study samples and design provides additional insights about how classic and atypical antipsychotics might compare (Table 27–2).

In phase I of CATIE, 1,460 patients with schizophrenia were assigned to treatment with either an FGA (perphenazine) or one of four SGAs (risperidone, olanzapine, quetiapine, and ziprasidone), and duration of treatment on the originally assigned medication was assessed over an 18-month period. After control for important variables, no differences in rates of all-cause discontinuation between perphenazine and various SGAs were noted; in fact, no significant differences were observed with reference to symptomatology, cognition, social function, or motor side effects. In band I of CUtLASS, 227 patients with psychotic illness (75% of patients with schizophrenia) were assigned to treatment with either an FGA (one of 11) or an SGA (one of 4), and quality of life was assessed after 12 months of treatment. No difference in quality of life or any other outcome measure was noted between patients assigned to the two groups. Results of these two studies appear to indicate that there are no differences in effectiveness between classic and atypical antipsychotics. Although a variety of methodological issues have been discussed with reference to these studies, one key attribute that should be noted is the fact that study inclusion/exclusion criteria and logistics led to patients in both studies being at low risk for EPS. Baseline EPS ratings of patients in both studies were low. It was in the context of this study sample that the two studies did not discern any advantage for SGAs over FGAs. Given that the essential distinction between SGAs and FGAs is based on the lower liability of atypical antipsychotics to cause EPS (Figure 27–3), the two studies had low assay sensitivity in regard to this difference; in fact, neither study detected any difference in EPS rates or anticholinergic use between classic and atypical antipsychotics.

What CATIE and CUtLASS tell us is that avoiding EPS and anticholinergic use during effective antipsychotic therapy may explain the broader spectrum of efficacy sometimes observed with atypical versus classic antipsychotic agents. The lower risk of tardive dyskinesia observed with SGAs also appears to be driven by these agents' greater ability to achieve an equivalent antipsychotic effect without EPS. The principal advantage of SGAs over FGAs thus appears to be the greater ease of the former in providing an adequate antipsychotic effect without causing EPS or requiring use of an anticholinergic to treat or prevent EPS. In patients at high risk for developing EPS, this difference is magnified, whereas in patients at low risk for developing EPS, this difference is minimized. In a substantial proportion of patients, however, this difference will likely be meaningful, and an antipsychotic effect without EPS can be achieved with less difficulty (because of the broader window; Figure 27–

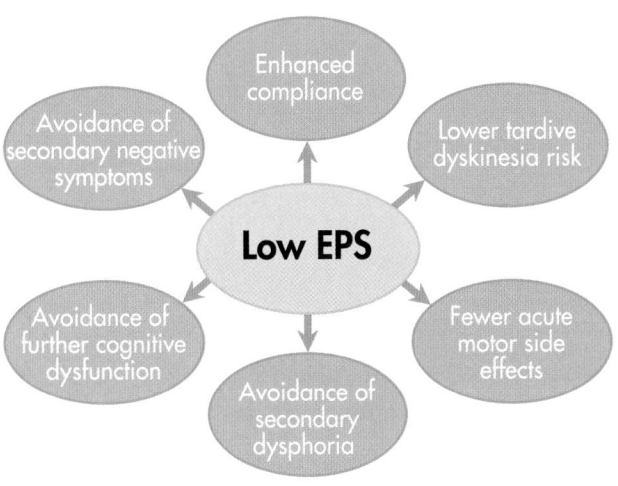

FIGURE 27–3. Clinical benefits of low extrapyramidal side effect (EPS) risk.

4) with an SGA rather than an FGA. It is true that previous industry-sponsored studies magnified the SGA–FGA difference by utilizing high doses of the high-potency agent haloperidol as the FGA comparator and that this difference is smaller when more temperate doses of lower-potency FGAs are utilized. It is equally true that these differences were minimized in CATIE and CUtLASS by sample characteristics of low risk of EPS. The findings from CATIE and CUtLASS confirm broadly held clinical impressions that different agents are associated with different adverse effects, which can make it challenging to achieve maximum efficacy while also maximizing safety and tolerability. However, it is these very differences among the antipsychotic agents, along with heterogeneity in individual response and vulnerabilities, that may allow optimization of antipsychotic treatment. Different agents at different doses may provide the best balance for individual patients.

Substance-Induced Psychosis

As noted previously, conventional agents can reverse the psychosis associated with acute and chronic amphetamine intoxication as well as that associated with cocaine use. However, the risk of acute dystonia must be considered in these populations, as dopamine receptor downregulation is common, resulting in greater sensitivity to rapid D_2 blockade. Results in treatment of psychosis secondary to drugs acting in nondopaminergic mechanisms (such as hallucinogens) are less satisfactory, although there may be some role for the classic antipsychotics in treating phencyclidine (PCP) psychosis.

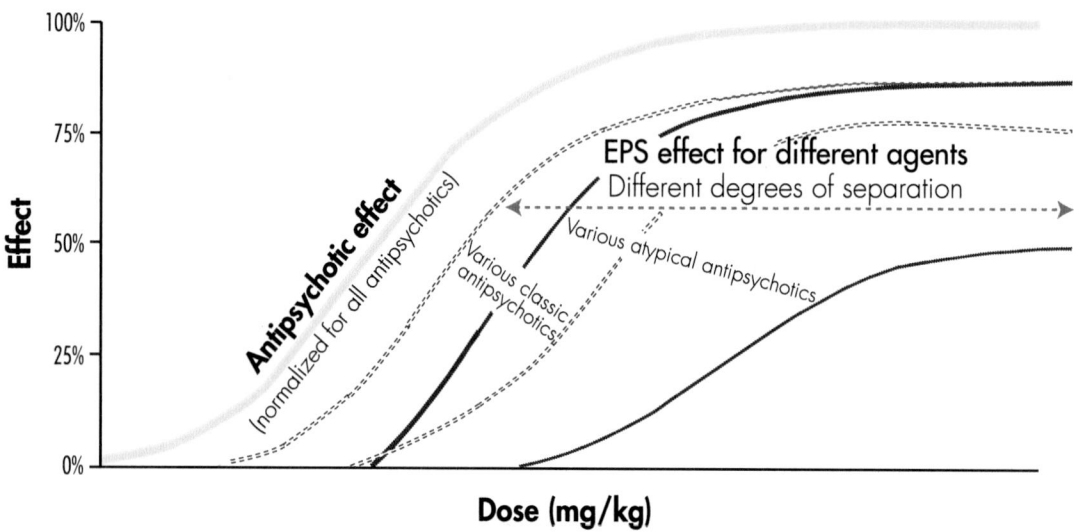

FIGURE 27–4. Dose–response curves of classic versus atypical antipsychotic agents for antipsychotic effects versus extrapyramidal side effects (EPS).

Source. Adapted from Jibson and Tandon 1998.

Personality Disorders

Although any personality disorder can be associated with transient psychotic features emerging under stressful conditions, Cluster B disorders are most often associated with this phenomenon. Treatment for the transient psychotic episodes has included short-term use of a high-potency antipsychotic. Although many symptoms of personality disorders may be amenable to such pharmacological treatment, long-term conventional antipsychotic treatment has not been recommended, since core personality structure is largely resistant to pharmacological therapy and there is a risk of tardive dyskinesia with long-term conventional antipsychotic therapy.

Affective Disorders

The utility of antipsychotic agents in the treatment of affective disorders with psychotic features is well known. However, their utility in the treatment of nonpsychotic depression is described as well. When profoundly negative views of oneself, the world, and the future become severe, the boundaries between psychotic and nonpsychotic depression can become blurred. Several conventional antipsychotics (such as thioridazine) are FDA approved for the treatment of depression and anxiety without overt psychosis. However, they are rarely used for this purpose anymore because of the availability of other, more effective, and better-tolerated agents. The utility of conventional agents as adjuncts to mood stabilizers in the treat-

ment of patients with bipolar spectrum disorders has been well described, both in the acute management of mania and in the maintenance of severe and psychotic bipolar disorder. However, the newer atypical antipsychotics have largely replaced conventional antipsychotics in the management of bipolar disorder.

Tourette's Syndrome

The tics present within Tourette's syndrome are believed to be due to a hyperdopaminergic state that is amenable to treatment by dopamine receptor antagonists. Pimozide is the only conventional antipsychotic with this indication, which is its only FDA-approved indication.

Huntington's Disease

Although there is no cure for Huntington's disease, the psychosis and choreiform movements associated with this disease may be ameliorated by dopamine receptor antagonism. Several conventional antipsychotics carry FDA indications for treatment of this disease.

Nausea, Emesis, and Hiccups

The lower-potency antipsychotics exert a potent antiemetic effect through histamine$_1$ (H$_1$) receptor antagonism. This effect is closely related to their original role in reducing perioperative stress and emesis. Many well-known antiemetics, such as promethazine (Phenergan), are phenothiazines with a short-chain substitution. In addition, chlorpromazine is approved as oral, intramuscular, or intravenous therapy of intractable hiccups, depending on severity.

Side Effects and Toxicology

As noted earlier, it is the side-effect profile that serves to differentiate the conventional antipsychotics from one another rather than their efficacy in treating psychosis. They serve as antagonists at four major neurotransmitter receptor systems in the CNS: the dopamine type 2 receptor family (D_2, D_3, and D_4), muscarinic cholinergic receptors (M_1), α-adrenergic receptors (a_1 and α_2), and histamine receptors (H_1) (Table 27–3).

Their therapeutic response in ameliorating the positive symptoms of schizophrenia is believed to be due to D_2 blockade in the mesolimbic dopamine tract (Table 27–4). Blockade of D_2 receptors in the mesocortical, nigrostriatal, and tuberoinfundibular systems leads to the tract-related side effects described earlier in this chapter (see section "Mechanism of Action"). Lower-potency agents, such as chlorpromazine, require higher doses to achieve therapeutic efficacy and therefore have a greater effect on other receptor systems. They have more antihistaminergic, anticholinergic, and antiadrenergic actions. However, they have fewer D_2-related side effects because of their lower affinity to D_2 receptors and relatively high anticholinergic activity. Higher-potency agents, such as haloperidol, produce more D_2-related movement disorders and prolactin elevation but otherwise have a cleaner side-effect profile, having fewer anticholinergic, antiadrenergic, and antihistaminergic side effects. Anticholinergic action often leads to dry mouth (xerostomia), blurred vision (mydriasis), constipation, urinary retention, sinus tachycardia, prolonged QRS interval, confusion, impaired cognition, paralytic ileus, exacerbation of open-angle glaucoma, and drowsiness. Antagonism of $\alpha1$-adrenergic receptors is associated with orthostatic hypotension, QTc prolongation, reflex tachycardia, dizziness, incontinence, and sedation. Antagonism of α_2 receptors can be associated with retrograde ejaculation and priapism. Antagonism of H_1 receptors leads to sedation, drowsiness, and weight gain. The frequencies of adverse reactions of classic antipsychotic agents are summarized in Table 27–5.

Cognitive Side Effects

CNS side effects of conventional antipsychotics can be subclassified into cognitive and neuromuscular side effects. Cognitive effects include sedation, confusion, disturbed concentration, memory impairment, and delirium. Antihistaminergic and anticholinergic actions lead to the sedation and slowed mentation. These effects, which are most pronounced in the lower-potency agents (e.g., chlorpromazine), are most severe earlier in treatment, with some tolerance developing over time. Anticholinergic delirium is the most common cause of medication-induced delirium. Since delirium results in high rates of morbidity and mortality (over 20% mortality), this potential side effect is important, especially in populations of individuals who are more sensitive to anticholinergic medications, such as the elderly. In addition, every antipsychotic—especially the low-potency drugs—can potentially lower the seizure threshold.

Extrapyramidal Side Effects

Neuromuscular CNS side effects are due to antagonism of D_2 receptors in the nigrostriatal dopaminergic pathway. Generally, antipsychotics manifest EPS when dopaminergic blockade exceeds 75%–80% of D_2 receptors. EPS effects are most frequent with the high-potency agents such as haloperidol.

Acute-Onset EPS

Acute-onset EPS include medication-induced parkinsonism, acute dystonia, and akathisia. *Antipsychotic-induced parkinsonism* occurs in 15% of patients after several weeks of treatment. It is more common in patients older than 40 years, although it can occur at any age. Symptoms are identical to those of Parkinson's disease and include muscle stiffness (lead-pipe rigidity), cogwheel rigidity, shuffling gait, stooped posture, drooling, bradykinesia, resting tremor, masked facies, and akinesia. Slowed, restricted movements of the body and face may be mistakenly diagnosed as being due to depression or the negative symptoms of schizophrenia. It is estimated that up to 10% of patients may experience an acute dystonic episode, which usually occurs within the first few hours or days of treatment. It is more common in men younger than 30 years and women younger than 25 years, in recent cocaine users, and when intramuscular doses of high-potency antipsychotics are used.

Dystonia is an acute sustained, painful muscular contraction that may manifest as either generalized or focal in effect on the musculature. Potential areas of involvement include the tongue (protrusions, twisting), jaw, neck (spasmodic retrocollis or torticollis), and back (opisthotonos). If the dystonia involves the eyes, it results in a symmetrical or unilateral upward lateral movement called

546	The American Psychiatric Publishing Textbook of Psychopharmacology, Fourth Edition

TABLE 27-3. Relative affinities of classic antipsychotics to various neurotransmitter receptors

	Chlorpromazine	Thioridazine	Perphenazine	Trifluoperazine	Fluphenazine	Thiothixene	Haloperidol	Loxapine	Molindone
D_1	High	—	High	High	High	Moderate	High	High	Low
D_2	High	Very high	Very high	Very high	Very high	Very high	Very high	Very high	Very high
D_3	Very high	Very high	Unknown	Unknown	Very high	Unknown	Very high	Unknown	Unknown
D_4	Very high	Very high	Unknown	High	Very high	Unknown	Very high	Very high	Low
H_1	High	High	Very high	Moderate	High	Very high	Low	High	Very low
M_1	High	High	Low	Low	Low	Low	Low	Moderate	None
α_1	Very high	Very high	High	High	High	Moderate	Low	High	Low
α_2	Moderate	Very high	Moderate	Low	Low	Moderate	Low	Low	Moderate
$5\text{-}HT_1$	Low	Low	Low	Low	Low	Low	Low	Low	Low
$5\text{-}HT_2$	Very high	Very high	Very high	Very high	Very high	Very high	High	Very high	Low

TABLE 27–4. Clinical implications of blockade of different receptors

RECEPTOR	POSSIBLE BENEFITS	POSSIBLE SIDE EFFECTS
Dopamine D_2	Antipsychotic effect, efficacy on positive symptoms, efficacy on agitation	EPS, dystonia, parkinsonism, akathisia, tardive dyskinesia Prolactin elevation and other endocrine effects, leading to sexual and menstrual dysfunction, galactorrhea, gynecomastia, and bone changes
Serotonin 5-HT_{2A}	Reduced EPS	Not definitely known
Serotonin 5-HT_{2C}	Not definitely known	Weight gain
Acetylcholine (muscarinic)	Reduced EPS	Central (memory impairment, confusion), cardiac (sinus tachycardia, other arrhythmias), and peripheral (blurred vision, dry mouth, constipation) Anticholinergic side effects
Histamine H_1		Sedation, weight gain
Noradrenergic alpha$_1$		Dizziness, postural hypotension

Note. EPS = extrapyramidal side effects.

an *oculogyric crisis*. Unlike previously mentioned dystonias, an oculogyric crisis can also occur late in treatment with antipsychotics. A laryngeal dystonia can result in sudden death secondary to a patient's inability to breathe. Resurgent dopamine activity in the basal ganglia that occurs when the CNS level of the antipsychotic begins to decrease is thought to be the mechanism of action. Dystonia can be extremely uncomfortable and frightening for patients and can lead to noncompliance with medication for fear of recurrence. Treatment of dystonia requires rapid diagnosis and intravenous administration of antihistaminergic or anticholinergic agents. Anticholinergic agents are often initiated with high-potency antipsychotics in an effort to avoid this side effect, but long-term use may increase the risk of developing tardive dyskinesia.

Akathisia is a subjective feeling of motor restlessness in which patients feel an irresistible urge to move continuously. It is described as an unpleasant sensation and may result in dysphoria. Akathisia can occur at any time during treatment and is the most prevalent EPS. It frequently leads to noncompliance with medications and is believed to increase suicide risk in some patients.

Late-Onset EPS

Tardive dyskinesia is characterized by a persistent syndrome of involuntary choreoathetoid movements of the head, limbs, and trunk. It generally takes at least 3–6 months of exposure to antipsychotics before the disorder develops. Perioral movements involving buccolingual masticatory musculature are the most common early manifestation of tardive dyskinesia.

Tardive dyskinesia has an estimated yearly incidence of 5% among adults and as high as 25% in the elderly who receive continuous conventional antipsychotic therapy and has been a major source of litigation in past psychiatric practice. The risk of developing tardive dyskinesia is reported to increase with age and to be higher in certain ethnic groups; female gender, presence of mood disorders, and early onset of EPS have also been associated with increased risk of tardive dyskinesia.

Tardive dyskinesia may be masked by continuing dopamine blockade and has a variable course following development. Over time, spontaneous resolution or improvement has been described in some individuals. There is no single effective treatment, although treatment with clozapine has been reported to improve symptoms. Tardive dyskinesia is thought to be secondary to upregulation of postsynaptic dopamine receptors in the basal ganglia secondary to long-term dopamine blockade. Cases of tardive dyskinesia have been described with every antipsychotic, although high-potency conventional agents are the most closely related causative agents. Other tardive syndromes include tardive dystonia, tardive akathisia, and tardive pain.

Neuroleptic Malignant Syndrome

Neuroleptic malignant syndrome (NMS) is a poorly understood syndrome that usually occurs within hours or days of initiation of antipsychotic treatment. This syndrome is characterized by muscular rigidity, hyperpyrexia (101–107°F), autonomic instability (hypo- or hypertension, tachycardia, diaphoresis, pallor), and altered con-

TABLE 27–5.   Incidence of adverse reactions to classic antipsychotics at therapeutic doses

	PHENOTHIAZINES						BUTYROPHENONE	DIBENZOXAZEPINE	DIHYDROINDOLE	DIPHENYLBUTYLPIPERIDINE	THIOXANTHENE
	CHLORPROMAZINE	MESORIDAZINE	THIORIDAZINE	FLUPHENAZINE	PERPHENAZINE	TRIFLUOPERAZINE	HALOPERIDOL	LOXAPINE	MOLINDONE	PIMOZIDE	THIOTHIXENE
Drowsiness, sedation	High	High	High	Low	Moderate	Low	Low	High	High	Moderate	Moderate
Insomnia, agitation	Low	Low	Low	Low	Low	Low	Moderate	Low	Low	Low	Moderate
Extrapyramidal effects											
Parkinsonism	Low–Moderate	Low–Moderate	Low	High	Moderate	Moderate–High	High	Moderate	Moderate–High	Moderate	High
Akathisia	Low	Moderate	Low	High	Moderate	High	High	Moderate	High	Moderate	High
Dystonic reactions	Low	Low	Low	High	Moderate	Moderate	High	Moderate	Moderate	Low	Low
Cardiovascular effects											
Orthostatic hypotension	High	High	High	Low	Low	Low–Moderate	Low	Moderate	Low	Low	Low
Tachycardia	Moderate	Moderate	High	Low	Low	Low	Low	Moderate	Low	Low	Low
ECG abnormalities	Moderate	Low	Moderate	Low	Low	Low	Low	Low	Low	Low	Low
Cardiac arrhythmias	Low	Moderate	Moderate	Low	Low	Low	Moderate	Low	Low	Low	Low
Anticholinergic effects	High	High	High	Low	Low	Low	Low	Moderate	Moderate	Low	Low
Endocrine effects											
Sexual dysfunction	Moderate	Moderate	High	Moderate	Moderate	Moderate	Moderate	Low	Moderate	Low	Low
Galactorrhea	Moderate	Moderate	Moderate	High	Moderate	Moderate	High	Moderate	Moderate	Low	Low
Weight gain	High	High	High	Moderate	Moderate	Moderate	Low	Moderate	Low	Low	Moderate

TABLE 27–5. Incidence of adverse reactions to classic antipsychotics at therapeutic doses *(continued)*

	PHENOTHIAZINES						BUTYRO-PHENONE	DIBENZ-OXAZEPINE	DIHYDRO-INDOLE	DIPHENYL-BUTYLPIPERI-DINE	THIO-XANTHENE
	CHLORPROM-AZINE	MESORID-AZINE	THIORID-AZINE	FLUPHEN-AZINE	PERPHEN-AZINE	TRIFLUO-PERAZINE	HALO-PERIDOL	LOXAPINE	MOLINDONE	PIMOZIDE	THIOTHIXENE
Skin reactions											
Photosensitivity	Moderate	Low	Moderate	Low	Low	Low	Low	Low	Low	Low	Low
Rashes	Moderate	Low	Moderate	Low	Low	Low	Low	Low	Low	Low	Low
Pigmentation	High	Low	Low	Low	Low	Low	Low	Low	Low	Low	Low
Ocular effects											
Lenticular pigmentation	Low	Low	Low	Low	Low	Low	Low	Low	Low	Low	Low
Pigmentary retinopathy	Low	Low	Moderate	Low	Low	Low	Low	Low	Low	Low	Low
Other											
Blood dyscrasias	Low–Moderate	Low	Low	Low	Low	Low	Low	Low	Low	Low	Low
Hepatic disorder	Low	Low	Low	Low	Low	Low	Low	Low	Low	Low	Low
Seizures	Moderate	Moderate	Moderate	Low	Low	Low	Low	Low	Low	Low	Low

sciousness. NMS has an estimated incidence of 0.02%–2% and carries a mortality rate of 20%–30%. Death often occurs secondary to dysrhythmias, renal failure secondary to rhabdomyolysis, aspiration pneumonia, or respiratory failure. Laboratory findings include elevated creatine phosphokinase (CPK), elevated white blood cell count, elevated liver enzymes, myoglobinemia, and myoglobinuria. The syndrome can last up to 10–14 days.

Treatment requires immediate discontinuation of the offending antipsychotic and supportive care with aggressive intravenous hydration. In the past, mild cases of NMS were treated with intravenous bromocriptine, while more severe cases were treated with intravenous dantrolene. However, evidence-based studies of NMS treatment have never been performed because of its infrequent occurrence.

NMS is more common in men than in women and occurs more often within the summer months. Risk factors include dehydration, poor nutrition, presence of mood disorders or organic brain syndromes, rapid titration, use of physical restraints, and intramuscular usage. Although onset of NMS is possible at any point during treatment, a significant proportion of the cases of NMS manifest during the first 2 weeks of antipsychotic treatment.

Cardiac Effects

α-Adrenergic antagonism is associated with orthostatic hypotension with reflex tachycardia, with tolerance possibly developing later in the treatment course. Orthostasis is important because of an increase in falls and related injuries. Serious hypotension should never be treated with epinephrine, since this hypotension is mediated through intense α receptor blockade and diffuse vascular dilation. Administration of epinephrine may only exacerbate this problem by causing further vascular dilation through its β receptor stimulation. If necessary, agents such as norepinephrine should be used, as this type of agent will stimulate only α-adrenergic receptors, reversing vasodilation.

Recent studies involving several conventional antipsychotics have drawn attention to the risk of cardiac dysrhythmias, which is especially prominent with use of lower-potency conventional antipsychotics. High dosage, rapid titration, intramuscular administration, and especially intravenous administration may be associated with a lengthening of the QRS or QTc intervals, with resulting risk of serious dysrhythmias such as torsades de pointes and ventricular fibrillation. Recent studies involving thioridazine have raised concerns about piperidine anti-

psychotics and have led to a decrease in their use, despite an infrequent incidence of fatal dysrhythmias in clinical practice. In reality, torsades de pointes is rarely encountered during treatment with conventional antipsychotics, although some speculate that a syndrome of unexplained sudden death described with all conventional antipsychotics may be related to sudden dysrhythmias.

Gastrointestinal Side Effects

As expected, the anticholinergic actions of conventional agents include dry mouth, nausea, vomiting, and constipation that can progress to paralytic ileus. Antihistaminergic action is associated with medication-related weight gain, which greatly increases the patient's risk of developing diabetes.

Cholestatic jaundice is a hypersensitivity reaction described with the aliphatic phenothiazines, especially chlorpromazine (incidence of 0.1%). This reaction typically manifests during the first 1–2 months of treatment and presents with nausea, malaise, fever, pruritus, abdominal pain, and jaundice, with resulting elevations in levels of bilirubin and alkaline phosphatase. This condition rarely lasts more than 2–4 weeks after discontinuation.

Weight Gain, Diabetes Mellitus, and Dyslipidemia

With the introduction of atypical antipsychotics, several of which cause significant weight gain, there is renewed awareness of the metabolic side effects associated with antipsychotic therapy such as obesity, elevated cholesterol and triglyceride levels, and an increased risk of diabetes mellitus. These metabolic changes increase the risk of ischemic heart disease and contribute to the increased mortality observed in schizophrenia. Antihistaminergic action is associated with medication-related weight gain, which greatly increases the patient's risk of developing diabetes. Diabetes is currently described as a worldwide epidemic. Serotonin 5-HT$_{2C}$ receptor blockade also significantly contributes to weight gain; anticholinergic and 5-HT$_{2A}$ antagonism may also contribute. There are significant differences among FGAs with reference to their propensity to cause these metabolic adverse effects. Molindone is the least likely to cause weight gain, whereas thioridazine and chlorpromazine are among the most likely to do so. In general, high-potency agents cause less weight gain and related metabolic adverse effects than low-potency agents do.

Genitourinary Side Effects

Renal effects secondary to blockade of M_1 receptors include urinary hesitancy or retention that can lead to a comparable increase in urinary tract infections in both genders. As mentioned previously, antagonism of tuberoinfundibular dopaminergic tracts increases prolactin secretion. Hyperprolactinemia causes both endocrine and sexual side effects, including gynecomastia, galactorrhea, diminished libido, erectile dysfunction, amenorrhea, decreased bone density, menstrual irregularities, infertility, delayed ovulation, anorgasmia, and possibly increased risk of breast cancer.

Sexual difficulties, including erectile dysfunction, retrograde ejaculation (due to blockade of α_2-adrenergic receptors), anorgasmia, and occasionally priapism, can also occur.

Hematological Side Effects

Hematological effects of conventional antipsychotics include transient leukopenia (white blood cell [WBC] count <3,500/mm^3), which is common but not usually problematic, and agranulocytosis (WBC count <500/mm^3), a life-threatening problem. Agranulocytosis occurs most often during the first 3 months of treatment, with an incidence of 1 in 500,000. It is more common in white women older than 40 years. The mortality rate related to this agranulocytosis may be as high as 30%. Aliphatic and piperidine phenothiazines are the most common causal agents among the conventional antipsychotics. Rarely, thrombocytopenic or nonthrombocytopenic purpura, hemolytic anemia, and pancytopenia may occur.

Ocular Side Effects

In addition to direct anticholinergic effects such as blurred vision (mydriasis and cycloplegia) and exacerbation of open-angle glaucoma, direct optic toxicity has been described. The conventional antipsychotics are associated with several kinds of optical pathology, including pathology of the lens, cornea, and retina.

Lenticular opacities have been reported with some phenothiazines, including perphenazine, chlorpromazine, and thioridazine. An irreversible increase in retinal pigmentation has been described with thioridazine when high dosages are used (>800 mg/day). This retinal pigmentation, which can progress even after drug discontinuation, can lead to reduced visual acuity and even blindness. Early symptoms include poor night vision and secondary nocturnal confusion. Two reports of ocular pathology in young schizophrenic inpatients and outpatients who were treated predominantly with the older antipsychotics demonstrated a high rate of overall ocular pathology (82%) and a much higher rate of lenticular opacities (22%–26%) than the general population in the third decade of life (0.2%). The high rate of lenticular opacities in patients with schizophrenia is striking and may be due in part to antipsychotic treatment but is also related to other known risk factors, such as diabetes, smoking, exposure to ultraviolet radiation, stress, and facial trauma.

Dermatological Side Effects

Cutaneous side effects of conventional antipsychotics involve hypersensitivity rashes—most commonly maculopapular erythematous rashes of the trunk, face, neck, and extremities—and photosensitivity reactions that can lead to severe sunburn. Care must be taken with injectable versions of many antipsychotics because of direct dermatological toxicity if the skin or subcutaneous layers are exposed. Prolonged use of chlorpromazine can lead to bluegray discoloration in body areas exposed to sunlight.

Adverse Effects in Special Populations

In general, there have been few controlled studies of conventional antipsychotics within the pediatric population and almost none during pregnancy and the peripartum period. Currently, with the availability of atypical antipsychotics, most of the conventional agents have fallen into disuse in pediatric populations. The only conventional antipsychotic agent FDA approved for use during childhood is pimozide, for the indication of Tourette's syndrome.

It is ethically problematic to design controlled studies involving pediatric populations and women during pregnancy because of the long-term and serious side effects associated with conventional agents. However, safety concerns in the peripartum mother sometimes require the use of antipsychotics to ameliorate psychosis (whether it was preexisting or developed peripartum), delirium, and extremes of affective syndromes. Potential threats of the drugs to the mother, fetus, and/or children must be carefully weighed against the potentially life-threatening nature of severe psychiatric pathology. Although no formal drug trials have been performed, haloperidol has been the most widely used antipsychotic in the peripartum period, with the best empirical track record of safety during that time. However, one must be mindful that haloperidol has been shown to cross the placenta and to be present within breast milk. Also, animal models have demonstrated complications such as decreased gestational size and infant withdrawal syndromes. Chlorpromazine should not be used during pregnancy, due to a relatively worse empirical side-effect profile, including gray baby syndrome. Use of antipsychotics during pregnancy should be undertaken only with careful consideration of the risks, benefits, and alternatives with the obstetrical specialist who is managing the remainder of the patient's prenatal care.

Geriatric populations pose a special challenge because of the increased sensitivity to all side effects of antipsychotics, impaired hepatic and renal metabolism of these agents, increased risk of delirium, increased use of other medications, and increased risk of tardive dyskinesia. Annual incidence of tardive dyskinesia in the elderly seems to increase exponentially with age and is estimated to be as high as 10-fold greater than the incidence in younger patients. Increasing permeability of the blood–brain barrier with age and an increase in adverse side effects both necessitate much lower dosing of conventional antipsychotics, as well as routine consideration of taper and discontinuation of these agents. Alternative means of managing elderly patients, such as other medical, behavioral, and environmental means of management, should be sought on a continuing basis. If antipsychotic therapy is still required, cautious utilization and diligent monitoring are essential.

Summary of Side Effects

The antagonistic action of the conventional antipsychotics on D_2 receptors in the nigrostriatal, mesocortical, and tuberoinfundibular tracts, as well as blockade of adrenergic, histaminic, and muscarinic cholinergic receptors, produces many undesirable side effects involving multiple body systems. The lower-potency agents cause more peripheral side effects and less dopaminergic tract–related pathology, while the reverse is true of the higher-potency agents.

Drug–Drug Interactions

Careful consideration of a patient's existing drug regimen should be given prior to the initiation of antipsychotic therapy. Except under very special circumstances, antipsychotics should be used in monotherapy, after selection of the appropriate agent. Clear rationales should be provided, and target symptoms should be identified and monitored routinely. Oral forms of medications should be used whenever possible, and the patient's medical condition should be routinely monitored and patients should have physical exams regularly.

Protein Binding

Since conventional antipsychotics are tightly protein bound, care must be taken when these medications are administered with other highly protein-bound medications. Mutual displacement of medications such as phenytoin, digoxin, warfarin, and valproate could lead to a short-term increase in serum levels of these drugs and of the conventional antipsychotic, with a long-term decrease to subtherapeutic levels through increased elimination.

Cytochrome P450 Inhibition

As mentioned previously, conventional antipsychotics are primarily hepatically metabolized through the cytochrome P450 2D6 and 3A4 enzymes. In addition, each inhibits the 2D6 enzyme to some degree. Care must be taken when these agents are coadministered with such potent 2D6 inhibitors as fluoxetine, paroxetine, cimetidine, erythromycin, and certain class IC antiarrhythmics, such as quinidine. Similarly, potent 3A4 inhibitors, such as nefazodone, fluoxetine, fluvoxamine, and ketoconazole, should be used with care. Inhibitors of 2D6 and 3A4, as well as competitive substrates, should be used carefully with conventional antipsychotics because of their potential to increase plasma levels and subsequent side effects. Also, consideration should be given when other drugs that are primarily metabolized by 2D6 are coadministered with conventional agents, because of their potential to increase serum levels of these drugs, including tricyclic antidepressants, selective serotonin reuptake inhibitors, some antiarrhythmics, and several β-blockers. CYP1A2, induced by nicotine and inhibited by estrogen, plays a role in metabolizing some antipsychotics. The complexity of these and other potential drug interactions requires a psychiatrist who is familiar with general medicine if these medicines are to be used competently and safely. Needless patient suffering and lawsuits are the only alternative.

Other Interactions

A syndrome of neurotoxic encephalopathy has been described on coadministration of lithium with haloperidol or thioridazine. Care should be taken if these agents are coadministered, especially in individuals older than 50 years.

Conclusion

Despite the presence of some serious side effects, the conventional antipsychotics revolutionized the practice of psychiatry and the treatment of the severely mentally ill throughout the world. They remain effective agents despite their burdensome side-effect profiles. However, as time progresses, newer atypical antipsychotics appear to have eclipsed these agents to a large extent, as newer short-acting intramuscular and depot formulations have been introduced. It is estimated that less than 10% of current antipsychotic prescriptions in the United States are for conventional agents. The recognition of weight gain and related metabolic adverse effects in conjunction with atypical antipsychotic therapy, along with the results of CATIE and CUtLASS indicating little difference in effectiveness between classic and atypical agents, has reinvigorated interest in conventional agents. As the metabolic profiles of both classic and atypical agents are better elucidated, it is conceivable that there may be a resurgence in the use of classic agents if they are found to provide a more benign metabolic profile than atypical agents. Motor side effects and the narrower antipsychotic–EPS dose window will continue to be limiting factors.

As models of psychosis and antipsychotics are further refined, additional neurotransmitter systems will be addressed in the pathology of schizophrenia and psychosis. Unfortunately, early attempts to treat schizophrenia and reduce side effects by blocking a single neurotransmitter system were unsuccessful. The next generation of drugs following atypical antipsychotics will likely address glutamatergic and cholinergic systems to target cognitive deficits and certain neurophysiological aberrations, such as poor prepulse inhibition. Clearly, much work remains, as the enigma of psychopathology of the human mind is unraveled. Conventional antipsychotics will always be remembered for their vital role as the foundation of antipsychotic pharmacotherapy and the main impetus for the remarkable neuropharmacological progress in psychiatric neuroscience over the second half of the twentieth century. They retain an important, if limited, role in our antipsychotic armamentarium in the first decade of the twenty-first century.

References

Carlsson A, Lindqvist M: Effect of chlorpromazine or haloperidol on formation of 3-methoxytyramine and normetanephrine in mouse brain. Acta Pharmacol Toxicol 20:140–144, 1963

Travis AS: Paul Ehrlich: a hundred years of chemotherapy—1891–1991. The Biochemist 13:5, 1991

Suggested Reading

Arana G, Rosenbaum J: Handbook of Psychiatric Drug Therapy. Philadelphia, PA, Lippincott Williams & Wilkins, 2000

Constantine RC, Tandon R: Antipsychotics equivalent? CUtLASS renews the debate. Curr Psychiatry 6:58–78, 2006

Correll CU, Leucht S, Kane JM: Lower risk of tardive dyskinesia associated with second-generation antipsychotics: a systematic review. Am J Psychiatry 161:414–425, 2004

Glazer WM: Review of incidence studies of tardive dyskinesia associated with typical antipsychotics. J Clin Psychiatry 61 (suppl):15–20, 2000

Janicak PA, Davis JM, Preskorn SH, et al: Principles and Practice of Psychopharmacotherapy, 4th Edition. Philadelphia, PA, Lippincott Williams & Wilkins, 2006

Jibson MD, Tandon R: New atypical antipsychotic medications. J Psychiatr Res 32:215–228, 1998

Jeste DV, Lacro JP, Palmer B, et al: Incidence of tardive dyskinesia in early stages of low-dose treatment with typical neuroleptics in older patients. Am J Psychiatry 156:309–311, 1999

Jones PB, Davies L, Barnes TR, et al: Randomized controlled trial of effect on quality of life of second-generation versus first-generation antipsychotic drugs in schizophrenia. Arch Gen Psychiatry 63:1079–1087, 2006

Kapur S, Seeman P: Does fast dissociation from the dopamine D2 receptor explain the action of atypical antipsychotics? A new hypothesis. Am J Psychiatry 158:360–369, 2001

Lee JW: Catatonic variants, hyperthermic extrapyramidal reactions, and subtypes of neuroleptic malignant syndrome. Ann Clin Psychiatry 19:9–16, 2007

Lieberman JA, Stroup ST, McEvoy JP, et al: Effectiveness of antipsychotic drugs in patients with chronic schizophrenia. N Engl J Med 353:1209–1233, 2005

Maxmen J, Ward N: Psychotropic Drugs Fast Facts, 2nd Edition. New York, WW Norton, 1995

McCarty CA, Wood CA, Fu CL, et al: Schizophrenia, psychotropic medications, and cataract. Ophthalmology 106:683–687, 1999

Meyer JM, Nasrallah HA (eds): Medical Illness and Schizophrenia. Washington, DC, American Psychiatric Publishing, 2003

Nasrallah HA: CATIE's surprises: in antipsychotics' standoff, were there winners or losers? Curr Psychiatry 5:11–19, 2006

Nasrallah HA, Smeltzer D: Contemporary Diagnosis and Management of the Patient with Schizophrenia. Newtown, PA, Handbooks in Health Care Company, 2002

Rosenheck R, Stroup ST, Keefe RS, et al: Study samples key to assessing risk: the authors reply. Curr Psychiatry 6:3–19, 2007

Sachdev PS: Neuroleptic-induced movement disorders: an overview. Psychiatr Clin North Am 28:255–274, 2005

Sadock BJ, Sadock V (eds): Comprehensive Textbook of Psychopharmacology. Philadelphia, PA, Lippincott Williams & Wilkins, 2000

Smith D, Pantelis S, McGrath J, et al: Ocular abnormalities in chronic schizophrenia: clinical implications. Aust N Z J Psychiatry 31:252–256, 1997

Stahl SM: Essential Psychopharmacology. New York, Cambridge University Press, 1996

Tandon R, Constantine RC: The biggest surprise finding of CATIE and the important clinical pearl it reveals: avoiding EPS is the key to realizing "atypical benefits." Curr Psychiatry 5:35–45, 2006

Tandon R, Targum SD, Nasrallah HA, et al: Strategies for maximizing clinical effectiveness in the treatment of schizophrenia. J Psychiatr Pract 12:348–363, 2006

Tandon R, Moller H-J, Belmaker RH, et al: World Psychiatric Association Pharmacopsychiatry Section statement on comparative effectiveness of antipsychotics in the treatment of schizophrenia. Schizophr Res 100:20–38, 2008

CHAPTER 28

Clozapine

Stephen R. Marder, M.D.

Donna A. Wirshing, M.D.

History and Discovery

Clozapine has played a critical role in the history of therapeutics for psychosis. When clozapine was initially developed in the 1960s (following its synthesis in 1958 in Switzerland), there was skepticism as to whether an agent that barely caused catalepsy in rodents could be an effective antipsychotic. According to Hippius (1999), there was limited enthusiasm for this drug because it was inconsistent with the "neuroleptic dogma" that extrapyramidal side effects (EPS) were an essential feature of an antipsychotic agent. Nevertheless, Hippius and others challenged this dogma and supported clozapine's development in Germany. As a result, clozapine was eventually marketed in a number of countries in Europe.

Enthusiasm about clozapine's unique profile turned to despair when it was reported that 13 patients in Finland developed agranulocytosis during treatment with clozapine and that 8 of these patients died (Griffith and Saamerli 1975). This led to a near-halt in research on clozapine and attempts to switch patients to other agents. However, some individuals demonstrated substantial deterioration when they were switched (Hippius 1999). These patients were changed back to clozapine and carefully monitored with regular white blood cell (WBC) counts. It was subsequently confirmed that clozapine-induced agranulocytosis was reversible. If clozapine was discontinued before patients developed infections, the drug could be readministered safely (Honigfeld et al. 1998). Moreover, studies revealed that clozapine was particularly effective for patients who were severely ill and for patients who had failed to respond to treatment with conventional antipsychotics.

These observations led to attempts to gain approval for clozapine in the United States for patients who failed to respond to other antipsychotics. This resulted in a multicenter study (Kane et al. 1988; described in greater detail later in this chapter) in which severely ill inpatients with a history of poor responsiveness to at least three antipsychotics were assigned to a 6-week comparison of either clozapine or chlorpromazine with benztropine. Clozapine was significantly more effective on a broad range of psychopathology that included both positive and negative symptoms. This breadth of improvement suggested not only that clozapine was more effective than chlorpromazine but also that it was qualitatively different. Another study (Claghorn et al. 1987) evaluated the effectiveness of clozapine and chlorpromazine in patients with either tardive dyskinesia or EPS. This report also found that clozapine was superior in a broad range of psychopathology. The completion of these studies was instrumental in the approval of clozapine by the U.S. Food and Drug Administration (FDA) in 1990. Approval in the United States was followed by its introduction in a number of other countries.

The discovery that clozapine was an effective antipsychotic with minimal EPS led to a reassessment of models for developing antipsychotic agents. This reassessment, in turn, led to the later development of a new generation of antipsychotics. Moreover, attempts to understand clozapine's mechanism of action have had important effects on current views of the pharmacology of schizophrenia.

Structure-Activity Relations

Clozapine belongs to the group of tricyclic antipsychotics known as the dibenzepines. This group is characterized by a seven-member central ring (Figure 28–1). The antipsychotic dibenzepines include a loxapine-like group of compounds (the dibenzoxazepines) and a clozapine-like group (the dibenzodiazepines). Substitutions in the clozapine group resulted in the development of both quetiapine and olanzapine.

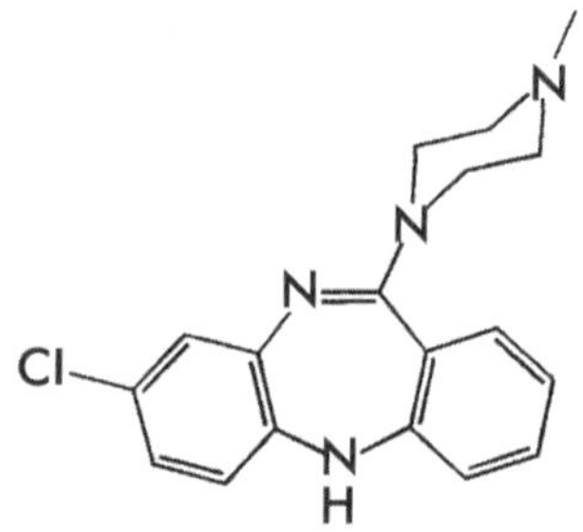

FIGURE 28–1. Chemical structure of clozapine.

Pharmacological Profile

Animal behavioral models have been of limited use in schizophrenia. The primary problem is that there is not a well-accepted animal model for psychopathology in schizophrenia. A number of models—including latent inhibition of the conditioned response, prepulse inhibition, and P_{50} gating—are being studied, and these models suggest unique properties of clozapine that may be clinically relevant. The models used in the development of antipsychotics over the years were empirical models based on dopamine blockade. Criteria for antipsychotic action included the ability of the agent to cause catalepsy at higher doses as well as its antagonism of stereotypies in animals resulting from the administration of amphetamine. Although clozapine meets neither of these criteria, it does block the conditioned avoidance response, suggesting that it has antipsychotic activity.

One model of schizophrenia is based on the theory that individuals with the disorder are impaired in their ability to filter out irrelevant internal or external stimuli. Clinically, patients may describe the experience of being inundated by an excess of stimulation. One method of studying impairments of gating employs a paradigm known as prepulse inhibition (PPI) of the startle reflex. PPI uses a stimulus, such as a puff of air aimed at the eye, that evokes a startle response. The prepulse is a weak stimulus that is presented just prior to the stimulus that elicits a startle. The insertion of the prepulse inhibits the startle response. The usefulness of this model is supported by the observation that in comparison with healthy control subjects, patients with schizophrenia (as well as those with other psychiatric illnesses) demonstrate decreased PPI. Moreover, these PPI deficits correlate with the severity of thought disorder and psychotic symptoms (Braff et al. 1999).

The PPI model can be used in both rodents and humans. Moreover, as a model of gating disturbances, it has face validity. In rodents, dopamine receptor agonists,

serotonin$_2$ (5-HT$_2$) receptor agonists, N-methyl-D-aspartate (NMDA) receptor antagonists, and isolation rearing can result in impairment of PPI (Geyer et al. 2001). Clozapine—as well as other antipsychotics—restores PPI in rats treated with apomorphine (Swerdlow and Geyer 1993) as well as rats treated with the NMDA antagonist ketamine (Swerdlow et al. 1998). In addition, clozapine restores PPI in rats exposed to social isolation (Varty and Higgins 1995). In patients with schizophrenia, clozapine was superior to typical antipsychotics in normalizing PPI (Kumari et al. 1999).

Pharmacokinetics and Disposition

Peak plasma levels of clozapine are reached approximately 2 hours after oral administration. The elimination half-life is about 12 hours. Patients will usually reach steady-state plasma concentrations in less than 1 week. The coadministration of highly protein-bound drugs may lead to increased free clozapine levels, although the total (free plus bound) levels may be unchanged. Clozapine's volume of distribution is lower than that of other antipsychotic drugs but is nonetheless large, with a mean of 2.0–5.1 L/kg (range: 1.0–10.2 L/kg).

Clozapine undergoes extensive first-pass metabolism in the liver and gut. Although clozapine is predominately metabolized by cytochrome P450 (CYP) 1A2, CYP2D6 and CYP3A3 also contribute (Buur-Rasmussen and Brosen 1999).

Plasma concentrations of clozapine average about 10–80 ng/mL per mg of drug given per kg of weight. Thus, a typical daily dose of 300–400 mg (about 5 mg/kg) is associated with levels ranging between 200 and 400 ng/mL. However, there is considerable variability among patients treated with clozapine. This was demonstrated by Potkin et al. (1994), who administered 400 mg of clozapine to a group of patients and found a 45-fold variation in plasma concentrations. A number of studies focused on the clinical implications of this variation in plasma concentrations. These studies, when taken together, indicate that patients are more likely to do well when their levels are greater than 350 ng/mL (Bell et al. 1998; Kronig et al. 1995; D.D. Miller 1996; D.D. Miller et al. 1994; Potkin et al. 1994). If patients have not responded after 6 weeks with a plasma level of 250 ng/mL, the clinician should increase the level to approximately 350 ng/mL. High levels, such as 600 ng/mL, are not associated with a greater likelihood of improvement than are moderate levels, and they may be associated with a higher incidence of side effects. Therefore, patients with high levels and side effects may benefit from having the dosage reduced. In interpreting plasma concentrations of clozapine, it is important for clinicians to consider if the laboratory is reporting just the parent drug or clozapine plus norclozapine. If it is the combination, levels will be higher.

Mechanism of Action

The explanation for clozapine's unique effectiveness remains controversial. As mentioned earlier, clozapine was the first agent to challenge the dogma that antipsychotic efficacy required high levels of EPS. There are a number of characteristics of clozapine that could explain how it can reduce psychosis without causing EPS.

Clozapine's low incidence of EPS could be explained by its low dopamine$_2$ (D$_2$) receptor occupancy at therapeutic doses. Studies using positron emission tomography (PET) with selective D$_2$ receptor ligands, such as raclopride, make it possible to determine the proportion of D$_2$ receptors that are occupied by an antipsychotic in a particular individual at a particular time. These studies found that conventional antipsychotics are effective when approximately 80% of receptors are occupied (Farde et al. 1992). Higher levels of occupancy may increase EPS, but they do not result in greater efficacy. In contrast, clozapine is effective when it occupies 20%–67% of D$_2$ receptors. This observation may explain two important properties of clozapine: its tendency to cause very little EPS and the suggestion that its effectiveness is associated with something more than just D$_2$ receptor occupancy.

It has also been suggested that clozapine's properties are associated with its combination of relatively low affinity for D$_2$ receptors and high affinity for other receptors, including 5-HT$_{2A}$, 5-HT$_{1C}$, adrenergic, and cholinergic receptors. Most of the attention has focused on clozapine's high ratio of 5-HT$_{2A}$ to D$_2$ receptors, because this property is shared by nearly all of the other second-gener-

ation antipsychotics (SGAs). Moreover, serotonin can modulate dopamine neurons in the substantia nigra, which in turn may decrease EPS. Clozapine also has a very high affinity for the dopamine$_4$ (D$_4$) receptor. The D$_4$ receptor is widely distributed in the cortex and less so in striatal areas. However, other agents with high D$_4$ receptor activity have failed to demonstrate antipsychotic activity.

Another theory—supported by both Seeman (2002) and Kapur and Seeman (2001)—hypothesizes that the lack of EPS with clozapine and other SGAs is related to their fast dissociation from the D$_2$ receptor. Conventional antipsychotics tend to bind more tightly to dopamine receptors than to dopamine itself. Nearly all of the SGAs, including clozapine, bind more loosely and tend to come off the receptor more readily in the presence of dopamine. As a result, these newer agents may block these receptors more transiently, coming off the receptor to permit more normal dopamine transmission. Another approach to understanding the mechanism of action of clozapine is based on the finding that acute administration of conventional antipsychotic drugs to rodents leads to an increase in the firing of dopamine neurons in the substantia nigra and the ventral tegmental area. However, after 3 weeks of treatment with these agents, there is a decrease in the number of firing dopamine neurons in both of these areas. This prolonged decrease in firing has been referred to as *depolarization inactivation*. Inactivation in the ventral tegmental area has been used to explain the sustained therapeutic effectiveness of these agents, and inactivation in the substantia nigra has been used to explain EPS. Clozapine—together with other SGAs—causes inactivation in the ventral tegmental area, but not in the substantia nigra (Chiodo and Bunney 1983), suggesting that these agents have different effects in these two brain areas.

Indications and Efficacy

Acute Schizophrenia and Schizoaffective Disorder

Because of its side-effect profile, clozapine is the only available antipsychotic that should not be administered as a first-line agent for schizophrenia or schizoaffective disorder. However, this does not mean that clozapine is ineffective in these disorders. Early trials comparing clozapine with haloperidol and chlorpromazine indicated that clozapine was at least as effective as the other agents for acutely psychotic patients. In the chlorpromazine comparison (Fischer-Cornelssen and Ferner 1976), the advantages were most apparent for the more severely ill patients. The comparison with haloperidol (Honigfeld et al. 1984) was carried out in a more severely ill group of patients and found a substantial advantage for clozapine. A report by Shopsin et al. (1979) compared clozapine, chlorpromazine, and placebo in 31 newly admitted patients with acute illness. Clozapine was found to be superior to both chlorpromazine and placebo. Taken together, these early studies indicate that clozapine is effective for treatment of a broad range of individuals with acute psychosis. In China, for example, clozapine is commonly prescribed as a first-line antipsychotic for acute schizophrenia.

Treatment-Refractory Schizophrenia

As noted above, early studies suggested that clozapine was particularly effective in patients with more severe treatment-refractory forms of schizophrenia. This was important when it was discovered that clozapine was associated with a risk of agranulocytosis. Given that clozapine was viewed as an agent that might be helpful for patients who had failed to respond to other antipsychotics, a study was designed to test whether there was a role for clozapine in this population. The result was the design of a multicenter study comparing clozapine with chlorpromazine in severely ill patients with treatment-refractory schizophrenia (Kane et al. 1988). Treatment-refractory illness was characterized on the basis of a history of drug nonresponsiveness and a failure to improve during a 6-week trial of up to 60 mg of haloperidol. Clozapine resulted in greater improvement in nearly every dimension of psychopathology. Clozapine-treated patients were less depressed and less anxious. In addition, they demonstrated substantial improvements in Brief Psychiatric Rating Scale (BPRS) items that measured emotional withdrawal, motor retardation, and blunted affect. These items may reflect the negative symptoms of schizophrenia and suggest that clozapine is more effective than conventional antipsychotics in treating negative symptoms. Thirty percent of the clozapine-treated patients met stringent improvement criteria, compared with only 4% of those treated with chlorpromazine. However, this study was only 6 weeks in duration and may have underestimated the proportion of patients who improved with clozapine treatment.

Other studies suggest that the proportion of patients improving with clozapine treatment will be higher if clozapine is continued for a longer time. For example, a 16-week trial by Pickar et al. (1992) found a 38% improvement rate. A more recent report (Kane et al. 2001) found

that 60% of patients with treatment-refractory illness improved after a 29-week trial on clozapine.

The early studies of clozapine focused on individuals who had been unresponsive to first-generation antipsychotics (FGAs) and had subsequently been switched to clozapine. There are a number of reasons to suspect that the proportions of patients responding to clozapine are lower if patients had previously been treated with other SGAs. First, failure to respond to an FGA may result from an inability to tolerate an adequate dose because of EPS. In addition, a number of studies suggest that patients who fail to respond to FGAs may improve if they are changed to an SGA other than clozapine. However, comparisons of clozapine and SGAs have yielded results that can be difficult to interpret. For example, some studies comparing risperidone (Bondolfi et al. 1998) or olanzapine (Bitter et al. 2004; Tollefson et al. 2001) with clozapine in patients with treatment-refractory illness suggested that these agents had similar efficacy. Other studies (Azorin et al. 2001; Breier et al. 1999) suggested advantages for clozapine. Volavka et al. (2002) compared clozapine, risperidone, olanzapine, and haloperidol in patients with suboptimal responses to FGAs. The study showed advantages for the SGAs over haloperidol on total Positive and Negative Syndrome Scale (PANSS) scores. Effect sizes for improvement were largest for olanzapine and clozapine, smallest for haloperidol, and intermediate for risperidone. Clozapine was more effective than the other medications for negative symptoms.

Two large trials compared clozapine with SGAs in patients with treatment-resistant illness. In the United States, the National Institute of Mental Health (NIMH) Clinical Antipsychotic Trials of Intervention Effectiveness (CATIE) compared clozapine with risperidone, olanzapine, or quetiapine in patients with schizophrenia who had failed to respond in an earlier phase of the study because of a lack of efficacy (Stroup et al. 2006). Clozapine was administered open label, whereas the other antipsychotics were administered double-blind. Patients assigned to clozapine had the lowest discontinuation rates, with 56% of patients on clozapine discontinuing treatment, compared with 71% on olanzapine, 86% on risperidone, and 93% on quetiapine. Clozapine-treated patients also showed greater symptom improvements than those receiving the other agents. Another trial in the UK, the Cost Utility of the Latest Antipsychotic Drugs in Schizophrenia Study—band 2 (CUtLASS-2) (Lewis et al. 2006), randomly assigned 136 patients who had responded poorly to two prior antipsychotics to either clozapine or an SGA selected prior to the randomization. Patients who received clozapine demonstrated greater improvement than those on the comparison drugs.

Chakos et al. (2001) conducted a review and meta-analysis of studies comparing the efficacy and tolerability of clozapine with that of FGAs and other SGAs in treatment-resistant schizophrenia. Clozapine was superior to FGAs, but findings for other SGAs were inconclusive. (However, this study was carried out prior to CATIE and CUtLASS-2, both of which supported superior efficacy for clozapine.) Despite clozapine's advantages, a significant number of patients with treatment-refractory illness do not respond to clozapine. The Chakos et al. (2001) meta-analysis found that in most studies, fewer than half of the patients with treatment-resistant illness responded to clozapine. Additionally, many patients who do respond favorably to clozapine continue to have significant symptoms that impair their functioning in the community.

Taken together, these studies—particularly CATIE and CUtLASS-2—indicate that clozapine has an important role in the treatment of patients who have failed to respond to either FGAs or other SGAs. Clozapine's advantages are clearest in patients who have failed to respond to FGAs but are still apparent in those who have had an inadequate response to other SGAs. Because clozapine is associated with a risk of agranulocytosis and other side effects (summarized later in this chapter under "Side Effects and Toxicology"), patients should probably receive a trial of one or two other SGAs before receiving a trial of clozapine. Clinical guidelines (Lehman et al. 2004a, 2004b; Marder et al. 2002; A.L. Miller et al. 2004) differ to a minor degree on the number of trials that should precede a trial with clozapine, but most recommend at least two agents, one of which is an SGA. There is a consensus that patients should not be considered to have treatment-refractory illness until they have received an adequate trial with clozapine.

Hostile and Aggressive Behavior in Schizophrenia

Clozapine may have other advantages for patients with schizophrenia. A number of studies suggest that clozapine may decrease hostility and aggression, compared with other agents. In a study of 157 inpatients (Citrome et al. 2001), clozapine resulted in greater reductions in the hostility item from the PANSS than did the FGAs and other SGAs. A study by Chengappa et al. (2003) found significant reductions in the rates of seclusion and restraint in schizophrenia patients who received clozapine during the first 3 years after its introduction. Other randomized trials have consistently found that patients treated with clozapine experience less hostility and fewer aggressive behaviors than patients on comparators (Essock et al. 2000; Kane et al. 1988). These findings suggest that clozapine may be of particular benefit to patients with treatment-refractory illness who demonstrate hostile and aggressive behaviors.

Schizophrenia Patients at High Risk for Suicide

Clozapine may also be a preferred agent for patients with schizophrenia who are at a higher risk for suicide. Large epidemiological studies have found that mortality from suicide is reduced among individuals taking clozapine (Reid et al. 1998; Walker et al. 1997). Meltzer and Okayli (1995) followed patients who were changed to clozapine and found a reduction in the number of serious suicide attempts as well as in expressed depression and hopelessness. The most convincing study was a comparison of clozapine and olanzapine in 980 patients with schizophrenia who were considered at risk for suicide. In that study, clozapine was more effective in reducing the risk of suicide (Meltzer 2002).

Clozapine may also have advantages for patients with polydipsia–hyponatremia syndrome (Canuso and Goldman 1999). These patients tend to intoxicate themselves through excessive water drinking. Hyponatremia may result in seizures.

Schizophrenia With Comorbid Substance Abuse

Although the effectiveness of clozapine in patients with comorbid substance abuse has not been demonstrated in randomized, controlled trials, there is some supporting evidence from naturalistic studies. One retrospective study (Green et al. 2003) found that patients treated with clozapine were more likely than those treated with risperidone to abstain from alcohol and cannabis use. A prospective study (Green et al. 2007) found that patients treated with clozapine were often able to reduce their substance abuse. This finding was supported by other prospective studies (Brunette et al. 2006; Drake et al. 2000), indicating that clozapine is effective for reducing substance abuse.

Supplemental Antipsychotic Treatment in Partial Responders to Clozapine

A number of studies have evaluated augmentation strategies for individuals who are partial responders to clozapine. Paton et al. (2007) reviewed open and randomized, controlled trials in which partial responders to clozapine received supplemental treatment with another antipsychotic. Among the controlled trials, three used risperidone as the supplementing agent and one used sulpiride. The two studies with a duration of greater than 10 weeks favored augmentation, whereas the briefer studies did not.

Maintenance Therapy in Schizophrenia

Clozapine use has largely been confined to patients with treatment-refractory schizophrenia. As a result, clozapine has not been studied in the traditional relapse prevention trial in which patients who are stable are randomly assigned to either clozapine or a comparator. Nevertheless, there are substantial data supporting the long-term effectiveness of clozapine. Breier et al. (2000) evaluated the outcomes of 30 patients with schizophrenia who were treated with clozapine for 1 year. Patients taking clozapine experienced fewer relapses and rehospitalizations than they did in the year prior to being changed to clozapine. A study in the state hospitals in Connecticut compared patients who were assigned to clozapine with patients who were maintained on their usual antipsychotics (Essock et al. 2000). Although clozapine did not result in a greater likelihood of hospital discharge, patients who were treated with clozapine had a higher likelihood of remaining in the community following discharge. This finding supports the observation that clozapine is associated with a reduced risk of relapse, compared with a conventional antipsychotic.

A study from the U.S. Department of Veterans Affairs (VA) Cooperative Studies Program compared haloperidol and clozapine in patients with treatment-refractory schizophrenia (Rosenheck et al. 1997). This study was not designed as a relapse prevention trial, but rather as a comparison of the two agents in individuals who were poor responders to conventional therapy. However, the 1-year study is somewhat informative about the usefulness of the two drugs in patients living in the community. Fifty-seven percent of the patients taking clozapine completed the study, compared with only 28% of the patients taking haloperidol (P<0.001). Using 20% improvement on the PANSS as the criterion for response, the investigators found that 42% of patients treated with clozapine and 31% of patients treated with haloperidol were responders (P=0.09). In addition, clozapine-treated patients had fewer mean days of hospitalization (143.8 days) compared with haloperidol-treated patients (168.1 days; P=0.03).

These studies are encouraging for a number of reasons. First, the VA study (Rosenheck et al. 1997) addressed the issue of whether clozapine's advantage in relapse prevention is only an effect of the monitoring system for agranulocytosis—that is, does the requirement for weekly blood tests act as a means of assuring compliance? Because the clozapine-treated and haloperidol-treated patients had the same blood monitoring, the advantage of clozapine appears to be an intrinsic effect of the drug. Also, clozapine is a drug that has its own discomforting side effects, including sedation, hypersalivation, constipation, and hypotension. These studies indicate that patients in long-term treatment are able to tolerate these effects.

Mania in Bipolar Disorder

Given that all available antipsychotics are effective in reducing manic symptoms, it is not surprising that clozapine is effective in bipolar mania. However, accumulating evidence suggests that clozapine is particularly effective for manic symptoms that are not responsive to other agents. McElroy et al. (1991) were among the first to observe clozapine's unique effects in patients with bipolar disorder. Subsequent studies have confirmed clozapine's effectiveness as monotherapy and as a supplementation medication for mania. In an open-label randomized trial in acutely manic patients (Barbini et al. 1997), clozapine was as effective as chlorpromazine and had a more rapid onset. Suppes et al. (1999) randomly assigned patients with schizoaffective and bipolar illnesses to either supplemental clozapine or treatment as usual during a 1-year open-label trial. Among both schizoaffective and bipolar patients, those treated with clozapine demonstrated greater improvements. Other prospective open-label studies (Calabrese et al. 1996; Green et al. 2000) confirmed clozapine's effectiveness in refractory bipolar illness. Although the available data support clozapine's effectiveness in mania, none of these trials has been double blind.

Depression With Psychotic Features

Limited evidence suggests that clozapine is effective as monotherapy and as an adjunctive treatment for patients with major depression with psychotic features. This evidence is currently confined to case reports with relatively small numbers of cases (Ranjan and Meltzer 1996; Rothschild 1996).

Psychosis in Parkinson's Disease

Psychosis with delusions and hallucinations occurs in approximately 25% of patients with Parkinson's disease (Wolters and Berendse 2001). These symptoms frequently appear in patients who are receiving dopaminomimetic drugs but may also occur as a result of a cholinergic deficit. Three double-blind studies (French Clozapine Parkinson Study Group 1999; Jones and Stoukides 1992; Parkinson Study Group 1999; Pollak et al. 2004) found that clozapine at doses as low as 25–50 mg was effective in reducing psychotic symptoms. Moreover, these doses were not associated with an increase in tremor and rigidity. A report from the American Academy of Neurology (Miyasaki et al. 2006) recommended clozapine as a preferred agent for psychosis in Parkinson's disease.

Schizophrenia in Children and Adolescents

Two randomized, controlled trials from the NIMH have evaluated the effectiveness of clozapine in childhood-onset schizophrenia. The first (Kumra et al. 1996) compared clozapine and haloperidol in individuals with a mean age of about 14 years who had done poorly on FGAs. Clozapine was superior for both positive and negative symptoms. A more recent double-blind study (Shaw et al. 2006) compared clozapine and olanzapine in subjects with a mean age of about 12 years. The results from this study were less clear. Although there were substantial differences favoring clozapine, the differences were only statistically significant for negative symptoms. The small sample ($n = 12$ for clozapine and $n = 13$ for olanzapine) was a limiting factor for obtaining statistical significance. Both studies found that this younger population appeared to be particularly vulnerable to clozapine's side effects. Nevertheless, these studies suggest an important role for clozapine in younger patients with schizophrenia with refractory symptoms.

Side Effects and Toxicology

Hematological Effects

The side effects of clozapine make it one of the most challenging medications for psychiatrists to prescribe. The main factor that limits its use is the potential serious side effect of agranulocytosis. Agranulocytosis is defined as a drop in absolute neutrophil count (ANC) to levels below 500/mm^3. In 1975, there were 17 cases of agranulocytosis in Finland, and widespread use of the medication for the treatment of schizophrenia was temporarily halted (Amsler et al. 1977; de la Chapelle et al. 1977). Agranulocytosis is a potentially lethal side effect that occurs in less than 1% of patients treated in the United States (Alvir et al. 1993). In the United States, all patients who

are taking clozapine are entered into a national registry. Through the national registry, patients are prescribed the medication only if their WBC count shows no signs of clinically meaningful suppression (Honigfeld 1996). In a review of the morbidity and mortality of clozapine-treated patients (Honigfeld et al. 1998) over a 5-year period, 99,502 patients were registered through the Clozaril National Registry. Of these, 2,931 (2.95%) patients developed leukopenia (WBC count = 3,500/mm^3), and 382 (0.38%) patients developed agranulocytosis (ANC < 500/mm^3). Twelve of the cases of agranulocytosis (0.012%) were fatal. These findings contrast with the 1%–2% cumulative incidence expected from the premarketing experience with clozapine. In the United States, 1,743 patients received the drug in premarketing trials. In addition, this estimate was based on trials in Europe performed in the 1970s and 1980s (Honigfeld et al. 1998). The encouraging report by Honigfeld et al. (1998) supports the monitoring system for clozapine as an adequate measure to prevent agranulocytosis.

The rates of clozapine-induced agranulocytosis in other parts of the world are similar to the rate in the United States (Gaszner et al. 2002; Helmchen 1989; Jungi et al. 1977). However, it is unclear what the rates are in parts of the world where generic medication is used and no registry exists. The onset of agranulocytosis occurs most often during the first 6 months of treatment and is usually marked by a gradual fall in WBC count, often over several weeks. A precipitous fall within 1 week can occur but is much less common (Honigfeld et al. 1998). Thus, patients must be monitored with weekly blood cell counts for the first 6 months and every 2 weeks thereafter. Various investigators have tried to determine whether there are predictors of clozapine-induced agranulocytosis. Our group and others examined the possibility that agranulocytosis is immune mediated and thus preceded by eosinophilia. However, such a relationship has not been supported by our study or by others (Ames et al. 1996; Hummer et al. 1994). It has been observed that patients of Ashkenazi Jewish origin (Lieberman et al. 1990) are overrepresented among the cases of agranulocytosis, prompting researchers to examine whether there may exist a genetic predisposition for a particular immunohistocompatibility complex and/or immune response (Dettling et al. 2001). No clear relationship has been found, although speculations about human leukocyte antigen (HLA) types have been made, particularly HLA B38, in American Jews of Ashkenazi origin who develop agranulocytosis (Lieberman et al. 1990). In contrast, one Israeli study, composed of patients with non-Ashkenazi background, did not support this relationship (Meged et al. 1999).

When clozapine treatment is discontinued upon identification of marked leukopenia, patients usually recover within 14–24 days and without any long-term consequences. However, rechallenging patients who have experienced agranulocytosis almost always leads to reoccurrence of the problem. The onset of the second episode is more aggressive than the first. In nine patients who were known to be rechallenged, the average time to onset was 10 weeks shorter (14 weeks) than the first episode (24 weeks) (Safferman et al. 1992). Agranulocytosis has been successfully treated by discontinuing the medication, providing supportive measures, and administering granulocyte colony–stimulating factor, a medication that is commonly prescribed to patients with medical illnesses that precipitate WBC count suppression (Raison et al. 1994; Weide et al. 1992; Wickramanayake et al. 1995).

When clozapine first appeared on the market, mandatory monitoring of WBC levels each week was recommended for all patients taking clozapine. In January 2006, Novartis and the FDA notified clinicians of modifications to the recommended monitoring schedule for patients receiving clozapine (available at: www.pharma.us.novartis.com/product/pi/pdf/Clozaril.pdf).

Under the new monitoring guidelines, when a patient begins clozapine treatment, he or she must have a baseline WBC count of no less than 3,500/mm^3 and an ANC of no less than 2,000/mm^3. Weekly WBC and ANC levels must be taken for 6 months, at which time the frequency can be reduced to every 2 weeks, provided that treatment and monitoring have not been interrupted and WBC counts and ANCs have been within acceptable ranges. After 1 year, monitoring can be reduced to monthly blood tests. There are specific recommendations for intensified monitoring following discontinuation of clozapine therapy, particularly if therapy is interrupted because of blood dyscrasias.

Cardiac Effects

Well-known side effects of clozapine on the cardiovascular system include tachycardia and orthostatic hypotension. Tachycardia is thought to be attributable to the anticholinergic activity of the medication, whereas hypotension is due to α-adrenergic blockade. Reports of clozapine-associated myocarditis and cardiomyopathy have raised concern that clozapine may be associated with other forms of cardiovascular toxicity. In January 2002, Novartis reported that there had been 213 cases of myo-

carditis, 85% of which occurred at recommended dosages of clozapine within the first 2 months of therapy. The presence of eosinophilia in many of the reported cases indicates that an immunoglobulin E (IgE)–mediated hypersensitivity reaction may be involved (Killian et al. 1999). Novartis (2002) also reported 178 cases of clozapine-associated cardiomyopathy, 80% of which occurred in patients younger than 50 years. Almost 20% of the incidents resulted in death, an alarming figure that may reflect delay in diagnosis and treatment. The detection of cardiac toxicity is particularly challenging, because its manifestations (tachycardia, fatigue, and orthostatic hypotension) are frequently observed in clozapine-treated patients, particularly when alterations in dosage are made (Lieberman and Safferman 1992). The poor specificity of signs for cardiac toxicity demands that patients with any personal or family history of heart disease be identified, and the threshold for medical evaluation of patients developing respiratory and cardiovascular symptoms must be low (Wooltorton 2002). The etiology of the myocarditis and cardiomyopathy remains unclear at this time.

Sudden death has been associated with both conventional antipsychotic treatment and treatment of patients with clozapine. A thorough review of the literature examining reports from 1970 to 2004 of cardiac side effects in patients on clozapine concluded that clozapine is associated with a low risk (0.015%–0.188%) of potentially fatal myocarditis or cardiomyopathy (Merrill and Goff 2005). The cause of the sudden death is unclear; it is probably secondary to ventricular arrhythmia and may be associated with sudden increases in clozapine dosage.

Double-blind clinical trials of antipsychotic medications given to manage agitated behavior in elderly patients with dementia supported the notion that a greater risk of sudden death is associated with use of these medications in older populations. As a result, the labeling of all antipsychotics, including clozapine, was updated to include a boxed warning of this risk. In 2006, the FDA issued a reminder that off-label use of clozapine for dementia-related psychosis in elderly patients is associated with an increased risk of sudden death. It is extremely important when raising the dosage of clozapine that incremental changes do not exceed 50 mg every 2 days (Worm et al. 1993). Clinicians must weigh the potential superb clinical benefit of clozapine against these cardiac risks. We recommend that an electrocardiogram be performed prior to initiation of clozapine.

For hypotension caused by clozapine, we also recommend a slow upward titration of the medication and monitoring of orthostatic vital signs during the first weeks of therapy. Patients should be educated about the risk of orthostatic hypotension and should be taught to rise slowly from supine positions. Concomitant treatment with β-blocking agents may be necessary for persistent tachycardia. However, the use of β-blockers may exacerbate the hypotensive effects of clozapine and should be used cautiously.

Metabolic Effects

Weight Gain

The metabolic side effects of clozapine are prominent (Henderson 2001; D. A. Wirshing et al. 1998, 1999). Weight gain has been observed in both premarketing and postmarketing trials (Henderson 2001; Simpson and Varga 1974). In patients observed in various clinical trials in our laboratory, the average weight gain in a 6-month period with clozapine treatment was 6.9±0.8 kg. Allison et al. (1999) performed a meta-analysis of the weight-gain data in short-term trials of medications. The average weight gain observed with clozapine was 4.45 kg, which exceeded the weight gain observed with all of the other medications in the study, including the conventional agent thioridazine (3.19 kg), a medication known for its weight-gain liability. The weight gain observed with clozapine seems to occur for a prolonged period of time—up to 40 weeks. In one naturalistic study, Henderson (2001) observed patients in a clozapine clinic for 5 years and noted weight gain occurring for up to 46 months in some patients.

Body mass index (BMI; expressed in kg/m^2), which takes into account a patient's weight relative to his or her height, and waist-to-hip ratio (WHR) are important parameters to measure, because they both are predictors of cardiovascular risk. Obesity is defined as a BMI of 27 kg/ m^2. Waist measurements of 102 cm (or >40 inches) in men and 88 cm (or >35 inches) in women are indicative of the metabolic syndrome and are strong predictors of diabetes and other medical complications, including heart disease and sleep apnea (D. A. Wirshing et al. 2002a, 2002c). Deposition of weight in the abdomen, in excess of weight on the hips (highly correlated with the development of diabetes), can also be assessed with the WHR. Frankenburg et al. (1998) examined BMI and WHR in 42 patients treated with clozapine. The majority of patients experienced increases in both of these parameters. In females, the authors observed an average WHR of 0.8 after 37 months of clozapine therapy, with a significant average increase in BMI from 23.2 to 29.1 kg/m^2 ($P=0.001$). Male subjects also gained weight and body mass. After 39

months of clozapine therapy, the average WHR in males was 0.93, with a significant average increase in BMI, from 26.4 to 29.7 kg/m2 ($P<0.001$). Both males and females in the sample became obese.

Phase II of CATIE provided an opportunity to compare weight gain among patients assigned to clozapine, olanzapine, risperidone, and quetiapine (McEvoy et al. 2006). The numbers of patients assessed in the analyses were small, with only 45 patients in the clozapine group, 17 in the olanzapine group, 14 in the quetiapine group, and 14 in the risperidone group. Although the differences in weight gain among these agents were not statistically significant, they were interesting, with patients on clozapine gaining a mean of 0.5 lb per month, compared with 1.0 lbs on olanzapine, −0.4 lb on quetiapine, and 0.5 lb on risperidone.

Researchers have tried to determine predictors of clozapine-associated weight gain. Of concern is that adolescents may be among the most vulnerable to this side effect. Theisen et al. (2001a, 2001b) reported that the prevalence of obesity in adolescent patients taking clozapine was 64% ($n=69$). Others have speculated that clozapine-associated weight gain may be genetically determined, and several candidate genes are being explored (Basile et al. 2001). Numerous neurotransmitters and receptors are affected by clozapine. Specifically, we noted a logarithmic association between clozapine-associated weight gain and its effect on the histamine$_1$ (H$_1$) system (D. A. Wirshing et al. 1999). Other researchers have speculated that clozapine interferes with metabolism by interrupting the feedback loop between leptin, a hormone produced by adipose cells that should signal satiety to the brain, and neuropeptide Y, a peptide that is thought to stimulate appetite. Instead, patients treated with clozapine have been observed to have elevated levels of leptin (Bromel et al. 1998; Kraus et al. 1999; Melkersson and Hulting 2001).

Diabetes

The weight gain observed with clozapine can place patients at risk for significant health problems. Diabetes is naturally the most concerning potential sequela of this weight gain. Numerous case reports have linked clozapine with new-onset diabetes (D. A. Wirshing et al. 1998). In Henderson's (2001) naturalistic study of 81 patients observed over a 5-year time period, 36.6% of the patients developed diabetes. The prevalence of diabetes in the United States is estimated to be approximately 7%, with another 7% of cases undiagnosed. Koller et al. (2001) published the largest series of case reports submitted voluntarily to the FDA MedWatch Program. The report revealed that there were 2,424 new-onset cases, 54 of which were cases of diabetic exacerbations and 80 of which were cases of diabetic ketoacidosis, a potentially life-threatening condition. The average age of the patients in the report was 40±12 years, and the male-to-female ratio was 2:1. Diabetes usually occurred within 6 months of starting clozapine. In our review of the peer-reviewed case literature, there seemed to be a preponderance of African Americans and males (D.A. Wirshing et al. 1998). As noted by Popli et al. (1997), there is a higher prevalence of non-insulin-dependent diabetes in African Americans compared with Caucasians in the United States, and this is likely the result of both nutritional factors and impaired access to health care. The significance of the overrepresentation of males is unclear but may reflect some hormonal interaction with glucose metabolism (Andersson et al. 1994)—or, more likely, selection bias, in which fewer women are placed on novel drugs.

We reviewed the charts of 590 patients taking antipsychotic medications and found statistically significant shifts in blood glucose among patients treated with clozapine and olanzapine, but not among patients treated with risperidone and quetiapine (D.A. Wirshing et al. 2002a). Sernyak et al. (2002) published a study examining the records of more than 30,000 patients in a VA database and found that the prevalence of the diagnosis of diabetes was higher among patients treated with novel antipsychotic medications than among patients treated with conventional agents. In particular, clozapine, olanzapine, and quetiapine were associated with much higher rates of diabetes than were conventional agents for all age ranges, whereas risperidone was not associated with a higher diabetes prevalence. The etiology of diabetes in clozapine-treated patients remains unclear. The most likely mechanism is that clozapine-associated weight gain causes an increase in insulin resistance.

However, weight gain is often, although not always, seen in patients treated with novel antipsychotics who develop new-onset diabetes, although a literature review spanning the years 1975–2006 by Newcomer (2006) concluded that antipsychotic medication–associated adiposity is the main culprit in the development of diabetes. Thus, one potential mechanism of diabetes induction is an increase in adiposity that, in turn, leads to insulin insensitivity, glucose intolerance, and, if sufficiently severe, diabetes. This notion is supported by results from a small study by Yazici et al. (1998), who found that clozapine increased blood glucose, insulin, and C peptide, which suggests that glucose intolerance was due to increased insulin resistance. It is also speculated that clozapine directly af-

fects beta cells of the pancreas (D.A. Wirshing et al. 1998). Recent evidence from animal studies suggests that clozapine dysregulates glucose metabolism by directly impairing the reaction of islet cells to glucose stimulation (Sasaki et al. 2006). Thus, the etiology of diabetes may be independent of adiposity, instead reflecting a direct effect of muscarinic blockade on the pancreatic islet cells.

Much of the information concerning the association of clozapine and diabetes mellitus is based on case reports, retrospective chart reviews, naturalistic studies, and cross-sectional studies. Although definitive studies have yet to be reported, the evidence is growing that clozapine may significantly impair glucose metabolism and increase the risk of diabetes in patients with schizophrenia. Diabetic ketoacidosis, although occurring infrequently, is of concern because of the risk of death. Patients treated with clozapine should be routinely screened for diabetes and other metabolic abnormalities, including raised lipid levels. Patients with risk factors for diabetes should be monitored more closely. Reports and clinical experience suggest that in a case of atypical antipsychotic–associated diabetes or diabetic ketoacidosis, discontinuation of the antipsychotic agent may result in reversal of the hyperglycemia and diabetes. During clozapine therapy, we recommend monitoring fasting glucose, cholesterol, and lipids at baseline and every 6 months thereafter.

Prevention of weight gain with clozapine, through nutrition and diet counseling, is recommended. Caloric restriction and exercise for 30 minutes per day should be recommended. Screening questions by physicians that we find useful include the following: "Have you noticed if your belt or pants size has changed?" "Have you noticed an increase in thirst or urinary frequency?" We strongly recommend weighing patients at each visit and monitoring blood pressure.

Dyslipidemias

Compelling data indicate that clozapine treatment is associated with dyslipidemias. Ghaeli and Dufresne (1996) performed a retrospective review of data from 24 male and 15 female patients treated with clozapine and 13 male and 15 female patients treated with typical antipsychotics (primarily high-potency agents). All patients had been taking these agents for at least 1 year. Age and gender of the patient, concomitant medications taken, and antipsychotic dosages were used as covariates in the analyses. Patients taking clozapine demonstrated significantly higher triglyceride levels than did patients taking typical agents (mean triglyceride level of 264.6 mg/dL for patients in the clozapine group vs. 149.8 mg/dL for patients taking typical agents; *P*<0.001). A retrospective chart review by Gaulin et al. (1999) compared 117 patients taking clozapine with 45 patients taking haloperidol. The study found significant increases in triglyceride levels for both men and women taking clozapine—a mean increase from 184.6 mg/dL to 273.4 mg/dL for men (*P*<0.01) and from 164.9 mg/dL to 223.3 mg/dL for women (*P*<0.05).

Spivak et al. (1999) reported on a retrospective data from 70 patients being treated with clozapine for 6 months. They observed a significant increase in triglyceride levels from 69.6 mg/dL prior to the initiation of clozapine to 77.3 mg/dL just 6 months after initiation (*P*< 0.05). This suggests not only that clozapine can increase triglyceride levels but also that it can do so over a relatively short period of time. Another prospective sample of 8 clozapine-treated patients showed an 11% increase in triglyceride levels (*P*<0.05) after 12 weeks of clozapine therapy at an average dosage of 352 mg/day. No significant changes in total cholesterol, low-density lipoprotein (LDL) cholesterol, or high-density lipoprotein (HDL) cholesterol were observed (Dursun et al. 1999). More recently, patients who received clozapine in phase II of CATIE demonstrated greater elevations in both triglycerides and cholesterol than patients on olanzapine, risperidone, or quetiapine (McEvoy et al. 2006). However, these differences were not statistically significant.

Our group published the first study to compare multiple SGAs (clozapine, risperidone, olanzapine, and quetiapine) against each other and against the typical agents fluphenazine and haloperidol in their propensity to affect lipid parameters (D. A. Wirshing et al. 2002a). This study was a retrospective review of the charts of 215 patients taking antipsychotics (clozapine, olanzapine, risperidone, quetiapine, haloperidol, or fluphenazine). Lipid data from 2.5 years before and after initiation of the target antipsychotic were collected. Covariates used in the analysis included age of patient, duration of antipsychotic treatment, concomitant use of other medications that could affect lipids, and initial laboratory values. Patients receiving clozapine or olanzapine demonstrated statistically significant increases in triglyceride levels compared with the other groups. Triglyceride levels increased by more than 30% for patients taking clozapine or olanzapine, compared with only a 19% increase for patients taking risperidone; patients taking haloperidol or fluphenazine developed decreases in triglyceride levels.

The clinical implications of these findings are thought-provoking—for example, could triglyceride elevation account for the beneficial psychiatric effect of

these medications through stabilization of neuronal membranes? Some authors have suggested that changes in triglycerides may actually affect serotonergic activity. Diebold et al. (1998) postulated that elevated triglyceride levels cause increases in brain cell membrane fluidity, which in turn lead to increased presynaptic reuptake of serotonin and decreased postsynaptic serotonergic function. This effect on triglycerides may enhance the ability of SGA medications such as clozapine to inhibit serotonergic activity and thus may contribute to their mechanism of action (Kingsbury et al. 2001). Studies have also shown correlations between elevations in triglyceride levels and changes in mood. For example, increases in triglyceride levels have been shown to be associated with decreased hostility (Diebold et al. 1998). Spivak et al. (1998) observed that patients taking clozapine who developed increases in triglycerides also demonstrated decreases in aggression and suicidal behavior in comparison with patients taking typical antipsychotics, although the difference was not significant (*P*=0.07). Muldoon et al. (1990) reviewed numerous randomized clinical trials that focused on reducing lipid levels for primary prevention of coronary artery disease. They concluded that the risk of death due to accidents, suicide, or violence was significantly higher in patients with reduced lipid levels (*P*=0.004).

The overall impact of clozapine—and of virtually all other antipsychotic medications—on lipids, glucose, and obesity may result in an increase in the prevalence of the metabolic syndrome. The term *metabolic syndrome* describes a set of risk factors for diabetes, heart disease, and cerebrovascular disease. According to the National Cholesterol Education Program and American Diabetes Association criteria (Lamberti et al. 2006; Meyer et al. 2006), metabolic syndrome is defined as the presence of three or more of the following:

- Waist circumference >102 cm for men and >88 cm for women
- Fasting blood triglyceride level ≥150 mg/dL
- HDL cholesterol level <40 mg/dL for men and <50 mg/dL for women
- Blood pressure ≥130 mm Hg systolic or ≥85 mm Hg diastolic
- Fasting blood glucose level ≥100 mg/dL

To examine whether the medical consequences of obesity may offset the lifesaving benefits gained from clozapine's potentially decreased suicide rate, Fontaine et al. (2001), using mathematical modeling, estimated that 492 suicide deaths per 100,000 schizophrenia patients would be prevented over 10 years with the use of clozapine. This was compared with an estimated 416 additional deaths due to antipsychotic-induced weight gain. Although this estimate is mathematically based and somewhat controversial, these investigators suggest that the lives saved by clozapine may essentially be offset by the deaths associated with weight gain. Thus, it behooves physicians prescribing clozapine to monitor weight, glucose, and lipids—we recommend obtaining measurements at the onset of therapy and every 6 months thereafter—to assist in minimizing the increased risks for coronary artery disease to which our patients are already predisposed.

In 2004, in response to growing concern that the majority of antipsychotic medications may be associated with weight gain and other metabolic changes, the American Diabetes Association and other groups published a set of guidelines for monitoring weight, glucose, and lipids (American Diabetes Association et al. 2004). Also in 2004, a very comprehensive literature review was conducted by Marder et al. (2004) to provide guidance to clinicians regarding monitoring of weight, glucose, lipids, and other parameters of physical health in patients with schizophrenia. Labeling changes were made for all antipsychotic medications, including clozapine, regarding these metabolic risk factors.

Seizures

A well-known risk of clozapine treatment is the risk for seizures, which are thought to occur in 5%–10% of patients treated with this medication (Welch et al. 1994). The cause of seizures is unclear, but it is generally thought that rapid escalations in dosage and possibly high plasma levels of clozapine may account for the development of seizures (Klimke and Klieser 1995). Clozapine-associated seizures occur most often at dosages greater than 600 mg/day. The relationship between clozapine plasma levels and seizures is somewhat inconsistent in the literature (Simpson and Cooper 1978; Vailleau et al. 1996). Some speculations as to whether the therapeutic efficacy of clozapine lies in its ability to induce subcortical seizure-like activity have been put forth by Stevens and colleagues (Stevens 1995; Stevens et al. 1996), who proposed that the amino acid neurotransmitter system might include naturally occurring anticonvulsants that suppress signal transduction and ultimately lead to information-processing deficits. According to this hypothesis, the emergence of electroencephalogram (EEG) abnormalities would correspond to an increase in signal transduction and improved information processing.

In addition to seizure risk, several researchers have observed that EEG abnormalities, such as slowing, occur in the majority of patients treated with clozapine (Welch et al. 1994). Slowing may be attributable to the anticholinergic activity of this medication. Because patients with schizophrenia often have EEG abnormalities (some estimated rates are 25%), it is unclear whether a baseline EEG would predict whether a particular patient would develop seizures when given clozapine. On the basis of their experience with clozapine in treating patients with refractory illness, Welch et al. (1994) proposed guidelines that recommend increased monitoring for patients with abnormal baseline EEGs. Our own experience leads us to recommend obtaining a baseline EEG when initiating clozapine treatment in patients who have a history of possible head injury, loss of consciousness, or other risk factors for seizures. In cases where EEG abnormalities are found, we still believe that clozapine treatment is warranted, but it would be best if treatment were initiated with prophylactic anticonvulsant medication.

The anticonvulsant agents sodium valproate, gabapentin, and topiramate have been used successfully to treat clozapine-induced seizures (Navarro et al. 2001; Toth and Frankenburg 1994; Usiskin et al. 2000). Topiramate has an advantage over sodium valproate in that it is associated with very little weight gain. In cases in our clinic where patients have developed seizures while taking clozapine, we institute rapid loading with anticonvulsant medication and temporarily discontinue the clozapine treatment. We then slowly reintroduce and retitrate the clozapine once the patient is taking an adequate dose of anticonvulsant medication.

Constipation

A truly problematic consequence of clozapine's anticholinergic activity is its propensity to cause significant constipation. This can be a difficult side effect to manage in severely mentally ill individuals, who may not complain about the problem until a medical emergency, such as acute bowel obstruction, occurs. In institutional settings and in prisons, where patients may have little access to exercise and where monitoring of patients' fluid intake is not performed, constipation from clozapine can be serious or even fatal (Drew and Herdson 1997; Hayes and Gibler 1995; Levin et al. 2002). Typically, constipation can be avoided by proactive modifications in patients' diets and education about adequate fluid intake and exercise. The medical treatment that we favor is prophylactic therapy with sorbitol. We are less inclined to recommend treatments involving bulking agents, particularly in the setting of poor fluid intake. High-fiber diets can also be beneficial.

Other Side Effects

Sedation is one of the most difficult and common side effects of clozapine to manage. Patients often do not want their doses increased in the setting of increased sedation and will complain of sedation as one of the most annoying consequences of clozapine treatment (Angermeyer et al. 2001). In our experience, sedation is usually the limiting factor controlling both the rate at which the dosage of clozapine can be increased and the maximum dosage the patient can tolerate. However, no rigorous studies have been published.

There have been several reports of respiratory arrest or depression during the early stages of treatment with clozapine (Novartis 2002). Two of the patients who experienced respiratory arrest were concomitantly taking benzodiazepines.

Sialorrhea is a commonly reported side effect of clozapine (occurring in over 50% of patients) that can be problematic for patients. The etiology of sialorrhea is unclear, but the condition does not seem to be caused by the dopamine blockade. It may be mediated through α-adrenergic receptor blockade. Case series and small pilot studies indicate that treating sialorrhea with antiadrenergic agents, such as the clonidine patch, or anticholinergic agents, such as benztropine and intranasal ipratropium bromide, may be successful (Calderon et al. 2000). We generally recommend that patients sleep with a towel on their pillow, as this side effect seems to be most bothersome during the night. Unfortunately, the use of concomitant antiadrenergic or anticholinergic agents adds to the potential side-effect burdens of hypotension and constipation, respectively.

Neuroleptic malignant syndrome (NMS), a syndrome of unknown etiology that includes hyperthermia, autonomic instability, and severe rigidity, has been reported in several patients treated with clozapine (Anderson and Powers 1991). The etiology of NMS that occurs in the context of clozapine use, as well as that occurring with use of conventional antipsychotics, remains unclear.

Hepatotoxicity has been reported with clozapine, especially in the setting of polypharmacy (Macfarlane et al. 1997; W. Wirshing et al. 1997). Asymptomatic elevation of transaminase levels was observed most commonly, affecting between 30% and 50% of patients treated with clozapine. Icteric hepatitis was uncommonly seen in Mac-

farlane et al.'s (1997) review of clozapine-related hepatotoxicity and was noted in 84 of 136,000 patients (0.06%). Fatal acute fulminant hepatitis has been documented in 2 patients (0.001%). Although serious toxicity is rare, prescribers of clozapine should be aware of its hepatotoxic potential.

Sexual side effects, including priapism and impotence, have been reported with clozapine. Urinary retention and bladder dysfunction can also result from clozapine. In a study surveying patients' sexual side effects, we found that clozapine-treated patients actually had fewer sexual complaints than patients on other antipsychotic medications (prolixin and risperidone) (D. A. Wirshing et al. 2002b).

Although this daunting array of side effects—along with the management of the risk of agranulocytosis—makes the treatment of patients with clozapine complex, it is common for patients to report a sense of relief from the dysphoric moods they experienced while taking conventional drugs. Additionally, the freedom from EPS may account for the enhanced sense of well-being in patients treated with clozapine.

Drug–Drug Interactions

As previously mentioned, clozapine is predominately metabolized by cytochrome P450 (CYP) 1A2, although CYP2D6 and CYP3A3 also contribute to its metabolism (Buur-Rasmussen and Brosen 1999). Smoking, which induces CYP1A2, lowers clozapine plasma levels. Fluvoxamine, a potent inhibitor of CYP1A2, dramatically increases plasma levels of clozapine (Heeringa et al. 1999), and on occasion, adverse effects are seen (Koponen et al. 1996). This phenomenon can lead to clozapine intoxication in patients receiving high doses of fluvoxamine. Other reports suggest that inhibitors of CYP2D6, including paroxetine and fluoxetine, can elevate clozapine levels (Joos et al. 1997; Spina et al. 1998).

Conclusion

Clozapine maintains an important place in the treatment of severe psychosis. Side effects, including agranulocytosis, seizures, sedation, and weight gain, make it the most difficult antipsychotic to prescribe. As a result, clozapine should be reserved for patients who have failed to respond to other SGAs. The difficulty in administering clozapine has led many patients and their clinicians to resist its use. This is unfortunate, because patients should never be deemed "treatment refractory" or "partial responders" until they have received an adequate trial of clozapine.

References

Allison DB, Mentore JL, Heo M, et al: Antipsychotic-induced weight gain: a comprehensive research synthesis. Am J Psychiatry 156:1686–1696, 1999

Alvir JM, Lieberman JA, Safferman AZ, et al: Clozapine-induced agranulocytosis. Incidence and risk factors in the United States. N Engl J Med 329:162–167, 1993

American Diabetes Association; American Psychiatric Association; American Association of Clinical Endocrinologists; North American Association for the Study of Obesity: Consensus development conference on antipsychotic drugs and obesity and diabetes. Diabetes Care 27:596–601, 2004

Ames D, Wirshing WC, Baker RW, et al: Predictive value of eosinophilia for neutropenia during clozapine treatment. J Clin Psychiatry 57:579–581, 1996

Amsler HA, Teerenhovi L, Barth E, et al: Agranulocytosis in patients treated with clozapine. A study of the Finnish epidemic. Acta Psychiatr Scand 56:241–488, 1977

Anderson ES, Powers PS: Neuroleptic malignant syndrome associated with clozapine use. J Clin Psychiatry 52:102–104, 1991

Andersson B, Marin P, Lissner L, et al: Testosterone concentrations in women and men with NIDDM. Diabetes Care 17:405–411, 1994

Angermeyer MC, Loffler W, Muller P, et al: Patients' and relatives' assessment of clozapine treatment. Psychol Med 31:509–517, 2001

Azorin JM, Spiegel R, Remington G, et al: A double-blind comparative study of clozapine and risperidone in the management of severe chronic schizophrenia. Am J Psychiatry 158:1305–1313, 2001

Barbini B, Scherillo P, Benedetti F, et al: Response to clozapine in acute mania is more rapid than that of chlorpromazine. Int Clin Psychopharmacol 12:109–112, 1997

Basile VS, Masellis M, McIntyre RS, et al: Genetic dissection of atypical antipsychotic-induced weight gain: novel preliminary data on the pharmacogenetic puzzle. J Clin Psychiatry 62 (suppl 23):45–66, 2001

Bell R, McLaren A, Galanos J, et al: The clinical use of plasma clozapine levels. Aust N Z J Psychiatry 32:567–574, 1998

Bitter I, Dossenbach MR, Brook S, et al: Olanzapine versus clozapine in treatment-resistant or treatment-intolerant schizophrenia. Prog Neuropsychopharmacol Biol Psychiatry 28:173–180, 2004

Bondolfi G, Dufour H, Patris M, et al: Risperidone versus clozapine in treatment-resistant chronic schizophrenia: a randomized double-blind study. The Risperidone Study Group. Am J Psychiatry 155:499–504, 1998

Braff DL, Swerdlow NR, Geyer MA: Symptom correlates of prepulse inhibition deficits in male schizophrenic patients. Am J Psychiatry 156:596–602, 1999

Breier AF, Malhotra AK, Su TP, et al: Clozapine and risperidone in chronic schizophrenia: effects on symptoms, parkinsonian side effects, and neuroendocrine response. Am J Psychiatry 156:294–298, 1999

Breier A, Buchanan R, Irish D, et al: Clozapine treatment of outpatients with schizophrenia: outcome and long-term response patterns, 1993. Psychiatr Serv 51:1249–1253, 2000

Bromel T, Blum WF, Ziegler A, et al: Serum leptin levels increase rapidly after initiation of clozapine therapy. Mol Psychiatry 3:76–80, 1998

Brunette MF, Drake RE, Xie H, et al: Clozapine use and relapses of substance use disorder among patients with co-occurring schizophrenia and substance use disorders. Schizophr Bull 32:637–643, 2006

Buur-Rasmussen B, Brosen K: Cytochrome P450 and therapeutic drug monitoring with respect to clozapine. Eur Neuropsychopharmacol 9:453–459, 1999

Calabrese JR, Kimmel SE, Woyshville MJ, et al: Clozapine for treatment-refractory mania. Am J Psychiatry 153:759–764, 1996

Calderon J, Rubin E, Sobota WL: Potential use of ipratropium bromide for the treatment of clozapine-induced hypersalivation: a preliminary report. Int Clin Psychopharmacol 15:49–52, 2000

Canuso CM, Goldman MB: Clozapine restores water balance in schizophrenic patients with polydipsia-hyponatremia syndrome. J Neuropsychiatry Clin Neurosci 11:86–90, 1999

Chakos M, Lieberman J, Hoffman E, et al: Effectiveness of second-generation antipsychotics in patients with treatment-resistant schizophrenia: a review and meta-analysis of randomized trials. Am J Psychiatry 158:518–526, 2001

Chengappa KN, Goldstein JM, Greenwood M, et al: A post hoc analysis of the impact on hostility and agitation of quetiapine and haloperidol among patients with schizophrenia. Clin Ther 25:530–541, 2003

Chiodo LA, Bunney BS: Typical and atypical neuroleptics: differential effects of chronic administration on the activity of A9 and A10 midbrain dopaminergic neurons. J Neurosci 3:1607–1619, 1983

Citrome L, Volavka J, Czobor P, et al: Effects of clozapine, olanzapine, risperidone, and haloperidol on hostility among patients with schizophrenia. Psychiatr Serv 52:1510–1514, 2001

Claghorn J, Honigfeld G, Abuzzahab FS Sr, et al: The risks and benefits of clozapine versus chlorpromazine. J Clin Psychopharmacol 7:377–384, 1987

de la Chapelle A, Kari C, Nurminem M, et al: Clozapine-induced agranulocytosis: a genetic and epidemiologic study. Hum Genet 37:183–194, 1977

Dettling M, Cascorbi I, Roots I, et al: Genetic determinants of clozapine-induced agranulocytosis: recent results of HLA subtyping in a non-Jewish Caucasian sample. Arch Gen Psychiatry 58:93–94, 2001

Diebold K, Michel G, Schweizer J, et al: Are psychoactive-drug-induced changes in plasma lipid and lipoprotein levels of significance for clinical remission in psychiatric disorders? Pharmacopsychiatry 31:60–67, 1998

Drake RE, Xie H, McHugo GJ, et al: The effects of clozapine on alcohol and drug use disorders among patients with schizophrenia. Schizophr Bull 26:441–449, 2000

Drew L, Herdson P: Clozapine and constipation: a serious issue. Aust N Z J Psychiatry 31:149–150, 1997

Dursun SM, Szemis A, Andrews H, et al: The effects of clozapine on levels of total cholesterol and related lipids in serum of patients with schizophrenia: a prospective study. J Psychiatry Neurosci 24:453–455, 1999

Essock SM, Frisman LK, Covell NH, et al: Cost-effectiveness of clozapine compared with conventional antipsychotic medication for patients in state hospitals. Arch Gen Psychiatry 57:987–994, 2000

Farde L, Nordstrom AL, Wiesel FA, et al: Positron emission tomographic analysis of central D and D1 and D2 dopamine receptor occupancy in patients treated with classical neuroleptics and clozapine. Relation to extrapyramidal side effects. Arch Gen Psychiatry 49:538–544, 1992

Fischer-Cornelssen KA, Ferner UJ: An example of European multicenter trials: multispectral analysis of clozapine. Psychopharmacol Bull 12:34–39, 1976

Fontaine KR, Heo M, Harrigan EP, et al: Estimating the consequences of anti-psychotic induced weight gain on health and mortality rate. Psychiatry Res 101:277–288, 2001

Frankenburg FR, Zanarini MC, Kando J, et al: Clozapine and body mass change. Biol Psychiatry 32:718–721, 1998

French Clozapine Parkinson Study Group: Clozapine in drug-induced psychosis in Parkinson's disease. Lancet 353:2041–2042, 1999

Gaszner P, Makkos Z, Kosza P, et al: Agranulocytosis during clozapine therapy. Prog Neuropsychopharmacol Biol Psychiatry 26:603–607, 2002

Gaulin BD, Markowitz JS, Caley CF, et al: Clozapine-associated elevation in serum triglycerides. Am J Psychiatry 156:1270–1272, 1999

Geyer MA, Krebs-Thomson K, et al: Pharmacological studies of prepulse inhibition models of sensorimotor gating deficits in schizophrenia: a decade in review. Psychopharmacology (Berl) 156(2–3):117–154, 2001

Ghaeli P, Dufresne RL: Serum triglyceride levels in patients treated with clozapine. Am J Health Syst Pharm 53:2079–2081, 1996

Green AI, Tohen M, Patel JK, et al: Clozapine in the treatment of refractory psychotic mania. Am J Psychiatry 157:982–986, 2000

Green AI, Burgess ES, Dawson R, et al: Alcohol and cannabis use in schizophrenia: effects of clozapine vs risperidone. Schizophr Res 60:81–85, 2003

Green AI, Drake RE, Brunette MF, et al: Schizophrenia and co-occurring substance use disorder. Am J Psychiatry 164:402–408, 2007

Griffith RW, Saamerli K: Clozapine and agranulocytosis. Lancet 2(7936):657, 1975

Hayes G, Gibler B: Clozapine-induced constipation. Am J Psychiatry 152:298, 1995

Heeringa M, Beurskens R, Schouten W, et al: Elevated plasma levels of clozapine after concomitant use of fluvoxamine. Pharm World Sci 21:243–244, 1999

Helmchen H: Clinical experience with clozapine in Germany. Psychopharmacology (Berl) 99 (suppl):S80–S83, 1989

Henderson D: Clozapine: diabetes mellitus, weight gain, and lipid abnormalities. J Clin Psychiatry 62 (suppl 23):39–44, 2001

Hippius H: A historical perspective of clozapine. J Clin Psychiatry 60 (suppl 12):22–23, 1999

Honigfeld G: Effects of the clozapine national registry system on incidence of deaths related to agranulocytosis. Psychiatr Serv 47:52–56, 1996

Honigfeld G, Patin J, Singer J: Clozapine: antipsychotic activity in treatment-resistant schizophrenics. Adv Ther 1:77–97, 1984

Honigfeld G, Arellano F, Sethi J, et al: Reducing clozapine-related morbidity and mortality: 5 years of experience with the Clo-zaril National Registry. J Clin Psychiatry 59 (suppl 3):3–7, 1998

Hummer M, Kurz M, Barnas C, et al: Clozapine-induced transient white blood count disorders. J Clin Psychiatry 55:429–432, 1994

Jones KM, Stoukides CA: Clozapine in treatment of Parkinson's disease. Ann Pharmacother 26:1386–1377, 1992

Joos AA, Konig F, Frank UG, et al: Dose-dependent pharmacokinetic interaction of clozapine and paroxetine in an extensive metabolizer. Pharmacopsychiatry 30:266–270, 1997

Jungi WF, Fischer J, Senn HJ, et al: [Frequent cases of agranulocytosis due to clozapine (leponex) in eastern Switzerland.] Schweiz Med Wochenschr 107:1861–1864, 1977

Kane J, Honigfeld G, Singer J, et al: Clozapine for the treatment-resistant schizophrenic. A double-blind comparison with chlorpromazine. Arch Gen Psychiatry 45:789–796, 1988

Kane JM, Marder SR, Schooler NR, et al: Clozapine and haloperidol in moderately refractory schizophrenia. A 6-month randomized and double-blind comparison. Arch Gen Psychiatry 58:965–972, 2001

Kapur S, Seeman P: Does fast dissociation from the dopamine D2 receptor explain the action of atypical antipsychotics? a new hypothesis. Am J Psychiatry 158:360–369, 2001

Killian JG, Kerr K, Lawrence C, et al: Myocarditis and cardiomyopathy associated with clozapine. Lancet 354(9193):1841–1845, 1999

Kingsbury SJ, Fayek M, Trufasiu D, et al: The apparent effects of ziprasidone on plasma lipids and glucose. J Clin Psychiatry 62:347–349, 2001

Klimke A, Klieser E: [The atypical neuroleptic clozapine (Leponex)—current knowledge and recent clinical aspects.] Fortschr Neurol Psychiatr 63:173–193, 1995

Koller E, Schneider B, Bennett K, et al: Clozapine-associated diabetes. Am J Med 111:716–723, 2001

Koponen HJ, Leinonen E, Lepola U: Fluvoxamine increases the clozapine serum levels significantly. Eur Neuropsychopharmacol 6:69–71, 1996

Kraus T, Haack M, Schuld A, et al: Body weight and leptin plasma levels during treatment with antipsychotic drugs, patients with anorexia have low leptin levels. Am J Psychiatry 156:312–314, 1999

Kronig MH, Munne RA, Szymanski S, et al: Plasma clozapine levels and clinical response for treatment-refractory schizophrenic patients. Am J Psychiatry 152:179–182, 1995

Kumari V, Soni W, Sharma T: Normalization of information processing deficits in schizophrenia with clozapine. Am J Psychiatry 156:1046–1051, 1999

Kumra S, Frazier JA, Jacobsen LK, et al: Childhood-onset schizophrenia. A double-blind clozapine-haloperidol comparison. Arch Gen Psychiatry 53:1090–1097, 1996

Lamberti JS, Olson D, Crilly JF, et al: Prevalence of the metabolic syndrome among patients receiving clozapine. Am J Psychiatry 163:1273–1276, 2006

Lehman AF, Kreyenbuhl J, Buchanan RW, et al: The Schizophrenia Patient Outcomes Research Team (PORT): updated treatment recommendations 2003. Schizophr Bull 30:193–217, 2004a

Lehman AF, Lieberman JA, Dixon LB, et al: Practice guideline for the treatment of patients with schizophrenia, second edition. Am J Psychiatry 161 (2 suppl):1–56, 2004b

Levin TT, Barrett J, Mendelowitz A: Death from clozapine-induced constipation: case report and literature review. Psychosomatics 43:71–73, 2002

Lewis SW, Barnes TR, Davies L, et al: Randomized controlled trial of effect of prescription of clozapine versus other second-generation antipsychotic drugs in resistant schizophrenia. Schizophr Bull 32:715–723, 2006

Lieberman JA, Safferman AZ: Clinical profile of clozapine: adverse reactions and agranulocytosis. Psychiatr Q 63:51–70, 1992

Lieberman JA, Yunis J, Egea E, et al: HLA-B38, DR4, DQw3 and clozapine-induced agranulocytosis in Jewish patients with schizophrenia. Arch Gen Psychiatry 47:945–948, 1990

Macfarlane B, Davies S, Mannan K, et al: Fatal acute fulminant liver failure due to clozapine: a case report and review of clozapine-induced hepatotoxicity. Gastroenterology 112:1707–1709, 1997

Marder SR, Essock SM, Miller AL, et al: The Mount Sinai conference on the pharmacotherapy of schizophrenia. Schizophr Bull 28:5–16, 2002

Marder SR, Essock SM, Miller AL, et al: Physical health monitoring of patients with schizophrenia. Am J Psychiatry 161:1334–1349, 2004

McElroy SL, Dessain EC, Pope HG Jr, et al: Clozapine in the treatment of psychotic mood disorders, schizoaffective disorder, and schizophrenia. J Clin Psychiatry 52:411–414, 1991

McEvoy JP, Lieberman JA, Stroup TS, et al: Effectiveness of clozapine versus olanzapine, quetiapine, and risperidone in patients with chronic schizophrenia who did not respond to prior atypical antipsychotic treatment. Am J Psychiatry 163:600–610, 2006

Meged S, Stein D, Sitrota P, et al: Human leukocyte antigen typing, response to neuroleptics, and clozapine-induced agranulocytosis in Jewish Israeli schizophrenic patients. Int Clin Psychopharmacol 14:305–312, 1999

Melkersson K, Hulting AL: [Antipsychotic drugs can affect hormone balance: weight gain, blood lipid disturbances and diabetes are important.] Lakartidningen 98:5462–5464, 5467–5469, 2001

Meltzer HY: Suicidality in schizophrenia: a review of the evidence for risk factors and treatment options. Curr Psychiatry Rep 4:279–283, 2002

Meltzer HY, Okayli G: Reduction of suicidality during clozapine treatment of neuroleptic-resistant schizophrenia: impact on risk-benefit assessment. Am J Psychiatry 152:183–190, 1995

Merrill DB, Goff DC: Adverse cardiac effects associated with clozapine. J Clin Psychopharmacol 25:32–41, 2005

Meyer J, Loh C, Leckband SG, et al: Prevalence of the metabolic syndrome in veterans with schizophrenia. J Psychiatr Pract 12:5–10, 2006

Miller AL, Hall CS, Buchanan RW, et al: The Texas Medication Algorithm Project antipsychotic algorithm for schizophrenia: 2003 update. J Clin Psychiatry 65:500–508, 2004

Miller DD: The clinical use of clozapine plasma concentrations in the management of treatment-refractory schizophrenia. Ann Clin Psychiatry 8:99–109, 1996

Miller DD, Fleming F, Holman TL, et al: Plasma clozapine concentrations as a predictor of clinical response: a follow-up study. J Clin Psychiatry 55 (suppl B):117–121, 1994

Miyasaki JM, Shannon K, Voon V, et al: Practice parameter: evaluation and treatment of depression, psychosis, and dementia in Parkinson disease (an evidence-based review): report of the Quality Standards Subcommittee of the American Academy of Neurology. Neurology 66:996–1002, 2006

Muldoon MF, Manuck SB, Matthews KA: Lowering cholesterol concentrations and mortality: a quantitative review of primary prevention trials. BMJ 301(6747):309–314, 1990

Navarro V, Pons A, Romero A, et al: Topiramate for clozapine-induced seizures. Am J Psychiatry 158:968–969, 2001

Newcomer JW: Medical risk in patients with bipolar disorder and schizophrenia. J Clin Psychiatry 67(11):e16, 2006

Novartis: Clozaril (clozapine) tablets: prescribing information. Hanover, NJ, Novartis Pharmaceuticals, July 2002

Parkinson Study Group: Low-dose clozapine for the treatment of drug-induced psychosis in Parkinson's disease. N Engl J Med 340:757–763, 1999

Paton C, Whittington C, Barnes TR: Augmentation with a second antipsychotic in patients with schizophrenia who partially respond to clozapine: a meta-analysis. J Clin Psychopharmacol 27:198–204, 2007

Pickar D, Owen RR, Litman RE, et al: Clinical and biologic response to clozapine in patients with schizophrenia. Crossover comparison with fluphenazine. Arch Gen Psychiatry 49:345–353, 1992

Pollak P, Tison F, Rascol O, et al: Clozapine in drug induced psychosis in Parkinson's disease: a randomised, placebo controlled study with open follow up. J Neurol Neurosurg Psychiatry 75:689–695, 2004

Popli AP, Konicki PE, Jurjus GJ, et al: Clozapine and associated diabetes mellitus. J Clin Psychiatry 58:108–111, 1997

Potkin SG, Bera R, Gulasekaram B, et al: Plasma clozapine concentrations predict clinical response in treatment resistant schizophrenia. J Clin Psychiatry 55 (9, suppl B):117–121, 1994

Raison CL, Guze BH, Kissell RL, et al: Successful treatment of clozapine-induced agranulocytosis with granulocyte colony-stimulating factor. J Clin Psychopharmacol 14:285–286, 1994

Ranjan R, Meltzer HY: Acute and long-term effectiveness of clozapine in treatment-resistant psychotic depression. Biol Psychiatry 40:253–258, 1996

Reid WH, Mason M, Hogan T: Suicide prevention effects associated with clozapine therapy in schizophrenia and schizoaffective disorder. Psychiatr Serv 49:1029–1033, 1998

Rosenheck R, Cramer J, Xu W, et al: A comparison of clozapine and haloperidol in hospitalized patients with refractory schizophrenia. Department of Veterans Affairs Cooperative Study Group on Clozapine in Refractory Schizophrenia. N Engl J Med 337:809–815, 1997

Rothschild AJ: Management of psychotic, treatment-resistant depression. Psychiatr Clin North Am 19:237–252, 1996

Safferman AZ, Lieberman JA, Alvir JM, et al: Rechallenge in clozapine-induced agranulocytosis (letter). Lancet 339(8804):1296–1297, 1992

Sasaki N, Iwase M, Uchizono Y, et al: The atypical antipsychotic clozapine impairs insulin secretion by inhibiting glucose metabolism and distal steps in rat pancreatic islets. Diabetologia 49:2930–2938, 2006

Seeman P: Atypical antipsychotics: mechanism of action. Can J Psychiatry 47:27–38, 2002

Sernyak MJ, Leslie DL, Alarcon RD, et al: Association of diabetes mellitus with use of atypical neuroleptics in the treatment of schizophrenia. Am J Psychiatry 159:561–566, 2002

Shaw P, Sporn A, Gogtay N, et al: Childhood-onset schizophrenia: a double-blind, randomized clozapine-olanzapine comparison. Arch Gen Psychiatry 63:721–730, 2006

Shopsin B, Klein H, Aaronsom M, et al: Clozapine, chlorpromazine, and placebo in newly hospitalized, acutely schizophrenic patients: a controlled, double-blind comparison. Arch Gen Psychiatry 36:657–664, 1979

Simpson GM, Cooper TA: Clozapine plasma levels and convulsions. Am J Psychiatry 135:99–100, 1978

Simpson GM, Varga E: Clozapine—a new antipsychotic agent. Curr Ther Res Clin Exp 16:679–686, 1974

Spina E, Avenoso A, Facciola G, et al: Effect of fluoxetine on the plasma concentrations of clozapine and its major metabolites in patients with schizophrenia. Int Clin Psychopharmacol 13:141–145, 1998

Spivak B, Roitman S, Vered Y, et al: Diminished suicidal and aggressive behavior, high plasma norepinephrine levels, and serum triglyceride levels in chronic neuroleptic-resistant schizophrenic patients maintained on clozapine. Clin Neuropharmacol 21:245–250, 1998

Spivak B, Lamschtein C, Talmon Y, et al: The impact of clozapine treatment on serum lipids in chronic schizophrenic patients. Clin Neuropharmacol 22:98–101, 1999

Stevens JR: Clozapine: the yin and yang of seizures and psychosis. Biol Psychiatry 37:425–426, 1995

Stevens JR, Denney D, Szot P, et al: Kindling with clozapine: behavioral and molecular consequences. Epilepsy Res 26:295–304, 1996

Stroup TS, Lieberman JA, McEvoy JP, et al: Effectiveness of olanzapine, quetiapine, risperidone, and ziprasidone in patients with chronic schizophrenia following discontinuation of a previous atypical antipsychotic. Am J Psychiatry 163:611–622, 2006

Suppes T, Webb A, Paul B, et al: Clinical outcome in a randomized 1-year trial of clozapine versus treatment as usual for patients with treatment-resistant illness and a history of mania. Am J Psychiatry 156:1164–1169, 1999

Swerdlow NR, Geyer MA: Clozapine and haloperidol in an animal model of sensorimotor gating deficits in schizophrenia. Pharmacol Biochem Behav 44:741–744, 1993

Swerdlow NR, Bakshi V, et al: Seroquel, clozapine and chlorpromazine restore sensorimotor gating in ketamine-treated rats. Psychopharmacology (Berl) 140:75–80, 1998

Theisen FM, Cichon S, Linden A, et al: Clozapine and weight gain. Am J Psychiatry 158:816, 2001a

Theisen F, Linden A, Geller F, et al: Prevalence of obesity in adolescent and young adult patients with and without schizophrenia and in relationship to antipsychotic medication. J Psychiatr Res 35:339–345, 2001b

Tollefson GD, Birkett MA, Kiesler GM, et al: Double-blind comparison of olanzapine versus clozapine in schizophrenic patients clinically eligible for treatment with clozapine. Biol Psychiatry 49:52–63, 2001

Toth P, Frankenburg FR: Clozapine and seizures: a review. Can J Psychiatry 39:236–238, 1994

Usiskin SI, Nicolson R, Lenane M, et al: Gabapentin prophylaxis of clozapine-induced seizures. Am J Psychiatry 157:482–483, 2000

Vailleau JL, Jeanny B, Chomard P, et al: [Importance of determining clozapine plasma level in follow-up of schizophrenic patients.] Encephale 22:103–109, 1996

Varty GB, Higgins GA: Examination of drug-induced and isolation-induced disruptions of prepulse inhibition as models to screen antipsychotic drugs. Psychopharmacology (Berl) 122:15–26, 1995

Volavka J, Czobor P, Sheitman B, et al: Clozapine, olanzapine, risperidone, and haloperidol in the treatment of patients with chronic schizophrenia and schizoaffective disorder. Am J Psychiatry 159:255–262, 2002

Walker AM, Lanzall LL, Arellano F, et al: Mortality in current and former users of clozapine. Epidemiology 8:671–677, 1997

Weide R, Koppler H, Heymanns J, et al: Successful treatment of clozapine induced agranulocytosis with granulocyte–colony-stimulating factor (G-CSF). Br J Haematol 80:557–559, 1992

Welch J, Manschreck T, Redmond D: Clozapine-induced seizures and EEG changes. J Neuropsychiatry Clin Neurosci 6:250–256, 1994

Wickramanayake PD, Scheid C, Josting A, et al: Use of granulocyte colony-stimulating factor (filgrastim) in the treatment of non-cytotoxic drug-induced agranulocytosis. Eur J Med Res 1:153–156, 1995

Wirshing DA, Spellberg BJ, Erhart SM, et al: Novel antipsychotics and new onset diabetes. Biol Psychiatry 44:778–783, 1998

Wirshing DA, Wirshing WC, Kysar L, et al: Novel antipsychotics: comparison of weight gain liabilities. J Clin Psychiatry 60:358–363, 1999

Wirshing DA, Boyd J, Meng LR: The effects of novel antipsychotics on glucose and lipid levels. J Clin Psychiatry 63:856–865, 2002a

Wirshing DA, Pierre JM, Marder SR, et al: Sexual side effects of novel antipsychotic medications. Schizophr Res 56:25–30, 2002b

Wirshing DA, Pierre JM, Wirshing WC: Sleep apnea associated with antipsychotic-induced obesity. J Clin Psychiatry 63:369–370, 2002c

Wirshing W, Ames D, Bisheff S, et al: Hepatic encephalopathy associated with combined clozapine and divalproex sodium treatment. J Clin Psychopharmacol 17:120–121, 1997

Wolters EC, Berendse HW: Management of psychosis in Parkinson's disease. Curr Opin Neurol 14:499–504, 2001

Wooltorton E: Antipsychotic clozapine (Clozaril): myocarditis and cardiovascular toxicity. CMAJ 166:1185–1186, 2002

Worm K, Kringsholm B, Steentoft A: Clozapine cases with fatal, toxic or therapeutic concentrations. Int J Legal Med 106:115–118, 1993

Yazici KM, Erbas T, Yazici AH, et al: The effect of clozapine on glucose metabolism. Exp Clin Endocrinol Diabetes 106:475–477, 1998

CHAPTER 29

Olanzapine

Jacob S. Ballon, M.D.

Donna A. Wirshing, M.D.

S. Charles Schulz, M.D.

History and Discovery

The story of specific antipsychotic medications for patients with schizophrenia and other severe psychiatric illnesses began in the early 1950s, when chlorpromazine was first given to psychotic patients in France (Delay and Bernitzer 1952). The antipsychotic qualities of this compound, as well as its "tranquilizing" effect, were dramatic and substantial. Studies performed around the world during the 1950s showed the usefulness of this new compound and the others that followed. As is well known, multicenter trials of antipsychotic medications found that the approved medications were substantially and significantly better than placebo (Cole et al. 1964). Furthermore, despite the range of chemical structures, the clinical effects were similar. In addition, the need to investigate the new medications for psychiatric illness led to improved clinical trial methodology for the field. During the 1960s, randomized and placebo-controlled trials became the standard for assessing the new medications for schizophrenia. These trials led to the neuroleptic medications becoming the standard somatic treatment for schizophrenia.

However, over time, the adverse effects of the neuroleptic medications began to be recognized as more troublesome (Table 29–1). For example, most patients complained of iatrogenic parkinsonism, dystonias, slowed thinking, blunted affect, akathisia, and tardive dyskinesia. These side effects were uncomfortable for patients

taking the neuroleptic medications and, in many cases, led to poor adherence with treatment.

In addition to the adverse effects of the neuroleptic medications, continued research of the neuroleptics indicated that a substantial number of patients were not fully treated (Angrist and Schulz 1990). Therefore, the field had the problem of an intervention that was not useful for all patients and was uncomfortable to take for many patients whose symptoms did respond.

Studies with the first atypical antipsychotic medication, clozapine, began in the late 1960s, although the compound was initially discovered in 1961. This interesting agent led to decreases in symptoms of psychosis without causing movement disorder side effects. Trials were moving forward in Europe (Povlsen et al. 1985) and the United States (Shopsin et al. 1979) when reports of agranulocytosis resulting in the death of some subjects first appeared (Amster et al. 1977). These unfortunate outcomes stopped research of clozapine essentially in its tracks. However, the hope for the development of an atypical antipsychotic medication did not die with these early studies of clozapine. Eventually, clozapine was approved as a treatment of last resort for schizophrenia, and its use must be accompanied by rigorous medical follow-up (Kane et al. 1988).

Concurrent with this research, investigators at Eli Lilly were screening numerous compounds for psychotropic properties. In 1990, the company applied for and received a patent for the compound olanzapine. It is interesting to

TABLE 29–1.   Shortcomings of traditional antipsychotic medications

Significant response in only 60%–70% of patients
Movement disorder side effects
Dystonia
Parkinsonism
Tardive dyskinesia
Akathisia
Slowed thinking ("cognitive parkinsonism")
Secondary negative symptoms

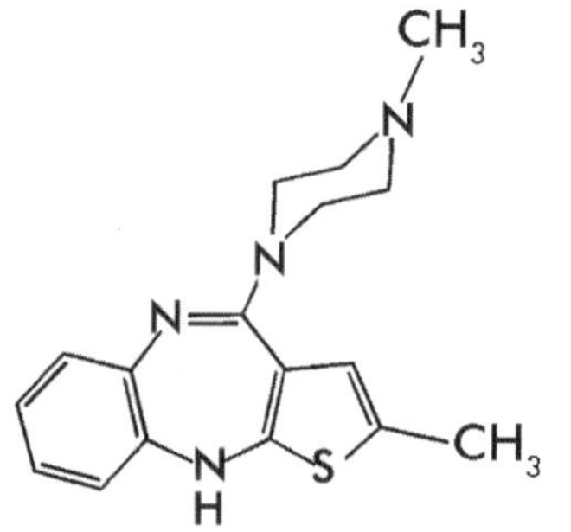

FIGURE 29–1.   Chemical structure of olanzapine.

note that the new compound had many structural similarities to clozapine and was thought to have potential for schizophrenia, mania, and anxiety.

Olanzapine was first given to patients with schizophrenia in 1995 (Baldwin and Montgomery 1995). The patients in the study had a substantial decrease in their symptoms while receiving 5–30 mg/day of the compound. The authors noted a low degree of extrapyramidal side effects (EPS), although concern was raised for elevation of liver enzymes, as one patient had to discontinue the study for that reason.

The initial testing of olanzapine had useful results and led to a program of four pivotal trials of olanzapine. These first four controlled studies examined the differences between olanzapine (10 mg/day fixed dose) and placebo (Beasley et al. 1996a), olanzapine and haloperidol or placebo (Beasley et al. 1996b), olanzapine (low, medium, or high dose) and olanzapine 1.0 mg/day or haloperidol 15 mg/day (Beasley et al. 1997), and olanzapine and haloperidol in a large international study (Tollefson et al. 1997). The positive results for olanzapine led to U.S. Food and Drug Administration (FDA) approval in 1997 and then widespread use in the United States and around the world.

Structure–Activity Relations

Olanzapine is a thiobenzodiazepine derivative (Figure 29–1) that bears a close structural resemblance to clozapine. The formal chemical name of olanzapine is 2-methyl-4-(4-methyl-1-piperazinyl)-10H-thieno[2,3-b] [1,5]benzodiazepine. Structurally, it differs from clozapine by two additional methyl groups and the lack of a chloride moiety. This similarity leads to a relative similarity in the in vitro receptor binding profiles. According to the package insert, olanzapine is known to have a high affinity for selective dopaminergic, serotonergic (5-HT), histaminer-gic (H), and α-adrenergic receptors, with weaker affinity for muscarinic (M) receptors and weak activity at benzodiazepine (BZD), γ-aminobutyric acid type A (GABA$_A$), and β-adrenergic receptors (Eli Lilly 2006).

Pharmacological Profile

In vitro and preclinical behavioral studies of olanzapine predicted significant antipsychotic activity with a low propensity to induce EPS. Because clozapine is the prototype for second-generation antipsychotic action, similarity to its effects relative to those of classic antipsychotics is evidence for the "atypicality" of comparator compounds such as olanzapine.

One possible mechanism for lowering risk for EPS is nonselective dopamine receptor binding. Classic antipsychotics selectively block D$_2$-like (D$_2$, D$_3$, and D$_4$) receptors over D$_1$-like (D$_1$ and D$_5$) receptors—for example, haloperidol has a D$_2$-to-D$_1$ binding ratio of 25:1. Clozapine nonselectively binds all five dopamine receptor subtypes, with a D$_2$-to-D$_1$ ratio of 0.7:1, whereas olanzapine is only partially selective for the D$_2$-like group, with a D$_2$-to-D$_1$ ratio of approximately 3:1, intermediate between those of haloperidol and clozapine.

Antipsychotics have traditionally been most effective in treating the positive symptoms of schizophrenia, including delusions, hallucinations, and the agitation brought on by these symptoms. The hallmark of second-generation or atypical antipsychotics is a decreased propensity to cause EPS. "Atypicality" has generally been used to refer to agents with reduced risk of EPS. Olanzapine has a low tendency to induce catalepsy, once regarded as a marker of antipsychotic efficacy but now seen as an indicator of a drug's likelihood of producing EPS (Fu et al. 2000).

In animal models predictive of antipsychotic efficacy, olanzapine produces effects indicating dopamine antagonism, with a low propensity to produce EPS. For example, in rats, olanzapine reduces climbing behavior induced by apomorphine and antagonizes stimulant-induced hyperactivity, both characteristic of antipsychotic effect. The ratio of the dose needed to produce catalepsy to the dose needed to inhibit conditioned avoidance, another model for atypical efficacy, is higher for olanzapine than for conventional agents, a circumstance that also denotes "atypicality" (Moore 1999).

Another potential mechanism whereby dopamine antagonists may exert antipsychotic effects with minimal EPS is through selective activity in the A10 dopaminergic tracts from the ventral tegmentum to mesolimbic areas compared with effects antagonizing the A9 nigrostriatal projections that mediate EPS. Olanzapine in chronic administration, like clozapine, selectively inhibits firing of A10 neurons without significant inhibition of A9 tracts (Stockton and Rasmussen 1996a). The nigrostriatal tract has often been implicated in EPS, whereas the limbic system has been associated with the positive symptoms of schizophrenia. Olanzapine shows increased c-fos activity in the nucleus accumbens relative to the dorsolateral striatum, thus demonstrating selective blockade of the mesolimbic dopamine tract compared with the nigrostriatal tract (Robertson and Fibiger 1996).

The current leading theory regarding atypicality relates to the fleeting effects of atypical antipsychotics at the D_2 receptor, coupled with regional selectivity of these compounds (Seeman 2002). The $5\text{-}HT_{2A}$ receptor in the nigrostriatal tract was once theorized to provide increased dopaminergic activity in that tract, thus sparing one from the parkinsonism frequently seen with conventional antipsychotics. However, this theory of atypicality is generally falling out of favor. Whereas olanzapine shows higher affinity for $5\text{-}HT_{2A}$ receptors than for D_2 receptors, the tight binding of serotonergic neurons does not show any influence on dopamine receptor blockade, and olanzapine still has a dopamine receptor saturation that is sufficient to produce antipsychotic activity and, at high enough doses, also strong enough to cause EPS (Kapur et al. 1998, 1999). Olanzapine has been shown to have a D_2 receptor occupancy saturation that is between that of clozapine and haloperidol and may be responsible for a decreased risk of EPS (Tauscher et al. 1999). However, as the current second-generation antipsychotic medications have substantially differing effects at all of these targets thought to play a role in atypicality, consensus is not there regarding the true rationale for atypicality compared to the first-generation antipsychotics (Farah 2005).

Amphetamine administration in rats is often used as a model for psychosis. The sympathomimetic activity and dopamine release provide a target for testing antipsychotic medications. Olanzapine disrupts the activity of amphetamines in rats (Gosselin et al. 1996). Olanzapine was shown in a rat model to decrease dopamine release in the A10 dopaminergic neurons of the ventral tegmentum greater than the A9 dopaminergic neurons of the striatum after chronic administration and after an amphetamine challenge (Stockton and Rasmussen 1996a, 1996b). Olanzapine does not induce catalepsy in rats at doses needed for antipsychotic efficacy.

Another model of psychosis in rats is the administration of the glutamatergic N-methyl-D-aspartic acid (NMDA) receptor antagonist phencyclidine (PCP). Chronic PCP use in humans is associated with similar symptoms to schizophrenia, including negative symptoms, thus making it a putative model for schizophrenia (Krystal et al. 1994). Second-generation antipsychotics have been shown to enhance glutamatergic neurotransmission in pyramidal cells of the prefrontal cortex compared with first-generation antipsychotics (Ninan et al. 2003a). Olanzapine has been shown to decrease the hyperactivity of NMDA receptors under chronic PCP administration, which may have a bearing on the effect on negative symptoms (Ninan et al. 2003b). With chronic administration, glutamatergic activity continues to be affected by olanzapine (Jardemark et al. 2000). Despite these findings, olanzapine has no direct affinity for the NMDA receptor (Stephenson and Pilowsky 1999).

Effects on other systems show that olanzapine has a broad range of neurotransmitter effects. Although olanzapine has potent muscarinic M_{1-5} receptor affinity in vitro (another contributor to putative anti-EPS effects), in practice few patients have anticholinergic side effects that are clinically significant. α_1-Adrenergic and H_1 histaminergic antagonism contribute to the adverse-effect profile of orthostatic hypotension (α_1), sedation (H_1), and possibly weight gain (H_1). Olanzapine has little or no effect on α_2- and β-adrenergic, H_2, nicotinic, GABA, opioid, sigma, or benzodiazepine receptors.

Pharmacokinetics and Disposition

Olanzapine is well absorbed after oral administration, with peak concentrations in most people occurring 4–6 hours after ingestion (Kassahun et al. 1997). Approximately 40% of a given dose undergoes first-pass metabolism and therefore does not reach the systemic circulation, and food has little effect on olanzapine's bioavailability (Callaghan et al. 1999; Eli Lilly 2006; Kassahun et al. 1997).

Two bioequivalent oral formulations of olanzapine are currently available: a standard oral tablet and an oral disintegrating tablet. The oral disintegrating tablets are intended for swallowing and absorption through the gut; however, sublingual administration has also been favored by some. Markowitz et al. (2006) discovered that while the oral disintegrating preparation of olanzapine is more quickly absorbed than a standard oral tablet, it is absorbed at an equal rate if taken sublingually or if swallowed conventionally. In either case, the onset of action with the oral dissolving tablet is faster than with the standard oral tablet. After a 12.5-mg oral dose of ^{14}C-labeled olanzapine, approximately 57% of the radiocarbon was recovered in urine and 30% in feces. In vitro studies suggest that olanzapine is approximately 93% protein bound, binding primarily to albumin and α_1-acid glycoprotein (Kassahun et al. 1997).

Olanzapine is also available as an intramuscular preparation, intended for treatment of the acute agitation typically seen in schizophrenia or acute manic episodes of bipolar disorder. The peak plasma concentration is typically reached between 15 and 45 minutes after administration. The potency of intramuscular olanzapine is nearly five times greater than that of orally administered drug, based on plasma levels. Clinical antipsychotic onset with intramuscular olanzapine is evident within 2 hours of administration, with benefits lasting for at least 24 hours (Kapur et al. 2005).

Olanzapine is currently being tested in a long-acting injectable preparation composed of a dihydrate form of olanzapine pamoate. As a dihydrate molecule, it is less soluble in water than a monohydrate and thus has the longer half-life required for a depot formulation. This formulation is currently being evaluated in studies with a dosage schedule of once every 4 weeks (Mamo et al. 2008).

Finally, olanzapine is available in a combined preparation with fluoxetine. The olanzapine–fluoxetine combination (OFC) tablet provides fixed doses of olanzapine and fluoxetine to enhance adherence to a regimen that includes both an antipsychotic agent and an antidepressant. Overall, there are few pharmacokinetic differences from adding fluoxetine to olanzapine, and those present are generally related to cytochrome P450 (CYP) 2D6 inhibition. There is no change in the overall half-life of olanzapine. While there are minor yet statistically significant differences in the concentration of olanzapine when taken in combination with fluoxetine, these changes are not clinically significant and do not change the side-effect profile of olanzapine (Gossen et al. 2002).

Olanzapine is extensively metabolized to multiple metabolites but primarily to 10-N-glucuronide and 4'-N-desmethylolanzapine (Macias et al. 1998). After long-term administration, average plasma concentrations for these metabolites are 44% and 30% of olanzapine concentrations, respectively (Callaghan et al. 1999). Other metabolites include 4'-N-oxide olanzapine and 2-hydroxymethyl olanzapine (Kassahun et al. 1997). In vitro studies assessing the oxidative metabolism of olanzapine suggest that CYP1A2 is the enzyme primarily responsible for the formation of 4'-N-desmethylolanzapine, flavin-containing monooxygenase-3 (FMO3) is responsible for the formation of 4'-N-oxide olanzapine, and CYP2D6 is the primary enzyme responsible for the formation of 2-hydroxymethyl olanzapine (Ring et al. 1996b). Although CYP1A2 appears to be a major route of metabolism, olanzapine clearance in one study was not significantly correlated with salivary paraxanthine-to-caffeine ratio (thought to be a measure of CYP1A2 activity) (Hagg et al. 2001). Another analysis, however, found that the 4'-N-desmethylolanzapine–to–olanzapine plasma metabolic ratio significantly correlated with olanzapine clearance (Callaghan et al. 1999). Olanzapine pharmacokinetic parameters do not differ significantly between extensive and poor metabolizers of CYP2D6 (see Hagg et al. 2001).

Olanzapine shows linear pharmacokinetics within the recommended dosage range (Aravagiri et al. 1997; Bergstrom et al. 1995; Callaghan et al. 1999). Peak mean olanzapine concentrations after 8 days of olanzapine at 7.5 mg/day in 12 healthy males (11 smokers) were 18.3 ng/mL. Mean half-life was 36 hours, mean clearance was 29.4 L/hour, mean volume of distribution was 19.2 L/kg, and area under the concentration-time curve over 24 hours (AUC_{0-24}) was 333 ng*hour/mL. The half-lives of the two major metabolites (4'-N-desmethylolanzapine and 10-N-glucuronide) were 92.6 and 39.6 hours, respectively, and their AUC_{0-24} were 57 ng*hour/mL and 112 ng*hour/mL (Macias et al. 1998). Other analyses also have found the mean half-life of olanzapine to be approximately 30 hours and the mean apparent clearance to be approximately 25 L/hour (Callaghan et al. 1999; Eli Lilly 2006; Kassahun et al. 1997). Once-daily administration of olanzapine produces steady-state concentrations in about a week that are approximately twofold higher than concentrations after single doses (Callaghan et al. 1999). An in vitro study suggested that olanzapine may be an intermediate substrate of P-glycoprotein (Boulton et al. 2002). In a recent study, Mitchell et al. (2006) compared the pharmacokinetics of a 10- to 20-mg olanzapine dosage with that of a 30- to 40-mg dosage. Both dosages showed similar pharmacokinetic profiles and general tolerability, although akathisia was noted to be slightly higher in the high-dose group.

The clearance of olanzapine is generally decreased in women. Clearance of olanzapine is approximately 25%–30% lower in women than in men, based on results of population pharmacokinetic analyses (Callaghan et al. 1999; Patel et al. 1995, 1996). A study of 20 male and 7 female patients with schizophrenia receiving olanzapine also found that women had higher trough concentrations (29 ng/mL vs. 19 ng/mL) after receiving 1 week of olanzapine 12.5 mg/day; they continued to have higher plasma concentrations than men after the dosage was increased to 25 mg/day, with average week 8 plasma concentrations of 65 ng/mL and 35 ng/mL in women and men, respectively (Kelly et al. 1999). Despite the differences in clearance and plasma levels, there is no difference between sexes in incidence of EPS or other movement disorders (Aichhorn et al. 2006).

Olanzapine's pharmacokinetics in the elderly and in children have been noted to differ from that in adults. In the elderly, olanzapine clearance is approximately 30% lower than in younger individuals, and the half-life is approximately 50% longer (Callaghan et al. 1999; Patel et al. 1995). A study of eight children and adolescents (ages 10–18 years) found pharmacokinetic parameters similar to those reported in nonsmoking adults, with an average T_{max} (time required to reach the maximal plasma concentration) of 4.7 hours, an average apparent oral clearance of 9.6 L/hour, and an average half-life of 37.2 hours (Grothe et al. 2000). In this study, patients could receive olanzapine dosages of up to 20 mg/day. The highest concentrations were seen when smaller-sized patients received dosages greater than 10 mg/day; therefore, dosing should take into consideration the size of the child.

Impairment in either hepatic or renal function has not been associated with altered olanzapine disposition. In a study of four healthy individuals and eight patients with hepatic cirrhosis, no significant differences in olanzapine pharmacokinetics were found, although urinary concentrations of olanzapine 10-N-glucuronide were increased in patients with cirrhosis (Callaghan et al. 1999). A study comparing olanzapine pharmacokinetics in six subjects with normal renal function, six subjects with renal failure who received an olanzapine dose 1 hour before hemodialysis, and six subjects with renal failure who received an olanzapine dose during their 48-hour interdialytic interval did not find any significant differences. In subjects receiving olanzapine 1 hour before hemodialysis, olanzapine was not detected in the dialysis fluid, suggest-ing that hemodialysis does not remove significant quantities of olanzapine. These data suggest that olanzapine dosage does not need to be adjusted in patients with renal or hepatic disease (Callaghan et al. 1999).

Mechanism of Action

In discussing the mechanism of action for olanzapine in the treatment of schizophrenia, it should be noted that there is no established molecular mechanism to unify the symptoms of schizophrenia. No precise animal or in vitro model for the illness exists, nor is there a consensus on the precise etiology or pathophysiology. Numerous neurochemical hypotheses exist, including abnormalities in dopaminergic, glutamatergic, serotonergic, and other systems such as neurotensin (Boules et al. 2007) and neuregulin (Benzel et al. 2007). Furthermore, other theories about the etiology and pathophysiology of schizophrenia include the possibility of abnormal development of the brain resulting in postulated changes in the relation of one part of the brain to the other (e.g., the prefrontal cortex to limbic areas) (Weinberger 1987). Further complicating these theories of pathophysiology of schizophrenia has been the understanding of the multiple different types of receptors for the same neurotransmitters that exist in the brain. Therefore, it is no longer possible to simply discuss hypotheses such as increased dopamine as a comprehensive theory for the etiology of schizophrenia.

Despite the caveats noted above regarding the rudimentary knowledge of the nature of schizophrenia, it is important to note that all approved antipsychotic medications have an important effect on the dopaminergic system, largely through the blockade of D_2 receptors (Kapur and Remington 2001). Even though there are substantial differences in affinities to the D_2 receptor among the traditional antipsychotic medications and the atypical antipsychotics, they all are full antagonists or are partial agonists at the D_2 receptor. Of interest is the evolving research indicating the importance for blockade of other receptors by the atypical antipsychotic medication class. As these systems have been investigated in the neuropsychopharmacology of schizophrenia, evidence is emerging that the action of second-generation antipsychotics, and olanzapine specifically, may improve different parts of the schizophrenia syndrome through effects on 5-HT receptors, by multiple-receptor binding, by region-specific and more fleeting binding to dopamine receptors, by effects on glutamate neurotransmission, and perhaps by influence on neuroprotein neurotransmitters. Each of these specific ideas for the mechanism of action of olanzapine is discussed in order.

As has been noted in the section on history of the development of olanzapine, innovations in the production of antipsychotic medications that cause fewer movement side effects have been a major advance clinically. One of the first theories about the mechanism of atypicality was the 5-HT–dopamine antagonist hypothesis (Meltzer et al. 1989). By comparing the ratio of 5-HT_{2A} to dopamine receptor blockade, these groups showed that the agents with greater relative 5-HT receptor blockade were in the atypical group, whereas those with greater relative dopamine receptor blockade were more likely to be in the typical group. Both in vitro and in vivo studies have clearly reported that olanzapine has a substantially greater ability to block 5-HT_{2A} receptors than dopamine receptors (Kapur et al. 1998).

For several years, psychopharmacological research on schizophrenia focused on finding drugs that block specific receptors. In the area of schizophrenia, medications such as pimozide, which has very few nondopaminergic properties, were thought to focus on the specific etiology and pathophysiology of schizophrenia. Therefore, it was somewhat surprising that the first atypical antipsychotic medicine, clozapine, was a multiple-receptor blocker. As noted earlier in this chapter, olanzapine has many similarities to clozapine in its chemical structure as well as its receptor-blocking profile. Therefore, investigators have indicated that perhaps the multiple receptor–blocking properties of olanzapine are significant in its atypical antipsychotic effects. Blockade of dopamine receptors, 5-HT receptors, and histamine receptors, and perhaps other neurochemical properties as well, may be the result of the multiple receptor–blocking capabilities of the compound (Bymaster et al. 1999).

In clinical investigations with positron emission tomography (PET) imaging, Kapur et al. (1998) showed that olanzapine at a wide range of doses blocks a high percentage (95% or greater) of 5-HT_{2A} receptors and blocks dopamine receptors in a dose-dependent fashion—crossing the putative antipsychotic blockade line at doses commonly used to diminish psychotic symptoms of schizophrenia. This study indicated that olanzapine's primary mechanism was related to the blockade of dopamine receptors, and additionally noted that olanzapine showed stronger affinity for 5-HT_{2A} receptors than for dopamine receptors at all dosage ranges.

In addition to considering individual neurotransmitters, it has been noted that each neurotransmitter has multiple types of receptors. For dopamine, there are cur-

rently five different receptors that are grouped into two families (D_1 and D_5 vs. D_2, D_3, and D_4). Work by Casey (1993) with nonhuman primates found that there may be regionally specific characteristics of the atypical antipsychotic medications compared with the typical compounds. These regionally specific characteristics of receptors and the observation that antipsychotic medications such as olanzapine have regionally specific activity may explain the ability of atypical compounds to decrease psychotic symptoms without causing movement disorders (Stockton and Rasmussen 1996a). Such regional selectivity is supported by molecular biology studies, such as those by Robertson and Fibiger (1996), which have reported increases of c-fos expression, which is regionally specific for the caudate area of the brain.

A more compelling hypothesis regarding the atypicality of olanzapine has emerged from the in vivo PET scanning work being performed in a series of experiments at the University of Toronto and in Sweden. Results of the initial PET scanning studies of patients receiving clozapine indicated that there was atypical dopamine receptor binding (Farde and Nordstrom 1992; Farde et al. 1992; Kapur et al. 2000). The group subsequently found similar results for quetiapine and, to some degree, olanzapine (Kapur et al. 1998). The authors indicated that the successful reduction of psychotic symptoms in schizophrenic patients without movement disorder side effects may be the result of a "fast off" property of some of the atypical antipsychotic medications. They argued that for medicines that block the dopamine receptor but leave that receptor quickly, there may be an effect at the receptor to decrease psychosis but that a "physiological" dopamine activity at the receptor remains. Thus, for olanzapine, as likely also with clozapine and quetiapine, this may contribute to the treatment of schizophrenia while causing fewer EPS at standard doses. From a clinical view, it is important to note that at higher dosages of olanzapine (30 mg/day), higher dopamine receptor blockade is seen, and movement disorder side effects, such as akathisia, are more likely to occur.

In recent years, there has been substantial interest in the role of glutamate, an excitatory neurotransmitter, in the pathophysiology of schizophrenia (see, e.g., Javitt and Zukin 1991; Krystal et al. 1994; Lahti et al. 1995). This theory is supported by the psychotomimetic properties of glutamate antagonists such as phencyclidine and ketamine. These NMDA receptor antagonists lead to a group of behaviors that often have closer parallels to schizophrenia than do those of the dopamine sympathomimetic agents, in both mice and humans. Clinical trial evidence points to the usefulness of glutamatergic agonists (e.g., D-cycloserine) in treating schizophrenia (Goff et al. 1995). People with schizophrenia have been shown to have decreased glutamine synthetase and glutamate dehydrogenase in the prefrontal cortex, thus impacting the glutamate-to-glutamine conversion (Burbaeva et al. 2003). A current strategy under investigation involves administration of compounds such as D-cycloserine to patients. When glutamatergic agents have been given to patients with schizophrenia, there has generally been a measurable improvement in cognition and a decrease in negative symptoms, unless clozapine (a glutamatergic partial agonist) is present (Evins et al. 2000). However, no measurable decrease in the positive symptoms of the illness has occurred. Thus far, glutamatergic agonists have shown mixed results, although further research on the NMDA receptor, as well as on glycine transport antagonists, is in progress (Javitt 2006). Recent studies have also shown that LY2140023, a metabotropic glutamate receptor agonist, may be effective in treating schizophrenia. In a Phase II trial comparing LY2140023 with olanzapine and placebo, LY2140023 produced improvement in positive and negative symptoms, as measured by the Positive and Negative Syndrome Scale (PANSS), and had rates of EPS and weight gain similar to those of placebo (Patil et al. 2007).

One way of examining the possible effect of olanzapine on glutamatergic measures was addressed in a study of rats with isolation-induced disruption of prepulse inhibition. Prepulse inhibition, a measure of sensory motor gating, is believed to be abnormal in patients with schizophrenia. In a study by Bakshi et al. (1998), both quetiapine and olanzapine reversed the isolation-induced prepulse inhibition deficit. Because there is a connection between NMDA antagonists and prepulse inhibition, this finding is evidence of olanzapine's effect on the glutamatergic system. Glutamine synthetase–like proteins (GSLP) and glutamate dehydrogenase have also been seen to be significantly higher in schizophrenia patients. Burbaeva et al. (2006) have shown that patients with a higher amount of GSLP in the platelets tend to respond more quickly to medication and specifically that olanzapine treatment alters the amounts of these peptides, further enhancing its antipsychotic properties.

Utilizing magnetic resonance spectroscopy (MRS), Goff et al. (2002) have shown a more direct measure of olanzapine on patients' glutamate levels. They found that after a switch from conventional antipsychotic medications to olanzapine, serum glutamate levels increased appreciably. Brain glutamate levels, however, did not increase. Further examination indicated that in the patients whose negative symptoms improved, brain glutamate concentrations increased.

The neuropeptide neurotensin also has been explored for its role in the pathophysiology of schizophrenia (Nemeroff et al. 1983), with several findings supporting an association of neurotensin with the symptoms of schizophrenia. Such findings include the close anatomical association between neurotensin and other neurotransmitter systems that have been implicated in schizophrenia, changes in neurotensin brain levels in animals when antipsychotic medications have been administered, and similarities between the effects of centrally administered neurotensin and the effects of antipsychotic medications. The effect of olanzapine and other antipsychotics on the neurotensin system has been investigated by using molecular biology techniques. After assessing neurotensin messenger RNA (mRNA) in the rat brain, the investigators reported increases in neurotensin mRNA when olanzapine was administered. The pattern of neurotensin changes seen with olanzapine was different from the pattern seen with haloperidol. These results are more similar to the results seen with the antipsychotic medication clozapine and show the effect of olanzapine on another system with importance in schizophrenia (Binder et al. 2001; Radke et al. 1998).

In summary, regarding the mechanism of action of olanzapine, a second-generation antipsychotic with well-demonstrated efficacy for psychosis in patients with schizophrenia, research indicates an effect on dopamine, acetylcholine, histamine, 5-HT (with greater affinity for 5-HT receptors than for dopamine receptors). glutamate, and neurotensin. Other effects are in the process of being evaluated. These effects have been measured by both biochemical assay and MRS and have been demonstrated in both human and animal models of the illness. At this time, dopamine receptor–blocking capabilities appear to be a necessary but not sufficient characteristic of an antipsychotic medication. The other studied mechanisms, when taken in total, may be the factors leading to olanzapine's broad efficacy and side-effect profile.

Indications and Efficacy

To be prescribed in the United States, a medication must be approved by the FDA for a specific indication. This initial approval is based on an assessment of efficacy and safety requiring multiple tests of a medication compared with placebo and at least two studies demonstrating efficacy compared with placebo. In the case of olanzapine, its original indication was for psychosis. Currently, it has multiple indications, including schizophrenia, acute mania or mixed states in bipolar disorder, and as monotherapy or combination therapy in the maintenance treatment of bipolar disorder. The olanzapine–fluoxetine combination (OFC) has an FDA indication for bipolar depression. Intramuscular olanzapine carries an indication for acute agitation in schizophrenia and bipolar mania. Once a medication has received an FDA indication, physicians are able to use that medication off label for other theorized indications. Olanzapine has been studied, and at times used with limited evidence, in several other illnesses. In this section, we present the evidence base that supports the use of olanzapine for its FDA-indicated usages as well as for other off-label usages.

Schizophrenia

As noted earlier, olanzapine was originally developed as a medication with potential for treating schizophrenia, mania, and anxiety. During the 1990s, significant energy was focused on the development of antipsychotic medications with new actions such that patients could have a reduction of psychosis with fewer side effects, especially neurological side effects. To gain FDA approval for the treatment of schizophrenia, olanzapine was tested in four pivotal studies to assess the compound for efficacy, safety, and dose ranging. The earliest testing of olanzapine was an assessment of olanzapine in doses of 5–30 mg following an initial starting dose of 10 mg. Brief Psychiatric Rating Scale (BPRS) scores were reduced substantially for the participants in the study, and EPS were low (Baldwin and Montgomery 1995). These encouraging results led to further studies and pointed to a dose range to be tested.

Efficacy Studies

The first pivotal study examined a dose of 10 mg of olanzapine. The study showed that 10 mg of olanzapine was statistically significantly superior to placebo on objective rating scales (Beasley et al. 1996a). The next step was a dose-ranging study of olanzapine compared with haloperidol and placebo. The dosage ranges were 1) low (5 ± 2.5 mg/day), 2) medium (10 ± 2.5 mg/day), and 3) high (15 ± 2.5 mg/day). Haloperidol was dosed to 15 ± 2.5 mg/day. The medium and high doses of olanzapine and haloperidol led to significant improvements compared with placebo (Beasley et al. 1996b). Tollefson and Sanger (1997), after analysis of these early data, pointed out that the effect on negative symptoms by olanzapine was independent of movement disorders.

Another large international multicenter trial used a flexible dosing strategy to show a statistical superiority of olanzapine over haloperidol. In this study, patients were started on olanzapine or haloperidol at dosages ranging from 5 to 20 mg/day. Ultimately, patients received olanzapine 13 mg/day compared with haloperidol 11.8 mg/day (Tollefson et al. 1997).

The third pivotal study included an interesting arm—olanzapine 1 mg/day—in comparison to low-, medium-, and high-dose olanzapine and haloperidol (15 ± 5 mg/day). This study established the statistical efficacy of low- and high-dose olanzapine compared with 1 mg/day of olanzapine (Beasley et al. 1997).

The group of studies described above led to the approval of olanzapine for psychosis (later changed to schizophrenia). Several other studies have reinforced olanzapine's efficacy for the treatment of schizophrenia. Coupled with its efficacy and substantially fewer movement disorder side effects, olanzapine has become an important addition to the armamentarium of the psychiatrist treating schizophrenia. Leucht et al. (1999) reported that olanzapine was statistically more effective than placebo (moderate effect) and also more effective than haloperidol (small effect) on global schizophrenia symptomatology.

Olanzapine has shown superiority to haloperidol in several comparison studies. In a double-blind, placebo-controlled trial, it was shown to be modestly superior to haloperidol in improving cognitive functioning (Purdon et al. 2000). Its superiority was again demonstrated in a study of patients with prominent negative symptoms. Followed for 1 year, the olanzapine group and the risperidone group performed modestly better than the haloperidol group (Gurpegui et al. 2007). In a randomized, controlled trial versus haloperidol, 31.3% of olanzapine-treated patients showed an improvement in cognitive symptoms at study endpoint, compared with 12.5% for the haloperidol group (Lindenmayer et al. 2007). Despite these findings, other studies have shown no difference between olanzapine and haloperidol in effects on cognitive symptoms in schizophrenia patients with treatment-resistant illness (Buchanan et al. 2005).

A large National Institute of Mental Health (NIMH)–funded trial was recently completed that sought to compare the atypical antipsychotics olanzapine, risperidone, quetiapine, and ziprasidone with perphenazine in order to understand the efficacy and side-effect profiles of the newer versus older antipsychotic medications (Lieberman et al. 2005). The study, Clinical Antipsychotic Trials of Intervention Effectiveness (CATIE), was designed to provide a double-blind yet reasonably naturalistic way for clinicians to treat patients, using the time to discontinuation as a primary outcome variable. This outcome was intended to provide an estimate of overall efficacy and morbidity on a particular medication, as it was considered likely that patients would discontinue the medication if it was not working for any particular reason. Although the study design and its findings have at times been controversial, olanzapine demonstrated the longest time to discontinuation in the trial, based on all-cause discontinuation. Olanzapine had the highest rate of discontinuation due to metabolic complications such as weight gain, while perphenazine had the highest rate of discontinuation for EPS. Overall, however, the discontinuation rate was high for all medications, with nearly 75% of patients changing medications within the 18-month study duration. Much has been written since the initial findings were published, including analyses of cost-effectiveness (Rosenheck et al. 2006), psychosocial functioning (Swartz et al. 2007), and switching of medications (Essock et al. 2006), as well as numerous editorials about the treatment implications from the study and about the methodology of the study design.

The pharmacoeconomics of using olanzapine in the treatment of schizophrenia are complicated. Rosenheck et al. (2003) have demonstrated that in pharmacoeconomic studies, olanzapine and haloperidol differentiate from each other. In these studies, haloperidol is accompanied by prophylactic benztropine to ward off EPS. When the cost-effectiveness of olanzapine and the other atypical antipsychotics was evaluated in the CATIE, perphenazine came out as the most cost-effective of the medications studied (Rosenheck et al. 2006). The general equality of efficacy among the medications, at least with respect to rehospitalization rates, as well as the decreased cost for the older medication, is partially responsible for this difference. Additionally, the metabolic consequences of olanzapine treatment become significant when one considers the overall total cost for the medication within the entire health care system, as the increased rates of diabetes and associated medical conditions can cost thousands of dollars per year in associated medication, hospitalization, medical tests, and lost productivity. However, because the older antipsychotics carry a higher risk of neurological side effects, adherence to medications becomes relevant, and maintenance on medication is crucial to preventing relapse and expensive hospitalizations.

Schizophrenia is not always responsive to traditional antipsychotic medication treatment. Clozapine was shown to be superior to chlorpromazine in treating schizophrenia that is refractory to other medications, and this led to its approval for traditional antipsychotic medication failures (Kane et al. 1988). However, clozapine has a unique and potentially more dangerous side-effect profile, with a rigorous associated treatment regimen, which can make it a difficult medication to use. Assessment of olanzapine for this difficult-to-treat patient group did not indicate usefulness for the treatment-refractory group in a stringent nonresponder protocol (Conley et al. 1998). However, in an Eli Lilly–sponsored double-blind, noninferiority multicenter trial, olanzapine was shown to lower PANSS scores similarly to clozapine, although superiority of one agent over another was not addressed in this study design (Tollefson et al. 2001). A second phase of the CATIE examined the use of clozapine in patients with treatment-refractory illness and found that clozapine was a superior treatment for patients in which failure with other atypical medications had occurred, based on the time to discontinuation (McEvoy et al. 2006).

Olanzapine has often been linked to improvements in the negative symptoms and cognitive symptoms of schizophrenia, although perhaps with less potency than for the positive symptoms. Negative and cognitive symptoms often do not respond to conventional antipsychotics and have even been shown to worsen, particularly if an adjunctive anticholinergic medication is used for treatment of EPS. The efficacy of olanzapine for negative symptoms was first reported by Tollefson et al. (1997), following completion of a large double-blind trial of olanzapine and haloperidol. A factor analytic model was used to determine the effect of olanzapine on negative symptoms, separate from the effect on positive symptoms. When all symptom improvements were taken into consideration, olanzapine-treated subjects had greater improvement in negative symptoms on both the Scale for the Assessment of Negative Symptoms (SANS) and the BPRS negative symptom subscore. In a flexible-dose comparison between risperidone and olanzapine in patients followed for 1 year, olanzapine-treated patients showed significantly greater improvement on SANS scores than did risperidone-treated patients (Alvarez et al. 2006). Interestingly, in a study by researchers from Eli Lilly that followed patients taking either quetiapine or olanzapine for 6 months, the two groups showed similar improvements on the SANS at study completion (Kinon et al. 2006). In a study comparing olanzapine and amisulpride, there was also no difference between the two medications, and only low-dose olanzapine outperformed placebo, with higher-dose olanzapine (20 mg) and amisulpride (150 mg) not showing a statistical benefit on the SANS (Lecrubier et al. 2006).

Cognitive functioning is the most important prognostic indicator for schizophrenia (Green 2006). In a 1-year comparison of olanzapine with risperidone, both groups showed modest benefits on a cognitive function battery (Gurpegui et al. 2007). In a study conducted over a 1-year period by Eli Lilly researchers in Spain, olanzapine showed greater benefit on social functioning than did risperidone, as assessed by scores on the Social Functioning Scale (SFS). The greatest difference was in occupation/employment, but improvements were also seen in measures of independence, social engagement, and recreation (Ciudad et al. 2006).

Olanzapine is indicated for the treatment of schizophrenia; however, studies leading to FDA approval are designed to include only patients between the ages of 18 and 65 years. Therefore, usefulness of olanzapine for young people with schizophrenia and patients older than 65 years was not addressed in the early studies. In a recent systematic review of the literature in children, second-generation antipsychotics were shown to be beneficial overall for targeting psychotic symptoms, although there is still a need for research on the long-term safety profile of these agents (Jensen et al. 2007). To inform clinicians about the use of olanzapine in adolescents with schizophrenia, Findling et al. (2003) performed an open-label study of olanzapine using outcome measures from the PANSS and Clinical Global Impressions (CGI) Scale. In the 16 adolescent patients studied, there was a statistically significant reduction in PANSS-rated symptoms, and further exploration of the PANSS subscales found an effect on positive, negative, and general symptoms. The patients ended the study receiving an average olanzapine dosage of 12.4 mg/day, which was similar to the dosage used in many adult schizophrenic patients. A double-blind, flexible-dose study conducted in North Carolina demonstrated similar efficacy for risperidone, olanzapine, and haloperidol in psychotic young people (Sikich et al. 2004). In an NIMH-sponsored trial of adolescents with treatment-refractory schizophrenia, clozapine and olanzapine were compared. While clozapine showed a modestly more consistent pattern of symptom alleviation, particularly for negative symptoms, more side effects were noted in the clozapine group (Shaw et al. 2006).

The use of olanzapine in a population considered to be at risk for schizophrenia but not yet meeting full symptom criteria was evaluated in a double-blind multicenter study. The olanzapine group demonstrated a decreased rate of conversion to psychosis compared with the placebo group, although the difference did not quite reach statistical significance. However, a number of factors, including high dropout rates in both groups, lack of a systematic method for diagnosing Axis I disorders, and the method of patient selection, limited the generalizability and reliability of the findings (McGlashan et al. 2006). The number needed to treat, a measure of effect size, was 4.5 in this study; thus, early medication treatment may benefit some patients. Nonetheless, given the long-term side-effect consequences of antipsychotics, much further refinement, including greater precision in identifying appropriate candidates for treatment, is required before presyndromal medication therapy can be considered to be evidence based.

At the other end of the age spectrum, olanzapine has been tested in the treatment of several syndromes in the elderly. Further discussion of the use of olanzapine in dementia will follow in a separate subsection. Special challenges are involved in treating any disorder in elderly individuals, and schizophrenia or other psychosis is no exception. An early presentation of data reported a comparison of olanzapine with haloperidol in elderly psychotic patients. This report noted a decrease in symptoms for the olanzapine-treated patients, but the reduction was not statistically greater than in the haloperidol-treated patients. Notably, more movement disorder side effects were seen in the haloperidol group (Reams et al. 1998). The movement disorder results are important for the elderly, because they are at high risk for tardive dyskinesia. A more recent study of a group of older patients with chronic schizophrenia actually showed a statistical advantage for olanzapine (Barak et al. 2002). For a broad group of psychotic patients, Hwang et al. (2003) reported reduction in BPRS symptoms in 94 acutely ill patients, some with organic psychosis, thus illustrating the usefulness of olanzapine in this older patient group. As in any treatment with the elderly, special care must be taken for cardiovascular complications. With olanzapine, orthostatic hypotension, oversedation, and thus the risk of falls must be factored into the dosing decision (Gareri et al. 2006).

Treatment Approaches

Early studies of olanzapine assessed dosages ranging from 5 to 30 mg/day. When olanzapine was initially released, it was recommended that it be started at a dosage of 10 mg/day—frequently as a bedtime dose. Subsequently, clinicians have used average dosages higher than 10 mg/day (e.g., approximately 13 mg/day). In the CATIE, the average daily dose in the flexible-dose segment (available doses were 7.5, 15.0, 22.5, and 30.0 mg) was 20.1 mg (Lieberman et al. 2005). For inpatient use, clinicians often will give patients 5 mg of olanzapine in the morning and 10 mg at bedtime (Schulz 1999). Some patients appear to have an inadequate response to olanzapine at the recommended doses, so clinicians have assessed the usefulness of olanzapine at dosages above the recommended 20 mg/day. Many inpatient clinicians employ a loading strategy with olanzapine, particularly in patients presenting with agitation, using up to 40 mg/day for the first 2 days and gradually decreasing the dose to a goal of 20–30 mg/day (Baker et al. 2003; Brooks et al. 2008). While sedation and hypotension must be watched for in any individual patient, increased rates of those side effects were not seen in a study comparing the loading dose strategy with conventional 10-mg/day dosing (Baker et al. 2003).

Typically, agitated patients are best treated with the rapid-dissolving preparation of olanzapine. Given their faster onset of action compared with the conventional pill form and their decreased risk for "cheeking" of the medication, rapid-dissolving tablets are preferable in the acute setting, particularly when some sedation is also needed. When patients are severely agitated, use of injectable olanzapine is often necessary. The intramuscular preparation also has a rapid onset of action, similar to that of dissolvable tablets, and a certainty of delivery that is imperative in an acute emergency. The injectable preparation has been shown to be superior to placebo at doses of 10 mg and as effective as haloperidol, with significantly fewer side effects (Breier et al. 2002). Case reports, however, caution against use of olanzapine in conjunction with intramuscular lorazepam because of hypotension (Zacher and Roche-Desilets 2005).

Empirical studies of a "lowest effective dose" of olanzapine for long-term maintenance have not been performed, so clinical judgment regarding dose is needed at all stages of treatment. For schizophrenia, combinations of medications are sometimes helpful. As can be seen throughout this chapter, olanzapine has been tested in combination with antidepressant and mood-stabilizing compounds in patients with mood disorders. Therefore, these combinations in schizophrenic patients appear safe and appropriate when used judiciously.

Bipolar Disorder and Major Depressive Disorder

In the past, before the introduction of atypical antipsychotic medications, it was well known that traditional antipsychotic medications were useful in the treatment of mania. Medications such as chlorpromazine and haloperidol could rapidly reduce agitation and excitement as well as diminish the psychotic symptoms of mania, when present. Early studies with clozapine indicated that this atypical agent was even useful in reducing symptoms of

bipolar disorder refractory to previous mood stabilizer and traditional antipsychotic medication treatment (Calabrese et al. 1996). An assessment of the effect of olanzapine on symptoms of schizoaffective disorder provided a rationale for studying olanzapine in bipolar patients. The schizoaffective patients were identified as part of a larger study. When the results for the schizoaffective disorder patients were analyzed, those patients who received olanzapine had a superior outcome, compared with patients who received haloperidol, on many, but not all, measures (Tran et al. 1999).

Therefore, a series of studies was conducted to assess the efficacy and safety of olanzapine in the treatment of bipolar disorder. The first controlled study was a comparison of olanzapine with placebo in a 21-day study that used objective rating scales (Tohen et al. 1999). The dosage of olanzapine could be adjusted between 5 and 20 mg/day. An analysis of the Young Mania Rating Scale (YMRS) showed a significant score reduction for patients taking olanzapine compared with those taking placebo. Of interest in treating bipolar patients, no difference was seen in the outcomes for depression; therefore, olanzapine did not lead to depression. It is also well known that bipolar patients are sensitive to the potential of movement disorders from antipsychotic medications. In this study, EPS were not more frequent in the olanzapine-treated patients than in the patients taking placebo (Tohen et al. 1999). These findings were confirmed by a second pivotal study showing an advantage of olanzapine over placebo (Tohen et al. 2000). An open-label follow-up (49 weeks) added valuable information, especially noting that decreases in YMRS scores continued. For the longer term, depression scores also improved. Importantly, for the patients who were exposed to olanzapine at a mean dosage of approximately 14 mg/day, no cases of tardive dyskinesia occurred (Sanger et al. 2001).

An important question of practical interest is how olanzapine compares with conventional mood stabilizers such as lithium or valproic acid. The first study to approach this question, which was a small pilot study ($N = 30$ patients), compared olanzapine with lithium. No difference was found between BPRS and Mania Scale scores; patients in both groups showed significant improvement (Berk et al. 1999).

In a larger double-blind trial conducted by Eli Lilly, olanzapine was compared with lithium in the maintenance treatment of bipolar disorder (mixed or manic) (Tohen et al. 2005). In the study, patients were stabilized on a combination of lithium and olanzapine and then randomly assigned to receive one or the other for

52 weeks. In the noninferiority analysis, olanzapine was shown to prevent depression relapse as well as lithium, and in fact it had a lower rate of mixed or manic relapse over the 52-week follow-up. Weight gain was higher in the olanzapine group (Tohen et al. 2005).

Further studies confirmed the equivalent efficacy of olanzapine and the most widely used anticonvulsant mood stabilizer, divalproex (Tohen et al. 2002). In this 3-week study, olanzapine was found to be superior to placebo in reducing mania ratings (YMRS). More recently, another comparison of the two compounds confirmed no differences in treatment outcome but did note more sedation and weight gain in the olanzapine group (Zajecka et al. 2002). The group of studies focusing on olanzapine's use in treating mania that showed reduction of manic as well as psychotic symptoms led to the approval of olanzapine by the FDA for the treatment of manic symptoms. Mean dosages of olanzapine used in monotherapy appear similar to those used in schizophrenia: 13 mg/day. For acute mania, a recent study has shown the usefulness of intramuscular olanzapine in treating agitated bipolar patients (Meehan et al. 2001).

Olanzapine has also been shown in several studies to be an effective adjunctive agent. In another study conducted by the group at Eli Lilly, olanzapine was found to reduce suicidal ideation in bipolar patients when added to a regimen that included lithium or valproic acid (Houston et al. 2006).

The treatment of bipolar depression is often complicated. Monotherapy with antidepressants is associated with an increased risk of switching into mania. Olanzapine packaged with fluoxetine—the olanzapine–fluoxetine combination (OFC)—has been studied in the treatment of depression in bipolar disorder. In an 8-week double-blind trial conducted by Eli Lilly, OFC was compared against olanzapine monotherapy and placebo in patients with bipolar I disorder in a depressed phase. While both treatments were more effective than placebo, OFC was significantly more effective than either olanzapine or placebo in treating depressive symptoms. OFC-treated patients showed greater improvement in mood compared with olanzapine-treated patients by the fourth week of the study (Tohen et al. 2003). Benefits were also seen in the subjects' health-related quality of life (Shi et al. 2004). OFC was also recently compared with lamotrigine in a 7-week study (Brown et al. 2006). Although OFC demonstrated a statistical separation from lamotrigine by the first week, it is difficult to make a full comparison in such a short study. As lamotrigine requires slow titration to decrease the risk of serious rash, it was received at the target

dose (200 mg/day) only for the last 2 weeks of the study, whereas the OFC dosage could be titrated to therapeutic levels much more quickly. Although the rapid titration of OFC is helpful when a more urgent approach is required, further study is needed to determine whether OFC's greater benefits persist once lamotrigine has had an opportunity to remain at a therapeutic dose for a longer period of time (Brown et al. 2006). Rates of treatment-emergent mania with OFC were low and did not significantly differ from rates with placebo or olanzapine monotherapy (Amsterdam and Shults 2005; Tohen et al. 2003).

Patients with schizophrenia frequently have symptoms of depression, whereas others may appear to be depressed secondary to negative symptoms and the use of typical antipsychotic medications (Siris et al. 2000). This serious problem was addressed by Tollefson et al. (1998a, 1998b), who examined the results of olanzapine pivotal trials in order to assess the effect of olanzapine on symptoms of depression in schizophrenic patients. In the Tollefson et al. (1998b) study, they used a path analysis to control for negative symptoms and EPS. They found a statistically significantly greater effect of olanzapine on depression compared with placebo, and at medium (10±2.5 mg/day) and high dosages, reductions in BPRS Anxiety/Depression scale scores were similar to those seen with haloperidol. For subjects with higher depression scores, olanzapine was statistically superior to haloperidol. These results demonstrate that olanzapine may have a useful effect in this patient group and suggest that further exploration of the potential for olanzapine in treating depressive mood disorders is warranted.

The tricyclic antidepressants, selective serotonin reuptake inhibitors (SSRIs), and serotonin–norepinephrine reuptake inhibitors (SNRIs) are all effective treatments for depression compared with placebo, but not all patients' symptoms respond to these agents. These patients with treatment-refractory illness present a substantial challenge to clinicians and investigators alike. Augmentation strategies, including lithium, liothyronine, and other medications, have been tried with limited success and risks of side effects. OFC has been studied in treatment-refractory major depressive disorder. Thase et al. (2007) conducted a study comparing OFC against olanzapine or fluoxetine monotherapy in patients who had failed to respond to at least two prior trials with antidepressants. In the pooled analysis, which separated the subjects into two groups (group 1 had failed previous treatment with an SSRI; group 2 had failed previous treatment with an agent other than an SSRI), OFC showed improvement over olanzapine or fluoxetine monotherapy on the Montgomery-Åsberg Depression Rating Scale (MADRS). Although the difference was not significant for group 1 alone, it was significant for group 2 (Thase et al. 2007). In a double-blinded trial sponsored by Eli Lilly that compared olanzapine, fluoxetine, OFC, and venlafaxine, all treatments showed similar rates of efficacy (Corya et al. 2006).

Another significant challenge in treating mood disorders is developing a strategy for patients who have major depression with psychotic features. Earlier work by Spiker et al. (1985) had indicated greater efficacy for a combination of antipsychotics and antidepressants over each administered alone. Because olanzapine has low levels of EPS compared with typical antipsychotics and has a positive effect on mood in schizophrenic patients (Tollefson et al. 1998a, 1998b), it would be a good candidate for depression with psychosis. In an open-label study, olanzapine monotherapy produced a significant reduction in symptoms of both depression and psychosis (measured by the Scale for the Assessment of Positive Symptoms). Again, it must be pointed out that this was an early pilot study, and no comparisons with other treatments were made (for an update on the overall significance of and approach to major depression with psychotic features, see Schatzberg 2003).

In summary, the newer atypical antipsychotic medications have found a role in treating not only mania but also depression. Olanzapine has demonstrated efficacy in both acute and maintenance phases of bipolar disorder, and when combined in the OFC formulation has shown benefit in treating depression in bipolar I disorder. Particularly in cases where psychosis is prominent with mania, olanzapine is a reasonable first-line agent, although consideration must be given to the potential metabolic consequences. In depression, olanzapine has been studied primarily in treatment-refractory cases, and given its metabolic side-effect profile, it is most appropriate for use in such cases.

Dementia-Related Agitation and Psychosis

Olanzapine is often used in an off-label manner for the treatment of dementia. Alzheimer's disease, the most prevalent form of dementia in the Western world, is characterized by progressive memory loss, decreased executive functioning, and deficits in language and visuospatial skills. However, Alzheimer's disease is also frequently accompanied by psychotic and mood symptoms, such as depression, paranoia, and hallucinations. In Lewy body dementia, visual hallucinations are a common manifestation, along with parkinsonism and autonomic instability.

Frontotemporal dementia is characterized by disinhibition and euphoria, along with memory loss and changes in motor function (Bird and Miller 2005). Olanzapine and other antipsychotic medications are typically used off-label for treatment of the neuropsychiatric manifestations of dementia. As elderly people are generally more sensitive to the EPS and tardive dyskinesia associated with first-generation antipsychotic medications, the second-generation medications are often preferred when antipsychotics are needed.

A large placebo-controlled trial of olanzapine in Alzheimer's patients showed that the lower dosages of olanzapine (5–10 mg/day) were significantly better than placebo in treating target symptoms of agitation, hallucinations, and delusions (Street et al. 2000, 2001). However, the treatment of dementia-related psychosis is complicated. The FDA recently mandated placement of a black box warning on the prescribing information of antipsychotic medications calling attention to the increased risk of death, primarily from cardiovascular and infectious complications. According to the warning, second-generation antipsychotic use over a 10-week period carries a 1.6- to 1.7-fold increased risk of mortality based on data from 17 placebo-controlled trials of atypical antipsychotics in dementia-related psychosis. The warning does not differentiate medications and has subsequently been extended to apply to first-generation antipsychotics as well. In a recent Cochrane review of atypical antipsychotic use in agitation associated with dementia, both risperidone and olanzapine were shown to effectively treat the agitation but were associated with an increased risk of stroke, even at olanzapine doses of less than 10 mg/day (Ballard and Waite 2006). However, the finding of increased stroke risk with antipsychotics, and the necessity of the black box warning, remains controversial, as several large population-based studies have reported conflicting results (Gill et al. 2005; Herrmann and Lanctot 2005; Herrmann et al. 2004; Layton et al. 2005; Schneider et al. 2006a). Ultimately, clinical judgment and thorough documentation are important, as in certain situations the hazards of untreated psychotic agitation may outweigh the potential risks of treatment.

Several studies have examined olanzapine in the treatment of dementia without agitation (Brooks and Hoblyn 2007). A placebo-controlled multicenter trial conducted by researchers at Eli Lilly evaluated olanzapine at low fixed doses (1.0, 2.5, 5.0, and 7.5 mg/day) in the treatment of dementia-related psychosis (De Deyn et al. 2004). Although olanzapine did not separate from placebo on the primary outcome measure, Hallucinations and Delusions of the Neuropsychiatric Inventory—Nursing Home edition (NPI/NH), improvements were seen in each of the dosage groups studied. All patients who received dosages of 2.5 mg/day or greater were initially started on 2.5 mg/day, with the dosage titrated upward by 2.5 mg/week (as indicated based on their assigned study group), and there was an overall difference from placebo in the acute phase of the study, suggesting that a 2.5-mg dose was an effective starting dose in the more acute setting. On some secondary outcome measures, the greatest improvement was seen with the highest olanzapine dosage (7.5 mg/day), suggesting that for some patients, an increase to 7.5 mg/day is beneficial. Because no higher dosages were used in the study, it is unclear whether continuing to increase the dosage would lead to greater efficacy (De Deyn et al. 2004).

In treatment of cognitive decline, acetylcholine has been the focus of treatments aimed at protecting people with dementia from undergoing as rapid a deterioration as they would naturally. Cholinesterase inhibitors have been used on that basis. Olanzapine may have beneficial effects on prefrontal cortex cholinergic and serotonergic neurons that may facilitate acetylcholine release to that region. However, in a double-blind study conducted by researchers at Eli Lilly, olanzapine was shown to worsen cognitive functioning, as assessed on the Alzheimer's Disease Assessment Scale for Cognition (ADAS-Cog), and there was no statistical difference between the olanzapine and placebo groups in scores on the Clinician's Interview-Based Impression of Change (CIBIC) scale (Kennedy et al. 2005). Patients in the olanzapine group also showed worsening on the Mini-Mental State Examination (MMSE). Previous studies have found little to no benefit on cognition from olanzapine treatment in nonagitated patients with dementia (De Deyn et al. 2004; Street et al. 2000).

The CATIE studies described earlier also had an Alzheimer's disease component in which olanzapine, risperidone, and quetiapine were compared with placebo for the treatment of psychosis and agitation in outpatients (Schneider et al. 2006b). Patients were included if they had psychotic symptoms and lived either in an assisted living facility or at home, but were excluded for skilled nursing needs or primary psychotic disorders. Patients who were to receive cholinesterase inhibitors or antidepressants were also excluded from the study. Like the schizophrenia portion of CATIE, the primary outcome variable was time to discontinuation. No difference was found among the groups in time to discontinuation, and no benefit was seen on the Clinical Global Impressions of Change (CGI-C). The average time to discontinuation

ranged between 5 and 8 weeks among the treatments. Discontinuation because of lack of efficacy occurred sooner for placebo or quetiapine than for risperidone or olanzapine. Side effects such as parkinsonism, sedation, and higher body mass index were all increased with the study medications over placebo (Schneider et al. 2006b).

Overall, there are limited data to support the effectiveness of atypical antipsychotics in the treatment of dementia. Risks for worsened cognitive function and metabolic concerns must be considered when use of antipsychotic medications is contemplated. Nonetheless, there are times when behavioral consequences and patient safety require more aggressive treatment, and antipsychotic medication may be warranted. Ultimately, a painstaking evaluation of the risk–benefit ratio of antipsychotic medications must precede any decision to prescribe these agents, in both the acute and the long-term time frames. Further study is needed, however, regarding the use of second-generation antipsychotic medications in this population (Schneider et al. 2006a).

Borderline Personality Disorder

Borderline personality disorder is a severe psychiatric illness that afflicts nearly 1% of the population (Torgersen et al. 2001). It is well known to clinicians that symptoms of affective lability, self-injurious behavior, and impulse/aggression action patterns make this patient group difficult to treat. Patients with borderline personality disorder are often taking several medications of various classes, including mood stabilizers, antidepressants, and antipsychotics. Based on earlier studies indicating that low doses of traditional antipsychotic medications may be useful for borderline personality disorder (Goldberg et al. 1986; Soloff et al. 1986), Schulz et al. (1999) reported on an open-label study that found that olanzapine led to a substantial decrease in Symptom Checklist–90 symptoms, as well as on objective measures of impulsivity and aggression. Of the patients entered in the trial, 9 of 11 (82%) completed the study. The design of the trial allowed for early flexible dosing, and the subjects ended the 8-week trial taking olanzapine at an average dosage of approximately 7.5 mg/day, usually at bedtime. Zanarini and Frankenburg (2001) extended this open-label trial and showed superiority of olanzapine over placebo in a longer-term (26-week) study. This interesting study of only women indicated that lower dosages (5 mg/day) of olanzapine can be useful and are associated with only minimal weight gain.

In a study comparing olanzapine, fluoxetine, and OFC in women with borderline personality disorder, olanzapine monotherapy was found to be more effective in treating the depressive symptoms of borderline personality disorder than either fluoxetine or OFC, as assessed on the MADRS. Additionally, olanzapine was superior to fluoxetine in treating symptoms of impulsivity and aggression, as measured by the Overt Aggression Scale (OAS). Weight gain was seen in a greater percentage of olanzapine-treated patients than of fluoxetine-treated patients (Zanarini et al. 2004).

Dialectical behavioral therapy (DBT) is a mainstay of current treatment for borderline personality disorder. In a double-blind, placebo-controlled trial, olanzapine was studied as an adjunctive agent in patients receiving DBT. Impulsive and aggressive behaviors were found to be lower in the group that received olanzapine than in the placebo group. The average olanzapine dosage in the trial was 8.8 mg/day. Statistically significant levels of weight gain and dyslipidemia were observed in the olanzapine group compared with the placebo group (Soler et al. 2005). Therefore, with consideration for side effects, olanzapine may be helpful for a broader range of illnesses, particularly when used in conjunction with psychotherapy.

Anorexia Nervosa

Anorexia nervosa is a common and severe psychiatric illness that may well have the highest mortality of all mental disorders. Among the symptoms of this illness is severe restriction of food intake, leading to low weight; however, patients also have psychotic-like levels of self-perception of body size and appearance and unusual ideas about food and metabolism. Some investigators have begun to explore the possibility that olanzapine may help with this patient group. Initially, reports were largely from pilot studies, including case series, but data are now emerging from small controlled trials.

In an open-label trial, 17 patients hospitalized for anorexia nervosa were given olanzapine in conjunction with concurrent cognitive-behavioral therapy (CBT) and DBT group treatment (Barbarich et al. 2004). Olanzapine was initiated at a dosage of 1.25–5.00 mg/day, with upward titration as needed, balancing sedation and side effects with efficacy. Although patients showed improvement in weight as well as in Beck Depression Inventory (BDI) and Spielberger State-Trait Anxiety Inventory (STAI) scores, the lack of a control group limits the validity of these results (Barbarich et al. 2004).

Because olanzapine has weight gain as a significant side effect, the utility of that effect and the mechanism behind it have become a target for research. Ghrelin and leptin are hormones associated with satiety. In a double-blind, placebo-controlled trial, olanzapine was given concurrently with CBT in patients with anorexia, and ghrelin and leptin levels were assessed over 3 months. While both the olanzapine patients and the placebo patients gained weight, there was no statistical difference between groups in the amount of weight gained, nor in leptin or ghrelin levels, which remained unchanged over the course of the study (Brambilla et al. 2007).

In addition to severe distortions of body image, people with anorexia nervosa often have ruminations and obsessions about their bodies and food intake that can lead to significant distress as well as morbidity and mortality in the illness. In a pilot study in Australia, olanzapine was compared with chlorpromazine in a flexible-dose trial. Based on assessments with self-report instruments, olanzapine demonstrated a benefit for the obsessive ruminations seen in anorexia (Mondraty et al. 2005).

As the newer second-generation antipsychotic olanzapine continues to be tried in illnesses beyond psychosis, its potential benefit in anorexia will be followed up closely. Even though olanzapine has the side effects noted in other sections of this chapter, this illness is of such severity that further investigation of a possible role for olanzapine in its treatment is warranted.

Obsessive-Compulsive Disorder

Obsessive-compulsive disorder (OCD) is characterized by repetitive thoughts and behaviors that are often disabling and are difficult to treat. Affecting up to 2%–3% of the population, OCD has a very high prevalence and is the fourth most common psychiatric condition. Because nearly half of patients do not respond to conventional treatments with SSRIs, augmentation strategies are often sought. A significant portion of patients with OCD have comorbid psychosis. Second-generation antipsychotics had a number needed to treat of 4.5 to achieve a 35% reduction in Yale-Brown Obsessive Compulsive Scale (Y-BOCS) score, according to a systematic review (Bloch et al. 2006). Olanzapine was first evaluated as an adjunctive agent in several open-label trials and case series (Bogetto et al. 2000; D'Amico et al. 2003; Francobandiera 2001; Koran et al. 2000). In a small double-blind, placebo-controlled augmentation study (Bystritsky et al. 2004) in patients who had failed to respond to conventional treatment with serotonin reuptake inhibitors, the olanzapine-augmentation group showed a statistically significant decrease of 4 points on the Y-BOCS compared with the placebo group, which showed a slight gain in Y-BOCS score over the 6-week study duration. Subjects could be on any serotonin reuptake inhibitor, and the dosing of olanzapine was flexible (average dosage = 11 mg/day). In another double-blind, placebo-controlled augmentation trial, patients who were taking fluoxetine 40 mg, generally considered a low dose for treatment of OCD, were randomly assigned to augmentation with either olanzapine (up to 10 mg/day) or placebo and followed for 6 weeks. In this study, there was no statistical difference between the groups; however, that could be attributed to the relatively low dose of fluoxetine used in the study and the high rate of response in the placebo group (Shapira et al. 2004). In an open-label study, subjects received olanzapine augmentation in addition to a serotonergic reuptake inhibitor and were followed for 1 year. Those who evidenced benefit at 12 weeks tended to continue to show a benefit when assessed at 1 year. Subjects with comorbid bipolar disorder showed the greatest response and demonstrated improvement in MADRS scores as well (Marazziti et al. 2005).

Olanzapine has also been studied in Gilles de la Tourette syndrome (GTS), a disorder characterized by motor and vocal tics and frequently including obsessive and compulsive symptoms. Olanzapine has been noted in case reports to have benefit in treatment of the obsessive-compulsive features, as well as the tics (Van den Eynde et al. 2005). In a small (N = 4) double-blind, placebo-controlled crossover trial, olanzapine was compared with pimozide for the treatment of GTS. Olanzapine demonstrated positive effects at 5-mg and 10-mg doses, compared with pimozide doses of 2 mg or 4 mg, over 52 weeks (Onofrj et al. 2000). However, given the small sample size of this study, further research is needed to support a potential role for olanzapine in GTS.

Overall, olanzapine has demonstrated benefit as an adjunctive agent in the treatment of several anxiety disorders. In OCD and GTS, there have been open-label studies that have shown benefit, and in small double-blind studies, there have been generally positive, although ultimately equivocal, results. Further research, including head-to-head trials and more long-term studies, is needed to fully evaluate the efficacy of olanzapine and other second-generation antipsychotic medications in OCD (Ballon et al. 2007).

Posttraumatic Stress Disorder

Posttraumatic stress disorder (PTSD) is a clinically significant disorder with symptoms of reexperiencing a traumatic event, avoidance of situations associated with the trauma, and increased arousal. To qualify for the diagnosis, a patient must have experienced or witnessed a serious event that threatened injury or death or threatened physical integrity (American Psychiatric Association 2000). Clinical observations of such patients show that they have periods of insomnia, nightmares, perceptual disturbances, sensory illusions, and suspiciousness. Some clinicians have noted nonspecific psychotic comorbidities. To date, SSRIs have been frequently used for PTSD, but there is no sole pharmacological standard of treatment. Not surprisingly, olanzapine has been assessed for symptoms of PTSD. As in some of the other disorders discussed in this chapter, the early data are limited and in pilot form.

The first study examined olanzapine in a double-blind, placebo-controlled study (2:1 randomization, olanzapine to placebo) at dosages ranging up to 20 mg/day. The research group reported no difference from placebo in this study but noted a high rate of placebo response (Butterfield et al. 2001). In the same year, a case series reported significant symptom reduction in the Clinician-Administered PTSD Scale, as well as in depression and anxiety scale (Hamilton Rating Scale for Depression and Hamilton Anxiety Scale) scores. In this relatively short (8-week) study, olanzapine was found to be helpful in this group of patients with combat-related trauma.

A third study examined the effect of olanzapine as an augmentation to SSRIs in patients not fully responsive to that treatment. This strategy is similar to that reported by Shelton et al. (2001) for refractory depression. Olanzapine or placebo was added to the patients' SSRI treatment. Active medication treatment led to statistically significantly greater reduction in PTSD symptoms, as assessed by PTSD scales, as well as in symptoms of anxiety and depression (Stein et al. 2002).

These early studies have similarities to the others for borderline personality disorder and anorexia nervosa in that some success is noted in difficult-to-treat patient groups. Further controlled trials are needed to determine whether olanzapine's use for these indications is supported by an evidence base beyond the theoretical and anecdotal rationales currently used. Again, in the clinical arena, the treating psychiatrist would need to weigh the evidence and alternative treatments before proceeding.

Side Effects and Toxicology

The adverse effects of olanzapine in clinical use are consistent with the preclinical studies predicting few neurological effects. EPS, as manifested by dystonic reactions and parkinsonism, are uncommon, although these may be seen in patients who are sensitive to antipsychotics, such as patients with Parkinson's disease. In Phase II and III clinical trials, olanzapine-treated groups generally showed an improvement in EPS from baseline, reflecting the fact that most of the subjects had previously taken typical neuroleptics. In a large multinational comparison study (Tollefson et al. 1997), olanzapine produced fewer treatment-emergent neurological adverse effects than haloperidol for parkinsonism (14% vs. 38%) and akathisia (12% vs. 40%). In another study (Volavka et al. 2002), antiparkinsonian agents were prescribed to 13% of both clozapine- and olanzapine-treated subjects, compared with 32% of risperidone-treated patients.

The reduction of EPS is predictive of decreased risk of tardive dyskinesia, the most problematic of the common adverse effects of classic neuroleptics. To date, the accumulated experience with atypical antipsychotics indicates that tardive dyskinesia is 10- to 15-fold less common, at an annual rate of 0.52% of olanzapine-treated patients compared with 7.45% of haloperidol-treated patients, based on pooled data from long-term comparison trials (Beasley et al. 1999).

A major adverse effect found during treatment with olanzapine is weight gain. This is a serious concern because persons with schizophrenia are more likely than the general population to be obese, and weight gain may contribute to nonadherence to antipsychotic treatment, leading to increased risk for relapse. With the decrease in neurological side effects with second-generation antipsychotic agents, metabolic effects have emerged as a major risk for patients and a focus of consideration for clinicians. The relative degree of weight gain associated with first- and second-generation antipsychotics was studied in a comprehensive meta-analysis by Allison et al. (1999). Estimates of weight change associated with standardized doses over 10 weeks were calculated from published data from 81 studies. Clozapine produced the greatest weight gain (4.45 kg), followed by olanzapine (4.15 kg). By comparison, risperidone was associated with a gain of 2.1 kg, haloperidol was associated with a gain of 1.08 kg, and patients lost 0.74 kg while taking placebo. In long-term treatment, 30%–50% of patients may gain more than 7% of body weight, with low pretreatment weight and good clinical response associated with more weight gain.

Efforts involving use of other pharmacotherapies to combat weight gain have largely been unsuccessful. Sibutramine, an SNRI, has been shown to be an effective weight-loss agent and has been tested as an adjunct to behavioral modification for management of olanzapine- and clozapine-induced weight gain in double-blind, placebo-controlled trials. In the olanzapine study (Henderson et al. 2005), there was an average 8-pound weight loss compared with placebo, while in the clozapine study (Henderson et al. 2007), there was no statistical difference from placebo. Unfortunately, there have been case reports of sibutramine-induced psychosis (Rosenbohm et al. 2007; Taflinski and Chojnacka 2000), so its use in the psychotic disorder population must be carefully monitored. Other agents, including H_2 antagonists such as famotidine, have also been studied. In a double-blind trial in first-episode patients, famotidine given prophylactically had no benefit in preventing weight gain (Poyurovsky et al. 2004). Additionally, a trial of fluoxetine in first-episode schizophrenia patients yielded the same results (Poyurovsky et al. 2002). Small studies have shown modest positive results with the SNRI reboxetine (Poyurovsky et al. 2003) and the H_2 antagonist nizatidine (Atmaca et al. 2003).

A recent post hoc analysis of first-episode patients in Spain indicated that use of the orally disintegrating formulation of olanzapine might result in decreased weight gain (Arranz et al. 2007). This hypothesis was first proposed by de Haan et al. (2004) in a report of a small nonrandomized study in which adolescents switched from conventional olanzapine to sublingual dissolvable olanzapine lost an average of 6.6 kg in 16 weeks. The authors suggested that differential effects on serotonergic receptors in the gut, particularly at the pylorus, might be responsible for their findings, but larger randomized studies are needed on this topic.

Small studies using metformin, an agent known to decrease hepatic glucose output, have tested the possibility that it may help patients either lose weight or remain at the same weight while receiving olanzapine or other second-generation antipsychotics. In a double-blind, placebo-controlled trial (Baptista et al. 2006), patients were given 10 mg of olanzapine and randomly assigned to receive either metformin or placebo for 14 weeks. No differences between groups were seen in body mass index or waist circumference. There was a modest improvement in overall glucose levels and in measures of glucose homeostasis (homeostasis model assessment for insulin resistance [HOMA-IR]), but no change was seen in lipid levels. A follow-up study conducted by the same group (Baptista et al. 2007) demonstrated similar results, although in the second study, small differences in weight gain between the groups were found, with the metformin group losing an average of 1.5 kg and showing decreased leptin levels, while the placebo group maintained a consistent weight. In a double-blind, placebo-controlled trial in adolescents who had gained weight after 1 year of treatment with a second-generation antipsychotic (olanzapine, risperidone, or quetiapine), the addition of metformin resulted in statistical differences in waist circumference, body mass index, and overall weight gain (Klein et al. 2006). HOMA-IR scores were significantly decreased, and the number of subjects requiring referral for a glucose tolerance test was reduced, among the subjects who received metformin. These equivocal results suggest that further research is needed on adjunctive agents to help with the metabolic complications often seen with olanzapine.

Weight gain is an even greater concern in the treatment of children and adolescents, who may be exposed to medication for a longer time and are concerned with body image. After 12 weeks of treatment with olanzapine, hospitalized adolescent patients gained 7.2±6.3 kg, approximately twice the weight gain experienced by those taking risperidone; 19 of 21 patients (90%) gained more than 7% of their body weight (Ratzoni et al. 2002). These findings in patients younger than 18 years have been confirmed by Findling et al. (2003), who reported an average 6.5-kg weight gain in their assessment of schizophrenic patients over 8 weeks.

Concurrently with the attention to weight gain with second-generation antipsychotics, other metabolic effects have been noted. Reports of glucose intolerance, hyperglycemia, hyperlipidemia, diabetes, and diabetic ketoacidosis have surfaced, mostly associated with clozapine and olanzapine therapy. Cases reported to the FDA Drug Surveillance System and published cases of olanzapine-associated diabetes and hyperglycemia were reviewed by Koller and Doriswamy (2002). Two hundred eighty-nine cases were identified, of which 225 (78%) were new-onset diabetes, 100 (35%) involved ketosis or acidosis, and 23 (8%) patients died. Most cases developed within 6 months of initiation of olanzapine therapy. Many cases occurred in the first month of therapy, indicating that weight gain alone did not mediate the occurrence of diabetes-related problems. On the basis of the temporal relation between metabolic changes and the introduction and withdrawal of olanzapine, the young age of patients affected, and the number of reports, the authors concluded that the data suggested that olanzapine was causally related to the development or worsening of diabetes. A similar conclusion about clozapine and diabetes was reported earlier (Koller et al. 2001). Because case studies and reports by clinicians to regulatory agencies may reflect reporting bias, controlled studies comparing the development of metabolic disorders are needed to clarify whether these are related to the underlying psychosis,

causally related to drug treatment in general, or specifically related to individual agents.

Studies that used large health system databases have been published linking use of antipsychotics with subsequent diagnoses of diabetes or use of hypoglycemic agents. These studies show increased risk of development of type 2 diabetes following the use of olanzapine and clozapine relative to the use of risperidone or typical antipsychotics or compared with matched untreated persons (Gianfrancesco et al. 2002; Koro et al. 2002a; Sernyak et al. 2002).

While olanzapine has been associated with weight gain and type 2 diabetes, there have also been reports of diabetic ketoacidosis (DKA), a condition more often associated with type 1 diabetes mellitus. These reports first appeared in the literature in 1999 (Gatta et al. 1999; Goldstein et al. 1999; Lindenmayer and Patel 1999). In a review of 45 published cases of DKA associated with atypical antipsychotic medications, 42% of cases were related to olanzapine, 44% were related to clozapine, and 6% each were related to risperidone and quetiapine (Jin et al. 2004). The onset of DKA was not associated with weight gain, though 80% of the patients were overweight prior to initiating treatment. The overall incidence of DKA is unknown; however, given the potential morbidity and mortality associated with this acute condition, close monitoring is critical, as DKA was the first presenting sign of diabetes in 42% of reported cases and generally required an intensive care unit admission. In a review of California Medicaid data on cases of risperidone- and olanzapine-associated DKA, Ramaswamy et al. (2007) found a higher incidence of DKA for olanzapine than for risperidone and noted that the risk increased with duration of treatment with olanzapine.

Another metabolic adverse effect seen with olanzapine is the development of dyslipidemia, often in association with weight gain. In a large British patient database, olanzapine conferred a fivefold increase in the rates of dyslipidemia over an untreated control condition and a threefold increase over conventional antipsychotics, whereas risperidone did not increase the risk (Koro et al. 2002b).

Sedation is frequent at the start of therapy with olanzapine but diminishes as patients develop tolerance for this side effect. In long-term treatment, the incidence of sedation is about 15%, similar to that of haloperidol. Anticholinergic effects occur during treatment but at rates only slightly higher than those of placebo, and they rarely lead to treatment discontinuation. Mild elevations of liver enzymes may be seen in some patients, but these are stable or decline over time without progression to hepatic dysfunction. Prolactin elevations observed during olanzapine treatment occur early in the course of treatment, and levels are much lower than those seen with risperidone or classic antipsychotic treatment. However, prolactin concentrations may exceed normal levels in patients taking 30 mg/day or more of olanzapine. Leukopenia is rare and occurs at a rate similar to that seen with other typical and atypical antipsychotics, but olanzapine does not cause agranulocytosis, even in patients who developed this effect while taking clozapine. In animal toxicology studies and in clinical trials, no QTc prolongation was observed, and other cardiovascular effects are rarely of clinical importance.

In summary, olanzapine is a well-tolerated antipsychotic agent with a low rate of EPS and diminished risk for tardive dyskinesia. Weight gain is common and can lead to discontinuation by choice or by clinician decision because of long-term health concerns. Patients should be monitored for the development of type II diabetes and dyslipidemia. Studies addressing weight gain are progressing, and new strategies may emerge in the near future.

Drug–Drug Interactions

Olanzapine is metabolized primarily via glucuronidation and via oxidation by CYP1A2 (see section "Pharmacokinetics and Disposition" earlier in this chapter). Other drugs that affect the activity of these metabolic pathways would therefore be expected to affect olanzapine pharmacokinetics. Indeed, drugs that inhibit CYP1A2 activity have been shown to decrease olanzapine clearance, thereby increasing olanzapine plasma concentrations.

Fluvoxamine, a known inhibitor of CYP1A2, has been shown to inhibit olanzapine metabolism in several studies. A study of 10 healthy male smokers receiving 11 days of fluvoxamine administration (50–100 mg) resulted in an 84% increase in maximal olanzapine concentrations (C_{max}) and a 119% increase in AUC_{0-24} compared with olanzapine administered with placebo. In this study, olanzapine clearance decreased 50%, and apparent volume of distribution decreased approximately 45%. The C_{max} of olanzapine's metabolite 4'-N-desmethylolanzapine decreased 64%, and its AUC_{0-24} decreased 77%. No change in half-life was observed in either olanzapine or 4'-N-desmethylolanzapine, suggesting that fluvoxamine inhibited olanzapine's first-pass metabolism (Maenpaa et al. 1997). Another study found that in a population of patients receiving olanzapine, those also receiving fluvoxamine ($n = 21$) had, on average, a 2.3-fold higher concentration per

dose ratio than did those not receiving fluvoxamine ($n = 144$) (Weigmann et al. 2001). A separate case report indicated that a patient who discontinued ciprofloxacin (also a CYP1A2 inhibitor) while receiving olanzapine experienced an approximately twofold decrease in olanzapine concentrations (Markowitz and DeVane 1999).

Fluoxetine and imipramine, although not known to be significant inhibitors of CYP1A2, when coadministered with olanzapine have been associated with statistically significant but small changes in olanzapine pharmacokinetics. Coadministration of fluoxetine resulted in a 15% decrease in olanzapine clearance and an 18% increase in C_{max}, with no significant difference in the half-life of olanzapine (Callaghan et al. 1999). Coadministration of imipramine resulted in an approximately 14% increase in olanzapine C_{max} and a non–statistically significant increase in AUC of 19% (Callaghan et al. 1997).

Inducers of the CYP1A2 enzyme increase olanzapine clearance, thereby decreasing olanzapine systemic exposure. Carbamazepine, an inducer of several CYP enzymes (including 1A2), affects olanzapine disposition. A study in healthy volunteers showed that 18 days of carbamazepine therapy (200 mg twice daily) resulted in significantly higher clearance (32.6 vs. 47.6 L/hour) and apparent volume of distribution (1,190 vs. 1,400 L/kg) but significantly lower C_{max} (11.7 vs. 8.8 µg/L), AUC (336 vs. 223 h*µg/L), and half-life (26.0 vs. 20.8 hours) after a single 10-mg dose of olanzapine (Lucas et al. 1998). In one case report, the discontinuation of carbamazepine was associated with a 114% increase in olanzapine concentrations (Licht et al. 2000).

Smoking, also known to induce CYP1A2, can affect olanzapine disposition. A study comparing 19 male smokers with 30 male nonsmokers found that olanzapine clearance in smokers was 23% higher than that in nonsmokers (Callaghan et al. 1999). A population pharmacokinetic analysis of 910 patients receiving olanzapine found that clearance among nonsmokers was 37% lower in men and 48% lower in women than it was in the corresponding group of smokers (Patel et al. 1996). A smaller analysis of healthy volunteers also found higher drug clearances among smokers (Patel et al. 1995). The polycyclic aromatic hydrocarbons in cigarette smoke are responsible for inducing the aryl hydrocarbon hydroxylases and thus lead to enzymatic induction (Desai et al. 2001). Thus, dosage adjustments might be needed when a patient who smokes is placed in a smoke-free inpatient unit, even if adequate nicotine replacement is provided.

A recent study suggested that probenecid, a nonspecific inhibitor of uridine diphosphoglucuronate-glucuronosyltransferase (UDPGT), can affect the disposition of a single 5-mg olanzapine dose. Following probenecid administration, a statistically significant increase of 19% occurred in olanzapine C_{max}, an increase of 26% occurred in olanzapine AUC ($P=0.002$), and an increase of 57% occurred in the absorption rate constant, indicating a faster rate of absorption. Clearance was not significantly altered by probenecid coadministration. Because probenecid may also inhibit the P-glycoprotein efflux transporter, this alternative mechanism may be contributing to this drug interaction (Markowitz et al. 2002). It is not known whether other UDPGT inhibitors also will affect olanzapine disposition, although in vitro testing with valproic acid did not show an interaction (Eli Lilly 2006).

In vitro studies suggest that olanzapine does not significantly inhibit the activity of the CYP enzymes 1A2, 3A, 2D6, 2C9, or 2C19 (Ring et al. 1996a). In vivo studies suggest that olanzapine does not affect the disposition of aminophylline (Macias et al. 1998), diazepam, alcohol, imipramine (Callaghan et al. 1997), warfarin, biperiden, or lithium (Callaghan et al. 1999; Demolle et al. 1995).

Conclusion

After review of the research focused on olanzapine, it is clear that this compound, which has been approved for use in the United States since 1997, has wide utility and is a step forward from the traditional antipsychotic medications. In addition to the positive effect on a broad group of symptoms of schizophrenia, olanzapine has now been approved for treatment of mania, both acute and long term, in bipolar disorder. Recent research has shown that there may be benefit to disorders beyond psychosis (e.g., borderline personality disorder, anorexia, PTSD, OCD, Tourette's syndrome) with olanzapine. The extension of uses of olanzapine is in many ways allowed by the low rates of movement disorders. The lack of dystonia, parkinsonism, and tardive dyskinesia leads to greater acceptability in chronic schizophrenia and has encouraged clinicians and investigators to find patients earlier in the course of their illness, thus reducing the duration of untreated psychosis and perhaps decreasing the number of patients who develop psychosis (McGlashan et al. 2003). The low rate of movement disorders has been a major factor in moving forward with treatment of mood disorders and nonpsychotic illnesses.

As noted in the section on side effects, olanzapine is not free of adverse effects, even though they are outside the movement disorder arena. Weight gain and metabolic disturbances are of significant concern and are the objects of intense research—in areas of both pathophysiology and prevention/treatment.

In addition to providing better treatment for schizophrenia and other disorders, olanzapine's actions in the brain have provided new avenues of research in the exploration of pathophysiology of psychiatric disease. As noted earlier in this chapter, olanzapine's effects on glutamate measures and neurotensin may open new avenues of treatment.

In conclusion, olanzapine is a psychotropic medication that was first approved for the treatment of psychosis related to schizophrenia. It has become a widely used medication for schizophrenia as well as other disorders. As noted, metabolic side effects are of concern and are the object of intense research. The future holds significant interest for understanding side effects, learning more about the effect of olanzapine on different syndromes, and gaining knowledge about the pathophysiology of psychiatric disease.

References

Aichhorn W, Whitworth AB, Weiss EM, et al: Second-generation antipsychotics: is there evidence for sex differences in pharmacokinetic and adverse effect profiles? Drug Saf 29:587–598, 2006

Allison D, Mentore JL, Heo M, et al: Antipsychotic-induced weight gain: a comprehensive research synthesis. Am J Psychiatry 156:1686–1696, 1999

Alvarez E, Ciudad A, Olivares JM, et al: A randomized, 1-year follow-up study of olanzapine and risperidone in the treatment of negative symptoms in outpatients with schizophrenia. J Clin Psychopharmacol 26:238–249, 2006

American Psychiatric Association: Diagnostic and Statistical Manual of Mental Disorders, Fourth Edition, Text Revision. Washington, DC, American Psychiatric Association, 2000

Amster HA, Teerenhovi L, Barth E: Agranulocytosis in patients treated with clozapine. Acta Psychiatr Scand 56:241–248, 1977

Amsterdam JD, Shults J: Comparison of fluoxetine, olanzapine, and combined fluoxetine plus olanzapine initial therapy of bipolar type I and type II major depression—lack of manic induction. J Affect Disord 87:121–130, 2005

Angrist B, Schulz SC: The Neuroleptic-Nonresponsive Patient. Washington, DC, American Psychiatric Press, 1990

Aravagiri M, Ames D, Wirshing WC, et al: Plasma level monitoring of olanzapine in patients with schizophrenia: determination by high-performance liquid chromatography with electrochemical detection. Ther Drug Monit 19:307–313, 1997

Arranz B, San L, Duenas RM, et al: Lower weight gain with the orally disintegrating olanzapine than with standard tablets in first-episode never treated psychotic patients. Hum Psychopharmacol 22:11–15, 2007

Atmaca M, Kuloglu M, Tezcan E, et al: Nizatidine treatment and its relationship with leptin levels in patients with olanzapine-induced weight gain. Hum Psychopharmacol 18:457–461, 2003

Baker RW, Kinon BJ, Maguire GA, et al: Effectiveness of rapid initial dose escalation of up to forty milligrams per day of oral olanzapine in acute agitation. J Clin Psychopharmacol 23:342–348, 2003

Bakshi VP, Swerdlow NR, Braff DL, et al: Reversal of isolation rearing-induced deficits in prepulse inhibition by Seroquel and olanzapine. Biol Psychiatry 43:436–445, 1998

Baldwin DS, Montgomery SA: First clinical experience with olanzapine (LY 170053): results of an open-label safety and dose-ranging study in patients with schizophrenia. Int Clin Psychopharmacol 10:239–244, 1995

Ballard C, Waite J: The effectiveness of atypical antipsychotics for the treatment of aggression and psychosis in Alzheimer's disease. Cochrane Database Syst Rev (1):CD003476, 2006

Ballon JS, Boyd JA, Wirshing DA: Stress and anxiety: treatment with second-generation antipsychotic drugs, in Encyclopedia of Stress, 2nd Edition, Vol 3. Fink G, Editor-in-Chief. Oxford, UK, Academic Press, 2007, pp 587–590

Baptista T, Martinez J, Lacruz A, et al: Metformin for prevention of weight gain and insulin resistance with olanzapine: a double-blind placebo-controlled trial. Can J Psychiatry 51:192–196, 2006

Baptista T, Rangel N, Fernandez V, et al: Metformin as an adjunctive treatment to control body weight and metabolic dysfunction during olanzapine administration: a multicentric, double-blind, placebo-controlled trial. Schizophr Res 93:99–108, 2007

Barak Y, Shamir E, Zemishlani H, et al: Olanzapine vs. haloperidol in the treatment of elderly chronic schizophrenic patients. Prog Neuropsychopharmacol Biol Psychiatry 26:1199–1202, 2002

Barbarich NC, McConaha CW, Gaskill J, et al: An open trial of olanzapine in anorexia nervosa. J Clin Psychiatry 65:1480–1482, 2004

Beasley CM Jr, Sanger T, Satterlee W, et al: Olanzapine versus placebo: results of a double-blind, fixed-dose olanzapine trial. Psychopharmacology (Berl) 124:159–167, 1996a

Beasley CM Jr, Tollefson G, Tran P, et al: Olanzapine versus placebo and haloperidol: acute phase results of the North American double-blind olanzapine trial. Neuropsychopharmacology 14:111–123, 1996b

Beasley CM Jr, Hamilton SH, Crawford AM, et al: Olanzapine versus haloperidol: acute phase results of the international double-blind olanzapine trial. Eur Neuropsychopharmacol 7:125–137, 1997

Beasley CM, Dellva MA, Tamura RN, et al: Randomised double-blind comparison of the incidence of tardive dyskinesia in patients with schizophrenia during long-term treatment with olanzapine or haloperidol. Br J Psychiatry 174:23–30, 1999

Benzel I, Bansal A, Browning BL, et al: Interactions among genes in the ErbB-Neuregulin signalling network are associated with increased susceptibility to schizophrenia. Behav Brain Funct 3:31, 2007

Bergstrom RF, Callaghan JT, Cerimele BJ, et al: Pharmacokinetics of olanzapine in elderly and young (abstract). Pharm Res 12 (9, suppl):S358, 1995

Berk M, Ichim L, Brook S: Olanzapine compared to lithium in mania: a double-blind randomized controlled trial. Int Clin Psychopharmacol 14:339–343, 1999

Binder EB, Kinkead B, Owens MJ, et al: The role of neurotensin in the pathophysiology of schizophrenia and the mechanism of action of antipsychotic drugs. Biol Psychiatry 50:856–872, 2001

Bird TD, Miller BL: Alzheimer's disease and other dementias, in Harrison's Principles of Internal Medicine, 16th Edition. Edited by Kasper DL, Braunwald E, Fauci AS, et al. New York, McGraw-Hill, 2005, pp 2393–2406

Bloch MH, Landeros-Weisenberger A, Kelmendi B, et al: A systematic review: antipsychotic augmentation with treatment refractory obsessive-compulsive disorder. Mol Psychiatry 11:622–632, 2006

Bogetto F, Bellino S, Vaschetto P, et al: Olanzapine augmentation of fluvoxamine-refractory obsessive-compulsive disorder (OCD): a 12-week open trial. Psychiatry Res 96:91–98, 2000

Boules M, Shaw A, Fredrickson P, et al: Neurotensin agonists: potential in the treatment of schizophrenia. CNS Drugs 21:13–23, 2007

Boulton DW, DeVane CL, Liston HL, et al: In vitro P-glycoprotein affinity for atypical and conventional antipsychotics. Life Sci 71:163–169, 2002

Brambilla F, Monteleone P, Maj M: Olanzapine-induced weight gain in anorexia nervosa: involvement of leptin and ghrelin secretion? Psychoneuroendocrinology 32:402–406, 2007

Breier A, Meehan K, Kirkett M, et al: A double-blind, placebo-controlled dose-response comparison of intramuscular olanzapine and haloperidol in the treatment of acute agitation in schizophrenia. Arch Gen Psychiatry 59:441–448, 2002

Brooks JO, Hoblyn JC: Neurocognitive costs and benefits of psychiatric medication in older adults: invited review. J Geriatr Psychiatr Neurol 20:199–214, 2007

Brooks JO, Karnik N, Hoblyn JC: High initial dosing of olanzapine for stabilization of acute agitation a retrospective case series. J Pharm Technol 24:7–11, 2008

Brown EB, McElroy SL, Keck PE Jr, et al: A 7-week, randomized, double-blind trial of olanzapine/fluoxetine combination versus lamotrigine in the treatment of bipolar I depression. J Clin Psychiatry 67:1025–1033, 2006

Buchanan RW, Ball MP, Weiner E, et al: Olanzapine treatment of residual positive and negative symptoms. Am J Psychiatry 162:124–129, 2005

Burbaeva GS, Boksha IS, Tereshkina EB, et al: Effect of olanzapine treatment on platelet glutamine synthetase-like protein and glutamate dehydrogenase immunoreactivity in schizophrenia. World J Biol Psychiatry 7:75–81, 2006

Burbaeva GS, Boksha IS, Turishcheva MS, et al: Glutamine synthetase and glutamate dehydrogenase in the prefrontal cortex of patients with schizophrenia. Prog Neuropsychopharmacol Biol Psychiatry 27:675–680, 2003

Butterfield MI, Becker ME, Connor KM, et al: Olanzapine in the treatment of post-traumatic stress disorder: a pilot study. Int Clin Psychopharmacol 16:197–203, 2001

Bymaster FP, Nelson DL, DeLapp NW, et al: Antagonism by olanzapine of dopamine D1, serotonin2, muscarinic, histamine H1 and alpha1-adrenergic receptors in vitro. Schizophr Res 37:107–122, 1999

Bystritsky A, Ackerman DL, Rosen RM, et al: Augmentation of serotonin reuptake inhibitors in refractory obsessive-compulsive disorder using adjunctive olanzapine: a placebo-controlled trial. J Clin Psychiatry 65:565–568, 2004

Calabrese JR, Kimmel SE, Woyshville MJ, et al: Clozapine for treatment-refractory mania. Am J Psychiatry 153:759–764, 1996

Callaghan JT, Cerimele BJ, Kassahun KJ, et al: Olanzapine: interaction study with imipramine. J Clin Pharmacol 37:971–978, 1997

Callaghan JT, Bergstrom RF, Ptak LR, et al: Olanzapine: pharmacokinetic and pharmacodynamic profile. Clin Pharmacokinet 37:177–193, 1999

Casey DE: Serotonergic and dopaminergic aspects of neuroleptic-induced extrapyramidal syndromes in nonhuman primates. Psychopharmacology (Berl) 112:S55–S59, 1993

Ciudad A, Olivares JM, Bousono M, et al: Improvement in social functioning in outpatients with schizophrenia with prominent negative symptoms treated with olanzapine or risperidone in a 1 year randomized, open-label trial. Prog Neuropsychopharmacol Biol Psychiatry 30:1515–1522, 2006

Cole JO, Goldberg SC, Klerman GL: Phenothiazine in treatment of acute schizophrenia. Arch Gen Psychiatry 10:246–261, 1964

Conley RR, Tamminga CA, Bartko JJ, et al: Olanzapine compared with chlorpromazine in treatment-resistant schizophrenia. Am J Psychiatry 155:914–920, 1998

Corya SA, Williamson D, Sanger TM, et al: A randomized, double-blind comparison of olanzapine/fluoxetine combination, olanzapine, fluoxetine, and venlafaxine in treatment-resistant depression. Depress Anxiety 23:364–372, 2006

D'Amico G, Cedro C, Muscatello MR, et al: Olanzapine augmentation of paroxetine-refractory obsessive-compulsive disorder. Prog Neuropsychopharmacol Biol Psychiatry 27:619–623, 2003

De Deyn PP, Carrasco MM, Deberdt W, et al: Olanzapine versus placebo in the treatment of psychosis with or without associated behavioral disturbances in patients with Alzheimer's disease. Int J Geriatr Psychiatry 19:115–126, 2004

de Haan L, van Amelsvoort T, Rosien K, et al: Weight loss after switching from conventional olanzapine tablets to orally disintegrating olanzapine tablets. Psychopharmacology (Berl) 175:389–390, 2004

Delay J, Bernitzer P: Le traitment des psychoses par une methode neuroleptique derivee de l'hibernotherapie, in Congres de Medecins Alienistes et Neurologistes de France. Edited by Ossa PC. Paris, Masson, 1952, pp 497–502

Demolle D, Onkelinx C, Miller-Oerlinghausen B: Interaction between olanzapine and lithium in healthy male volunteer (abstract 486). Therapie 50 (suppl), 1995

Desai HD, Seabolt J, Jann MW: Smoking in patients receiving psychotropic medications: a pharmacokinetic perspective. CNS Drugs 15:469–494, 2001

Eli Lilly: Zyprexa (olanzapine) tablets: prescribing information. Indianapolis, IN, Eli Lilly, 2006

Essock SM, Covell NH, Davis SM, et al: Effectiveness of switching antipsychotic medications. Am J Psychiatry 163:2090–2095, 2006

Evins AE, Fitzgerald SM, Wine L, et al: Placebo-controlled trial of glycine added to clozapine in schizophrenia. Am J Psychiatry 157:826–828, 2000

Farah A: Atypicality of atypical antipsychotics. Prim Care Companion J Clin Psychiatry 7:268–274, 2005

Farde L, Nordstrom AL: PET analysis indicates atypical central dopamine receptor occupancy in clozapine-treated patients. Br J Psychiatry 17 (suppl):30–33, 1992

Farde L, Nordstrom AL, Wiesel FA, et al: Positron emission tomographic analysis of central D1 and D2 dopamine receptor occupancy in patients treated with classical neuroleptics and clozapine: relation to extrapyramidal side effects. Arch Gen Psychiatry 49:538–544, 1992

Findling RL, McNamara NK, Youngstrom EA, et al: A prospective, open-label trial of olanzapine in adolescents with schizophrenia. J Am Acad Child Adolesc Psychiatry 42:170–175, 2003

Francobandiera G: Olanzapine augmentation of serotonin uptake inhibitors in obsessive-compulsive disorder: an open study. Can J Psychiatry 46:356–358, 2001

Fu Y, Zhu ZT, Chen LJ, et al: Behavioral characteristics of olanzapine: an atypical neuroleptic. Acta Pharmacol Sin 21:329–334, 2000

Gareri P, De Fazio P, De Fazio S, et al: Adverse effects of atypical antipsychotics in the elderly: a review. Drugs Aging 23:937–956, 2006

Gatta B, Rigalleau V, Gin H: Diabetic ketoacidosis with olanzapine treatment. Diabetes Care 22:1002–1003, 1999

Gianfrancesco FD, Grogg AL, Mahmoud RA, et al: Differential effects of risperidone, olanzapine, clozapine, and conventional antipsychotics on type 2 diabetes: findings from a large health plan database. J Clin Psychiatry 63:920–930, 2002

Gill SS, Rochon PA, Herrmann N, et al: Atypical antipsychotic drugs and risk of ischaemic stroke: population based retrospective cohort study. BMJ 330:445, 2005

Goff DC, Tsai G, Manoach DS, et al: Dose-finding trial of D-cycloserine added to neuroleptics for negative symptoms in schizophrenia. Am J Psychiatry 152:1213–1215, 1995

Goff DC, Hennen J, Lyoo IK, et al: Modulation of brain and serum glutamatergic concentrations following a switch from conventional neuroleptics to olanzapine. Biol Psychiatry 51:493–497, 2002

Goldberg SC, Schulz SC, Schulz PM, et al: Borderline and schizotypal personality disorders treated with low-dose thiothixene vs placebo. Arch Gen Psychiatry 43:680–686, 1986

Goldstein LE, Sporn J, Brown S, et al: New-onset diabetes mellitus and diabetic ketoacidosis associated with olanzapine treatment. Psychosomatics 40:438–443, 1999

Gosselin G, Oberling P, Di Scala G: Antagonism of amphetamine-induced disruption of latent inhibition by the atypical antipsychotic olanzapine in rats. Behav Pharmacol 7:820–826, 1996

Gossen D, de Suray JM, Vandenhende F, et al: Influence of fluoxetine on olanzapine pharmacokinetics. AAPS PharmSci 4(2):E11, 2002

Green MF: Cognitive impairment and functional outcome in schizophrenia and bipolar disorder. J Clin Psychiatry 67(10):e12, 2006

Grothe DR, Calis KA, Jacobsen L, et al: Olanzapine pharmacokinetics in pediatric and adolescent inpatients with childhood-onset schizophrenia. J Clin Psychopharmacol 20:220–225, 2000

Gurpegui M, Alvarez E, Bousono M, et al: Effect of olanzapine or risperidone treatment on some cognitive functions in a one-year follow-up of schizophrenia outpatients with prominent negative symptoms. Eur Neuropsychopharmacol 17:725–734, 2007

Hagg S, Spigset O, Lakso HA, et al: Olanzapine disposition in humans is unrelated to CYP1A2 and CYP2D6 phenotypes. Eur J Clin Pharmacol 57:493–497, 2001

Henderson DC, Copeland PM, Daley TB, et al: A double-blind, placebo-controlled trial of sibutramine for olanzapine-associated weight gain. Am J Psychiatry 162:954–962, 2005

Henderson DC, Fan X, Copeland PM, et al: A double-blind, placebo-controlled trial of sibutramine for clozapine-associated weight gain. Acta Psychiatr Scand 115:101–105, 2007

Herrmann N, Lanctot KL: Do atypical antipsychotics cause stroke? CNS Drugs 19:91–103, 2005

Herrmann N, Mamdani M, Lanctot KL: Atypical antipsychotics and risk of cerebrovascular accidents. Am J Psychiatry 161:1113–1115, 2004

Houston JP, Ahl J, Meyers AL, et al: Reduced suicidal ideation in bipolar I disorder mixed-episode patients in a placebo-controlled trial of olanzapine combined with lithium or divalproex. J Clin Psychiatry 67:1246–1252, 2006

Hwang J, Yang CH, Lee TW, et al: The efficacy and safety of olanzapine for the treatment of geriatric psychosis. J Clin Psychopharmacol 23:113–118, 2003

Jardemark KE, Liang X, Arvanov V, et al: Subchronic treatment with either clozapine, olanzapine or haloperidol produces a hyposensitive response of the rat cortical cells to N-methyl-D-aspartate. Neuroscience 100:1–9, 2000

Javitt DC, Zukin SR: Recent advances in the phencyclidine model of schizophrenia. Am J Psychiatry 148:1301–1308, 1991

Javitt DC: Is the glycine site half saturated or half unsaturated? Effects of glutamatergic drugs in schizophrenia patients. Curr Opin Psychiatry 19:151–157, 2006

Jin H, Meyer JM, Jeste DV: Atypical antipsychotics and glucose dysregulation: a systematic review. Schizophr Res 71:195–212, 2004

Jensen PS, Buitelaar J, Pandina GJ, et al: Management of psychiatric disorders in children and adolescents with atypical antipsychotics: a systematic review of published clinical trials. Eur Child Adolesc Psychiatry 16:104–120, 2007

Kane J, Honigfeld G, Singer J, et al: Clozapine for the treatment-resistant schizophrenic: a double-blind comparison with chlorpromazine. Arch Gen Psychiatry 45:789–796, 1988

Kapur S, Remington G: Dopamine D(2) receptors and their role in atypical antipsychotic action: still necessary and may even be sufficient. Biol Psychiatry 50:873–883, 2001

Kapur S, Zipursky RB, Remington G, et al: 5-HT2 and D2 receptor occupancy of olanzapine in schizophrenia: a PET investigation. Am J Psychiatry 155:921–928, 1998

Kapur S, Zipursky RB, Remington G: Clinical and theoretical implications of 5-HT2 and D2 receptor occupancy of clozapine, risperidone, and olanzapine in schizophrenia. Am J Psychiatry 156:286–293, 1999

Kapur S, Zipursky R, Jones C, et al: A positron emission tomography study of quetiapine in schizophrenia: a preliminary finding of an antipsychotic effect with only transiently high dopamine D2 receptor occupancy. Arch Gen Psychiatry 57:553–559, 2000

Kapur S, Arenovich T, Agid O, et al: Evidence for onset of antipsychotic effects within the first 24 hours of treatment. Am J Psychiatry 162:939–946, 2005

Kassahun K, Mattiuz E, Nyhart E Jr, et al: Disposition and biotransformation of the antipsychotic agent olanzapine in humans. Drug Metab Dispos 25:81–93, 1997

Kelly DL, Conley RR, Tamminga CA: Differential olanzapine plasma concentrations by sex in a fixed-dose study. Schizophr Res 40:101–104, 1999

Kennedy J, Deberdt W, Siegal A, et al: Olanzapine does not enhance cognition in non-agitated and non-psychotic patients with mild to moderate Alzheimer's dementia. Int J Geriatr Psychiatry 20:1020–1027, 2005

Kinon BJ, Noordsy DL, Liu-Seifert H, et al: Randomized, double-blind 6-month comparison of olanzapine and quetiapine in patients with schizophrenia or schizoaffective disorder with prominent negative symptoms and poor functioning. J Clin Psychopharmacol 26:453–461, 2006

Klein DJ, Cottingham EM, Sorter M, et al: A randomized, double-blind, placebo-controlled trial of metformin treatment of weight gain associated with initiation of atypical antipsychotic therapy in children and adolescents. Am J Psychiatry 163:2072–2079, 2006

Koller E, Doriswamy PM: Olanzapine-associated diabetes mellitus. Pharmacotherapy 22:841–845, 2002

Koller E, Schneider B, Bennett K, et al: Clozapine-associated diabetes. Am J Med 111:716–723, 2001

Koran LM, Ringold AL, Elliott MA: Olanzapine augmentation for treatment-resistant obsessive-compulsive disorder. J Clin Psychiatry 61:514–517, 2000

Koro C, Fedder DO, L'Italien GL, et al: Assessment of independent effect of olanzapine and risperidone on risk of diabetes among patients with schizophrenia: population based nested case-control study. BMJ 325:243, 2002a

Koro C, Fedder DO, L'Italien GL, et al: An assessment of the independent effects of olanzapine and risperidone exposure on the risk of hyperlipidemia in schizophrenic patients. Arch Gen Psychiatry 59:1021–1026, 2002b

Krystal JH, Karper LP, Seibyl JP, et al: Subanesthetic effects of the noncompetitive NMDA antagonist, ketamine, in humans: psychotomimetic, perceptual, cognitive, and neuroendocrine responses. Arch Gen Psychiatry 51:199–214, 1994

Lahti AC, Koffel B, LaPorte D, et al: Subanesthetic doses of ketamine stimulate psychosis in schizophrenia. Neuropsychopharmacology 13:9–19, 1995

Layton D, Harris S, Wilton LV, et al: Comparison of incidence rates of cerebrovascular accidents and transient ischaemic attacks in observational cohort studies of patients prescribed risperidone, quetiapine or olanzapine in general practice in England including patients with dementia. J Psychopharmacol 19:473–482, 2005

Lecrubier Y, Quintin P, Bouhassira M, et al: The treatment of negative symptoms and deficit states of chronic schizophrenia: olanzapine compared to amisulpride and placebo in a 6-month double-blind controlled clinical trial. Acta Psychiatr Scand 114:319–327, 2006

Leucht S, Pitschel-Walz G, Abraham D, et al: Efficacy and extrapyramidal side-effects of the new antipsychotics olanzapine, quetiapine, risperidone, and sertindole compared to conventional antipsychotics and placebo: a meta-analysis of randomized controlled trials. Schizophr Res 35:51–68, 1999

Licht RW, Olesen OV, Friis P, et al: Olanzapine serum concentrations lowered by concomitant treatment with carbamazepine. J Clin Psychopharmacol 20:110–112, 2000

Lieberman JA, Stroup TS, McEvoy JP, et al: Effectiveness of antipsychotic drugs in patients with chronic schizophrenia. N Engl J Med 353:1209–1223, 2005

Lindenmayer JP, Patel R: Olanzapine-induced ketoacidosis with diabetes mellitus. Am J Psychiatry 156:1471, 1999

Lindenmayer JP, Khan A, Iskander A, et al: A randomized controlled trial of olanzapine versus haloperidol in the treatment of primary negative symptoms and neurocognitive deficits in schizophrenia. J Clin Psychiatry 68:368–379, 2007

Lucas RA, Gilfillan DJ, Bergstrom RF: A pharmacokinetic interaction between carbamazepine and olanzapine. Eur J Clin Pharmacol 54:639–643, 1998

Macias WL, Bergstrom RF, Cerimele BJ, et al: Lack of effect of olanzapine on the pharmacokinetics of a single aminophylline dose in healthy men. Pharmacotherapy 18:1237–1248, 1998

Maenpaa J, Wrighton S, Bergstrom R, et al: Pharmacokinetic (PK) and pharmacodynamic (PD) interactions between fluvoxamine and olanzapine (abstract). Clin Pharmacol Ther 61:225, 1997

Mamo D, Kapur S, Keshavan M, et al: D(2) Receptor occupancy of olanzapine pamoate depot using positron emission tomography: an open-label study in patients with schizophrenia. Neuropsychopharmacology 33:298–304, 2008

Marazziti D, Pfanner C, Dell'Osso B, et al: Augmentation strategy with olanzapine in resistant obsessive compulsive disorder: an Italian long-term open-label study. J Psychopharmacol 19:392–394, 2005

Markowitz JS, DeVane CL: Suspected ciprofloxacin inhibition of olanzapine resulting in increased plasma concentration. J Clin Psychopharmacol 19:289–291, 1999

Markowitz JS, Devane CL, Liston HL, et al: The effects of probenecid on the disposition of risperidone and olanzapine in healthy volunteers. Clin Pharmacol Ther 71:30–38, 2002

Markowitz JS, DeVane CL, Malcolm RJ, et al: Pharmacokinetics of olanzapine after single-dose oral administration of standard tablet versus normal and sublingual administration of an orally disintegrating tablet in normal volunteers. J Clin Pharmacol 46:164–171, 2006

McEvoy JP, Lieberman JA, Stroup TS, et al: Effectiveness of clozapine versus olanzapine, quetiapine, and risperidone in patients with chronic schizophrenia who did not respond to prior atypical antipsychotic treatment. Am J Psychiatry 163:600–610, 2006

McGlashan T, Zipursky RB, Perkins DO, et al: Olanzapine versus placebo treatment of the schizophrenia prodrome: one year results (abstract). Schizophr Res 60 (suppl):295, 2003

McGlashan TH, Zipursky RB, Perkins D, et al: Randomized, double-blind trial of olanzapine versus placebo in patients prodromally symptomatic for psychosis. Am J Psychiatry 163:790–799, 2006

Meehan K, Zhang F, David S, et al: A double-blind, randomized comparison of the efficacy and safety of intramuscular injections of olanzapine, lorazepam, or placebo in treating acutely agitated patients diagnosed with bipolar mania. J Clin Psychopharmacol 21:389–397, 2001

Meltzer HY, Matsubara S, Lee JC: Classification of typical and atypical antipsychotic drugs on the basis of dopamine D1, D2 and serotonin2 pKi values. J Pharmacol Exp Ther 251:238–246, 1989

Mitchell M, Riesenberg R, Bari MA, et al: A double-blind, randomized trial to evaluate the pharmacokinetics and tolerability of 30 or 40 mg/d oral olanzapine relative to 20 mg/d oral olanzapine in stable psychiatric subjects. Clin Ther 28:881–892, 2006

Mondraty N, Birmingham CL, Touyz S, et al: Randomized controlled trial of olanzapine in the treatment of cognitions in anorexia nervosa. Australas Psychiatry 13:72–75, 2005

Moore NA: Behavioural pharmacology of the new generation of antipsychotic agents. Br J Psychiatry 174 (suppl 138):5–11, 1999

Nemeroff CB, Youngblood WW, Manberg PJ, et al: Regional brain concentrations of neuropeptides in Huntington's chorea and schizophrenia. Science 221:972–975, 1983

Ninan I, Jardemark KE, Wang RY: Differential effects of atypical and typical antipsychotic drugs on N-methyl-D-aspartate- and electrically evoked responses in the pyramidal cells of the rat medial prefrontal cortex. Synapse 48:66–79, 2003a

Ninan I, Jardemark KE, Wang RY: Olanzapine and clozapine but not haloperidol reverse subchronic phencyclidine-induced functional hyperactivity of N-methyl-D-aspartate receptors in pyramidal cells of the rat medial prefrontal cortex. Neuropharmacology 44:462–472, 2003b

Onofrj M, Paci C, D'Andreamatteo G, et al: Olanzapine in severe Gilles de la Tourette syndrome: a 52-week double-blind crossover study vs low-dose pimozide. J Neurol 247:443–446, 2000

Patel BR, Kurtz DL, Callaghan JT, et al: Effects of smoking and gender on population pharmacokinetics of olanzapine (OL) in a phase III clinical trial (abstract). Pharm Res 13 (9, suppl): S408, 1996

Patel BR, Nyhart EH, Callaghan JT, et al: Combined population pharmacokinetic analysis of olanzapine in healthy volunteers (abstract). Pharm Res 12:S360, 1995

Patil ST, Zhang L, Martenyi F, et al: Activation of mGlu2/3 receptors as a new approach to treat schizophrenia: a randomized phase 2 clinical trial. Nat Med 13:1102–1107, 2007

Povlsen J, Noring U, Fog R: Tolerability and therapeutic effect of clozapine for up to 12 years. Acta Psychiatr Scand 7:176–185, 1985

Poyurovsky M, Pashinian A, Gil-Ad I, et al: Olanzapine-induced weight gain in patients with first-episode schizophrenia: a double-blind, placebo-controlled study of fluoxetine addition. Am J Psychiatry 159:1058–1060, 2002

Poyurovsky M, Isaacs I, Fuchs C, et al: Attenuation of olanzapine-induced weight gain with reboxetine in patients with schizophrenia: a double-blind, placebo-controlled study. Am J Psychiatry 160:297–302, 2003

Poyurovsky M, Tal V, Maayan R, et al: The effect of famotidine addition on olanzapine-induced weight gain in first-episode schizophrenia patients: a double-blind placebo-controlled pilot study. Eur Neuropsychopharmacol 14:332–336, 2004

Purdon SE, Jones BD, Stip E, et al: Neuropsychological change in early phase schizophrenia during 12 months of treatment with olanzapine, risperidone, or haloperidol. The Canadian Collaborative Group for Research in Schizophrenia. Arch Gen Psychiatry 57:249–258, 2000

Radke JM, Owens MJ, Ritchie JC, et al: Atypical antipsychotic drugs selectively increase neurotensin efflux in dopamine terminal regions. Proc Natl Acad Sci U S A 95:11462–11464, 1998

Ramaswamy K, Kozma CM, Nasrallah H: Risk of diabetic ketoacidosis after exposure to risperidone or olanzapine. Drug Saf 30:589–599, 2007

Ratzoni G, Gothelf D, Brand-Gothelf A, et al: Weight gain associated with olanzapine and risperidone in adolescent patients: a comparative prospective study. J Am Acad Child Adolesc Psychiatry 41:337–343, 2002

Reams S, Sanger TM, Beasley CM: Olanzapine in the treatment of elderly patients with schizophrenia and related psychotic disorders. Schizophr Res 29:151–152, 1998

Ring BJ, Binkley SN, Vandenbranden M, et al: In vitro interaction of the antipsychotic agent olanzapine with human cytochromes P450 CYP2C9, CYP2C19, CYP2D6 and CYP3A. Br J Clin Pharmacol 41:181–186, 1996a

Ring BJ, Catlow J, Lindsay TJ, et al: Identification of the human cytochromes P450 responsible for the in vitro formation of the major oxidative metabolites of the antipsychotic agent olanzapine. J Pharmacol Exp Ther 276:658–666, 1996b

Robertson GS, Fibiger HC: Effects of olanzapine on regional c-fos expression in rat forebrain. Neuropsychopharmacology 14:105–110, 1996

Rosenbohm A, Bux CJ, Connemann BJ: Psychosis with sibutramine. J Clin Psychopharmacol 27:315–317, 2007

Rosenheck R, Perlick D, Bingham S, et al: Effectiveness and cost of olanzapine and haloperidol in the treatment of schizophrenia: a randomized controlled trial. Department of Veterans Affairs Cooperative Study Group on the Cost-Effectiveness of Olanzapine. JAMA 290:2693–2702, 2003

Rosenheck RA, Leslie DL, Sindelar J, et al: Cost-effectiveness of second-generation antipsychotics and perphenazine in a randomized trial of treatment for chronic schizophrenia. Am J Psychiatry 163:2080–2089, 2006

Sanger T, Grundy S, Gibson PJ, et al: Long-term olanzapine therapy in the treatment of bipolar I disorder: an open-label continuation phase study. J Clin Psychiatry 62:273–281, 2001

Schatzberg AF: New approaches to managing psychotic depression. J Clin Psychiatry 64 (suppl 1):19–23, 2003

Schneider LS, Dagerman K, Insel PS: Efficacy and adverse effects of atypical antipsychotics for dementia: meta-analysis of randomized, placebo-controlled trials. Am J Geriatr Psychiatry 14:191–210, 2006a

Schneider LS, Tariot PN, Dagerman KS, et al: Effectiveness of atypical antipsychotic drugs in patients with Alzheimer's disease. N Engl J Med 355:1525–1538, 2006b

Schulz SC: Pharmacologic treatment of schizophrenia. Psychiatr Clin North Am 6:51–71, 1999

Schulz SC, Camlin KL, Berry SA, et al: Olanzapine safety and efficacy in patients with borderline personality disorder and comorbid dysthymia. Biol Psychiatry 46:1429–1435, 1999

Seeman P: Atypical antipsychotics: mechanism of action. Can J Psychiatry 47:27–38, 2002

Sernyak M, Leslie DL, Alarcon RD, et al: Association of diabetes mellitus with use of atypical neuroleptics in the treatment of schizophrenia. Am J Psychiatry 159:561–566, 2002

Shapira NA, Ward HE, Mandoki M, et al: A double-blind, placebo-controlled trial of olanzapine addition in fluoxetine-refractory obsessive-compulsive disorder. Biol Psychiatry 55:553–555, 2004

Shaw P, Sporn A, Gogtay N, et al: Childhood-onset schizophrenia: a double-blind, randomized clozapine-olanzapine comparison. Arch Gen Psychiatry 63:721–730, 2006

Shelton RC, Tollefson GD, Tohen M, et al: A novel augmentation strategy for treating resistant major depression. Am J Psychiatry 158:131–134, 2001

Shi L, Namjoshi MA, Swindle R, et al: Effects of olanzapine alone and olanzapine/fluoxetine combination on health-related quality of life in patients with bipolar depression: secondary analyses of a double-blind, placebo-controlled, randomized clinical trial. Clin Ther 26:125–134, 2004

Shopsin B, Klein H, Aaronsom M, et al: Clozapine, chlorpromazine, and placebo in newly hospitalized, acutely schizophrenic patients: a controlled, double-blind comparison. Arch Gen Psychiatry 36:657–664, 1979

Sikich L, Hamer RM, Bashford RA, et al: A pilot study of risperidone, olanzapine, and haloperidol in psychotic youth: a double-blind, randomized, 8-week trial. Neuropsychopharmacology 29:133–145, 2004

Siris S, Pollack S, Bermanzohn P, et al: Adjunctive imipramine for a broader group of post-psychotic depressions in schizophrenia. Schizophr Res 44:187–192, 2000

Soler J, Pascual JC, Campins J, et al: Double-blind, placebo-controlled study of dialectical behavior therapy plus olanzapine for borderline personality disorder. Am J Psychiatry 162:1221–1224, 2005

Soloff P, George A, Nathan RS, et al: Progress in pharmacotherapy of borderline disorders. Arch Gen Psychiatry 43:691–697, 1986

Spiker DG, Weiss JC, Dealy RS, et al: The pharmacological treatment of delusional depression. Am J Psychiatry 142:430–436, 1985

Stein MB, Kline NA, Matloff JL: Adjunctive olanzapine for SSRI-resistant combat-related PTSD: a double-blind, placebo-controlled study. Am J Psychiatry 159:1777–1779, 2002

Stephenson C, Pilowsky LS: Psychopharmacology of olanzapine: a review. Br J Psychiatry 174 (suppl 38):52–58, 1999

Stockton ME, Rasmussen K: Electrophysiological effects of olanzapine, a novel atypical antipsychotic, on A9 and A10 dopamine neurons. Neuropsychopharmacology 14:97–105, 1996a

Stockton ME, Rasmussen K: Olanzapine, a novel atypical antipsychotic, reverses d-amphetamine-induced inhibition of midbrain dopamine cells. Psychopharmacology 124:50–56, 1996b

Street JS, Clark WS, Gannon KS, et al: Olanzapine treatment of psychotic and behavioral symptoms in patients with Alzheimer disease in nursing care facilities: a double-blind, randomized, placebo-controlled trial. The HGEU Study Group. Arch Gen Psychiatry 57:968–976, 2000

Street JS, Clark WS, Kadam DL, et al: Long-term efficacy of olanzapine in the control of psychotic and behavioral symptoms in nursing home patients with Alzheimer's dementia. Int J Geriatr Psychiatry 16 (suppl 1):S62–S70, 2001

Swartz MS, Perkins DO, Stroup TS, et al: Effects of antipsychotic medications on psychosocial functioning in patients with chronic schizophrenia: findings from the NIMH CATIE study. Am J Psychiatry 164:428–436, 2007

Taflinski T, Chojnacka J: Sibutramine-associated psychotic episode. Am J Psychiatry 157:2057–2058, 2000

Tauscher J, Kufferle B, Asenbaum S, et al: In vivo 123I IBZM SPECT imaging of striatal dopamine-2 receptor occupancy in schizophrenic patients treated with olanzapine in comparison to clozapine and haloperidol. Psychopharmacology (Berl) 141:175–181, 1999

Thase ME, Corya SA, Osuntokun O, et al: A randomized, double-blind comparison of olanzapine/fluoxetine combination, olanzapine, and fluoxetine in treatment-resistant major depressive disorder. J Clin Psychiatry 68:224–236, 2007

Tohen M, Sanger TM, McElroy SL, et al: Olanzapine versus placebo in the treatment of acute mania. Olanzapine HGEH Study Group. Am J Psychiatry 156:702–709, 1999

Tohen M, Jacobs TG, Grundy SL, et al: Efficacy of olanzapine in acute bipolar mania: a double-blind, placebo-controlled study. The Olanzapine HGGW Study Group. Arch Gen Psychiatry 57:841–849, 2000

Tohen M, Baker RW, Altshuler LL, et al: Olanzapine versus divalproex in the treatment of acute mania. Am J Psychiatry 159:1011–1017, 2002

Tohen M, Vieta E, Calabrese J, et al: Efficacy of olanzapine and olanzapine-fluoxetine combination in the treatment of bipolar I depression. Arch Gen Psychiatry 60:1079–1088, 2003

Tohen M, Greil W, Calabrese JR, et al: Olanzapine versus lithium in the maintenance treatment of bipolar disorder: a 12-month, randomized, double-blind, controlled clinical trial. Am J Psychiatry 162:1281–1290, 2005

Tollefson GD, Sanger TM: Negative symptoms: a path analytic approach to a double-blind, placebo- and haloperidol-controlled clinical trial with olanzapine. Am J Psychiatry 154:466–474, 1997

Tollefson GD, Beasley CM Jr, Tran PV, et al: Olanzapine versus haloperidol in the treatment of schizophrenia and schizoaffective and schizophreniform disorders: results of an international collaborative trial. Am J Psychiatry 154:457–465, 1997

Tollefson GD, Sanger TM, Beasley CM, et al: A double-blind, controlled comparison of the novel antipsychotic olanzapine vs haloperidol or placebo on anxious and depressive symptoms accompanying schizophrenia. Biol Psychiatry 43:803–810, 1998a

Tollefson GD, Sanger TM, Lu Y, et al: Depressive signs and symptoms in schizophrenia: a prospective blinded trial of olanzapine and haloperidol. Arch Gen Psychiatry 55:250–258, 1998b

Tollefson GD, Birkett MA, Kiesler GM, et al: Double-blind comparison of olanzapine versus clozapine in schizophrenic patients clinically eligible for treatment with clozapine. Biol Psychiatry 49:52–63, 2001

Torgersen S, Kringlen E, Cramer V: The prevalence of personality disorders in a community sample. Arch Gen Psychiatry 58:590–596, 2001

Tran PV, Tollefson GD, Sanger TM, et al: Olanzapine versus haloperidol in the treatment of schizoaffective disorder: acute and long-term therapy. Br J Psychiatry 174:15–22, 1999

Van den Eynde F, Naudts KH, De Saedeleer S, et al: Olanzapine in Gilles de la Tourette syndrome: beyond tics. Acta Neurol Belg 105:206–211, 2005

Volavka J, Czobor P, Sheitman B, et al: Clozapine, olanzapine, risperidone, and haloperidol in the treatment of patients with chronic schizophrenia and schizoaffective disorder. Am J Psychiatry 159:255–262, 2002

Weigmann H, Gerek S, Zeisig A, et al: Fluvoxamine but not sertraline inhibits the metabolism of olanzapine: evidence from a therapeutic drug monitoring service. Ther Drug Monit 23:410–413, 2001

Weinberger DR: Implications of normal brain development for the pathogenesis of schizophrenia. Arch Gen Psychiatry 44:660–669, 1987

Zacher JL, Roche-Desilets J: Hypotension secondary to the combination of intramuscular olanzapine and intramuscular lorazepam. J Clin Psychiatry 66:1614–1615, 2005

Zajecka JM, Weisler R, Sachs G, et al: A comparison of the efficacy, safety, and tolerability of divalproex sodium and olanzapine in the treatment of bipolar disorder. J Clin Psychiatry 63:1148–1155, 2002

Zanarini MC, Frankenburg FR: Olanzapine treatment of female borderline personality disorder patients: a double-blind, placebo-controlled pilot study. J Clin Psychiatry 62:849–854, 2001

Zanarini MC, Frankenburg FR, Parachini EA: A preliminary, randomized trial of fluoxetine, olanzapine, and the olanzapine-fluoxetine combination in women with borderline personality disorder. J Clin Psychiatry 65:903–907, 2004

CHAPTER 30

Quetiapine

Peter F. Buckley, M.D.
Adriana E. Foster, M.D.

History and Discovery

Quetiapine is a second-generation antipsychotic (SGA) developed and subsequently marketed by AstraZeneca. In preclinical trials, quetiapine showed both the features associated with antipsychotic efficacy and a low rate of motor effects (Goldstein 1999; Nemeroff et al. 2002). The Phase III placebo-controlled clinical trials necessary for product registration confirmed this preclinical impression and demonstrated that quetiapine was efficacious in treating the manifestations of psychosis (Arvanitis and Miller 1997; Small et al. 1997). Of note, these studies also reported a low rate of treatment-emergent extrapyramidal side effects (EPS) with quetiapine use across a wide range of dosages that was comparable to the rate among placebo recipients. Quetiapine was approved in 1997 by the U.S. Food and Drug Administration (FDA) for the treatment of schizophrenia. Approval for use in Europe and in other countries worldwide has followed. Further clinical trials in patients with mania (McIntyre et al. 2005; Vieta et al. 2005) and patients with bipolar depression (Calabrese et al. 2005; Thase et al. 2006) led the FDA to approve additional indications for quetiapine's use in the acute and maintenance treatment of bipolar disorder. Most recently, the FDA has also approved a slow-release formulation of quetiapine for the treatment of schizophrenia (Kahn et al. 2007; Möller et al. 2007; Peuskens et al. 2007). Quetiapine is an established antipsychotic with broad efficacy and good tolerability, particularly with respect to EPS (Miodownik and Lerner 2006).

Structure–Activity Relations

Quetiapine is an SGA of the dibenzothiazepine class. It has a complex neuropharmacology, with binding at brain receptors of several classes (Goldstein 1999). Its binding profile, in comparison with that of several other antipsychotics, is shown in Table 30–1. Of considerable interest is the fact that quetiapine has a relatively low binding profile for dopamine type 2 (D_2) receptors (Kapur et al. 2000a, 2000b; Kufferle et al. 1997; Seeman and Tallerico 1998; Stephenson et al. 2000). Indeed, considering the idea that an antipsychotic needs to occupy 60% or more of D_2 receptors in order to be clinically efficacious (Kapur et al. 2000b), quetiapine's low D_2 binding—typically approximately 30%—is noteworthy.

In attempting to reconcile this apparently subtherapeutic D_2 receptor antagonism with the well-recorded efficacy of quetiapine as an antipsychotic, Kapur and colleagues proposed an elegant *kiss and run hypothesis* for quetiapine's mechanisms of action (Kapur et al. 2000a). In a series of studies, they found that when D_2 receptor occupancy with quetiapine was measured with positron emission tomography (PET) at shorter intervals (4 hours and 6 hours) than the conventional 12 hours after the last dose was taken, quetiapine did indeed show high D_2 occupancy. They found that in contrast to other antipsychotics, quetiapine had a more rapid "run-off" from D_2 receptors; that is, there was rapid dissociation of the D_2 receptors (Kapur et al. 2000a). This was proposed to account for the discrepancy between observations of clinical potency and pharmacodynamic subthreshold receptor

TABLE 30–1. Comparative receptor binding profile of quetiapine[a]

	QUETIAPINE[a]	ZIPRASIDONE[a]	RISPERIDONE[a]	OLANZAPINE[a]	CLOZAPINE[a]	ARIPIPRAZOLE[b]
D_2	+	+++	+++	++	+	+++[b]
$5\text{-}HT_{2A}$	+	+++	++++	+++	+++	+++
$5\text{-}HT_{2C}$	−	++++	+++	+++	++	++
$5\text{-}HT_{1A}$	+	+++[b]	+	−	+	+++[b]
$5\text{-}HT_{1D}$[c]	−	+++	+	+	−	−
α_1-adrenergic	++	++	+++	++	+++	++
M_1	++	−	−	+++	+++	−
H_1	+++	++	++	+++	+++	++
$5\text{-}HT$/NE reuptake[d]						
$5\text{-}HT$	−	++	−	−	−	++
NE	+	+	−	−	+	−

Note.   ++++ = Very high affinity; +++ = high affinity; ++ = moderate affinity; + = low affinity; − = negligible affinity; D_2 = dopamine type 2 receptors; H_1 = histaminergic type 1 receptors; $5\text{-}HT$ = 5-hydroxytryptamine (serotonin); $5\text{-}HT_{2A}$ = serotonin type 2A receptors; M_1 = muscarinic type 1 receptors; NE = norepinephrine.
[a]All information from human studies unless noted otherwise.
[b]Partial agonist.
[c]Bovine binding affinity.
[d]In rat synaptosomes.

Source.   Schmidt AW, Lebel LA, Howard HR Jr, et al: "Ziprasidone: A Novel Antipsychotic Agent With a Unique Human Receptor Binding Profile." *European Journal of Pharmacology* 425:197–201, 2001. Otsuka Pharmaceutical Co: Abilify (aripiprazole) full prescribing information. August 2008.

binding. This kiss-and-run theory is also put forward to explain the consistent observation of low rates of EPS and lack of increased prolactin levels during treatment with quetiapine (Nemeroff et al. 2002).

Quetiapine also, like clozapine, has strong binding at 5-hydroxytryptamine (serotonin) type 2 receptors (5-HT$_2$ receptors). This profile contrasts with its relatively weak affinity for other subclasses of the serotonin receptor family (Goldstein 1999). Quetiapine also has strong affinity for α_1-noradrenergic receptors. This antagonism may relate to its propensity to induce postural hypotension—especially during rapid dose titration. Additionally, quetiapine has strong antagonism at histamine type 1 (H$_1$) receptors. This most likely relates to its sedative effect. Weight gain during quetiapine therapy may also emanate from H$_1$ receptor antagonism. However, this structure–activity relationship is less clear than the association between H$_1$ antagonism and sedation.

Relatively less is known about quetiapine's effects on other aspects of neurochemistry that are thought to be of relevance (but not central) to antipsychotic activity. Some studies have shown that SGAs can induce brain cell proliferation (*neurogenesis*) in experimental animals (Lieberman et al. 2006). The evidence for quetiapine in this regard is sparse. Also, little is known about the effect of quetiapine on brain neurotrophins. One study (Xu et al. 2002) reported that quetiapine could reverse reductions in levels of brain-derived neurotrophic factor in an animal model. There is accumulating evidence that other SGAs may also increase brain neurotrophins (Buckley et al. 2007).

Pharmacokinetics and Disposition

Quetiapine is absorbed in the gastrointestinal tract, and its absorption is unaffected by food. Peak blood levels are achieved in about 2 hours, and effective plasma levels are sustained for approximately 6 hours (DeVane and Nemeroff 2001). This provides the basis for the usual clinical regimen of twice-daily dosing. However, Chengappa et al. (2003b) conducted a short-term trial comparing once-daily dosing versus twice-daily dosing in patients with schizophrenia or schizoaffective disorder. The dosing profiles were equivalent in terms of efficacy and tolerability. Using PET, Mamo et al. (2008) found comparable plasma levels and D$_2$ receptor occupancy between the immediate-release and the extended-release formulation.

Quetiapine is metabolized by cytochrome P450 (CYP) 3A4 to inactive metabolites. Although genetic variations are not clearly described for the CYP3A4 enzyme, drug interactions with inhibitors and inducers of CYP3A4 are likely to be clinically significant. The anticonvulsants carbamazepine and phenytoin are common examples of CYP3A4 inducers, and in their presence quetiapine doses may need to be increased due to accelerated drug clearance (Potkin et al. 2002a, 2002b; Strakowski et al. 2002). Ritonavir, erythromycin, ketoconazole, and nefazodone are potent inhibitors of CYP3A4, and their use requires caution when they are coadministered with quetiapine; while they are used, doses of quetiapine should be lowered (de Leon et al. 2005; Wong et al. 2001).

In 2007, the FDA approved an extended-release (XR) formulation of quetiapine for the treatment of schizophrenia on the basis of results from clinical trials (Kahn et al. 2007; Lindenmayer et al. 2008). These studies compared the efficacy and tolerability of XR and regular immediate-release (IR) formulations. Overall, the results of these studies indicate that quetiapine XR given once daily (at dosages of 400–800 mg/day) is effective for the treatment of schizophrenia. The XR formulation appears to have efficacy comparable to that of the IR formulation. The XR formulation was also similar in tolerability to the IR formulation in clinical trials, with perhaps some marginal benefit in causing less sedation. Quetiapine is excreted in the kidneys and is not affected by gender or smoking status (Thyrum et al. 2000). The metabolism of quetiapine is reduced by approximately 30% with advancing age (Goldstein 1999).

Indications and Efficacy

Quetiapine currently has the following FDA-approved indications:

- Schizophrenia
- Bipolar disorder

There are also reports of quetiapine's efficacy in treating other conditions, such as mood disorders in children and anxiety disorders, obsessive-compulsive disorder (OCD), and Parkinson's disease in adults. These uses have not been approved by the FDA. As a result of its use in the FDA indications and also in several unapproved circumstances, quetiapine is the most frequently prescribed antipsychotic in the United States at the time of writing. In this section of the chapter, we describe results of pivotal and recent studies of quetiapine for its FDA-approved indications. For completeness's sake and in recognition of quetiapine's use in nonapproved conditions, we also provide an account of some studies of subjects with other conditions. The use of any medication (in this case quetiapine) in situations that are not FDA-approved indications is not recommended for clinical practice.

Schizophrenia

The pivotal product registration trials and early trials of quetiapine (Arvanitis and Miller 1997; Borison et al. 1996; Copolov et al. 2000; King et al. 1998; Peuskens and Link 1997; Small et al. 1997) demonstrated that quetiapine is an efficacious antipsychotic for the treatment of schizophrenia. In the United States, short-term (6-week) trials compared quetiapine and placebo using quetiapine dosages of either 250 mg/day or 750 mg/day (Small et al. 1997) or daily dosages of 75 mg, 150 mg, 300 mg, or 750 mg (Arvanitis and Miller 1997); the latter trial also compared quetiapine and haloperidol. Similar to registration trials of other antipsychotics, these studies established a range of effective dosages for quetiapine. However, they provided no clear evidence of a dose-dependent increase in efficacy (although post hoc analyses have suggested that higher doses of quetiapine are more efficacious). Additionally, because of the wide range of dosages used in these studies, the initial dosing recommendations for quetiapine in schizophrenia patients were unclear and were further complicated by a slow titration pattern. As a result, clinicians tended to favor the lower end of the quetiapine dosing range.

Subsequent studies helped refine quetiapine dosing strategies. Clinicians are also now using higher doses of quetiapine that are, on average, more consistent with those used in recent studies. Emsley et al. (2000) conducted a fixed-dose comparison trial of quetiapine at 600 mg/day versus haloperidol at 20 mg/day. The drugs had similar efficacy in this 8-week trial of patients who were a priori deemed "partial responders." More recent studies have shown that the titration of quetiapine can be quicker than heretofore considered. Pae et al. (2007) compared a rapid titration strategy (beginning at 200 mg/day, increasing to 800 mg/day by day 4) with a more conventional dosing strategy (50 mg/day on day 1, up to 400 mg/day by day 5). The two groups fared equally well in terms of tolerability during this 14-day study. The higher-dose, more rapid titration strategy had a marginal advantage in overall efficacy. Information on the use of high dosages (>800 mg/day) of quetiapine is very limited. Pierre et al. (2005) reported on quetiapine's efficacy in a sample of treatment-

refractory schizophrenic patients at dosages of up to 1,200 mg/day. More fixed-dose comparison studies with quetiapine are needed to assist clinicians in further refining their dosing strategies with this agent.

Although two meta-analyses cast doubt on quetiapine's efficacy with respect to first-generation antipsychotics (FGAs; Davis et al. 2003; Geddes et al. 2000), most studies comparing quetiapine with haloperidol or chlorpromazine report that the agents have similar efficacy in treating schizophrenia (Emsley et al. 2000; Peuskens and Link 1997; Small et al. 1997). Given that today most clinicians in the United States select one of the SGAs, comparisons between quetiapine and other SGAs are perhaps more meaningful. Several studies have been published that inform this consideration. A 4-month open-label trial of quetiapine and risperidone in a heterogeneous patient population—although predominantly subjects with schizophrenia and related psychotic disorders—showed overall comparability between the two agents (Mullen et al. 2001). Zhong et al. (2006) reported on an 8-week comparative trial of quetiapine and risperidone in a chronic schizophrenia patient population. The average quetiapine dosage was 525 mg/day and the average risperidone dosage was 5.2 mg/day. The drugs proved similar in efficacy. Quetiapine-treated patients had fewer EPS, lower prolactin levels, and fewer sexual side effects. Weight gain was similar in both treatment groups. Quetiapine was more sedating and was more frequently associated with dry mouth than was risperidone. Another study comparing quetiapine and risperidone, a 6-month study, reported better efficacy with risperidone (Potkin et al. 2006). Quetiapine was associated with more polypharmacy in that study. Kinon et al. (2006) reported on a 6-month double-blind comparative trial of quetiapine and olanzapine. Quetiapine-treated patients were less likely to complete the study. Relapse rates were comparable overall in the two treatment groups. More weight gain occurred in olanzapine recipients. As yet, no studies have directly compared quetiapine with either ziprasidone or aripiprazole in the treatment of schizophrenia.

The most extensive comparative evaluation of quetiapine and other SGAs comes from the Clinical Antipsychotic Trials of Intervention Effectiveness (CATIE) schizophrenia studies. In the phase I study, in which the effectiveness of several antipsychotics was examined over 18 months, more quetiapine-treated patients than olanzapine-treated patients had discontinued treatment by 18 months (78% vs. 64%), and a similar (not statistically significant) trend was seen in comparisons of quetiapine versus risperidone, ziprasidone, or perphenazine (Lieberman et al. 2005). In the phase II study of efficacy pathways for patients with persistent symptoms, discontinuation rates favored clozapine and olanzapine over risperidone and quetiapine (McEvoy et al. 2006). The results from the tolerability pathways were more mixed, with similar efficacy observed between quetiapine and other agents (Stroup et al. 2007). The findings relating to quetiapine's relative adverse-effects profile in this formative study are presented later in this chapter (see "Side Effects and Toxicology"). Another interesting analysis from the CATIE schizophrenia studies (Stroup et al. 2007) examined how those patients originally assigned to the perphenazine arm of the phase I study fared. In this analysis, switching to quetiapine was more efficacious than switching to any of the other agents. Much of the efficacy and tolerability differences among agents observed in the CATIE schizophrenia studies have been attributed to differential dosing profiles.

An analogous comparative trial of quetiapine, risperidone, and olanzapine was conducted with patients experiencing their first episode of psychosis—the Comparison of Atypicals in First Episode Psychosis (CAFÉ) study. Here, discontinuation rates were similar with all three drugs over the course of the 1-year trial (McEvoy et al. 2007). The comparative dosing profiles for quetiapine, risperidone, and olanzapine in the CAFÉ study and the CATIE schizophrenia study, referenced against the FDA-approved dosages, are shown in Table 30–2.

The use of quetiapine in patients with prodromal features of schizophrenia has not yet been studied. Little is known about quetiapine's efficacy in treatment-refractory patients. In a subanalysis of more severely ill patients in an 8-week comparative trial of quetiapine and haloperidol, quetiapine showed a small benefit over haloperidol (Buckley et al. 2004). The open-label observational study by Pierre et al. (2005) also showed some benefit for quetiapine at high doses in treatment-refractory patients.

Sacchetti et al. (2004) reported a 50% response rate in a small sample of patients who had been refractory to prior treatment with FGAs.

Information on the long-term efficacy of quetiapine is limited. Open-label follow-up in extension studies for up to 4 years has shown sustained efficacy, with the average dosage of quetiapine recorded at 450 mg/day (Buckley et al. 2004). A recently conducted 6-month placebo-controlled study of quetiapine (the new XR formulation) in schizophrenia patients showed a clinically beneficial effect on relapse prevention (Peuskens et al. 2007). Several studies have demonstrated improvements in cognitive performance during quetiapine therapy in patients with schizophrenia (Sax et al. 1998; Velligan et al. 2002, 2003).

Mood Disorders

There is evidence that quetiapine is an effective and well-tolerated antipsychotic for treating patients with bipolar mania and bipolar depression. Initial evidence for mood effects were derived from observations on mood assessment items in the pivotal schizophrenia trials. In one of the pivotal product registration trials evaluating quetiapine (Small et al. 1997), both high and low doses of quetiapine were significantly better than placebo in improving Brief Psychiatric Rating Scale (BPRS) measures of mood disturbance in patients with schizophrenia (Goldstein 1999). In an analysis of another pivotal trial comparing five dosages of quetiapine in patients with schizophrenia (Arvanitis and Miller 1997), patients receiving 150 mg/day showed significant improvement in BPRS-derived measures of mood. In the Quetiapine Experience with Safety and Tolerability (QUEST) study, quetiapine was compared with risperidone in a 4-month open-label, flexible-dose trial (Mullen et al. 2001). This study included patients with schizophrenia, schizoaffective disor-

TABLE 30–2. Antipsychotic dosages used in CATIE and CAFÉ studies versus FDA-approved dosages: quetiapine, olanzapine, and risperidone

	CATIE (CHRONIC) MEAN MODAL DOSAGE (MG/DAY)	CAFÉ (FIRST EPISODE) MEAN MODAL DOSAGE (MG/DAY)	FDA-APPROVED DOSAGE RANGE (MG/DAY)
Olanzapine	20.1	11.7	5–20
Risperidone	3.9	2.4	1–16
Quetiapine	543.4	506.0	25–800

Higher dosages may be required to achieve efficacy in chronic versus first-episode schizophrenia.

Note. CAFÉ = Comparison of Atypicals in First Episode Psychosis; CATIE = Clinical Antipsychotic Trials of Intervention Effectiveness; FDA = U.S. Food and Drug Administration.

Source. Data derived from McEvoy et al. 2007 (CAFÉ) and Lieberman et al. 2005 (CATIE).

der, bipolar disorder, and depression. At week 16 the mean dosage of quetiapine was 317 mg/day, and the mean dosage of risperidone was 4.5 mg/day. Mean improvement on the Hamilton Rating Scale for Depression was significantly greater in quetiapine recipients than in risperidone recipients.

More recent studies have confirmed that quetiapine is efficacious for the acute treatment of mania and bipolar depression. In short-term placebo-controlled trials, quetiapine as a monotherapy reduced symptoms of mania. Quetiapine has also been assessed as an add-on agent with either lithium or valproic acid. Calabrese et al. (2005) and Thase et al. (2006) have studied quetiapine in patients with bipolar depression. In an 8-week trial, Calabrese et al. (2005) compared two dosages of quetiapine (300 mg/day and 600 mg/day) versus placebo. Both dosages were efficacious, with improvements observed across the full range of depressive and anxiety symptoms. Fifty-eight percent of patients met a priori criteria for treatment response. Additionally, this antidepressant effect was observed with a once-daily dosage regimen. In a subsequent similar study of the same two dosages (300 mg/day and 600 mg/day; Thase et al. 2006), quetiapine was again compared with placebo in an 8-week trial in patients with bipolar depression. Again, both dosages of quetiapine showed efficacy across a broad range of depressive symptoms. These two studies led to FDA approval of quetiapine for treating bipolar depression. Furthermore, Dorée et al. (2007) recently reported that in a pilot study ($n=20$) quetiapine was an efficacious augmenting agent for major depression. There is also emerging information that quetiapine's metabolite may have mood-regulating effects (Goldstein et al. 2007).

Other Conditions and Patient Populations

The two studies on bipolar depression cited above (Calabrese et al. 2005; Thase et al. 2006) also showed improvements in anxiety symptoms with quetiapine. Additionally, the sedative/calming effect of quetiapine is well described in a variety of product registration trials (Buckley et al. 2007; Chengappa et al. 2003a). Thus, there is interest in whether quetiapine may be helpful in treating anxiety states, and off-label use of quetiapine in patients with anxiety disorders has been reported. This is a complicated issue. A clinical trial of quetiapine to treat anxiety disorders is ongoing (www.clinicaltrials.gov). There is also published information from a small study showing that quetiapine reduces symptoms of both anxiety and posttraumatic stress disorder (Hamner et al. 2003).

Information has also been published on the use of quetiapine as an augmenting agent with selective serotonin reuptake inhibitors in treating OCD (Dell'Osso et al. 2006; Denys et al. 2007). Dell'Osso et al. (2006) showed that quetiapine provided benefit in a small case series of patients with OCD. Denys et al. (2007) analyzed published augmentation studies in OCD patients and found that quetiapine augmentation was efficacious and, interestingly, was more efficacious in patients who were receiving lower doses of a selective serotonin reuptake inhibitor (SSRI) than in those receiving higher SSRI doses.

Quetiapine appears to be an effective treatment for children with schizophrenia or bipolar disorder (Barzman et al. 2006; DelBello et al. 2007; McConville et al. 2000). DelBello et al. (2007) recently reported therapeutic effects of quetiapine in a cohort of children who showed subsyndromal symptoms and were at risk for bipolar disorder but who did not actually meet diagnostic threshold criteria for a bipolar diagnosis. Quetiapine is also used more broadly for treating agitation in children (Findling et al. 2007).

Quetiapine has also been used in elderly populations. McManus et al. (1999) reported baseline and 12-week data for 151 elderly patients (mean age, 76.8 years) who were treated in a 1-year open-label trial of quetiapine. Seventy percent of patients had some organic condition, predominantly Alzheimer's disease, with the majority of remaining patients having a diagnosis of a functional psychosis such as schizophrenia, schizoaffective disorder, or delusional disorder. Fifty-two percent of all patients achieved a 20% or greater decline in BPRS total score. Quetiapine was well tolerated at a mean dosage of 100 mg/day. Zhong et al. (2007) reported a 10-week study comparing two dosages of quetiapine (100 mg/day and 200 mg/day) versus placebo in nursing home residents with dementia and agitation. Quetiapine at 100 mg/day was not efficacious, whereas quetiapine at 200 mg/day was efficacious for treating agitation. Quetiapine (100 mg/day) was also compared with risperidone (1.0 mg/day), olanzapine (5.5 mg/day), and placebo over 36 weeks in the CATIE Alzheimer's disease study (Schneider et al. 2006). This is the largest comparative study to date of the relative efficacy and tolerability of antipsychotics in elderly patients with Alzheimer's disease and related dementias. Overall, no effect was seen with any of the agents, and no differences were seen between the agents in terms of time to discontinuation of treatment for any reason.

Several neuropsychiatric conditions, the most notable being Parkinson's disease, are associated with the emergence of transient or sometimes persistent psychotic symptoms (Juncos 1999). The management of Parkinson's disease is further complicated by hallucinations associated with levodopa therapy. Older antipsychotics were effective in relieving psychotic symptoms in these patients, but their use also aggravated the disease. Quetiapine may be a preferred treatment in patients with Parkinson's disease (Friedman 2003; Friedman et al. 1998; Juncos 1999; Targum and Abbott 2000). In a 24-week study of quetiapine in 29 patients with Parkinson's disease (mean age, 73 years), Juncos (1999) observed that treatment with quetiapine at a mean dosage of 62.5 mg/day improved psychosis without causing deterioration in motor function. Menza et al. (1999) reported similar results using quetiapine at dosages of 12.5–150 mg/day in three patients with Parkinson's disease whose medication was switched from clozapine to quetiapine. In another study, 25 patients with Parkinson's disease were switched from either clozapine or olanzapine to quetiapine; 17 (68%) of the patients were switched to quetiapine without a worsening of psychosis (Friedman et al. 1998). Targum and Abbott (2000) reported that quetiapine stopped visual hallucinations in 6 of 10 patients with Parkinson's disease, but delusions were less responsive to treatment. In a study by Merims et al. (2006), both clozapine and quetiapine showed efficacy in treating psychosis in Parkinson's disease patients. Clozapine was marginally more efficacious but was associated with a high adverse-effect burden.

Agitation is a core aspect of several conditions. There is, of course, no FDA-approved drug for treating agitation, and use of antipsychotics for nonapproved clinical indications is strongly discouraged. Nevertheless, antipsychotics have been used to manage agitation in a variety of circumstances. Currier et al. (2006) reported an interesting study of quetiapine in agitated patients in the emergency room. Here, Currier and colleagues reported that quetiapine could be used as an acute antiagitation agent if the dose titration is judicious. Postural hypotension was observed in this study. Other studies of quetiapine and agitation reflect post hoc analyses of clinical trials and report benefits in treating hostility both in adults with schizophrenia (Chengappa et al. 2003a) or bipolar disorder (Buckley et al. 2007) and in children with conditions associated with disruptive, hostile behaviors (Barzman et al. 2006; Findling et al. 2007).

Side Effects and Toxicology

To illustrate the profile of adverse effects that are typically seen with quetiapine, we have reproduced herein the results from a recent clinical trial of 8 weeks' duration (Zhong et al. 2006) in which schizophrenic patients received an average quetiapine dosage of 525 mg/day (Table 30–3). Overall, quetiapine was well tolerated in this study, and only 6% of patients discontinued treatment due to adverse effects. The most commonly recorded side effects of quetiapine treatment in this study were somnolence (26% of patients), headache (15%), weight gain (14%), dizziness (14%), and dry mouth (12%).

Somnolence is a common side effect of quetiapine that most likely relates to its antihistaminergic effects. It occurs early in treatment and generally decreases over time. It may persist in some patients, however. It may also cause patients to stop taking their medication, because sedation is generally a poorly tolerated side effect. In the bipolar depression study by Calabrese et al. (2005), somnolence was observed in 24% of patients receiving quetiapine at a dosage of 300 mg/day and in 27% of patients receiving 600 mg/day. Dizziness is another troublesome side effect when it occurs. It may be associated with postural hypotension—an effect that is of even greater concern. Sometimes, like sedation, this can cause discontinuation of quetiapine therapy.

There is growing concern about antipsychotic-induced weight gain and metabolic disturbances (Allison et al. 1999; Brooke et al. 2009; Newcomer et al. 2002). Quetiapine is associated with weight gain, although current evidence indicates that neither the frequency nor the magnitude of the weight gain effect is as great as that seen with clozapine or olanzapine. On the other hand, the weight-effects profile of quetiapine is not as favorable as that of either ziprasidone or aripiprazole (Brooke et al. 2009). The lack of data on long-term maintenance treatment with quetiapine makes it hard to quantify its weight-effects liability with robust objectivity over the course of illness (Brooke et al. 2009).

In a report of open-label extension studies of patients with schizophrenia who continued taking quetiapine for up to 18 months, patients experienced on average a 1.74-kg increase over their baseline weight (Brecher et al. 2000). Weight gain was most pronounced—and, conversely, least pronounced—in those who were underweight and markedly obese, respectively. This is consistent with a lower body mass index being a predictor for weight gain in genetic studies of weight gain in schizophrenic patients (Müller and Kennedy 2006). In the 8-week comparative study by Zhong et al. (2006), weight gain that was clinically significant (a 7.7% increase above baseline weight) was observed in 10.4% of patients receiving quetiapine and in 10.5% of patients receiving ris-

TABLE 30–3. Comparative side-effect profile of quetiapine versus risperidone: adverse effects present in ≥5% of patients in an 8-week study

ADVERSE EFFECT	QUETIAPINE (N=338; MEDIAN DOSAGE, 525 MG/DAY)	RISPERIDONE (N=334; MEDIAN DOSAGE, = 5.2 MG/DAY)	P VALUE[a]
	N (%)	N (%)	
Somnolence	89 (26.3)	66 (19.7)	0.044
Headache	51 (15.1)	56 (16.7)	0.599
Weight gain	48 (14.2)	45 (13.4)	0.824
Dizziness	48 (14.2)	32 (9.6)	0.0737
Dry mouth	41 (12.1)	17 (5.1)	<0.01
Dyspepsia	22 (6.5)	26 (7.8)	0.552
Nausea	21 (6.2)	22 (6.6)	0.876
Pain	21 (6.2)	24 (7.2)	0.536
Asthenia	17 (5.0)	14 (4.2)	0.714
Agitation	17 (5.0)	10 (3.0)	0.238
Pharyngitis	15 (4.4)	24 (7.2)	0.140
Akathisia	13 (3.8)	28 (8.4)	0.016
Vomiting	13 (3.8)	18 (5.4)	0.364
Dystonia	1 (0.3)	18 (5.4)	<0.001

[a]Fisher exact test, unadjusted.

Source.   Adapted from Zhong KX, Sweitzer DE, Hamer RM, et al: "Comparison of Quetiapine and Risperidone in the Treatment of Schizophrenia: A Randomized, Double-Blind, Flexible-Dose, 8-Week Study." *Journal of Clinical Psychiatry* 67:1093–1103, 2006.

peridone. The average weight gain was 1.6 kg for quetiapine recipients and 2.12 kg for risperidone recipients. In the phase I CATIE schizophrenia study, quetiapine had a moderate effect on weight (and other aspects of the metabolic profile) compared with the other agents in that major study (Lieberman et al. 2005). Those data are shown in Table 30–4. In the first-episode CAFÉ study, quetiapine had a more favorable weight-effects profile than did olanzapine or risperidone. Fifty percent of patients taking quetiapine gained weight, compared with 80% of those taking olanzapine and 58% of those taking risperidone. Interestingly, females taking quetiapine were less likely than males to gain weight in this 1-year study of patients treated for their first episode of psychosis (J.K. Patel, P.F. Buckley, S. Woolson, et al., "Metabolic Profiles of Second-Generation Antipsychotics in Early Psychosis: Findings From the CAFE Study" (submitted for publication), October 2008). It is also important to consider quetiapine's propensity to induce weight gain among bipolar patients (especially because these patients may also be taking lithium or valproic acid). In the BOLDER (BipOLar DEpRession) study of patients with bipolar depression

(Calabrese et al. 2005), 9% of patients receiving quetiapine at a dosage of 600 mg/day and 8.5% of patients receiving 300 mg/day had a 7% or greater increase in weight. The average weight gains for quetiapine-treated patients in this study were 1.6 kg and 1.0 kg for the 600-mg/day and 300-mg/day groups, respectively.

We have less information on other aspects of quetiapine's metabolic effects, in part because only recently conducted studies have included careful measurements of fasting glucose and lipid levels. In the bipolar depression study by Calabrese et al. (2005), the mean increases in glucose levels at study endpoint were 6 mg/dL and 3 mg/dL with quetiapine dosages of 600 mg/day and 300 mg/day, respectively. In the comparative study of quetiapine and risperidone in the treatment of schizophrenia (Zhong et al. 2006), the mean increases in fasting glucose levels from baseline to study endpoint were 1.8 mg/dL with quetiapine and 5.6 mg/dL with risperidone. The metabolic profile of quetiapine appeared moderate in the phase I CATIE schizophrenia study (see Table 30–4). Meyer and Stahl (2009) examined the biology of and reviewed the available data concerning distinct metabolic

TABLE 30–4. Comparative metabolic profiles of antipsychotics in the phase I CATIE schizophrenia trial: change from baseline

	OLANZAPINE	QUETIAPINE	PERPHENAZINE	RISPERIDONE	ZIPRASIDONE	P VALUE
Weight gain >7%, n/total N (%)	92/307 (30)	49/305 (16)	29/243 (12)	42/300 (14)	12/161 (7)	<0.001
Weight change (lb), mean±SE	9.4±0.9	1.1±0.9	−2.0±1.1	0.8±0.9	−1.6±1.1	<0.001
Blood glucose change (mg/dL), exposure-adjusted mean±SE	13.7±2.5	7.5±2.5	5.4±2.8	6.6±2.5	2.9±3.4	0.59
Glycosylated Hb (%), exposure-adjusted mean±SE	0.40±0.07	0.04±0.08	0.09±0.09	0.07±0.08	0.11±0.09	0.01
Cholesterol (mg/dL), exposure-adjusted mean±SE	9.4±2.4	6.6±2.4	1.5±2.7	−1.3±2.4	−8.2±3.2	<0.001
Triglycerides (mg/dL), exposure-adjusted mean±SE	40.5±8.9	21.2±9.2	9.2±10.1	−2.4±9.1	−16.5±12.2	<0.001

Note. Hb = hemoglobin; SE = standard error.

P values for laboratory values and for the change in weight are based on ranked analysis of covariance with adjustment for whether patient had an exacerbation in the preceding 3 months and the duration of exposure to the study drug in phase I. Mean values for metabolic factors (other than weight change) were also adjusted for duration of exposure to study drug.

Source. Adapted from Lieberman JA, Stroup TS, McEvoy JP, et al, Clinical Antipsychotic Trials of Intervention Effectiveness (CATIE) Investigators: "Effectiveness of Antipsychotic Drugs in Patients With Chronic Schizophrenia." *New England Journal of Medicine* 353:1209–1223, 2005.

profiles in the context of antipsychotic therapy. New-comer et al. (2009) have presented data from a euglyce-mic clamp study of quetiapine. They found little evidence of insulin insensitivity, although it was noteworthy that there was a small signal of raised triglyceride levels in this study. This was also found in another recent naturalistic study (de Leon et al. 2007). Overall, quetiapine appears to carry a risk of causing weight gain and other metabolic disturbances. This risk appears to be variable in patients, and it is not as pronounced as the risk with either cloza-pine or olanzapine. The results of an intriguing study in which the addition of quetiapine to clozapine resulted in lower rates of diabetes (Reinstein et al. 1999) have not been replicated.

Two side-effect characteristics that distinguish que-tiapine from other SGAs and from FGAs are its low rates of prolactin elevation and low rates of EPS. Consistently, quetiapine is associated with a low risk of raising prolactin levels (Hamner et al. 1996; Lieberman et al. 2005; Small et al. 1997; Zhong et al. 2006). In the quetiapine versus risperidone schizophrenia study (Zhong et al. 2006), mean prolactin levels were reduced by 11.5 mg/mL in quetiapine-treated patients, whereas they were increased by 35.5 mg/mL in risperidone-treated patients. Similar ef-fects on prolactin levels were observed with quetiapine in both the CATIE and CAFÉ schizophrenia studies (Lie-berman et al. 2005; McEvoy et al. 2007).

The low-EPS advantage of quetiapine is compelling and consistent across studies. Indeed, in the SPECTRUM switch study (Larmo et al. 2005), switching to quetiapine from either an FGA or an SGA was associated with a ro-bust reduction in EPS. This low propensity for EPS was also seen in the bipolar depression studies (Calabrese et al. 2005; Thase et al. 2006). Moreover, quetiapine's EPS advantage has propelled it to the status of being the agent of choice among neurologists who treat psychosis in pa-tients with Parkinson's disease.

The potential of quetiapine to induce cataracts is still unknown. The relationship of antipsychotic therapy in general to cataract formation is unclear (Isaac et al. 1991; Johnson 1998). A large pragmatic trial that includes reg-ular specialist ophthalmological examinations to investi-gate the incidence of cataract formation during therapy with quetiapine is nearing completion (www.clinical-trials.gov). It is hoped that this study will shed new light on the issue. At present it appears that most clinicians do not obtain specialist eye examinations when prescribing quetiapine.

Abnormalities in thyroid hormone levels were a con-cern that emanated from early trials of quetiapine (Ar-vanitis and Miller 1997). This no longer appears to be a clinically meaningful risk, and recent studies have not shown any consistent evidence of thyroid dysfunction with quetiapine use (Kelly and Conley 2006).

Quetiapine's prescribing information (AstraZeneca 2008a, 2008b) possesses a warning similar to that required in the prescribing information of many other antipsychot-ics concerning cardiovascular risks. These potential car-diac risks, especially prolongation of the QTc interval (the ventricular depolarization and repolarization phase, or QT phase, of the electrocardiogram corrected for heart rate), have been comprehensively reviewed by Glassman and Bigger (2001). However, there is no evidence of any heightened QTc risk with quetiapine (Lieberman et al. 2005). It is also suggested that quetiapine might have abuse potential (Pierre et al. 2005; Pinta and Taylor 2007). Given that it is used more broadly than other SGAs, this observation merits further consideration and vigilance.

Overall, the adverse-effect profile of the XR formula-tion is similar to that of the IR formulation. As is the case with all SGAs, there is little information about the effects of quetiapine during pregnancy. A prospective study by McKenna et al. (2005) studied a sample of pregnant women in Canada, Israel, and England treated with SGAs, which was matched to a comparison group of pregnant women who were not exposed to these agents. Among them were 36 women treated with quetiapine. The preg-nancy outcomes in the exposed and comparison groups were not significantly different, with the exceptions of the rate of low birthweight, which was 10% in exposed babies versus 2% in the comparison group ($P=0.05$), and the rate of therapeutic abortions, which was 9.9% in exposed women versus 1.3% in the comparison group ($P=0.003$). Atypical antipsychotics as a group did not appear to be as-sociated with an increased risk for major malformations. Yaeger et al. (2006) reported that among 39 prospectively identified cases of fetal exposure to quetiapine, including the 36 in the study by McKenna et al. (2005), no congen-ital malformations were found.

Conclusion

Quetiapine is now a well-established and widely pre-scribed antipsychotic. There is strong evidence for effi-cacy in all current FDA-approved indications: the treat-ment of schizophrenia and bipolar disorder. This agent is also used extensively under circumstances not approved by the FDA (off-label use), and evidence for efficacy in some of these uses is reviewed (but *not* endorsed clinically) in this chapter. Major clinical trials of quetiapine for several unapproved uses are ongoing (www.clinicaltrials.com). Quetiapine possesses a particularly favorable profile with respect to D_2 receptor antagonism–related side effects. Its low propensity to cause EPS is well established, and studies have consistently shown that quetiapine does not appear to elevate prolactin levels. These two differential tolerability advantages are important when considering whether a patient might benefit from switching from his or her current medication to quetiapine (Weiden and Buckley 2007). On the other hand, the weight-gain effects and metabolic profile of quetiapine are of concern. However, the weight and metabolic risks have yet to be clearly determined for quetiapine relative to other SGAs. Based on current evidence, it appears to have an intermediate position among the SGAs with respect to metabolic risk. Overall, quetiapine represents a useful addition to the psychopharmocological armamentarium, with established efficacy and a broadly favorable tolerability profile.

References

Allison DB, Mentore JL, Heo M, et al: Antipsychotic-induced weight gain: a comprehensive research synthesis. Am J Psychiatry 156:1686–1696, 1999

Arvanitis LA, Miller BG: Multiple fixed doses of "Seroquel" (quetiapine) in patients with acute exacerbation of schizophrenia: a comparison with haloperidol and placebo. The Seroquel Trial 13 Study Group. Biol Psychiatry 42:233–246, 1997

AstraZeneca Pharmaceuticals: Seroquel (quetiapine fumarate) tablets, full prescribing information. July 2008a

AstraZeneca Pharmaceuticals: Seroquel XR (quetiapine fumarate) extended-release tablets, full prescribing information. July 2008b

Barzman DH, DelBello MP, Adler CM, et al: The efficacy and tolerability of quetiapine versus divalproex for the treatment of impulsivity and reactive aggression in adolescents with co-occurring bipolar disorder and disruptive behavior disorder(s). J Child Adolesc Psychopharmacol 16:665–670, 2006

Borison RL, Arvanitis LA, Miller BG: ICI 204,636, an atypical antipsychotic: efficacy and safety in a multicenter, placebo-controlled trial in patients with schizophrenia. US Seroquel Study Group. J Clin Psychopharmacol 16:158–169, 1996

Brecher M, Rak IW, Melvin K, et al: The long-term effect of quetiapine ("Seroquel") monotherapy on weight in patients with schizophrenia. International Journal of Psychiatry in Clinical Practice 4:287–291, 2000

Brooke JO III, Chang HS, Krasnykh O: Metabolic risks in older adults receiving second-generation antipsychotic medication. Curr Psychiatry Rep 11:33–40, 2009

Buckley PF, Goldstein JM, Emsley RA: Efficacy and tolerability of quetiapine in poorly responsive, chronic schizophrenia. Schizophr Res 66:143–150, 2004

Buckley PF, Paulsson B, Brecher M: Treatment of agitation and aggression in bipolar mania: efficacy of quetiapine. J Affect Disord 100 (suppl 1):S33–S43, 2007

Calabrese JR, Keck PE Jr, Macfadden W, et al: A randomized, double-blind, placebo-controlled trial of quetiapine in the treatment of bipolar I or II depression. Am J Psychiatry 162:1351–1360, 2005

Chengappa KN, Goldstein JM, Greenwood M, et al: A post hoc analysis of the impact on hostility and agitation of quetiapine and haloperidol among patients with schizophrenia. Clin Ther 25:530–541, 2003a

Chengappa KN, Parepally H, Brar JS, et al: A random-assignment, double-blind, clinical trial of once- vs twice-daily administration of quetiapine fumarate in patients with schizophrenia or schizoaffective disorder: a pilot study. Can J Psychiatry 48:187–194, 2003b

Copolov DL, Link CG, Kowalcyk B: A multicenter, double-blind randomized comparison of quetiapine (ICI 204,636, "Seroquel") and haloperidol in schizophrenia. Psychol Med 30:95–105, 2000

Currier GW, Trenton AJ, Walsh PG, et al: A pilot, open-label safety study of quetiapine for treatment of moderate psychotic agitation in the emergency setting. J Psychiatr Pract 12:223–228, 2006

Davis JM, Chen N, Glick ID: A meta-analysis of the efficacy of second-generation antipsychotics. Arch Gen Psychiatry 60:553–564, 2003

de Leon J, Armstrong SC, Cozza KL: The dosing of atypical antipsychotics. Psychosomatics 46:262–273, 2005

de Leon J, Susce MT, Johnson M, et al: A clinical study of the association of antipsychotics with hyperlipidemia. Schizophr Res 92:95–102, 2007

DelBello MP, Adler CM, Whitsel RM, et al: A 12-week single-blind trial of quetiapine for the treatment of mood symptoms in adolescents at high risk for developing bipolar I disorder. J Clin Psychiatry 68:789–795, 2007

Dell'Osso B, Mundo E, Altamura AC: Quetiapine augmentation of selective serotonin reuptake inhibitors in treatment-resistant obsessive-compulsive disorder: a six-month follow-up case series. CNS Spectr 11:879–883, 2006

Denys D, Fineberg N, Carey PD, et al: Quetiapine addition in obsessive-compulsive disorder: is treatment outcome affected by type and dose of serotonin reuptake inhibitors? Biol Psychiatry 61:412–414, 2007

DeVane CL, Nemeroff CB: Clinical pharmacokinetics of quetiapine: an atypical antipsychotic. Clin Pharmacokinet 40:509–522, 2001

Dorée JP, Des Rosiers J, Lew V, et al: Quetiapine augmentation of treatment-resistant depression: a comparison with lithium. Curr Med Res Opin 23:333–341, 2007

Emsley RA, Raniwalla J, Bailey PJ, et al: A comparison of the effects of quetiapine ("Seroquel") and haloperidol in schizophrenic patients with a history of and a demonstrated, partial response to conventional antipsychotic treatment. PRIZE Study Group. Int Clin Psychopharmacol 15:121–131, 2000

Findling RL, Reed MD, O'Riordan MA, et al: A 26-week open-label study of quetiapine in children with conduct disorder. J Child Adolesc Psychopharmacol 17:1–9, 2007

Friedman JH: Atypical antipsychotics in the EPS-vulnerable patient. Psychoneuroendocrinology 28 (suppl 1):39–51, 2003

Friedman JH, Goldstein S, Jacques C: Substituting clozapine for olanzapine in psychiatrically stable Parkinson's disease patients: results of an open label pilot study. Clin Neuropharmacol 21:285–288, 1998

Geddes J, Freemantle N, Harrison P, et al: Atypical antipsychotics in the treatment of schizophrenia: systematic overview and meta-regression analysis. BMJ 321:1371–1376, 2000

Glassman AH, Bigger JT Jr: Antipsychotic drugs: prolonged QTc interval, torsades de pointes, and sudden death. Am J Psychiatry 158:1774–1782, 2001

Goldstein JM: Quetiapine fumarate (Seroquel): a new atypical antipsychotic. Drugs Today (Barc) 35:193–210, 1999

Goldstein JM, Christoph G, Grimm S, et al: Unique mechanism of action for the antidepressant properties of the atypical antipsychotic quetiapine. Presented at the annual meeting of the American Psychiatric Association, San Diego, CA, May 19–24, 2007

Hamner MB, Arvanitis LA, Miller BG, et al: Plasma prolactin in schizophrenia subjects treated with Seroquel (ICI 204, 636). Psychopharmacol Bull 32:107–110, 1996

Hamner MB, Deitsch SE, Brodrick PS, et al: Quetiapine treatment in patients with posttraumatic stress disorder: an open trial of adjunctive therapy. J Clin Psychopharmacol 23:15–20, 2003

Isaac NE, Walker AM, Jick H, et al: Exposure to phenothiazine drugs and risk of cataract. Arch Ophthalmol 109:256–260, 1991

Johnson GJ: Limitations of epidemiology in understanding pathogenesis of cataracts. Lancet 351:925–926, 1998

Juncos JL: Management of psychotic aspects of Parkinson's disease. J Clin Psychiatry 60 (suppl 8):42–53, 1999

Kahn RS, Schulz SC, Palazov VD, et al. Efficacy and tolerability of once-daily extended release quetiapine fumarate in acute schizophrenia; a randomized, double-blind, placebo-controlled study. J Clin Psychiatry 68:832–842, 2007

Kapur S, Zipursky R, Jones C, et al: A positron emission tomography study of quetiapine in schizophrenia: a preliminary finding of an antipsychotic effect with only transiently high dopamine D2 receptor occupancy. Arch Gen Psychiatry 57:553–559, 2000a

Kapur S, Zipursky R, Jones C, et al: Relationship between dopamine D2 occupancy, clinical response, and side effects: a double-blind PET study of first-episode schizophrenia. Am J Psychiatry 157:514–520, 2000b

Kelly DL, Conley RR: A randomized double-blind 12-week study of quetiapine, risperidone or fluphenazine on sexual functioning in people with schizophrenia. Psychoneuroendocrinology 31:340–346, 2006

King DJ, Link CG, Kowalcyk B: A comparison of bid and tid dose regimens of quetiapine (Seroquel) in the treatment of schizophrenia. Psychopharmacology (Berl) 137:139–146, 1998

Kinon BJ, Noordsy DL, Liu-Seifert H, et al: Randomized, double-blind 6-month comparison of olanzapine and quetiapine in patients with schizophrenia or schizoaffective disorder with prominent negative symptoms and poor functioning. J Clin Psychopharmacol 26:453–461, 2006

Kufferle B, Tauscher J, Asenbaum S, et al: IBZM SPECT imaging of striatal dopamine-2 receptors in psychotic patients treated with the novel antipsychotic substance quetiapine in comparison to clozapine and haloperidol. Psychopharmacology (Berl) 133:323–328, 1997

Larmo I, de Nayer A, Windhager E, et al: Efficacy and tolerability of quetiapine in patients with schizophrenia who switched from haloperidol, olanzapine or risperidone. Hum Psychopharmacol 20:573–581, 2005

Lieberman JA, Stroup TS, McEvoy JP, et al: Effectiveness of antipsychotic drugs in patients with chronic schizophrenia. N Engl J Med 353:1209–1223, 2005

Lieberman JA, Malaspina D, Jarskog LF: Preventing clinical deterioration in the course of schizophrenia: the potential for neuroprotection. CNS Spectr 11 (suppl):10–13, 2006

Lindenmayer JP, Brown D, Liu S, et al: The efficacy and tolerability of once-daily extended release quetiapine fumarate in hospitalized patients with acute schizophrenia: a 6-week randomized, double-blind, placebo-controlled study. Psychopharmacol Bull 41:11–35, 2008

Mamo DC, Uchida H, Vitcu I, et al. Quetiapine extended-release versus immediate-release formulation: a positron emission tomography study. J Clin Psychiatry 69:81–86, 2008

McConville BJ, Arvanitis LA, Thyrum PT, et al: Pharmacokinetics, tolerability, and clinical effectiveness of quetiapine fumarate: an open-label trial in adolescents with psychotic disorders. J Clin Psychiatry 61:252–260, 2000

McEvoy JP, Lieberman JA, Stroup TS, et al: Effectiveness of clozapine versus olanzapine, quetiapine, and risperidone in patients with chronic schizophrenia who did not respond to prior atypical antipsychotic treatment. Am J Psychiatry 163:600–610, 2006

McEvoy JP, Lieberman JA, Perkins DO, et al: Efficacy and tolerability of olanzapine, quetiapine, and risperidone in the treatment of early psychosis: a randomized, double-blind 52-week comparison. Am J Psychiatry 164:1050–1060, 2007

McIntyre RS, Brecher M, Paulsson B, et al: Quetiapine or haloperidol as monotherapy for bipolar mania—a 12-week, double-blind, randomized, parallel-group, placebo-controlled trial. Eur Neuropsychopharmacol 15:573–585, 2005

McKenna K, Koren G, Tetelbaum M, et al: Pregnancy outcome of women using atypical antipsychotic drugs: a prospective comparative study. J Clin Psychiatry 66:444–449, 2005

McManus DQ, Arvanitis LA, Kowalcyk BB: Quetiapine, a novel antipsychotic: experience in elderly patients with psychotic disorders. Seroquel Trial 48 Study Group. J Clin Psychiatry 60:292–298, 1999

Menza MM, Palermo B, Mark M: Quetiapine as an alternative to clozapine in the treatment of dopamimetic psychosis in patients with Parkinson's disease. Ann Clin Psychiatry 11:141–144, 1999

Merims D, Balas M, Peretz C, et al: Rater-blinded, prospective comparison: quetiapine versus clozapine for Parkinson's disease psychosis. Clin Neuropharmacol 29:331–337, 2006

Meyer JM, Stahl SM: The metabolic syndrome and schizophrenia. Acta Psychiatr Scand 119:4–14, 2009

Miodownik C, Lerner V: Quetiapine: efficacy, tolerability and safety in schizophrenia. Expert Rev Neurother 6:983–992, 2006

Möller H, Johnson S, Meulien D, et al: Once-daily quetiapine sustained release (SR) is effective and well tolerated in patients with schizophrenia switched from the same total daily dose of quetiapine immediate release (IR). Schizophr Bull 33:449, 2007

Mullen J, Jibson MD, Sweitzer D: A comparison of the relative safety, efficacy, and tolerability of quetiapine and risperidone in outpatients with schizophrenia and other psychotic disorders: the quetiapine experience with safety and tolerability (QUEST) study. Clin Ther 23:1839–1854, 2001

Müller D, Kennedy JL: Genetics of antipsychotic weight gain in schizophrenia. Pharmacogenomics 7:863–887, 2006

Nemeroff CB, Kinkead B, Goldstein J: Quetiapine: preclinical studies, pharmacokinetics, drug interactions, and dosing. J Clin Psychiatry 63 (suppl 13):5–11, 2002

Newcomer JW, Haupt DW, Fucetola R, et al: Abnormalities in glucose regulation during antipsychotic treatment of schizophrenia. Arch Gen Psychiatry 59:337–345, 2002

Newcomer JW, Ratner RE, Eriksson JW, et al: A 24-week multicenter, open-label, randomized study to compare changes in glucose metabolism in patients with schizophrenia receiving treatment with olanzapine, quetiapine and risperidone. J Clin Psychiatry (in press; 2009)

Pae CU, Kim JJ, Lee Cu, et al: Rapid versus conventional initiation of quetiapine in the treatment of schizophrenia: a randomized, parallel-group trial. J Clin Psychiatry 68:399–405, 2007

Peuskens J, Link CG: A comparison of quetiapine and chlorpromazine in the treatment of schizophrenia. Acta Psychiatr Scand 96:265–273, 1997

Peuskens JC, Trivedi JK, Malyarov S, et al: A randomized, placebo-controlled relapse-prevention study with once-daily quetiapine sustained release in patients with schizophrenia. Schizophr Bull 33:453, 2007

Pierre JM, Wirshing DA, Wirshing WC, et al: High-dose quetiapine in treatment refractory schizophrenia. Schizophr Res 73:373–375, 2005

Pinta ER, Taylor RE: Quetiapine addiction? Am J Psychiatry 164:174–175, 2007

Potkin SG, Thyrum PT, Alva G, et al: Effect of fluoxetine and imipramine on the pharmacokinetics and tolerability of the antipsychotic quetiapine. J Clin Psychopharmacol 22:174–182, 2002a

Potkin SG, Thyrum PT, Alva G, et al: The safety and pharmacokinetics of quetiapine when coadministered with haloperidol, risperidone, or thioridazine. J Clin Psychopharmacol 22:121–130, 2002b

Potkin SG, Gharabawi GM, Greenspan AJ, et al: A double-blind comparison of risperidone, quetiapine and placebo in patients with schizophrenia experience an acute exacerbation requiring hospitalization. Schizophr Res 85:254–265, 2006

Reinstein M, Sirotovskaya L, Jones L, et al: Effect of clozapine-quetiapine combination therapy on weight and glycaemic control. Clin Drug Investig 18:99–104, 1999

Sacchetti E, Panariello A, Regini C, et al: Quetiapine in hospitalized patients with schizophrenia refractory to treatment with first-generation antipsychotics: a 4-week, flexible-dose, single-blind, exploratory, pilot trial. Schizophr Res 29:325–331, 2004

Sax KW, Strakowski SM, Keck PE Jr: Attentional improvement following quetiapine fumarate treatment in schizophrenia. Schizophr Res 33:151–155, 1998

Schneider LS, Tariot PN, Dagerman KS, et al: Effectiveness of atypical antipsychotic drugs in patients with Alzheimer's disease. N Engl J Med 355:1525–1538, 2006

Seeman P, Tallerico T: Antipsychotic drugs which elicit little or no parkinsonism bind more loosely than dopamine to brain D2 receptors, yet occupy high levels of these receptors. Mol Psychiatry 3:123–134, 1998

Small JG, Hirsch SR, Arvanitis LA, et al: Quetiapine in patients with schizophrenia: a high- and low-dose double-blind comparison with placebo. Arch Gen Psychiatry 54:549–557, 1997

Stephenson CM, Bigliani V, Jones HM, et al: Striatal and extrastriatal D(2)/D(3) dopamine receptor occupancy by quetiapine in vivo: [(123)I]-epidepride single photon emission tomography (SPET) study. Br J Psychiatry 177:408–415, 2000

Strakowski SM, Keck PE Jr, Wong YW, et al: The effect of multiple doses of cimetidine on the steady-state pharmacokinetics of quetiapine in men with selected psychotic disorders. J Clin Psychopharmacol 22:201–205, 2002

Stroup TS, Lieberman JA, McEvoy JP, et al: Effectiveness of olanzapine, quetiapine, and risperidone in patients with chronic schizophrenia after discontinuing perphenazine: a CATIE study. Am J Psychiatry 164:415–427, 2007

Targum SD, Abbott JL: Efficacy of quetiapine in Parkinson's patients with psychosis. J Clin Psychopharmacol 20:54–60, 2000

Thase ME, Macfadden W, Weisler RH, et al: Efficacy of quetiapine monotherapy in bipolar I and II depression: a double-blind, placebo-controlled study (the BOLDER II study). J Clin Psychopharmacol 26:600–609, 2006

Thyrum PT, Wong YW, Yeh C: Single-dose pharmacokinetics of quetiapine in subjects with renal or hepatic impairment. Prog Neuropsychopharmacol Biol Psychiatry 24:521–533, 2000

Velligan DI, Newcomer J, Pultz J, et al: Does cognitive function improve with quetiapine in comparison to haloperidol? Schizophr Res 53:239–248, 2002

Velligan DI, Prihoda TJ, Sui D, et al: The effectiveness of quetiapine vs conventional antipsychotics in improving cognitive and functional outcomes in standard treatment settings. J Clin Psychiatry 64:524–531, 2003

Vieta LN, Mullen J, Brecher M, et al: Quetiapine monotherapy for mania associated with bipolar disorder; combined analysis of two international, double-blind, randomized, placebo-controlled studies. Curr Med Res Opin 21:923–934, 2005

Weiden PJ, Buckley PF: Reducing the burden of side effects during long-term antipsychotic therapy: the role of "switching" medications. J Clin Psychiatry 68:14–23, 2007

Wong YW, Yeh C, Thyrum PT: The effects of concomitant phenytoin administration on the steady-state pharmacokinetics of quetiapine. J Clin Psychopharmacol 21:89–93, 2001

Xu H, Qing H, Lu W, et al: Quetiapine attenuates the immobilization stress-induced decrease of brain-derived neurotrophic factor expression in rat hippocampus. Neurosci Lett 321(1–2):65–68, 2002

Yaeger DD, Smith HG, Altshuler LL: Atypical antipsychotics in the treatment of schizophrenia during pregnancy and the postpartum. Am J Psychiatry 163:2064–2070, 2006

Zhong KX, Sweitzer DE, Hamer RM, et al: Comparison of quetiapine and risperidone in the treatment of schizophrenia: a randomized, double-blind, flexible-dose, 8-week study. J Clin Psychiatry 67:1093–1103, 2006

Zhong KX, Tariot PN, Mintzer J, et al: Quetiapine to treat agitation in dementia: a randomized, double-blind, placebo-controlled study. Curr Alzheimer Res 4:81–93, 2007

CHAPTER 31

Aripiprazole

Zafar A. Sharif, M.D.

Jeffrey A. Lieberman, M.D.

History and Discovery

Aripiprazole is a dihydroquinolinone antipsychotic agent. Chemically, it is unrelated to phenothiazine, butyrophenone, thienobenzodiazepine, or other antipsychotic agents. Pharmacologically, it exhibits a novel mechanism of action, combining partial agonist activity at dopamine$_2$ (D$_2$), dopamine$_3$ (D$_3$), and serotonin$_{1A}$ (5-HT$_{1A}$) receptors with antagonist activity at serotonin$_{2A}$ (5-HT$_{2A}$) and D$_2$ receptors (Burris et al. 2002; Jordan et al. 2002). The development and approval of aripiprazole represent a significant event in the history of antipsychotic agents, as it potentially represents another significant innovation following the introduction of first-generation, or typical, antipsychotic drugs and second-generation, or atypical, antipsychotic drugs in the pharmacology and mechanism of action of therapeutic agents for psychotic disorders.

Although effective in alleviating psychotic symptoms and preventing their recurrence, the typical agents are ineffective in up to 40% of patients with schizophrenia. Even in patients who respond, typical antipsychotics lack efficacy against the negative symptoms of schizophrenia, such as anhedonia and apathy. The typical agents are also associated with a considerable burden of extrapyramidal side effects (EPS) and other side effects, including tardive dyskinesia and hyperprolactinemia. Among patients with first-episode schizophrenia, parkinsonian side effects have been identified as a predictor of discontinuation of antipsychotic treatment (Robinson et al. 2002).

The atypical agents are partially effective against negative as well as positive symptoms and are also associated with fewer EPS. Nevertheless, individual atypical agents are associated with side effects such as weight gain, hyperprolactinemia, QTc prolongation, and alterations in glucose and lipid levels (Allison et al. 1999; Glassman and Bigger 2001; Koro et al. 2002a, 2002b; McIntyre et al. 2001). These side effects may reduce patient adherence to treatment and so increase the long-term risk of acute schizophrenic relapse (Fleischhacker et al. 1994; Kurzthaler and Fleischhacker 2001). They may also be associated with harmful medical sequelae.

The development of aripiprazole was guided by prevailing hypotheses of the etiology of schizophrenia. The dopamine (DA) hypothesis (Seeman and Niznik 1990) proposes that abnormalities in dopaminergic neurotransmission in the brain cause the symptoms of schizophrenia. In its current form, the DA hypothesis suggests that schizophrenia involves a biphasic disturbance in dopaminergic pathways, leading to altered function in different anatomical regions (Davis et al. 1991; Pycock et al. 1980; Weinberger 1987). According to this model, underactivity of the mesocortical dopaminergic pathway leads to hypodopaminergic activity in the frontal cortex, whereas overactivity in the mesolimbic pathway causes increased dopaminergic neurotransmission. The latter is presumed to cause positive or psychotic symptoms, while the former is believed to underlie negative symptoms and cognitive impairment. Another influential hypothesis suggests that the activity of dopaminergic pathways is modulated by serotonergic neurons that project from the raphe nuclei to the corpus striatum and the frontal cortex. In the striatum, serotonin release inhibits DA, while in

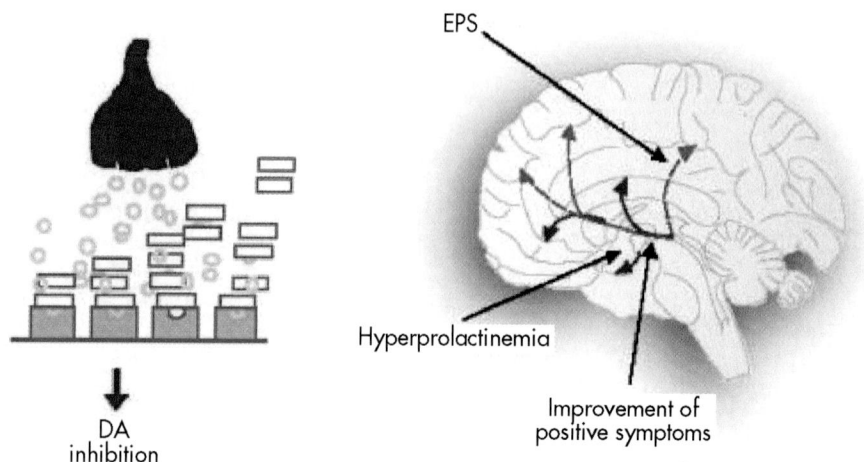

FIGURE 31–1.   Conventional dopamine (DA) antagonist activity: effect on positive symptoms, extrapyramidal side effects (EPS), and prolactin levels.

the frontal cortex it has a modulatory effect on pyramidal neurons and can affect glutamate release.

These hypotheses help to explain several features of typical and atypical antipsychotic agents. All these agents behave as full D_2 antagonists. Their actions in the mesolimbic pathway would therefore be expected to benefit patients with schizophrenia by reducing positive symptoms. D_2 antagonism in the other dopaminergic pathways would, however, be expected to cause unwanted side effects, including exacerbation of negative symptoms (mesocortical pathways), EPS and tardive dyskinesia (nigrostriatal tract), and hyperprolactinemia (tuberoinfundibular pathway) (Figure 31–1).

Similarly, the serotonin (5-HT) hypothesis may help to explain why the atypical agents, which have antagonist activity at 5-HT_{2A} receptors, are associated with fewer EPS and do not exacerbate (and, in fact, partially alleviate) negative symptoms and cognitive impairment (Leysen et al. 1993; Millan 2000; Rao and Möller 1994; Richelson 1999).

On the basis of aripiprazole's unique pharmacodynamic profile—partial agonist activity (rather than full antagonist activity) at both dopaminergic (D_2; Burris et al. 2002) and serotonergic (5-HT_{1A}; Jordan et al. 2002) receptors, and full antagonist activity at 5-HT_{2A} receptors (McQuade et al. 2002)—it was anticipated that aripiprazole treatment would be associated with a reduced burden of unwanted D_2 antagonist activity in the mesocortical, nigrostriatal, and tuberoinfundibular pathways—the activity associated with some of the side effects of typical and atypical antipsychotic agents (Figure 31–2).

Structure–Activity Relations

Aripiprazole is 7-[4-(4-[2,3-dichlorophenyl]-1-piperazinyl)butoxy]-3,4-dihydrocarbostyril (Figure 31–3), a dihydroquinolinone.

Pharmacological Profile

Aripiprazole exhibits potent partial agonist activity at D_2 (Burris et al. 2002) and 5-HT_{1A} (Jordan et al. 2002) receptors, together with potent antagonist activity at 5-HT_{2A} receptors. It also has high affinity for D_3 receptors; moderate affinity for dopamine$_4$ (D_4), serotonin$_{2C}$ (5-HT_{2C}), serotonin$_7$ (5-HT_7), α_1-adrenergic, and histamine$_1$ (H_1) receptors and the serotonin reuptake site (SERT); and negligible affinity for cholinergic muscarinic receptors (Table 31–1). The active metabolite of aripiprazole, dehydroaripiprazole, exhibits a similar affinity at D_2 receptors and has not been shown to have a pharmacological profile that is clinically significantly different from that of the parent compound.

Pharmacokinetics and Disposition

Aripiprazole is available for oral administration as tablets in strengths of 2, 5, 10, 15, 20, and 30 mg. The effective dose range is 10–30 mg/day for schizophrenia patients and 15–30 mg/day for bipolar I disorder patients. A rapidly disintegrating oral formulation of aripiprazole is available in 10-mg and 15-mg strengths. In addition, aripiprazole is

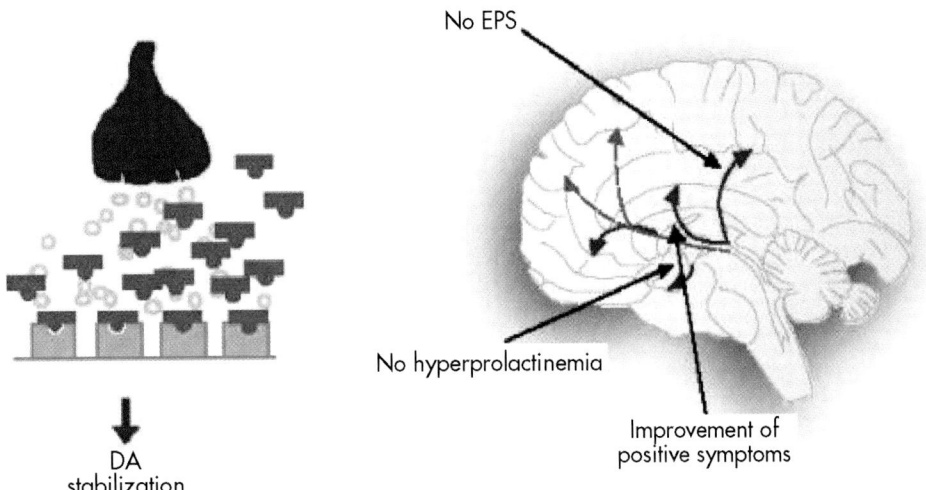

No EPS

No hyperprolactinemia

Improvement of positive symptoms

DA stabilization

FIGURE 31–2. Dopamine (DA) partial agonist activity: effect on positive symptoms, extrapyramidal side effects (EPS), and prolactin levels.

available in a 1-mg/mL nonrefrigerated oral solution. Aripiprazole is taken once daily with or without food and is well absorbed after oral administration, with peak plasma concentrations occurring within 3–5 hours. Absolute oral bioavailability is 87%. An injectable form of aripiprazole for intramuscular (IM) use to provide rapid control of agitation in adults with schizophrenia or bipolar mania was approved by the U.S. Food and Drug Administration (FDA) in September 2006. Aripiprazole injection is available in single-dose, ready-to-use vials containing 9.75 mg aripiprazole in 1.3 mL of diluent (7.5 mg/mL); the recommended initial dose is 9.75 mg IM. Time to the peak plasma concentration is 1–3 hours after IM injection, and the absolute bioavailability of a 5-mg injection is 100%. The mean maximum concentration achieved after an IM dose is on average 19% higher than the maximum plasma concentration (C_{max}) of the oral tablet. While the systemic exposure over 24 hours is generally similar for aripiprazole administered as an IM injection and as an oral tablet, the aripiprazole area under the curve (AUC) in the first 2 hours after an IM injection is 90% greater than the AUC after the same dose in a tablet (Otsuka Pharmaceutical 2008).

In plasma, aripiprazole and its major metabolite, dehydroaripiprazole, are both more than 99% bound to proteins, primarily albumin. Aripiprazole is extensively distributed outside the vascular system, and human studies demonstrating dose-dependent occupancy of D_2 receptors have confirmed that aripiprazole penetrates the brain. Elimination half-lives for aripiprazole and dehydroaripiprazole are 75 hours and 94 hours, respectively.

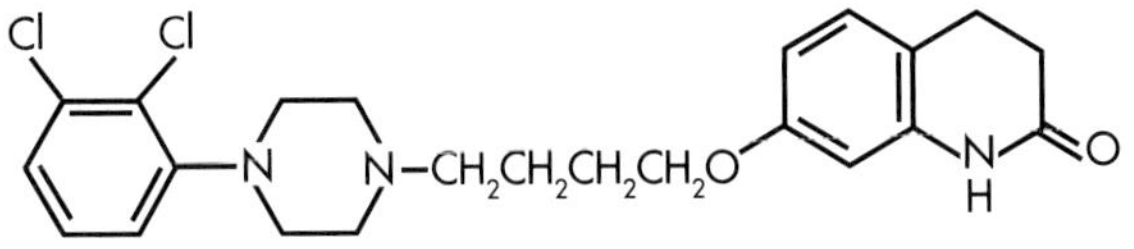

FIGURE 31–3. Chemical structure of aripiprazole.

Aripiprazole is metabolized primarily in the liver. Two hepatic cytochrome P450 (CYP) enzymes, 2D6 and 3A4, catalyze dehydrogenation to dehydroaripiprazole. Therefore, coadministration with inducers or inhibitors of these CYP enzymes may require dosage adjustment of aripiprazole. The active metabolite accounts for 40% of drug exposure, but the predominant circulating moiety is the parent drug. Aripiprazole does not undergo direct glucuronidation and is not a substrate for the following CYP enzymes: 1A1, 1A2, 2A6, 2B6, 2C8, 2C9, 2C19, and 2E1. Interactions with inhibitors or inducers of these enzymes, or with chemicals related to cigarette smoke, are therefore unlikely to occur.

Patient demographic characteristics have not been shown to have any clinically significant impact on the pharmacokinetics of aripiprazole. In general, dosing does not need to be adjusted in respect of a patient's age, gender, race, smoking status, or hepatic or renal function.

Following a single oral dose of ^{14}C-labeled aripiprazole, approximately 25% and 55% of the administered radioactivity were recovered in the urine and feces, respectively. Less than 1% of unchanged aripiprazole was excreted in the urine, and approximately 18% of the oral dose was recovered unchanged in the feces.

TABLE 31–1. Receptor-binding profile of aripiprazole

RECEPTOR TYPE	K_i (NM)
Dopaminergic	
D_1	265
D_2[a]	0.34
D_3	0.8
D_4	44
D_5	95
Serotonergic	
5-HT_{1A}[b]	1.7
5-HT_{2A}	3.4
5-HT_{2C}	15
5-HT_6	214
5-HT_7	39
SERT	98
Histaminic	
H_1	61
Adrenergic	
a_1[c]	57
	IC_{50} (NM)
Muscarinic[c]	>1,000

Note. SERT = serotonin reuptake site.

Source. Adapted from McQuade RD, Burris KD, Jordan S, et al.: "Aripiprazole: A Dopamine–Serotonin System Stabilizer." *International Journal of Neuropsychopharmacology* 5 (Suppl 1): S176, 2002, with the following exceptions:

[a]Burris KD, Molski TF, Xu C, et al.: "Aripiprazole, A Novel Antipsychotic, Is a High Affinity Partial Agonist at Human Dopamine D_2 Receptors." *Journal of Pharmacology and Experimental Therapeutics* 302: 381–389, 2002.

[b]Jordan S, Koprivica V, Chen R, et al.: "The Antipsychotic Aripiprazole Is a Potent, Partial Agonist at the Human 5-HT_{1A} Receptor." *European Journal of Pharmacology* 441:137–140, 2002.

[c]Abilify (Aripiprazole) Tablets. Full Prescribing Information. Tokyo, Otsuka Pharmaceutical Co., Ltd., November 2008.

Mechanism of Action

Aripiprazole has partial agonist activity at D_2 receptors, a feature that distinguishes it from all other currently available antipsychotics, which are full D_2 antagonists. In vitro studies in D_2 receptors in rat striatal membranes (A. Inoue et al. 1997) and rat anterior pituitary slices (T. Inoue et al. 1996) showed that aripiprazole acts as an antagonist when coadministered in the presence of a DA agonist. In other in vitro studies using cloned D_2 receptors from either rat (Lawler et al. 1999) or human (Burris et al. 2002), aripiprazole dose-dependently inhibited isoproterenol-stimulated cyclic adenosine monophosphate (cAMP) synthesis. In these studies, aripiprazole acted as an agonist in the absence of DA, although its maximal agonist activity was less than that of DA, a full agonist.

The activity of aripiprazole at D_2 receptors has also been studied in animal models of schizophrenia (Kikuchi et al. 1995). Aripiprazole exhibits DA antagonist activity in an animal model of hyperdopaminergic activity. In the intact rat with repetitive stereotyped behavior (stereotypy) induced by apomorphine, aripiprazole inhibits stereotypy and locomotion (Kikuchi et al. 1995). This agent may therefore be expected to inhibit hyperdopaminergic activity in the mesolimbic pathway of patients with schizophrenia and so, like other available agents, provide antipsychotic efficacy against the positive symptoms of schizophrenia. On the other hand, in animal models of hypodopaminergic activity, such as the reserpinized rat, aripiprazole has D_2 receptor agonist activity. Because aripiprazole may display either D_2 antagonist activity under hyperdopaminergic conditions or D_2 agonist activity under hypodopaminergic conditions, this agent may be less likely than other antipsychotics to cause excessive D_2 antagonism.

Aripiprazole may offer further therapeutic benefits through modulation of central serotonergic pathways. Preclinical studies showed that aripiprazole has antagonist activity at 5-HT_{2A} receptors (McQuade et al. 2002), a feature that has been associated with reductions in EPS (Meltzer 1999) and negative symptoms. In vitro studies also have shown that aripiprazole has partial agonist activity at 5-HT_{1A} receptors (Jordan et al. 2002), a feature that has been associated with improvement in negative, cognitive, depressive, and anxiety symptoms (Millan 2000).

Other receptor activity may explain some of the side effects of aripiprazole; for example, nausea/vomiting may be explained by its DA agonist effects, whereas orthostatic hypotension and mild sedation/weight gain are likely related to its antagonist activity at α_1-adrenergic and H_1 receptors, respectively.

Indications and Efficacy

In the United States, aripiprazole is approved by the FDA for: acute and maintenance treatment of schizophrenia in adults and in adolescents 13–17 years of age; for acute and maintenance treatment of manic and mixed episodes associated with bipolar I disorder with or without psychotic features in adults and pediatric patients 10–17 years of age; as adjunctive therapy to either lithium or valproate for the acute treatment of manic and mixed episodes associated with bipolar I disorder with or without psychotic features in adults and pediatric patients 10–17 years of age; and as an adjunctive therapy to antidepressants for the acute treatment of major depressive disorder in adults. Additionally, aripiprazole injection is indicated for the acute treatment of agitation associated with schizophrenia or bipolar disorder (manic or mixed) in adults (Otsuka Pharmaceutical 2008).

The efficacy of aripiprazole as a treatment for acute relapse of schizophrenia was demonstrated in four short-term (4-week) double-blind, placebo-controlled studies. Among these was a pivotal Phase III parallel-group multicenter study with four treatment arms comparing aripiprazole (15 mg or 30 mg) with placebo (Kane et al. 2002). Haloperidol (10 mg/day) was used as an active control to confirm the study population's responsiveness to antipsychotic therapy. The total group of patients who were randomized to treatment ($N=414$) comprised 282 patients with schizophrenia and 132 with schizoaffective disorder. Compared with placebo, aripiprazole at either dose produced statistically significant improvements from baseline in the following psychometric scores: Positive and Negative Syndrome Scale (PANSS)—Total, PANSS positive subscale, PANSS-derived Brief Psychiatric Rating Scale (BPRS)—Core, Clinical Global Impression (CGI)–Severity of Illness, and CGI–Improvement. Aripiprazole 15 mg also significantly improved PANSS negative score compared with placebo. Both doses of aripiprazole produced measurable improvement rapidly, with improvement from placebo detectable on psychometric scales by week 2. This trial suggests that at doses of 15 mg and 30 mg, aripiprazole provides effective symptom control in patients with acute relapse of schizophrenia.

Similar findings emerged from another pivotal short-term multicenter Phase III study involving 404 inpatients with an acute relapse of schizophrenia or schizoaffective disorder (Potkin et al. 2003). Patients were randomly assigned to aripiprazole 20 mg, aripiprazole 30 mg, risperidone 6 mg, or placebo for 4 weeks. Compared with placebo, aripiprazole at both doses and risperidone treatment produced statistically significant improvements in scores on standard scales designed to measure antipsychotic efficacy. Likewise, responder rates (with response defined as a score of 1 or 2 on the CGI–Improvement) for both doses of aripiprazole and for risperidone were significantly higher than those for placebo. This study showed that aripiprazole at doses of 20 mg and 30 mg was significantly more effective than placebo.

The antipsychotic efficacy of aripiprazole in acute relapse of schizophrenia was also demonstrated in two Phase II dose-ranging studies, both of which used haloperidol as an active control. In one study, 307 patients with an acute relapse of schizophrenia were randomized to aripiprazole 2 mg, 10 mg, or 30 mg daily or haloperidol 10 mg/day (Daniel et al. 2000). All three doses of aripiprazole produced improvements in efficacy measures from baseline, and the 30-mg dose produced statistically significant improvement compared with placebo on all illness scores, including CGI–Severity, BPRS–Total, BPRS–Core, PANSS–Total, and PANSS positive and negative subscales. Similarly, in a Phase II dose-titrating study, aripiprazole 5–30 mg was superior to placebo in improving BPRS–Total, BPRS–Core, CGI–Severity, and PANSS–Total scores (Petrie et al. 1997).

Results from the three 4-week fixed-dose studies discussed above were pooled for analysis with those of an additional 6-week placebo-controlled, fixed-dose study of aripiprazole at doses of 10 mg, 15 mg, and 20 mg (Lieberman et al. 2002). The pooled analysis involving 898 patients randomized to aripiprazole showed that at all investigated doses greater than 2 mg, aripiprazole exhibited antipsychotic efficacy superior to placebo. Onset of efficacy was rapid, with improvement on psychometric scores detectable within 1 week of starting treatment. These pooled efficacy results demonstrate that doses of 10–30 mg represent an effective therapeutic range for aripiprazole treatment.

The antipsychotic efficacy of aripiprazole in patients with schizophrenia has been further confirmed in two long-term double-blind, randomized, controlled multicenter trials. A 26-week placebo-controlled study in 310 patients with chronic stable schizophrenia investigated the efficacy of aripiprazole 15 mg in relapse prevention (Pigott et al. 2003). Patients who had been symptomatically stable on other antipsychotic medications for 3 months or longer were taken off these medications and randomly assigned to aripiprazole 15 mg or placebo for up to 26 weeks and observed for relapse (defined as a score of ≥5 [minimally worse] on the CGI–Improvement, a score of ≥5 [moderately severe] on the hostility or uncooperativeness items of the PANSS, or a ≥20% increase in the PANSS–Total score). Aripiprazole treatment significantly increased the time to relapse and resulted in significantly fewer relapses at endpoint compared with placebo (34% vs. 57%). From week 6 of therapy, PANSS–Total and PANSS positive subscale scores were significantly more improved with aripiprazole than with placebo.

Another study evaluated the long-term efficacy of aripiprazole when treatment was maintained for up to 52 weeks (Kasper et al. 2003). Patients with acute relapse of schizophrenia (N=1,294) were randomized to aripiprazole 30 mg/day (n=861) or haloperidol 10 mg/day (n=433). Significantly more aripiprazole-treated patients were still taking the medication and were responding to treatment at weeks 8, 26, and 52 than were haloperidol-treated patients. Both treatments produced sustained improvements in the PANSS–Total and PANSS positive subscale scores from baseline. However, aripiprazole produced significantly greater improvements in negative and depressive symptoms at weeks 26 and 52 and was associated with significantly lower scores on all EPS assessments compared with haloperidol.

The efficacy of aripiprazole monotherapy in antipsychotic-resistant schizophrenia was evaluated in a 6-week double-blind, randomized trial in 300 patients who had failed to improve in a prospective 4- to 6-week open trial with olanzapine or risperidone (Kane et al. 2007). Subjects were randomly assigned to aripiprazole (15–30 mg/day) or perphenazine (8–64 mg/day). After 6 weeks, there was no statistical difference between the two groups on efficacy measures; 27% of aripiprazole-treated patients and 25% of perphenazine-treated patients were classified as responders (≥30% improvement from baseline or CGI–Improvement score of 1 or 2). Compared with aripiprazole, perphenazine was associated with a higher rate of EPS and elevated serum prolactin.

The efficacy of aripiprazole in the treatment of schizophrenia in pediatric patients (ages 13–17 years) was evaluated in a 6-week placebo-controlled trial of outpatients who met DSM-IV (American Psychiatric Association 1994) criteria for schizophrenia and had a PANSS score ≥70 at baseline (Findling et al. 2008). In this trial comparing two fixed doses of aripiprazole (10 mg/day or 30 mg/day) with placebo, aripiprazole was titrated starting from 2 mg/day to the target dose in 5 days in the 10 mg/day treatment arm and in 11 days in the 30 mg/day treatment arm. Of 302 patients, 85% completed the 6-week study. Both aripiprazole doses showed statistically significant differences from placebo in reduction in PANSS–Total score; the 30 mg/day dose was not shown to be more efficacious than the 10 mg/day dose. Adverse events occurring in more than 5% of either aripiprazole group and with a combined incidence at least twice the rate for placebo were extrapyramidal disorder, somnolence, and tremor. Mean body weight changes were −0.8, 0.0, and

0.2 kg for placebo, aripiprazole 10 mg, and aripiprazole 30 mg, respectively

The efficacy of aripiprazole in the treatment of acute manic episodes was established in two 3-week placebo-controlled trials in hospitalized patients who met DSM-IV criteria for bipolar I disorder with manic or mixed episodes (Keck et al. 2003; Sachs et al. 2006). These trials included patients with and without psychotic features and with and without a rapid-cycling course. The primary instrument used for assessing manic symptoms was the Young Mania Rating Scale (YMRS), an 11-item clinician-rated scale traditionally used to assess the degree of manic symptomatology. A key secondary instrument included the Clinical Global Impression–Bipolar (CGI-BP) scale. In both trials (n=268; n−248), aripiprazole was started at 30 mg/day, but the dosage could be reduced to 15 mg/day on the basis of efficacy and tolerability. Aripiprazole was superior to placebo in the reduction of YMRS total score and CGI-BP Severity of Illness score (mania). In a third large randomized, double-blind trial involving 347 patients (Vieta et al. 2005), aripiprazole was compared with haloperidol in the treatment of acute bipolar mania over a 12-week period. Significantly more patients remained in treatment and were classified as responders (>50% reduction in YMRS score from baseline) at week 12 for aripiprazole (49.7%) than for haloperidol (28.4%). EPS adverse events were more frequent with haloperidol than with aripiprazole (62.7% vs. 24.0%).

The efficacy of adjunctive aripiprazole with concomitant lithium or valproate in the treatment of manic or mixed episodes was established in a 6-week placebo-controlled study (N=384) with a 2-week lead-in mood stabilizer monotherapy phase in adult patients who met DSM-IV criteria for bipolar I disorder. This study included patients with manic or mixed episodes and with or without psychotic features. Patients were initiated on open-label lithium or valproate at therapeutic serum levels and remained on stable doses for 2 weeks. At the end of 2 weeks, patients demonstrating inadequate response to lithium or valproate (YMRS total score ≥16 and ≤25% improvement on the YMRS total score) were randomized to receive either aripiprazole (15 mg/day with an increase to 30 mg/day as early as day 7) or placebo as adjunctive therapy with open-label lithium or valproate. In the 6-week placebo-controlled phase, adjunctive aripiprazole starting at 15 mg/day with concomitant lithium or valproate (in a therapeutic range of 0.6–1.0 mEq/L or 50–125 µg/mL, respectively) was superior to lithium or valproate with adjunctive placebo in the reduction of the YMRS total score and CGI-BP Severity of Illness score (mania). Seventy-one percent of the patients coadministered valproate and 62% of the patients coadministered lithium were on 15 mg/day at the 6-week endpoint.

Aripiprazole monotherapy was also evaluated in the treatment of nonpsychotic depressive episodes associated with bipolar I disorder. The results of two identically designed 8-week randomized, double-blind, placebo-controlled multicenter studies were reported by Thase et al. (2008). Patients were randomly assigned to placebo or aripiprazole (initiated at 10 mg/day, then flexibly dosed at 5–30 mg/day based on clinical effect and tolerability). The primary endpoint was mean change from baseline to week 8 (last observation carried forward [LOCF]) in the Montgomery-Åsberg Depression Rating Scale (MADRS) total score. Although statistically significant differences were observed during weeks 1–6, aripiprazole did not achieve statistical significance versus placebo at week 8 in either study in the change in MADRS total score (primary endpoint). In addition, despite early statistical separation on the Clinical Global Impressions Bipolar Version Severity of Illness–Depression score (key secondary endpoint), aripiprazole was not superior to placebo at endpoint. Aripiprazole was associated with a higher incidence of akathisia, insomnia, nausea, fatigue, restlessness, and dry mouth versus placebo. More patients discontinued with aripiprazole versus placebo in both studies. Thus, aripiprazole monotherapy as dosed in this study design was not significantly more effective than placebo in the treatment of bipolar depression at endpoint (Thase et al. 2008).

To evaluate the long-term effectiveness of aripiprazole in delaying relapse in bipolar I disorder patients, a trial was conducted in patients meeting DSM-IV criteria for bipolar I disorder with a recent manic or mixed episode who had been stabilized on open-label aripiprazole and who had maintained a clinical response for at least 6 weeks (Keck et al. 2006). The first phase of this trial was an open-label stabilization period in which inpatients and outpatients were clinically stabilized (YMRS score ≤10 and MADRS score ≤13) and then maintained on open-label aripiprazole (15 or 30 mg/day, with a starting dose of 30 mg/day) for at least 6 consecutive weeks. One hundred sixty-one outpatients were then randomized in a double-blind fashion to either the same dose of aripiprazole they were on at the end of the stabilization and maintenance period or a switch to placebo and were then monitored for manic or depressive relapse. During the randomization phase, aripiprazole was superior to placebo on time to the number of combined affective relapses (manic plus depressive), the primary outcome measure for this study. The majority of these relapses were due to manic rather

than depressive symptoms. Aripiprazole-treated patients had significantly fewer relapses than placebo-treated patients (25% vs. 43%). Aripiprazole was superior to placebo in delaying the time to manic relapse but did not differ from placebo in delaying time to depressive relapse. Significant weight gain (≥7% increase from baseline) was seen in 13% of the aripiprazole patients and none of the placebo patients. An examination of population subgroups did not reveal any clear evidence of differential responsiveness on the basis of age and gender; however, there were insufficient numbers of patients in each of the ethnic groups to adequately assess intergroup differences.

The efficacy of aripiprazole in the treatment of bipolar I disorder in pediatric patients (ages 10–17 years) was evaluated in a 4-week placebo-controlled trial of outpatients ($N = 296$) who met DSM-IV criteria for bipolar I disorder manic or mixed episodes with or without psychotic features and had a YMRS score ≥20 at baseline. This double-blind, placebo-controlled trial compared two fixed doses of aripiprazole (10 mg/day or 30 mg/day) against placebo. The aripiprazole dose was started at 2 mg/day, which was increased to 5 mg/day after 2 days and to the target dose in 5 days in the 10 mg/day treatment arm and in 13 days in the 30 mg/day treatment arm. Both doses of aripiprazole were superior to placebo in change from baseline to week 4 on the YMRS total score. Although maintenance efficacy in pediatric patients has not been systematically evaluated, maintenance efficacy can be extrapolated from adult data, along with comparisons of aripiprazole pharmacokinetic parameters in adult and pediatric patients (Otsuka Pharmaceutical 2008).

Aripiprazole is also available in an injectable formulation for IM administration. The efficacy of aripiprazole injection in controlling acute agitation was evaluated in three short-term (24-hour) randomized, double-blind, placebo-controlled studies in patients with schizophrenia (Andrezina et al. 2006; Tran-Johnson et al. 2007) and patients with bipolar disorder (manic or mixed) (Zimbroff et al. 2007), involving a total of 1,086 patients. The effectiveness of aripiprazole injection in controlling agitation was measured in these studies using several instruments, including the PANSS Excited Component (PANSS EC) and CGI–I scale. The primary efficacy measure used for assessing signs and symptoms of agitation was the change from baseline in the PANSS EC at 2 hours' postinjection. PANSS EC includes five items: poor impulse control, tension, hostility, uncooperativeness, and excitement. Aripiprazole injection was statistically superior to placebo ($P < 0.05$) in all three studies, as measured with the PANSS EC. In the two studies in agitated patients with schizophrenia, injectable aripiprazole and IM haloperidol were compared with placebo. The injectable formulations of aripiprazole and haloperidol were both superior to placebo. In the study in agitated bipolar I disorder (manic or mixed) patients, aripiprazole injection and lorazepam injection were compared with placebo. Both active agents were superior to placebo. FDA-approved dosage preparations are as follows: 5.25 mg/0.7 mL, 9.75 mg/1.3 mL, and 15 mg/2.0 mL. The recommended initial dose of aripiprazole injection is 9.75 mg.

De Deyn et al. (2005) compared the efficacy, safety, and tolerability of aripiprazole against placebo in patients with psychosis associated with Alzheimer's disease (AD). This 10-week double-blind multicenter study randomized 208 outpatients (mean age = 81.5 years) with AD-associated psychosis to aripiprazole (n = 106) or placebo (n = 102). The initial aripiprazole dose of 2 mg/day was titrated upward (5, 10, or 15 mg/day) according to efficacy and tolerability. Evaluations included the Neuropsychiatric Inventory (NPI) Psychosis subscale and the BPRS, adverse event (AE) reports, EPS rating scales, and body weight measurement. Overall, 172 patients (83%) completed the study. The mean aripiprazole dose at study endpoint was 10.0 mg/day. The NPI Psychosis subscale score showed improvements in both groups (aripiprazole, −6.55; placebo, −5.52; $P = 0.17$ at endpoint). Aripiprazole-treated patients showed significantly greater improvements from baseline in BPRS Psychosis and BPRS–Core subscale scores at endpoint compared with placebo-treated patients. Somnolence was mild and was not associated with falls or accidental injury. There were no significant differences from placebo in EPS scores or in clinically significant electrocardiogram abnormalities, vital signs, or weight.

In another double-blind, multicenter study (Mintzer et al. 2007), 487 institutionalized patients with psychosis associated with AD were randomized to placebo or aripiprazole, 2, 5 or 10 mg/day. Primary efficacy assessment was the mean change from baseline to week 10 on the Neuropsychiatric Inventory–Nursing Home (NPI-NH) version Psychosis Subscale score. Aripiprazole 10 mg/day showed significantly greater improvements than placebo on the NPI-NH Psychosis Subscale (−6.87 vs. −5.13; $P = 0.013$) by analysis of covariance; CGI-S (−0.72 vs. −0.46; $P = 0.031$); BPRS Total (−7.12 vs. −4.17; $P = 0.030$); and NPI-NH Psychosis response rate (65% vs. 50%; $P = 0.019$). Aripiprazole 5 mg/day showed significant improvements versus placebo on BPRS and Cohen-Mansfield Agitation Inventory (CMAI) scores. Aripiprazole 2 mg/day was not efficacious. Four cases of cerebrovascular

adverse events were reported in the aripiprazole 10 mg/day group, two in the 5-mg group, and one in the 2-mg group. No cerebrovascular adverse events were reported in the placebo group.

In 2005, the FDA issued a black box warning for second-generation antipsychotics based on increased mortality rates (4.5% vs. 2.6%) observed in patients with dementia-related psychosis treated with second-generation antipsychotics as compared with placebo over a modal duration treatment period of 10 weeks. This warning was extended in June 2008 to include all older conventional antipsychotic agents. No antipsychotic is currently approved in the United States for treating the behavioral and psychotic symptoms that frequently accompany dementia.

Nickel et al. (2006) conducted a double-blind, placebo-controlled study in 52 subjects (43 women and 9 men) meeting criteria for borderline personality disorder who were randomly assigned in a 1:1 ratio to 15 mg/day of aripiprazole (n = 26) or placebo (n = 26) for 8 weeks. Significant changes in scores on most scales of the Symptom Checklist (SCL-90-R), on the Hamilton Rating Scale for Depression (Ham-D), on the Hamilton Anxiety Scale (Ham-A), and on all scales of the State-Trait Anger Expression Inventory were observed in subjects treated with aripiprazole after 8 weeks. The improvements noted at 8 weeks of therapy were maintained at 18-month follow-up (Nickel et al. 2007).

Because of aripiprazole's partial DA agonist activity, there has been substantial interest in evaluating the utility of aripiprazole in reducing cravings and drug use in cocaine-, alcohol-, and amphetamine-abusing patients and as an augmentation strategy in patients with treatment-resistant depression. Tiihonen et al. (2007) conducted a study in individuals meeting DSM-IV criteria for intravenous amphetamine dependence (N = 53) who were randomly assigned to receive aripiprazole (15 mg/day), slow-release methylphenidate (54 mg/day), or placebo for 20 weeks. The study was terminated prematurely because of unexpected results of interim analysis. Contrary to the hypothesized result, patients who received aripiprazole treatment had significantly more amphetamine-positive urine samples than did patients in the placebo group, whereas patients who received methylphenidate had significantly fewer amphetamine-positive urine samples than patients who had received placebo. Studies in cocaine-abusing subjects are ongoing.

In a study in alcoholic patients (Anton et al. 2008) the efficacy and safety of aripiprazole was compared with placebo in a 12-week double-blind multicenter trial in 295 patients with alcohol dependence according to DSM-IV criteria. Patients were randomly assigned to treatment with aripiprazole (initiated at 2 mg/day and titrated to a maximum dose of 30 mg/day at day 28) or placebo after minimum 3 day abstinence during the screening period. The primary efficacy measure was percentage of days abstinent over 12 weeks. Discontinuations (40.3% vs. 26.7%) and treatment-related adverse events (82.8% vs. 63.6%) were higher with aripiprazole than with placebo. Mean percentage of days abstinent was similar between aripiprazole and placebo (58.7% vs. 63.3%; $P=0.227$). Percentage of subjects without a heavy drinking day and the time to first drinking day were also comparable between groups, although the aripiprazole group had fewer drinks per drinking day (4.4 vs. 5.5 drinks; $P<0.001$). The aripiprazole group showed a larger decrease in percentage carbohydrate-deficient transferrin, a biomarker of heavy alcohol consumption at weeks 4 (-14.91% vs. -2.23%; $P=0.02$) and 8 (-16.92% vs. -5.33%; $P=0.021$), although not at week 12 (-9.06% vs. -4.12%; $P=0.298$). At study endpoint, aripiprazole-treated subjects reported more positive subjective treatment effects and less overall severity of alcohol dependence than placebo-treated subjects. Although there was no difference between aripiprazole and placebo on the primary endpoint, effects on the secondary outcomes suggest that further study of aripiprazole for treatment of alcohol dependence may be warranted at lower doses (Anton et al. 2008).

The efficacy of aripiprazole in the adjunctive treatment of major depressive disorder was demonstrated in two identical short-term (6-week) placebo-controlled trials of adult patients meeting DSM-IV criteria for major depressive disorder who had had an inadequate response to prior antidepressant therapy (1 to 3 courses) in the current episode. In both studies, a 7- to 28-day screening phase was followed by an 8-week prospective antidepressant treatment phase and a 6-week double-blind adjunctive treatment phase. During prospective antidepressant treatment, patients received one of several antidepressants (escitalopram, fluoxetine, paroxetine controlled-release, sertraline, or venlafaxine extended-release), each with single-blind adjunctive placebo. Patients with incomplete response (defined as <50% improvement on the 17-item version of the Hamilton Rating Scale for Depression [Ham-D-17], a final Ham-D-17 score >14, and a Clinical Global Impressions Improvement rating of no better than minimal improvement) continued on the antidepressant and were randomly assigned to double-blind adjunctive placebo or adjunctive aripiprazole (2–15 mg/day with potent CYP2D6 inhibitors fluoxetine or pa-

roxetine; 2–20 mg/day with all other antidepressants). The primary efficacy measure was mean change from end of prospective treatment to end of double-blind treatment (LOCF) in MADRS total score (analysis of covariance). A key secondary outcome was the Sheehan Disability Scale (SDS), a 3-item self-rated instrument used to assess the impact of depression on three domains of functioning (work/school, social life, and family life), with each item scored from 0 (not at all) to 10 (extreme).

In the first trial (Berman et al. 2007), a total of 178 patients were randomly assigned to adjunctive placebo and 184 to adjunctive aripiprazole in the double-blind adjunctive treatment phase. The mean change in MADRS total score was significantly greater with adjunctive aripiprazole (-8.8) than with adjunctive placebo (-5.8; $P<0.001$). Adverse events that occurred in 10% or more of patients with adjunctive placebo or adjunctive aripiprazole were akathisia (4.5% vs. 23.1%), headache (10.8% vs. 6.0%), and restlessness (3.4% vs. 14.3%). Discontinuations due to adverse events were low with adjunctive placebo (1.7%) and adjunctive aripiprazole (2.2%); only one adjunctive aripiprazole–treated patient discontinued because of akathisia. About 1% of placebo recipients and 7.1% of aripiprazole recipients experienced weight gain of 7% or greater from baseline.

In the second trial (Marcus et al. 2008), 190 patients were randomly assigned to adjunctive placebo and 191 to adjunctive aripiprazole. The mean change in MADRS total score was significantly greater with adjunctive aripiprazole than with placebo (-8.5 vs. -5.7; $P=0.001$). Remission rates were significantly greater with adjunctive aripiprazole than placebo (25.4% vs. 15.2%; $P=0.016$) as were response rates (32.4% vs. 17.4%; $P<0.001$). The mean SDS total score—the key secondary outcome measure—improved significantly more with adjunctive aripiprazole than with adjunctive placebo at endpoint (-1.3 vs. -0.7; $P=0.012$). Adverse events occurring in 10% or more of patients with adjunctive placebo or aripiprazole were akathisia (4.2% vs. 25.9%), headache (10.5% vs. 9.0%), and fatigue (3.7% vs. 10.1%). Incidence of adverse events leading to discontinuation was low (adjunctive placebo [1.1%] vs. adjunctive aripiprazole [3.7%]). By the last study visit, continuing akathisia was reported in 25 (51%) of the 49 patients who had ever reported this symptom. Furthermore, the majority of akathisia (n = 38/49; 78%) was first reported during the first 3 weeks of treatment. Akathisia, at its maximum, was generally mild (n = 12/49; 25%) or moderate (n = 33/49; 67%) in severity, with few patients reporting akathisia as severe (n = 4/49; 8%). For those subjects whose akathisia resolved during the study (n = 24), 58% (n = 14/24) received dosage reduction and 42% (n = 10/24) received no intervention. Mean (SE) weight gain in the adjunctive aripiprazole group (1.47±0.16 kg) was significantly greater than the placebo group (0.42±0.17 kg; P<0.001; LOCF). Weight gain of 7% or greater from baseline occurred in 0% of adjunctive placebo–treated patients and 3.4% of adjunctive aripiprazole–treated patients (P=0.031).

These scientifically rigorous studies confirmed initial observations from case reports, retrospective chart reviews, and small open-label trials of the utility of aripiprazole in augmenting antidepressants in patients with major depressive disorder and led to the FDA approval for this indication in late 2007.

Side Effects and Toxicology

The safety and tolerability of antipsychotic therapy are important aspects of schizophrenia management, as they have an impact on treatment adherence and so on patients' risk of relapse and quality of life. Specific side effects seen with some antipsychotics, such as weight gain and hyperprolactinemia, may also have long-term implications for patient health.

A pooled analysis of safety and tolerability data from the five short-term studies (Marder et al. 2003; Stock et al. 2002) showed that aripiprazole treatment was well tolerated. The most commonly reported adverse events with aripiprazole were headache, insomnia, agitation, and anxiety; these were also the most frequently reported events in the placebo, haloperidol, and risperidone groups. The incidence of adverse events was similar in the aripiprazole and placebo groups. Akathisia, somnolence, and EPS were more common among patients receiving haloperidol than those receiving aripiprazole, while akathisia, somnolence, and tachycardia were more frequent in the risperidone group than in the aripiprazole group. The adverse-event profile of aripiprazole did not vary according to patient characteristics of age, gender, and race, and no deaths were reported during the short-term studies. Data from the four fixed-dose studies showed that somnolence was the only adverse event seen with aripiprazole that was possibly dose-related. The overall incidence of somnolence with aripiprazole, however, was similar to that seen with placebo and lower than that seen with other active treatments. Objective rating scale assessments were used to assess changes in parkinsonian symptoms (Simpson-Angus Scale [SAS]), dyskinesias (Abnormal Involuntary Movement Scale [AIMS]), and akathisia (Barnes Akathi-

sia Rating Scale [BAS]). SAS scores with aripiprazole did not differ significantly from those with placebo, whereas AIMS scores improved significantly from baseline with aripiprazole compared with placebo. Aripiprazole did not produce consistent dose-dependent changes in BAS scores. Haloperidol produced significant increases in SAS and BAS scores over placebo. Rates of discontinuation due to adverse events were similar among the groups: 9.4% with placebo, 8.0% with haloperidol, and 7.3% with aripiprazole (Otsuka Pharmaceutical 2008). According to the product labeling for aripiprazole in the United States, treatment-emergent adverse events reported with aripiprazole in short-term trials of patients with schizophrenia (up to 6 weeks) or bipolar disorder (up to 3 weeks) that occurred at an incidence greater than or equal to 10% and greater than placebo, respectively, included headache (30% vs. 25%), anxiety (20% vs. 17%), insomnia (19% vs. 14%), nausea (16% vs. 12%), vomiting (12% vs. 6%), dizziness (11% vs. 8%), constipation (11% vs. 7%), dyspepsia (10% vs. 8%), and akathisia (10% vs. 4%). A similar adverse-event profile was observed in a 26-week trial in schizophrenia except for a higher incidence of tremor (aripiprazole 8% vs. placebo 2%).

The most frequently reported adverse events with aripiprazole injection were headache (aripiprazole 12% vs. placebo 7%), nausea (aripiprazole 9% vs. placebo 3%), dizziness (aripiprazole 8% vs. placebo 5%), and somnolence (aripiprazole 7% vs. placebo 4%). In the three aripiprazole injection trials, the safety profile was comparable to that of placebo regarding the incidence of EPS, akathisia, or dystonia. The incidence of akathisia-related adverse events with aripiprazole injection was 2% (vs. 0% for placebo), while the incidence of dystonia with aripiprazole injection was less than 1% (vs. 0% for placebo). In addition, the incidence of QTc prolongation was also comparable between aripiprazole injection and placebo.

Weight gain is another adverse event of concern seen with some antipsychotic treatments, as it is associated with noncompliance (Allison et al. 1999), and excessive weight gain and obesity are linked to an increased risk of morbidity and mortality from heart disease, hypertension, and diabetes (Aronne 2001). Minimal changes in mean body weight were observed with aripiprazole treatment in short-term studies (pooled data, +0.71 kg) (Marder et al. 2003) and long-term studies (26-week: −1.26 kg; 52-week: +1.05 kg) (Kasper et al. 2003; Pigott et al. 2003).

Olanzapine and aripiprazole were compared on their propensity to cause weight gain and other metabolic disturbances in a 26-week randomized, double-blind multicenter trial in patients with DSM-IV schizophrenia who were in acute relapse and required hospitalization (Mc-Quade et al. 2004). Significant weight gain was defined as more than 7% increase in body weight from baseline. Three hundred seventeen patients were randomly assigned to aripiprazole ($n = 156$) or olanzapine ($n = 161$). By week 26, 37% of olanzapine-treated patients had experienced significant weight gain, compared with 14% of aripiprazole-treated patients ($P < .001$). Statistically significant differences in mean weight change were observed between treatments beginning at week 1 and sustained throughout the study. At week 26, there was a mean weight loss of 1.37 kg (3.04 lb) with aripiprazole compared with a mean increase of 4.23 kg (9.40 lb) with olanzapine among patients who remained on therapy ($P < 0.001$). Changes in fasting plasma levels of total cholesterol, high-density lipoprotein cholesterol, and triglycerides were significantly different in the two treatment groups, with worsening of the lipid profile among patients treated with olanzapine.

Aripiprazole treatment was not associated with increases in prolactin levels during short- or long-term studies (in fact, prolactin levels were shown to be slightly decreased by aripiprazole). Patients receiving aripiprazole treatment also showed decreases in mean QTc interval that were similar to those seen in patients who were receiving placebo in short-term studies (4.4 msec vs. 3.5 msec), as well as a low incidence of QTc increase ≥ 30 msec (aripiprazole: 4.3%; placebo: 5.5%). Aripiprazole was not associated with significant increases in QTc interval in long-term studies. Aripiprazole treatment was not associated with adverse changes in glucose or lipid levels during short- or long-term studies.

Overall, aripiprazole treatment is associated with a low incidence of EPS-related symptoms and with minimal or no effects on weight gain, QTc interval, or circulating levels of cholesterol, glucose, and prolactin. Treatment with aripiprazole may reduce the burden of antipsychotic-associated side effects, which is expected to improve patient adherence and reduce the risk of acute relapse.

Drug–Drug Interactions

Aripiprazole is metabolized primarily by the hepatic cytochrome P450 enzymes 2D6 and 3A4, so it has the potential to interact with other substrates for these enzymes. Inducers of these enzymes may increase clearance and so lower blood levels of aripiprazole, whereas inhibitors of 3A4 or 2D6 may inhibit elimination and so increase blood

levels of aripiprazole. In vivo studies showed decreased levels of aripiprazole and dehydroaripiprazole in the plasma when aripiprazole was coadministered with carbamazepine, a cytochrome P450 3A4 inducer. The aripiprazole dose should therefore be increased when the drug is administered concomitantly with carbamazepine. In vivo studies coadministering aripiprazole and ketoconazole (a 3A4 inhibitor) or quinidine (a 2D6 inhibitor) suggest that the aripiprazole dose should be reduced when aripiprazole is administered with strong 3A4 or 2D6 inhibitors.

Aripiprazole is not a substrate for the cytochrome P450 enzymes 1A1, 1A2, 2A6, 2B6, 2C8, 2C9, 2C19, or 2E1 and so is unlikely to interact with inhibitors or inducers of these enzymes. Specific studies have demonstrated no clinically important interactions of aripiprazole with famotidine, valproate, lithium, dextromethorphan, warfarin, or omeprazole. Aripiprazole exhibits α_1-adrenergic receptor antagonist activity and so may enhance the effects of certain antihypertensive agents.

Conclusion

Aripiprazole is a novel antipsychotic agent that combines partial agonist activity at D_2 receptors with partial agonist activity at $5\text{-}HT_{1A}$ receptors and antagonist activity at $5\text{-}HT_{2A}$ receptors. This makes aripiprazole the first agent that is not a full D_2 antagonist to show rapid and sustained antipsychotic activity, and it may be considered the first partial DA agonist combined with 5-HT-stabilizing properties.

Short-term and long-term clinical trials in adult and pediatric patients with schizophrenia and bipolar I disorder have demonstrated that aripiprazole combines sustained antipsychotic and mood-stabilizing efficacy with an excellent safety and tolerability profile. Additional augmentation trials have confirmed the utility of aripiprazole in alleviating depressive symptomatology in patients with major depressive disorder who have not achieved adequate symptom relief with antidepressants alone. In general, aripiprazole treatment is associated with a low liability for EPS, QTc interval prolongation, prolactin elevation, weight gain, or disturbances of glucose or lipid metabolism. This combination of efficacy, safety, and tolerability suggests that aripiprazole has the potential to improve treatment adherence and decrease relapse rates and so represents an important new option for both acute and long-term treatment of schizophrenia and bipolar I disorder and as an adjunct to antidepressants in major depressive disorder.

References

Allison DB, Mentore JL, Heo M, et al: Antipsychotic-induced weight gain: a comprehensive research synthesis. Am J Psychiatry 156:1686–1696, 1999

American Psychiatric Association: Diagnostic and Statistical Manual of Mental Disorders, 4th Edition. Washington, DC, American Psychiatric Association, 1994

American Psychiatric Association: Diagnostic and Statistical Manual of Mental Disorders, 4th Edition, Text Revision. Washington, DC, American Psychiatric Association, 2000

Andrezina R, Josiassen RC, Marcus RN, et al: Intramuscular aripiprazole for the treatment of acute agitation in patients with schizophrenia or schizoaffective disorder: a double-blind, placebo-controlled comparison with intramuscular haloperidol. Psychopharmacology 188:281–292, 2006

Anton RF, Kranzler H, Breder C, et al: A randomized, multicenter, double-blind, placebo-controlled study of the efficacy and safety of aripiprazole for the treatment of alcohol dependence. J Clin Psychopharmacol 28:5–12, 2008

Aronne LJ: Epidemiology, morbidity, and treatment of overweight and obesity. J Clin Psychiatry 62 (suppl):13–22, 2001

Berman RM, Marcus RN, Swanink R, et al: The efficacy and safety of aripiprazole as adjunctive therapy in major depressive disorder: a multicenter, randomized, double-blind, placebo-controlled study. J Clin Psychiatry 68:843–853, 2007

Burris KD, Molski TF, Xu C, et al: Aripiprazole, a novel antipsychotic, is a high affinity partial agonist at human dopamine D_2 receptors. J Pharmacol Exp Ther 302:381–389, 2002

Daniel DG, Saha AR, Ingenito G, et al: Aripiprazole, a novel antipsychotic: overview of a phase II study result (abstract). Int J Neuropsychopharmacol 3 (suppl):S157, 2000

Davis KL, Kahn RS, Ko G, et al: Dopamine in schizophrenia: a review and reconceptualization. Am J Psychiatry 148:1474–1486, 1991

De Deyn P, Jeste DV, Swanink R, et al: Aripiprazole for the treatment of psychosis in patients with Alzheimer's disease: a randomized, placebo-controlled study. J Clin Psychopharmacol 25:463–467, 2005

Findling RL, Robb A, Nyilas M, et al: A multiple-center, randomized, double-blind, placebo-controlled study of oral aripiprazole for treatment of adolescents with schizophrenia. Am J Psychiatry 165:1432–1441, 2008

Fleischhacker WW, Meise U, Gunther V, et al: Compliance with antipsychotic drug treatment: influence of side effects. Acta Psychiatr Scand Suppl 382:11–15, 1994

Glassman AH, Bigger JT Jr: Antipsychotic drugs: prolonged QTc interval, torsades de pointes, and sudden death. Am J Psychiatry 158:1774–1782, 2001

Inoue A, Miki S, Seto M, et al: Aripiprazole, a novel antipsychotic drug, inhibits quinpirole-evoked GTPase activity but does not up-regulate dopamine D_2 receptor following repeated treatment in the rat striatum. Eur J Pharmacol 321:105–111, 1997

Inoue T, Domae M, Yamada K, et al: Effects of the novel antipsychotic agent 7-(4-[(2,3-dichlorophenyl)-1-piperazinyl] butyloxy)-3,4-dihydro-2 (1H)-quinolinone (OPC-14597) on prolactin release from the rat anterior pituitary gland. J Pharmacol Exp Ther 277:137–143, 1996

Jordan S, Koprivica V, Chen R, et al: The antipsychotic aripiprazole is a potent, partial agonist at the human 5-HT1A receptor. Eur J Pharmacol 441:137–140, 2002

Kane JM, Carson WH, Saha AR, et al: Efficacy and safety of aripiprazole and haloperidol vs placebo in patients with schizophrenia and schizoaffective disorder. J Clin Psychiatry 63:763–771, 2002

Kane JM, Meltzer HY, Carson WH Jr, et al: Aripiprazole for treatment-resistant schizophrenia: results of a multicenter, randomized, double-blind, comparison study versus perphenazine. J Clin Psychiatry 68:213–223, 2007

Kasper S, Lerman MN, McQuade RD, et al: Efficacy and safety of aripiprazole vs. haloperidol for long-term maintenance treatment following acute relapse of schizophrenia. Int J Neuropsychopharmacol 6:325–337, 2003

Keck PE Jr, Marcus R, Tourkodimitris S, et al: A placebo-controlled, double-blind study of the efficacy and safety of aripiprazole in patients with acute bipolar mania. Am J Psychiatry 160:1651–1658, 2003

Keck PE Jr, Calabrese JR, McQuade RD, et al: A randomized, double-blind, placebo-controlled 26-week trial of aripiprazole in recently manic patients with bipolar I disorder. J Clin Psychiatry 67:626–637, 2006

Kikuchi T, Tottori K, Uwahodo Y, et al: 7-{4-[4-(2,3-dichlorophenyl)-1-piperazinyl]butyloxy}-3,4-dihydro-2 (1H)-quinolinone (OPC-14597), a new putative antipsychotic drug with both presynaptic dopamine autoreceptor agonistic activity and postsynaptic D_2 receptor antagonist activity. J Pharmacol Exp Ther 274:329–336, 1995

Koro CE, Fedder DO, L'Italien GJ, et al: An assessment of the independent effects of olanzapine and risperidone exposure on the risk of hyperlipidemia in schizophrenic patients. Arch Gen Psychiatry 59:1021–1026, 2002a

Koro CE, Fedder DO, L'Italien GJ, et al: Assessment of independent effect of olanzapine and risperidone on risk of diabetes among patients with schizophrenia: population based nested case-control study. BMJ 325:243, 2002b

Kurzthaler I, Fleischhacker WW: The clinical implications of weight gain in schizophrenia. J Clin Psychiatry 62 (suppl):32–37, 2001

Lawler CP, Prioleau C, Lewis MM, et al: Interactions of the novel antipsychotic aripiprazole (OPC-14597) with dopamine and serotonin receptor subtypes. Neuropsychopharmacology 20:612–627, 1999

Leysen JE, Janssen PMF, Schotte A, et al: Interaction of antipsychotic drugs with neurotransmitter receptor sites in vitro and in vivo in relation to pharmacological and clinical role of 5-HT$_2$ receptors. Psychopharmacology (Berl) 112 (suppl):S40–S54, 1993

Lieberman J, Carson WH, Saha AR, et al: Meta-analysis of the efficacy of aripiprazole in schizophrenia. Int J Neuropsychopharmacol 5 (suppl):S186, 2002

Marcus RN, McQuade RD, Carson WH, et al: The efficacy and safety of aripiprazole as adjunctive therapy in major depressive disorder: a second multicenter, randomized, double-blind, placebo-controlled study. J Clin Psychopharmacol 28:156–165, 2008

Marder SR, McQuade RD, Stock E, et al: Aripiprazole in the treatment of schizophrenia: safety and tolerability in short-term placebo-controlled trials. Schizophr Res 61:123–136, 2003

McIntyre RS, McCann SM, Kennedy SH: Antipsychotic metabolic effects: weight gain, diabetes mellitus, and lipid abnormalities. Can J Psychiatry 46:273–281, 2001

McQuade RD, Burris KD, Jordan S, et al: Aripiprazole: a dopamine-serotonin system stabilizer (abstract). Int J Neuropsychopharmacol 5 (suppl):S176, 2002

McQuade RD, Stock E, Marcus R, et al: A comparison of weight change during treatment with olanzapine or aripiprazole: results from a randomized, double-blind study. J Clin Psychiatry 65 (suppl):47–56, 2004

Meltzer HY: The role of serotonin in antipsychotic drug action. Neuropsychopharmacology 21 (suppl):106S–115S, 1999

Millan MJ: Improving the treatment of schizophrenia: focus on serotonin (5-HT)$_{1A}$ receptors. J Pharmacol Exp Ther 295:853–861, 2000

Mintzer JE, Tune LE, Breder CD, et al: Aripiprazole for the treatment of psychoses in institutionalized patients with Alzheimer dementia: a multicenter, randomized, double-blind, placebo-controlled assessment of three fixed doses. Am J Geriatr Psychiatry 15:918–931, 2007

Nickel MK, Muehlbacher M, Nickel C, et al: Aripiprazole in the treatment of patients with borderline personality disorder: a double-blind, placebo-controlled study. Am J Psychiatry 163:833–838, 2006

Nickel MK, Loew TH, Gil FP: Aripiprazole in treatment of borderline patients, part II: an 18-month follow-up. Psychopharmacology 191:1023–1026, 2007

Otsuka Pharmaceutical: Abilify (Aripiprazole) tablets: prescribing information. Tokyo, Japan, Otsuka Pharmaceutical Co, 2008. Available at: http://www.abilify.com/pdf/pi.aspx. Accessed January 5, 2009.

Petrie JL, Saha AR, McEvoy JP: Aripiprazole, a new novel atypical antipsychotic: phase II clinical trial result (abstract). Eur Neuropsychopharmacol 7 (suppl):S227, 1997

Pigott TA, Carson WH, Saha AR, et al: Aripiprazole for the prevention of relapse in stabilized patients with chronic schizophrenia: a placebo-controlled 26-week study. J Clin Psychiatry 64:1048–1056, 2003

Potkin SG, Saha AR, Kujawa MJ, et al: Aripiprazole, an antipsychotic with a novel mechanism of action, and risperidone vs placebo in patients with schizophrenia and schizoaffective disorder. Arch Gen Psychiatry 60:681–690, 2003

Pycock CJ, Kerwin RW, Carter CJ: Effect of lesion of cortical dopamine terminals on subcortical dopamine receptors in rats. Nature 286:74–76, 1980

Rao ML, Möller HJ: Biochemical findings of negative symptoms in schizophrenia and their positive relevance to pharmacologic treatment. Neuropsychobiology 30:160–164, 1994

Richelson E: Receptor pharmacology of neuroleptics: relation to clinical effects. J Clin Psychiatry 60 (suppl):5–14, 1999

Robinson DG, Woerner MG, Alvir JM, et al: Predictors of medication discontinuation by patients with first-episode schizophrenia and schizoaffective disorder. Schizophr Res 57:209–219, 2002

Sachs G, Sanchez R, Marcus R, et al: Aripiprazole in the treatment of acute manic or mixed episodes in patients with bipolar I disorder: a 3-week placebo-controlled study. J Psychopharmacol 20:536–546, 2006

Seeman P, Niznik HB: Dopamine receptors and transporters in Parkinson's disease and schizophrenia. FASEB J 4:2737–2744, 1990

Stock E, Marder SR, Saha AR, et al: Safety and tolerability meta-analysis of aripiprazole in schizophrenia (abstract). Int J Neuropsychopharmacol 5 (suppl):S185, 2002

Thase ME, Jonas A, Khan A, et al: Aripiprazole monotherapy in nonpsychotic bipolar I depression: results of 2 randomized, placebo-controlled studies. J Clin Psychopharmacol 28:13–20, 2008

Tiihonen J, Kuoppasalmi K, Fohr J, et al: A comparison of aripiprazole, methylphenidate, and placebo for amphetamine dependence. Am J Psychiatry 164:160–162, 2007

Tran-Johnson TK, Sack DA, Marcus RN, et al: Efficacy and safety of intramuscular aripiprazole in patients with acute agitation: a randomized, double-blind, placebo-controlled trial. J Clin Psychiatry 68:111–119, 2007

Vieta E, Bourin M, Sanchez R, et al: Effectiveness of aripiprazole vs. haloperidol in acute bipolar mania: double-blind, randomised, comparative 12-week trial. Br J Psychiatry 187:235–242, 2005

Weinberger DR: Implications of normal brain development for the pathogenesis of schizophrenia. Arch Gen Psychiatry 44:660–669, 1987

Zimbroff DL, Marcus RN, Manos G, et al: Management of acute agitation in patients with bipolar disorder: efficacy and safety of intramuscular aripiprazole. J Clin Psychopharmacol 27:171–176, 2007

CHAPTER 32

Risperidone and Paliperidone

Donald C. Goff, M.D.

History and Discovery

A decade before clozapine was approved for marketing in the United States, Janssen Pharmaceuticals established a program to examine the potential role of serotonergic agents in schizophrenia. Early interest in serotonergic agents stemmed from a preclinical literature demonstrating that both behavioral effects of dopamine agonists and haloperidol-induced catalepsy could be modulated by serotonin$_2$ (5-HT$_2$) antagonists; in addition, the early butyrophenone derivative pipamperone, which was observed to reduce agitation and improve social activity in patients with severe depression, was found to possess primarily 5-HT$_2$ antagonist activity (Ansoms et al. 1977; Leysen et al. 1978).

In 1981, Janssen Pharmaceuticals developed setoperone, a 5-HT$_2$ antagonist with weak dopamine$_2$ (D$_2$) antagonism that displayed antipsychotic effects and efficacy for negative symptoms in a preliminary open trial (Ceulemans et al. 1985). Janssen Pharmaceuticals additionally synthesized a selective 5-HT$_{2A}$ and 5-HT$_{2C}$ antagonist, ritanserin, which was shown to decrease extrapyramidal side effects (EPS) when combined with haloperidol in rat studies. Ritanserin also was active in animal models of anxiety (Colpaert and Meert 1985; Meert and Colpaert 1986) and partially ameliorated behavioral effects of lysergic acid diethylamide (LSD) (Colpaert and Meert 1985). In placebo-controlled trials in patients with chronic schizophrenia, addition of ritanserin to conventional antipsychotics improved negative symptoms and EPS (Bersani et al. 1990; Duinkerke et al. 1993; Gelders 1989; Reyntjens et al. 1986). Concluding that 5-HT$_2$ antagonism might improve efficacy of D$_2$ blockers, particu-

larly for negative symptoms, and reduce EPS, but that it was not sufficiently effective as monotherapy, Paul Janssen and colleagues undertook development of risperidone, which combined potent 5-HT$_{2A}$ and D$_2$ blockade.

After extensive preclinical characterization (Janssen et al. 1988), risperidone was first studied in clinical trials in 1986 and received U.S. Food and Drug Administration (FDA) approval for marketing in the United States in 1994. By the time risperidone became available to clinicians, the prominence of theories attributing 5-HT$_2$ enhancement of D$_2$ antagonism as a primary mechanism for clozapine's atypical properties (Meltzer et al. 1989), and the evidence from registration trials of reduced EPS and greater efficacy compared with high-dose haloperidol, resulted in considerable enthusiasm for the first of the "serotonin–dopamine antagonists." Risperidone was rapidly incorporated into clinical practice in the United States, where within 2 years it became the most frequently prescribed antipsychotic agent. In 2003, risperidone microspheres (Consta) received FDA approval as the first long-acting injectable second-generation antipsychotic. In December 2006, Janssen Pharmaceuticals introduced paliperidone (9-hydroxyrisperidone), the active metabolite of risperidone, formulated as an extended-release tablet marketed under the brand name Invega. A depot preparation, paliperidone palmitate, is currently in late-stage development.

Pharmacological Profile

Risperidone, or 3-[2-(4-[6-fluoro-1,2-benzisoxazol-3-yl]-1-piperidinyl)ethyl]-6,7,8,9-tetrahydro-2-methyl-4H-pyrido[1,2-a]pyrimidin-4-one, is a benzisoxazole deriva-

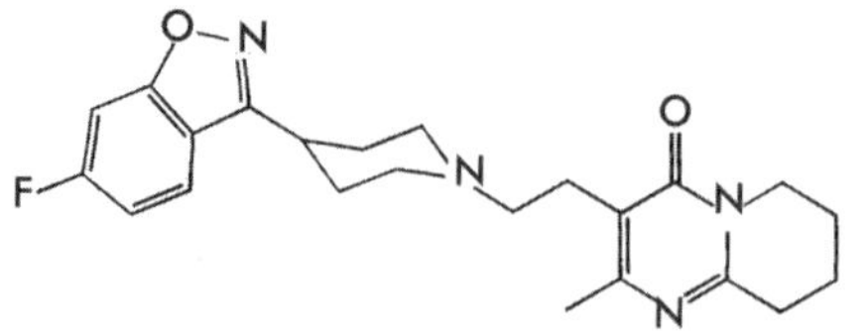

FIGURE 32–1.   Chemical structure of risperidone.

tive (Figure 32–1) characterized by very high affinity for 5-HT_{2A} and moderately high affinity for D_2, H_1, and α_1- and α_2-adrenergic receptors. In vitro, the affinity of risperidone for 5-HT_{2A} receptors is roughly 10- to 20-fold greater than for D_2 receptors (Leysen et al. 1994; Schotte et al. 1996); in vivo binding to rat striatal D_2 receptors occurs at a dose 10 times higher than does binding to 5-HT_{2A} receptors (Leysen et al. 1994). The affinity for 5-HT_{2A} receptors is more than 100-fold greater than for other serotonin receptor subtypes. The active metabolite 9-hydroxyrisperidone has a similar receptor affinity profile. Both risperidone and 9-hydroxyrisperidone display high affinities for 5-HT_{2A} receptors in rat brain tissue and for cloned human receptors expressed in COS-7 cells (Leysen et al. 1994). Risperidone binds to 5-HT_{2A} receptors with approximately 20-fold greater affinity than clozapine and 170-fold greater affinity than haloperidol (Leysen et al. 1994).

The affinity of risperidone for D_2 receptors is approximately 50-fold greater than that of clozapine and approximately 20%–50% that of haloperidol (Leysen et al. 1994) (Table 32–1). Binding affinity for D_2 receptors was similar in rat mesolimbic and striatal tissue and in the long and short forms of cloned human D_2 receptors expressed in embryonic kidney cells (Leysen et al. 1993a). The affinities of risperidone and 9-hydroxyrisperidone for dopamine$_4$ (D_4) and D_1 receptors are similar to those of clozapine and haloperidol (Leysen et al. 1994). Risperidone has essentially no affinity for muscarinic acetylcholine receptors and modest histaminergic H_1 activity, whereas 9-hydroxyrisperidone minimally binds to H_1 receptors. Unlike haloperidol, risperidone does not bind to sigma sites (Leysen et al. 1994). However, compared with other agents, risperidone has a relatively high affinity for α_2-adrenergic receptors, which is substantially greater than that of clozapine or any conventional agent and which approaches the affinity of phentolamine (Richelson 1996). The affinity of risperidone for α_1-adrenergic receptors is roughly comparable to that of chlorpromazine and approximately 5 to 10 times greater than that of clozapine (Leysen et al. 1993b; Richelson 1996). The me-

dian effective dose (ED_{50}) of risperidone required to inhibit D_2-mediated apomorphine-induced stereotypies in rats is 0.5 mg/kg; at this dose, approximately 40% of D_2 receptors are occupied, as are 80% of 5-HT_{2A} receptors, 50% of H_1 receptors, 38% of α_1-adrenergic receptors, and 10% of α_2-adrenergic receptors (Leysen et al. 1994).

Several groups have studied the occupancy of D_2 and 5-HT_2 receptors in patients with schizophrenia, employing positron emission tomography (PET) or single-photon emission computed tomography (SPECT) ligand-binding techniques. Kapur et al. (1999) used PET to measure D_2 occupancy with ^{11}C-labeled raclopride and 5-HT_2 occupancy with ^{18}F-labeled setoperone in patients with chronic schizophrenia maintained on a stable clinician-determined dose of risperidone. The PET was performed 12–14 hours after the last dose of risperidone. Occupancy of D_2 receptors ranged from 63% to 89%; 50% occupancy was calculated to occur with a daily risperidone dose of 0.8 mg. Patients treated with risperidone (6 mg/day) exhibited a mean D_2 occupancy of 79%, which was consistent with the mean occupancy of 82% that was previously reported by Nyberg et al. (1999) and would be expected to exceed the putative threshold for EPS in some patients. A similar degree of D_2 occupancy was calculated to occur with olanzapine at approximately 30 mg daily (Kapur et al. 1999). A maximal 5-HT_2 occupancy of greater than 95% was achieved with risperidone at daily doses as low as 2–4 mg. In a small sample of patients treated biweekly for at least 10 weeks with risperidone microspheres (Consta), Remington et al. (2006) found that the 25-mg dose produced a mean D_2 occupancy of 54% (preinjection) and 71% (postinjection), whereas the 50-mg dose produced occupancy levels of 65% (preinjection) and 74% (postinjection).

Preclinical characterization of risperidone in rats revealed more potent antiserotonergic activity, compared with ritanserin, in all tests (Janssen et al. 1988). For example, in reversal of tryptophan-induced effects in rats, risperidone was 6.4 times more potent than ritanserin for reversal of peripheral 5-HT_2-mediated effects and 2.4 times more potent for reversal of centrally mediated 5-HT_2 effects (Janssen et al. 1988). Risperidone was also found to completely block discrimination of LSD, in contrast to the partial attenuation observed with ritanserin (Meert et al. 1989). Although risperidone demonstrated activity in all dopamine-mediated tests, the dose–response pattern differed from that of haloperidol (Janssen et al. 1988). The two drugs were roughly equipotent for inhibition of certain dopamine effects, such as amphetamine-induced oxygen hyperconsumption, whereas the dose of risperidone necessary to cause pronounced cata-

TABLE 32–1. Receptor-binding affinities (K_i values, in nM) of risperidone (versus haloperidol and clozapine) in rat

	RISPERIDONE	**HALOPERIDOL**	**CLOZAPINE**
Dopaminergic			
D_2	3.1	1.2	152
D_1	536	430	570
Serotonergic			
$5\text{-}HT_{2A}$	0.16	27	3.3
$5\text{-}HT_{1A}$	420	1,500	145
Adrenergic			
α_1	2.4	19	24
α_2	7.5	>10,000	159
H_1 histaminergic	2.1	4,400	0.78
Muscarinic	>10,000	4,400	33

Source. Adapted from Leysen et al. 1993b.

lepsy in rats was 18-fold higher than that of haloperidol (Janssen et al. 1988). Risperidone depressed vertical and horizontal activity in rats at a dose 2–3 times greater than that of haloperidol but required doses more than 30 times greater than those of haloperidol to depress small motor movements (Megens et al. 1988).

Pharmacokinetics and Disposition

Risperidone is rapidly absorbed after oral administration, with peak plasma levels achieved within 1 hour (Heykants et al. 1994). In early Phase I studies, risperidone demonstrated linear pharmacokinetics at dosages between 0.5 and 25 mg/day (Mesotten et al. 1989; Roose et al. 1988). After a single dose of the extended-release formulation of paliperidone (Invega), serum concentrations gradually increase until a maximum concentration is achieved approximately 24 hours after ingestion. Absorption of paliperidone is increased by approximately 50% when taken with a meal compared with the fasted state. Extended-release paliperidone also demonstrates dose-proportional pharmacokinetics within the recommended dosing range (3–12 mg/day). Risperidone microspheres do not begin to release appreciable amounts of drug until 3 weeks after injection and continue to release drug for approximately 4 weeks, with maximal drug release occurring after about 5 weeks. Risperidone is 90% plasma protein bound, whereas 9-hydroxyrisperidone (paliperidone) is 74% plasma protein bound (Borison 1994). The absolute bioavailability of risperidone is about 100%; that of extended-release paliperidone is about 28%.

Risperidone is metabolized by hydroxylation of the tetrahydropyridopyrimidinone ring at the seven and nine positions and by oxidative N-dealkylation (Mannens et al. 1993). The most important metabolite, 9-hydroxyrisperidone, accounts for up to 31% of the dose excreted in the urine and has a receptor affinity profile similar to that of the parent compound. Because hydroxylation of risperidone is catalyzed by cytochrome P450 (CYP) 2D6, the half-life of the parent compound varies according to the relative activity of this enzyme. In "extensive metabolizers," which include about 90% of Caucasians and as many as 99% of Asians, the half-life of risperidone is approximately 3 hours. In healthy subjects, approximately 60% of 9-hydroxyrisperidone is excreted unchanged in the urine, and the remainder is metabolized by at least four different pathways (dealkylation, hydroxylation, dehydrogenation, and benzisoxazole scission), none of which accounts for more than 10% of the total. The terminal half-life of 9-hydroxyrisperidone (and of extended-release paliperidone) is 23 hours. "Poor metabolizers" metabolize risperidone primarily via oxidative pathways; the half-life may exceed 20 hours. In extensive metabolizers, radioactivity from ^{14}C-labeled risperidone is not detectable in plasma 24 hours after a single dose, whereas 9-hydroxyrisperidone accounts for 70%–80% of radioactivity. In poor metabolizers, risperidone is primarily responsible for radioactivity after 24 hours. In the U.S. multicenter registration trial, the correlations between risperidone dose and serum risperidone and 9-hydroxyrisperidone concentrations were 0.59 and 0.88, respectively (Anderson et al. 1993).

Mechanism of Action

As previously discussed, risperidone was developed specifically to exploit the apparent pharmacological advantages of combining 5-HT_2 antagonism with D_2 blockade. Selective 5-HT_{2A} antagonists administered alone have demonstrated activity in several animal models suggestive of antipsychotic effect, including blockade of both amphetamine- and phencyclidine (PCP)–induced locomotor activity (Schmidt et al. 1995). Dizocilpine-induced disruption of prepulse inhibition is also blocked by 5-HT_{2A} antagonists, suggesting that sensory gating deficits characteristic of schizophrenia and perhaps resulting from glutamatergic dysregulation might also benefit from the 5-HT_2 antagonism of risperidone (Varty et al. 1999). The disruption of prepulse inhibition by dizocilpine (MK-801, a noncompetitive N-methyl-D-aspartate [NMDA] antagonist) is attenuated by atypical antipsychotics, but not by conventional D_2 blockers (Geyer et al. 1990). From a study in which the selective 5-HT_{2A} antagonist M100907 was added to low-dose raclopride (a selective D_2 blocker), Wadenberg et al. (1998) concluded that 5-HT_{2A} antagonism facilitates D_2 antagonist blockade of conditioned avoidance, another behavioral model associated with antipsychotic efficacy, but does not block conditioned avoidance when administered alone.

One mechanism by which risperidone, paliperidone, and similar atypical agents might produce enhanced efficacy for negative symptoms and cognitive deficits and reduced risk for EPS is via 5-HT_{2A} receptor modulation of dopamine neuronal firing and cortical dopamine release. Prefrontal dopaminergic hypoactivity has been postulated to underlie negative symptoms and cognitive deficits in schizophrenia (Goff and Evins 1998); both clozapine and ritanserin have been shown to increase dopamine release in prefrontal cortex, whereas haloperidol does not (Busatto and Kerwin 1997). Following 21 days of administration, risperidone, but not haloperidol, continued to increase dopamine turnover in the dorsal striatum and prefrontal cortex (Stathis et al. 1996). Ritanserin has been shown to enhance midbrain dopamine cell firing by blocking a tonic inhibitory serotonin input (Ugedo et al. 1989). Ritanserin also normalized ventral tegmental dopamine neuron firing patterns in rats after hypofrontality was induced by experimental cooling of the frontal cortex (Svensson et al. 1989).

Svensson et al. (1995) have performed a series of elegant studies examining the impact of atypical antipsychotics on ventral tegmental dopamine firing patterns disrupted by glutamatergic NMDA receptor antagonists. In healthy human subjects, administration of the NMDA antagonist ketamine is widely regarded as a promising model for several clinical aspects of schizophrenia, including psychosis, negative symptoms, and cognitive deficits (Goff and Coyle 2001; Krystal et al. 1994). In rats, administration of the NMDA channel blockers dizocilpine or PCP increased burst firing of ventral tegmental dopamine neurons predominately projecting to limbic structures but reduced firing of mesocortical tract dopamine neurons and disrupted firing patterns. Administration of ritanserin and clozapine preferentially enhanced firing of dopamine neurons with cortical projections, and when added to a D_2 blocker, ritanserin increased dopamine release in prefrontal cortex. In addition to modulating ventral tegmental dopamine neuron firing, risperidone also blocks 5-HT_2 receptors on inhibitory γ-aminobutyric acid (GABA)-ergic interneurons, which could also influence activity of cortical pyramidal neurons that are regulated by these local inhibitory circuits (Gellman and Aghajanian 1994).

In placebo-controlled clinical trials, 5-HT_2 antagonists have reduced antipsychotic-induced parkinsonism and akathisia (Duinkerke et al. 1993; Poyurovsky et al. 1999). This effect may reflect 5-HT_{2A} antagonist effects upon nigrostriatal dopamine release. When combined with haloperidol, selective 5-HT_2 antagonists increase dopamine metabolism in the striatum and prevent an increase in D_2 receptor density, thereby possibly reducing the effects of D_2 receptor blockade and dopamine supersensitivity (Saller et al. 1990). These agents do not affect dopamine metabolism in the absence of D_2 blockade.

The relative importance of 5-HT_2 antagonist activity in producing atypical characteristics is the subject of debate. As argued by Kapur and Seeman (2001) and Seeman (2002), most atypical antipsychotic agents have dissociation constants for the D_2 receptor that are larger than the dissociation constant of dopamine. This "loose binding" to the D_2 receptor may allow displacement by endogenous dopamine and may contribute to a reduced liability for EPS and hyperprolactinemia. Unique among atypical agents, risperidone is "tightly bound" to the D_2 receptor, with a dissociation constant smaller than that of dopamine (Seeman 2002). A model for atypical antipsychotic mechanisms that emphasizes D_2 dissociation constants would predict that the apparent atypicality of risperidone, compared with that of haloperidol, reflects the reduced D_2 occupancy achieved by more favorable dosing rather than the intrinsic pharmacological characteristics of risperidone. According to some binding data, a comparable clinical dosage of haloperidol would be approximately 4 mg/day, rather than 20 mg/day as used in the North American multicenter registration trial (Kapur et al. 1999). Consistent with this view, benefits of risperidone for negative symptoms and EPS were less apparent when compared with lower doses of haloperidol or with lower-potency conventional agents (see "Indications and Efficacy" section later in this chapter) than when compared with high-dose haloperidol (20 mg/day).

An additional mechanism possibly contributing to the enhanced efficacy of risperidone and paliperidone is their considerable α-adrenergic antagonism. In a placebo-controlled augmentation trial, Litman et al. (1996) demonstrated significant improvement in psychosis and negative symptoms with the α_2-adrenergic antagonist idazoxan when it was added to conventional antipsychotics. Idazoxan has been shown to increase dopamine levels in the rat medial prefrontal cortex (Hertel et al. 1999). In aged rats (Haapalinna et al. 2000) and in patients with frontal dementias (Coull et al. 1996), α_2-adrenergic blockers have also been reported to improve cognitive functioning. Svensson et al. (1995) found that prazosin, an α_1 antagonist, inhibited both behavioral activation and the increase in mesolimbic dopamine release produced by PCP or MK-801.

In summary, risperidone and paliperidone possess at least two mechanisms that may confer atypical characteristics. 5-HT$_{2A}$ antagonism partially protects against D$_2$ antagonist–induced neurological side effects and may improve negative symptoms and cognitive functioning via modulation of mesocortical dopamine activity. In addition, blockade of adrenoceptors may further increase prefrontal cortical activity and could enhance antipsychotic efficacy by modulation of mesolimbic dopamine activity. Unlike other atypical agents, risperidone and paliperidone do not differ from conventional agents in their dissociation constant for the D$_2$ receptor; this feature perhaps accounts for the risk of EPS at high doses, as well as their greater propensity to cause hyperprolactinemia.

Indications and Efficacy

Risperidone is approved by the FDA for the treatment of schizophrenia, bipolar mania, and irritability associated with autism. In August 2007, the indication for schizophrenia was extended to include adolescents ages 13–17 years, and the bipolar mania indication was extended to include children 10–17 years of age. Risperidone microspheres (Consta long-acting injection) and extended-release paliperidone (Invega) are approved for the treatment of schizophrenia.

Schizophrenia

Clinical Trial Results for Risperidone

In the two North American registration trials (Chouinard et al. 1993; Marder and Meibach 1994), a total of 513 patients with chronic schizophrenia were randomly assigned to an 8-week double-blind, fixed-dose, placebo-controlled comparison of risperidone (2, 6, 10, or 16 mg/day) or haloperidol (20 mg/day). Risperidone dosages of 6, 10, and 16 mg/day produced significantly greater reductions, as compared with haloperidol, in each of the five domains of the Positive and Negative Syndrome Scale (PANSS), derived by principal-components analysis (Marder et al. 1997), and significantly higher response rates, defined as a 20% reduction in the PANSS total score. Effect sizes representing the difference in change scores between risperidone (6 mg/day) and haloperidol, although statistically significant, were uniformly small by Cohen's classification system (Cohen 1988): negative symptoms 0.31; positive symptoms 0.26; disorganized thoughts 0.22; uncontrolled hostility/excitement 0.29; and anxiety/depression 0.30 (Table 32–2). Severity of EPS was greater with haloperidol than with risperidone; further statistical analysis suggested that differences in EPS rates did not significantly influence the differences in PANSS subscale ratings (Marder et al. 1997). In fact, risperidone (10 and 16 mg/day) produced improvements in negative symptoms equivalent to those seen with risperidone (6 mg/day), despite increased EPS at the higher dosages of risperidone.

When risperidone (1, 4, 8, 12, and 16 mg/day) was compared with haloperidol (10 mg/day) in a large 8-week European trial involving 1,362 subjects with schizophrenia (Peuskens 1995), PANSS subscale change scores indicated preferential response to daily risperidone doses of 4 and 8 mg. However, neither the risperidone group taken as a whole nor individual risperidone doses achieved significantly better outcomes than haloperidol (10 mg/day) on any measure except for EPS, suggesting that the degree of the clinical superiority of risperidone, compared with haloperidol, may be dependent on the dosing of the comparator.

In the National Institute of Mental Health–funded Clinical Antipsychotic Trials of Intervention Effectiveness (CATIE; Stroup et al. 2003), 1,432 patients with chronic schizophrenia were randomly assigned to double-blind, flexibly dosed treatment for 18 months with risperidone, olanzapine, quetiapine, ziprasidone, or the conventional antipsychotic comparator perphenazine. Clinicians could adjust the dosage of each drug by prescribing 1–4 capsules daily; risperidone capsules contained 1.5 mg, and

TABLE 32–2.   Effect sizes on Positive and Negative Syndrome Scale (PANSS) symptom dimensions: North American trials (*N*=513)

| | ADJUSTED MEAN CHANGE SCORES | | | RISPERIDONE 6 MG/DAY | |
	PLACEBO	RISPERIDONE 6 MG/DAY	HALOPERIDOL	EFFECT SIZE VS. PLACEBO	EFFECT SIZE VS. HALOPERIDOL
PANSS total	–3.8	–18.6	–5.1	0.53	0.31
Negative	0.2	–3.4	–0.1	0.27	0.26
Positive	0.9	–5.7	–2.3	0.48	0.22
Disorganized thought	0.1	–4.6	–0.2	0.43	0.24
Hostility/excitement	0.2	–2.5	–0.1	0.47	0.29
Anxiety/depression	–0.1	–2.5	–0.6	0.36	0.30

Source.   Adapted from Marder et al. 1997.

the mean daily dose administered in the study was 3.9 mg. Based on the primary outcome measure, time to all-cause discontinuation, risperidone was less effective than olanzapine (mean dosage = 20 mg/day) and comparable in effectiveness to perphenazine (mean dosage = 21 mg/day) and the other atypical agents (Lieberman et al. 2005). Although differences in rates of dropout due to intolerance did not reach statistical significance, risperidone consistently was the best-tolerated drug, particularly in subjects who had failed their first-assigned drug due to intolerance.

Whereas the superior efficacy of risperidone for acute symptom reduction, compared with haloperidol, is quite broad (but of relatively small magnitude) and may be determined in part by the haloperidol dose, efficacy for prevention of relapse appears to be of a substantially greater relative magnitude. For example, Csernansky et al. (2002) randomly assigned 365 patients with stable schizophrenia or schizoaffective disorder to clinician-determined flexible dosing with risperidone or haloperidol for a minimum of 1 year. Kaplan-Meier estimates of the risk of relapse at the end of the study were 34% with risperidone, compared with 60% with haloperidol, a highly significant difference (*P* = 0.001).

Several studies have indicated that risperidone may significantly enhance cognitive functioning, particularly verbal working memory, compared with haloperidol (Green et al. 1997). More recently, in a large double-blind, flexibly dosed 3-month trial in first-episode schizophrenia patients, risperidone (mean dosage = 3.2 mg/day) produced a modest, although statistically significant, improvement in the composite cognitive score compared with haloperidol (mean dosage = 2.9 mg/day) (Harvey et al. 2005). Another large double-blind trial examined cognitive effects in chronic schizophrenia patients treated for

52 weeks with risperidone (mean dosage = 5.2 mg/day), olanzapine (12.3 mg/day), and haloperidol (8.2 mg/day) (Keefe et al. 2006). No difference between treatments was found in improvement on the composite cognitive score, although risperidone and olanzapine were superior to haloperidol in a secondary analysis of completers (Keefe et al. 2006). No significant differences in cognitive effects were found among risperidone, perphenazine, or the other atypical antipsychotics in the CATIE (Keefe et al. 2007).

Risperidone has been found to be well tolerated and effective in subgroups of patients with schizophrenia, including first-episode patients and elderly patients. In a 4-month double-blind trial comparing risperidone (mean dosage = 3.9 mg/day) and olanzapine (mean dosage = 11.8 mg/day) in 112 first-episode patients, both treatments were well tolerated, with an overall completion rate of 72% (Robinson et al. 2006). Response rates did not differ significantly between risperidone (54%) and olanzapine (44%), although patients who responded to risperidone were significantly more likely to retain their response. Experience with patients with treatment-resistant schizophrenia has been less consistent. In the U.S. multicenter registration study, Marder and Meibach (1994) found that patients who were presumed to have failed to respond to conventional agents, on the basis of a history of hospitalization for at least 6 months prior to study entry, did not respond to haloperidol (20 mg/day) but did display significant response to risperidone (6 and 16 mg/day), compared with placebo. Wirshing et al. (1999) reported significant improvement with risperidone (6 mg/day), compared with haloperidol (15 mg/day), during a 4-week fixed-dose trial in 67 patients with schizophrenia and histories of treatment resistance. However, the difference between treatments was lost during a subsequent 4-week flexible-dose phase in which the mean risperidone dosage was increased to 7.5 mg/day and the mean haloperidol dosage was increased to 19.4 mg/day. Bondolfi et al. (1998) reported comparable significant improvement with risperidone (mean dosage = 6.4 mg/day) and clozapine (mean dosage = 292 mg/day) in a randomized, double-blind trial involving 86 patients with schizophrenia described as resistant or intolerant to conventional antipsychotics by history. In a large open trial, risperidone produced significantly higher response rates than did haloperidol in 184 patients with histories of poor response (Bouchard et al. 2000). The relative superiority of risperidone over haloperidol steadily increased over time, reaching a maximum at the conclusion of the 12-month study. In contrast, Volavka et al. (2002) found no difference between high-dose risperidone (8–16 mg/day) and haloperidol (10–20 mg/day) in patients established by history to be treatment resistant to conventional antipsychotics. In the CATIE, risperidone was more effective than quetiapine but did not differ from olanzapine and ziprasidone in patients who discontinued their first-assigned atypical antipsychotic medication due to lack of efficacy (Stroup et al. 2006). In contrast, patients who discontinued perphenazine (for any reason) subsequently did better on quetiapine or olanzapine than they did on risperidone (Stroup et al. 2007).

Clinical Trial Results for Paliperidone

Extended-release paliperidone (Invega) at dosages of 6, 9, and 12 mg/day was more effective than placebo in a 6-week trial in acutely ill schizophrenia patients (Kane et al. 2007). In a flexibly dosed trial, extended-release paliperidone (9–15 mg/day) significantly reduced relapse compared with placebo (Kramer et al. 2007). The long-acting risperidone microsphere (Consta) formulation at fixed doses of 25 mg, 50 mg, and 75 mg administered biweekly was also superior in efficacy to placebo in a 12-week trial (Kane et al. 2003). In a 52-week study, treatment with risperidone microspheres was associated with low relapse rates; the incidence of relapse was 21.6% with the 25-mg dose and 14.9% with the 50-mg dose administered every 2 weeks (Simpson et al. 2006). In an open-label pilot trial of risperidone microspheres administered at a dose of 50 mg every 4 weeks, the 1-year relapse rate was estimated to be 22.4% (Gharabawi et al. 2007).

Affective Disorders

Six controlled trials of 3–4 weeks' duration that included a total of 1,343 patients have examined the efficacy of risperidone as monotherapy or in combination with a mood stabilizer for the acute treatment of bipolar mania (Rendell et al. 2006). As monotherapy and in combination, risperidone was more effective than placebo and comparable to haloperidol (Rendell et al. 2006). Risperidone's comparative efficacy in long-term prevention of relapse in bipolar disorder has not been established (Rendell and Geddes 2006).

Risperidone 1–2 mg/day was evaluated as an adjunct to antidepressant therapy in a 4-week placebo-controlled trial in 174 antidepressant-resistant patients with major depression recruited from 19 primary care and psychiatric centers (Mahmoud et al. 2007). Risperidone significantly lowered ratings of depressive symptoms compared with placebo. Remission rates were 25% with risperidone versus 11% with placebo (*P* = 0.004). Risperidone was well tolerated, with an 81% completion rate (vs. 88% with placebo).

Autism

Risperidone was also studied in a large 8-week placebo-controlled trial in 101 children (ages 5–17 years) with autism accompanied by severe tantrums, aggression, or self-injurious behavior (McCracken et al. 2002). Flexible dosing with risperidone (range = 0.5–3.5 mg/day; mean dosage = 1.2 mg/day) resulted in a mean reduction of 57% in irritability, compared with a decrease of 14% in the placebo group, and the response rate was 69% with risperidone versus 12% with placebo. In a study of 32 children (ages 5–17 years) treated for 4 months with open-label risperidone (mean dosage = 2 mg/day), those who continued treatment with risperidone during the second study arm, an 8-week double-blind substitution trial, had much lower relapse rates than patients switched to placebo (Research Units on Pediatric Psychopharmacology Autism Network 2005). Risperidone at a mean dosage of 2 mg/day was also found to be effective compared with placebo in a study of 31 adults with autism or pervasive developmental disorder (McDougle et al. 1998). In these studies, risperidone improved irritability and behavioral problems associated with autism but was not effective for social or language deficits. Risperidone at a dosage of 0.02–0.06 mg/kg was found to be well tolerated and effective for disruptive behaviors in children with low intelligence (intelligence quotient [IQ] between 36 and 84) in a 6-week placebo-controlled trial (Aman et al. 2002).

Other Disorders

In a 4-week placebo-controlled trial in 417 patients with generalized anxiety disorder, anxiety symptoms improved to a similar degree in both the placebo and the risperidone groups (Pandina et al. 2007). Risperidone was highly effective for obsessive-compulsive disorder symptoms in a 6-week placebo-controlled trial in 36 adults prospectively confirmed to be refractory to treatment with a selective serotonin reuptake inhibitor (McDougle et al. 2000). Symptoms of anxiety and depression also responded to risperidone compared with placebo. Fifty percent of risperidone-treated patients responded (mean dosage = 2.2 mg/day), compared with 0% in the placebo group.

Side Effects and Toxicology

Risperidone shares class warnings with other atypical antipsychotics in the United States, including the risks of tardive dyskinesia, neuroleptic malignant syndrome, and hyperglycemia and diabetes, as well as the risk of increased mortality in elderly patients with dementia-related psychosis. However, risperidone generally has been very well tolerated in clinical trials. In the U.S. multicenter trial reported by Marder and Meibach (1994), only headache and dizziness were significantly more frequent with risperidone (6 mg/day), compared with placebo, whereas the group receiving risperidone (16 mg/day) treatment also reported more EPS and dyspepsia than did the group receiving placebo (Table 32–3). Fatigue, sedation, accommodation disturbances, orthostatic dizziness, palpitations or tachycardia, weight gain, diminished sexual desire, and erectile dysfunction displayed a statistically significant relationship to risperidone dose, although most were not significantly elevated compared with placebo. In a flexible-dose relapse prevention study reported by Csernansky et al. (2002), no side effects were more frequent with risperidone, compared with haloperidol, although risperidone produced significantly greater weight gain. In a flexibly dosed, placebo-controlled trial of risperidone for children with disruptive behavior, risperidone (mean dosage = 1.2 mg/day) produced more somnolence, headache, vomiting, dyspepsia, weight gain, and prolactin elevation than did placebo; most side effects were rated mild to moderate and did not adversely affect compliance (Aman et al. 2002).

Weight gain with risperidone is intermediate—that is, the degree of weight gain is between that associated with agents like molindone and ziprasidone, which appear to be relatively weight neutral, and that associated with agents like clozapine, olanzapine, and low-potency phenothiazines. In a meta-analysis of controlled trials, Allison et al. (1999), using a random effects model, estimated the mean weight gain at 10 weeks with risperidone to be 2.0 kg,

compared with 0.5 kg with haloperidol, 3.5 kg with olanzapine, and 4.0 kg with clozapine. Although determining the risk for hyperglycemia is complex, and results of studies have not been completely consistent, it appears that risperidone does not produce insulin resistance and dyslipidemia to the degree associated with olanzapine and clozapine (American Diabetes Association et al. 2004; Henderson et al. 2006; Lieberman et al. 2005). In the CATIE, risperidone was associated with the lowest rate of discontinuation due to side effects (Lieberman et al. 2005). Risperidone treatment resulted in a mean 0.4-lb weight gain per month, compared with 2.0 lbs with olanzapine, 0.5 lb with quetiapine, and a mean monthly weight loss of 0.2 lb with perphenazine and 0.3 lb with ziprasidone.

Mesotten et al. (1989) reported the results of a safety trial involving 17 inpatients with psychosis in which, following a washout of previous medication, risperidone was started at 10 mg/day, and the dosage was then increased weekly by 5 mg/day to a maximum of 25 mg/day. Despite extremely high doses, sedation was the only prominent side effect. Although risperidone does not bind significantly to muscarinic cholinergic receptors, transient dry mouth, blurred vision, and urinary retention were observed in individual subjects. Palpitations occurred in 2 subjects. Heart rate significantly increased during the trial, and blood pressure slightly decreased; however, no cases of significant hypotension were reported. An endocrine battery, including plasma triiodothyronine, thyroid-stimulating hormone, growth hormone, prolactin, follicle-stimulating hormone, luteinizing hormone, and cortisol levels, was performed, and only prolactin was found to be affected.

Extrapyramidal Side Effects

Significant reductions in EPS with risperidone, compared with high-dose haloperidol, were a consistent finding in the North American trials (Chouinard et al. 1993; Marder and Meibach 1994). Measurement of EPS in the placebo group was complicated because 25% of the subjects were taking depot antipsychotics prior to enrollment. Risperidone produced significantly fewer parkinsonian side effects than did haloperidol (20 mg/day), based on several measures, including self-report, change scores on the Extrapyramidal Symptom Rating Scale (ESRS), and use of anticholinergic medication. Patients receiving risperidone (2 and 6 mg/day) did not differ from the group receiving placebo in mean ratings of parkinsonism and in the use of anticholinergic medication. Parkinsonism

TABLE 32–3. Side effects reported by patients with schizophrenia receiving placebo, risperidone, or haloperidol in the U.S. multicenter trial

	PERCENTAGE OF PATIENTS			
	PLACEBO (*N*=66)	RISPERIDONE 6 MG (*N*=64)	RISPERIDONE 16 MG (*N*=64)	HALOPERIDOL (*N*=66)
Insomnia	9.1	12.5	9.4	12.1
Agitation	7.6	10.9	12.5	16.7
Anxiety	1.5	7.8	4.7	1.5
Nervousness	1.5	6.3	1.6	0
Somnolence	0	3.1	9.4[a]	4.5
Extrapyramidal side effects	10.6	10.9	25.0[a]	25.8[a]
Headache	4.5	15.6[a]	9.4	7.6
Dizziness	0	9.4[a]	10.9[b]	0
Dyspepsia	4.5	9.4	6.3	4.5
Vomiting	1.5	6.3	6.3	3.0
Nausea	0	6.3	3.1	1.5
Constipation	0	1.6	6.3	1.5
Rhinitis	6.1	15.6	6.3	4.5
Coughing	1.5	9.4	3.1	3.0
Sinusitis	1.5	6.3	1.6	0
Fever	0	6.3	3.1	1.5
Tachycardia	0	4.7	6.3	1.5

[a]$P<0.05$ versus placebo.
[b]$P<0.01$ versus placebo.

Source. Adapted from Marder and Meibach 1994.

change scores were significantly correlated with the risperidone dosage ($r=0.94$); however, risperidone (16 mg/day) was associated with fewer parkinsonian side effects than was haloperidol. Dystonia occurred in six of the patients treated with risperidone (1.7%) versus two of the patients treated with haloperidol (2.4%). Dystonia rates did not differ between treatment groups, and the rates did not exhibit a relationship to risperidone dosage.

In the large European multicenter trial, maximum ratings of parkinsonism, hyperkinesias, and dystonia were greater with haloperidol (10 mg/day) than with all dosages of risperidone (maximum of 12 mg/day), and anticholinergic dosing was accordingly higher in the group treated with haloperidol (Peuskens 1995). Similarly, in a flexible-dose comparison of risperidone (mean dosage=4.9 mg/day) and haloperidol (mean dosage=11.7 mg/day) for prevention of relapse, EPS rates and use of anticholinergic medication significantly favored the group taking risperidone (Csernansky et al. 2002). However, in a smaller double-blind, flexible-dose trial comparing risperidone (5–15 mg/day) and the moderate-potency conventional agent perphenazine (16–48 mg/day) in 107 patients, no difference in EPS rates was observed (Hoyberg et al. 1993), indicating that the potency of the comparator agent may in part determine the relative benefit of risperidone for EPS. Of interest, in a study of low-dose risperidone (mean dosage=1.16 mg/day) in children with behavioral disorders, ratings of EPS did not differ between risperidone and placebo (Aman et al. 2002). No differences in EPS ratings were found between any treatment groups in the CATIE (Lieberman et al. 2005), although discontinuation rates due to EPS significantly differed, with perphenazine producing the highest discontinuation rate (8%) and olanzapine (2%), risperidone (3%), and quetiapine (3%) producing the lowest.

The experience with tardive dyskinesia (TD) in patients treated with risperidone has been quite promising. Jeste et al. (1999) randomly treated 122 elderly patients with low-dose haloperidol (median dose = 1 mg) versus risperidone (median dose = 1 mg). The very high rates of treatment-emergent TD typically found in geriatric patients make this sample a sensitive assay for TD risk. After 9 months, treatment-emergent TD rates were 30% with haloperidol versus less than 5% with risperidone. Risperidone was also noted to decrease dyskinetic movements, compared with haloperidol, in a Canadian multicenter trial reported by Chouinard et al. (1993), and it was associated with a treatment-emergent TD rate of 0.6%, compared with a rate of 2.7% with haloperidol, in a relapse prevention trial reported by Csernansky et al. (2002).

Hyperprolactinemia

Unlike other atypical antipsychotic agents, risperidone substantially increases serum prolactin levels—in some studies, to a greater degree than does haloperidol (Kearns et al. 2000; Markianos et al. 1999). The relationship between serum prolactin concentrations and clinical side effects remains somewhat unclear, however. Kleinberg et al. (1999) analyzed combined results from the North American and European multicenter registration trials, which included plasma prolactin concentrations from 841 patients and clinical ratings of symptoms associated with hyperprolactinemia from 1,884 patients. Mean prolactin levels significantly correlated with risperidone dosage; risperidone 6 mg/day produced elevations roughly comparable to those seen with haloperidol 20 mg/day and significantly higher than those seen with haloperidol 10 mg/day. The combined incidence of amenorrhea and galactorrhea in women, which varied between 8% and 12%, was similar for all dosages of risperidone and haloperidol (10 mg/day). Because symptom frequencies were available only for 14 women treated with placebo, comparisons with placebo were not informative. Sexual dysfunction or gynecomastia occurred in 15% of men treated with risperidone (4–6 mg/day), compared with 14% of men treated with haloperidol (10 mg/day) and 8% of men in the placebo group. Compared with placebo, ejaculatory dysfunction was significantly more frequent only in the group treated with risperidone (12–16 mg/day). Mean plasma prolactin levels were not significantly related to clinical side effects for either men or women. Decreased libido also did not differ between treatment groups and did not correlate with plasma prolactin levels. In the CATIE, prolactin levels increased by a mean of 15.4 ng/mL with risperidone, compared with a 0.4-ng/mL mean elevation with perphenazine and decreases of 4.5–9.3 ng/mL with the other atypical agents (Lieberman et al.

2005). Despite having significantly higher serum prolactin concentrations, patients treated with risperidone did not report significantly higher rates of sexual dysfunction, gynecomastia, galactorrhea, or irregular menses.

Two reports of clinical trials with extended-release paliperidone have indicated low levels of prolactin-related side effects (1% and 4%) (Kane et al. 2007; Kramer et al. 2007). However, in the one publication that reported prolactin levels, substantial increases in mean plasma prolactin concentrations were observed (males: 17.4 ng/mL at baseline to 45.3 ng/mL at week 6; females: 38.0 ng/mL to 124.5 ng/mL) (Kane et al. 2007). Two preliminary studies with risperidone found that plasma prolactin concentrations correlated with 9-hydroxyrisperidone (paliperidone) concentrations and not with risperidone concentrations (Melkersson 2006; Troost et al. 2007). The ratio of 9-hydroxyrisperidone levels to risperidone levels also correlated with prolactin concentration (Troost et al. 2007); in agreement with this finding, rapid metabolizers of CYP2D6 were found to have higher prolactin concentrations than poor metabolizers (Troost et al. 2007). Because of the difficulty in establishing dose equivalence between risperidone and paliperidone in clinical trials, it is not clear whether the two drugs differ in their potential to elevate prolactin. Additional studies are needed to compare prolactin elevations with the two drugs.

Cardiovascular Effects

Because of relatively high affinities for adrenoreceptors, risperidone would be expected to produce orthostatic hypotension. However, by following a 3- to 7-day dosage escalation schedule, initial postural hypotension and tachycardia have been avoided in clinical trials, with only rare cases of hypotension and syncope reported (Chouinard et al. 1993; Marder and Meibach 1994). Risperidone has very modest effects on cardiac conduction. No significant prolongation of the QTc interval was detected at dosages of up to 25 mg/day in early safety trials, and no relationship between QTc interval and risperidone dose was apparent (Mesotten et al. 1989). In the CATIE, risperidone was associated with the least QTc prolongation (mean 0.2 msec) and quetiapine with the greatest (mean 5.9 msec), although differences were not statistically significant (Lieberman et al. 2005). A mean 10-msec prolongation of the QTc, measured after peak absorption of risperidone (16 mg/day), was found in a study comparing atypical and typical antipsychotic agents, according to data filed with the FDA by Pfizer Inc. (Harrigan et al. 2004). Reported overdoses with risperidone have generally been benign, with moderate QT prolongation and no serious cardiac complications (Brown et al. 1993; Lo Vecchio et al. 1996).

Drug–Drug Interactions

Because CYP2D6 status affects the half-life of risperidone and the relative ratio of risperidone to 9-hydroxyrisperidone in plasma, the total serum concentration of the "active moiety," or risperidone plus 9-hydroxyrisperidone, may be significantly increased with addition of a CYP2D6 inhibitor (e.g., fluoxetine) in rapid metabolizers but not in poor metabolizers (Bondolfi et al. 2002; Spina et al. 2002). Paliperidone plasma concentrations are not influenced by CYP2D6 status, nor are paliperidone plasma concentrations likely to be affected by drug–drug interactions. It is possible that the addition of a CYP2D6 inhibitor (e.g., fluoxetine) could decrease risperidone-induced prolactin elevation by increasing the ratio of risperidone to 9-hydroxyrisperidone (Troost et al. 2007).

Conclusion

Risperidone was the first antipsychotic agent developed specifically to exploit the clinical advantages of combined D_2 and 5-HT_{A2} antagonism. α-Adrenergic antagonism additionally may contribute to the antipsychotic and cognitive-enhancing effects of risperidone. Risperidone is generally quite well tolerated, producing only moderate weight gain and mild sedation. Initial dosage titration is necessary to prevent orthostatic blood pressure changes and dizziness, although this may be less necessary with extended-release paliperidone. EPS are dose related, but their incidence at dosages less than or equal to 6 mg/day has not significantly differed from placebo. Risperidone substantially elevates prolactin levels, although the relationship between plasma prolactin concentrations and clinical symptoms is complex; prolactin-related side effects have not been detected in several studies of risperidone and paliperidone despite considerable prolactin elevation. The efficacy of risperidone is well established; compared with high-dose haloperidol, risperidone (6 mg/day) is significantly more effective for all five symptom clusters derived from the PANSS. Although it is broadly more effective, the magnitude of difference in effect size is not large for individual symptom clusters. At a dosage of 3.9 mg/day, risperidone did not differ from perphenazine in rates of discontinuation due to lack of effectiveness in the CATIE (Lieberman et al. 2005). Perhaps most im-

pressive has been evidence indicating that risperidone is substantially more effective than haloperidol in preventing relapse. Evidence of enhanced cognitive functioning with risperidone, with particular benefits for verbal memory, is encouraging, although also of a relatively modest magnitude. The availability of risperidone microspheres (Consta), the first long-acting injectable atypical agent, represents an important advance with the potential both to improve compliance and to minimize peak serum drug concentrations associated with oral dosing. While extended-release paliperidone also produces more uniform serum concentrations and avoids the variability associated with CYP2D6 status, the possibility of greater prolactin elevation with this formulation requires further study.

References

Allison DB, Mentore JL, Heo M, et al: Antipsychotic-induced weight gain: a comprehensive research synthesis. Am J Psychiatry 156:1686–1696, 1999

Aman MG, De Smedt G, Derivan A, et al: Double-blind, placebo-controlled study of risperidone for the treatment of disruptive behaviors in children with subaverage intelligence. Am J Psychiatry 159:1337–1346, 2002

American Diabetes Association, American Psychiatric Association, American Association of Clinical Endocrinologists, et al: Consensus development conference on antipsychotic drugs and diabetes and obesity. Diabetes Care 27:596–601, 2004

Anderson CB, True JE, Ereshefsky L, et al: Risperidone dose, plasma levels, and response. Presentation at the 146th annual meeting of the American Psychiatric Association, San Francisco, CA, May 22–27, 1993

Ansoms C, Backer-Dierick GD, Vereecken JL: Sleep disorders in patients with severe mental depression: double-blind placebo-controlled evaluation of the value of pipamperone (Dipiperon). Acta Psychiatr Scand 55:116–122, 1977

Bersani G, Grispini A, Marini S: 5-HT2 antagonist ritanserin in neuroleptic-induced parkinsonism: a double-blind comparison with orphenadrine and placebo. Clin Neuropharmacol 13:500–506, 1990

Bondolfi G, Dufour H, Patris M, et al: Risperidone versus clozapine in treatment-resistant chronic schizophrenia: a randomized double-blind trial. Am J Psychiatry 155:499–504, 1998

Bondolfi G, Eap CB, Bertschy G, et al: The effect of fluoxetine on the pharmacokinetics and safety of risperidone in psychotic patients. Pharmacopsychiatry 35:50–56, 2002

Borison RL: Risperidone: pharmacokinetics. J Clin Psychiatry 12:46–48, 1994

Bouchard R-H, Merette C, Pourcher E, et al: Longitudinal comparative study of risperidone and conventional neuroleptics for treating patients with schizophrenia. J Clin Psychopharmacol 20:295–304, 2000

Brown K, Levy H, Brenner C, et al: Overdose of risperidone. Ann Emerg Med 22:1908–1910, 1993

Busatto FG, Kerwin RW: Perspectives on the role of serotonergic mechanisms in the pharmacology of schizophrenia. J Psychopharmacol 11:3–12, 1997

Ceulemans D, Gelders Y, Hoppenbrouwers M, et al: Effect of serotonin antagonism in schizophrenia: a pilot study with setoperone. Psychopharmacology (Berl) 85:329–332, 1985

Chouinard G, Jones B, Remington G, et al: A Canadian multicenter placebo-controlled study of fixed doses of risperidone and haloperidol in the treatment of chronic schizophrenic patients. J Clin Psychopharmacol 13:25–40, 1993

Cohen J: Statistical Power Analysis for the Behavioral Sciences, 2nd Edition. Hillsdale, NJ, Lawrence Erlbaum, 1988

Colpaert FC, Meert TF: Behavioral and 5-HT antagonist effects of ritanserin: pure and selective antagonist effects of LSD discrimination in the rat. Psychopharmacology 86:45–54, 1985

Coull JT, Sahakian BJ, Hodges JR: The alpha 2 antagonist idazoxan remediates certain attentional and executive dysfunction in patients with dementia of frontal type. Psychopharmacology (Berl) 123:239–249, 1996

Csernansky JG, Mahmoud R, Brenner R: A comparison of risperidone and haloperidol for the prevention of relapse in patients with schizophrenia. N Engl J Med 346:16–22, 2002

Duinkerke SJ, Botter PA, Jansen AAI, et al: Ritanserin, a selective 5-HT2/1c antagonist, and negative symptoms in schizophrenia: a placebo-controlled double blind trial. Br J Psychiatry 163:451–455, 1993

Gelders YG: Thymosthenic agents, a novel approach in the treatment of schizophrenia. Br J Psychiatry 155 (suppl 5):33–36, 1989

Gellman RL, Aghajanian GK: Serotonin 2 receptor-mediated excitation of interneurons in piriform cortex: antagonism by atypical antipsychotic drugs. Neuroscience 58:515–525, 1994

Geyer MA, Swerdlow NR, Mansbach RS, et al: Startle response models of sensorimotor gating, and habituation deficits in schizophrenia. Brain Res 25:485–498, 1990

Gharabawi GM, Gearhart NC, Lasser RA, et al: Maintenance therapy with once-monthly administration of long-acting injectable risperidone in patients with schizophrenia or schizoaffective disorder: a pilot study of an extended dosing interval. Ann Gen Psychiatry 6:3, 2007

Goff DC, Coyle JT: The emerging role of glutamate in the pathophysiology and treatment of schizophrenia. Am J Psychiatry 158:1367–1377, 2001

Goff D, Evins A: Negative symptoms in schizophrenia: neurobiological models and treatment response. Harv Rev Psychiatry 6:59–77, 1998

Green M, Marshall B, Wirshing W, et al: Does risperidone improve verbal working memory in treatment-resistant schizophrenia? Am J Psychiatry 154:799–804, 1997

Haapalinna A, Sirvio J, MacDonald E: The effects of a specific alpha(2)-adrenoceptor antagonist, atipamezole, on cognitive performance and brain neurochemistry in aged Fisher 344 rats. Eur J Pharmacol 387:141–150, 2000

Harrigan EP, Miceli JJ, Anziano R, et al: A randomized evaluation of the effects of six antipsychotic agents on QTc, in the absence and presence of metabolic inhibition. J Clin Psychopharmacol 24:62–69, 2004

Harvey PD, Rabinowitz J, Eerdekens M, et al: Treatment of cognitive impairment in early psychosis: a comparison of risperidone and haloperidol in a large long-term trial. Am J Psychiatry 162:1888–1895, 2005

Henderson DC, Copeland PM, Borba CP, et al: Glucose metabolism in patients with schizophrenia treated with olanzapine or quetiapine: a frequently sampled intravenous glucose tolerance test and minimal model analysis. J Clin Psychiatry 67:789–797, 2006

Hertel P, Fagerquist M, Svensson TH: Enhanced cortical dopamine output and antipsychotic-like effects of raclopride by a2 adrenergic blockade. Science 286:105–107, 1999

Heykants J, Huang ML, Mannens G, et al: The pharmacokinetics of risperidone in humans: a summary. J Clin Psychiatry 55 (suppl):13–17, 1994

Hoyberg O, Fensbo C, Remvig J, et al: Risperidone versus perphenazine in the treatment of chronic schizophrenic patients with acute exacerbations. Acta Psychiatr Scand 88:395–402, 1993

Janssen PAJ, Niemegeers CJE, Awouters F, et al: Pharmacology of risperidone (R 64 766), a new antipsychotic with serotonin-S2 and dopamine D2-antagonist properties. J Pharmacol Exp Ther 244:685–693, 1988

Jeste DV, Lacro JP, Bailey A, et al: Lower incidence of tardive dyskinesia with risperidone compared to haloperidol in older patients. J Am Geriatr Soc 47:716–719, 1999

Kane JM, Eerdekens M, Lindenmayer JP, et al: Long-acting injectable risperidone: efficacy and safety of the first long-acting atypical antipsychotic. Am J Psychiatry 160:1125–1132, 2003

Kane J, Canas F, Kramer M, et al: Treatment of schizophrenia with paliperidone extended-release tablets: a 6-week placebo-controlled trial. Schizophr Res 90:147–161, 2007

Kapur S, Seeman P: Does fast dissociation from the dopamine D2 receptor explain the action of atypical antipsychotics? a new hypothesis. Am J Psychiatry 158:360–369, 2001

Kapur S, Zipursky R, Remington G: Clinical and theoretical implications of 5-HT2 and D2 occupancy of clozapine, risperidone and olanzapine in schizophrenia. Am J Psychiatry 156:286–293, 1999

Kearns A, Goff DC, Hayden D, et al: Risperidone-associated hyperprolactinemia. Endocr Pract 6:425–429, 2000

Keefe RS, Young CA, Rock SL, et al: One-year double-blind study of the neurocognitive efficacy of olanzapine, risperidone, and haloperidol in schizophrenia. Schizophr Res 81:1–15, 2006

Keefe RS, Bilder RM, Davis SM, et al: Neurocognitive effects of antipsychotic medications in patients with chronic schizophrenia in the CATIE Trial. Arch Gen Psychiatry 64:633–647, 2007

Kleinberg DL, Davis JM, deCoster R, et al: Prolactin levels and adverse events in patients treated with risperidone. J Clin Psychopharmacol 19:57–61, 1999

Kramer M, Simpson G, Maciulis V, et al: Paliperidone extended-release tablets for prevention of symptom recurrence in patients with schizophrenia: a randomized, double-blind, placebo-controlled study. J Clin Psychopharmacol 27:6–14, 2007

Krystal JH, Karper LP, Seibyl JP, et al: Subanesthetic effects of the noncompetitive NMDA antagonist, ketamine, in humans: psychotomimetic, perceptual, cognitive, and neuroendocrine responses. Arch Gen Psychiatry 51:199–214, 1994

Leysen JE, Niemegeers CJE, Tollenaere JP: Serotonergic component of neuroleptic receptors. Nature 272:168–171, 1978

Leysen JE, Gommeren W, Mertens J: Comparison of in vitro binding properties of a series of dopamine antagonists and agonists for cloned human dopamine D2S and D2L receptors and for D2 receptors in rat striatal and mesolimbic tissues, using

[125I]2-iodospiperone. Psychopharmacology (Berl) 110:27–36, 1993a

Leysen JE, Janssen PMF, Schotte A, et al: Interaction of antipsychotic drugs with neurotransmitter receptor sites in vitro and in vivo in relation to pharmacological and clinical effects: role of 5-HT2 receptors. Psychopharmacology (Berl) 112:S40–S54, 1993b

Leysen JE, Janssen PMF, Megens AAHP, et al: Risperidone: a novel antipsychotic with balanced serotonin-dopamine antagonism, receptor occupancy profile, and pharmacologic activity. J Clin Psychiatry 55 (suppl 5):5–12, 1994

Lieberman JA, Stroup TS, McEvoy JP, et al: Effectiveness of antipsychotic drugs in patients with chronic schizophrenia. Clinical Antipsychotic Trials of Intervention Effectiveness (CATIE) Investigators. N Engl J Med 353:1209–1223, 2005

Litman RE, Su T-P, Potter WZ, et al: Idazozan and response to typical neuroleptics in treatment-resistant schizophrenia. Br J Psychiatry 168:571–579, 1996

Lo Vecchio FL, Hamilton RJ, Hoffman RJ: Risperidone overdose (letter). Am J Emerg Med 14:95–96, 1996

Mahmoud RA, Pandina GJ, Turkoz I, et al: Risperidone for treatment-refractory major depressive disorder: a randomized trial. Ann Intern Med 147:593–602, 2007

Mannens G, Huang M-L, Meuldermans W: Absorption, metabolism and excretion of risperidone in humans. Drug Metab Dispos 21:1134–1141, 1993

Marder SR, Meibach RC: Risperidone in the treatment of schizophrenia. Am J Psychiatry 151:825–835, 1994

Marder S, Davis J, Chouinard G: The effects of risperidone on the five dimensions of schizophrenia derived by factor analysis: combined results of the North American trials. J Clin Psychiatry 58:538–546, 1997

Markianos M, Hatzimanolis J, Lykouras L: Gonadal axis hormones in male schizophrenic patients during treatment with haloperidol and after switch to risperidone. Psychopharmacology (Berl) 143:270–272, 1999

McCracken JT, McGough J, Shah B, et al: Risperidone in children with autism and serious behavioral problems. Research Units on Pediatric Psychopharmacology Autism Network. N Engl J Med 347:314–321, 2002

McDougle CJ, Holmes JP, Carlson DC, et al: A double-blind, placebo-controlled study of risperidone in adults with autistic disorder and other pervasive developmental disorders. Arch Gen Psychiatry 55:633–641, 1998

McDougle CJ, Epperson CN, Pelton GH, et al: A double-blind, placebo-controlled study of risperidone addition in serotonin reuptake inhibitor-refractory obsessive-compulsive disorder. Arch Gen Psychiatry 57:794–801, 2000

Meert TF, Colpaert FC: Effects of S2-antagonists in two conflict procedures that involve exploratory behavior. Psychopharmacology (Berl) 89:S23, 1986

Meert TF, de Haes P, Janssen PA: Risperidone (R 64 766), a potent and complete LSD antagonist in drug discrimination by rats. Psychopharmacology (Berl) 97:206–212, 1989

Megens AA, Awouters FHL, Niemegeers CJE: Differential effects of the new antipsychotic risperidone on large and small motor movements in rats: a comparison with haloperidol. Psychopharmacology (Berl) 95:493–496, 1988

Melkersson KI: Prolactin elevation of the antipsychotic risperidone is predominantly related to its 9-hydroxy metabolite. Hum Psychopharmacol 21:529–532, 2006

Meltzer HY, Bastani B, Ramirez L, et al: Clozapine: new research on efficacy and mechanism of action. Eur Arch Psychiatry Neurol Sci 238:332–339, 1989

Mesotten F, Suy E, Pietquin M, et al: Therapeutic effect and safety of increasing doses of risperidone (R 64766) in psychotic patients. Psychopharmacology (Berl) 99:445–449, 1989

Nyberg S, Eriksson B, Oxenstierna G, et al: Suggested minimal effective dose of risperidone based on PET-measured D2 and 5-HT2A receptor occupancy in schizophrenic patients. Am J Psychiatry 156:869–875, 1999

Pandina GJ, Canuso CM, Turkoz I, Kujawa M, Mahmoud RA. Adjunctive risperidone in the treatment of generalized anxiety disorder: a double-blind, prospective, placebo-controlled, randomized trial. Psychopharmacol Bull 40:41–57, 2007

Peuskens J: Risperidone in the treatment of patients with chronic schizophrenia: a multi-national, multi-centre, double-blind, parallel-group study versus haloperidol. Br J Psychiatry 166:712–726, 1995

Poyurovsky M, Shardorodsky M, Fuchs C, et al: Treatment of neuroleptic-induced akathisia with the 5-HT2 antagonist mianserin. Double-blind, placebo-controlled study. Br J Psychiatry 174:238–242, 1999

Remington G, Mamo D, Labelle A, et al: A PET study evaluating dopamine D2 receptor occupancy for long-acting injectable risperidone. Am J Psychiatry 163:396–401, 2006

Rendell JM, Geddes JR: Risperidone in long-term treatment for bipolar disorder. Cochrane Database Syst Rev (4):CD004999, 2006

Rendell JM, Gijsman HJ, Bauer MS, et al: Risperidone alone or in combination for acute mania. Cochrane Database Syst Rev (1):CD004043, 2006

Research Units on Pediatric Psychopharmacology Autism Network: Risperidone treatment of autistic disorder: longer-term benefits and blinded discontinuation after 6 months. Am J Psychiatry 162:1361–1369, 2005

Reyntjens A, Gelders YG, Hoppenbrouwers M-LJA, et al: Thymostenic effects of ritanserin (R55 667), a centrally active serotonin-S2 receptor blocker. Drug Dev Res 8:205–211, 1986

Richelson E: Preclinical pharmacology of neuroleptics: focus on new generation compounds. J Clin Psychiatry 57:S4–S11, 1996

Robinson DG, Woerner MG, Napolitano B, et al: Randomized comparison of olanzapine versus risperidone for the treatment of first-episode schizophrenia: 4-month outcomes. Am J Psychiatry 163:2096–2102, 2006

Roose K, Gelders YG, Heylen S: Risperidone (R64766) in psychotic patients: a first clinical therapeutic exploration. Acta Psychiatr Belg 88:233–241, 1988

Saller CF, Czupryna MJ, Salama AI: 5-HT2 receptor blockade by ICI 169,369 and other 5-HT2 antagonists modulates the effects of D-2 dopamine receptor blockade. J Pharmacol Exp Ther 253:1162–1170, 1990

Schmidt CJ, Sorensen SM, Kehne JH: The role of 5-HT2A receptors in antipsychotic activity. Life Sci 56:2209–2222, 1995

Schotte A, Janssen P, Gommeren W, et al: Risperidone compared with new and reference antipsychotic drugs-in vitro and in vivo receptor binding. Psychopharmacology (Berl) 124:57–73, 1996

Seeman P: Atypical antipsychotics: mechanism of action. Can J Psychiatry 47:27–38, 2002

Simpson GM, Mahmoud RA, Lasser RA, et al: A 1-year double-blind study of 2 doses of long-acting risperidone in stable patients with schizophrenia or schizoaffective disorder. J Clin Psychiatry 67:1194–1203, 2006

Spina E, Avenoso A, Scordo MG, et al: Inhibition of risperidone metabolism by fluoxetine in patients with schizophrenia: a clinically relevant pharmacokinetic drug interaction. J Clin Psychopharmacol 22:419–423, 2002

Stathis P, Antoniou K, Papadopoulou-Daifotis Z, et al: Risperidone: a novel antipsychotic with many "atypical" properties? Psychopharmacology (Berl) 127:181–186, 1996

Stroup TS, McEvoy JP, Swartz MS, et al: The National Institute of Mental Health Clinical Antipsychotic Trials of Intervention Effectiveness (CATIE) project: schizophrenia trial design and protocol development. Schizophr Bull 29:15–31, 2003

Stroup TS, Lieberman JA, McEvoy JP, et al: Effectiveness of olanzapine, quetiapine, risperidone, and ziprasidone in patients with chronic schizophrenia following discontinuation of a previous atypical antipsychotic. Am J Psychiatry 163:611–622, 2006

Stroup TS, Lieberman JA, McEvoy JP, et al: Effectiveness of olanzapine, quetiapine, and risperidone in patients with chronic schizophrenia after discontinuing perphenazine: a CATIE study. Am J Psychiatry 164:415–427, 2007

Svensson TH, Tung C-S, Grenhoff J: The 5-HT2 antagonist ritanserin blocks the effect of pre-frontal cortex inactivation on rat A10 dopamine neurons in vivo. Acta Physiol Scand 136:497–498, 1989

Svensson TH, Mathe JM, Andersson JL, et al: Mode of action of atypical neuroleptics in relation to the phencyclidine model of schizophrenia: role of 5-HT2 receptor and alpha1-adrenoreceptor antagonism. J Clin Psychopharmacol 15:S11–S18, 1995

Troost PW, Lahuis BE, Hermans MH, et al: Prolactin release in children treated with risperidone: impact and role of CYP2D6 metabolism. J Clin Psychopharmacol 27:52–57, 2007

Ugedo L, Grenhoff J, Svensson TH: Ritanserin, a 5-HT2 receptor antagonist, activates midbrain dopamine neurons by blocking serotonergic inhibition. Psychopharmacology (Berl) 98:45–50, 1989

Varty GB, Bakshi VP, Geyer MA: M100907, a serotonin 5-HT2A receptor antagonist and putative antipsychotic, blocks dizocilpine-induced prepulse inhibition deficits in Sprague-Dawley and Wistar rats. Neuropsychopharmacology 20:311–321, 1999

Volavka J, Czobor P, Sheitman B, et al: Clozapine, olanzapine, risperidone, and haloperidol in the treatment of patients with chronic schizophrenia and schizoaffective disorder. Am J Psychiatry 159:255–262, 2002

Wadenberg ML, Hicks PB, Richter JT, et al: Enhancement of antipsychotic properties of raclopride in rats using the selective serotonin 2A receptor antagonist MDL 100907. Biol Psychiatry 44:508–515, 1998

Wirshing DA, Barringer DMJ, Green MF, et al: Risperidone in treatment-refractory schizophrenia. Am J Psychiatry 156:1374–1379, 1999

CHAPTER 33

Ziprasidone

John W. Newcomer, M.D.

Elise M. Fallucco, M.D.

History and Discovery

Ziprasidone (CP-88059) is an atypical, or *second-genera-tion*, antipsychotic agent that has demonstrated activity for treating positive, negative, cognitive, and affective symptoms of schizophrenia and schizoaffective disorder and for treating mania and mixed states in bipolar disorder, with limited adverse extrapyramidal, sedative, anticholinergic, and cardiometabolic effects. Ziprasidone was first synthesized on the Pfizer Central Research campus in Groton, Connecticut. Both the oral and intramuscular formulations of this antipsychotic were initially part of a new drug application for the treatment of psychotic disorders submitted to the U.S. Food and Drug Administration (FDA) under the product name Zeldox in 1997. Because of concerns regarding an observed increase in the mean duration of the QT interval, an electrocardiographic measure of the ventricular depolarization and repolarization phases of cardiac conduction, the application was not initially approved. Further studies, designed in collaboration with the FDA, quantified the limited extent of this effect seen with ziprasidone compared with the effect seen with other agents in wide use; these studies established an approvable level of safety for ziprasidone with respect to cardiac conduction and a benchmark for the approach to evaluating drug effects on the QT interval that has subsequently been applied to other agents evaluated by the FDA. The FDA approved oral ziprasi-done in February 2001 under the trade name Geodon for the treatment of schizophrenia. The intramuscular formulation received FDA approval in 2002 for the treatment of acute agitation due to schizophrenia. In August 2004, oral ziprasidone received FDA approval for the treatment of bipolar mania, including manic and mixed episodes. At the time of writing, ziprasidone has received regulatory approval and is available in over 70 countries, usually under the trade name Zeldox, with more than 1.08 million patient-years of drug exposure.

Pharmacological Profile

Neuropharmacology and Receptor-Binding Profile

Ziprasidone, or 5-[2-[4-(1,2-benzisothiazol-3-yl)-1-piperazinyl]ethyl]-6-chloro-1,3-dihydro-2H-indol-2-one, is a novel benzisothiazolylpiperazine antipsychotic (Figure 33–1) with a unique structure and combination of receptor- and transporter-binding properties that distinguish it from other atypical/second-generation antipsychotics (Table 33–1) (Richelson and Souder 2000; Shapiro et al. 2003; Weiner et al. 2004).

Ziprasidone is a potent antagonist at dopamine type 2 (D_2) receptors but possesses inverse agonist activity at 5-hydroxytryptamine (serotonin) type 2A receptors (5-HT$_{2A}$ receptors). D_2 receptor antagonism is thought

Dr. John Newcomer would like to thank Glennon M. Floyd and Amber Spies for editorial assistance on this chapter.

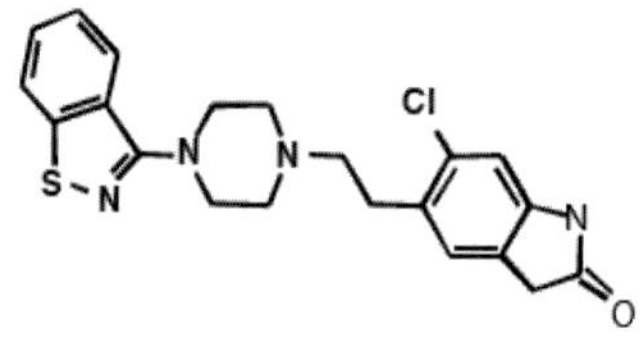

FIGURE 33–1. Chemical structure of ziprasidone.

to be a key mechanism underlying efficacy for the treatment of psychotic symptoms (Kapur and Remington 2001); positron emission tomography (PET) studies have shown that clinical antipsychotic response to ziprasidone is predicted by occupancy of at least 60% of striatal D_2 receptors. D_2 antagonism is also associated with potential liability for extrapyramidal side effects (EPS). However, ziprasidone's inverse agonist activity at $5\text{-}HT_{2A}$ receptors disinhibits dopamine neurotransmission in the nigrostriatal, mesocortical, and tuberoinfundibular pathways (Kapur and Remington 1996; Schmidt et al. 2001); this reduces liability for EPS compared with antipsychotics with unopposed D_2 antagonism and potentially contributes to therapeutic effects. Increased dopamine activity in the prefrontal cortex is putatively linked to efficacy in improving the negative and cognitive symptoms of schizophrenia (Stahl and Shayegan 2003). Enhanced dopaminergic transmission in the tuberoinfundibular pathway minimizes the potential effect of D_2 receptor antagonism on prolactin secretion. Ziprasidone's relatively high in vitro $5\text{-}HT_{2A}/D_2$ receptor affinity ratio, compared with that of other second-generation antipsychotics, predicts both a low liability for EPS and potential therapeutic benefits for negative symptoms (Altar et al. 1986).

Ziprasidone exhibits antagonist activity at $5\text{-}HT_{1D}$ and $5\text{-}HT_{2C}$ receptors, and unique (among second-generation antipsychotics) agonist activity at $5\text{-}HT_{1A}$ receptors (see Table 33–1) (DeLeon et al. 2004; Schmidt et al. 2001). The $5\text{-}HT_{1A}$ affinity is comparable to that of buspirone, an agent with antidepressant and anxiolytic properties (Mazei et al. 2002), suggesting a mechanism that may contribute to observed beneficial effects on affective, cognitive, and negative symptoms in schizophrenia and schizoaffective disorder (Diaz-Mataix et al. 2005; Ichikawa et al. 2001; Millan 2000; Rollema et al. 2000; Sumiyoshi et al. 2003; Tauscher et al. 2002). Blockade of $5\text{-}HT_{2C}$ receptors disinhibits both dopamine and norepinephrine neurons in the cortex, an effect that could contribute to improvements in cognitive and affective abnormalities (Bremner et al. 2003; Bymaster et al. 2002; Mazei et al. 2002; Stahl 2003). Although $5\text{-}HT_{2C}$ antagonist

activity is potentially predictive of weight gain liability, based, for example, on a $5\text{-}HT_{2C}$ knockout mouse model of obesity (Tecott et al. 1995), clinically significant predictive effects of $5\text{-}HT_{2C}$ antagonist activity on the weight gain risk associated with antipsychotic drugs have not been reliably detected (Kroeze et al. 2003), and the weight gain risk associated with ziprasidone is among the lowest of any currently available antipsychotic (Allison et al. 1999b). Potent antagonism at $5\text{-}HT_{1D}$ receptors has been proposed to potentially mediate antidepressant and anxiolytic effects (Briley and Moret 1993; Zorn et al. 1998).

Another unique feature of ziprasidone is its relatively high affinity for serotonin and norepinephrine transporters (Seeger et al. 1995; Tatsumi et al. 1999). In vitro, ziprasidone demonstrates dose-dependent reuptake inhibition of serotonin and norepinephrine transport, with effects ranging up to those of imipramine and amitriptyline (Schmidt et al. 2001), suggesting potential antidepressant activity. In vivo, the clinical significance of ziprasidone's monoaminergic reuptake inhibition may be limited by plasma protein binding or be clinically relevant only at higher than currently recommended daily dosages. Monoaminergic reuptake inhibition is associated with hippocampal neurogenesis, suggesting potential value in countering the neuronal cell loss observed in both affective illness and schizophrenia (Arango et al. 2001; Duman 2004; Thome et al. 1998). Relevant to this activity, treatment with ziprasidone and risperidone has been associated with an increase in cortical gray matter volume (Garver et al. 2005).

Ziprasidone has a low affinity for histaminergic$_1$ (H_1), muscarinic$_1$ (M_1), and α_1-noradrenergic receptors. Among the biogenic amine receptors, H_1 antagonist activity is the largest predictor of weight gain liability (Figure 33–2) (Kroeze et al. 2003). H_1 antagonist activity is also predictive of sedative effects, which are potentially undesirable for patients aiming to maximize cognitive performance and social, occupational, and community engagement. Low affinity for α_1-adrenergic receptors predicts a lower likelihood of orthostatic hypotension and sedation with ziprasidone than with commonly used antipsychotics with potent α_1-adrenergic antagonist activity. Low affinity for M_1 receptors predicts a low risk for anticholinergic side effects such as dry mouth, blurry vision, urinary retention, constipation, confusion, and memory impairment.

Ziprasidone's complex neuropharmacology provides explanatory support for observed treatment effects on psychotic and affective symptoms of schizophrenia, schizoaffective disorder, and bipolar disorder and for its favorable

TABLE 33–I. Binding affinities of atypical antipsychotics (compared with haloperidol) for human receptors and rat transporters

	HALOPERIDOL	CLOZAPINE	OLANZAPINE	RISPERIDONE	QUETIAPINE	ZIPRASIDONE	ARIPIPRAZOLE
Binding affinities associated with potential therapeutic effects (mean pKi, nM)							
D_2 receptors	1.4	130	20	2.2	180	3.1	0.4
5-HT$_{1A}$ receptors	3,600	140	2,100	210	230	2.5	4.4
5-HT$_{1B/1D}$ receptors	>5,000	1,700	530	170	>5,100	2.0	68
5-HT$_{2A}$ receptors	120	8.9	3.3	0.29	220	0.39	3.4
5-HT$_{2C}$ receptors	4,700	17	10	10	1,400	1.72	15
5-HT uptake transporters	1,800	3,900	>15,000	1,400	>18,000	53	98
NE uptake transporters	5,500	390	2,000	28,000	680	48	2,090
Binding affinities associated with potential adverse effects (mean pKi, nM)							
H_1 receptors	440	1.8	2.8	19	8.7	47	61
M_1 receptors	1,600	1.8	4.7	2,800	100	5,100	>10,000
α_1-adrenoceptors	4.7	4.0	54	1.4	15	13	57
α_2-adrenoceptors	1,200	33	170	5.1	1,000	310	74

Note. D_2 = dopamine$_2$ receptor; H_1 = histamine$_1$ receptor; 5-HT = 5-hydroxytryptamine (serotonin); M_1 = muscarinic$_1$ receptor; NE = norepinephrine.

Source. DeLeon et al. 2004; Kroeze et al. 2003; Richelson and Souder 2000; Schmidt et al. 2001; Shapiro et al. 2003; Stahl and Shayegan 2003; Weiner et al. 2004.

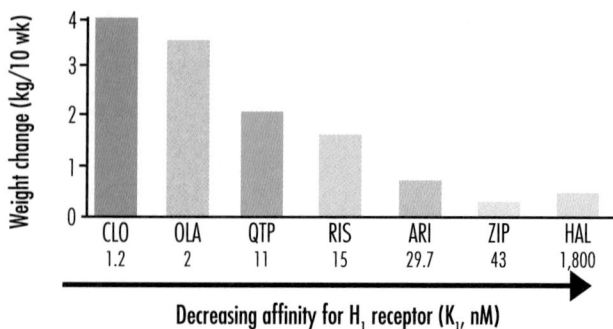

FIGURE 33–2. Histamine₁ (H₁) receptor affinity predicts antipsychotic-induced weight gain.

ARI = aripiprazole; CLO = clozapine; HAL = haloperidol; K_1 = binding affinity; OLA = olanzapine; QTP = quetiapine; RIS = risperidone; ZIP = ziprasidone.
Source. Adapted from Kroeze et al. 2003.

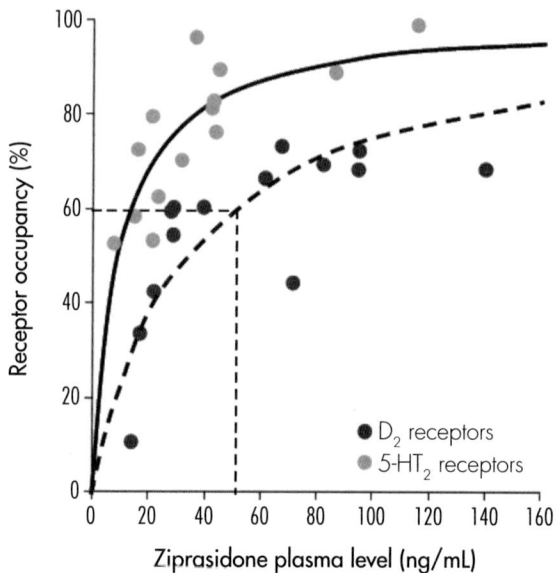

FIGURE 33–3. Relationship between dopamine₂ (D₂) and serotonin₂ (5-HT₂) receptor occupancy and ziprasidone plasma levels in 16 patients with schizophrenia or schizoaffective disorder receiving therapeutic dosages of ziprasidone.

Dotted straight lines represent minimal D₂ receptor occupancy and plasma concentration that would be expected to be associated with a clinical antipsychotic response, corresponding to a ziprasidone dosage of approximately 120 mg/day.
Source. Adapted from Mamo et al. 2004.

tolerability profile including minimal extrapyramidal and metabolic side effects (Stahl and Shayegan 2003).

Positron Emission Tomography Studies

An in vivo PET study (Mamo et al. 2004) examining the affinity of ziprasidone for dopamine (D₂) and serotonin (5-HT₂) receptors observed that optimal D₂ receptor occupancy occurs at the high end of the initially recommended dosage range. In this study, the ziprasidone plasma concentration associated with 50% of maximal D₂ receptor occupancy was more than twice the plasma concentration associated with 50% of maximal 5-HT₂ receptor occupancy. Using an imaging protocol where 60% or greater D₂ dopamine receptor occupancy is generally predictive of antipsychotic activity, approximately 60% D₂ occupancy was observed in relation to plasma concentrations equivalent to those attained with a dosage at or above 120 mg/day. These results, consistent with clinical trial results discussed later in this chapter (see "Indications and Efficacy"), strongly suggest that antipsychotic activity with ziprasidone is most commonly associated with dosages of 120 mg/day or greater (Figure 33–3).

Dosing Recommendations

In addition to the PET data, accumulating evidence from clinical trials (discussed below) suggests that ziprasidone dosing targets should be higher than initially recommended. In the United States, it was initially recommended that ziprasidone treatment in patients with schizophrenia be initiated at a dosage of 20 mg twice daily and then titrated at no less than 2-day intervals to a max-

imal dosage of 80 mg twice daily (Pfizer Inc. 2008). In contrast, more recent FDA approval of ziprasidone for the treatment of bipolar mania includes a recommendation that treatment be initiated at 40 mg twice daily with a more rapid titration; on the second day of treatment, the dosage should be increased to 60 or 80 mg twice daily and should subsequently be adjusted on the basis of toleration and efficacy within the 40- to 80-mg twice-daily range.

A review of short-term trials of ziprasidone (Kane 2003) concluded that daily dosages of 120–160 mg are more effective than lower dosages in the treatment of acute schizophrenia and also are associated with lower rates of medication discontinuation. A more recent 6-month prospective, observational, naturalistic, uncontrolled study performed in Spain also found that dosages greater than 120 mg/day were associated with a lower risk of discontinuation for any cause (Arango et al. 2007). As a corollary, another European observational multicenter trial found that both initial and overall underdosing are associated with high discontinuation rates (Kudla et al. 2007). In a pooled analysis of both flexible-dose and fixed-dose studies (N = 2,174), greater efficacy was observed in patients who received an initial dosage of 80 mg/day than in patients who received an initial dosage of 40 mg/day (Murray et al. 2004). Reported clinical experience with ziprasidone has also suggested the need for dosages greater than 160 mg/day in selected patients (Harvey and Bowie 2005; Nemeroff et al. 2005).

Finally, two large observational database analyses support the other lines of evidence suggesting that higher dosages of ziprasidone are associated with better treatment outcomes than lower dosages (Joyce et al. 2006; Mullins et al. 2006). Both studies used prescription refills as an indicator of prescription adherence, a key measure of treatment continuation and overall effectiveness. Joyce et al. (2006) examined the files of more than 1,000 commercially insured patients with schizophrenia or schizoaffective disorder and concluded that an initial daily dosage of 120–160 mg was associated with a significantly lower risk of discontinuation at 6 months than an initial daily dosage of 60–80 mg. Mullins et al. (2006), evaluating a sample of more than 1,000 Medicaid recipients with schizophrenia, similarly concluded that patients receiving an initial dosage of 120–160 mg daily had lower rates of medication discontinuation than patients receiving an initial dosage of 20–60 mg daily. Taken together, results from receptor occupancy studies, clinical trials, and pharmacoepidemiological analyses provide support for the conclusion that initiation and treatment with ziprasidone dosages greater than 120 mg/day are more likely to be effective than lower dosages in the treatment of schizophrenia and schizoaffective disorder.

Pharmacokinetics and Disposition

Absorption and Distribution

Based on evidence of enhanced absorption in the presence of food, it is recommended that ziprasidone be taken with meals. Administration with food increases absorption by more than 50%, giving ziprasidone an oral bioavailability of approximately 60% (Pfizer Inc. 2008). Maximal plasma concentration (C_{max}) is achieved in 3.7–4.7 hours and reaches 45–139 μg/L in healthy volunteers receiving 20–60 mg twice daily, and steady-state serum concentrations occur within 1–3 days of twice-daily dosing (Hamelin et al. 1998; Miceli et al. 2000c). In contrast to oral administration, intramuscular administration of ziprasidone results in 100% bioavailability. A therapeutic plasma level is reached within 10 minutes, and C_{max} is achieved within 30 minutes of administration of a 20-mg dose (Pfizer Inc. 2008).

The mean apparent volume of distribution of ziprasidone is 1.5 L/kg (Pfizer Inc. 2008), which is lower than that of many other antipsychotic drugs. Given the wider potential for unwanted interactions with various intracellular targets that has been observed with lipophilic drugs having a high volume of distribution (Dwyer et al. 1999), this may be a favorable attribute for ziprasidone and other similar compounds. Ziprasidone is more than 99% bound to plasma proteins. However, in vitro binding studies indicate that it does not alter the protein binding of two highly protein-bound drugs, warfarin and propranolol, neither do these two drugs interfere with the protein binding of ziprasidone, suggesting that these types of drug interactions are unlikely.

Metabolism and Elimination

Ziprasidone is extensively metabolized with a mean terminal elimination half-life of approximately 7 hours after oral administration within the recommended clinical dosage range (Pfizer Inc. 2008). The elimination half-life of intramuscular ziprasidone is less than 3 hours with a single dose (Brook et al. 2000). Ziprasidone is cleared primarily via three metabolic pathways to yield four major circulating metabolites (Figure 33–4). Elimination occurs primarily through hepatic metabolism, with less than one-third of metabolic clearance mediated via cytochrome P450 (CYP)–catalyzed oxidation and approximately two-thirds via reduction of the parent compound by aldehyde oxidase to dihydroziprasidone, which then undergoes S-methylation. The current published literature reports no commonly encountered clinically significant pharmacological inhibitors of aldehyde oxidase, suggesting limited real-world potential for drug–drug interactions that would alter the clinical activity of ziprasidone (Obach et al. 2004).

Additional secondary metabolic pathways include N-dealkylation (via CYP enzymes 3A4 and 1A2) and direct S-oxidation (via CYP3A4) (Beedham et al. 2003; Prakash et al. 2000). S-methyl-dihydroziprasidone is the only active metabolite, with lower D_2 receptor affinity and no significant binding to H_1, M_1, or α_1- and α_2-adrenergic receptors. A small amount of the parent compound is excreted unchanged in the urine (<1%) and feces (<4%).

There are no clinically significant age- or gender-related differences in the pharmacokinetics of oral ziprasidone (Pfizer Inc. 2008). Hepatic impairment might be expected to increase the area under the time–concentration curve (AUC). A multiple-dose study (Everson et al. 2000) comparing subjects with clinically significant

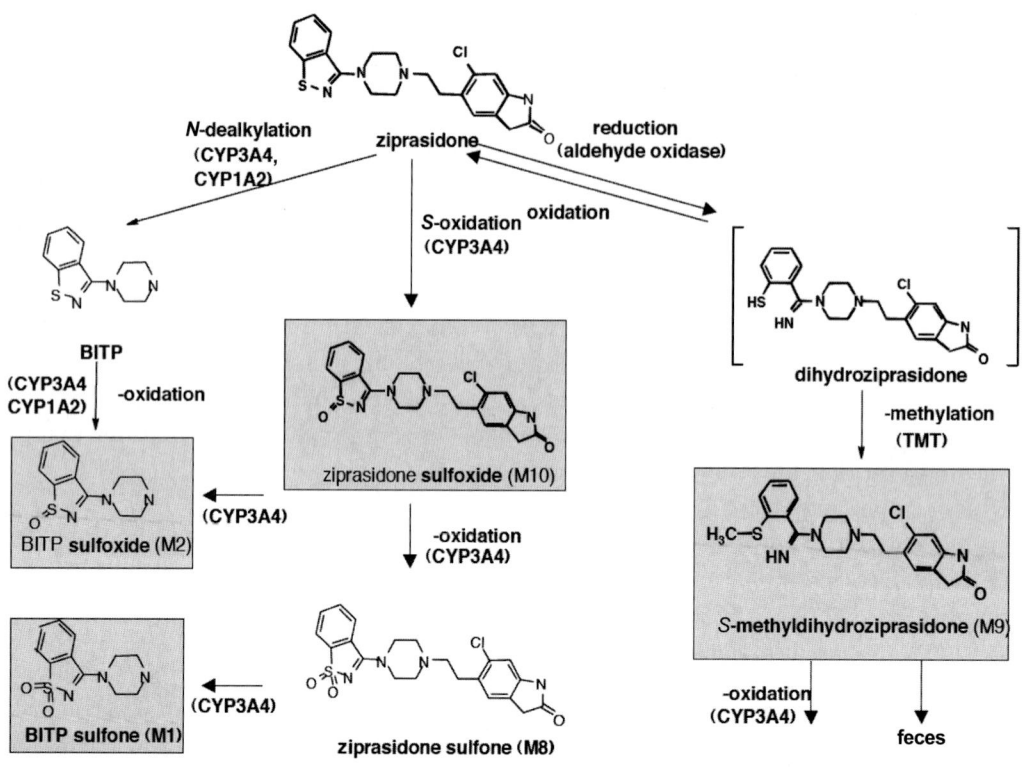

FIGURE 33–4.   Major metabolic pathways of ziprasidone.

BITP = benzisothiazole piperazine; CYP = cytochrome P450; M = metabolite; TMT = thiol methyltransferase.

Source.   Adapted from U.S. Food and Drug Administration Pharmacological Drugs Advisory Committee: Briefing Document for Ziprasidone Mesylate for Intramuscular Injection (Figure 2 [Metabolism of Ziprasidone in Humans: Proposed Metabolic Pathways to Major Circulating Metabolites], p. 5). February 15, 2001. Available at: http://www.fda.gov/ohrms/dockets/ac/01/briefing/3685b2_01_pfizer.pdf.

(Childs-Pugh Class A and B) cirrhosis versus healthy control subjects indicated that 12 hours after administration of ziprasidone, the AUC was 13% and 34% greater in subjects with Childs-Pugh Class A and B cirrhosis, respectively, than in matched control subjects, suggesting that dose adjustments are generally not mandatory for patients with hepatic impairment. Impairment in renal function is unlikely to significantly alter the pharmacokinetics of oral ziprasidone, suggesting that ziprasidone would not be removed by hemodialysis (Pfizer Inc. 2008). Intramuscular ziprasidone has not been systematically evaluated in the elderly or in patients with hepatic or renal impairment. Intramuscular ziprasidone contains a cyclodextrin excipient that is cleared by renal filtration; thus, it should be administered with caution to patients with impaired renal function (Pfizer Inc. 2008).

Impact of Food on Pharmacokinetics

Recent pharmacokinetic studies examined ziprasidone bioavailability under fasting conditions and after eating food with varying caloric and fat composition to better understand effects of food intake on drug availability (Lombardo et al. 2007). In an open-label, nonrandomized, six-way crossover study, healthy adults received single doses of ziprasidone under fasting conditions and then under fed conditions with a standard meal of 800–1,000 calories. Serum ziprasidone levels were measured immediately prior to drug administration and at multiple scheduled time points up to 72 hours following drug administration. Ziprasidone exhibited linear pharmacokinetics in fed subjects, but nonlinear pharmacokinetics in fasting subjects. Dose-proportional increases in ziprasidone AUC and C_{max} were observed under fed but not fasting conditions. C_{max} was significantly higher in fed states than in fasting states at doses of 40 mg (63% higher) and 80 mg (97% higher). Results from two additional open-label crossover studies further clarified the factors regulating drug bioavailability (Lombardo et al. 2007). Results indicated that 1) significantly greater absorption is achieved during administration with a meal of at least 500 calories and 2) absorption is not significantly influenced by the fat content of the meal. These studies suggest that the administration of ziprasidone with food provides linear pharmacokinetics and optimal absorption, supporting predictable symptom control. In addition, the results suggest that total meal bulk sufficient to slow gastric and duodenal transit time (e.g., a bowl of oatmeal), rather than fat content or specific calorie counts, may be the key factor contributing to reliable dose-dependent drug absorption with meals.

Drug–Drug Interactions

A study of in vitro enzyme inhibition (Pfizer Inc. 2008) indicated that ziprasidone has little inhibitory effect on CYP1A2, CYP2C9, CYP2C19, CYP2D6, and CYP3A4 and is thus unlikely to interfere with the metabolism of other medications relying on these enzymes for clearance. In vivo studies indicated that ziprasidone has no effect on the pharmacokinetics of lithium, estrogen, progesterone, or dextromethorphan (Pfizer Inc. 2008). As noted above (in "Metabolism and Elimination" subsection), less than one-third of ziprasidone clearance is mediated by CYP-catalyzed oxidation and, based on this, one would not anticipate a substantial change in ziprasidone AUC during coadministration with CYP3A4 inhibitors or inducers. Aldehyde oxidase–mediated reduction of ziprasidone to its dihydro- metabolite constitutes the primary metabolic pathway for ziprasidone. As also noted above, currently no clinically significant pharmacological inhibitors of aldehyde oxidase are commonly encountered, which suggests that ziprasidone has limited potential for drug–drug interactions that would alter its clinical activity (Obach et al. 2004).

Consistent with this prediction, coadministration with ketoconazole, a potent CYP3A4 inhibitor, results in only a modest increase in ziprasidone AUC (33%) and C_{max} (34%) (Miceli et al. 2000b), while coadministration with carbamazepine, an inducer of 3A4, results in modest reductions in ziprasidone AUC (44%) and C_{max} (39%) (Miceli et al. 2000a). For comparison, a threefold increase in quetiapine C_{max} is observed during coadministration with ketoconazole, and a significant decrease in quetiapine C_{max} occurs during coadministration with CYP3A4 inducers (AstraZeneca 2008). Furthermore, coadministration with CYP2D6 inhibitors has no effect on ziprasidone plasma levels, whereas antipsychotics such as aripiprazole and risperidone exhibit a significant increase in plasma concentrations when coadministered with CYP2D6 inhibitors. Coadministration of ziprasidone with

lithium results in no significant change, in steady-state lithium levels (Apseloff et al. 2000) and commonly used antacids and cimetidine do not significantly alter ziprasidone pharmacokinetics (Pfizer Inc. 2008).

Indications and Efficacy

Schizophrenia and Schizoaffective Disorder

Acute Treatment

Ziprasidone is indicated for the acute treatment of schizophrenia and schizoaffective disorder. Its efficacy in the treatment of hospitalized patients with acute schizophrenia or schizoaffective disorder has been demonstrated in a series of double-blind, placebo-controlled trials of 4–6 weeks' duration (Daniel et al. 1999; Kane 2003; P. Keck et al. 1998; P.E. Keck et al. 2001). Additional randomized, double-blind, short-term (4- to 8-week) treatment studies using active antipsychotic agent comparators have indicated that ziprasidone has efficacy comparable to that of haloperidol, risperidone, and olanzapine for the treatment of positive symptoms and overall psychopathology (Addington et al. 2004; Goff et al. 1998; Simpson et al. 2004a). In a pooled analysis of four placebo-controlled, short-term trials and three active-comparator trials, Murray et al. (2004) demonstrated that ziprasidone dosages of at least 120 mg/day, in comparison with lower dosages, are associated with a more rapid and favorable response in overall psychopathology as well as a lower discontinuation rate due to inadequate clinical response, suggesting the importance of rapid titration to at least 120 mg/day in patients with acute schizophrenia (Kane 2003; McCue et al. 2006).

Suboptimal dosing, titration, and administration of ziprasidone may have negatively impacted its performance in some clinical trials. Some clinical trials included efficacy data for dosages that would now be consider suboptimal (i.e., <120 mg/day), while other studies used prolonged titration of ziprasidone, only reaching a therapeutic dosage 1 week or more into the study. Clinical trials conducted before the release of the recent pharmacokinetic data by Lombardo et al. (2007) may not have been designed to ensure that ziprasidone was administered with food for optimal oral absorption. For example, one small randomized, open-label trial ($N=327$) by McCue et al. (2006) compared the effectiveness of haloperidol, aripiprazole, olanzapine, quetiapine, risperidone, and ziprasidone for a minimum of 3 weeks as measured by duration of inpatient hospitalization. Although all six antipsychotics demonstrated comparable changes in Brief Psychiatric Rating Scale (BPRS) scores, treatment with haloperidol, olanzapine, and risperidone was associated with shorter hospital stays than treatment with aripiprazole, quetiapine, and ziprasidone. This study used slow, gradual titration of ziprasidone, so many patients did not obtain an optimal dosage of ziprasidone (e.g., 80 mg twice daily) until 1 week or more into this short-term study, suggesting an explanation for the longer duration of hospitalization in ziprasidone recipients despite achieving comparable improvement in BPRS scores.

Another approach to evaluating the comparative efficacy of first- and second-generation antipsychotics is the use of meta-analysis. A series of meta-analyses has found no clear or consistent differences among the atypical antipsychotics, either when comparing agents within the same class or when comparing second-generation with first-generation antipsychotics (Bagnall et al. 2003; Geddes et al. 2000; Leucht et al. 1999; Srisurapanont and Maneeton 1999; Tandon and Fleischhacker 2005). One meta-analysis of randomized, controlled trials by Davis et al. (2003) suggested that some atypical antipsychotics (i.e., clozapine, risperidone, olanzapine, and amisulpride) were significantly more efficacious than first-generation antipsychotics, whereas in this analysis the efficacy of ziprasidone was not observed to be statistically significantly better than that of first-generation antipsychotics. It is important to note that this meta-analysis excluded data relating to low dosages of other antipsychotics (olanzapine <11 mg/day and risperidone <4 mg/day), but included data on ziprasidone dosages as low as 80 mg/day. In addition, the Davis et al. meta-analysis included relatively few studies of ziprasidone (4 studies as compared with 31 studies of clozapine, 22 studies of risperidone, and 14 studies of olanzapine), making it more difficult to show statistical significance with this agent. In a subsequent analysis of data from four major meta-analyses plus additional data from head-to-head comparisons of agents in randomized, controlled clinical trials, Tandon and Fleischhacker (2005) found that all of the second-generation antipsychotics including ziprasidone were statistically equivalent in terms of efficacy.

It should be noted that meta-analyses involving ziprasidone are challenged by the same limitations incurred by the original study designs. These early study limitations included problems related to inadequate dosing and/or dose titration and administration without food. Although meta-analyses provide useful information, a need remains for head-to-head comparator studies with flexible doses and appropriate dosage ranges to ad-

dress whether specific antipsychotic drugs exhibit preferential benefit–risk ratios in relevant patient populations.

Debate continues about potential explanations for why some studies find differences in acute efficacy among the second-generation antipsychotics and other studies do not, with limited evidence suggesting that study sponsorship might occasionally contribute to a biased study design (e.g., sponsors might design a study using suboptimal dosing or titration of a comparator) (Lexchin et al. 2003). Based on the totality of available evidence, it is our opinion that there is currently no compelling overall evidence to support propositions that clinically significant differences (i.e., differences that are not explainable by lack of equipotent dosing with respect to D_2 antagonist activity) exist in the intrinsic efficacy of second-generation antipsychotics for the treatment of positive psychotic symptoms in patients with schizophrenia or schizoaffective disorder, with the exception of the superior efficacy for positive symptoms of clozapine in well-defined populations of patients with treatment-resistant illness.

With respect to drug effects on total psychopathology, beyond specific effects for positive symptoms, it is important to note that in general, when the less sedating antipsychotics compete in head-to-head comparisons with more sedating agents, they tend to face challenges in conventionally designed randomized, double-blind trials. When the acute state under study also involves agitation and insomnia, less sedating medications (e.g., ziprasidone) may be at a disadvantage with respect to ratings for these additional symptoms. Although conventional study designs allow "as needed" access to adjunctive benzodiazepines, the as-needed approach carries a potential for underutilization that may fail to fully level the playing field with respect to sedative effects in the competing treatment arms. Conventional study designs will continue to present challenges for the growing list of novel antipsychotic agents under development that, like ziprasidone, are at the less sedating end of the spectrum of currently available agents. The key question is whether it is desirable to continue to rely on study designs that favor more sedating agents, given that this will tend to favor agents with higher levels of intrinsic antihistaminic, antimuscarinic, or anti–α_1-adrenergic activity, encouraging the development of medications with predictable short- and longer-term adverse-event liabilities.

Maintenance Therapy

The maintenance efficacy of ziprasidone in treating schizophrenia and schizoaffective disorder has been studied in a series of double-blind and open-label extension trials (Arato et al. 2002; Hirsch et al. 2002; Kane et al. 2003; Schooler 2003; Simpson et al. 2002, 2004b). These studies indicate that long-term therapy with ziprasidone maintains clinical response and is effective in preventing relapse. The majority of efficacy and effectiveness studies for ziprasidone can be divided into specific categories based on what the studies were designed to assess:

1. Maintenance of effect: patients who meet acute response criteria are randomized to stay on the current medication or switch to a comparator treatment
2. Relapse prevention: stable patients defined in terms of remission or level of symptom control are randomly assigned to ziprasidone versus a control condition and are compared by time to achievement of relapse criteria
3. Long-term response: symptomatic patients are compared by improvements in clinical symptom response
4. Clinical effectiveness: so-called effectiveness trials use endpoints such as time to drug discontinuation as a marker for clinical effectiveness

Maintenance of effect.   In two maintenance-of-effect trials, patients with schizophrenia or schizoaffective disorder with a demonstrated acute response to treatment (defined as a ≥20% decrease in Positive and Negative Syndrome Scale [PANSS] for schizophrenia total score and a Clinical Global Impression [CGI] Scale score of ≤2) were randomly assigned to receive either ziprasidone or a comparator antipsychotic agent for at least 26 weeks (Addington et al. 2003; Schooler 2003; Simpson et al. 2002, 2005). The ziprasidone treatment groups in both studies demonstrated significant improvements from baseline in overall psychopathology, as measured by mean changes in symptom ratings using PANSS total, PANSS negative subscale, Brief Psychiatric Rating Scale–Depression Factor (BPRSd), and CGI–Severity (CGI-S) scores. These improvements were comparable to those seen in the olanzapine (Simpson et al. 2005) and risperidone (Addington et al. 2003) treatment groups.

Relapse prevention.   To evaluate the efficacy of ziprasidone for relapse prevention, the Ziprasidone Extended Use in Schizophrenia study enrolled stable inpatients with chronic schizophrenia and randomly assigned participants to 1 year of treatment with ziprasidone 40 mg/day (n=72), 80 mg/day (n=68), or 160 mg/day (n=67) or placebo (n=71), with a planned primary Kaplan-Meier analysis of time to relapse (Arato et al. 2002). Stability

was defined by symptom level but this was short of strict definitions of remission. In this study, all three dosages of ziprasidone were superior to placebo in the prevention of relapse. In addition, a penultimate-observation-carried-forward analysis (in which the last visit prior to relapse is excluded) was performed to filter out clinical worsening associated with relapse that might otherwise obscure symptom response trends during the rest of maintenance therapy (O'Connor and Schooler 2003), which indicated that nonrelapsing patients treated with ziprasidone experienced modest symptomatic improvement during maintenance treatment. This study, like a number of other studies of other antipsychotic agents in schizophrenia patients, was limited by the relatively high level of attrition observed in all groups over the year of treatment.

Long-term response to treatment in symptomatic patients.   A number of long-term double-blind trials designed to examine the efficacy of ziprasidone in symptomatic patients with schizophrenia have been performed (Breier et al. 2005; Hirsch et al. 2002; Kinon et al. 2006a; Simpson et al. 2004a, 2005). Investigators (Hirsch et al. 2002) have compared the efficacy of ziprasidone (n=148) and haloperidol (n=153) in a 28-week double-blind trial of stable outpatients with schizophrenia with prominent negative symptoms. In this study, ziprasidone and haloperidol were similarly efficacious in reducing overall psychopathology, with an advantage for ziprasidone in the percentage of patients classified as negative symptom responders. Breier et al. (2005) conducted a 28-week study of ziprasidone and olanzapine in outpatients as well as inpatients (N=548) with active symptoms. In this study, olanzapine treatment was associated with greater improvement from baseline in total psychopathology scores (PANSS total, the primary efficacy measure) than ziprasidone and a higher rate of criterion-level response to treatment. Simpson et al. (2004a) conducted a 6-week double-blind, parallel-design flexible-dose comparison (N=269) of ziprasidone (n=136) and olanzapine (n=133) where at least minimal responders (CGI-I score ≤2 or ≥20% reduction in PANSS total score) were enrolled in a 6-month double-blind continuation trial (Simpson et al. 2005). In both the 6-week and the 6-month analyses, no differences between the treatment groups were detected on any primary (e.g., BPRS total, CGI severity) or secondary (e.g., PANSS total, CGI-I) measures.

Factors contributing to the apparent differences in study results may include differences in study design. Breier et al. (2005) randomly assigned symptomatic inpatients and outpatients, whereas Simpson et al. (2004a) enrolled symptomatic inpatients at baseline for the 6-week trial and patients with at least minimal response into the subsequent 6-month trial. Breier et al. (2005) used a higher mean daily dosage of olanzapine (15.3 mg) and a lower mean daily dosage of ziprasidone (116.0 mg) in comparison with the Simpson et al. (2004a, 2005) studies, which used relatively lower mean daily dosages of olanzapine (11.3 mg and 12.6 mg, respectively) and relatively higher mean daily dosages of ziprasidone (129.9 mg and 135.2 mg, respectively). Breier et al. (2005) also employed a prolonged titration of ziprasidone, along with the lower dosage, increasing the likelihood of initial and sustained underdosing of ziprasidone.

In another comparison study of ziprasidone and olanzapine, Kinon et al. (2006a) evaluated their efficacy in schizophrenia and schizoaffective disorder patients with prominent depressive symptoms ($N = 394$). They detected greater improvement in PANSS total scores in the olanzapine group, using a last-observation-carried-forward analysis. However, no significant difference in PANSS total scores between olanzapine and ziprasidone treatment was detected using an alternative mixed-effects model for repeated measures (MMRM) analysis. The MMRM analysis notably uses all observed data to adjust for changes related to dropouts and may offer a more robust approach to the analysis of treatment effects in clinical trials when missing data occur (Mallinckrodt et al. 2003).

Effectiveness trials.   There have been a number of ziprasidone effectiveness trials, with use of various definitions for *effectiveness*. The Clinical Antipsychotic Trials of Intervention Effectiveness (the CATIE studies, funded by the National Institute of Mental Health [NIMH]) included a long-term, double-blind, randomized study of patients with schizophrenia ($N = 1,493$; Lieberman et al. 2005). Phase I of the CATIE schizophrenia study compared ziprasidone, olanzapine, quetiapine, risperidone, and perphenazine on the primary endpoint of time to discontinuation for lack of efficacy or for any cause. Because of the timing of its FDA approval, ziprasidone was added to the study after enrollment had begun for all other treatment arms; this resulted in a smaller sample size for the ziprasidone treatment arm.

The primary analysis for the phase I study detected significant differences in time to discontinuation across the treatment groups overall. The longest time to discontinuation was in the olanzapine group. In the total study sample, no significant differences were seen in the time to discontinuation between the ziprasidone and olanzapine treatment groups, nor between the ziprasidone group and

other antipsychotic treatment groups. Although a subanalysis that was restricted to the overall study cohort of patients who enrolled after ziprasidone became available indicated a higher rate of discontinuation with ziprasidone treatment than with olanzapine, this was not significant after a planned adjustment for multiple comparisons. After adjusting the data for multiple comparisons, the investigators found no significant differences between ziprasidone and olanzapine or the other antipsychotics in the analyses of all-cause discontinuations and discontinuations due to lack of efficacy.

Several considerations in this complex study are worth mentioning. Relatively few patients who entered the CATIE schizophrenia study were currently (i.e., prior to study entry) taking the relatively newly available medication, ziprasidone, compared with the number of patients taking the other antipsychotic medications in the trial. This resulted in a larger proportion of patients assigned to the ziprasidone treatment arm who were just starting to take a new medication and discontinuing their prior treatment, compared with patients in other treatment arms. For example, 23% of subjects randomly assigned to olanzapine treatment were already receiving olanzapine monotherapy as their ongoing treatment, requiring no medication discontinuation or new drug initiation as a result of their random assignment to the study arm. Supplemental analysis of phase I CATIE data by Essock et al. (2006) indicated the overall importance, in terms of subsequent discontinuation rates, of whether randomized subjects were switching medications or whether the study design allowed them to continue receiving their prior treatment. A significantly higher rate of subsequent discontinuation was observed in patients who actually made a medication switch compared with those who were randomly assigned to stay with the same medication they had been taking prior to the trial. This effect of switching medications may therefore favor treatment arms with a larger percentage of "nonswitchers" (i.e., olanzapine and risperidone recipients in the CATIE phase I study, in which nonswitching was allowed). In a reanalysis of phase I CATIE data that excluded those patients randomly assigned to continue taking the antipsychotic that they were already taking at baseline, Essock et al. (2006) found that differences between rates of discontinuation in the ziprasidone group and rates in the other antipsychotic groups were attenuated, and no statistically significant differences were observed.

Further evidence regarding the effectiveness of ziprasidone was anticipated from the phase II CATIE study. Subjects enrolled in the phase I study consisted of a population that included some patients with unremitted illness and some patients with treatment-refractory illness (Meltzer and Bobo 2006), not undesirably increasing the likelihood that subjects would discontinue treatment in phase I and move on to phase II of the CATIE study. However, the CATIE study hypothesized that patients who discontinued phase I due to lack of efficacy would tend to enter the phase IIE *efficacy arm*, which included clozapine, while those who discontinued phase I due to intolerability would tend to enter the phase IIT *tolerability arm*, which included ziprasidone (Stroup et al. 2006). Instead, a substantial percentage of patients who discontinued phase I due to lack of efficacy chose not to enter the IIE arm of the study, possibly due to reluctance to receive treatment with clozapine, and instead entered the IIT arm. From this larger-than-expected sample of phase IIT subjects, those randomly assigned to the ziprasidone group received a mean modal dosage of 116 mg/day, with only about one-third of those treated receiving the maximal allowed dosage of 160 mg/day and about 60% receiving 120 mg/day or less, and there were no study-specified requirements or instructions regarding administration of the drug with food. In this setting, ziprasidone, like quetiapine, was associated with a shorter time to all-cause discontinuation of treatment than risperidone or olanzapine. In the subset of the sample that entered phase II due to lack of tolerability in phase I (rather than lack of efficacy), no differences in all-cause discontinuation rates were observed between the treatment arms.

The ZEISIG study (Ziprasidone Experience in Schizophrenia in Germany/Austria) investigated the effectiveness of ziprasidone as measured by discontinuation rates and mean changes of the BPRS total in moderately ill and reasonably stable patients ($N=276$) with schizophrenia or schizoaffective disorder (Kudla et al. 2007). Approximately 60% of subjects discontinued ziprasidone prematurely, most within the first 4 weeks of study treatment. In study completers, ziprasidone was associated with significant improvements in BPRS total score. The relatively high rate of discontinuation may be explained in part by the planned dosing strategy. In this study, ziprasidone use was initiated at a low dosage of 40 mg/day, which is now known to be associated with higher discontinuation rates and shorter durations of therapy compared with higher dosages (Joyce et al. 2006; Mullins et al. 2006). As in other studies, the maximal dosage allowed was 160 mg/day, which may be insufficient for some patients (Harvey and Bowie 2005; Nemeroff et al. 2005).

Arango et al. (2007), of the Ziprasidone in Spain Study Group, examined the effectiveness of ziprasidone

($n=1,022$ in the primary analysis sample) as measured by response rate (defined as a $\geq 30\%$ reduction in the PANSS total score). Nearly half of the patients experienced the defined level of clinical response, and patients overall had significant and clinically relevant mean reductions in both the PANSS total score and the positive, negative, and general psychopathology subscale scores (effect sizes were 1.60, 1.83, 0.62, and 1.40, respectively). Ziprasidone dosages of greater than 120 mg/day were associated with a lower risk of discontinuation for any cause.

Kinon et al. (2006b) published a post hoc pooled analysis of clinical trials from the Eli Lilly database using treatment discontinuation rates as a measure of effectiveness. An additional long-term effectiveness study (Ascher-Svanum et al. 2006) using time to all-cause discontinuation as a measure of effectiveness, and a naturalistic treatment setting, is available. In both cases, small numbers of subjects in the ziprasidone arms (e.g., 25 subjects), compared with hundreds or more subjects in comparative arms, limit the interpretation of results and conclusions with respect to ziprasidone.

Efficacy by Symptom Type

Efficacy for cognitive symptoms of schizophrenia.
The effect of ziprasidone on cognitive function in schizophrenia patients has been evaluated by a battery of cognitive tests that were included in a double-blind olanzapine comparator study that evaluated changes at 6 weeks and 6 months (Harvey et al. 2004, 2006a). Antipsychotic treatment with ziprasidone and with olanzapine both resulted in significant cognitive improvements from baseline in attention memory, working memory, motor speed, and executive functions, with olanzapine also associated with improvement in verbal fluency. Further improvements in both treatment groups were observed from the end of 6 weeks to the 6-month assessment time point on verbal learning, executive functioning, and verbal fluency, with no differences between treatment groups. A similar magnitude of improvement was seen with each agent, with the exception of verbal fluency. It should be noted that despite improvements, a substantial proportion of patients studied continued to experience clinically significant cognitive impairment posttreatment. Neuropsychological improvements in general are not related to clinical changes (Harvey et al. 2006b).

Recent data from the CATIE schizophrenia study indicate that treatment with all of the antipsychotics tested (i.e., ziprasidone, perphenazine, olanzapine, risperidone, and quetiapine) was associated with a small but significant improvement in neurocognition after 2 months of treatment (Keefe et al. 2007). There was no significant difference between ziprasidone and the other antipsychotics. Neurocognitive improvement predicted a longer time to treatment discontinuation, independent of symptom improvement, in patients treated with quetiapine or ziprasidone.

Efficacy for affective symptoms.   Ziprasidone has been hypothesized to be a promising treatment for affective disorders, based on its unique in vitro potency as a serotonin and norepinephrine reuptake inhibitor comparable to that of known antidepressants (see "Neuropharmacology and Receptor-Binding Profile" section above). If this effect translates to antidepressant activity in vivo, it could be useful in reducing the likelihood of treatment-emergent depression, an outcome in approximately 10%–20% of patients with bipolar or schizoaffective disorder treated with first-generation antipsychotics or olanzapine (Kohler and Lallart 2002; Tohen et al. 2000, 2001, 2003). Addressing the question of ziprasidone's potential antidepressant efficacy in schizophrenia patients with comorbid affective symptoms, data can be examined from randomized, double-blind, placebo-controlled clinical trials (Daniel et al. 1999; P. Keck et al. 1998; P.E. Keck et al. 2001) and from double-blind, head-to-head trials comparing ziprasidone to risperidone or olanzapine (Kane 2003). The results of placebo-controlled studies (Daniel et al. 1999; P. Keck et al. 1998) suggest that treatment of schizophrenia and schizoaffective disorder with ziprasidone is associated with significant improvement in comorbid depressive symptoms, based on intent-to-treat analyses, but sometimes only in the subset of patients with higher levels of baseline depression. The baseline severity of depressive symptoms in these studies tends to be relatively mild, so subgroups of patients with more pronounced comorbid depressive symptoms at baseline were also analyzed; the antidepressant effect of ziprasidone is larger than that of placebo in these analyses. In the two active-comparator studies, improvement in depression and anxiety symptoms in patients receiving ziprasidone was comparable to the improvement in olanzapine recipients but greater than the improvement in risperidone recipients. A smaller study (Kinon et al. 2006a) compared the efficacy of olanzapine and ziprasidone over 24 weeks in the treatment of schizophrenia or schizoaffective disorder patients with prominent depressive symptoms. Both treatment groups had significant improvements in depressive symptoms for the first 8 weeks, with olanzapine-treated patients showing significantly greater improvements in depressive symptoms at study endpoint. However, the interpretation of this study is limited by that fact that a substantial number of patients (52.8% of $N = 394$ at study entry) received concurrent treatment with non-standardized antidepressants. These overall results provide preliminary evidence suggesting that ziprasidone, like some other antipsychotic agents, may be effective in treating comorbid depressive symptoms in patients with schizophrenia and schizoaffective disorder.

Efficacy for social deficits and improvement in quality of life.   To date, the NIMH CATIE study is the largest trial examining the effect of ziprasidone and other antipsychotics on psychosocial functioning in patients with schizophrenia (Swartz et al. 2007). This study used the Quality of Life Scale, a widely used clinician-rated measurement (Heinrichs et al. 1984), to assess changes in social functioning, interpersonal relationships, vocational functioning, and psychological well-being. One-third of the patients in the phase I study antipsychotic treatment groups made modest improvements on the Quality of Life Scale from baseline to the 12-month endpoint (average effect size, 0.19 standard deviation units), with no significant differences between the agents.

The effect of ziprasidone on social functioning has also been evaluated using the prosocial subscale of the PANSS, including items related to active and passive social avoidance, emotional withdrawal, stereotypical thinking, and suspiciousness (Purnine et al. 2000). In three separate but related studies from one group, stable patients taking either conventional antipsychotics, olanzapine, or risperidone were switched to ziprasidone and followed for 6 weeks with ratings of safety, efficacy, and effectiveness (Weiden et al. 2003b). Six weeks of treatment with ziprasidone in all three prior-treatment groups resulted in significant improvement on the PANSS prosocial subscale (Loebel et al. 2004). The interpretation of results as being specific to ziprasidone use, rather than being simply an effect of extended, closely monitored treatment, is complicated by the absence of a control condition other than the prior-treatment baseline ratings.

Treatment-Resistant Schizophrenia

The efficacy of ziprasidone for treatment-resistant schizophrenia was evaluated in a 12-week double-blind chlorpromazine comparator study ($N = 306$ patients), with treatment-resistant status defined by failure to achieve criterion-level response after 6 weeks of prospective treatment with haloperidol (Kane et al. 2005). The mean daily dosage of ziprasidone at study endpoint was approximately 154 mg, compared with a mean daily chlorpromazine dosage of approximately 744 mg. Treatment with ziprasidone produced significantly greater improvement at endpoint in PANSS negative subscale scores compared with chlorpromazine. In addition, ziprasidone treatment was associated with a 1.3-fold higher likelihood of achieving a 50% reduction in BPRS total score compared with chlorpromazine treatment.

Switching From Other Antipsychotics

As discussed above, evidence suggests that the efficacy of ziprasidone is comparable to that of other atypical and conventional antipsychotics during both acute and maintenance treatment of schizophrenia and schizoaffective disorder. Subsequent sections provide evidence to support the safety, particularly the cardiometabolic safety, of ziprasidone compared with other antipsychotics (see "Side Effects and Toxicology" section). These results support interest in the clinical outcomes associated with switching from antipsychotic treatment with other agents to treatment with ziprasidone.

Three open-label, medication-switching studies evaluated the effect of switching to ziprasidone on measures of efficacy, safety, and tolerability, as well as the effect of different titration schedules on the outcome (Weiden et al. 2003b). In each study, patients were randomly assigned to one of three switching strategies to be completed in 1 week:

1. Immediate discontinuation of the previous antipsychotic and immediate starting of ziprasidone the next day
2. Lowering the dose of the previous antipsychotic by half while simultaneously starting ziprasidone
3. Overlapping the start of ziprasidone with the full dosage of the prior antipsychotic and then gradually reducing the prior antipsychotic dosage after 4 days of ziprasidone therapy.

For all switching strategies, the starting dosage of ziprasidone was 80 mg/day (40 mg twice daily), with subsequent dosage adjustments based on clinical judgment. In one study, patients taking high-potency conventional antipsychotics (N = 108) were switched to ziprasidone. In the second study, patients (N = 58) were switched from risperidone to ziprasidone. In the third study, patients (N = 104) were switched from olanzapine to ziprasidone. Discontinuation rates were low in all three studies, ranging

from 2%–6% for lack of efficacy to 6%–9% for adverse events. In study completers, statistically significant improvements were observed on PANSS total, PANSS positive subscale, PANSS negative subscale, and BPRSd total scores. Different switching strategies were not associated with a different likelihood of trial completion or different magnitude of clinical response. The absence of active or placebo control subjects in this set of studies, in combination with the similarly favorable response profile, limits the interpretation of results with respect to changes in psychiatric symptoms associated with the change in medications.

Bipolar Disorder

Acute Mania

Ziprasidone has received regulatory approval (e.g., by the FDA) for the acute treatment of bipolar mania, with efficacy for acute mania demonstrated in two double-blind, placebo-controlled trials, each 3 weeks in duration, in patients with bipolar I disorder (P. E. Keck et al. 2003b; Potkin et al. 2005). In both studies, onset of action was rapid (within 48 hours) and sustained through 3 weeks of treatment in patients with bipolar mania or bipolar mixed states, with or without psychotic symptoms (results of P. E. Keck et al. [2003b] are shown in Figure 33–5). At endpoint, approximately half of the treated patients from both studies met response criteria for mania (≥50% reduction in Mania Rating Scale [MRS] scores).

A growing number of placebo-controlled trials evaluating the efficacy of short-term monotherapy with various atypical antipsychotics, including ziprasidone, olanzapine, risperidone, quetiapine, and aripiprazole, have demonstrated comparable improvement in symptoms of mania (Bowden et al. 2005; Hirschfeld et al. 2004; P. E. Keck et al. 2003a, 2003b; Khanna et al. 2005; McIntyre et al. 2005; McQuade et al. 2003; Potkin et al. 2005; Sachs et al. 2006; Smulevich et al. 2005; Tohen et al. 1999, 2000; Weisler et al. 2003). Two recent large meta-analyses of randomized, placebo-controlled trials have examined the relative efficacy of various atypical antipsychotics for the adjunctive treatment of mania (Perlis et al. 2006; Scherk et al. 2007). Although the statistical results of the two meta-analyses are similar, the authors of each study interpreted the results somewhat differently. Perlis et al. (2006) concluded that add-on therapy with atypical antipsychotics (ziprasidone, olanzapine, quetiapine, and risperidone) conferred an additional benefit over monotherapy with a traditional mood stabilizer in reducing

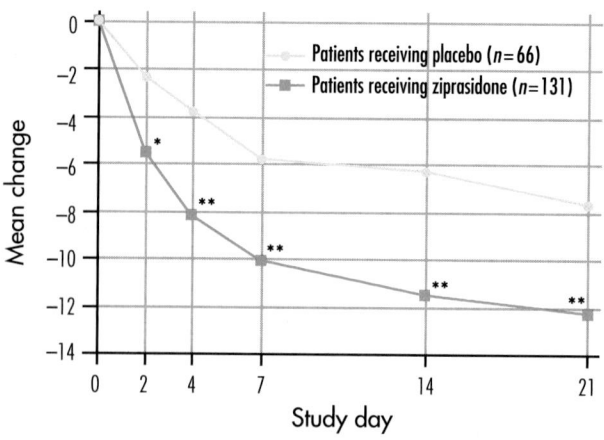

FIGURE 33–5. Effect of ziprasidone on mania: rating scale scores in patients with bipolar disorder receiving 21-day randomized treatment with ziprasidone or placebo.

*P<0.003 (F test), placebo-treated patients versus ziprasidone-treated patients.

**P<0.001 (F test), placebo-treated patients and ziprasidone-treated patients (P<0.001, F test).

Source. Adapted from P.E. Keck et al. 2003b.

manic symptoms, with no difference in efficacy among the drugs. Scherk et al. (2007) also concluded that atypical antipsychotics as a group were significantly superior to placebo as adjunctive treatment for mania, but that ziprasidone and other individual agents may not be significantly superior to placebo in the adjunctive treatment of manic symptoms. Although regulatory approvals for the individual agents have supported the efficacy and safety of a number of individual antipsychotics for the acute treatment of mania, including ziprasidone (which is also approved for the acute treatment of mixed states), prospective, head-to-head comparator trials may be required to clarify whether differences suggested by some meta-analyses are clinically meaningful or are related to differences in study design or methodology.

Maintenance Treatment

Two 52-week open-label extension studies support the safety, tolerability, and sustained efficacy of ziprasidone as maintenance treatment for bipolar disorder (P.E. Keck et al. 2004; Weisler et al. 2004). P.E. Keck et al. (2004) reported that treatment with ziprasidone (n=127; mean daily dosage, 123 mg) was associated with significantly lower MRS and CGI-S scores compared with baseline, beginning as early as the first week. Overall, improvements in manic symptoms achieved during acute treatment continued to consolidate during maintenance treatment with ziprasidone. During 52 weeks of treatment, only 6% of patients discontinued ziprasidone use due to relapse of mania. Similarly, only 4% of patients discontinued due to a clinical switch into depression. An important caveat regarding these results is the high rate of attrition observed by the end of 1 year, which is consistent with long-term studies involving other atypical antipsychotics but which limits the full interpretation of results. Similar results were observed in a separate extension study of adjunctive ziprasidone therapy (mean daily dosage, 92.6 mg) by Weisler et al. (2004); this study reported a mean improvement from baseline in MRS scores at all points throughout the study (Patel and Keck 2006).

Treatment-Resistant Depression

Although there have been no randomized studies, small uncontrolled studies have prompted interest in the efficacy of ziprasidone for treatment-resistant depression (Barbee et al. 2004; Jarema 2007; Papakostas et al. 2004). Papakostas et al. (2004) reported the results of a small study of 20 patients with major depression resistant to treatment with selective serotonin reuptake inhibitors (SSRIs). Open-label treatment with ziprasidone for 6 weeks, adjunctive to ongoing SSRI treatment, was evaluated with an intent-to-treat analysis that identified 10 treatment responders (defined as having a ≥50% decrease in depressive symptoms as measured by the Ham-D-17). In a smaller retrospective chart review (Barbee et al. 2004), in which only 5 of 10 patients were exposed to ziprasidone for at least 6 weeks, 1 patient met criteria for being a treatment responder (requiring ratings of "very much improved"). Randomized studies are needed to evaluate the efficacy and safety of ziprasidone for patients with treatment-resistant depression.

Agitation

The efficacy of intramuscular ziprasidone for the treatment of agitated psychosis has been demonstrated in two randomized, double-blind trials (2 mg im vs. 20 mg or 10 mg im, respectively, with up to three more doses allowed as needed at 4-hour or 2-hour intervals, respectively), leading to regulatory approval by the FDA (Daniel et al. 2001; Lesem et al. 2001). Treatment with single 10- or 20-mg doses leads to rapid reductions in symptom severity, with most patients having remission of agitation within 1 hour of dosing. Treatment with intramuscular ziprasidone is associated with a relatively low rate of concomitant benzodiazepine use (<20%). Sequential use of intramuscular ziprasidone followed by oral ziprasidone for the treatment of acute psychotic agitation has demonstrated superior efficacy, compared with sequential use of intramuscular and oral haloperidol, in two 7-day randomized, open-label trials (Brook et al. 2000; Swift et al. 1998) as well as in a 6-week randomized, single-blind, flexible-dose study (Brook et al. 2005). Clinical improvement occurred more rapidly than with haloperidol in one study, and as quickly as 30 minutes after the first intramuscular administration of ziprasidone (Swift et al. 1998). Cumulative data from these studies indicate that intramuscular ziprasidone can rapidly control agitation and psychotic symptoms and provide greater mean improvements in acute agitation than seen with intramuscular haloperidol (e.g., greater mean improvements in BPRS total score, agitation, and CGI-S score) (Brook 2003).

One uncontrolled prospective study of 21 patients (Barak et al. 2006) and a retrospective chart review of 35 cases (Kohen et al. 2005) evaluated the safety and efficacy of intramuscular ziprasidone for treatment of acute psychotic agitation in the elderly; both suggested that ziprasidone is effective and well tolerated in the elderly. Larger controlled studies are necessary to confirm these results and the safety of ziprasidone in this patient population.

Pediatric Patients

Ziprasidone has not to date been approved by the FDA for use in children or adolescents, and published data concerning the safety and efficacy of ziprasidone use in children and adolescents remain limited. To date, there has been one randomized, controlled trial of ziprasidone in children and adolescents (ages 10–17 years) with bipolar disorder (Versavel et al. 2005). In this study, treatment with ziprasidone was associated with improvement in mania and overall psychopathology. Two retrospective chart reviews of hospitalized children and adolescents reported that intramuscular ziprasidone demonstrated efficacy in the treatment of acute agitation and aggression (Staller 2004) and that intramuscular ziprasidone was as effective as intramuscular olanzapine in pediatric patients (Khan and Mican 2006). Two additional small studies suggested that ziprasidone may reduce tic severity in children and adolescents with Tourette's syndrome (Sallee et al. 2006) and may improve symptoms of aggression, agitation, and irritability in children and adolescents with autism (McDougle et al. 2002).

Side Effects and Toxicology

Ziprasidone has a favorable tolerability profile based on both short- and long-term clinical trials (Daniel 2003; Pfizer Inc. 2004). The four most common treatment-related adverse events associated with oral ziprasidone in short-term premarketing, placebo-controlled trials for schizophrenia were somnolence (14%), EPS (14%), nausea (10%), and constipation (9%) (Pfizer Inc. 2008). In subsequent clinical trials, treatment with ziprasidone was associated with a low occurrence of adverse events, most of which were considered mild to moderate in severity (Arango et al. 2007; Arato et al. 2002; Lieberman 2007; Nemeroff et al. 2005; Weiden et al. 2002, 2003b). In addition to the comprehensive listing of potential adverse events available in the full U.S. prescribing information (USPI) (Pfizer Inc. 2008), published case reports offer accounts of various rare adverse events that may be associated with the use of ziprasidone (Akkaya et al. 2006; Kaufman et al. 2006; Miodownik et al. 2005; Murty et al. 2002; Villanueva et al. 2006). Intramuscular ziprasidone shows a favorable tolerability profile similar to that of oral ziprasidone. In premarketing trials, the most common side effects of intramuscular ziprasidone (those with an incidence of >5% and an incidence greater than that seen in placebo recipients) were somnolence (20%), headache (13%), and nausea (12%) (Pfizer Inc. 2008). Pooled data from more recent clinical trials of intramuscular ziprasidone indicate that most treatment-related adverse events were mild to moderate in severity, with the most common side effects being headache, nausea, dizziness, insomnia, anxiety, and pain at the injection site (Daniel 2003; Zimbroff et al. 2002). Ziprasidone is considered a Category C drug in pregnancy. Although some specific developmental effects have been noted in animal studies at dosages ranging from 0.5 to 8.0 times the maximal recommended human dosage (Pfizer Inc. 2008), there are as yet no similar reports of such effects in humans. The reader is advised to consult the current USPI for a detailed listing of potential adverse drug effects identified in the regulatory approval process and postmarketing surveillance.

The FDA recently required the addition of black box warnings in the USPI regarding an increased risk of mortality associated with the use of both atypical and conventional antipsychotics used in elderly patients with dementia-related psychosis. Observed causes of death have been varied, and the mechanism of any drug effect in schizophrenia remains uncertain (Pfizer Inc. 2008). In particular, it remains unclear to what extent these uncontrolled observations of increased mortality are due to specific drug effects or to the advanced medical risk characteristics of patients with dementia or delirium who tend to receive these medications (Farber et al. 2000; Rochon et al. 2008). Regulatory interest in drug effects on cerebrovascular risk (i.e., risk of stroke) in the elderly, in contrast to generalized considerations of cardiovascular risk factors (e.g., myocardial infarction and stroke) discussed below (see "Metabolic Adverse Events" and "Cardiac Conduction, Including Ventricular Depolarization and Repolarization"), has also been focused on some atypical antipsychotics. Studies including those by Street et al. (2000), Wooltorton (2002), and De Deyn et al. (2004) have suggested that olanzapine and risperidone treatment may be associated with an increase in the risk of cerebrovascular adverse events and mortality. Again, possible mechanisms underlying hypothesized effects remain unclear, with some evidence suggesting that patient characteristics other than the specific antipsychotic used may be more significant predictors of cerebrovascular event risk than any drug-specific effects (Finkel et al. 2005).

Clinical experience with ziprasidone in the years following initial U.S. approval has suggested that a small subgroup of patients may experience insomnia or what has been characterized as *activation* or *akathisia* soon after initiation of treatment (Nemeroff et al. 2005). These presentations have been described as transient manifestations of anxiety, restlessness, insomnia, increased energy, or hypomania-like symptoms, occurring most commonly at what is now considered the lower end of the dosage range. Anecdotal reports suggest that starting dosages of 120 mg/day or greater and more rapid dose titration can substantially reduce the incidence of these clinical presentations (Weiden et al. 2002). These anecdotal clinical observations are consistent with controlled experimental evidence indicating that a significantly lower rate of discontinuation occurs in patients who begin ziprasidone therapy at higher dosages (120–160 mg/day) than in patients who receive initial dosages of 80 mg/day or less (Joyce et al. 2006). Several mechanisms may explain these observations:

- First, ziprasidone, like some of the other newer antipsychotics and many under development, is less intrinsically sedating than many other antipsychotics in current widespread use (e.g., due to less H_1 receptor antagonism), so that patients initiating ziprasidone treatment after months or years of receiving a different, more sedating therapy may experience initial difficulties adjusting to the new level of dosing time–specific (e.g., at bedtime) or around-the-clock sedation.

- Second, as discussed above (see "Pharmacological Profile" and "Indications and Efficacy" sections earlier in chapter) many patients have been treated with ziprasidone at doses that were insufficient to achieve optimal D_2 receptor blocking, leading to undertreatment of the underlying illness compared with what might have been achieved with an appropriately dosed prior therapy.

- Furthermore, ziprasidone underdosing with respect to D_2 receptor binding can produce a well-understood but unwanted pharmacodynamic situation with respect to the differential balance of 5-HT_{2C} receptor antagonism relative to D_2 receptor antagonism. As illustrated in Figure 33–3, using ziprasidone doses at the lower end of the clinical dosage range can allow 5-HT_2 receptors to reach 50% of maximal receptor occupancy or more, well before clinically significant levels of D_2 occupancy are achieved (Mamo et al. 2004). 5-HT_{2C} antagonist activity at this level disinhibits cortical monoaminergic neurotransmission (e.g., dopamine release), which, in the absence of sufficient D_2 blockade, may lead to clinically relevant excess monoaminergic neurotransmission (Bonaccorso et al. 2002; Pozzi et al. 2002).

Clinicians commonly address these potential issues through appropriate dosing and through the transient, targeted use of concomitant medication strategies (e.g., adjunctive benzodiazepine treatment) for relevant patients starting new treatment in the acute inpatient setting or for stable outpatients needing a smooth transition to new therapy.

Two other areas of potential adverse drug effects deserve further discussion: drug effects on risk for EPS and drug effects on cardiometabolic risk factors (e.g., changes in weight, plasma lipids, and glucose). These adverse-event domains are notable as areas of considerable clinical and research interest. For example, drug effects on EPS and cardiometabolic risk factors such as weight and plasma lipid level changes were the only side effect categories observed to contribute to differential rates of treatment discontinuation in the primary analysis of the NIMH-funded phase I CATIE study (Lieberman et al. 2005).

Extrapyramidal Side Effects

Short-term trials indicate that treatment with ziprasidone is associated a measurably larger incidence of EPS than treatment with placebo (Pfizer Inc. 2008; Potkin et al. 2005). In contrast, data from a 52-week trial (Arato et al.

2002) indicate that the incidence of abnormal movement disorders during treatment with ziprasidone is comparable to the incidence during placebo treatment. Other long-term studies suggest a low (<6%) incidence of treatment-related EPS (Arango et al. 2007; Kudla et al. 2007). Both active-comparator studies and medication-switching studies suggest that ziprasidone is associated with fewer EPS than risperidone (Addington et al. 2003; Weiden et al. 2003a, 2003b) or conventional antipsychotics (Hirsch et al. 2002; Weiden et al. 2003a, 2003b). Comparing ziprasidone and olanzapine, a drug with intrinsic antimuscarinic activity as well as 5-HT$_2$ receptor antagonist activity, one direct comparison study indicates that treatment with olanzapine is associated with fewer EPS (Kinon et al. 2006a), whereas two other direct comparison studies (Breier et al. 2005; Simpson et al. 2002) and one medication-switching study (Weiden et al. 2003b) have reported that both drugs exhibit a similar liability for EPS. With respect to akathisia, one comparison study indicates that less akathisia occurs with olanzapine use (Breier et al. 2005), whereas another study suggests no difference in akathisia rates with olanzapine versus ziprasidone (Kinon et al. 2006a). Results from phase I and phase II of the large-scale CATIE trial suggest no significant differences between ziprasidone, perphenazine, olanzapine, quetiapine, and risperidone in the incidence of EPS and akathisia (Lieberman 2007; Lieberman et al. 2005; Stroup et al. 2006). However, the perphenazine arm in the CATIE study was restricted to patients who did not already have tardive dyskinesia, suggesting a possible selection bias toward patients less likely to experience EPS. Despite this advantage, the perphenazine group still had the highest rate of dropouts due to EPS, suggesting along with other lines of evidence that clinically meaningful EPS are more common in patients treated with conventional agents like perphenazine.

Intramuscular ziprasidone has been tolerated at dosages of up to 80 mg/day with a low liability for EPS (Daniel 2003; Daniel et al. 2001; Lesem et al. 2001). Both intramuscular ziprasidone use and sequential intramuscular/oral ziprasidone use are associated with a lower incidence of treatment-related movement disorders than intramuscular haloperidol use (Swift et al. 1998; Zimbroff et al. 2002) and sequential intramuscular/oral haloperidol use (Brook et al. 2000, 2005). Although the results of controlled experimental studies indicate a generally low risk of EPS with ziprasidone, there have been several uncontrolled observational reports of EPS-related adverse events co-occurring with ziprasidone treatment and, in many cases, concomitant treatment with other agents

(Dew and Hughes 2004; Duggal 2007; M.E. Keck et al. 2004; Mason et al. 2005; Papapetropoulos et al. 2005; Ramos et al. 2003; Rosenfield et al. 2007; Weinstein et al. 2006; Yumru et al. 2006; Ziegenbein et al. 2003).

Metabolic Adverse Events

Adverse medication effects on modifiable risk factors for cardiovascular disease and type 2 diabetes mellitus have become an important topic of clinical, research, and regulatory concern, based in part on the increased prevalence of these disease states and associated premature mortality observed in patients with major mental disorders like schizophrenia and bipolar disorder (Brown 1997; Brown et al. 2000; Colton and Manderscheid 2006; Harris and Barraclough 1998; Hennekens et al. 2005; Joukamaa et al. 2001; Osby et al. 2000, 2001). Modifiable cardiometabolic risk factors include obesity, hyperglycemia, dyslipidemia, hypertension, and smoking, all prevalent conditions in patients with major mental disorders, with substantial evidence that primary and secondary prevention approaches are underutilized in these patients (Allison et al. 1999a; Brown et al. 2000; Druss and Rosenheck 1998; Druss et al. 2000, 2001; Frayne et al. 2005; Hippisley-Cox et al. 2007; McEvoy et al. 2005; Nasrallah et al. 2006; Newcomer and Hennekens 2007). In particular, use of recommended monitoring of changes in weight and in plasma glucose and lipid levels during antipsychotic treatment has heightened interest in cardiometabolic risk effects that may go undetected during the course of treatment (American Diabetes Association 2004; Morrato et al. 2008). All currently available antipsychotic medications are associated with a risk of weight gain, as well as potential adverse effects on plasma glucose and lipid levels, although there is substantial variability in the magnitude of these effects across individual agents (Casey et al. 2004; Eli Lilly 2008; "Eli Lilly updates label warning for Zyprexa" 2007; Newcomer 2005). Potential adverse treatment effects on body weight can be predicted to increase the risk for cardiovascular disease as well as for conditions like type 2 diabetes, commonly involving corresponding, measurable increases in insulin resistance, dyslipidemia, and hyperglycemia (Fontaine et al. 2001; Haupt et al. 2007; Koro et al. 2002a, 2002b).

Treatment with ziprasidone is associated with a relatively small risk of clinically significant increases in body weight. An analysis of available studies with this agent and other antipsychotics, both first- and second-generation antipsychotics (Allison et al. 1999b), estimated a 0.04-kg weight gain over a 10-week treatment period with ziprasidone, identifying ziprasidone as having one of the lowest estimated effects on body weight of those analyzed. In a 6-week randomized, controlled trial in patients with acute exacerbations of schizophrenia or schizoaffective disorder, treatment with ziprasidone 80 mg/day produced a median increase in body weight of 1 kg, compared with no change in median weight with ziprasidone 160 mg/day or placebo (Daniel et al. 1999). In a 28-week study of outpatients with schizophrenia, mean changes in body weight from baseline to endpoint were similar during treatment with ziprasidone (+0.31 kg) and haloperidol (+0.22 kg) (Hirsch et al. 2002). In a 28-week study comparing the effects of ziprasidone and olanzapine, ziprasidone-treated patients experienced a small decrease in mean body weight (−1.12 kg) compared with a statistically and clinically different 3.06-kg mean increase in body weight observed with olanzapine treatment (Hardy et al. 2003; Kinon et al. 2006a). Reductions in body weight were also associated with ziprasidone treatment in the 1-year Ziprasidone Extended Use in Schizophrenia study of patients with chronic, stable schizophrenia (Arato et al. 2002); this study reported mean decreases from baseline of 2.7 kg, 3.2 kg, and 2.9 kg reported with 40 mg/day, 80 mg/day, and 160 mg/day dosages of ziprasidone, respectively, compared with a 3.6-kg decrease observed with placebo treatment. Results from the phase I and phase IIT CATIE studies provide further confirmation that treatment with ziprasidone has a low intrinsic risk for producing clinically significant weight gain, with 6%–7% of ziprasidone recipients demonstrating a 7% or greater increase from baseline body weight compared with, for example, 27%–30% of olanzapine recipients (Lieberman 2007; Stroup et al. 2006). In the phase I CATIE study, ziprasidone treatment was associated with a mean reduction in body weight of 0.14 kg (0.3 lb) per month of treatment, compared with a mean increase of 0.91, 0.23, and 0.18 kg/month (2.0, 0.5, and 0.4 lb/month) during treatment with olanzapine, quetiapine, and risperidone, respectfully, the other atypical antipsychotics tested (Lieberman et al. 2005).

It is important to note that the ranking of weight gain liability for individual medications appears to apply in patients being treated for their first psychotic episode or during early drug exposure but perhaps not during chronic treatment, although there have been fewer studies in this area and initial courses of treatment can clearly be associated with greater weight gain than subsequent courses of treatment (McEvoy et al. 2007). In addition, chronically treated patients switching treatment from a medication with greater weight gain liability to a medication with less weight gain liability are likely to lose body weight in relation to that medication change, an effect that likely underlies the mean reductions in weight noted in some of the trials with ziprasidone discussed above. The magnitude of change in body weight during treatment with ziprasidone varies as a function of the weight gain liability of the prior treatment: the greatest potential for weight loss is associated with switching from previous treatments with the greatest weight gain liability (Weiden et al. 2008). For example, 6 weeks of ziprasidone therapy was associated with statistically significant decreases in mean body weight from baseline in patients switched from olanzapine (−1.8 kg) and from risperidone (−0.9 kg), whereas patients switched from high-potency conventional antipsychotics such as haloperidol experienced a small increase in weight (+0.3 kg) (Weiden et al. 2008). The 1-year extension of this medication-switching study indicated that weight loss was progressive and persistent throughout the 1-year period for patients who switched from olanzapine (−9.8 kg, or 10.3% of baseline body weight) and from risperidone (−6.9 kg, or 7.8% of baseline) (Figure 33–6; Weiden et al. 2008). Another study found similar significant decreases in weight in patients treated for 6 months with ziprasidone who were switched from olanzapine (−7.0 kg) and from risperidone (−2.2 kg) (Montes et al. 2006).

Ziprasidone's effects on plasma glucose and lipid levels are best understood as a function of treatment-related changes in adiposity. Whereas some antipsychotics, such as clozapine and olanzapine, have been reported to produce adiposity-independent effects on insulin sensitivity, and related changes in glucose and lipid metabolism, ziprasidone has demonstrated no similar adiposity-independent effects in this same experimental paradigm (Houseknecht et al. 2007). In general, increases in adiposity are associated with decreases in insulin sensitivity in individuals taking or not taking antipsychotic medications, with reduced insulin sensitivity leading to increased risk for hyperglycemia, dyslipidemia, and other adverse changes in cardiometabolic risk indicators (Haupt et al. 2007; Newcomer and Haupt 2006).

Ziprasidone's relatively low risk for drug-related increases in weight is therefore not surprisingly associated with a low risk for adverse effects on plasma lipids and other metabolic indices. Both short- and long-term studies have shown little significant adverse effect of ziprasidone on glucose levels, plasma insulin levels, insulin resistance, or fasting and nonfasting lipid levels (Daniel et al. 1999; Glick et al. 2001; Rettenbacher et al. 2006; Simpson et al. 2004a, 2005) in contrast to the degree of adverse

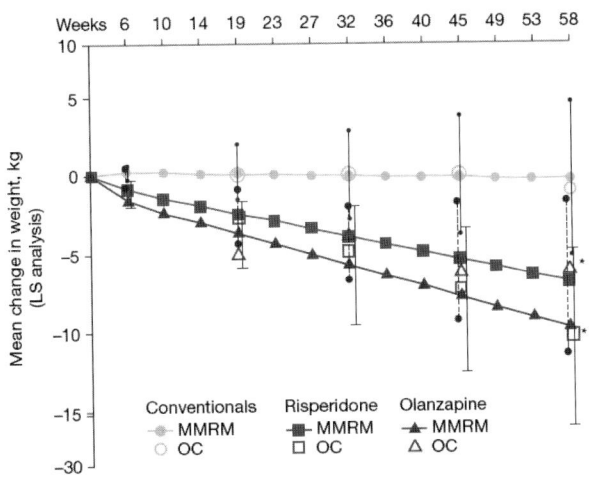

FIGURE 33–6. Time course of weight change over 58 weeks after switching to ziprasidone.

Previous treatments were conventional antipsychotics (line with circles; n=71), risperidone (line with squares; n=43), or olanzapine (line with triangles; n=71). Individual observed cases within each treatment group are also shown (circle = conventional agent: baseline weight, 198 lb [90 kg]; square = risperidone: baseline weight, 194.9 lb [88.6 kg]; triangle = olanzapine: baseline weight, 210.3 lb [95.6 kg]).

LS=least-squares analysis; MMRM=mixed-model repeated measures analysis; OC=observed case analysis.

*P<0.01 versus baseline (MMRM and OC).

Source. Adapted from Weiden PJ, Newcomer JW, Loebel AD, et al.: "Long-Term Changes in Weight and Plasma Lipids During Maintenance Treatment With Ziprasidone." *Neuropsychopharmacology* 33:985–994, 2008 (Figure 1, p. 988).

effects detected with some active comparators. For example, olanzapine treatment can produce statistically significant increases in fasting glucose and insulin levels (Glick et al. 2001; Hardy et al. 2003; Simpson et al. 2002, 2005) as well as fasting lipids and insulin resistance calculated by homeostasis model assessment (Simpson et al. 2004a, 2005). In the CATIE phase I study, olanzapine-treated patients demonstrated drug exposure–adjusted mean increases in blood glucose (+13.7±2.5 mg/dL) and glycosylated hemoglobin (hemoglobin A$_{1c}$ [HbA$_{1c}$]) (+0.4±0.07%), plasma triglycerides (+40.5±8.9 mg/dL), and total cholesterol (+9.4±2.4 mg/dL), whereas ziprasidone treatment was associated with minimal drug exposure–adjusted mean increases in blood glucose (+2.9±3.4 mg/dL) and HbA$_{1c}$ (+0.11±0.09%), and decreases in plasma triglycerides (−16.5±12.2 mg/dL) and total cholesterol (−8.2±3.2 mg/dL) (Lieberman 2007). In the CATIE phase IIT study, olanzapine-treated patients again had the greatest drug exposure–adjusted mean increases in HbA$_{1c}$ (+0.97±0.3%), triglycerides (+94.1±21.8 mg/dL),

and total cholesterol (+17.5±5.2 mg/dL), with quetiapine treatment associated with drug exposure–adjusted mean increases in blood glucose (+1.2±6.0 mg/dL) and HbA$_{1c}$ (+0.61±0.3%), glucose (+13.8±5.9 mg/dL), triglycerides (+39.3±22.1 mg/dL), and total cholesterol (+6.5±5.3 mg/dL). In contrast, ziprasidone-treated patients in CATIE phase IIT showed minimal drug exposure–adjusted mean increases in blood glucose (+0.8±5.6 mg/dL) and HbA$_{1c}$ (+0.46±0.3%) and decreases in triglycerides (−3.5±20.9 mg/dL) and total cholesterol (−10.7±5.1 mg/dL) (Stroup et al. 2006).

Similar to the effect of prior treatment conditions on changes in weight during treatment with ziprasidone, improvements in plasma lipid levels observed in the CATIE study can best be understood as the effect of switching from a previous treatment that is associated with larger adverse effects on lipid metabolism to a treatment with minimal adverse effects. Weiden et al. (2003a) noted that ziprasidone treatment was associated with significant decreases from baseline in both median nonfasting triglyceride levels and median nonfasting total cholesterol levels at the end of the 6-week treatment period in patients whose prior medication was olanzapine or risperidone, with minimal change following prior treatment with high-potency conventional agents like haloperidol. Notably, the reductions in lipids observed in this study occurred within the first 6 weeks of initiating treatment with ziprasidone, with substantial reductions in total cholesterol (>20 mg/dL) and plasma triglycerides (78 mg/dL) in the patients previously treated with olanzapine. In the 12-month extension of this study, the reductions achieved in the initial weeks following the switch from prior treatment were sustained during continued treatment with ziprasidone (Weiden et al. 2008).

Cardiac Conduction, Including Ventricular Depolarization and Repolarization

Some medications, including psychotropics, can increase the duration of the QTc interval (the QT interval corrected for heart rate). Basic research suggests plausible mechanisms by which an increase in the QTc interval could increase the risk of sudden cardiac death, and clinical investigations suggest that certain small subgroups of the general population may have an increased risk of sudden cardiac death, for example, those with a family history of congenital long-QT syndrome (>500 msec) and those who concomitantly use drugs that markedly increase the QTc interval (e.g., by >60 msec) via either pharmacokinetic or pharmacodynamic interactions

(Montanez et al. 2004). This has understandably led to regulatory interest in drug effects on the QTc interval. It should be noted that epidemiological studies in the general population suggest that modest prolongations of the QTc interval are not a risk factor for cardiovascular mortality or sudden death, so any risk in the general population of modest QTc prolongations is likely to be small and difficult to detect reliably (Montanez et al. 2004). Compared with risks like obesity, hypercholesterolemia, diabetes, hypertension, physical inactivity, or cigarette smoking, each with well-characterized effects in the general population, modest QTc prolongations are not a comparable risk factor for cardiovascular mortality or sudden death in the general population.

Against this background, thioridazine was recently required to add to its prescribing information a black box warning related to its QTc interval–prolonging effects, following decades of use. Other conventional antipsychotics, including haloperidol, are also associated with some risk of QTc prolongation (Gury et al. 2000; O'Brien et al. 1999). Investigators (Glassman and Bigger 2001) have estimated the rate of occurrence of torsades de pointes with conventional antipsychotics as "10–15 such events in 10,000 person-years of observation" (p. 1774). Ziprasidone, like some other antipsychotic agents, can induce orthostatic hypotension, particularly early in treatment exposure, which can lead to transient tachycardia, dizziness, or syncope (Swainston Harrison and Scott 2006). However, tachycardia has been observed to be infrequent and as common in patients treated with ziprasidone as in those treated with placebo (Swainston Harrison and Scott 2006). Tachycardia and syncope related to hypotension are to be distinguished from ventricular arrhythmias that can rarely occur in relation to QTc prolongation.

Ziprasidone treatment has been demonstrated to result in a modestly increased risk of QTc prolongation (Pfizer Inc. 2008). This QTc prolongation at C_{max} (mean increase, >15 msec) is 9–14 msec greater than that seen with risperidone, olanzapine, quetiapine, or haloperidol but approximately 14 msec less than that seen with thioridazine. Unlike the case with thioridazine, the modest effect of ziprasidone on the QTc interval is not worsened by the presence of commonly encountered inhibitors of drug metabolism. In clinical trials of ziprasidone monotherapy that report QTc changes as well as in case reports of ziprasidone overdosing (with doses up to 12,800 mg), there has been no evidence of any significant clinical sequelae such as torsades de pointes or sudden death (Arato et al. 2002; Arbuck 2005; Daniel 2003; Gomez-Criado et al. 2005; Harrigan et al. 2004; Insa Gómez and Gutiérrez

Casares 2005; Levy et al. 2004; Lieberman 2007; Miceli et al. 2004; Montanez et al. 2004; Nemeroff et al. 2005; Taylor 2003; Weiden et al. 2002, 2003a). This is consistent with analyses of large population samples, which have failed to demonstrate any association between QTc duration and either cardiovascular or all-cause mortality (Goldberg et al. 1991). Rare cases of torsades de pointes have been reported in patients being treated with multiple medications including ziprasidone, but the incidence of these events appears to be below the known prevalence of torsades de pointes in community-based population samples (Heinrich et al. 2006). The USPI suggests that clinicians should nonetheless be cognizant of this potential risk and be aware of circumstances that may increase risk for the occurrence of torsades de pointes and/or sudden death in association with the use of any drugs that can prolong the QTc interval. Such circumstances include bradycardia, hypokalemia, or hypomagnesemia; concomitant use of other medications known to cause clinically significant QT prolongation (although an additive effect with ziprasidone has not been established); and presence of congenital long-QT syndrome. The USPI further states that ziprasidone should not be used in patients with significant cardiovascular conditions, such as uncompensated heart failure or a cardiac arrhythmia, or in those who have had a recent acute myocardial infarction or persistent QTc measurements of greater than 500 msec, and the prudent clinician might consider employing the same caution with many other antipsychotic and psychotropic medications currently in use.

Conclusion

Ziprasidone is the fourth atypical antipsychotic following clozapine to become available in the United States. This agent has a unique pharmacological profile with the highest $5\text{-HT}_{2A}/D_2$ affinity ratio of currently available agents, potent serotonin and norepinephrine reuptake inhibition activity, agonist activity at 5-HT_{1A} receptors, and clinically relevant antagonist activity at various 5-HT_2 receptor subtypes. Ziprasidone has demonstrated rapid-onset and sustained efficacy for the treatment of schizophrenia, schizoaffective disorder, and bipolar mania, with promising evidence of favorable mood, cognitive, and prosocial effects. It is now available in an intramuscular formulation for the treatment of acute agitated psychoses.

Ziprasidone has a highly favorable safety and tolerability profile with limited potential for drug–drug and drug–disease interactions, critical issues for a patient population that generally has a high burden of medical comorbidity and is commonly exposed to complex polypharmacy. The adverse-effect profile of ziprasidone is particularly noteworthy in areas that are key to safety and tolerability in patients with major mental disorders such as schizophrenia and bipolar disorder, including low drug-related risk for EPS and minimal effects on cardiometabolic risk factors like obesity and dyslipidemia. As a fuller understanding of the cumulative risks associated with prolonged antipsychotic treatment develops, along with the risks and benefits of various commonly used adjunctive medications, it is likely that clinicians will increasingly appreciate individual medications with a wide spectrum of therapeutic activity and a favorable safety profile that support long-term use and optimize both medical and psychiatric outcomes.

References

Addington D, Pantelis C, Dineen M, et al: Ziprasidone vs risperidone in schizophrenia: 52 weeks' comparison. Poster presented at the annual meeting of the American Psychiatric Association, San Francisco, CA, May 17–22, 2003

Addington DE, Pantelis C, Dineen M, et al: Efficacy and tolerability of ziprasidone versus risperidone in patients with acute exacerbation of schizophrenia or schizoaffective disorder: an 8-week, double-blind, multicenter trial. J Clin Psychiatry 65:1624–1633, 2004

Akkaya C, Sarandol A, Sivrioglu EY, et al: A patient using ziprasidone with polydipsia, seizure, hyponatremia and rhabdomyolysis. Prog Neuropsychopharmacol Biol Psychiatry 30:1535–1538, 2006

Allison DB, Fontaine KR, Heo M, et al: The distribution of body mass index among individuals with and without schizophrenia. J Clin Psychiatry 60:215–220, 1999a

Allison DB, Mentore JL, Heo M, et al: Antipsychotic-induced weight gain: a comprehensive research synthesis. Am J Psychiatry 156:1686–1696, 1999b

Altar CA, Wasley AM, Neale RF, et al: Typical and atypical antipsychotic occupancy of D2 and S2 receptors: an autoradiographic analysis in rat brain. Brain Res Bull 16:517–525, 1986

American Diabetes Association: Consensus development conference on antipsychotic drugs and obesity and diabetes. Diabetes Care 27:596–601, 2004

Apseloff G, Mullet D, Wilner KD, et al: The effects of ziprasidone on steady-state lithium levels and renal clearance of lithium. Br J Clin Pharmacol 49 (suppl 1):61S–64S, 2000

Arango C, Kirkpatrick B, Koenig J: At issue: stress, hippocampal neuronal turnover, and neuropsychiatric disorders. Schizophr Bull 27:477–480, 2001

Arango C, Gomez-Beneyto M, Brenlla J, et al: A 6-month prospective, observational, naturalistic, uncontrolled study to evaluate the effectiveness and tolerability of oral ziprasidone in patients with schizophrenia. Eur Neuropsychopharmacol 17:456–463, 2007

Arato M, O'Connor R, Meltzer HY: A 1-year, double-blind, placebo-controlled trial of ziprasidone 40, 80 and 160 mg/day in chronic schizophrenia: the Ziprasidone Extended Use in Schizophrenia (ZEUS) study. Int Clin Psychopharmacol 17:207–215, 2002

Arbuck DM: 12,800-mg ziprasidone overdose without significant ECG changes. Gen Hosp Psychiatry 27:222–223, 2005

Ascher-Svanum H, Zhu B, Faries D, et al: Time to discontinuation of atypical versus typical antipsychotics in the naturalistic treatment of schizophrenia. BMC Psychiatry 6:8, 2006

AstraZeneca Pharmaceuticals: Seroquel (quetiapine fumarate) tablets, full prescribing information. July 2008

Bagnall AM, Jones L, Ginnelly L, et al: A systematic review of atypical antipsychotic drugs in schizophrenia. Health Technol Assess 7:1–193, 2003

Barak Y, Mazeh D, Plopski I, et al: Intramuscular ziprasidone treatment of acute psychotic agitation in elderly patients with schizophrenia. Am J Geriatr Psychiatry 14:629–633, 2006

Barbee JG, Conrad EJ, Jamhour NJ: The effectiveness of olanzapine, risperidone, quetiapine, and ziprasidone as augmentation agents in treatment-resistant major depressive disorder. J Clin Psychiatry 65:975–981, 2004

Beedham C, Miceli JJ, Obach RS: Ziprasidone metabolism, aldehyde oxidase, and clinical implications. J Clin Psychopharmacol 23:229–232, 2003

Bonaccorso S, Meltzer HY, Li Z, et al: SR46349-B, a 5-HT(2A/2C) receptor antagonist, potentiates haloperidol-induced dopamine release in rat medial prefrontal cortex and nucleus accumbens. Neuropsychopharmacology 27:430–441, 2002

Bowden CL, Grunze H, Mullen J, et al: A randomized, double-blind, placebo-controlled efficacy and safety study of quetiapine or lithium as monotherapy for mania in bipolar disorder. J Clin Psychiatry 66:111–121, 2005

Breier A, Berg PH, Thakore JH, et al: Olanzapine versus ziprasidone: results of a 28-week double-blind study in patients with schizophrenia. Am J Psychiatry 162:1879–1887, 2005

Bremner JD, Vythilingam M, Ng CK, et al: Regional brain metabolic correlates of alpha-methylparatyrosine-induced depressive symptoms: implications for the neural circuitry of depression. JAMA 289:3125–3134, 2003

Briley M, Moret C: Neurobiological mechanisms involved in antidepressant therapies. Clin Neuropharmacol 16:387–400, 1993

Brook S: Intramuscular ziprasidone: moving beyond the conventional in the treatment of acute agitation in schizophrenia. J Clin Psychiatry 64 (suppl 19):13–18, 2003

Brook S, Lucey JV, Gunn KP: Intramuscular ziprasidone compared with intramuscular haloperidol in the treatment of acute psychosis. Ziprasidone IM Study Group. J Clin Psychiatry 61:933–941, 2000

Brook S, Walden J, Benattia I, et al: Ziprasidone and haloperidol in the treatment of acute exacerbation of schizophrenia and schizoaffective disorder: comparison of intramuscular and oral formulations in a 6-week, randomized, blinded-assessment study. Psychopharmacology (Berl) 178:514–523, 2005

Brown S: Excess mortality of schizophrenia: a meta-analysis. Br J Psychiatry 171:502–508, 1997

Brown S, Inskip H, Barraclough B: Causes of the excess mortality of schizophrenia. Br J Psychiatry 177:212–217, 2000

Bymaster FP, Katner JS, Nelson DL, et al: Atomoxetine increases extracellular levels of norepinephrine and dopamine in prefrontal cortex of rat: a potential mechanism for efficacy in attention deficit/hyperactivity disorder. Neuropsychopharmacology 27:699–711, 2002

Casey DE, Haupt DW, Newcomer JW, et al: Antipsychotic-induced weight gain and metabolic abnormalities: implications for increased mortality in patients with schizophrenia. J Clin Psychiatry 65:4–18, 2004

Colton CW, Manderscheid RW: Congruencies in increased mortality rates, years of potential life lost, and causes of death among public mental health clients in eight states. Prev Chronic Dis 3:A42, 2006

Daniel DG: Tolerability of ziprasidone: an expanding perspective. J Clin Psychiatry 64 (suppl 19):40–49, 2003

Daniel DG, Zimbroff DL, Potkin SG, et al: Ziprasidone 80 mg/day and 160 mg/day in the acute exacerbation of schizophrenia and schizoaffective disorder: a 6-week placebo-controlled trial. Ziprasidone Study Group. Neuropsychopharmacology 20:491–505, 1999

Daniel DG, Potkin SG, Reeves KR, et al: Intramuscular (IM) ziprasidone 20 mg is effective in reducing acute agitation associated with psychosis: a double-blind, randomized trial. Psychopharmacology (Berl) 155:128–134, 2001

Davis JM, Chen N, Glick ID: A meta-analysis of the efficacy of second-generation antipsychotics. Arch Gen Psychiatry 60:553–564, 2003

De Deyn PP, Carrasco MM, Deberdt W, et al: Olanzapine versus placebo in the treatment of psychosis with or without associated behavioral disturbances in patients with Alzheimer's disease. Int J Geriatr Psychiatry 19:115–126, 2004

DeLeon A, Patel NC, Crismon ML: Aripiprazole: a comprehensive review of its pharmacology, clinical efficacy, and tolerability. Clin Ther 26:649–666, 2004

Dew RE, Hughes D: Acute dystonic reaction with moderate-dose ziprasidone. J Clin Psychopharmacol 24:563–564, 2004

Diaz-Mataix L, Scorza MC, Bortolozzi A, et al: Involvement of 5-HT1A receptors in prefrontal cortex in the modulation of dopaminergic activity: role in atypical antipsychotic action. J Neurosci 25:10831–10843, 2005

Druss BG, Rosenheck RA: Mental disorders and access to medical care in the United States. Am J Psychiatry 155:1775–1777, 1998

Druss BG, Bradford DW, Rosenheck RA, et al: Mental disorders and use of cardiovascular procedures after myocardial infarction. JAMA 283:506–511, 2000

Druss BG, Bradford WD, Rosenheck RA, et al: Quality of medical care and excess mortality in older patients with mental disorders. Arch Gen Psychiatry 58:565–572, 2001

Duggal HS: Ziprasidone-induced acute laryngeal dystonia. Prog Neuropsychopharmacol Biol Psychiatry 31:970; author reply 31:971, 2007

Duman RS: Depression: a case of neuronal life and death? Biol Psychiatry 56:140–145, 2004

Dwyer DS, Pinkofsky HB, Liu Y, et al: Antipsychotic drugs affect glucose uptake and the expression of glucose transporters in PC12 cells. Prog Neuropsychopharmacol Biol Psychiatry 23:69–80, 1999

Eli Lilly: Zyprexa (olanzapine tablets), Zyprexa (intramuscular olanzapine for injection), and Zyprexa Zydis (olanzapine orally disintegrating tablets), full prescribing information. August 2008. Available at: http://pi.lilly.com/us/zyprexa-pi.pdf. Accessed December 30, 2008.

Eli Lilly updates label warning for Zyprexa to better inform on side-effects. October 5, 2007. Available at: http://www.schizophrenia.com/sznews/archives/005617.html. Accessed December 30, 2008.

Essock SM, Covell NH, Davis SM, et al: Effectiveness of switching antipsychotic medications. Am J Psychiatry 163:2090–2095, 2006

Everson G, Lasseter KC, Anderson KE, et al: The pharmacokinetics of ziprasidone in subjects with normal and impaired hepatic function. Br J Clin Pharmacol 49 (suppl 1):21S–26S, 2000

Farber NB, Rubin EH, Newcomer JW, et al: Increased neocortical neurofibrillary tangle density in subjects with Alzheimer disease and psychosis. Arch Gen Psychiatry 57:1165–1173, 2000

Finkel S, Kozma C, Long S, et al: Risperidone treatment in elderly patients with dementia: relative risk of cerebrovascular events versus other antipsychotics. Int Psychogeriatr 17:617–629, 2005

Fontaine KR, Heo M, Harrigan EP, et al: Estimating the consequences of anti-psychotic induced weight gain on health and mortality rate. Psychiatry Res 101:277–288, 2001

Frayne SM, Halanych JH, Miller DR, et al: Disparities in diabetes care: impact of mental illness. Arch Intern Med 165:2631–2638, 2005

Garver DL, Holcomb JA, Christensen JD: Cerebral cortical gray expansion associated with two second-generation antipsychotics. Biol Psychiatry 58:62–66, 2005

Geddes J, Freemantle N, Harrison P, et al: Atypical antipsychotics in the treatment of schizophrenia: systematic overview and meta-regression analysis. BMJ 321:1371–1376, 2000

Glassman AH, Bigger JT Jr: Antipsychotic drugs: prolonged QTc interval, torsade de pointes, and sudden death. Am J Psychiatry 158:1774–1782, 2001

Glick ID, Romano SJ, Simpson G, et al: Insulin resistance in olanzapine- and ziprasidone-treated patients: results of a double-blind, controlled 6-week trial. Paper presented at the annual meeting of the American Psychiatric Association, New Orleans, LA, May 5–10, 2001

Goff DC, Posever T, Herz L, et al: An exploratory haloperidol-controlled dose-finding study of ziprasidone in hospitalized patients with schizophrenia or schizoaffective disorder. J Clin Psychopharmacol 18:296–304, 1998

Goldberg RJ, Bengtson J, Chen ZY, et al: Duration of the QT interval and total and cardiovascular mortality in healthy persons (The Framingham Heart Study experience). Am J Cardiol 67:55–58, 1991

Gomez-Criado MS, Bernardo M, Florez T, et al: Ziprasidone overdose: cases recorded in the database of Pfizer-Spain and literature review. Pharmacotherapy 25:1660–1665, 2005

Gury C, Canceil O, Iaria P: Antipsychotic drugs and cardiovascular safety: current studies of prolonged QT interval and risk of ventricular arrhythmia [in French]. Encephale 26:62–72, 2000

Hamelin BA, Allard S, Laplante L, et al: The effect of timing of a standard meal on the pharmacokinetics and pharmacodynamics of the novel atypical antipsychotic agent ziprasidone. Pharmacotherapy 18:9–15, 1998

Hardy TA, Poole-Hoffmann V, Lu Y, et al: Fasting glucose and lipid changes in patients with schizophrenia treated with olanzapine or ziprasidone. Poster presented at the annual meeting of the American College of Neuropsychopharmacology, San Juan, PR, December 7–11, 2003

Harrigan EP, Miceli JJ, Anziano R, et al: A randomized evaluation of the effects of six antipsychotic agents on QTc, in the absence and presence of metabolic inhibition. J Clin Psychopharmacol 24:62–69, 2004

Harris EC, Barraclough B: Excess mortality of mental disorder. Br J Psychiatry 173:11–53, 1998

Harvey PD, Bowie CR: Ziprasidone: efficacy, tolerability, and emerging data on wide-ranging effectiveness. Expert Opin Pharmacother 6:337–346, 2005

Harvey PD, Siu CO, Romano S: Randomized, controlled, double-blind, multicenter comparison of the cognitive effects of ziprasidone versus olanzapine in acutely ill inpatients with schizophrenia or schizoaffective disorder. Psychopharmacology (Berl) 172:324–332, 2004

Harvey PD, Bowie CR, Loebel A: Neuropsychological normalization with long-term atypical antipsychotic treatment: results of a six-month randomized, double-blind comparison of ziprasidone vs. olanzapine. J Neuropsychiatry Clin Neurosci 18:54–63, 2006a

Harvey PD, Green MF, Bowie C, et al: The dimensions of clinical and cognitive change in schizophrenia: evidence for independence of improvements. Psychopharmacology (Berl) 187:356–363, 2006b

Haupt DW, Fahnestock PA, Flavin KA, et al: Adiposity and insulin sensitivity derived from intravenous glucose tolerance tests in antipsychotic-treated patients. Neuropsychopharmacology 32:2561–2569, 2007

Heinrich TW, Biblo LA, Schneider J: Torsades de pointes associated with ziprasidone. Psychosomatics 47:264–268, 2006

Heinrichs DW, Hanlon TE, Carpenter WT Jr: The Quality of Life Scale: an instrument for rating the schizophrenic deficit syndrome. Schizophr Bull 10:388–398, 1984

Hennekens CH, Hennekens AR, Hollar D, et al: Schizophrenia and increased risks of cardiovascular disease. Am Heart J 150:1115–1121, 2005

Hippisley-Cox J, Parker C, Coupland CA, et al: Inequalities in the primary care of coronary heart disease patients with serious mental health problems: a cross-sectional study. Heart 93:1256–1262, 2007

Hirsch SR, Kissling W, Bauml J, et al: A 28-week comparison of ziprasidone and haloperidol in outpatients with stable schizophrenia. J Clin Psychiatry 63:516–523, 2002

Hirschfeld RM, Keck PE Jr, Kramer M, et al: Rapid antimanic effect of risperidone monotherapy: a 3-week multicenter, double-blind, placebo-controlled trial. Am J Psychiatry 161:1057–1065, 2004

Houseknecht KL, Robertson AS, Zavadoski W, et al: Acute effects of atypical antipsychotics on whole-body insulin resistance in rats: implications for adverse metabolic effects. Neuropsychopharmacology 32:289–297, 2007

Ichikawa J, Ishii H, Bonaccorso S, et al: 5-HT(2A) and D(2) receptor blockade increases cortical DA release via 5-HT(1A) receptor activation: a possible mechanism of atypical antipsychotic-induced cortical dopamine release. J Neurochem 76:1521–1531, 2001

Insa Gómez FJ, Gutiérrez Casares JR: Ziprasidone overdose: cardiac safety. Actas Esp Psiquiatr 33:398–400, 2005

Jarema M: Atypical antipsychotics in the treatment of mood disorders. Curr Opin Psychiatry 20:23–29, 2007

Joukamaa M, Heliövaara M, Knekt P, et al: Mental disorders and cause-specific mortality. Br J Psychiatry 179:498–502, 2001

Joyce AT, Harrison DJ, Loebel AD, et al: Effect of initial ziprasidone dose on length of therapy in schizophrenia. Schizophr Res 83:285–292, 2006

Kane JM: Oral ziprasidone in the treatment of schizophrenia: a review of short-term trials. J Clin Psychiatry 64 (suppl 19):19–25, 2003

Kane JM, Berg PH, Thakore J, et al: Olanzapine versus ziprasidone: results of the 28-week double-blind study in patients with schizophrenia [abstract]. J Psychopharmacol 17:A50, 2003

Kane J, Khanna S, Giller E, et al: Ziprasidone's long-term efficacy in treatment-refractory schizophrenia. Poster presented at the International Congress on Schizophrenia Research, Savannah, GA, April 2–6, 2005

Kapur S, Remington G: Serotonin-dopamine interaction and its relevance to schizophrenia. Am J Psychiatry 153:466–476, 1996

Kapur S, Remington G: Dopamine D(2) receptors and their role in atypical antipsychotic action: still necessary and may even be sufficient. Biol Psychiatry 50:873–883, 2001

Kaufman KR, Stern L, Mohebati A, et al: Ziprasidone-induced priapism requiring surgical treatment. Eur Psychiatry 21:48–50, 2006

Keck ME, Müller MB, Binder EB, et al: Ziprasidone-related tardive dyskinesia. Am J Psychiatry 161:175–176, 2004

Keck P Jr, Buffenstein A, Ferguson J, et al: Ziprasidone 40 and 120 mg/day in the acute exacerbation of schizophrenia and schizoaffective disorder: a 4-week placebo-controlled trial. Psychopharmacology (Berl) 140:173–184, 1998

Keck PE Jr, Reeves KR, Harrigan EP: Ziprasidone in the short-term treatment of patients with schizoaffective disorder: results from two double-blind, placebo-controlled, multicenter studies. J Clin Psychopharmacol 21:27–35, 2001

Keck PE Jr, Marcus R, Tourkodimitris S, et al: A placebo-controlled, double-blind study of the efficacy and safety of aripiprazole in patients with acute bipolar mania. Am J Psychiatry 160:1651–1658, 2003a

Keck PE Jr, Versiani M, Potkin S, et al: Ziprasidone in the treatment of acute bipolar mania: a three-week, placebo-controlled, double-blind, randomized trial. Am J Psychiatry 160:741–748, 2003b

Keck PE Jr, Potkin S, Warrington L, et al: Efficacy and safety of ziprasidone in bipolar disorder: short- and long-term data. Poster presented at the annual meeting of the American Psychiatric Association, New York, May 1–6, 2004

Keefe RS, Bilder RM, Davis SM, et al: Neurocognitive effects of antipsychotic medications in patients with chronic schizophrenia in the CATIE trial. Arch Gen Psychiatry 64:633–647, 2007

Khan SS, Mican LM: A naturalistic evaluation of intramuscular ziprasidone versus intramuscular olanzapine for the management of acute agitation and aggression in children and adolescents. J Child Adolesc Psychopharmacol 16:671–677, 2006

Khanna S, Vieta E, Lyons B, et al: Risperidone in the treatment of acute mania: double-blind, placebo-controlled study. Br J Psychiatry 187:229–234, 2005

Kinon BJ, Lipkovich I, Edwards SB, et al: A 24-week randomized study of olanzapine versus ziprasidone in the treatment of schizophrenia or schizoaffective disorder in patients with prominent depressive symptoms. J Clin Psychopharmacol 26:157–162, 2006a

Kinon BJ, Liu-Seifert H, Adams DH, et al: Differential rates of treatment discontinuation in clinical trials as a measure of treatment effectiveness for olanzapine and comparator atypical antipsychotics for schizophrenia. J Clin Psychopharmacol 26:632–637, 2006b

Kohen I, Preval H, Southard R, et al: Naturalistic study of intramuscular ziprasidone versus conventional agents in agitated elderly patients: retrospective findings from a psychiatric emergency service. Am J Geriatr Pharmacother 3:240–245, 2005

Kohler CG, Lallart EA: Postpsychotic depression in schizophrenia patients. Curr Psychiatry Rep 4:273–278, 2002

Koro CE, Fedder DO, L'Italien GJ, et al: Assessment of independent effect of olanzapine and risperidone on risk of diabetes among patients with schizophrenia: population based nested case-control study. BMJ 325:243, 2002a

Koro CE, Fedder DO, L'Italien GJ, et al: An assessment of the independent effects of olanzapine and risperidone exposure on the risk of hyperlipidemia in schizophrenic patients. Arch Gen Psychiatry 59:1021–1026, 2002b

Kroeze WK, Hufeisen SJ, Popadak BA, et al: H1-histamine receptor affinity predicts short-term weight gain for typical and atypical antipsychotic drugs. Neuropsychopharmacology 28:519–526, 2003

Kudla D, Lambert M, Domin S, et al: Effectiveness, tolerability, and safety of ziprasidone in patients with schizophrenia or schizoaffective disorder: results of a multi-centre observational trial. Eur Psychiatry 22:195–202, 2007

Lesem MD, Zajecka JM, Swift RH, et al: Intramuscular ziprasidone, 2 mg versus 10 mg, in the short-term management of agitated psychotic patients. J Clin Psychiatry 62:12–18, 2001

Leucht S, Pitschel-Walz G, Abraham D, et al: Efficacy and extrapyramidal side-effects of the new antipsychotics olanzapine, quetiapine, risperidone, and sertindole compared to conventional antipsychotics and placebo: a meta-analysis of randomized controlled trials. Schizophr Res 35:51–68, 1999

Levy WO, Robichaux-Keene NR, Nunez C: No significant QTc interval changes with high-dose ziprasidone: a case series. J Psychiatr Pract 10:227–232, 2004

Lexchin J, Bero LA, Djulbegovic B, et al: Pharmaceutical industry sponsorship and research outcome and quality: systematic review. BMJ 326:1167–1170, 2003

Lieberman JA: Effectiveness of antipsychotic drugs in patients with chronic schizophrenia: efficacy, safety and cost outcomes of CATIE and other trials. J Clin Psychiatry 68:e04, 2007

Lieberman JA, Stroup TS, McEvoy JP, et al: Effectiveness of antipsychotic drugs in patients with chronic schizophrenia. N Engl J Med 353:1209–1223, 2005

Loebel A, Siu C, Romano S: Improvement in prosocial functioning after a switch to ziprasidone treatment. CNS Spectr 9:357–364, 2004

Lombardo I, Alderman J, Preskorn S, et al: Effect of food on absorption of ziprasidone. Abstract of poster presented at the International Congress on Schizophrenia Research, March 28–April 1, 2007, Colorado Springs, CO. Schizophr Bull 33:475–476, 2007

Mallinckrodt CH, Sanger TM, Dube S, et al: Assessing and interpreting treatment effects in longitudinal clinical trials with missing data. Biol Psychiatry 53:754–760, 2003

Mamo D, Kapur S, Shammi CM, et al: A PET study of dopamine D2 and serotonin 5-HT2 receptor occupancy in patients with schizophrenia treated with therapeutic doses of ziprasidone. Am J Psychiatry 161:818–825, 2004

Mason MN, Johnson CE, Piasecki M: Ziprasidone-induced acute dystonia. Am J Psychiatry 162:625–626, 2005

Mazei MS, Pluto CP, Kirkbride B, et al: Effects of catecholamine uptake blockers in the caudate-putamen and subregions of the medial prefrontal cortex of the rat. Brain Res 936:58–67, 2002

McCue RE, Waheed R, Urcuyo L, et al: Comparative effectiveness of second-generation antipsychotics and haloperidol in acute schizophrenia. Br J Psychiatry 189:433–440, 2006

McDougle CJ, Kem DL, Posey DJ: Case series: use of ziprasidone for maladaptive symptoms in youths with autism. J Am Acad Child Adolesc Psychiatry 41:921–927, 2002

McEvoy JP, Meyer JM, Goff DC, et al: Prevalence of the metabolic syndrome in patients with schizophrenia: baseline results from the Clinical Antipsychotic Trials of Intervention Effectiveness (CATIE) schizophrenia trial and comparison with national estimates from NHANES III. Schizophr Res 80:19–32, 2005

McEvoy JP, Lieberman JA, Perkins DO, et al: Efficacy and tolerability of olanzapine, quetiapine, and risperidone in the treatment of early psychosis: a randomized, double-blind 52-week comparison. Am J Psychiatry 164:1050–1060, 2007

McIntyre RS, Brecher M, Paulsson B, et al: Quetiapine or haloperidol as monotherapy for bipolar mania—a 12-week, double-blind, randomised, parallel-group, placebo-controlled trial. Eur Neuropsychopharmacol 15:573–585, 2005

McQuade RD, Marcus R, Sanchez R: Aripiprazole vs placebo in acute mania: safety and tolerability pooled analysis. Poster presented at the International Conference on Bipolar Disorder, Pittsburgh, PA, June 12–14, 2003

Meltzer HY, Bobo WV: Interpreting the efficacy findings in the CATIE study: what clinicians should know. CNS Spectr 11:14–24, 2006

Miceli JJ, Anziano RJ, Robarge L, et al: The effect of carbamazepine on the steady-state pharmacokinetics of ziprasidone in healthy volunteers. Br J Clin Pharmacol 49 (suppl 1):65S–70S, 2000a

Miceli JJ, Smith M, Robarge L, et al: The effects of ketoconazole on ziprasidone pharmacokinetics—a placebo-controlled crossover study in healthy volunteers. Br J Clin Pharmacol 49 (suppl 1):71S–76S, 2000b

Miceli JJ, Wilner KD, Hansen RA, et al: Single- and multiple-dose pharmacokinetics of ziprasidone under non-fasting conditions in healthy male volunteers. Br J Clin Pharmacol 49 (suppl 1): 5S–13S, 2000c

Miceli JJ, Murray S, Sallee FR, et al: Pharmacokinetic and pharmacodynamic QTc profile of oral ziprasidone in pediatric and adult subjects following single-dose administration. Poster presented at the annual meeting of the American Psychiatric Association, New York, May 1–6, 2004

Millan MJ: Improving the treatment of schizophrenia: focus on serotonin (5-HT)(1A) receptors. J Pharmacol Exp Ther 295:853–861, 2000

Miodownik C, Hausmann M, Frolova K, et al: Lithium intoxication associated with intramuscular ziprasidone in schizoaffective patients. Clin Neuropharmacol 28:295–297, 2005

Montanez A, Ruskin JN, Hebert PR, et al: Prolonged QTc interval and risks of total and cardiovascular mortality and sudden death in the general population: a review and qualitative overview of the prospective cohort studies. Arch Intern Med 164:943–948, 2004

Montes JM, Rodriguez JL, Balbo E, et al: Improvement in antipsychotic-related metabolic disturbances in patients with schizophrenia switched to ziprasidone. Prog Neuropsychopharmacol Biol Psychiatry 31:383–388, 2006

Morrato EH, Newcomer JW, Allen RR, et al: Prevalence of baseline serum glucose and lipid testing in users of second-generation antipsychotic drugs: a retrospective, population-based study of Medicaid claims data. J Clin Psychiatry 69:316–322, 2008

Mullins CD, Shaya FT, Zito JM, et al: Effect of initial ziprasidone dose on treatment persistence in schizophrenia. Schizophr Res 83:277–284, 2006

Murray S, Mandel FS, Loebel A: Optimal initial dosing of ziprasidone: clinical trial data. Poster presented at the annual meeting of the American Psychiatric Association. New York, May 1–6, 2004

Murty RG, Mistry SG, Chacko RC: Neuroleptic malignant syndrome with ziprasidone. J Clin Psychopharmacol 22:624–626, 2002

Nasrallah HA, Meyer JM, Goff DC, et al: Low rates of treatment for hypertension, dyslipidemia and diabetes in schizophrenia: data from the CATIE schizophrenia trial sample at baseline. Schizophr Res 86:15–22, 2006

Nemeroff CB, Lieberman JA, Weiden PJ, et al: From clinical research to clinical practice: a 4-year review of ziprasidone. CNS Spectr 10 (suppl):s1–s20, 2005

Newcomer JW: Second-generation (atypical) antipsychotics and metabolic effects: a comprehensive literature review. CNS Drugs 19 (suppl 1):1–93, 2005

Newcomer JW, Haupt DW: The metabolic effects of antipsychotic medications. Can J Psychiatry 51:480–491, 2006

Newcomer JW, Hennekens CH: Severe mental illness and risk of cardiovascular disease. JAMA 298:1794–1796, 2007

Obach RS, Huynh P, Allen MC, et al: Human liver aldehyde oxidase: inhibition by 239 drugs. J Clin Pharmacol 44:7–19, 2004

O'Brien JM, Rockwood RP, Suh KI: Haloperidol-induced torsade de pointes. Ann Pharmacother 33:1046–1050, 1999

O'Connor R, Schooler NR: Penultimate observation carried forward (POCF): a new approach to analysis of long-term symptom change in chronic relapsing conditions. Schizophr Res 60:319–320, 2003

Osby U, Correia N, Brandt L, et al: Mortality and causes of death in schizophrenia in Stockholm county, Sweden. Schizophr Res 45:21–28, 2000

Osby U, Brandt L, Correia N, et al: Excess mortality in bipolar and unipolar disorder in Sweden. Arch Gen Psychiatry 58:844–850, 2001

Papakostas GI, Petersen TJ, Nierenberg AA, et al: Ziprasidone augmentation of selective serotonin reuptake inhibitors (SSRIs) for SSRI-resistant major depressive disorder. J Clin Psychiatry 65:217–221, 2004

Papapetropoulos S, Wheeler S, Singer C: Tardive dystonia associated with ziprasidone. Am J Psychiatry 162:2191, 2005

Patel NC, Keck PE Jr: Ziprasidone: efficacy and safety in patients with bipolar disorder. Expert Rev Neurother 6:1129–1138, 2006

Perlis RH, Welge JA, Vornik LA, et al: Atypical antipsychotics in the treatment of mania: a meta-analysis of randomized, placebo-controlled trials. J Clin Psychiatry 67:509–516, 2006

Pfizer Inc.: Dear Healthcare Practitioner letter, August 2004. Available at: http://www.fda.gov/medwatch/SAFETY/2004/GeodonDearDoc.pdf. Accessed December 30, 2008.

Pfizer Inc.: Geodon (ziprasidone HCl) capsules and Geodon (ziprasidone mesylate) for injection, full prescribing information. June 2008

Potkin SG, Keck PE Jr, Segal S, et al: Ziprasidone in acute bipolar mania: a 21-day randomized, double-blind, placebo-controlled replication trial. J Clin Psychopharmacol 25:301–310, 2005

Pozzi L, Acconcia S, Ceglia I, et al: Stimulation of 5-hydroxytryptamine (5-HT(2C)) receptors in the ventrotegmental area inhibits stress-induced but not basal dopamine release in the rat prefrontal cortex. J Neurochem 82:93–100, 2002

Prakash C, Kamel A, Cui D, et al: Identification of the major human liver cytochrome P450 isoform(s) responsible for the formation of the primary metabolites of ziprasidone and prediction of possible drug interactions. Br J Clin Pharmacol 49 (suppl 1):35S–42S, 2000

Purnine DM, Carey KB, Maisto SA, et al: Assessing positive and negative symptoms in outpatients with schizophrenia and mood disorders. J Nerv Ment Dis 188:653–661, 2000

Ramos AE, Shytle RD, Silver AA, et al: Ziprasidone-induced oculogyric crisis. J Am Acad Child Adolesc Psychiatry 42:1013–1014, 2003

Rettenbacher MA, Ebenbichler C, Hofer A, et al: Early changes of plasma lipids during treatment with atypical antipsychotics. Int Clin Psychopharmacol 21:369–372, 2006

Richelson E, Souder T: Binding of antipsychotic drugs to human brain receptors focus on newer generation compounds. Life Sci 68:29–39, 2000

Rochon PA, Normand SL, Gomes T, et al: Antipsychotic therapy and short-term serious events in older adults with dementia. Arch Intern Med 168:1090–1096, 2008

Rollema H, Lu Y, Schmidt AW, et al: 5-HT(1A) receptor activation contributes to ziprasidone-induced dopamine release in the rat prefrontal cortex. Biol Psychiatry 48:229–237, 2000

Rosenfield PJ, Girgis RR, Gil R: High-dose ziprasidone-induced acute dystonia. Prog Neuropsychopharmacol Biol Psychiatry 31:546–547, 2007

Sachs G, Sanchez R, Marcus R, et al: Aripiprazole in the treatment of acute manic or mixed episodes in patients with bipolar I disorder: a 3-week placebo-controlled study. J Psychopharmacol 20:536–546, 2006

Sallee FR, Miceli JJ, Tensfeldt T, et al: Single-dose pharmacokinetics and safety of ziprasidone in children and adolescents. J Am Acad Child Adolesc Psychiatry 45:720–728, 2006

Scherk H, Pajonk FG, Leucht S: Second-generation antipsychotic agents in the treatment of acute mania: a systematic review and meta-analysis of randomized controlled trials. Arch Gen Psychiatry 64:442–455, 2007

Schmidt AW, Lebel LA, Howard HR Jr, et al: Ziprasidone: a novel antipsychotic agent with a unique human receptor binding profile. Eur J Pharmacol 425:197–201, 2001

Schooler NR: Maintaining symptom control: review of ziprasidone long-term efficacy data. J Clin Psychiatry 64 (suppl 19):26–32, 2003

Seeger TF, Seymour PA, Schmidt AW, et al: Ziprasidone (CP-88,059): a new antipsychotic with combined dopamine and serotonin receptor antagonist activity. J Pharmacol Exp Ther 275:101–113, 1995

Shapiro DA, Renock S, Arrington E, et al: Aripiprazole, a novel atypical antipsychotic drug with a unique and robust pharmacology. Neuropsychopharmacology 28:1400–1411, 2003

Simpson G, Weiden P, Pigott TA, et al: Ziprasidone vs olanzapine in schizophrenia: 6-month continuation study. Eur Neuropsychopharmacol 12 (suppl):S310, 2002

Simpson GM, Glick ID, Weiden PJ, et al: Randomized, controlled, double-blind multicenter comparison of the efficacy and tolerability of ziprasidone and olanzapine in acutely ill inpatients with schizophrenia or schizoaffective disorder. Am J Psychiatry 161:1837–1847, 2004a

Simpson GM, Weiden PJ, Loebel A, et al: Ziprasidone: long-term post-switch efficacy in schizophrenia. Poster presented at the annual meeting of the American Psychiatric Association, New York, May 1–6, 2004b

Simpson GM, Weiden P, Pigott T, et al: Six-month, blinded, multicenter continuation study of ziprasidone versus olanzapine in schizophrenia. Am J Psychiatry 162:1535–1538, 2005

Smulevich AB, Khanna S, Eerdekens M, et al: Acute and continuation risperidone monotherapy in bipolar mania: a 3-week placebo-controlled trial followed by a 9-week double-blind trial of risperidone and haloperidol. Eur Neuropsychopharmacol 15:75–84, 2005

Srisurapanont M, Maneeton N: Comparison of the efficacy and acceptability of atypical antipsychotic drugs: a meta-analysis of randomized, placebo-controlled trials. J Med Assoc Thai 82:341–346, 1999

Stahl SM: Neurotransmission of cognition, part 2: selective NRIs are smart drugs: exploiting regionally selective actions on both dopamine and norepinephrine to enhance cognition. J Clin Psychiatry 64:110–111, 2003

Stahl SM, Shayegan DK: The psychopharmacology of ziprasidone: receptor-binding properties and real-world psychiatric practice. J Clin Psychiatry 64 (suppl 19):6–12, 2003

Staller JA: Intramuscular ziprasidone in youth: a retrospective chart review. J Child Adolesc Psychopharmacol 14:590–592, 2004

Street JS, Clark WS, Gannon KS, et al: Olanzapine treatment of psychotic and behavioral symptoms in patients with Alzheimer disease in nursing care facilities: a double-blind, randomized, placebo-controlled trial. The HGEU Study Group. Arch Gen Psychiatry 57:968–976, 2000

Stroup TS, Lieberman JA, McEvoy JP, et al: Effectiveness of olanzapine, quetiapine, risperidone, and ziprasidone in patients with chronic schizophrenia following discontinuation of a previous atypical antipsychotic. Am J Psychiatry 163:611–622, 2006

Sumiyoshi T, Jayathilake K, Meltzer HY: The effect of melperone, an atypical antipsychotic drug, on cognitive function in schizophrenia. Schizophr Res 59:7–16, 2003

Swainston Harrison T, Scott LJ: Ziprasidone: a review of its use in schizophrenia and schizoaffective disorder. CNS Drugs 20:1027–1052, 2006

Swartz MS, Perkins DO, Stroup TS, et al: Effects of antipsychotic medications on psychosocial functioning in patients with chronic schizophrenia: findings from the NIMH CATIE study. Am J Psychiatry 164:428–436, 2007

Swift RH, Harrigan EP, van Kammen DP: A comparison of fixed-dose intramuscular (IM) ziprasidone with flexible-dose IM haloperidol. Poster presented at the annual meeting of the American Psychiatric Association, Toronto, ON, Canada, May 30–June 4, 1998

Tandon R, Fleischhacker WW: Comparative efficacy of antipsychotics in the treatment of schizophrenia: a critical assessment. Schizophr Res 79:145–155, 2005

Tatsumi M, Jansen K, Blakely RD, et al: Pharmacological profile of neuroleptics at human monoamine transporters. Eur J Pharmacol 368:277–283, 1999

Tauscher J, Kapur S, Verhoeff NP, et al: Brain serotonin 5-HT(1A) receptor binding in schizophrenia measured by positron emission tomography and [11C]WAY-100635. Arch Gen Psychiatry 59:514–520, 2002

Taylor D: Ziprasidone in the management of schizophrenia: the QT interval issue in context. CNS Drugs 17:423–430, 2003

Tecott LH, Sun LM, Akana SF, et al: Eating disorder and epilepsy in mice lacking 5-HT2c serotonin receptors. Nature 374:542–546, 1995

Thome J, Foley P, Riederer P: Neurotrophic factors and the maldevelopmental hypothesis of schizophrenic psychoses: review article. J Neural Transm 105:85–100, 1998

Tohen M, Sanger TM, McElroy SL, et al: Olanzapine versus placebo in the treatment of acute mania. Olanzapine HGEH Study Group. Am J Psychiatry 156:702–709, 1999

Tohen M, Jacobs TG, Grundy SL, et al: Efficacy of olanzapine in acute bipolar mania: a double-blind, placebo-controlled study. The Olanzapine HGGW Study Group. Arch Gen Psychiatry 57:841–849, 2000

Tohen M, Zhang F, Keck PE, et al: Olanzapine versus haloperidol in schizoaffective disorder, bipolar type. J Affect Disord 67:133–140, 2001

Tohen M, Goldberg JF, Gonzalez-Pinto Arrillaga AM, et al: A 12-week, double-blind comparison of olanzapine vs haloperidol in the treatment of acute mania. Arch Gen Psychiatry 60:1218–1226, 2003

Versavel M, DelBello MP, Ice K, et al: Ziprasidone dosing study in pediatric patients with bipolar disorder, schizophrenia or schizoaffective disorder [abstract]. Neuropsychopharmacology 30 (suppl):S122, 2005

Villanueva N, Markham-Abedi C, McNeely C, et al: Probable association between ziprasidone and worsening hypertension. Pharmacotherapy 26:1352–1357, 2006

Weiden PJ, Iqbal N, Mendelowitz AJ, et al: Best clinical practice with ziprasidone: update after one year of experience. J Psychiatr Pract 8:81–97, 2002

Weiden PJ, Daniel DG, Simpson G, et al: Improvement in indices of health status in outpatients with schizophrenia switched to ziprasidone. J Clin Psychopharmacol 23:595–600, 2003a

Weiden PJ, Simpson GM, Potkin SG, et al: Effectiveness of switching to ziprasidone for stable but symptomatic outpatients with schizophrenia. J Clin Psychiatry 64:580–588, 2003b

Weiden PJ, Newcomer JW, Loebel AD, et al: Long-term changes in weight and plasma lipids during maintenance treatment with ziprasidone. Neuropsychopharmacology 33:985–994, 2008

Weiner DM, Meltzer HY, Veinbergs I, et al: The role of M1 muscarinic receptor agonism of N-desmethylclozapine in the unique clinical effects of clozapine. Psychopharmacology (Berl) 177:207–216, 2004

Weinstein SK, Adler CM, Strakowski SM: Ziprasidone-induced acute dystonic reactions in patients with bipolar disorder. J Clin Psychiatry 67:327–328, 2006

Weisler R, Dunn J, English P: Ziprasidone in adjunctive treatment of acute bipolar mania: double-blind, placebo-controlled trial. Poster presented at the annual meeting of the Institute on Psychiatric Services, Boston, MA, Oct 29–Nov 2, 2003

Weisler R, Warrington L, Dunn J: Adjunctive ziprasidone in bipolar mania: short- and long-term data. Biol Psychiatry 55 (suppl):43S, 2004

Wooltorton E: Risperidone (Risperdal): increased rate of cerebrovascular events in dementia trials. CMAJ 167:1269–1270, 2002

Yumru M, Savas HA, Selek S, et al: Acute dystonia after initial doses of ziprasidone: a case report. Prog Neuropsychopharmacol Biol Psychiatry 30:745–747, 2006

Ziegenbein M, Schomerus G, Kropp S: Ziprasidone-induced Pisa syndrome after clozapine treatment. J Neuropsychiatry Clin Neurosci 15:458–459, 2003

Zimbroff DL, Brook S, Benattia I: Safety and tolerability of IM ziprasidone: review of clinical trial data. Poster presented at the annual meeting of the American Psychiatric Association, Philadelphia, PA, May 18–23, 2002

Zorn SH, Bebel LA, Schmidt AW, et al: Pharmacological and neurochemical studies with the new antipsychotic ziprasidone, in Interactive Monoaminergic Basis of Brain Disorders. Edited by Palomo T, Beninger R, Archer T. Madrid, Spain, Editorial Sintesis, 1998, pp 377–394

CHAPTER 34

Drugs to Treat Extrapyramidal Side Effects

Joseph K. Stanilla, M.D.

George M. Simpson, M.D.

Extrapyramidal Side Effects

History

The discovery of the therapeutic properties of chlorpromazine (Delay and Deniker 1952; Laborit et al. 1952) was soon followed by the description of its tendency to produce extrapyramidal side effects (EPS) that were indistinguishable from classical Parkinson's syndrome. A debate soon arose regarding the relationship between EPS and therapeutic efficacy. Flügel (1953) suggested that a therapeutic response from chlorpromazine required the development of EPS. Haase (1954) postulated that the neuroleptic dose that produced minimal subclinical rigidity and hypokinesis (i.e., the "neuroleptic threshold") was the minimal neuroleptic dose necessary for therapeutic antipsychotic effect and that it was manifested by micrographic handwriting changes. Other investigators also reported that EPS were necessary for therapeutic efficacy (see Denham and Carrick 1960; Karn and Kasper 1959).

Brooks (1956), on the other hand, suggested that "signs of parkinsonism heralded the particular effect being sought" (p. 1122) but that "the therapeutic effects were not dependent on extrapyramidal dysfunction. On the contrary, alleviation of such dysfunction, as soon as it occurred, sped the progress of recovery" (p. 1122). The need to develop EPS for therapeutic efficacy was also questioned by others. The differences in opinion regarding EPS and neuroleptic efficacy were partially attribut-

able to differences in the definitions of EPS and in the methodologies of the studies (Chien and DiMascio 1967).

Haase's concept—that mild subclinical EPS manifested by handwriting changes were indicative of a therapeutic dose—was demonstrated in studies that found no difference in therapeutic response at doses beyond the neuroleptic threshold (Angus and Simpson 1970a; G.M. Simpson et al. 1970). Patients treated with doses beyond the neuroleptic threshold received significantly larger doses of medication without further therapeutic benefit. This finding has been discussed more fully (Baldessarini et al. 1988) and has been replicated (McEvoy et al. 1991).

When clozapine was first developed in 1960, it sparked little interest as a potential antipsychotic. Many investigators believed that EPS were necessary for antipsychotic effect, and clozapine appeared not to produce EPS. Even after studies showed that clozapine possessed antipsychotic activity, interest regarding commercial development was still limited. The hesitancy on the part of the pharmaceutical company was related to the belief held by many members of the psychiatric community—that is, that a drug could not have antipsychotic effect without producing EPS (Hippius 1989).

In contrast, the current goal in the development of new antipsychotic medications is to replicate the EPS profile of clozapine and to develop antipsychotics that do not produce EPS. This situation essentially brings the story of EPS full circle.

The terms used to name and characterize antipsychotic medications have also evolved. The term *tranquilizer* was initially introduced to characterize the psychic effects of reserpine. The term *neuroleptic*, derived from Greek and meaning "to clasp the neuron," was introduced to describe chlorpromazine and the extrapyramidal effects that it produced (Delay et al. 1952). Until clozapine was approved for use, all commercially available drugs with antipsychotic properties possessed the following neuroleptic properties: blocking apomorphine and amphetamine-induced stereotypy; antagonizing the conditioned avoidance response; and producing catalepsy, elevated serum prolactin levels, and EPS. For that reason, all antipsychotic drugs were referred to as *neuroleptics*. With the subsequent development of clozapine and other antipsychotic drugs that possess reduced EPS profiles, the term *neuroleptic* no longer correctly categorizes all drugs with antipsychotic effects; therefore, the term *antipsychotic* is more accurate and more preferable.

Severe EPS can have a significantly negative effect on treatment outcome by contributing to poor compliance and exacerbation of psychiatric symptoms (Van Putten et al. 1981). Akathisia, in particular, is associated with poor clinical outcome (Levinson et al. 1990; Van Putten et al. 1984), increased violence (Keckich 1978), and even suicide (Shear et al. 1983). The presence of EPS early in treatment may place a patient at increased risk of developing tardive dyskinesia (TD) (Saltz et al. 1991). Orofacial TD may have a negative effect on the social acceptability of patients, even though they are often unaware of the movements (Boumans et al. 1994). Laryngeal dystonia can adversely affect speech, breathing, and swallowing (Feve et al. 1995; Khan et al. 1994) and can be potentially life-threatening (Koek and Pi 1989). Clearly, EPS are significant, need to be assessed, and should be minimized so that the overall treatment and health of patients may be optimized.

Types

Four types of EPS have been delineated, and the treatment of each type should be individualized. Acute dystonic reactions (ADRs) are generally the first EPS to appear and are often the most dramatic (Angus and Simpson 1970b). *Dystonias* are involuntary sustained or spasmodic muscle contractions that cause abnormal twisting or rhythmical movements and/or postures. ADRs tend to occur suddenly and generally involve muscles of the head and neck (as in torticollis, facial grimacing, or oculogyric crisis). Nearly 90% of all ADRs occur within

4 days of antipsychotic initiation or dosage increase, and virtually 100% of all ADRs occur by day 10 (Singh et al. 1990; Sramek et al. 1986). Although tardive dystonia can occur after this period, movements occurring beyond this time frame are much less likely to be ADRs. Instead, other conditions, including seizures, need to be considered.

Akathisia is the second type of EPS to appear. Akathisia, meaning "inability to sit," consists of both an objective restless movement and a subjective feeling of restlessness that the patient experiences as the need to move. It may be difficult for a patient to explain the sensation of akathisia, and the diagnosis can be missed. At times, patients may display the classical movements of akathisia, but they may not have the subjective distress—a condition that has been termed *pseudoakathisia*, which may be a type of tardive syndrome (Barnes 1990).

The third type of EPS, (pseudo)parkinsonism, is virtually indistinguishable from classical Parkinson's syndrome. The symptoms include a generalized slowing of movement (akinesia), masked facies, rigidity (including cogwheeling rigidity), resting tremor, and hypersalivation. Parkinsonism generally occurs after a few weeks or more of neuroleptic treatment. Akinesia needs to be differentiated from primary depression and the blunted affect of schizophrenia (Rifkin et al. 1975).

Tardive syndromes make up the fourth group of EPS. TD, although clearly associated with the use of antipsychotic medications, was actually described prior to the advent of antipsychotics (G.M. Simpson 2000). TD consists of irregular stereotypical movements of the mouth, face, and tongue and choreoathetoid movements of the fingers, arms, legs, and trunk. It tends to occur after months to years of use of antipsychotic medications. Patients frequently have no awareness of the abnormal movements. The lack of awareness may be related to frontal lobe dysfunction (Sandyk et al. 1993).

Tardive dystonia, a variant of TD, also generally emerges months to years after treatment with antipsychotics (Burke et al. 1982) Unlike in ADRs, the movements associated with tardive dystonia tend to be persistent and more resistant to medical treatment (Kang et al. 1988).

Incidence

Ayd (1961) was the first to report the incidence of EPS, noting an overall incidence of 39%, with 21% demonstrating akathisia, 15% demonstrating parkinsonism, and only 2% having ADRs. Varying rates of occurrence, including much higher incidences of ADRs, have been reported since that time. A prospective study found that the range of incidence of ADRs was between 17% and 38%, with the higher rate occurring with haloperidol (Sramek et al. 1986). In general, higher prevalence rates for all types of EPS occur at higher doses and with higher-potency antipsychotics. In a series of surveys of 721 patients with schizophrenia conducted over 10 years, Mc-Creadie (1992) found that the point prevalence was 27% for parkinsonism, 23% for akathisia or pseudoakathisia, and 29% for TD. Forty-four percent of patients had no movement disorder. A 10-year prospective study found that the overall incidence of TD within a group remained fairly stable—30% at baseline, 37% at 5 years, and 32% at 10 years (Gardos et al. 1994).

Data from the Clinical Antipsychotic Trials of Intervention Effectiveness (CATIE) studies found the presence of probable TD by Schooler-Kane criteria in 212 (15%) of 1,460 subjects (D.D. Miller et al. 2005). Tardive dystonia has been reported to occur in 1%–2% of patients taking antipsychotic medications (Yassa et al. 1986).

Extrapyramidal movements have been reported to occur in 17%–29% of neuroleptic-naive patients with schizophrenia (Caligiuri et al. 1993; Chatterjee et al. 1995). This finding raises questions regarding the role of antipsychotics in the etiology of TD (see G.M. Simpson et al. 1981).

These data refer to first-generation typical antipsychotics. Data from the CATIE trials include subjects treated with second-generation atypical antipsychotics as well as typical antipsychotics. The presence of probable TD by Schooler-Kane criteria was found in 212 of 1,460 subjects (15%), which is lower than rates noted above (D.D. Miller et al. 2005). The incidence for all types of EPS has been shown to be less with the second-generation atypical antipsychotics.

Etiology

The exact mechanisms involved in the production of EPS are not known. Control of motor activity apparently involves an interaction between nigrostriatal dopaminergic, intrastriatal cholinergic, and γ-aminobutyric acid (GABA)–ergic neurons (Côté and Crutcher 1991). Extrapyramidal movements of parkinsonism and dystonia classically have been thought to result from antipsychotic blockade of dopaminergic nigrostriatal tracts, resulting in a relative increase in cholinergic activity (Snyder et al. 1974). Drugs that either decrease cholinergic activity or increase dopaminergic activity reduce EPS, presumably by restoring the two systems to their previous equilibrium, as demonstrated in ADRs in monkeys (Casey et al. 1980).

This feature is the basis for the use of anticholinergics in the treatment of EPS.

The etiology of TD is thought to result from more complex changes, which include increased dopamine receptor sensitivity following prolonged dopamine blockade (Gerlach 1977). The production of EPS probably involves more complex interactions of other factors and receptor types, which have become the subject of investigation.

Decreased serum calcium has been associated with increased EPS. Calcium is involved in the function of the cholinergic system and in the metabolism of dopamine (Kuny and Binswanger 1989), and antipsychotic drugs bind to the calcium-dependent activator of several enzyme systems. (Calmodulin has been studied by el-Defrawi and Craig [1984].)

GABA may have an effect on EPS through inhibitory feedback on the dopaminergic system. Reduced GABA synthesis and reduced GABA levels have been found with TD (Gunne et al. 1984; Thaker et al. 1987). The effect of GABA on ADRs is not as clear. ADRs in baboons were found to be increased by drugs that increased GABA levels, as well as by drugs that decreased GABA (Casey et al. 1980).

β-Adrenergic mechanisms may be involved in TD, akathisia, and tremor (Wilbur et al. 1988). Clozapine is a potent α_1-adrenergic receptor antagonist in the brain, causing α_1 receptor upregulation and increased noradrenergic metabolism, factors that may affect the EPS profile of clozapine (Baldessarini et al. 1992).

Free radicals, possibly produced by chronic neuroleptic use, have been proposed as contributors to the development of neuropathic damage and TD. Vitamin E, as an antioxidant that binds free radicals, has been suggested as a treatment for TD by limiting the process (Cadet et al. 1986). Levels of lipid peroxides, theoretically produced by free radicals, have not been found to correlate with TD (McCreadie et al. 1995), nor have changes in levels correlated with treatment with vitamin E, although it was noted that these changes could be occurring centrally (Corrigan et al. 1993).

A somewhat related theory suggests that increased iron levels in the basal ganglia may contribute to TD because of the involvement of iron in the production of free radicals (Ben-Shachar and Youdim 1987). However, neuroimaging and pathological studies have not demonstrated increased iron levels on a consistent basis (Elkashef et al. 1994).

The metabolism of antipsychotics may contribute to EPS. Haloperidol, when given intravenously, has a much lower incidence of EPS than when it is used orally or intramuscularly, even when given at extremely high doses. Haloperidol is metabolized to reduced haloperidol in the liver. When administered intravenously, haloperidol enters the central nervous system (CNS) before metabolites are produced. It has been proposed that dopamine$_2$ (D$_2$) receptor saturation by haloperidol, rather than by reduced haloperidol, could account for the difference in EPS production (Menza et al. 1987).

More recent investigations of clozapine and other novel antipsychotics have focused on dopamine and serotonin (5-HT) receptors (Kapur and Remington 1996). Clozapine, olanzapine, quetiapine, risperidone, and ziprasidone are potent serotonin$_{2A}$ (5-HT$_{2A}$) receptor antagonists and relatively weaker D$_2$ antagonists, compared with typical antipsychotics. They all have a reduced EPS profile, compared with typical antipsychotics (Meltzer 1999).

Typical antipsychotics initially increase dopamine synthesis, turnover, and release in the striatum of baboons (Meldrum et al. 1977). This increased dopamine production reaches a maximum 1–5 hours after a single neuroleptic injection, which corresponds in time with the development of ADRs in baboons. During chronic treatment (up to 11 days), there is a marked diminution in the capacity of the antipsychotics to provoke an increased turnover of dopamine. Chronic haloperidol treatment causes decreased striatal dopaminergic neurotransmission and upregulation of postsynaptic D$_2$ receptors (Ichikawa and Meltzer 1991). In contrast, chronic clozapine treatment causes a slight *increase* in striatal dopaminergic neurotransmission and no changes in D$_2$ receptors. This has recently also been demonstrated in humans (Silvestri et al. 2000). These differences may partly explain the lack of occurrence of EPS and TD with clozapine and perhaps also with the other novel antipsychotics.

Dopamine$_1$ (D$_1$) receptor antagonists have a lower EPS potential than do traditional D$_2$ antipsychotics in nonhuman primates (Coffin et al. 1989). Patients who were clinical responders to antipsychotics and who had lower D$_2$ receptor occupancy by positron emission tomography (PET) analysis were found to have a lower incidence of EPS. Patients treated with clozapine had lower D$_2$ receptor occupancy than patients treated with typical antipsychotics (Farde et al. 1992). The balanced D$_1$/D$_2$ receptor function may prevent development of EPS and TD (Gerlach and Hansen 1992).

The rate of dissociation from the D$_2$ receptor may be as important as the degree of D$_2$ blockade, with regard to EPS. Novel antipsychotics have a faster dissociation rate

from the D$_2$ receptor than do traditional antipsychotics (Kapur and Seeman 2001).

The high ratio of serotonin$_2$ (5-HT$_2$) receptor blockade to striatal D$_2$ receptor blockade that occurs with clozapine may account for clozapine's lack of EPS (Meltzer et al. 1989). Evidence suggests that decreasing serotonergic neurotransmission reverses or prevents catalepsy induced by D$_2$ receptor blockade (Meltzer and Nash 1991).

Clozapine also has a high affinity for dopamine$_3$ (D$_3$) and dopamine$_4$ (D$_4$) receptors (Sokoloff et al. 1990; Van Tol et al. 1991). The binding of clozapine to these receptors has also been proposed as a possible mechanism involved in the favorable EPS profile of clozapine.

Rating

Investigations of treatment for EPS led to the need to develop instruments to evaluate and quantify them. An initial EPS scale was shown to have both clinical validity and high interrater reliability, but it did not adequately assess salivation and tremor (G.M. Simpson et al. 1964). Scores were low, despite obvious and disabling tremor or salivation that required treatment with antiparkinson medication. Subsequently, the scale was expanded to 10 items (rated on a five-point scale), including tremor and salivation (G.M. Simpson and Angus 1970). This scale has good psychometric properties and is simple to use and score. It has been modified for outpatient use by eliminating the leg rigidity item and by replacing head dropping with head rotation. Studies using this scale have shown that scores correlate with the dosages and plasma levels of an antipsychotic. The scale is widely used in clinical trials and can be completed by nurses for the routine monitoring of neuroleptic treatment.

The Simpson-Angus Scale does not include a direct rating for bradykinesia or akinesia. Mindham (1976) modified the scale to include an item for lack of facial expression. Additional rating scales for EPS have since been developed, including the Chouinard Extrapyramidal Rating Scale (Chouinard et al. 1980), Targeting of Abnormal Kinetic Effects (TAKE) Scale (Wojcik et al. 1980), St. Hans Rating Scale for Extrapyramidal Syndromes (Gerlach et al. 1993), and Dyskinesia Identification System Condensed User Scale (DISCUS; Kalachnik and Sprague 1993).

The Modified Simpson-Angus Scale includes a single item for rating akathisia. More comprehensive scales have been devised specifically to rate akathisia, including the Barnes Akathisia Rating Scale (Barnes 1989), Hillside Akathisia Scale (Fleischhacker et al. 1989), and

Prince Henry Hospital Akathisia Rating Scale (PHH Scale; Sachdev 1994).

Scales have also been developed for the assessment of dyskinetic movements. These include the Abnormal Involuntary Movement Scale (AIMS; Guy 1976) and the Simpson/Rockland Scale (G.M. Simpson et al. 1979).

Instrumental devices have been developed for the assessment of EPS, and several have been shown to correlate with clinical scales (Büchel et al. 1995). Instrumental devices have the advantage of increased reliability of quantitative measures, primarily through the elimination of subjective error associated with clinical raters; however, instrumental devices also have disadvantages. They often require greater patient cooperation than do clinical scales. They may require physical contact with the subject, which can affect measurements. They often evaluate a limited area, unlike clinical scales, which evaluate a patient in multiple areas as well as globally. As of this writing, clinical scales generally can be considered to have better global clinical validity with greater ease of use, while instrumental measures provide greater reliability (Büchel et al. 1995).

Anticholinergic Medications

Trihexyphenidyl

History and Discovery

Antiparkinsonian medications are drugs that have primarily been used to treat EPS and include anticholinergic, antihistaminic, and dopaminergic agents (Table 34–1).

Trihexyphenidyl, a synthetic analogue of atropine, was introduced as benzhexol hydrochloride in 1949. It was found to be effective in the treatment of Parkinson's disease in a study of 411 patients (Doshay et al. 1954). Thereafter, it was also used to treat neuroleptic-induced parkinsonism (NIP) (Rashkis and Smarr 1957).

Structure–Activity Relations

Trihexyphenidyl, a tertiary-amine analogue of atropine, is a competitive antagonist of acetylcholine and other muscarinic agonists that compete for a common binding site on muscarinic receptors (Yamamura and Snyder 1974). It exerts little blockade at nicotinic receptors (Timberlake et al. 1961). Trihexyphenidyl and all drugs in this class are referred to as anticholinergic, antimuscarinic, or atropine-like drugs. As a tertiary amine, it readily crosses the blood–brain barrier (Brown and Taylor 1996).

Pharmacological Profile

The pharmacological properties of trihexyphenidyl are qualitatively similar to those of atropine and other anticholinergic drugs, although trihexyphenidyl acts primarily centrally, with few peripheral effects and little sedation. In the eye, anticholinergic drugs block both the sphincter muscle of the iris, causing the pupil to dilate (mydriasis), and the ciliary muscle of the lens, preventing accommodation and causing cycloplegia. In the heart, anticholinergic drugs usually produce a mild tachycardia through vagal blockade at the sinoatrial node pacemaker, although a mild slowing can occur. In the gastrointestinal tract, anticholinergic drugs reduce gut motility and salivary and gastric secretions. Salivary secretion is particularly sensitive and can be completely abolished. In the respiratory system, anticholinergic agents reduce secretions and can produce mild bronchodilatation. Anticholinergics inhibit the activity of sweat glands and mildly decrease contractions in the urinary and biliary tracts (Brown and Taylor 1996).

Pharmacokinetics and Disposition

Peak concentration for trihexyphenidyl is reached 1–2 hours after oral administration, and its half-life is 10–12 hours (Cedarbaum and McDowell 1987). As a tertiary amine, it crosses the blood–brain barrier to enter the CNS.

Mechanism of Action

The presumed mechanism of action of trihexyphenidyl for treatment of EPS is the blockade of intrastriatal cholinergic activity, which is relatively increased, compared with nigrostriatal dopaminergic activity, which has become decreased by antipsychotic blockade. The blockade of cholinergic activity returns the system to its previous equilibrium.

Indications and Efficacy

Anticholinergic agents were reported to have been effective treatment for NIP from open empirical trials (Medina et al. 1962; Rashkis and Smarr 1957). Eventually, controlled trials were conducted, with most involving comparisons only with different anticholinergics and not with placebo. Despite the limited evidence of efficacy against placebo, anticholinergic agents became the mainstay of treatment for NIP, and they remain so today.

Trihexyphenidyl has U.S. Food and Drug Administration (FDA) approval for treatment of all forms of parkinsonism, including NIP. Daily doses of 5–30 mg have been used in studies of trihexyphenidyl in the treatment of Parkinson's disease and NIP. Much higher dosages (up to

TABLE 34–1. Pharmacological agents for the treatment of neuroleptic-induced parkinsonism and acute dystonic reactions

COMPOUND	RELATIVE EQUIVALENCE (MG)[a]	ROUTE	AVAILABILITY	DOSING	DOSAGE RANGE (MG/DAY)
Anticholinergic					
Trihexyphenidyl	2	Oral	Tablets: 2, 5 mg Elixir: 2 mg/mL Sequels: 5 mg (sustained release)	qd–bid	2–30
Benztropine (Cogentin)	1	Oral Injectable	Tablets: 0.5, 1, 2 mg Ampules: 1 mg/mL (2 mL)	qd–bid Every 30 minutes (until symptom relief)	1–12 2–8
Biperiden (Akineton)[b]	2	Oral Injectable	Tablets: 2 mg Ampules: 5 mg/mL (1 mL)[b]	qd–tid Every 30 minutes (until symptom relief)	2–24 2–8
Procyclidine (Kemadrin)	2	Oral	Tablets: 5 mg (scored)	bid–tid	5–20
Antihistaminic					
Diphenhydramine (Benadryl)	50	Oral Injectable	Tablets: 25, 50 mg Ampules: 50 mg/mL (1 mL, 10 mL) Syringe (prefilled): 1 mL	bid–qd	50–200
Dopaminergic					
Amantadine (Symmetrel)	N/A	Oral	Tablets: 100 mg Syrup: 50 mg/5 mL	qd–bid	100–300

Note. N/A=not applicable; qd=once daily; bid=twice daily; tid=three times daily.
[a]Adapted from Klett and Caffey 1972.
[b]No longer available as an injectable in the United States.

75 mg/day) have been used for the treatment of primary dystonia. However, the benefits of high doses have been limited by the adverse effects on cognition and memory (Jabbari et al. 1989; Taylor et al. 1991). Side effects correlate with blood levels, but efficacy does not (Burke and Fahn 1985). The individual therapeutic dose must be determined empirically and can vary widely.

Side Effects and Toxicology

Peripheral side effects. The peripheral side effects of trihexyphenidyl result from parasympathetic muscarinic blockade, and they occur in a consistent hierarchy among different organs. They are qualitatively similar to the side effects of atropine and other anticholinergic drugs, but they are quantitatively less because of the reduced peripheral activity of trihexyphenidyl (Brown 1990).

Anticholinergic drugs initially depress salivary and bronchial secretions and sweat production. Reduced salivation produces dry mouth and contributes to the high incidence of dental caries among patients with chronic psychi-

atric problems (Winer and Bahn 1967). Treatment for this condition is unsatisfactory, and chewing sugar-free gum or sucking on hard candy is limited by the need for constant use. Reduced sweating can contribute to heat prostration and heat stroke, particularly in warmer ambient temperatures. The next physiological effects occur in the eyes and heart. Pupillary dilatation and inhibition of accommodation in the eye lead to photophobia and blurred vision. Attacks of acute glaucoma can occur in susceptible subjects with narrow-angle glaucoma, although this is relatively uncommon. Vagus nerve blockade leads to increased heart rate and is more apparent in patients with high vagal tone (usually younger males). The next effects are inhibition of urinary bladder function and bowel motility, which can produce urinary retention, constipation, and obstipation. Sufficiently high doses of anticholinergics will inhibit gastric secretion and motility (Brown and Taylor 1996).

Central side effects. Memory disturbance is the most common central side effect of anticholinergic medications because memory is dependent on the cholinergic system (Drachman 1977). Patients with underlying brain pathology are more susceptible to memory disturbance (Fayen et al. 1988). Patients with chronic psychiatric conditions often have a decreased ability to express themselves, making evaluation of memory more difficult; therefore, subtle memory changes can be missed or attributed to the underlying illness. Memory disturbances have been identified in patients with Parkinson's disease treated with anticholinergics (Yahr and Duvoisin 1968), even in some patients receiving only small doses (Stephens 1967). Patients receiving an antipsychotic and benztropine demonstrated significantly increased overall scores on the Wechsler Memory Scale when benztropine was withdrawn (Baker et al. 1983).

Anticholinergic toxicity produces restlessness, irritability, disorientation, hallucinations, and delirium. Elderly patients are at increased risk for both memory loss and toxic delirium, even at very low anticholinergic doses, because of the natural loss of cholinergic neurons with aging (Perry et al. 1977). Toxic doses can produce a clinical situation identical to atropine poisoning, including fixed dilated pupils, flushed face, sinus tachycardia, urinary retention, dry mouth, and fever. This condition can proceed to coma, cardiorespiratory collapse, and death.

Drug–Drug Interactions

There may be increased anticholinergic effects, including side effects, when trihexyphenidyl or any anticholinergic is combined with amantadine. Anticholinergic side effects are also much more likely to occur when drugs with anticholinergic properties are combined.

Anticholinergic effect on antipsychotic blood levels. Some investigators have suggested that anticholinergic medications can affect antipsychotic blood levels. However, a review of this subject suggests that the available data are too limited to reach a definite conclusion on this matter. The best studies indicate that anticholinergic drugs do not affect antipsychotic blood levels or, at most, that they lower these levels only transiently (McEvoy 1983).

Anticholinergic effect on antipsychotic activity. Haase and Janssen (1965) reported from open studies that when anticholinergic drugs are added to antipsychotic drugs given at the neuroleptic threshold, rigidity, hypokinesia, and therapeutic effects disappear but psychopathology worsens. Other studies have demonstrated no change or an improvement in scores of psychopathology, with the addition of anticholinergics (Hanlon et al. 1966; G.M. Simpson et al. 1980).

Anticholinergic Abuse

Anticholinergic drugs may be abused for their euphoriant and hallucinogenic effects, and they may be combined with street drugs for enhanced effect (Crawshaw and Mullen 1984). Patients with a history of substance abuse are more likely to abuse anticholinergics (Wells et al. 1989). Cases of abuse have been reported with all anticholinergics, but trihexyphenidyl apparently is the anticholinergic most likely to be abused (MacVicar 1977). Theoretically, one anticholinergic should be as effective as another, although an idiosyncratic response is possible. The potential for abuse needs to be considered, particularly in patients with a history of substance abuse.

Benztropine

History and Discovery

Benztropine was synthesized by uniting the tropine portion of atropine with the benzhydryl portion of diphenhydramine hydrochloride. Benztropine was found to be effective in the treatment of 302 patients with Parkinson's disease (Doshay 1956). The best results in the control of rigidity, contracture, and tremor were obtained at doses of 1–4 mg qd for older patients and 2–8 mg qd for younger ones. Doses of 15–30 mg qd caused excessive flaccidity in some patients, who became unable to lift their arms or raise their heads off the bed. Subsequently, benztropine was found to be effective for the treatment of NIP (Karn and Kasper 1959).

Structure–Activity Relations

Benztropine is a tertiary amine with activity similar to that of trihexyphenidyl, and as a tertiary amine, it enters the CNS.

Pharmacological Profile

Benztropine has the pharmacological properties of an anticholinergic and an antihistaminic; however, it produces less sedation (in experimental animals) than does diphenhydramine.

Pharmacokinetics and Disposition

Little is known about the pharmacokinetics of benztropine. A correlation between serum anticholinergic levels and the presence of EPS has been demonstrated (Tune and Coyle 1980). There is little correlation between the total daily dose of benztropine and the serum anticholinergic level, with the serum activity for a given dose varying 100-fold between subjects. When treated with increased doses of anticholinergics, patients with EPS demonstrated increased serum anticholinergic activity and decreased EPS. Relatively small increments in the oral dose of an anticholinergic drug can result in significant nonlinear increases in serum anticholinergic activity levels. Benztropine has a long-acting effect and can be given once or twice a day.

Indications and Efficacy

Benztropine has FDA approval for the treatment of all forms of parkinsonism, including NIP. Total daily doses of 1–8 mg have generally been used to treat NIP.

Mechanism of Action, Side Effects, and Drug–Drug Interactions

The mechanisms of action and the drug interactions for benztropine are similar to those of trihexyphenidyl. The side effects of these two drugs are also similar, but the degree of sedation produced by benztropine may be less (Doshay 1956). Although not yet confirmed in double-blind studies, this reported difference in sedation might account for the fact that trihexyphenidyl is reportedly the anticholinergic drug more likely to be abused.

Biperiden

Biperiden is an analogue of trihexyphenidyl that has greater peripheral anticholinergic activity than trihexyphenidyl and greater activity against nicotinic receptors (Timberlake et al. 1961). Biperiden is well absorbed from the gastrointestinal tract. Its metabolism, though not completely understood, involves hydroxylation in the liver. Its activity, pharmacological profile, and side effects are similar to those of other anticholinergics. It has FDA approval for use in the treatment of all forms of parkinsonism, including NIP. Total daily doses of 2–24 mg have been used in studies of biperiden for the treatment of parkinsonism and NIP.

Procyclidine

Procyclidine is an analogue of trihexyphenidyl (Schwab and Chafetz 1955). Its activity, pharmacology, and side effects are similar to those of other anticholinergics. There is little information about its pharmacokinetics. Procyclidine has FDA approval for use in treating all forms of parkinsonism, including NIP. Total daily doses of 5–30 mg have been used in studies of procyclidine for the treatment of parkinsonism and NIP.

Antihistaminic Medications

Diphenhydramine

History and Discovery

Antihistaminic agents have been used for the treatment of Parkinson's disease. Diphenhydramine, one of the first antihistamines developed and used clinically (Bovet 1950), has been the primary antihistamine studied in the treatment of EPS. Although some antihistamines may be effective, other antihistamines have not been systematically studied for the treatment of EPS.

Structure–Activity Relations

All drugs referred to as antihistamines are reversible competitive inhibitors of histamine at the H_1 receptor. Some antihistamines also inhibit the action of acetylcholine at the muscarinic receptor. It is believed that central muscarinic blockade, rather than histaminic blockade, is responsible for the therapeutic effect of antihistamines for EPS. Ethanolamine antihistamines (diphenhydramine, dimenhydrinate, and carbinoxamine maleate) have the greatest anticholinergic activity, and ethylenediamine antihistamines have the least anticholinergic activity. Antihistamines such as terfenadine and astemizole have no anticholinergic activity, while many of the remaining antihistamines have very mild anticholinergic activity (Babe and Serafin 1996).

Pharmacological Profile

Antihistamines inhibit the constrictor action of histamine on respiratory smooth muscle. They restrict the vasoconstrictor and vasodilatory effects of histamine on vascular smooth muscle and block histamine-induced capillary permeability. Antihistamines with CNS activity are depressants, producing diminished alertness, slowed reaction times, and somnolence. They can also block motion sickness. Antihistaminic drugs with anticholinergic activity also possess mild antimuscarinic pharmacological properties similar to those of other atropine-like drugs (Babe and Serafin 1996).

Pharmacokinetics and Disposition

Diphenhydramine is well absorbed from the gastrointestinal tract. Peak concentrations occur 2–3 hours after oral administration. Its therapeutic effects usually last 4–6 hours, and it has a half-life of 3–9 hours. Diphenhydramine is widely distributed throughout the body, and as a tertiary amine, it enters the CNS. Age does not affect its pharmacokinetics. It undergoes demethylations in the liver and is then oxidized to carboxylic acid (Paton and Webster 1985).

Mechanism of Action

Diphenhydramine possesses some anticholinergic activity, which is believed to be the basis for its effect in diminishing EPS.

Indications and Efficacy

Diphenhydramine has FDA approval for parkinsonism, including NIP, in the elderly and for mild cases in other age groups. It is probably not as efficacious for treating EPS as are pure anticholinergic drugs, but it may be better tolerated in patients bothered by anticholinergic side effects, such as geriatric patients. Diphenhydramine also tends to be more sedating than anticholinergics, which can also be beneficial for some patients. The dosage generally ranges from 50 to 400 mg/day, given in divided doses.

Diphenhydramine also has indications for multiple other conditions that are unrelated to EPS.

Side Effects and Toxicology

The primary side effect of diphenhydramine is sedation. Although other antihistamines may cause gastrointestinal distress, diphenhydramine has a low incidence of such an effect. Drying of the mouth and respiratory passages can occur. In general, the toxic effects are similar to those of trihexyphenidyl and of other anticholinergics.

Drug–Drug Interactions

Diphenhydramine has no reported interactions with other drugs, but it has an additive depressant effect when used in combination with alcohol or with other CNS depressants.

Dopaminergic Medications

Amantadine

History and Discovery

Anticholinergic side effects and inadequate treatment response eventually led to the investigation of other agents to treat EPS. Initially, both methylphenidate and intravenous caffeine were investigated as treatments for NIP.

Neither agent achieved general use, despite apparent efficacy (Brooks 1956; Freyhan 1959).

Amantadine is an antiviral agent that is effective against A2 (Asian) influenza (Wingfield et al. 1969). It was unexpectedly found to produce symptomatic improvement in patients with Parkinson's disease (Parkes et al. 1970; Schwab et al. 1969), and soon thereafter, it was reported to be effective for NIP (Kelly and Abuzzahab 1971).

Structure–Activity Relations

Amantadine is a water-soluble tricyclic amine. It binds to the M2 protein, a membrane protein that functions as an ion channel on the influenza A virus (Hay 1992). Its activity in reducing EPS is not known, although it has been shown to have activity at glutamate receptors (Stoof et al. 1992).

Pharmacological Profile

Amantadine is effective in preventing and treating illness from influenza A virus. It also reduces the symptoms of parkinsonism.

Pharmacokinetics and Disposition

In young healthy subjects, amantadine is slowly and well absorbed from the gastrointestinal tract, with unchanged oral bioavailability over the dose range of 50–300 mg. It reaches steady state in 4–7 days. Plasma concentrations (0.12–1.12 µg/mL) may have some correlation with improvement in EPS (Greenblatt et al. 1977; Pacifici et al. 1976). Amantadine has relatively constant blood levels and a long duration of action (Aoki et al. 1979) and is excreted unchanged by the kidneys. Its half-life for elimination is about 16 hours, which is prolonged in elderly patients and in patients with impaired renal function (Hayden et al. 1985).

Mechanism of Action

Amantadine inhibits viral replication by binding to the M2 protein on the viral membrane and inhibiting replication (Hay 1992). Its mechanism of action as an antiparkinson agent is less clear. It has no anticholinergic activity in tests on animals, being only 1/209,000th as potent as atropine (Grelak et al. 1970). It appears to cause the release of dopamine and other catecholamines from intraneuronal storage sites in an amphetamine-like mechanism. It has also been shown to have activity at glutamate receptors, which may contribute to its antiparkinsonian effect (Stoof et al. 1992). Amantadine has preferential selectivity for central catecholamine neurons (Grelak et al. 1970; Strömberg et al. 1970).

Indications and Efficacy

Amantadine has undergone more extensive investigation than have anticholinergic agents with regard to the efficacy of EPS. Most studies, though not all, found amantadine to be equal in efficacy to benztropine or biperiden in the treatment of parkinsonism (DiMascio et al. 1976; Fann and Lake 1976; Konig et al. 1996; Silver et al. 1995; Stenson et al. 1976). Some studies found amantadine to be more effective than benztropine (Merrick and Schmitt 1973) or effective for EPS that are refractory to benztropine (Gelenberg 1978). However, other studies found that amantadine was inferior to benztropine (Kelly et al. 1974), no more effective than placebo (Mindham et al. 1972), or unable to control EPS when used to replace an anticholinergic agent (McEvoy et al. 1987). The varying results can be attributed to differing methodologies and patient populations. The conclusion that can be drawn from these studies is that amantadine is an effective drug for treating parkinsonism but that there are no clear data to support its use prior to using anticholinergic agents. Most of the studies were of short duration, and in patients with Parkinson's disease, amantadine appears to lose efficacy after several weeks (Mawdsley et al. 1972; Schwab et al. 1972). Similar studies evaluating the long-term efficacy of amantadine have not been conducted for EPS.

Amantadine has also been evaluated for the treatment of akathisia, but in only a small number of patients. The conclusion from these studies is that amantadine is probably not effective for treating akathisia (Fleischhacker et al. 1990).

Amantadine has FDA approval for the treatment of NIP and Parkinson's disease/syndrome, as well as for the treatment and prophylaxis of influenza A respiratory illness. Dosages of 100–300 mg/day are used for the treatment of NIP, and plasma concentrations may have some correlation with improvement.

Side Effects and Toxicology

At dosages of 100–300 mg/day, amantadine does not produce adverse effects as readily as do anticholinergic medications. Side effects of amantadine result from CNS stimulation, with symptoms including irritability, tremor, dysarthria, ataxia, vertigo, agitation, reduced concentration, hallucinations, and delirium (Postma and Tilburg 1975). Hallucinations are often visual. Side effects are more likely to occur in elderly patients and in patients with reduced renal function (Borison 1979; Ing et al. 1979). Toxic effects are directly related to elevated amantadine serum levels (>1.5 μg/mL). Resolution of toxic symptoms is dependent on renal clearance and may require dialysis in extreme cases, although less than 5% of amantadine is removed by dialysis.

Patients with congestive heart failure or peripheral edema should be monitored because of amantadine's ability to increase the availability of catecholamines. Long-term use of amantadine may produce livedo reticularis in the lower extremities from the local release of catecholamines and resulting vasoconstriction (Cedarbaum and Schleifer 1990). Amantadine should be used with caution in patients with seizures because of possible increased seizure activity. Amantadine is embryotoxic and teratogenic in animals, but there are no well-controlled studies in women regarding teratogenicity.

Drug–Drug Interactions

There are no reported interactions between amantadine and other drugs. There may be increased anticholinergic side effects when amantadine is used in combination with an anticholinergic agent.

β-Adrenergic Receptor Antagonists

History and Discovery

Propranolol was reported to be effective for the treatment of restless legs syndrome (Ekbom's syndrome; Ekbom 1965), which resembles the physical movements of akathisia (Strang 1967). Later it was reported to be effective in the treatment of neuroleptic-induced akathisia (Kulik and Wilbur 1983; Lipinski et al. 1983). Subsequently, other β-blockers have also been investigated for the treatment of akathisia.

Structure–Activity Relations

Competitive β-adrenergic receptor antagonism is the property common to all β-blockers. β-Blockers are distinguished by the additional properties of their relative affinity for β_1 and β_2 receptors (selectivity), lipid solubility, intrinsic β-adrenergic receptor *agonist* activity, blockade of β receptors, capacity to induce vasodilation, and general pharmacokinetic properties (Hoffman and Lefkowitz 1996). β-Blockers with high lipid solubility readily cross the blood–brain barrier.

TABLE 34–2. Beta-blockers investigated in the treatment of akathisia

COMPOUND	B₁ BLOCKADE	B₂ BLOCKADE	LIPID SOLUBILITY	EFFECTIVE FOR EPS	DOSAGE RANGE (MG/DAY)
Propranolol (Inderal)	++	++	++++	Yes	20–120
Nadolol (Corgard)	++	++	+	Yes	40–80
Metoprolol (Lopressor)	++	0 at low doses; + at high doses	++	Yes	~300
Pindolol (Visken)	++	++	++	Yes	5
Atenolol (Tenormin)	++	0	0	No	50–100
Betaxolol (Kerlone)	++	0	+++	Yes	5–20
Sotalol (Betapace, Sorine)	++	++	0	No	40–80

Note. EPS = extrapyramidal side effects.
Source. Adapted from Hoffman and Lefkowitz 1996.

Pharmacological Profile

The major pharmacological effects of β-blockers involve the cardiovascular system. β-Blockers slow the heart rate and decrease cardiac contractility; however, these effects are modest in a normal heart. In the lung, they can cause bronchospasm, although, again, there is little effect in normal lungs. They block glycogenolysis, preventing production of glucose during hypoglycemia (Hoffman and Lefkowitz 1996). β-Blockers affect lipid metabolism by preventing release of free fatty acids while elevating triglycerides (N.E. Miller 1987). In the CNS, they produce fatigue, sleep disturbance (insomnia and nightmares), and CNS depression (see Drayer 1987; Gengo et al. 1987).

Pharmacokinetics and Disposition

All β-blockers, except atenolol and nadolol, are well absorbed from the gastrointestinal tract (McDevitt 1987). All β-blockers undergo metabolism in the liver. Propranolol and metoprolol undergo significant first-pass effect, with bioavailability as low as 25%. Large interindividual variation (as much as 20-fold) leads to wide variation in clinically therapeutic doses (Hoffman and Lefkowitz 1996). Metabolites appear to have limited β-receptor antagonistic activity. The degree to which a particular β-blocker enters the CNS is related directly to its lipid solubility (Table 34–2).

Mechanism of Action

The exact mechanism of action of β-blockers in the treatment of EPS is unclear. The existence of a noradrenergic pathway from the locus coeruleus to the limbic system has been proposed as a modulator involved in symptoms of

TD, akathisia, and tremor (Wilbur et al. 1988). It appears that lipid solubility and the corresponding ability to enter the CNS are the most important factors determining the efficacy of a β-blocker in treating akathisia and perhaps other types of EPS (Adler et al. 1991).

Indications and Efficacy

β-Blockers have FDA approval primarily for cardiovascular indications, and propranolol is also indicated for familial essential tremor, but there are no FDA-approved indications for the treatment of any type of EPS.

β-Blockers have been studied primarily for the treatment of akathisia. Both nonselective (β₁ and β₂ antagonism) and selective (β₁ antagonism) β-blockers have been reported to be efficacious. The studies have generally been for short periods of time, involving small numbers of patients who were often receiving varying combinations of additional antiparkinsonian agents or benzodiazepines to which β-blockers had been added (Fleischhacker et al. 1990). From these studies, it is difficult to draw any firm conclusions, but β-blockers probably have some efficacy in the treatment of akathisia. The maximum benefit for propranolol occurred at 5 days (Fleischhacker et al. 1990). Betaxolol may be the β-blocker of choice in patients with lung disease and smokers because of its β₁ selectivity at lower dosages (5–10 mg/day).

In addition to essential tremor, β-blockers have also been reported to be beneficial for the tremor of Parkinson's disease (Foster et al. 1984) and lithium-induced tremor (Gelenberg and Jefferson 1995). However, for neuroleptic-induced tremor, propranolol was found to be not any better than placebo (Metzer et al. 1993), which could be an indication of a difference in etiologies for the different tremors.

Side Effects and Toxicology

The side effects of β-blockers result from β receptor blockade. β_2 Blockade of bronchial smooth muscle produces bronchospasm. Individuals with normal lung function are unlikely to be affected, but smokers and others with lung disease can develop serious breathing difficulties. β-Blockers can contribute to heart failure in susceptible individuals, such as those with compensated heart failure, acute myocardial infarction, or cardiomegaly. Abrupt cessation of β-blockers can also exacerbate coronary heart disease in susceptible patients, producing angina or, potentially, myocardial infarction (for details, see Hoffman and Lefkowitz 1996).

In individuals with normal heart function, bradycardia produced by β-blockers is insignificant; however, in patients with conduction defects or when combined with other drugs that impair cardiac conduction, β-blockers can contribute to serious conduction problems.

β-Blockers can block the tachycardia associated with hypoglycemia, eliminating this warning sign in patients with diabetes. β_2 Blockade also can inhibit glycogenolysis and glucose mobilization, interfering with recovery from hypoglycemia (Hoffman and Lefkowitz 1996).

β-Blockers can impair exercise performance and produce fatigue, insomnia, and major depression. However, the development of major depression probably only occurs in individuals with a predisposition to developing depression.

Drug–Drug Interactions

β-Blockers can have significant interactions with other drugs. Chlorpromazine in combination with propranolol may increase the blood levels of both drugs. Additive effects on cardiac conduction and blood pressure can occur when β-blockers are combined with drugs having similar effects (e.g., calcium channel blockers). Phenytoin, phenobarbital, and rifampin increase the clearance of propranolol. Cimetidine increases propranolol blood levels by decreasing hepatic metabolism. Theophylline clearance is reduced by propranolol. Aluminum salts (antacids), cholestyramine, and colestipol may reduce the absorption of β-blockers (Hoffman and Lefkowitz 1996).

Benzodiazepines

History and Discovery

Diazepam was initially shown to be effective in the treatment of restless legs syndrome (Ekbom's syndrome), which resembles the physical movements of akathisia (Ekbom 1965). Subsequently, diazepam, lorazepam, and clonazepam were reported to be beneficial for neuroleptic-induced akathisia (Adler et al. 1985; Donlon 1973; Kutcher et al. 1987). Clonazepam has also been reported to be beneficial for drug-induced dystonia (O'Flanagan 1975) and TD (Thaker et al. 1987).

Mechanism of Action

All benzodiazepines promote the binding of GABA to $GABA_A$ receptors, magnifying the effects of GABA. The mechanism of action regarding improvement of EPS is unknown, but it may be related to the augmentation of inhibitory GABAergic effect (Hobbs et al. 1996). For a complete discussion of the properties of benzodiazepines, see Chapter 24.

Indications and Efficacy

Benzodiazepines have FDA approval for their use in treating anxiety disorders, agoraphobia, insomnia, management of alcohol withdrawal, anesthetic premedication, seizure disorders, and skeletal muscle relaxation; however, there is no approval for its use in treating any type of EPS. As noted above, a few initial reports have indicated that benzodiazepines are beneficial for the treatment of akathisia. Other studies have also reported similar benefit (Bartels et al. 1987; Braude et al. 1983; Gagrat et al. 1978; Horiguchi and Nishimatsu 1992; Kutcher et al. 1989; Pujalte et al. 1994).

Clonazepam has also been reported to be effective in the treatment of TD (Bobruff et al. 1981; Thaker et al. 1990). Doses of 1–10 mg were used in the first study, although the optimal dosage was found to be 4 mg/day, with many patients unable to tolerate higher dosages. In the second study, dosages of 2–4.5 mg/day were used, and tolerance developed after 5–8 months.

Although some of the studies were limited by short duration and by the small number of subjects also receiving other antiparkinsonian agents, the overall conclusion was that benzodiazepines probably have some efficacy in the treatment of akathisia and TD. However, the potential problems associated with the chronic use of benzodiazepines (i.e., tolerance and abuse) need to be kept in mind.

Lorazepam (intermediate-acting) and clonazepam (long-acting) are the two primary benzodiazepines that have been studied in the treatment of EPS. Because of its long duration of action, clonazepam can often be given once a day. Lorazepam has the advantage of having no active metabolites, which eliminates potential side effects and toxicity.

Botulinum Toxin

History and Discovery

Botulinum toxin, produced by *Clostridium botulinum*, causes botulism when ingested. The first clinical use of the toxin was in the treatment of childhood strabismus (Scott 1980). The first focal dystonia treated was blepharospasm (Elston 1988). Botulinum toxin has been subsequently used to treat a number of other conditions associated with excessive muscle activity, including neuroleptic-induced dystonias (Hughes 1994).

Structure–Activity Relations

There are seven immunologically distinct botulinum toxins (L.L. Simpson 1981). Type A is the primary type used clinically (Hambleton 1992). Type F and possibly type B also have clinical utility, but they have much shorter durations of action (≤3 weeks, compared with ≥3 months for type A) (Borodic et al. 1996). The toxin is quantified by bioassay and is expressed as mouse units, which refers to the dose that is lethal to 50% of animals following intraperitoneal injection (Quinn and Hallet 1989).

Pharmacological Profile

Botulinum toxin binds to cholinergic motor nerve terminals, preventing release of acetylcholine and producing a functionally denervated muscle. The prevention of acetylcholine release occurs within a few hours, but the clinical effect does not occur for 1–3 days. The innervation gradually becomes restored, although the number and/or size of active muscle fibers is reduced (Odergren et al. 1994).

Pharmacokinetics and Disposition

After binding to the presynaptic nerve terminal, the toxin is taken into the nerve cell and is metabolized. When antibodies are present, the toxin is metabolized by immunological processes.

Mechanism of Action

Botulinum toxin acts presynaptically to prevent the release of acetylcholine at the neuromuscular junction. This produces a functional chemical denervation and paralysis of the muscle. When botulinum toxin is used clinically, the aim is to reduce the excessive muscle activity without producing significant weakness (Hughes 1994).

Indications and Efficacy

The FDA has approved the use of botulinum toxin for strabismus, blepharospasm, and other facial nerve disorders (see Jankovic and Brin 1991). Botulinum toxin has been used to treat focal neuroleptic-induced dystonias that may occur as part of TD, including laryngeal dystonia (Blitzer and Brin 1991) and refractory torticollis (Kaufman 1994). For laryngeal dystonia, the toxin is injected percutaneously through the cricothyroid membrane into the thyroarytenoid muscle bilaterally. The response rate is 80%–90%, and the effect lasts 3–4 months and sometimes longer. Botulinum treatment of tardive cervical dystonia has been found to be effective; the observed improvement is similar to the improvement seen in the treatment of idiopathic cervical dystonia, although patients with tardive cervical dystonia required higher doses (Brashear et al. 1998).

Side Effects and Toxicology

The major potential side effect of botulinum toxin is focal weakness in the muscle group injected—an effect that is usually dose dependent. This effect is generally temporary, given the mechanism of action. Transient weakness can occur through diffusion of the toxin into surrounding noninjected muscles (Hughes 1994).

Antibodies to the toxin can occur and thus can prevent a therapeutic response, particularly during subsequent treatments. The two main factors that apparently contribute to the development of antibodies are receiving a dose of the toxin for the first time at an early age and total cumulative dose (Jankovic and Schwartz 1995). Some patients with antibodies will respond to other botulinum serotypes, such as type F (Greene and Fahn 1993). Local skin reactions can also occur. Some degree of muscle atrophy is apparent in injected muscles (Hughes 1994). Reinnervation usually takes place over the course of 3–4 months (Odergren et al. 1994).

There are no known contraindications. Because the effect on the fetus is unknown, use of the toxin is not recommended during pregnancy. In conditions in which there are neuromuscular junction disorders, such as myasthenia gravis, patients could theoretically experience increased weakness. The long-term effects are unknown (Hughes 1994).

Drug–Drug Interactions

There are no known interactions of botulinum toxin with other drugs.

Vitamin E (α-Tocopherol)

History and Discovery

The existence of vitamin E was postulated in 1922, at which time it appeared that rats required an unknown dietary supplement to sustain pregnancy. That supplement, vitamin E (α-tocopherol), was eventually isolated from wheat germ oil (Evans et al. 1936). Vitamin E deficiency in animals leads to several specific diseases; however, in humans, there is little evidence of any specific metabolic effects or illnesses. Despite the paucity of evidence for its benefit, vitamin E has been used over the years to treat multiple conditions, including infertility, various menstrual disorders, neurological and muscular disorders, and anemias (Marcus and Coulston 1996).

Vitamin E was proposed as a treatment for TD after it was noted that a neurotoxin in rats induced an irreversible movement disorder and axonal damage similar to that caused by vitamin E deficiency. It was proposed that chronic neuroleptic use might produce free radicals, which would contribute to neurological damage and TD, and that the antioxidant effect of vitamin E could attenuate the damage (Cadet et al. 1986).

Pharmacological Profile

In humans, symptoms of vitamin E deficiency are not very common, and they almost always result from malabsorption (Bieri and Farrell 1976). The only consistent laboratory finding is that subjects with low serum vitamin E levels demonstrate increased hemolysis of erythrocytes exposed to oxidizing agents (Leonard and Losowsky 1967). In addition, patients with glucose-6-phosphate dehydrogenase deficiency may have improved erythrocyte survival when treated with large doses (Corash et al. 1980).

Side Effects and Toxicology

Side effects are minimal when vitamin E is given orally. High levels of vitamin E can exacerbate bleeding abnormalities that are associated with vitamin K deficiency. Dosages of up to 3,200 mg/day in studies for other conditions have been used without significant adverse effects (Kappus and Diplock 1992). The only known drug interactions are with vitamin K (when it is being given for a deficiency) and bleeding abnormalities and possibly with oral anticoagulants. High doses of vitamin E can exacerbate the coagulation abnormalities in both cases and therefore are contraindicated (Kappus and Diplock 1992).

Indications and Efficacy

The only known indication for vitamin E is treatment of vitamin E deficiency, which almost always results from malabsorption syndromes or abnormal transport, such as with abetalipoproteinemia. In most cases, other vitamins and nutrients are also deficient; therefore, symptoms may not be the result of only vitamin E deficiency. Supplementation in children has been shown to be effective for the neurological symptoms resulting from malabsorption and vitamin E deficiency in chronic cholestasis (Sokol et al. 1993). Apparently, there is also a rare condition of spinocerebellar degeneration caused by deficiency without malabsorption (Sokol 1988).

Early studies of vitamin E treatment of TD demonstrated a range of results from general benefit (Adler et al. 1993; Dabiri et al. 1994; Lohr et al. 1988) to benefit only in subjects with TD of less than 5 years' duration (Egan et al. 1992; Lohr and Caligiuri 1996) to no benefit (Schmidt et al. 1991; Shriqui et al. 1992).

Subsequently, a major prospective randomized trial treated 158 subjects with TD for up to 2 years with d-vitamin E (1,600 IU/day) or placebo (Adler et al. 1999). There were no significant effects of vitamin E on total scores or subscale scores for the AIMS, on electromechanical measures of dyskinesia, or on scores for four other scales measuring dyskinesia. The authors concluded that there was no evidence for efficacy of vitamin E in the treatment of TD (Adler et al. 1999). The use of vitamin E supplementation is not without risk. A meta-analysis of high-dosage vitamin E supplementation trials showed a statistically significant relationship between vitamin E dosage and all-cause mortality, with increased risk of dosages greater than 150 IU/day (E.R. Miller et al. 2005). Given the lack the data demonstrating consistent effectiveness for TD, we do not recommend that vitamin E be used for this purpose.

Treatment of Extrapyramidal Side Effects

Acute Dystonic Reactions

Intramuscular anticholinergics are the treatment of choice for ADRs. Benztropine 2 mg or diphenhydramine 50–100 mg generally will produce complete resolution within 20–30 minutes, with a second dose repeated after 30 minutes if there is not a complete recovery. Benztropine has been shown to resolve ADRs in less time than diphenhydramine (Lee 1979). Starting a standing dose of an antiparkinsonian agent afterward is generally not necessary. ADRs do not recur, unless large doses of high-potency antipsychotics are being used or unless the dose is increased. A more complete discussion of prophylaxis is given below.

Parkinsonism and Akathisia

The initial steps in treatment of parkinsonism (Table 34–3) and of akathisia (referred to here as EPS) are identical: evaluating the dose and type of antipsychotic. It has been shown that an increase in dose beyond the neuroleptic threshold will not produce any greater therapeutic benefit but will increase EPS (Angus and Simpson 1970a; Baldessarini et al. 1988; McEvoy et al. 1991). It has also been demonstrated that EPS frequently can be eliminated with a reduction in dosage or a change to a lower-potency antipsychotic (Braude et al. 1983; Stratas et al. 1963).

If this approach does not resolve EPS, or if a lower-potency antipsychotic cannot be substituted, the addition of an anticholinergic drug is the next step. Maximum therapeutic response occurs in 3–10 days, with more severe EPS taking a longer time to respond (DiMascio et al. 1976; Fann and Lake 1976). The anticholinergic dose should be increased until EPS are alleviated or until an unacceptable degree of anticholinergic side effects is obtained. Akathisia frequently does not respond as well to anticholinergic medications and amantadine as do parkinsonism and ADRs (DiMascio et al. 1976). Akathisia is more likely to be responsive to anticholinergic agents if symptoms of parkinsonism are also present (Fleischhacker et al. 1990).

If EPS remain uncontrolled, amantadine can be either added to the regimen or substituted as a single agent. The next step would be the addition of a benzodiazepine or a β-blocker, although there are fewer data supporting both of these treatments.

In the case of severe EPS, the antipsychotic should be temporarily stopped, because severe EPS may be a risk factor for the development of neuroleptic malignant syndrome (Levinson and Simpson 1986).

Additional drugs have been studied or suggested as treatments for akathisia. The data supporting the use of amantadine for the treatment of akathisia are limited. Clonidine has been studied in a small number of patients, but its benefit was limited by sedation and hypotension (Fleischhacker et al. 1990). Sodium valproate was reported to have had no significant effect on akathisia and was found to increase parkinsonism (Friis et al. 1983).

TABLE 34–3.   Treatment of parkinsonism

STEP	ACTION
1	Reduce dose of antipsychotic, if clinically possible.
2	Substitute a lower-potency antipsychotic, or carry out step 8.
3	Add an anticholinergic agent.
4	Titrate anticholinergic to maximum dose tolerable.
5	Add amantadine in combination with anticholinergic or as a single agent.
6	Add a benzodiazepine or a β-blocker.
7	In severe cases of EPS, stop antipsychotic temporarily and repeat process, beginning with step 3.
8	Substitute antipsychotic with atypical antipsychotic or clozapine.

Iron supplementation has been suggested as a possible treatment for akathisia (Blake et al. 1986). A review of this subject concluded that iron supplements would, at best, have no effect on akathisia but that they could potentially worsen the condition and promote further long-term damage (Gold and Lenox 1995). Iron supplementation therefore should not be considered a treatment for akathisia and should not be given indiscriminately.

Atypical Antipsychotics for Treatment of Parkinsonism and Akathisia

Patients treated with clozapine were found to have significantly less parkinsonism than patients treated with the combination of chlorpromazine and an antiparkinsonian agent (benztropine) (Kane et al. 1988). The prevalence and incidence of akathisia have also been shown to be less in patients treated with clozapine than in patients treated with typical antipsychotics (Chengappa et al. 1994; Kurz et al. 1995; Stanilla et al. 1995). Subsequently, the new atypical antipsychotics (risperidone, olanzapine, quetiapine, ziprasidone, and aripiprazole) have also been shown to produce less EPS than haloperidol. Paliperidone extended release was compared with placebo and found to have a comparable incidence of EPS.

At lower doses, risperidone usually does not produce significant parkinsonism, but unlike clozapine, it can produce significant parkinsonism at higher doses (Chouinard et al. 1993). In initial studies comparing risperidone with haloperidol, the extrapyramidal scores for patients receiving risperidone were not significantly different from the scores of patients receiving placebo at 6 mg qd. Risperidone can cause ADRs, and patients with severe EPS at baseline were more likely to develop EPS when treated with risperidone (G.M. Simpson and Lindenmayer 1997). Subsequent studies have confirmed a reduced level of EPS with risperidone, compared with haloperidol (Csernansky et al. 2002). In general, risperidone has also been shown to produce less akathisia than haloperidol (Wirshing et al. 1999).

Olanzapine has been shown to have an antipsychotic effect comparable to that of haloperidol while producing less dystonia, parkinsonism, and akathisia (Tollefson et al. 1997). The reduced incidence of EPS occurred across the entire therapeutic dosage range of 5–24 mg/day. Olanzapine has subsequently been shown to produce less parkinsonism and akathisia, compared with haloperidol, in patients with treatment-resistant schizophrenia (Breier and Hamilton 1999) and in patients with first-episode psychosis (Sanger et al. 1999). Olanzapine has also been shown to have similar rates of EPS and akathisia, compared with chlorpromazine, but without the need for any antiparkinsonian drugs (see Conley et al. 1998).

Quetiapine has been found to have antipsychotic activity comparable to haloperidol at doses ranging from 150 to 750 mg/day while producing parkinsonism at a level similar to that produced by placebo across the entire dosage range (Arvanitis and Miller 1997; Small et al. 1997). For most patients, there were no significant changes in AIMS scores at baseline and in scores at the end of a 6-week period of treatment.

A double-blind, dose-ranging trial comparing ziprasidone with haloperidol found comparable antipsychotic effect at higher dosages of ziprasidone. Concomitant benztropine use at any time during the study was less frequent with the highest dosage (160 mg/day) of ziprasidone (15%) than with haloperidol (53%) (Goff et al. 1998). Studies of ziprasidone found no significant differences in baseline-to-endpoint mean changes in Simpson-Angus Scale and AIMS scores with placebo or ziprasidone (40–160 mg/day) (Keck et al. 2001).

Aripiprazole was found to be comparable to risperidone in antipsychotic effect while producing EPS comparable to those seen with placebo (Kane et al. 2002; Potkin et al. 2003).

The most recent antipsychotic to gain FDA approval in the United States is paliperidone extended release (ER). Paliperidone ER was found to have an incidence of EPS nearly comparable to placebo (7% vs. 3%) at a dosage range of 3–15 mg/day (Kramer et al. 2007).

A study comparing 150 patients who were treated with either risperidone or olanzapine found that a statis-

tically significantly smaller percentage of patients treated with olanzapine (25.3%) required anticholinergic treatment than did patients treated with risperidone (45.3%) (Egdell et al. 2000). Another study involving 377 patients comparing risperidone with olanzapine found EPS to be similar in both groups (24% and 20%, respectively) and of low severity (Conley and Mahmoud 2001).

Comparisons between clozapine and risperidone have found a reduced incidence of EPS for clozapine (Azorin et al. 2001). A study comparing the incidence of EPS produced by clozapine, risperidone, and typical antipsychotics found a hierarchy in the production of EPS, with clozapine producing the fewest EPS, followed by risperidone and then the typical antipsychotics (C.H. Miller et al. 1998).

In general, the novel antipsychotics have a reduced incidence of EPS compared with high-potency typical antipsychotics. Data from the CATIE study suggest that the difference in incidence of EPS with an atypical antipsychotic may not be as great when compared with a moderate-potency typical antipsychotic.

The difference in the incidence of EPS between an atypical antipsychotic and a typical antipsychotic has generally involved the comparison of a high-potency typical, specifically haloperidol. Data from the CATIE studies showed that there was no clinically significant difference in the incidence of parkinsonian symptoms and akathisia between the atypical agents and a moderate-potency typical agent, perphenazine. Although a statistically significantly greater number of perphenazine-treated subjects than of atypical-treated subjects discontinued treatment because of EPS (8% vs. 2%–4%), the incidence was low and of limited clinical significance.

In the past, if a patient receiving a typical antipsychotic developed severe parkinsonism or akathisia and did not respond to antiparkinsonian treatment, the recommended strategy was to switch to an atypical antipsychotic. Now, the recommendation can be made to consider the use of a less potent typical antipsychotic as one of the options for treatment, along with possibly changing to an atypical.

For patients with severe refractory EPS who have not responded to standard treatments, the use of clozapine specifically to treat the EPS is indicated (Casey 1989). This is particularly true for akathisia, given its significant negative correlation with the outcome of schizophrenia. This is also true for patients who do not have any psychotic symptoms, if the EPS are judged to be severe enough to be disabling or potentially life-threatening, such as laryngeal dystonia.

Tardive Dyskinesia and Tardive Dystonia

Historically, TD has been refractory to treatment, which explains the large number of drugs employed in attempts to alleviate the condition. Treatments investigated have included, but are not limited to, noradrenergic antagonists (propranolol and clonidine), antagonists of dopamine and other catecholamines, dopamine agonists, catecholamine-depleting drugs (reserpine and tetrabenazine), GABAergic drugs, cholinergic drugs (deanol, choline, and lecithin), catecholaminergic drugs (Kane et al. 1992), calcium channel blockers (Cates et al. 1993), and selective monoamine oxidase inhibitors (selegiline) (Goff et al. 1993). Based on the investigations of the above drugs, the American Psychiatric Association Task Force on TD concluded that there is no consistently effective treatment for TD (Kane et al. 1992).

There are inherent difficulties in evaluating the effects of any treatment for TD. These include the variability of clinical raters (Bergen et al. 1984), placebo response (Sommer et al. 1994), and the diurnal and longitudinal variability of TD (Hyde et al. 1995; Stanilla et al. 1996). The degree of improvement needs to be greater than the sum of the above variations in order to demonstrate an actual benefit.

The first step in evaluating TD is to determine the type of antipsychotic agent that is being used. If a typical antipsychotic is necessary, it is important to use the lowest dose possible (G.M. Simpson 2000). Second, if anticholinergic antiparkinsonian medications are being used, the patient should be gradually weaned from these medications and the medications then discontinued. Anticholinergic medications will make, in contrast to their effect on other extrapyramidal movements, TD movements worse (see Greil et al. 1984; Jeste and Wyatt 1982).

Some drugs have been shown to have some benefit in the treatment of TD, but they have limitations. Clonazepam has been reported to reduce the movements of TD for up to 9 months, although tolerance to the benefits developed (Thaker et al. 1990). Additional limitations are the inherent problems associated with chronic use of a benzodiazepine. Botulinum toxin is beneficial for treating localized tardive dystonias, particularly laryngeal and cervical dystonias (Hughes 1994). The injections need to be repeated every 3–6 months, and botulinum toxin is not a general treatment for TD. Vitamin E has not consistently been shown to be beneficial in all studies, and a large long-term double-blind study found no benefit for vitamin E compared with placebo (Adler et al. 1999).

Tardive dystonia also tends to be resistant to treatment; however, unlike TD, it may respond to anticholinergic medications (Wojcik et al. 1991) and to reserpine (Kang et al. 1988).

Atypical Antipsychotics for Treatment of Tardive Dyskinesia

Clozapine has been shown to decrease the symptoms of TD (G.M. Simpson and Varga 1974; G.M. Simpson et al. 1978), with the greatest improvement occurring in cases of severe TD and tardive dystonia (Lieberman et al. 1991). These findings have been replicated and suggest that clozapine is unlikely to cause TD (Chengappa et al. 1994; Kane et al. 1993). The disadvantages to clozapine are the potential side effects of agranulocytosis and seizures and the need for regular blood monitoring.

Three possible mechanisms for clozapine's benefit have been proposed. First, clozapine may suppress TD movements in a fashion similar to that of typical antipsychotics. Second, TD may improve spontaneously, given that the typical antipsychotics are no longer present to cause or sustain TD. Such improvement occurs in some patients when antipsychotics are withdrawn. Third, clozapine may have an active therapeutic effect on TD (Lieberman et al. 1991), but the issue remains to be clarified. In some patients, TD movements have recurred on withdrawal of clozapine.

More data demonstrating the potential benefit of the other novel antipsychotics in the prevention and treatment of TD are being reported. A prospective study examined the incidence of emergent dyskinesia in middle-aged to elderly patients (mean age 66 years) being treated with haloperidol and low-dose risperidone (mean total daily dose of 1 mg). The patients treated with risperidone were significantly less likely to develop TD (Jeste et al. 1999). A double-blind prospective study comparing 397 stable patients with schizophrenia who were switched to either risperidone or haloperidol and followed for at least a year found that only 1 of the patients receiving risperidone developed dyskinetic movements, compared with 5 of the patients receiving haloperidol (Csernansky et al. 2002).

In a prospective double-blind study of patients with schizophrenia being treated with either olanzapine or haloperidol and followed for up to 2.6 years, there was a significantly decreased risk for the development of TD with olanzapine. The 1-year risk was 0.52% for olanzapine and 7.45% for haloperidol (Beasley et al. 1999).

The data regarding the effect of quetiapine, ziprasidone, aripiprazole, and paliperidone on TD are more limited; however, any drug that is less likely to produce EPS is probably less likely to produce TD.

The best treatment for TD is prevention. Of the 1,460 subjects involved in the CATIE study, D.D. Miller et al. (2005) found 212 to have probable TD by Schooler-Kane criteria. They found that subjects with TD were older, had a longer duration of receiving antipsychotic medications, and were more likely to have been receiving a conventional antipsychotic and an anticholinergic agent. They also found that substance abuse significantly predicted TD, as well as subjects with higher ratings of psychopathology, parkinsonian symptoms, and akathisia (D.D. Miller et al. 2005).

Patients with TD who are taking typical antipsychotics are candidates for switching to an atypical antipsychotic. In the case of severe TD or dystonia that has been unresponsive to other treatment, the use of clozapine is indicated (G.M. Simpson 2000).

Prophylaxis of Extrapyramidal Side Effects

Prophylactic use of antiparkinsonian agents to prevent EPS is a common, but not completely accepted, practice. Most controlled prospective studies regarding prophylactic use of antiparkinsonian medication have shown that prophylaxis can be beneficial for certain patients who are at high risk but that it is *not* beneficial in routine use across all patient groups (Hanlon et al. 1966; Sramek et al. 1986). Studies that have demonstrated a greater general benefit across all groups have involved the use of very high doses of antipsychotics. Several retrospective studies have also demonstrated that there is a limited need for prophylaxis of EPS (Swett et al. 1977). The retrospective studies that demonstrated a greater benefit from prophylaxis also involved the use of high antipsychotic dosages (Keepers et al. 1983; Stern and Anderson 1979). The prophylactic use of antiparkinsonian medication is not routinely indicated for all patients but should be reserved for those patients at high risk of developing ADRs.

The risk factors for developing ADRs include younger age (<35 years), higher doses of antipsychotic, higher potency of antipsychotic, intramuscular route of delivery, (possibly) male gender (Sramek et al. 1986), and history of ADRs from a similar antipsychotic (Keepers and Casey 1991). The use of cocaine has been suggested as a possible risk factor (van Harten et al. 1998; see Table 34–4 for summary).

Dosages that have been used for prophylaxis are 1–4 mg/day for benztropine, 5–15 mg/day for trihexyphenidyl, and 75–150 mg/day for diphenhydramine, although the dose required to achieve prophylaxis is highly variable for each individual and can only be determined by trial and

TABLE 34–4. Risk factors leading to acute dystonic reactions

High-potency neuroleptics
  Haloperidol
  Fluphenazine
  Trifluoperazine
High dose
Younger age (<35 years of age)[a]
Intramuscular route of delivery
Previous dystonic reaction to similar neuroleptic and dose
Male sex?

[a]Approaches 100% at ages <20 years

error (Moleman et al. 1982; Sramek et al. 1986). Serious anticholinergic side effects, such as acute urinary retention or paralytic ileus, can occur even in a young patient; therefore, high doses of anticholinergics cannot be used with impunity, even for short periods.

Prophylactic anticholinergics for ADRs need only be used for a limited time because 85%–90% of ADRs occur within the first 4 days of treatment, and the incidence drops to nearly zero after 10 days (Keepers et al. 1983; Singh et al. 1990; Sramek et al. 1986). After 10 days, anticholinergics can be weaned slowly while the patient is being observed for development of parkinsonism or akathisia.

Depot Antipsychotics

In patients receiving depot antipsychotics, prophylactic anticholinergics also only need to be used for patients at high risk of developing ADRs (Idzorek 1976). However, the onset and characterization of EPS may be different in people receiving depot antipsychotics, including more bizarre dystonic reactions (G.M. Simpson 1970). The buildup of antipsychotic levels with depot antipsychotics can lead to the development of EPS at later stages of treatment; therefore, an ongoing evaluation is necessary. Some patients receiving fluphenazine decanoate were found to experience EPS only between days 3 and 10 following injection (McClelland et al. 1974).

Duration of Treatment

Withdrawal Studies

Studies investigating the withdrawal of antiparkinsonian agents have demonstrated that not all subjects redevelop EPS, a serendipitous finding noted when only 20% of patients withdrawn from benztropine in preparation for a trial of a new antiparkinsonian agent developed recurrent parkinsonian symptoms. This led to the suggestion that antiparkinsonian agents should be withdrawn after 2 months and that their use should only be resumed in patients who develop EPS again (Cahan and Parrish 1960).

Subsequently, other withdrawal studies have been conducted that revealed wide-ranging rates of EPS recurrence. Differences in rates of recurrence are related to the varying methodologies involved in the studies, including methods of rating and the initial reason for treatment with anticholinergics—prophylaxis or active treatment (Ananth et al. 1970). The types, dosages, and combinations of antipsychotics used—the same factors that contribute to the initial development of EPS—have also been major factors in determining reoccurrence rates (Baker et al. 1983; McClelland et al. 1974). In addition, there are inherent difficulties in evaluating EPS, including the role of psychological factors and placebo effect (Ekdawi and Fowke 1966; G.M. Simpson et al. 1972; St. Jean et al. 1964).

Almost all anticholinergic withdrawal studies have involved abrupt withdrawal of the anticholinergic medications. Abrupt, compared with gradual, withdrawal is more likely to result in a return of EPS. Gradual withdrawal studies have demonstrated that a large percentage (up to 90%) of patients can be completely withdrawn from anticholinergic medications without developing EPS, while the remaining patients can have their EPS controlled with a considerably reduced dose (Double et al. 1993; Ungvari et al. 1999).

Withdrawal Syndrome

Almost all anticholinergic withdrawal studies have involved abrupt withdrawal of the anticholinergic medications. Specific studies to evaluate the effect of cholinergic sensitization by anticholinergic agents on the subsequent development of EPS following withdrawal of the anticholinergic agent have not been done. There is evidence that sensitization can take place and contribute to EPS and other symptoms. Some patients with no symptoms of EPS prior to treatment with anticholinergics did develop EPS on withdrawal of the anticholinergics (Klett and Caffey 1972; G.M. Simpson et al. 1965). Withdrawal symptoms of nausea, vomiting, diaphoresis, sebaceous secretion, and restlessness can occur following withdrawal of any psychotropic with anticholinergic properties (Luchins et al. 1980). These symptoms are most likely the result of cholinergic rebound and perhaps sensitization following removal of the cholinergic blockade of the drug (G.M.

Simpson et al. 1965). Abrupt clozapine withdrawal can produce agitation, delirium, and severe choreoathetoid movements, which are also probably the result of cholinergic rebound related to the very high antimuscarinic activity of clozapine (Stanilla et al. 1997).

The potential for cholinergic sensitization with the use of anticholinergic agents is significant because EPS following withdrawal may initially be more severe but may diminish over time without treatment. Potential cholinergic sensitization leading to subsequent EPS is also a reason for limiting the routine use of prophylactic anticholinergic agents.

The conclusion that can be drawn from the withdrawal studies is that patients are more likely to develop EPS on withdrawal of antiparkinsonian agents if the risk factors for developing EPS are present. If these risk factors are minimized, the rate of EPS recurrence is lowered.

In patients who experience a reoccurrence of EPS, the EPS generally reappear within 2 weeks and control is easily reestablished (Klett and Caffey 1972). Patients respond rapidly and often require smaller doses of antiparkinsonian medications for control while continuing to take the same dose of antipsychotic (McClelland et al. 1974).

It needs to be emphasized that the withdrawal of antiparkinsonian agents should be conducted slowly and gradually over weeks or months, not abruptly, as was done in the reported studies. Patients should be evaluated for recurrence of EPS following a partial dose reduction of the antiparkinsonian agent. This process should be continued until the antiparkinsonian agent is completely withdrawn or until the lowest dose for maintenance control is achieved.

Conclusion

The unique properties of chlorpromazine and other similarly active agents in ameliorating psychotic symptoms and producing parkinsonian side effects were described in the early 1950s by French psychiatrists. Theories soon arose regarding the relationship between these two properties. The recognition of the benefits of reducing Parkinson-like side effects led to investigations of methods to reduce EPS and to the development of instruments to measure EPS. The debate regarding the routine and prophylactic use of antiparkinsonian agents has continued since that time. It appears that prophylactic antiparkinsonian agents need to be used in some situations, but probably less frequently and for briefer periods of time than has generally been the practice. The trend toward the use of lower dosages of antipsychotics should also lead to a decreased need for the use of antiparkinsonian agents. Finally, the advent of atypical antipsychotic agents has opened a new chapter in both the treatment and prevention of EPS and suggests that, in the future, EPS will be less of a problem than they have been in the past.

A summary of an American Psychiatric Association Task Force report on TD suggested that "[a] deliberate and sustained effort must be made to maintain patients on the lowest effective amount of drug and to keep the treatment regimen as simple as possible" (Baldessarini et al. 1980, p. 1168) and to discontinue anticholinergic drugs as soon as possible. Apart from a greater emphasis on avoiding the initial use of antiparkinsonian agents, this statement remains valid.

References

Adler L, Angrist B, Peselow E, et al: Efficacy of propranolol in neuroleptic-induced akathisia. J Clin Psychopharmacol 5:164–166, 1985

Adler LA, Angrist B, Weinreb H, et al: Studies on the time course and efficacy of β-blockers in neuroleptic-induced akathisia and the akathisia of idiopathic Parkinson's disease. Psychopharmacol Bull 27:107–111, 1991

Adler LA, Peselow E, Rotrosen J, et al: Vitamin E treatment of tardive dyskinesia. Am J Psychiatry 150:1405–1407, 1993

Adler LA, Rotrosen J, Edson R, et al: Vitamin E treatment for tardive dyskinesia. Veterans Affairs Cooperative Study #394 Study Group. Arch Gen Psychiatry 56:836–841, 1999

Ananth JV, Horodesky S, Lehmann HE, et al: Effect of withdrawal of antiparkinsonian medication on chronically hospitalized psychiatric patients. Laval Med 41:934–938, 1970

Angus JWS, Simpson GM: Handwriting changes and response to drugs—a controlled study. Acta Psychiatr Scand Suppl 21:28–37, 1970a

Angus JWS, Simpson GM: Hysteria and drug-induced dystonia. Acta Psychiatr Scand Suppl 21:52–58, 1970b

Aoki FY, Sitar DS, Ogilvie RI: Amantadine kinetics in healthy young subjects after long-term dosing. Clin Pharmacol Ther 26:729–736, 1979

Arvanitis LA, Miller BG: Multiple fixed doses of "Seroquel" (quetiapine) in patients with acute exacerbation of schizophrenia: a comparison with haloperidol and placebo. The Seroquel Trial 13 Study Group. Biol Psychiatry 42:233–246, 1997

Ayd FJ: A survey of drug-induced extrapyramidal reactions. JAMA 175:1054–1060, 1961

Azorin JM, Spiegel R, Remington G, et al: A double-blind comparative study of clozapine and risperidone in the management of severe chronic schizophrenia. Am J Psychiatry 158:1305–1313, 2001

Babe KS, Serafin WE: Histamine, bradykinin, and their antagonists, in Goodman and Gilman's The Pharmacological Basis of Therapeutics, 9th Edition. Edited by Hardman JG, Limbird LE, Molinoff PB, et al. New York, McGraw-Hill, 1996, pp 581–600

Baker LA, Cheng LY, Amara IB: The withdrawal of benztropine mesylate in chronic schizophrenic patients. Br J Psychiatry 143:584–590, 1983

Baldessarini RJ, Cole JO, Davis JM, et al: Tardive dyskinesia: summary of a task force report of the American Psychiatric Association. Am J Psychiatry 137:1163–1172, 1980

Baldessarini RJ, Cohen BM, Teicher MH: Significance of neuroleptic dose and plasma level in the pharmacological treatment of psychoses. Arch Gen Psychiatry 45:79–91, 1988

Baldessarini RJ, Huston-Lyons D, Campbell A, et al: Do central antiadrenergic actions contribute to the atypical properties of clozapine? Br J Psychiatry 160 (suppl 17):12–16, 1992

Barnes TRE: A rating scale for drug-induced akathisia. Br J Psychiatry 1564:672–676, 1989

Barnes TR: Movement disorder associated with antipsychotic drugs: the tardive syndromes. Int Rev Psychiatry 2:355–366, 1990

Bartels M, Heide K, Mann K, et al: Treatment of akathisia with lorazepam: an open clinical trial. Pharmacopsychiatry 20:51–53, 1987

Beasley CM, Dellva MA, Tamura RN, et al: Randomised double-blind comparison of the incidence of tardive dyskinesia in patients with schizophrenia during long-term treatment with olanzapine or haloperidol. Br J Psychiatry 174:23–30, 1999

Ben-Shachar D, Youdim MB: Neuroleptic-induced dopamine receptor supersensitivity and tardive dyskinesia may involve altered brain iron metabolism (abstract). Br J Pharmacol 90 (suppl):95, 1987 (Abstract presented at the proceedings of the British Pharmacological Society, December 17–19, 1986)

Bergen JA, Griffiths DA, Rey JM, et al: Tardive dyskinesia: fluctuating patient or fluctuating rater. Br J Psychiatry 144:498–502, 1984

Bieri JG, Farrell PM: Vitamin E. Vitam Horm 34:31–75, 1976

Blake DR, William AC, Pall H, et al: Iron and akathisia (letter). BMJ 292:1393, 1986

Blitzer A, Brin MF: Laryngeal dystonia: a series with botulinum toxin therapy. Ann Otol Rhinol Laryngol 100:85–89, 1991

Bobruff A, Gardos G, Tarsy D, et al: Clonazepam and phenobarbital in tardive dyskinesia. Am J Psychiatry 138:189–193, 1981

Borison RL: Amantadine-induced psychosis in a geriatric patient with renal disease. Am J Psychiatry 136:111–112, 1979

Borodic G, Johnson E, Goodnough M, et al: Botulinum toxin therapy, immunologic resistance, and problems with available materials. Neurology 46:26–29, 1996

Boumans CE, de Mooij KJ, Koch PA, et al: Is the social acceptability of psychiatric patients decreased by orofacial dyskinesia. Schizophr Bull 20:339–344, 1994

Bovet D: Introduction to antihistamine agents and antergan derivatives. Ann N Y Acad Sci 50:1089–1126, 1950

Brashear A, Ambrosius WT, Eckert GJ, et al: Comparison of treatment of tardive dystonia and idiopathic cervical dystonia with botulinum toxin type A. Mov Disord 13:158–161, 1998

Braude WM, Barnes TR, Gore SM: Clinical characteristics of akathisia: a systematic investigation of acute psychiatric inpatient admissions. Br J Psychiatry 143:139–150, 1983

Breier A, Hamilton SH: Comparative efficacy of olanzapine and haloperidol for patients with treatment-resistant schizophrenia (comment appears in Biol Psychiatry 45:383–384, 1999). Biol Psychiatry 45:403–411, 1999

Brooks GW: Experience with use of chlorpromazine and reserpine in psychiatry with special reference to the significance and management of extrapyramidal dysfunction. N Engl J Med 254:1119–1123, 1956

Brown JH: Atropine, scopolamine, and related antimuscarinic drugs, in Goodman and Gilman's The Pharmacological Basis of Therapeutics, 8th Edition. Edited by Gilman AG, Rall TW, Nies AS, et al. New York, Pergamon, 1990, pp 150–165

Brown JH, Taylor P: Muscarinic receptor agonists and antagonists, in Goodman and Gilman's The Pharmacological Basis of Therapeutics, 9th Edition. Edited by Hardman JG, Limbird LE, Molinoff PB, et al. New York, McGraw-Hill, 1996, pp 141–160

Büchel C, de Leon J, Simpson GM, et al: Oral tardive dyskinesia: validation of a measuring device using digital image processing. Psychopharmacology (Berl) 117:162–165, 1995

Burke RE, Fahn S: Serum trihexyphenidyl levels in the treatment of torsion dystonia. Neurology 35:1066–1069, 1985

Burke RE, Fahn S, Jankovic J, et al: Tardive dystonia: late-onset and persistent dystonia caused by antipsychotic drugs. Neurology 32:1335–1346, 1982

Cadet JL, Lohr J, Jeste D: Free radicals and tardive dyskinesia (letter). Trends Neurosci 9:107–108, 1986

Cahan RB, Parrish DD: Reversibility of drug-induced parkinsonism. Am J Psychiatry 116:1022–1023, 1960

Caligiuri MP, Lohr JB, Jeste DV: Parkinsonism in neuroleptic-naive schizophrenic patients. Am J Psychiatry 150:1343–1348, 1993

Casey DE: Clozapine: neuroleptic-induced EPS and tardive dyskinesia. Psychopharmacology (Berl) 99:S47-S53, 1989

Casey DE, Gerlach J, Christensson E: Dopamine, acetylcholine, and GABA effects in acute dystonia in primates. Psychopharmacologia 70:83–87, 1980

Cates M, Lusk K, Wells BG: Are calcium-channel blockers effective in the treatment of tardive dyskinesia? Ann Pharmacother 27:191–196, 1993

Cedarbaum JM, McDowell FH: Sixteen-year follow-up of 100 patients begun on levodopa in 1968: emerging problems, in Advances in Neurology, Vol 45: Parkinson's Disease. Edited by Yahr MD, Bergmann KJ. New York, Raven, 1987, pp 469–472

Cedarbaum JM, Schleifer LS: Drugs for Parkinson's disease, spasticity, and acute muscle spasms, in Goodman and Gilman's The Pharmacological Basis of Therapeutics, 8th Edition. Edited by Gilman AG, Rall TW, Nies AS, et al. New York, Pergamon, 1990, pp 463–484

Chatterjee A, Chakos M, Koreen A, et al: Prevalence and clinical correlates of extrapyramidal signs and spontaneous dyskinesia in never-medicated schizophrenic patients. Am J Psychiatry 152:1724–1729, 1995

Chengappa KN, Shelton MD, Baker RW, et al: The prevalence of akathisia in patients receiving stable doses of clozapine. J Clin Psychiatry 55:142–145, 1994

Chien CP, DiMascio A: Drug-induced extrapyramidal symptoms and their relations to clinical efficacy. Am J Psychiatry 123:1490–1498, 1967

Chouinard G, Ross-Chouinard A, Annable L, et al: Extrapyramidal symptom rating scale. Poster presented at the annual meeting of the Canadian College of Neuropsychopharmacology, Edmonton, AB, Canada, May 12–13, 1980. Can J Neurol Sci 7:233, 1980

Chouinard G, Jones B, Remington G, et al: A Canadian multicenter placebo-controlled study of fixed doses of risperidone and haloperidol in the treatment of chronic schizophrenic pa-

tients (erratum appears in J Clin Psychopharmacol 13:149, 1993). J Clin Psychopharmacol 13:25–40, 1993

Coffin VL, Latranyi MB, Chipkin RE: Acute extrapyramidal syndrome in Cebus monkeys: development medicated by dopamine D2 but not D1 receptors. J Pharmacol Exp Ther 249:769–774, 1989

Conley RR, Mahmoud R: A randomized double-blind study of risperidone and olanzapine in the treatment of schizophrenia or schizoaffective disorder (erratum appears in Am J Psychiatry 158:1759, 2001). Am J Psychiatry 158:765–774, 2001

Conley RR, Tamminga CA, Bartko JJ, et al: Olanzapine compared with chlorpromazine in treatment-resistant schizophrenia. Am J Psychiatry 155:914–920, 1998

Corash L, Spielberg S, Bartsocas C, et al: Reduced chronic hemolysis during high-dose vitamin E administration in Mediterranean-type glucose-6-phosphate dehydrogenase deficiency. N Engl J Med 303:416–420, 1980

Corrigan FM, van Rhijn AG, MacKay AVP, et al: Vitamin E treatment of tardive dyskinesia (letter). Am J Psychiatry 150:991–992, 1993

Côté L, Crutcher MD: The basal ganglia, in Principles of Neural Science, 3rd Edition. Edited by Kandel ER, Schwartz JH, Jessell TM. New York, Elsevier, 1991, pp 647–659

Crawshaw JA, Mullen PE: A study of benzhexol abuse. Br J Psychiatry 145:300–303, 1984

Csernansky JG, Mahmoud R, Brenner R: A comparison of risperidone and haloperidol for the prevention of relapse in patients with schizophrenia. N Engl J Med 346:16–22, 2002

Dabiri LM, Pasta D, Darby JK, et al: Effectiveness of vitamin E for treatment of long-term tardive dyskinesia. Am J Psychiatry 151:925–926, 1994

Delay J, Deniker P: Trente-huit cas de psychoses traitrées par la cure prolongée et continue de 4560 RP. Léme Congrès des Alién, et Neurol de Langue Française, Luxembourg, 21–27 juillet 1952. [Thirty-eight cases of psychoses treated with a long and continued course of 4560 RP. The Congress of the French Language for Alienists and Neurologists, Luxembourg, 21–27 July 1952.] Paris, Masson et Cie, 1952, pp 503–513

Delay J, Deniker P, Harl JM: [Therapeutic method derived from hiberno-therapy in excitation and agitation states.] Annales Medico-Psychologiques (Paris) 110:267–273, 1952

Denham J, Carrick JEL: Therapeutic importance of extrapyramidal phenomena evoked by a new phenothiazine. Am J Psychiatry 116:927–928, 1960

DiMascio A, Bernardo DL, Greenblatt DJ, et al: A controlled trial of amantadine in drug-induced extrapyramidal disorders. Arch Gen Psychiatry 33:599–602, 1976

Donlon PT: The therapeutic use of diazepam for akathisia. Psychosomatics 14:222–225, 1973

Doshay LJ: Five-year study of benztropine (Cogentin) methanesulfonate: outcome in three hundred two cases of paralysis agitans. JAMA 162:1031–1034, 1956

Doshay LJ, Constable K, Zier A: Five year follow-up of treatment with trihexyphenidyl (Artane): outcome in four hundred and eleven cases of paralysis agitans. JAMA 154:1334–1336, 1954

Double DB, Warren GC, Evans M, et al: Efficacy of maintenance use of anticholinergic agents. Acta Psychiatr Scand 88:381–384, 1993

Drachman DA: Memory and cognitive function in man: does the cholinergic system have a specific role? Neurology 27:783–790, 1977

Drayer DE: Lipophilicity, hydrophilicity, and the central nervous system side effects of beta blockers. Pharmacotherapy 7:87–91, 1987

Egan MF, Hyde TM, Albers GW, et al: Treatment of tardive dyskinesia with vitamin E. Am J Psychiatry 149:773–777, 1992

Egdell ET, Andersen SW, Johnstone BM, et al: Olanzapine versus risperidone: a prospective comparison of clinical and economic outcomes in schizophrenia. Pharmacoeconomics 18:567–579, 2000

Ekbom KA: [Restless legs]. Lakartidningen 62:2376–2378, 1965

Ekdawi MY, Fowke R: A controlled trial of anti-Parkinson drugs in drug-induced parkinsonism. Br J Psychiatry 112:633–636, 1966

el-Defrawi MH, Craig TJ: Neuroleptics, extrapyramidal symptoms, and serum calcium levels. Compr Psychiatry 25:539–545, 1984

Elkashef AM, Egan MF, Frank JA, et al: Basal ganglia iron in tardive dyskinesia: an MRI study. Biol Psychiatry 35:16–21, 1994

Elston J: Botulinum toxin treatment of blepharospasm. Adv Neurol 50:579–581, 1988

Evans HM, Emerson OH, Emerson GA: The isolation from wheat germ oil of an alcohol, α-tocopherol, having properties of vitamin E. J Biol Chem 113:329–332, 1936

Fann WE, Lake CR: Amantadine versus trihexyphenidyl in the treatment of neuroleptic-induced parkinsonism. Am J Psychiatry 133:940–943, 1976

Farde L, Nordström AL, Wiesel FA, et al: Positron emission tomographic analysis of central D1 and D2 dopamine receptor occupancy in patients treated with classical neuroleptics and clozapine: relation to extrapyramidal side effects. Arch Gen Psychiatry 49:538–544, 1992

Fayen M, Goldman MB, Moulthrop MA, et al: Differential memory function with dopaminergic versus anticholinergic treatment of drug-induced extrapyramidal symptoms. Am J Psychiatry 145:483–486, 1988

Feve A, Angelard B, Lacau St. Guily J: Laryngeal tardive dyskinesia. J Neurol 242:455–459, 1995

Fleischhacker W, Bergmann KJ, Perovich R, et al: The Hillside akathisia scale: a new rating instrument for neuroleptic-induced akathisia, parkinsonism and hyperkinesia. Psychopharmacol Bull 25:222–226, 1989

Fleischhacker WW, Roth SD, Kane JM: The pharmacologic treatment of neuroleptic-induced akathisia. J Clin Psychopharmacol 10:12–21, 1990

Flügel F: [Clinical observations on the effect of the phenothiazine derivative megaphen on psychic disorders in children.] Med Klin 48:1027–1029, 1953

Foster NL, Newman RP, LeWitt, et al: Peripheral beta-adrenergic blockade treatment of parkinsonian tremor. Ann Neurol 16:505–508, 1984

Freyhan FA: Therapeutic implications of differential effects of new phenothiazine compounds. Am J Psychiatry 115:577–585, 1959

Friis T, Christensen TR, Gerlach J: Sodium valproate and biperiden in neuroleptic-induced akathisia, parkinsonism and hyperkinesia: a double-blind crossover study with placebo. Acta Psychiatr Scand 67:178–187, 1983

Gagrat D, Hamilton J, Belmaker RH: Intravenous diazepam in the treatment of neuroleptic-induced acute dystonia and akathisia. Am J Psychiatry 135:1232–1233, 1978

Gardos G, Case DE, Cole JO, et al: Ten-year outcome of tardive dyskinesia. Am J Psychiatry 151:836–841, 1994

Gelenberg AJ: Amantadine in the treatment of benztropine refractory extrapyramidal disorders induced by antipsychotic drugs. Curr Ther Res Clin Exp 23:375–380, 1978

Gelenberg AJ, Jefferson JW: Lithium tremor. J Clin Psychiatry 56:283–287, 1995

Gengo FM, Huntoon L, McHugh WB: Lipid-soluble and water-soluble beta-blockers: comparison of the central nervous system depressant effect. Arch Intern Med 147:39–43, 1987

Gerlach J: The relationship between parkinsonism and tardive dyskinesia. Am J Psychiatry 134:781–784, 1977

Gerlach J, Hansen L: Clozapine and D1/D2 antagonism in extrapyramidal functions. Br J Psychiatry 160 (suppl 17):34–37, 1992

Gerlach J, Korsgaard S, Clemmesen P, et al: The St. Hans Rating Scale for Extrapyramidal Syndromes: reliability and validity. Acta Psychiatr Scand 87:244–252, 1993

Goff DC, Renshaw PF, Sarid-Segal O, et al: A placebo-controlled trial of selegiline (L-deprenyl) in the treatment of tardive dyskinesia. Biol Psychiatry 33:700–706, 1993

Goff DC, Posever T, Herz L, et al: An exploratory haloperidol-controlled dose-finding study of ziprasidone in hospitalized patients with schizophrenia or schizoaffective disorder. J Clin Psychopharmacol 18:296–304, 1998

Gold R, Lenox RH: Is there a rationale for iron supplementation in the treatment of akathisia? A review of the evidence. J Clin Psychiatry 56:476–483, 1995

Greenblatt DJ, DiMascio A, Harmatz JS, et al: Pharmacokinetics and clinical effects of amantadine in drug-induced extrapyramidal symptoms. J Clin Pharmacol 17:704–708, 1977

Greene PE, Fahn S: Use of botulinum toxin type F injections to treat torticollis in patients with immunity to botulinum toxin type A. Mov Disord 8:479–483, 1993

Greil W, Haag H, Rossnagl G, et al: Effect of anticholinergics on tardive dyskinesia: a controlled discontinuation study. Br J Psychiatry 145:304–310, 1984

Grelak RP, Clark R, Stump JM, et al: Amantadine-dopamine interaction: possible mode of action in parkinsonism. Science 169:203–204, 1970

Gunne LM, Häggström JE, Sjöquist B: Association with persistent neuroleptic-induced dyskinesia of regional changes in brain GABA synthesis. Nature 309:347–349, 1984

Guy W: ECDEU Assessment Manual for Psychopharmacology, Revised Edition. Washington, DC, U.S. Department of Health, Education, and Welfare, 1976

Haase HJ: [The presentation and meaning of the psychomotor Parkinson syndrome during long-term treatment with megaphen, also known as Largactil.] Nervenarzt 25:486–492, 1954

Haase HJ, Janssen PAJ: The Action of Neuroleptic Drugs. Chicago, IL, Year Book Medical, 1965

Hambleton P: Clostridium botulinum toxins: a general review of involvement in disease, structure, mode of action and preparation for clinical use. J Neurol 239:16–20, 1992

Hanlon TE, Schoenrich C, Freinek W, et al: Perphenazine–benztropine mesylate treatment of newly admitted psychiatric patients. Psychopharmacologia 9:328–339, 1966

Hay AJ: The action of amantadine against influenza A viruses: inhibition of the M2 ion channel protein. Semin Virol 3:21–30, 1992

Hayden FG, Minocha A, Spyker DA, et al: Comparative single dose pharmacokinetics of amantadine hydrochloride and rimantadine hydrochloride in young and elderly adults. Antimicrob Agents Chemother 28:216–221, 1985

Hippius H: The history of clozapine. Psychopharmacology (Berl) 99 (suppl):S3–S5, 1989

Hobbs WR, Rall TW, Verdoorn TA: Hypnotics and sedatives; ethanol, in Goodman and Gilman's The Pharmacological Basis of Therapeutics, 9th Edition. Edited by Hardman JG, Limbird LE, Molinoff PB, et al. New York, McGraw-Hill, 1996, pp 361–396

Hoffman BB, Lefkowitz RJ: Catecholamines, sympathomimetic drugs, and adrenergic receptor antagonists, in Goodman and Gilman's The Pharmacological Basis of Therapeutics, 9th Edition. Edited by Hardman JG, Limbird LE, Molinoff PB, et al. New York, McGraw-Hill, 1996, pp 199–248

Horiguchi J, Nishimatsu O: Usefulness of antiparkinsonian drugs during neuroleptic treatment and the effect of clonazepam on akathisia and parkinsonism occurred after antiparkinsonian drug withdrawal: a double-blind study. Jpn J Psychiatry Neurol 46:733–739, 1992

Hughes AJ: Botulinum toxin in clinical practice. Drugs 48:888–893, 1994

Hyde TM, Egan MF, Brown RJ, et al: Diurnal variation in tardive dyskinesia. Psychiatry Res 56:53–57, 1995

Ichikawa J, Meltzer HY: Differential effects of repeated treatment with haloperidol and clozapine on dopamine release and metabolism in the striatum and the nucleus accumbens. J Pharmacol Exp Ther 256:348–357, 1991

Idzorek S: Antiparkinsonian agents and fluphenazine decanoate. Am J Psychiatry 133:80–82, 1976

Ing TS, Daugirdas JT, Soung LS, et al: Toxic effects of amantadine in patients with renal failure. CMAJ 120:695–698, 1979

Jabbari B, Scherokman B, Gunderson CH, et al: Treatment of movement disorders with trihexyphenidyl. Mov Disord 4:202–212, 1989

Jankovic J, Brin MF: Therapeutic uses of botulinum toxin. N Engl J Med 324:1186–1194, 1991

Jankovic J, Schwartz K: Response and immunoresistance to botulinum toxin injections. Neurology 45:1743–1746, 1995

Jeste DV, Wyatt RJ: Therapeutic strategies against tardive dyskinesia. Two decades of experience. Arch Gen Psychiatry 39:803–816, 1982

Jeste DV, Lacro JP, Bailey A, et al: Lower incidence of tardive dyskinesia with risperidone compared with haloperidol in older patients. J Am Geriatr Soc 47:716–719, 1999

Kalachnik JE, Sprague RL: The Dyskinesia Identification System Condensed User Scale (DISCUS): reliability, validity, and a total score cut-off for mentally ill and mentally retarded populations. J Clin Psychol 49:177–189, 1993

Kane J, Honigfeld G, Singer J, et al: Clozapine for the treatment-resistant schizophrenic, double-blind comparison with chlorpromazine. Arch Gen Psychiatry 45:789–796, 1988

Kane JM, Jeste DV, Barnes TRE, et al: Treatment of tardive dyskinesia, in Tardive Dyskinesia: A Task Force Report of the American Psychiatric Association. Washington, DC, American Psychiatric Association, 1992, pp 103–120

Kane JM, Werner MG, Pollack S, et al: Does clozapine cause tardive dyskinesia? J Clin Psychiatry 54:327–330, 1993

Kane JM, Carson WH, Saha AR, et al: Efficacy and safety of aripiprazole and haloperidol versus placebo in patients with schizophrenia and schizoaffective disorder. J Clin Psychiatry 63:763–771, 2002

Kang UJ, Burke RE, Fahn S: Tardive dystonia. Adv Neurol 50:415–429, 1988

Kappus H, Diplock AT: Tolerance and safety of vitamin E: a toxicological position report. Free Radic Biol Med 13:55–74, 1992

Kapur S, Remington GJ: Serotonin-dopamine interaction and its relevance to schizophrenia. Am J Psychiatry 153:466–476, 1996

Kapur S, Seeman P: Does fast dissociation from the dopamine D2 receptor explain the action of the atypical antipsychotics? A new hypothesis. Am J Psychiatry 158:360–369, 2001

Karn WN, Kasper S: Pharmacologically induced Parkinsonlike signs as index of the therapeutic potential. Dis Nerv Syst 20:119–122, 1959

Kaufman DM: Use of botulinum toxin injections for spasmodic torticollis of tardive dystonia. J Neuropsychiatry Clin Neurosci 6:50–53, 1994

Keck PE Jr, Reeves KR, Harrigan EP: Ziprasidone in the short-term treatment of patients with schizoaffective disorder: results from two double-blind, placebo-controlled multicenter studies. J Clin Psychopharmacology 21:27–35, 2001

Keckich WA: Violence as a manifestation of akathisia. JAMA 240:2185, 1978

Keepers GA, Casey DE: Use of neuroleptic-induced extrapyramidal symptoms to predict future vulnerability to side effects. Am J Psychiatry 148:85–89, 1991

Keepers GA, Clappison VJ, Casey DE: Initial anticholinergic prophylaxis for neuroleptic-induced extrapyramidal syndromes. Arch Gen Psychiatry 40:1113–1117, 1983

Kelly JT, Abuzzahab FS: The antiparkinson properties of amantadine in drug-induced parkinsonism. J Clin Pharmacol 11:211–214, 1971

Kelly JT, Zimmermann RL, Abuzzahab FS Sr, et al: A double-blind study of amantadine hydrochloride versus benztropine mesylate in drug-induced parkinsonism. Pharmacology 12:65–73, 1974

Khan R, Jampala VC, Dong K, et al: Speech abnormalities in tardive dyskinesia. Am J Psychiatry 151:760–762, 1994

Klett CJ, Caffey E: Evaluating the long-term need for antiparkinsonian drugs by chronic schizophrenics. Arch Gen Psychiatry 26:374–379, 1972

Koek RJ, Pi EH: Acute laryngeal dystonic reactions to neuroleptics. Psychosomatics 30:359–364, 1989

Konig P, Chwatal K, Havelec L, et al: Amantadine versus biperiden: a double-blind study of treatment efficacy in neuroleptic extrapyramidal movement disorders. Neuropsychobiology 33:80–84, 1996

Kramer M, Simpson, GM, Maciulis V, et al: Paliperidone extended-release tablets for prevention of symptom recurrence in patients with schizophrenia: a randomized, double-blind, placebo-controlled study. J Clin Psychopharmacol 27:6–14, 2007

Kulik AV, Wilbur R: Case report of propranolol (Inderal) pharmacotherapy for neuroleptic-induced akathisia and tremor. Prog Neuropsychopharmacol Biol Psychiatry 7:223–225, 1983

Kuny S, Binswanger U: Neuroleptic-induced extrapyramidal symptoms and serum calcium levels. Pharmacopsychiatry 21:67–70, 1989

Kurz M, Hummer M, Oberbauer H, et al: Extrapyramidal side effects of clozapine and haloperidol. Psychopharmacology (Berl) 118:52–56, 1995

Kutcher SP, Mackenzie S, Galarraga W, et al: Clonazepam treatment of adolescents with neuroleptic-induced akathisia (letter). Am J Psychiatry 144:823–824, 1987

Kutcher S, Williamson P, MacKenzie S, et al: Successful clonazepam treatment of neuroleptic-induced akathisia in older adolescents and young adults: a double-blind, placebo-controlled study. J Clin Psychopharmacol 9:403–406, 1989

Laborit H, Huguenard P, Alluaume R: [A new vegetative stabilizer (4560 RP).] Presse Med 60:206–208, 1952

Lee A-S: Treatment of drug-induced dystonic reactions. JACEP 8(11):453–457, 1979

Leonard PJ, Losowsky MS: Relationship between plasma vitamin E level and peroxide hemolysis test in human subjects. Am J Clin Nutr 20:795–798, 1967

Levinson DF, Simpson GM: Neuroleptic-induced extrapyramidal symptoms with fever: heterogeneity of the "neuroleptic malignant syndrome." Arch Gen Psychiatry 43:839–848, 1986

Levinson DF, Simpson GM, Singh H, et al: Fluphenazine dose, clinical response, and extrapyramidal symptoms during acute treatment. Arch Gen Psychiatry 47:761–768, 1990

Lieberman JA, Saltz BL, Johns CA, et al: The effects of clozapine on tardive dyskinesia. Br J Psychiatry 158:503–510, 1991

Lipinski JF, Zubenko GS, Barreira P, et al: Propranolol in the treatment of neuroleptic-induced akathisia. Lancet 1:685–686, 1983

Lohr JB, Caligiuri MP: A double-blind placebo-controlled study of vitamin E treatment of tardive dyskinesia. J Clin Psychiatry 57:167–173, 1996

Lohr JB, Cadet JL, Lohr MA, et al: Vitamin E in the treatment of tardive dyskinesia: the possible involvement of free radical mechanisms. Schizophr Bull 14:291–296, 1988

Luchins DJ, Freed WJ, Wyatt RJ: The role of cholinergic supersensitivity in the medical symptoms associated with the withdrawal of antipsychotic drugs. Am J Psychiatry 137:1395–1398, 1980

MacVicar K: Abuse of antiparkinsonian drugs by psychiatric patients. Am J Psychiatry 134:809–811, 1977

Marcus R, Coulston AM: Fat-soluble vitamins: vitamins A, K, and E, in Goodman and Gilman's The Pharmacological Basis of Therapeutics, 9th Edition. Edited by Hardman JG, Limbird LE, Molinoff PB, et al. New York, McGraw-Hill, 1996, pp 1573–1590

Mawdsley C, Williams IR, Pullar IA, et al: Treatment of parkinsonism by amantadine and levodopa. Clin Pharmacol Ther 13:575–583, 1972

McClelland HA, Blessed G, Bhate S, et al: The abrupt withdrawal of antiparkinsonian drugs in schizophrenic patients. Br J Psychiatry 124:151–159, 1974

McCreadie RG: The Nithsdale schizophrenia surveys: an overview. Soc Psychiatry Psychiatr Epidemiol 27:40–45, 1992

McCreadie RG, MacDonald E, Wiles D, et al: The Nithsdale schizophrenia surveys, XIV: plasma lipid peroxide and serum vitamin E levels in patients with and without tardive dyskinesia, and in normal subjects. Br J Psychiatry 167:610–617, 1995

McDevitt DG: Comparison of pharmacokinetic properties of beta-adrenoceptor blocking drugs. Eur Heart J 8 (suppl M):9–14, 1987

McEvoy JP: The clinical use of anticholinergic drugs as treatment for extrapyramidal side effects of neuroleptic drugs. J Clin Psychopharmacol 3:288–302, 1983

McEvoy JP, McCue M, Freter S: Replacement of chronically administered anticholinergic drugs by amantadine in outpatient management of chronic schizophrenia. Clin Ther 9:429–433, 1987

McEvoy JP, Hogarty GE, Steingard S: Optimal dose of neuroleptic in acute schizophrenia: a controlled study of the neuroleptic threshold and higher haloperidol dose. Arch Gen Psychiatry 48:739–745, 1991

Medina C, Kramer MD, Kurland AA: Biperiden in the treatment of phenothiazine-induced extrapyramidal reactions. JAMA 182:1127–1129, 1962

Meldrum BS, Anlezark GM, Marsden CD: Acute dystonia as an idiosyncratic response to neuroleptics in baboons. Brain 100:313–326, 1977

Meltzer HY: The role of serotonin in antipsychotic drug action. Neuropsychopharmacology 21 (suppl 2):S106–S115, 1999

Meltzer HY, Nash JF: Effects of antipsychotic drugs on serotonin receptors. Pharmacol Rev 43:587–604, 1991

Meltzer HY, Matsubara S, Lee JC: Classification of typical and atypical antipsychotic drugs on the basis of dopamine D1, D2 and serotonin2 pKi values. J Pharmacol Exp Ther 251:238–246, 1989

Menza MA, Murray GB, Holmes VF, et al: Decreased extrapyramidal symptoms with intravenous haloperidol. J Clin Psychiatry 48:278–280, 1987

Merrick EM, Schmitt P: A controlled study of the clinical effects of amantadine hydrochloride (Symmetrel). Curr Ther Res 15:552–558,1973

Metzer WS, Paige SR, Newton JE: Inefficacy of propranolol in attenuation of drug-induced parkinsonian tremor. Mov Disord 8:43–46, 1993

Miller CH, Mohr F, Umbricht D, et al: The prevalence of acute extrapyramidal signs and symptoms in patients treated with clozapine, risperidone, and conventional antipsychotics. J Clin Psychiatry 59:69–75, 1998

Miller DD, McEvoy JP, Davis SM, et al: Clinical correlates of tardive dyskinesia in schizophrenia: baseline data from the CATIE schizophrenia trial. Schizophr Res 80:33–43, 2005

Miller ER, Pastor-Barriuso R, Dalal D, et al: Meta-analysis: high-dosage vitamin E supplementation may increase all-cause mortality. Ann Intern Med 142:37–46, 2005

Miller NE: Effects of adrenoceptor-blocking drugs on plasma lipoprotein concentrations. Am J Cardiol 60:17E–23E, 1987

Mindham RHS: Assessment of drugs in schizophrenia. Assessment of drug-induced extrapyramidal reactions and of drugs given for their control. Br J Clin Pharmacol 3 (suppl 2):395–400, 1976

Mindham RHS, Gaind R, Anstee BH, et al: Comparison of amantadine, orphenadrine, and placebo in the control of phenothiazine-induced parkinsonism. Psychol Med 2:406–413, 1972

Moleman P, Schmitz PJM, Ladee GA: Extrapyramidal side effects and oral haloperidol: an analysis of explanatory patient and treatment characteristics. J Clin Psychiatry 43:492–496, 1982

Odergren T, Tollback A, Borg J: Electromyographic single motor unit potentials after repeated botulinum toxin treatments in cervical dystonia. Electroencephalogr Clin Neurophysiol 93:325–329, 1994

O'Flanagan PM: Clonazepam in the treatment of drug-induced dyskinesia. BMJ 1(5952):269–270, 1975

Pacifici GM, Nardini M, Ferrari P, et al: Effect of amantadine on drug-induced parkinsonism: relationship between plasma levels and effect. Br J Clin Pharmacol 3:883–889, 1976

Parkes JD, Zilkha KJ, Calver DM, et al: Controlled trial of amantadine hydrochloride in Parkinson's disease. Lancet 1(7641):259–262, 1970

Paton DM, Webster DR: Clinical pharmacokinetics of H1 receptor antagonists (the antihistamines). Clin Pharmacokinet 10:477–497, 1985

Perry EK, Perry RH, Blessed G, et al: Necropsy evidence of central cholinergic deficits in senile dementia (letter). Lancet 1(8004):189, 1977

Postma JU, Tilburg VW: Visual hallucinations and delirium during treatment with amantadine (Symmetrel). J Am Geriatr Soc 23:212–215, 1975

Potkin SG, Saha AR, Kujawa MJ, et al: Aripiprazole, an antipsychotic with a novel mechanism of action, and risperidone vs placebo in patients with schizophrenia and schizoaffective disorder. Arch Gen Psychiatry 60:681–690, 2003

Pujalte D, Bottaï T, Huë B, et al: A double-blind comparison of clonazepam and placebo in the treatment of neuroleptic-induced akathisia. Clin Neuropharmacol 17:236–242, 1994

Quinn N, Hallet M: Dose standardisation of botulinum toxin (letter) (erratum appears in Lancet 1[8646]:1092, 1989). Lancet 1(8644):964, 1989

Rashkis HA, Smarr ER: Protection against reserpine-induced "Parkinsonism" (clinical note). Am J Psychiatry 113:1116, 1957

Rifkin A, Quitkin F, Klein DF: Akinesia, a poorly recognized drug-induced extrapyramidal behavioral disorder. Arch Gen Psychiatry 32:672–674, 1975

Sachdev P: A rating scale for acute drug-induced akathisia: development, reliability, and validity. Biol Psychiatry 35:263–271, 1994

Saltz BL, Woerner MG, Kane JM, et al: Prospective study of tardive dyskinesia incidence in the elderly. JAMA 266:2402–2406, 1991

Sandyk R, Kay SR, Awerbuch GI: Subjective awareness of abnormal involuntary movements in schizophrenia. Int J Neurosci 69:1–20, 1993

Sanger TM, Lieberman JA, Tohen M, et al: Olanzapine versus haloperidol treatment in first-episode psychosis. Am J Psychiatry 156:79–87, 1999

Schmidt M, Meister P, Baumann P: Treatment of tardive dyskinesias with vitamin E. Eur Psychiatry 6:201–207, 1991

Schwab RS, Chafetz ME: Kemadrin in the treatment of parkinsonism. Neurology 5:273–277, 1955

Schwab RS, England AC, Poskanzer DC, et al: Amantadine in the treatment of Parkinson's disease. JAMA 208:1160–1170, 1969

Schwab RS, Poskanzer DC, England AC Jr, et al: Amantadine in Parkinson's disease. Review of more than two years' experience. JAMA 222:792–795, 1972

Scott AB: Botulinum toxin injections into extra ocular muscles as an alternative to strabismus surgery. Ophthalmology 87:1044–1049, 1980

Shear MK, Frances A, Weiden P: Suicide associated with akathisia and depot fluphenazine treatment. J Clin Psychopharmacol 3:235–236, 1983

Shriqui CL, Bradwejn J, Annable L, et al: Vitamin E in the treatment of tardive dyskinesia: a double-blind placebo-controlled study. Am J Psychiatry 149:391–393, 1992

Silver H, Geraisy N, Schwartz M: No difference in the effect of biperiden and amantadine on parkinsonian- and tardive dyskinesia-type involuntary movements: a double-blind crossover, placebo-controlled study in medicated chronic schizophrenic patients (erratum appears in J Clin Psychiatry 56:435, 1995). J Clin Psychiatry 56:167–170, 1995

Silvestri S, Seeman MV, Negrete JC, et al: Increased dopamine D2 receptor binding after long-term treatment with antipsychotics in humans: a clinical PET study. Psychopharmacologia 152:174–180, 2000

Simpson GM: Long-acting antipsychotic agents and extrapyramidal side effects. Dis Nerv Syst 31 (suppl):12–14, 1970

Simpson GM: The treatment of tardive dyskinesia and tardive dystonia. J Clin Psychiatry 61 (suppl 4):39–44, 2000

Simpson GM, Angus JWS: A rating scale for extrapyramidal side effects. Acta Psychiatr Scand 212:11–19, 1970

Simpson GM, Lindermayer JP: Extrapyramidal symptoms in patients treated with risperidone. J Clin Psychopharmacol 17:194–201, 1997

Simpson GM, Varga E: Clozapine—a new antipsychotic agent. Curr Ther Res 18:679–868, 1974

Simpson GM, Amuso D, Blair JH, et al: Phenothiazine-produced extrapyramidal system disturbance. Arch Gen Psychiatry 10:199–208, 1964

Simpson GM, Amin M, Kunz E: Withdrawal effects of phenothiazines. Compr Psychiatry 6:347–351, 1965

Simpson GM, Krakov L, Mattke D, et al: A controlled comparison of the treatment of schizophrenic patients when treated according to the neuroleptic threshold or by clinical judgment. Acta Psychiatr Scand Suppl 212:38–43, 1970

Simpson GM, Beckles D, Isalski Z, et al: Some methodological considerations in the evaluation of drug-induced extrapyramidal disorders: a study of X10–029, a new morphanthridine derivative. J Clin Pharmacol 12:142–152, 1972

Simpson GM, Lee JH, Shrivastava RK: Clozapine in tardive dyskinesia. Psychopharmacologia 56:75–80, 1978

Simpson GM, Lee JH, Zoubok B, et al: A rating scale for tardive dyskinesia. Psychopharmacologia 64:171–179, 1979

Simpson GM, Cooper TB, Bark N, et al: Effect of antiparkinsonian medications on plasma levels of chlorpromazine. Arch Gen Psychiatry 37:205–208, 1980

Simpson GM, Pi EH, Sramek JJ Jr: Adverse effects of antipsychotic agents. Drugs 21:138–151, 1981

Simpson LL: The origin, structure, and pharmacologic activity of botulinum toxin. Pharmacol Rev 33:155–188, 1981

Singh H, Levinson DF, Simpson GM, et al: Acute dystonia during fixed-dose neuroleptic treatment. J Clin Psychopharmacol 10:389–396, 1990

Small JG, Hirsch SR, Arvanitis LA, et al: Quetiapine in patients with schizophrenia. A high- and low-dose double-blind comparison with placebo. Arch Gen Psychiatry 54:549–557, 1997

Snyder S, Greenberg D, Yamamura HI: Anti-schizophrenic drugs and brain cholinergic receptors. Arch Gen Psychiatry 31:58–61, 1974

Sokol RJ: Vitamin E deficiency and neurologic disease. Annu Rev Nutr 8:351–373, 1988

Sokol RJ, Butler-Simon N, Conner C, et al: Multicenter trial of d-alpha-tocopherol polyethylene glycol 1000 succinate for treatment of vitamin E deficiency in children with chronic cholestasis. Gastroenterology 104:1727–1735, 1993

Sokoloff P, Giros B, Martres MP, et al: Molecular cloning and characterization of a novel dopamine receptor (D3) as a target for neuroleptics. Nature 347:146–151, 1990

Sommer BR, Cohen BM, Satlin A, et al: Changes in tardive dyskinesia symptoms in elderly patients treated with ganglioside GM1 or placebo. J Geriatr Psychiatry Neurol 7:234–237, 1994

Sramek JJ, Simpson GM, Morrison RL, et al: Anticholinergic agents for prophylaxis of neuroleptic-induced dystonic reactions: a prospective study. J Clin Psychiatry 47:305–309, 1986

St. Jean A, Donald MW, Ban TA: Uses and abuses of antiparkinsonian medication. Am J Psychiatry 120:801–803, 1964

Stanilla JK, Nair C, de Leon J, et al: Clozapine does not produce akathisia or parkinsonism. Poster presented at the 34th annual meeting of the American College of Neuropsychopharmacology, San Juan, Puerto Rico, December 11–15, 1995

Stanilla JK, Büchel C, Alarcon J, et al: Diurnal and weekly variation of tardive dyskinesia measured by digital image processing. Psychopharmacology (Berl) 124:373–376, 1996

Stanilla JK, de Leon J, Simpson GM: Clozapine withdrawal resulting in delirium with psychosis: a report of three cases. J Clin Psychiatry 58:252–255, 1997

Stenson RL, Donlon PT, Meyer JE: Comparison of benztropine mesylate and amantadine HCL in neuroleptic-induced extrapyramidal symptoms. Compr Psychiatry 17:763–768, 1976

Stephens DA: Psychotoxic effects of benzhexol hydrochloride (Artane). Br J Psychiatry 113:213–218, 1967

Stern TA, Anderson WH: Benztropine prophylaxis of dystonic reactions. Psychopharmacologia 61:261–262, 1979

Stoof JC, Booij J, Drukarch B: Amantadine as N-methyl-d-aspartic acid receptor antagonist: new possibilities for therapeutic applications? Clin Neurol Neurosurg 94:S4–S6, 1992

Strang RR: The symptom of restless legs. Med J Aust 24:1211–1213, 1967

Stratas NE, Phillips RD, Walker PA, et al: A study of drug induced parkinsonism. Dis Nerv Syst 24:180, 1963

Strömberg U, Svensson TH, Waldeck B: On the mode of action of amantadine. J Pharm Pharmacol 22:959–962, 1970

Swett C, Cole JO, Shapiro S, et al: Extrapyramidal side effects in chlorpromazine recipients. Arch Gen Psychiatry 34:942–943, 1977

Taylor AE, Lang AE, Saint-Cyr JA, et al: Cognitive processes in idiopathic dystonia treated with high-dose anticholinergic therapy: implications for treatment strategies. Clin Neuropharmacol 14:62–77, 1991

Thaker GK, Tamminga CA, Alphs LD, et al: Brain gamma-aminobutyric acid abnormality in tardive dyskinesia: reduction in cerebrospinal fluid GABA levels and therapeutic response to GABA agonist treatment. Arch Gen Psychiatry 44:522–529, 1987

Thaker GK, Nguyen JA, Strauss ME, et al: Clonazepam treatment of tardive dyskinesia: a practical GABAmimetic strategy. Am J Psychiatry 147:445–451, 1990

Timberlake WH, Schwab RS, England AC Jr: Biperiden (Akineton) in parkinsonism. Arch Neurol 5:560–564, 1961

Tollefson GD, Beasley CM Jr, Tran PV, et al: Olanzapine versus haloperidol in the treatment of schizophrenia and schizoaffective and schizophreniform disorders: results of an international collaborative trial. Arch Gen Psychiatry 54:457–465, 1997

Tune L, Coyle JT: Serum levels of anticholinergic drugs in treatment of acute extrapyramidal side effects. Arch Gen Psychiatry 37:293–297, 1980

Ungvari GS, Chiu HF, Lam LC, et al: Gradual withdrawal of long-term anticholinergic antiparkinson medication in Chinese patients with chronic schizophrenia. J Clin Psychopharmacol 19:141–148, 1999

van Harten PN, van Trier JC, Horwitz EH, et al: Cocaine as a risk factor for neuroleptic-induced acute dystonia. J Clin Psychiatry 59:128–130, 1998

Van Putten T, May PR, Marder SR, et al: Subjective response to antipsychotic drugs. Arch Gen Psychiatry 38:187–190, 1981

Van Putten TR, May PR, Marder SR: Response to antipsychotic medication: the doctor's and the consumer's view. Am J Psychiatry 141:16–19, 1984

Van Tol H, Bunzow J, Guan H, et al: Cloning of the gene for a human dopamine D4 receptor with high affinity for the antipsychotic clozapine. Nature 350:610–614, 1991

Wells BG, Marken PA, Rickman LA, et al: Characterizing anticholinergic abuse in community mental health. J Clin Psychopharmacol 9:431–435, 1989

Wilbur R, Kulik FA, Kulik AV: Noradrenergic effects in tardive dyskinesia, akathisia and pseudoparkinsonism via the limbic system and basal ganglia. Prog Neuropsychopharmacol Biol Psychiatry 12:849–864, 1988

Winer JA, Bahn S: Loss of teeth with antidepressant drug therapy. Arch Gen Psychiatry 16:239–240, 1967

Wingfield WL, Pollack D, Grunert RR: Therapeutic efficacy of amantadine HCl and rimantadine HCl in naturally occurring influenza A2 respiratory illness in man. N Engl J Med 281:579–584, 1969

Wirshing DA, Marshall BD Jr, Green MF, et al: Risperidone in treatment-refractory schizophrenia. Am J Psychiatry 156:1374–1379, 1999

Wojcik J, Gelenberg A, La Brie RA, et al: Prevalence of tardive dyskinesia in an outpatient population. Compr Psychiatry 21:370–379, 1980

Wojcik JD, Falk WE, Fink JS, et al: A review of 32 cases of tardive dystonia (see comments). Am J Psychiatry 148:1055–1059, 1991

Yahr MD, Duvoisin RC: Medical therapy of parkinsonism. Modern Treatment 5:283–300, 1968

Yamamura HI, Snyder SH: Muscarinic cholinergic receptor binding in the longitudinal muscle of the guinea pig ileum with [3H]quinuclidinyl benzilate. Mol Pharmacol 10:861–867, 1974

Yassa R, Nair V, Dimitry R: Prevalence of tardive dystonia. Acta Psychiatr Scand 73:629–633, 1986

Drugs for Treatment of Bipolar Disorder

CHAPTER 35

Lithium

Marlene P. Freeman, M.D.

Christopher B. Wiegand, M.D.

Alan J. Gelenberg, M.D.

History and Discovery

First used in the 1800s as a medicinal treatment, lithium was touted for a wide range of medical woes—including gout and neurological and gastrointestinal ailments—and was used as a table salt substitute and even sold in bottled beverages (El-Mallakh and Jefferson 1999). After noting its sedating properties in animals, Cade (1949) first described the successful treatment of mania with lithium salts. The U.S. Food and Drug Administration (FDA) approved lithium for use in treating acute mania in 1970 and for the prophylaxis of bipolar disorder 4 years later (Jefferson and Greist 1977). However, lithium did not come onto the market easily in the United States. Pharmaceutical companies were reluctant to produce this inexpensive drug that they could not patent (Kline 1973).

Lithium has stood the test of time. Despite a growing number of choices for the treatment of bipolar disorder, lithium remains a cost-effective and efficacious treatment. Baldessarini and Tondo (2000) questioned whether lithium has remained stable in efficacy across the decades. Analyzing 11 controlled and 13 open studies of lithium treatment, as well as their own data, they concluded that lithium's efficacy has remained constant but that some clinical research settings may serve a more complex and refractory patient population than the population typically seen in psychiatric practice.

Wyatt et al. (2001) computed the savings from lithium use during the years 1970 and 1991, estimating that more than $8 million was saved annually, after consideration of treatment costs, lost earnings, and lost productivity. Lithium is still a highly cost-effective treatment for bipolar disorder (Chisholm et al. 2005). In contrast to most other medications for bipolar disorder, lithium is available generically and is relatively inexpensive. The pharmaceutical industry spends considerable funds for research and marketing for drugs still on patent, and therefore lithium has achieved an orphan status, with little incentive for private funding of studies with lithium (Rosenthal 2001).

> Lithium is effective and well tolerated, especially at moderate serum lithium concentrations.... One factor that may be responsible for lithium's fall from grace among clinicians and patients is its status as an "orphan" or "poor relative." Since lithium is cheap and unpatented, no wealthy drug company has any interest in demonstrating its merits as a mood stabilizer. There are no lavishly catered all-star symposia at major psychiatric meetings to sing the praises of this humble salt. And when did you last see a pen, notepad, calendar, or trinket with "Lithium" embossed on it? Finally, lithium is regarded as old news and, as such, is less appealing to psychiatric researchers eager to make their mark on the field. (Rosenthal 2001, p. 973)

Structure–Activity Relations

Lithium is the lightest alkali metal and a monovalent cation, and it shares some properties with sodium, potassium, and calcium (Baldessarini 1996; Ward et al. 1994). It is the third element of the periodic table. Substitution or competition with other cations may contribute to its effects (Ward et al. 1994).

Pharmacological Profile

Lithium is minimally protein bound, does not undergo biotransformation, and is renally eliminated (Kilts 2000). The narrow therapeutic index necessitates careful drug monitoring. Lithium appears to affect multiple neurotransmitter systems and affects second-messenger systems such as cyclic adenosine monophosphate (cAMP) and cyclic guanosine monophosphate (cGMP) (Ward et al. 1994).

Pharmacokinetics and Disposition

Lithium is available in multiple preparations, including lithium carbonate tablets and capsules, lithium citrate, and slow-release forms (Jefferson et al. 1983). Lithium is absorbed from the gastrointestinal tract and renally excreted unchanged in approximately 24 hours (Baldessarini and Tarazi 2001). Peak plasma concentrations are reached within 1–2 hours with rapid-release preparations and 4–5 hours after sustained-release formulations (Finley et al. 1995). Brain levels, as measured by in vivo nuclear magnetic resonance, are highest 0–2 hours after peak serum concentrations are achieved (Komoroski et al. 1993). Lithium is not protein bound and is evenly distributed in total body water space (Jermain et al. 1991). Lithium excretion is controlled by osmotic factors and is a function of renal sufficiency (Birch et al. 1980). Steady-state concentrations are achieved within 4–5 days (Keck and McElroy 2002).

Mechanism of Action

Despite extensive research, the exact mechanism of action of lithium as a mood stabilizer has yet to be elucidated. The importance of defining lithium's mechanism of action is twofold: 1) to shed light on the disorder's etiology and 2) to open up investigation into new treatments for bipolar disorder (Phiel and Klein 2001). Multiple theories, based on animal models and limited studies in humans, have been proposed; those with the most compelling evidence are reviewed here.

Eventually, an integrated theory of lithium's action will be necessary because it has numerous physiological effects. Ikonomov and Manji (1999) have offered the "initiation and adaptation paradigm" as a nicely integrated view of lithium's actions: lithium has both immediate short-term effects and effects that emerge only after long-term treatment. They propose that the immediate effects eventually cause downstream changes in gene expression.

Inositol Depletion

There has been much focus on the role of the inositol cycle in the clinical effects of lithium. Lithium is a noncompetitive inhibitor of inositol monophosphatase, depleting free inositol within 5 days of treatment initiation (Berridge et al. 1989). These changes last for 3–4 weeks after lithium's discontinuation (Moore et al. 1997). Depletion of free inositol can lead to effects on neurotransmitter and second-messenger systems linked to the inositol cycle. For example, adrenergic, serotonergic, and cholinergic receptor subtypes are coupled to the cycle via G proteins, and the cycle in turn regulates protein kinase C action, which appears to be influenced by lithium treatment in mania (Hahn et al. 2005). Lithium decreases levels of protein kinase C isoenzymes in the frontal cortex and hippocampus, two areas of the brain known to be involved in the pathophysiology of mood disorders (Drevets et al. 1997; Ketter et al. 1997; Manji et al. 1993, 1999; Rajkowska et al. 1999).

Berridge et al. (1989) suggested that lithium, because it is a noncompetitive inhibitor of inositol monophosphatase, only affects *activated* systems via the inositol-depletion mechanism; basal functioning of the cycle is not affected. This would account for lithium's profound effects on mood in bipolar and depressive disorders and its relatively minor effects on mood in control subjects (Judd 1979).

Lithium affects rearing behavior in rats, which is reversible by inositol administration. Also, administration of inositol inhibits the epileptogenic effects of pilocarpine challenge after lithium administration in rats (Belmaker et al. 1996). Of note, depression is associated with low cerebrospinal fluid inositol levels in humans (Barkai et al. 1978). Exogenous inositol can alleviate depression (Levine et al. 1993, 1995) and panic attacks (Benjamin et al. 1995). Belmaker et al. (1996) suggested a complex "pendulum" relationship between inositol and lithium, which may be a basis for understanding lithium's antimanic and antidepressant effects.

In rats and humans, inositol attenuates some of the side effects of lithium, particularly polyuria (Bersudsky et al. 1993; Geisler et al. 1972) resulting from either lithium's effects on the inositol cycle or inositol's osmotic effects (P.A. Garcia and Burg 1991). Death due to lithium toxicity in rats is not prevented by inositol administration, suggesting a different mechanism (Belmaker et al. 1996).

Glycogen Synthase Kinase Inhibition

Lithium inhibits glycogen synthase kinase–3 (GSK-3) (Klein and Melton 1996; Li et al. 2007). Valproic acid also inhibits GSK-3, making this theory attractive because it involves a common mechanism in two known mood stabilizers (G. Chen et al. 1999). GSK-3 is an inhibitor of the Wnt protein signaling pathway, which affects neuronal signal transduction. Lithium thus would be predicted to mimic Wnt signaling (Phiel and Klein 2001). Wnt signaling stimulates a cascade of events that leads to stimulation of protein kinase C activity (Grahame-Smith 1998; Williams and Harwood 2000). Thus, lithium's actions on both the inositol cycle and the GSK-3 signaling pathway lead to a common effect on protein kinase C.

Wnt signaling, which is inhibited by and in turn inhibits GSK-3 activity, also causes axonal remodeling in mouse cerebellar cells (Hall et al. 2000). GSK-3 activity elevation can cause breakdown of catenins, which can cause structural changes in cytoskeleton (Cotter et al. 1998). β-Catenin produces changes in gene expression that are related to cytoskeletal structures. Lithium stabilizes cytoskeleton structures (Williams and Harwood 2000).

Lithium's Effects on Neurotransmitter Systems

Perhaps because of its effects on second-messenger systems, lithium brings about changes in all of the major neurotransmitter systems in the brain. Chronic administration of lithium in mice increases and stabilizes glutamate uptake. This could, in part, explain lithium's antimanic effect because it results in overall reduction of an excitatory neurotransmitter (Dixon and Hokin 1998). Lithium also normalizes low cerebrospinal fluid γ-aminobutyric acid levels in bipolar subjects (see Berrettini et al. 1983, 1986).

Lithium enhances norepinephrine and serotonin function in the central nervous system, which could explain its antidepressant effects (Price et al. 1990; Schildkraut et al. 1969; D.N. Stern et al. 1969). Of particular interest is lithium's confirmed antagonistic action at serotonin$_{1A}$ (5-HT$_{1A}$) and serotonin$_{1B}$ (5-HT$_{1B}$) autoreceptors (Haddjeri et al. 2000; Massot et al. 1999); such action would increase serotonin availability in the synaptic cleft (Shaldubina et al. 2001). Clinically, 5-HT$_{1A}$ may be involved in alleviation of depression, and 5-HT$_{1B}$ receptors may play a role in the regulation of sleep, sensorimotor inhibition, and locomotor activity (Monti et al. 1995; Sipes and Geyer 1996).

Lithium, Mood Disorders, and Circadian Rhythms

Bipolar disorder and depression are associated with disturbances in the body's natural rhythms; the most clinically evident of these is the disruption of the sleep–wake cycle, but the temperature cycle, cortisol cycle, and others are also affected (Hallonquist et al. 1986; Healy and Waterhouse 1995). Associated with such changes is a decoupling of the major and minor oscillators located in the hypothalamus, which in healthy subjects work in a synchronized fashion. Lithium administration causes the oscillators to resynchronize (DeMet and Chicz-Demet 1987; Klemfuss 1992). The mechanism by which resynchronization occurs is unknown; it is likely *not* via the inositol depletion mechanism (Lakin-Thomas 1992, 1993). Also, a cause–effect relation has not been established for circadian rhythm abnormalities and mood disorders; the changes seen in circadian rhythms could be a cause of bipolar disorder and/or unipolar depression or could be an effect of the disease process.

Indications and Efficacy

Bipolar Disorder

Acute Mania

Cade (1949) first published data on the efficacy of lithium in mania more than half a century ago. As we begin the twenty-first century, lithium remains one of the most efficacious treatments for bipolar disorder.

Lithium versus placebo.   Lithium has been shown to be more efficacious than placebo in acute mania in randomized trials (Bowden et al. 1994, 2005; Goodwin et al. 1969; Maggs 1963; Schou et al. 1954; Stokes et al. 1971). Analysis of response rates in these studies indicates that lithium was at least somewhat efficacious in the treatment of mania in 87 of 124 patients (70%) (Keck et al. 2000).

Lithium versus typical antipsychotics. In studies that used various designs, lithium was more effective than chlorpromazine and other traditional antipsychotic medications in the treatment of acute mania. In a review of studies, Goodwin and Zis (1979) found lithium efficacious in at least 70% of patients, as defined by remission or marked improvement. Lithium also worked more quickly than typical antipsychotics and was better tolerated (Takahashi et al. 1975). In addition, patients with psychotic symptoms during a manic episode tend to have a better response to lithium prophylactic treatment than do those without psychosis (see Rosenthal et al. 1979).

In a 3-week double-blind study of lithium, haloperidol, and their combination for acute mania, patients who received haloperidol or haloperidol plus lithium had more significant improvement than did those who received lithium alone (Garfinkel et al. 1980). The combination of lithium and haloperidol was as well tolerated as haloperidol alone. In patients with schizoaffective disorder, lithium was as effective as chlorpromazine in acute mania (Brockington et al. 1978). More recently, Segal et al. (1998) reported that inpatients with acute mania responded equally well to lithium, haloperidol, and risperidone. Lithium has been used as a comparator in trials versus atypical (second-generation) antipsychotic medications, but these studies primarily assess the efficacy of the antipsychotic in a non-inferiority approach rather than demonstrate significant differences between lithium and the atypicals. To date, there is no obvious effect-size difference between any agent and lithium for antimanic effects. By and large, antipsychotics appear to work faster. Most probably, genetic variables mediate the likelihood and magnitude of treatment response to different agents in different patients, so although we can detect no overall efficacy differences, for individual patients there are likely great differences.

Lithium versus calcium channel blockers. Lithium appears superior to verapamil in the treatment of mania (Walton et al. 1996).

Lithium versus electroconvulsive therapy. Small et al. (1988) compared the effects of lithium with those of electroconvulsive therapy (ECT) for acute mania. Patients who received ECT had significantly more improvement during the first 2 months of treatment than did those who received lithium carbonate, especially those with mixed mania. After 8 weeks, no significant differences were found between the groups.

In a retrospective chart review, Black et al. (1987) found that a significantly greater percentage of patients who received ECT (78%) had "marked improvement" than those who received lithium, either "adequately or inadequately" (62%, 56%). Almost 70% of the patients who did not respond to lithium experienced "marked improvement" after treatment with ECT.

Lithium versus anticonvulsants. Double-blind, randomized studies have suggested that carbamazepine and lithium are equally effective for acute mania (Lerer et al. 1987; Small et al. 1991). However, neither trial included a placebo arm. Swann et al. (1999) reported that for patients who had experienced a greater number of previous episodes, divalproex was more effective than lithium for acute mania, as determined by a 3-week double-blind study. For patients with a history of fewer episodes, lithium had no significantly different effect compared with divalproex in acute mania. Bowden et al. (1994) reported that both lithium and divalproex sodium were significantly more effective than placebo in the treatment of acute mania. Almost one-third of the patients receiving either lithium or divalproex dropped out of the study secondary to lack of efficacy, compared with approximately half of the patients who received placebo.

In a meta-analysis of the efficacy of lithium, valproate, and carbamazepine in mania, no significant differences in efficacy were found among the three groups (Emilien et al. 1996). Only some of the included studies were placebo controlled. Anticonvulsants were generally better tolerated than lithium. Neurological abnormalities may predict a better response to anticonvulsants than to lithium in mania. Patients with electroencephalogram abnormalities are more likely to respond to valproate than to lithium (Reeves et al. 2001). One double-blind study suggested that lamotrigine may be as effective as lithium for acute mania (Ichim et al. 2000).

Mixed mania, the co-occurrence of mania with depression, may predict a poor response to lithium. In a double-blind study of acute mania, depressive symptoms were associated with a poorer response to lithium (Swann et al. 1997). Other predictors of a poor antimanic response to lithium include rapid cycling and substance abuse (Dunner and Fieve 1974; Goodwin and Jamison 1990; Himmelhoch et al. 1976).

Rapid efficacy is desirable in a mood stabilizer, and rapid administration of lithium has been preliminarily studied. Lynn et al. (1971) discussed lithium "loading" for acute mania. More recently, Keck et al. (2001) assessed the safety and efficacy of rapid lithium administration in the treatment of acute mania; in an open-label study of 15 inpatients, 20 mg/kg/day appeared well tolerated and efficacious for acute mania.

Bipolar Depression

Lithium is a first-line treatment for acute bipolar depression (Compton and Nemeroff 2000). In 2004, an expert consensus report found lithium monotherapy to be both a preferred initial medication for mild to moderate depression in bipolar I disorder and a component of an initial medication regimen in severe nonpsychotic and psychotic depression in bipolar I disorder (Keck et al. 2004). The American Psychiatric Association's (2002) "Practice Guideline for the Treatment of Patients With Bipolar Disorder" states that the first-line treatment for bipolar depression is pharmacotherapy with either lithium or lamotrigine, with the former approach as the better-supported option.

Placebo-controlled studies of lithium in bipolar depression generally have reported efficacy. Goodwin and Jamison (1990) analyzed the placebo-controlled trials that have been completed in bipolar depression and found that 79% of the bipolar patients in those trials had either a complete or a partial response to lithium. Placebo-controlled trials that show the efficacy of lithium in bipolar depression include those by Baron et al. (1975), Donnelly et al. (1978), Fieve et al. (1968), Goodwin et al. (1969, 1972), Greenspan et al. (1970), Mendels (1975), and Noyes et al. (1974). These studies generally were small (involving between 3 and 40 patients [Goodwin et al. 1972]). One study, by Stokes et al. (1971), did not show a significant benefit of lithium over placebo, but lithium was administered for only a 10-day period in that trial.

Suicide: Is Lithium Protective?

Twenty-five percent to 50% of bipolar patients attempt suicide during their lifetime (Compton and Nemeroff 2000). On average, studies of deaths among individuals with bipolar disorder indicate that 19% complete suicide (see Goodwin and Jamison 1990). In an analysis of studies of lithium treatment (Schou 1998), patients treated with lithium had a lower overall mortality rate than bipolar patients in general. Schou (1998) studied a population of approximately 2,000 patients who received lithium and found that these patients did not have a significantly higher suicide rate than the general population. After discontinuation of the lithium, the mortality rate increased. Fewer patients attempted or committed suicide while treated prophylactically with lithium than when they were not.

Also, Tondo et al. (1997) reviewed studies of the use of lithium in the treatment of major mood disorders; these included 28 studies that involved more than 17,000 pa-

tients. Risks of completed and attempted suicides were 8.6-fold higher in patients who were not given lithium compared with those who were. They also found increased rates of suicide after lithium discontinuation (Baldessarini et al. 1999). The risk of suicide with lithium discontinuation may be decreased with gradual discontinuation. Lithium may have a specific antisuicidal effect in addition to mood-stabilizing properties (Aherns and Muller-Oerlinghausen 2001). In addition to a marked reduction in suicide attempts in lithium responders, lithium seems to reduce suicide attempts independent of classification of clinical response (i.e., excellent, moderate, poor).

In meta-analyses of studies of lithium treatment in major mood disorders, Tondo et al. (2001) and Baldessarini et al. (2006) found significantly lower suicide risk for subjects who were receiving treatment with lithium. However, Coryell et al. (2001) conducted a case–control study in which patients with major mood disorders who completed or attempted suicide were matched with control subjects who were receiving similar treatment (antidepressant and/or mood-stabilizing medication). The patients who committed suicide were slightly less likely to be using lithium, but the difference was not statistically significant.

Methodological problems exist in the studies that have examined lithium and suicide risk, and large-scale prospective studies are necessary for definitive recommendations to inform treatment decisions (Gelenberg 2001).

Prophylaxis and Maintenance

Once the diagnosis of bipolar disorder is established, a patient will be afflicted for the rest of his or her lifetime, with ongoing risks of relapse and recurrence. Therefore, prophylactic or maintenance therapy is often considered after the resolution of an acute mood episode. Lithium is the best-studied drug for this indication.

Tondo et al. (2001) found lithium effective in long-term use (more than 1 year) in decreasing frequency of mood episodes and "time ill" in patients with bipolar I and bipolar II disorders. Benefits of lithium treatment were not significantly different among patients with psychosis or mixed episodes, rapid cycling, or more classic forms. There was no decrease in efficacy with long-term use. Early commencement of lithium therapy and a diagnosis of bipolar II disorder may predict a better course of illness (Tondo et al. 1998).

Rosenthal et al. (1979) also found that psychotic symptoms during manic episodes predicted a good response to lithium prophylaxis in bipolar I patients. The chronological pattern of illness also may predict response to lithium prophylaxis: the pattern mania–depression–euthymia is associated with better response than depression–mania or rapid-cycling bipolar disorder (Maj 1990). Additionally, a poorer response after 1 year of lithium therapy is associated with poor response to lithium within the first 6 months, more severe episodes, higher ratio of manic episodes to depressive episodes, and being unmarried (Yazici et al. 1999).

Kulhara et al. (1999) found that only 24% of the patients with bipolar disorder followed up in a lithium clinic were free of mood episodes while receiving lithium prophylaxis (duration of monitoring: average = 11 years, range = 2–27 years). Noncompliance and/or subtherapeutic lithium blood levels (<0.4 mEq/L), high number of psychosocial stressors, higher number of depressive episodes before lithium treatment, and poor social supports may predict poorer response to lithium prophylaxis (Kulhara et al. 1999). Patients had significantly fewer mood episodes after starting lithium.

Starting lithium early in the course of illness predicts a better response to treatment (Franchini et al. 1999). Time of onset of lithium prophylaxis was significantly related to outcome of lithium treatment ($P<0.001$), after polarity, sex, age at onset, duration of illness, and duration of lithium prophylaxis were accounted for.

Psychotic symptoms during a manic episode also have been associated with better response to lithium prophylaxis (Rosenthal et al. 1979).

Lithium appears superior to carbamazepine in the prophylactic treatment of classic bipolar I disorder. Denicoff et al. (1997) compared the efficacy of lithium, carbamazepine, and their combination in the prophylactic treatment of bipolar disorder. Patients were randomly assigned to double-blind treatment for 1 year with lithium or carbamazepine, experienced a crossover to the other drug in the second year, and received a combination of the two in the third year. Thirty-one percent failed to complete a full year of lithium therapy because of lack of efficacy, 37% failed to complete a full year of carbamazepine therapy because of lack of efficacy, and 24% failed to complete a full year of combination therapy because of lack of efficacy. Lithium was more effective than carbamazepine for prophylaxis of mania; patients with rapid cycling did poorly with either monotherapy (28% responded to lithium, compared with 19% to carbamazepine), and patients with rapid cycling did significantly better on the combination of the two drugs than on either alone.

In a randomized study, Kleindienst and Greil (2000) found that lithium was superior to carbamazepine in treating classic mania, but carbamazepine was more efficacious for nonclassic features, such as mixed episodes and comorbidity.

In a comparison of lithium, divalproex, and placebo in a 1-year treatment study of patients with bipolar I disorder after recovery from an index manic episode, Bowden et al. (2000) found that median times to 50% survival without mood episode were 40 weeks for divalproex, 24 weeks for lithium, and 28 weeks for placebo, although the differences were not statistically significant. Patients who received divalproex remained in treatment significantly longer than did those who received lithium. Calabrese et al. (2005) found similarly high rates of relapse in patients with rapid-cycling bipolar disorder randomly assigned to either lithium or valproate monotherapy (56% and 50% relapse rates, respectively). In patients with mixed or manic episodes who responded to cotreatment with lithium and olanzapine, investigators conducted a double-blind, randomized maintenance trial of lithium versus olanzapine (Tohen et al. 2005). Recurrence rates were similar between groups, with 38.8% of those on lithium and 30.0% on olanzapine experiencing relapse, with similar prophylaxis for depressive episodes among treatments and some advantage for prevention of mania and mixed episodes with olanzapine.

The combination of lithium and valproate also has been studied as maintenance therapy for bipolar disorder: the two may work synergistically (Solomon et al. 1998).

Quitkin et al. (1981) assessed the efficacy of lithium with and without the antidepressant imipramine in the prophylaxis of bipolar I disorder. Few depressive episodes occurred in either group, and the risk of mania increased with the addition of imipramine. Most relapses occurred in the first 6 months of treatment.

Maintenance dosing.   To be effective in prophylaxis, lithium must be administered daily. Lithium administration every other day is not as effective as daily dosing (Jensen et al. 1995). Perry et al. (1984) formulated tables to assist in the determination of maintenance dosage requirements, based on 24-hour serum lithium levels after the administration of a 1,200-mg test dose. Once-daily dosing at bedtime yields higher brain-to-serum ratios of lithium levels than twice-daily dosing schedules (Soares et al. 2001). Investigators have observed substantial variation in brain lithium levels among individuals with similar serum lithium levels (Gonzalez et al. 1993).

Unipolar Depression

Analysis of five controlled trials of lithium augmentation for unipolar depression found significant improvement in 56%–96% of patients (Austin et al. 1991; Heit and Nemeroff 1998; Heninger et al. 1983; Kantor et al. 1986; Schopf et al. 1989; Stein and Bernadt 1993; Zusky et al. 1988). In treatment-refractory depression, open-label data support the addition of lithium to antidepressants, including tricyclics, trazodone, and selective serotonin reuptake inhibitors (SSRIs) (De Montigny et al. 1981, 1983, 1985; Dinan 1993; Fontaine et al. 1991; Price et al. 1986). Double-blind studies support the use of lithium for augmentation of tricyclics, monoamine oxidase inhibitors (MAOIs), trazodone, and SSRIs (Baumann et al. 1996; Fava et al. 1994; Heninger et al. 1983; Joffe et al. 1993; Kantor et al. 1986; Katona et al. 1995; Nierenberg et al. 2006; Schopf et al. 1989; Zusky et al. 1988). In the large Sequenced Treatment Alternatives to Relieve Depression (STAR*D) multisite trial, 15.9% of subjects who did not experience remission with citalopram monotherapy and another medication trial experienced remission after the addition of lithium (Nierenberg et al. 2006).

Time of onset of lithium action as an adjunct to antidepressants remains unclear. Also, new studies are needed to determine the appropriate duration of treatment with lithium augmentation and the appropriate serum lithium levels (Heit and Nemeroff 1998).

Personality Disorders

In a double-blind crossover study, Rifkin et al. (1972) studied lithium and placebo in patients with "emotionally unstable character disorder," consisting of "short mood swings, both depressive and hypomanic, lasting hours to a few days" as well as "chronically maladaptive behavior." Patients were significantly more likely to show improvement while receiving treatment with lithium. LaWall and Wesselius (1982) reported five cases in which patients with borderline personality disorder (DSM-III; American Psychiatric Association 1980) showed clinical improvement with lithium treatment.

Aggression and Impulsivity

In placebo-controlled trials of adults without bipolar disorder, lithium has been effective for aggressive behavior (Worrall et al. 1975). Lithium reduced the frequency of aggressive episodes in patients with mental retardation, per retrospective chart reviews (Luchins and Dojka 1989; Spreat et al. 1989) and prospective double-blind, pla-

cebo-controlled clinical trial data (Craft et al. 1987). Both open-label and double-blind, placebo-controlled data have found lithium to be effective in reducing aggression in children with conduct disorder (Campbell et al. 1995; Malone et al. 1994, 2000). There may be broad public health implications for the relation between lithium and aggression. In one study, counties with higher lithium levels in drinking water had lower rates of suicide, homicide, and rape than did counties with lower lithium levels (Schrauzer and Shrestha 1990). Lithium treatment has been demonstrated to decrease impulsive gambling in individuals with bipolar spectrum disorders (Hollander et al. 2005).

Anxiety

Information on the use of lithium in anxiety disorders is limited. Open-label (Van der Kolk 1983) and case-report (Forster et al. 1995; Kitchner and Greenstein 1985) data suggest efficacy in posttraumatic stress disorder. Case reports support a role for lithium in treating refractory panic disorder (Feder 1988) and obsessive-compulsive disorder (Golden et al. 1988; T. A. Stern and Jenike 1983). However, two controlled trials failed to demonstrate efficacy for lithium in the treatment of obsessive-compulsive disorder (McDougle et al. 1991; Pigott et al. 1991).

Use in Special Populations

Children and Adolescents

Lithium is FDA approved for the treatment of bipolar disorder in adolescents (Ryan et al. 1999). Lithium has a large effect size in the open-label treatment of acute mania or mixed episodes in children and adolescents (Kowatch et al. 2000). Geller et al. (1998a) conducted a randomized trial of lithium for adolescents with bipolar disorder and secondary substance abuse and found that lithium was significantly more efficacious than placebo for both bipolar disorder and substance abuse. Geller et al. (1998b) found no significant differences in treatment outcomes between lithium and placebo in a double-blind trial of prepubertal major depression. In an open study of lithium for bipolar depression in adolescents with bipolar I disorder, investigators found a large effect size and noted response and remission rates of 48% and 30%, respectively (Patel et al. 2006). Findling et al. (2005) conducted a randomized, double-blind maintenance trial of lithium versus divalproex in children 5–17 years of age who were initially stabilized for mania/hypomania on a combination of lithium and divalproex. They observed similar time to relapse with both treatments.

Saliva and serum lithium levels have been correlated in children receiving lithium maintenance treatment, and monitoring of saliva levels may someday play a role in monitoring lithium levels (Spencer et al. 1990). After weight and serum lithium levels were controlled for, younger age is associated with more side effects (Campbell et al. 1991).

The Elderly

S.T. Chen et al. (1999) retrospectively assessed the response of patients at least 55 years old with mania to either lithium or valproate. Overall, significantly more patients improved with lithium, especially in cases of classic mania, whereas the two drugs had similar results when considering only the cases of mixed mania. They also found the therapeutic range for elderly patients to be similar to that for younger adults: ≥ 0.8 mmol/L.

Despite possibly greater efficacy, lithium may cause more side effects and be more costly in the elderly. Although a year's supply of lithium costs less than divalproex, these savings were offset by higher annual laboratory costs (Conney and Kaston 1999). The lithium group also experienced more adverse events, further increasing medical expenditures. Elderly patients with neurological or other medical conditions may respond less well to and experience more side effects from lithium than from anticonvulsant mood stabilizers (McDonald and Nemeroff 1996). Elderly patients may respond less well to lithium augmentation for refractory unipolar depression, and older age may predict increased incidence of side effects (Flint and Rifat 1994). On the basis of pharmacokinetic differences, Hardy et al. (1987) suggested that elderly patients may require up to one-third or one-half less lithium than younger patients. However, Slater et al. (1984) did not find a correlation between age and required lithium dosage in adults.

Medical comorbidity may be a consideration in elderly patients. Volume depletion, use of nonsteroidal anti-inflammatory drugs, and use of thiazide diuretics can increase lithium levels (Stoudemire et al. 1990). Also, patients with kidney disease receiving hemodialysis do not eliminate lithium other than through dialysis. Lithium should only be given after a dialysis treatment and need not be given daily (Stoudemire et al. 1990).

Lithium appears to have neuroprotective effects, decreasing oxidative damage, and could play a role in the prevention of neurocognitive decline in aging, although

the clinical implications of this remain to be determined (Bachmann et al. 2005; Cui et al. 2007; Shao et al. 2005; Tsaltas et al. 2007). Animal models suggest lithium may prevent Alzheimer's disease by inhibition of GSK-3 and its effect on tau protein phosphorylation and role in neurofibrillary tangle formation (Engle et al. 2006; Phiel et al. 2003; Su et al. 2004; Yoshida et al. 2006). In addition to neuroprotective effects, lithium appears to exert neurotrophic factors and aid in neurogenesis as demonstrated in animal models (G. Chen et al. 2000).

Pregnant/Lactating Women

The risks and benefits of lithium treatment must be carefully assessed in the context of pregnancy and breast feeding. Data suggest that lithium exposure during pregnancy is less harmful than experts believed in past decades. In an analysis of published studies of lithium exposure during pregnancy, the association between lithium use and teratogenicity appeared weaker than was assumed in the 1970s (L.S. Cohen et al. 1994). Ebstein's anomaly, a cardiac malformation, was in the past thought to be a relatively high risk of lithium use in the first trimester of pregnancy (Weinstein and Goldfield 1975). In Ebstein's anomaly, a dysplastic tricuspid valve may yield tricuspid regurgitation, and clinical manifestations include cyanosis and atrial tachyarrhythmias. The condition can be surgically treated. In fact, although the overall risk of Ebstein's anomaly may be higher with lithium use than without, because the condition is quite rare in the general population (1 per 20,000 live births), prevalence associated with lithium use is still low. First-trimester exposure to lithium results in 0.05%–0.1% prevalence of Ebstein's anomaly, and relative risk is 10–20 compared with the general population (L.S. Cohen and Rosenbaum 1998). By comparison, this risk is substantially lower than the risk of neural tube defects with some anticonvulsants used for mood stabilization.

Many mood stabilizers are potentially teratogenic (see Llewellyn et al. 1998). For example, up to 5% prevalence of neural tube defects or other neurological problems is reported with valproate exposure during the first trimester (Viguera and Cohen 1998). Reports have suggested that overall lithium is not a high-risk teratogen. For example, in a prospective study of women who took lithium during the first trimester ($N = 148$) and control subjects matched for age, rates of major malformations did not differ between the lithium and control groups (2.8% and 2.4%, respectively), although women in the lithium group were significantly more likely to be smokers (Jacobson et al.

1992). The authors concluded that pregnant women with mood disorders may continue taking lithium, provided that adequate screening of level II ultrasounds and fetal echocardiography are performed. Maternal serum α-fetoprotein screening is also recommended for women taking mood stabilizers during pregnancy (American Psychiatric Association 2002). Also, in a cohort study ($N = 350$), 7% of the women who used lithium early in pregnancy had infants with cardiac defects, although none had Ebstein's anomaly (Kallen and Tandberg 1983). However, there was no statistically significant difference between delivery outcome with lithium and that with other psychotropics.

Lithium today is considered a first-line alternative for the treatment of bipolar disorder during pregnancy. However, many women may want to discontinue psychotropic medications during pregnancy. Viguera et al. (2000) found that rates of relapse were similar in pregnant and nonpregnant women but higher in the postpartum period. During the postpartum period, significantly more women experienced a relapse after lithium discontinuation (followed by 40 weeks of euthymia) compared with nonpregnant patients matched for time after discontinuation (70% vs. 24%). Despite continued treatment with lithium, three of nine (33%) women who were maintained on lithium during pregnancy experienced a relapse postpartum, underscoring the high risk of postpartum relapse in women with bipolar disorder. This high risk has led to experts in the field recommending prophylactic treatment with a mood stabilizer for postpartum women (L.S. Cohen et al. 1995). Newport et al. (2005) studied lithium levels in maternal blood and umbilical cord blood and found that lithium equilibrates across the placenta. They observed that infants with higher lithium levels experienced more neonatal complications and suggested withholding lithium therapy 24–48 hours before an anticipated delivery to minimize risk to the baby.

Despite a general paucity of documented adverse effects to breast-feeding infants of mothers taking lithium, the American Academy of Pediatrics has contraindicated lithium use in breast-feeding women (Chaudron and Jefferson 2000). As reviewed by Chaudron and Jefferson (2000), lithium is passed on to breast-feeding infants and is found in breast milk and infant serum. Concentration in breast milk ranges from 24% to 72% of maternal serum concentration. A wide range of infant serum levels has been reported (5%–200% of mother's level), and two cases of adverse events in breast-feeding infants have been published. Burt et al. (2001) found documentation of only 13 infants exposed to lithium in breast milk—4 had no adverse effects; clinical status was not reported for

8; and 1 infant who was exposed both in utero and while breast feeding had serious adverse reactions, including cyanosis, heart murmur, and hypotonia (Tunnessen and Hertz 1972). Viguera et al. (2007) recently assessed babies who were breast fed while their mothers were treated with lithium monotherapy for bipolar disorder. They assessed 10 mother–baby pairs. Serum lithium levels in the babies ranged from 0.09 to 0.3 mEq/L (mean 0.16). Transient elevations in infant thyroid-stimulating hormone (TSH), blood urea nitrogen (BUN), and creatinine level were observed without evident long-term effects. They recommended that breast feeding in the context of lithium therapy may be considered reasonable for a healthy infant when the mother's bipolar disorder is clinically stable, lithium monotherapy or a simple medication regimen is being utilized, and the pediatrician supports breast feeding while the mother is treated with lithium. They recommend monitoring of serum lithium, TSH, BUN, and creatinine level in the infant immediately postpartum, 4–6 weeks after delivery, and then every 8–12 weeks while the mother is breast feeding.

Side Effects and Toxicology

> Psychological issues ultimately proved far more important than side effects in my prolonged resistance to lithium. I simply did not want to believe that I needed to take medication. I had become addicted to my high moods…. I couldn't give them up. (Jamison 1995, pp. 98–99)

Laboratory Monitoring

Before lithium therapy is started, medical history should be obtained, as well as baseline renal laboratory tests (BUN, creatinine level), thyroid function tests, and an electrocardiogram for patients older than 40 years (American Psychiatric Association 2002). The American Psychiatric Association practice guideline suggests that renal function should be assessed every 2–3 months and thyroid function tested once or twice during the first 6 months of treatment. After the first 6 months, renal laboratory tests and thyroid function tests should be monitored every 6–12 months or whenever clinically indicated (American Psychiatric Association 2002).

Side Effects

Cognitive side effects and weight gain have been reported to be the most disturbing side effects to patients receiving lithium maintenance treatment, whereas self-reported noncompliance was mostly associated with effects on cognition and coordination (Gitlin et al. 1989). Weight gain may be a greater risk for patients who are obese before commencement of lithium treatment, compared with normal-weight individuals (Bowden et al. 2006). Keck et al. (1996) reported that 64% of the patients hospitalized for bipolar disorder were noncompliant within the month prior to admission. Lack of compliance was associated with mania severity and polypharmacy (Keck et al. 1996). Most patients who receive treatment with lithium will experience signs or symptoms of toxicity at some time (Groleau 1994). However, a minority (27.8%) of patients with excessive levels of lithium (≥ 1.5 mmol/L) manifested symptoms of toxicity when hospitalized (Webb et al. 2001). Women and the elderly were most likely to have excessive levels.

Neurotoxicity

Neurotoxicity, delirium, and encephalopathy have been reported with lithium use. Specific populations have been noted to be at higher risk. Also, certain circumstances such as concomitant ECT or other psychotropics—especially neuroleptics—have been implicated in increasing the risk of such adverse effects of lithium treatment. West and Meltzer (1979) reported five cases in which patients experienced severe neurotoxic reactions, with lithium levels ranging from 0.75 to 1.7 mEq/L, and suggested that those with greater levels of psychotic symptomatology and anxiety may be at higher risk for neurotoxic reactions.

Neurotoxic reactions are potentially irreversible. Permanent neurological deficits have been reported after episodes of lithium intoxication (Apte and Langston 1983; Donaldson and Cuningham 1983). These have included deficits in recent memory, ataxia, and movement disorders. Early hemodialysis may help prevent permanent sequelae. Donaldson and Cuningham (1983) also reported persistent neurological sequelae of lithium toxicity involving multiple sites within the nervous system. Himmelhoch et al. (1980) found a greater incidence of neurotoxicity secondary to lithium treatment in the elderly. Squire et al. (1980) reported that lithium treatment may adversely affect fine motor skills. In a double-blind, placebo-controlled crossover study ($N=16$), patients were given lithium or placebo for 2 weeks after a washout period and were then crossed over to placebo or lithium, respectively. Neuropsychiatric test results showed a slowing of performance rate. Stoll et al. (1996) reported a case series in which 7 patients who experienced lithium-associated cognitive deficits improved when switched to treatment with divalproex sodium.

Productivity and Creativity

Reports on the effects of lithium on associative productivity and creativity are inconsistent. Shaw et al. (1986) assessed 28 outpatients receiving chronic lithium treatment. Euthymic patients who had received chronic lithium treatment completed a protocol consisting of 2 weeks of lithium treatment and 2 weeks of placebo. Patients had been treated with lithium for an average of 9.4 years and had average lithium levels of 0.80±0.23 mEq/L. During the lithium phase of the study, patients had significantly lower mean associations and lower idiosyncratic associations compared with the placebo phase. Kocsis et al. (1993) also found lower associative productivity in patients during lithium treatment when compared with placebo. However, an anecdotal report by Schou (1979) did not indicate a negative effect of lithium on creativity and productivity. In a study of 24 bipolar artists treated with lithium, 12 reported increased artistic productivity, 6 reported unaltered productivity, and 6 reported lowered artistic productivity.

Tremor

A fine postural tremor affects between 4% and 65% of the patients who receive lithium (Gelenberg and Jefferson 1995). The tremor may decrease with time; a severe tremor may indicate toxicity. Elimination of caffeine may actually worsen tremor because renal lithium clearance can be reduced with reduction of caffeine intake (Jefferson 1988). Lithium tremor, which resembles essential tremor, may worsen with age.

Thyroid Function

In a chart review of 135 patients who received maintenance treatment with lithium, 38% were found to have abnormal thyroid function tests (thyroid-stimulating hormone and/or free thyroxine index), with an association between these laboratory abnormalities and length of time on lithium (Fagiolini et al. 2006). In another retrospective study of 209 patients who received lithium, Kirov (1998) found that 14.9% of the females and 3.4% of the males developed hypothyroidism. Female patients and those older than 50 years were more likely to develop hypothyroidism. Some reports suggested that clinical hypothyroidism with lithium use may not exceed the prevalence in the general population (Bocchetta et al.

2001). Other reports suggested that subclinical hypothyroidism is more frequent (Lombardi et al. 1993). A family history of thyroid disease may lead to earlier onset of hypothyroidism that occurs with lithium use (Kusalic and Engelsmann 1999). Haggerty et al. (1990) found that the rate of antithyroid antibodies in patients with mood disorders is unrelated to lithium exposure.

Renal Complications

Lithium treatment may lead to renal tubular damage, although clinically significant renal morbidity is rare (Gitlin 1999). Risk factors for lithium-related renal complications include polypharmacy, episodes of lithium intoxication, and concurrent medical illnesses (Gitlin 1999). Patients taking lithium may experience polyuria as a result of impairment in renal concentrating ability. Although uncommon, renal structural changes are possible (Gitlin 1999). Diabetes insipidus, caused by unresponsiveness of the kidneys to antidiuretic hormone, occurs in approximately 10% of the patients who receive long-term lithium therapy (Bendz and Aurell 1999). Treatment for diabetes insipidus may include thiazides or amiloride.

Acute renal failure after lithium intoxication has been reported (Fenves et al. 1984). Acute lithium intoxication may result in histopathological kidney changes, but little change is seen in patients without acute episodes of lithium intoxication, and glomerular function and renal clearance are preserved during long-term treatment with therapeutic dosages (Hetmar 1988). Renal function may be evaluated by measuring serum creatinine every 2–3 months initially and then annually or semiannually in stable patients (American Psychiatric Association 2002). In an assessment of 207 patients treated with lithium (between 1 and 30 years), no cases of renal insufficiency were observed (Kallner and Petterson 1995). Studies in rats have indicated that dietary potassium supplementation may reduce the risk of renal insults.

Cardiac Changes

Lithium intoxication has been reported to cause cardiac alterations, including sinus bradycardia and sinus node dysfunction (Steckler 1994). Sinus node dysfunction is more prevalent in patients who have been taking lithium for at least a year when compared with age-matched control subjects, although clinically significant dysfunction is uncommon (Rosenqvist et al. 1993). Also, cases of atrioventricular block in patients treated with therapeutic lithium levels have been reported (Martin and Piascik 1985). Electrocardiographic T wave changes, as well as ventricular irritability, may occur (Mitchell and Mackenzie 1982). In healthy male volunteers, administration of lithium was shown to cause a reduction in T wave amplitude without clinically significant effects on cardiac function (Dumovic et al. 1980). In patients with clinical indications for lithium use, cardiovascular disease does not preclude the possibility of lithium use. Dosage adjustment and frequent cardiac monitoring are essential for the safe use of lithium in patients with cardiac disease (Tilkian et al. 1976). Because of the risk of sinus node dysfunction and other cardiac effects, careful monitoring of the pulse and electrocardiographic monitoring are recommended in patients older than 50 years (Roose et al. 1979).

Sexual Functioning

Aizenberg et al. (1996) assessed sexual function in euthymic male patients ($N = 35$) with bipolar or schizoaffective disorder who received treatment with lithium monotherapy. Sexual side effects most frequently reported were reduced sexual thoughts (22.9%), diminished waking erections (17.1%), and loss of erections during coitus (20%). Lithium levels were unrelated to levels of sexual satisfaction. Cases have been reported of decreased libido and erectile dysfunction associated with lithium use (Blay et al. 1982). However, Ghadirian et al. (1992) found that sexual side effects with lithium were related to concomitant benzodiazepine use. A conceivable mechanism for sexual effects of lithium may be increased serotonergic neurotransmission (Price et al. 1989).

Drug–Drug Interactions

Lithium and Other Mood Stabilizers

Polypharmacy is common in the treatment of bipolar disorder, and lithium is commonly used in combination with other mood stabilizers. Multiple mood stabilizers can be synergistic, but polypharmacy may introduce an increased risk of adverse reactions (Freeman and Stoll 1998; Lenox et al. 1996). The combination of lithium and valproate is a strategy in the treatment of mania refractory to monotherapy with either lithium or valproate (Frances et al. 1996). Double-blind, placebo-controlled data support that lithium plus valproate is more effective in relapse prevention than lithium alone (Solomon et al. 1997). The combination appears to confer benefit in mania, bipolar depression, and rapid cycling (Mitchell et al. 1994; Schaff et al. 1993; Sharma and Persad 1992; Sharma et al. 1993). Interactions may include additive side effects, such as sedation, tremor, or weight gain, but the pharmacokinetics of lithium are not altered by the addition of valproate (Granneman et al. 1996).

Lithium and carbamazepine also have been combined for bipolar disorder refractory to lithium alone (Frances et al. 1996) and may confer a more rapid antimanic effect than lithium alone for some patients (Di Costanzo and Schifano 1991; Kramlinger and Post 1989). This combination is better tolerated than and at least as effective as the combination of lithium and a typical antipsychotic (Shukla et al. 1985; Small et al. 1995). The combination also may work synergistically in the prophylaxis of mood episodes (Kishimoto 1992). Neurotoxicity, especially in patients with central nervous system deficits, may be an increased risk with the combination of lithium and carbamazepine (Chaudhry and Waters 1983; Shukla et al. 1984). Neurotoxic and other adverse reactions have been associated with the concomitant administration of lithium with calcium channel blockers (Dubovsky et al. 1987; Finley et al. 1995; Helmuth et al. 1989; Wright and Jarrett 1991).

Although many investigators have reported the safe and efficacious results of combining lithium and typical antipsychotics (Baastrup et al. 1976; Bigelow et al. 1981; Carman et al. 1981; Garfinkel et al. 1980; Ghadirian et al. 1989; Goldney and Spence 1986; Juhl et al. 1977; Krishna et al. 1978; Loew 1986; Miller and Menninger 1987; Perenyi et al. 1983), use of lithium with "typicals" may increase the occurrence of side effects, including neurotoxicity and even tardive dyskinesia (Byrne et al. 1994; W.J. Cohen and Cohen 1974; Dinan and Kohen 1989; Loudon and Waring 1976; Mani et al. 1996; Mann et al. 1983; Marhold et al. 1974; Menes et al. 1980; Miller et al. 1986; Perenyi et al. 1984; Spring 1979; Spring and Frankel 1981). Goodwin and Jamison (1990) recommended that when incorporating a typical antipsychotic into a regimen of lithium therapy, the antipsychotic should be used in lower doses and the lithium levels should be maintained below 1.0 mEq/L.

The use of lithium with atypical antipsychotics also may result in adverse reactions. Clozapine and lithium, when used concomitantly, have been reported to be efficacious for refractory bipolar disorder (Fuchs 1994; Puri et al. 1995; Suppes et al. 1994), but adverse reactions, including diabetic ketoacidosis, neuroleptic malignant syndrome, and neurological side effects, also have been reported (Blake et al. 1992; G. Garcia et al. 1994; Lemus et al. 1989; Peterson and Byrd 1996; Pope et al. 1986). Some investigators have reported safe and effective use of risperidone and lithium (Ghaemi et al. 1997; Tohen et al.

1996), although adverse effects, including fever, increased white blood cell counts and creatine phosphokinase levels, and delirium, also have been reported (B. Chen and Cardasis 1996; Swanson et al. 1995).

Preliminary data suggest that the combination of lithium and olanzapine is efficacious and well tolerated in acute mania (Madhusoodanan et al. 2000; Sanger et al. 2001). Gabapentin is also used adjunctively in the treatment of bipolar disorder, and because gabapentin has no known drug interactions, it is likely safe with lithium use (Frye et al. 1998; Vollmer et al. 1986). Benzodiazepines are not especially problematic when used with lithium. Sachs et al. (1990a, 1990b) reported that benzodiazepines can be used successfully instead of antipsychotic medications in some patients with bipolar disorder. Others have shown that clonazepam and lorazepam are efficacious and well tolerated with lithium in the treatment of acute mania (Adler 1986; Modell et al. 1985).

Lithium and Antidepressants

Lithium is often used concomitantly with antidepressants in the treatment of bipolar depression and refractory unipolar depression. Serotonin syndrome—a constellation of mental status and behavioral changes (either agitation or sedation), motor symptoms (restlessness, weakness, hyperreflexia, or ataxia), and autonomic dysfunction (nausea and/or vomiting, dizziness, sweating, fever) (Lejoyeux et al. 1994)—has been reported with the use of lithium and serotonergic antidepressants, including fluoxetine (Karle and Bjorndal 1995; Muly et al. 1993), paroxetine (Sobanski et al. 1997), venlafaxine (Mekler and Woggon 1997), and fluvoxamine (Ohman and Spigset 1993). Retrospective evaluation of clinical records by Fagiolini et al. (2001) suggested the development of serotonin syndrome in 4 of 17 (24%) patients receiving the combination of lithium and paroxetine.

Lithium and Electroconvulsive Therapy

Patients who undergo concurrent ECT and lithium treatment may experience neurotoxic reactions, which include delirium and memory deficits (Ayd 1981; DePaulo et al. 1982; El-Mallakh 1988; Jefferson et al. 1987; Mielke et al. 1984). Additionally, Small et al. (1980) retrospectively compared adverse reactions of patients who received concurrent lithium and ECT with those of patients who received ECT alone. The group that received both ECT and lithium experienced more memory loss than did the group undergoing ECT without lithium treatment. However, Himmelhoch and Neil (1980) found similar outcomes in 21 patients receiving ECT and lithium and in age- and sex-matched control subjects receiving ECT alone. They did not find differences in adverse reactions, including post-ECT confusion. To minimize adverse reactions, Ayd (1981) recommended that lithium be discontinued at least 2 days prior to ECT and restarted 2–3 days after the last treatment.

Lithium and Nonpsychotropic Medications

When lithium is used with concurrent nonsteroidal anti-inflammatory drugs, signs and symptoms of toxicity and lithium levels must be monitored more carefully because nonsteroidal anti-inflammatory drugs increase the risk of toxicity (Johnson et al. 1993). Because lithium excretion relies on renal clearance, diuretic medications may affect lithium levels, depending on their site of action. Thiazide diuretics trigger a compensatory increase in reabsorption in the proximal tubule and lead to elevations in lithium levels, whereas loop diuretics do not promote lithium reabsorption and do not greatly affect lithium levels (Finley et al. 1995). Osmotic diuretics enhance lithium excretion and may serve to counteract lithium toxicity, and either no change or a slight increase in lithium levels has been reported with potassium-sparing diuretics. Angiotensin-converting enzyme inhibitors may raise lithium levels (DasGupta et al. 1992; Finley et al. 1996). Serum lithium levels may increase in the context of sodium restriction (Bennett 1997).

Conclusion

Lithium is an important option in the evidence-based rational treatment of bipolar disorder. Bipolar disorder is a mental illness that affects between 1% and 5% of the population (Akiskal et al. 2000). Bipolar disorder causes significant morbidity and mortality, and the diagnosis of bipolar disorder carries a high risk for suicide. Of patients with bipolar disorder, 25%–50% attempt suicide and an estimated 19% complete suicide (Goodwin and Jamison 1990).

Lithium has been shown to be effective for acute mania and bipolar depression and as a prophylactic treatment for bipolar disorder. Some data suggest that conditions such as comorbid neurological illness and mixed episodes favor other mood stabilizers rather than lithium. Evidence also suggests that lithium can play a role in the treatment of refractory unipolar depression, aggression, and personality disorders. Lithium may be less risky than anticonvulsants in pregnancy. We seek new treatments in our field and hope that they will be more efficacious and better tolerated than our "old" medications. At present, lithium remains an important treatment option.

References

Adler LW: Mixed bipolar disorder responsive to lithium and clonazepam. J Clin Psychiatry 47:49–50, 1986

Aherns B, Muller-Oerlinghausen B: Does lithium exert an independent antisuicidal effect? Pharmacopsychiatry 34:132–136, 2001

Aizenberg D, Sigler M, Zemishlani Z, et al: Lithium and male sexual function in affective patients. Clin Neuropharmacol 19:515–519, 1996

Akiskal HS, Bourgeois ML, Angst J, et al: Re-evaluating the prevalence of and diagnostic composition within the broad clinical spectrum of bipolar disorders. J Affect Disord 59 (suppl):S5–S30, 2000

American Psychiatric Association: Diagnostic and Statistical Manual of Mental Disorders, 3rd Edition. Washington, DC, American Psychiatric Association, 1980

American Psychiatric Association: Practice guideline for the treatment of patients with bipolar disorder (revision). Am J Psychiatry 159 (suppl):1–50, 2002

Apte SN, Langston JW: Permanent neurological deficits due to lithium toxicity. Ann Neurol 13:453–455, 1983

Austin MPV, Souza FGM, Goodwin GM: Lithium augmentation in antidepressant-resistant patients: a quantitative analysis. Br J Psychiatry 159:510–514, 1991

Ayd FJ: Lithium-ECT induced cerebral toxicity. Int Drug Ther Newsl 16:21–23, 1981

Baastrup PC, Hollnagel P, Sorensen R, et al: Adverse reactions in treatment with lithium carbonate and haloperidol. JAMA 236:2645–2646, 1976

Bachmann RF, Schloesser RJ, Gould TD, et al: Mood stabilizers target cellular plasticity and resilience cascades: implications for the development of novel therapeutics. Mol Neurobiol 32:173–202, 2005

Baldessarini RJ: Drugs and the treatment of psychiatric disorders: depression and mania, in Goodman and Gilman's The Pharmacological Basis of Therapeutics, 9th Edition. Edited by Hardman JG, Limbird LE. New York, McGraw-Hill, 1996, pp 431–459

Baldessarini RJ, Tarazi FI: Drugs and the treatment of psychiatric disorders: psychosis and mania, in Goodman and Gilman's The Pharmacological Basis of Therapeutics, 10th Edition. Edited by Hardman JG, Limbird LE. New York, McGraw-Hill, 2001, pp 485–520

Baldessarini RJ, Tondo L: Does lithium treatment still work? Evidence of stable responses over three decades. Arch Gen Psychiatry 57:187–190, 2000

Baldessarini RJ, Tondo L, Viguera A: Discontinuing lithium maintenance treatment in bipolar disorders: risks and implications. Bipolar Disord 1:17–24, 1999

Baldessarini RJ, Tondo L, Davis P, et al: Decreased risk of suicides and attempts during long-term lithium treatment: a meta-analytic review. Bipolar Disord 5:625–639, 2006

Barkai IA, Dunner DL, Gross HA, et al: Reduced myo-inositol levels in cerebrospinal fluid from patients with affective disorder. Biol Psychiatry 13:65–72, 1978

Baron M, Gerson ES, Rudy V, et al: Lithium carbonate response in depression: prediction by unipolar/bipolar illness, average-evoked response, catechol-O-methyl transferase, and family history. Arch Gen Psychiatry 32:1107–1111, 1975

Baumann P, Nil R, Souche A, et al: A double-blind, placebo-controlled study of citalopram with and without lithium in the treatment of therapy-resistant depressive patients: a clinical, pharmacokinetic, and pharmacogenetic investigation. J Clin Psychopharmacol 16:307–314, 1996

Belmaker RH, Bersudsky Y, Agam G, et al: How does lithium work on manic depression? Clinical and psychological correlates of the inositol theory. Annu Rev Med 47:47–56, 1996

Bendz H, Aurell M: Drug-induced diabetes insipidus: incidence, prevention and management. Drug Saf 21:449–456, 1999

Benjamin J, Levine J, Fux M, et al: Inositol treatment for panic disorder: a double-blind placebo-controlled crossover trial. Am J Psychiatry 152:1084–1086, 1995

Bennett WM: Drug interactions and consequences of sodium restriction. Am J Clin Nutr 65:678–681, 1997

Berrettini WH, Nurnberger JI Jr, Hare T, et al: Reduced plasma and CSF γ-aminobutyric acid in affective illness: effect of lithium carbonate. Biol Psychiatry 18:185–194, 1983

Berrettini WH, Nurnberger JI Jr, Hare T, et al: CSF GABA in euthymic manic-depressive patients and controls. Biol Psychiatry 21:842–844, 1986

Berridge MJ, Downes CP, Hanley RR: Neural and developmental action of lithium: a unifying hypothesis. Cell 59:411–419, 1989

Bersudsky Y, Vinnitsky I, Grisaru N, et al: The effect of inositol on lithium-induced polyuria-polydipsia in rats and humans. Hum Psychopharmacol 7:403–407, 1993

Bigelow LB, Weinberger DR, Wyatt RJ: Synergism of combined lithium-neuroleptic therapy: a double-blind, placebo-controlled case study. Am J Psychiatry 138:81–83, 1981

Birch NJ, Greenfield AA, Hullin RP: Pharmacodynamic aspects of long-term prophylactic lithium. Int Pharmacopsychiatry 15:91–98, 1980

Black DW, Winokur G, Nasrallah A: Treatment of mania: a naturalistic study of electroconvulsive therapy versus lithium in 438 patients. J Clin Psychiatry 48:132–139, 1987

Blake LM, Marks RC, Luchins DJ: Reversible neurologic symptoms with clozapine and lithium. J Clin Psychopharmacol 12:297–299, 1992

Blay SL, Ferraz MP, Calil HM: Lithium-induced male sexual impairment: two case reports. J Clin Psychiatry 43:497–498, 1982

Bocchetta A, Mossa P, Velluzzi F, et al: Ten-year follow-up of thyroid function in lithium patients. J Clin Psychopharmacol 21:594–598, 2001

Bowden CL, Brugger AM, Swann AC, et al: Efficacy of divalproex vs lithium and placebo in the treatment of acute mania. JAMA 271:918–924, 1994

Bowden CL, Calabrese JR, McElroy SL, et al: A randomized, placebo-controlled 12-month trial of divalproex and lithium in treatment of outpatients with bipolar I disorder. Arch Gen Psychiatry 57:481–489, 2000

Bowden CL, Grunze H, Mullen J, et al: A randomized, double-blind, placebo-controlled efficacy and safety study of quetiapine or lithium as monotherapy for mania in bipolar disorder. J Clin Psychiatry 66:111–121, 2005

Bowden CL, Calabrese JR, Ketter KA, et al: Impact of lamotrigine and lithium on weight in obese and nonobese patients with bipolar I disorder. Am J Psychiatry 163:1199–1201, 2006

Brockington IF, Kendell RE, Kellett JM, et al: Trials of lithium, chlorpromazine and amitriptyline in schizoaffective patients. Br J Psychiatry 133:162–168, 1978

Burt VK, Suri R, Altshuler L, et al: The use of psychotropic medications during breast-feeding. Am J Psychiatry 158:1001–1009, 2001

Byrne A, Zibin T, Chimich W, et al: Severe hypotension associated with combined lithium and chlorpromazine therapy: a case report and a review. Can J Psychiatry 39:294–296, 1994

Cade JF: Lithium salts in the treatment of psychotic excitement. Med J Aust 36:349–352, 1949

Calabrese JR, Shelton MD, Rapport DJ, et al: A 20-month, double-blind, maintenance trial of lithium versus divalproex in rapid-cycling bipolar disorder. Am J Psychiatry 162:2152–2161, 2005

Campbell M, Silva RR, Kafantaris V, et al: Predictors of side effects associated with lithium administration in children. Psychopharmacol Bull 27:373–380, 1991

Campbell M, Adams PB, Small AM, et al: Lithium in hospitalized aggressive children with conduct disorder: a double-blind and placebo-controlled study. J Am Acad Child Adolesc Psychiatry 34:445–453, 1995

Carman JS, Bigelow LB, Wyatt RJ: Lithium combined with neuroleptics in chronic schizophrenic and schizoaffective patients. J Clin Psychiatry 42:124–128, 1981

Chaudhry RP, Waters BG: Lithium and carbamazepine interaction: possible neurotoxicity. J Clin Psychiatry 44:30–31, 1983

Chaudron LH, Jefferson JW: Mood stabilizers during breastfeeding: a review. J Clin Psychiatry 61:79–90, 2000

Chen B, Cardasis W: Delirium induced by lithium and risperidone combination. Am J Psychiatry 153:1233–1234, 1996

Chen G, Huang LD, Jiang YM, et al: The mood stabilizing agent valproate inhibits the activity of glycogen synthase kinase 3. J Neurochem 72:1327–1330, 1999

Chen G, Rajkowska G, Du F, et al: Enhancement of hippocampal neurogenesis by lithium. J Neurochem 75:1729–1734, 2000

Chen ST, Altshuler LL, Melnyk KA, et al: Efficacy of lithium vs valproate in the treatment of mania in the elderly: a retrospective study. J Clin Psychiatry 60:181–186, 1999

Chisholm D, van Ommeren M, Ayuso-Mateos JL, et al: Cost-effectiveness of clinical interventions for reducing the global burden of bipolar disorder. Br J Psychiatry 187:559–567, 2005

Cohen LS, Rosenbaum JF: Psychotropic drug use during pregnancy: weighing the risks. J Clin Psychiatry 59:18–28, 1998

Cohen LS, Friedman JM, Jefferson JW, et al: A reevaluation of risk of in utero exposure to lithium. JAMA 271:146–150, 1994

Cohen LS, Sichel DA, Robertson LM, et al: Postpartum prophylaxis for women with bipolar disorder. Am J Psychiatry 152:1641–1645, 1995

Cohen WJ, Cohen NH: Lithium carbonate, haloperidol, and irreversible brain damage. JAMA 230:1283–1287, 1974

Compton MT, Nemeroff CB: The treatment of bipolar depression. J Clin Psychiatry 61 (suppl):57–67, 2000

Conney J, Kaston B: Pharmacoeconomic and health outcome comparison of lithium and divalproex in a VA geriatric nursing home population: influence of drug-related morbidity on total cost of treatment. Am J Manag Care 5:197–204, 1999

Coryell W, Arndt S, Turvey C, et al: Lithium and suicidal behavior in major affective disorder: a case-control study. Acta Psychiatr Scand 104:193–197, 2001

Cotter D, Kerwin R, al-Sarraji S, et al: Abnormalities of Wnt signaling in schizophrenia: evidence for neurodevelopmental abnormality. Neuroreport 9:1379–1383, 1998

Craft M, Ismail IA, Krishnamurti D, et al: Lithium in the treatment of aggression in mentally handicapped patients: a double-blind trial. Br J Psychiatry 150:685–689, 1987

Cui J, Shao L, Young LT, Wang JF: Role of glutathione in neuroprotective effects of mood stabilizing drugs lithium and valproate. Neuroscience 144:1447–1453, 2007

DasGupta K, Jefferson JW, Kobak KA, et al: The effect of enalapril on serum lithium levels in healthy men. J Clin Psychiatry 53:398–400, 1992

De Montigny C, Grunberg F, Mayer A, et al: Lithium induces rapid relief of depression in tricyclic antidepressant drug non-responders. Br J Psychiatry 138:252–256, 1981

De Montigny C, Cournoyer G, Morissette R, et al: Lithium carbonate addition in tricyclic antidepressant-resistant unipolar depression: correlations with the neurobiologic actions of tricyclic antidepressant drugs and lithium ion on the serotonin system. Arch Gen Psychiatry 40:11327–11334, 1983

De Montigny C, Elie R, Caille G: Rapid response to the addition of lithium in iprindole-resistant unipolar depression: a pilot study. Am J Psychiatry 142:220–223, 1985

DeMet E, Chicz-DeMet A: Effects of psychoactive drugs on circadian rhythms. Psychiatr Ann 17:682–688, 1987

Denicoff KD, Smith-Jackson EE, Disney ER, et al: Comparative prophylactic effect of lithium, carbamazepine, and the combination in bipolar disorder. J Clin Psychiatry 58:470–478, 1997

DePaulo JR, Folstein MF, Correa EI: The course of delirium due to lithium intoxication. J Clin Psychiatry 43:447–449, 1982

Di Costanzo E, Schifano F: Lithium alone or in combination with carbamazepine for the treatment of rapid-cycling bipolar affective disorder. Acta Psychiatr Scand 83:456–459, 1991

Dinan T: Lithium augmentation in sertraline-resistant depression: a preliminary dose-response study. Acta Psychiatr Scand 88:300–301, 1993

Dinan T, Kohen D: Tardive dyskinesia in bipolar affective disorder: relationship to lithium therapy. Br J Psychiatry 155:55–57, 1989

Dixon JF, Hokin LE: Lithium acutely inhibits and chronically up-regulates and stabilizes glutamate uptake by presynaptic nerve endings in mouse cerebral cortex. Proc Natl Acad Sci U S A 95:8363–8368, 1998

Donaldson IM, Cuningham J: Persisting neurologic sequela of lithium carbonate therapy. Arch Neurol 40:747–751, 1983

Donnelly EF, Goodwin FK, Waldman IN, et al: Prediction of antidepressant responses to lithium. Am J Psychiatry 135:552–556, 1978

Drevets WC, Price JL, Simpson JR Jr, et al: Subgenual prefrontal cortex abnormalities in mood disorders. Nature 38:824–827, 1997

Dubovsky SL, Franks RD, Allen S: Verapamil: a new antimanic drug with potential interactions with lithium. J Clin Psychiatry 48:371–372, 1987

Dumovic P, Burrows GD, Chamberlain K, et al: Effect of therapeutic dosage of lithium on the heart. Br J Clin Pharmacol 9:599–604, 1980

Dunner DL, Fieve RR: Clinical factors in lithium prophylaxis failure. Arch Gen Psychiatry 30:229–233, 1974

El-Mallakh RS: Complications of concurrent lithium and electroconvulsive therapy: a review of clinical material and theoretical considerations. Biol Psychiatry 23:595–601, 1988

El-Mallakh RS, Jefferson JW: Prethymoleptic use of lithium. Am J Psychiatry 156:129, 1999

Emilien G, Maloteau JM, Seghers A, et al: Lithium compared to valproic acid and carbamazepine in the treatment of mania: a statistical meta-analysis. Eur Neuropsychopharmacol 6:245–252, 1996

Engle T, Goni-Oliver P, Lucas JJ, et al: Chronic lithium administration to FTDP-17 tau and GSK-3beta overexpressing mice prevents tau hyperphosphorylation and neurofibrillary tangle formation, but pre-formed neurofibrillary tangles do not revert. J Neurochem 99:1445–1455, 2006

Fagiolini A, Buysse DJ, Frank E, et al: Tolerability of combined treatment with lithium and paroxetine in patients with bipolar disorder and depression. J Clin Psychopharmacol 21:474–478, 2001

Fagiolini A, Kupfer DJ, Scott J, et al: Hypothyroidism in patients with bipolar I disorder treated primarily with lithium. Epidemiol Psichiatr Soc 15:123–127, 2006

Fava M, Rosenbaum JF, McGrath PJ, et al: Lithium and tricyclic augmentation of fluoxetine treatment for resistant major depression: a double-blind, controlled study. Am J Psychiatry 151:1372–1374, 1994

Feder R: Lithium augmentation of clomipramine (letter). J Clin Psychiatry 49:458, 1988

Fenves AZ, Emmett M, White MG: Lithium intoxication associated with acute renal failure. South Med J 77:1472–1474, 1984

Fieve RR, Platman SR, Plutchik RR: The use of lithium in affective disorders, I: acute endogenous depression. Am J Psychiatry 125:79–83, 1968

Findling RL, McNamara NK, Youngstrom EA, et al: Double-blind 18-month trial of lithium versus divalproex maintenance treatment in pediatric bipolar disorder. J Am Acad Child Adolesc Psychiatry 44:409–417, 2005

Finley P, Warner M, Peabody C: Clinical relevance of drug interactions with lithium. Clin Pharmacokinet 29:172–191, 1995

Finley PR, O'Brien JG, Coleman RW: Lithium and angiotensin-converting enzyme inhibitors: evaluation of a potential interaction. J Clin Psychopharmacol 16:68–71, 1996

Flint AJ, Rifat SL: A prospective study of lithium augmentation in antidepressant-resistant geriatric depression. J Clin Psychopharmacol 14:353–356, 1994

Fontaine R, Ontiveros A, Elie R, et al: Lithium carbonate augmentation of desipramine and fluoxetine in refractory depression. Biol Psychiatry 29:946–948, 1991

Forster PL, Schoenfeld FB, Marmar CR, et al: Lithium for irritability in post-traumatic stress disorder. J Trauma Stress 8:143–149, 1995

Frances A, Docherty JP, Kahn DA: Treatment of bipolar disorder. J Clin Psychiatry 57 (suppl):5–58, 1996

Franchini L, Zanardi R, Smeraldi E, et al: Early onset of lithium prophylaxis as a predictor of good long-term outcome. Eur Arch Psychiatry Clin Neurosci 249:227–230, 1999

Freeman MP, Stoll AL: Mood stabilizers in combination: a review of safety and efficacy. Am J Psychiatry 155:12–21, 1998

Frye MA, Kimbrell TA, Dunn RT, et al: Gabapentin does not alter single-dose lithium pharmacokinetics. J Clin Psychopharmacol 18:461–464, 1998

Fuchs DC: Clozapine treatment of bipolar disorder in a young adolescent. J Am Acad Child Adolesc Psychiatry 33:1299–1302, 1994

Garcia G, Crismon M, Dorson P: Seizures in two patients after the addition of lithium to a clozapine regimen. J Clin Psychopharmacol 14:426–428, 1994

Garcia PA, Burg MB: Renal medullary organic osmolytes. Physiol Rev 71:1081–1115, 1991

Garfinkel PE, Stancer HC, Persad E: A comparison of haloperidol, lithium carbonate and their combination in the treatment of mania. J Affect Disord 2:279–288, 1980

Geisler A, Wraae O, Olesen OV: Adenyl cyclase activity in kidneys of rats with lithium-induced polyuria. Acta Pharmacol Toxicol 31:203–208, 1972

Gelenberg AJ: Can lithium help to prevent suicide? (editorial) Acta Psychiatr Scand 104:161, 2001

Gelenberg AJ, Jefferson JW: Lithium tremor. J Clin Psychiatry 56:283–287, 1995

Geller B, Cooper TB, Sun K, et al: Double-blind and placebo-controlled study of lithium for adolescent bipolar disorders with secondary substance dependency. J Am Acad Child Adolesc Psychiatry 37:171–178, 1998a

Geller B, Cooper TB, Zimerman B, et al: Lithium for prepubertal depressed children with family history predictors of future bipolarity: a double-blind, placebo-controlled study. J Affect Disord 51:165–175, 1998b

Ghadirian AM, Nair NP, Schwartz G: Effect of lithium and neuroleptic combination on lithium transport, blood pressure, and weight in bipolar patients. Biol Psychiatry 26:139–144, 1989

Ghadirian AM, Annable L, Belanger MC: Lithium, benzodiazepines, and sexual function in bipolar patients. Am J Psychiatry 149:801–805, 1992

Ghaemi SN, Sachs GS, Baldassano CF, et al: Acute treatment of bipolar disorder with adjunctive risperidone in outpatients. Can J Psychiatry 42:196–199, 1997

Gitlin M: Lithium and the kidney: an updated review. Drug Saf 20:231–243, 1999

Gitlin MJ, Cochran SD, Jamison KR: Maintenance lithium treatment: side effects and compliance. J Clin Psychiatry 50:127–131, 1989

Golden RN, Morris JE, Sack DA: Combined lithium-tricyclic treatment of obsessive-compulsive disorder. Biol Psychiatry 23:181–185, 1988

Goldney RD, Spence ND: Safety of the combination of lithium and neuroleptic drugs. Am J Psychiatry 143:882–884, 1986

Gonzalez RG, Guimaraes AR, Sachs GS, et al: Measurement of human brain lithium in vivo by MR spectroscopy. Am J Neuroradiol 14:1027–1037, 1993

Goodwin FK, Jamison KR: Manic Depressive Illness. New York, Oxford University Press, 1990

Goodwin FK, Zis AP: Lithium in the treatment of mania: comparisons with neuroleptics. Arch Gen Psychiatry 36:840–844, 1979

Goodwin FK, Murphy DL, Bunny WF: Lithium carbonate treatment in depression and mania: a longitudinal double-blind study. Arch Gen Psychiatry 21:486–496, 1969

Goodwin FK, Murphy DL, Dunner DL, et al: Lithium response in unipolar versus bipolar depression. Am J Psychiatry 129:44–47, 1972

Grahame-Smith DG: Disorder of synaptic homeostasis as a cause of depression and a target for treatment, in Antidepressant Therapy at the Dawn of the Third Millennium. Edited by Briley M, Montgomery S. London, Martin Dunitz, 1998, pp 111–140

Granneman GR, Schneck DW, Cavanaugh JH, et al: Pharmacokinetic interactions and side effects resulting from concomitant administration of lithium and divalproex sodium. J Clin Psychiatry 57:204–206, 1996

Greenspan K, Schildkraut JJ, Gordon EK, et al: Catecholamine metabolism in affective disorders, III: MHPG and other catecholamine metabolites in patients treated with lithium carbonate. J Psychiatr Res 7:171–182, 1970

Groleau G: Lithium toxicity. Emerg Med Clin North Am 12:511–531, 1994

Haddjeri N, Szabo ST, De Montigny C, et al: Increased tonic activation of rat forebrain 5-HT(1A) receptors by lithium addition to antidepressant treatments. Neuropsychopharmacology 22:346–356, 2000

Haggerty JJ Jr, Evans DL, Golden RN, et al: The presence of antithyroid antibodies in patients with affective and nonaffective psychiatric disorders. Biol Psychiatry 27:51–60, 1990

Hahn CG, Umapathy, Wang HY, et al: Lithium and valproic acid treatments reduce PKC activation and receptor–G protein coupling in platelets of bipolar manic patients. J Psychiatr Res 39:355–363, 2005

Hall AC, Lucas FR, Salinas PC: Axonal remodeling and synaptic differentiation in the cerebellum is regulated by Wnt-7a signaling. Cell 100:525–535, 2000

Hallonquist JD, Goldberg MA, Brandes JS: Affective disorders and circadian rhythms. Can J Psychiatry 31:259–272, 1986

Hardy BG, Shulman KI, Mackenzie SE, et al: Pharmacokinetics of lithium in the elderly. J Clin Psychopharmacol 7:153–158, 1987

Healy D, Waterhouse JM: The circadian system and the therapeutics of the affective disorders. Pharmacol Ther 65:241–263, 1995

Heit S, Nemeroff CB: Lithium augmentation of antidepressants in treatment-refractory depression. J Clin Psychiatry 59 (suppl): 28–33, 1998

Helmuth D, Ljaljevic Z, Ramirez L, et al: Choreoathetosis induced by verapamil and lithium treatment. J Clin Psychopharmacol 9:454–455, 1989

Heninger GR, Charney DS, Sternberg DE: Lithium carbonate augmentation of antidepressant treatment. Arch Gen Psychiatry 40:1335–1342, 1983

Hetmar O: The impact of long-term lithium treatment on renal function and structure. Acta Psychiatr Scand Suppl 345:85–89, 1988

Himmelhoch JM, Neil JF: Lithium therapy in combination with other forms of treatment, in Handbook of Lithium Therapy. Edited by Johnson FN. Lancaster, England, MTP Press, 1980, pp 51–67

Himmelhoch JM, Mulla D, Neil JF, et al: Incidence and significance of mixed affective states in a bipolar population. Arch Gen Psychiatry 33:1062–1066, 1976

Himmelhoch JM, Neil JK, May SJ, et al: Age, dementia, dyskinesias, and lithium response. Am J Psychiatry 137:941–945, 1980

Hollander E, Pallanti S, Allan A, et al: Does sustained-release lithium reduce impulsive gambling and affective instability versus placebo in pathological gamblers with bipolar spectrum disorders? Am J Psychiatry 162:137–145, 2005

Ichim L, Berk M, Brook S: Lamotrigine compared with lithium in mania: a double-blind randomized controlled trial. Ann Clin Psychiatry 12:5–10, 2000

Ikonomov OC, Manji HK: Molecular mechanisms underlying mood stabilization in manic-depressive illness: the phenotype challenge. Am J Psychiatry 156:1506–1514, 1999

Jacobson SJ, Jones K, Johnson K, et al: Prospective multicentre study of pregnancy outcome after lithium exposure during first trimester. Lancet 339:530–533, 1992

Jamison KR: An Unquiet Mind. New York, Alfred A Knopf, 1995

Jefferson JW: Lithium tremor and caffeine intake: two cases of drinking less and shaking more. J Clin Psychiatry 49:72–73, 1988

Jefferson JW, Greist JH: Primer of Lithium Therapy. Baltimore, MD, Williams & Wilkins, 1977

Jefferson JW, Greist JH, Ackerman DL: Lithium Encyclopedia for Clinical Practice. Washington, DC, American Psychiatric Press, 1983

Jefferson JW, Greist JH, Ackerman DL, et al: Lithium Encyclopedia for Clinical Practice, 2nd Edition. Washington, DC, American Psychiatric Press, 1987

Jensen HV, Plenge P, Mellerup ET, et al: Lithium prophylaxis of manic-depressive disorder: daily lithium dosing schedule versus every second day. Acta Psychiatr Scand 92:69–74, 1995

Jermain DM, Crismon ML, Martin ES 3rd: Population pharmacokinetics of lithium. Clin Pharm 10:376–381, 1991

Joffe RT, Singer W, Levitt AJ, et al: A placebo-controlled comparison of lithium and triiodothyronine augmentation of tricyclic antidepressants in unipolar refractory depression. Arch Gen Psychiatry 50:387–393, 1993

Johnson AG, Seideman P, Day RO: Adverse drug interactions with nonsteroidal anti-inflammatory drugs (NSAIDs): recognition, management and avoidance. Drug Saf 8:99–127, 1993

Judd LL: Effects of lithium on mood, cognition, and personality function in normal subjects. Arch Gen Psychiatry 36:860–865, 1979

Juhl RP, Tsuang MT, Perry PJ: Concomitant administration of haloperidol and lithium carbonate in acute mania. Dis Nerv Syst 38:675–676, 1977

Kallen B, Tandberg A: Lithium and pregnancy: a cohort study on manic-depressive women. Acta Psychiatr Scand 68:134–139, 1983

Kallner G, Petterson U: Renal, thyroid and parathyroid function during lithium treatment: laboratory tests in 207 people treated for 1–30 years. Acta Psychiatr Scand 91:48–51, 1995

Kantor D, McNevin S, Leichner P, et al: The benefit of lithium carbonate adjunct in refractory depression. Am J Psychiatry 31:416–418, 1986

Karle J, Bjorndal F: Serotonergic syndrome in combination therapy with lithium and fluoxetine. Ugeskr Laeger 157:1204–1205, 1995

Katona CLE, Abou-Saleh MT, Harrison DA, et al: Placebo-controlled study of lithium augmentation of fluoxetine and lofepramine. Br J Psychiatry 166:80–86, 1995

Keck PE Jr, McElroy SL: Clinical pharmacodynamics and pharmacokinetics of antimanic and mood-stabilizing medications. J Clin Psychiatry 63 (suppl):3–11, 2002

Keck PE Jr, McElroy SL, Strakowski SM, et al: Factors associated with pharmacologic noncompliance in patients with mania. J Clin Psychiatry 57:292–297, 1996

Keck PE Jr, Mendlwicz J, Calabrese JR, et al: A review of randomized, controlled clinical trials in acute mania. J Affect Disord 59:S31–S37, 2000

Keck PE Jr, Strakowski SM, Hawkins JM, et al: A pilot study of rapid lithium administration in the treatment of acute mania. Bipolar Disord 3:68–72, 2001

Keck PE Jr, Perlis RH, Otto MW, et al: The Expert Consensus Guidelines: treatment of bipolar disorder 2004. Postgrad Med Special Report (December):1–120, 2004

Ketter TA, George MS, Kimbrell TA, et al: Neuroanatomical models and brain imaging studies in bipolar disorder, in Biological Models and Their Clinical Application. Edited by Young JT, Joffe RT. New York, Marcel Dekker, 1997, pp 179–217

Kilts CD: In vivo imaging of the pharmacodynamics and pharmacokinetics of lithium. J Clin Psychiatry 61:41–46, 2000

Kirov G: Thyroid disorders in lithium-treated patients. J Affect Disord 50:33–40, 1998

Kishimoto A: The treatment of affective disorder with carbamazepine: prophylactic synergism of lithium and carbamazepine combination. Prog Neuropsychopharmacol Biol Psychiatry 16:483–493, 1992

Kitchner I, Greenstein R: Low dose lithium carbonate in the treatment of posttraumatic stress disorder: brief communication. Mil Med 150:378–381, 1985

Klein PS, Melton DA: A molecular mechanism for the effect of lithium on development. Proc Natl Acad Sci U S A 93:8455–8459, 1996

Kleindienst N, Greil W: Differential efficacy of lithium and carbamazepine in the prophylaxis of bipolar disorder: results of the MAP study. Neuropsychobiology 42 (suppl):2–10, 2000

Klemfuss H: Rhythms and the pharmacology of lithium. Pharmacol Ther 56:53–78, 1992

Kline NS: A narrative account of lithium usage in psychiatry, in Lithium: Its Role in Psychiatric Research and Treatment. Edited by Gershon S, Shopsin B. New York, Plenum, 1973, pp 5–24

Kocsis JH, Shaw ED, Stokes PE, et al: Neuropsychological effects of lithium discontinuation. J Clin Psychopharmacol 13:268–275, 1993

Komoroski RA, Newton JE, Sprigg JR, et al: In vivo 7Li nuclear magnetic resonance study of lithium pharmacokinetics and chemical shift imaging in psychiatric patients. Psychiatry Res 50:67–76, 1993

Kowatch RA, Suppes T, Carmody TJ, et al: Effect size of lithium, divalproex sodium, and carbamazepine in children and adolescents with bipolar disorder. J Am Acad Child Adolesc Psychiatry 39:713–720, 2000

Kramlinger K, Post R: Adding lithium carbonate to carbamazepine: antimanic efficacy in treatment-resistant mania. Acta Psychiatr Scand 79:378–385, 1989

Krishna NR, Taylor MA, Abrams R: Combined haloperidol and lithium carbonate in treating manic patients. Compr Psychiatry 19:119–120, 1978

Kulhara P, Basu D, Mattoo SK, et al: Lithium prophylaxis of recurrent bipolar affective disorder: long-term outcome and its psychosocial correlates. J Affect Disord 54:87–96, 1999

Kusalic M, Engelsmann F: Effect of lithium maintenance therapy on thyroid and parathyroid function. J Psychiatry Neurosci 24:227–233, 1999

Lakin-Thomas PL: Phase resetting of the *Neurospora crassa* circadian oscillator: effects of inositol depletion on sensitivity to light. J Biol Rhythms 7:227–239, 1992

Lakin-Thomas PL: Evidence against a direct role for inositol phosphate metabolism in the circadian oscillator and the blue-light signal transduction pathway in *Neurospora crassa*. Biochem J 292:813–818, 1993

LaWall JS, Wesselius CL: The use of lithium carbonate in borderline patients. J Psychiatr Treat Eval 4:265–267, 1982

Lejoyeux M, Ades J, Rouillon F: Serotonin syndrome: incidence, symptoms and treatment. CNS Drugs 2:132–143, 1994

Lemus C, Lieberman J, Johns C: Myoclonus during treatment with clozapine and lithium: the role of serotonin. Hillside J Clin Psychiatry 11:127–130, 1989

Lenox RH, McNamara RK, Watterson JM, et al: Myristoylated alanine-rich C kinase substrate (MARCKS): a molecular target for the therapeutic action of mood stabilizers in the brain? J Clin Psychiatry 57 (suppl):23–31, 1996

Lerer B, Moore N, Meyendorff E, et al: Carbamazepine versus lithium in mania: a double-blind study. J Clin Psychiatry 48:89–93, 1987

Levine J, Gonsalves M, Babur I, et al: Inositol 6 g daily may be effective in depression but not in schizophrenia. Hum Psychopharmacol 8:49–53, 1993

Levine J, Barak Y, Gonsalves M, et al: A double-blind controlled trial of inositol treatment in depression. Am J Psychiatry 152:792–794, 1995

Li X, Friedman AB, Zhu W, et al: Lithium regulates glycogen synthase kinase-3beta in human peripheral blood mononuclear cells: implication in the treatment of bipolar disorder. Biol Psychiatry 61:216–222, 2007

Llewellyn A, Stowe ZN, Strader JR: The use of lithium and management of women with bipolar disorder during pregnancy and lactation. J Clin Psychiatry 59:57–64, 1998

Loew MR: Rapid cycling disorders and the role of combined lithium and haloperidol decanoate. Can J Psychiatry 31:877–878, 1986

Lombardi G, Panza N, Biondi B, et al: Effects of lithium treatment on hypothalamic-pituitary-thyroid axis: a longitudinal study. J Endocrinol Invest 16:259–263, 1993

Loudon JB, Waring H: Toxic reactions to lithium and haloperidol (letter). Lancet 2:1088, 1976

Luchins DJ, Dojka D: Lithium and propranolol in aggression and self-injurious behavior in the mentally retarded. Psychopharmacol Bull 25:372–375, 1989

Lynn EJ, Satloff A, Tinling DC: Mania and the use of lithium: a three-year study. Am J Psychiatry 127:96–100, 1971

Madhusoodanan S, Brenner R, Suresh P, et al: Efficacy and tolerability of olanzapine in elderly patients with psychotic disorders: a prospective study. Ann Clin Psychiatry 12:11–18, 2000

Maggs R: Treatment of manic illness with lithium carbonate. Br J Psychiatry 109:56–65, 1963

Maj M: Clinical prediction of response to lithium prophylaxis in bipolar patients: the importance of the previous pattern of course of the illness. Clin Neuropharmacol 13:S66–S70, 1990

Malone RP, Luebbert J, Pena-Ariet M, et al: The Overt Aggression Scale in a study of lithium in aggressive conduct disorder. Psychopharmacol Bull 30:215–218, 1994

Malone RP, Delaney MA, Luebbert JF, et al: A double-blind placebo-controlled study of lithium in hospitalized aggressive children and adolescents with conduct disorder. Arch Gen Psychiatry 57:649–654, 2000

Mani J, Tandel S, Shah P, et al: Prolonged neurological sequelae after combination treatment with lithium and antipsychotic drugs. J Neurol Neurosurg Psychiatry 60:350–351, 1996

Manji HK, Etcheberrigaray R, Chen G, et al: Lithium decreases membrane-associated protein kinase C in hippocampus: selectivity for the alpha isozyme. J Neurochem 61:2303–2310, 1993

Manji HK, Bebchuk JM, Moore GJ, et al: Modulation of CNS signal transduction pathways and gene expression by mood stabilizing agents: therapeutic implications. J Clin Psychiatry 60 (suppl):27–39, 1999

Mann SC, Greenstein RA, Eilers R: Early onset of severe dyskinesia following lithium-haloperidol treatment. Am J Psychiatry 140:1385–1386, 1983

Marhold J, Zimanova J, Lachman M, et al: To the incompatibility of haloperidol with lithium salts. Activitas Nervosa Superior (Praha) 16:199–200, 1974

Martin CA, Piascik MT: First-degree A-V block in patients on lithium carbonate. Can J Psychiatry 30:114–116, 1985

Massot O, Rousselle JC, Fillion MP, et al: 5-HT1B receptors: a novel target for lithium: possible involvement in mood disorders. Neuropsychopharmacology 21:533–541, 1999

McDonald WM, Nemeroff CB: The diagnosis and treatment of mania in the elderly. Bull Menninger Clin 60:174–196, 1996

McDougle CJ, Price LH, Goodman WK, et al: A controlled trial of lithium augmentation in fluvoxamine-refractory obsessive-compulsive disorder: lack of efficacy. J Clin Psychopharmacol 11:175–184, 1991

Mekler G, Woggon B: A case of serotonin syndrome caused by venlafaxine and lithium. Pharmacopsychiatry 30:272–273, 1997

Mendels J: Lithium in the treatment of depressive states, in Lithium Research and Therapy. Edited by Johnson FN. New York, Academic Press, 1975, pp 43–62

Menes C, Burra P, Hoaken P: Untoward effects following combined neuroleptic-lithium therapy: cardiac arrhythmias and seizure. Can J Psychiatry 25:573–576, 1980

Mielke DH, Winstead DK, Goethe JW: Multiple-monitored electroconvulsive therapy: safety and efficacy in elderly depressed patients. J Am Geriatr Soc 32:180–182, 1984

Miller F, Menninger J: Lithium-neuroleptic neurotoxicity is dose dependent. J Clin Psychopharmacol 7:89–91, 1987

Miller F, Menninger J, Whitcup S: Lithium-neuroleptic neurotoxicity in the elderly bipolar patient. J Clin Psychopharmacol 6:176–178, 1986

Mitchell JE, Mackenzie TB: Cardiac effects of lithium therapy in man: a review. J Clin Psychiatry 43:47–51, 1982

Mitchell P, Withers K, Jacobs G, et al: Combining lithium and sodium valproate for bipolar disorder. Aust NZ J Psychiatry 28:141–143, 1994

Modell JG, Lenox RH, Weiner S: Inpatient clinical trial of lorazepam for the management of manic agitation. J Clin Psychopharmacol 5:109–113, 1985

Monti JM, Monti D, Jantos H, et al: Effects of selective activation of the 5-HT1B receptor with CP-94,253 on sleep and wakefulness in the rat. Neuropharmacology 34:1647–1651, 1995

Moore GJ, Bebchuk JM, Manji HK: Proton MRS in manic depressive illness: monitoring of lithium induced modulation of brain myo-inositol. Soc Neurosci 23:335–336, 1997

Muly EC, McDonald W, Steffens D, et al: Serotonin syndrome produced by a combination of fluoxetine and lithium. Am J Psychiatry 150:1565, 1993

Nierenberg AA, Fava M, Trivedi MH, et al: A comparison of lithium and T3 augmentation following two failed medication treatments for depression: a STAR*D report. Am J Psychiatry 163:1519–1530, 2006

Newport DJ, Viguera AC, Beach AJ, et al: Lithium placental passage and obstetrical outcome: implications for clinical management during late pregnancy. Am J Psychiatry 162:2162–2170, 2005

Noyes R Jr, Dempsey GM, Blum A, et al: Lithium treatment of depression. Compr Psychiatry 15:187–193, 1974

Ohman R, Spigset O: Serotonin syndrome induced by fluvoxamine–lithium interaction. Pharmacopsychiatry 26:263–264, 1993

Patel NC, DelBello MP, Bryan HS, et al: Open-label lithium for the treatment of adolescents with bipolar depression. J Am Acad Child Adolesc Psychiatry 45:289–297, 2006

Perenyi A, Rihmer Z, Banki C: Parkinsonian symptoms with lithium, lithium-neuroleptic, and lithium-antidepressant treatment. J Affect Disord 5:171–177, 1983

Perenyi A, Szucs R, Frecska E: Tardive dyskinesia in patients receiving lithium maintenance therapy. Biol Psychiatry 19:1573–1578, 1984

Perry PJ, Alexander B, Prince RA, et al: Prospective evaluation of two lithium maintenance dose schedules. J Clin Psychopharmacol 4:242–246, 1984

Peterson GA, Byrd SL: Diabetic ketoacidosis from clozapine and lithium cotreatment. Am J Psychiatry 153:737–738, 1996

Phiel CJ, Klein PS: Molecular targets of lithium action. Annu Rev Pharmacol Toxicol 41:789–813, 2001

Phiel CJ, Wilson CA, Lee VM, et al: GSK-3alpha regulates production of Alzheimer's disease amyloid-beta peptides. Nature 423:435–439, 2003

Pigott TA, Pato MT, L'Heureux F, et al: A controlled comparison of adjuvant lithium carbonate or thyroid hormone in clomipramine-treated patients with obsessive-compulsive disorder. J Clin Psychopharmacol 11:242–248, 1991

Pope HG Jr, Cole JO, Choras PT, et al: Apparent neuroleptic malignant syndrome with clozapine and lithium. J Nerv Ment Dis 174:493–495, 1986

Price LH, Charney DX, Heninger GR: Variability of response to lithium augmentation in refractory depression. Am J Psychiatry 143:1387–1392, 1986

Price LH, Charney DS, Delgado PL, et al: Lithium treatment and serotonergic function. Arch Gen Psychiatry 46:13–19, 1989

Price LH, Charney DS, Delgado PL, et al: Lithium and serotonin function: implications for the serotonin hypothesis of depression. Psychopharmacology (Berl) 100:3–12, 1990

Puri BK, Taylor DG, Alcock ME: Low-dose maintenance clozapine treatment in the prophylaxis of bipolar disorder. Br J Clin Pract 49:333–334, 1995

Quitkin FM, Kane J, Rifkin A, et al: Prophylactic lithium carbonate with and without imipramine for bipolar I patients. Arch Gen Psychiatry 38:902–907, 1981

Rajkowska G, Miguel-Hidalgo JJ, Wei J, et al: Morphometric evidence for neuronal and glial prefrontal cell pathology in major depression. Biol Psychiatry 45:1085–1098, 1999

Reeves RR, Struve FA, Patrick G: Does EEG predict response to valproate versus lithium in patients with mania. Ann Clin Psychiatry 13:69–73, 2001

Rifkin A, Quitkin F, Carrillo C, et al: Lithium carbonate in emotionally unstable character disorder. Arch Gen Psychiatry 27:519–523, 1972

Roose SP, Nurnberger JI, Dunner DL, et al: Cardiac sinus node dysfunction during lithium treatment. Am J Psychiatry 136:804–806, 1979

Rosenqvist M, Bergfeldt L, Aili H, et al: Sinus node dysfunction during long-term lithium treatment. Br Heart J 70:371–375, 1993

Rosenthal NE: Lithium: an orphan drug (editorial). Arch Gen Psychiatry 58:973, 2001

Rosenthal NE, Rosenthal LN, Stallone F, et al: Psychosis as a predictor of response to lithium maintenance treatment in bipolar affective disorder. J Affect Disord 1:237–245, 1979

Ryan ND, Bhatara VS, Perel JM: Mood stabilizers in children and adolescents. J Am Acad Child Adolesc Psychiatry 38:529–536, 1999

Sachs GS, Rosenbaum JF, Jones L: Adjunctive clonazepam for maintenance treatment of bipolar affective disorder. J Clin Psychopharmacol 10:42–47, 1990a

Sachs GS, Weilburg JB, Rosenbaum JF: Clonazepam vs neuroleptics as adjuncts to lithium maintenance. Psychopharmacol Bull 26:137–143, 1990b

Sanger TM, Grundy SL, Gibson PJ, et al: Long-term olanzapine therapy in the treatment of bipolar I disorder: an open-label continuation phase study. J Clin Psychiatry 62:273–281, 2001

Schaff M, Fawcett J, Zajecka J: Divalproex sodium in the treatment of refractory affective disorders. J Clin Psychiatry 38:137–139, 1993

Schildkraut JJ, Logue MA, Dodge GA: The effect of lithium salts on the turnover and metabolism of norepinephrine in the rat brain. Psychopharmacologia 14:135–141, 1969

Schopf J, Baumann P, Lemarchand T, et al: Treatment of endogenous depressions resistant to tricyclic antidepressants of related drugs by lithium addition: results of a placebo-controlled double-blind study. Pharmacopsychiatry 22:183–187, 1989

Schou M: Artistic productivity and lithium prophylaxis on manic-depressive illness. Br J Psychiatry 135:97–103, 1979

Schou M: The effect of prophylactic lithium treatment on mortality and suicidal behavior: a review for clinicians. J Affect Disord 50:253–259, 1998

Schou M, Juel-Nielson N, Stromgren E: The treatment of manic psychoses by administration of lithium salts. J Neurol Neurosurg Psychiatry 17:250–260, 1954

Schrauzer GN, Shrestha KP: Lithium in drinking water and the incidences of crimes, suicides, and arrests related to drug addictions. Biol Trace Elem Res 25:105–113, 1990

Segal J, Berk M, Brook S: Risperidone compared with both lithium and haloperidol in mania: a double-blind randomized controlled trial. Clin Neuropharmacol 21:176–180, 1998

Shaldubina A, Agam G, Belmaker RH: The mechanism of lithium action: state of the art, ten years later. Prog Neuropsychopharmacol Biol Psychiatry 25:855–866, 2001

Shao L, Young RT, Wang JF: Chronic treatment with mood stabilizers lithium and valproate prevents excitotoxicity by inhibiting oxidative stress in rat cerebral cortical cells. Biol Psychiatry 58:879–884, 2005

Sharma V, Persad E: Augmentation of valproate with lithium in a case of rapid cycling affective disorder. Can J Psychiatry 37:584–585, 1992

Sharma V, Persad E, Mazmanian D, et al: Treatment of rapid cycling bipolar disorder with combination therapy of valproate and lithium. Can J Psychiatry 38:137–139, 1993

Shaw ED, Mann JJ, Stokes PE, et al: Effects of lithium carbonate on associative productivity and idiosyncrasy in bipolar patients. Am J Psychiatry 143:1166–1169, 1986

Shukla S, Godwin CD, Long LEB, et al: Lithium-carbamazepine neurotoxicity and risk factors. Am J Psychiatry 141:1604–1606, 1984

Shukla S, Cook BL, Miller MG: Lithium-carbamazepine versus lithium-neuroleptic prophylaxis in bipolar illness. J Affect Disord 9:219–222, 1985

Sipes TE, Geyer MA: Functional behavioral homology between rat 5-HT1B and guinea pig 5-HT1D receptors in the modulation of prepulse inhibition of startle. Psychopharmacology 122:231–237, 1996

Slater V, Milanes F, Talcott V, et al: Influence of age on lithium therapy. South Med J 77:153–158, 1984

Small JG, Kellams JJ, Milstein V: Complications with electroconvulsive treatment combined with lithium. Biol Psychiatry 12:103–112, 1980

Small JG, Klapper MH, Kellams JJ, et al: Electroconvulsive treatment compared with lithium in the management of manic states. Arch Gen Psychiatry 45:727–732, 1988

Small JG, Klapper MH, Milstein V, et al: Carbamazepine compared with lithium in the treatment of mania. Arch Gen Psychiatry 48:915–921, 1991

Small JG, Klapper MH, Marhenke JD, et al: Lithium combined with carbamazepine in the treatment of mania. Psychopharmacol Bull 31:265–272, 1995

Soares JC, Boada F, Spencer S, et al: Brain lithium concentrations in bipolar disorder patients: preliminary (7)Li magnetic resonance studies at 3 T. Biol Psychiatry 49:437–443, 2001

Sobanski T, Bagli M, Laux G, et al: Serotonin syndrome after lithium add-on medication to paroxetine. Pharmacopsychiatry 30:106–107, 1997

Solomon DA, Ryan CE, Keitner GI, et al: A pilot study of lithium carbonate plus divalproex sodium for the continuation and maintenance treatment of patients with bipolar I disorder. J Clin Psychiatry 58:95–99, 1997

Solomon DA, Keitner GI, Ryan CE, et al: Lithium plus valproate as maintenance polypharmacy for patients with bipolar I disorder: a review. J Clin Psychopharmacol 18:38–49, 1998

Spencer EK, Campbell M, Adams P, et al: Saliva and serum lithium monitoring in hospitalized children. Psychopharmacol Bull 26:239–243, 1990

Spreat S, Behar D, Reneski B, et al: Lithium carbonate for aggression in mentally retarded persons. Compr Psychiatry 30:505–511, 1989

Spring G: Neurotoxicity with combined use of lithium and thioridazine. J Clin Psychiatry 40:135–138, 1979

Spring G, Frankel M: New data on lithium and haloperidol incompatibility. Am J Psychiatry 138:818–821, 1981

Squire LR, Judd LL, Janowsky DS, et al: Effects of lithium carbonate on memory and other cognitive functions. Am J Psychiatry 137:1042–1046, 1980

Steckler TL: Lithium- and carbamazepine-associated sinus node dysfunction: nine-year experience in a psychiatric hospital. J Clin Psychopharmacol 14:336–339, 1994

Stein G, Bernadt B: Lithium augmentation therapy in tricyclic-resistant depression. Br J Psychiatry 162:634–640, 1993

Stern DN, Fieve RR, Neff NH, et al: The effect of lithium chloride administration on brain and heart norepinephrine turnover rates. Psychopharmacologia 14:315–322, 1969

Stern TA, Jenike MA: Treatment of obsessive-compulsive disorder with lithium carbonate. Psychosomatics 24:671–673, 1983

Stokes PE, Shamoian CA, Stoll PM, et al: Efficacy of lithium as acute treatment of manic depressive illness. Lancet 1:1319–1325, 1971

Stoll AL, Locke CA, Vuckovic A, et al: Lithium-associated cognitive and functional deficits reduced by a switch to divalproex sodium: a case series. J Clin Psychiatry 57:356–359, 1996

Stoudemire A, Moran MG, Fogel BS: Psychotropic drug use in the medically ill. Psychosomatics 21:377–391, 1990

Su Y, Ryder J, Li B, et al: Lithium, a common drug for bipolar disorder treatment, regulates amyloid-beta precursor protein processing. Biochemistry 43:6899–6908, 2004

Suppes T, Phillips KA, Judd CR: Clozapine treatment of nonpsychotic rapid cycling bipolar disorder: a report of three cases. Biol Psychiatry 136:338–340, 1994

Swann AC, Bowden CL, Morris D, et al: Depression during mania: treatment response to lithium or divalproex. Arch Gen Psychiatry 54:37–42, 1997

Swann AC, Bowden CL, Calabrese JR, et al: Differential effect of number of previous episodes of affective disorder on response to lithium or divalproex in acute mania. Am J Psychiatry 156:1264–1266, 1999

Swanson CL Jr, Price WA, McEvoy JP: Effects of concomitant risperidone and lithium treatment (letter). Am J Psychiatry 152:1096, 1995

Takahashi R, Sakuma A, Itoh K, et al: Comparison of efficacy of lithium carbonate and chlorpromazine in mania: report of collaborative study group on treatment of mania in Japan. Arch Gen Psychiatry 32:1310–1318, 1975

Tilkian AG, Schroeder JS, Kao JJ, et al: The cardiovascular effects of lithium in man: a review of the literature. Am J Med 61:665–670, 1976

Tohen M, Zarate CA Jr, Centorrino F, et al: Risperidone in the treatment of mania. J Clin Psychiatry 57:249–253, 1996

Tohen M, Greil W, Calabrese JR, et al: Olanzapine versus lithium in the maintenance treatment of bipolar disorder: a 12-month, randomized, double-blind, controlled clinical trial. Am J Psychiatry 162:1281–1290, 2005

Tondo L, Jamison KR, Baldessarini RJ: Effect of lithium maintenance on suicidal behavior in major mood disorders. Ann N Y Acad Sci 836:339–351, 1997

Tondo L, Baldessarini RJ, Hennen J, et al: Lithium maintenance treatment of depression and mania in bipolar I and II disorders. Am J Psychiatry 155:638–645, 1998

Tondo L, Hennen J, Baldessarini RJ: Lower suicide risk with long-term lithium treatment in major affective illness: a meta-analysis. Acta Psychiatr Scand 104:163–172, 2001

Tsaltas E, Kontis D, Boulougouris V, et al: Enhancing effects of chronic lithium on memory in the rat. Behav Brain Res 177:51–60, 2007

Tunnessen WW, Hertz CG: Toxic effects of lithium in newborn infants: a commentary. J Pediatr 81:804–807, 1972

Van der Kolk BA: Psychopharmacologic issues in posttraumatic stress disorder. Hosp Community Psychiatry 34:683–691, 1983

Viguera AC, Cohen LS: The course and management of bipolar disorder during pregnancy. Psychopharmacol Bull 34:339–346, 1998

Viguera AC, Nonacs R, Cohen LS, et al: Risk of recurrence of bipolar disorder in pregnant and nonpregnant women after discontinuing lithium maintenance. Am J Psychiatry 157:179–184, 2000

Viguera AC, Newport DJ, Ritchie J, et al: Lithium in breastmilk and nursing infants: clinical implications. Am J Psychiatry 164:342–345, 2007

Vollmer KO, Von Hodenberg A, Kolle EU: Pharmacokinetics and metabolism of gabapentin in rat, dog, and man. Arzneimittelforschung 36:830–839, 1986

Walton SA, Berk M, Brook S: Superiority of lithium over verapamil in mania: a randomized, controlled, single-blind trial. J Clin Psychiatry 57:543–546, 1996

Ward ME, Musa MN, Bailey L: Clinical pharmacokinetics of lithium. J Clin Pharmacol 34:280–285, 1994

Webb A, Solomon DA, Ryan C: Lithium levels and toxicity among hospitalized patients. Psychiatr Serv 52:229–231, 2001

Weinstein MR, Goldfield MD: Cardiovascular malformations with lithium use during pregnancy. Am J Psychiatry 132:529–531, 1975

West AP, Meltzer HY: Paradoxical lithium neurotoxicity: a report of 5 cases and a hypothesis about risk for neurotoxicity. Am J Psychiatry 136:963–966, 1979

Williams RS, Harwood AJ: Lithium therapy and signal transduction. Trends Pharmacol Sci 21:61–64, 2000

Worrall EP, Moody JP, Naylor GJ: Lithium in non-manic-depressives: antiaggressive effect and red blood cell lithium values. Br J Psychiatry 126:464–468, 1975

Wright B, Jarrett D: Lithium and calcium channel blockers: possible neurotoxicity. Biol Psychiatry 30:635–636, 1991

Wyatt RJ, Henter ID, Jamison JC: Lithium revisited: savings brought about by the use of lithium, 1970–1991. Psychiatr Q 72:149–166, 2001

Yazici O, Kora K, Ucok A, et al: Predictors of lithium prophylaxis in bipolar patients. J Affect Disord 55:133–142, 1999

Yoshida S, Maeda M, Kaku S, et al: Lithium inhibits stress-induced changes in tau phosphorylation in the mouse hippocampus. J Neural Transm 113:1803–1814, 2006

Zusky PM, Biederman J, Rosenbaum JF, et al: Adjunct low dose lithium carbonate in lithium-resistant depression: a placebo-controlled study. J Clin Psychopharmacol 8:120–124, 1988

Valproate

Charles L. Bowden, M.D.

History and Discovery

Valproic acid was first synthesized by Burton in the United States in 1882 and subsequently was used as an organic solvent. The drug's antiepileptic properties were discovered serendipitously by Meunier in 1963 in France. Meunier used valproic acid as a vehicle for other compounds that were being screened for antiepileptic activity. He found that compounds that did not have antiepileptic properties when administered alone inhibited seizure activity when dissolved in valproic acid and concluded that the antiepileptic activity was due to the solvent, valproic acid, rather than to the test drugs (Bowden and McElroy 1995; Fariello and Smith 1989; Meunier et al. 1975).

Valproate was the first alternative mood stabilizer to be studied, with Lambert's first research published in 1966 (Lambert et al. 1966). Valproate was first introduced as an antiepileptic in France in 1967. It has been used in Holland and Germany since 1968 and in the United Kingdom since 1973, and it became available in the United States in 1978. An enteric-coated formulation, divalproex sodium, was introduced to the U.S. market in 1983. A formulation consisting of a capsule containing coated particles of divalproex sodium was introduced in 1989. An extended-release formulation of divalproex was approved for migraine in 2001 and mania in 2006. Valproate was approved for treatment of mania in the United States in 1995. Valproate, either as divalproex or as other formulations, is now approved for treatment of mania in most developed countries.

Structure–Activity Relations

Valproic acid (dipropylacetic acid) is an eight-carbon, branched-chain carboxylic acid that is structurally distinct from other antiepileptic and psychotropic compounds (Bocci and Beretta 1976; Levy et al. 2002) (Figure 36–1). Although straight-chain acids have little or no antiepileptic activity, other branched-chain carboxylic acids have potencies similar to that of valproate in antagonizing pentylenetetrazole-induced seizures. However, increasing the number of carbon atoms to nine introduces marked sedative properties. The primary amide of valproic acid, valpromide, has been reported to be about twice as potent as the parent compound.

Pharmacological Profile

Valproate blocks pentylenetetrazole-induced and maximal electroshock seizures in a variety of animals and suppresses secondarily generalized seizures without affecting focal activity in chemically lesioned animals (Fariello and Smith 1989). Valproate also has antikindling properties,

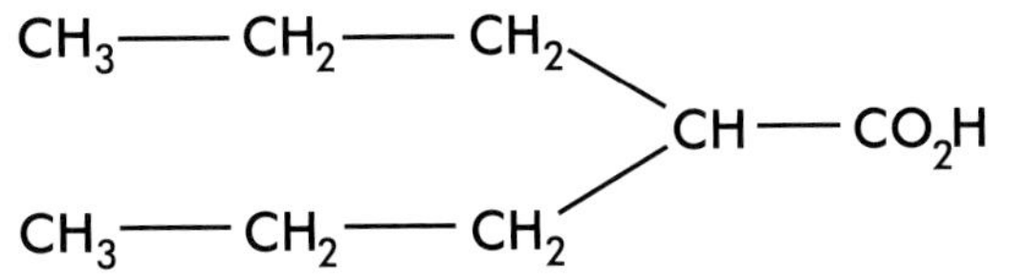

$$CH_3 - CH_2 - CH_2 \diagdown$$
$$CH - CO_2H$$
$$CH_3 - CH_2 - CH_2 \diagup$$

FIGURE 36–1. Chemical structure of valproic acid (2-propyl-pentanoic acid).

preventing the spread of epileptiform activity in cats without affecting focal seizures (Leveil and Nanquet 1977).

Studies in epilepsy and bipolar disorder indicate that divalproex causes a reduction in plasma levels of γ-aminobutyric acid (GABA) and that plasma GABA levels positively correlate with the degree of improvement in manic symptomatology (Brennan et al. 1984; Emrich et al. 1981). Animal studies also indicate that chronic valproate increases the expression of mRNA encoding the 67-kilodalton isoform of glutamate decarboxylase (GAD_{67}) in the brain, thereby facilitating GABAergic transmission (Tremolizzo et al. 2002). Valproate is incorporated into neuronal membranes in a saturable manner and appears to displace naturally occurring branched-chain phospholipids (Siafaka-Kapadai et al. 1998). Chronic valproate reduces protein kinase C (PKC) activity in manic patients (Hahn et al. 2005). Elevated PKC activity has been associated with manic patients and in animal models for mania (Einat and Manji 2006). Valproate inhibits glycogen synthase kinase 3 (GSK-3) at concentrations present therapeutically. The effect is indirect, linked to its capability to upregulate gene expression through inhibition of histone deacetylase (Harwood and Agam 2003). In laboratory animals, valproate activates the extracellular signal-regulated kinase (ERK) pathway (Einat et al. 2003). Valproate increases the expression of the cytoprotective protein B-cell lymphoma/leukemia-2 gene (bcl-2) in the central nervous system in vivo and in cells of human neuronal origin (Gray et al. 2003). Valproate provided antioxidant effects, reversing early DNA damage caused by amphetamine in an animal model of mania (Andreazza et al. 2007). Valproate and lithium both reduce inositol biosynthesis. However, the mechanism of valproate action is unique, resulting from decreased myo-inositol 1-phosphate synthase inhibition (Shaltiel et al. 2004). Valproate and lithium both lengthen the period of circadian rhythms and increase arrhythmicity in Drosophila. This action of the two drugs is of interest given recent data implicating sets of genes associated with circadian rhythmicity in bipolar disorders (Dokucu et al. 2005). Therapeutic doses of either valproate or lithium increase the antiapoptotic protein bcl-2 in anterior cingulate cortex, potentially providing a buffer against the destructive effects of increased intracellular Ca^{2+} in bipolar disorder (Quiroz et al. 2008).

Despite primary differences in the initial modes of action of valproate and lithium, it is noteworthy that valproate and lithium have substantial overlapping effects on neuronal systems involved in maintaining mood stability and alertness that have not been observed in studies of similar systems with carbamazepine or atypical antipsychotic drugs. Whereas several of the above-reviewed systems are impacted by both lithium and valproate, only valproate inhibits histone deacetylase, which in turn results in a gradual increase in the phosphorylation of Akt and GSK-3β (Harwood and Agam 2003). Valproate enhances acetylated histone content, thereby preventing methionine-induced reelin promoter hypermethylation and normalizing behavioral responses in a mouse model for schizophrenia-like behavior (Tremolizzo et al. 2005). Recent study of valproate as a cancer chemotherapeutic agent may also be stimulated by its effects on cell proliferation through inhibition of histone deacetylase (Andratschke et al. 2001).

Valproate increased corticotropin-releasing factor (CRF) mRNA expression in the cortex and reduced CRF type 1 receptor (CRF_1) binding in the amygdala and cortex of nonstressed rats, suggesting that one of valproate's effects in the brain is to dampen tone in this pathway, which is associated with stress-linked psychopathology (Gilmor et al. 2003).

Pharmacokinetics and Disposition

Valproate is commercially available in the United States in five oral preparations: 1) divalproex sodium, an enteric-coated, stable-coordination compound containing equal proportions of valproic acid and sodium valproate in a 1:1 molar ratio; 2) valproic acid; 3) sodium valproate; 4) divalproex sodium sprinkle capsule (containing coated particles of divalproex sodium), which can be ingested intact or pulled apart and contents sprinkled on food; and 5) an extended-release form of divalproex that provides once-daily dosing and a substantially flatter peak-to-trough ratio. Sodium valproate is available for intravenous use and, as such, has been demonstrated to provide reduction in manic symptoms within 1 day or less (Grunze et al. 1999). Valproate can also be compounded in suppository form for rectal administration. The valproate ion is the common compound in plasma.

The bioavailability of valproate approaches 100% with all preparations (Levy et al. 2002; Penry and Dean 1989; Wilder 1992). All preparations taken orally, except divalproex sodium, are rapidly absorbed after oral ingestion. Sodium valproate and valproic acid attain peak serum concentrations within 2 hours. Divalproex sodium reaches peak serum concentrations within 3–8 hours. The extended-release form of divalproex has an earlier onset of absorption than divalproex sodium regular-release tablets and approximately a 20% smaller difference in trough

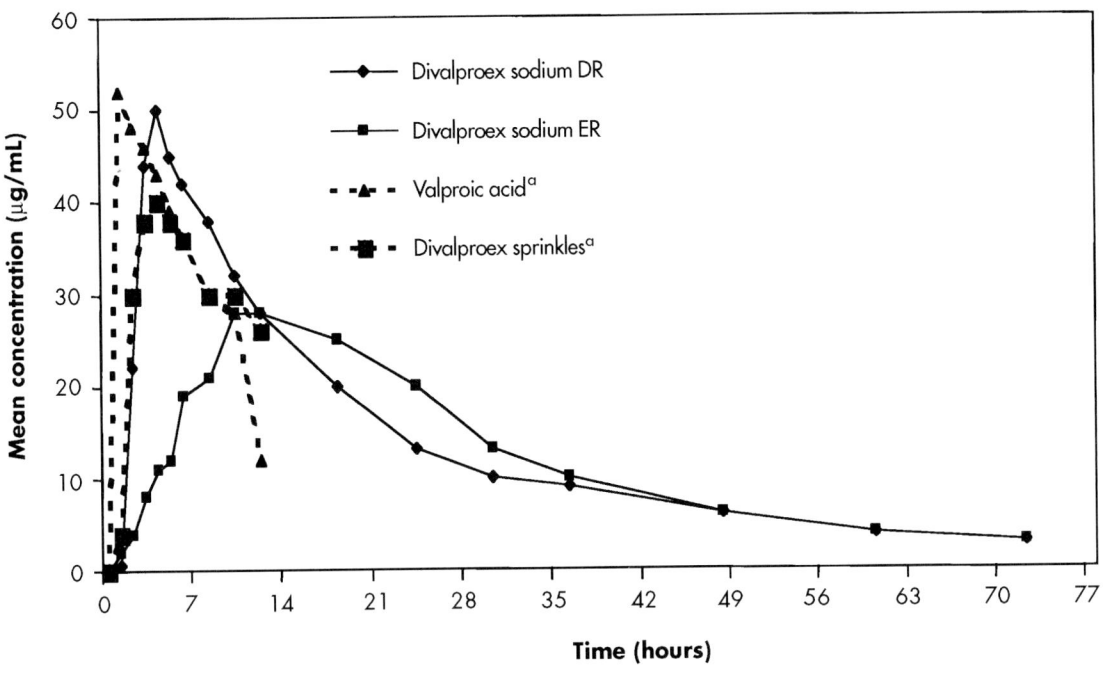

FIGURE 36–2. Mean plasma valproate concentrations with different formulations.

[a]Data derived from different studies after 500-mg doses.

DR = delayed-release; ER = extended-release.

Source. Abbott Laboratories, data on file.

and peak serum levels than regular-release divalproex (Figure 36–2). Absorption can also be delayed if the drug is taken with food.

Valproate is highly protein bound, predominantly to serum albumin and proportional to the albumin concentration. Although patients with low levels of albumin have a higher fraction of unbound drug, the steady-state level of total drug is not altered. Only the unbound drug crosses the blood–brain barrier and is bioactive. Thus, when valproate is displaced from protein-binding sites through drug interactions, the total drug concentration may not change; however, the pharmacologically active unbound drug does increase and may produce signs and symptoms of toxicity. Moreover, when the plasma concentration of valproate increases in response to increased dosing, the amount of unbound (active) valproate increases disproportionately and is metabolized, with an apparent increase in clearance of total drug, yielding lower-than-expected total plasma concentrations (Levy et al. 2002; Wilder 1992) (Figure 36–3). In addition, valproate protein binding is increased by low-fat diets and decreased by high-fat diets. Because of lower serum protein levels, women and elderly patients will generally have a higher proportion of the active free moiety.

The concentration range generally required for good clinical effect in mania is approximately 45 to 125 µg/mL

(Bowden et al. 1996). Patients who tolerate higher serum levels, up to around 125 µg/mL, may have greater improvement (Allen et al. 2006). One open report suggests that patients with bipolar II conditions and cyclothymia may respond to serum valproate concentrations of less than 50 µg/mL (Jacobsen 1993).

Valproate is metabolized primarily in the liver by glucuronidation. In addition, oxidative pathways yield a large number of metabolites, some of which have antiepileptic and/or toxic effects (Bocci and Beretta 1976; Levy et al. 2002; Penry and Dean 1989; Wilder 1992) (Figure 36–4). The oxidative pathways are mitochondrial β-oxidation to 3-hydroxyvalproate, 3-oxo-valproate, and 2-en-valproate; and the cytochrome P450 microsomal metabolism to the toxic 4-en- and 2,4-en metabolites. Less than 3% of valproate is excreted unchanged in the urine and feces. Valproate's elimination half-life is typically 5–20 hours and can be altered by agents that affect the mitochondrial and/or microsomal enzyme systems responsible for its metabolism.

Treatment with valproate for bipolar disorder is usually begun at a dosage of 15–20 mg/kg/day. The drug can be "orally loaded" at 20–30 mg/kg/day in patients with acute mania to induce more rapid response. The dosage of valproate is increased according to the patient's response

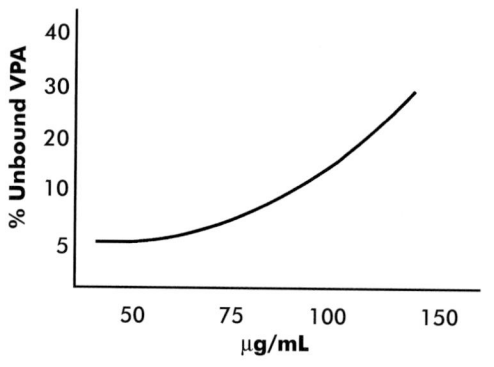

FIGURE 36–3. Total valproate (VPA) concentrations.

As the total concentration of VPA increases, protein-binding sites become saturated, and the percentage of unbound to bound VPA increases.
Source. Reprinted from Wilder BJ: "Pharmacokinetics of Valproate and Carbamazepine." *Journal of Clinical Psychopharmacology* 12 (1, suppl):64S–68S, 1992. Used with permission.

VPA →(mitochondrial β-oxidation)→ 3-OH-VPA, 3-OXO-VPA, Δ^2VPA*

* Active anticonvulsant—Long $t_{1/2}$

VPA →(microsomal P450 pathway)→ Δ^4 VPA and other inactive metabolites, $\Delta^{2,4}$VPA

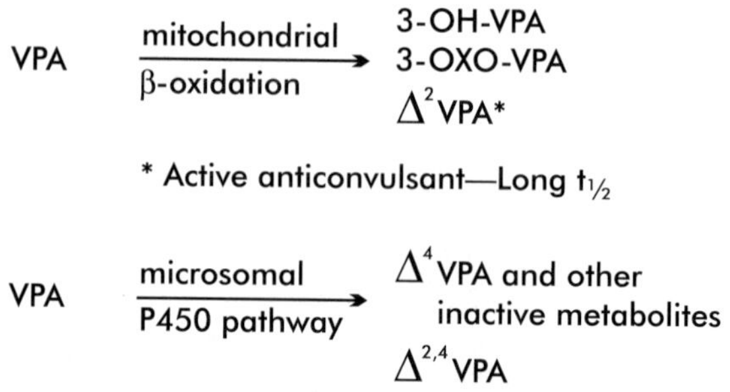

FIGURE 36–4. Two pathways for metabolism of valproate (VPA).

VPA is metabolized within the mitochondria by the β-oxidative pathway, which metabolizes medium- and long-chain fatty acids. This is the major metabolic pathway used in patients taking VPA as monotherapy. VPA is also metabolized by the microsomal cytochrome P450 pathway, which occurs outside the mitochondria; metabolism via this pathway is increased when VPA is administered in combination with enzyme-inducing drugs (e.g., carbamazepine). 3-OH-VPA = 3-hydroxyvalproate; 3-OXO-VPA = 3-oxo-valproate; Δ^2 VPA = 2-en-valproate metabolite; Δ^4 VPA = 4-en-valproate metabolite; $\Delta^{2,4}$ VPA = 2,4-en-valproate metabolite; $t_{1/2}$ = half-life.
Source. Reprinted from Wilder BJ: "Pharmacokinetics of Valproate and Carbamazepine." *Journal of Clinical Psychopharmacology* 12 (1, suppl):64S–68S, 1992. Used with permission.

and side effects, usually by 250–500 mg/day every 1–3 days, to serum concentrations of 45–125 µg/mL. Of note, sedation, increased appetite, and reduction in white blood count and platelet count all become more frequent at serum concentrations above 100 µg/mL (Bowden 2000). During maintenance treatment, bipolar I patients whose serum levels were between 75 and 100 µg/mL had significantly longer time to intervention for a developing mood episode than did patients with serum levels either lower or higher than this range (Keck et al. 2005).

Indications and Efficacy

The indications for valproate that are currently recognized by the U.S. Food and Drug Administration (FDA) are for the treatment of manic episodes associated with bipolar disorder; for sole and adjunctive therapy in the treatment of simple and complex absence seizures; for adjunctive therapy in multiple seizure types, including absence seizures; and for prophylaxis of migraine. Controlled studies have also shown that valproate is effective in prevention of recurrence of mania in bipolar disorder (Tohen et al. 2003) and in prolongation of the depression-free period compared with lithium (Gyulai et al. 2003). Controlled studies additionally indicate that valproate is effective in generalized epilepsies, including generalized tonic–clonic and myoclonic seizures, as well as in secondarily generalized tonic–clonic seizures, infantile spasms, photosensitive epilepsy, and febrile seizures (Bourgeois 1989; Rimmer and Richens 1985).

Use in Bipolar Disorder

Acute Bipolar Mania

Numerous open studies and controlled trials (five placebo-controlled, one haloperidol-controlled, one lithium-controlled, and one placebo- and lithium-controlled) indicate that valproate is effective in the treatment of acute mania (Bowden et al. 1994; McElroy et al. 1993). In the controlled trials (Bowden et al. 1994, 2006; Brennan et al. 1984; Emrich et al. 1985; Freeman et al. 1992; McElroy et al. 1996; Pope et al. 1991), valproate was superior to placebo and comparable to lithium and haloperidol in the short-term treatment of acute mania. The most recent placebo-controlled study indicated that patients with more severe manic symptoms experienced greater benefits from valproate relative to placebo compared with patients with milder manic symptomatology (Bowden et al. 2006). In these studies, the antimanic response to valproate occurred as early as 5 days following initiation of treatment.

In an open-label, rater-blind study of valproate administration via an oral loading dosage of 20 mg/kg/day to 19 patients with acute mania, 10 (53%) of the patients had a significant response within 5 days of treatment, with minimal side effects (Keck et al. 1993). Similarly, in a controlled comparison study with haloperidol, divalproex administered at 20 mg/kg/day produced rapid antimanic and antipsychotic effects comparable to those of haloperidol (McElroy et al. 1996). Valproate and carbamazepine were compared in a small (*n* = 30) blinded, randomized study in acute mania (Vasudev et al. 2000). Valproate provided greater reduction in mania scores, produced earlier response, and was associated with fewer adverse effects than carbamazepine.

Intravenous valproate infused as 600 mg over 20 minutes yielded rapid improvement in 4 of 5 manic patients (Grunze et al. 1999). In the aggregate, studies of the past decade have extended the evidence of the efficacy of valproate and the breadth of circumstances in which it can be effectively employed. The area of weakness in studies for valproate, as well as other antimanic agents, is that there have been only open case series for patients with hypomania or cyclothymia (Jacobsen 1993).

Adjunctive Regimens in Mania

Valproate has been studied in an add-on design in mania with consistent evidence that addition either of valproate to an antipsychotic (Muller-Oerlinghausen et al. 2000) or of an antipsychotic (olanzapine, quetiapine, risperidone, haloperidol) to valproate (or lithium) resulted in approximately 20% higher rates of antimanic response than with the antipsychotic or valproate alone (Tohen et al. 2002; Yatham 2003, 2005).

Patients treated with valproate plus lithium were significantly less likely to relapse over the course of a year than were patients treated with lithium. Side effects were more common with the combination regimen (Solomon et al. 1997).

One of the combination studies enrolled both patients who had received treatment with either valproate or lithium at an adequate dose for 2 weeks or longer and were still manic and patients who were manic without treatment, in which case both risperidone or haloperidol and either lithium or valproate were started concurrently. No advantage for the combination treatment occurred in the cotherapy group, whereas patients who had demonstrated unresponsiveness to valproate or lithium showed the advantage of the add-on therapy. The results suggest that in most circumstances combination therapy should be limited to patients who fail to respond to a relatively short period of adequate treatment with a first drug before adding the second (Sachs et al. 2002).

Maintenance Treatment of Bipolar Disorder

Several recent studies address the question of maintenance of effect in mania. A 12-week randomized, blinded comparison of valproate and olanzapine showed equivalent efficacy on mania for the two treatments (Zajecka et al. 2002). A 47-week study of the two drugs reported low rates of completion for both treatments (15% vs. 16%), with earlier symptomatic remission with olanzapine but equivalent efficacy for the two drugs over the remaining portion of the study. For both drugs, patients who were in remission at the end of week 3 of treatment were significantly more likely to complete the 47-week trial than those not in remission (divalproex: 26.2% vs. 11.1%; olanzapine: 20.3% vs. 10.6%; *P* = 0.001). This finding indicates that acute treatment response to a drug (either valproate or olanzapine) during a manic episode is predictive of effective treatment with the same drug in maintenance therapy. In both studies, weight gain was greater with olanzapine than with divalproex, and divalproex was associated with a significant reduction in cholesterol levels, compared with an increase in cholesterol levels with olanzapine (Tohen et al. 2003; Zajecka et al. 2002).

One large (*n* = 372) double-blind, placebo-controlled maintenance monotherapy study of valproate has been published (Bowden et al. 2000). Patients who recovered with open treatment with either divalproex or lithium were randomly assigned to maintenance treatment with divalproex, lithium, or placebo. The divalproex group did not differ significantly from the placebo group in time to any mood episode (*P* = 0.06), in part because the rate of relapse into mania with placebo was lower than anticipated. On most secondary outcome measures, divalproex was superior to placebo, with lower rates of discontinuation for either any recurrent mood episode or a depressive episode (Bowden 2004). Divalproex was superior to lithium on some comparisons, including longer duration of successful prophylaxis in the study and less deterioration in depressive symptom scores. Among the subset of patients treated with divalproex in the open acute phase, those subsequently randomized to divalproex had significantly longer times to recurrence of any mood episode (*P* = 0.05) or a depressive episode (*P* = 0.03), and the proportion of patients who completed the 1-year study without developing either a manic or a depressive episode was significantly higher for divalproex than for placebo (41% vs. 13%; *P* = 0.01). This is the only study published to date that has allowed a statistical test of the relationship between acute-episode response to treatment and maintenance treatment outcomes (Bowden et al. 2000). A secondary post hoc review of the study employing relative risk analysis found that patients treated with divalproex were significantly less likely than those treated with placebo to have prematurely left the study because of a mood episode (relative risk [RR]=0.63, 95% confidence interval [CI]=0.44–0.90) (Macritchie et al. 2001). A post hoc analysis of time to any mood episode or early discontinuation for any reason, a measure of effectiveness that has been incorporated in recent maintenance studies in bipolar disorder, indicated a significant advantage for divalproex over lithium ($P>0.004$) (Bowden 2003a).

A randomized open comparison of valpromide (the primary amide of valproic acid) and lithium for an 18-month period reported good efficacy for both drugs, with somewhat more favorable results among valpromide-treated patients (Lambert and Venaud 1992). The mean number of recurrent affective episodes per patient during the maintenance period was 0.61 in the lithium-treated group and 0.51 in the valpromide-treated group.

A separate study comparing valproate and lithium in a randomized, blinded trial of rapid-cycling patients reported that only one-quarter of patients enrolled met criteria for an acute bimodal response to either drug, with fewer than 25% of those randomized retaining benefits without relapse for the 20-month maintenance period. The results indicate that monotherapy regimens with either mood stabilizer are unlikely to be effective in any more than a small minority of rapid-cycling patients (Calabrese et al. 2005).

Acute Bipolar Depression

An 8-week randomized, placebo-controlled, blinded study reported that divalproex-treated subjects experienced significantly greater improvement than placebo-treated patients in both depressive and anxious symptomatology, based on Hamilton Rating Scale for Depression (Ham-D) and Hamilton Anxiety Scale (Ham-A) scores (Davis et al. 2005). In a 6-week randomized, blinded study in bipolar depression, divalproex was superior to placebo, with a large effect size advantage (Cohen's $d=0.81$). Primary improvement was on core mood symptoms rather than on anxiety or insomnia (Ghaemi et al. 2007). In an 8-week double-blind study of bipolar I or II depressed patients, 43% of patients treated with divalproex recovered, compared with 27% of patients treated with placebo. However, change in the total Ham-D score did not differ significantly between divalproex and placebo, although the depressed mood item favored divalproex at weeks 2, 4, and 5 (Sachs et al. 2001). In a 1-year randomized, double-blind study of initially manic bipolar patients, divalproex was more effective than lithium or placebo in delaying time to clinical depression. In those subjects who developed depression, divalproex plus paroxetine or sertraline

was superior to either antidepressant alone in treatment of the depression (Gyulai et al. 2003).

In summary, several relatively small studies suggest some antidepressant properties for valproate both in acute depression and in prophylaxis; however, adequately powered studies have not yet been conducted.

Bipolar Disorder in Children and Adolescents

Open trials of valproate report moderate to marked improvement in manic youth ages 8–18 years (Deltito et al. 1998; Mandoki 1993; Papatheodorou and Kutcher 1993; Wagner et al. 2002). Kowatch et al. (2000) studied 42 bipolar I manic patients (ages 9–18 years) who were treated for 6 weeks with divalproex, lithium, or carbamazepine in a randomized open study. Overall, 61% achieved 50% or greater improvement, which did not differ significantly across the groups. The effect size for improvement was greater for divalproex-treated patients than for lithium-treated or carbamazepine-treated patients (divalproex = 1.63, lithium = 1.06, carbamazepine = 1.00). A 6-month open study of valproate as monotherapy for 34 pediatric subjects with mixed mania reported high treatment completion rates and effectiveness of the drug (Pavuluri et al. 2005). Because the available data are limited to findings from open trials, valproate's comparative efficacy and effectiveness remain to be established.

One double-blind, randomized, placebo-controlled study has been conducted in youth ages 8–10 years who met criteria for oppositional defiant disorder or conduct disorder and had experienced temper and mood liability but did not meet the full criteria for bipolar disorder. By the end of phase 1, 8 of 10 patients who received divalproex had responded, compared with none on placebo. Of the 15 patients who completed both phases, 12 had superior responses to divalproex (Donovan et al. 2000).

Bipolar Disorder in the Elderly

Open trials (Narayan and Nelson 1997; Risinger et al. 1994) and one randomized, placebo-controlled study (Porsteinsson et al. 2001) reported benefits of valproate for irritable, agitated symptoms of dementia and for mania in elderly patients with bipolar disorder (Kahn et al. 1988; McFarland et al. 1990). The studies are difficult to summarize, as the authors did not utilize consistent terminology to report the behavioral disturbances of interest. For example, the terms *behavioral disturbance, aggression, agitation, hostility,* and *impulsivity* have all been used to describe effects of valproate on a symptom set that deals with the hyperactive and irritable dimensions of mania in the elderly (Narayan and Nelson 1997; Tariot et al. 1998). In a randomized, blinded study of 56 nursing home patients with agitation and dementia treated with either placebo or individualized doses of divalproex, when several covariates were taken into account, the drug/placebo difference in Brief Psychiatric Rating Scale Agitation scores became statistically significant ($P = 0.05$). Sixty-eight percent of patients on divalproex were rated as showing reduced agitation on the Clinical Global Impression Scale, versus 52% on placebo ($P = 0.06$ in the adjusted analysis). Side effects occurred in 68% of the divalproex group versus 33% of the placebo group ($P = 0.03$) and were generally rated as mild. This placebo-controlled study, despite some limitations, suggests possible short-term efficacy, tolerability, and safety of divalproex for agitation in dementia and supports further placebo-controlled studies (Porsteinsson et al. 2001). Patients with dementia are most frequently institutionalized for agitation and behavioral disturbances. A smaller randomized, placebo-controlled study using a fixed dose (valproate 480 mg/day) that may have been inadequate failed to find any difference between valproate and placebo groups.

Bipolar Disorder With Alcoholism

Bipolar disorder is often associated with comorbid substance use disorders, particularly alcoholism. In the largest prospective, blinded, placebo-controlled study, 59 bipolar I patients with alcohol dependence were treated with lithium carbonate and psychosocial interventions for 24 weeks, with half randomly assigned to receive adjunctive valproate. The addition of valproate was associated with significantly fewer heavy drinking days, fewer drinks per heavy drinking day, and fewer drinks per drinking day. Higher serum valproate concentrations were correlated with improved alcohol use outcomes. Both manic and depressive symptoms improved equivalently (Salloum et al. 2005).

In a 12-week double-blind, placebo-controlled trial, divalproex was associated with a significantly smaller percentage of individuals relapsing to heavy drinking, but there were no significant differences in other alcohol-related outcomes. There were significantly greater decreases in irritability in the divalproex-treated group and a trend toward greater decreases on measures of lability and verbal assault. There were no significant between-group differences on measures of impulsivity (Brady et al. 2002).

Bipolar Disorder Comorbid With Borderline Personality Disorder

Frankenburg and Zanarini (2002) conducted a placebo-controlled, double-blind study of divalproex sodium in 30 female subjects ages 18–40 years who met Revised Diagnostic Interview for Borderlines (Zanarini et al. 1989) and DSM-IV (American Psychiatric Association 1994) criteria for borderline personality disorder and DSM-IV criteria for bipolar II disorder. Subjects were randomly assigned to divalproex or placebo in a 2:1 manner. Treatment duration was 6 months. Divalproex was significantly superior to placebo in diminishing interpersonal sensitivity and anger/hostility as well as overall aggression. Adverse effects were infrequent (Frankenburg and Zanarini 2002).

Potential Predictors of Positive Response to Valproate Versus Lithium

Mixed mania. Patients treated with divalproex who had mixed manic presentations had greater improvement in manic symptoms with divalproex than with lithium treatment in two randomized studies, one of which was placebo controlled (Bowden 1995; Freeman et al. 1992; Swann et al. 1997). Patients with mixed manic and pure manic symptoms who received divalproex had equivalent improvement, thereby indicating a lack of differential effectiveness of divalproex for the two subtypes (Swann et al. 1997). By contrast, during maintenance treatment, patients with mixed mania had equivalent responses to divalproex or lithium, with evidence of higher adverse effects as a function of illness features of mixed mania, compared with rates of adverse effects in patients with euphoric mania (Bowden et al. 2005). The results suggest that mixed manic states require more complex regimens than monotherapies for effective long-term management.

Mania with irritability. Results from a large randomized, double-blind study of manic patients showed that valproate was significantly superior to placebo in reducing symptoms of hostility, whereas lithium was not. Similarly, among patients with an irritable subtype of mania, divalproex reduced overall manic symptomatology, whereas lithium did not. By contrast, both valproate and lithium were effective in reducing impulsivity and hyperactivity (Swann et al. 2002). These results are consistent with studies of valproate for irritability in patients with personality disorders and for secondary manic states (Hollander et al. 2003; Kavoussi and Coccaro 1998; Noaghiul et al. 1998).

Irritability in manic patients has been associated with greater likelihood of response to divalproex than to lithium (Swann et al. 2002) and carbamazepine (Vasudev et al. 2000). Irritability has been the most consistently differentiating symptom favoring divalproex benefit in patients with disorders other than bipolar disorder—namely, Cluster B personality disorders (including borderline personality disorder) and schizophrenia (Casey et al. 2003; Frankenburg and Zanarini 2002; Hollander et al. 2003; Swann et al. 2002).

Prior nonresponse to lithium.   Manic patients with a history of nonresponse to lithium who were randomly assigned to divalproex showed significantly greater improvement than patients who were randomized to lithium (Bowden et al. 1994). These data are consistent with reports of the efficacy of divalproex among patients selected for nonresponse to lithium (Pope et al. 1991).

High lifetime number of episodes.   Divalproex was significantly more effective than lithium among manic patients with more than 10 episodes of illness (Swann et al. 1999) or more than 2 depressive episodes (Swann et al. 2000).

Rapid cycling.   One blinded, randomized study reported that manic patients with a rapid-cycling illness course showed improvement in manic symptoms that was similar to the improvement seen in the entire patient cohort (Chamberlain et al. 1987).

In an open study of valproate in patients with rapid-cycling bipolar I or II disorder who were followed for a mean of 17.2 months, 52 of 58 (90%) had a marked or moderate antimanic response, 88 of 94 (94%) had a prophylactic antimanic response, 13 of 15 (87%) had an acute anti–mixed state response, and 17 of 18 (94%) had a prophylactic anti–mixed state response (Calabrese et al. 1993). A comparison of bipolar I rapid-cycling patients treated with divalproex, lithium, or the combination found that both drugs were highly effective acutely among patients entering into a manic episode but only moderately effective among initially depressed patients (Calabrese et al. 2005). As discussed in the section on maintenance treatment, a longer-term maintenance study comparing divalproex and lithium reported low rates of response (both acute and sustained) for both treatments (Calabrese et al. 2005). Although reasons for the somewhat discrepant responses reported by the same group of investigators are not clear, in the aggregate the data suggest that rapid-cycling bipolar disorder is difficult to treat effectively with any monotherapy regimen.

In a double-blind, placebo-controlled trial of valproate in acutely manic bipolar patients, the 12 patients whose symptoms responded to valproate did not differ with respect to frequency of rapid cycling from the 5 valproate-treated patients who showed no response (McElroy et al. 1991).

Migraine in bipolar disorder.   The prevalence of migraine is increased in persons with bipolar disorder, particularly bipolar II disorders. Valproate has been shown to be effective in the prophylaxis of migraine. The dosage of valproate is lower for migraine than for bipolar disorders, generally in the range of 500–1,000 mg/day (Freitag et al. 2002).

Other Potential Uses

Cotherapy in Schizophrenia

The use of valproate among patients with schizophrenia has increased, with one report indicating that over a third received valproate during hospitalization (Citrome et al. 2000; Wassef et al. 2000, 2001). A 4-week randomized, double-blind study of 242 schizophrenic patients who received risperidone or olanzapine alone, or divalproex plus the antipsychotic drug, indicated significantly greater improvement in Positive and Negative Syndrome Scale (PANSS)—Total and PANSS positive subscale scores among combination therapy patients from day 3 through day 21, but not at day 28. Platelet count was lower with combination therapy, and cholesterol levels increased with olanzapine or risperidone, compared with the significantly lower levels seen with antipsychotic plus divalproex. Weight gain did not differ between olanzapine and divalproex plus olanzapine; weight gain was greater with divalproex plus risperidone (7.5 pounds) than with risperidone (4.2 pounds) (Casey et al. 2003). A small ($n=12$) randomized, blinded study also indicated greater global improvement and improvement in negative symptoms for patients who were receiving divalproex plus haloperidol than for those who were receiving haloperidol alone (Wassef et al. 2000). Divalproex appeared to be effective as adjunctive therapy for schizoaffective disorder in a retrospective study of 20 patients with schizoaffective disorder, bipolar type (Bogan et al. 2000).

Substance Use Disorders

Open-label studies have demonstrated the efficacy of valproic acid in reducing both cocaine craving and rates of relapse. The rate of relapse to cocaine in 55 patients treated with valproic acid was related to serum levels: patients who had serum levels of >50 µg/ml had lower rates of relapse as compared to those whose levels were <50 µg/ml. A direct relationship was also noted between serum levels and a decrease in number of days of cocaine use and improved levels of subjective functioning (Myrick et al. 2003).

Mania Secondary to Head Trauma or Organic Brain Syndromes

Evidence suggesting that secondary or complicated mania responds well to valproate is mixed. In an open study of 56 valproate-treated patients with mania, response was associated with the presence of nonparoxysmal abnormalities on the electroencephalogram but not with neurological soft signs or abnormalities on computed axial tomography scans of brain (McElroy et al. 1988). Nevertheless, there was a trend for responders to have histories of closed-head injury antedating the onset of their affective symptoms (Pope et al. 1988). Furthermore, case reports described successful valproate treatment of organic brain syndromes with affective features (Kahn et al. 1988) and mental retardation in patients with bipolar disorder or bipolar symptoms (Kastner et al. 1990; Sovner 1989).

Impulsive Aggression

Valproate has been reported to be effective in reducing impulsive aggression among patients with personality disorders. In the one randomized, placebo-controlled, double-blind study that has been reported, 249 patients with Cluster B personality disorders, intermittent explosive disorder, or posttraumatic stress disorder were treated for 12 weeks with divalproex or placebo. Divalproex did not differ from placebo among all subjects, but among the 96 Cluster B patients, aggression and irritability scores were improved significantly over the course of the study (Hollander et al. 2003). These results are consistent with smaller open trials of valproate for impulsive aggression (Kavoussi and Coccaro 1998).

Side Effects and Toxicology

Valproate has been extensively used over several decades; thus, its adverse-effect profile is well characterized (DeVane 2003; Prevey et al. 1996). Patients treated for epilepsy are more likely to experience adverse events than patients being treated for migraine or mania, consequent to generally higher doses of valproate and more complex drug regimens in epilepsy (DeVane 2003). In a large 1-year placebo-controlled study in bipolar disorder, tremor and reported weight gain were the only symptoms more commonly seen with divalproex than placebo (Prevey et al. 1996).

Gastrointestinal Effects

The most common gastrointestinal effects include nausea, vomiting, diarrhea, dyspepsia and anorexia. These are dose dependent, are usually encountered at the start of treatment, and are often transient (DeVane 2003). Immediate-release formulations of valproate are more likely to cause adverse events compared with the extended-release and enteric-coated formulations (Horn and Cunanan 2003; Zarate et al. 2000).

Tremor

Tremor consequent to valproate resembles benign essential tremor and is more frequently seen in patients with seizure disorder than in patients with bipolar disorder (DeVane 2003). Tremor may respond to a reduction in dosage or treatment with propranolol. Extended-release or enteric-coated formulations may lessen the frequency of tremor (Wilder et al. 1983; Zarate et al. 2000).

Sedation

Mild to moderate sedation is common, usually at the initiation of treatment. This adverse event is dose dependent and may be minimized by dosage reduction, slower titration, use of extended-release formulations, and taking all medication at bedtime.

Hair Loss

Loss of hair can occur with valproate, possibly consequent to chelation of trace metals by valproate in the intestines and to its effects on histone deacetylase, which result in interference with rapidly dividing cells. As with many other characteristic side effects, lowering dosage can control this effect in some patients. Valproate ingestion should be spaced several hours before or after ingestion of vitamin preparations, supplemental zinc, folate, and biotin, which appear able to reverse this adverse effect in some patients (Bowden 2003b; Hurd et al. 1984).

Pancreatitis

Valproate is associated with infrequent idiosyncratic acute pancreatitis. In three migraine trials, the rates of elevation of amylase were similar between the valproate and placebo groups (Pellock et al. 2002). Therefore, precautionary amylase levels provide little benefit in predicting pancreatitis. Psychiatrists should be guided by clinical symptoms of pancreatitis.

Hematological Effects

Leukopenia and thrombocytopenia are directly related to higher valproate serum level, usually ≥100 µg/mL (Acharya and Bussel 1996). Thrombocytopenia is usually mild and rarely associated with bleeding complications. Management consists of dosage reduction. Platelet counts below 75,000/mm (Casey et al. 2003) should also be regularly reassessed, since levels below this are more often associated with bruising or bleeding.

Hepatotoxicity

The risk of liver toxicity is largely limited to patients younger than 2 years of age, because hepatic function is immature until age 2. In long-term study of divalproex, full-dosage regimens for 1 year were associated with improvements in laboratory indices of hepatic function, and no hepatotoxicity was reported in the 187 patients treated with divalproex (Bowden et al. 2000). Similar results were reported in a 47-week study of divalproex in bipolar disorder (Tohen et al. 2003).

A risk factor for the development of hepatotoxicity is the concomitant administration of anticonvulsants such as carbamazepine, which cause induction of enzymes involved in the metabolism of valproate, leading to increased concentrations of an active and hepatotoxic metabolite, 2-propyl-4-pentenoic acid.

Weight Gain

Weight gain of 3–24 pounds is seen in 3%–20% of patients treated with valproic acid over a time course that has ranged from 3 to 12 months (Bowden 2003b). In a 47-week study, divalproex (dosage range = 500–2,500 mg/day) resulted in less weight gain in manic and mixed-manic patients than olanzapine (1.22 kg vs. 2.79 kg) (Tohen et al. 2003). In a 3-week trial in manic patients, weight gain as a side effect was seen in 10% of valproate-treated patients and in 25% of olanzapine-treated patients (Zajecka et al. 2002). Valproate serum levels greater than 125 µg/mL are more likely to cause weight gain than those below this level (Bowden et al. 2000). If increased appetite and weight gain occur, valproate dosage should be lowered so long as clinical effectiveness is maintained, or alternatively should be discontinued and replaced by regimens without risks of weight gain.

Cognitive Dulling

Valproate has infrequent adverse effects on cognitive functioning, and it improves cognition in some patients (Prevey et al. 1996). In a 20-week randomized, observer-blinded, parallel-group trial, the addition of valproate to carbamazepine resulted in improvement on short-term verbal memory (Aldenkamp et al. 2000). No adverse cognitive effects with the use of valproate were seen in a group of elderly patients (mean age = 77 years) (Craig and Tallis 1994).

Lipid-Lowering Effects

Several studies indicate that valproate reduces total cholesterol and low-density lipoprotein (LDL) and high-density lipoprotein (HDL) cholesterol levels and protects against the adverse effects of some antipsychotic drugs on lipid function. An open case series found no changes in lipid profiles in children receiving long-term valproate (Geda et al. 2002). Valproate significantly lowered total and LDL cholesterol in comparison with phenobarbital and carbamazepine in a study of children with epilepsy (Ylmaz et al. 2001). In a 47-week study in manic and mixed-manic patients, valproate reduced cholesterol levels (Tohen et al. 1995). In patients with schizophrenia, valproate adjunctive to olanzapine or risperidone resulted in lowered cholesterol levels (Casey et al. 2003). The cholesterol-lowering effect of valproate is apparent even in short 3-week trials in acute mania. For the full sample in the randomized, blinded study, total cholesterol decreased significantly more in the divalproex group than in the placebo group (−13.47 mg/dL vs. −2.46 mg/dL; P=0.001). Stratification by baseline total cholesterol levels (≥200 mg/dL vs. <200 mg/dL) indicated that reduction with divalproex compared with placebo was limited to the stratum with higher mean baseline values (−18.6mg/dL vs. −6.5 mg/dL, respectively) (Bowden et al. 2006). In a 12-week comparison of divalproex and olanzapine in bipolar disorder patients, cholesterol and LDL levels fell with valproate use, compared with significant increases in olanzapine-treated patients (Zajecka and Weisler 2000).

Polycystic Ovarian Syndrome

Polycystic ovarian syndrome (PCOS) occurs in 4%–12% of women and is the leading cause of ovulatory infertility. PCOS appears to have a higher incidence in women with epilepsy; PCOS was found in 20% of 50 women with temporal lobe epilepsy and in 25% of 20 women with complex partial seizures, most of whom were unmedicated (Ernst and Goldberg 2002).

The prevalence of menstrual disturbances is high in women with bipolar disorder, irrespective of medication received, probably representing a dysfunction of the hypothalamic-pituitary-gonadal axis. A study of 10 lithium-treated, 10 valproate-treated, and 2 carbamazepine-treated women with bipolar disorder found a high frequency of menstrual dysfunction in all groups. Ultrasound identified an increased number of ovarian follicles in 1 of the lithium-treated patients but no increases in any valproate-treated patient. PCOS did not occur in any of the patients. Hormonal assessment of estrone, luteinizing hormone, follicle-stimulating hormone, testosterone, and dehydroepiandrosterone (DHEA) yielded no abnormal values in any patient (Rasgon et al. 2000).

In the cross-sectional National Institute of Mental Health Systematic Treatment Enhancement Program for Bipolar Disorder (STEP-BD) program, new-onset menstrual cycle irregularities and hyperandrogenism occurred in 10.5% of 86 women treated with valproate as a component of their prior treatment regimen before entering the STEP-BD study (Joffe et al. 2006a). A follow-up study of 7 women who had developed valproate-associated PCOS reported that PCOS reproductive features remitted in 3 of the 4 patients who discontinued valproate and persisted in all 3 patients who remained on valproate (Joffe et al. 2006b). No changes in polycystic ovarian morphology were associated with valproate in either study.

A study evaluating four groups of women with epilepsy—an untreated group, a carbamazepine-treated group, a valproate-treated group, and a group receiving more than one antiepileptic agent—found no differences in rates of PCOS among the drug-treated groups (Bauer et al. 2000). Valproate did not alter endocrine measures indicative of PCOS in a 12- to 15-month study in rhesus monkeys (Ferin et al. 2003). Obesity may be a mechanistic pathway whereby valproate (and potentially other drugs) predisposes women to PCOS. It is advisable to treat weight gain as a risk factor for possible development of PCOS and intervene as needed to avoid clinically significant weight gain.

Use During Pregnancy and Lactation

Birth Defects

Valproate is associated with an increased incidence of birth defects, including neural tube defects, craniofacial anomalies, limb abnormalities, and cardiovascular anomalies, if infants are exposed to valproic acid in the first 10 weeks of gestation (Kinrys et al. 2003; Samren et al. 1997). Neural tube defects, the most serious of the congenital anomalies, occur in 1%–4% of such infants. Prenatal exposure to valproate prior to the closure of the neural tube, during the fourth of week of gestation, leads to a prevalence of spina bifida in 1%–2% of infants, a 10–20 times greater rate than in the general population (Kinrys et al. 2003). Most of the available data involved patients with epilepsy, who are generally treated with higher doses of valproate than the doses employed for bipolar disorder and migraine and who are often concurrently treated with other teratogenic anticonvulsants (Bowden 2003b). The risk of malformations is increased with higher dosages and higher serum levels of valproate, as well as with concomitant use of other anticonvulsants (due to higher concentration of 2-propyl-4-pentenoic acid, a teratogenic agent); is possibly decreased with supplemental folic acid; and is definitely reduced with lower dosages of valproate (Bowden 2003b). Because alternate treatment strategies lacking teratogenic risk may work to effectively manage bipolar symptoms, valproate should generally be discontinued if conception is desired and during the early course of pregnancy if it occurs.

Breast-Feeding

Valproate is minimally present in breast milk. Piontek et al. (2000) reported that among six mother–infant pairs, serum valproate levels in the infants ranged from 0.9% to 2.3% of the mother's serum level, with absolute serum levels of 0.7–1.56 µg/mL. The valproate concentration in an infant was 1.5% of the maternal concentration (Wisner and Perel 1998).

Overdose

Regarding overdose, recovery from coma has occurred with serum valproate concentrations of greater than 2,000 µg/mL. In addition, serum valproate concentrations have been reduced by hemodialysis and hemoperfusion, and valproate-induced coma has been reversed with naloxone (Rimmer and Richens 1985). It is generally not necessary to perform routine blood monitoring of hematological and hepatic function in patients receiving valproate (Willmore et al. 1991). Superior to routine laboratory screening is educating the patient about the signs and symptoms of organ system dysfunction and instructing the patient to report these symptoms if they occur, in conjunction with careful monitoring of the patient's clinical status.

Drug–Drug Interactions

Because valproate is highly protein bound and extensively metabolized by the liver, a number of potential drug–drug interactions may occur with other protein-bound or metabolized drugs (Fogel 1988; Levy et al. 2002;

Rall and Schleifer 1985; Rimmer and Richens 1985). Thus, free fraction concentrations of valproate in serum can be increased and valproate toxicity can be precipitated by coadministration of other highly protein-bound drugs (e.g., aspirin) that can displace valproate from its protein-binding sites.

Because valproate tends to inhibit drug oxidation—it is the only major antiepileptic that does not induce hepatic microsomal enzymes—serum concentrations of a number of metabolized drugs can be increased by the coadministration of valproate. Valproate has been reported to increase serum concentrations of phenobarbital, phenytoin, and tricyclic antidepressants. Conversely, the metabolism of valproate can be increased, and valproate serum concentrations subsequently decreased, by coadministration of microsomal enzyme–inducing drugs such as carbamazepine. Drugs that inhibit metabolism may increase valproate concentrations in serum. Fluoxetine, for instance, has been reported to boost valproate concentrations (Sovner and Davis 1991).

The competitive inhibition by valproate of excretion of lamotrigine via glucuronidation requires that lamotrigine be started at a lower dosage, usually 25 mg every other day, and increased more cautiously. Steady-state dosage of lamotrigine used with valproate is also generally lower, but not in all patients.

Conclusion

The broad spectrum of efficacy in bipolar spectrum disorders and generally good tolerability of valproate make it a foundation of treatment for many patients with bipolar disorders. For optimal results, most patients should be treated with a formulation that permits single daily dosing and has the lowest peak-to-trough serum level, which in the United States currently is extended-release divalproex. Although onset of action of valproate is prompt with loading-dose strategies, given the paramount importance of tolerability and adherence of bipolar patients to long-term treatment regimens, gradual dosage increase is preferable for all but severely manic states.

During maintenance treatment, it is often important to reduce dosage if adverse effects persist. Valproate alleviates and is prophylactic principally for manic symptoms, although prophylactic benefits for depression are now relatively well established. A history of many episodes or current irritability may be a particularly strong indicator of a favorable response to valproate. Although some patients may have acute and sustained remission

with valproate monotherapy, many patients are more effectively treated with combinations, including other mood stabilizers and adjunctive medications. All current medications with established or putative roles can be combined with valproate.

Although valproate is now approved for mania in most countries, well-designed studies that advance clinical knowledge continue to be conducted with this drug. Additionally, scientific information coming from studies in patients with migraine, epilepsy, and other psychiatric disorders will continue to provide useful, reliable information, especially regarding prescribing practices and adverse-effect profiles and management.

References

Acharya S, Bussel JB: Hematologic toxicity of sodium valproate. J Pediatr Neurol 14:303–307, 1996
Aldenkamp AP, Baker G, Mulder OG, et al: A multicenter, randomized clinical study to evaluate the effect on cognitive function of topiramate compared with valproate as add-on therapy to carbamazepine in patients with partial-onset seizures. Epilepsia 41:1167–1178, 2000
Allen MH, Hirschfeld RM, Wozniak PJ, et al: Linear relationship of valproate serum concentration to response and optimal serum levels for acute mania. Am J Psychiatry 163:272–275, 2006
American Psychiatric Association: Diagnostic and Statistical Manual of Mental Disorders, 4th Edition. Washington, DC, American Psychiatric Association, 1994
Andratschke N, Grosu AL, Molis M, et al: Perspectives in the treatment of malignant gliomas in adults. Anticancer Res 21:3541–3550, 2001
Andreazza AC, Frey BN, Stertz L, et al: Effects of lithium and valproate on DNA damage and oxidative stress markers in an animal model of mania. Bipolar Disord 9:16, 2007
Bauer J, Jarre A, Klingmüller D, et al: Polycystic ovary syndrome in patients with focal epilepsy: a study in 93 women. Epilepsy Res 41:163–167, 2000
Bocci U, Beretta G: Esperienze sugli alcoolisti e tossicomania con dipropilacetate di sodio. Lavoro Neuropsichiatrico 58:51–61, 1976
Bogan AM, Brown ES, Suppes T: Efficacy of divalproex therapy for schizoaffective disorder. J Clin Psychopharmacol 20:520–522, 2000
Bourgeois B: Valproate: clinical use, in Antiepileptic Drugs, 3rd Edition. Edited by Levy RH, Dreifuss FE, Mattson RH, et al. New York, Raven, 1989, pp 633–642
Bowden CL: Predictors of response to divalproex and lithium. J Clin Psychiatry 56:25–30, 1995
Bowden CL: Valproate in mania, in Bipolar Medications: Mechanisms of Action. Edited by Manji HK, Bowden CL, Belmaker RH. Washington, DC, American Psychiatric Press, 2000, pp 357–365
Bowden CL: Acute and maintenance treatment with mood stabilizers. Int J Neuropsychopharmacol 6:269–275, 2003a
Bowden CL: Valproate. Bipolar Disord 5:189–202, 2003b

Bowden CL: Relationship of acute mania symptomatology to maintenance treatment response. Curr Psychiatry Rep 6:473–477, 2004

Bowden CL, McElroy SL: History of the development of valproate for treatment of bipolar disorder. J Clin Psychiatry 56:3–5, 1995

Bowden CL, Brugger AM, Swann AC, et al: Efficacy of divalproex vs lithium and placebo in the treatment of mania. JAMA 271:918–924, 1994

Bowden CL, Janicak PG, Orsulak P, et al: Relation of serum valproate concentration to response in mania. Am J Psychiatry 153:765–770, 1996

Bowden CL, Calabrese JR, McElroy SL, et al: A randomized, placebo-controlled 12-month trial of divalproex and lithium in treatment of outpatients with bipolar I disorder. Divalproex Maintenance Study Group. Arch Gen Psychiatry 57:481–489, 2000

Bowden CL, Collins MA, McElroy SL, et al: Relationship of mania symptomatology to maintenance treatment response with divalproex, lithium or placebo. Neuropsychopharmacology 30:323–330, 2005

Bowden CL, Swann AC, Calabrese JR, et al: A randomized, placebo-controlled, multicenter study of valproex sodium extended release in the treatment of acute mania. J Clin Psychiatry 67:1501–1510, 2006

Brady KT, Myrick H, Henderson S, et al: The use of divalproex in alcohol relapse prevention: a pilot study. Drug Alcohol Depend 67:323–330, 2002

Brennan MJW, Sandyk R, Borseek D: Use of sodium-valproate in the management of affective disorders: basic and clinical aspects, in Anticonvulsants in Affective Disorders. Edited by Emrich HM, Okuma T, Muller AA. Amsterdam, The Netherlands, Excerpta Medica, 1984, pp 56–65

Calabrese JR, Woyshville MJ, Kimmel SE, et al: Predictors of valproate response in bipolar rapid cycling. J Clin Psychopharmacol 13:280–283, 1993

Calabrese JR, Shelton MD, Rapport DJ, et al: A 20-month, double-blind, maintenance trial of lithium versus divalproex in rapid-cycling bipolar disorder. Am J Psychiatry 162:2152–2161, 2005

Casey DE, Daniel DG, Wassef AA, et al: Effect of divalproex combined with olanzapine or risperidone in patients with an acute exacerbation of schizophrenia. Neuropsychopharmacology 28:182–192, 2003

Chamberlain B, Ervin FR, Pihl RO, et al: The effect of raising or lowering tryptophan levels on aggression in vervet monkeys. Pharmacol Biochem Behav 28:503–510, 1987

Citrome L, Levine J, Allingham B: Changes in use of valproate and other mood stabilizers for patients with schizophrenia from 1994 to 1998. Psychiatr Serv 51:634–638, 2000

Craig I, Tallis R: Impact of valproate and phenytoin on cognitive function in elderly patients: results of a single-blind randomized comparative study. Epilepsia 35:381–390, 1994

Davis LL, Bartolucci A, Petty F: Divalproex in the treatment of bipolar depression: a placebo-controlled study. J Affect Disord 85:259–266, 2005

Deltito JA, Levitan J, Damore J, et al: Naturalistic experience with the use of divalproex sodium on an in-patient unit for adolescent psychiatric patients. Acta Psychiatr Scand 97:236–240, 1998

DeVane CL: Pharmacokinetics, drug interactions and tolerability of valproate. Psychopharmacol Bull 37 (suppl):25–42, 2003

Dokucu M, Yu L, Taghert P: Lithium- and valproate-induced alterations in circadian locomotor behavior in Drosophila. Neuropsychopharmacology 30:2216–2224, 2005

Donovan SJ, Stewart JW, Nunes EV, et al: Divalproex treatment for youth with explosive temper and mood lability: a double-blind, placebo-controlled crossover design. Am J Psychiatry 157:818–820, 2000

Einat H, Manji HK: Cellular plasticity cascades: genes-to-behavior pathways in animal models of bipolar disorder. Biol Psychiatry 59:1160–1171, 2006

Einat H, Yuan P, Gould TD, et al: The role of the extracellular signal-regulated kinase signaling pathway in mood modulation. J Neurosci 23:7311–7316, 2003

Emrich HM, von Zerssen DKW, Moller HJ: On a possible role of GABA in mania: therapeutic efficacy of sodium valproate. Adv Biochem Psychopharmacol 26:287–296, 1981

Emrich HM, Dose M, von Zerssen D: The use of sodium valproate, carbamazepine, and oxcarbazepine in patients with affective disorders. J Affect Disord 8:243–250, 1985

Ernst CL, Goldberg JF: The reproductive safety profile of mood stabilizers, atypical antipsychotics, and broad-spectrum psychotropics. J Clin Psychiatry 63 (suppl):42–55, 2002

Fariello R, Smith MC: Valproate: mechanisms of action, in Antiepileptic Drugs, 3rd Edition. Edited by Levy RH, Dreifuss FE, Mattson RH, et al. New York, Raven, 1989, pp 567–575

Ferin M, Morrell M, Xiao E, et al: Endocrine and metabolic responses to long-term monotherapy with the antiepileptic drug valproate in the normally cycling rhesus monkey. J Clin Endocrinol Metab 88:2908–2915, 2003

Fogel BS: Combining anticonvulsants with conventional psychopharmacologic agents, in Use of Anticonvulsants in Psychiatry: Recent Advances. Edited by McElroy SL, Pope HG Jr. Clifton, NJ, Oxford Health Care, 1988, pp 77–94

Frankenburg FR, Zanarini MC: Divalproex sodium treatment of women with borderline personality disorder and bipolar II disorder: a double-blind placebo-controlled pilot study. J Clin Psychiatry 63:442–446, 2002

Freeman TW, Clothier JL, Pazzaglia P, et al: A double-blind comparison of valproate and lithium in the treatment of acute mania. Am J Psychiatry 149:108–111, 1992

Freitag FG, Collins SD, Carlson HA, et al: A randomized trial of divalproex sodium extended-release tablets in migraine prophylaxis. Neurology 58:1652–1659, 2002

Geda G, Casken H, Icagasioglu D: Serum lipids with B-12 and folic acid levels in children receiving long term valproate therapy. Acta Neurol Belg 102:122–126, 2002

Ghaemi NS, Gilmer WS, Goldberg JF, et al. Divalproex in the treatment of acute bipolar depression: a preliminary double-blind, randomized, placebo-controlled pilot study. J Clin Psychiatry 68:1840–1844, 2007

Gilmor M, Skelton K, Nemeroff C, et al: The effects of chronic treatment with the mood stabilizers valproic acid and lithium on corticotrophin-releasing factor neuronal systems. J Pharmacol Exp Ther 305:434–439, 2003

Gray NA, Zhou R, Du J, et al: The use of mood stabilizers as plasticity enhancers in the treatment of neuropsychiatric disorders. J Clin Psychiatry 64 (suppl):3–17, 2003

Grunze H, Erfurth A, Amann B, et al: Intravenous valproate loading in acutely manic and depressed bipolar I patients. J Clin Psychopharmacol 19:303–309, 1999

Gyulai L, Bowden CL, McElroy SL, et al: Maintenance efficacy of divalproex in the prevention of bipolar depression. Neuropsychopharmacology 28:1374–1382, 2003

Hahn CG, Umapathy, Wagn HY, et al: Lithium and valproic acid treatments reduce PKC activation and receptor-G protein coupling in platelets of bipolar manic patients. J Psychiatr Res 39:35–63, 2005

Harwood AJ, Agam G: Search for a common mechanism of mood stabilizers. Biochem Pharmacol 66:179–189, 2003

Hollander E, Tracy KA, Swann AC, et al: Divalproex in the treatment of impulsive aggression: efficacy in Cluster B personality disorders. Neuropsychopharmacology 28:1186–1197, 2003

Horn RL, Cunanan C: Safety and efficacy of switching psychiatric patients from a delayed-release to an extended-release formulation of divalproex sodium. J Clin Psychopharmacol 23:176–181, 2003

Hurd RW, Van Rinsvelt HA, Wilder BJ, et al: Selenium, zinc, and copper changes with valproic acid: possible relation to drug side effects. Neurology 34:1393–1395, 1984

Jacobsen FM: Low dose valproate: a new treatment for cyclothymia, mild rapid cycling disorders, and premenstrual syndrome. J Clin Psychiatry 54:229–234, 1993

Joffe H, Cohen LS, Suppes T, et al: Valproate is associated with new-onset oligoamenorrhea with hyperandrogenism in women with bipolar disorder. Biol Psychiatry 59:1078–1086, 2006a

Joffe H, Cohen LS, Suppes T, et al: Longitudinal follow-up of reproductive and metabolic features of valproate-associated polycystic ovarian syndrome features: a preliminary report. Biol Psychiatry 60:1378–1381, 2006b

Kahn D, Stevenson E, Douglas CJ: Effect of sodium valproate in three patients with organic brain syndromes. Am J Psychiatry 145:1010–1011, 1988

Kastner T, Friedman DL, Plummer AT, et al: Valproic acid for the treatment of children with mental retardation and mood symptomatology. Pediatrics 86:467–472, 1990

Kavoussi RJ, Coccaro EF: Divalproex sodium for impulsive aggressive behavior in patients with personality disorder. J Clin Psychiatry 59:676–680, 1998

Keck PE Jr, McElroy SL, Tugrul KC, et al: Valproate oral loading in the treatment of acute mania. J Clin Psychiatry 54:305–308, 1993

Keck PE Jr, Bowden CL, Meinhold JM, et al: Relationship between serum valproate and lithium levels and efficacy and tolerability in bipolar maintenance therapy. Int J Psychiatry Clin Pract 9:271–277, 2005

Kinrys G, Pollack MH, Simon NM, et al: Valproic acid for the treatment of social anxiety disorder. Int Clin Psychopharmacol 18:169–172, 2003

Kowatch RA, Suppes T, Carmody TJ, et al: Effect size of lithium, divalproex sodium, and carbamazepine in children and adolescents with bipolar disorder. J Am Acad Child Adolesc Psychiatry 39:713–720, 2000

Lambert PA, Venaud G: Comparative study of valpromide versus lithium as prophylactic treatment in affective disorders. Nervure 5:57–65, 1992

Lambert PA, Cavaz G, Borselli S, et al: Action neuropsychotrope d'un nouvel anti-epileptique: le depamide. Ann Med Psychol 1:707–710, 1966

Leveil V, Nanquet R: A study of the action of valproic acid on the kindling effect. Epilepsia 18:229–234, 1977

Levy RH, Mattson RH, Meldrum BS, et al (eds): Antiepileptic Drugs, 5th Edition. New York, Lippincott Williams & Wilkins, 2002

Macritchie KA, Geddes JR, Scott J, et al: Valproic acid, valproate and divalproex in the maintenance treatment of bipolar disorder. Cochrane Database Syst Rev (3):CD003196, 2001

Mandoki MW: Valproate-lithium combination and verapamil as treatments of bipolar disorder in children and adolescents (abstract). Neuropsychopharmacology 9 (suppl):183S, 1993

McElroy SL, Pope HG Jr, Keck PE Jr: Treatment of psychiatric disorders with valproate: a series of 73 cases. Psychiatrie Psychobiologie 3:81–85, 1988

McElroy SL, Keck PE, Pope HG, et al: Correlates of antimanic response to valproate. Psychopharmacol Bull 27:127–133, 1991

McElroy SL, Keck PE, Tugrul KC, et al: Valproate as a loading treatment in acute mania. Neuropsychobiology 27:146–149, 1993

McElroy SL, Keck PE, Stanton SP, et al: A randomized comparison of divalproex oral loading versus haloperidol in the initial treatment of acute psychotic mania. J Clin Psychiatry 57:142–146, 1996

McFarland BH, Miller MR, Straumfjord AA: Valproate use in the older manic patient. J Clin Psychiatry 51:479–481, 1990

Meunier H, Carraz G, Meunier V, et al: Proprietes pharmacodynamiques de l'acide n-propylacetique. Therapie 18:435–438, 1975

Muller-Oerlinghausen B, Retzow A, Henn FA, et al: Valproate as an adjunct to neuroleptic medication for the treatment of acute episodes of mania: a prospective, randomized, double-blind, placebo-controlled, multicenter study. J Clin Psychopharmacol 20:195–203, 2000

Myrick H, Malcolm R, Raymond A: The use of antiepileptics in the treatment of addictive disorders. Prim Psychiatry 10:59–63, 2003

Narayan N, Nelson J: Treatment of dementia with behavioral disturbance using divalproex or a combination of divalproex and a neuroleptic. J Clin Psychiatry 58:351–354, 1997

Noaghiul S, Narayan M, Nelson JC: Divalproex treatment of mania in elderly patients. Am J Geriatr Psychiatry 6:257–262, 1998

Papatheodorou G, Kutcher SP: Divalproex sodium treatment in late adolescent and young adult acute mania. Psychopharmacol Bull 29:213–219, 1993

Pavuluri MN, Henry DB, Carbray JA, et al: Divalproex sodium for pediatric mixed mania: a 6-month prospective trial. Bipolar Disord 7:266–273, 2005

Pellock JM, Wilder BJ, Deaton R, et al: Acute pancreatitis coincident with valproate use: a critical review. Epilepsia 43:1421–1424, 2002

Penry JK, Dean JC: The scope and use of valproate in epilepsy. J Clin Psychiatry 50 (suppl):17–22, 1989

Piontek CM, Baab S, Peindl KS, et al: Serum valproate levels in 6 breastfeeding mother-infant pairs. J Clin Psychiatry 61:170–172, 2000

Pope HG Jr, McElroy SL, Satlin A, et al: Head injury, bipolar disorder, and response to valproate. Compr Psychiatry 29:34–38, 1988

Pope HG Jr, McElroy SL, Keck PE Jr, et al: Valproate in the treatment of acute mania: a placebo-controlled study. Arch Gen Psychiatry 48:62–68, 1991

Porsteinsson AP, Tariot PN, Erb R, et al: Placebo-controlled study of divalproex sodium for agitation in dementia. Am J Geriatr Psychiatry 9:58–66, 2001

Prevey ML, Delaney RC, Cramer JA, et al: Effect of valproate on cognitive functioning: comparison with carbamazepine. The Department of Veteran Affairs Epilepsy Cooperative Study 264 Group. Arch Neurol 53:1008–1016, 1996

Quiroz JA, Gray NA, Kato T, et al: Mitchondrially mediated plasticity in the pathophysiology and treatment of bipolar disorder. Neuropsychopharmacology 33:2551–2565, 2008

Rall TW, Schleifer LS: Drugs effective in the therapy of the epilepsies, in Goodman and Gilman's The Pharmacological Basis of Therapeutics, 7th Edition. Edited by Gilman AG, Goodman LS, Rall TW. New York, Macmillan, 1985, pp 446–472

Rasgon NL, Altshuler LL, Gudeman D, et al: Medication status and polycystic ovary syndrome in women with bipolar disorder: a preliminary report. J Clin Psychiatry 61:173–178, 2000

Rimmer E, Richens A: An update on sodium valproate. Pharmacotherapy 5:171–184, 1985

Risinger RC, Risby ED, Risch SC: Safety and efficacy of divalproex sodium in elderly bipolar patients (letter). J Clin Psychiatry 55:215, 1994

Sachs GS, Collins MA, Altshuler LL, et al: Divalproex sodium versus placebo for treatment of bipolar depression. Paper presented at annual meeting of the American College of Neuropsychopharmacology, San Juan, PR, December 2001

Sachs G, Grossman F, Okamoto A, et al: Risperidone plus mood stabilizer versus placebo plus mood stabilizer for acute mania of bipolar disorder: a double-blind comparison of efficacy and safety. Am J Psychiatry 159:1146–1154, 2002

Salloum IM, Cornelius JR, Daley DC, et al: Efficacy of valproate maintenance in patients with bipolar disorder and alcoholism: a double-blind placebo-controlled study. Arch Gen Psychiatry 62:37–45, 2005

Samren EB, Duijn CM, Koch S, et al: Maternal use of antiepileptic drugs and the risk of major congenital malformations: a joint European prospective study of human teratogens associated with maternal epilepsy. Epilepsia 38:981–990, 1997

Shaltiel G, Shamir A, Shapiro J, et al: Valproate decreases inositol biosynthesis. Biol Psychiatry 56:868–874, 2004

Siafaka-Kapadai A, Patiris M, Bowden C, et al: Incorporation of [3H]-valproic acid into lipids in GT1–7 neurons. Biochem Pharmacol 56:207–212, 1998

Solomon DA, Ryan CE, Keitner GI, et al: A pilot study of lithium carbonate plus divalproex sodium for the continuation and maintenance treatment of patients with bipolar I disorder. J Clin Psychiatry 58:95–99, 1997

Sovner R: The use of valproate in the treatment of mentally retarded persons with typical and atypical bipolar disorders. J Clin Psychiatry 50:40–43, 1989

Sovner R, Davis JM: A potential drug interaction between fluoxetine and valproic acid (letter). J Clin Psychopharmacol 11:389, 1991

Swann AC, Bowden CL, Morris D, et al: Depression during mania: treatment response to lithium or divalproex. Arch Gen Psychiatry 54:37–42, 1997

Swann AC, Bowden CL, Calabrese JR, et al: Differential effect of number of previous episodes of affective disorder on response to lithium or divalproex in acute mania. Am J Psychiatry 156:1264–1266, 1999

Swann AC, Bowden CL, Calabrese JR, et al: Mania: differential effects of previous depressive and manic episodes on response to treatment. Acta Psychiatr Scand 101:444–451, 2000

Swann AC, Bowden CL, Calabrese JR, et al: Pattern of response to divalproex, lithium, or placebo in four naturalistic subtypes of mania. Neuropsychopharmacology 26:530–536, 2002

Tariot PN, Erb R, Podgorski CA, et al: Efficacy and tolerability of carbamazepine for agitation and aggression in dementia. Am J Psychiatry 155:54–61, 1998

Tohen M, Baldessarini RJ, Zarate C et al: Blood dyscrasias with carbamazepine and valproate: a pharmacological study of 2,228 patients at risk. Am J Psychiatry 152:413–418, 1995

Tohen M, Chengappa KNR, Suppes T, et al: Efficacy of olanzapine in combination with valproate or lithium in the treatment of mania in patients partially nonresponsive to valproate or lithium monotherapy. Arch Gen Psychiatry 59:62–69, 2002

Tohen M, Ketter TA, Zarate CA: Olanzapine versus divalproex sodium for the treatment of acute mania and maintenance of remission: a 47 week study. Am J Psychiatry 160:1263–1271, 2003

Tremolizzo L, Carboni G, Ruzicka WB, et al: An epigenetic mouse model for molecular and behavioral neuropathologies related to schizophrenia vulnerability. Proc Natl Acad Sci U S A 99:17095–17100, 2002

Tremolizzo L, Doueiri MS, Dong E, et al: Valproate corrects the schizophrenia-like epigenetic behavioral modifications induced by methionine in mice. Biol Psychiatry 57:500–509, 2005

Vasudev K, Goswami U, Kohli K: Carbamazepine and valproate monotherapy: feasibility, relative safety and efficacy, and therapeutic drug monitoring in manic disorder. Psychopharmacology 150:15–23, 2000

Wagner KD, Weller EB, Carlson GA, et al: An open-label trial of divalproex in children and adolescents with bipolar disorder. J Am Acad Child Adolesc Psychiatry 41:1224–1230, 2002

Wassef AA, Dott SG, Harris A, et al: Randomized, placebo-controlled pilot study of divalproex sodium in the treatment of acute exacerbations of chronic schizophrenia. J Clin Psychopharmacol 20:357–361, 2000

Wassef AA, Hafiz NG, Hampton D, et al: Divalproex sodium augmentation of haloperidol in hospitalized patients with schizophrenia: clinical and economic implications. J Clin Psychopharmacol 21:21–26, 2001

Wilder BJ: Pharmacokinetics of valproate and carbamazepine. J Clin Psychopharmacol 12 (suppl):64S–68S, 1992

Wilder BJ, Karas BJ, Penry JK, et al: Gastrointestinal tolerance of divalproex sodium. Neurology 33:808–811, 1983

Willmore LJ, Triggs WJ, Pellock JM: Valproate toxicity: risk-screening strategies. J Child Neurol 6:3–6, 1991

Wisner KL, Perel JM: Serum levels of valproate and carbamazepine in breastfeeding mother-infant pairs. J Clin Psychopharmacol 18:167–169, 1998

Yatham LN: Efficacy of atypical antipsychotics in mood disorders. J Clin Psychopharmacol 23:S9–S14, 2003

Yatham LN: Atypical antipsychotics for bipolar disorder. Psychiatr Clin North Am 28:325–347, 2005

Ylmaz E, Dosan Y, Gurgoze MK, et al: Serum lipid changes during anticonvulsant treatment in epileptic children. Acta Neurol Belg 101:217–220, 2001

Zajecka J, Weisler R: Divalproex sodium vs olanzapine for the treatment of mania in bipolar disorder. Presented at the 39th Annual Meeting of the American College of Neuropsychopharmacology, San Juan, Puerto Rico, December 2000

Zajecka J, Weisler R, Sachs G, et al: A comparison of the efficacy, safety and tolerability of divalproex sodium and olanzapine in the treatment of bipolar disorder. J Clin Psychiatry 63:1148–1155, 2002

Zanarini MC, Gunderson JG, Frankenburg FR, et al: The Revised Diagnostic Interview for Borderlines: discriminating BPD from other Axis II disorders. J Personal Disord 3:10–18, 1989

Zarate CA Jr, Tohen M, Narendran R, et al: The adverse effect profile and efficacy of divalproex sodium compared with valproic acid: a pharmacoepidemiology study. J Clin Psychiatry 60:232–236, 2000

CHAPTER 37

Carbamazepine and Oxcarbazepine

Terence A. Ketter, M.D.

Po W. Wang, M.D.

Robert M. Post, M.D.

Pharmacotherapy of bipolar disorder is a complex and rapidly evolving field. The development of new treatments has helped to refine concepts of illness subtypes and generated important new management options. Although the mood stabilizers—the first-line agents lithium, valproate, and lamotrigine and the alternative agents carbamazepine (CBZ) and oxcarbazepine (OXC)—are considered the primary medications for bipolar disorder, antipsychotics, antidepressants, anxiolytics, and a new generation of anticonvulsants are commonly combined with mood stabilizers in clinical settings (American Psychiatric Association 2002; Ketter 2005; Suppes et al. 2005). These diverse medications have varying pharmacodynamics, pharmacokinetics, drug–drug interactions, and adverse effects, thus offering not only new therapeutic opportunities but also a variety of new potential pitfalls.

Therefore, clinicians are challenged with integrating complex data regarding efficacy and adverse-effect spectra with pharmacological properties in their efforts to provide safe, effective state-of-the-art pharmacotherapy for patients with bipolar disorder. In this chapter, we review the preclinical and clinical pharmacology of CBZ and its analog OXC. In the past, CBZ was considered an alternative to lithium and valproate rather than a first-line intervention in the treatment of bipolar disorder (American Psychiatric Association 2002) in view of methodological limitations of early studies of efficacy in bipolar disorder, complexity of use because of adverse effects and drug–

drug interactions, and lack of U.S. Food and Drug Administration (FDA) indication for the treatment of bipolar disorder. However, evidence of the efficacy of a proprietary CBZ extended-release formulation (Equetro) in two randomized, double-blind, placebo-controlled, parallel-group studies in bipolar disorder patients with acute manic and mixed episodes (Weisler et al. 2004, 2005) has addressed methodological concerns and led to CBZ's receiving an indication for the treatment of acute manic and mixed episodes in patients with bipolar disorder. Importantly, in selected patients, CBZ and OXC may offer efficacy and tolerability that are favorable compared with first-line therapies and thus can be important treatment options for some individuals with bipolar disorders. In particular, CBZ's low propensity to cause the weight gain and metabolic problems seen with some other agents may lead clinicians to reassess its role in the management of patients with bipolar disorder (Ketter et al. 2005). Although OXC appears easier to use than CBZ, use of OXC remains limited by the lack of compelling data regarding its efficacy in bipolar disorder.

History and Discovery

CBZ, as one of the initial alternatives to lithium and older antipsychotics, has played an important role in the development of therapeutic interventions for bipolar disorder (Post et al. 2007). Lithium was reported by Cade (1949) to be effective in acute mania and saw widespread use in

Europe by the 1960s, but in view of safety concerns (risk of toxicity), it was only approved for the treatment of acute mania in the United States in 1970. CBZ was developed in 1957 by J.R. Geigy AG in Europe, and its efficacy in epilepsy and paroxysmal pain was appreciated by the 1960s and in bipolar disorder by the early 1970s (Takezaki and Hanaoka 1971). As with lithium, marketing of CBZ in the United States was delayed because of safety concerns (risk of blood dyscrasias), and CBZ was thus not approved for the treatment of epilepsy in adults until 1974, in children older than 6 years until 1978, and without age limitation until 1987.

The first-generation antipsychotic chlorpromazine was approved for the treatment of acute mania in the United States in 1973. The next year, lithium received a maintenance indication for the treatment of bipolar disorder. Thus, in the 1970s, acute mania was managed primarily with lithium and first-generation antipsychotics. Lithium proved dramatically effective in classic euphoric mania but had limitations, which included the need for initial titration and a clinically significant response latency. In addition, lithium proved less effective in patients with mixed or dysphoric mania, rapid cycling, greater numbers of previous episodes, mood-incongruent delusions, or concurrent substance abuse than in those with classic bipolar disorder (Ketter and Wang 2002). The response latency and the spectrum of efficacy limitations of lithium resulted in the common practice of concurrently administering first-generation antipsychotics in acute mania. However, first-generation antipsychotics had adverse effects that imposed substantial limitations, as mood disorder patients appeared to be at even greater risk than schizophrenia patients for acute extrapyramidal side effects (Nasrallah et al. 1988) and tardive dyskinesia (Kane and Smith 1982). In addition, these agents appeared to have unimodal (antimanic but not antidepressant) activity in bipolar disorder in that they could exacerbate the depressive component of the illness (Ahlfors et al. 1981).

These limitations of lithium and first-generation antipsychotics led investigators to explore other treatment options for bipolar disorder. On the basis of early reports of favorable psychotropic profiles in epilepsy patients and preliminary observations in mood disorders, systematic investigations of CBZ (Ballenger and Post 1978) and valproate commenced, and these anticonvulsants emerged as effective in acute mania, even in subtypes associated with lithium resistance. Thus, CBZ and then valproate were increasingly used off label for bipolar disorder in the 1980s and early 1990s, respectively. The CBZ analog OXC was anecdotally reported as useful in bipolar disor-

der in the 1980s (Müller and Stoll 1984) but was not marketed in the United States for the treatment of epilepsy until 2000.

Because of economic concerns such as patent protection limitations and the high cost of obtaining FDA approval, a CBZ indication for bipolar disorder was not initially sought in the United States but was obtained from agencies in Canada, Japan, Australia, and several European countries. The development of divalproex, a well-tolerated proprietary valproate formulation, allowed the patent protection necessary to make seeking an FDA indication for bipolar disorder economically feasible. The FDA's approval of divalproex for the treatment of acute mania in 1994, lack of major safety concerns, and relative ease of use were important factors in divalproex use overtaking that of CBZ and even lithium by the late 1990s. In addition, divalproex's efficacy in acute mania was considered better established than that of CBZ, because the pivotal trials for obtaining the divalproex mania indication were conducted with contemporary randomized, parallel, double-blind, placebo-controlled paradigms (Bowden et al. 1994; Pope et al. 1991), whereas early controlled CBZ studies in bipolar disorder used alternative (e.g., active comparator and on–off–on) designs, as described later in this chapter (see section "Indications and Efficacy"). Despite the limitations in the controlled maintenance data for both drugs, CBZ and divalproex were considered mood stabilizers along with lithium.

The emergence of and evidence of the efficacy of a proprietary CBZ extended-release formulation (Equetro) in two randomized, double-blind, placebo-controlled studies in patients with acute manic and mixed episodes (Weisler et al. 2004, 2005) led to an FDA indication in late 2004 for this CBZ formulation in the treatment of acute manic and mixed episodes in patients with bipolar disorder.

OXC was approved for the treatment of epilepsy in the United States in 2000, in the setting of the development of several new anticonvulsants in the 1990s. The new anticonvulsants appear to have heterogeneous psychotropic profiles (Ketter et al. 2003), with only OXC thus far showing benefit in some controlled (albeit small) trials in acute mania (Emrich 1990) and lamotrigine in the prophylaxis of and (to a lesser extent) acute treatment of bipolar depression. As with CBZ, economic concerns such as patent protection limitations and the high cost of obtaining FDA approval are substantial barriers to seeking an OXC indication for acute mania in the United States. Because of its greater ease of use, OXC is considered by some to be an important alternative to CBZ

(American Psychiatric Association 2002). However, use of OXC remains limited by the lack of compelling data regarding its efficacy in bipolar disorder.

Structure–Activity Relations

CBZ is an iminostilbine derivative with a dibenzazepine nucleus. CBZ's tricyclic nucleus appears to relate more to local anesthetic and antihistaminic actions than to anticonvulsant actions. In contrast, the carbamyl (carboxamide) group at position 5 appears related to substantial anticonvulsant effects. CBZ's 5-carboxamide substituent, in contrast to the 5-aryl substituent of imipramine, appears to account for CBZ's markedly different effects compared with those of imipramine, as described below. OXC differs structurally from CBZ only in that it has a ketone substitution at the 10,11-position, and as noted below, the bulk of the evidence thus far suggests that this structural similarity is paralleled by a mechanistic similarity.

Pharmacological Profile

CBZ and OXC have a preclinical anticonvulsant profile similar to that of phenytoin and less broad than that of valproate or lamotrigine. Thus, CBZ and OXC, like phenytoin, valproate, and lamotrigine, are effective in the maximal electroshock model of generalized tonic and/or clonic seizures, and like phenytoin but unlike valproate and lamotrigine, they are not effective in the pentylenetetrazole model of absence seizures. CBZ and OXC, like phenytoin, valproate, and lamotrigine, are effective in blocking seizures resulting from amygdala kindling (a model of partial seizures). However, CBZ and OXC, like phenytoin and lamotrigine but unlike valproate, fail to block kindling development (a model of epileptogenesis).

As expected from their preclinical profiles, CBZ and OXC, like phenytoin, valproate, and lamotrigine, are effective in partial seizures with and without secondary generalization, and like phenytoin but unlike valproate and lamotrigine, they are ineffective in absence seizures. CBZ and OXC also have analgesic effects and thus are effective in trigeminal neuralgia.

Pharmacokinetics and Disposition

Carbamazepine

CBZ is available in the United States as a proprietary product (Tegretol) marketed for epilepsy by Novartis

Pharmaceuticals Corporation in suspension (100 mg/5 mL), chewable tablets (100 mg), nonchewable tablets (200 mg), and extended-release (Tegretol XR) tablets (100-, 200-, and 400-mg) ("Tegretol" 2008). An additional proprietary extended-release formulation marketed for epilepsy as Carbatrol (by Shire US Inc.) and for bipolar disorder as Equetro (by Validus Pharmaceuticals) is available in 100-, 200-, and 300-mg capsules ("Carbatrol" 2008; "Equetro" 2008). Intramuscular and depot formulations are not available. CBZ is also available in generic formulations. Differences have been observed in the bioavailability of proprietary and generic formulations (Meyer et al. 1992).

CBZ is extensively metabolized, with only about 3% excreted unchanged in the urine. The main metabolic pathway of CBZ (to its active 10,11-epoxide, CBZ-E) appears to be mediated primarily by cytochrome P450 (CYP) 3A3/4 (Figure 37–1, top), with a minor contribution by CYP2C8 (Kerr et al. 1994). This epoxide pathway accounts for about 40% of CBZ disposition and an even greater proportion in patients with induced epoxide pathway metabolism (presumably via CYP3A3/4 induction) (Faigle and Feldmann 1995). Although a genetic polymorphism has been observed for CYP2C8 (Wrighton and Stevens 1992), this probably does *not* account for the variability observed in CBZ disposition, in view of the minor role of this isoform. The frequency distribution of CBZ kinetic parameters is unimodal, consistent with CYP3A3/4 (which lacks genetic polymorphism) being the crucial isoform. With enzyme induction (of the epoxide pathway, presumably via CYP3A3/4 induction), formation of CBZ-E triples, its subsequent transformation to the inactive diol (CBZ-D) doubles, and thus the ratio of CBZ-E to CBZ increases (Eichelbaum et al. 1985). Other pathways include aromatic hydroxylation (25%), which is apparently mediated by CYP1A2 and not induced concurrently with the epoxide pathway, and glucuronide conjugation of the carbamoyl side chain (15%) by uridine diphosphoglucuronosyltransferase (UGT), presumably primarily by UGT2B7 (Staines et al. 2004). These other pathways yield inactive metabolites.

CBZ has erratic absorption and a bioavailability of about 80%. CBZ should not be exposed to humidity, because this can cause solidification and decrease bioavailability (Nightingale 1990). It is about 75% bound to plasma proteins and has a moderate volume of distribution (about 1 L/kg). Before autoinduction of the epoxide pathway, the half-life of CBZ is about 24 hours, and the clearance is about 25 mL/minute. However, after autoinduction (2–4 weeks into therapy), the half-life falls to

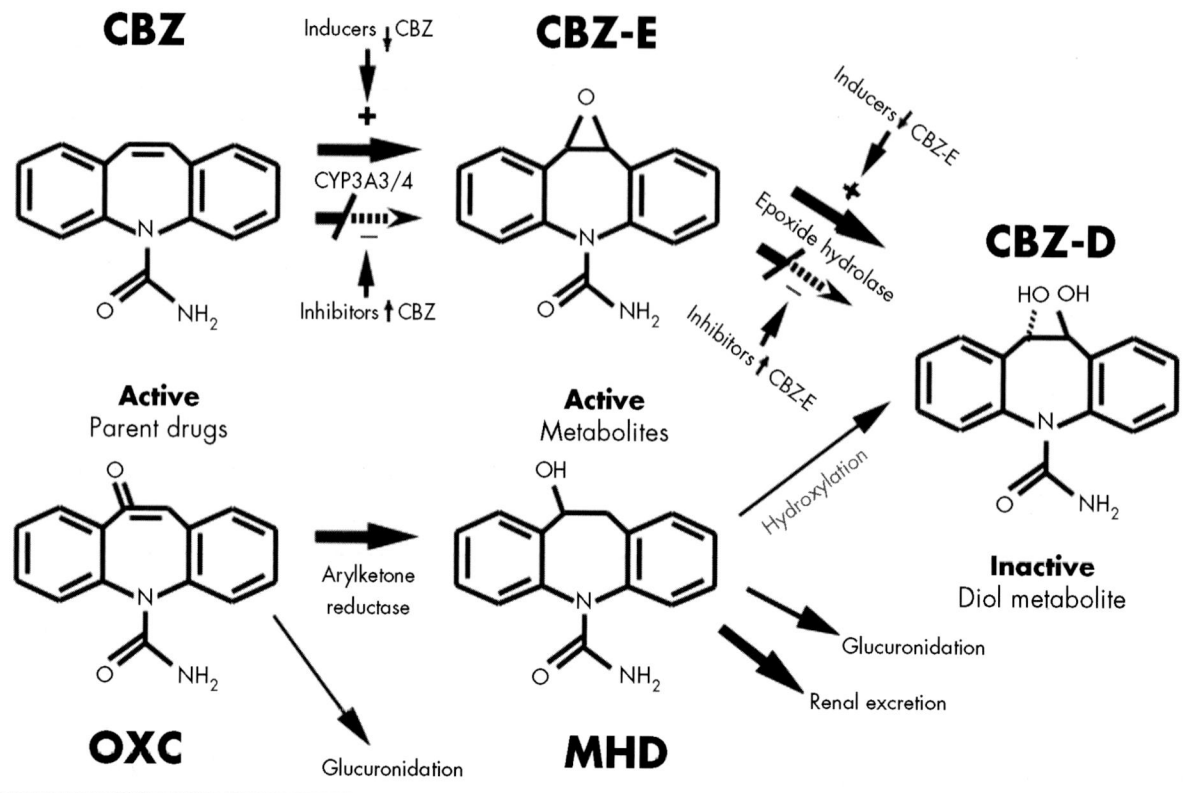

FIGURE 37–1.   Carbamazepine and oxcarbazepine metabolism.

CBZ = carbamazepine; CBZ-D = carbamazepine-10,11-dihydro-dihydroxide; CBZ-E = carbamazepine-10,11-epoxide; CYP3A3/4 = cytochrome P450 3A3/4 isoenzyme; MHD = monohydroxy derivative; OXC = oxcarbazepine.
+ = indicates enzyme induction; – = indicates enzyme inhibition.

about 8 hours, and clearance rises to about 75 mL/minute. This may require dosage adjustment to maintain adequate blood concentrations and therapeutic effects. The active CBZ-E metabolite has a half-life of about 6 hours and is converted to an inactive diol (CBZ-D) by epoxide hydrolase. The extended-release CBZ formulations available in the United States given twice a day yield steady-state CBZ concentrations similar to those seen with the immediate-release formulation given four times a day (Garnett et al. 1998; Thakker et al. 1992).

In the treatment of acute mania, two divergent clinical needs influence the rate of dosage titration. First, there is a pressing need for rapid control of the manic syndrome, which suggests that faster titration to higher doses could provide more rapid attainment of sufficient serum concentrations, potentially yielding quicker onset not only of nonspecific sedation but also of specific antimanic effects. On the other hand, there is a need to not excessively burden patients with the increased adverse effects associated with overly rapid escalation of CBZ dosage. Such adverse effects include neurotoxicity (sedation, diplopia, and ataxia) and gastrointestinal disturbances

that not only can complicate acute management but also may lead patients to develop negative perceptions about the adverse effects of CBZ that later interfere with their adherence to prophylactic therapy. Thus, although a loading-dose strategy may be tolerated and effective in the treatment of mania with valproate (Keck et al. 1993), the potential for neurotoxic adverse effects limits such an approach with CBZ.

Nonetheless, in the inpatient therapy of mania, CBZ is commonly started at 400–800 mg/day in divided doses, with the dosage increased as tolerated (by 200 mg/day every 1–4 days) to provide clinical efficacy. In recent controlled studies, a beaded extended-release capsule formulation was started at 200 mg twice per day and titrated by daily increments of 200 mg to final dosages as high as 1,600 mg/day (Weisler et al. 2004, 2005). Titration of dosage against adverse effects is more important than blood concentrations, which usually reach between 4 and 12 µg/mL (17 and 51 µM/L), and there does not appear to be a close blood concentration–efficacy relationship for CBZ in treating either seizure or mood disorders. Usual dosages are 800–1,600 mg/day given in up to three or four divided doses with the immediate-release formulation. Extended-release formulations permit two divided doses per day, and most mood disorder patients may even be able to take the entire daily dose at bedtime. Although this strategy is convenient, it may not be feasible in some individuals because of neurotoxicity at peak serum concentrations, which occurs about 4–8 hours after ingesting CBZ. CBZ has fairly rapid onset of antimanic efficacy, in some comparisons similar to that of neuroleptics. Thus, lack of clinical improvement after 7–10 days may be an indication that augmentation or alternative strategies should be considered.

In a recent report of open extension therapy after controlled acute mania studies, beaded extended-release capsule CBZ was started at 200 mg twice per day and titrated by increments of 200 mg every 3 days (versus every day in the acute studies) to final dosages as high as 1,600 mg/day (Ketter et al. 2004). This approach decreased the incidence of central nervous system (dizziness, somnolence, ataxia), digestive (nausea, vomiting), and dermatological (pruritus) adverse effects by about 50%. Euthymic or depressed patients tend to tolerate aggressive initiation less well than do manic patients. Thus, in less acute situations such as the initiation of prophylaxis or adjunctive use, CBZ is often started at 100–200 mg/day and increased (as necessary and tolerated) by 200 mg/day every 4–7 days. Even this gradual initiation may result in adverse effects. Thus, starting with 50 mg (half of a chewable 100-mg tablet) at bedtime and increasing the dosage by 50 mg every 4 days may provide better tolerability. Moreover, doses of CBZ initially associated with adverse effects during the first 2 weeks of therapy may be readily used after 1 month of therapy, once autoinduction of CBZ metabolism has decreased serum CBZ concentrations (Cereghino 1975) and accommodation and tolerance to adverse effects such as sedation have occurred. Target dosages are commonly between 600 and 1,200 mg/day, yielding serum levels from 4 to 12 μg/mL, with the higher portion of the range used acutely, and lower doses used in prophylaxis or adjunctive therapy. In a CBZ versus lithium maintenance study, serum trough CBZ concentrations were maintained at 4–12 μg/mL, with a mean of 6.4 μg/mL (Greil et al. 1997). In another CBZ versus lithium maintenance study, serum trough CBZ concentrations were maintained at 4 to 12 μg/mL, with a mean of 7.7 μg/mL (Denicoff et al. 1997).

Because CBZ dosage and serum and cerebrospinal fluid concentrations fail to correlate with psychotropic efficacy (Post 1989; Post et al. 1983a, 1984a), it is common practice to gradually increase CBZ dosage as tolerated, monitoring both adverse effects and clinical efficacy, un-til therapeutic efficacy is adequate, adverse effects supervene, or serum concentrations exceed 12 μg/mL. The 4- to 12-μg/mL serum CBZ concentration range from use in epilepsy may be considered as a broad target, and CBZ serum concentrations may be used as checks for pharmacokinetic problems. The active CBZ-E metabolite can yield therapeutic and adverse effects similar to those of CBZ but is not detected in conventional CBZ assays. Thus, the unwary clinician may misinterpret the significance of therapeutic or adverse effects associated with low or moderate serum CBZ concentrations.

Cerebrospinal fluid CBZ-E (but not CBZ) concentrations may correlate with degree of clinical improvement in patients with mood disorders (Post et al. 1983a, 1984a, 1984c). Clinical improvement in depressed patients may tend to correlate with serum CBZ-E (but not CBZ) concentration and serum CBZ-E to CBZ ratio. This ratio may suggest a possible relationship between clinical response and the degree of enzyme induction.

In responders, a dose–response relationship may be evident, so that slowly increasing CBZ doses to maximize response in the absence of significant adverse effects is a clinically useful strategy. However, if there is no hint of therapeutic response at moderate doses, it is unlikely that pushing to very high doses will be beneficial.

Oxcarbazepine

OXC is available in the United States as a proprietary product (Trileptal) manufactured by Novartis Pharmaceuticals Corporation in a 300-mg/5-mL suspension and in 150-, 300-, and 600-mg tablets ("Trileptal" 2008). Extended-release, intramuscular, and depot formulations are not available.

OXC is 96% absorbed, and the modest effect of food on OXC kinetics does not appear to be of therapeutic consequence (Degen et al. 1994). OXC is 60% bound to plasma proteins. Like CBZ, OXC has complex metabolism (see Figure 37–1, bottom). Thus, OXC is rapidly reduced to an active monohydroxy derivative (MHD) by cytosol arylketone reductase. The MHD is 40% bound to plasma proteins, has a moderate volume of distribution (about 0.8 L/kg), and has a half-life of about 9 hours. OXC is eliminated primarily in the form of MHD (70%) and MHD glucuronide conjugates (20%), with small portions (10%) in the form of OXC glucuronide conjugates and CBZ-D. OXC does not cause autoinduction and yields substantially less heteroinduction than does CBZ. Thus, as described below, drug–drug interactions are less problematic with OXC than with CBZ (Baruzzi et al. 1994).

In epilepsy patients, OXC is commonly started at 600 mg/day and increased weekly by 600 mg/day, with final dosages commonly ranging between 900 and 2,400 mg/day in two divided doses, yielding serum concentrations of approximately 13–35 µg/mL (50–140 µM/L) (Johannessen et al. 2003; "Trileptal" 2008). In bipolar disorder patients, OXC, like CBZ, is titrated to clinical desired effect as tolerated, with the serum concentration range used in epilepsy considered as a broad target and with OXC serum concentrations used as checks for pharmacokinetic problems. For patients taking CBZ, equipotent doses of OXC range from 1.2 to 1.5 times the CBZ dose. In an early small, double-blind, on–off–on acute mania trial, the mean OXC dose was 1,886 mg/day (range 1,800–2,100) (Emrich et al. 1983). In small active-comparator multicenter studies in acute mania, mean OXC dosages were 2,400 mg/day and 1,400 mg/day in comparison with haloperidol and lithium, respectively (Emrich 1990). In a recent pediatric acute mania study, OXC was increased every 2 days by 300 mg/day to a maximum of 900–2,400 mg/day, with mean dosages of 1,200 mg/day and 2,040 mg/day in children and adolescents, respectively, but therapeutic effects did not exceed that of placebo (Wagner et al. 2006).

Mechanisms of Action

CBZ and OXC have not only structural but also mechanistic similarities. However, these agents have such a diversity of biochemical effects that linking these mechanisms to their varying clinical actions presents a considerable challenge.

Carbamazepine

As noted above, although CBZ has a tricyclic structure like imipramine's, the two agents have markedly different neurochemical, hepatic, and clinical effects. Thus, CBZ, unlike imipramine, lacks major effects on monoamine reuptake or high affinity for histaminergic or cholinergic receptors and, unlike many antidepressants, fails to downregulate β-adrenergic receptors. Also, CBZ, unlike antipsychotics, does not block dopamine receptors. However, CBZ has a wide range of other cellular and intracellular effects, as described below.

One way to consider CBZ's diverse actions is from the perspective of commonalities with and dissociations from the actions of the other mood stabilizers, lithium and valproate. CBZ shares a few mechanistic commonalities with both of these mood stabilizers in that all three agents in-crease limbic γ-aminobutyric acid type B ($GABA_B$) receptors, decrease GABA and dopamine turnover, inhibit inositol transport, and weakly inhibit calcium influx by an N-methyl-D-aspartate (NMDA)–mediated effect in preclinical studies. Chronic (but not acute) lithium, CBZ, and valproate increase hippocampal (but not frontal, thalamic, or striatal) $GABA_B$ (but not $GABA_A$) receptors in rats (Motohashi 1992; Motohashi et al. 1989) and decrease GABA turnover in rodents (Bernasconi 1982; Bernasconi and Martin 1979; Bernasconi et al. 1984), suggesting that hippocampal $GABA_B$ receptor mechanisms and decreased GABA turnover could be important in medications that stabilize mood.

However, CBZ shares some actions with valproate but not lithium, and shares other actions with lithium but not valproate. Thus, CBZ, like valproate but unlike lithium, decreases glutamate and aspartate release by blocking sodium channels, decreases somatostatin-like immunoreactivity, and increases potassium efflux and serum L-tryptophan. CBZ, like lithium but unlike valproate, decreases serum levothyroxine, cyclic adenosine monophosphate (cAMP), and cyclic guanosine monophosphate (cGMP) and increases serotonin and substance P neurotransmission. CBZ differs from both lithium and valproate in that it has effects at peripheral-type benzodiazepine receptors, blocks adenosine A_1 receptors, increases G protein–stimulating alpha subunits ($G_s\alpha$) and inositol monophosphatase (IMPase), and decreases G protein–inhibitory alpha subunits ($G_i\alpha$).

In contrast, CBZ may lack certain intracellular actions shared by valproate and lithium, such as increasing expression of the cytoprotective protein bcl-2 and transcription factor AP-1 binding and decreasing glycogen synthase kinase-3 beta (GSK-3β), protein kinase C (PKC), and myristoylated alanine-rich C kinase substrate (MARCKS). CBZ appears to lack additional intracellular signaling actions seen with lithium but not valproate, such as decreasing G protein coupling to phosphatidylinositol (PI) and adenylate cyclase, phospholipase C, and inositol and increasing intracellular calcium, as well as increasing basal and decreasing stimulated cAMP. CBZ also lacks other actions seen with lithium but not valproate, such as having effects on neuropeptide Y or glucocorticoid type II receptors or decreasing calcium influx or α_2-adrenergic neurotransmission. CBZ appears to lack some actions seen with valproate but not lithium, such as increasing microtubule-associated protein (MAP) kinase, decreasing GABA catabolism, and increasing GABA release.

In one three-way mechanistic dissociation, lithium decreased, CBZ increased, and valproate did not change

IMPase (Vadnal and Parthasarathy 1995). CBZ's mixture of mechanistic commonalities with and dissociations from lithium and valproate is consistent with the view that CBZ's clinical effects in bipolar disorder may overlap with but are not identical to those of lithium and valproate.

Another potentially useful way of considering CBZ's diverse mechanisms is from the perspective of onset of action (Post 1988). Thus, CBZ cellular actions with acute onset that might parallel the time course of clinical anticonvulsant effects include decreasing sodium influx and glutamate release, increasing potassium conductance, and acting on peripheral benzodiazepine and α_2-adrenergic receptors. Acute $GABA_B$ receptor actions like those of baclofen may relate to the rapid onset of clinical analgesic effects. Acute or subchronic actions such as increasing striatal cholinergic neurotransmission; decreasing adenylate cyclase activity stimulated by dopamine, norepinephrine and serotonin; and decreasing turnover of dopamine, norepinephrine, and GABA may be pertinent to clinical antimanic effects. Finally, actions requiring chronic administration may be most closely related to clinical antidepressant effects. These include increasing serum and urinary free cortisol, free tryptophan, substance P sensitivity, and adenosine A_1 receptors and decreasing cerebrospinal somatostatin-like immunoreactivity.

Oxcarbazepine

Less is known about OXC mechanisms than about CBZ mechanisms. The bulk of the evidence thus far suggests that OXC's structural similarity to CBZ is paralleled by mechanistic similarity (Ambrosio et al. 2002). For example, OXC, like CBZ, appears to decrease sodium (Benes et al. 1999; Wamil et al. 1994) and calcium (Stefani et al. 1995) influx, glutamate release (Ambrosio et al. 2001), and serum thyroxine (T_4) concentrations (Isojarvi et al. 2001b); increase potassium conductance (McLean et al. 1994) and dopaminergic neurotransmission (Joca et al. 2000); and block adenosine A_1 receptors (Deckert et al. 1993). However, there may be some mechanistic dissociations, particularly given OXC's and CBZ's marked differences in degree of hepatic enzyme induction. For example, OXC appears to be a less potent modulator of voltage-gated calcium channels compared with CBZ (Schmutz et al. 1994; Stefani et al. 1997). The general OXC–CBZ mechanistic overlap is consistent with the hypothesis that OXC and CBZ have similar effects in bipolar disorder, which is consistent with preliminary clinical observations but remains to be established in large controlled clinical studies.

Indications and Efficacy

Seizure Disorders and Trigeminal Neuralgia

In the United States, CBZ is approved by the FDA as monotherapy for the treatment of trigeminal neuralgia and complex partial, generalized tonic–clonic, and mixed seizure disorders ("Carbatrol" 2008; "Tegretol" 2008). OXC is approved for the treatment of partial seizures as monotherapy in adults and as adjunctive therapy in adults and children older than 4 years ("Trileptal" 2008). CBZ and OXC appear to have overlapping anticonvulsant effects, with similar efficacy in patients with newly diagnosed epilepsy (Dam et al. 1989). However, there may be dissociations. For example, switching to OXC may be effective in patients with inadequate responses or intolerable adverse effects with CBZ (Beydoun et al. 2000; Van Parys and Meinardi 1994), and adding OXC may yield efficacy in patients with inadequate responses to CBZ (Barcs et al. 2000; Glauser et al. 2000). In contrast to valproate and lamotrigine, which are approved first-line medications for bipolar disorder, CBZ and OXC are generally considered alternative agents in the management of bipolar disorder (American Psychiatric Association 2002), based on the studies reviewed below.

Acute Mania

Twenty-three controlled studies have investigated CBZ and OXC efficacy in acute mania (Table 37–1) (Ballenger and Post 1978; D. Brown et al. 1989; Desai et al. 1987; Emrich 1990; Emrich et al. 1985; Goncalves and Stoll 1985; Grossi et al. 1984; Klein et al. 1984; Lenzi et al. 1986; Lerer et al. 1987; Lusznat et al. 1988; Möller et al. 1989; Müller and Stoll 1984; Okuma et al. 1979, 1989, 1990; Post et al. 1987; Small et al. 1991; Stoll et al. 1986; Wagner et al. 2006; Weisler et al. 2004, 2005; Zhang et al. 2007). In these studies, there is more compelling evidence for CBZ efficacy (18 studies including 594 patients receiving CBZ) than for OXC efficacy (5 studies including 119 patients receiving OXC).

Two recent trials, which found a proprietary CBZ beaded extended-release capsule formulation (Equetro) superior to placebo, are of particular interest because they used a randomized, double-blind, placebo-controlled paradigm (Weisler et al. 2004, 2005) and yielded an FDA indication for the treatment of acute manic and mixed episodes in patients with bipolar disorder.

These recent reports are consistent with multiple earlier studies using placebo–drug–placebo, active-compara-

TABLE 37–1. Carbamazepine (CBZ) and oxcarbazepine (OXC) in acute mania: 23 double-blind studies

Study	Design	CBZ/OXC (N)	Comparator (N)	Duration (days)	CBZ/OXC response	Comparator response
Weisler et al. 2004	CBZ vs. PBO	101	103	21	42%	22%
Weisler et al. 2005	CBZ vs. PBO	122	117	21	61%	29%
Zhang et al. 2007	CBZ vs. PBO	41	21	84	88%	57%
Wagner et al. 2006	OXC vs. PBO	55	55	42	42%	26%
Ballenger and Post 1978; Post et al. 1987	PBO–CBZ–PBO	19	—	11–56	63%	Frequent relapse
Emrich et al. 1985	PBO–OXC–PBO	7	—	Varied	67%	—
Klein et al. 1984	CBZ vs. PBO adjunct (HAL)	14	13	35	71%	54%
Müller and Stoll 1984; Goncalves and Stoll 1985	CBZ vs. PBO adjunct (HAL)	6	6	21	CBZ>PBO	—
Desai et al. 1987	CBZ vs. PBO adjunct (Li)	5	5	28	CBZ>PBO	—
Möller et al. 1989	CBZ vs. PBO adjunct (HAL)	11	9	21	CBZ=PBO	—
Okuma et al. 1989	CBZ vs. PBO adjunct (NL)	82	80	28	48%	30%
Okuma et al. 1979	CBZ vs. NL (CPZ)	32	28	21–35	66%	54%
Grossi et al. 1984	CBZ vs. NL (CPZ)	18	19	21	67%	76%
Emrich 1990	OXC vs. NL (HAL)	19	19	14	OXC=HAL	—
Stoll et al. 1986	CBZ vs. NL (HAL) adjunct (CPZ)	14	18	21	86%	67%
D. Brown et al. 1989	CBZ vs. NL (HAL) adjunct (CPZ)	8	9	28	75%	33%
Müller and Stoll 1984	OXC vs. NL (HAL) adjunct (HAL)	10	10	14	OXC=HAL	—
Lerer et al. 1987	CBZ vs. Li	14	14	28	29%	79%
Small et al. 1991	CBZ vs. Li	24	24	56	33%	33%
Emrich 1990	OXC vs. Li	28	24	14	OXC=Li	—
Lenzi et al. 1986	CBZ vs. Li adjunct (CPZ)	11	11	19	73%	73%
Lusznat et al. 1988	CBZ vs. Li adjunct (CPZ, HAL)	22	22	42	CBZ=Li	—
Okuma et al. 1990	CBZ vs. Li adjunct (NL)	50	51	28	62%	59%
Total		**713**	**658**			
Response rates[a]	CBZ/OXC monotherapy				55% (237/433)	
	NL monotherapy					64% (30/47)
	Li monotherapy					50% (19/38)
	PBO monotherapy					28% (83/296)

TABLE 37–1. Carbamazepine (CBZ) and oxcarbazepine (OXC) in acute mania: 23 double-blind studies *(continued)*

STUDY	DESIGN	CBZ/OXC (N)	COMPARATOR (N)	DURATION (DAYS)	CBZ/OXC RESPONSE	COMPARATOR RESPONSE
Response rates[a]	CBZ/OXC adjunctive				59% (106/179)	
	NL adjunctive					**56%** (15/27)
	Li adjunctive					**61%** (38/62)
	PBO adjunctive					**33%** (31/93)

Note. CBZ=carbamazepine; CPZ=chlorpromazine; HAL=haloperidol; Li=lithium; NL=neuroleptic; NS=not stated; OXC=oxcarbazepine; PBO=placebo.
[a]Weighted means of patients with response data.

tor (lithium or neuroleptics), and adjunctive (compared with placebo, lithium, or neuroleptics added to lithium or neuroleptics) designs. Thus, across studies that used diverse paradigms (see Table 37–1), overall antimanic response rates were generally comparable to those seen with lithium or neuroleptics or in other studies with valproate (Ketter 2005). Taken together, this collection of clinical trials provides substantial evidence for the acute antimanic efficacy of CBZ and preliminary evidence for the acute antimanic efficacy of OXC. For CBZ, this current body of existing data appears greater than that initially considered by the FDA in approving lithium for the treatment of acute mania.

Improvement appears to occur across the entire manic syndrome and does not seem to be due to nonspecific sedative properties, in that patients often show dramatic clinical improvement in the absence of marked sedation. Because CBZ and OXC are frequently used in combination with other medications in the acute treatment of mania, knowledge of CBZ's extensive and OXC's more limited drug–drug interactions (as described later in this chapter) is often required to achieve optimal outcomes.

Acute Depression

There are limited controlled data regarding the acute antidepressant effects of CBZ, and no published controlled studies of the antidepressant effects of OXC (Table 37–2). Although CBZ appears to have weaker antidepressant than antimanic properties, some evidence suggests that it may provide antidepressant benefit in about one-third of treatment-resistant patients (Neumann et al. 1984; Post et al. 1986; Small 1990), and in a Chinese study, CBZ yielded a response rate closer to two-thirds in non-treatment-resistant patients (Zhang et al. 2007). Unfortu-

nately, most of these studies are limited by the use of small samples of heterogeneous (both bipolar and unipolar) and highly treatment-resistant patients. Nevertheless, double-blind off–on–off–on observations and a randomized, double-blind, placebo-controlled trial have provided evidence of individual responsiveness in at least a subgroup of depressed bipolar patients.

Prophylaxis

Findings from a series of 16 double-blind, randomized, open randomized, or otherwise partially controlled studies (Ballenger and Post 1978; Bellaire et al. 1988; Cabrera et al. 1986; Coxhead et al. 1992; Denicoff et al. 1997; Di Costanzo and Schifano 1991; Elphick et al. 1988; Greil et al. 1997; Hartong et al. 2003; Kishimoto and Okuma 1985; Lusznat et al. 1988; Mosolov 1991; Okuma et al. 1981; Placidi et al. 1986; Post et al. 1983b; Watkins et al. 1987; Wildgrube 1990) are consistent with a very substantial open literature suggesting that CBZ may be effective in preventing bipolar manic and depressive episodes when administered as long-term prophylaxis, either alone or in combination with lithium, in patients who previously had not responded to lithium (Table 37–3). CBZ may have equal *prophylactic* antidepressant and antimanic efficacy, in contrast to its less potent *acute* antidepressant versus antimanic effects. In contrast, there are only sparse data regarding the efficacy of OXC in the prophylaxis of episodes in patients with bipolar disorder.

In one study, the overall analysis suggested that maintenance treatment was more effective with lithium than with CBZ (Greil et al. 1997), but subsequent analysis revealed subgroup differences. Thus, maintenance treatment was more effective with lithium than with CBZ in patients with "classic" bipolar disorder (bipolar I disorder

TABLE 37–2. Carbamazepine (CBZ) in acute depression: four controlled studies

STUDY	DESIGN	CBZ (N)	COMPARATOR (N)	DURATION (DAYS)	CBZ RESPONSE	COMPARATOR RESPONSE
Post et al. 1986	PBO–CBZ–PBO (24 BP, 11 UP)	35	35	Median 45	34%	—
Zhang et al. 2007	CBZ vs. PBO	47	23	84	64%	35%
Small 1990	CBZ/CBZ+Li vs. Li (4 BP, 24 UP)	NS	NS	28	32%	13%
Neumann et al. 1984	CBZ vs. TMI (5 BP, 5 UP)	5	5	28	CBZ=TMI	—

Note. BP=bipolar; CBZ=carbamazepine; Li=lithium; NS=not stated; PBO=placebo; TMI=trimipramine; UP=unipolar.

with no mood-incongruent delusions or comorbidity) but tended to be more effective with CBZ than with lithium in patients with "nonclassic" bipolar disorder (bipolar II disorder, bipolar disorder not otherwise specified, bipolar disorder with mood-incongruent delusions or comorbidity) (Greil et al. 1998).

In another study, maintenance treatment appeared to be more effective with lithium than with CBZ in patients with no more than 6 months' prior exposure to either agent (Hartong et al. 2003). However, this advantage was offset by more early discontinuations in the lithium group, so that similar proportions (about one-third) of lithium-treated and CBZ-treated patients completed 2 years with no episode. Patients on lithium compared to CBZ tended to have a somewhat greater risk of episodes in the first 3 months and markedly less risk of episodes after the first 3 months, with a recurrence risk of only 10% per year with lithium after the first 3 months. Patients on CBZ had a more consistent rate of relapse/recurrence of about 40% per year.

Some CBZ prophylaxis trials have been criticized due to methodological limitations (D.J. Murphy et al. 1989), but such difficulties are common in maintenance studies. For example, apparently due in part to methodological limitations, divalproex and lithium failed to separate from placebo on the primary efficacy measure in a 1-year maintenance study (Bowden et al. 2000). Taken together, the randomized, placebo-controlled, placebo–drug–placebo, and lithium comparator studies and trials in patients with rapid-cycling or lithium-resistant illness constitute substantial evidence for the efficacy of CBZ (Prien and Gelenberg 1989). CBZ may be effective in some individuals with valproate-resistant illness (Post et al. 1984b), and the CBZ plus valproate combination may be effective in patients who show little or no response to either agent alone (Keck et al. 1992; Ketter et al. 1992).

In a retrospective study, although 22 of 34 (65%) patients with treatment-resistant bipolar disorder responded to primarily adjunctive open CBZ acutely, when patients were assessed 3–4 years later, only 7 of 34 (21%) and 2 of 34 (6%) were considered probable and clear responders, respectively (Frankenburg et al. 1988). Post et al. (1990) have suggested that loss of CBZ prophylactic efficacy over time may be related to a unique form of contingent tolerance. In these instances, the optimal algorithm for recapturing CBZ response has not been determined. However, techniques such as switching to another treatment regimen with a different mechanism of action or returning later to CBZ (after a period of not taking CBZ) are worth considering, based on case reports and anecdotal observations. Systematic clinical trials are required to better determine the efficacy of these and other approaches for recapturing CBZ response.

Response Predictors

Predictors of CBZ and OXC response have not been adequately elucidated. CBZ appears to be effective in patients with a history of lithium unresponsiveness or intolerance (Okuma et al. 1979; Post et al. 1987). Nonclassic bipolar disorder (Greil et al. 1998; Small et al. 1991) and stable or decreasing episode frequency (Post et al. 1990) have been reported to be associated with CBZ response. Studies have indicated that patients with a history of affective illness in first-degree relatives may have preferential responses to lithium, whereas the converse may be the case for CBZ (Ballenger and Post 1978; Post et al. 1987). Himmelhoch and colleagues (Himmelhoch 1987; Himmelhoch and Garfinkel 1986) have suggested that patients with comorbid neurological or substance abuse problems and inadequate lithium responses might respond to CBZ or valproate. Preliminary observations

TABLE 37–3. Carbamazepine (CBZ) and oxcarbazepine (OXC) in prophylaxis of bipolar disorder: 16 controlled or quasi-controlled studies

STUDY	DESIGN	CBZ (N)	COMPARATOR (N)	DURATION (YEARS)	CBZ/OXC RESPONSE	COMPARATOR RESPONSE
Okuma et al. 1981	CBZ vs. PBO (B, R)	12	10	1	60%	22%
Ballenger and Post 1978; Post et al. 1983b	CBZ vs. PBO (B, M)	7	7	1.7	86%	—
Placidi et al. 1986	CBZ vs. Li (B, R)	20	16	≤3	67%	67%
Watkins et al. 1987	CBZ vs. Li (B, R)	19	18	1.5	84%	83%
Lusznat et al. 1988	CBZ vs. Li (B, R)	16	15	≤1	56%	29%
Coxhead et al. 1992	CBZ vs. Li (B, R)	13	15	1	54%	47%
Bellaire et al. 1988	CBZ vs. Li (R)	46	52	1	CBZ=Li	—
Greil et al. 1997	CBZ vs. Li (R)	70	74	2.5	45%	65%
Hartong et al. 2003	CBZ vs. Li (R)	50	44	2	58%	73%
Di Costanzo and Schifano 1991	CBZ+Li vs. Li (R)	8	8	≤5	CBZ+Li>Li	—
Mosolov 1991	CBZ vs. Li (R?)	30	30	≥1	73%	70%
Cabrera et al. 1986	OXC vs. Li (R)	4	6	≤22	75%	100%
Elphick et al. 1988	CBZ vs. Li (B, C)	8	11	0.75	38%	73%
Denicoff et al. 1997	CBZ vs. Li (B, C)	46	50	1	33%	55%
Kishimoto and Okuma 1985	CBZ vs. Li (C)	18	18	≥2	CBZ>Li	—
Wildgrube 1990	OXC vs. Li (NR)	8	7	≤33	33%	67%
Total		**375**	**373**			
Response rates[a]	CBZ/OXC				54% (165/303)	
	Li					64% (185/286)
	PBO					22% (2/9)

Note. B=blind; C=crossover; CBZ=carbamazepine; Li=lithium; M=mirror image; NR=not randomized; OXC=oxcarbazepine; PBO=placebo; R=randomized.
[a]Weighted means of patients with response data.

indicate that baseline cerebral (left insula) hypermetabolism may be a marker of CBZ response (Ketter et al. 1999).

There are varying reports with respect to the relationships between CBZ response and dysphoric manic presentations (Lusznat et al. 1988; Post et al. 1989) and illness severity (Post et al. 1987; Small et al. 1991). Although several investigators have suggested that psychosensory symptoms (which have been hypothesized to be due to limbic dysfunction) may indicate preferential response to CBZ and other anticonvulsants, such a relationship has not been observed in acute therapy, and the relationship to prophylactic response remains to be delineated.

Antidepressant responses to CBZ may be seen in patients with more severe depression, more discrete depressive episodes, less chronicity, and greater decreases in serum T_4 concentrations with CBZ (Post et al. 1991, 1986).

Although the initial studies of Post et al. (1987) and Okuma et al. (1981; Okuma 1983) indicated that some rapid-cycling patients were responsive to CBZ, other investigators found less robust results (Dilsaver et al. 1993; Joyce 1988). As with lithium, later studies by Okuma (1993) reported a lower CBZ maintenance response rate in rapid-cycling compared with non-rapid-cycling illness. However, even these rapid-cycling patients had a CBZ response rate (40%) that was higher than the rates reported for other agents in other studies. Denicoff et al. (1997) also observed that patients with a history of rapid cycling had a lower CBZ maintenance response rate compared with those without such a history (19% vs. 54%).

Side Effects and Toxicology

Baseline evaluation of bipolar disorder patients includes not only psychosocial assessment but also general medical evaluation, in view of the risk of medical processes, which could confound diagnosis or influence management decisions, and the risk of adverse effects, which may occur with treatment. Assessment commonly includes history; physical examination; complete blood count with differential and platelets; renal, hepatic, and thyroid function; toxicology; pregnancy tests; and other chemistries and electrocardiogram as clinically indicated (American Psychiatric Association 2002). Such evaluation provides baseline values for parameters that influence decisions about choice of medication and intensity of clinical and laboratory monitoring.

Carbamazepine

CBZ adverse effects appear to have substantial impact on the utility of CBZ in the treatment of bipolar disorder. For example, in a retrospective study, 12 of 55 (22%) patients with treatment-resistant psychotic disorders (including 34 with bipolar disorder) discontinued primarily adjunctive open CBZ in the first 2 months because of adverse effects (Frankenburg et al. 1988). Also, in a randomized, double-blind crossover maintenance study, significantly more patients receiving CBZ (10 of 46, 22%) than those receiving lithium (2 of 50, 4%) discontinued the drug early because of adverse effects (Denicoff et al. 1997). In a randomized open maintenance study, although nonsignificantly more CBZ (9 of 70, 13%) than lithium (4 of 74, 5%) patients discontinued early because of adverse effects, significantly more CBZ (26 of 33, 79%) than lithium (20 of 51, 39%) patients who completed the study were free of adverse effects (Greil et al. 1997). Thus, adverse effects requiring discontinuation may occur more commonly with CBZ than with other drugs, particularly during acute therapy if CBZ is rapidly introduced. However, some patients may tolerate CBZ better than other agents, particularly during longer-term treatment, as CBZ appears to have a low propensity to cause adverse effects such as weight gain and metabolic disturbance that can limit the utility of some other agents (Ketter et al. 2005).

CBZ has several common dose-related adverse effects that can generally be minimized by attention to drug–drug interactions and gradual titration of dosage or reversed by decreasing dosage. At high doses, patients can develop neurotoxicity with sedation, ataxia, diplopia, and nystagmus, particularly early in therapy before autoinduction and the development of some tolerance to CBZ's central nervous system adverse effects occur. However, in contrast to neuroleptic treatment, CBZ therapy is not associated with extrapyramidal adverse effects. Because there is wide interindividual variation in susceptibility to adverse effects at any given concentration, it is most useful clinically to titrate doses against each patient's adverse effects rather than targeting a fixed dosage or serum concentration range.

Dizziness, ataxia, or diplopia emerging 1–2 hours after an individual dose is often a sign that the adverse-effect threshold has been exceeded and that dosage redistribution (spreading out the dose or giving more of the dosage at bedtime) or dosage reduction may be required. Use of extended-release formulations can also attenuate CBZ peak serum concentrations, enhancing tolerability.

The United States prescribing information for carbamazepine includes black box warnings regarding the risks of aplastic anemia (16 per million patient-years) and agranulocytosis (48 per million patient-years), as well as serious dermatological reactions and the HLA-B*1502 allele. Other warnings include the risks of teratogenicity, and increased intraocular pressure due to mild anticholinergic activity. Thus, CBZ can yield hematological (benign leukopenia, benign thrombocytopenia), dermatological (benign rash), electrolyte (asymptomatic hyponatremia), and hepatic (benign transaminase elevations) problems. Much less commonly, CBZ can yield analogous serious problems. For example, mild leukopenia and benign rash occur in as many as 1 of 10 patients, with the slight possibility that these usually benign phenomena are heralding malignant aplastic anemia and Stevens-Johnson syndrome/toxic epidermal necrolysis, seen in approximately 1 per 100,000 and 1 to 6 per 10,000 patients, respectively (Kramlinger et al. 1994; Tohen et al. 1995). Recent evidence indicates that the risk of serious rash may be 10 times as high in some Asian countries and strongly linked to the HLA-B*1502 allele. Thus, the United States prescribing information states that individuals of Asian descent should be genetically tested before initiating carbamazepine therapy. An individual who is HLA-B*1502 positive should not be treated with CBZ unless the benefit clearly outweighs the risk. In view of the risk of rare but serious decreases in blood counts, it is important to alert patients to seek immediate medical evaluation if they develop signs and symptoms of possible hematological reactions, such as fever, sore throat, oral ulcers, petechiae, and easy bruising or bleeding. Hematological monitoring needs to be intensified in patients with low or marginal leukocyte counts, and CBZ is generally discontinued if the leukocyte count falls below 3,000/mm^3 or the granulocyte count below 1,000/mm^3.

In early 2008, the FDA released an alert regarding increased risk of suicidality (suicidal behavior or ideation) in patients with epilepsy as well as psychiatric disorders for 11 anticonvulsants (including CBZ and OXC). In the FDA's analysis, anticonvulsants compared with placebo yielded approximately twice the risk of suicidality (0.43% vs. 0.22%). The relative risk for suicidality was higher in patients with epilepsy than in patients with psychiatric disorders. As of late 2008, a class warning regarding this risk had not yet been added to the United States prescribing information for anticonvulsants, but it is anticipated that this may occur.

In the instance of benign leukopenia, the addition of lithium can increase the neutrophil count back toward normal (Kramlinger and Post 1990), but this strategy is not likely to be helpful for the suppression of red cells or platelets, which is likely to be indicative of a more problematic process.

Rash presenting with systemic illness or involvement of the eyes, mouth, or bladder (dysuria) constitutes a medical emergency, and CBZ should be discontinued immediately and the patient assessed emergently. For more benign presentations, CBZ is generally discontinued, as there is little ability to predict which rashes will progress to more severe, potentially life-threatening problems. However, in rare instances of resistance to all medications except CBZ, a repeat trial of CBZ with a course of prednisone has usually been well tolerated (J.M. Murphy et al. 1991; Vick 1983). If there is evidence of systemic allergy, fever, or malaise, prednisone is less likely to be helpful. A substantial number of patients with CBZ-induced rashes may not have a rash on reexposure (even without prednisone coverage), but if a rash again develops, it usually appears more rapidly than in the first occurrence. Only 25%–30% of the patients who develop a rash while taking CBZ also develop a rash (cross-sensitivity) with OXC.

Due to the risk of rare hepatitis, patients should be advised to seek medical evaluation immediately if they develop malaise, abdominal pain, or other marked gastrointestinal symptoms. In general, CBZ (like other anticonvulsants) is discontinued if liver function tests exceed three times the upper limit of the normal range (Martinez et al. 1993).

CBZ may affect cardiac conduction and should be used with caution in patients with cardiac disorders such as heart block. A baseline electrocardiogram is worth considering if the patient has a positive cardiac history.

Conservative laboratory monitoring during CBZ therapy includes baseline studies and reevaluation of complete blood count, differential, platelets, and hepatic indices initially at 2, 4, 6, and 8 weeks, and then every 3 months (American Psychiatric Association 1994, 2002). Most of the serious hematological reactions occur in the first 3 months of therapy (Tohen et al. 1995). In contemporary clinical practice, somewhat less focus is placed on scheduled monitoring; instead, monitoring as clinically indicated (e.g., when a patient becomes ill with a fever) is emphasized. Patients who have abnormal or marginal indices at any point merit careful scheduled and clinically indicated monitoring. The United States prescribing information for the beaded extended-release capsule CBZ formulation that was recently approved for the treatment of acute mania includes monitoring baseline complete blood count, platelets, ±reticulocytes, ±serum iron, and hepatic function tests; closely monitoring patients with low or decreased white blood cell count or platelets; and considering discontinuation of CBZ if there is evidence of bone marrow depression ("Equetro" 2008). Serum CBZ concentrations are typically assessed at steady state and then as clinically indicated (e.g., by inefficacy or adverse effects).

Dividing or reducing doses, moving doses in relation to mealtimes, and changing formulations can attenuate CBZ-induced gastrointestinal disturbances. CBZ suspension may have more proximal absorption and thus exacerbate upper gastrointestinal (nausea and vomiting) or attenuate lower gastrointestinal (diarrhea) adverse effects. The reverse holds for extended-release preparations.

Weight gain and obesity are important clinical concerns in the management of bipolar disorder. Medications and the hyperphagia, hypersomnia, and anergy commonly seen in bipolar depression can contribute to this important obstacle to optimal outcomes. CBZ is less likely than lithium (Coxhead et al. 1992; Denicoff et al. 1997) or valproate (Mattson et al. 1992) to yield weight gain. In one study, CBZ caused weight gain in depressed (but not manic) patients, an effect that seemed to be related to the degree of relief of depression (Joffe et al. 1986b). Nevertheless, in view of its relatively favorable effect on weight, CBZ may provide an important alternative to other mood stabilizers for patients who struggle with weight gain and obesity.

CBZ can induce hyponatremia that may be tolerated well by some younger patients but can be particularly problematic in the elderly. If confusion develops in an elderly patient, serum sodium should be assessed. In rare instances water intoxication and seizures can occur. In some cases, hyponatremia can be effectively counteracted with the addition of lithium or the antibiotic demeclocycline (Ringel and Brick 1986).

CBZ increases plasma high-density lipoprotein (HDL) (O'Neill et al. 1982) and total cholesterol (D.W. Brown et al. 1992) concentrations. However, because the ratio of HDL to total cholesterol does not change (O'Neill et al. 1982), CBZ-induced increases in total cholesterol are not likely to be clinically problematic in regard to atherosclerosis (D.W. Brown et al. 1992).

CBZ decreases serum T_4, free T_4 index, and, less consistently, triiodothyronine (T_3) (Bentsen et al. 1983; Connell et al. 1984; Haidukewych and Rodin 1987; Joffe et al. 1986a) but does not substantially alter serum thyroid-binding globulin, reverse T_3, basal thyroid-stimulating hormone (TSH) concentrations (Bentsen et al. 1983; Connell et al. 1984), or somatic basal metabolic rates (Herman et al. 1991). In contrast to lithium, the TSH response to thyrotropin-releasing hormone is blunted (Joffe et al. 1986a) or unaltered (Connell et al. 1984) with CBZ therapy, and clinical hypothyroidism during treatment with CBZ is exceedingly rare.

CBZ is teratogenic (Pregnancy Category D) and is associated with low birth weight, craniofacial deformities, digital hypoplasia, and (in approximately 3% of exposures) spina bifida (Jones et al. 1989; Rosa 1991). For the latter, folate supplementation may attenuate the risk, and fetal ultrasound studies may allow early detection. In rare patients with severe mood disorders, clinicians may determine in consultation with a gynecologist that the benefits of treating with CBZ outweigh the risks in comparison with other treatment options (Sitland-Marken et al. 1989).

CBZ is present in breast milk at concentrations about half those present in maternal blood but may not accumulate in fetal blood (Froescher et al. 1984; Kuhnz et al. 1983; Pynnönen et al. 1977; Shimoyama et al. 2000). Clinicians may prefer to avoid the putative risks of exposing infants to CBZ in breast milk (Frey et al. 2002) and discourage breast-feeding in women taking CBZ ("Carbatrol" 2008; "Tegretol" 2008).

Oxcarbazepine

Adverse effects may limit the use of OXC, as with CBZ. In a retrospective study, adverse events were noted in one-third of 947 epilepsy patients (Friis et al. 1993). However, OXC may have tolerability advantages over CBZ, in part perhaps related to the absence of the CBZ-E metabolite.

For example, in a 1-year randomized, double-blind study of 235 patients with newly diagnosed epilepsy, OXC monotherapy yielded fewer severe adverse effects than CBZ monotherapy (Dam et al. 1989). OXC and valproate may have similar tolerability; in a 1-year randomized, double-blind study of 249 patients with newly diagnosed epilepsy, monotherapy with these agents had similar rates of adverse effects (Christe et al. 1997). Importantly, OXC yielded anticonvulsant effects similar to those of CBZ and valproate in the above-mentioned studies.

Much less is known about the tolerability of OXC in bipolar disorder patients. In randomized, double-blind studies of monotherapy for acute mania, the proportions of patients experiencing adverse effects were lower with OXC 2,400 mg/day (2 of 19, 10%) than with high-dose haloperidol 42 mg/day (7 of 19, 37%) and were not statistically different with OXC 1,400 mg/day (8 of 29, 28%) compared with lithium 1,100 mg/day (5 of 27, 19%) (Emrich 1990). A retrospective study of open OXC in acutely manic inpatients found that by the time of discharge, only 6 of 200 (3%) had discontinued the medication because of adverse effects (3 due to hyponatremia) or potential drug–drug interactions (3 due to concomitant treatment with hormonal contraceptives) (Reinstein et al. 2002). However, in another retrospective study of primarily depressed patients with treatment-resistant bipolar disorder, 7 of 13 (54%) patients discontinued primarily adjunctive OXC because of adverse effects (Ghaemi et al. 2002).

OXC appears to yield less neurotoxicity and rash than CBZ. In a retrospective study of 947 epilepsy patients, OXC adverse effects most frequently involved the central nervous system and included dizziness, sedation, and fatigue, each of which was noted in 6% of patients (Friis et al. 1993). Rash was seen in 6% of patients, half of whom had previously experienced CBZ allergic reactions. About 75% of patients with a rash on CBZ will tolerate OXC. Importantly, OXC has not been associated with blood dyscrasias, lacks a boxed warning in the prescribing information, and does not appear to require hematological monitoring.

As noted earlier for CBZ, in early 2008 the FDA released an alert regarding increased risk of suicidality (suicidal behavior or ideation) in patients with epilepsy as well as psychiatric disorders for 11 anticonvulsants (including OXC and CBZ). As of late 2008, a class warning regarding this risk had not yet been added to the United States prescribing information for anticonvulsants, but it is anticipated that this may occur.

OXC, like CBZ, may produce transaminase elevations and gastrointestinal adverse effects but is associated with less weight gain than valproate (Rattya et al. 1999). In addition, OXC may have less impact on lipids than does CBZ; in 12 male patients with epilepsy, switching to OXC from CBZ yielded decreased serum total cholesterol (but not HDL cholesterol or triglyceride) concentrations (Isojarvi et al. 1994).

Hyponatremia occurs with OXC (Friis et al. 1993) and may be the main adverse effect that occurs more commonly than with CBZ. In one study of 10 male epileptic patients who switched to OXC monotherapy from CBZ monotherapy, mean serum sodium concentrations decreased—in 2 of 10 (20%), below the reference range (Isojarvi et al. 2001a). However, clinically significant hyponatremia is less common than asymptomatic hyponatremia. In a retrospective study of inpatients with acute mania, OXC yielded serum sodium concentrations below the reference range in 24 of 200 (12%), but only 3 of 200 (1.5%) discontinued as a result of hyponatremia with serum sodium less than 125 mmol/L (Reinstein et al. 2002).

In comparison with CBZ, OXC has less impact on blood concentrations of thyroid and sex hormones, likely because of its less marked hepatic enzyme induction. In one study, only 24% of 29 male epileptic patients taking OXC—versus 45% of 40 taking CBZ—had low serum total and/or free T_4 (but not T_3 and thyrotropin) concentrations (Isojarvi et al. 2001b). In addition, male epileptic patients taking CBZ (but not those taking OXC) had decreased serum dehydroepiandrosterone sulfate concentrations (Rattya et al. 2001). Switching to OXC from CBZ in male epileptic patients yielded increased serum dehydroepiandrosterone sulfate concentrations (Isojarvi et al. 1995). In healthy male volunteers, higher ($\geq$900 mg/day) but not lower (<900 mg/day) dosages of OXC appeared to yield increased levels of testosterone and gonadotropins (Larkin et al. 1991). Importantly, as noted below (see "Drug–Drug Interactions"), OXC induction of female hormone metabolism is sufficient to decrease the efficacy of hormonal contraceptives (Fattore et al. 1999; Klosterskov Jensen et al. 1992).

OXC, in contrast to CBZ, has not to date been associated with congenital malformations in humans (FDA Pregnancy Category C). This could be merely related to fewer OXC exposures. However, the absence of the CBZ-E metabolite could render OXC less teratogenic; in mice, CBZ-E (but not OXC) yielded two- to fourfold increases in malformations compared with placebo (Bennett et al. 1996). As with CBZ, in rare patients with severe mood disorders, clinicians may determine in consultation with a gynecologist that the benefits of treating with OXC out-

weigh the risks in comparison with other treatment options.

OXC is present in breast milk, and as with CBZ, clinicians may prefer to avoid the putative risks of exposing infants to OXC in breast milk and discourage breast-feeding in women taking OXC ("Trileptal" 2008).

Drug–Drug Interactions

Combination therapy is common in bipolar disorder, with up to two-thirds of patients receiving more than one medication (Kupfer et al. 2002). Patients with treatment-resistant illness may require a stepped-care approach (Figure 37–2) and appear to be receiving increasingly complex medication regimens (Frye et al. 2000). CBZ and, to a lesser extent, OXC have clinically significant drug–drug interactions, which increase the complexity of managing patients with bipolar disorder.

Carbamazepine

The pharmacokinetic properties of CBZ are typical of older enzyme-inducing anticonvulsants used by neurologists but atypical among medications prescribed by psychiatrists and necessitate special care when treating patients concurrently with other medications (Ketter et al. 1991a, 1991b). Three major principles appear to contribute importantly to CBZ drug–drug interactions:

1. **CBZ is a robust inducer of catabolic enzymes (including CYP3A3/4) and decreases the serum concentrations of many medications, including CBZ itself (Table 37–4).** CBZ induces not only CYP3A3/4 and conjugation but also presumably other cytochrome P450 isoforms that remain to be characterized. Thus, CBZ decreases the serum concentrations not only of CBZ itself (autoinduction) but also of many other medications (heteroinduction). CBZ-induced decreases in serum concentrations of certain concurrent medications can render them ineffective (see Table 37–4). Moreover, if CBZ is discontinued (or, in some instances, if replaced with OXC), serum concentrations of these other medications can increase, potentially leading to adverse effects.

2. **CBZ metabolism (which is primarily by CYP3A3/4) can be inhibited by certain enzyme inhibitors, yielding increases in serum CBZ concentrations and CBZ intoxication (Table 37–5; see Figure 37–1, top).** Autoinduction makes CBZ particularly vulnerable to the effects of enzyme inhibitors. Thus, a variety of

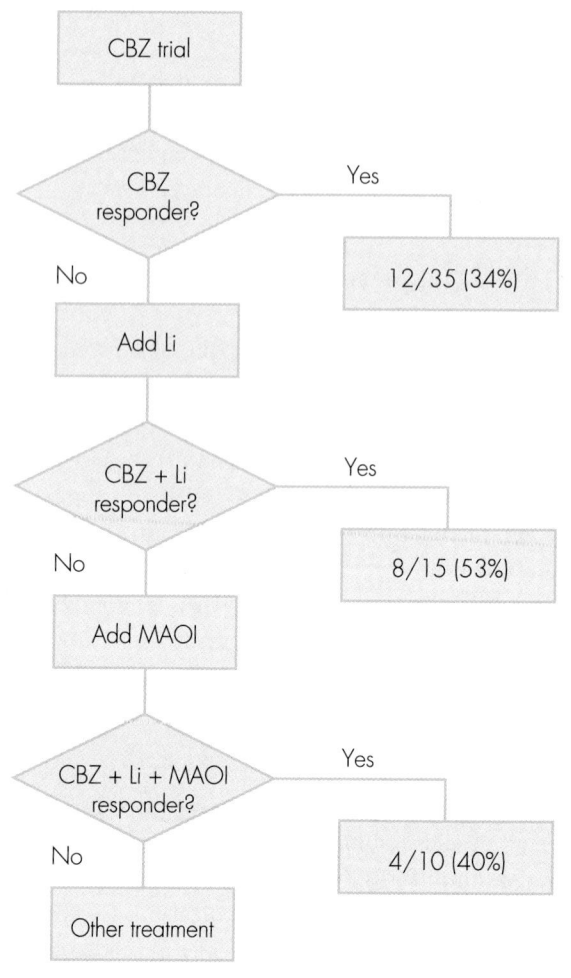

FIGURE 37–2. Stepped-care approach to bipolar depression.

Composite schema of results from three different studies in which patients with bipolar depression received carbamazepine (CBZ) monotherapy (Post et al. 1986), lithium (Li) added to CBZ (Kramlinger and Post 1989b), and a monoamine oxidase inhibitor (MAOI) added to CBZ±Li (Ketter et al. 1995b). Each successive intervention yielded additional efficacy.

agents that inhibit CYP3A3/4 can yield increased serum CBZ concentrations and intoxication (see Table 37–5; see Figure 37–1, top).

3. **CBZ has an active epoxide (CBZ-E) metabolite (see Figure 37–1, top).** Valproate inhibits epoxide hydrolase, yielding increased serum CBZ-E (but not CBZ) concentrations and intoxication (see Table 37–5). Free CBZ may also increase because of valproate-induced displacement of CBZ protein binding.

Thus, CBZ has a wide variety of pharmacokinetic drug–drug interactions that are in excess of and different from those seen with lithium or valproate. Knowledge of

CBZ drug–drug interactions is crucial in effective management, and patients should be instructed to consult their pharmacist when prescribed other medications by other physicians. Advances in molecular pharmacology have characterized the specific cytochrome P450 isoforms responsible for metabolism of various medications. This may allow clinicians to anticipate and avoid pharmacokinetic drug–drug interactions and thus provide more effective combination pharmacotherapies. Below, we review CBZ drug interactions with other medications, with agents of particular interest in the management of mood disorders indicated in **boldface** type. The reader interested in detailed reviews of CBZ drug–drug interactions may find these in other articles (Ketter et al. 1991a, 1991b).

Interactions With Mood Stabilizers

The combination of CBZ plus lithium is frequently used in bipolar disorder and may provide additive or synergistic antimanic (Kramlinger and Post 1989a) and antidepressant (Kramlinger and Post 1989b) effects. The combination is generally well tolerated, with merely additive neurotoxicity (McGinness et al. 1990), which can be minimized by gradual dose escalation. Pharmacokinetic interactions between these drugs do not occur, because lithium is excreted by the kidney, with no hepatic metabolism. Adverse effects of lithium and CBZ can be either additive or complementary, so that combination therapy decreases the serum concentrations of thyroid hormones in an additive fashion (Kramlinger and Post 1990), whereas lithium-induced increases in leukocytes and neutrophils override the common benign decreases in these indices seen with CBZ (Kramlinger and Post 1990). However, there is no evidence that lithium can alter the course of the rare severe bone marrow suppression caused by CBZ (Joffe and Post 1989). Also, the diuretic effect of lithium overrides the antidiuretic effect of CBZ (Klein 1987). Thus, CBZ will not reverse lithium-induced diabetes insipidus, but lithium attenuates CBZ-induced hyponatremia (Klein 1987; Vieweg et al. 1987).

Reports suggest that the CBZ plus **valproate** combination not only is tolerated but also may show psychotropic synergy (Keck et al. 1992; Ketter et al. 1992; Tohen et al. 1994). However, the effective use of these two medications together requires a thorough knowledge of their drug interactions, which can be simplified into the general principle that usual doses of CBZ should be reduced. Valproate inhibits CBZ metabolism (Macphee et al. 1988) and also displaces CBZ from plasma proteins, in-

TABLE 37–4. Drugs whose serum concentrations are DECREASED by carbamazepine (and oxcarbazepine)

Antidepressants
Bupropion
Citalopram
Mirtazapine
Sertraline
Tricyclics

Antipsychotics
Aripiprazole
Chlorpromazine (?)
Clozapine
Fluphenazine (?)
Haloperidol
Olanzapine
Quetiapine
Risperidone
Thiothixene (?)
Ziprasidone (?)

Anxiolytics/sedatives
Alprazolam (?)
Buspirone
Clonazepam
Eszopiclone (?)
Midazolam

Stimulants
Methylphenidate
Modafinil

Anticonvulsants
Carbamazepine
Ethosuximide
Felbamate
Lamotrigine
Levetiracetam (?)
Oxcarbazepine
Phenytoin
Primidone
Tiagabine
Topiramate
Valproate
Zonisamide

Analgesics
Alfentanil
Buprenorphine
Fentanyl (?)
Levobupivacaine
Methadone
Tramadol

Anticoagulants
Warfarin

Anti-infectives
Caspofungin
Delavirdine
Doxycycline
Praziquantel
Protease inhibitors

Dihydropyridine CCBs
Felodipine
Nimodipine

Immunosuppressants
Cyclosporine (?)
Sirolimus
Tacrolimus

Muscle relaxants
Atracurium
Cisatracurium
Doxacurium
Mivacurium
Pancuronium
Pipercuronium
Rocuronium
Vecuronium

Steroids
Dexamethasone
Hormonal contraceptives
Mifepristone
Prednisolone

Others
Paclitaxel
Quinidine
Repaglinide
Theophylline (?)
Thyroid hormones

Note. **Boldface italic** type indicates that serum concentration of the medication may decrease to a clinically significant extent not only with carbamazepine but also with oxcarbazepine, hindering efficacy of the agent.
CCBs=calcium channel blockers; (?)=Unclear clinical significance.

creasing the free CBZ fraction that is active and available to be metabolized (Macphee et al. 1988; Moreland et al. 1984). Depending on which effect predominates, total serum CBZ concentrations can rise (Moreland et al. 1984) or fall (Rambeck et al. 1987) or remain unchanged (Brodie et al. 1983; Kutt et al. 1985; Macphee et al. 1988). Valproate inhibits epoxide hydrolase, increasing the se-

rum CBZ-E concentration, at times without altering the total serum CBZ concentration (Brodie et al. 1983; Rambeck et al. 1987).

Thus, these interactions can potentially confound clinicians, because patients can have neurotoxicity due to elevated serum CBZ-E or free CBZ concentrations despite having therapeutic serum total CBZ concentrations

TABLE 37–5. Drugs that INCREASE serum concentrations of carbamazepine (but not oxcarbazepine)

Antidepressants	Calcium channel blockers
Fluoxetine	Diltiazem
Fluvoxamine	Verapamil
Nefazodone	
	Hypolipidemics
	Gemfibrozil
Anti-infectives	Nicotinamide
Isoniazid	
Quinupristin/dalfopristin	
	Others
	Acetazolamide
Azole antifungals	Cimetidine
Fluconazole	Danazol
Itraconazole	Grapefruit juice
Ketoconazole	Omeprazole
	d-Propoxyphene
Macrolide antibiotics	Ritonavir
Clarithromycin	Ticlopidine (?)
Erythromycin	Valproate (increases CBZ-E)
Troleandomycin	

Note. (?) = Unclear clinical significance.

(Kutt et al. 1985). CBZ decreases serum valproate concentrations (Kondo et al. 1990), and its discontinuation can yield increased serum valproate concentrations and toxicity (Jann et al. 1988). CBZ enzyme induction also increases the formation of the active valproate metabolite, 2-propyl-4-pentenoic acid (4-ene-valproate) (Kondo et al. 1990), which may be hepatotoxic and also may add to teratogenicity (Nau and Loscher 1986; Scheffner et al. 1988). Although fatal hepatitis in infants treated with combinations of valproate with other anticonvulsants is of great concern (Scheffner et al. 1988), the risk of combined therapy is much lower in adults (Dreifuss et al. 1989). As a general rule, clinicians should clinically monitor patients receiving the CBZ plus valproate combination for adverse effects and consider decreasing the CBZ dose in advance (because of the expected displacement of CBZ from plasma proteins and increase in CBZ-E) and possibly increasing the valproate dose (because of expected CBZ-induced decrements in valproate).

CBZ increases **lamotrigine** metabolism and approximately halves blood lamotrigine concentrations. Thus, lamotrigine doses can be doubled with this combination.

In addition, CBZ combined with lamotrigine may have additive neurotoxicity, probably due to a pharmacodynamic interaction. CBZ even appears to affect **OXC** metabolism; in patients with epilepsy, CBZ yielded decreased serum MHD concentrations (McKee et al. 1994).

Interactions With Antidepressants

Antidepressants are commonly combined with mood stabilizers in the treatment of bipolar disorder. Because CBZ can increase metabolism of some antidepressants, and because some antidepressants can inhibit CBZ metabolism, dosage adjustments may be necessary in combination therapy.

Selective serotonin reuptake inhibitors (SSRIs) have fewer adverse effects than do older antidepressants, but paroxetine and fluoxetine potently inhibit CYP2D6 (but not CYP1A2), and fluvoxamine inhibits CYP1A2 (but not CYP2D6). The atypical antidepressant nefazodone, norfluoxetine, and to a lesser extent fluvoxamine appear to inhibit CYP3A4 (Brosen 1994). **Fluoxetine** (Grimsley et al. 1991; Pearson 1990), **fluvoxamine** (Fritze et al. 1991), and **nefazodone** (Ashton and Wolin 1996; Laroudie et al. 2000; Roth and Bertschy 2001) have been reported to inhibit CBZ metabolism, causing increased CBZ concentrations and toxicity, although evidence to the contrary also has emerged for fluoxetine and fluvoxamine (Spina et al. 1993). Viloxazine (Pisani et al. 1984, 1986) and perhaps trazodone (Romero et al. 1999) can also increase CBZ levels.

Taken together, these observations suggest that fluoxetine, fluvoxamine, and nefazodone may increase CBZ concentrations, possibly by inhibition of CYP3A4. In addition, parkinsonian symptoms have been reported after addition of fluoxetine to CBZ (Gernaat et al. 1991). In contrast, sertraline (Rapeport et al. 1996), paroxetine (Andersen et al. 1991), citalopram (Moller et al. 2001), and mirtazapine (Sitsen et al. 2001) do not appear to alter CBZ metabolism. CBZ appears to decrease serum concentrations of racemic **citalopram,** including those of the active enantiomer **escitalopram** (Steinacher et al. 2002). CBZ also appears to induce the metabolism of **mirtazapine** (Sitsen et al. 2001), **mianserin** (Eap et al. 1999), **sertraline** (Khan et al. 2000; Pihlsgard and Eliasson 2002), and to some extent trazodone (Otani et al. 1996), but not viloxazine (Pisani et al. 1986). The combination of CBZ with mirtazapine is of potential concern given that mirtazapine has been associated with rare agranulocytosis, and CBZ could induce metabolism of this drug, decreasing plasma mirtazapine concentrations.

Patients receiving CBZ and **bupropion** have extremely low serum bupropion concentrations and high hydroxybupropion (metabolite) concentrations (Ketter et al. 1995a). Because hydroxybupropion is active, the clinical impact of this dramatic decrease in the bupropion-to-hydroxybupropion ratio is probably not problematic, and the combination of CBZ and bupropion may often be effective and well tolerated.

Theoretical grounds have been stated for concern about combining CBZ with monoamine oxidase inhibitors (MAOIs) ("Carbatrol" 2008; "Tegretol" 2008; Thweatt 1986). CBZ may increase rather than decrease serum levels of transdermal selegiline and its metabolites ("Emsam" 2008), and higher CBZ doses were needed in five patients taking tranylcypromine than in four taking phenelzine to yield similar serum CBZ concentrations (Barklage et al. 1992). However, case reports (Joffe et al. 1985; Yatham et al. 1990) and a series of 10 patients (Ketter et al. 1995b) suggest that the addition of phenelzine or tranylcypromine to CBZ may be well tolerated, does not affect CBZ pharmacokinetics, and may provide relief of resistant depressive symptoms in some patients. However, the antituberculosis drug isoniazid, which is also an MAOI, increases CBZ levels.

CBZ appears to induce the metabolism of **tricyclic antidepressants (TCAs),** including amitriptyline (Leinonen et al. 1991), nortriptyline (Brosen and Kragh-Sorensen 1993), imipramine (C.S. Brown et al. 1990), desipramine (Baldessarini et al. 1988), doxepin (Leinonen et al. 1991), and clomipramine (De la Fuente and Mendlewicz 1992), so that if patients fail to respond to standard doses of TCAs, TCA and metabolite concentrations should be checked. CBZ-induced decreases in tertiary-amine TCA concentrations could be mediated by CYP3A4 induction, because this isoenzyme (as well as CYP1A2 and CYP2D6) has been implicated in the *N*-demethylation of imipramine but not desipramine (Lemoine et al. 1993; Ohmori et al. 1993). The mechanism of possible CBZ induction of secondary-amine TCA metabolism remains to be determined. Spina et al. (1994) suggested that induction of CYP2D6 (the isoenzyme responsible for TCA 2-hydroxylation) may be the operative process, although no other medication has been observed to definitely yield significant induction of this isoenzyme.

Interactions With Antipsychotics

Combinations of antipsychotics with mood stabilizers are commonly required in treatment of severe mania (American Psychiatric Association 2002). Newer antipsychotics are preferred over older antipsychotics in the management of bipolar disorder because of their better tolerability (American Psychiatric Association 2002). CBZ can be used effectively in combination with antipsychotics, although clinicians need to be aware of potential drug–drug interactions.

CBZ increases **haloperidol** metabolism (Ereshefsky et al. 1986; Jann et al. 1989; Kahn et al. 1990), dramatically lowering its blood concentrations. Haloperidol metabolism is complex (Tsang et al. 1994), and the mechanism of CBZ induction of this metabolism remains to be determined. Some patients have improvement in psychiatric status or fewer neuroleptic adverse effects during combination treatment, while others show deterioration in psychiatric status (Jann et al. 1989; Kahn et al. 1990). Neurotoxicity possibly related to receiving the combination of CBZ and haloperidol has been very rarely reported (Brayley and Yellowlees 1987). There is weaker evidence that CBZ may increase the metabolism of other first-generation antipsychotic agents, including fluphenazine (Ereshefsky et al. 1986; Jann et al. 1989), chlorpromazine (Raitasuo et al. 1994), and thiothixene (Ereshefsky et al. 1986), but not thioridazine (Tiihonen et al. 1995), and that loxapine, chlorpromazine, and amoxapine may increase CBZ-E concentrations (Pitterle and Collins 1988). Thioridazine does not yield clinically significant changes in serum CBZ or CBZ-E concentrations (Spina et al. 1990). Also, animal studies suggest that promazine, chlorpromazine, perazine, chlorprothixene, and flupenthixol may increase CBZ concentrations (Daniel et al. 1992). In view of the above, serum antipsychotic medication concentrations should be checked if patients fail to respond to standard dosages of antipsychotic agents during combination therapy with CBZ.

Combination of **clozapine** with CBZ is not recommended in view of the hypothetical possibility of synergistic bone marrow suppression ("Carbatrol" 2008; "Tegretol" 2008). However, these drugs have been used in combination in some European centers, one of which reported that CBZ decreases clozapine (a CYP2D6 substrate [Fischer et al. 1992]) concentrations (Raitasuo et al. 1993). Thus, clinicians wishing to combine a psychotropic anticonvulsant with clozapine should consider valproate, lamotrigine, or another anticonvulsant rather than CBZ, except under unusual circumstances.

CBZ increases metabolism of **olanzapine** (Linnet and Olesen 2002; Lucas et al. 1998), **risperidone** (Ono et al. 2002; Spina et al. 2000; Yatham et al. 2003), **quetiapine** (Grimm et al. 2006), **aripiprazole** (Physicians' Desk Reference 2008), and ziprasidone (Miceli et al. 2000). Although the clinical significance of CBZ-induced decreases in ziprasidone serum concentrations remains to be determined, CBZ interactions with other atypical antipsychotics can be clinically significant. For example, in a recent acute mania combination therapy study, CBZ decreased serum risperidone plus active metabolite concentrations by 40%, interfering with antipsychotic efficacy (Yatham et al. 2003). In another combination therapy study, CBZ yielded lower-than-expected blood olanzapine concentrations, and even though this was addressed in part by more aggressive olanzapine dosage, the efficacy of the olanzapine plus CBZ combination was still not significantly better than that of CBZ monotherapy in the treatment of acute mania (Tohen et al. 2008). In two patients, quetiapine appeared to increase CBZ-E levels (Fitzgerald and Okos 2002). The effects of clozapine, olanzapine, risperidone, ziprasidone, and aripiprazole on CBZ pharmacokinetics remain to be established.

Interactions With Anxiolytics and Sedatives

CBZ is commonly administered along with **benzodiazepines** in patients with bipolar disorder, with merely additive central nervous system (e.g., sedation, ataxia) adverse effects. Indeed, contemporary controlled CBZ trials routinely permit some adjunctive benzodiazepine (e.g., lorazepam) administration (Weisler et al. 2004, 2005). However, CBZ may decrease serum concentrations of clonazepam (Lai et al. 1978; Yukawa et al. 2001), alprazolam (Arana et al. 1988; Furukori et al. 1998), clobazam (Levy et al. 1983), and midazolam (Backman et al. 1996), potentially decreasing the efficacy of these agents. CBZ-induced decreases in certain benzodiazepine concentrations could be mediated by induction of CYP3A4, as this isoenzyme has been implicated in the metabolism of clonazepam (Seree et al. 1993), triazolam (Kronbach et al. 1989), midazolam (Gascon and Dayer 1991; Kronbach et al. 1989), and possibly alprazolam (Greenblatt et al. 1993; von Moltke et al. 1993). The newer hypnotics eszopiclone and zolpidem may have drug interactions with CBZ, as these agents appear to be more susceptible than zaleplon to drugs that induce CYP3A4 (Drover 2004). On the other hand, clonazepam (Lander et al. 1975; Lehtovaara et al. 1978) and clobazam (Goggin and Callaghan 1985; Munoz et al. 1990) appear to have variable effects on CBZ metabolism. Of interest, CBZ may be effective in ameliorating benzodiazepine withdrawal symptoms (Ries et al. 1989).

Interactions With Stimulants

The use of stimulants in bipolar disorder is circumscribed largely because of concerns about the risk of abuse and mood destabilization. CBZ appears to decrease serum concentrations of methylphenidate and modafinil.

Interactions With Calcium Channel Blockers

Of clear clinical importance, elevated serum CBZ concentrations and neurotoxicity have been reported during concurrent treatment with the nondihydropyridines **verapamil** and **diltiazem,** but not the dihydropyridines nifedipine (Brodie and MacPhee 1986; Price and DiMarzio 1988) and nimodipine. (This is easily remembered by the "N" rule: Not Nifedipine or Nimodipine.) These observations are consistent with the finding that verapamil and diltiazem, but not nifedipine, inhibit the hepatic oxidative metabolism of various drugs (Hunt et al. 1989). Preliminary observations also indicate that the dihydropyridine nimodipine may not substantially influence CBZ kinetics and that the addition of CBZ to nimodipine may yield therapeutic synergy (Pazzaglia et al. 1993, 1998).

Enzyme-inducing anticonvulsants such as CBZ appear to decrease serum concentrations of **dihydropyridines** such as nimodipine (Tartara et al. 1991) and felodipine (Capewell et al. 1988; Zaccara et al. 1993), presumably by induction of CYP3A4, given that this isoenzyme mediates metabolism of nimodipine, felodipine, nifedipine, and nicardipine, as well as a variety of other dihydropyridines (Guengerich et al. 1991).

Interactions With Substances of Abuse

In view of the high comorbidity of bipolar disorder and alcohol abuse, knowledge of interactions between ethanol and CBZ is of clinical utility. Ethanol is a CYP2E1 substrate (Gonzalez et al. 1991) and inducer (Hansson et al. 1990). Although ethanol and CBZ do not have pharmacokinetic interactions (Dar et al. 1989; Pynnönen et al. 1978) (presumably because of their metabolism by different CYP families), CBZ attenuates alcohol withdrawal symptoms (Malcolm et al. 1989), a potentially useful property given the risk of alcohol abuse in bipolar disorder patients. Combination therapy with disulfiram and CBZ is well tolerated and does not cause clinically significant changes in serum CBZ and CBZ-E concentrations (Krag et al. 1981).

Tobacco smoking (which induces CYP1A [Guengerich 1992]) does not alter CBZ metabolism (Bachmann et al. 1990), and CBZ does not alter caffeine (a CYP1A2 substrate [Fuhr et al. 1992]) pharmacokinetics (Wietholtz et al. 1989).

Preliminary clinical studies suggested that CBZ attenuated acute cocaine effects and seizures and possibly cocaine craving (Halikas et al. 1989; Kuhn et al. 1989;

Sherer et al. 1990), but later controlled studies generally failed to support these observations (Cornish et al. 1995; Kranzler et al. 1995; Montoya et al. 1994).

Interactions With Anticonvulsants

As noted above, CBZ induces the metabolism of **carbamazepine** (autoinduction) and **oxcarbazepine** (McKee et al. 1994), as well as the mood-stabilizing anticonvulsants **valproate** and **lamotrigine.** CBZ also induces the metabolism of several older anticonvulsants, including ethosuximide, phenytoin, and primidone. Moreover, CBZ induces the metabolism of multiple newer anticonvulsants, including felbamate, **topiramate** (Sachdeo et al. 1996), tiagabine (Samara et al. 1998), **zonisamide** (Ojemann et al. 1986), and possibly levetiracetam (May et al. 2003), but not gabapentin (Radulovic et al. 1994) or pregabalin (Brodie et al. 2005). In contrast, none (aside from felbamate) of these newer anticonvulsants yields clinically significant changes in CBZ pharmacokinetics (Brodie et al. 2005; Gidal et al. 2005; Gustavson et al. 1998; McKee et al. 1994; Radulovic et al. 1994; Ragueneau-Majlessi et al. 2004; Sachdeo et al. 1996). However, the anticonvulsants phenytoin, phenobarbital, primidone, methsuximide, and felbamate decrease serum CBZ concentrations. In addition, CBZ may have a pharmacodynamic interaction with levetiracetam (Sisodiya et al. 2002).

Interactions With Nonpsychotropic Drugs

Drug–drug interactions between CBZ and other (nonpsychotropic) drugs are also of substantial clinical importance. CBZ induces metabolism of diverse medications, raising the possibility of undermining the efficacy of steroids such as **hormonal contraceptives,** dexamethasone, prednisolone, and mifepristone. In women taking CBZ, oral contraceptive preparations need to contain at least 50 μg of ethinylestradiol, levonorgestrel implants are contraindicated because of cases of contraceptive failure, and medroxyprogesterone injections need to be given every 10 rather than 12 weeks (Crawford 2002). CBZ also induces metabolism of **methylxanthines** such as theophylline and aminophylline; antibiotics such as **doxycycline;** antivirals such as **protease inhibitors; neuromuscular blockers** such as pancuronium, vecuronium, and doxacurium; analgesics such as **methadone; immunosuppressants** such as sirolimus and tacrolimus; and the anticoagulants **warfarin** and possibly dicumarol (see Table 37–4).

Similarly, a variety of medications can increase serum CBZ concentrations and yield clinical toxicity, including **isoniazid, azole antifungals** such as ketoconazole, **mac-**rolide antibiotics** such as erythromycin and clarithromycin, **protease inhibitors** such as ritonavir and nelfinavir, **hypolipidemics** such as gemfibrozil and nicotinamide, and the carbonic anhydrase inhibitor **acetazolamide** (see Table 37–5). In addition, other medications such as cisplatin and doxorubicin may decrease serum CBZ levels, potentially yielding inefficacy.

Oxcarbazepine

In contrast to CBZ, OXC has fewer clinically significant drug–drug interactions. Differences in three major areas appear to contribute importantly to differences between OXC and CBZ drug–drug interactions:

1. **OXC is only a modest to moderate enzyme (CYP3A4) inducer, which yields clinically significant decreases in serum concentrations of some medications (see Table 37–4).** OXC yields minor enzyme heteroinduction (but not autoinduction), which is clearly less robust than that seen with CBZ. For example, in healthy male volunteers, measures of enzyme activity such as antipyrine metabolism and urinary 6-β-hydroxycortisol excretion concentrations were unaltered with OXC (Larkin et al. 1991), and in male epileptic patients, switching to OXC from CBZ yielded decreased antipyrine clearance (Isojarvi et al. 1994). In some instances, OXC compared to CBZ induction is substantially less robust, so that switching from OXC to CBZ (or vice versa) will make adjustments of doses of other medications necessary. The extent of OXC induction of metabolism of other drugs is often clinically insignificant but is clinically significant for hormonal contraceptives. Serum concentrations of some of the medications (in **_boldface italic_** type) listed in Table 37–4 may decrease to a clinically significant extent with OXC, hindering efficacy of such agents. OXC decreases serum concentrations of female hormones, presumably mediated by heteroinduction of CYP3A, sufficiently to compromise the efficacy of hormonal contraceptives (Fattore et al. 1999) and to require higher doses. In contrast, induction of conjugation is more limited, yielding only modest clinical effects on clearance of drugs such as valproate and lamotrigine. Finally, OXC inhibits CYP2C19 (Tripp et al. 1996) and thus may increase serum phenytoin concentrations.

2. **OXC metabolism (which is primarily by arylketone reductase) generally is not susceptible to enzyme inhibitors.** The absence of autoinduction and the robust actions of cytosol reductases that mediate conversion

to MHD appear to render OXC metabolism not susceptible to the common phenomenon of inhibition by other agents seen with CBZ. Thus, the medications listed in Table 37–5 that can elevate serum CBZ concentrations and yield neurotoxicity do NOT appear to have such interactions with OXC.

3. **OXC has an active (MHD) metabolite (see Figure 37–1, bottom middle).** However, MHD metabolism, unlike CBZ-E catabolism, is not inhibited by valproate, presumably due to the lack of involvement of epoxide hydrolase in MHD disposition. Thus, coadministration of valproate does NOT yield toxicity related to increased MHD.

Interactions With Mood Stabilizers

OXC, in contrast to CBZ, does not induce valproate metabolism. In patients with epilepsy, OXC did not significantly alter valproate (or CBZ) area under the concentration–time curve (McKee et al. 1994), and switching to OXC from CBZ yielded increased serum total valproate concentration-to-dose ratios and increased valproate-related adverse effects (Battino et al. 1992). Also, in rats, valproate did not significantly alter OXC pharmacokinetic parameters (Matar et al. 1999).

OXC, in comparison with CBZ, also appears to have less robust effects on **lamotrigine** metabolism; in women with epilepsy, OXC was associated with a 29% and CBZ a 54% decrease in serum lamotrigine concentrations (May et al. 1999). The clinical significance of this interaction remains to be established and could vary across patients (Theis et al. 2005). Lamotrigine does not appear to alter OXC pharmacokinetics (Theis et al. 2005). A possible pharmacodynamic interaction has been reported with OXC and lamotrigine (Sabers and Gram 2000).

In addition, **carbamazepine** induces OXC metabolism, yielding decreased serum MHD concentrations (McKee et al. 1994). The presence or absence of pharmacokinetic interactions between OXC and lithium remains to be established.

Interactions With Antidepressants

OXC, in contrast to CBZ, may not robustly induce citalopram metabolism; switching to OXC from CBZ in two patients yielded increased serum citalopram concentrations (Leinonen et al. 1996).

Interactions With Antipsychotics

OXC, unlike CBZ, may not robustly induce antipsychotic metabolism; switching to OXC from CBZ in six patients

with schizophrenia or organic psychosis who were taking haloperidol, chlorpromazine, or clozapine yielded 50%–200% increases in serum neuroleptic concentrations and additional extrapyramidal symptoms (Raitasuo et al. 1994). OXC does not cause clinically significant alterations in serum olanzapine or risperidone concentrations (Rosaria Muscatello et al. 2005).

Interactions With Anxiolytics and Sedatives

OXC may decrease serum concentrations of **benzodiazepines.**

Interactions With Calcium Channel Blockers

OXC appears to decrease serum concentrations of **dihydropyridine** calcium channel blockers (which are CYP3A4 substrates) to some extent. Although OXC reduced felodipine area under the concentration–time curve by 28% in healthy volunteers, this effect was much smaller than that previously reported with CBZ (Zaccara et al. 1993). In a retrospective study, 16 inpatients with acute mania who were taking calcium channel blockers had no clinically significant changes in blood pressure when treated with concurrent OXC (Reinstein et al. 2002).

Interactions With Nonpsychotropic Drugs

OXC, compared with CBZ, also appears to have fewer interactions with nonpsychotropic drugs. Thus, neither the CYP3A4 inhibitor erythromycin (Keranen et al. 1992a) nor the heteroinhibitor cimetidine (Keranen et al. 1992b) appears to alter OXC pharmacokinetics in healthy volunteers. Also, OXC does not appear to robustly induce warfarin metabolism; in healthy volunteers receiving steady-state warfarin, OXC did not significantly alter prothrombin time (Kramer et al. 1992).

However, as noted earlier in this chapter, OXC appears to have a clinically significant interaction with **hormonal contraceptives;** in healthy female volunteers, OXC appeared to decrease ethinylestradiol and levonorgestrel derived from hormonal contraceptives by up to about 50% (Fattore et al. 1999; Klosterskov Jensen et al. 1992).

OXC, like CBZ, may decrease serum concentrations of the analgesic buprenorphine, the anticancer agent paclitaxel, and the antidiabetic agent repaglinide. As previously noted, OXC also yields decreases in serum concentrations of the dihydropyridine calcium channel blocker felodipine (which is also a CYP3A4 substrate). In contrast to CBZ, the CYP3A4 inhibitor erythromycin and the antidepressant viloxazine do not yield clinically significant increases in serum OXC concentrations.

OXC may modestly decrease serum concentrations of topiramate (May et al. 2002) and levetiracetam (May et al. 2003). In addition, the anticonvulsants **CBZ**, phenytoin, phenobarbital, and primidone may induce OXC metabolism. Finally, OXC can increase serum phenytoin concentrations, presumably by inhibiting the activity of CYP2C19.

Conclusion

In the past, because of lack of an FDA indication, complexity of use, and methodological concerns regarding earlier efficacy studies, CBZ was generally considered an alternative rather than a first-line intervention in bipolar disorder. However, the recent approval of a proprietary CBZ beaded extended-release capsule formulation (Equetro) for the treatment of acute manic and mixed episodes in patients with bipolar disorder and the low propensity of CBZ to cause weight gain and metabolic problems seen with some other agents may lead clinicians to reassess its role in the management of patients with bipolar disorder (Ketter et al. 2005). This long-acting preparation in some patients with bipolar disorder can be given as a single nighttime dose, which will enhance compliance and minimize daytime side effects.

OXC, compared with CBZ, has more limited evidence of efficacy in bipolar disorder but has enhanced tolerability and fewer drug–drug interactions. For example, with CBZ (but not OXC), common benign leukopenia is difficult to distinguish from what may be a harbinger of the very rare serious aplastic anemia, and patients and caregivers need to monitor carefully for symptoms of this adverse effect. In addition, CBZ (and to a lesser extent OXC) in combination therapy induces metabolism of other drugs, sometimes undermining their efficacy unless doses are adjusted. Also, other drugs (such as erythromycin or verapamil) can inhibit CBZ (but not OXC) metabolism, causing CBZ toxicity. Instructing patients to alert their other caregivers and pharmacists that they are receiving CBZ may help avoid drug interactions. Informing patients of several of the common interactions can further assist in the warning process, as other practitioners may inadvertently introduce commonly used drugs such as erythromycin with the attendant risk of CBZ toxicity.

CBZ and OXC are important treatment options for bipolar disorder patients who experience inadequate responses to or unacceptable adverse effects with lithium and valproate. Awareness of CBZ and OXC pharmacology and potential drug–drug interactions will provide cli-

nicians with the opportunity to enhance outcomes when managing bipolar disorder with these agents.

References

Ahlfors UG, Baastrup PC, Dencker SJ, et al: Flupenthixol decanoate in recurrent manic-depressive illness: a comparison with lithium. Acta Psychiatr Scand 64:226–237, 1981
Ambrosio AF, Silva AP, Malva JO, et al: Inhibition of glutamate release by BIA 2-093 and BIA 2-024, two novel derivatives of carbamazepine, due to blockade of sodium but not calcium channels. Biochem Pharmacol 61:1271–1275, 2001
Ambrosio AF, Soares-Da-Silva P, Carvalho CM, et al: Mechanisms of action of carbamazepine and its derivatives, oxcarbazepine, BIA 2-093, and BIA 2-024. Neurochem Res 27:121–130, 2002
American Psychiatric Association: Practice guideline for the treatment of patients with bipolar disorder. Am J Psychiatry 151:1–36, 1994
American Psychiatric Association: Practice guideline for the treatment of patients with bipolar disorder (revision). Am J Psychiatry 159:1–50, 2002
Andersen BB, Mikkelsen M, Vesterager A, et al: No influence of the antidepressant paroxetine on carbamazepine, valproate and phenytoin. Epilepsy Res 10:201–204, 1991
Arana GW, Epstein S, Molloy M, et al: Carbamazepine-induced reduction of plasma alprazolam concentrations: a clinical case report. J Clin Psychiatry 49:448–449, 1988
Ashton AK, Wolin RE: Nefazodone-induced carbamazepine toxicity (letter). Am J Psychiatry 153:733, 1996
Bachmann KA, Nunlee M, Martin M, et al: The use of single sample clearance estimates to probe hepatic drug metabolism: handprinting the influence of cigarette smoking on human hepatic drug metabolism. Xenobiotica 20:537–547, 1990
Backman JT, Olkkola KT, Ojala M, et al: Concentrations and effects of oral midazolam are greatly reduced in patients treated with carbamazepine or phenytoin. Epilepsia 37:253–257, 1996
Baldessarini RJ, Teicher MH, Cassidy JW, et al: Anticonvulsant cotreatment may increase toxic metabolites of antidepressants and other psychotropic drugs (letter). J Clin Psychopharmacol 8:381–382, 1988
Ballenger JC, Post RM: Therapeutic effects of carbamazepine in affective illness: a preliminary report. Comm Psychopharmacol 2:159–175, 1978
Barcs G, Walker EB, Elger CE, et al: Oxcarbazepine placebo-controlled, dose-ranging trial in refractory partial epilepsy. Epilepsia 41:1597–1607, 2000
Barklage NE, Jefferson JW, Margolis D: Do monoamine oxidase inhibitors alter carbamazepine blood levels? (letter). J Clin Psychiatry 53:258, 1992
Baruzzi A, Albani F, Riva R: Oxcarbazepine: pharmacokinetic interactions and their clinical relevance. Epilepsia 35 (suppl 3):S14–S19, 1994
Battino D, Croci D, Granata T, et al: Changes in unbound and total valproic acid concentrations after replacement of carbamazepine with oxcarbazepine. Ther Drug Monit 14:376–379, 1992
Bellaire W, Demish K, Stoll KD: Carbamazepine versus lithium in prophylaxis of recurrent affective disorder (abstract). Psychopharmacology (Berl) 96:287, 1988

Benes J, Parada A, Figueiredo AA, et al: Anticonvulsant and sodium channel-blocking properties of novel 10,11-dihydro-5H-dibenz[b,f]azepine-5-carboxamide derivatives. J Med Chem 42:2582–2587, 1999

Bennett GD, Amore BM, Finnell RH, et al: Teratogenicity of carbamazepine-10,11-epoxide and oxcarbazepine in the SWV mouse. J Pharmacol Exp Ther 279:1237–1242, 1996

Bentsen KD, Gram L, Veje A: Serum thyroid hormones and blood folic acid during monotherapy with carbamazepine or valproate: a controlled study. Acta Neurol Scand 67:235–241, 1983

Bernasconi R: The GABA hypothesis of affective illness: influence of clinically effective antimanic drugs on GABA turnover, in Basic Mechanisms in the Action of Lithium. Proceedings of a Symposium, Bavaria, Oct 4–6, 1981. Edited by Emrich HM, Aidenhoff JB, Lux HD. Amsterdam, Elsevier Science, 1982, pp 183–192

Bernasconi R, Martin P: Effects of antiepileptic drugs on the GABA turnover rate (abstract 251). Naunyn Schmiedebergs Arch Pharmacol 307:R63, 1979

Bernasconi R, Hauser K, Martin P, et al: Biochemical aspects of the mechanism of action of valproate, in Anticonvulsants in Affective Disorders. Edited by Emrich HM, Okuma T, Müller AA. Amsterdam, Elsevier Science, 1984, pp 14–32

Beydoun A, Sachdeo RC, Rosenfeld WE, et al: Oxcarbazepine monotherapy for partial-onset seizures: a multicenter, double-blind, clinical trial. Neurology 54:2245–2251, 2000

Bowden CL, Brugger AM, Swann AC, et al: Efficacy of divalproex vs lithium and placebo in the treatment of mania. The Depakote Mania Study Group. JAMA 271:918–924, 1994

Bowden CL, Calabrese JR, McElroy SL, et al: A randomized, placebo-controlled 12-month trial of divalproex and lithium in treatment of outpatients with bipolar I disorder. Divalproex Maintenance Study Group [see comments]. Arch Gen Psychiatry 57:481–489, 2000

Brayley J, Yellowlees P: An interaction between haloperidol and carbamazepine in a patient with cerebral palsy. Aust N Z J Psychiatry 21:605–607, 1987

Brodie MJ, Forrest G, Rapeport WG: Carbamazepine 10,11 epoxide concentrations in epileptics on carbamazepine alone and in combination with other anticonvulsants. Br J Clin Pharmacol 16:747–749, 1983

Brodie MJ, MacPhee GJ: Carbamazepine neurotoxicity precipitated by diltiazem. BMJ 292:1170–1171, 1986

Brodie MJ, Wilson EA, Wesche DL, et al: Pregabalin drug interaction studies: lack of effect on the pharmacokinetics of carbamazepine, phenytoin, lamotrigine, and valproate in patients with partial epilepsy. Epilepsia 46:1407–1413, 2005

Brosen K: Isozyme specific metabolism and interactions in psychopharmacology (abstract S-107–472), in 19th Congress of Collegium Internationale Neuro-Psychopharmacologicum, Washington, June 27–July 1, 1994. Neuropsychopharmacology 10 (3S, part 1):491S, 1994

Brosen K, Kragh-Sorensen P: Concomitant intake of nortriptyline and carbamazepine. Ther Drug Monit 15:258–260, 1993

Brown CS, Wells BG, Cold JA, et al: Possible influence of carbamazepine on plasma imipramine concentrations in children with attention deficit hyperactivity disorder. J Clin Psychopharmacol 10:359–362, 1990

Brown D, Silverstone T, Cookson J: Carbamazepine compared to haloperidol in acute mania. Int Clin Psychopharmacol 4:229–238, 1989

Brown DW, Ketter TA, Crumlish J, et al: Carbamazepine-induced increases in total serum cholesterol: clinical and theoretical implications. J Clin Psychopharmacol 12:431–437, 1992

Cabrera JF, Muhlbauer HD, Schley J, et al: Long-term randomized clinical trial of oxcarbazepine vs lithium in bipolar and schizoaffective disorders: preliminary results. Pharmacopsychiatry 19:282–283, 1986

Cade JFJ: Lithium salts in the treatment of psychotic excitement. Med J Aust 14:349–352, 1949

Capewell S, Freestone S, Critchley JA, et al: Reduced felodipine bioavailability in patients taking anticonvulsants. Lancet 2(8609):480–482, 1988

Carbatrol (carbamazepine extended-release) package insert. Physicians' Desk Reference, 62nd Edition. Montvale, NJ, Thomson PDR, 2008

Cereghino JJ: Serum carbamazepine concentration and clinical control, in Advances in Neurology. Edited by Penry JK, Daly DD. New York, Raven, 1975, pp 309–330

Christe W, Kramer G, Vigonius U: A double-blind controlled clinical trial: oxcarbazepine vs sodium valproate in adults with newly diagnosed epilepsy. Epilepsy Res 26:451–460, 1997

Connell JM, Rapeport WG, Gordon S, et al: Changes in circulating thyroid hormones during short-term hepatic enzyme induction with carbamazepine. Eur J Clin Pharmacol 26:453–456, 1984

Cornish JW, Maany I, Fudala PJ, et al: Carbamazepine treatment for cocaine dependence. Drug Alcohol Depend 38:221–227, 1995

Coxhead N, Silverstone T, Cookson J: Carbamazepine versus lithium in the prophylaxis of bipolar affective disorder. Acta Psychiatr Scand 85:114–118, 1992

Crawford P: Interactions between antiepileptic drugs and hormonal contraception. CNS Drugs 16:263–272, 2002

Dam M, Ekberg R, Loyning Y, et al: A double-blind study comparing oxcarbazepine and carbamazepine in patients with newly diagnosed, previously untreated epilepsy. Epilepsy Res 3:70–76, 1989

Daniel W, Janczar L, Danek L, et al: Pharmacokinetic interaction between carbamazepine and neuroleptics after combined prolonged treatment in rats. Naunyn Schmiedebergs Arch Pharmacol 345:598–605, 1992

Dar MS, Hardee M, Ganey T: Brain adenosine modulation of behavioral interactions between ethanol and carbamazepine in mice. Alcohol 6:297–301, 1989

De la Fuente JM, Mendlewicz J: Carbamazepine addition in tricyclic antidepressant-resistant unipolar depression. Biol Psychiatry 32:369–374, 1992

Deckert J, Berger W, Kleopa K, et al: Adenosine A1 receptors in human hippocampus: inhibition of [3H]8-cyclopentyl-1,3-dipropylxanthine binding by antagonist drugs. Neurosci Lett 150:191–194, 1993

Degen PH, Flesch G, Cardot JM, et al: The influence of food on the disposition of the antiepileptic oxcarbazepine and its major metabolites in healthy volunteers. Biopharm Drug Dispos 15:519–526, 1994

Denicoff K, Smith-Jackson E, Disney E, et al: Comparative prophylactic efficacy of lithium, carbamazepine, and the combination in bipolar disorder. J Clin Psychiatry 58:470–478, 1997

Desai NG, Gangadhar BN, Channabasavanna SM, et al: Carbamazepine hastens therapeutic action of lithium in mania (abstract), in Proceedings of the International Conference on

New Directions in Affective Disorders, Jerusalem, Israel, 1987, p 97

Di Costanzo E, Schifano F: Lithium alone or in combination with carbamazepine for the treatment of rapid-cycling bipolar affective disorder. Acta Psychiatr Scand 83:456–459, 1991

Dilsaver SC, Swann AC, Shoaib AM, et al: The manic syndrome: factors which may predict a patient's response to lithium, carbamazepine and valproate. J Psychiatry Neurosci 18:61–66, 1993

Dreifuss FE, Langer DH, Moline KA, et al: Valproic acid hepatic fatalities, II: US experience since 1984. Neurology 39:201–207, 1989

Drover DR: Comparative pharmacokinetics and pharmacodynamics of short-acting hypnosedatives: zaleplon, zolpidem and zopiclone. Clin Pharmacokinet 43:227–238, 2004

Eap CB, Yasui N, Kaneko S, et al: Effects of carbamazepine coadministration on plasma concentrations of the enantiomers of mianserin and of its metabolites. Ther Drug Monit 21:166–170, 1999

Eichelbaum M, Tomson T, Tybring G, et al: Carbamazepine metabolism in man: induction and pharmacogenetic aspects. Clin Pharmacokinet 10:80–90, 1985

Elphick M, Lyons F, Cowen PJ: Low tolerability of carbamazepine in psychiatric patients may restrict its clinical usefulness. J Psychopharmacol 2:1–4, 1988

Emrich HM: Studies with (Trileptal) oxcarbazepine in acute mania. Int Clin Psychopharmacol 5:83–88, 1990

Emrich HM, Altmann H, Dose M, et al: Therapeutic effects of GABA-ergic drugs in affective disorders. A preliminary report. Pharmacol Biochem Behav 19:369–372, 1983

Emrich HM, Dose M, von Zerssen D: The use of sodium valproate, carbamazepine and oxcarbazepine in patients with affective disorders. J Affect Disord 8:243–250, 1985

Emsam (transdermal selegiline) package insert. Physicians' Desk Reference, 62nd Edition. Montvale, NJ, Thomson PDR, 2008

Equetro (carbamazepine beaded extended-release capsule) package insert. Physicians' Desk Reference, 62nd Edition. Montvale, NJ, Thomson PDR, 2008

Ereshefsky L, Jann MW, Saklad SR, et al: Bioavailability of psychotropic drugs: historical perspective and pharmacokinetic overview. J Clin Psychiatry 47:6–15, 1986

Faigle JW, Feldmann KF: Carbamazepine: chemistry and biotransformation, in Antiepileptic Drugs, 4th Edition. Edited by Levy RH, Mattson RH, Meldrum BS. New York, Raven, 1995, pp 499–513

Fattore C, Cipolla G, Gatti G, et al: Induction of ethinylestradiol and levonorgestrel metabolism by oxcarbazepine in healthy women. Epilepsia 40:783–787, 1999

Fischer V, Vogels B, Maurer G, et al: The antipsychotic clozapine is metabolized by the polymorphic human microsomal and recombinant cytochrome P450 2D6. J Pharmacol Exp Ther 260:1355–1360, 1992

Fitzgerald BJ, Okos AJ: Elevation of carbamazepine-10,11-epoxide by quetiapine. Pharmacotherapy 22:1500–1503, 2002

Frankenburg FR, Tohen M, Cohen BM, et al: Long-term response to carbamazepine: a retrospective study. J Clin Psychopharmacol 8:130–132, 1988

Frey B, Braegger CP, Ghelfi D: Neonatal cholestatic hepatitis from carbamazepine exposure during pregnancy and breast feeding. Ann Pharmacother 36:644–647, 2002

Friis ML, Kristensen O, Boas J, et al: Therapeutic experiences with 947 epileptic out-patients in oxcarbazepine treatment. Acta Neurol Scand 87:224–227, 1993

Fritze J, Unsorg B, Lanczik M: Interaction between carbamazepine and fluvoxamine. Acta Psychiatr Scand 84:583–584, 1991

Froescher W, Eichelbaum M, Niesen M, et al: Carbamazepine levels in breast milk. Ther Drug Monit 6:266–271, 1984

Frye MA, Ketter TA, Leverich GS, et al: The increasing use of polypharmacotherapy for refractory mood disorders: 22 years of study. J Clin Psychiatry 61:9–15, 2000

Fuhr U, Doehmer J, Battula N, et al: Biotransformation of caffeine and theophylline in mammalian cell lines genetically engineered for expression of single cytochrome P450 isoforms. Biochem Pharmacol 43:225–235, 1992

Furukori H, Otani K, Yasui N, et al: Effect of carbamazepine on the single oral dose pharmacokinetics of alprazolam. Neuropsychopharmacology 18:364–369, 1998

Garnett WR, Levy B, McLean AM, et al: Pharmacokinetic evaluation of twice-daily extended-release carbamazepine (CBZ) and four-times-daily immediate-release CBZ in patients with epilepsy. Epilepsia 39:274–279, 1998

Gascon MP, Dayer P: In vitro forecasting of drugs which may interfere with the biotransformation of midazolam. Eur J Clin Pharmacol 41:573–578, 1991

Gernaat HB, Van de Woude J, Touw DJ: Fluoxetine and parkinsonism in patients taking carbamazepine (letter). Am J Psychiatry 148:1604–1605, 1991

Ghaemi NS, Ko JY, Katzow JJ: Oxcarbazepine treatment of refractory bipolar disorder: a retrospective chart review. Bipolar Disord 4:70–74, 2002

Gidal BE, Baltes E, Otoul C, et al: Effect of levetiracetam on the pharmacokinetics of adjunctive antiepileptic drugs: a pooled analysis of data from randomized clinical trials. Epilepsy Res 64:1–11, 2005

Glauser T, Nigro M, Sachdeo R, et al: Adjunctive therapy with oxcarbazepine in children with partial seizures. Oxcarbazepine Pediatric Study Group. Neurology 54:2237–2244, 2000

Goggin T, Callaghan N: Blood levels of clobazam and its metabolites and therapeutic effect, in Clobazam: Human Psychopharmacology and Clinical Applications (International Congress and Symposium Series, No 74). Edited by Hindmarch I, Stonier PD, Trimble MR. London, Royal Society of Medicine, 1985, pp 149–153

Goncalves N, Stoll KD: [Carbamazepine in manic syndromes: a controlled double-blind study.] Nervenarzt 56:43–47, 1985

Gonzalez FJ, Ueno T, Umeno M, et al: Microsomal ethanol oxidizing system: transcriptional and posttranscriptional regulation of cytochrome P450, CYP2E1. Alcohol Alcohol Suppl 1:97–101, 1991

Greenblatt DJ, von Moltke LL, Harmatz JS, et al: Alprazolam pharmacokinetics, metabolism, and plasma levels: clinical implications. J Clin Psychiatry 54:4–11, 1993

Greil W, Ludwig-Mayerhofer W, Erazo N, et al: Lithium versus carbamazepine in the maintenance treatment of bipolar disorders—a randomised study. J Affect Disord 43:151–161, 1997

Greil W, Kleindienst N, Erazo N, et al: Differential response to lithium and carbamazepine in the prophylaxis of bipolar disorder. J Clin Psychopharmacol 18:455–460, 1998

Grimm SW, Richtand NM, Winter HR, et al: Effects of cytochrome P450 3A modulators ketoconazole and carbamazepine on quetiapine pharmacokinetics. Br J Clin Pharmacol 61:58–69, 2006

Grimsley SR, Jann MW, Carter JG, et al: Increased carbamazepine plasma concentrations after fluoxetine coadministration. Clin Pharmacol Ther 50:10–15, 1991

Grossi E, Sacchetti E, Vita A, et al: Carbamazepine versus chlorpromazine in mania: a double-blind trial, in Anticonvulsants in Affective Disorders. Edited by Emrich HM, Okuma T, Müller AA. Amsterdam, Excerpta Medica, 1984, pp 177–187

Guengerich FP, Brian WR, Iwasaki M, et al: Oxidation of dihydropyridine calcium channel blockers and analogues by human liver cytochrome P-450 IIIA4. J Med Chem 34:1838–1844, 1991

Guengerich FP: Characterization of human cytochrome P450 enzymes. FASEB J 6:745–748, 1992

Gustavson LE, Cato A 3rd, Boellner SW, et al: Lack of pharmacokinetic drug interactions between tiagabine and carbamazepine or phenytoin. Am J Ther 5:9–16, 1998

Haidukewych D, Rodin EA: Chronic antiepileptic drug therapy: classification by medication regimen and incidence of decreases in serum thyroxine and free thyroxine index. Ther Drug Monit 9:392–398, 1987

Halikas J, Kemp K, Kuhn K, et al: Carbamazepine for cocaine addiction? (letter) Lancet 1(8638):623–624, 1989

Hansson T, Tindberg N, Ingelman-Sundberg M, et al: Regional distribution of ethanol-inducible cytochrome P450 IIE1 in the rat central nervous system. Neuroscience 34:451–463, 1990

Hartong EG, Moleman P, Hoogduin CA, et al: Prophylactic efficacy of lithium versus carbamazepine in treatment-naive bipolar patients. J Clin Psychiatry 64:144–151, 2003

Herman R, Obarzanek E, Mikalauskas KM, et al: The effects of carbamazepine on resting metabolic rate and thyroid function in depressed patients. Biol Psychiatry 29:779–788, 1991

Himmelhoch JM: Cerebral dysrhythmia, substance abuse, and the nature of secondary affective illness. Psychiatric Annals 17:710–727, 1987

Himmelhoch JM, Garfinkel ME: Sources of lithium resistance in mixed mania. Psychopharmacol Bull 22:613–620, 1986

Hunt BA, Self TH, Lalonde RL, et al: Calcium channel blockers as inhibitors of drug metabolism. Chest 96:393–399, 1989

Isojarvi JI, Pakarinen AJ, Rautio A, et al: Liver enzyme induction and serum lipid levels after replacement of carbamazepine with oxcarbazepine. Epilepsia 35:1217–1220, 1994

Isojarvi JI, Pakarinen AJ, Rautio A, et al: Serum sex hormone levels after replacing carbamazepine with oxcarbazepine. Eur J Clin Pharmacol 47:461–464, 1995

Isojarvi JI, Huuskonen UE, Pakarinen AJ, et al: The regulation of serum sodium after replacing carbamazepine with oxcarbazepine. Epilepsia 42:741–745, 2001a

Isojarvi JI, Turkka J, Pakarinen AJ, et al: Thyroid function in men taking carbamazepine, oxcarbazepine, or valproate for epilepsy. Epilepsia 42:930–934, 2001b

Jann MW, Fidone GS, Israel MK, et al: Increased valproate serum concentrations upon carbamazepine cessation. Epilepsia 29:578–581, 1988

Jann MW, Fidone GS, Hernandez JM, et al: Clinical implications of increased antipsychotic plasma concentrations upon anticonvulsant cessation. Psychiatry Res 28:153–159, 1989

Joca SR, Skalisz L, Beijamini V, et al: The antidepressive-like effect of oxcarbazepine: possible role of dopaminergic neurotransmission. Eur Neuropsychopharmacol 10:223–228, 2000

Joffe RT, Post RM: Lithium and carbamazepine-induced agranulocytosis (letter). Am J Psychiatry 146:404, 1989

Joffe RT, Post RM, Ballenger JC, et al: Neuroendocrine effects of carbamazepine in patients with affective illness. Epilepsia 27:156–160, 1986a

Joffe RT, Post RM, Uhde TW: Effect of carbamazepine on body weight in affectively ill patients. J Clin Psychiatry 47:313–314, 1986b

Joffe RT, Post RM, Uhde TW: Lack of pharmacokinetic interaction of carbamazepine with tranylcypromine (letter). Arch Gen Psychiatry 42:738, 1985

Johannessen SI, Battino D, Berry DJ, et al: Therapeutic drug monitoring of the newer antiepileptic drugs. Ther Drug Monit 25:347–363, 2003

Jones KL, Lacro RV, Johnson KA, et al: Pattern of malformations in the children of women treated with carbamazepine during pregnancy. N Engl J Med 320:1661–1666, 1989

Joyce PR: Carbamazepine in rapid cycling bipolar affective disorder. Int Clin Psychopharmacol 3:123–129, 1988

Kahn EM, Schulz SC, Perel JM, et al: Change in haloperidol level due to carbamazepine—a complicating factor in combined medication for schizophrenia. J Clin Psychopharmacol 10:54–57, 1990

Kane JM, Smith JM: Tardive dyskinesia: prevalence and risk factors, 1959 to 1979. Arch Gen Psychiatry 39:473–481, 1982

Keck P Jr, McElroy SL, Vuckovic A, et al: Combined valproate and carbamazepine treatment of bipolar disorder. J Neuropsychiatry Clin Neurosci 4:319–322, 1992

Keck PE Jr, McElroy SL, Tugrul KC, et al: Valproate oral loading in the treatment of acute mania. J Clin Psychiatry 54:305–308, 1993

Keranen T, Jolkkonen J, Jensen PK, et al: Absence of interaction between oxcarbazepine and erythromycin. Acta Neurol Scand 86:120–123, 1992a

Keranen T, Jolkkonen J, Klosterskov-Jensen P, et al: Oxcarbazepine does not interact with cimetidine in healthy volunteers. Acta Neurol Scand 85:239–242, 1992b

Kerr BM, Thummel KE, Wurden CJ, et al: Human liver carbamazepine metabolism: role of CYP3A4 and CYP2C8 in 10,11-epoxide formation. Biochem Pharmacol 47:1969–1979, 1994

Ketter TA: Advances in the Treatment of Bipolar Disorder. Washington, DC, American Psychiatric Publishing, 2005

Ketter TA, Wang PW: Predictors of treatment response in bipolar disorders: evidence from clinical and brain imaging studies. J Clin Psychiatry 63:21–25, 2002

Ketter TA, Post RM, Worthington K: Principles of clinically important drug interactions with carbamazepine, part I. J Clin Psychopharmacol 11:198–203, 1991a

Ketter TA, Post RM, Worthington K: Principles of clinically important drug interactions with carbamazepine, part II. J Clin Psychopharmacol 11:306–313, 1991b

Ketter TA, Pazzaglia PJ, Post RM: Synergy of carbamazepine and valproic acid in affective illness: case report and review of the literature. J Clin Psychopharmacol 12:276–281, 1992

Ketter TA, Jenkins JB, Schroeder DH, et al: Carbamazepine but not valproate induces bupropion metabolism. J Clin Psychopharmacol 15:327–333, 1995a

Ketter TA, Post RM, Parekh PI, et al: Addition of monoamine oxidase inhibitors to carbamazepine: preliminary evidence of safety and antidepressant efficacy in treatment-resistant depression. J Clin Psychiatry 56:471–475, 1995b

Ketter TA, Kimbrell TA, George MS, et al: Baseline cerebral hypermetabolism associated with carbamazepine response, and hypometabolism with nimodipine response in mood disorders. Biol Psychiatry 46:1364–1374, 1999

Ketter TA, Wang PW, Becker OV, et al: The diverse roles of anticonvulsants in bipolar disorders. Ann Clin Psychiatry 15:95–108, 2003

Ketter TA, Kalali AH, Weisler RH: A 6-month, multicenter, open-label evaluation of beaded, extended-release carbamazepine capsule monotherapy in bipolar disorder patients with manic or mixed episodes. J Clin Psychiatry 65:668–673, 2004

Ketter TA, Akiskal HS, Keck PE Jr, et al: Reassessing carbamazepine in the treatment of bipolar disorder: clinical implications of new data. CNS Spectr 10:1–13, 2005

Khan A, Shad MU, Preskorn SH: Lack of sertraline efficacy probably due to an interaction with carbamazepine. J Clin Psychiatry 61:526–527, 2000

Kishimoto A, Okuma T: Antimanic and prophylactic effects of carbamazepine in affective disorders (abstract 506.4), in 4th World Congress of Biological Psychiatry, September 8–13, 1985, p 363

Klein E, Bental E, Lerer B, et al: Carbamazepine and haloperidol v placebo and haloperidol in excited psychoses: a controlled study. Arch Gen Psychiatry 41:165–170, 1984

Klein EM: Lithium and carbamazepine therapy in a patient with manic depressive illness: clinical effects, interactions and side effects. Isr J Psychiatry Relat Sci 24:295–298, 1987

Klosterskov Jensen P, Saano V, Haring P, et al: Possible interaction between oxcarbazepine and an oral contraceptive. Epilepsia 33:1149–1152, 1992

Kondo T, Otani K, Hirano T, et al: The effects of phenytoin and carbamazepine on serum concentrations of mono-unsaturated metabolites of valproic acid. Br J Clin Pharmacol 29:116–119, 1990

Krag B, Dam M, Angelo H, et al: Influence of disulfiram on the serum concentration of carbamazepine in patients with epilepsy. Acta Neurol Scand 63:395–398, 1981

Kramer G, Tettenborn B, Klosterskov Jensen P, et al: Oxcarbazepine does not affect the anticoagulant activity of warfarin. Epilepsia 33:1145–1148, 1992

Kramlinger KG, Post RM: Adding lithium carbonate to carbamazepine: antimanic efficacy in treatment-resistant mania. Acta Psychiatr Scand 79:378–385, 1989a

Kramlinger KG, Post RM: The addition of lithium to carbamazepine: antidepressant efficacy in treatment-resistant depression. Arch Gen Psychiatry 46:794–800, 1989b

Kramlinger KG, Post RM: Addition of lithium carbonate to carbamazepine: hematological and thyroid effects. Am J Psychiatry 147:615–620, 1990

Kramlinger KG, Phillips KA, Post RM: Rash complicating carbamazepine treatment. J Clin Psychopharmacol 14:408–413, 1994

Kranzler HR, Bauer LO, Hersh D, et al: Carbamazepine treatment of cocaine dependence: a placebo-controlled trial. Drug Alcohol Depend 38:203–211, 1995

Kronbach T, Mathys D, Umeno M, et al: Oxidation of midazolam and triazolam by human liver cytochrome P450IIIA4. Mol Pharmacol 36:89–96, 1989

Kuhn KL, Halikas JA, Kemp KD: Carbamazepine treatment of cocaine dependence in methadone maintenance patients with dual opiate-cocaine addiction. NIDA Res Monogr 95:316–317, 1989

Kuhnz W, Jager-Roman E, Rating D, et al: Carbamazepine and carbamazepine-10,11-epoxide during pregnancy and postnatal period in epileptic mother and their nursed infants: pharmacokinetics and clinical effects. Pediatric Pharmacology (New York) 3:199–208, 1983

Kupfer DJ, Frank E, Grochocinski VJ, et al: Demographic and clinical characteristics of individuals in a bipolar disorder case registry. J Clin Psychiatry 63:120–125, 2002

Kutt H, Solomon G, Peterson H, et al: Accumulation of carbamazepine epoxide caused by valproate contributing to intoxication syndromes. Neurology 35:286–287, 1985

Lai AA, Levy RH, Cutler RE: Time-course of interaction between carbamazepine and clonazepam in normal man. Clin Pharmacol Ther 24:316–323, 1978

Lander CM, Eadie M, Tyrer J: Interactions between anticonvulsants. Proc Australian Assoc Neurologists 12:111–116, 1975

Larkin JG, McKee PJ, Forrest G, et al: Lack of enzyme induction with oxcarbazepine (600 mg daily) in healthy subjects. Br J Clin Pharmacol 31:65–71, 1991

Laroudie C, Salazar DE, Cosson JP, et al: Carbamazepine-nefazodone interaction in healthy subjects. J Clin Psychopharmacol 20:46–53, 2000

Lehtovaara R, Bardy A, Hari R, et al: Sodium valproate and clonazepam interactions with phenytoin and carbamazepine, in Advances in Epileptology. Edited by Meinardi H, Rowan AJ. Amsterdam, Swets & Zeitlinger, 1978, pp 269–270

Leinonen E, Lillsunde P, Laukkanen V, et al: Effects of carbamazepine on serum antidepressant concentrations in psychiatric patients. J Clin Psychopharmacol 11:313–318, 1991

Leinonen E, Lepola U, Koponen H: Substituting carbamazepine with oxcarbazepine increases citalopram levels: a report on two cases. Pharmacopsychiatry 29:156–158, 1996

Lemoine A, Gautier JC, Azoulay D, et al: Major pathway of imipramine metabolism is catalyzed by cytochromes P-450 1A2 and P-450 3A4 in human liver. Mol Pharmacol 43:827–832, 1993

Lenzi A, Lazzerini F, Grossi E, et al: Use of carbamazepine in acute psychosis: a controlled study. J Int Med Res 14:78–84, 1986

Lerer B, Moore N, Meyendorff E, et al: Carbamazepine versus lithium in mania: a double-blind study. J Clin Psychiatry 48:89–93, 1987

Levy RH, Lane EA, Guyot M, et al: Analysis of parent drug-metabolite relationship in the presence of an inducer. Application to the carbamazepine-clobazam interaction in normal man. Drug Metab Dispos Biol Fate Chem 11:286–292, 1983

Linnet K, Olesen OV: Free and glucuronidated olanzapine serum concentrations in psychiatric patients: influence of carbamazepine comedication. Ther Drug Monit 24:512–517, 2002

Lucas RA, Gilfillan DJ, Bergstrom RF: A pharmacokinetic interaction between carbamazepine and olanzapine: observations on possible mechanism. Eur J Clin Pharmacol 54:639–643, 1998

Lusznat RM, Murphy DP, Nunn CM: Carbamazepine vs lithium in the treatment and prophylaxis of mania. Br J Psychiatry 153:198–204, 1988

Macphee GJ, Mitchell JR, Wiseman L, et al: Effect of sodium valproate on carbamazepine disposition and psychomotor profile in man. Br J Clin Pharmacol 25:59–66, 1988

Malcolm R, Ballenger JC, Sturgis ET, et al: Double-blind controlled trial comparing carbamazepine to oxazepam treatment of alcohol withdrawal. Am J Psychiatry 146:617–621, 1989

Martinez P, Gonzalez de Etxabarri S, Ereno C, et al: [Acute severe hepatic insufficiency caused by carbamazepine]. Rev Esp Enferm Dig 84:124–126, 1993

Matar KM, Nicholls PJ, Bawazir SA, et al: Effect of valproic acid on the pharmacokinetic profile of oxcarbazepine in the rat. Pharm Acta Helv 73:247–250, 1999

Mattson RH, Cramer JA, Collins JF: A comparison of valproate with carbamazepine for the treatment of complex partial seizures and secondarily generalized tonic-clonic seizures in adults. The Department of Veterans Affairs Epilepsy Cooperative Study No. 264 Group. N Engl J Med 327:765–771, 1992

May TW, Rambeck B, Jurgens U: Influence of oxcarbazepine and methosuximide on lamotrigine concentrations in epileptic patients with and without valproic acid comedication: results of a retrospective study. Ther Drug Monit 21:175–181, 1999

May TW, Rambeck B, Jurgens U: Serum concentrations of topiramate in patients with epilepsy: influence of dose, age, and comedication. Ther Drug Monit 24:366–374, 2002

May TW, Rambeck B, Jurgens U: Serum concentrations of levetiracetam in epileptic patients: the influence of dose and comedication. Ther Drug Monit 25:690–699, 2003

McGinness J, Kishimoto A, Hollister LE: Avoiding neurotoxicity with lithium-carbamazepine combinations. Psychopharmacol Bull 26:181–184, 1990

McKee PJ, Blacklaw J, Forrest G, et al: A double-blind, placebo-controlled interaction study between oxcarbazepine and carbamazepine, sodium valproate and phenytoin in epileptic patients. Br J Clin Pharmacol 37:27–32, 1994

McLean MJ, Schmutz M, Wamil AW, et al: Oxcarbazepine: mechanisms of action. Epilepsia 35:S5–S9, 1994

Meyer MC, Straughn AB, Jarvi EJ, et al: The bioinequivalence of carbamazepine tablets with a history of clinical failures. Pharm Res 9:1612–1616, 1992

Miceli JJ, Anziano RJ, Robarge L, et al: The effect of carbamazepine on the steady-state pharmacokinetics of ziprasidone in healthy volunteers. Br J Clin Pharmacol 49:65S–70S, 2000

Möller HJ, Kissling W, Riehl T, et al: Double-blind evaluation of the antimanic properties of carbamazepine as a comedication to haloperidol. Prog Neuropsychopharmacol Biol Psychiatry 13:127–136, 1989

Moller SE, Larsen F, Khant AZ, et al: Lack of effect of citalopram on the steady-state pharmacokinetics of carbamazepine in healthy male subjects. J Clin Psychopharmacol 21:493–499, 2001

Montoya ID, Levin FR, Fudala P, et al: A double-blind comparison of carbamazepine and placebo treatment of cocaine dependence. NIDA Res Monogr 141:435, 1994

Moreland TA, Chang SL, Levy RH: Mechanisms of interaction between sodium valproate and carbamazepine in the rhesus monkey and in the isolated perfused rat liver, in Metabolism of Antiepileptic Drugs. Edited by Levy RH, Pitlick WH, Eichelbaum M, et al. New York, Raven, 1984, pp 53–60

Mosolov SN: [Comparative effectiveness of preventive use of lithium carbonate, carbamazepine and sodium valproate in affective and schizoaffective psychoses]. Zh Nevrol Psikhiatr Im S S Korsakova 91:78–83, 1991

Motohashi N: GABA receptor alterations after chronic lithium administration: comparison with carbamazepine and sodium valproate. Prog Neuropsychopharmacol Biol Psychiatry 16:571–579, 1992

Motohashi N, Ikawa K, Kariya T: GABAB receptors are up-regulated by chronic treatment with lithium or carbamazepine: GABA hypothesis of affective disorders? Eur J Pharmacol 166:95–99, 1989

Müller AA, Stoll KD: Carbamazepine and oxcarbazepine in the treatment of manic syndromes: studies in Germany, in Anticonvulsants in Affective Disorders. Edited by Emrich HM, Okuma T, Müller AA. Amsterdam, Excerpta Medica, 1984, pp 139–147

Munoz JJ, De Salamanca RE, Diaz-Obregon C, et al: The effect of clobazam on steady state plasma concentrations of carbamazepine and its metabolites. Br J Clin Pharmacol 29:763–765, 1990

Murphy DJ, Gannon MA, McGennis A: Carbamazepine in bipolar affective disorder (letter). Lancet 2(8672):1151–1152, 1989

Murphy JM, Mashman J, Miller JD, et al: Suppression of carbamazepine-induced rash with prednisone. Neurology 41:144–145, 1991

Nasrallah HA, Churchill CM, Hamdan-Allan GA: Higher frequency of neuroleptic-induced dystonia in mania than in schizophrenia. Am J Psychiatry 145:1455–1456, 1988

Nau H, Loscher W: Pharmacologic evaluation of various metabolites and analogs of valproic acid: teratogenic potencies in mice. Fundam Appl Toxicol 6:669–676, 1986

Neumann J, Seidel K, Wunderlich HP: Comparative studies of the effect of carbamazepine and trimipramine in depression, in Anticonvulsants in Affective Disorders. Edited by Emrich HM, Okuma T, Müller AA. Amsterdam, Excerpta Medica, 1984, pp 160–166

Nightingale SL: From the Food and Drug Administration (letter). JAMA 263:1896, 1990

O'Neill B, Callaghan N, Stapleton M, et al: Serum elevation of high density lipoprotein (HDL) cholesterol in epileptic patients taking carbamazepine or phenytoin. Acta Neurol Scand 65:104–109, 1982

Ohmori S, Takeda S, Rikihisa T, et al: Studies on cytochrome P450 responsible for oxidative metabolism of imipramine in human liver microsomes. Biol Pharm Bull 16:571–575, 1993

Ojemann LM, Shastri RA, Wilensky AJ, et al: Comparative pharmacokinetics of zonisamide (CI-912) in epileptic patients on carbamazepine or phenytoin monotherapy. Ther Drug Monit 8:293–296, 1986

Okuma T: Therapeutic and prophylactic effects of carbamazepine in bipolar disorders. Psychiatr Clin North Am 6:157–174, 1983

Okuma T: Effects of carbamazepine and lithium on affective disorders. Neuropsychobiology 27:138–145, 1993

Okuma T, Inanaga K, Otsuki S, et al: Comparison of the antimanic efficacy of carbamazepine and chlorpromazine: a double-blind controlled study. Psychopharmacology 66:211–217, 1979

Okuma T, Inanaga K, Otsuki S, et al: A preliminary double-blind study on the efficacy of carbamazepine in prophylaxis of manic-depressive illness. Psychopharmacology (Berl) 73:95–96, 1981

Okuma T, Yamashita I, Takahashi R, et al: A double-blind study of adjunctive carbamazepine versus placebo on excited states of schizophrenic and schizoaffective disorders. Acta Psychiatr Scand 80:250–259, 1989

Okuma T, Yamashita I, Takahashi R, et al: Comparison of the antimanic efficacy of carbamazepine and lithium carbonate by double-blind controlled study. Pharmacopsychiatry 23:143–150, 1990

Ono S, Mihara K, Suzuki A, et al: Significant pharmacokinetic interaction between risperidone and carbamazepine: its relationship with CYP2D6 genotypes. Psychopharmacology (Berl) 162:50–54, 2002

Otani K, Ishida M, Kaneko S, et al: Effects of carbamazepine coadministration on plasma concentrations of trazodone and its active metabolite, m-chlorophenylpiperazine. Ther Drug Monit 18:164–167, 1996

Pazzaglia PJ, Post RM, Ketter TA, et al: Preliminary controlled trial of nimodipine in ultra-rapid cycling affective dysregulation. Psychiatry Res 49:257–272, 1993

Pazzaglia PJ, Post RM, Ketter TA, et al: Nimodipine monotherapy and carbamazepine augmentation in patients with refractory recurrent affective illness. J Clin Psychopharmacol 18:404–413, 1998

Pearson HJ: Interaction of fluoxetine with carbamazepine (letter). J Clin Psychiatry 51:126, 1990

Physicians' Desk Reference, 62nd Edition. Montvale, NJ, Thomson PDR, 2008

Pihlsgard M, Eliasson E: Significant reduction of sertraline plasma levels by carbamazepine and phenytoin. Eur J Clin Pharmacol 57:915–916, 2002

Pisani F, Narbone MC, Fazio A, et al: Effect of viloxazine on serum carbamazepine levels in epileptic patients. Epilepsia 25:482–485, 1984

Pisani F, Fazio A, Oteri G, et al: Carbamazepine-viloxazine interaction in patients with epilepsy. J Neurol Neurosurg Psychiatry 49:1142–1145, 1986

Pitterle ME, Collins DM: Carbamazepine-10–11-epoxide evaluation associated with coadministration of loxapine or amoxapine (abstract). Epilepsia 29:654, 1988

Placidi GF, Lenzi A, Lazzerini F, et al: The comparative efficacy and safety of carbamazepine versus lithium: a randomized, double-blind 3-year trial in 83 patients. J Clin Psychiatry 47:490–494, 1986

Pope HG Jr, McElroy SL, Keck PE Jr, et al: Valproate in the treatment of acute mania: a placebo-controlled study. Arch Gen Psychiatry 48:62–68, 1991

Post RM: Time course of clinical effects of carbamazepine: implications for mechanisms of action. J Clin Psychiatry 49:35–48, 1988

Post RM: Carbamazepine treatment of bipolar affective disorder, in Directions in Psychiatry, Vol 9, Lesson 19. New York, Hatherleigh, 1989, pp 1–12

Post RM, Uhde TW, Ballenger JC, et al: Carbamazepine and its -10,11-epoxide metabolite in plasma and CSF: relationship to antidepressant response. Arch Gen Psychiatry 40:673–676, 1983a

Post RM, Uhde TW, Ballenger JC, et al: Prophylactic efficacy of carbamazepine in manic-depressive illness. Am J Psychiatry 140:1602–1604, 1983b

Post RM, Ballenger JC, Uhde TW, et al: Efficacy of carbamazepine in manic-depressive illness: implications for underlying mechanisms, in Neurobiology of Mood Disorders. Edited by Post RM, Ballenger JC. Baltimore, MD, Williams & Wilkins, 1984a, pp 777–816

Post RM, Berrettini W, Uhde TW, et al: Selective response to the anticonvulsant carbamazepine in manic-depressive illness: a case study. J Clin Psychopharmacol 4:178–185, 1984b

Post RM, Uhde TW, Wolff EA: Profile of clinical efficacy and side effect of carbamazepine in psychiatric illness: relationship to blood and CSF levels of carbamazepine and its 10,11-epoxide metabolite. Acta Psychiatr Scand Suppl 313:104–120, 1984c

Post RM, Uhde TW, Roy-Byrne PP, et al: Antidepressant effects of carbamazepine. Am J Psychiatry 143:29–34, 1986

Post RM, Uhde TW, Roy-Byrne PP, et al: Correlates of antimanic response to carbamazepine. Psychiatry Res 21:71–83, 1987

Post RM, Rubinow DR, Uhde TW, et al: Dysphoric mania: clinical and biological correlates. Arch Gen Psychiatry 46:353–358, 1989

Post RM, Leverich GS, Rosoff AS, et al: Carbamazepine prophylaxis in refractory affective disorders: a focus on long-term follow-up. J Clin Psychopharmacol 10:318–327, 1990

Post RM, Altshuler LL, Ketter TA, et al: Antiepileptic drugs in affective illness: clinical and theoretical implications. Adv Neurol 55:239–277, 1991

Post RM, Ketter TA, Uhde T, et al: Thirty years of clinical experience with carbamazepine in the treatment of bipolar illness: principles and practice. CNS Drugs 21:47–71, 2007

Price WA, DiMarzio LR: Verapamil-carbamazepine neurotoxicity (letter). J Clin Psychiatry 49:80, 1988

Prien RF, Gelenberg AJ: Alternatives to lithium for preventive treatment of bipolar disorder. Am J Psychiatry 146:840–848, 1989

Pynnönen S, Kanto J, Sillanpaa M, et al: Carbamazepine: placental transport, tissue concentrations in foetus and newborn, and level in milk. Acta Pharmacologica et Toxicologica 41:244–253, 1977

Pynnönen S, Björkquist SE, Pekkarinen A: The pharmacokinetics of carbamazepine in alcoholics, in Advances in Epileptology. Edited by Meinardi H, Rowan AJ. Amsterdam, Swets & Zeitlinger, 1978, pp 285–290

Radulovic LL, Wilder BJ, Leppik IE, et al: Lack of interaction of gabapentin with carbamazepine or valproate. Epilepsia 35:155–161, 1994

Ragueneau-Majlessi I, Levy RH, Bergen D, et al: Carbamazepine pharmacokinetics are not affected by zonisamide: in vitro mechanistic study and in vivo clinical study in epileptic patients. Epilepsy Res 62:1–11, 2004

Raitasuo V, Lehtovaara R, Huttunen MO: Carbamazepine and plasma levels of clozapine (letter). Am J Psychiatry 150:169, 1993

Raitasuo V, Lehtovaara R, Huttunen MO: Effect of switching carbamazepine to oxcarbazepine on the plasma levels of neuroleptics: a case report. Psychopharmacology (Berl) 116:115–116, 1994

Rambeck B, May T, Juergens U: Serum concentrations of carbamazepine and its epoxide and diol metabolites in epileptic patients: the influence of dose and comedication. Ther Drug Monit 9:298–303, 1987

Rapeport WG, Williams SA, Muirhead DC, et al: Absence of a sertraline-mediated effect on the pharmacokinetics and pharmacodynamics of carbamazepine. J Clin Psychiatry 57:20–23, 1996

Rattya J, Vainionpaa L, Knip M, et al: The effects of valproate, carbamazepine, and oxcarbazepine on growth and sexual maturation in girls with epilepsy. Pediatrics 103:588–593, 1999

Rattya J, Turkka J, Pakarinen AJ, et al: Reproductive effects of valproate, carbamazepine, and oxcarbazepine in men with epilepsy. Neurology 56:31–36, 2001

Reinstein MD, Sonnenberg JG, Mohan SC, et al: Oxcarbazepine: review of 200 subjects treated for mania in a hospital setting. Paper presented at 155th annual meeting of the American Psychiatric Association, Philadelphia, PA, May 18–23, 2002

Ries RK, Roy-Byrne PP, Ward NG, et al: Carbamazepine treatment for benzodiazepine withdrawal. Am J Psychiatry 146:536–537, 1989

Ringel RA, Brick JF: Perspective on carbamazepine-induced water intoxication: reversal by demeclocycline. Neurology 36:1506–1507, 1986

Romero AS, Delgado RG, Pena MF: Interaction between trazodone and carbamazepine. Ann Pharmacother 33:1370, 1999

Rosa FM: Spina bifida in infants of women treated with carbamazepine during pregnancy. N Engl J Med 324:674–677, 1991

Rosaria Muscatello M, Pacetti M, Cacciola M, et al: Plasma concentrations of risperidone and olanzapine during coadministration with oxcarbazepine. Epilepsia 46:771–774, 2005

Roth L, Bertschy G: Nefazodone may inhibit the metabolism of carbamazepine: three case reports. Eur Psychiatry 16:320–321, 2001

Sabers A, Gram L: Newer anticonvulsants: comparative review of drug interactions and adverse effects. Drugs 60:23–33, 2000

Sachdeo RC, Sachdeo SK, Walker SA, et al: Steady-state pharmacokinetics of topiramate and carbamazepine in patients with epilepsy during monotherapy and concomitant therapy. Epilepsia 37:774–780, 1996

Samara EE, Gustavson LE, El-Shourbagy T, et al: Population analysis of the pharmacokinetics of tiagabine in patients with epilepsy. Epilepsia 39:868–873, 1998

Scheffner D, Konig S, Rauterberg-Ruland I, et al: Fatal liver failure in 16 children with valproate therapy. Epilepsia 29:530–542, 1988

Schmutz M, Brugger F, Gentsch C, et al: Oxcarbazepine: preclinical anticonvulsant profile and putative mechanisms of action. Epilepsia 35 (suppl 5):S47–S50, 1994

Seree EJ, Pisano PJ, Placidi M, et al: Identification of the human and animal hepatic cytochromes P450 involved in clonazepam metabolism. Fundam Clin Pharmacol 7:69–75, 1993

Sherer MA, Kumor KM, Mapou RL: A case in which carbamazepine attenuated cocaine "rush" (letter). Am J Psychiatry 147:950, 1990

Shimoyama R, Ohkubo T, Sugawara K: Monitoring of carbamazepine and carbamazepine 10,11-epoxide in breast milk and plasma by high-performance liquid chromatography. Ann Clin Biochem 37:210–215, 2000

Sisodiya SM, Sander JW, Patsalos PN: Carbamazepine toxicity during combination therapy with levetiracetam: a pharmacodynamic interaction. Epilepsy Res 48:217–219, 2002

Sitland-Marken PA, Rickman LA, Wells BG, et al: Pharmacologic management of acute mania in pregnancy. J Clin Psychopharmacol 9:78–87, 1989

Sitsen J, Maris F, Timmer C: Drug-drug interaction studies with mirtazapine and carbamazepine in healthy male subjects. Eur J Drug Metab Pharmacokinet 26:109–121, 2001

Small JG: Anticonvulsants in affective disorders. Psychopharmacol Bull 26:25–36, 1990

Small JG, Klapper MH, Milstein V, et al: Carbamazepine compared with lithium in the treatment of mania. Arch Gen Psychiatry 48:915–921, 1991

Spina E, Amendola D'Agostino AM, Ioculano MP, et al: No effect of thioridazine on plasma concentrations of carbamazepine and its active metabolite carbamazepine-10,11-epoxide. Ther Drug Monit 12:511–513, 1990

Spina E, Avenoso A, Pollicino AM, et al: Carbamazepine coadministration with fluoxetine or fluvoxamine. Ther Drug Monit 15:247–250, 1993

Spina E, Avenoso A, Campo G, et al: Phenobarbital induces the CYP2D6-mediated 2-hydroxylation of desipramine. Presentation at the 19th Congress of Collegium Internationale Neuro-

Psychopharmacologicum, Washington, DC, June 27–July 1, 1994

Spina E, Avenoso A, Facciola G, et al: Plasma concentrations of risperidone and 9-hydroxyrisperidone: effect of comedication with carbamazepine or valproate. Ther Drug Monit 22:481–485, 2000

Staines AG, Coughtrie MW, Burchell B: N-glucuronidation of carbamazepine in human tissues is mediated by UGT2B7. J Pharmacol Exp Ther 311:1131–1137, 2004

Stefani A, Pisani A, De Murtas M, et al: Action of GP 47779, the active metabolite of oxcarbazepine, on the corticostriatal system, II: modulation of high-voltage-activated calcium currents. Epilepsia 36:997–1002, 1995

Stefani A, Spadoni F, Bernardi G: Voltage-activated calcium channels: targets of antiepileptic drug therapy? Epilepsia 38:959–965, 1997

Steinacher L, Vandel P, Zullino DF, et al: Carbamazepine augmentation in depressive patients non-responding to citalopram: a pharmacokinetic and clinical pilot study. Eur Neuropsychopharmacol 12:255–260, 2002

Stoll KD, Bisson HE, Fischer E, et al: Carbamazepine versus haloperidol in manic syndromes—first report of a multicentric study in Germany, in Biological Psychiatry 1985. Edited by Shagass C. Amsterdam, Elsevier, 1986, pp 332–334

Suppes T, Dennehy EB, Hirschfeld RM, et al: The Texas Implementation of Medication Algorithms: update to the algorithms for treatment of bipolar I disorder. J Clin Psychiatry 66:870–886, 2005

Takezaki H, Hanaoka M: The use of carbamazepine (Tegretol) in the control of manic-depressive psychosis and other manic-depressive states. Clinical Psychiatry 13:173–183, 1971

Tartara A, Galimberti CA, Manni R, et al: Differential effects of valproic acid and enzyme-inducing anticonvulsants on nimodipine pharmacokinetics in epileptic patients. Br J Clin Pharmacol 32:335–340, 1991

Tegretol (carbamazepine) package insert. Physicians' Desk Reference, 62nd Edition. Montvale, NJ, Thomson PDR, 2008

Thakker KM, Mangat S, Garnett WR, et al: Comparative bioavailability and steady state fluctuations of Tegretol commercial and carbamazepine OROS tablets in adult and pediatric epileptic patients. Biopharm Drug Dispos 13:559–569, 1992

Theis JG, Sidhu J, Palmer J, et al: Lack of pharmacokinetic interaction between oxcarbazepine and lamotrigine. Neuropsychopharmacology 30:2269–2274, 2005

Thweatt RE: Carbamazepine/MAOI interaction (letter). Psychosomatics 27:538, 1986

Tiihonen J, Vartiainen H, Hakola P: Carbamazepine-induced changes in plasma levels of neuroleptics. Pharmacopsychiatry 28:26–28, 1995

Tohen M, Castillo J, Pope H Jr, et al: Concomitant use of valproate and carbamazepine in bipolar and schizoaffective disorders. J Clin Psychopharmacol 14:67–70, 1994

Tohen M, Castillo J, Baldessarini RJ, et al: Blood dyscrasias with carbamazepine and valproate: a pharmacoepidemiological study of 2,228 patients at risk. Am J Psychiatry 152:413–418, 1995

Tohen M, Bowden CL, Smulevich AB, et al: Olanzapine plus carbamazepine vs carbamazepine alone in treating manic episodes. Br J Psychiatry 192:135–143, 2008

Trileptal (oxcarbazepine) package insert. Physicians' Desk Reference, 62nd Edition. Montvale, NJ, Thomson PDR, 2008

Tripp SL, Hundal J, Kapeghian JC, et al: Evaluation of oxcarbazepine and its mono-hydroxy metabolite (GP 47779) for potential drug interactions in vitro. Presentation at the annual meeting of the American Epilepsy Society, San Francisco, CA, December 7–10, 1996

Tsang MW, Shader RI, Greenblatt DJ: Metabolism of haloperidol: clinical implications and unanswered questions (editorial). J Clin Psychopharmacol 14:159–162, 1994

Vadnal R, Parthasarathy R: Myo-inositol monophosphatase: diverse effects of lithium, carbamazepine, and valproate. Neuropsychopharmacology 12:277–285, 1995

Van Parys JA, Meinardi H: Survey of 260 epileptic patients treated with oxcarbazepine (Trileptal) on a named-patient basis. Epilepsy Res 19:79–85, 1994

Vick NA: Suppression of carbamazepine-induced skin rash with prednisone (letter). N Engl J Med 309:1193–1194, 1983

Vieweg V, Glick JL, Herring S, et al: Absence of carbamazepine-induced hyponatremia among patients also given lithium. Am J Psychiatry 144:943–947, 1987

von Moltke LL, Greenblatt DJ, Harmatz JS, et al: Alprazolam metabolism in vitro: studies of human, monkey, mouse, and rat liver microsomes. Pharmacology 47:268–276, 1993

Wagner KD, Kowatch RA, Emslie GJ, et al: A double-blind, randomized, placebo-controlled trial of oxcarbazepine in the treatment of bipolar disorder in children and adolescents. Am J Psychiatry 163:1179–1186, 2006

Wamil AW, Schmutz M, Portet C, et al: Effects of oxcarbazepine and 10-hydroxycarbamazepine on action potential firing and generalized seizures. Eur J Pharmacol 271:301–308, 1994

Watkins SE, Callender K, Thomas DR, et al: The effect of carbamazepine and lithium on remission from affective illness. Br J Psychiatry 150:180–182, 1987

Weisler RH, Kalali AH, Ketter TA: A multicenter, randomized, double-blind, placebo-controlled trial of extended-release carbamazepine capsules as monotherapy for bipolar disorder patients with manic or mixed episodes. J Clin Psychiatry 65:478–484, 2004

Weisler RH, Keck PE Jr, Swann AC, et al: Extended-release carbamazepine capsules as monotherapy for acute mania in bipolar disorder: a multicenter, randomized, double-blind, placebo-controlled trial. J Clin Psychiatry 66:323–330, 2005

Wietholtz H, Zysset T, Kreiten K, et al: Effect of phenytoin, carbamazepine, and valproic acid on caffeine metabolism. Eur J Clin Pharmacol 36:401–406, 1989

Wildgrube C: Case studies on prophylactic long-term effects of oxcarbazepine in recurrent affective disorders. Int Clin Psychopharmacol 5:89S–94S, 1990

Wrighton SA, Stevens JC: The human hepatic cytochromes P450 involved in drug metabolism. Crit Rev Toxicol 22:1–21, 1992

Yatham LN, Barry S, Mobayed M, et al: Is the carbamazepine-phenelzine combination safe? (letter) Am J Psychiatry 147:367, 1990

Yatham LN, Grossman F, Augustyns I, et al: Mood stabilisers plus risperidone or placebo in the treatment of acute mania. International, double-blind, randomised controlled trial. Br J Psychiatry 182:141–147, 2003

Yukawa E, Nonaka T, Yukawa M, et al: Pharmacoepidemiologic investigation of a clonazepam-carbamazepine interaction by mixed effect modeling using routine clinical pharmacokinetic data in Japanese patients. J Clin Psychopharmacol 21:588–593, 2001

Zaccara G, Gangemi PF, Bendoni L, et al: Influence of single and repeated doses of oxcarbazepine on the pharmacokinetic profile of felodipine. Ther Drug Monit 15:39–42, 1993

Zhang ZJ, Kang WH, Tan QR, et al: Adjunctive herbal medicine with carbamazepine for bipolar disorders: a double-blind, randomized, placebo-controlled study. J Psychiatr Res 41:360–369, 2007

CHAPTER 38

Gabapentin and Pregabalin

Mark A. Frye, M.D.

Katherine Marshall Moore, M.D.

Gabapentin

Anticonvulsants have long been used in the treatment of certain psychiatric conditions. As exemplified by the U.S. Food and Drug Administration (FDA) indications for divalproex sodium, carbamazepine, and lamotrigine in the acute and maintenance phases of bipolar disorder (Yatham et al. 2002), anticonvulsants are widely viewed as valid alternatives to, and in some cases preferred over, the conventional first-line psychopharmacotherapy choices of lithium and antipsychotics. Early observations of enhanced general well-being in epileptic patients treated with anticonvulsants, as well as various early hypotheses of kindling and sensitization proposed as models of affective illness progression (Weiss and Post 1998), have promoted controlled investigations of anticonvulsant drugs as potential mood-stabilizing agents.

Gabapentin is FDA approved for the adjunctive treatment of complex partial epilepsy with and without generalization and for the management of postherpetic neuralgia in adults. A retrospective review of five placebo-controlled trials of gabapentin in more than 700 patients with refractory partial seizure disorder additionally supported the concept of improvement in general well-being, prompting controlled investigation of the drug in primary psychiatric conditions (Dimond et al. 1996).

Pharmacological Profile and Mechanism of Action

The mechanism of gabapentin's anticonvulsant and psychotropic action is not fully understood. Gabapentin was originally developed as a γ-aminobutyric (GABA) analog. As reviewed by Taylor et al. (1998), GABA is the major inhibitory neurotransmitter in the cerebral cortex. Gabapentin does not act as a GABA precursor, agonist, or antagonist. Preclinical studies have suggested that gabapentin increases brain and intracellular GABA by an amino acid active transporter at the blood–brain barrier and multiple enzymatic regulatory mechanisms, respectively. For example, in vitro studies have shown that gabapentin increased the activity of glutamic acid decarboxylase, which is the enzyme that converts glutamate to GABA (Taylor et al. 1992). Conversely, gabapentin has been shown to inhibit GABA-transaminase (GABA-T), which is the enzyme primarily responsible for GABA catabolism (Loscher et al. 1991). Glutamate metabolism is also modulated by gabapentin. In vitro studies have demonstrated that gabapentin inhibits branched-chain amino acid aminotransferase (BCAA-T), an enzyme responsible for glutamate synthesis (Hutson et al. 1998), and activates glutamate dehydrogenase, an enzyme primarily involved in glutamate catabolism (Goldlust et al. 1995).

These enzymatic regulatory mechanisms that suggest an increased synthesis and decreased degradation of GABA are clinically relevant. Several, but not all, studies have reported decreased levels of cerebrospinal fluid (Gerner et al. 1996; Gold et al. 1980; Roy et al. 1991), plasma (Petty et al. 1990), and magnetic resonance (MR) spectroscopic GABA (Sanacora et al. 1999) in patients with affective illness in comparison with healthy controls. Furthermore, increased MR spectroscopic occipital GABA concentrations have been reported with serotonin reuptake inhibitor treatment in depressed patients (Sanacora et al. 2002) and gabapentin treatment in patients with complex partial epilepsy (Petroff et al. 1996).

Gabapentin has also been shown to bind to the α_2 subunit receptor of brain voltage-dependent calcium channels, which may relate to the subsequent inhibition of monoaminergic transmission (Schlicker et al. 1985). There is no known direct activity at the dopamine, serotonin, benzodiazepine, or histamine receptors. However, gabapentin has been reported to increase whole-blood levels of serotonin in healthy controls (Rao et al. 1988). These potentially important mechanisms of action have not been tested formally in psychiatric patient populations.

Pharmacokinetics and Disposition

All bioavailability, distribution, and elimination parameters are based on the gabapentin molecule itself, as there is no active metabolite. Gabapentin exhibits nonlinear bioavailability most likely related to an active saturable L-amino acid transport carrier present in gut and blood–brain barrier (McLean 1999). There is no evidence of plasma protein binding, hepatic metabolism, or cytochrome P450 (CYP) autoinduction. Elimination half-life is 6–8 hours, with a recommended three-times-a-day dosing strategy. Gabapentin is eliminated from systemic circulation unchanged by renal excretion. Patients with compromised renal function will show evidence of reduced gabapentin clearance.

Indications and Efficacy

Epilepsy

Gabapentin currently is FDA approved as an adjunctive treatment for partial seizures with and without secondary generalization in adults with epilepsy ("Neurontin" 2006). This indication was based on controlled evaluations of gabapentin at daily doses of 600–1,800 mg. Additional research has reported efficacy and tolerability for gabapentin monotherapy at daily dosages up to 4,800 mg in patients with refractory epilepsy (Beydoun et al. 1998). There is no established therapeutic plasma level for seizure control. Gabapentin has a highly desirable side-effect profile. Only mild side effects (sedation, dizziness, and ataxia) have been commonly reported.

Nonepilepsy Neurological Conditions

Neuropathic pain. On the basis of two placebo-controlled studies (Rice et al. 2001; Rowbotham et al. 1998), gabapentin has received FDA approval for use in the management of postherpetic neuralgia in adults. Gabapentin has also been systemically evaluated in diabetic neuropathy (Backonja et al. 1998).

The initial postherpetic neuralgia (Rowbotham et al. 1998) and diabetic neuropathy (Backonja et al. 1998) studies were randomized, double-blind, placebo-controlled, parallel-group multicenter investigations with three phases of evaluation. The first phase identified the subject population (patients with diabetic neuropathy of 1–5 years' duration [Backonja et al. 1998] or postherpetic neuralgia of 3 months' duration [Rowbotham et al. 1998]). The 8-week double-blind phases consisted of a 4-week step titration (week 1, 900 mg; week 2, 1,800 mg; week 3, 2,400 mg; and week 4, 3,600 mg) and a 4-week fixed-dose period wherein the dose that was effective and tolerable from the titration phase was held constant. There were no differences in demographics or rates of dropout because of inefficacy or adverse events between the gabapentin group and the placebo group.

Among the 229 postherpetic neuralgia patients (Rowbotham et al. 1998), greater pain reduction occurred with gabapentin, noted as early as week 2 and maintained throughout the entire study period. Similarly, secondary measures of mood such as depression, anger–hostility, fatigue–inertia, and physical functioning were more effectively treated with gabapentin than with placebo. Eighty-three percent of the gabapentin group was maintained on the 2,400-mg daily dose, and 65% were maintained on the 3,600-mg daily dose.

Among the 165 diabetic neuropathy patients (Backonja et al. 1998), greater pain reduction (as measured with an 11-point Likert scale) occurred with gabapentin than with placebo; this difference was statistically significant as early as week 2 of the blind titration phase and remained significant for the duration of the 8-week study. The difference was also clinically relevant, as demonstrated by significant reductions in sleep interference related to pain and improved quality of life. Gabapentin appeared to be well tolerated, as 67% of the patient group maintained a maximum dose of 3,600 mg. The most common side effects noted with greater frequency in the gabapentin group were dizziness and somnolence.

Finally, a 7-week placebo-controlled study evaluated gabapentin (1,800 or 2,400 mg/day in three divided doses) in 334 patients with postherpetic neuralgia (Rice et al. 2001). Pain was significantly reduced with both gabapentin doses, with similar improvements in sleep. The improvement in pain score was noted as early as week 1 and was maintained throughout the study.

Movement disorders. Controlled investigations of gabapentin have been conducted in several movement disorders. These studies, albeit controlled, were much smaller than the neuropathic pain studies mentioned in the prior section but included amyotrophic lateral sclerosis (ALS) (Miller et al. 1996), essential tremor (Ondo et al. 2000; Pahwa et al. 1998), and parkinsonism (Olson et al. 1997).

In a study of 152 patients with ALS, patients were randomly assigned to a 2,400-mg daily dose of gabapentin or placebo for 6 months. Decline in muscle strength, the primary outcome measure, was slower in the gabapentin-treated patients than in the placebo-treated patients (Miller et al. 1996).

Controlled studies of gabapentin for essential tremor have reported mixed results. The first 2-week controlled study showed no difference between gabapentin 1,800 mg/day and placebo for treatment of essential tremor (Pahwa et al. 1998). A second 6-week controlled study evaluating two gabapentin dosages—1,800 mg/day and 3,600 mg/day—in patients with essential tremor found significant improvements in self-report scores, observed tremor scores, and activities of daily living scores in patients randomly assigned to gabapentin compared with patients who received placebo (Ondo et al. 2000).

In a 1-month double-blind, placebo-controlled evaluation of gabapentin in 19 patients with advanced parkinsonism, gabapentin at a mean daily total dose of 1,200 mg was superior to placebo in reducing rigidity, bradykinesia, and tremor, as measured by the United Parkinson's Disease Rating Scale (Olson et al. 1997). The authors pointed out that the rigidity and bradykinesia improvements were independent of tremor improvement.

Migraine headache. The comorbidity of migraine headache disorder and bipolar disorder is highly prevalent and clinically significant (Mahmood et al. 1999). Anticonvulsants, both for their anticonvulsant mood-stabilizing effects and for their migraine prophylactic properties, appear to be ideal in this patient population. A study by Mathew et al. (2001) suggested that gabapentin is an effective agent for migraine prophylaxis. One hundred forty-three patients with migraine (with and without aura) participated in this three-phase controlled evaluation of gabapentin. Phase 1 was a 4-week single-blind pla-

cebo period during which baseline migraine headache frequency was established. Phase 2 was a 4-week double-blind, placebo-controlled, flexible-dose titration period during which patients received gabapentin dosages of up to 2,400 mg/day. Phase 3 was an 8-week double-blind, placebo-controlled period during which the dosage of gabapentin was held constant. Patients randomly assigned to 2,400 mg/day gabapentin had significant reductions in migraine attacks in comparison with placebo-treated patients. Dropout rates were higher with gabapentin and were primarily related to drowsiness and somnolence.

Anxiety Disorders

Gabapentin has been shown in a number of animal models to exhibit a dose-dependent anxiolytic response (Singh et al. 1996). Open-trial investigations have reported positive results with add-on gabapentin in the treatment of generalized anxiety disorder (Pollack et al. 1998), panic disorder (Pollack et al. 1998), and refractory obsessive-compulsive disorder (Cora-Locatelli et al. 1998). Two controlled investigations of gabapentin in social phobia (Pande et al. 1999) and panic disorder (Pande et al. 2000b) suggest anxiolytic activity.

Pande et al. (1999) investigated gabapentin in a 14-week randomized, double-blind, placebo-controlled two-site study of 69 outpatients with DSM-IV (American Psychiatric Association 1994)–confirmed social phobia. All patients were required to have a score of 50 or higher on the Liebowitz Social Anxiety Scale (LSAS) at baseline. Reduction in the LSAS score served as the primary outcome measure. In the 69 patients randomly assigned to the intent-to-treat analysis, gabapentin was more effective than placebo in reducing social anxiety symptoms. The dosage range for gabapentin was 900–3,600 mg/day, with 56% of patients responding to and tolerating the maximum daily dosage of 3,600 mg. Dizziness and dry mouth were significantly more common in patients treated with gabapentin.

The second study was an 8-week randomized, placebo-controlled six-site monotherapy study of 103 patients with DSM-IV–confirmed panic disorder with or without agoraphobia (Pande et al. 2000b). Subjects had been experiencing at least one panic attack per week for 3 weeks prior to study entry. Gabapentin was dosed flexibly between 600 and 3,600 mg/day. The primary outcome measure was a decrease in the Panic and Agoraphobia Scale (PAS) score. The two groups had no differences in demographic profile or dropout rate. In the intent-to-treat analysis, no difference in PAS score reduction was seen between patients randomly assigned to gabapentin and those given placebo. In a post hoc stratification between high (≥20) and low (<20) PAS symptom severity, patients with high symptom severity randomly assigned to gabapentin had a greater baseline-to-endpoint decrease in the PAS score than did those randomly assigned to placebo. Somnolence, headache, dizziness, infection, asthenia, and ataxia were more common in gabapentin-treated patients.

Bipolar Disorder

Given the demonstrated role of the FDA-approved anticonvulsants in the treatment of bipolar disorder, it was inevitable that there should be interest in evaluating gabapentin's utility as a mood stabilizer. Numerous case reports and open trials, encompassing more than 400 patients with a pooled response rate between 65% and 70%, have been reviewed elsewhere (Frye et al. 2000; Yatham et al. 2002).

One double-blind, placebo-controlled outpatient study evaluated add-on gabapentin for the treatment of bipolar I disorder with manic, hypomanic, or mixed symptoms (Pande et al. 2000a). The first phase of the study involved a 2-week single-blind, placebo lead-in wherein doses of the subject's primary mood stabilizer (lithium or valproate) could be adjusted to maximal clinical benefit and minimum threshold of therapeutic level (i.e., lithium level of 0.5 mmol/L, valproate level >50 μg/mL). The second phase of the study was a 10-week double-blind phase in which subjects were randomly assigned to either gabapentin, dosed flexibly between 600 and 3,600 mg/day (three-times-a-day dosing) or placebo. In the intent-to-treat population, 117 subjects were randomized; no differences in demographic profile or dropout rate were found between the two groups. The primary outcome measure—total decreased score on the Young Mania Rating Scale—was significantly different between groups in favor of add-on placebo. In a post hoc analysis, lithium adjustments in the single-blind, placebo lead-in phase were made more frequently in the placebo group than in the gabapentin group; most of these adjustments (9 of 12; 75%) consisted of a dosage increase. This fact suggests either a strong placebo response or the effect of maximizing lithium blood levels to achieve a greater antimanic response. Of the gabapentin-treated patients who had drug levels measured, nearly 20% had plasma gabapentin levels that were undetectable.

The second controlled study was a 6-week double-blind, placebo-controlled crossover comparative trial of gabapentin monotherapy, lamotrigine monotherapy, and placebo in 35 inpatients with refractory mood disorder (Frye et al. 2000; Obrocea et al. 2002). The primary outcome measure was a score of very much or much improved on the Clinical Global Impressions Scale; in the preliminary analysis (Frye et al. 2000) and final analysis (Obrocea et al. 2002), gabapentin demonstrated no better treatment response than placebo in a group of patients with highly refractory bipolar (primarily rapid-cycling) disorder.

There appears to be a marked contrast between the pooled results of the uncontrolled observations (generally positive) and the results of the controlled studies (generally negative). The important limitations of the controlled investigations include placebo response versus maximizing lithium response in the placebo group, lack of rigorous compliance assessment, and a monotherapy study design in a cohort of patients with primarily rapid-cycling, treatment-refractory illness.

Substance Abuse and Withdrawal

Although benzodiazepines remain the gold standard for alcohol withdrawal, mood-stabilizing anticonvulsants such as divalproex sodium and carbamazepine are clearly alternatives and possibly preferred treatments for alcohol-abusing bipolar patients (Malcolm et al. 2001). Gabapentin has been shown to decrease excitability and convulsions in animal models of alcohol withdrawal (Watson et al. 1997). The lack of hepatic metabolism, CYP enzyme induction, protein binding, or addictive potential makes gabapentin a potentially useful compound in this patient population.

The potential of gabapentin for treating alcohol withdrawal was considered after initial positive reports emerged (Bozikas et al. 2002). One study demonstrated a similar efficacy to phenobarbital in treating alcohol withdrawal (Mariani et al. 2006), although another controlled trial did not substantiate gabapentin's benefit over placebo (Bonnet et al. 2003). This latter study involved 61 inpatients admitted for a 1-week alcohol detoxification and randomly assigned to gabapentin (400 mg four times daily) or placebo. The primary outcome measure was the amount of rescue medication (clomethiazole; 1 capsule = 192 mg) required during the first 24 hours (6.2 capsules for gabapentin and 6.1 capsules for placebo). In a post hoc analysis (Bonnet et al. 2007), there was a significant increase in the Profile of Mood States (POMS) vigor subscore in the gabapentin group versus the placebo group; this was particularly robust in patients with comorbid mild depression.

Despite the conflicting results for gabapentin's efficacy in alcohol withdrawal, there is increasing recognition of its therapeutic benefit for the sleep disturbance component of alcohol withdrawal syndrome. Low-dose gabapentin (mean dose = 900 mg) in the treatment of alcohol withdrawal, in comparison with trazodone, was associated with greater improvement in sleep problems, as assessed with the Sleep Problems Questionnaire (Karam-Hage and Brower 2003). As well, in patients with a history of multiple previous alcohol withdrawals, gabapentin, in comparison with lorazepam, was associated with significant reductions in self-report sleep disturbances and daytime sleepiness (Malcolm et al. 2007).

One 4-week placebo-controlled, randomized, double-blind study evaluated gabapentin in alcohol abuse relapse prevention (Furieri and Nakamura-Palacios 2007). After detoxification, 60 alcohol-dependent men who had been consuming, on average, 17 drinks per day for the preceding 3 months were randomly assigned to gabapentin (300 mg twice daily) or placebo. The gabapentin group showed a significant reduction in both the number of drinks per day and the percentage of heavy drinking days. In addition to an increase in the percentage of days abstinent, the gabapentin group reported a significant reduction in craving for alcohol, specifically automaticity of drinking.

Side Effects and Toxicology

Gabapentin has a highly desirable side-effect profile that has been remarkably consistent among the controlled studies of diverse disease states. Sedation, drowsiness, and dizziness always have been reported, and ataxia, dry mouth, infection, and asthenia have been reported in at least one placebo-controlled study.

Adverse events caused by gabapentin have been few but have important psychiatric implications. Gabapentin-induced hypomania and mania have been reported (Leweke et al. 1999; Short and Cooke 1995). The controlled mania study did not report data on percentage of the patients with exacerbation of mania secondary to gabapentin treatment (Pande et al. 2000a). Gabapentin also has been associated with aggression, both in pediatric epilepsy (Wolf et al. 1996) and in adult mania (Pinninti and Mahajan 2001).

Gabapentin has a broad therapeutic index and appears to be safe in overdose. The broadness of the therapeutic index is most likely related to its nonlinear bioavailability secondary to a saturable transport carrier (McLean 1999).

Drug–Drug Interactions

Given its lack of hepatic metabolism, CYP autoinduction, and minimal plasma protein binding, gabapentin has been shown not to affect levels of anticonvulsant drugs; similarly, gabapentin pharmacokinetics were unchanged with hepatically metabolized anticonvulsants ("Neurontin" 2006). Gabapentin's renal excretion, however, does pose potential risk when the drug is used concomitantly with lithium.

Although the therapeutic index with gabapentin is large, that is not the case with lithium. In a single 600-mg lithium dose pharmacokinetic study, there was no difference in maximal lithium concentration (Li C_{max}), time to reach C_{max}, or area under the curve in 13 patients receiving steady-state gabapentin (mean dose = 3,645.15 ± 931.5 mg) compared with those receiving steady-state placebo (Frye et al. 1998). It is important to emphasize that this study was in a patient population with normal renal function; cases of reversible renal impairment associated with gabapentin have been reported (Grunze et al. 1998).

Summary for Gabapentin

Controlled studies of gabapentin clearly have suggested its efficacy in several medical conditions, including complex partial epilepsy, postherpetic neuropathy, diabetic neuropathy, and migraine prophylaxis. Conclusions are less clear, either because of positive controlled studies of a small sample size or because of negative studies in alcohol abuse/dependence relapse prevention, ALS, essential tremor, parkinsonism, social phobia, and panic disorder. Gabapentin's role as a mood stabilizer is not clearly established. Gabapentin has a favorable pharmacokinetic profile, with particular advantage in patients with compromised hepatic function. Its minimal drug–drug interactions, low risk of toxicity, and favorable side-effect profile make it a useful addition to the pharmacopoeia.

Pregabalin

Pregabalin is an anticonvulsant drug approved by the FDA for the adjunctive treatment of partial-onset seizures in adults. It is also approved for the treatment of neuropathic pain associated with diabetic peripheral neuropathy, postherpetic neuralgia, and fibromyalgia. Like many of the newer anticonvulsant agents, pregabalin has been evaluated in carefully controlled studies for possible utility in neurological and psychiatric conditions other than primary epilepsy.

Pharmacological Profile and Mechanism of Action

Pregabalin, like gabapentin, is a structural analog of the inhibitory neurotransmitter GABA. Pregabalin has shown greater potency than gabapentin in preclinical models of epilepsy, pain, and anxiety (Hamandi and Sander 2006). Although pregabalin is a GABA structural analog, it has no clinically significant effect at either the GABA$_A$ or GABA$_B$ receptor and is not converted metabolically into GABA or a GABA agonist (Kavoussi 2006). Furthermore, pregabalin does not bind to any serotonergic, dopaminergic, or glutamatergic receptors. It is known that pregabalin does bind to the $\alpha_2\delta$ subunit of the presynaptic voltage-gated calcium channel and that this binding results in a decrease in excitatory neurotransmitter release (Dooley et al. 2002; Kavoussi 2006). In contrast to other GABA reuptake inhibitory anticonvulsants (e.g., tiagabine) or anticonvulsants that modulate enzymatic activity related to GABA production (e.g., vigabatrin), pregabalin does not have any direct GABA reuptake–inhibitory effects or GABA transaminase–inhibiting effects.

Pharmacokinetics and Disposition

Pregabalin exhibits linear pharmacokinetics. Pregabalin is not associated with any significant protein binding or hepatic metabolism. Pregabalin oral bioavailability is greater than 90% and independent of dose. Steady-state plasma levels are generally achieved within 24–48 hours. Administration with food has no clinically significant effect on the extent of absorption or on elimination. The elimination half-life of the drug is approximately 6.5 hours (Montgomery 2006). Pregabalin is highly lipophilic and does not bind to plasma protein and, therefore, readily crosses the blood–brain barrier. Pregabalin is primarily renally excreted. There are no active metabolites. Pregabalin does not induce or inhibit CYP enzymes, nor do CYP enzyme inhibitors alter its pharmacokinetics as a consequence. Because of its renal elimination, dosage adjustment is required in patients with renal impairment.

Indications and Efficacy

Epilepsy

Several placebo-controlled studies have evaluated pregabalin in the treatment of patients with refractory partial

epilepsy (Elger et al. 2005; Hamandi and Sander 2006). Response rates for pregabalin dosed at 600 mg/day were similar to those reported in other trials of antiepileptic drugs in refractory epilepsy. The study by Elger et al. (2005) showed that pregabalin administered in either fixed or flexible doses was highly effective and generally well tolerated as add-on therapy for partial seizures with or without secondary generalization.

Nonepilepsy Neurological Conditions

Postherpetic neuralgia.   Four placebo-controlled studies have evaluated pregabalin for postherpetic neuropathic pain (Dworkin et al. 2003; Freynhagen et al. 2005; Sabatowski et al. 2004; Van Seventer et al. 2006). The first study (Dworkin et al. 2003) was an 8-week parallel-group, double-blind, placebo-controlled, randomized multicenter trial of patients with postherpetic neuralgia, who received either pregabalin 600 mg/day (300 mg/day if reduced creatinine clearance) or placebo. The primary efficacy measure was mean pain ratings using an 11-point numerical pain rating scale kept in a daily diary. At study endpoint, there was a significant decrease in mean pain scores for patients treated with pregabalin compared with placebo. The superior pain relief with pregabalin was identified as early as day 2 and was maintained throughout the 8 weeks of double-blind treatment. In a second study (Freynhagen et al. 2005), patients with chronic postherpetic neuralgia or diabetic peripheral neuropathy were randomly assigned to placebo, flexible-dose pregabalin titrated upward to a maximum dosage of 600 mg/day, or fixed-dose pregabalin at 300 mg/day for the first week followed by 600 mg/day for the remaining 11 weeks. Both flexible- and fixed-dose pregabalin significantly reduced endpoint mean pain scores and were significantly superior to placebo in improving pain-related sleep interference. In a third study, Van Seventer et al. (2006) evaluated pregabalin (150, 300, or 600 mg/day in bid dosing) or placebo in 370 patients with postherpetic neuralgia. Pregabalin provided significant dose-proportional pain relief at endpoint, different from placebo. Sleep interference in all pregabalin groups was significantly improved at endpoint. Similar results were obtained in the Sabatowski et al. (2004) study, which reported improvement in sleep and mood disturbance in patients treated with pregabalin. In total, these four studies showed benefit in pain reduction, sleep improvement, and mood associated with pregabalin treatment. The most common side effects were dizziness, peripheral edema, weight gain, and somnolence. The pain-reduction benefits, in comparison with placebo, were noted early in the clinical trial and were sustained for the duration of the study.

Diabetic peripheral neuropathy. Freeman et al. (2008) conducted a pooled analysis of data from seven published randomized, placebo-controlled trials encompassing 400 patients with diabetic peripheral neuropathy. The primary outcome measure was change from baseline to endpoint in mean pain score from patients' daily pain diaries. With three-times-daily administration, all pregabalin dosages (150, 300, and 600-mg/day) significantly reduced pain and pain-related sleep interference in comparison with placebo. With twice-daily administration, only the 600-mg/day dosage showed efficacy. Pregabalin's pain-reducing and sleep-improving properties appeared to be positively correlated with dose, with the greatest effect observed in patients treated with 600 mg/day.

Fibromyalgia

Pregabalin is the first medication to receive an FDA indication for the treatment of fibromyalgia. Fibromyalgia is a common chronic pain disorder characterized by widespread diffuse musculoskeletal pain and tenderness frequently accompanied by significant psychiatric comorbidity, including fatigue, sleep disturbance, and mood and anxiety disorders. Classifications of disease severity for fibromyalgia have been published by the American College of Rheumatology (Wolfe et al. 1990). Prevalence estimates for fibromyalgia are 2% of the U.S. population, with rates higher in adult women than in men (Arnold et al. 2007).

Two placebo-controlled acute-treatment studies (Crofford et al. 2005; Mease et al. 2008) and one placebo-controlled relapse prevention study (Crofford et al. 2008) have evaluated pregabalin in the treatment of patients with fibromyalgia. In the first, an 8-week double-blind, randomized, placebo-controlled study of pregabalin (150, 300, and 450 mg/day) versus placebo, the 450-mg daily dose significantly reduced the average severity of pain in comparison with placebo (Crofford et al. 2005). Sleep improvement was noted at both the 300- and the 450-mg daily dosages. Dizziness and somnolence were the most frequent adverse events. Arnold et al. (2007), in recognition of the large overlap of psychiatric comorbidity in fibromyalgia, conducted a post hoc analysis of the Crofford et al. (2005) study to assess symptoms of anxiety and depression and their impact on pregabalin treatment. Of 529 patients who had enrolled in pregabalin treatment for fibromyalgia, significantly more patients endorsed anxiety symptoms (71%) than endorsed depressive symptoms (56%). Improvement in pain symptoms with pregabalin versus placebo did not depend on baseline anxiety or depression; in fact, 75% of the pain reduction was not explained by improvements in mood and/or anxiety.

The second 13-week double-blind, placebo-controlled multicenter study randomly assigned 748 patients with fibromyalgia to receive either placebo or pregabalin dosages of 300, 450, or 600 mg/day (twice-daily dosing) (Mease et al. 2008). The primary outcome measure was symptomatic relief of pain associated with fibromyalgia, as measured by a mean pain score from an 11-point numeric rating scale (0 = no pain; 10 = worst possible pain) from patients' daily diaries. Patients in all pregabalin groups showed statistically significant improvement in endpoint mean pain score. Compared with the placebo group, all pregabalin treatment groups showed statistically significant improvement in sleep.

Finally, the FREEDOM (Fibromyalgia Relapse Evaluation and Efficacy for Durability Of Meaningful relief) study evaluated pregabalin in a 6-month double-blind, placebo-controlled design (Crofford et al. 2008). This study included an initial 6-week open-label phase followed by a 26-week double-blind treatment with ongoing pregabalin or blind substitution to placebo. The primary outcome measure was time to loss of therapeutic response, defined as a less than 30% reduction in pain or worsening of symptoms of fibromyalgia. More than 1,000 patients entered the open-label phase, with 287 being randomly assigned to placebo and 279 to pregabalin. Time to loss of therapeutic response was significantly greater for the pregabalin group than for the placebo group, with Kaplan-Meier estimates of time to event showing that half of the placebo group had relapsed by day 19, whereas half of the pregabalin group had still not lost response by trial end. At the end of the double-blind phase, 61% of the placebo-treated patients had lost therapeutic response, compared with only 32% of the pregabalin-treated patients.

These three placebo-controlled studies in the acute or relapse prevention phase in patients with fibromyalgia mark a substantial advance in clinical trial design of novel uses of anticonvulsants and represent a milestone in the first FDA-approved treatment for fibromyalgia.

Anxiety Disorders

Generalized anxiety disorder. Four placebo-controlled studies have evaluated pregabalin in generalized anxiety disorder (Montgomery et al. 2006; Pande et al. 2003; Pohl et al. 2005; Rickels et al. 2005). In the first study (Pande et al. 2003), 276 patients with generalized anxiety disorder were randomly assigned to pregabalin 150 or 600 mg/day, lorazepam 6 mg/day, or placebo. The 6-week trial included a 1-week placebo lead-in, 4 weeks of blind treatment, and a 1-week taper. The primary efficacy outcome measure was the endpoint Hamilton Anxiety Scale (Ham-A) score. The mean baseline-to-endpoint decrease in Ham-A total score in all three active-treatment groups (pregabalin 150 mg/day, pregabalin 600 mg/day, and lorazepam 6 mg/day) was significantly greater than the decrease in the placebo group. Percentages of subjects who met a secondary outcome measure, a reduction of 50% or greater in the Ham-A score, were significantly higher in the pregabalin 600-mg/day group (46%) and the lorazepam group (61%) than in the placebo group (27%). There were no significant differences in response rates by either definition between patients receiving pregabalin 150 mg/day and patients receiving placebo.

In the second study by Pohl et al. (2005), twice-daily versus three-times-daily dosing of pregabalin was evaluated in a 6-week double-blind, placebo-controlled study. In this study, 250 patients with generalized anxiety disorder were randomly assigned to pregabalin 100 mg twice daily, 200 mg twice daily, 150 mg three times daily, or placebo. Mean improvement in the Ham-A total score was significantly greater with pregabalin at all doses than with placebo. Pairwise comparisons of twice-daily versus three-times-daily dosing found no significant differences in outcome. All three pregabalin groups showed significantly greater improvement in comparison with placebo at endpoint.

In the third study by Rickels et al. (2005), 454 patients with generalized anxiety disorder were randomly assigned in a 4-week design to pregabalin 300 mg/day, 450 mg/day, or 600 mg/day; alprazolam 1.5 mg/day; or placebo. The primary outcome measure was change from baseline to endpoint in the total Ham-A score. In comparison with the placebo group, all treatment groups showed significantly greater reductions in mean Ham-A total score at last-observation-carried-forward (LOCF) analysis. A significantly higher proportion of patients in the pregabalin (all dosages) and alprazolam groups than in the placebo group met the endpoint response criterion of 50% or greater reduction in Ham-A total score. The response rate for the 300-mg/day pregabalin group (61%) was significantly higher than that for the alprazolam group (43%).

In the only pregabalin study with an active antidepressant comparator, Montgomery et al. (2006) randomly assigned 421 patients with generalized anxiety disorder to 6 weeks of double-blind treatment with pregabalin (400 or 600 mg/day), venlafaxine (75 mg/day), or placebo. The primary outcome measure was change in the Ham-A total score from baseline to LOCF analysis. Pregabalin (both dosages) and venlafaxine produced significantly greater improvement in the Ham-A total score than did placebo. Patients receiving pregabalin 400 mg/day experienced significant improvement in all primary and secondary outcome measures in comparison with those receiving placebo. Rates of discontinuation associated with adverse events were highest in the venlafaxine group (20.4%), followed by the pregabalin 600 mg/day (13.6%), pregabalin 400 mg/day (6.2%), and placebo (9.9%) groups. These studies, taken together, contributed to the approval of pregabalin in Europe for generalized anxiety disorder.

Social anxiety disorder.   In the one study by Pande et al. (2004), 135 patients with social anxiety disorder were randomly assigned to 10 weeks of double-blind treatment with either pregabalin (low dose: 150 mg/day; high dose: 600 mg/day) or placebo. The primary outcome measure was change from baseline to endpoint in the LSAS total score. Patients randomly assigned to pregabalin 600 mg/day showed significant decreases in LSAS total score compared with those receiving placebo. Significant differences between high-dose pregabalin and placebo were also noted on several secondary measures, including the LSAS subscales total fear, avoidance, social fear, and social avoidance. Low-dose pregabalin (150 mg/day) was not significantly better than placebo. Somnolence and dizziness were the most frequently reported adverse events.

Substance Abuse and Withdrawal

As previously noted, pregabalin has no hepatic metabolism and is excreted essentially unchanged in the urine. This pharmacokinetic profile is ideal for patients with alcohol abuse or dependence who have elevated transaminases but need safe, efficacious treatment for symptoms of alcohol withdrawal. One preclinical study highlighted the potential use of pregabalin and its anticonvulsant, analgesic, anxiolytic properties in a mouse model of alcohol dependence (Becker et al. 2006). Controlled clinical studies of pregabalin in alcohol-dependent patients are encouraged.

Side Effects and Toxicology

In general, the side effects commonly occurring with pregabalin treatment have been mild and not associated with a severity sufficient to warrant drug discontinuation. The most frequently reported symptoms have been dizziness, sedation, dry mouth, edema, blurred vision, weight gain, and concentration difficulty. In controlled clinical trials with pregabalin, significant weight gain (a gain of 7% or more over baseline) was observed in 9% of patients treated with pregabalin, compared with 2% of patients treated with placebo. Pregabalin treatment does not appear to be associated with significant changes in heart rate, blood pressure, respirations, or electrocardiogram measures. Peripheral edema has occurred in a small percentage of patients, but only in rare circumstances has it been identified as severe.

Available preclinical and clinical data suggest that pregabalin has very low abuse liability and is unlikely to produce significant physical dependence. There have been postmarketing reports of angioedema and hypersensitivity in patients treated with pregabalin (Pfizer 2006).

Drug–Drug Interactions

Pregabalin does not induce or inhibit CYP enzymes, nor do CYP enzyme inhibitors alter its pharmacokinetics as a consequence. Therefore, hepatic and CYP drug–drug interactions are not relevant when pregabalin is part of a complex polypharmacotherapy regimen. Because of the drug's renal elimination, dosage adjustment is required for patients with renal impairment. To date, no pharmacokinetic drug–drug interactions have been identified. There is some literature to suggest that there can be an additive cognitive impairment when pregabalin is taken in conjunction with oxycodone and that pregabalin may potentiate the effects of lorazepam and alcohol (Pfizer 2006).

Summary for Pregabalin

Controlled studies of pregabalin clearly have suggested its efficacy in complex partial epilepsy, postherpetic neuropathy, diabetic neuropathy, fibromyalgia, generalized anxiety disorder, and social anxiety disorder. Like gabapentin, pregabalin has a favorable pharmacokinetic profile, with particular advantages in patients with compromised hepatic function. Its minimal drug–drug interactions, low risk of toxicity, and favorable side-effect profile make it a useful addition to the pharmacopoeia.

Conclusion

There is increasing interest in the use of anticonvulsant drugs in mood and anxiety disorders. Controlled studies are needed to further assess specific patient populations and disease states that can benefit from these agents.

References

American Psychiatric Association: Diagnostic and Statistical Manual of Mental Disorders, 4th Edition. Washington, DC, American Psychiatric Association, 1994

Arnold LM, Crofford LJ, Martin SA, et al: The effect of anxiety and depression on improvements in pain in a randomized, controlled trial of pregabalin for treatment of fibromyalgia. Pain Medicine 8:633–638, 2007

Backonja M, Beydoun A, Edwards KR, et al: Gabapentin for the symptomatic treatment of painful neuropathy in patients with diabetes mellitus. JAMA 280:1831–1836, 1998

Becker HC, Myrick H, Veatch LM: Pregabalin is effective against behavioral and electrographic seizures during alcohol withdrawal. Alcohol Alcohol 4:399–406, 2006

Beydoun A, Fakhoury T, Nasreddine W, et al: Conversion to high dose gabapentin monotherapy in patients with medically refractory partial epilepsy. Epilepsia 39:188–193, 1998

Bonnet U, Banger M, Leweke FM, et al: Treatment of acute alcohol withdrawal with gabapentin: results from a controlled two-center trial. J Clin Psychopharmacol 23:514–519, 2003

Bonnet U, Specka M, Leweke FM, et al: Gabapentin's acute effect on mood profile—a controlled study on patients with alcohol withdrawal. Prog Neuropsychopharmacol Biol Psychiatry 31:434–438, 2007

Bozikas V, Petrikis P, Gamvrula K, et al: Treatment of alcohol withdrawal with gabapentin. Prog Neuropsychopharmacol Biol Psychiatry 26:197–199, 2002

Cora-Locatelli G, Greenburg BD, Martin JD, et al: Gabapentin augmentation for fluoxetine-treated patients with obsessive-compulsive disorder. J Clin Psychiatry 59:480–481, 1998

Crofford LJ, Rowbotham MC, Mease PJ, et al: Pregabalin for the treatment of fibromyalgia syndrome: results of a randomized, double-blind, placebo-controlled trial. Pregabalin 1008–105 Study Group. Arthritis Rheum 52:1264–1273, 2005

Crofford LJ, Mease PJ, Simpson SL, et al: Fibromyalgia Relapse Evaluation and Efficacy for Durability Of Meaningful Relief (FREEDOM): a 6-month, double-blind, placebo-controlled trial with pregabalin. Pain 136:419–431, 2008

Dimond KR, Pande AC, Lamoreaux L, et al: Effect of gabapentin (Neurontin) on mood and well-being in patients with epilepsy. Prog Neuropsychopharmacol Biol Psychiatry 20:407–417, 1996

Dooley DJ, Donovan CM, Meder WP, et al: Preferential action of gabapentin and pregabalin at P/Q-type voltage-sensitive calcium channels: inhibition of K+-evoked [3H]-norepinephrine release from rat neocortical slices. Synapse 45:171–190, 2002

Dworkin RH, Corbin AE, Young JP, et al: Pregabalin for the treatment of postherpetic neuralgia: a randomized, placebo-controlled trial. Neurology 60:1274–1283, 2003

Elger CE, Brodie MJ, Anhut H, et al: Pregabalin add-on treatment in patients with partial seizures: a novel evaluation of flexible-dose and fixed-dose treatment in a double-blind, placebo-controlled study. Epilepsia 46:1926–1935, 2005

Freeman R, Durso-Decruz E, Emir B: Efficacy, safety, and tolerability of pregabalin treatment of painful diabetic peripheral neuropathy: findings from 7 randomized controlled trials across a range of doses. Diabetes Care 31:1448–1454, 2008

Freynhagen R, Strojek K, Griesing T, et al: Efficacy of pregabalin in neuropathic pain evaluated in a 12-week randomized, double-blind, multicentre, placebo-controlled trial of flexible and fixed dose regimens. Pain 115:254–263, 2005

Frye MA, Kimbrell TA, Dunn RT, et al: Gabapentin does not alter single-dose lithium pharmacokinetics. J Clin Psychopharmacol 18:461–464, 1998

Frye MA, Ketter TA, Kimbrell TA, et al: A placebo-controlled study of lamotrigine and gabapentin monotherapy in refractory mood disorders. J Clin Psychopharmacol 20:607–614, 2000

Furieri FA, Nakamura-Palacios EM: Gabapentin reduces alcohol consumption and craving: a randomized, double-blind, placebo-controlled trial. J Clin Psychiatry 11:1691–1700, 2007

Gerner RH, Fairbanks L, Anderson GM, et al: Plasma levels of GABA and panic disorder. Psychiatry Res 63:223–225, 1996

Gold BI, Bowers MB, Roth RH, et al: GABA levels in CSF of patients with psychiatric disorders. Am J Psychiatry 137:362–364, 1980

Goldlust A, Su T, Welty DF, et al: Effects of the anticonvulsant drug gabapentin on enzymes in the metabolic pathways of glutamate and GABA. Epilepsy Res 22:1–11, 1995

Grunze H, Dittert S, Bungert M, et al: Renal impairment as a possible side effect of gabapentin: a single case report. Neuropsychobiology 38:198–199, 1998

Hamandi K, Sander JW: Pregabalin: a new antiepileptic drug for refractory epilepsy. Seizure 15:73–78, 2006

Hutson SM, Berkich D, Drown P, et al: Role of branched-chain aminotransferase isoenzymes and gabapentin in neurotransmitter metabolism. J Neurochem 71:863–874, 1998

Karam-Hage M, Brower KJ: Open pilot study of gabapentin versus trazodone to treatment insomnia in alcoholic outpatients. Psychiatry Clin Neurosci 57:542–544, 2003

Kavoussi R: Pregabalin: from molecule to medicine. Eur Neuropsychopharmacol 16:S128–S133, 2006

Leweke FM, Bauer J, Elger CE: Manic episode due to gabapentin treatment. Br J Psychiatry 175:291, 1999

Loscher W, Honack D, Taylor CP: Gabapentin increased aminooxyacetic acid-induced GABA accumulation in several regions of rat brain. Neurosci Lett 128:150–154, 1991

Pfizer: Lyrica (pregabalin) tablets: prescribing information. New York, Pfizer, 2006

Mahmood T, Romans S, Silverstone T: Prevalence of migraine in bipolar disorder. J Affect Disord 99:239–241, 1999

Malcolm R, Myrick H, Brady KT, et al: Update on anticonvulsants for the treatment of alcohol withdrawal. Am J Addict 10 (suppl):16–23, 2001

Malcolm R, Myrick LH, Veatch LM, et al: Self-reported sleep, sleepiness, and repeated alcohol withdrawals: a randomized, double blind, controlled comparison of lorazepam vs gabapentin. J Clin Sleep Med 3:24–32, 2007

Mariani JJ, Rosenthal RN, Tross S, et al: A randomized, open-label, controlled trial of gabapentin and phenobarbital in the treatment of alcohol withdrawal. Am J Addict 15:76–84, 2006

Mathew NT, Rapoport A, Saper J, et al: Efficacy of gabapentin in migraine prophylaxis. Headache 41:119–128, 2001

McLean MJ: Gabapentin in the management of convulsive disorders. Epilepsia 40 (suppl 6):S39–S50, 1999

Mease PJ, Russell J, Arnold LM, et al: A randomized, double-blind, placebo-controlled phase III trial of pregabalin in the treatment of patients with fibromyalgia. J Rheumatol 35:502–514, 2008

Miller RG, Moore D, Young LA, et al: Placebo-controlled trial of gabapentin in patients with ALS. Neurology 47:1383–1388, 1996

Montgomery SA: Pregabalin for the treatment of generalised anxiety disorder. Expert Opin Pharmacother 7:2139–2154, 2006

Montgomery SA, Tobias K, Zornberg GL, et al: Efficacy and safety of pregabalin in the treatment of generalized anxiety disorder: a 6-week, multicenter, randomized, double-blind, placebo-controlled comparison of pregabalin and venlafaxine. J Clin Psychiatry 67:771–782, 2006

Neurontin (gabapentin) package insert. Physicians' Desk Reference, 60th Edition. Montvale, NJ, Medical Economics Company, 2006

Obrocea GV, Dunn RM, Frye MA, et al: Clinical predictors of response to lamotrigine and gabapentin monotherapy in refractory affective disorders. Biol Psychiatry 51:253–260, 2002

Olson W, Gruenthal M, Muller ME, et al: Gabapentin for parkinsonism: a double-blind, placebo-controlled, cross-over trial. Am J Med 102:60–66, 1997

Ondo W, Hunter C, Vuong KD, et al: Gabapentin for essential tremor: a multiple-dose, double-blind, placebo controlled trial. Mov Disord 15:678–682, 2000

Pahwa R, Lyons K, Hubble JP, et al: Double-blind controlled trial of gabapentin in essential tremor. Mov Disord 13:465–467, 1998

Pande AC, Davidson JRT, Jefferson JW, et al: Treatment of social phobia with gabapentin: a placebo-controlled study. J Clin Psychopharmacol 19:341–348, 1999

Pande AC, Crockatt JG, Janney CA, et al: Gabapentin in bipolar disorder: a placebo-controlled trial of adjunctive therapy. Gabapentin Bipolar Disorder Study Group. Bipolar Disord 2(3 pt 2):249–255, 2000a

Pande AC, Pollack MH, Crockatt J, et al: Placebo-controlled study of gabapentin treatment of panic disorder. J Clin Psychopharmacol 20:467–471, 2000b

Pande AC, Crockatt JG, Feltner DE, et al: Pregabalin in generalized anxiety disorder: a placebo-controlled trial. Am J Psychiatry 160:533–540, 2003

Pande AC, Feltner DE, Jefferson JW, et al: Efficacy of the novel anxiolytic pregabalin in social anxiety disorder: a placebo-controlled, multicenter study. J Clin Psychopharmacol 24:141–149, 2004

Petroff OA, Rothman Dl, Behar KL, et al: The effect of gabapentin on brain gamma-aminobutyric acid in patients with epilepsy. Ann Neurol 39:95–99, 1996

Petty F, Kraemer GL, Dunnam D, et al: Plasma GABA in mood disorders. Psychopharmacol Bull 26:157–161, 1990

Pinninti NR, Mahajan DS: Gabapentin-associated aggression. J Neuropsychiatry Clin Neurosci 13:424–429, 2001

Pohl RB, Feltner DE, Rieve RR, et al: Efficacy of pregabalin in the treatment of generalized anxiety disorder: double-blind, placebo-controlled comparison of BPI versus TID dosing. J Clin Psychopharmacology 25:151–158, 2005

Pollack MH, Matthews M, Scott EL: Gabapentin as a potential treatment for anxiety disorders. Am J Psychiatry 155:992–993, 1998

Rao ML, Clarenbach P, Vahlensieck M, et al: Gabapentin augments whole blood serotonin in healthy young men. J Neural Transm 73:129–134, 1988

Rice AS, Maton S, Postherpetic Neuralgia Study Group: Gabapentin in postherpetic neuralgia: a randomised, double blind, placebo controlled study. Pain 94:215–224, 2001

Rickels K, Pollack MH, Feltner DE, et al: Pregabalin for treatment of generalized anxiety disorder: a 4-week, multicenter, double-blind, placebo-controlled trial of pregabalin and alprazolam. Arch Gen Psychiatry 62:1022–1030, 2005

Rowbotham M, Harden N, Stacey B, et al: Gabapentin for the treatment of postherpetic neuralgia. JAMA 280:1837–1842, 1998

Roy A, Dejong J, Ferraro T: CSF GABA in depressed patients and normal controls. Psychol Med 21:613–618, 1991

Sabatowski R, Gálvez R, Cherry DA, et al: Pregabalin reduces pain and improves sleep and mood disturbances in patients with post-herpetic neuralgia: results of a randomised, placebo-controlled clinical trial. Pain 109:26–35, 2004

Sanacora G, Mason GF, Rothman DL, et al: Reduced cortical gamma-aminobutyric acid levels in depressed patients determined by proton magnetic resonance spectroscopy. Arch Gen Psychiatry 56:1043–1047, 1999

Sanacora G, Mason GF, Rothman DL, et al: Increased occipital cortex GABA concentrations in depressed patients after therapy with selective serotonin reuptake inhibitors. Am J Psychiatry 159:663–665, 2002

Schlicker E, Reimann W, Gothert M: Gabapentin decreases monoamine release without affecting acetylcholine release in the brain. Arzneimittelforschung 35:1347–1349, 1985

Short C, Cooke L: Hypomania induced by gabapentin. Br J Psychiatry 167:549, 1995

Singh L, Field MJ, Ferris P, et al: The antiepileptic agent gabapentin (Neurontin) processes anxiolytic-like and antinociceptive actions that are reversed by D-serine. Psychopharmacology 127:1–9, 1996

Taylor CP, Vartanina MG, Andruszkiewiewicz R, et al: 3-alkyl GABA and 3-alkylglutamic acid analogues: two new classes of anticonvulsants agents. Epilepsy Res 11:103–110, 1992

Taylor CP, Gee NS, Su TZ, et al: A summary of mechanistic hypotheses of gabapentin pharmacology. Epilepsy Res 29:233–249, 1998

Van Seventer R, Feister HA, Young JP, et al: Efficacy and tolerability of twice-daily pregabalin for treating pain and related sleep interference in postherpetic neuralgia: a 13-week randomized trial. Curr Med Res Opin 222:375–384, 2006

Watson WP, Robinson E, Little HJ: The novel anticonvulsant gabapentin protects against both convulsant and anxiogenic aspects of the ethanol withdrawal syndrome. Neuropsychopharmacology 36:1369–1375, 1997

Weiss SR, Post RM: Kindling: separate vs shared mechanisms in affective disorders and epilepsy. Neuropsychobiology 38:167–180, 1998

Wolf SM, Shinnar S, Kang H et al: Gabapentin toxicity in children manifesting as behavioral changes. Epilepsia 36:1203–1205, 1996

Wolfe F, Smythe HA, Yunus MB, et al: The American College of Rheumatology 1990 Criteria for the Classification of Fibromyalgia: report of the Multicenter Criteria Committee. Arthritis Rheum 33:160–172, 1990

Yatham LN, Kusumakar V, Calabrese JR, et al: Third generation anticonvulsants in bipolar disorder: a review of efficacy and summary of clinical recommendations. J Clin Psychiatry 63:275–283, 2002

CHAPTER 39

Lamotrigine

David E. Kemp, M.D.

David J. Muzina, M.D.

Keming Gao, M.D., Ph.D.

Joseph R. Calabrese, M.D.

History and Discovery

The initial premise in evaluating lamotrigine as an anticonvulsant was that it might possess sufficient dihydrofolate reductase inhibition to decrease folate activity, a mechanism known to reduce epileptic effects. Although its antifolate properties were only modest, anticonvulsant effects were significant. During the clinical development of lamotrigine as a treatment for intractable seizures, improved mood in lamotrigine-treated patients was anecdotally reported (Jawad et al. 1989; Smith et al. 1993). Indeed, antiepileptic drugs (AEDs) have been described as a heterogeneous class of medications with a diverse range of utility in psychiatry with variable effects on mood (Muzina et al. 2005).

In 1993, Smith et al. evaluated mood state and quality of life among patients taking AEDs. Using a crossover design, the investigators administered add-on lamotrigine to 81 epileptic patients who were already receiving either enzyme-inducing AEDs ($n = 56$) or both enzyme inducers and valproate ($n = 25$). The principal variable of interest was seizure frequency; among the secondary response variables were subjective reports of anxiety, depression, self-esteem, mastery, and happiness. Although no difference was found in the levels of depression reported by patients receiving lamotrigine and those receiving placebo, lamotrigine-treated patients reported significantly higher levels of happiness on the Affect Balance Scale (Bradburn 1969) and an improvement in perceived internal locus of control according to a self-reported mastery scale (Pearlin and Schooler 1978). There was no correlation between perceived happiness and changes in seizure frequency or severity. Thus, the investigators concluded that lamotrigine has an effect on mood independent of its antiepileptic effect (Smith et al. 1993).

Structure–Activity Relations

Lamotrigine (3,5-diamino-6-[2,3-dichlorophenyl]-1,2,4-triazine, $C_9H_7Cl_2N_5$) is an AED of the phenyltriazine class that is chemically unrelated to hepatic enzyme inducers (e.g., carbamazepine) and enzyme inhibitors (e.g., valproic acid) (Figure 39–1). The reduction of dihydrofolate to tetrahydrofolate via inhibition of dihydrofolate reductase may result in the inhibition of nucleic acid and protein synthesis, secondary disruption of neural structure and function, and tertiary disruption of mood. However, as noted above, the correlation between inhibition of folic acid production and antiepileptic activity was found to be low, so the structure–activity relationship of lamotrigine with respect to antiseizure activity is unknown. Similarly, there are no published data clearly linking the structure of lamotrigine to its empirical mood-stabilizing properties.

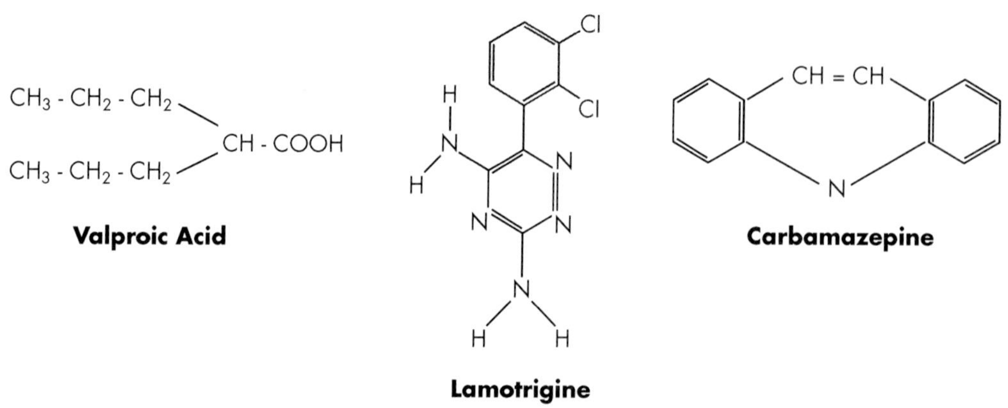

FIGURE 39–1.   Chemical structure of lamotrigine, with chemical structures of valproic acid and carbamazepine for comparison.

Pharmacological Profile

Lamotrigine has not been shown to inhibit the reuptake of norepinephrine, dopamine, or serotonin. Although it exerts inhibitory effects at the serotonin$_3$ (5-HT$_3$) receptor, this activity is weak and unlikely to contribute to its therapeutic profile. Lamotrigine does not exhibit high binding affinity to adrenergic (α_1, α_2, β), dopamine (D$_1$, D$_2$), γ-aminobutyric acid (GABA), histamine (H$_1$), opioid (κ or σ), or muscarinic (M$_1$, M$_2$) acetylcholine receptors. Like phenytoin, lamotrigine inhibits use-dependent Na$^+$ channels, allowing continued normal depolarizations but suppressing paroxysmal burst firing encountered in seizures and hypoxic insult. It exhibits neuroprotective effects through inhibiting glutamate release secondary to ischemia, but it does not inhibit N-methyl-D-aspartate (NMDA)–induced depolarizations.

Pharmacokinetics and Disposition

Oral lamotrigine is rapidly absorbed with negligible first-pass metabolism. Peak plasma concentrations are reached in approximately 2–4 hours, and its half-life is approximately 25 hours (GlaxoSmithKline 2007). Bioavailability is not altered by food, and the chewable tablets are equivalent in the rate and extent of absorption as compared to the compressed tablets. Lamotrigine is approximately 55% bound to plasma proteins and is unlikely to significantly interact with drugs that are highly protein bound. Metabolism is primarily achieved by competitive glucuronic acid conjugation. The principal product is an inactive lamotrigine-2-N-glucuronide conjugate, found predominantly in urine and to a lesser extent

in feces. Ten percent of lamotrigine is excreted unchanged. At steady-state concentrations, the pharmacokinetics of lamotrigine are linear within a dosage range of 100–700 mg/day (Leach et al. 1995). The clearance of lamotrigine is reduced in the setting of renal insufficiency and hepatic disease. Race also appears to affect the clearance of lamotrigine, with rates 25% lower in nonwhites than in whites.

There is growing awareness that perturbations in lamotrigine levels occur during pregnancy. Ohman et al. (2000) first reported data from nine pregnant epileptic women, revealing marked elevations in maternal plasma lamotrigine levels during the first 2 weeks postpartum. Lamotrigine levels increased by as much as 170% from levels taken at the time of delivery. Pennell et al. (2004) extended upon this finding in a sample of 14 women treated with lamotrigine monotherapy throughout pregnancy and during the postpartum period. The authors observed an increasing magnitude of lamotrigine clearance during each trimester, reaching a peak of 330% of baseline clearance by week 32 gestational age. Plasma levels were noted to rapidly return to normal during the first few postpartum weeks. The increase in clearance during pregnancy presumably reflects an increase in gonadal steroid production (Pennell 2003) and primary metabolism through hepatic glucuronidation.

In newborns of mothers receiving lamotrigine, extensive placental transfer of drug has been found to occur, with umbilical cord concentrations approaching those of maternal serum (Ohman et al. 2000). Nursing infants demonstrate plasma lamotrigine concentrations approximately 23%–50% of maternal levels. Any adverse effects to neonates that may result from lamotrigine exposure through breast-feeding are not well characterized.

Mechanism of Action

The mechanism by which lamotrigine exerts its therapeutic psychotropic effects is not clear but is presumed to be associated with its antiepileptic activity. Given this presumption, it is the use- and voltage-dependent inhibition of voltage-activated sodium channels (Xie and Hagan 1998) that best characterize lamotrigine's mechanism of action. In addition to sodium channel inhibition, lamotrigine demonstrates inhibition of glutamine-induced repetitive burst firing in cultured rat cortical neurons (Miller et al. 1986) and cultured spinal cord neurons (Cheung et al. 1992). Initial, but not subsequent, stimuli of burst-firing wavetrains are comparatively unimpeded by high-concentration lamotrigine (Cheung et al. 1992; Miller et al. 1986). This effect is attenuated by hyperpolarization. Subsequent stimuli in the wavetrains show attenuation, as evidenced by frequency-dependent inhibition of Na^+ receptor flux (Cheung et al. 1992; Lang and Wang 1991; Lang et al. 1993; Miller et al. 1986). Together, these data support the concept of lamotrigine-induced inhibition of Na^+ flux at presynaptic use- and voltage-sensitive sodium channels. The inhibition appears to be greatest in paroxysmally depolarized (rapidly firing) neurons. This is significant, because paroxysmal discharge produced by neuronally, physically, or chemically induced kindling has been generally accepted as a model of the induction and propagation of cortical seizure activity (Ayala et al. 1970). In a complementary manner, kindling has also been proposed as a potential contributor to mood cycling in bipolar disorder (Post et al. 1984). According to the kindling theory, the progression of bipolar episodes evolves from being reactive and triggered by environmental life stressors to occurring spontaneously. More worrisome, this process may contribute to a treatment-refractory course of illness (Post et al. 2001). Mechanistically, preferential attenuation of paroxysmal wavetrains could permit normal neuronal activity to continue unimpeded but still suppress seizure activity and affective instability. However, this hypothesis is limited in its ability to explain the more enduring mood-stabilizing effects that occur apart from bursts of paroxysmal electrical discharges.

In addition to inhibitory activity on sodium channels, there is also evidence for antagonistic action by lamotrigine on N-type Ca^{++} channels in rat cortical neurons and CA1/CA3 regions of guinea pig hippocampal slices (Stefani et al. 1996; von Wegerer et al. 1997). Given prior reports ascribing modest antimanic effects to calcium channel blockers, the mechanism of calcium channel blockade

may also contribute to lamotrigine's thymoleptic properties (Dubovsky 1993).

Antiglutamatergic action is another means by which lamotrigine may function as a mood stabilizer. The presynaptic inhibitory effects of lamotrigine on voltage- and use-sensitive sodium channels, calcium channels, and potassium channels (Grunze et al. 1998) are believed to result in decreased release of the excitatory amino acid glutamate. In humans, support for lamotrigine's antiglutamatergic action includes an ability to reduce perceptual abnormalities induced by the NMDA receptor antagonist ketamine (Anand et al. 2000). Yet blockade of glutamate release is independent of any NMDA affinity, as lamotrigine-associated antagonism of NMDA-induced depolarizations or other NMDA-linked stimuli has not been reported in animal models (Harrison and Simmonds 1985). Lamotrigine's ability to inhibit veratrine-induced glutamate and aspartate release (Leach et al. 1986) may translate clinically into greater activation and alertness, accounting for its observed ability to stabilize mood from below baseline.

Mechanisms unlikely to account for lamotrigine's clinical efficacy in bipolar depression and ability to provide prophylaxis against recurring mood episodes include activity at GABAergic, serotonergic, and other monoaminergic receptors. Lamotrigine does not have robust monoamine oxidase inhibitor activity for either the A or B isoforms (Southam et al. 2005), nor does lamotrigine have high affinity for $GABA_A$ or $GABA_B$ receptors. At the 5-HT_3 receptor, only weak inhibitory effects have been reported. Although there were no alterations in 5-HT_{1A} receptor function after 1 week of lamotrigine administration to healthy male volunteers (Shiah et al. 1998), there is preliminary evidence in animals to show that postsynaptic 5-HT_{1A} receptors may be affected by lamotrigine (Bourin et al. 2005). In this regard, lamotrigine appears to function more similarly to valproate and carbamazepine than to lithium. Although the mechanisms are not completely understood, support for potential neuroprotective effects of lamotrigine come from studies of rat hippocampal CA1 cells, where the agent reduced cell damage resulting from global cerebral ischemia (Crumrine et al. 1997) and decreased hippocampal neuronal loss after pretreatment with lamotrigine (Maj et al. 1998).

Indications and Efficacy

Lamotrigine is indicated for adjunctive antiepileptic therapy in adults with partial seizures and in patients with generalized seizures secondary to Lennox-Gastaut syndrome. The most recently approved indication is for adjunctive use in primary and generalized tonic-clonic seizures in adults and pediatric patients (≥2 years of age).

In 2003, lamotrigine became the first medication since lithium to be granted U.S. Food and Drug Administration (FDA) approval for use in the maintenance treatment of bipolar I disorder to delay the time to occurrence of new mood episodes. Olanzapine, aripiprazole, and quetiapine have subsequently received this indication for bipolar disorder.

Maintenance Therapy in Bipolar I Disorder

Two large randomized, double-blind, parallel-group, placebo-controlled multicenter studies led to the approval of lamotrigine as a maintenance therapy in bipolar I disorder (Bowden et al. 2003; Calabrese et al. 2003). Both of these paired studies included a screening phase of up to 2 weeks; an 8- to 16-week open-label phase during which lamotrigine was initiated as adjunctive or monotherapy and other psychotropic drugs were discontinued; and an 18-month double-blind phase during which patients received lamotrigine, lithium, or placebo as maintenance therapy. The primary efficacy variable in both studies was time to intervention for any mood episode.

One of the studies (Bowden et al. 2003) evaluated subjects who were or had recently been in a manic, hypomanic, or mixed state. The other study (Calabrese et al. 2003) examined subjects who were or had recently been depressed.

Both lamotrigine and lithium were significantly superior to placebo on time to intervention for any mood episode ($P=0.018$ for previously manic; $P=0.029$ for previously depressed). Lamotrigine-treated patients showed longer survival-in-study times than did control subjects ($P=0.03$ for formerly manic; $P=0.003$ for formerly depressed). Lithium-treated formerly depressed patients also showed longer survival-in-study times relative to control subjects ($P=0.022$), and there was a nonsignificant trend for lithium-treated formerly manic patients to show longer in-study survival as well ($P=0.07$). Lamotrigine, but not lithium, was superior to placebo at prolonging the time to a depressive episode ($P=0.015$ for previously manic; $P=0.047$ for previously depressed). Lithium, but not lamotrigine, was superior to placebo at prolonging the time to a manic, hypomanic, or mixed episode ($P=0.006$ for previously manic; $P=0.026$ for previously depressed). There was no evidence in these studies of worsening manic or depressive symptoms or of accelerated cycling frequency during lamotrigine treatment.

In contrast to both individual maintenance studies, a pooled analysis of these two clinical trials conducted by Goodwin et al. (2004) found lithium and lamotrigine to be statistically superior to placebo at prolonging the time to intervention for a manic, hypomanic, or mixed episode ($P=0.034$ for lamotrigine vs. placebo; $P≤0.001$ for lithium vs. placebo). However, lamotrigine, but not lithium, remained the only compound that was statistically superior to placebo at prolonging the time to intervention for a depressive episode ($P=0.009$ for lamotrigine vs. placebo; $P=0.120$ for lithium vs. placebo).

In the interpretation of maintenance-phase data, it is important to distinguish between efficacy in relapse prevention and pure prophylactic efficacy (Ghaemi et al. 2004). Mood episodes of the same polarity as the index episode that occur during the initial 2 months following recovery are generally regarded as *relapses*. As such, this period is termed the acute recovery phase. Alternatively, mood episodes that occur beyond this phase during the period of remission are regarded as *recurrences*. To test the pure maintenance efficacy of lamotrigine, Calabrese et al. (2006) conducted a post hoc analysis of the two double-blind 18-month maintenance trials that compared lamotrigine and lithium against placebo. In their analysis, all subjects were excluded who experienced a relapse to a mood episode of the same polarity as the index episode within 90 or 180 days of randomization. After subjects who relapsed to a mood episode within 90 days of randomization were excluded, data were available from 167 lamotrigine-treated patients, 131 lithium-treated patients, and 133 placebo-treated patients. Lamotrigine and lithium were both more effective than placebo at delaying the time to intervention for a mood episode ($P=0.02$ for lamotrigine; $P=0.010$ for lithium). Similar results were found when patients who relapsed to a mood episode of the same polarity as their index episode within 180 days of randomization were excluded. When overall survival in the study until dropout for any reason was examined, only lamotrigine was significantly more effective than placebo ($P=0.002$ for lamotrigine; $P=0.098$ for lithium). Because these results are consistent with the primary analyses of the independent studies that included patients who potentially relapsed into their index episode, the findings indicate that lamotrigine and lithium possess true maintenance efficacy.

Acute Treatment of Bipolar Depression

Evaluation of lamotrigine's spectrum of activity was prompted by early reports of putative psychotropic efficacy in patients with epilepsy as summarized above. To replicate and extend preliminary open-label prospective findings suggesting moderate to marked efficacy in depression, hypomania, and mixed states (Calabrese et al. 1999a), a series of multicenter double-blind, placebo-controlled studies was completed. The first study in this series was conducted to evaluate the efficacy and safety of two doses of lamotrigine compared with placebo in the acute treatment of a major depressive episode in 195 patients with bipolar I disorder (Calabrese et al. 1999b). Outpatients received lamotrigine (50 or 200 mg/day) or placebo as monotherapy for 7 weeks. Psychiatric evaluations, including the Hamilton Rating Scale for Depression (Ham-D), the Montgomery-Åsberg Depression Rating Scale (MADRS), the Mania Rating Scale (MRS), and the Severity of Illness and Improvement subscales of the Clinical Global Impression Scale (CGI-S and CGI-I, respectively), were completed at 4 days and then weekly. Lamotrigine at a dosage of 200 mg/day demonstrated significant antidepressant efficacy on the MADRS, Ham-D Item 1, CGI-S, and CGI-I compared with placebo. Improvements were seen as early as week 3. Lamotrigine at a dosage of 50 mg/day approached significance compared with placebo on several efficacy measures. The proportion of patients exhibiting a marked response on the CGI-I was 51%, 41%, and 26% for the lamotrigine 200 mg/day, lamotrigine 50 mg/day, and placebo groups, respectively. The rate of switching was not significantly different between lamotrigine (4.6%–5.4%) and placebo (5%) without concurrent psychotropic medication. Of 65 subjects randomly assigned to placebo, 3% cycled into hypomania, 0% into mania, and less than 1% into mixed states. Of 129 patients randomly assigned to lamotrigine, less than 1% cycled into hypomania, 3% into mania, and less than 1% into mixed states. These data suggest that lamotrigine monotherapy is an efficacious and well-tolerated treatment for bipolar depression and that the switch rate associated with the use of lamotrigine does not exceed that typically seen in the natural course of the illness.

Although there is expert consensus that lamotrigine is effective for acute bipolar depression and confirmation with one adequately powered placebo-controlled trial (Calabrese et al. 1999b), there have been four randomized, parallel-group, placebo-controlled monotherapy trials of lamotrigine that have failed to separate from placebo (Calabrese et al. 2008). These include a 10-week flexible-dose (100–400 mg) study of patients with bipolar I or II disorder, an 8-week fixed-dose (200 mg) study of patients with bipolar II disorder, and two 8-week fixed-dose (200 mg) studies of patients with bipolar I disorder. In none of the four studies were significant improvements over placebo observed on the 17- and 31-item Ham-D, MADRS, CGI-S, or CGI-I. The effect sizes of the primary and secondary endpoints for these four studies were small, suggesting that insufficient numbers of subjects may have been randomized to detect a significant treatment effect. In contrast to the study demonstrating superiority of lamotrigine over placebo in treating acute bipolar depression, the placebo response rates in these four studies were variably high.

To clarify the effects of lamotrigine in acute bipolar depression, Geddes et al. (2009) conducted a systematic meta-analysis of individual patient data from 1,072 participants in all five randomized, controlled trials comparing lamotrigine with placebo. The pooled analysis showed that more patients treated with lamotrigine than with placebo responded on both the Ham-D and the MADRS ($P = 0.002$). However, the advantage over placebo was larger in more severely depressed patients.

Rapid-Cycling Bipolar Disorder

Calabrese et al. (2000) conducted a large study in rapid-cycling bipolar disorder consisting of two phases: an 8- to 12-week open-label preliminary phase and a 26-week randomized phase. Subjects who met criteria for mood stabilization at the end of the preliminary phase were stratified for type I and II bipolar disorder and then randomly assigned to flexible-dose lamotrigine (100–500 mg/day) or placebo to compare the efficacy of lamotrigine monotherapy with that of placebo in preventing mood episodes and to evaluate the safety of lamotrigine in this population. Three hundred twenty-six subjects were enrolled into the preliminary phase, and 182 subjects were randomly assigned to receive placebo ($n = 89$) or lamotrigine ($n = 93$). The difference between the treatment groups in time to additional pharmacotherapy for a developing or fully developed mood episode did not achieve statistical significance. However, overall survival time in the study (i.e., time to dropout for any reason) was significantly different between the treatment groups in favor of lamotrigine ($P = 0.036$). When patients with bipolar I and II subtypes were compared, lamotrigine-treated bipolar II disorder patients demonstrated a significantly longer median survival of 17 weeks compared with a median of 7 weeks for placebo-treated patients ($P = 0.015$). This study was the first long-term prospective placebo-controlled evaluation of a maintenance treatment in a large population of patients diagnosed with rapid-cycling bipolar disorder. The results suggest that lamotrigine is particularly useful for the prevention of mood episodes in bipolar II disorder. This is likely due to the predominance of depressive symptoms in bipolar II patients.

Lamotrigine Comparator Trials

To date, only two compounds are FDA approved for the treatment of acute bipolar depression: an olanzapine–fluoxetine combination (OFC) and quetiapine. To compare efficacy with an established agent for managing bipolar depression, a head-to-head randomized, double-blind, parallel-group study of lamotrigine and OFC was conducted over 7 weeks in patients with bipolar I disorder in an acute depressive phase (E.B. Brown et al. 2006). The study randomly assigned 410 subjects to either lamotrigine (titrated to 200 mg/day; $n = 205$) or OFC (6/25, 6/50, 12/25, or 12/50 mg/day; $n = 205$). Rates of response, defined as a $\geq 50\%$ reduction in MADRS total score, did not differ significantly between lamotrigine (59.7%) and OFC (68.8%; $P = 0.073$). When a MADRS score of ≤ 12 was used to define remission, no significant differences were observed in the remission rate between lamotrigine (49.2%) and OFC (56.4%; $P = 0.181$), nor were there differences in the time to remission ($P = 0.072$). However, when improvement on the individual rating scales was compared, OFC-treated subjects showed greater decreases in the MADRS total score ($P = 0.002$) and Young Mania Rating Scale total score ($P = 0.001$) compared with lamotrigine-treated subjects. Although overall response and remission rates were comparable between the active agents, interesting differences did emerge in regard to tolerability profiles. Adverse-event rates of suicidal and self-injurious behavior were more common among patients treated with lamotrigine (3.4%) compared with OFC (0.5%; $P = 0.037$). However, significant differences in mean change from baseline to endpoint for clinically relevant laboratory results favored treatment with lamotrigine on measures such as hemoglobin A1c, prolactin, total cholesterol, high-density lipoprotein cholesterol, low-density lipoprotein cholesterol, and triglyceride levels. Importantly, the incidence of potentially clinically relevant weight gain, defined as a $\geq 7\%$ increase in body weight, in OFC-treated patients was 23.4%, compared with 0% with lamotrigine ($P < 0.001$). As anticipated for a treatment trial comparing two active treatments, the effect size was modest between treatment arms (0.26).

Although lamotrigine is not indicated for the treatment of acute bipolar I depression, the similarity of its response and remission rates to those seen with OFC, an agent granted FDA approval, provide a rationale for la-

motrigine's use in the acutely depressed phase of bipolar disorder, especially for patients at risk for weight gain or adverse metabolic effects. One explanation for the greater improvement on MADRS scores, but not overall response or remission rates, among OFC-treated patients may pertain to the tolerability profile of olanzapine. Side effects such as sedation or weight gain may be driving improvement on standardized rating scale measurements of insomnia or appetite loss, rather than a true antidepressant mechanism. This may place agents with a clean tolerability profile, such as lamotrigine, at a disadvantage.

An add-on trial comparing lamotrigine with placebo has also been conducted in the treatment of bipolar I and II depression (van der Loos et al. 2006). All patients were required to be taking lithium maintained at a therapeutic blood level (0.6–1.2 mmol/L) prior to randomization to lamotrigine ($n = 64$) or placebo ($n = 60$). Subjects were treated for 8 weeks and assessed for response using the MADRS (primary outcome measure) and the Clinical Global Impression Scale–Bipolar Version (CGI-BP; Spearing et al. 1997). The change from baseline to endpoint on the MADRS was significantly greater in lamotrigine-treated subjects (15.38) compared with those receiving placebo (11.03; $P = 0.024$). A higher percentage of patients responded to add-on lamotrigine (51.6%) compared with placebo (31.7%; $P = 0.030$), although no difference was observed in the rate of response based on the CGI-BP (64.1% for lamotrigine vs. 48.3% for placebo; $P = 0.103$). A randomized, double-blind pilot trial has also compared lamotrigine ($n = 10$) and citalopram ($n = 10$) as an add-on to lithium, divalproex, or carbamazepine for bipolar I or II depression (Schaffer et al. 2006). MADRS scores decreased to a similar degree for patients taking citalopram (-10.6, SD = 8.6) as for patients taking lamotrigine (-5.0, SD = 10; $P = 0.21$). There was one case of adverse switch into hypomania in each treatment arm.

A summary of the 16 randomized, controlled multicenter trials involving lamotrigine in the treatment of mood disorders is represented in Table 39–1.

Alternative Clinical Applications

Case studies and open-label reports have been published supporting further investigation of lamotrigine for use in the treatment of myriad disorders and behavioral symptoms, including depersonalization disorder (Sierra et al. 2006), impulsive behavior (Daly and Fatemi 1999); Alzheimer's disease (Tekin et al. 1998), aggression in dementia (Devarajan and Dursun 2000), borderline personality disorder (Pinto and Akiskal 1998), posttraumatic

TABLE 39–1. Summary of multicenter randomized, controlled trials of lamotrigine in mood disorders

Study (protocol number)	Mood state	Bipolar subtype	Study type	Dose	Duration	Response or overall efficacy
Calabrese et al. 1999b (602)	Bipolar depression	I	Acute monotherapy	LTG 200 mg/day (n=63) LTG 50 mg/day (n=66) PBO (n=65)	7 weeks	Ham-D: NS MADRS: LTG>PBO CGI-I: LTG>PBO
Calabrese et al. 2008 (603)	Bipolar depression	I and II	Acute monotherapy	LTG 100–400 mg/day (n=103) PBO (n=103)	10 weeks	NS
Calabrese et al. 2008 (SCA 40910)	Bipolar depression	I	Acute monotherapy	LTG 200 mg/day (n=133) PBO (n=124)	8 weeks	NS
Calabrese et al. 2008 (SCA 100223)	Bipolar depression	II	Acute monotherapy	LTG 200 mg/day (n=111) PBO (n=124)	8 weeks	MADRS: NS Ham-D: NS CGI-I responders: LTG>PBO
Calabrese et al. 2008 (SCA 30924)	Bipolar depression	I	Acute monotherapy	LTG 200 mg/day (n=131) PBO (n=128)	8 weeks	NS
E. B. Brown et al. 2006	Bipolar depression	I	Acute monotherapy	LTG 200 mg/day (n=205) OFC up to 12/50 mg/day (n=205)	7 weeks	MADRS: OFC>LTG CGI-S: OFC>LTG
van der Loos et al. 2006	Bipolar depression	I or II	Acute, add-on therapy	LTG 200 mg/day (N=64) PBO (N=60)	8 weeks	MADRS: LTG>PBO CGI-I: NS
Calabrese et al. 2003 (605)	Bipolar depression (index episode)	I	Maintenance monotherapy following open stabilization	LTG 50, 200, or 400 mg/day (n=221) Li 0.8–1.1 mEq/L (n=121) PBO (n=121)	76 weeks	LTG>PBO Li>PBO
Bowden et al. 2000 (609)	Mania	I	Acute monotherapy	LTG 50 mg/d (n=84) Li 0.8–1.3 mEq/L (n=36) PBO (n=95)	3 weeks	NS
Bowden et al. 2000 (610)	Mania	I	Acute, add-on therapy	LTG 200 mg/day (n=74) Li 0.7–1.3 mEq/L (n=78) PBO (n=77)	6 weeks	LTG: NS Li>PBO
Bowden et al. 2003 (606)	Mania (index episode)	I	Maintenance monotherapy following open stabilization	LTG 100–400 mg/day (n=59) Li 0.8–1.1 mEq/L (n=46) PBO (n=70)	76 weeks	LTG>PBO Li>PBO
GlaxoSmithKline Study* (611)	Rapid cycling	I and II	Prophylaxis, add-on therapy	LTG 100–500 mg/day (n=68) PBO (n=69)	32 weeks	NS

TABLE 39–1.   Summary of multicenter randomized, controlled trials of lamotrigine in mood disorders (*continued*)

STUDY (PROTOCOL NUMBER)	MOOD STATE	BIPOLAR SUBTYPE	STUDY TYPE	DOSE	DURATION	RESPONSE OR OVERALL EFFICACY
Calabrese et al. 2000 (614)	Rapid cycling	I and II	Maintenance monotherapy following open stabilization	LTG 100–500 mg/day (n=92) PBO (n=88)	26 weeks	LTG>PBO for BP II
Laurenza et al. 1999 (613)	Unipolar depression	N/A	Acute monotherapy	LTG 200 mg/day (n=142) Desipramine 200 mg/day (n=147) PBO (n=145)	8 weeks	Ham-D: NS MADRS: NS CGI-S: LTG>PBO
DeVeaugh-Geiss et al. 2000 (20022)	Unipolar depression	N/A	Acute monotherapy	LTG 200 mg/day (n=74) PBO (n=75)	7 weeks	NS
DeVeaugh-Geiss et al. 2000 (20025)	Unipolar depression	N/A	Acute monotherapy	LTG 200 mg/day (n=151) PBO (n=150)	7 weeks	NS

*=data on file, GlaxoSmithKline

BP I=bipolar I disorder; BP II=bipolar II disorder; CGI-I=Clinical Global Impression–Improvement Scale; CGI-S=Clinical Global Impression–Severity Scale; Ham-D=Hamilton Rating Scale for Depression; Li=lithium; LTG=lamotrigine; MADRS=Montgomery-Åsberg Depression Rating Scale; N/A=not applicable; NS=not statistically significant (*P*≥0.05); OFC=olanzapine–fluoxetine combination; PBO=placebo.

stress disorder (Hertzberg et al. 1999), treatment-resistant unipolar depression (Gabriel 2006), alcohol (Rubio et al. 2006) and cocaine dependence (E.S. Brown et al. 2006) comorbid with bipolar disorder, schizoaffective disorder (Erfurth et al. 1998b), Rett syndrome (Stenbom et al. 1998), self-injurious behavior in the profoundly mentally retarded (Davanzo and King 1996), refractory schizophrenia (coadministered with clozapine [Saba et al. 2002]), and decreased consciousness with impaired cognition in severe brain injury (Showalter and Kimmel 2000).

Dosing

The recommended titration schedule for lamotrigine added to valproate in adult patients begins at 25 mg every other day for 14 days, advances to 25 mg daily for 14 days, and then increases by 50 mg daily beginning each of the fifth and sixth week of treatment, reaching a target dose of 100 mg daily (Table 39–2). Titration of adjunctive lamotrigine in the presence of an enzyme inducer begins at 50 mg daily for 14 days, advances to 100 mg daily (divided doses) for 14 days, to a target dosage of 400 mg daily (Table 39–3). There are no published data supporting greater efficacy of lamotrigine in the treatment of bipolar disorder at dosages greater than 200 mg/day. Additionally, there is no clear association between serum levels of lamotrigine and measures of affective response.

Side Effects and Toxicity

In trials of epileptic patients who received adjunctive or monotherapy lamotrigine, the spectrum of reported side effects included dizziness, headache, diplopia, nausea, and ataxia (Messenheimer et al. 1998). In controlled monotherapy trials in mood disorders, lamotrigine has been associated with headache, changes in sleep habits, nausea, and dizziness (Bowden et al. 2004). Although the prevalence of rash in mood disorder randomized trials did not exceed that of placebo, rash is generally recognized as the side effect most likely to significantly complicate lamotrigine's clinical use (see "Rash" subsection below).

A unique feature of lamotrigine in comparison with other agents used in the management of bipolar disorder is its weight-neutral tolerability profile. Among 583 patients with bipolar disorder treated with lamotrigine, lithium, or placebo for 52 weeks, a pooled analysis showed that the percentage of patients with a greater than 7% increase in weight or change in weight did not differ between those treated with lamotrigine and those treated

TABLE 39–2. Recommended titration schedule for lamotrigine for patients with bipolar disorder taking valproate

Week	Dosage
Weeks 1 and 2	25 mg every other day
Weeks 3 and 4	25 mg daily
Week 5	50 mg daily
Week 6	100 mg daily
Week 7	100 mg daily

The usual maintenance dosage when lamotrigine is added to valproate is 100 mg/day.
Source. Adapted from GlaxoSmithKline 2007.

with lithium or placebo (Sachs et al. 2006). A higher percentage of lamotrigine-treated subjects than of lithium-treated subjects lost more than 7% of their body weight. A post hoc analysis revealed that nonobese patients taking lamotrigine are unlikely to experience a change in weight. However, obese patients are significantly more likely to lose weight with lamotrigine and to gain weight with lithium (Bowden et al. 2006).

Clinical case reports made since the release of lamotrigine have included rare associations with Tourette's syndrome (Lombroso 1999); obsessionality in the form of intrusive, repetitive phrases (Kemp et al. 2007); nephritis with colitis (Fervenza et al. 2000); eosinophilic hepatitis (Fix et al. 2006); visual loss due to cicatrizing conjunctivitis (McDonald and Favilla 2003); female sexual dysfunction (Erfurth et al. 1998a); lupus erythematosus (Sarzi-Puttini et al. 2000); stupor (Sbei and Campellone 2001); and hyponatremia in patients with diabetes insipidus (Mewasingh et al. 2000). Hypersensitivity reactions (multiorgan failure/dysfunction, hepatic abnormalities, disseminated intravascular coagulation) have also occurred with lamotrigine use.

Rash

Incidence and Prevalence

In early epilepsy trials, rash led to hospitalization and treatment discontinuation or Stevens-Johnson syndrome in 0.3% of adults treated with lamotrigine. During the controlled phase of 12 multicenter trials, no cases of serious rash occurred in lamotrigine-treated subjects (Calabrese et al. 2002). Among 1,955 patients treated with lamotrigine in an open-label setting, there was 1 case of mild Stevens-Johnson syndrome and 2 cases of serious

TABLE 39–3.   Recommended titration schedule for lamotrigine when used as monotherapy and when added to an enzyme-inducing antiepileptic drug regimen* (without valproate)

	FOR PATIENTS NOT TAKING AN ENZYME-INDUCING ANTIEPILEPTIC DRUG REGIMEN* AND NOT TAKING VALPROATE	FOR PATIENTS TAKING AN ENZYME-INDUCING ANTIEPILEPTIC DRUG REGIMEN* AND NOT TAKING VALPROATE
Weeks 1 and 2	25 mg daily	50 mg daily
Weeks 3 and 4	50 mg daily	100 mg/day (in two divided doses)
Week 5	100 mg daily	200 mg daily (in two divided doses)
Week 6	200 mg daily	300 mg daily (in two divided doses)
Usual maintenance dosage	200 mg daily	400 mg daily (in two divided doses)

*Carbamazepine, phenytoin, phenobarbital, primidone, and rifampin have been shown to increase the apparent clearance of lamotrigine.
Source.   Adapted from GlaxoSmithKline 2007.

rash. Both cases of serious rash resolved uneventfully upon lamotrigine discontinuation, with one case requiring additional treatment with oral steroids.

The annual incidence of serious drug-based skin reactions associated with lamotrigine was highest in 1993 (4.2%) but steadily declined and had stabilized by 1998 (0.02%). This is likely attributable to the manufacturer's dosage revision in 1994, which advised a more protracted titration schedule (Calabrese et al. 2002; Messenheimer et al. 1998). It is well documented that the risk of rash is heightened in children younger than 12 years, by the coadministration of valproic acid, or by exceeding the recommended initial dosage or rate of dosage escalation of lamotrigine.

Clinical Management

The most common lamotrigine-associated rash is an exanthematic maculopapular or morbilliform eruption that is benign. However, a clinically similar eruption may be associated with more rare and serious systemic hypersensitivity reactions (Guberman et al. 1999). Thus, all patients who develop a rash during the first few months of lamotrigine therapy should be instructed to hold the next dose and immediately seek medical consultation. The greatest risk of rash appears to be during the first 8 weeks of treatment. A rash during the first 5 days of therapy is usually due to a nondrug cause.

Figure 39–2 presents a decision-making algorithm for the management of benign and serious rashes. A serious lamotrigine rash is usually confluent with prominent facial and neck involvement. The rash may be tender or have a purpuric or hemorrhagic appearance. It is accompanied or preceded by fever, malaise, pharyngitis, anorexia, or lymphadenopathy (Guberman et al. 1999).

Rashes with any feature(s) suggestive of a serious reaction necessitate immediate drug cessation, followed by monitoring for hepatic, renal, and hematological involvement. Tavernor et al. (1995) reported successfully restarting patients on lamotrigine after mild isolated rash; however, retitration should progress slowly and begin at 5–12.5 mg/day. Patients should not be rechallenged if they have had a serious rash, such as a reaction associated with systemic symptoms or internal toxicity (Besag et al. 2000). Because immune tolerance to lamotrigine is lost following interruption of dosage for more than 1 week, patients should be instructed to resume lamotrigine at the prior initial start-up dose and gradually titrate upward whenever therapy has been interrupted for more than a few days.

To explore whether the incidence of dermatological reactions could be mitigated by adherence to a series of dermatological precautions, Ketter et al. (2006) led an intervention study that randomly assigned patients to usual precautionary care versus dermatological precautionary care prior to initiation of lamotrigine therapy. Outpatients 13 years of age and older received 12 weeks of open-label lamotrigine and were instructed not to exceed the recommended initial dosage or dosage-escalation schedule. Those in the dermatological precautions group were instructed not to ingest new food, receive immunizations, or use new conditioners, cosmetics, soaps, detergents, or fabric softeners and to reduce exposure to poison ivy. Among 1,139 subjects enrolled into the trial, none experienced a serious rash. The incidence of nonserious rash did not differ between the usual care group (8.8%) and those advised to follow dermatological precautions (8.6%).

Attention must be drawn to the black box warning in the prescribing information, which instructs prescribers

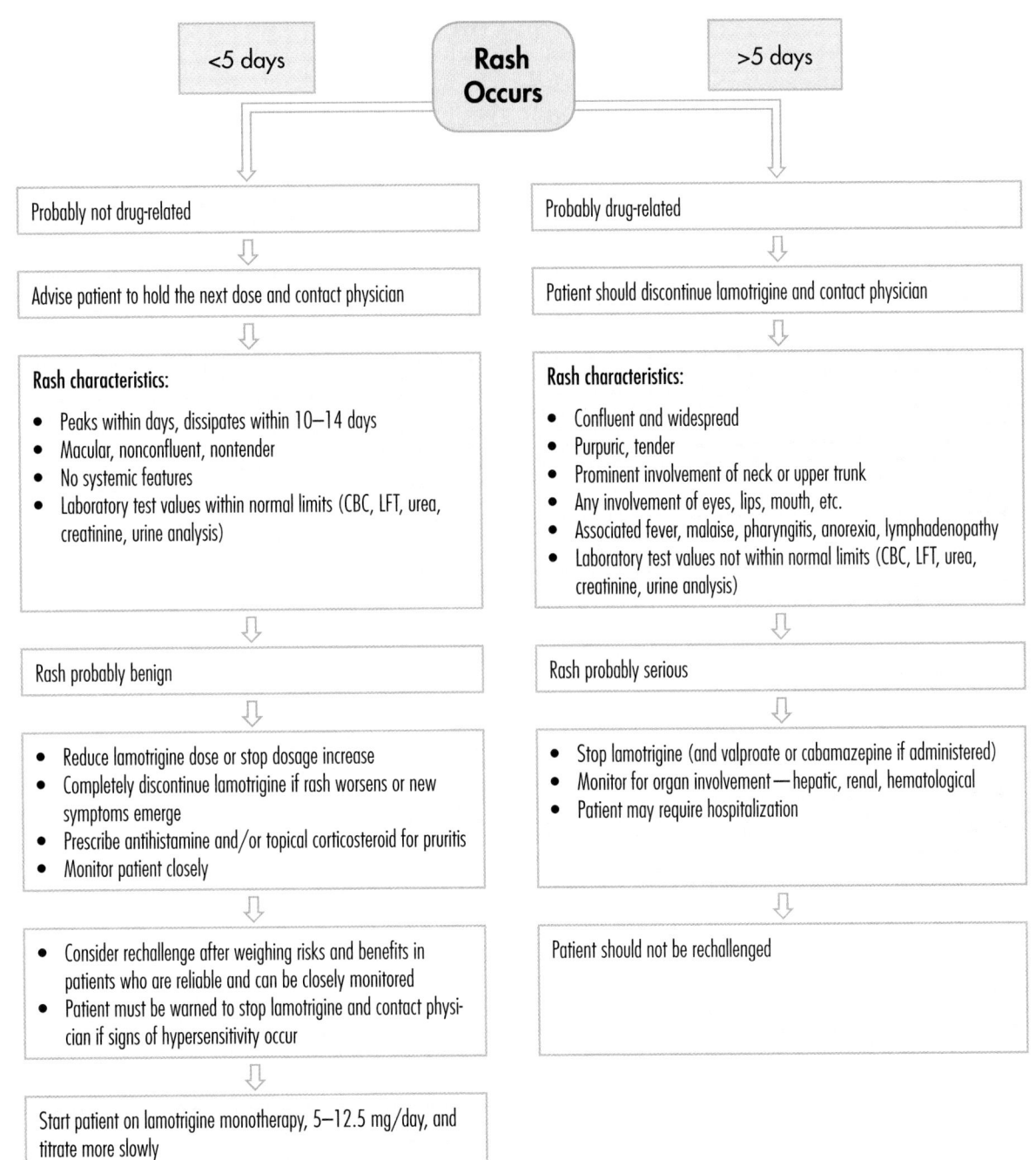

FIGURE 39–2. Clinical management of rash related to lamotrigine treatment.

CBC = complete blood count; LFT = liver function test.

Source. Reprinted from Calabrese JR, Sullivan JR, Bowden CL, et al: "Rash in Multicenter Trials of Lamotrigine in Mood Disorders: Clinical Relevance and Management." *Journal of Clinical Psychiatry* 63:1012–1019, 2002. Copyright 2000, Physicians Postgraduate Press. Used with permission.

to ordinarily discontinue lamotrigine "at the first sign of rash, unless the rash is clearly not drug related" because "it is not possible to predict reliably which rashes will prove to be serious or life threatening" (GlaxoSmithKline 2007).

Overdose

Among 493 cases of lamotrigine toxicity in overdose, the majority of patients (52.1%) experienced no toxic clinical effects (Lofton and Klein-Schwartz 2004). Common symptoms included drowsiness, vomiting, nausea, ataxia, dizziness, and tachycardia. Rare cases of coma, seizures, heart conduction delay, and respiratory depression have been reported in overdose. Some ingestions of lamotrigine involving quantities up to 15 grams have been fatal.

Use During Pregnancy

Lamotrigine may represent an option for women with bipolar disorder during pregnancy due to its favorable tolerability profile and maintenance effects against bipolar depression. An observational study by Newport et al. (2008) examined risk of illness recurrence in pregnant women with stable bipolar disorder who continued lamotrigine treatment during pregnancy ($n=10$) versus those who discontinued mood stabilizer therapy during pregnancy ($n=16$). The risk of illness recurrence was 3.3 times lower when lamotrigine was continued (30.0% recurrence [3/10] vs. 100% recurrence [16/16] when patients discontinued mood stabilizers; $P<0.0001$; odds ratio = 23.2; 95% confidence interval = 1.5–366). A reduced risk of depressive recurrence, as well as of manic or hypomanic recurrence, was observed with continued lamotrigine treatment. It remains unclear, however, whether lamotrigine carries a lower risk of major teratogenic defects compared with other mood-stabilizing medications.

Potential adverse effects to the developing fetus of mothers receiving lamotrigine are beginning to emerge upon examination of data from international pregnancy registries (Cunnington and Tennis 2004; Holmes et al. 2006). As with any mood stabilizer, lamotrigine use during pregnancy represents an inherent dilemma for clinicians and expectant mothers, who must balance the risks associated with untreated bipolar disorder with the potential for occurrence of major congenital malformations. During treatment with valproate or carbamazepine, neural tube defects are estimated to occur in 1%–5% of neonates after first-trimester exposure. However, the risk for malformations with newer antiepileptic drugs, including lamotrigine, is less well characterized. Preliminary data from the North American Antiepileptic Drug Pregnancy Registry suggests a possible association between first-trimester exposure to lamotrigine monotherapy and cleft lip and/or cleft palate (Holmes et al. 2006). The documented oral clefts were not part of a syndrome that included other birth defects. A total of 5 cases of oral cleft occurred among 564 pregnant women, resulting in a total prevalence of 8.9 cases per 1,000. This contrasts with 0.37 per 1,000 cases in an unexposed group, representing a 24-fold increase in risk. As this association requires confirmation from other prospectively collected registries or ongoing research, the validity of the findings are uncertain. An International Lamotrigine Registry, maintained by GlaxoSmithKline since 1992, recorded a total of 14 congenital malformations among 414 outcomes (2.9%) involving a first-trimester monotherapy exposure (Cunnington and Tennis 2004). This is similar to the background risk of 2%–3% for congenital malformations in the general population. Likewise, a more recent population-based case–control study found no evidence of increased risk for orofacial clefts relative to other malformations due to lamotrigine monotherapy (Dolk et al. 2008). Lamotrigine is listed as Pregnancy Category C in terms of teratogenic effects.

Drug–Drug Interactions

Lamotrigine is not known to inhibit the activity of the cytochrome P450 2D6 enzyme. However, the addition of adjunctive lamotrigine to enzyme inducers such as carbamazepine, phenytoin, primidone, and phenobarbital decreases lamotrigine plasma concentrations by approximately 40%–50% (Hahn et al. 2004). The inducing effect of oxcarbazepine is approximately half that of carbamazepine (Weintraub et al. 2005). Because lamotrigine is nearly exclusively metabolized by glucuronidation, the introduction of adjunctive valproate (an enzyme inhibitor) results in immediate and successful competition for metabolism, with resultant increases in half-life. The steady-state half-life for lamotrigine in the presence of valproate is 69.6 hours (Yau et al. 1992), compared with a multidose mean half-life of 25.4 hours with lamotrigine monotherapy (GlaxoSmithKline 2007). Mixed results have been found on the composite effect of administering lamotrigine in combination with valproate plus an enzyme-inducing antiepileptic drug. Some studies have found no difference in lamotrigine clearance from that associated with monotherapy (May et al. 1996), while others have found the inhibitory effects of valproate to predominate, resulting in lower lamotrigine clearance (May et al. 1996; Weintraub et al. 2005).

Evidence has emerged that oral contraceptives containing estrogen have the potential to decrease serum concentrations of lamotrigine by up to 64% (Sabers et al. 2001, 2003). During the long-term treatment of bipolar disorder, use of ethinyl estradiol–containing compounds may require an increase in the maintenance dose of lamotrigine by as much as twofold over the recommended target maintenance dose. Conversely, stopping estrogen-containing oral contraceptives, including during the "pill-free" week, may increase lamotrigine levels to a clinically significant range. It appears that progestogen-only compounds do not influence lamotrigine levels, regardless of whether administered by the oral, intramuscular, subdermal, or intrauterine modes (Reimers et al. 2005). Despite the potential for increased metabolism of lamotrigine when used in combination with oral contraceptives, the manufacturer does not recommend any dosage adjustments to the initial titration schedule.

Conclusion

The mechanism by which lamotrigine achieves its therapeutic effect in the treatment of bipolar disorder is unknown. However, its discovery has provided investigators with a novel AED for empirical validation in the routine treatment of bipolar disorder. Although initial results from trials of lamotrigine in the treatment of mania were unfavorable, subsequent maintenance studies have provided compelling data to show that lamotrigine prevents the recurrence of mood episodes and displays antidepressant efficacy, albeit most convincingly for the prophylaxis against depression in contrast to the acute diminution of depression. Even with its ability to stabilize mood from below baseline, lamotrigine appears to have a switch rate to mania or hypomania that is similar to treatment with placebo. Lamotrigine's neutral effects on body weight and favorable side-effect profile make it appealing for use in patients with comorbid metabolic syndrome or when other treatments have resulted in poor tolerability. At present, lamotrigine remains the only AED mood stabilizer with more established efficacy in the depressed illness phase than in mania or hypomania. Future controlled investigations should determine whether lamotrigine is effective in comorbid populations, such as individuals with substance use disorders, where it may act to both stabilize mood and decrease drug consumption. Trials are also needed to explore the use of lamotrigine in combination with other mood stabilizers or atypical antipsychotics, providing insight into whether combination treatment is superior to monotherapy in preventing mood relapse and recurrence.

References

Anand A, Charney DS, Oren DA, et al: Attenuation of the neuropsychiatric effects of ketamine with lamotrigine: support for hyperglutamatergic effects of N-methyl-D-aspartate receptor antagonists. Arch Gen Psychiatry 57:270–276, 2000

Ayala G, Matsumoto H, Gumnit R: Excitability changes and inhibitory mechanisms in neurocortical neurons during seizures. J Neurophysiol 33:73–85, 1970

Besag F, Ng G, Pool F: Successful re-introduction of lamotrigine after initial rash. Seizure 9:282–286, 2000

Bourin M, Masse F, Hascoet M: Evidence for the activity of lamotrigine at 5-HT(1A) receptors in the mouse forced swimming test. J Psychiatry Neurosci 30:275–282, 2005

Bowden CL, Calabrese JR, Ascher J, et al: Spectrum of efficacy of lamotrigine in bipolar disorder: overview of double-blind, placebo-controlled studies. Presented at the American College of Neuropsychopharmacology (ACNP) Annual Meeting, San Juan, PR, December 2000

Bowden CL, Calabrese JR, Sachs G, et al: A placebo-controlled 18-month trial of lamotrigine and lithium maintenance treatment in recently manic or hypomanic patients with bipolar I disorder. Arch Gen Psychiatry 60:392–400, 2003

Bowden CL, Asnis GM, Ginsberg LD, et al: Safety and tolerability of lamotrigine for bipolar disorder. Drug Saf 27:173–184, 2004

Bowden CL, Calabrese JR, Ketter TA, et al: Impact of lamotrigine and lithium on weight in obese and nonobese patients with bipolar I disorder. Am J Psychiatry 163:1199–1201, 2006

Bradburn NM: The Structure of Psychological Well-Being. Chicago, IL, Alpine, 1969

Brown EB, McElroy SL, Keck PE Jr, et al: A 7-week, randomized, double-blind trial of olanzapine/fluoxetine combination versus lamotrigine in the treatment of bipolar I depression. J Clin Psychiatry 67:1025–1033, 2006

Brown ES, Perantie DC, Dhanani N, et al: Lamotrigine for bipolar disorder and comorbid cocaine dependence: a replication and extension study. J Affect Disord 93:219–222, 2006

Calabrese JR, Bowden CL, McElroy SL, et al: Spectrum of activity of lamotrigine in treatment-refractory bipolar disorder. Am J Psychiatry 156:1019–1023, 1999a

Calabrese JR, Bowden CL, Sachs GS, et al: A double-blind placebo-controlled study of lamotrigine monotherapy in outpatients with bipolar I depression. J Clin Psychiatry 60:79–88, 1999b

Calabrese JR, Suppes T, Bowden C, et al: A double-blind, placebo-controlled, prophylaxis study of lamotrigine in rapid-cycling bipolar disorder. J Clin Psychiatry 61:841–850, 2000

Calabrese JR, Sullivan JR, Bowden CL, et al: Rash in multicenter trials of lamotrigine in mood disorders: clinical relevance and management. J Clin Psychiatry 63:1012–1019, 2002

Calabrese JR, Bowden CL, Sachs G, et al: A placebo-controlled 18-month trial of lamotrigine and lithium maintenance treatment in recently depressed patients with bipolar I disorder. J Clin Psychiatry 64:1013–1024, 2003

Calabrese JR, Goldberg JF, Ketter TA, et al: Recurrence in bipolar I disorder: a post hoc analysis excluding relapses in two double-blind maintenance studies. Biol Psychiatry 59:1061–1064, 2006

Calabrese JR, Huffman RF, White RL, et al: Lamotrigine in the acute treatment of bipolar depression: results of five double-blind, placebo-controlled clinical trials. Bipolar Disord 10:323–333, 2008

Cheung H, Kamp D, Harris E: An in vitro investigation of the action of lamotrigine on neuronal voltage-activated sodium channels. Epilepsy Res 13:107–112, 1992

Crumrine RC, Bergstrand K, Cooper AT, et al: Lamotrigine protects hippocampal CA1 neurons from ischemic damage after cardiac arrest. Stroke 28:2230–2236, 1997

Cunnington M, Tennis P: International Lamotrigine Pregnancy Registry Scientific Advisory Committee: Lamotrigine and the risk of malformations in pregnancy. Neurology 64:955–960, 2004

Daly K, Fatemi S: Lamotrigine and impulse behavior. Can J Psychiatry 44:395–396, 1999

Davanzo P, King B: Open trial of lamotrigine in the treatment of self-injurious behavior in an adolescent with profound mental retardation. J Child Adolesc Psychopharmacol 6:273–279, 1996

Devarajan S, Dursun S: Aggression in dementia with lamotrigine treatment. Am J Psychiatry 157:1178, 2000

DeVeaugh-Geiss J, Ascher J, Brook S, et al: Safety and tolerability of lamotrigine in controlled monotherapy trials in mood disorders. Presented at the American College of Neuropsychopharmacology (ACNP) Annual Meeting, San Juan, PR, December 2000

Dolk H, Jentink J, Loane M, et al: Does lamotrigine use in pregnancy increase orofacial cleft risk relative to other malformations? Neurology 71:714–722, 2008

Dubovsky SL: Calcium antagonists in manic-depressive illness. Neuropsychobiology 27:184–192, 1993

Erfurth A, Amann BA, Grunze H: Female genital disorder as adverse symptom of lamotrigine treatment: a serotonergic effect? Neuropsychobiology 38:200–201, 1998a

Erfurth A, Walden J, Grunze H: Lamotrigine in the treatment of schizoaffective disorder. Neuropsychobiology 38:204–205, 1998b

Fervenza FC, Kanakiriya S, Kunau RT, et al: Acute granulomatous interstitial nephritis and colitis in anticonvulsant hypersensitivity syndrome associated with lamotrigine treatment. Am J Kidney Dis 36:1034–1040, 2000

Fix OK, Peters MG, Davern TJ: Eosinophilic hepatitis caused by lamotrigine. Clin Gastroenterol Hepatol 4:xxvi, 2006

Gabriel A: Lamotrigine adjunctive treatment in resistant unipolar depression: an open, descriptive study. Depress Anxiety 23:485–488, 2006

Geddes JR, Calabrese JR, Goodwin GM: Lamotrigine for treatment of bipolar depression: an independent meta-analysis and meta-regression of individual patient data from 5 randomized trials. Br J Psychiatry Br J Psychiatry 194:4–9, 2009

Ghaemi SN, Pardo RB, Hsu DJ: Strategies for preventing the recurrence of bipolar disorder. J Clin Psychiatry 65 (suppl):16–23, 2004

GlaxoSmithKline: Lamictal (lamotrigine) prescribing information. Research Triangle Park, NC, GlaxoSmithKline, May 2007. Available at: http://us.gsk.com/products/assets/us_lamictal.pdf

Goodwin GM, Bowden CL, Calabrese JR, et al: A pooled analysis of 2 placebo-controlled 18-month trials of lamotrigine and lithium maintenance in bipolar I disorder. J Clin Psychiatry 65:432–441, 2004

Grunze H, von Wegerer J, Greene RW, et al: Modulation of calcium and potassium currents by lamotrigine. Neuropsychobiology 38:131–138, 1998

Guberman A, Besag F, Brodie M, et al: Lamotrigine-associated rash: risk/benefit considerations in adults and children. Epilepsia 40:985–991, 1999

Hahn CG, Gyulai L, Baldassano CF, et al: The current understanding of lamotrigine as a mood stabilizer. J Clin Psychiatry 65:791–804, 2004

Harrison N, Simmonds M: Quantitative studies on some antagonists of N-methyl-D-aspartate in slices of rat cerebral cortex. Br J Pharmacol 84:381–391, 1985

Hertzberg M, Butterfield M, Feldman M, et al: A preliminary study of lamotrigine for the treatment of posttraumatic stress disorder. Biol Psychiatry 45:1226–1229, 1999

Holmes LB, Wyszynski DF, Baldwin EJ, et al: Increased risk for nonsyndromic cleft palate among infants exposed to lamotrigine during pregnancy. Birth Defects Res A Clin Mol Teratol 76:318, 2006

Jawad S, Richens A, Goodwin G, et al: Controlled trial of lamotrigine (Lamictal) for refractory partial seizures. Epilepsia 30:656–663, 1989

Kemp DE, Gilmer WS, Fleck J, et al: An association of intrusive, repetitive phrases with lamotrigine treatment in bipolar II disorder. CNS Spectr 12:106–111, 2007

Ketter TA, Greist JH, Graham JA, et al: The effect of dermatologic precautions on the incidence of rash with addition of lamotrigine in the treatment of bipolar I disorder: a randomized trial. J Clin Psychiatry 67:400–406, 2006

Lang D, Wang C: Lamotrigine and phenytoin interactions on ionic channels present in N4TG1 and GH3 clonal cells. Soc Neurosci Abs 17:1256, 1991

Lang D, Wang C, Cooper B: Lamotrigine, phenytoin, and carbamazepine interactions on the sodium current present in N4TG1 mouse neuroblastoma cells. J Pharmacol Exp Ther 266:829–835, 1993

Laurenza A, Asnis G, Beaman M, et al: A double-blind, placebo-controlled study supporting the efficacy of lamotrigine in unipolar depression. Bipolar Disord 1 (suppl):39–40, 1999

Leach MJ, Marden CM, Miller AA: Pharmacological studies on lamotrigine, a novel potential antiepileptic drug, II: neurochemical studies on the mechanism of action. Epilepsia 27:490–497, 1986

Leach MJ, Lees G, Riddall DR: Lamotrigine: mechanisms of action, in Antiepileptic Drugs, 4th Edition. Edited by Levy RH, Mattson RH, Meldrum BS. New York, Raven, 1995, pp 861–869

Lofton AL, Klein-Schwartz W: Evaluation of lamotrigine toxicity reported to poison control centers. Ann Pharmacother 38:1811–1815, 2004

Lombroso C: Lamotrigine-induced tourettism. Neurology 52:1191–1194, 1999

Maj R, Fariello RG, Ukmar G, et al: PNU-151774E protects against kainate-induced status epilepticus and hippocampal lesions in the rat. Eur J Pharmacol 359:27–32, 1998

May TW, Rambeck B, Jurgens U: Serum concentrations of lamotrigine in epileptic patients: the influence of dose and comedication. Ther Drug Monit 18:523–531, 1996

McDonald MA, Favilla I: Visual loss in a patient with lamotrigine-induced cicatrizing conjunctivitis. Clin Exp Ophthalmol 31:541–543, 2003

Messenheimer JA, Mullens EL, Giorgi L, et al: Safety review of adult clinical trial experience with lamotrigine. Drug Saf 18:281–296, 1998

Mewasingh L, Aylett S, Kirkham F, et al: Hyponatraemia associated with lamotrigine in cranial diabetes insipidus. Lancet 356:656, 2000

Miller AA, Wheatley P, Sawyer DA, et al: Pharmacological studies on lamotrigine, a novel antiepileptic drug: anticonvulsant profile in mice and rats. Epilepsia 27:483–489, 1986

Muzina DJ, Elhaj O, Gajwani P, et al: Lamotrigine and antiepileptic drugs as mood stabilizers in bipolar disorder. Acta Psychiatr Scand 111 (suppl):21–28, 2005

Newport DJ, Stowe ZN, Viguera AC, et al: Lamotrigine in bipolar disorder: efficacy during pregnancy. Bipolar Disord 10:432–436, 2008

Ohman I, Vitols S, Tomson T: Lamotrigine in pregnancy: pharmacokinetics during delivery, in the neonate, and during lactation. Epilepsia 41:709–713, 2000

Pearlin L, Schooler C: The structure of coping. J Health Soc Behav 19:2–21, 1978

Pennell PB: Antiepileptic drug pharmacokinetics during pregnancy and lactation. Neurology 61:S35–S42, 2003

Pennell PB, Newport DJ, Stowe ZN, et al: The impact of pregnancy and childbirth on the metabolism of lamotrigine. Neurology 62:292–295, 2004

Pinto O, Akiskal H: Lamotrigine as a promising approach to borderline personality: an open case series without DSM-IV major mood disorder. J Affect Disord 51:333–343, 1998

Post R, Weiss S, Pert A: Differential effects of carbamazepine and lithium on sensitization and kindling. Prog Neuropsychopharmacol Biol Psychiatry 8:425–434, 1984

Post R, Nolen WA, Kupka RW, et al: The Stanley Foundation Bipolar Network, I: rationale and methods. Br J Psychiatry Suppl 41:S169–S176, 2001

Reimers A, Helde G, Brodtkorb E: Ethinyl estradiol, not progestogens, reduces lamotrigine serum concentrations. Epilepsia 46:1414–1417, 2005

Rubio G, Lopez-Munoz F, Alamo C: Effects of lamotrigine in patients with bipolar disorder and alcohol dependence. Bipolar Disord 8:289–293, 2006

Saba G, Dumortier G, Kalalou K, et al: Lamotrigine-clozapine combination in refractory schizophrenia: three cases. J Neuropsychiatry Clin Neurosci 14:1, 2002

Sabers A, Buchholt J, Uldall P, et al: Lamotrigine plasma levels reduced by oral contraceptives. Epilepsy Res 47:151–154, 2001

Sabers A, Ohman I, Christensen J, et al: Oral contraceptives reduce lamotrigine plasma levels. Neurology 26:570–571, 2003

Sachs G, Bowden CL, Calabrese JR, et al: Effects of lamotrigine and lithium on body weight during maintenance treatment of bipolar I disorder. Bipolar Disord 8:175–181, 2006

Sarzi-Puttini P, Panni B, Cazzola M, et al: Lamotrigine-induced lupus. Lupus 9:555–557, 2000

Sbei M, Campellone J: Stupor from lamotrigine toxicity. Epilepsia 42:1082–1083, 2001

Schaffer A, Zucker P, Levitt A: Randomized, double-blind pilot trial comparing lamotrigine versus citalopram for the treatment of bipolar depression. J Affect Disord 96:95–99, 2006

Shiah IS, Yatham LN, Lam RW, et al: Effects of lamotrigine on the 5-HT1A receptor function in healthy human males. J Affect Disord 49:157–162, 1998

Showalter P, Kimmel D: Stimulation of consciousness and cognition after severe brain injury. Brain Inj 14:997–1001, 2000

Sierra M, Baker D, Medford N, et al: Lamotrigine as an add-on treatment for depersonalization disorder: a retrospective study of 32 cases. Clin Neuropharmacol 29:253–258, 2006

Smith D, Chadwick D, Baker G, et al: Seizure severity and the quality of life. Epilepsia 34 (suppl):S31–S35, 1993

Southam E, Pereira R, Stratton SC, et al: Effect of lamotrigine on the activities of monoamine oxidases A and B in vitro and on monoamine disposition in vivo. Eur J Pharmacol 519:237–245, 2005

Spearing MK, Post RM, Leverich GS, et al: Modification of the Clinical Global Impressions (CGI) scale for use in bipolar illness (BP): the CGI-BP. Psychiatry Res 73:159–171, 1997

Stefani A, Spadoni F, Sinischali A, et al: Lamotrigine inhibits Ca2+ currents in cortical neurons: functional implications. Eur J Pharmacol 307:113–116, 1996

Stenbom Y, Tonnby B, Hagberg B: Lamotrigine in Rett syndrome: treatment experience from a pilot study. Eur Child Adolesc Psychiatry 7:49–52, 1998

Tavernor S, Wong I, Newton R, et al: Rechallenge with lamotrigine after initial rash. Seizure 4:67–71, 1995

Tekin S, Aykut-Bingol C, Tanridag T, et al: Antiglutamatergic therapy in Alzheimer's disease: effects of lamotrigine. J Neural Transm 105:295–303, 1998

van der Loos M, Nolen WA, Vieta E, et al: Lamotrigine as add-on to lithium in bipolar depression. Presented at the fifth European Stanley Conference on Bipolar Disorder, Barcelona, Spain, October 2006

von Wegerer J, Hesslinger B, Berger M, et al: A calcium antagonistic effect of the new antiepileptic drug lamotrigine. Eur Neuropsychopharmacol 7:77–78, 1997

Weintraub D, Buchsbaum R, Resor SR Jr, et al: Effect of antiepileptic drug comedication on lamotrigine clearance. Arch Neurol 62:1432–1436, 2005

Xie X, Hagan RM: Cellular and molecular actions of lamotrigine: possible mechanisms of efficacy in bipolar disorder. Neuropsychobiology 38:119–130, 1998

Yau M, Wargin W, Wolf K, et al: Effect of valproate on the pharmacokinetics of lamotrigine at steady state. Epilepsia 33 (suppl):82, 1992

CHAPTER 40

Topiramate

Susan L. McElroy, M.D.

Paul E. Keck Jr., M.D.

History and Discovery

Topiramate is a derivative of the naturally occurring monosaccharide D-fructose. It was originally synthesized to be a structural analog of fructose-1,6-diphosphatase as part of a project to develop agents that inhibit gluconeogenesis by inhibiting the enzyme fructose-1,6-biphosphatase (Shank et al. 2000). To date, however, it has not been shown by clinical evidence to have direct hypoglycemic activity. Topiramate contains a sulfamate moiety. The structural resemblance of this moiety to the sulfonamide moiety in the established antiepileptic drug acetazolamide prompted researchers to evaluate topiramate for possible anticonvulsant effects. Topiramate subsequently was shown to have potent anticonvulsant properties in a broad range of preclinical epilepsy models (Shank et al. 2000).

The drug's efficacy in patients with epilepsy was established in the early 1990s. These studies also showed that topiramate had a favorable pharmacokinetic profile, had a high therapeutic index, was not associated with hematological or hepatic abnormalities, did not require routine serum concentration monitoring, and was associated with anorexia and weight loss (rather than appetite stimulation and weight gain like some other antiepileptic drugs) (Langtry et al. 1997). Topiramate was approved by the U.S. Food and Drug Administration (FDA) for the treatment of epilepsy in 1996. It was approved for migraine prevention in adults in 2004.

Reports appearing in the late 1990s of the drug having potential beneficial effects in bipolar disorder led Johnson and Johnson Pharmaceutical Research and Development

(PRD), the discoverer and manufacturer of topiramate, to conduct a large clinical study program of topiramate in the treatment of acute bipolar mania (McElroy and Keck 2004). Controlled trials of the drug in bipolar adults with manic symptoms failed to demonstrate significant separation between the topiramate and placebo groups (Chengappa et al. 2006; Kushner et al. 2006). However, topiramate has been shown to be efficacious in placebo-controlled trials in several neuropsychiatric conditions often comorbid with bipolar disorder, including, in addition to migraine, binge-eating disorder (BED), bulimia nervosa, alcohol dependence, borderline personality disorder (BPD), psychotropic-associated weight gain, and obesity.

Structure–Activity Relations

Topiramate is a sulfamate-substituted monosaccharide derived from D-fructose (Figure 40–1). As such, it is structurally distinct from other antiepileptic medications. Its sulfamate moiety is essential for its pharmacological activity (Shank et al. 2000). It has been postulated that topiramate's multiple pharmacological properties (which are discussed in the following section) are regulated by protein phosphorylation. Specifically, it has been hypothesized that topiramate interacts with voltage-activated sodium channels, γ-aminobutyric acid (GABA) type A ($GABA_A$) receptors, α-amino-3-hydroxy-5-methyl-isoxazole-4-propionic acid (AMPA)/kainate glutamate receptors, and high-voltage-activated calcium channels via formation of hydrogen bonds between proton-accepting oxygens in its sulfamate moiety and proton donor groups

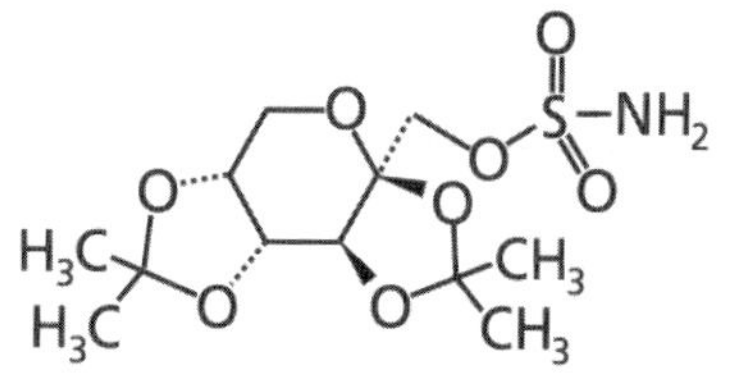

FIGURE 40–1.   Chemical structure of topiramate.

in tetrapeptide sequences in the latter (Shank et al. 2000).

Pharmacological Profile

Topiramate has multiple pharmacological properties that may contribute to its anticonvulsant effects, as well as its therapeutic effects in other neuropsychiatric disorders (Langtry et al. 1997; Rho and Sankar 1999; Rosenfeld 1997; Shank et al. 2000; White 2002, 2005; White et al. 2007). First, topiramate inhibits voltage-gated sodium channels in a voltage-sensitive, use-dependent manner and thus suppresses action potentials associated with sustained repetitive cell firing (Kawasaki et al. 1998; Shank et al. 2000).

Second, topiramate increases brain GABA levels, possibly by activating a site on the GABA$_A$ receptor, thereby enhancing the inhibitory chloride ion influx mediated by the GABA$_A$ receptor and potentiating GABA-evoked currents (Kuzniecky et al. 1998; Petroff et al. 2001; Simeone et al. 2006). Because this action is not blocked by the benzodiazepine antagonist flumazenil, it is thought that topiramate exerts this effect via an interaction with the GABA$_A$ receptor that is not modulated by benzodiazepines (White et al. 2000). This action may also be sensitive to GABA concentrations and GABA$_A$ receptor subunit composition (Simeone et al. 2006).

Third, topiramate antagonizes glutamate receptors of the AMPA/kainate subtype and may selectively inhibit glutamate receptor 5 (GluR$_5$) kainate receptors (Kaminski et al. 2004). It has essentially no effect on glutamate N-methyl-D-aspartate (NMDA) receptors. AMPA/kainate receptors mediate fast excitatory postsynaptic potentials responsible for excitatory neurotransmission; blockade of kainate-evoked currents decreases neuronal excitability.

Fourth, topiramate negatively modulates high-voltage-activated calcium channels (Zhang et al. 2000). Of note, Shank et al. (2000) proposed that topiramate's combined effects on voltage-activated sodium channels,

GABA$_A$ receptors, AMPA/kainate receptors, and high-voltage-activated calcium channels are unique as compared with those of other antiepileptic drugs. Indeed, Schiffer et al. (2001) found that pretreatment with topiramate inhibited nicotine-induced increases in mesolimbic extracellular dopamine and norepinephrine but not serotonin. They hypothesized that this property was a result of the drug's ability to affect both GABAergic and glutamatergic function.

Fifth, topiramate has weak inhibitory actions against some carbonic anhydrase isoenzymes, including subtypes II and VI. Carbonic anhydrase is essential for the generation of GABA$_A$-mediated depolarizing responses. By inhibiting carbonic anhydrase, topiramate has been shown to reversibly reduce the GABA$_A$-mediated depolarizing responses evoked by either synaptic stimulation or pressure application of GABA (but not to modify GABA$_A$-mediated hyperpolarizing postsynaptic potentials) (Herrero et al. 2002). As a result of the effects of carbonic anhydrase inhibition on intracellular pH, topiramate also may activate a potassium conductance (Herrero et al. 2002).

Finally, topiramate has been shown to have a number of other properties. These include an interaction with glycine receptor channels (Mohammadi et al. 2005), effects on mitochondrial permeability (Kudin et al. 2004), and antikindling properties in some animal models (Wauguier and Zhou 1996).

Pharmacokinetics and Disposition

Topiramate has a favorable pharmacokinetic profile (Bialer et al. 2004; Doose and Streeter 2002; Langtry et al. 1997; Rosenfeld 1997; Shank et al. 2000). It is rapidly and almost completely absorbed after oral administration, with bioavailability estimated to be about 80%. Peak plasma concentrations are reached within 2–4 hours. Plasma concentration increases in proportion to dose over the pharmacologically relevant dose range.

The volume of distribution of topiramate is inversely proportional to the dose, with the drug distributed primarily to body water. It is minimally protein-bound (9%–17%).

Topiramate is minimally metabolized by the liver in the absence of hepatic enzyme–inducing drugs. It inhibits cytochrome P450 (CYP) enzyme 2C19 but not other hepatic CYP enzymes. Topiramate is excreted mostly unchanged (approximately 70%) in the urine. The nonrenal (hepatic) clearance of topiramate increases two- to threefold when the drug is administered with hepatic enzyme–inducing drugs such as carbamazepine and phenytoin. Six minor metabolites have been identified (Shank et al. 2000).

Topiramate's elimination half-life is 19–25 hours, with linear pharmacokinetics in the dose range of 100–1,200 mg. The pharmacokinetics of topiramate in children are similar to those in adults, except that clearance is 50% higher, resulting in 33% lower plasma concentrations. Moderate or severe renal failure is associated with reduced renal clearance and increased elimination half-life of topiramate. Moderate or severe liver impairment is associated with clinically insignificant increased plasma concentrations of the drug.

Mechanism of Action

Although the mechanism of topiramate's anticonvulsant action is unknown, it has been hypothesized to be due to some combination of the drug's multiple pharmacological properties (Rho and Sankar 1999; Shank et al. 2000; White 2002, 2005; White et al. 2007).

As discussed, these include state-dependent blockade of voltage-activated sodium channels, enhancement of GABA activity at the $GABA_A$ receptor via interaction with a nonbenzodiazepine receptor site, antagonism of the AMPA/kainate glutamate receptor, antagonism of high-voltage-activated calcium channels, and inhibition of carbonic anhydrase. For example, the drug's anticonvulsant profile, as well as its benefits in substance use and eating disorders, has been hypothesized to be due to its dual actions on the GABAergic and glutamatergic systems (Johnson et al. 2003, 2005; McElroy et al. 2003, 2007b; Rho and Sankar 1999; Schiffer et al. 2001). By contrast, carbonic anhydrase inhibition is thought by some not to play a large role in topiramate's anticonvulsant properties despite acetazolamide's clinical efficacy as an antiepileptic because of topiramate's much weaker potency as an inhibitor (Rho and Sankar 1999). Others, however, have suggested that topiramate's inhibition of carbonic anhydrase contributes to its anticonvulsant properties via reduction of $GABA_A$-mediated depolarizing responses and/or activation of a potassium conductance (Herrero et al. 2002).

Indications and Efficacy

FDA-Approved Indications

Topiramate is currently indicated by the FDA as initial monotherapy in patients 10 years of age and older with partial-onset or primary generalized tonic-clonic seizures; as adjunctive therapy for adults and pediatric patients ages 2–16 years with partial-onset seizures or primary generalized tonic-clonic seizures; and in patients 2 years of age and older with seizures associated with Lennox-Gastaut syndrome (van Passel et al. 2006). It is also indicated for the prophylaxis of migraine headache in adults (Brandes 2005; Bussone et al. 2006).

Other Indications

Topiramate is not currently approved by the FDA for use in the treatment of any psychiatric disorder. Because the drug was widely used off-label in the treatment of bipolar disorder after it came to market (see subsection "Bipolar Disorder" below), Johnson and Johnson PRD, the discoverer of topiramate, conducted a large study program of topiramate in adults with acute bipolar mania. These placebo-controlled studies failed to demonstrate a significant benefit of topiramate over placebo on the Young Mania Rating Scale (YMRS) (Chengappa et al. 2001a; Kushner et al. 2006; McElroy and Keck 2004). In contrast, a placebo-controlled trial in pediatric mania, which was prematurely discontinued in the aftermath of the failed adult trials, did show significant efficacy results favoring topiramate based on a retrospective analysis of 56 patients (DelBello et al. 2005).

Topiramate has been studied in the treatment of a variety of other neuropsychiatric disorders, many of which co-occur with bipolar disorder. Data from placebo-controlled clinical trials suggest that topiramate is efficacious in BED with obesity (McElroy et al. 2003, 2007b), bulimia nervosa (Hedges et al. 2003; Hoopes et al. 2003; C. Nickel et al. 2005b), alcohol dependence (Johnson et al. 2003, 2007), psychotropic-induced weight gain (Ko et al. 2005; M.K. Nickel et al. 2005b), obesity (McElroy et al. 2008), and neuropathic pain (Raskin et al. 2004). These and other studies will be reviewed below.

Bipolar Disorder

Five randomized, placebo-controlled studies have shown that topiramate monotherapy is not efficacious in the short-term treatment of acute manic or mixed episodes in adults with bipolar I disorder (Kushner et al. 2006; McElroy and Keck 2004). All five studies used week 3 as the primary endpoint; in addition, three studies had a week 12 secondary endpoint, two studies had lithium comparator groups, and all trials measured weight as a secondary outcome. Analyses of the 3-week data from all five trials were consistent. In each trial, the primary efficacy outcome—

the change from baseline to week 3 in the YMRS score—failed to show a statistically significant separation between topiramate and placebo. There was also no drug–placebo separation in the three trials with week 12 data. By contrast, in the two trials in which lithium was used, lithium did show statistical superiority to placebo. Topiramate, however, showed significant separation from placebo in weight loss, whereas lithium was associated with statistically significant weight gain.

Similarly, in the only placebo-controlled study of adjunctive topiramate in bipolar disorder, 287 outpatients experiencing a manic or mixed episode (by DSM-IV [American Psychiatric Association 1994] criteria) and a YMRS score ≥18 while taking therapeutic levels of valproate or lithium showed similar reductions (40%) in baseline YMRS scores for both topiramate and placebo after 12 weeks (Chengappa et al. 2006). Topiramate, however, was again associated with significant weight loss as compared to placebo.

Despite the negative results of the adult acute mania trials, numerous clinical reports suggest that topiramate may have a role in the management of bipolar disorder. In the only placebo-controlled study of topiramate in pediatric bipolar I disorder, 56 children and adolescents (6–17 years) with manic or mixed episodes were randomly assigned to topiramate ($n = 29$) or placebo ($n = 27$) for 4 weeks (DelBello et al. 2005). Initially designed to enroll approximately 230 subjects, the study was prematurely discontinued when the adult mania trials were negative. Decrease in mean YMRS score from baseline to final visit using last observation carried forward (LOCF) was not statistically different between treatment groups (-9.7 ± 9.65 for topiramate vs. -4.7 ± 9.79 for placebo, $P = 0.152$). However, a post hoc repeated-measures linear regression model of the primary efficacy analysis showed a statistically significant difference in the slopes of the linear mean profiles ($P = 0.003$).

No placebo-controlled study of topiramate has yet been done in acute bipolar depression. Results from an 8-week single-blind comparison trial in which 36 outpatient adults with bipolar depression were randomly assigned to receive either topiramate (mean dosage = 176 mg/day; range = 50–300 mg/day) or bupropion SR (sustained release) (mean dosage = 250 mg/day; range = 100–400 mg/day) suggested that the drug might have antidepressant properties in some bipolar patients (McIntyre et al. 2002). The percentage of patients meeting a priori response criteria (50% or greater decrease from baseline in mean total score on the 17-item Hamilton Rating Scale for Depression [Ham-D]) was significant for both topiramate (56%) and bupropion SR (59%). There were no cases of manic switching with either drug. Moreover, numerous open-label reports have described patients with milder forms of bipolarity (i.e., "soft" bipolar spectrum disorders), including those with mixed states or rapid cycling, that respond to topiramate (McElroy and Keck 2004; McElroy et al. 2000; McIntyre et al. 2005).

Finally, a number of open-label reports have described the successful topiramate treatment of bipolar disorder with various comorbid psychiatric or general medical disorders ("complicated" bipolar disorder). Comorbid psychiatric conditions in which improvement was seen included alcohol abuse; anxiety disorders such as obsessive-compulsive disorder (OCD) and posttraumatic stress disorder (PTSD); eating disorders such as bulimia nervosa, BED, and anorexia nervosa; impulse-control disorders; and catatonia (Barzman and DelBello 2006; Guille and Sachs 2002; Huguelet and Morand-Collomb 2005; McDaniel et al. 2006; McElroy et al. 2008; Shapira et al. 2000). Comorbid general medical conditions in which improvement was seen included obesity, psychotropic-induced weight gain, type 2 diabetes mellitus, tremor, and Tourette's disorder (Chengappa et al. 2001b; Guille and Sachs 2002; McIntyre et al. 2005; Vieta et al. 2002).

These observations call for controlled studies of topiramate in pediatric bipolar disorder, acute bipolar depression, bipolar II disorder and other "softer" forms of bipolar disorder, and complicated bipolar disorder. No controlled maintenance or prophylactic treatment studies of topiramate in bipolar disorder have yet been completed.

Depressive Disorders

In the only controlled study of topiramate in a depressive disorder, 64 females with DSM-IV recurrent major depressive disorder were randomly assigned to topiramate ($n = 32$) or placebo ($n = 32$) for 10 weeks (C. Nickel et al. 2005a). Topiramate was superior to placebo in reducing depressive and anger symptoms (as assessed by the Ham-D [$P = 0.02$] and the State-Trait Anger Expression Inventory [STAXI; $P < 0.001$ on all scales]), respectively, and on most scales of the SF-36 Health Survey (all Ps between 0.15 and 0.001). The reduction in expression of anger correlated significantly with changes on the Ham-D. Five subjects (2 topiramate, 3 placebo) were lost to follow-up. Weight loss was greater in the topiramate group by 4.2 kg ($P < 0.001$). All subjects tolerated topiramate well, and there were no suicidal events.

Psychotic Disorders

Two randomized, placebo-controlled studies of topiramate targeting psychopathology in psychotic disorders have been conducted. In the first, 26 patients with treatment-resistant schizophrenia had topiramate (gradually increased to 300 mg/day) or placebo added to their ongoing treatment (clozapine, olanzapine, risperidone, or quetiapine) over two 12-week crossover treatment periods (Tiihonen et al. 2005). In the intent-to-treat analysis, topiramate was superior to placebo in reducing general psychopathological symptoms as assessed by the Positive and Negative Syndrome Scale (PANSS), but no significant improvement was observed in positive or negative symptoms.

In the second study, 48 patients with schizoaffective disorder, bipolar type, were randomly assigned in a 2:1 ratio (favoring topiramate) to 8 weeks of double-blind treatment with topiramate (100–400 mg/day) or placebo (Chengappa et al. 2007). Patients who had achieved ≥20% decrease from baseline in their PANSS total scores were given the opportunity to continue for an additional 8 weeks of double-blind treatment. Study medication dosage was continued unchanged from the earlier 8-week study period. Adjunctive topiramate (nearly 275 mg/day) did not show increased efficacy relative to placebo on the PANSS (the primary outcome measure) or on any of the secondary outcome measures. Topiramate-treated patients lost significantly more body weight than did placebo-treated patients, but they also experienced higher rates of paresthesias, sedation, word-finding difficulty, sleepiness, and forgetfulness.

Case reports regarding topiramate's effectiveness as an adjunct treatment in schizophrenia have been inconsistent, with improvement, no change, and deterioration in clinical state all being described (Citrome 2008). However, there are several case reports of the successful use of topiramate to treat catatonia in patients with chronic psychotic disorders (McDaniel et al. 2006).

Eating Disorders

Five randomized, placebo-controlled studies have shown that topiramate reduces binge eating and excessive body weight in 640 subjects with bulimia nervosa (n = 2 studies, 99 subjects) or BED (n = 3 studies, 541 subjects). In the first study in bulimia nervosa, a 10-week trial in 69 subjects, topiramate (median dosage = 100 mg/day; range = 25–400 mg/day) was superior to placebo in reducing the frequency of binge and purge days (days during which at least one binge-eating or purging episode occurred; P = 0.004); de-

creasing scores on the bulimia/uncontrollable overeating (P = 0.005), body dissatisfaction (P = 0.007), and drive for thinness (P = 0.002) subscales of the Eating Disorder Inventory; decreasing scores on the bulimia/food preoccupation (P = 0.019) and dieting (P = 0.031) subscales of the Eating Attitudes Test; and reducing body weight (mean decrease of 1.8 kg for topiramate vs. 0.2 kg mean increase for placebo; P = 0.004) (Hedges et al. 2003; Hoopes et al. 2003). Binge-eating/purging remission rates were 32% for topiramate and 6% for placebo (P = NS). Dropout rates were 34% for topiramate and 47% for placebo. In the second study, 60 subjects with DSM-IV bulimia nervosa for at least 12 months received 10 weeks of topiramate (titrated to 250 mg/day in the sixth week) (n = 30) or placebo (n = 30) (C. Nickel et al. 2005b). Topiramate was associated with significant decreases in binge/purge frequency (defined as a >50% reduction; 37% for topiramate and 3% for placebo), body weight (difference in weight loss between the 2 groups = 3.8 kg), and all of the SF-36 Health Survey scales (all Ps < 0.001). Five (17%) subjects on topiramate and 6 (20%) subjects on placebo were dropouts.

In the first controlled study in BED, 61 subjects with DSM-IV BED and obesity (defined as a body mass index [BMI] ≥30) received topiramate (n = 30) or placebo (n = 31) for 14 weeks (McElroy et al. 2003). Topiramate was significantly superior to placebo in reducing binge frequency, as well as global severity of illness, obsessive-compulsive features of binge-eating symptoms, body weight, and BMI. Topiramate-treated subjects experienced a 94% reduction in binge frequency and a mean weight loss of 5.9 kg, whereas placebo-treated subjects experienced a 46% reduction in binge frequency and a mean weight loss of 1.2 kg. The dropout rate, however, was high—14 (47%) subjects receiving topiramate and 12 (39%) subjects receiving placebo failed to complete the trial.

The second controlled study of topiramate in BED was a multicenter trial in which subjects with DSM-IV BED and ±3 binge-eating days per week, a BMI ranging from 30 kg/m² to 50 kg/m², and no current psychiatric disorders or substance abuse were randomly assigned in a 1:1 ratio to topiramate or placebo for 16 weeks (McElroy et al. 2007b). Of 407 subjects enrolled, 13 failed to meet inclusion criteria; 95 topiramate and 199 placebo subjects were therefore evaluated for efficacy. Topiramate significantly reduced binge-eating days per week (−3.5±1.9 vs. −2.5±2.1), binge episodes per week (−5±4.3 vs. −3.4±3.8), weight (−4.5±5.1 kg vs. 0.2±3.2 kg), and BMI (−1.6±1.8 kg/m² vs. 0.1±1.2 kg/m²) compared with placebo (all Ps < 0.001). The drug also significantly decreased measures of obsessive-compulsive symptoms, impulsivity, hunger, and disability. Fifty-eight percent of topiramate-treated subjects achieved remission compared with 29% of placebo-treated subjects ($P<0.001$). Discontinuation rates were 30% in each group; adverse events were the most common reason for topiramate discontinuation (16%; placebo, 8%).

The third controlled study of topiramate in BED was another multicenter trial in which 73 patients with BED and obesity were randomly assigned to 19 sessions of cognitive-behavior therapy in conjunction with topiramate ($n=37$) or placebo ($n=36$) for 21 weeks (Claudino et al. 2007). Compared with patients given placebo, patients given topiramate showed a significantly greater rate of reduction in weight, the primary outcome measure, over the course of treatment ($P<0.001$). Topiramate recipients also showed a significant weight loss (−6.8 kg) relative to placebo recipients (−0.9 kg). Rates of reduction of binge frequencies and scores on the Binge Eating Scale and BDI did not differ between the groups, but a greater percentage of topiramate-treated patients (31 of 37) than of placebo-treated patients (22 of 36) attained remission of binge eating ($P=0.03$). There was no difference between groups in completion rates, although one topiramate recipient withdrew because of an adverse effect.

In open studies, topiramate has also been reported to have long-term therapeutic effects in BED with obesity; to reduce symptoms of BED, bulimia nervosa, and anorexia nervosa with comorbid mood disorders; and to reduce nocturnal eating and overweight in patients with night-eating syndrome and sleep-related eating disorders (Guille and Sachs 2002; McElroy et al. 2008; Winkelman 2006). However, there is a report of topiramate possibly "triggering" a recurrent episode of anorexia nervosa in a woman with epilepsy and several reports of eating disorder patients misusing the drug to lose weight (McElroy et al. 2008).

Substance Use Disorders

Four randomized, placebo-controlled studies suggest that topiramate may have therapeutic effects in alcohol, cocaine, and nicotine dependence. Two studies examined topiramate in alcohol dependence. In the first, 150 subjects with alcohol dependence were randomly assigned to topiramate ($n=75$; up to 300 mg/day) or placebo ($n=75$) for 12 weeks (Johnson et al. 2003). All subjects received compliance enhancement therapy. At study end, subjects receiving topiramate, compared with those on placebo, had 2.88 (95% CI=−4.50 to −1.27) fewer drinks per day ($P=0.0006$), 3.10 (95% CI=−4.88 to −1.31) fewer drinks

per drinking day ($P=0.0009$), 27.6% fewer heavy drinking days ($P=0.0003$), 26.2% more days abstinent ($P=0.0003$), and a log plasma gamma-glutamyl transferase (GGT) ratio of 0.07 (−0.11 to −0.02) less ($P=0.0046$). Changes in craving were also significantly greater with topiramate than with placebo. In the second study, 371 subjects were randomly assigned to topiramate (up to 300 mg) or placebo, along with a weekly compliance enhancement intervention, at 16 sites for 14 weeks (Johnson et al. 2007). Topiramate was significantly superior to placebo in reducing the percentage of heavy drinking days and other drinking outcomes, such as drinks per drinking day, percentage of days abstinent, and log plasma GGT ratio (all $Ps≤0.002$).

In the study in cocaine dependence, 40 subjects were randomly assigned to topiramate (titrated gradually over 8 weeks to 200 mg/day) or placebo for 13 weeks (Kampman et al. 2004). Topiramate-treated subjects were more likely to be abstinent from cocaine after week 8 compared with placebo-treated subjects ($P=0.01$). They were also more likely to achieve 3 weeks of continuous abstinence from cocaine ($P=0.05$).

In the first of two controlled studies in smoking cessation, topiramate ($n=45$) was superior to placebo ($n=49$) in 94 male and female subjects with comorbid alcohol dependence (Johnson et al. 2005). This study was a subgroup analysis of the first controlled study of topiramate in alcohol dependence (Johnson et al. 2003). In the second study, the drug ($n=43$) was superior to placebo ($n=44$) for smoking cessation in male ($n=38$), but not female ($n=49$), subjects who had no associated psychopathology (Anthenelli et al. 2008).

There have also been case reports of the successful use of topiramate in opiate and benzodiazepine withdrawal, but these uses will need to be evaluated in placebo-controlled trials (Michopoulos et al. 2006; Zullino et al. 2004).

Anxiety Disorders

Topiramate has been evaluated in one controlled study of PTSD. Thirty-eight patients with non-combat-related PTSD were randomly assigned to flexible doses of topiramate (median dosage=150 mg/day, range=25–400 mg/day) or placebo for 12 weeks (Tucker et al. 2007). No significant difference was found on the primary efficacy measure, the total Clinician-Administered PTSD Scale (CAPS) score. However, significant or near significant effects were found in favor of topiramate on the eight-item Treatment Outcome PTSD scale (TOP-8) (decrease in overall severity 68% vs. 41.6%; $P=0.025$) and endpoint Clinical Global Impression Scale—Improvement (CGI-I) scores (1.9±1.2 vs. 2.6±1.1; *P*=0.055).

Open-label studies suggest that topiramate may have therapeutic effects in generalized social phobia and OCD (Mula et al. 2007). In contrast, there are case reports of patients experiencing panic attacks apparently induced by topiramate (Damsa et al. 2006).

Borderline Personality Disorder

Three placebo-controlled studies, all conducted by the same group, have evaluated topiramate in DSM-IV-defined BPD. In the first, 29 female subjects were randomly assigned in a 2:1 ratio to topiramate (*n*=21, analysis based on 19) or placebo (*n*=10) for 8 weeks (M.K. Nickel et al. 2004). Topiramate dosage was increased to 250 mg/day over 6 weeks. At study end, significant improvement on four subscales of the STAXI (state–anger, trait–anger, anger–out, and anger–control) was observed for topiramate compared with placebo. In the second study, 42 male subjects with BPD received topiramate (*n*=22) or placebo (*n*=20) for 8 weeks (M.K. Nickel et al. 2005a). Similar to the study in females, significant improvement on the same four subscales on the STAXI was found for topiramate compared with placebo. In the third study, 56 women with BPD received topiramate (*n*=28) or placebo (*n*=28) for 10 weeks (Loew et al. 2006). Topiramate was titrated to 200 mg/day over 6 weeks and then held constant. Topiramate was superior to placebo on the somatization, interpersonal sensitivity, anxiety, hostility, phobic anxiety, and Global Severity Index subscales of the Symptom Checklist (SCL-90-R) (all *P*s<0.001); all eight scales of the SF-36 Health Survey (all *P*s<0.01); and four of eight scales of the Inventory of Interpersonal Problems (all *P*s<0.001). Four patients (1 on topiramate, 3 on placebo) dropped out. In all three studies, topiramate was associated with significantly greater weight loss then placebo. It was also well tolerated, and there were no psychotic or suicidal adverse events.

Psychotropic-Associated Weight Gain

Two placebo-controlled studies suggest that topiramate reduces antipsychotic-induced weight gain in schizophrenia. In one study, 66 inpatients with schizophrenia receiving antipsychotic medication and "carrying excess weight" were randomly assigned to topiramate 100 mg/day, topiramate 200 mg/day, or placebo for 12 weeks (Ko et al. 2005). Body weight, BMI, and waist and hip circumference decreased significantly in the topiramate 200 mg/day group compared with the topiramate 100 mg/day and pla-

cebo groups. Scores on the Clinical Global Impression Scale—Severity of Illness (CGI-S) and the Brief Psychiatric Rating Scale (BPRS) were also significantly decreased, but the decreases were not thought to be clinically meaningful. In the other study, 43 women with mood or psychotic disorders who had gained weight while receiving olanzapine were given topiramate (*n*=25) or placebo (*n*=18) for 10 weeks (Nickel et al. 2005b). Weight loss was significantly greater (by 5.6 kg) in the topiramate group. Topiramate-treated subjects also experienced significantly greater improvement in measures of health-related quality of life and psychological impairment.

One placebo-controlled study and two randomized comparison trials suggest that topiramate may be superior to placebo and at least as effective as bupropion and sibutramine in psychotropic-associated weight gain in bipolar patients. In the controlled study in bipolar I manic or mixed patients receiving lithium or valproate, adjunctive topiramate was ineffective for manic symptoms but was associated with significantly greater reductions in body weight compared with placebo (−2.5 vs. 0.2 kg, respectively; *P*<0.001) and BMI (−0.84 vs. 0.07 kg/m², respectively; *P*<0.001) (Chengappa et al. 2006). In a single-blind comparator trial in 36 outpatients with bipolar depression, adjunctive bupropion and topiramate showed similar rates of antidepressant response (59% vs. 56%), but topiramate was associated with a greater mean weight loss (5.8 kg vs. 1.2 kg) (McIntyre et al. 2002). In a 24-week open-label, flexible-dose comparison trial, 46 euthymic outpatients with a bipolar disorder (types I, II, or not otherwise specified [NOS]) who had a BMI ≥30 kg/m², or a BMI ≥27 with obesity-related medical comorbidities, and psychotropic-associated weight gain (defined as a weight gain of 10 lbs [4.5 kg] since initiation of their current psychotropic regimen) were randomly assigned to receive topiramate (*n*=28; 25–600 mg/day) or sibutramine (*n*=18; 5–15 mg/day) for 24 weeks (McElroy et al. 2007a). Patients receiving either drug lost comparable amounts of weight (2.8±3.5 kg for topiramate and 4.1±5.7 kg for sibutramine) and displayed similar rates of weight loss (0.82 kg/week and 0.85 kg/week, respectively). However, only 4 (22%) patients receiving sibutramine and 6 (21%) patients receiving topiramate completed the trial. In addition, the attrition patterns for the two drugs were different, with patients discontinuing topiramate doing so early in treatment and patients discontinuing sibutramine doing so throughout treatment.

Several open-label, prospective trials suggest that initiating treatment with the combination of topiramate with either risperidone or olanzapine may successfully stabilize mood in patients with bipolar disorder while preventing weight gain (Bahk et al. 2005; Vieta et al. 2003, 2004). Finally, topiramate has also been used to treat weight gain in patients with major depression receiving antidepressants, patients with anxiety disorders receiving selective serotonin reuptake inhibitors, and patients with autism receiving antipsychotics (McElroy et al. 2008).

Obesity

Nine randomized, placebo-controlled trials have evaluated topiramate (Astrup et al. 2004; Bray et al. 2003; Eliasson et al. 2007; Stenlöf et al. 2007; Tonstad et al. 2005; Toplak et al. 2007; Tremblay et al. 2007; Wilding et al. 2004) or a controlled-release (CR) formulation of topiramate (Rosenstock et al. 2007) for weight loss in subjects with obesity. In one study, subjects were required to have comorbid essential hypertension (Tonstad et al. 2005); in four studies, subjects were required to have concurrent type 2 diabetes (Eliasson et al. 2007; Rosenstock et al. 2007; Stenlöf et al. 2007; Toplak et al. 2007). In all nine studies, topiramate was superior to placebo for weight loss at all doses (range 64–400 mg/day) and at all endpoints (range 28 weeks to 1 year) evaluated. The four long-term studies (duration 40 weeks to 1 year) showed that topiramate was associated with weight loss that increased up to 1 year without plateauing (Astrup et al. 2004; Eliasson et al. 2007; Stenlöf et al. 2007; Wilding et al. 2004). In the study of topiramate in obese subjects with comorbid hypertension, there were significant decreases in diastolic, but not systolic, blood pressure in the two groups receiving topiramate compared with the placebo group. In the four studies of topiramate in obese subjects with comorbid type 2 diabetes, topiramate-treated patients showed significant decreases in glycosylated hemoglobin (Hb_{A1c}) compared with placebo-treated patients.

Neuropathic Pain and Other Neurological Conditions

Five randomized, placebo-controlled studies of topiramate in painful diabetic neuropathy have produced mixed results. Three similarly designed trials in 1,259 subjects with moderate or extreme pain evaluating topiramate at 100 mg, 200 mg, or 400 mg/day did not find statistical separation on the 100-mm Visual Analog Scale (VAS) after 18–22 weeks of treatment (Thienel et al. 2004). Across all studies, 24% of topiramate-treated subjects and 8% of placebo-treated subjects discontinued treatment due to adverse events; groups did not differ in the occurrence of serious adverse events.

The other two controlled studies showed separation between topiramate and placebo in 345 subjects (Raskin et al. 2004). In the larger trial ($N=323$), subjects with a pain visual analog (PVA) scale score of at least 40 (on a scale of 0 [no pain] to 100 mm [worst possible pain]) were given topiramate (up to 400 mg/day; $n=214$) or placebo ($n=109$) for 12 weeks (Raskin et al. 2004). Topiramate was associated with significantly greater reductions in the PVA scale score ($P=0.038$), the worst pain intensity score ($P=0.003$), and sleep disruption ($P=0.020$). Topiramate also reduced body weight (−2.6 vs. +0.2 kg for placebo; $P<0.001$) without disrupting glycemic control.

Regarding other neurological conditions, topiramate has been shown superior to placebo in controlled trials in preventing pediatric migraine (Winner et al. 2005) and treating essential tremor (Ondo et al. 2006). Open data suggest that topiramate may have beneficial effects in cluster headache (Pascual et al. 2007).

Side Effects and Toxicology

The side-effect profile of topiramate may vary with the patient's illness, mood state, and concomitant medications. The most common side effects of topiramate in the initial dose-ranging studies in patients with epilepsy when used in combination with other antiepileptic drugs at dosages of 200–1,000 mg/day were related to the central nervous system and included dizziness, somnolence, psychomotor slowing, nervousness, paresthesias, ataxia, difficulty with memory, difficulty with concentration or attention, confusion, and speech disorders or related speech problems (Langtry et al. 1997; Shorvon 1996). Other side effects were nystagmus, depression, nausea, diplopia, abnormal vision, anorexia, language problems, and tremor. When used as monotherapy in patients with epilepsy, the most common side effects were dizziness, anxiety, paresthesias, insomnia, somnolence, myalgia, anorexia, nausea, dyspepsia, and diarrhea. The most common side effects of topiramate in the large registration trials for migraine (which used total daily doses of 50, 100, and 200 mg) were paresthesias, fatigue, memory difficulties, concentration/attention problems, and mood problems (Bussone et al. 2006). In the monotherapy trials in adult mania, paresthesias, decreased appetite, dry mouth, and weight loss were more common with topiramate than placebo (Kushner et al. 2006). In the adolescent mania trial, the most common adverse events occurring with topiramate were decreased appetite, nausea, diarrhea, paresthesias, somnolence, insomnia, and rash (DelBello et al. 2005). In the obesity trials, events related to the central or peripheral nervous systems or to psychiatric disorders were most commonly reported (Rosenstock et al. 2007). These included paresthesias; fatigue; difficulty with attention, concentration and/or memory; taste perversion; and anorexia. Overall, paresthesias and cognitive complaints are the most troublesome adverse events (van Passel et al. 2006).

The central nervous system and gastrointestinal effects of topiramate are usually mild to moderate in severity and often decrease or resolve with time or dosage reduction (Meador et al. 2003; Shorvon 1996). Also, they may be minimized by slow titration of topiramate dosage (Biton et al. 2001). However, topiramate may be associated with more cognitive impairment than some of the other new antiepileptic drugs (Martin et al. 1999; Meador et al. 2003).

Infrequent but serious side effects of topiramate include nephrolithiasis, an ocular syndrome of acute myopia with secondary angle-closure glaucoma, oligohydrosis and hyperthermia, and metabolic acidosis (van Passel et al. 2006). The incidence of nephrolithiasis has been estimated to be 1.5% (Shorvon 1996). In the epilepsy trials, more than 75% of the patients who developed renal stones elected to continue treatment with topiramate (Reife et al. 2000). Nephrolithiasis is thought to be related to topiramate exerting carbonic anhydrase inhibition in the kidney (Welch et al. 2006).

The secondary angle-closure glaucoma associated with topiramate is characterized by acute onset of bilateral blurred vision and ocular pain (Fraunfelder and Fraunfelder 2004; Fraunfelder et al. 2004). Ophthalmological findings include bilateral myopia, conjunctival hyperemia, anterior chamber shallowing, and increased intraocular pressure. Most cases have occurred within 1 month of topiramate initiation and fully resolve with drug discontinuation. Peripheral iridectomy or laser iridotomy are not effective. The syndrome has been attributed to sulfamate-induced ciliary body edema.

There were no clinically relevant changes in hepatic, renal, or hematological parameters in the registration trials of topiramate, and laboratory monitoring was initially thought not to be required (Reife et al. 2000; Sachdeo and Karia 2002). In addition, no treatment-related changes in physical or neurological examinations (except body weight loss; see next paragraph), in the electrocardiogram, or in ophthalmological or audiometric test results were noted. However, as a carbonic anhydrase inhibitor, topiramate reduces serum bicarbonate levels, and it is believed that this is the mechanism underlying reports of

reversible metabolic acidosis in some patients (Sachdeo and Karia 2002; van Passel et al. 2006; Welch et al. 2006). It is now recommended that baseline and periodic serum bicarbonate levels be measured in patients receiving topiramate. A case of liver failure in a young woman with epilepsy after addition of topiramate to carbamazepine (Bjoro et al. 1998) and a case of significant liver enzyme elevation in another young woman with bipolar disorder and obesity after addition of topiramate to divalproex sodium, benztropine, risperidone, clonazepam, and an oral contraceptive (Doan and Clendenning 2000) have been reported. To date, no cases of liver failure have been reported with topiramate monotherapy.

A growing concern is the psychiatric adverse-event profile of antiepileptic drugs in patients with epilepsy, including whether such drugs cause suicidality and psychosis. Although some data suggest that a subgroup of epilepsy patients may be susceptible to such psychiatric adverse events, other data indicate that topiramate may be associated with depression in epilepsy patients, especially during rapid titration (Mula and Sander 2007). There are also isolated reports of the drug inducing mood and anxiety symptoms in psychiatric patients (Damsa et al. 2006; Klufas and Thompson 2001). Moreover, one obesity study reported eight (6.2%) suicidal-related events occurring in topiramate-treated subjects versus none in placebo-treated subjects (Rosenstock et al. 2007).

Body weight loss in patients enrolled in clinical trials for epilepsy was reported as an adverse event in 7% of the patients receiving topiramate 200–400 mg/day and 13% of the patients receiving topiramate 600–1,000 mg/day, compared with 3% of the placebo-treated patients (Reife et al. 2000). Weight loss was associated with anorexia and was more common in heavier patients. Degree of weight loss was dose related; mean weight loss was 1.1 kg in patients receiving less than 200 mg/day of topiramate and 5.9 kg in patients receiving 800 mg/day or more (Langtry et al. 1997). Weight reduction usually plateaued after 15–18 months of treatment (Rosenfeld et al. 1997b).

Drug–Drug Interactions

Although topiramate is minimally metabolized by the liver, its clearance can be increased by the coadministration of hepatic enzyme–inducing drugs (Bialer et al. 2004; Gidal 2002; Langtry et al. 1997; Rosenfeld et al. 1997a; van Passel et al. 2006). Thus, carbamazepine and phenytoin may substantially decrease topiramate levels. Conversely, topiramate has mild enzyme-inducing properties and may enhance metabolism of ethinyl estradiol. Available data suggest that at topiramate doses of 200 mg/day or lower, this induction is insignificant, but at doses greater than 200 mg/day, induction becomes dose dependent and occurs to a great extent (Bialer et al. 2004). Women taking combination oral contraceptive agents therefore need to be counseled about this potential interaction.

There have been reports of topiramate causing increased lithium levels (Abraham and Owen 2004). This effect appears to be rarely clinically significant. Indeed, pharmacokinetic studies suggest that topiramate may slightly decrease serum lithium concentrations (Bialer et al. 2004).

Conclusion

Five controlled monotherapy trials and one adjunctive therapy trial indicate that topiramate is not efficacious in the treatment of acute bipolar mania in adults. However, clinical reports suggest that topiramate may be effective in other aspects of bipolar disorder, including juvenile mania, bipolar depression, "soft" forms of bipolar spectrum disorder, and bipolar disorder with comorbid conditions. Moreover, placebo-controlled trials suggest that topiramate is efficacious in binge-eating disorder, bulimia nervosa, alcohol dependence, borderline personality disorder, psychotropic-induced weight gain, and obesity. Further controlled clinical trials of topiramate in mood, eating, substance use, and personality disorders are needed to more clearly delineate its role as a psychotropic agent.

References

Abraham G, Owen J: Topiramate can cause lithium toxicity. J Clin Psychopharmacol 24:565–567, 2004

American Psychiatric Association: Diagnostic and Statistical Manual of Mental Disorders, 4th Edition. Washington, DC, American Psychiatric Association, 1994

Anthenelli RM, Blom TJ, McElroy SL, et al: Preliminary evidence for gender-specific effects of topiramate as a potential aid to smoking cessation. Addiction 103:687–694, 2008

Astrup A, Caterson I, Zelissen P, et al: Topiramate: long-term maintenance of weight loss induced by low-calorie diet in obese subjects. Obes Res 12:1658–1669, 2004

Bahk WM, Shin YC, Woo J, et al: Topiramate and divalproex in combination with risperidone for acute mania: a randomized open-label study. Prog Neuropsychopharmacol Biol Psychiatry 29, 115–121, 2005

Barzman DH, DelBello MP: Topiramate for co-occurring bipolar disorder and disruptive behavior disorders (letter). Am J Psychiatry 163:1451–1452, 2006

Bialer M, Doose DR, Murthy B, et al: Pharmacokinetic interactions of topiramate. Clin Pharmacokinet 43:763–780, 2004

Biton V, Edwards KR, Montouris GD, et al: Topiramate titration and tolerability. Ann Pharmacother 35:173–179, 2001

Bjoro K, Gjerstad L, Oystein B, et al: Topiramate and fulminant liver failure (letter). Lancet 352:1119, 1998

Brandes JL: Practical use of topiramate for migraine prevention. Headache Suppl 1:S66–73, 2005

Bray GA, Hollander P, Klein S, et al: A 6-month randomized, placebo-controlled, dose-ranging trial of topiramate for weight loss in obesity. Obes Res 11:722–733, 2003

Bussone G, Usai S, D'Amico D: Topiramate in migraine prophylaxis: data from a pooled analysis and open-label extension study. Neurol Sci 27 (suppl 2):159–163, 2006

Chengappa KN, Gershon S, Levine J: The evolving role of topiramate among other mood stabilizers in the management of bipolar disorder. Bipolar Disord 3:215–232, 2001a

Chengappa [Roy Chengappa] KN, Levine J, Rathore D, et al: Long-term effects of topiramate on bipolar mood instability, weight change and glycemic control: a case-series. European Psychiatry 16:186–190, 2001b

Chengappa [Roy Chengappa] KN, Schwarzman LK, Hulihan JF, et al: Adjunctive topiramate therapy in patients receiving a mood stabilizer for bipolar I disorder: a randomized, placebo-controlled trial. J Clin Psychiatry 67:1698–1706, 2006

Chengappa [Roy Chengappa] KN, Kupfer DJ, Parepally H, et al: A placebo-controlled, random-assignment, parallel-group pilot study of adjunctive topiramate for patients with schizoaffective disorder, bipolar type. Bipolar Disord 9:609–617, 2007

Citrome L: Antiepileptics in the treatment of schizophrenia, in Antiepileptic Drugs to Treat Psychiatric Disorders. Edited by McElroy SL, Keck PE Jr, Post RM. New York, Informa Healthcare, 2008, pp 187–206

Claudino AM, de Oliveira IR, Appolinario JC, et al: Double-blind, randomized, placebo-controlled trial of topiramate plus cognitive-behavior therapy in binge-eating disorder. J Clin Psychiatry 68:1324–1332, 2007

Damsa C, Warczyk S, Cailhol L, et al: Panic attacks associated with topiramate. J Clin Psychiatry 67:326–327, 2006

DelBello MP, Findling RL, Kushner S, et al: A pilot controlled trial of topiramate for mania in children and adolescents with bipolar disorder. J Am Acad Child Adolesc Psychiatry 44:539–547, 2005

Doan RJ, Clendenning M: Topiramate and hepatotoxicity (letter). Can J Psychiatry 45:937–938, 2000

Doose DR, Streeter AJ: Topiramate: chemistry, biotransformation, and pharmacokinetics, in Antiepileptic Drugs, 5th Edition. Edited by Levy RH, Mattson RH, Meldrum BS, et al. Philadelphia, PA, Lippincott Williams & Wilkins, 2002, pp 727–734

Eliasson B, Gudbjörnsdottir S, Cederholm J, et al: Weight loss and metabolic effects of topiramate in overweight and obese type 2 diabetic patients: randomized double-blind placebo-controlled trial. Int J Obes (Lond) 31:1140–1147, 2007

Fraunfelder FW, Fraunfelder FT: Adverse ocular drug reactions recently identified by the National Registry of Drug-Induced Ocular Side Effects. Ophthalmology 111:1275–1279, 2004

Fraunfelder FW, Fraunfelder FT, Keates EU: Topiramate-associated acute, bilateral, secondary angle-closure glaucoma. Ophthalmology 111:109–111, 2004

Gidal BE: Topiramate: drug interactions, in Antiepileptic Drugs, 5th Edition. Edited by Levy RH, Mattson RH, Meldrum BS, et al. Philadelphia, PA, Lippincott Williams & Wilkins, 2002, pp 735–739

Guille C, Sachs G: Clinical outcome of adjunctive topiramate treatment in a sample of refractory bipolar patients with comorbid conditions. Prog Neuropsychopharmacol Biol Psychiatry 26:1035–1039, 2002

Hedges DW, Reimherr FW, Hoopes SP, et al: Treatment of bulimia nervosa with topiramate in a randomized, double-blind, placebo-controlled trial, part 2: improvement in psychiatric measures. J Clin Psychiatry 64:1449–1454, 2003

Herrero AL, Del Olmo N, González-Escalada JR, et al: Two new actions of topiramate: inhibition of depolarizing GABAA-mediated responses and activation of a potassium conductance. Neuropharmacology 42:210–220, 2002

Hoopes SP, Reimherr FW, Hedges DW, et al: Part I. Topiramate in the treatment of bulimia nervosa: a randomized, double-blind, placebo-controlled trial. J Clin Psychiatry 64:1335–1341, 2003

Huguelet P, Morand-Collomb S: Effect of topiramate augmentation on two patients suffering from schizophrenia or bipolar disorder with comorbid alcohol abuse. Pharmacol Res 52:392–394, 2005

Johnson BA, Ait-Daoud N, Bowden CL, et al: Oral topiramate for treatment of alcohol dependence: a randomized controlled trial. Lancet 361:1677–1685, 2003

Johnson BA, Ait-Daoud N, Akhtar FZ, et al: Use of oral topiramate to promote smoking abstinence among alcohol-dependent smokers: a randomized controlled trial. Arch Intern Med 165:1600–1605, 2005

Johnson BA, Rosenthal N, Capece JA, et al: Topiramate for treating alcohol dependence: a randomized controlled trial. JAMA 298:1641–1651, 2007

Kaminski RM, Banerjee M, Rogawski MA: Topiramate selectively protects against seizures induced by ATPA, a GluR5 kainate receptor agonist. Neuropharmacology 46:1097–1104, 2004

Kampman KM, Pettinati H, Lynch KG, et al: A pilot trial of topiramate for the treatment of cocaine dependence. Drug Alcohol Depend 75:233–240, 2004

Kawasaki H, Tancredi V, D'Arcangelo G, et al: Multiple actions of the novel anticonvulsant drug topiramate in the rat subiculum in vitro. Brain Res 807(1–2):125–134, 1998

Klufas A, Thompson D: Topiramate-induced depression (letter). Am J Psychiatry 158:1736, 2001

Ko YH, Joe SH, Jung IK, et al: Topiramate as an adjuvant treatment with atypical antipsychotics in schizophrenic patients experiencing weight gain. Clin Neuropharmacol 28:169–175, 2005

Kudin AP, Debska-Vielhaber G, Vielhaber S, et al: The mechanism of neuroprotection by topiramate in an animal model of epilepsy. Epilepsia 45:1478–1487, 2004

Kushner SF, Khan A, Lane R, et al: Topiramate monotherapy in the management of acute mania: results of four double-blind placebo-controlled trials. Bipolar Disord 8:15–27, 2006

Kuzniecky R, Hetherington H, Ho S, et al: Topiramate increases cerebral GABA in healthy humans. Neurology 51:627–629, 1998

Langtry HD, Gillis JC, Davis R: Topiramate: a review of its pharmacodynamic and pharmacokinetic properties and clinical efficacy in the management of epilepsy. Drugs 54:752–773, 1997

Loew TH, Nickel MK, Muehlbacher M, et al: Topiramate treatment for women with borderline personality disorder: a dou-

ble-blind, placebo-controlled study. J Clin Psychopharmacol 26:61–66, 2006

Martin R, Kuzniecky R, Ho S, et al: Cognitive effects of topiramate, gabapentin, and lamotrigine in healthy young adults. Neurology 52:321–327, 1999

McDaniel WW, Spiegel DR, Sahota AK: Topiramate effect in catatonia: a case series. J Neuropsychiatry Clin Neurosci 18:234–238, 2006

McElroy SL, Keck PE Jr: Topiramate, in American Psychiatric Publishing Textbook of Psychopharmacology, 3rd Edition. Edited by Schatzberg AF, Nemeroff CB. Washington, DC, American Psychiatric Publishing, 2004, pp 627–636

McElroy SL, Suppes T, Keck PE Jr, et al: Open-label adjunctive topiramate in the treatment of bipolar disorders. Biol Psychiatry 47:1025–1033, 2000

McElroy SL, Arnold LA, Shapira AN, et al: Topiramate in the treatment of binge eating disorder associated with obesity: a randomized, placebo controlled trial (erratum in: Am J Psychiatry 160:612, 2003). Am J Psychiatry 160:255–261, 2003

McElroy SL, Frye MA, Altshuler LL, et al: A 24-week, randomized, controlled trial of adjunctive sibutramine versus topiramate in the treatment of weight gain in overweight or obese patients with bipolar disorders. Bipolar Disord 9:426–434, 2007a

McElroy SL, Hudson JI, Capece JA, et al: Topiramate for the treatment of binge eating disorder associated with obesity: a placebo-controlled study. Biol Psychiatry 61:1039–1048, 2007b

McElroy SL, Guerdjikova A, Keck PE Jr, et al: Antiepileptic drugs in obesity, psychotropic-associated weight gain, and eating disorders, in Antiepileptic Drugs to Treat Psychiatric Disorders. Edited by McElroy SL, Keck PE Jr, Post RM. New York, Informa Healthcare, 2008, pp 283–309

McIntyre RS, Mancini DA, McCann S, et al: Topiramate versus bupropion SR when added to mood stabilizer therapy for the depressive phase of bipolar disorder: a preliminary single-blind study. Bipolar Disord 4:207–213, 2002

McIntyre RS, Riccardelli R, Binder C, et al: Open-label adjunctive topiramate in the treatment of unstable bipolar disorder. Can J Psychiatry 50:415–422, 2005

Meador KJ, Loring DW, Hulihan JF, et al: Differential cognitive and behavioral effects of topiramate and valproate. Neurology 60:1483–1488, 2003

Michopoulos I, Douzenis A, Christodoulou C, et al: Topiramate use in alprazolam addiction. World J Biol Psychiatry 7:265–267, 2006

Mohammadi B, Krampfl K, Cetinkaya C, et al: Interaction of topiramate with glycine receptor channels. Pharmacol Res 51:587–592, 2005

Mula M, Sander JW: Negative effects of antiepileptic drugs on mood in patients with epilepsy. Drug Saf 30:555–567, 2007

Mula M, Pini S, Cassano GB: The role of anticonvulsant drugs in anxiety disorders: a critical review of the evidence. J Clin Psychopharmacol 27:263–272, 2007

Nickel C, Lahmann C, Tritt K, et al: Topiramate in the treatment of depressive and anger symptoms in female depressive patient: a randomized, double-blind, placebo-controlled study. J Affect Disord 87:243–252, 2005a

Nickel C, Tritt K, Muehlbacher M, et al: Topiramate treatment in bulimia nervosa patients: a randomized, double-blind, placebo-controlled trial. Int J Eat Disord 38:295–300, 2005b

Nickel MK, Nickel C, Mitterlehner FO, et al: Topiramate treatment of aggression in female borderline personality disorder patients: a double-blind, placebo-controlled study. J Clin Psychiatry 65:1515–1519, 2004

Nickel MK, Nickel C, Kaplan P, et al: Treatment of aggression with topiramate in male borderline patients: a double-blind, placebo-controlled study. Biol Psychiatry 57:495–499, 2005a

Nickel MK, Nickel C, Muehlbacher M, et al: Influence of topiramate on olanzapine-related adiposity in women: a random, double-blind, placebo-controlled study. J Clin Psychopharmacol 25:211–217, 2005b

Ondo WG, Jankovic J, Connor GS, et al: Topiramate in essential tremor: a double-blind, placebo-controlled trial. Neurology 66:672–677, 2006

Pascual J, Láinez MJ, Dodick D, et al: Antiepileptic drugs for the treatment of chronic and episodic cluster headache: a review. Headache 47:81–89, 2007

Petroff OA, Hyder F, Rothman DL, et al: Topiramate rapidly raises brain GABA in epilepsy patients. Epilepsia 42:543–548, 2001

Raskin P, Donofrio PD, Rosenthal NR, et al: Topiramate vs placebo in painful diabetic neuropathy: analgesic and metabolic effects. Neurology 63:865–873, 2004

Reife R, Pledger G, Wu S-C: Topiramate as add-on therapy: pooled analysis of randomized controlled trials in adults. Epilepsia 41 (suppl 1):S66–S71, 2000

Rho JM, Sankar R: The pharmacologic basis of antiepileptic drug action. Epilepsia 40:1471–1483, 1999

Rosenfeld WE: Topiramate: a review of preclinical, pharmacokinetic, and clinical data. Clin Ther 19:1294–1308, 1997

Rosenfeld WE, Doose DR, Walker SA, et al: Effect of topiramate on the pharmacokinetics of an oral contraceptive containing norethindrone and ethinyl estradiol in patients with epilepsy. Epilepsia 38:317–323, 1997a

Rosenfeld WE, Kanner A, Jacobson M, et al: Topiramate and concomitant weight loss (abstract). Epilepsia 38 (suppl 8):98, 1997b

Rosenstock J, Hollander P, Gadde KM, et al: A randomized, double-blind, placebo-controlled multicenter study to assess the efficacy and safety of topiramate controlled-release in the treatment of obese, type 2 diabetic patients. Diabetes Care 30:1480–1486, 2007

Sachdeo RC, Karia RM: Topiramate: adverse effects, in Antiepileptic Drugs, 5th Edition. Edited by Levy RH, Mattson RH, Meldrum BS, et al. Philadelphia, PA, Lippincott Williams & Wilkins, 2002, pp 760–764

Schiffer WK, Gerasimov MR, Marsteller DA, et al: Topiramate selectively attenuates nicotine induced increases in monoamine release. Synapse 42:196–198, 2001

Shank RP, Gardocki JF, Streeter AJ, et al: An overview of the preclinical aspects of topiramate: pharmacology, pharmacokinetics, and mechanism of action. Epilepsia 41 (suppl 1):S3–S9, 2000

Shapira NA, Goldsmith TD, McElroy SL: Treatment of binge-eating disorder with topiramate: a clinical case series. J Clin Psychiatry 61:368–372, 2000

Shorvon SD: Safety of topiramate: adverse events and relationships to dosing. Epilepsia 37 (suppl 2):S18–S22, 1996

Simeone TA, Wilcox KS, White HS: Subunit selectivity of topiramate modulation of heteromeric GABA(A) receptors. Neuropharmacology 50:845–857, 2006

Stenlöf K, Rössner S, Vercruysse F, et al: Topiramate in the treatment of obese subjects with drug-naive type 2 diabetes. Diabetes Obes Metab 9:360–368, 2007

Thienel U, Neto W, Schwabe SK, et al: Topiramate in painful diabetic polyneuropathy: findings from three double-blind placebo-controlled trials. Acta Neurol Scand 110:221–231, 2004

Tiihonen J, Halonen P, Wahlbeck K, et al: Topiramate add-on in treatment-resistant schizophrenia: a randomized, double-blind, placebo-controlled, crossover trial. J Clin Psychiatry 66:1012–1015, 2005

Tonstad S, Tykarski A, Weissgarten J, et al: Efficacy and safety of topiramate in the treatment of obese subjects with essential hypertension. Am J Cardiol 96:243–251, 2005

Toplak H, Hamann A, Moore R, et al: Efficacy and safety of topiramate in combination with metformin in the treatment of obese subjects with type 2 diabetes: a randomized, double-blind, placebo-controlled study. Int J Obesity 31:138–146, 2007

Tremblay A, Chaput J-P, Bérubé S, et al: The effect of topiramate on energy balance in obese men: a 6-month double-blind randomized placebo-controlled study with a 6-month open-label extension. Eur J Clin Pharmacol 63:123–134, 2007

Tucker P, Trautman RP, Wyatt DB, et al: Efficacy and safety of topiramate monotherapy in civilian posttraumatic stress disorder: a randomized, double-blind, placebo-controlled study. J Clin Psychiatry 68:201–206, 2007

van Passel L, Arif H, Hirsch LJ: Topiramate for the treatment of epilepsy and other nervous system disorders. Expert Rev Neurother 6:19–31, 2006

Vieta E, Torrent C, Garcia-Ribas G, et al: Use of topiramate in treatment-resistant bipolar spectrum disorders. J Clin Psychopharmacol 22:431–435, 2002

Vieta E, Goikolea JM, Olivares JM, et al: 1-year follow-up of patients treated with risperidone and topiramate for a manic episode. J Clin Psychiatry 64:834–839, 2003

Vieta E, Sanchez-Moreno J, Goikolea JM, et al: Effects on weight and outcome of long-term olanzapine-topiramate combination treatment in bipolar disorder. J Clin Psychopharmacol 24:374–378, 2004

Wauguier A, Zhou S: Topiramate: a potent anticonvulsant in the amygdala-kindled rat. Epilepsy Res 24:73–77, 1996

Welch BJ, Graybeal D, Moe OW, et al: Biochemical and stone-risk profiles with topiramate treatment. Am J Kidney Dis 48:555–563, 2006

White HS: Topiramate: mechanisms of action, in Antiepileptic Drugs, 5th Edition. Edited by Levy RH, Mattson RH, Meldrum BS, et al. Philadelphia, PA, Lippincott Williams & Wilkins, 2002, pp 719–726

White HS: Molecular pharmacology of topiramate: managing seizures and preventing migraine. Headache 45 (suppl 1):S48–S56, 2005

White HS, Brown SD, Woodhead JH, et al: Topiramate modulates GABA-evoked currents in murine cortical neurons by a non-benzodiazepine mechanism. Epilepsia 41 (suppl 1):S17–S20, 2000

White HS, Smith MD, Wilcox KS: Mechanisms of action of antiepileptic drugs. Int Rev Neurobiol 81:85–110, 2007

Wilding J, Gaal L, Rissanan A, et al: A randomized double-blind placebo-controlled study of the long-term efficacy and safety of topiramate in the treatment of obese subjects. Int J Obes Relat Metab Disord 28:1399–1410, 2004

Winkelman JW: Efficacy and tolerability of open-label topiramate in the treatment of sleep-related eating disorder: a retrospective case series. J Clin Psychiatry 67:1729–1734, 2006

Winner P, Pearlman EM, Linder SL, et al: Topiramate for migraine prevention in children: a randomized, double-blind, placebo-controlled trial. Headache 45:1304–1312, 2005

Zhang X, Velumian AA, Jones OT, et al: Modulation of high voltage-activated calcium channels in dentate granule cells by topiramate. Epilepsia 41 (suppl 1):S52–S60, 2000

Zullino DF, Krenz S, Zimmerman G, et al: Topiramate in opiate withdrawal—comparison with clonidine and with carbamazepine/mianserin. Subst Abus 25:27–33, 2004

Other Agents

CHAPTER 41

Cognitive Enhancers

Frank W. Brown, M.D.

Disruption of cholinergic neurotransmission and excitatory amino acids is correlated with the development of cognitive impairment and, specifically, Alzheimer's disease (Mesulam 2004). Multiple mechanisms exist that may account for the progression of cognitive impairment, including those related to cholinesterase, N-methyl-D-aspartate, vascular disease, and oxidative damage (Aisen and Davis 1994; Bartus et al. 1982; Behl 1999; Behl et al. 1992; Jick et al. 2000; Kalaria et al. 1996; Selkoe 2000; Terry and Buccafusco 2003; Wolozin et al. 2000). An outcome of the disruption of many neurotransmitter systems, cognitive impairment may occur at any time during the disease process as synaptic plasticity becomes impaired, degrading the efficiency of neuronal transmission (Malik et al. 2007). It is intuitive that the earliest intervention prior to irreversible disease progression is optimal. Currently, it is unknown when the irreversible disease processes begin; no specific markers have been identified that could guide clinicians to initiate prophylactic treatment prior to the development of cognitive or behavioral manifestations.

Cognitive enhancer is a general term that denotes a pharmacological or nutraceutical intervention that improves cognitive functioning in an impaired or normal brain by reversing or delaying underlying neuropathological changes within the brain or by modulating the existing neurochemistry to facilitate a desired performance differential. The molecular pathogenesis of cognitive impairment is not fully understood; thus, an ideal pharmacological agent has been difficult to develop. No single agent developed to date is ideally suited for this task; however, several agents have shown beneficial results. In this chapter, I review the established and the most promising potential cognitive enhancers.

Cholinesterase-Related Therapies

Impairment of cholinergic neurotransmission, especially in the hippocampus and cerebral cortex, has been clearly established over the last 30 years as a significant factor in the clinical signs of cognitive impairment, including those of Alzheimer's disease (Davies and Maloney 1976; Mesulam 2004; Whitehouse et al. 1982). Butyrylcholinesterase (BChE) and acetylcholinesterase (AChE) are the two main types of cholinesterase present in the brain. The development of AChE inhibitors (AChEIs) to increase acetylcholine levels in the brain for enhanced synaptic transmission has been successful, with marginal positive clinical outcomes to date (Birks 2006; Thompson et al. 2004). Four AChEIs have been marketed in the United States for cognitive therapy: tacrine, donepezil, rivastigmine, and galantamine. These pharmaceuticals are primarily for symptomatic relief and have limited current value in stopping or reversing the disease process, although research into subtle neurotrophic and neuroprotective effects of these agents proceeds (Murphy et al. 2006). A significant number of AChEI nonresponders exists (Jones 2003). Improvements in cognitive functioning have been shown with AChEIs without major differences in their efficacy (Birks 2006; Seltzer 2006; Thompson et al. 2004). The major side effects of AChEIs are gastrointestinal.

Recommendations

Tacrine is no longer recommended for routine clinical use. Donepezil, rivastigmine, and galantamine are recommended with or without other cognitive enhancers (e.g., memantine) (Table 41–1). Tolerability is improved by

TABLE 41–1.   Recommended cholinesterase inhibitors

	DONEPEZIL (ARICEPT)	RIVASTIGMINE (EXELON)	GALANTAMINE (RAZADYNE)
Cholinesterase inhibition	AChE >> BChE	AChE and BChE	AChE > BChE
Elimination half-life	70 hours	2 hours	6–8 hours
AChE inhibitor type	Piperidine based	Carbamyl derivative	Tertiary alkaloid
Type of inhibition	Reversible, noncompetitive	Reversible (slow)	Reversible, competitive, nicotinic modulation
Titration schedule	5 mg/day for 4–6 weeks; 10 mg/day thereafter	1.5 mg twice daily, increasing by 1.5 mg every 2 weeks, or 4.6-mg skin patch daily for at least 4 weeks, then 9.5-mg skin patch daily	4 mg twice daily, increasing by 4 mg per dose every 4 weeks up to 24 mg daily total; extended-release form available for once-daily dosing
Target dose per day	5 or 10 mg	6, 9, or 12 mg, divided dose, or 9.5-mg skin patch daily	16 or 24 mg, divided dose
Major side effects	Nausea, vomiting, diarrhea, anorexia, headache, bradycardia, abdominal pain, nightmares; consider 5 mg/day in patients with moderate to severe renal disease	Nausea, vomiting, diarrhea, anorexia, headache, abdominal pain, weight loss; consider lower dose (6 mg daily orally or 4.6-mg skin patch daily) in patients with moderate to severe renal or hepatic disease	Same as rivastigmine; 16 mg/day maximum in patients with moderate renal or hepatic disease; contraindicated with severe renal or hepatic disease
Formulations	Tablets (oral, disintegrating)	Tablets, oral solution, skin patch	Tablets, oral suspension, extended-release tablets

Note.   >=greater than; >>=much greater than; AChE=acetylcholinesterase; BChE=butyrylcholinesterase.

slow dosage titration. All cholinesterase inhibitors have significant potential for side effects; it is difficult to determine whether one AChEI has a significantly better side-effect profile than another AChEI, given individual patients' variability. Switching AChEIs can be a reasonable treatment strategy if lack of efficacy or tolerability is an issue.

Tacrine

Tacrine, a first-generation AChEI and BChE inhibitor (BChEI), is rarely used today due to its (reversible) hepatotoxicity, drug–drug interactions, and the four-times-daily dosing schedule required to achieve adequate central nervous system concentrations for cognitive enhancement. Tacrine is available in an oral tablet formulation. Dosing begins with 40 mg/day given in four 10-mg doses, with titration upward every 4 weeks by 10 mg per dose to a maximal dosage of 160 mg/day (four 40-mg doses). The use of tacrine requires monitoring of liver enzymes.

Indole-tacrine heterodimers are being developed as dual-site AChEIs that would also inhibit β-amyloid peptide aggregation. Early studies indicated a net reduction of β-peptide plaque formation in an animal model (Muñoz-Ruiz et al. 2005). The simultaneous targeting of multiple recep-

tor sites, reduction of amyloid burden, and other neuroprotective modulations are the major mechanisms of combination therapy. Combination therapy approaches likely represent the future for the field of cognitive enhancers.

Donepezil

Donepezil, a piperidine-based, reversible, noncompetitive AChEI with a plasma half-life of about 70 hours, was approved for the treatment of mild to moderate Alzheimer's disease in the United States in 1996 and for severe Alzheimer's disease in 2006. Donepezil is given once daily in 5-mg or 10-mg doses; 5-mg therapy is only slightly less effective than 10-mg therapy and can be an appropriate regimen, especially when tolerability is an issue (Birks and Harvey 2006).

Donepezil has shown benefit in treating mild, moderate, and severe Alzheimer's disease (Birks and Harvey 2006; Wallin et al. 2007) and is currently being studied for efficacy in patients with mild cognitive impairment (Chen et al. 2006; Seltzer 2007). A recent meta-analysis of pooled data on the use of donepezil indicated caution is warranted in its use to treat mild cognitive impairment due to modest treatment effects with significant side effects (Birks and Flicker 2006).

In addition to Alzheimer's disease patients, Parkinson's disease, multiple sclerosis, and vascular dementia patients have benefited from donepezil therapy (Aarsland et al. 2002; Black et al. 2003; Blasko et al. 2004; Christodoulou et al. 2006; Leroi et al. 2004; Rowan et al. 2007; Seltzer 2007; Wilkinson et al. 2003). The use of donepezil as pretreatment in electroconvulsive therapy (ECT) has also been studied; patients who received donepezil prior to ECT have shown significantly faster recovery of cognitive deficits in the post-ECT period (Jyoti et al. 2006).

Rivastigmine

Rivastigmine, a carbamyl derivative, is a slowly reversible AChEI and BChEI with an elimination half-life of about 2 hours. It was approved in 2000 for use in the United States to treat mild to moderate dementia of Alzheimer's disease and Parkinson's disease. Rivastigmine inhibits the G1 isoenzyme of AChE selectively up to four times more potently than it does the G4 isoenzyme (Enz et al. 1993). This unique compound with its BChEI properties has been postulated to be of greater benefit than other AChEIs in the treatment of Alzheimer's disease because BChE activity increases in the hippocampus and cortex while AChE activity diminishes (Tasker et al. 2005); to date, this has not been conclusively shown to be of clinical significance. However, as a therapy involving multiple target receptor sites, this agent does have a theoretical advantage over single-target approaches. A rivastigmine skin patch received U.S. Food and Drug Administration approval in 2007; gastrointestinal side effects are reduced in frequency with this drug delivery system.

Rivastigmine is initiated at 1.5 mg taken twice daily; the dosage is increased by 1.5 mg every 2 weeks to a daily maximum of 6–12 mg divided into two doses. Transdermal therapy is initiated at one 4.6-mg skin patch applied daily for at least 4 weeks, at which time the dosage may be increased to the 9.5-mg daily patch.

Galantamine

Galantamine hydrobromide, a tertiary alkaloid, is a specific, competitive, and reversible AChEI with a plasma half-life of 6–8 hours that was first marketed in the United States in 2001 as a treatment of mild to moderate dementia of Alzheimer's disease. Galantamine is unique in that it modulates neuronal nicotinic receptors (Coyle and Kershaw 2001). Whether this nicotinic receptor modulation imparts any significant clinical benefit in disease modification remains unknown. The optimal dosage range is 16–24 mg/day. The extended-release formulation for once-daily dosing has similar efficacy and side effects as the twice-daily dosing formulation. Pooled data from trials in patients with mild cognitive impairment have shown significantly higher rates of death due to bronchial carcinoma/sudden death, cerebrovascular disorder/syncope, myocardial infarction, and suicide in the galantamine treatment groups (Cusi et al. 2007; Loy and Schneider 2006); follow-up studies are under way to clarify these findings. One double-blind, placebo-controlled trial of galantamine with antipsychotic medication in the treatment of subjects with schizophrenia did not show significant benefit, although the trend was toward improvement in several cognitive domains (Lee et al. 2007).

Other Agents

Physostigmine

Physostigmine, a reversible inhibitor of BChE and AChE, is poorly tolerated due to multiple gastrointestinal side effects, especially nausea and vomiting, and has a very short half-life. Physostigmine is inactivated within approximately 2 hours due to hydrolysis. An evaluation of 15 studies using physostigmine showed only marginal clinical efficacy and significant adverse side effects even with controlled-release formulations (Coelho and Birks 2001).

Huperzine Alpha

Huperzine alpha (more commonly known as huperzine A) is sold in the United States as a dietary supplement for cognitive enhancement. It was first isolated from club moss (*Huperzia serrata*) as a sesquiterpene alkaloid and is a slow, reversible inhibitor of AChE. Huperzine A has been shown to significantly improve memory in Alzheimer's disease patients with only limited side effects to date (Zangara 2003; Z. Zhang et al. 2002). It is believed to have neuroprotective effects by reducing neuronal cell death caused by glutamate (Ved et al. 1997). The combination of other AChEIs with huperzine A may exacerbate gastrointestinal side effects; patients' usage of this over-the-counter supplement should be monitored, especially if other AChEIs are considered for treatment.

Metrifonate

Metrifonate, a long-acting irreversible cholinesterase inhibitor, was tested in clinical trials, but further development was discontinued after a higher-than-expected incidence of neuromuscular dysfunction and respiratory paralysis was found. Metrifonate recipients with Alzheimer's disease showed significant cognitive improvement compared with placebo recipients at most dosages (50–80 mg/day) (Lopez-Arrieta and Schneider 2006).

Nicotinic Receptor Agonists

Selective and nonselective neuronal nicotinic receptor agonists have shown statistically significant cognitive enhancement in young, healthy subjects and in subjects with Alzheimer's disease (Dunbar et al. 2007; Newhouse et al. 1997, 2001; Potter et al. 1999; Sunderland et al. 1988). Some prior research using nicotine skin patches to improve attention in Alzheimer's disease patients has been conducted with limited efficacy shown (White and Levin 1999). Other studies have shown that chronic administration of nicotine using skin patches did improve cognitive functioning in Alzheimer's disease patients (Rusted et al. 2000). The use of selective neuronal nicotinic receptor agonists is an intuitive combination therapy with AChEIs for cognitive enhancement; research continues in this developing area.

N-Methyl-D-Aspartate–Related Therapy

Glutamate is an agonist of kainate, N-methyl-D-aspartate (NMDA), and α-amino-3-hydroxy-5-methyl-4-isoxazole propionic acid (AMPA) receptors. Neuronal plasticity of memory and learning is influenced by glutamate's direct modulation of the NMDA postsynaptic receptor; glutamate acts as an excitatory neurotransmitter activating the NMDA receptor. Glutamate excess results in neurotoxicity affecting cognitive functioning (Koch et al. 2005).

Recommendations

Memantine appears to reduce the level of cognitive impairment in patients with moderate to severe Alzheimer's disease. Memantine in combination with an AChEI is an appropriate consideration for improvement in cognition and behavior.

Memantine

Memantine is a noncompetitive NMDA receptor antagonist approved in the United States for treating moderate to severe Alzheimer's disease. The NMDA receptor modulates memory function. Memantine may prevent neurotoxicity due to its low-affinity antagonism of glutamate, which has been linked to neurodegeneration and excitotoxicity (Lipton and Rosenberg 1994). Memantine has been shown to be effective in reducing the level of cogni-

tive impairment in patients with moderate to severe Alzheimer's disease (Bullock 2006; Reisberg et al. 2003). Memantine is available in tablets and as an oral solution; dosing should be adjusted for patients with moderate or severe renal impairment. It is recommended that memantine be initiated at a dosage of 5 mg/day for 1 week, increasing weekly by 5 mg/day up to a target dosage of 20 mg/day. Memantine is generally given in twice-daily doses, although the elimination half-life ranges from 60 to 80 hours.

Memantine Combination Therapy

Memantine in combination with an AChEI has been shown to improve cognitive domains significantly and to improve behavioral dyscontrol (agitation/aggression, eating/appetite, irritability/lability) (Cummings et al. 2006; Tariot et al. 2004). Given the disruption of multiple neurotransmitter systems and pathways in Alzheimer's disease and other cognitive disorders, the use of adjunctive cognition-enhancing medications is understandable (Grossberg et al. 2006). The specific neurobiological deficit(s) that any pharmacological or nutraceutical intervention may impact should be considered.

Vascular and Inflammation-Related Therapies

Major known modifiable risk factors for vascular cognitive impairment (with or without dementia) include diabetes mellitus, hypertension, cardiac ischemia, atrial fibrillation, smoking, hyperlipidemia, and peripheral vascular disease (Desmond et al. 1993; Rockwood et al. 1997). Controversial risk factors include hyperhomocysteinemia. Established vascular treatment interventions have included low-dose aspirin and other antiplatelet agents, anticoagulation agents, antihypertensives, aggressive management of diabetes mellitus, carotid endarterectomy for selected patients, and the treatment of hyperlipidemia. There is a significant overlap of patients with vascular cognitive impairment and those with Alzheimer's disease (Gearing et al. 1995; O'Brien 1994). Cholinergic receptors (muscarinic and nicotinic) are known modulators of cerebral blood flow (Schwarz et al. 1999; W. Zhang et al. 1998). Ischemia-induced NMDA stimulation may further cognitive impairment.

A meta-analysis of four randomized, placebo-controlled studies of AChEIs to treat vascular dementia—two with donepezil and two with galantamine—showed statistically significant cognitive enhancement even though the treatment effect was less than what has been observed in

Alzheimer's disease patients (Birks and Flicker 2007). In addition, the authors analyzed pooled results from memantine studies and found statistically significant improvement of cognitive functioning with memantine treatment in patients with vascular impairment similar to that seen with the AChEIs (Birks and Flicker 2007). A Cochrane review indicated that donepezil in doses of either 5 mg or 10 mg improves both functional ability and cognitive symptoms in patients with mild to moderate vascular cognitive impairment; donepezil was well tolerated in this analysis (Malouf and Birks 2004). A more recent Cochrane review of the use of galantamine to treat vascular cognitive impairment showed statistically significant results in terms of cognition and executive function with galantamine versus placebo in one study but not in a second study that had fewer subjects; gastrointestinal side effects were noted to be higher in galantamine recipients (Craig and Birks 2006).

Recommendations

AChEIs appear to have a valid role in the treatment of vascular cognitive impairment. Combination therapy is an important consideration, especially with other known vascular risk modifiers including aspirin, other NSAIDs, and CDP-choline. Randomized, controlled trials do not currently support the use of aspirin or other NSAIDs for the treatment of vascular cognitive impairment. The active use of statins for the prevention and treatment of vascular cognitive impairment is currently not well supported by the literature; however, research with statins remains very active in this pursuit.

Statins

β-Amyloid formation and accumulation may be modulated by cholesterol. The Cardiovascular Health Study results indicated that the use of statins (3-hydroxy-3-methylglutaryl coenzyme A [HMG-CoA] reductase inhibitors) was associated with a decrease in cognitive decline that was not attributed to the lowering of serum cholesterol levels (Bernick et al. 2005). Some epidemiological investigations also suggest that the progression of cognitive decline decreases with statin use (Rockwood et al. 2002; Wolozin et al. 2000). Studies to date are not conclusive about the benefit of statins for the long-term treatment of vascular cognitive impairment, however. In a post hoc analysis of pooled data from three placebo-controlled, double-blind studies of patients with Alzheimer's disease who were treated with galantamine or galantamine plus a statin, galantamine was associated with significant benefits in cognitive functioning, whereas the use of statins and

galantamine did not result in a significant improvement, only a small positive improvement (Winblad et al. 2007).

CDP-Choline

Cytidine 5'-diphosphocholine (CDP-choline), or citicoline, has shown mixed results regarding its potential benefit in the treatment of cognitive impairment (Cohen et al. 2003; Secades and Lorenzo 2006). CDP-choline is an intermediate in the production of phospholipids of cell membranes. Impairment in phospholipids leads to cell function loss and has been shown to be a factor in cerebral ischemia (Klein 2000). A Cochrane review of 14 studies indicated a positive benefit of CDP-choline on memory and behavior (Fioravanti and Yanagi 2005). CDP-choline may have antiplatelet aggregation effects and cholinergic modulation effects and may increase dopamine synthesis in selected brain regions (Secades and Lorenzo 2006).

Aspirin

Strong data have not yet emerged supporting the cognitive benefits of aspirin usage to treat vascular cognitive impairment (Kang et al. 2007; Whalley and Mowat 2007). Aspirin remains a cornerstone first-line intervention for decreasing potential cardiovascular comorbidity. As such, aspirin may have a future role as a combination therapy with cognitive enhancers; future longitudinal research will help clarify this position.

Other Nonsteroidal Anti-Inflammatory Drugs

Other nonsteroidal anti-inflammatory drugs (NSAIDs) provide a neuroprotective effect and affect amyloid pathology (H. Hao et al. 2005; Siskou et al. 2007; Weggen et al. 2001). A specific role for their use in the treatment of cognitive impairment has not been well established. Significant gastrointestinal side effects remain a concern for long-term usage. Active research continues on novel anti-inflammatory derivatives that have desired properties with limited side effects (Siskou et al. 2007).

Antioxidant-Related Therapies

Antioxidant-related treatment for cognitive impairment remains poorly supported by placebo-controlled, double-blind studies. Although this may be a potential combination therapy modality, further research is required before endorsing specific treatment recommendations with current antioxidants.

Ginkgo Biloba

Ginkgo biloba could be classified within several potential treatment categories, including antioxidants, nutraceuticals, cholinergic agents, and vasodilators. *Ginkgo biloba* extract is currently marketed in the United States as a food supplement. Studies have shown potential benefit in using ginkgo to delay the progression of cognitive impairment or to enhance survival rates in humans and animal models (Andrieu et al. 2003; Dartigues et al. 2007; Naik et al. 2006). A review based on Cochrane meta-analyses showed a significant cognitive benefit of ginkgo only with pooled results (Kurz and Van Baelen 2004). Although the use of ginkgo appears to have a definite positive benefit in patients with cognitive impairment, most studies have shown marginal significance. The recommended dosage range is 120–240 mg/day.

Vitamins and Carotenoids

Vitamin E (including tocopherols and tocotrienols), vitamin C, and carotenoids are accepted agents with known antioxidant properties. Vitamin E is believed to act as a peroxyl radical scavenger. Reports of its benefit in treating patients with cognitive impairment are mixed, with some studies showing a delay in the progression of Alzheimer's disease symptoms (Engelhart et al. 2002; Sano et al. 1997). Vitamin E can affect blood coagulation and has potential cardiovascular side effects. The research on the efficacy of vitamin C as an antioxidant for treating cognitive impairment is currently less supportive. Carotenoids have a potential role as free radical scavengers; however, current research has not shown a significant time delay in the progression of cognitive impairment with their use. Combination therapy for cognitive impairment may well incorporate judicious amounts of vitamins and carotenoids as future research delineates the specific role of these agents in managing free radicals.

Other Agents

Currently, no recommendations for use of the following agents as monotherapy or combination therapy can be made.

Secretase Inhibitors

The use of secretase inhibitors is one of the approaches to reduce the β-amyloid protein load in the aging brain. The β-amyloid precursor protein is cleaved by proteases; the major proteases are β-secretase and γ-secretase and, to a lesser extent, α-secretase (Hamaguchi et al. 2006).

Mice models using a β-secretase inhibitor have shown reduced levels of β-amyloid protein (Asai et al. 2006). Inhibition of γ-secretase can have an impact on the familial expression of Alzheimer's disease through the genetic influence of presenilin and presenilin-2. However, each of these secretases may impact multiple protein substrates, in which case a nonspecific β- or γ-secretase inhibitor may yield major unwanted side effects (Hamaguchi et al. 2006). Secretase inhibition remains an active area of research and has the potential to have a major impact on the treatment of cognitive impairment.

Tramiprosate

Tramiprosate is a small-molecule glycosaminoglycan compound that inhibits the development of β-amyloid plaque formation, thus reducing neurotoxic effects (Geerts 2004, Molecule of the month 2006). Tramiprosate failed to show significantly better efficacy than placebo in Phase III clinical trials. Agents that prevent amyloid production or amyloid aggregation would have great utility in preventing the progression of Alzheimer's disease. Research targeting neuropathological substrates is exploring tau phosphorylation, apoptosis, formation of neurofibrillary tangles, amyloid production, and amyloid aggregation to develop pharmaceuticals with the potential to prevent and treat cognitive impairment, especially Alzheimer's disease.

Modafinil

Modafinil is marketed in the United States as a wakefulness-promoting drug. Minimal cognition-enhancing effects have been noted in low-dose (100-mg) treatment in non-sleep-deprived, middle-age subjects (Randall et al. 2004). Clinicians have used modafinil for the treatment of apathy associated with Alzheimer's disease. Modafinil is not recommended as monotherapy or in combination therapy for cognitive enhancement based on the current literature.

Hormone Replacement Therapy

Hormone replacement with estrogen-related compounds is not recommended at this time. For women in early perimenopause, hormone replacement therapy may provide an initial benefit for preventing cognitive decline. Once the clinical symptoms of Alzheimer's disease are present, however, studies have shown that estrogen replacement may have negative effects on sustained cognitive performance (Thal et al. 2003). However, recent research in elderly primates indicates that early intervention with estrogen replacement can significantly benefit the structural and functional integrity of key brain sites by enabling synaptic plasticity (J. Hao et al. 2007). Research on the use of hormone replacement therapy for the prevention and treatment of cognitive impairment in perimenopausal women remains active.

Nutraceuticals

To date, randomized, placebo-controlled studies of nutraceutical and herbal treatments for cognitive impairment are limited. Animal studies and limited human studies are of interest but yet not conclusive about the treatments' benefits in humans. Agents of interest include *Rubia cordifolia* root, sage (*Salvia lavandulaefolia*), rosemary (*Rosmarinus officinalis*), and lemon balm (*Melissa officinalis*) (Kennedy and Scholey 2006; Patil et al. 2006). Sage has been shown to improve immediate word recall in healthy young adults (Tildesley et al. 2003). Various compounds found in these agents have been shown to have AChE and BChE inhibitory properties, possess anti-inflammatory and antioxidant properties, and modulate muscarinic and nicotinic receptors (Kennedy and Scholey 2006). L-theanine, an amino acid found in green tea, has shown limited cognition-enhancing effects (Nathan et al. 2006). If further randomized, placebo-controlled studies show even a modest beneficial effect, these agents would have potential in combination therapy for the prevention and treatment of Alzheimer's disease and other types of cognitive impairment. Prior to recommending any of these agents, clarity with regard to the expected target system is important because combination therapy with existing AChEIs could cause profound exacerbation of side effects.

Dehydro-3-Epiandrosterone

Dehydro-3-epiandrosterone (DHEA), including the sulfated ester form, is an adrenal hormone with potential neuroprotective effects and the ability to enhance glutamate's effects. Research results are mixed concerning the potential benefit of DHEA for the treatment of cognitive impairment. Case reports suggest improvement in cognition with DHEA usage. DHEA supplementation has been suggested to have a direct negative effect on cognition (Parsons et al. 2006). A recent Cochrane review of three studies did not find a beneficial effect of DHEA supplementation in a population without dementia; however, the authors noted a need for long-term studies with an adequate number of subjects (Evans et al. 2006). DHEA may have a transient effect on cognitive functioning but not provide sustained cognitive improvement (Wolkowitz et al. 2003).

General Compounds

Aniracetam has been shown to improve cognitive impairment from traumatic brain injury to a rat model even after a delay of up to 11 days (Baranova et al. 2006). Piracetam, a cyclic derivative of γ-aminobutyric acid, has mild beneficial cognitive effects on memory and learning (Winnicka et al. 2005). In animal models, unifiram has been shown to induce acetylcholine release and act as a cognition-enhancing agent (Martini et al. 2005).

Immunomodulatory Agents

Antiamyloid immunization may provide one of the greatest opportunities to prevent β-amyloid deposition. Immunization strategies generally focus on active or passive immunization and direct central nervous system delivery of anti–amyloid beta antibodies. Active immunization with β-amyloid antibodies can reduce plaque formation (Lemere et al. 2006; Solomon 2006). Passive immunization with monoclonal antibodies or preparations of immunoconjugates shows promise for treating cognitive impairment due to Alzheimer's disease and may be safer than active immunization (Geylis and Steinitz 2006; Solomon 2007). Active and passive immunization may cause microhemorrhages, and further research continues to seek safer vaccines. Reversal of plaque load occurred in mutant mice after active immunization with β-peptide (Games et al. 2000; Schenk et al. 1999). However, during early human trials, meningoencephalitis occurred in up to 5% of the subjects, causing the study to be halted. The occurrence of meningoencephalitis may have been caused by excessive cell-mediated immunity (Asuni et al. 2006). Further research into the potential use of vaccine-driven immunomodulatory approaches is warranted.

Conclusion

The molecular pathogenesis of nerve cell death remains elusive, especially as it relates to the onset and progression of cognitive impairment. Alzheimer's disease and other types of cognitive impairment represent a wide spectrum of neurosystem dysfunction, and no single treatment modality yet found is sufficient to address the global apoptosis and degeneration that occur. Due to the multiple types of neurochemical and substructure dysfunction occurring in cognitive impairment, multiple-drug interventions will likely be required (Siskou et al. 2007; Sunderland et al. 1992).

Future studies will explore second-messenger modulation, inhibition of the synthesis of β-amyloid using a mimic of the prion protein to inhibit β-secretase cleavage of the amyloid precursor protein, amyloid plaque sheet breakers, AMPA receptor modulators, and the role of σ_1-receptor agonists and selective neuronal nicotinic receptor agonists (Parkin et al. 2007; Rose et al. 2005; Sarter 2006). Currently, the AChEIs and memantine are appropriate choices for slowing the progression of cognitive impairment. Several other promising agents are likely to become available within the next few years.

References

Aarsland D, Laake K, Larsen JP, et al: Donepezil for cognitive impairment in Parkinson's disease: a randomized controlled study. J Neurol Neurosurg Psychiatry 72:708–712, 2002

Aisen PS, Davis KL: Inflammatory mechanisms in Alzheimer's disease: implications for therapy. Am J Psychiatry 151:1105–1113, 1994

Andrieu S, Gillette S, Amouyal K, et al: Association of Alzheimer's disease onset with ginkgo biloba and other symptomatic cognitive treatments in a population of women aged 75 years and older from the EPIDOS study. J Gerontol A Biol Sci Med Sci 58A:M372–M377, 2003

Asai M, Hattori C, Iwata N, et al: The novel beta-secretase inhibitor KMI-429 reduces amyloid B peptide production in amyloid precursor protein transgenic and wild-type mice. J Neurochem 96:533–540, 2006

Asuni AA, Boutajangout A, Scholtzova H, et al: Vaccination of Alzheimer's model mice with Abeta derivative in alum adjuvant reduces Abeta burden without microhemorrhages. Eur J Neurosci 24:2530–2542, 2006

Baranova AI, Whiting MD, Hamm RJ: Delayed, post-injury treatment with aniracetam improves cognitive performance after traumatic brain injury in rats. J Neurotrauma 23:1233–1240, 2006

Bartus RT, Dean RL, Beer B, et al: The cholinergic hypothesis of geriatric memory dysfunction. Science 217:408–414, 1982

Behl C: Vitamin E and other antioxidants in neuroprotection. Int J Vitam Nutr Res 69:213–219, 1999

Behl C, Davis J, Cole GM, et al: Vitamin E protects nerve cells from amyloid beta protein toxicity. Biochem Biophys Res Commun 186:944–950, 1992

Bernick C, Katz R, Smith NL, et al: Statins and cognitive function in the elderly: the Cardiovascular Health Study. Neurology 65:1388–1394, 2005

Birks J: Cholinesterase inhibitors for Alzheimer's disease. Cochrane Database Syst Rev (1):CD005593, 2006

Birks J, Flicker L: Donepezil for mild cognitive impairment. Cochrane Database Syst Rev (3):CD006104, 2006

Birks J, Flicker L: Investigational treatment for vascular cognitive impairment. Expert Opin Investig Drugs 16:647–658, 2007

Birks J, Harvey RJ: Donepezil for dementia due to Alzheimer's disease. Cochrane Database Syst Rev (1):CD001190, 2006

Black S, Roman GC, Geldmacher DS, et al: Efficacy and tolerability of donepezil in vascular dementia: positive results of a 24-week, multicenter, international, randomized, placebo-controlled clinical trial. Stroke 34:2323–2330, 2003

Blasko I, Bodner T, Knaus G, et al: Efficacy of donepezil treatment in Alzheimer patients with and without subcortical vascular lesions. Pharmacology 72:1–5, 2004

Bullock R: Efficacy and safety of memantine in moderate-to-severe Alzheimer disease: the evidence to date. Alzheimer Dis Assoc Disord 20:23–29, 2006

Chen X, Magnotta VA, Duff K, et al: Donepezil effects on cerebral blood flow in older adults with mild cognitive deficits. J Neuropsychiatry Clin Neurosci 18:178–185, 2006

Christodoulou C, Melville P, Scherl WF, et al: Effects of donepezil on memory and cognition in multiple sclerosis. J Neurol Sci 245:127–136, 2006

Coelho F, Birks J: Physostigmine for Alzheimer's disease. Cochrane Database Syst Rev (2):CD001499, 2001

Cohen RA, Browndyke JN, Moser DJ, et al: Long-term citicoline (cytidine diphosphate choline) use in patients with vascular dementia: neuroimaging and neuropsychological outcomes. Cerebrovascular Dis 16:199–204, 2003

Coyle J, Kershaw P: Galantamine, a cholinesterase inhibitor that allosterically modulates nicotinic receptors: effects on the course of Alzheimer's disease. Biol Psychiatry 49:289–299, 2001

Craig D, Birks J: Galantamine for vascular cognitive impairment. Cochrane Database Syst Rev (1):CD004746, 2006

Cummings JL, Schneider E, Tariot PN, et al: Behavioral effects of memantine in Alzheimer disease patients receiving donepezil treatment. Neurology 67:57–63, 2006

Cusi C, Cantisani T, Celani M, et al: Galantamine for Alzheimer's disease and mild cognitive impairment. Neuroepidemiology 28:116–117, 2007

Dartigues JF, Carcaillon L, Helmer C, et al: Vasodilators and nootropics as predictors of dementia and mortality in the PAQUID cohort. J Am Geriatr Soc 55:395–399, 2007

Davies P, Maloney AFJ: Selective loss of central cholinergic neurons in Alzheimer's disease (letter). Lancet 2:1403, 1976

Desmond DW, Tatemichi TK, Paik M, et al: Risk factors for cerebrovascular disease as correlates of cognitive function in a stroke-free cohort. Arch Neurol 50:162–166, 1993

Dunbar G, Boeijinga PH, Demazieres A, et al: Effects of TC-1734 (AZD3480), a selective neuronal nicotinic receptor agonist, on cognitive performance and the EEG of young healthy male volunteers. Psychopharmacology (Berl) 191:919–929, 2007

Engelhart MJ, Geerlings MI, Ruitenberg A, et al: Dietary intake of antioxidants and risk of Alzheimer disease. JAMA 287:3223–3229, 2002

Enz A, Amstutz R, Boddeke H, et al: Brain selective inhibition of acetylcholinesterase: a novel approach to therapy for Alzheimer's disease. Prog Brain Res 98:431–438, 1993

Evans JG, Malouf R, Huppert F, et al: Dehydroepiandrosterone (DHEA) supplementation for cognitive function in healthy elderly people. Cochrane Database Syst Rev (4):CD006221, 2006

Fioravanti M, Yanagi M: Cytidinediphosphocholine (CDP-choline) for cognitive and behavioral disturbances associated with chronic cerebral disorders in the elderly. Cochrane Database Syst Rev (2):CD000269, 2005

Games D, Bard F, Grajeda H, et al: Prevention and reduction of AD-type pathology in PDAPP mice immunized with A beta 1–42. Ann N Y Acad Sci 920:274–284, 2000

Gearing M, Mirra SS, Hedreen JC, et al: The Consortium to Establish a Registry for Alzheimer's Disease (CERAD): part X: neuropathology confirmation of the clinical diagnosis of Alzheimer's disease. Neurology 45:461–466, 1995

Geerts H: NC-531 (Neurochem). Curr Opin Investig Drugs 5:95–100, 2004

Geylis V, Steinitz M: Immunotherapy of Alzheimer's disease (AD): from murine models to anti-amyloid beta (Abeta) human monoclonal antibodies. Autoimmun Rev 5:33–39, 2006

Grossberg GT, Edwards KR, Zhao Q: Rationale for combination therapy with galantamine and memantine in Alzheimer's disease. J Clin Pharmacol 46:17S–26S, 2006

Hamaguchi T, Ono K, Yamada M: Anti-amyloidogenic therapies: strategies for prevention and treatment of Alzheimer's disease. Cell Mol Life Sci 63:1538–1552, 2006

Hao H, Wang G, Sun J: Enantioselective pharmacokinetics of ibuprofen and involved mechanisms. Drug Metab Rev 37:215–234, 2005

Hao J, Rapp PR, Janssen WG, et al: Interactive effects of age and estrogen on cognition and pyramidal neurons in monkey prefrontal cortex. Proc Natl Acad Sci U S A 104:11465–11470, 2007

Jick H, Zornberg GL, Jick SS, et al: Statins and the risk of dementia. Lancet 356:1627–1631, 2000

Jones RW: Have cholinergic therapies reached their clinical boundary in Alzheimer's disease? Int J Geriatr Psychiatry 18:S7–S13, 2003

Jyoti P, Kotwai A, Prabhu HRA: Therapeutic and prophylactic utility of the memory-enhancing drug donepezil hydrochloride on cognition of patients undergoing electroconvulsive therapy: a randomized controlled trial. J ECT 22:163–168, 2006

Kalaria RN, Cohen DL, Premkumar DR: Cellular aspects of the inflammatory response in Alzheimer's disease. Neurodegeneration 5:497–503, 1996

Kang JH, Cook N, Manson JA, et al: Low dose aspirin and cognitive function in the Women's Health Study cognitive cohort. BMJ 334:987, 2007

Kennedy DO, Scholey AB: The psychopharmacology of European herbs with cognition-enhancing properties. Curr Pharm Des 12:4613–4623, 2006

Klein J: Membrane breakdown in acute and chronic neurodegeneration: focus on choline-containing phospholipids. J Neural Transm 107:1027–1063, 2000

Koch HJ, Uyanik G, Fischer-Barnicol D: Memantine: a therapeutic approach in treating Alzheimer's and vascular dementia. Curr Drug Targets CNS Neurol Disord 4:499–506, 2005

Kurz A, Van Baelen B: Ginkgo biloba compared with cholinesterase inhibitors in the treatment of dementia: a review based on meta-analyses by the Cochrane collaboration. Dement Geriatr Cogn Disord 18:217–226, 2004

Lee SW, Lee JG, Lee BJ, et al: A 12-week, double-blind, placebo-controlled trial of galantamine adjunctive treatment to conventional antipsychotics for the cognitive impairments in chronic schizophrenia. Int Clin Psychopharmacol 22:63–68, 2007

Lemere CA, Maier M, Jiang L, et al: Amyloid-beta immunotherapy for the prevention and treatment of Alzheimer disease: lessons from mice, monkeys, and humans. Rejuvenation Res 9:77–84, 2006

Leroi I, Brandt J, Reich SG, et al: Randomized placebo-controlled trial of donepezil in cognitive impairment in Parkinson's disease. Int J Geriatr Psychiatry 19:1–8, 2004

Lipton SA, Rosenberg PA: Excitatory amino acids as a final common pathway for neurologic disorders. N Engl J Med 330:613–622, 1994

Lopez-Arrieta JM, Schneider L: Metrifonate for Alzheimer's disease. Cochrane Database Syst Rev (2):CD003155, 2006

Loy C, Schneider L: Galantamine for Alzheimer's disease and mild cognitive impairment. Cochrane Database Syst Rev (1):CD001747, 2006

Malik R, Sangwan A, Saihgal R, et al: Towards better brain management: nootropics. Curr Med Chem 14:123–131, 2007

Malouf R, Birks J: Donepezil for vascular cognitive impairment. Cochrane Database Syst Rev (1):CD004395, 2004

Martini E, Ghelardini C, Bertucci C, et al: Enantioselective synthesis and preliminary pharmacological evaluation of the enantiomers of unifiram (DM232), a potent cognition-enhancing agent. Med Chem 1:473–480, 2005

Mesulam M: The cholinergic lesion of Alzheimer's disease: pivotal factor or side show? Learn Mem 11:43–49, 2004

Molecule of the month: tramiprosate. Drug News Perspect 19:64, 2006

Muñoz-Ruiz P, Rubio L, Garcia-Palomero E, et al: Design, synthesis, and biological evaluation of dual binding site acetylcholinesterase inhibitors: new disease-modifying agents for Alzheimer's disease. J Med Chem 48:7223–7233, 2005

Murphy KJ, Foley AG, O'Connell AW, et al: Chronic exposure of rats to cognition enhancing drugs produces a neuroplastic response identical to that obtained by complex environment rearing. Neuropsychopharmacology 31:90–100, 2006

Naik SR, Pilgaonkar VW, Panda VS: Neuropharmacological evaluation of Ginkgo biloba phytosomes in rodents. Phytother Res 20:901–905, 2006

Nathan PJ, Lu K, Gray M, et al: The neuropharmacology of L-theanine (N-ethyl-L-glutamine): a possible neuroprotective and cognitive enhancing agent. J Herb Pharmacother 6:21–30, 2006

Newhouse PA, Potter A, Levin ED: Nicotinic system involvement in Alzheimer's and Parkinson's diseases: implications for therapeutics. Drugs Aging 11:206–228, 1997

Newhouse PA, Potter A, Kelton M, et al: Nicotinic treatment of Alzheimer's disease. Biol Psychiatry 49:268–278, 2001

O'Brien MD: How does cerebrovascular disease cause dementia? Dementia 5:133–136, 1994

Parkin ET, Watt NT, Hussain I, et al: Cellular prion protein regulates beta-secretase cleavage of the Alzheimer's amyloid precursor protein. Proc Natl Acad Sci U S A 104:11062–11067, 2007

Parsons TD, Kratz KM, Thompson E, et al: DHEA supplementation and cognition in postmenopausal women. Int J Neurosci 116:141–155, 2006

Patil RA, Jagdale SC, Kasture SB: Antihyperglycemic, antistress and nootropic activity of roots of Rubia cordifolia Linn. Indian J Exp Biol 44:987–992, 2006

Potter A, Corwin J, Lang J, et al: Acute effects of the selective cholinergic channel activator (nicotinic agonist) ABT-418 in Alzheimer's disease. Psychopharmacology (Berl) 142:334–342, 1999

Randall DC, Fleck NL, Shneerson JM, et al: The cognitive-enhancing properties of modafinil are limited in non-sleep-deprived middle-aged volunteers. Pharmacol Biochem Behav 77:547–555, 2004

Reisberg B, Doody R, Stoffler A, et al: Memantine in moderate-to-severe Alzheimer's disease. N Engl J Med 348:1333–1341, 2003

Rockwood K, Ebly E, Hachinski V, et al: Presence and treatment of vascular risk factors in patients with vascular cognitive impairment. Arch Neurol 54:33–39, 1997

Rockwood K, Kirkland S, Hogan DB, et al: Use of lipid-lowering agents, indication bias, and the risk of dementia in community-dwelling elderly people. Arch Neurol 59:223–227, 2002

Rose GM, Hopper A, De Vivo M, et al: Phosphodiesterase inhibitors for cognitive enhancement. Curr Pharm Des 11:3329–3334, 2005

Rowan E, McKeith IG, Saxby BK, et al: Effects of donepezil on central processing speed and attentional measures in Parkinson's disease with dementia and dementia with Lewy bodies. Dement Geriatr Cogn Disord 23:161–167, 2007

Rusted JM, Caulfield D, King L, et al: Moving out of the laboratory: does nicotine improve everyday attention? Behav Pharmacol 11:621–629, 2000

Sano M, Ernesto C, Thomas RG, et al: A controlled trial of selegiline, alpha-tocopherol, or both as treatment for Alzheimer's disease. The Alzheimer's Disease Cooperative Study. N Engl J Med 336:1216–1222, 1997

Sarter M: Preclinical research into cognition enhancers. Trends Pharmacol Sci 27:602–608, 2006

Schenk D, Barbour R, Dunn W, et al: Immunization with amyloid-beta attenuates Alzheimer-disease-like pathology in the PDAPP mouse. Nature 400:173–177, 1999

Schwarz RD, Callahan MJ, Coughenour LL, et al: Milameline (CI-979/RU35926): a muscarinic receptor agonist with cognition-activating properties: biochemical and in vivo characterization. J Pharmacol Exp Ther 29:812–822, 1999

Secades JJ, Lorenzo JL: Citicoline: Pharmacological and clinical review, 2006 update. Methods Find Exp Clin Pharmacol 27:S1–S56, 2006

Selkoe DJ: Toward a comprehensive theory for Alzheimer's disease: hypothesis: Alzheimer's disease is caused by the cerebral accumulation and cytotoxicity of amyloid beta-protein. Ann N Y Acad Sci 924:17–25, 2000

Seltzer B: Cholinesterase inhibitors in the clinical management of Alzheimer's disease: importance of early and persistent treatment. J Int Med Res 34:339–347, 2006

Seltzer B: Donepezil: an update. Expert Opin Pharmacother 8:1011–1023, 2007

Siskou IC, Rekka EA, Kourounakis AP, et al: Design and study of some novel ibuprofen derivatives with potential nootropic and neuroprotective properties. Bioorg Med Chem 15:951–961, 2007

Solomon B: Alzheimer's disease immunotherapy: from in vitro amyloid immunomodulation to in vivo vaccination. J Alzheimers Dis 9:433–438, 2006

Solomon B: Clinical immunologic approaches for the treatment of Alzheimer's disease. Expert Opin Investig Drugs 16:819–828, 2007

Sunderland T, Tariot PN, Newhouse PA: Differential responsivity of mood, behavior, and cognition to cholinergic agents in elderly neuropsychiatric populations. Brain Res 472:371–389, 1988

Sunderland T, Molchan S, Lawlor B, et al: A strategy of "combination chemotherapy" in Alzheimer's disease: rationale and preliminary results with physostigmine plus deprenyl. Int Psychogeriatr 4:291–309, 1992

Tariot PN, Farlow MR, Grossberg GT, et al: Memantine treatment in patients with moderate to severe Alzheimer's disease already receiving donepezil: a randomized controlled trial. JAMA 291:317–324, 2004

Tasker A, Perry EK, Ballard CG: Butyrylcholinesterase: impact on symptoms and progression of cognitive impairment. Expert Rev Neurother 5:101–106, 2005

Terry AV, Buccafusco JJ: The cholinergic hypothesis of age and Alzheimer's disease-related cognitive deficits: recent challenges and their implications for novel drug development. J Pharmacol Exp Ther 306:821–827, 2003

Thal LJ, Thomas RG, Mulnard R, et al: Estrogen levels do not correlate with improvement in cognition. Arch Neurol 60:209–212, 2003

Thompson S, Lanctot KL, Herrmann N: The benefits and risks associated with cholinesterase inhibitor therapy in Alzheimer's disease. Expert Opin Drug Saf 3:425–440, 2004

Tildesley NT, Kennedy DO, Perry EK, et al: Salvia lavandulaefolia (Spanish sage) enhances memory in healthy young volunteers. Pharmacol Biochem Behav 75:669–674, 2003

Ved HS, Koenig ML, Dave JR, et al: Huperzine A, a potential therapeutic agent for dementia, reduces neuronal cell death caused by glutamate. Neuroreport 8:963–968, 1997

Wallin AK, Andreasen N, Eriksson S, et al: Donepezil in Alzheimer's disease: what to expect after 3 years of treatment in a routine clinical setting. Dement Geriatr Cogn Disord 23:150–160, 2007

Weggen S, Eriksen JL, Das P, et al: A subset of NSAIDs lower amyloidogenic Abeta42 independently of cyclooxygenase activity. Nature 414:212–216, 2001

Whalley LJ, Mowat DH: Aspirin and cognitive function. BMJ 334:961–962, 2007

White HK, Levin ED: Four-week nicotine skin patch treatment effects on cognitive performance in Alzheimer's disease. Psychopharmacology (Berl) 143:158–165, 1999

Whitehouse PJ, Price DL, Struble RG, et al: Alzheimer's disease and senile dementia: loss of neurons in the basal forebrain. Science 215:1237–1239, 1982

Wilkinson D, Doody R, Helme R, et al: Donepezil in vascular dementia: a randomized, placebo-controlled study. Neurology 61:479–486, 2003

Winblad B, Jelic V, Kershaw P, et al: Effects of statins on cognitive function in patients with Alzheimer's disease in galantamine clinical trials. Drugs Aging 24:57–61, 2007

Winnicka K, Tomasiak M, Bielawska A: Piracetam—an old drug with novel properties? Acta Pol Pharm 62:405–409, 2005

Wolkowitz OM, Kramer JH, Reus VI, et al: DHEA treatment of Alzheimer's disease: a randomized, double-blind, placebo-controlled study. Neurology 60:1071–1076, 2003

Wolozin B, Kellman W, Ruosseau P, et al: Decreased prevalence of Alzheimer disease associated with 3-hydroxy-3-methyglutaryl coenzyme A reductase inhibitors. Arch Neurol 57:1439–1443, 2000

Zangara A: The psychopharmacology of huperzine A: an alkaloid with cognitive enhancing and neuroprotective properties of interest in the treatment of Alzheimer's disease. Pharmacol Biochem Behav 75:675–686, 2003

Zhang W, Edvinsson L, Lee TJ: Mechanism of nicotine-induced relaxation in the porcine basilar artery. J Pharmacol Exp Ther 284:790–797, 1998

Zhang Z, Wang X, Chen Q, et al: Clinical efficacy and safety of huperzine alpha in treatment of mild to moderate Alzheimer disease, a placebo-controlled, double-blind, randomized trial [in Chinese]. Zhonghua Yi Xue Za Zhi 82:941–944, 2002

CHAPTER 42

Sedative-Hypnotics

Seiji Nishino, M.D., Ph.D.

Kazuo Mishima, M.D., Ph.D.

Emmanuel Mignot, M.D., Ph.D.

William C. Dement, M.D., Ph.D.

In this chapter, we examine some of the pharmacological properties of benzodiazepines, barbiturates, and other sedative-hypnotic compounds. Sedative drugs moderate excitement, decrease activity, and induce calmness, whereas hypnotic drugs produce drowsiness and facilitate the onset and maintenance of a state that resembles normal sleep in its electroencephalographic characteristics. Although these agents are central nervous system (CNS) depressants, they usually produce therapeutic effects at doses that are far lower than those that cause coma and generalized depression of the CNS.

Some sedative-hypnotic drugs retain other therapeutic uses as muscle relaxants (especially benzodiazepines), antiepileptic agents, or preanesthetic medications. Although benzodiazepines are used widely as antianxiety drugs, whether their effect on anxiety is truly distinct from their effect on sleepiness remains unconfirmed.

Sedative-hypnotics are also important drugs to neuroscientists. These substances modulate basic behaviors such as arousal and response to stress. With increasing understanding of the molecular structure of the γ-aminobutyric acid type A ($GABA_A$) receptor, the cellular mechanisms of these compounds' mode of action have become elucidated. Further understanding of their mode of action could thus help to elucidate neurochemical and neurophysiological control of these behaviors.

Benzodiazepines

History and Discovery

Benzodiazepines were first synthesized in the 1930s but were not systematically evaluated until 20 years later. The introduction of chlorpromazine and meprobamate, which had sedative effects in animals, in the early 1950s, led to the decade of development of sophisticated in vivo pharmacological screening methods that were used to identify the sedative properties of benzodiazepines. More than 3,000 benzodiazepines have been synthesized since chlordiazepoxide, which was synthesized by Sterbach in 1957, was introduced into clinical medicine. About 40 of them are in clinical use.

Several drugs chemically unrelated to the benzodiazepines have been shown to have sedative-hypnotic effects with a benzodiazepine-like profile, and these drugs have been determined to act via the benzodiazepine binding site on $GABA_A$ receptor.

Most of the benzodiazepines currently on the market were selected for their high anxiolytic potential relative to CNS depression. Nevertheless, all benzodiazepines have sedative-hypnotic properties to various degrees, and some compounds that facilitate sleep have been used as hypnotics.

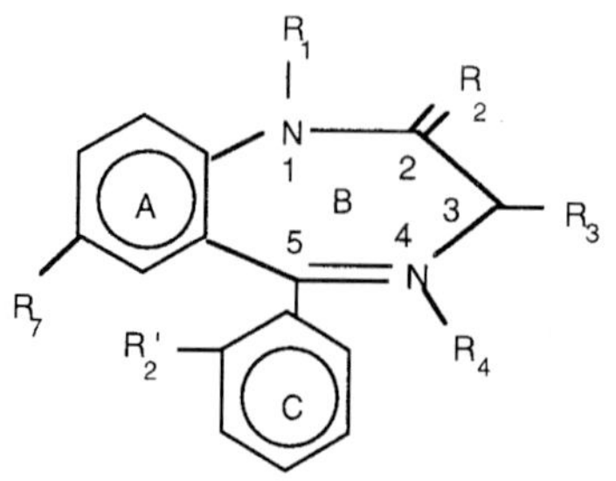

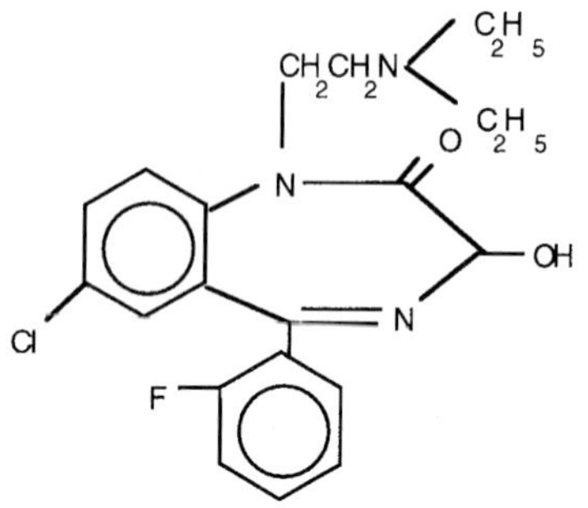

Flurazepam

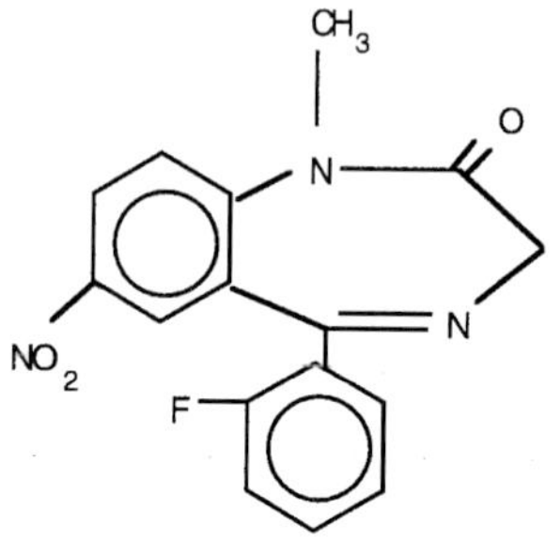

Flunitrazepam

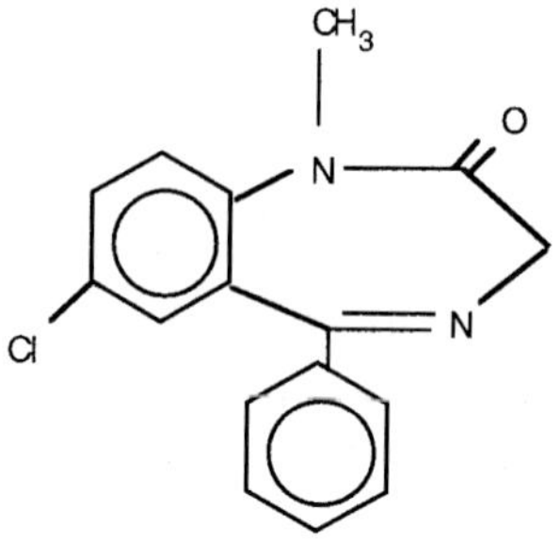

Diazepam

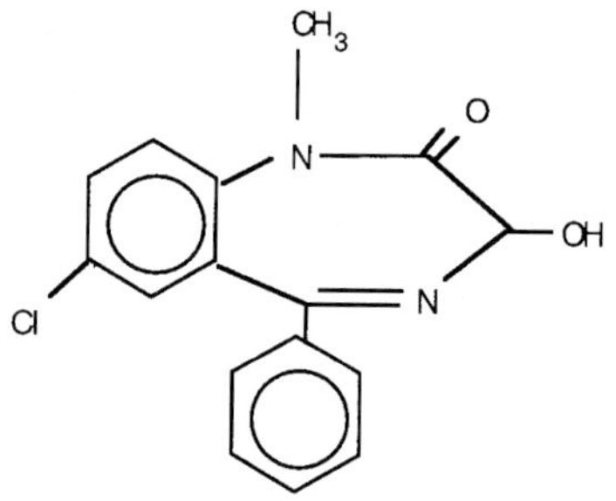

Temazepam

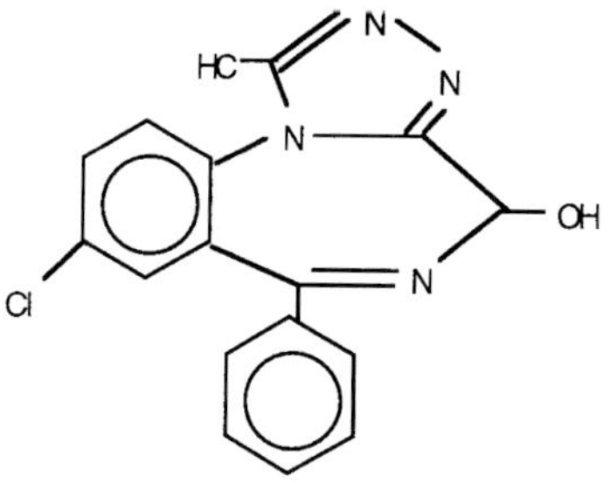

Triazolam

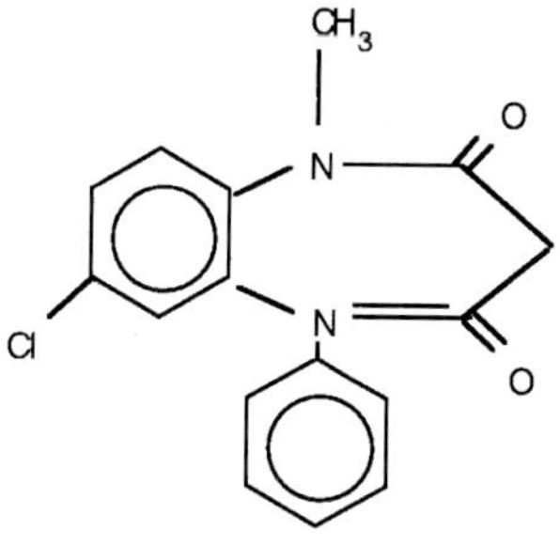

Clobazam

FIGURE 42–1. Chemical structures of some commonly used benzodiazepines.

Mainly because of their remarkably low capacity to produce fatal CNS depression, benzodiazepines have displaced barbiturates as sedative-hypnotic agents.

Structure–Activity Relations

The term *benzodiazepine* refers to the portion of the structure composed of benzene rings (*A* in Figure 42–1) fused to a seven-membered diazepine ring (*B*). However, most of the older benzodiazepines contain a 5-aryl substituent (*C*) and a 1,4-diazepine ring, and the term has come to mean 1,4-benzodiazepines.

A substituent (most often chloride) at position 7 is essential for biological activity. A carbonyl at position 2 enhances activity and is generally present. Most of the newest products also substitute the 2 position, as with flurazepam. These general features are important for the metabolic fate of the compounds. Because the 7 and 2 positions of the molecule are resistant to all major degradative pathways, many of the metabolites retain substantial pharmacological activity.

Pharmacological Profile

Benzodiazepines share anticonvulsant and sedative-hypnotic effects with the barbiturates. In addition, they have a remarkable ability to reduce anxiety and aggression (Cook and Sepinwall 1975). In the mammalian CNS, two subtypes of benzodiazepine omega (ω) receptors have been pharmacologically recognized. Benzodiazepine ω_1 (or BZ1) receptors are sensitive to β-carbolines, imidazopyridines (e.g., zolpidem), and triazolopyridazines. Benzodiazepine ω_2 (or BZ2) receptors have low affinity for these ligands and relatively high affinity for benzodiazepines. Benzodiazepine ω_1 sites are enriched in the cerebellum, whereas ω_2 sites are mostly present in the spinal cord, and both receptor subtypes are found in the cerebral cortex and hippocampus. Benzodiazepine ω_1 and ω_2 receptor subtypes are also located peripherally in adrenal chromaffin cells.

Another subtype, ω_3, was identified and is commonly labeled as the *peripheral benzodiazepine receptor subtype* because of its distribution on glial cell membranes in nonnervous tissues such as adrenal, testis, liver, heart, and kidney. The subtype was later detected in the CNS, especially on the mitochondrial membrane and not in association with GABA$_A$ receptors (Gavish et al. 1992). The ω_3 receptor subtype has high affinity for benzodiazepines and isoquinoline carboxamides (Awad and Gavish 1987). The functional role of this receptor is unknown, but it may be involved in the biosynthesis and mediation of the sedative-hypnotic effects of some neuroactive steroids (pregnenolone, dehydroepiandrosterone [DHEA], allopregnanolone, tetrahydrodeoxycorticosterone) (Edgar et al. 1997; Friess et al. 1996; Rupprecht et al. 1996). Neurosteroids modulate GABA$_A$-mediated transmission through an allosteric mechanism that is distinct from that of benzodiazepines and barbiturates. By stimulation of ω_3 receptors with agonists, cholesterol is transferred from intracellular stores in mitochondria and becomes available to the mitochondrial P450 cholesterol-side-chain-cleavage (P450scc), and neurosteroid biosynthesis begins (Papadopoulos et al. 2001). Benzodiazepine ω_3 receptor subtypes also may serve as mitochondrial membrane stabilizers and protect against pathologically induced mitochondrial and cell toxicity (Papadopoulos et al. 2001).

The GABA$_A$ receptor is a ligand-gated ion channel that mediates fast synaptic neurotransmission in the CNS. When the GABA$_A$ receptor is occupied by GABA or GABA agonists such as muscimol, the chloride channels open and chloride ions diffuse into the cell. Schmidt et al. (1967) first reported that diazepam could potentiate the inhibitory effects of GABA on the spinal cord in cats. Later, it was shown that the effect of diazepam could be abolished if the endogenous content of GABA was depleted. These findings established that diazepam (and related benzodiazepines) did not act directly through GABA but modulated inhibitory transmission through the GABA$_A$ receptor in some other way. It was subsequently reported that benzodiazepines bind specifically to neural elements in the mammalian brain with high affinity and that an excellent correlation exists between drug affinities for these specific binding sites and in vivo pharmacological potencies (Möhler and Okada 1977; Squires and Braestrup 1977).

The binding of a benzodiazepine to this receptor site is enhanced in the presence of GABA or a GABA agonist, thereby suggesting that a functional (but independent) relationship exists between the GABA$_A$ receptor and the benzodiazepine receptor (Tallman et al. 1978). Barbiturates (and to some extent alcohol) also seem to produce anxiolytic and sedative effects at least partly by facilitating GABAergic transmission (see section "Barbiturates" in this chapter). This common action for chemically unrelated compounds can be explained by the ability of these compounds to stimulate specific sites on the GABA$_A$ receptor.

The benzodiazepines bind with high affinity to their binding sites so that the action of GABA on its receptor is allosterically enhanced. GABA can produce stronger postsynaptic inhibition in the presence of a benzodiazepine. Benzodiazepine agonists are assumed to potentiate only ongoing physiologically initiated actions of GABA (at GABA$_A$ receptors), whereas barbiturates are thought to cause inhibition at all GABAergic synapses regardless of their physiological activity. In addition, barbiturates appear to increase the duration of the open state of the chloride channel, whereas benzodiazepines increase the frequency of channel openings with little effect on duration (Twyman et al. 1989). These fundamental differences between the allosteric effects of benzodiazepines within the GABA$_A$ receptor and the conducive effects of barbiturates on the chloride ion channel may explain why low doses of barbiturates have a pharmacological profile similar to that of benzodiazepines, whereas high doses of barbiturates cause a profound and sometimes fatal suppression of brain synaptic transmission. Note that selective GABA$_A$ agonists, such as muscimol, have no sedative or anxiolytic properties; thus, the whole GABA$_A$–benzodiazepine receptor complex must be involved to possess sedative-hypnotic properties.

Molecular Mechanism of GABA$_A$–Benzodiazepine Receptor Interaction

The structure of the GABA$_A$–benzodiazepine receptor complex has been elucidated by the cloning of all the implicated subunit genes and the study of the corresponding encoded proteins. The GABA$_A$ receptor is a pentameric protein consisting of five subunits, which forms a rosette surrounding a transmembrane ion channel pore for Cl$^-$ (Figure 42–2). The GABA$_A$ receptor in humans includes the following known subunits: α_1–α_6, β_1–β_4, γ_1–γ_4, δ, ε,

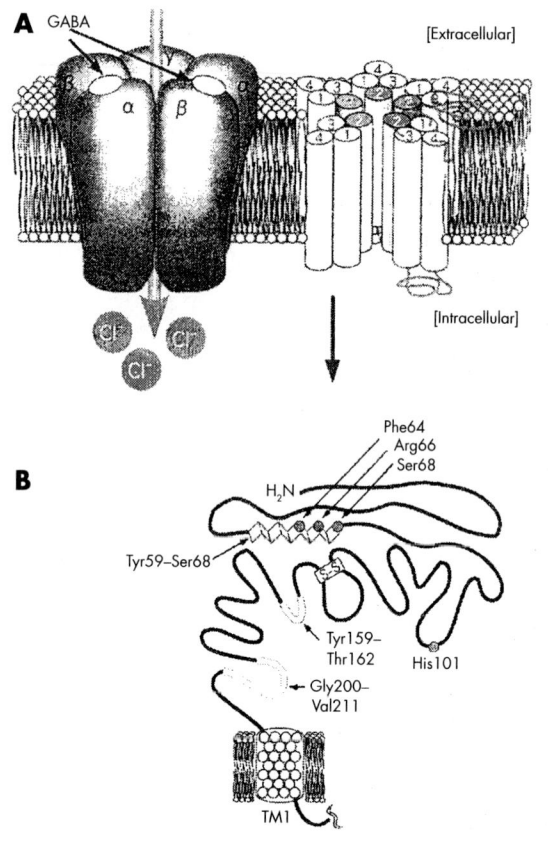

FIGURE 42–2. The GABA$_A$–benzodiazepine receptor complex.

(A) Schematic model of the mammalian γ-aminobutyric acid type A (GABA$_A$) receptor embedded in the cell membrane, representatively possessing the α, β, and γ subunits (2:2:1). The binding of two molecules of GABA to the action site composed of α and β subunits causes the opening of the chloride channel pore, and the chloride ions diffuse into the cell. Each subunit comprises four transmembrane domains (TM1–TM4). The ion channel pore consists of TM2 of five subunits with a rosette formation. **(B)** Structure of the α$_1$ subunit, with amino acid sequence, indicating amino acid residues implicated in GABA and benzodiazepine binding domains.
Source.   Modified from Ueno et al. 2001.

π, and τ (7 kinds of subunits, 18 isoforms total) (Mehta and Ticku 1999). Two alternatively spliced versions of the γ$_2$ subunit, γ$_{2S}$ and γ$_{2L}$, are also known to exist (Kofuji et al. 1991).

Despite many studies, the physiological and neuroanatomical processes mediating benzodiazepine action on the GABA$_A$ receptor complex remain poorly understood. One reason is that the GABAergic system is the most widespread of all inhibitory neurotransmitters and could be involved in many circuits responsive to various effects of benzodiazepine agonists. In addition, the various subtypes of GABA$_A$ receptor have different ligand affinity

and channel functions in response to benzodiazepine agonists. These subtypes of GABA$_A$ are broadly distributed in various brain areas to form a mosaic of receptor subtypes (Wisden and Stephens 1999), making it difficult to understand the functional mechanisms of interaction of benzodiazepine agonists on the GABA$_A$-ergic system from the physiological point of view (Rudolph et al. 1999). However, recent site-directed mutagenesis and gene knock-in techniques have identified several important findings about the benzodiazepine action sites on GABA$_A$ receptors and their physiological functions.

It is postulated that the binding of GABA to N-terminal extracellular domains of α and β subunits causes conformational changes within the subunits. Ion channel pores subsequently open, and Cl$^-$ flows across the neuronal membrane, resulting in neuronal inhibition (Amin and Weiss 1993; Boileau et al. 1999; Sigel et al. 1992; Smith and Olsen 1994) (see Figure 42–2). The extracellular domains of the α and γ subunits, which consist of about 220 amino acids in the N-terminal region, also have been shown to bind GABA and benzodiazepines. Pharmacologically classified ω$_1$ and ω$_2$ receptors are now thought to correspond to GABA$_A$ receptors possessing the α$_1$ and α$_2$ subunits and the α$_3$ and α$_5$ subunits, respectively.

Extracellular benzodiazepine binding sites on these subunits consist of several divided portions; His101, Tyr159–Thr162, and Gly200–Val211 on α$_1$ subunits, as well as Lys41–Trp82 and Arg114–Asp161 on γ$_2$ subunits, are essential to the formation of the binding pockets (Boileau et al. 1998). Most strikingly, His101 is a critical residue for diazepam to exhibit its sedative effect (Crestani et al. 2001; Low et al. 2000; McKernan et al. 2000; Rudolph et al. 1999). Knock-in mice with displacement of His101Arg are insensitive to benzodiazepine-induced allosteric modulation of the complex but have preserved physiological regulation by GABA (Rudolph et al. 1999). These knock-in mice failed to be sedated by diazepam but retained other effects of diazepam, such as anxiolytic-like, myorelaxant, motor-impairing, and ethanol-potentiating effects. This suggests the possibility that the sedative action of the benzodiazepine is mediated through GABA$_A$ receptors possessing the α$_1$ subunit. It is also noteworthy that His101Arg knock-in mice responded to diazepam and showed similar sleep changes as wild-type mice do, despite the lack of its sedative response in these animals (Tobler et al. 2001). Thus, hypnotic and sedative effects by benzodiazepines may be mediated via different subtypes, with hypnotic effects involving GABA$_A$ receptors possessing subunits other than α$_1$ (i.e., α$_2$, α$_3$, or α$_5$) (Tobler et al. 2001).

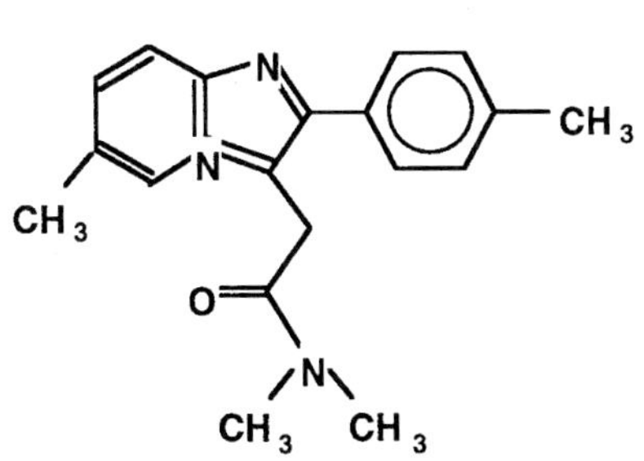

FIGURE 42-3. Three nonbenzodiazepine hypnotics—zolpidem (an imidazopyridine), zopiclone (a cyclopyrrolone), and zaleplon (a pyrazolopyrimidine)—have been shown to be useful sedative-hypnotics with benzodiazepine-like profiles.

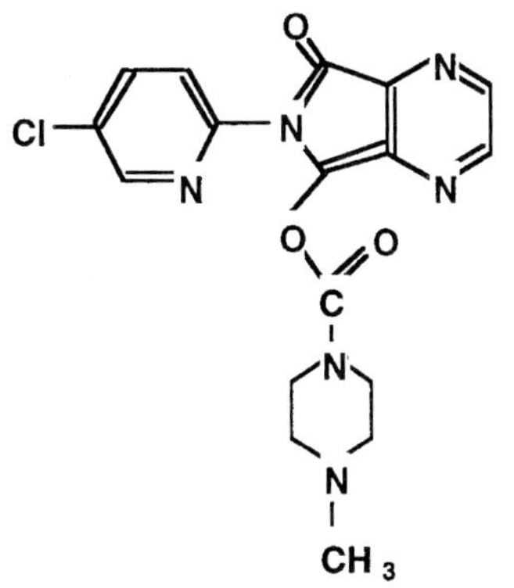

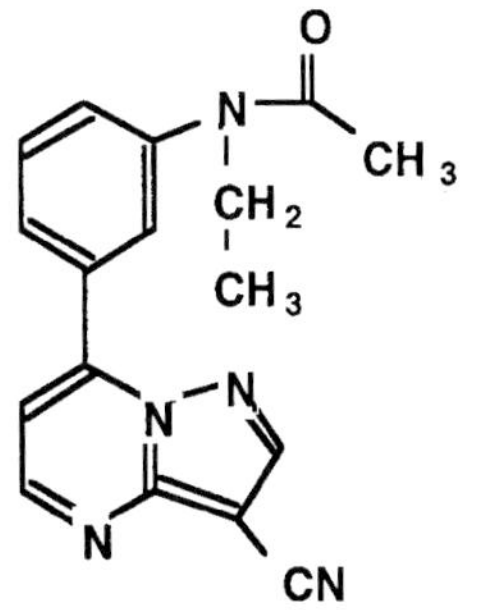

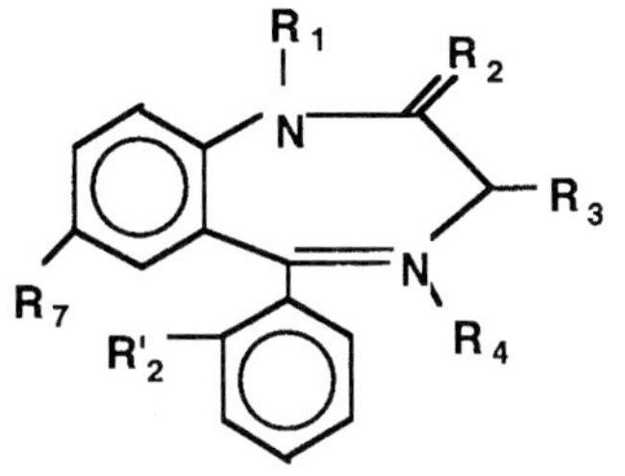

Nonbenzodiazepine Hypnotics (Acting on the Benzodiazepine Receptor)

Until about 1980, it was widely accepted that the benzodiazepine structure was a prerequisite for the anxiolytic profile and for benzodiazepine receptor recognition and binding. However, more recently, three chemically unrelated drugs—the imidazopyridine zolpidem, the cyclopyrrolone zopiclone (and its S[+]-enantiomer, eszopiclone), and the pyrazolopyrimidine zaleplon—have been shown to be useful sedative-hypnotics with benzodiazepine-like profiles (Figure 42–3). Other chemical classes of drugs that are structurally dissimilar to the benzodiazepines (e.g., triazolopyridazines) but act through the benzodiazepine receptor also have been developed and have anxiolytic activity in humans.

Nonbenzodiazepine hypnotics have a pharmacological profile slightly different from that of classic benzodiazepines. For example, zolpidem binds selectively to ω_1 (the 50% inhibitory concentration [IC$_{50}$] ratio for ω_1/ω_2

is nearly 1:10) and has sedative-hypnotic properties relative to other properties such as anxiolytic activity or muscle relaxation. Zolpidem and zopiclone have short half-lives (3 hours and 6 hours, respectively). These drugs were originally thought not to appreciably affect the rapid eye movement (REM) sleep pattern, whereas the quality of slow-wave sleep (SWS) may be slightly increased (Jovanovic and Dreyfus 1983; Shlarf 1992). Rebound effects (insomnia, anxiety), which are commonly seen following withdrawal of short-acting benzodiazepines, are minimal for zolpidem and zopiclone. These compounds also induce little respiratory depression and have less abuse potential than common clinical benzodiazepine hypnotics. However, much longer clinical trials are needed to show whether the imidazopyridines or cyclopyrrolones have any significant advantages over the short- to medium-half-life benzodiazepines in the treatment of insomnia. Eszopiclone, the active stereoisomer of zopiclone with longer half-life, was recently approved by the U.S. Food and Drug Administration (FDA). The drug was claimed to help for sleep maintaining as well as for sleep induction. Because the compound induces little tolerance, it is suitable for long-term use.

Zaleplon (N-[3-(3-cyanopyrazolo[1,5-a]pyrimidin-7-yl)phenyl]-N-ethylacetamide), a pyrazolopyrimidine, also has been developed as a novel nonbenzodiazepine hypnotic (see Figure 42–3). Clinical trials have shown that zaleplon is a well-tolerated, safe, rapidly acting, and effective sedative with advantages over lorazepam with respect to unwanted cognitive and psychomotor impairments (Allen et al. 1993; Beer et al. 1994).

Thanks to an increased understanding of the molecular structure of the $GABA_A$ receptor and its functional correlates, several pharmaceutical companies are also currently developing subtype-selective $GABA_A$ receptor agonists, such as for α_1, α_3, and α_4 (selective extrasynaptic $GABA_A$ receptor agonist) subtypes. Preclinical and clinical studies of these compounds suggested hypnotic effects, and hypnotic uses of some of these are likely to be approved within few years.

Benzodiazepine Antagonists, Partial Agonists, and Inverse Agonists

As knowledge of the relation between the structure of benzodiazepine receptor ligands and their pharmacological properties has increased, potent receptor agonists that stimulate the receptor and produce pharmacological effects qualitatively similar to those of classic benzodiazepines have been developed. *Antagonists*, which block the effects of the agonists without having any effects themselves, and *partial agonists*, drugs that have a mixture of agonistic and antagonistic properties, also have been introduced (Haefley 1988). Partial agonists may be particularly important to develop in the future as sedative-hypnotics that lack common side effects such as ataxia and amnesia.

At the molecular level, benzodiazepine *agonists* are defined as drugs that induce a conformational change in the receptor that produces functional consequences in terms of cellular changes, whereas *antagonists* occupy only the binding site. Braestrup and Nielsen (1986) found that a group of nonbenzodiazepine compounds, the β-carbolines, not only antagonized the action of the full agonists but also had intrinsic activity themselves. These compounds are called *benzodiazepine inverse agonists* because they have biological effects exactly opposite to those of the pure agonists while also having intrinsic activity like that of agonists. Their effects are blocked by antagonists; thus, the benzodiazepine receptor is particularly unique in that it has a bidirectional function (Figure 42–4).

Natural Ligands for Benzodiazepine Receptors in the Brain

The presence of benzodiazepine receptors in the brain suggests that natural ligands modulate GABAergic transmission through these sites. Small amounts of benzodiazepines, such as diazepam and desmethyldiazepam, can be detected in human and animal tissues. This finding was confirmed with human brain tissue samples that had been stored since the 1940s before the first synthesis of benzodiazepines (see Sangameswaran et al. 1986 for details). These benzodiazepines most likely originate from plants, such as wheat, corn, potatoes, or rice, and the levels that are detected are too low to be pharmacologically active (e.g., diazepam, <1 ng/g; desmethyldiazepam, 0.5 ng/g).

Other endogenous benzodiazepine-like substances with neuromodulatory effects probably exist in mammals. Endogenous ligands named *diazepam binding inhibitors*, or *endozepines*, that bind to the benzodiazepine site on the $GABA_A$-ergic receptor complex have been identified and are being isolated with biochemical purification protocols (Costa and Guidotti 1991; Marquardt et al. 1986; Rothstein et al. 1992). Their intrinsic action, like that of diazepam, is to potentiate $GABA_A$ receptor–mediated neurotransmission by acting as positive allosteric modulators of this receptor. Endozepines are present in the brain at pharmacologically active concentrations and may play a role both physiologically (e.g., regulation of memory, sleep, and learning) and pathologically (e.g., in panic attacks or hepatic encephalopathy) (Mullen et al. 1990; Nutt et al. 1990). Finally, endozepines have been involved in a newly described neurological condition, *idiopathic recurring stupor*, which is characterized by recurrent episodes of stupor or coma in the absence of any known toxic, metabolic, or structural brain damage. In this condition, the concentrations of endozepines are greatly increased in the plasma of affected individuals, and stupor can be interrupted by injections of flumazenil, a benzodiazepine antagonist. Thus, further knowledge of the roles of endozepines in physiological and pathological processes should be forthcoming once these endogenous ligands have been isolated and characterized (Rothstein et al. 1992).

Pharmacokinetics and Disposition

Benzodiazepines are generally absorbed rapidly and completely. Plasma binding is high (e.g., about 98% for diazepam). Benzodiazepines are very lipophilic (except for oxazepam), and penetration into the brain is rapid. For

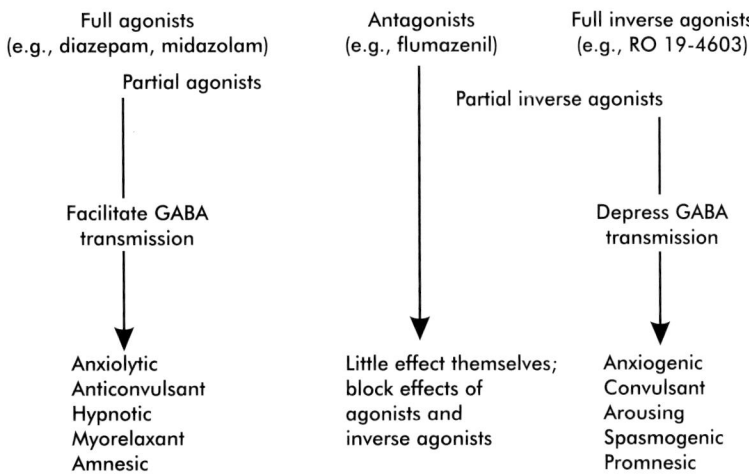

FIGURE 42–4. Properties of the various types of benzodiazepine receptor ligands.

GABA = γ-aminobutyric acid.

rapid onset of action, diazepam is available as an emulsion that is administered intravenously for rapid control of epilepsy; midazolam is a water-soluble benzodiazepine suitable for intravenous injection.

The major metabolic pathways for the 1,4-benzodiazepines are shown in Figure 42–5. Medazepam is metabolized to diazepam, which is *N*-desmethylated to desmethyldiazepam. Chlordiazepoxide is also partly converted to desmethyldiazepam. Clorazepate is transformed to desmethyldiazepam.

Desmethyldiazepam is a critical metabolite for biological activity because of its long half-life of more than 72 hours. Because diazepam's half-life is about 36 hours, the concentration of its desmethyl derivative soon exceeds that of diazepam during chronic administration. Desmethyldiazepam undergoes oxidation to oxazepam, which (like its 3-hydroxy analog temazepam) is rapidly conjugated with glucuronic acid and excreted.

Among the various benzodiazepines, triazolam has a particularly short half-life (<4 hours), and flurazepam and nitrazepam both have long half-lives. A major active metabolite of flurazepam, *N*-desalkylflurazepam, has a very long half-life of about 100 hours.

Because benzodiazepines are often prescribed for long periods, their long-term pharmacokinetics are particularly important. Concentrations of diazepam and desmethyldiazepam reach a plateau after a few weeks. Diazepam concentrations may then decline somewhat without much change in the concentration of the desmethyl metabolite.

Although benzodiazepines can stimulate liver metabolism in some animals, induction is of little clinical significance in humans.

Regarding the pharmacokinetics of nonbenzodiazepine hypnotics, no (or only weak) active metabolites exist for the compounds currently available.

Effects on Stages of Sleep

The hypnotic effects of benzodiazepines (and nonbenzodiazepine hypnotics described in this section) have been suggested to result from the inhibitory effects of the GABAergic system on the raphe and locus coeruleus monoaminergic ascending arousal systems, but this hypothesis may only partially explain their action. Magnocellular regions of the basal forebrain and the preoptic areas have been recognized as important sites for SWS regulation (Szymusiak 1995). Neurons that are selectively active during SWS have been described in these structures, most typically in the ventrolateral preoptic areas (Saper et al. 2001; Sherin et al. 1996). These neurons contain GABA and galanin, an inhibitory peptide, and project to the main components of the ascending arousal system, such as the raphe and locus coeruleus and brain stem cholinergic nuclei (Saper et al. 2001). The ventrolateral preoptic nucleus also sends a dense inhibitory projection to the tuberomammillary histaminergic nucleus, another important wake-promoting system (see Saper et al. 2001; Sherin et al. 1996). Benzodiazepines may thus indirectly modulate these wake-active monoaminergic neurotransmission to promote their hypnotic effects.

Another important site of action for benzodiazepines might be the suprachiasmatic nucleus (SCN). In SCN-lesioned animals, benzodiazepine treatment does not induce sleep (Edgar et al. 1993), but the hypnotic effect is restored if the SCN-lesioned animal is sleep deprived before

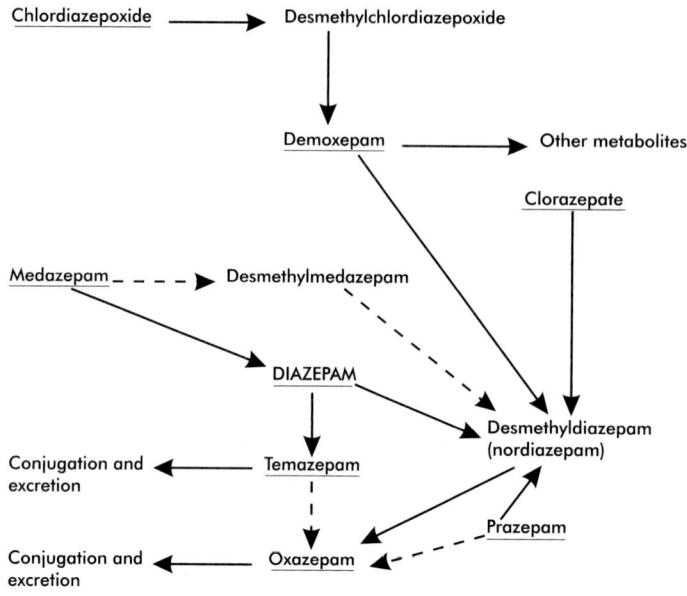

FIGURE 42–5.   Metabolic pathways for the principal 1,4-benzodiazepines.

Solid and *broken arrows* denote major and minor pathways, respectively; commercially available drugs are underscored. Flurazepam, fluni-trazepam, nitrazepam, and triazolam have separate metabolic pathways.

drug administration. Benzodiazepines thus may facilitate the release of a sleep debt accumulated during wakefulness rather than produce de novo sleep (Mignot et al. 1992).

The effects of benzodiazepines on sleep architectures are well known. Most benzodiazepines decrease sleep latency, especially when first used, and diminish the number of awakenings (Table 42–1). All benzodiazepines increase time spent in stage 2 sleep. Benzodiazepines also affect the quality of the SWS pattern. Thus, stages 3 and 4 sleep are suppressed and remain so during the period of drug administration. The decrease in stage 4 sleep is accompanied by a reduction in nightmares.

Most benzodiazepines increase REM latency. The time spent in REM sleep is usually shortened; however,

the reduction in percentage of REM sleep is minimal because the number of cycles of REM sleep usually increases late in the sleep time. Despite the shortening of SWS and REM sleep, the net effect of administration of benzodiazepines is usually an increase in total sleep time, so that the individual feels that the quality of sleep has improved. Furthermore, the hypnotic effect is greatest in subjects with the shortest baseline total sleep time.

If the benzodiazepine is discontinued after 3–4 weeks of nightly use, a considerable rebound in the amount and density of REM sleep and SWS may occur. However, this is not a consistent finding.

Because long-acting benzodiazepine hypnotics impair daytime performance and increase the risk of falls in geri-

TABLE 42–1.   Comparative properties of benzodiazepines and barbiturates on sleep parameters

	BENZODIAZEPINES	BARBITURATES
Total sleep time	↑ tolerance with short-acting agents	↑ rapid tolerance
Stage 2, %	↑	↑
Slow-wave sleep (stages 3 and 4), %	↓	↓ (slight)
REM latency	↑	↑
REM, %	↓ (slight)	↓
Withdrawal	Rebound insomnia with short-acting agents Carryover effectiveness with long-acting agents REM rebound (slight)	REM rebound Rebound decrease in stage 2 and total sleep time

Note.   REM = rapid eye movement sleep.

atric patients, several shorter-acting compounds have been introduced and are the preferred choice for elderly patients (see section "General Considerations in the Pharmacological Treatment of Insomnia" later in this chapter). However, it has since been found that short-acting benzodiazepines induce rebound insomnia (a worsening of sleep difficulty beyond baseline levels on discontinuation of a hypnotic) (Kales et al. 1979), rebound anxiety, anterograde amnesia, and even paradoxical rage (Figure 42–6). Many other factors, such as the subtype of insomnia being treated and the dosage and duration of treatment, are also important in explaining the occurrence of these specific side effects that may also be observed with other benzodiazepines. Nevertheless, enthusiasm for shorter-acting compounds has been tempered.

Indications and Efficacy

Benzodiazepines are the drug treatment of choice in the management of anxiety, insomnia, and stress-related conditions. Although none of the currently available compounds has any significant advantage over the others, some drugs can be selected to match the patient's symptom patterns to the pharmacokinetics of the various drugs. If a patient has a persistently high level of anxiety, one of the precursors of desmethyldiazepam such as diazepam or clorazepate is most appropriate. Patients with fluctuating anxiety may prefer to take shorter-acting compounds, such as oxazepam or lorazepam, when stressful circumstances occur or are expected. The indications of nonbenzodiazepine hypnotics are equivalent to those of benzodiazepine hypnotics but may be more specific depending on the pharmacological property of each compound.

An ideal hypnotic should induce sleep rapidly without producing sedation the next day. Both flurazepam and nitrazepam have inappropriately long half-lives as hypnotics unless a persistent anxiolytic effect is desired the next day (see Figure 42–6). Even in such situations, diazepam given as one dose at night may be preferable. Oxazepam penetrates too slowly for a dependable hypnotic effect (slow onset of action). Both lorazepam and temazepam are appropriate treatments for insomnia, but the dosages available are quite high (Table 42–2). Triazolam is the shortest-acting hypnotic available. When very small doses of benzodiazepines (which were assumed to have no significant hypnotic action) are administered to patients with insomnia, sleep quality often improves greatly, and usually it is not necessary to use a benzodiazepine at a hypnotic dose as a first-choice treatment.

Benzodiazepines can increase the frequency of apnea and exacerbate oxygen desaturation in healthy subjects and in subjects with chronic bronchitis (Geddes et al. 1976). Although many reports suggest that benzodiazepines are safe in patients with obstructive sleep apnea,

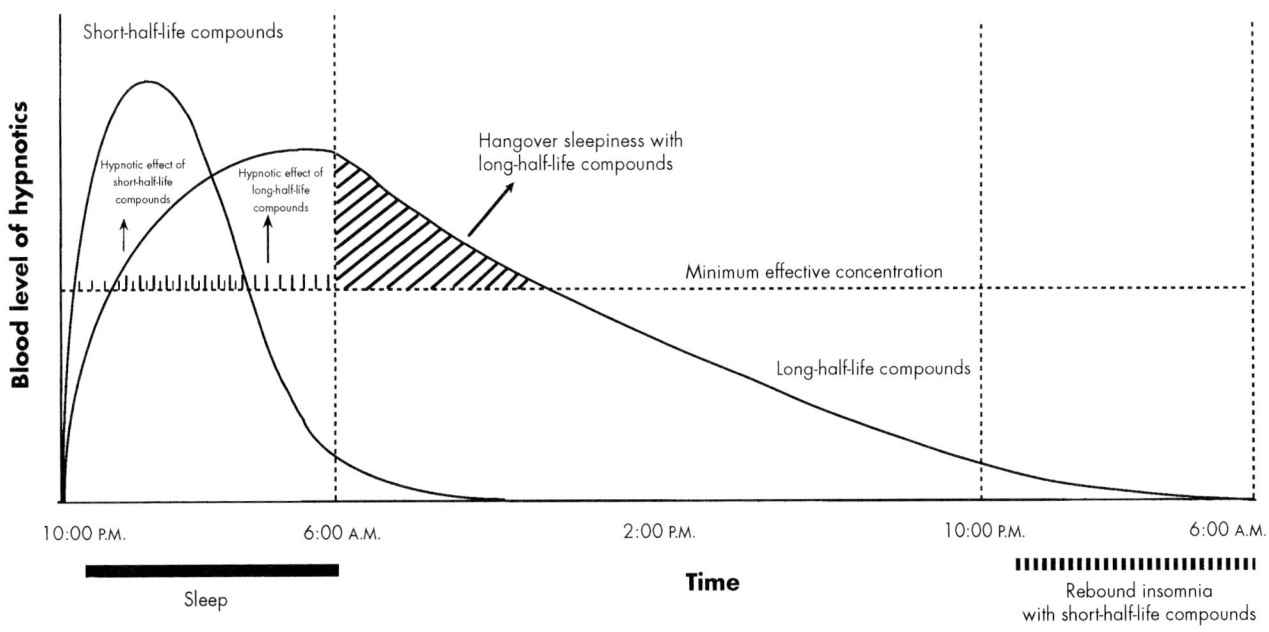

FIGURE 42–6. Duration of action of hypnotics and hangover and rebound insomnia.

Hypnotics with long half-lives may impair daytime performance the day after drug administration, whereas short-acting compounds may induce rebound insomnia on discontinuation.

TABLE 42–2. Pharmacokinetic properties of the most commonly used (in the United States) hypnotic compounds acting on the benzodiazepine receptors

Hypnotic compounds	Usual dose (mg)	T_{MAX} (hours)[a]	Half-life (hours)[b]	Active metabolites
Benzodiazepines				
Flurazepam (Dalmane)	15–30	0.5–1.0	48–150	N-Desalkylflurazepam
Quazepam (Doral)	7.5–15	2	48–120	2-Oxoquazepam, N-dealkyl-2-oxoquazepam
Estazolam (ProSom)	1–2	4.9	18–30	1-Oxoestazolam
Temazepam (Restoril)	15–30	1.5	8–20	None
Triazolam (Halcion)	0.125–0.25	1.3	2–6	None
Nonbenzodiazepines				
Zolpidem (Ambien)	5–10	0.8	1.5–2.4	None
Zopiclone	3.75–7.5	1.5	5–6	N-Oxide zopiclone (weak agonist)
Eszopiclone (Lunesta)	1–3	1	6–9	S-Desmethylzopiclone (weak agonist)
Zaleplon (Sonata)	5–20	1.0	1.0–2.5	None

[a]T_{max} is the time required to reach the maximal plasma concentration.
[b]Half-life is the time required by the body to metabolize or inactivate half the amount of a substrate taken.

other authors disagree, and it seems wise to avoid hypnotics in patients with severe sleep apnea. One of the only other contraindications is myasthenia gravis, a condition in which muscle relaxation with benzodiazepines can exacerbate muscle atonia.

Benzodiazepines have many indications other than sleep induction and anxiolysis, such as epilepsy (see Chapter 24, "Benzodiazepines"). Lorazepam and diazepam can be used for relaxation procedures, preoperative medication, and sedation during minor operations and investigations, often causing retrograde amnesia, a side effect that is sometimes desirable in this indication. Benzodiazepines have been used to manage alcohol withdrawal because cross-tolerance usually exists with alcohol, but large doses are often needed to suppress the withdrawal syndrome.

Side Effects and Toxicology

When a benzodiazepine is taken at high doses, tiredness, drowsiness, and profound feelings of detachment are common but can be minimized by a careful dose adjustment. Headache, dizziness, ataxia, confusion, and disorientation are less common except in the elderly. A marked potentiation of the depressant effect of alcohol occurs. Other less common side effects include weight gain, skin rash, menstrual irregularities, impairment of sexual function, and, very rarely, agranulocytosis.

Although otherwise asymptomatic subjects clearly show mental impairment with benzodiazepines, the situation with anxious patients is more complex. Because anxiety itself interferes with mental performance, alleviation of anxiety may result in improved functioning, which more than compensates for the direct drug-related decrement. The effects in some patients may be complicated and unpredictable, even at low dosages.

Because the safety of benzodiazepines in early pregnancy is not established, they should be avoided unless absolutely necessary. Diazepam is secreted in breast milk and may make the infant sleepy, unresponsive, and slow to feed.

Overdose

The benzodiazepines are extremely widely prescribed, so it is not surprising that they are used in many suicide attempts. For adults, overdoses of benzodiazepines reportedly are not fatal unless alcohol or other psychotropic drugs are taken simultaneously. Typically, the patient falls asleep but is arousable and wakes after 24–48 hours. Treatment is supportive. A stomach pump is usually more punitive than therapeutic, and dialysis is usually useless because of high plasma binding.

Tolerance and Dependence

Dependence, both psychological and physical, occurs with benzodiazepines as with other sedative-hypnotics.

Abrupt discontinuation results in withdrawal phenomena such as anxiety, agitation, restlessness, and tension, which are usually delayed for several days because of the long half-life of the major metabolite, desmethyldiazepam. Even with the normal dose, some patients have withdrawal effects. The fact that some patients gradually increase the dose suggests tolerance, but increases in dose are sometimes related to particularly stressful crises.

Psychological dependence is also common, based on the high incidence of repeated prescriptions, but it is mild, and the drug-seeking behavior is much less persistent than with barbiturates.

Barbiturates

History and Discovery

Before 1900, a few agents, such as bromide, chloral hydrate, paraldehyde, urethane, and sulfonal, were used as sedatives and hypnotics. Barbital, one of the derivatives of barbituric acid, was introduced in 1903 and soon became extremely popular in clinical medicine because of its sleep-inducing and anxiolytic effects (Maynert 1965). In 1912, phenobarbital was introduced. In addition to its use as a sedative-hypnotic, phenobarbital has become one of the most important pharmacological treatments for epilepsy. Since then, more than 2,500 barbiturate analogs have been synthesized, about 50 of which have been made commercially available and only 20 of which remain on the market.

The success of the partial separation of anticonvulsant from sedative-hypnotic properties led to the development of nonsedative anticonvulsants such as phenytoin in the late 1930s and trimethadione in the early 1940s. The success of barbiturates as sedative-hypnotics was largely overshadowed by the discovery of benzodiazepines in the late 1960s. With pharmacological properties very similar to those of barbiturates, these compounds have a much safer pharmacological profile. Thus, benzodiazepines have replaced barbiturates in many incidents, especially for psychiatric conditions in which suicide is a possibility.

Structure–Activity Relations

Barbituric acid (2,4,6-trihexahydroxypyrimidine) is the parent compound of all barbiturates. This basic structure lacks CNS depressant activity, and the addition of two alkyl groups at position 5 is needed to confer sedative activity (Figure 42–7).

The barbituric acid derivatives do not dissolve readily in water but are quite soluble in nonpolar solvents, a feature shared with most other organic compounds that depress the CNS. In general, structural changes that increase liposolubility also decrease these compounds' duration of action, decrease latency to onset of activity, accelerate metabolic degradation, and often increase hypnotic potency.

Derivatives with large aliphatic groups at position 5 have greater activity than do those with methyl groups but shorter duration of action. However, groups with more than seven carbons lose their hypnotic activity and tend to exhibit convulsant activity. Methylation of the 1-N atom increases liposolubility and shortens duration of action, and desmethylation may increase the duration of action (Rall 1990).

Pharmacological Profile and Mechanism of Action

The main effects of barbiturates are sedation, sleep induction, and anesthesia. Some of the barbiturates, such as phenobarbital, also have selective anticonvulsant properties. The mechanisms of action of barbiturates are complex and still not fully understood. Nonanesthetic doses of barbiturates preferentially suppress polysynaptic responses. Pertinent to their sedative-hypnotic effects is the fact that the mesencephalic reticular activating system is extremely sensitive to these drugs (Killam 1962). The synaptic site of inhibition is either postsynaptic (e.g., at the level of cortical and cerebellar pyramidal cells and in the cuneate nucleus, substantia nigra, and thalamus relay neurons) or presynaptic (e.g., in the spinal cord). This inhibition occurs only at synapses where physiological inhibition is GABAergic but not glycinergic or monoaminergic. Thus, barbiturates, like benzodiazepines, specifically potentiate GABA-mediated inhibitory processes in the brain. However, it remains unclear whether all of the effects of barbiturates are entirely mediated by GABAergic mechanisms.

Barbiturates do not displace benzodiazepines from their binding sites; instead, barbiturates enhance benzodiazepine binding by increasing the affinity of the receptor for benzodiazepines (Leeb-Lundberg et al. 1980). They also enhance the binding of GABA and its agonists to specific binding sites (Asano and Ogasawara 1981). These effects are almost completely dependent on the presence of chloride or other anions that are known to permeate the chloride channels associated with the GABA receptor complex, and they are competitively antagonized by picro-

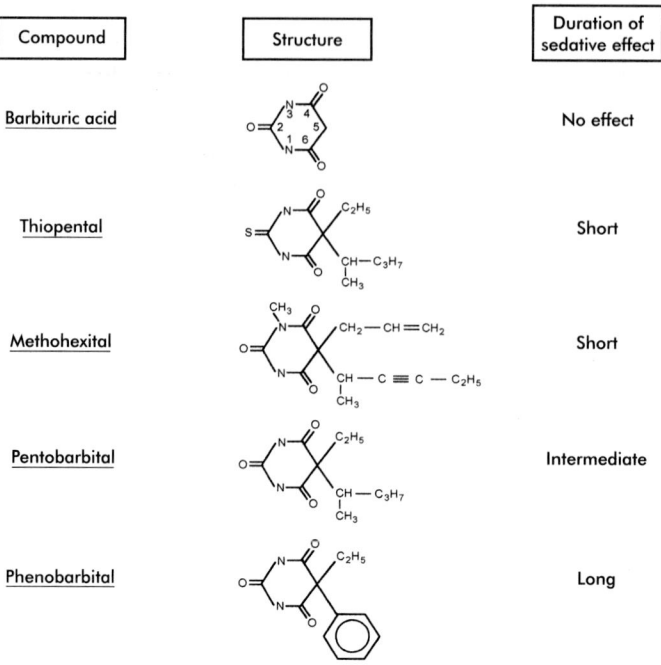

FIGURE 42–7.   Structure–activity relations among barbiturates.

toxin (a convulsant) (Olsen et al. 1978). Taken together, these observations suggest that the macromolecular complex composed of $GABA_A$-ergic receptors, chloride ionophores, and binding sites for benzodiazepines (ω site) is also an important site of action for a depressant.

Although both barbiturates and benzodiazepines can potentiate the GABA-induced increase in chloride conductance, barbiturates appear to increase the duration of the open state of chloride channels that are regulated by $GABA_A$-ergic receptors. In contrast, benzodiazepines increase the frequency of channel openings with little effect on the duration. Barbiturates may prolong the activation of the channel by acting directly on the ion channel (Enna and Möhler 1987; Richter and Holman 1982).

The molecular correlations of the barbiturate-acting sites on the $GABA_A$ receptor are also studied. The Tyr-Gly-Tyr sequence in the β subunit is undoubtedly important for the binding of GABA and other direct receptor agonists (Amin and Weiss 1993), as is Phe64 in the α_1 subunit (Smith and Olsen 1995). However, neither the Tyr-Gly-Tyr sequence in β, the Phe64 sequence in α, nor the His101 sequence (which is important for the action of benzodiazepines) in α is of vital importance to barbiturate function (Amin and Weiss 1993). Some reports suggest that the β subunit alone may form a site for barbiturates (Sanna et al. 1995). Although there is still much to be known, new molecular experimental approaches hold great promise for resolving the most important pharma-

cological questions regarding which molecular species are important for the anticonvulsant, sedative, anesthetic, and toxic actions of the barbiturates.

Pharmacokinetics and Disposition

For hypnotic use, barbiturates usually are administered orally. Barbiturates are rapidly absorbed in the stomach, and their absorption decreases when the stomach is full. Because sodium salts are rapidly dissolved, they are more rapidly absorbed than free acids.

Barbiturates are metabolized mainly in the liver. Oxidation of the larger of the two side chains at position 5 is a major catabolic pathway. It generally produces inactive polar metabolites that are rapidly excreted in the urine (Rall 1990). Changes in liver function can markedly alter the rate at which these compounds are inactivated. Chronic administration leads to pharmacokinetic tolerance, even when low or infrequent doses of barbiturates are used (see section "Drug–Drug Interactions" later in this chapter).

The rate of penetration of barbiturates into the CNS varies according to their lipophilicity. In general, liposolubility decreases latency to onset of action and duration of action. Thiopental, for example, enters the CNS rapidly and is used to rapidly induce anesthesia; barbitone crosses into the brain so slowly that it is inappropriate as a hypnotic drug.

Effects on Stages of Sleep

Barbiturates decrease sleep latency; however, they also slightly increase fast electroencephalogram (EEG) activity during sleep. Barbiturates decrease body movement during sleep. Stage 2 sleep increases, whereas stage 3 and stage 4 SWS generally decreases, except in some patients with anxiety and in patients who are addicted to barbiturates (see Table 42–1). REM sleep latency is prolonged, and both the total time spent in REM sleep and the number of REM cycles are diminished. With repeated nighttime administration of barbiturates, drug tolerance to the effects on sleep occurs in a few days. Discontinuation of barbiturates may lead to insomnia and disrupted sleep patterns (with a decrease in stage 2 sleep) and increases in REM sleep (Kay et al. 1976).

Indications and Efficacy

Although clinical trials have shown that the barbiturates have sedative and hypnotic properties, barbiturates generally compare poorly with benzodiazepines. The patient feels "drugged" the next day, and there is always the risk of fatal overdose because of the depressant effect on respiration. Barbiturates suppress respiration, and the therapeutic dose of barbiturates may cause fatal respiratory depression in patients with sleep apnea. Patients with sleep apnea should therefore avoid taking barbiturates. Because of these risks, many clinicians have stopped using barbiturates as hypnotics and sedatives (one exception is in the treatment of severe psychomotor excitation) and prescribe them only as anticonvulsants.

Barbiturates also have been administered intravenously to facilitate patient interviews (i.e., amobarbital interview). This technique is also helpful in 1) mobilizing the stuporous catatonic patient, 2) aiding the diagnosis of intellectual impairment, and 3) lessening disturbance associated with previous negative experiences (i.e., abreactions).

Barbiturates are contraindicated in patients with porphyria because they enhance porphyrin synthesis. Liver function should be checked before and during drug administration. Liver dysfunction can significantly prolong the sedative effects of these drugs and may lead to fatal overdose.

Side Effects and Toxicology

In treating many patients who are prescribed barbiturates, it is difficult to control symptoms without causing oversedation. Patients typically oscillate between anxiety and torpor. Mental performance is often impaired, and patients should not drive or operate dangerous machinery.

Patients whose conditions have been stabilized for years with barbiturates must be considered drug dependent. Withdrawal leads to anxiety, agitation, trembling, and, frequently, convulsions. Substitution with a benzodiazepine that can be withdrawn more easily later is often successful.

In some patients, barbiturates repeatedly produce excitement rather than depression (paradoxical excitement), and the patients may appear to be intoxicated.

Hypersensitive reactions (especially of the skin) may occur, and cases of megaloblastic anemia have been reported.

Overdose

An overdose of barbiturates leads to fatal respiratory and cardiovascular depression. Suicide attempts frequently involve overdoses of barbiturates, taken either alone or in combination with alcohol or other psychotropic drugs, particularly tricyclic antidepressants. These suicide attempts, unfortunately, are often successful. Depending on local factors such as proximity to a hospital and expertise of staff for intensive emergency care, death occurs in 0.5%–10% of these cases. Severe poisoning results at 10 times the hypnotic dose, and twice that amount may be fatal.

Tolerance and Dependence

Tolerance to barbiturates occurs rapidly and is a result of both pharmacokinetic factors (e.g., liver enzyme induction) and pharmacodynamic factors (e.g., neuronal adaptation to chronic drug administration). Cross-tolerance develops to alcohol, gas anesthetics, and other sedatives, including benzodiazepines.

Psychological dependence (i.e., drug-seeking behavior) is common. Patients typically visit several physicians to obtain more barbiturates. Physical dependence may be induced by dosages of 500 mg/day. Intoxication may occur, as evidenced by impaired mental functioning, emotional instability, and neurological signs. Abrupt discontinuation after high doses is likely to induce convulsions and delirium. After normal doses, withdrawal phenomena include anxiety, insomnia, restlessness, agitation, tremor, muscle twitching, nausea and vomiting, orthostatic hypotension, and weight loss.

Drug–Drug Interactions

Barbiturates used with other CNS depressants can cause severe depression. Ethanol is the drug most frequently used, and interactions with antihistaminic compounds are also common. Monoamine oxidase inhibitors and methylphenidate also increase the CNS depressant effect of barbiturates.

Barbiturates may increase the activity of hepatic microsomal enzymes two- to threefold. Clinically, this change is particularly important for patients who are also receiving metabolic competitors such as warfarin or digitoxin, for which careful control of plasma concentrations is vital (Rall 1990).

Other Sedative-Hypnotic Compounds

Alcohol-Type Hypnotics and Gamma-Hydroxybutyrate

The alcohol-type hypnotics include the chloral derivatives, of which chloral hydrate, clomethiazole, and ethchlorvynol are still used occasionally in the elderly. Chloral hydrate is metabolized to another active sedative-hypnotic—trichloroethanol. These drugs have short half-lives (about 4–6 hours) and decrease sleep latency and number of awakenings; SWS is slightly depressed, but overall REM sleep time is largely unaffected. Chloral hydrate and its metabolite have an unpleasant taste and frequently cause epigastric distress and nausea. Undesirable side effects include light-headedness, ataxia, and nightmares. Chronic use of these drugs can lead to tolerance and occasionally to physical dependence. As with barbiturates, overdosage can lead to respiratory and cardiovascular depression, and therapeutic use of these drugs has largely been superseded by the use of benzodiazepines.

γ-Hydroxybutyrate (GHB) is a hypnotic agent that has been used mostly in the treatment of insomnia in narcoleptic patients (Scrima et al. 1990). It is rarely used in other indications and is frequently abused by athletes because of its SWS-promoting effects, with resulting increases in growth hormone secretion (Chin et al. 1992); it is also abused because of its euphoric effects (Chin et al. 1992). GHB was classified as a schedule I controlled substance in March 2000 in the United States, but in July 2002, its sodium salt form, sodium oxybate (Xynem), was approved for the treatment of narcolepsy. Nighttime administration of GHB reduces excessive daytime sleepiness associated with narcolepsy. Although the compound is structurally related to GABA, its mode of action involves specific non-GABAergic binding sites and a potent inhibitory effect on dopaminergic transmission (Vayer et al. 1987). The compound promotes SWS and REM sleep (Lapierre et al. 1990), but its effects on sleep architecture

are short-lasting, and repeated administration usually is necessary during the night. GHB is also used for the treatment of cataplexy of narcolepsy, but the mechanisms of GHB's effect on cataplexy remain unknown.

Antihistamines

Antihistamines, such as promethazine, diphenhydramine, and doxylamine, are sometimes prescribed as sleep inducers. They decrease sleep latency but do not increase total sleep time (see Reite et al. 1997). These compounds are especially useful for patients who cannot sleep well because of acute allergic reactions or itching. Sedative antihistamines also may be prescribed for those persons who tend to abuse psychoactive drugs, because sedative antihistamines have not been shown to have abuse potential. Rapid tolerance is a problem.

In April 2008, the FDA approved the filing of a new drug application for doxepin hydrochloride, a tricyclic antidepressant with histaminergic$_1$ (H$_1$) antagonism, for the treatment of insomnia (marketed under the trade name Silenor). Doxepin (as Sinequan) has been used for more than 40 years for the treatment of depression, but hypnotic effects at low doses (3–6 mg) were also reported. Doxepin reduces wake after sleep onset (WASO) and prolongs sleep time. Several other selective H$_1$ blockers and H$_1$ reverse agonists are also under development for hypnotic uses.

Melatonin

Melatonin is a neurohormone produced by the pineal gland during the dark phase of the day–night cycle. In animals, melatonin has been implicated in the circadian regulation of sleep and in the seasonal control of reproduction. Studies suggest that melatonin administration may have some therapeutic effects in various disturbances of circadian rhythmicity, such as jet lag (Arendt et al. 1987), shift work (Folkard et al. 1993), non-24-hour sleep–wake cycle in blind subjects (Arendt et al. 1988), and delayed–sleep phase insomnia (Dahlitz et al. 1991), an effect associated with few side effects (e.g., headaches or nausea). High doses of melatonin (3–100 mg), which increase serum melatonin levels far beyond the normal nocturnal range, have been suggested to produce hypnotic effects in humans. Lower and more physiological doses of melatonin (e.g., 0.3 mg) also might be active, but the data available to date are less convincing.

In humans, the production of melatonin during the dark period declines with age; this effect parallels declines in sleep quantity and quality (Van Coevorden et al. 1991), especially in elderly persons with insomnia (Haimov et al. 1994; Mishima et al. 2001). These results seemingly suggest that deficiency in nocturnal melatonin secretion might contribute to disrupted sleep in the elderly; thus, in this population, insomnia is a particularly attractive indication for melatonin. Indeed, some studies reported favorable effects with supplementary administration of melatonin in elderly persons with sleep maintenance disturbances (Garfinkel et al. 1995; Haimov et al. 1995). However, several recent studies reported contradictory findings indicating no significant relation between physiological melatonin secretion levels and sleep maintenance parameters (Hughes et al. 1998; Lushington et al. 1998; Youngstedt et al. 1998; Zeitzer et al. 1999) as well as no significant therapeutic effect of melatonin replacement on sleep maintenance in elderly persons with insomnia (Hughes et al. 1998).

One of the difficulties in establishing therapeutic efficacy of melatonin is its short half-life (20–30 minutes). Bedtime melatonin administration reduces sleep latency but has few objective effects on sleep architecture. It is also unclear whether the hypnotic effect of a physiological or pharmacological dose is a direct effect on sleep, an indirect effect on circadian timing that subsequently gates the release of sleep, or both. Finally, very few double-blind, placebo-controlled studies have been done, and most current reports are confounded by strong placebo effects in the context of a melatonin fad. Melatonin might be an effective hypnotic in some indications, but better controlled studies are needed to establish efficacy in specific indications. The purity of the products sold in health food stores is also a problem, and the long-term effects of melatonin administration in humans are unknown.

There are at least three subtypes of melatonin receptors with high (MT_1) and low (MT_2 and MT_3) affinities for this ligand (Dubocovich 1995; Dubocovich et al. 2003; Morgan et al. 1994). MT_1 receptors are high-affinity receptors that fall into the G protein–coupled receptor superfamily; binding of melatonin to these receptors results in inhibition of adenylate cyclase activity in target cells (Ebisawa et al. 1994). The MT_1 receptor is further divided into two subclasses, MT_{1a} and MT_{1b} (Reppert et al. 1994, 1995). The localization of the MT_{1a} receptor in the SCN and median eminence in humans and rodents suggests that this receptor is essential for circadian regulation and reproduction, whereas the MT_{1b} receptor is localized mainly in the retina. The MT_3 receptor appears almost exclusively in the gut. MT_2 receptors are coupled to phosphoinositol hydrolysis. Activation of MT_3 receptors inhibits leukotriene B_4–induced leukocyte adhesion and

decreases intraocular pressure (Dubocovich et al. 2003). The functional importance of MT_{1b}, MT_2, and MT_3 remains unclear.

Ramelteon, a melatonin receptor agonist with both high affinity for melatonin MT_1 and MT_2 receptors and selectivity over the MT_3 receptor, and with a longer half-life than melatonin, has recently been approved by the FDA for long-term treatment of insomnia, particularly for delayed sleep onset. Ramelteon does not show any appreciable binding to $GABA_A$ receptors, which are associated with anxiolytic, myorelaxant, and amnesic effects. Ramelteon has not been demonstrated to produce dependence and has shown no potential for abuse, and the withdrawal and rebound insomnia typically seen with other GABA modulators are not present.

Animal studies demonstrated that sleep-enhancing effects of ramelteon are not associated with reduction in REM sleep (Miyamoto et al. 2004). It is currently the only nonscheduled prescription drug for the treatment of insomnia available in the United States. Ramelteon has no appreciable affinity for receptors that bind neuropeptides, cytokines, serotonin, dopamine, norepinephrine, acetylcholine, and opiates. It also does not interfere with the activity of a number of selected enzymes in a standard panel. The activity of ramelteon at the MT_1 and MT_2 receptors, especially on the SCN, is believed to contribute to its sleep-promoting properties, as these receptors, acted upon by endogenous melatonin, are thought to be involved in the maintenance of the circadian rhythm underlying the normal sleep–wake cycle.

The biological action of melatonin is similar to that of ramelteon. No published studies have indicated whether ramelteon is more or less safe or effective than melatonin, a much less expensive drug widely available in the United States without a prescription. Several other MT_1/MT_2 receptor agonists are under development.

A prolonged-release formulation of melatonin (marketed under the trade name Circadin) was approved by the European Commission in June 2007 as monotherapy for the short-term treatment of primary insomnia characterized by poor-quality sleep in patients 55 years and older (Lemoine et al. 2007).

Thalidomide

Thalidomide is a unique hypnotic compound that deserves special mention. The compound was first introduced as a sleep-inducing agent in the 1950s but was rapidly withdrawn after reports of secondary fetal malformations. In the 1960s, thalidomide was found to be surprisingly effective in the treatment of severe granulomatous skin complications associated with leprosy (e.g., erythema nodosum). Since then, thalidomide has been reintroduced to treat various conditions that involve pathological immune reactions (e.g., graft-versus-host disease, lupus) and pharyngeal ulcerations in patients with AIDS (see Kaplan 1994). In patients with leprosy and AIDS, thalidomide inhibited the production of tumor necrosis factor–α (TNF-α). The efficacy of thalidomide in multiple myeloma was reported in the medical literature in 1999 (Desikan et al. 1999). In 2006, the FDA granted accelerated approval for thalidomide in combination with dexamethasone for the treatment of newly diagnosed multiple myeloma.

Together with GHB and ramelteon, thalidomide increases REM sleep and SWS (Frederickson et al. 1977; Kaitin 1985) (benzodiazepines and barbiturates decrease REM sleep and deep SWS). Thalidomide does not bind to or enzymatically modify any neurotransmitter systems known to be involved in the regulation of sleep (e.g., histamine, serotonin, benzodiazepine, excitatory amino acids, and GABA) (Kanbayashi et al. 1996). Thalidomide thus may affect sleep through neuroimmune interactions in the brain, because TNF-α and other cytokines secreted by microglia in the brain have been reported to be endogenous sleep-modulating substances (Krueger et al. 1995). Thalidomide inhibits TNF-α gene expression in the brain and in peripheral tissue such as spleen (Nishino et al. 2005). When administered to TNF-α knockout mice, thalidomide enhanced SWS in these animals, but REM enhancement was not observed (Nishino et al. 2005), suggesting that REM enhancement but not SWS enhancement of thalidomide is dependent on inhibition of TNF-α. Thalidomide analogs with hypnotic effects and/or immunomodulatory effects without any teratogenic effects in animals are available for experimental use but have never been developed for clinical use. Thalidomide thus remains a unique and powerful pharmacological tool in studying the regulation of normal and abnormal sleep, which could lead to the development of new hypnotic agents.

General Considerations in the Pharmacological Treatment of Insomnia

Insomnia is a subjective complaint of insufficient, inadequate, or nonrestorative sleep (Buysse and Reynolds 1990; see also Chapter 60, "Treatment of Insomnia"). Disturbances in daytime functioning, such as fatigue, mood disturbances, and impaired performance, result from inadequate sleep. Insomnia is a common symptom. In 1983, a survey indicated that 35% of the general population reported having trouble sleeping in the past year, and 17% considered their problem serious (Mellinger et al. 1985). In the same survey, 7.1% of the population had used a hypnotic in the past year (Mellinger et al. 1985).

Insomnia is a symptom that must be explored clinically before treatment is initiated. Sleep disturbances often indicate a larger psychiatric problem, such as depression. As mentioned above, a complaint of insomnia is also common with old age, especially in an institutional setting. In other cases, environmental factors (e.g., noise) and associated sleep disorders (periodic leg movements, sleep apneas, parasomnias) may be involved.

A useful initial approach to the patient with insomnia is to consider the duration of the complaint. Insomnia can occur as a transient (1–2 days), short-term (more than a few days to a few months), or chronic disturbance (several months or even years). The duration of insomnia not only suggests its cause (Table 42–3) but also provides some guidance on how to use hypnotics.

Transient insomnias are typically caused by an environmental acute stressor, jet lag, or shift work. In this indication, pharmacotherapy with benzodiazepine hypnotics or other hypnotics has no risks because dependence on the treatment is unlikely to develop when the therapy lasts less than a week to 10 days.

Short-term (a few days to a few months) insomnias are particularly important to recognize because they may evolve into chronic psychophysiological insomnia if untreated or inadequately treated. Typically, patients develop insomnia during a stressful period of their lives (e.g., work or personal difficulties). The condition frequently worsens if untreated, and the patient worries excessively about his or her sleep, which evolves into a behaviorally learned, chronic insomnia that does not resolve once the stressful period is over. In this indication, the daily use of benzodiazepine hypnotics is also dangerous because it may lead to tolerance and dependence. Reassurance regarding the favorable resolution of the stressful event is important, and the patient should be instructed to use hypnotic medications intermittently (e.g., every few days, as needed) to avoid the development of tolerance. An education in sleep hygiene (not taking naps even when very tired, having regular wake-up times, avoiding caffeine and alcohol) is also important to reduce the possibility of evolution into a chronic problem.

Chronic insomnia should first be evaluated with a sleep log of a 2-week period. Most commonly, some degree of sleep-state misperception is present, and patients

TABLE 42–3. Nosological classification of insomnia (International Classification of Sleep Disorders diagnostic criteria)

CATEGORY	PERCENTAGE OF PATIENTS WITH CORRESPONDING DIAGNOSIS[a]	DESCRIPTION
Psychophysiological	15	Transient or persistent insomnia that develops as a result of psychological factors, physiological tension/arousal, and negative conditioning
Idiopathic insomnia	<5	Insomnia and daytime dysfunction, which begin in childhood and continue into adulthood
Associated with sleep-induced respiratory impairment	5–10	Frequent respiratory pauses or hypoxia (e.g., sleep apnea, alveolar hypoventilation) that leads to brief arousals during the night
Associated with periodic leg movements and restless legs	12	Repetitive, stereotyped jerking leg movements or unpleasant dysesthesias in legs on falling asleep, which frequently interrupt sleep
Associated with psychiatric disorders	35	Insomnia associated with behavioral symptoms and underlying biological disturbances of psychiatric disorders (including mood, anxiety, psychotic, and personality disorders)
Associated with neurological disorders	~5	Insomnia associated with neurological disorders, such as cerebral degenerative disorders, dementia, and parkinsonism
Associated with other medical disorders	~5	Insomnia associated with other medical disorders, such as nocturnal cardiac ischemia, chronic obstructive pulmonary disease, and sleep-related asthma; sleep is expected to improve when the underlying condition is treated
Associated with chronic drugs and alcohol	12	Insomnia associated with use of, tolerance to, or withdrawal from CNS-active agents, including stimulants, sedative-hypnotics, and alcohol
Sleep-state misperception	5–10	Subjective insomnia complaint that is not substantiated by polysomnography
Transient sleep–wake disorders[b]	NA	Rapid time zone change (jet lag) or schedule or work shift change results in symptoms of insomnia during new, desired sleep hours and sleepiness during new, desired wake hours
Persistent sleep–wake disorders[b]	NA	A frequently changing sleep–wake schedule, delayed or advanced sleep-phase syndrome, non-24-hour sleep–wake pattern, or irregular sleep–wake pattern results in symptoms of insomnia during desired sleep hours and sleepiness during desired wake hours

Note. CNS = central nervous system; NA = not available.
[a]Estimated from approximately 2,000 patients with a diagnosed disorder of initiating and maintaining sleep by 20 centers; contributed by the Association of Sleep Disorders Centers National Case Series (Coleman 1983).
[b]These diagnoses are classified as circadian rhythm sleep disorders in the International Classification of Sleep Disorders diagnostic criteria (American Sleep Disorders Association 1990).
Source. Adapted from Buysse and Reynolds 1990.

with insomnia greatly exaggerate the complaint (i.e., they sleep more than they claim and take less time to fall asleep than they report). In most cases, insomnia has developed as a result of psychological factors and negative conditioning, as mentioned above. In rare cases, insomnia began in childhood and has persisted into adulthood (idiopathic insomnia). In chronic insomnia, improved sleep hygiene and various behavioral techniques that aim to reduce negative conditioning (stimulus control therapy), sleep restriction, and phototherapy are often helpful on a long-term basis, but these methods are successful only if the patient is motivated and if specialized clinical supervision is available. Drug use is most appropriate in patients whose sleep disturbance is clearly causing some daytime dysfunction. If the clinician decides to use pharmacotherapy, it is always helpful to start with the lowest dose of hypnotic possible (hypnotic medications are frequently overdosed) to reduce the risk of tolerance and dependence and to try to avoid daily use.

Insomnia also can be classified on the basis of individual clinical features—that is, as sleep initiation, sleep maintenance, or termination (early-morning awakening). In this context, the most important pharmacological properties to consider when selecting a hypnotic for treatment are how quickly it acts and how long the effects last (see Table 42–2 for commonly used compounds). The rate of absorption is the most critical factor determining onset of action. T_{max} (time required to reach the maximal plasma concentration) is the pharmacological parameter that best predicts onset of action. After absorption, hypnotics are distributed to various organs; distribution and drug elimination influence the duration of action. The elimination half-life (see Table 42–2) usually provides a good first estimate of the duration of action for drugs that have comparable absorption and distribution profiles. Hypnotics with long duration of action are helpful for patients who have difficulty both initiating and maintaining sleep. One advantage of these long-acting compounds is that rebound insomnia is often delayed and milder if the drug has to be withdrawn (see Figure 42–6). Patients who have difficulty initiating sleep might prefer short-acting compounds; however, for these compounds, it may be necessary, paradoxically, to switch to longer-acting hypnotics before withdrawal of all hypnotic treatment.

The importance of determining whether insomnia is the symptom of an underlying neuropsychiatric condition must be emphasized (see Table 42–3). For depression, trazodone (25–50 mg), amitriptyline (10 mg), trimipramine (25–50 mg), or doxepin (25–50 mg) can be used as a hypnotic or in combination with another hypnotic. Most persons with schizophrenia also have persistent insomnia (initiation and maintenance of sleep), and phenothiazines, such as chlorpromazine, thioridazine, and levomepromazine, are effective therapies. When psychotic symptoms are associated with insomnia, butyrophenones, such as haloperidol, also can be used. For insomnia associated with anxiety disorders, hypnotics supplemented with anxiolytics can be used, and this treatment may prevent rebound insomnia and its related anxiety.

Sleep disturbances are very frequent complaints in old age, and treatment must be initiated carefully in this population (see Chapter 65, "Treatment During Late Life"). About 12% of the United States population is older than 60 years, and this segment of the population receives 35%–40% of all sedative-hypnotic prescriptions (Gottlieb 1990).

Before starting pharmacological therapy, all possible causes of insomnia should be examined (i.e., psychophysiological; associated with drugs and alcohol; due to disturbance of the sleep–wake cycle; associated with periodic leg movements, sleep apnea, or other physical or psychiatric conditions). Before selecting a specific hypnotic, the clinician should consider its pharmacological properties and side-effect profile, the patient's medical health and medical history, and the patient's history of sedative-hypnotic use. The special case of melatonin has been discussed earlier in this chapter. Hypnotics or their active metabolites often accumulate during chronic use in elderly patients, and this accumulation may cause cognition problems, disorientation, confusion, and, occasionally, falls. Hypnotics with short or intermediate half-lives are thus recommended, and the lowest dose possible should be used. Compounds with a short half-life, such as triazolam or zolpidem, may be effective for problems with sleep initiation and sleep fragmentation. Zolpidem has little muscle relaxant effect and may be preferable. Compounds with an intermediate hypnotic profile, such as estazolam and temazepam, are also reported to be effective in elderly patients. Hypnotics with intermediate half-lives may alter daytime performance and memory to a lesser extent and are not as likely to induce rebound insomnia after withdrawal as are regular hypnotics.

Conclusion

The mechanism of action of most currently available hypnotics (benzodiazepines, barbiturates, alcohol, and recent nonbenzodiazepine hypnotics) involves a modulatory effect of GABAergic activity. These compounds stimulate GABAergic transmission by acting on the $GABA_A$–benzodiazepine–Cl^- macromolecular complex, known to contain multiple modulatory binding sites and many receptor subtypes. This recently discovered molecular diversity within the macromolecular complex suggests that new GABAergic hypnotic compounds with subtype selectivity may have better side-effect profiles.

Other non-GABAergic hypnotics, including mostly sedative antidepressants, antihistamines, and melatonin and melatonin receptor agonists, are viable strategies in the treatment of insomnia, especially because these hypnotics may lack some of the hampering side effects often seen with classical GABAergic hypnotics, such as abuse potential and amnesic effects. Their prescription, as with the prescription of other regular benzodiazepine-like hypnotic compounds, should be guided by the knowledge that insomnia is a heterogeneous condition that should be explored clinically before any pharmacological treatment is initiated.

References

Allen D, Curran HV, Lader M: The effects of single doses of CL284,846, lorazepam, and placebo on psychomotor and memory function in normal male volunteers. Eur J Clin Pharmacol 45:313–320, 1993

American Sleep Disorders Association: The International Classification of Sleep Disorders: Diagnostic and Coding Manual. Rochester, MN, American Sleep Disorders Association, 1990

Amin J, Weiss DS: GABAA receptor needs two homologous domains of the beta-subunit for activation by GABA but not by pentobarbital. Nature 366:565–569, 1993

Arendt J, Aldhous M, Marks V, et al: Some effects of jet-lag and their alleviation by melatonin. Ergonomics 30:1379–1393, 1987

Arendt J, Aldhous M, Wright J: Synchronisation of a disturbed sleep-wake cycle in a blind man by melatonin treatment. Lancet 1(8588):772–773, 1988

Asano T, Ogasawara N: Chloride-dependent stimulation of GABA and benzodiazepine receptor binding by pentobarbital. Brain Res 225:212–216, 1981

Awad M, Gavish M: Binding of [3H]Ro 5–4864 and [3H]PK 11195 to cerebral cortex and peripheral tissues of various species: species differences and heterogeneity in peripheral benzodiazepine binding sites. J Neurochem 49:1407–1414, 1987

Beer B, Ieni JR, Wu WH, et al: A placebo-controlled evaluation of single, escalating doses of CL 284,846, a non-benzodiazepine hypnotic. J Clin Pharmacol 34:335–344, 1994

Boileau AJ, Kucken AM, Evers AR, et al: Molecular dissection of benzodiazepine binding and allosteric coupling using chimeric gamma-aminobutyric acidA receptor subunits. Mol Pharmacol 53:295–303, 1998

Boileau AJ, Evers AR, Davis AF, et al: Mapping the agonist binding site of the GABAA receptor: evidence for a beta-strand. J Neurosci 19:4847–4854, 1999

Braestrup C, Nielsen M: Benzodiazepine binding in vivo and efficacy, in Benzodiazepine/GABA Receptors and Chloride Channels: Structural and Functional Properties. Edited by Olsen RW, Venter JC. New York, Alan R Liss, 1986, pp 167–184

Buysse DJ, Reynolds CF III: Insomnia, in Handbook of Sleep Disorders. Edited by Thorpy MJ. New York, Marcel Dekker, 1990, pp 375–433

Chin M, Kreutzer RA, Dyer JL: Acute poisoning from gamma-hydroxybutyrate in California. West J Med 156:380–384, 1992

Coleman RM: Diagnosis, treatment, and follow-up of about 8,000 sleep/wake disorder patients, in Sleep/Wake Disorders: National History, Epidemiology, and Long Term Evolution. Edited by Guilleminault C, Lugarese E. New York, Raven, 1983, pp 29–35

Cook L, Sepinwall J: Behavioral analysis of the effects and mechanisms of action of benzodiazepines. Adv Biochem Psychopharmacol 14:1–28, 1975

Costa E, Guidotti A: Diazepam binding inhibitor (DBI): a peptide with multiple biological actions. Life Sci 49:325–344, 1991

Crestani F, Low K, Keist R, et al: Molecular targets for the myorelaxant action of diazepam. Mol Pharmacol 59:442–445, 2001

Dahlitz M, Alvarez B, Vignan J, et al: Delayed sleep phase syndrome response to melatonin. Lancet 337:1121–1124, 1991

Desikan R, Munshi N, Zeldis J, et al: Activity of thalidomide (THAL) in multiple myeloma (MM) confirmed in 180 patients with advanced disease (abstract). Blood 94 (suppl 1):603a–603a, 1999

Dubocovich ML: Melatonin receptors: are there multiple subtypes? Trends Pharmacol Sci 16:50–56, 1995

Dubocovich ML, Rivera-Bermudez MA, Gerdin MJ, et al: Molecular pharmacology, regulation and function of mammalian melatonin receptors. Front Biosci 8:d1093–d1108, 2003

Ebisawa T, Karne S, Lerner MR, et al: Expression cloning of a high-affinity melatonin receptor from Xenopus dermal melanophores. Proc Natl Acad Sci U S A 91:6133–6137, 1994

Edgar DM, Dement WC, Fuller CA: Effect of SCN-lesions on sleep in squirrel monkeys: evidence for opponent processes in sleep-wake regulation. J Neurosci 13:1065–1079, 1993

Edgar DM, Seidel WF, Gee KW, et al: CCD-3693: an orally bioavailable analog of the endogenous neuroactive steroid, pregnanolone, demonstrates potent sedative hypnotic action in the rat. J Pharmacol Exp Ther 282:420–429, 1997

Enna SJ, Möhler H: Gamma-aminobutyric acid (GABA) receptors and their association with benzodiazepine recognition sites, in Psychopharmacology: The Third Generation of Progress. Edited by Meltzer HY. New York, Raven, 1987, pp 265–272

Folkard S, Arendt J, Clark M: Can melatonin improve shift workers' tolerance of the night shift? Some preliminary findings. Chronobiol Int 10:315–320, 1993

Frederickson RC, Slater IH, Dusenberrry WE: A comparison of thalidomide and pentobarbital—new methods for identifying novel hypnotic drugs. J Pharmacol Exp Ther 203:240–251, 1977

Friess E, Lance M, Holster F: The effects of "neuroactive" steroids upon sleep in human and rats (abstract). J Sleep Res 5:S69, 1996

Garfinkel D, Laudon M, Nof D, et al: Improvement of sleep quality in elderly people by controlled-release melatonin. Lancet 346:541–544, 1995

Gavish M, Katz Y, Bar-Ami S, et al: Biochemical, physiological, and pathological aspects of the peripheral benzodiazepine receptor. J Neurochem 58:1589–1601, 1992

Geddes DM, Rudorf M, Saunders KB: Effect of nitrazepam and flurazepam on the ventilatory response to carbon dioxide. Thorax 31:548–551, 1976

Gottlieb GL: Sleep disorders and their management: special considerations in the elderly. Am J Med 88:29S–33S, 1990

Haefley W: Partial agonists of the benzodiazepine receptor: from animal data to results in patients, in Chloride Channels and Their Modulation by Neurotransmission and Drugs. Edited by Biggio G, Costa E. New York, Raven, 1988, pp 275–292

Haimov I, Laudon M, Zisapel N, et al: Sleep disorders and melatonin rhythms in elderly people. BMJ 309:167, 1994

Haimov I, Lavie P, Lauden M, et al: Melatonin treatment of sleep onset insomnia in the elderly. Sleep 18:598–603, 1995

Hughes RJ, Sack RL, Lewy AJ: The role of melatonin and circadian phase in age-related sleep-maintenance insomnia: assessment in a clinical trial of melatonin replacement. Sleep 21:52–68, 1998

Jovanovic UJ, Dreyfus JF: Polygraphical sleep recording in insomniac patients under zopiclone or nitrazepam. Pharmacology 27 (suppl 2):136–145, 1983

Kaitin KI: Effects of thalidomide and pentobarbital on neuronal activity in the preoptic area during sleep and wakefulness in the cat. Psychopharmacology (Berl) 85:47–50, 1985

Kales A, Shlarf MB, Kales JD, et al: Rebound insomnia: a potential hazard following withdrawal of certain benzodiazepines. JAMA 241:1691–1695, 1979

Kanbayashi T, Nishino S, Tafti M, et al: Thalidomide, a hypnotic with immune modulating properties, increases cataplexy in canine narcolepsy. Neuroreport 12:1881–1886, 1996

Kaplan G: Cytokine regulation of disease progression in leprosy and tuberculosis. Immunobiology 191:564–568, 1994

Kay DC, Blackburn AB, Buckingham JA, et al: Human pharmacology of sleep, in Pharmacology of Sleep. Edited by Williams RL, Karakan I. New York, Wiley, 1976, pp 83–210

Killam K: Drug action on the brainstem reticular formation. Pharmacol Rev 14:175–224, 1962

Kofuji P, Wang JB, Moss SJ, et al: Generation of two forms of the gamma-aminobutyric acidA receptor gamma 2-subunit in mice by alternative splicing. J Neurochem 56:713–715, 1991

Krueger JM, Takahashi S, Kapas L: Cytokines in sleep regulation. Adv Neuroimmunol 5:171–188, 1995

Lapierre O, Montplaisir J, Lamarre M, et al: The effect of gamma-hydroxybutyrate on nocturnal and diurnal sleep of normal subjects: further consideration on REM sleep-triggering mechanisms. Sleep 13:24–30, 1990

Leeb-Lundberg F, Snowman A, Olsen RW: Barbiturate receptor sites are coupled to benzodiazepine receptors. Proc Natl Acad Sci U S A 77:7467–7472, 1980

Lemoine P, Nir T, Laudon M, et al: Prolonged-release melatonin improves sleep quality and morning alertness in insomnia patients aged 55 years and older and has no withdrawal effects. J Sleep Res 16:372–380, 2007

Low K, Crestani F, Keist R, et al: Molecular and neuronal substrate for the selective attenuation of anxiety. Science 290:131–134, 2000

Lushington K, Lack L, Kennaway DJ, et al: 6-Sulfatoxymelatonin excretion and self-reported sleep in good sleeping controls and 55–80-year-old insomniacs. J Sleep Res 7:75–83, 1998

Marquardt H, Todaro GJ, Shoyab M: Complete amino acid sequences of bovine and human endozepines: homology with rat diazepam binding inhibitor. J Biol Chem 261:9727–9731, 1986

Maynert EW: Sedative and hypnotics, II: barbiturates, in Drill's Pharmacology in Medicine. Edited by DiPalma IR. New York, McGraw-Hill, 1965, pp 188–209

McKernan RM, Rosahl TW, Reynolds DS, et al: Sedative but not anxiolytic properties of benzodiazepines are mediated by the GABAA receptor alpha1 subtype. Nature Neuroscience 3:587–592, 2000

Mehta AK, Ticku MK: An update on GABAA receptors. Brain Res Brain Res Rev 29:196–217, 1999

Mellinger GD, Balter MB, Uhlenhuth EH: Insomnia and its treatment: prevalence and correlates. Arch Gen Psychiatry 42:225–232, 1985

Mignot E, Edgar DM, Miller JD, et al: Strategies for the development of new treatments in sleep disorders medicine, in Target Receptors for Anxiolytics and Hypnotics: From Molecular Pharmacology to Therapeutics. Edited by Mendelwicz J, Ra-

cagni G, Karger AG. Basel, Switzerland, Karger, 1992, pp 129–150

Mishima K, Okawa M, Shimizu T, et al: Diminished melatonin secretion in the elderly caused by insufficient environmental illumination. J Clin Endocrinol Metab 86:129–134, 2001

Miyamoto M, Nishikawa H, Doken Y, et al: The sleep-promoting action of ramelteon (TAK-375) in freely moving cats. Sleep 27:1319–1325, 2004

Möhler H, Okada T: Benzodiazepine receptor: demonstration in the central nervous system. Science 198:849–851, 1977

Morgan PJ, Barrett P, Howell HE, et al: Melatonin receptors: localization, molecular pharmacology and physiological significance. Neurochem Int 24:101–146, 1994

Mullen KD, Szauter KM, Kaminsky-Russ K: "Endogenous" benzodiazepine activity in physiological fluids of patients with hepatic encephalopathy. Lancet 336:81–83, 1990

Nishino S, Shiba T, Mishima K, et al: REM sleep enhancing effect of thalidomide is dependent on the availability of TNFalpha. Sleep 28:A18 (Abstract Supplement), 2005

Nutt DJ, Glue P, Lawson C, et al: Flumazenil provocation of panic attacks. Arch Gen Psychiatry 47:917–925, 1990

Olsen RW, Tick MK, Miller T: Dihydropicotoxine binding to crayfish muscle sites possibly related to gamma-aminobutyric acid receptor ionophores. Mol Pharmacol 14:381 390, 1978

Papadopoulos V, Amri H, Li H, et al: Structure, function and regulation of the mitochondrial peripheral-type benzodiazepine receptor. Therapie 56:549–556, 2001

Rall TR: Hypnotics and sedatives: ethanol, in The Pharmacological Basis of Therapeutics, 8th Edition. Edited by Gilman AG, Rall TW, Niles AS, et al. New York, Pergamon, 1990, pp 345–382

Reite M, Ruddy J, Nagel K: Concise Guide to Evaluation and Management of Sleep Disorders, 2nd Edition. Washington, DC, American Psychiatric Press, 1997

Reppert SM, Weaver DR, Ebisawa T: Cloning and characterization of a mammalian melatonin receptor that mediates reproductive and circadian responses. Neuron 13:1177–1185, 1994

Reppert SM, Godson C, Mahle CD, et al: Molecular characterization of a second melatonin receptor expressed in human retina and brain: the Mel1b melatonin receptor. Proc Natl Acad Sci U S A 92:8734–8738, 1995

Richter JA, Holman JR Jr: Barbiturates: their in vivo effects and potential biochemical mechanisms. Prog Neurobiol 18:275–319, 1982

Rothstein JD, Guidotti A, Tinuper P, et al: Endogenous benzodiazepine receptor ligands in idiopathic recurring stupor. Lancet 340:1002–1004, 1992

Rudolph U, Crestani F, Benke D, et al: Benzodiazepine actions mediated by specific gamma-aminobutyric acidA receptor subtypes. Nature 401:796–800, 1999

Rupprecht R, Hauser CAE, Trapp T, et al: Neurosteroids: molecular mechanisms of action and psychopharmacological significance. J Steroid Biochem Mol Biol 56:163–168, 1996

Sangameswaran L, Fales HM, Friedrich P, et al: Purification of a benzodiazepine from bovine brain and detection of benzodiazepine-like immunoreactivity in human brain. Proc Natl Acad Sci U S A 83:9236–9240, 1986

Sanna E, Garau F, Harris RA: Novel properties of homomeric b1 g-aminobutyric acid type A receptors: actions of the anesthetics propofol and pentobarbital. Mol Pharmacol 47:213–217, 1995

Saper CB, Chou TC, Scammell TE: The sleep switch: hypothalamic control of sleep and wakefulness. Trends Neurosci 24:726–731, 2001

Schmidt RF, Vogel ME, Zimmermann M: Effect of diazepam on presynaptic inhibition and other spinal reflexes. Naunyn Schmiedebergs Arch Pharmacol 258:69–82, 1967

Scrima L, Hartman PG, Johnson FH, et al: The effects of gamma-hydroxybutyrate on the sleep of narcolepsy patients: a double-blind study. Sleep 13:479–490, 1990

Sherin JE, Shiromani PJ, McCarley RW, et al: Activation of ventrolateral preoptic neurons during sleep. Science 271:216–219, 1996

Shlarf MB: Pharmacology of classic and novel hypnotic drugs, in Target Receptors for Anxiolytics and Hypnotics: From Molecular Pharmacology to Therapeutics. Edited by Mendelwicz J, Racagni G. Basel, Switzerland, Karger, 1992, pp 109–116

Sigel E, Baur R, Kellenberger S, et al: Point mutations affecting antagonist affinity and agonist dependent gating of GABAA receptor channels. EMBO J 11:2017–2023, 1992

Smith GB, Olsen RW: Identification of a [3H]muscimol photoaffinity substrate in the bovine gamma-aminobutyric acidA receptor alpha subunit. J Biol Chem 269:20380–20387, 1994

Smith GB, Olsen RW: Functional domains of GABAA receptors. Trends Neurosci 16:162–167, 1995

Squires RF, Braestrup C: Benzodiazepine receptors in rat brain. Nature 266:732–734, 1977

Szymusiak R: Magnocellular nuclei of the basal forebrain: substrates of sleep and arousal regulation. Sleep 18:478–500, 1995

Tallman JF, Thomas JW, Gllager DW: GABAergic modulation of benzodiazepine binding site sensitivity. Nature 274:383–385, 1978

Tobler I, Kopp C, Deboer T, et al: Diazepam-induced changes in sleep: role of the alpha 1 GABA(A) receptor subtype. Proc Natl Acad Sci U S A 98:6464–6469, 2001

Twyman RE, Rogers CJ, Macdonald RL: Differential regulation of gamma-aminobutyric acid receptor channels by diazepam and phenobarbital. Ann Neurol 25:213–220, 1989

Ueno S, Minami K, Yanagihara N: [Structure and function of GABAA receptors: recent studies by site-directed mutagenesis] (in Japanese). Protein, Nucleic Acid, and Enzyme 46:2042–2051, 2001

Van Coevorden A, Mockel J, Laurent E, et al: Neuroendocrine rhythms and sleep in aging men. Am J Physiol 260:651–661, 1991

Vayer P, Mandel P, Maitre M: Gamma-hydroxybutyrate, a possible neurotransmitter. Life Sci 41:1547–1557, 1987

Wisden W, Stephens DN: Towards better benzodiazepines. Nature 401:751–752, 1999

Youngstedt SD, Kripke DF, Elliott JA: Melatonin excretion is not related to sleep in the elderly. J Pineal Res 24:142–145, 1998

Zeitzer JM, Daniels JE, Duffy JF, et al: Do plasma melatonin concentrations decline with age? Am J Med 107:432–436, 1999

CHAPTER 43

Psychostimulants and Wakefulness-Promoting Agents

Christos A. Ballas, M.D.

Dwight L. Evans, M.D.

David F. Dinges, Ph.D.

Amphetamine, first discovered in 1887, and the subsequently developed stimulants have been used in clinical psychiatry with varying results. Beyond their use for attention-deficit/hyperactivity disorder (ADHD), they have been used for symptomatic relief based on their effects on mood and hedonic drive. Research into the use of stimulants as adjunctive agents in the treatment of specific symptoms and syndromes has been increasing. Evaluation of new medications, such as modafinil and armodafinil, which are classified as wakefulness-promoting agents, has further heightened interest in a possible therapeutic role for such agents in treatment of neurobehavioral disorders. Various common adjunctive psychotherapeutic uses for stimulants, such as depression, have not been well researched, while other indications, such as narcolepsy, are backed by considerable clinical data. Nonetheless, much more data are needed on the safety and efficacy of traditional psychostimulants as well as the newer agents in the treatment of psychiatric disorders. In this chapter, we review the pharmacology of these medications and their indications (Tables 43–1 and 43–2).

Amphetamines

Structure–Activity Relations

Structurally, amphetamine is phenylisopropylamine. Ultimate pharmacological action is determined by alterations to any of the three basic parts of the amphetamine molecule.

Amine Changes

In terms of affecting clinical utility, substitution at the amine group is the most common alteration. Methamphetamine (both L and D isomers), which is characterized by an additional methyl group attached to the amine, making it a secondary substituted amine, is more potent than amphetamine. Likewise, N-hydroxyamphetamine, a minor metabolite of amphetamine, is more potent than unsubstituted amphetamine. Usefully, one may think of the amine group as enhancing stimulant-like properties. Nevertheless, it may have the reverse effect on the hallucinogenic properties of entactogens, as described later in this section.

This chapter is dedicated to our late colleague Martin P. Szuba, M.D. The substantive review and evaluation for this chapter were supported by Air Force Office of Scientific Research (AFOSR) grant F49620-00-1-0266 (D.F.D.) and National Aeronautics and Space Administration (NASA) cooperative agreement NCC 9-58 with the National Space Biomedical Research Institute (D.F.D.).

TABLE 43–1.   FDA classifications of psychostimulants and wakefulness-promoting agents

	SCHEDULE	APPROVED FOR	TYPE OF MEDICATION	ABUSE POTENTIAL
Amphetamine	II	ADHD, narcolepsy	Anorexiant/stimulant	Black box warning
Lisdexamfetamine	II	ADHD	Stimulant	Black box warning
Methylphenidate	II	ADHD, narcolepsy	Anorexiant/stimulant ("Mild stimulant")	Black box warning
Modafinil	IV	Excessive daytime sleepiness associated with narcolepsy, OSAHS, and SWSD	Wakefulness-promoting agent	Reinforcing
Armodafinil	IV	Excessive daytime sleepiness associated with narcolepsy, OSAHS, and SWSD	Wakefulness-promoting agent	Reinforcing

Note.   ADHD=attention-deficit/hyperactivity disorder; OSAHS=obstructive sleep apnea/hypopnea syndrome; SWSD=shift work sleep disorder; FDA=U.S. Food and Drug Administration.
Source.   Adapted from *Physicians' Desk Reference*, 60th Edition. Montvale, NJ, Medical Economics Company, 2006.

Isopropyl Changes

An intact isopropyl side chain appears to be needed in order to maintain the potency of amphetamine. For example, changing the propyl to an ethyl chain creates phenyl-ethylamine, an endogenous neuroamine (and metabolite of the monoamine oxidase inhibitor [MAOI] phenelzine), which has mood- and energy-enhancing properties but less potency and a much shorter half-life than amphetamine (Janssen et al. 1999).

Aromatic Changes

Substitutions on the phenyl group are associated with a decrease in amphetamine-like properties. Interestingly, reduction of the phenyl to a cyclohexyl ring reduces the potency, but not the efficacy, of amphetamine properties. Unlike changes at the amine or isopropyl level, additions to the aromatic ring substantially alter the effects of the compound. The most common changes at the aromatic ring are of the methoxy type and are associated with hallucinogenic properties. For example, adding a para-methoxy group (paramethoxyamphetamine) creates a hallucinogen. The street drug referred to as "Ecstasy" (3,4-methyl-enedioxy-N-methylamphetamine, or MDMA) is built on a methamphetamine backbone, with a dimethoxy ring extending from the aromatic group. If this hallucinogen is instead designed without the methyl group on the terminal amine, making it a primary amine (i.e., 3,4-methyl-enedioxy-N-amphetamine or MDA), as is the case with the street drug referred to as "Love," the hallucinogenic potency and duration are further increased. Consequently, substitution at the terminal amine clearly increases am-

phetamine-like properties. However, the agents MDMA, MDA, and the ethylated form (3,4-methylenedioxy-N-ethylamphetamine, or MDE) are referred to collectively as *entactogens* to distinguish them from simple stimulants or hallucinogens.

Stereospecificity

Recently, there has been renewed interest in drugs that are pure stereoisomers, as opposed to racemic mixtures, especially with the recent release of dexmethylphenidate (the dextro isomer of methylphenidate) and escitalopram (the levo isomer of citalopram). In the case of amino acids and sugars, only one stereoisomer (the L amino acid and the D sugar, respectively) is used by the body. It is erroneously assumed that the comparable situation exists for medications (i.e., that only one isomer is biologically active). This is an oversimplification, however. For example, with respect to amphetamine isomers, it is true that the dextro form (i.e., dextro isomer, or dextroamphetamine) is almost twice as potent as the levo form (i.e., levo isomer, or levoamphetamine) in promoting wakefulness, but they are of equal potency in reducing cataplexy and rapid eye movement (REM) sleep (Nishino and Mignot 1997). Similarly, whereas the dextro isomer has a more potent effect on dopamine efflux than does the levo isomer form, they are equally potent in promoting norepinephrine efflux (Kanbayashi et al. 2000). The effect on dopamine reuptake is, like the effect on efflux, stereospecific; inhibition in rat brain, striatum, and hypothalamus has been found to be markedly different between the two isomers (Ferris and Tang 1979). This is not surprising, given that dopamine efflux and reuptake may be mediated by the

TABLE 43–2.   Amphetamine and methylphenidate preparations

STIMULANT	TIME TO EFFECT	PEAK (HOURS)	DURATION (HOURS)	DOSING
Amphetamine preparations				
Adderall[a]	~1 hour	3	6–9	bid
Adderall XR	1–2 hours	7	6–10	qd (or bid)
Dexedrine	1 hour	3	4–6	bid or tid
Dexedrine Spansules	1 hour	4	6–10	qd or bid
Desoxyn (methamphetamine)	40 minutes	1–3	4–24	qd, bid, or tid
Vyvanse (lisdexamfetamine)	~1 hour	2	9	qd
Methylphenidate preparations				
Methylphenidate	15–30 minutes	1–2	4–5	bid or tid
Focalin (dexmethylphenidate)	15–30 minutes	1–2	4–5	bid or tid
Ritalin SR (tablet)	1–2 hours	5	8	qd or bid
Concerta[b]	1–2 hours	6–8	12	qd or bid
Metadate-CD[c]	1 hour	Biphasic: 1–2 and 4–5	6–8	qd or bid

Note.   qd = once daily; bid = twice daily; tid = three times daily.

[a]Amphetamine/dextroamphetamine, 1:3 ratio.

[b]Laser hole in capsule allows passage of drug; osmotically active push layer expels drug.

[c]Rapid-release and continuous-release beads give biphasic response.

same transport mechanism (see subsection "Mechanism of Action" later in this section). There does not appear to be any difference in the enantiomeric specificity of amphetamine to monoamine oxidase A or B (Robinson 1985).

Amphetamine stereospecificity is not generalizable across other amphetamine compounds. For example, both individual isomers of MDMA, as well as the racemic mixture, have the same potency in reinforcement (Meyer et al. 2002). MDE, by contrast, appears to have an (*R*)-mediated neurotoxicity and an (*S*)-mediated entactogenic specificity. The (*S*) isomer induces more euphoria, while the (*R*) isomer induces more depression (Spitzer et al. 2001). Because many of these studies have been done in animals, it remains to be seen if the stereospecificity of these compounds will be detectable or important in humans.

The clinical utility of stereospecificity is unclear. Urine levels of the levo isomer have been used to measure compliance in amphetamine-addicted patients prescribed dextroamphetamine for maintenance or detoxification; the logic is that the more levo isomer present in urine, the less compliance (George and Braithwaite 2000).

Perhaps the most clinically useful difference between amphetamine isomers involves their differential effects on reinforcement. Studies in rats have shown that the dextro isomer is four times more potent than the levo isomer in promoting lever pressing for intracranial stimulation (Hunt and Atrens 1992). However, that pure dextro-

amphetamine is better for the treatment of ADHD than, for example, the mixed salts of dextroamphetamine/amphetamine is neither obvious nor conclusively shown. In addition, the overall greater potency of the dextro form to central actions suggests that this form may have a higher potential for abuse.

Methamphetamine, differing from amphetamine by the presence of a methyl group, is more rapidly absorbed into the central nervous system (CNS) and possesses a longer half-life (approximately 20 hours). The increased toxicity of methamphetamine is believed to be due to a combination of its rapid absorption into the CNS, its potency in causing dopamine and glutamate release, and through a mechanism similar to neuronal apoptosis. The toxicity of methamphetamine is mediated via the mitochondria by the generation of free radicals (Choi et al. 2002)—a process inhibited by both glutathione and L-carnitine (Virmani et al. 2002) (see subsection "Side Effects and Toxicology" later in this section).

Pharmacological Profile

Amphetamines are noncatecholamine, sympathomimetic amines with CNS stimulant activity that causes catecholamine efflux and inhibits the reuptake of these neurotransmitters (see subsection "Mechanism of Action" later in this section).

Pharmacokinetics and Disposition

Amphetamines are highly lipid soluble and achieve peak levels in approximately 2 hours. Because of this lipid solubility, amphetamines have rapid distribution into tissues and transit across the blood–brain barrier. The protein binding is highly variable, but the average volume of distribution, or V_d, is 5 L/kg.

Because amphetamine is a weak base, much of its elimination can be altered. In general, the half-life is approximately 16–30 hours. If the urine is acidified, excretion can be increased to approximately 60% of the unaltered amphetamine in 48 hours. Alkalinizing the urine, however, can drive the elimination almost totally through a metabolic pathway (deamination).

On average, 30% of amphetamine is excreted unchanged, although the dextro isomer is more rapidly excreted. Another 20% (or substantially more, depending on the pH of the urine) of amphetamine is deaminated to phenylacetone and, to a trivial extent, parahydroxyamphetamine. Phenylacetone is in turn oxidized to benzoic acid and excreted as hippuric acid. A small but likely clinically insignificant metabolism (hydroxylation) occurs through the cytochrome P450 (CYP) 2D6 isoenzyme (see subsection "Drug–Drug Interactions" later in this section).

Mechanism of Action

The classic mechanism of action of amphetamines involves rapid diffusion directly into neuron terminals; through dopamine and norepinephrine transporters, amphetamine enters vesicles, causing release of dopamine and norepinephrine. The release of these neurotransmitters into the synapse mediates some of the psychological and motoric effects of amphetamine, including euphoria, increased energy, and locomotor activation.

However, the actual mechanism of action of amphetamine appears to be more complex than simply promoting dopamine or norepinephrine efflux. This is most notably observed with respect to dopamine. Release of dopamine is a two-step process: 1) release from the vesicles into the presynaptic terminal and then 2) release from the presynaptic terminal into the synaptic cleft. Although amphetamine rapidly caused the release of dopamine from the vesicles into the presynaptic terminal, in knockout mice lacking an intact dopamine transporter (DAT), dopamine was not released into the synaptic cleft, thus showing that the role of the DAT is the rate-limiting step in the effects of amphetamine (Jones et al. 1998). This finding led to the further discovery that the

DAT functions in a bidirectional manner; its transport of amphetamine from extracellular space into the presynaptic terminal both diminishes the amount of dopamine that is taken back into the presynaptic terminal and catalyzes a reaction promoting the outward transport of dopamine from the presynaptic membrane to the synaptic cleft (Jones et al. 1999).

The dopaminergic effects of amphetamines are opposite those found for the norepinephrine transporter (NET). Knockout mice lacking the NET were supersensitive to the locomotor stimulation of amphetamine. It appears that in the absence of norepinephrine transport, there is no feedback control on amphetamine-induced dopaminergic function (Xu et al. 2000). The primacy of dopamine in the effects of amphetamine is similarly revealed by the observation that amphetamine decreases γ-aminobutyric acid (GABA)–ergic transmission in the striatum through stimulation of dopamine$_2$ (D_2) receptors (Centonze et al. 2002). This likely represents an important, albeit not yet quantified, contribution to the psychostimulant effects of amphetamines.

One hypothesis concerning how amphetamines paradoxically suppress or reduce hyperactivity in certain patient populations has been dispelled. It was believed that at certain therapeutic doses (which are in actuality low doses compared with those that produce locomotor activation and stereotypy), amphetamines bind to presynaptic autoreceptors and prevent neurotransmission. This belief has not been supported; results from a 2001 study showed that at doses as low as 0.2 mg/kg (even lower than traditional therapeutic doses), amphetamine still had low affinity for the autoreceptor and was much more potent at the postsynaptic site (Ruskin et al. 2001). It appears that the mechanism of putative paradoxical effects of amphetamine administered at low doses remains to be identified.

With respect to the anorectic effects of amphetamines, the role of hypothalamic neuropeptide Y (NPY), a potent stimulant of appetite, is being considered as a possible mechanism. In ordinary circumstances, the anorectic effects of amphetamines are seen on the first day, but tolerance to this appetite suppressant effect quickly develops. It has been reported that the level of hypothalamic NPY markedly decreases on the first day of amphetamine administration but then quickly returns to normal. This tolerance was abolished with a daily dose of NPY antisense treatment (which effectively blocks the expression of the NPY gene) (Kuo et al. 2001).

Precisely how amphetamines enhance waking cognitive functions is not known. A repeated finding is increased activity in the brain, whether measured as regional cerebral blood flow in positron emission tomography (PET) scans (Mattay et al. 1996) or as activated voxels in functional magnetic resonance imaging (Uftring et al. 2001). In a given task, the brain regions that are active during amphetamine administration are those that are also active during placebo administration; in other words, amphetamine did not activate new brain areas to produce its effect (Uftring et al. 2001). A more controversial but quite impressive discovery in the PET study by Mattay et al. (1996) was that whereas amphetamine increased cerebral blood flow in task-specific regions, it decreased blood flow in those regions not needed in the task, forming the basis for the hypothesis that amphetamine acts in a "neural network–specific" manner. Methylphenidate showed similar effects in a study of 11 children with attention-deficit disorder. The drug increased perfusion in the mesencephalon but decreased it in motor and sensory areas (Lou et al. 1984). Caffeine, by contrast, does not appear to have this region-specific effect but instead affects cerebral blood flow more globally (Cameron et al. 1990).

Side Effects and Toxicology

The side effects of amphetamines are predictable relative to their sympathomimetic pharmacology. The most common effects are nervousness, agitation, and decreased sleep. Serious adverse consequences have been observed with amphetamines, including arrhythmias, hyperpyrexia, rhabdomyolysis, and convulsions. Death, although uncommon, generally occurs only after the manifestation of one of these symptoms. Hallucinosis and psychosis are frequent complications of injected or inhaled amphetamines but uncommon with oral intoxication.

Methamphetamine is more frequently associated with complications; because of its higher toxicity, it is not clear whether severe complications are dose dependent. For example, in a retrospective study of methamphetamine-related deaths in a large city, methamphetamine use was significantly associated with a higher risk of coronary artery disease, as well as a higher rate of subarachnoid hemorrhage, although it was of course impossible to determine whether the subjects were first-time users or chronic abusers (Karch et al. 1999). Of particular note in this study, however, was that blood levels of methamphetamine did not differ between the group in which methamphetamine was judged to be the cause of death and the group in which methamphetamine was detected but judged not to be related to the cause of death, suggesting that these toxicities are not necessarily dose dependent. Similarly, in one 5-year study, methamphetamine ac-

counted for 43% of rhabdomyolysis cases in an emergency department setting. Methamphetamine rhabdomyolysis was associated with substantially higher creatine phosphokinase (CPK) values (mean = 12,439 U/L) (Richards et al. 1999). In addition, hyperthermia is a common cause of death and may in fact be the cause of rhabdomyolysis (Callaway and Clark 1994). Thus, in contrast to the relative safety of oral amphetamines, methamphetamine carries greater risks.

Methamphetamine is more neurotoxic than amphetamine; it can cause destruction of dopaminergic neurons in the basal ganglia and, thus, is widely suspected to increase the likelihood of future parkinsonism (Guilarte 2001). Although it is commonly believed that MDMA ("Ecstasy") is primarily toxic to serotonergic neurons (Sprague et al. 1998), evidence shows that it is also toxic to dopaminergic neurons (Ricaurte et al. 2002).

Methamphetamine appears to increase free radicals and causes mitochondrial damage and decreased adenosine triphosphate (ATP) synthesis. In dopaminergic neurons, the neurotoxicity is mediated by formation of peroxynitrite, which can be reduced by antioxidants or L-carnitine (Virmani et al. 2002). L-Carnitine is needed to transport long-chain fatty acids into the mitochondria for fatty acid oxidation, preventing the generation of free radicals and peroxynitrite. MDMA appears also to decrease glutathione and vitamin E (in brain), and mice deficient in vitamin E were found to have greater susceptibility to both MDMA neurotoxicity and hepatic necrosis, further supporting a free radical mechanism for toxicity (Johnson et al. 2002).

Seizures are fairly common in amphetamine abuse scenarios, especially with the more potent methamphetamine and hallucinogenic analogs. Some differences are seen in the phenotype of seizures from different stimulants. Methamphetamine produced the longest seizure, and cocaine produced the shortest; however, although phenytoin effectively prevented cocaine seizures, it had no effect on methamphetamine seizures, which could be prevented only by diazepam and valproate. MDMA was unique in that it produced a secondary clonic phase after the initial seizure (Hanson et al. 1999). It should be noted that the most common complication of MDMA is seizures (Zagnoni and Albano 2002); thus, MDMA always should be suspected in new-onset seizures in patients of the appropriate demographic.

Stimulant psychosis—often referred to as *paranoid psychosis*—is also common in amphetamine abuse scenarios because of the overwhelming presentation of the eponymous symptom. Visual hallucinations are also disproportionately common with amphetamine psychosis; in contrast, disorientation and thought disorder, which are more common in schizophrenia, are rarely seen (Angrist et al. 1974). Psychosis is often seen together with stereotypy. In humans, stereotypy can take many forms but usually is expressed as pacing, searching, or examining minute details.

Traditionally, stimulants have been contraindicated in patients with tics because stimulants are believed to worsen tics; the prescribing information notes that dextroamphetamine exacerbates motor and phonic tics and Tourette's syndrome (GlaxoSmithKline 2006). This relation is not consistently found (Law and Schachar 1999) and is discussed in further detail below

The U.S. Food and Drug Administration (FDA) has added a black box warning to all stimulant medications, describing the risks of heart-related problems, especially sudden death in those with prior cardiac disease; stroke; and increased blood pressure and heart rate. Additionally, the warning describes the risk of new mental problems, especially bipolar disorder, hostility, or psychosis.

Drug–Drug Interactions

A comprehensive review found that drug interactions with amphetamine were mostly pharmacodynamic in nature (Markowitz and Patrick 2001); however, because a small portion of amphetamine's metabolism occurs via CYP2D6, those drugs that inhibit 2D6 metabolism can, theoretically, have the effect of increasing the plasma level of amphetamines. This is generally not a significant effect with therapeutic doses of amphetamines; however, more severe reactions are possible with the inhibition of CYP2D6 metabolism of MDMA (Ramamoorthy et al. 2002) and paramethoxyamphetamine (Kraner et al. 2001), which are more toxic compounds. Only two reported cases of serotonin syndrome have been associated with amphetamine and venlafaxine or citalopram use (Prior et al. 2002).

Lisdexamfetamine

Lisdexamfetamine dimesylate, a prodrug that on absorption is metabolized to dextroamphetamine and L-lysine, was approved in 2007 for the treatment of ADHD. Food does not affect absorption of lisdexamfetamine; however, as with all amphetamines, acidification of the urine results in more rapid clearance.

Two small studies in children found good efficacy and tolerability for lisdexamfetamine in the treatment of ADHD. A 4-week randomized, double-blind, forced-dose, parallel-group study compared lisdexamfetamine 30, 50, or 70 mg with placebo in children (ages 6–12 years) with ADHD (Biederman et al. 2007b). Efficacy, as measured by the ADHD Rating Scale–Version IV (ADHD-RS-IV), the Conners Parent Rating Scale (CPR), and the Clinical Global Impression of Improvement scale, was statistically superior to placebo for all doses tested. A randomized, double-blind, placebo-controlled crossover study compared lisdexamfetamine with placebo and mixed amphetamine salts extended-release (Adderall XR) in 52 children (ages 6–12 years) with ADHD in an analog classroom setting (Biederman et al. 2007a). The study found comparable efficacy and safety for the active medications and superiority over placebo as measured by CGI and Swanson, Kotkin, Agler, M-Flynn, and Pelham (SKAMP)–Deportment scores.

In 420 adults, a 4-week forced-dose study (30, 50, and 70 mg) found lisdexamfetamine to have significantly greater efficacy over placebo as measured by ADHD-RS scores. Human liability studies have also found lower abuse-related drug-liking scores compared with immediate-release D-amphetamine at equivalent doses (Najib 2009).

Methylphenidate

Structure–Activity Relations

Although methylphenidate has two chiral centers, only one contributes to its clinical effect. The D- and L-threo enantiomers are in a racemic mixture, although a single-isomer form of methylphenidate, dexmethylphenidate [(R,R)-(+)], is currently being marketed under the brand name Focalin. There are some differences in the pharmacological parameters of the two isomers, as described in the following subsection.

Pharmacokinetics and Disposition

Methylphenidate is almost totally absorbed on oral administration (as is the single isomer dexmethylphenidate), although it is absorbed at a faster rate in the presence of food (Chan et al. 1983). Methylphenidate has low protein binding (15%) and is fairly short acting; the effects last approximately 4 hours, with a half-life of 3 hours. The primary means of clearance is through the urine, in which 90% is excreted.

There is a substantial albeit likely clinically insignificant difference in the metabolism of the two isomers of methylphenidate. If the racemic mixture is given intravenously, there is no difference in urine D- or L-methylphenidate levels, and there is no difference in the metabolite isomer levels, D- and L-ritalinic acid. However, if a racemic mixture is given orally, urine D-methylphenidate levels are 10 times that of L-methylphenidate levels, whereas levels of L-ritalinic acid are almost three times greater than those of D-ritalinic acid (Srinivas et al. 1992, 1993). This difference can be explained by the fact that L-methylphenidate, but not D-methylphenidate, undergoes significant first-pass metabolism (by de-esterification) to L-ritalinic acid.

Mechanism of Action

Although it is both a norepinephrine and a dopamine reuptake inhibitor, methylphenidate appears to exert its effects primarily through its action on dopamine neurobiology. It blocks the DAT and increases extracellular dopamine. The amount of extracellular dopamine increase varies greatly among individuals depending on the extent of both DAT blockade and baseline dopamine release. It is hypothesized, therefore, that methylphenidate will be more potent in someone with a high baseline level of dopamine release (Volkow et al. 2001).

Because of studies showing that the dextro isomer is a more potent locomotor activator than the levo isomer and that there is no difference between the levo form and placebo in improving attention (Challman and Lipsky 2000), it is at times proposed that the levo form is thus entirely inactive in the human body. This is not wholly accurate, however, because there are differences in isomer binding among brain regions. For example, the dextro form binds stereoselectively in the striatum and basal ganglia, whereas the levo form binds nonspecifically throughout the brain (Challman and Lipsky 2000).

Side Effects and Toxicology

The common side effects of methylphenidate are similar to those of amphetamine and include nervousness, insomnia, and anorexia, as well as dose-related systemic effects such as increased heart rate and blood pressure. Overdose may lead to seizures, dysrhythmias, or hyperthermia (Klein-Schwartz 2002). At therapeutic doses, discontinuation symptoms tend to be slight, but with chronic abuse, symptoms similar to those in amphetamine withdrawal, including lethargy, depression, and paranoia, can occur (Klein-Schwartz 2002).

Although worry over the possibility that methylphenidate worsens tics is common, controlled trials indicate that this concern may be unfounded (Castellanos et al. 1997; Law and Schachar 1999). At least one such controlled study found that in children with comorbid tic disorder, tic severity was no worse with methylphenidate than with placebo until approximately 12 weeks, at which point the tic severity actually improved with methylphenidate (Tourette's Syndrome Study Group 2002).

To date, no evidence has shown that methylphenidate is carcinogenic. Surprisingly, it has been observed that in both rats and humans, the incidence of certain cancers is lower than expected (Dunnick and Hailey 1995). There are case reports of growth impairment in children, possibly due to an effect on growth hormone secretion (Holtkamp et al. 2002), although numerous studies have not found such an effect on growth (Kramer et al. 2000; Lahat et al. 2000; Toren et al. 1997).

The FDA has added a black box warning to all stimulant medications, describing the risks of heart-related problems, especially sudden death in those with prior cardiac disease; stroke; and increased blood pressure and heart rate. Additionally, the warning describes the risk of new mental problems, especially bipolar disorder, hostility, or psychosis.

Drug–Drug Interactions

Although theoretically a substrate of CYP2D6, methylphenidate was found not to have any significant metabolism in humans via this enzyme (DeVane et al. 2000). This is likely because the vast majority of methylphenidate metabolism occurs at first pass and outside of the liver. The prescribing information (Novartis 2007) does cite methylphenidate's potential ability to inhibit the metabolism of coumadin, some antiepileptics, and tricyclic antidepressants (TCAs), and thus caution should be observed. However, a review found that methylphenidate is relatively safe and has minimal substantial drug–drug interactions, with the exception of concomitant MAOI use (Markowitz and Patrick 2001).

Modafinil

Modafinil is the first FDA-designated "wakefulness-promoting agent." Modafinil is approved by the FDA for the treatment of excessive sleepiness associated with narcolepsy, sleep apnea, and residual sleepiness after standard treatment for shift work sleep disorder (Cephalon Inc. 2008). As described below, modafinil does little to prevent or alter sleep when one is trying to do so; however, it appears to permit more stable wakefulness (i.e., reduced sleep propensity) when one is attempting to stay awake in the presence of elevated sleep pressure.

Structure–Activity Relations

Modafinil (2-[(diphenylmethyl)sulfinyl]acetamide) exists in racemic form. Both stereoisomers appear to have the same activity in animals.

Pharmacokinetics and Disposition

Modafinil, the primary metabolite of adrafinil, lacks adrafinil's terminal amide hydroxyl group (Figure 43–1). It also lacks many of the side effects found in adrafinil, such as increased liver enzymes, anxiety, and stomach pain. Modafinil is rapidly absorbed but slowly cleared. It has fairly high protein binding (60%) and a V_d of 0.8 L/kg. Its half-life is 11–14 hours.

The metabolism of modafinil is complex. In contrast to excretion of amphetamines, less than 10% of modafinil is excreted unchanged. For reasons not understood, the dextro isomer is cleared three times faster than the levo isomer, and females clear modafinil faster than do males (Wong et al. 1999a). This sex difference was not observed to correspond to differences in efficacy or tolerability. Armodafinil, although named after the (R) isomer, is properly levorotatory (i.e., L-(R)-modafinil) and is thus the longer-acting isomer.

Up to 60% of modafinil is converted into modafinil acid and modafinil sulfone, both of which are inactive. Metabolism is primarily via CYP3A4/5. It has been reported that modafinil also has in vitro capacity to induce CYP3A4 (Robertson et al. 2000), especially gastrointestinal 3A4. A clinically significant reduction of triazolam has been reported (Robertson et al. 2002).

Mechanism of Action

The precise mechanism by which modafinil exerts its wakefulness-promoting effect in patients with excessive sleepiness due to narcolepsy is not yet known. Human narcolepsy is associated with a loss of hypocretin cells in the lateral hypothalamus. Modafinil, given its efficacy in narcolepsy, is not surprisingly observed to increase c-fos activity of hypocretin cells, as well as in the tuberomammillary nucleus (which is primarily histaminergic), striatum, and cingulate cortex at higher doses (Scammell et al. 2000). The precise mechanism of action for modafinil's effects on sleepiness in narcolepsy remains to be determined. Additionally, in rats, an increase in histamine release in the anterior hypothalamus is seen (Ishizuka et al. 2003). Interestingly, humans with narcolepsy have decreased levels of histamine in the cerebrospinal fluid; this, along with the c-fos activity in the histaminergic tubero-

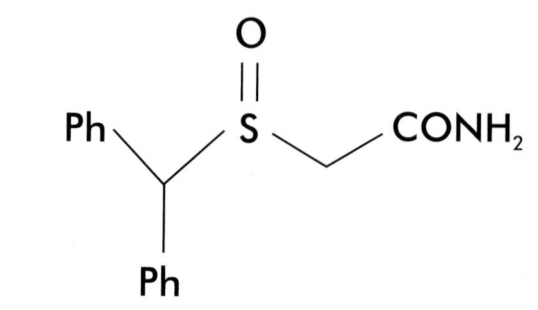

FIGURE 43–1.   Chemical structure of modafinil.

mammillary nucleus, suggests a histaminergic mechanism (Mignot and Nishino 2005). However, modafinil's wakefulness-promoting effects were not decreased in histamine knockout mice (Bonaventure et al. 2007).

It may be easier to describe the pathways by which modafinil does *not* exert its effects. Modafinil only weakly binds to the DAT and causes a smaller release of dopamine compared with other stimulants. Dopaminergic mechanisms that are affected by traditional stimulants, such as amphetamine, are not thought to account for the wakefulness induced by modafinil. However, in DAT knockout mice, modafinil had no wakefulness-promoting effects (Wisor et al. 2001), suggesting that its mechanism of action may involve some feature of dopamine transport that is necessary for its efficacy. Furthermore, all agents that inhibit dopaminergic function and suppress the effects of stimulants in the form of dopamine$_1$ (D$_1$) blockade, D$_2$ blockade, and tyrosine hydroxylase blockade were found to have no effect on modafinil (Simon et al. 1995). A recent in vitro study found that modafinil blocked norepinephrine reuptake in the ventrolateral preoptic nucleus—a putative sleep-promoting center (Gallopin et al. 2004; Saper and Scammell 2004). Norepinephrine ordinarily inhibits sleep-promoting neurons in this area, thereby inhibiting sleep; modafinil therefore increases this inhibition of sleep.

Despite modafinil's having no affinity for α receptors, central $α_1$ blockers such as prazosin have been reported to block modafinil's wakefulness-promoting action (Duteil et al. 1990). It may be the absence of modafinil's effect on catecholamine levels that explains the lack of rebound sedation that commonly occurs after amphetamine usage.

Modafinil appears to increase glutamate and suppress GABA in the posterior hypothalamus (Ferraro et al. 1999) and medial preoptic area (Ferraro et al. 1996) (as well as increasing glutamate in the hippocampus and ventral thalamus [Ferraro et al. 1997]), a finding consistent with promotion of increased wakefulness.

What may be an important aspect of the pharmacology of modafinil is its lack of effect on the neuroendocrine system. A comparison of healthy volunteers who were sleep deprived for 36 hours with those who received modafinil during sleep deprivation found no difference in cortisol, melatonin, or growth hormone levels (Brun et al. 1998). Modafinil has been reported to increase body temperature in healthy adults undergoing sleep deprivation (Bourdon et al. 1994); however, the increase appears slight (0.15–0.2°C) and does not appear to be disproportionately increased (relative to placebo) by exercise even during sustained wakefulness (McLellan et al. 2002).

Side Effects and Toxicology

Modafinil appears to be well tolerated, with the most frequent side effects being headache and nausea. Side effects have been found to increase with doses from 100 to 600 mg, and very high doses (800 mg) have been found to be associated with higher rates of tachycardia and hypertension (Wong et al. 1999b). In Phase III trials, three patients with a history of mitral valve prolapse or left ventricular hypertrophy had transient ischemic changes on electrocardiogram; one patient taking 300 mg/day for almost a month had a 9-second asystole. One patient with chronic sleep deprivation taking 600 mg/day for several days experienced auditory hallucinations and paranoia, which quickly resolved after discontinuation of the modafinil. Overall, only 5% of the patients in Phase III trials discontinued modafinil because of side effects (Cephalon Inc. 2008).

Modafinil appears to be fairly safe in high doses. Reports indicate that 32 patients have safely taken 1,000 mg/day for more than 50 days; one individual safely took 1,200 mg/day for 21 consecutive days. Two patients took 4,000 mg and 4,500 mg, respectively, at once and experienced only transient (<24 hours) agitation, insomnia, and mild elevations in heart rate and blood pressure (Cephalon Inc. 2008). There have been no reports of seizures with modafinil. However, because modafinil has become clinically available only relatively recently, the results of clinical trials on its safety and efficacy are limited relative to those for many other stimulants. It is anticipated that more published data on modafinil will become available in the coming years.

During the recent attempts to have modafinil approved for ADHD, concern arose over the possibility that modafinil may have a risk of Stevens-Johnson syndrome. Three cases of drug-induced rash were reported during clinical trials (U.S. Food and Drug Administration 2007).

In the first, a 7-year-old Asian boy who was concomitantly taking amoxicillin for an upper respiratory tract infection developed rash 16 days after starting modafinil, which by day 23 progressed to what was believed to be Stevens-Johnson syndrome. It was not clear whether this rash was due to the modafinil or to the amoxicillin. The second case involved a girl who developed a maculopapular rash that resolved with antihistamines. In the third case, an 8-year-old boy developed fever, blisters on lips, and rash on cheeks 14 days after initiating modafinil therapy. There was insufficient evidence to diagnose the rash, nor was it clear to the panel that the rash was related to modafinil.

The package insert describes a risk of "serious rash, including Stevens-Johnson syndrome," in adults and children and cautions that modafinil is not indicated for children. The insert cites a rash incidence of 0.8% in pediatric patients, with one case of possible Stevens-Johnson syndrome and one case of multiorgan hypersensitivity reported, and concludes with the statement that although there are no known predictive factors, and that benign rashes do occur, modafinil should be discontinued if rash develops.

Drug–Drug Interactions

As described earlier in this section, modafinil induces CYP3A4/5 and thus conceivably could lower the plasma concentrations of medications with substantial 3A4/5 metabolism. However, it is not clear if this induction is substantial only on the gastrointestinal cytochrome and is thus relevant only for other drugs undergoing significant first-pass metabolism.

Modafinil inhibits CYP2C19 in vitro (Robertson et al. 2000). It is prudent to assume that the effect of modafinil on the cytochrome system is not well characterized and to be vigilant for these potential drug–drug interactions.

Armodafinil

Armodafinil, properly L-(R)-modafinil (or (−)-(R)-modafinil), is the longer-acting isomer of racemic modafinil. In 2007, it received FDA approval for the same indications as modafinil—specifically, excessive sleepiness associated with narcolepsy; obstructive sleep apnea/hypopnea syndrome (OSAHS) as an adjunct to standard treatment; and shift work sleep disorder (SWSD).

Armodafinil and racemic modafinil give comparable peak plasma concentrations, although the peak for armodafinil occurs later than that for modafinil and is maintained for 6–14 hours postdose (Dinges et al. 2006).

Although no human equivalence studies have been performed, it appears that in rats, 100 mg/kg armodafinil was equally efficacious to 1 mg/kg D-methamphetamine. In keeping with the differential pharmacology and effects, this comparable dose did not affect locomotor activity or body temperature. While there were no differences in rebound sleep parameters such as latency to consolidated sleep, a greater proportion of time was spent in non-REM sleep with D-methamphetamine than armodafinil—which was not different from placebo. Similarly, brief awakenings, another measure of rebound hypersomnolence, were suppressed with D-methamphetamine but not with armodafinil (Wisor et al. 2006).

Published data on armodafinil are minimal. At the time this chapter was finalized, a MEDLINE search on the term "armodafinil" returned 11 citations, only 6 of which were actual studies. Two 12-week double-blind studies using armodafinil 150 mg as an adjunct to continuous positive airway pressure (CPAP), both in patients who were otherwise stable except for some residual sleepiness (Hirshkowitz et al. 2006) and in patients who were still symptomatic (Roth et al. 2006), found improvements in wakefulness measures. Armodafinil also significantly improved the quality of episodic secondary memory (i.e., the ability to recall unrehearsed information). Whether this effect was due directly to the medication, to improved wakefulness, or to decreased hypoxia (as a function of being more awake) is unclear. However, armodafinil did not adversely affect the CPAP or any other physiological parameters.

A 12-week double-blind study of armodafinil in narcolepsy found improvements similar to those seen with modafinil. These included improved wakefulness (as measured by the Maintenance of Wakefulness Test), improved Clinical Global Impression of Change (CGI-C) scores, and improvement in memory and attention. Armodafinil 150 mg and 250 mg were similarly effective (Harsh et al. 2006).

In SWSD, armodafinil 150 mg/day was tested versus placebo in a 12-week study, showing significant prolongation of time to sleep onset and an improvement in overall clinical condition by CGI-C. Armodafinil had no effect on daytime sleep polysomnography (Roth et al. 2005).

Clinical Uses of Stimulants and Wakefulness-Promoting Agents

Although stimulants have been used for many years in a number of clinical scenarios, double-blind, randomized, controlled trials examining their safety, efficacy, and effectiveness in neurobehavioral disorders other than ADHD are relatively rare. Most of the support for their use comes from open-label studies and case series. Randomized trials on modafinil for neurobehavioral disorders with symptoms of sleepiness and fatigue are beginning to be published.

Attention-Deficit/Hyperactivity Disorder

Several double-blind, placebo-controlled studies have shown the efficacy of stimulants for ADHD, and their use is well investigated in both adults and children (Greenhill et al. 2002; Wilens et al. 2002). Recent studies are aimed at showing superiority of one preparation relative to another, although this approach is not always fruitful; for example, one study comparing various single-dose amphetamine preparations with one another and with placebo over 8 weeks found that they were all superior to placebo; however, immediate-release amphetamines had a faster onset but shorter duration of action; spansules, although much slower to take effect than the others, lasted several hours longer (James et al. 2001).

With respect to individual stimulants, all appear to be equally efficacious in the treatment of ADHD, but they have been reported to have different time courses. In a double-blind, double-control (placebo and methylphenidate) study, the mixed amphetamine salts of Adderall were found to exert their effects rapidly but to dissipate quickly over the course of the day, although Adderall lasted longer than methylphenidate (Swanson et al. 1998). Interestingly, higher doses of Adderall lasted longer than lower doses, indicating a dose-dependent effect in duration of action not found with methylphenidate. Thus, although stimulants may appear to be of equal efficacy overall, there is considerable variability in individual response to each stimulant.

The decision to choose amphetamines or methylphenidate for the treatment of ADHD is often based on the clinician's preference and degree of experience with the medication. At least one important blinded, crossover study found that in performance tasks, both drugs were generally equally efficacious (Efron et al. 1997). Some studies have investigated electroencephalogram (EEG) correlates that may predict response to methylphenidate or amphetamine. One study comparing good and poor responders to methylphenidate found that those who responded well had higher levels of cortical hypoarousal, showing increases in theta activity and decreases in alpha and beta activity (Clarke et al. 2002b); this is similar to the findings of another group, which suggested that methylphenidate acts by increasing arousal (Loo et al. 1999). With respect to amphetamine, good responders had EEG features more typical of those seen in younger children, indicating that those persons who had a good response to dexamphetamine were more maturationally delayed (Clarke et al. 2002a).

Modafinil is not FDA approved for the treatment of ADHD. A 4-week double-blind study with an 8-week open-label extension found modafinil to be efficacious across all ADHD rating subscales for the duration of the open-label extension (Boellner et al. 2006). Interestingly, 10% of the 220 children studied lost an average of 3 kg, while 4% gained the same. Another such double-blind study found significant efficacy with dosages of 300 mg/day, although heavier children (<30 kg) required 400 mg/day (Biederman et al. 2006). A pooled analysis of three trials (638 patients) found modafinil had similar and impressive improvements in ADHD scales between stimulant-naive and prior-stimulant subgroups, relative to placebo (Wigal et al. 2006). As in other studies, insomnia and headache were the most common, but infrequent, side effects. A 9-week trial (Biederman et al. 2005) found that almost half of patients (mean age 10 years, mean dose 368 mg) were much or very much improved; and efficacy was seen in both inattentive and hyperactive subgroups and both school and home ratings. In this study, weights did not change significantly. Some small but controlled trials (Rugino and Samsock 2003; Turner et al. 2004) found efficacy with modafinil, and in one study (Taylor and Russo 2000) equivalence to dextroamphetamine. However, because of modafinil's apparent low abuse and dependence potential, its use is potentially of interest, but controlled clinical trials are needed to establish any benefit it may have for ADHD. Modafinil is currently indicated only for the treatment of excessive sleepiness associated with narcolepsy, OSAHS, and SWSD.

Stroke and Traumatic Brain Injury

The results from studies on the effects of stimulants in patients who had strokes and traumatic brain injury are mixed. Although small early studies showed some superiority of amphetamine to placebo in improving motor function poststroke (Crisostomo et al. 1988; Walker-Batson et al. 1995), a double-blind study found that 10 mg/day of amphetamine combined with physiotherapy in geriatric stroke patients was not superior to placebo plus physiotherapy in improving activities of daily living or motor function 5 weeks later (Sonde et al. 2001). Neither was amphetamine found to be superior to placebo in improving somatosensory training outcomes (Knecht et al. 2001).

In contrast, relative to placebo, dextroamphetamine 10 mg/day significantly improved language recovery in poststroke aphasic patients when immediately coupled with a session of speech therapy; this effect was seen as quickly as within 1 week (Walker-Batson et al. 2001). A recent review lamented the lack of good data in brain-injured patients but did note that available data suggest that the bulk of stimulant efficacy may lie with its improvements in mood and cognitive processing (Whyte et al. 2002).

Although there is a dearth of placebo-controlled studies, there are some interesting reports in which stimulants were compared with antidepressants in patients with poststroke depression. One such study, comparing methylphenidate with TCAs, found similar and significant response to both drugs, although the stimulant worked faster (Lazarus et al. 1994).

Modafinil has been reported to have some therapeutic efficacy in one type of brain injury. Two double-blind studies by the same group (Saletu et al. 1990, 1993) found modafinil effective in improving cognition and accelerating improvement in patients with alcoholic brain syndrome.

The very limited available evidence for the efficacy of certain psychostimulants and modafinil in functional recovery from certain types of brain injury is promising, but much more work needs to be done in this area.

Cocaine and Stimulant Abuse Treatment

It may not be surprising that a double-blind study showed sustained-release dextroamphetamine to be superior to placebo in reducing cocaine use (Grabowski et al. 2001). However, a similarly designed study by the same authors did not find this effect with methylphenidate (Grabowski et al. 1997) (or risperidone [Grabowski et al. 2000]). The implications of this are not obvious. It may suggest that methylphenidate is not as addictive or reinforcing as either cocaine or amphetamine and thus cannot substitute for either of them. This could be because of the slower clearance of methylphenidate from the brain relative to cocaine (Volkow et al. 1995) or, more likely, because the rate at which methylphenidate blocks the DAT is slower than the rate that cocaine blocks it and thus the same subjective "high" is not produced (Volkow et al. 1999). On the other hand, a small open trial found that methylphenidate was effective in cocaine abusers with comorbid ADHD (Levin et al. 1998), suggesting that such individuals may be "self-medicating" with cocaine. A double-blind, placebo-controlled study found that modafinil did not increase the euphoria or craving for cocaine; it may, in fact, have blunted the euphoria (Dackis et al. 2003). A more recent double-blind, placebo-controlled study of 62 patients found that modafinil-treated patients had a longer duration of cocaine abstinence (>3 weeks), with no dropouts due to adverse events (Dackis et al. 2005). Most recently, a 48-day double-blind trial found that under controlled laboratory conditions, modafinil significantly attenuated self-administration and effects of cocaine (Hart et al. 2008). These preliminary investigations suggest that further exploration of modafinil's utility in cocaine abuse treatment is warranted.

Alcohol Dependence

Basic research suggests that amphetamine appears to have an unexpected effect in alcohol abuse disorders. In rats, amphetamines reduced alcohol consumption during choice trials; this reduction was specific to alcohol intake, because amphetamine administration had no effect on rodents' intake of water (Yu et al. 1997). This effect of amphetamine on alcohol consumption may involve the neurobiology of reward systems. Much more research is needed to identify the mechanisms by which stimulants affect alcohol intake.

Narcolepsy

Stimulants have traditionally been used for the treatment of excessive sleepiness associated with narcolepsy. Narcolepsy is characterized by excessive sleepiness that is typically associated with cataplexy and other REM sleep phenomena such as sleep paralysis and hypnagogic hallucinations. Modafinil's approval for treatment of excessive sleepiness in narcolepsy was based on substantial evidence from large multicenter clinical trials (Broughton et al. 1997; U.S. Modafinil in Narcolepsy Multicenter Study Group 1998, 2000). Modafinil is less disruptive of sleep than amphetamines and is rated as having a lower abuse potential (Shelton et al. 1995) (see Table 43–1). A recent study found that taking an extra dose (200 mg) at midday improved wakefulness in patients with narcolepsy without causing insomnia at night (J.R. Schwartz et al. 2004). Importantly, cataplexy—the sudden occurrence of muscle weakness in association with experiencing laughter, anger, or surprise—is responsive to amphetamines but not to modafinil (Shelton et al. 1995).

Fatigue

The use of stimulants for the treatment of fatigue syndromes may seem intuitive, but evidence from large-scale controlled clinical trials to warrant this use is scant. In one of the only double-blind, placebo-controlled studies, men with HIV, depression, and fatigue had significantly less fatigue with dextroamphetamine (73% response) (Wagner and Rabkin 2000). Tolerance, dependence, and abuse were not observed even through a 6-month open phase. A double-blind study of methylphenidate and pemoline in a similar group of 144 patients with HIV who had severe fatigue found both stimulants effective in improving fatigue and quality of life (Breitbart et al. 2001).

Two controlled trials (Adler et al. 2003; Hogl et al. 2002) found modafinil effective in reducing excessive sleepiness in Parkinson's disease. Open-label studies of modafinil for fatigue in multiple sclerosis (Rammohan et al. 2002) and myotonic dystrophy (Damian et al. 2001) are suggestive of modafinil's utility in management of fatigue. A small double-blind crossover study in myotonic dystrophy found reduction in fatigue but no improvement in activity measures (Wintzen et al. 2007). This would be consistent with modafinil's rather selective effect on wakefulness and minimal impact on motor or autonomic parameters. In the same vein, a study of 98 patients with fibromyalgia found that low doses of modafinil (mean 160 mg) substantially reduced fatigue (T.L. Schwartz et al. 2007).

Obstructive Sleep Apnea

There are two placebo-controlled studies of modafinil in the treatment of residual sleepiness in patients with obstructive sleep apnea (OSA) (Kingshott et al. 2001; Pack et al. 2001). The studies show modafinil's efficacy in treating the residual daytime sleepiness experienced by some OSA patients who were compliant in their use of CPAP treatment.

Importantly, modafinil's use was studied in—and should be limited to—the treatment of OSA only after CPAP has been instigated and maximized. OSA carries significant cardiovascular risks if the airway collapse during sleep is not treated appropriately with CPAP and related therapies. It is conceivable that lessened daytime sleepiness from use of modafinil might fool the patient into thinking that CPAP is unnecessary, thus posing a risk via the untreated underlying OSA disorder.

Obesity

That amphetamines are anorectic is well known; however, the extent of the effect may be overstated. Bray and Greenway (1999) summarized the studies of obesity treatments, wherein they cited a large review of more than

200 short-term (3 months) double-blind studies of various noradrenergic agents, including amphetamine and amphetamine derivatives. Patients taking stimulants were twice as likely as those taking placebo to lose 1 lb/week; however, the percentage of patients who lost 3 lb/week was quite small (10%). The mean difference between drug and placebo weight losses was 0.5 lb/week. Bray and Greenway (1999) also noted that long-term (>14 weeks) double-blind studies with amphetamine proper have not been done, but the noradrenergic drugs diethylpropion and phentermine were associated with significantly more weight loss than was placebo. However, few studies were done (five total), and they had small sample sizes (10–36 people in each study), making the results difficult to interpret. A small study found that high doses of amphetamine (30 mg) decreased overall caloric intake but did so primarily through a decrease in fat consumption; carbohydrate consumption actually increased (Foltin et al. 1995). This mild effect on appetite is important when considering the use of stimulants in elderly patients who lack both energy and motivation and have poor appetite.

Depression

No controlled trials have investigated the use of stimulants in depression to date. Most of the evidence for stimulant utility in depression derives from case series. The bulk of the current evidence derives from case series by Feighner et al. (1985) and Fawcett et al. (1991), which suggested the efficacy of stimulants combined with MAOIs and MAOI/TCA combinations, as well as their safety in not causing hypertensive or hyperthermic crises, and case series by Stoll et al. (1996) and Metz and Shader (1991), in which a combination of stimulant and selective serotonin reuptake inhibitor (SSRI) was used. Another case series argued for amphetamine's ability to augment an antidepressant effect in patients with only partial response, although the effects were, not unexpectedly, primarily in improving fatigue and apathy (Masand et al. 1998).

In an open-label trial of depressed cancer patients, both amphetamine and methylphenidate were reported to improve depressive symptoms to the same extent, and effects were seen within 2 days. In this series, stimulants did not cause anorexia; in fact, they improved appetite in more than half of the patients studied (Olin and Masand 1996), suggesting that these agents are not contraindicated solely on the basis of concerns about anorexia.

In a recent review, Orr and Taylor (2007) noted the paucity of high-quality data and suggested a possible role for stimulants in depression, particularly as adjunctive agents, in specific patient subgroups.

The utility of modafinil in depressive states is still not well characterized, the majority of evidence being either anecdotal or retrospective. More work is likely forthcoming, but there are two studies that bear some examination. The mood-altering properties of modafinil were studied in 32 normal volunteers, in a double-blind, crossover, inpatient study (Taneja et al. 2007). Modafinil had positive results on general mood, especially on alertness and energy measures, but also had a negative effect on feeling calm (i.e., increased anxiety). Whether similar divergent effects would be found in depression remains to be seen.

A double-blind, placebo-controlled trial (Dunlop et al. 2007) examining the effects of modafinil initiated at the outset of treatment with an SSRI in depressed patients with fatigue found no difference in the primary outcome measure of the Epworth Sleepiness Scale, but some improvement in the hypersomnia items of the 31-item Hamilton Rating Scale for Depression. However, power to detect differences was limited by premature termination of the study. Two subjects (both on SSRIs) developed suicidal ideation in their respective second weeks of treatment with modafinil; one required hospitalization. While it is not clear what role modafinil played—post hoc analysis of the suicide item in the rating scales showed no difference from the placebo group—continued vigilance in this area is recommended. Two other controlled trials (DeBattista et al. 2003; Fava et al. 2005) and two openlabel trials (DeBattista et al. 2001; Menza et al. 2000) suggest that modafinil may have some utility as an augmentation agent to antidepressants in depressed patients with fatigue or excessive sleepiness. Further study is needed.

Conclusion

The safety and efficacy of stimulants for the treatment of ADHD have been established. Modafinil and armodafinil are also firmly established as efficacious as wakefulness-promoting agents in narcolepsy, sleep apnea, and shift work sleep disorder. The utility of these drugs in other areas is being examined. Although there is intense interest in the potential use of stimulants and modafinil in other psychiatric and neurobehavioral conditions, controlled studies on their safety and efficacy are limited. It is unclear why stimulants have not been extensively investigated for clinical utility over the years, except for the treatment of ADHD. The approval of armodafinil, as the newest of the wakefulness-promoting compounds, may perhaps spur further research. Well-designed large-scale controlled trials are needed to define and characterize the role of stimulants and modafinil in various psychiatric illnesses. It is hoped that this will be an area of continued interest and development, from the elucidation of the molecular mechanisms of stimulants and modafinil to the demonstration through controlled trials of their potential clinical safety and benefits.

References

Adler CH, Caviness JN, Hentz JG, et al: Randomized trial of modafinil for treating subjective daytime sleepiness in patients with Parkinson's disease. Mov Disord 18:287–293, 2003

Angrist BM, Sathananthan G, Wilk S, et al: Amphetamine psychosis: behavioral and biochemical aspects. J Psychiatr Res 11:13–23, 1974

Biederman J, Swanson JM, Wigal SB, et al: Efficacy and safety of modafinil film-coated tablets in children and adolescents with attention-deficit/hyperactivity disorder: results of a randomized, double-blind, placebo-controlled, flexible-dose study. Pediatrics 116:e777–e784, 2005

Biederman J, Swanson JM, Wigal SB, et al: A comparison of once-daily and divided doses of modafinil in children with attention-deficit/hyperactivity disorder: a randomized, double-blind, and placebo-controlled study. Modafinil ADHD Study Group. J Clin Psychiatry 67:727–735, 2006

Biederman J, Boellner SW, Childress A, et al: Lisdexamfetamine dimesylate and mixed amphetamine salts extended-release in children with ADHD: a double-blind, placebo-controlled, crossover analog classroom study. Biol Psychiatry 62:970–976, 2007a

Biederman J, Krishnan S, Zhang Y, et al: Efficacy and tolerability of lisdexamfetamine dimesylate (NRP-104) in children with attention-deficit/hyperactivity disorder: a phase III multicenter, randomized, double-blind, forced-dose, parallel-group study. Clin Ther 29:450–463, 2007b

Boellner SW, Earl CQ, Arora S: Modafinil in children and adolescents with attention-deficit/hyperactivity disorder: a preliminary 8-week, open-label study. Curr Med Res Opin 22:2457–2465, 2006

Bonaventure P, Letavic M, Dugovic C, et al: Histamine H3 receptor antagonists: from target identification to drug leads. Biochem Pharmacol 73:1084–1096, 2007

Bourdon L, Jacobs I, Bateman WA, et al: Effect of modafinil on heat production and regulation of body temperatures in cold-exposed humans. Aviat Space Environ Med 65:999–1004, 1994

Bray GA, Greenway FL: Current and potential drugs for treatment of obesity. Endocrinol Rev 20:805–875, 1999

Breitbart W, Rosenfeld B, Kaim M, et al: A randomized, double-blind, placebo-controlled trial of psychostimulants for the treatment of fatigue in ambulatory patients with human immunodeficiency virus disease. Arch Intern Med 161:411–420, 2001

Broughton RJ, Fleming JA, George CF, et al: Randomized, double-blind, placebo-controlled crossover trial of modafinil in the treatment of excessive daytime sleepiness in narcolepsy. Neurology 49:444–451, 1997

Brun J, Chamba G, Khalfallah Y, et al: Effect of modafinil on plasma melatonin, cortisol and growth hormone rhythms, rectal temperature and performance in healthy subjects during a 36 h sleep deprivation. J Sleep Res 7:105–114, 1998

Callaway CW, Clark RF: Hyperthermia in psychostimulant overdose. Ann Emerg Med 24:68–76, 1994

Cameron OG, Modell JG, Hariharan M: Caffeine and human cerebral blood flow: a positron emission tomography study. Life Sci 47:1141–1146, 1990

Castellanos FX, Giedd JN, Elia J, et al: Controlled stimulant treatment of ADHD and comorbid Tourette's syndrome: effects of stimulant and dose. J Am Acad Child Adolesc Psychiatry 36:589–596, 1997

Centonze D, Picconi B, Baunez C, et al: Cocaine and amphetamine depress striatal GABAergic synaptic transmission through D2 dopamine receptors. Neuropsychopharmacology 26:164–175, 2002

Cephalon Inc.: Provigil (modafinil) tablets: prescribing information. Frazer, PA, Cephalon, Inc., March 2008. Available at: http://www.provigil.com. Accessed December 2008.

Challman TD, Lipsky JJ: Methylphenidate: its pharmacology and uses. Mayo Clin Proc 75:711–721, 2000

Chan YP, Swanson JM, Soldin SS, et al: Methylphenidate hydrochloride given with or before breakfast, II: effects on plasma concentration of methylphenidate and ritalinic acid. Pediatrics 72:56–59, 1983

Choi HJ, Yoo TM, Chung SY, et al: Methamphetamine-induced apoptosis in a CNS-derived catecholaminergic cell line. Mol Cells 13:221–227, 2002

Clarke AR, Barry RJ, McCarthy R, et al: EEG differences between good and poor responders to methylphenidate and dexamphetamine in children with attention-deficit/hyperactivity disorder. Clin Neurophysiol 113:194–205, 2002a

Clarke AR, Barry RJ, McCarthy R, et al: EEG differences between good and poor responders to methylphenidate in boys with the inattentive type of attention-deficit/hyperactivity disorder. Clin Neurophysiol 113:1191–1198, 2002b

Crisostomo EA, Duncan PW, Propst M, et al: Evidence that amphetamine with physical therapy promotes recovery of motor function in stroke patients. Ann Neurol 23:94–97, 1988

Dackis CA, Lynch KG, Yu E, et al: Modafinil and cocaine: a double-blind, placebo-controlled drug interaction study. Drug Alcohol Depend 70:29–37, 2003

Dackis CA, Kampman KM, Lynch KG, et al: A double-blind, placebo-controlled trial of modafinil for cocaine dependence. Neuropsychopharmacology 30:205–211, 2005

Damian MS, Gerlach A, Schmidt F, et al: Modafinil for excessive daytime sleepiness in myotonic dystrophy. Neurology 56:794–796, 2001

DeBattista C, Solvason HB, Kendrick E, et al: Modafinil as an adjunctive agent in the treatment of fatigue and hypersomnia associated with major depression, in New Research Program and Abstracts of the 154th Annual Meeting of the American Psychiatric Association, May 9, 2001, New Orleans, LA, USA Abstract NR532, 144, 2001

DeBattista C, Doghramji K, Menza MA, et al: Adjunct modafinil for the short-term treatment of fatigue and sleepiness in patients with major depressive disorder: a preliminary double-blind, placebo-controlled study. J Clin Psychiatry 64:1057–1064, 2003

DeVane CL, Markowitz JS, Carson SW, et al: Single-dose pharmacokinetics of methylphenidate in CYP2D6 extensive and poor metabolizers. J Clin Psychopharmacol 20:347–349, 2000

Dinges DF, Arora S, Darwish M, et al: Pharmacodynamic effects on alertness of single doses of armodafinil in healthy subjects during a nocturnal period of acute sleep loss. Curr Med Res Opin 22:159–167, 2006

Dunlop BW, Crits-Christoph P, Evans DL, et al: Coadministration of modafinil and a selective serotonin reuptake inhibitor from the initiation of treatment of major depressive disorder with fatigue and sleepiness: a double-blind, placebo-controlled study. J Clin Psychopharmacol 27:614–619, 2007

Dunnick JK, Hailey JR: Experimental studies on the long-term effects of methylphenidate hydrochloride. Toxicology 103:77–84, 1995

Duteil J, Rambert FA, Pessonnier J, et al: Central alpha 1-adrenergic stimulation in relation to the behaviour stimulating effect of modafinil: studies with experimental animals. Eur J Pharmacol 180:49–58, 1990

Efron D, Jarman F, Barker M: Methylphenidate versus dexamphetamine in children with attention deficit hyperactivity disorder: a double-blind, crossover trial. Pediatrics 100:E6, 1997

Fava M, Thase ME, DeBattista C: A multicenter, placebo-controlled study of modafinil augmentation in partial responders to selective serotonin reuptake inhibitors with persistent fatigue and sleepiness. J Clin Psychiatry 66:85–93, 2005

Fawcett J, Kravitz HM, Zajecka JM, et al: CNS stimulant potentiation of monoamine oxidase inhibitors in treatment-refractory depression. J Clin Psychopharmacol 11:127–132, 1991

Feighner JP, Herbstein J, Damlouji N: Combined MAOI, TCA, and direct stimulant therapy of treatment-resistant depression. J Clin Psychiatry 46:206–209, 1985

Ferraro L, Tanganelli S, O'Connor WT, et al: The vigilance promoting drug modafinil decreases GABA release in the medial preoptic area and in the posterior hypothalamus of the awake rat: possible involvement of the serotonergic 5-HT3 receptor. Neurosci Lett 220:5–8, 1996

Ferraro L, Antonelli T, O'Connor WT, et al: The antinarcoleptic drug modafinil increases glutamate release in thalamic areas and hippocampus. Neuroreport 8:2883–2887, 1997

Ferraro L, Antonelli T, Tanganelli S, et al: The vigilance promoting drug modafinil increases extracellular glutamate levels in the medial preoptic area and the posterior hypothalamus of the conscious rat: prevention by local GABAA receptor blockade. Neuropsychopharmacology 20:346–356, 1999

Ferris RM, Tang FL: Comparison of the effects of the isomers of amphetamine, methylphenidate and deoxypipradol on the uptake of l-[3H]norepinephrine and [3H]dopamine by synaptic vesicles from rat whole brain, striatum and hypothalamus. J Pharmacol Exp Ther 210:422–428, 1979

Foltin RW, Kelly TH, Fischman MW: Effect of amphetamine on human macronutrient intake. Physiol Behav 58:899–907, 1995

Gallopin T, Luppi PH, Rambert FA, et al: Effect of the wake-promoting agent modafinil on sleep-promoting neurons from the ventrolateral preoptic nucleus: an in vitro pharmacologic study. Sleep 27:19–25, 2004

George S, Braithwaite RA: Using amphetamine isomer ratios to determine the compliance of amphetamine abusers prescribed Dexedrine. J Anal Toxicol 24:223–227, 2000

GlaxoSmithKline: Dexedrine (dextroamphetamine) SPANSULE sustained-release capsules and tablets: prescribing information. Research Triangle Park, NC, GlaxoSmithKline, June 2006. Available at: http://www.fda.gov/medWatch/SAFETY/2006/Dexedrine_PI.pdf. Accessed December 2008.

Grabowski J, Roache JD, Schmitz JM, et al: Replacement medication for cocaine dependence: methylphenidate. J Clin Psychopharmacol 17:485–488, 1997

Grabowski J, Rhoades H, Silverman P, et al: Risperidone for the treatment of cocaine dependence: randomized, double-blind trial. J Clin Psychopharmacol 20:305–310, 2000

Grabowski J, Rhoades H, Schmitz J, et al: Dextroamphetamine for cocaine-dependence treatment: a double-blind randomized clinical trial. J Clin Psychopharmacol 21:522–526, 2001

Greenhill LL, Pliszka S, Dulcan MK, et al; American Academy of Child and Adolescent Psychiatry: Practice parameter for the use of stimulant medications in the treatment of children, adolescents, and adults. J Am Acad Child Adolesc Psychiatry 41 (2 suppl):26S–49S, 2002

Guilarte TR: Is methamphetamine abuse a risk factor in parkinsonism? Neurotoxicology 22:725–731, 2001

Hanson GR, Jensen M, Johnson M, et al: Distinct features of seizures induced by cocaine and amphetamine analogs. Eur J Pharmacol 377:167–173, 1999

Harsh JR, Hayduk R, Rosenberg R, et al: The efficacy and safety of armodafinil as treatment for adults with excessive sleepiness associated with narcolepsy. Curr Med Res Opin 22:761–774, 2006

Hart CL, Haney M, Vosburg SK, et al: Smoked cocaine self-administration is decreased by modafinil. Neuropsychopharmacology 33:761–768, 2008

Hirshkowitz M, Black JE, Wesnes K, et al: Adjunct armodafinil improves wakefulness and memory in obstructive sleep apnea/hypopnea syndrome. Respir Med 101:616–627, 2006

Hogl B, Saletu M, Brandauer E, et al: Modafinil for the treatment of daytime sleepiness in Parkinson's disease: a double-blind, randomized, crossover, placebo-controlled polygraphic trial. Sleep 25:905–909, 2002

Holtkamp K, Peters-Wallraf B, Wüller S, et al: Methylphenidate-related growth impairment. J Child Adolesc Psychopharmacol 12:55–61, 2002

Hunt GE, Atrens DM: Reward summation and the effects of pimozide, clonidine, and amphetamine on fixed-interval responding for brain stimulation. Pharmacol Biochem Behav 42:563–577, 1992

Ishizuka T, Sakamoto Y, Sakurai T, et al: Modafinil increases histamine release in the anterior hypothalamus of rats, Neurosci Lett 339:143–146, 2003

James RS, Sharp WS, Bastain TM, et al: Double-blind, placebo-controlled study of single-dose amphetamine formulations in ADHD. J Am Acad Child Adolesc Psychiatry 40:1268–1276, 2001

Janssen PA, Leysen JE, Megens AA, et al: Does phenylethylamine act as an endogenous amphetamine in some patients? Int J Neuropsychopharmacol 2:229–240, 1999

Johnson EA, Shvedova AA, Kisin E, et al: d-MDMA during vitamin E deficiency: effects on dopaminergic neurotoxicity and hepatotoxicity. Brain Res 933:150–163, 2002

Jones SR, Gainetdinov RR, Wightman RM, et al: Mechanisms of amphetamine action revealed in mice lacking the dopamine transporter. J Neurosci 18:1979–1986, 1998

Jones SR, Joseph JD, Barak LS, et al: Dopamine neuronal transport kinetics and effects of amphetamine. J Neurochem 73:2406–2414, 1999

Kanbayashi T, Honda K, Kodama T, et al: Implication of dopaminergic mechanisms in the wake-promoting effects of amphetamine: a study of D- and L-derivatives in canine narcolepsy. Neuroscience 99:651–659, 2000

Karch SB, Stephens BG, Ho CH: Methamphetamine-related deaths in San Francisco: demographic, pathologic, and toxicologic profiles. J Forens Sci 44:359–368, 1999

Kingshott RN, Vennelle M, Coleman EL, et al: Randomized, double-blind, placebo-controlled crossover trial of modafinil in the treatment of residual excessive daytime sleepiness in the sleep apnea/hypopnea syndrome. Am J Respir Crit Care Med 163:918–923, 2001

Klein-Schwartz W: Abuse and toxicity of methylphenidate. Curr Opin Pediatr 14:219–223, 2002

Knecht S, Imai T, Kamping S, et al: D-amphetamine does not improve outcome of somatosensory training. Neurology 57:2248–2252, 2001

Kramer JR, Loney J, Ponto LB, et al: Predictors of adult height and weight in boys treated with methylphenidate for childhood behavior problems. J Am Acad Child Adolesc Psychiatry 39:517–524, 2000

Kraner JC, McCoy DJ, Evans MA, et al: Fatalities caused by the MDMA-related drug paramethoxyamphetamine (PMA). J Anal Toxicol 25:645–648, 2001

Kuo DY, Hsu CT, Cheng JT: Role of hypothalamic neuropeptide Y (NPY) in the change of feeding behavior induced by repeated treatment of amphetamine. Life Sci 70:243–251, 2001

Lahat E, Weiss M, Ben-Shlomo A, et al: Bone mineral density and turnover in children with attention-deficit hyperactivity disorder receiving methylphenidate. J Child Neurol 15:436–439, 2000

Law SF, Schachar RJ: Do typical clinical doses of methylphenidate cause tics in children treated for attention-deficit hyperactivity disorder? J Am Acad Child Adolesc Psychiatry 38:944–951, 1999

Lazarus LW, Moberg PJ, Langsley PR, et al: Methylphenidate and nortriptyline in the treatment of poststroke depression: a retrospective comparison. Arch Phys Med Rehabil 75:403–406, 1994

Levin FR, Evans SM, McDowell DM, et al: Methylphenidate treatment for cocaine abusers with adult attention-deficit/hyperactivity disorder: a pilot study. J Clin Psychiatry 59:300–305, 1998

Loo SK, Teale PD, Reite ML: EEG correlates of methylphenidate response among children with ADHD: a preliminary report. Biol Psychiatry 45:1657–1660, 1999

Lou HC, Henriksen L, Bruhn P: Focal cerebral hypoperfusion in children with dysphasia and/or attention deficit disorder. Arch Neurol 41:825–829, 1984

Markowitz JS, Patrick KS: Pharmacokinetic and pharmacodynamic drug interactions in the treatment of attention-deficit hyperactivity disorder. Clin Pharmacokinet 40:753–772, 2001

Masand PS, Anand VS, Tanquary JF: Psychostimulant augmentation of second generation antidepressants: a case series. Depress Anxiety 7:89–91, 1998

Mattay VS, Berman KF, Ostrem JL, et al: Dextroamphetamine enhances "neural network-specific" physiological signals: a positron-emission tomography rCBF study. J Neurosci 16:4816–4822, 1996

McLellan TM, Ducharme MB, Canini F, et al: Effects of modafinil on core body temperature during sustained wakefulness and exercise in a warm environment. Aviat Space Environ Med 73:1079–1088, 2002

Menza MA, Kaufman KR, Castellanos A: Modafinil augmentation of antidepressant treatment in depression. J Clin Psychiatry 61:378–381, 2000

Metz A, Shader RI: Combination of fluoxetine with pemoline in the treatment of major depressive disorder. Int Clin Psychopharmacol 6:93–96, 1991

Meyer A, Mayerhofer A, Kovar K, et al: Rewarding effects of the optical isomers of 3,4-methylenedioxy-methylamphetamine ("Ecstasy") and 3,4-methylenedioxy-ethylamphetamine ("Eve") measured by conditioned place preference in rats. Neurosci Lett 330:280–284, 2002

Mignot E, Nishino S: Emerging therapies in narcolepsy-cataplexy. Sleep 28:754–763, 2005

Najib J: The efficacy and safety profile of lisdexamfetamine dimesylate, a prodrug of d-amphetamine, for the treatment of attention-deficit/hyperactivity disorder in children and adults. Clin Ther 31:142–176, 2009

Nishino S, Mignot E: Pharmacological aspects of human and canine narcolepsy. Prog Neurobiol 52:27–78, 1997

Novartis: Ritalin LA (methylphenidate hydrochloride) extended-release capsules: prescribing information. East Hanover, NJ, Novartis, April 2007. Available at: http://www.pharma.us.novartis.com/product/pi/pdf/ritalin_la.pdf. Accessed December 2008.

Olin J, Masand P: Psychostimulants for depression in hospitalized cancer patients. Psychosomatics 37:57–62, 1996

Orr K, Taylor D: Psychostimulants in the treatment of depression: a review of the evidence. CNS Drugs 21:239–257, 2007

Pack AI, Black JE, Schwartz JR, et al: Modafinil as adjunct therapy for daytime sleepiness in obstructive sleep apnea. Am J Respir Crit Care Med 164:1675–1681, 2001

Prior FH, Isbister GK, Dawson AH, et al: Serotonin toxicity with therapeutic doses of dexamphetamine and venlafaxine. Med J Aust 176:240–241, 2002

Ramamoorthy Y, Yu AM, Suh N, et al: Reduced (+/–)-3,4-methylenedioxymethamphetamine ("Ecstasy") metabolism with cytochrome P450 2D6 inhibitors and pharmacogenetic variants in vitro. Biochem Pharmacol 63:2111–2119, 2002

Rammohan KW, Rosenberg JH, Lynn DJ, et al: Efficacy and safety of modafinil (Provigil) for the treatment of fatigue in multiple sclerosis: a two centre phase 2 study. J Neurol Neurosurg Psychiatry 72:179–183, 2002

Ricaurte GA, Yuan J, Hatzidimitriou G, et al: Severe dopaminergic neurotoxicity in primates after a common recreational dose regimen of MDMA ("ecstasy"). Science 297:2260–2263, 2002

Richards JR, Johnson EB, Stark RW, et al: Methamphetamine abuse and rhabdomyolysis in the ED: a 5-year study. Am J Emerg Med 17:681–685, 1999

Robertson P, DeCory HH, Madan A, et al: In vitro inhibition and induction of human hepatic cytochrome P450 enzymes by modafinil. Drug Metab Dispos 28:664–671, 2000

Robertson P Jr, Hellriegel ET, Arora S, et al: Effect of modafinil on the pharmacokinetics of ethinyl estradiol and triazolam in healthy volunteers. Clin Pharmacol Ther 71:46–56, 2002

Robinson JB: Stereoselectivity and isoenzyme selectivity of monoamine oxidase inhibitors. Enantiomers of amphetamine, N-methylamphetamine and deprenyl. Biochem Pharmacol 34:4105–4108, 1985

Roth T, Czeisler CA, Walsh JK, et al: Randomized, double-blind, placebo-controlled study of armodafinil for the treatment of excessive sleepiness associated with chronic shift work sleep disorder [abstract no. 161]. Neuropsychopharmacology 30:S140, 2005

Roth T, White D, Schmidt-Nowara W, et al: Effects of armodafinil in the treatment of residual excessive sleepiness associated with obstructive sleep apnea/hypopnea syndrome: a 12-week, multicenter, double-blind, randomized, placebo-controlled study in nCPAP-adherent adults. Clin Ther 28:689–706, 2006

Rugino TA, Samsock TC: Modafinil in children with attention-deficit hyperactivity disorder. Pediatr Neurol 29:136–142, 2003

Ruskin DN, Bergstrom DA, Shenker A, et al: Drugs used in the treatment of attention-deficit/hyperactivity disorder affect postsynaptic firing rate and oscillation without preferential dopamine autoreceptor action. Biol Psychiatry 49:340–350, 2001

Saletu B, Saletu M, Grunberger J, et al: On the treatment of the alcoholic organic brain syndrome with an alpha-adrenergic agonist modafinil: double-blind, placebo-controlled clinical, psychometric and neurophysiological studies. Prog Neuropsychopharmacol Biol Psychiatry 14:195–214, 1990

Saletu B, Saletu M, Grunberger J, et al: Treatment of the alcoholic organic brain syndrome: double-blind, placebo-controlled clinical, psychometric and electroencephalographic mapping studies with modafinil. Neuropsychobiology 27:26–39, 1993

Saper CB, Scammell TE: Modafinil: a drug in search of a mechanism. Sleep 27:11–12, 2004

Scammell TE, Estabrooke IV, McCarthy MT, et al: Hypothalamic arousal regions are activated during modafinil-induced wakefulness. J Neurosci 20:8620–8628, 2000

Schwartz JR, Nelson MT, Schwartz ER, et al: Effects of modafinil on wakefulness and executive function in patients with narcolepsy experiencing late-day sleepiness. Clin Neuropharmacol 27:74–79, 2004

Schwartz TL, Rayancha S, Rashid A, et al: Modafinil treatment for fatigue associated with fibromyalgia. J Clin Rheumatol 13:52, 2007

Shelton J, Nishino S, Vaught J, et al: Comparative effects of modafinil and amphetamine on daytime sleepiness and cataplexy of narcoleptic dogs. Sleep 18:817–826, 1995

Simon P, Hemet C, Ramassamy C, et al: Non-amphetaminic mechanism of stimulant locomotor effect of modafinil in mice. Eur Neuropsychopharmacol 5:509–514, 1995

Sonde L, Nordstrom M, Nilsson CG, et al: A double-blind placebo-controlled study of the effects of amphetamine and physiotherapy after stroke. Cerebrovasc Dis 12:253–257, 2001

Spitzer M, Franke B, Walter H, et al: Enantio-selective cognitive and brain activation effects of N-ethyl-3,4-methylenedioxyamphetamine in humans. Neuropharmacology 41:263–271, 2001

Sprague JE, Everman SL, Nichols DE: An integrated hypothesis for the serotonergic axonal loss induced by 3,4-methylenedioxymethamphetamine. Neurotoxicology 19:427–441, 1998

Srinivas NR, Hubbard JW, Korchinski ED, et al: Stereoselective urinary pharmacokinetics of dl-threo-methylphenidate and its major metabolite in humans. J Pharm Sci 81:747–749, 1992

Srinivas NR, Hubbard JW, Korchinski ED, et al: Enantioselective pharmacokinetics of dl-threo-methylphenidate in humans. Pharm Res 10:14–21, 1993

Stoll AL, Pillay SS, Diamond L, et al: Methylphenidate augmentation of serotonin selective reuptake inhibitors: a case series. J Clin Psychiatry 57:72–76, 1996

Swanson JM, Wigal S, Greenhill LL, et al: Analog classroom assessment of Adderall in children with ADHD. J Am Acad Child Adolesc Psychiatry 37:519–526, 1998

Taneja I, Haman K, Shelton RC, et al: A randomized, double-blind, crossover trial of modafinil on mood. J Clin Psychopharmacol 27:76–79, 2007

Taylor FB, Russo J: Efficacy of modafinil compared to dextroamphetamine for the treatment of attention deficit hyperactivity disorder in adults. J Child Adolesc Psychopharmacol 10:311–320, 2000

Tourette's Syndrome Study Group: Treatment of ADHD in children with tics: a randomized controlled trial. Neurology 58:527–536, 2002

Toren P, Silbergeld A, Eldar S, et al: Lack of effect of methylphenidate on serum growth hormone (GH), GH-binding protein, and insulin-like growth factor I. Clin Neuropharmacol 20:264–269, 1997

Turner DC, Clark L, Dowson J, et al: Modafinil improves cognition and response inhibition in adult attention-deficit/hyperactivity disorder. Biol Psychiatry 55:1031–1040, 2004

Uftring SJ, Wachtel SR, Chu D, ct al: An fMRI study of the effect of amphetamine on brain activity. Neuropsychopharmacology 25:925–935, 2001

U.S. Food and Drug Administration: Provigil (Modafinil): Follow-up to Hypersensitivity Reactions in the Pediatric Population. Pediatric Advisory Committee. November 28, 2007. Available at: http://www.fda.gov/ohrms/dockets/AC/07/slides/2007-4325s2_12_Modafinil,%20Villalba,%20MD%20(FDA).pdf. Accessed December 2008.

U.S. Modafinil in Narcolepsy Multicenter Study Group: Randomized trial of modafinil for the treatment of pathological somnolence in narcolepsy. Ann Neurol 43:88–97, 1998

U.S. Modafinil in Narcolepsy Multicenter Study Group: Randomized trial of modafinil as a treatment for the excessive daytime somnolence of narcolepsy. Neurology 54:1166–1175, 2000

Virmani A, Gaetani F, Imam S, et al: The protective role of L-carnitine against neurotoxicity evoked by drug of abuse, methamphetamine, could be related to mitochondrial dysfunction. Ann N Y Acad Sci 965:225–232, 2002

Volkow ND, Ding YS, Fowler JS, et al: Is methylphenidate like cocaine? Studies on their pharmacokinetics and distribution in the human brain. Arch Gen Psychiatry 52:456–463, 1995

Volkow ND, Fowler JS, Wang GJ: Imaging studies on the role of dopamine in cocaine reinforcement and addiction in humans. J Psychopharmacol 13:337–345, 1999

Volkow ND, Wang G, Fowler JS, et al: Therapeutic doses of oral methylphenidate significantly increase extracellular dopamine in the human brain. J Neurosci 21:RC121, 2001

Wagner GJ, Rabkin R: Effects of dextroamphetamine on depression and fatigue in men with HIV: a double-blind, placebo-controlled trial. J Clin Psychiatry 61:436–440, 2000

Walker-Batson D, Smith P, Curtis S, et al: Amphetamine paired with physical therapy accelerates motor recovery after stroke: further evidence. Stroke 26:2254–2259, 1995

Walker-Batson D, Curtis S, Natarajan R, et al: A double-blind, placebo-controlled study of the use of amphetamine in the treatment of aphasia. Stroke 32:2093–2098, 2001

Whyte J, Vaccaro M, Grieb-Neff P, et al: Psychostimulant use in the rehabilitation of individuals with traumatic brain injury. J Head Trauma Rehabil 17:284–299, 2002

Wigal SB, Biederman J, Swanson JM, et al: Efficacy and safety of modafinil film-coated tablets in children and adolescents with or without prior stimulant treatment for attention-deficit/hyperactivity disorder: pooled analysis of 3 randomized, double-blind, placebo-controlled studies. Prim Care Companion J Clin Psychiatry 8:352–360, 2006

Wilens TE, Spencer TJ, Biederman J: A review of the pharmacotherapy of adults with attention-deficit/hyperactivity disorder. J Atten Disord 5:189–202, 2002

Wintzen AR, Lammers GJ, van Dijk JG: Does modafinil enhance activity of patients with myotonic dystrophy? A double-blind placebo-controlled crossover study. J Neurol 254:26–28, 2007

Wisor JP, Nishino S, Sora I, et al: Dopaminergic role in stimulant-induced wakefulness. J Neurosci 21:1787–1794, 2001

Wisor JP, Dement WC, Aimone L, et al: Armodafinil, the R-enantiomer of modafinil: wake-promoting effects and pharmacokinetic profile in the rat. Pharmacol Biochem Beh 85:492–499, 2006

Wong YN, King SP, Simcoe D, et al: Open-label, single-dose pharmacokinetic study of modafinil tablets: influence of age and gender in normal subjects. J Clin Pharmacol 39:281–288, 1999a

Wong YN, Simcoe D, Hartman LN, et al: A double-blind, placebo-controlled, ascending-dose evaluation of the pharmacokinetics and tolerability of modafinil tablets in healthy male volunteers. J Clin Pharmacol 39:30–40, 1999b

Xu F, Gainetdinov RR, Wetsel WC, et al: Mice lacking the norepinephrine transporter are supersensitive to psychostimulants. Nat Neurosci 3:465–471, 2000

Yu YL, Fisher H, Sekowski A, et al: Amphetamine and fenfluramine suppress ethanol intake in ethanol-dependent rats. Alcohol 14:45–48, 1997

Zagnoni PG, Albano C: Psychostimulants and epilepsy. Epilepsia 43 (suppl 2):28–31, 2002

Electroconvulsive Therapy

William M. McDonald, M.D.

Thomas W. Meeks, M.D.

W. Vaughn McCall, M.D., M.S.

Charles F. Zorumski, M.D.

Over the past 70 years, electroconvulsive therapy (ECT) has been proven to be one of the most effective somatic treatments for mood disorders (Abrams 1992). Although the serendipitous discovery of psychotropic medications such as chlorpromazine and iproniazid in the 1950s revolutionized psychiatric treatment, clinicians and researchers soon recognized the limitations of psychotropic medications and ECT remained an important therapeutic alternative. The continued use of ECT has provided support for ECT-related research, including exploration of clinical indications, techniques to maximize efficacy and minimize toxicity (especially cognitive and cardiac side effects), and therapeutic mechanisms of action. In this chapter, we review the history of ECT, the preclinical and clinical data on the mechanism of action of ECT, and the relevant literature related to efficacy. We also provide practical guidelines for the administration of ECT, including the efficacy of ECT in treating various psychiatric disorders as well as appropriate patient selection, stimulus settings and electrode placement, pretreatment medical evaluation, and management of the patient during acute, continuation, and maintenance courses of ECT. Finally, we outline an overview of some recent developments to treat depression with nonconvulsive stimuli such as transcranial magnetic stimulation (TMS).

History of ECT

The development of ECT occurred at a time when few somatic treatments were available for psychiatric disorders and physicians were desperately attempting to find treatments for severely ill psychotic patients. The first attempts at inducing therapeutic seizures in such patients were performed chemically. In 1935, Manfred Sakel (1900–1957) induced hypoglycemic episodes in psychiatric patients (using insulin shock therapy) while in the same year Lazlo Meduna (1896–1964) injected patients with pentylenetetrazol to induce convulsions in order to treat psychosis. Three years later, the Italian psychiatrists Ugo Cerletti (1877–1963) and Lucio Bini (1908–1964) used electroshock treatments to induce seizures. This treatment proved safer and easier to administer than chemically induced seizures and replaced other methods of inducing seizures.

Modern psychopharmacology developed with the discovery of lithium (1949) and iproniazid (1957) for the treatment of mood disorders and the synthesis of the first antipsychotic, chlorpromazine (1952); the first tricyclic antidepressant, imipramine (1959); and the first benzodiazepine, chlordiazepoxide (1960). The development of psychotropic medications was associated with a decline in the use of ECT from the 1960s to the 1980s. However, in the 1980s, the use of ECT began to increase, and more than 36,000 patients received ECT in 1986, the last year a national survey on its use was conducted (Thompson et al. 1994). Recent studies in Canada and Denmark have demonstrated relatively stable rates of ECT utilization over the last 15–30 years (Munk-Olsen et al. 2006; Rapoport et al. 2006). Since the 1980s, the safety of ECT has improved significantly with the introduction of sophisticated cardiopulmonary and electroencephalographic monitoring, better anesthetic agents, and the adoption of the brief-pulse stimulus machine. Today, ECT is arguably the fastest, most effective treatment for mood disorders. ECT is possibly the safest procedure performed under general anesthesia, with a mortality rate reported at 0.002% (Abrams 1997).

Yet, despite these advances, the availability and use of ECT varies dramatically in different parts of the United States. A 1988 study of ECT usage rates in 317 metropolitan areas reported a wide variation (from 0.4 to 81.2 patients per 10,000 population), and 36% of the sampled areas did not have ECT available as a treatment (Hermann et al. 1995). The strongest predictors of ECT use were the number of psychiatrists, number of primary care physicians, and number of private hospital beds per capita. The stringency of state regulations restricting ECT was negatively associated with its use.

Studies in other countries, including Great Britain, Spain, and Ireland, have shown a similar pattern of variation in rates of ECT use (Bertolín-Guillén et al. 2006; Latey and Fahy 1985; Pippard and Ellam 1981). Although it is unclear whether such differences represent overuse of ECT in some areas or underuse of ECT in other areas, great variability in the use of other medical and surgical procedures has been hypothesized to result from a lack of consensus in the medical community regarding the appropriate use and efficacy of a particular medical procedure (Wennberg et al. 1982). ECT is clearly one of the most controversial procedures in medicine, with widely varying beliefs about the safety and efficacy of the procedure among the lay public and medical students (Walter et al. 2002), as well as psychiatrists and other mental health professionals (Janicak et al. 1985). In the Irish study, one of the most important variables in the availability of ECT was whether the psychiatrist had a favorable attitude toward ECT (Latey and Fahy 1985). The availability of ECT was more closely related to the physician's perceptions of the procedure than to the data indicating the potential benefits of the somatic treatment. Unfortunately, this often leads to a significant lack of access to ECT. Ongoing education of physicians and the public may improve the availability of ECT to all who might benefit from it.

In the United States, middle and upper socioeconomic groups receive ECT more frequently than do lower socioeconomic groups (Babigian and Guttmacher 1984; Kramer 1985), possibly because ECT is used more often in private hospitals than in public hospitals (Thompson and Blaine 1987). Private hospitals have fewer regulations governing ECT use, better financial reimbursement, and a higher percentage of patients with mood disorders that respond to ECT (Hermann et al. 1995). As with many medical treatments, financial incentives have shifted ECT toward the outpatient setting, although this is also because of improved safety and increased use of continuation and maintenance courses of ECT.

Older adults receive ECT more often than do younger patients (Kramer 1985; Thompson et al. 1994), although a 1992 National Institutes of Health (NIH) consensus panel found that ECT was underused as a treatment for late-life depression ("NIH Consensus Conference" 1992). A survey of older adults with Medicare insurance showed that the overall rate of ECT use increased nearly 30% from 1987 to 1992, particularly among women, white people, and disabled persons (Rosenbach et al. 1997). There are several reasons that women may be overrepresented in ECT populations including the greater prevalence of depression in women and the fact that women live longer than men. Racial differences among patients receiving ECT may be related to the above-mentioned socioeconomic factors or to differing cultural beliefs about ECT or psychiatric illnesses. White people are more likely to receive ECT than black people (Breakey and Dunn 2004), and the paucity of information on ECT use in the growing Hispanic American population has been highlighted (Euba and Saiz 2006; Major 2005).

Mechanism of Action of ECT

Despite extensive clinical use of ECT for more than 60 years and unequivocal documented efficacy, its mechanism of action remains poorly understood. Theories have ranged from psychological and psychodynamic concepts to theories involving neurotransmitter changes, neuroendocrine effects, alterations in intracellular signaling pathways, and changes in gene expression (Sackeim 1994). Some theories are easy to discard. For example, there is no convincing evidence that ECT causes structural brain damage or that the memory-impairing effects of ECT are associated with clinical improvement (Devanand et al. 1994; R.D. Weiner 1984).

Most serious efforts to understand the mechanisms of ECT have focused on changes in neurotransmitter systems and intracellular biochemical processes (for reviews, see Fochtmann 1994; Newman et al. 1998; Nutt and Glue 1993). Researchers have identified changes possibly leading to therapeutic benefits at cellular and neural system levels using neurochemical information about ECT from studies of electroconvulsive shock (ECS) in rodents. Repeated seizures, whether electrically induced or spontaneous, clearly result in short- and long-term changes in brain function. The assumption is that the effects of repeated generalized seizures in animals reflect the effects of ECT in patients with psychiatric disorders (Lerer et al. 1984).

An alternative strategy is to examine the effects of ECT on central nervous system (CNS) processes for which there is better mechanistic understanding. The assumption is that the effects of ECT on CNS processes are related to the known antidepressive effects of other treatments including psychotherapy, pharmacotherapy, and newer brain stimulation techniques such as deep brain stimulation and TMS. Advances in understanding the neurocircuitry and cellular changes associated with major psychiatric disorders offer hope in defining the effects of ECT and are likely to be important. Although all of these strategies have weaknesses, the anticonvulsant hypothesis described below explains both the effects of ECT on an intracellular level and the efficacy of ECT in relation to the anticonvulsant medications used to treat mood disorders.

Anticonvulsant Hypothesis

One of the most popular theories defining the mechanism of action of ECT is that the antidepressive efficacy is directly correlated with the anticonvulsant effect of ECT. That is, the therapeutic effect of ECT is proportional to an increase in the seizure threshold during ECT; successive ECT treatments cause both an increase in seizure threshold and a decrease in seizure duration (Sackeim 1999). This theory focuses on changes in neurotransmitter systems and intracellular biochemical processes and is supported by preclinical data of the effect of ECT in modulating the seizure threshold.

γ-Aminobutyric acid (GABA) is the predominant inhibitory transmitter in the brain and is a target for multiple anticonvulsant drugs (e.g., barbiturates, benzodiazepines). Data from animal studies demonstrate increases in the threshold for bicuculline- and pentylenetetrazole-induced seizures following a series of ECS treatments (Nutt et al. 1981; Plaznik et al. 1989). Because bicuculline and pentylenetetrazole act by inhibiting GABA type A ($GABA_A$) receptors, these findings suggest that ECT results in changes in GABAergic inhibition. In addition,

GABA levels increase in certain CNS regions after ECS (Green et al. 1982), and there is evidence from magnetic resonance spectroscopy that ECT increases GABA levels in the occipital cortex in humans (Sanacora et al. 2003). These changes in GABA levels suggest that an increase in tonic inhibition may occur after repeated seizures, and effects on GABA-mediated tonic inhibition are increasingly recognized as an important aspect of several neuroactive drugs (Farrant and Nusser 2005). Changes in the $GABA_A$ receptor–chloride channels that are the primary postsynaptic GABA receptors are less certain (Fochtmann 1994), although it is clear that different receptor subtypes contribute to tonic and phasic (synaptic) inhibition. There is also evidence that ECS enhances the function of $GABA_B$ receptors that mediate presynaptic and postsynaptic inhibition (Lloyd et al. 1985), and this is likely to contribute to an overall depression of CNS excitation.

An interesting finding in rodents is that repeated seizures cause the release of an anticonvulsant substance into cerebrospinal fluid. Anticonvulsant activity can be transferred to treatment-naive animals by intracerebroventricular injections of cerebrospinal fluid from animals that have experienced seizures (Tortella and Long 1985, 1988). Tortella et al. (1989) summarized evidence that the anticonvulsant substance is likely to be an endogenous opioid and that treatment with naloxone, an opiate receptor antagonist, blocked the anticonvulsant effects of ECS. There is also evidence that upregulation of delta (δ) opioid receptor binding sites (e.g., sites for D-alanine-D-leucine enkephalin) occurs after repeated seizures (Hitzemann et al. 1987). Whether similar changes occur in humans is speculative, and, to date, efforts to lengthen ECT-induced seizures using naloxone have not been successful (Prudic et al. 1999; Rasmussen and Pandurangi 1999).

Efforts to identify anticonvulsant mechanisms in ECT must account for changes in both seizure threshold and duration because different mechanisms may govern the two processes. Of note is the finding that adenosine is released extracellularly during seizures and may play a role in seizure termination. Adenosine is an important inhibitory neuromodulator that acts on several receptor types. Adenosine A_1 receptors are upregulated in the cortex after ECS, but not in the hippocampus or striatum (Gleiter et al. 1989). Clinically, adenosine receptor antagonists such as caffeine and theophylline prolong ECT-induced seizures (Hinkle et al. 1987), with less effect on seizure threshold (McCall et al. 1993a). Furthermore, theophylline use has been associated with prolonged seizures and status epilepticus during ECT (Rasmussen and Zorumski

1993). These observations suggest that release of adenosine, and perhaps increased sensitivity of certain adenosine receptors, may contribute to decreases in seizure duration during ECT, although caffeine and theophylline have other effects that could influence excitability including phosphodiesterase inhibition and release of calcium from intracellular stores (Sawynok and Yaksh 1993).

Much of the focus in studying anticonvulsant mechanisms of ECT has centered on changes in neural inhibition after repeated seizures. It is also important to consider how ECT influences excitation, particularly the glutamate system, which serves as the predominant mode of fast excitatory transmission in the CNS. Seizures are accompanied by acute release of glutamate, but we have little information about the effects of repeated seizures on glutamate release, uptake, and receptors. Although the brain damage that accompanies status epilepticus appears to result, in part, from excessive activation of N-methyl-D-aspartate (NMDA)–type glutamate receptors (Clifford et al. 1989), seizure-related brain damage typically requires more than 20 minutes of continuous activity and is therefore unlikely to be relevant to ECT (Devanand et al. 1994; Gruenthal et al. 1986). Furthermore, there is evidence that repeated use of ECS actually prevents seizure-related brain damage in some animal models of status epilepticus (Kondratyev et al. 2001). Repeated ECS treatments increase levels of messenger RNA (mRNA) for the NR2A and NR2B subunits of the NMDA receptor and decrease levels of mRNA for the metabotropic receptor mGluR5b in dentate gyrus and the CA1 hippocampal region (Watkins et al. 1998). These effects are transient and the mRNA levels return to control values within 48 hours. Other studies suggest that repeated ECS treatments decrease NMDA receptor function by altering the potency of glycine for its regulatory site on NMDA receptors, an effect that could diminish the ability of glycine to promote opening of the NMDA ion channel by glutamate (Paul et al. 1994; Petrie et al. 2000).

Effects of Antidepressant Medications and ECT on Mood Disorders: Possible Shared Mechanisms

The efficacy of anticonvulsants as mood stabilizers supports the anticonvulsant hypothesis; this hypothesis is appealing in that it can explain the therapeutic effects of ECT in treating both mania and depression (Sackeim 1994, 1999). Yet most antidepressants are not anticonvulsants, and researchers have investigated other possible mechanisms of action that ECT and antidepressant med-

ications may have in common to elucidate the therapeutic effects of ECT.

There are a number of common threads in the neurotransmitter changes induced by ECT and antidepressant medications. ECT, like antidepressant pharmacotherapy, has been reported to normalize hypothalamic-pituitary-adrenal axis perturbations associated with major depression (Yuuki et al. 2005). However, a more productive area of research has focused on determining how a course of ECT affects biogenic amines. Of interest is the finding that certain antidepressants cause β_1-adrenergic receptor subsensitivity, and similar effects have been observed with ECS (Nutt and Glue 1993). ECS has multiple other effects on the adrenergic system, including increased norepinephrine turnover, increased α_1-adrenergic receptor sensitivity, and possibly decreased presynaptic α_2-adrenergic receptor sensitivity. ECS also enhances the function of the serotonin system, producing increased behavioral responses to serotonin agonists and possibly increases in 5-hydroxytryptamine type 2 (5-HT$_2$) receptor binding in the cerebral cortex (Fochtmann 1994; Nutt and Glue 1993; Sackeim 1994). The latter effect was initially observed in rodents and differs from changes induced by chronic use of antidepressant drugs. Studies in nonhuman primates question the rodent results and provide evidence that ECS diminishes 5-HT$_2$ binding in the cortex (Strome et al. 2005). Thus, 5-HT$_2$ downregulation, like β-adrenergic receptor subsensitivity, may be a mechanism common to several antidepressive treatments.

An emerging trend in research on antidepressive mechanisms is the effect of antidepressive treatments on glutamatergic and GABAergic neurotransmission. In particular, a decrease in the function of NMDA receptors appears to be a mechanism shared by several antidepressive treatments, including ECS (Petrie et al. 2000). In the case of ECS, effects on NMDA receptors appear to be mediated by changes in the glycine regulatory site on the ligand-gated ion channels. There is also evidence that ketamine, a noncompetitive NMDA receptor antagonist, has acute antidepressive properties (Berman et al. 2000; Zarate et al. 2006). Coupled with the possibility that untimely NMDA receptor activation may contribute to ECT-induced anterograde memory problems, the antidepressive effects of ketamine raise the possibility that ketamine or other NMDA receptor–blocking anesthetics may be preferred agents for use during ECT.

One of the more intriguing avenues of research for understanding the effects of ECT is the neurocircuitry of mood regulation and depression. This circuitry involves connections between and within regions of the prefrontal cortex, anterior cingulate gyrus, subgenual prefrontal cortex, anterior thalamus, and more traditional limbic structures (the hippocampus and amygdala) (Drevets 2000; Seminowicz et al. 2004). There is now evidence of structural changes including cell loss (loss of glia and possibly neurons) in several of these regions in patients with unipolar as well as bipolar mood disorders (Harrison 2002). It also appears that different antidepressive treatments may differentially affect metabolism in the neurocircuitry. Effective treatment with paroxetine appears to increase metabolism in frontal regions while decreasing metabolism in the hippocampus, whereas cognitive-behavioral therapy has the opposite effects (Goldapple et al. 2004; Seminowicz et al. 2004). ECT, in contrast, diminishes metabolism in both the prefrontal cortex and the hippocampus (Nobler et al. 2001). Although it is too early to draw firm conclusions about these observations, it is intriguing that chronic deep brain stimulation targeted toward the subgenual prefrontal region appears to be effective in a small sample of patients with treatment-resistant chronic depression (Mayberg et al. 2005), further implicating neurocircuitry changes in the biology of depression.

In addition to the imaging results noted above, there is evidence that several antidepressive treatments, including ECS, have neurotrophic effects and result in neurogenesis in the dentate gyrus of adult rodents (Madsen et al. 2000; Malberg et al. 2000; B. W. Scott et al. 2000). These effects may result from changes in brain-derived neurotrophic factor (BDNF) and the receptor tyrosine kinase (TRK_B) through which BDNF exerts its actions, as well as from the treatment's effects on the adenylate cyclase intracellular signaling system, including cyclic adenosine monophosphate (cAMP) response element–binding protein (CREB), a downstream effector (Duman and Vaidya 1998; Nestler et al. 2002; Schloss and Henn 2004). Other evidence suggests that new neurons produced in the dentate gyrus of adult rodents have the properties of functional neurons and participate in synaptic transmission (Song et al. 2002), suggesting that antidepressive treatments, including ECT, may ultimately enhance hippocampal function. Hippocampal changes also appear to include increases in angiogenesis and possibly blood flow in specific subregions of the hippocampus (Hellsten et al. 2005; Newton et al. 2006).

Whether effects on neurogenesis are important to the therapeutic effects of ECT and other antidepressive treatments remains speculative, although elegant studies in rodents provide evidence that neurogenesis is important to at least some behavioral effects of medications (Santarelli et al. 2003). It is uncertain whether similar neurotrophic

effects occur with ECT in humans. However, studies using magnetic resonance spectroscopy to monitor regional changes in the glutamate-to-glutamine ratio (called *Glx*), a marker of local intracellular excitatory transmitter metabolism (Hasler et al. 2007), indicate that depressed subjects have low Glx values that increase to normal values with effective ECT (Michael et al. 2003; Pfleiderer et al. 2003). Changes in Glx in depressed patients treated with ECT may reflect alterations in glial function in the circuitry underlying depression.

Recent efforts to identify mechanisms contributing to the effects of ECT and antidepressant drugs have included the use of microarrays to study gene expression in multiple brain regions. Although these studies are in their infancy, some evidence indicates that rapidly acting treatments like ECT cause changes primarily in the catecholaminergic system, whereas treatments that act more slowly, like fluoxetine, act predominantly on the serotonergic system. These studies also show strong effects of ECT on BDNF and transcripts encoding proteins involved in hippocampal synaptic plasticity (Conti et al. 2007). Follow-up studies examining the effects of ECT on protein expression and downstream functioning will be important in determining their relevance to ECT's clinical actions.

Efficacy of ECT

Depression

Indications

The summary statement by the American Psychiatric Association Task Force on Electroconvulsive Therapy (2001) and research over the past 30 years (Abrams 1992; Fink 1979; O'Connor et al. 2001; Petrides et al. 2001) have confirmed that ECT is an effective treatment for depression in more than 80% of patients with treatment-resistant unipolar major depression or bipolar disorder. A meta-analysis of randomized, controlled trials (RCTs) performed by the UK ECT Review Group (2003) confirmed the following about the efficacy of ECT for major depression:

- ECT is more efficacious than sham ECT (shown in six RCTs; effect size, 0.91).
- ECT is more efficacious than antidepressant pharmacotherapy (18 RCTs; effect size, 0.80).
- Aspects of ECT associated with a positive response include higher total dose and bilateral electrode place-

ment (although many studies likely underdosed patients with unilateral ECT).

It is noteworthy, however, that several of these studies compared the response rates in patients receiving ECT with the response rates in patients receiving subtherapeutic doses of antidepressants.

Given these data, ECT should no longer be considered a treatment of last resort but a potential first-line treatment when a rapid clinical response is essential in severely ill patients (e.g., those with active suicidal ideation, malignant catatonia, or a compromised medical condition related to depression such as dehydration or malnutrition), when the patient has a history of a positive response to ECT, or when the patient and family request ECT over other treatment options. ECT generally exerts its antidepressive effects more rapidly that pharmacotherapy does, and recent research has confirmed a rapid resolution of suicidal ideation with ECT (Kellner et al. 2005; Patel et al. 2006). Beale and Kellner (2000) argued that the use of ECT after multiple failed medication trials does not take into account the tolerability and efficacy of modern ECT and may lead to needless suffering on the part of the patient. They pointed out that antidepressive treatment algorithms place ECT as a tertiary treatment (e.g., Rush and Thase 1997) instead of recommending that ECT practitioners be consulted early in the treatment process to determine whether ECT would be appropriate therapy. Surveys show that patients who have received ECT rate it as a highly effective treatment (Parker et al. 2001), and that 85% of patients who have received ECT would agree to a second course of ECT if needed (Bernstien et al. 1998). ECT-related relief of depressive symptoms has also been associated with long-term improvements in health-related quality of life, an increasingly important outcome measure in medical research (McCall et al. 2006).

Predictors of Response

Clinical predictors of response to ECT have not been consistent across studies. Potential positive predictors of response include increasing age (Dombrovski et al. 2005; O'Connor et al. 2001) and the presence of psychotic or catatonic symptoms (Birkenhager et al. 2005; Buchan et al. 1992; Petrides et al. 2001). Several studies have reported that patients with longer current episodes of depression (Dombrovski et al. 2005; Prudic et al. 1996) or personality disorders (e.g., borderline personality disorder) (Feske et al. 2004; Parker et al. 2001) are less likely to respond to ECT. Patients with depression complicated by

dysthymia (i.e., double depression) appear to respond to ECT to the same extent that patients without dysthymia do (Prudic et al. 1993). Attempts to link subtypes of depression (e.g., melancholic vs. atypical, unipolar depression vs. depression associated with bipolar disorder) to the likelihood of ECT response have generally failed to reveal differences. However, response by session 3 of ECT may predict long-term efficacy in relieving depression (Tsuchiyama et al. 2005).

Medication resistance also has correlated with a failure to respond to ECT. Patients who had failed to respond to treatment with one or more antidepressants before receiving ECT responded less favorably to ECT than did patients who had not failed to respond to medication (Devanand et al. 1991; Dombrovski et al. 2005; Prudic et al. 1990; Sackeim et al. 1990). This was true for resistance to the heterocyclic antidepressants but not to the selective serotonin reuptake inhibitors (SSRIs) or monoamine oxidase inhibitors (MAOIs) (Prudic et al. 1996).

To date, the most consistent biological marker for ECT response has been increased frontal delta activity (i.e., postictal depression) shown on the electroencephalogram (EEG) after ECT (Mayur 2006; Sackeim et al. 1996), which is associated with decreased cerebral blood flow in the immediate postictal period (Nobler et al. 1994). More sophisticated methods of EEG analysis (e.g., nonlinear analysis) may hold promise in helping to discern electroencephalographic predictors of the antidepressive efficacy of ECT (Mayur 2006).

Coffey et al. (1989) described a greater number of structural abnormalities observed on magnetic resonance imaging (MRI) scans of the brain (e.g., deep white matter, basal ganglia, and periventricular hyperintensities) in elderly depressed patients referred for ECT, compared with age-matched control subjects. These preexisting structural brain abnormalities may predispose elderly depressed patients to a less favorable response to ECT (Hickie et al. 1995; Steffens et al. 2001), although case reports indicate that ECT may be helpful in the treatment of depression after a stroke (Currier et al. 1992).

Mania

Early anecdotal reports as well as more recent case studies suggest that ECT is beneficial in the treatment of mania associated with bipolar disorder and delirious mania (Fink 2001b, 2006). ECT also has been shown to be effective in patients with treatment-resistant mixed mood disorders (Gruber et al. 2000). Given the benefit of anticonvulsant medications in treating mania and the evidence that ECT may exert its therapeutic effect by raising the seizure threshold (Sackeim 1999), we have a theoretical basis for assuming that ECT is effective in the treatment of mania. Since 1970, several retrospective studies have confirmed the efficacy of ECT in patients with mania, with approximately two-thirds of patients showing marked clinical improvement (Mukherjee et al. 1994). In a prospective, controlled trial, Small et al. (1988) compared the efficacy of ECT with that of lithium in the treatment of mania. Patients who received ECT improved more during the first 8 weeks of treatment than did patients who received lithium. Nevertheless, after 8 weeks of treatment, ECT and lithium were comparable in efficacy. In addition, patients with mixed symptoms of depression and mania responded particularly well to ECT. Catatonia may be especially common in patients with bipolar disorder, and this represents another scenario in which ECT may offer advantages in efficacy and rapidity of response versus pharmacotherapy (Taylor and Fink 2003). Challenges specific to treating mania with ECT include the following:

- Concomitant use of anticonvulsants, which may interfere with seizure induction in ECT
- Reports of prolonged seizures and delirium when ECT is given with lithium (Sartorius et al. 2005), although other authors have reported safe coadministration of ECT and lithium (Dolenc and Rasmussen 2005)
- Decreased likelihood that manic (vs. depressed) patients will voluntarily consent to ECT treatment

Despite a rapid increase in studies evaluating alternative antimania medications, including newer anticonvulsants and the atypical antipsychotics, there is a lack of research comparing the potential benefits of ECT in the acute and maintenance treatment of bipolar disorder (Fink 2001b; Keck et al. 2000). This is regrettable given the advantages of ECT as a true mood stabilizer that can effectively treat both the manic and the depressed phases of the illness. ECT has been given safely to children with intractable mania (Hill et al. 1997) and to patients with dementia and comorbid mania (McDonald and Thompson 2001). ECT also may have an important role in the treatment of mania during pregnancy, given the potential teratogenic effects of many anticonvulsant medications as well as the potential harm to both the mother and the fetus from a prolonged affective episode.

Controversy persists over whether unilateral ECT is as effective as bilateral ECT in the treatment of mania. Unfortunately, studies comparing unilateral and bilateral ECT in the treatment of mania have reported neither the amount of electrical charge used nor the percentage by which the electrical stimulus exceeded the seizure threshold. Daly et al. (2001) compared 228 patients with bipolar disorder or unipolar depression who were randomly assigned to ECT conditions that differed in electrode placement and stimulus intensity. They found that the bipolar patients had a rapid response to both unilateral and bilateral ECT and did not differ from the unipolar patients in either the rate of response or the response to unilateral or bilateral ECT. ECT also has been shown to be efficacious in the treatment of mixed mania (Ciapparelli et al. 2001). Future research is certainly needed to clarify the role of ECT in the treatment of mania, although clear evidence indicates that ECT is an effective treatment and should be included in any algorithm of therapy for treatment-resistant or severely disabling mania.

Schizophrenia

With the introduction of clozapine and the atypical antipsychotics, ECT has become a third-line treatment for schizophrenia, although it continues to have an important role in the treatment of an acute psychotic episode, catatonic schizophrenia, and neuroleptic malignant syndrome. Although the mechanism of action of ECT in treating psychosis has received much less attention than the mechanism of its antidepressant effects, a possible mechanism of ECT's antipsychotic effects has been inferred from the therapeutic action of ECT in patients with phencyclidine-induced psychosis (Dinwiddie et al. 1988). One of the major actions of phencyclidine and related drugs (e.g., ketamine) is the blocking of open channels for NMDA receptors. Phencyclidine-induced channel blocking is voltage dependent and long lived, with the ion channel closing around the phencyclidine molecule (MacDonald et al. 1991). Relief of channel blocks requires NMDA ion channels to open at depolarized membrane potentials (Huettner and Bean 1988). Thus, neuronal membrane depolarization and glutamate receptor binding are important for allowing phencyclidine to exit the channel. Although it is not certain that blocking of NMDA channels causes phencyclidine-induced psychosis, it is interesting that ECT-induced seizures have the requisite effects to relieve the channel block. During a seizure, neurons depolarize (via synaptic excitation and action potential firing) and glutamate is released at synapses. These events together would be expected to relieve phencyclidine-induced blockage and could provide a rationale for the effectiveness of ECT. As a corollary, this mechanism would also lead to the prediction that the use of ketamine for anesthesia during ECT should be associated with a low incidence of ketamine-induced psychosis.

Fink and Sackeim (1996) reviewed the use of ECT in the treatment of schizophrenia and cautiously noted that most studies examining the efficacy of ECT in treating schizophrenia do not meet current standards for scientific methodology. Nonetheless, the authors concluded that ECT is a highly effective treatment for psychosis and that it should be considered, particularly for patients with schizophrenia and an initial psychotic episode, symptoms of agitation, increased psychomotor activity, delirium, or delusions. The authors also concluded that ECT is effective in treating schizophrenia when catatonia, prominent affective symptoms, or positive symptoms of psychosis (e.g., hallucinations) are present. They speculated that the use of ECT early in the course of schizophrenia may decrease the progressive, debilitating effects of the illness.

ECT combined with neuroleptics has been shown to be more effective than ECT or neuroleptics alone in treating schizophrenia (Friedel 1986; Gujavarty et al. 1987; Klapheke 1993; Sajatovic and Meltzer 1993). A recent meta-analysis of the four most methodologically sound studies of ECT augmentation to antipsychotics for treating schizophrenia concluded that ECT offers a modest but significant benefit (equivalent to 5 points on the Brief Psychiatric Rating Scale) compared with neuroleptic therapy alone (Painuly and Chakrabarti 2006). The effects are apparent in the first several weeks of treatment but appear to diminish with prolonged treatment. Interestingly, all of these studies were conducted in India, where the use of ECT to treat schizophrenia appears to be more common than it is in the United States. Notably, open-label studies and case studies suggest that ECT may be safe and helpful in combination with clozapine, another treatment typically reserved for more treatment-refractory illness (Havaki-Kontaxaki et al. 2006). ECT combined with neuroleptic therapy may also be effective in the management of aggressive behavior in patients with schizophrenia (Hirose et al. 2001) and for maintenance treatment of schizophrenia (Chanpattana et al. 1999b).

The recommendations of the American Psychiatric Association Task Force on Electroconvulsive Therapy (2001) state that ECT is an effective treatment for schizophrenia in the following clinical conditions: 1) during acute onset of symptoms, 2) when the catatonic subtype of schizophrenia is present, and 3) when there is a history of a positive response to ECT. Not surprisingly, patients with an affective component (i.e., schizoaffective patients) also respond more favorably to ECT than do schizophrenic patients without subsyndromal affective

disorders. In addition, ECT represents a potentially life-saving intervention for patients with neuroleptic malignant syndrome that does not respond to more conservative treatments (e.g., supportive care or pharmacotherapy). Clearly, there is a need for further research related to the role of ECT in treating schizophrenia.

Parkinson's Disease

ECT has been shown to be effective treatment for the motor symptoms of Parkinson's disease (Faber and Trimble 1991; Kellner et al. 1994; Rasmussen and Abrams 1991), and a recent meta-analysis of five studies confirmed that ECT acutely improves global motor functioning in patients with this disease (Fregni et al. 2005). These reports have included patients with and without psychiatric illnesses; ECT improves the motor symptoms of Parkinson's disease independently of its effects on the patient's mood. Because antimuscarinic drugs are useful in treating parkinsonism, the effects of ECT on central muscarinic systems may be relevant (Fochtmann 1988). However, ECT also alters central dopaminergic systems that are involved in the pathophysiology of Parkinson's disease (Fochtmann 1994). Acutely, ECS increases dopamine levels in the frontal cortex and striatum and has variable effects on basal dopamine levels. Furthermore, dopamine autoreceptor sensitivity is diminished after ECS, an effect that would tend to augment dopamine release. There is also evidence that dopamine$_1$ (D_1) receptor agonists increase the stimulation of adenylate cyclase after ECS. However, after ECS, D_1 receptor binding is increased in the substantia nigra (Fochtmann et al. 1989), but not in the striatum (Nowak and Zak 1989).

Favorable predictors of response include advanced age, severe disability (on–off syndromes), and painful dyskinesias. Reduction in the symptoms of Parkinson's disease tends to occur during the first several sessions of ECT. However, the effects of ECT are not permanent and usually last from several days to several months, although prolonged improvement has been reported in a few patients. Maintenance ECT also has been shown to be effective for up to 4 years in treating the motor symptoms of Parkinson's disease (Aarsland et al. 1997; Wengel et al. 1998).

Because of the increased risk for ECT-induced interictal delirium in patients with Parkinson's disease (or any neurological disease such as Alzheimer's disease or neurological condition such as impairment caused by a stroke), careful consideration must be given to the amount of electrical charge administered, the electrode placement used, and the frequency of treatments (Figiel et al. 1991). The delirium associated with ECT in patients with Parkinson's disease can be significantly reduced without losing effectiveness by doing the following:

- Using right-unilateral ECT with an initial electrical stimulus approximately 3.5 times the seizure threshold
- Administering ECT treatments every 3–4 days
- Withholding the dose of levodopa on the morning of ECT
- Discontinuing ECT until the cognitive impairment completely resolves if any impairment in attention or orientation develops, then restarting ECT at a lower electrical charge

Other Illnesses

ECT can be a life-saving treatment for patients with catatonia regardless of the etiology, including catatonia resulting from a medical disease (e.g., lupus erythematosus), neuroleptic malignant syndrome, schizophrenia, bipolar disorder, and unipolar depression (Fink 1994, 1997).

Limited evidence suggests that ECT may relieve symptoms associated with obsessive-compulsive disorder (OCD) (Maletzky et al. 1994; Thomas and Kellner 2003) and schizophrenia complicated by OCD (Lavin and Halligan 1996). Because it raises the seizure threshold, ECT can interrupt status epilepticus (Fink et al. 1999; Lisanby et al. 2001a) and treat intractable seizures (Griesemer et al. 1997; Regenold et al. 1998). ECT also has been shown to be safe and effective in the treatment of comorbid mood disorders in patients with closed head injuries (Kant et al. 1999), dementia (McDonald and Thompson 2001), and mental retardation (Aziz et al. 2001; Fink 2001a; Friedlander and Solomons 2002; Gabriel 1998; van Waarde et al. 2001). ECT may exert some analgesic effects independent of its effects on mood, as evidenced in a recent trial with positive results using ECT to treat fibromyalgia (Usui et al. 2006).

ECT Use During Pregnancy

During pregnancy, ECT may be an effective, safe treatment for women with bipolar disorder or major depression and is recommended by the American Psychiatric Association (1994) practice guidelines as a possible first-line treatment for pregnant women with mood disorders. ECT has been safely used in all three trimesters of pregnancy (Rabheru 2001), although prospective, controlled studies of ECT use in pregnancy are lacking. Miller's (1994) review of more than 400 cases of women treated with ECT during pregnancy failed to identify a consistent pattern of complications; more recent case reports have associated

ECT with premature labor (Bhatia et al. 1999; Echevarría Moreno et al. 1998). The risks of and risk management strategies for administering ECT during pregnancy have been reviewed by Rabheru (2001).

The treatment of mania during pregnancy can be particularly difficult given the reported teratogenicity of several antimania medications. Although early case reports suggested that lithium use in the first trimester is associated with an increased risk of cardiac anomalies, more recent prospective, case–control studies have shown only weak teratogenic effects (L.S. Cohen et al. 1994). Carbamazepine and valproic acid are both associated with neural tube defects (Oakeshott and Hunt 1994). Many of the other medications, including atypical antipsychotics, benzodiazepines, and antidepressants, have less clear effects on the fetus. Yet the complications of untreated or partially treated bipolar disorder endanger both the mother and the fetus and include poor compliance with neonatal care, impaired judgment, substance abuse, poor nutrition and self-care, and depression with suicide attempts (Miller 2001).

Stimulus Dosing in ECT for Treatment of Depression

Questions about the proper management of the electrical stimulus have been central to the science and practice of ECT since the inception of the treatment. Cerletti and Bini modeled ECT on the success of pharmacologically induced convulsive therapy and assumed that the stimulus should be convulsive. Interestingly, the first ECT session in 1938 involved two subconvulsive stimulations before Cerletti and Bini increased the stimulus intensity to produce a convulsion (Endler 1988). Thus, the first ECT session was a "titrated" ECT session involving the serial application of increasing stimulus intensities passing from the subconvulsive range through the convulsive threshold. Issues in stimulus dosing that have been considered since that time include the following:

- Whether the stimulus should be subconvulsive or convulsive
- What the optimal stimulus waveform is
- If a convulsive stimulus is desired, to what degree the stimulus intensity should be in excess of the convulsive threshold
- Which physiological parameters, if any, provide useful feedback to continuously refine stimulus dosing throughout the ECT course

Convulsive, Subconvulsive, and Sham Stimulation

The use of nonconvulsive electrical stimulation to treat psychiatric disorders preceded the introduction of ECT by decades. Most of the treatments involved administering static electricity to parts of the body including but not limited to the head (Grover 1924). The availability of commercial ECT devices did not lead to the immediate replacement of subconvulsive stimulation with convulsive stimulation. Instead, some practitioners used the devices to deliver lengthy (several minutes long) subconvulsive cranial stimulation. However, it became clear that subconvulsive stimulation was associated with a *poorer* outcome than conventional psychotherapy in psychoneurotic patients, and the practice of treating patients with subconvulsive stimuli decreased (Hargrove et al. 1953). Now, many years later, the use of rapid-rate transcranial magnetic stimulation (rTMS) has re-opened the question of whether subconvulsive stimuli are an effective treatment for depression; these data are reviewed in a later section (see "Transcranial Magnetic Stimulation and Subconvulsive Stimuli").

The elements of modified ECT (including muscle relaxation and general anesthesia) were described early in the history of ECT. The wide-scale adoption of these modifications raised new questions as to whether seizure is central to the antidepressive efficacy of ECT or whether anesthesia alone would be just as effective. The Northwick Park trial (Johnstone et al. 1980) and the Leicestershire trial (Brandon et al. 1984) are examples of two "sham" ECT studies in which anesthesia alone was compared with real ECT. It was convincingly demonstrated that real ECT is more efficacious, especially for the most severe forms of depression (Brandon et al. 1984; Johnstone et al. 1980). The efficacy of ECT was clearly linked to the production of a seizure. Neither the use of anesthesia alone without the electrical stimulus nor the use of subconvulsive stimuli appears to have real merit in the treatment of depression.

Stimulus Waveform

Given that a convulsive stimulus is necessary for the antidepressive effects of ECT, a nearly infinite number of variations are available for formulating the stimulus waveform. The earliest ECT devices delivered a sinusoidal stimulus. Other waveforms available on early ECT devices included the "chopped" sine wave, the unidirectional pulse square wave, and the alternating brief-pulse square wave. Al-

though some investigators had a suspicion that sine wave stimuli might produce slightly better antidepressive effects than did brief-pulse stimuli, that suspicion was mitigated by a randomized study showing that sine wave ECT produced more memory side effects than brief-pulse ECT, irrespective of the placement of the stimulating electrode (R.D. Weiner et al. 1986). This finding of greater cognitive side effects with sine wave ECT was recently replicated in an efficacy study using a prospective cohort design, which showed that compared with brief-pulse stimulation, sine wave stimulation was associated with a slowing of reaction time that persisted for at least 6 months after ECT (Sackeim et al. 2007). The more severe cognitive side effects produced by sinusoidal stimuli may be explained by the slower rise time for each sine wave cycle as compared with the brief-pulse cycle. Consequent to the slower rise time, much of the sine wave stimulus is subconvulsive and thus presumably adds nothing to the therapeutic effect of ECT, adding only to cognitive side effects. The steep rise in the brief-pulse waveform allows for the entire stimulus to be above the convulsive threshold (suprathreshold). Because much of the sine wave stimulus is nonproductive, being in the subconvulsive range, it would be predicted that brief-pulse stimuli would be more efficient, requiring a stimulus of smaller magnitude to produce a seizure. *Standard* brief-pulse stimuli are defined by pulse duration of 1–2 milliseconds, while *ultrabrief*-pulse stimuli are defined by pulse duration of 0.25–0.50 milliseconds.

In 1980, Weiner showed that standard brief-pulse stimuli could provoke a seizure with only one-third of the energy required with sine wave stimuli (Weiner 1980). In the last decade, standard brief-pulse ECT devices replaced sine wave devices in the United States (Farah and McCall 1993). New devices using ultrabrief-pulse stimuli have the advantage of improving the efficiency of seizure induction. Abrams (2002) estimated that it takes only about 0.25 milliseconds to initiate neuronal depolarization, and wider pulse widths are inefficient and waste electrical charge. The total energy output of these ultrabrief-pulse modalities is the same as the total energy output of the standard brief-pulse widths; thus, as the stimulus pulse widths are shortened, the stimulus trains are lengthened. Ultrabrief-pulse widths may have an advantage because shorter pulse widths and longer pulse trains have been shown to elicit seizures with a smaller electrical charge and therefore may have fewer cognitive side effects (Sackeim et al. 2001b). Similarly, decreasing the frequency of pulses with a corresponding lengthening of the stimulus train will improve the efficiency of seizure induction (Kotresh et al. 2004).

Magnitude of the Stimulus Dose

The consensus regarding the need for convulsive (as opposed to subconvulsive) stimuli and brief-pulse waveforms would seem to make stimulus dosing in ECT a straightforward process, except for the question of the degree to which the stimulus should exceed the convulsive threshold. For years, ECT practitioners were satisfied that the answer to this question was found in the work of Ottosson (1962), who compared routine ECT with ECT modified by pretreatment with intravenous lidocaine. He found that seizures induced by lidocaine-modified ECT were shorter than those induced by routine ECT and observed an inverse relationship between seizure duration and antidepressive effect. From this work, it was widely accepted that stimulus doses producing seizures lasting at least 25 seconds have an antidepressive effect (American Psychiatric Association Task Force on Electroconvulsive Therapy 1978).

Initially, ECT was administered using bilateral (typically bitemporal) electrode placement. In 1949, Goldman introduced right-unilateral ECT and placed stimulating electrodes over the right hemisphere rather than the mesial temporal lobes in an attempt to decrease the direct stimulation of language areas and decrease cognitive side effects. Although right-unilateral ECT was associated with fewer cognitive side effects, most studies showed that bilateral ECT had a marked therapeutic advantage over unilateral ECT for depression (d'Elia and Raotma 1975).

The clinical wisdom that bilateral ECT was more effective than right-unilateral ECT in treating depression came into question with the groundbreaking work of Sackeim's research group. Sackeim et al. (1993) reported that when the magnitude of the electrical stimulus was just barely above the convulsive threshold, ECT with right-unilateral electrode placement was not efficacious, despite the production of electrographic seizures typically in excess of 25 seconds. However, as the electrical dose was progressively increased, response rates in right-unilateral ECT improved significantly and approached those of bilateral ECT. In contrast, bilateral ECT was fully efficacious with stimuli minimally above or 2.5 times the seizure threshold, but excess memory side effects accrued at the higher stimulus dose.

The dose–response relationship of right-unilateral ECT holds true to the extent that the stimulus exceeds the convulsive threshold for a given patient, but is not related to the absolute magnitude of the stimulus dose. The efficacy of right-unilateral ECT follows a nearly linear relationship to the degree that the stimulus dose exceeds the seizure threshold, at least through 12 times the seizure threshold (McCall et al. 2000). This relationship is analogous to the pharmacological treatment of depression with tricyclic antidepressants: serum blood levels are more important than the absolute oral dose in determining both efficacy and side effects.

These findings led to the following conclusions:

- With standard brief-pulse stimulation delivered with right-unilateral electrode placement, the stimulus should be substantially above the convulsive threshold in order to ensure the effectiveness of ECT.
- With standard brief-pulse stimulation delivered with bilateral electrode placement, the stimulus should not be excessively above the convulsive threshold, in order to avoid undue cognitive side effects.

The convulsive threshold varies by a factor of at least 40 in large patient samples; thus, the mean threshold for a group of patients is useless for individual cases (Sackeim et al. 1991). It is clear that the convulsive threshold is related to age, sex, race, choice of stimulating electrode placement, and, perhaps, cranial dimensions (Chung 2006; Colenda and McCall 1996; McCall et al. 1993b; Sackeim et al. 1991). Still, these factors predict only a small amount of the variance in the convulsive threshold, and statistical models to predict the convulsive threshold, including age-based dosing approaches, fare poorly (Colenda and McCall 1996; Tiller and Ingram 2006).

Seizure Morphology

The report of Sackeim et al. (1993) that threshold right-unilateral ECT produced seizures of 25 seconds or longer without antidepressive efficacy cast into doubt the clinical wisdom that the stimulus dose was therapeutic if the electrographic seizure lasted at least 25 seconds. Investigators have sought to find a physiological marker of treatment adequacy to replace seizure duration. The most promising candidate is seizure morphology. Ottosson (1962) reported that lidocaine changed the shape of ECT seizures and affected their duration, although the first finding is largely overlooked. Lidocaine-modified seizures, in addition to being less efficacious than standard ECT seizures, were characterized by loss of spike activity and poor postictal suppression.

This finding has been extended by evidence that seizure morphology varies with ECT techniques. That is, greater seizure intensity correlates with ECT techniques that progress from lower efficacy (with right-unilateral electrode placement and low stimulus intensity) to higher efficacy (with bilateral placement and high stimulus intensity) (Krystal et al. 1993). Electrode placement and stimulus intensity have independent and additive effects on seizure morphology. Seizures of greater intensity are characterized by higher peak ictal amplitudes, greater stereotypy of the ictal discharge, greater symmetry and coherence between the left and right cerebral hemispheres, and more profound postictal suppression. Preliminary evidence suggests that greater seizure intensity is predictive of a greater likelihood of response and/or faster response (McCall et al. 1995; Nobler et al. 1993).

The natural extension of this reasoning leads to the hope that seizure morphology could guide decisions about stimulus intensity as the course of ECT progresses. For example, if seizure intensity is poor in the middle of the treatment course, then the treatment technique should be changed (by switching electrode placement and/or increasing the stimulus intensity) in order to optimize the clinical outcome. Manufacturers of ECT devices now incorporate automated measures of seizure intensity onto the ECT chart recorder, and the accompanying owner's manual instructs the practitioner to increase the stimulus intensity if the seizure morphology appears to be degraded. The unstated implication is that poor seizure morphology is a problem and that increasing the stimulus intensity will fix the problem. This instruction might have merit if stimulus intensity were the primary determinant of seizure morphology, but other factors, such as age, baseline convulsive threshold, and other intrinsic patient factors likely play an equal role in determining seizure expression (McCall et al. 1996, 1998). For example, greater seizure durations coupled with greater seizure regularity as shown by electroencephalography at the second ECT session are predictive of a better antidepressive outcome at the conclusion of the ECT course, and this relationship is independent of the choice of stimulus electrode placement (Rosenquist et al. 2007).

Poor seizure morphology (e.g., in older patients with high seizure thresholds) is little influenced by increasing the stimulus intensity above 2.5 times the seizure threshold. Therefore, it is premature to recommend stimulus dosing on the basis of seizure morphology. The importance of seizure morphology in predicting clinical outcome is far from being understood, and more work is needed to make it a practical tool for governing ECT technique. Peak heart rate has been proposed as an alternative physiological measure of treatment adequacy, with higher heart rates perhaps indicating better clinical out-

comes (Swartz 2000). Again, this approach has yet to be widely accepted.

Integrating the Science of Stimulus Dosing With the Choice of Electrode Placement

Estimating the Convulsive Threshold

The recent advances in knowledge pertaining to stimulus dosing lead to the conclusion that standard brief-pulse, right-unilateral ECT should be initiated with a stimulus known to be at least five times the seizure threshold, while standard brief-pulse, bilateral ECT should be initiated with a stimulus about 50% above the seizure threshold. Choosing between these two strategies requires consideration of both efficacy and side effects. An indirect comparison was made by Stoppe et al. (2006) in a study of older depressed patients randomly assigned to receive fixed high doses of either right-unilateral ECT ($n=17$) or bilateral ECT ($n=22$). Although the failure of this study to dose according to a known seizure threshold makes the cognitive findings difficult to evaluate, it did show similar remission rates with right-unilateral ECT (88%) and bilateral ECT (68%), suggesting that efficacy need not be compromised by choosing right-unilateral placement.

McCall et al. (2000) conducted the first randomized comparison of low-dose (1.5 times the seizure threshold) bilateral ECT ($n=37$) versus high-dose (8 times the seizure threshold) right-unilateral ECT ($n=40$). Again, depression remission rates were not significantly different with right-unilateral electrode placement (60%) versus bilateral placement (73%), and memory effects were likewise similar. This study can be criticized for having insufficient power to detect small but meaningful effects. That concern was addressed in a subsequent study by Haskett et al. (2007) contrasting 339 patients randomly assigned to receive either standard brief-pulse, right-unilateral ECT administered at 6 times the seizure threshold or bilateral ECT administered at 1.5 times the seizure threshold. Although differences between the treatments' antidepressive effects were again indistinguishable, the extent of autobiographical memory loss was greater in the bilateral group. This study solidifies the position of high-dose right-unilateral ECT as the preferred initial strategy. Even if patients fail to respond to an initial approach using right-unilateral electrode placement, increasing the stimulus intensity with right-unilateral ECT is associated with a subsequent antidepressant response equal to the response obtained after switching to bilateral ECT, with fewer cognitive side effects (Tew et al. 2002).

The bulk of the evidence thus suggests that it is desirable to set the stimulus dose as a proportion of the convulsive threshold; the convulsive threshold of each patient should be known, preferably by measuring convulsive threshold early in the ECT course. The most accurate means of measuring the convulsive threshold for a given patient is empirical observation: giving intentionally subconvulsive stimuli at the first treatment; then, in the same session, administering successively larger stimuli until a seizure is produced. This stimulus "titration" technique defines the convulsive threshold for each patient. This approach applies to right-unilateral and bilateral electrode placement.

If ECT practitioners agree with the above reasoning and use this stimulus dosing technique, they should ascertain the convulsive threshold at the first ECT session. However, some ECT researchers have argued against titration of stimulus doses with unilateral ECT and instead have encouraged practitioners to use fixed high doses of unilateral ECT (Abrams 2002) or fixed moderate doses of bilateral ECT (Kellner 2001). In fact, a survey of ECT practitioners in 1993 showed that only a minority performed titration of the stimulus dose (Farah and McCall 1993). The reasons for this are unclear, but possible explanations include concerns that 1) the subconvulsive stimulation inherent in stimulus titration might be medically dangerous, 2) subconvulsive stimulation might add to memory side effects, or 3) production of a barely suprathreshold seizure with right-unilateral placement would constitute ineffective treatment, thus rendering the first treatment a wasted effort.

It is true that subconvulsive stimulation transiently slows the heart rate, and that if subconvulsive stimulation is given to patients who have received a β-blocker and no anticholinergic drug, there is risk of substantial asystole (McCall et al. 1994). On the other hand, atropine pretreatment eliminates this risk. The possibility of excess acute cognitive side effects with subconvulsive stimuli has been examined and discounted (Prudic et al. 1994). The possibility of a sluggish antidepressive response when stimulus doses are titrated to a level moderately above the seizure threshold in combination with right-unilateral electrode placement, however, is a real concern. A prospective, randomized trial in elderly depressed subjects showed that a titrated, moderately suprathreshold dosing strategy with right-unilateral electrode placement produced a slower antidepressive response than did fixed high stimulus doses with right-unilateral electrode placement (McCall et al. 1995). Similar results were seen in a naturalistic comparison of young adults receiving titrated,

right-unilateral ECT at 2–3 times the seizure threshold versus right-unilateral ECT at a fixed high dose (Ward et al. 2006). Interpretation of these studies is made more difficult by differences between the treatment groups (titrated vs. fixed doses; moderate vs. high doses). At the very least, however, it is clear that different dosing strategies affect the antidepressive outcome of right-unilateral ECT, even when the doses being compared are substantially above the convulsive threshold.

Alternatives to Estimating the Convulsive Threshold

Abrams (2002) suggested that the most efficient method of administering right-unilateral ECT is to use 100% of the maximum device capacity and a pulse width of 0.25–0.50 milliseconds and recommended changing to bilateral ECT if the patient does not improve sufficiently. However, insufficient data support the routine use of ultrabrief-pulse widths (Fink 2002), and the use of stimulus titration to establish a dose relative to the seizure threshold would potentially decrease cognitive problems while ensuring an adequate seizure (Rasmussen 2002). Alternatively, twice-weekly bilateral ECT could be initiated using the half-age method (Abrams 2002). In the half-age method, the age of the patient is divided by 2; the resulting number is the percentage of the device's maximal output with which the patient is first treated (e.g., a 50-year-old would be treated at 25% of the machine's maximal output). Kellner (2001) recommended an alternative fixed-dose strategy that involves starting with 75% of maximal output for right-unilateral ECT and 30%–60% of maximal output for bilateral ECT.

Our recommendations for stimulus dosing are made with the following two caveats:

1. Recommendations can be made only in regard to treating major depression, as it is unknown whether dosing strategies for patients with other diagnoses should be the same as those for treating depression.
2. Dosing recommendations can be made only in the context of the chosen electrode placement and the patient's clinical condition.

It is clear that a supraconvulsive stimulus is necessary to obtain an antidepressive effect with right-unilateral ECT. It is unclear whether any supraconvulsive stimulus would have equivalent antidepressive efficacy with bilateral electrode placement, but a stimulus of at least 2.5 times the convulsive threshold is required with right-unilateral ECT in most patients.

Choosing an Electrode Placement and Stimulus Dose

Those patients with the most serious complications of major depression (i.e., active suicidal behavior in the hospital, catatonia, or food refusal) merit an approach most likely to yield quick antidepressive results. In such circumstances, bilateral ECT with a relatively high fixed stimulus dose (e.g., 50% of the machine's maximal output) could be justified; stimulus dose titration would not be required because concern about cognitive side effects becomes a purely secondary issue, based on the severity of the patient's clinical status. However, whether fixed high-dose right-unilateral ECT could provide an equally fast and effective response needs to be examined.

In contrast, a depressed patient in whom medication has failed but who is otherwise not in urgent need of treatment may be an appropriate candidate for right-unilateral ECT at 5–6 times the seizure threshold, especially if cognitive side effects are a concern or if the patient is being treated in an outpatient setting. The patient can start with right-unilateral ECT and after five or six treatments change to bilateral ECT if he or she has not had an adequate response. Other special situations favoring titrated right-unilateral ECT include the treatment of depressed patients with comorbid dementia or other neurological conditions such as Parkinson's disease. The treatment of these patients should minimize even transient memory side effects and may include starting at a very conservative unilateral dose (i.e., 3.5 times the seizure threshold) and increasing the dose as tolerated.

Other dosing strategies, such as titrated bilateral or fixed high-dose right-unilateral ECT, occupy the strategic middle ground between titrated right-unilateral and fixed-dose bilateral ECT for patients whose condition is of intermediate acuity. One promising area of research is the development of bifrontal ECT, which has the potential for providing the efficacy of bilateral ECT with a cognitive side-effect profile similar to that of right-unilateral ECT. In bifrontal ECT, the electrodes are placed 5 cm above the lateral angle of each orbit in a line parallel to the sagittal plane in order to directly stimulate the frontal lobes, which have been implicated in the pathology of major depression (Nobler et al. 2000) and response to ECT (Nobler et al. 1993). Compared with bilateral and right-unilateral ECT, bifrontal ECT would potentially spare the temporal lobes and decrease cognitive side effects. Preliminary research has shown that bifrontal ECT is comparable in efficacy to bilateral ECT, and preliminary evidence indicates that bifrontal ECT (at either the seizure threshold or 1.5 times the seizure threshold) has fewer cognitive side effects than bilateral ECT (Bailine et al. 2000; Lawson et al. 1990; Letemendia et al. 1993; Ranjkesh et al. 2005). A retrospective chart review of 76 patients found that bilateral ECT was more effective than bifrontal ECT with modestly increased side effects (Bakewell et al. 2004).

In a study comparing right-unilateral and bifrontal ECT, Heikman et al. (2002) randomly assigned 24 depressed patients to receive high-dose right-unilateral ECT (at 5 times the seizure threshold), moderate-dose right-unilateral ECT (at 2.5 times the seizure threshold), or low-dose bifrontal ECT (just above the seizure threshold). Among the 22 patients who completed the study, depression remitted in 7 of 8 patients (88%) treated with high-dose right-unilateral ECT, compared with just 3 of 7 patients (43%) each in the groups treated with moderate-dose right-unilateral and low-dose bifrontal ECT (the difference was not statistically significant). All three groups were similar in terms of cognitive changes measured by the Mini-Mental State Exam (Folstein et al. 1975), it is difficult to know exactly when bifrontal ECT should be used in a clinical ECT service, because the research is lagging behind clinical practice (C.K. Loo et al. 2006). A multisite study funded by the National Institute of Mental Health is under way using more sophisticated cognitive testing and outcome measures to determine whether bifrontal ECT is a viable alternative to high-dose right-unilateral or bilateral ECT.

ECT Techniques

Pretreatment Medical Evaluation

Although no medical condition is an absolute contraindication for ECT, several clinical conditions may increase the risk of complications from ECT:

- Recent myocardial infarction or unstable cardiac conditions
- Any illness that increases intracranial pressure (e.g., brain tumor)
- Recent cerebral infarction, particularly hemorrhagic infarction
- Aneurysm or vascular malformation
- American Society of Anesthesiology physical status classification level 4 or 5
- Severe pulmonary disease

When treating high-risk patients with ECT, clinicians must evaluate the effects of ECT on cerebral and cardiac physiology and review data from the extant ECT literature to help develop individual risk–benefit ratios (American Psychiatric Association Task Force on Electroconvulsive Therapy 2001; Applegate 1997; Bader et al. 1995; Krystal and Coffey 1997; Weisberg et al. 1991; Zwil et al. 1992). All patients should undergo a thorough medical and neuropsychiatric review before beginning ECT. Particular emphasis should be placed on diseases affecting the CNS and the cardiovascular system. The pre-ECT evaluation should include a physical examination, detailed neurological examination, mental status examination, medical history, and review of systems. The patient's mental status should be evaluated before initiation of ECT and monitored closely before administration of ECT at every session thereafter.

The baseline screening should include some basic laboratory tests (blood count and electrolytes) and an electrocardiogram. Clinicians should obtain a chest X ray for patients with pulmonary disease. Spine films should be considered for patients with a history of back pain, positive findings on physical examination, or medical conditions that may affect the skeletal system. Even patients who are recovering from surgery to repair a broken hip can be safely treated with ECT if appropriate doses of succinylcholine are used to ensure adequate relaxation. The greatest risks for fractures are in the recovery room if the patient has significant postictal confusion and agitation, and during the acute ECT course when patients, particularly the elderly and those with Parkinson's disease, are at increased risk for falling.

Information obtained about the patient's neuropsychiatric history should include the following:

- Complications from anesthesia (including a family or personal history of malignant hyperthermia)
- Dementia or other neurological disease
- Any symptoms on neurological examination suggestive of increased intracranial pressure (e.g., severe headaches, new-onset incontinence, or gait ataxia) or primary neurological disease (e.g., lateralizing neurological deficits)

Based on the patient's examination, brain imaging may be ordered before ECT. Some (Kellner 1996) have called for a reevaluation of the common practice of obtaining brain imaging for all patients prior to ECT. Kellner argues that with proper screening, the number of patients with significant CNS findings on imaging who

have normal neurological examination findings is very low, and the expense of routine screening is high.

The clinician also must assess the patient's cardiovascular status, including evidence for dyspnea on exertion, angina, orthopnea, or conditions that might increase the risk of coronary artery disease (e.g., hyperlipidemia, hypercholesterolemia, poorly controlled hypertension, obesity, or diabetes). ECT in some ways represents a cardiac stress test, with an abrupt rise in the heart rate and blood pressure occurring after the stimulus. Therefore, one of the most important screens to determine whether a patient can tolerate ECT is accurately assessing exercise tolerance. This can be accomplished by asking questions such as the number of stairs a patient can climb without becoming short of breath. Patients with evidence of coronary artery disease can be screened with a relatively inexpensive treadmill test establishing a peak heart rate of approximately 120. However, ECT patients with severe depression are typically sedentary, elderly, and often unable to tolerate even minimal physical activity. Many would be unable to complete a treadmill test; more expensive tests, such as a persantine thallium stress test, can be substituted when appropriate.

Establishing a working relationship with a cardiologist is an essential part of developing an ECT service. Often the consulting cardiologist is asked to "clear a patient for ECT" without understanding exactly what effects ECT would have on the patient's cardiovascular system. A significant acute risk to the patient undergoing ECT is the potential for a cardiovascular event, and optimizing the management of cardiovascular disease before and during ECT can decrease this risk. Inviting the consulting cardiologist to observe the ECT procedure and including the cardiologist in discussions with both the patient and the family help ensure that all the involved parties make informed decisions regarding the relative risk–benefit ratio of the procedure.

Finally, informed consent should be obtained from all patients before ECT. Patients deemed to be incompetent may require the appointment of a legal guardian for consent. States vary in the legal regulations governing the use of involuntary ECT.

Medications Used During ECT

Patients should have nothing by mouth the night before their treatment and should limit the number of medications, and water needed to swallow the medications, on the morning of ECT to cardiac medications (except lidocaine), pulmonary medications (except theophylline), and glaucoma medications (except cholinesterase inhibitors, e.g., echothiophate). Given that the patient's oral intake is restricted, clinicians should also consider withholding any diuretics until after the treatment depending on the patient's cardiac status.

It is recommended that theophylline be discontinued and inhalers substituted and brought to the ECT suite to be given immediately prior to the treatment. Theophylline has been associated with status epilepticus during ECT (Devanand et al. 1988). A case review of ECT use in patients with asthma was recently published, noting its overall good safety (Mueller et al. 2006). Patients with glaucoma who are receiving echothiophate should be switched to another medication because echothiophate can potentially interact with succinylcholine and prolong the apneic period. The same is potentially true for the cholinesterase inhibitors used to treat Alzheimer's disease—tacrine, donepezil, rivastigmine, and galantamine—although there are no data to determine whether this interaction is clinically significant. In fact, a preliminary study reported the successful and safe use of donepezil to mitigate cognitive side effects associated with ECT (Prakash et al. 2006).

In diabetic patients, hypoglycemic medications are usually withheld on the morning of treatment to minimize the risk of hypoglycemia in a patient who is taking nothing by mouth. The patient's blood sugar level should be checked before ECT, and hyperglycemia or hypoglycemia should be treated appropriately. An ECT treatment will result in a modest short-term increase in the patient's blood sugar. In general, patients with epilepsy or mania should continue taking their anticonvulsants during ECT. If difficulty arises in eliciting seizures, decreasing the dose of the anticonvulsant can be considered. Lunde et al. (2006) recently summarized reports of ECT use in persons with epilepsy and recommendations for its safe use in this population.

In the past, it was recommended in the United States that all psychotropic medications be discontinued prior to beginning ECT. In other countries, it is common practice to continue using antidepressants during ECT (Royal College of Psychiatrists 1995). Available data are mixed regarding the use of antidepressants concurrently with ECT. Previous studies in the 1950s and 1960s suggested a possible better response to ECT in patients receiving tricyclic antidepressants (Dunlop 1960; Kay et al. 1970; Sargant 1961). Later studies also suggested that the response to ECT may be superior when combined with tricyclic antidepressant use but not with the use of SSRIs (Lauritzen et

al. 1996; Nelson and Benjamin 1989). Further research is needed to clarify this issue. When neuroleptic agents are necessary to control agitation or psychotic symptoms, a high-potency neuroleptic or an atypical antipsychotic medication is preferable to minimize any hypotension that may develop during ECT. Antipsychotics are generally continued during ECT treatment of persons with primary psychotic disorder (e.g., schizophrenia or schizoaffective disorder).

Concerns have been raised over whether MAOIs can be used safely with anesthesia. Although some clinicians still recommend caution and a 7- to 14-day washout period before proceeding with ECT, extensive reported experience with MAOIs and ECT has documented few significant problems (American Psychiatric Association Task Force on Electroconvulsive Therapy 2001; Dolenc et al. 2004).

Lithium usually is discontinued at least 48 hours before ECT because a potentially increased risk of delirium and cognitive impairment during ECT has been reported with its use (Ahmed and Stein 1987; Small 1990; Small et al. 1980). In more recent studies, however, the use of lithium was not associated with increased confusion in acute (Jha et al. 1996; Mukherjee 1993) or maintenance (J. T. Stewart 2000) ECT.

Benzodiazepines can interfere with the induction of a seizure during ECT, thereby decreasing the efficacy of the treatments (Jha and Stein 1996). As a result, benzodiazepine doses should be reduced to the lowest possible or eliminated before ECT. Patients taking benzodiazepines should be receiving a stable dose for 24–48 hours before ECT in order to reduce the risk of prolonged seizures or status epilepticus during ECT. Flumazenil, a competitive benzodiazepine antagonist, at a dose of 0.4–0.5 mg, has been effective in maintaining seizures without decreasing efficacy in patients who could not be withdrawn from benzodiazepines prior to ECT (Krystal et al. 1998).

ECT Administration

ECT sessions usually are scheduled for the morning. The patient's bladder should be emptied before treatment. Patients should not eat or drink for at least 6–8 hours before receiving the treatment. Famotidine or ranitidine is given the night before and the morning of ECT to neutralize the patient's gastric contents. Alternatively, sodium citrate can be given the morning of the treatment and will have an effect within 5–10 minutes. The ECT treatment team consists of a psychiatrist, an anesthesiologist (or nurse anesthetist), and a nursing team that is specially trained in ECT. The ECT treatment area should have resuscitative equipment available in case a medical emergency arises.

The historically standard anesthetic agent is methohexital, a short-acting barbiturate with minimal anticonvulsant effects. Methohexital is given in a dose of approximately 0.75–1.0 mg/kg; one alternative is propofol, given in a dose of approximately 0.75–1.50 mg/kg. Methohexital has been used more commonly because of its effectiveness and safety record. Concerns regarding the use of propofol include that it induces shorter seizures than methohexital—with propofol, some patients will not achieve a seizure lasting more than 20 seconds—and increases the number of missed seizures (i.e., delivery of an electrical stimulus without induction of a seizure) (Swaim et al. 2006). However, seizure duration has not been correlated with clinical efficacy, and trials comparing the use of methohexital versus propofol have not shown significant differences in the antidepressive efficacy of ECT (Avramov et al. 1995) based on the anesthetic agent.

Etomidate (0.15–0.3 mg/kg) can be used instead of propofol and is associated with significantly longer seizures (Bergsholm et al. 1996; Stadtland et al. 2002) and, in one retrospective naturalistic study, was associated with a significantly shorter treatment course (Swaim et al. 2006). Another strategy that is suggested by the results of one small randomized trial is to use remifentanil, an ultrafast-acting opioid that is used to induce and maintain anesthesia, in addition to propofol. That study found that adding remifentanil had no adverse anesthetic or cardiovascular effects and patients receiving the combination anesthesia had significantly longer seizures than those receiving propofol alone (Vishne et al. 2005).

Immediately after the patient is anesthetized, a muscle relaxant is administered intravenously. Succinylcholine, at doses of 0.75–1.50 mg/kg, is a widely used depolarizing blocking agent. In patients with musculoskeletal disease, a nondepolarizing agent can be considered. Anticholinergic agents, such as atropine or glycopyrrolate, are used to prevent ECT-induced bradycardia and to minimize airway secretions. Glycopyrrolate does not cross the blood–brain barrier and therefore may be associated with less postictal confusion than atropine in the elderly. An anticholinergic agent always should be used in conjunction with a β-blocker to control the ECT-induced rise in blood pressure and heart rate. Atropine (0.4–1.0 mg) or glycopyrrolate (0.2–0.4 mg) can be given either intramuscularly 30 minutes before the ECT treatment or intravenously at the time of treatment.

The choice of electrode placement was discussed previously (see "Integrating the Science of Stimulus Dosing With the Choice of Electrode Placement"). Regardless of the electrode placement selected, meticulous care should be taken to ensure that the electrodes are properly applied. The scalp should be cleansed and prepared with a saline solution and conductive gel. The electrodes should be adequately spaced to prevent excess shunting of the electrical stimulus and to prevent skin burns. With bilateral ECT, electrodes are placed frontotemporally, with the center of each electrode approximately 1 inch (2.54 cm) above the center of an imaginary line, the endpoints of which are the tragus of the ear and the external canthus of the eye. With unilateral ECT, d'Elia electrode placement is the safest and most effective placement (R.D. Weiner and Coffey 1986). In this technique, one electrode is placed over the nondominant frontotemporal area, and the other electrode is placed high on the nondominant centroparietal scalp, just lateral to the midline vertex. The treating physician may choose to either titrate the first seizure stimulus dose or use fixed-dose ECT.

The patient is oxygenated by positive-pressure ventilation from the onset of anesthesia until spontaneous respiration is resumed. In addition, the patient is monitored with a pulse oximeter and should have his or her blood pressure and heart rate continuously monitored. Before the electrical stimulus is administered, a rubber bite block is inserted into the patient's mouth.

Regarding dosing of the electrical stimulus, the titration or *method-of-limits* approach uses a table with incremental increases in the electrical energy to determine the minimal amount of energy necessary to produce a seizure of at least 25 seconds as monitored by electroencephalography. Typically, a seizure lasting 30–90 seconds occurs during treatment. Seizures lasting longer than 3 minutes should be terminated by administering an anticonvulsant (e.g., a second dose of methohexital or a benzodiazepine). Inflating a blood pressure cuff on the right ankle before the muscle relaxant is administered allows the clinician to monitor the motor manifestations of the seizure. Patients usually are alert and oriented 20–45 minutes after receiving an ECT treatment.

If no seizure is elicited by the electrical stimulus, a detailed reevaluation should be performed. Often, immediately re-treating the patient with a higher stimulus charge is effective in producing a seizure. Medication use should be reviewed, and anticonvulsant and benzodiazepine doses should be reduced or discontinued, before subsequent ECT treatments. In situations that do not allow the reduction of benzodiazepine doses, flumazenil, a benzodiazepine antagonist, can be used to help produce seizures.[1] Reducing the methohexital dose to the lowest effective level and using vigorous hyperventilation are other relatively easy steps that can be taken to aid in producing a seizure. Some patients who are sensitive to pain at the intravenous site (particularly when an intravenous line is inserted in a small peripheral vein) may be given intravenous lidocaine as a local anesthetic just prior to administering general anesthesia; if possible, however, lidocaine should be omitted because it can shorten the seizure length. If these methods are not effective, switching methohexital to etomidate, which should have less of an effect on the seizure threshold, may be considered (Bergsholm et al. 1996; Folk et al. 2000; Stadtland et al. 2002).

Caffeine sodium benzoate (usual dose, 120–140 mg) may be administered intravenously during ECT to maintain adequate seizure duration (Coffey et al. 1987). Caffeine appears to lengthen seizure duration during ECT without lowering the seizure threshold (McCall et al. 1993a). At present, it is not known whether caffeine augments the antidepressive effects of ECT or increases the speed of response to ECT. Theoretically, caffeine would have little therapeutic effect on unilateral ECT because the length of the seizure is less important than the degree to which the seizure stimulus exceeds the seizure threshold. Caffeine use during ECT should be reserved for patients who are having short seizures during ECT and who cannot tolerate higher stimulus doses.

Conversely, if the seizure is too long (>180 seconds), the seizure can be terminated using additional intravenous methohexital, propofol, or midazolam. Seizure length is inversely correlated with age and is particularly longer in young women. Propofol can be used as the anesthetic agent to shorten the seizure length (Bailine et al. 2003).

Frequency and Number of Treatments

The American Psychiatric Association Task Force on Electroconvulsive Therapy (2001) recommends that an ECT course be completed when a plateau in response occurs. No convincing data support that additional treatments beyond this point reduce the rate of relapse after ECT (Barton et al. 1973). In addition, the Task Force recommendations imply that rather than having clinicians predetermine the number of ECT sessions, the patient's clinical status during the course of ECT should dictate the number of treatments given.

Shapira et al. (2000) have shown that ECT administered twice weekly is as effective as treatments administered three times a week. One advantage of a more frequent treatment schedule is a faster rate of response. On the other hand, a disadvantage is the potential development of cognitive side effects. Given these observations, it is recommended that the frequency of ECT treatments be tailored to the individual patient's needs. For example, a patient with a life-threatening illness will benefit from a faster rate of response and should be given more frequent treatments. In patients for whom the risk of cognitive side effects from ECT is a particular concern (e.g., those with Alzheimer's disease, Parkinson's disease, or severe frontal lobe or caudate hyperintensities shown on a brain MRI scan, as well as those receiving outpatient or bilateral ECT), a less frequent ECT treatment schedule is certainly a reasonable choice.

Management of ECT-Related Side Effects

Postictal Agitation

Postictal agitation can be a significant practical problem in ECT, with the potential for causing injury to both the patient and the nursing staff caring for the patient (Augoustides et al. 2002). Postictal agitation is difficult to predict in an individual patient but is likely to reoccur if it occurs with the initial treatment. Postictal agitation must be differentiated from status epilepticus and is clearly distinguished by the random flailing movements of the patient in contrast to the rhythmic convulsions of a seizure and by the fact that the patient does not lose consciousness or demonstrate the fixed gaze of a patient experiencing a grand mal seizure.

Several strategies exist for treating postictal agitation, and most involve intravenous access. Midazolam or methohexital will often sedate the patient and can be very effective. Additionally, propofol can be used to manage postictal agitation (O'Reardon et al. 2006). Intravenous haloperidol has been associated with ventricular ec-

---

[1] When flumazenil is administered to counter benzodiazepine use, it should be given immediately after seizure induction because the patient may experience sudden symptoms of benzodiazepine withdrawal. After the seizure has terminated, intravenous midazolam should be given because flumazenil has a longer half-life than methohexital and the patient may experience withdrawal on emergence from the anesthesia.

topy (Greene et al. 2000) and should only be used in patients with cardiac monitors. The intramuscular atypical antipsychotic medications can be just as effective, with a more benign cardiac profile.

Preventive measures can also be taken, including additional preoperative medication and changing the way ECT is administered to reduce the chance of postictal agitation in future treatments. First, the use of a dissolvable atypical antipsychotic medication such as olanzapine or risperidone 5–10 minutes prior to ECT can be very effective and does not require administration of any additional liquids. Second, current drug use should be reviewed. Lithium has been associated with postictal agitation (el-Mallakh 1988) and should be discontinued throughout the ECT course or withheld the night and morning of ECT treatments. Carbidopa has also been associated with postictal delirium and should be withheld the morning of ECT treatment (Nymeyer and Grossberg 1997). Postictal agitation may be associated with increased serum lactate levels, and some have argued that increasing the succinylcholine dose to decrease ictal muscle activity and subsequent rises in serum lactate levels can decrease postictal agitation (Auriacombe et al. 2000). Another strategy may therefore be to increase the succinylcholine dose if any muscle movement is present during the seizure. However, care should be taken because another potential cause of postictal agitation is the patient awakening from anesthesia with latent paralysis of the respiratory muscles. Patients describe this as frightening and may question continuing ECT.

The data on the effect of switching from bilateral to unilateral ECT in order to decrease postictal agitation are unclear (Augoustides et al. 2002); the success of this approach is probably dependent on several factors including ECT dosage and the patient's age.

Interictal Delirium

Interictal delirium develops during a course of ECT and persists on days when the patient does not receive a treatment. This side effect is observed primarily in elderly patients and increases in incidence with advancing age (Figiel et al. 1990). ECT-induced interictal delirium is associated with prolonged hospitalization and an increased risk of falls. Among the elderly, additional risk factors for interictal delirium are 1) Parkinson's disease, 2) Alzheimer's disease, 3) one or more cardiovascular risk factors, and 4) preexisting structural changes in the caudate nucleus observed on brain scans. Patients who develop postictal confusion are likely to have greater retrograde am-

nesia in the weeks and months after ECT (Sobin et al. 1995).

The incidence of delirium during a course of ECT can vary dramatically depending on the ECT technique used. As a rule, ECT-induced interictal delirium is a short-lived, reversible side effect if identified early. Once it has been identified, ECT treatments should be withheld until the delirium resolves. Subsequent treatments should be administered less frequently and/or at a lower electrical charge.

Cardiovascular Side Effects

ECT is associated with an increased risk of cardiovascular complications in elderly patients who have, or who are at risk for, cardiovascular disease. Studies have found widely varying rates of cardiac complications in the elderly receiving ECT. The retrospective design of the studies, the lack of continuous cardiovascular monitoring, and the different definitions of what constitutes a cardiac complication probably account for the discrepancies in the results. Despite the inconsistencies, most studies have found a correlation between cardiac complications and age. ECT often produces transient systemic hypertension and abrupt transitions in cardiac rate, which can result in myocardial ischemia or arrhythmias. The increased incidence of cardiac complications among elderly patients is probably associated with the increased rate of preexisting cardiac conditions such as hypertension, coronary artery disease, and arrhythmias. On the basis of these observations, several authors have recommended the use of prophylactic cardiac medications to dampen cardiovascular responses during ECT in elderly patients who have (or are at risk for) cardiovascular disease.

Research has now documented that labetalol (a medication with both α- and β-adrenergic–blocking activity), esmolol (a shorter-acting β-blocker), and nifedipine (a calcium channel–blocking agent with vasodilating effects) can be safely used to attenuate the cardiac response during ECT (Cattan et al. 1990; Figiel et al. 1994; McCall et al. 1991; Stoudemire et al. 1990; Zielinski et al. 1993). Nicardipine (a shorter-acting calcium channel blocker) is routinely substituted for nifedipine because it can be given intravenously and has a shorter half-life.

It is recommended that adequate doses of an anticholinergic medication (intravenous atropine or glycopyrrolate) be used to prevent bradycardia whenever β-blockers are used during ECT. To help prevent ECT-induced hypotension, it is additionally recommended that all patients be adequately hydrated before undergoing ECT. If patients experience significant orthostatic hypotension in the recovery room, labetalol can be switched to the shorter-acting pure β-blocker esmolol.

The anesthetic agent propofol has been shown to have lesser cardiovascular effects than methohexital and can be used in patients with preexisting cardiac conditions requiring an attenuated hemodynamic response during treatment (Bailine et al. 2003). As noted earlier, the trade-off is a shortening of the seizure length with the use of propofol (see "ECT Administration" subsection).

Cognitive Side Effects

The greatest area of concern about ECT among the lay public, patients, and their families is the potential development of adverse cerebral and cognitive changes. The medical community's concerns about cognitive side effects and the negative images of ECT in the media also are important factors in determining the availability of ECT. The technique by which ECT is administered determines the incidence and severity of cognitive side effects that may develop during a course of ECT. Specifically, electrode placement, the type of electrical waveform, the intensity of the electrical stimulus, and the frequency of ECT sessions determine the type and severity of cognitive side effects from ECT. Preexisting structural brain changes and medical illness, advancing age, and concomitant administration of certain psychotropic medications also may be factors. It is important to recognize that depression itself (especially late-life depression) often causes cognitive deficits, such that successful treatment of depression with ECT may actually improve some aspects of cognition in certain patients. Hihn et al. (2006) showed that prefrontally mediated aspects of cognition, such as attention and immediate encoding, improved during ECT treatment of depression, whereas long-term memory functions remained impaired.

The memory loss attributed to ECT is typically anterograde and retrograde and has a temporal gradient, being more profound around the time of treatment and continuing several weeks after the ECT course (American Psychiatric Association Task Force on Electroconvulsive Therapy 2001; Sackeim 2000). The retrograde memory loss extends to months before the treatment. In most patients the anterograde memory loss clears quickly after ECT, but the retrograde memory loss can be permanent in some patients and may even extend to years before the ECT. Clearly, the degree of amnesia incurred during a course of ECT is greater with bilateral ECT than with unilateral ECT (Lisanby et al. 2000) and increases

with the number of treatments administered and the stimulus intensity (Sackeim et al. 2000). Although unilateral ECT is associated with fewer memory problems, the cognitive deficits that occur show a dose relationship and increase as the stimulus dose is increased to 8–12 times the seizure threshold (McCall et al. 2000). Research comparing bilateral and unilateral ECT has not addressed the important question of whether right-unilateral ECT given at a dose of 10–12 times the seizure threshold would cause more cognitive side effects than bilateral ECT that is minimally above or 1.5 times the seizure threshold.

Sine wave stimulus produces greater amnestic deficits than does a brief- or ultrabrief-pulse stimulus. Furthermore, Sackeim et al. (1991, 1993) reported that within a specific waveform, the magnitude by which an electrical dose exceeds the seizure threshold (rather than the absolute electrical dose) is related to the severity of cognitive defects that develop during ECT. In a prospective, naturalistic longitudinal study of cognitive outcomes in depressed patients treated with ECT at seven facilities in the New York City metropolitan area (Sackeim et al. 2007), sine wave stimulation resulted in pronounced slowing of reaction time, both immediately and 6 months following ECT. As expected, bilateral ECT resulted in more severe and persistent retrograde amnesia than right-unilateral ECT. The researchers found that several clinical variables also were associated with post-ECT memory problems, including older age, lower premorbid intellectual function, and female sex. In addition, Shapira et al. (2000) reported that twice-weekly treatments produced less cognitive impairment than did treatments administered three times a week.

The causes of the memory disturbance associated with ECT are thus multifactorial and likely include the effects of anesthetic drugs, electrode placement, stimulus waveform, generalized seizures, and electrical dose (Sackeim et al. 2007). Progress in understanding the neural mechanisms underlying memory makes it possible to consider how neurotransmitter changes might contribute to ECT-induced memory dysfunction. Muscarinic cholinergic receptors participate in some forms of memory, and antimuscarinic drugs are associated with memory impairment in humans (Krueger et al. 1992). In animals, the effects of ECS on central muscarinic systems have been variable (Fochtmann 1994). However, some studies suggest that ECS treatments diminish muscarinic binding in the cortex and hippocampus. Twenty-four hours after a series of ECS-induced seizures, decreases in levels of mRNA for M_1 and M_3 muscarinic receptors are seen in the hippocampus, although mRNA levels are significantly higher 28 days after the last seizure (Mingo et al. 1998). Other studies indicate that behavioral responses to muscarinic agonists are diminished after ECS and that brain choline acetyltransferase and acetylcholine levels are decreased (Nutt and Glue 1993). These findings suggest that alterations in muscarinic neurotransmission may contribute to memory impairment.

Long-term, use-dependent plasticity of glutamatergic synapses appears to play a major role in memory processing in the CNS, and disruption of this plasticity could contribute to anterograde amnesia. The term *long-term potentiation* (LTP) typically refers to a persistent enhancement of glutamate-mediated transmission that follows repeated high-frequency synapse use, and LTP is a potential synaptic memory mechanism. Repeated ECS treatments disrupt the induction of LTP and produce memory impairment in animals (Anwyl et al. 1987; C. Stewart and Reid 1993), suggesting a possible tie to anterograde memory problems.

Several ECS-induced changes, including effects on muscarinic and adrenergic neurotransmission, could contribute to the disruption of LTP. The enhanced inhibition that may contribute to the anticonvulsant effects of ECT could play a role because these inhibitory systems modulate efficacy at glutamatergic synapses. The release of glutamate during a seizure may also contribute to memory impairment. In many CNS regions, the induction of LTP depends on NMDA receptors. However, untimely activation of NMDA receptors before delivery of a stimulus that usually induces LTP results in LTP inhibition, a process broadly referred to as *metaplasticity*. Metaplasticity may result from activation of certain intercellular messengers, such as nitric oxide, or from the activation of phosphatases that alter the phosphorylation of key synaptic proteins (Zorumski and Izumi 1993). Longer-term effects of ECS on basal synaptic transmission or NMDA receptor function could also contribute to memory impairment (Petrie et al. 2000). To date, there is little clinical evidence favoring any of these mechanisms in ECT-induced memory impairment, although several avenues are worth pursuing. There is some interesting evidence that verbal memory improves when an anesthetic agent that blocks NMDA receptors, ketamine, is used rather than etomidate, a GABAergic anesthetic (Krystal et al. 2003; McDaniel et al. 2006). There is also evidence that propofol, an agent that enhances GABAergic transmission but also partially inhibits NMDA receptors at anesthetic concentrations, may have beneficial effects on memory following ECT compared with thiopental (Butterfield et al. 2004).

Effects on Cerebral Physiology

Immediately after an ECT treatment, the EEG shows generalized slowing of brain wave activity. This slowing tends to increase and persist longer after successive treatments. After a course of ECT is completed, slow-wave activity gradually decreases, and EEGs show a reversion to baseline activity within 3 months (R.D. Weiner et al. 1986). Rarely, electroencephalographic abnormalities may persist for more than 3 months. Prior electroencephalographic abnormalities may increase the risk for developing prolonged abnormalities after ECT, but the clinical significance of these abnormalities is unknown.

Electrically induced seizures in animals and humans have been shown to produce transient increases in permeability of the blood–brain barrier (Laursen et al. 1991). These findings are consistent with a brain MRI study in which increased T1 relaxation times were observed after ECT (A.I. Scott et al. 1990). Laursen et al. (1991) reported that the ECT-induced increase in blood–brain barrier permeability is associated with increased stimulus intensity and an increased number of ECT treatments. In addition, Bolwig et al. (1977) were able to reduce changes in blood–brain barrier permeability during ECT by blocking ECT-induced hypertensive response with high-spinal anesthesia. Because a disturbed blood–brain barrier may predispose some patients to ECT-induced neurological complications, research is needed to examine the ways that ECT-induced changes in blood–brain barrier permeability can be minimized, such as by attenuating the ECT-induced cardiovascular response or by reducing the amount of the stimulus charge.

The combination of increased carbon dioxide production, decreased pH, and systemic hypertension that occurs with ECS treatment can cause the cerebral blood flow to increase to 300% of baseline measurements and the cerebral metabolic rate to increase by 200% (Ingvar 1986). The transient increase in cerebral blood flow results in a sharp rise in both intracranial and intraocular pressure (Maltbie et al. 1980). Both the cerebral blood flow (Saito et al. 1995) and the cerebral metabolic rate (Ackermann et al. 1986) return to baseline values during the postictal period. Methods that limit the accumulation of carbon dioxide in the bloodstream, such as forced hyperventilation, or that attenuate the increase in blood pressure tend to diminish the rise in intracranial pressure associated with ECT.

Does ECT Cause Brain Damage?

Human autopsy studies of patients who have received ECT have shown no convincing evidence of irreversible brain damage when ECT was administered with current techniques (Devanand et al. 1994; R.D. Weiner 1984). These findings are supported by a brain MRI study in which no significant structural brain changes were found immediately or 6 months after the completion of ECT (Coffey et al. 1991). In a study of six depressed patients, cerebrospinal fluid markers of neuronal/glial degeneration (τ protein, neurofilament, and S-100 β protein) were measured before and after a successful course of ECT and showed no biochemical evidence of neuronal/glial damage or blood–brain barrier dysfunction (Zachrisson et al. 2000).

Minor Complications

Patients often report nausea and headaches after ECT; these complaints usually are easily treated and do not appear to be related to electrode placement or stimulus dose (Devanand et al. 1995). The exact incidence of nausea is not known; estimates indicate that approximately one-quarter of patients complain of some nausea (Gomez 1975). Treatments for nausea include prochlorperazine, metoclopramide, and ondansetron. If effective, they can be given prior to ECT on subsequent treatments. The anesthetic propofol can also be substituted for etomidate or methohexital to reduce post-ECT nausea and vomiting (Bailine et al. 2003).

The incidence of ECT-induced headaches is also unknown; however, some estimates are that up to 45% of patients have headaches after ECT (Devanand et al. 1995; S.J. Weiner et al. 1994). Acetaminophen or nonsteroidal anti-inflammatory agents, including intravenous ketorolac, usually are effective. The etiology of the ECT headache is unclear, but a vascular process (S.J. Weiner et al. 1994) has been suggested, and sumatriptan can also be effective (Fantz et al. 1998). Patients who have a history of migraine headaches should be given their migraine medication before ECT; prophylactic treatment with these agents immediately prior to the ECT treatment usually is effective in reducing the severity of post-ECT headaches.

Prophylactic Somatic Treatment After Acute Response to ECT

Although the short-term therapeutic benefits of ECT are clearly established, the 6-month relapse rate after ECT to treat depression remains high (Bourgon and Kellner 2000). The debate over appropriate prophylactic treatment for patients with an acute response to ECT has focused on the clinical decision to either continue therapy with antidepressant medications or initiate maintenance ECT. Confusion in this area persists because of the lack of controlled studies comparing the efficacy of antidepressants with that of maintenance ECT.

Most study designs have been naturalistic. O'Leary and Lee (1996) evaluated the 7-year mortality and hospital readmission rates in the Nottingham ECT cohort of patients hospitalized for major depression and found that the risk of death was double the risk in the general population, and the probability of not being readmitted was 0.79 at 16 weeks and only 0.27 over the 7-year follow-up period. Delusions were the most important clinical characteristic predicting relapse. Two studies (Aronson et al. 1987; Spiker et al. 1985) evaluated adult patients after an acute course of ECT for psychotic depression and found a combined relapse rate of 68% ($n=53$) at 1 year. Spiker et al. (1985) reported a 1-year relapse rate of 50% in patients with delusional depression who initially responded to an acute course of ECT. Aronson et al. (Aronson et al. 1987) followed patients with delusional depression who had responded to either medication or ECT and found that 80% of the medication-responsive patients and 95% of the ECT-responsive patients relapsed in the first year after hospitalization. These studies did not compare the adequacy of the initial (pre-ECT) medication trial or the continuation medication trial.

In a prospective, naturalistic study of 347 depressed patients at seven hospitals, Prudic et al. (2004) found that between 30% and 47% of patients met criteria for remission at the end of their acute course of ECT. In the 24-week follow-up period, 64% of remitters relapsed. Among those patients who did not achieve remission during the acute course, only 23% had sustained remission during the 6-month follow-up period.

Sackeim et al. (1990) followed 58 patients for 1 year after ECT and found a differential relapse rate of 64% in those with major depression (with and without psychotic features) in whom an adequate pre-ECT medication trial had failed. In contrast, the relapse rate in patients who did not receive an adequate pre-ECT antidepressant trial was only 32%. Other clinical and demographic factors, including the presence of delusions, were not significant in predicting relapse. The adequacy of the post-ECT maintenance medication did not correlate with relapse rates. However, as in the studies cited above, maintenance medications post-ECT were not standardized, and evaluation of the pre-ECT medication trial was retrospective.

The conclusion of this study is intuitively appealing: Patients whose symptoms do not respond to antidepressant medication before ECT are those most likely to relapse with maintenance medication. With relapse occurring in almost two-thirds of such patients within 1 year after ECT, the relapse rate is alarmingly high.

In a prospective, randomized, double-blind trial, Sackeim et al. (2001a) compared three maintenance strategies: placebo, nortriptyline (target steady-state level, 75–125 ng/mL), and nortriptyline plus lithium (target steady-state level, 0.5–0.9 mEq/L). Over the 24-week trial, the depression relapse rate was 84% with placebo, 60% with nortriptyline, and 39% with nortriptyline plus lithium, indicating a statistically significant advantage for combination therapy. In another prospective study, Shapira et al. (1995) found that patients who responded to an acute course of ECT and subsequently received maintenance therapy with lithium for 6 months had a relapse rate of only 36%. Of the 22 patients, the 8 who relapsed did so in the first 13 weeks. Several clinical factors were associated with relapse; these included a shorter duration of the index depressive episode, an additional depressive episode in the 12 months prior to ECT, and, again, failure of an adequate trial of antidepressant therapy before the ECT course.

Lauritzen et al. (1996) randomly assigned patients with major depression who were receiving ECT to also receive either paroxetine 30 mg, imipramine 150 mg, or placebo and to continue the medication treatment after they had responded to ECT. In the continuation phase of the study, paroxetine was superior to both imipramine and placebo in preventing relapse: 65% of the placebo recipients relapsed, compared with 30% of the patients treated with imipramine and 10% of the patients treated with paroxetine.

The elderly are particularly prone to increased disability from depression and form a substantial proportion of patients in an acute ECT program. Data from naturalistic studies confirm that the relapse rates for elderly patients treated with ECT are high. These rates have varied from 21% within 6 months (Karlinsky and Shulman 1984) to 50% (10 of 20 patients) within 1 year (Murphy 1983). A naturalistic study that followed 94 patients over 3 years after an acute course of ECT noted a rehospitalization rate of 44% (Stoudemire et al. 1994). Of the 10 patients in the Murphy study who did not relapse within 1 year, 1 developed dementia and 4 died; thus, only 5 of the 20 elderly patients were well 1 year after ECT. These studies indicate that the elderly are at risk for relapse after acute ECT. However, two small studies in adolescent popula-

tions showed that younger patients also have high relapse rates: 40% within 1 year (D. Cohen et al. 1997) and 38% within 3 years (Moise and Petrides 1996).

Studies, primarily in the 1980s, have focused on finding a biological marker that would predict relapses after ECT; the possible markers included nonsuppression of cortisol in response to a challenge dose of dexamethasone (in the dexamethasone suppression test, or DST), blunted thyrotropin response to thyrotropin-releasing hormone (TRH; in the TRH stimulation test), and shortened rapid eye movement latency on a sleep EEG. These studies had many methodological flaws, including the fact that most of the studies were retrospective reviews, had nonblinded raters and a small number of subjects, and used nonstandardized follow-up treatment after ECT. Given these limitations, preliminary evidence suggests that patients who continue to show a biological marker consistent with depression after responding to ECT (e.g., a positive DST result) are at increased risk for relapse. In Bourgon and Kellner's (2000) review, six of the nine studies in which the DST was used, two of the four studies in which the TRH test was used, and the one sleep study in which shortened rapid eye movement latency was used showed that persistent abnormalities in these biological markers after ECT are predictive of relapse.

Continuation/Maintenance ECT

The high relapse rates of depression in patients receiving antidepressant medications after a successful course of ECT have led clinicians to use alternative therapies, such as continuation/maintenance ECT, in patients who are at high risk for recurrence of their mood disorder. *Continuation ECT* is defined as ECT for up to 6 months after the acute ECT course (i.e., aimed at relapse prevention). Continuation ECT is differentiated from *maintenance ECT*, which is defined as ECT that continues for more than 6 months after the initial course (i.e., aimed at recurrence prevention). In this chapter, the term *prophylactic ECT* is used to refer to any ECT treatments given as continuation or maintenance therapy. Many of the studies reviewed here do not differentiate patients receiving continuation ECT from those receiving maintenance ECT, although treatment indications, side effects, and outcomes may be different for the two types of prophylactic ECT.

According to clinical guidelines, candidates for prophylactic ECT include patients who have recurring affective episodes that are responsive to ECT and/or who are resistant to, intolerant of, or noncompliant with antidepressant medications (American Psychiatric Association

Task Force on Electroconvulsive Therapy 2001). Prophylactic ECT strategies are increasingly being used to treat major depression and bipolar disorder in patients thought to be at high risk for relapse. A 1985 survey of private psychiatric hospitals showed that 64% of the hospitals that provided ECT also provided prophylactic ECT (Levy and Albrecht 1985). Kramer (1987) found a similar pattern of use in a survey of ECT practitioners, with 59% of the 86 respondents using prophylactic ECT, primarily for recurrent depression.

Several theories have been advanced to explain the potential effectiveness of prophylactic ECT versus medication:

1. Bourne and Long (1954) suggested that patients with psychotic depression may become "convulsion dependent" such that they need to be tapered from ECT to prevent relapse.
2. Prophylactic ECT has a different mechanism of action than antidepressants, and patients with medication-resistant illness do respond to an acute course of ECT. The corollary is that patients who respond preferentially to ECT may have lower relapse rates with prophylactic ECT than with medication.
3. Prophylactic ECT may not provide a better therapeutic benefit than medication at all. Rather, the benefit may be the result of better treatment compliance in the groups receiving ECT than in those receiving maintenance medication.

Most reports of relapse rates in patients receiving prophylactic ECT include only those patients who were compliant and presented for their treatments. As Clarke et al. (1989) pointed out, when patients receiving continuation ECT do not complete 6 months of treatment, relapse rates approach the 50% rate seen in patients receiving maintenance medication. Thus, future studies of ECT need to include both compliant and noncompliant patients in their outcome measures.

A recent case study of an elderly woman with recurrent psychotic depression receiving maintenance ECT showed a correlation between resolution of cerebral hypoperfusion and a treatment response to her depressive symptoms (Suzuki et al. 2006). At baseline, the patient demonstrated anterior cerebral hypoperfusion on single photon emission computed tomography (SPECT), which did not change 12 days after the first course of ECT. After the acute ECT course she continued to have residual depressive symptoms. Two weeks later she experienced a relapse, but her condition improved again after a second

course of acute ECT. The hypoperfusion improved after the second course of ECT and resolved completely after 2 years of maintenance ECT. This case report is particularly interesting given the data by Prudic et al. (2004) demonstrating the relationship between residual depressive symptoms and relapse. Another case study, of two patients, found that cerebral blood flow and metabolic rates were no different than in control subjects prior to ECT, but that at the end of a successful continuation course of ECT, cerebral blood flow and metabolic activity in the prefrontal cortex had decreased (Conca et al. 2003), which is consistent with findings about changes in cerebral activity in response to an acute course of ECT (e.g., Nobler et al. 2001).

Most of the information on the use of prophylactic ECT has come from case reports and retrospective case series. The more recent studies have a naturalistic design with relatively few subjects, but they generally describe a marked decrease in the number of hospitalizations, the number of days spent in the hospital, and depressive symptoms; an increase in functional status; and stable cognitive functioning for the period of continuation ECT (Clarke et al. 1989; Decina et al. 1987; Fox 2001; Gagne et al. 2000; Kramer 1999; Russell et al. 2003; Thienhaus et al. 1990; Thornton et al. 1990). These positive results extend to elderly depressed patients (Dubin et al. 1992; H. Loo et al. 1991), patients with bipolar disorder (Husain et al. 1993; Nascimento et al. 2006; Sienaert and Peuskens 2006; Tsao et al. 2004; Vanelle et al. 1994), schizophrenic patients (Shimizu et al. 2007; Suzuki et al. 2006), and patients with Parkinson's disease (Faber and Trimble 1991; Shulman 2003). A moderately sized study of treatment-resistant schizophrenia patients who were responsive to acute treatment with a combination of ECT plus antipsychotic medication found that these individuals fared better with the combination of continuation ECT plus the antipsychotic medication than with either treatment alone (Chanpattana et al. 1999a).

In a prospective study, Clarke et al. (1989) used continuation ECT in 27 patients who received an acute course of ECT to treat major depression because of a history of medication intolerance or resistance. The rate of rehospitalization was six times lower (8%) in patients who completed a 5-month course of continuation ECT than in patients who did not complete the protocol (47%). Swoboda et al. (2001) prospectively followed 13 patients diagnosed with major depression and 8 patients who had schizoaffective disorder who were administered maintenance ECT and compared them with controls who received maintenance pharmacotherapy alone. The maintenance ECT group had a significantly lower rate of rehospitalization at 1 year than control subjects, although the schizoaffective patients had a poorer outcome overall than patients with major depression. The largest prospective study of continuation ECT to date included 184 patients who were randomly assigned to receive either maintenance pharmacotherapy with a combination of lithium and nortriptyline or continuation ECT for 6 months; both treatments had limited efficacy, with more than half of patients in each group either relapsing or dropping out of the study (Kellner et al. 2006). Although these results were disappointing, the efficacy of continuation ECT was being compared with that of the "gold standard" of nortriptyline and lithium, and both treatments were superior to placebo (using historical placebo controls) or follow-up with monotherapy. There are few other prospective studies and/or controlled trials of continuation or maintenance ECT.

Studies that have evaluated the side effects of maintenance ECT on memory are limited. A retrospective study of 18 patients receiving maintenance ECT for 3–10 months showed minimal memory side effects and an excellent clinical response (Abraham et al. 2006). Three patients (17%) had slightly impaired memory, which improved to normal, and one patient experienced severe memory problems in the third month and discontinued treatment. Another study found no difference in the neuropsychological functioning of 13 patients receiving maintenance pharmacotherapy and 11 patients receiving maintenance ECT after an acute course of ECT (Vothknecht et al. 2003). A telephone screening system for evaluating cognitive side effects of maintenance ECT has been proposed that successfully identified a patient with significant deficits the day after an ECT treatment (Datto et al. 2001). This type of monitoring would be practical for evaluating patients receiving maintenance ECT in both clinical and research settings.

Guidelines for the use of prophylactic ECT unfortunately remain vague, primarily because of the paucity of data on which to base guidelines. Monroe (1991) delineated the contradiction of the increasing use of prophylactic ECT and the lack of research defining the parameters of administering the treatments and their potential side effects and contraindications. More recently, the National Institute for Clinical Excellence (NICE) Technology Appraisal's "Guidance on the Use of Electroconvulsive Therapy" questioned the use of continuation and maintenance ECT because of the lack of empirical evidence. From their examination of the data, the authors concluded that ECT is "not recommended as a mainte-

nance therapy in depressive illness" (NICE 2003). Other researchers have challenged this conclusion, pointing out that the typical patient receiving continuation or maintenance ECT has chronic relapsing depression that has failed to respond to multiple medication trials (Frederikse et al. 2006). In fairness, it should be pointed out that the NICE report was published before the above-cited studies by Prudic et al. (2004) and Kellner et al. (2006), two prospective studies supporting the use of continuation ECT.

Patients Who May Benefit From Prophylactic ECT

Patients who receive prophylactic ECT after an acute course of ECT usually fall into one of three categories:

1. Patients whose illness has failed to respond to previous trials of medications and are therefore relatively medication resistant
2. Patients who are severely ill (e.g., psychotic or suicidal)
3. Patients who cannot tolerate the side effects of antidepressant medications, because of either concomitant medical illness or a personal sensitivity to antidepressants' side effects, or who are noncompliant with their medication

These groups overlap and include patients who, because of their own experience or the experiences of acquaintances or relatives, prefer ECT to the traditional somatic treatments.

Patients Who Have Failed to Respond to Previous Trials of Medication

A significant minority of patients with major depression are relatively medication resistant despite adequate medication trials (trials of antidepressants with adequate doses and length of treatment to elicit a response). Sackeim et al. (1990) noted that the most important factor in relapse after an acute course of ECT that enables a patient to achieve remission is whether the patient participated in an adequate medication trial prior to ECT. The relapse rate in the 6 months following ECT was found to be twofold higher in patients who had participated in an adequate medication trial than in those who had not (Sackeim et al. 1990). Shapira et al. (1995) also found that patients who had received adequate previous treatment with pharmacotherapy relapsed post-ECT (while receiving lithium maintenance therapy) at a significantly higher rate than did patients who had not received adequate prior medication. Interestingly, Grunhaus et al. (1990) reported a relapse rate of only 17% in patients in whom a previous medication trial had failed and who received up to 12 weeks of prophylactic ECT after a successful initial course of ECT.

Patients in whom an adequate medication trial failed before ECT was initiated should be informed of the risk of relapse and given the option of receiving continuation ECT for 6 months, followed by maintenance medication. The clinical decision of whether to continue ECT beyond 6 months should be made on an individual basis, weighing the risks (primarily the cognitive effects of ongoing ECT vs. the risk of suicide or recurrent psychosis if the patient relapses while taking medication) and benefits (the long-term effects of a period of mood stability).

Patients Who Are Severely Ill

Some researchers have found that the 1-year relapse rate in patients with psychotic depression treated with medication alone may be as high as 95% (Aronson et al. 1987; Spiker et al. 1985). Petrides et al. (1994) retrospectively examined the records of patients with delusional depression treated with prophylactic ECT and found the relapse rate at 1 year to be only 42%. They compared their findings with those from the study by Aronson et al. (1987). Both patient groups were drawn from the same institution, although prophylactic ECT was not available at the time that Aronson et al. (1987) reported relapse rates of 95% in patients with delusional depression who were taking antidepressants. Vanelle et al. (1994) prospectively administered maintenance ECT, often with concomitant antipsychotic medication, approximately once a month for 1 year to a group of patients with psychotic depression and found full or partial remission in 80% of the patients. Grunhaus et al. (1990) also found an excellent clinical response in patients with psychotic depression who were administered prophylactic ECT. Prophylactic ECT may therefore be a viable option in patients with delusional depression and should be discussed with these patients and their families.

Patients Who Cannot Tolerate the Side Effects of Antidepressant Medications or Who Are Noncompliant With Their Medication

Most patients who cannot tolerate the side effects of antidepressant medications because of either concomitant medical illness or a personal sensitivity to antidepressants' side effects can benefit from trying maintenance medication after a successful course of ECT. Many patients who are acutely ill may be extremely sensitive to

the side effects of medications but may tolerate the same medication once they have responded to acute treatment with ECT. Conditions associated with depression, such as malnutrition and dehydration, may worsen the orthostatic hypotension caused by tricyclic antidepressants. In a patient with agitated depression, minimal activation from the SSRIs may be experienced as extreme agitation. Once the depressive episode has remitted, patients usually can tolerate an additional trial of medication. Patients who are noncompliant with their antidepressant medication should be evaluated on an individual basis and, after discussions with the patient and the family, the risks and benefits of prophylactic ECT should be weighed against those of an additional medication trial.

Guidelines for Prophylactic ECT

Treatment Parameters

The electrode placement and dose parameters used in the initial course of ECT are maintained during continuation and maintenance ECT. Retrospective reviews have not found that stimulus placement affects the clinical outcome (Petrides et al. 1994), although no systematic studies have compared unilateral and bilateral placement in prophylactic ECT. Since seizure threshold can increase during acute treatment because of the frequency of treatments, the threshold would be expected to decrease during prophylactic ECT. In one small study the threshold was shown to decrease significantly when the treatments were separated by 60 days or more (Wild et al. 2004).

Few guidelines exist on what frequency of prophylactic ECT is optimal to maintain mood stability. The intervals between courses of continuation ECT in the studies reviewed vary from 3–5 weeks (H. Loo et al. 1991) to 4–8 weeks (Thienhaus et al. 1990). Other clinicians argue that treatments should be gradually tapered from once a week to once a month, depending on clinical response (Aronson et al. 1987; Clarke et al. 1989; Matzen et al. 1988). Kramer (1987) surveyed 51 clinicians in 24 states and found the frequency and duration of maintenance ECT to vary from as often as two treatments per week to once every 3–4 weeks for 30 months to one treatment every 6 months for 60 months to as long as 48 years. In Kramer's survey, clinicians described continuing ECT until the patient was asymptomatic for a predetermined period ranging from 1 month to 2 years.

Grunhaus et al. (1990) assessed individual patients' clinical histories and assigned them to receive either abbreviated continuation ECT (once or twice a week for 4–12 weeks) or full continuation ECT (gradually tapering

ECT frequency to once a month over 3 months and continuing ECT once a month for 6 months). Abbreviated continuation ECT was used when symptoms were unresponsive to medication after the index depressive episode and lasted more than 12 months, or when the patient relapsed after a successful course of ECT or had difficulties tolerating continuation pharmacotherapy. Full continuation ECT was used in patients who relapsed after a successful course of ECT despite adequate pharmacotherapy. Among 10 patients, these researchers found an excellent response in 6 (5 of 6 patients receiving abbreviated continuation therapy; 1 of 4 patients receiving full continuation therapy), particularly in those with delusional depression.

In their prospective study, Vanelle et al. (1994) administered maintenance ECT with an average frequency of once every 3.5–3.9 weeks for 1 year and found that 64% of the patients ($n=22$) needed shorter intervals between treatments to prevent a recurrence of their depressive disorders. The patients who required a shorter interval were older and had a longer duration of illness. Vanelle et al. (1994) posited that the older patients may have had a shorter time to relapse, a suggestion that is consistent with data showing that older patients tend to have accelerated mood cycles (Zis et al. 1980). Others have suggested tapering the ECT treatments from once a week for 4 weeks to once every 2 weeks for 4 weeks and then to once monthly for 4–6 months (Fox 2001).

Treatment Considerations

The greatest risk of relapse after ECT is within the first few months after acute treatment (Clarke et al. 1989; Sackeim et al. 1990; Shapira et al. 1995). During this crucial period, many patients and their families describe a recurrence of symptoms of depression when prophylactic ECT treatment intervals are extended by even a few days. This pattern of response has resulted in the development of a continuation ECT protocol in which treatment intervals are extended in increments—from once a week for the first four treatments to every 10 days for the next three treatments and then to every 2 weeks for the final 4 months. During the initial 6 months of prophylactic ECT, treatments are not extended beyond every 2 weeks. If a patient becomes symptomatic, the treatment interval is again shortened until the patient is clinically stable. Usually this requires an additional 3–4 treatments and not a full acute course of 6–10 treatments. The patient then resumes the longest ECT treatment interval during which he or she remained healthy.

Patients are encouraged to continue ECT for at least 6 months. In the final month of continuation ECT, treatment with an antidepressant is initiated. However, which antidepressant drugs can be safely and effectively used during continuation ECT requires further study. For patients who relapse quickly after continuation ECT ends, maintenance ECT should be considered.

Informed Consent

Individual hospital policies and state laws dictate the procedure for obtaining informed consent. The administration of prophylactic ECT on an outpatient basis is subject to the same guidelines that apply to the ambulatory surgery service in the treating hospital. In general, the same policies governing consent for the initial ECT course apply to the prophylactic course of ECT. The consent procedures have been reviewed extensively elsewhere (Abrams 1997; American Psychiatric Association Task Force on Electroconvulsive Therapy 2001). A new consent should be obtained before each course of prophylactic ECT, when a patient changes from inpatient to outpatient status, and at least every 6 months. The physician also should document at the beginning of each ECT course (i.e., at the time of the consent) the justification for the prophylactic ECT.

Cognitive Complications

Few data exist on the cognitive changes that patients experience while receiving repeated ECT treatments over a period of months to years. Most of the available reports in which prophylactic ECT has been used describe only minor subjective complaints (e.g., Fox 2001). Grunhaus et al. (1990) reported that the patients in their study experienced minor memory difficulties (recent recall and names) that resolved within 6–8 months. Patients in the study by Vanelle et al. (1994) (mean age, 70 ± 13 years) described either no subjective memory problems ($n=8$) or minor subjective cognitive complaints ($n=14$). Petrides et al. (1994) noted only minor subjective memory problems in 30 patients (mean age, 52 ± 15 years) who received an average of seven continuation ECT treatments over 2 months. Thienhaus et al. (1990) found stable cognitive function (as measured on the Mini-Mental State Exam) in six elderly patients (mean age, 71 ± 5 years) receiving prophylactic ECT for 1–5 years. A naturalistic 1-year study of 20 persons receiving maintenance ECT found no global cognitive decline over the course of the study (Rami et al. 2004).

Transcranial Magnetic Stimulation and Subconvulsive Stimuli

To date, there are a number of subconvulsive treatments for depression including TMS, vagus nerve stimulation (VNS), and deep brain stimulation, all of which hold promise both for the treatment of depression and for elucidating the underlying biology of depression.

These treatments bring into question the axiom that subconvulsive stimuli cannot be therapeutic. Prototypes of the modern subconvulsive brain stimulation devices were first developed by Pollacsek and Beer in 1903. These colleagues of Sigmund Freud used electromagnetic currents to stimulate cortical neurons, but it was not until 80 years later that Barker developed modern TMS equipment (Barker et al. 1985) and research began to focus on the effects of TMS on psychiatric disorders. TMS equipment is relatively simple and uses capacitors to store an electrical charge. The charge is then discharged through a coil and produces a magnetic field that lasts from 100 to 200 milliseconds. When placed over the skull, the magnetic field passes unimpeded into the brain, stimulating the underlying brain regions; TMS can be used to assess both motor function (Homberg et al. 1991) and other complex brain functions such as speech (Epstein et al. 1996) and visual information processing (Beckers and Zeki 1995). Early preclinical studies of TMS in rats showed that TMS had effects similar to those of ECS in behavioral models of depression, including enhancement of apomorphine-induced stereotypy, reduction of immobility in the Porsolt swim test, and increases in seizure threshold on subsequent stimulation (Fleischmann et al. 1995; Lisanby and Belmaker 2000).

Rapid-Rate Transcranial Magnetic Stimulation

Within a decade of the development of modern TMS equipment, TMS was being used to treat depression and schizophrenia (Grisaru et al. 1994; Hoflich et al. 1993; Kolbinger et al. 1995). These studies used TMS coils that were nonfocal, and the antidepressive effects were limited. Additional work by George et al. (1995) provided the impetus for a renewal in TMS research in mood disorders. These studies used rTMS—repetitive or rapid-rate TMS—to apply multiple stimuli in one session and target treatment to the prefrontal cortex, an area that has been shown to be important in the response to ECT (Nobler et al. 2001). Imaging studies have demonstrated a response

to rTMS based on changing metabolic patterns in the frontal cortex (Kimbrell et al. 1999). Yet the magnitude of the response to rTMS is rarely more than a 50% decline in the depression rating scales (e.g., clinical criteria for response), and few patients meet the criteria for clinical remission (or an absolute value for a scale that indicates no evidence of depression). A meta-analysis noted that although rTMS was clearly superior to sham stimulation and the effect size was moderate (effect size = 0.81 [95% confidence interval = 0.42–1.20; $P < 0.001$]), the clinical significance was modest (Holtzheimer et al. 2001).

Studies comparing rTMS and ECT have shown that the efficacy of rTMS is equivalent to that of ECT for the treatment of major depression (Grunhaus et al. 2000; Janicak et al. 2002). A combination of ECT and rTMS has been shown to be as efficacious as ECT alone (Pridmore 2000) and could potentially produce fewer side effects. Some researchers have pointed out that studies comparing ECT and rTMS have had unusually low response rates in the ECT treatment arms, suggesting possible underdosing of ECT (Euba 2005; Kellner et al. 2002; Schulze-Rauschenbach et al. 2005). A recent study found rTMS less efficacious than "a standard ECT course" for relieving acute symptoms of depression, without appreciable differences in cognitive side effects (Eranti et al. 2007).

Recent data from an industry-sponsored trial demonstrated a modest effect for rTMS in the treatment of depression. In this study, 301 medication-free patients participated in a double-blind multisite study using sham stimulation in control subjects (O'Reardon et al. 2007). The response rate at week 4 was significant, indicating a 50% decline in depression scores for approximately 18% of patients in the active treatment group versus 11% of those in the sham control group (and 24% vs. 12% at week 6). The remission rates at week 6, but not at week 4, were also significant (14% vs. 5%). In October 2008, the U.S. Food and Drug Administration (FDA) approved the use of rTMS for treatment of patients with depression who have failed to respond to an antidepressant treatment trial.

rTMS clearly has several advantages over ECT. rTMS requires no anesthesia, is easy to administer, and has only transient, mild cognitive side effects. Furthermore, rTMS does not have the negative stigma associated with ECT. Yet some physicians question whether the subconvulsive stimuli of rTMS can have an antidepressive effect comparable to that of ECT (Swartz 1997). A technique called *magnetic seizure therapy* has been developed as another alternative to ECT, combining the therapeutic effect of a seizure with the more focused stimulation of rTMS (Lisanby et al. 2001b, 2001c). Magnetic seizure therapy initiates a tonic–clonic seizure using a magnetic stimulator that focuses on a specific area of the brain and delivers a peak electrical charge that is comparable to that of an ECT treatment. The potential advantage of magnetic seizure therapy is that the maximum voltage can be focused on an area associated with a therapeutic benefit (e.g., the prefrontal cortex) and spare areas associated with debilitating side effects (e.g., the hippocampus). Magnetic seizure therapy offers the opportunity to target areas for stimulation and has some advantages over ECT, which affects multiple cortical and subcortical areas. Work in this area is ongoing and still in the preliminary stages.

Vagus Nerve Stimulation

Approved by the FDA for use in patients with treatment-resistant epilepsy, VNS therapy exerts its effect by applying intermittent subconvulsive electrical stimulation to the left vagus nerve. The left vagus nerve has autonomic connections to limbic and cortical areas known to be involved in mood regulation (George et al. 2000; Nemeroff et al. 2006), and as previously discussed, a putative effect of ECT is to act as an anticonvulsant (Sackeim 1999) (see "Anticonvulsant Hypothesis" subsection). Studies of the effect of VNS on mood regulation in a small sample of patients with epilepsy demonstrated a trend toward mood improvements (Elger et al. 2000) or showed a positive effect on mood that was no different from that seen in a group of epilepsy patients treated with anticonvulsant medications alone (Harden et al. 1999, 2000). However, a 10-week open pilot study of 60 depressed nonepileptic patients showed a response rate of 31% and a remission rate of 15% (Rush et al. 2000; Sackeim et al. 2001c), and the initial treatment response continued over the following 2 years (Nahas et al. 2005).

These pilot data served as the basis for a larger multicenter trial with 222 patients (Rush et al. 2005a). The study design included a 2-week single-blind recovery period after implantation (during which patients received no stimulation), followed by 10 weeks of masked active VNS treatment or sham treatment. At 10 weeks, response rates were 15% for the active treatment group ($n=112$) and 10% for the sham treatment group ($n=110$) ($P=0.251$). Although this study did not yield definitive evidence of short-term efficacy for adjunctive VNS in patients with treatment-resistant depression, the subjects were then followed for a year in a naturalistic study in which they had stimulator adjustments and could have their medication changed or receive other treatments for depression (Rush

et al. 2005b). These caveats should be kept in mind when considering that the 1-year response rate was 27% (55/202) and the remission rate was 16% (32/202). The patients showed significant improvement when compared with a matched control group of patients with similar treatment-resistant depression who were receiving only medication (George et al. 2005). The FDA considered these data and approved VNS therapy for treatment-resistant depression, although it required the patients receiving VNS to be followed to determine the long-term treatment response.

Comparison With ECT

Although rTMS and VNS provide therapeutic alternatives for patients with depression, neither provides the efficacy of ECT. The response to ECT is remarkable given the data that more than 80% of depressed patients may achieve remission despite multiple medication failures. However, ECT is expensive, has been stigmatized, and has significant side effects, including long-term memory loss. Furthermore, after responding to an initial course of ECT, patients face a relapse rate of up to 60% within 6 months while receiving antidepressant medication. Prophylactic ECT to prevent relapse and remission is a viable and cost-effective option (McDonald et al. 1998) but can be difficult to implement, given the time demands and potential side effects. Time constraints may also hinder the use of rTMS, which, although it requires no anesthesia, is easy to administer, and has only transient, mild cognitive side effects, can be impractical because the patient is required to come in 5 days a week for up to 6 weeks. Disadvantages of VNS are that it is expensive and requires surgery and adjustments of the stimulator.

Like ECT, pharmacotherapy, and psychotherapy, both rTMS and VNS are relatively nonspecific: the treatment effects target areas of the brain and circuits involved in depression, rather than specific nuclei and nodes. This lack of specificity may be an advantage in that major depression is a relatively nonspecific disease that includes diagnoses as disparate as postpartum depression and depression secondary to stroke. The lack of specificity may also account for the suboptimal response to treatment with antidepressant drugs in patients with major depression. (This point was recently highlighted by the Sequenced Treatment Alternatives to Relieve Depression [STAR*D] trial, which found a 37% remission rate in patients treated with a selective serotonin reuptake inhibitor [Rush et al. 2006].)

Deep Brain Stimulation

Deep brain stimulation is the most highly focused treatment for depression—it is the treatment that most specifically targets the neural networks involved in depression—and has shown promise as a subconvulsive stimulus. It has been used in treatment-refractory Parkinson's disease and was the direct result of preclinical research that outlined the neural circuits and underlying positive and negative feedback loops integral to the Parkinson's disease process. Understanding this circuitry enabled surgeons to place a small electrical stimulator in specific subcortical nuclei including the subthalamic nucleus and internal globus pallidus to redirect neural stimuli and treat that disease with remarkable success (Rodriguez-Oroz et al. 2005). With advances in neuroimaging, the neural networks underlying depression have been further defined and targets for deep brain stimulation have been identified.

In an open study, Mayberg et al. (2005) demonstrated that bilateral high-frequency stimulation of white matter tracts adjacent to the subgenual cingulate cortex produced a treatment response in four of six patients with highly treatment-resistant depression. In fact, five of the six patients had failed to respond to ECT, but after 6 months of deep brain stimulation, half of the patients were in remission. The treatment was well tolerated and correlated with regional blood flow changes in areas of the dorsolateral prefrontal cortex, subgenual cingulate, and anterior cingulate, which are hypothesized to be integral to the development of depression.

The further development of research tools such as genomics and neuroradiology may help improve our understanding of the neural targets in the treatment of depression (Holtzheimer and Nemeroff 2006). If successful, treatments with specific neural targets may replace ECT, particularly for patients who need long-term maintenance ECT or for the minority of patients who fail to respond to an acute course of ECT.

Conclusion

More than 70 years have passed since ECT was first used in the treatment of psychiatric disorders. The lack of rigorous scientific studies during the early use of ECT contributed to the controversy that developed over its use. A significant stigma remains associated with ECT. This stigma is related more to past perceptions of ECT and portrayals of ECT in the media than to its current use. No medical treatment is as effective in treating a debilitating, life-threatening illness and yet associated with such a negative public image. Despite the ongoing controversy, ECT continues to be an extremely important tool in the treatment of several psychiatric disorders. The increased use of ECT in outpatient settings and as a prophylactic treatment for depression has been shown to be both effective and cost-efficient compared with medication. Alternative strategies such as rTMS have recently attracted increasing interest as possible replacements for ECT, but these treatments are clearly still in the investigational phase. For patients with severe, treatment-resistant depression, ECT remains the gold standard.

References

Aarsland D, Larsen JP, Waage O, et al: Maintenance electroconvulsive therapy for Parkinson's disease. Convuls Ther 13:274–277, 1997

Abraham G, Milev R, Delva N, et al: Clinical outcome and memory function with maintenance electroconvulsive therapy: a retrospective study. J ECT 22.43–45, 2006

Abrams R: Electroconvulsive Therapy, 2nd Edition. New York, Oxford University Press, 1992

Abrams R: The mortality rate with ECT. Convuls Ther 13:125–127, 1997

Abrams R: Stimulus titration and ECT dosing. J ECT 18:3–9; discussion, 14–15, 2002

Ackermann RF, Engel J Jr, Baxter L: Positron emission tomography and autoradiographic studies of glucose utilization following electroconvulsive seizures in humans and rats. Ann N Y Acad Sci 462:263–269, 1986

Ahmed SK, Stein GS: Negative interaction between lithium and ECT. Br J Psychiatry 151:419–420, 1987

American Psychiatric Association: Practice guideline for the treatment of patients with bipolar disorder. Am J Psychiatry 151:1–36, 1994

American Psychiatric Association Task Force on Electroconvulsive Therapy: Electroconvulsive Therapy: Report of the Task Force on Electroconvulsive Therapy of the American Psychiatric Association. Washington, DC, American Psychiatric Association Press, 1978

American Psychiatric Association Task Force on Electroconvulsive Therapy: The Practice of Electroconvulsive Therapy: Recommendations for Treatment, Training and Privileging, Task Force Report on ECT, 2nd Edition. Washington, DC, American Psychiatric Association, 2001

Anwyl R, Walshe J, Rowan M: Electroconvulsive treatment reduces long-term potentiation in rat hippocampus. Brain Res 435:377–379, 1987

Applegate RJ: Diagnosis and management of ischemic heart disease in the patient scheduled to undergo electroconvulsive therapy. Convuls Ther 13:128–144, 1997

Aronson TA, Shukla S, Hoff A: Continuation therapy after ECT for delusional depression: a naturalistic study of prophylactic treatments and relapse. Convuls Ther 3:251–259, 1987

Augoustides JG, Greenblatt E, Abbas MA, et al: Clinical approach to agitation after electroconvulsive therapy: a case report and literature review. J ECT 18:213–217, 2002

Auriacombe M, Reneric JP, Usandizaga D, et al: Post-ECT agitation and plasma lactate concentrations. J ECT 16:263–267, 2000

Avramov MN, Husain MM, White PF: The comparative effects of methohexital, propofol, and etomidate for electroconvulsive therapy. Anesth Analg 81:596–602, 1995

Aziz M, Maixner DF, DeQuardo J, et al: ECT and mental retardation: a review and case reports. J ECT 17:149–152, 2001

Babigian HM, Guttmacher LB: Epidemiologic considerations in electroconvulsive therapy. Arch Gen Psychiatry 41:246–253, 1984

Bader GM, Silk KR, Dequardo JR, et al: Electroconvulsive therapy and intracranial aneurysm. Convuls Ther 11:139–143, 1995

Bailine SH, Rifkin A, Kayne E, et al: Comparison of bifrontal and bitemporal ECT for major depression. Am J Psychiatry 157:121–123, 2000

Bailine SH, Petrides G, Doft M, et al: Indications for the use of propofol in electroconvulsive therapy. J ECT 19:129–132, 2003

Bakewell CJ, Russo J, Tanner C, et al: Comparison of clinical efficacy and side effects for bitemporal and bifrontal electrode placement in electroconvulsive therapy. J ECT 20:145–153, 2004

Barker AT, Jalinous R, Freeston IL: Non-invasive magnetic stimulation of human motor cortex (letter). Lancet 1(8437):1106–1107, 1985

Barton JL, Mehta S, Snaith RP: The prophylactic value of extra ECT in depressive illness. Acta Psychiatr Scand 49:386–392, 1973

Beale MD, Kellner CH: ECT in treatment algorithms: no need to save the best for last. J ECT 16:1–2, 2000

Beckers G, Zeki S: The consequences of inactivating areas V1 and V5 on visual motion perception. Brain 118:49–60, 1995

Bergsholm P, Swartz CM, Conrad M: Anesthesia in electroconvulsive therapy and alternatives to barbiturates. Psychiatr Ann 26:709–712, 1996

Berman RM, Cappiello A, Anand A, et al: Antidepressant effects of ketamine in depressed patients. Biol Psychiatry 47:351–354, 2000

Bernstien HJ, Beale MD, Burns CM: Patient attitudes about ECT after treatment. Psychiatr Ann 28:524–527, 1998

Bertolín-Guillén JM, Peiró-Moreno S, Hernández-de-Pablo ME: Patterns of electroconvulsive therapy use in Spain. Eur Psychiatry 21:463–470, 2006

Bhatia SC, Baldwin SA, Bhatia SK: Electroconvulsive therapy during the third trimester of pregnancy. J ECT 15:270–274, 1999

Birkenhager TK, van den Broek WW, Mulder PG, et al: One-year outcome of psychotic depression after successful electroconvulsive therapy. J ECT 21:221–226, 2005

Bolwig TG, Hertz MM, Westergaard E: Acute hypertension causing blood-brain barrier breakdown during epileptic seizures. Acta Psychiatr Scand 56:335–342, 1977

Bourgon LN, Kellner CH: Relapse of depression after ECT: a review. J ECT 16:19–31, 2000

Bourne H, Long MB: Convulsion dependence. Lancet 2(6850):1193–1196, 1954

Brandon S, Cowley P, McDonald C, et al: Electroconvulsive therapy: results in depressive illness from the Leicestershire trial. Br Med J (Clin Res Ed) 288:22–25, 1984

Breakey WR, Dunn GJ: Racial disparity in the use of ECT for affective disorders. Am J Psychiatry 161:1635–1641, 2004

Buchan H, Johnstone E, McPherson K, et al: Who benefits from electroconvulsive therapy? Combined results of the Leicester and Northwick Park trials. Br J Psychiatry 160:355–359, 1992

Butterfield NN, Graf P, Macleod BA, et al: Propofol reduces cognitive impairment after electroconvulsive therapy. J ECT 20:3–9, 2004

Cattan RA, Barry PP, Mead G, et al: Electroconvulsive therapy in octogenarians. J Am Geriatr Soc 38:753–758, 1990

Chanpattana W, Chakrabhand ML, Kongsakon R, et al. Short-term effect of combined ECT and neuroleptic therapy in treatment-resistant schizophrenia. J ECT 129–139, 1999a

Chanpattana W, Chakrabhand ML, Sackeim HA, et al: Continuation ECT in treatment-resistant schizophrenia: a controlled study. J ECT 15:178–192, 1999b

Chung KF: Determinants of seizure threshold of electroconvulsive therapy in Chinese. J ECT 22:100–102, 2006

Ciapparelli A, Dell'Osso L, Tundo A, et al: Electroconvulsive therapy in medication-nonresponsive patients with mixed mania and bipolar depression. J Clin Psychiatry 62:552–555, 2001

Clarke TB, Coffey CE, Hoffman GW, et al: Continuation therapy for depression using outpatient electroconvulsive therapy. Convuls Ther 5:330–337, 1989

Clifford DB, Zorumski CF, Olney JW: Ketamine and MK-801 prevent degeneration of thalamic neurons induced by focal cortical seizures. Exp Neurol 105:272–279, 1989

Coffey CE, Weiner RD, Hinkle PE, et al: Augmentation of ECT seizures with caffeine. Biol Psychiatry 22:637–649, 1987

Coffey CE, Figiel GS, Djang WT, et al: White matter hyperintensity on magnetic resonance imaging: clinical and neuroanatomic correlates in the depressed elderly. J Neuropsychiatry Clin Neurosci 1:135–144, 1989

Coffey CE, Weiner RD, Djang WT, et al: Brain anatomic effects of electroconvulsive therapy: a prospective magnetic resonance imaging study. Arch Gen Psychiatry 48:1013–1021, 1991

Cohen D, Paillère-Martinot ML, Basquin M: Use of electroconvulsive therapy in adolescents. Convuls Ther 13:25–31, 1997

Cohen LS, Friedman JM, Jefferson JW, et al: A reevaluation of risk of in utero exposure to lithium. JAMA 271:146–150, 1994

Colenda CC, McCall WV: A statistical model predicting the seizure threshold for right unilateral ECT in 106 patients. Convuls Ther 12:3–12, 1996

Conca A, Prapotnik M, Peschina W, et al: Simultaneous pattern of rCBF and rCMRGlu in continuation ECT: case reports. Psychiatry Res 124:191–198, 2003

Conti B, Maier R, Barr AM, et al: Region-specific transcriptional changes following the three antidepressant treatments electro convulsive therapy, sleep deprivation and fluoxetine. Mol Psychiatry 12:167–189, 2007

Currier MB, Murray GB, Welch CC: Electroconvulsive therapy for post-stroke depressed geriatric patients. J Neuropsychiatry Clin Neurosci 4:140–144, 1992

Daly JJ, Prudic J, Devanand DP, et al: ECT in bipolar and unipolar depression: differences in speed of response. Bipolar Disord 3:95–104, 2001

Datto CJ, Levy S, Miller DS, et al: Impact of maintenance ECT on concentration and memory. J ECT 17:170–174, 2001

Decina P, Guthrie EB, Sackeim HA, et al: Continuation ECT in the management of relapses of major affective episodes. Acta Psychiatr Scand 75:559–562, 1987 d'Elia G, Raotma H: Is unilateral ECT less effective than bilateral ECT? Br J Psychiatry 126:83–89, 1975

Devanand DP, Decina P, Sackeim HA, et al: Status epilepticus following ECT in a patient receiving theophylline. J Clin Psychopharmacol 8:153, 1988

Devanand DP, Sackeim HA, Prudic J: Electroconvulsive therapy in the treatment-resistant patient. Psychiatr Clin North Am 14:905–923, 1991

Devanand DP, Dwork AJ, Hutchinson ER, et al: Does ECT alter brain structure? Am J Psychiatry 151:957–970, 1994

Devanand DP, Fitzsimons L, Prudic J, et al: Subjective side effects during electroconvulsive therapy. Convuls Ther 11:232–240, 1995

Dinwiddie S, Drevets WC, Smith DR: Treatment of phencyclidine-associated psychosis with ECT. Convuls Ther 4:230–235, 1988

Dolenc TJ, Rasmussen KG: The safety of electroconvulsive therapy and lithium in combination: a case series and review of the literature. J ECT 21:165–170, 2005

Dolenc TJ, Habl SS, Barnes RD, et al: Electroconvulsive therapy in patients taking monoamine oxidase inhibitors. J ECT 20:258–261, 2004

Dombrovski AY, Mulsant BH, Haskett RF, et al: Predictors of remission after electroconvulsive therapy in unipolar major depression. J Clin Psychiatry 66:1043–1049, 2005

Drevets WC: Functional anatomical abnormalities in limbic and prefrontal cortical structures in major depression. Prog Brain Res 126:413–431, 2000

Dubin WR, Jaffe R, Roemer R, et al: The efficacy and safety of maintenance ECT in geriatric patients. J Am Geriatr Soc 40:706–709, 1992

Duman RS, Vaidya VA: Molecular and cellular actions of chronic electroconvulsive seizures. J ECT 14:181–193, 1998

Dunlop E: Combination of antidepressants with electroshock therapy. Dis Nerv Syst 21:513–514, 1960

Echevarría Moreno M, Martin Muñoz J, Sanchez Valderrabanos J, et al: Electroconvulsive therapy in the first trimester of pregnancy. J ECT 14:251–254, 1998

Elger G, Hoppe C, Falkai P, et al: Vagus nerve stimulation is associated with mood improvements in epilepsy patients. Epilepsy Res 42:203–210, 2000

el-Mallakh RS: Complications of concurrent lithium and electroconvulsive therapy: a review of clinical material and theoretical considerations. Biol Psychiatry 23:595–601, 1988

Endler NS: The origins of electroconvulsive therapy (ECT). Convuls Ther 4:5–23, 1988

Epstein CM, Lah JJ, Meador K, et al: Optimum stimulus parameters for lateralized suppression of speech with magnetic brain stimulation. Neurology 47:1590–1593, 1996

Eranti S, Mogg A, Pluck G, et al: A randomized, controlled trial with 6-month follow-up of repetitive transcranial magnetic stimulation and electroconvulsive therapy for severe depression. Am J Psychiatry 164:73–81, 2007

Euba R: ECT in depression. Br J Psychiatry 187:487, 2005

Euba R, Saiz A: A comparison of the ethnic distribution in the depressed inpatient population and in the electroconvulsive therapy clinic. J ECT 22:235–236, 2006

Faber R, Trimble MR: Electroconvulsive therapy in Parkinson's disease and other movement disorders. Mov Disord 6:293–303, 1991

Fantz RM, Markowitz JS, Kellner CH: Sumatriptan for post-ECT headache. J ECT 14:272–274, 1998

Farah A, McCall WV: Electroconvulsive therapy stimulus dosing: a survey of contemporary practices. Convuls Ther 9:90–94, 1993

Farrant M, Nusser Z: Variations on an inhibitory theme: phasic and tonic activation of GABA(A) receptors. Nat Rev Neurosci 6:215–229, 2005

Feske U, Mulsant BH, Pilkonis PA, et al: Clinical outcome of ECT in patients with major depression and comorbid borderline personality disorder. Am J Psychiatry 161:2073–2080, 2004

Figiel GS, Coffey CE, Djang WT, et al: Brain magnetic resonance imaging findings in ECT-induced delirium. J Neuropsychiatry Clin Neurosci 2:53–58, 1990

Figiel GS, Hassen MA, Zorumski C, et al: ECT-induced delirium in depressed patients with Parkinson's disease. J Neuropsychiatry Clin Neurosci 3:405–411, 1991

Figiel GS, McDonald L, LaPlante R: Cardiovascular complications of ECT (letter). Am J Psychiatry 151:790–791, 1994

Fink M: Convulsive Therapy: Theory and Practice. New York, Raven, 1979

Fink M: Indications for the use of ECT. Psychopharmacol Bull 30:269–275; discussion, 30:276–280, 1994

Fink M: Catatonia, in Contemporary Behavioral Neurology. Edited by Trimble MR, Cummings JL. Oxford, UK, Butterworth-Heinemann, 1997, pp 289–309

Fink M: The broad clinical activity of ECT should not be ignored (letter). J ECT 17:233–235, 2001a

Fink M: Treating bipolar affective disorder: ECT is effective (letter). BMJ 322:365–366, 2001b

Fink M: Move on! (commentary). J ECT 18:11–13, 2002

Fink M: ECT in therapy-resistant mania: does it have a place? Bipolar Disord 8:307–309, 2006

Fink M, Sackeim HA: Convulsive therapy in schizophrenia? Schizophr Bull 22:27–39, 1996

Fink M, Kellner CH, Sackeim HA: Intractable seizures, status epilepticus, and ECT. J ECT 15:282–284, 1999

Fleischmann A, Prolov K, Abarbanel J, et al: The effect of transcranial magnetic stimulation of rat brain on behavioral models of depression. Brain Res 699:130–132, 1995

Fochtmann LJ: A mechanism for the efficacy of ECT in Parkinson's disease. Convuls Ther 4:321–327, 1988

Fochtmann LJ: Animal studies of electroconvulsive therapy: foundations for future research. Psychopharmacol Bull 30:321–444, 1994

Fochtmann LJ, Cruciani R, Aiso M, et al: Chronic electroconvulsive shock increases D-1 receptor binding in rat substantia nigra. Eur J Pharmacol 167:305–306, 1989

Folk JW, Kellner CH, Beale MD, et al: Anesthesia for electroconvulsive therapy: a review. J ECT 16:157–170, 2000

Folstein MF, Folstein SE, McHugh PR: "Mini-mental state": a practical method for grading the cognitive state of patients for the clinician. J Psychiatr Res 12:189–198, 1975

Fox HA: Extended continuation and maintenance ECT for long-lasting episodes of major depression. J ECT 17:60–64, 2001

Frederikse M, Petrides G, Kellner C: Continuation and maintenance electroconvulsive therapy for the treatment of depressive illness: a response to the National Institute for Clinical Excellence report. J ECT 22:13–17, 2006

Fregni F, Simon DK, Wu A, et al: Non-invasive brain stimulation for Parkinson's disease: a systematic review and meta-analysis of the literature. J Neurol Neurosurg Psychiatry 76:1614–1623, 2005

Friedel RO: The combined use of neuroleptics and ECT in drug resistant schizophrenic patients. Psychopharmacol Bull 22:928–930, 1986

Friedlander RI, Solomons K: ECT: use in individuals with mental retardation. J ECT 18:38–42, 2002

Gabriel A: ECT continuation and maintenance in a patient with psychosis and mental disability (letter). Can J Psychiatry 43:305–306, 1998

Gagne GG Jr, Furman MJ, Carpenter LL, et al: Efficacy of continuation ECT and antidepressant drugs compared to long-term antidepressants alone in depressed patients. Am J Psychiatry 157:1960–1965, 2000

George MS, Wassermann EM, Williams WA, et al: Daily repetitive transcranial magnetic stimulation (rTMS) improves mood in depression. Neuroreport 6:1853–1856, 1995

George MS, Sackeim HA, Marangell LB, et al: Vagus nerve stimulation: a potential therapy for resistant depression? Psychiatr Clin North Am 23:757–783, 2000

George MS, Rush AJ, Marangell LB, et al: A one-year comparison of vagus nerve stimulation with treatment as usual for treatment-resistant depression. Biol Psychiatry 58:364–373, 2005

Gleiter CH, Deckert J, Nutt DJ, et al: Electroconvulsive shock (ECS) and the adenosine neuromodulatory system: effect of single and repeated ECS on the adenosine A1 and A2 receptors, adenylate cyclase, and the adenosine uptake site. J Neurochemistry 52:641–646, 1989

Goldapple K, Segal Z, Garson C, et al: Modulation of cortical-limbic pathways in major depression: treatment-specific effects of cognitive behavior therapy. Arch Gen Psychiatry 61:34–41, 2004

Goldman D: Brief stimulus electric shock therapy. J Nerv Ment Dis 110:36–45, 1949

Gomez J: Subjective side-effects of ECT. Br J Psychiatry 127:609–611, 1975

Green AR, Sant K, Bowdler JM, et al: Further evidence for a relationship between changes in GABA concentration in rat brain and enhanced monoamine-mediated behavioural responses following repeated electroconvulsive shock. Neuropharmacology 21:981–984, 1982

Greene YM, McDonald WM, Duggan J, et al: Ventricular ectopy associated with low-dose intravenous haloperidol and electroconvulsive therapy. J ECT 16:309–311, 2000

Griesemer DA, Kellner CH, Beale MD, et al: Electroconvulsive therapy for treatment of intractable seizures: initial findings in two children. Neurology 49:1389–1392, 1997

Grisaru N, Yarovslavsky U, Arbarbanel J, et al: Transcranial magnetic stimulation in depression and schizophrenia. Eur Neuropsychopharmacol 4:287–288, 1994

Grover BB: Handbook of Electrotherapy for Practitioners and Students. Philadelphia, PA, Davis, 1924

Gruber NP, Dilsaver SC, Shoaib AM, et al: ECT in mixed affective states: a case series. J ECT 16:183–188, 2000

Gruenthal M, Armstrong DR, Ault B, et al: Comparison of seizures and brain lesions produced by intracerebroventricular kainic acid and bicuculline methiodide. Exp Neurol 93:621–630, 1986

Grunhaus L, Pande A, Haskett R: Full and abbreviated courses of electroconvulsive therapy. Convuls Ther 6:130–138, 1990

Grunhaus L, Dannon PN, Schreiber S, et al: Repetitive transcranial magnetic stimulation is as effective as electroconvulsive therapy in the treatment of nondelusional major depressive disorder: an open study. Biol Psychiatry 47:314–324, 2000

Gujavarty K, Greenberg L, Fink M: Electroconvulsive therapy and neuroleptic medication in therapy-resistant positive-symptom psychosis. Convuls Ther 3:185–195, 1987

Harden CL, Pulver MC, Nikolov B, et al: Effect of vagus nerve stimulation on mood in adult epilepsy patients (abstract). Neurology 52 (suppl 2):A238–P03122, 1999

Harden CL, Pulver MC, Ravdin LD, et al: A pilot study of mood in epilepsy patients treated with vagus nerve stimulation. Epilepsy Behav 1(2):93–99, 2000

Hargrove EA, Bennett AE, Ford FR: The value of subconvulsive electrostimulation in the treatment of some emotional disorders. Am J Psychiatry 8:612–616, 1953

Harrison PJ: The neuropathology of primary mood disorder. Brain 125:1428–1449, 2002

Haskett RF, Rosenquist PB, McCall WV, et al: The role of antidepressant medications during ECT: new findings from OPT-ECT (Meeting Abstracts: 2007 ACT/ISTS Scientific Program). J ECT 23:56, 2007

Hasler G, van der Veen JW, Tumonis T, et al: Reduced prefrontal glutamate/glutamine and gamma-aminobutyric acid levels in major depression determined using proton magnetic resonance spectroscopy. Arch Gen Psychiatry 64:193–200, 2007

Havaki-Kontaxaki BJ, Ferentinos PP, Kontaxakis VP, et al: Concurrent administration of clozapine and electroconvulsive therapy in clozapine-resistant schizophrenia. Clin Neuropharmacol 29:52–56, 2006

Heikman P, Kalska H, Katila H, et al: Right unilateral and bifrontal electroconvulsive therapy in the treatment of depression: a preliminary study. J ECT 18:26–30, 2002

Hellsten J, West MJ, Arvidsson A, et al: Electroconvulsive seizures induce angiogenesis in adult rat hippocampus. Biol Psychiatry 58:871–878, 2005

Hermann RC, Dorwart RA, Hoover CW, et al: Variation in ECT use in the United States. Am J Psychiatry 152:869–875, 1995

Hickie I, Scott E, Mitchell P, et al: Subcortical hyperintensities on magnetic resonance imaging: clinical correlates and prognostic significance in patients with severe depression. Biol Psychiatry 37:151–160, 1995

Hihn H, Baune BT, Michael N, et al: Memory performance in severely depressed patients treated by electroconvulsive therapy. J ECT 22:189–195, 2006

Hill MA, Courvoisie H, Dawkins K, et al: ECT for the treatment of intractable mania in two prepubertal male children. Convuls Ther 13:74–82, 1997

Hinkle PE, Coffey CE, Weiner RD, et al: Use of caffeine to lengthen seizures in ECT. Am J Psychiatry 144:1143–1148, 1987

Hirose S, Ashby CR Jr, Mills MJ: Effectiveness of ECT combined with risperidone against aggression in schizophrenia. J ECT 17:22–26, 2001

Hitzemann RJ, Hitzemann BA, Blatt S, et al: Repeated electroconvulsive shock: effect on sodium dependency and regional distribution of opioid-binding sites. Mol Pharmacol 31:562–566, 1987

Hoflich G, Kasper S, Hufnagel A, et al: Application of transcranial magnetic stimulation in the treatment of drug-resistant major depression. Hum Psychopharmacol 8:361–365, 1993

Holtzheimer PE 3rd, Nemeroff CB: Advances in the treatment of depression. NeuroRx 3:42–56, 2006

Holtzheimer PE 3rd, Russo J, Avery DH: A meta-analysis of repetitive transcranial magnetic stimulation in the treatment of depression. Psychopharmacol Bull 35:149–169, 2001

Homberg V, Stephan KM, Netz J: Transcranial stimulation of motor cortex in upper motor neurone syndrome: its relation to the motor deficit. Electroencephalogr Clin Neurophysiol 81:377–388, 1991

Huettner JE, Bean BP: Block of N-methyl-D-aspartate-activated current by the anticonvulsant MK-801: selective binding to open channels. Proc Natl Acad Sci U S A 85:1307–1311, 1988

Husain MM, Meyer DE, Muttakin MH, et al: Maintenance ECT for treatment of recurrent mania (letter). Am J Psychiatry 150:985, 1993

Ingvar M: Cerebral blood flow and metabolic rate during seizures: relationship to epileptic brain damage. Ann N Y Acad Sci 462:194–206, 1986

Janicak PG, Mask J, Trimakas KA, et al: ECT: an assessment of mental health professionals' knowledge and attitudes. J Clin Psychiatry 46:262–266, 1985

Janicak PG, Dowd SM, Martis B, et al: Repetitive transcranial magnetic stimulation versus electroconvulsive therapy for major depression: preliminary results of a randomized trial. Biol Psychiatry 51:659–667, 2002

Jha A, Stein G: Decreased efficacy of combined benzodiazepines and unilateral ECT in treatment of depression. Acta Psychiatr Scand 94:101–104, 1996

Jha AK, Stein GS, Fenwick P: Negative interaction between lithium and electroconvulsive therapy—a case-control study. Br J Psychiatry 168:241–243, 1996

Johnstone EC, Deakin JF, Lawler P, et al: The Northwick Park electroconvulsive therapy trial. Lancet 2(8208–8209):1317–1320, 1980

Kant R, Coffey CE, Bogyi AM: Safety and efficacy of ECT in patients with head injury: a case series. J Neuropsychiatry Clin Neurosci 11:32–37, 1999

Karlinsky H, Shulman KI: The clinical use of electroconvulsive therapy in old age. J Am Geriatr Soc 32:183–186, 1984

Kay DW, Fahy T, Garside RF: A seven-month double bind trial of amitriptyline and diazepam in ECT-treated depressed patients. Br J Psychiatry. 117:667–671, 1970

Keck PE Jr, Mendlwicz J, Calabrese JR, et al: A review of randomized, controlled clinical trials in acute mania. J Affect Disord 59 (suppl 1):S31–S37, 2000

Kellner CH: The CT scan (or MRI) before ECT: a wonderful test has been overused. Convuls Ther 12:79–80, 1996

Kellner CH: Towards the modal ECT treatment. J ECT 17:1–2, 2001

Kellner CH, Beale MD, Pritchett JT, et al: Electroconvulsive therapy and Parkinson's disease: the case for further study. Psychopharmacol Bull 30:495–500, 1994

Kellner CH, Husain M, Petrides G, et al: Comment on "Repetitive transcranial magnetic stimulation versus electroconvulsive therapy for major depression: preliminary results of a randomized trial" (comment). Biol Psychiatry 52:1032–1033, 2002

Kellner CH, Fink M, Knapp R, et al: Relief of expressed suicidal intent by ECT: a consortium for research in ECT study. Am J Psychiatry 162:977–982, 2005

Kellner CH, Knapp RG, Petrides G, et al: Continuation electroconvulsive therapy vs pharmacotherapy for relapse prevention in major depression: a multisite study from the Consortium for Research in Electroconvulsive Therapy (CORE). Arch Gen Psychiatry 63:1337–1344, 2006

Kimbrell TA, Little JT, Dunn RT, et al: Frequency dependence of antidepressant response to left prefrontal repetitive transcranial magnetic stimulation (rTMS) as a function of baseline cerebral glucose metabolism. Biol Psychiatry 46:1603–1613, 1999

Klapheke M: Combining ECT and antipsychotic agents: benefits and risks. Convuls Ther 9:241–255, 1993

Kolbinger HM, Hoflich G, Hufnagel A, et al: Transcranial magnetic stimulation (TMS) in the treatment of major depression: a pilot study. Hum Psychopharmacol 10:305–310, 1995

Kondratyev A, Sahibzada N, Gale K: Electroconvulsive shock exposure prevents neuronal apoptosis after kainic acid-evoked status epilepticus. Brain Res Mol Brain Res 91:1–13, 2001

Kotresh S, Girish K, Janakiramaiah N, et al: Effect of ECT stimulus parameters on seizure physiology and outcome. J ECT 20:10–12, 2004

Kramer BA: Use of ECT in California, 1977–1983. Am J Psychiatry 142:1190–1192, 1985

Kramer BA: Maintenance ECT: a survey of practice. Convuls Ther 3:260–268, 1987

Kramer BA: A naturalistic review of maintenance ECT at a university setting. J ECT 15:262–269, 1999

Krueger RB, Sackeim HA, Gamzu ER. Pharmacological treatment of the cognitive side effects of ECT: a review. Psychopharmacol Bull 28:409–424, 1992

Krystal AD, Coffey CE: Neuropsychiatric considerations in the use of electroconvulsive therapy. J Neuropsychiatry Clin Neurosci 9:283–292, 1997

Krystal AD, Weiner RD, McCall WV, et al: The effects of ECT stimulus dose and electrode placement on the ictal electroencephalogram: an intraindividual crossover study. Biol Psychiatry 34:759–767, 1993

Krystal AD, Coffey CE, Weiner RD, et al: Changes in seizure threshold over the course of electroconvulsive therapy affect therapeutic response and are detected by ictal EEG ratings. J Neuropsychiatry Clin Neurosci 10:178–186, 1998

Krystal AD, Weiner RD, Dean MD, et al: Comparison of seizure duration, ictal EEG, and cognitive effects of ketamine and methohexital anesthesia with ECT. J Neuropsychiatry Clin Neurosci 15:27–34, 2003

Latey RH, Fahy TJ: Electroconvulsive therapy in the Republic of Ireland 1982: a summary of findings. Br J Psychiatry 147:438–439, 1985

Lauritzen L, Odgaard K, Clemmesen L, et al: Relapse prevention by means of paroxetine in ECT-treated patients with major depression: a comparison with imipramine and placebo in medium-term continuation therapy. Acta Psychiatr Scand 94:241–251, 1996

Laursen H, Gjerris A, Bolwig TG, et al: Cerebral edema and vascular permeability to serum proteins following electroconvulsive shock in rats. Convuls Ther 7:237–244, 1991

Lavin MR, Halligan P: ECT for comorbid obsessive-compulsive disorder and schizophrenia. Am J Psychiatry 153:1652–1653, 1996

Lawson JS, Inglis J, Delva NJ, et al: Electrode placement in ECT: cognitive effects. Psychol Med 20:335–344, 1990

Lerer B, Weiner RD, Belmaker RH: ECT: Basic Mechanisms. Washington, DC, American Psychiatric Association, 1984

Letemendia FJ, Delva NJ, Rodenburg M, et al: Therapeutic advantage of bifrontal electrode placement in ECT. Psychol Med 23:349–360, 1993

Levy SD, Albrecht E: Electroconvulsive therapy: a survey of use in the private psychiatric hospital. J Clin Psychiatry 46:125–127, 1985

Lisanby SH, Belmaker RH: Animal models of the mechanisms of action of repetitive transcranial magnetic stimulation (RTMS): comparisons with electroconvulsive shock (ECS). Depress Anxiety 12:178–187, 2000

Lisanby SH, Maddox JH, Prudic J, et al: The effects of electroconvulsive therapy on memory of autobiographical and public events. Arch Gen Psychiatry 57:581–590, 2000

Lisanby SH, Bazil CW, Resor SR, et al: ECT in the treatment of status epilepticus. J ECT 17:210–215, 2001a

Lisanby SH, Luber B, Sackeim HA, et al: Deliberate seizure induction with repetitive transcranial magnetic stimulation in nonhuman primates. Arch Gen Psychiatry 58:199–200, 2001b

Lisanby SH, Schlaepfer TE, Fisch HU, et al: Magnetic seizure therapy of major depression. Arch Gen Psychiatry 58:303–305, 2001c

Lloyd KG, Thuret F, Pilc A: Upregulation of gamma-aminobutyric acid (GABA) B binding sites in rat frontal cortex: a common action of repeated administration of different classes of antidepressants and electroshock. J Pharmacol Exp Ther 235:191–199, 1985

Loo CK, Schweitzer I, Pratt C: Recent advances in optimizing electroconvulsive therapy (review). Aust N Z J Psychiatry 40:632–638, 2006

Loo H, Galinowski A, De Carvalho W, et al: Use of maintenance ECT for elderly depressed patients (letter). Am J Psychiatry 148:810, 1991

Lunde ME, Lee EK, Rasmussen KG: Electroconvulsive therapy in patients with epilepsy. Epilepsy Behav 9:355–359, 2006

MacDonald JF, Bartlett MC, Mody I, et al: Actions of ketamine, phencyclidine and MK-801 on NMDA receptor currents in cultured mouse hippocampal neurones. J Physiol 432:483–508, 1991

Madsen TM, Treschow A, Bengzon J, et al: Increased neurogenesis in a model of electroconvulsive therapy. Biol Psychiatry 47:1043–1049, 2000

Major K: Latinos and electroconvulsive therapy: implications for treatment, research, and reform in Texas and beyond. Ethical Hum Psychol Psychiatry 7:159–166, 2005

Malberg JE, Eisch AJ, Nestler EJ, et al: Chronic antidepressant treatment increases neurogenesis in adult rat hippocampus. J Neurosci 20:9104–9110, 2000

Maletzky B, McFarland B, Burt A: Refractory obsessive compulsive disorder and ECT. Convuls Ther 10:34–42, 1994

Maltbie AA, Wingfield MS, Volow MR, et al: Electroconvulsive therapy in the presence of brain tumor: case reports and an evaluation of risk. J Nerv Ment Dis 168:400–405, 1980

Matzen TA, Martin RL, Watt TJ, et al: The use of maintenance electroconvulsive therapy for relapsing depression. Jefferson Journal of Psychiatry 6:52–58, 1988

Mayberg HS, Lozano AM, Voon V, et al: Deep brain stimulation for treatment-resistant depression. Neuron 45:651–660, 2005

Mayur P: Ictal electroencephalographic characteristics during electroconvulsive therapy: a review of determination and clinical relevance. J ECT 22:213–217, 2006

McCall WV, Shelp FE, Weiner RD, et al: Effects of labetalol on hemodynamics and seizure duration during ECT. Convuls Ther 7:5–14, 1991

McCall WV, Reid S, Rosenquist P, et al: A reappraisal of the role of caffeine in ECT. Am J Psychiatry 150:1543–1545, 1993a

McCall WV, Shelp FE, Weiner RD, et al: Convulsive threshold differences in right unilateral and bilateral ECT. Biol Psychiatry 34:606–611, 1993b

McCall WV, Reid S, Ford M: Electrocardiographic and cardiovascular effects of subconvulsive stimulation during titrated right unilateral ECT. Convuls Ther 10:25–33, 1994

McCall WV, Farah A, Reboussin DM, et al: Comparison of the efficacy of titrated moderate-dose and fixed, high-dose right unilateral ECT in elderly patients. Am J Geriatr Psychiatry 3:317–324, 1995

McCall WV, Robinette GD, Hardesty D: Relationship of seizure morphology to the convulsive threshold. Convuls Ther 12:147–151, 1996

McCall WV, Sparks W, Jane J, et al: Variation of ictal electroencephalographic regularity with low-, moderate-, and high-dose stimuli during right unilateral electroconvulsive therapy. Biol Psychiatry 43:608–611, 1998

McCall WV, Reboussin DM, Weiner RD, et al: Titrated moderately suprathreshold vs fixed high-dose right unilateral electroconvulsive therapy: acute antidepressant and cognitive effects. Arch Gen Psychiatry 57:438–444, 2000

McCall WV, Prudic J, Olfson M, et al: Health-related quality of life following ECT in a large community sample. J Affect Disord 90:269–274, 2006

McDaniel WW, Sahota AK, Vyas BV, et al: Ketamine appears associated with better word recall than etomidate after a course of 6 electroconvulsive therapies. J ECT 22:103–106, 2006

McDonald WM, Thompson TR: Treatment of mania in dementia with electroconvulsive therapy. Psychopharmacol Bull 35:72–82, 2001

McDonald WM, Phillips VL, Figiel GS, et al: Cost-effective maintenance treatment of resistant geriatric depression. Psychiatric Annals 28:47–52, 1998

Michael N, Erfurth A, Ohrmann P, et al: Metabolic changes within the left dorsolateral prefrontal cortex occurring with electroconvulsive therapy in patients with treatment resistant unipolar depression. Psychol Med 33:1277–1284, 2003

Miller LJ: Psychiatric medication during pregnancy: understanding and minimizing risks. Psychiatr Ann 24:69–75, 1994

Miller LJ: Psychiatric disorders during pregnancy, in Psychological Aspects of Women's Health Care: The Interface Between Psychiatry and Obstetrics and Gynecology. Edited by Stotland NL, Stewart DE. Washington, DC, American Psychiatric Press, 2001, pp 51–66

Mingo NS, Cottrell GA, Mendonca A, et al: Amygdala-kindled and electroconvulsive seizures alter hippocampal expression of the m1 and m3 muscarinic cholinergic receptor genes. Brain Res 810:9–15, 1998

Moise FN, Petrides G: Case study: electroconvulsive therapy in adolescents. J Am Acad Child Adolesc Psychiatry 35:312–318, 1996

Monroe RRJ: Maintenance electroconvulsive therapy. Psychiatr Clin North Am 14:947–960, 1991

Mueller PS, Schak KM, Barnes RD, et al: Safety of electroconvulsive therapy in patients with asthma. Neth J Med 64:417–421, 2006

Mukherjee S: Combined ECT and lithium therapy. Convuls Ther 9:274–284, 1993

Mukherjee S, Sackeim HA, Schnur DB: Electroconvulsive therapy of acute manic episodes: a review of 50 years' experience. Am J Psychiatry 151:169–176, 1994

Munk-Olsen T, Laursen TM, Videbech P, et al: Electroconvulsive therapy: predictors and trends in utilization from 1976 to 2000. J ECT 22:127–132, 2006

Murphy E: The prognosis of depression in old age. Br J Psychiatry 142, 111–119, 1983

Nahas Z, Marangell LB, Husain MM, et al: Two-year outcome of vagus nerve stimulation (VNS) for treatment of major depressive episodes. J Clin Psychiatry 66:1097–1104, 2005

Nascimento AL, Appolinario JC, Segenreich D, et al: Maintenance electroconvulsive therapy for recurrent refractory mania. Bipolar Disord 8:301–303, 2006

National Institute for Clinical Excellence (NICE): Guidance on the Use of Electroconvulsive Therapy (Technology Appraisal 59). London, UK, National Institute for Clinical Excellence, 2003

Nelson JP, Benjamin L: Efficacy and safety of combined ECT and tricyclic antidepressant therapy in the treatment of depressed geriatric patients. Convuls Ther 5:321–329, 1989

Nemeroff CB, Mayberg HS, Krahl SE, et al: VNS therapy in treatment-resistant depression: clinical evidence and putative neurobiological mechanisms. Neuropsychopharmacology 31:1345–1355, 2006

Nestler EJ, Barrot M, DiLeone RJ, et al: Neurobiology of depression. Neuron 34:13–25, 2002

Newman ME, Gur E, Shapira B, et al: Neurochemical mechanisms of action of ECS: evidence from in vivo studies. J ECT 14:153–171, 1998

Newton SS, Girgenti MJ, Collier EF, et al: Electroconvulsive seizure increases adult hippocampal angiogenesis in rats. Eur J Neurosci 24:819–828, 2006

NIH Consensus Conference. Diagnosis and treatment of depression in late life. JAMA 268:1018–1024, 1992

Nobler MS, Sackeim HA, Solomou M, et al: EEG manifestations during ECT: effects of electrode placement and stimulus intensity. Biol Psychiatry 34:321–330, 1993

Nobler MS, Sackeim HA, Prohovnik I, et al: Regional cerebral blood flow in mood disorders, III: treatment and clinical response. Arch Gen Psychiatry 51:884–897, 1994

Nobler MS, Luber B, Moeller JR, et al: Quantitative EEG during seizures induced by electroconvulsive therapy: relations to treatment modality and clinical features, I: global analyses. J ECT 16:211–228, 2000

Nobler MS, Oquendo MA, Kegeles LS, et al: Decreased regional brain metabolism after ECT. Am J Psychiatry 158:305–308, 2001

Nowak G, Zak J: Repeated electroconvulsive shock (ECS) enhances striatal D-1 dopamine receptor turnover in rats. Eur J Pharmacol 167:307–308, 1989

Nutt DJ, Glue P: The neurobiology of ECT: animal studies, in The Clinical Science of Electroconvulsive Therapy. Edited by Coffey CE. Washington, DC, American Psychiatric Association, 1993, pp 213–234

Nutt DJ, Cowen PJ, Green AR: Studies on the post-ictal rise in seizure threshold. Eur J Pharmacol 71:287–295, 1981

Nymeyer L, Grossberg GT: Delirium in a 75-year-old woman receiving ECT and levodopa. Convuls Ther 13:114–116, 1997

Oakeshott P, Hunt G: Prevention of neural tube defects. Lancet 343:123, 1994

O'Connor MK, Knapp R, Husain M, et al: The influence of age on the response of major depression to electroconvulsive therapy: a C.O.R.E. report. Am J Geriatr Psychiatry 9:382–390, 2001

O'Leary DA, Lee AS: Seven year prognosis in depression: mortality and readmission risk in the Nottingham ECT cohort. Br J Psychiatry 169:423–429, 1996

O'Reardon JP, Takieddine N, Datto CJ, et al: Propofol for the management of emergence agitation after electroconvulsive therapy: review of a case series. J ECT 22:247–252, 2006

O'Reardon JP, Solvason HB, Janicak PG, et al: Efficacy and safety of transcranial magnetic stimulation in the acute treatment of major depression: a multisite randomized controlled trial. Biol Psychiatry 62:1208–1216, 2007

Ottosson JO: Seizure characteristics and therapeutic efficiency in electroconvulsive therapy: an analysis of the antidepressant efficiency of grand mal and lidocaine-modified seizures. J Nerv Ment Dis 135:239–251, 1962

Painuly N, Chakrabarti S: Combined use of electroconvulsive therapy and antipsychotics in schizophrenia: the Indian evidence: a review and a meta-analysis. J ECT 22:59–66, 2006

Parker G, Roy K, Wilhelm K, et al: Assessing the comparative effectiveness of antidepressant therapies: a prospective clinical practice study. J Clin Psychiatry 62:117–125, 2001

Patel M, Patel S, Hardy DW, et al: Should electroconvulsive therapy be an early consideration for suicidal patients? J ECT 22:113–115, 2006

Paul IA, Nowak G, Layer RT, et al: Adaptation of the N-methyl-D-aspartate receptor complex following chronic antidepressant treatments. J Pharmacol Exp Ther 269:95–102, 1994

Petrides G, Dhossche D, Fink M, et al: Continuation ECT: relapse prevention in affective disorders. Convuls Ther 10:189–194, 1994

Petrides G, Fink M, Husain MM, et al: ECT remission rates in psychotic versus nonpsychotic depressed patients: a report from CORE. J ECT 17:244–253, 2001

Petrie RX, Reid IC, Stewart CA: The N-methyl-D-aspartate receptor, synaptic plasticity, and depressive disorder: a critical review. Pharmacol Ther 87:11–25, 2000

Pfleiderer B, Michael N, Erfurth A, et al: Effective electroconvulsive therapy reverses glutamate/glutamine deficit in the left anterior cingulum of unipolar depressed patients. Psychiatry Res 122:185–192, 2003

Pippard J, Ellam L: Electroconvulsive Treatment in Great Britain, 1980. London, Gaskell, 1981

Plaznik A, Kostowski W, Stefanski R: The influence of antidepressive treatment on GABA-related mechanisms in the rat hippocampus: behavioral studies. Pharmacol Biochem Behav 33:749–753, 1989

Prakash J, Kotwal A, Prabhu H: Therapeutic and prophylactic utility of the memory-enhancing drug donepezil hydrochloride on cognition of patients undergoing electroconvulsive therapy: a randomized controlled trial. J ECT 22:163–168, 2006

Pridmore S: Substitution of rapid transcranial magnetic stimulation treatments for electroconvulsive therapy treatments in a course of electroconvulsive therapy. Depress Anxiety 12:118–123, 2000

Prudic J, Sackeim HA, Devanand DP: Medication resistance and clinical response to electroconvulsive therapy. Psychiatry Res 31:287–296, 1990

Prudic J, Sackeim HA, Devanand DP, et al: The efficacy of ECT in double depression. Depression 1:38–44, 1993

Prudic J, Sackeim HA, Devanand DP, et al: Acute cognitive effects of subconvulsive electrical stimulation. Convuls Ther 10:4–24, 1994

Prudic J, Haskett RF, Mulsant B, et al: Resistance to antidepressant medications and short-term clinical response to ECT. Am J Psychiatry 153:985–992, 1996

Prudic J, Fitzsimons L, Nobler MS, et al: Naloxone in the prevention of the adverse cognitive effects of ECT: a within-subject, placebo controlled study. Neuropsychopharmacology 21:285–293, 1999

Prudic J, Olfson M, Marcus SC, et al: Effectiveness of electroconvulsive therapy in community settings. Biol Psychiatry 55:301–312, 2004

Rabheru K: The use of electroconvulsive therapy in special patient populations. Can J Psychiatry 46:710–719, 2001

Rami L, Bernardo M, Boget T, et al: Cognitive status of psychiatric patients under maintenance electroconvulsive therapy: a one-year longitudinal study. J Neuropsychiatry Clin Neurosci 16:465–471, 2004

Ranjkesh F, Barekatain M, Akuchakian S: Bifrontal versus right unilateral and bitemporal electroconvulsive therapy in major depressive disorder. J ECT 21:207–210, 2005

Rapoport MJ, Mamdani M, Herrmann N: Electroconvulsive therapy in older adults: 13-year trends. Can J Psychiatry 51:616–619, 2006

Rasmussen K: Commentaries: stimulus titration and ECT dosing. J ECT 18:10–11, 2002

Rasmussen K, Abrams R: Treatment of Parkinson's disease with electroconvulsive therapy. Psychiatr Clin North Am 14:925–933, 1991

Rasmussen KG, Pandurangi AK: Naloxone fails to prolong seizure length in ECT. J ECT 15:258–261, 1999

Rasmussen KG, Zorumski CF: Electroconvulsive therapy in patients taking theophylline. J Clin Psychiatry 54:427–431, 1993

Regenold WT, Weintraub D, Taller A: Electroconvulsive therapy for epilepsy and major depression. Am J Geriatr Psychiatry 6:180–183, 1998

Rodriguez-Oroz MC, Obeso JA, Lang AE, et al: Bilateral deep brain stimulation in Parkinson's disease: a multicentre study with 4 years follow-up. Brain 128:2240–2249, 2005

Rosenbach ML, Hermann RC, Dorwart RA: Use of electroconvulsive therapy in the Medicare population between 1987 and 1992. Psychiatr Serv 48:1537–1542, 1997

Rosenquist PB, Kimball JN, McCall WV: Prediction of antidepressant response in both 2.25 X threshold RUL and fixed high dose RUL ECT. J ECT 23:55, 2007

Royal College of Psychiatrists: The ECT Handbook: The Second Report of the Royal College of Psychiatrists' Special Committee on ECT. Edited by Freeman CP. London, Royal College of Psychiatrists, 1995

Rush AJ, Thase ME: Strategies and tactics in the treatment of chronic depression. J Clin Psychiatry 58 (suppl 13):14–22, 1997

Rush AJ, George MS, Sackeim HA, et al: Vagus nerve stimulation (VNS) for treatment-resistant depressions: a multicenter study. Biol Psychiatry 47:276–286, 2000

Rush AJ, Marangell LB, Sackeim HA, et al: Vagus nerve stimulation for treatment-resistant depression: a randomized, controlled acute phase trial. Biol Psychiatry 58:347–354, 2005a

Rush AJ, Sackeim HA, Marangell LB, et al: Effects of 12 months of vagus nerve stimulation in treatment-resistant depression: a naturalistic study. Biol Psychiatry 58:355–363, 2005b

Rush AJ, Trivedi MH, Wisniewski SR, et al: Acute and longer-term outcomes in depressed outpatients requiring one or several treatment steps: a STAR*D report. Am J Psychiatry 163:1905–1917, 2006

Russell JC, Rasmussen KG, O'Connor MK, et al: Long-term maintenance ECT: a retrospective review of efficacy and cognitive outcome. J ECT 19:4–9, 2003

Sackeim HA: Central issues regarding the mechanisms of action of electroconvulsive therapy: directions for future research. Psychopharmacol Bull 30:281–308, 1994

Sackeim HA: The anticonvulsant hypothesis of the mechanisms of action of ECT: current status. J ECT 15:5–26, 1999

Sackeim HA: Memory and ECT: from polarization to reconciliation (editorial). J ECT 16:87–96, 2000

Sackeim HA, Prudic J, Devanand DP, et al: The impact of medication resistance and continuation pharmacotherapy on relapse following response to electroconvulsive therapy in major depression. J Clin Psychopharmacol 10:96–104, 1990

Sackeim HA, Devanand DP, Prudic J: Stimulus intensity, seizure threshold, and seizure duration: impact on the efficacy and safety of electroconvulsive therapy. Psychiatr Clin North Am 14:803–843, 1991

Sackeim HA, Prudic J, Devanand DP, et al: Effects of stimulus intensity and electrode placement on the efficacy and cognitive effects of electroconvulsive therapy. N Engl J Med 328:839–846, 1993

Sackeim HA, Luber B, Katzman GP, et al: The effects of electroconvulsive therapy on quantitative electroencephalograms: relationship to clinical outcome. Arch Gen Psychiatry 53:814–824, 1996

Sackeim HA, Luber B, Moeller JR, et al: Electrophysiological correlates of the adverse cognitive effects of electroconvulsive therapy. J ECT 16:110–120, 2000

Sackeim HA, Haskett RF, Mulsant BH, et al: Continuation pharmacotherapy in the prevention of relapse following electroconvulsive therapy: a randomized controlled trial. JAMA 285:1299–1307, 2001a

Sackeim HA, Prudic J, Nobler MS, et al: Ultra-brief pulse ECT and the affective and cognitive consequences of ECT. J ECT 17:77, 2001b

Sackeim HA, Rush AJ, George MS, et al: Vagus nerve stimulation (VNS) for treatment-resistant depression: efficacy, side effects, and predictors of outcome. Neuropsychopharmacology 25:713–728, 2001c

Sackeim HA, Prudic J, Fuller R, et al: The cognitive effects of electroconvulsive therapy in community settings. Neuropsychopharmacology 32:244–254, 2007

Saito S, Yoshikawa D, Nishihara F, et al: The cerebral hemodynamic response to electrically induced seizures in man. Brain Res 673:93–100, 1995

Sajatovic M, Meltzer HY: The effect of short-term electroconvulsive treatment plus neuroleptics in treatment-resistant schizophrenia and schizoaffective disorder. Convuls Ther 9:167–175, 1993

Sanacora G, Mason GF, Rothman DL, et al: Increased cortical GABA concentrations in depressed patients receiving ECT. Am J Psychiatry 160:577–579, 2003

Santarelli L, Saxe M, Gross C, et al: Requirement of hippocampal neurogenesis for the behavioral effects of antidepressants. Science 301:805–809, 2003

Sargant W: Drugs in the treatment of depression. Br Med J 1:225–227, 1961

Sartorius A, Wolf J, Henn FA: Lithium and ECT—concurrent use still demands attention: three case reports. World J Biol Psychiatry 6:121–124, 2005

Sawynok J, Yaksh TL: Caffeine as an analgesic adjuvant: a review of pharmacology and mechanisms of action. Pharmacol Rev 45:43–85, 1993

Schloss P, Henn FA: New insights into the mechanisms of antidepressant therapy. Pharmacol Ther 102:47–60, 2004

Schulze-Rauschenbach SC, Harms U, Schlaepfer TE, et al: Distinctive neurocognitive effects of repetitive transcranial magnetic stimulation and electroconvulsive therapy in major depression. (See comments in Br J Psychiatry 187:386 [author reply, 386–387]; 187:487 [author reply, 488]; and 187:487–488 [author reply, 488], 2005.) Br J Psychiatry 186:410–416, 2005

Scott AI, Douglas RH, Whitfield A, et al: Time course of cerebral magnetic resonance changes after electroconvulsive therapy. Br J Psychiatry 156:551–553, 1990

Scott BW, Wojtowicz JM, Burnham WM: Neurogenesis in the dentate gyrus of the rat following electroconvulsive shock seizures. Exp Neurol 165:231–236, 2000

Seminowicz DA, Mayberg HS, McIntosh AR, et al: Limbic-frontal circuitry in major depression: a path modeling metanalysis. Neuroimage 22:409–418, 2004

Shapira B, Gorfine M, Lerer B: A prospective study of lithium continuation therapy in depressed patients who have responded to electroconvulsive therapy. Convuls Ther 11:80–85, 1995

Shapira B, Tubi N, Lerer B: Balancing speed of response to ECT in major depression and adverse cognitive effects: role of treatment schedule. J ECT 16:97–109, 2000

Shimizu E, Imai M, Fujisaki M, et al: Maintenance electroconvulsive therapy (ECT) for treatment-resistant disorganized schizophrenia. Prog Neuropsychopharmacol Biol Psychiatry 31:571–573, 2007

Shulman RB: Maintenance ECT in the treatment of PD. Therapy improves psychotic symptoms, physical function. Geriatrics 58:43–45, 2003

Sienaert P, Peuskens J: Electroconvulsive therapy: an effective therapy of medication-resistant bipolar disorder. Bipolar Disord 8:304–306, 2006

Small JG: Anticonvulsants in affective disorders. Psychopharmacol Bull 26:25–36, 1990

Small JG, Kellams JJ, Milstein V, et al: Complications with electroconvulsive treatment combined with lithium. Biol Psychiatry 15:103–112, 1980

Small JG, Klapper MH, Kellams JJ, et al: Electroconvulsive treatment compared with lithium in the management of manic states. Arch Gen Psychiatry 45:727–732, 1988

Sobin C, Sackeim HA, Prudic J, et al: Predictors of retrograde amnesia following ECT. Am J Psychiatry 152:995–1001, 1995

Song HJ, Stevens CF, Gage FH: Neural stem cells from adult hippocampus develop essential properties of functional CNS neurons. Nat Neurosci 5:438–445, 2002

Spiker DG, Stein J, Rich CL: Delusional depression and electroconvulsive therapy: one year later. Convuls Ther 1:167–172, 1985

Stadtland C, Erfurth A, Ruta U, et al: A switch from propofol to etomidate during an ECT course increases EEG and motor seizure duration. J ECT 18:22–25, 2002

Steffens DC, Conway CR, Dombeck CB, et al: Severity of subcortical gray matter hyperintensity predicts ECT response in geriatric depression. J ECT 17:45–49, 2001

Stewart C, Reid I: Electroconvulsive stimulation and synaptic plasticity in the rat. Brain Res 620:139–141, 1993

Stewart JT: Lithium and maintenance ECT. J ECT 16:300–301, 2000

Stoppe A, Louza M, Rosa M, et al: Fixed high-dose electroconvulsive therapy in the elderly with depression: a double-blind, randomized comparison of efficacy and tolerability between unilateral and bilateral electrode placement. J ECT 22:92–99, 2006

Stoudemire A, Knos G, Gladson M, et al: Labetalol in the control of cardiovascular responses to electroconvulsive therapy in high-risk depressed medical patients. J Clin Psychiatry 51:508–512, 1990

Stoudemire A, Hill CD, Dalton ST, et al: Rehospitalization rates in older depressed adults after antidepressant and electroconvulsive therapy treatment. J Am Geriatr Soc 42:1282–1285, 1994

Strome EM, Clark CM, Zis AP, et al: Electroconvulsive shock decreases binding to 5-HT2 receptors in nonhuman primates: an in vivo positron emission tomography study with [18F]setoperone. Biol Psychiatry 57:1004–1010, 2005

Suzuki K, Awata S, Takano T, et al: Resolution of SPECT-determined anterior cerebral hypoperfusion correlated with maintenance ECT-derived improvement in residual symptoms in a case of late-life psychotic depression. Clin Nucl Med 31:253–255, 2006

Swaim JC, Mansour M, Wydo SM, et al: A retrospective comparison of anesthetic agents in electroconvulsive therapy. J ECT 22:243–246, 2006

Swartz CM: Subconvulsive magnetic brain stimulation no replacement for ECT [letter]. Am J Psychiatry 154:716–717, 1997

Swartz CM: Physiological response to ECT stimulus dose. Psychiatry Res 97:229–235, 2000

Swoboda E, Conca A, Konig P, et al: Maintenance electroconvulsive therapy in affective and schizoaffective disorder. Neuropsychobiology 43:23–28, 2001

Taylor MA, Fink M: Catatonia in psychiatric classification: a home of its own. Am J Psychiatry 160:1233–1241, 2003

Tew JD Jr, Mulsant BH, Haskett RF, et al: A randomized comparison of high-charge right unilateral electroconvulsive therapy and bilateral electroconvulsive therapy in older depressed patients who failed to respond to 5 to 8 moderate-charge right unilateral treatments. J Clin Psychiatry 63:1102–1105, 2002

Thienhaus OJ, Margletta S, Bennet JA: A study of the clinical efficacy of maintenance ECT. J Clin Psychiatry 51:141–144, 1990

Thomas SG, Kellner CH: Remission of major depression and obsessive-compulsive disorder after a single unilateral ECT. J ECT 19:50–51, 2003

Thompson JW, Blaine JD: Use of ECT in the United States in 1975 and 1980. Am J Psychiatry 144:557–562, 1987

Thompson JW, Weiner RD, Myers CP: Use of ECT in the United States in 1975, 1980, and 1986. Am J Psychiatry 151:1657–1661, 1994

Thornton JE, Mulsant BH, Dealy R, et al: A retrospective study of maintenance electroconvulsive therapy in a university-based psychiatric practice. Convuls Ther 2:121–129, 1990

Tiller JW, Ingram N: Seizure threshold determination for electroconvulsive therapy: stimulus dose titration versus age-based estimations. Aust N Z J Psychiatry 40:188–192, 2006

Tortella FC, Long JB: Endogenous anticonvulsant substance in rat cerebrospinal fluid after a generalized seizure. Science 228:1106–1108, 1985

Tortella FC, Long JB: Characterization of opioid peptide-like anticonvulsant activity in rat cerebrospinal fluid. Brain Res 456:139–146, 1988

Tortella FC, Long JB, Hong JS, et al: Modulation of endogenous opioid systems by electroconvulsive shock. Convuls Ther 5:261–273, 1989

Tsao CI, Jain S, Gibson RH, et al: Maintenance ECT for recurrent medication-refractory mania. J ECT 20:118–119, 2004

Tsuchiyama K, Nagayama H, Yamada K, et al: Predicting efficacy of electroconvulsive therapy in major depressive disorder. Psychiatry Clin Neurosci 59:546–550, 2005

UK ECT Review Group: Efficacy and safety of electroconvulsive therapy in depressive disorders: a systematic review and meta-analysis. Lancet 361:799–808, 2003

Usui C, Doi N, Nishioka M, et al: Electroconvulsive therapy improves severe pain associated with fibromyalgia. Pain 121:276–280, 2006

van Waarde JA, Stolker JJ, van der Mast RC: ECT in mental retardation: a review. J ECT 17:236–243, 2001

Vanelle JM, Loo H, Galinowski A, et al: Maintenance ECT in intractable manic-depressive disorders. Convuls Ther 10:195–205, 1994

Vishne T, Aronov S, Amiaz R, et al: Remifentanil supplementation of propofol during electroconvulsive therapy: effect on seizure duration and cardiovascular stability. J ECT 21:235–238, 2005

Vothknecht S, Kho KH, van Schaick HW, et al: Effects of maintenance electroconvulsive therapy on cognitive functions. J ECT 19:151–157, 2003

Walter G, McDonald A, Rey JM, et al: Medical student knowledge and attitudes regarding ECT prior to and after viewing ECT scenes from movies. J ECT 18:43–46, 2002

Ward WK, Lush P, Kelly M, et al: A naturalistic comparison of two right unilateral electroconvulsive therapy dosing protocols: 2–3X seizure threshold versus fixed high-dose. Psychiatry Clin Neurosci 60:429–433, 2006

Watkins CJ, Pei Q, Newberry NR: Differential effects of electroconvulsive shock on the glutamate receptor mRNAs for NR2A, NR2B and mGluR5b. Brain Res Mol Brain Res 61:108–113, 1998

Weiner RD: ECT and seizure threshold: effects of stimulus wave form and electrode placement. Biol Psychiatry 15:225–241, 1980

Weiner RD: Does electroconvulsive therapy cause brain damage? Behav Brain Sci 7:1–53, 1984

Weiner RD, Coffey CE: Minimizing therapeutic differences between bilateral and unilateral nondominant ECT. Convuls Ther 2:261–265, 1986

Weiner RD, Rogers HJ, Davidson JR, et al: Effects of stimulus parameters on cognitive side effects. Ann N Y Acad Sci 462:315–325, 1986

Weiner SJ, Ward TN, Ravaris CL: Headache and electroconvulsive therapy. Headache 34:155–159, 1994

Weisberg LA, Elliott D, Mielke D: Intracerebral hemorrhage following electroconvulsive therapy. Neurology 41:1849, 1991

Wengel SP, Burke WJ, Pfeiffer RF, et al: Maintenance electroconvulsive therapy for intractable Parkinson's disease. Am J Geriatr Psychiatry 6:263–269, 1998

Wennberg JE, Barnes BA, Zubkoff M: Professional uncertainty and the problem of supplier-induced demand. Soc Sci Med 16:811–824, 1982

Wild B, Eschweiler GW, Bartels M: Electroconvulsive therapy dosage in continuation/maintenance electroconvulsive therapy: when is a new threshold titration necessary? J ECT 20:200–203, 2004

Yuuki N, Ida I, Oshima A, et al: HPA axis normalization, estimated by DEX/CRH test, but less alteration on cerebral glucose metabolism in depressed patients receiving ECT after medication treatment failures. Acta Psychiatr Scand 112:257–265, 2005

Zachrisson OC, Balldin J, Ekman R, et al: No evident neuronal damage after electroconvulsive therapy. Psychiatry Res 96:157–165, 2000

Zarate CA Jr, Singh JB, Carlson PJ, et al: A randomized trial of an N-methyl-D-aspartate antagonist in treatment-resistant major depression. Arch Gen Psychiatry 63:856–864, 2006

Zielinski RJ, Roose SP, Devanand DP, et al: Cardiovascular complications of ECT in depressed patients with cardiac disease. Am J Psychiatry 150:904–909, 1993

Zis AP, Grof P, Webster M, et al: Prediction of relapse in recurrent affective disorder. Psychopharmacol Bull 16:47–49, 1980

Zorumski CF, Izumi Y: Nitric oxide and hippocampal synaptic plasticity. Biochem Pharmacol 46:777–785, 1993

Zwil AS, McAllister TW, Price TR: Safety and efficacy of ECT in depressed patients with organic brain disease: review of a clinical experience. Convuls Ther 8:103–109, 1992

PART III

Clinical Psychobiology and Psychiatric Syndromes

David J. Kupfer, M.D., Section Editor

CHAPTER 45

Neurobiology of Mood Disorders

Charles F. Gillespie, M.D., Ph.D.

Steven J. Garlow, M.D., Ph.D.

Elisabeth B. Binder, M.D., Ph.D.

Alan F. Schatzberg, M.D.

Charles B. Nemeroff, M.D., Ph.D.

Introduction and Historical Context

The search for the biological substrates of affective disorders spans many centuries. Indeed, Hippocrates (460–357 B.C.) speculated that melancholia emerged when environmental conditions, such as the alignment of the planets, caused the spleen to secrete black bile, which then darkened the mood. During the next 2,000 years, few significant contributions to our understanding of mood disorders emerged until Robert Burton's *Anatomy of Melancholy* (1621). Positing that depressed people often "are born of melancholy parents," Burton anticipated the genetic underpinnings of melancholia as well as other factors in the pathogenesis of depression, including alcohol, diet, and biological rhythms. Through his careful longitudinal observations, Emil Kraepelin (1856–1926) was subsequently able to detect a genetic contribution to manic-depressive illness. Kraepelin also hypothesized that other constitutional factors resulted in specific brain abnormalities in manic-depressive patients, although postmortem tissue studies were unrevealing.

Adolf Meyer (1866–1950), at Johns Hopkins University, attempted to integrate psychological and biological theories of mental illness. Coining the term *psychobiology*, he speculated that depression was the result of genetic or biological factors, with additional effects of the environment after birth. Influenced by the work of Freud and other contemporaries, Meyer also emphasized the importance of current life stressors in the generation of depressive symptoms.

Investigation into the pathophysiological basis of psychiatric illness retreated with the preeminence of psychoanalytic theory and practice during the immediate post–World War II era. Biological theories reemerged in the 1950s after the introduction of the effective antipsychotic agent chlorpromazine and were further fostered by the introduction of effective antidepressants. Furthermore, the biogenic amine hypothesis (attributed to Joseph Schildkraut, John Davis, and William Bunney, with additional contributions by Alec Coppen and I.P. Lapin) posited that major depression was caused by a deficiency in central nervous system (CNS) concentration or receptor

This research was supported by National Institutes of Health (NIH) grants MH-42088 and MH-52899 to Charles B. Nemeroff, M.D., Ph.D., and NIH grant NCRRM01-RR00039 to Emory University.

function of the neurotransmitters norepinephrine (NE), epinephrine, and dopamine (DA) or the indoleamine serotonin (5-hydroxytryptamine [5-HT]).

American investigators during the 1960s, including Schildkraut (1965) and Bunney and Davis (1965), developed a variation of the biogenic amine hypothesis—the catecholamine hypothesis. The catecholamine hypothesis of affective disorders proposes that some types of depression are associated with a relative deficiency of catecholamines, particularly NE, in the CNS, whereas mania is associated with a relative overabundance of catecholamines. Substantial data have accumulated, however, documenting the contributions of other putative neurotransmitters in the maintenance of mood.

As American investigators during the 1960s focused on the importance of NE in the pathogenesis of abnormal mood states, European researchers—Alec Coppen (1968) in England and Lapin and Oxenkrug (1969) in the Soviet Union—turned their attention to the CNS serotonergic system. They proposed that a deficiency in serotonergic neuronal function produced depressive symptoms. This hypothesis was bolstered by the observations of Åsberg et al. (1976b) that a sizable subgroup of depressed patients had low cerebrospinal fluid (CSF) concentrations of 5-hydroxyindoleacetic acid (5-HIAA) and moreover that this subgroup was at greater risk for attempting or committing suicide, particularly by violent means. The association between indices of reduced 5-HT turnover and impulsive violent behavior was consistently replicated in several studies (Roy et al. 1989; Träskman et al. 1981; Van Praag 1982), although it does not appear to be specific to depression (V.M. Linnoila and Virkkunen 1992; Virkkunen et al. 1994).

In the 1970s, Janowsky et al. (1972) proposed a variation in the catecholamine hypothesis: they suggested that a relative increase or decrease in CNS cholinergic activity is associated with depression or mania, respectively.

Concurrent with the aforementioned work, psychiatrists repeatedly observed disturbances in mood in patients with clinical endocrinopathies. Indeed, hypercortisolemia was first noted as a feature of major depression in the late 1950s. During the 1970s, great strides were made in the understanding of the neuroendocrine mechanisms underlying major depression, including perturbations of the hypothalamic-pituitary-adrenal (HPA) and the hypothalamic-pituitary-thyroid (HPT) axes. Carroll's group demonstrated that 40%–50% of patients with endogenous depression show resistance to dexamethasone-induced HPA axis suppression, in the now well-known

dexamethasone suppression test (DST) (W.A. Brown et al. 1979; Carroll et al. 1968b). Prange and colleagues detected abnormalities in the HPT axis in patients with major depression (Prange et al. 1972) and also reported that augmentation of antidepressant treatment with the thyroid hormone triiodothyronine (T_3) was effective (Prange et al. 1969).

The biogenic amine hypotheses also arose in part from pharmacological interventions and observation of their effects on mood. Reserpine, a rauwolfia alkaloid antihypertensive agent, produces depressive symptoms in many patients, presumably resulting from depletion of biogenic amines from CNS neurons. The mood-elevating action of monoamine oxidase inhibitors (MAOIs) was discovered by the chance observation of the effects of iproniazid, a drug originally developed to treat tuberculosis. Imipramine, a tricyclic compound related to chlorpromazine and originally designed to treat schizophrenia, was demonstrated to be an effective antidepressant. Tricyclic antidepressants (TCAs) not only block the reuptake of NE and 5-HT into presynaptic neurons but also are muscarinic cholinergic receptor antagonists. Shopsin et al. (1975, 1976) found that administration of p-chlorophenylalanine, an inhibitor of 5-HT synthesis, reversed the antidepressant action of imipramine, as well as tranylcypromine, an MAOI. Interest in the mechanistic role of serotonergic systems in depression was further stimulated by the introduction of selective serotonin reuptake inhibitors (SSRIs) (e.g., fluoxetine) in the late 1980s. During the 1990s and the initial part of the present century, advances in molecular biology have made possible the structural characterization and cloning of several 5-HT receptors, as well as of the serotonin transporter (5-HTT).

More recently, research examining the role of developmental stress, trauma, and gene–environment interactions in the etiology of particular subtypes of depression and other forms of psychopathology (Caspi et al. 2003; Chapman et al. 2004; Dube et al. 2001; Heim et al. 2000; Kaufman et al. 2006; Kendler et al. 2001b; McCauley et al. 1997) and medical illness (Batten et al. 2004; Caspi et al. 2006; Danese et al. 2007; Dong et al. 2004; Felitti et al. 1998; R.D. Goodwin and Davidson 2005; R.D. Goodwin and Stein 2004; Lissau and Sorensen 1994; G.D. Smith et al. 1998) has had a large impact on mood disorders research and is clearly a burgeoning area for understanding relationships between environmental and genetic risks with respect to medical and psychiatric comorbidity.

Clinically, mood disorders are syndromal illnesses characterized by symptomatology suggestive of the disruption of a variety of brain regions/neural systems within the CNS. These include the frontal cortex, cingulate, hippocampus, striatum, amygdala, and hypothalamus that together participate in the regulation of mood, sleep, motivation, energy balance, and cognition (Nestler et al. 2002). This view is supported by a very large body of multidisciplinary research using state-of-the-art genetics and molecular neurobiology, biomarkers, responses to physiological challenge tests, structural and functional imaging, psychological testing, and postmortem studies. These data, however, suggest that mood disorders are not likely to be diseases resulting solely from dysfunction of a single gene, brain region, or neurotransmitter system. Rather, mood disorders likely represent distinct disorders with overlapping phenomenology and pathophysiology. Subtypes of depression likely differ with respect to allelic patterns of genetic vulnerability (or resilience), changes in gene regulation, and abnormal signaling at the cellular and systems levels within the CNS and between the CNS and other organ systems of the body—in short, they are systemic diseases (Belmaker and Agam 2008; Manji et al. 2001; Mayberg 1997; Nemeroff 2002; Nestler et al. 2002). In this chapter, we provide an overview of research examining the neuroendocrinology, neurochemistry, neuroimmunology, genetics, and brain imaging alterations of patients with mood disorders.

Epidemiology

Over the past 30 years, epidemiological studies of the major mood disorders have reported considerable variation in the prevalence rates of depression and bipolar mood disorder. This variability may be explained by the differing methodology of these surveys: the sampling of the populations at risk, the particular diagnostic system used, the method for obtaining information about symptoms, and the time when information was obtained (Weissman et al. 1992).

Most recently, the National Comorbidity Survey Replication (NCSR) reported the following 12-month prevalence rates of mood disorders based on DSM-IV-TR (American Psychiatric Association 2000) criteria: major depression (6.7%), dysthymia (1.5%), and bipolar I and II disorder (2.6%) (Kessler et al. 2005). Of the mood disorders, major depressive disorder is the most common psychiatric disorder (Kessler et al. 2003). In the United States, the lifetime prevalence of depression is nearly 17% (Kessler et al. 2005). Worldwide, depression remains a leading cause of disability (Murray and Lopez 1996; WHO World Mental Health Survey Consortium 2004).

The Neuroendocrine Axes

Several psychiatric disorders, including the major mood disorders, are associated with specific highly reproducible neuroendocrine alterations. Conversely, certain endocrine disorders (e.g., hypothyroidism and Cushing's disease) are associated with higher-than-expected rates of psychiatric morbidity. Neuroendocrine abnormalities have long been thought to provide a unique "window to the brain," revealing clues about the pathophysiology of specific CNS neurotransmitter systems in the particular psychiatric disorder under study. This so-called neuroendocrine window strategy is based on an extensive literature that indicates that the secretion of the peripheral endocrine organs is largely controlled by their respective pituitary trophic hormone. This pituitary hormone secretion, in turn, is controlled primarily by the secretion of the hypothalamic release and release-inhibiting hormones. Unipolar depression (and to a lesser extent bipolar disorder) is associated with multiple endocrine alterations, specifically of the hypothalamic-pituitary-adrenal/thyroid/growth hormone axes. In addition, a continually growing body of evidence indicates that components of the neuroendocrine axes, such as corticotropin-releasing hormone (CRH), may themselves directly contribute to mood symptomatology.

Hypothalamic-Pituitary-Adrenal Axis

Excess secretion of cortisol (Carpenter and Bunney 1971; Gibbons and McHugh 1962) and its metabolites (Sachar et al. 1970) was first observed in depressed patients more than 40 years ago. Moreover, the prominent presence of depression and anxiety in patients with endocrinopathies affecting the HPA axis such as Cushing's disease or syndrome (Dorn et al. 1995, 1997) in conjunction with the observation of increased secretion of cortisol in healthy patients exposed to stress contributed in part to the development of the stress–diathesis model of depression (Figure 45–1). This model hypothesizes that individual predisposition to excess reactivity of the neural and endocrine stress response systems plays a seminal role in susceptibility to depression. The presence of acute or prolonged stress in vulnerable individuals is thus believed to play a significant role in both the onset and relapse of certain forms of depression and may also contribute to the burden of medical illness in patients with depression (E.S. Brown et al. 2004). A wide variety of abnormalities of HPA axis function have been identified in patients with unipolar depression and bipolar disorder and are described below.

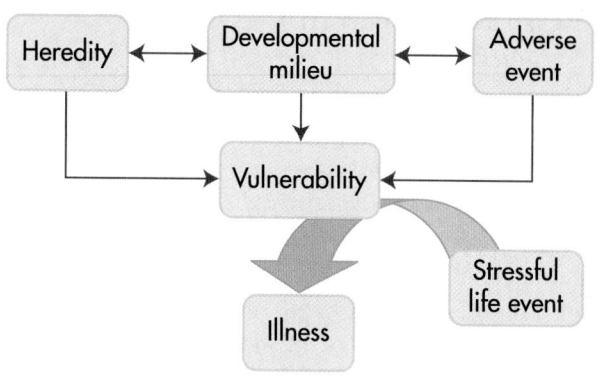

FIGURE 45-1. Stress–diathesis model of depression.

Functional Organization of the HPA Axis

The discovery of CRH (Vale et al. 1981) greatly accelerated research into the biology of stress and helped clarify the organization of the HPA axis, a collection of neural and endocrine structures that function collectively to facilitate the adaptive response to stress. Parvocellular neurons of the paraventricular nucleus (PVN) of the hypothalamus project to the median eminence where they secrete CRH into the primary plexus of blood vessels that comprise the hypothalamo-hypophyseal portal system (Swanson et al. 1983). The secreted CRH is then transported to the anterior pituitary gland, where it activates CRH_1 receptors on pituitary corticotrophs, resulting in increased secretion of adrenocorticotrophic hormone (ACTH). ACTH released from the anterior pituitary into the systemic circulation subsequently stimulates the production and release of cortisol from the adrenal cortex by activation of type 2 melanocortin receptors. Two glucocorticoid-responsive receptors, the mineralocorticoid receptor (MR) and the glucocorticoid receptor (GR), have been identified within the brain (Joels and de Kloet 1994). MRs have a high affinity for glucocorticoids and are restricted within the brain to limbic structures such as the septum, hippocampus, and amygdala where they regulate basal activity of the HPA axis (Jacobson and Sapolsky 1991). In contrast, GRs have a lower affinity for glucocorticoids than MRs and are distributed throughout the brain but are densely concentrated within the limbic system, parvocellular division of the PVN, pituitary, and ascending monoaminergic projection neurons. With elevated activity of the HPA axis, circulating levels of cortisol increase and the lower-affinity GRs become occupied, leading to suppression of HPA axis activity through effects at the hip-

pocampus, PVN, and pituitary (de Kloet et al. 1991). Mechanistically, these effects appear to be nongenomic and may act by triggering secretion of endocannabinoids from CRH-containing cells of the PVN. Endocannabinoids released from the PVN act through type 1 cannabinoid receptors to dampen the activity of glutamatergic afferents to the PVN, which subsequently reduces the neural outflow of the PVN (Di et al. 2003). Feedback inhibition, mediated in part by activity of MRs and GRs at multiple anatomical sites within the CNS, thus reduces stress-induced activation of the HPA axis and limits excess secretion of glucocorticoids, effectively dampening the stress response (Jacobson and Sapolsky 1991).

In addition to its major role in the regulation of the HPA axis, CRH is widely distributed in areas of the brain outside the hypothalamus, including the amygdala, septum, bed nucleus of the stria terminalis, and cerebral cortex (Swanson et al. 1983), where it functions, along with the hypothalamic CRH system, as a neurotransmitter in coordinating the behavioral, autonomic, endocrine, and immune responses to stress (Arborelius et al. 1999). Two CRH receptor subtypes (CRH_1 and CRH_2), both coupled positively to the production of adenylate cyclase (Chalmers et al. 1996), appear to mediate divergent effects of CRH on behavior (Heinrichs et al. 1997). CRH_1 receptors are broadly distributed within the CNS and have a high affinity for CRH. Decreased activity of CRH_1 receptors is associated with reduced anxiety in animal models. CRH_2 receptors are broadly distributed throughout the brain, overlapping topographically with CRH_1 receptors. CRH_2 receptors display a lower affinity for CRH than CRH_1 receptors and likely utilize urocortin as their endogenous ligand. However, in contrast to CRH_1 receptors, reduced activity of CRH_2 receptors results in increased anxiety in animal models.

Injection of CRH into the CNS of laboratory animals initiates changes in the activity of the autonomic nervous system that result in the elevation of peripheral catecholamines, reduced gastrointestinal activity, increased heart rate, and elevated blood pressure. Furthermore, behavioral changes such as disturbed sleep, diminished food intake, reduced grooming, decreased reproductive behavior, and enhanced fear conditioning, similar to those observed in humans with depression, also occur following direct CNS administration of CRH (Dunn and Berridge 1990; Owens and Nemeroff 1991) and are reduced by pretreatment with CRH receptor antagonists (Gutman et al. 2003; Heinrichs et al. 1995).

Corticotropin-Releasing Hormone and HPA Axis Pathophysiology

Cortisol and the dexamethasone suppression test. The DST, a test originally designed to aid in the diagnosis of Cushing's syndrome, was one of the first endocrine challenge tests to be studied in psychiatric patients. Studies of patients with mood disorders using the DST provided some of the first evidence of abnormal HPA axis function in depression (Table 45–1). The DST consists of the administration of a low dose (1 mg) of the synthetic glucocorticoid dexamethasone at 2300 h followed by measurement of plasma cortisol concentrations at two or three time points the following day. Dexamethasone acts at the level of the anterior pituitary corticotrophs to reduce the secretion of ACTH, resulting in a decrease in the synthesis and release of cortisol from the adrenal cortex. Failure to suppress plasma cortisol concentrations after dexamethasone administration suggests impaired feedback regulation and hyperactivity of the HPA axis.

A large percentage of drug-free patients with major depression fail to suppress secretion of cortisol following administration of dexamethasone, a finding known as dexamethasone nonsuppression (Carroll et al. 1968a), suggesting the use of DST nonsuppression as a biological marker for depression (Carroll 1982). DST nonsuppression status and hypercortisolemia are both common in depression but certainly not universal. Meta-analyses have revealed that DST nonsuppression status is most commonly found in patients with psychotic depression or mixed bipolar states, as previously reported by several investigators (Evans and Nemeroff 1983; Schatzberg et al. 1984) and that DST nonsuppression status generally predicts a more severe course of illness (Arana et al. 1985). Additional data, also procured using meta-analysis, have provided further support to the relationship between hypercortisolemia and psychotic depression as assessed with the DST (Nelson and Davis 1997). Finally, data derived from meta-analysis (S.C. Ribeiro et al. 1993) confirmed that 1) baseline DST status was not predictive of response to treatment, 2) DST nonsuppression status was associated with poor response to placebo, and 3) posttreatment DST nonsuppression was a significant risk factor for relapse and poor outcome, as initially reported by Greden et al. (1980) and confirmed by Nemeroff and Evans (1984). The prognostic utility of the DST with respect to suicide remains unclear. Some data suggest that DST nonsuppression is predictive of future completed suicide (Coryell and Schlesser 2001), whereas other data suggest that it is not (Black et al. 2002).

TABLE 45–1. Alterations in hypothalamic-pituitary-adrenal (HPA) axis activity in unipolar depression

Increased corticotropin-releasing hormone (CRH) in cerebrospinal fluid[a,b]

Blunted corticotropin and β-endorphin response to CRH stimulation[a]

Decreased density of CRH receptors in frontal cortex of suicide victims

Diminished hippocampal volume

Enlarged pituitary gland in depressed patients[b]

Enlarged adrenal gland in depressed patients[b] and suicide victims

Increased corticotropin production during depression

Elevated secretion of corticotropin and cortisol in depressed patients with a history of early life stress

Increased cortisol production during depression[a]

Nonsuppression of plasma glucocorticoid, corticotropin, and β-endorphin after dexamethasone administration[a]

Increased urinary free cortisol concentrations

[a]State-dependent.
[b]Significantly correlated to postdexamethasone cortisol concentrations.

Substantial rates of DST nonsuppression have been reported in patients with a variety of other DSM Axis I and Axis II diagnoses (Baxter et al. 1984; Gerner and Gwirtsman 1981; Hubain et al. 1986), calling into question its specificity as a diagnostic test. However, the greatest contribution of the DST was to serve as an impetus for subsequent studies exploring the underlying pathophysiology of the HPA axis in depression.

Corticotropin-releasing hormone and depression. A large body of data using markers such as CSF CRH concentrations, postmortem brain CRH concentrations, CRH mRNA expression, and CRH receptor autoradiography has accumulated suggesting that the abnormal activity of the HPA axis often observed in depressed patients (Plotsky et al. 1998) is due, in part, to hypersecretion of CRH (Arborelius et al. 1999). Elevated CSF concentrations of CRH have repeatedly been reported in patients with depression (Hartline et al. 1996; Nemeroff et al. 1984), as well as in combat veterans with posttraumatic stress disorder (PTSD) (Baker et al. 1999; Bremner et al. 1997a). In addition, the transcription (Raadsheer et al. 1995) as well as expression (Raadsheer et al. 1994) of CRH is increased in postmortem tissue in patients with depression. Furthermore, postmortem studies of individuals who have committed suicide have revealed elevated concentrations of CSF CRH (Arato et al. 1989), decreased expression of CRH_1 receptor mRNA within the frontal cortex (Merali et al. 2004), and increased CRH concentrations and decreased density of CRH receptors within the frontal cortex in comparison with control subjects (Merali et al. 2006; Nemeroff et al. 1988). Successful treatment of depression using either electroconvulsive therapy (Nemeroff et al. 1991) or fluoxetine (De Bellis et al. 1993b) has been shown to reduce the high pretreatment concentrations of CSF CRH. By contrast, persistent elevations of CSF CRH in symptomatically improved depressed patients are associated with early relapse of depression (Banki et al. 1992).

Considerable data support the hypothesis that the dysregulation of the HPA axis observed in depression is a state, rather than a trait, phenomenon. In this context, state dependence implies the presence of pathophysiological phenomena that are related to a particular phase of illness rather than being constitutively present (i.e., trait based). In depressed hypercortisolemic patients, plasma and urinary free cortisol concentrations (Sachar et al. 1970), DST nonsuppression status (Arana et al. 1985), blunting of the ACTH response to CRH infusion (Amsterdam et al. 1988), dexamethasone–CRH test results (Ising et al. 2005; Nickel et al. 2003), hypersecretion of CRH (Nemeroff et al. 1991), and adrenal hypertrophy (Rubin et al. 1995) all normalize following resolution of clinical symptoms.

HPA axis pathophysiology in specific mood disorders. *Major depression with psychotic features.* Patients with psychotic depression demonstrate hyperactivity of the HPA axis along with the highest rates of DST nonsuppression (Evans et al. 1983; Schatzberg et al. 1983). Distinct patterns of HPA axis abnormalities have been observed in depressed patients with and without psychotic features. Posener et al. (2000) reported that nonpsychotic depressed patients exhibited a lower 24-hour cortisol amplitude compared with depressed patients with psychosis, whereas patients with psychotic features had an increased 24-hour mean corticotropin secretion compared with depressed patients without psychosis. Subsequent studies have also identified disturbances between HPA axis function and the circadian timing system in patients with psychotic depression (Keller et al. 2006). In a study examining the relationship between cognition and the diurnal variation of cortisol in patients with depression, higher afternoon cortisol levels and a higher rate of errors of commission on a test of verbal memory were found in patients with psychotic depression as compared

with patients with nonpsychotic depression (Belanoff et al. 2001b; Gomez et al. 2006). Hypercortisolemia has also been associated with cognitive impairment in schizophrenia and schizoaffective disorder as well (Walder et al. 2000). The glucocorticoid antagonist mifepristone (RU-486) has been suggested to be an efficacious treatment for psychotic depression (Belanoff et al. 2001a, 2002; A.H. Young 2006; A.H. Young et al. 2004) as well as treatment-refractory Cushing's disease (Chu et al. 2001).

Nonpsychotic major depression. Depressed patients without psychosis may have either decreased or normal activity of the HPA axis (Posener et al. 2000), whereas depressed patients who have a history of childhood adversity show elevated secretion of ACTH and cortisol in response to a laboratory stress test (Heim et al. 2000) as well as neuroendocrine challenge tests, including the dexamethasone–CRH test (Heim et al. 2001, 2008). Appreciating the presence of childhood trauma in patients with depression may be integral to their treatment because a multisite treatment study found that patients with chronic depression with a history of trauma during childhood responded preferentially to treatment with a form of cognitive-behavioral therapy (CBT) developed for chronic depression compared with the antidepressant nefazodone (Nemeroff et al. 2003). This suggests that particular subtypes of depression may require different approaches to treatment.

Bipolar disorder. Alterations of the HPA axis also have been documented in patients with bipolar affective disorder (Daban et al. 2005; Kiriike et al. 1988) (Table 45–2). Increased HPA axis activity has been associated with mixed manic states (Evans and Nemeroff 1983; R.R. Krishnan et al. 1983; Swann et al. 1992), mania (Godwin et al. 1984; Linkowski et al. 1994), and depression in rapid-cycling patients (Kennedy et al. 1989). In addition, the enhanced salivary cortisol response to waking may represent an ongoing tendency to abnormal cortisol regulation in clinically well, lithium-responsive bipolar patients, indicating the presence of enduring HPA dysregulation (Deshauer et al. 2003). Similarly, abnormal findings using the combined dexamethasone–CRH test have been reported in both remitted and nonremitted patients with bipolar disorder, suggesting its use as a potential trait marker in bipolar disorder (Watson et al. 2004, 2005). Furthermore, the offspring of parents with bipolar disorder have increased basal HPA axis activity through normal psychosocial stress reactivity (Ellenbogen et al. 2004, 2006). One molecular target for heritable predispo-

TABLE 45–2. Alterations in hypothalamic-pituitary-adrenal (HPA) axis activity in bipolar disorder

Increased plasma cortisol concentrations

Blunted diurnal variation of plasma cortisol concentrations

Increased cortisol in cerebrospinal fluid

Nonsuppression of plasma glucocorticoid concentrations after dexamethasone administration

sition to altered HPA reactivity and possibly mood disorder is the GR. Both unipolar and bipolar depressed patients as well as the first-degree relatives of bipolar probands demonstrate reduced expression of GR-α mRNA (Matsubara et al. 2006) as well as alteration of a number of intracellular signaling cascades in lymphocytes (Spiliotaki et al. 2006).

Hypothalamic-Pituitary-Thyroid Axis

Functional Organization of the HPT Axis

The discovery of the tripeptide thyrotropin-releasing hormone (TRH) in 1970 (Burgus et al. 1970; Nair et al. 1970) facilitated expanded understanding of the regulation of the HPT axis. Like CRH, TRH is widely distributed within extrahypothalamic regions of the brain where it acts as a neurotransmitter quite distinct from its role as a hypothalamic–hypophysiotropic hormone. Also similar to CRH, TRH is released by parvocellular neurons of the hypothalamic paraventricular nucleus, whose fibers project to the median eminence where they secrete TRH into the hypothalamo-hypophyseal portal system (Greer 1952; Swanson and Kuypers 1980). TRH is then transported to the anterior pituitary where it acts upon TRH receptors located on pituitary thyrotrophs to cause the release of thyroid-stimulating hormone (TSH), also known as thyrotropin. TSH released from the pituitary is trans-

TABLE 45–3. Alterations in hypothalamic-pituitary-thyroid (HPT) axis activity in unipolar depression

Increased thyrotropin-releasing hormone (TRH) in cerebrospinal fluid

Decreased nocturnal plasma thyroid-stimulating hormone (TSH) concentrations

Blunted or exaggerated TSH response to TRH stimulation

Decreased ΔΔTSH (difference between 11:00 P.M. change in TSH [ΔTSH] and 8:00 A.M. ΔTSH after TRH administration)

Presence of antithyroid microsomal and/or antithyroglobulin antibodies

ported within the systemic circulation to the thyroid gland where activation of TSH receptors results in increased iodine uptake, follicle cell metabolism, and the release of the two major thyroid hormones, T_3 and thyroxine (T_4). Once released into the general circulation, T_3 and T_4 are bound to plasma proteins, including transthyretin and thyroxine-binding globulin. Thyroid hormones regulate a wide variety of metabolic activities and provide negative feedback at the level of the hypothalamus and pituitary to regulate, respectively, the release of TRH and TSH.

Mood Disorders and Pathophysiology of the HPT Axis

Unipolar depression. Several lines of inquiry are indicative of dysregulation of the HPT axis in depression (Table 45–3). Elevated CSF TRH concentrations have been reported in depressed patients (Banki et al. 1988; Kirkegaard et al. 1979), although there is one discordant report (Roy et al. 1994). In addition, reduction of the mean and peak amplitudes of the 24-hour TSH secretion cycle in depressed patients suggests the presence of chronobiological dysfunction within the HPT axis (Duval et al. 1990, 1996). Furthermore, a multitude of studies using a standardized TRH stimulation test in depressed patients with normal thyroid function have consistently revealed a blunted TSH response (Esposito et al. 1997; Nemeroff and Evans 1989), suggesting downregulation of pituitary TRH receptors perhaps in response to hypersecretion of hypothalamic TRH. Alternatively, thyroid hormones may not be effectively transported to the CNS in patients with depression. Reduced CSF concentrations of transthyretin, which is essential for the transport of thyroid hormone across the blood–brain barrier, have been reported in patients with depression (Hatterer et al. 1993; G.M. Sullivan et al. 1999). Clinically, there have been reports that thyroid hormone supplementation, primarily with T_3, is an effective augmentation strategy in the treatment of depression (Aronson et al. 1996; Iosifescu et al. 2005), although again discordant reports have appeared (Appelhof et al. 2004). Recently, a double-blind, placebo-controlled multisite trial of T_3 augmentation of sertraline treatment of depression demonstrated clear efficacy of this augmentation strategy (Cooper-Kazaz et al. 2007). Our group failed to demonstrate any advantage of T_3 coadministration with sertraline compared with placebo in depressed patients in terms of speed of onset or magnitude of antidepressant response (Garlow et al. 2007). One major difference between these two studies is

TABLE 45–4. Grades of hypothyroidism

GRADE	T_3, T_4	BASAL TSH	TSH RESPONSE TO TRH	ANTITHYROID ANTIBODIES
I	Decreased	Increased	Increased	Often present
II	Normal	Increased	Increased	Often present
III	Normal	Normal	Increased	Often present
IV	Normal	Normal	Normal	Present

Note. T_3 = triiodothyronine; T_4 = thyroxine; TRH = thyrotropin-releasing hormone; TSH = thyroid-stimulating hormone.

the dose of sertraline; in the former, the mean dose was considerably lower than in the latter.

Depressed patients have also been repeatedly shown to have a higher-than-expected occurrence of symptomless autoimmune thyroiditis (Table 45–4), as defined by the abnormal presence of circulating thyroid antimicrosomal or antithyroglobulin antibodies (M.S. Gold et al. 1982; Nemeroff et al. 1985). Depressed women with symptomless autoimmune thyroiditis and diffuse nontoxic goiter were more likely to have a reduced response to TRH administration than were depressed women without thyroid disease (Bunevicius et al. 1996). Moreover, the incidence of symptomless autoimmune thyroiditis is higher (i.e., 50%) in depressed patients who are DST nonsuppressors (Haggerty et al. 1987). These patients may be designated as having grade IV hypothyroidism; they have positive antithyroid antibodies but normal T_3, T_4, TSH, and TRH-induced TSH response (Haggerty et al. 1990).

Bipolar disorder. Abnormalities of the HPT axis (e.g., hypothyroidism) also have been reported in patients with bipolar disorder (Table 45–5), as indicated by an exaggerated TSH response to TRH and elevated basal plasma concentrations of TSH (Haggerty et al. 1987; Loosen and Prange 1982). In fact, two groups have reported a higher prevalence rate of hypothyroidism (grades I, II, and III) in bipolar patients who experience rapid cycling of their mood than in bipolar patients who do not (Bauer and

TABLE 45–5. Alterations in hypothalamic-pituitary-thyroid (HPT) axis activity in bipolar disorder

Blunted plasma thyroid-stimulating hormone (TSH) response to thyrotropin-releasing hormone (TRH) stimulation

Exaggerated plasma TSH response to TRH stimulation

Blunted or absent nocturnal surge in plasma TSH concentration

Presence of antithyroid microsomal and/or antithyroglobulin antibodies

Whybrow 1990a; Cowdry et al. 1983). Other abnormalities of the thyroid axis, including a blunted TSH response to TRH, a blunted or absent nocturnal surge in concentrations of plasma TSH (Sack et al. 1988; Souetre et al. 1988), and a higher-than-expected prevalence of antithyroid microsomal or antithyroglobulin antibodies (Lazarus et al. 1986; Myers et al. 1985), have been documented in bipolar patients (see Table 45–4). The presence of antithyroid antibodies often observed in patients with bipolar disorder is apparently not a result of lithium treatment (Kupka et al. 2002), but lithium may exacerbate the process (Calabrese et al. 1985; Dang and Hershman 2002), and autoimmune thyroiditis may form part of the component genetic vulnerability for bipolar disorder (Vonk et al. 2007). Thyroid hormone supplementation has been suggested to be an effective adjunctive treatment for bipolar disorder because hypothyroidism is frequently observed in patients with bipolar disorder (Bauer and Whybrow 1990a, 1990b; Cowdry et al. 1983). As predictors of treatment response, lower free T_4 indices and higher plasma TSH concentrations have been significantly associated with longer times to remission in patients with bipolar disorder (Cole et al. 2002; Fagiolini et al. 2006).

Hypothalamic-Pituitary–Growth Hormone Axis

Functional Organization of the HPGH Axis

Growth hormone (GH) is synthesized and secreted from the somatotrophs of the anterior pituitary. Its secretion is modulated by two hypothalamic–hypophysiotropic hormones, growth hormone–releasing hormone (GHRH, or growth hormone–releasing factor [GRF]) and somatostatin (growth hormone release–inhibiting hormone [GH-RIH], or somatotropin release–inhibiting factor [SRIF]) as well as by the classical monoamine neurotransmitters (e.g., DA, NE, and 5-HT) that innervate the GRF-containing neurons. Located primarily in the arcuate nucleus of the hypothalamus, GRF stimulates the synthesis and release of GH (Flament-Durand 1980). Inhibition of GH release is mediated primarily by SRIF, which is found predominantly in the paraventricular nucleus of the hypothalamus (Flament-Durand 1980). However, unlike GRF, SRIF is also widely distributed in extrahypothalamic brain regions, including the cerebral cortex, hippocampus, and amygdala. Both GRF and SRIF are released from nerve terminals in the median eminence and transported via the hypothalamic–hypophysiotropic portal system to act on the GH-producing somatotrophs of the anterior pituitary.

Release of GH is stimulated by L-dopa (Boyd et al. 1970), a DA precursor, and by apomorphine, a centrally active DA receptor agonist (Lal et al. 1975). GH release also occurs following the administration of the 5-HT precursors L-tryptophan and 5-hydroxytryptophan (5-HTP) (Imura et al. 1973; Muller et al. 1974). The 5-HT receptor antagonists methysergide and cyproheptadine attenuate the GH response to hypoglycemia (Toivola et al. 1972). Under normal basal conditions, GH is secreted in pulses that are highest during the initial hours of the night (Finkelstein et al. 1972).

Mood Disorders and Pathophysiology of the HPGH Axis

Mood disorders have been reported to be associated with multiple alterations in GH secretion (Table 45–6). Nocturnal GH secretion is diminished in depressed patients (Schilkrut et al. 1975), whereas in both unipolar and bipolar depressed patients, daylight GH secretion is exaggerated (Mendlewicz et al. 1985). Furthermore, multiple studies have reported a marked attenuation of the GH response to clonidine, an α_1-adrenergic receptor agonist, and, to a lesser extent, apomorphine, a D_2 and D_3 dopamine receptor agonist, in depressed and bipolar patients (Charney et al. 1982; Checkley et al. 1981; Matussek et al. 1980; Siever et al. 1982). Blunting of noradrenergic agonist–stimulated GH secretion has been observed during mania as well (Dinan et al. 1991). Dexamethasone-induced GH secretion is also significantly decreased in depressed patients (Thakore and Dinan 1994).

GH response to stimulation by GRF has been scrutinized in depressed patients in a limited number of studies, and the results are somewhat discordant. Three research groups have reported a diminished GH response to GRF in depressed patients (Contreras et al. 1996; Lesch et al. 1987a, 1987b; S.C. Risch et al. 1988). However, K.R. Krishnan et al. (1988) found minimal differences between depressed patients and nondepressed control subjects in

TABLE 45–6. Alterations in hypothalamic–growth hormone axis activity in depression

Decreased nocturnal growth hormone secretion in depressed patients

Increased daylight growth hormone secretion (unipolar and bipolar depressed patients)

Decreased growth hormone response to challenge with clonidine and apomorphine

Decreased growth hormone response to growth hormone–releasing factor

Decreased somatostatin in cerebrospinal fluid that is inversely correlated with postdexamethasone plasma cortisol concentrations

GH plasma concentrations following GRF stimulation. These conflicting findings could be explained by various other factors that can influence the GH response to GRF, including gender, age, menstrual cycle, plasma glucocorticoid or somatomedin concentrations, and body weight (Casanueva et al. 1988, 1990; K.R. Krishnan et al. 1988).

Somatostatin (SRIF), the tetradecapeptide hypothalamic GHRIH, inhibits secretion of both CRH and corticotropin (M.R. Brown et al. 1984; Heisler et al. 1982; Richardson and Schonbrunn 1981). In several studies, CSF SRIF concentrations have been reported to be reduced in depressed patients (Agren and Lundqvist 1984; Bissette et al. 1986; Gerner and Yamada 1982; Rubinow et al. 1983) and are inversely correlated with postdexamethasone plasma cortisol concentrations (Rubinow 1986). In fact, exogenous glucocorticoids reduce CSF SRIF concentrations (Wolkowitz et al. 1987). Glucocorticoids likely inhibit the activity of somatostatinergic neurons within the anterior and paraventricular hypothalamus because dexamethasone administration stimulates GH release in nondepressed control subjects (Casanueva et al. 1990).

Hypothalamic-Pituitary-Gonadal Axis

Functional Organization of the HPG Axis

Like the HPA and HPT axes, the HPG axis is organized in a "hierarchical" fashion. Driven by a pulse generator in the arcuate nucleus of the hypothalamus, gonadotropin-releasing hormone (GnRH) secretion occurs in a pulsatile fashion (Knobil 1990). GnRH acts upon the gonadotrophs in the anterior pituitary, releasing luteinizing hormone (LH) and follicle-stimulating hormone (FSH) (Midgley and Jaffe 1971). Fluctuations in LH concentrations in the peripheral circulation are used as an indirect measure of GnRH secretory pulses (Clarke and Cummins 1982) largely because peripheral plasma concentrations of GnRH, like those of TRH and CRH, cannot easily be reliably measured (Meller et al. 1997). In the follicular phase of the menstrual cycle, LH pulses of nearly constant amplitude occur with regular frequency, approximately every 1–2 hours (Reame et al. 1984). In the luteal phase, LH pulse amplitude (reflecting GnRH secretion) is more variable, with pulse frequency declining to one pulse every 2–6 hours (Jaffe et al. 1990). Through negative feedback, gonadal steroids inhibit the secretion of GnRH from the hypothalamus, as well as the secretion of LH and FSH from the anterior pituitary. GnRH secretion is also inhibited by CRH (Jaffe et al. 1990) and β-endorphin (Ferin and Van de Wiele 1984).

Mood Disorders and Pathophysiology of the HPG Axis

Despite the higher incidence of depression in women and the increased occurrence of depression during and after menopause, data are relatively limited on HPG axis function in patients with mood disorders (Table 45–7).

In early studies, no significant differences were reported in plasma concentrations of LH and FSH in depressed postmenopausal women compared with nondepressed matched control subjects (Sachar et al. 1972). However, in a later study, plasma LH concentrations were reported to be decreased in depressed postmenopausal women compared with matched control subjects (Brambilla et al. 1990). Furthermore, depressed *premenopausal* women show increased amplitude pulses of LH in a nonrhythmic fashion in comparison with nondepressed women of similar age (Meller et al. 1997).

Rather than measure baseline plasma levels of the pituitary gonadotropins in depressed patients, other investigators have studied the response of the pituitary to exogenous administration of GnRH. Normal LH and FSH responses to a supraphysiological dose of GnRH (i.e., 250 μg) have been reported in depressed male and female (pre- and postmenopausal) patients (Winokur et al. 1982), whereas a decreased LH response to a lower dose of GnRH (150 μg) has been reported in pre- and postmenopausal depressed patients (Brambilla et al. 1990). In a depressed cohort including both sexes (analyses of men and premenopausal vs. postmenopausal depressed women were not separately performed), no change in baseline or TRH/luteinizing hormone–releasing hormone (LHRH)–stimulated LH or FSH concentrations (200 μg TRH and 100 μg LHRH combined, intravenously) was observed

TABLE 45–7. Alterations of the hypothalamic-pituitary-gonadal axis in depression

Decreased plasma luteinizing hormone concentrations in depressed postmenopausal women

Increased amplitude of nonrhythmic luteinizing hormone pulses in depressed premenopausal women

Decreased luteinizing hormone response to gonadotropin-releasing hormone challenge test in depressed postmenopausal women

DST nonsuppression more common in depressed premenopausal women

(Unden et al. 1988). Notably, plasma LH concentrations have been reported to be increased in individuals who have recovered from a manic episode—possibly a trait phenomenon (Whalley et al. 1987).

Many measures of HPA, HPT, and human GH axis activity do not appear to fluctuate predictably during the menstrual cycle (Leibenluft et al. 1994; E. A. Young et al. 2001). However, estrogen and progesterone do exert important actions on certain components of the HPA axis in women. Estrogen stimulates production of corticosteroid-binding globulin, thereby decreasing concentrations of unbound and physiologically available cortisol, whereas progesterone functions as a glucocorticoid receptor antagonist. In postmenopausal depressed women, DST nonsuppression is more common and occurs with lower plasma cortisol concentrations in comparison with premenopausal depressed women. Thus, ovarian steroids may play a protective role in depressed premenopausal women against elevated circulating glucocorticoid levels as might occur during episodes of major depression (E. A. Young 1995). It is interesting to note that lower follicular-phase mean plasma estradiol levels and a shorter half-life of LH have been reported among depressed women compared with age-matched control subjects (E. A. Young et al. 2000). Additional research on the HPG axis in depression is warranted.

Neurotransmitter Systems

Monoaminergic Neurotransmitters

Serotonin

5-HT is an indoleamine neurotransmitter derived enzymatically from tryptophan and produced in neurons of the rostral and caudal raphe nuclei. Projections originating from the raphe are widespread and innervate a variety of forebrain structures including the hypothalamus, amygdala, basal ganglia, thalamus, hippocampus, cingulate cortex, and prefrontal cortex (Azmitia and Gannon 1986). Fourteen 5-HT receptors, localized on both pre- and postsynaptic elements, have now been identified and include members of the ionotropic as well as metabotropic receptor gene superfamilies (Baez et al. 1995). Following release from synaptic terminals, 5-HT is removed from extracellular fluid by the 5-HTT, located on the presynaptic terminal, and is either repackaged into synaptic vesicles or degraded by monoamine oxidase (MAO).

Several lines of evidence (Table 45–8) suggest a role for deficient 5-HT signaling in depression (Owens and Nemeroff 1994; Purselle and Nemeroff 2003; S.C. Risch and Nemeroff 1992; Vergne and Nemeroff 2006). Low CSF concentrations of the major metabolite of serotonin, 5-HIAA, have repeatedly been found in depressed (Åsberg et al. 1976a, 1976b) and suicidal (Åsberg et al. 1976b; Mann et al. 1996) patients. In addition, acute experimental depletion of tryptophan in patients with remitted depression who had responded to SSRIs has been found to rapidly precipitate recurrence of depression (Booij et al. 2002; K.A. Smith et al. 1997). 5-HTT binding, as measured by functional brain imaging techniques, is reduced in the CNS of depressed patients (Malison et al. 1998; Oquendo et al. 2007; Perry et al. 1983) as well as in postmortem tissue of individuals who have committed suicide (Mann et al. 2000; Stanley et al. 1982), although discordant findings have appeared (Little et al. 1997).

Although there are 14 5-HT receptor subtypes, both 5-HT_{2A} and 5-HT_{2C} have arguably received the most scrutiny in depression (Stahl 1998), although abnormalities in other 5-HT receptor subtypes in depressed patients have been identified, most notably the 5-HT_{1A} receptor (Drevets et al. 1999). Indeed, an increased density of 5-HT_2 receptors is found in the prefrontal cortex and amygdala of untreated suicide victims compared with control subjects (Hrdina et al. 1993), suggesting a possible compensatory upregulation of 5-HT_2 receptor density as a consequence of reduced synaptic concentrations of 5-HT. Similarly, elevation of 5-HT_2 receptor binding on platelets differentiates suicidal from nonsuicidal depressed patients (Bakish et al. 1997), and a reduction in platelet 5-HT_2 receptor binding in antidepressant-treated patients is associated with clinical improvement in depression (Biegon et al. 1987, 1990) in antidepressant-treated patients. Other investigators, however, have reported discordant results with respect to platelet 5-HT_2 receptor binding (Bakish et al. 1997), as well as CNS 5-HT_2 receptor binding (Biver et al. 1997) as a marker of

TABLE 45–8. Alterations in the serotonergic system in depression

Decreased plasma tryptophan concentrations

Decreased cerebrospinal fluid (CSF) 5-hydroxyindoleacetic acid (5-HIAA)

Increased CSF 5-HIAA in psychotic depression

Increased postsynaptic 5-HT_2 receptors

Decreased brain and platelet [^{3}H]imipramine binding

Decreased brain and platelet [^{3}H]paroxetine binding

Blunted prolactin response to fenfluramine

Decreased serotonin transporter (5-HTT) binding in the midbrain of depressed patients (on [^{123}I]- β-CIT)

Note. [^{123}I]-β-CIT = ^{123}I-labeled 2-β-carbomethoxy-3-β-(4-iodophenyl) tropane.

improvement of depressive symptoms or as a marker of depression itself (Meyer et al. 1999). Finally, and perhaps most importantly, a large body of data supports the use of SSRIs, which act primarily by increasing synaptic levels of 5-HT, as first-line agents in the treatment of depression (Nemeroff 2007).

Norepinephrine

NE is a catecholamine neurotransmitter derived enzymatically from tyrosine and produced in neurons of the locus coeruleus (LC) and, to a lesser extent, the lateral tegmental nuclei. Projections originating from the LC innervate a variety of forebrain structures including the cerebral cortex, thalamus, cerebellar cortex, hippocampus, hypothalamus, and amygdala (Moore and Bloom 1979). NE acts through activation of alpha (α) and beta (β) adrenergic receptors. Following release from central synaptic terminals, NE is taken up into the presynaptic element by the norepinephrine transporter (NET) and is either repackaged into synaptic vesicles or degraded by MAO. Within the peripheral nervous system, NE is released from terminals of the sympathetic nervous system, as well as from the adrenal medulla.

Although the database may not be as large or diverse as for 5-HT, findings (Table 45–9) derived from studies of NE turnover, experimental NE depletion, and antidepressant efficacy implicate NE in the pathophysiology and treatment of depression (Ressler and Nemeroff 2001). Elevated CSF concentrations of the major NE metabolite, 3-methoxy-4-hydroxyphenylglycol (MHPG), have been observed in depressed patients, as well as in those with mania and schizoaffective disorder, in some studies (Schildkraut 1965) but not others (De Bellis et al. 1993a). In the latter

TABLE 45–9. Alterations in the noradrenergic system in depression

Increased or decreased 3-methoxy-4-hydroxyphenylglycol (MHPG)

Increased α_2-adrenergic binding in platelets

Blunted growth hormone response to clonidine

Increased β-adrenergic receptors in postmortem brain of suicide victims

Downregulation of β-adrenergic receptors after treatment with antidepressants

study, MHPG levels were found to decline in the subset of patients with depression following treatment with an SSRI, fluoxetine, and subsequent symptom reduction (De Bellis et al. 1993a). Additional studies have confirmed that successful SSRI treatment of depression results in decreased CSF MHPG concentrations (Sheline et al. 1997). In contrast, concentrations of NE and its metabolites have been found to be increased in the plasma (Louis et al. 1975; Roy et al. 1988; Veith et al. 1994; Wyatt et al. 1971) and urine (Roy et al. 1986, 1988) of depressed patients. Depressed patients as a group demonstrate higher baseline plasma NE concentrations compared with control subjects and following orthostatic challenge; melancholic depressed patients exhibit higher plasma NE concentrations than do nonmelancholic depressed patients or healthy control subjects (Roy et al. 1987). Furthermore, depressed DST nonsuppressors have higher basal and cold-stimulated plasma NE levels than do depressed DST suppressors (Roy et al. 1987), suggesting that differences in depressive subtype or severity of mood symptoms may increase noradrenergic activity. Similar to the above-described studies of SSRI treatment on concentrations of CSF MHPG, treatment of depressed patients with TCAs results in decreased plasma (Charney et al. 1981) and urinary concentrations of (Golden et al. 1988; M. Linnoila et al. 1982, 1986) NE metabolites. The validity of plasma or urine concentrations of NE or its metabolites compared with CSF measures as an index of CNS NE circuit activity has long been a subject of intense debate.

In addition to data on NE and NE metabolite turnover, experimental depletion of NE in depressed patients treated with an NE reuptake inhibitor (e.g., desipramine) can precipitate relapse of depression (Charney 1998), as can experimental depletion of catecholamines (which depletes both NE and DA) in euthymic, unmedicated patients with a history of depression (R.M. Berman et al. 1999). Furthermore, suicide victims have been found to

exhibit increased activity of the rate-limiting enzyme in NE synthesis, tyrosine hydroxylase (TH), within the LC in postmortem tissue studies (Ordway 1997), suggestive of high NE turnover in severely depressed patients with compensatory upregulation of TH. Endocrine challenge tests conducted in unmedicated depressed patients using clonidine, an α_2-adrenergic agonist, demonstrate blunting of the normally robust GH response to such adrenergic stimulation (Matussek et al. 1980; Siever et al. 1982, 1992). Finally, a large body of clinical data supports the efficacy of relatively selective NE reuptake inhibitors, such as reboxetine and desipramine, in the treatment of depression (Nemeroff 2007).

Dopamine

DA, the direct precursor to NE, is a catecholamine neurotransmitter in its own right. Within the CNS, dopaminergic neurons are organized into three major systems anatomically (Moore and Bloom 1978): 1) the nigroneostriatal system, which plays a key role in the regulation of movement, originates within the pigmented cells of the substantia nigra pars compacta, and its fibers project rostrally into the corpus striatum; 2) the mesolimbic/mesocortical system is a key regulator of limbic and cortical neural activity and originates within the A10 cell group of the ventral tegmental area (VTA), and its fibers project to numerous limbic structures (mesolimbic system) and the prefrontal cortex (mesocortical system); 3) the tuberoinfundibular system originates within the A12 cells of the arcuate nucleus of the hypothalamus, and its fibers project to the median eminence where released DA acts at the anterior pituitary to inhibit the secretion of prolactin. DA acts through several subtypes of G protein–coupled receptors and, similar to other monoamines, is taken up by the dopamine transporter (DAT) on the presynaptic terminal. Like 5-HT and NE, DA is catabolized by MAO if not repackaged into vesicles for subsequent release.

Dopamine and mood disorders. DA has been implicated in the pathogenesis of depression (Table 45–10) on the basis of metabolite and radioligand data both in postmortem tissue and in patients using functional brain imaging. CSF concentrations of the major DA metabolite homovanillic acid (HVA) (Reddy et al. 1992; Roy et al. 1992) as well as urinary concentrations of 3,4-dihydroxyphenylacetic acid (DOPAC) (Roy et al. 1986) are decreased in patients with depression and may also be associated with suicidal behavior (Roy et al. 1992). In addition, a recent report confirmed and extended the

TABLE 45–10. Alterations in the dopaminergic system in depression

Decreased CSF concentrations of homovanillic acid and urinary concentrations of 3,4-dihydroxyphenylacetic acid in patients with depression

Reduced dopaminergic activity within the caudate, putamen, and nucleus accumbens of depressed patients with affective flattening and psychomotor retardation as measured by [^{18}F]-fluorodopa PET imaging

Reduced dopaminergic activity in the CNS of depressed patients (PET imaging) and suicide victims (postmortem autoradiography)

Decreased levels of serum dopamine β-hydroxylase activity, higher concentrations of plasma dopamine and increased CSF concentrations of homovanillic acid in patients with psychotic depression

Note. CNS=central nervous system; CSF=cerebrospinal fluid; PET=positron emission tomography.

original observations of M. Martinot et al. (2001), in which altered dopaminergic activity, as measured with [^{18}F]fluorodopa positron emission tomography (PET), within the caudate, putamen, and nucleus accumbens of depressed patients with affective flattening and psychomotor retardation was noted (Bragulat et al. 2007). Furthermore, PET studies of the DAT as well as of radiolabeled DOPA uptake in depressed patients (Meyer et al. 2001), in concert with postmortem autoradiography studies in suicide victims (Klimek et al. 2002), collectively indicate reduced activity of DA neurons in depressed patients. This is concordant with the relatively high rate of comorbidity of depression in patients with Parkinson's disease (McDonald et al. 2003), a disorder characterized by DA neuronal degeneration and depression. Finally, preliminary data suggest that DA$_{2/3}$ receptor agonists such as pramipexole or ropinirole may be effective in the treatment of bipolar depression (Goldberg et al. 2004; Zarate et al. 2004b).

Dopamine beta-hydroxylase and mood disorders. The enzyme dopamine β-hydroxylase (DBH) catalyzes the conversion of DA to NE. Preclinical research suggests a major role for DBH in the biological response to antidepressants (Cryan et al. 2004). Compared with nonpsychotic depressed patients, depressed patients with psychotic symptoms have been reported to have lower levels of serum DBH activity and higher concentrations of plasma DA, as well as increased concentrations of CSF and plasma HVA (Aberg-Wistedt et al. 1985; Devanand et al. 1985; Schatzberg et al. 1985a; Sweeney et al. 1978).

Several studies have measured DBH activity in major psychiatric disorders, including schizophrenia and mood disorders. However, results generally have been consistent only for patients with unipolar psychotic depression, who have been reported to have reduced serum DBH activity. Sapru et al. (1989) reported lower serum DBH activity in patients with psychotic major depression compared with control subjects, with no differences between patients with schizophrenia, bipolar disorder (manic phase), or nonpsychotic major depression. Indeed, diminished DBH activity has been hypothesized to be a risk factor for developing psychotic depression, and investigations into allelic variants influencing DBH activity are ongoing (Cubells and Zabetian 2004; Cubells et al. 2002).

Several studies have suggested that dopaminergic activity may be increased, at least partially, as a result of increased adrenocortical activity. Glucocorticoids induce tyrosine hydroxylase, the rate-limiting enzyme in the biosynthesis of DA and NE. The administration of dexamethasone can significantly increase plasma free DA and HVA concentrations in healthy control subjects (Rothschild et al. 1984; Wolkowitz et al. 1985), and the administration of corticosterone or dexamethasone to rats significantly increases central dopaminergic activity (Rothschild et al. 1985; Wolkowitz et al. 1986). Schatzberg et al. (1985a) have hypothesized that the glucocorticoids' enhancement of dopaminergic activity may underlie the development of psychosis in depressed patients.

Monoamine Oxidase

Platelet MAO activity has been studied as a possible biological marker in mood disorders (Table 45–11). Bipolar probands and their relatives have been reported to exhibit decreased platelet MAO activity in comparison with unipolar patients or control subjects (Leckman et al. 1977; Samson et al. 1985). Reduced platelet MAO activity is found primarily in bipolar I, not in bipolar II, sub-

TABLE 45–11. Alterations of monoamine oxidase (MAO) activity in depression

Platelet MAO activity higher in patients with psychotic depression compared with nonpsychotic depressed patients and healthy control subjects

High platelet MAO activity correlated with elevated urinary free cortisol and DST nonsuppression

Elevated MAO-A activity within the CNS of depressed patients as measured by PET imaging

Note. CNS=central nervous system; DST=dexamethasone suppression test; PET=positron emission tomography.

jects (Samson et al. 1985). Although studies have suggested that MAO activity is under strong genetic control and is linked to affective pathology, these results have not been widely replicated (Maubach et al. 1981). Interestingly, Schatzberg et al. (1987) reported that MAO activity was significantly higher in patients with psychotic depression than in patients with nonpsychotic depression or in healthy control subjects.

High platelet MAO activity has been found to correlate with elevated urinary free cortisol concentrations and DST nonsuppression (Agren and Oreland 1982; Schatzberg et al. 1985b). This association between high platelet MAO activity and DST nonsuppression has been replicated by several groups (Meltzer et al. 1988; Pandey et al. 1992). Recently, PET methods have been used to reveal elevated MAO-A activity within the CNS of depressed patients relative to nondepressed patients, suggesting that intracerebral elevations of MAO-A may contribute to depression (Meyer et al. 2006).

Excitatory and Inhibitory Amino Acid Neurotransmitters

Glutamate

Glutamate is the major excitatory neurotransmitter within the CNS and is critically involved in learning and memory formation by both its release as a conventional neurotransmission and its role in the regulation of synaptic plasticity (Derkach et al. 2007; Gillespie and Ressler 2005; Rao and Finkbeiner 2007). These effects are mediated by a large variety of glutamate receptor subtypes that have been identified. They include three major groups of excitatory ionotropic receptors—the N-methyl-D-aspartate (NMDA) receptor, the α-amino-3-hydroxy-5-methylisoxazole-4-propionic acid (AMPA) receptor, and the kainate receptor—and a group of metabotropic glutamate receptors (mGluRs).

Increasing evidence suggests a role for glutamate in the biology of mood disorders (Table 45–12) (Kugaya and Sanacora 2005). Several investigators have reported elevated levels of either serum or plasma glutamate concentrations in depressed patients (Altamura et al. 1993; J.S. Kim et al. 1982; Mauri et al. 1998), although discordant results have also been reported (Maes et al. 1998). Whether circulating glutamate levels are in any way representative of CNS glutamatergic function remains unclear. A reduced density of NMDA–glycine binding sites within the brains of both suicide victims (Nowak et al. 1995) and patients with major depression or bipolar dis-

TABLE 45–12. Alterations of the glutamatergic system in depression and bipolar disorder

Reduced density of NMDA/glycine binding sites within the brains of suicide victims and patients with major depression and bipolar disorder

Reduced neuronal nitric oxide synthase immunoreactivity within the locus coeruleus of depressed patients

Elevated concentrations of the glutamate receptor subunit, NR2C, within the locus coeruleus of depressed patients

Note. NMDA = N-methyl-D-aspartate.

order has been reported (Nudmamud-Thanoi and Reynolds 2004). In addition, reduced neuronal nitric oxide synthase immunoreactivity (Karolewicz et al. 2004) and elevated concentrations of the glutamate receptor subunit, NR2C (Karolewicz et al. 2005), have been reported in the locus coeruleus of depressed patients indicating substantial alterations in glutamatergic tone.

Several agents that either directly or indirectly modulate glutamatergic neurotransmission have been reported to exert therapeutic effects in patients with depression. Nearly 50 years ago, the NMDA partial agonist D-cycloserine (Hood et al. 1989), originally used as an antibiotic in the treatment of tuberculosis, was reported to be effective in the treatment of the vegetative symptoms of depression in patients with tuberculosis (Crane 1959, 1961). D-Cycloserine has also been found to be effective as an adjunctive treatment for behavior therapy in patients with anxiety disorders (Davis et al. 2006; Hofmann et al. 2006; Ressler et al. 2004). Anecdotal reports (Goforth and Holsinger 2007; Kudoh et al. 2002) and placebo-controlled studies (R.M. Berman et al. 2000) have suggested that the NMDA receptor antagonist ketamine may also have efficacy in the treatment of depression. Lamotrigine is an anticonvulsant believed to inhibit the release of glutamate through actions on several different ion channels. It is effective in the prevention of depressive episodes in patients with bipolar disorder (Bowden et al. 2003; Calabrese et al. 1999, 2003; G.M. Goodwin et al. 2004). Finally, riluzole, a purported modulator of glutamatergic neurotransmission (Doble 1996; Iwasaki et al. 2002), may be effective in the treatment of depression (Sanacora et al. 2007; Zarate et al. 2004a, 2005).

Gamma-Aminobutyric Acid

γ-Aminobutyric acid (GABA) functions as the major inhibitory neurotransmitter within the CNS (Akerman and Cline 2007; Mehta and Ticku 1999; Michels and

Moss 2007; Schousboe and Waagepetersen 2007). GABA receptors have been identified throughout the CNS; in addition to its role as a neurotransmitter, GABA also plays a central role during development and neurogenesis (Barker et al. 1998). GABA is a major regulator of many CNS functions and affects a variety of other neurotransmitter systems as well in facilitating the interplay of both "fast" and "slow" synaptic transmission (Greengard 2001).

Three types of GABA receptors, $GABA_A$, $GABA_B$, and $GABA_C$, have been identified. $GABA_A$ receptors are ionotropic receptors coupled to chloride ion channels and are associated with benzodiazepine binding sites (Mehta and Ticku 1999; Michels and Moss 2007). $GABA_B$ receptors, activated by drugs such as baclofen, are metabotropic receptors associated with G proteins and the regulation of potassium channels (Kornau 2006; Ulrich and Bettler 2007). $GABA_C$ receptors, the least common form of GABA receptor, are ionotropic receptors and have been found within the midbrain and retina (Enz 2001; Johnston et al. 2003).

There is some evidence that GABAergic neurotransmission may be altered in mood disorders (Table 45–13) (Kugaya and Sanacora 2005; Sanacora and Saricicek 2007; Tunnicliff and Malatynska 2003). The role of the GABAergic system in the pathophysiology of certain forms of epilepsy has been extensively studied, as has its role in the mechanism of action of antiepileptic drugs (White et al. 2007). The anticonvulsants valproic acid and carbamazepine were serendipitously noted to have a mood-stabilizing effect, decreasing the intensity and frequency of manic and perhaps depressive phases of bipolar disorder. All antimanic agents (including lithium) have been suggested to stabilize mood in part by increasing GABAergic transmission, leading to the hypothesis that a relative GABA deficiency plays a role in mania (Bernasconi 1982).

B.I. Gold et al. (1980) reported that CSF GABA concentrations in depressed patients were significantly lower than in nondepressed control subjects (this finding has been replicated in several studies); GABA plasma concentrations are reduced in depressed patients as well (Petty and Schlesser 1981; Petty and Sherman 1984). Honig et al. (1988) reported that GABA concentrations in brain tissue from patients undergoing cingulotomy for intractable depression were inversely correlated with severity of depression. Healthy subjects with a first-degree relative with a history of major depression appear to have lower plasma GABA concentrations in comparison with subjects without such a family history (Bjork et al. 2001).

TABLE 45–13. Alterations of the GABAergic system in depression

Cerebrospinal fluid GABA concentrations are lower in depressed patients compared with nondepressed control subjects.

Healthy first-degree relatives of patients with a history of major depression have lower plasma concentrations of GABA compared with subjects without such a family history.

Note. GABA = γ-aminobutyric acid.

Of note, low plasma concentrations of GABA are not specific to patients with mood disorders, as they have also been observed in patients with alcoholism (Petty 1994).

Acetylcholine

In the 1970s, Janowsky et al. (1972) proposed that a relative increase or decrease in CNS cholinergic activity in comparison with noradrenergic activity is associated with depression or mania, respectively. Although the adrenergic–cholinergic balance hypothesis appears incomplete in the face of increasing data on the preeminent role of alterations in serotonergic, dopaminergic, and CRHergic neurotransmission in major depression, the importance of cholinergic mechanisms in some forms of depression is supported by both preclinical and clinical observations.

In certain animal models of depression (e.g., the forced-swim model), the administration of cholinesterase inhibitors such as physostigmine is "depressogenic" (McKinney 1984), whereas muscarinic receptor antagonists reverse the effects of such "procholinergic" agents. More convincing evidence of the importance of acetylcholine in the maintenance of mood is the induction of depressed mood following administration of physostigmine or cholinergic agonists (e.g., arecoline) in euthymic control subjects (El-Yousef et al. 1973), unipolar depressed patients (Janowsky and Risch 1984), and bipolar manic patients (Janowsky and Risch 1984).

If cholinergic mechanisms contribute in some manner to the pathophysiology of major depression, then anticholinergic drugs should be effective antidepressants. Although physostigmine-induced dysphoria may be reversed with atropine (El-Yousef et al. 1973), there is no evidence that anticholinergic medications possess antidepressant properties (Janowsky and Risch 1984). Moreover, antidepressants, including the SSRIs, have little affinity for muscarinic cholinergic receptors yet are effective antidepressants. Sitaram et al. (1984) proposed that primary affective illness (specifically bipolar disorder) may be characterized by a state-independent cholinergic hypersensitivity in conjunction with a state-dependent noradrenergic supersensitivity (during late depression and early mania), which returns to normal during remission. They administered arecoline intravenously during the second non–rapid eye movement (NREM) sleep period of the night, which resulted in a more rapid onset of rapid eye movement (REM) sleep in currently depressed as well as remitted patients in comparison with control subjects. This research group has replicated this finding of supersensitive cholinergic responses in patients with major depressive disorder (Dube et al. 1985; Jones et al. 1985). These findings also suggest that cholinergic sensitivity may play a key role in the pathogenesis of depression.

Brain-Derived Neurotrophic Factor

Brain-derived neurotrophic factor (BDNF) is a protein that plays a substantial role in the regulation of neuronal survival and the differentiation and function within the developing and adult CNS, and it also serves important regulatory roles in short- and long-term synaptic plasticity (Bramham 2007; Poo 2001). These effects appear to be mediated, in part, by the activity of the tyrosine kinase B receptor (TrkB, encoded by the *NTRK2* locus) on which BDNF acts. Functionally, BDNF appears to be important in episodic as well as emotion-related memory. Preclinical research using animal models of fear conditioning indicates a central role for BDNF and the TrkB receptor in the development of fear-related memory (Berton et al. 2006; Chhatwal et al. 2006; Rattiner et al. 2004, 2005). Clinical research with humans has identified a functional polymorphism within the BDNF gene that impacts hippocampal function and episodic memory (Egan et al. 2003).

The complex relationship that exists between stress and mood disorders may be mediated in part by the activity of BDNF and other neurotrophic factors (Table 45–14) (Duman and Monteggia 2006; Schmidt and Duman 2007) that ultimately may provide a window for the development of novel antidepressants (Berton and Nestler 2006), although discordant views have appeared (Groves 2007). In rodent models, stress has been found to decrease BDNF mRNA expression within the hippocampus using restraint (M.A. Smith et al. 1995a, 1995b), maternal deprivation (Roceri et al. 2002), and social defeat (Tsankova et al. 2006) paradigms, among others. Notably, reductions in the concentrations of other neurotrophic factors, including nerve growth factor (Ueyama et al. 1997), vascular endothelial growth factor (VEGF), and VEGF receptors (Heine et al. 2005), are also produced by stress as well.

TABLE 45–14. Alterations of the brain-derived neurotrophic factor system in depression

Postmortem studies of depressed suicide victims exhibit decreased hippocampal BDNF expression.

Increased hippocampal BDNF immunoreactivity is observed in depressed patients treated with antidepressants.

Downregulation of the extracellular regulated kinase pathway is seen in completed suicides.

Variety of antidepressant treatments used in humans increase the expression of hippocampal BDNF and block stress-induced downregulation of BDNF expression.

Note. BDNF = brain-derived neurotrophic factor.

Postmortem studies of depressed suicide victims have demonstrated decreased hippocampal BDNF expression (Dwivedi et al. 2003; Karege et al. 2005). Increased hippocampal BDNF-like immunoreactivity in depressed patients treated with antidepressants (B. Chen et al. 2001) has been observed as well as downregulation of the extracellular regulated kinase (ERK) pathway, a major signaling pathway utilized by BDNF (Dwivedi et al. 2001, 2007) in completed suicides. Serum BDNF concentrations are decreased in depressed patients (Karege et al. 2002; Shimizu et al. 2003) and appear to normalize after antidepressant treatment (Aydemir et al. 2005; Gervasoni et al. 2005; Gonul et al. 2005).

The effects of stress appear to be regionally specific within the CNS. Restraint stress increases BDNF expression within the hypothalamus and pituitary (M.A. Smith et al. 1995a). An intriguing finding in regard to the relationship between stress, depression, and BDNF is that antidepressant treatments used in humans, including acute sleep disruption (Fujihara et al. 2003) as well as long-term administration of various antidepressants or repeated electroconvulsive treatments (Nibuya et al. 1995), increase the expression of hippocampal BDNF and block the downregulation of BDNF expression observed in response to restraint (Nibuya et al. 1995) or social defeat (Tsankova et al. 2006) stress paradigms or corticosterone treatment (Dwivedi et al. 2006). Experiments using BDNF knockout mice suggest that BDNF may also play a role in gender differences observed in depressive behavior and that the behavioral effects of antidepressants are at least partially dependent on BDNF (Monteggia et al. 2007).

One possible mediator of the effects of BDNF may be the cyclic adenosine monophosphate (cAMP) response element binding protein (CREB). Chronic, but not acute, administration of a variety of antidepressants, including 5-HT- and NE-selective reuptake inhibitors, increases the expression of hippocampal CREB mRNA in rats. In contrast, chronic administration of other psychotropic drugs does not lead to this effect, highlighting the pharmacological specificity of these effects (Nibuya et al. 1996). At the genomic level, one possible mechanism for the effects of antidepressants is chromatin modification by way of histone remodeling. Indeed, social defeat induces repressive BDNF promoter histone methylation, which is reversed by histone acetylation in the presence of chronic imipramine treatment (Tsankova et al. 2006).

Neuroimaging Studies

Frontal and Prefrontal Cortex

A number of studies using a variety of imaging modalities have identified functional abnormalities within the frontal and prefrontal cortex of patients with unipolar depression (Table 45–15) and bipolar disorder (Table 45–16). Compared with nondepressed individuals, patients with unipolar depression have a lateralized decrease in activity in the left lateral prefrontal cortex repeatedly documented by PET and single photon emission computed tomography (SPECT) investigations (Baxter et al. 1985, 1989; Bench et al. 1992; Dolan et al. 1992, 1993; Hurwitz et al. 1990; J.L. Martinot et al. 1990; Navarro et al. 2002), although this finding is apparently not specific to depression and has been seen in patients with schizophrenia (Barch et al. 2003; K.F. Berman et al. 1988; Dolan et al. 1993; Weinberger et al. 1986), depressed patients with Parkinson's disease (Ring et al. 1994) or traumatic brain injury (Jorge et al. 2004), and patients with other neurological diseases with depression as a secondary outcome (Mayberg 1994). Similarly, structural magnetic resonance imaging (MRI) studies have revealed prefrontal cortex abnormalities in unipolar depression, including reduced left subgenual prefrontal cortex volume (Botteron et al. 2002), increased lesion density in medial orbital prefrontal white matter (MacFall et al. 2001), and decreased medial orbitofrontal cortical volume (Ballmaier et al. 2004; Bremner et al. 2002; Lacerda et al. 2004; Monkul et al. 2007). Reductions in left prefrontal gray matter volume have also been reported in patients with bipolar disorder (Lopez-Larson et al. 2002).

Using patients with major depression, changes in prefrontal activity were initially associated with impaired cognition (Aizenstein et al. 2005; Bench et al. 1993; Okada et al. 2003). Metabolic changes observed in depressed patients normalize on recovery from depression,

TABLE 45–15. Abnormalities of the frontal and prefrontal cortex in unipolar depression by neuroimaging

Decreased activity within the left prefrontal cortex using both PET and SPECT methods that normalizes upon recovery from depression

Reduced left subgenual prefrontal cortex volume

Increased lesion density in medial orbital frontal white matter that correlates with depression severity in elderly depressed patients

Decreased medial orbitofrontal cortical volume in patients with remitted major depression

Note. PET = positron emission tomography; SPECT = single photon emission computed tomography.

suggesting that the lateralized reduction in left prefrontal activity may be a state, rather than trait, marker for depression (Bench et al. 1995; Navarro et al. 2002; Schaefer et al. 2006). Since then, use of functional imaging of the prefrontal response in various visual imagery provocation paradigms has enabled the differentiation of depressed unipolar patients with and without anger attacks (Dougherty et al. 2004), anhedonic symptoms in unipolar patients (Keedwell et al. 2005a, 2005b), and response to valenced social imagery in unipolar depressed patients (Schaefer et al. 2006; Wang et al. 2006). Furthermore, depressed bipolar patients may be distinguished from depressed unipolar patients on the basis of subcortical and ventral prefrontal cortical responses to positive and negative emotional expressions (Lawrence et al. 2004). Additionally, imaging studies using nondepressed subjects have demonstrated a significant effect of genotype on the coupling of ventromedial prefrontal and amygdala activation following exposure to aversive imagery (Heinz et al. 2005). Consistent with the foregoing data, a recently reported stereotactic meta-analysis using pooled imaging data supports repeated findings of abnormal brain activation in depression within regions of the brain that represent the substrate for normal emotional experience in healthy subjects (Steele et al. 2007).

TABLE 45–16. Abnormalities of the frontal and prefrontal cortex in bipolar disorder by neuroimaging

Reduced left prefrontal gray matter volume in patients with bipolar disorder

Depressed bipolar patients differentiated from depressed unipolar patients on subcortical and ventral prefrontal cortical responses to positive and negative emotional expression

Subgenual Cingulate

The subgenual cingulate (Cg25) has received considerable attention in studies of patients with mood disorders (Table 45–17). Brain imaging studies (Brody et al. 2001; Drevets 1999; Mayberg 1994) suggested the importance of limbic–cortical pathways in the pathogenesis of major depression. Additional research (Mayberg et al. 1999; Seminowicz et al. 2004) demonstrated the importance of Cg25 in the modulation of acute sadness and response to antidepressant treatment, indicative of a role for Cg25 in the regulation of negative affect states. Cg25 possesses descending projections to a variety of brain regions (brain stem, hypothalamus, and insula) implicated in regulating neurovegetative and motivational states associated with depression (Barbas et al. 2003; Freedman et al. 2000; Jurgens and Muller-Preuss 1977; Ongur et al. 1998). Furthermore, a number of pathways link Cg25 to the orbitofrontal, medial prefrontal, and anterior and posterior cingulate cortices, providing a means through which autonomic and homeostatic processes influence learning, reward, and motivation (Barbas et al. 2003; Carmichael and Price 1996; Haber 2003; Vogt and Pandya 1987). Decreased activity of Cg25 has been associated with positive clinical response to a diverse variety of antidepressant treatments (Dougherty et al. 2003; Goldapple et al. 2004; Mayberg et al. 2000; Mottaghy et al. 2002; Nobler et al. 2001). More recently, deep brain stimulation (DBS) of Cg25, originally developed for the treatment of Parkinson's disease (Benabid 2003), has been shown to produce significant clinical benefits for patients with treatment-resistant depression (Mayberg et al. 2005).

Hippocampus

Owing to its major role in the regulation of both stress and learning, the hippocampus has been a major focus of neuroanatomical studies in patients with depression (Table 45–18). Functionally, the hippocampus plays a central

TABLE 45–17. Abnormalities of the subgenual cingulate in depression by neuroimaging

Neural activity in Cg25 correlates with experimental induction of acute sadness.

Decreased activity of Cg25 correlates with a positive clinical response to several different antidepressant treatments.

Deep brain stimulation of Cg25 produces clinical improvement in patients with treatment-resistant depression.

Note.   Cg25=subgenual cingulate.

TABLE 45–18. Abnormalities of the hippocampus in depression by neuroimaging

Reduced hippocampal volume is found in some, but not all, patients with depression as well as those with other neuropsychiatric illnesses such as posttraumatic stress disorder.

In patients with hippocampal atrophy, the extent of atrophy correlates positively with the duration of depression.

Small hippocampal size may be a risk factor for depression.

Exposure to traumatic stress during childhood or adulthood is associated with decreased hippocampal volume.

Depression associated with childhood traumatic stress is associated with hippocampal atrophy, whereas depression without childhood traumatic stress is not.

role in adaptation to stress because of its seminal role in the regulation of HPA axis activity, as well as the registration of explicit memory and learning context. Furthermore, the hippocampus is a remarkably plastic structure, being a major site of neurogenesis in the adult brain while also possessing a well-demonstrated vulnerability to stress. Neurons of the CA3 region exhibit a loss of dendritic spines, reduced dendritic branching, and impaired neurogenesis in response to stress exposure (Duman and Monteggia 2006; Fuchs and Gould 2000; Nestler et al. 2002).

Hippocampal vulnerability to stress may, in part, be a consequence of its high concentration of type I and type II corticosteroid receptors that enable the hippocampus to exert an inhibitory role on activity of the HPA axis (Jacobson and Sapolsky 1991). Prolonged exposure to high concentrations of corticosteroids during stress results in hippocampal damage in rodents (Magarinos and McEwen 1995a, 1995b; Magarinos et al. 1997) and nonhuman primates (Magarinos et al. 1996; Sapolsky et al. 1990; Uno et al. 1989, 1994). In humans, bilateral hippocampal atrophy has been observed in patients with Cushing's syndrome, in whom the extent of hippocampal atrophy correlates with the magnitude of corticosteroid hypersecretion (Starkman et al. 1992).

Reduced hippocampal size has been documented in a wide variety of neuropsychiatric disorders (Geuze et al. 2005). With respect to mood disorders, reduced hippocampal volume has been found in some (Bremner et al. 2000; Frodl et al. 2002b; Sheline 1996) but not all (Rusch et al. 2001; Vakili et al. 2000) studies of patients with unipolar depression (Campbell and Macqueen 2004). In patients with a history of depression who also have hippocampal atrophy, the extent of atrophy is greater in patients with a higher total lifetime duration of depression (Sheline et al. 1996, 1999). The finding of reduced hippocampal volume in patients with remitted unipolar depression (Neumeister et al. 2005) has raised the possibility that small hippocampal size may be a risk factor for depression.

Exposure to traumatic stress, either early in life or during adulthood, is associated with loss of hippocampal volume and has been documented in individuals with combat-induced (Bremner et al. 1995; Vythilingam et al. 2005), childhood abuse–related (Bremner et al. 1997b, 2003), and chronic (Kitayama et al. 2005) PTSD as well as those with dissociative identity disorder (Vermetten et al. 2006). Similarly, patients with a history of early-life stress or trauma and depression also have been found to have decreased hippocampal volume (Driessen et al. 2000; Stein et al. 1997). Vythilingam et al. (2002) reported that depressed women with a history of childhood sexual abuse, but not depressed women without such a history, had a reduction in hippocampal volume compared with control subjects, suggesting that previous reports of reduced hippocampal size in patients with depression may in fact be secondary to childhood trauma rather than to depression per se.

Basal Ganglia

Vulnerability to affective dysfunction might derive from disruption of connections between the basal ganglia or from interruption of pathways connecting the basal ganglia to other parts of the brain, specifically the limbic system and prefrontal cortex (Alexander et al. 1986; K.R. Krishnan 1991). A substantial preclinical literature suggests a major role for the nucleus accumbens/ventral striatum and ventral tegmental area in the motivational and hedonic components of mood disorders (Nestler and Carlezon 2006).

Initial imaging investigations into the role of the basal ganglia focused on metabolic and volumetric comparisons between different populations of mood disorder patients and healthy control subjects. These studies have used a variety of imaging modalities and have identified structural and functional abnormalities within components of the basal ganglia of patients with unipolar depression (Table 45–19) and bipolar disorder (Table 45–20). For example, a PET study measuring neural activity of different brain regions of manic and euthymic patients with bipolar disorder showed increased activity in the head of the left caudate as well as in the left dorsal anterior cingulate among subjects with symptoms of mania (Blumberg et al. 2000). PET and functional magnetic resonance imaging (fMRI) studies of patients with major de-

TABLE 45–19. Abnormalities of the basal ganglia in unipolar depression by neuroimaging

Decreased left caudate activity in depressed patients with psychomotor retardation compared with depressed patients with anxiety and healthy control subjects

Behavioral response to feedback associated with abnormal activity within the medial caudate and ventromedial orbitofrontal cortex

Correlation between psychomotor–anhedonia symptoms and decreased activity of the anteroventral caudate and putamen during nonemotional auditory task

Reduced activation of the right putamen in response to facial expressions of increasing happiness

Reduced bilateral ventral striatal activation in response to positive stimuli that correlates with the extent of anhedonia in depressed patients

pression found that left caudate activity was lower in depressed patients with psychomotor retardation compared with depressed patients with anxiety and healthy control subjects (M. Martinot et al. 2001). In a structural MRI study of patients with bipolar disorder compared with matched healthy control subjects, the age of the patients and length of illness correlated with respectively larger left globus pallidus and smaller left putamen volumes (Brambilla et al. 2001).

Several imaging studies are consistent with deficient responsiveness of frontostriatal circuits of depressed patients. Elliott et al. (1998) reported that the behavioral response to feedback in depressed patients is associated with an abnormal neural response within the medial caudate and ventromedial orbitofrontal cortex. Building on this finding, other investigators (Dunn et al. 2002) reported a correlation between the psychomotor–anhedonia symptom cluster of the Beck Depression Inventory

TABLE 45–20. Abnormalities of the basal ganglia in bipolar disorder by neuroimaging

Increased activity of the head of the left caudate and the left dorsal anterior cingulate in manic patients using positron emission tomography methods

Increased volume of the left globus pallidus and decreased volume of the left putamen correlates with the age of bipolar patients and the length of illness

Increased subcortical and ventral prefrontal cortical response to positive and negative emotional expressions

Increased metabolic activity in the caudate and ventral striatum of medicated depressed bipolar II patients and decreased metabolism within the anteroventral caudate and putamen in subjects performing a nonemotional auditory task. Depressed patients have also been found to exhibit reduced activation of the right putamen in response to facial expressions of increasing happiness (Surguladze et al. 2005). Furthermore, in comparison with healthy control subjects and unipolar depressed patients, bipolar patients demonstrate increased subcortical and ventral prefrontal cortical responses to both positive and negative emotional expressions (Lawrence et al. 2004). Epstein et al. (2006) used a functional imaging paradigm to examine the ventral striatal responses to positive and negative stimuli in depressed patients. Depressed subjects exhibited reduced bilateral ventral striatal activation in response to positive stimuli, and this decrease was correlated with reduced interest/pleasure in, and performance of, activities. More recently, increased metabolic activity has been reported in the caudate and ventral striatum of medicated depressed bipolar II patients (Mah et al. 2007).

Amygdala

The amygdala is known to play a significant role in the processing of emotions and affectively charged stimuli (Davidson et al. 2002). For example, Isenberg et al. (1999) found significantly greater bilateral amygdala activation during both the response to and the perception of emotionally charged stimuli when compared with non–emotionally charged stimuli. Several imaging studies of patients with mood disorders have focused on elucidating the association between mood alterations and abnormalities in the amygdala (Table 45–21) as well as other structures (Leppanen 2006; Phan et al. 2004). An initial report found that increased resting metabolism within the right amygdala of depressed patients is predictive of negative affect (Abercrombie et al. 1998). Subsequent fMRI investigation using a masked face paradigm found relative increased activity of the left amygdala among depressed patients that normalized with antidepressant treatment (Sheline et al. 2001). Similarly, increased activation of the left amygdala in depressed adolescents using evocative face viewing has been associated with poor memory for faces relative to healthy and anxious control subjects (Roberson-Nay et al. 2006). In addition to the response to valenced visual stimuli, the amygdala also responds differentially to both positive and negative words (Hamann and Mao 2002). Using PET methodologies, Drevets et al. (2002) reported that left amygdala metabolism was increased and positively correlated with stress-induced plasma cortisol concentrations in subjects with unipolar

TABLE 45–21. Abnormalities of the amygdala in unipolar depression and bipolar disorder by neuroimaging

Increased activity of left amygdala during evocative face viewing and normalization with antidepressant treatment in unipolar depressed patients

Increased activity of left amygdala positively correlated with stress-induced plasma cortisol in unipolar and bipolar depressed patients

Bilateral increases in amygdala volume in first-episode, but not recurrent, major depression

In depression, sustained amygdala processing in response to negative information possibly correlated with self-reported rumination

Anticipation of aversive stimuli increases activation of the extended amygdala in women with major depression

Decreased density of amygdala serotonin transporter (5-HTT) in unipolar and bipolar depressed patients

Structural imaging studies have identified bilateral increases in amygdala volume in patients during the first episode of major depression (Frodl et al. 2002a; Lange and Irle 2004), although not in patients with recurrent depression (Frodl et al. 2003). Increased right amygdala volume has been reported in women with depression and a history of suicidality (Monkul et al. 2007). Decreased amygdala volume (Rosso et al. 2005) and blunted amygdala activation have been reported in children with depression (Thomas et al. 2001). Sustained activation of the amygdala observed in unipolar depressed patients relative to nondepressed control subjects in response to negative information correlates with self-reported rumination (Siegle et al. 2002), as well as personal relevance rating of words (Siegle et al. 2007). Anticipation of aversive stimuli increases activation of the extended amygdala in women with major depression compared with healthy control subjects (Abler et al. 2007).

Serotonin may play a central role in modulating amygdala activity during emotional information processing (Hariri and Holmes 2006). Genomic imaging studies using nondepressed subjects have demonstrated a significant effect of 5-HTT genotype on the response of the amygdala to fearful stimuli (Hariri et al. 2002); the coupling of ventromedial prefrontal, cingulate, and amygdala activation (Heinz et al. 2005; Pezawas et al. 2005); and the response to tryptophan depletion in patients with remitted depression (Neumeister et al. 2006). Short-term administration of the SSRI citalopram to nondepressed subjects alters amygdala reactivity to nonconscious threat stimuli (Harmer et al. 2006), and amygdala reactivity may be influenced partially by the density of amygdala 5-HT_{1A} receptors (Fisher et al. 2006). Depressed patients, both bipolar and unipolar, have decreased 5-HTT density within the amygdala (Oquendo et al. 2007).

Thalamus

It is unclear whether thalamic volumes are altered in patients with mood disorders (Table 45–22). A structural imaging study comparing patients with bipolar disorder, patients with unipolar depression, and healthy control subjects found no differences between groups with respect to thalamic volume (Caetano et al. 2001). Consistent with this finding, several previous studies also failed to show differences in thalamic volumes of patients with mood disorders compared with healthy control subjects (Buchsbaum et al. 1997; K.R. Krishnan et al. 1993; Strakowski et al. 1993). Alternatively, other studies have found smaller thalamic volumes in patients with bipolar disorder and unipolar depression (Dasari et al. 1999; Dupont et al. 1995). Interestingly, in a PET study, decreased glucose metabolism in the thalamus was reported in patients with unipolar depression (Buchsbaum et al. 1997).

Pituitary

Relatively few imaging studies have measured pituitary volumes in patients with mood disorders (Table 45–23). Pituitary volumes were reported to be larger in patients with major depression (16 with unipolar depression and 3 with bipolar depression) in comparison with healthy control subjects (K.R. Krishnan et al. 1991). In a study of psychiatric inpatients, of whom 20 had unipolar depression, a positive correlation was found between postdexamethasone plasma cortisol concentrations and pituitary volume (Axelson et al. 1992). In contrast, in a study examining the association between seasonal depression and pituitary volumes, no significant difference in pituitary volumes was found between acutely depressed patients and healthy control subjects (Schwartz et al. 1997). In a study of patients with bipolar disorder, patients with unipolar depression, and healthy control subjects, no differences in pituitary volumes were observed between patients with unipolar depression and control subjects; however, significantly smaller pituitary volumes were found in the patients with bipolar disorder (Sassi et al. 2001). In a more recent study, pituitary volumes did not differ between pediatric bipolar patients and control subjects (H.H. Chen et al. 2004).

Inflammation, Depression, and Stress

A growing body of evidence suggests that systemic inflammation may contribute to the pathophysiology of mood disorders (Table 45–24). Inflammation is a key component of the adaptive response to stress (Chrousos 1995). Acute stress results in secretion of proinflammatory cytokines (Elenkov et al. 2005; Glaser and Kiecolt-Glaser 2005; McEwen 1998), peripheral secretion of acute-phase proteins such as fibrinogen and C reactive protein that promote infection resistance and tissue repair, and induction of nuclear factor kappa B (NF-κB), a candidate mediator for some of the CNS effects related to the inflammatory response (Bierhaus et al. 2003). The latter is also a potentially important mediator in synaptic development within the central and peripheral nervous systems (Gutierrez et al. 2005). Another component of the adaptive response to acute stress is increased HPA axis activity and its end product, the increased secretion of glucocorticoids, that act on intracellular signaling pathways that help to terminate the inflammatory response after cessation of acute stress (Chrousos 1995). This relationship between the HPA axis and systemic in-

TABLE 45–22. Abnormalities of the thalamus in unipolar depression and bipolar disorder by neuroimaging

The relation between thalamic abnormalities and mood disorders remains unclear.

Smaller thalamic volumes may be associated with bipolar disorder and unipolar depression.

Decreased metabolism in the thalamus may be associated with unipolar depression.

TABLE 45–23. Abnormalities of the pituitary in unipolar depression and bipolar disorder by neuroimaging

Pituitary volumes may be increased in patients with bipolar and unipolar depression.

Postdexamethasone plasma cortisol concentrations appear to be positively correlated with pituitary volumes among unipolar depressed patients.

No significant correlation has been found between seasonal depression and pituitary volumes.

Few studies have examined the relation between pituitary volume and mood disorders.

TABLE 45–24.   Inflammation and depression

Systemic inflammation may play a key role in the etiology of a number of common medical diseases, including diabetes, cardiovascular disease, and depression.

Nuclear factor kappa B is a candidate mediator for some of the CNS effects related to the inflammatory response.

Administration of proinflammatory cytokines to laboratory animals results in behavioral and neurovegetative symptoms that are similar to those observed in patients with depression.

Clinical research in humans has identified a number of proinflammatory cytokines that are elevated in patients with depression.

Humans treated with interferon-α, which promotes the release of IL-6, IL-1β, and TNF-α, commonly develop symptoms of depression.

Patients with a history of childhood trauma have an elevated risk not only for depression but also for a variety of common chronic medical diseases.

A graded relationship exists between childhood maltreatment and elevations in plasma inflammatory markers in adulthood.

Depressed male patients with a history of early-life stress demonstrate an increased inflammatory response to acute psychosocial stress.

Note.   CNS = central nervous system; IL = interleukin; TNF-α = tumor necrosis factor–alpha.

flammation may be especially relevant to mood disorders in view of the findings that patients with a history of early-life stress have an impaired capacity to regulate the HPA axis in the presence of psychosocial stress (Heim et al. 2000) as well as an increase in inflammatory cytokines, suggesting that control of the inflammatory response may be impaired as well.

A diverse and growing database indicates that systemic inflammation may play a key role in the etiology of a number of common medical diseases including diabetes (Wellen and Hotamisligil 2005), cardiovascular disease (Willerson and Ridker 2004), cancer (Li et al. 2005), and depression (Evans et al. 2005; Maes 1999; Raison et al. 2006) (see Table 45–24). Administration of proinflammatory cytokines to laboratory animals results in a pattern of behavioral and neurovegetative symptoms known as "sickness behavior" that is similar to the depression observed in human patients and includes psychomotor slowing, fatigue, elevated pain sensitivity, disrupted sleep, and anxiety (Kent et al. 1992). Clinical research in humans has identified an array of proinflammatory cytokines including interleukin (IL)-6, IL-1β, and tumor necrosis factor–alpha (TNF-α) (Alesci et al. 2005; Kahl et al. 2005; Miller et al. 2002; Musselman et al. 2001b; Penninx et al.

2003) and inflammatory markers such as C reactive protein (Danner et al. 2003; Ford and Erlinger 2004; Kahl et al. 2005; Miller et al. 2002; Panagiotakos et al. 2004; Penninx et al. 2003) that are elevated in patients with depression. Humans treated with interferon-α, which promotes the release of IL-6, IL-1β, and TNF-α, commonly develop symptoms of depression, and a significant subset of these individuals fulfill diagnostic criteria for an episode of major depression (Musselman et al. 2001a; Raison et al. 2005), which may be effectively treated with SSRIs (Musselman et al. 2001a).

Inflammation may be particularly relevant to three populations of depressed patients: those with treatment-resistant depression (Maes 1999; Sluzewska et al. 1997), those with chronic medical illness comorbid with depression (Evans et al. 2005), and those with depression associated with early-life stress (Danese et al. 2007; Pace et al. 2006). In some patients, exposure to trauma or stressful childhood experiences may be a variable connecting risk for depression, chronic medical illness, and inflammation. Thus, patients with childhood trauma have an elevated risk not only for depression (Kendler et al. 2004), which is often chronic in course (Hayden and Klein 2001; Kaplan and Klinetob 2000; Lara et al. 2000), but also for a variety of common, chronic, and progressive medical diseases including coronary artery disease (R.D. Goodwin and Stein 2004). Elevated levels of inflammatory markers including C reactive protein, fibrinogen, and IL-6 are associated with psychosocial risk factors for cardiovascular disease (Ranjit et al. 2007), and a graded relationship exists between childhood maltreatment and elevations in plasma C reactive protein concentrations in adulthood (Danese et al. 2007). Moreover, depressed male patients with a history of early-life stress demonstrate an increased inflammatory response to acute psychosocial stress (Pace et al. 2006).

Genetic Studies of Mood Disorders

Major depressive disorder and bipolar disorder are both, in part, heritable illnesses (Table 45–25). Heritability estimates for major depression based on estimates from twin studies range from 40% to 50% with respect to major depressive disorder (Bierut et al. 1999; Kendler et al. 1993, 2001a; McGuffin et al. 1991, 1996; P.F. Sullivan et al. 2000; Torgersen 1986) and as high as 85% to 93% for bipolar disorder (Kieseppa et al. 2004; McGuffin et al. 2003). Genetic influences on resilience to depression may be as important as the genetic influence on vulnerability to depression (Rijsdijk et al. 2003). Adoption studies also fee and Price 2007; Lee and Lupski 2006; N. J. Risch 2000).

TABLE 45–25. Genetics and mood disorders

Family, twin, linkage, and association studies support a strong role for genetic liability with respect to risk for depression.

Mood disorders are complex (as opposed to Mendelian or single-gene) genetic diseases involving multiple and variably penetrant genes with individually variable modes of inheritance.

Interactions between individual genes and the environment are likely to play an important role in the etiology of unipolar depression and bipolar disorder.

Genetic influences on both resilience and risk for the development of mood disorders are developing areas of investigation in psychiatric genetics.

support the notion of a substantial genetic component of risk for major depression (Cadoret 1978; Mendlewicz and Rainer 1977; Wender et al. 1986) and bipolar disorder (Wender et al. 1986). Family studies indicate that the relative risk ratio for major depression probands is 2%–3% (Gershon et al. 1982; Maier et al. 1992; Weissman et al. 1984), whereas risk for the development of bipolar disorder among first-degree relatives of bipolar probands ranges from 5% to 12% (Alda 1997). When the scope of risk is expanded to include the development of any form of mood disorder, risk for first-degree relatives of bipolar probands increases to 20% to 25% (Smoller and Finn 2003). Finally, risk for the development of major mood disorder (unipolar or bipolar) is increased by exposure to detrimental environmental factors such as childhood abuse and neglect or other forms of early-life stress that promote vulnerability to major depression (Kendler et al. 2002, 2004) and bipolar disorder (Neria et al. 2005).

The mode of inheritance for major depression (Marazita et al. 1997; Moldin et al. 1991; Price et al. 1987) and bipolar disorder (Nurnberger and Foroud 2000) is unclear. Historically, genetic research on mood disorders has focused on the use of single gene models that likely do not apply to major depression, bipolar disorder, or other psychiatric illnesses. Like many common medical illnesses such as hypertension, coronary artery disease, and diabetes mellitus, mood disorders as clinical syndromes likely evolve from the differential contribution of multiple variably penetrant genes with differing modes of inheritance and whose expression is likely influenced by environmental exposures and possibly architectural changes within the genome such as genomic rearrangement or copy number variation. As a consequence, major depression, types I and II bipolar disorder, and other forms of mood disorder such as minor depression, dysthymia, and cyclothymia may be termed *complex* genetic diseases (Baron 2001; Jaf-

The term *complex* stands in distinction to classic genetic diseases such as Huntington's disease or phenylketonuria, often referred to as Mendelian disorders (in honor of the Augustinian monk Gregor Mendel), in which mutations of a single gene are entirely or largely responsible for a particular disease. Within the context of complex genetic disease, additive and multiplicative, rather than purely dominant or recessive, models of genetic risk may be useful in dissecting the genetic contribution to major depression and bipolar disorder (Orstavik et al. 2007; Rijsdijk et al. 2003) as well as other forms of psychiatric disease (Comings 2001).

Candidate Gene Studies

An enormous body of research examining candidate genes for mood disorders and other psychiatric illnesses exists. Much of this research has focused on attempting to identify candidate genes whose allelic variants are thought to predict differences in risk for categorical diagnosis of major depression or quantitative differences in depressive symptomatology either alone, as genetic main effects, or in concert with the environment. In some cases, these variants are single nucleotide polymorphisms (SNPs) that alter the regulation of the gene or the structure of the protein that it codes for, whereas in other cases the gene variants may be structural alterations within the genome such as variable number tandem repeats (VNTRs) that alter the function of the gene they reside within, or the investigated variants may themselves just be markers of so far unknown genetic variation close by. Some of the more well-known genes that have been investigated include the 5-HTT gene (Caspi et al. 2003; Chorbov et al. 2007; Kaufman et al. 2006; Kendler et al. 2005), the BDNF gene (Kaufman et al. 2006), the glucocorticoid receptor chaperone protein gene *FKBP5* (Binder et al. 2004; Lekman et al. 2008; Willour et al. 2008), and the type 1 corticotropin-releasing hormone receptor gene (Bradley et al. 2008; Licinio et al. 2004).

The candidate gene literature for psychiatric disease is complex, and the frequently discordant results between well-designed studies of candidate genes make interpretation of the literature challenging (Caspi et al. 2003; Chorbov et al. 2007). Comprehensive review of this literature is beyond the scope of this chapter (but see Craddock and Forty 2006; Kato 2007; Levinson 2006 for useful reviews). Some continuing areas of intense discussion include the phenotypic description of psychiatric disease (Bearden et al. 2004; Craddock and Forty 2006) and putatively related endophenotypes (Bearden and Freimer 2006; Cannon and Keller 2006; Hasler et al. 2004), measurement of gene–environment interactions and correlations (Craddock and Forty 2006; Eaves 2006; Jaffee and Price 2007), epigenetic influences on the genome (Mill and Petronis 2007), statistical issues related to multiple comparisons (Abecasis et al. 2005; Sabatti et al. 2003), and study replication criteria (Chanock et al. 2007).

Association studies investigating individual candidate genes differ fundamentally from linkage studies in that they generate a hypothesis that a particular gene, or region of a gene, plays a central role in some component of the pathophysiology of a disease. Historically, candidate genes for association studies have been chosen on the basis of linkage data or a biological rationale for how a particular gene may contribute to the production, maintenance, or relapse of the disease under investigation. We provide a brief selected review of candidate gene studies in mood disorders below.

Serotonin

The 5-HTT gene, *SLC6A4* (Lesch et al. 1993), has repeatedly been implicated as an important candidate gene in association studies conducted with depressed patients. Several polymorphisms have been described for this gene. A common functional polymorphism in the 5′ promoter region of *SLC6A4*, referred to as the 5-HTT gene–linked polymorphic region (5-HTTLPR), consists of a repetitive region containing 16 imperfect repeat units of 22 bp, located ~1,000 bp upstream of the transcriptional start site (Heils et al. 1996; Lesch and Mossner 1998) (for more detail, see Chapter 3 in this volume, "Genetics and Genomics"). The 5-HTTLPR has been associated with different basal activity of the transporter, most likely related to differential transcriptional activity (Gelernter et al. 1999). The long variant (L allele) of this polymorphism has been shown to lead to higher serotonin reuptake by the transporter in vitro. However, a PET study could not identify differences in serotonin transporter binding potential by 5-HTTLPR genotype in healthy control subjects or patients with major depression (Parsey et al. 2006). Other potentially functional polymorphisms include a VNTR polymorphism located within intron 3 as well as several nonsynonymous SNPs in the coding region (for a review, see Hahn and Blakely 2002). The latter polymorphisms have been less studied in psychiatric genetics, while for the 5-HTTLPR, well over 400 association studies are listed in PubMed to date. The effects of this polymorphism on response to SSRI treatment have been investigated by

a number of studies, and a recent meta-analysis by Serretti et al. (2007) indicates that the L allele may be associated with a beneficial response profile. However, this finding could not be replicated in the large Sequenced Treatment Alternatives to Relieve Depression (STAR*D) trial, and some evidence suggests that this association with treatment response may be carried by an increased risk for side effects in individuals carrying the short variant (S allele) (Kraft et al. 2007; Murphy et al. 2004).

A large number of studies have investigated the association of this polymorphism with unipolar and bipolar depression as well as suicide. Several meta-analyses on this topic seem to support an involvement of this polymorphism in bipolar disorder and suicide attempts, albeit with odds ratios less than 1.2 for bipolar disorder (Anguelova et al. 2003; Cho et al. 2005; Lasky-Su et al. 2005; Li and He 2007; Lin and Tsai 2004; Lotrich and Pollock 2004). Associations with unipolar depression are more controversial and are likely dependent on gene–environment interactions that are now well validated for this polymorphism. Using a large well-characterized cohort in New Zealand, Caspi et al. (2003) demonstrated that exposure to stress in childhood, in concert with a particular 5-HTTLPR genotype, predicts depressive symptoms in adulthood. This finding has now been replicated in a series of studies (Eley et al. 2004; Grabe et al. 2005; Kaufman et al. 2004; Sjoberg et al. 2006; Wilhelm et al. 2006). Twin-study replications (Kendler et al. 2005) and nonreplications (Gillespie et al. 2005) of this finding have also been reported, as have been findings in twins that are discordant with respect to the genotype of risk (Chorbov et al. 2007) but concordant with respect to an effect of stress and genotype on depressive symptomatology. The gene–environment interactions with this polymorphism have been the first well-established interactions of this kind in the genetics of mood disorders.

HPA Axis–Related Genes

As described in the previous section, a large and diverse body of evidence indicates a substantial role for HPA axis dysregulation in depression. Licinio et al. (2004) identified a unique haplotype within the *CRHR1* gene, which codes for the CRH$_1$ receptor, that predicts antidepressant response in Mexican Americans, and this has been replicated in a Chinese sample (Liu et al. 2007). Furthermore, associations with major depression have also been reported for this gene (Liu et al. 2006).

More recently, Bradley et al. (2008) reported data, ascertained from a large sample of heavily traumatized inner-city African Americans, identifying SNPs as well as haplotypes within the *CRHR1* gene that predict scores on the Beck Depression Inventory as a function of trauma exposure. Interestingly, gene–environment interactions of this gene with lifetime stress have also been reported for suicide attempts in males (Wasserman et al. 2008). SNPs of the *FKBP5* gene, which codes for a cochaperone of the glucocorticoid receptor, also have been reported to predict antidepressant response and the response to the dexamethasone–CRH stimulation test by Binder et al. (2004) in two independent European samples, and this was replicated in the STAR*D sample (Lekman et al. 2008). Interestingly, while the results for association with unipolar depression are controversial (Binder—negative, Lekman—positive), a recently published family study shows evidence for association of *FKBP5* with bipolar disorder (Willour et al. 2008), and a recently published association study provides evidence that *FKBP5* SNPs interact with severity of child abuse to predict PTSD symptoms in adults (Binder et al. 2008).

Brain-Derived Neurotrophic Factor

As described earlier in the chapter, BDNF may play a key role in synaptic maintenance and neurotransmission and thus participate in the biology of mood disorders. More recently, the BDNF Val66Met polymorphism has also emerged as a factor moderating risk for stress-sensitive diseases such as diabetes mellitus (Krabbe et al. 2007) and systemic lupus erythematosus (Oroszi et al. 2006).

Strauss et al. (2004, 2005) as well as others (Geller et al. 2004) have identified an association between BDNF genotype and childhood-onset mood disorder. Similar studies examining associations between polymorphisms of the BDNF receptor TrkB (*NTRK2*) and childhood-onset mood disorder have been negative (Adams et al. 2005). Examining children for risk of depression in a more elaborate study, Kaufman et al. (2006) reported data suggesting that particular variants of the 5-HTT gene and the Met allele of the BDNF Val66Met polymorphism in the context of early-life stress influence the development of depression in children. Notably, these variants only confer risk for depression in the presence of a history of childhood maltreatment, and positive experiences in childhood offset this risk. Similar findings, with respect to the effects of stressful life events on risk for depression as a function of 5-HTT and Val66Met genotype, have been reported in a sample of geriatric Korean patients (J.M. Kim et al. 2007). Other investigators have reported associations between the Val66Met polymorphism and risk

for major depression (L. Ribeiro et al. 2007; Schumacher et al. 2005). Alternatively, other reports (Iga et al. 2007) indicate an association between Val66Met genotype and psychosis or suicidal behavior, but not major depression, in a Japanese population.

In addition to studies indicating risk for depression in the setting of early-life stress with respect to BDNF Val66Met genotype, other investigators have examined the relationship between BDNF and bipolar disorder. Several groups (Geller et al. 2004; Neves-Pereira et al. 2002; Sklar et al. 2002) report positive associations between BDNF genotype and bipolar disorder, although discordant results exist (Green et al. 2006; Oswald et al. 2004). More recently, a meta-analysis of pooled data was unable to provide evidence to support an association between the Val66Met polymorphism and bipolar disorder (Kanazawa et al. 2007).

One way that variability within BDNF may influence the development of depression is regulation of the reactivity of the HPA axis. Preliminary data exist indicating that homozygous carriers of the Met/Met genotype demonstrate significantly higher HPA axis activity during the DEX/CRH test than patients carrying the Val/Val or Val/Met genotype (ACTH, cortisol) (Schule et al. 2006). Consistent with this is a recent report that smaller hippocampal volumes were observed for depressed patients and for control subjects carrying the Met BDNF allele compared with subjects homozygous for the Val BDNF allele (Frodl et al. 2007).

Whole-Genome Association Studies

The recent introduction of technological platforms for whole-genome association (WGA) studies provides an opportunity to rapidly identify allelic variants of novel candidate genes for further investigation without theoretical bias (for a review, see Chapter 3 in this volume, "Genetics and Genomics"). Within the literature of psychiatric genetics, WGA studies have begun to appear, and at present there are reports for Alzheimer's disease (Coon et al. 2007), schizophrenia (Lencz et al. 2007), and bipolar disorder (Baum et al. 2008; Wellcome Trust Case Control Consortium 2007). Candidate gene studies to evaluate the initial findings from these reports are currently under way.

Conclusion

In this chapter we have provided an overview of research findings on the biology of mood disorders. However, the central question of what variables drive the pathophysiology of mood disorders remains unanswered. Since the last edition of this textbook, research examining the role of developmental stress, trauma, and genetic risk in the etiology of mood disorders has grown considerably. These findings have enriched our understanding of the biological relationships between environmental and genetic risks for mood disorders. Interpretation of seemingly disparate findings from the continuously growing number of individual biological studies is challenging, but over time, integration of these findings will form an overarching understanding of these complex disorders.

References

Abecasis GR, Ghosh D, Nichols TE: Linkage disequilibrium: ancient history drives the new genetics. Hum Hered 59:118–124, 2005

Abercrombie HC, Schaefer SM, Larson CL, et al: Metabolic rate in the right amygdala predicts negative affect in depressed patients. Neuroreport 9:3301–3307, 1998

Aberg-Wistedt A, Wistedt B, Bertilsson L: Higher CSF levels of HVA and 5-HIAA in delusional compared to nondelusional depression. Arch Gen Psychiatry 42:925–926, 1985

Abler B, Erk S, Herwig U, et al: Anticipation of aversive stimuli activates extended amygdala in unipolar depression. J Psychiatr Res 41:511–522, 2007

Adams JH, Wigg KG, King N, et al: Association study of neurotrophic tyrosine kinase receptor type 2 (NTRK2) and childhood-onset mood disorders. Am J Med Genet B Neuropsychiatr Genet 132:90–95, 2005

Agren H, Lundqvist G: Low levels of somatostatin in human CSF mark depressive episodes. Psychoneuroendocrinology 9:233–248, 1984

Agren H, Oreland L: Early morning awakening in unipolar depressives with higher levels of platelet MAO activity. Psychiatry Res 7:245–254, 1982

Aizenstein HJ, Butters MA, Figurski JL, et al: Prefrontal and striatal activation during sequence learning in geriatric depression. Biol Psychiatry 58:290–296, 2005

Akerman CJ, Cline HT: Refining the roles of GABAergic signaling during neural circuit formation. Trends Neurosci 30:382–389, 2007

Alda M: Bipolar disorder: from families to genes. Can J Psychiatry 42:378–387, 1997

Alesci S, Martinez PE, Kelkar S, et al: Major depression is associated with significant diurnal elevations in plasma interleukin-6 levels, a shift of its circadian rhythm, and loss of physiological complexity in its secretion: clinical implications. J Clin Endocrinol Metab 90:2522–2530, 2005

Alexander GE, Delong MR, Strick PL: Parallel organization of functionally segregated circuits linking basal ganglia and cortex. Annu Rev Neurosci 9:357–381, 1986

Altamura CA, Mauri MC, Ferrara A, et al: Plasma and platelet excitatory amino acids in psychiatric disorders. Am J Psychiatry 150:1731–1733, 1993

American Psychiatric Association: Diagnostic and Statistical Manual of Mental Disorders, 4th Edition, Text Revision. Washington, DC, American Psychiatric Association, 2000

Amsterdam JD, Maislin G, Winokur A, et al: The oCRF test before and after clinical recovery from depression. J Affect Disord 14:213–222, 1988

Anguelova M, Benkelfat C, Turecki G: A systematic review of association studies investigating genes coding for serotonin receptors and the serotonin transporter, II: suicidal behavior. Mol Psychiatry 8:646–653, 2003

Appelhof BC, Brouwer JP, van Dyck R, et al: Triiodothyronine addition to paroxetine in the treatment of major depressive disorder. J Clin Endocrinol Metab 89:6271–6276, 2004

Arana GW, Baldessarini RJ, Ornsteen M: The dexamethasone suppression test for diagnosis and prognosis in psychiatry. Arch Gen Psychiatry 42:1193–1204, 1985

Arato M, Banki CM, Bissette G, et al: Elevated CSF CRF in suicide victims. Biol Psychiatry 25:355–359, 1989

Arborelius L, Owens MJ, Plotsky PM, et al: The role of corticotropin-releasing factor in depression and anxiety disorders. J Endocrinol 160:1–12, 1999

Aronson R, Offman HJ, Joffe RT, et al: Triiodothyronine augmentation in the treatment of refractory depression. A meta-analysis. Arch Gen Psychiatry 53:842–848, 1996

Åsberg M, Thorén P, Träskman L, et al: "Serotonin depression"—a biochemical subgroup within the affective disorders? Science 191:478–483, 1976a

Åsberg M, Träskman L, Thorén P: 5-HIAA in the cerebrospinal fluid: a biochemical suicide predictor? Arch Gen Psychiatry 33:1193–1197, 1976b

Axelson DA, Doraiswamy PM, Boyko OB, et al: In vivo assessment of pituitary volume using MRI and systemic stereology: relationship to dexamethasone suppression test results in patients with affective disorder. Psychiatry Res 46:63–70, 1992

Aydemir O, Deveci A, Taneli F: The effect of chronic antidepressant treatment on serum brain-derived neurotrophic factor levels in depressed patients: a preliminary study. Prog Neuropsychopharmacol Biol Psychiatry 29:261–265, 2005

Azmitia EC, Gannon PJ: The primate serotonergic system: a review of human and animal studies and a report on Macaca fascicularis. Adv Neurol 43:407–468, 1986

Baez M, Kursar JD, Helton LA, et al: Molecular biology of serotonin receptors. Obes Res 3 (suppl 4):441S–447S, 1995

Baker DG, West SA, Nicholson WE, et al: Serial CSF corticotropin-releasing hormone levels and adrenocortical activity in combat veterans with posttraumatic stress disorder. Am J Psychiatry 156:585–588, 1999

Bakish D, Cavazzoni P, Chudzik J, et al: Effects of selective serotonin reuptake inhibitors on platelet serotonin parameters in major depressive disorder. Biol Psychiatry 41:184–190, 1997

Ballmaier M, Toga AW, Blanton RE, et al: Anterior cingulate, gyrus rectus, and orbitofrontal abnormalities in elderly depressed patients: an MRI-based parcellation of the prefrontal cortex. Am J Psychiatry 161:99–108, 2004

Banki CM, Bissette G, Arato M, et al: Elevation of immunoreactive CSF TRH in depressed patients. Am J Psychiatry 145:1526–1531, 1988

Banki CB, Karmacsi L, Bissette G, et al: CSF corticotropin-releasing hormone and somatostatin in major depression: response to antidepressant treatment and relapse. Eur Neuropsychopharmacol 2:107–113, 1992

Barbas H, Saha S, Rempel-Clower N, et al: Serial pathways from primate prefrontal cortex to autonomic areas may influence emotional expression. BMC Neurosci 4:25, 2003

Barch DM, Sheline YI, Csernansky JG, et al: Working memory and prefrontal cortex dysfunction: specificity to schizophrenia compared with major depression. Biol Psychiatry 53:376–384, 2003

Barker JL, Behar T, Li YX, et al: GABAergic cells and signals in CNS development. Perspect Dev Neurobiol 5:305–322, 1998

Baron M: The search for complex disease genes: fault by linkage or fault by association? Mol Psychiatry 6:143–149, 2001

Batten SV, Aslan M, Maciejewski PK, et al: Childhood maltreatment as a risk factor for adult cardiovascular disease and depression. J Clin Psychiatry 65:249–254, 2004

Bauer MS, Whybrow PC: Rapid cycling bipolar affective disorder, I: association with grade I hypothyroidism. Arch Gen Psychiatry 47:427–432, 1990a

Bauer MS, Whybrow PC: Rapid cycling bipolar affective disorder, II: treatment of refractory rapid cycling with high-dose levothyroxine: a preliminary study. Arch Gen Psychiatry 47:435–447, 1990b

Baum AE, Akula N, Cabanero M, et al: A genome-wide association study implicates diacylglycerol kinase eta (DGKH) and several other genes in the etiology of bipolar disorder. Mol Psychiatry 13:197–207, 2008

Baxter L, Edell W, Gerner R, et al: Dexamethasone suppression test and Axis I diagnoses of inpatients with DSM-III borderline personality disorder. J Clin Psychiatry 45:150–153, 1984

Baxter LR, Phelps MC, Mazziotta JC, et al: Cerebral metabolic rates for glucose in mood disorders studied with positron emission tomography (PET) and (F-18)-fluoro-2-deoxyglucose (FDG). Arch Gen Psychiatry 42:441–447, 1985

Baxter LR, Schwartz JM, Phelps ME, et al: Reduction of prefrontal cortex glucose metabolism common to three types of depression. Arch Gen Psychiatry 46:243–250, 1989

Bearden CE, Freimer NB: Endophenotypes for psychiatric disorders: ready for primetime? Trends Genet 22:306–313, 2006

Bearden CE, Reus VI, Freimer NB: Why genetic investigation of psychiatric disorders is so difficult. Curr Opin Genet Dev 14:280–286, 2004

Belanoff JK, Flores BH, Kalezhan M, et al: Rapid reversal of psychotic depression using mifepristone. J Clin Psychopharmacol 21:516–521, 2001a

Belanoff JK, Kalehzan M, Sund B, et al: Cortisol activity and cognitive changes in psychotic major depression. Am J Psychiatry 158:1612–1616, 2001b

Belanoff JK, Rothschild AJ, Cassidy F, et al: An open label trial of C-1073 (mifepristone) for psychotic major depression. Biol Psychiatry 52:386–392, 2002

Belmaker RH, Agam G: Major depressive disorder. N Engl J Med 358:55–68, 2008

Benabid AL: Deep brain stimulation for Parkinson's disease. Curr Opin Neurobiol 13:696–706, 2003

Bench CJ, Friston KJ, Brown RG, et al: The anatomy of melancholia: focal abnormalities of cerebral blood flow in major depression. Psychol Med 22:607–615, 1992

Bench CJ, Friston KJ, Brown RG, et al: Regional cerebral blood flow in depression measured by positron emission tomography: the relationship with clinical dimensions. Psychol Med 23:579–590, 1993

Bench CJ, Frackowiak RSJ, Dolan RJ: Changes in regional cerebral blood flow on recovery from depression. Psychol Med 25:247–251, 1995

Berman KF, Illowsky BP, Weinberger DR: Physiological dysfunction of dorsolateral prefrontal cortex in schizophrenia, IV: further evidence for regional and behavioral specificity. Arch Gen Psychiatry 45:616–622, 1988

Berman RM, Narasimhan M, Miller HL, et al: Transient depressive relapse induced by catecholamine depletion: potential phenotypic vulnerability marker? Arch Gen Psychiatry 56:395–403, 1999

Berman RM, Cappiello A, Anand A, et al: Antidepressant effects of ketamine in depressed patients. Biol Psychiatry 47:351–354, 2000

Bernasconi R: The GABA hypothesis of affective illness: influence of clinically effective antimanic drugs on GABA turnover, in Basic Mechanisms in the Action of Lithium. Edited by Emrich HM, Aldenhoff JB, Lux HD. Amsterdam, Elsevier, 1982, pp 183–192

Berton O, Nestler EJ: New approaches to antidepressant drug discovery: beyond monoamines. Nat Rev Neurosci 7:137–151, 2006

Berton O, McClung CA, Dileone RJ, et al: Essential role of BDNF in the mesolimbic dopamine pathway in social defeat stress. Science 311:864–868, 2006

Biegon A, Weizman A, Karp L, et al: Serotonin 5-HT2 receptor binding on blood platelets—a peripheral marker for depression? Life Sci 41:2485–2492, 1987

Biegon A, Essar N, Israeli M, et al: Serotonin 5-HT2 receptor binding on blood platelets as a state dependent marker in major affective disorder. Psychopharmacology (Berl) 102:73–75, 1990

Bierhaus A, Wolf J, Andrassy M, et al: A mechanism converting psychosocial stress into mononuclear cell activation. Proc Natl Acad Sci U S A 100:1920–1925, 2003

Bierut LJ, Heath AC, Bucholz KK, et al: Major depressive disorder in a community-based twin sample: are there different genetic and environmental contributions for men and women? Arch Gen Psychiatry 56:557–563, 1999

Binder EB, Salyakina D, Lichtner P, et al: Polymorphisms in FKBP5 are associated with increased recurrence of depressive episodes and rapid response to antidepressant treatment. Nat Genet 36:1319–1325, 2004

Binder EB, Bradley RG, Liu W, et al: Association of FKBP5 polymorphisms and childhood abuse with risk of posttraumatic stress disorder symptoms in adults. JAMA 299:1291–1305, 2008

Bissette G, Widerlov E, Walleus H, et al: Alterations in cerebrospinal fluid concentrations of somatostatin-like immunoreactivity in neuropsychiatric disorders. Arch Gen Psychiatry 43:1148–1151, 1986

Biver F, Wikler D, Lotstra F, et al: Serotonin 5-HT2 receptor imaging in major depression: focal changes in orbito-insular cortex. Br J Psychiatry 171:444–448, 1997

Bjork JM, Moeller FG, Kramer GL, et al: Plasma GABA levels correlate with aggressiveness in relatives of patients with unipolar depressive disorder. Psychiatry Res 101:131–136, 2001

Black DW, Monahan PO, Winokur G: The relationship between DST results and suicidal behavior. Ann Clin Psychiatry 14:83–88, 2002

Blumberg HP, Stern E, Martinez D, et al: Increased anterior cingulate and caudate activity in bipolar mania. Biol Psychiatry 48:1045–1052, 2000

Booij L, Van der Does W, Benkelfat C, et al: Predictors of mood response to acute tryptophan depletion. A reanalysis. Neuropsychopharmacology 27:852–861, 2002

Botteron KN, Raichle ME, Drevets WC, et al: Volumetric reduction in left subgenual prefrontal cortex in early onset depression. Biol Psychiatry 51:342–344, 2002

Bowden CL, Calabrese JR, Sachs G, et al: A placebo-controlled 18-month trial of lamotrigine and lithium maintenance treatment in recently manic or hypomanic patients with bipolar I disorder. Arch Gen Psychiatry 60:392–400, 2003

Boyd AE, Levovitz HE, Pfeiffer JB: Stimulation of growth hormone secretion by L-dopa. N Engl J Med 283:1425–1429, 1970

Bradley RG, Binder EB, Epstein MP, et al: Influence of child abuse and trauma on adult depression is moderated by the corticotropin releasing hormone receptor gene. Arch Gen Psychiatry 65:190–200, 2008

Bragulat V, Paillere-Martinot ML, Artiges E, et al: Dopaminergic function in depressed patients with affective flattening or with impulsivity: [18F]fluoro-L-dopa positron emission tomography study with voxel-based analysis. Psychiatry Res 154:115–124, 2007

Brambilla F, Maggioni M, Ferrari E, et al: Tonic and dynamic gonadotropin secretion in depressive and normothymic phases of affective disorders. Psychiatry Res 32:229–239, 1990

Brambilla F, Harenski K, Nicoletti MA, et al: Anatomical MRI study of basal ganglia in bipolar disorder patients. Psychiatry Res 106:65–80, 2001

Bramham CR: Control of synaptic consolidation in the dentate gyrus: mechanisms, functions, and therapeutic implications. Prog Brain Res 163:453–471, 2007

Bremner JD, Randall P, Scott TM, et al: MRI-based measurement of hippocampal volume in combat-related posttraumatic stress disorder. Am J Psychiatry 152:973–981, 1995

Bremner JD, Licinio J, Darnell A, et al: Elevated CSF corticotropin-releasing factor concentrations in posttraumatic stress disorder. Am J Psychiatry 154:624–629, 1997a

Bremner JD, Randall P, Vermetten E, et al: MRI-based measurement of hippocampal volume in posttraumatic stress disorder related to childhood physical and sexual abuse: a preliminary report. Biol Psychiatry 41:23–32, 1997b

Bremner JD, Narayan M, Anderson ER, et al: Hippocampal volume reduction in major depression. Am J Psychiatry 157:115–117, 2000

Bremner JD, Vythilingam M, Vermetten E, et al: Reduced volume of orbitofrontal cortex in major depression. Biol Psychiatry 51:273–279, 2002

Bremner JD, Vythilingam M, Vermetten E, et al: MRI and PET study of deficits in hippocampal structure and function in women with childhood sexual abuse and posttraumatic stress disorder. Am J Psychiatry 160:924–932, 2003

Brody AL, Barsom MW, Bota RG, et al: Prefrontal-subcortical and limbic circuit mediation of major depressive disorder. Semin Clin Neuropsychiatry 6:102–112, 2001

Brown ES, Varghese FP, McEwen BS: Association of depression with medical illness: does cortisol play a role? Biol Psychiatry 55:1–9, 2004

Brown MR, Rivier C, Vale W, et al: Central nervous system regulation of adrenocorticotropin secretion: role of somatostatins. Endocrinology 114:1546–1549, 1984

Brown WA, Johnson R, Mayfield D: 24-Hour dexamethasone suppression test in a clinical setting: relationship to diagnosis, symptoms and responses to treatment. Am J Psychiatry 136:543–547, 1979

Buchsbaum MS, Someya T, Teng CY, et al: Neuroimaging bipolar illness with positron emission tomography and magnetic resonance imaging. Psychiatric Annals 27:489–495, 1997

Bunevicius R, Lasas L, Kazanavicius G, et al: Pituitary responses to thyrotropin releasing hormone stimulation in depressed women with thyroid gland disorders. Psychoneuroendocrinology 21:631–639, 1996

Bunney WE Jr, Davis M: Norepinephrine in depressive reactions. Arch Gen Psychiatry 13:483–494, 1965

Burgus R, Dunn TF, Desiderio D, et al: Characterization of ovine hypothalamic hypophysiotropic TSH-releasing factor. Nature 226:321–325, 1970

Cadoret RJ: Evidence for genetic inheritance of primary affective disorder in adoptees. Am J Psychiatry 135:463–466, 1978

Caetano SC, Sassi R, Brambilla P, et al: MRI study of thalamic volumes in bipolar and unipolar patients and healthy individuals. Psychiatry Res 108:161–168, 2001

Calabrese JR, Gulledge AD, Hahn K, et al: Autoimmune thyroiditis in manic-depressive patients treated with lithium. Am J Psychiatry 142:1318–1321, 1985

Calabrese JR, Bowden CL, Sachs GS, et al: A double-blind placebo-controlled study of lamotrigine monotherapy in outpatients with bipolar I depression. Lamictal 602 Study Group. J Clin Psychiatry 60:79–88, 1999

Calabrese JR, Bowden CL, Sachs G, et al: A placebo-controlled 18-month trial of lamotrigine and lithium maintenance treatment in recently depressed patients with bipolar I disorder. J Clin Psychiatry 64:1013–1024, 2003

Campbell S, Macqueen G: The role of the hippocampus in the pathophysiology of major depression. J Psychiatry Neurosci 29:417–426, 2004

Cannon TD, Keller MC: Endophenotypes in the genetic analyses of mental disorders. Annu Rev Clin Psychol 2:267–290, 2006

Carmichael ST, Price JL: Connectional networks within the orbital and medial prefrontal cortex of macaque monkeys. J Comp Neurol 371:179–207, 1996

Carpenter W, Bunney W: Adrenal cortical activity in depressive illness. Am J Psychiatry 128:31–40, 1971

Carroll BJ: Use of the dexamethasone test in depression. J Clin Psychiatry 43:44–50, 1982

Carroll BJ, Martin FI, Davies B: Pituitary-adrenal function in depression. Lancet 1(7556):1373–1374, 1968a

Carroll BJ, Martin FI, Davies B: Resistance to suppression by dexamethasone of plasma 11-O.H.C.S. levels in severe depressive illness. BMJ 3:285–287, 1968b

Casanueva FF, Burguera S, Tome M, et al: Depending on the time of administration, dexamethasone potentiates or blocks growth hormone-releasing hormone-induced growth hormone release in man. Neuroendocrinology 47:46–49, 1988

Casanueva FF, Burguera S, Murais C, et al: Acute administration of corticoids: a new and peculiar stimulus of growth hormone secretion in man. J Clin Endocrinol Metab 70:234–237, 1990

Caspi A, Sugden K, Moffitt TE, et al: Influence of life stress on depression: moderation by a polymorphism in the 5-HTT gene. Science 301:386–389, 2003

Caspi A, Harrington H, Moffitt TE, et al: Socially isolated children 20 years later: risk of cardiovascular disease. Arch Pediatr Adolesc Med 160:805–811, 2006

Chalmers DT, Lovenberg TW, Grigoriadis DE, et al: Corticotrophin-releasing factor receptors: from molecular biology to drug design. Trends Pharmacol Sci 17:166–172, 1996

Chanock SJ, Manolio T, Boehnke M, et al: Replicating genotype-phenotype associations. Nature 447:655–660, 2007

Chapman DP, Whitfield CL, Felitti VJ, et al: Adverse childhood experiences and the risk of depressive disorders in adulthood. J Affect Disord 82:217–225, 2004

Charney DS: Monoamine dysfunction and the pathophysiology and treatment of depression. J Clin Psychiatry 59 (suppl 14):11–14, 1998

Charney DS, Heninger GR, Sternberg DE, et al: Plasma MHPG in depression: effects of acute and chronic desipramine treatment. Psychiatry Res 5:217–229, 1981

Charney DS, Henninger GR, Sternberg DE, et al: Adrenergic receptor sensitivity in depression: effects of clonidine in depressed patients and healthy controls. Arch Gen Psychiatry 39:290–294, 1982

Checkley SA, Slade AP, Shur E: Growth hormone and other responses to clonidine in patients with endogenous depression. Br J Psychiatry 138:51–55, 1981

Chen B, Dowlatshahi D, MacQueen GM, et al: Increased hippocampal BDNF immunoreactivity in subjects treated with antidepressant medication. Biol Psychiatry 50:260–265, 2001

Chen HH, Nicoletti M, Sanches M, et al: Normal pituitary volumes in children and adolescents with bipolar disorder: a magnetic resonance imaging study. Depress Anxiety 20:182–186, 2004

Chhatwal JP, Stanek-Rattiner L, Davis M, et al: Amygdala BDNF signaling is required for consolidation but not encoding of extinction. Nat Neurosci 9:870–872, 2006

Cho HJ, Meira-Lima I, Cordeiro Q, et al: Population-based and family based studies on the serotonin transporter gene polymorphisms and bipolar disorder: a systematic review and meta-analysis. Mol Psychiatry 10:771–781, 2005

Chorbov VM, Lobos EA, Todorov AA, et al: Relationship of 5-HTTLPR genotypes and depression risk in the presence of trauma in a female twin sample. Am J Med Genet B Neuropsychiatr Genet 144B:830–833, 2007

Chrousos GP: The hypothalamic-pituitary-adrenal axis and immune-mediated inflammation. N Engl J Med 332:1351–1362, 1995

Chu JW, Matthias DF, Belanoff J, et al: Successful long-term treatment of refractory Cushing's disease with high-dose mifepristone (RU 486). J Clin Endocrinol Metab 86:3568–3573, 2001

Clarke IJ, Cummins JT: The temporal relationship between gonadotropin releasing hormone (GnRH) and luteinizing hormone (LH) secretion in ovariectomized ewes. Endocrinology 111:1737–1739, 1982

Cole DP, Thase ME, Mallinger AG, et al: Slower treatment response in bipolar depression predicted by lower pretreatment thyroid function. Am J Psychiatry 159:116–121, 2002

Comings DE: Clinical and molecular genetics of ADHD and Tourette syndrome. Two related polygenic disorders. Ann N Y Acad Sci 931:50–83, 2001

Contreras F, Navarro MA, Menchon JM, et al: Growth hormone response to growth hormone releasing hormone in non-delusional and delusional depression and healthy controls. Psychol Med 26:301–307, 1996

Coon KD, Myers AJ, Craig DW, et al: A high-density whole-genome association study reveals that APOE is the major susceptibility gene for sporadic late-onset Alzheimer's disease. J Clin Psychiatry 68:613–618, 2007

Cooper-Kazaz R, Apter JT, Cohen R, et al: Combined treatment with sertraline and liothyronine in major depression: a randomized, double-blind, placebo-controlled trial. Arch Gen Psychiatry 64:679–688, 2007

Coppen A: Depressive states and indolealkylamines, in Advances in Pharmacology, Vol 6. Edited by Garattini S, Shore PA. New York, Academic Press, 1968, pp 283–291

Coryell W, Schlesser M: The dexamethasone suppression test and suicide prediction. Am J Psychiatry 158:748–753, 2001

Cowdry RW, Wehr TA, Zis AP, et al: Thyroid abnormalities associated with rapid-cycling bipolar illness. Arch Gen Psychiatry 40:414–420, 1983

Craddock N, Forty L: Genetics of affective (mood) disorders. Eur J Hum Genet 14:660–668, 2006

Crane G: Cycloserine as an antidepressant agent. Am J Psychiatry 115:1025–1026, 1959

Crane G: The psychotropic use of cycloserine: a new use of an antibiotic. Compr Psychiatry 2:51–59, 1961

Cryan JF, O'Leary OF, Jin SH, et al: Norepinephrine-deficient mice lack responses to antidepressant drugs, including selective serotonin reuptake inhibitors. Proc Natl Acad Sci U S A 101:8186–8191, 2004

Cubells JF, Zabetian CP: Human genetics of plasma dopamine beta-hydroxylase activity: applications to research in psychiatry and neurology. Psychopharmacology (Berl) 174:463–476, 2004

Cubells JF, Price LH, Meyers BS, et al: Genotype-controlled analysis of plasma dopamine beta-hydroxylase activity in psychotic unipolar major depression. Biol Psychiatry 51:358–364, 2002

Daban C, Vieta E, Mackin P, et al: Hypothalamic-pituitary-adrenal axis and bipolar disorder. Psychiatr Clin North Am 28:469–480, 2005

Danese A, Pariante CM, Caspi A, et al: Childhood maltreatment predicts adult inflammation in a life-course study. Proc Natl Acad Sci U S A 104:1319–1324, 2007

Dang AH, Hershman JM: Lithium-associated thyroiditis. Endocr Pract 8:232–236, 2002

Danner M, Kasl SV, Abramson JL, et al: Association between depression and elevated C-reactive protein. Psychosom Med 65:347–356, 2003

Dasari M, Friedman L, Jesberger J, et al: A magnetic resonance imaging study of the thalamic area in adolescent patients with either schizophrenia or bipolar disorder as compared to healthy controls. Psychiatry Res 91:155–162, 1999

Davidson RJ, Pizzagalli D, Nitschke JB, et al: Depression: perspectives from affective neuroscience. Annu Rev Psychol 53:545–574, 2002

Davis M, Ressler K, Rothbaum BO, et al: Effects of D-cycloserine on extinction: translation from preclinical to clinical work. Biol Psychiatry 60:369–375, 2006

De Bellis MD, Geracioti TD Jr, Altemus M, et al: Cerebrospinal fluid monoamine metabolites in fluoxetine-treated patients with major depression and in healthy volunteers. Biol Psychiatry 33:636–641, 1993a

De Bellis MD, Gold PW, Geracioti TD Jr, et al: Association of fluoxetine treatment with reductions in CSF concentrations of corticotropin-releasing hormone and arginine vasopressin in patients with major depression. Am J Psychiatry 150:656–657, 1993b

de Kloet ER, Joels M, Oitzl M, et al: Implication of brain corticosteroid receptor diversity for the adaptation syndrome concept. Methods Achiev Exp Pathol 14:104–132, 1991

Derkach VA, Oh MC, Guire ES, et al: Regulatory mechanisms of AMPA receptors in synaptic plasticity. Nat Rev Neurosci 8:101–113, 2007

Deshauer D, Duffy A, Alda M, et al: The cortisol awakening response in bipolar illness: a pilot study. Can J Psychiatry 48:462–466, 2003

Devanand DP, Bowers MB, Hoffman FJ, et al: Elevated plasma homovanillic acid in depressed females with melancholia and psychosis. Psychiatry Res 15:1–4, 1985

Di S, Malcher-Lopes R, Halmos KC, et al: Nongenomic glucocorticoid inhibition via endocannabinoid release in the hypothalamus: a fast feedback mechanism. J Neurosci 23:4850–4857, 2003

Dinan TG, Yatham LN, O'Keane VO, et al: Blunting of noradrenergic-stimulated growth hormone release in mania. Am J Psychiatry 148:936–938, 1991

Doble A: The pharmacology and mechanism of action of riluzole. Neurology 47:S233–S241, 1996

Dolan RJ, Bench CJ, Brown RG, et al: Regional cerebral blood flow abnormalities in depressed patients with cognitive impairment. J Neurol Neurosurg Psychiatry 55:768–773, 1992

Dolan RJ, Bench CJ, Liddle PF, et al: Dorsolateral prefrontal cortex dysfunction in the major psychoses: symptom or disease specificity? J Neurol Neurosurg Psychiatry 56:1290–1294, 1993

Dong M, Giles WH, Felitti VJ, et al: Insights into causal pathways for ischemic heart disease: adverse childhood experiences study. Circulation 110:1761–1766, 2004

Dorn LD, Burgess ES, Dubbert B, et al: Psychopathology in patients with endogenous Cushing's syndrome: "atypical" or melancholic features. Clin Endocrinol (Oxf) 43:433–442, 1995

Dorn LD, Burgess ES, Friedman TC, et al: The longitudinal course of psychopathology in Cushing's syndrome after correction of hypercortisolism. J Clin Endocrinol Metab 82:912–919, 1997

Dougherty DD, Weiss AP, Cosgrove GR, et al: Cerebral metabolic correlates as potential predictors of response to anterior cingulotomy for treatment of major depression. J Neurosurg 99:1010–1017, 2003

Dougherty DD, Rauch SL, Deckersbach T, et al: Ventromedial prefrontal cortex and amygdala dysfunction during an anger induction positron emission tomography study in patients with major depressive disorder with anger attacks. Arch Gen Psychiatry 61:795–804, 2004

Drevets WC: Prefrontal cortical-amygdalar metabolism in major depression. Ann N Y Acad Sci 877:614–637, 1999

Drevets WC, Frank E, Price JC, et al: PET imaging of serotonin 1A receptor binding in depression. Biol Psychiatry 46:1375–1387, 1999

Drevets WC, Price JL, Bardgett ME, et al: Glucose metabolism in the amygdala in depression: relationship to diagnostic subtype and plasma cortisol levels. Pharmacol Biochem Behav 71:431–447, 2002

Driessen M, Herrmann J, Stahl K, et al: Magnetic resonance imaging volumes of the hippocampus and the amygdala in women with borderline personality disorder and early traumatization. Arch Gen Psychiatry 57:1115–1122, 2000

Dube S, Kumar N, Ettedgui E, et al: Cholinergic REM induction response: separation of anxiety and depression. Biol Psychiatry 20:408–418, 1985

Dube SR, Anda RF, Felitti VJ, et al: Childhood abuse, household dysfunction, and the risk of attempted suicide throughout the life span: findings from the adverse childhood experiences study. JAMA 286:3089–3096, 2001

Duman RS, Monteggia LM: A neurotrophic model for stress-related mood disorders. Biol Psychiatry 59:1116–1127, 2006

Dunn AJ, Berridge CW: Physiological and behavioral responses to corticotropin-releasing factor administration: is CRF a mediator of anxiety or stress responses? Brain Res Brain Res Rev 15:71–100, 1990

Dunn RT, Kimbrell TA, Ketter TA, et al: Principal components of the Beck Depression Inventory and regional cerebral metabolism in unipolar and bipolar depression. Biol Psychiatry 51:387–399, 2002

Dupont RM, Jernigan TL, Heindel W, et al: Magnetic resonance imaging and mood disorders: localization of white matter and other subcortical abnormalities. Arch Gen Psychiatry 52:747–755, 1995

Duval F, Macher JP, Mokrani MC: Difference between evening and morning thyrotropin responses to protirelin in major depressive episode. Arch Gen Psychiatry 47:443–448, 1990

Duval F, Mokrani M-C, Crocq M-A, et al: Effect of antidepressant medication on morning and evening thyroid function tests during a major depressive episode. Arch Gen Psychiatry 53:833–840, 1996

Dwivedi Y, Rizavi HS, Roberts RC, et al: Reduced activation and expression of ERK1/2 MAP kinase in the post-mortem brain of depressed suicide subjects. J Neurochem 77:916–928, 2001

Dwivedi Y, Rizavi HS, Conley RR, et al: Altered gene expression of brain-derived neurotrophic factor and receptor tyrosine kinase B in postmortem brain of suicide subjects. Arch Gen Psychiatry 60:804–815, 2003

Dwivedi Y, Rizavi HS, Pandey GN: Antidepressants reverse corticosterone-mediated decrease in brain-derived neurotrophic factor expression: differential regulation of specific exons by antidepressants and corticosterone. Neuroscience 139:1017–1029, 2006

Dwivedi Y, Rizavi HS, Teppen T, et al: Aberrant extracellular signal-regulated kinase (ERK) 5 signaling in hippocampus of suicide subjects. Neuropsychopharmacology 32:2338–2350, 2007

Eaves LJ: Genotype × environment interaction in psychopathology: fact or artifact? Twin Res Hum Genet 9:1–8, 2006

Egan MF, Kojima M, Callicott JH, et al: The BDNF val66met polymorphism affects activity-dependent secretion of BDNF and human memory and hippocampal function. Cell 112:257–269, 2003

Elenkov IJ, Iezzoni DG, Daly A, et al: Cytokine dysregulation, inflammation and well-being. Neuroimmunomodulation 12:255–269, 2005

Eley TC, Sugden K, Corsico A, et al: Gene-environment interaction analysis of serotonin system markers with adolescent depression. Mol Psychiatry 9:908–915, 2004

Ellenbogen MA, Hodgins S, Walker CD: High levels of cortisol among adolescent offspring of parents with bipolar disorder: a pilot study. Psychoneuroendocrinology 29:99–106, 2004

Ellenbogen MA, Hodgins S, Walker CD, et al: Daytime cortisol and stress reactivity in the offspring of parents with bipolar disorder. Psychoneuroendocrinology 31:1164–1180, 2006

Elliott R, Sahakian BJ, Michael A, et al: Abnormal neural response to feedback on planning and guessing tasks in patients with unipolar depression. Psychol Med 28:559–571, 1998

El-Yousef M, Janowsky DS, Davis JM, et al: Induction of severe depression in marijuana intoxicated individuals. Br J Addict 68:321–325, 1973

Enz R: GABAC receptors: a molecular view. Biol Chem 382:1111–1122, 2001

Epstein J, Pan H, Kocsis JH, et al: Lack of ventral striatal response to positive stimuli in depressed versus normal subjects. Am J Psychiatry 163:1784–1790, 2006

Esposito S, Prange AJ Jr, Golden RN: The thyroid axis and mood disorders: overview and future prospects. Psychopharmacol Bull 33:205–217, 1997

Evans DL, Nemeroff CB: The dexamethasone suppression test in mixed bipolar disorder. Am J Psychiatry 140:615–617, 1983

Evans DL, Burnett GB, Nemeroff CB: The dexamethasone suppression test in the clinical setting. Am J Psychiatry 140:586–589, 1983

Evans DL, Charney DS, Lewis L, et al: Mood disorders in the medically ill: scientific review and recommendations. Biol Psychiatry 58:175–189, 2005

Fagiolini A, Kupfer DJ, Scott J, et al: Hypothyroidism in patients with bipolar I disorder treated primarily with lithium. Epidemiol Psichiatr Soc 15:123–127, 2006

Felitti VJ, Anda RF, Nordenberg D, et al: Relationship of childhood abuse and household dysfunction to many of the leading causes of death in adults. The Adverse Childhood Experiences (ACE) Study. Am J Prev Med 14:245–258, 1998

Ferin M, Van de Wiele R: Endogenous opioid peptides and the control of the menstrual cycle. Eur J Obstet Gynecol Reprod Biol 18:365–373, 1984

Finkelstein JW, Roffwarg HP, Boyar RM, et al: Age-related changes in the twenty-four-hour spontaneous secretion of growth hormone. J Clin Endocrinol Metab 35:665–670, 1972

Fisher PM, Meltzer CC, Ziolko SK, et al: Capacity for 5-HT1A-mediated autoregulation predicts amygdala reactivity. Nat Neurosci 9:1362–1363, 2006

Flament-Durand J: The hypothalamus: anatomy and functions. Acta Psychiatr Belg 80:364–375, 1980

Ford DE, Erlinger TP: Depression and C-reactive protein in US adults: data from the Third National Health and Nutrition Examination Survey. Arch Intern Med 164:1010–1014, 2004

Freedman LJ, Insel TR, Smith Y: Subcortical projections of area 25 (subgenual cortex) of the macaque monkey. J Comp Neurol 421:172–188, 2000

Frodl T, Meisenzahl E, Zetzsche T, et al: Enlargement of the amygdala in patients with a first episode of major depression. Biol Psychiatry 51:708–714, 2002a

Frodl T, Meisenzahl E, Zetzsche T, et al: Hippocampal changes in patients with a first episode of major depression. Am J Psychiatry 159:1112–1118, 2002b

Frodl T, Meisenzahl EM, Zetzsche T, et al: Larger amygdala volumes in first depressive episode as compared to recurrent major depression and healthy control subjects. Biol Psychiatry 53:338–344, 2003

Frodl T, Schule C, Schmitt G, et al: Association of the brain-derived neurotrophic factor Val66Met polymorphism with reduced hippocampal volumes in major depression. Arch Gen Psychiatry 64:410–416, 2007

Fuchs E, Gould E: Mini-review: in vivo neurogenesis in the adult brain: regulation and functional implications. Eur J Neurosci 12:2211–2214, 2000

Fujihara H, Sei H, Morita Y, et al: Short-term sleep disturbance enhances brain-derived neurotrophic factor gene expression in rat hippocampus by acting as internal stressor. J Mol Neurosci 21:223–232, 2003

Garlow SJ, Dunlop B, Ninan PT, et al: Addition of triiodothyronine (T3) to sertraline does not impact treatment response in patients with major depressive disorder. American College of Neuropsychopharmacology Abstracts, 2007

Gelernter J, Cubells JF, Kidd JR, et al: Population studies of polymorphisms of the serotonin transporter protein gene. Am J Med Genet 88:61–66, 1999

Geller B, Badner JA, Tillman R, et al: Linkage disequilibrium of the brain-derived neurotrophic factor Val66Met polymorphism in children with a prepubertal and early adolescent bipolar disorder phenotype. Am J Psychiatry 161:1698–1700, 2004

Gerner RH, Gwirtsman HE: Abnormalities of dexamethasone suppression test and urinary MHPG in anorexia nervosa. Am J Psychiatry 138:650–653, 1981

Gerner RH, Yamada T: Altered neuropeptide concentrations in cerebrospinal fluid of psychiatric patients. Brain Res 238:298–302, 1982

Gershon ES, Hamovit J, Guroff JJ, et al: A family study of schizoaffective, bipolar I, bipolar II, unipolar, and normal control probands. Arch Gen Psychiatry 39:1157–1167, 1982

Gervasoni N, Aubry JM, Bondolfi G, et al: Partial normalization of serum brain-derived neurotrophic factor in remitted patients after a major depressive episode. Neuropsychobiology 51:234–238, 2005

Geuze E, Vermetten E, Bremner JD: MR-based in vivo hippocampal volumetrics, II: findings in neuropsychiatric disorders. Mol Psychiatry 10:160–184, 2005

Gibbons JL, McHugh PR: Plasma cortisol in depressive illness. J Psychiatr Res 1:162–171, 1962

Gillespie CF, Ressler KJ: Glutamate and emotional learning: translational perspectives. CNS Spectr 10:831–839, 2005

Gillespie NA, Whitfield JB, Williams B, et al: The relationship between stressful life events, the serotonin transporter (5-HTTLPR) genotype and major depression. Psychol Med 35:101–111, 2005

Glaser R, Kiecolt-Glaser JK: Stress-induced immune dysfunction: implications for health. Nat Rev Immunol 5:243–251, 2005

Godwin CD, Greenberg LB, Shukla S: Predictive value of the dexamethasone suppression test in mania. Am J Psychiatry 141:1610–1612, 1984

Goforth HW, Holsinger T: Rapid relief of severe major depressive disorder by use of preoperative ketamine and electroconvulsive therapy. J ECT 23:23–25, 2007

Gold BI, Bowers MB, Roth RH, et al: GABA levels in CSF of patients with psychiatric disorders. Am J Psychiatry 137:362–364, 1980

Gold MS, Pottash AC, Extein I: "Symptomless" autoimmune thyroiditis in depression. Psychiatry Res 6:261–269, 1982

Goldapple K, Segal Z, Garson C, et al: Modulation of cortical-limbic pathways in major depression: treatment-specific effects of cognitive behavior therapy. Arch Gen Psychiatry 61:34–41, 2004

Goldberg JF, Burdick KE, Endick CJ: Preliminary randomized, double-blind, placebo-controlled trial of pramipexole added to mood stabilizers for treatment-resistant bipolar depression. Am J Psychiatry 161:564–566, 2004

Golden RN, Markey SP, Risby E, et al: Antidepressants reduce whole-body NE turnover while enhancing 6-hydroxymelatonin output. Arch Gen Psychiatry 45:150–154, 1988

Gomez RG, Fleming SH, Keller J, et al: The neuropsychological profile of psychotic major depression and its relation to cortisol. Biol Psychiatry 60:472–478, 2006

Gonul AS, Akdeniz F, Taneli F, et al: Effect of treatment on serum brain-derived neurotrophic factor levels in depressed patients. Eur Arch Psychiatry Clin Neurosci 255:381–386, 2005

Goodwin GM, Bowden CL, Calabrese JR, et al: A pooled analysis of 2 placebo-controlled 18-month trials of lamotrigine and lithium maintenance in bipolar I disorder. J Clin Psychiatry 65:432–441, 2004

Goodwin RD, Davidson JR: Self-reported diabetes and posttraumatic stress disorder among adults in the community. Prev Med 40:570–574, 2005

Goodwin RD, Stein MB: Association between childhood trauma and physical disorders among adults in the United States. Psychol Med 34:509–520, 2004

Grabe HJ, Lange M, Wolff B, et al: Mental and physical distress is modulated by a polymorphism in the 5-HT transporter gene interacting with social stressors and chronic disease burden. Mol Psychiatry 10:220–224, 2005

Greden JF, Albala AA, Haskett RF, et al: Normalization of dexamethasone suppression test: a laboratory index of recovery from endogenous depression. Biol Psychiatry 15:449–458, 1980

Green EK, Raybould R, Macgregor S, et al: Genetic variation of brain-derived neurotrophic factor (BDNF) in bipolar disorder: case-control study of over 3000 individuals from the UK. Br J Psychiatry 188:21–25, 2006

Greengard P: The neurobiology of slow synaptic transmission. Science 294:1024–1030, 2001

Greer MA: The role of the hypothalamus in the control of thyroid function. J Clin Endocrinol Metab 12:1259–1268, 1952

Groves JO: Is it time to reassess the BDNF hypothesis of depression? Mol Psychiatry 12:1079–1088, 2007

Gutierrez H, Hale VA, Dolcet X, et al: NF-kappaB signalling regulates the growth of neural processes in the developing PNS and CNS. Development 132:1713–1726, 2005

Gutman DA, Owens MJ, Skelton KH, et al: The corticotropin-releasing factor1 receptor antagonist R121919 attenuates the behavioral and endocrine responses to stress. J Pharmacol Exp Ther 304:874–880, 2003

Haber SN: The primate basal ganglia: parallel and integrative networks. J Chem Neuroanat 26:317–330, 2003

Haggerty JJ, Simon JS, Evans DL, et al: Relationship of serum TSH concentration and antithyroid antibodies to diagnosis and DST response in psychiatric inpatients. Am J Psychiatry 144:1491–1493, 1987

Haggerty JJ, Evans DL, Golden RN, et al: The presence of anti-thyroid antibodies in patients with affective and non-affective psychiatric disorders. Biol Psychiatry 27:51–60, 1990

Hahn MK, Blakely RD: Monoamine transporter gene structure and polymorphisms in relation to psychiatric and other complex disorders. Pharmacogenomics J 2:217–235, 2002

Hamann S, Mao H: Positive and negative emotional verbal stimuli elicit activity in the left amygdala. Neuroreport 13:15–19, 2002

Hariri AR, Holmes A: Genetics of emotional regulation: the role of the serotonin transporter in neural function. Trends Cogn Sci 10:182–191, 2006

Hariri AR, Mattay VS, Tessitore A, et al: Serotonin transporter genetic variation and the response of the human amygdala. Science 297:400–403, 2002

Harmer CJ, Mackay CE, Reid CB, et al: Antidepressant drug treatment modifies the neural processing of nonconscious threat cues. Biol Psychiatry 59:816–820, 2006

Hartline KM, Owens MJ, Nemeroff CB: Postmortem and cerebrospinal fluid studies of corticotropin-releasing factor in humans. Ann N Y Acad Sci 780:96–105, 1996

Hasler G, Drevets WC, Manji HK, et al: Discovering endophenotypes for major depression. Neuropsychopharmacology 29:1765–1781, 2004

Hatterer JA, Herbert J, Hidaka C, et al: CSF transthyretin in patients with depression. Am J Psychiatry 150:813–815, 1993

Hayden EP, Klein DN: Outcome of dysthymic disorder at 5-year follow-up: the effect of familial psychopathology, early adversity, personality, comorbidity, and chronic stress. Am J Psychiatry 158:1864–1870, 2001

Heils A, Teufel A, Petri S, et al: Allelic variation of human serotonin transporter gene expression. J Neurochem 66:2621–2624, 1996

Heim C, Newport DJ, Heit S, et al: Pituitary-adrenal and autonomic responses to stress in women after sexual and physical abuse in childhood. JAMA 284:592–597, 2000

Heim C, Newport DJ, Bonsall R, et al: Altered pituitary-adrenal axis responses to provocative challenge tests in adult survivors of childhood abuse. Am J Psychiatry 158:575–581, 2001

Heim C, Mletzko T, Purselle D, et al: The dexamethasone/corticotropin-releasing factor test in men with major depression: role of childhood trauma. Biol Psychiatry 63:398–405, 2008

Heine VM, Zareno J, Maslam S, et al: Chronic stress in the adult dentate gyrus reduces cell proliferation near the vasculature and VEGF and Flk-1 protein expression. Eur J Neurosci 21:1304–1314, 2005

Heinrichs SC, Menzaghi F, Merlo Pich E, et al: The role of CRF in behavioral aspects of stress. Ann N Y Acad Sci 771:92–104, 1995

Heinrichs SC, Lapsansky J, Lovenberg TW, et al: Corticotropin-releasing factor CRF1, but not CRF2, receptors mediate anxiogenic-like behavior. Regul Pept 71:15–21, 1997

Heinz A, Braus DF, Smolka MN, et al: Amygdala-prefrontal coupling depends on a genetic variation of the serotonin transporter. Nat Neurosci 8:20–21, 2005

Heisler S, Reisine T, Hook V, et al: Somatostatin inhibits multireceptor stimulation of cyclic AMP formation and adrenocorticotropin secretion in mouse pituitary tumor cells. Proc Natl Acad Sci U S A 79:6502–6507, 1982

Hofmann SG, Meuret AE, Smits JA, et al: Augmentation of exposure therapy with D-cycloserine for social anxiety disorder. Arch Gen Psychiatry 63:298–304, 2006

Honig A, Bartlett JR, Bouras N, et al: Amino acid levels in depression: a preliminary investigation. J Psychiatr Res 22:159–164, 1988

Hood WF, Compton RP, Monahan JB: D-cycloserine: a ligand for the N-methyl-D-aspartate coupled glycine receptor has partial agonist characteristics. Neurosci Lett 98:91–95, 1989

Hrdina PD, Demeter E, Vu TB, et al: 5-HT uptake sites and 5-HT2 receptors in brain of antidepressant-free suicide victims/depressives: increase in 5-HT2 sites in cortex and amygdala. Brain Res 614:37–44, 1993

Hubain PP, Simonnet MP, Mendlewicz J: The dexamethasone suppression test in affective illnesses and schizophrenia: relationship with psychotic symptoms. Neuropsychobiology 16:57–60, 1986

Hurwitz TA, Clark C, Murphy E, et al: Regional cerebral glucose metabolism in major depressive disorder. Can J Psychiatry 35:684–688, 1990

Iga J, Ueno S, Yamauchi K, et al: The Val66Met polymorphism of the brain-derived neurotrophic factor gene is associated with psychotic feature and suicidal behavior in Japanese major depressive patients. Am J Med Genet B Neuropsychiatr Genet 144B:1003–1006, 2007

Imura H, Nakai Y, Hoshimi T: Effect of 5-hydroxytryptophan (5-HTP) on growth hormone and ACTH release in man. J Clin Endocrinol Metab 36:204–206, 1973

Iosifescu DV, Nierenberg AA, Mischoulon D, et al: An open study of triiodothyronine augmentation of selective serotonin reuptake inhibitors in treatment-resistant major depressive disorder. J Clin Psychiatry 66:1038–1042, 2005

Isenberg N, Silbersweig D, Engelien A, et al: Linguistic threat activates the human amygdala. Proc Natl Acad Sci U S A 96:10456–10459, 1999

Ising M, Kunzel HE, Binder EB, et al: The combined dexamethasone/CRH test as a potential surrogate marker in depression. Prog Neuropsychopharmacol Biol Psychiatry 29:1085–1093, 2005

Iwasaki Y, Ikeda K, Kinoshita M: Molecular and cellular mechanism of glutamate receptors in relation to amyotrophic lateral sclerosis. Curr Drug Targets CNS Neurol Disord 1:511–518, 2002

Jacobson L, Sapolsky R: The role of the hippocampus in feedback regulation of the hypothalamic-pituitary-adrenocortical axis. Endocr Rev 12:118–134, 1991

Jaffe RB, Plosker S, Marshall L, et al: Neuromodulatory regulation of gonadotropin-releasing hormone pulsatile discharge in women. Am J Obstet Gynecol 163:1727–1731, 1990

Jaffee SR, Price TS: Gene–environment correlations: a review of the evidence and implications for prevention of mental illness. Mol Psychiatry 12:432–442, 2007

Janowsky DS, Risch SC: Cholinomimetic and anticholinergic drugs used to investigate an acetylcholine hypothesis of affective disorder and stress. Drug Dev Res 4:125–142, 1984

Janowsky DS, el-Yousef MK, Davis JM, et al: A cholinergic-adrenergic hypothesis of mania and depression. Lancet 2(7778):573–577, 1972

Joels M, de Kloet ER: Mineralocorticoid and glucocorticoid receptors in the brain. Implications for ion permeability and transmitter systems. Prog Neurobiol 43:1–36, 1994

Johnston GA, Chebib M, Hanrahan JR, et al: GABA(C) receptors as drug targets. Curr Drug Targets CNS Neurol Disord 2:260–268, 2003

Jones D, Kelwala S, Bell J, et al: Cholinergic REM sleep induction response correlation with endogenous major depressive type. Psychiatry Res 14:99–110, 1985

Jorge RE, Robinson RG, Moser D, et al: Major depression following traumatic brain injury. Arch Gen Psychiatry 61:42–50, 2004

Jurgens U, Muller-Preuss P: Convergent projections of different limbic vocalization areas in the squirrel monkey. Exp Brain Res 29:75–83, 1977

Kahl KG, Rudolf S, Stoeckelhuber BM, et al: Bone mineral density, markers of bone turnover, and cytokines in young women with borderline personality disorder with and without comorbid major depressive disorder. Am J Psychiatry 162:168–174, 2005

Kanazawa T, Glatt SJ, Kia-Keating B, et al: Meta-analysis reveals no association of the Val66Met polymorphism of brain-derived neurotrophic factor with either schizophrenia or bipolar disorder. Psychiatr Genet 17:165–170, 2007

Kaplan MJ, Klinetob NA: Childhood emotional trauma and chronic posttraumatic stress disorder in adult outpatients with treatment-resistant depression. J Nerv Ment Dis 188:596–601, 2000

Karege F, Perret G, Bondolfi G, et al: Decreased serum brain-derived neurotrophic factor levels in major depressed patients. Psychiatry Res 109:143–148, 2002

Karege F, Vaudan G, Schwald M, et al: Neurotrophin levels in post-mortem brains of suicide victims and the effects of antemortem diagnosis and psychotropic drugs. Brain Res Mol Brain Res 136:29–37, 2005

Karolewicz B, Szebeni K, Stockmeier CA, et al: Low nNOS protein in the locus coeruleus in major depression. J Neurochem 91:1057–1066, 2004

Karolewicz B, Stockmeier CA, Ordway GA: Elevated levels of the NR2C subunit of the NMDA receptor in the locus coeruleus in depression. Neuropsychopharmacology 30:1557–1567, 2005

Kato T: Molecular genetics of bipolar disorder and depression. Psychiatry Clin Neurosci 61:3–19, 2007

Kaufman J, Yang BZ, Douglas-Palumberi H, et al: Social supports and serotonin transporter gene moderate depression in maltreated children. Proc Natl Acad Sci U S A 101:17316–17321, 2004

Kaufman J, Yang BZ, Douglas-Palumberi H, et al: Brain-derived neurotrophic factor-5-HTTLPR gene interactions and environmental modifiers of depression in children. Biol Psychiatry 59:673–680, 2006

Keedwell PA, Andrew C, Williams SC, et al: A double dissociation of ventromedial prefrontal cortical responses to sad and happy stimuli in depressed and healthy individuals. Biol Psychiatry 58:495–503, 2005a

Keedwell PA, Andrew C, Williams SC, et al: The neural correlates of anhedonia in major depressive disorder. Biol Psychiatry 58:843–853, 2005b

Keller J, Flores B, Gomez RG, et al: Cortisol circadian rhythm alterations in psychotic major depression. Biol Psychiatry 60:275–281, 2006

Kendler KS, Neale MC, Kessler RC, et al: The lifetime history of major depression in women: reliability of diagnosis and heritability. Arch Gen Psychiatry 50:863–870, 1993

Kendler KS, Gardner CO, Neale MC, et al: Genetic risk factors for major depression in men and women: similar or different heritabilities and same or partly distinct genes? Psychol Med 31:605–616, 2001a

Kendler KS, Thornton LM, Gardner CO: Genetic risk, number of previous depressive episodes, and stressful life events in predicting onset of major depression. Am J Psychiatry 158:582–586, 2001b

Kendler KS, Gardner CO, Prescott CA: Toward a comprehensive developmental model for major depression in women. Am J Psychiatry 159:1133–1145, 2002

Kendler KS, Kuhn JW, Prescott CA: Childhood sexual abuse, stressful life events and risk for major depression in women. Psychol Med 34:1475–1482, 2004

Kendler KS, Kuhn JW, Vittum J, et al: The interaction of stressful life events and a serotonin transporter polymorphism in the prediction of episodes of major depression: a replication. Arch Gen Psychiatry 62:529–535, 2005

Kennedy SH, Tighe S, McVey G, et al: Melatonin and cortisol "switches" during mania, depression, and euthymia in a drug-free bipolar patient. J Nerv Ment Dis 177:300–303, 1989

Kent S, Bluthe RM, Kelley KW, et al: Sickness behavior as a new target for drug development. Trends Pharmacol Sci 13:24–28, 1992

Kessler RC, Berglund P, Demler O, et al: The epidemiology of major depressive disorder: results from the National Comorbidity Survey Replication (NCS-R). JAMA 289:3095–3105, 2003

Kessler RC, Berglund P, Demler O, et al: Lifetime prevalence and age-of-onset distributions of DSM-IV disorders in the National Comorbidity Survey Replication. Arch Gen Psychiatry 62:593–602, 2005

Kieseppa T, Partonen T, Haukka J, et al: High concordance of bipolar I disorder in a nationwide sample of twins. Am J Psychiatry 161:1814–1821, 2004

Kim JM, Stewart R, Kim SW, et al: Interactions between life stressors and susceptibility genes (5-HTTLPR and BDNF) on depression in Korean elders. Biol Psychiatry 62:423–428, 2007

Kim JS, Schmid-Burgk W, Claus D, et al: Increased serum glutamate in depressed patients. Arch Psychiatr Nervenkr 232:299–304, 1982

Kiriike N, Izumiya Y, Nishiwaki S, et al: TRH test and DST in schizoaffective mania, mania, and schizophrenia. Biol Psychiatry 24:415–422, 1988

Kirkegaard CJ, Faber J, Hummer L, et al: Increased levels of TRH in cerebrospinal fluid from patients with endogenous depression. Psychoneuroendocrinology 4:227–235, 1979

Kitayama N, Vaccarino V, Kutner M, et al: Magnetic resonance imaging (MRI) measurement of hippocampal volume in posttraumatic stress disorder: a meta-analysis. J Affect Disord 88:79–86, 2005

Klimek V, Schenck JE, Han H, et al: Dopaminergic abnormalities in amygdaloid nuclei in major depression: a postmortem study. Biol Psychiatry 52:740–748, 2002

Knobil E: The GnRH pulse generator. Am J Obstet Gynecol 163:1721–1727, 1990

Kornau HC: GABA(B) receptors and synaptic modulation. Cell Tissue Res 326:517–533, 2006

Krabbe KS, Nielsen AR, Krogh-Madsen R, et al: Brain-derived neurotrophic factor (BDNF) and type 2 diabetes. Diabetologia 50:431–438, 2007

Kraft JB, Peters EJ, Slager SL, et al: Analysis of association between the serotonin transporter and antidepressant response in a large clinical sample. Biol Psychiatry 61:734–742, 2007

Krishnan KR: Organic bases of depression in the elderly. Annu Rev Med 42:261–266, 1991

Krishnan KR, Manepalli AN, Ritchie JC, et al: Growth hormone-releasing factor stimulation test in depression. Am J Psychiatry 145:190–192, 1988

Krishnan KR, Doraiswamy PM, Lurie SN, et al: Pituitary size in depression. J Clin Endocrinol Metab 72:256–259, 1991

Krishnan KR, McDonald WM, Doraiswamy PM, et al: Neuroanatomical substrates of depression in the elderly. Eur Arch Psychiatry Clin Neurosci 243:41–46, 1993

Krishnan RR, Maltbie AA, Davidson JR: Abnormal cortisol suppression in bipolar patients with simultaneous manic and depressive symptoms. Am J Psychiatry 140:203–205, 1983

Kudoh A, Takahira Y, Katagai H, et al: Small-dose ketamine improves the postoperative state of depressed patients. Anesth Analg 95:114–118, 2002

Kugaya A, Sanacora G: Beyond monoamines: glutamatergic function in mood disorders. CNS Spectr 10:808–819, 2005

Kupka RW, Nolen WA, Post RM, et al: High rate of autoimmune thyroiditis in bipolar disorder: lack of association with lithium exposure. Biol Psychiatry 51:305–311, 2002

Lacerda AL, Keshavan MS, Hardan AY, et al: Anatomic evaluation of the orbitofrontal cortex in major depressive disorder. Biol Psychiatry 55:353–358, 2004

Lal S, Martin JB, de la Vega C, et al: Comparison of the effect of apomorphine and L-dopa on serum growth hormone levels in man. Clin Endocrinol (Oxf) 4:277–285, 1975

Lange C, Irle E: Enlarged amygdala volume and reduced hippocampal volume in young women with major depression. Psychol Med 34:1059–1064, 2004

Lapin IP, Oxenkrug GF: Intensification of the central serotonergic process as a possible determinant of thymoleptic effect. Lancet 1(7586):132–136, 1969

Lara ME, Klein DN, Kasch KL: Psychosocial predictors of the short-term course and outcome of major depression: a longitudinal study of a nonclinical sample with recent-onset episodes. J Abnorm Psychol 109:644–650, 2000

Lasky-Su JA, Faraone SV, Glatt SJ, et al: Meta-analysis of the association between two polymorphisms in the serotonin transporter gene and affective disorders. Am J Med Genet B Neuropsychiatr Genet 133:110–115, 2005

Lawrence NS, Williams AM, Surguladze S, et al: Subcortical and ventral prefrontal cortical neural responses to facial expressions distinguish patients with bipolar disorder and major depression. Biol Psychiatry 55:578–587, 2004

Lazarus JH, McGregor AM, Ludgate M, et al: Effect of lithium carbonate therapy on thyroid immune status in manic depressive patients: a prospective study. J Affect Disord 11:155–160, 1986

Leckman JF, Gershon ES, Nichols AS, et al: Reduced MAO activity in first-degree relatives of individuals with bipolar affective disorders: a preliminary report. Arch Gen Psychiatry 34:601–606, 1977

Lee JA, Lupski JR: Genomic rearrangements and gene copy-number alterations as a cause of nervous system disorders. Neuron 52:103–121, 2006

Leibenluft E, Fiero PL, Rubinow DR: Effects of the menstrual cycle on dependent variables in mood disorder research. Arch Gen Psychiatry 51:761–781, 1994

Lekman M, Laje G, Charney D, et al: The FKBP5 gene in depression and treatment response—an association study in the Sequenced Treatment Alternatives to Relieve Depression (STAR*D) cohort. Biol Psychiatry 63:1103–1110, 2008

Lencz T, Morgan TV, Athanasiou M, et al: Converging evidence for a pseudoautosomal cytokine receptor gene locus in schizophrenia. Mol Psychiatry 12:572–580, 2007

Leppanen JM: Emotional information processing in mood disorders: a review of behavioral and neuroimaging findings. Curr Opin Psychiatry 19:34–39, 2006

Lesch KP, Mossner R: Genetically driven variation in serotonin uptake: is there a link to affective spectrum, neurodevelopmental, and neurodegenerative disorders? Biol Psychiatry 44:179–192, 1998

Lesch KP, Laux G, Erb A, et al: Attenuated growth hormone response to growth hormone RH in major depressive disorder. Biol Psychiatry 22:1495–1499, 1987a

Lesch KP, Laux G, Pfuller H, et al: Growth hormone response to GH-releasing hormone in depression. J Clin Endocrinol Metab 65:1278–1281, 1987b

Lesch KP, Wolozin BL, Estler HC, et al: Isolation of a cDNA encoding the human brain serotonin transporter. J Neural Transm 91:67–72, 1993

Levinson DF: The genetics of depression: a review. Biol Psychiatry 60:84–92, 2006

Li D, He L: Meta-analysis supports association between serotonin transporter (5-HTT) and suicidal behavior. Mol Psychiatry 12:47–54, 2007

Li Q, Withoff S, Verma IM: Inflammation-associated cancer: NF-kappaB is the lynchpin. Trends Immunol 26:318–325, 2005

Licinio J, O'Kirwan F, Irizarry K, et al: Association of a corticotropin-releasing hormone receptor 1 haplotype and antidepressant treatment response in Mexican-Americans. Mol Psychiatry 9:1075–1082, 2004

Lin PY, Tsai G: Association between serotonin transporter gene promoter polymorphism and suicide: results of a meta-analysis. Biol Psychiatry 55:1023–1030, 2004

Linkowski P, Kerkhofs M, Van Onderbergen A, et al: The 24-hour profiles of cortisol, prolactin, and growth hormone secretion in mania. Arch Gen Psychiatry 51:616–624, 1994

Linnoila M, Karoum F, Calil HM, et al: Alteration of norepinephrine metabolism with desipramine and zimelidine in depressed patients. Arch Gen Psychiatry 39:1025–1028, 1982

Linnoila M, Guthrie S, Lane EA, et al: Clinical studies on norepinephrine metabolism: how to interpret the numbers. Psychiatry Res 17:229–239, 1986

Linnoila VM, Virkkunen M: Aggression, suicidality and serotonin. J Clin Psychiatry 53 (suppl):46–51, 1992

Lissau I, Sorensen TI: Parental neglect during childhood and increased risk of obesity in young adulthood. Lancet 343:324–327, 1994

Little KY, McLauglin DP, Ranc J, et al: Serotonin transporter binding sites and mRNA levels in depressed persons committing suicide. Biol Psychiatry 41:1156–1164, 1997

Liu Z, Zhu F, Wang G, et al: Association of corticotropin-releasing hormone receptor1 gene SNP and haplotype with major depression. Neurosci Lett 404:358–362, 2006

Liu Z, Zhu F, Wang G, et al: Association study of corticotropin-releasing hormone receptor1 gene polymorphisms and antidepressant response in major depressive disorders. Neurosci Lett 414:155–158, 2007

Loosen PT, Prange AJ Jr: Serum thyrotropin response to thyrotropin-releasing hormone in psychiatric patients: a review. Am J Psychiatry 139:405–416, 1982

Lopez-Larson MP, DelBello MP, Zimmerman ME, et al: Regional prefrontal gray and white matter abnormalities in bipolar disorder. Biol Psychiatry 52:93–100, 2002

Lotrich FE, Pollock BG: Meta-analysis of serotonin transporter polymorphisms and affective disorders. Psychiatr Genet 14:121–129, 2004

Louis WJ, Doyle AE, Anavekar SN: Plasma noradrenaline concentration and blood pressure in essential hypertension, pheochromocytoma and depression. Clinical Science and Molecular Medicine 48(suppl):239S–242S, 1975

MacFall JR, Payne ME, Provenzale JE, et al: Medial orbital frontal lesions in late-onset depression. Biol Psychiatry 49:803–806, 2001

Maes M: Major depression and activation of the inflammatory response system. Adv Exp Med Biol 461:25–46, 1999

Maes M, Verkerk R, Vandoolaeghe E, et al: Serum levels of excitatory amino acids, serine, glycine, histidine, threonine, taurine, alanine and arginine in treatment-resistant depression: modulation by treatment with antidepressants and prediction of clinical responsivity. Acta Psychiatr Scand 97:302–308, 1998

Magarinos AM, McEwen BS: Stress-induced atrophy of apical dendrites of hippocampal CA3c neurons: comparison of stressors. Neuroscience 69:83–88, 1995a

Magarinos AM, McEwen BS: Stress-induced atrophy of apical dendrites of hippocampal CA3c neurons: involvement of glucocorticoid secretion and excitatory amino acid receptors. Neuroscience 69:89–98, 1995b

Magarinos AM, McEwen BS, Flugge G, et al: Chronic psychosocial stress causes apical dendritic atrophy of hippocampal CA3 pyramidal neurons in subordinate tree shrews. J Neurosci 16:3534–3540, 1996

Magarinos AM, Verdugo JM, McEwen BS: Chronic stress alters synaptic terminal structure in hippocampus. Proc Natl Acad Sci U S A 94:14002–14008, 1997

Mah L, Zarate CA Jr, Singh J, et al: Regional cerebral glucose metabolic abnormalities in bipolar II depression. Biol Psychiatry 61:765–775, 2007

Maier W, Lichtermann D, Minges J, et al: Schizoaffective disorder and affective disorders with mood-incongruent psychotic features: keep separate or combine? Evidence from a family study. Am J Psychiatry 149:1666–1673, 1992

Malison RT, Price LH, Berman R, et al: Reduced brain serotonin transporter availability in major depression as measured by [123I]-2 beta-carbomethoxy-3 beta-(4-iodophenyl)tropane and single photon emission computed tomography. Biol Psychiatry 44:1090–1098, 1998

Manji HK, Drevets WC, Charney DS: The cellular neurobiology of depression. Nat Med 7:541–547, 2001

Mann JJ, Malone KM, Psych MR, et al: Attempted suicide characteristics and cerebrospinal fluid amine metabolites in depressed inpatients. Neuropsychopharmacology 15:576–586, 1996

Mann JJ, Huang YY, Underwood MD, et al: A serotonin transporter gene promoter polymorphism (5-HTTLPR) and prefrontal cortical binding in major depression and suicide. Arch Gen Psychiatry 57:729–738, 2000

Marazita ML, Neiswanger K, Cooper M, et al: Genetic segregation analysis of early onset recurrent unipolar depression. Am J Hum Genet 61:1370–1378, 1997

Martinot JL, Hardy P, Feline A, et al: Left prefrontal glucose hypometabolism in the depressed state: a confirmation. Am J Psychiatry 147:1313–1317, 1990

Martinot M, Bragulat V, Artiges E, et al: Decreased presynaptic dopamine function in the left caudate of depressed patients with affective flattening and psychomotor retardation. Am J Psychiatry 158:314–316, 2001

Matsubara T, Funato H, Kobayashi A, et al: Reduced glucocorticoid receptor alpha expression in mood disorder patients and first-degree relatives. Biol Psychiatry 59:689–695, 2006

Matussek N, Ackenheil M, Hippius H, et al: Effects of clonidine on growth hormone release in psychiatric patients and controls. Psychiatry Res 2:25–36, 1980

Maubach M, Dieblod K, Fried W, et al: Platelet MAO activity in patients with affective psychosis and their first-degree relatives. Pharmacopsychiatry 14:87–93, 1981

Mauri MC, Ferrara A, Boscati L, et al: Plasma and platelet amino acid concentrations in patients affected by major depression and under fluvoxamine treatment. Neuropsychobiology 37:124–129, 1998

Mayberg HS: Frontal lobe dysfunction in secondary depression. J Neuropsychiatry Clin Neurosci 6:428–442, 1994

Mayberg HS: Limbic-cortical dysregulation: a proposed model of depression. J Neuropsychiatry Clin Neurosci 9:471–481, 1997

Mayberg HS, Liotti M, Brannan SK, et al: Reciprocal limbic-cortical function and negative mood: converging PET findings in depression and normal sadness. Am J Psychiatry 156:675–682, 1999

Mayberg HS, Brannan SK, Tekell JL, et al: Regional metabolic effects of fluoxetine in major depression: serial changes and relationship to clinical response. Biol Psychiatry 48:830–843, 2000

Mayberg HS, Lozano AM, Voon V, et al: Deep brain stimulation for treatment-resistant depression. Neuron 45:651–660, 2005

McCauley J, Kern DE, Kolodner K, et al: Clinical characteristics of women with a history of childhood abuse: unhealed wounds. JAMA 277:1362–1368, 1997

McDonald WM, Richard IH, DeLong MR: Prevalence, etiology, and treatment of depression in Parkinson's disease. Biol Psychiatry 54:363–375, 2003

McEwen BS: Protective and damaging effects of stress mediators. N Engl J Med 338:171–179, 1998

McGuffin P, Katz R, Rutherford J: Nature, nurture and depression: a twin study. Psychol Med 21:329–335, 1991

McGuffin P, Katz R, Watkins S, et al: A hospital-based twin register of the heritability of DSM-IV unipolar depression. Arch Gen Psychiatry 53:129–136, 1996

McGuffin P, Rijsdijk F, Andrew M, et al: The heritability of bipolar affective disorder and the genetic relationship to unipolar depression. Arch Gen Psychiatry 60:497–502, 2003

McKinney WT: Animal models of depression: an overview. Psychiatric Developments 2:77–96, 1984

Mehta AK, Ticku MK: An update on GABAA receptors. Brain Res Brain Res Rev 29:196–217, 1999

Meller WH, Zander KM, Crosby RD, et al: Luteinizing hormone pulse characteristics in depressed women. Am J Psychiatry 154:1454–1455, 1997

Meltzer HY, Lowy MT, Locascio JJ: Platelet MAO activity and the cortisol response to dexamethasone in major depression. Biol Psychiatry 24:129–142, 1988

Mendlewicz J, Rainier J: Adoption study supporting genetic transmission in manic-depressive illness. Nature 268:326–329, 1977

Mendlewicz J, Linkowski P, Kerkhofs M, et al: Diurnal hypersecretion of growth hormone in depression. J Clin Endocrinol Metab 60:505–512, 1985

Merali Z, Du L, Hrdina P, et al: Dysregulation in the suicide brain: mRNA expression of corticotropin-releasing hormone receptors and GABA(A) receptor subunits in frontal cortical brain region. J Neurosci 24:1478–1485, 2004

Merali Z, Kent P, Du L, et al: Corticotropin-releasing hormone, arginine vasopressin, gastrin-releasing peptide, and neuromedin B alterations in stress-relevant brain regions of suicides and control subjects. Biol Psychiatry 59:594–602, 2006

Meyer JH, Kapur S, Houle S, et al: Prefrontal cortex 5-HT2 receptors in depression: an [18F]setoperone PET imaging study. Am J Psychiatry 156:1029–1034, 1999

Meyer JH, Kruger S, Wilson AA, et al: Lower dopamine transporter binding potential in striatum during depression. Brain Imaging 12:4121–4125, 2001

Meyer JH, Ginovart N, Boovariwala A, et al: Elevated monoamine oxidase a levels in the brain: an explanation for the monoamine imbalance of major depression. Arch Gen Psychiatry 63:1209–1216, 2006

Michels G, Moss SJ: GABAA receptors: properties and trafficking. Crit Rev Biochem Mol Biol 42:3–14, 2007

Midgley AR Jr, Jaffe RB: Regulation of human gonadotropins: episodic fluctuation of LH during the menstrual cycle. J Clin Endocrinol Metab 33:962–969, 1971

Mill J, Petronis A: Molecular studies of major depressive disorder: the epigenetic perspective. Mol Psychiatry 12:799–814, 2007

Miller GE, Stetler CA, Carney RM, et al: Clinical depression and inflammatory risk markers for coronary heart disease. Am J Cardiol 90:1279–1283, 2002

Moldin SO, Reich T, Rice JP: Current perspectives on the genetics of unipolar depression. Behav Genet 21:211–242, 1991

Monkul ES, Hatch JP, Nicoletti MA, et al: Fronto-limbic brain structures in suicidal and non-suicidal female patients with major depressive disorder. Mol Psychiatry 12:360–366, 2007

Monteggia LM, Luikart B, Barrot M, et al: Brain-derived neurotrophic factor conditional knockouts show gender differences in depression-related behaviors. Biol Psychiatry 61:187–197, 2007

Moore RY, Bloom FE: Central catecholamine neuron systems: anatomy and physiology of the dopamine systems. Annu Rev Neurosci 1:129–169, 1978

Moore RY, Bloom FE: Central catecholamine neuron systems: anatomy and physiology of the norepinephrine and epinephrine systems. Annu Rev Neurosci 2:113–168, 1979

Mottaghy FM, Keller CE, Gangitano M, et al: Correlation of cerebral blood flow and treatment effects of repetitive transcranial magnetic stimulation in depressed patients. Psychiatry Res 115:1–14, 2002

Muller EE, Brambilla F, Cavagnini F, et al: Slight effect of l-tryptophan on growth hormone release in normal human subjects. J Clin Endocrinol Metab 39:1–5, 1974

Murphy GM Jr, Hollander SB, Rodrigues HE, et al: Effects of the serotonin transporter gene promoter polymorphism on mirtazapine and paroxetine efficacy and adverse events in geriatric major depression. Arch Gen Psychiatry 61:1163–1169, 2004

Murray CL, Lopez AD (eds): The Global Burden of Disease: Summary. Cambridge, MA, Harvard School of Public Health, 1996

Musselman DL, Lawson DH, Gumnick JF, et al: Paroxetine for the prevention of depression induced by high-dose interferon alfa. N Engl J Med 344:961–966, 2001a

Musselman DL, Miller AH, Porter MR, et al: Higher than normal plasma interleukin-6 concentrations in cancer patients with depression: preliminary findings. Am J Psychiatry 158:1252–1257, 2001b

Myers DH, Carter RA, Burns BH, et al: A prospective study of the effects of lithium on thyroid function and on the prevalence of antithyroid antibodies. Psychol Med 15:55–61, 1985

Nair RM, Barrett JF, Bowers CY, et al: Structure of porcine thyrotropin releasing hormone. Biochemistry 9:1103–1106, 1970

Navarro V, Gasto C, Lomena F, et al: Normalization of frontal cerebral perfusion in remitted elderly major depression: a 12 month follow-up SPECT study. Neuroimage 16:781–787, 2002

Nelson JC, Davis JM: DST studies in psychotic depression: a meta-analysis. Am J Psychiatry 154:1497–1503, 1997

Nemeroff CB: Recent advances in the neurobiology of depression. Psychopharmacol Bull 36 (suppl 2):6–23, 2002

Nemeroff CB: The burden of severe depression: a review of diagnostic challenges and treatment alternatives. J Psychiatr Res 41:189–206, 2007

Nemeroff CB, Evans DL: Correlation between the dexamethasone suppression test in depressed patients and clinical response. Am J Psychiatry 141:247–249, 1984

Nemeroff CB, Evans DL: Thyrotropin-releasing hormone (TRH), the thyroid axis, and affective disorder. Ann N Y Acad Sci 553:304–310, 1989

Nemeroff CB, Widerlov E, Bissette G, et al: Elevated concentrations of CSF corticotropin-releasing factor-like immunoreactivity in depressed patients. Science 226:1342–1344, 1984

Nemeroff CB, Simon JS, Haggerty JJ, et al: Antithyroid antibodies in depressed patients. Am J Psychiatry 142:840–843, 1985

Nemeroff CB, Owens MJ, Bissette G, et al: Reduced corticotropin-releasing factor (CRF) binding sites in the frontal cortex of suicides. Arch Gen Psychiatry 45:577–579, 1988

Nemeroff CB, Bissette G, Akil H, et al: Neuropeptide concentrations in the cerebrospinal fluid of depressed patients treated with electroconvulsive therapy: corticotropin-releasing factor, beta-endorphin and somatostatin. Br J Psychiatry 158:59–63, 1991

Nemeroff CB, Heim CM, Thase ME, et al: Differential responses to psychotherapy versus pharmacotherapy in patients with chronic forms of major depression and childhood trauma. Proc Natl Acad Sci U S A 100:14293–14296, 2003

Neria Y, Bromet EJ, Carlson GA, et al: Assaultive trauma and illness course in psychotic bipolar disorder: findings from the Suffolk county mental health project. Acta Psychiatr Scand 111:380–383, 2005

Nestler EJ, Carlezon WA Jr: The mesolimbic dopamine reward circuit in depression. Biol Psychiatry 59:1151–1159, 2006

Nestler EJ, Barrot M, DiLeone RJ, et al: Neurobiology of depression. Neuron 34:13–25, 2002

Neumeister A, Wood S, Bonne O, et al: Reduced hippocampal volume in unmedicated, remitted patients with major depression versus control subjects. Biol Psychiatry 57:935–937, 2005

Neumeister A, Hu XZ, Luckenbaugh DA, et al: Differential effects of 5-HTTLPR genotypes on the behavioral and neural responses to tryptophan depletion in patients with major depression and controls. Arch Gen Psychiatry 63:978–986, 2006

Neves-Pereira M, Mundo E, Muglia P, et al: The brain-derived neurotrophic factor gene confers susceptibility to bipolar disorder: evidence from a family based association study. Am J Hum Genet 71:651–655, 2002

Nibuya M, Morinobu S, Duman RS: Regulation of BDNF and trkB mRNA in rat brain by chronic electroconvulsive seizure and antidepressant drug treatments. J Neurosci 15:7539–7547, 1995

Nibuya M, Nestler EJ, Duman RS: Chronic antidepressant administration increases the expression of cAMP response element-binding protein (CREB) in rat hippocampus. J Neurosci 16:2365–2372, 1996

Nickel T, Sonntag A, Schill J, et al: Clinical and neurobiological effects of tianeptine and paroxetine in major depression. J Clin Psychopharmacol 23:155–168, 2003

Nobler MS, Oquendo MA, Kegeles LS, et al: Decreased regional brain metabolism after ECT. Am J Psychiatry 158:305–308, 2001

Nowak G, Ordway GA, Paul IA: Alterations in the N-methyl-D-aspartate (NMDA) receptor complex in the frontal cortex of suicide victims. Brain Res 675:157–164, 1995

Nudmamud-Thanoi S, Reynolds GP: The NR1 subunit of the glutamate/NMDA receptor in the superior temporal cortex in schizophrenia and affective disorders. Neurosci Lett 372:173–177, 2004

Nurnberger JI Jr, Foroud T: Genetics of bipolar affective disorder. Curr Psychiatry Rep 2:147–157, 2000

Okada G, Okamoto Y, Morinobu S, et al: Attenuated left prefrontal activation during a verbal fluency task in patients with depression. Neuropsychobiology 47:21–26, 2003

Ongur D, An X, Price JL: Prefrontal cortical projections to the hypothalamus in macaque monkeys. J Comp Neurol 401:480–505, 1998

Oquendo MA, Hastings RS, Huang YY, et al: Brain serotonin transporter binding in depressed patients with bipolar disorder using positron emission tomography. Arch Gen Psychiatry 64:201–208, 2007

Ordway GA: Pathophysiology of the locus coeruleus in suicide. Ann N Y Acad Sci 836:233–252, 1997

Oroszi G, Lapteva L, Davis E, et al: The Met66 allele of the functional Val66Met polymorphism in the brain-derived neurotrophic factor gene confers protection against neurocognitive dysfunction in systemic lupus erythematosus. Ann Rheum Dis 65:1330–1335, 2006

Orstavik RE, Kendler KS, Czajkowski N, et al: Genetic and environmental contributions to depressive personality disorder in a population-based sample of Norwegian twins. J Affect Disord 99:181–189, 2007

Oswald P, Del-Favero J, Massat I, et al: Non-replication of the brain-derived neurotrophic factor (BDNF) association in bipolar affective disorder: a Belgian patient-control study. Am J Med Genet B Neuropsychiatr Genet 129:34–35, 2004

Owens MJ, Nemeroff CB: Physiology and pharmacology of corticotropin-releasing factor. Pharmacol Rev 43:425–473, 1991

Owens MJ, Nemeroff CB: Role of serotonin in the pathophysiology of depression: focus on the serotonin transporter. Clin Chem 40:288–295, 1994

Pace TW, Mletzko TC, Alagbe O, et al: Increased stress-induced inflammatory responses in male patients with major depression and increased early life stress. Am J Psychiatry 163:1630–1633, 2006

Panagiotakos DB, Pitsavos C, Chrysohoou C, et al: Inflammation, coagulation, and depressive symptomatology in cardiovascular disease-free people: the ATTICA study. Eur Heart J 25:492–499, 2004

Pandey GN, Sharma RP, Janicak PG, et al: Monoamine oxidase and cortisol response in depression and schizophrenia. Psychiatry Res 44:1–8, 1992

Parsey RV, Hastings RS, Oquendo MA, et al: Effect of a triallelic functional polymorphism of the serotonin-transporter-linked promoter region on expression of serotonin transporter in the human brain. Am J Psychiatry 163:48–51, 2006

Penninx BW, Kritchevsky SB, Yaffe K, et al: Inflammatory markers and depressed mood in older persons: results from the Health, Aging and Body Composition study. Biol Psychiatry 54:566–572, 2003

Perry EK, Marshall EF, Blessed G, et al: Decreased imipramine binding in the brains of patients with depressive illness. Br J Psychiatry 142:188–192, 1983

Petty F: Plasma concentrations of gamma-aminobutyric acid (GABA) and mood disorders: a blood test for manic depressive disease? Clin Chem 40:296–302, 1994

Petty F, Schlesser MA: Plasma GABA in affective illness. J Affect Disord 3:339–343, 1981

Petty F, Sherman AD: Plasma GABA levels in psychiatric illness. J Affect Disord 6:131–138, 1984

Pezawas L, Meyer-Lindenberg A, Drabant EM, et al: 5-HTTLPR polymorphism impacts human cingulate-amygdala interactions: a genetic susceptibility mechanism for depression. Nat Neurosci 8:828–834, 2005

Phan KL, Wager TD, Taylor SF, et al: Functional neuroimaging studies of human emotions. CNS Spectr 9:258–266, 2004

Plotsky PM, Owens MJ, Nemeroff CB: Psychoneuroendocrinology of depression. Hypothalamic-pituitary-adrenal axis. Psychiatr Clin North Am 21:293–307, 1998

Poo MM: Neurotrophins as synaptic modulators. Nat Rev Neurosci 2:24–32, 2001

Posener JA, DeBattista C, Williams GH, et al: 24-Hour monitoring of cortisol and corticotrophin secretion in psychotic and nonpsychotic major depression. Arch Gen Psychiatry 57:755–760, 2000

Prange AJ Jr, Wilson IC, Rabon AM, et al: Enhancement of imipramine antidepressant activity by thyroid hormone. Am J Psychiatry 126:457–469, 1969

Prange AJ Jr, Wilson IC, Lara PP, et al: Effects of thyrotropin-releasing hormone in depression. Lancet 2(7785):999–1002, 1972

Price RA, Kidd KK, Weissman MM: Early onset (under age 30 years) and panic disorder as markers for etiologic homogeneity in major depression. Arch Gen Psychiatry 44:434–440, 1987

Purselle DC, Nemeroff CB: Serotonin transporter: a potential substrate in the biology of suicide. Neuropsychopharmacology 28:613–619, 2003

Raadsheer FC, Hoogendijk WJG, Stam FC, et al: Increased number of corticotropin-releasing hormone neurons in the hypothalamic paraventricular nuclei of depressed patients. Neuroendocrinology 60:436–444, 1994

Raadsheer FC, Van Heerikhuize JJ, Lucassen PJ, et al: Increased corticotropin-releasing hormone (CRH) mRNA in paraventricular nucleus of patients with Alzheimer's disease or depression. Am J Psychiatry 152:1372–1376, 1995

Raison CL, Borisov AS, Broadwell SD, et al: Depression during pegylated interferon-alpha plus ribavirin therapy: prevalence and prediction. J Clin Psychiatry 66:41–48, 2005

Raison CL, Capuron L, Miller AH: Cytokines sing the blues: inflammation and the pathogenesis of depression. Trends Immunol 27:24–31, 2006

Ranjit N, Diez-Roux AV, Shea S, et al: Psychosocial factors and inflammation in the multi-ethnic study of atherosclerosis. Arch Intern Med 167:174–181, 2007

Rao VR, Finkbeiner S: NMDA and AMPA receptors: old channels, new tricks. Trends Neurosci 30:284–291, 2007

Rattiner LM, Davis M, French CT, et al: Brain-derived neurotrophic factor and tyrosine kinase receptor B involvement in amygdala-dependent fear conditioning. J Neurosci 24:4796–4806, 2004

Rattiner L, Davis M, Ressler KJ: BDNF and amygdala-dependent learning. Neuroscientist 11:323–333, 2005

Reame N, Sauder SE, Kelch RP, et al: Pulsatile gonadotropin secretion during the human menstrual cycle: evidence for altered pulse frequency of gonadotropin releasing hormone secretion. J Clin Endocrinol Metab 59:328–337, 1984

Reddy PL, Khanna S, Subhash MN, et al: CSF amine metabolites in depression. Biol Psychiatry 31:112–118, 1992

Ressler KJ, Nemeroff CB: Role of norepinephrine in the pathophysiology of neuropsychiatric disorders. CNS Spectr 6:663–666, 670, 2001

Ressler KJ, Rothbaum BO, Tannenbaum L, et al: Cognitive enhancers as adjuncts to psychotherapy: use of D-cycloserine in phobic individuals to facilitate extinction of fear. Arch Gen Psychiatry 61:1136–1144, 2004

Ribeiro L, Busnello JV, Cantor RM, et al: The brain-derived neurotrophic factor rs6265 (Val66Met) polymorphism and depression in Mexican-Americans. Neuroreport 18:1291–1293, 2007

Ribeiro SC, Tandon R, Grunhaus L, et al: The DST as a predictor of outcome in depression: a meta-analysis. Am J Psychiatry 150:1618–1629, 1993

Richardson UI, Schonbrunn A: Inhibition of adrenocorticotropin secretion somatostatin in pituitary cells in culture. Endocrinology 108:281–284, 1981

Rijsdijk FV, Snieder H, Ormel J, et al: Genetic and environmental influences on psychological distress in the population: General Health Questionnaire analyses in UK twins. Psychol Med 33:793–801, 2003

Ring HA, Bench CJ, Trimble MR, et al: Depression in Parkinson's disease. A positron emission study. Br J Psychiatry 165:333–339, 1994

Risch NJ: Searching for genetic determinants in the new millennium. Nature 405:847–856, 2000

Risch SC, Ehlers C, Janowsky DS, et al: Human growth hormone releasing factor infusion effects on plasma growth hormone in affective disorder patients and normal controls. Peptides 9 (suppl 1):45–48, 1988

Risch SC, Nemeroff CB: Neurochemical alterations of serotonergic neuronal systems in depression. J Clin Psychiatry 53 (suppl):3–7, 1992

Roberson-Nay R, McClure EB, Monk CS, et al: Increased amygdala activity during successful memory encoding in adolescent major depressive disorder: an FMRI study. Biol Psychiatry 60:966–973, 2006

Roceri M, Hendriks W, Racagni G, et al: Early maternal deprivation reduces the expression of BDNF and NMDA receptor subunits in rat hippocampus. Mol Psychiatry 7:609–616, 2002

Rosso IM, Cintron CM, Steingard RJ, et al: Amygdala and hippocampus volumes in pediatric major depression. Biol Psychiatry 57:21–26, 2005

Rothschild AJ, Langlais PJ, Schatzberg AF, et al: Dexamethasone increases plasma free dopamine in man. J Psychiatr Res 18:217–223, 1984

Rothschild AJ, Langlais PJ, Schatzberg AF, et al: The effects of a single dose of dexamethasone on monoamine and metabolite levels in rat brain. Life Sci 36:2491–2501, 1985

Roy A, Pickar D, Douillet P, et al: Urinary monoamines and monoamine metabolites in subtypes of unipolar depressive disorder and normal controls. Psychol Med 16:541–546, 1986

Roy A, Guthrie S, Pickar D, et al: Plasma NE responses to cold challenge in depressed patients and normal controls. Psychiatry Res 21:161–168, 1987

Roy A, Pickar D, De Jong J, et al: Norepinephrine and its metabolites in cerebrospinal fluid, plasma and urine: relationship to

hypothalamic-pituitary-adrenal axis function in depression. Arch Gen Psychiatry 45:849–857, 1988

Roy A, De Jong J, Linnoila M: Cerebrospinal fluid monoamine metabolites and suicidal behavior in depressed patients. Arch Gen Psychiatry 46:609–612, 1989

Roy A, Karoum F, Pollack S: Marked reduction in indexes of dopamine metabolism among patients with depression who attempt suicide. Arch Gen Psychiatry 49:447–450, 1992

Roy A, Wolkowitz OM, Bissette G, et al: Differences in CSF concentrations of thyrotropin-releasing hormone in depressed patients and normal subjects: negative findings. Am J Psychiatry 151:600–602, 1994

Rubin RT, Phillips JJ, Sadow TF, et al: Adrenal gland volume in major depression: increase during the depressive episode and decrease with successful treatment. Arch Gen Psychiatry 52:213–218, 1995

Rubinow DR: Cerebrospinal fluid somatostatin and psychiatric illness. Biol Psychiatry 21:341–365, 1986

Rubinow DR, Gold PW, Post RM, et al: CSF somatostatin in affective illness. Arch Gen Psychiatry 40:409–412, 1983

Rusch BD, Abercrombie HC, Oakes TR, et al: Hippocampal morphometry in depressed patients and control subjects: relations to anxiety symptoms. Biol Psychiatry 50:960–964, 2001

Sabatti C, Service S, Freimer N: False discovery rate in linkage and association genome screens for complex disorders. Genetics 164:829–833, 2003

Sachar E, Hellman L, Fukushima D, et al: Cortisol production in depressive illness. Arch Gen Psychiatry 23:289–298, 1970

Sachar EJ, Schalch DS, Reichlin S, et al: Plasma gonadotrophins in depressive illness: a preliminary report, in Recent Advances in the Psychobiology of the Depressive Illnesses. Edited by Williams TA, Katz MM, Shield JA Jr. Washington, DC, U.S. Department of Health and Welfare, 1972, pp 229–233

Sack DA, James SP, Rosenthal NE, et al: Deficient nocturnal surge of TSH secretion during sleep and sleep deprivation in rapid-cycling bipolar illness. Psychiatry Res 23:179–191, 1988

Samson JA, Gudeman JE, Schatzberg AF, et al: Toward a biochemical classification of depressive disorders, VIII: platelet monoamine oxidase activity in subtypes of depressions. J Psychiatr Res 19:547–555, 1985

Sanacora G, Saricicek A: GABAergic contributions to the pathophysiology of depression and the mechanism of antidepressant action. CNS Neurol Disord Drug Targets 6:127–140, 2007

Sanacora G, Kendell SF, Levin Y, et al: Preliminary evidence of riluzole efficacy in antidepressant-treated patients with residual depressive symptoms. Biol Psychiatry 61:822–825, 2007

Sapolsky RM, Uno H, Rebert CS, et al: Hippocampal damage associated with prolonged stress exposure in primates. J Neurosci 9:2897–2902, 1990

Sapru MK, Rao BSSR, Channabasavana SM: Serum dopamine-beta-hydroxylase activity in classical subtypes of depression. Acta Psychiatr Scand 80:474–478, 1989

Sassi RB, Nicoletti M, Brambilla P, et al: Decreased pituitary volume in patients with bipolar disorder. Biol Psychiatry 50:271–280, 2001

Schaefer HS, Putnam KM, Benca RM, et al: Event-related functional magnetic resonance imaging measures of neural activity to positive social stimuli in pre- and post-treatment depression. Biol Psychiatry 60:974–986, 2006

Schatzberg AF, Rothschild AJ, Stahl JB, et al: The dexamethasone suppression test: identification of subtypes of depression. Am J Psychiatry 140:88–91, 1983

Schatzberg AF, Rothschild AJ, Bond TC, et al: The DST in psychotic depression: diagnostic and pathophysiologic implications. Psychopharmacol Bull 20:362–364, 1984

Schatzberg AF, Rothschild AJ, Gerson B, et al: Toward a biochemical classification of depressive disorders, IX: DST results and platelet MAO activity. Br J Psychiatry 146:633–637, 1985a

Schatzberg AF, Rothschild AJ, Langlais PJ, et al: A corticosteroid/dopamine hypothesis for psychotic depression and related states. J Psychiatr Res 19:57–64, 1985b

Schatzberg AF, Rothschild AJ, Langlais PJ, et al: Psychotic and nonpsychotic depressions, II: platelet MAO activity, plasma catecholamines, cortisol, and specific symptoms. Psychiatry Res 20:155–164, 1987

Schildkraut JJ: The catecholamine hypothesis of affective disorders: a review of supporting evidence. Am J Psychiatry 122:509–522, 1965

Schilkrut R, Chandra O, Osswald M, et al: Growth hormone during sleep and with thermal stimulation in depressed patients. Neuropsychobiology 1:70–79, 1975

Schmidt HD, Duman RS: The role of neurotrophic factors in adult hippocampal neurogenesis, antidepressant treatments and animal models of depressive-like behavior. Behav Pharmacol 18:391–418, 2007

Schousboe A, Waagepetersen HS: GABA: homeostatic and pharmacological aspects. Prog Brain Res 160:9–19, 2007

Schule C, Zill P, Baghai TC, et al: Brain-derived neurotrophic factor Val66Met polymorphism and dexamethasone/CRH test results in depressed patients. Psychoneuroendocrinology 31:1019–1025, 2006

Schumacher J, Jamra RA, Becker T, et al: Evidence for a relationship between genetic variants at the brain-derived neurotrophic factor (BDNF) locus and major depression. Biol Psychiatry 58:307–314, 2005

Schwartz PJ, Loe JA, Bash CN, et al: Seasonality and pituitary volume. Psychiatry Res 74:151–157, 1997

Seminowicz DA, Mayberg HS, McIntosh AR, et al: Limbic-frontal circuitry in major depression: a path modeling metanalysis. Neuroimage 22:409–418, 2004

Serretti A, Kato M, De Ronchi D, et al: Meta-analysis of serotonin transporter gene promoter polymorphism (5-HTTLPR) association with selective serotonin reuptake inhibitor efficacy in depressed patients. Mol Psychiatry 12:247–257, 2007

Sheline YI: Hippocampal atrophy in major depression: a result of depression-induced neurotoxicity? Mol Psychiatry 1:298–299, 1996

Sheline YI, Wang PW, Gado MH, et al: Hippocampal atrophy in recurrent major depression. Proc Natl Acad Sci U S A 93:3908–3913, 1996

Sheline Y, Bardgett ME, Csernansky JG: Correlated reductions in cerebrospinal fluid 5-HIAA and MHPG concentrations after treatment with selective serotonin reuptake inhibitors. J Clin Psychopharmacol 17:11–14, 1997

Sheline YI, Sanghavi M, Mintun MA, et al: Depression duration but not age predicts hippocampal volume loss in medically healthy women with recurrent major depression. J Neurosci 19:5034–5043, 1999

Sheline YI, Barch DM, Donnelly JM, et al: Increased amygdala response to masked emotional faces in depressed subjects re-

solves with antidepressant treatment: an fMRI study. Biol Psychiatry 50:651–658, 2001

Shimizu E, Hashimoto K, Okamura N, et al: Alterations of serum levels of brain-derived neurotrophic factor (BDNF) in depressed patients with or without antidepressants. Biol Psychiatry 54:70–75, 2003

Shopsin B, Gershon S, Goldstein M, et al: Use of synthesis inhibitors in defining a role for biogenic amines during imipramine treatment in depressed patients. Psychopharmacology Communications 1:239–249, 1975

Shopsin B, Friedman E, Gershon S: Parachlorophenylalanine reversal of tranylcypromine effects in depressed outpatients. Arch Gen Psychiatry 33:811–819, 1976

Siegle GJ, Steinhauer SR, Thase ME, et al: Can't shake that feeling: event-related fMRI assessment of sustained amygdala activity in response to emotional information in depressed individuals. Biol Psychiatry 51:693–707, 2002

Siegle GJ, Thompson W, Carter CS, et al: Increased amygdala and decreased dorsolateral prefrontal BOLD responses in unipolar depression: related and independent features. Biol Psychiatry 61:198–209, 2007

Siever LJ, Uhde TW, Silberman EK, et al: Growth hormone response to clonidine as a probe of noradrenergic receptor responsiveness in affective disorder patients and controls. Psychiatry Res 6:171–183, 1982

Siever LJ, Trestman RL, Coccaro EF, et al: The growth hormone response to clonidine in acute and remitted depressed male patients. Neuropsychopharmacology 6:165–177, 1992

Sitaram N, Gillin JC, Bunney WE Jr: Cholinergic and catecholaminergic receptor sensitivity in affective illness: strategy and theory, in Neurobiology of Mood Disorders. Edited by Post RM, Ballenger JC. Baltimore, MD, Williams & Wilkins, 1984, pp 519–528

Sjoberg RL, Nilsson KW, Nordquist N, et al: Development of depression: sex and the interaction between environment and a promoter polymorphism of the serotonin transporter gene. Int J Neuropsychopharmacol 9:443–449, 2006

Sklar P, Gabriel SB, McInnis MG, et al: Family based association study of 76 candidate genes in bipolar disorder: BDNF is a potential risk locus. Brain-derived neurotrophic factor. Mol Psychiatry 7:579–593, 2002

Sluzewska A, Sobieska M, Rybakowski JK: Changes in acute-phase proteins during lithium potentiation of antidepressants in refractory depression. Neuropsychobiology 35:123–127, 1997

Smith GD, Hart C, Blane D, et al: Adverse socioeconomic conditions in childhood and cause specific adult mortality: prospective observational study. BMJ 316:1631–1635, 1998

Smith KA, Fairburn CG, Cowen PJ: Relapse of depression after rapid depletion of tryptophan. Lancet 349:915–919, 1997

Smith MA, Makino S, Kim SY, et al: Stress increases brain-derived neurotrophic factor messenger ribonucleic acid in the hypothalamus and pituitary. Endocrinology 136:3743–3750, 1995a

Smith MA, Makino S, Kvetnansky R, et al: Stress and glucocorticoids affect the expression of brain-derived neurotrophic factor and neurotrophin-3 mRNAs in the hippocampus. J Neurosci 15:1768–1777, 1995b

Smoller JW, Finn CT: Family, twin, and adoption studies of bipolar disorder. Am J Med Genet C Semin Med Genet 123:48–58, 2003

Souetre E, Salvati E, Wehr TA, et al: Twenty-four hour profiles of body temperature and plasma TSH in bipolar patients during depression and during remission and in normal control subjects. Am J Psychiatry 145:1133–1137, 1988

Spiliotaki M, Salpeas V, Malitas P, et al: Altered glucocorticoid receptor signaling cascade in lymphocytes of bipolar disorder patients. Psychoneuroendocrinology 31:748–760, 2006

Stahl SM: Mechanism of action of serotonin selective reuptake inhibitors. Serotonin receptors and pathways mediate therapeutic effects and side effects. J Affect Disord 51:215–235, 1998

Stanley M, Virgilio J, Gershon S: Tritiated imipramine binding sites are decreased in the frontal cortex of suicides. Science 216:1337–1339, 1982

Starkman MN, Gebarski SS, Berent S, et al: Hippocampal formation volume, memory dysfunction, and cortisol levels of inpatients with Cushing's syndrome. Biol Psychiatry 32:756–765, 1992

Steele JD, Currie J, Lawrie SM, et al: Prefrontal cortical functional abnormality in major depressive disorder: a stereotactic meta-analysis. J Affect Disord 101:1–11, 2007

Stein MB, Koverola C, Hanna C, et al: Hippocampal volume in women victimized by childhood sexual abuse. Psychol Med 27:951–959, 1997

Strakowski SM, Wilson DR, Tohen M, et al: Structural brain abnormalities in first episode mania. Biol Psychiatry 33:602–609, 1993

Strauss J, Barr CL, George CJ, et al: Association study of brain-derived neurotrophic factor in adults with a history of childhood onset mood disorder. Am J Med Genet B Neuropsychiatr Genet 131:16–19, 2004

Strauss J, Barr CL, George CJ, et al: Brain-derived neurotrophic factor variants are associated with childhood-onset mood disorder: confirmation in a Hungarian sample. Mol Psychiatry 10:861–867, 2005

Sullivan GM, Hatterer JA, Herbert J, et al: Low levels of transthyretin in the CSF of depressed patients. Am J Psychiatry 156:710–715, 1999

Sullivan PF, Neale MC, Kendler KS: Genetic epidemiology of major depression: review and meta-analysis. Am J Psychiatry 157:1552–1562, 2000

Surguladze S, Brammer MJ, Keedwell P, et al: A differential pattern of neural response toward sad versus happy facial expressions in major depressive disorder. Biol Psychiatry 57:201–209, 2005

Swann AC, Stokes PE, Casper R, et al: Hypothalamic-pituitary-adrenocortical function in mixed and pure mania. Acta Psychiatr Scand 85:270–274, 1992

Swanson LW, Kuypers HG: The paraventricular nucleus of the hypothalamus: cytoarchitectonic subdivisions and organization of projections to the pituitary, dorsal vagal complex, and spinal cord as demonstrated by retrograde fluorescence double-labeling methods. J Comp Neurol 194:555–570, 1980

Swanson LW, Sawchenko PE, Rivier J, et al: Organization of ovine corticotropin-releasing factor immunoreactive cells and fibers in the rat brain: an immunohistochemical study. Neuroendocrinology 36:165–186, 1983

Sweeney D, Nelson C, Bowers M, et al: Delusional versus nondelusional depression: neurochemical differences. Lancet 2(8080):100–101, 1978

Thakore JH, Dinan TG: Subnormal growth hormone responses to acutely administered dexamethasone in depression. Clin Endocrinol (Oxf) 40:623–627, 1994

Thomas KM, Drevets WC, Dahl RE, et al: Amygdala response to fearful faces in anxious and depressed children. Arch Gen Psychiatry 58:1057–1063, 2001

Toivola PTK, Gale CC, Goodner CJ, et al: Central alpha-adrenergic regulation of growth hormone and insulin. Hormones 3:192–213, 1972

Torgersen S: Genetic factors in moderately severe and mild affective disorders. Arch Gen Psychiatry 43:222–226, 1986

Träskman L, Åsberg M, Bertilsson L, et al: Monoamine metabolites in CSF and suicidal behavior. Arch Gen Psychiatry 10:253–261, 1981

Tsankova NM, Berton O, Renthal W, et al: Sustained hippocampal chromatin regulation in a mouse model of depression and antidepressant action. Nat Neurosci 9:519–525, 2006

Tunnicliff G, Malatynska E: Central GABAergic systems and depressive illness. Neurochem Res 28:965–976, 2003

Ueyama T, Kawai Y, Nemoto K, et al: Immobilization stress reduced the expression of neurotrophins and their receptors in the rat brain. Neurosci Res 28:103–110, 1997

Ulrich D, Bettler B: GABAB receptors: synaptic functions and mechanisms of diversity. Curr Opin Neurobiol 17:298–303, 2007

Unden F, Ljunggren JG, Beck-Friis J, et al: Hypothalamic-pituitary-gonadal axis pulse detection. Am J Physiol 250:E486–E493, 1988

Uno H, Tarara R, Else JG, et al: Hippocampal damage associated with prolonged and fatal stress in primates. J Neurosci 9:1705–1711, 1989

Uno H, Eisele S, Sakai A, et al J: Neurotoxicity of glucocorticoids in the primate brain. Horm Behav 28:336–348, 1994

Vakili K, Pillay SS, Lafer B, et al: Hippocampal volume in primary unipolar major depression: a magnetic resonance imaging study. Biol Psychiatry 47:1087–1090, 2000

Vale W, Spiess J, Rivier C, et al: Characterization of a 41 residue ovine hypothalamic peptide that stimulates secretion of corticotropin of b-endorphin. Science 213:1394–1397, 1981

Van Praag HM: Depression, suicide, and the metabolites of serotonin in the brain. J Affect Disord 4:21–29, 1982

Veith RC, Lewis L, Linares OA, et al: Sympathetic nervous system activity in major depression: basal and desipramine-induced alterations in plasma NE kinetics. Arch Gen Psychiatry 51:411–422, 1994

Vergne DE, Nemeroff CB: The interaction of serotonin transporter gene polymorphisms and early adverse life events on vulnerability for major depression. Curr Psychiatry Rep 8:452–457, 2006

Vermetten E, Schmahl C, Lindner S, et al: Hippocampal and amygdalar volumes in dissociative identity disorder. Am J Psychiatry 163:630–636, 2006

Virkkunen M, Rawlings R, Tokola R, et al: CSF biochemistries, glucose metabolism, and diurnal activity rhythms in alcoholic, violent offenders, fire setters, and healthy volunteers. Arch Gen Psychiatry 51:20–27, 1994

Vogt BA, Pandya DN: Cingulate cortex of the rhesus monkey, II: cortical afferents. J Comp Neurol 262:271–289, 1987

Vonk R, van der Schot AC, Kahn RS, et al: Is autoimmune thyroiditis part of the genetic vulnerability (or an endophenotype) for bipolar disorder? Biol Psychiatry 62:135–140, 2007

Vythilingam M, Heim C, Newport J, et al: Childhood trauma associated with smaller hippocampal volume in women with major depression. Am J Psychiatry 159:2072–2080, 2002

Vythilingam M, Luckenbaugh DA, Lam T, et al: Smaller head of the hippocampus in Gulf War-related posttraumatic stress disorder. Psychiatry Res 139:89–99, 2005

Walder DJ, Walker EF, Lewine RJ: Cognitive functioning, cortisol release, and symptom severity in patients with schizophrenia. Biol Psychiatry 48:1121–1132, 2000

Wang L, LaBar KS, McCarthy G: Mood alters amygdala activation to sad distractors during an attentional task. Biol Psychiatry 60:1139–1146, 2006

Wasserman D, Sokolowski M, Rozanov V, et al: The CRHR1 gene: a marker for suicidality in depressed males exposed to low stress. Genes Brain Behav 7:14–19, 2008

Watson S, Gallagher P, Ritchie JC, et al: Hypothalamic-pituitary-adrenal axis function in patients with bipolar disorder. Br J Psychiatry 184:496–502, 2004

Watson S, Thompson JM, Malik N, et al: Temporal stability of the dex/CRH test in patients with rapid-cycling bipolar I disorder: a pilot study. Aust N Z J Psychiatry 39:244–248, 2005

Weinberger DR, Berman KF, Zec RF: Physiologic dysfunction of dorsolateral prefrontal cortex in schizophrenia, I: regional cerebral blood flow evidence. Arch Gen Psychiatry 43:114–124, 1986

Weissman MM, Gershon ES, Kidd KK, et al: Psychiatric disorders in the relatives of probands with affective disorders: the Yale University–National Institute of Mental Health Collaborative Study. Arch Gen Psychiatry 41:13–21, 1984

Weissman MM, Merikangas KR, Boyd JH: Epidemiology of affective disorders, in Psychiatry, Vol I. Edited by Michels R, Cavenar JO, Brodie HKH, et al. Philadelphia, PA, JB Lippincott, 1992, pp 1–14

Wellcome Trust Case Control Consortium: Genome-wide association study of 14,000 cases of seven common diseases and 3,000 shared controls. Nature 447:661–678, 2007

Wellen KE, Hotamisligil GS: Inflammation, stress, and diabetes. J Clin Invest 115:1111–1119, 2005

Wender PH, Kety SS, Rosenthal D, et al: Psychiatric disorders in the biological and adoptive families of adopted individuals with affective disorders. Arch Gen Psychiatry 43:923–929, 1986

Whalley LJ, Kutcher S, Blackwood DHR, et al: Increased plasma LH in manic-depressive illness: evidence of a state-independent abnormality. Br J Psychiatry 150:682–684, 1987

White HS, Smith MD, Wilcox KS: Mechanisms of action of antiepileptic drugs. Int Rev Neurobiol 81:85–110, 2007

WHO World Mental Health Survey Consortium: Prevalence, severity, and unmet need for treatment of for treatment of mental disorders in the World Health Organization World Mental Health Surveys. JAMA 291:2581–2590, 2004

Wilhelm K, Mitchell PB, Niven H, et al: Life events, first depression onset and the serotonin transporter gene. Br J Psychiatry 188:210–215, 2006

Willerson JT, Ridker PM: Inflammation as a cardiovascular risk factor. Circulation 109:II2–II10, 2004

Willour VL, Chen H, Toolan J, et al: Family-based association of FKBP5 in bipolar disorder. Mol Psychiatry 2008 Jan 8 [Epub ahead of print]

Winokur A, Amsterdam J, Caroff S, et al: Variability of hormonal responses to a series of neuroendocrine challenges in depressed patients. Am J Psychiatry 139:39–44, 1982

Wolkowitz OM, Sutton ME, Doran AR, et al: Dexamethasone increases plasma HVA but not MHPG in normal humans. Psychiatry Res 16:101–109, 1985

Wolkowitz O, Sutton M, Koulu M, et al: Chronic corticosterone administration in rats: behavioral and biochemical evidence of increased central dopaminergic activity. Eur J Pharmacol 122:329–338, 1986

Wolkowitz OM, Rubinow DR, Breier A, et al: Prednisone decreases CSF somatostatin in healthy humans: implications for neuropsychiatric illness. Life Sci 41:1929–1933, 1987

Wyatt RJ, Portnoy B, Kupfer DJ, et al: Resting plasma catecholamine concentrations in patients with depression and anxiety. Arch Gen Psychiatry 24:65–70, 1971

Young AH: Antiglucocorticoid treatments for depression. Aust N Z J Psychiatry 40:402–405, 2006

Young AH, Gallagher P, Watson S, et al: Improvements in neurocognitive function and mood following adjunctive treatment with mifepristone (RU-486) in bipolar disorder. Neuropsychopharmacology 29:1538–1545, 2004

Young EA: Glucocorticoid cascade hypothesis revisited: role of gonadal steroids. Depression 3:20–27, 1995

Young EA, Midgley AR, Carlson NE, et al: Alteration in the hypothalamic-pituitary-ovarian axis in depressed women. Arch Gen Psychiatry 57:1157–1162, 2000

Young EA, Carlson NE, Brown MB: Twenty-four-hour ACTH and cortisol pulsatility in depressed women. Neuropsychopharmacology 25:267–276, 2001

Zarate CA Jr, Payne JL, Quiroz J, et al: An open-label trial of riluzole in patients with treatment-resistant major depression. Am J Psychiatry 161:171–174, 2004a

Zarate CA Jr, Payne JL, Singh J, et al: Pramipexole for bipolar II depression: a placebo-controlled proof of concept study. Biol Psychiatry 56:54–60, 2004b

Zarate CA Jr, Quiroz JA, Singh JB, et al: An open-label trial of the glutamate-modulating agent riluzole in combination with lithium for the treatment of bipolar depression. Biol Psychiatry 57:430–432, 2005

CHAPTER 46

Neurobiology of Schizophrenia

Raquel E. Gur, M.D., Ph.D.

Steven E. Arnold, M.D.

Schizophrenia is a complex disorder defined by positive symptoms (hallucinations, delusions, thought disorder), negative symptoms (apathy, alogia, anhedonia, blunted affect), and deterioration of the patient's personal, social, and occupational functioning. Recent advances in elucidating the neurobiology of schizophrenia have capitalized on progress in clinical and basic neuroscience that has contributed to the integration of neurobiology with the clinical features of the disorder.

In this chapter, we highlight selected areas emphasizing recent progress and short-term future goals. Noteworthy advances link clinical and basic neuroscience research, address mechanisms underlying this challenging disorder, and have implications for treatment. Such progress includes strong evidence of selective cognitive deficits against a background of global impairment, aberrations in electrophysiological activity in response to sensory input, and abnormalities in brain anatomy and physiology through the application of structural and functional neuroimaging methods; a shift from examining the genetics of diagnostic categories to a focus on endophenotypic markers with parallel paradigms in humans and animals; identification of specific candidate genes from genome-wide scans and microarray technologies; evidence of cellular and molecular abnormalities in diverse brain regions; and a growing appreciation of schizophrenia as a life span neurodevelopmental disorder. Considered jointly, these advances establish a firm foundation for hypothesis-driven research that systematically examines core neurobiological abnormalities underlying schizophrenia.

When evaluating the body of data on the neurobiology of schizophrenia, two important questions deserve further consideration.

First, are the findings specific to schizophrenia? That is, are the brain abnormalities observed on multiple levels of analysis unique to schizophrenia, or do they characterize psychosis? Although the literature across the methods we summarize is limited regarding direct prospective comparisons between patients with schizophrenia and patients with bipolar disorder, overall it appears that patients with schizophrenia are distinct from those with bipolar disorder. Thus, despite commonality in some underlying affected brain systems, the extent and topography of aberrations observed differentiate schizophrenia from bipolar disorder.

Second, do the abnormalities observed relate to clinical subtypes as defined by DSM-IV-TR (American Psychiatric Association 2000) or to symptom dimensions such as positive and negative symptoms of schizophrenia? The literature, in general, suggests "a signature" across subtypes of schizophrenia and symptom dimensions, with some variability related to illness duration and severity. We are now at the cusp of advancing the understanding of brain circuitry that examines neurocognitive and affective processes that relate to social cognition in schizophrenia. As progress is made, it can guide novel therapeutics that target these deficits more directly.

Neurobehavioral Deficits

Impaired cognition in schizophrenia, leading to early conceptualizations of "dementia praecox" (Kraepelin 1919), is well recognized and fundamental to the disorder. While the clinical symptoms and course of the disorder are heterogeneous, most patients with schizophrenia exhibit cognitive deficits that are present at the onset of illness and persist following improvement in their psychosis. Neuropsychological studies have found impairments in multiple domains, including perception, attention, visuospatial abilities, language, memory, emotion, executive function, and coordination (Sharma and Harvey 1999). However, within this diffuse impairment, attention, working and episodic memory, and executive functioning are more severely impaired (Cornblatt and Keilp 1994; Heinrichs and Zakzanis 1998; Saykin et al. 1994). While neurocognitive measures have shown limited, albeit consistent, relation to clinical symptoms, they appear more closely related to functional outcome (Goldberg and Gold 1995; Green 1996; Green et al. 2000).

In addition to the relevance of neuropsychological measures to functioning and outcome, they have stimulated the investigation of their underlying neurobiology. Several brain systems are implicated by these deficits. The attention-processing circuitry includes brain stem–thalamo-striato-accumbens-temporal-hippocampal-prefrontal-parietal regions. Deficits in working memory implicate the dorsolateral prefrontal cortex, and the ventromedial temporal lobe is implicated in deficits in episodic memory. A dorsolateral-medial-orbital prefrontal cortical circuit mediates executive functions.

Relative to the extensive and well-documented cognitive deficits in schizophrenia, more recently, emotion-processing and olfaction deficits have also been noted. Clinically, emotional impairment is manifested in flat, blunted, inappropriate affect and in depression (Gur et al. 2006; Kohler et al. 2000b). Although these clinical features have been detailed as part of the disorder, the methodologies for neuroscience research have lagged behind research on cognition. Studies have reported emotion-processing deficits in identification, discrimination, and recognition of facial expressions (Kring and Neale 1996). Although these deficits may represent generalized cognitive impairment (Kerr and Neale 1993), they relate specifically to symptoms and neurobiological measures (Kohler et al. 2000a). Animal and human investigations have implicated the limbic system, primarily the amygdala, hypothalamus, and mesocorticolimbic dopaminergic systems, and cortical regions including orbitofrontal, dorsolateral prefrontal, temporal, and parts of the parietal cortex (LeDoux 2000).

Psychophysical studies of schizophrenia have described impairments in elementary sensory perceptual processing. Patients are impaired in their ability to detect and identify odors (Moberg et al. 1999). Olfactory deficits are present at the onset of illness, do not relate to disease severity or treatment, and are possibly progressive (Kopala et al. 1993). It is unclear whether the deficits are part of the generalized neurocognitive impairment (Moberg et al. 2006). The neuroanatomical differences noted in patients (Turetsky et al. 2000) suggest that olfactory bulb changes and medial temporal lobe abnormalities could mediate the observed behavioral aberrations. In the visual domain, abnormalities in elementary contrast sensitivity and functional dyslexia have been described (Butler and Javitt 2005; Kurylo et al. 2007; Revheim et al. 2006), and electrophysiological studies have suggested dysfunction of the thalamic lateral geniculate's magnocellular processing stream as playing a role in these deficits. In the auditory domain, deficits in tone discrimination and matching have been reported (Javitt et al. 2000), consistent with many electrophysiological studies and recent postmortem evidence of primary auditory cortex abnormality in schizophrenia (Sweet et al. 2007).

The application of neurobehavioral probes (Gur et al. 1992) in functional imaging studies has helped elucidate links between neurobehavioral deficits and the underlying brain dysfunction evident in schizophrenia. With these paradigms, we can examine the topography of brain activity in response to engagement in tasks in which deficits have been noted in patients. This provides "on-line" correlation between brain activity and performance in a way that permits direct examination of brain–behavior relations.

Electrophysiology

Event-related potentials (ERPs), coupled with specific stimulus events and cognitive tasks, enable monitoring of associated brain activity in real time. There is an extensive literature on ERP abnormalities in schizophrenia (Adler et al. 1982; Erwin et al. 1991; Grillon et al. 1991) including deficits in early preattentive stages of information processing and relatively late higher cortical processes. Aberrations in encoding of input may involve difficulty in screening out information and inhibiting responses to irrelevant stimuli. There may be reciprocal deficits in response facilitation to salient stimuli.

Various ERP indices have been examined in schizophrenia—including the P50 (Erwin et al. 1991; Freedman et al. 1991) and startle prepulse inhibition (PPI; Braff et al. 1992)—that suggest failure of inhibitory processes. Later potentials related to detection of deviant or novel stimuli, including the N100, mismatch negativity (MMN), and P300, also show abnormalities in schizophrenia. The N100 is an obligate response sensitive to the physical characteristics of a stimulus but not to its context. By contrast, the MMN is elicited by deviant or novel sounds presented amid repeated trains of identical tones. It reflects sensory or echoic memory processes that facilitate response to unexpected environmental changes. Auditory MMN originates in the auditory cortex and is N-methyl-D-aspartate (NMDA) sensitive (Javitt et al. 1996). A semblance of the MMN has been described in the hippocampus and thalamus as well (Alho 1995). The most widely studied late ERP is the P300 (Patel and Azzam 2005; Polich 2004). The P300 reflects higher-order processing of a deviant or novel stimulus that surpasses a threshold to elicit orienting (P3a) or matches with a consciously maintained working memory trace (P3b). Analogs of these ERPs have been established in rodents, allowing experimentation not feasible in humans. Latencies are shorter in rodents, but the P20, N40, MMN, and P120 in mice share stimulus and pharmacological response properties with the human P50, N100, MMN, and P3a, respectively (Connolly et al. 2003; Siegel et al. 2003; Umbricht et al. 2004).

The established ERP methods highlighted above examine latencies and amplitudes of averaged evoked responses. Newer measures, which characterize electroencephalogram (EEG) activity in terms of underlying constituent oscillations, more directly represent the synchronized activity of aggregate neuronal assemblies. Evoked oscillations (time- and phase-locked to stimulus) and induced oscillations (loosely time-locked, not phase-locked) are thought to reflect different dynamic neurophysiological processes (Pfurtscheller and Lopes da Silva 1999). Scalp-recorded evoked oscillations reflect the summed postsynaptic potentials of local assemblies of cortical pyramidal neurons. Induced oscillations reflect changes in the dynamic interactions within and among brain structures. These interactions may be subcorticocortical or corticocortical and may underlie dynamic processes such as long-range integration, feature binding, or memory formation (Bastiaansen and Hagoort 2003). Gamma (40 Hz) and theta (4–7 Hz) frequency oscillations, in particular, appear to be intrinsically involved in the processes of stimulus perception, integration, novelty detection, and recognition. Induced gamma oscillations are proposed to "bind" the spatially and temporally discrete neuronal representations of features of a complex stimulus (Bertrand and Tallon-Baudry 2000; Pantev et al. 1991). The growing literature on the gamma band suggests reduced oscillatory power and decreased phase synchrony in schizophrenia, associated with disturbances in the cognitive processes of feature binding and perceptual integration in both the visual (Spencer et al. 2003) and auditory modalities (Lee et al. 2003). Theta oscillations are observed consistently in the hippocampus, where long-term potentiation depends on the phase of the theta rhythm (Sederberg et al. 2003). Induced theta oscillations are also increased diffusely in the cortex during working memory tasks (Raghavachari et al. 2001) and frontally during orienting to novel stimuli. The theta literature in schizophrenia is limited. Notably, the neural mechanisms—glutamatergic and γ-aminobutyric acid (GABA)–ergic—that regulate both synchronized gamma and theta rhythms are implicated in the pathophysiology of schizophrenia. Thus, disturbances in glutamatergic and GABAergic function could provide the neurophysiological basis for impairments in sensory evoked potentials, MMN, and synchronized rhythmic EEG oscillations in schizophrenia.

Neuroimaging

Advances in neuroimaging technologies have created opportunities to examine schizophrenia as a brain disorder, and investigators have applied diverse methods to study brain structure and function (Gur et al. 2007a). With progress in quantitative computational anatomy methodologies we are at the cusp of an exciting era in neuroscience research that can capitalize on the ability to study the living brain with refined approaches both for hypothesis testing and for exploration. In vivo measurement is afforded by magnetic resonance imaging (MRI) examining neuroanatomy through structural MRI (sMRI), connectivity through diffusion tensor imaging (DTI), and neurochemistry through magnetic resonance spectroscopy (MRS). MRI also enables examination of brain physiology using functional MRI (fMRI) methods that measure changes in signal intensity attributable to cerebral blood flow. Other functional neuroimaging methods include positron emission tomography (PET), which enables measurement of local cerebral glucose metabolism, blood flow, and receptor function. Single photon computed emission tomography (SPECT) can also be used to measure cerebral perfusion and receptor function.

Structural Imaging

An extensive literature of whole-brain volume and specific regions of interest documents consistent morphometric differences between patients with schizophrenia and healthy people. Structural neuroimaging studies with MRI have highlighted diffuse reductions in cortical gray matter volumes as well as diverse but selective regional abnormalities in schizophrenia (Gur et al. 2000a, 2000b; Konick and Friedman 2001; Nelson et al. 1998; Shenton et al. 2001; Wright et al. 2000). Most consistent have been reports of ventricular enlargement and reduced volumes of temporal lobe, superior temporal gyrus, and medial temporal lobe structures. Somewhat less consistent have been reports of abnormal volumes of prefrontal cortex, parietal lobe, thalamus, basal ganglia, cerebellar vermis, and olfactory bulbs, among others regions. Differences in reported results can be attributed to methodologies applied. For example, morphometric prefrontal studies differed in magnetic field, scanning parameters, slice thickness and contiguity, image processing, and regions examined. Consequently, findings seem inconsistent, with some noting no differences between patients and healthy participants and others observing volume reduction in gray matter, white matter, or both tissue compartments. Relatively fewer studies have related subregional volumes to clinical or neurocognitive measures. These studies support the hypothesis that increased volume is associated with better performance (Antonova et al. 2004).

Automated methods for regional parcellation and voxel-based morphometry can now efficiently yield information on the entire brain, permitting validation of reported findings and identification of new possible regions. Such studies corroborate the region of interest approach showing gray matter density reductions in medial temporal lobes and the superior temporal gyrus (Honea et al. 2005). There are also replicated associations between superior temporal gyrus volume and positive symptoms and between medial temporal lobe volume reduction and memory impairment (Gur et al. 2007a). Furthermore, based on morphological parameters, it is possible to apply high-dimensional nonlinear pattern classification techniques to quantify the degree of separation of patients with schizophrenia and healthy control subjects. Such procedures enable testing the potential of sMRI as an aid to diagnosis. In a study of patients with schizophrenia and healthy control subjects, such a procedure demonstrated average classification accuracy of 82% for women and 85% for men (Davatzikos et al. 2005). While such automated methods are promising, further investigation is needed in their potential integration into diagnostic procedures.

The abnormalities evident in brain anatomy should be considered in relation to several potential confounding factors including illness chronicity, treatment with antipsychotic medications, and comorbid diagnosis such as substance abuse. The study of first-episode schizophrenia provides an opportunity to examine if morphometric abnormalities are evident early in the course of illness. A recent review of sMRI studies in first-episode schizophrenia confirms only a reduction in the volumes of the whole brain and of the hippocampus (Vita et al. 2006). There is therefore a need for additional studies of recent-onset patients to determine if other abnormalities are evident at that time or if they are progressive (Ho et al. 2003).

Distinguishing the effects of illness duration from the effects of ongoing antipsychotic treatment is likely impossible. Most MRI studies that examined the specific regions of interest also evaluated possible relationships with antipsychotic medications. An association with treatment has been reported for the basal ganglia, where an increase of up to 20% in the volume of the globus pallidus has been related to first-generation (typical) antipsychotic medication dose (Wright et al. 2000). For second-generation (atypical) antipsychotics, there is an insufficient body of literature to document specific effects on neuroanatomy. In addition, because substance abuse is so common in schizophrenia, the possible effects of such substances merit consideration. Alcohol abuse has diffuse effects on the brain, with greater impact on the prefrontal cortex than on the temporal lobe, which is the area with the greatest volume reduction in schizophrenia. Moreover, the volume abnormalities are present in patients with no history of alcohol abuse. The potential effect of other substances, such as cannabis, on brain structure is unclear, and volume reduction is evident in patients without a history of cannabis abuse.

The study of people at risk for schizophrenia is an additional strategy to evaluate vulnerability markers for the disorder. Early MRI studies that applied the region of interest approach focused on the amygdala and hippocampus. These found volume reduction in first-degree relatives compared with control subjects, with the family members showing a degree of volume reduction intermediate to that shown in patients and control subjects. Literature reviews and meta-analysis concluded that reduced hippocampal volumes were likely to be a vulnerability marker for schizophrenia (Boos et al. 2006; Lawrie et al. 2004).

Diffusion Tensor Imaging

DTI examines white matter integrity and is a more recent addition to structural measures. The availability of DTI enhances the ability to evaluate compartmental brain tissue abnormalities. Although gray matter volume deficits are more marked than white matter abnormalities in schizophrenia, reduced anisotropy, a measure of directionality of flow of water molecules in axons, providing an index of white matter integrity, is observed with DTI in multiple brain regions. The application of this rapidly developing technology is relatively new, and different approaches are used for data acquisition and analysis. Thus, a consistent literature in schizophrenia has yet to emerge. Abnormalities have been reported in interhemispheric connectivity, as well as in intrahemispheric connectivity among frontal, temporal, and occipital lobes via association fibers (Foong et al. 2002; Kubicki et al. 2005). It is possible that white matter structures may be disorganized in schizophrenia rather than reduced in size (Kanaan et al. 2005). With the growing efforts to understand brain development in infancy and childhood through the application of MRI technology (Giedd et al. 1999; Matsuzawa et al. 2001), the neuroimaging literature in schizophrenia is consistent with diffuse disruption of normal maturation.

Magnetic Resonance Spectroscopy

MRS is a noninvasive method for investigating brain metabolites. Most of this research has focused on investigating phosphorus (^{31}P MRS) and proton-containing metabolites (^{1}H MRS). Proton MRS metabolites such as *N*-acetylaspartate (NAA), which may provide a measure of neuronal integrity, are reduced in schizophrenia, especially in the hippocampus and frontal cortex (Steen et al. 2005). NAA reductions have been associated with decreased cortical volume and correlate with clinical features of the disorder, including illness duration, negative symptoms, and cognitive deficits (Keshavan et al. 2000; Stanley et al. 2000). Notably, NAA reductions have been observed in first-degree relatives of patients with schizophrenia and in prodromal cases and therefore may represent an indicator of vulnerability to the illness (Jessen et al. 2006; Tibbo et al. 2004).

^{31}P MRS studies in neuroleptic-naive first-episode patients suggest increased membrane breakdown with reduced membrane generation throughout the course of illness (Jensen et al. 2004; Stanley et al. 1995). Such changes are commonly evident during cell generation, synaptogenesis, and degeneration and may reflect diverse processes affecting the brain of patients with schizophrenia. Notably, adolescents at genetic risk for schizophrenia manifest membrane alterations similar to those observed in patients early in the course of illness.

Neuroreceptor Imaging

PET and SPECT provide an important avenue for examining in vivo neurochemistry. The investigation of receptor function with PET followed progress with in vitro binding measurements and autoradiography. Early ligand studies in schizophrenia examined primarily dopamine receptors, especially dopamine$_2$ (D$_2$). Results were somewhat inconsistent, most likely because of differences in patient populations, ligands, and modeling methods used (Andreasen et al. 1988). As neuroleptic-naive patients participated in such studies, the samples were still relatively small, with fewer than 20 patients per study. However, several reviews concluded that increases in both D$_2$ receptor density and affinity are present in schizophrenia.

A consistent literature has emerged indicating increased presynaptic dopaminergic turnover in schizophrenia. Such studies measured striatal fluorodopa uptake as an index of increased dopa decarboxylase activity and greater presynaptic dopamine turnover in the striatum. Increased activity of dopamine neurons in the striatum appears to be associated with clinical status and is more evident during acute exacerbations and presence of positive symptoms (Erritzoe et al. 2003). Such effects are consistent with studies of neuropharmacological stimulants, such as amphetamine, and cannot be attributed to antipsychotic medication, as approximately half the studies were conducted in medication-free (including neuroleptic naive) patients.

Increased striatal dopamine, most evident in patients with active psychotic symptoms, has been related to the positive symptoms of schizophrenia. More recently, neuroreceptor studies have related dopamine function to cognitive processes in schizophrenia. Cortical dopamine transmission via dopamine$_1$ (D$_1$) receptors may play a role in impaired working memory and negative symptoms (Abi-Dargham 2004), whereas striatal dopamine activity via D$_2$ receptors may modulate response inhibition, temporal organization, and motor performance (Cropley et al. 2006).

Receptor imaging by PET and SPECT allows investigation of in vivo targets for antipsychotic drug action (Talbott and Laruelle 2002). It is now known that extrapyramidal (parkinsonian) side effects of first-generation antipsychotic drugs result from high striatal D$_2$ receptor blockade (~75%), whereas second-generation

antipsychotic drugs produce therapeutic benefit in relation to modest and transient striatal D_2 receptor occupancy levels (~65%). These neuroimaging observations point to a rationale for the use of relatively low doses of first-generation antipsychotics and equivalent doses of second-generation antipsychotics (Tauscher and Kapur 2001), although use of neuroimaging to determine dosage ranges in a given patient is far from practical. Neuroreceptor PET and SPECT studies are valuable research tools that can help examine compounds that may regulate or stabilize dopamine, as well as nondopaminergic pathways—such as serotonin, glutamate, and GABA—that may offer promising targets for drug development.

Functional Imaging

The early emphasis on "hypofrontality" in schizophrenia has been refined. The transition from isotopic methods, such as PET, to fMRI for measuring regional brain activation has offered several advantages, including higher spatial and temporal resolution, noninvasiveness, lack of ionizing radiation, direct correlation with anatomical imaging, greater repeatability, and economy. Consequently, numerous studies have applied neurocognitive paradigms in fMRI aimed at dissecting complex behavior. Most of these studies have been in healthy people, applying the blood oxygenation level–dependent (BOLD) method using blocked designs and, in recent years, event-related paradigms. Diverse neurobehavioral probes have been applied in activation paradigms designed to elucidate the underlying brain circuitry in schizophrenia. Tasks applied have evaluated executive function, such as attention, abstraction, and working memory, as well as declarative and procedural memory, language, spatial, sensorimotor, and emotion processing.

A potential strength of activation studies is the ability to relate the extent of activation to performance obtained "on line." However, relative underactivation in patients who have difficulties performing a task may reflect either a deficit in underlying processes related to that task or a lack of engagement (Davidson and Heinrichs 2003; K. Hill et al. 2004). PET and fMRI studies that attempted to correct for patient impairment by balancing performance of patients and healthy control subjects often failed to find hypofrontality, and some even found hyperfrontality (Honea et al. 2005).

In two recent reviews, 12 N-back (working memory) fMRI studies and 18 episodic memory studies with PET or fMRI found hypofrontality in dorsolateral and inferolateral prefrontal cortex, respectively (Achim and Lepage

2005; Glahn et al. 2005). Hyperfrontality was also reported in medial areas, including the (dorsal) anterior cingulate. Antipsychotic medication is likely to normalize performance on these tasks and hypofrontality (Davis et al. 2005). Regarding the temporal lobe, studies noted increased temporal lobe cortical activity in SPECT and PET studies (Zakzanis et al. 2000), as well as bilateral reductions in perfusion in the medial temporal lobes. Perhaps a hypothesis that will incorporate these findings will evaluate the interaction between laterality and frontality. The relations between frontal and temporal activity merit further investigation and have been related to the hypothesis of decreased connectivity in schizophrenia (Stephan et al. 2006). PET, SPECT, and fMRI studies of disconnectivity are also supported by electrophysiological findings of reduced coherence and gamma asynchrony in schizophrenia (Uhlhaas et al. 2006).

The application of neurobehavioral probes during functional imaging studies has contributed to the effort to investigate involvement of defined neural systems in the pathophysiology of schizophrenia (Gur et al. 1992). Such neurobehavioral probes document deficits in performance associated with abnormal brain activation and implicate the ventromedial temporal lobe, prefrontal cortices, and limbic subcortical nuclei mediating memory, executive functioning, and attention. These systems are characterized by dynamic plasticity, high connectivity, and vulnerability to insult (Arnold and Trojanowski 1996c; Harrison 1999), consistent with the hypothesis that abnormal plasticity is a core neurobiological feature of schizophrenia. Such fundamental mechanisms of abnormal structural, molecular, or physiological plasticity should be evident throughout the central nervous system (CNS) but may be most prominently expressed in neural systems mediating the highly activity-dependent cognitive processes of attention, memory, and executive functioning.

Genetics

Schizophrenia is a heritable complex brain disorder. Although the mode of inheritance is unknown, the disorder likely results from multiple genes of variable effect interacting with environmental factors. Linkage for schizophrenia has been reported in several regions: 1q32–q41 (Hovatta et al. 1999), 5q31 (Schwab et al. 1997), 6p24–p22 (Straub et al. 1996; Wang et al. 1995), 6q25.2 (Lindholm et al. 2001), 6q13–q26 (Cao et al. 1997), 8p21 (Blouin et al. 1998), 8p23.3 (Suarez et al. 2006), 10p15–p11 (Faraone et al. 1998, 1999), 13q32 (Blouin et al.

1998), 10q22 (Fallin et al. 2003), 10q25.3–q26.3 (Williams et al. 2003), and 22q12–q13 (Brzustowicz et al. 2000; Pulver et al. 1994a, 1994b). While some independent samples have detected linkage in the same or overlapping regions (6p24–p22, 6q13–q26, 10p15–p11, 13q32, 22q12–q13), many have failed to do so (Blouin et al. 1998; Cao et al. 1997; Moises et al. 1995; Schwab et al. 1995a, 1995b, 1998). Lack of overlap may reflect false-positive results or genetic heterogeneity. A meta-analysis of 20 published genomewide scans revealed evidence for linkage on chromosome 2q (C.M. Lewis et al. 2003). Eleven additional loci had suggestive linkage. Because power to detect linkage is limited for genes of intermediate or small effect size (Risch and Merikangas 1996), these variable findings are not surprising. It is noteworthy that several of the genes identified are directly linked to glutamatergic presynaptic or postsynaptic functioning, and others can be indirectly linked.

Association studies have used primarily functional, rather than positional, candidate gene markers (Shirts and Nimgaonkar 2004). Recent studies report some consistent associations, possibly due to evaluation of positional candidate genes, such as *dysbindin, neuregulin 1,* and *G72* (Harrison and Weinberger 2005; Owen et al. 2005). The risk conferred by associated alleles is modest (odds ratio [OR] ~ 1.2). The primary risk alleles have not been identified at these genes. Because schizophrenia is phenotypically heterogeneous (Gottesman and Gould 2003), it may be helpful to identify variables correlated with liability. A complementary approach to dissecting the genetic architecture of schizophrenia is to examine the neurobiological traits associated with genetic susceptibility. Here the phenotype is not a clinical diagnosis but a neurobiologically defined trait. Given the heterogeneity of schizophrenia at the phenotypic and likely genotypic levels, analyzing neurobiological phenotypes may improve power by constraining some heterogeneity. Whereas an unequivocal clinical diagnosis may be difficult to establish, quantitative neurobiological phenotypes can be reliably measured in family members. Therefore, chromosomal regions showing inconsistent linkage results, or subthreshold LOD scores with the clinical phenotype, may yield stronger linkage to a neurobiological phenotype. The challenge is selection of informative endophenotypic markers that will efficiently lead to a mechanistic model of schizophrenia. The neurocognitive measures tap neural systems that can be directly studied with structural and functional neuroimaging.

The potential of neurocognitive measures as markers of genetic liability is suggested by the presence of interme-diate deficits in unaffected family members of schizophrenia probands (Calkins et al. 2005; Egan et al. 2001a; Thompson et al. 2005). Supporting an additive model, simplex families (those with one individual is affected) have less impairment than multiplex families (those with two or more individuals affected) in language processing (Shedlack et al. 1997), intelligence, verbal learning and memory, visual reproduction (Faraone et al. 2000), visual working memory (Tuulio-Henriksson et al. 2003), verbal learning, delayed visual recall, and perceptual–motor and pure motor speed (Hoff et al. 2005). These results are consistent with several recent reports showing significant heritability of these features (Gur et al. 2007b). Such findings support the role of neurocognitive measures in molecular genetic studies in healthy people (Burdick et al. 2006; de Frias et al. 2005; Plomin and Kosslyn 2001; Posthuma et al. 2005) and in schizophrenia (Bilder et al. 2002; Burdick et al. 2006; Hallmayer et al. 2005; Hennah et al. 2005; Szekeres et al. 2004).

As an example, one candidate gene that has been extensively reported on in the schizophrenia endophenotype literature is the gene encoding catechol-O-methyltransferase (COMT). Consistent with the role of COMT in controlling prefrontal cortex phasic dopamine levels (D. A. Lewis et al. 2001; Sesack et al. 1998; Weinberger et al. 2001), subjects with the COMT Val/Val genotype performed worse on executive functions (Egan et al. 2001b) and working memory (Goldberg et al. 2003) compared with those with other genotypes. However, subsequent studies suggest a more complex relationship (Tunbridge et al. 2006). Only 1–2 polymorphisms are typically analyzed at each locus, and we need to investigate additional polymorphisms and study their neurobiological context. Furthermore, studies that evaluate a specific cognitive domain and differential deficit require understanding of a profile (Saykin et al. 1991).

By providing quantitative measures of brain structure and function, neuroimaging has become the main approach to the study of brain and behavior in health and disease, fueling the nascent field of imaging genomics (Callicott and Weinberger 2003). Twin studies with sMRI reported heritability estimates greater than 0.90 for whole-brain volume, with lower heritability for regional volumes (Wright et al. 2002). In schizophrenia, the potential of volumetric measures as endophenotypic markers is suggested by reduced brain volume in unaffected siblings compared with control subjects (Gogtay et al. 2003; Staal et al. 2000) and reduced parahippocampal volume in multiplex, relative to simplex, healthy family members (Seidman et al. 2002). Molecular genetic studies with sMRI have observed smaller hippocampal volumes in Val/Val compared with Met/Met genotypes of *COMT* (Szeszko et al. 2005); an association of disrupted-in-schizophrenia 1 (*DISC1*)/translin-associated factor X (*TRAX*) haplotypes with schizophrenia and reduced prefrontal gray matter, which in turn were associated with impaired memory (Cannon et al. 2005); and reduced dorsolateral prefrontal cortex volume associated with regulator of G protein signaling 4 (*RGS4*) polymorphisms in first-episode schizophrenia patients (Prasad et al. 2005). The application of fMRI in genetic paradigms is more limited and has focused on the *COMT* Val/Met polymorphism and dorsolateral prefrontal cortex activation in healthy people and schizophrenia patients (Egan et al. 2001b; Winterer et al. 2004). Individuals homozygous for the Met allele showed diminished hippocampal engagement during performance of episodic memory encoding and retrieval compared with Val/Val subjects (Hariri et al. 2003). Such studies support use of multimodal imaging in genetic paradigms.

Neuropathology

Neuropathological studies of brain tissues from patients with schizophrenia have reported a wide variety of morphometric, cellular, subcellular, and molecular abnormalities in diverse brain regions. While many findings are controversial or require confirmation, common themes have emerged from the data. Among these themes are abnormal neurodevelopment, abnormal synaptic integrity and plasticity, glutamatergic and GABAergic system abnormalities, mitochondrial dysfunction, and abnormal white matter integrity. Notably, all of these abnormalities occur in the absence of any grossly observable evidence of neural injury or neurodegenerative lesions common in other brain diseases (Arnold et al. 1998).

Abnormal Neurodevelopment

While clinical and epidemiological findings present a compelling case for the role of abnormal neurodevelopment in schizophrenia, characterizing the cellular and molecular mechanism(s) by which this might occur has been a challenge. Neurons are born, migrate, and assume their mature phenotype, and the major axon pathways are laid down in a complex and highly orchestrated process during fetal development and early childhood (Arnold and Trojanowski 1996a, 1996b; Hatten 1999; Nowakowski and Rakic 1981). By the time schizophrenia is clinically expressed, typically in adolescence or young

adulthood, much of development has transpired. Limited numbers of new neurons continue to be generated in the adult human brain in certain areas (e.g., the dentate gyrus [Eriksson et al. 1998]), but their number is small and their functionality is still being investigated (Eisch 2002). In contrast, there is ongoing synaptogenesis and synaptic remodeling within all major axon terminal fields throughout life.

Aberrant neurodevelopment in schizophrenia has been inferred by findings from several postmortem research approaches. Among the earliest and most influential neuropathological findings of the modern era were reports of cytoarchitectural disorganization of hippocampal subfields and the entorhinal cortex, a limbic periallocortex intimately related to the hippocampus (Arnold et al. 1991a, 1991b; Conrad et al. 1991; Falkai et al. 1988; Jakob and Beckmann 1986, 1989, 1994; Kovelman and Scheibel 1984). Specific abnormalities have included misalignment of pyramidal cell neurons in ammonic subfields of the hippocampus, abnormal clustering and heterotopic displacement of neurons in the entorhinal cortex, and abnormalities in neuronal densities in different layers of the entorhinal cortex. Similar approaches in other corticolimbic regions, especially anterior cingulate cortex, also have revealed subtle cytoarchitectural differences in schizophrenia compared with control subjects (Benes and Bird 1987; Benes et al. 1992; Chana et al. 2003). However, not all of these findings have been replicated (Akil and Lewis 1997; Altshuler et al. 1987; Arnold et al. 1995; Benes et al. 1991; Krimer et al. 1997; Zaidel et al. 1997).

Another cytoarchitectural approach has been to map the number and position of interstitial white matter neurons lying deep to cerebrocortical gray matter. These neurons are considered to be remnants of the cortical subplate and are thought to reflect incomplete neuronal migration during brain development. Furthermore, because the subplate is important in directing the establishment of normal connectivity, disturbance of the subplate could lead to altered formation of connections. Several groups of investigators reported abnormal numbers or positions of neurons positive for nicotinamide adenine dinucleotide phosphate (NADPH)–diaphorase or microtubule-associated protein 2 (MAP2) within white matter of frontal, temporal, and parahippocampal cortices in schizophrenia, although the specific parameters of maldistribution varied among studies (Akbarian et al. 1993, 1996; Anderson et al. 1996; Kirkpatrick et al. 1999; Rioux et al. 2003).

To explain these phenomena, researchers have proposed that the migration of neurons from the subventricular zone to the appropriate cortical lamina during fetal development is disturbed, that select populations of neurons fail to survive, and/or that neurons fail to generate axonal and dendritic processes appropriately, thus altering their normal orientation or placement. Complex and concerted, generative and regressive neurobiological processes determine the ultimate cytoarchitecture of a given region. In addition to neuronal migration, a host of intrinsic signaling mechanisms responding to extrinsic growth factors and neurotransmitters influence neuron survival, morphology, neurite outgrowth, and patterns of synapse formation. Young neurons that fail to establish adequate synaptic connectivity and access to trophic factors do not survive. Furthermore, the spatial organization of neurons depends not only on the number of neurons that migrate to a particular position and survive but also on the neuropil space in which those neurons reside. Increases or decreases in this space due to its many cellular (e.g., dendritic, axonal, glial processes) and extracellular matrix constituents will affect the spatial distribution of neurons. This has been a major interpretation of reports of reductions in neuropil space in the dorsolateral prefrontal cortex in schizophrenia (Selemon et al. 1998). Finally, environmental factors during growth and development (e.g., infection, ischemic injury, trauma) as well as regressive changes that are part of normal aging may further alter the cytoarchitecture that is observed at postmortem examination.

Abnormal Synaptic Integrity and Plasticity

Synapses have been investigated by a variety of means in postmortem tissues in schizophrenia. At the ultrastructural level, studies described abnormalities in the densities and aggregation of synapses (Aganova and Uranova 1992; Kung et al. 1998; Soustek 1989), dendritic spine morphology and morphometry (Kolomeets and Uranova 1999; Roberts et al. 1996), axon terminal mitochondria (Kolomeets and Uranova 1999; Uranova et al. 1996), and various other changes in axospinous densities and morphologies (for a review, see Honer et al. 2000).

Abnormalities in dendritic arborization and dendritic spines have been reported. Golgi impregnation studies have described decreased spine densities in prefrontal and temporal cortices and in the hippocampus (Garey et al. 1998; Glantz and Lewis 1995; D.A. Lewis and Glantz 1997; Rosoklija et al. 2000), decreased densities of pyramidal basilar dendrites in prefrontal cortex pyramidal neurons (Broadbelt et al. 2002), and increased densities of dentate gyrus granule cell basilar and recurrent dendrites (Lauer et al. 2003). Another index of dendritic densities that has been used in schizophrenia is immuno-

labeling for the MAP2 that is selectively expressed in the somatodendritic domain of neurons. Several studies have reported a decrease in the density of MAP2 expression in the hippocampus and prefrontal cortex (Arnold et al. 1991b; Jones et al. 2002; Rosoklija et al. 1995, 2005), although other groups have not found this (Cotter et al. 2000; Law et al. 2004). Molecular components of dendritic spines have also been assessed in schizophrenia, with reports of decreased spinophilin messenger RNA (mRNA) in the hippocampus (Law et al. 2004) and decreased mRNA expression of members of the rhoGTPase family, especially Cdc42 and Duo, in dorsolateral prefrontal cortex (J.J. Hill et al. 2006).

Molecules enriched in axon terminals and the presynaptic machinery for neurotransmitter release have been examined in postmortem tissues using a variety of methods, including Western blotting, enzyme-linked immunosorbent assay (ELISA), immunohistochemistry, in situ hybridization, Northern blotting, and quantitative real-time polymerase chain reaction (qPCR), as well as gene expression microarrays. Among the many proteins that have been investigated are synaptic vesicle membrane docking and fusion proteins such as synaptophysin, synapsin, synaptosome-associated protein of 25,000 daltons (SNAP-25), complexins I and II, Rab3a, and syntaxin; synaptic plasticity proteins such as growth-associated protein 43 (GAP-43) and neural cell adhesion molecules (NCAMs); and neurotransmitter system–specific proteins such as vesicular glutamate transporters (VGluTs) and vesicular GABA transporters (VGATs). The regions most commonly examined have been the hippocampus, dorsolateral prefrontal cortex, anterior cingulate, thalamus, and, more recently, the superior temporal gyrus. Most studies reported significant decreases in presynaptic terminal markers, although this has not been without controversy (Eastwood and Harrison 2001; Harrison and Eastwood 2001; Honer and Young 2004; Honer et al. 2000; Mirnics et al. 2001; Sweet et al. 2007).

Glutamatergic and GABAergic System Abnormalities

The glutamate hypothesis of schizophrenia originated with the observations that dissociative anesthetics produce psychotic effects (Luby et al. 1959) and that the NMDA antagonists ketamine and phencyclidine induce schizophrenia-like psychosis and cognitive deficits (Javitt and Zukin 1991). Supporting data in schizophrenia include ketamine induction of eye-tracking abnormalities, impaired prepulse inhibition of the startle response, frontal hypometabolism, abnormal cortical ERPs, and enhanced subcortical dopamine release (Coyle 2004). Molecular neuropathological studies have produced complex and at times conflicting data on glutamatergic synapses in schizophrenia. Most have examined glutamate receptors, with the principal regions of interest being the hippocampus, prefrontal cortex, and thalamus. There are numerous findings of abnormal expression of NMDA receptor subunits NR1 and NR2B; the kainic acid receptor; α-amino-3-hydroxy-5-methyl-4-isoxazole-propionic acid (AMPA) receptors, phosphorylation of NR1; postsynaptic density proteins PSD95, SAP102, and SAP97; excitatory amino acid (EAA) transporters EAAT1 and EAAT2; and the N-acetyl-aspartyl-glutamate (NAAG)–degrading enzyme glutamate carboxypeptidase II (Coyle 2004; Dracheva et al. 2005; Harrison et al. 2003). Although it is currently difficult to weave these diverse findings into a coherent mechanism, the weight of the evidence indicates significant derangement in postsynaptic glutamatergic neurotransmission in schizophrenia.

Compared with data on glutamate, clinical evidence for major GABA involvement in schizophrenia is less compelling. However, substantial postmortem data indicate that GABA markers are abnormal (Benes and Berretta 2001; Blum and Mann 2002; D.A. Lewis et al. 2005; Wassef et al. 2003). In the hippocampus, prefrontal cortex, and elsewhere, there are reports of decreased expression of the GABA-producing enzyme glutamic acid decarboxylase67 (GAD67) mRNA and probably protein (but not GAD65), decreased GABA membrane transporter 1 (GAT1), decreased densities of nonpyramidal (presumably GABA) neurons, decreased calbindin-containing neurons, decreased parvalbumin mRNA, increased $GABA_A$ ligand binding, and increased $GABA_A$ α_1 mRNA levels. In an elegant and compelling set of experiments in localized microcircuitry of the prefrontal cortex, D.A. Lewis et al. (2005) provided evidence for a deficit of GAD67 mRNA expression in presynaptic GAT1 in chandelier interneurons and compensatory changes in postsynaptic $GABA_A$ receptors. They have suggested that these GABA changes may be relatively specific for the prefrontal cortex; however, a similarly detailed investigation has not been conducted elsewhere.

One interpretation of GABA deficits in schizophrenia is that GABA activity is secondarily downregulated due to decreased glutamatergic stimulation. Genetic data associating a growing number of glutamatergic genes with schizophrenia (Harrison and Weinberger 2005) are consistent with primary glutamatergic abnormalities. Other data indicating that a primary glutamate deficit could ac-

count for GABA abnormalities include evidence that administration of NMDA antagonists or surgical ablation of glutamatergic innervation to prefrontal cortex in rodents decreases GABA markers in prefrontal cortex (Cochran et al. 2003; Lipska et al. 2003; Paulson et al. 2003). However, other findings have suggested that GABA deficits are potentially primary (Addington et al. 2005; Caruncho et al. 2004; Guidotti et al. 2000; Hashimoto et al. 2005).

Mitochondrial Dysfunction

Mitochondrial metabolic pathways represent an emerging area of interest in postmortem studies of schizophrenia. Certainly, the long history of findings of brain metabolic abnormalities from PET, SPECT, and fMRI (see "Neuroimaging" section) provide indirect support for the notion that metabolic pathways are dysfunctional in the disease, and, conversely, psychosis and other psychiatric symptoms have been reported as presenting symptoms in bona fide mitochondrial diseases (Fattal et al. 2006).

Mitochondria are cellular organelles, which produce energy as adenosine triphosphate (ATP) via the electron transport chain and the oxidative phosphorylation system and help in the synthesis of other important cell constituents, including amino acids, phospholipids, and nucleotides. A few ultrastructural studies of postmortem tissues have described decreased densities and abnormal morphological profiles of mitochondria in limbic cortices, striatum, and substantia nigra (Kolomeets and Uranova 1999; Kung and Roberts 1999; Uranova et al. 1989). At the molecular level, Middleton et al. (2002) used complementary DNA (cDNA) microarrays to profile the expression of genes in a large number of metabolic pathways in the dorsolateral prefrontal cortex of subjects with schizophrenia and control subjects. They found consistent decreases in the expression levels of genes involved in five specific pathways: ornithine and polyamine metabolism, the mitochondrial malate shuttle system, the transcarboxylic acid cycle, aspartate and alanine metabolism, and ubiquitin metabolism. Prabakaran et al. (2004) used parallel gene expression microarray, proteomic, and metabolomic approaches to examine prefrontal cortex and reported 28 significantly downregulated metabolic pathways and 13 upregulated pathways in schizophrenia. Abnormal pathways included glycolytic and oxidative metabolism, intracellular and vesicle-mediated transport, and pathways involved in defense against reactive oxygen species. In a third microarray study, Iwamoto et al. (2005) reported a global downregulation in mitochondrial genes in schizophrenia and bipolar disorder, although they suggested that this was more related to antipsychotic medication than to disease. Targeted studies of mitochondrial metabolism have reported alterations in mitochondrial enzyme activities for cytochrome c oxidase, succinate dehydrogenase, and NADPH–cytochrome c reductase and mitochondrial complex I expression (Cavelier et al. 1995; Karry et al. 2004; Maurer et al. 2001; Prince et al. 1999; Whatley et al. 1996). While still relatively few, these promising studies indicate a need for increased investigation of mitochondrial metabolic pathways in schizophrenia.

Abnormal White Matter Integrity

Another relatively new area of neuropathological interest in schizophrenia has been oligodendroglia and myelin integrity in schizophrenia. White matter abnormalities have long been hypothesized in schizophrenia. As noted above, clinical neuroimaging and electrophysiological research have yielded evidence of poor functional connectivity between and within brain regions, and some sMRI studies have shown reductions in white matter volumes. Most recently, magnetic transfer and diffusion tensor MRI studies have reported abnormalities in axon membrane integrity and anisotropy.

Postmortem studies have found white matter–related abnormalities at cellular and molecular levels in schizophrenia. A seminal microarray study by Hakak et al. (2001) used a large oligonucleotide microarray to examine dorsolateral prefrontal cortex in an elderly cohort with highly chronic schizophrenia. Although abnormal expression of a variety of genes was reported, the authors were especially impressed with the decreased expression of oligodendroglial genes, including myelin-associated glycoprotein (MAG), 2′,3′-cyclic nucleotide 3′-phosphohydrolase (CNP), myelin and lymphocyte protein (MAL), gelsolin, erbB3, and transferrin. Subsequent studies with qPCR and in situ hybridization continued to find decreased myelin-related gene abnormalities in other samples and brain regions (Dracheva et al. 2006; McCullumsmith et al. 2007) as well as marginal decreases in CNP and MAG using immunohistochemistry (Flynn et al. 2003).

Cellular and subcellular abnormalities of white matter have also been reported. Ultrastructural studies have described decreased compaction of myelin sheath lamellae and abnormal inclusion bodies as well as signs of oligodendroglial degeneration in schizophrenia samples (Uranova et al. 2001). Cell counting studies have reported decreased densities and altered spatial distribution of oligodendroglia in white matter (Hof et al. 2003; Rajkowska et al. 2001).

Genes Associated With Schizophrenia: Implications for Neuropathology

As evident from the foregoing sections, the cellular and molecular neuropathological findings in schizophrenia are widespread in location, diverse in nature, and difficult to weave together mechanistically. Much more research needs to be done on multiple levels to advance our understanding of this complex and severe illness. However, recent advances in the genetics of schizophrenia provide some reason for optimism. In the past decade, associations between schizophrenia and a number of specific genes have been reported (for reviews, see Harrison and Weinberger 2005; O'Donovan and Owen 1996; Riley and Kendler 2006), suggesting molecular pathways and pathophysiological mechanisms that, at least theoretically, play diverse roles in the development and ongoing health of the nervous systems.

Among the most highly replicated susceptibility genes are *neuregulin-1*, *dysbindin*, and *DISC-1*, along with *COMT* discussed previously. While variations in each of these genes confers only a modest increase in risk for the disorder, their discovery nonetheless identifies candidate proteins and molecular pathways that may substantially contribute to the pathophysiology of schizophrenia. This opens the door to a functional genomics of schizophrenia. It is noteworthy that most of these genes play important roles in neurodevelopment, neurotransmission, and neuroplasticity.

Neuregulin-1 is a complex molecule with at least 15 different isoforms that have varied functions in the CNS (Buonanno and Fischbach 2001). Neuregulin-1 plays important roles in neurogenesis, neuronal migration, neuronal survival, axon and dendrite outgrowth, modulation of NMDA signaling via erbB4 receptors, and astroglia and oligodendroglia development via erbB3 receptors, among others. While levels of neuregulin-1 and erbB receptor expression do not appear to be abnormal in schizophrenia, markedly abnormal activation of neuregulin–erbB4 signaling has been found (Hahn et al. 2006).

Dysbindin protein has only recently been characterized (Benson et al. 2001; Li et al. 2003; Talbot et al. 2006). It is neuron-specific; widely distributed in the CNS; present in presynaptic vesicles, postsynaptic densities, neuronal cytoskeleton, and cell nucleus; and important in intracellular trafficking and vesicle formation. So far, dysbindin expression has been found to be decreased in the hippocampus and dorsolateral prefrontal cortex in schizophrenia and may at least in part affect presynaptic gluta-mate release (Numakawa et al. 2004; Talbot et al. 2004; Weickert et al. 2004).

DISC-1 has been characterized only recently also, after its association with schizophrenia was discovered (Ishi-zuka et al. 2006). *DISC-1* is preferentially expressed in the forebrain and has multiple isoforms with potential post-translational modifications. It is present in multiple sub-cellular compartments, including the actin and microtu-bule cytoskeletons, centrosomes, postsynaptic densities, mitochondria, and the nucleus. It appears to be important in the centrosome–dynein cascade and cyclic adenosine monophosphate (cAMP) signaling. While its expression level appears to be unaltered in schizophrenia, the expres-sion levels of important binding partners (i.e., fascicula-tion and elongation protein zeta-1 [FEZ1], lissencephaly 1 protein [LIS1], and nuclear distribution element–like [NUDEL]) are significantly reduced in schizophrenia (Lipska et al. 2006).

COMT is an enzyme involved in the clearance of cat-echolamines from synapses and thus could be involved in regulation of neurotransmission related to schizophrenia both in development and maturity (Craddock et al. 2006). A functional polymorphism involving the pres-ence of either valine or methionine at a specific codon af-fects the enzyme's activity. Variants with methionine have lower activity, and thus, people with two copies of the methionine allele may be expected to have higher dopamine and norepinephrine levels. Given the critical roles these neurotransmitters play in the development of the nervous system and mental functioning especially rel-evant to psychiatric illness, abnormal levels could have far-reaching cellular, molecular, and clinical effects.

Conclusion

Considerable advances with a range of technologies have been made in the efforts to advance the understanding of the neurobiology of schizophrenia. Elucidating the vital neurobiological mechanisms at play is a continuing chal-lenge. Given the complexity of the disorder, we do not ex-pect a single gene, pathological lesion, cellular, molecular or neurochemical abnormality, or even neural system to be nodal to schizophrenia. Indeed, abnormalities are evi-dent at many levels of neurobehavioral and neurophysio-logical processing and in multiple neural systems—from the cerebellum to diencephalon to diverse primary, asso-ciation, and limbic cortices to the olfactory bulb and epi-thelium. However, these diffuse abnormalities, which im-

plicate neurodevelopmental aberrations, are not fully expressed phenotypically until after brain development and maturation are largely completed.

The recognition that the underlying pathological pro-cesses of schizophrenia are present throughout the CNS suggests that there may be some core defects in neuro-transmission whereby the ability of neurons to respond to and process stimuli is curtailed. However, within the con-text of global abnormalities, some neural systems are dif-ferentially affected. Brain regions with greater vulnerabil-ity, such as the hippocampus, prefrontal cortex, and olfactory system, are dynamic and maintain a high degree of plasticity during brain maturation and thereafter. Thus, neuronal plasticity—evident in molecular, chemical, morphological, and physiological modifiability with neu-ral activity—is abnormal in schizophrenia. This may ulti-mately be manifested in the array of complex features that characterize schizophrenia. However, functions mediated through other neural systems, where greater plasticity is not required, show subtle abnormalities, and motor abili-ties, sensation, and autonomic functions are relatively spared.

These challenges are further compounded by the ab-sence of suitable animal models for the disorder as cur-rently phenotypically defined, buttressing the need to identify endophenotypes that can be studied in both hu-mans and animals. For example, sensorimotor gating and encoding can be characterized in animals and in humans. The identification of such endophenotypes in schizophre-nia that have counterparts in rodents enables investiga-tion of the genetic, molecular, biochemical, anatomical, and physiological aspects of these behaviors in ways not possible in the human. Findings from studies in rodents will continue to provide new information about these be-haviors and elucidate the effects of genetic, pharmacolog-ical, and behavioral manipulations, which can be pursued in humans. This top-down/bottom-up translational inter-change holds great promise for advancing our understand-ing of the pathophysiology of schizophrenia. As progress is made, we will be in a better position to relate neurobio-logical processes to major clinical phenotypic characteris-tics of schizophrenia with the hope of targeted therapeu-tics that enhance cognition and ameliorate the negative symptoms associated with poor outcome.

References

Abi-Dargham A: Do we still believe in the dopamine hypothesis? New data bring new evidence. Int J Neuropsychopharmacol 7 (suppl 1):S1–S5, 2004

Achim AM, Lepage M: Episodic memory-related activation in schizophrenia: meta-analysis. Br J Psychiatry 187:500–509, 2005

Addington AM, Gornick M, Duckworth J, et al: GAD1 (2q31.1), which encodes glutamic acid decarboxylase (GAD67), is associated with childhood-onset schizophrenia and cortical gray matter volume loss. Mol Psychiatry 10:581–588, 2005

Adler LE, Pachtman E, Frank RD, et al: Neurophysiological evidence for a defect in neuronal mechanisms involved in sensory gating in schizophrenia. Biol Psychiatry 17:639–654, 1982

Aganova EA, Uranova NA: Morphometric analysis of synaptic contacts in the anterior limbic cortex in the endogenous psychoses. Neurosci Behav Physiol 22:59–65, 1992

Akbarian S, Vinuela A, Kim JJ, et al: Distorted distribution of nicotinamide-adenine dinucleotide phosphate-diaphorase neurons in temporal lobe of schizophrenics implies anomalous cortical development. Arch Gen Psychiatry 50:178–187, 1993

Akbarian S, Kim JJ, Potkin SG, et al: Maldistribution of interstitial neurons in prefrontal white matter of the brains of schizophrenic patients. Arch Gen Psychiatry 53:425–436, 1996

Akil M, Lewis DA: Cytoarchitecture of the entorhinal cortex in schizophrenia. Am J Psychiatry 154:1010–1012, 1997

Alho K: Cerebral generators of mismatch negativity (MMN) and its magnetic counterpart (MMNm) elicited by sound changes. Ear Hear 16:38–51, 1995

Altshuler LL, Conrad A, Kovelman JH, et al: Hippocampal pyramidal cell orientation in schizophrenia. Arch Gen Psychiatry 44:1094–1098, 1987

American Psychiatric Association: Diagnostic and Statistical Manual of Mental Disorders, 4th Edition, Text Revision. Washington, DC, American Psychiatric Association, 2000

Anderson SA, Volk DW, Lewis DA: Increased density of microtubule associated protein 2-immunoreactive neurons in the prefrontal white matter of schizophrenic subjects. Schizophr Res 19:111–119, 1996

Andreasen NC, Carson R, Diksic M, et al: Workshop on schizophrenia, PET, and dopamine D2 receptors in the human neostriatum. Schizophr Bull 14:471–484, 1988

Antonova E, Sharma T, Morris R, et al: The relationship between brain structure and neurocognition in schizophrenia: a selective review. Schizophr Res 70:117–145, 2004

Arnold SE, Trojanowski JQ: Human fetal hippocampal development, I: cytoarchitecture, myeloarchitecture, and neuronal morphologic features. J Comp Neurol 367:274–292, 1996a

Arnold SE, Trojanowski JQ: Human fetal hippocampal development, II: the neuronal cytoskeleton. J Comp Neurol 367:293–307, 1996b

Arnold SE, Trojanowski JQ: Recent advances in the neuropathology of schizophrenia. Acta Neuropathologica 92:217–231, 1996c

Arnold SE, Hyman BT, Van Hoesen GW, et al: Some cytoarchitectural abnormalities of entorhinal cortex in schizophrenia. Arch Gen Psychiatry 48:625–632, 1991a

Arnold SE, Lee VM, Gur RE, et al: Abnormal expression of two microtubule-associated proteins (MAP2 and MAP5) in specific subfields of the hippocampal formation in schizophrenia. Proc Natl Acad Sci U S A 88:10850–10854, 1991b

Arnold SE, Franz BR, Gur RC, et al: Smaller neuron size in schizophrenia in hippocampal subfields that mediate cortical-hippocampal interactions. Am J Psychiatry 152:738–748, 1995

Arnold SE, Trojanowski JQ, Gur RE, et al: Absence of neurodegeneration and neural injury in the cerebral cortex in a sample of elderly patients with schizophrenia. Arch Gen Psychiatry 5:225–232, 1998

Bastiaansen M, Hagoort P: Event-induced theta responses as a window on the dynamics of memory. Cereb Cortex 39:967–992, 2003

Benes FM, Berretta S: GABAergic interneurons: implications for understanding schizophrenia and bipolar disorder. Neuropsychopharmacol 25:1–27, 2001

Benes FM, Bird ED: An analysis of the arrangement of neurons in the cingulate cortex of schizophrenic patients. Arch Gen Psychiatry 44:608–616, 1987

Benes FM, Sorensen I, Bird ED: Reduced neuronal size in posterior hippocampus of schizophrenic patients. Schizophr Bull 17:597–608, 1991

Benes FM, Sorensen I, Vincent SL, et al: Increased density of glutamate-immunoreactive vertical processes in superficial laminae in cingulate cortex of schizophrenic brain. Cereb Cortex 2:503–512, 1992

Benson MA, Newey SE, Martin-Rendon E, et al: Dysbindin, a novel coiled-coil-containing protein that interacts with the dystrobrevins in muscle and brain. J Biol Chem 276:24232–24241, 2001

Bertrand O, Tallon-Baudry C: Oscillatory gamma activity in humans: a possible role for object representation. Int J Psychophysiol 38:211–223, 2000

Bilder RM, Volavka J, Czobor P, et al: Neurocognitive correlates of the COMT Val(158)Met polymorphism in chronic schizophrenia. Biol Psychiatry 52:701–707, 2002

Blouin JL, Dombroski BA, Nath SK, et al: Schizophrenia susceptibility loci on chromosomes 13q32 and 8p21. Nat Genetics 20:70–73, 1998

Blum BP, Mann JJ: The GABAergic system in schizophrenia. Int J Neuropsychopharmacol 5:159–179, 2002

Boos HBM, Aleman A, Cahn W, et al: Brain volumes in relatives of patients with schizophrenia: a meta-analysis. Schizophr Res 81:41, 2006

Braff DL, Grillon C, Geyer MA: Gating and habituation of the startle reflex in schizophrenic patients. Arch Gen Psychiatry 49:206–215, 1992

Broadbelt K, Byne W, Jones LB: Evidence for a decrease in basilar dendrites of pyramidal cells in schizophrenic medial prefrontal cortex. Schizophr Res 58:75–81, 2002

Brzustowicz LM, Hodgkinson KA, Chow EW, et al: Location of a major susceptibility locus for familial schizophrenia on chromosome 1q21-q22. Science 288:678–682, 2000

Buonanno A, Fischbach GD: Neuregulin and ErbB receptor signaling pathways in the nervous system. Curr Opin Neurobiol 11:287–296, 2001

Burdick KE, Lencz T, Funke B, et al: Genetic variation in DTNBP1 influences general cognitive ability. Hum Mol Genet 15:1563–1568, 2006

Butler PD, Javitt DC: Early stage visual processing deficits in schizophrenia. Curr Opin Psychiatry 18:151–157, 2005

Callicott JH, Weinberger DR: Brain imaging as an approach to phenotype characterization for genetic studies of schizophrenia. Methods Mol Med 77:227–247, 2003

Calkins ME, Gur RC, Ragland JD, et al: Face recognition memory deficits and visual object memory performance in patients with schizophrenia and their relatives. Am J Psychiatry 162:1963–1966, 2005

Cannon TD, Hennah W, van Erp TG, et al: Association of DISC1/TRAX haplotypes with schizophrenia, reduced prefrontal gray matter, and impaired short- and long-term memory. Arch Gen Psychiatry 62:1205–1213, 2005

Cao Q, Martinez M, Zhang J, et al: Suggestive evidence for a schizophrenia susceptibility locus on chromosome 6q and a confirmation in an independent series of pedigrees. Genomics 43:1–8, 1997

Caruncho HJ, Dopeso-Reyes IG, Loza MI, et al: GABA, reelin, and the neurodevelopmental hypothesis of schizophrenia. Crit Rev Neurobiol 16:25–32, 2004

Cavelier L, Jazin EE, Eriksson I, et al: Decreased cytochrome-c oxidase activity and lack of age-related accumulation of mitochondrial DNA deletions in the brains of schizophrenics. Genomics 29:217–224, 1995

Chana G, Landau S, Beasley C, et al: Two-dimensional assessment of cytoarchitecture in the anterior cingulate cortex in major depressive disorder, bipolar disorder, and schizophrenia: evidence for decreased neuronal somal size and increased neuronal density. Biol Psychiatry 53:1086–1098, 2003

Cochran SM, Kennedy M, McKerchar CE, et al: Induction of metabolic hypofunction and neurochemical deficits after chronic intermittent exposure to phencyclidine: differential modulation by antipsychotic drugs. Neuropsychopharmacol 28:265–275, 2003

Connolly PM, Maxwell CR, Kanes SJ, et al: Inhibition of auditory evoked potentials and prepulse inhibition of startle in DBA/2J and DBA/2Hsd inbred mouse substrains. Brain Res 992:85–95, 2003

Conrad AJ, Abebe T, Austin R, et al: Hippocampal pyramidal cell disarray in schizophrenia as a bilateral phenomenon. Arch Gen Psychiatry 48:413–417, 1991

Cornblatt BA, Keilp JG: Impaired attention, genetics, and the pathophysiology of schizophrenia. Schizophr Bull 20:31–46, 1994

Cotter D, Wilson S, Roberts E, et al: Increased dendritic MAP2 expression in the hippocampus in schizophrenia. Schizophr Res 41:313–323, 2000

Coyle JT: The GABA-glutamate connection in schizophrenia: which is the proximate cause? Biochem Pharmacol 68:1507–1514, 2004

Craddock N, Owen MJ, O'Donovan MC: The catechol-O-methyl transferase (COMT) gene as a candidate for psychiatric phenotypes: evidence and lessons. Mol Psychiatry 11:446–458, 2006

Cropley VL, Fujita M, Innis RB, et al: Molecular imaging of the dopaminergic system and its association with human cognitive function. Biol Psychiatry 59:898–907, 2006

Davatzikos C, Shen D, Gur RC, et al: Whole brain morphometric study of schizophrenia reveals a spatially complex set of focal abnormalities. Arch Gen Psychiatry 62:1218–1227, 2005

Davidson LL, Heinrichs RW: Quantification of frontal and temporal lobe brain-imaging findings in schizophrenia: a meta-analysis. Psychiatry Res 122:69–87, 2003

Davis CE, Jeste DV, Eyler LT: Review of longitudinal functional neuroimaging studies of drug treatments in patients with schizophrenia. Schizophr Res 78:45–60, 2005

de Frias CM, Annerbrink K, Westberg L, et al: Catechol O-methyltransferase Val158Met polymorphism is associated with cognitive performance in nondemented adults. J Cogn Neurosci 17:1018–1025, 2005

Dracheva S, McGurk SR, Haroutunian V: mRNA expression of AMPA receptors and AMPA receptor binding proteins in the cerebral cortex of elderly schizophrenics. J Neurosci Res 79:868–878, 2005

Dracheva S, Davis KL, Chin B, et al: Myelin-associated mRNA and protein expression deficits in the anterior cingulate cortex and hippocampus in elderly schizophrenia patients. Neurobiol Dis 21:531–540, 2006

Eastwood SL, Harrison PJ: Synaptic pathology in the anterior cingulate cortex in schizophrenia and mood disorders.: a review and a Western blot study of synaptophysin, GAP-43 and the complexins. Brain Res Bull 55:569–578, 2001

Egan MF, Goldberg TE, Gscheidle T, et al: Relative risk for cognitive impairments in siblings of patients with schizophrenia. Biol Psychiatry 50:98–107, 2001a

Egan MF, Goldberg TE, Kolachana BS, et al: Effect of COMT Val108/158 Met genotype on frontal lobe function and risk for schizophrenia. PNAS 98:6917–6922, 2001b

Eisch AJ: Adult neurogenesis: implications for psychiatry. Prog Brain Res 138:315–342, 2002

Eriksson PS, Perfilieva E, Bjork-Eriksson T, et al: Neurogenesis in the adult human hippocampus. Nat Med 4:1313–1317, 1998

Erritzoe D, Talbot P, Frankle WG, et al: Positron emission tomography and single photon emission CT molecular imaging in schizophrenia. Neuroimaging Clin N Am 13:817–832, 2003

Erwin RJ, Mawhinney-Hee M, Gur RC, et al: Midlatency auditory evoked responses in schizophrenia. Biol Psychiatry 30:430–442, 1991

Falkai P, Bogerts B, Rozumek M: Limbic pathology in schizophrenia: the entorhinal region—a morphometric study. Biol Psychiatry 24:515–521, 1988

Fallin MD, Lasseter VK, Wolyniec PS, et al: Genomewide linkage scan for schizophrenia susceptibility loci among Ashkenazi Jewish families shows evidence of linkage on chromosome 10q22. Am J Hum Genet 73:601–611, 2003

Faraone SV, Matise T, Svrakic D, et al: Genome scan of European-American schizophrenia pedigrees: results of the NIMH Genetics Initiative and Millennium Consortium. Am J Med Genet 81:290–295, 1998

Faraone SV, Meyer J, Matise T, et al: Suggestive linkage of chromosome 10p to schizophrenia is not due to transmission ratio distortion. Am J Med Genet 88:607–608, 1999

Faraone SV, Seidman LJ, Kremen WS, et al: Neuropsychologic functioning among the nonpsychotic relatives of schizophrenic patients: the effect of genetic loading. Biol Psychiatry 48:120–126, 2000

Fattal O, Budur K, Vaughan AJ, et al: Review of the literature on major mental disorders in adult patients with mitochondrial diseases. Psychosomatics 47:1–7, 2006

Flynn SW, Lang DJ, Mackay AL, et al: Abnormalities of myelination in schizophrenia detected in vivo with MRI, and postmortem with analysis of oligodendrocyte proteins. Mol Psychiatry 8:811–820, 2003

Foong J, Symms MR, Barker GJ, et al: Investigating regional white matter in schizophrenia using diffusion tensor imaging. Neuroreport 13:333–336, 2002

Freedman R, Waldo M, Bickford-Wimer P, et al: Elementary neuronal dysfunction in schizophrenia. Schizophr Res 4:233–243, 1991

Garey LJ, Ong WY, Patel TS, et al: Reduced dendritic spine density on cerebral cortical pyramidal neurons in schizophrenia. J Neurol Neurosurg Psychiatry 65:446–453, 1998

Giedd JN, Blumenthal J, Jeffries NO, et al: Brain development during childhood and adolescence: a longitudinal MRI study. Nat Neurosci 2:861–863, 1999

Glahn DC, Ragland JD, Abramoff A, et al: Beyond hypofrontality: a quantitative meta-analysis of functional neuroimaging studies of working memory in schizophrenia. Hum Brain Mapp 25:60–69, 2005

Glantz LA, Lewis DA: Assessment of spine density on layer III pyramidal cells in the prefrontal cortex of schizophrenic subjects. Soc Neuroscience Abstracts 21:239, 1995

Gogtay N, Sporn A, Clasen LS, et al: Structural brain MRI abnormalities in healthy siblings of patients with childhood-onset schizophrenia. Am J Psychiatry 160:569–571, 2003

Goldberg TE, Gold JM: Neurocognitive functioning in patients with schizophrenia, in Psychopharmacology: The Fourth Generation of Progress. Edited by Bloom FE, Kupfer DJ. New York, Raven Press, 1995, pp 1245–1257

Goldberg TE, Egan MF, Gscheidle T, et al: Executive subprocesses in working memory: relationship to catechol-O-methyltransferase Val158Met genotype and schizophrenia. Arch Gen Psychiatry 60:889–896, 2003

Gottesman II, Gould TD: The endophenotype concept in psychiatry: etymology and strategic intentions. Am J Psychiatry 160:636–645, 2003

Green MF: What are the functional consequences of neurocognitive deficits in schizophrenia? Am J Psychiatry 153:321–330, 1996

Green MF, Kern RS, Braff DL, et al: Neurocognitive deficits and functional outcome in schizophrenia: are we measuring the "right stuff"? Schizophr Bull 26:119–136, 2000

Grillon C, Ameli R, Braff DL: Middle latency auditory evoked potentials (MAEPs) in chronic schizophrenics. Schizophr Res 5:61–66, 1991

Guidotti A, Auta J, Davis JM, et al: Decrease in reelin and glutamic acid decarboxylase67 (GAD67) expression in schizophrenia and bipolar disorder: a postmortem brain study. Arch Gen Psychiatry 57:1061–1069, 2000

Gur RC, Erwin RJ, Gur RE: Neurobehavioral probes for physiologic neuroimaging studies. Arch Gen Psychiatry 49:409–414, 1992

Gur RE, Cowell PE, Latshaw A, et al: Reduced dorsal and orbital prefrontal gray matter volumes in schizophrenia. Arch Gen Psychiatry 57:761–768, 2000a

Gur RE, Turetsky BI, Cowell PE, et al: Temporolimbic volume reductions in schizophrenia. Arch Gen Psychiatry 57:769–775, 2000b

Gur RE, Kohler CG, Ragland JD, et al: Flat affect in schizophrenia: Relation to emotion processing and neurocognitive measures. Schizophr Bull 32:279–287, 2006

Gur RE, Keshavan MS, Lawrie SM: Deconstructing psychosis with human brain imaging. Schizophr Bull 33:921–931, 2007a

Gur RE, Nimgaonkar VL, Almasy L, et al: Neurocognitive endophenotypes in a multiplex multigenerational family study of schizophrenia. Am J Psychiatry 164:813–819, 2007b

Hahn CG, Wang HY, Cho DS, et al: Altered neuregulin 1-erbB4 signaling contributes to NMDA receptor hypofunction in schizophrenia. Nat Med 12:824–828, 2006

Hakak Y, Walker JR, Li C, et al: Genome-wide expression analysis reveals dysregulation of myelination-related genes in chronic schizophrenia. Proc Natl Acad Sci U S A 98:4746–4751, 2001

Hallmayer JF, Kalaydjieva L, Badcock J, et al: Genetic evidence for a distinct subtype of schizophrenia characterized by pervasive cognitive deficit. Am J Hum Genet 77:468–476, 2005

Hariri AR, Goldberg TE, Mattay VS, et al: Brain-derived neurotrophic factor val66met polymorphism affects human memory-related hippocampal activity and predicts memory performance. J Neurosci 23:6690–6694, 2003

Harrison PJ: The neuropathology of schizophrenia: a critical review of the data and their interpretation. Brain 122:593–624, 1999

Harrison PJ, Eastwood SL: Neuropathological studies of synaptic connectivity in the hippocampal formation in schizophrenia. Hippocampus 11:508–519, 2001

Harrison PJ, Weinberger DR: Schizophrenia genes, gene expression, and neuropathology: on the matter of their convergence. Mol Psychiatry 10:40–68, 2005

Harrison PJ, Law AJ, Eastwood SL: Glutamate receptors and transporters in the hippocampus in schizophrenia. Ann N Y Acad Sci 1003:94–101, 2003

Hashimoto T, Bergen SE, Nguyen QL, et al: Relationship of brain-derived neurotrophic factor and its receptor TrkB to altered inhibitory prefrontal circuitry in schizophrenia. J Neurosci 25:372–383, 2005

Hatten ME: Central nervous system neuronal migration. Annu Rev Neurosci 22:511–539, 1999

Heinrichs RW, Zakzanis KK: Neurocognitive deficit in schizophrenia: a quantitative review of the evidence. Neuropsychology 12:426–445, 1998

Hennah W, Tuulio-Henriksson A, Paunio T, et al: A haplotype within the DISC1 gene is associated with visual memory functions in families with a high density of schizophrenia. Mol Psychiatry 10:1097–1103, 2005

Hill JJ, Hashimoto T, Lewis DA: Molecular mechanisms contributing to dendritic spine alterations in the prefrontal cortex of subjects with schizophrenia. Mol Psychiatry 11:557–566, 2006

Hill K, Mann L, Laws KR, et al: Hypofrontality in schizophrenia: a meta-analysis of functional imaging studies. Acta Psychiatr Scand 110:243–256, 2004

Ho BC, Andreasen NC, Nopoulos P, et al: Progressive structural brain abnormalities and their relationship to clinical outcome: a longitudinal magnetic resonance imaging study early in schizophrenia. Arch Gen Psychiatry 60:585–594, 2003

Hof PR, Haroutunian V, Friedrich VL, et al: Loss and altered spatial distribution of oligodendrocytes in the superior frontal gyrus in schizophrenia. Biol Psychiatry 53:1075–1085, 2003

Hoff AL, Svetina C, Maurizio AM, et al: Familial cognitive deficits in schizophrenia. Am J Med Genet B Neuropsychiatr Genet 133:43–49, 2005

Honea R, Crow TJ, Passingham D, et al: Regional deficits in brain volume in schizophrenia: a meta-analysis of voxel-based morphometry studies. Am J Psychiatry 162:2233–2245, 2005

Honer WG, Young CE: Presynaptic proteins and schizophrenia. Int Rev Neurobiol 59:175–199, 2004

Honer WG, Young C, Falkai P: Synaptic pathology, in The Neuropathology of Schizophrenia. Edited by Harrison PJ, Roberts GW. New York, Oxford University Press, 2000, pp 105–136

Hovatta I, Varilo T, Suvisaari J, et al: A genomewide screen for schizophrenia genes in an isolated Finnish subpopulation, suggesting multiple susceptibility loci. Am J Hum Genet 65:1114–1124, 1999

Ishizuka K, Paek M, Kamiya A, et al: A review of Disrupted-In-Schizophrenia-1 (DISC1): neurodevelopment, cognition, and mental conditions. Biol Psychiatry 59:1189–1197, 2006

Iwamoto K, Bundo M, Kato T: Altered expression of mitochondria-related genes in postmortem brains of patients with bipolar disorder or schizophrenia, as revealed by large-scale DNA microarray analysis. Hum Mol Genet 14:241–253, 2005

Jakob H, Beckmann H: Prenatal developmental disturbances in the limbic allocortex in schizophrenics. J Neural Transm 65:303–326, 1986

Jakob H, Beckmann H: Gross and histological criteria for developmental disorders in brains of schizophrenics. J Royal Soc Med 82:466–469, 1989

Jakob H, Beckmann H: Circumscribed malformation and nerve cell alterations in the entorhinal cortex of schizophrenics: pathogenetic and clinical aspects. J Neural Transm 98:83–106, 1994

Javitt DC, Zukin SR: Recent advances in the phencyclidine model of schizophrenia. Am J Psychiatry 148:1301–1308, 1991

Javitt DC, Steinschneider M, Schroeder C, et al: Role of cortical N-methyl-D-aspartate receptors in auditory sensory memory and mismatch negativity generation: implications of schizophrenia. Proc Natl Acad Sci U S A 93:11962–11967, 1996

Javitt DC, Shelley A, Ritter W: Associated deficits in mismatch negativity generation and tone matching in schizophrenia. Clin Neurophysiol 111:1733–1737, 2000

Jensen JE, Miller J, Williamson PC, et al: Focal changes in brain energy and phospholipid metabolism in first-episode schizophrenia: 31P-MRS chemical shift imaging study at 4 Tesla. Br J Psychiatry 184:409–415, 2004

Jessen F, Scherk H, Traber F, et al: Proton magnetic resonance spectroscopy in subjects at risk for schizophrenia. Schizophr Res 87:81–88, 2006

Jones LB, Johnson N, Byne W: Alterations in MAP2 immunocytochemistry in areas 9 and 32 of schizophrenic prefrontal cortex. Psychiatry Res 114:137–148, 2002

Kanaan RA, Kim JS, Kaufmann WE, et al: Diffusion tensor imaging in schizophrenia. Biol Psychiatry 58:921–929, 2005

Karry R, Klein E, Ben Shachar D: Mitochondrial complex I subunits expression is altered in schizophrenia: a postmortem study. Biol Psychiatry 55:676–684, 2004

Kerr SL, Neale JM: Emotion perception in schizophrenia: specific deficit or further evidence of generalized poor performance? J Abnorm Psychol 102:312–318, 1993

Keshavan MS, Stanley JA, Pettegrew JW: Magnetic resonance spectroscopy in schizophrenia: methodological issues and findings, part II. Biol Psychiatry 48:369–380, 2000

Kirkpatrick B, Conley RC, Kakoyannis A, et al: Interstitial cells of the white matter in the inferior parietal cortex in schizophrenia: an unbiased cell-counting study. Synapse 34:95–102, 1999

Kohler CG, Bilker W, Hagendoorn M, et al: Emotion recognition deficit in schizophrenia: association with symptomatology and cognition. Biol Psychiatry 48:127–136, 2000a

Kohler CG, Gur RC, Gur RE: Emotional processes in schizophrenia: a focus on affective states, in The Neuropsychology of Emotion. Edited by Borod JC. Oxford, UK, Oxford University Press, 2000b, pp 432–455

Kolomeets NS, Uranova NA: Synaptic contacts in schizophrenia: studies using immunocytochemical identification of dopaminergic neurons. Neurosci Behav Physiol 29:217–221, 1999

Konick LC, Friedman L: Meta-analysis of thalamic size in schizophrenia. Biol Psychiatry 49:28–38, 2001

Kopala LC, Clark C, Hurwitz T: Olfactory deficits in neuroleptic naive patients with schizophrenia. Schizophr Res 8:245–250, 1993

Kovelman JA, Scheibel AB: A neurohistological correlate of schizophrenia. Biol Psychiatry 19:1601–1621, 1984

Kraepelin E: Dementia Praecox and Paraphrenia. Edinburgh, Scotland, E & S Livingston, 1919

Krimer LS, Herman MM, Saunders RC, et al: A qualitative and quantitative analysis of the entorhinal cortex in schizophrenia. Cereb Cortex 7:732–739, 1997

Kring AM, Neale JM: Do schizophrenia patients show a disjunctive relationship among expressive, experiential, and psychophysiological components of emotion? J Abnorm Psychol 105:249–257, 1996

Kubicki M, Westin CF, McCarley RW, et al: The application of DTI to investigate white matter abnormalities in schizophrenia. Ann N Y Acad Sci 1064:134–148, 2005

Kung L, Conley R, Chute DJ, et al: Synaptic changes in the striatum of schizophrenic cases: a controlled postmortem ultrastructural study. Synapse 28:125–139, 1998

Kung L, Roberts RC: Mitochondrial pathology in human schizophrenic striatum: a postmortem ultrastructural study. Synapse 31:67–75, 1999

Kurylo DD, Pasternak R, Silipo G, et al: Perceptual organization by proximity and similarity in schizophrenia. Schizophr Res 95:205–214, 2007

Lauer M, Beckmann H, Senitz D: Increased frequency of dentate granule cells with basal dendrites in the hippocampal formation of schizophrenics. Psychiatry Res 12:89–97, 2003

Law AJ, Shannon Weickert C, Hyde TM, et al: Neuregulin-1 (NRG-1) mRNA and protein in the adult human brain. Neuroscience 127:125–136, 2004

Lawrie SM, Johnstone EC, Weinberger DR: Schizophrenia: From Neuroimaging to Neuroscience. Oxford, UK, Oxford University Press, 2004

LeDoux JE: Emotion circuits in the brain. Annu Rev Neurosci 23:155–184, 2000

Lee K-H, Williams L, Breakspear M, et al: Synchronous gamma activity: a review and contribution to an integrative neuroscience model of schizophrenia. Brain Res Rev 41:57–78, 2003

Lewis CM, Levinson DF, Wise LH, et al: Genome scan meta-analysis of schizophrenia and bipolar disorder, part II: schizophrenia. Am J Hum Genet 73:34–48, 2003

Lewis DA, Glantz LA: Specificity of decreased spine density on layer III pyramidal cells in schizophrenia. Schizophr Res 24:39, 1997

Lewis DA, Melchitzky DS, Sesack SR, et al: Dopamine transporter immunoreactivity in monkey cerebral cortex: regional, laminar, and ultrastructural localization. J Comp Neurol 432:119–136, 2001

Lewis DA, Hashimoto T, Volk DW: Cortical inhibitory neurons and schizophrenia. Nat Rev Neurosci 6:312–324, 2005

Li W, Zhang Q, Oiso N, et al: Hermansky-Pudlak syndrome type 7 (HPS-7) results from mutant dysbindin, a member of the biogenesis of lysosome-related organelles complex 1 (BLOC-1). Nat Genet 35:84–89, 2003

Lindholm E, Ekholm B, Shaw S, et al: A schizophrenia-susceptibility locus at 6q25, in one of the world's largest reported pedigrees. Am J Hum Genet 69:96–105, 2001

Lipska BK, Lerman DN, Khaing ZZ, et al: Gene expression in dopamine and GABA systems in an animal model of schizophrenia: effects of antipsychotic drugs. Eur J Neurosci 18:391–402, 2003

Lipska BK, Peters T, Hyde TM, et al: Expression of DISC1 binding partners is reduced in schizophrenia and associated with DISC1 SNPs. Hum Mol Genet 15:1245–1258, 2006

Luby ED, Cohen BD, Rosenbaum G, et al: Study of a new schizophrenomimetic drug: sernyl. AMA Arch Neurol Psychiatry 81:363–369, 1959

Matsuzawa J, Matsui M, Konishi T, et al: Age-related volumetric changes of brain gray and white matter in healthy infants and children. Cereb Cortex 11:335–342, 2001

Maurer I, Zierz S, Moller H: Evidence for a mitochondrial oxidative phosphorylation defect in brains from patients with schizophrenia. Schizophr Res 48:125–136, 2001

McCullumsmith RE, Gupta D, Beneyto M, et al: Expression of transcripts for myelination-related genes in the anterior cingulate cortex in schizophrenia. Schizophr Res 90:15–27, 2007

Middleton FA, Mirnics K, Pierri JN, et al: Gene expression profiling reveals alterations of specific metabolic pathways in schizophrenia. J Neurosci 22:2718–2729, 2002

Mirnics K, Middleton FA, Stanwood GD, et al: Disease-specific changes in regulator of G-protein signaling 4 (RGS4) expression in schizophrenia. Mol Psychiatry 6:293–301, 2001

Moberg PJ, Agrin, RN, Gur RE, et al: Olfactory dysfunction in schizophrenia: a qualitative and quantitative review. Neuropsychopharmacology 21:325–340, 1999

Moberg PJ, Arnold SE, Doty RL, et al: Olfactory functioning in schizophrenia: relationship to clinical, neuropsychological, and volumetric MRI measures. J Clin Exp Neuropsychol 28:1444–1461, 2006

Moises HW, Kristbjarnarson H, Yang L, et al: A two-stage genome-wide search for schizophrenia susceptibility genes. Psychiatr Genet 5:S33, 1995

Nelson MD, Saykin AJ, Flashman LA, et al: Hippocampal volume reduction in schizophrenia as assessed by magnetic resonance imaging: a meta-analytic study. Arch Gen Psychiatry 55:433–440, 1998

Nowakowski RS, Rakic P: The site of origin and route and rate of migration of neurons to the hippocampal region in the rhesus monkey. J Comp Neurol 196:129–154, 1981

Numakawa T, Yagasaki Y, Ishimoto T, et al: Evidence of novel neuronal functions of dysbindin, a susceptibility gene for schizophrenia. Hum Mol Genet 13:2699–2708, 2004

O'Donovan MC, Owen MJ: The molecular genetics of schizophrenia. Ann Med 28:541–546, 1996

Owen MJ, Craddock N, O'Donovan MC: Schizophrenia: genes at last? Trends Genet 21:518–525, 2005

Pantev C, Makeig S, Hoke M, et al: Human auditory evoked gamma-band magnetic fields. Proc Natl Acad Sci U S A 88:8996–9000, 1991

Patel SH, Azzam PN: Characterization of N200 and P300: selected studies of the event-related potential. Int J Med Sci 2:147–154, 2005

Paulson L, Martin P, Persson A, et al: Comparative genome- and proteome analysis of cerebral cortex from MK-801-treated rats. J Neurosci Res 71:526–533, 2003

Pfurtscheller G, Lopes da Silva FH: Event-related EEG/MEG synchronization and desynchronization: basic principles. Clin Neurophysiol 110:1842–1857, 1999

Plomin R, Kosslyn SM: Genes, brain and cognition. Nat Neurosci 4:1153–1154, 2001

Polich J: Clinical application of the P300 event-related brain potential. Phys Med Rehabil Clin N Am 15:133–161, 2004

Posthuma D, Luciano M, Geus EJ, et al: A genomewide scan for intelligence identifies quantitative trait loci on 2q and 6p. Am J Hum Genet 77:318–326, 2005

Prabakaran S, Swatton JE, Ryan MM, et al: Mitochondrial dysfunction in schizophrenia: evidence for compromised brain metabolism and oxidative stress. Mol Psychiatry 9:684–697, 2004

Prasad KM, Chowdari KV, Nimgaonkar VL, et al: Genetic polymorphisms of the RGS4 and dorsolateral prefrontal cortex morphometry among first episode schizophrenia patients. Mol Psychiatry 10:213–219, 2005

Prince JA, Blennow K, Gottfries CG, et al: Mitochondrial function is differentially altered in the basal ganglia of chronic schizophrenics. Neuropsychopharmacol 21:372–379, 1999

Pulver AE, Karayiorgou M, Lasseter VK, et al: Follow-up of a report of a potential linkage for schizophrenia on chromosome 22q12-q13.1, part 2. Am J Med Genet 54:44–50, 1994a

Pulver AE, Karayiorgou M, Wolyniec PS, et al: Sequential strategy to identify a susceptibility gene for schizophrenia: report of potential linkage on chromosome 22q12-q13.1, part 1. Am J Med Genetics 54:36–43, 1994b

Raghavachari S, Kahana MJ, Rizzuto DS, et al: Gating of human theta oscillations by a working memory task. J Neurosci 21:3175–3183, 2001

Rajkowska G, Halaris A, Selemon LD: Reductions in neuronal and glial density characterize the dorsolateral prefrontal cortex in bipolar disorder. Biol Psychiatry 49:741–752, 2001

Revheim N, Butler PD, Schechter I, et al: Reading impairment and visual processing deficits in schizophrenia. Schizophr Res 87:238–245, 2006

Riley B, Kendler KS: Molecular genetic studies of schizophrenia. Eur J Hum Genet 14:669–680, 2006

Rioux L, Nissanov J, Lauber K, et al: Distribution of microtubule-associated protein MAP2-immunoreactive interstitial neurons in the parahippocampal white matter in subjects with schizophrenia. Am J Psychiatry 160:149–155, 2003

Risch N, Merikangas K: The future of genetic studies of complex human diseases. Science 273:1516–1517, 1996

Roberts RC, Conley R, Kung L, et al: Reduced striatal spine size in schizophrenia: a postmortem ultrastructural study. Neuroreport 7:1214–1218, 1996

Rosoklija G, Kaufman MA, Liu D, et al: Subicular MAP-2 immunoreactivity in schizophrenia. Society for Neuroscience Abstracts 21:2126, 1995

Rosoklija G, Toomayan G, Ellis SP, et al: Structural abnormalities of subicular dendrites in subjects with schizophrenia and mood disorders: preliminary findings. Arch Gen Psychiatry 57:349–356, 2000

Rosoklija G, Keilip JG, Toomayan G: Altered subicular MAP2 immunoreactivity in schizophrenia. Prilozi 26:13–34, 2005

Saykin AJ, Gur RC, Gur RE, et al: Neuropsychological function in schizophrenia: selective impairment in memory and learning. Arch Gen Psychiatry 48:618–624, 1991

Saykin AJ, Shtasel DL, Gur RE, et al: Neuropsychological deficits in neuroleptic-naive, first-episode schizophrenic patients. Arch Gen Psychiatry 51:124–131, 1994

Schwab SG, Albus M, Hallmayer J, et al: Evaluation of a susceptibility gene for schizophrenia on chromosome 6p by multipoint affected sib-pair linkage analysis. Nat Genet 11:325–327, 1995a

Schwab SG, Lerer B, Albus M, et al: Potential linkage for schizophrenia on chromosome 22q12-q13: a replication study. Am J Med Genet 60:436–443, 1995b

Schwab SG, Eckstein GN, Hallmayer J, et al: Evidence suggestive of a locus on chromosome 5q31 contributing to susceptibility for schizophrenia in German and Israeli families by multipoint affected sib-pair linkage analysis. Mol Psychiatry 2:156–160, 1997

Schwab SG, Hallmayer J, Albus M, et al: Further evidence for a susceptibility locus on chromosome 10p14-p11 in 72 families with schizophrenia by nonparametric linkage analysis. Am J Med Genet 81:302–307, 1998

Sederberg PB, Kahana MJ, Howard MW, et al: Theta and gamma oscillations during encoding predict subsequent recall. J Neurosci 23:10809–10814, 2003

Seidman LJ, Faraone SV, Goldstein JM, et al: Left hippocampal volume as a vulnerability indicator for schizophrenia: a magnetic resonance imaging morphometric study of nonpsychotic first-degree relatives. Arch Gen Psychiatry 59:839–849, 2002

Selemon LD, Rajkowska G, Goldman-Rakic PS: Elevated neuronal density in prefrontal area 46 in brains from schizophrenic patients: application of a three-dimensional, stereologic counting method. J Comp Neurol 392:402–412, 1998

Sesack SR, Hawrylak VA, Matus C, et al: Dopamine axon varicosities in the prelimbic division of the rat prefrontal cortex exhibit sparse immunoreactivity for the dopamine transporter. J Neurosci 18:2697–2708, 1998

Sharma T, Harvey P (eds): Cognition in Schizophrenia. Oxford, UK, Oxford University Press, 1999

Shedlack K, Lee G, Sakuma M, et al: Language processing and memory in ill and well siblings from multiplex families affected with schizophrenia. Schizophr Res 25:43–52, 1997

Shenton ME, Dickey CC, Frumin M, et al: A review of MRI findings in schizophrenia. Schizophr Res 49:1–52, 2001

Shirts BH, Nimgaonkar V: The genes for schizophrenia: finally a breakthrough? Curr Psychiatry Rep 6:303–312, 2004

Siegel SJ, Connolly P, Liang Y, et al: Effects of strain, novelty, and NMDA blockade on auditory-evoked potentials in mice, Neuropsychopharmacol 28:675–682, 2003

Soustek Z: Ultrastructure of cortical synapses in the brain of schizophrenics. Zentralbl Allg Pathol 135:25–32, 1989

Spencer K, Nestor P, Niznikiewicz M, et al: Abnormal neural synchrony in schizophrenia. J Neurosci 23:7407–7411, 2003

Staal WG, Hulshoff Pol HE, Schnack HG, et al: Structural brain abnormalities in patients with schizophrenia and their healthy siblings. Am J Psychiatry 157:416–421, 2000

Stanley JA, Williamson PC, Drost DJ, et al: An in vivo study of the prefrontal cortex of schizophrenic patients at different stages of illness via phosphorus magnetic resonance spectroscopy. Arch Gen Psychiatry 52:399–406, 1995

Stanley JA, Pettegrew JW, Keshavan MS: Magnetic resonance spectroscopy in schizophrenia: methodological issues and findings, part I. Biol Psychiatry 48:357–368, 2000

Steen RG, Hamer RM, Lieberman JA: Measurement of brain metabolites by 1H magnetic resonance spectroscopy in patients with schizophrenia: a systematic review and meta-analysis. Neuropsychopharmacology 30:1949–1962, 2005

Stephan KE, Baldeweg T, Friston KJ: Synaptic plasticity and dysconnection in schizophrenia. Biol Psychiatry 59:929–939, 2006

Straub RE, MacLean CJ, Kendler KS: The putative schizophrenia locus on chromosome 6p: a brief overview of the linkage studies. Mol Psychiatry 1:89–92, 1996

Suarez BK, Duan J, Sanders AR, et al: Genomewide linkage scan of 409 European-ancestry and African American families with schizophrenia: suggestive evidence of linkage at 8p23.3-p21.2 and 11p13.1-q14.1 in the combined sample. Am J Hum Genet 78:315–333, 2006

Sweet RA, Bergen SE, Sun Z, et al: Anatomical evidence of impaired feedforward auditory processing in schizophrenia. Biol Psychiatry 61:854–864, 2007

Szekeres G, Keri S, Juhasz A, et al: Role of dopamine D3 receptor (DRD3) and dopamine transporter (DAT) polymorphism in cognitive dysfunctions and therapeutic response to atypical antipsychotics in patients with schizophrenia. Am J Med Genet B Neuropsychiatr Genet 124:1–5, 2004

Szeszko PR, Lipsky R, Mentschel C, et al: Brain-derived neurotrophic factor val66met polymorphism and volume of the hippocampal formation. Mol Psychiatry 10:631–636, 2005

Talbot K, Eidem WL, Tinsley CL, et al: Dysbindin-1 is reduced in intrinsic, glutamatergic terminals of the hippocampal formation in schizophrenia. J Clin Invest 113:1353–1363, 2004

Talbot K, Cho DS, Ong WY, et al: Dysbindin-1 is a synaptic and microtubular protein that binds brain snapin. Hum Mol Genet 15:3041–3054, 2006

Talbott PS, Laruelle M: The role of in vivo molecular imaging with PET and SPECT in the elucidation of psychiatric drug action and new drug development. Eur Neuropsychopharmacol 12:503–511, 2002

Tauscher J, Kapur S: Choosing the right dose of antipsychotics in schizophrenia: lessons from neuroimaging studies. CNS Drugs 15:671–678, 2001

Thompson JL, Watson JR, Steinhauer SR, et al: Indicators of genetic liability to schizophrenia: a sibling study of neuropsychological performance. Schizophr Bull 31:85–96, 2005

Tibbo P, Hanstock C, Valiakalayil A, et al: 3-T proton MRS investigation of glutamate and glutamine in adolescents at high genetic risk for schizophrenia. Am J Psychiatry 161:1116–1118, 2004

Tunbridge EM, Harrison PJ, Weinberger DR: Catechol-O-methyltransferase, cognition, and psychosis: Val(158)Met and beyond. Biol Psychiatry 60:141–151, 2006

Turetsky BI, Moberg PJ, Yousem DM, et al: Reduced olfactory bulb volume in patients with schizophrenia. Am J Psychiatry 157:828–830, 2000

Tuulio-Henriksson A, Arajarvi R, Partonen T, et al: Familial loading associates with impairment in visual span among healthy siblings of schizophrenia patients. Biol Psychiatry 54:623–628, 2003

Uhlhaas PJ, Linden DE, Singer W, et al: Dysfunctional long-range coordination of neural activity during Gestalt perception in schizophrenia. J Neurosci 26:8168–8175, 2006

Umbricht D, Vyssotky D, Latanov A, et al: Midlatency auditory event-related potentials in mice: comparison to midlatency auditory ERPs in humans. Brain Res 1019:189–200, 2004

Uranova NA, Klintzova AJ, Istomin VV, et al: The effects of amphetamine on synaptic plasticity in rat's medial prefrontal cortex. J Hirnforsch 30:45–50, 1989

Uranova NA, Casanova MF, DeVaughn NM, et al: Ultrastructural alterations of synaptic contacts and astrocytes in postmortem caudate nucleus of schizophrenic patients. Schizophr Res 22:81–83, 1996

Uranova N, Orlovskaya D, Vikhreva O, et al: Electron microscopy of oligodendroglia in severe mental illness. Brain Res Bull 55:597–610, 2001

Vita A, De Peri L, Silenzi C, et al: Brain morphology in first-episode schizophrenia: a meta-analysis of quantitative magnetic resonance imaging studies. Schizophr Res 82:75–88, 2006

Wang S, Sun CE, Walczak CA, et al: Evidence for a susceptibility locus for schizophrenia on chromosome 6pter-p22. Nat Genet 10:41–46, 1995

Wassef A, Baker J, Kochan LD: GABA and schizophrenia: a review of basic science and clinical studies. J Clin Psychopharmacol 23:601–640, 2003

Weickert CS, Straub RE, McClintock BW, et al: Human dysbindin (DTNBP1) gene expression in normal brain and in schizophrenic prefrontal cortex and midbrain. Arch Gen Psychiatry 61:544–555, 2004

Weinberger DR, Egan MF, Bertolino A, et al: Prefrontal neurons and the genetics of schizophrenia. Biol Psychiatry 50:825–844, 2001

Whatley SA, Curti D, Marchbanks RM: Mitochondrial involvement in schizophrenia and other functional psychoses. Neurochem Res 21:995–1004, 1996

Williams NM, Norton N, Williams H, et al: A systematic genome-wide linkage study in 353 sib pairs with schizophrenia. Am J Hum Genet 73:1355–1367, 2003

Winterer G, Coppola R, Goldberg TE, et al: Prefrontal broadband noise, working memory, and genetic risk for schizophrenia. Am J Psychiatry 161:490–500, 2004

Wright IC, Rabe-Hesketh S, Woodruff PW, et al: Meta-analysis of regional brain volumes in schizophrenia. Am J Psychiatry 157:16–25, 2000

Wright IC, Sham P, Murray RM, et al: Genetic contributions to regional variability in human brain structure: methods and preliminary results. Neuroimage 17:256–271, 2002

Zaidel DW, Esiri MM, Harrison PJ: Size, shape, and orientation of neurons in the left and right hippocampus: investigations of normal asymmetries and alterations in schizophrenia. Am J Psychiatry 154:812–818, 1997

Zakzanis KK, Poulin P, Hansen KT, et al: Searching the schizophrenic brain for temporal lobe deficits: a systematic review and meta-analysis. Psychol Med 30:491–504, 2000

CHAPTER 47

Neurobiology of Anxiety Disorders

Jonathan M. Amiel, M.D.

Sanjay J. Mathew, M.D.

Amir Garakani, M.D.

Alexander Neumeister, M.D.

Dennis S. Charney, M.D.

Our understanding of the neurobiological basis of fear and anxiety continues to improve at a rapid pace. The principal brain regions involved in processing and responding to anxiety are known, many neurochemical systems mediating responses to fearful stimuli have been identified, and new technologies are advancing the study of the interactions of these brain regions with one another. There is also active investigation regarding the relationship between genes and the environment in the development of chronically dysregulated anxiety with the hope that characterizing the neurobiology of anxiety will bring forth therapeutic advances that reduce the significant burden and long-term functional impairment associated with anxiety disorders.

In this chapter, we review preclinical and clinical data relevant to normal and pathological anxiety states. We begin with a brief summary of paradigms of fear learning. We then relate these preclinical paradigms with their neuroanatomical functional localization observed in animals models and more recently in humans with anxiety disorders. Subsequently, we present the major neurochemical systems mediating anxiety processes with a selection of supporting preclinical and clinical data. We then briefly describe findings specific to several of the individual anxiety disorders—panic disorder with and without agoraphobia, specific and social phobias, and posttraumatic stress

disorder (PTSD)—and we comment on the state of investigations into the genetic basis of anxiety. We conclude with some of the key questions that will drive future research investigations. The neural circuitry of generalized anxiety disorder (GAD) may be distinct from the disorders noted above (Coplan et al. 2006; Mathew et al. 2008), and will not be further addressed in this chapter. Likewise, although obsessive-compulsive disorder (OCD) is categorized as an anxiety disorder in DSM-IV-TR (American Psychiatric Association 2000), there appears to be sufficient symptomatic and epidemiological heterogeneity between OCD and the other anxiety disorders that it will not be addressed in this chapter (Hollander et al. 2007).

Neural Paradigms of Fear and Anxiety

Fear Learning Processes

Investigations into anxiety states depend on a heuristic by which an individual becomes frightened of a novel stimulus and develops means to avoid this stimulus and its implied danger. These means include forming a short-term memory of the stimulus and consolidating this fleeting memory into a long-term memory associated with an avoidant behavior. The retained memories are dynamic and, when evoked by subsequent experience, are subject to change including retention (reconsolidation) or deletion (extinction). Anxiety is the emotional response to new and remembered frightening stimuli.

Formal studies of fear learning processes date back to the experiments of the Russian physiologist Ivan Pavlov in the late nineteenth century. Pavlov's conditional reflex, an involuntary response that was conditionally based on prior experiences, formed the basis for the enduring fear learning paradigm of classical conditioning (Pavlov 1927). Pavlov observed that dogs have habitual responses to salient stimuli, such as salivating when presented with food. He then observed that animals exposed to a neutral stimulus, such as the sound of a bell, repeatedly paired with a salient stimulus would associate the two stimuli, and the environment in which they were trained, and enact the same habitual response whether presented with the salient stimulus, the neutral stimulus, or even just the environment in which they were trained. Thus, the dog that salivates when presented with food also salivates to the sound of a bell or when entering the training laboratory. The salient stimulus was termed an unconditioned stimulus (US), the neutral stimulus was termed the conditioned stimulus (CS), the habitual response to the US was termed the unconditioned response (UR), and the habitual response to the CS was termed the conditioned response (CR). The association of the CS with the US is learning by explicit cue, whereas the association of the CS with the training environment is learning by context.

The principles of classical conditioning apply to fear learning when the US is aversive and the UR includes the range of motor, autonomic, and endocrine behaviors of the fight-or-flight response. Whereas in healthy people fear learning allows for situational anticipation of danger and generates an adaptive and protective vigilance, people with anxiety disorders frequently mount this response to misinterpreted or neutral stimuli. These maladaptive hypervigilant responses, and their associated avoidant behaviors, are likely to be central to the "fear circuitry" anxiety disorders, including panic disorder, specific and social phobias, and PTSD.

Memory, Consolidation, and Reconsolidation

The conversion of experience into memory is called *consolidation* and relies on changes in synaptic affinity first proposed by the Spanish neuroanatomist Santiago Ramón y Cajal (1894). With brief stimulation, neuronal in-

terconnections transiently strengthen while stimulation of sufficient quantity and appropriate quality causes enduring changes in synaptic strength and structure (reviewed by Bailey et al. 2004). The brief and transient retention of memory is called *sensitization* and occurs due to enhancement of glutamatergic transmission via the α-amino-3-hydroxy-5-methylisoxazole-4-propionic acid (AMPA) receptor, while *long-term potentiation* (LTP) refers to the lasting changes in synaptic affinity in which persistent glutamatergic stimulation of the N-methyl-D-aspartate (NMDA) receptor initiates a signaling cascade ending in gene transcription and protein synthesis (reviewed in Malenka and Bear 2004).

The hippocampus and amygdala are key areas in which LTP and, therefore, consolidation, occur. This finding was particularly evident in the case of H.M., a young man who underwent bilateral medial temporal resections to treat his intractable epilepsy and after surgery experienced complete anterograde amnesia and, to a lesser degree, retrograde amnesia (Scoville and Milner 1957). Many animal models have replicated this clinical finding, and hippocampal LTP was recently documented in an in vivo mouse model (Whitlock et al. 2006).

As in Pavlov's experiments, stimuli that are pertinent, or salient, are more likely to be remembered than neutral events. Fear-inducing or emotion-evoking experiences generate a glucocorticoid and catecholamine flux, as we will describe below, which selectively enhances memory consolidation by activating the basolateral complex of the amygdala, an effect which can be blocked by administration of β-adrenoreceptor antagonists (Roozendaal et al. 2006). This paradigm holds true in humans, where memory for an emotional story is superior to memory for a nonemotional story (Cahill et al. 1994). A study showing increased noradrenergic activity after viewing an emotional story suggests that similar neurochemical signaling may be implicated (Southwick et al. 2002). However, clinical trials studying secondary prevention of PTSD with propranolol shortly after exposure to trauma have been equivocal (reviewed in Pitman and Delahanty 2005).

An interesting finding from the late 1960s suggested an additional level of complexity to memory mechanisms. Classically conditioned rats undergoing electroconvulsive shock, which reliably induces retrograde amnesia, 1 day after training (a long enough period of time for consolidation to have occurred) retained their training, but rats that were reexposed to the CS shortly before electroconvulsive treatment lost their conditioning (Misanin et al. 1968). This finding suggested that when retrieved, long-term memories are subject to modification and must undergo reconsolidation (reviewed in Riccio et al. 2006). Like consolidation, reconsolidation is enacted through a signaling cascade ending in protein synthesis, though these two processes employ independent and dissociable cellular processes (Lee at al. 2004).

Extinction

After Pavlov classically conditioned his dogs to salivate (UR) to the sound of a bell (CS), he found that repeated presentation of the bell (CS) in the absence of food (US) diminished the dogs' salivatory response in a process called *extinction* (Pavlov 1927). Rather than erasing the conditioning process from memory, extinction is a process of integrating new memory that may reverse with a change of context or renewed pairing with the US (Bouton 2004). Like consolidation, extinction involves a cell-signaling cascade and protein synthesis. Glutamatergic NMDA receptors in the amygdala play a key role, and extinction may be blocked by NMDA receptor antagonists like AP5 (Falls et al. 1992) or γ-aminobutyric acid (GABA), an effect that is reversible with D-cycloserine (DCS), an NMDA partial agonist (Akirav 2007).

Extinction is thought to occur by the medial prefrontal cortex's inhibiting the lateral amygdala under hippocampal modulation (Sotres-Bayon et al. 2006). Inactivation of the medial prefrontal cortex by surgical lesion (Milad and Quirk 2002) or local chemical blockade of protein synthesis disables extinction (Santini et al. 2004). Supporting this model, people with PTSD have been found to have depressed ventral medial prefrontal cortex activity during exposure to traumatic reminders (Bremner et al. 1999b).

Clinically, employing extinction to "de-link" neutral stimuli from aversive responses is an important goal of psychotherapy and pharmacotherapy of anxiety disorders. Small clinical trials have shown some benefits to augmenting exposure therapy or cognitive-behavioral therapy with medications to enhance the extinction learning process. In one trial, DCS combined with exposure therapy improved acrophobic symptoms early in treatment and maintained benefit at 3 months (Ressler et al. 2004). This benefit was not observed in the treatment of spider or snake phobias (Guastella et al. 2007a, 2007b). A recent trial of DCS given prior to exposure therapy in people with social anxiety disorder showed significant but modest effects in symptom severity, cognitive dysfunction, and functional impairment (Guastella et al. 2008). A number of larger trials of DCS in several of the anxiety disorders are currently under way.

Neuroanatomy of Fear and Anxiety

The neuroanatomical substrates of anxiety detect, process, modulate, and respond to fearful stimuli serially and in parallel with one another, with varying degrees of conscious awareness. Afferent structures are the visual, auditory, vestibular, gustatory, and somatosensory receptors that transmit stimuli to the thalamus. The thalamus distributes signals to brain stem nuclei for automatic reflexes, to the basolateral amygdala via a direct subcortical "short loop" for rapid processing, and to primary and associative sensory, insular, cingulate, and prefrontal cortices that feed back to the amygdala via an indirect "long loop" for higher-order processing and modulation (LeDoux 2000). Olfactory afferents bypass the thalamus and project directly to the entorhinal cortex and the amygdala. Viscerosensory afferents communicate primarily with the nucleus of the solitary tract in the brain stem that relays signals to the central nucleus of the amygdala. Primary sensory cortices and their related association areas form a reciprocal neural circuit with the amygdala and hippocampus by which continued processing, comparison, and learning take place. Expressions of fear are effected through the motor pathways and the neuroendocrine autonomic pathways involving the hypothalamus and pituitary glands, the bed nucleus of the stria terminalis (BNST) and the raphe nuclei, periaqueductal gray matter, and locus coeruleus of the brain stem. In normal function, this network of afferent, modulatory, and efferent pathways offers protection from physical and psychological threats. When dysregulated, pathological anxiety imposes undue behavioral inhibition and resultant decline in social functioning (Figure 47–1).

The existence of direct and indirect pathways to amygdalar activation via the short and long loops suggests that the amygdala integrates sensory information with previous experience to determine the significance of complex stimuli and trigger responses based on the determined value of the stimuli. The lasting changes that occur in the amygdala in response to fearful cues occur via LTP in the pathways involving AMPA and NMDA glutamate receptors, calcium fluxes, and protein synthesis described above (reviewed in LeDoux 2007). The pharmacological inhibition of glutamatergic tone and, to a lesser degree, calcium fluxes has been shown to reduce anxiety in several anxiety disorders (reviewed in Amiel and Mathew 2007; Balon and Ramesh 1996). Recent functional magnetic resonance imaging (MRI) studies of the processing of conscious and unconscious fearful images have implicated subspecificity within the amygdala,

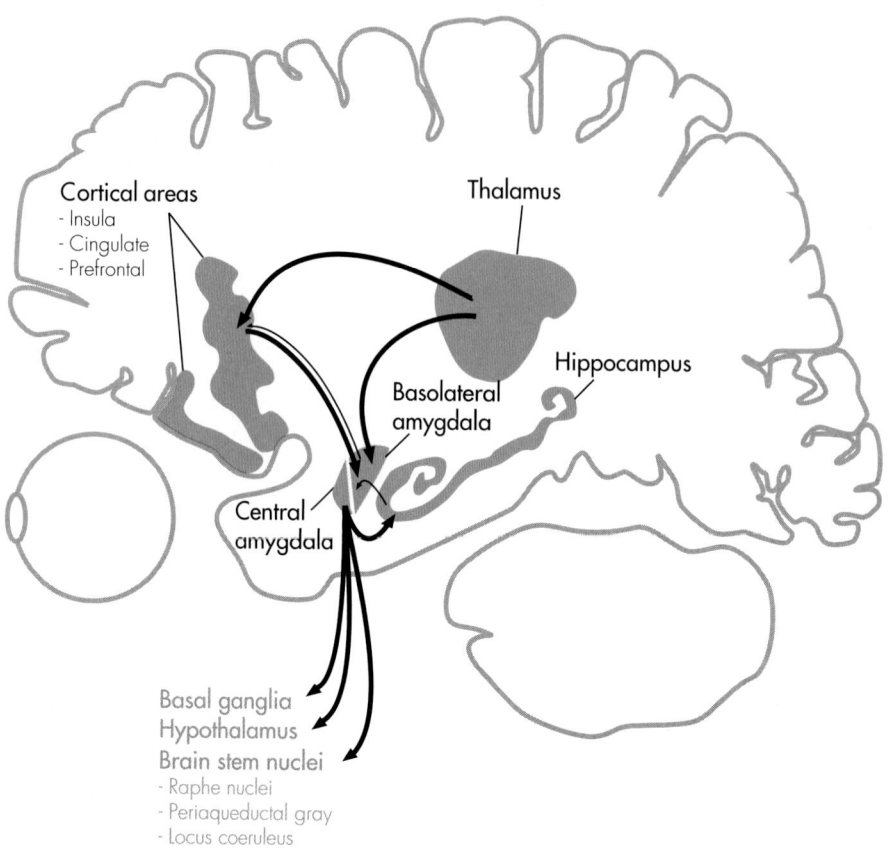

FIGURE 47-1.   Brain circuits implicated in fear and anxiety.

A major function of the amygdala is the integration of information from the thalamus and cortical regions into efferent signals (*thick arrows*). Integration of signals occurs in the basolateral amygdaloid complex, whereas efferent responses are mediated by the central nucleus. Reciprocal circuits to the cortex and the hippocampus are particularly relevant to affective modulation and contextual memory (*thin arrows*).

with conscious processing modulated in the dorsal amygdala and unconscious processing modulated in the basolateral complex (Etkin et al. 2004). In contrast, contextual fear learning also requires the recruitment of the hippocampus and the BNST (Walker and Davis 1997).

When fear-evoking stimuli are perceived and their processing and modulation do not result in inhibition of the stimulus, the efferent mechanisms of the anxiety–fear circuit generate a range of autonomic, neuroendocrine, and motor responses originally named by Walter Cannon (1915) as the fight-or-flight response. In particular, the lateral nucleus and intercalated cells of the amygdala engage the central nucleus that is the principal output of the amygdala (see Figure 47–1). The central nucleus activates the sympathetic nervous system via the lateral hypothalamus, the parasympathetic nervous system via the dorsal motor nucleus of the vagus nerve, the endogenous opioid system via the periaqueductal gray matter, and the major neurotransmitters of the central nervous system (norepinephrine, dopamine, serotonin, and acetylcholine) via

their brain stem nuclei (Schafe et al. 2001). The amygdala also engages the motor system through its connectivity with the motor cortex and the extrapyramidal corticostriatal-pallidal motor system (McDonald 1991). Interestingly, while the experience of an aversive stimulus generates motor activation, there is functional MRI evidence that anticipation of an aversive stimulus causes marked inhibition of primary motor cortex with reciprocal hyperactivity in the basal ganglia (Butler et al. 2007).

Neurochemistry and Genetics of Fear and Anxiety

The anatomical substrates for fear and anxiety described above interact via a diversity of neurochemical messengers. Acute stress triggers the release of these neurotransmitters and neuropeptides, enhancing attention, motor, and memory systems to defend against the present threat and to avoid it in the future. The body upregulates metabolic activity through a surge of catecholamines and glucocorticoids that synergistically increase oxygenation, channel blood flow to the brain and muscle, and make stored energy available. These neurochemical systems operate in a vast and complex network of excitatory, inhibitory, and modulatory circuits. In this section we review the major neurochemical systems that contribute to the fear response under conditions of acute and chronic stress. As anxiety disorders have estimated heritabilities ranging from 30% (Hettema et al. 2001) to 60% when factors of measurement error and gene–environment interactions are controlled (Kendler et al. 1999), we will also discuss data pertaining to genes encoding the receptors that participate in synaptic transmission and modulation of impulses. The heritable component of anxiety is undoubtedly polygenetic, and classical genetic findings that have yielded elegant pathophysiological mechanisms in fields such as oncology and immunology have been elusive.

Noradrenergic System

Noradrenaline/norepinephrine (NE) is a catecholamine that broadly activates cortical, subcortical, and cardiovascular systems via G protein–coupled adrenergic receptors. NE is synthesized from tyrosine peripherally in the adrenal medulla and postganglionic sympathetic efferents and centrally in the locus coeruleus. The locus coeruleus is a small blue-tinted pontine nucleus that constitutes the major noradrenergic cell body aggregate in the brain and is activated most notably in fear states by inputs from the amygdala and the lateral hypothalamus (reviewed in Charney and Drevets 2002). Noradrenergic stimulation of limbic and cortical regions is involved in the elaboration of adaptive responses to stress (Morilak et al. 2005).

Increased NE function accounts for many symptoms of pathological anxiety, such as panic attacks, insomnia, startle, and autonomic hyperarousal (Charney et al. 1987). Cerebrospinal fluid (CSF) NE concentrations are abnormally elevated in PTSD (Geracioti et al. 2001). Platelet α_2-adrenergic receptor density, platelet basal adenosine, isoproterenol, forskolin-stimulated cyclic adenosine monophosphate (cAMP) signal transduction, and basal platelet monoamine oxidase (MAO) activity were decreased in PTSD—findings hypothesized to reflect compensatory responses to chronically elevated NE release (reviewed in Southwick et al. 1999b).

Feedback inhibition appears to play a major role in the regulation of NE activity. Agonists of the presynaptic α_2-adrenergic receptor, including endogenous NE and epinephrine as well as drugs such as clonidine, inhibit the release of NE. α_2-adrenergic receptor antagonists such as yohimbine or idazoxan stimulate the release of NE. People with panic disorder are very sensitive to the anxiogenic effects of yohimbine (Charney et al. 1987). They also have exaggerated plasma 3-methoxy-4-hydroxyphenylglycol (MHPG), cortisol, and cardiovascular responses to the administration of this compound (Charney et al. 1992). People with combat-related PTSD exposed to yohimbine also were reported to have enhanced behavioral, biochemical, and cardiovascular responses (Southwick et al. 1999a). Children with anxiety disorders show greater anxiogenic responses to yohimbine than do nonanxious comparison children (Sallee et al. 2000). The responses to the α_2-adrenergic receptor agonist clonidine are also abnormal in people with panic disorder. Clonidine administration caused greater hypotension and decreases in plasma MHPG, and less sedation, in people with panic disorder than in control subjects (Uhde et al. 1988).

α_2-Adrenergic receptor antagonists have been found to sensitize the locus coeruleus such that excitatory stimuli generate increased responsiveness in the absence of an altered baseline activity, a phenomenon known as sensitization (Simson and Weiss 1988). Clinically, sensitization appears particularly relevant to symptoms of anxiety and PTSD such as tension, irritability, hypervigilance, and exaggerated startle reactivity. The hypothesis that sensitization is implicated in the development of pathological anxiety is supported by clinical studies indicating that repeated exposure to stress is an important risk factor for the development of anxiety disorders, particularly PTSD (Heim and Nemeroff 2001).

Investigation into polymorphisms of the adrenergic receptor has revealed an intriguing insight into the genetic predisposition for the development of pathological anxiety involving noradrenergic synapses. Healthy people homozygous for an in-frame deletion in a subtype of the α_2-adrenergic receptor (α_{2C}-Del322–325) show higher baseline NE levels and more sustained increases in NE levels, heart rate, and anxiety than do control subjects when exposed to yohimbine (Neumeister et al. 2005). A follow-up study of people with this polymorphism and with remitted major depressive disorder found altered recruitment of cortical and limbic brain regions compared with control subjects, suggesting that variability in NE function impacts emotional processing (Neumeister et al. 2006).

Corticotropin-Releasing Hormone

Corticotropin-releasing hormone (CRH) is a principal mediator of the stress response through its well-characterized indirect effects in activating the hypothalamic-pituitary-adrenal (HPA) axis and its lesser-known direct effects in the brain. CRH-containing neurons are located throughout the brain, including the central nucleus of the amygdala, prefrontal and cingulate cortices, BNST, nucleus accumbens, periaqueductal gray, and the noradrenergic locus coeruleus and serotonergic raphe nuclei (Steckler and Holsboer 1999). In response to stress, CRH levels rise and locally activate their target organs via regionally localized CRH_1 and CRH_2 receptors (Sanchez et al. 1999). Animal models studying the differences between CRH_1 and CRH_2 receptor activation suggest opposing function. Mice deficient in CRH_1 display decreased anxiety-like behavior and an impaired stress response (Bale et al. 2002). In contrast, CRH_2-deficient mice display increased anxiety-like behavior and are hypersensitive to stress (Bale et al. 2000; Coste et al. 2000). People with high levels of anxiety and depression, though not depression alone, and homozygous for a GAG haplotype in the CRH_1 locus, were found to respond more robustly to selective serotonin reuptake inhibitors than those without the same polymorphism (Licinio et al. 2004).

Stress-related CRH secretion inhibits a variety of neurovegetative functions such as food intake, sexual activity, and endocrine programs for growth and reproduction. Exposure to stress in early life can produce long-term elevation of CRH (i.e., exaggerated CRH release) and sensitization of CRH neurons to subsequent stress. The long-term response to heightened CRH is individual and may depend on the social environment, trauma history, and behavioral dominance (Strome et al. 2002). Early exposure of the hippocampus to elevated levels of CRH may be associated with hippocampal damage later in life (Brunson et al. 2001).

CSF concentrations of CRH in people with PTSD are increased relative to those in healthy control subjects (Baker et al. 1999). However, cortisol levels in these samples were not increased, as is the case in most PTSD studies. CSF CRH concentrations are not correlated with plasma cortisol (Baker et al. 1999). High levels of cortisol decrease hypothalamic CRH but increase CRH in areas such as the amygdala (Schulkin et al. 1998).

A number of CRH_1 receptor antagonists are currently being evaluated in preclinical and early clinical trials for their efficacy as anxiolytics and antidepressants and their utility in the treatment of substance abuse. Preclinical data show the promise of one of these compounds, R-121919, in treating symptoms of substance withdrawal (Funk et al. 2007). Although clinical data remain prelim-

inary, R-121919 also may have clinical utility in treating depression and anxiety (Ising and Holsboer 2007). These findings await replication in larger randomized trials.

Arginine Vasopressin

Like CRH, arginine vasopressin (AVP) is a major secretagogue of the HPA/stress system. AVP is produced by the parvicellular neurons of the hypothalamic paraventricular nucleus and secreted into the pituitary portal circulation from axon terminals projecting to the external zone of the median eminence. AVP release is triggered primarily by increasing serum osmolality, hypovolemia, hypotension, and hypoglycemia. AVP has corticotropin-releasing properties when administered alone in humans, a response that may depend on the ambient endogenous CRH level. Following the combination of AVP and CRH, a much greater corticotropin response is seen. The sensitivity of CRH and AVP transcription to glucocorticoid feedback apparently differs, and AVP-stimulated corticotropin secretion may be refractory to glucocorticoid feedback. AVP regulation of the HPA axis may therefore be critical for sustaining corticotropin responsiveness in the presence of high circulating glucocorticoid levels or supersensitive glucocorticoid receptors. Thus, in animals deficient for the CRH_1 receptor, there is a selective compensatory activation of the hypothalamic AVP system, which maintains basal corticotropin secretion and HPA activity. Similar response patterns have been observed following chronic stress, leading to a hypothesis that CRH plays a predominantly permissive role in HPA regulation but that AVP represents the dynamic mediator of corticotropin release.

Extrahypothalamic AVP-containing neurons also have been characterized in the rat, notably in the medial amygdala, where they project to limbic structures such as the lateral septum and the ventral hippocampus and are thought to act as neurotransmitters. Central AVP receptors include V_{1A} and V_{1B}, which are found in the septum, cortex, and hippocampus (Hernando et al. 2001). V_{1A} knockout mice were found to have reduced anxiety in tasks such as the elevated plus-maze and forced swim (Bielsky et al. 2004; Egashira et al. 2007), and conversely, mice overexpressing V_{1A} were found to be more anxious (Bielsky et al. 2005). Preclinical trials of V_{1B} receptor antagonists such as SSR149415 have been promising in showing anxiolytic and antidepressant effects of blocking the activity of AVP on these receptors (Griebel et al. 2002). There is work under way to develop these agents as antidepressants and anxiolytics (Serradeil–Le Gal et al. 2005).

Cortisol

Cortisol is a steroid hormone secreted by the zona fasciculata of the adrenal cortex. Under normal physiological conditions, cortisol levels peak just before awakening and reach a nadir soon after the onset of sleep. With stress, HPA axis activation causes an increase in serum cortisol levels (Morgan et al. 2000). Higher cortisol levels mobilize energy stores, inhibit activity of the growth and reproductive systems, and contain the immune response. Cortisol also may contribute to the recruitment of higher cortical functions to ensure arousal, vigilance, focused attention, rapid recall, and efficient memory encoding and storage. Preclinical data have shown that glucocorticoids can enhance amygdala activity (Charney et al. 1992; Makino et al. 1994), increase the effects of CRH on conditioned fear, and facilitate the encoding of emotion-related memory via an NE-dependent pathway (Roozendaal et al. 2006).

Although transiently elevated serum cortisol may serve adaptive purposes in combating fearful stimuli, long-term exposure to high levels of cortisol have significant deleterious effects, both peripherally and in the central nervous system. Under normal conditions, cortisol feeds back on hypothalamic receptors to inhibit further HPA activation. When this feedback system fails to inhibit cortisol secretion, excessive and sustained cortisol secretion causes hypertension, osteoporosis, immunosuppression, insulin resistance, dyslipidemia, dyscoagulation, atherosclerosis, and cardiovascular disease (Karlamangla et al. 2002). In the brain, a sustained increase in glucocorticoid levels impairs cell survival, alters metabolism and neuronal morphology, and adversely affects hippocampal-dependent cognitive and memory function (McEwen 2000).

There is inconsistent evidence regarding cortisol levels in people with anxiety disorders. People with PTSD generally have normal or decreased 24-hour serum and urine cortisol levels and in some studies have had increased intra-day variability in levels suggestive of increased adrenal reactivity with a reduced threshold for hypothalamic suppression, a finding consistent with pharmacological suppression data (reviewed in Yehuda 2006). A recent small study found that people with PTSD have higher CSF cortisol, which may represent a dissociation between peripheral and central levels (Baker et al. 2005). Similarly, HPA studies in people with panic disorder have yielded inconsistent results, but it appears that there exists a consistent HPA hyperreactivity to novel fear-provoking cues (Abelson et al. 2007).

Neuropeptide Y

Neuropeptide Y (NPY) is a 36–amino acid peptide found mostly in the locus coeruleus, hypothalamus, amygdala, hippocampus, basal ganglia, and midbrain nuclei. NPY is expressed under fearful conditions and appears to inhibit or contain the stress response (reviewed in Heilig 2004). Localized microinjections of NPY in the rat amygdala reduce anxiety and impair memory retention, whereas injections in the locus coeruleus are inhibitory (Flood et al. 1989; Heilig et al. 1989). NPY knockout rats demonstrate increased emotionality in the face of stress and impaired spatial learning (Thorsell et al. 2000), whereas rats in which NPY is overexpressed spend more time in open arms of mazes, implying decreased anxiety (Primeaux et al. 2005). The anxiolytic effects of NPY appear to be mediated in part by glutamate receptor ligands in a manner reversible by Y_1 and Y_2 receptor antagonists (Smiaowska et al. 2007).

The balance between NPY and CRH neurotransmission may be important to emotional responses to stress. NPY counteracts the anxiogenic effects of CRH, and a CRH antagonist blocks the anxiogenic effects of an NPY–Y_1 receptor antagonist. Brain regions that express CRH and CRH receptors also contain NPY and NPY receptors, and the functional effects are often opposite, especially at the level of the locus coeruleus, amygdala, and periaqueductal gray (reviewed in Kask et al. 2002). The reciprocal antagonism appears to be related to bidirectional GABAergic transmission in the BNST (Kash and Winder 2006).

Human studies have found that NPY levels are not significantly different in subjects with PTSD after combat or domestic violence (Morgan et al. 2003; Seedat et al. 2003). Soldiers who underwent distressing interrogation and were found to have clinically significant dissociation had elevated plasma NPY levels (Morgan et al. 2000) that were later found to correlate with improved performance (Morgan et al. 2002). This finding was reinforced by another study that showed that elevated NPY levels were associated with PTSD symptom improvement and may represent a biological correlate of resilience (Yehuda et al. 2006).

Galanin

Galanin is a 30–amino acid neuropeptide involved in emotion-related behaviors including cognition, nociception, sexual behavior, feeding, sleep, and reward (reviewed in Holmes and Picciotto 2006). In rodent studies, galanin collocates with the ascending monoamine systems and, consequently, is found in the locus coeruleus, the raphe nuclei, and the ventral tegmental area and inhibits monoamine, glutamate, and acetylcholine release via three known G protein–coupled receptors (Gal$_1$, Gal$_2$, and Gal$_3$) in the brain stem as well as its subcortical and cortical projections (reviewed in Karlsson and Holmes 2006).

Several preclinical studies have shown a role for galanin in modulating anxiety. Centrally administered galanin produced conflicting results in rats, with some studies showing anxiolytic effects (Bing et al. 1993) and others showing anxiogenic effects (Khoshbouei et al. 2002; Moller et al. 1999). In vivo microdialysis studies have shown that galanin is released in the amygdala in the context of stress and presynaptic α_2-adrenergic receptor blockade, independently of noradrenergic influence from the locus coeruleus (Barrera et al. 2006). In the hippocampus, local overexpression or administration of galanin impairs fear conditioning (Kinney et al. 2002), and Gal$_1$ receptor–deficient mice show increased anxiety-like behavior.

Preclinical pharmacological studies have shown anxiolytic and antidepressant effects of galanin receptor agonists. Galnon, a nonselective galanin receptor agonist, was shown to have anxiolytic properties reversible with M35, a nonselective galanin receptor antagonist (Rajarao et al. 2006). A similar finding was reported on a forced swim test with rats, suggesting an antidepressant effect of galanin as well (Kuteeva et al. 2007). However, two Gal$_3$ receptor antagonists, SNAP 37889 and SNAP 398299, were found to have anxiolytic and antidepressant properties in several animal models, such as forced swim and stress-induced hyperthermia (Swanson et al. 2005).

To date, only one known study has examined galanin in anxiety disorders. Women with panic disorder and two polymorphisms of the galanin gene were found to have more severe symptoms than women with other haplotypes, a finding that did not extend to the men tested (Unschuld et al. 2008). These findings, in light of the preclinical data reviewed above, suggest a potential role for agents modulating the galanin system in the treatment of anxiety.

Dopamine

Dopamine (DA) is a catecholamine involved in a number of emotional processes including reward, affect, and anxiety. Under conditions of acute stress, DA is released via mesocortical projections in the medial prefrontal cortex and, to a lesser degree, via subcortical projections in the nucleus accumbens and the basolateral amygdala. Stress causes DA to be released and metabolized in the medial

prefrontal cortex with an associated inhibition in meso-accumbens dopaminergic tone (King et al. 1997) via an amygdala-dependent pathway (Goldstein et al. 1996).

These inverse effects on the medial prefrontal cortex and the nucleus accumbens suggest an aversive subjective experience that may play a role in stress-induced depression. In the forced swimming test animal model for depression, mice vulnerable to stress-induced despair stopped swimming almost immediately and were found to have high mesocortical DA metabolism and low meso-accumbens DA metabolism compared with normal mice; these findings were reversed by either chemical lesioning of the medial prefrontal cortex or treatment with the tricyclic antidepressant clomipramine (Ventura et al. 2002). Interestingly, lesions of the medial prefrontal cortex inhibit extinction, a situation hypothesized to occur in PTSD (Morrow et al. 1999). Thus, excessive medial prefrontal cortex DA results in helplessness, while insufficient medial prefrontal cortex DA retards extinction, leading to the hypothesis that there exists an optimal range of medial prefrontal cortex DA activation necessary to preserve the reward function of the nucleus accumbens while maintaining the ability to extinguish conditioned emotional memories. These processes may be relevant to understanding the high mood disorder comorbidity observed across all the anxiety disorders.

Clinical research on DA function in anxiety disorders is relatively sparse. To date, investigations into serum and CSF levels of DA or its metabolites have not yielded convincing evidence of alterations in global DA activity. Recently, genetic analyses into polymorphisms of the major DA metabolizing enzyme catechol-O-methyltransferase (COMT) have suggested an association between specific polymorphisms and anxiety disorders. In one study, healthy women with the Val158Met COMT polymorphism were found to have higher levels of phobic anxiety (McGrath et al. 2004). A meta-analysis of six case–control studies of COMT polymorphisms did not replicate the Val158Met finding but did find an ethnicity effect, whereby white populations with the 158Val allele and Asian populations with the 158Met allele were found to have a higher incidence of panic disorder (Domschke et al. 2007).

Serotonin

Serotonin (5-HT) is a monoamine neurotransmitter with a diversity of neural, gastrointestinal, and cardiovascular functions. Under conditions of acute stress, regional increases in 5-HT turnover occur in the prefrontal cortex, nucleus accumbens, amygdala, and lateral hypothalamus (Kent et al. 2002). 5-HT release has both anxiogenic and anxiolytic effects, depending on the brain region involved and the receptor subtype activated. One theory is that 5-HT plays a dual role in anxiety, enhancing learned responses to distal threat through projections to the amygdala and the prefrontal cortex while inhibiting unconditioned responses to proximal threats through projections to the periaqueductal gray matter (reviewed in Graeff 2002). 5-HT stimulation of the 5-HT$_{2A}$ receptor is generally anxiogenic, whereas stimulation of the 5-HT$_{1A}$ receptor is generally anxiolytic (Graeff 2004).

Investigation into the function of the 5-HT$_{1A}$ receptor has yielded interesting insights into the role of 5-HT in anxiety. 5-HT$_{1A}$ is primarily inhibitory and is found as a presynaptic autoreceptor in the neurons of the raphe nuclei, whereas it is postsynaptic in the hippocampus, septum, and cortex. 5-HT$_{1A}$ knockout mice exhibit increased anxiety-like behaviors (Parks et al. 1998) which can be reversed if gene expression is conditionally inhibited in adulthood but not in early life (Gross et al. 2002). These findings imply that 5-HT$_{1A}$ receptor activity is required for normal development of the neural circuits regulating anxiety. Clinically, people with panic disorder and social anxiety disorder have a lower density of 5-HT$_{1A}$ receptors in limbic structures including the amygdala, raphe nuclei, and anterior cingulate gyrus (Lanzenberger et al. 2007; Neumeister et al. 2004). This finding was not replicated after exposure to stress in people with PTSD (Bonne et al. 2005).

The 5-HT transporter (5-HTT) and its encoding gene SCL6A4 also play a significant role in the neurobiology of anxiety. Polymorphisms of the SCL6A4 promoter 5-HT-TLPR encoding a short (S) or long (L) allele have been linked to mood and anxiety disorders. Carriers of the S allele have lower expression of 5-HTT, decreased 5-HT reuptake, and a higher incidence of anxious traits (Lesch et al. 1996), as well as increased amygdalar activation in response to fearful faces (Hariri et al. 2002, 2005). Children homozygous for the S allele are more shy than controls and may be more vulnerable to developing anxiety disorders later in life (Battaglia et al. 2005). The S allele also confers a depressive and anxious diathesis when combined with early-life stressors. Carriers of the S allele with a history of early-life stress have a higher incidence of depression and behavioral inhibition as children (Fox et al. 2005; Kaufman et al. 2004) and rates of depression as adults (Caspi et al. 2003). A significant number of negative studies also exist in which there is no association between the presence of the S allele, adverse life events, and

the incidence of anxiety disorders, confirming the multifactorial nature of the pathophysiology of anxiety.

Similarly, pharmacological dissection of serotonergic systems has not yet established the role of 5-HT in the pathogenesis of anxiety disorders. Panic disorder has been most closely studied, and pharmacological challenges with the 5-HT precursors L-tryptophan (Charney and Heninger 1986) and 5-hydroxytryptophan (DenBoer and Westenberg 1990) or the tryptophan depletion challenge (Goddard et al. 1994) failed to elicit or inhibit panic symptoms in people suffering from panic disorder compared with healthy controls. Fenfluramine, an agent triggering release of 5-HT, has been shown to be anxiogenic and stimulate the HPA axis in people with panic disorder (Targum and Marshall 1989). In sum, it appears that 5-HT dysfunction plays an indirect role in the pathogenesis of anxiety disorders through its modulatory effects on other neurotransmitter systems.

GABA and Benzodiazepines

GABA is the main inhibitory neurotransmitter of the central nervous system and binds to rapid ionotropic GABA$_A$ and GABA$_C$ receptors and slow metabotropic GABA$_B$ receptors most densely concentrated in the cortical gray matter (Bormann 2000). In general, GABAergic tone counteracts excitatory glutamatergic tone, and thus plays a major role in the pathophysiology and treatment of anxiety disorders (Nemeroff 2003). GABA$_A$ and GABA$_C$ receptors contain a chloride channel mediating neuronal hyperpolarization and consequent inhibition. The role of GABA$_B$ receptors is less clearly understood but appears to modulate excitatory transmission and LTP (Chang et al. 2003).

In general, agents that enhance GABA receptor activity are anxiolytic, while those that inhibit GABA receptors are anxiogenic. There are various mechanisms of GABA receptor enhancement and inhibition. Agents that mimic GABA or increase its synaptic concentrations include ethanol, valproate, gabapentin, tiagabine, vigabatrin, and some neurosteroids (reviewed in Kalueff and Nutt 2007). Benzodiazepine agents bind to distinct benzodiazepine (BDZ) receptors on GABA$_A$ receptors, potentiating and prolonging the synaptic actions of GABA binding by increasing the frequency of GABA-mediated chloride channel openings (Smith 2001). The physiological role of BDZ receptors is unknown. Although there is evidence of endogenous BDZ receptor agonists, or endozapines, in unusual conditions including idiopathic recurrent stupor (Tinuper et al. 1994) and hepatic encephalopathy (Cossar et al. 1997), attempts to characterize an endozapine as common as its receptor have been unsuccessful. It is possible that rather than serving a physiological function, the physiological function of the BDZ receptor site is as an intrinsic modulator of GABA receptor activity.

GABA$_A$ receptors contain a chloride channel mediating neuronal hyperpolarization and consequent inhibition. Specific subunits of the GABA$_A$ receptor have been implicated in anxiogenic and anxiolytic phenomena. Preclinical investigations using inverse agonists (Atack et al. 2006), selective agonists (Dias et al. 2005), and behavioral paradigms (Morris et al. 2006) have shown that the α_2 and α_3 subunits have a primary role in modulating anxiety. Furthermore, preclinical models of acute stress have revealed reduced BDZ receptor binding, as well as reduced amygdala and hippocampus expression of the α_2 subunit, which correlate with clinical neuroimaging findings of reduced BDZ receptor binding in people with panic disorder and PTSD (reviewed extensively in Kalueff and Nutt 2007).

Pharmacological modulation of the GABA receptor has revealed interesting findings regarding the role of the GABAergic system in anxiety. Administration of flumazenil, a BDZ receptor antagonist, provokes panic attacks in people with panic disorder, but not in healthy control subjects (Nutt et al. 1990) or in people with other anxiety disorders (reviewed in Nutt and Malizia 2001).

Glutamate

Glutamate is the principal excitatory neurotransmitter in the CNS and also a precursor to the inhibitory neurotransmitter GABA, in addition to its central roles in protein synthesis and metabolism. Glutamatergic networks mediate associative functions of the cortex and hippocampus, sensory relay operations of the hypothalamus, danger-processing functions of the amygdala, and motivation systems in the basal forebrain (Chambers et al. 1999). Glutamatergic neurotransmission is also central to CNS mechanisms of plasticity, such as long-term potentiation or depression and short-term potentiation (Sheng and Kim 2002). Stress-related glutamatergic hyperactivity of sufficient magnitude may lead to increased intracellular calcium levels and neuronal toxicity. Such effects are described in concert with increased glucocorticoid levels and adversely affect varied brain structures, notably hippocampi (Sapolsky 1996). Given the repeated descriptions of reduced hippocampal volume in PTSD, this attribute of glutamate is of particular interest.

Preclinical studies have shown that immediate increase in glutamate efflux in prefrontal cortex and hippocampus occurred after induction of acute stress (Bagley and Moghaddam 1997). NMDA receptors may mediate lasting increases in anxiety-like behavior brought on by the stress of predator exposure. Ketamine (an NMDA antagonist) administration at a subanesthetic dosage in humans induced alterations in identity and perception resembling dissociation, a symptom of PTSD and panic attacks. These phenomena were attenuated by administration of the glutamate antagonist lamotrigine (Anand et al. 2000).

Programmatic investigation into the clinical application of glutamate-modulating drugs for treating anxiety is under way. Small trials have suggested the efficacy of a range of medications including anticonvulsants and the glutamate release inhibitor riluzole (reviewed in Amiel and Mathew 2007). New drugs under investigation include agonists of presynaptic metabotropic glutamate receptors, glycine receptor antagonists, NMDA subtype selective antagonists, and glutamate glial transport blockers.

Neurosteroids

Steroids influence neuronal function through binding to intracellular receptors, which may act as transcription factors in the regulation of gene expression (reviewed in Rupprecht 2003). Several neurosteroids, particularly 3α-reduced metabolites of progesterone and deoxycorticosterone, modulate ligand-gated channels via nongenomic mechanisms (Strömberg et al. 2006). Neurosteroids enhance the function of GABA$_A$ receptors by interacting with NMDA receptors in the central nucleus of the amygdala (Wang et al. 2007) and appear to be anxiolytic in preclinical models (Vanover et al. 2000).

Neurosteroid production is postulated to counteract the negative effects of acute stress. In response to stress, levels of neurosteroids increase rapidly first in the brain and then in the blood. Clinical studies have found that pharmacologically induced panic attacks with cholecystokinin-tetrapeptide (CCK-4) or lactate are associated with decreased 3α-reduced neurosteroids in people with panic disorders, whereas healthy control subjects showed an increase in 3α,5α-tetrahydrodeoxyxortixosterone, also known as allopregnanolone (reviewed in Eser et al. 2006). These findings imply a decreased GABA tone in people with panic disorder.

Progesterone also has been found to be anxiolytic in animals and humans by upregulating allopregnanolone (Reddy et al. 2005) independently of classic progesterone receptors (Frye et al. 2006). Pregnant animals show a decrease in anxiety behaviors correlating with elevated levels of serum progesterone that is reversible with finasteride, an inhibitor of the enzyme 5-α-reductase responsible for the synthesis of allopregnanolone (de Brito-Faturi et al. 2006). Pregnancy has also been found to reduce anxiety and increase allopregnanolone in healthy women (Paoletti et al. 2006) and in women with panic disorder (reviewed in Hertzberg and Wahlbeck 1999). Other studies of serum progesterone metabolite levels in anxiety disorders have been inconsistent, though premenopausual women with PTSD were found to have reduced CSF allopregnanolone levels (Rasmusson et al. 2006).

Interestingly, drugs that are classically known as 5-HT reuptake inhibitors increase allopregnanolone levels at doses insufficient to block reuptake (Pinna et al. 2006). Further investigations into the interaction between 5-HT and neuropeptides may yield interesting new targets for novel pharmacotherapy of anxiety and affective disorders. The study of the anxiolytic and antidepressant effects of synthetic neurosteroids such as ganaxolone, now being tested in epilepsy, has been proposed (Eser et al. 2006).

Cholecystokinin

Cholecystokinin (CCK) is a neuropeptide, originally discovered in the gastrointestinal tract, found in high density in the cerebral cortex, amygdala, hippocampus, midbrain periaqueductal gray, substantia nigra, and raphe. Its major effect is anxiogenic, and it has important functional interactions with other systems implicated in fear and anxiety (reviewed in Harro 2006).

Rodent models have shown that CCK-like agents induce anxiety, whereas agents that block the effects of CCK are anxiolytic (Bourin and Dailly 2004; Hano et al. 1993). Furthermore, the panicogenic effects of cholecystokinin-tetrapeptide, a CCK_2 receptor agonist acting on the periaqueductal gray matter, are blocked by administration of LY-225910, a CCK_2 receptor antagonist (Bertoglio and Zangrossi 2005; Bertoglio et al. 2007; Netto and Guimaraes 2004; Zanoveli et al. 2004). Pharmacological challenge with CCK increases anxiety in people with panic disorder (Bradwejn et al. 1994) and PTSD (Kellner et al. 2000), but not in people with social phobia (Katzman et al. 2004). CCK antagonists, propranolol, and imipramine seem to reduce the anxiogenic effects of CCK (Bradwejn and Koszycki 1994), suggesting that CCK interacts with the NE system in a manner reversible by the β-adrenergic receptor–downregulating effects of impira-

mine. There is some evidence of CCK-B gene polymorphisms in subjects with panic disorder, suggesting a possible genetic vulnerability (Hösing et al. 2004).

Although these data suggest that CCK receptor antagonists have a role in the treatment of anxiety, placebo-controlled trials have not shown effects in panic disorder or generalized anxiety disorder (Adams et al. 1995; Goddard et al. 1999; Kramer et al. 1995; Pande et al. 1999; van Megen et al. 1997). Further elucidation of the receptor specificity, regional effects, and neurotransmitter system interactions of CCK may aid in the identification of therapeutic applications.

Endogenous Opioids

The endogenous opioids are a group of neuropeptides including endorphins, enkephalins, dynorphins, and orphanins/nociceptins that bind to opioid receptors. In particular, μ-opioid receptors are distributed throughout the brain and are found in higher concentrations in limbic regions including the amygdala, the periaqueductal gray matter, the ventral pallidum, and the cingulate gyrus (Lever 2007). Endogenous opioids have a role in nociception, social attachment, and reward.

Preclinical models have shown that uncontrollable stress induces significant analgesia (Fanselow 1986) and that reexposure to less intense shock in the acute period also results in analgesia (Madden et al. 1977), but that chronic unpredictable stress inhibits nociception, causing hyperalgesia (Pinto-Ribeiro et al. 2004). It also appears that endogenous opioids act on the periaqueductal gray matter in rat models of fear learning, which is blocked with naloxone, indicating that endogenous opioids may be important for extinction (Cole and McNally 2007). An antagonistic interaction with CCK has also been described (reviewed in Hebb et al. 2005).

Human correlates of endogenous opioid abnormalities related to anxiety have also been described. In people with PTSD, β-endorphin levels have been found to be decreased in plasma (Hoffman et al. 1989) but elevated in CSF (Baker et al. 1997). Combat veterans with PTSD were found to have naloxone-reversible pain insensitivity in comparison with combat veterans without PTSD (Pitman et al. 1990). Women who have suffered domestic violence show a correlation between stress-induced analgesia and the development of PTSD hyperarousal 3 months after the trauma (Nishith et al. 2002). Neuroimaging has shown that people with PTSD have increased activation of μ-opioid receptors in the anterior cingulate but decreased activation of these receptors in the amygdala and thalamus (Liberzon et al. 2007). Therapeutic trials have shown that treatment with opiates reduces the incidence of PTSD in hospitalized children by reducing separation anxiety (Saxe et al. 2006), and opioid antagonists reduce PTSD hyperarousal symptoms (Petrakis et al. 2007). In sum, it appears that endogenous opiates offer protection from unbearable pain during acute stress or danger, but that with chronic stress, a dysregulation of the endogenous opioid system occurs characterized by altered nociception and extinction.

Genetic investigations into the endogenous opioid system are preliminary, but individuals with high levels of worry and homozygous for the met158 polymorphism of the COMT allele were found to have regionally blunted μ-opioid response to pain and increased report of subjective pain and distress in comparison with heterozygotes (Zubieta et al. 2003).

Neurocircuitry of Specific Anxiety Disorders

Panic disorder, specific and social phobias, and PTSD share many mechanisms underlying fear and anxiety responses and may best represent the "fear-based" anxiety disorders. The regions most often implicated with psychopathology include the limbic, paralimbic, and sensory association areas. Below we review key findings in these disorders.

Panic Disorder

Panic disorder is characterized by recurrent, short-lived, but intense panic attacks and a continuous but more moderate type of anxiety (termed anticipatory anxiety). Studies in the "resting state" are assumed to represent the latter type of anxiety. Earlier resting-state studies initially found an asymmetry (left less than right) of blood flow and oxygen metabolism in the hippocampus and parahippocampal gyrus (for a review, see Charney and Drevets 2002). Abnormal glucose metabolism in this region, but with the opposite laterality (i.e., elevated metabolism in the left hippocampal/parahippocampal area), was reported in a more recent study (Sakai et al. 2005). However, decreased resting-state bilateral perfusion also was reported in lactate-sensitive subjects with panic disorder compared with control subjects.

Functional imaging of subjects with panic disorder also has been performed during experimentally induced panic attacks. Because states of extreme fear are also observed or induced in healthy control subjects, it is unknown if the neuroanatomy of panic attacks would be similar or different in healthy subjects and people with panic disorder. Regional cerebral blood flow (CBF) increases in the anterior insula, anteromedial cerebellum, and midbrain were observed after sodium lactate infusion–induced panic attacks in people with panic disorder. Anxiety attacks induced in healthy humans with cholecystokinin-tetrapeptide (CCK-4) also were associated with CBF increases in similar regions and the anterior cingulate cortex. Yohimbine administration increased medial frontal CBF in healthy control subjects but decreased relative prefrontal cortical perfusion in people with panic disorder relative to control subjects. People with panic disorder, but not healthy control subjects, had reductions in absolute measures of global CBF under CO_2 provocation (Ponto et al. 2002). In pentagastrin-induced panic attacks, hypoactivity in people with panic disorder, compared with control subjects, was found in the precentral gyrus, inferior frontal gyrus, right amygdala, and anterior insula. Hyperactivity in people with panic disorder was observed in the parahippocampal gyrus, superior temporal lobe, hypothalamus, anterior cingulate gyrus, and midbrain (Boshuisen et al. 2002). Positron emission tomography (PET) studies have shown that doxapram-induced paniclike states are associated with decreased prefrontal activity and increased amygdala and cingulate activation in people with panic disorder, but not in healthy control subjects, further supporting the model that prefrontal inhibition is important in attenuating anxiety (Garakani et al. 2007).

In a preliminary functional MRI study comparing people with panic disorder and healthy subjects during mental imagery of high anxiety states, people with panic disorder showed increased activity in the inferior frontal cortex, hippocampus, and anterior and posterior cingulate gyrus, extending into the orbitofrontal cortex and encompassing both hemispheres (Bystritsky et al. 2001). In the first report of functional MRI of spontaneous panic attack, a woman with panic disorder was found to have markedly increased activity in the right amygdala (Pfleiderer et al. 2007).

Only a few structural MRI studies have investigated morphometric or morphological abnormalities in panic disorder. Ontiveros et al. (1989) reported qualitative abnormalities of temporal lobe structure in panic disorder, although these findings have not been replicated. Vythilingam et al. (2000) reported that hippocampal volume did not differ between people with panic disorder and healthy control subjects, but the entire temporal lobe volume was reduced bilaterally in the people with panic disorder. However, this finding was difficult to interpret, because when normalized to whole-brain volume, the differences in temporal lobe measures between panic disorder and control samples had magnitudes of 2%. A volumetric MRI study found bilaterally reduced amygdala volumes in patient with panic disorder without associated differences in hippocampal or overall temporal lobe size (Massana et al. 2003). Neuroimaging studies found reduced BZD receptor binding in people with anxiety disorders (reviewed earlier in this chapter in the subsection "GABA and Benzodiazepines").

Phobias

The phobic response is phenomenologically similar to a panic attack. It has been imaged by acquiring blood flow scans while exposing people to their feared object (for review, see Charney and Drevets 2002). A progressive pattern of regional CBF responses was observed during successive scans. Perfusion initially increased in the lateral orbital/anterior insular cortex bilaterally, in the pregenual anterior cingulate cortex, and in the anteromedial cerebellum. During continued presentations of the phobic stimulus, the magnitude of the hemodynamic response diminished in the anterior insula and the medial cerebellum but increased in the left posterior orbital cortex. The CBF increase was inversely correlated with decreases in heart rate and anxiety ratings. In a PET [^{15}O]butanol study of people with simple spider phobia, phobic stimulation elevated regional CBF bilaterally in the secondary visual cortex compared with neutral stimulation but reduced regional CBF in the hippocampus and in the prefrontal, orbitofrontal, temporopolar, and posterior cingulate cortices (Pissiota et al. 2003). A recent functional MRI study (Paquette et al. 2003) reported reversal of phobic (spider) provocation increases in the dorsolateral prefrontal cortex (Brodmann area 10) and parahippocampal gyrus in people with simple phobia after clinically successful treatment with cognitive-behavioral therapy. These authors concluded that effective psychotherapeutic treatment (i.e., cognitive-behavioral therapy) can modify dysfunctional neural circuitry associated with pathological anxiety.

Several functional imaging studies have focused on social phobia. When speaking in public, people with social phobia had elevated CBF in the amygdaloid complex and reduced CBF in orbitofrontal and insular cortices and the temporal pole relative to comparison subjects (Tillfors et al. 2001). It is hypothesized that in social phobia, as in PTSD (see the following subsection, "Posttraumatic Stress Disorder"), exaggerated fear response is related to

an absence of cortical inhibition. Another study compared subjects with social phobia scanned either before or after speaking in public (Tillfors et al. 2002). In the anticipation group, increased CBF was found in the right dorsolateral prefrontal cortex, left inferior temporal cortex, and left amygdaloid–hippocampal region, and decreased CBF was found in the left temporal pole and bilaterally in the cerebellum. Anticipatory anxiety in people with social phobia may involve a fear network encompassing the amygdaloid–hippocampal region and prefrontal and temporal areas, much like the anticipatory anxiety neurocircuitry of people with panic disorder.

Another PET study by the same group (Furmark et al. 2002) reported that clinical improvement in social phobia, obtained by treatment with group psychotherapy or citalopram, was accompanied by similar decreases in provocation-induced regional CBF in the amygdala, hippocampus, and periamygdaloid, rhinal, and parahippocampal cortices. CBF in these regions decreased significantly more in responders compared with nonresponders, particularly in the right hemisphere. Tc-99m hexamethylpropyleneamine oxime ([^{99m}Tc]-HMPAO) single photon emission computed tomography (SPECT) was used to evaluate resting-state regional CBF ratios in a group of 15 people with social phobia before and after treatment with citalopram (Van der Linden et al. 2000). Regional CBF was significantly reduced in the anterior and lateral part of the left temporal cortex; the anterior, lateral, and posterior part of the left midfrontal cortex; and the left cingulum. Results from both treatment studies are conceptually and anatomically similar to those obtained from the above-described treatment studies in simple phobia and panic disorder, suggesting a mutual neurocircuitry for fear responses in diverse anxiety disorders.

Functional MRI studies have been useful in assessing regional brain activity in phobic individuals. In comparison with healthy control subjects, people with social phobia have larger increases of the amygdala (Stein et al. 2002) and anterior cingulate (Amir et al. 2005) blood oxygen level–dependent signal when viewing angry faces rather than happy faces. Arachnophobic individuals experiencing anticipatory anxiety have fMRI hyperactivation of anterior cingulate, insula, thalamus, and visual areas as well as the BNST (Straube et al. 2007). Interestingly, group exposure therapy was found to reduce amygala and insula hyperactivation in arachnophobic subjects over the course of treatment (Schienle et al. 2007). These findings are consistent with the hypothesis of a hyperactive limbic/amygdala response to anxiogenic stimuli in anxiety and stress-related disorders.

Posttraumatic Stress Disorder

Activation brain imaging studies comparing people with PTSD with healthy or trauma-exposed control subjects were expected to detect differences in the amygdala, hippocampus, and medial prefrontal cortex, because it was assumed that there was an exaggerated fear response in the absence of cortical inhibition. Amygdala activation was observed as PTSD subjects were compelled to reexperience trauma (Liberzon et al. 1999; Rauch et al. 1996; Shin et al. 1997). Other studies found no significant changes in amygdala CBF under similar conditions (Bremner et al. 1999a, 1999b; Shin et al. 1999). In contrast to the inconsistencies in amygdala activation, the pattern of CBF changes in the medial prefrontal cortex consistently differentiated between PTSD and healthy subjects, showing increased activation in the latter group (Bremner et al. 1999b; Shin et al. 1997, 1999).

In the infralimbic cortex, CBF decreased in subjects with combat-related PTSD but increased in matched, non-PTSD control subjects during exposure to combat-related stimuli (Bremner et al. 1999b). The findings of decreased anterior cingulate and increased amygdala function after traumatic recall have been interpreted as a failure of cortical inhibition of amygdala-mediated fear responses. Findings from two functional MRI studies support anterior cingulate hypofunction in PTSD, particularly in the emotional component of this structure. Reduced perfusion in the anterior cingulate in PTSD subjects compared with trauma-exposed control subjects was found after activation by the emotional Stroop test (Shin et al. 2001) and traumatic recall (Lanius et al. 2001). Given preclinical evidence that the anterior cingulate and infralimbic cortices play roles in extinguishing fear-conditioned responses (Milad and Quirk 2002), failure to activate the anterior cingulate cortex in PTSD suggests impairment of neural substrate mediation extinction in PTSD.

A preliminary functional MRI study found exaggerated amygdala response in PTSD subjects relative to trauma-matched control subjects during exposure to masked-fearful faces relative to masked-happy faces (Rauch et al. 2000). Because participants were only aware of seeing the mask, the increased activation of the amygdala can be understood as a "bottom-up" phenomenon, suggesting an inherent malfunction in the amygdala regardless of the presence or absence of cortical inhibition.

Structural imaging of hippocampal volume in PTSD was stimulated by preclinical studies reporting hippocampal neuronal loss and dendritic atrophy following expo-

sure to chemical or psychosocial stress (McEwen 1999). Structural MRI studies of PTSD have identified subtle reductions in the volume of the hippocampus in PTSD samples relative to healthy or traumatized, non-PTSD control samples (for review, see Hull 2002; Villarreal et al. 2002). These studies mainly investigated people with chronic PTSD, often associated with comorbid mental disorders, pharmacological treatment, and alcohol and substance abuse, although most studies attempted to control for these factors. However, Agartz et al. (1999) have shown that in the presence of alcohol abuse, the additional occurrence of PTSD has no added effect on hippocampal volume. De Bellis et al. (2000) reported a decrease in hippocampal volume in young adults with adolescent-onset alcohol use disorder.

A few studies did not report hippocampal reduction in PTSD. Prospective longitudinal studies of acute single civilian trauma survivors found no difference in hippocampal volume between healthy trauma survivors and people with PTSD at two time points as well as across time (for review, see Hull 2002). The difference in hippocampal volume in PTSD may apply to specific subtypes of the disorder (i.e., chronic vs. acute trauma), reflect chronic stress associated with long-term PTSD, or indicate a biological antecedent that may confer risk for developing PTSD.

Conclusion

Physiological and pathological anxiety likely represent a spectrum of hyperactivation of specific neurochemical axes and neuroanatomical circuits. There are significant genetic contributions to the anxiety diathesis, but undoubtedly the experience of fearful stimuli in the environment plays a major role in inducing, reinforcing, and sometimes generalizing the fear response. We have reviewed polymorphisms associated with clinical findings in the noradrenergic, HPA, dopaminergic, serotonergic, and endogenous opioid systems. There is also active investigation of the genetics of intracellular processes associated with learning and unlearning that will undoubtedly relate to the study of anxiety. In addition, explorations in the field of epigenetics, or nongenomic variations in gene expression and protein synthesis, are just beginning. Evolving technologies of gene arrays and automated screening, as well as the linkage of imaging modalities with genetic research, will offer new insights into the neurobiology of anxiety disorders.

In this chapter, we attempted to provide a framework for understanding these phenomena, linking potential and still largely hypothetical neural mechanisms derived from preclinical research to the neurobiological findings in people with anxiety disorders. We presented data showing an association among neurotransmitters, neuropeptides, and hormones and various states of anxiety. A neurocircuitry apparently shared by many anxiety disorders was illustrated. Several important questions are raised in light of this review:

- Are there qualitative differences in the neurocircuitry of fear and anxiety in pathological versus physiological anxiety?
- How do the neurobiological systems implicated in anxiety change over time and with new experiences?
- How do pharmacological and behavioral interventions alter the neurobiology of anxiety?
- Is the neurobiology of each DSM-IV-TR anxiety disorder distinct, or do they represent subtle variations of a shared etiology?

Continuing research into the epidemiology, genetics, neurochemistry, and functional anatomy of physiological anxiety, pathological anxiety, and the effect of therapeutic interventions will address these questions and inform clinical practice by supporting or refuting currently accepted nosologies and pharmacological and psychotherapeutic interventions.

References

Abelson JL, Khan S, Liberzon I, et al: HPA axis activity in patients with panic disorder: review and synthesis of four studies. Depress Anxiety 24:66–76, 2007

Adams JB, Pyke RE, Costa J, et al: A double-blind, placebo-controlled study of a CCK-B receptor antagonist, CI-988, in patients with generalized anxiety disorder. J Clin Psychopharmacol 15:428–34, 1995

Agartz I, Momenan R, Rawlings RR, et al: Hippocampal volume in patients with alcohol dependence. Arch Gen Psychiatry 56:356–363, 1999

Akirav I: NMDA Partial agonist reverses blocking of extinction of aversive memory by GABA(A) agonist in the amygdala. Neuropsychopharmacology 32:542–550, 2007

American Psychiatric Association: Diagnostic and Statistical Manual of Mental Disorders, 4th Edition, Text Revision. Washington, DC, American Psychiatric Association, 2000

Amiel JM, Mathew SJ: Glutamate and anxiety disorders. Curr Psychiatry Rep 9:278–283, 2007

Amir N, Klumpp H, Elias J, et al: Increased activation of the anterior cingulate cortex during processing of disgust faces in individuals with social phobia. Biol Psychiatry 57:975–981, 2005

Anand A, Charney DS, Oren DA, et al: Attenuation of the neuropsychiatric effects of ketamine with lamotrigine: support for hyperglutamatergic effects of N-methyl-D-aspartate receptor antagonists. Arch Gen Psychiatry 57:270–276, 2000

Atack JR, Wafford KA, Tye SJ, et al: TPA023 [7-(1,1-dimethylethyl)-6-(2-ethyl-2H-1,2,4-triazol-3-ylmethoxy)-3-(2-fluorophenyl)-1,2,4-triazolo[4,3-b]pyridazine], an agonist selective for alpha2- and alpha3-containing GABAA receptors, is a nonsedating anxiolytic in rodents and primates. J Pharmacol Exp Ther 316:410–422, 2006

Bagley J, Moghaddam B: Temporal dynamics of glutamate efflux in the prefrontal cortex and in the hippocampus following repeated stress: effects of pretreatment with saline or diazepam. Neuroscience 77:65–73, 1997

Bailey CH, Kandel ER, Si K: The persistence of long-term memory: a molecular approach to self-sustaining changes in learning-induced synaptic growth. Neuron 44:49–57, 2004

Baker DG, West SA, Orth DN, et al: Cerebrospinal fluid and plasma beta endorphin in combat veterans with posttraumatic stress disorder. Psychoneuroendocrinology 22:517–529, 1997

Baker DG, West SA, Nicholson WE, et al: Serial CSF corticotropin-releasing hormone levels and adrenocortical activity in combat veterans with posttraumatic stress disorder. Am J Psychiatry 156:585–588, 1999

Baker DG, Ekhator NN, Kasckow JW: Higher levels of basal serial CSF cortisol in combat veterans with posttraumatic stress disorder. Am J Psychiatry 162:992–994, 2005

Bale TL, Contarino A, Smith GW, et al: Mice deficient for corticotrophin-releasing hormone receptor-2 display anxiety-like behavior and are hypersensitive to stress. Nat Genet 24:410–414, 2000

Bale TL, Picetti R, Contarino A, et al: Mice deficient for both corticotropin-releasing factor receptor 1 (CRFR1) and CRFR2 have an impaired stress response and display sexually dichotomous anxiety-like behavior. J Neurosci 22:193–199, 2002

Balon R, Ramesh C: Calcium channel blockers for anxiety disorders? Ann Clin Psychiatry 8:215–220, 1996

Barrera G, Hernandez A, Poulin JF, et al: Galanin-mediated anxiolytic effect in rat central amygdala is not a result of corelease from noradrenergic terminals. Synapse 59:27–40, 2006

Battaglia M, Ogliari A, Zanoni A: Influence of the serotonin transporter promoter gene and shyness on children's cerebral responses to facial expressions. Arch Gen Psychiatry 62:85–94, 2005

Bertoglio LJ, Zangrossi H Jr: Involvement of dorsolateral periaqueductal gray cholecystokinin-2 receptors in the regulation of a panic-related behavior in rats. Brain Res 1059:46–51, 2005

Bertoglio LJ, de Bortoli VC, Zangrossi H Jr: Cholecystokinin-2 receptors modulate freezing and escape behaviors evoked by the electrical stimulation of the rat dorsolateral periaqueductal gray. Brain Res 1156:133–138, 2007

Bielsky IF, Hu SB, Szegda KL, et al: Profound impairment in social recognition and reduction in anxiety-like behavior in vasopressin V1a receptor knockout mice. Neuropsychopharmacology 29:483–493, 2004

Bielsky IF, Hu SB, Ren X, et al: The V1a vasopressin receptor is necessary and sufficient for normal social recognition: a gene replacement study. Neuron 47:503–513, 2005

Bing O, Moller C, Engel JA, et al: Anxiolytic-like action of centrally administered galanin. Neurosci Lett 164:17–20, 1993

Bonne O, Bain E, Neumeister A, et al: No change in serotonin type 1A receptor binding in patients with posttraumatic stress disorder. Am J Psychiatry 162:383–385, 2005

Bormann J: The "ABC" of GABA receptors. Trends Pharmacol Sci 21:16–19, 2000

Boshuisen ML, Ter Horst GJ, Paans A, et al: rCBF differences between panic disorder patients and control subjects during anticipatory anxiety and rest. Biol Psychiatry 52:126–135, 2002

Bourin M, Dailly E: Cholecystokinin and panic disorder. Acta Neuropsychiatr 16:85–93, 2004

Bouton ME: Context and behavioral processes in extinction. Learn Mem 11:485–494, 2004

Bradwejn J, Koszycki D: Imipramine antagonism of the panicogenic effects of cholecystokinin tetrapeptide in panic disorder patients. Am J Psychiatry 151:261–263, 1994

Bradwejn J, Koszycki D, Couetoux du Tetre A, et al: The panicogenic effects of CCK-4 are antagonized by L-365–260, a CCK receptor antagonist, in patients with panic disorder. Arch Gen Psychiatry 51:486–493, 1994

Bremner JD, Narayan M, Staib LH, et al: Neural correlates of memories of childhood sexual abuse in women with and without posttraumatic stress disorder. Am J Psychiatry 156:1787–1795, 1999a

Bremner JD, Staib LH, Kaloupek D, et al: Neural correlates of exposure to traumatic pictures and sound in Vietnam combat veterans with and without posttraumatic stress disorder: a positron emission tomography study. Biol Psychiatry 45:806–816, 1999b

Brunson KL, Eghbal-Ahmadi M, Bender R, et al: Long-term, progressive hippocampal cell loss and dysfunction induced by early life administration of corticotropin-releasing hormone reproduce the effects of early life stress. Proc Natl Acad Sci U S A 98:8856–8861, 2001

Butler T, Pan H, Tuescher O et al: Human fear-related motor neurocircuitry. Neuroscience 150:1–7, 2007

Bystritsky A, Pontillo D, Powers M, et al: Functional MRI changes during panic anticipation and imagery exposure. Neuroreport 12:3953–3967, 2001

Cahill L, Prins B, Weber M, et al: Beta-adrenergic activation and memory for emotional events. Nature 371:702–704, 1994

Canon WB: Bodily Changes in Pain, Hunger, Fear and Rage: An Account of Recent Research Into the Function of Emotional Excitement. New York, Appleton, 1915

Caspi A, Sugden K, Moffitt TE, et al: Influence of life stress on depression: moderation by a polymorphism in the 5-HTT gene. Science 301:386–389, 2003

Chambers RA, Bremner JD, Moghaddam B, et al: Glutamate and post-traumatic stress disorder: toward a psychobiology of dissociation. Semin Clin Neuropsychiatry 4:274–281, 1999

Chang L, Cloak CC, Ernst T: Magnetic resonance spectroscopy studies of GABA in neuropsychiatric disorders. J Clin Psychiatry 64 (suppl 3):7–14, 2003

Charney DS, Drevets WD: Neurobiological basis of anxiety disorders, in Neuropsychopharmacology: The Fifth Generation of Progress. Edited by Davis KL, Charney D, Coyle JT, et al. Baltimore, MD, Lippincott Williams & Wilkins, 2002, pp 901–930

Charney DS, Heninger GR: Serotonin function in panic disorders: The effects of intravenous tryptophan in healthy subjects and panic disorder patients before and after alprazolam treatment. Arch Gen Psychiatry 43:1059–1065, 1986

Charney DS, Woods SW, Goodman WK, et al: Neurobiological mechanisms of panic anxiety: biochemical and behavioral correlates of yohimbine-induced panic attacks. Am J Psychiatry 144:1030–1036, 1987

Charney DS, Woods SW, Krystal JH, et al: Noradrenergic neuronal dysregulation in panic disorder: the effects of intravenous yohimbine and clonidine in panic disorder patients. Acta Psychiatr Scand 86:273–282, 1992

Cole S, McNally GP: Opioid receptors mediate direct predictive fear learning: evidence from one-trial blocking. Learn Mem 14:229–235, 2007

Coplan JD, Mathew SJ, Mao X, et al: Decreased choline and creatine concentrations in centrum semiovale in patients with generalized anxiety disorder: relationship to IQ and early trauma. Psychiatry Res 147:27–39, 2006

Cossar JA, Hayes PC, O'Carroll RE: Benzodiazepine-like substances and hepatic encephalopathy: implications for treatment. CNS Drugs 8:91–101, 1997

Coste SC, Kesterson RA, Heldwein KA, et al: Abnormal adaptations to stress and impaired cardiovascular function in mice lacking corticotrophin-releasing hormone receptor-2. Nat Genet 24:403–409, 2000

De Bellis MD, Clark DB, Beers SR, et al: Hippocampal volume in adolescent-onset alcohol use disorders. Am J Psychiatry 157:737–744, 2000

de Brito-Faturi C, Teixeira-Silva F, Leite JR: The anxiolytic effect of pregnancy in rats is reversed by finasteride. Pharmacol Biochem Behav 85:569–574, 2006

DenBoer JA, Westenberg HGM: Behavioral, neuroendocrine, and biochemical effects of 5-hydroxytryptophan administration in panic disorder. Psychiatry Res 31:367–378, 1990

Dias R, Sheppard WF, Fradley RL, et al: Evidence for a significant role of alpha 3-containing GABAA receptors in mediating the anxiolytic effects of benzodiazepines. J Neurosci 25:10682–10688, 2005

Domschke K, Deckert J, O'donovan MC, et al: Meta-analysis of COMT val158met in panic disorder: ethnic heterogeneity and gender specificity. Am J Med Genet 144:667–673, 2007

Egashira N, Tanoue A, Matsuda T, et al: Impaired social interaction and reduced anxiety-related behavior in vasopressin V1a receptor knockout mice. Behav Brain Res 178:123–127, 2007

Eser D, Romeo E, Baghai TC: Neuroactive steroids as modulators of depression and anxiety. Neuroscience 138:1041–1048, 2006

Etkin A, Klemenhagen KC, Dudman JT, et al: Individual differences in trait anxiety predict the response of the basolateral amygdala to unconsciously processed fearful faces. Neuron 44:1043–1055, 2004

Falls WA, Miserendino MJ, Davis M: Extinction of fear-potentiated startle: blockade by infusion of an NMDA antagonist into the amygdala. J Neurosci 12:854–863, 1992

Fanselow MS: Conditioned fear-induced opiate analgesia: a competing motivational state theory of stress analgesia. Ann N Y Acad Sci 467:40–54, 1986

Flood JF, Baker ML, Hernande WN, et al: Modulation of memory processing by neuropeptide Y varies with brain injection site. Brain Res 503:73–82, 1989

Fox NA, Nichols KE, Henderson HA, et al: Evidence for a gene-environment interaction in predicting behavioral inhibition in middle childhood. Psychol Sci 16:921–926, 2005

Funk CK, Zorrilla EP, Lee MJ, at al: Corticotropin-releasing factor 1 antagonists selectively reduce ethanol self-administration in ethanol-dependent rats. Biol Psychiatry 61:78–86, 2007

Frye CA, Sumida K, Dudek BC, et al: Progesterone's effects to reduce anxiety behavior of aged mice do not require actions via intracellular progestin receptors. Psychopharmacology (Berl) 186:312–322, 2006

Furmark T, Tillfors M, Marteinsdottir I, et al: Common changes in cerebral blood flow in patients with social phobia treated with citalopram or cognitive-behavioral therapy. Arch Gen Psychiatry 59:425–433, 2002

Garakani A, Buchsbaum MS, Newmark RE, et al: The effect of doxapram on brain imaging in patients with panic disorder. Eur Neuropsychopharmacol 17:672–686, 2007

Geracioti TD Jr, Baker DG, Ekhator NN, et al: CSF norepinephrine concentrations in posttraumatic stress disorder. Am J Psychiatry 158:1227–1230, 2001

Goddard AW, Sholomskas DE, Augeri FM, et al: Effects of tryptophan depletion in panic disorders. Biol Psychiatry 36:775–777, 1994

Goddard AW, Woods SW, Money R, et al: Effects of the CCK(B) antagonist CI-988 on responses to mCPP in generalized anxiety disorder. Psychiatry Res 85:225–240, 1999

Goldstein LE, Rasmusson AM, Bunney BS, et al: Role of the amygdala in the coordination of behavioral, neuroendocrine, and prefrontal cortical monoamine responses to psychological stress in the rat. J Neurosci 16:4787–4798, 1996

Graeff FG: On serotonin and experimental anxiety. Psychopharmacology (Berl) 163:467–476, 2002

Graeff FG: Serotonin, the periaqueductal gray and panic. Neurosci Biobehav Rev 28:239–259, 2004

Griebel G, Simiand J, Serradeil-Le Gal C, et al: Anxiolytic- and antidepressant-like effects of the non-peptide vasopressin V1b receptor antagonist, SSR149415, suggest an innovative approach for the treatment of stress-related disorders. Proc Natl Acad Sci U S A 99:6370–6375, 2002

Gross C, Zhuang X, Stark K, et al: Serotonin1A receptor acts during development to establish normal anxiety-like behaviour in the adult. Nature 416:396–400, 2002

Guastella AJ, Dadds MR, Lovibond PF, et al: A randomized controlled trial of the effect of D-cycloserine on exposure therapy for spider fear. J Psychiatr Res 41:466–471, 2007a

Guastella AJ, Lovibond PF, Dadds MR, et al: A randomized controlled trial of the effect of D-cycloserine on extinction and fear conditioning in humans. Behav Res Ther 45:663–672, 2007b

Guastella AJ, Richardson R, Lovibond PF, et al: A randomized controlled trial of D-cycloserine enhancement of exposure therapy for social anxiety disorder. Biol Psychiatry 63:544–549, 2008

Hano J, Vasar E, Bradwejn J: Cholecystokinin in animal and human research on anxiety. Trends Pharmacol Sci 14:244–249, 1993

Hariri AR, Mattay VS, Tessitore A, et al: Serotonin transporter genetic variation and the response of the human amygdala. Science 297:400–403, 2002

Hariri AR, Drabant EM, Munoz KE, et al: A susceptibility gene for affective disorders and the response of the human amygdala. Arch Gen Psychiatry 62:146–152, 2005

Harro J: CCK and NPY as anti-anxiety treatment targets: promises, pitfalls, and strategies. Amino Acids 31:215–230, 2006

Hebb AL, Poulin JF, Roach SP, et al: Cholecystokinin and endogenous opioid peptides: interactive influence on pain, cognition, and emotion. Prog Neuropsychopharmacol Biol Psychiatry 29:1225–1238, 2005

Heilig M, Soderpalm B, Engel J, et al: Centrally administered neuropeptide Y produces anxiolytic-like effects in animal anxiety models. Psychopharmacology 98:524–529, 1989

Heilig M: The NPY system in stress, anxiety and depression. Neuropeptides 38:213–224, 2004

Heim C, Nemeroff CB: The role of childhood trauma in the neurobiology of mood and anxiety disorders: preclinical and clinical studies. Biol Psychiatry 49:1023–1039, 2001

Hernando F, Schoots O, Lolait SJ, et al: Immunohistochemical localization of the vasopressin V1b receptor in the rat brain and pituitary gland: anatomical support for its involvement in the central effects of vasopressin. Endocrinology 142:1659–1668, 2001

Hertzberg T, Wahlbeck K: The impact of pregnancy and puerperium on panic disorder: a review. J Psychosom Obstet Gynaecol 20:59–64, 1999

Hettema JM, Neale MC, Kendler KS: A review and meta-analysis of the genetic epidemiology of anxiety disorders. Am J Psychiatry 158:1568–1578, 2001

Hoffman L, Burges Watson P, Wilson G, et al: Low plasma beta-endorphin in post-traumatic stress disorder. Aust N Z J Psychiatry 23:269–273, 1989

Hollander E, Kim S, Khanna S, et al: Obsessive-compulsive disorder and obsessive-compulsive spectrum disorders: diagnostic and dimensional issues. CNS Spectr 12 (suppl 3):5–13, 2007

Holmes A, Picciotto MR: Galanin: a novel therapeutic target for depression, anxiety disorders and drug addiction. CNS Neurol Disord Drug Targets 5:225–232, 2006

Hösing VG, Schirmacher A, Kuhlenbäumer G, et al: Cholecystokinin- and cholecystokinin-B-receptor gene polymorphisms in panic disorder. J Neural Transm Suppl 68:147–156, 2004

Hull AM: Neuroimaging findings in post-traumatic stress disorder. Br J Psychiatry 181:102–110, 2002

Ising M, Holsboer F: CRH-sub-1 receptor antagonists for the treatment of depression and anxiety. Exp Clin Psychopharmacol 15:519–528, 2007

Kalueff AV, Nutt DJ: Role of GABA in anxiety and depression. Depress Anxiety 24:495–517, 2007

Karlamangla AS, Singer BH, McEwen BS, et al: Allostatic load as a predictor of functional decline. MacArthur studies of successful aging. J Clin Epidemiol 55:696–710, 2002

Karlsson RM, Holmes A: Galanin as a modulator of anxiety and depression and as a therapeutic agent for affective disease. Amino Acids 31:231–239, 2006

Kash TL, Winder DG: Neuropeptide Y and corticotropin-releasing factor bi-directionally modulate inhibitory synaptic transmission in the bed nucleus of the stria terminalis. Neuropharmacology 51:1013–1022, 2006

Kask A, Harro J, von Horsten S, et al: The neurocircuitry and receptor subtypes mediating anxiolytic-like effects of neuropeptide Y. Neurosci Biobehav Rev 26:259–283, 2002

Katzman MA, Koszycki D, Bradwejn J: Effects of CCK-tetrapeptide in patients with social phobia and obsessive-compulsive disorder. Depress Anxiety 20:51–58, 2004

Kaufman J, Yang BZ, Douglas-Palumberi H, et al: Social supports and serotonin transporter gene moderate depression in maltreated children. Proc Natl Acad Sci U S A 101:17316–17321, 2004

Kellner M, Wiedemann K, Yassouridis A, et al: Behavioral and endocrine response to cholecystokinin tetrapeptide in patients with posttraumatic stress disorder. Biol Psychiatry 47:107–111, 2000

Kendler KS, Karkowski LM, Prescott CA: Fears and phobias: reliability and heritability. Psychol Med 29:539–553, 1999

Kent JM, Mathew SJ, Gorman JM: Molecular targets in the treatment of anxiety. Biol Psychiatry 52:1008–1030, 2002

Khoshbouei H, Cecchi M, Morilak DA: Modulatory effects of galanin in the lateral bed nucleus of the stria terminalis on behavioral and neuroendocrine responses to acute stress. Neuropsychopharmacology 27:25–34, 2002

King D, Zigmond MJ, Finlay JM: Effects of dopamine depletion in the medial prefrontal cortex on the stress-induced increase in extracellular dopamine in the nucleus accumbens core and shell. Neuroscience 77:141–153, 1997

Kinney JW, Starosta G, Holmes A, et al: Deficits in trace cued fear conditioning in galanin-treated rats and galanin-overexpressing transgenic mice. Learn Mem 9:178–190, 2002

Kramer MS, Cutler NR, Ballenger JC, et al: A placebo-controlled trial of L-365,260, a CCKB antagonist, in panic disorder. Biol Psychiatry 37:462–466, 1995

Kuteeva E, Wardi T, Hokfelt T, et al: Galanin enhances and a galanin antagonist attenuates depression-like behaviour in the rat. Eur Neuropsychopharmacol 17:64–69, 2007

Lanius RA, Williamson PC, Densmore M, et al: Neural correlates of traumatic memories in posttraumatic stress disorder: a functional MRI investigation. Am J Psychiatry 158:1920–1922, 2001

Lanzenberger, RR, Mitterhauser M, Spindelegger C, et al: Reduced serotonin-1A receptor binding in social anxiety disorder. Biol Psychiatry 61:1081–1089, 2007

LeDoux JE: Emotion circuits in the brain. Annu Rev Neurosci 23:155–184, 2000

LeDoux JE: The amygdala. Curr Biol 17:R868–R874, 2007

Lee JL, Everitt BJ, Thomas KL: Independent cellular processes for hippocampal memory consolidation and reconsolidation. Science 304:839–843, 2004

Lesch KP, Bengel D, Heils A, et al: Association of anxiety-related traits with a polymorphism in the serotonin transporter gene regulatory region. Science 274:1527–1531, 1996

Lever JR: PET and SPECT imaging of the opioid system: receptors, radioligands and avenues for drug discovery and development. Curr Pharm Des 13:33–49, 2007

Liberzon I, Taylor SF, Amdur R, et al: Brain activation in PTSD in response to trauma-related stimuli. Biol Psychiatry 45:817–826, 1999

Liberzon I, Taylor SF, Phan KL, et al: Altered central micro-opioid receptor binding after psychological trauma. Biol Psychiatry 61:1030–1038, 2007

Licinio J, O'Kirwan F, Irizarry K, et al: Association of a corticotropin-releasing hormone receptor 1 haplotype and antidepressant treatment response in Mexican Americans. Mol Psychiatry 9:1075–1082, 2004

Madden J, Akil H, Patrick RL, et al: Stress induced parallel changes in central opioid levels and pain responsiveness in the rat. Nature 265:358–360, 1977

Makino S, Gold PW, Schulkin J: Corticosterone effects on corticotropin-releasing hormone mRNA in the central nucleus of the amygdala and the parvocellular region of the paraventricular nucleus of the hypothalamus. Brain Res 640:105–112, 1994

Malenka RC, Bear MF: LTP and LTD: an embarrassment of riches. Neuron 44:5–21, 2004

Massana G, Serra-Grabulosa JM, Salgado-Pineda P, et al: Amygdalar atrophy in panic disorder patients detected by volumetric magnetic resonance imaging. Neuroimage 19:80–90, 2003

Mathew SJ, Price RB, Mao X, et al: Hippocampal N-acetylaspartate concentration and response to riluzole in generalized anxiety disorder. Biol Psychiatry 63:891–898, 2008

McDonald AJ: Topographical organization of amygdaloid projections to the caudatoputamen, nucleus accumbens, and related striatal-like areas of the rat brain. Neuroscience 44:15–33, 1991

McEwen BS: Stress and hippocampal plasticity. Annu Rev Neurosci 22:105–122, 1999

McEwen BS: Effects of adverse experiences for brain structure and function. Biol Psychiatry 48:721–731, 2000

McGrath M, Kawachi I, Ascherio A, et al: Association between catechol-O-methyltransferase and phobic anxiety. Am J Psychiatry 161:1703–1705, 2004

Milad MR, Quirk GJ: Neurons in medial prefrontal cortex signal memory for fear extinction. Nature 420:70–74, 2002

Misanin JR, Miller RR, Lewis DJ: Retrograde amnesia produced by electroconvulsive shock after reactivation of a consolidated memory trace. Science 160:554–555, 1968

Moller C, Sommer W, Thorsell A, et al: Anxiogenic-like action of galanin after intra-amygdala administration in the rat. Neuropsychopharmacology 21:507–512, 1999

Morgan CA 3rd, Wang S, Southwick SM, et al: Plasma neuropeptide-Y concentrations in humans exposed to military survival training. Biol Psychiatry 47:902–909, 2000

Morgan CA 3rd, Rasmusson AM, Wang S, et al: Neuropeptide-Y, cortisol, and subjective distress in humans exposed to acute stress replication and extension of previous report. Biol Psychiatry 52:136–142, 2002

Morgan CA 3rd, Rasmusson AM, Winters B, et al: Trauma exposure rather than posttraumatic stress disorder is associated with reduced baseline plasma neuropeptide-Y levels. Biol Psychiatry 54:1087–1091, 2003

Morilak DA, Barrera G, Echevarria DJ, et al: Role of brain norepinephrine in the behavior response to stress. Prog Neuropsychopharmacol Biol Psychiatry 29:1214–1224, 2005

Morris HV, Dawson GR, Reynolds DS, et al: Both alpha2 and alpha3 GABAA receptor subtypes mediate the anxiolytic properties of benzodiazepine site ligands in the conditioned emotional response paradigm. Eur J Neurosci 23:2495–2504, 2006

Morrow BA, Elsworth JD, Rasmusson AM, et al: The role of mesoprefrontal dopamine neurons in the acquisition and expression of conditioned fear in the rat. Neuroscience 92:553–564, 1999

Nemeroff CB: The role of GABA in the pathophysiology and treatment of anxiety disorders. Psychopharmacol Bull 37:133–146, 2003

Netto CF, Guimaraes FS: Anxiogenic effect of cholecystokinin in the dorsal periaqueductal gray. Neuropsychopharmacology 29:101–107, 2004

Neumeister A, Bain E, Nugent AC, et al: Reduced serotonin type 1A receptor binding in panic disorder. J Neurosci 24:589–591, 2004

Neumeister A, Charney DS, Belfer I, et al: Sympathoneural and adrenomedullary functional effects of alpha2C-adrenoreceptor gene polymorphism in healthy humans. Pharmacogenet Genomics 15:143–149, 2005

Neumeister A, Drevets WC, Belfer I, et al: Effects of a alpha 2C-adrenoreceptor gene polymorphism on neural responses to facial expressions in depression. Neuropsychopharmacology 31:1750–1756, 2006

Nishith P, Griffin MG, Poth TL: Stress-induced analgesia: prediction of posttraumatic stress symptoms in battered versus non-battered women. Biol Psychiatry 51:867–874, 2002

Nutt DJ, Glue P, Lawson CW, et al: Flumazenil provocation of panic attacks: evidence for altered benzodiazepine receptor sensitivity in panic disorders. Arch Gen Psychiatry 47:917–925, 1990

Nutt DJ, Malizia AL: New insights into the role of the GABAA-benzodiazepine receptor in psychiatric disorder. Br J Psychiatry 179:390–396, 2001

Ontiveros A, Fonaine R, Breton G: Correlation of severity of panic disorder and neuroanatomical changes on magnetic resonance imaging. J Neuropsychiatry Clin Neurosci 1:404–408, 1989

Pande AC, Greiner M, Adams JB, et al: Placebo-controlled trial of the CCK-B antagonist, CI-988, in panic disorder. Biol Psychiatry 46:860–862, 1999

Paoletti AM, Romagnino S, Contu R, et al: Observational study on the stability of the psychological status during normal pregnancy and increased blood levels of neuroactive steroids with GABA-A receptor agonist activity. Psychoneuroendocrinology 31:485–492, 2006

Paquette V, Levesque J, Mensour B, et al: "Change the mind and you change the brain": effects of cognitive-behavioral therapy on the neural correlates of spider phobia. Neuroimage 18:401–409, 2003

Parks C, Robinson P, Sibille E, et al: Increased anxiety of mice lacking the serotonin 1A receptor. Proc Natl Acad Sci U S A 95:10734–10739, 1998

Pavlov IP: Conditioned Reflexes. London, Oxford University Press, 1927

Petrakis I, Ralevski E, Nich C, et al: Naltrexone and disulfiram in patients with alcohol dependence and current depression. J Clin Psychopharmacol 27:160–165, 2007

Pfleiderer B, Zinkirciran S, Arolt V, et al: fMRI amygdala activation during a spontaneous panic attack in a patient with panic disorder. World J Biol Psychiatry 8:269–272, 2007

Pinna G, Costa E, Guidotti A: Fluoxetine and norfluoxetine stereospecifically and selectively increase brain neurosteroid content at doses that are inactive on 5-HT reuptake. Psychopharmacology (Berl) 186:362–372, 2006

Pinto-Ribeiro F, Almeida A, Pêgo JM, at al: Chronic unpredictable stress inhibits nociception in male rats. Neurosci Lett 359:73–76, 2004

Pissiota A, Frans O, Michelgård A, et al: Amygdala and anterior cingulate cortex activation during affective startle modulation: a PET study of fear. Eur J Neurosci 18:1325–1331, 2003

Pitman RK, Delahanty DL: Conceptually driven pharmacologic approaches to acute trauma. CNS Spectr 10:99–106, 2005

Pitman RK, van der Kolk BA, Orr SP, et al: Naloxone reversible analgesic response to combat-related stimuli in posttraumatic stress disorder. Arch Gen Psychiatry 47:541–544, 1990

Ponto LL, Kathol RG, Kettelkamp R, et al: Global cerebral blood flow after CO_2 inhalation in normal subjects and patients with panic disorder determined with [15O]water and PET. J Anxiety Disord 16:247–258, 2002

Primeaux SD, Wilson SP, Cusick MC, et al: Effects of altered amygdalar neuropeptide Y expression on anxiety-related behaviors. Neuropsychopharmacology 30:1589–1597, 2005

Rajarao J, Potestio L, Malberg J, et al: In vitro and in vivo pharmacological characterization of galanin and galnon. FASEB J 20:A686, 2006

Ramón y Cajal S: The Croonian lecture: la fine structure des centres nerveux. Proc Royal Soc London 55:444–468, 1894

Rasmusson AM, Pinna G, Paliwal P, et al: Decreased cerebrospinal fluid allopregnanolone levels in women with posttraumatic stress disorder. Biol Psychiatry 60:704–713, 2006

Rauch SL, van der Kolk BA, Fisler RE, et al: A symptom provocation study of posttraumatic stress disorder using positron emission tomography and script-driven imagery. Arch Gen Psychiatry 53:380–387, 1996

Rauch SL, Whalen PJ, Shin LM, et al: Exaggerated amygdala response to masked facial stimuli in posttraumatic stress disorder: a functional MRI study. Biol Psychiatry 47:769–776, 2000

Reddy DS, O'Malley BW, Rogawski MA: Anxiolytic activity of progesterone in progesterone receptor knockout mice. Neuropharmacology 48:14–24, 2005

Ressler KJ, Rothbaum BO, Tanenbaum L, et al: Cognitive enhancers as adjuncts to psychotherapy: use of D-cycloserine in phobic individuals to facilitate extinction of fear. Arch Gen Psychiatry 61:1136–1144, 2004

Riccio DC, Millin PM, Bogart AR: Reconsolidation: a brief history, a retrieval view, and some recent issues. Learn Mem 13:536–544, 2006

Roozendaal B, Okuda S, Van der Zee EA, et al: Glucocorticoid enhancement of memory requires arousal-induced noradrenergic activation in the basolateral amygdala. Proc Natl Acad Sci U S A 103:6741–6746, 2006

Rupprecht R: Neuroactive steroids: mechanisms of action and neuropsychopharmacological properties. Psychoneuroendocrinology 28:139–168, 2003

Sakai Y, Kumano H, Nishikawa M, et al: Cerebral glucose metabolism associated with a fear network in panic disorder. Neuroreport 16:927–931, 2005

Sallee FR, Sethuraman G, Sine L, et al: Yohimbine challenge in children with anxiety disorders. Am J Psychiatry 157:1236–1242, 2000

Sanchez MM, Young LJ, Plotsky PM, et al: Autoradiographic and in situ hybridization localization of corticotrophin-releasing factor 1 and 2 receptors in nonhuman primate brain. J Comp Neurol 408:365–377, 1999

Santini E, Ge H, Ren K, et al: Consolidation of fear extinction requires protein synthesis in the medial prefrontal cortex. J Neurosci 24:5704–5710, 2004

Sapolsky RM: Why stress is bad for your brain. Science 273:749–750, 1996

Saxe G, Geary M, Bedard K, et al: Separation anxiety as a mediator between acute morphine administration and PTSD symptoms in injured children. Ann N Y Acad Sci 1071:41–45, 2006

Schafe GE, Nader K, Blair HT, et al: Memory consolidation of Pavlovian fear conditioning: a cellular and molecular perspective. Trends Neurosci 24:540–546, 2001

Schienle A, Schäfer A, Hermann A, et al: Symptom provocation and reduction in patients suffering from spider phobia: an fMRI study on exposure therapy. Eur Arch Psychiatry Clin Neurosci 257:486–493, 2007

Schulkin J, Gold PW, McEwen BS: Induction of corticotropin-releasing hormone gene expression by glucocorticoids: implications for understanding the states of fear and anxiety and allostatic load. Psychoneuroendocrinology 23:219–243, 1998

Scoville WB, Milner B: Loss of recent memory after bilateral hippocampal lesions. J Neurol Neurosurg Psychiatry 20:11–21, 1957

Seedat S, Stein MB, Kennedy CM, et al: Plasma cortisol and neuropeptide Y in female victims of intimate partner violence. Psychoneuroendocrinology 28:796–808, 2003

Serradeil-Le Gal C, Wagnon J 3rd, Tonnerre B, et al: An overview of SSR149415, a selective nonpeptide vasopressin V(1b) receptor antagonist for the treatment of stress-related disorders. CNS Drug Rev 11:53–68, 2005

Sheng M, Kim MJ: Postsynaptic signaling and plasticity mechanisms. Science 298:776–780, 2002

Shin LM, McNally RJ, Kosslyn SM, et al: A positron emission tomographic study of symptom provocation in PTSD. Ann N Y Acad Sci 821:521–523, 1997

Shin LM, McNally RJ, Kosslyn SM, et al: Regional cerebral blood flow during script-driven imagery in childhood sexual abuse-related PTSD: a PET investigation. Am J Psychiatry 156:575–584, 1999

Shin LM, Whalen PJ, Pitman RK, et al: An fMRI study of anterior cingulate function in posttraumatic stress disorder. Biol Psychiatry 50:932–942, 2001

Simson PE, Weiss JM: Altered activity of the locus coeruleus in an animal model of depression. Neuropsychopharmacology 1:287–295, 1988

Smiaowska M, Wieroska JM, Domin H, et al: The effect of intrahippocampal injection of group II and III metabotropic glutamate receptor agonists on anxiety: the role of neuropeptide Y. Neuropsychopharmacology 32:1242–1250, 2007

Smith TA: Type A gamma-aminobutyric acid (GABAA) receptor subunits and benzodiazepine binding: significance to clinical syndromes and their treatment. Br J Biomed Sci 58:111–121, 2001

Sotres-Bayon F, Cain CK, LeDoux JE. Brain mechanisms of fear extinction: historical perspectives on the contribution of prefrontal cortex. Biol Psychiatry 60:329–336, 2006

Southwick SM, Morgan CA 3rd, Charney DS, et al: Yohimbine use in a natural setting: effects on posttraumatic stress disorder. Biol Psychiatry 46:442–444, 1999a

Southwick SM, Paige S, Morgan CA 3rd, et al: Neurotransmitter alterations in PTSD: catecholamines and serotonin. Semin Clin Neuropsychiatry 4:242–248, 1999b

Southwick SM, Davis M, Horner B, et al: Relationship of enhanced norepinephrine activity during memory consolidation to enhanced long-term memory in humans. Am J Psychiatry 159:1420–1422, 2002

Steckler T, Holsboer F: Corticotropin-releasing hormone receptor subtypes and emotion. Biol Psychiatry 46:1480–1508, 1999

Stein MB, Goldin PR, Sareen J, et al: Increased amygdala activation to angry and contemptuous faces in generalized social phobia. Arch Gen Psychiatry 59:1027–1034, 2002

Straube T, Mentzel HJ, Miltner WH: Waiting for spiders: brain activation during anticipatory anxiety in spider phobics. Neuroimage 37:1427–1436, 2007

Strömberg J, Haage D, Taube M, et al: Neurosteroid modulation of allopregnanolone and GABA effect on the GABA-A receptor. Neuroscience 143:73–81, 2006

Strome EM, Wheler GH, Higley JD, et al: Intracerebroventricular corticotropin-releasing factor increases limbic glucose metabolism and has social context-dependent behavioral effects in nonhuman primates. Proc Natl Acad Sci U S A 99:15749–15754, 2002

Swanson CJ, Blackburn TP, Zhang X, et al: Anxiolytic- and antidepressant-like profiles of the galanin-3 receptor (Gal3) antagonists SNAP 37889 and SNAP 398299. Proc Natl Acad Sci U S A 102:17489–17494, 2005

Targum SD, Marshall LE: Fenfluramine provocation of anxiety in patients with panic disorder. Psychiatry Res 28:295–306, 1989

Thorsell A, Michalkiewicz M, Dumont Y, et al: Behavioral insensitivity to restraint stress, absent fear suppression of behavior and impaired spatial learning in transgenic rats with hippocampal neuropeptide Y overexpression. Proc Natl Acad Sci U S A 97:12852–12857, 2000

Tillfors M, Furmark T, Marteinsdottir I, et al: Cerebral blood flow in subjects with social phobia during stressful speaking tasks: a PET study. Am J Psychiatry 158:1220–1226, 2001

Tillfors M, Furmark T, Marteinsdottir I, et al: Cerebral blood flow during anticipation of public speaking in social phobia: a PET study. Biol Psychiatry 52:1113–1119, 2002

Tinuper P, Montagna P, Plazzi G, et al: Idiopathic recurring stupor. Neurology 44:621–625, 1994

Uhde TW, Joffe RT, Jimerson DC, et al: Normal urinary free cortisol and plasma MHPG in panic disorder: clinical and theoretical implications. Biol Psychiatry 23:575–585, 1988

Unschuld PG, Ising M, Erhardt A, et al: Polymorphisms in the galanin gene are associated with symptom-severity in female patients suffering from panic disorder. J Affect Disord 105:177–184, 2008

van der Linden G, van Heerden B, Warwick J, et al: Functional brain imaging and pharmacotherapy in social phobia: single photon emission computed tomography before and after treatment with the selective serotonin reuptake inhibitor citalopram. Prog Neuropsychopharmacol Biol Psychiatry 24:419–438, 2000

van Megen HJ, Westenberg HG, den Boer JA, et al: The cholecystokinin-B receptor antagonist CI-988 failed to affect CCK-4 induced symptoms in panic disorder patients. Psychopharmacology (Berl) 129:243–248, 1997

Vanover KE, Rosenzweig-Lipson S, Hawkinson JE, et al: Characterization of the anxiolytic properties of a novel neuroactive steroid, Co 2-6749 (GMA-839; WAY-141839; 3alpha, 21-dihydroxy-3beta-trifluoromethyl-19-nor-5beta-pregnan-20-one), a selective modulator of gamma-aminobutyric acid(A) receptors. J Pharmacol Exp Ther 295:337–345, 2000

Ventura R, Cabib S, Puglisi-Allegra S: Genetic susceptibility of mesocortical dopamine to stress determines liability to inhibition of mesoaccumbens dopamine and to behavioral "despair" in a mouse model of depression. Neuroscience 115:999–1007, 2002

Villarreal G, Hamilton DA, Petropoulos H, et al: Reduced hippocampal volume and total white matter volume in posttraumatic stress disorder. Biol Psychiatry 52:119–125, 2002

Vythilingam M, Anderson ER, Goddard A, et al: Temporal lobe volume in panic disorder—a quantitative magnetic resonance imaging study. Psychiatry Res 99:75–82, 2000

Walker DL, Davis M: Double dissociation between the involvement of the bed nucleus of the stria terminalis and the central nucleus of the amygdala in startle increases produced by conditioned versus unconditioned fear. J Neurosci 17:9375–9383, 1997

Wang C, Marx CE, Morrow AL, et al: Neurosteroid modulation of GABAergic neurotransmission in the central amygdala: a role for NMDA receptors. Neurosci Lett 415:118–123, 2007

Whitlock JR, Heynen AJ, Shuler MG, et al: Learning induces long-term potentiation in the hippocampus. Science 313:1093–1097, 2006

Yehuda R: Advances in understanding neuroendocrine alterations in PTSD and their therapeutic implications. Ann N Y Acad Sci 1071:137–166, 2006

Yehuda R, Brand S, Yang R: Plasma neuropeptide Y concentrations in combat exposed veterans: relationship to trauma exposure, recovery from PTSD, and coping. Biol Psychiatry 59:660–663, 2006

Zanoveli JM, Netto CF, Guimarães FS, et al: Systemic and intra-dorsal periaqueductal gray injections of cholecystokinin sulfated octapeptide (CCK-8s) induce a panic-like response in rats submitted to the elevated T-maze. Peptides 25:1935–1941, 2004

Zubieta JK, Heitzeg MM, Smith YR, et al: COMT val158met genotype affects mu-opioid neurotransmitter responses to a pain stressor. Science 299:1240–1243, 2003

CHAPTER 48

Neurobiology of Alzheimer's Disease

Albert A. Davis, B.S.

James J. Lah, M.D., Ph.D.

Allan I. Levey, M.D., Ph.D.

Of the broad spectrum of brain diseases that can produce dementia, Alzheimer's disease (AD) is the most common. AD is a devastating disorder characterized by progressive loss of memory and intellectual abilities, affecting more than 40% of individuals older than 85 years of age. The remarkable increase in disease prevalence that has accompanied the growth of the oldest segment of the population has heightened public awareness and accelerated research efforts to understand the disease. AD has been recognized as a clinical and neuropathological entity for more than 100 years, but specific therapies were unavailable until the development of the first cholinesterase inhibitor, tacrine, about 20 years ago. Since that time, several new cholinesterase inhibitors have been approved for the treatment of AD patients, and novel therapies, such as the N-methyl-D-aspartate (NMDA) receptor antagonist memantine, have shown modest benefit in improving cognitive function in patients with AD. Common clinical practice has also embraced the use of high-dose vitamin E as an antioxidant that may provide some neuroprotective benefit. Research on AD funded by the government, private foundations, and the pharmaceutical industry commits billions of dollars annually for achieving better understanding of the disease and for de-veloping more effective treatments. These efforts will inevitably lead to continued improvement in clinical practice in the coming years.

AD is complex, with multiple genetic components, risk factors, neuropathological features, and theories of pathogenesis. This chapter provides an update on our current understanding of the biological basis of the disease and background for understanding the anticipated rapid changes in the clinical approach to AD. Because our understanding of AD is still evolving, it is difficult to predict the form of future clinical applications. Some of these will certainly be surprising. However, the most dramatic advances and changes in clinical management of AD are likely to emerge from the rational development of treatments to modify the basic mechanisms of disease. With this in mind, we begin this chapter by reviewing well-established neuropathological and neurochemical changes observed in AD. These abnormalities are particularly relevant for understanding the rationale for the use of cholinesterase inhibitors and other drugs for ameliorating cognitive, emotional, and behavioral symptoms. Next we examine epidemiological studies that have revealed several risk factors for AD and have offered clues to potentially important mechanisms in disease pathogenesis

The authors are grateful to Dr. Marla Gearing for providing photomicrographs and for critical reading of the text.

and possible prevention. AD genetics is a rapidly expanding field, and some of the more salient observations are noted here. We conclude the chapter by considering several theories of AD etiopathogenesis as well as future directions of research and disease therapy. This discussion will certainly require modification and refinement as new research findings emerge. However, these theories provide the rationale for most of the current efforts to develop new therapies that will produce a significant impact on preventing, halting, or perhaps reversing the disease process.

Pathology

The primary pathological hallmarks of AD, described a century ago by Alois Alzheimer (1906), consist of senile (neuritic) plaques and neurofibrillary tangles (Figure 48–1). These morphological changes, which are visible on silver-stained specimens, provide important clues to the biology of AD. *Neuritic plaques* are complex structures that consist of extracellular aggregates of the amyloid-beta (Aβ) peptide, surrounded by swollen dystrophic neurites and infiltrated by microglia and reactive astrocytes. *Neurofibrillary tangles* are intracellular accumulations of hyperphosphorylated tau, a cytoskeleton-associated protein organized in disease states as paired helical filaments. Grossly, there is often atrophy of the frontal, parietal, and temporal lobes in brains with AD. The medial temporal lobe structures, including the amygdala, hippocampus, and entorhinal cortex, are usually markedly shrunken. While atrophy is not specific to AD, the areas of atrophy reflect the selective vulnerability of certain brain regions and correspond to the microscopic accumulation of plaques and tangles.

In addition to plaques and tangles, other pathological changes are visible in the AD brain (Terry et al. 1994). Amyloid deposition in leptomeningeal blood vessel walls, known as *amyloid angiopathy*, results in increased frequency of lobar hemorrhages. *Neuropil threads* are short neuronal processes that are marked by silver stains, thioflavin, and tau immunoreactivity, found mostly in cortical regions associated with tangle pathology. *Hirano bodies* are rod-like filaments composed of actin and other microfilaments, most commonly occurring in pyramidal neurons in the hippocampus. *Granulovacuolar degeneration*, detectable by the appearance of large cytoplasmic membrane-delimited vacuoles, is often found in the same regions. These vacuoles also contain cytoskeleton-associated proteins. All of the pathological lesions occur in "normal" aging to a limited extent, but they occur much more frequently in the hippocampus, neocortex, and other areas in AD.

Cellular and synaptic alterations also occur in AD. There is a loss of large neurons, particularly in layer II of the entorhinal cortex, pyramidal neurons in layers III and V of neocortex, cholinergic neurons in the basal forebrain, and in select subcortical nuclei. Loss of synapses is an important change because this pathology presumably results in the disconnection of cortical association areas. Indeed, of all pathological alterations measured to date, synapse loss best correlates with cognitive deficits. There are also a variety of intracellular changes in endomembranous compartments. For example, the biosynthetic machinery, including the Golgi apparatus, is shrunken (Salehi et al. 1994), and there is an expansion of endosomal compartments (Cataldo et al. 1995, 1996; Nixon 2005). Endosomal changes occur early in the disease, even at preclinical stages in vulnerable neurons, and appear to be intimately associated with genetic factors in AD.

The wide variety of pathological changes raises questions about their sequence of occurrence; that is, a more complete understanding of the disease's pathogenesis rests on the identification of the primary changes that cause the disease versus the secondary changes that occur in later stages of neurodegeneration. This key issue remains unresolved. Moreover, it is possible that there may be several distinct mechanisms that are capable of initiating the pathogenic cascade. For example, genetic studies indicate that mutations in several genes (*amyloid precursor protein* [APP], *presenilin 1* [PSEN1], and *presenilin 2* [PSEN2]) are sufficient to initiate disease and that polymorphisms in other genes can accelerate the process. Ultimately, the development of strategies to modify the course or to prevent the disease demands understanding of the mechanisms by which genetic and environmental factors interact to cause disease. These factors are further discussed in the sections that follow. Advances in understanding the biology of all phases of AD will impact drug development. In particular, the improved understanding of the neurochemical changes has opened the door for the first successful attempts to develop efficacious drugs.

Neurochemistry and Neuropharmacology

Numerous studies have examined the neurochemical changes that occur in the brains of individuals with AD. The most consistent changes involve loss of cholinergic, serotonergic, and glutamatergic markers (Bowen and

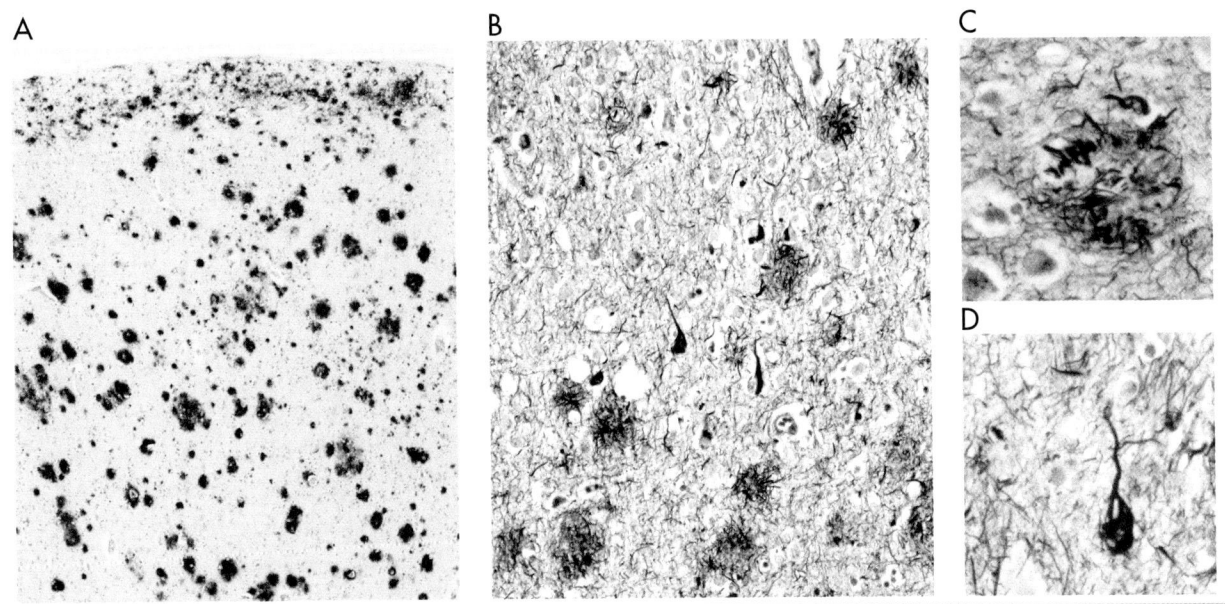

FIGURE 48-1. Pathological hallmarks of Alzheimer's disease.

(A) Low-magnification view of cerebral cortex showing multiple Aβ-immunopositive plaques. (B) Higher magnification of a Bielschowsky silver stain showing argyrophilic amyloid plaques (*arrow*) and neurofibrillary tangles (*arrowhead*) in cerebral cortex. (C) High-magnification view of a single neuritic plaque. The central core of the plaque contains amyloid peptides that are surrounded by a clear halo and then swollen silver-positive dystrophic neurites. (D) High-magnification view of a neurofibrillary tangle.

Francis 1990). The acetylcholine and serotonin neurons are located in the basal forebrain and upper brain stem, respectively, and their degeneration results in the loss of ascending modulatory effects on neocortical and hippocampal function. In contrast, the loss of glutamate, the primary excitatory neurotransmitter, reflects degeneration of cortical pyramidal neurons.

Abundant evidence suggests that the clinical syndrome involves failed neurotransmission at cholinergic synapses in neocortex and hippocampus (Coyle et al. 1983). This concept is based on numerous observations. First, presynaptic cholinergic markers are decreased in neocortex and hippocampus in AD, and they have been found to correlate with dementia severity (Bowen and Francis 1990; Davies and Maloney 1976). Second, basal forebrain neurons, which provide the majority of cholinergic innervation to the neocortex and hippocampus, degenerate in AD (Whitehouse et al. 1982). Third, basal forebrain lesions or pharmacological blockade of muscarinic acetylcholine receptors (mAChR) impairs learning, memory, and attention (Bartus et al. 1982; Damasio et al. 1985; Drachman 1977). Fourth, clinical trials of acetylcholinesterase (AChE) inhibitors show improved cognition and quality of life, reduced behavioral problems, and delayed institutionalization (Cummings and Cole 2002; Dooley and Lamb 2000; Knopman et al. 1996; Lamb and Goa 2001; Olin and Schneider 2002). Finally, brains from Parkinson's disease patients treated chronically with antimuscarinic drugs show increased AD neuropathology compared to brains from untreated or acutely treated patients (Perry et al. 2003).

Perturbations in specific cholinergic markers seem to occur at different stages of the disease (Mufson et al. 2003). For example, the numbers of neurons in the basal forebrain that express choline acetyltransferase (ChAT) and vesicular acetylcholine transporter (VAChT) are not altered in cases of mild cognitive impairment (MCI; a prodrome of clinically defined AD) or even in the early stages of AD (Gilmor et al. 1999). However, the numbers of basal forebrain neurons expressing p75[NTR], a low-affinity neurotrophin receptor (NTR), are significantly decreased in both AD and MCI (Mufson et al. 2002). These findings have been suggested to reflect a phenotypic alteration in cholinergic basal forebrain neurons that precedes absolute neuron loss, and they highlight the importance of developing neuroprotective strategies that could be utilized, even after symptoms emerge, to prevent or slow the degeneration of cholinergic and other neurons. There are also complex changes in cortical markers of cholinergic neurotransmission. In early stages, ChAT, the rate-limiting enzyme for acetylcholine synthesis, is not decreased (Davis et al. 1999; DeKosky et al. 2002). As the disease progresses, however, the activity of ChAT, together with AChE (the degradative enzyme for acetyl-

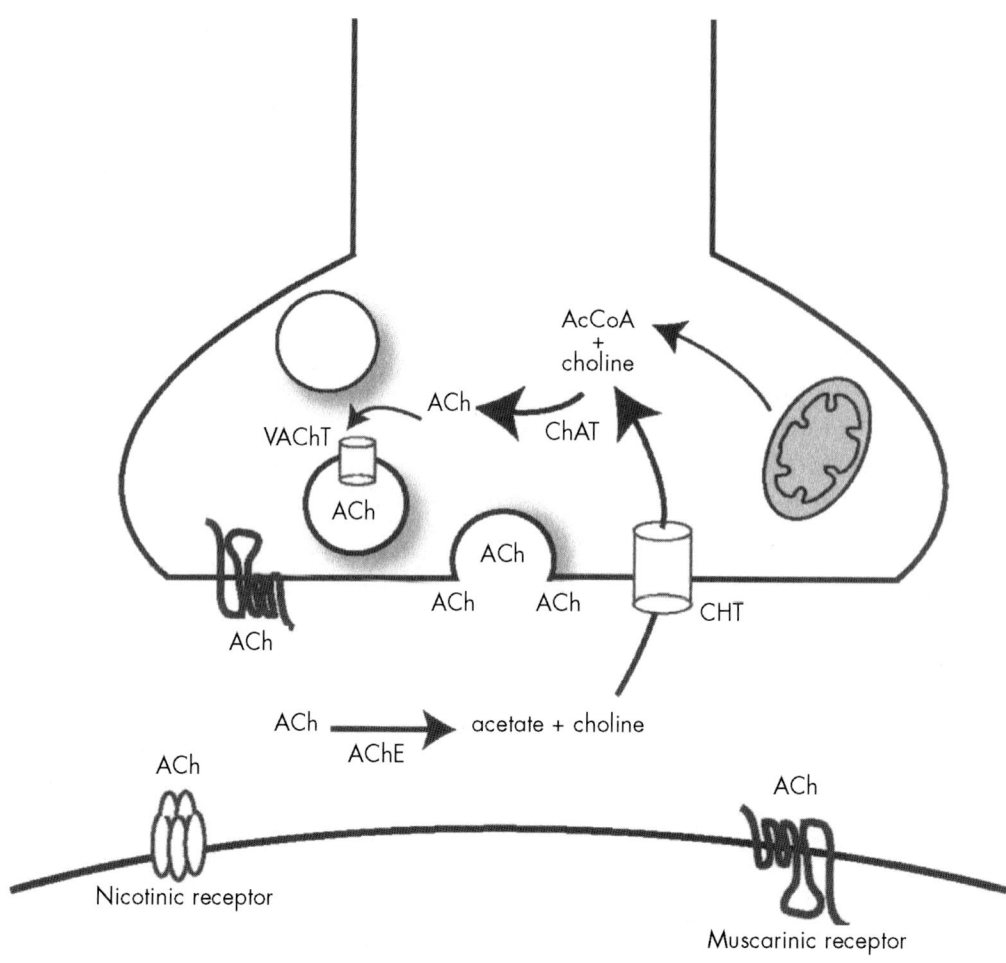

FIGURE 48–2.   Molecular basis of cholinergic neurotransmission.

Acetylcholine (ACh) is synthesized in the nerve terminal cytoplasm and is incorporated into synaptic vesicles via the vesicular acetylcholine transporter (VAChT). Upon nerve impulse, cholinergic vesicles release ACh into the synaptic cleft, where the transmitter binds to pre- and postsynaptic muscarinic and nicotinic receptor subtypes. Transmission is terminated by the rapid hydrolysis of ACh by acetylcholinesterase (AChE). The degradation product choline is recycled into the terminal by the high-affinity choline transporter (CHT). This reuptake process is a key regulated and rate-limiting step in ACh synthesis. AcCoA = acetyl coenzyme A.

choline), diminishes. Of interest, molecules selectively present in cholinergic nerve terminals in cortex, including ChAT, VAChT (responsible for packaging acetylcholine into synaptic vesicles), and the high-affinity choline transporter (responsible for the uptake of choline), seem to increase, suggesting compensatory changes in surviving terminals. The diversity of molecules involved in different aspects of cholinergic transmission (Figure 48–2) provides a variety of potential strategies for reducing the dysfunction of cholinergic systems in AD.

AChE inhibitors are currently the primary symptomatic treatment for AD. There are different types of cholinesterase enzymes, including an AChE and a butyrylcholinesterase type, both of which degrade acetylcholine. AChE is the primary enzyme expressed by neurons, and complete disruption of the gene for this enzyme in mice re-

sults in the overactivity of cholinergic systems in both brain and peripheral nervous system. Moreover, mice deficient in AChE display significant changes in the levels, cellular distribution, and function of muscarinic acetylcholine receptors, phenomena that may antagonize the potential benefit of cholinesterase inhibitors (Volpicelli-Daley et al. 2003a, 2003b). The goal of cholinesterase inhibition in humans is to prevent the degradation of acetylcholine once it is released from surviving cholinergic nerve terminals. The typical degree of AChE inhibition achievable with available drugs is only about 30% (Kuhl et al. 2000), which provides one explanation for their modest efficacy. However, because the same activity is essential for cholinergic function in the gut and in other organs receiving autonomic innervation, more complete inhibition would likely increase the side effects that already limit the dosing of cholinesterase inhibitors. In addition, cardiac and neuromuscular blockade are major concerns with more potent and irreversible drugs that inhibit acetylcholine breakdown.

Although AChE inhibitors provide an important advance, they are limited by the above considerations. The development of compounds that bind directly to cholinergic receptors is an alternative approach to enhancing cholinergic transmission. Moreover, the discovery of families of mAChR (Bonner et al. 1987; Peralta et al. 1987) and nicotinic receptor (Sargent 1993) subtypes may enable the development of selective drugs to overcome many of the side effects associated with AChE inhibitors and nonselective agonists. Receptor subtypes often have opposing actions; therefore, targeting one subtype produces more robust effects (Bymaster et al. 1998; Farber et al. 1995). Most studies have focused on mAChRs, because this receptor family has better-defined roles in central cholinergic transmission and functions, such as learning and memory (Bartus et al. 1982; Coyle et al. 1983). The nicotinic receptors also play an important role in cognition and neurodegenerative disease (Romanelli et al. 2007). Thus, selective drugs targeted at receptor subtypes offer hope for better cholinergic-based therapies for AD and other disorders involving central cholinergic systems.

The mAChR family consists of five distinct subtypes, M_1–M_5, encoded by different genes and all expressed in the brain. The M_1, M_2, and M_4 receptors are the most abundant subtypes. Their precise roles in central cholinergic function and their potential for AD treatments remain uncertain (Levey 1996), but several lines of evidence suggest that M_1 may be a key target. M_1 is the most abundant receptor in the cortex and hippocampus; it is postsynaptic on pyramidal neurons and plays an important role in enhancing glutamatergic transmission via NMDA receptors (Marino et al. 1998). M_1 also activates protein kinase pathways involved in the long-term changes in gene expression that underlie learning and memory (Berkeley et al. 2001). There is some loss of M_1 receptor protein and high-affinity states involving coupling to G proteins (Flynn et al. 1991, 1995). M_2 is the primary autoreceptor on cholinergic terminals in cortical structures, and it is also present on inhibitory interneurons. Loss of M_2 receptors in AD probably involves both neuronal populations. M_4, the most abundant receptor in the striatum, is a presynaptic heteroreceptor on commissural projections in cortex, suggesting that it is involved in the regulation of excitatory associational connections. Of interest, this subtype is increased in AD.

Subtype-selective agonists and antagonists have been difficult to develop, but they remain promising. One of the first relatively selective M_1 agonists, xanomeline, showed significant clinical efficacy in a double-blind multicenter study (Bodick et al. 1997). Some of the most remarkable benefits were in the reduction of agitation, delusions, and hallucinations, providing evidence that the cholinergic system plays an important role in behavior as well as in cognition. Subsequent studies of cholinesterase inhibitors have reinforced this idea (Cummings and Cole 2002) and have provided a rationale for long-term treatment and use of these agents in later stages of AD. In addition to their potential benefit in ameliorating symptoms, direct-acting muscarinic receptor agonists may also alter the course of the disease. Several preclinical studies have established distinct roles of muscarinic receptor subtypes in regulating amyloidogenesis, and an M_1 muscarinic agonist reduced both amyloid plaque and neurofibrillary tangle pathology in a transgenic mouse model of AD (Caccamo et al. 2006). In human studies, M_1 agonist treatment reduced cerebrospinal fluid (CSF) amyloid levels (Hock et al. 2003). In addition, postmortem analysis of Lewy body dementia cases treated with cholinesterase inhibitors showed significantly less amyloid pathology than cases examined prior to the advent of these drugs (Ballard et al. 2007). While these studies suggest that cholinergic treatment has the potential to be disease modifying, the therapeutic potential of drugs selective for cholinergic receptor subtypes remains to be determined.

Neurochemical alterations in serotonin, norepinephrine, and glutamate also have important therapeutic implications for AD. Serotonin plays a key role in mood and anxiety disorders, which commonly coexist with dementia in AD. Selective serotonin reuptake inhibitors are frequently used for these patients and have demonstrated efficacy. There is a loss of noradrenergic neurons in the locus coeruleus in AD, although the significance of this change and its implications for therapeutic intervention are only beginning to be systematically investigated. Preclinical studies have suggested that noradrenergic neurotransmission may have a role in disease modification. For example, locus coeruleus degeneration exacerbated amyloid pathology, behavioral deficits, and neuron loss in a transgenic mouse model of AD, suggesting that loss of noradrenergic neurotransmission may be a contributing factor in the development or progression of AD (Heneka et al. 2006). Drugs that modulate glutamatergic transmission also have potential utility for the cognitive and behavioral symptoms of AD. In addition, since excitotoxicity may play some role in the neurodegenerative process, such drugs could potentially be neuroprotective. Ampakines, a class of drugs that modulate amino-3-hydroxy-5-

methyl-4-isoxazole propionic acid (AMPA) subtypes of glutamate receptors, are under development. Memantine, a noncompetitive NMDA antagonist, is now approved for the treatment of AD in the United States. Although clinical trials of high-affinity NMDA antagonists have been hindered by serious side effects, memantine seems to be well tolerated. Recent clinical trials indicate a significant benefit of this drug in AD patients, particularly with respect to language and memory domains (Peskind et al. 2006; Pomara et al. 2007).

Risk Factors and Clues to the Biology of Alzheimer's Disease

Aging is the biggest risk factor for AD, and the prevalence of AD doubles about every 5 years after age 65 years, increasing to about 40% by age 85 years. This relationship has contributed to speculations that AD is simply accelerated aging (rather than a disease) and that everyone would develop AD if they lived long enough. However, the risk may actually decline after age 90 years (Lautenschlager et al. 1996), indicating that AD is not an inevitable result of aging. Because age alone is insufficient to cause the disease, other risk factors must therefore interact with the aging process (Table 48–1). Of the many factors that have been examined, retrospective studies indicate that individuals with severe traumatic brain injury have a higher-than-expected incidence of AD pathology (Jellinger et al. 2001). Head injury also seems to interact with genetic predisposition (ApoE ε4) to decrease the age at AD onset (Mayeux et al. 1995; Schofield et al. 1997). Down syndrome is another well-established risk factor. Virtually all Down syndrome patients who are older than 40 years of age exhibit the hallmark neuropathology of AD (Karlinsky 1986). However, clinically evident AD is less common. There is also an increased risk for mothers of children with Down syndrome (Schupf et al. 2001).

Several studies suggest that education (D.A. Evans et al. 1997; Katzman 1993; Stern et al. 1994) and early cognitive and linguistic abilities (Snowdon et al. 1996; Whalley et al. 2000) correlate with decreased risk for AD. In many studies, a higher level of education is associated with a lower risk of developing AD (D.A. Evans et al. 1997; Katzman 1993; Stern et al. 1994). Participation in other activities that require cognitive ability is also associated with a lower risk of AD (Wilson et al. 2002). One possible explanation is that people who are more intelligent and healthy have a higher "cerebral reserve" and thus do not manifest signs of dementia until more brain tissue is dam-

aged. In a longitudinal study of AD in a group of nuns, linguistic ability in early life strongly predicted cognitive abilities in old age (Snowdon et al. 1996). In addition, neuropathological analysis has documented significant correlations between low idea density in early-life autobiographies and neuropathological signs of AD (Riley et al. 2005). Similarly, in a Scottish study, lower performance on childhood school tests was associated with increased late-life dementia (Whalley et al. 2000). Despite obvious limitations in these types of correlational studies, the strength of the associations raises the intriguing possibility that developmental mechanisms or early education may play a role in the development of AD in late life.

Epidemiological studies indicate that AD is more common in women, and initial reports suggested that postmenopausal estrogen replacement is associated with a lower incidence of AD. There is experimental evidence that estrogen may modify the production of Aβ peptide (Xu et al. 1998), linking the epidemiological data with a potential biological mechanism. Additional studies of hormone replacement therapy have produced conflicting data. In the Women's Health Initiative Memory Study (WHIMS), both estrogen plus progestin and estrogen therapy alone were found to be associated with an increased risk of developing dementia (Shumaker et al. 2003, 2004). However, the Cache County Study found that hormone replacement therapy is associated with a lower risk of late-onset AD in a manner dependent on the duration of exposure. In this study, women taking hormone replacement therapy for more than 10 years showed the greatest reduction of AD risk (Zandi et al. 2002). The observed gender bias may reflect biological factors underlying disease susceptibility or, alternatively, the greater longevity of females (Hebert et al. 2001). Other gender-specific factors may exist, however. For example, the offspring of a father with AD have a 1.4-fold greater risk than if the mother was affected (Lautenschlager et al. 1996). Despite an increasing understanding of the interaction between hormones and the risk of dementia, the precise role of gender in AD pathogenesis remains to be clarified.

Epidemiological studies have revealed patterns of medication use associated with altered risk of AD, including exposure to nonsteroidal anti-inflammatory drugs (NSAIDs) and 3-hydroxy-3-methylglutaryl coenzyme A reductase inhibitors (statins). The magnitude of the reduced risk associated with NSAIDs, estrogen, or statins is similar, ranging from ~30% to 80%. As with any epidemiological study, a variety of biases are possible, and results do not imply a causal relationship. Nevertheless, several epidemiological investigations, including one

TABLE 48–1. Risk factors for developing Alzheimer's disease (AD)

CATEGORY	FACTOR	INFLUENCE ON AD RISK
Life events	Aging	Risk increases with increasing age
	Early-life linguistic ability	Decreases risk
	Traumatic brain injury	Increases risk
Genetics	Down syndrome	Greatly increases risk
	ApoE ε4	Increases risk
Sex	Female vs. male	Females have increased risk
	Estrogen replacement	Sustained estrogen replacement may lower risk
Diet/medication	Vitamin/nutrient supplementation	Vitamins C and E may be protective
	Nonsteroidal anti-inflammatory drug use	Decreases risk
	Statin use	Decreases risk
Cardiovascular risk factors	Hypercholesterolemia	Increases risk
	Hypertension	Increases risk
	Elevated plasma homocysteine	Increases risk
	Diabetes mellitus	Increases risk

large prospective population-based study, have found the relative risk of AD to be lower with long-term use of NSAIDs (in t' Veld et al. 2001). Thus far, only two small prospective clinical trials of NSAIDs have indicated a protective effect in AD. Notably, all trials involving selective cyclo-oxygenase-2 (COX-2) inhibitors have been negative, a finding that may shed light on the biological mechanism by which certain nonselective anti-inflammatory agents exert their protective effect (Aisen et al. 2003; McGeer and McGeer 2007).

There is accumulating evidence that some NSAIDs modulate the activity of the γ-secretase enzyme independently of their effect on cyclo-oxygenase enzymes, and Phase II clinical trials have shown that the Aβ42-lowering drug R-flurbiprofen may have cognitive and behavioral benefits in AD. It is unclear whether NSAIDs will ultimately prove to be beneficial in AD, but because these medications have serious potential side effects, the evidence to date does not warrant recommendations for use as a primary treatment for AD. Epidemiological studies have also shown that statins are associated with a significantly lower relative risk of AD (Jick et al. 2000; Rockwood et al. 2002; Wolozin et al. 2000) and that the association seems specific, compared with the use of other lipid-lowering agents and cardiovascular drugs. Given that hypercholesterolemia is a potential risk factor for developing AD (Kivipelto et al. 2001; Notkola et al. 1998), the data linking statin use and decreased risk of AD strengthen the biological relationship between cholesterol homeostasis and

AD. The results of additional research, including ongoing multicenter clinical trials, will ultimately determine the role for statins in the growing armamentarium of AD therapies. Taken together, these associations provide potential insights into the biology of AD. Specifically, they implicate hormones, inflammation, and cholesterol as relevant factors for further study in the pathogenesis of the disease.

It has been postulated that several lifestyle factors, including dietary habits, physical activity, and leisure activities (Scarmeas et al. 2001), play a role in the development of AD. Dietary intake of several vitamins and nutrients has been studied. Subclinical deficiencies of vitamin B_6, vitamin B_{12}, and folate are associated with poorer cognitive function in the elderly, and AD patients tend to have lower levels of these vitamins (Clarke et al. 1998; H.X. Wang et al. 2001). These vitamins are essential cofactors in the generation of donor methyl groups, which in turn are necessary for the biosynthesis of numerous neural components, such as neurotransmitters and myelin. Therefore, mild defects in the methyl donor pathway might have subtle effects on neuronal function and viability. Alternatively (or additively), the deleterious effects of B vitamin or folate deficiency may be mediated by elevated homocysteine, a metabolite of the methyl donor pathway. Homocysteine causes vascular damage and has been linked to ischemic changes in the brain, as well as in other organs. Beginning several years before diagnosis, patients with AD have elevated homocysteine levels (Seshadri et al. 2002), regardless of vitamin B_{12}/folate status.

This observation adds to the growing connection between vascular disease and AD (Kivipelto et al. 2001). Vitamin D deficiency, a common disorder among the elderly, has been recently linked with poor cognitive performance in participants of a study of memory and aging (Wilkins et al. 2006). The antioxidant vitamins C and E have been associated with reduced risk of AD (Engelhart et al. 2002). Despite an initial finding that vitamin E slows disease progression in patients with AD (Sano et al. 1997), another study demonstrated that vitamin E had no apparent effect on progression from MCI to AD, even among high-risk subjects (ApoE ε4 positive) (Petersen et al. 2005). However, major differences in the study populations may have influenced the outcomes. AD has also been linked to dietary fat intake—namely, with higher levels of total and saturated fat and cholesterol and with lower levels of fish oils, which contain polyunsaturated fats. While it is not clear exactly how these dietary factors impact the development and progression of AD, if the associations are confirmed in clinical trials, which are currently under way, specific nutritional interventions may be warranted as a means of preventing or slowing the onset of disease.

The effects of ethanol and smoking remain unclear. Heavy ethanol use produces a characteristic dementia syndrome that shares some features with AD. Of interest, several studies have found that moderate consumption of red wine was associated with a decreased risk of AD (Luchsinger et al. 2004; Orgogozo et al. 1997). Moderate ethanol intake has been linked to improved cardiovascular health, which may account for this effect. Conflicting evidence exists regarding the effects of smoking. Some studies have found an increased incidence of AD in smokers, which could be caused by the well-established deleterious effects of smoking on cardiovascular health. Other studies have observed that smokers have a lower risk of AD. Although surprising, this latter observation might be attributable to the stimulatory effects of nicotine at nicotinic acetylcholine receptors.

In addition, decreased leisure activity in midlife is a risk factor for AD (Scarmeas et al. 2001). Although people who remain active may be enhancing their cerebral reserve, it is also possible that decreased leisure activity is an early sign of subclinical cognitive impairment.

Genetics

AD is a complex genetic disease. Multiple genes are associated with the disease, with mutations in some genes linked to fully penetrant cases with autosomal dominant inheritance and polymorphisms in other genes linked to disease risk. To date, four genes—APP, PSEN1, PSEN2, and APOE—have been consistently linked to AD in studies around the world (Blacker and Tanzi 1998; Selkoe and Podlisny 2002). Many other genes have been associated with AD in only a few studies and/or remain controversial, and these genes will not be discussed here unless otherwise specified. It is clear that several other genes with strong links to AD remain to be identified. The diversity of genes and other factors result in two major presentations of illness: familial and sporadic.

Less than 5% of all cases of AD are familial—mostly with an early onset (i.e., younger than 65 years)—and they seem to follow an autosomal dominant mode of inheritance. In these families, mutations in three distinct genes—APP on chromosome 21, PSEN1 on chromosome 14, and PSEN2 on chromosome 1—have been linked to the affected individuals. Although important for understanding the biology of AD, APP mutations are extremely rare. PSEN1 mutations account for the majority of the familial cases with early-onset disease. Although APP and PSEN1 mutations are linked exclusively to families with early onset, some families with PSEN2 mutations exhibit symptom onset in their late 60s or 70s, suggesting that the pathogenic mechanisms are less severe. PSEN2 mutations are mostly associated with descendants of Volga Germans. Collectively, APP, PSEN1, and PSEN2 mutations account for most families with autosomal dominant AD, but for at least 30% of familial cases, other responsible genes remain to be elucidated (Liddell et al. 2001).

The vast majority of AD cases are termed sporadic, in that they do not have a definite familial clustering or linkage to a known disease-causing mutation. However, in many of these cases, careful family histories suggest that relatives have been affected, indicating contributions from genetic factors. For example, about one-third of sporadic AD cases are associated with a positive family history (Rosen et al. 2007). Only one gene, APOE, has been reproducibly associated with AD risk in virtually all populations and studies. The APOE genotype is not causative (as in the case of the autosomal dominant APP, PSEN1, and PSEN2 mutations), but inheritance of different alleles is significantly associated with a modified risk of AD. APOE exists as three allelic variants (ε2, ε3, and ε4), and inheritance of the APOE4 allele confers a greater risk of AD. Individuals who are homozygous for APOE4 have a substantially greater risk of developing AD than individuals with no APOE4 alleles (APOE 2/2, 2/3, or 3/3 genotype), and individuals with a single APOE4 allele (APOE 2/4 or 3/4) have an intermediate risk (Chartier-Harlin et al. 1994; Corder et al. 1993; Saunders et al. 1993). The age at disease onset is lower among AD patients who possess an *APOE4* allele (Corder et al. 1993; Tsai et al. 1994). These genetic associations strongly suggest that the *APOE* genotype plays an important contributing role in the development of sporadic AD.

In addition to *APOE4*, there are likely to be many other genes that contribute to AD susceptibility, albeit with lesser influence on risk. It has been difficult to identify these other genes because of the smaller degree of risk associated with them. However, numerous genetic association studies have examined many other candidate genes for the risk of sporadic or late-onset AD, and some positive associations have been reported. Polymorphisms in the *SORL1* gene, which encodes the neuronal receptor LR11/sorLA, have recently been associated with AD in multiple populations (J.H. Lee et al. 2007; Rogaeva et al. 2007). Given the strong biological evidence for the role of this receptor in AD pathogenesis (Andersen et al. 2005; Offe et al. 2006; Scherzer et al. 2004), further research is warranted to elucidate the pathogenic mechanisms of genetic variants of *SORL1*. Interest in genes with potential biological plausibility has increased, particularly those linked to mechanisms such as inflammation (interleukin 1 [IL-1] and α-macroglobulin) and amyloidogenesis (nicastrin, insulin-degrading enzyme, and neprilysin). However, almost all of these studies have been underpowered, and the results have not been reliably confirmed in multiple studies using large independent populations. Nonetheless, abundant evidence suggests that several other genes contribute to the risk of sporadic AD. Undoubtedly, additional genetic factors will be identified in the near future, providing new clues to the pathogenesis of the disease. As knowledge of genetic associations in AD continues to grow, it will be important to integrate this information in a systematic manner. A recent meta-analysis has catalogued all published studies of genetic associations in AD and has made this information publicly available in a continuously updated online forum (Bertram et al. 2007). Coordinated efforts such as this will undoubtedly catalyze rapid progress in the understanding of this disease as well as treatment strategies.

Theories of Etiopathogenesis

The cause of most cases of AD remains unknown. As discussed above, autosomal dominant single-gene mutations in *APP*, *PSEN1*, and *PSEN2* are sufficient to cause disease in a small percentage of cases, but even in these familial cases, the relationship between mutant genes and neuro-

degeneration is not completely understood. Postmortem observations in brains with AD, including changes in neurotransmitter systems, accumulation of amyloid plaques, intraneuronal neurofibrillary tangles, inflammatory changes, increased oxidative stress, mitochondrial dysfunction, and reactivation of cell cycle–related gene products, have spawned numerous theories regarding the etiopathogenesis of AD. It is likely that many of these observations reflect different aspects of disease initiation and progression, and one of the key goals in AD research is to develop a unifying theory that accurately identifies the triggering event(s) and explains the relationship between apparently distinct elements of disease biology and neuropathology. Achievement of this daunting task will provide a foundation for developing rational therapeutic approaches for treating patients with AD at different stages of illness.

Although a complete discussion of all of the theories of the pathogenesis of AD is beyond the scope of this chapter, the amyloid cascade hypothesis has gained increasing support in recent years and merits more detailed discussion. It should be understood that whereas this is the theory currently favored by many investigators, the hypothesis is not proven. Indeed, evolution and refinement of the hypothesis are quite likely. Nevertheless, it does have considerable value in establishing a rationale for developing and testing potential therapies. In addition to the amyloid hypothesis, other theories have particular relevance for current clinical practice. The involvement of cholinergic systems was discussed earlier, and the roles of inflammation and oxidative injury in the pathogenesis of AD are discussed briefly below.

Amyloid Cascade Hypothesis

Since its identification as the primary component of senile plaques in 1984, the Aβ peptide and its precursor molecule, amyloid-β precursor protein (APP), have been the targets of intense research interest. The importance of these molecules in the pathogenesis of AD is supported by neuropathological observations and a variety of experimental data. As noted previously, amyloid-containing senile plaques are invariably present in the brains of patients with AD. More recently, characterization of genes associated with early-onset familial AD (*APP*, *PSEN1*, and *PSEN2*) and late-onset sporadic AD (*APOE*) has strengthened the notion that abnormal metabolism of Aβ plays a central role in disease pathogenesis.

The amyloid hypothesis of AD proposes that amyloid production and accumulation play the central role in initiating a cascade of events that leads to cellular dysfunction, neuron loss, and eventual clinical disease manifestations. Downstream effects may involve cytoskeletal dysfunction, inflammation, oxidative injury, neuronal apoptosis, and other mechanisms that result in neurodegeneration, but a critical tenet of the hypothesis is that abnormal Aβ metabolism represents the principal triggering event. An important corollary to this hypothesis is that interventions that reduce the production and deposition of amyloid may provide an effective means of ameliorating symptoms, halting progression, and possibly preventing disease. The amyloid cascade hypothesis has become widely accepted, and most current efforts to develop new therapies for AD directly or indirectly target this mechanism (Hardy and Selkoe 2002).

Mechanisms of Amyloidogenesis

Production of Aβ from APP is regulated by three enzymes (α-, β-, and γ-secretases) (Figure 48–3). Initial cleavage by α-secretase precludes A production by cleaving APP within the Aβ domain. Alternatively, cleavage by β-secretase, followed by γ-secretase activity, produces Aβ. Although the predominant Aβ species is a peptide that is 40 amino acids in length (Aβ40), a slightly longer form (42 amino acids [Aβ42]) seems to have particular pathogenic significance. Because of its biophysical properties, Aβ42 is substantially more fibrillogenic than Aβ40 (Barrow and Zagorski 1991; Burdick et al. 1992; Knauer et al. 1992), and it is believed that extracellular aggregation of Aβ42 provides a nidus on which additional Aβ deposition and plaque formation can occur. Pathological examination of brains with AD suggests that Aβ42 is present at early stages of amyloid deposition in diffuse plaques, whereas Aβ40 is prominent in mature neuritic plaques (Iwatsubo et al. 1994). The physiological significance of Aβ42 was highlighted by the recognition that pathogenic mutations in PSEN1 and PSEN2 invariably increase the production of Aβ42, relative to Aβ40 (Borchelt et al. 1996; Citron et al. 1997; Duff et al. 1996; Scheuner et al. 1996; Tomita et al. 1997). To date, more than 125 distinct mutations in PSEN1 and PSEN2 have been reported in human pedigrees associated with autosomal dominant familial AD. All of these mutations enhance the production of the longer form of the Aβ peptide, suggesting that overproduction of Aβ42 plays an important role in the pathogenesis of aggressive early-onset forms of AD.

Intense research efforts have yielded rapid advances in our understanding of the mechanisms mediating Aβ production. The enzyme responsible for β-secretase cleavage of APP has been identified (Hussain et al. 1999; Vassar et al. 1999; Yan et al. 1999). Beta-site APP cleaving enzyme (BACE) represents the primary β-secretase activity in brain tissue, and initial results from BACE knockout mice suggested that disruption of BACE expression could drastically reduce brain Aβ production without causing significant developmental problems or toxicity in adult animals (Cai et al. 2001; Luo et al. 2001; Roberds et al. 2001). However, a recent study has documented that deletion of BACE in mice results in hypomyelination of peripheral nerves (Willem et al. 2006), raising concerns about potential side effects of BACE inhibitors. Nevertheless, pharmacological inhibitors of BACE are under active development and may represent a viable therapeutic approach to AD. It is important to note that BACE is a member of a conserved family of membrane-bound aspartic proteases of unknown functions (Lin et al. 2000; Turner et al. 2002). The existence of these related enzymes poses uncertain risks, and the potential usefulness of β-secretase inhibitors will depend greatly on the ability to design pharmacological agents capable of specifically inhibiting brain β-secretase activity without affecting the biological activity of related enzymes.

The discovery of γ-secretase as a complex of multiple proteins, including presenilin, represents a critical advance in the understanding of APP processing and has presented an additional avenue of therapeutic intervention for AD (Edbauer et al. 2003; Kimberly et al. 2003). As discussed above, pathogenic mutations in PSEN1 and PSEN2 alter γ-secretase cleavage of APP, resulting in enhanced production of the longer (42-amino-acid) Aβ. The precise mechanism by which mutations alter APP cleavage remains unclear, but presenilin appears to be involved in the active site of the enzyme. Pivotal observations in PSEN1 knockout mice revealed dramatic reduction in Aβ production (De Strooper et al. 1998). Subsequently, it was recognized that two highly conserved aspartate residues in PS1 and PS2 are critical for γ-secretase activity, suggesting the possibility that presenilins might possess intrinsic protease activity (Wolfe et al. 1999). In addition, transition-state enzyme inhibitors modeled on the γ-secretase active site seem to physically interact with presenilin (Esler et al. 2000; Y.M. Li et al. 2000; Shearman et al. 2000). The structure of presenilins, which contain multiple membrane-spanning domains, is distinctly unusual for aspartyl proteases. The γ-secretase complex is tightly regulated and appears to require coordinated expression for normal maturation and stability of the components (Periz and Fortini 2004).

Presenilins appear to play an essential role in the final cleavage step that produces Aβ, presenting another po-

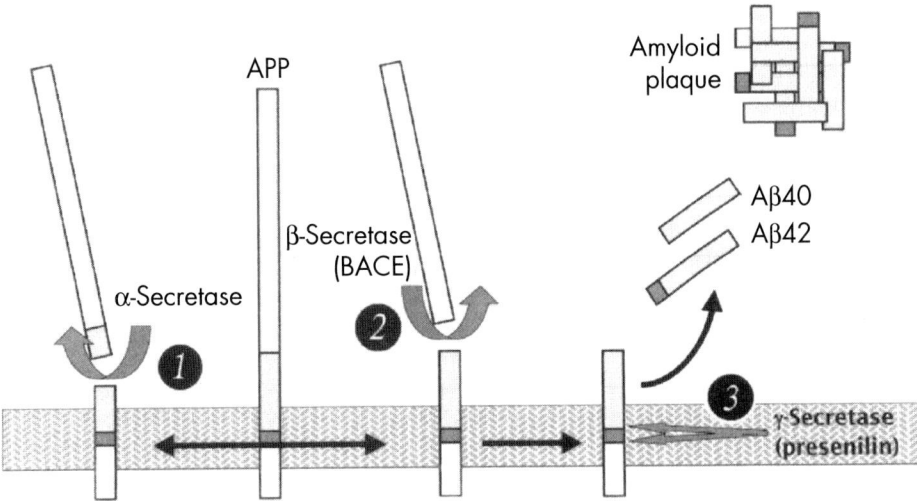

FIGURE 48–3. Proteolytic cleavage of amyloid precursor protein (APP) and amyloidogenesis.

The APP molecule is metabolized via alternate pathways with distinct cleavages. A nonamyloidogenic pathway involves an α-secretase cleavage (1) within the Aβ peptide sequence (lightly shaded), shedding an N-terminal ectodomain. Degradation of the membrane-bound C-terminus does not produce Aβ, because part of the peptide sequence has been cleaved. In contrast, Aβ is produced via the amyloidogenic pathway involving sequential cleavages by β-secretase (2) and γ-secretase (3). Presenilin is a necessary component for γ-secretase activity. The final γ-secretase cleavage releases Aβ peptides of predominantly 40–42 amino acids. The longer 42-residue peptide is more toxic and hydrophobic, and it seeds aggregation into extracellular deposits of amyloid plaques. BACE = beta-site APP cleaving enzyme.

tential target for new therapeutic agents. Unlike BACE, however, loss of *PSEN1* has clearly detrimental effects in animal models. Targeted gene disruption and loss of *PSEN1* in knockout mice result in a late embryonic lethal phenotype associated with severe developmental defects (Shen et al. 1997). These effects arise from an unexpected link between γ-secretase activity and Notch, a receptor that plays a critical role in cell fate decisions during development. In addition to APP, presenilin and γ-secretase regulate the proteolytic processing of a growing list of important molecules, including Notch, erb4, the epidermal growth factor (EGF) receptor, the p75[NTR] low-affinity neurotrophin receptor, and many others (De Strooper et al. 1999; Jung et al. 2003; H.J. Lee et al. 2002; Struhl and Greenwald 1999; Weihofen et al. 2002; Ye et al. 1999). These additional functions present a serious challenge for developing γ-secretase inhibitors as potential therapeutic agents for AD. Nevertheless, γ-secretase inhibitors are still undergoing clinical trials, and improved understanding of presenilin function may reveal effective approaches for disrupting γ-secretase activity in a brain- and APP-specific manner.

Mechanisms of Amyloid-Beta Peptide Clearance

Aβ production from APP has been studied more intensively than perhaps any other process in protein biochem-

istry. The other half of the equation, the clearance of Aβ, has received less attention but may be equally important in regulating Aβ. The mechanisms responsible for amyloid degradation and clearance are not fully understood, but several metallopeptidases, including the insulin-degrading enzyme (IDE), are known to have Aβ-degrading activity (Kurochkin 2001; Qiu et al. 1998). Of interest, the *IDE* gene is present on chromosome 10q, near a region of linkage with late-onset AD. While results from genetic analyses have varied (Abraham et al. 2001; Bertram et al. 2000), current findings support both genetic and functional links between IDE and AD pathogenesis (Bertram et al. 2007; Kim et al. 2007). Administration of thiorphan, a potent inhibitor of the neprilysin family of zinc metalloproteinases, increased Aβ deposition in rat brain (Carson and Turner 2002; Iwata et al. 2000). Abnormalities in endosomal–lysosomal function may also be relevant to Aβ-degrading activity in neurons. These changes are among the earliest neuropathological changes present in AD brains, visible in presymptomatic individuals at high risk of developing AD, and they appear to be fundamentally linked to APP expression (Cataldo et al. 2000, 2003; Troncoso et al. 1998). Although genetic evidence from familial AD pedigrees associated with *APP*, *PSEN1*, and *PSEN2* mutations identifies abnormal production of Aβ as a pivotal mechanism in disease pathogenesis, abnormal degradation and clearance of amyloid may be an equally important mechanism in sporadic cases of AD.

As noted above, the *APOE* gene exists in three different allelic forms (ε2, ε3, and ε4), and the ε4 allele has been shown to be an important risk factor for sporadic late-onset AD. Studies of this gene have revealed a number of potential links to amyloidogenesis. The apoE protein is present in amyloid deposits, and plaque burden is increased in individuals with AD possessing ε4 alleles (Gearing et al. 1995; Rebeck et al. 1993; Schmechel et al. 1993). One possible explanation for this may be that the apoE4 protein isoform enhances the deposition of fibrillar Aβ peptides (Castano et al. 1995; K.C. Evans et al. 1995; Wisniewski et al. 1994). Interaction between Aβ and apoE4 may promote extracellular amyloid deposition and trigger the cascade of events leading to the development of AD (Wisniewski et al. 1994). An alternative means by which apoE may influence amyloidogenesis involves a brain apoE receptor called low-density lipoprotein (LDL) receptor–related protein (LRP) (Kounnas et al. 1995). This receptor mediates internalization of apoE-containing lipid particles, and through its interaction with α_2-macroglobulin, LRP can also mediate clearance of Aβ (Kang et al. 2000; Shibata et al. 2000). The LDL- and sortilin-related receptor LR11/SorLA has recently been shown to modulate amyloidogenesis, presumably by regulating APP traffic through endosomal compartments (Andersen et al. 2005; Offe et al. 2006). Since LR11/SorLA is also an apoE receptor, this represents yet another possible mechanism by which apoE may influence AD development and progression. As noted above, variants in *SORL1*, the gene that encodes LR11/SorLA, are associated with late-onset AD in multiple populations (J.H. Lee et al. 2007; Rogaeva et al. 2007). Further investigation is warranted to fully determine the cell biological significance of this receptor in normal neuronal function and disease states, but its identification represents a major advance in understanding the basis of late-onset AD, the most common form of the illness.

The appearance of dense deposits of amyloid in senile plaques produces the impression that they are static lesions. However, evidence from transgenic mouse models of AD suggests that extracellular amyloid may be much more dynamic than previously believed. Examination of plaque formation in live animals indicates that plaques can form rapidly, disrupting the architecture of dendrites in their vicinity. Remarkably, administration of anti-Aβ antibodies to plaque-forming mice results in rapid clearance of amyloid plaques and restoration of normal dendritic morphology (Lombardo et al. 2003; Spires et al.

2005). In addition, vaccination to induce production of anti-Aβ antibodies has shown a dramatic ability to prevent or reverse the accumulation of amyloid plaques in animal models (Morgan et al. 2000). These observations suggest that the induction of immunity to Aβ may be a viable treatment for AD. The first clinical trial employing this approach was halted because of safety concerns and the development of encephalitis in some patients receiving the Aβ vaccine, but the notion of promoting amyloid clearance as a potential treatment strategy remains viable. Of particular note, participants in the original trial who were good antibody responders had better outcomes than placebo-treated patients in cognitive as well as pathological assessments (Fox et al. 2005; Gilman et al. 2005). Furthermore, cognitive improvement was correlated with antibody titer, suggesting a direct relationship between anti-Aβ immune response and favorable clinical outcome. Several humanized anti-Aβ monoclonal antibodies are currently being tested, and vaccine and passive immunization strategies designed to minimize adverse side effects are under way in early phases of human clinical trials.

Inflammation and Alzheimer's Disease

Inflammation is a key component of AD (Eikelenboom et al. 2000; McGeer and McGeer 2001a; McGeer et al. 2006). In fact, the presence of an inflammatory response is a key feature that distinguishes the pathological neuritic plaque from the benign diffuse plaque. Neuritic plaques are surrounded by activated astrocytes and microglia, the resident immune cells of the central nervous system. Activated complement, including membrane attack complexes, is prominent on damaged neurons and dystrophic neurites. A classical antibody-mediated pathway or an alternative antibody-independent pathway can activate complement, but brains from patients with AD do not show increased antibodies or T cells, indicating that a specific immune response is not responsible for complement activation. The most likely trigger for complement activation in AD is Aγ itself. Several inflammatory proteins are also elevated in AD. These include C-reactive protein, amyloid P, α_2-macroglobulin, intercellular adhesion molecule–1 (ICAM-1), and proinflammatory cytokines, such as IL-1, interleukin 6 (IL-6), and tumor necrosis factor–α (TNF-α). Many of these proteins can influence APP expression and processing, and many associate with Aβ in plaques. Genetic polymorphisms in proinflammatory genes, including IL-1, TNF-α, and α_2-macroglobulin, have been associated (albeit inconsistently) with an increased likelihood of developing AD or an earlier age at disease onset (McGeer and McGeer 2001b).

The role of anti-inflammatory agents in the treatment of AD remains unclear. In numerous epidemiological studies, the use of NSAIDs was suggested to prevent or delay AD (in t' Veld et al. 2001; Stewart et al. 1997). However, randomized trials with NSAIDs (as well as with other anti-inflammatory agents, such as COX-2 inhibitors and steroids) have shown little benefit. Because the strongest association of NSAIDs in epidemiological studies is with drug exposure that is at least 2–3 years before disease onset, it is possible that anti-inflammatory agents may have a protective role only at earlier preclinical stages of AD. In addition, the lack of positive outcomes in prospective anti-inflammatory drug trials may also reflect inappropriate choice of drugs or suboptimal dosages. Numerous biochemical and transgenic mouse model studies now support the hypothesis that some, but not all, NSAIDs lower Aβ42 by directly modulating the activity of γ-secretase in a manner independent of their action on COX-1 and COX-2 (Eriksen et al. 2003; Weggen et al. 2001, 2003). Considering this, it may be important to consider alternative mechanisms other than COX inhibition (such as γ-secretase regulation) when selecting anti-inflammatory drugs for human AD trials.

Aging, Oxidative Injury, and Mitochondrial Dysfunction

Oxidative injury is caused by the reaction of free radicals with cellular components. The major source of oxygen-containing free radicals is incomplete reduction of oxygen by the mitochondrial electron transport chain. Oxygen free radicals are highly reactive and can damage cellular lipids, proteins, and DNA. The brain is particularly susceptible to oxidative injury for several reasons: high oxygen consumption; increased levels of transition metals, which act as catalysts for free radical generation; low levels of endogenous antioxidants; and an abundance of polyunsaturated lipids, which are more prone to free radical modification.

Extensive evidence supports a role for oxidative damage in AD. Numerous studies have shown higher levels of oxidized lipids, proteins, and DNA in brains from AD patients. Of significance, oxidative damage is highest in brain areas that are most heavily affected in AD (e.g., neocortex and hippocampus) and lowest in areas that are spared (e.g., cerebellum) (Praticò 2002). Neurofibrillary tangles and amyloid plaques show signs of oxidative in-

jury. Oxidative damage may play a central role in the formation of these pathological hallmarks by promoting protein cross-linking and aggregation. The cytotoxic effect of Aβ is mediated by reactive oxygen species; antioxidants can attenuate amyloid-induced neuronal cell death in vitro (Markesbery 1999). Oxidative injury also increases with normal aging, providing a possible explanation for the association between aging and AD.

Is oxidative stress a key player in disease etiology, or is it merely a secondary effect of neuronal damage? Increasing evidence implies that oxidative damage may be an early event (Beal 2005). In AD brains, healthy neurons in vulnerable brain areas have increased amounts of 8-hydroxy-guanosine (8-OHG), a marker of recent oxidative damage (Smith et al. 2000). In contrast, neurons with neurofibrillary tangles have low levels of 8-OHG, implying that oxidative injury precedes tangle formation. In transgenic mouse models of AD, mice expressing a mutant form of *APP* show increased lipid peroxidation months before amyloid deposits are first detected (Praticò et al. 2001). Strikingly, loss of one allele of the manganese superoxide dismutase (*MnSOD*) gene significantly increases amyloid plaque deposition in APP transgenic mice (F. Li et al. 2004). Potential sources of early oxidative stress include mitochondrial dysfunction and changes in cytoplasmic transition metals like copper and zinc.

The role of oxidative stress in AD has implications for both disease diagnosis and treatment. Increased levels of oxidized lipid metabolites are detectable in the CSF, serum, and urine of patients with AD. Levels of one metabolite, an isomer of prostaglandin F2, are elevated in the CSF of patients with mild cognitive impairment, a condition that progresses to AD in 50% of cases (Praticò et al. 2002). Thus, detection of increased oxidative stress may be useful for the diagnosis of existing or future AD. Antioxidants may also play an important role in AD therapy. Observations from the Cache County Study Group have indicated reduced risk of AD among participants taking vitamin C and E supplements, and better cognitive performance was noted among participants who reported a diet rich in antioxidants (Wengreen et al. 2007; Zandi et al. 2004). However, data from controlled clinical trials have been mixed. The antioxidants vitamin E and selegiline have been shown to slow disease progression by 6–12 months in patients with moderate AD (Sano et al. 1997). However, another recent trial found no benefit from vitamin E in preventing the development of AD in patients with mild cognitive impairment (Petersen et al. 2005). Additional trials with more potent antioxidants are also in progress.

Future Directions

Although much progress has been made toward understanding the biological basis of AD, it is clear that further advances are required to identify individuals at risk and develop effective treatments to prevent or reverse disease progression. As is the case with other neurodegenerative diseases, early detection is paramount to the success of treatment of AD. In the past 5 years, exciting progress has been made in the development of molecular probes and imaging techniques to monitor the development and progression of AD neuropathology in living human subjects. As these technologies improve, they will permit earlier and more accurate diagnosis of AD and enable scientists and clinicians to evaluate the efficacy of treatments. The identification of biomarkers specific for AD will aid tremendously in the development of screening tools that can be used efficiently to detect the early stages of AD in the general population. It is also becoming clear that AD has a substantial genetic component (distinct from the small percentage of "familial" AD cases that are attributable to known genes), and the elucidation of new AD-associated genes will certainly improve the ability of the medical community to counsel and treat those at increased risk of developing the disease.

The treatments for AD are evolving from a strategy of neurotransmitter replacement (via inhibition of AChE) to therapies that target discrete molecular events in the disease pathogenesis. Ongoing research in Aβ immunotherapy and clearance, neuroprotective and antioxidant agents, and compounds designed to modulate endogenous signaling pathways promises to revolutionize the way AD is approached as an illness. Consequently, it can be expected that the results of AD therapies will soon move beyond modest amelioration of symptoms, providing tangible improvements in cognitive function, memory formation and retrieval, and interpersonal behavior.

Finally, the pace of basic science research into AD continues to gain momentum. The accumulation of knowledge of the pathophysiological basis of AD will serve to guide future diagnostic and treatment modalities, and the importance of continued investigation cannot be overstated.

Conclusion

Since Alzheimer's observations, more than 100 years ago, of the pathological hallmarks of the disease that would later bear his name, tremendous progress has been made

in the many areas reviewed in this chapter. Remarkably, the pace of discovery into the biological basis of AD continues to accelerate. Inevitably, perspectives on the findings presented here will change as new discoveries are made. Exciting progress can be anticipated on several fronts. Genes at several chromosomal loci linked to AD will likely be identified in the near future. The study of the biology of the gene products will yield insights into the basic biological processes at play in the disease. The role of diet and environmental factors in AD will continue to evolve, and the roles of gene–environment interactions will follow. Existing theories of etiopathogenesis undoubtedly will be modified, and new theories will arise.

We can also safely anticipate that the improved understanding of the biology of AD will have a huge impact on clinical practice. New insights into the biology of AD will help in the identification of biomarkers and in the development of novel strategies to aid in early diagnosis and guide therapy. The neuropharmacology for this disease will continue to shift from an approach based on simple neurotransmitter replacement to one that capitalizes on the multiplicity of receptors and signaling pathways to develop more effective and better-tolerated medications to ameliorate symptoms. Moreover, the neuropharmacology will evolve together with the knowledge of etiopathogenesis to focus on new disease-modifying therapies.

References

Abraham R, Myers A, Wavrant-DeVrieze F, et al: Substantial linkage disequilibrium across the insulin-degrading enzyme locus but no association with late-onset Alzheimer's disease. Hum Genet 109:646–652, 2001

Aisen PS, Schafer KA, Grundman M, et al: Effects of rofecoxib or naproxen vs placebo on Alzheimer disease progression: a randomized controlled trial. JAMA 289:2819–2826, 2003

Alzheimer A: Uber einen eigenartigen schweren Erkrankungsprozeff der Hirnrinde. Neurologisches Centralblatt 23:1129–1136, 1906

Andersen OM, Reiche J, Schmidt V, et al: Neuronal sorting protein-related receptor sorLA/LR11 regulates processing of the amyloid precursor protein. Proc Natl Acad Sci U S A 102:13461–13466, 2005

Ballard CG, Chalmers KA, Todd C, et al: Cholinesterase inhibitors reduce cortical Abeta in dementia with Lewy bodies. Neurology 68:1726–1729, 2007

Barrow CJ, Zagorski MG: Solution structures of beta peptide and its constituent fragments: relation to amyloid deposition. Science 253:179–182, 1991

Bartus RT, Dean RL 3rd, Beer B, et al: The cholinergic hypothesis of geriatric memory dysfunction. Science 217:408–414, 1982

Beal MF: Oxidative damage as an early marker of Alzheimer's disease and mild cognitive impairment. Neurobiol Aging 26:585–586, 2005

Berkeley JL, Gomeza J, Wess J, et al: M1 muscarinic acetylcholine receptors activate extracellular signal-regulated kinase in CA1 pyramidal neurons in mouse hippocampal slices. Mol Cell Neurosci 18:512–524, 2001

Bertram L, Blacker D, Mullin K, et al: Evidence for genetic linkage of Alzheimer's disease to chromosome 10q. Science 290:2302–2303, 2000

Bertram L, McQueen MB, Mullin K, et al: Systematic meta-analyses of Alzheimer disease genetic association studies: the AlzGene database. Nat Genet 39:17–23, 2007

Blacker D, Tanzi RE: The genetics of Alzheimer disease: current status and future prospects. Arch Neurol 55:294–296, 1998

Bodick NC, Offen WW, Levey AI, et al: Effects of xanomeline, a selective muscarinic receptor agonist, on cognitive function and behavioral symptoms in Alzheimer disease. Arch Neurol 54:465–473, 1997

Bonner TI, Buckley NJ, Young AC, et al: Identification of a family of muscarinic acetylcholine receptor genes. Science 237:527–532, 1987

Borchelt DR, Thinakaran G, Eckman CB, et al: Familial Alzheimer's disease-linked presenilin 1 variants elevate Abeta1–42/1–40 ratio in vitro and in vivo. Neuron 17:1005–1013, 1996

Bowen D, Francis P: Neurochemistry, neuropharmacology, and aetiological factors in Alzheimer's disease. Semin Neurosci 2:101–108, 1990

Burdick D, Soreghan B, Kwon M, et al: Assembly and aggregation properties of synthetic Alzheimer's A4/beta amyloid peptide analogs. J Biol Chem 267:546–554, 1992

Bymaster FP, Carter PA, Peters SC, et al: Xanomeline compared to other muscarinic agents on stimulation of phosphoinositide hydrolysis in vivo and other cholinomimetic effects. Brain Res 795:179–190, 1998

Caccamo A, Oddo S, Billings LM, et al: M1 receptors play a central role in modulating AD-like pathology in transgenic mice. Neuron 49:671–682, 2006

Cai H, Wang Y, McCarthy D, et al: BACE1 is the major beta-secretase for generation of Abeta peptides by neurons. Nat Neurosci 4:233–234, 2001

Carson JA, Turner AJ: Beta-amyloid catabolism: roles for neprilysin (NEP) and other metallopeptidases? J Neurochem 81:1–8, 2002

Castano EM, Prelli F, Wisniewski T, et al: Fibrillogenesis in Alzheimer's disease of amyloid beta peptides and apolipoprotein E. Biochem J 306(Pt 2):599–604, 1995

Cataldo AM, Barnett JL, Berman SA, et al: Gene expression and cellular content of cathepsin D in Alzheimer's disease brain: evidence for early up-regulation of the endosomal-lysosomal system. Neuron 14:671–680, 1995

Cataldo AM, Hamilton DJ, Barnett JL, et al: Properties of the endosomal-lysosomal system in the human central nervous system: disturbances mark most neurons in populations at risk to degenerate in Alzheimer's disease. J Neurosci 16:186–199, 1996

Cataldo AM, Peterhoff CM, Troncoso JC, et al: Endocytic pathway abnormalities precede amyloid beta deposition in sporadic Alzheimer's disease and Down syndrome: differential effects of APOE genotype and presenilin mutations. Am J Pathol 157:277–286, 2000

Cataldo AM, Petanceska S, Peterhoff CM, et al: App gene dosage modulates endosomal abnormalities of Alzheimer's disease in a segmental trisomy 16 mouse model of down syndrome. J Neurosci 23:6788–6792, 2003

Chartier-Harlin MC, Parfitt M, Legrain S, et al: Apolipoprotein E, epsilon 4 allele as a major risk factor for sporadic early and late-onset forms of Alzheimer's disease: analysis of the 19q13.2 chromosomal region. Hum Mol Genet 3:569–574, 1994

Citron M, Westaway D, Xia W, et al: Mutant presenilins of Alzheimer's disease increase production of 42-residue amyloid beta-protein in both transfected cells and transgenic mice. Nat Med 3:67–72, 1997

Clarke R, Smith AD, Jobst KA, et al: Folate, vitamin B12, and serum total homocysteine levels in confirmed Alzheimer disease. Arch Neurol 55:1449–1455, 1998

Corder EH, Saunders AM, Strittmatter WJ, et al: Gene dose of apolipoprotein E type 4 allele and the risk of Alzheimer's disease in late onset families. Science 261:921–923, 1993

Coyle JT, Price DL, DeLong MR: Alzheimer's disease: a disorder of cortical cholinergic innervation. Science 219:1184–1190, 1983

Cummings JL, Cole G: Alzheimer disease. JAMA 287:2335–2338, 2002

Damasio AR, Graff-Radford NR, Eslinger PJ, et al: Amnesia following basal forebrain lesions. Arch Neurol 42:263–271, 1985

Davies P, Maloney AJ: Selective loss of central cholinergic neurons in Alzheimer's disease. Lancet 2(8000):1403, 1976

Davis KL, Mohs RC, Marin D, et al: Cholinergic markers in elderly patients with early signs of Alzheimer disease. JAMA 281:1401–1406, 1999

De Strooper B, Saftig P, Craessaerts K, et al: Deficiency of presenilin-1 inhibits the normal cleavage of amyloid precursor protein. Nature 391:387–390, 1998

De Strooper B, Annaert W, Cupers P, et al: A presenilin-1-dependent gamma-secretase-like protease mediates release of Notch intracellular domain. Nature 398:518–22, 1999

DeKosky ST, Ikonomovic MD, Styren SD, et al: Upregulation of choline acetyltransferase activity in hippocampus and frontal cortex of elderly subjects with mild cognitive impairment. Ann Neurol 51:145–155, 2002

Dooley M, Lamb HM: Donepezil: a review of its use in Alzheimer's disease. Drugs Aging 16:199–226, 2000

Drachman DA: Memory and cognitive function in man: does the cholinergic system have a specific role? Neurology 27:783–790, 1997

Duff K, Eckman C, Zehr C, et al: Increased amyloid-beta42(43) in brains of mice expressing mutant presenilin 1. Nature 383:710–713, 1996

Edbauer D, Winkler E, Regula JT, et al: Reconstitution of gamma-secretase activity. Nat Cell Biol 5:486–488, 2003

Eikelenboom P, Rozemuller AJ, Hoozemans JJ, et al: Neuroinflammation and Alzheimer disease: clinical and therapeutic implications. Alzheimer Dis Assoc Disord 14 (suppl 1):S54–S61, 2000

Engelhart MJ, Geerlings MI, Ruitenberg A, et al: Dietary intake of antioxidants and risk of Alzheimer disease. JAMA 287:3223–3229, 2002

Eriksen JL, Sagi SA, Smith TE, et al: NSAIDs and enantiomers of flurbiprofen target gamma-secretase and lower Abeta 42 in vivo. J Clin Invest 112:440–449, 2003

Esler WP, Kimberly WT, Ostaszewski BL, et al: Transition-state analogue inhibitors of gamma-secretase bind directly to presenilin-1. Nat Cell Biol 2:428–434, 2000

Evans DA, Hebert LE, Beckett LA, et al: Education and other measures of socioeconomic status and risk of incident Alzheimer disease in a defined population of older persons. Arch Neurol 54:1399–1405, 1997

Evans KC, Berger EP, Cho CG, et al: Apolipoprotein E is a kinetic but not a thermodynamic inhibitor of amyloid formation: implications for the pathogenesis and treatment of Alzheimer disease. Proc Natl Acad Sci U S A 92:763–767, 1995

Farber SA, Nitsch RM, Schulz JG, et al: Regulated secretion of beta-amyloid precursor protein in rat brain. J Neurosci 15:7442–7451, 1995

Flynn DD, Weinstein DA, Mash DC: Loss of high-affinity agonist binding to M1 muscarinic receptors in Alzheimer's disease: implications for the failure of cholinergic replacement therapies. Ann Neurol 29:256–262, 1991

Flynn DD, Ferrari-DiLeo G, Mash DC, et al: Differential regulation of molecular subtypes of muscarinic receptors in Alzheimer's disease. J Neurochem 64:1888–1891, 1995

Fox NC, Black RS, Gilman S, et al: Effects of Abeta immunization (AN1792) on MRI measures of cerebral volume in Alzheimer disease. Neurology 64:1563–1572, 2005

Gearing M, Schneider JA, Robbins RS, et al: Regional variation in the distribution of apolipoprotein E and A beta in Alzheimer's disease. J Neuropathol Exp Neurol 54:833–841, 1995

Gilman S, Koller M, Black RS, et al: Clinical effects of Abeta immunization (AN1792) in patients with AD in an interrupted trial. Neurology 64:1553–1562, 2005

Gilmor ML, Erickson JD, Varoqui H, et al: Preservation of nucleus basalis neurons containing choline acetyltransferase and the vesicular acetylcholine transporter in the elderly with mild cognitive impairment and early Alzheimer's disease. J Comp Neurol 411:693–704, 1999

Hardy J, Selkoe DJ: The amyloid hypothesis of Alzheimer's disease: progress and problems on the road to therapeutics. Science 297:353–356, 2002

Hebert LE, Scherr PA, McCann JJ, et al: Is the risk of developing Alzheimer's disease greater for women than for men? Am J Epidemiol 153:132–136, 2001

Heneka MT, Ramanathan M, Jacobs AH, et al: Locus ceruleus degeneration promotes Alzheimer pathogenesis in amyloid precursor protein 23 transgenic mice. J Neurosci 26:1343–1354, 2006

Hock C, Maddalena A, Raschig A, et al: Treatment with the selective muscarinic m1 agonist talsaclidine decreases cerebrospinal fluid levels of A beta 42 in patients with Alzheimer's disease. Amyloid 10:1–6, 2003

Hussain I, Powell D, Howlett DR, et al: Identification of a novel aspartic protease (Asp 2) as beta-secretase. Mol Cell Neurosci 14:419–427, 1999

in t' Veld BA, Ruitenberg A, Hofman A, et al: Nonsteroidal anti-inflammatory drugs and the risk of Alzheimer's disease. N Engl J Med 345:1515–1521, 2001

Iwata N, Tsubuki S, Takaki Y, et al: Identification of the major Abeta1–42 degrading catabolic pathway in brain parenchyma: suppression leads to biochemical and pathological deposition. Nat Med 6:143–150, 2000

Iwatsubo T, Odaka A, Suzuki N, et al: Visualization of A beta 42(43) and A beta 40 in senile plaques with end-specific A beta monoclonals: evidence that an initially deposited species is A beta 42(43). Neuron 13:45–53, 1994

Jellinger KA, Paulus W, Wrocklage C, et al: Effects of closed traumatic brain injury and genetic factors on the development of Alzheimer's disease. Eur J Neurol 8:707–710, 2001

Jick H, Zornberg GL, Jick SS, et al: Statins and the risk of dementia. Lancet 356:1627–1631, 2000

Jung KM, Tan S, Landman N, et al: Regulated intramembrane proteolysis of the p75 neurotrophin receptor modulates its association with the TrkA receptor. J Biol Chem 278:42161–42169, 2003

Kang DE, Pietrzik CU, Baum L, et al: Modulation of amyloid beta-protein clearance and Alzheimer's disease susceptibility by the LDL receptor-related protein pathway. J Clin Invest 106:1159–1166, 2000

Karlinsky H: Alzheimer's disease in Down's syndrome: a review. J Am Geriatr Soc 34:728–734, 1986

Katzman R: Education and the prevalence of dementia and Alzheimer's disease. Neurology 43:13–20, 1993

Kim M, Hersh LB, Leissring MA, et al: Decreased catalytic activity of the insulin-degrading enzyme in chromosome 10-linked Alzheimer disease families. J Biol Chem 282:7825–7832, 2007

Kimberly WT, LaVoie MJ, Ostaszewski BL, et al: Gamma-secretase is a membrane protein complex comprised of presenilin, nicastrin, Aph-1, and Pen-2. Proc Natl Acad Sci U S A 100:6382–6387, 2003

Kivipelto M, Helkala EL, Laakso MP, et al: Midlife vascular risk factors and Alzheimer's disease in later life: longitudinal, population based study. BMJ 322:1447–51, 2001

Knauer MF, Soreghan B, Burdick D, et al: Intracellular accumulation and resistance to degradation of the Alzheimer amyloid A4/beta protein. Proc Natl Acad Sci U S A 89:7437–7441, 1992

Knopman D, Schneider L, Davis K, et al: Long-term tacrine (Cognex) treatment: effects on nursing home placement and mortality, Tacrine Study Group. Neurology 47:166–177, 1996

Kounnas MZ, Moir RD, Rebeck GW, et al: LDL receptor-related protein, a multifunctional ApoE receptor, binds secreted beta-amyloid precursor protein and mediates its degradation. Cell 82:331–340, 1995

Kuhl DE, Minoshima S, Frey KA, et al: Limited donepezil inhibition of acetylcholinesterase measured with positron emission tomography in living Alzheimer cerebral cortex. Ann Neurol 48:391–395, 2000

Kurochkin IV: Insulin-degrading enzyme: embarking on amyloid destruction. Trends Biochem Sci 26:421–425, 2001

Lamb HM, Goa KL: Rivastigmine: a pharmacoeconomic review of its use in Alzheimer's disease. Pharmacoeconomics 19:303–318, 2001

Lautenschlager NT, Cupples LA, Rao VS, et al: Risk of dementia among relatives of Alzheimer's disease patients in the MIRAGE study: what is in store for the oldest old? Neurology 46:641–650, 1996

Lee HJ, Jung KM, Huang YZ, et al: Presenilin-dependent gamma-secretase-like intramembrane cleavage of ErbB4. J Biol Chem 277:6318–6323, 2002

Lee JH, Cheng R, Schupf N, et al: The association between genetic variants in SORL1 and Alzheimer disease in an urban, multi-ethnic, community-based cohort. Arch Neurol 64:501–506, 2007

Levey AI: Muscarinic acetylcholine receptor expression in memory circuits: implications for treatment of Alzheimer disease. Proc Natl Acad Sci U S A 93:13541–13546, 1996

Li F, Calingasan NY, Yu F, et al: Increased plaque burden in brains of APP mutant MnSOD heterozygous knockout mice. J Neurochem 89:1308–1312, 2004

Li YM, Xu M, Lai MT, et al: Photoactivated gamma-secretase inhibitors directed to the active site covalently label presenilin 1. Nature 405:689–694, 2000

Liddell MB, Lovestone S, Owen MJ: Genetic risk of Alzheimer's disease: advising relatives. Br J Psychiatry 178:7–11, 2001

Lin X, Koelsch G, Wu S, et al: Human aspartic protease memapsin 2 cleaves the beta-secretase site of beta-amyloid precursor protein. Proc Natl Acad Sci U S A 97:1456–1460, 2000

Lombardo JA, Stern EA, McLellan ME, et al: Amyloid-beta antibody treatment leads to rapid normalization of plaque-induced neuritic alterations. J Neurosci 23:10879–10883, 2003

Luchsinger JA, Tang MX, Siddiqui M, et al: Alcohol intake and risk of dementia. J Am Geriatr Soc 52:540–546, 2004

Luo Y, Bolon B, Kahn S, et al: Mice deficient in BACE1, the Alzheimer's beta-secretase, have normal phenotype and abolished beta-amyloid generation. Nat Neurosci 4:231–232, 2001

Marino MJ, Rouse ST, Levey AI, et al: Activation of the genetically defined m1 muscarinic receptor potentiates N-methyl-D-aspartate (NMDA) receptor currents in hippocampal pyramidal cells. Proc Natl Acad Sci U S A 95:11465–11470, 1998

Markesbery WR: The role of oxidative stress in Alzheimer disease. Arch Neurol 56:1449–1452, 1999

Mayeux R, Ottman R, Maestre G, et al: Synergistic effects of traumatic head injury and apolipoprotein-epsilon 4 in patients with Alzheimer's disease. Neurology 45(3 Pt 1):555–557, 1995

McGeer PL, McGeer EG: Inflammation, autotoxicity and Alzheimer disease. Neurobiol Aging 22:799–809, 2001a

McGeer PL, McGeer EG: Polymorphisms in inflammatory genes and the risk of Alzheimer disease. Arch Neurol 58:1790–1792, 2001b

McGeer PL, McGeer EG: NSAIDs and Alzheimer disease: epidemiological, animal model and clinical studies. Neurobiol Aging 28:639–647, 2007

McGeer PL, Rogers J, McGeer EG: Inflammation, anti-inflammatory agents and Alzheimer disease: the last 12 years. J Alzheimers Dis 9 (3 suppl):271–276, 2006

Morgan D, Diamond DM, Gottschall PE, et al: A beta peptide vaccination prevents memory loss in an animal model of Alzheimer's disease. Nature 408:982–985, 2000

Mufson EJ, Ma SY, Dills J, et al: Loss of basal forebrain P75(NTR) immunoreactivity in subjects with mild cognitive impairment and Alzheimer's disease. J Comp Neurol 443:136–153, 2002

Mufson EJ, Ginsberg SD, Ikonomovic MD, et al: Human cholinergic basal forebrain: chemoanatomy and neurologic dysfunction. J Chem Neuroanat 26:233–242, 2003

Nixon RA: Endosome function and dysfunction in Alzheimer's disease and other neurodegenerative diseases. Neurobiol Aging 26:373–382, 2005

Notkola IL, Sulkava R, Pekkanen J, et al: Serum total cholesterol, apolipoprotein E epsilon 4 allele, and Alzheimer's disease. Neuroepidemiology 17:14–20, 1998

Offe K, Dodson SE, Shoemaker JT, et al: The lipoprotein receptor LR11 regulates amyloid beta production and amyloid precursor protein traffic in endosomal compartments. J Neurosci 26:1596–1603, 2006

Olin J, Schneider L: Galantamine for Alzheimer's disease. Cochrane Database Syst Rev (3):CD001747, 2002

Orgogozo JM, Dartigues JF, Lafont S, et al: Wine consumption and dementia in the elderly: a prospective community study in the Bordeaux area. Rev Neurol (Paris) 153:185–192, 1997

Peralta EG, Ashkenazi A, Winslow JW, et al: Distinct primary structures, ligand-binding properties and tissue-specific expression of four human muscarinic acetylcholine receptors. Embo J 6:3923–3929, 1987

Periz G, Fortini ME: Functional reconstitution of gamma-secretase through coordinated expression of presenilin, nicastrin, Aph-1, and Pen-2. J Neurosci Res 77:309–322, 2004

Perry EK, Kilford L, Lees AJ, et al: Increased Alzheimer pathology in Parkinson's disease related to antimuscarinic drugs. Ann Neurol 54:235–238, 2003

Peskind ER, Potkin SG, Pomara N, et al: Memantine treatment in mild to moderate Alzheimer disease: a 24-week randomized, controlled trial. Am J Geriatr Psychiatry 14:704–715, 2006

Petersen RC, Thomas RG, Grundman M, et al: Vitamin E and donepezil for the treatment of mild cognitive impairment. N Engl J Med 352:2379–2388, 2005

Pomara N, Ott BR, Peskind E, et al: Memantine treatment of cognitive symptoms in mild to moderate Alzheimer disease: secondary analyses from a placebo-controlled randomized trial. Alzheimer Dis Assoc Disord 21:60–64, 2007

Praticò D: Alzheimer's disease and oxygen radicals: new insights. Biochem Pharmacol 63:563–567, 2002

Praticò D, Uryu K, Leight S, et al: Increased lipid peroxidation precedes amyloid plaque formation in an animal model of Alzheimer amyloidosis. J Neurosci 21:4183–4187, 2001

Praticò D, Clark CM, Liun F, et al: Increase of brain oxidative stress in mild cognitive impairment: a possible predictor of Alzheimer disease. Arch Neurol 59:972–976, 2002

Qiu WQ, Walsh DM, Ye Z, et al: Insulin-degrading enzyme regulates extracellular levels of amyloid beta-protein by degradation. J Biol Chem 273:32730–32738, 1998

Rebeck GW, Reiter JS, Strickland DK, et al: Apolipoprotein E in sporadic Alzheimer's disease: allelic variation and receptor interactions. Neuron 11:575–580, 1993

Riley KP, Snowdon DA, Desrosiers MF, et al: Early life linguistic ability, late life cognitive function, and neuropathology: findings from the Nun Study. Neurobiol Aging 26:341–347, 2005

Roberds SL, Anderson J, Basi G, et al: BACE knockout mice are healthy despite lacking the primary beta-secretase activity in brain: implications for Alzheimer's disease therapeutics. Hum Mol Genet 10:1317–1324, 2001

Rockwood K, Kirkland S, Hogan DB, et al: Use of lipid-lowering agents, indication bias, and the risk of dementia in community-dwelling elderly people. Arch Neurol 59:223–227, 2002

Rogaeva E, Meng Y, Lee JH, et al: The neuronal sortilin-related receptor SORL1 is genetically associated with Alzheimer disease. Nat Genet 39:168–177, 2007

Romanelli MN, Gratteri P, Guandalini L, et al: Central nicotinic receptors: structure, function, ligands, and therapeutic potential. ChemMedChem 2:746–767, 2007

Rosen AR, Steenland NK, Hanfelt J, et al: Evidence of shared risk for Alzheimer's disease and Parkinson's disease using family history. Neurogenetics 8:263–270, 2007

Salehi A, Lucassen PJ, Pool CW, et al: Decreased neuronal activity in the nucleus basalis of Meynert in Alzheimer's disease as suggested by the size of the Golgi apparatus. Neuroscience 59:871–880, 1994

Sano M, Ernesto C, Thomas RG, et al: A controlled trial of selegiline, alpha-tocopherol, or both as treatment for Alzheimer's disease. The Alzheimer's Disease Cooperative Study. N Engl J Med 336:1216–1222, 1997

Sargent PB: The diversity of neuronal nicotinic acetylcholine receptors. Annu Rev Neurosci 16:403–443, 1993

Saunders AM, Strittmatter WJ, Schmechel D, et al: Association of apolipoprotein E allele epsilon 4 with late-onset familial and sporadic Alzheimer's disease. Neurology 43:1467–1472, 1993

Scarmeas N, Levy G, Tang MX, et al: Influence of leisure activity on the incidence of Alzheimer's disease. Neurology 57:2236–2242, 2001

Scherzer CR, Offe K, Gearing M, et al: Loss of apolipoprotein E receptor LR11 in Alzheimer disease. Arch Neurol 61:1200–1205, 2004

Scheuner D, Eckman C, Jensen M, et al: Secreted amyloid beta-protein similar to that in the senile plaques of Alzheimer's disease is increased in vivo by the presenilin 1 and 2 and APP mutations linked to familial Alzheimer's disease. Nat Med 2:864–870, 1996

Schmechel DE, Saunders AM, Strittmatter WJ, et al: Increased amyloid beta-peptide deposition in cerebral cortex as a consequence of apolipoprotein E genotype in late-onset Alzheimer disease. Proc Natl Acad Sci U S A 90:9649–9653, 1993

Schofield PW, Tang M, Marder K, et al: Alzheimer's disease after remote head injury: an incidence study. J Neurol Neurosurg Psychiatry 62:119–124, 1997

Schupf N, Kapell D, Nightingale B, et al: Specificity of the fivefold increase in AD in mothers of adults with Down syndrome. Neurology 57:979–984, 2001

Selkoe DJ, Podlisny MB: Deciphering the genetic basis of Alzheimer's disease. Annu Rev Genomics Hum Genet 3:67–99, 2002

Seshadri S, Beiser A, Selhub J, et al: Plasma homocysteine as a risk factor for dementia and Alzheimer's disease. N Engl J Med 346:476–483, 2002

Shearman MS, Beher D, Clarke EE, et al: L-685,458, an aspartyl protease transition state mimic, is a potent inhibitor of amyloid beta-protein precursor gamma-secretase activity. Biochemistry 39:8698–8704, 2000

Shen J, Bronson RT, Chen DF, et al: Skeletal and CNS defects in Presenilin-1-deficient mice. Cell 89:629–639, 1997

Shibata M, Yamada S, Kumar SR, et al: Clearance of Alzheimer's amyloid-ss(1–40) peptide from brain by LDL receptor-related protein-1 at the blood-brain barrier. J Clin Invest 106:1489–1499, 2000

Shumaker SA, Legault C, Rapp SR, et al: Estrogen plus progestin and the incidence of dementia and mild cognitive impairment in postmenopausal women: the Women's Health Initiative Memory Study: a randomized controlled trial. JAMA 289:2651–2662, 2003

Shumaker SA, Legault C, Kuller L, et al: Conjugated equine estrogens and incidence of probable dementia and mild cognitive impairment in postmenopausal women: Women's Health Initiative Memory Study. JAMA 291:2947–2958, 2004

Smith MA, Rottkamp CA, Nunomura A, et al: Oxidative stress in Alzheimer's disease. Biochim Biophys Acta 1502:139–144, 2000

Snowdon DA, Kemper SJ, Mortimer JA, et al: Linguistic ability in early life and cognitive function and Alzheimer's disease in late life. Findings from the Nun Study. JAMA 275:528–532, 1996

Spires TL, Meyer-Luehmann M, Stern EA, et al: Dendritic spine abnormalities in amyloid precursor protein transgenic mice demonstrated by gene transfer and intravital multiphoton microscopy. J Neurosci 25:7278–7287, 2005

Stern Y, Gurland B, Tatemichi TK, et al: Influence of education and occupation on the incidence of Alzheimer's disease. JAMA 271:1004–1010, 1994

Stewart WF, Kawas C, Corrada M, et al: Risk of Alzheimer's disease and duration of NSAID use. Neurology 48:626–632, 1997

Struhl G, Greenwald I: Presenilin is required for activity and nuclear access of Notch in Drosophila. Nature 398:522–525, 1999

Terry R, Masliah E, Hansen LA: Structural basis of cognitive alterations, in Alzheimer Disease. Edited by Terry R, Katzman RD, Bick KL. New York, Raven, 1994, pp 179–196

Tomita T, Maruyama K, Saido TC, et al: The presenilin 2 mutation (N141I) linked to familial Alzheimer disease (Volga German families) increases the secretion of amyloid beta protein ending at the 42nd (or 43rd) residue. Proc Natl Acad Sci U S A 94:2025–2030, 1997

Troncoso JC, Cataldo AM, Nixon RA, et al: Neuropathology of preclinical and clinical late-onset Alzheimer's disease. Ann Neurol 43:673–676, 1998

Tsai MS, Tangalos EG, Petersen RC, et al: Apolipoprotein E: risk factor for Alzheimer disease. Am J Hum Genet 54:643–649, 1994

Turner RT 3rd, Loy JA, Nguyen C, et al: Specificity of memapsin 1 and its implications on the design of memapsin 2 (beta-secretase) inhibitor selectivity. Biochemistry 41:8742–8746, 2002

Vassar R, Bennett BD, Babu-Khan S, et al: Beta-secretase cleavage of Alzheimer's amyloid precursor protein by the transmembrane aspartic protease BACE. Science 286:735–741, 1999

Volpicelli-Daley LA, Duysen EG, Lockridge O, et al: Altered hippocampal muscarinic receptors in acetylcholinesterase-deficient mice. Ann Neurol 53:788–796, 2003a

Volpicelli-Daley LA, Hrabovska A, Duysen EG, et al: Altered striatal function and muscarinic cholinergic receptors in acetylcholinesterase knockout mice. Mol Pharmacol 64:1309–1316, 2003b

Wang HX, Wahlin A, Basun H, et al: Vitamin B(12) and folate in relation to the development of Alzheimer's disease. Neurology 56:1188–1194, 2001

Weggen S, Eriksen JL, Das P, et al: A subset of NSAIDs lower amyloidogenic Abeta42 independently of cyclooxygenase activity. Nature 414:212–216, 2001

Weggen S, Eriksen JL, Sagi SA, et al: Evidence that nonsteroidal anti-inflammatory drugs decrease amyloid beta 42 production by direct modulation of gamma-secretase activity. J Biol Chem 278:31831–31837, 2003

Weihofen A, Binns K, Lemberg MK, et al: Identification of signal peptide peptidase, a presenilin-type aspartic protease. Science 296:2215–2218, 2002

Wengreen HJ, Munger RG, Corcoran CD, et al: Antioxidant intake and cognitive function of elderly men and women: the Cache County Study. J Nutr Health Aging 11:230–237, 2007

Whalley LJ, Starr JM, Athawes R, et al: Childhood mental ability and dementia. Neurology 55:1455–1459, 2000

Whitehouse PJ, Price DL, Struble RG, et al: Alzheimer's disease and senile dementia: loss of neurons in the basal forebrain. Science 215:1237–1239, 1982

Wilkins CH, Sheline YI, Roe CM, et al: Vitamin D deficiency is associated with low mood and worse cognitive performance in older adults. Am J Geriatr Psychiatry 14:1032–1040, 2006

Willem M, Garratt AN, Novak B, et al: Control of peripheral nerve myelination by the beta-secretase BACE1. Science 314:664–666, 2006

Wilson RS, Mendes De Leon CF, Barnes LL, et al: Participation in cognitively stimulating activities and risk of incident Alzheimer disease. JAMA 287:742–748, 2002

Wisniewski T, Castaño EM, Golabek A, et al: Acceleration of Alzheimer's fibril formation by apolipoprotein E in vitro. Am J Pathol 145:1030–1035, 1994

Wolfe MS, Xia W, Ostaszewski BL, et al: Two transmembrane aspartates in presenilin-1 required for presenilin endoproteolysis and gamma-secretase activity. Nature 398:513–517, 1999

Wolozin B, Kellman W, Ruosseau P, et al: Decreased prevalence of Alzheimer disease associated with 3-hydroxy-3-methyglutaryl coenzyme A reductase inhibitors. Arch Neurol 57:1439–1443, 2000

Xu H, Gouras GK, Greenfield JP, et al: Estrogen reduces neuronal generation of Alzheimer beta-amyloid peptides. Nat Med 4:447–451, 1998

Yan R, Bienkowski MJ, Shuck ME, et al: Membrane-anchored aspartyl protease with Alzheimer's disease beta-secretase activity. Nature 402:533–537, 1999

Ye Y, Lukinova N, Fortini ME: Neurogenic phenotypes and altered Notch processing in Drosophila Presenilin mutants. Nature 398:525–529, 1999

Zandi PP, Carlson MC, Plassman BL, et al: Hormone replacement therapy and incidence of Alzheimer disease in older women: the Cache County Study. JAMA 288:2123–2129, 2002

Zandi PP, Anthony JC, Khachaturian AS, et al: Reduced risk of Alzheimer disease in users of antioxidant vitamin supplements: the Cache County Study. Arch Neurol 61:82–88, 2004

CHAPTER 49

Neurobiology of Substance Abuse and Addiction

Ashley P. Kennedy, B.S.

Clinton D. Kilts, Ph.D.

Drug addiction is characterized by pathological motivation for drug-seeking and -use behaviors associated with the inability to inhibit such behaviors in spite of their clear adverse consequences (Kalivas and Volkow 2005). These features are clinically operationalized as a diagnosis of drug dependence based on an individual's fulfilling at least three of seven criteria defined by DSM-IV-TR (American Psychiatric Association 2000). The authors conform to the position (O'Brien et al. 2006) that drug *addiction* rather than *dependence* is more appropriate in referring to this maladaptive behavioral disorder and refer to drug dependence only when referring to clinical populations defined by DSM-IV-TR criteria. Drug addiction represents a major public health concern due to its high population prevalence, associated suffering and disability, and limited efficacy of extant therapies to promote recovery and relapse prevention. Understanding the underlying neurobiology of drug abuse and addiction offers the best promise to control drug addiction by identifying the bases of risk for addiction and targeting intervention strategies, uncoupling relapse from its precipitants, and minimizing the personal and social burden of addiction. This chapter represents a critical review of the current state of this understanding and a synthesis of knowledge into present and future directives for managing drug abuse and addiction. The treatment here of this topic is not meant to be comprehensive, but rather focuses on the

authors' prioritization of those scientific areas of discovery that are perceived to be most relevant to curbing drug addiction. Attempts have been made to direct interested readers to more exhaustive treatments of less prioritized areas of addiction research findings.

Using a theoretical model of the addiction process (Figure 49–1), this review focuses on the neurobiological events that underlie the transition from initial drug use to addiction, the events that maintain its enduring nature, and the events that underlie the immense socioeconomic costs of being drug addicted. This stage model is introduced, and several examples of population stratifying factors that alter a simple neurobiological explanation are discussed. Next, the major tools of neurobiological investigation of the addiction process are discussed. The neurobiology of the acquisition/transition stage of the addiction process is then discussed, as well as its modulation by genetic, environmental, and neurodevelopmental factors. A major section of this chapter deals with the burgeoning neurobiology of the chronically relapsing nature of drug addiction and focuses on contrasting the three major precipitants of relapse. This section is followed by a discussion of the little-studied neurobiology of the immense socioeconomic costs of end-stage drug addiction and of the relapse prevention and recovery goals of addiction therapies. Finally, a closing, brief discussion of perceived future directions for addiction neuroscience research is provided.

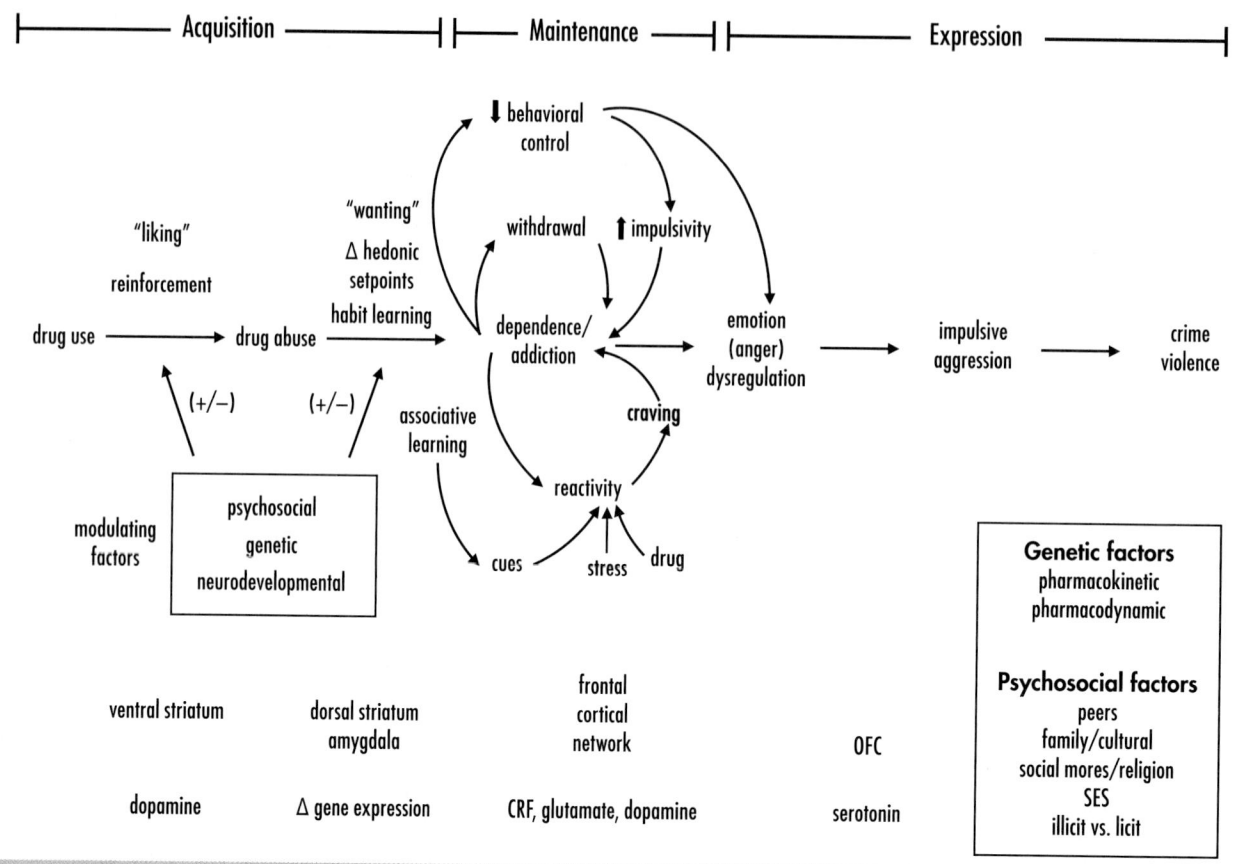

FIGURE 49–1. Theoretical model of the causes and consequences of drug addiction.

A three-stage model is proposed that entails the addiction process from initial drug use, the transition to chronic drug abuse and addiction, the chronically relapsing nature of addiction, and the social and personal costs of end-stage addiction. The roles of learning, memory, reward sensitivity, and emotion regulation are highlighted. Factors that positively and negatively modulate the addiction acquisition stage are shown. *Psychosocial* factors include the influence of peers, family, cultural variables, social and religious beliefs, socioeconomic status, drug attitudes, and the illicit versus licit nature of the drug of abuse. *Genetic* factors include allelic and haplotypic variation for genes regulating cognitive functions, drug pharmacokinetics and pharmacodynamics, and personality traits. *Neurodevelopmental* factors include risks posed by the adolescent period and by childhood maltreatment. Brain anatomical and neurotransmitter substrates are proposed for the different stages of the addiction process. CRF=corticotropin-releasing factor; OFC=orbitofrontal cortex; SES=socioeconomic status.

The Drug Addiction Process

The organization of this discussion of the neurobiology of drug abuse and addiction is based on a now-common view of addiction as a multistage process (see Figure 49–1).

This theoretical framework involves an addiction process that extends from initial drug use to the long-term consequences of end-stage addiction and focuses on the three stages of acquisition of the addicted state, its maintenance as a chronically relapsing state, and the long-term personal and social sequelae or consequences of end-stage drug addiction. In this model, drug abuse acquisition and subsequent addiction are mediated by a transition of drug incentives from reinforcing to habit-based effects associated with altered reward sensitivity, which is positively and negatively modulated by multiple factors, and mediated by maladaptive alterations in patterns of neural activity in striatal and frontal cortical areas and their modes of functional connectivity. In this model, the chronically relapsing nature of the addicted state is maintained by pathological motivations for drug-related behaviors unchecked by a diminished behavioral control that are precipitated by conditioned drug cues, stress, and the drug itself, as well as drug motivation related to a wish to relieve aversive drug withdrawal states. The concept of drug addiction as a disorder of too much gas related to the drug-seeking and -use behaviors associated with too little brakes to stop such behavior is an increasingly used analogy. While less studied as a component of the addiction process, the neurobiology of the social and personal expression of drug addiction is considered here, as these factors underlie the immense socioeconomic costs of addiction. The neurobiology of the drug addiction process is complex and includes numerous population stratifying factors. Noteworthy among these are differences due to the sex of the individuals and their racial and ethnic backgrounds. Although it is beyond the scope of this discussion to treat these factors in detail, we offer the following, as any discussion of the neurobiology of drug abuse and addiction is incomplete without considering these important variables.

Sex Differences in the Addiction Process

There are prominent differences between the sexes in the clinical presentation and neurobiology of drug addiction. While such differences are often described as gender differences, we adhere to their distinction as being based on the categorical distinction between men and women rather than the gender dimension of masculine and feminine characteristics. Whereas drug abuse and addiction are problems often attributed to men, and males have been the focus of the majority of drug abuse research, women are also clearly affected. However, significant sex differences are apparent in the patterns of drug abuse and addiction. It has been suggested that sex differences in behavioral responses to drugs render women more susceptible to drug addiction than men (Lynch et al. 2002; Quiñones-Jenab 2006). Cocaine-dependent men and women display differing clinical characteristics in that women are more likely to have an earlier age at onset of cocaine use than men, women tend to use more cocaine on more days in a given month and take less time to become addicted following initial drug use compared with men, and women enter treatment earlier and present a greater severity of abuse when admitted to treatment programs (Griffin et al. 1989; Kosten et al. 1993; R.D. Weiss et al. 1997). Cocaine-dependent women also demonstrate greater depressive symptomatology and severity of family/social problems, while men are more likely to have antisocial personality disorders (Dudish and Hatsukami 1996; Elman et al. 2001; Griffin et al. 1989; Kosten et al. 1993; R.D. Weiss et al. 1997). Although clinical studies imply that cocaine-dependent women are more negatively affected by cocaine than are men, it has been demonstrated that women relative to men have better treatment outcomes in remaining cocaine abstinent at 6-month follow-up (Kosten et al. 1993; R.D. Weiss et al. 1997). McKay et al. (1996) also determined that women are more likely to seek help after relapsing, whereas men engage in self-justification after relapsing.

Differences between the sexes in the neurobiology of relapse to drug seeking and use behaviors are increasingly apparent. Cocaine-dependent men and women activate different regions of the brain when exposed to drug- and stress-related cues. Clinical research studies have demonstrated that women compared to men have higher levels of drug craving when exposed to drug cues (Elman et al. 2001; Robbins et al. 1999). Women and men exhibit different patterns of neural activation in response to conditioned cocaine cues, which suggests that drug cue–induced relapse involves differing neural pathways in men and women (Kilts et al. 2001, 2004). Cocaine craving in women was associated with less activation of the amygdala, insula, ventral cingulate cortex, and orbitofrontal cortex and greater activation of the anterior cingulate cortex compared with men. Cocaine-dependent women, compared to their male counterparts, showed greater stress-induced activation of the inferior frontal cortex, left insula, dorsal anterior cingulate cortex, and right posterior cingulate cortex (C.S. Li et al. 2005). These results are consistent with the contention that women exhibit less cocaine addiction–related pathology of the frontal cortex than do men (Chang et al. 1999; Levin et al. 1994).

Racial and Ethnic Differences in the Addiction Process

Racial and ethnic differences in socioeconomic status and cultural acceptance contribute to a differing exposure and vulnerability to a host of social problems, with one of the most problematic being drug abuse and addiction. For some drug addictions, the personal and social costs of drug addiction are disproportionately greater for blacks and Hispanics relative to their white counterparts (Wallace 1999). For example, African Americans and Hispanics represent the majority of arrests and incarceration for drug-related crimes in the United States (King and Mauer 2002). Stratifying factors such as allele frequency for risk genes, personality characteristics, substance use among family members and friends, level of drug availability, and neighborhood poverty can all influence drug abuse and addiction in various populations (Wallace 1999). Elevated risk can also be attributed to racial and ethnic group differences in socioeconomic factors such as income, net worth, employment, and poverty. Social frameworks and the neighborhood environment can also be disadvantageous as blacks and Hispanics are more likely to live in rural and urban areas of concentrated poverty (Jones-Webb et al. 1997). A recent functional magnetic resonance imaging (fMRI) study compared African American and white smoking populations and demonstrated that differences in the brain response to smoking cues exist between African American and white smokers (Okuyemi et al. 2006). This difference in the neural representation of relapse suggests racial group differences in the neurobiology of nicotine addiction that, further, may contribute to differences in the effectiveness of drug addiction treatments for individuals of different racial and ethnic backgrounds. Increasingly recognized differences in risk factors for drug abuse and addiction related to racial and ethnic backgrounds warrant a greater future emphasis on these complex population variables when characterizing the neurobiology of drug addiction. Such research is necessary to define, identify, and study high-risk populations for drug addiction.

Neuroscientific Approaches to the Drug Addiction Process

The neuroscience of drug abuse and addiction represents a rapidly advancing edge in the larger field of discovery related to the biological bases of psychiatric disorders. Much of this recent scientific progress is attributable to the evolving tools and technologies available to addiction researchers and their complementary use. Here we focus on two such tools or technologies: animal models and in vivo neuroimaging approaches.

Animal Models

Animal models of normal and abnormal human behavior have value as simpler, more accessible analogs of complex, inaccessible human conditions. Animal models of the drug addiction process represent arguably the best validated, most widely used animal models of psychiatric disorders. The interested reader should consult Shalev et al. (2002) for a more thorough description of animal models of the drug addiction process. There are numerous animal behavioral models that have been developed and used extensively to elucidate the human drug addiction process. Here we consider the condition place preference (CPP) paradigm and the reinstatement model. The CPP paradigm models the ability of contextual cues associated with drug states to provoke drug-seeking behavior as a function of their properties as rewards (Calcagnetti and Schechter 1993; Schechter and Calcagnetti 1998). The CPP paradigm is based on classical (Pavlovian) conditioning, as contextual cues acquire secondary reinforcing (conditioned stimulus [CS]) properties through their temporal pairing with a psychoactive drug that functions as an unconditioned stimulus (US) (Calcagnetti and Schechter 1993). In this model, a drug is administered to an animal immediately before placement in an environment with distinctive contextual stimuli (olfactory, visual, tactile). Drug-seeking behavior related to the reinforcing property of a drug is then subsequently assessed by the animal's preference for the drug-paired versus unpaired environment expressed in time spent in each environment.

As discussed below, drug addiction is characterized by the high rate of relapse related to drug-seeking and -use behaviors. The reinstatement animal model of relapse represents a critical tool in attempts to characterize the neural mechanisms of relapse and the development of medications promoting relapse prevention in addicted human populations. In the self-administration version of the reinstatement procedure, drug addiction–related relapse refers to the precipitated resumption of drug seeking after extinction of drug-reinforced responding (Epstein et al. 2006; Fuchs et al. 2003; Lynch et al. 2002; Shaham et al. 2003). In reinstatement, operant responding (e.g., lever pressing) resulting in drug self-administration is extinguished after a period of drug availability. Following extinction, noncontingent presentation of the previously self-administered drug (Shaham et al. 2003) or exposure to conditioned drug cues or stressors reinstates responding (Brown and Erb 2007; de Wit and Stewart 1981; Fuchs et al. 1998; Goddard and Leri 2006; Meil and See 1996; Shelton et al. 2004; Worley et al. 1994). The similarity of these relapse precipitants between the animal model and human drug addiction renders significant face validity to the reinstatement model (Epstein et al. 2006). The model also has good predictive validity and unestablished but building construct validity as an animal model of relapse associated with addiction (Epstein et al. 2006). Reinstatement can also be modeled using the CPP paradigm in which CPP is induced by drug administration, extinguished, and then reinstated by drug-priming injections (Mueller and Stewart 2000). Thus, the drug reinstatement model in animals has important and valid utility in exploring the factors underlying relapse in drug-addicted individuals.

Although animal behavioral models represent valuable tools in exploring the acquisition and maintenance of human drug addiction, genetic animal models provide further insights into the brain mechanisms involved in the acquisition and maintenance of drug addiction. Cocaine blocks the activity of neuronal plasma membrane transporters for dopamine (DAT [dopamine transporter]) as well as serotonin (SERT [serotonin transporter]) and norepinephrine (NET [norepinephrine transporter]) (Kuhar et al. 1991). Genetic models of transgenic knockout mice for these transporters have been studied extensively in establishing the role of each monoamine transporter in the neuropharmacology of cocaine. DAT knockout mice self-administer cocaine and exhibit cocaine-induced CPP (Giros et al. 1996; Medvedev et al. 2005; Rocha et al. 1998; Sora et al. 1998). Knockouts of SERT and NET also display cocaine reward or reinforcement (Sora et al. 1998; Xu et al. 2000). Mice with no DAT and either no or one SERT gene copy display no cocaine-induced CPP (Hall et al. 2002; Shen et al. 2004; Sora et al. 2001). This example suggests that DAT inhibition is not solely required for the reinforcing effects of cocaine. Animal genetic models represent powerful tools in the study of the drug addiction process.

In Vivo Molecular, Anatomical, and Functional Neuroimaging

The development of in vivo neuroimaging technologies such as positron emission tomography (PET), single photon emission computed tomography (SPECT), and magnetic resonance imaging (MRI) has dramatically altered the study of the relationship between the brain and behavior. These technologies have furnished important, novel insights into the neurobiology of the addiction process; specific examples are provided in other sections of this chapter.

The radiometric imaging procedures PET and SPECT represent scanners designed to provide two-dimensional and three-dimensional localizations of photon emissions resulting from radionuclide decay for radiopharmaceuticals that react with or bind to brain proteins involved in the regulation of neurotransmission. Such proteins include enzymes, receptors, and transporters. Although the number of valid PET radioligands that satisfy the requisite affinity, selectivity, metabolic stability, binding site kinetics, and physicochemical properties is limited, the strength of this imaging modality lies in the potential diversity of brain "functions" that can be imaged. Images of neurotransmitter receptor density and occupancy, neurotransmitter release, neurotransmitter synthesis, and metabolic and blood flow corollaries of neural activity in human and nonhuman primates and in small animals have been acquired in support of drug addiction research.

As a nonradiometric imaging technology, MRI also offers multimodal imaging opportunities based on the spatial tuning using gradient coils of the behavior of protons in a large magnetic main field. Optimized pulse sequences permit the acquisition of MRI of hemodynamic corollaries of neural activity, of brain gray and white matter, and of neurochemicals. Images of brain gray and white matter support morphometric and morphological magnetic resonance imaging (mMRI) of the roles of altered brain anatomy in the drug addiction process. For example, drug addiction has been linked to abnormal patterns of regional gray and white matter volumes or densities in the brain of drug-dependent individuals using voxel-based morphometry (VBM). Cocaine- and alcohol-dependent individuals had decreased gray matter densities in the amygdala, frontal cortex, orbitofrontal cortex, cingulate gyrus, temporal cortex, cerebellum, and premotor cortex when compared with control individuals (Franklin et al. 2002; Matochik et al. 2003; Mechtcheriakov et al. 2007; Sim et al. 2007). Numerous examples of the application of in vivo functional neuroimaging approaches such as fMRI and PET to the investigation of the neurobiology of the drug addiction process are discussed in subsections of this chapter; fewer illustrations of the application of magnetic resonance spectroscopy (MRS) are also provided. These examples illustrate the argument that in vivo brain imaging technologies have led to unparalleled advances in the understanding of the neural basis of the acquisition and maintenance of human drug addiction.

The Acquisition of Addiction

Many individuals experiment with drugs of abuse. For many and perhaps all such drugs, their activation of the mesolimbic dopamine projections to the ventral striatum plays a pivotal role in their reinforcing effects (Abi-Dargham et al. 2003; Rodd-Henricks et al. 2002; Volkow et al. 1997), resulting in further experimentation. However, while exact numbers are lacking, only a small percentage of individuals who try drugs of abuse proceed to the compulsive and uncontrolled abuse that characterizes addiction. Individuals comprising this minority share a predisposition that is generally attributed to genetic or environmental factors and their interactions.

The neurobiology of the transition by some susceptible individuals from drug abuse to addiction has been best informed by animal models of drug self-administration. Rats given extended versus limited access to cocaine or heroin self-administration exhibit an escalation of drug intake and an enhanced reinstatement of extinguished drug-seeking behavior by the systemic administration of the self-administered drug—responses that represent well-accepted symptoms of human drug addiction (Ferrario et al. 2005; Knackstedt and Kalivas 2007; Koob and Kreek 2007; Lenoir and Ahmed 2007). Whether this transition occurs in the presence or absence of behavioral sensitization of drug effects remains controversial (Ferrario et al. 2005; Knackstedt and Kalivas 2007; Lenoir and Ahmed 2007). The specific neuroadaptations that underlie this transition include empirical and theoretical accounts of altered striatal and prefrontal cortex circuits. One model attributes the acquisition of addiction to a synaptic reorganization of the core subdivision of the nucleus accumbens that results in a pathological increase in the incentive value of drugs (Ferrario et al. 2005). Another model emphasizes an allostatic decrease in reward system responsivity as the mechanism of escalated drug intake (Ahmed and Koob 2005). A third model emphasizes a neural transition from prefrontal cortical to striatal control over drug-seeking and drug-use behavior and a progression from ventral to more dorsal divisions of the striatum (Everitt and Robbins 2005). The significance of the dorsal striatum and its dopaminergic innervations to the transition from drug use to abuse to addiction is supported by their demonstrated roles in habit formation in humans and animal models (Faure et al. 2005; Yin et al. 2004).

In addition to striatal and frontal cortex involvement in the acquisition of drug addiction, other brain areas code the associative learning and memories reflecting the conditioning of the reinforcing actions of drugs of abuse with the environmental and other contexts of drug use that promote further conditioned drug abuse. Inactivation of the basolateral amygdala disrupts the learning of the conditioned reinforcing effects of drug-paired stimuli (Kruzich and See 2001). The well-recognized role of the hippocampus in the formation and processing of contextual memories (Holland and Bouton 1999) suggests its involvement in the formation and retrieval of cognitive representations of contextual memories of drug reinforcement. The critical role of the dorsal hippocampus and its projections in the ventral subiculum in the drug cue–induced reinstatement of drug-seeking behavior (Fuchs et al. 2005; Sun and Rebec 2003; Zhao et al. 2006) supports their involvement in the retrieval of associative memories of drug reinforcement. However, the dorsal subiculum may have a selective role in the formation of contextual memories of drug reinforcement as its transient inactivation during conditioning blocked the acquisition of drug-seeking induced by drug-paired stimuli in the reinstatement model (Martin-Fardon et al. 2008). Collective insights from animal models yield a neurobiology of the acquisition of drug-addicted states that includes the engagement of limbic, striatal, and prefrontal cortex areas in drug-related behavioral reinforcement and learning and memory processes that imbue drug-related stimuli with incentive motivation, rewarding, contextual, and habitual properties.

Genetic Influences

Human studies of the neurobiology of the transition from drug use to abuse and addiction have focused more on the roles played by genetic and environmental risk factors (see Figure 49–1). Environmental and genetic factors contribute to individual differences in vulnerability to initiating use of drugs of abuse and in vulnerability to the shift from drug use to addiction (Goldman et al. 2005). Drug addictions represent some of the most heritable psychiatric disorders. Heritabilities differ for different drug addictions, ranging from moderate values (0.39) for hallucinogens to high heritabilities (0.72) for cocaine (Goldman et al. 2005). Estimated heritabilities for the initiation and use of drugs of abuse are typically lower than those for addiction (M.D. Li et al. 2003). The obvious questions are what exactly is being inherited by individuals and populations that enhances the risk for drug use and addiction, and what are the relative contributions of genetic and environmental factors to the observed heritabilities? The genetic determinants of drug abuse and addiction include the regulation of pharmacodynamic and pharmacokinetic processes that determine drug sensitivity and the genetic regulation of intermediate cognitive, personality, and other phenotypes that influence the addiction process (Goldman et al. 2005). The neurobiological corollaries of the genetics of addiction that confer vulnerability for, and protection from, drug abuse and addiction are in an early stage of identification. The emerging field of "imaging genetics" (Meyer-Lindenberg and Weinberger 2006) is based on the use of in vivo neuroimaging approaches to define the neurobiology mediating the influence of genetic variation on the expression of normal and abnormal human behavior. These approaches provide clues as to what is being inherited in the form of identified gene influences on brain morphology and morphometrics, task-related brain activity, functional and anatomical connectivity between brain areas comprising neural circuits and pathways, and the expression and occupancy of neurotransmitter receptors, transporters, and enzymes.

Due to the demonstrated roles of neurotransmitter alterations in the addiction process, variations in genes that regulate neurotransmission have been the primary focus of efforts to identify addiction-related genes. Quantitative trait locus (QTL) analyses of ethanol-related behaviors including preference and sensitivity to withdrawal and sedation in mice implicate gene clusters harboring the γ-aminobutyric acid A (GABA$_A$) receptor (Crabbe et al. 1999). While a detailed discussion of the neurobiology of genetic risk for drug abuse and addiction is beyond the scope of this chapter, we offer the following as examples of the impact of, and insights from, early approaches.

Dopamine-related genes have been implicated in the addiction process, particularly functional polymorphisms for genes encoding catechol-O-methyltransferase (COMT), the human dopamine transporter (DAT1), and the D$_2$ and D$_4$ dopamine receptors (DRD2 and DRD4, respectively). The level of expression of D$_2$ receptors in the prefrontal cortex as defined by [^{11}C]raclopride PET imaging determines the subjective experience of pleasure following the administration of methylphenidate and presumably other psychostimulants (Volkow et al. 2005). Interindividual differences in the structure or expression of genes involved in dopaminergic neurotransmission (e.g., DRD2) could account for some of the genetically mediated variability in substance abuse behaviors in humans (Uhl et al. 1993). Allelic variation for the DRD2 Taq1 restriction fragment length polymorphism (RFLP) regulates the craving response to conditioned drug cues associated with nicotine (Erblich et al. 2005) and heroin (Y. Li et al. 2006) addiction. Recent [^{11}C]raclopride PET imaging studies indicate that variable number of tandem repeat (VNTR) polymorphisms in the DAT1 and DRD4 genes, and a single nucleotide polymorphism (SNP) in the COMT gene, regulate the release of ventral striatal dopamine in response to cigarette smoking, with the response inversely related to cigarette craving (Brody et al. 2006). Many studies also suggest that SLC6A3, the gene that encodes DAT, has a genetic link with cocaine addiction (Haile et al. 2007). Individual variation in dopamine-related genes may thus regulate individual differences in acquisition of drug addiction and risk for relapse.

The genetic regulation of cognitive functions related to the addiction process, or of personality traits that modulate risk for drug abuse and addiction, represents another source of the observed heritability of addictive disorders (Kreek et al. 2005). Personality traits such as impulsivity, risk taking, and novelty seeking are associated with drug addiction (Moeller et al. 2001) and with risk for drug abuse and addiction (Dawe and Loxton 2004; Kreek et al. 2005). These traits are regulated by serotonin-related genes that encode the brain isoform of tryptophan hydroxylase (TPH2) (Zhou et al. 2005) and the serotonin transporter (SERT) (Gerra et al. 2005). Allelic variation of the TPH2 gene (TPH2) and the SERT gene (5-HTTLPR) regulates the neural response to demands for cognitive and affective processing (Canli et al. 2008; Herrmann et al.

2007). Similarly, cognitive functions related to the addiction process, such as inhibitory executive control, the processing of incentives and rewards, and delay discounting, have a neurobiology that is profoundly influenced by polymorphic variation in genes regulating dopamine neurotransmission. Putative functional polymorphisms in COMT and DAT1 additively regulate the neural basis of reward sensitivity (Yacubian et al. 2007) and thus, potentially, vulnerability to drug abuse and addiction. Importantly, genes that regulate pharmacodynamic, pharmacokinetic, and cognitive functions and personality traits exhibit epistatic gene–gene interactions that convey multiplicative contributions to risk for drug abuse and addiction in allele carriers (Yacubian et al. 2007).

Environmental Influences

Genetic factors explain, on average, only about half of the total variability in drug addiction, with the remaining variability influenced by environmental factors. Also, genetic risk may be differentially expressed in the presence versus absence of particular environmental conditions (Lessov et al. 2004). Environmental factors that can contribute to drug abuse and addiction include psychosocial factors such as socioeconomic status, peer influence, and family dissension and early-life adversity such as physical, sexual, and emotional abuse and/or neglect (see Figure 49–1). More than half of drug abusers entering addiction treatment report a history of childhood physical or sexual abuse (Pirard et al. 2005). High rates of childhood maltreatment (e.g., childhood physical, sexual, and emotional abuse and/or neglect) have been associated with drug abuse and addiction (Simpson and Miller 2002). Studies also suggest that relationships between drug use and abuse and childhood maltreatment are stronger in women (Hyman et al. 2005; MacMillan et al. 2001). Childhood maltreatment was also associated with a younger age of first cocaine use and a greater lifetime severity of drug use (Hyman et al. 2006). Women also typically had more instances of sexual and emotional abuse and overall childhood maltreatment, while in men emotional abuse was the main type of abuse reported. Recent findings suggest that having a history of childhood maltreatment may influence how recently abstinent cocaine-dependent individuals experience and cope with stress, a recognized relapse factor (Hyman et al. 2007). Cocaine-dependent individuals have a higher incidence of trauma and comorbid posttraumatic stress disorder (PTSD) (Back et al. 2000). The neurobiology of childhood abuse and neglect is intimately intertwined with the neurobiology of drug abuse and addiction. For instance, the observation that childhood maltreatment is associated with a persistent, perhaps permanent, sensitization of the endocrine and autonomic response to stress (Heim et al. 2000) implies a related sensitization of drug-addicted individuals with childhood maltreatment histories to stress-induced relapse. The impossibility of understanding the neurobiology of the acquisition of drug addiction without appreciating the genetic and environmental determinants of individual differences in the risk for abuse and addiction and in the response to addiction therapies is increasingly obvious.

Neurodevelopmental Influences

Adolescence is a time of high-risk behavior and increased exploration. The neurodevelopmental period of adolescence represents typically the first experimentation with drugs of abuse and is associated with an increased risk to develop drug addiction in adulthood (see Figure 49–1). Adolescents typically exhibit higher rates of experimental drug use and abuse disorders than adults (Chambers et al. 2003). Recognized risk factors for adolescent drug abuse include early marijuana and cigarette use, deviant behavior, negative family interactions, poor parent–child communication, school disengagement, family drug problems, drug availability, and prodrug attitudes and intentions (Ellickson and Morton 1999; Kliewer and Murrelle 2007). Adolescence also represents a critical period for factors such as parental support or nonfamily mentors to exert their durable protective effects on drug abuse and addiction. Adolescence is a critical period for maturation of neurobiological processes that underlie higher cognitive functions and social and emotional behavior (Yurgelun-Todd 2007). Functional neuroimaging studies indicate that brain regions that underlie attention, reward evaluation, affective discrimination, response inhibition, and goal-directed behavior undergo structural and functional organization throughout late childhood and early adulthood (Bjork et al. 2004; Galvan et al. 2006; Yurgelun-Todd 2007). The vulnerability of adolescents to drug abuse and addiction may reflect the delayed brain maturation of executive processes of behavioral regulation relative to those that encode incentive valuation. Adolescents, relative to children and adults, exhibited increased nucleus accumbens activity relative to prefrontal cortex activity during reward valuation, whereas the orbitofrontal cortex response was similar to that of children and less than that of adults (Galvan et al. 2006). Greater motivational drives for rewards, coupled with an immature neu-

ral mechanism of inhibitory control, could predispose adolescents to impulsive actions and risky behaviors including experimentation with drugs of abuse (Chambers et al. 2003). Elucidating the developmental timing of the neural processing of incentive valuation, goal representation, delay discounting, response inhibition, and other behaviors related to the addiction process using technologies such as fMRI over the adolescent period would clearly inform the pathogenesis of substance use disorders and inform intervention strategies for preventing drug abuse and other high-risk behaviors in youth.

Relapse to Drug-Seeking and Drug-Use Behaviors

Drug addiction in treatment-seeking individuals is associated with high rates of recidivism (O'Brien 1997). Attentional and motivational responses to conditioned drug cues represent powerful precipitants of relapse in drug-addicted individuals (Kalivas and Volkow 2005). There has been scant research focusing on identifying neural markers of relapse in drug-dependent human populations, in spite of the clear value of such predictors to defining relapse risk and treatment prognosis. A recent fMRI study in treatment-completing methamphetamine-dependent subjects examined the relationship between the magnitude of the distributed neural response to a decision-making task and the incidence of relapse over a 1-year follow-up interval (Paulus et al. 2005). Lower task-related activation of the right middle frontal gyrus, middle temporal gyrus, and posterior cingulate cortex best predicted time to relapse. These predictive neural responses suggest their representation of deficit functions related to decision making that bias individuals for relapse.

The process of relapse to drug-seeking and -use behavior is multidetermined, with at least three putative precipitants that are recognized in drug-addicted human subjects and reliably modeled in reinstatement versions of animal drug self-administration paradigms (Figure 49–2). The formation of learned associations between drug-use reminders, or cues, and the euphoria or "high" associated with drug use underlies the pathological motivations for drug seeking and use that define relapse due to *conditioned drug cues* (Figure 49–2A). Such cues are diverse in nature and include exteroceptive stimuli, such as persons, places, or sensory cues, as well as interoceptive stimuli, such as mood states. The experience of *stress* represents a second well-recognized precipitant of relapse (Figure 49–2B). *Drug use itself* is also recognized as a precipitant of motivation for further drug abuse in the form of drug bingeing (Figure 49–2C). The interested reader should consult Epstein et al. (2006) for a thoughtful discussion of the validity of the reinstatement procedure as an animal model of drug relapse.

The human motivational state for drug use that propels drug-seeking behavior is often referred to as "craving." Empirically, drug craving is defined by subjective measures of self-rated intensities of craving, using Likert or other scales, or by objective measures of craving-related arousal, such as skin conductance, heart rate, blood pressure, or pupil diameter. The following describes research findings related to the functional neuroanatomy and neurochemistry of precipitated drug craving defined by animal models or human neuroimaging studies. While often assumed, the true relationship between craving and relapse is complex and only modestly established at this time (Epstein et al. 2006). It is also noteworthy that a neuroanatomy of precipitated drug seeking based on the collected findings from even a single animal model is less than definitive as different means of probing the involvement of a given brain area (e.g., tetrodotoxin, receptor antagonists or agonists, lesions) yield conflicting outcomes (Bossert et al. 2005). As such, the following discussion of the neurobiology of relapse comparing the drug-seeking condition defined by the reinstatement animal model and human drug craving defined in the laboratory should be critically considered.

Relapse Related to Conditioned Drug Cues

In drug-dependent subjects, exposure to drug-related stimuli (e.g., drug paraphernalia, drug-taking environment) elicits intense craving and increases the probability of relapse even following prolonged abstinence (Childress et al. 1988; Ehrman et al. 1992; Jaffe et al. 1989; Johnson et al. 1998). The neural representation of conditioned cue–induced drug craving has been explored in the reinstatement model in rats, in which a conditioned stimulus (e.g., a light) that was paired with access to cocaine in a self-administration paradigm reinstates drug-seeking behavior (i.e., lever pressing) following extinction of the drug access contingency of the lever. Understandably, there is considerable overlap of affected brain regions with brain regions thought to be involved in appetitive conditioning and the retrieval of conditioned associations (Kelley et al. 2005; See 2002; Thomas and Everitt 2001). A combination of results from lesioning and pharmacological inactivation studies, intracerebral microdialysis, electrophysiology, and molecular markers of neu-

ronal activity implicates the amygdala (Hayes et al. 2003; Thomas and Everitt 2001), the anterior cingulate and orbitofrontal cortex (McLaughlin and See 2003), and the dorsal (Ito et al. 2002) and ventral (Ghitza et al. 2003) striatum in the drug motivational response to conditioned drug cues (Figure 49–2A).

Beyond their use in elucidating the neuroanatomy of conditioned cue–induced drug craving, animal models have uniquely contributed to our understanding of the specific neurotransmitters involved in the coupling of drug-predictive stimuli with drug-seeking behavior. Conditioned drug cues are associated with glutamate release in the nucleus accumbens and dopamine release in the amygdala, nucleus accumbens, dorsal striatum, and prefrontal cortex (Ito et al. 2002; Phillips et al. 2003; Vanderschuren et al. 2005; F. Weiss et al. 2000) (see Figure 49–2A). It is noteworthy that the neuroanatomy and neurobiology of drug seeking precipitated by conditioned drug cues differs when the drug-paired cue is a discrete cue, discriminative cue, or contextual cue (Bossert et al. 2005). Interested readers should consult Kalivas and Volkow (2005) or Bossert et al. (2005) for more elaborated models of the roles of alterations in cellular signaling, receptor translocation, and cell morphology in the neural basis of the relapse process.

In vivo functional neuroimaging approaches have provided novel insights into the distributed patterns of neural processing that transduce the experience of conditioned drug-use reminders into drug craving and relapse in human drug addicts. Here, a clear challenge has been to capture the neural response to drug cues within the nonnaturalistic environment of a PET, SPECT, or MRI scanner for drug-use reminders that are highly individualized and context-dependent. In response to these challenges in experimental design, researchers have devised generalized drug cues represented by videotape and still images of drug-use behavior, the handling of drug paraphernalia, individualized drug cues in the form of the mental imagery of personal drug use guided by autobiographical scripts, and compound drug cues represented by virtual reality environments. Additional experimental design challenges are posed by the need to document and quantify the induced drug motivational state and to compare it to responses to control conditions that correct for sensory, motor, attentional, mnemonic, and other features of cue processing. The combination of subjective self-ratings of the intensity of drug-use urges and of corollary emotional states with objective psychophysiological measures (heart rate, skin conductance, pupil diameter, or respiratory rate) of craving-related arousal has emerged

(A) Cue-induced relapse

Human

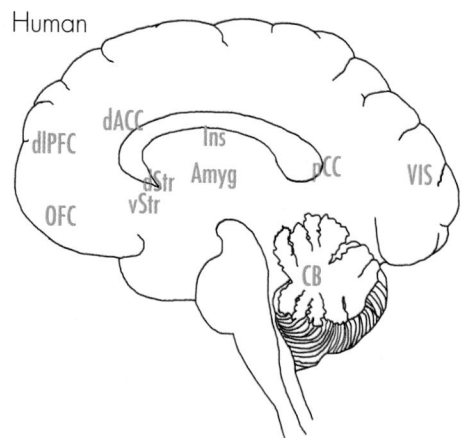

Rodent model

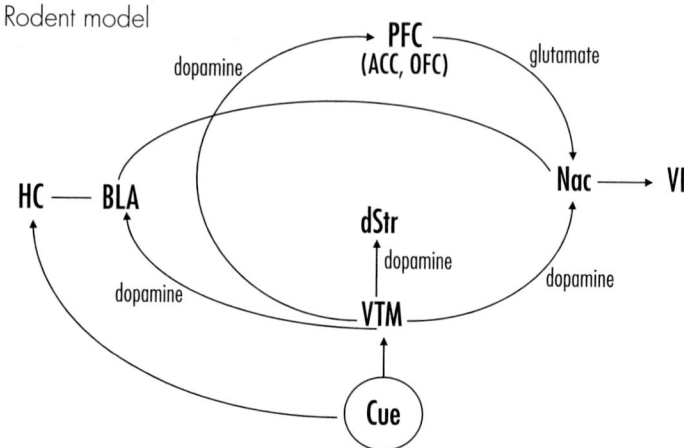

(B) Stress-induced relapse

Human

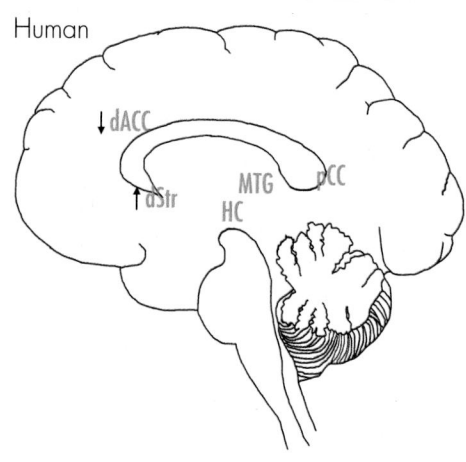

Rodent model

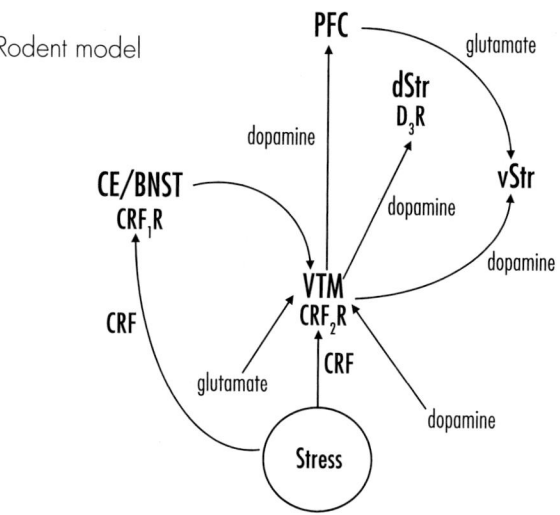

(C) Drug-induced relapse

Human

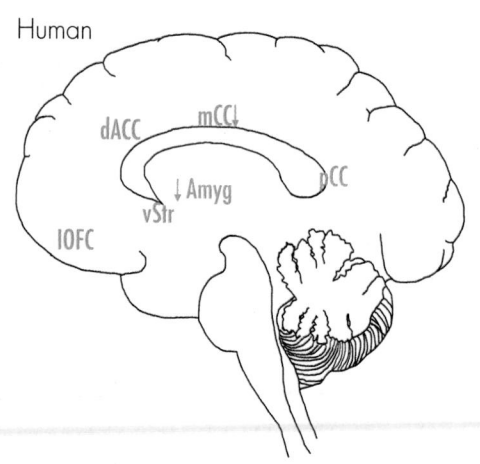

Rodent model

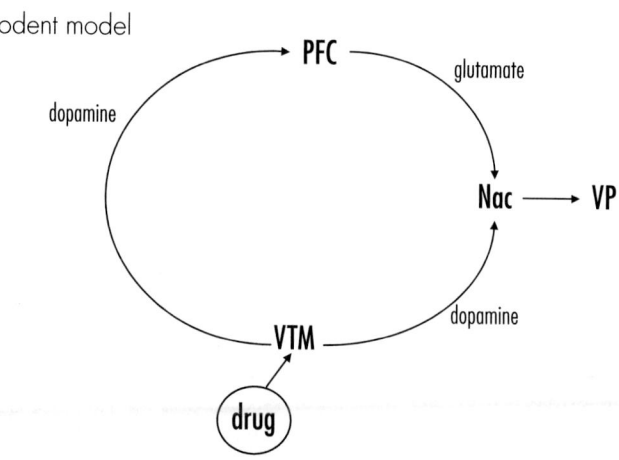

FIGURE 49–2. Models of neurobiological mechanisms of relapse to drug seeking and drug use (*opposite*).
To elucidate the emerging neurobiology of mechanisms of relapse to drug-seeking and -use behaviors associated with drug addiction, we consider and compare three potential precipitants of relapse: conditioned drug-use reminders or cues (**A, Cue-induced relapse model**), stress (**B, Stress-induced relapse model**), and use/administration of the drug itself (**C, Drug-induced relapse model**). For each model presented, the neuroanatomical areas and neurotransmitter mechanisms involved (as defined by investigation of the reinstatement animal model of relapse) are shown *on the right*, and the distributed neural processing associated with experiencing the relapse precipitant (as defined by human in vivo functional neuroimaging studies in males) is shown *on the left*. It should be emphasized that these neurobiological mechanisms reflect major but not all research findings and represent an as-yet-incomplete characterization of the mechanisms of relapse. Therefore, strict comparisons of the underlying mechanisms between the three relapse precipitants should be done with caution.
ACC=anterior cingulate cortex; Amyg=amygdala; BLA=basolateral amygdaloid nucleus; BNST=bed nucleus of the stria terminalis; CB=cerebellum; CE=central amygdaloid nucleus; CRF=corticotropin-releasing factor; CRF_1R=corticotropin-releasing factor 1 receptor; CRF_2R=corticotropin-releasing factor 2 receptor; D_3R=D_3 dopamine receptor; dACC=dorsal anterior cingulate cortex; dlPFC=dorsolateral prefrontal cortex; dStr=dorsal striatum; HC=hippocampus; Ins=insula; lOFC=left orbitofrontal cortex; mCC=middle cingulate cortex; MTG=medial temporal gyrus; Nac=nucleus accumbens; OFC=orbitofrontal cortex; pCC=posterior cingulate cortex; PFC=prefrontal cortex; VIS=visual cortex; VP=ventral pallidum; vStr=ventral striatum; VTM=ventral tegmentum.

as a best approach to defining and quantifying cue-induced drug craving. Implementing the ideal control condition(s) has been a more elusive aspect of experimental design. Finally, the characteristics of the sample of drug-dependent individuals studied represents a critical determinant of the neural response to drug cues. Features such as age, sex (Kilts et al. 2004), duration of drug abstinence, treatment enrollment (Wilson et al. 2003), specific drug dependency, expectancy of drug availability (McBride et al. 2006; Wertz and Sayette 2001), comorbid psychiatric illness or drug dependencies, or experiences of recent stress or early-life adversities critically modulate the neural processing of conditioned drug cues. The interested reader should consult Kilts et al. (2001) for a more detailed treatment of experimental approaches to the use of in vivo functional neuroimaging technology to define the neurobiology of the drug motivational state.

The neurobiology of cue-induced craving in drug-addicted human subjects exhibits many parallels with findings from the reinstatement animal model (see Figure 49–2A). First, [^{11}C]raclopride PET imaging studies of cocaine abusers demonstrated that the occupancy of D_2 receptors in the human dorsal (but not ventral) striatum was increased by exposure to cocaine cues (Volkow et al. 2006; Wong et al. 2006), and imaging of alcoholic subjects has revealed increased D_2 receptor occupancy in both striatal subdivisions in response to exposure to alcohol cues (Heinz et al. 2004). This cue response presumably reflects a cue-induced increase in dorsal striatal dopamine release and was positively correlated with both the intensity of self-reported cocaine craving and the severity of addiction-related functional impairment. Conditioned cocaine cues increase dorsal striatal dopamine release in cocaine-dependent human subjects and animal models of cocaine self-administration, implicating this cue response

in the processing of cues as reward predictors and as a biomarker of the habitual nature of addiction. Second, the distributed neural response to drug cues in drug-dependent human subjects involves many of the same brain areas implicated by the response to discrete drug-paired stimuli in rats.

Figure 49–2 presents a summary of human study findings across diverse experimental approaches. Brain areas activated by the passive or active processing of conditioned drug cues include the anterior and posterior cingulate cortex, amygdala, ventral striatum, insula, orbitofrontal cortex, dorsolateral prefrontal cortex, cerebellum, and visual cortex (Anderson et al. 2006; Bonson et al. 2002; Childress et al. 1999; Daglish et al. 2001; Garavan et al. 2000; Grant et al. 1996; Heinz et al. 2004; Kilts et al. 2001, 2004; Maas et al. 1998; Wexler et al. 2001). The results of correlational and other approaches to data analysis, expanded experimental designs (e.g., the inclusion of attempts to volitionally inhibit the craving response), and comparisons of localized brain responses with other imaging studies furnish plausible inferences of the roles of each neural activation site to the complex state of conditioned drug craving and relapse. Consistent drug cue–induced activation of the amygdala may reflect the motivational evaluation of emotional and other associations to drug cues (Kilts et al. 2004). Cue-induced activation of the dorsal anterior cingulate cortex (dACC) may reflect the computation of conditional drug probabilities (Kilts et al. 2004) and the related processing of response conflict due to drug nonavailability in the scanner context. Greater dACC activation to drug cues may reflect an adaptive regulatory role that dampens the drug cue evaluative functions of brain areas mediating their sensory and motivational processing when drug availability is low or when drug use is resisted (Brody et al. 2007; Kilts et al.

2004). The dorsolateral prefrontal cortex activation by drug cues may reflect the access to mental representations of drug use and/or the engagement of executive control of drug-related behaviors signaled by the dACC response. Cue-induced activation of the insula may reflect the access of somatic representations of drug states and/or the aversive properties of experiencing drug motivation in the absence of availability. Activation of the ventral striatum by drug cues may reflect the processing of the strong incentive motivational property of drug cues, while activation of the precommissural dorsal striatum may reflect the retrieval of motor cognitions related to habits of drug abuse. These findings suggest a complex relationship between the experiencing of drug-use reminders and motivation for drug abuse. The interested reader should consult Kilts et al. (2001) for a more thorough description of the human functional brain imaging studies and their designs that have investigated the neural response to conditioned drug cues in diverse drug addictions.

Much has been learned about the neurobiology of conditioned drug craving from animal model and human studies. In several instances this knowledge has driven the development of novel treatments for drug addiction. As an example, the findings that the reinstatement of drug-seeking behavior by conditioned drug cues in rats was related to deficits in frontal–striatal glutamate signaling that was rescued by stimulation of the cysteine–glutamate exchanger by administration of the cysteine prodrug N-acetylcysteine (Zhou and Kalivas 2008) led to the demonstration that N-acetylcysteine administration reduces the urge to use cocaine provoked by drug cues in cocaine-dependent human subjects (LaRowe et al. 2007).

Relapse Related to Stressful Events

Stress is another factor that can precipitate intense drug wanting or craving. The neural representation of stress-induced drug craving has been explored in the reinstatement model in rats in which stressors (typically footshock) reinstate drug-seeking behavior (i.e., lever pressing) following extinction of the drug access contingency of the lever. In this animal model, stress-induced drug-seeking behavior shares many of the neural substrates associated with cue-induced drug seeking including the midbrain ventral tegmentum, prefrontal cortex, and dorsal and ventral striatum (Figure 49–2B).

A glutamatergic projection from the prefrontal cortex to the ventral striatum has been proposed as a final common pathway for the precipitation of drug seeking by stress, conditioned drug cues, or the drug itself (Kalivas

and Volkow 2005). The neural pathways associated with stress- and drug cue–induced drug seeking are, however, distinct in other ways (Shalev et al. 2002). Unlike cue-induced drug seeking, stress-primed drug seeking does not involve the basolateral amygdala (McFarland et al. 2004), but rather engages the bed nucleus of the stria terminalis and other brain areas comprising the extended amygdala (Shaham et al. 2002). Stress and drug cues exhibit additive effects on drug seeking related to their shared activation of the corticotropin-releasing factor (CRF) system (Liu and Weiss 2002). However, the role of CRF signaling in stress-induced relapse is particularly important and related to multiple actions at CRF_1 and CRF_2 receptors regulating dopamine and glutamate release in midbrain and forebrain elements of drug motivational pathways (Wang et al. 2007) (see Figure 49–2B).

Recent evidence supports the relatedness of stress-related increases in drug craving to cocaine relapse outcomes in cocaine-dependent individuals (Sinha et al. 2006). The intensity of stress-induced increases in drug craving and hypothalamic-pituitary-adrenal (HPA) axis responses predicted a shorter time to relapse and higher amounts of cocaine use per occasion, respectively. Recent in vivo functional neuroimaging studies have also provided novel insights into the distributed patterns of neural processing that transduce the experience of acute stress into drug craving and relapse in drug-addicted human subjects. In studies employing script-guided mental imagery as a means of exposure to a stressor in a scanner environment, a mixed-sex sample of cocaine-dependent subjects exhibited decreased activation in paralimbic (anterior cingulate) and limbic (hippocampus) regions and increased activation in the dorsal striatal region in response to stress relative to comparison subjects (Sinha et al. 2005) (see Figure 49–2B). The dorsal striatal response scaled with the intensity of stress-induced cocaine craving. The implication of these findings is that stress diminishes responses associated with the self-regulation of affect- and drug-related behaviors and activates the habit pattern of compulsive drug abuse (Sinha et al. 2005). As discussed previously, a comparison of male and female cocaine-addicted subjects supported significant differences between the sexes in the neural response to a stressor, in spite of equivalent anxiety and craving responses (Sinha et al. 2005). Compared with males, cocaine-dependent females exhibited greater paralimbic and left frontal responses, suggesting activation of greater conflict detection and response inhibition in reacting to stress. The functional neuroanatomy of stress-induced drug craving in drug-addicted humans is critically uninformed, as drug dependencies other than cocaine have not been examined and the dependence of observed neural responses on the nature of the acute stress and its interaction with prior and early-life stress has not been defined.

In contrast to the extensive research conducted in animal models, the comparative neurobiology of drug cue–induced and stress-induced drug craving in human addicts has been little explored. A comparison of script-guided mental imagery paradigms indicated that drug cue and stress imagery in cocaine-dependent subjects similarly activated the HPA and autonomic components of the stress response system (Sinha et al. 2003). Findings from the reinstatement animal model indicate that stress-induced and drug cue–induced drug-seeking behavior exhibits an additive interaction (F. Weiss 2005). A recent fMRI study in cocaine-dependent men demonstrated a greater drug cue–induced activation of the posterior cingulate and parietal cortex response in the presence versus absence of an acute stressor (anticipation of electric shock) (Duncan et al. 2007). These results indicate that stress and conditioned drug cues interact to augment drug-seeking behavior and that stress may provoke relapse by activating brain areas involved in processing the incentive and attention biasing properties of drug-use reminders.

Much has been learned about the neurobiology of stress-induced drug craving from animal model and human studies. In several instances this knowledge has driven the development of novel treatments for drug addiction. As an example, the demonstration in rats that activation of α_2-adrenergic receptors by the administration of lofexidine or clonidine attenuated footshock-induced reinstatement of cocaine or heroin seeking (Erb et al. 2000; Shaham et al. 2002) led to the subsequent preliminary demonstration that lofexidine attenuates stress-induced drug craving and promotes drug abstinence rates in opiate-addicted subjects (Sinha et al. 2006).

Relapse Related to Drug Use

The neural representation of drug-induced drug craving has been explored in the reinstatement model in rats in which noncontingent administration of the self-administered drug reinstates drug-seeking behavior (i.e., lever pressing) following extinction of the drug access contingency of the lever. This drug-primed reinstatement of drug seeking has been observed for cocaine, heroin, alcohol, and nicotine self-administration; generalizes to other members of the same pharmacological class; exhibits cross-reinstatement for drugs from different classes than

the self-administered drug; and is positively correlated in its magnitude with the priming dose (Shalev et al. 2002). Like stress- and drug cue–induced reinstatement of drug seeking, drug-primed reinstatement involves the prefrontal cortex and its glutamatergic projections to the nucleus accumbens (Bossert et al. 2005; Kalivas and Volkow 2005; McFarland and Kalivas 2001) (Figure 49–2C).

However, evidence from animal models indicates that drug-induced relapse differs neurobiologically from relapse precipitated by conditioned drug cues or stress. While the prefrontal cortex is consistently implicated in the reinstatement of drug seeking, different subregions of the medial prefrontal cortex appear to be involved in drug-induced, drug cue–induced, and stress-induced reinstatement (Capriles et al. 2003; Fuchs et al. 2004). Temporally, mice exhibited a transient (<2 months) drug-primed reinstatement of methamphetamine-seeking behavior following extinction, while cue-induced reinstatement was persistent (>5 months), suggesting the involvement of differing neuroadaptations for the two relapse factors (Yan et al. 2007).

Human in vivo functional neuroimaging studies have examined the neural responses associated with subjective drug abuse experiences, including drug craving. The neurobiology of drug craving, as elucidated through in vivo functional neuroimaging of cocaine's effects in drug-addicted human subjects, also exhibits clear parallels with findings from research paradigms employing the reinstatement animal model of relapse (see Figure 49–2C). Passive delivery of cocaine to cocaine-dependent subjects produced experiences of "high" that were temporally correlated with fMRI responses in the ventral tegmentum, dorsal striatum, and anterior and posterior cingulate cortices, whereas experiences of craving correlated with activity in the ventral striatum, anterior and posterior cingulate cortices, parahippocampal gyrus, and amygdala (negative correlation) (Breiter et al. 1997). A more recent fMRI study examining the neural correlates of "high" and craving during cocaine self-administration noted that self-reported craving correlated positively with activity in the anterior cingulate cortex, ventral striatum, and lateral orbitofrontal cortex, whereas cocaine-induced "high" correlated negatively with activity in the same brain regions (Risinger et al. 2005). Cocaine-induced craving was negatively correlated with activity in the middle cingulate cortex and thalamus. A related PET study noted that methylphenidate-induced craving in cocaine-addicted individuals was also associated with activation of the orbitofrontal cortex (Kalivas and Volkow 2005). These convergent findings indicate that the drug motivational state precipitated by noncontingent and contingent drug administration is transduced by the distributed activation of limbic, paralimbic, and striatal brain areas involved in incentive processing/valuation, cognitive control, and habit learning.

Neural Substrates Underlying the Association of Drug Addiction With Impulsive Aggression and Violence

Many of the neuroadaptive responses to prolonged drug intake are enduring and persist even following long periods of drug abstinence. Drug-addicted individuals are vulnerable to relapse for years after initiating and maintaining abstinence. This section deals with the social neuroscience of drug addiction, specifically the impact of end-stage drug addiction on the perception of social signals, the organization of reciprocal social responses, and the regulation of antisocial behavior. Is there a neurobiology of the social cost of drug addiction? A recent characterization of the prevalence and population estimates of violent behavior among individuals with DSM-IV-TR psychiatric disorders demonstrated that substance use disorders were by far the most significant contributors to the public health burden of violent behavior (Pulay et al. 2008). This discussion will focus on the neurobiology of the specific social cost due to the association of drug abuse with escalation of aggression and violence in some drug cultures (Boles and Miotto 2003; Fals-Stewart et al. 2003; Hoaken and Stewart 2003). The introduction of crack cocaine in an urban area in the 1980s was marked not so much by drug arrests as by crimes of assault and emergency room data related to the corollary escalation of aggression and violence. The economic costs of crime related to drug abuse and addiction are enormous. A large proportion of violent and property crimes in the United States involve drugs of abuse. Costs associated with medical care, property loss, future earnings, and adjudication, and pain and suffering associated with drug-related crime exceed $200 billion per year in the United States (Miller et al. 2006). Emergency room studies indicate that 35%–40% of injuries are associated with illicit drug use that is confirmed by toxicology (Vitale and van de Mheen 2006), particularly in association with intentional violent crime (Macdonald et al. 2003). Complex, multifactorial relationships exist between aggressive behavior and drug abuse and addiction that are moderated by situational and personal variables (Ousey and Lee 2004). This stage of the addiction process constitutes the greatest social and personal cost of addiction, yet, paradoxically, has been the least studied and characterized (see Figure 49–1). Key to understanding the escalation of interpersonal aggression and violence associated with some drug addictions is an understanding of its neurobiology in valid animal models and human populations.

Initial insights into the neural substrates of the association of drug addiction with impulsive aggression and violence were provided by the relationship between anger traits (Goldstein et al. 2005) and anger states (Drexler et al. 2000) with decreased neural activity in the lateral orbitofrontal cortex of cocaine-addicted men. These findings suggest that the behavioral regulatory roles of the orbitofrontal cortex and other brain areas are compromised in cocaine addiction, resulting in unchecked impulsive aggression in response to anger-provoking situations. These associations, however, lack the social context necessary to establish a relationship between experiences of anger, inhibitory control failures, and aggressive behavior in drug-addicted populations. Currently, these relationships may be best explored by the combination of in vivo functional neuroimaging technology and game behavior to define the neural responses of drug-addicted individuals to aggressive and affiliative behaviors emitted by playing partners in ongoing social dyadic interactions (Rilling et al. 2002). Such simulated social interactions in the context of game behavior offer novel insights into the impact of state (e.g., drug withdrawal) and trait (e.g., personality, race/ethnicity) variables on the brain response to real-world prosocial and antisocial behaviors. For example, using an iterated prisoner's dilemma game, Rilling et al. (2007) demonstrated that individuals scoring higher on psychopathic traits (versus those scoring lower on such traits) employed a more interpersonally aggressive game strategy that was associated with blunted amygdala responses to unreciprocated cooperation, consistent with less aversive conditioning to these social outcomes. High psychopathy trait scores were also associated with blunted anterior cingulate and dorsolateral prefrontal cortex responses when subjects chose to defect on their playing partners, a finding consistent with lesser conflict and cognitive control related to such antisocial behaviors. A game-based study of reactive aggression in a general population sample indicated that the decision to act aggressively was associated with paralimbic cortex activation consistent with conflict between emotional motivations to act and cognitive control processes regulating the tendency to act impulsively (Kramer et al. 2007). It would seem of significant interest whether drug addiction is associated with diminished functional activation and/or connectivity in brain areas involved in monitoring or resolving emotional conflict or in implementing cognitive control in response to a stimulus or opportunity for impulsive aggression. The further study of at-risk populations using game-based elicitation of aggression and functional neuroimaging would be useful in exploring a cause-versus-effect explanation of observed neural processing deficits associated with impulsive aggression.

Drug Addiction Treatment Outcome

Currently used therapies promoting recovery and relapse prevention in drug-addicted individuals are largely behavioral approaches such as 12-Step programs, cognitive-behavioral therapy (CBT), contingency management, and cognitive skills training (Carroll and Onken 2005). Indeed, behavioral therapies for drug addiction represent arguably the oldest, most prevalent forms of behavioral therapy in medicine. These approaches attempt to thwart the addiction process at multiple levels (Table 49–1).

Despite the fact that such treatments for drug addiction have long been recognized to be efficacious, surprisingly little research effort has been directed toward examination of the neurobiology underlying treatment-related recovery, relapse prevention, and predictors of treatment response versus nonresponse. This virtual absence of neuroscientific investigation of the efficacy and effectiveness of addiction therapies is related to the fact that the scientific rigor of controlled clinical trial designs has only recently been applied to addiction behavioral therapies (Carroll and Onken 2005) and thus, empirical evidence of their absolute and relative efficacy remains largely unestablished. However, a brief consideration of the primarily cognitive underpinnings of major addiction therapies (see Table 49–1) illustrates that fact that they seek to engage the processes of incentive valuation, learning, memory, and inhibitory control that are currently highly active areas of human neuroscience research in non-drug-addicted individuals. Therefore, immense opportunities exist to pair addiction therapies with longitudinal functional neuroimaging studies to define the specific ways in which the brain changes when relapse prevention occurs and to define neural predictors of relapse.

As a relapse prevention therapy, CBT targets the extinction of conditioned drug associations as a means of dissociating cocaine-related cues and intense drug motivations. CBT helps cocaine-dependent individuals "relearn" a distinct association or contingency between conditioned drug cues and drug-seeking and -use behaviors.

TABLE 49–1. Stages of the addiction process targeted by addiction therapies

Decrease the incentive motivational value of the drug (U.S. devaluation)

Increase the willful control of drug-related behavior

Increase the salience and motivational value of nondrug reinforcers

Inhibit conditioned responses to drug-predictive stimuli

Source. Adapted from Kalivas and Volkow 2005.

CBT is based on the tenet that learning processes play an important role in the acquisition and maintenance of drug addiction and that these same learning processes can be used to help individuals reduce their drug use (Carroll 2002). CBT focuses on treating substance abuse as a learned behavior that can be modified by fostering the motivation for drug abstinence, coping with drug cravings, and enhancing drug refusal skills (Carroll et al. 1994). Components of CBT include a functional analysis of drug use in which the patient identifies thoughts, feelings, and circumstances before and after drug use and skills training through which subjects learn strategies for modifying these behaviors, moods, or cognitions. CBT has proven efficacy in the treatment of drug-dependent populations (Covi et al. 2002; Maude-Griffin et al. 1998) and may have long-term durability in promoting drug abstinence (Carroll et al. 1994).

In contingency management, patients receive incentives or rewards for meeting addiction treatment goals (e.g., negative urine drug screen). Contingency management is based on operant conditioning in which behavior that is followed by positive consequences is more likely to be repeated (Carroll and Onken 2005). Several studies utilizing contingency management have demonstrated the efficacy of voucher-based incentives contingent on the patient providing a drug-free urine sample in reducing drug use, enhancing treatment retention, and maintaining cocaine abstinence (Higgins et al. 2000, 2003; Petry et al. 2004).

Twelve-Step recovery programs such as Alcoholics Anonymous are spiritually based in which drug-dependent individuals relinquish power over their addiction by yielding to a higher power. The literature contains limited evidence supporting the efficacy of 12-Step programs; however, 12-Step group participation in a given month predicted less cocaine use in the next month, and patients who increased their 12-Step group participation during the first 3 months of treatment had significantly less cocaine use and lower addiction-related functional impairments (R.D. Weiss et al. 2005).

Exploring the neural basis of response to extant addiction therapies arguably represents the most impacting future area of neuroscientific exploration targeting the reduction of the occurrence and costs of drug addiction.

Future Directions

The immense social, economic, and public health costs of drug abuse and addiction have been little checked by government interdiction policies. The "war on drugs" would be unquestionably advanced by programs of evidence-based prevention and treatment enabled by a more concise and comprehensive understanding of the neurobiology of the stages of the drug addiction process. Such an understanding demands the merger of the fields of social, affective, cognitive, cultural, behavioral, and molecular neuroscience to address the many and diverse driving mechanisms behind this complex process. In this chapter, the specific areas of emphasis on the neurobiology of the addiction process reflect not only a review of the corpus of relevant research findings but also the authors' opinions as to the needed areas of neuroscientific investigation from which a comprehensive and translationally significant understanding of the addiction process would be derived. Defining the influence of differences due to sex or to racial or ethnic background on the neurobiology of drug addiction is deemed imperative. Defining the neurobiology of largely neglected areas of crime and violence related to drug addiction and of response to addiction behavioral therapies is also of high priority. Innovative research approaches to treatment such as the exploration of the use of neurofeedback supported by real-time fMRI (deCharms et al. 2005; Weiskopf et al. 2004) of responses to relapse precipitants are needed. Much has been learned but much more research knowledge is needed to enable science, rather than interdiction policies, to lead the "war on drugs."

References

Abi-Dargham A, Kegeles LS, Martinez D, et al: Dopamine mediation of positive reinforcing effects of amphetamine in stimulant-naive healthy volunteers: results from a large cohort. Eur Neuropsychopharmacol 13:459–468, 2003

Ahmed SH, Koob GF: Transition to drug addiction: a negative reinforcement model based on an allostatic decrease in reward function. Psychopharmacology (Berl) 180:473–490, 2005

American Psychiatric Association: Diagnostic and Statistical Manual of Mental Disorders, 4th Edition, Text Revision. Washington, DC, American Psychiatric Association, 2000

Anderson CM, Maas LC, Frederick B, et al: Cerebellar vermis involvement in cocaine-related behaviors. Neuropsychopharmacology 31:1318–1326, 2006

Back S, Dansky BS, Coffey S, et al: Cocaine dependence with and without post traumatic stress disorder: a comparison of substance use, trauma history, and psychiatric comorbidity. Am J Addict 9:51–62, 2000

Bjork JM, Knutson B, Fong GW, et al: Incentive-elicited brain activation in adolescents: similarities and difference from young adults. J Neurosci 24:1793–1802, 2004

Boles SM, Miotto K: Substance abuse and violence: a review of the literature. Aggress Violent Behav 8:155–174, 2003

Bonson KR, Grant SJ, Contoreggi CS, et al: Neural systems and cue-induced cocaine craving. Neuropsychopharmacology 26:376–386, 2002

Bossert JM, Ghitza UE, Lu L, et al: Neurobiology of relapse to heroin and cocaine seeking: an update and clinical implications. Eur J Pharmacol 526:36–50, 2005

Breiter HC, Gollub RL, Weisskoff RM, et al: Acute effects of cocaine on human brain activity and emotion. Neuron 19:591–611, 1997

Brody AL, Mandelkern MA, Olmstead RE, et al: Gene variants of brain dopamine pathways and smoking-induced dopamine release in the ventral caudate/nucleus accumbens. Arch Gen Psychiatry 63:808–816, 2006

Brody AL, Mandelkern MA, Olmstead RE, et al: Neural substrates of resisting craving during cigarette cue exposure. Biol Psychiatry 62:642–651, 2007

Brown ZJ, Erb S: Footshock stress reinstates cocaine seeking in rats after extended post-stress delays. Psychopharmacology (Berl) 195:61–70, 2007

Calcagnetti DJ, Schechter MD: Extinction of cocaine-induced place approach in rats—a validation of the biased conditioning procedure. Brain Res Bull 30:695–700, 1993

Canli T, Congdon E, Todd Constable R, et al: Additive effects of serotonin transporter and tryptophan hydroxylase-2 gene variation on neural correlates of affective processing. Biol Psychol 79:118–125, 2008

Capriles N, Rodaros D, Sorge RE, et al: A role for the prefrontal cortex in stress- and cocaine-induced reinstatement of cocaine seeking in rats. Psychopharmacology (Berl) 168:66–74, 2003

Carroll KM: Therapy Manuals for Drug Addiction: A Cognitive-Behavioral Approach: Treating Cocaine Addiction. (DHHS Publ No 02-4308). Rockville, MD, National Institute on Drug Abuse, 2002

Carroll KM, Onken LS: Behavioral therapies for drug abuse. Am J Psychiatry 162:1452–1460, 2005

Carroll KM, Rounsaville BJ, Nich C, et al: One-year follow-up of psychotherapy and pharmacotherapy for cocaine dependence: delayed emergence of psychotherapy effects. Arch Gen Psychiatry 51:989–997, 1994

Chambers RA, Taylor JR, Potenza MN: Developmental neurocircuitry of motivation in adolescence: a critical period of addiction vulnerability. Am J Psychiatry 160:1041–1052, 2003

Chang L, Ernst T, Strickland T, et al: Gender effects on persistent cerebral metabolite changes in the frontal lobes of abstinent cocaine users. Am J Psychiatry 156:716–722, 1999

Childress AR, McLellan AT, Ehrman R, et al: Classically conditioned responses in opioid and cocaine dependence: a role in relapse? NIDA Res Monogr 84:25–43, 1988

Childress AR, Mozley PD, McElgin W, et al: Limbic activation during cue-induced cocaine craving. Am J Psychiatry 156:11–18, 1999

Covi L, Hess JM, Schroeder JR, et al: A dose response study of cognitive behavioral therapy in cocaine abusers. J Subst Abuse Treat 23:191–197, 2002

Crabbe JC, Phillips TJ, Buck KJ, et al: Identifying genes for alcohol and drug sensitivity: recent progress and future directions. Trends Neurosci 22:173–179, 1999

Daglish MRC, Weinstein A, Malizia AL, et al: Changes in regional cerebral blood flow elicited by craving memories in abstinent opiate-dependent subjects. Am J Psychiatry 158:1680–1686, 2001

Dawe S, Loxton NJ: The role of impulsivity in the development of substance use and eating disorders. Neurosci Biobehav Rev 28:343–351, 2004

deCharms RC, Maeda F, Glover GH, et al: Control over brain activation and pain learned by using real-time functional MRI. Proc Natl Acad Sci U S A 102:18626–18631, 2005

de Wit H, Stewart J: Reinstatement of cocaine-reinforced responding in the rat. Psychopharmacology (Berl) 75:134–143, 1981

Drexler K, Schweitzer JB, Quinn CK, et al: Neural activity related to anger in cocaine-dependent men: a possible link to violence and relapse. Am J Addict 9:331–339, 2000

Dudish SA, Hatsukami DK: Gender differences in crack users who are research volunteers. Drug Alcohol Depend 42:55–63, 1996

Duncan E, Boshoven W, Harenski K, et al: An fMRI study of the interaction of stress and cocaine cues on cocaine craving in cocaine-dependent men. Am J Addict 16:174–182, 2007

Ehrman RN, Robbins SJ, Childress AR, et al: Conditioned responses to cocaine-related stimuli in cocaine abuse patients. Psychopharmacology (Berl) 107:523–529, 1992

Ellickson PL, Morton SC: Identifying adolescents at risk for hard drug use: racial/ethnic variations. J Adolesc Health 25:382–395, 1999

Elman I, Karlsgodt KH, Gastfriend DR: Gender differences in cocaine craving among non-treatment-seeking individuals with cocaine dependence. Am J Drug Alcohol Abuse 27:193–202, 2001

Epstein DH, Preston KL, Stewart J: Toward a model of drug relapse: an assessment of the validity of the reinstatement procedure. Psychopharmacology (Berl) 189:1–16, 2006

Erb S, Hitchcott PK, Rajabi H, et al: Alpha-2 adrenergic agonists block stress-induced reinstatement of cocaine seeking. Neuropsychopharmacology 23:138–150, 2000

Erblich J, Lerman C, Self DW, et al: Effects of dopamine D2 receptor (DRD2) and transporter (SLC6A3) polymorphisms on smoking cue-induced cigarette craving among African American smokers. Mol Psychiatry 10:407–414, 2005

Everitt BJ, Robbins TW: Neural systems of reinforcement for drug addiction: from actions to habits to compulsion. Nat Neurosci 8:1481–1489, 2005

Fals-Stewart W, Golden J, Schumacher JA: Intimate partner violence and substance use: a longitudinal day-to-day examination. Addict Behav 28:1555–1574, 2003

Faure A, Haberland U, Condé F, et al: Lesion to the nigrostriatal dopamine system disrupts stimulus-response habit formation. J Neurosci 25:2771–2780, 2005

Ferrario CR, Gorny G, Crombag HS, et al: Neural and behavioral plasticity associated with the transition from controlled to escalated cocaine use. Biol Psychiatry 58:751–759, 2005

Franklin TR, Acton PD, Maldjian JA, et al: Decreased gray matter concentration in the insular, orbitofrontal, cingulate, and temporal cortices of cocaine patients. Biol Psychiatry 51:134–142, 2002

Fuchs RA, Tran-Nguyen LT, Specio SE, et al: Predictive validity of the extinction/reinstatement model of drug craving. Psychopharmacology (Berl) 135:151–160, 1998

Fuchs RA, See RS, Middaugh LD: Conditioned stimulus-induced reinstatement of extinguished cocaine seeking in C57BL/6 mice: a mouse model of drug relapse. Brain Res 973:99–106, 2003

Fuchs RA, Evans A, Parker MP, et al: Differential involvement of orbitofrontal cortex subregions in conditioned cue-induced and cocaine-primed reinstatement of cocaine seeking in rats. J Neurosci 24:6600–6610, 2004

Fuchs RA, Evans KA, Ledford CC, et al: The role of the dorsomedial prefrontal cortex, basolateral amygdala, and dorsal hippocampus in contextual reinstatement of cocaine seeking in rats. Neuropsychopharmacology 30:296–309, 2005

Galvan A, Hare TA, Parra CE, et al: Earlier development of the accumbens relative to orbitofrontal cortex might underlie risk-taking behavior in adolescents. J Neurosci 26:6885–6892, 2006

Garavan H, Pakiewicz J, Bloom A, et al: Cue-induced cocaine craving: neuroanatomical specificity for drug users and drug stimuli. Am J Psychiatry 157:1789–1798, 2000

Gerra G, Garofano L, Castaldini L, et al: Serotonin transporter promoter polymorphism genotype is associated with temperament, personality traits and illegal drugs use among adolescents. J Neural Transm 112:1397–1410, 2005

Ghitza UE, Fabbricatore AT, Prokopenko V, et al: Persistent cue-evoked activity of accumbens neurons after prolonged abstinence from self-administered cocaine. J Neurosci 23:7239–7245, 2003

Giros B, Jaber M, Jones SR, et al: Hyperlocomotion and indifference to cocaine and amphetamine in mice lacking the dopamine transporter. Nature 379:606–612, 1996

Goddard B, Leri F: Reinstatement of conditioned reinforcing properties of cocaine-conditioned stimuli. Pharmacol Biochem Behav 83:540–546, 2006

Goldman D, Oroszi G, Ducci F: The genetics of addictions: uncovering the genes. Nat Rev Genet 6:521–531, 2005

Goldstein RZ, Alia-Klein N, Leskovjan AC, et al: Anger and depression in cocaine addiction: association with the orbitofrontal cortex. Psychiatry Res 138:13–22, 2005

Grant S, London ED, Newlin DB, et al: Activation of memory circuits during cue-elicited cocaine craving. Proc Natl Acad Sci U S A 93:12040–12045, 1996

Griffin ML, Weiss RD, Mirin SM, et al: A comparison of male and female cocaine abusers. Arch Gen Psychiatry 46:122–126, 1989

Haile CN, Kosten TR, Kosten TA: Genetics of dopamine and its contributions to cocaine addiction. Behav Genet 37:119–145, 2007

Hall FS, Li XF, Sora I, et al: Cocaine mechanisms: enhanced cocaine, fluoxetine and nisoxetine place preference following monoamine transporter depletions. Neuroscience 115:153–161, 2002

Hayes RJ, Vorel SR, Spector J, et al: Electrical and chemical stimulation of the basolateral complex of the amygdala reinstates cocaine-seeking behavior in the rat. Psychopharmacology (Berl) 168:75–83, 2003

Heim C, Newport DJ, Heit S, et al: Pituitary-adrenal and autonomic responses to stress in women after sexual and physical abuse in childhood. JAMA 284:592–597, 2000

Heinz A, Siessmeier T, Wrase J, et al: Correlation between dopamine D2 receptors in the ventral striatum and central processing of alcohol cues and craving. Am J Psychiatry 161:1783–1789, 2004

Herrmann MJ, Huter T, Müller F, et al: Additive effects of serotonin transporter and tryptophan hydroxylase-2 gene variation on emotional processing. Cereb Cortex 17:1160–1163, 2007

Higgins ST, Wong CJ, Badger GJ, et al: Contingent reinforcement increases cocaine abstinence during outpatient treatment and 1 year of follow-up. J Consult Clin Psychol 68:64–72, 2000

Higgins ST, Sigmon SC, Wong CJ, et al: Community reinforcement therapy for cocaine-dependent outpatients. Arch Gen Psychiatry 60:1043–1052, 2003

Hoaken PMS, Stewart SH: Drugs of abuse and the elicitation of human aggressive behavior. Addict Behav 28:1533–1554, 2003

Holland PC, Bouton ME: Hippocampus and context in classical conditioning. Curr Opin Neurobiol 9:195–202, 1999

Hyman SM, Garcia M, Kemp K, et al: A gender specific psychometric analysis of the early trauma inventory short form in cocaine dependent adults. Addict Behav 30:847–852, 2005

Hyman SM, Garcia M, Sinha R: Gender specific associations between types of childhood maltreatment and the onset, escalation, and severity of substance use in cocaine dependent adults. Am J Drug Alcohol Abuse 32:655–664, 2006

Hyman SM, Paliwal P, Sinha R: Childhood maltreatment, perceived stress, and stress-related coping in recently abstinent cocaine dependent adults. Psychol Addict Behav 21:233–238, 2007

Ito R, Dalley JW, Robbins TW, et al: Dopamine release in the dorsal striatum during cocaine-seeking behavior under the control of a drug-associated cue. J Neurosci, 22:6247–6253, 2002

Jaffe JH, Cascella NG, Kumor KM, et al: Cocaine-induced cocaine craving. Psychopharmacology (Berl) 97:59–64, 1989

Johnson BA, Chen YR, Schmitz J, et al: Cue-reactivity in cocaine-dependent subjects: effects of cue type and cue modality. Addict Behav 23:7–15, 1998

Jones-Webb R, Snowden L, Herd D, et al: Alcohol-related problems among black, Hispanic and white men: the contribution of neighborhood poverty. J Stud Alcohol 58:539–545, 1997

Kalivas PW, Volkow ND: The neural basis of addiction: a pathology of motivation and choice. Am J Psychiatry 162:1403–1413, 2005

Kelley AE, Schiltz CA, Landry CF: Neural systems recruited by drug- and food-related cues: studies of gene activation in corticolimbic regions. Physiol Behav 86:11–14, 2005

Kilts CD, Schweitzer JB, Quinn CK, et al: Neural activity related to drug craving in cocaine addiction. Arch Gen Psychiatry 58:334–341, 2001

Kilts CD, Gross RE, Ely TD, et al: The neural correlated of cue-induced craving in cocaine-dependent women. Am J Psychiatry 161:233–241, 2004

King RS, Mauer M: Distorted priorities: drug offenders in state prisons. Washington, DC, The Sentencing Project, September 2002. Available at: http://www.sentencingproject.org/pdfs/9038.pdf. Accessed December 2008.

Kliewer W, Murrelle L: Risk and protective factors for adolescent substance use: findings from a study in selected central American countries. J Adolesc Health 40:448–455, 2007

Knackstedt LA, Kalivas PW: Extended access to cocaine self-administration enhances drug-primed reinstatement but not behavioral sensitization. J Pharmacol Exp Ther 322:1103–1109, 2007

Koob G, Kreek MJ: Stress, dysregulation of drug reward pathways, and the transition to drug dependence. Am J Psychiatry 164:1149–1159, 2007

Kosten TA, Gawin FH, Kosten TR, et al: Gender differences in cocaine use and treatment response. J Subst Abuse Treat 10:63–66, 1993

Kramer UM, Jansma H, Tempelmann C, et al: Tit-for-tat: the neural basis of reactive aggression. Neuroimage 38:203–211, 2007

Kreek MJ, Nielsen DA, Butelman ER, et al: Genetic influences on impulsivity, risk taking, stress responsivity and vulnerability to drug abuse and addiction. Nat Neurosci 8:1450–1457, 2005

Kruzich PJ, See RE: Differential contributions of the basolateral and central amygdala in the acquisition and expression of conditioned relapse to cocaine-seeking behavior. J Neurosci 21:RC155, 2001

Kuhar MJ, Ritz MC, Boja JW: The dopamine hypothesis of the reinforcing properties of cocaine. Trends Neurosci 14:299–302, 1991

LaRowe SD, Myrick H, Hedden S, et al: Is cocaine desire reduced by n-acetylcysteine? Am J Psychiatry 164:1115–1117, 2007

Lenoir M, Ahmed SH: Heroin-induced reinstatement is specific to compulsive heroin use and dissociable from heroin reward and sensitization. Neuropsychopharmacology 32:616–624, 2007

Lessov CN, Swan GE, Ring HZ, et al: Genetics and Drug Use as a Complex Phenotype. Subst Use Misuse 39:1515–1569, 2004

Levin JM, Holman BL, Mendelson JH, et al: Gender differences in cerebral perfusion in cocaine abuse-technetium-99m-HMPAO SPECT study of drug-abusing women. J Nucl Med 35:1902–1909, 1994

Li CS, Kosten TR, Sinha R: Sex differences in brain activation during stress imagery in abstinent cocaine users: a functional magnetic resonance imaging study. Biol Psychiatry 57:487–494, 2005

Li MD, Cheng R, Ma JZ, et al: A meta-analysis of estimated genetic and environmental effects on smoking behavior in male and female adult twins. Addiction 98:23–31, 2003

Li Y, Shao C, Zhang D, et al: The effect of dopamine D2, D5 receptor and transporter (SLC6A3) polymorphisms on the cue-elicited heroin craving in Chinese. Am J Med Genet B Neuropsychiatr Genet 141:269–273, 2006

Liu X, Weiss F: Additive effect of stress and drug cues on reinstatement of ethanol seeking: exacerbation by history of dependence and role of concurrent activation of corticotropin-releasing factor and opioid mechanisms. J Neurosci 22:7856–7861, 2002

Lynch WJ, Roth ME, Carroll ME: Biological basis of sex differences in drug abuse: preclinical and clinical studies. Psychopharmacology (Berl) 164:121–137, 2002

Maas LC, Lukas SE, Kaufman MJ, et al: Functional magnetic resonance imaging of human brain activation during cue-induced cocaine craving. Am J Psychiatry 155:124–126, 1998

Macdonald S, Anglin-Bodrug K, Mann RE, et al: Injury risk associated with cannabis and cocaine use. Drug Alcohol Depend 72:99–115, 2003

MacMillan HL, Fleming JE, Streiner DL, et al: Childhood abuse and lifetime psychopathology in a community sample. Am J Psychiatry 158:1878–1883, 2001

Martin-Fardon R, Ciccocioppo R, Aujla H, et al: The dorsal subiculum mediates the acquisition of conditioned reinstatement of cocaine-seeking. Neuropsychopharmacology 33:1827–1834, 2008

Matochik JA, London ED, Eldreth DA, et al: Frontal cortical tissue composition in abstinent cocaine abusers: a magnetic resonance imaging study. Neuroimage 19:1095–1102, 2003

Maude-Griffin PM, Hohenstein JM, Humfleet GL, et al: Superior efficacy of cognitive-behavioral therapy for urban crack cocaine abusers: main and matching effects. J Consult Clin Psychol 66:832–837, 1998

McBride D, Barrett SP, Kelly JT, et al: Effects of expectancy and abstinence on the neural response to smoking cues in cigarette smokers: an fMRI study. Neuropsychopharmacology 31:2728–2738, 2006

McFarland K, Kalivas PW: The circuitry mediating cocaine-induced reinstatement of drug-seeking behavior. J Neurosci 21:8655–8663, 2001

McFarland K, Davidge SB, Lapish CC, et al: Limbic and motor circuitry underlying footshock-induced reinstatement of cocaine-seeking behavior. J Neurosci 24:1551–1560, 2004

McKay JR, Rutherford MJ, Cacciola JS, et al: Gender differences in the relapse experience of cocaine patients. J Nerv Ment Dis 184:616–622, 1996

McLaughlin J, See RE: Selective inactivation of the dorsomedial prefrontal cortex and the basolateral amygdala attenuates conditioned-cued reinstatement of extinguished cocaine-seeking behavior in rats. Psychopharmacology (Berl) 168:57–65, 2003

Mechtcheriakov S, Brenneis C, Egger K, et al: A widespread distinct pattern of cerebral atrophy in patients with alcohol addiction revealed by voxel-based morphometry. Neurol Neurosurg Psychiatry 78:610–614, 2007

Medvedev IO, Gainetdinov R, Sotnikova TD, et al: Characterization of conditioned place preference to cocaine in congenic dopamine transporter knockout female mice. Psychopharmacology (Berl) 180:408–413, 2005

Meil WM, See RE: Conditioned cues responding following prolonged withdrawal from self-administered cocaine in rats: an animal model of relapse. Behav Pharmacol 7:754–763, 1996

Meyer-Lindenberg A, Weinberger DR: Intermediate phenotypes and genetic mechanisms of psychiatric disorders. Nat Rev Neurosci 7:818–827, 2006

Miller TR, Levy DT, Cohen MA, et al: Costs of alcohol and drug-involved crime. Prev Sci 7:333–342, 2006

Moeller FG, Dougherty DM, Barratt ES, et al: The impact of impulsivity on cocaine use and retention in treatment. J Subst Abuse Treat 21:193–198, 2001

Mueller D, Stewart J: Cocaine-induced conditioned place preference: reinstatement by priming injections of cocaine after extinction. Behav Brain Res 115:39–47, 2000

O'Brien CP: A range of research-based pharmacotherapies for addiction. Science 278:66–70, 1997

O'Brien CP, Volkow N, Li TK: What's in a word? Addiction versus dependence in DSM-V. Am J Psychiatry 163:764–765, 2006

Okuyemi KS, Powell JN, Savage CR, et al: Enhanced cue-elicited brain activation in African American compared with Caucasian smokers: an fMRI study. Addict Biol 11:97–106, 2006

Ousey GC, Lee MR: Investigating the connections between race, illicit drug markets, and lethal violence, 1984–1997. Journal of Research in Crime and Delinquency 41:352–383, 2004

Paulus MP, Tapert SF, Schuckit MA: Neural activation patterns of methamphetamine-dependent subjects during decision making predict relapse. Arch Gen Psychiatry 62:761–768, 2005

Petry NM, Tedford J, Austin M, et al: Prize reinforcement contingency management for treating cocaine abusers: how low can we go, and with whom? Addiction 99:349–360, 2004

Phillips PEM, Stuber GD, Heien ML, et al: Subsecond dopamine release promotes cocaine seeking. Nature 422:614–618, 2003

Pirard S, Sharona E, Kanga SK, et al: Prevalence of physical and sexual abuse among substance abuse patients and impact on treatment outcomes. Drug Alcohol Depend 78:57–64, 2005

Pulay AJ, Dawson DA, Hasin DS, et al: Violent behavior and DSM-IV psychiatric disorders: results from the national epidemiologic survey on alcohol and related conditions. J Clin Psychiatry 69:12–22, 2008

Quiñones-Jenab V: Why are women from Venus and men from Mars when they abuse cocaine? Brain Res 1126:200–203, 2006

Rilling JK, Gutman DA, Zeh TR, et al: A neural basis for social cooperation. Neuron 35:395–405, 2002

Rilling JK, Glenn AL, Jairam MA, et al: Neural correlates of social cooperation and non-cooperation as a function of psychopathy. Biol Psychiatry 61:1260–1271, 2007

Risinger RC, Salmeron BJ, Ross TJ, et al: Neural correlates of high and craving during cocaine self-administration using BOLD fMRI. Neuroimage 26:1097–1108, 2005

Robbins SJ, Ehrman RN, Childress AR, et al: Comparing levels of cocaine cue reactivity in male and female outpatients. Drug Alcohol Depend 53:223–230, 1999

Rocha B, Fumagalli F, Gainetdinov R, et al: Cocaine self-administration in dopamine transporter knockout mice. Nat Neurosci 1:132–137, 1998

Rodd-Henricks ZA, McKinzie DL, Li TK: Cocaine is self-administered into the shell but not the core of the nucleus accumbens of Wistar rats. J Pharmacol Exp Ther 303:1216–1226, 2002

Schechter MD, Calcagnetti DJ: Continued trends in the conditioned place preference literature from 1992 to 1996, inclusive, with a cross-indexed bibliography. Neurosci Biobehav Rev 22:827–846, 1998

See RE: Neural substrates of conditioned-cued relapse to drug-seeking behavior. Pharmacol Biochem Behav 71:517–529, 2002

Shaham Y, Erb S, Stewart J: Stress-induced drug seeking to heroin and cocaine in rats: a review. Brain Res Rev 33:13–33, 2002

Shaham Y, Shalev U, Lu L, et al: The reinstatement model of drug relapse: history, methodology and major findings. Psychopharmacology (Berl) 168:3–20, 2003

Shalev U, Grimm JW, Shaham Y: Neurobiology of relapse to heroin and cocaine seeking: a review. Pharmacol Rev 54:1–42, 2002

Shelton KL, Hendrick E, Beardsley PM: Interaction of noncontingent cocaine and contingent drug-paired stimuli on cocaine reinstatement. Eur J Clin Pharmacol 497:35–40, 2004

Shen H, Hagino Y, Kobayashi H, et al: Regional differences in extracellular dopamine and serotonin assessed by in vivo microdialysis in mice lacking dopamine and/or serotonin transporters. Neuropsychopharmacology 29:1790–1799, 2004

Sim ME, Lyoo IK, Streeter CC, et al: Cerebellar gray matter volume correlated with duration of cocaine use in cocaine-dependent subjects. Neuropsychopharmacology 32:2229–2237, 2007

Simpson TL, Miller WR: Concomitance between childhood sexual and physical abuse and substance abuse problems: a review. Clin Psychol Rev 22:27–77, 2002

Sinha R, Talih M, Malison R, et al: Hypothalamic-pituitary-adrenal axis and sympatho-adreno-medullary responses during stress-induced and drug cue-induced cocaine craving states. Psychopharmacology (Berl) 170:62–72, 2003

Sinha R, Lacadie C, Skudlarski P, et al: Neural activity associated with stress-induced cocaine craving: a functional magnetic resonance imaging study. Psychopharmacology (Berl) 183:171–180, 2005

Sinha R, Garcia M, Paliwal P, et al: Stress-induced cocaine craving and hypothalamic-pituitary-adrenal responses are predictive of cocaine relapse outcomes. Arch Gen Psychiatry 63:324–331, 2006

Sora I, Wichems C, Takahashi N, et al: Cocaine reward models: conditioned place preference can be establish in dopamine- and in serotonin-transporter knockout mice. Proc Natl Acad Sci U S A 95:7699–7704, 1998

Sora I, Hall FS, Andrews AM, et al: Molecular mechanisms of cocaine reward: combined dopamine and serotonin transporter knockouts eliminates cocaine place preference. Proc Natl Acad Sci U S A 98:5300–5305, 2001

Sun W, Rebec GV: Lidocaine inactivation of ventral subiculum attenuates cocaine-seeking behavior in rats. J Neurosci 23:10258–10264, 2003

Thomas KL, Everitt BJ: Limbic-cortical-ventral striatal activation during retrieval of a discrete cocaine-associated stimulus: a cellular imaging study with gamma protein kinase C expression. J Neurosci 21:2526–2535, 2001

Uhl G, Blum K, Noble E, et al: Substance abuse vulnerability and D2 receptor genes. Trends Neurosci 16:83–88, 1993

Vanderschuren LJ, Di Cano P, Everitt BJ: Involvement of the dorsal striatum in cue-controlled cocaine seeking. J Neurosci 25:8665–8670, 2005

Vitale S, van de Mheen D: Illicit drug use and injuries: a review of emergency room studies. Drug Alcohol Depend 82:1–9, 2006

Volkow ND, Wang G-J, Fischman MW, et al: Relationship between subjective effects of cocaine and dopamine transporter occupancy. Nature 186:827–830, 1997

Volkow ND, Wang G-J, Ma Y, et al: Activation of orbital and medial prefrontal cortex by methylphenidate in cocaine-addicted subjects but not in controls: relevance to addiction. J Neurosci 25:3932–3939, 2005

Volkow ND, Wang G-J, Telang F, et al: Cocaine cues and dopamine in dorsal striatum: mechanism of craving in cocaine addiction. J Neurosci 26:6583–6588, 2006

Wallace JM: The social ecology of addiction: race, risk, and resilience. Pediatrics 103:1122–1127, 1999

Wang B, You ZB, Rice KC, et al: Stress-induced relapse to cocaine seeking: roles for the CRF2 receptor and CRF-binding protein in the ventral tegmental area of the rat. Psychopharmacology (Berl) 193:283–294, 2007

Weiskopf N, Mathiak K, Bock SW, et al: Principles of a brain-computer interface (BCI) based on real-time functional magnetic resonance imaging (fMRI). IEEE Trans Biomed Eng 51:966–970, 2004

Weiss F: Neurobiology of craving, conditioned reward and relapse. Curr Opin Pharmacol 5:9–19, 2005

Weiss F, Maldonado-Vlaar CS, Parsons LH, et al: Control of cocaine-seeking behavior by drug-associated stimuli in rats: effects on recovery of extinguished operant-responding and extracellular dopamine levels in amygdala and nucleus accumbens. Proc Natl Acad Sci U S A 97:4321–4326, 2000

Weiss RD, Martinez-Raga J, Griffin ML, et al: Gender differences in cocaine dependent patients: a 6 month follow-up study. Drug Alcohol Depend 44:35–40, 1997

Weiss RD, Griffin ML, Gallop RJ, et al: The effect of 12-step self-help group attendance and participation on drug use outcomes among cocaine-dependent patients. Drug Alcohol Depend 77:177–184, 2005

Wertz JM, Sayette MA: A review of the effects of perceived drug use opportunity of self-reported urge. Exp Clin Psychopharmacol 9:3–13, 2001

Wexler BE, Gottschalk CH, Fulbright RK, et al: Functional magnetic resonance imaging of cocaine craving. Am J Psychiatry 158:86–95, 2001

Wilson SJ, Sayette MA, Fiez JA: Prefrontal responses to drug cues: a neurocognitive analysis. Nat Neurosci 7:211–214, 2003

Wong DF, Kuwabara H, Schretlen DJ, et al: Increased occupancy of dopamine receptors in human striatum during cue-elicited cocaine craving. Neuropsychopharmacology 31:2716–2727, 2006

Worley CM, Valadez A, Schenk S: Reinstatement of extinguished cocaine-taking behavior by cocaine and caffeine. Pharmacol Biochem Behav 48:217–221, 1994

Xu F, Gainetdinov RR, Wessel WC, et al: Mice lacking the norepinephrine transporter are supersensitive to psychostimulants. Nat Neurosci 3:465–471, 2000

Yacubian J, Sommer T, Schroeder K, et al: Gene-gene interaction associated with neural reward sensitivity. Proc Natl Acad Sci U S A 104:8125–8130, 2007

Yan Y, Yamada K, Nitta A, et al: Transient drug-primed but persistent cue-induced reinstatement of extinguished methamphetamine-seeking behavior in mice. Behav Brain Res 177:261–268, 2007

Yin HH, Knowlton BJ, Balleine BW: Lesions of dorsolateral striatum preserve outcome expectancy but disrupt habit formation in instrumental learning. Eur J Neurosci 19:181–189, 2004

Yurgelun-Todd D: Emotional and cognitive changes during adolescence. Curr Opin Neurobiol 17:251–257, 2007

Zhao Y, Dayas CV, Aujla H, et al: Activation of group II metabotropic glutamate receptors attenuates both stress and cue-induced ethanol-seeking and modulates c-fos expression in the hippocampus and amygdala. J Neurosci 26:9967–9974, 2006

Zhou W, Kalivas PW: N-acetylcysteine reduces extinction responding and induces enduring reductions in cue- and heroin-induced drug-seeking. Biol Psychiatry 63:338–340, 2008

Zhou Z, Roy A, Lipsky R, et al: Haplotype-based linkage of tryptophan hydroxylase 2 to suicide attempt, major depression, and cerebrospinal fluid 5-hydroxyindoleacetic acid in 4 populations. Arch Gen Psychiatry 62:1109–1118, 2005

CHAPTER 50

Neurobiology of Eating Disorders

Walter H. Kaye, M.D.

Michael A. Strober, Ph.D.

Anorexia nervosa (AN) and bulimia nervosa (BN) are disorders characterized by aberrant patterns of feeding behavior and weight regulation and disturbances in attitudes and perceptions toward body weight and shape. The distinguishing features of AN are an inexplicable fear of weight gain, unrelenting obsession with fatness, and extreme cachexia, to which the person appears strikingly indifferent. In BN, the differentiating characteristics are binge eating of variable frequency and intensity, usually emerging after a period of dieting and which may or may not have been associated with weight loss, and either self-induced vomiting or some other means of compensation for the excess of food that is consumed. Unlike in AN, weight does not decrease to dangerously low levels. In most people affected with BN, feeding patterns are disrupted and satiety may be impaired. However, although abnormally low body weight is an exclusion for the diagnosis of BN, a significant proportion of persons affected with this illness have a prior history of AN (Eddy et al. 2007).

AN and BN are cross-transmitted in families (Strober et al. 2000), often transform from one subtype to another over the course of the illness (Eddy et al. 2002; Milos et al. 2005), and share common traits and liability factors (Lilenfeld et al. 2000). Moreover, studies in the literature have often not clearly distinguished subtypes. In addition, state-related influences of malnutrition and weight loss (which tend to be worse in AN) have confounded symptoms and neurobiological measures. Thus, as we move through this chapter, rather than dividing our discussion of the two conditions along strictly categorical lines, we will highlight where they overlap and how they diverge.

The clinical distinction between AN and BN of obvious importance is that of emaciation, and while temperamental features of inhibition, restraint, and conformity are especially prominent in AN (Strober 1980), there are many areas of overlap and commonality. Persons with either condition have pathological overconcern with weight and shape, and common to both AN and BN are low self-esteem, perfectionism, depression, and anxiety (Fairburn et al. 1997, 1999). The diagnostic labels are misleading, too, as individuals with AN rarely have complete suppression of appetite but rather exhibit a motivated, and more often than not ego-syntonic, resistance to feeding drives while eventually becoming preoccupied with food and eating rituals to the point of obsession. Similarly, persons with BN, rather than suffering from a primary pathological drive to overeat, have a seemingly relentless drive to restrain their food intake, an extreme fear of weight gain, and a distorted view of their actual body size and shape. Loss of control of normative feeding patterns usually occurs intermittently and typically only some time after the onset of dieting behavior. Furthermore, episodes of binge eating ultimately develop in a significant proportion of people with AN (Halmi et al. 1991), and some 3%–5% of those starting out with BN will eventually develop AN (Fichter and Quadflieg 2007; Milos et al. 2005). Thus, because restrained eating behavior and dysfunctional cognitions relating weight and shape to self-concept are shared by patients with both of these syndromes, and because diagnostic crossover is not unusual, it has been argued that AN and BN share at least some risk and liability factors in common.

The etiology of AN and BN is presumed to be complex and multiply influenced by developmental, social, and biological processes (Treasure and Campbell 1994), the exact nature of which remain poorly understood. Certainly, cultural attitudes toward standards of physical attractiveness have relevance, but it is unlikely that sociocultural influences in pathogenesis are preeminent. First, dieting behavior and the drive toward thinness are unusually common in industrialized countries throughout the world, yet AN and BN affect only an estimated 0.3%–0.7%, and 1.7%–2.5%, respectively, of females in the general population. Moreover, numerous, seemingly unambiguous descriptions of AN date from the middle of the nineteenth century (Treasure and Campbell 1994), suggesting that factors other than the modern social milieu play a more powerful causal role. Second, these syndromes, AN in particular, have a relatively stereotypical clinical presentation, sex distribution, and age at onset, supporting the plausibility of intrinsic biological vulnerabilities.

Clinical Phenomenology and Disease Course

Following the points above, variations in feeding behavior have been the basis for subdividing AN into diagnostic subgroups that have been shown to differ in other psychopathological characteristics (Garner et al. 1985). In the restricting subtype of AN, subnormal body weight is sustained by unremitting food avoidance, whereas in the bulimic subtype, there is comparable weight loss and malnutrition, yet the illness course is punctuated by intermittent episodes of binge eating. Interestingly, individuals with this binge subtype exhibit other dyscontrol phenomena, including histories of self-harm, affective and behavioral disorder, substance abuse, and overt family conflict in comparison to those with the restricting subtype. Regardless of subtype, individuals with AN are characterized by marked perfectionism, harm avoidance, low novelty seeking, conformity, and obsessionality, most of which appear in advance of the onset of weight loss and which tend to persist even after long-term weight recovery, indicating that they are not merely epiphenomena of acute malnutrition or disordered eating behavior (Casper 1990; Srinivasagam et al. 1995; Strober 1980).

Individuals with BN remain at normal body weight, although many aspire to preferred weights far below the range of normalcy for their age and height. The core fea-

tures of BN include repeated episodes of binge eating followed by compensatory self-induced vomiting, laxative abuse, or pathologically extreme exercise, as well as abnormal concern with weight and shape. DSM-IV-TR (American Psychiatric Association 2000) specifies a distinction within this group between those individuals with BN who engage in self-induced vomiting or laxative, diuretic, or enema abuse (purging type) and those who exhibit other forms of compensatory action such as fasting or exercise (nonpurging type). Beyond these differences, it has been speculated (Vitousek and Manke 1994) that there are two clinically divergent subgroups of individuals with BN: a so-called multi-impulsive type in which bulimia occurs in conjunction with more pervasive difficulties in behavioral self-regulation and affective instability, and a second type whose distinguishing features include self-effacing behaviors, dependence on external rewards, and extreme compliance. Individuals with BN of the multi-impulsive type are far more likely to have histories of substance abuse, and they characteristically display other impulse-control problems, such as shoplifting and self-injurious behaviors. Considering these differences, it has been postulated that multi-impulsive BN individuals rely on binge eating and purging as a means of regulating intolerable states of tension, anger, and fragmentation, whereas individuals of the latter type have binge episodes precipitated through dietary restraint, with compensatory behaviors maintained through reduction of guilty feelings associated with fears of weight gain.

For most who are affected, AN is a protracted disease; roughly 50%–70% of affected individuals will eventually have reasonably complete resolution of the illness, but the time to achieve this state is, for the most part, quite lengthy. Thus, a significant proportion of persons with AN express subthreshold levels of illness that wax and wane in severity long into adulthood, with some individuals having a chronic, wholly unremitting course, and with 5%–10% of those affected eventually dying from complications of the disease or from suicide. For BN, the course trajectory is somewhat different. Rather than continuously presenting symptoms that persist for years without periods of full recovery, follow-up studies of 5–10 years in duration show that 50% of BN individuals have recovered while nearly 20% continue to meet full syndromal criteria for BN (Keel and Mitchell 1997). The typical course pattern is one of unpredictable vacillation between periods of restricted food intake, gorging, and vomiting, one that will wax and wane over the course of several years.

Family Epidemiology and Genetics

Family and Twin Studies

Findings from systematic case–control studies (Lilenfeld et al. 1998; Strober et al. 2000) suggest a 7- to 12-fold increase in the prevalence of AN and BN in relatives of eating disorder probands compared with never-ill control subjects. These significant familial recurrence risks of AN and BN provide impressive evidence of the transmissibility of both phenotypes.

Twin studies of AN and BN are still few in number, but evidence to date suggests greater resemblance among monozygotic twins relative to dizygotic twins for both AN and BN, with 58%–76% of the variance in AN (Klump et al. 2001a; Wade et al. 2000) and 54%–83% of the variance in BN (Bulik et al. 1998; Kendler et al. 1991) accounted for by additive genetic factors, estimates that accord with those found in studies of schizophrenia and bipolar disorder.

In accord with previous discussion of clinical overlap and longitudinal continuities, AN and BN appear to have familial liabilities shared in common. Convergent findings from family and twin studies indicate an increased coaggregation of AN and BN among relatives of AN and BN probands (Lilenfeld et al. 1998; Strober et al. 2000; Walters and Kendler 1995), suggesting both unique and common familially transmitted causative elements.

In this vein, the transmitted liability to eating disorders may express a more diffuse phenotype of continuous traits. In support of this model of transmitted vulnerability is strong evidence of the heritability of disordered eating attitudes, weight preoccupation, dissatisfaction with weight and shape, dietary restraint, binge eating, and self-induced vomiting in the general population, with 32%–72% of the variance in these behavioral features potentially accounted for by additive genetic factors (Klump et al. 2000b; Rutherford et al. 1993; Sullivan et al. 1998; Wade et al. 1998, 1999). In addition, subthreshold forms of eating disorders have also been shown to coaggregate in families with full-syndrome AN and BN (Strober et al. 2000), lending added support to the idea of a continuum of transmitted liability in at-risk families manifesting a broad spectrum of eating disorder phenotypes.

That risk is mediated by developmental processes is supported by recent data (Klump et al. 2000b, 2007) from the Minnesota Twin Family Study, which examined the effects of age and pubertal status on the heritability of eating attitudes and behaviors. In the first of these studies (Klump et al. 2000b), the differential influence of genetic versus environmental effects was compared in 11-year-old twins ($n = 680$) and 17-year-old twins ($n = 602$). Whereas genetic influence on weight preoccupation and overall eating pathology was negligible for the younger age cohort, more than half of the variance in these attitudes and behaviors could be accounted for by genetic factors in the 17-year-old cohort. The follow-up analysis of the data set (Klump et al. 2007), in which the younger cohort was subdivided by pubertal status, revealed a more powerful effect of puberty than of age per se, suggesting a potential role of pubertal ovarian steroid activity in activating genes of etiological importance in eating disorders.

Genetic Findings

Comprehensive genomic studies of AN and BN remain sparse. The first genomewide search for potential disease susceptibility genes in AN (Kaye et al. 2000) was an international collaboration that applied a nonparametric allele-sharing linkage analysis to data from 192 kindreds with at least one affected relative pair with AN and related eating disorders, including BN (Grice et al. 2002). Although evidence for linkage in the entire sample was negligible, an analysis using a narrow affection status model composed only of relatives with restricting-type AN generated a peak multipoint nonparametric linkage score of 3.45 in the 1p33–36 region. In a further analysis (B. Devlin et al. 2002), two variables incorporated as covariates into the linkage analysis—drive for thinness and obsessionality—yielded several regions of suggestive linkage, one close to genomewide significance on another region of chromosome 1 (logarithm of odds [LOD] score = 3.46). Although considered preliminary, these initial findings suggest genetic heterogeneity in eating disorders and the potential value of applying more refined genomic analyses on large samples of AN subjects.

A growing number of studies using a case–control design have examined the potential association of various candidate genes with AN and BN (see reviews by Klump et al. 2001b; Tozzi et al. 2002). Evidence linking AN and BN to monoamine functioning (see below) has led researchers to target serotonin-related (5-HT$_{2A}$, 5-HT1$_{D\beta}$, 5-HTT, 5-HT$_7$, tryptophan hydroxylase receptor) and dopamine-related (D$_3$, D$_4$) genes, but findings to date have been inconsistent or negative. Our group has followed up the initial report of linkage of restricting AN to the chromosome 1p region (Grice et al. 2002), with evidence of significant association with two genes under this linkage peak, the 5-HT$_{1D}$ (HTR1D) and delta opioid (OPRD1) receptors, along with the dopamine receptor on chromosome 11 (Bergen et al. 2003), and a British group has reported a confirmation of the HTR1D and OPRD1 association in a case–control study (Brown et al. 2007).

The presumptive role of atypicalities in feeding and energy expenditure in the pathophysiology of AN and BN has led researchers to examine genes related to these processes. Findings suggest possible associations between AN and the UCP-2/UCP-3 gene (Campbell et al. 1999), the estrogen receptor β gene (Rosenkranz et al. 1998), and the gene for agouti-related protein (Vink et al. 2001), but here, too, no consistently replicated evidence for association with either AN or BN has accrued to date.

Association studies of BN are scant, with one study (Bulik et al. 2003) reporting significant linkage on chromosome 10p and another (Steiger et al. 2005) suggesting that the short (S) allele in the promoter region of the 5-HTT gene may confer risk for affective and behavior dysregulation among persons with BN.

In general, the results in this area to date argue convincingly for the importance of characterizing the latent phenotypic structure underlying these conditions and the application of more refined covariate and quantitative trait locus models of genomewide association and linkage analyses (Bacanu et al. 2005; Bulik et al. 2005) in the search for genes of potential relevance.

Associations With Other Behavioral Phenotypes

As noted, a variety of behavioral symptoms and traits occurs prominently in people with AN. Accordingly, several family and twin studies have examined the covariation between eating disorders and various other psychiatric conditions. These studies have been reviewed in detail (Lilenfeld et al. 1998; Strober et al. 2000). With regard to major affective illness, studies of AN probands have yielded familial risk estimates in the range of 7%–25%, with relative risk estimates in studies employing healthy control subjects in the range of 2.1–3.4. Likewise, studies of BN probands have shown, with rare exception, that their first-degree relatives are several times more likely to develop affective disorders than are relatives of control subjects (Mangweth et al. 2003). Several recent twin and family studies support this conclusion, as both found evidence for shared as well as unique genetic influences on major depression in both AN and BN (Kendler et al. 1995; Wade et al. 2000). In short, and lending further support to the notion of shared liability in AN and BN, both conditions often co-occur with major mood/anxiety disorders, which likewise cluster in family members.

An interesting potential discontinuity is with regard to substance use disorders. Although several studies (Kaye et al. 1996; Schuckit et al. 1996) found no evidence of cross-transmission of BN and substance use disorder in families, and twin data (Kendler et al. 1995) have shown that the genes influencing susceptibility to alcoholism were independent of those underlying BN risk, one recent study suggests some sharing of genetic influences that confer risk to drug use disorder and BN (Baker et al. 2007).

Independent familial transmission of obsessive-compulsive disorder (OCD) and both AN and BN was recently found in a controlled family study of eating disorders (Lilenfeld et al. 1998). By contrast, shared transmission was found between broadly defined AN and BN and various anxiety disorder phenotypes (Miller et al. 1998), and a genetic correlation has been reported between BN and both phobia and panic disorder (Kendler et al. 1995). Preliminary data also suggest common familial transmission of AN and obsessive-compulsive personality disorder (OCPD) (Lilenfeld et al. 1998; Strober et al. 2007). These results point in the general direction of linking genetic risk factors for various anxiety-related phenomena to susceptibility to eating disorders.

Neurobiology of Eating Disorders

Overview

The assumed absence of confounding nutritional influences in recovered eating-disordered women suggests that persistent psychobiological abnormalities and atypical behaviors might be trait related and etiopathogenetic. Investigators (Casper 1990; Kaye et al. 1998; Srinivasagam et al. 1995; Strober 1980; Wagner et al. 2006a) have found that many women who were in long-term recovery from AN and BN have persistence of anxiety, harm avoidance, perfectionism, and obsessional behaviors. Moreover, persons recovered from AN and BN often express associated eating disorder psychological symptoms, including ineffectiveness, drive for thinness, and significant psychopathology related to eating habits. Therefore, persistence of certain features after recovery raises the question of whether a disturbance of such behaviors may in fact occur premorbidly and contribute to the pathogenesis of AN and BN.

The role of biology in the etiology of AN has been proposed for many decades (Treasure and Campbell 1994). New understandings of the neurotransmitter modulation of appetitive behaviors have raised the question of whether such disturbances cause eating disorders (Fava et al. 1989; Morley and Blundell 1988). Moreover, technologies that permit direct measurement of complex brain functions and their relationships to behavior are shedding new light on the pathophysiology of these disorders.

Imaging Studies

It is well known that ill subjects with AN have enlarged ventricles and sulci widening (see review by Ellison and Foong 1998). Proton magnetic resonance spectroscopy (^{1}H-MRS) revealed reduced lipid signals in the frontal white matter and occipital gray matter and was associated with decreased body mass index (BMI) (Roser et al. 1999). Whether these abnormalities persist to a lesser degree after weight restoration is less certain, since some studies show persistent alterations (Katzman et al. 1996) but other studies show normalization of gray and white matter after recovery in AN and BN (Wagner et al. 2006b).

I. Gordon et al. (1997) found that 13 of 15 ill AN subjects studied had unilateral temporal lobe hypoperfusion that persisted after weight restoration. A later study (Chowdhury et al. 2001) found that adolescent AN subjects had unilateral temporoparietal and frontal lobe hypoperfusion. Kuruoglu et al. (1998), studying two ill AN patients, found bilateral hypoperfusion in frontal, temporal, and parietal regions that normalized after 3 months of remission. Takano et al. (2001) found hypoperfusion in the medial prefrontal cortex and anterior cingulate and hyperperfusion in the thalamus and amygdalo–hippocampal complex. Rastam et al. (2001) found temporoparietal and orbitofrontal hypoperfusion in ill and recovered AN subjects. Fewer studies have assessed glucose metabolism using positron emission tomography (PET). Delvenne et al. (1995) studied ill AN subjects who, in comparison with control subjects, had frontal and parietal hypometabolism that normalized with weight gain. More recently, single photon emission computed tomography (SPECT) studies of resting blood flow in restricting-type AN patients before and after weight restoration have suggested reduced blood flow in the anterior cingulate in both state conditions, compared with control subjects (Kojima et al. 2005a). Few brain imaging studies have examined BN subjects, but findings from several groups (Andreason et al. 1992; Delvenne et al. 1999; Nozoe et al. 1995; Wu et al. 1990) have raised the possibility of frontal or temporal alterations and hemispheric asymmetry.

In summary, these studies show temporal, frontal, parietal, and cingulate region disturbances in AN subjects, both when ill and after various degrees of recovery. Although these studies show some consistency, particularly in terms of temporal involvement, it should be noted that the numbers of subjects in each study tended to be small, and definitions of subgroups and states of illness were often inconsistent. Small sample sizes and irregular definitions make it difficult to know whether these are lateralizing findings or there are differences between subtypes of eating disorders. The meaning of these findings is open to interpretation. At the least, they suggest that regions of the brain involved in the modulation of mood, cognition, impulse control, and decision making may be altered in AN and BN.

Body Image Distortion

A most puzzling symptom of AN is the severe and intense body image distortion, in which emaciated individuals perceive themselves as fat. Wagner et al. (2003) confronted AN patients and age-matched healthy control subjects with their own digitally distorted body images as well as images of a different person using a computer-based video technique. These studies reported a hyperresponsiveness in brain areas belonging to the frontal visual system and the attention network (Brodmann area 9) as well as the inferior parietal lobule (Brodmann area 40), including the anterior part of the intraparietal sulcus. Bailer et al. (2004) reported negative relationships between 5-HT$_{2A}$ receptor activity and the Eating Disorder Inventory Drive for Thinness scale in the left parietal cortex and other regions. Uher et al. (2005) showed a cohort of women (9 with BN, 13 with AN, and 18 healthy controls) line drawings of female bodies and found that the subjects with eating disorders had reduced hemodynamic response in the right parietal (Brodmann area 40) cortex. It is intriguing to raise the possibility that parietal disturbances may contribute to body image distortion. Theoretically, body image distortion might be related to the syndrome of neglect (Mesulam 1981), which may be coded in parietal, frontal, and cingulate regions that assign motivational relevance to sensory events. It is well known that lesions in the right parietal cortex not only may result in denial of illness or anosognosia, somatoparaphrenia, and numerous misidentification syndromes but also may produce experiences of disorientation of body parts and body image distortion. It has long been recognized that the parietal cortex mediates perceptions of the body and its activity in physical space (Gerstmann 1924). Recent work extends this concept to suggest that the parietal lobe contributes to the experience of being an "agent" of one's own actions (Farrar et al. 2003).

Appetitive Regulation

Individuals with AN and those who have had lifetime diagnoses of both AN and BN (AN-BN) tend to have negative mood states and dysphoric temperament. There is evidence that there is a dysphoria reducing character to dietary restraint in AN (Kaye et al. 2003; Strober 1995; Vitousek and Manke 1994) and binge/purge behaviors in BN (Abraham and Beaumont 1982; Johnson and Larson 1982; Kaye et al. 1986). This would suggest some interaction between pathways regulating appetitive behaviors and emotions. In fact, imaging studies support this hypothesis. When emaciated and malnourished AN individuals are shown pictures of food, they display abnormal activity in the insula and orbitofrontal cortex as well as in mesial temporal, parietal, and anterior cingulate cortex (Ellison et al. 1998; C.M. Gordon et al. 2001; Naruo et al. 2000; Nozoe et al. 1993, 1995; Uher et al. 2004). In addition, studies using SPECT, PET (with ^{15}O), or functional magnetic resonance imaging (fMRI) found that when subjects ill with AN ate food or were exposed to food, they showed activation in temporal regions and often experienced increased anxiety (Ellison et al. 1998; C.M. Gordon et al. 2001; Naruo et al. 2000; Nozoe et al. 1993). Those results could be consistent with anxiety provocation and related amygdala activation and with the notion that the emotional value of an experience is stored in the amygdala (LeDoux 2003). Uher et al. (2003) used pictures of food and nonfood aversive emotional stimuli and fMRI to assess ill and recovered AN subjects. Food stimulated medial prefrontal and anterior cingulate cortex in both recovered and ill AN subjects but lateral prefrontal regions only in the recovered group. The prefrontal cortex, anterior cingulate cortex, and cerebellum were more highly activated after food intake in recovered AN subjects compared with both control subjects and subjects chronically ill with AN. This finding suggested that higher anterior cingulate cortex and medial prefrontal cortex activity in both ill and recovered AN women compared with controls may be a trait marker for AN.

A recent study (Wagner et al. 2008) used fMRI to investigate the effect of administration of nutrients. In comparison with controls, recovered AN subjects had a significantly reduced fMRI signal response to the blind administration of sucrose or water in the insula, anterior cingulate, and striatal regions. For controls, self-ratings of pleasantness of the sugar taste were positively correlated to the signal response in the insula, anterior cingulate, and ventral and dorsal putamen. By contrast, recovered AN individuals failed to show any relationship in these regions to self-ratings of pleasant response to a sucrose taste. A large literature shows that the anterior insula and associated gustatory cortex respond not only to the taste and physical properties of food but also to its rewarding properties (O'Doherty et al. 2001; Schultz et al. 2000; Small et al. 2001). Insular inputs to the ventrolateral striatum are hypothesized to mediate behaviors involving eating, particularly of highly palatable, high-energy foods (Kelley et al. 2002). AN subjects tend to avoid high-calorie, high-palatability food. In theory, this is consistent with abnormal responses of insula–striatal circuits that are hypothesized to mediate behavioral responses to the incentive value of food.

Implications

Do individuals with AN have an insular disturbance specifically related to gustatory modulation or a more generalized disturbance related to the integration of interoceptive stimuli? This is of interest because the insula is thought to play an important role in processing interoceptive information (Craig 2002). Interoception, which can be defined as the sense of the physiological condition of the entire body, has long been thought to be critical for self-awareness, because it provides the link between cognitive and affective processes and the current body state. Aside from taste, interoceptive information includes sensations such as temperature, touch, muscular and visceral sensations, vasomotor flush, air hunger, and others (Paulus and Stein 2006). It remains to be determined which altered insula function contributes to symptoms in AN, such as disturbed self-awareness (e.g., ego-syntonic denial and impaired central coherence), lack of recognition of the effects of starvation and pain tolerance, and perhaps body image distortions. Finally, it is possible that AN individuals have reduced insula and striatal "reward" response to palatable foods. Because food may lack reward value or may be paradoxically anxiolytic for individuals with AN, they may not be able to respond to normal homeostatic mechanisms that drive hunger, thus becoming emaciated.

Studies of Neurotransmitters

Neuropeptides

The past decade has witnessed accelerating basic research on the role of neuropeptides in the regulation of feeding behavior and obesity. The mechanisms for controlling food intake involve a complicated interplay between peripheral systems (including gustatory stimulation, gastrointestinal peptide secretion, and vagal afferent nerve responses) and central nervous system (CNS) neuropeptides and/or monoamines. Thus, studies in animals show that neuropeptides—such as cholecystokinin, the endogenous opioids (e.g., β-endorphin), and neuropeptide Y—regulate the rate, duration, and size of meals, as well as macronutrient selection (Morley and Blundell 1988; Schwartz et al. 2000). In addition to regulating eating behavior, a number of CNS neuropeptides participate in the regulation of neuroendocrine pathways. Thus, clinical studies have evaluated the possibility that CNS neuropeptide alterations may contribute to dysregulated secretion of gonadal hormones, cortisol, thyroid hormones, and growth hormone in the eating disorders (Jimerson et al. 1998; Stoving et al. 1999).

While there are relatively few studies to date, most of the neuroendocrine and neuropeptide alterations apparent during symptomatic episodes of AN and BN tend to normalize after recovery. This observation suggests that most of the disturbances are consequences rather than causes of malnutrition, weight loss, and altered meal patterns. Still, an understanding of these neuropeptide disturbances may shed light on why many people with AN or BN cannot easily "reverse" their illness. In AN, malnutrition may contribute to a downward spiral sustaining and perpetuating the desire for more weight loss and dieting. Symptoms such as increased satiety, obsessions, and dysphoric mood may be exaggerated by these neuropeptide alterations and thus contribute to the downward spiral. Additionally, mutual interactions between neuropeptide, neuroendocrine, and neurotransmitter pathways may contribute to the constellation of psychiatric comorbidity often observed in these disorders. Even after weight gain and normalized eating patterns, many individuals who have recovered from AN or BN have physiological, behavioral, and psychological symptoms that persist for extended periods of time. Menstrual cycle dysregulation, for example, may persist for some months after weight restoration. In the following sections we provide a brief overview of studies of neuropeptides in AN and BN.

Corticotropin-Releasing Hormone

When underweight, patients with AN have increased plasma cortisol secretion that is thought to be at least in part a consequence of hypersecretion of endogenous corticotropin-releasing hormone (CRH) (Gold et al. 1986; Kaye et al. 1987b; Licinio et al. 1996; Walsh et al. 1987). Given that the plasma and cerebrospinal fluid (CSF) measures return toward normal, it appears likely that activation of the hypothalamic-pituitary-thyroid axis is precipi-

tated by weight loss. The observation of increased CRH activity is of great theoretical interest in AN, given that intracerebroventricular CRH administration in experimental animals produces many of the physiological and behavioral changes associated with AN, including markedly decreased eating behavior (Glowa and Gold 1991).

Opioid Peptides

Studies in laboratory animals raise the possibility that altered endogenous opioid activity might contribute to pathological feeding behavior in eating disorders because opioid agonists generally increase, and opioid antagonists decrease, food intake (Morley et al. 1985). State-related reductions in concentrations of CSF β-endorphin and related opiate concentrations have been found in both underweight AN and ill BN subjects (Brewerton et al. 1992; Kaye et al. 1987a; Lesem et al. 1991). In contrast, using the T lymphocyte as a model system, Brambilla et al. (1995a) found elevated β-endorphin levels in AN, although the levels were normal in BN. If β-endorphin activity is a facilitator of feeding behavior, then reduced CSF concentrations could reflect decreased central activity of this system, which then maintains or facilitates inhibition of feeding behavior in the eating disorders.

Neuropeptide Y and Peptide YY

Neuropeptide Y (NPY) and peptide YY (PYY) are of considerable theoretical interest, because they have potent endogenous effects on feeding behavior within the CNS (Kalra et al. 1991; Morley et al. 1985; Schwartz et al. 2000). Underweight individuals with AN have been shown to have elevated CSF levels of NPY but normal levels of PYY (Kaye et al. 1990b). Clearly, elevated NPY does not result in increased feeding in underweight AN individuals; however, the possibility that increased NPY activity underlies the obsessive and paradoxical interest in dietary intake and food preparation is a hypothesis worth exploring. On the other hand, CSF levels of NPY and PYY have been reported to be normal in women with BN when measured while subjects were acutely ill. Although levels of PYY increased above normal when subjects were reassessed after 1 month of abstinence from bingeing and vomiting, levels of the peptides were similar to control values in long-term recovered individuals (Gendall 1999).

More recently, it has been reported that the plasma concentration of NPY was lower in patients with AN than in control subjects, whereas patients with BN had elevated NPY levels (Baranowska et al. 2000). Other data indicate that basal plasma PYY levels in AN are similar to or elevated in comparison with control values, with variability in postprandial PYY responses also noted across studies (Germain et al. 2007; Misra et al. 2006; Nakahara et al. 2007; Otto et al. 2007; Stock et al. 2005). Initial studies indicate that basal plasma PYY levels in BN are similar to control values but that the postprandial response is significantly blunted in the patient group (Kojima et al. 2005b; Monteleone et al. 2005). Additional research will be needed to assess the potential behavioral correlates of these findings.

Cholecystokinin

Cholecystokinin (CCK) is a peptide secreted by the gastrointestinal system in response to food intake. Release of CCK is thought to be one means of transmitting satiety signals to the brain by way of vagal afferents (Gibbs et al. 1973). In parallel to its role in satiety in rodents, exogenously administered CCK reduces food intake in humans. The preponderance of data suggests that patients with BN, in comparison with control subjects, have diminished release of CCK following ingestion of a standardized test meal (M.J. Devlin et al. 1997; Geracioti and Liddle 1988; Phillipp et al. 1991; Pirke et al. 1994). Measurements of basal CCK values in blood lymphocytes and in CSF also appear to be decreased in patients with BN (Brambilla et al. 1995a; Lydiard et al. 1993). It has been suggested that the diminished CCK response to a meal may play a role in diminished postingestive satiety observed in BN. The CCK response in bulimic patients was found to return toward normal following treatment (Geracioti and Liddle 1988).

Studies of CCK in AN have yielded less consistent findings. Some studies have found elevations in basal levels of plasma CCK (Phillipp et al. 1991; Tamai et al. 1993), as well as increased peptide release following a test meal (Harty et al. 1991; Phillipp et al. 1991). One study found that blunting of CCK response to an oral glucose load normalized in AN patients after partial restoration of body weight (Tamai et al. 1993). Other studies have found that measures of CCK function in AN were similar to or lower than control values (Baranowska et al. 2000; Brambilla et al. 1995b; Geracioti et al. 1992; Pirke et al. 1994). Further studies are needed to evaluate the relationship between altered CCK regulation and other indices of abnormal gastric function in symptomatic BN and AN patients (Geliebter et al. 1992).

Leptin

Leptin, the protein product of the *ob* gene, is secreted predominantly by adipose tissue cells and acts in the CNS to decrease food intake, thus regulating body fat stores. In rodent models, defects in the leptin coding sequence resulting in leptin deficiency or defects in leptin receptor function are associated with obesity. In humans, serum and CSF concentrations of leptin are positively correlated with fat mass in individuals across a broad range of body weight. Obesity in humans is not thought to be a result of leptin deficiency per se, although rare genetic deficiencies in leptin production have been associated with familial obesity.

Underweight patients with AN have consistently been found to have significantly reduced serum leptin concentrations in comparison with normal-weight control subjects (Baranowska et al. 2001; Grinspoon et al. 1996; Hebebrand et al. 1995; Mantzoros et al. 1997). Based on studies in laboratory animals, it has been suggested that low leptin levels may contribute to amenorrhea and other hormonal changes in the disorder (Mantzoros et al. 1997). Although the reduction in fasting serum leptin levels in AN is correlated with reduction in BMI, there has been some discussion of the possibility that leptin levels in patients with AN may be higher than expected based on the extent of weight loss (Frederich et al. 2002; Jimerson 2002). Mantzoros et al. (1997) reported an elevated CSF-to-serum leptin ratio in AN patients compared with control subjects, suggesting that the proportional decrease in leptin levels with weight loss is greater in serum than in CSF. A longitudinal investigation during refeeding in patients with AN showed that CSF leptin concentrations reach normal values before full weight restoration, possibly as a consequence of the relatively rapid and disproportionate accumulation of fat during refeeding (Mantzoros et al. 1997). This finding led the authors to suggest that premature normalization of leptin concentration might contribute to difficulty in achieving and sustaining a normal weight in AN. Plasma and CSF leptin levels appear to be similar to control values in long-term recovered AN subjects (Gendall 1999).

More recent studies indicate that patients with BN, in comparison with carefully matched control subjects, have significantly decreased leptin concentrations in serum samples obtained after an overnight fast (Baranowska et al. 2001; Brewerton et al. 2000). Initial findings in individuals who have achieved sustained recovery from BN, compared with control subjects with closely matched percentages of body fat, suggest that serum leptin levels remain decreased. This finding may be related to evidence for a persistent decrease in activity in the hypothalamic-pituitary-thyroid axis in long-term recovered BN individuals. These alterations could be associated with decreased metabolic rate and a tendency toward weight gain, contributing to the preoccupation with body weight characteristic of BN.

Ghrelin

Intracerebroventricular injections of the gut-related peptide ghrelin strongly stimulated feeding in rats and increased body weight gain. When administered to healthy human volunteers, ghrelin results in increased hunger and food intake (Wren et al. 2001). In addition, it has been reported that fasting plasma ghrelin concentrations in humans are negatively correlated with BMI (Shiiya et al. 2002; Tanaka et al. 2002), percentage body fat, and fasting leptin and insulin concentrations (Tschop et al. 2001). As recently reviewed, a number of studies have shown elevation in circulating ghrelin levels in AN, with a return to normal levels as patients regain weight (Jimerson and Wolfe 2006). Further research is needed to explore the possible existence of ghrelin resistance in cachectic states related to the eating disorders.

Studies comparing fasting plasma ghrelin concentrations in patients with BN and healthy controls have yielded variable results (Jimerson and Wolfe 2006). It is of interest, however, that the postprandial decrease in ghrelin levels appears to be blunted in patients with BN (Kojima et al. 2005b; Monteleone et al. 2005), consistent with other evidence for diminished satiety responses in the disorder.

Monoamine Systems

There is an abundance of evidence that individuals with AN and BN have disturbances of monoamine function in the ill state. While less well studied, monoamine disturbances appear to persist after recovery.

Dopamine

Altered dopamine activity has been found among ill AN and BN individuals. Homovanillic acid (HVA), the major metabolite of dopamine in humans, was decreased in CSF of underweight AN subjects (Kaye et al. 1984). Although ill subjects with BN, as a group, have normal CSF levels of HVA, several studies have shown significant reductions of CSF HVA levels in BN patients with high binge frequency (Jimerson et al. 1992; Kaye et al. 1990a). Individuals with AN have altered frequency of functional polymorphisms of dopamine D_2 receptor genes that might affect receptor transcription and translation efficiency (Bergen et al. 2005) and impaired visual discrimination

learning (Lawrence 2003), a task thought to reflect dopamine signaling function. CNS dopamine metabolism may explain differences in symptoms between AN, AN-BN, and BN subjects. Our group (Kaye et al. 1999) found that recovered AN subjects had significantly reduced concentrations of CSF HVA in comparison with recovered AN-BN or BN women. A PET imaging study (Frank et al. 2005) found recovered AN subjects had increased binding of D_2 and D_3 receptors in the anteroventral striatum. Dopamine neuronal function has been associated with motor activity (Kaye et al. 1999) and with optimal response to reward stimuli (Montague et al. 2004; Schultz 2004). Individuals with AN have stereotyped and hyperactive motor behavior and anhedonic and restrictive personalities.

Serotonin

5-HT pathways play an important role in postprandial satiety. Treatments that increase intrasynaptic 5-HT or that directly activate 5-HT receptors tend to reduce food consumption, whereas interventions that dampen 5-HT neurotransmission or block receptor activation reportedly increase food consumption and promote weight gain (Blundell 1984; Leibowitz and Shor-Posner 1986). Moreover, CNS 5-HT pathways have been implicated in the modulation of mood, impulse regulation and behavioral constraint, and obsessionality, and they affect a variety of neuroendocrine systems.

There has been considerable interest in the role that 5-HT may play in AN and BN (Brewerton 1995; Jimerson et al. 1990; Kaye and Weltzin 1991; Kaye et al. 1998; Steiger et al. 2005; Treasure and Campbell 1994). In part, this interest derives from study findings of alterations in 5-HT metabolism in AN and BN. When underweight, individuals with AN have a significant reduction in basal concentrations of the serotonin metabolite 5-hydroxyindolacetic acid (5-HIAA) in the CSF compared with healthy control subjects, as well as blunted plasma prolactin response to drugs with 5-HT activity and reduced ^{3}H-imipramine binding. Together, these findings suggest reduced serotonergic activity, although this may arise secondarily to reductions in dietary supplies of the 5-HT–synthesizing amino acid tryptophan. By contrast, CSF concentrations of 5-HIAA are reported to be elevated in long-term weight-recovered AN individuals. These contrasting findings of reduced and heightened serotonergic activity in acutely ill and long-term recovered AN individuals, respectively, may seem counterintuitive; however, since dieting lowers plasma tryptophan levels in otherwise healthy women (Anderson et al. 1990), resumption of normal eating in individuals with AN may unmask intrinsic abnormalities in serotonergic systems that mediate certain core behavioral or temperamental underpinnings of risk and vulnerability.

Considerable evidence also exists for a dysregulation of serotonergic processes in BN. Examples include blunted prolactin response to the 5-HT receptor agonists *m*-chlorophenylpiperazine (m-CPP), 5-hydroxytryptophan, and *dl*-fenfluramine and enhanced migraine-like headache response to m-CPP challenge. Acute perturbation of serotonergic tone by dietary depletion of tryptophan has been linked to increased food intake and mood irritability in individuals with BN compared with healthy control subjects. Also, as in AN, women with long-term recovery from BN have been shown to have elevated CSF concentrations of 5-HIAA as well as reduced platelet binding of paroxetine (Steiger et al. 2005).

Serotonin and Behavior

There is an extensive literature associating the serotonergic systems and fundamental aspects of behavioral inhibition (Geyer 1996; Soubrie 1986). Reduced CSF 5-HIAA levels are associated with increased impulsivity and aggression in humans and nonhuman primates, whereas increased CSF 5-HIAA levels are related to behavioral inhibition (Fairbanks et al. 2001; Westergaard et al. 2003). Thus, it is of interest that women who had recovered from AN and BN showed elevated CSF 5-HIAA concentrations. Behaviors found after recovery from AN and BN, such as obsessionality with symmetry and exactness, anxiety, and perfectionism, tend to be opposite in character to behaviors displayed by people with low 5-HIAA levels. Together, these studies contribute to a growing literature suggesting that reduced CSF 5-HIAA levels are related to behavioral undercontrol, whereas increased CSF 5-HIAA concentrations may be related to behavioral overcontrol.

The possibility of a common vulnerability for BN and AN may seem puzzling, given the well-recognized differences in behavior in these disorders. However, studies suggest that AN and BN have a shared etiological vulnerability—that is, there is a familial aggregation of a range of eating disorders in relatives of probands with either BN or AN, and these two disorders are highly comorbid in twin studies. BN responds to 5-HT-specific medications. Few controlled trials of 5-HT-specific medication have been done in AN, and it remains uncertain whether there is a beneficial response. Both disorders have high levels of harm

avoidance (Klump et al. 2000a), a personality trait hypothesized to be related to increased 5-HT activity. These data raise the possibility that a disturbance of 5-HT activity may create a vulnerability for the expression of a cluster of symptoms that are common to both AN and BN. Other factors that are *independent* of a vulnerability for the development of an eating disorder may contribute to the development of eating disorder subgroups. For example, people with restricting-type AN have extraordinary self-restraint and self-control. The risk for obsessive-compulsive *personality* disorder is elevated only in this subgroup and in their families and shows a shared transmission with restricting-type AN (Lilenfeld et al. 1998). In other words, an additional vulnerability for behavioral overcontrol and rigid and inflexible mood states, combined with a vulnerability for an eating disorder, may result in restricting-type AN.

The contribution of 5-HT to specific human behaviors remains uncertain. 5-HT has been postulated to contribute to temperament or personality traits such as harm avoidance (Cloninger 1987) and behavioral inhibition (Soubrie 1986) or to categorical dimensions such as OCD (Barr et al. 1992), anxiety and fear (Charney et al. 1990), and depression (Grahame-Smith 1992), as well as satiety for food consumption. It is possible that separate components of 5-HT neuronal systems (i.e., different pathways or receptors) are coded for such specific behaviors. However, that may not be consistent with the neurophysiology of 5-HT neuronal function.

PET Studies Using 5-HT Receptor Radioligands

The marriage of PET imaging with selective neurotransmitter radioligands has resulted in a technology permitting new insights into regional binding and specificity of 5-HT and dopamine neurotransmission in vivo in humans and their relationship to behaviors.

The 5-HT$_{1A}$ autoreceptor is located presynaptically on 5-HT somatodendritic cell bodies in the raphe nucleus, where it functions to decrease 5-HT neurotransmission (Staley et al. 1998). High densities of postsynaptic 5-HT$_{1A}$ exist in the hippocampus, septum, amygdala, and entorhinal and frontal cortex, where they serve to mediate the effects of released 5-HT. Studies in animals and humans implicate the 5-HT$_{1A}$ receptor in anxiety (File et al. 2000) and depression and/or suicide (Mann 1999). Pharmacological and knockout studies implicate the 5-HT$_{1A}$ receptor in the modulation of anxiety (Gross et al. 2002). Bailer et al. (2007) reported that ill AN individuals had a 50%–70% increase in 5-HT$_{1A}$ receptor–binding potential in subgenual, mesial temporal, orbitofrontal, and raphe brain regions, as well as in prefrontal, lateral temporal, anterior cingulate, and parietal regions. Increased 5-HT$_{1A}$ postsynaptic activity has been reported in ill BN subjects (Tiihonen et al. 2004). Recovered binge-eating/purging–type AN subjects and BN subjects (Bailer et al. 2005; W. Kaye, unpublished data, March 2008) showed significant (20%–40%) increases in 5-HT$_{1A}$ receptor binding potential in these same regions compared with healthy control subjects (Bailer et al. 2005). By contrast, recovered restricting-type AN women showed no difference in 5-HT$_{1A}$ receptor binding potential compared with control subjects (Bailer et al. 2005).

AN and BN are frequently comorbid with depression and anxiety disorders. However, reduced 5-HT$_{1A}$ receptor binding potential has been found in ill (Drevets et al. 1999; Sargent et al. 2000) and recovered (Bhagwagar et al. 2004) depressed subjects, as well as in a primate model for depression (Shively et al. 2006). Parsey et al. (2005) found no difference in carbonyl-[11C]WAY100635 binding potential in major depressive disorder, although a subgroup of never-medicated subjects had elevated carbonyl-[11C]WAY-100635 binding potential. Recent studies have found reduced [11C]WAY100635 binding potential in social phobia (Lanzenberger et al. 2007) and panic disorder (Neumeister et al. 2004). These findings suggest that AN and BN, anxiety, and depression share disturbances of common neuronal pathways but are etiologically different.

Postsynaptic 5-HT$_{2A}$ receptors, which are present at high densities in the cerebral cortex and other regions of rodents and humans (Burnet et al. 1997; Saudou and Hen 1994), are of interest because they have been implicated in the modulation of feeding and mood as well as in selective serotonin reuptake inhibitor response (Bailer et al. 2004; Bonhomme and Esposito 1998; De Vry and Schreiber 2000; Simansky 1996; Stockmeier 1997). Ill AN subjects were found to have normal 5-HT$_{2A}$ receptor binding potential values in one study (Bailer et al. 2007) and reduced binding potential in another study (Audenaert et al. 2003) in the left frontal, bilateral parietal, and occipital cortex. After recovery, individuals with restricting-type AN had reduced 5-HT$_{2A}$ receptor binding potential in mesial temporal and parietal cortical areas as well as in subgenual and pregenual cingulate cortex (Frank et al. 2002). Similarly, recovered binge-eating/purging–type AN women had reduced 5-HT$_{2A}$ receptor binding potential in the left subgenual cingulate, left parietal, and right occipital cortex (Bailer et al. 2004), and recovered BN women had reduced [18F]altanserin binding potential relative to controls in the orbitofrontal region (Kaye et al. 2001).

The PET imaging studies in ill and recovered AN and BN subjects described above found significant correlations between harm avoidance and binding for the 5-HT$_{1A}$, 5-HT$_{2A}$, and dopamine D$_2$/D$_3$ receptors in mesial temporal and other limbic regions. Bailer et al. (2004) found that recovered AN-BN subjects showed a positive relationship between [18F]altanserin binding potential in the left subgenual cingulate and mesial temporal cortex and harm avoidance. For ill AN subjects, [18F]altanserin binding potential was positively related to harm avoidance in the supragenual cingulate, frontal, and parietal regions. 5-HT$_{2A}$ receptor binding and harm avoidance were shown to be negatively correlated in the frontal cortex in healthy subjects (Moresco et al. 2002) and in the prefrontal cortex in patients who attempted suicide (van Heeringen et al. 2003). Clinical and epidemiological studies have consistently shown that one or more anxiety disorders occur in the majority of people with AN or BN (Godart et al. 2002; Kaye et al. 2004; Kendler et al. 1995; Walters and Kendler 1995). Silberg and Bulik (2005), using twins, found a unique genetic effect that influences liability to early anxiety and eating disorder symptoms. When a lifetime anxiety disorder is present, the anxiety most commonly occurs first in childhood, preceding the onset of AN or BN (Bulik et al. 1997; Deep et al. 1995; Godart et al. 2000). Anxiety and harm avoidance remain elevated after recovery from AN, AN-BN, and BN (Wagner et al. 2006a), even if individuals never had a lifetime anxiety disorder diagnosis (Kaye et al. 2004). Finally, anxiety (Spielberger et al. 1970) and harm avoidance from Cloninger's Temperament and Character Inventory (Cloninger et al. 1994) have been a robust signal in genetic studies (Bacanu et al. 2005). In summary, the premorbid onset and the persistence of anxiety and harm avoidance symptoms after recovery suggest these are traits that contribute to the pathogenesis of AN and BN. The PET imaging data suggest that such behaviors are related to disturbances of 5-HT and dopamine neurotransmitter function in limbic and executive pathways.

This technology holds the promise of a new era of understanding the complexity of neuronal systems in human behavior. For example, postsynaptic 5-HT$_{1A}$ receptors (Celada et al. 2001; Richer et al. 2002; Sibille et al. 2000; Szabo and Blier 2001) have downstream effects and interactions with other neuronal systems, such as norepinephrine, glutamate, and γ-aminobutyric acid (GABA). Enhanced 5-HT$_{1A}$ activity in AN and BN may cause or reflect an altered balance between these neuronal systems. Moreover, 5-HT$_{1A}$ receptors interact with other 5-HT receptors such as 5-HT$_{2A}$ (Martin et al. 1997;

Szabo and Blier 2001). 5-HT$_{1A}$ postsynaptic receptors mediate locus coeruleus firing through 5-HT transmission at 5-HT$_{2A}$ receptors (Szabo and Blier 2001). Theoretically, increased 5-HT$_{1A}$ and reduced 5-HT$_{2A}$ postsynaptic receptor activity in AN might result in an increase in noradrenergic neuron firing (Szabo and Blier 2001). Moreover, postsynaptic 5-HT$_{1A}$ receptors hyperpolarize and 5-HT$_{2A}$ receptors depolarize layer V pyramidal neurons (Martin-Ruiz et al. 2001). In AN, synergistic effects of these receptors, which are collocated on pyramidal neurons, may reduce pyramidal neuronal excitability.

In summary, these PET–radioligand studies confirm that altered 5-HT neuronal pathway activity persists after recovery from AN and BN and support the possibility that these psychobiological alterations might contribute to traits, such as increased anxiety, that may contribute to a vulnerability to develop an eating disorder.

Conclusion

There remain daunting challenges to the investigation of neurobiological mediators of risk and clinical pathology in AN and BN. To what extent abnormalities detected are consequences of pathological eating behavior, malnutrition, or their long-term sequelae remains speculative. Data on the functional status of these neurobiological systems are too sparse to allow for definitive conclusions regarding the possible etiological significance of differences reported between individuals with eating disorders and healthy control subjects.

Clearly, many of the alterations in neuropeptide and monoaminergic function in eating disorders are state dependent; however, given the effects of these systems on mood, anxiety, memory organization, and body physiology, these alterations may well have significant pathogenic influences, both sustaining and exacerbating certain psychological and cognitive elements of these syndromes. Thus, neurobiologically mediated effects may be contributing factors to the frequently long-term, pernicious, and self-sustaining course of illness, at least in many patients. These associations, although speculative, nevertheless underscore the importance of aggressive and sustained treatment of both the nutritional and the behavioral/psychological elements of the syndromes to allow for stabilization and possible normalization of neuropeptidergic and monoaminergic functions.

Still, several lines of evidence from family and twin research, premorbid and retrospective data, and studies with recovered individuals suggest that traits, perhaps re-

lated to 5-HT modulation of anxiety and perfectionistic obsessiveness, create a susceptibility for some people to develop an eating disorder. Adolescence is a time of transition, where individuals leave the security of their home environment and must learn to balance immediate and long-terms needs and goals in order to achieve independence. For such individuals, learning to flexibly interact and master complex and mixed cultural and societal messages and pressures, or cope with stress, may be difficult and overwhelming, exacerbating underlying traits of harm avoidance and a desire to perfectly achieve.

To a large extent, current treatments for AN and BN have been based on therapies developed for other psychiatric disorders. While these are effective to some degree, particularly for BN, many individuals with AN and BN remain ill for many years and have only partial resolution of symptoms with treatment. Thus, there is a substantial need to understand how neurobiological risk factors contribute to symptoms, as well as the interaction of temperament with the environment, in order to develop specific and more effective therapy for these disorders.

References

Abraham S, Beaumont P: How patients describe bulimia or binge eating. Psychol Med 12:625–635, 1982

American Psychiatric Association: Diagnostic and Statistical Manual of Mental Disorders, 4th Edition, Text Revision. Washington, DC, American Psychiatric Association, 2000

Anderson IM, Parry-Billings M, Newsholme EA, et al: Dieting reduces plasma tryptophan and alters brain 5-HT function in women. Psychol Med 20:785–791, 1990

Andreason PJ, Altemus M, Zametkin AJ, et al: Regional cerebral glucose metabolism in bulimia nervosa. Am J Psychiatry 149:1506–1513, 1992

Audenaert K, Van Laere K, Dumont F, et al: Decreased 5-HT2a receptor binding in patients with anorexia nervosa. J Nucl Med 44:163–169, 2003

Bacanu S, Bulik C, Klump K, et al: Linkage analysis of anorexia and bulimia nervosa cohorts using selected behavioral phenotypes as quantitative traits or covariates. Am J Med Genet B Neuropsychiatr Genet 139:61–68, 2005

Bailer UF, Price JC, Meltzer CC, et al: Altered 5-HT2A receptor binding after recovery from bulimia-type anorexia nervosa: relationships to harm avoidance and drive for thinness. Neuropsychopharmacology 29:1143–1155, 2004

Bailer UF, Frank GK, Henry SE, et al: Altered brain serotonin 5-HT1A receptor binding after recovery from anorexia nervosa measured by positron emission tomography and [11C]WAY100635. Arch Gen Psychiatry 62:1032–1041, 2005

Bailer UF, Frank G, Henry S, et al: Exaggerated 5-HT1A but normal 5-HT2A receptor activity in individuals ill with anorexia nervosa. Biol. Psychiatry 61:1090–1099, 2007

Baker JH, Mazzeo SE, Kendler KS: Association between broadly defined bulimia nervosa and drug use disorders: common genetic and environmental influences. Int J Eat Disord 40:673–678, 2007

Baranowska B, Radzikowska M, Wasilewska-Dziubinska E, et al: Disturbed release of gastrointestinal peptides in anorexia nervosa and in obesity. Diabet Obes Metab 2:99–103, 2000

Baranowska B, Wolinska-Witort E, Wasilewska-Dziubinska E, et al: Plasma leptin, neuropeptide Y (NPY) and galanin concentrations in bulimia nervosa and in anorexia nervosa. Neuroendocrinol Lett 22:356–358, 2001

Barr LC, Goodman WK, Price LH, et al: The serotonin hypothesis of obsessive compulsive disorder: implications of pharmacologic challenge studies. J Clin Psychiatry 53 (suppl):17–28, 1992

Bergen AW, van den Bree MBM, Yeager M, et al: Serotonin 1D (HRT1D) and delta opioid (OPRD1) receptor locus sequence variation is significantly associated with anorexia nervosa. Mol Psychiatry 8:397–406, 2003

Bergen A, Yeager M, Welch R, et al: Association of multiple DRD2–141 polymorphism with anorexia nervosa. Neuropsychopharmacology 30:1703–1710, 2005

Bhagwagar Z, Rabiner E, Sargent P, et al: Persistent reduction in brain serotonin1A receptor binding in recovered depressed men measured by positron emission tomography with [11C]WAY-100635. Mol Psychiatry 9:386–392, 2004

Blundell JE: Serotonin and appetite. Neuropharmacology 23:1537–1551, 1984

Bonhomme N, Esposito E: Involvement of serotonin and dopamine in the mechanism of action of novel antidepressant drugs: a review. J Clin Psychopharmacol 18:447–454, 1998

Brambilla F, Brunetta M, Draisci A, et al: T-lymphocyte cholecystokinin-8 and beta-endorphin in eating disorders, II: bulimia nervosa. Psychiatry Res 59:51–56, 1995a

Brambilla F, Brunetta M, Peirone A, et al: T-lymphocyte cholecystokinin-8 and beta-endorphin concentrations in eating disorders, I: anorexia nervosa. Psychiatry Res 59:43–50, 1995b

Brewerton TD: Toward a unified theory of serotonin dysregulation in eating and related disorders. Psychoneuroendocrinology 20:561–590, 1995

Brewerton TD, Lydiard RB, Laraia MT, et al: CSF beta-endorphin and dynorphin in bulimia nervosa. Am J Psychiatry 149:1086–1090, 1992

Brewerton TD, Lesem MD, Kennedy A, et al: Reduced plasma leptin concentration in bulimia nervosa. Psychoneuroendocrinology 25:649–658, 2000

Brown K, Bujac S, Mann E, et al: Further evidence of association of OPDR1 and HTR1D polymorphisms with susceptibility to anorexia nervosa. Biol Psychiatry 61:367–373, 2007

Bulik CM, Sullivan PF, Fear JL, et al: Eating disorders and antecedent anxiety disorders: a controlled study. Acta Psychiatr Scand 96:101–107, 1997

Bulik CM, Sullivan PF, Kendler KS: Heritability of binge-eating and broadly defined bulimia nervosa. Biol Psychiatry 44:1210–1218, 1998

Bulik CM, Devlin B, Bacanu SA, et al: Significant linkage on chromosome 10p in families with bulimia nervosa. Am J Hum Genet 72:200–207, 2003

Bulik C, Bacanu S, Klump K, et al: Selection of eating-disorder phenotypes for linkage analysis. Am J Med Genet B Neuropsychiatr Genet 139:81–87, 2005

Burnet PW, Eastwood SL, Harrison PJ: [3H]WAY-100635 for 5-HT1A receptor autoradiography in human brain: a comparison with [3H]8-OH-DPAT and demonstration of increased binding in the frontal cortex in schizophrenia. Neurochem Int 30:565–574, 1997

Campbell DA, Sundaramurthy D, Gordon D, et al: Association between a marker in the UCP-2/UCP-3 gene cluster and genetic susceptibility to anorexia nervosa. Mol Psychiatry 4:68–70, 1999

Casper RC: Personality features of women with good outcome from restricting anorexia nervosa. Psychosom Med 52:156–170, 1990

Celada P, Puig MV, Casanovas JM, et al: Control of dorsal raphe serotonergic neurons by the medial prefrontal cortex: involvement of serotonin-1A, GABAA, and glutamate receptors. J Neurosci 21:9917–9929, 2001

Charney DS, Woods SW, Krystal JH, et al: Serotonin function and human anxiety disorders. Ann N Y Acad Sci 600:558–572, 1990

Chowdhury U, Gordon I, Lask B: Neuroimaging and anorexia nervosa. J Am Acad Child Adolesc Psychiatry 40:738, 2001

Cloninger CR: A systematic method for clinical description and classification of personality variants. A proposal. Arch Gen Psychiatry 44:573–588, 1987

Cloninger CR, Przybeck TR, Svrakic DM, et al: The Temperament and Character Inventory (TCI): A Guide to its Development and Use. St Louis, MO, Center for Psychobiology of Personality, Washington University, 1994

Craig AD: How do you feel? Interoception: the sense of the physiological condition of the body. Nat Rev Neurosci 3:655–666, 2002

De Vry J, Schreiber R: Effects of selected serotonin 5-HT(1) and 5-HT(2) receptor agonists on feeding behavior: possible mechanisms of action. Neurosci Biobehav Rev 24:341–353, 2000

Deep AL, Nagy LM, Weltzin TE, et al: Premorbid onset of psychopathology in long-term recovered anorexia nervosa. Int J Eat Disord 17:291–297, 1995

Delvenne V, Lotstra F, Goldman S, et al: Brain hypometabolism of glucose in anorexia nervosa: a PET scan study. Biol Psychiatry 37:161–169, 1995

Delvenne V, Goldman S, De Maertelaer V, et al: Brain glucose metabolism in eating disorders assessed by positron emission tomography. Int J Eat Disord 25:29–37, 1999

Devlin B, Bacanu S-A, Klump KL, et al: Linkage analysis of anorexia nervosa incorporating behavioral covariates. Hum Mol Genet 11:689–696, 2002

Devlin MJ, Walsh BT, Guss JL, et al: Postprandial cholecystokinin release and gastric emptying in patients with bulimia nervosa. Am J Clin Nutr 65:114–120, 1997

Drevets WC, Frank E, Price JC, et al: PET imaging of serotonin 1A receptor binding in depression. Biol Psychiatry 46:1375–1387, 1999

Eddy KT, Keel PK, Dorer DJ, et al: Longitudinal comparison of anorexia nervosa subtypes. Int J Eat Disord 31:191–201, 2002

Eddy KT, Dorer DJ, Franko DL, et al: Should bulimia nervosa be subtyped by history of anorexia nervosa? A longitudinal validation. Int J Eat Disord 40 (suppl):S67–S71, 2007

Ellison ZR, Foong J: Neuroimaging in eating disorders, in Neurobiology in the Treatment of Eating Disorders. Edited by Hoek HW, Treasure JL, Katzman MA. Chichester, UK, Wiley, 1998, pp 255–269

Ellison Z, Foong J, Howard R, et al: Functional anatomy of calorie fear in anorexia nervosa. Lancet 352:1192, 1998

Fairbanks L, Melega W, Jorgensen M, et al: Social impulsivity inversely associated with CSF 5-HIAA and fluoxetine exposure in vervet monkeys. Neuropsychopharmacology 24:370–378, 2001

Fairburn CG, Welch SL, Doll HA, et al: Risk factors for bulimia nervosa. A community-based case-control study. Arch Gen Psychiatry 54:509–517, 1997

Fairburn CG, Cooper JR, Doll HA, et al: Risk factors for anorexia nervosa: three integrated case-control comparisons. Arch Gen Psychiatry 56:468–476, 1999

Farrar C, Franck N, Georgieff N, et al: Modulating the experience of agency: a positron emission tomography study. Neuroimage 18:324–333, 2003

Fava M, Copeland PM, Schweiger U, et al: Neurochemical abnormalities of anorexia nervosa and bulimia nervosa. Am J Psychiatry 146:963–971, 1989

Fichter M, Quadflieg N: Long-term stability of eating disorder diagnoses. Int J Eating Disord 40 (suppl):S61–S66, 2007

File SE, Kenny PJ, Cheeta S: The role of the dorsal hippocampal serotonergic and cholinergic systems in the modulation of anxiety. Pharmacol Biochem Behav 66:65, 2000

Frank GK, Kaye WH, Meltzer CC, et al: Reduced 5-HT2A receptor binding after recovery from anorexia nervosa. Biol Psychiatry 52:896–906, 2002

Frank G, Bailer UF, Henry S, et al: Increased dopamine D2/D3 receptor binding after recovery from anorexia nervosa measured by positron emission tomography and [11C]raclopride. Biol Psychiatry 58:908–912, 2005

Frederich R, Hu S, Raymond N, et al: Leptin in anorexia nervosa and bulimia nervosa: importance of assay technique and method of interpretation. J Lab Clin Med 139:72–79, 2002

Garner DM, Garfinkel PE, O'Shaughnessy M: The validity of the distinction between bulimia with and without anorexia nervosa. Am J Psychiatry 142:581–587, 1985

Geliebter A, Melton PM, McCray RS, et al: Gastric capacity, gastric emptying, and test-meal intake in normal and bulimic women. Am J Clin Nutr 56:656–661, 1992

Gendall K: Leptin, neuropeptide Y, and peptide YY in long-term recovered eating disorder patients. Biol Psychiatry 46:292–299, 1999

Geracioti TD Jr, Liddle RA: Impaired cholecystokinin secretion in bulimia nervosa. N Engl J Med 319:683–688, 1988

Geracioti TD Jr, Liddle RA, Altemus M, et al: Regulation of appetite and cholecystokinin secretion in anorexia nervosa. Am J Psychiatry 149:958–961, 1992

Germain N, Galusca B, Le Roux C, et al: Constitutional thinness and lean anorexia nervosa display opposite concentrations of peptide YY, glucagon-line peptide 1, ghrelin, and leptin. Am J Clin Nutr 85:957–971, 2007

Gerstmann J: Fingeragnosie: eine umschriebene Storung der Orientierung am eigenen Korper. Wien Klinische Wochenschr 37:1010–1013, 1924

Geyer MA: Serotonergic functions in arousal and motor activity. Behav Brain Res 73:31, 1996

Gibbs J, Young RC, Smith GP: Cholecystokinin decreases food intake in rats. J Comp Physiol Psychol 84:488–495, 1973

Glowa JR, Gold PW: Corticotropin releasing hormone produces profound anorexigenic effects in the rhesus monkey. Neuropeptides 18:55–61, 1991

Godart NT, Flament MF, Lecrubier Y, et al: Anxiety disorders in anorexia nervosa and bulimia nervosa: co-morbidity and chronology of appearance. Eur Psychiatry 15:38–45, 2000

Godart NT, Flament MF, Perdereau F, et al: Comorbidity between eating disorders and anxiety disorders: a review. Int J Eat Disord 32:253–270, 2002

Gold PW, Gwirtsman H, Avgerinos PC, et al: Abnormal hypothalamic-pituitary-adrenal function in anorexia nervosa. Pathophysiologic mechanisms in underweight and weight-corrected patients. N Engl J Med 314:1335–1342, 1986

Gordon CM, Dougherty DD, Fischman AJ, et al: Neural substrates of anorexia nervosa: a behavioral challenge study with positron emission tomography. J Pediatr 139:51–57, 2001

Gordon I, Lask B, Bryant-Waugh R, et al: Childhood-onset anorexia nervosa: towards identifying a biological substrate. Int J Eat Disord 22:159–165, 1997

Grahame-Smith DG: Serotonin in affective disorders. Int Clin Psychopharmacol 6 (suppl 4):5–13, 1992

Grice DE, Halmi KA, Fichter M, et al: Evidence for a susceptibility gene for anorexia nervosa on chromosome 1. Am J Hum Genet 70:787–792, 2002

Grinspoon S, Gulick T, Askari H, et al: Serum leptin levels in women with anorexia nervosa. J Clin Endocrinol Metab 81:3861–3863, 1996

Gross C, Zhuang X, Stark K, et al: Serotonin1A receptor acts during development to establish normal anxiety-like behaviour in the adult. Nature 416:396–400, 2002

Halmi KA, Eckert E, Marchi P, et al: Comorbidity of psychiatric diagnoses in anorexia nervosa. Arch Gen Psychiatry 48:712–718, 1991

Harty RF, Pearson PH, Solomon TE, et al: Cholecystokinin, vasoactive intestinal peptide and peptide histidine methionine responses to feeding in anorexia nervosa. Regul Pept 36:141–150, 1991

Hebebrand J, van der Heyden J, Devos R, et al: Plasma concentrations of obese protein in anorexia nervosa. Lancet 346:1624–1625, 1995

Jimerson DC: Leptin and the neurobiology of eating disorders. J Lab Clin Med 139:70–71, 2002

Jimerson D, Wolfe B: Psychobiology of eating disorders, in Annual Review of Eating Disorders: Part 2. Edited by Wonderlich SMJ, de Zwaan M, Steiger H. Oxford, UK, Radcliffe Publishing, 2006, pp 1–15

Jimerson DC, Lesem MD, Kaye WH, et al: Eating disorders and depression: is there a serotonin connection? Biol Psychiatry 28:443–454, 1990

Jimerson DC, Lesem MD, Kaye WH, et al: Low serotonin and dopamine metabolite concentrations in cerebrospinal fluid from bulimic patients with frequent binge episodes. Arch Gen Psychiatry 49:132–138, 1992

Jimerson DC, Wolfe BE, Naab S: Anorexia nervosa and bulimia nervosa, in Textbook of Pediatric Neuropsychiatry. Edited by Coffey CE, Brumback RA. Washington, DC, American Psychiatric Press, 1998, pp 563–578

Johnson C, Larson R: Bulimia: an analysis of mood and behavior. Psychosom Med 44:341–351, 1982

Kalra SP, Dube MG, Sahu A, et al: Neuropeptide Y secretion increases in the paraventricular nucleus in association with increased appetite for food. Proc Natl Acad Sci U S A 88:10931–10935, 1991

Katzman DK, Lambe EK, Mikulis DJ, et al: Cerebral gray matter and white matter volume deficits in adolescent girls with anorexia nervosa. J Pediatr 129:794–803, 1996

Kaye WH, Weltzin TE: Serotonin activity in anorexia and bulimia nervosa: relationship to the modulation of feeding and mood. J Clin Psychiatry 52 (suppl):41–48, 1991

Kaye WH, Ebert MH, Raleigh M, et al: Abnormalities in CNS monoamine metabolism in anorexia nervosa. Arch Gen Psychiatry 41:350–355, 1984

Kaye WH, Gwirtsman HE, George DT, et al: Relationship of mood alterations to bingeing behaviour in bulimia. Br J Psychiatry 149:479–485, 1986

Kaye WH, Berrettini WH, Gwirtsman HE, et al: Reduced cerebrospinal fluid levels of immunoreactive pro-opiomelanocortin related peptides (including beta-endorphin) in anorexia nervosa. Life Sci 41:2147–2155, 1987a

Kaye WH, Gwirtsman HE, George DT, et al: Elevated cerebrospinal fluid levels of immunoreactive corticotropin-releasing hormone in anorexia nervosa: relation to state of nutrition, adrenal function, and intensity of depression. J Clin Endocrinol Metab 64:203–208, 1987b

Kaye WH, Ballenger JC, Lydiard RB, et al: CSF monoamine levels in normal-weight bulimia: evidence for abnormal noradrenergic activity. Am J Psychiatry 147:225–229, 1990a

Kaye WH, Berrettini W, Gwirtsman H, et al: Altered cerebrospinal fluid neuropeptide Y and peptide YY immunoreactivity in anorexia and bulimia nervosa. Arch Gen Psychiatry 47:548–556, 1990b

Kaye WH, Lilenfeld LR, Plotnicov K, et al: Bulimia nervosa and substance dependence: association and family transmission. Alcohol Clin Exp Res 20:878–881, 1996

Kaye WH, Greeno CG, Moss H, et al: Alterations in serotonin activity and psychiatric symptomatology after recovery from bulimia nervosa. Arch Gen Psychiatry 55:927–935, 1998

Kaye WH, Frank GK, McConaha C: Altered dopamine activity after recovery from restricting-type anorexia nervosa. Neuropsychopharmacology 21:503–506, 1999

Kaye WH, Lilenfeld LR, Berrettini WH, et al: A search for susceptibility loci for anorexia nervosa: methods and sample description. Biol Psychiatry 47:794–803, 2000

Kaye WH, Frank GK, Meltzer CC, et al: Altered serotonin 2A receptor activity in women who have recovered from bulimia nervosa. Am J Psychiatry 158:1152–1155, 2001

Kaye WH, Barbarich NC, Putnam K, et al: Anxiolytic effects of acute tryptophan depletion in anorexia nervosa. Int J Eat Disord 33:257–267, 2003

Kaye W, Bulik C, Thornton L, et al: Comorbidity of anxiety disorders with anorexia and bulimia nervosa. Am J Psychiatry 161:2215–2221, 2004

Keel PK, Mitchell JE: Outcome in bulimia nervosa. Am J Psychiatry 154:313–321, 1997

Kelley AE, Bakshi VP, Haber S, et al: Opioid modulation of taste hedonics within ventral striatum. Physiol Behav 76:365–377, 2002

Kendler KS, MacLean C, Neale M, et al: The genetic epidemiology of bulimia nervosa. Am J Psychiatry 148:1627–1637, 1991

Kendler KS, Walters EE, Neale MC, et al: The structure of the genetic and environmental risk factors for six major psychiatric disorders in women. Phobia, generalized anxiety disorder, panic disorder, bulimia, major depression, and alcoholism. Arch Gen Psychiatry 52:374–383, 1995

Klump KL, Bulik CM, Pollice C, et al: Temperament and character in women with anorexia nervosa. J Nerv Ment Dis 188:559–567, 2000a

Klump KL, McGue M, Iacono WG: Age differences in genetic and environmental influences on eating attitudes and behaviors in preadolescent and adolescent female twins. J Abnorm Psychol 109:239–251, 2000b

Klump KL, McGue M, Iacono WG: Genetic and environmental influences on anorexia nervosa syndromes in a population-based sample of twins. Psychol Med 31:737–740, 2001a

Klump KL, Miller KB, Keel PK, et al: Genetic and environmental influences on anorexia nervosa syndromes in a population-based twin sample. Psychol Med 31:737–740, 2001b

Klump K, Perkins P, Alexandra Burt S, et al: Puberty moderates genetic influences on disordered eating. Psychol Med 37:627–634, 2007

Kojima S, Nagai N, Nakabeppu Y: Comparison of regional cerebral blood flow in patients with anorexia nervosa before and after weight gain. Psychiatry Res 140:251–258, 2005a

Kojima S, Nakahara T, Nagai N, et al: Altered ghrelin and peptide YY responses to meals in bulimia nervosa. Clin Endocrinol (Oxf) 62:74–78, 2005b

Kuruoglu AC, Kapucu O, Atasever T, et al: Technetium-99m-HMPAO brain SPECT in anorexia nervosa. J Nucl Med 39:304–306, 1998

Lanzenberger R, Mitterhauser M, Spindelegger C, et al: Reduced serotonin-1A receptor binding in social anxiety disorder. Biol Psychiatry 61:1081–1089, 2007

Lawrence A: Impaired visual discrimination learning in anorexia nervosa. Appetite 20:85–89, 2003

LeDoux J: The emotional brain, fear, and the amygdala. Cell Mol Neurobiol 23:727–738, 2003

Leibowitz SF, Shor-Posner G: Brain serotonin and eating behavior. Appetite 7:1–14, 1986

Lesem MD, Berrettini W, Kaye WH, et al: Measurement of CSF dynorphin A 1–8 immunoreactivity in anorexia nervosa and normal-weight bulimia. Biol Psychiatry 29:244–252, 1991

Licinio J, Wong ML, Gold PW: The hypothalamic-pituitary-adrenal axis in anorexia nervosa. Psychiatry Res 62:75–83, 1996

Lilenfeld LR, Kaye WH, Greeno CG, et al: A controlled family study of anorexia nervosa and bulimia nervosa: psychiatric disorders in first-degree relatives and effects of proband comorbidity. Arch Gen Psychiatry 55:603–610, 1998

Lilenfeld LR, Stein D, Bulik CM, et al: Personality traits among currently eating disordered, recovered and never ill first-degree female relatives of bulimic and control women. Psychol Med 30:1399–1410, 2000

Lydiard RB, Brewerton TD, Fossey MD, et al: CSF cholecystokinin octapeptide in patients with bulimia nervosa and in normal comparison subjects. Am J Psychiatry 150:1099–1101, 1993

Mangweth B, Hudson J, Pope H, et al: Family study of the aggregation of eating disorders and mood disorders. Psychol Med 33:1319–1323, 2003

Mann JJ: Role of the serotonergic system in the pathogenesis of major depression and suicidal behavior. Neuropsychopharmacology 21:99S–105S, 1999

Mantzoros C, Flier JS, Lesem MD, et al: Cerebrospinal fluid leptin in anorexia nervosa: correlation with nutritional status and potential role in resistance to weight gain. J Clin Endocrinol Metab 82:1845–1851, 1997

Martin-Ruiz R, Puig MV, Celada P, et al: Control of serotonergic function in medial prefrontal cortex by serotonin-2A receptors through a glutamate-dependent mechanism. J Neurosci 21:9856–9866, 2001

Martin ER, Kaplan NL, Weir BS: Tests for linkage and association in nuclear families. Am J Hum Genet 61:439–448, 1997

Mesulam M: A cortical network for directed attention and unilateral neglect. Ann Neurol 10:309–325, 1981

Miller KB, Klump KL, Keel PK, et al: A population-based twin study of anorexia and bulimia nervosa: heritability and shared transmission with anxiety disorders. Eating Disorders Research Society Meeting, Boston, MA, 1998

Milos G, Spindler A, Schnyder U, et al: Instability of eating disorder diagnoses: prospective study. Br J Psychiatry 187:573–578, 2005

Misra M, Miller K, Tsai P, et al: Elevated peptide YY levels in adolescent girls with anorexia nervosa. J Clin Endocrinol Metab 91:1027–1033, 2006

Montague R, Hyman S, Cohen J: Computational roles for dopamine in behavioural control. Nature 431:760–767, 2004

Monteleone P, Martiadis V, Rigamonti A, et al: Investigation of peptide YY and ghrelin responses to a test meal in bulimia nervosa. Biol Psychiatry 57:926–931, 2005

Moresco FM, Dieci M, Vita A, et al: In vivo serotonin 5HT2A receptor binding and personality traits in healthy subjects: a positron emission tomography study. Neuroimage 17:1470–1478, 2002

Morley JE, Blundell JE: The neurobiological basis of eating disorders: some formulations. Biol Psychiatry 23:53–78, 1988

Morley JE, Levine AS, Gosnell BA, et al: Peptides and feeding. Peptides 6:181–192, 1985

Nakahara T, Kojima S, Tanaka M, et al: Incomplete restoration of the secretion of ghrelin and PYY compared to insulin after food ingestion following weight gain in anorexia nervosa. J Psych Res 41:814–820, 2007

Naruo T, Nakabeppu Y, Sagiyama K, et al: Characteristic regional cerebral blood flow patterns in anorexia nervosa patients with binge/purge behavior. Am J Psychiatry 157:1520–1522, 2000

Neumeister A, Brain E, Nugent A, et al: Reduced serotonin type 1A receptor binding in panic disorder. J Neurosci 24:589–591, 2004

Nozoe S, Naruo T, Nakabeppu Y, et al: Changes in regional cerebral blood flow in patients with anorexia nervosa detected through single photon emission tomography imaging. Biol Psychiatry 34:578–580, 1993

Nozoe S, Naruo T, Yonekura R, et al: Comparison of regional cerebral blood flow in patients with eating disorders. Brain Res Bull 36:251–255, 1995

O'Doherty J, Rolls ET, Francis S, et al: Representation of pleasant and aversive taste in the human brain. J Neurophysiol 85:1315–1321, 2001

Otto B, Cuntz U, Otto C, et al: Peptide YY release in anorectic patients after liquid meal. Appetite 48:301–304, 2007

Parsey RV, Oquendo MA, Ogden RT, et al: Altered serotonin 1A binding in major depression: a [carbonyl-C-11]WAY100635 positron emission tomography study. Biol Psychiatry 59:106–113, 2005

Paulus M, Stein MB: An insular view of anxiety. Biol Psychiatry 60:383–387, 2006

Phillipp E, Pirke KM, Kellner MB, et al: Disturbed cholecystokinin secretion in patients with eating disorders. Life Sci 48:2443–2450, 1991

Pirke KM, Kellner MB, Friess E, et al: Satiety and cholecystokinin. Int J Eating Disord 15:63–69, 1994

Rastam M, Bjure J, Vestergren E, et al: Regional cerebral blood flow in weight-restored anorexia nervosa: a preliminary study. Dev Med Child Neurol 43:239–242, 2001

Richer M, Hen R, Blier P: Modification of serotonin neuron properties in mice lacking 5-HT1A receptors. Eur J Pharmacol 435:195–203, 2002

Rosenkranz K, Hinney A, Ziegler A, et al: Systematic mutation screening of the estrogen receptor beta gene in probands of different weight extremes: identification of several genetic variants. J Clin Endocrinol Metab 83:4524–4527, 1998

Roser W, Bubl R, Buergin D, et al: Metabolic changes in the brain of patients with anorexia and bulimia nervosa as detected by proton magnetic resonance spectroscopy. Int J Eat Disord 26:119–136, 1999

Rutherford J, McGuffin P, Katz RJ, et al: Genetic influences on eating attitudes in a normal female twin population. Psychol Med 23:425–436, 1993

Sargent PA, Kjaer KH, Bench CJ, et al: Brain serotonin1A receptor binding measured by positron emission tomography with [11C]WAY-100635: effects of depression and antidepressant treatment. Arch Gen Psychiatry 57:174–180, 2000

Saudou F, Hen R: 5-Hydroxytryptamine receptor subtypes in vertebrates and invertebrates. Neurochem Int 25:503–532, 1994

Schuckit MA, Tipp JE, Anthenelli RM, et al: Anorexia nervosa and bulimia nervosa in alcohol-dependent men and women and their relatives. Am J Psychiatry 153:74–82, 1996

Schultz W: Neural coding of basic reward terms of animal learning theory, game theory, microeconomics and behavioural ecology. Science 14:139–147, 2004

Schultz W, Tremblay L, Hollerman JR: Reward processing in primate orbitofrontal cortex and basal ganglia. Cereb Cortex 10:272–284, 2000

Schwartz MW, Woods SC, Porte D Jr, et al: Central nervous system control of food intake. Nature 404:661–671, 2000

Shiiya T, Nakazato M, Mizuta M, et al: Plasma ghrelin levels in lean and obese humans and the effect of glucose on ghrelin secretion. J Endocrinol Metab 87:240–244, 2002

Shively C, Friedman D, Gage H, et al: Behavioral depression and positron emission tomography-determined serotonin 1A receptor binding potential in cynomolgus monkeys. Arch Gen Psychiatry 63:396–403, 2006

Sibille E, Pavlides C, Benke D, et al: Genetic inactivation of the serotonin(1A) receptor in mice results in downregulation of major GABA(A) receptor alpha subunits, reduction of GABA(A) receptor binding, and benzodiazepine-resistant anxiety. J Neurosci 20:2758–2765, 2000

Silberg J, Bulik C: Developmental association between eating disorders symptoms and symptoms of depression and anxiety in juvenile twin girls. J Child Psychol Psychiatry 46:1317–1326, 2005

Simansky KJ: Serotonergic control of the organization of feeding and satiety. Behav Brain Res 73:37–42, 1996

Small D, Zatorre R, Dagher A, et al: Changes in brain activity related to eating chocolate: from pleasure to aversion. Brain 124:1720–1733, 2001

Soubrie P: Reconciling the role of central serotonin neurons in human and animal behavior. Behav Brain Sci 9:319, 1986

Spielberger CD, Gorsuch RL, Lushene RE: STAI Manual for the State Trait Anxiety Inventory. Mountain View, CA, Consulting Psychologists Press, 1970

Srinivasagam NM, Kaye WH, Plotnicov KH, et al: Persistent perfectionism, symmetry, and exactness after long-term recovery from anorexia nervosa. Am J Psychiatry 152:1630–1634, 1995

Staley J, Malison R, Innis R: Imaging of the serotonergic system: interactions of neuroanatomical and functional abnormalities of depression. Biol Psychiatry 44:534–549, 1998

Steiger H, Richardson J, Israel M, et al: Reduced density of platelet-binding sites for [3H]paroxetine in remitted bulimic women. Neuropsychopharmacology 30:1028–1032, 2005

Stock S, Leichner P, Wong A, et al: Ghrelin, peptide YY, glucose-dependent insulinotropic polypeptide, and hunger responses to a mixed meal in anorexic, obese, and control female adolescents. J Clin Endocrinol Metab 90:2161–2168, 2005

Stockmeier CA: Neurobiology of serotonin in depression and suicide. Ann N Y Acad Sci 836:220–232, 1997

Stoving RK, Hangaard J, Hansen-Nord M, et al: A review of endocrine changes in anorexia nervosa. J Psychiatr Res 33:139–152, 1999

Strober M: Personality and symptomatological features in young, nonchronic anorexia nervosa patients. J Psychosom Res 24:353–359, 1980

Strober M: Family genetic perspectives on anorexia nervosa and bulimia nervosa, in Eating Disorders and Obesity: A Comprehensive Handbook. Edited by Brownell K, Fairburn C. New York, Guilford, 1995, pp 212–218

Strober M, Freeman R, Lampert C, et al: Controlled family study of anorexia nervosa and bulimia nervosa: evidence of shared liability and transmission of partial syndromes. Am J Psychiatry 157:393–401, 2000

Strober M, Freeman R, Lampert C, et al: The association of anxiety disorders and obsessive compulsive personality disorder with anorexia nervosa: evidence from a family study with discussion of nosological and neurodevelopmental implications. Int J Eat Disord 40 (suppl):S46–S51, 2007

Sullivan PF, Bulik CM, Kendler KS: The epidemiology and classification of bulimia nervosa. Psychol Med 28:599–610, 1998

Szabo ST, Blier P: Serotonin (1A) receptor ligands act on norepinephrine neuron firing through excitatory amino acid and GABA(A) receptors: a microiontophoretic study in the rat locus coeruleus. Synapse 42:203–212, 2001

Takano A, Shiga T, Kitagawa N, et al: Abnormal neuronal network in anorexia nervosa studied with I-123-IMP SPECT. Psychiatry Research: Neuroimaging 107:45–50, 2001

Tamai H, Takemura J, Kobayashi N, et al: Changes in plasma cholecystokinin concentrations after oral glucose tolerance test in anorexia nervosa before and after therapy. Metab Clin Exp 42:581–584, 1993

Tanaka M, Naruo T, Muranaga T, et al: Increased fasting plasma ghrelin levels in patients with bulimia nervosa. Eur J Endocrinol 146:R1–R3, 2002

Tiihonen J, Keski-Rahkonen A, Lopponen M, et al: Brain serotonin 1A receptor binding in bulimia nervosa. Biol Psychiatry 55:871, 2004

Tozzi F, Bergen AW, Bulik CM: Candidate gene studies in eating disorders. Psychopharmacol Bull 36:60–90, 2002

Treasure J, Campbell I: The case for biology in the aetiology of anorexia nervosa. Psychol Med 24:3–8, 1994

Tschop M, Wawarta R, Reiepl R, et al: Postprandial decrease of circulating human ghrelin levels. J Endocrinol Invest 24:RC19–RC21, 2001

Uher R, Brammer M, Murphy T, et al: Recovery and chronicity in anorexia nervosa: brain activity associated with differential outcomes. Biol Psychiatry 54:934–942, 2003

Uher R, Murphy T, Brammer M, et al: Medial prefrontal cortex activity associated with symptom provocation in eating disorders. Am J Psychiatry 161:1238–1246, 2004

Uher R, Murphy T, Friederich HC, et al: Functional neuroanatomy of body shape perception in healthy and eating-disordered women. Biol Psychiatry 58:990–997, 2005

van Heeringen C, Audenaert K, Van Laere K, et al: Prefrontal 5-HT2a receptor binding index, hopelessness and personality characteristics in attempted suicide. J Affect Disord 74:149–158, 2003

Vink T, Hinney A, van Elburg AA, et al: Association between an agouti-related protein gene polymorphism and anorexia nervosa. Mol Psychiatry 6:325–328, 2001

Vitousek K, Manke F: Personality variables and disorders in anorexia nervosa and bulimia nervosa. J Abnorm Psychol 103:137–147, 1994

Wade T, Martin NG, Tiggemann M: Genetic and environmental risk factors for the weight and shape concerns characteristic of bulimia nervosa. Psychol Med 28:761–771, 1998

Wade T, Neale MC, Eaves LJ, et al: A genetic analysis of the eating and attitudes associated with bulimia nervosa: dealing with the problem of ascertainment. Behav Genet 29:1–10, 1999

Wade TD, Bulik CM, Neale M, et al: Anorexia nervosa and major depression: shared genetic and environmental risk factors. Am J Psychiatry 157:469–471, 2000

Wagner A, Ruf M, Braus DF, et al: Neuronal activity changes and body image distortion in anorexia nervosa. Neuroreport 14:2193–2197, 2003

Wagner A, Barbarich N, Frank G, et al: Personality traits after recovery from eating disorders: do subtypes differ? Int J Eat Disord 39:276–284, 2006a

Wagner A, Greer P, Bailer U, et al: Normal brain tissue volumes after long-term recovery in anorexia and bulimia nervosa. Biol Psychiatry 59:291–293, 2006b

Wagner A, Aizenstein H, Frank GK, et al: Altered insula response to a taste stimulus in individuals recovered from restricting-type anorexia nervosa. Neuropsychopharmacology 33:513–523, 2008

Walsh BT, Roose SP, Katz JL, et al: Hypothalamic-pituitary-adrenal-cortical activity in anorexia nervosa and bulimia. Psychoneuroendocrinology 12:131–140, 1987

Walters EE, Kendler KS: Anorexia nervosa and anorexic-like syndromes in a population-based female twin sample. Am J Psychiatry 152:64–71, 1995

Westergaard G, Suomi S, Chavanne T, et al: Physiological correlates of aggression and impulsivity in free-ranging female primates. Neuropsychopharmacology 28:1045–1055, 2003

Wren A, Seal L, Cohen M, et al: Ghrelin enhances appetite and increases foot intake in humans. J Clin Endocrinol Metab 86:5992–5995, 2001

Wu JC, Hagman J, Buchsbaum MS, et al: Greater left cerebral hemisphere metabolism in bulimia assessed by positron emission tomography. Am J Psychiatry 147:309–312, 1990

CHAPTER 51

Neurobiology of Personality Disorders

Royce Lee, M.D.

Emil F. Coccaro, M.D.

The personality disorders as represented in the DSM-IV-TR (American Psychiatric Association 2000) and ICD-10 (World Health Organization 1992) classification systems are characterized by trait-like disturbances in emotion, cognition, and social function. As a group, they share the important commonalities of chronic course with early onset, relative preservation of intelligence, and absence of gross neurological deficit. In order to summarize the neurobiological literature, we have chosen a heuristic organization that emphasizes the location of "lesion" of personality disorder within neural networks mediating mental activity. This is opposed to a model that locates the lesion in *personality*, phenomenology (Siever and Davis 1991), or molecules. All of these are equally valid as heuristics. The advantage of this approach is that it allows a novel, useful reorganization of the existing database, characterized by a close relationship between the identified neurobiological abnormalities and a neurobiologically plausible brain-based model.

We propose that three principal neurobiological processes may be affected lastingly in personality disorder: 1) representation, the working memory process whereby information about the environment is accurately held in biological neural networks; 2) metarepresentation, multidimensional representations of aspects of the self, the environment, and others that permit self-consciousness and social interaction; and 3) motivation and emotion, the process by which discrepancy between an internal moti-

vational state and current state is registered by neurotransmitter- and/or neuropeptide-mediated feedback loops.

This model is clearly not complete, nor is it intended to propose the existence of three biologically discrete categories of personality disorder. Its value is that it facilitates organization of recent findings regarding the neurobiology of personality disorder into a model of mind–brain operations that will remain compatible with rapid advances in the neurosciences in the near future.

What Is a Neurobiology of Personality Disorders?

There is no question that the brain mediates normal and abnormal mental activity. However, it is fair to ask if speaking of a *neurobiology* of personality disorders is a *category mistake*, a mixture of incompatible forms of knowledge. On the one hand, there is general agreement that some aspects of personality disorder (e.g., anxiety proneness, impulsivity) are validly modeled by genetically based, molecularly mediated *traits* that are preserved across cultures (Yamagata et al. 2006). Such traits can be biologically and behaviorally modeled in nonhuman animals. This approach is firmly validated by the remarkable preservation of the molecular building blocks of brain and nervous function throughout evolution and across species, as exemplified by the similarity of amino acid sequences for neurotransmitters, neuropeptides, and associated receptor systems across phylogenies. Alterations of these systems bias behavior and mentation *probabilistically*. This molecularly based, dimensional *trait* perspective has proven to be of value in reducing the complexity of brain and behavioral relationships. However, the dimensional trait perspective does not account for other important features of personality disorder (e.g., suicide, self-injury, social dysfunction) that do not yet have animal model equivalents and to date are most readily studied in human volunteers, using techniques such as behavioral measurements, electrophysiology, functional neuroimaging, and quantitative assay of biological specimens. It is assumed that these complex phenomena develop over time, with interaction between genes and environment, and involve decision-making processes. It is not yet clear if these represent trait-like dimensions, or if there are clear demarcations between abnormality and normality. As has been pointed out by Kendler (2005), overly strict biological reductionism is an insufficient approach, insofar as the complexity of the molecular determinants is more than matched by the complexity of neuronal networks that have developed in interaction with the environment. However, personality disorders are still clearly biological in the sense that their symptoms are mediated by dysfunction in neuronal networks located in the brain. Definitive progress will eventually depend on our ability to adequately model the biological neural networks and developmental processes that underlie what has traditionally been understood in psychiatry in psychological or *folk psychological* terms.

A heuristic approach to organizing the existing database is justified by the lack of certainty that existing personality disorder categories truly carve "at nature's joints." The most recent behavioral genetic studies confirm the existence of complex genetic relationships *between and within* the Cluster A, B, and C disorders as currently defined (Fogelson et al. 2007; Kendler et al. 2007; Reichborn-Kjennerud et al. 2007; Torgersen et al. 2008). The results are too complex to summarize here, but they simultaneously *confirm some* and *dispute other* cluster, dimensional, and categorical attempts at personality disorder description. An important conclusion of this work is that speaking of the neurobiology of any given specific Axis II disorder is premature without the caveat that the current Axis II nosology contains heterogeneity and overlap. Thus, becoming overly focused on differences and similarities between disorders (e.g., antisocial vs. borderline personality disorder) could result in conclusions that are invalid due to invalid premises.

Representation

The process whereby information regarding the environment is represented in symbolic form by electrophysiological activity in biological neural networks is known as *representation*. Abnormalities in representation are the prominent feature of schizotypal personality disorder, but stress may cause transient abnormal representation in the Cluster B disorders as well.

Representation is mediated by reverberant neural activity (i.e., oscillations) over widely distributed and highly interconnected networks of pyramidal cells and associated neurons. Persistence of activity in networked circuits of corticothalamic and cortico-cortico neurons can sustain a neural representation even after the original stimulus is no longer present. If the representation concerns an environmental stimulus, the corresponding areas of primary and secondary sensory cortex mediate representation of sensory information, but other brain regions are also activated in the process. For example, verbal working memory tasks are associated with activation of parietal and cerebellar brain regions, in addition to prefrontal and temporal regions (Paulesu et al. 1993). To what extent neural resources are utilized for the representation of a stimulus is partially determined by the salience of the stimulus. The *anticipated* reward value of a stimulus is reflected in the gain of delay activity (persistent activity) of the dorsolateral prefrontal cortex (Postle 2006; Sawaguchi and Yamane 1999), although not all information processed in the brain necessarily passes through circuits in the dorsolateral prefrontal cortex. Thus, working memory processes are shaped by the interaction of attention and representation (Fuster 2006).

It is useful here to review the biological building blocks of working memory before moving on to abnormalities associated with personality disorder. Synchronization of network oscillations is regulated by fast-spiking γ-aminobutyric acid (GABA) neurons, which are in turn modulated by glutamate inputs. Network oscillations facilitate information transfer across different brain regions, and according to the *global workspace theory*, their synchronization is important for the binding of disparate aspects of a stimulus in conscious awareness. According to the Cohen-Braver-Brown hypothesis (Cohen et al. 2002), dopamine plays a key role in modulating the activity of oscillating cortical circuits. An optimal balance of tonic (D_1) and phasic (D_2) dopaminergic tone shapes the signal-to-noise characteristics of information flow in the prefrontal cortical neural networks. Tonic D_1 receptor stimulation stabilizes neural network activity around attractors. Phasic "bursts" of D_2 receptor stimulation in the striatum reset prefrontal cortical neural networks and open a subcortical, striatal "gate" for salient information. D_1 and D_2 functions are interrelated, with D_1 tone restraining D_2 activity. The end result of low D_1 tone according to the computation model is reduced signal-to-noise ratio, instability of neural network state, and aberrant assignment of salience to information. This may be apparent to an outside observer as increased distractibility and unreliable or invalid salience being attributed to stimuli. It may also be measured by an observer as eye-tracking abnormalities. The reason for this is that tracking of a moving object in space with the eyes requires working memory "buffers" to constantly update and store visual information and eye movement position.

Abnormalities in the Neurobiology of Representation in Schizotypal Personality Disorder

It is of great interest then that schizotypal personality disorder has been associated with eye-tracking abnormalities (Siever et al. 1991) and that eye-tracking abnormalities are correlated with the dimensional severity of psychotic-like and schizotypal-like characteristics (Siever et al. 1984). Confirmation of connections between eye-tracking abnormalities and schizotypy comes from follow-up studies of visual and auditory attention/working memory (Condray and Steinhauer 1992; Harvey et al. 1996; Lees Roitman et al. 1997; Siever 1985). Neurophysiological studies have found disturbed neural network function during working memory tasks in schizotypal personality disorder, in the form of diminished slow negative potential magnitude (or contingent negative variation) (Klein et al. 1999). Additionally, electroencephalographic activity in the theta-band, believed to correspond to memory-related representational processes and originating from the hippocampal generators, has been found to be decreased in patients with schizotypal personality disorder versus controls (Lazarev 1998).

As dopamine receptor blockade is essential for anti-psychotic drug efficacy, dopamine is a candidate neurotransmitter mediator of psychosis and working memory breakdown. Homovanillic acid (HVA), the product of dopamine metabolism, is measurable in the cerebrospinal fluid (CSF) and may serve as an index of brain dopamine activity. CSF HVA levels are positively related to severity of psychotic-like symptoms in schizotypal personality disorder (Siever et al. 1991), as has been found in schizophrenia (Pickar et al. 1990). Elevated brain HVA concentration may reflect diminished D_1 receptor activity; D_1 receptors are more widely expressed in the brain relative to D_2 or other dopamine receptors, and administration of D_1 receptor antagonists is associated with increased local HVA concentration (See et al. 1991). As dopamine receptors are most densely expressed in the striatum, dysfunction in this brain region may be related to dopaminergic problems. Lower left and right caudate nucleus volumes have been found in schizotypal personality disorder subjects compared with normal control subjects (Levitt et al. 2002). Consistent with this, schizotypal personality disorder patients exhibit lower resting regional glucose metabolism in the caudate, as compared with patients with schizophrenia or normal control subjects (Shihabuddin et al. 2001). Structural and functional regional findings in the putamen mirror those of the caudate, with schizotypal personality disorder associated with decreased putamen size (Shihabuddin et al. 2001) and resting metabolism (Buchsbaum et al. 1992), although increased putamen resting glucose metabolism is also reported (Shihabuddin et al. 2001). In general, these findings are consistent with underlying abnormalities in striatal structure and function, and they support the plausibility of a dopamine-related functional deficit in striatal gating of information in schizotypal personality disorder.

It would be premature to conclude that there is a localized striatal or frontal "lesion" underlying schizotypal personality disorder, however. The neural circuits implicated in working memory deficits in schizotypal personality disorder are widely distributed across the brain and include the frontal, temporal, and parietal cortex (Koenigsberg et al. 2005). Additionally, brain structural differences between schizotypal personality disorder subjects and controls implicate a wider circuit that includes the temporal lobes and thalamus (Dickey et al. 2002). In summary, a significant body of work describes abnormal function and structure of widely distributed neural circuits involved in working memory and representational processes. Dopamine plays a key role in these processes, and indices of abnormal dopamine function have been associated with schizotypal personality disorder. Other biological factors such as GABA and glutamate are also likely to play a role in dysfunctional representational processes in schizotypal personality disorder but have not yet been extensively studied.

Genetics of Cluster A Personality Disorders

Schizotypal personality disorder is more prevalent among first-degree relatives of persons with schizophrenia. This relationship to schizophrenia seems to be specific to schizotypal personality disorder, as it is present only in diminished form with paranoid, schizoid, and avoidant personality disorder and is absent with borderline personality disorder (BPD) (Fogelson et al. 2007; Kendler et al. 1993). It is thought that the trait of schizotypy is conserved because of the increase in fitness that accompanies some aspects of it, such as creative nonconformity (Nettle 2006) on the behavioral level or neural network complexity on the molecular level (Burns 2004). High heritability (72%) has been found for dimensional measures for schizotypy. Molecular genetics studies confirm shared susceptibility between schizotypal personality disorder and schizophrenia (Fanous et al. 2007). Schizotypy has been associated with a high-activity catechol-O-methyltransferase (COMT) genotype in a single study (Schurhoff et al. 2007), as well as a functional polymorphism of the neuroregulin-1 (NG1) gene (Lin et al. 2005). However, the field is still quite far from understanding the molecular determinants of schizotypy.

Metarepresentation

Disturbed self-concept, empathy, social attribution, and social interaction are critical aspects of personality disorder that are mediated in brain neuron networks by metarepresentation (sometimes referred to as metacognition). Metarepresentation refers to the symbolic representation of the self in the context of its environment. The environment is not merely the physical environment but could include "meta" spaces such as a social environment. Metarepresentational abnormalities include visuospatial processing deficits (BPD), aberrant social cognition (in nearly all personality disorders), and deficiencies in self-awareness (alexithymia, poor self-concept, and inaccurate sense of social worth, primarily in borderline, narcissistic, histrionic, dependent, and avoidant personality disorder).

In addition to the working memory processes of the prefrontal cortex, metarepresentation additionally relies on analog and digital-like computational processes native to the parietal cortex (Tudusciuc and Nieder 2007). Neural networks in these regions are specialized in multimodal sensory and object processing and visuospatial processing, as well as the processing of symbolic objects (i.e., mathematics and language). Importantly, representation of the

position of the self in physical space is dependent on intact parietal function, as lesions here result in the rapid decay of the sense of one's own body position. Movement-related proprioceptive information can refresh the sense of the body in space, but the information rapidly decays until movement occurs again (Arzy et al. 2006a).

All available evidence points toward overlapping neural circuits involved in the processing of the body in physical space and in "social" space. So-called mirror neurons in the parietal lobe respond automatically to the body movements of the self *and* others and reflect the importance of the parietal lobe in social communication, as well as the automatic parallel structure of social cognitive processing. It is not yet clear to what degree these processes are automatic or require effortful attention (reviewed in Satpute and Lieberman 2006). Preliminary findings suggest that at least some portion of metarepresentational processes that mediate social cognition is automatic. Examples include temporoparietal alpha-band electroencephalographic activity evoked during human social interaction and parietal neuron spiking in socializing nonhuman primates (Fujii et al. 2007). Effortful social cognition, such as empathy or accurate attribution, is likewise associated with the activity of the parietal cortex (Fogassi et al. 2005), although prefrontal regions may be necessary for processing of emotion-related information (Saxe 2006). Self-consciousness is another form of metarepresentation that similarly relies on distributed networks that include the frontal, temporal, and parietal brain regions. Intact function of the parietal precuneus may be a *necessary* condition for self-consciousness, as deactivation of the precuneus with anesthetic agents is characterized specifically by a temporary loss of high-order representation of body or self (Cavanna and Trimble 2006; Maquet et al. 1999). Dissociative episodes can be marked by disturbed awareness of one's own body. It is of interest then that stimulation of the temporoparietal junction results in out-of-body experiences similar to those experienced during intense episodes of depersonalization (Arzy et al. 2006b).

Cholinergic neurons from the substantia inominata/nucleus basalis magnocellularis enervate the frontal and parietal cortex. Disruption of the cholinergic neurons of the parietal cortex is associated with impaired attention and learning, in the absence of deficits in classical conditioning, suggesting a role for these parietal neurons in effortful learning (Thiel et al. 2005). Serotonin (5-HT) is also important in the development and function of the parietal cortex. During in utero and infant development, serotonin is a powerful signal for cortical development. Disrupted 5-HT metabolism results in the poorly differentiated laminar cortical barrels (Osterheld-Haas and Hornung 1996), with severe deficits in the development of sensory and cognitive capacities related to the type of cortex affected. Less dramatic variations in 5-HT metabolism, in the form of genetic polymorphisms of the 5-HT transporter and/or monoamine oxidase A enzyme, probably exert their greatest effect during neural development. In adulthood, 5-HT alters signal-to-noise characteristics of pyramidal cell networks, and administration of fluoxetine grossly increases the metabolic rate of the parietal cortex (Buchsbaum et al. 1997).

It is established that metarepresentational capacities are shaped by gene–environment interaction. Biologically informed neural network models confirm the importance of parietal and frontal lobe interactions in shaping development (Edin et al. 2007). The development of visuospatial working memory ability in humans over the first two decades of life is paralleled by age-related changes in frontoparietal network activations during visuospatial working memory performance (Kwon et al. 2002); the protracted time course of this development suggests that the process is complex. Accordingly, connectivity between frontal and parietal lobes has been shown to increase in early childhood and continue to increase through adolescence, as measured by diffusion tensor imaging (DTI) (Olesen et al. 2003). It is biologically plausible that disruptions in normative processes such as abnormal parental care or exposure to environmental toxins could derail optimal development. As an example, in animals early-life environment has been demonstrated to affect the expression of parietal serotonin$_{2A}$ (5-HT$_{2A}$) receptor mRNA (Vazquez et al. 2000).

Parietal Lobe Dysfunction in Borderline Personality Disorder

Patients with BPD have difficulties with visual memory and visuospatial abilities in the absence of gross deficits of executive function (Beblo et al. 2006b). This raises the possibility that in addition to frontolimbic connectivity (see below), BPD may be associated with abnormal frontoparietal connectivity. Electrophysiological evidence corroborating deficits in frontoparietal connectivity includes findings of decreased P300 amplitude to novel stimuli in a multitude of event-related potential (ERP) studies (reviewed in Boutros et al. 2003) and decreased gamma frequency range neural synchrony of posterior cortical regions during early phases of stimulus processing (Williams et al. 2006). Criminal psychopaths have also been found to have decreased amplitude of late (>300 msec) positivity

over parietal electrodes to novel stimuli (Howard and McCullagh 2007), suggesting that this abnormal parietal neural synchronization may underlie the known overlap between borderline and antisocial personality disorder.

In addition to the electrophysiological abnormalities, BPD has been consistently linked to structural and functional parietal findings. Patients with BPD compared with matched controls have smaller parietal lobe volume (Irle et al. 2005) and diminished resting parietal metabolic rate (Lange et al. 2005; Lepping and Swinton 2004). During tasks designed to stress cortical circuits, BPD patients show exaggerated parietal metabolism (Beblo et al. 2006a; Schnell et al. 2007). This is interpretable as a compensatory mechanism for decreased processing efficiency. Parietal serotonergic function may be impaired as well, as there is evidence of decreased parietal metabolic activation following pharmacochallenge with the 5-HT releasing agent fenfluramine in BPD (Soloff et al. 2000).

Disturbances in Awareness

Dissociation is perhaps the most dramatic disturbance of metarepresentation, in which the experience of the self is disturbed. Dissociation usually occurs during a stressful experience and is most closely associated with BPD. Although dissociation is usually associated with psychopathology, it can also be evoked in healthy individuals, although without the same level of severity. Evidence suggests that the tendency to dissociate is heritable (Jang et al. 1998) and is associated with emotion dysregulation and suspiciousness (de Ruiter et al. 2007). Thus, its neurobiology should be tractable to investigation.

States of stress and high arousal are characterized by glutamatergic, dopaminergic, and noradrenergic hyperactivity that may impair prefrontal cortical information-processing ability. Dopamine and norepinephrine function are thought to exhibit an inverted U-shaped relationship with prefrontal cortical information-processing capacity. It has been hypothesized that dissociation permits learning during an otherwise overwhelmed, dysfunctional state (de Ruiter et al. 2007), or it may serve to decrease arousal by modulating neural function in the prefrontal, limbic, and parietal brain regions, in much the same way that hypnosis decreases pain perception by modulating brain function (Roder et al. 2007). On the other hand, dissociation does not always occur in reaction to stress. In depersonalization disorder, individuals may feel dissociated in the absence of stress, and during these episodes, metabolism is increased in the right parietal lobe (Simeon et al. 2000).

Individuals with depersonalization disorder, like patients with BPD, also show deficits in visuospatial information processing, with deficits in visual working memory and spatial reasoning. Therefore, individuals prone to dissociation may have an underlying parietal cortex vulnerability or faulty connectivity with the parietal cortex. This vulnerability could manifest itself at baseline with subtle difficulties in visual working memory; under stress, the vulnerability may be unmasked in a breakdown in metarepresentation of the self or even in representation of the environment. We do not yet know whether the underlying biological abnormalities also affect self-awareness in social cognition (e.g., representation of one's own social value). However, a lack of awareness of one's actual social worth is manifested in narcissistic and antisocial personality disorder as overestimation of one's self-worth and contempt for others. In BPD and histrionic personality disorder, it is manifested by contempt for the self and dependency on others. Very little attention has been paid to why these seemingly opposite tendencies occur in genetically related disorders and whether this phenomenon represents a sexually dimorphic expression of a common neurobiological problem.

Perfectionism

Perfectionism is a psychological tendency to hold the self or others to an unnatural standard with respect to performance, beauty, or other attributes. It is most closely associated with obsessive-compulsive personality disorder (OCPD) (Halmi et al. 2005), especially when OCPD is comorbid with an eating disorder or obsessive-compulsive disorder (OCD) (Coles et al. 2008). Abnormal dopaminergic function is implicated in perfectionism. OCPD has been associated with polymorphisms of the dopamine D_3 receptor gene (Light et al. 2006). The association is plausible, as stimulation of the striatal D_3 receptors can cause compulsive, repetitive behavior. The severity of perfectionist traits in eating disorders has been associated with DRD4 polymorphisms (Bachner-Melman et al. 2007). Dopaminergic abnormalities would be expected to heighten approach/avoidance conflicts that occur during evaluation of self or others. Such a process would in theory result in behavioral manifestations of perfectionism. 5-HT dysfunction may also play a role. By inhibiting reversal learning, serotonergic deficits may contribute to the narrow focus on seemingly arbitrary or inappropriate goals (Clarke et al. 2007). Further work is necessary to explore specific relationships between serotonergic function and perfectionism in OCPD.

Motivation and Emotion

Disturbances in brain-based motivational and emotion systems result in some of the most self-destructive symptoms of personality disorder, such as suicidality, self-injury, violence, and reckless behavior. Psychological conceptualizations of emotion have tended to emphasize the subjective experience of affect and how this is mediated by brain activity. Although useful, this emphasis runs the danger of placing a hidden observer in an infinitely receding phrenological conception of brain function and when overemphasized results in a conceptual and clinical dead end. Neural network models of brain function focus on the more tractable issue of *feedback systems for control*. Hence, E. T. Rolls (2000) defined emotion is an internal motivational state transiently evoked by positive or negative reinforcers. The experience of affect provides motivation for motor behavior, whether it is appropriate and/or adaptive or not. So-called *primary reinforcers* include stimuli with intrinsic negative or positive survival significance (e.g., the pleasant taste of palatable food). So-called *secondary reinforcers* are more complex, involving multidimensional representations (e.g., a context of perceived social threat). Thus, emotional processes involve the modification of representations of the reinforcement value of an attended stimulus (e.g., the appetitive aspects of the odor of food) by a continuously updated representation, or metarepresentation, of motivational state (e.g., nutritional need). Thus, both emotion and motivation are slightly different aspects of a complex system that has evolved to guide decision making and behavior.

Circuits that traverse, among other brain regions, the amygdala and orbitofrontal cortex are necessary to be able to update the reinforcement value of a stimulus held in working memory with new information. Circuits including the medial prefrontal cortex, orbitofrontal cortex, insula, amygdala, bed nucleus of the stria terminalis, parietal lobes, and cerebellum are involved in the maintenance of internal motivational states and affect. Induction of such subjective states can predictably bias the interpretation of internal and external stimuli and thus have a strong but *probabilistic* effect on motor response. Abstract representations of motivational state are mediated by hypothalamic and brain stem networks. Within these structures, neuropeptides such as corticotropin-releasing hormone (CRH), vasopressin, and oxytocin play important signaling roles. Disruption of normal neuropeptide signaling results in abnormal development and severe dysregulation of motivated behaviors such as

feeding, sex, and attachment. Neuropeptide signaling appears to play a *deterministic* role on behavior. Sometimes, but not necessarily always, these modifications can be accompanied by the induction of a subjective state (e.g., hunger). Finally, working memory and metarepresentation are both implicated in emotion in motivation, as these processes require reinforcement information to be sustained and processed.

All three of the monoamine neurotransmitters (serotonin, norepinephrine, and dopamine) have receptors in frontal cortical and limbic brain regions. Stimulation of monoamine receptors with a change in synaptic monoamine neurotransmitter level alters the input gain and output gain of information-processing circuits of predominantly pyramidal cell neurons in the cortex. This permits systematic and coordinated adjustment of the signal-to-noise properties of neuronal networks in the cortex. The resulting change in information processing can thus have effects on emotion and motivation. When monoamines are altered by a drug or medication, an artificial state is induced. It is important to remember that usually the brain stem nuclei coordinate changes in monoamine neurotransmitter drive in concert with changes in internal motivational state. Stimulation of monoamine receptors in brain regions such as the hypothalamus can also alter neuropeptide release, and neuropeptides can have more direct effects on emotion and motivation. Finally, monoamine receptor stimulation of brain stem structures may stimulate autoreceptors, which may have global effects on monoamine function. Thus, it is not surprising that altering any one of the three monoamines with psychotropic drugs can reliably alter emotional state. Dopamine powerfully affects the striatum and can thus directly the hedonic quality of stimuli and can quickly affect the motor response to motivational states. Norepinephrine powerfully stimulates the amygdala, prefrontal cortex, and hypothalamus and thus can cause arousal. Even in phylogenetically distant animals such as the mollusk, 5-HT release is involved in the regulation of approach and avoidance behaviors (Inoue et al. 2004). 5-HT is complex in its actions, with phasic-like serotonergic function being implicated in states of high arousal and heightened emotionality and tonic-like serotonergic function being implicated in the regulation of other biological systems such as the hypothalamic-pituitary-adrenal (HPA) axis and dopaminergic function in the striatum and cortex. Additionally, modulation of 5-HT by proserotonergic drugs is known to facilitate reward processing (Vollm et al. 2006).

Nonmonoamine neurotransmitters are also implicated in the neurobiology of abnormal emotion in person-ality disorder. These include the excitatory neurotransmitters (glutamate), inhibitory neurotransmitters (GABA), and the neuropeptides (vasopressin, oxytocin, cholecystokinin, CRH, thyroid hormone).

We have selected four common symptoms of personality disorder that reflect disrupted emotion/motivation systems: 1) impulsivity, 2) aggression, 3) affective instability, and 4) suicide. It is clear that the underlying neurobiology of these "symptoms" overlap, and so it is not surprising that when one is present, the chance of finding others is high.

Impulsivity, Serotonin, and the Orbitofrontal Cortex

Although the term *impulsivity* is sometimes casually employed to describe recklessness, a more careful accounting provides better insight into the underlying process of impulsivity. The ability to delay gratification (or tolerate frustration) relies on delay discounting, mediated by the so-called delay neurons of the orbitofrontal cortex. These neurons encode the time-decay function of the reinforcement value of a stimulus. In general, future rewards are devalued relative to immediate rewards. The steepness of the time-decay function may be modulated by intense motivational states, and thus the steepness probabilistically affects a motor response. Consistent with an underlying orbitofrontal cortex–based defect in the representation of time-delayed reinforcement value, patients with BPD exhibit an abnormal sense of elapsed time (Berlin and Rolls 2004) that is actually more accelerated even than in patients with orbitofrontal cortex lesions. Patients with antisocial personality disorder also show acceleration of time estimation, and this deficit is accompanied by either higher amplitude or faster rise time of the Contingent Negative Variation, a slow (>300 msec) negatively sloped change in cortical electrical field potential over the frontal cortex (Bauer 2001). It is possible that this behavioral abnormality is related to abnormal ventral prefrontal structural connectivity (Rüsch et al. 2007), functional connectivity (New et al. 2007), or function (Soloff et al. 2003).

Impulsivity related to intolerance of frustration can be conceptualized as a manifestation of so-called frustrative nonreward, the phenomenon of increased arousal and appetitive behavior in response to surprising or inconsistent reinforcement. Frustrative nonreward is an aversive state. It is associated with hypothalamic-pituitary activation (Lyons et al. 2000), as well as noradrenergic activation. Indeed, severity of impulsivity is correlated with sensitiv-

ity to frustrative nonreward (Douglas and Parry 1994). As frustrative nonreward involves the neural circuits controlling appetitive behavior, it is abolished by depletion of dopamine, which is released in response to reward availability (Taghzouti et al. 1985). Trait impulsivity is also linked to dopamine, as individuals with higher trait impulsivity show greater sensitization of dopamine release in the ventral striatum, dorsal caudate nucleus, and putamen, as measured by [^{11}C]raclopride binding (Boileau et al. 2006). Additionally, genetic polymorphisms of COMT and DRD2 (the gene encoding the D$_4$ dopamine receptor) predict impulsivity-related personality traits (Reuter et al. 2006). Impulsive reward-sensitive individuals are more likely to experience frustrative nonreward (Corr 2002). 5-HT has been demonstrated to have a constraining effect on impulsivity. It is possible that personality disorder patients high in impulsivity may thus have deficiencies in serotonergic modulation of the aversive aspects of frustrative nonreward and consequently have greater difficulty suppressing appetitive behaviors even when they are harmful. Impulsive BPD patients have higher availability of the 5-HT transporter in the hypothalamus and brain stem, as measured by [I^{123}]ADAM (2-([2-([dimethyl-amino]methyl)phenyl]thio)), a 5-HT transporter–specific radioactive ligand (Koch et al. 2007). They may also have lower 5-HT synthesis capacity in the medial prefrontal gyrus, anterior cingulate gyrus, temporal gyrus, and striatum, as evidenced by a brain PET imaging using the tryptophan precursor tracer α-[^{11}C] methyl-L-tryptophan (α-[^{11}C]MTrp) (Leyton et al. 2001). Increased 5-HT transporter availability and decreased 5-HT synthesis could result in a relative hyposerotonergic state, which in turn could decrease frustration tolerance or increase frustrative nonreward, thereby contributing to impulsivity.

While impulsivity in BPD is linked to emotion dysregulation, some manifestations of impulsivity may be linked to emotional underarousal and insensitivity to negative reinforcement. In psychopathic individuals with antisocial personality disorder, impulsivity has been linked to decreased trait anxiety (Fowles 2000) and decreased skin conductance (sympathetic underarousal). These deficits most likely reflect inadequate or abnormal reactivity of limbic and prefrontal neuronal networks. This has been demonstrated as decreased blood oxygen level–dependent (BOLD) signal response in limbic and prefrontal networks following exposure to arousing and aversive stimuli (Birbaumer et al. 2005). In contrast to impulsivity, deceitful aspects of psychopathy may be related to increased, rather than decreased, serotonergic function, as measured by prolactin response to fenfluramine (Dolan

and Anderson 2003). These findings would predict that augmenting serotonergic function with medications would not be expected to alter deceitful aspects of psychopathy. On the other hand, knowledge of subsensitivity to punishment and anxiety, and relative hypersensitivity to reward, may be utilized in the treatment of individuals with substance abuse disorders, many of whom exhibit psychopathic traits (Messina et al. 2003).

Aggression

Aggression encountered in personality disorder is typically classified as impulsive versus nonimpulsive. There is little evidence of a biological distinction between the two subtypes, but the most systematic work has focused on so-called impulsive, reactive, or affective aggression. Impulsive aggression in personality disorder is typically encountered in patients with Cluster A or B disorders. Impulsive aggressive episodes do not typically result in homicide but may result in injury, property damage, or reputation damage. By definition, they cause dysfunction in social relationships. Triggers for acts of impulsive aggression are usually either agonistic social interactions or frustration. Neuropeptides such as CRH, vasopressin, and oxytocin play an important role as mediators of change in social motivational state. Monoamines, as reviewed above, are important in mediating emotional reactivity (anger, contempt) and in processes related to impulsivity (frustrative nonreward). Thus, impulsive aggression represents a complex phenomenon, concatenating social behavior, emotion, and impulsivity.

A considerable amount of research has focused on the finding of low 5-HT metabolite levels in abnormal aggression. A simple correlation between 5-HT "level" and aggression is probably invalid, given the complexity of 5-HT's role in a wide range of neural functions. 5-HT levels in the brain are at their lowest during rapid eye movement sleep, but are acutely and phasically released in the brain during agonistic social encounters between conspecifics. Interestingly, prefrontal cortical levels of 5-HT and 5-hydroxyindoleacetic acid (5-HIAA) decrease preceding an aggressive attack (van Erp and Miczek 2000), suggesting that regardless of what happens after an aggressive encounter, low prefrontal 5-HT remains a risk factor for aggressive behavior. In total, these data suggest that low 5-HT in prefrontal cortical circuits may prime an aggressive response, while elevated 5-HT levels during agonistic encounters reflect 5-HT released during motor activity. Early human studies found reduced levels of CSF 5-HIAA to be associated with aggression and suicidal behavior (Brown

et al. 1979) and impulsive homicide (Linnoila et al. 1983), although not all studies to date have found an inverse relationship between CSF 5-HIAA and aggression (Balaban et al. 1996). CSF 5-HIAA provides an incomplete picture of serotonergic function, and thus other indices have been examined. Fenfluramine, which is an agonist at the 5-HT_{2A} and/or 5-HT_{2C} receptor site, has been used extensively to study postsynaptic 5-HT receptor function by measuring the pituitary prolactin response to fenfluramine challenge (Coccaro et al. 1996; Park and Cowen 1995). Coccaro et al. (1989) found that aggression was correlated with decreased prolactin response to fenfluramine in personality disorder subjects. The correlation of decreased responsiveness of the serotonergic system with impulsive aggression has been replicated in personality disorder subjects (Stein et al. 1996), in antisocial violent offenders (O'Keane et al. 1992), and in primates (Botchin et al. 1993) and remains one of the most replicated findings in biological and clinical psychiatric research.

A separate strand of research has focused on the role of the prefrontal cortex in impulsive aggression. Aggressive personality disorder individuals have reduced resting state metabolism in the orbitofrontal cortex and right temporal lobe (Goyer et al. 1994). These metabolic abnormalities may be related to an underlying structural abnormality in neural circuits residing in prefrontal cortical gray matter, which is reduced in volume in aggressive antisocial personality disorder individuals (Raine et al. 2000). Impulsive aggressive individuals have exaggerated amygdala blood flow *increases* and orbitofrontal blood flow *decreases* in response to passive viewing of angry facial expressions (Coccaro et al. 2007). As impulsive aggression has previously been associated with difficulty in correctly identifying angry and disgusted facial expressions (Best et al. 2002), this suggests that the increased amygdala blood flow response measured by functional magnetic resonance imaging (fMRI) during viewing of angry faces may reflect inefficiency in neural network processing, in line with resting state and structural study findings. Findings of disturbed structure of inferior frontal white tracts in impulsive, hostile BPD (with comorbid attention-deficit/hyperactivity disorder [ADHD]) patients provide confirmatory evidence of abnormal prefrontal cortex neuronal network architecture as a biological risk factor (Rüsch et al. 2007).

Uniting findings of the serotonergic deficits with prefrontal cortex deficits, several studies now have found serotonergic abnormalities on the brain regional level. Administration of 5-HT receptor agonists in impulsive aggressive individuals results in blunted metabolic activa-

tions in orbitofrontal, ventromedial, parietal, and cingulate cortex (New et al. 2002; Siever et al. 1999; Soloff et al. 2000). Putting these findings together, the following interpretations are plausible. The first possibility is that 5-HT receptor subsensitivity in the prefrontal cortex may reflect decreased dynamic range of 5-HT-related neuronal function, and this in turn contributes to aggressive behavior. The second possibility is that aggressive behavior, or other high arousal states, results in compensatory blunting of postsynaptic serotonergic function. Arguing for the validity of the first interpretation and a causal role for serotonergic dysfunction in aggression is the finding that treatment with selective serotonin reuptake inhibitor (SSRI) drugs such as fluoxetine has been shown to *decrease* aggression in personality disorder patients (Coccaro et al. 1997). Additionally, treatment with fluoxetine is associated with increased resting orbitofrontal cortical metabolism, as measured by positron emission tomography (PET) imaging (New et al. 2004), with some evidence of greater efficacy in patients who carry the L allele versus the less potent S allele of the 5-HT transporter (Silva et al. 2007).

Animal studies have clearly implicated vasopressin as a neuropeptide mediator of aggressive behavior (Ferris et al. 1994). Coccaro et al. (1998) found that resting CSF vasopressin level correlated directly with life history measures of aggression in personality disordered subjects, whereas CSF oxytocin correlates inversely (unpublished data). Although in rodents vasopressin has been demonstrated to directly affect aggressive behavior, it also affects nonaggressive social behaviors such as flank marking. Thus, vasopressin appears to modulate social motivation, above and beyond its effects on aggressive behavior.

Social motivation shares with emotion the representation of an internal motivational state (affiliation and/or dominance) and is highly conserved in vertebrates. The ability to use visual information regarding spatial position as feedback regarding social dominance is confirmed even in fish (Grosenick et al. 2007). Metarepresentation of the social environment may rely on circuits that originally served in the metarepresentation of spatial self–other relationships. As an example, the spatial position of an individual bird in a flock can powerfully predict feeding success and protection from predators (Krause 1994). Finally, the internal motivational state may itself be shifted by hormonal factors into new configurations, such as the effect of testosterone on dominance (Gould and Ziegler 2007) or menstrual cycle–related changes on sexual desire. Incentive-driven social behavior probably relies on the same limbic neurocircuitry that guides other incentive-driven behaviors, as is illustrated by the effect of

amygdala lesions on dominance status (Bauman et al. 2006). Further work needs to be done in order to better understand how changes in social motivational state may alter impulsive aggression.

Affective Instability, Frontolimbic Brain Function, and Acetylcholine

In BPD, affective instability is manifest as excessive mood lability and stress reactivity. In histrionic personality disorder, it is manifest as shallow, shifting affect. In comparison with affective disorder patients, affective instability in BPD patients shows more circadian variability and a more random distribution of mood changes (Cowdry et al. 1991) rather than fluctuations between depressive and elated affects (Larsen and Diener 1985).

Psychophysiological data help to confirm that at least some portion of the affective instability of BPD represents excessive reactivity to stressful stimuli, and not simply a reporting bias or willful social manipulation. In response to startling noise bursts, individuals with BPD exhibit an enhanced startle reflex (Ebner-Priemer et al. 2005). Additionally, the induction of an aroused negative mood state potentiates startle magnitude to a greater degree in BPD patients versus controls (Hazlett et al. 2007). Given that the brain stem and spinal cord basis of the startle reflex is subject to top-down modulation by prefrontal and limbic circuits, these findings are suggestive of disinhibition of the startle reflex by either limbic hyperreactivity or deficient prefrontal cortical control.

Neuroimaging studies have focused on abnormalities of the limbic system. BPD has been associated with decreased left amygdala volume (Driessen et al. 2000; Tebartz van Elst et al. 2007), as well as decreased hippocampal volume (Brambilla et al. 2004). Decreased hippocampal volume has also been associated with history of childhood trauma (Vythilingam et al. 2002) and dissociative identity disorder with posttraumatic stress disorder (Vermetten et al. 2006), raising the possibility that exposure to traumatic stress may cause or magnify a structural brain defect. Given the high rates of abuse and neglect in the childhood history of many patients with Cluster B disorders, this is an important question for future research. Although the amygdala may be smaller than normal in some BPD patients, it appears to be *functionally hyperreactive* during tasks of emotion processing (Minzenberg et al. 2007), especially in response to emotionally ambiguous contexts (Schnell et al. 2007). Because of the importance of reciprocal connections between frontal and limbic brain regions in control and communication, structural

and functional connectivity has been investigated in BPD. DTI of white matter microstructure has revealed aberrant white matter tracts in the inferior prefrontal cortex in patients diagnosed with comorbid BPD and ADHD (Rüsch et al. 2007), suggestive of connectivity abnormalities within prefrontal circuits, between prefrontal and limbic circuits, or between thalamus and prefrontal cortex. A major shortcoming of this work is its lack of clinical applicability (as of yet) and its nonspecificity with regard to personality disorder versus affective or anxiety disorder.

Cholinergic neuronal activity in limbic neural circuits is important for information processing and plasticity. Administration of anticholinergic drugs interferes with emotion-related memory processes (Kamboj and Curran 2006a). Anticholinergic drugs have also been found to selectively impair the recognition of anger and disgust (Kamboj and Curran 2006b). Challenge with cholinergic agents causes limbic activation, which can be detected by changes in limbic blood flow and corresponding induction of mood states of fear and euphoria (Ketter et al. 1997). Following challenge with physostigmine, a procholinergic drug, patients with BPD show more severe depressive mood changes compared with other personality disorder patients. Furthermore, the severity of the depressive response was greater in patients with prominent affective instability (Steinberg et al. 1997).

5-HT plays in an important role in cortical information processing and also in constraining the intensity of limbic and hypothalamic stress reactivity. BPD has been associated with 5-HT-related genetic polymorphisms, including the S allele of the 5-HT transporter (Steiger et al. 2005), and polymorphisms encoding high activity of the monoamine oxidase (MAO) gene (Ni et al. 2007). Serotonergic abnormalities have been linked to affective symptoms. 5-HT$_{2A}$ receptor binding is greater in BPD patients with a history of depression, suggesting a role for the 5-HT$_{2A}$ receptor in at least depressive mood changes (Soloff et al. 2007). Patients with histrionic personality disorder, who exhibit rapidly shifting affects, have increased loudness dependence of auditory evoked potentials (AEPs), which is inversely related to serotonergic tone in the cortex (Wang et al. 2006). Further work needs to be done regarding the uniqueness of association of 5-HT-related genetic polymorphisms with personality disorder versus other disorders.

Studies of the hypothalamic-pituitary axis in BPD have found inconsistent results. Data from studies of the dexamethasone suppression test (Beeber et al. 1984; Sternbach et al. 1983) and the thyrotropin-releasing hor-

mone (TRH) stimulation test (Kavoussi et al. 1993) have been inconclusive. These results highlight the biological heterogeneity of the existing categorical groups and suggest that BPD is not as closely associated with HPA axis abnormalities as is affective disorder. On the other hand, central CSF CRH levels are positively related to the severity of early-life parental abuse and neglect in personality disorder (Lee et al. 2005, 2006). This could be of considerable importance, given the inordinately high rates of history of abuse and/or neglect across personality disorder diagnoses. Additionally, it is consistent with preclinical investigation findings that central CRH drive is lastingly affected by early-life disruption of parental care (Coplan et al. 1996; Plotsky and Meaney 1993) and with evidence of peripheral downregulation of pituitary sensitivity to exogenous CRH from our laboratory (unpublished data) and other laboratories in non–personality disorder populations (Heim et al. 1998). What is the consequence of increased central CRH drive as a result of early-life trauma on the brain and behavior? Given the known effect of administering exogenous CRH on inhibiting socialization in primates (Strome et al. 2002), we would postulate that increased CRH drive would induce a form of social anhedonia, which is partially supported by our finding of an association of paranoid personality disorder with elevated CSF CRH (Lee et al. 2006). Although CRH plays a physiological role in normal behavior that provides phenotypic plasticity during times of stress, decreased dynamic range of CRH systems would render the system inflexible to the environment. This work would suggest that CRH receptor antagonists could be of value in the treatment of paranoid anxiety, as is found in paranoid personality disorder. In summary, it seems that dysregulation of the HPA axis in the Cluster B personality disorders may reflect either underlying affective disorder or exposure to trauma.

Suicide

A mechanistic neurobiological understanding of suicide remains out of reach. Most of the work to date has been an effort to identify biological correlates of psychosocial risk factors. A limited amount of data suggests that self-injurious behavior in personality disorder patients is related to serotonergic abnormalities. New et al. (1997) found that suicidal and self-injurious behavior was associated with blunted prolactin and cortisol responses to D,L-fenfluramine. In a separate study, those with both impulsive and premeditative self-injury were found to have blunted prolactin response to D-fenfluramine compared with normal subjects, suggesting postsynaptic 5-HT receptor downreg-

ulation (Herpertz et al. 1995). However, several recent studies have implicated increased 5-HT_{2A} receptor binding in suicide and impulsivity, including studies of patients with BPD (Soloff et al. 2007). These results support a possible antisuicide effect of chronic antidepressant treatment and/or atypical antipsychotic drugs.

Suicide victims have increased CRH and vasopressin immunoreactivity in the brain, implicating biological mediators of emotional or social motivation in successful suicide (Merali et al. 2006). This important finding provides biological confirmation of data from psychological autopsies of suicide victims; recent social stress is a potent risk factor for suicide. The mechanism whereby environmental stress and the ensuing stress response increase the probability of a suicidal act is not yet identified.

Predictions and Limitations of the Model

One important prediction of our model is that a problem with representation would go on to affect complex processes that rely on representation, such as metarepresentation and/or motivation. The clinical implication would be that patients with working memory deficits might also be expected to additionally exhibit social or emotional deficits. This notion is supported by the high rates of Axis I–Axis II comorbidity in the clinic and the tendency for these comorbidities to occur across cluster categories. The other important clinical implication is that the circuits that are affected in personality disorder are the same circuits that are affected in Axis I disorders such as schizophrenia, anxiety, and depression. This is reflected in ubiquitous Axis I–Axis II comorbidity.

Another important prediction of our model is that the array of neurobiological deficits in clinical patients may be quite complex, and simple models of personality psychopathology based on "limbic hyperreactivity" or "hypofrontality" fail to account for prominent symptom classes such as disturbed sense of self or dissociative symptoms. With regard to these specific symptoms, there may be some benefit in looking outside psychiatry in fields such as learning disorders, which have focused on the parietal cortex as a biological mediator and so-called *metacognition* for therapeutic approaches. Although it is often stated that emotional lability is *the cause* of the unstable sense of self and others found in the Cluster B personality disorders, this has not actually been proven to be true. We would argue that it is plausible that the opposite mechanism may be equally valid, that inaccurate or distorted social cognition/motivation could result in emotional instability. This remains a testable hypothesis.

A model should be able to make quantitative predictions. Our model is clearly not yet quantitative, although it is compatible with a computational approach. For this reason, it remains a *heuristic* model of personality disorder. Brain/neuron-based computational models of personality disorder are not yet available for research purposes but may prove to be useful, if not *absolutely necessary*, to develop more sophisticated, reliable, and effective approaches to neuropsychopharmacology in this population.

Finally, we have also not focused on precise mechanisms of development and change. Although the current emphasis on regional functional brain imaging has resulted in canonization of the lesion model of psychopathology, time may prove this overemphasis to have limits. Careful examination of the literature also reports *positive* changes in personality disorder–related behavior after frontal head injuries (Labbate et al. 1997). Findings such as these call into question the validity of lesion-based models. They also suggest that not-yet-identified compensatory mechanisms in neural network function, rather than restoration of a "lesion," may play a role in both spontaneous (without therapeutic intervention) or therapeutically induced remission from personality disorder.

Conclusion

Meaningful progress in our understanding of the neurobiology of personality disorders brings hope that in the near future this understanding will result in substantive progress in treating these disorders. Clinicians recognize that these disorders can represent serious mental illness, with potentially crippling disability, disproportional public health care expenditure, and tremendous suffering. That progress in our understanding of the neurobiology of personality disorder comes in parallel with growing sophistication of both the basic and clinical neurosciences means that old conceptualizations must be challenged and tested. One advantage of a non-symptom-based heuristic is that the conceptual dissonance caused by the natural overlap of Axis I and Axis II disorders is deemphasized. In other words, this model highlights the biological overlap between these two subclasses of disorders. While previous symptom-based heuristics remain valid, we hope that this one raises new and fruitful questions.

References

American Psychiatric Association: Diagnostic and Statistical Manual of Mental Disorders, 4th Edition, Text Revision. Washington, DC, American Psychiatric Association, 2000

Arzy S, Overney LS, Landis T, et al: Neural mechanisms of embodiment: asomatognosia due to premotor cortex damage. Arch Neurol 63:1022–1025, 2006a

Arzy S, Thut G, Mohr C, et al: Neural basis of embodiment: distinct contributions of temporoparietal junction and extrastriate body area. J Neurosci 26:8074–8081, 2006b

Bachner-Melman R, Lerer E, Zohar AH, et al: Anorexia nervosa, perfectionism, and dopamine D4 receptor (DRD4). Am J Med Genet B Neuropsychiatr Genet 144B:748–756, 2007

Balaban E, Alper JS, Kasamon YL: Mean genes and the biology of aggression: a critical review of recent animal and human research. J Neurogenet 11:1–43, 1996

Bauer LO: Antisocial personality disorder and cocaine dependence: their effects on behavioral and electroencephalographic measures of time estimation. Drug Alcohol Depend 63:87–95, 2001

Bauman MD, Toscano JE, Mason WA, et al: The expression of social dominance following neonatal lesions of the amygdala or hippocampus in rhesus monkeys (Macaca mulatta). Behav Neurosci 120:749–760, 2006

Beblo T, Driessen M, Mertens M, et al: Functional MRI correlates of the recall of unresolved life events in borderline personality disorder. Psychol Med 36:845–856, 2006a

Beblo T, Saavedra AS, Mensebach C, et al: Deficits in visual functions and neuropsychological inconsistency in borderline personality disorder. Psychiatry Res 145:127–135, 2006b

Beeber AR, Kline MD, Pies RW, et al: Dexamethasone suppression test in hospitalized depressed patients with borderline personality disorder. J Nerv Ment Dis 172:301–303, 1984

Berlin HA, Rolls ET: Time perception, impulsivity, emotionality, and personality in self-harming borderline personality disorder patients. J Personal Disord 18:358–378, 2004

Best M, Williams JM, Coccaro EF: Evidence for a dysfunctional prefrontal circuit in patients with an impulsive aggressive disorder. Proc Natl Acad Sci U S A 99:8448–8453, 2002

Birbaumer N, Veit R, Lotze M, et al: Deficient fear conditioning in psychopathy: a functional magnetic resonance imaging study. Arch Gen Psychiatry 62:799–805, 2005

Boileau I, Dagher A, Leyton M, et al: Modeling sensitization to stimulants in humans: an [11C]raclopride/positron emission tomography study in healthy men. Arch Gen Psychiatry 63:1386–1395, 2006

Botchin MB, Kaplan JR, Manuck SB, et al: Low versus high prolactin responders to fenfluramine challenge: marker of behavioral differences in adult male cynomolgus macaques. Neuropsychopharmacology 9:93–99, 1993

Boutros NN, Torello M, McGlashan TH: Electrophysiological aberrations in borderline personality disorder: state of the evidence. J Neuropsychiatry Clin Neurosci 15:145–154, 2003

Brambilla P, Soloff PH, Sala M, et al: Anatomical MRI study of borderline personality disorder patients. Psychiatry Res 131:125–133, 2004

Brown GL, Goodwin FK, Ballenger JC, et al: Aggression in humans correlates with cerebrospinal fluid amine metabolites. Psychiatry Res 1:131–139, 1979

Buchsbaum MS, Potkin SG, Siegel BV, et al: Striatal metabolic rate and clinical response to neuroleptics in schizophrenia. Arch Gen Psychiatry 49:966–974, 1992

Buchsbaum MS, Wu J, Siegel BV, et al: Effect of sertraline on regional metabolic rate in patients with affective disorder. Biol Psychiatry 41:15–22, 1997

Burns JK: An evolutionary theory of schizophrenia: cortical connectivity, metarepresentation, and the social brain. Behav Brain Sci 27:831–885, 2004

Cavanna AE, Trimble MR: The precuneus: a review of its functional anatomy and behavioural correlates. Brain 129:564–583, 2006

Clarke HF, Walker SC, Dalley JW, et al: Cognitive inflexibility after prefrontal serotonin depletion is behaviorally and neurochemically specific. Cereb Cortex 17:18–27, 2007

Coccaro EF, Siever LJ, Klar HM, et al: Serotonergic studies in patients with affective and personality disorders: correlates with suicidal and impulsive aggressive behavior. Arch Gen Psychiatry 46:587–599, 1989

Coccaro EF, Kavoussi RJ, Oakes M, et al: 5-HT2a/2c receptor blockade by amesergide fully attenuates prolactin response to d-fenfluramine challenge in physically healthy human subjects. Psychopharmacology (Berl) 126:24–30, 1996

Coccaro EF, Kavoussi RJ, Hauger RL: Serotonin function and antiaggressive responses to fluoxetine: a pilot study. Biol Psychiatry 42:546–552, 1997

Coccaro EF, Kavoussi RK, Hauger RL, et al: Cerebrospinal fluid vasopressin: correlates with aggression and serotonin function in personality disordered subjects. Arch Gen Psychiatry 55:708–714, 1998

Coccaro EF, McCloskey MS, Fitzgerald DA, et al: Amygdala and orbitofrontal reactivity to social threat in individuals with impulsive aggression. Biol Psychiatry 62:168–178, 2007

Cohen JD, Braver TS, Brown JW: Computational perspectives on dopamine function in prefrontal cortex. Curr Opin Neurobiol 12:223–229, 2002

Coles ME, Pinto A, Mancebo MC, et al: OCD with comorbid OCPD: a subtype of OCD? J Psychiatr Res 42:289–296, 2008

Condray R, Steinhauer SR: Schizotypal personality disorder in individuals with and without schizophrenic relatives: similarities and contrasts in cognitive functioning. Schizophr Res 7:33–41, 1992

Coplan JD, Andrews MW, Rosenblum L, et al: Persistent elevations of cerebrospinal fluid concentrations of corticotropin releasing factor in adult nonhuman primates exposed to early life stressors: implications for the pathophysiology of mood and anxiety disorders. Proc Natl Acad Sci U S A 93:1619–1623, 1996

Corr PJ: JA Gray's reinforcement sensitivity theory and frustrative nonreward: a theoretical note on expectancies in reactions to rewarding stimuli. Personality and Individual Differences 32:1247–1253, 2002

Cowdry RW, Gardner DL, O'Leary KM, et al: Mood variability: a study of four groups. Am J Psychiatry 148:1505–1511, 1991

de Ruiter MB, Veltman DJ, Phaf RH, et al: Negative words enhance recognition in nonclinical high dissociators: an fMRI study. Neuroimage 37:323–334, 2007

Dickey CC, McCarley RW, Shenton ME: The brain in schizotypal personality disorder: a review of structural MRI and CT findings. Harv Rev Psychiatry 10:1–15, 2002

Dolan MC, Anderson IM: The relationship between serotonergic function and the Psychopathy Checklist: Screening Version. J Psychopharmacol 17:216–222, 2003

Douglas VI, Parry PA: Effects of reward and nonreward on frustration and attention in attention deficit disorder. J Abnorm Child Psychol 22:281–302, 1994

Driessen M, Herrmann J, Stahl K, et al: Magnetic resonance imaging volumes of the hippocampus and the amygdala in women with borderline personality disorder and early traumatization. Arch Gen Psychiatry 57:1115–1122, 2000

Ebner-Priemer UW, Badeck S, Beckmann C, et al: Affective dysregulation and dissociative experience in female patients with borderline personality disorder: a startle response study. J Psychiatr Res 39:85–92, 2005

Edin F, Macoveanu J, Olesen P, et al: Stronger synaptic connectivity as a mechanism behind development of working memory-related brain activity during childhood. J Cogn Neurosci 19:750–760, 2007

Fanous AH, Neale MC, Aggen SH, et al: A longitudinal study of personality and major depression in a population-based sample of male twins. Psychol Med 37:1163–1172, 2007

Ferris CF, Delville Y, Irvin RW, et al: Septo-hypothalamic organization of a stereotyped behavior controlled by vasopressin in golden hamsters. Physiol Behav 55:755–759, 1994

Fogassi L, Ferrari PF, Gesierich B, et al: Parietal lobe: from action organization to intention understanding. Science 308:662–667, 2005

Fogelson DL, Neuchterlein KH, Asarnow RA, et al: Avoidant personality disorder is a separable schizophrenia-spectrum personality disorder even when controlling for the presence of paranoid and schizotypal personality disorders. The UCLA family study. Schizophr Res 91:192–199, 2007

Fowles DC: Electrodermal hyporeactivity and antisocial behavior: does anxiety mediate the relationship? J Affect Disord 61:177–189, 2000

Fujii N, Hihara S, Iriki A: Dynamic social adaptation of motion-related neurons in primate parietal cortex. PLoS ONE 2:e397, 2007

Fuster JM: The cognit: a network model of cortical representation. Int J Psychophysiol 60:125–132, 2006

Gould L, Ziegler TE: Variation in fecal testosterone levels, intermale aggression, dominance rank and age during mating and post-mating periods in wild adult male ring-tailed lemurs (Lemur catta). Am J Primatol 69:1325–1339, 2007

Goyer PF, Andreason PJ, Semple WE, et al: Positron-emission tomography and personality disorders. Neuropsychopharmacology 10:21–28, 1994

Grosenick L, Clement TS, Fernald RD: Fish can infer social rank by observation alone. Nature 445:429–432, 2007

Halmi KA, Tozzi F, Thornton LM, et al: The relation among perfectionism, obsessive-compulsive personality disorder and obsessive-compulsive disorder in individuals with eating disorders. Int J Eat Disord 38:371–374, 2005

Harvey PD, Keefe RSE, Mitropoulou V: Attentional markers of vulnerability to schizophrenia: performance of patients with schizotypal and nonschizotypal personality disorders. Psychiatry Res 60:49–56, 1996

Hazlett EA, Speiser LJ, Goodman M, et al: Exaggerated affect-modulated startle during unpleasant stimuli in borderline personality disorder. Biol Psychiatry 62:250–255, 2007

Heim C, Ehlert U, Hanker JP, et al: Abuse-related posttraumatic stress disorder and alterations of the hypothalamic-pituitary-adrenal axis in women with chronic pelvic pain. Psychosom Med 60:309–318, 1998

Herpertz SC, Steinmeyer SM, Marx D, et al: The significance of aggression and impulsivity for self-mutilative behavior. Pharmacopsychiatry 28 (suppl 2):64–72, 1995

Howard R, McCullagh P: Neuroaffective processing in criminal psychopaths: brain event-related potentials reveal task-specific anomalies. J Personal Disord 21:322–339, 2007

Inoue T, Inokuma Y, Watanabe S, et al: In vitro study of odor-evoked behavior in a terrestrial mollusk. J Neurophysiol 91:372–381, 2004

Irle E, Lange C, Sachsse U: Reduced size and abnormal asymmetry of parietal cortex in women with borderline personality disorder. Biol Psychiatry 57:173–182, 2005

Jang KL, Paris J, Zweig-Frank H, et al: Twin study of dissociative experience. J Nerv Ment Dis 186:345–351, 1998

Kamboj SK, Curran HV: Neutral and emotional episodic memory: global impairment after lorazepam or scopolamine. Psychopharmacology (Berl) 188:482–488, 2006a

Kamboj SK, Curran HV: Scopolamine induces impairments in the recognition of human facial expressions of anger and disgust. Psychopharmacology (Berl) 185:529–535, 2006b

Kavoussi RJ, Coccaro EF, Klar H, et al: The TRH-stimulation test in DSM-III personality disorder. Biol Psychiatry 34:234–239, 1993

Kendler KS: Toward a philosophical structure for psychiatry. Am J Psychiatry 162:433–440, 2005

Kendler KS, McGuire M, Gruenberg AM, et al: The Roscommon Family Study, III: schizophrenia-related personality disorders in relatives. Arch Gen Psychiatry 50:781–788, 1993

Kendler KS, Myers J, Torgersen S, et al: The heritability of cluster A personality disorders assessed by both personal interview and questionnaire. Psychol Med 37:655–665, 2007

Ketter TA, Malow BA, Post RM, et al: Psychiatric effects of felbamate. J Neuropsychiatry Clin Neurosci 9:118–119, 1997

Klein C, Berg P, Rockstroh B, et al: Topography of the auditory P300 in schizotypal personality. Biol Psychiatry 45:1612–1621, 1999

Koch W, Schaaff N, Popperl G, et al: [I-123] ADAM and SPECT in patients with borderline personality disorder and healthy control subjects. J Psychiatry Neurosci 32:234–240, 2007

Koenigsberg HW, Buchsbaum MS, Buchsbaum BR, et al: Functional MRI of visuospatial working memory in schizotypal personality disorder: a region-of-interest analysis. Psychol Med 35:1019–1030, 2005

Krause J: Differential fitness returns in relation to spatial position in groups. Biol Rev Camb Philos Soc 69:187–206, 1994

Kwon H, Reiss AL, Menon V: Neural basis of protracted developmental changes in visuo-spatial working memory. Proc Natl Acad Sci U S A 99:13336–13341, 2002

Labbate LA, Warden D, Murray GB: Salutary change after frontal brain trauma. Ann Clin Psychiatry 9:27–30, 1997

Lange C, Kracht L, Herholz K, et al: Reduced glucose metabolism in temporo-parietal cortices of women with borderline personality disorder. Psychiatry Res 139:115–126, 2005

Larsen RJ, Diener E: A multitrait-multimethod examination of anhedonic level and emotional intensity. Pers Individ Diff 6:631–636, 1985

Lazarev VV: On the intercorrelation of some frequency and amplitude parameters of the human EEG and its functional significance. Communication II: neurodynamic imbalance in endogenous asthenic-like disorders. Int J Psychophysiol 29:227–289, 1998

Lee R, Geracioti TD Jr, Kasckow JW, et al: Childhood trauma and personality disorder: positive correlation with adult CSF corticotropin-releasing factor concentrations. Am J Psychiatry 162:995–997, 2005

Lee RJ, Gollan J, Kasckow J, et al: CSF corticotropin-releasing factor in personality disorder: relationship with self-reported parental care. Neuropsychopharmacology 31:2289–2295, 2006

Lees Roitman SE, Cornblatt BA, Bergman A, et al: Attentional functioning in schizotypal personality disorder. Am J Psychiatry 154:655–660, 1997

Lepping P, Swinton M: [Borderline personality disorder associated with psychotic symptoms and parietal lobe abnormalities]. Psychiatr Prax 31:96–99, 2004

Levitt JJ, McCarley RW, Dickey CC, et al: MRI study of caudate nucleus volume and its cognitive correlates in neuroleptic-naive patients with schizotypal personality disorder. Am J Psychiatry 159:1190–1197, 2002

Leyton M, Okazawa H, Diksic M, et al: Brain Regional alpha-[11C]methyl-L-tryptophan trapping in impulsive subjects with borderline personality disorder. Am J Psychiatry 158:775–782, 2001

Light KJ, Joyce PR, Luty SE, et al: Preliminary evidence for an association between a dopamine D3 receptor gene variant and obsessive-compulsive personality disorder in patients with major depression. Am J Med Genet B Neuropsychiatr Genet 141B:409–413, 2006

Lin HF, Liu YL, Liu CM, et al: Neuregulin 1 gene and variations in perceptual aberration of schizotypal personality in adolescents. Psychol Med 35:1589–1598, 2005

Linnoila M, Virkkunen M, Scheinin M, et al: Low cerebrospinal fluid 5-hydroxyindoleacetic acid concentration differentiates impulsive from nonimpulsive violent behavior. Life Sci 33:2609–2614, 1983

Lyons DM, Fong KD, Schrieken N, et al: Frustrative nonreward and pituitary-adrenal activity in squirrel monkeys. Physiol Behav 71:559–563, 2000

Maquet P, Faymonville ME, Degueldre C, et al: Functional neuroanatomy of hypnotic state. Biol Psychiatry 45:327–333, 1999

Merali Z, Kent P, Du L, et al: Corticotropin-releasing hormone, arginine vasopressin, gastrin-releasing peptide, and neuromedin B alterations in stress-relevant brain regions of suicides and control subjects. Biol Psychiatry 59:594–602, 2006

Messina N, Farabee D, Rawson R: Treatment responsivity of cocaine-dependent patients with antisocial personality disorder to cognitive-behavioral and contingency management interventions. J Consult Clin Psychol 71:320–329, 2003

Minzenberg MJ, Fan J, New AS, et al: Fronto-limbic dysfunction in response to facial emotion in borderline personality disorder: an event-related fMRI study. Psychiatry Res 155:231–243, 2007

Nettle D: Schizotypy and mental health amongst poets, visual artists, and mathematicians. J Res Pers 40:876–890, 2006

New AS, Trestman RL, Mitropoulou V, et al: Serotonergic function and self-injurious behavior in personality disorder patients. Psychiatry Res 69:17–26, 1997

New AS, Hazlett EA, Buchsbaum MS, et al: Blunted prefrontal cortical 18fluorodeoxyglucose positron emission tomography response to meta-chlorophenylpiperazine in impulsive aggression. Arch Gen Psychiatry 59:621–629, 2002

New AS, Buchsbaum MS, Hazlett EA, et al: Fluoxetine increases relative metabolic rate in prefrontal cortex in impulsive aggression. Psychopharmacology (Berl) 176(3–4):451–458, 2004

New AS, Hazlett EA, Buchsbaum MS, et al: Amygdala-prefrontal disconnection in borderline personality disorder. Neuropsychopharmacology 32:1629–1640, 2007

Ni X, Sicard T, Bulgin N, et al: Monoamine oxidase a gene is associated with borderline personality disorder. Psychiatr Genet 17:153–157, 2007

O'Keane V, Loloney E, O'Neil H, et al: Blunted prolactin responses to d-fenfluramine challenge in sociopathy: evidence for subsensitivity of central serotonergic function. Br J Psychiatry 160:643–646, 1992

Olesen PJ, Nagy Z, Westerberg H, et al: Combined analysis of DTI and fMRI data reveals a joint maturation of white and gray matter in a fronto-parietal network. Brain Res Cogn Brain Res 18:48–57, 2003

Osterheld-Haas MC, Hornung JP: Laminar development of the mouse barrel cortex: effects of neurotoxins against monoamines. Exp Brain Res 110:183–195, 1996

Park SB, Cowen P: Effect of pindolol on prolactin response to D-fenfluramine. Psychopharmacology (Berl) 118:471–474, 1995

Paulesu E, Frith CD, Frackowiak RS: The neural correlates of the verbal component of working memory. Nature 362:342–345, 1993

Pickar D, Breier A, Hsiao JK, et al: Cerebrospinal fluid and plasma monoamine metabolites and their relation to psychosis. Arch Gen Psychiatry 47:641–648, 1990

Plotsky PM, Meaney MJ: Early, postnatal experience alters hypothalamic corticotropin-releasing factor (CRF) mRNA, median eminence CRF content and stress-induced release in adult rats. Brain Res Mol Brain Res 18:195–200, 1993

Postle BR: Working memory as an emergent property of the mind and brain. Neuroscience 139:23–38, 2006

Raine A, Lencz T, Bihrle S, et al: Reduced prefrontal gray volume and autonomic deficits in antisocial personality disorder. Arch Gen Psychiatry 57:119–127, 2000

Reichborn-Kjennerud T, Czajkowski N, Neale MC, et al: Genetic and environmental influences on dimensional representations of DSM-IV cluster C personality disorders: a population-based multivariate twin study. Psychol Med 37:645–653, 2007

Reuter M, Schmitz A, Corr P, et al: Molecular genetics support Gray's personality theory: the interaction of COMT and DRD2 polymorphisms predicts the behavioural approach system. Int J Neuropsychopharmacol 9:155–166, 2006

Roder CH, Michal M, Overbeck G, et al: Pain response in depersonalization: a functional imaging study using hypnosis in healthy subjects. Psychother Psychosom 76:115–121, 2007

Rolls ET: Précis of The brain and emotion. Behav Brain Sci 23:177–191, 2000

Rüsch N, Weber M, Il'yasov KA, et al: Inferior frontal white matter microstructure and patterns of psychopathology in women with borderline personality disorder and comorbid attention-deficit hyperactivity disorder. Neuroimage 35:738–747, 2007

Satpute AB, Lieberman MD: Integrating automatic and controlled processes into neurocognitive models of social cognition. Brain Res 1079:86–97, 2006

Sawaguchi T, Yamane I: Properties of delay-period neuronal activity in the monkey dorsolateral prefrontal cortex during a spatial delayed matching-to-sample task. J Neurophysiol 82:2070–2080, 1999

Saxe R: Uniquely human social cognition. Curr Opin Neurobiol 16:235–239, 2006

Schnell K, Dietrich T, Schnitker R, et al: Processing of autobiographical memory retrieval cues in borderline personality disorder. J Affect Disord 97:253–259, 2007

Schurhoff F, Szoke A, Chevalier F, et al: Schizotypal dimensions: an intermediate phenotype associated with the COMT high activity allele. Am J Med Genet B Neuropsychiatr Genet 144:64–68, 2007

See RE, Sorg BA, Chapman MA, et al: In vivo assessment of release and metabolism of dopamine in the ventrolateral striatum of awake rats following administration of dopamine D1 and D2 receptor agonists and antagonists. Neuropharmacology 30(12A):1269–1274, 1991

Shihabuddin L, Buchsbaum M, Hazlett E, et al: Striatal size and relative glucose metabolic rate in schizotypal personality disorder and schizophrenia. Arch Gen Psychiatry 58:877–884, 2001

Siever LJ: Biological markers in schizotypal personality disorder. Schizophr Bull 11:564–575, 1985

Siever LJ, Davis KL: Psychobiological perspective on the personality disorders. Am J Psychiatry 148:1647–1658, 1991

Siever LJ, Coursey RD, Alterman IS: Impaired smooth pursuit eye movement: vulnerability marker for schizotypal personality disorder in a normal volunteer population. Am J Psychiatry 141:1560–1566, 1984

Siever LJ, Amin F, Coccaro EF, et al: Plasma homovanillic acid in schizotypal personality disorder. Am J Psychiatry 148:1246–1248, 1991

Siever LJ, Buchsbaum MS, New AS, et al: d,l-Fenfluramine response in impulsive personality disorder assessed with [18F]-fluorodeoxyglucose positron emission tomography. Neuropsychopharmacology 20:413–423, 1999

Silva H, Iturra P, Solari A, et al: Serotonin transporter polymorphism and fluoxetine effect on impulsiveness and aggression in borderline personality disorder. Actas Esp Psiquiatr 35:387–392, 2007

Simeon D, Guralnik O, Hazlett EA, et al: Feeling unreal: a PET study of depersonalization disorder. Am J Psychiatry 157:1782–1788, 2000

Soloff PH, Meltzer CC, Greer PJ, et al: A fenfluramine-activated FDG-PET study of borderline personality disorder. Biol Psychiatry 47:540–547, 2000

Soloff PH, Meltzer CC, Becker C, et al: Impulsivity and prefrontal hypometabolism in borderline personality disorder. Psychiatry Res 123:153–163, 2003

Soloff PH, Price JC, Meltzer CC, et al: 5HT2A receptor binding is increased in borderline personality disorder. Biol Psychiatry 62:580–587, 2007

Steiger H, Joober R, Israel M, et al: The 5HTTLPR polymorphism, psychopathologic symptoms, and platelet [3H]paroxetine binding in bulimic syndromes. Int J Eat Disord 37:57–60, 2005

Stein D, Trestman RL, Mitropoulou V: Impulsivity and serotonergic function in compulsive personality disorder. J Neuropsychiatry Clin Neurosci 8:393–398, 1996

Steinberg BJ, Trestman R, Mitropoulou V, et al: Depressive response to physostigmine challenge in borderline personality disorder patients. Neuropsychopharmacology 17:264–273, 1997

Sternbach HA, Fleming J, Extein I: The dexamethasone suppression and thyrotropin-releasing hormone tests in depressed borderline patients. Psychoneuroendocrinology 8:459–462, 1983

Strome EM, Wheler GH, Higley JD, et al: Intracerebroventricular corticotropin-releasing factor increases limbic glucose metabolism and has social context-dependent behavioral effects in nonhuman primates. Proc Natl Acad Sci U S A 99:15749–15754, 2002

Taghzouti K, Le Moal M, Simon H: Enhanced frustrative nonreward effect following 6-hydroxydopamine lesions of the lateral septum in the rat. Behav Neurosci 99:1066–1073, 1985

Tebartz van Elst L, Ludaescher P, Thiel T, et al: Evidence of disturbed amygdalar energy metabolism in patients with borderline personality disorder. Neurosci Lett 417:36–41, 2007

Thiel CM, Zilles K, Fink GR: Nicotine modulates reorienting of visuospatial attention and neural activity in human parietal cortex. Neuropsychopharmacology 30:810–820, 2005

Torgersen S, Czajkowski N, Jacobson K, et al: Dimensional representations of DSM-IV cluster B personality disorders in a population based sample of Norwegian twins: a multivariate study. Psychol Med 14:1–9, 2008

Tudusciuc O, Nieder A: Neuronal population coding of continuous and discrete quantity in the primate posterior parietal cortex. Proc Natl Acad Sci U S A 104:14513–14518, 2007

van Erp AM, Miczek KA: Aggressive behavior, increased accumbal dopamine, and decreased cortical serotonin in rats. J Neurosci 20:9320–9325, 2000

Vazquez DM, Lopez JF, Van Hoers H, et al: Maternal deprivation regulates serotonin 1A and 2A receptors in the infant rat. Brain Res 855:76–82, 2000

Vermetten E, Schmahl C, Lindner S, et al: Hippocampal and amygdalar volumes in dissociative identity disorder. Am J Psychiatry 163:630–636, 2006

Vollm B, Richardson P, McKie S, et al: Serotonergic modulation of neuronal responses to behavioural inhibition and reinforcing stimuli: an fMRI study in healthy volunteers. Eur J Neurosci 23:552–560, 2006

Vythilingam M, Heim C, Newport J, et al: Childhood trauma associated with smaller hippocampal volume in women with major depression. Am J Psychiatry 159:2072–2080, 2002

Wang W, Wang Y, Fu X, et al: Cerebral information processing in personality disorders, I: intensity dependence of auditory evoked potentials. Psychiatry Res 141:173–183, 2006

Williams LM, Sidis A, Gordon E, et al: "Missing links" in borderline personality disorder: loss of neural synchrony relates to lack of emotion regulation and impulse control. J Psychiatry Neurosci 31:181–188, 2006

World Health Organization: The ICD-10 Classification of Mental and Behavioural Disorders: Clinical Descriptions and Diagnostic Guidelines. Geneva, Switzerland, World Health Organization, 1992

Yamagata S, Suzuki A, Ando J, et al: Is the genetic structure of human personality universal? A cross-cultural twin study from North America, Europe, and Asia. J Pers Soc Psychol 90:987–998, 2006

CHAPTER 52

Neurobiology of Childhood Disorders

Daniel S. Pine, M.D.

Mental health sciences witnessed a paradigm shift in the late twentieth century through the influence of three research themes. First, a focus on biology emerged following changes in psychiatric nomenclature and psychopharmacology. Second, advances in neuroscience provided heretofore unseen insights on the relationship between neural and information-processing functions, paving the way for a clinical neuroscience approach to mental illness. Third, the school of developmental psychopathology emerged, based on the recognition that most chronic mental illnesses have their roots in childhood. The current chapter, which focuses on the biology of childhood mental disorders, integrates these three themes. Given the breadth of work in each area, let alone the combination of the three, this chapter cannot provide a comprehensive review. Rather, I summarize major themes while providing illustrative examples from research on specific disorders.

In this chapter I present data on nine families of disorders: 1) pervasive developmental disorders (PDDs) such as autism, 2) schizophrenia and other psychoses, 3) learning disorders such as dyslexia, 4) disruptive behavior disorders (DBDs) and attention-deficit/hyperactivity disorder (ADHD), 5) bipolar disorder, 6) major depressive disorder (MDD), 7) obsessive-compulsive disorder (OCD) and Tourette's syndrome, 8) posttraumatic stress disorder (PTSD), and 9) pediatric anxiety disorders. Aspects of clinical presentation and therapeutics are reviewed in other chapters.

The chapter unfolds in four sections. The first section presents principles that provide a framework within which current biological research can be placed. The second section reviews current approaches in genetics research, which raises questions on the manner in which genes ultimately influence behavior emerging in a developmental context. In the third section, data on information-processing functions are reviewed, considering data from cognitive and affective neuroscience. These data suggest that specific neural information-processing pathways might provide the conduit through which genes sculpt behavior as genes interact with the environment. The final section reviews data on brain circuitry structure, function, and modulation, with a strong focus on brain imaging.

Integration of Developmental Psychopathology and Biology

Virtually all chronic mental disorders are conceptualized as disorders of brain maturation. This view emerged from an integration of research in epidemiology and neuroscience. From the epidemiological perspective, the school of developmental psychopathology recognizes that diverse behaviors show consistent, robust patterns of change as children mature through adolescence (Rutter et al. 2006). Marked individual variability results from differences in the timing of these changes, revealing child-specific risks. From the neuroscience perspective, adult patterns of information processing emerge from development, since the immature brain is uniquely susceptible to both genetic and environmental influences (Nelson et al. 2002). Individual variability reflects variations in the timing of these influences. Together, this literature suggests that chronic psychiatric disorders emerge from the effects of genes and the environment on brain development.

Despite the insights emerging from these breakthroughs, research on the biology of pediatric mental disorders has proceeded less quickly than research on adult mental disorders. This discrepancy has resulted from many factors, including the dearth of experienced researchers, the complex ethical issues confronting efforts to launch such studies, and the inherent difficulty of assessing both behavior and biology in the context of development. Due to these limitations, enthusiasm has emerged from avenues outside of biological research with children.

Epidemiology

Developmental psychopathology, as a distinct theoretical school, emerged following changes in psychiatric nomenclature in the 1970s. The advent of a standard nosology set the stage for longitudinal and family-based research. Armed with new assessment techniques, large cohorts of children received serial, standardized psychiatric assessments over time, beginning in the school age years and spanning into adulthood. Three key insights emerged from this work:

1. Longitudinal community-based research demonstrated the surprisingly high prevalence of pediatric mental disorders, revealing as many as a third of individuals to be affected before adulthood (Rutter et al. 2006). Interestingly, many common conditions were shown to be transient in children followed longitudinally, whereas rarer disorders, such as the PDDs, typically were persistent. Nevertheless, the roots of chronic psychopathology were shown to lie both in rare, persistent disorders and in the exceedingly common, typically transient conditions, such as the anxiety disorders. Longitudinal studies showed that most adult mental disorders arose in individuals who had manifest psychopathology as children, typically in the most common forms of pediatric mental illnesses. This truism held for virtually all forms of psychopathology.

2. Longitudinal family-based research confirmed these observations while establishing the familial nature of mental illnesses. Again, for most psychopathology, including PDDs, psychosis, mood disorders, anxiety dis-

orders, and DBDs, disorders were shown to be developmental and family based (Caspi and Moffitt 2006; Dickstein and Leibenluft 2006; Merikangas et al. 1999; Rutter 2005; Weissman et al. 2006). Offspring of adults with various mental syndromes face a high risk for psychiatric illness. Moreover, even in children free of overt psychopathology, signs of risk are manifest in patterns of information processing (Merikangas et al. 1999). Finally, manifestations of risk change developmentally. For example, offspring of parents with MDD might show high rates of anxiety as opposed to MDD, whereas offspring of parents with bipolar disorder might show high rates of MDD rather than mania (Dickstein and Leibenluft 2006). As some children of MDD parents with anxiety disorders mature, they manifest MDD, whereas some children of parents with bipolar disorder ultimately manifest bipolar disorder (Rutter et al. 2006).

3. A focus on risk factors for mental illness emphasized the need for research on biology. Although longitudinal studies established the clear relationship between social risk factors (e.g., poverty) and psychopathology, a surprisingly high number of children were resilient (Rutter 2000). The recognition of marked individual differences in susceptibility to risk raised questions on the role of biology in the modulation of risk. Moreover, some biological factors were shown to predispose toward pediatric mental illness even in the absence of social risks. Initial work emphasized the strong relationship between epilepsy and mental disorders, particularly the PDDs (Rutter 2005). These observations soon extended to a wealth of other neurological conditions, such as brain injury manifesting either in overt developmental delays or in more subtle indicators of brain dysfunction. With continued refinements, epidemiological research extended to focus on ever-subtler developmental influences. This included research relating teratology, such as from maternal smoking, to pediatric DBDs, as well as studies linking various perinatal immunological or nutritional compromises to psychosis (Rutter et al. 2006). Finally, findings from work that focused on very young children, a group thought to be particularly susceptible to environmental and social influences, further contributed to this focus on early biology. Temperamental profiles, such as behavioral inhibition, were identified in these studies. Such profiles were ultimately shown to be stable across many environments, influenced by genes, and associated with biological profiles (Fox et al. 2005).

Developmental Neuroscience

Advances in developmental neuroscience proceeded in parallel with advances in clinical conceptualization. Considerable work prior to the 1980s had established the importance of developmental events for the foundation of healthy neurological function. Some of the strongest evidence in this regard focused on relatively extreme manipulations involving events that seemed relatively removed from those implicated in developmental psychopathology. For example, work on the visual system firmly established the presence of age-related differences in susceptibility to alterations in environmental input: complete deprivation of visual input to one eye early in life produced long-term robust effects on visual function. Similarly profound deprivations in early-life social experience had demonstrated the malleability of emotional functioning. Work in the final decades of the twentieth century revealed the broader applicability of the developmental neuroscience approach. Even relatively subtle variations in developmental events were shown to produce robust changes in behavior that appeared relevant to emerging views of psychopathology.

One relevant example emerged through research using relatively subtle manipulations of the rearing environment (Meaney 2001). This work demonstrated long-term effects on emotional systems. Much of the early work in this area relied on experiments with rodents, where pups and dams were separated for brief periods of time. Such manipulations produce lifelong alterations in the pups' response to stress. The robust, replicable nature of these findings facilitated work on the neural architecture mediating these effects: changes in glucocorticoid receptor biology, with reverberating effects on measures of information processing and threat-response behavior, instantiated in the hypothalamic-pituitary-adrenal (HPA) axis, the medial temporal lobe, and the prefrontal cortex (PFC). As this work continued, the molecular underpinnings were revealed, involving epigenetics. Finally, studies in both humans and nonhuman primates began to demonstrate parallel effects and associations (Gross and Hen 2004). Enthusiasm for extensions to research on the biology of pediatric mental disorders soon followed.

Another relevant example emerged from work on genetic manipulations in mice. Research throughout the 1980s had firmly established the modulatory role of serotonin (5-hydroxytryptamine; 5-HT) over complexly organized high-level behaviors, such as those engaged by threats and danger (Gross and Hen 2004). For example, deletion of the 5-HT type 1A (5-HT$_{1A}$) receptor in the mouse altered the threshold for engaging in these behav-

iors. Further research elucidated the developmental context in which these effects emerge: 5-HT$_{1A}$ receptor deletion in the mature mouse produced no detectable effects on threat-response behavior, whereas transient deletion only in the immature mouse produced a long-lasting effect well into adulthood, even in mice with transiently abnormal 5-HT$_{1A}$ activity as juveniles and normal 5-HT$_{1A}$ profiles as adults. As with work on the HPA axis, studies in primates complemented these findings. Given the role of the amygdala in rodent fear, for example, studies in nonhuman primates examined developmental influences on amygdala function. This work showed that the effects of amygdala lesions on fear varied as a function of development (Prather et al. 2001). As work from these and other projects accumulated, enthusiasm for extensions to developmental psychopathology grew.

Endophenotypes

Initial attempts to integrate findings from clinical and basic science called attention to significant hurdles complicating such integrative research. Primary among these were questions on the validity of clinical phenotypes. Initial questions arose from limitations in the assessment techniques, related to complications in combining information from multiple informants and the need to ground assessments of pathology in understandings of normal variations in behavior. However, even after these problems were solved, major questions on phenotypes persisted. For example, studies in the PDDs found that relatively few relatives of children with autism manifest overt diagnoses of autism, yet such relatives often manifest subtle variants of core symptoms in autism, such as mild problems in language or social relatedness (Rutter 2005). Similarly, studies in MDD found that many children at high-risk for MDD were free of psychopathology but exhibited subtle subclinical perturbations in their responses to threats or rewards (Grillon et al. 2005). These observations elucidated the need for alternative approaches to phenotype classification in children, given demonstrations of changing manifestations in risk across the life span.

A focus on endophenotypes provided the opportunity to ground classifications of children in emerging understandings of neuroscience (Gottesman and Gould 2003). Thus, potential endophenotypes were selected based on understandings of brain–behavior relationships. As the sophistication of these understandings grew, the applicability of this perspective increased, ushering in new frameworks for the conceptualization of developmental psychopathology and its relationship to biology.

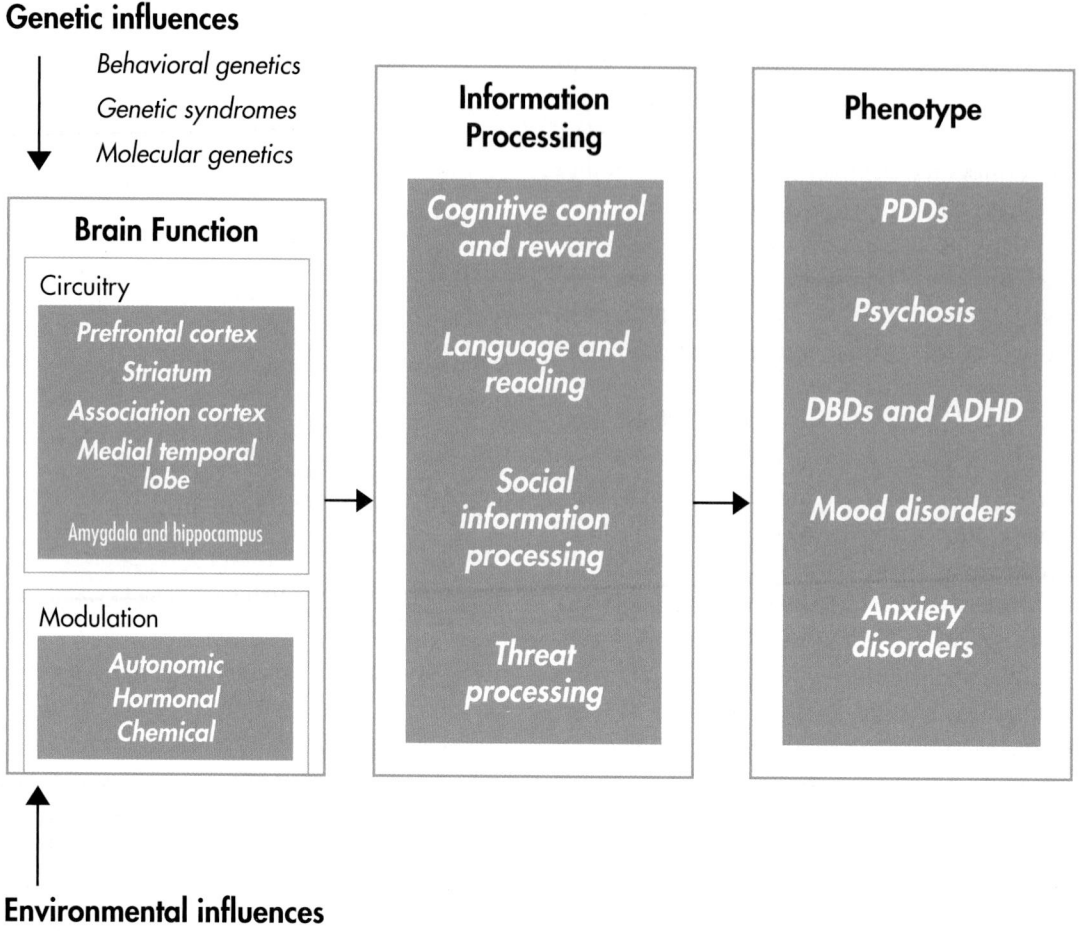

FIGURE 52–1.   A conceptual framework for biological research.

This figure illustrates a framework in which to place current research on the biology of pediatric mental syndromes. The framework attempts to link understandings of brain function to clinical categorization by examining the relationship between variations in brain function and specific information-processing functions. ADHD = attention-deficit/hyperactivity disorder; DBDs = disruptive behavior disorders; PDDs = pervasive developmental disorders.

Current Frameworks

Figure 52–1 illustrates one current framework for conceptualizing the biological correlates of pediatric mental illnesses. Material covered in the remainder of this chapter can be organized around this figure. Thus, the origins of mental illness are shown on the left side of this figure, where genetic and environmental events impinge on development, ultimately through effects on brain development. In this framework, considering individual disorders, distinct genetic and environmental effects produce effects on distinct but overlapping neural circuits, accounting for the specific manifestations of pediatric psychopathologies. For some conditions, these effects are likely to be overwhelmingly genetic, at least in their earliest inception. For other conditions, these effects are likely to involve stronger environmental components.

A major challenge is to map the manner in which variations in brain function (shown on the left side of the figure) give rise to variations in psychopathology, represented as phenotypes (shown on the right side of the figure). For studies in juveniles, the magnitude of this challenge is particularly large, given the need to delineate a constantly changing relationship between brain function and behavior. One approach delineates brain–phenotype relationships by focusing on measures of information processing, as depicted in the middle box of Figure 52–1. Research that connects elements of information processing (the middle box in the figure) to the clinical phenotypes (the box on the right) capitalizes on the success of neuroscience research linking understanding of brain function and information processing, thus connecting the middle and the left boxes in Figure 52–1. Taken together, this research allows clinical–neuroscience integration.

The remainder of this chapter reviews the manner in which ongoing research on childhood mental disorders maps relationships between genes and the environment, through measures of brain function and associated information-processing profiles, onto clinical phenotypes. This review is organized around three sections. For the first two sections, the review focuses more on aspects of methodology than on specific pediatric mental disorders, discussing findings in specific disorders only for illustrative purposes. Thus, the initial section, on genetics, focuses more on available methods than on findings in one or another disorder. Similarly, the next section, on information processing, focuses on the four cognitive domains depicted in the middle box of Figure 52–1 linked to distinct neural circuitry function, again without comprehensively reviewing findings in specific disorders. Greater depth is provided, however, in the final section ("Brain Function"). Given the promise of brain imaging, this section summarizes findings across diverse clinical domains, considering conditions broadly grouped into five categories: PDDs; psychosis; DBDs and ADHD; mood disorders; and anxiety disorders.

Ultimately, this work is likely to lead to conceptual changes, as nomenclature moves toward classifications based on pathophysiology. Scientific and practical complications limit efforts to ground such research in studies of juveniles. Nevertheless, evidence delineating the importance of the developmental approach emphasizes the importance of addressing these complications.

Genetics

As indicated in Figure 52–1, three research areas document genetic influences on developmental psychopathology: behavioral genetics, specific genetic syndromes, and molecular genetics.

Behavioral Genetics

Observations of strong, consistent familial aggregation encouraged efforts to identify genetic and environmental correlates of psychopathology. As with most research on pathophysiology, this work began with studies based in adults. Such work showed that retrospectively assessed factors operating in childhood modulated the impact of genetic and environmental effects on risk for psychopathology. This generated enthusiasm for implementing such studies directly in children.

Initial results in children have demonstrated both commonalities with and differences from findings of re-

search in adults. As in adult disorders, wide variability exists for the pediatric mental disorders in the contributions of environmental and genetic effects. Thus, some disorders, particularly PDDs and ADHD, have been shown to be overwhelmingly genetic, whereas most common disorders are influenced heavily by nonshared environmental effects (Thapar and Rutter 2008). Certain DBDs have emerged as the rare examples of conditions with strong shared environmental influences. As in adults, these data emphasize the importance of genetic and environmental contributions.

Findings in children have also generated novel insights, relative to studies in adults. For example, genetic contributions to a disorder in adulthood (e.g., MDD) might be shared with genetic contributions to a different type of disorder in childhood (e.g., anxiety) (Thapar and Rutter 2008). Alternatively, some disorders classified as nosologically similar might exhibit distinct genetics, such as has been shown for some forms of conduct disorder. Behavioral genetics research in juveniles has also benefited from the opportunity to directly assess environmental contributors to psychopathology, going beyond indirect statistical measures. Such work has emphasized the role of gene–environment interactions, operating in a developmental context, to shape risk for many of the more common disorders (Thapar and Rutter 2008). These include DBDs, mood disorders, and anxiety disorders.

Genetic Syndromes

Interest in molecular genetics has been stimulated further by research demonstrating behavioral correlates of developmental syndromes associated with specific genetic alterations. Some chromosomal syndromes either are relatively common (e.g., Down syndrome) or are associated with extreme alterations in behavior (e.g., Lesch-Nyhan syndrome). With these conditions, focus on the psychiatric concomitants emerged shortly after the syndromes were first described, and these features were attributed at least partially to consequences of intellectual disability, given its recognized role in shaping risk for psychopathology. Accordingly, few implications emerged for understandings of psychopathology as typically manifested in the community.

More recently, continued advance in molecular genetics techniques has generated interest in a wider array of developmental syndromes and their relevance for psychopathology in the community (Thapar and Rutter 2008). For these conditions, insights on gene–behavior associations have begun to broadly shape thinking on developmental psychopathology. For example, deletion at chromosome band 22q11.2 gives rise to velocardiofacial syndrome (VCF), which manifests in cutaneous, cardiac, and neurological changes. VCF is associated with a high risk for psychosis, generating interest in the role of genes lying within this region of chromosome 22. Suggestive findings in adult patients with schizophrenia, in the absence of VCF, increase interest in this area, as do recent brain imaging studies on neural correlates of VCF. Similarly, William syndrome results from a deletion on the long arm of chromosome 7 (band 7q11.23). This syndrome also presents with a unique behavioral pattern, characterized by intellectual deficits and high levels of anxiety but surprisingly high levels of sociability. Here, too, findings using brain imaging technology raise questions on the role of chromosome 7 in the regulation of social experience in behavior.

For these two syndromes, VCF and William syndrome, the presence of intellectual deficits raises questions about the role of indirect mechanisms contributing to the observed psychiatric profiles. However, studies in other single-gene disorders that typically manifest in childhood, such as 21-α-hydroxylase deficiency, have generated further interest in understanding the role of specific genes in shaping behavior across development (Ernst et al. 2007). As reviewed elsewhere (Thapar and Rutter 2008), considerable other research in a range of genetic disorders has delineated the promise of this approach. Finally, other work in sporadically appearing cases of conditions that are typically highly familial has informed targeted focusing on specific genes, as illustrated in recent work on Tourette's syndrome (Abelson et al. 2005). Alternatively, work in highly familial forms of language dysfunction also has led to the identification of novel genes.

Molecular Genetics

Much like research among adults, studies in children have begun to rely on the techniques of both genetic linkage and genetic association to delineate the role of specific genes in relatively common psychiatric disorders ascertained in the community or the mental health clinic. As a rule, work using the technique of genetic association generally has fared better in generating replicated findings, though suggestive findings have emerged from linkage studies focused on PDDs and dyslexia. Reviews of these findings can be found elsewhere (Faraone and Khan 2006; Gupta and State 2007; Swanson et al. 2007; Thapar and Rutter 2008).

The best-replicated work in genetic association derives from studies of ADHD, where research in many thousands of patients implicates genes for various monoamines in the disorder (Faraone and Khan 2006; Swanson et al. 2007). As with all association studies, work on ADHD is facilitated by research on pathophysiology implicating one or another pathway in the disorder, where the robust efficacy of psychostimulants has provided important clues. Associations with both the dopamine$_4$ (D$_4$) receptor and the dopamine transporter appear reasonably well replicated.

Similarly strong evidence has emerged in association studies of PDDs and OCD, with work on 5-HT genetics extending earlier studies on 5-HT neurochemistry and therapeutics in both of these disorders (Gupta and State 2007). For other disorders, findings generally are less well established. Nevertheless, a steady stream of biological clues has provided many targets for a range of clinical phenotypes in children. Thus, brain-derived neurotrophic factor has been implicated in pediatric MDD; the glutamate transporter gene solute carrier family 1, member 1 (SLC1A1) gene has been implicated in OCD; and various 5-HT–related or HPA-related genes have been implicated in one or another anxiety phenotype.

Across genetic research on children, the magnitude of association generally has been small, rarely increasing the risk for one or another psychopathology by more than twofold (Thapar and Rutter 2008). This suggests that pediatric mental illnesses arise from complex cascades of genetic and environmental events. Such realizations have encouraged efforts to map these specific cascades, as exemplified by recent work on gene–gene interactions in risk for adverse reactions to trauma and by recent work on gene–environment interactions in risk for DBDs and MDD. For example, Caspi and colleagues mapped one such interaction in research conducted with the so-called Dunedin cohort from New Zealand, one of the best-characterized longitudinal, epidemiological samples (Caspi and Moffitt 2006). In this cohort, environmental risk for conduct problems and associated DBDs was modulated by genetic variation in the gene for monoamine oxidase A, a gene that had been selected for study based on earlier work in a family with a rare deletion of this gene. Such findings have generated enthusiasm more broadly in efforts to map the complex way in which individual genetic and environmental events shape risk.

Information Processing

The current framework rests heavily on research examining information processing, because studies in this area play a unique role in the integration of research on brain function and phenotypes, as shown in Figure 52–1. Work in this area relies heavily on studies from the fields of cognitive and affective neuroscience. Tools from these fields index observable variations in behavior, and these behaviors are selected based on knowledge of the underlying neural architecture and associated information-processing functions. If variations in these behaviors can be linked to clinically relevant phenotypes, it is possible to bridge research on brain function and its influence by genes or the environment with research on clinical phenotypes. Moreover, this research can be based in a developmental context, allowing changes in such behaviors to be mapped to changes in associated brain function.

Given the explosion of work in this area, the current chapter cannot exhaustively summarize all aspects of the relevant work. Rather, I highlight illustrative examples where information-processing functions with known neural architecture have been most consistently linked to childhood mental disorders. This section focuses on the four information-processing functions delineated in Figure 52–1: cognitive control and reward, language and reading, social information processing, and threat processing. For each of these four functions, the section summaries prior research on the neural architecture of each function before highlighting key findings relating the function to psychopathology.

Cognitive Control and Reward

Research on choice behaviors in the context of competing goal demands implicates a specific neural circuit in decision making. Much of this work relies on experimental paradigms in which a subject must make a difficult choice, perhaps because one or another response is rendered prepotent due to the rapid pace of the task or because the appropriate choice is ambiguous, as exemplified by the "stop" task, various Go/No-Go paradigms, and the flanker tasks. In these tasks, behavior is thought to be regulated by components of the PFC that represent aspects of the task's rules, whereas interactions between the PFC and striatum facilitate efforts to adjust behavior when task contingencies change (Blair et al. 2005). This occurs, for example, on events with high conflict, such as "stop" trials on the stop task. Children with a select group of pediatric psychopathologies exhibit perturbations on these tasks, providing a strong foundation for integration of clinical and research perspectives in these disorders. Thus, this research implicates PFC–striatal dysfunction in ADHD, PDDs, and OCD while distinguishing these conditions from non-OCD anxiety disorders or MDD, where performance is intact (Nigg 2007; Swanson et al. 2007).

The affective salience of these so-called cognitive control tasks can be augmented by manipulating the costs and benefits of one or another decision. For example, a subject might be rewarded on a select series of trials for a correct response or punished on other trials for an incorrect response. The difficulty of the task can be increased by focusing on a child's ability to alter responses as task contingencies change. Figure 52–2 illustrates one such task, based on the so-called response reversal paradigm, wherein a subject is required to select one of two objects to obtain rewards in the context of continually changing contingencies (Budhani et al. 2007). This task engages brain systems that facilitate adaptive behavior required when task rules change, such as when contingencies reverse. As shown in the figure, in the context of the need to reverse choices, these paradigms influence activity in medial PFC. Other work shows that children with DBDs and related disorders perform poorly on such tasks (Blair et al. 2005; Nigg 2007; van Goozen et al. 2007). Thus, through the use of these and other manipulations, considerable research implicates PFC–striatal circuitry in reward-related behaviors, ADHD, trauma, and mood disorders.

Language and Reading

The effects of brain lesions on cognition generated early interest in elucidating relevant neural pathways. The development of language abilities and the development of reading abilities represent two of the most significant aspects of cognitive development, and considerable work in cognitive neuroscience examines the underlying circuitry.

Research on language development has pursued diverse avenues. One set of studies extended observations in children with specific language impairment. This condition is hypothesized to result from a relatively specific deficit in decoding subtle temporal variations in phonemes. Consistent with this possibility, focused training designed to compensate for this specific deficit was shown to remedy the language deficit in some children (Tallal and Gaab 2006). In other work, children with unusual familial forms of language dysfunction were found to exhibit a unique neural and molecular profile (Vargha-Khadem et al. 2005).

Research on both normal and abnormal reading abilities, as manifested in developmental reading disorder or dyslexia, has followed similarly divergent pathways. Considerable work with typically developing children has iso-

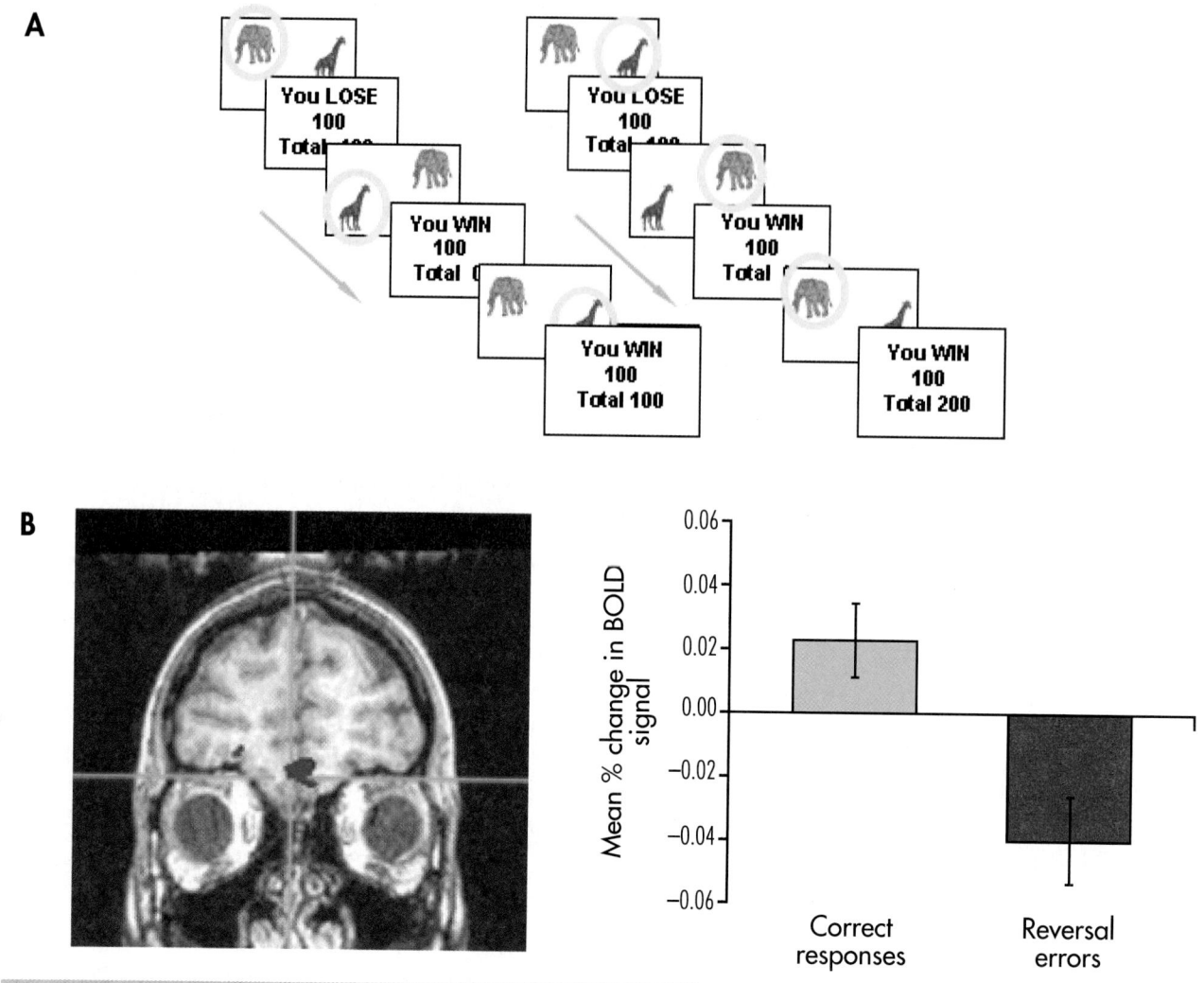

FIGURE 52–2.   Response reversal and the medial prefrontal cortex.

This figure shows details of a probabilistic response reversal task **(A).** In this task, subjects begin by trying to select a rewarded target (e.g., the giraffe) while avoiding a punished target (e.g., the elephant). Following acquisition of this "giraffe-reward" rule, the contingencies change in the reversal phase of the task. Functional magnetic resonance imaging **(B)** demonstrates that during this learning-related process, decreased engagement of the medial prefrontal cortex (PFC) occurs in trials when adult subjects commit errors by failing to learn the new "elephant-reward" rule. Deficient medial PFC engagement on such tasks in some pediatric mental syndromes might reflect a role for perturbed medial PFC function in the condition. BOLD = blood oxygenation level–dependent.

Source.   (A) Reprinted from Finger EC, Marsh AA, Mitchell DG, et al: "Abnormal Ventromedial Prefrontal Cortex Function in Children With Psychopathic Traits During Reversal Learning." *Archives of General Psychiatry* 65:586–594, 2008. Copyright 2008, American Medical Association. Used with permission.

(B) Reprinted from Budhani S, Marsh AA, Pine DS, et al: "Neural Correlates of Response Reversal: Considering Acquisition." *Neuroimage* 34:1754–1765, 2007. Copyright 2007, Elsevier. Used with permission.

lated the cognitive processes that provide foundations for successful reading. This work has delineated the typical development timing during which these processes mature, as well as the complex collection of brain regions required (Joseph et al. 2001). This provides a rich backdrop against which to place dyslexia. A parallel series of studies implicates specific processes in reading disorders (Joseph et al. 2001). As with the work on specific language im-

pairment, these insights have provided novel insights on treatments. Such treatments have been tailored to correct relatively specific core underlying deficits in the relevant psychological process. In emerging work, this model of developing remedial training after identifying a specific deficit in a relatively pure cognitive disorder has been extended to other disorders, such as ADHD, that are less typically considered purely cognitive conditions.

Social Information Processing

Perturbations in social relationships represent core features of many disorders. Recent developments implicate specific neural circuitry in the regulation of human interaction, providing a rich context in which to place research on developmental psychopathologies. In this area, the most consistent findings emerge in studies of PDDs, DBDs, traumatic exposure, and bipolar disorder.

Major disruptions in social relatedness represent one of the three key features of PDDs, along with deficits in language and stereotypical behaviors. Given the profound nature of clinical deficits, it should come as no surprise that children with PDDs also exhibit deficits on social neuroscience paradigms (Rutter 2005). For example, one set of studies, which relied on examinations of eye-scanning patterns, showed that individuals with PDDs attend to distinctly different social cues compared with healthy individuals, with very large effect size differences (Volkmar et al. 2004). Similarly, individuals with PDDs also have been shown to exhibit deficits on so-called theory-of-mind tasks that require the decoding of complex social motivations of peers. Both areas rely on relatively complex aspects of social information processing. Studies of more elementary processes, such as the labeling of face emotions, also have revealed deficits in children with PDDs.

Although perturbed social information processing might be expected in PDDs, other syndromes associated with less severe social deficits also have been linked to poor ability to decode social signals. Such deficits are likely to arise from many different pathways, as they have been found in children exposed to traumatic circumstances, which might lead to environmentally mediated deficiencies, as well as in children with psychopathy, a condition where the deficit in social processing is thought to result from genes (Blair et al. 2005). Children with bipolar disorder also show such deficits (Leibenluft et al. 2003). Of note, these deficits are relatively specific to this family of conditions; children with ADHD, other DBDs, anxiety disorders, and MDD show no such deficits.

Threat Processing

Research on threat processing has benefited from advances in affective neuroscience, a field focused specifically on the role of emotionally salient events in regulating the processing of information. Threats have been shown to heavily influence many aspects of behavior, through effects on diverse information-processing functions. Some of the most consistent findings have emerged in research finding that threats show a greater capacity than neutral material to influence attention (Pine 2007). For example, threats are recognized more quickly than neutral stimuli in some paradigms, whereas they interfere more strongly than neutral stimuli in other paradigms. These effects have been mapped to specific neural circuits encompassing the amygdala and PFC. Most importantly, these paradigms have been used to differentiate children with various psychopathologies, particularly the anxiety disorders, in which threats exhibit a particularly marked effect on attention. This work has generated interest in the use of other paradigms, co-opted from basic science, which require coordinated engagement of the amygdala and PFC. For example, considerable work suggests that anxiety disorders reflect a perturbation in processes related to fear conditioning and extinction.

Work on other disorders emphasizes the effects of threats or other emotional stimuli on processes distinct from attention. For example, in work on MDD, effects appear larger in memory than in attention paradigms. Similarly, work on bipolar disorder has documented a range of perturbations in threat-response behavior.

Brain Function

As shown in Figure 52–1, knowledge of brain function derives from research in two areas: functioning of relevant brain circuitry and modulation of this circuitry through autonomic, hormonal, and chemical influences. For studies in children, some of the most promising insights linking brain function to clinical phenotypes have emerged through research using brain imaging to examine circuitry. Research on modulation of circuitry has provided less profound influences on current clinical thinking. As a result, in the first portion of this section on brain function, I only briefly summarize research on brain circuitry modulation, whereas in the remainder of the section I provide a more detailed review of imaging studies in specific developmental psychopathologies. This review delineates relevant findings by focusing on normal development and the five classes of disorders illustrated on the right side of Figure 52–1, depicted as groups of phenotypes: PDDs, psychosis, DBDs and ADHD, mood disorders, and anxiety disorders.

Modulation of Circuitry

Autonomic, hormonal, and monoamine systems modulate activity in key neural systems, either when chemicals act directly on neural structures or when chemicals enable communication among components of circuitry-based feedback loops. These modulatory influences can be assessed by measuring variations in peripheral physiological indices. Considerable work in children relies on these measures, given ethical constraints on more invasive measures. Nevertheless, this chapter only briefly summarizes these findings. Work on modulation of circuitry has had a less profound influence on current clinical thinking than brain imaging research in recent years, because measures derived from imaging provide a more direct index, relative to measures of autonomic, hormonal, or monoamine system modulation, of neural system function associated with mental illnesses.

Autonomic Activity

Activity in the sympathetic and parasympathetic systems is influenced by the amygdala and associated systems. As a result, considerable work has attempted to infer the nature of individual differences in amygdala function through an examination of individual differences in autonomic parameters. Probably the most consistent findings in this area have emerged from research on the association between low heart rate and conduct problems in children (van Goozen et al. 2007). This association is thought to reflect blunted amygdala sensitivity to punishment cues, consistent with current models of some DBDs. Conversely, other work has linked elevated heart rate to various forms of pediatric anxiety, including behavioral inhibition, viewing these associations as a sign of amygdala hypersensitivity to threat (Fox et al. 2005; Pine 2007). Because these differences in heart rate could arise from differences in either parasympathetic or sympathetic systems, other work has used spectral analysis of heart period variability to draw inferences specifically on parasympathetic regulation. Findings in this area generally have been less consistent than findings linking differences in heart rate to differences in pediatric psychopathology.

Beyond work on cardiac activity, other research links childhood psychopathology to respiratory perturbation, extending work on the biology of adult panic disorder. Here, a consistent association has emerged between respiratory dysregulation and pediatric separation anxiety disorder, consistent with other work linking separation anxiety and panic disorders (Pine 2007). Of note, pediatric social anxiety disorder involves normal respiratory regulation, suggesting that individual anxiety disorders display unique biology.

While findings in this area have generated consistent interest in biological correlates, recent work has focused more closely on cognitive neuroscience than autonomic

physiology. This provides a more direct measure of activity in neural systems that are thought to mediate observed associations between autonomic physiology and psychopathology.

Hypothalamic-Pituitary-Adrenal Axis

Interest in the association between pediatric mental illness and HPA axis function follows from work relating variations in HPA activity of the rat pup to lifelong emotional response patterns (Gunnar 2003). As with work on autonomic function, the most consistent association has emerged in studies of DBDs, where a subgroup of children has been shown to exhibit low cortisol levels, possibly through the effects of the early-life rearing environment (Gunnar 2003; van Goozen et al. 2007). Consistent with this possibility, a recent randomized, controlled trial demonstrated an association between changes in DBD symptoms and increases in HPA axis activity (Brotman et al. 2007). Each of these findings is thought to reflect perturbed amygdala-based regulation of HPA axis activity. On the other hand, many other areas of research have found inconsistent associations between HPA axis activity and pediatric psychopathology. For example, work in MDD has found less consistent associations in children and adolescents, relative to the associations found in adults. This contributes to some questions on the utility of further work focused on the HPA axis in the absence of concomitant direct assessment of underlying brain system function.

Monoamine Function

Two findings have stimulated interest in monoamine function. First, considerable work implicates monoamines in adult disorders, and the developmental conceptualization of these adult psychopathologies encourages efforts to link pediatric syndromes to monoamine dysfunction. Second, effective psychotropic agents exert robust effects on monoamine systems. Despite consistent enthusiasm, it has been more difficult to implement work in children than in adults, given the limited availability of ethically permissible measures of central monoaminergic function.

Efficacy data in pediatric mood and anxiety disorders have generated interest in the serotonin (5-HT) and norepinephrine systems. The superior efficacy of the selective serotonin reuptake inhibitors compared with the tricyclic antidepressants has generated considerable interest (Emslie and Mayes 2001). Some suggest that the differing neurochemical profiles of these medication classes support a stronger role for 5-HT than for norepinephrine in pediatric syndromes targeted by antidepressants. Consistent with these suggestions, relatively few studies have documented associations between pediatric mental illnesses and individual differences in norepinephrine system functioning, although some work implicates the norepinephrine system in pediatric anxiety disorders (Pine 2007).

Considerable research implicates 5-HT dysfunction in pediatric mental syndromes. This includes most consistently PDDs, MDD, and DBDs (Birmaher and Heydl 2001; Rutter 2005; van Goozen et al. 2007). Work in this area has relied on a wealth of techniques, including assessment of peripheral 5-HT–related parameters such as whole-blood 5-HT or platelet 5-HT receptor profiles, cerebrospinal fluid 5-HT metabolite levels, and neuroendocrine assessment following administration of 5-HT agonists. One of the major questions emerging from this work examines the degree to which development impinges on the 5-HT–behavior association in humans, as it does in rodents and primates. Some physiology data suggest the presence of human developmental variation (van Goozen et al. 2007), and this is consistent with data documenting age-related changes in the adverse effects of treatment with selective serotonin reuptake inhibitors (Emslie and Mayes 2001). Nevertheless, it remains unclear how to extend such findings, given that positron emission tomography techniques that are currently used in research on 5-HT correlates of adult psychopathology are poorly suited for research with juveniles.

Work on the dopamine system has also generated consistent interest. The robust efficacy of the psychostimulants in ADHD and other DBDs indirectly implicates dopamine dysfunction in these conditions, as do the genetic association studies reviewed above. Preliminary positron emission tomography studies have provided further support (van Goozen et al. 2007). Work in this area also is relevant for developmental conceptualizations of psychosis, which is rare before puberty, and of substance abuse, which typically intensifies in adolescence. Consistent with these age-related changes in risk, which have been attributed to maturation of the dopamine system, pharmacological studies have documented developmental changes in the response to dopamine challenge across the period around puberty (Spear 2000). Moreover, this work is also relevant for current models of psychosis implicating interactions between the dopamine system and glutamate systems. Much like developmental changes for dopamine response, the response to glutamate manipulations also has shown robust age-related changes (Olney

2003). Taken together, these data implicate developmental changes in the dopamine and glutamate systems, and their interactions, in developmental changes in risk for various mental disorders. However, as with work on the 5-HT system, complications in assessment of dopamine or glutamate function in children place limits on the degree to which future research can explore the neural basis of such developmental changes.

Brain Function: Circuitry Assessed With Brain Imaging

In many ways, biological research on childhood mental disorders has only recently begun to come of age, with advances in brain imaging techniques. For the first time, these advances have allowed a direct assessment of neural structure and functions in children with levels of temporal and spatial resolution appropriate for extensions to developmental work in animal models. This final section provides examples illustrating the manner in which brain imaging research facilitates integration of basic and clinical research.

Relevant examples have emerged from research in diverse areas, including both normal and pathological variations in behavior, utilizing diverse techniques, including structural and functional magnetic resonance imaging approaches (sMRI and fMRI), magnetic resonance spectroscopy (MRS), event-related potentials (ERPs), and quantitative electroencephalography. As with summaries of research in other areas, the current summary does not provide an exhaustive review but rather illustrates the manner in which research in specific clinical areas provides a bridge to findings emerging both from basic science research in rodents or nonhuman primates and from cognitive or affective neuroscience research in humans. I have organized this review in six sections, beginning with a summary of findings on normal development, followed by a review of key findings in the five clinical domains depicted in Figure 52–1.

Normal Development

The ability to directly visualize brain development has strengthened interest in developmental aspects of psychopathology. Recently emerging data chart robust changes in brain structure and function that extend from early childhood through late adolescence. These data support the view emerging from epidemiological studies that most chronic psychopathologies are disorders of brain development. These data also resonate with data in cognitive neuroscience delineating the developmental trajectories for specific information-processing functions.

Much of the interest in neural development comes from sMRI findings demonstrating robust regional variations across development in the architecture of gray and white matter. These variations follow three basic trends (Sowell et al. 2004; Steinberg et al. 2006; Toga and Thompson 2003):

1. Consistent with postmortem work in humans and basic science studies in nonhuman primates, human brain development as shown in sMRI exhibits a clear trend to progress from primary sensory or motor cortices, which mature early, to association cortices, which mature late. This is also reflected in the spatial posterior-to-anterior gradient on which the progression from primary to association cortex is arranged.
2. Human brain development shows a general trend for a plateau of gray matter volume in childhood, with a progressive reduction through adolescence in tandem with a parallel increase in white matter volume. Taken together, these two trends lead to a progressive increase in the white-to-gray-matter volume ratio, consistent with a growing emphasis on integrative functions in the nervous system with maturation.
3. This general trend of a decrease in gray matter volume does not occur in all brain areas, as circuitry involving frontotemporal association cortices involved in linguistic maturation shows an opposite trend of increasing gray matter volume.

Taken together, these findings have generated considerable interest in mapping the relationships that such structural changes show with various measures of brain function, as manifested in direct measures of functional activity, as well as measures manifested in the environment, either on neuropsychological tests or in everyday experience.

Data from fMRI studies in developing humans generally confirm findings in sMRI studies (Nelson et al. 2002). Although far fewer studies rely on fMRI than sMRI, trends in fMRI research support the view of brain maturation as a process that extends well through late adolescence, with particularly later maturation of association cortices. Considerable interest has focused on functional aspects of medial temporal, striatal, and PFC development, given evidence from studies of behavior and sMRI studies suggesting these regions exhibit protracted development (Steinberg et al. 2006). Although many questions remain, the weight of the data suggests that each of these regions undergoes protracted development.

Pervasive Developmental Disorders

Current theories of PDD pathophysiology have been informed by data emerging using virtually every imaging modality. Together, this work extends insights emerging from other findings in epidemiology and cognitive neuroscience research. For example, early epidemiological studies raised questions on gross patterns of brain development in autism, based on perturbations in early-life head growth; sMRI studies confirmed that these differences in head growth are reflected in patterns of brain growth while also noting many regionally specific alterations in brain development in the cerebellum, amygdala, and other regions where one would expect perturbations, based on findings in cognitive neuroscience (Rutter 2005). These prior findings in cognitive neuroscience have generated specific interest in functional aspects of brain regions implicated in the regulation of social experience.

Ongoing fMRI research also successfully extends this work. For example, eye-movement data implicating perturbed attention control when processing social stimuli are consistent with fMRI studies documenting abnormal engagement of the amygdala, fusiform gyrus, and other components of neural circuitry implicated in the assessment of social significance (Volkmar et al. 2004). Similarly, cognitive neuroscience findings documenting perturbed abilities at imitation in PDDs have been extended through fMRI studies documenting abnormal engagement of so-called mirror-neuron systems implicated in imitation. Such fMRI work has unique advantages related to the excellent spatial resolution of the technique. However, the findings have also been extended through research using ERPs, with their superior spatial resolution, demonstrating the time course over which social processing dysfunction in PDDs manifests. Taken together, this work has generated considerable enthusiasm for refining our understandings of PDD pathophysiology by grounding these understandings in knowledge of neural development.

Psychosis

Data in child-onset schizophrenia uniquely demonstrate the advantages afforded by longitudinal examination of brain development, as is possible with sMRI. A central question emerging from early theories of psychosis focuses on contributions of static and dynamic neural developmental processes in changing manifestations of the illness. One of the most influential theories had suggested that a static temporal lesion interacts with dynamic changes in PFC structure emerging at adolescence to unmask a latent risk for psychosis. sMRI allows repeated as-

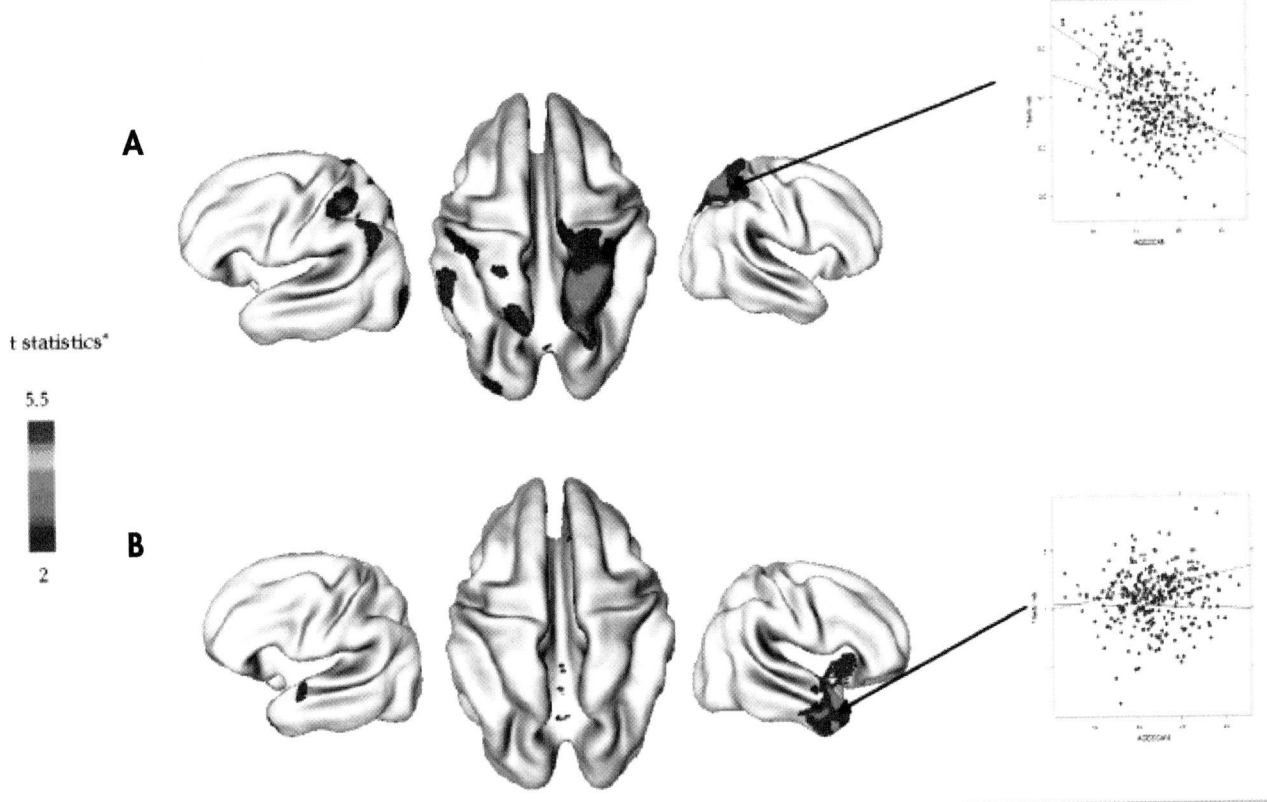

t statistics*

5.5

2

FIGURE 52–3.   Changes in cerebral cortex in childhood-onset schizophrenia.

Serial acquisition of structural magnetic resonance imaging data was used to map portions of the cerebral cortex (shown in scatterplots on the right side of the figure). Patients with childhood-onset schizophrenia (COS {●}) show distinct changes in brain structure relative to healthy peers (control subjects {●}). **Part A** shows normalization in posterior regions in COS patients; **part B** shows divergence from control subjects in anterior regions.

*A false discovery rate procedure was used to determine the threshold for significance at $t = 2$. No covariates were included in the model.

Source.   Reprinted from Greenstein D, Lerch J, Shaw P, et al.: "Childhood Onset Schizophrenia: Cortical Brain Abnormalities as Young Adults." *Journal of Child Psychology and Psychiatry* 47:1003–1012, 2006. Copyright 2006, Wiley-Blackwell. Used with permission.

sessment of brain structure across developmental periods with precise spatial localization of relevant static or changing morphology (Greenstein et al. 2006). This provides an assessment of the degree to which the structures of specific brain regions change and adapt as children develop and show changing manifestations of the illness. Figure 52–3 illustrates the possibilities inherent with this technique, revealing the degree to which specific brain regions show distinct developmental topographies in typically developing children and children with schizophrenia. These findings document very large differences between children with overt manifestations of schizophrenia and healthy children. The demonstrable utility of this approach raises essential questions on applications to other forms of psychosis. For example, using this approach, it may be possible to capture emerging patterns of neural changes that place children at risk for psychosis before the full manifestation of pathological clinical syn-

dromes. This may provide unique insights for both identification of at-risk individuals and targeted treatments designed to disrupt the ongoing pathological process before it has become fully entrenched.

Disruptive Behavior Disorders and ADHD

As with research on PDDs, work on DBDs and ADHD has relied on virtually every suitable imaging modality in research that directly extends findings generated in cognitive neuroscience. Without question, more research considers aspects of ADHD than DBDs, but important insights are beginning to emerge on differences among these disorders, each of which shows strong relationships in family-based and longitudinal research.

In research on ADHD, the most consistent approach extends findings emerging from research on cognitive control and reward processing. Studies in this area implicate a distributed neural circuit in the condition, encompassing the PFC as it connects with the striatum and cerebellum. sMRI studies provide some support for theories that implicate this circuitry in ADHD (Nigg 2007). However, overall reduction in brain volume represents a more consistent finding than selective reductions in these specific regions, independent of the more general reduction in brain volume. fMRI research provides more consistent support in that consistent dysfunction in the striatum and in the medial and ventral PFC emerges in this work, which supports findings from cognitive neuroscience research (Nigg 2007; Swanson et al. 2007). Data emerging from ERP research further refine understandings of the manner in which this circuit might be perturbed. Due to the superior temporal resolution of this technique, ERP data generate insights on the role of each PFC subregion and the striatum in perturbed cognitive control. As these findings have been steadily accumulating, questions have arisen concerning the degree to which one or another finding in brain imaging relates specifically to risk for ADHD, to overt manifestations associated with severity of the disorder, or to long-term trajectories of ADHD symptoms. The clinical utility of imaging approaches would be enhanced if data could be mapped onto distinct aspects of ADHD risk, presentation, or trajectory. Emerging data suggest that this may be possible.

Beyond research on ADHD, research data in other DBDs suggest that brain imaging measures might allow a refined categorization of behavior disorders (Blair et al. 2005; van Goozen et al. 2007). Although considerable research documents parallels in the neural correlates of ADHD and DBDs, emerging findings also suggest that a subgroup of children with DBDs can be differentiated from other children with DBDs and children with ADHD, based on functional aspects of brain circuitry engaged by emotionally salient events. One relevant theory in this respect suggests that a unique subgroup of children with DBDs exhibits a particularly poor prognosis and an unusually strong genetic component to their disorder (Blair et al. 2005). Current theory suggests that this profile is reflected in patterns of amygdala–PFC function during the evaluation of emotionally salient stimuli. Emerging brain imaging work generates findings generally consistent with this theory. As with work on ADHD, continued refinements of this approach may provide novel means for classifying pediatric DBDs based on associated neural circuitry dysfunction.

Mood Disorders

Data from cognitive neuroscience studies in pediatric bipolar disorder implicate two information-processing

functions in the condition: cognitive control and social information processing. Given knowledge on neural correlates of these information-processing functions, data from brain imaging studies are consistent with these findings in cognitive neuroscience. Specifically, cognitive control has been linked to functional aspects of frontostriatal circuitry. Both sMRI and fMRI studies in pediatric bipolar disorder implicate this circuit in the condition (Dickstein and Leibenluft 2006; Leibenluft et al. 2003; Rich et al. 2006). Similarly, social information processing has been linked to amygdala function. Again, findings from sMRI and fMRI studies in pediatric bipolar disorder also support findings in cognitive neuroscience. Reduced amygdala volume in pediatric bipolar disorder is probably the best-replicated finding emerging from all of the imaging work in any pediatric mood disorder. Moreover, fMRI studies find evidence of enhanced amygdala activation, specifically under conditions where deficits in social information processing manifest.

Considerable controversy surrounds the diagnosis of pediatric bipolar disorder. Ideally, emerging findings in brain imaging will provide some insights helpful in resolving this controversy. Although imaging work is only beginning to speak to issues of classification, some evidence suggests that future work in this area may be helpful in refining understandings of bipolar phenotypes. Figure 52–4 illustrates one relevant finding using ERP technology (Rich et al. 2007). Much of the controversy in nomenclature concerns the classification of children presenting with marked irritability and hyperarousal in the absence of classic symptoms of mania, particularly distinct periods of elevated mood. Figure 52–4 shows that children presenting with these features can be differentiated from children with classic presentations of mania, whereas other findings from the same study also show that these children can be differentiated, using other ERP measures, from healthy peers as well as from children with classic bipolar presentations.

Imaging work on MDD also has generated consistent findings, again extending findings that have emerged from cognitive neuroscience studies based in the laboratory. Deficits in reward-related processes represent one of the most consistent correlates of MDD, in juveniles as well as in adults. Emerging fMRI data implicate perturbed striatal function in this information-processing profile (Forbes et al. 2006). Similarly, perturbations in memory, particularly for emotional stimuli, represent a second consistently manifested correlate of MDD across the age span. Considerable imaging work implicates the amygdala in emotional modulation of memory. Consistent with these

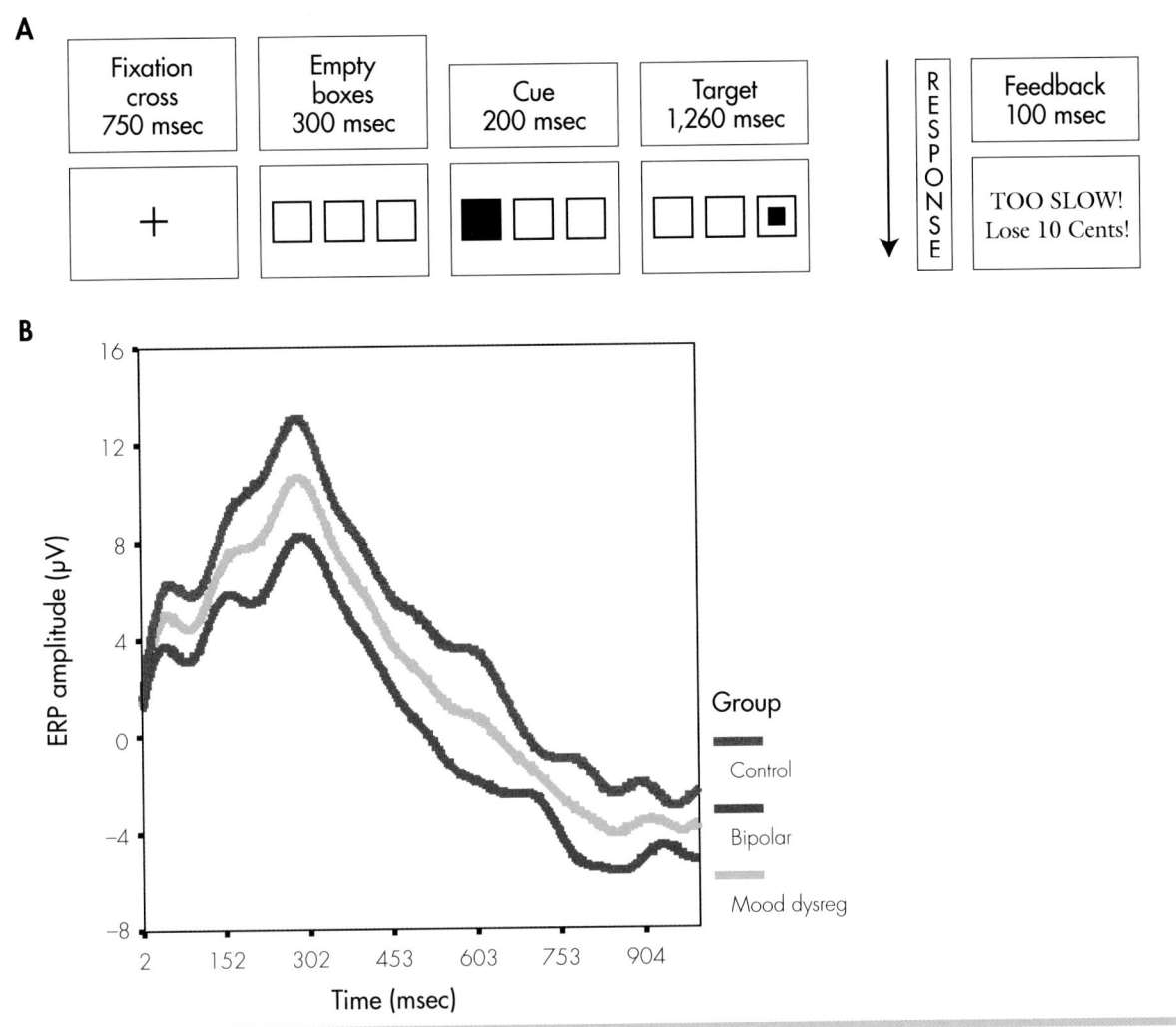

FIGURE 52–4. Event-related potentials in pediatric bipolar disorder.

This figure shows P3 event-related potential (ERP) amplitude at the parietal Pz site during performance of a frustrating task. The task, which requires subjects to quickly identify a target, is made quite difficult, leading to frustration through frequent incorrect responses **(A).** As shown in **B,** when patients with bipolar disorder (*n*=35; blue) make errors, ERP amplitude, phase-locked to these errors, is significantly lower than in both healthy peers (*n*=26; red) (*P*<0.01) and peers with severe mood dysregulation but without bipolar disorder (*n*=21; green) (*P*<0.05). *Source.*   Rich et al. 2007.

data in healthy subjects, as well as with evidence of abnormal emotional memory in MDD, emerging imaging work suggests that emotional memory perturbations in adolescents with MDD are associated with amygdala-based dysfunction (Roberson-Nay et al. 2006). Such amygdala hypersensitivity has been attributed to increased afferent input from PFC-based glutamatergic neurons, possibly leading to excitotoxic processes over time. This view is supported by demonstrations of reduced amygdala volume in both pediatric and adult MDD.

Anxiety Disorders

Available imaging data demonstrate potential circuitry-based differences in the correlates of distinct pediatric

anxiety disorders, consistent with data from family-based and longitudinal research. These data document one set of abnormalities in OCD, another set in pediatric PTSD, and a third set in other pediatric anxiety disorders.

Unique aspects of pediatric OCD relate to the distinct associations with basal ganglia dysfunction in OCD, dysfunction that is also thought to occur in other syndromes, such as Tourette's syndrome, that exhibit longitudinal and familial associations with OCD. Consistent with this view, the few available sMRI and MRS studies in pediatric OCD implicate perturbed frontostriatal circuitry in the condition (Rosenberg and Hanna 2000). Thus, pediatric OCD has been linked to altered striatal volumes, although the nature of these alterations varies across studies, as well as to signs of altered glutamate transmission. These findings are consistent with data in both ADHD and Tourette's syndrome, where other signs of altered basal ganglia dysfunction emerge.

Pediatric PTSD, in contrast, has been most consistently linked to abnormalities in specific components of the corpus callosum and PFC (De Bellis 2001). Neuroanatomical studies have documented reduced volume in various components of the corpus callosum, with the most consistent data implicating middle and posterior portions of this structure, contrasting with data in other disorders, such as OCD, where different regions show volume reductions. Relatively consistent findings have also emerged in research on the PFC, where various components show volume reductions. Other regions implicated include various aspects of posterior association cortex, such as the superior temporal gyrus, the pituitary, and the cerebellum, as well as overall reductions in brain size. Unlike in research on adult PTSD and in other anxiety disorders, however, medial temporal lobe structure and function generally appear intact in pediatric PTSD—despite a wealth of research attempting to document abnormalities in this region, based on the theoretical importance of this structure.

Finally, considerable research in anxiety disorders besides PTSD and OCD has documented abnormalities in brain circuitry encompassing the PFC and medial temporal cortex. As reviewed elsewhere (Pine 2007), six studies have used face-viewing paradigms with fMRI to examine amygdala function in children with these conditions or behavioral inhibition, a major risk factor for these conditions. Five of the six studies documented signs of enhanced amygdala response to evocative faces, consistent with considerable work in adults with social phobia and with research linking both pediatric anxiety disorders and behavioral inhibition to adult social phobia. Other notable findings in these six studies include evidence of perturbed PFC activation as well as dysfunctional connectivity between the amygdala and PFC, findings that, again, are consistent with data from studies in adults.

Future Directions

As delineated in the current review, the stage has been set for major breakthroughs in research on the biology of pediatric mental disorders. The emerging advances in genetics, cognitive neuroscience, and brain imaging have provided the field with heretofore-unanticipated tools. These tools allow developmental scientists to chart brain–behavior relationships, and their underlying un-

folding through genetic and environmental influences, in young children as they pass through each stage of development. The greatest excitement for future directions concerns applications of these tools. Thus, in each of the various clinical domains, considerable work remains to be done. Longitudinal research in young children is needed, documenting genetic and environmental influences on specific neural circuits and their chemical modulation. The development of these specific neural circuits must be mapped to specific information-processing functions, as delineated in cognitive and affective neuroscience. Finally, this mapping of brain function to information-processing indices must be linked to current conceptualizations of phenotypes.

Conclusion

The importance of biological research on childhood disorders has emerged largely from findings in epidemiology, basic science, and biological research among adults. Thus, epidemiology research has demonstrated the strong longitudinal and family-based associations between pediatric and adult mental disorders. Findings in basic science and in biological research among adults suggest that these associations between childhood and adult psychiatric syndromes emerge through the effects of perturbed brain development. This suggests that better knowledge about the nature of such developmental perturbations may provide novel avenues for treatments that interrupt processes contributing to chronic psychiatric disorders early in the pathophysiological process. However, realization of this goal will require the field to enhance understandings of the relationship between biological factors and development through studies implemented directly in children.

References

Abelson JF, Kwan KY, O'Roak BJ, et al: Sequence variants in SLITRK1 are associated with Tourette's syndrome. Science 310:317–320, 2005

Birmaher B, Heydl P: Biological studies in depressed children and adolescents. Int J Neuropsychopharmacol 4:149–157, 2001

Blair J, Mitchell D, Blair K: The Psychopath: Emotion and the Brain. Malden, MA, Blackwell Publishing, 2005

Brotman LM, Gouley KK, Huang KY, et al: Effects of a psychosocial family-based preventive intervention on cortisol response to a social challenge in preschoolers at high risk for psychopathology. Arch Gen Psychiatry 64:1172–1179, 2007

Budhani S, Marsh AA, Pine DS, et al: Neural correlates of response reversal: considering acquisition. Neuroimage 34:1754–1765, 2007

Caspi A, Moffitt TE: Gene-environment interactions in psychiatry: joining forces with neuroscience. Nat Rev Neurosci 7:583–590, 2006

De Bellis MD: Developmental traumatology: the psychobiological development of maltreated children and its implications for research, treatment, and policy. Dev Psychopathol 13:539–564, 2001

Dickstein DP, Leibenluft E: Emotion regulation in children and adolescents: boundaries between normalcy and bipolar disorder. Dev Psychopathol 18:1105–1131, 2006

Emslie GJ, Mayes TL: Mood disorders in children and adolescents: psychopharmacological treatment. Biol Psychiatry 49:1082–1090, 2001

Ernst M, Maheu FS, Schroth E, et al: Amygdala function in adolescents with congenital adrenal hyperplasia: a model for the study of early steroid abnormalities. Neuropsychologia 45:2104–2113, 2007

Faraone SV, Khan SA: Candidate gene studies of attention-deficit/hyperactivity disorder. J Clin Psychiatry 67 (suppl 8):13–20, 2006

Forbes EE, May JC, Siegle GJ, et al: Reward-related decision making in pediatric major depression: an fMRI study. J Child Psychol Psychiatry 47:1031–1040, 2006

Fox NA, Henderson HA, Marshall PJ, et al: Behavioral inhibition: linking biology and behavior within a developmental framework. Annu Rev Psychol 56:235–262, 2005

Gottesman II, Gould TD: The endophenotype concept in psychiatry: etymology and strategic intentions. Am J Psychiatry 160:636–645, 2003

Greenstein D, Lerch J, Shaw P, et al: Childhood onset schizophrenia: cortical brain abnormalities as young adults. J Child Psychol Psychiatry 47:1003–1012, 2006

Grillon C, Warner V, Hille J, et al: Families at high and low risk for depression: a three-generation startle study. Biol Psychiatry 57:953–960, 2005

Gross C, Hen R: The developmental origins of anxiety. Nat Rev Neurosci 5:545–552, 2004

Gunnar MR: Integrating neuroscience and psychological approaches in the study of early experiences. Ann N Y Acad Sci 1008:238–247, 2003

Gupta AR, State MW: Recent advances in the genetics of autism. Biol Psychiatry 61:429–437, 2007

Joseph J, Noble K, Eden G: The neurobiological basis of reading. J Learn Disabil 34:566–579, 2001

Leibenluft E, Charney DS, Pine DS: Researching the pathophysiology of pediatric bipolar disorder. Biol Psychiatry 53:1009–1020, 2003

Meaney MJ: Maternal care, gene expression, and the transmission of individual differences in stress reactivity across generations. Annu Rev Neurosci 24:1161–1192, 2001

Merikangas KR, Avenevoli S, Dierker L, et al: Vulnerability factors among children at risk for anxiety disorders. Biol Psychiatry 46:1523–1535, 1999

Nelson CA, Bloom FE, Cameron JL, et al: An integrative, multidisciplinary approach to the study of brain-behavior relations in the context of typical and atypical development. Dev Psychopathol 14:499–520, 2002

Nigg J: What Causes ADHD? New York, Guilford, 2007

Olney JW: Excitotoxicity, apoptosis and neuropsychiatric disorders. Curr Opin Pharmacol 3:101–109, 2003

Pine DS: Research review: a neuroscience framework for pediatric anxiety disorders. J Child Psychol Psychiatry 48:631–648, 2007

Prather MD, Lavenex P, Mauldin-Jourdain ML, et al: Increased social fear and decreased fear of objects in monkeys with neonatal amygdala lesions. Neuroscience 106:653–658, 2001

Rich BA, Vinton DT, Roberson-Nay R, et al: Limbic hyperactivation during processing neutral facial expressions in children with bipolar disorder. Proc Natl Acad Sci U S A 103:8900–8905, 2006

Rich BA, Schmajuk M, Perez-Edgar KE, et al: Different psychophysiological and behavioral responses elicited by frustration in pediatric bipolar disorder and severe mood dysregulation. Am J Psychiatry 164:309–317, 2007

Roberson-Nay R, McClure EB, Monk CS, et al: Increased amygdala activity during successful memory encoding in adolescent major depressive disorder: an fMRI study. Biol Psychiatry 60:966–973, 2006

Rosenberg DR, Hanna GL: Genetic and imaging strategies in obsessive-compulsive disorder: potential implications for treatment development. Biol Psychiatry 48:1210–1222, 2000

Rutter M: Psychosocial influences: critiques, findings, and research needs. Dev Psychopathol 12:375–405, 2000

Rutter M: Autism research: lessons from the past and prospects for the future. J Autism Dev Disord 35:241–257, 2005

Rutter M, Kim-Cohen J, Maughan B: Continuities and discontinuities in psychopathology between childhood and adult life. J Child Psychol Psychiatry 47:276–295, 2006

Sowell ER, Thompson PM, Leonard CM, et al: Longitudinal mapping of cortical thickness and brain growth in normal children. J Neurosci 24:8223–8231, 2004

Spear LP: The adolescent brain and age-related behavioral manifestations. Neurosci Biobehav Rev 24:417–463, 2000

Steinberg L, Dahl R, Keating D, et al: The study of developmental psychopathology in adolescence: integrating affective neuroscience with the study of context, in Developmental Psychopathology, 2nd Edition, Vol 2: Developmental Neuroscience. Edited by Cicchetti D, Cohen DJ. Hoboken, NJ, Wiley, 2006, pp 710–741

Swanson JM, Kinsbourne M, Nigg J, et al: Etiologic subtypes of attention-deficit/hyperactivity disorder: brain imaging, molecular genetic and environmental factors and the dopamine hypothesis. Neuropsychol Rev 17:39–59, 2007

Tallal P, Gaab N: Dynamic auditory processing, musical experience and language development. Trends Neurosci 29:382–390, 2006

Thapar A, Rutter M: Genetics, in Rutter's Child and Adolescent Psychiatry, 5th Edition. Edited by Rutter M, Bishop D, Pine DS, et al. Malden, MA, Blackwell Publishing, 2008, pp 339–358

Toga AW, Thompson PM: Temporal dynamics of brain anatomy. Annu Rev Biomed Eng 5:119–145, 2003

van Goozen SH, Fairchild G, Snoek H, et al: The evidence for a neurobiological model of childhood antisocial behavior. Psychol Bull 133:149–182, 2007

Vargha-Khadem F, Gadian DG, Copp A, et al: FOXP2 and the neuroanatomy of speech and language. Nat Rev Neurosci 6:131–138, 2005

Volkmar FR, Lord C, Bailey A, et al: Autism and pervasive developmental disorders. J Child Psychol Psychiatry 45:135–170, 2004

Weissman MM, Wickramaratne P, Nomura Y, et al: Offspring of depressed parents: 20 years later. Am J Psychiatry 163:1001–1008, 2006

PART IV

Psychopharmacological Treatment

David L. Dunner, M.D., Section Editor

Treatment of Depression

Catherine Bresee, M.S.

Jennifer Gotto, M.D.

Mark Hyman Rapaport, M.D.

Changes in Conceptualization of Depressive Disorders

The past 20 years have seen a shift in the way psychiatrists conceptualize depressive disorders. This evolution in our thinking has been stimulated by the results of epidemiological studies and of long-term clinical follow-up studies, investigations of spectrum disorders, advances in biological psychiatry, and results of large clinically focused national trials. In the past, major depressive disorder was viewed as episodic and self-limited. However, longitudinal observations of patients treated for major depressive disorder show that after recovery from an index episode of major depression, patients remain symptomatic about 60% of the remainder of their lives with another episode of major depression, minor depressive disorder, or subsyndromal symptoms of depression (Judd et al. 1998a). Data from the National Institute of Mental Health (NIMH) Collaborative Depression Study demonstrated that the recurrence rates of major depressive disorder are extraordinarily high over time: 60% at 5 years of follow-up, 75% at 10 years, and 87% at 15 years (Keller et al. 1982, 1984, 1992; Kupfer 1991).

Thus, the majority of people with major depressive disorder can be conceptualized as having a chronic illness with a dynamic course. This view of depression as a chronic and frequently recurring illness is a major paradigm shift. A second major shift in our thinking about major depressive disorder has revolved around the ten-sion between conceptualizing the "depressions" as several discrete disorders (e.g., major depressive disorder, dysthymia, double depression, minor depression) versus considering major depressive disorder as part of a spectrum of mood disorders. In this schema, an individual may traverse over time between meeting criteria for major depressive disorder and meeting criteria for euthymia, minor depression, or subsyndromal depressive symptoms (Judd et al. 1998b; Maddux and Rapaport 2004).

Current epidemiological and clinical outcome data support the postulate that major depressive disorder is part of a fluid spectrum of depressive disorders. The presence of depressive symptoms—be they symptoms of subsyndromal depression or minor depression or residual symptoms after partially successful treatment—carries significant risks for psychosocial disability, increases the risk for chronicity, and is associated with greater medical comorbidity, greater health care utilization, greater risk for recurrence, and greater risk for suicide (Akiskal et al. 1997; Judd and Akiskal 2000; Rapaport et al. 2002; Wells et al. 1989). The results of preliminary clinical trials suggest that both minor depressive disorder and subsyndromal depressive disorder are responsive to treatment with either pharmacotherapy or focused brief psychotherapies (Maddux and Rapaport 2004; Rapaport et al. 2002). This paradigm shift has profound implications for how we conceptualize the goals for treatment of major depressive disorder. In the past, the goals of treatment were the acute amelioration of the most troublesome symptoms of major depressive disorder: a 50% response on an objective measure of the severity of depression was defined as a successful outcome. Now the goal of treatment for an episode of major depressive disorder is the complete eradication of depressive symptoms. Asymptomatic status is defined as the elimination of all signs and symptoms of depression and a return to normal functioning (Judd and Akiskal 2000; Judd et al. 1998b).

Another significant advance that has modified our conceptualization of major depressive disorder and its treatment is the NIMH-funded Sequenced Treatment Alternatives to Relieve Depression (STAR*D) study. This study is the largest and most authoritative investigation of the efficacy of an evidence-based approach to the acute treatment of major depressive disorder. Results from the STAR*D study (Trivedi et al. 2006d) indicate that only 28% of patients remit even with a systematic, ratings-guided initial trial with a selective serotonin reuptake inhibitor (SSRI). The majority of patients required a stepwise application of treatments with increasingly aggressive augmentation or treatment-switching strategies to attain remission (Rush et al. 2006b). At 6-month naturalistic follow-up, the patients who remitted earlier in their course of treatment and those with less resistant depression (i.e., those who remitted with level 1 or level 2 treatment [see study description in the "Acute Treatment" section]) were less likely to have relapsed at follow-up. This supports the idea that early successful treatment focused on remission gives the patient the best opportunity for long-term success. Further large-scale studies are needed to inform not only our continued understanding of acute therapy for depressive disorders but also our knowledge of what strategies are most effective during the continuation and maintenance phases of therapy.

The development and refinement of imaging techniques, preclinical models, molecular genetic techniques, and computational techniques are leading to a marked increase in our knowledge about the biological underpinnings of depressive disorders. At this time, we have not been able to link our phenotypic investigations of the course and prognosis of depressive disorders with specific biological processes; however, our knowledge of the neuroanatomical circuits that are abnormal in some patients with depressive disorders is rapidly expanding (Goldapple et al. 2004; Kennedy et al. 2001; Mayberg et al. 2000). This knowledge combined with fundamental advances in animal model development, molecular biology, and whole-genome scanning techniques in genetics will markedly alter our understanding of the biology of mood disorders in the future (Nemeroff and Vale 2005; Perlis 2007).

In summary, major depressive disorder is a chronic illness with symptoms that fluctuate over a continuum of severity. Even the mildest form of depression, subsyndromal depression, is associated with both psychosocial morbidity and a risk for developing major depressive disorder (Beekman et al. 1997; Fergusson et al. 2005; Fogel et al. 2006; Hermens et al. 2004; Judd et al. 1994; Rieckmann et al. 2006). The goal of treatment of all forms of depression needs to be the return to an asymptomatic state of the patient's prior "normal" functioning. Thus, the treatment of patients with major depressive disorder requires aggressive and varied therapies that may need to continue for years, if not indefinitely.

Epidemiology

Prevalence of Depressive Disorders

Major depressive disorder is one of the most common medical disorders affecting adults in the world (Lopez and Murray 1998). In the United States the lifetime prevalence of major depression for men is 9% and 17% for women (Hasin et al. 2005), while the lifetime prevalence of dysthymia is 4% for men and 8% for women (Kessler et al. 1994). The lifetime prevalence of minor depression is 10% for individuals between the ages of 15 and 54 years (Kessler et al. 1997). For persons 65 years and older, the 1-month point prevalence of minor depression is 13%, which is twice the prevalence of major depressive disorder for this age group (Judd and Akiskal 2002; McCusker et al. 2005). The lifetime prevalence for subsyndromal depression is 11.8% for the general population (Goldney et al. 2004; Judd et al. 1994).

Risk Factors for Depressive Disorders

Several risk factors seem to increase a person's vulnerability to developing a depressive disorder. The vulnerability factors for which the greatest preponderance of evidence exists suggesting that they might increase the risk include female sex, age, a family history of a mood disorder, a history of trauma, and comorbid medical and psychiatric conditions.

A significant body of evidence indicates that the sex of an individual is an important risk factor for the development of depressive disorders. Prior to puberty the prevalence of depression is equal in boys and girls. However, beginning with puberty, women demonstrate a twofold increase in the prevalence of major depressive disorder (Weissman and Klerman 1977). This trend is seen across countries and ethnic groups (Weissman et al. 1996). The difference in prevalence rates between men and women is not easily understood. It has been postulated that the difference may in part be explained by the role of changes in levels of β-estradiol in the genesis of depression. Data suggest that there may be specific periods of the life cycle when a woman may be at greater risk of developing a mood disorder, such as during pregnancy and postpartum (Burt and Stein 2002; Joffe et al. 2002). It has also been speculated that this difference in prevalence rates may reflect the complex interplay between an intrinsic biological vulnerability, societal pressures, and a style of coping that more readily seeks help.

Age is another risk factor in the development of depressive disorders; the onset of major depressive disorder increases dramatically beginning in adolescence (12–16 years of age) and continuing through the age of about 44 years (Hasin et al. 2005). The mean age at onset has been reported to be 30 years, whereas the mean age at the start of treatment is 33.5 years of age, reflecting the amount of time depression often goes undiagnosed or untreated. In elderly populations, risk factors for depression are slightly different and include female sex, low socioeconomic status, bereavement, prior depression, medical comorbidity, disability, cognitive deterioration, and vascular disease (Helmer et al. 2004). The elderly are at risk for a "downward spiral" that can occur when disability or cognitive impairment leads to depressive symptoms, depressive symptoms increase disability, and so on. Depression in the elderly affects psychosocial function, health care utilization, quality of life, work productivity, risk for suicide, and medical compliance and outcome.

A family history of psychiatric illness is among the most profound risk factors for the development of an episode of major depressive disorder (Reinherz et al. 2003). No one gene has been clearly identified as a cause of major depression, and it may be concluded that depressive disorders are likely polygenetic in nature. This might further explain the heterogeneity of the disease and treatment response. New research has demonstrated that genetics coupled with environmental conditions may contribute to the development of depression. The work led by Caspi et al. (2003) and verified by others (Cervilla et al. 2007; Kendler et al. 2005) indicates that depressive responses to traumatic life events are modulated by genetic makeup. Individuals who carry two short alleles at the serotonin transporter (5-HTT) gene are more likely to develop depression after a stressful event than those with one or two long alleles. Other studies have found that genetic variants in the dopamine transporter (Elo-

vainio et al. 2007) or enzymes responsible for polyamine catabolism (Sequeira et al. 2006) may be implicated as a risk factor for the development of depression.

Prolonged exposure to severe traumatic events in childhood has been linked to future depressive episodes. Trauma such as sexual abuse or the loss of a parent that occurs at a critical developmental period can result in permanent alteration of the hypothalamic-pituitary-adrenal (HPA) axis. It is recognized that individuals with depression, particularly those exposed to early trauma, have altered stress responses (Gillespie and Nemeroff 2005; Heim et al. 2000; Nemeroff and Vale 2005). Some individuals with major depressive disorder have altered HPA axis activity with elevated circulating levels of cortisol, hypersecretion of corticotropin-releasing hormone, and adrenal hypertrophy, which normalize after resolution of depressive symptoms (Nemeroff and Vale 2005).

Other clinical and demographic variables have been linked to an increased risk of developing depressive disorders. These include stressful life events such as the death of a loved one, divorce, or job loss. Certain personality characteristics also may predispose an individual to develop a mood disorder. Individuals who score higher on measures of neuroticism, interpersonal dependency, or external locus of control may be vulnerable to stressful life events precipitating a major depressive episode (Hirschfeld et al. 1983; Paykel et al. 1996). Investigations suggesting that certain cultural groups may be at increased risk of a mood disorder (Native Americans) and that other cultural groups may have greater inherent resilience (Asian and Hispanic groups) are an area of renewed interest (Hasin et al. 2005). Further investigation of the role that intrinsic cultural differences may play, not only in the presentation of major depressive disorder but also in the protection against depressive symptoms, is warranted (Harris 2004).

Many medical illnesses are comorbid with major depressive disorder (Table 53–1). Cancer, acquired immunodeficiency syndrome, respiratory disease, cardiovascular disease, Parkinson's disease, and stroke are associated with an increased risk for depression. An interesting bidirectional relationship exists between depression and cardiovascular disease. For example, depression is a risk factor for a future cerebrovascular accident, and stroke is a well-documented risk factor for depression. Although there are little data on prevalence rates, an acute myocardial infarction is a risk factor for depression. Some studies suggest that depression is common among cardiac patients, with 40%–50% of cardiac patients having mild, moderate, or major depressive symptoms and women be-

TABLE 53–1.   Medical conditions often comorbid with major depressive disorder

INFECTIOUS	METABOLIC	NEUROLOGICAL	GENERAL MEDICAL
Encephalitis	Addison's disease	Brain tumor	Alcohol or sedative withdrawal
Hepatitis	Cushing's disease	Dementia, cortical	Arthritis
HIV/AIDS	Diabetes	Dementia, subcortical	Cancer
Influenza	Hyponatremia	Huntington's disease	Cardiovascular disease
Meningitis	Nutritional deficiencies	Migraine headaches	Chronic pain syndromes
Mononucleosis	Pituitary dysfunction	Multiple sclerosis	Cocaine or stimulant withdrawal
Pneumonia	Renal disease	Parkinson's disease	Connective tissue diseases
Postviral syndrome	Thyroid disease	Poststroke syndrome	Fibromyalgia
Syphilis		Seizure disorders	Heavy metal poisoning
Tuberculosis		Traumatic brain injury	Irritable bowel syndrome
Urinary tract infection			Liver failure
			Menopause
			Myocardial infarction
			Premenstrual syndrome
			Pulmonary disease
			Selenium toxicity
			Sleep disturbance

Note.   AIDS=acquired immunodeficiency syndrome; HIV=human immunodeficiency virus.

ing more likely to be depressed than men (Drago et al. 2007). The presence of moderate or major depression following myocardial infarction increases the risk for death by 3.5 times (Glassman and Shapiro 1998). Depression is also associated with rehospitalization and mortality in patients with heart failure.

Major depressive disorder is highly comorbid with other psychiatric disorders such as anxiety, dementia, schizophrenia, and substance abuse. In primary care settings, more than 75% of patients with diagnosed depression also present with an anxiety disorder (Olfson et al. 1997). Patients with depression and anxiety have more chronic and severe illness, greater occupational and psychosocial impairment, and, when the comorbidity is unrecognized, a greater rate of psychiatric hospitalization and suicide attempts (Hirschfeld 2001). Fifty percent of schizophrenic patients have comorbid depression. When present with schizophrenia, depression is an additional risk factor for suicide and decreased social and performance status (Ginsberg et al. 2005). The rate of major depressive disorder in Alzheimer's disease patients is between 20% and 40%. Diagnosing depression in Alzheimer's disease may be complicated by the overlap between symptoms of dementia and those of depression: loss of motivation, social withdrawal, isolation, and apathy are common to both disorders. Persons with dementia may have difficulty verbalizing subjective feelings such as sadness or hopelessness. Therefore, observable behavioral signs and symptoms such as irritability, social withdrawal, worsened functional impairment, and agitation may be more reliable indicators of the presence of a mood disorder in patients with Alzheimer's disease. There seems to be a complex relationship between depression and dementia: the presence of depression may be a harbinger of dementia, and dementia seems to be a risk factor for depression (Potter and Steffens 2007). Substance abuse is also highly comorbid with depressive disorders. Estimates of the prevalence of depressive disorders in patients with alcohol dependence is 15%–67%; for patients with cocaine addiction the prevalence is 33%–53%, and for patients with opiate dependence the lifetime rate of affective disorders ranges from 16% to 75% (Nunes 2003). Symptoms of substance withdrawal (cocaine, methamphetamine, alcohol) do overlap with symptoms of depression, but the type and severity tend to be distinctly different (Rapaport et al. 1993).

In summary, the exploration of factors that influence vulnerability and resilience has been complicated by the heterogeneity of depressive disorders. Despite this obstacle, it is clear that certain moderating factors have been identified that increase the risk of developing a depressive disorder. These include female sex, aging, family history, childhood trauma, certain personality styles, stressful life events, and presence of other psychiatric and medical illnesses.

Disability and Costs Associated With Depressive Illnesses

Major depressive disorder is associated with significant disease burden, exceeding that of cerebrovascular diseases and cancer. It is the leading cause of years lived with disability worldwide for young adults (Lopez et al. 2006). Psychosocial disability progresses along a gradient parallel to the increasing severity of depressive symptoms (Judd et al. 2000; Kessler et al. 1997). People with subsyndromal depressive symptoms and depressive disorder have higher disability ratings for social and role functioning than patients with hypertension, diabetes, arthritis, gastrointestinal problems, or back problems (Rapaport et al. 2002). Depressed persons rate themselves as having worse health and spend more days in bed than patients with many other chronic medical conditions including arthritis, diabetes, and lung disease (Wells et al. 1989). Even patients with minimal symptoms or subsyndromal depression have functional impairment more akin to that seen in patients with major depression than in nondepressed control subjects (Beekman et al. 2002). Thus, patients with depressive disorders have decreased income, productivity, physical functioning, and health status and more days spent in bed than control populations (Judd et al. 1996; Maddux and Rapaport 2004).

The costs associated with major depressive disorder are staggering. For individuals 18–65 years of age, 85% of the cost of depressive disorders is due to lost productivity (Smit et al. 2006). It is estimated that depressive disorders cost employers in the United States $44 billion in productivity annually. Twenty percent of this financial burden is due to absenteeism, with 80% of this loss due to *presenteeism*; that is, a worker is well enough to come to work but unable to perform the job efficiently (Stewart et al. 2003). Thus, although individuals who are mildly depressed may appear to be functional, subtle impairments in abilities have a significant impact on productivity.

Depressive disorders are also prevalent and incur significant societal costs in the elderly (Cuijpers et al. 2004; Horowitz et al. 2005). In contradistinction to the costs in younger adults, the costs associated with major depressive disorder and other forms of depression in the elderly are primarily driven by increased health care utilization, medical disease burden, and mortality.

The greatest "cost" associated with depressive disorders is the increased likelihood that an individual suffering from a depressive disorder will commit suicide. According to the Centers for Disease Control and Prevention, suicide is the eleventh leading cause of death in the United States: approximately 32,000 known suicides were identified in the 2005 census. In that year the overall suicide rate was almost double the homicide rate in the United States (11.05 per 100,000 vs. 5.9 per 100,000). Suicide is the second leading cause of death for individuals between the ages of 25 and 34 years and the third leading cause of death for young people between the ages of 15 and 24 years. Eighty percent of people who commit suicide are male. Suicide is more common in white than Hispanic or black individuals. Statistical risk factors for suicide include being male, being white, being single, having been hospitalized for a suicide attempt or having any history of a previous attempt, having a family history of suicide, and abusing substances. Women are more likely to attempt suicide, whereas men are more likely to complete it. In fact, longitudinal 40-year data from F. Angst et al. (2002) suggested that the 17.7% of the Zurich community cohort of people with a diagnosis of major depressive disorder committed suicide.

The elderly constitute a special at-risk group for successful completion of suicide. People older than 65 years constitute only 13% of the population and yet are responsible for 18% of all suicides: this is the highest suicide rate for any age group. Risk factors for suicide among older individuals are slightly different than the factors among younger individuals; for older individuals they include social isolation, physical illness, divorced or widowed status, and male sex (U.S. Department of Health and Human Services 2001). Older individuals who attempt suicide usually employ more lethal means (guns, drug overdoses) than younger individuals do.

It is clear that early identification and vigorous treatment are essential to decrease the likelihood that an individual with a depressive disorder who is suicidal will take his or her life (Clayton and Auster 2008). Despite recent guidance from the U.S. Food and Drug Administration (FDA) suggesting that suicidal thoughts and behavior among individuals younger than 25 years may increase during the first 10 days after starting an antidepressant, and despite a recent report based on the STAR*D database that found an association between two ionotropic glutamate receptor genes (*GRIA3* and *GRIK2*) and an increased risk of SSRI-induced suicidal thoughts, the vast majority of data suggest that antidepressant medication decreases suicidal thoughts and lowers rates of suicide

TABLE 53-2.   DSM-IV-TR criteria for major depressive episode

A. Five (or more) of the following symptoms have been present during the same 2-week period and represent a change from previous functioning; at least one of the symptoms is either (1) depressed mood or (2) loss of interest or pleasure.

>   **Note:**   Do not include symptoms that are clearly due to a general medical condition, or mood-incongruent delusions or hallucinations.

>   (1) depressed mood most of the day, nearly every day, as indicated by either subjective report (e.g., feels sad or empty) or observation made by others (e.g., appears tearful).   **Note:** In children and adolescents, can be irritable mood.

>   (2) markedly diminished interest or pleasure in all, or almost all, activities most of the day, nearly every day (as indicated by either subjective account or observation made by others)

>   (3) significant weight loss when not dieting or weight gain (e.g., a change of more than 5% of body weight in a month), or decrease or increase in appetite nearly every day.   **Note:** In children, consider failure to make expected weight gains.

>   (4) insomnia or hypersomnia nearly every day

>   (5) psychomotor agitation or retardation nearly every day (observable by others, not merely subjective feelings of restlessness or being slowed down)

>   (6) fatigue or loss of energy nearly every day

>   (7) feelings of worthlessness or excessive or inappropriate guilt (which may be delusional) nearly every day (not merely self-reproach or guilt about being sick)

>   (8) diminished ability to think or concentrate, or indecisiveness, nearly every day (either by subjective account or as observed by others)

>   (9) recurrent thoughts of death (not just fear of dying), recurrent suicidal ideation without a specific plan, or a suicide attempt or a specific plan for committing suicide

B. The symptoms do not meet criteria for a mixed episode.

C. The symptoms cause clinically significant distress or impairment in social, occupational, or other important areas of functioning.

D. The symptoms are not due to the direct physiological effects of a substance (e.g., a drug of abuse, a medication) or a general medical condition (e.g., hypothyroidism).

E. The symptoms are not better accounted for by bereavement (i.e., after the loss of a loved one, the symptoms persist for longer than 2 months or are characterized by marked functional impairment, morbid preoccupation with worthlessness, suicidal ideation, psychotic symptoms, or psychomotor retardation).

completion (R. D. Gibbons et al. 2005; Henriksson and Isacsson 2006; Laje et al. 2007; Rich and Isacsson 1997; Søndergård et al. 2006). These observations are supported by the longitudinal work of J. Angst et al. (2005), who found that treatment with antidepressants, lithium, and clozapine reduced the number of suicides in their cohort. They observed that long-term treatment, particularly combined treatment, was associated with reduced overall mortality over 40-year follow-up. Taken as a whole, these data suggest that suicidal ideation with intent and planning must be considered a medical emergency that merits the same type of diligent care that a physician would give to other emergent conditions like a myocardial infarction.

Definition of Depressive Illness

Beginning with DSM-III (American Psychiatric Association 1980), American psychiatry made the transition to descriptive nosology. The hallmarks of DSM-IV (Ameri-

can Psychiatric Association 1994) nosology for depressive illness are the requirement that a constellation of signs or symptoms be present for a minimum length of time and that they induce some type of measurable functional impairment. For the diagnosis of *major depressive episode*, an individual must have experienced, over a single 2-week period, one of two "gatekeeper" symptoms—feeling sad/"blue" or having anhedonia—plus four additional symptoms. These symptoms must cause substantial functional impairment or disability, cannot be due a concomitant medical or substance use disorder, and must persist every day for a significant portion of the day. DSM-IV-TR (American Psychiatric Association 2000a) criteria for major depressive episode are presented in Table 53–2.

DSM-IV-TR allows the clinician to categorize the severity of the depressive disorder as *mild* (symptoms barely meet the threshold for diagnosing the disorder and are not associated with significant impairment), *moderate* (symptoms and functional impairment are somewhere between mild and severe), or *severe* (several symptoms in excess of those required to make the diagnosis are present, and symptoms markedly impair the individual's functioning). The current nosology classifies psychotic depression as *major depressive disorder, severe, with psychotic features*, rather than as a distinct entity. DSM-IV-TR also provides specifiers to characterize the current depressive episode, the two most significant being "with melancholic features" and "with atypical features." DSM-IV-TR criteria for the melancholic features specifier and for dysthymic disorder are presented in Tables 53–3 and 53–4, respectively.

DSM-IV-TR provides two other major categorizations for unipolar depressive disorders: *dysthymic disorder* and *depressive disorder not otherwise specified*. (The cardinal features of dysthymic disorder are presented in Table 53–4.) In order to be classified as having dysthymic disorder, an individual may not meet the threshold criteria for major depressive disorder during the first 2 years of illness and cannot be better characterized as having *major depressive disorder, chronic*, or *major depressive disorder, in partial remission*. Dysthymic disorder is thought to have an early and insidious onset. Most patients who are seen in clinical settings seek treatment because of a major depressive

TABLE 53–3. DSM-IV-TR criteria for melancholic features specifier

Specify if:

With melancholic features (can be applied to the current or most recent major depressive episode in major depressive disorder and to a major depressive episode in bipolar I or bipolar II disorder only if it is the most recent type of mood episode)

A. Either of the following, occurring during the most severe period of the current episode:

(1) loss of pleasure in all, or almost all, activities

(2) lack of reactivity to usually pleasurable stimuli (does not feel much better, even temporarily, when something good happens)

B. Three (or more) of the following:

(1) distinct quality of depressed mood (i.e., the depressed mood is experienced as distinctly different from the kind of feeling experienced after the death of a loved one)

(2) depression regularly worse in the morning

(3) early morning awakening (at least 2 hours before usual time of awakening)

(4) marked psychomotor retardation or agitation

(5) significant anorexia or weight loss

(6) excessive or inappropriate guilt

TABLE 53–4. DSM-IV-TR criteria for 300.4 dysthymic disorder

A. Depressed mood for most of the day, for more days than not, as indicated either by subjective account or observation by others, for at least 2 years. **Note:** In children and adolescents, mood can be irritable and duration must be at least 1 year.

B. Presence, while depressed, of two (or more) of the following:

(1) poor appetite or overeating

(2) insomnia or hypersomnia

(3) low energy or fatigue

(4) low self-esteem

(5) poor concentration or difficulty making decisions

(6) feelings of hopelessness

C. During the 2-year period (1 year for children or adolescents) of the disturbance, the person has never been without the symptoms in criteria A and B for more than 2 months at a time.

D. No major depressive episode has been present during the first 2 years of the disturbance (1 year for children and adolescents); i.e., the disturbance is not better accounted for by chronic major depressive disorder, or major depressive disorder, in partial remission.

Note: There may have been a previous major depressive episode provided there was a full remission (no significant signs or symptoms for 2 months) before development of the dysthymic disorder. In addition, after the initial 2 years (1 year in children or adolescents) of dysthymic disorder, there may be superimposed episodes of major depressive disorder, in which case both diagnoses may be given when the criteria are met for a major depressive episode.

E. There has never been a manic episode, a mixed episode, or a hypomanic episode, and criteria have never been met for cyclothymic disorder.

F. The disturbance does not occur exclusively during the course of a chronic psychotic disorder, such as schizophrenia or delusional disorder.

G. The symptoms are not due to the direct physiological effects of a substance (e.g., a drug of abuse, a medication) or a general medical condition (e.g., hypothyroidism).

H. The symptoms cause clinically significant distress or impairment in social, occupational, or other important areas of functioning.

Specify if:

Early onset: if onset is before age 21 years

Late onset: if onset is age 21 years or older

Specify (for most recent 2 years of dysthymic disorder):

With atypical features

disorder that has become superimposed on dysthymia. These cases of *double depression* tend to be challenging to treat and have a worse prognosis than uncomplicated major depression.

The category *depressive disorder not otherwise specified* has been used as a catchall for the presence of signs and symptoms of depression that do not meet criteria for major depressive disorder, dysthymia, or one of the adjustment disorders. Minor depressive disorder and subsyndromal depressive disorder fall within the rubric of depressive disorder not otherwise specified in DSM-IV-TR. More recent work has demonstrated that minor depressive disorder is associated with significant disability, morbidity, and impairment (Howland et al. 2008; Judd and Akiskal 2000; Judd et al. 1994; Rapaport and Judd 1998; Rapaport et al. 2002). In contradistinction to major depressive disorder, minor depressive disorder is characterized mostly by affective and cognitive symptoms such as sadness, loss of pleasure/enjoyment, irritable mood, anxious mood, pessimism, difficulty concentrating, lack of involvement, and fatigue. This constellation of symptoms has been demonstrated to be stable and persistent in individuals with minor depression (Rapaport et al. 2002). The research criteria for minor depressive disorder in the appendix of DSM-IV-TR exclude individuals who have had a prior episode of major depressive disorder. However, research suggests that this is unnecessarily restrictive; subjects with and without a prior history of major depressive disorder have identical demographic and clinical presentations, severity of illness, and acute treatment response (Howland et al. 2008; Judd et al. 2004; Rapaport et al. 2002).

A number of different definitions of subsyndromal depressive disorder have been discussed in the literature. For many investigators, subsyndromal depressive disorder is thought to be equivalent to minor depressive disorder. However, Judd et al. (1994) suggested that subsyndromal depressive disorder be defined as the presence of any of two or more associated symptoms of depression: problems with sleep, appetite, concentration, or suicidal thinking without the presence of sadness or anhedonia. Although there is no consensus about the diagnosis of subsyndromal depression at this time, the presence of signs and symptoms associated with depression has negative prognostic value. Such individuals are at greater risk of developing an episode of minor or major depressive disorder within the next year (Judd et al. 1994, 1997).

In conclusion, the definitions of the syndromes that constitute the spectrum of unipolar mood disorders will continue to evolve with our understanding of the neurobiology of what we call mood disorders.

Neurobiology of Depression

Depressive disorders have many features that clearly indicate a complex neurobiological component to the disease state. The discovery in the 1950s of antidepressant pharmacological therapies provided the initial evidence of an underlying biochemical alteration in depressed patients. Studies in genomics and imaging and the identification of neural pathways involved have advanced our knowledge. As a result, several complementary but distinct lines of investigation into the neurobiology of depression have begun to take hold.

Depression has for many years been predominantly hypothesized to be marked by a depletion of monoamine neurotransmitters, specifically norepinephrine, serotonin, and dopamine. The involvement of monoamines in mood alterations was first documented in the 1950s with the observation that individuals treated with high doses of reserpine, an antihypertensive agent that depletes the brain of monoamines, developed depression (Freis 1954). Later studies of monoamine depletion were developed to investigate the direct effects of monoamines on mood. Because monoamines are synthesized from essential amino acid precursors tryptophan (for serotonin) and tyrosine (for norepinephrine and dopamine), a transient depletion can be achieved by ingesting a tryptophan-free or tyrosine-free amino acid mixture. In healthy individuals, depressed mood has been noted after tryptophan or tyrosine depletion in some studies, although more marked results are found in subjects with a family history of mood disorders or in drug-free subjects in remission from depression (Ruhe et al. 2007). Although depletion studies have never induced levels of clinical depression in healthy individuals or increased depressive symptoms in clinically ill patients not taking medication, what has been intriguing is that subjects with major depression who responded to SSRIs relapsed after serotonin depletion (Delgado et al. 1990). These results suggest that patients who are clinically ill with major depression have deficits in brain monoamine concentrations and that these deficits play a modulatory role with other systems that have a more direct role in the symptoms of depression.

As our understanding has grown about the mechanism of action of antidepressant therapies, more attention has been given to the neurotransmitter systems involving glutamate and γ-aminobutyric acid (GABA). Evidence for the role of these neurotransmitter systems in depression comes from studies of therapies that have been shown to target the *N*-methyl-D-aspartate (NMDA) class of glutamate receptors, specifically lamotrigine, ketamine, and amantadine (Pittenger et al. 2007), and anti-convulsant therapies, which have a GABAergic route of action. Studies have demonstrated alterations of these systems in subjects with depression. One postmortem gene expression study demonstrated that the brains of sui-cide victims suffering from major depression had down-regulation of the spermidine/spermine N1-acetyltrans-ferase (SSAT) gene, which was subsequently linked to the presence of an allelic variant (Sequeira et al. 2006). SSAT is the rate-limiting enzyme for the catabolism of polyamines, which in turn regulate the NMDA receptors. Furthermore, a meta-analysis of the body of studies per-formed revealed that cerebrospinal fluid levels of GABA in subjects with depression are significantly lower than levels in nondepressed control subjects (Petty et al. 1993).

Depression is also marked by dysregulation of other important systems. External stressful stimuli are known to be a major risk factor for a depressive episode, and de-pressed individuals are often characterized with altered biological responses to stress. This is likely due to dysreg-ulation and overstimulation of the HPA axis (Gertsik and Poland 2004; Holsboer 1995). Early studies (Brown and Shuey 1980; Carroll 1982; Coppen et al. 1983) found that in a large percentage of unmedicated individuals with de-pression, secretion of the stress hormone cortisol is not suppressed after dexamethasone administration, a condi-tion known as *dexamethasone nonsuppression*. Dexametha-sone is a synthetic glucocorticoid and acts at the level of the anterior pituitary corticotrophs to reduce the secre-tion of adrenocorticotropic hormone (ACTH), which in turn decreases the production of cortisol in the adrenal cortex. Dexamethasone nonsuppression therefore indi-cates impairments in the feedback mechanisms of the HPA axis. Correspondingly, elevated levels of circulating cortisol have been reported in subjects with depression (J. L. Gibbons and McHugh 1962; Rubin et al. 1987). This impairment of HPA axis regulation has been traced upstream to dysregulation of corticotropin-releasing hor-mone (CRH), a hypothalamic hormone that controls the release of ACTH (Holsboer 2000). Depressed individuals have higher CRH neuronal activity (Raadsheer et al. 1994) and display a blunted ACTH and cortisol response to infusion of synthetic CRH (Gispen-de Wied et al. 1993; Gold et al. 1986). This global hyperactivity of the stress response in depressed individuals has been demon-strated to be a characteristic of the current depressed state, because the remission of clinical symptoms induces a normalization of responses to dexamethasone or CRH along with normalization of plasma cortisol levels (Am-

sterdam et al. 1988; Arana et al. 1985; Sachar et al. 1970). Dysregulation of the HPA axis activity and higher rates of depression are more prominent in individuals exposed to childhood trauma or abuse (Bremne and Vermetten 2001), suggesting that hyperactivity of the HPA axis dur-ing critical periods of brain development leads to higher rates of depression later in life.

This cascade of alterations in the HPA axis, and sub-sequent increase in glucocorticoids, is thought to be re-sponsible for the structural and functional changes seen in the limbic structures of depressed individuals. In vivo magnetic resonance imaging studies demonstrate hippo-campal shrinkage in depressed patients relative to healthy control subjects (Campbell et al. 2004; Videbech and Ravnkilde 2004). Although the exact mechanism of this loss of hippocampal volume is unknown, it is presumably through cell death, cell atrophy, and/or reduction in neurogenesis. Successful antidepressant therapy has been shown to increase cellular proliferation (Duman 2004; Warner-Schmidt and Duman 2006), and chronic stress induces the converse, giving further credence to the neurobiological component of depression.

Taken together, these observed alterations in mono-amines and other neurotransmitters, in the HPA axis function, and in neuronal plasticity can be conceptualized as a state of depressive illnesses rather than a trait of the illnesses. Given that successful clinical therapies often re-verse these trends, one has to ask, What is the underlying cause? It is clear that a familial predisposition to depres-sion is present, lending support to the idea of a genetic component to depression. Ongoing research has failed to pinpoint a specific genetic anomaly, which is likely due to the heterogeneity of the disorder and the additive role that environmental factors play in triggering depressive episodes in individuals who may be genetically predis-posed to depression. However, with the advent of high-throughput technology, such as whole-genome sequenc-ing and single nucleotide polymorphism detection, spe-cific genetic trends have been demonstrated.

Some very positive studies point to polymorphisms of the *5-HTT* gene (Caspi et al. 2003; Kendler et al. 2005) that may modulate the sensitivity of individuals to stress-ful life events. Additional work has implicated allelic polymorphisms in glucocorticoid receptors (Binder et al. 2004; Brouwer et al. 2006; van Rossum et al. 2006) and CRH receptors (Liu et al. 2007; Papiol et al. 2007). Most interesting has been the discovery that there exist sub-populations of depressed individuals with genetic anom-alies in the *5-HTT* gene who have a higher risk of de-veloping adverse side effects to SSRI treatment than individuals without those anomalies (Hu et al. 2007; Smits et al. 2007a). A study was conducted to determine whether genetic prescreening for a variant in the *5-HTT* gene to identify which class of antidepressants would be best suited for each subject's course of treatment would lead to better treatment outcomes (Smits et al. 2007b). Positive results were minor, however, and the costs involved suggest that the gains made were unsubstantial. One clear genetic variation that has been demonstrated as clinically valuable is alteration in the gene for the cytochrome P450 enzyme CYP2D6, a liver enzyme involved in drug metabolism. Individuals may have normal, intermediate, or poor metabolism rates depending on whether they carry no alleles, one allele, or two alleles. This trait has been seized on as a potential aid in properly dosing patients, and the FDA has approved use of a test to aid physicians in genetic testing (Roche Pharmaceuticals 2008).

Other studies have begun to examine the contribution of the immune system and cytokines in major depressive disorder, suggesting a new avenue for therapeutic alternatives. Cytokines are a heterogeneous group of signaling and regulatory molecules produced by immunocompetent cells, and generally are categorized as proinflammatory or anti-inflammatory. The proinflammatory cytokines interferon alfa and interferon gamma have potent antiviral and immunomodulatory properties and are used to treat various forms of cancer and hepatitis C (Adams et al. 1984; Borgstrom et al. 1982; Meyers 1999). These cytokine therapies have been noted to be accompanied by depressed behavioral effects that can be significantly reduced by pretreatment with paroxetine (Capuron et al. 2002; Musselman et al. 2001), thus supporting the cytokine theory of depression. Furthermore, individuals with depressive disorders have higher plasma concentrations of the proinflammatory cytokines interleukin 1 (IL-1) and interleukin 6 (IL-6) than do nondepressed individuals, and concentrations correlate with the severity of depressive symptoms (Maes 1995, 1999). Some studies have demonstrated that the immune system is in an activated state in subjects with depressive disorders (Kling et al. 2007; Maes et al. 1995; Schiepers et al. 2005; Sluzewska et al. 1996). Although the precise role that cytokines play in depression is difficult to elucidate, continued research in this direction is warranted.

As presented in greater detail in other chapters of this book (see Chapter 45, "Neurobiology of Mood Disorders"), it is clear that our understanding of the biological underpinnings of depressive disorders is rapidly increasing. In the future the combination of advances in molecular medicine, imaging, and data analysis will begin to clarify the relationship between what currently appear to be disparate biological findings.

Evaluation of Depression

Context

The setting of the psychiatric assessment is important in that it provides a context that defines the focus of the encounter and therefore the content of the examination. For example, the assessment of the depressed patient in the emergency room is very different from the assessment of the depressed patient in the office, and that is very different from the assessment within a general hospital setting. The assessment of a depressed person in the emergency room focuses on a rapid, yet thoughtful, determination of safety and appropriate disposition—that is, does this person require hospitalization or is treatment in a less restrictive environment more appropriate? To expedite the determination of disposition in the emergency room, the evaluation focuses on issues of safety, suicidal thinking, future orientation, stability of social supports, housing, and recent drug and alcohol use. This assessment should also include a review of recent life events and potential precipitating stressors. Collateral information from family, friends, and outside physicians is helpful in determining the appropriate level of care.

In the office setting, it is possible to carry out a more traditional and complete initial examination. This includes a detailed review of the patient's signs and symptoms of depression, any comorbid medical or psychiatric disorders, and the patient's psychiatric history. A family history of psychiatric illness is very important. The focus of the initial evaluation is on establishing rapport, determining a working diagnosis, and developing an initial treatment plan.

In contrast, when a psychiatrist is acting as a consultant in a general hospital setting, the assessment has a different focus. Because either the illness itself or a treatment intervention may have provoked the episode requiring hospitalization, the consultant needs to carefully review the current medical chart. The stress of the hospitalization, bereavement, delirium, or a head injury may mimic a depressive disorder in an individual hospitalized in an acute care setting. Somatic symptoms such as pain, constipation, insomnia, and nausea frequently stimulate angry behavior or exacerbate a sense of helplessness in a patient. The amelioration of such somatic concerns may decrease the intensity of depressive symptoms in the hospital setting. Thus, the goals of the consultant in a

TABLE 53–5. Medications that may cause depression

Acyclovir	Clonidine	Metoclopramide
Alcohol	Cocaine (withdrawal)	Metrizamide
Amantadine	Contraceptives	Metronidazole
α methyldopa	Corticosteroids	NSAIDs
Amphetamines (withdrawal)	Cycloserine	Opiates
Anabolic steroids	Dapsone	Pentazocine
Anticonvulsants	Digitalis	Pergolide
Antihistamines	Disopyramide	Phenylpropanolamine
Antineoplastic agents	Disulfiram	Physostigmine
Antipsychotic medications	Estrogens	Prazosin
Baclofen	Ethambutol	Progestins, implanted
Barbiturates	Fluoroquinolone antibiotics	Reserpine
Benzodiazepines	Guanethidine	Statins
β-adrenergic blockers	Interferon alfa	Sulfonamides
Bromocriptine	Isotretinoin	Thiazide diuretics
Calcium channel blockers	Levodopa	
Cimetidine	Mefloquine	

Note. NSAIDs = nonsteroidal anti-inflammatory drugs.

general hospital setting are to determine a working diagnosis and intervention plan, to communicate this to the primary care team, to facilitate its implementation, and to establish a plan for follow-up after discharge.

Initial Evaluation and Differential Diagnosis

Although all psychiatrists have been trained in the appropriate approach to initial examination and differential diagnosis, unfortunately many times patients are misdiagnosed because components of the diagnostic assessment have been inadvertently omitted. It is important to remember that a complete initial diagnostic assessment should include not only the history of the present illness but also a complete assessment of current and past comorbid psychiatric conditions, a family medical and psychiatric history, and a social and developmental history. Frequently, busy practitioners forget to ask about early childhood trauma or sexual trauma. Performing a formal mental status examination may be particularly important if one is assessing either an older person with a depressive disorder or someone with significant medical comorbidities.

One needs to either contact the primary care physician or consider performing a medical history and a physical examination for patients with a new onset of major depressive disorder. Many medical conditions, medications, and substances (alcohol, benzodiazepines, barbitu-

rates) can cause depressive symptoms, as shown in Tables 53–1 and 53–5.

Rating Scales

One of the greatest challenges psychiatry and psychology have faced is quantifying the impact of psychiatric illness and therapies on a patient's life. Most practitioners do not establish baseline levels of symptom severity and do not systematically measure the changes in symptoms caused by their interventions. Some have worried that introducing scales to systematically assess symptom severity would contaminate the therapeutic process; however, this postulate has fallen out of favor. As the biology of depressive disorders is beginning to be elucidated and depressive disorders are being recognized as syndromes related to brain dysfunction, it is imperative for practitioners to employ a more rigorous approach to assessment and treatment. With "pay for performance" standards coming to psychiatry in the near future, employing standardized assessments will place the practitioner ahead of the curve in demonstrating the effectiveness of his or her treatment interventions.

Objective measurement of signs and symptoms of depressive disorders facilitates a more rational approach to treatment. These assessments provide accurate delineation of the severity of baseline signs and symptoms of depression. Thus, as was done in the STAR*D study, the clinician can use follow-up assessments to guide therapeutic decisions. Ratings also can be used as a tool to engage patients in their therapy and as an ongoing component of psychoeducation about depressive disorders.

The most commonly employed ratings (Table 53–6) evaluate the severity and frequency of specific symptoms associated with depression. These items' scores are usually summed into a composite score that represents the overall severity of the syndrome. The rating scales can be divided into two large groups: clinician-rated scales and self-report scales. For many years the field of psychiatry has placed greater value on clinician-rated scales. Proponents of clinician-rated scales suggest that they are more objective because the clinician is an unbiased observer, judging the severity and frequency of the symptoms (Carroll et al. 1973). Some favor clinician-rated measures because they allow the interviewer an opportunity to ask the patient follow-up questions and elicit sufficient data to ensure the accuracy of an answer. However, such ratings are highly dependent on the skill of the interviewer and the interviewer's fidelity to the intent and structure of the instrument. Proponents of patient-rated measures argue that a patient can provide a unique and valuable perspective to the assessment of his or her illness. Critics have raised legitimate concerns about self-reporting bias (Carroll et al. 1973); such bias could take the form of symptom minimization or symptom exaggeration. Furthermore, the presence of a negative cognitive schema might lead patients to minimize the extent of improvement that occurs early in therapy. Yet self-report assessments can be an important tool to enhance self-monitoring as the patient begins to "buy in" to therapy and adherence.

Clinician-Rated Scales

Three clinician-rated scales are commonly used to assess the severity of major depressive disorder: the Hamilton Rating Scale for Depression (Ham-D), the Montgomery-Åsberg Depression Rating Scale (MADRS), and the Inventory of Depressive Symptoms (IDS). These are described below:

1. The initial Ham-D was a 17-item scale developed by Max Hamilton in the United Kingdom while he worked with inpatients with primarily endogenous major depressive disorder (Hamilton 1960, 1967). When the scale was first published, it was suggested that the interview would usually require 45–60 minutes to perform (Hamilton 1960). This scale became a

TABLE 53–6.   Rating scales for symptoms of depression

Clinician-rated scales

Hamilton Rating Scale for Depression

Montgomery-Åsberg Depression Rating Scale

Inventory of Depressive Symptoms

Self-report scales

Zung Self-Rating Depression Scale

Beck Depression Inventory

Public Health Questionnaire–9

Quick Inventory of Depressive Symptoms–Self-Report

Rating scales for work and functioning

Endicott Work Productivity Scale

Work and Social Adjustment Scale

Sheehan Disability Scale

Rating scales for quality of life

Medical Outcome Survey

Quality of Life Enjoyment and Satisfaction Questionnaire

Quality of Well-Being Scale

Quality of Life in Depression Scale

mainstay of depression research, and a variety of iterations emerged: 21-, 24-, 25-, 28-, and 31-item forms of the Ham-D (Ham-D-21, Ham-D-24, etc.). Shorter forms of the original Ham-D have also been proposed that are thought to measure the "core features" of depression, but these have not been widely accepted by clinicians. Other attempts to refine the Ham-D have included the development of structured interviews. The most popularly accepted form is the Structured Interview Guide for the Ham-D (SIGH-D; Williams 1988), but that has recently been supplanted by the GRID-Ham-D, which systematically measures the severity and frequency of symptoms (Tabuse et al. 2007). Thus, the Ham-D is a commonly used clinician-rated scale with multiple refinements that has been frequently employed in research settings.

2. The MADRS (Montgomery and Åsberg 1979) was developed to be sensitive to the potential benefits of pharmacological interventions. It is shorter than the standard Ham-D-17 and does not contain as many items measuring somatic concerns or anxiety. Items are rated from 0 to 6, with two items not having the benefit of a specific series of descriptors to anchor them to the rest of the scale. This is a reliable and well-validated scale (Khan et al. 2004).

3. The IDS has both clinician-rated and self-report forms. The clinician-rated form has 30 items that are rated 0–3. This scale includes cognitive signs and symptoms of depression as well as the DSM-IV symptoms (Rush et al. 1986; Trivedi et al. 2004). It has been well validated. The IDS clinician-rated scale also comes in an abbreviated form, the Quick Inventory of Depressive Symptoms (Rush et al. 2003). This version rates all of the DSM-IV signs and symptoms of depression from 0 to 3. It is well validated and was one of the primary outcome measures in the STAR*D study (Rush et al. 2006a; Trivedi et al. 2004).

Self-Report Scales

A wide array of self-report measures are available for patients and clinicians to consider:

1. One of the first measures developed was the Zung Self-Rating Depression Scale (Zung 1965). This 20-item scale, with ratings from 1 to 4, measures the severity of depressive symptoms. As is the case with the Ham-D, the scale was developed prior to the advent of DSM-III, so some features of the scale are not as closely aligned with our current nosology as the more recently developed self-report measures (Guy 1976).
2. A second self-rating scale commonly employed, particularly in psychology, is the Beck Depression Inventory (BDI; A. T. Beck and Beamesderfer 1974). The BDI is a byproduct of A. T. Beck's descriptive, theoretical, and treatment work investigating cognitions and depression. It is a well-validated and commonly employed measure that focuses primarily on the more cognitive aspects of depression.
3. Another instrument, which has been gaining greater acceptance as a patient-rated measurement of major depressive disorder, is the Public Health Questionnaire–9. This questionnaire consists of the first nine items of the larger Public Health Questionnaire that was developed as an assessment tool for studying primary care patients (Kroenke et al. 2001). The nine symptoms are 1) depressed mood, 2) anhedonia, 3) appetite change, 4) sleep disturbance, 5) psychomotor change, 6) loss of energy, 7) feelings of worthlessness/guilt, 8) diminished concentration, and 9) suicide.

    Each item is scaled from absent (a score of 0) to present nearly every day (a score of 3). This instrument is well validated and has been used to longitudinally follow the course of illness because it is possible to assess the presence or absence of symptoms (Cannon et al.

2007; Kroenke et al. 2001). However, this instrument does not directly measure the intensity of symptoms.
4. A fourth patient-rated measure that is widely used is the Quick Inventory of Depressive Symptoms–Self-Report (QIDS-SR; Rush et al. 2003). This instrument correlates highly with the clinician-rated version. It includes assessments of intensity and frequency and covers all the cardinal signs and symptoms of major depressive disorder outlined in DSM-IV. This measure is easy for both clinicians and patients to use (Trivedi et al. 2004).

Self-report measures of work and functioning. If one is to reconceptualize major depressive disorder, symptoms are only part of the syndrome. Major depressive disorder impacts the individual's physical health, ability to function, interactions with significant others, interactions with family members, and quality of life. Thus, it is important to quantify not only the severity of symptoms but also the impact of the syndrome on other aspects of the patient's life. There are three readily available self-report measures of work and functioning that the clinician can ask the patient to complete:

1. One of the best-validated instruments is the Endicott Work Productivity Scale (Endicott and Nee 1997). Although this has the advantage of being well validated and complete, it has the disadvantage of being relatively time-consuming for the patient to use.
2. A second scale that has been validated, and that is very easy to use, is the Work and Social Adjustment Scale (Mundt et al. 2002). It consists of five Likert scales that measure an individual's perception of work and social functioning.
3. The Sheehan Disability Scale (Leon et al. 1992) is another simple and widely accepted approach to assessing disability. This 3-item Likert scale measures dysfunction at work, in social settings, and with family members. It is very easy to perform, is reliable, and has high patient acceptance.

Measurements of Quality of Life

Measurement of quality of life has been increasingly recognized as an important component for the treatment of psychiatric illnesses. There are several widely used instruments that measure aspects of quality of life, as described below:

1. The most widely accepted instrument, employed in both psychiatry and medicine in general, is the Med-

ical Outcome Survey. The versions most commonly used are the three Short Form (SF) instruments: SF-36, SF-12, and SF-4 (Ware and Sherbourne 1992; Ware et al. 1996). The advantage of these scales is that they are widely used, so there is a vast amount of data available validating them in a variety of conditions. The disadvantage of the Medical Outcome Survey is that it is relatively insensitive to change with symptom improvement. This is due to the scoring algorithm, which truncates the range of the scale.

2. The second instrument that has been commonly used in a variety of trials is the Quality of Life Enjoyment and Satisfaction Questionnaire (Q-LES-Q). The Q-LES-Q is available in both a long form and a one-page summary form, which is the most commonly used version of the questionnaire (Endicott et al. 1993; Rapaport et al. 2005). This scale has 14 items that are rated from 1 to 5 and summed to create a total score. There are also two general items; one is general life satisfaction, and the other assesses satisfaction with medication the patient is taking. The short form of the Q-LES-Q is well validated and takes less than 5 minutes to complete.

3. An instrument that is available in both an interview form and a self-report form is the Quality of Well-Being Scale (QWB) (Kaplan 1993; Kaplan and Anderson 1990). This scale has been developed and validated across many medical and psychiatric conditions. The QWB allows one to get a measure of quality-adjusted life-years. The intent of such a scale is to measure the impact of an illness or a number of illnesses on an individual's overall fitness.

4. An additional instrument that has been reported in the depression literature is the Quality of Life in Depression Scale (Hunt and McKenna 1992). Although this is a well-validated instrument, it does not allow one to generalize the impact of illness on quality-of-life dysfunction beyond major depressive disorder.

5. A less formal but ecologically valid approach is to elicit from the patient the three symptoms or life problems that are most debilitating for the patient at the time of initial assessment. These can be symptoms or signs of depressive disorder, functional impairment, or problems affecting quality of life. The patient is then asked to assess his or her symptoms/problems daily. In our practice at Cedars-Sinai Medical Center, we have called this approach the *most troubling symptoms model* for monitoring care.

During the initial interview, the patient and therapist collaboratively identify and quantify life problems related to the mood disorder on a Likert scale of 1–10. This approach has several strong points. First, if the patient assesses his or her condition daily, it facilitates the engagement of the patient in therapy, because the patient is monitoring problems that he or she has identified as significant. Second, it allows the patient to know that the physician truly hears what the patient's complaints and concerns are. This enhances the therapeutic relationship and adherence to therapy. Third, this being a fine-grained approach to assessing on a daily basis the severity of problems that the patient has identified, it allows the patient and the clinician to discern subtle changes that frequently are missed when patients are assessed weekly or less frequently. This approach facilitates rational discussion between the patient and the clinician about the patient's condition and, when necessary, the need to alter the treatment course. This has proven to be a simple yet effective technique for monitoring both the severity of the illness and the impact of the illness on the patient's life.

In summary, it is clear that a systematic assessment of the signs and symptoms of an illness, as well as the impact of the illness on other aspects of the patient's life, is necessary to maximize the opportunity for treatment gains. The use of either clinician-rated or self-report measures enables physicians to objectively monitor the course of treatment and the benefits of interventions and is essential for the optimal care of the patient.

Treatment Options

The treatment of major depressive disorder is now commonly conceptualized to have three phases: acute treatment, continuation treatment, and maintenance treatment (Frank et al. 1991b). The overall goal of acute treatment is remission. Thus, during acute treatment the patient is vigorously treated with pharmacotherapy, psychotherapy, or a combination of both until all symptoms of the depressive disorder have been eliminated. It is thought that remission is associated with the restoration, over time, of the individual's quality of life and functioning. The consequences of not achieving remission have been discussed previously in this chapter (see "Changes in Conceptualization of Depressive Disorders" and "Disability and Costs Associated With Depressive Illnesses"). They include an increased risk of treatment resistance (Judd et al. 1998b; Paykel et al. 1995), persistence of psychosocial dysfunction (Miller et al. 1998), an increased risk of morbidity and mortality from medical illnesses (Murray and Lopez 1997), and an increased risk of suicide. The focus of continuation treatment is to protect the patient against a relapse back into the current episode of major depressive disorder. Studies have demonstrated clearly that if treatment is discontinued after the acute phase, more than half of individuals will have a relapse of major depressive disorder (Thase 1999). The goal of maintenance therapy is to prevent a recurrence or new episode of major depressive disorder. Because major depressive disorder is a chronic and recurrent illness for most individuals, full-dose maintenance therapy is essential in order to minimize the risk for and the number of future episodes (Bump et al. 2001; Prien et al. 1984).

Antidepressant Medications

Under ideal circumstances, the choice of an antidepressant medication is a collaborative process between the physician and the patient. Considerations that need to be weighed by the physician and patient can be broadly grouped as patient preferences, pharmacodynamic concerns, and pharmacokinetic concerns. Particularly in the age of direct-to-consumer advertising and the Internet, many patients take an active approach to their pharmacotherapy. Patients either have searched the Internet for information about treatment options for major depressive disorder or have been influenced by the advertisements that they see on television. Thus, many patients come to the initial appointment with their own biases and beliefs about what would be the best treatment option. However, a variety of other patient-related variables may come into play when selecting an antidepressant medication including side effects (especially sexual side effects, weight gain, and insomnia), dietary restrictions, and ease of use (Table 53–7). Addressing these issues with the patient is important to enhance adherence to therapy. Other patient-specific factors that need to be taken into account are the patient's prior history of response to a medication or a family history of response to a certain class of medications. This may influence both the patient and the physician regarding the choice of medication to treat the current depressive episode.

Although we have not been able to discern distinct biological subtypes, pharmacogenetics (discussed in more detail below) has now developed to the point that it can inform our therapeutic decisions. The specific pharmacodynamic properties of an agent certainly need to be taken into account when identifying the appropriate medication for an individual. Although the tricyclic antidepressants

and the monoamine oxidase inhibitors have a long history of proven efficacy, these classes of agents have fallen out of favor because of their side-effect profiles. The majority of commonly used antidepressants (see Table 53–7) work via one or more mechanisms: 1) inhibition of serotonin reuptake, 2) inhibition of the reuptake of both serotonin and norepinephrine, 3) stimulation of noradrenergic and dopaminergic activity, or 4) α_2 antagonism of noradrenergic and serotonergic neurons. Physicians now can use knowledge about the pharmacodynamics of agents to influence a treatment choice. For example, a clinician is visited by a 50-year-old white male with chronic, persistent depression. The patient is currently complaining of diarrhea and persistent symptoms of depression despite medication with sertraline at a dosage of 200 mg/day. In taking the patient's history, the clinician learns that the patient has had persistent problems with diarrhea and lack of treatment response with three other SSRIs and with both of the FDA-approved serotonin–norepinephrine reuptake inhibitors. In this case, use of an agent like mirtazapine might be preferable.

The pharmacokinetic profile of the agent is another variable that needs to be taken into account in selecting an antidepressant medication. As would be expected, antidepressants differ in their protein binding, rate and mechanism of elimination, half-life, lipophilicity, and effects on other metabolic pathways. Therefore, it is important to carefully determine what other medications the patient may be taking. Drug–drug interactions may increase blood levels of concomitant medications, and at times those interactions can be unpleasant or even life-threatening.

In summary, the choice of initial antidepressant medication is ideally a collaborative decision-making process between the patient and the physician. It requires an understanding of the patient's preferences, family history, prior treatment history, and current medical conditions; any current medications he or she may be taking; the side-effect profile of the proposed agent; and the pharmacokinetic and pharmacodynamic properties of the compound. Engagement of the patient in this decision-making process is more likely to enhance adherence to the medication regimen.

Pharmacogenetics

There has been recent attention on the field of pharmacogenetics—the concept of tailoring drug therapy to a patient's genetic makeup (Perlis 2007). Currently, tests are available commercially to screen for allelic variation in

TABLE 53–7. Antidepressant medications

Type	Drug (Trade name)	Daily Dosing	Pharmacology	Side Effects and Other Concerns
TCA	Amitriptyline (Elavil)	75–300 mg	Inhibits reuptake of 5-HT and NE	Dry mouth, urinary retention, sedation, constipation, weight gain, hypotension, quinidine-like effect on heart conduction
SSRI	Fluoxetine (Prozac) Sertraline (Zoloft) Paroxetine (Paxil) Citalopram (Celexa) Escitalopram (Lexapro)	20–80 mg 25–200 mg 10–60 mg 10–60 mg 5–20 mg	Inhibits reuptake of 5-HT	Sexual dysfunction, nausea, diarrhea, insomnia, agitation, tremors, dizziness, rare hyponatremia, rare bruising, discontinuation syndrome, drug–drug interactions
SNRI	Venlafaxine (Effexor) Duloxetine (Cymbalta)	37.5–400 mg 30–120 mg	Inhibits reuptake of 5-HT and NE	Nausea, insomnia, sedation, sexual dysfunction, sweating, hypertension, discontinuation syndrome
MAOI	Phenelzine (Nardil) Tranylcypromine (Parnate)	45–75 mg 30–60 mg	Irreversibly inhibits MAO from breaking down into NE, 5-HT, and dopamine	Hypotension, weight gain, sedation, dry mouth, sexual dysfunction, dietary restrictions, risk of hypertensive crisis, life-threatening drug–drug interactions
	Selegiline (Emsam [transdermal])	20, 30, or 40 mg	At recommended doses, does not inhibit gut MAO-A	Weight gain, sedation
Atypical	Mirtazapine (Remeron)	15–45 mg	Improves 5-HT and NE tone: α_2 presynaptic blocker on NE and 5-HT neurons Blocks 5-HT$_{2A}$, 5-HT$_{2C}$, and 5-HT$_3$ Blocks H$_1$	Weight gain, sedation, abnormal dreams, dry mouth, hypotension, constipation, rare agranulocytosis
	Bupropion (Wellbutrin)	75–450 mg in three divided doses (maximal single dose, 150 mg) SR 200–450 mg in two divided doses XL 150–450 mg daily	Blocks reuptake of NE Increases dopamine in frontal cortex Blocks dopamine transporter pump	Agitation, restless insomnia, weight loss, anorexia, sweating, headache, tremor, hypertension, rare seizures
	Trazodone (Desyrel)	100–450 mg	Blocks 5-HT$_{2A}$ Blocks 5-HT reuptake	Orthostatic hypotension, nausea, dry mouth, dizziness, rare priapism, occasional sinus bradycardia

Note. 5-HT = 5-hydroxytryptamine (serotonin); 5-HT$_{2A}$ = 5-HT type 2A receptor; H$_1$ = histamine type 1 receptor; MAO = monoamine oxidase; MAO-A = monoamine oxidase isozyme A; MAOI = monoamine oxidase inhibitor; NE = norepinephrine; SNRI = serotonin–norepinephrine reuptake inhibitor; SR = sustained release; SSRI = selective serotonin reuptake inhibitor; TCA = tricyclic antidepressant; XL = extended release.

the CYP450 genes (Roche Diagnostics, Switzerland). These tests purportedly would allow the physician to select an antidepressant dose based on some knowledge of how the medication will be metabolized and possibly eliminated. This application has limitations given that many other factors are involved in drug metabolism besides a patient's genetic makeup, such as smoking status, diet, concurrent treatment therapies, and other environmental and physiological factors.

Other genetic variations that have been demonstrated to be associated with depression or response to therapy include variation in the gene for SSAT—an enzyme responsible for the metabolism of polyamines (Sequeira et al. 2006)—and genetic variation in CRH (Liu et al. 2007; Papiol et al. 2007) or glucocorticoid receptors (Binder et al. 2004; Brouwer et al. 2006; van Rossum et al. 2006), components of the stress response system. These variations may also prove useful in the future for tailoring pharmacological treatments to individual patients.

Of all other genetic variations, the gene encoding 5-HTT (the serotonin transporter) has been the most widely studied. Individuals who carry a specific polymorphic variation are genetically vulnerable to developing depression when exposed to trauma early in life (Caspi et al. 2003; Kendler et al. 2005). Testing for *5-HTT* genetic variation has been used to identify which class of antidepressants should be used to begin treatment (Smits et al. 2007b). In this study, results were positive in that when genetic testing was used to predict the best type of antidepressant to prescribe, 65% of the screened patients were in remission 6 weeks later, compared with 60% of non–genetically screened patients. Future pretreatment genetic testing must be evaluated on a wider scale and must also include a cost assessment. Nevertheless, other studies have demonstrated that such pretreatment genetic screening for the *5-HTT* variation may aid in determining a patient's vulnerability to side effects of pharmacological treatment (Hu et al. 2007; Smits et al. 2007a).

Somatic Therapies

Five somatic therapies have been investigated to various degrees either as monotherapies or as adjuvant therapies for treatment-resistant depression: electroconvulsive therapy (ECT), vagus nerve stimulation (VNS), repetitive transcranial magnetic stimulation (rTMS), deep brain stimulation (DBS), and light therapy. ECT is the best studied of the somatic interventions. It is clearly one of the treatments of choice for individuals with treat-

ment-resistant depression. Although the mechanism of action of ECT is still not well understood, it is a safe and efficacious treatment. In repeated studies, ECT has been found to be more efficacious than placebo (sham ECT) and more efficacious than pharmacotherapy for treatment-resistant patients. (For a review of ECT data from the United Kingdom, see UK ECT Review Group 2003.)

VNS was initially developed for the treatment of epilepsy. In 2005 it was approved by the FDA for use in treatment-resistant depression. The basis of this approval was a study in which patients with resistant depression who received adjunctive VNS therapy demonstrated statistically significantly greater improvement in both remission rates and response rates than comparably ill patients who did not receive VNS therapy (George et al. 2005). One of the key findings to emerge from these studies of VNS is that its effect may be cumulative and one may not see the full benefit of VNS stimulation until 9–12 months after treatment is begun (Sackeim et al. 2007; Schlaepfer et al. 2008). The most common side effects of VNS therapy are a voice tremor, cough, dyspnea, and neck soreness.

rTMS was first identified as a treatment for depression by a group of NIMH researchers (George et al. 1995). Since that time, several smaller studies have supported the finding that rTMS may be an effective treatment for major depressive disorder (for reviews, see Couturier 2005; George et al 2007). The results of a recent 21-site study that compared rTMS with sham treatment over the left dorsolateral prefrontal cortex indicated a response rate of 24.5% in the depressed group versus 15.1% in the control group (O'Reardon et al. 2007). These findings led to the recent FDA approval of rTMS for the treatment of depression.

DBS is an FDA-approved treatment for severe, intractable Parkinson's disease. It was used in a small open-label study by Mayberg et al. (2005) in which six patients with intractable treatment-resistant depression had electrodes implanted in the subgenual cingulate cortex. At 6-month follow-up, four of the six subjects were judged to be treatment responders.

Older literature suggested that phototherapy might be an effective augmentation therapy for individuals with certain forms of depressive disorders (Kripke 1981; Lewy and Sack 1986). This has been best studied in patients with seasonal affective disorder. Light therapy for 90 minutes per day has been able to effectively treat, and also prevent the development of, depressive disorder (Even et al. 2007; Westrin and Lam 2007). Light boxes are employed by some clinicians to augment typical antidepressant responses.

In summary, at this time few somatic therapies have demonstrated efficacy for treatment-resistant depression. Two approaches are FDA approved, ECT and VNS, and at least three other somatic therapies show potential benefits. It is clear that more work needs to be done investigating somatic options for patients with treatment-resistant depression.

Alternative Therapies

There is a panoply of alternative therapies that are being investigated both as monotherapies and in conjunction with more traditional forms of psychotherapy or pharmacotherapy. The best investigated alternative therapy is exercise. Evidence suggests that exercise performed a minimum of three times a week, the equivalent of walking 2 miles at a pace of 20 minutes per mile or faster, is associated with a significant decrease in symptoms of depression. Preliminary work studying the acute effects of exercise as a monotherapy or as an augmentation strategy suggests that exercise causes a sustained decrease in depressive mood ratings (Antunes et al. 2005; Osei-Tutu and Campagna 2005; Trivedi et al. 2006b, 2006c).

Data investigating the efficacy of massage therapy for the treatment of depressive disorders come mostly from open studies. In these studies, massage seems to decrease measures of depression and anxiety (Field et al. 1996). Yoga is an alternative therapy that has been investigated in small studies contrasting yoga with both pharmacotherapy and ECT. In these small acute trials, yoga did cause a significant decrease in measures of depression (Janakiramaiah et al. 2000; Pilkington et al. 2005) Acupuncture has not yet been demonstrated to have efficacy as an adjuvant therapy or as monotherapy for major depressive disorder. Both a recent Cochrane analysis and recently published results of a large sham-controlled study suggest that acupuncture may not be effective as a treatment for depressive disorders (Allen et al. 2006; Smith and Hay 2005).

Several alternatives to traditional pharmacotherapy show promise. The best studied natural products are St. John's wort, S-adenosyl-L-methionine, and omega-3 fatty acids (Conklin et al. 2007; M. Fava et al. 2005; Mischoulon and Fava 2002; Murck et al. 2005; Stahl et al. 2008). At this time, all three of these treatments show promise and are under investigation in large NIMH-funded trials.

In summary, although there is burgeoning interest in the use of nontraditional somatic and pharmacotherapeutic treatments for major depressive disorder, these therapies require significantly more rigorous investigation.

Psychotherapy for Major Depressive Disorder

Just as our concept of major depressive disorder has evolved over the last few decades, so has our understanding of the goals of treatment and the length of time required for effective treatment. As recently as the 1980s and early 1990s, there was a schism between psychotherapists and practitioners of pharmacotherapy. The field of psychiatry was caught in a miasma of arguments where disciples argued about the relative merits of psychotherapy versus pharmacotherapy (American Psychiatric Association 2000b; Elkin et al. 1989; Jacobson and Hollon 1996). Fortunately, we have made a transition to focus on helping patients attain remission, maintain remission, restore functioning, and enhance quality of life. Controlled studies have demonstrated that psychotherapy, pharmacotherapy, and combined treatment all have a valuable role to play in achieving these goals (Hollon et al. 2005; Keller et al. 2000; Otto et al. 2005).

At this time, practitioners and researchers involved in the study of psychotherapy for major depressive disorder face a variety of issues. Some of the questions that are currently being investigated, and for which we do not have definitive answers, are the following:

- Are there certain patients who are more responsive to psychotherapy than others? If so, are there certain patient characteristics that would predict whether an individual would be more responsive to cognitive-behavioral therapy (CBT) than to some other evidence-based form of psychotherapy such as interpersonal psychotherapy (IPT)?
- What are the attributes of the people who are most likely to benefit from combined therapy?
- If combined therapy is used, must both forms of therapy be continued after a response is achieved in order to sustain the response?
- Evidence-based psychotherapies require much greater participation by the patient, homework assignments, and much more effort than pharmacotherapy. Thus, it is reasonable to ask, are patients willing to accept psychotherapy?
- Another challenge is, how can academic institutions successfully disseminate evidence-based psychotherapies?
- A related challenge is, how can one ensure that therapists are truly adherent to the key principles of the therapy? It is clear that treatment success, to a signifi-

cant extent, is based on the fidelity of the practitioner to the model.

- An ever-pressing issue is, will insurers and society adequately compensate individuals to perform these time-intensive psychotherapies?

Cognitive-Behavioral Therapy

CBT comprises a constellation of interventions that target, to varying degrees, maladaptive or critical thinking and behavioral patterns that are destructive, such as inactivity, avoidance, and social withdrawal. A great deal of the initial theory and research validating cognitive therapy was performed by Aaron Beck. He was the first to cogently develop and articulate a cognitive model of depression, and he employed rigorous observational research techniques to study the efficacy of his postulated interventions (A.T. Beck et al. 1979). Key to this model is the observation that depressed individuals have negative mental self-representations of the world, themselves, and their future. He postulated that these representations negatively biased information processing. This led him to develop a short-term structured, collaborative, problem-focused, intervention that involves teaching patients cognitive and behavioral skills to combat depression (A.T. Beck et al. 1979).

One of the key components of CBT is helping patients identify "automatic thoughts"—the negative, depressogenic cognitions that pervade a depressed individual's thinking. By monitoring and recording these thoughts, patients can begin to get a sense of how their thoughts stimulate unpleasant feelings, sensations, and maladaptive behaviors. This allows a patient to learn to evaluate both the accuracy and the value of automatic thoughts and create an environment in which he or she learns to empirically test the accuracy of these thoughts. In the process of doing so, the patient begins to generate balanced and more adaptive cognitions (e.g., "There are many things that I do well in my life"). An important aspect of the cognitive model of depression is the presence of negative self-schemata, that is, feelings of being worthless or helpless (J.S. Beck 1995; Feldman 2007; Jacobson et al. 1996; Kuyken et al. 2007).

The second component of most forms of CBT is the development of behaviorally oriented interventions to target specific symptoms and to enhance rewarding experiences. Interventions like *behavioral activation* can be focused to eliminate target symptoms like inertia or social withdrawal. Another type of behavioral intervention that is commonly employed in CBT is the teaching of problem-solving skills. This entails the breaking down of tasks that feel overwhelming into smaller discrete, manageable goals. An important component of problem-solving skills training is the development of decision-making skills that help individuals formulate a model for weighing the pros and cons of a situation (Feldman 2007; Kuyken et al. 2007).

A number of modifications of classical CBT for depression are currently being investigated and are gaining significant attention. These include the use of behavioral activation as a stand-alone intervention for depression and the development of therapies that promote psychological well-being and that target cognitive reactivity (i.e., the tendency to respond to sad moods with more negative thinking) (Dimidjian et al. 2006). Well-being therapy is based on a theoretical model by Ryff (1989) that emphasizes the promotion of mental health and not merely the amelioration of mental illness. Thus, patients engaged in this therapy become aware of periods of well-being and challenge automatic thoughts and behaviors that interrupt such periods of pleasant emotions (G.A. Fava 1999). Another form of CBT that has become increasingly popular incorporates mindfulness-based interventions into CBT. It can be done either in individual settings or as part of group CBT treatment. This goal of this mindfulness-based approach is to enable patients to become "decentered" with regard to depressogenic thoughts and see them as mental events rather than as accurate reflections of their reality or core aspects of themselves (Kabat-Zinn 1990; Segal et al. 2002). A third form of cognitively based psychotherapy that has gained acceptance in the research community and increasing acceptance in the clinical community is the cognitive-behavioral analysis system of psychotherapy (CBASP). This was initially designed as a treatment for chronic depression that targets problematic interpersonal patterns and uses situational analysis to challenge maladaptive thinking processes (McCullough 2000). One of the key differences between traditional CBT and CBASP is the integration of concepts of transference reactions into the therapy itself (Butler et al. 2006).

This has been an exciting decade of development for CBT. Both the theoretical framework and practice of cognitively based therapies continue to be refined and modified by researchers. This suggests that cognitive-behavioral psychotherapy will play an increasingly important role in the treatment of depression.

Efficacy of CBT. The overwhelming majority of studies investigating the efficacy of CBT for major depressive disorder are outpatient studies. (The few inpatient studies that have been performed usually combined CBT with pharmacotherapy, and the results of these studies are equivocal [de Jong-Meyer et al. 1996; Hautzinger et al. 1996; Miller et al. 1989a, 1989b].) Meta-analyses suggest that CBT and medication are equally effective in the acute treatment of major depressive disorder (DeRubeis et al. 1999). This is a change from the results of an earlier study, which indicated that CBT was as efficacious as imipramine for treatment of mild and moderate depression but less efficacious for severe forms of depressive disorder (Elkin et al. 1995). This perception was promulgated by the initial analyses of the NIMH Treatment of Depression Collaborative Research Program. These findings were influential in the American Psychiatric Association (2000b) practice guideline recommendation that pharmacotherapy should be the first-line treatment for more severe depression.

CBT with either pharmacotherapy or psychotherapy is also effective for the treatment of moderate to severe depressive disorders, as demonstrated by DeRubeis et al. in a meta-analysis (DeRubeis et al. 1999) and an NIMH-funded clinical trial (DeRubeis et al. 2005). Behavioral activation therapy also has been found to be comparable to medication for the treatment of moderate to severe depression (Dimidjian et al. 2006). Data from one continuation study suggest that patients who receive CBT are more likely to maintain their remission status (with no more than three booster sessions of CBT during the 12-month continuation phase) than patients who responded to acute treatment with medication followed by discontinuation of medication (Hollon et al. 2005). Of course the flaw with many of the early studies is they did not follow the now commonly accepted tenet that appropriate pharmacotherapy requires sustained pharmacotherapy beyond the acute treatment period. Recent data from the NIMH-sponsored University of Pennsylvania–Vanderbilt University–Rush University treatment collaborative show that 1-year relapse rates were equivalent for individuals treated with CBT with up to three optional booster sessions and those maintained on medication over 1 year of follow-up (Hollon et al. 2005).

The number of well-performed studies that have combined antidepressant treatments with CBT is relatively limited. The studies performed to date suggest that there may be a slight advantage for combined treatment over either treatment alone. One very thoughtful large multisite study investigated the use of combined treatment consisting of nefazodone plus CBASP (a therapy for chronic depression that also has elements of IPT) versus CBASP alone or nefazodone alone. In this study, the effect sizes of combined treatment were significantly greater than the effect sizes of either treatment alone (Keller et al. 2000). The size of this study allowed the authors to perform additional analyses to examine whether specific factors might identify those patients best suited for a specific therapy. Secondary analyses of this data set determined that patients with a history of childhood trauma responded better to CBASP, either alone or in combination, than to monotherapy with medication.

Several studies have used some form of CBT either to augment antidepressants' effects or to attempt to treat residual symptoms (G.A. Fava et al. 1997; McPherson et al. 2005; Nemeroff et al. 2003). In the STAR*D study, augmentation of citalopram monotherapy with CBT and augmentation with pharmacological agents produced similar response rates; however, subjects receiving CBT augmentation tended to respond more slowly than those receiving pharmacological augmentation (Thase et al. 2007). CBT has also been used by investigators to treat residual symptoms of depressive disorders (G.A. Fava et al. 2004; Paykel et al. 1999); these studies suggest that adding CBT is more effective than continuing management with medication alone. Furthermore, follow-up evaluation of patients suggests that CBT augmentation may decrease the rate of relapse over time.

In summary, the data suggest that CBT is an effective first-line treatment for individuals with major depressive disorder. Furthermore, CBT may have an important role in facilitating remission for those who have residual symptoms of depression after adequate pharmacotherapy. Intriguing preliminary data suggest that CBT may play a powerful role in decreasing the risk of a relapse or recurrence of major depressive disorder. However, more research is needed.

Interpersonal Psychotherapy

IPT is a brief form of individual psychotherapy that focuses on one of four problem areas during acute treatment: grief, role transitions, role disputes, and interpersonal deficits. Acute therapy is tailored to the patient's specific presenting problems. IPT has been demonstrated to be an efficacious acute treatment both for outpatients and, more recently, for inpatients with major depressive disorder (Frank et al. 1990, 1991a; Luty et al. 2007; Reynolds et al. 1999; Schramm et al. 2007). The majority of studies investigating IPT as a monotherapy have been performed with outpatients. These studies demonstrated that IPT is an efficacious treatment for individuals with recurrent depressive disorder, older individuals with depression, and women with major depressive disorder

(Frank et al. 1990, 1991a; Luty et al. 2007; Reynolds et al. 1999). A study of inpatients with either major depressive disorder or bipolar II disorder (in the depressed phase of their illness) reported that the combination of 5 weeks of intensive IPT plus medication was more efficacious than medication and treatment as usual (Schramm et al. 2007). The group receiving combined therapy with IPT was more likely to sustain response and remission at 3-month follow-up than individuals in the medication management group without IPT. However, at 1-year follow-up, the two groups had comparable relapse rates (Schramm et al. 2007).

Ellen Frank and colleagues have been responsible for some of the most thoughtful work investigating the efficacy of IPT as a monotherapy, in combination with pharmacotherapy, and, most recently, as a maintenance therapy. The focus of maintenance IPT is broader than the focus of acute therapy because the goal is to prevent recurrence and to consolidate the gains made in therapy by augmenting the competencies and strengths achieved during acute IPT. Thus, the focus of maintenance IPT is to reinforce skills in coping with interpersonal life events in the four traditionally identified problem areas (grief, role transitions, role disputes, and interpersonal deficits). In a recent study designed to assess the treatment frequency necessary to prevent relapse into depression, Frank et al. (2007) reported that monthly booster sessions were as efficacious as twice-a-month booster sessions in preventing relapse for women who had been responsive to acute IPT as a monotherapy. However, maintenance IPT monotherapy was not efficacious as a relapse prevention technique for women who had initially required pharmacotherapy combined with IPT to achieve remission.

In conclusion, the data are clear that both CBT and IPT can be efficacious as monotherapies for the treatment of major depressive disorder. Growing data suggest that these psychotherapies may be effective not only in the acute treatment of depression but also in the maintenance treatment of depressive disorders. However, we are still not sure how to match the therapy to a specific patient. There is some indication that patients with avoidant or more passive personality styles may be less successfully treated with IPT than with CBT (Joyce et al. 2007). However, crucial issues limit the effectiveness of both of these psychotherapies: patient acceptance (Thase et al. 2007; Wisniewski et al. 2007), therapist training and fidelity to the techniques (Shaw et al. 1999), and public policy that limits reimbursement. Until we have dealt with these challenges, the dissemination and acceptance of evidence-based psychotherapies will be relatively limited.

Treatment Approaches

Acute Treatment

The goal of acute treatment of an individual with major depressive disorder is to identify a medication or psychotherapy that is effective and treat the individual vigorously enough to help him or her achieve remission. Recently, most of our understanding of acute treatment has been derived from Phase II and Phase III industry-sponsored studies of antidepressants. Many of these short-term studies were designed to differentiate an investigational compound from placebo. The goal of these trials was not to achieve disease remission but rather to demonstrate that the investigational compound was more efficacious than a placebo compound.

For many years, researchers have looked at the concept of *response*, defined as a 50% drop from baseline ratings of depression, as an indicator of an appropriate acute treatment trial. In most of these short-term studies, active treatment with psychotherapy, pharmacotherapy, or combined treatment was associated with a 60%–70% rate of response. However, it is now believed that remission rather than merely response is the appropriate goal for acute treatment (M. Fava et al. 2003). The majority of studies reporting remission rates have been short-term industry-sponsored trials that involved garden-variety depressive disorders and showed that approximately one-third of individuals achieve remission within 6–10 weeks of treatment. This finding was corroborated by the recent reports from the STAR*D study (Rush et al. 2006b), which showed that approximately 36% of patients achieved remission (as defined by QIDS-SR) with aggressive and vigorous treatment with citalopram.

The major question that has plagued the field of psychiatry has been what to do after an initial treatment intervention is not successful in achieving remission. The STAR*D study is the first large-scale investigation of mood disorders that has systematically attempted to answer this and other key questions. Patients who did not respond to treatment with citalopram were offered the option of allowing the physician to determine the next treatment, switching to another medication or to CBT monotherapy, or augmenting citalopram with psychotherapy or CBT (Rush et al. 2004). The majority of patients wanted to control their treatment course and elected to either switch medications or join the augmentation group (Wisniewski et al. 2007). Patients who chose the switch option were randomly assigned to receive either sustained-release bupropion, sertraline, or extended-release venlafaxine. In this study, it did not matter whether a patient was switched to a medication within the same class as the one that he or she was receiving previously (SSRIs) or to a medication with a different mechanism of action: all response rates were approximately 30% (Rush et al. 2006c).

In the medication arm of the augmentation group, individuals treated with citalopram had either bupropion or buspirone used as the augmenting agent. Again, the remission rates were essentially equivalent regardless of the agent used and were approximately 30% (Trivedi et al. 2006a). In the next level of the treatment algorithm (level 3), patients who did not meet remission criteria, and were willing to continue, again had the opportunity to switch medications, this time to either mirtazapine or nortriptyline, or to augment citalopram with lithium or triiodothyronine. The remission rates at this level ended up being approximately 13% no matter which treatment strategy was chosen. Individuals who still did not meet remission criteria, and who were willing to continue to participate in the study, were randomly assigned to receive either tranylcypromine or mirtazapine plus extended-release venlafaxine (level 4). By this time, the study, which had initially enrolled over 3,000 patients, had less than 100 patients in each arm of the trial. Remission rates for patients participating in this fourth step of the trial were approximately 13%. Thus, for individuals who were willing to participate through all four steps of the treatment algorithm used in the STAR*D study, the overall accumulative rate was 67% (Rush et al. 2006b).

The STAR*D study represents a significant advance in our knowledge about the acute treatment of major depressive disorder. Its strengths include the fact that it recruited subjects from both primary care and specialty clinics who were seeking treatment for major depressive disorder. Another strength of this study is the fact that there were few exclusion criteria, so this represented a real clinical sample. An acknowledged challenge faced by the investigators was the fact that it was not possible to truly perform a double-blind, placebo-controlled study. This study begins to answer some very important questions. The results from the study suggest that a switch in medication provides essentially the same remission rate as augmentation therapy. This has important clinical implications for patients, particularly as more and more medications become generic. A second important observation of this study is that a switch within a class of antidepressants was as efficacious as a switch between classes of agents. For many individuals, this seems counterintuitive; however, it may reflect the heterogeneity of depressive

disorders or the fact that medications, even within the same class, have subtle but possibly important pharmacodynamic and pharmacokinetic differences. A third important finding in this study is that as patients progressed further through the algorithm for treatment resistance, remission rates declined. This suggests that we need a wider array of treatment options than those studied in the STAR*D study to maximize the likelihood of remission.

Two interesting papers have come out as part of the second wave of STAR*D publications. The first covers the part of the study that investigated the efficacy of CBT for patients who did not respond initially to citalopram. Regardless of whether subjects switched to CBT alone or used it as an augmentation strategy, approximately 30% of individuals attained remission. These individuals generally took longer to reach remission than those who had opted for medication as either a switch from or augmentation to citalopram (Thase et al. 2007).

The second recently published STAR*D paper reported 12-month follow-up data (Rush et al. 2006b). The three major findings were as follows:

1. Individuals who did not attain remission were very likely to relapse into an episode of major depressive disorder within 6 months.
2. Even when individuals did achieve remission, two-thirds of those who met remission criteria acutely experienced a significant exacerbation of symptoms over the next 6 months.
3. The patients most likely to have an exacerbation were those who required multiple treatment attempts in order to reach remission (i.e., those entering levels 3 and 4 of the STAR*D algorithm).

The STAR*D study is a good first step toward the systematic approach of investigating treatment options for patients who are nonresponsive to an initial antidepressant therapy. There are, of course, many treatment options that were not selected to be part of this trial. They include augmentation with dopamine agonists (amantadine, pergolide, ropinirole, and pramipexole), psychostimulants (methylphenidate, dextroamphetamine, and modafinil), and natural products. Most of these agents have been used primarily in small or uncontrolled studies. The largest body of evidence suggesting efficacy is from studies with the atypical antipsychotic medications. A recent meta-analysis of 10 randomized, double-blind, controlled trials demonstrated superior response and remission rates for atypical antipsychotic medication augmentation of FDA-approved antidepressants versus placebo augmentation

(Papakostas et al. 2007). Aripiprazole has received FDA approval as an augmenting agent in patients who do not respond to SSRI or serotonin–norepinephrine reuptake inhibitor (SNRI) monotherapy. In general, more rigorous large-scale studies of these atypical antipsychotic agents are warranted.

In conclusion, only 30% of clinical patients vigorously respond to the first treatment approach tried during the acute phase of treatment. After an initial intervention has failed, it is important to carefully reassess the patient. It is important to reconfirm the diagnosis of major depressive disorder to assure oneself that all potential comorbidities have been identified and that one has taken a careful trauma history. In particular, subsyndromal forms of post-traumatic stress disorder and occult problems with alcohol and substance use disorders frequently confound the initial treatment of an episode of depression. It is also important to ensure that the patient is truly medically stable because neoplasms, vitamin deficiencies, and even certain infections and dementing disorders may initially masquerade as a depressive disorder. Another important variable to consider is the patient's commitment to getting well. Is the patient truly compliant with the proposed treatment measurement, be it psychotherapy or pharmacotherapy? When the physician is assured that the course has not been complicated by any of the above-mentioned confounding factors, it is reasonable to pursue an alternative approach to treatment. It is fortunate that with recently published data from the STAR*D study, we now have a stronger foundation for selecting second- and third-line treatment options for a patient whose depression is resistant to the initial treatment approach.

Continuation Treatment

The understanding for the need for continuation treatment evolved out of the series of consensus meetings sponsored by the MacArthur Foundation that were held to review the data about the course and treatment options for major depressive disorder. These meetings led to a series of papers suggesting that major depressive disorder is not a time-limited event for many people but rather a chronic and continuous syndrome that requires more than acute treatment (Frank et al. 1991b; Kupfer 1991). The goals of the continuation treatment phase include the following:

1. The prevention of relapse into an episode of major depressive disorder
2. A consolidation of gains made during acute treatment in terms of symptom reduction

3. The enhancement of quality of life and functioning of the patient

The need for continuation therapy has been documented in hundreds of trials investigating therapy after acute treatment. Thase (1999) estimated that the risk of relapse is at least 50% when pharmacotherapy is discontinued after acute treatment. Although there is no consensus about the time required for continuation treatment, most investigators and clinicians consider between 4 and 9 months of treatment, at the same intensity used in acute treatment, to be a minimal length of time for continuation therapy (Melfi et al. 1998).

Some interesting data suggest that combined therapy may facilitate continued remission; specifically, the combination of psychotherapy and pharmacotherapy may be beneficial (G.A. Fava et al. 1994). At this time, two studies have investigated the need to continue an augmentation therapy that was initially beneficial. Rapaport et al. (2006) studied the value of continuation therapy with risperidone added to antidepressant monotherapy for patients who were resistant to monotherapy but who entered remission with augmentation therapy. In this study, the relapse rates were identical for individuals randomly assigned to continue receiving antidepressants plus augmentation therapy versus those who received antidepressants plus a placebo. Bauer et al. (2000) investigated the value of continued lithium augmentation in patients with resistant depression and reported that continuation therapy with lithium decreased the relapse rate more than placebo augmentation.

Currently, we have more questions than answers about the best approach to treatment during the continuation phase. We do not yet know the appropriate length of time for continuation treatment, nor do we know what the best strategies are if a patient's condition begins to worsen during continuation treatment. However, it is clear that continuation treatment benefits patients by protecting against recurrence of the initial episode of depression and by allowing a consolidation of gains that impact not only symptom control but also quality of life and functioning.

Maintenance Treatment

A growing body of literature suggests that many individuals with major depressive disorder, a chronic and recurrent illness, require maintenance treatment. At this time, we are unable to biologically predict who will require maintenance or lifelong therapy. However, a series of risk factors have emerged indicating which patients may require maintenance therapy; they include the following:

1. A lifetime history of three or more episodes of major depressive disorder
2. The presence of double depression
3. At least two severe episodes of major depressive disorder within the past 5 years
4. Depressive disorders that are complicated by comorbid substance use or anxiety disorders
5. An age greater than 60 years at the onset of major depressive disorder

Most of these predictors come from longitudinal data gleaned from the NIMH Collaborative Depression Study (Keller and Berndt 2002).

The largest body of data about the value of maintenance therapy has come from two large studies that were performed at the University of Pittsburgh. The first study, by Frank et al. (1990), investigated the efficacy of maintenance with pharmacotherapy, psychotherapy, and combined therapy for adults who had had three or more episodes of major depressive disorder. In this study, the pharmacotherapies, both alone and in combination with ITP, were more successful than ITP alone or placebo. A second analysis from this study (Kupfer et al. 1992) demonstrated that individuals maintained the response to pharmacotherapy when the dosage was kept at the same level used during the acute treatment phase, and attempts to decrease the medication level by 50% led to relapse into major depressive disorder. Reynolds et al. (1999) published the results of a study with a very similar design, with elderly patients with recurrent major depressive disorder. In this study, both pharmacotherapy and psychotherapy maintenance therapies were efficacious in preventing a new episode of depression. There also have been interesting studies investigating the efficacy of fluoxetine, paroxetine, and extended-release venlafaxine as maintenance therapies. These studies also suggest that maintenance therapy is valuable for people with major depressive disorder (Dombrovski et al. 2007; Keller et al. 2007a, 2007b).

As is the case with continuation therapy, there are many unanswered questions regarding maintenance therapy. At this time, no studies have demonstrated what techniques to use if an individual's condition worsens during maintenance therapy. Another question is whether there are certain individuals who might not require lifelong maintenance therapy. A theoretical issue is the concept that medication may "poop out" and become less ef-

fective over time (Zimmerman and Thongy 2007). Although it is clear that some patients lapse into a new episode of depression despite the use of maintenance medication, it is not at all clear what the reasons for relapse are. To date, no careful studies have investigated the role of depressive disorders' progression and the need to alter pharmacotherapies. Just as individuals with hypertension, myocardial disease, or diabetes frequently need to have their treatment modified over a period of time, patients with major depressive disorder may need modifications over the course of treatment. We do not know whether this represents a lack of effectiveness of existing pharmacotherapies or the interaction of the aging body with progression of a diseased state.

In summary, although it is clear that maintenance therapy for depression is beneficial to our patients and their families, a great deal more investigation is needed about the necessary length of treatment, what to do when someone's condition worsens, and the underlying biology of the illness and the patient's response to therapy.

Conclusion

Over the past decade we have seen remarkable advances in our knowledge about the etiology, pathophysiology, and course of major depressive disorder and the prognosis for patients. The general consensus is that most people with major depressive disorder have a chronic lifelong condition that will wax and wane over time. An increasing body of evidence supports the postulate that some people with major depressive disorder have a disease that varies in presentation and symptom severity after the initial episode. Many people seem to traverse between having a full-blown episode of major depressive disorder and experiencing residual symptoms of depression, euthymia, minor depression, or new depressive symptoms. If the current evidence is correct, it suggests that our treatment approaches must be broadened to take into account both the chronic nature of the illness and its varied presentation. The implications for treatment are twofold: 1) we need to treat people until they achieve complete remission, and 2) we need to consider continuation and maintenance treatment for far more people than we have previously.

Although the field has made significant progress with information from the STAR*D trial, there are many important unanswered questions. We have limited data about the persistence of remission even after vigorous acute treatment. Only one study has investigated the need for continuation augmentation therapy, and that study suggested that it was not of significant value (Rapaport et al. 2006). No studies have addressed how patients whose condition worsens during continuation or maintenance therapy should be managed. However, the future is bright because of advances in basic biological investigations of depression. Imaging data are beginning to clearly define specific brain regions that seem to be altered in certain individuals with major depressive disorder. Preclinical studies are elucidating the roles of the function of a variety of neurotransmitter and neurohormonal systems in the pathogenesis of depression, including the noradrenergic system, the serotonergic system, the HPA axis, the immune system, and the NMDA system. Thus, with advances in preclinical animal models, clinical research, and genetics, we will begin to identify specific disorders that fall within the current rubric of major depressive disorder. This biologically informed approach to treatment will allow us to develop better and more personalized treatment plans.

References

Adams F, Quesada JR, Gutterman JU: Neuropsychiatric manifestations of human leukocyte interferon therapy in patients with cancer. JAMA 252:938–941, 1984

Akiskal HS, Judd LL, Gillin JC, et al: Subthreshold depressions: clinical and polysomnographic validation of dysthymic, residual and masked forms. J Affect Disord 45:53–63, 1997

Allen JJ, Schnyer RN, Chambers AS, et al: Acupuncture for depression: a randomized controlled trial. J Clin Psychiatry 67:1665–1673, 2006

American Psychiatric Association: Diagnostic and Statistical Manual of Mental Disorders, 3rd Edition. Washington, DC, American Psychiatric Association, 1980

American Psychiatric Association: Diagnostic and Statistical Manual of Mental Disorders, 4th Edition. Washington, DC, American Psychiatric Association, 1994

American Psychiatric Association: Diagnostic and Statistical Manual of Mental Disorders, 4th Edition, Text Revision. Washington, DC, American Psychiatric Association, 2000a

American Psychiatric Association: Practice guideline for the treatment of patients with major depressive disorder (revision). Am J Psychiatry 157 (4 suppl):1–45, 2000b

Amsterdam JD, Maislin G, Winokur A, et al: The oCRH stimulation test before and after clinical recovery from depression. J Affect Disord 14:213–222, 1988

Angst F, Stassen HH, Clayton PJ, et al: Mortality of patients with mood disorders: follow-up over 34–38 years. J Affect Disord 68:167–181, 2002

Angst J, Angst F, Gerber-Werder R, et al: Suicide in 406 mood-disorder patients with and without long-term medication: a 40 to 44 years' follow-up. Arch Suicide Res 9:279–300, 2005

Antunes HK, Stella SG, Santos RF, et al: Depression, anxiety and quality of life scores in seniors after an endurance exercise program. Rev Bras Psiquiatr 27:266–271, 2005

Arana GW, Baldessarini RJ, Ornsteen M: The dexamethasone suppression test for diagnosis and prognosis in psychiatry: commentary and review. Arch Gen Psychiatry 42:1193–1204, 1985

Beck AT, Beamesderfer A: Assessment of depression: the depression inventory. Mod Probl Pharmacopsychiatry 7:151–169, 1974

Beck AT, Rush AJ, Shaw BF, et al: Cognitive Therapy of Depression. New York, Guilford, 1979

Beck JS: Cognitive Therapy: Basics and Beyond. New York, Guilford, 1995

Beekman AT, Deeg DJ, Braam AW, et al: Consequences of major and minor depression in later life: a study of disability, well-being and service utilization. Psychol Med 27:1397–1409, 1997

Beekman AT, Geerlings SW, Deeg DJ, et al: The natural history of late-life depression: a 6-year prospective study in the community. Arch Gen Psychiatry 59:605–611, 2002

Binder EB, Salyakina D, Lichtner P, et al: Polymorphisms in FKBP5 are associated with increased recurrence of depressive episodes and rapid response to antidepressant treatment. Nat Genet 36:1319–1325, 2004

Borgstrom S, von Eyben FE, Flodgren P, et al: Human leukocyte interferon and cimetidine for metastatic melanoma. N Engl J Med 307:1080–1081, 1982

Bremne JD, Vermetten E: Stress and development: behavioral and biological consequences. Dev Psychopathol 13:473–489, 2001

Brouwer JP, Appelhof BC, van Rossum EF, et al: Prediction of treatment response by HPA-axis and glucocorticoid receptor polymorphisms in major depression. Psychoneuroendocrinology 31:1154–1163, 2006

Brown WA, Shuey I: Response to dexamethasone and subtype of depression. Arch Gen Psychiatry 37:747–751, 1980

Bump GM, Mulsant BH, Pollock BG, et al: Paroxetine versus nortriptyline in the continuation and maintenance treatment of depression in the elderly. Depress Anxiety 13:38–44, 2001

Burt VK, Stein K: Epidemiology of depression throughout the female life cycle. J Clin Psychiatry 63 (suppl 7):9–15, 2002

Butler AC, Chapman JE, Forman EM, et al: The empirical status of cognitive-behavioral therapy: a review of meta-analyses. Clin Psychol Rev 26:17–31, 2006

Campbell S, Marriott M, Nahmias C, et al: Lower hippocampal volume in patients suffering from depression: a meta-analysis. Am J Psychiatry 161:598–607, 2004

Cannon DS, Tiffany ST, Coon H, et al: The PHQ-9 as a brief assessment of lifetime major depression. Psychol Assess 19:247–251, 2007

Capuron L, Gumnick JF, Musselman DL, et al: Neurobehavioral effects of interferon-alpha in cancer patients: phenomenology and paroxetine responsiveness of symptom dimensions. Neuropsychopharmacology 26:643–652, 2002

Carroll BJ: The dexamethasone suppression test for melancholia. Br J Psychiatry 140:292–304, 1982

Carroll BJ, Fielding JM, Blashki TG: Depression rating scales: a critical review. Arch Gen Psychiatry 28:361–366, 1973

Caspi A, Sugden K, Moffitt TE, et al: Influence of life stress on depression: moderation by a polymorphism in the 5-HTT gene. Science 301:386–389, 2003

Cervilla JA, Molina E, Rivera M, et al: The risk for depression conferred by stressful life events is modified by variation at the serotonin transporter 5HTTLPR genotype: evidence from the

Spanish PREDICT-Gene cohort. Mol Psychiatry 12:748–755, 2007

Clayton P, Auster T: Strategies for the prevention and treatment of suicidal behavior. Focus 6:15–21, 2008

Conklin SM, Manuck SB, Yao JK, et al: High omega-6 and low omega-3 fatty acids are associated with depressive symptoms and neuroticism. Psychosom Med 69:932–934, 2007

Coppen A, Abou-Saleh M, Milln P, et al: Dexamethasone suppression test in depression and other psychiatric illness. Br J Psychiatry 142:498–504, 1983

Couturier JL: Efficacy of rapid-rate repetitive transcranial magnetic stimulation in the treatment of depression: a systematic review and meta-analysis. J Psychiatry Neurosci 30:83–90, 2005

Cuijpers P, de Graaf R, van Dorsselaer S: Minor depression: risk profiles, functional disability, health care use and risk of developing major depression. J Affect Disord 79:71–79, 2004

de Jong-Meyer R, Hautzinger M, Rudolf GAE, et al: The effectiveness of antidepressants and cognitive-behavioral therapy combined in patients with endogenous depression: results of analyses of variance regarding main and secondary outcome criteria [in German]. Z Klin Psychol 25:93–109, 1996

Delgado PL, Charney DS, Price LH, et al: Serotonin function and the mechanism of antidepressant action: reversal of antidepressant-induced remission by rapid depletion of plasma tryptophan. Arch Gen Psychiatry 47:411–418, 1990

DeRubeis RJ, Gelfand LA, Tang TZ, et al: Medications versus cognitive behavior therapy for severely depressed outpatients: mega-analysis of four randomized comparisons. Am J Psychiatry 156:1007–1013, 1999

DeRubeis RJ, Hollon SD, Amsterdam JD, et al: Cognitive therapy vs medications in the treatment of moderate to severe depression. Arch Gen Psychiatry 62:409–416, 2005

Dimidjian S, Hollon SD, Dobson KS, et al: Randomized trial of behavioral activation, cognitive therapy, and antidepressant medication in the acute treatment of adults with major depression. J Consult Clin Psychol 74:658–670, 2006

Dombrovski AY, Lenze EJ, Dew MA, et al: Maintenance treatment for old-age depression preserves health-related quality of life: a randomized, controlled trial of paroxetine and interpersonal psychotherapy. J Am Geriatr Soc 55:1325–1332, 2007

Drago S, Bergerone S, Anselmino M, et al: Depression in patients with acute myocardial infarction: influence on autonomic nervous system and prognostic role: results of a five-year follow-up study. Int J Cardiol 115:46–51, 2007

Duman RS: Depression: a case of neuronal life and death? Biol Psychiatry 56:140–145, 2004

Elkin I, Gibbons RD, Shea MT, et al: Initial severity and differential treatment outcome in the National Institute of Mental Health Treatment of Depression Collaborative Research Program. J Consult Clin Psychol 63:841–847, 1995

Elkin I, Shea MT, Watkins JT, et al: National Institute of Mental Health Treatment of Depression Collaborative Research Program: general effectiveness of treatments. Arch Gen Psychiatry 46:971–982; discussion 983, 1989

Elovainio M, Jokela M, Kivimaki M, et al: Genetic variants in the DRD2 gene moderate the relationship between stressful life events and depressive symptoms in adults: cardiovascular risk in young Finns study. Psychosom Med 69:391–395, 2007

Endicott J, Nee J: Endicott Work Productivity Scale (EWPS): a new measure to assess treatment effects. Psychopharmacol Bull 33:13–16, 1997

Endicott J, Nee J, Harrison W, et al: Quality of Life Enjoyment and Satisfaction Questionnaire: a new measure. Psychopharmacol Bull 29:321–326, 1993

Even C, Schröder CM, Friedman S, et al: Efficacy of light therapy in nonseasonal depression: a systematic review. J Affect Disord 108:11–23, 2007

Fava GA: Well-being therapy: conceptual and technical issues. Psychother Psychosom 68:171–179, 1999

Fava GA, Grandi S, Zielezny M, et al: Cognitive behavioral treatment of residual symptoms in primary major depressive disorder. Am J Psychiatry 151:1295–1299, 1994

Fava GA, Savron G, Grandi S, et al: Cognitive-behavioral management of drug-resistant major depressive disorder. J Clin Psychiatry 58:278–282; quiz 283–284, 1997

Fava GA, Ruini C, Rafanelli C, et al: Six-year outcome of cognitive behavior therapy for prevention of recurrent depression. Am J Psychiatry 161:1872–1876, 2004

Fava M, Rush AJ, Trivedi MH, et al: Background and rationale for the sequenced treatment alternatives to relieve depression (STAR*D) study. Psychiatr Clin North Am 26:457–494, 2003

Fava M, Alpert J, Nierenberg AA, et al: A double-blind, randomized trial of St John's wort, fluoxetine, and placebo in major depressive disorder. J Clin Psychopharmacol 25:441–447, 2005

Feldman G: Cognitive and behavioral therapies for depression: overview, new directions, and practical recommendations for dissemination. Psychiatr Clin North Am 30:39–50, 2007

Fergusson DM, Horwood LJ, Ridder EM, et al: Subthreshold depression in adolescence and mental health outcomes in adulthood. Arch Gen Psychiatry 62:66–72, 2005

Field T, Ironson G, Scafidi F, et al: Massage therapy reduces anxiety and enhances EEG pattern of alertness and math computations. Int J Neurosci 86:197–205, 1996

Fogel J, Eaton WW, Ford DE: Minor depression as a predictor of the first onset of major depressive disorder over a 15-year follow-up. Acta Psychiatr Scand 113:36–43, 2006

Frank E, Kupfer DJ, Perel JM, et al: Three-year outcomes for maintenance therapies in recurrent depression. Arch Gen Psychiatry 47:1093–1099, 1990

Frank E, Kupfer DJ, Wagner EF, et al: Efficacy of interpersonal psychotherapy as a maintenance treatment of recurrent depression: contributing factors. Arch Gen Psychiatry 48:1053–1059, 1991a

Frank E, Prien RF, Jarrett RB, et al: Conceptualization and rationale for consensus definitions of terms in major depressive disorder: remission, recovery, relapse, and recurrence. Arch Gen Psychiatry 48:851–855, 1991b

Frank E, Kupfer DJ, Buysse DJ, et al: Randomized trial of weekly, twice-monthly, and monthly interpersonal psychotherapy as maintenance treatment for women with recurrent depression. Am J Psychiatry 164:761–767, 2007

Freis ED: Mental depression in hypertensive patients treated for long periods with large doses of reserpine. N Engl J Med 251:1006–1008, 1954

George MS, Wassermann EM, Williams WA, et al: Daily repetitive transcranial magnetic stimulation (rTMS) improves mood in depression. Neuroreport 6:1853–1856, 1995

George MS, Rush AJ, Marangell LB, et al: A one-year comparison of vagus nerve stimulation with treatment as usual for treatment-resistant depression. Biol Psychiatry 58:364–373, 2005

George MS, Nahas Z, Borckardt JJ, et al: Brain stimulation for the treatment of psychiatric disorders. Curr Opin Psychiatry 20:250–254; discussion 247–249, 2007

Gertsik L, Poland RE: Psychoneuroendocrinology, in Textbook of Psychopharmacology. Edited by Schatzberg A, Nemeroff CB. Washington, DC, American Psychiatric Press, 2004, pp 115–129

Gibbons JL, McHugh PR: Plasma cortisol in depressive illness. J Psychiatr Res 1:162–171, 1962

Gibbons RD, Hur K, Bhaumik DK, et al: The relationship between antidepressant medication use and rate of suicide. Arch Gen Psychiatry 62:165–172, 2005

Gillespie CF, Nemeroff CB: Hypercortisolemia and depression. Psychosom Med 67 (suppl 1):S26–S28, 2005

Ginsberg DL, Schooler NR, Buckley PF, et al: Optimizing treatment of schizophrenia: enhancing affective/cognitive and depressive functioning. CNS Spectr 10:1–13; discussion 14–15, 2005

Gispen-de Wied CC, Kok FW, Koppeschaar HP, et al: Stimulation of the pituitary-adrenal system with graded doses of CRH and low dose vasopressin infusion in depressed patients and healthy subjects: a pilot study. Eur Neuropsychopharmacol 3:533–541, 1993

Glassman AH, Shapiro PA: Depression and the course of coronary artery disease. Am J Psychiatry 155:4–11, 1998

Gold PW, Loriaux DL, Roy A, et al: Responses to corticotropin-releasing hormone in the hypercortisolism of depression and Cushing's disease: pathophysiologic and diagnostic implications. N Engl J Med 314:1329–1335, 1986

Goldapple K, Segal Z, Garson C, et al: Modulation of cortical-limbic pathways in major depression: treatment-specific effects of cognitive behavior therapy. Arch Gen Psychiatry 61:34–41, 2004

Goldney RD, Fisher LJ, Dal Grande E, et al: Subsyndromal depression: prevalence, use of health services and quality of life in an Australian population. Soc Psychiatry Psychiatr Epidemiol 39:293–298, 2004

Guy W: ECDEU assessment manual for psychopharmacology. Rockville, MD, U.S. Department of Health, Education, and Welfare, Public Health Service, Alcohol, Drug Abuse, and Mental Health Administration, National Institute of Mental Health, Psychopharmacology Research Branch, Division of Extramural Research Programs, 1976

Hamilton M: A rating scale for depression. J Neurol Neurosurg Psychiatry 23:56–62, 1960

Hamilton M: Development of a rating scale for primary depressive illness. Br J Soc Clin Psychol 6:278–296, 1967

Harris PA: The impact of age, gender, race, and ethnicity on the diagnosis and treatment of depression. J Manag Care Pharm 10 (2 suppl):S2–S7, 2004

Hasin DS, Goodwin RD, Stinson FS, et al: Epidemiology of major depressive disorder: results from the National Epidemiologic Survey on Alcoholism and Related Conditions. Arch Gen Psychiatry 62:1097–1106, 2005

Hautzinger M, de Jong-Meyer R, Treiber R, et al: Efficacy of cognitive behavior therapy, pharmacotherapy, and the combination of both in non-melancholic, unipolar depression [in German]. Z Klin Psychol 25:130–145, 1996

Heim C, Newport DJ, Heit S, et al: Pituitary-adrenal and autonomic responses to stress in women after sexual and physical abuse in childhood. JAMA 284:592–597, 2000

Helmer C, Montagnier D, Pérès K: Descriptive epidemiology and risk factors of depression in the elderly [in French]. Psychol Neuropsychiatr Vieil 2 (suppl 1):S7–S12, 2004

Henriksson S, Isacsson G: Increased antidepressant use and fewer suicides in Jämtland county, Sweden, after a primary care educational programme on the treatment of depression. Acta Psychiatr Scand 114:159–167, 2006

Hermens ML, van Hout HP, Terluin B, et al: The prognosis of minor depression in the general population: a systematic review. Gen Hosp Psychiatry 26:453–462, 2004

Hirschfeld RM: The comorbidity of major depression and anxiety disorders: recognition and management in primary care. Prim Care Companion J Clin Psychiatry 3:244–254, 2001

Hirschfeld RM, Klerman GL, Clayton PJ, et al: Personality and depression: empirical findings. Arch Gen Psychiatry 40:993–998, 1983

Hollon SD, DeRubeis RJ, Shelton RC, et al: Prevention of relapse following cognitive therapy vs medications in moderate to severe depression. Arch Gen Psychiatry 62:417–422, 2005

Holsboer F: Neuroendocrinology of mood disorders, in Psychopharmacology: The Fourth Generation of Progress. Edited by Bloom FE, Kupfer DJ. New York, Raven, 1995, pp 957–971

Holsboer F: The corticosteroid receptor hypothesis of depression. Neuropsychopharmacology 23:477–501, 2000

Horowitz A, Reinhardt JP, Kennedy GJ: Major and subthreshold depression among older adults seeking vision rehabilitation services. Am J Geriatr Psychiatry 13:180–187, 2005

Howland RH, Schettler PJ, Rapaport MH, et al: Clinical features and functioning of patients with minor depression. Psychother Psychosom 77:384–389, 2008

Hu XZ, Rush AJ, Charney D, et al: Association between a functional serotonin transporter promoter polymorphism and citalopram treatment in adult outpatients with major depression. Arch Gen Psychiatry 64:783–792, 2007

Hunt SM, McKenna SP: The QLDS: a scale for the measurement of quality of life in depression. Health Policy 22:307–319, 1992

Jacobson NS, Hollon SD: Cognitive-behavior therapy versus pharmacotherapy: now that the jury's returned its verdict, it's time to present the rest of the evidence. J Consult Clin Psychol 64:74–80, 1996

Jacobson NS, Dobson KS, Truax PA, et al: A component analysis of cognitive-behavioral treatment for depression. J Consult Clin Psychol 64:295–304, 1996

Janakiramaiah N, Gangadhar BN, Naga Venkatesha Murthy PJ, et al: Antidepressant efficacy of Sudarshan Kriya Yoga (SKY) in melancholia: a randomized comparison with electroconvulsive therapy (ECT) and imipramine. J Affect Disord 57:255–259, 2000

Joffe H, Hall JE, Soares CN, et al: Vasomotor symptoms are associated with depression in perimenopausal women seeking primary care. Menopause 9:392–398, 2002

Joyce PR, McKenzie JM, Carter JD, et al: Temperament, character and personality disorders as predictors of response to interpersonal psychotherapy and cognitive-behavioural therapy for depression. Br J Psychiatry 190:503–508, 2007

Judd LL, Akiskal HS: Delineating the longitudinal structure of depressive illness: beyond clinical subtypes and duration thresholds. Pharmacopsychiatry 33:3–7, 2000

Judd LL, Akiskal HS: The clinical and public health relevance of current research on subthreshold depressive symptoms to elderly patients. Am J Geriatr Psychiatry 10:233–238, 2002

Judd LL, Rapaport MH, Paulus MP, et al: Subsyndromal symptomatic depression: a new mood disorder? J Clin Psychiatry 55 (suppl):18–28, 1994

Judd LL, Paulus MP, Wells KB, et al: Socioeconomic burden of subsyndromal depressive symptoms and major depression in a sample of the general population. Am J Psychiatry 153:1411–1417, 1996

Judd LL, Akiskal HS, Paulus MP: The role and clinical significance of subsyndromal depressive symptoms (SSD) in unipolar major depressive disorder. J Affect Disord 45:5–17; discussion 17–18, 1997

Judd LL, Akiskal HS, Maser JD, et al: A prospective 12-year study of subsyndromal and syndromal depressive symptoms in unipolar major depressive disorders. Arch Gen Psychiatry 55:694–700, 1998a

Judd LL, Akiskal HS, Maser JD, et al: Major depressive disorder: a prospective study of residual subthreshold depressive symptoms as predictor of rapid relapse. J Affect Disord 50(2–3):97–108, 1998b

Judd LL, Akiskal HS, Zeller PJ, et al: Psychosocial disability during the long-term course of unipolar major depressive disorder. Arch Gen Psychiatry 57:375–380, 2000

Judd LL, Rapaport MH, Yonkers KA, et al: Randomized, placebo-controlled trial of fluoxetine for acute treatment of minor depressive disorder. Am J Psychiatry 161:1864–1871, 2004

Kabat-Zinn J: Full Catastrophe Living: Using the Wisdom of Your Body and Mind to Face Stress, Pain, and Illness. New York, Delacorte Press, 1990

Kaplan RM: Quality of life assessment for cost/utility studies in cancer. Cancer Treat Rev 19 (suppl A):85–96, 1993

Kaplan RM, Anderson JP: An integrated approach to quality of life assessments: the general health policy model, in Quality of Life in Clinical Studies. Edited by Spilker B. New York, Raven, 1990, pp 131–149

Keller MB, Berndt ER: Depression treatment: a lifelong commitment? Psychopharmacol Bull 36 (suppl 2):133–141, 2002

Keller MB, Shapiro RW, Lavori PW, et al: Relapse in major depressive disorder: analysis with the life table. Arch Gen Psychiatry 39:911–915, 1982

Keller MB, Klerman GL, Lavori PW, et al: Long-term outcome of episodes of major depression: clinical and public health significance. JAMA 252:788–792, 1984

Keller MB, Lavori PW, Mueller TI, et al: Time to recovery, chronicity, and levels of psychopathology in major depression: a 5-year prospective follow-up of 431 subjects. Arch Gen Psychiatry 49:809–816, 1992

Keller MB, McCullough JP, Klein DN, et al: A comparison of nefazodone, the cognitive behavioral-analysis system of psychotherapy, and their combination for the treatment of chronic depression. N Engl J Med 342:1462–1470, 2000

Keller MB, Trivedi MH, Thase ME, et al: The Prevention of Recurrent Episodes of Depression with Venlafaxine for Two Years (PREVENT) Study: outcomes from the acute and continuation phases. Biol Psychiatry 62:1371–1379, 2007a

Keller MB, Trivedi MH, Thase ME, et al: The Prevention of Recurrent Episodes of Depression with Venlafaxine for Two Years (PREVENT) Study: outcomes from the 2-year and combined maintenance phases. J Clin Psychiatry 68:1246–1256, 2007b

Kendler KS, Kuhn JW, Vittum J, et al: The interaction of stressful life events and a serotonin transporter polymorphism in the prediction of episodes of major depression: a replication. Arch Gen Psychiatry 62:529–535, 2005

Kennedy SH, Evans KR, Kruger S, et al: Changes in regional brain glucose metabolism measured with positron emission tomography after paroxetine treatment of major depression. Am J Psychiatry 158:899–905, 2001

Kessler RC, McGonagle KA, Zhao S, et al: Lifetime and 12-month prevalence of DSM-III-R psychiatric disorders in the United States: results from the National Comorbidity Survey. Arch Gen Psychiatry 51:8–19, 1994

Kessler RC, Zhao S, Blazer DG, et al: Prevalence, correlates, and course of minor depression and major depression in the National Comorbidity Survey. J Affect Disord 45(1–2):19–30, 1997

Khan A, Brodhead AE, Kolts RL: Relative sensitivity of the Montgomery-Asberg depression rating scale, the Hamilton depression rating scale and the Clinical Global Impressions rating scale in antidepressant clinical trials: a replication analysis. Int Clin Psychopharmacol 19:157–160, 2004

Kling MA, Alesci S, Csako G, et al: Sustained low-grade pro-inflammatory state in unmedicated, remitted women with major depressive disorder as evidenced by elevated serum levels of the acute phase proteins C-reactive protein and serum amyloid A. Biol Psychiatry 62:309–313, 2007

Kripke DF: Photoperiodic mechanisms for depression and its treatment, in Biological Psychiatry. Edited by Perris C, Struwe G, Jansson B. Elsevier-North Holland Biomedical Press, 1981, pp 1249–1252

Kroenke K, Spitzer RL, Williams JB: The PHQ-9: validity of a brief depression severity measure. J Gen Intern Med 16:606–613, 2001

Kupfer DJ: Long-term treatment of depression. J Clin Psychiatry 52 (suppl):28–34, 1991

Kupfer DJ, Frank E, Perel JM, et al: Five-year outcome for maintenance therapies in recurrent depression. Arch Gen Psychiatry 49:769–773, 1992

Kuyken W, Dalgleish T, Holden ER: Advances in cognitive-behavioural therapy for unipolar depression. Can J Psychiatry 52:5–13, 2007

Laje G, Paddock S, Manji H, et al: Genetic markers of suicidal ideation emerging during citalopram treatment of major depression. Am J Psychiatry 164:1530–1538, 2007

Leon AC, Shear MK, Portera L, et al: Assessing impairment in patients with panic disorder: the Sheehan Disability Scale. Soc Psychiatry Psychiatr Epidemiol 27:78–82, 1992

Lewy AJ, Sack RL: Light therapy and psychiatry. Proc Soc Exp Biol Med. 183:11–18, 1986

Liu Z, Zhu F, Wang G, et al: Association study of corticotropin-releasing hormone receptor1 gene polymorphisms and antidepressant response in major depressive disorders. Neurosci Lett 414:155–158, 2007

Lopez AD, Murray CC: The global burden of disease, 1990–2020. Nat Med 4:1241–1243, 1998

Lopez AD, Mathers CD, Ezzati M, et al: Global and regional burden of disease and risk factors, 2001: systematic analysis of population health data. Lancet 367:1747–1757, 2006

Luty SE, Carter JD, McKenzie JM, et al: Randomised controlled trial of interpersonal psychotherapy and cognitive-behavioural therapy for depression. Br J Psychiatry 190:496–502, 2007

Maddux RE, Rapaport MH: Psychopharmacology and psychotherapy of subsyndromal depressions, in Handbook of Chronic Depression: Diagnosis and Therapeutic Management. Edited by Alpert JE, Fava M. New York, Informa Healthcare, 2004, pp 183–206

Maes M: Evidence for an immune response in major depression: a review and hypothesis. Prog Neuropsychopharmacol Biol Psychiatry 19:11–38, 1995

Maes M: Major depression and activation of the inflammatory response system, in Cytokines, Stress, and Depression. Edited by Dantzer R, Wollman EE, Yirmiya R. New York, Kluwer Academic/Plenum, 1999, pp 25–46

Maes M, Meltzer HY, Bosmans E, et al: Increased plasma concentrations of interleukin-6, soluble interleukin-6, soluble interleukin-2 and transferrin receptor in major depression. J Affect Disord 34:301–309, 1995

Mayberg HS, Brannan SK, Tekell JL, et al: Regional metabolic effects of fluoxetine in major depression: serial changes and relationship to clinical response. Biol Psychiatry 48:830–843, 2000

Mayberg HS, Lozano AM, Voon V, et al: Deep brain stimulation for treatment-resistant depression. Neuron 45:651–660, 2005

McCullough JP: Treatment for Chronic Depression: Cognitive Behavioral Analysis System of Psychotherapy. New York, Guilford, 2000

McCusker J, Cole M, Dufouil C, et al: The prevalence and correlates of major and minor depression in older medical inpatients. J Am Geriatr Soc 53:1344–1353, 2005

McPherson S, Cairns P, Carlyle J, et al: The effectiveness of psychological treatments for treatment-resistant depression: a systematic review. Acta Psychiatr Scand 111:331–340, 2005

Melfi CA, Chawla AJ, Croghan TW, et al: The effects of adherence to antidepressant treatment guidelines on relapse and recurrence of depression. Arch Gen Psychiatry 55:1128–1132, 1998

Meyers CA: Mood and cognitive disorders in cancer patients receiving cytokine therapy, in Cytokines, Stress, and Depression. Edited by Dantzer R, Wollman EE, Yirmiya R. New York, Kluwer Academic/Plenum, 1999, pp 75–81

Miller IW, Norman WH, Keitner GI, et al: Cognitive-behavioral treatment of depressed inpatients. Behav Ther 20:25–47, 1989a

Miller IW, Norman WH, Keitner GI: Cognitive-behavioral treatment of depressed inpatients: six- and twelve-month follow-up. Am J Psychiatry 146:1274–1279, 1989b

Miller IW, Keitner GI, Schatzberg AF, et al: The treatment of chronic depression, part 3: psychosocial functioning before and after treatment with sertraline or imipramine. J Clin Psychiatry 59:608–619, 1998

Mischoulon D, Fava M: Role of S-adenosyl-L-methionine in the treatment of depression: a review of the evidence. Am J Clin Nutr 76:1158S–1161S, 2002

Montgomery SA, Åsberg M: A new depression scale designed to be sensitive to change. Br J Psychiatry 134:382–389, 1979

Mundt JC, Marks IM, Shear MK, et al: The Work and Social Adjustment Scale: a simple measure of impairment in functioning. Br J Psychiatry 180:461–464, 2002

Murck H, Fava M, Alpert J, et al: Hypericum extract in patients with MDD and reversed vegetative signs: re-analysis from data of a double-blind, randomized trial of hypericum extract, fluoxetine, and placebo. Int J Neuropsychopharmacol 8:215–221, 2005

Murray CJ, Lopez AD: Alternative projections of mortality and disability by cause 1990–2020: Global Burden of Disease Study. Lancet 349:1498–1504, 1997

Musselman DL, Lawson DH, Gumnick JF, et al: Paroxetine for the prevention of depression induced by high-dose interferon alfa. N Engl J Med 344:961–966, 2001

Nemeroff CB, Vale WW: The neurobiology of depression: inroads to treatment and new drug discovery. J Clin Psychiatry 66 (suppl 7):5–13, 2005

Nemeroff CB, Heim CM, Thase ME, et al: Differential responses to psychotherapy versus pharmacotherapy in patients with chronic forms of major depression and childhood trauma. Proc Natl Acad Sci U S A 100:14293–14296, 2003

Nunes EV: Substance abuse and depression. Paper presented at the annual meeting of the American Psychiatric Association, San Francisco, CA, May 2003

Olfson M, Fireman B, Weissman MM, et al: Mental disorders and disability among patients in a primary care group practice. Am J Psychiatry 154:1734–1740, 1997

O'Reardon JP, Solvason HB, Janicak PG, et al: Efficacy and safety of transcranial magnetic stimulation in the acute treatment of major depression: a multisite randomized controlled trial. Biol Psychiatry 62:1208–1216, 2007

Osei-Tutu KB, Campagna PD: The effects of short- vs long-bout exercise on mood, VO2max, and percent body fat. Prev Med 40:92–98, 2005

Otto MW, Smits JAJ, Reese HE: Combined psychotherapy and pharmacotherapy for mood and anxiety disorders in adults: review and analysis. Clinical Psychology: Science and Practice 12:72–86, 2005

Papakostas GI, Shelton RC, Smith J, et al: Augmentation of antidepressants with atypical antipsychotic medications for treatment-resistant major depressive disorder: a meta-analysis. J Clin Psychiatry 68:826–831, 2007

Papiol S, Arias B, Gasto C, et al: Genetic variability at HPA axis in major depression and clinical response to antidepressant treatment. J Affect Disord 104:83–90, 2007

Paykel ES, Ramana R, Cooper Z, et al: Residual symptoms after partial remission: an important outcome in depression. Psychol Med 25:1171–1180, 1995

Paykel ES, Cooper Z, Ramana R, et al: Life events, social support and marital relationships in the outcome of severe depression. Psychol Med 26:121–133, 1996

Paykel ES, Scott J, Teasdale JD, et al: Prevention of relapse in residual depression by cognitive therapy: a controlled trial. Arch Gen Psychiatry 56:829–835, 1999

Perlis RH: Pharmacogenetic studies of antidepressant response: how far from the clinic? Psychiatr Clin North Am 30:125–138, 2007

Petty F, Kramer GL, Hendrickse W: GABA and depression, in Biology of Depressive Disorders, Part A: A Systems Perspective. Edited by Mann JJ, Kupler DJ. New York, Plenum, 1993, pp 79–108

Pilkington K, Kirkwood G, Rampes H, et al: Yoga for depression: the research evidence. J Affect Disord 89:13–24, 2005

Pittenger C, Sanacora G, Krystal JH: The NMDA receptor as a therapeutic target in major depressive disorder. CNS Neurol Disord Drug Targets 6:101–115, 2007

Potter GG, Steffens DC: Contribution of depression to cognitive impairment and dementia in older adults. Neurologist 13:105–117, 2007

Prien RF, Kupfer DJ, Mansky PA, et al: Drug therapy in the prevention of recurrences in unipolar and bipolar affective disorders: report of the NIMH Collaborative Study Group comparing lithium carbonate, imipramine, and a lithium carbonate-imipramine combination. Arch Gen Psychiatry 41:1096–1104, 1984

Raadsheer FC, Hoogendijk WJ, Stam FC, et al: Increased numbers of corticotropin-releasing hormone expressing neurons in the hypothalamic paraventricular nucleus of depressed patients. Neuroendocrinology 60:436–444, 1994

Rapaport MH, Judd LL: Minor depressive disorder and subsyndromal depressive symptoms: functional impairment and response to treatment. J Affect Disord 48:227–232, 1998

Rapaport MH, Tipp JE, Schuckit MA: A comparison of ICD-10 and DSM-III-R criteria for substance abuse and dependence. Am J Drug Alcohol Abuse 19:143–151, 1993

Rapaport MH, Judd LL, Schettler PJ, et al: A descriptive analysis of minor depression. Am J Psychiatry 159:637–643, 2002

Rapaport MH, Clary C, Fayyad R, et al: Quality-of-life impairment in depressive and anxiety disorders. Am J Psychiatry 162:1171–1178, 2005

Rapaport MH, Gharabawi GM, Canuso CM, et al: Effects of risperidone augmentation in patients with treatment-resistant depression: results of open-label treatment followed by double-blind continuation. Neuropsychopharmacology 31:2505–2513, 2006

Reinherz HZ, Paradis AD, Giaconia RM, et al: Childhood and adolescent predictors of major depression in the transition to adulthood. Am J Psychiatry 160:2141–2147, 2003

Reynolds CF 3rd, Frank E, Perel JM, et al: Nortriptyline and interpersonal psychotherapy as maintenance therapies for recurrent major depression: a randomized controlled trial in patients older than 59 years. JAMA 281:39–45, 1999

Rich CL, Isacsson G: Suicide and antidepressants in south Alabama: evidence for improved treatment of depression. J Affect Disord 45:135–142, 1997

Rieckmann N, Burg MM, Gerin W, et al: Depression vulnerabilities in patients with different levels of depressive symptoms after acute coronary syndromes. Psychother Psychosom 75:353–361, 2006

Roche Pharmaceuticals: AmpliChip® CYP450 Test. Available at: http://www.roche.com/products/product-details.htm?type=product&id=17. Accessed December 2008.

Rubin RT, Poland RE, Lesser IM, et al: Neuroendocrine aspects of primary endogenous depression, I: cortisol secretory dynamics in patients and matched controls. Arch Gen Psychiatry 44:328–336, 1987

Ruhe HG, Mason NS, Schene AH: Mood is indirectly related to serotonin, norepinephrine and dopamine levels in humans: a meta-analysis of monoamine depletion studies. Mol Psychiatry 12:331–359, 2007

Rush AJ, Giles DE, Schlesser MA, et al: The Inventory for Depressive Symptomatology (IDS): preliminary findings. Psychiatry Res 18:65–87, 1986

Rush AJ, Trivedi MH, Ibrahim HM, et al: The 16-Item Quick Inventory of Depressive Symptomatology (QIDS), clinician rating (QIDS-C), and self-report (QIDS-SR): a psychometric evaluation in patients with chronic major depression. Biol Psychiatry 54:573–583, 2003

Rush AJ, Fava M, Wisniewski SR, et al: Sequenced treatment alternatives to relieve depression (STAR*D): rationale and design. Control Clin Trials 25:119–142, 2004

Rush AJ, Bernstein IH, Trivedi MH, et al: An evaluation of the Quick Inventory of Depressive Symptomatology and the Hamilton Rating Scale for Depression: a Sequenced Treatment Alternatives to Relieve Depression trial report. Biol Psychiatry 59:493–501, 2006a

Rush AJ, Trivedi MH, Wisniewski SR, et al: Acute and longer-term outcomes in depressed outpatients requiring one or several treatment steps: a STAR*D report. Am J Psychiatry 163:1905–1917, 2006b

Rush AJ, Trivedi MH, Wisniewski SR, et al: Bupropion-SR, sertraline, or venlafaxine-XR after failure of SSRIs for depression. N Engl J Med 354:1231–1242, 2006c

Ryff CD: Happiness is everything, or is it?: explorations on the meaning of psychological well-being. J Pers Soc Psychol 57:1069–1081, 1989

Sachar EJ, Hellman L, Fukushima DK, et al: Cortisol production in depressive illness: a clinical and biochemical clarification. Arch Gen Psychiatry 23:289–298, 1970

Sackeim HA, Brannan SK, Rush AJ, et al: Durability of antidepressant response to vagus nerve stimulation (VNS). Int J Neuropsychopharmacol 10:817–826, 2007

Schiepers OJ, Wichers MC, Maes M: Cytokines and major depression. Prog Neuropsychopharmacol Biol Psychiatry 29:201–217, 2005

Schlaepfer TE, Frick C, Zobel A, et al: Vagus nerve stimulation for depression: efficacy and safety in a European study. Psychol Med 38:651–661, 2008

Schramm E, van Calker D, Dykierek P, et al: An intensive treatment program of interpersonal psychotherapy plus pharmacotherapy for depressed inpatients: acute and long-term results. Am J Psychiatry 164:768–777, 2007

Segal Z, Teasdale J, Williams M: Mindfulness-Based Cognitive Therapy for Depression. New York, Guilford, 2002

Sequeira A, Gwadry FG, Ffrench-Mullen JM, et al: Implication of SSAT by gene expression and genetic variation in suicide and major depression. Arch Gen Psychiatry 63:35–48, 2006

Shaw BF, Elkin I, Yamaguchi J, et al: Therapist competence ratings in relation to clinical outcome in cognitive therapy of depression. J Consult Clin Psychol 67:837–846, 1999

Sluzewska A, Rybakowski J, Bosmans E, et al: Indicators of immune activation in major depression. Psychiatry Res 64:161–167, 1996

Smit F, Cuijpers P, Oostenbrink J, et al: Costs of nine common mental disorders: implications for curative and preventive psychiatry. J Ment Health Policy Econ 9:193–200, 2006

Smith CA, Hay PP: Acupuncture for depression. Cochrane Database Syst Rev (2):CD004046, 2005

Smits K, Smits L, Peeters F, et al: Serotonin transporter polymorphisms and the occurrence of adverse events during treatment with selective serotonin reuptake inhibitors. Int Clin Psychopharmacol 22:137–143, 2007a

Smits KM, Smits LJ, Schouten JS, et al: Does pretreatment testing for serotonin transporter polymorphisms lead to earlier effects of drug treatment in patients with major depression? A decision-analytic model. Clin Ther 29:691–702, 2007b

Søndergård L, Kvist K, Lopez AG, et al: Temporal changes in suicide rates for persons treated and not treated with antidepressants in Denmark during 1995–1999. Acta Psychiatr Scand 114:168–176, 2006

Stahl LA, Begg DP, Weisinger RS, et al: The role of omega-3 fatty acids in mood disorders. Curr Opin Investig Drugs 9:57–64, 2008

Stewart WF, Ricci JA, Chee E, et al: Cost of lost productive work time among US workers with depression. JAMA 289:3135–3144, 2003

Tabuse H, Kalali A, Azuma H, et al: The new GRID Hamilton Rating Scale for Depression demonstrates excellent inter-rater reliability for inexperienced and experienced raters before and after training. Psychiatry Res 153:61–67, 2007

Thase ME: Redefining antidepressant efficacy toward long-term recovery. J Clin Psychiatry 60 (suppl 6):15–19, 1999

Thase ME, Friedman ES, Biggs MM, et al: Cognitive therapy versus medication in augmentation and switch strategies as second-step treatments: a STAR*D report. Am J Psychiatry 164:739–752, 2007

Trivedi MH, Rush AJ, Ibrahim HM, et al: The Inventory of Depressive Symptomatology, Clinician Rating (IDS-C) and Self-Report (IDS-SR), and the Quick Inventory of Depressive Symptomatology, Clinician Rating (QIDS-C) and Self-Report (QIDS-SR) in public sector patients with mood disorders: a psychometric evaluation. Psychol Med 34:73–82, 2004

Trivedi MH, Fava M, Wisniewski SR, et al: Medication augmentation after the failure of SSRIs for depression. N Engl J Med 354:1243–1252, 2006a

Trivedi MH, Greer TL, Grannemann BD, et al: Exercise as an augmentation strategy for treatment of major depression. J Psychiatr Pract 12:205–213, 2006b

Trivedi MH, Greer TL, Grannemann BD, et al: TREAD: TReatment with Exercise Augmentation for Depression: study rationale and design. Clin Trials 3:291–305, 2006c

Trivedi MH, Rush AJ, Wisniewski SR, et al: Evaluation of outcomes with citalopram for depression using measurement-based care in STAR*D: implications for clinical practice. Am J Psychiatry 163:28–40, 2006d

UK ECT Review Group: Efficacy and safety of electroconvulsive therapy in depressive disorders: a systematic review and meta-analysis. Lancet 361:799–808, 2003

U.S. Department of Health and Human Services: National strategy for suicide prevention. A collaborative effort of SAMHSA, CDC, NIH, HRSA, HIS. 2001. Available at: http://mental-health.samhsa.gov/suicideprevention/elderly.asp. Accessed December 2, 2008.

van Rossum EF, Binder EB, Majer M, et al: Polymorphisms of the glucocorticoid receptor gene and major depression. Biol Psychiatry 59:681–688, 2006

Videbech P, Ravnkilde B: Hippocampal volume and depression: a meta-analysis of MRI studies. Am J Psychiatry 161:1957–1966, 2004

Ware JE Jr, Sherbourne CD: The MOS 36-item short-form health survey (SF-36), I: conceptual framework and item selection. Med Care 30:473–483, 1992

Ware J Jr, Kosinski M, Keller SD: A 12-Item Short-Form Health Survey: construction of scales and preliminary tests of reliability and validity. Med Care 34:220–233, 1996

Warner-Schmidt JL, Duman RS: Hippocampal neurogenesis: opposing effects of stress and antidepressant treatment. Hippocampus 16:239–249, 2006

Weissman MM, Klerman GL: Sex differences and the epidemiology of depression. Arch Gen Psychiatry 34:98–111, 1977

Weissman MM, Bland RC, Canino GJ, et al: Cross-national epidemiology of major depression and bipolar disorder. JAMA 276:293–299, 1996

Wells KB, Stewart A, Hays RD, et al: The functioning and well-being of depressed patients: results from the Medical Outcomes Study. JAMA 262:914–919, 1989

Westrin A, Lam RW: Long-term and preventative treatment for seasonal affective disorder. CNS Drugs 21:901–909, 2007

Williams JB: A structured interview guide for the Hamilton Depression Rating Scale. Arch Gen Psychiatry 45:742–747, 1988

Wisniewski SR, Fava M, Trivedi MH, et al: Acceptability of second-step treatments to depressed outpatients: a STAR*D report. Am J Psychiatry 164:753–760, 2007

Zimmerman M, Thongy T: How often do SSRIs and other new-generation antidepressants lose their effect during continuation treatment? Evidence suggesting the rate of true tachyphylaxis during continuation treatment is low. J Clin Psychiatry 68:1271–1276, 2007

Zung WWK: A self-rating depression scale. Arch Gen Psychiatry 12:371–379, 1965

CHAPTER 54

Treatment of Bipolar Disorder

Paul E. Keck Jr., M.D.

Susan L. McElroy, M.D.

Bipolar disorder is a common, recurrent, often severe psychiatric illness that, without adequate treatment, is associated with high rates of morbidity and mortality (Goodwin and Jamison 2007). In the Global Burden of Disease survey, bipolar disorder was the sixth leading cause of disability worldwide in 1990 and, without improved access to treatment, was projected to remain so well into this century (Murray and Lopez 1996). Morbidity from bipolar disorder often extends well beyond manic, hypomanic, mixed, and depressive episodes. Full recovery of functioning can lag many months behind symptomatic improvement, and repeated episodes can lead to lasting functional impairment (Judd et al. 2005). Recent naturalistic outcome studies indicate that many patients with bipolar disorder spend protracted periods of time neither well nor syndromally ill but rather suffering from chronic subsyndromal, especially depressive, symptoms (Judd et al. 2002, 2003). Bipolar disorder is also among the most heritable of all medical illnesses (Goodwin and Jamison 2007).

The goals of treatment of bipolar disorder are similar to those of management of many chronic illnesses: rapid, complete remission of acute episodes; prevention of further episodes; suppression of subsyndromal symptoms; and optimization of functional outcome and quality of life (Keck et al. 2001). However, the treatment of bipolar disorder is often complicated. Although classified as a mood disorder, bipolar disorder is also characterized by disturbances of behavior, cognition, and perception. Thus, suc-

cessful treatment requires that these multiple symptom domains be addressed. Treatment is further complicated by the diversity of illness presentation (e.g., pattern, frequency, and severity of episodes; presence of psychosis, comorbid illnesses, acute or chronic environmental stressors) and course among individuals. Some medications have particular efficacy in one phase of illness but not in another, and some may actually increase the likelihood of precipitating a reciprocal mood episode.

The treatment of bipolar disorder has traditionally been divided into the management of acute manic, mixed, and depressive episodes and the prevention of further episodes and symptoms (Hirschfeld et al. 2002). Rush (1999) conceptualized a "strategies and tactics" approach to the management of major depressive disorder, with principles of pharmacotherapy that are readily applicable to bipolar disorder (Table 54–1). In this chapter we review strategies (i.e., what treatments to choose) and tactics (i.e., how to implement these strategies once chosen and what dose and duration of the chosen medication are to be used) for treating bipolar disorder, drawing primarily on data from randomized, controlled trials. Where such data are lacking, strategies based on data from open trials, naturalistic studies, and expert consensus guidelines are included. The treatment of bipolar disorder in children and adolescents is covered elsewhere in this book (see Chapter 63 in this volume, "Treatment of Child and Adolescent Disorders," by Wagner and Pliszka).

TABLE 54–1.   Treatment principles for bipolar disorder

Individually tailor guidelines.

Use proven treatments first.

Select best medication that is

   Safe and tolerable.

   Easiest to use (for the patient).

   Easiest to manage (for the physician).

Aim for symptom remission, not just response.

Measure symptomatic outcome.

Remember that no medication is a panacea.

Do not give up.

Recognize that psychosocial restoration follows symptom relief.

Interpersonal, family, educational, and social rhythm–targeted psychotherapies can help.

More chronic illness may respond more slowly.

Source. Adapted from Rush AJ: "Strategies and Tactics in the Management of Maintenance Treatment for Depressed Patients." *Journal of Clinical Psychiatry* 60 (Supplement 14):21–26, 1999.

Formulation and Implementation of a Treatment Plan

Patients with bipolar disorder enter into treatment at various phases of illness. Regardless of illness phase, treatment begins with a thorough diagnostic assessment (Hirschfeld et al. 2002). In addition to the clinical features of bipolar disorder described in DSM-IV-TR (American Psychiatric Association 2000), patients with bipolar disorder also commonly experience symptoms of anxiety, impulsivity, recklessness, elevated libido, poor insight, inattention, and sensory hyperacuity during manic or mixed episodes (Keck et al. 2001).

Bipolar disorder frequently presents with depressive episodes. A family history of bipolar disorder or early age at onset of depression should raise diagnostic questions about bipolar disorder in an individual presenting for treatment of depression. Studies suggest that 15%–30% of patients treated for apparent major depressive disorder in outpatient settings subsequently receive a diagnosis of bipolar I or II disorder (Manning et al. 1997, 1998). The Mood Disorder Questionnaire (MDQ) is a 13-item self-report screening instrument for bipolar disorder that has been successfully tested in psychiatric clinics (Hirschfeld et al. 2000) and in the general population (Hirschfeld 2002). Bipolar disorder is associated with elevated rates of substance use, anxiety, eating, attention-deficit/hyperac-

tivity, and impulse-control disorders and migraine (Birmaher et al. 2002; McElroy et al. 2001). Thus, the presence of these illnesses should be assessed in patients with bipolar disorder, and conversely, bipolar disorder should be assessed in patients presenting with these other illnesses. Other elements of a complete psychiatric evaluation are summarized in the American Psychiatric Association's (1995) "Practice Guideline for Psychiatric Evaluation of Adults."

The American Psychiatric Association's revised "Practice Guideline for the Treatment of Patients With Bipolar Disorder" (Hirschfeld et al. 2002) lists a number of other important elements in the treatment of patients with bipolar disorder (Table 54–2). Evaluation of safety of the patient and others and determination of the appropriate treatment setting are essential because of the risks of suicide, recklessness, and violence associated with mood episodes (Lopez et al. 2001) (Table 54–3). Establishing and maintaining a treatment alliance are early and ongoing goals to facilitate patient and family education, treatment adherence, and identification of precipitants and prodromal symptoms. Monitoring treatment response and providing illness education can be enhanced by using the Life-Chart Method (Denicoff et al. 2002) or other similar longitudinal self-assessments. In addition, a number of well-validated rating scales exist for monitoring mood symptoms in patients with bipolar disorder cross-sectionally. These include the Young Mania Rating Scale (R.C. Young et al. 1978) for manic symptoms and the Montgomery-Åsberg Depression Rating Scale (Montgomery and Åsberg 1979) for depressive symptoms, among others. Because bipolar disorder can lead to disability and varying degrees of functional impairment in all aspects of life, specific psychotherapeutic and rehabilitation interventions may be needed.

Definitions: What Is a Mood Stabilizer?

The treatment of bipolar disorder is among the most challenging of all treatments for psychiatric illnesses for a variety of reasons, one of which is that some agents effective in the treatment of one pole can exacerbate or cause a switch into another pole. Goodwin and Jamison (2007) have defined *mood stabilizer* as an agent that demonstrates efficacy in the acute treatment of both mania and depression, as well as in the prevention of both types of mood episodes (ideal definition) or an agent that is efficacious in two of these three aspects of treatment (strict definition).

TABLE 54–2. Clinical components of the management of bipolar disorder

Perform a diagnostic evaluation.

Evaluate the safety of the patient and others and determine a treatment setting.

Establish and maintain a therapeutic alliance.

Monitor treatment response.

Provide education to the patient and significant others.

Enhance treatment compliance.

Promote awareness of stress and regular patterns of activity and sleep.

Work with the patient to anticipate and address early signs of relapse.

Evaluate and manage functional impairments.

Source.   Reprinted from Hirschfeld RMA, Bowden CL, Gitlin MJ, et al.: "Practice Guideline for the Treatment of Patients With Bipolar Disorder (Revision)." *American Journal of Psychiatry* 159 (Supplement):1–50, 2002. Copyright 2002, American Psychiatric Association. Used with permission.

In this chapter, we use the term *mood stabilizer* according to the strict definition. To date, there is no ideal agent, although data from randomized, controlled trials suggest that lithium and olanzapine probably come closest.

Treatment of Acute Bipolar Manic and Mixed Episodes

Manic and mixed episodes are medical emergencies and frequently require treatment in a hospital to ensure safety of patients and those around them. The primary goal of treatment of manic and mixed episodes is rapid symptom reduction, followed by full remission of symptoms and restoration of psychosocial and vocational functioning (Hirschfeld et al. 2002). These are straightforward goals, but tailoring treatment to specific patients requires consideration of presenting symptoms and their severity (e.g., presence or absence of psychosis, manic or mixed episode, proximal frequency of episodes).

Pharmacotherapy is the cornerstone of treatment of acute manic and mixed episodes and of bipolar disorder in general. A number of medications have demonstrated efficacy in the treatment of acute manic and mixed episodes (Table 54–4). Lithium, divalproex, carbamazepine, olanzapine, risperidone, quetiapine, ziprasidone, aripiprazole, haloperidol, and chlorpromazine have shown efficacy as monotherapy in the treatment of acute mania in randomized, placebo-controlled trials (McElroy and Keck 2000;

TABLE 54–3. Characteristics to evaluate in an assessment of suicide risk in patients with bipolar disorder

Presence of suicidal or homicidal ideation, intent, or plans

Access to means for suicide and the lethality of those means

Presence of command hallucinations, other psychotic symptoms, or severe anxiety

Presence of alcohol or substance use

History and seriousness of previous attempts

Family history of or recent exposure to suicide

Source.   Adapted from American Psychiatric Association: "Practice Guideline for the Treatment of Patients With Major Depressive Disorder (Revision)." *American Journal of Psychiatry* 157 (Supplement):1–45, 2000. Copyright 2000, American Psychiatric Association; Hirschfeld RMA, Bowden CL, Gitlin MJ, Keck PE, Perlis RH, Suppes T, Thase ME: "Practice Guideline for the Treatment of Patients With Bipolar Disorder (Revision)." *American Journal of Psychiatry* 159 (Supplement):1–50, 2002. Copyright 2002, American Psychiatric Association. Used with permission.

Perlis et al. 2006c). Although these agents typically produce rates of response (defined as ≥50% reduction in manic symptoms from baseline to endpoint) of approximately 50% in short-term (3- to 4-week) trials, relatively few patients (<25%) actually achieve remission of symptoms within these time intervals while receiving monotherapy with any of these agents. Thus, use of combination therapy is common in clinical practice to improve response and remission rates (Suppes et al. 2005). For example, a number of studies comparing combination treatment with an antipsychotic and lithium or valproate demonstrated superior acute response rates with combination therapy compared with monotherapy (Scherk et al. 2007).

Lithium

Lithium has been a mainstay of treatment for acute mania for more than 50 years, with superior efficacy compared with placebo (Goodwin et al. 1969; Maggs 1963; Schou et al. 1954; Stokes et al. 1971) and comparable efficacy compared with divalproex (Bowden et al. 1994), carbamazepine (Lerer et al. 1987; Small et al. 1991), risperidone (Segal et al. 1998), olanzapine (Berk et al. 1999), quetiapine (Bowden et al. 2005), aripiprazole (Keck et al. 2007), and typical antipsychotics (Garfinkel et al. 1980; Johnson et al. 1976; Platman 1970; Prien et al. 1972; Shopsin et al. 1975; Spring et al. 1970; Takahashi et al. 1975). Lithium exerted improvement in psychotic as well as manic symptoms in these trials. Patients with elated or classic manic

TABLE 54–4.   Evidence-based treatment of acute mania

TREATMENT	NUMBER OF POSITIVE MONOTHERAPY RCTs
Lithium	18
Valproate	9
Carbamazepine	2
Aripiprazole	5
Olanzapine	8
Quetiapine	4
Risperidone	5
Ziprasidone	3
Chlorpromazine	4
Haloperidol	3
ECT	3

Note.   ECT = electroconvulsive therapy; RCTs = randomized, controlled trials.

symptoms (Bowden 1995) and relatively few lifetime mood episodes (Swann et al. 1999) appear to have better response rates to lithium than do patients with mixed episodes, rapid cycling (Dunner and Fieve 1974; McElroy et al. 1992), and numerous prior mood episodes.

Lithium response for acute mania can be maximized by titrating to plasma concentrations at the upper end of the therapeutic range (1.0–1.4 mmol/L) as tolerated (Stokes et al. 1976). In randomized, controlled trials, significant clinical improvement usually was reported within 7–14 days among responders (Keck and McElroy 2001). Preliminary data also suggest that the rate of lithium titration may affect response. Goldberg et al. (1998) found that the rapidity of antimanic effect of any mood stabilizer (lithium, valproate, carbamazepine) was proportional to the rate of titration to therapeutic plasma concentrations. Lithium is generally well tolerated during acute treatment, and dosages needed to produce acute antimanic effects may be higher than those needed for maintenance treatment (Bowden 1998). Common side effects associated with acute treatment with lithium include nausea, vomiting, tremor, somnolence, weight gain, and cognitive slowing.

Antiepileptics

Divalproex

Divalproex and related formulations of valproic acid had superior efficacy compared with placebo (Bowden et al.

1994, 2006; Brennan et al. 1984; Emrich et al. 1981; Pope et al. 1991) and comparable efficacy compared with lithium (Bowden et al. 1994; T. W. Freeman et al. 1992), haloperidol (McElroy et al. 1996), and olanzapine (Zajecka et al. 2002) in randomized, controlled acute treatment trials of bipolar manic or mixed episodes. Olanzapine was superior to divalproex in mean reduction of manic symptoms and in proportion of patients in remission at study completion in a second head-to-head comparison trial (Tohen et al. 2002a). Muller-Oerlinghausen et al. (2000) found that the combination of valproate and typical antipsychotics produced significantly lower mean antipsychotic doses and higher response rates compared with placebo added to typical antipsychotics in patients with acute mania.

Unlike lithium, valproate has a comparatively wide therapeutic index. Acute antimanic response is correlated with plasma concentrations between 50 and 125 mg/L, with some evidence of greater response at the upper end of the therapeutic range (Allen et al. 2006; Zajecka et al. 2002). Some patients may require plasma concentrations greater than 125 mg/L, but side effects become progressively more prevalent above this level. Divalproex can be administered at a therapeutic starting dosage of 20–30 mg/kg/day in inpatients with good tolerability, and some evidence indicates a more rapid response than with gradual titration from a lower (e.g., 750 mg/day) starting dose (Hirschfeld et al. 1999; Keck et al. 1993; McElroy et al. 1996; Zajecka et al. 2002).

Divalproex is generally well tolerated during treatment of acute manic or mixed episodes. Common side effects include somnolence, nausea, vomiting, tremor, weight gain, and cognitive slowing. Enteric-coated and extended-release formulations (the latter requiring a 20% dosage increase to yield plasma concentrations equivalent to those with immediate-release formulations) have improved tolerability compared with valproic acid formulations. Rare serious adverse events include pancreatitis, thrombocytopenia, significant hepatic transaminase elevation, hyperammonemic encephalopathy in patients with urea cycle disorders, and hepatic failure.

Carbamazepine and Oxcarbazepine

Until recently, there was a paucity of data from well-designed randomized, controlled trials of carbamazepine in the treatment of mania. However, an extended-release formulation of carbamazepine was superior to placebo in two large randomized, placebo-controlled multicenter trials (Weisler et al. 2004b, 2005). These findings replicated earlier results from a placebo-controlled crossover trial (Ballenger and Post 1978) and comparison studies against lithium (Lerer et al. 1987; Small et al. 1991) and chlorpromazine (Grossi et al. 1984; Okuma et al. 1979). In one small comparison study, valproate was more effective than carbamazepine (Vasudev et al. 2000). Common side effects of carbamazepine include diplopia, blurred vision, ataxia, somnolence, fatigue, and nausea. Less common side effects include rash, mild leukopenia and thrombocytopenia, and hyponatremia. Rare serious adverse events include agranulocytosis, aplastic anemia, thrombocytopenia, hepatic failure, pancreatitis, and exfoliative dermatitis.

Oxcarbazepine, in contrast to carbamazepine, does not induce its own metabolism, has a lower rate of side effects, and generally has good tolerability (Emrich 1991). Two small randomized, controlled trials of oxcarbazepine in acute mania found oxcarbazepine to be comparable in efficacy to haloperidol and lithium (Emrich 1991; Muller and Stoll 1984). However, both trials were confounded by the use of adjunctive antimanic medications during the trials, and the studies were too small to detect potential differences in efficacy. In the only large randomized, placebo-controlled multicenter trial of oxcarbazepine in acute mania to date, a 7-week study in children and adolescents, oxcarbazepine was not superior to placebo in reduction of manic symptoms (Wagner et al. 2006). Thus, the use of oxcarbazepine in acute bipolar mania has not been substantiated based on evidence from clinical studies but rather is based on putative similarities in mechanism of action with carbamazepine and improved tolerability.

Antipsychotics

Typical (First-Generation) Antipsychotics

Chlorpromazine (Klein 1967) and haloperidol (McIntyre et al. 2005) were superior to placebo in randomized, controlled trials. Typical antipsychotics bear the burden of neurological and neuroendocrinological side effects and may increase the risk of postmanic depressive episodes (Koukopoulos et al. 1980). Thus, typical antipsychotics are commonly regarded as antimanic but not mood-stabilizing agents.

Atypical (Second-Generation) Antipsychotics

The atypical antipsychotics olanzapine, risperidone, quetiapine, ziprasidone, and aripiprazole all have demonstrated efficacy in the treatment of acute bipolar mania in at least two randomized, placebo-controlled trials.

Olanzapine was found to be superior to placebo (Tohen et al. 1999, 2000), superior or equal in efficacy to divalproex (Tohen et al. 2002a; Zajecka et al. 2002), and comparable to lithium (Berk et al. 1999; Niufan et al. 2007), risperidone (Perlis et al. 2006a), and haloperidol (Tohen et al. 2003a) in mean reduction of manic and mixed symptoms in 3- to 4-week monotherapy trials. Adjunctive treatment with olanzapine was superior to placebo in patients who were inadequately responsive to lithium or divalproex monotherapy (Tohen et al. 2002b).

In the haloperidol comparison trial, olanzapine was significantly more likely to improve depressive symptoms during the treatment of manic and mixed episodes (Tohen et al. 2003a). In the two placebo-controlled trials, the rate of response was faster with an initial starting dosage of 15 mg/day (Tohen et al. 2000) compared with 10 mg/day (Tohen et al. 1999). Baker et al. (2003) reported significant improvement in agitation in manic patients within 24 hours with the use of rapid initial dosage escalation (20–40 mg/day) compared with usual titration. The intramuscular formulation of olanzapine has also been studied in the treatment of manic agitation (Meehan et al. 2001). In this study, an intramuscular olanzapine dose of 10 mg produced significant improvement compared with placebo and numerically greater improvement compared with intramuscular lorazepam 2 mg at 2 hours following administration. From these studies, it appears that acute antimanic response to olanzapine may be more rapid in patients treated with higher initial doses, with dosage administration in proportion to the degree of psychomotor agitation. In short-term studies, the most common side effects associated with olanzapine were somnolence, constipation, dry mouth, increased appetite, weight gain, and orthostatic hypotension.

Risperidone was superior to placebo (Hirschfeld et al. 2004; Khanna et al. 2005) and comparable to olanzapine (Perlis et al. 2006a), haloperidol (Smulevich et al. 2005), and lithium (Segal et al. 1998) in mean reduction of manic and mixed symptoms as monotherapy in 3- to 4-week trials. Risperidone was superior to placebo as adjunctive therapy with lithium or divalproex in one placebo-controlled trial (Sachs et al. 2002), but not in a second placebo-controlled trial in combination with lithium, divalproex, or carbamazepine (Yatham et al. 2003). However, because this latter study included patients receiving carbamazepine, it is possible that risperidone plasma concentrations may have been significantly reduced in these patients, limiting risperidone's efficacy. The rate of extrapyramidal side effects associated with risperidone was low when the drug was administered at average dosages up to

4 mg/day (Hirschfeld et al. 2004; Sachs et al. 2002; Yatham et al. 2003) but not when administered at average dosages of 6 mg/day or greater (Khanna et al. 2005; Segal et al. 1998). In short-term trials, other commonly occurring side effects included prolactin elevation, akathisia, somnolence, dyspepsia, and nausea.

Quetiapine was superior to placebo as monotherapy in two 12-week studies in adult patients (Bowden et al. 2005; McIntyre et al. 2005) and was comparable to lithium in a 4-week study in adult patients (Li et al. 2008) and to divalproex in adolescents with bipolar mania (Del-Bello et al. 2006). Similarly, quetiapine was superior to placebo as adjunctive treatment with lithium or divalproex (DelBello et al. 2002; Sachs et al. 2004; Yatham et al. 2004). In two placebo-controlled trials, lithium (Bowden et al. 2005) and haloperidol (McIntyre et al. 2005) were included as active comparators. There were no significant differences in efficacy among patients receiving quetiapine, lithium, or haloperidol, although the trials were not powered to detect such a difference if one existed. The mean modal dose of quetiapine associated with antimanic efficacy in most studies was approximately 600 mg/day (Vieta et al. 2005b). The most common side effects from quetiapine in monotherapy trials were headache, dry mouth, constipation, weight gain, somnolence, and dizziness.

Ziprasidone was superior to placebo (mean dose 120–130 mg/day) in two 3-week monotherapy trials in adult patients (Keck et al. 2003b; Potkin et al. 2005) and comparable to haloperidol in a 12-week trial (Ramey et al. 2003). Ziprasidone was not superior to placebo as adjunctive treatment with lithium in a study designed to prove superior onset of action by 2 weeks of treatment (Weisler et al. 2004a). However, ziprasidone was superior to placebo in reduction of manic symptoms at day 4 in this adjunctive trial. Ziprasidone appears to have dose-related antimanic efficacy within the therapeutic range of 80–160 mg/day. Ziprasidone-related side effects in monotherapy trials included headache, somnolence, extrapyramidal signs, akathisia, and dizziness. The intramuscular (IM) formulation of ziprasidone has also been studied in the treatment of manic agitation (Daniel et al. 2001; Lesem et al. 2001). In these studies, ziprasidone 10–20 mg IM produced significant improvement compared with ziprasidone 2 mg IM at 0.5–4 hours following administration.

Aripiprazole had significantly greater efficacy in the reduction of manic symptoms compared with placebo in three 3-week trials (Keck et al. 2003a, 2007; Sachs et al. 2006) and comparable efficacy with haloperidol (Vieta et

al. 2005a) and lithium (Keck et al. 2009) in adequately powered 12-week comparison trials. Aripiprazole was initiated at 15 or 30 mg/day. Common side effects associated with aripiprazole in the placebo-controlled trials were headache, nausea, vomiting, constipation, insomnia, and akathisia.

In the studies of atypical antipsychotics reviewed above, there were no significant differences in response between patients with or without psychotic features or between patients with manic or mixed episodes among all agents, with the exception of trials of quetiapine, many of which excluded mixed patients. Lastly, the prototypical atypical agent clozapine has been reported to have substantial efficacy in a number of large case series of patients with treatment-refractory mania (Calabrese et al. 1996; Green et al. 2000) but has not been studied in placebo-controlled trials in mania.

Electroconvulsive Therapy

Electroconvulsive therapy (ECT) is an important treatment option for manic patients with severe, psychotic, or catatonic symptoms. ECT was superior in efficacy to lithium (Small et al. 1988) and the combination of lithium and haloperidol (Mukherjee et al. 1994) in prospective comparison studies. In the lithium comparison trial (Small et al. 1988), the presence of depressive symptoms at baseline was the strongest predictor of ECT response. In addition, ECT in combination with chlorpromazine was superior to sham ECT and chlorpromazine (Sikdar et al. 1994). Although these were small studies, their findings are consistent with those of other naturalistic studies of ECT in the treatment of acute mania (Black et al. 1984; Thomas and Reddy 1982). There is a risk of neurotoxicity in patients receiving ECT while also receiving lithium; thus, lithium should be discontinued when ECT is administered (Hirschfeld et al. 2002).

Psychotherapy

Psychotherapeutic interventions in patients with acute mania focus on establishing and maintaining a therapeutic alliance, improving insight, monitoring treatment response, and providing the initial elements of education about bipolar disorder and its manifestations to patients and their families (Hirschfeld et al. 2002). As manic symptoms remit, more attention can be paid to further education, promoting awareness of stressors and sleep hygiene, identifying harbingers of relapse, and assessing need for rehabilitation services.

TABLE 54–5. Criteria for minimum adequate trials of antimanic agents

MEDICATION	DEFINITIVE (3-WEEK TRIAL)	PROBABLE (2-WEEK TRIAL)
Lithium	≥0.8 mmol/L	≥0.7 mmol/L
Valproate	≥75 µg/mL	≥50 µg/mL
Carbamazepine	≥800 mg/day	≥600 mg/day
Haloperidol	≥0.2 mg/kg/day	≥0.1 mg/kg/day
Chlorpromazine	≥500 mg/day	≥300 mg/day
Olanzapine	≥15 mg/day	≥10 mg/day
Ziprasidone	≥120 mg/day	≥80 mg/day
Risperidone	≥5 mg/day	≥4 mg/day
Quetiapine	≥600 mg/day	≥400 mg/day
Aripiprazole	≥30 mg/day	≥15 mg/day

Source. Adapted from Keck PE Jr, McElroy SL: "Definition, Evaluation, and Management of Treatment Refractory Mania." *Psychopharmacology Bulletin* 35:130–148, 2001. Copyright 2001, MedWorks Media. Used with permission.

Novel Treatments

The new atypical antipsychotics paliperidone, asenapine, and bifeprunox and new antiepileptics such as zonisamide, levetiracetam, and acamprosate are being studied as potential antimanic agents. Among these agents, the only randomized, controlled trial reported to date compared asenapine (mean dosage = 18 mg/day), olanzapine (mean dosage = 16 mg/day), and placebo over 3 weeks (Hirschfeld et al. 2007). Both treatment groups displayed comparable reductions in manic symptoms, and both were superior to placebo. By contrast, a number of potential antimanic agents have not demonstrated convincing efficacy in randomized, controlled trials. These include gabapentin (Frye et al. 2000; Pande et al. 2000), lamotrigine (Anand et al. 1999; Frye et al. 2000), topiramate (Kushner et al. 2006), and verapamil (Janicak et al. 1998; Walton et al. 1996).

In two short-term pilot trials, the protein kinase C inhibitor tamoxifen was superior to placebo in reduction of manic symptoms (Yildiz-Yesiloglu 2007; Zarate et al. 2007). The benzodiazepines lorazepam and clonazepam have been studied in a number of randomized, controlled trials in acute mania (Chou et al. 1999) but have not been demonstrated to exert specific antimanic effects. Nevertheless, adjunctive use of benzodiazepines to treat anxiety, insomnia, and agitation in manic patients is often therapeutic.

Monotherapy Versus Combination Therapy of Acute Bipolar Manic and Mixed Episodes

The data reviewed above provide evidence of the efficacy of specific agents administered for adequate treatment trials at therapeutic doses (Table 54–5). Monotherapy with an antimanic agent represents one of two initial options, primarily for patients with less severe manic symptoms. However, combination therapy has generally been demonstrated to have greater and more rapid efficacy than monotherapy (Scherk et al. 2007). Combination therapy may be a particularly useful option in patients with severe manic symptoms or psychosis.

To date, mainly combinations of antipsychotics in conjunction with lithium, valproate, and/or carbamazepine have been studied. The efficacy of combinations of lithium, valproate, or carbamazepine versus monotherapy with these agents has not been studied in randomized, controlled trials, although anecdotal evidence suggests that these combinations may have greater efficacy than either agent alone (M.P. Freeman and Stoll 1998). Similarly, there are no data to date to suggest that other than standard therapeutic doses of agents used in combination therapy are needed.

Treatment of Acute Bipolar Depressive Episodes

For many patients with bipolar disorder, depressive episodes or chronic waxing and waning subsyndromal depressive symptoms dominate their course of illness and constitute a major source of disability (Judd et al. 2002, 2003; Perlis et al. 2006b). In addition, suicide is a substantial risk of untreated bipolar depression. Thus, the goal of treatment of bipolar depression is full remission of symptoms (Hirschfeld et al. 2002). This straightforward goal is complicated by the limited efficacy of many mood stabilizers in bipolar depression (Zornberg and Pope 1993), often requiring the adjunctive use of unimodal antidepressants with the attendant risk of cycle acceleration or switching (Table 54–6). Moreover, there are very little data indicating that the addition of antidepressants to mood stabilizers is more effective than utilization of mood stabilizers alone in alleviating acute bipolar depressive symptoms (Sachs et al. 2007). To date, only quetiapine and combination olanzapine–fluoxetine have indications for the treatment of acute bipolar I depression.

Special Considerations in Bipolar Depression

Antidepressants and the Problem of Switching

The decision to recommend administration or avoidance of antidepressants often means attempting to walk a therapeutic razor's edge between alleviating depression and triggering mood switching. Thus, recent data regarding the protective effect of mood stabilizers against antidepressant-associated switching and the incidence of switching among antidepressants are important to weigh in these decisions. Until recently, most treatment guidelines recommended avoiding antidepressants and relying on mood stabilizers alone in mild to moderate bipolar depression, and when administering antidepressants for severe or persistent bipolar depression, they recommended withdrawing them as quickly as possible after remission (Ghaemi et al. 2001; Sachs et al. 2000). These recommendations were based on reported antidepressant-associated switch rates, which ranged widely, from 10% to 70% (Thase and Sachs 2000).

Many estimates of the incidence of antidepressant-associated switching were based on naturalistic studies that did not control for the switch rate associated with the illness itself. The switch rates reported in recent randomized, controlled acute treatment (i.e., 6–8 weeks) trials of lamotrigine (Calabrese et al. 1999), quetiapine (Calabrese et al. 2005a; Thase et al. 2006), and olanzapine monotherapy (Tohen et al. 2003c) and of combinations of paroxetine with lithium (Nemeroff et al. 2001), lithium with valproate (L. T. Young et al. 2000), and fluoxetine with olanzapine (Tohen et al. 2003c) ranged from 3% to 8%. In addition, Post et al. (2001) reported a switch rate of 14% (8% hypomania, 6% mania) in a 10-week acute treatment trial comparing bupropion, venlafaxine, and sertraline in combination with mood stabilizers. The switch rate with venlafaxine was significantly higher than that with the other agents (Post et al. 2006),

TABLE 54–6. Evidence-based treatment of acute bipolar I depression

TREATMENT	NUMBER OF POSITIVE RCTs
Monotherapy	
Quetiapine	2
Lamotrigine	2
Olanzapine	1
Lithium	8
Divalproex	1
Carbamazepine	2
Combination therapy	
Olanzapine–fluoxetine	1

Note. RCTs = randomized, controlled trials.

a finding consistent with an earlier report by Vieta et al. (2002), who also found a higher switch rate in patients receiving venlafaxine compared with paroxetine. Thus, with newer antidepressant medications administered in conjunction with mood stabilizers, switch rates appear to be low (Peet and Peters 1995), although switch rates may be slightly higher with dual serotonin and norepinephrine reuptake inhibitors such as venlafaxine. These data are also consistent with the results of several naturalistic studies that found that concomitant administration of mood stabilizers with antidepressants cut the risk of switching by about half (Boerlin et al. 1998; Bottlender et al. 2001). The risk of switching appears to be greater in patients with bipolar I depression than in those with bipolar II depression (Altshuler et al. 2006).

Mood Stabilizers as Antidepressants

Most randomized, controlled trials of bipolar depression involved patients with bipolar I disorder. When bipolar II patients were included, their response usually was not reported separately, except in the quetiapine trials, in which quetiapine was superior to placebo in reduction of depression symptoms in both bipolar I and II patients (Calabrese et al. 2005a; Thase et al. 2006). It is not clear whether patients with bipolar II depression require treatment with a mood stabilizer (Thase and Sachs 2000), although most recommendations suggest that mood stabilizers also form the cornerstone of treatment for patients with bipolar II disorder. Treatment with a mood-stabilizing medication, if a patient is not already receiving one, is usually the first-line treatment for bipolar depression, because the inherent risk of switching is likely to be less with a mood stabilizer alone than with an antidepressant alone or with a combination of a mood stabilizer and antidepressant.

Lithium

Eight of nine placebo-controlled trials conducted in the 1960s and 1970s in patients with bipolar I and II disorders found lithium superior to placebo in acute bipolar depression (reviewed in Zornberg and Pope 1993). In an analysis of five studies in which it was possible to distinguish "unequivocal" lithium responders from patients who displayed partial but incomplete improvement in depression, Zornberg and Pope (1993) found that 36% had an unequivocal response, compared with 79% who had at least partial benefit. The antidepressant efficacy of lithium also was examined in two studies of paroxetine added to mood stabilizers for bipolar depression (Nemeroff et al. 2001; L.T. Young et al. 2000). Nemeroff et al. (2001) found that patients receiving lithium at plasma concentrations greater than 0.8 mEq/L showed no antidepressant benefit from the addition of paroxetine or imipramine compared with placebo. In contrast, patients receiving lithium at concentrations less than or equal to 0.8 mEq/L showed significant antidepressant benefit from the addition of paroxetine compared with placebo. These data confirm earlier impressions that maximizing lithium levels in patients already receiving lithium, or titrating to levels greater than 0.8 mEq/L when initiating lithium, is important to ensure an adequate trial of lithium for bipolar depression. L.T. Young et al. (2000) found that adding an alternative mood stabilizer (lithium or valproate) to the regimen of patients receiving therapeutic doses of a mood stabilizer but experiencing breakthrough depressive episodes was as effective as adding the antidepressant paroxetine. Although this study was too small ($N=27$) to detect drug–drug differences in efficacy, the mood stabilizer–mood stabilizer combination was not as well tolerated as the mood stabilizer–antidepressant combination, and the only patient who switched did so during this treatment arm.

Atypical Antipsychotics

Quetiapine

Quetiapine (300 mg and 600 mg/day) was superior to placebo in reduction of depressive symptoms in two large 8-week multicenter trials involving outpatients with bipolar I and II depression (Calabrese et al. 2005a; Thase et al. 2006). Patients receiving quetiapine also demonstrated greater improvement in secondary measures of sleep and anxiety compared with patients receiving placebo. There

was no significant difference in efficacy between the two quetiapine dosage groups. However, the rate of side effects was lower in the 300 mg/day groups compared with the 600 mg/day groups. Switch rates were low (3%–4%) across all treatment groups and were not significantly different among the quetiapine and placebo groups.

Olanzapine and Olanzapine–Fluoxetine Combination

Olanzapine and the combination of olanzapine and fluoxetine (OFC) were superior to placebo in reducing depressive symptoms in an 8-week trial of 833 patients with bipolar I depression (Tohen et al. 2003c). However, the OFC was superior not only to placebo throughout the trial but also to olanzapine for weeks 4–8. There were no significant differences in switch rates (6%–7%) among the three groups. Brown et al. (2006) compared OFC with lamotrigine (titrated to 200 mg/day) in a 7-week comparison trial in outpatients with bipolar I depression. Patients receiving OFC displayed greater reduction in depressive symptoms compared with patients receiving lamotrigine, although the lamotrigine group may have had a greater response with a longer trial, given the need for gradual lamotrigine titration. Switch rates were not significantly different between the two groups.

Antiepileptics

Lamotrigine

In an initial large 7-week randomized, placebo-controlled trial, lamotrigine (at 50 mg/day and 200 mg/day) was superior to placebo in patients with bipolar I depression (Calabrese et al. 1999). Switch rates (3%–8%) were not significantly different among the three groups. A second large placebo-controlled, parallel-group, flexible-dose trial involving patients with bipolar I and II depression did not find a significant advantage for lamotrigine over placebo (Bowden 2001). However, in a post hoc analysis, lamotrigine was superior to placebo in bipolar I patients. Frye et al. (2000) found lamotrigine superior to placebo in improving depression in a double-blind crossover trial in patients with treatment-refractory rapid-cycling bipolar I and II disorders. Lamotrigine was superior to placebo when added to lithium in an 8-week trial in patients with breakthrough depressive episodes (van der Loos and Nolen 2007). Common side effects of lamotrigine in these studies included headache, nausea, infection, and xerostomia. The risk of serious rash from lamotrigine can be reduced by carefully adhering to Physicians' Desk Reference–recommended titration schedules, but patients should be warned of the risk of rash and the need to report it immediately.

Carbamazepine

In two small controlled trials of patients with treatment-refractory bipolar depression, response to carbamazepine was superior to placebo (Post et al. 1986) and lithium (Small 1990). The results of these initial intriguing findings have not been followed up by large placebo-controlled, parallel-group trials.

Divalproex

Two small randomized, placebo-controlled trials of divalproex in the treatment of acute bipolar depression yielded opposite findings. Sachs and Collins (2001) did not find divalproex to be superior to placebo in one pilot trial, whereas Davis et al. (2005) found divalproex superior to placebo in reduction of depressive and anxiety symptoms in a later pilot study. As with carbamazepine, the results of these initial findings have not been followed up by large placebo-controlled, parallel-group trials.

Antidepressants

There is a relative dearth of randomized, controlled trials of antidepressants as monotherapy or in combination with mood stabilizers in bipolar depression (Ghaemi et al. 2001). Thase and Sachs (2000, p. 558) emphasized that "not a single antidepressant medication, nor even a particular class of antidepressant, has been demonstrated to be effective in at least two adequately powered, placebo-controlled clinical trials." Thus, with a thin evidence base, current recommendations regarding the use of antidepressants in conjunction with mood stabilizers for acute bipolar I depression tend toward the conservative (i.e., avoid antidepressants if possible). However, some general impressions can be gleaned from the available clinical trials. First, switch rates of newer antidepressants in short-term trials, in general, appear to be lower than those associated with tricyclic antidepressants (TCAs) in older studies (Thase and Sachs 2000). Second, among all of the antidepressants studied, the most substantial evidence for efficacy rests with the monoamine oxidase inhibitor (MAOI) tranylcypromine (Himmelhoch et al. 1991), but safety concerns often eliminate this agent from first-line therapy choices (Hirschfeld et al. 2002). Bupropion (Sachs et al. 1994) and selective serotonin reuptake inhibitors (SSRIs) (Nemeroff et al. 2001; L.T. Young et al. 2000) are common first-line agents administered in conjunction with mood stabilizers.

Electroconvulsive Therapy

ECT had significantly greater efficacy than MAOIs, TCAs, or placebo in several randomized, controlled trials in patients with bipolar depression (reviewed in Zornberg and Pope 1993). ECT may be particularly indicated for patients with severe, psychotic, or catatonic symptoms.

Psychotherapy

There are very few randomized, controlled trials of any form of psychotherapy for patients with acute bipolar depression. Cognitive-behavioral and interpersonal therapy have demonstrated efficacy in the treatment of unipolar major depression, but these modalities have been examined only in very small preliminary studies in patients with bipolar depression, thus far without conclusive findings (Cole et al. 2002; Zaretsky et al. 1999).

Novel Treatments

As in the treatment of acute bipolar manic and mixed episodes, there is considerable interest in the potential efficacy of new atypical antipsychotics and antiepileptic agents in the treatment of acute bipolar depression. With the exceptions of olanzapine, quetiapine, aripiprazole, lamotrigine, and gabapentin, these agents have not yet been well studied in randomized, controlled trials in the depressed phase of the illness. In two placebo-controlled trials, aripiprazole-treated patients did not display significantly greater improvement in depressive symptoms compared with patients receiving placebo at the 8-week study endpoint (Thase et al. 2008). Shelton and Stahl (2004) conducted a small pilot study comparing adjunctive treatment with risperidone, paroxetine, or the combination added to a mood stabilizer in outpatients with bipolar I or bipolar II depression. There were no significant differences in efficacy among the three treatment groups, but the study was limited by its small sample size ($N=30$). McIntyre et al. (2002) found comparable efficacy for topiramate (mean dosage = 176 mg/day) and bupropion sustained-release (mean dosage = 250 mg/day) in an 8-week single-blind comparison trial in 36 patients with bipolar depression receiving mood stabilizers. No switches occurred in either treatment group.

Among other novel treatment approaches, two preliminary placebo-controlled adjunctive trials examined the efficacy and safety of the dopamine D_2/D_3 receptor agonist pramipexole in the treatment of patients with bipolar I and bipolar II depression (Goldberg et al. 2004; Zarate et al. 2004). In both trials, patients receiving pramipexole added to mood stabilizers had significantly greater reductions in depressive symptoms and significantly greater response rates compared with those receiving placebo. Switch rates did not differ significantly from those with placebo.

Stoll et al. (1999) reported significant global improvement in depressive symptoms in patients receiving omega-3 fatty acids compared with placebo. These findings were not replicated in a second placebo-controlled trial (Keck et al. 2006b).

Monotherapy Versus Combination Therapy of Acute Bipolar Depressive Episodes

The "mood stabilizer first" approach has guided most recommendations regarding the acute treatment of patients with bipolar I depression (Thase and Sachs 2000). This approach is supported by at least three lines of evidence: 1) randomized, controlled trials have demonstrated the inherent antidepressant activity of at least some mood stabilizers (lithium, lamotrigine, olanzapine, quetiapine); 2) mood stabilizer monotherapy appears to carry a lower switch risk as compared with mood stabilizer–antidepressant combination therapy; 3) protection against switching can be implemented if the mood stabilizer alone is not adequate and an antidepressant is needed. Lithium, lamotrigine, quetiapine, and olanzapine are mood stabilizers with demonstrated efficacy as monotherapy in acute bipolar depression.

Combination therapy with an antidepressant and a mood stabilizer is an important option in two clinical groups: patients who do not respond adequately to mood stabilizer monotherapy and patients who have moderate to severe bipolar depression (Hirschfeld et al. 2002). Among antidepressant options, paroxetine, fluoxetine, venlafaxine, bupropion, and tranylcypromine are the most well studied in randomized, controlled trials and appear to have a lower switch risk in comparison with TCAs. Although no randomized, controlled trials of pharmacotherapy of psychotic bipolar depression have been conducted, mood stabilizer–antidepressant–antipsychotic and atypical antipsychotic–antidepressant combinations are common clinical approaches (Keck et al. 2004).

Maintenance Treatment

Bipolar disorder is a recurrent lifelong illness in more than 90% of the patients who experience a manic episode (Goodwin and Jamison 2007). Because of the high risk of recurrence and morbidity associated with mood episodes

and interepisode symptoms, maintenance treatment is usually recommended after a single manic episode (Hirschfeld et al. 2002). The goals of maintenance treatment include prevention of syndromal relapse and subsyndromal symptoms, optimization of functioning, and prevention of suicide. As with bipolar depression, there are a limited number of randomized, controlled trials of maintenance treatment of bipolar disorder on which to base treatment recommendations (Table 54–7).

Lithium

Lithium is the most extensively studied medication in the maintenance treatment of bipolar disorder. Data from randomized, placebo-controlled trials conducted in the 1960s and 1970s indicated that lithium protected against relapse, with a fourfold lower risk compared with placebo at 6-month and 1-year follow-up intervals (Keck et al. 2000). Lithium was superior to placebo in preventing relapse into mania in two randomized, controlled parallel-group trials lasting 18 months (Bowden et al. 2003; Calabrese et al. 2003).

Lithium may also reduce the risk of suicide in bipolar disorder beyond that predicted by the successful prevention of mood episode recurrences (Baldessarini et al. 2003). Moreover, this risk reduction appears to exceed that of treatment by divalproex (Goodwin et al. 2003).

A number of predictors of poor response to lithium maintenance treatment have been identified. These include rapid cycling, multiple prior mood episodes, negative family history of mood disorder, co-occurring alcohol or substance use disorder, and episode sequence of depression–mania–euthymia (Bowden 1995).

The optimal maintenance lithium serum concentration is an important consideration in successful maintenance treatment. Maintenance lithium serum concentrations usually are lower than those required to produce acute antimanic efficacy (Bowden 1998). Studies by Gelenberg et al. (1989) and Keller et al. (1992) found a

TABLE 54–7. Evidence-based maintenance treatment of bipolar disorder

TREATMENT	NUMBER OF POSITIVE RCTs
Lithium	8
Lamotrigine	2
Olanzapine	3
Aripiprazole	1

Note. RCTs = randomized, controlled trials.

serum level–response relationship, with levels of 0.4–0.6 mEq/L being associated with 2.6 times the relapse rate and a significantly greater likelihood of experiencing sub-syndromal symptoms, compared with levels of 0.8 mEq/L or higher. There was also a serum level–side effect re-lationship, with patients at higher levels experiencing significantly higher rates of side effects, often leading to discontinuation. Perlis et al. (2002), in yet another re-analysis of the Gelenberg et al. (1989) data, reported that an abrupt drop in serum lithium levels, whether due to random reassignment or to nonadherence, was the most powerful predictor of relapse. In a comprehensive review of this issue, Baldessarini et al. (2002) concluded that lev-els of 0.6–0.7 mEq/L appear to provide the best efficacy–tolerability range for most patients. The optimal lithium level for many patients will be the level that balances re-lapse prevention and suppression of subsyndromal symp-toms against minimization of bothersome day-to-day side effects.

Antiepileptics

Lamotrigine

Two large 18-month placebo-controlled maintenance trials comparing lamotrigine (200–400 mg/day) with lith-ium (0.8–1.1 mEq/L) found lamotrigine, but not lithium, superior to placebo in preventing depressive episodes (Bowden et al. 2003; Calabrese et al. 2003). In contrast, lithium, but not lamotrigine, was superior to placebo in preventing manic episodes. Taken together, the results of these two studies suggest that the combination of lithium and lamotrigine might be especially useful in preventing both manic and depressive episodes, although this re-mains to be established in a randomized, controlled trial. Of the nearly 1,200 patients who received lamotrigine in these trials, 9% had benign rash (morbilliform or exan-thematous eruptions), compared with 8% of the 1,056 pa-tients receiving placebo. When patients who received lamotrigine during the open-label run-in phase of the studies were included in the analysis, the total incidence of rash was 13%, with two cases of serious rash requiring hospitalization (Calabrese 2002).

Calabrese et al. (2000) conducted a 6-month placebo-controlled relapse prevention study of lamotrigine (mean dose, 288 mg/day) in 182 patients with rapid-cycling bipo-lar I and II disorders. There was no significant difference between the lamotrigine and placebo treatment groups in time to need for additional medications for recurrent mood symptoms. However, there was a trend in favor of la-motrigine over placebo specifically in bipolar II patients.

Divalproex

In the only randomized, placebo-controlled maintenance trial of divalproex in bipolar I disorder, there was no sig-nificant difference in the time to development of any mood episode among patients receiving divalproex, lith-ium, or placebo (Bowden et al. 2000). A number of un-foreseen methodological limitations in this trial compli-cated the interpretation of its results. In patients who received divalproex for treatment of the index manic epi-sode in an open treatment period prior to randomization, divalproex was superior to placebo in early termination due to any mood episode (29% vs. 50%) during the subse-quent year. This is a clinically relevant observation, since it supports the efficacy of maintaining patients who re-spond to divalproex for a manic episode. Divalproex was also compared with olanzapine in a 47-week blinded maintenance trial (Tohen et al. 2003b) described earlier. Calabrese et al. (2005b) compared divalproex with lith-ium in a 20-month study of patients with rapid-cycling bi-polar disorder and found comparable relapse rates in both treatment groups.

There are no data regarding the optimal maintenance valproic acid concentration for bipolar disorder. Current practice usually consists of titrating to therapeutic serum concentrations (50–125 µg/mL) and, as with lithium, bal-ancing relapse and subsyndromal symptom prevention against minimization of side effects (Hirschfeld et al. 2002). Treatment with valproate appears to pose an in-creased risk of polycystic ovarian syndrome (PCOS), al-though the relationship between PCOS and weight gain as a possible mechanism is unclear (Hirschfeld et al. 2002).

Carbamazepine

Although a number of studies have examined the efficacy of carbamazepine in the maintenance treatment of bipo-lar disorder, most of these studies yielded results that were difficult to interpret on methodological grounds (Dar-dennes et al. 1995). Two studies compared carbamazepine with lithium. In the first study, there were no significant differences in relapse rates after 1 year between lithium (31%) and carbamazepine (37%) (Denicoff et al. 1997). In the second trial, lithium was superior to carbamazepine on a number of outcome measures at 2.5 years of treat-ment (Greil et al. 1997). There are no data regarding se-rum level–response relationships for carbamazepine maintenance therapy. Denicoff et al. (1997) found that patients receiving the combination of carbamazepine and lithium in the third year of their trial had a better response than patients receiving either agent alone. Greil et al. (1997) found that patients with atypical symptoms (e.g., psychosis) responded better to carbamazepine than to lithium (Greil et al. 1998).

Therapeutic Monitoring of Lithium, Valproate, and Carbamazepine

Once lithium treatment is established at therapeutic plasma concentrations, recommendations for monitoring patients receiving lithium maintenance treatment include creatinine level and thyroid function test, along with a lithium level at least every 6 months initially (Hirschfeld et al. 2002). Thyroid function testing should be especially considered in patients with rapid cycling. Similarly, in patients receiving valproate maintenance treatment, recommendations for ongoing monitoring include obtaining a valproic acid level, hepatic function tests, and complete blood count (CBC) with platelet count approximately every 6 months (Hirschfeld et al. 2002). For carbamazepine, CBC and hepatic function tests are recommended approximately every 3 months (Hirschfeld et al. 2002).

Atypical Antipsychotics

Olanzapine

Olanzapine was comparable to divalproex in a 47-week comparison trial (Tohen et al. 2003b) and to lithium in a 1-year comparison trial (Tohen et al. 2005). Olanzapine received an indication for maintenance treatment in bipolar disorder based on superiority over placebo in prevention of manic and depressive episodes over 48 weeks (Tohen et al. 2006). The combination of olanzapine and lithium or divalproex was superior to placebo and lithium or divalproex in relapse prevention over 18 months in patients who had initially responded to the active combination acutely (Tohen et al. 2002b) and then were rerandomized (Tohen et al. 2004). This is a very clinically relevant finding, since it suggests that patients who respond acutely to olanzapine in combination with lithium or divalproex in the treatment of a manic episode have a lower risk of relapse by staying on such a combination. However, patients in the combination therapy group had twice the weight gain of patients in the monotherapy group.

Aripiprazole

Aripiprazole was superior to placebo in preventing manic relapse over a 6-month follow-up period in patients with bipolar disorder who were initially stabilized on aripiprazole monotherapy for an acute manic or mixed episode (Keck et al. 2006a). There was no significant difference between treatment with aripiprazole and placebo in relapse into depressive episodes; however, the overall low relapse rate into depression of this trial may have been due to the inclusion of patients whose index episodes were manic or mixed, and not depressed.

Electroconvulsive Therapy

The use of ECT in the maintenance treatment of bipolar disorder has never been studied systematically in a randomized, controlled trial. However, a number of naturalistic studies suggest that maintenance ECT may be a useful treatment alternative for patients who are inadequately responsive to pharmacotherapy (Schwartz et al. 1995; Vanelle et al. 1994).

Psychotherapy

Most patients with bipolar disorder experience a common cluster of psychological problems stemming directly from the illness (Table 54–8). A number of specific psychosocial interventions as adjuncts to mood stabilizer therapy have been shown to improve the long-term outcome of bipolar disorder (reviewed in Rizvi and Zaretsky 2007). The best-studied interventions include educational, interpersonal, family, and cognitive-behavioral therapies. Randomized, controlled trials conducted over 1- to 2-year follow-up periods support the efficacy of cognitive-behavioral therapy (Lam et al. 2005), family-focused and related forms of therapy (Clarkin et al. 1990, 1998; Miklowitz et al. 2003; Rea et al. 2003), interpersonal and social rhythm therapy (Frank et al. 2005), and group psychoeducation (Colom et al. 2003) in reducing or delaying mood episode recurrence, increasing treatment adherence, and improving functioning. Family-focused, interpersonal, and social rhythm therapy were all associated with delaying time to depressive episode relapse compared with brief treatment (Miklowitz et al. 2007). Only one study, of cognitive-behavioral therapy, found no significant benefit overall after 1 year, although post hoc analysis suggested that patients with fewer than 12 lifetime episodes benefited (Scott et al. 2006).

Novel Treatments

Quetiapine, ziprasidone, risperidone, and paliperidone, as well as new antiepileptics, may be potential long-term mood-stabilizing agents but have yet to be studied in ran-

TABLE 54–8.   Common psychological issues associated with bipolar disorder

Emotional consequences of manic, mixed, and depressive episodes

Acceptance of and coping with an often chronic mental illness

Effects of stigmatization

Developmental delays or deviations

Fears of recurrence and resulting inhibitions

Interpersonal challenges: marriage, family, pregnancy, child-rearing

Academic and occupational problems

Legal, social, and emotional problems arising from reckless, impulsive, withdrawn, or violent behavior

Source.   Adapted from Hirschfeld RMA, Bowden CL, Gitlin MJ, et al.: "Practice Guideline for the Treatment of Patients With Bipolar Disorder (Revision)." *American Journal of Psychiatry* 159 (Supplement):1–50, 2002. Copyright 2002, American Psychiatric Association. Used with permission.

domized, controlled trials. Clozapine was more effective than "treatment as usual" (combinations of mood stabilizers and typical antipsychotics) in a 1-year study in patients with treatment-refractory bipolar and schizoaffective disorder (bipolar subtype) (Suppes et al. 1999) and represents an important treatment option for patients unresponsive to conventional agents.

Treatment Considerations

Monotherapy Versus Combination Therapy

Mood Stabilizers

The optimal pharmacological maintenance treatment of bipolar disorder requires titration of any single mood-stabilizing medication to eradicate subsyndromal symptoms and prevent relapse. However, outcome assessments from randomized, controlled trials and naturalistic studies indicate that only a minority of patients with bipolar disorder experience optimal benefit (no relapse or recurrences, minimal to no subsyndromal symptoms) from monotherapy with any single mood stabilizer. Combination therapy is therefore frequently necessary and is commonplace in clinical practice. Unfortunately, very few studies have addressed specific mood stabilizer combinations, their relative therapeutic advantages, and their tolerability. As described earlier (see "Maintenance Treatment" section earlier in chapter), the combination of olanzapine with lithium or divalproex was significantly

more likely to prevent relapse compared with lithium or divalproex (with placebo) in patients initially responsive to the combination (Tohen et al. 2004). In the only other study reported, Solomon et al. (1997) compared the efficacy of lithium alone versus the combination of lithium and divalproex for 1 year in 12 patients. The combination significantly reduced the risk of recurrence of mania or depression but was associated with more side effects. Thus, the clinical practice of combining mood stabilizers has greatly outstripped the limited data available from formal studies. Combinations of lithium and divalproex, lithium and carbamazepine, and divalproex and carbamazepine; triple therapy with all three agents; and lithium and/or divalproex with atypical antipsychotics, antidepressants, and lamotrigine have all been reported in case series to be useful maintenance treatment strategies (M.P. Freeman and Stoll 1998).

Mood Stabilizers With Antidepressants

Most recommendations regarding the duration of antidepressant treatment (in conjunction with a mood stabilizer) in patients with bipolar depression suggest prompt discontinuation of antidepressants after remission of depression (Ghaemi et al. 2001). Limiting antidepressant exposure is intended to reduce the risk of switching or cycling. However, discontinuation of antidepressants during maintenance therapy may also increase the risk of depressive relapse. Two studies involving different cohorts of bipolar patients treated naturalistically found that termination of antidepressants was associated with a two- to threefold increased risk of depressive relapse after 1 year (Altshuler et al. 2001, 2003). In contrast, antidepressant continuation was not significantly associated with an increased risk of mania. The results of these two studies suggest that the use of antidepressants in combination with mood stabilizers to prevent recurrence of bipolar depression may be indicated and necessary for many patients, particularly patients without a history of or risk factors for rapid cycling (e.g., substance use disorder, thyroid disease). The optimal duration of antidepressant maintenance treatment and possible predictors of switch versus depressive relapse require further study.

Rapid Cycling

Rapid cycling, the occurrence of four or more mood episodes within 12 months (Dunner and Fieve 1974), poses a special challenge. Among mood stabilizers, divalproex and atypical antipsychotics appear to have greater efficacy than lithium in patients with rapid cycling. Lamotrigine is also a treatment option based on the study by Frye et al. (2000), although its long-term benefit in rapid cycling may be limited to bipolar II rather than bipolar I disorder (Calabrese et al. 2000). Because very few randomized, controlled trials are available to inform treatment decisions, most recommendations are empirical. Combinations of mood stabilizers (e.g., lithium and divalproex, divalproex and atypical antipsychotics, lithium and lamotrigine) are often recommended (Hirschfeld et al. 2002).

Co-Occurring Psychiatric Disorders

Among the major psychiatric disorders, bipolar disorder has the highest comorbidity rate (McElroy et al. 2001). Co-occurring psychiatric disorders can affect treatment recommendations, but to date very few studies have specifically addressed the acute and long-term treatment of patients with bipolar disorder and psychiatric comorbidity. In a 6-month placebo-controlled trial in female patients with bipolar II disorder and borderline personality disorder, divalproex was superior to placebo in reducing measures of interpersonal sensitivity, anger, hostility, and aggression (Frankenberg and Zanarini 2002). Lithium was superior to placebo in patients with bipolar spectrum disorder and co-occurring pathological gambling in a 10-week trial (Hollander et al. 2005). Improvement in gambling severity was correlated with improvement in manic symptoms. Salloum et al. (2005) conducted a 24-week placebo-controlled trial of adjunctive divalproex in patients with bipolar I disorder and co-occurring alcohol dependence who were also receiving lithium and psychosocial treatment. Patients receiving divalproex had significantly fewer days of heavy drinking and showed a trend toward fewer drinks per heavy drinking day in comparison with patients receiving placebo. Lastly, Weiss et al. (2007) compared a specifically developed form of integrated group therapy for patients with bipolar disorder and concurrent substance dependence with group counseling in patients on mood stabilizers over 20 weeks and found significantly fewer days of substance use in the integrated therapy group during treatment and at 3-month posttreatment follow-up.

Mood Stabilizers and Bipolar-Specific Psychotherapy

From the evidence reviewed above regarding the efficacy of several different forms of psychotherapy specifically developed and operationalized for patients with bipolar disorder, it is clear that the combination of one of these forms of psychotherapy with maintenance pharmacotherapy is superior to pharmacotherapy alone in reducing the risk of relapse and recurrence.

Conclusion

There have been substantial advances in the pharmacological treatment of bipolar disorder in the past decade. A number of medications have demonstrated efficacy in the treatment of acute mania in placebo-controlled trials, either as monotherapy or as an adjunct to mood stabilizers. In addition, data are available for the first time indicating that combination therapy with an antipsychotic and a mood stabilizer is more rapidly effective, with better overall response rates in acute mania, than either mood stabilizers or antipsychotics alone.

The treatment of bipolar depression remains one of the most understudied aspects of the illness. The "mood stabilizer first" strategy and combined use of mood stabilizers and antidepressants in moderate to severe bipolar depression are common approaches.

Most patients with bipolar disorder require treatment with more than one medication during the course of their illness. The efficacy of combination strategies is only now receiving close scrutiny. Recent studies suggest that the use of combinations of antidepressants and mood stabilizers as maintenance treatment for some patients to prevent depressive relapse may be important.

The role and efficacy of different types of psychotherapy at different phases of illness management in bipolar disorder are now becoming clearly established. These components of treatment are important in educating patients and families, improving insight and treatment adherence, enhancing coping skills, and dealing with the sequelae of mood symptoms and episodes—and, it is hoped, improving functioning and outcome. Treatment advances in bipolar disorder are finally occurring rapidly. Artfully bringing these treatments to patients with bipolar disorder is both the challenge and the reward of helping people manage this illness.

References

Allen MH, Hirschfeld RMA, Wozniak PJ, et al: Linear relationship of valproate serum concentration to response and optimal serum levels for acute mania. Am J Psychiatry 163:272–275, 2006

Altshuler LL, Kiriakos L, Calcagno J, et al: The impact of antidepressant discontinuation versus antidepressant continuation on 1-year risk for relapse of bipolar depression: a retrospective chart review. J Clin Psychiatry 62:612–616, 2001

Altshuler LL, Suppes T, Black DO, et al: Impact of antidepressant discontinuation after acute bipolar depression remission on rates of depressive relapse at 1-year follow-up. Am J Psychiatry 160:1252–1262, 2003

Altshuler LL, Suppes T, Black DO, et al: Lower switch rate in depressed patients with bipolar II than bipolar I disorder treated adjunctively with second-generation antidepressants. Am J Psychiatry 163:313–315, 2006

American Psychiatric Association: Practice guideline for psychiatric evaluation of adults. Am J Psychiatry 152 (11 suppl): 53–80, 1995

American Psychiatric Association: Diagnostic and Statistical Manual of Mental Disorders, 4th Edition, Text Revision. Washington, DC, American Psychiatric Association, 2000

Anand A, Oren DA, Berman RM: Lamotrigine treatment of lithium failure in outpatient mania: a double-blind, placebo-controlled trial. Third International Conference on Bipolar Disorder. Pittsburgh, PA, June 1999

Baker RW, Kinon BJ, Maguire GA, et al: Effectiveness of rapid initial dose escalation of up to forty milligrams per day of oral olanzapine in acute agitation. J Clin Psychopharmacol 23:342–348, 2003

Baldessarini RJ, Tondo L, Hennen J, et al: Is lithium still worth using? An update of selected recent research. Harvard Rev Psychiatry 10:59–75, 2002

Baldessarini RJ, Tondo L, Hennen J: Lithium treatment and suicide risk in major affective disorders: update and new findings. J Clin Psychiatry 64 (suppl 50):44–52, 2003

Ballenger JC, Post RM: Therapeutic effects of carbamazepine in affective illness: a preliminary report. Commun Psychopharmacol 2:159–175, 1978

Berk M, Ichim L, Brook S: Olanzapine compared to lithium in mania: a double-blind randomized controlled trial. Int Clin Psychopharmacol 14:339–343, 1999

Birmaher B, Kennah A, Brent D, et al: Is bipolar disorder specifically associated with panic disorder in youths? J Clin Psychiatry 63:414–419, 2002

Black DW, Winokur G, Nasrallah A: Treatment of mania: a naturalistic study of electroconvulsive therapy versus lithium in 438 patients. J Clin Psychiatry 48:132–139, 1984

Boerlin HL, Gitlin MJ, Zoellner LA, et al: Bipolar depression and antidepressant-induced mania: a naturalistic study. J Clin Psychiatry 59:374–379, 1998

Bottlender R, Rudolf D, Strauss A, et al: Mood stabilizers reduce the risk for developing antidepressant-induced maniform states in acute treatment of bipolar I depressed patients. J Affect Disord 63:79–83, 2001

Bowden CL: Predictors of response to divalproex and lithium. J Clin Psychiatry 56 (suppl):25–30, 1995

Bowden CL: Treatment of bipolar disorder, in Textbook of Psychopharmacology, 2nd Edition. Edited by Schatzberg AF, Nemeroff CB. Washington, DC, American Psychiatric Press, 1998, pp 733–745

Bowden CL: Novel treatments for bipolar disorder. Exp Opin Investig Drugs 10:661–671, 2001

Bowden CL, Brugger AM, Swann AC, et al: Efficacy of divalproex vs lithium and placebo in the treatment of mania. JAMA 271:918–924, 1994

Bowden CL, Calabrese JR, McElroy SL, et al: Efficacy of divalproex versus lithium and placebo in maintenance treatment of bipolar disorder. Arch Gen Psychiatry 57:481–489, 2000

Bowden CL, Calabrese JR, Sachs GS, et al: A placebo-controlled 18-month trial of lamotrigine and lithium maintenance treatment in recently manic or hypomanic patients with bipolar I disorder. Arch Gen Psychiatry 60:392–400, 2003

Bowden CL, Grunze H, Mullen J, et al: A randomized, double-blind, placebo-controlled efficacy and safety study of quetiapine or lithium as monotherapy for mania in bipolar disorder. J Clin Psychiatry 66:111–121, 2005

Bowden CL, Swann AD, Calabrese JR, et al: A randomized, placebo-controlled, multicenter study of divalproex sodium extended release in the treatment of acute mania. J Clin Psychiatry 67:1501–1510, 2006

Brennan MJW, Sandyk R, Borsook D: Use of sodium valproate in the management of affective disorders: basic and clinical aspects, in Anticonvulsants in Affective Disorders. Edited by Emrich HM, Okuma T, Muller AA. Amsterdam, Excerpta Medica, 1984, pp 56–65

Brown E, McElroy SL, Keck PE Jr, et al: A 7-week, randomized, double-blind trial of olanzapine/fluoxetine combination versus lamotrigine in the treatment of bipolar I depression. J Clin Psychiatry 67:1025–1033, 2006

Calabrese JR: Clinical Relevance and Management of Bipolar Disorders: Weighing Benefits Versus Risks (Presentations in Focus). New York, Medical Education Network, 2002

Calabrese JR, Kimmel SE, Woyshville MJ, et al: Clozapine for treatment-refractory mania. Am J Psychiatry 153:759–764, 1996

Calabrese JR, Bowden CL, Sachs GS, et al: A double-blind placebo-controlled study of lamotrigine monotherapy in outpatients with bipolar I depression. J Clin Psychiatry 60:79–88, 1999

Calabrese JR, Suppes T, Bowden CL, et al: A double-blind, placebo-controlled, prophylaxis study of lamotrigine in rapid-cycling bipolar disorder. J Clin Psychiatry 61:841–850, 2000

Calabrese JR, Bowden CL, Sachs GS, et al: A placebo-controlled 18-month trial of lamotrigine and lithium maintenance treatment in recently depressed patients with bipolar I disorder. J Clin Psychiatry 64:1013–1024, 2003

Calabrese JR, Keck PE Jr, Macfadden W, et al: A randomized, double-blind, placebo-controlled trial of quetiapine in the treatment of bipolar I or II depression. Am J Psychiatry 162:1351–1360, 2005a

Calabrese JR, Shelton MD, Rapport DJ, et al: A 20-month, double-blind, maintenance trial of lithium versus divalproex in rapid-cycling bipolar disorder. Am J Psychiatry 162:2152–2161, 2005b

Chou JC, Czobor P, Charles O, et al: Acute mania: haloperidol dose and augmentation with lithium or lorazepam. J Clin Psychopharmacol 19:500–505, 1999

Clarkin JF, Glick ID, Haas GL, et al: A randomized clinical trial of inpatient family intervention, V: results for affective disorders. J Affect Disord 18:17–28, 1990

Clarkin JF, Carpenter D, Hull J, et al: Effects of psychoeducational intervention for married patients with bipolar disorder and their spouses. Psychiatr Serv 49:531–533, 1998

Cole DP, Thase ME, Mallinger AG, et al: Slower treatment response in bipolar depression predicted by lower pretreatment thyroid function. Am J Psychiatry 159:116–121, 2002

Colom F, Vieta E, Martinez-Aran A, et al: A randomized trial on the efficacy of group psychoeducation in the prophylaxis of recurrences in bipolar patients whose disease is in remission. Arch Gen Psychiatry 60:402–407, 2003

Daniel DG, Potkin SG, Reeves KR, et al: Intramuscular (IM) ziprasidone 20 mg is effective in reducing acute agitation associated with psychosis: a double-blind, randomized trial. Psychopharmacology (Berl) 155:128–134, 2001

Dardennes R, Even C, Bange F: Comparison of carbamazepine and lithium in the prophylaxis of bipolar disorders. A meta-analysis. Br J Psychiatry 166:375–381, 1995

Davis LL, Bartolucci A, Petty F: Divalproex in the treatment of bipolar depression: a placebo-controlled study. J Affect Disord 85:259–266, 2005

DelBello MP, Schwiers ML, Rosenberg HL, et al: A double-blind, randomized, placebo-controlled study of quetiapine as adjunctive treatment for adolescent mania. J Am Acad Child Adolesc Psychiatry 41:1216–1223, 2002

DelBello MP, Kowatch RA, Adler CM, et al: A double-blind randomized pilot study comparing quetiapine and divalproex for adolescent mania. J Am Acad Child Adolesc Psychiatry 45:305–313, 2006

Denicoff KD, Smith-Jackson EE, Disney ER, et al: Comparative prophylactic efficacy of lithium, carbamazepine, and the combination in bipolar disorder. J Clin Psychiatry 58:470–478, 1997

Denicoff KD, Ali SO, Sollinger AB, et al: Utility of the daily prospective National Institute of Mental Health Life-Chart Method (NIMH-LCM-p) ratings in clinical trials of bipolar disorder. Depress Anxiety 15:1–9, 2002

Dunner DL, Fieve RR: Clinical factors in lithium carbonate prophylaxis failure. Arch Gen Psychiatry 30:229–233, 1974

Emrich HM: Studies of oxcarbazepine (Trileptal) in acute mania. Int J Clin Psychopharmacol 5:83–88, 1991

Emrich HM, von Zerssen D, Kissling W: On a possible role of GABA in mania: therapeutic efficacy of sodium valproate, in GABA and Benzodiazepine Receptors. Edited by Costa E, Dicharia G, Gessa GL. New York, Raven Press, 1981, pp 287–296

Frank E, Kupfer DJ, Thase ME, et al: Two-year outcomes for interpersonal and social rhythm therapy in individuals with bipolar I disorder. Arch Gen Psychiatry 62:996–1004, 2005

Frankenberg FR, Zanarini MC: Divalproex sodium treatment of women with borderline personality disorder and bipolar II disorder: a double-blind placebo-controlled trial. J Clin Psychiatry 63:442–446, 2002

Freeman MP, Stoll AL: Mood stabilizer combinations: a review of safety and efficacy. Am J Psychiatry 155:12–21, 1998

Freeman TW, Clothier JL, Pazzaglia P, et al: A double-blind comparison of valproate and lithium in the treatment of acute mania. Am J Psychiatry 149:108–111, 1992

Frye MA, Ketter TA, Kimbrell TA, et al: A placebo-controlled study of lamotrigine and gabapentin monotherapy in refractory mood disorders. J Clin Psychopharmacol 20:607–614, 2000

Garfinkel PE, Stancer HC, Persad E: A comparison of haloperidol, lithium and their combination in the treatment of mania. J Affect Disord 2:279–288, 1980

Gelenberg AJ, Kane JM, Keller MB, et al: Comparison of standard and low serum levels of lithium for maintenance treatment of bipolar disorder. N Engl J Med 321:1489–1493, 1989

Ghaemi SN, Lenox MS, Baldessarini RJ: Effectiveness and safety of long-term antidepressant treatment of bipolar disorder. J Clin Psychiatry 62:565–569, 2001

Goldberg JF, Garno JL, Leon AC, et al: Rapid titration of mood stabilizers predicts remission from mixed or pure mania in bipolar patients. J Clin Psychiatry 59:151–158, 1998

Goldberg JF, Burdick KE, Endick CJ: Preliminary randomized, double-blind, placebo-controlled trial of pramipexole added to mood stabilizers for treatment-resistant bipolar depression. Am J Psychiatry 161:564–566, 2004

Goodwin FK, Jamison KR: Manic-Depressive Illness: Bipolar Disorders and Recurrent Depression. New York, Oxford University Press, 2007

Goodwin FK, Murphy DL, Bunney WE Jr: Lithium carbonate treatment of depression and mania: a longitudinal double-blind study. Arch Gen Psychiatry 21:486–496, 1969

Goodwin FK, Fireman B, Simon GE: Suicide risk in bipolar disorder during treatment with lithium and divalproex. JAMA 290:486–496, 2003

Green AI, Tohen M, Patel JK, et al: Clozapine in the treatment of refractory psychotic mania. Am J Psychiatry 157:982–986, 2000

Greil W, Ludwig-Mayerhofer W, Erazo N: Lithium versus carbamazepine in the maintenance treatment of bipolar disorders—a randomized study. J Affective Disord 43:151–161, 1997

Greil W, Kleindienst N, Erazo N, et al: Differential response to lithium and carbamazepine in the prophylaxis of bipolar disorder. J Clin Psychopharmacol 18:455–460, 1998

Grossi E, Sacchetti E, Vita A: Carbamazepine versus chlorpromazine in mania: a double-blind trial, in Anticonvulsants in Affective Disorders. Edited by Emrich HM, Okuma T, Muller AA. Amsterdam, Excerpta Medica, 1984, pp 177–187

Himmelhoch JM, Thase ME, Mallinger AG, et al: Tranylcypromine versus imipramine in anergic bipolar depression. Am J Psychiatry 148:910–916, 1991

Hirschfeld RMA: The Mood Disorder Questionnaire: a simple, patient-rated screening instrument for bipolar disorder. Prim Care Companion J Clin Psychiatry 4:9–11, 2002

Hirschfeld RMA, Allen MH, McEvoy JP, et al: Safety and tolerability of oral loading divalproex sodium in acutely manic bipolar patients. J Clin Psychiatry 60:815–818, 1999

Hirschfeld RMA, Williams JBW, Spitzer RL, et al: Development and validation of a screening instrument for bipolar spectrum disorder: the Mood Disorder Questionnaire. Am J Psychiatry 157:1873–1875, 2000

Hirschfeld RMA, Bowden CL, Gitlin MJ, et al: Practice guideline for the treatment of patients with bipolar disorder (revision). Am J Psychiatry 159 (suppl):1–50, 2002

Hirschfeld RMA, Keck PE Jr, Kramer M, et al: Rapid antimanic effect of risperidone monotherapy: a 3-week multicenter, double-blind, placebo-controlled trial. Am J Psychiatry 161:1057–171, 2004

Hirschfeld RMA, Panagides J, Alphs L, et al: Asenapine in acute mania: a randomized, double-blind, placebo- and olanzapine-controlled trial, in Abstracts of the 160th Annual Meeting of the American Psychiatric Association #333, San Diego, CA, May 21, 2007

Hollander E, Pallanti S, Allen A, et al: Does sustained-release lithium reduce impulsive gambling and affective instability versus placebo in pathological gamblers with bipolar spectrum disorder? Am J Psychiatry 162:137–145, 2005

Janicak PG, Sharma RP, Pandey G, et al: Verapamil for the treatment of acute mania: a double-blind, placebo-controlled trial. Am J Psychiatry 155:972–973, 1998

Johnson G, Gershon S, Burdock EI, et al: Comparative effects of lithium and chlorpromazine in the treatment of acute manic states. Br J Psychiatry 119:267–276, 1976

Judd LL, Akiskal HS, Schettler PJ, et al: The long-term natural history of the weekly symptomatic status of bipolar I disorder. Arch Gen Psychiatry 59:530–537, 2002

Judd LL, Akiskal HS, Schettler PJ, et al: A prospective investigation of the natural history of the long-term weekly symptomatic status of bipolar II disorder. Arch Gen Psychiatry 60:261–269, 2003

Judd LL, Akiskal HS, Schettler PJ, et al: Psychosocial disability in the course of bipolar I and II disorders: a prospective, comparative, longitudinal study. Arch Gen Psychiatry 62:1322–1330, 2005

Keck PE Jr, McElroy SL: Definition, evaluation, and management of treatment refractory mania. Psychopharmacol Bull 35:130–148, 2001

Keck PE Jr, McElroy SL, Tugrul KC, et al: Valproate oral loading in the treatment of acute mania. J Clin Psychiatry 54:305–308, 1993

Keck PE Jr, Welge JA, Strakowski SM, et al: Placebo effect in randomized, controlled maintenance studies of patients with bipolar disorder. Biol Psychiatry 47:756–765, 2000

Keck PE Jr, McElroy SL, Arnold LM: Bipolar disorder. Psychiatr Clin North Am 85:645–661, 2001

Keck PE Jr, Marcus R, Tourkodimitris S, et al: A placebo-controlled, double-blind study of the efficacy and safety of aripiprazole in patients with acute bipolar mania. Am J Psychiatry 160:1651–1658, 2003a

Keck PE Jr, Versiani M, Potkin S, et al: Ziprasidone in the treatment of acute bipolar mania: a three-week, placebo-controlled, double-blind, randomized trial. Am J Psychiatry 160:741–748, 2003b

Keck PE Jr, Perlis RH, Otto MW, et al: The Expert Consensus Guidelines Series. Treatment of Bipolar Disorder 2004. A Postgraduate Medicine Special Report. Minneapolis, MN, McGraw-Hill, 2004, pp 1–108

Keck PE Jr, Calabrese JR, McQuade RD, et al: A randomized, double-blind, placebo-controlled 26-week trial of aripiprazole in recently manic patients with bipolar I disorder. J Clin Psychiatry 67:626–637, 2006a

Keck PE Jr, Mintz J, McElroy SL, et al: Double-blind, randomized, placebo-controlled trials of eicosapentanoic acid in the treatment of bipolar depression and rapid cycling bipolar disorder. Biol Psychiatry 60:1020–1022, 2006b

Keck PE Jr, Calabrese JR, McIntyre RS, et al: Aripiprazole monotherapy for maintenance therapy in bipolar I disorder: a 100-week, double-blind study versus placebo. J Clin Psychiatry 68:1480–1491, 2007

Keck PE Jr, Sanchez R, Torbeyns A, Marcus RN, McQuade RD, Forbes A: Aripiprazole monotherapy in the treatment of acute bipolar I mania: a randomized, placebo- and lithium-controlled study. J Affect Disord 112:36–49, 2009

Keller MB, Lavori PW, Kane JM: Subsyndromal symptoms in bipolar disorder: a comparison of standard and low serum levels of lithium. Arch Gen Psychiatry 49:371–376, 1992

Khanna S, Vieta E, Lyons B, et al: Risperidone in the treatment of acute mania: double-blind, placebo-controlled study. Br J Psychiatry 187:229–234, 2005

Klein DF: Importance of psychiatric diagnosis in prediction of clinical drug effects. Arch Gen Psychiatry 16:118–126, 1967

Koukopoulos A, Reginaldi D, Laddomada P: Course of manic-depressive cycle and changes caused by treatments. Pharmakopsychiatrie Neuropsychopharmakologie 13:156–167, 1980

Kushner SF, Khan A, Lane R: Topiramate monotherapy in the management of acute mania: results of four double-blind placebo-controlled trials. Bipolar Disord 8:15–27, 2006

Lam DH, Hayward P, Watkins ER, et al: Relapse prevention in patients with bipolar disorder: cognitive therapy outcomes after 2 years. Am J Psychiatry 162:324–329, 2005

Lerer B, Moore N, Meyendorff E, et al: Carbamazepine versus lithium in mania: a double-blind study. J Clin Psychiatry 48:89–93, 1987

Lesem MD, Zajecka JM, Swift RH, et al: Intramuscular ziprasidone 2 mg versus 10 mg in the short-term management of agitated psychotic patients. J Clin Psychiatry 62:12–18, 2001

Li H, Ma C, Wang G, et al: Response and remission rates in Chinese patients with bipolar mania treated for 4 weeks with either quetiapine or lithium: a randomized and double-blind study. Curr Med Res Opin 24:1–10, 2008

Lopez P, Mosquera F, de Leon J, et al: Suicide attempts in bipolar patients. J Clin Psychiatry 62:963–966, 2001

Maggs R: Treatment of manic illness with lithium carbonate. Br J Psychiatry 109:56–65, 1963

Manning JS, Haykal RF, Connor PD: On the nature of depressive and anxious states in family practice residency setting: the high prevalence of bipolar II and related disorders in a cohort followed longitudinally. Compr Psychiatry 38:102–108, 1997

Manning JS, Connor PD, Sahai A: The bipolar spectrum: a review of current concepts and implications for the management of depression in primary care. Arch Fam Med 6:63–71, 1998

McElroy SL, Keck PE Jr: Pharmacological agents for the treatment of acute bipolar mania. Biol Psychiatry 48:539–557, 2000

McElroy SL, Keck PE Jr, Pope HG Jr: Clinical and research implications of the diagnosis of dysphoric or mixed mania or hypomania. Am J Psychiatry 149:1633–1644, 1992

McElroy SL, Keck PE Jr, Stanton SP, et al: A randomized comparison divalproex oral loading versus haloperidol in the initial treatment of acute psychotic mania. J Clin Psychiatry 57:142–146, 1996

McElroy SL, Altshuler LL, Suppes T, et al: Axis I psychiatric comorbidity and its relationship to historical illness variables in 288 patients with bipolar disorder. Am J Psychiatry 158:420–426, 2001

McIntyre RS, Mancini DA, McCann S, et al: Topiramate versus bupropion SR when added to mood stabilizer therapy for the depressive phase of bipolar disorder: a preliminary single-blind study. Bipolar Disord 4:207–213, 2002

McIntyre RS, Brecher M, Paulsson B, et al: Quetiapine or haloperidol as monotherapy for bipolar mania—a 12-week, double-blind, randomized, parallel-group, placebo-controlled trial. Eur Neuropsychopharmacol 15:573–585, 2005

Meehan K, Zhang F, David S, et al: A double-blind, randomized comparison of the efficacy and safety of intramuscular injections of olanzapine, lorazepam, or placebo in treating acutely agitated patients diagnosed with bipolar mania. J Clin Psychiatry 21:389–397, 2001

Miklowitz DJ, George GL, Richards JA, et al: A randomized, controlled study of family focused psychoeducation and pharmacotherapy in outpatient management of bipolar disorder. Arch Gen Psychiatry 60:904–912, 2003

Miklowitz DJ, Otto MW, Frank E, et al: Psychosocial treatments for bipolar depression. A 1-year randomized trial from the Systematic Treatment Enhancement Program. Arch Gen Psychiatry 64:419–427, 2007

Montgomery SA, Åsberg M: A new depression scale designed to be sensitive to change. Br J Psychiatry 134:382–389, 1979

Mukherjee S, Sackeim HA, Schnur DB: Electroconvulsive therapy of acute manic episodes: a review of 50 years' experience. Am J Psychiatry 151:169–176, 1994

Muller AA, Stoll KD: Carbamazepine and oxcarbazepine in the treatment of manic syndromes: studies in Germany, in Anticonvulsants in Affective Disorders. Edited by Emrich HM, Okuma T, Muller AA. Amsterdam, Excerpta Medica, 1984, pp 134–147

Muller-Oerlinghausen B, Retzow A, Henn FA, et al: Valproate as an adjunct to neuroleptic medication for the treatment of acute episodes of mania: a prospective, randomized, double-blind, placebo-controlled, multicenter study. J Clin Psychopharmacol 20:195–203, 2000

Murray CJL, Lopez AD: The Global Burden of Disease: Summary. Cambridge, MA: Harvard University Press, 1996

Nemeroff CB, Evans DL, Gyulai L, et al: Double-blind, placebo-controlled comparison of imipramine and paroxetine in the treatment of bipolar depression. Am J Psychiatry 62:906–912, 2001

Niufan F, Tohen M, Qiuqing A, et al: Olanzapine versus lithium in the acute treatment of bipolar mania: a double-blind, randomized, controlled trial. J Affect Disord 23:117–122, 2007

Okuma T, Inanaga K, Otsuki S, et al: Comparison of the antimanic efficacy of carbamazepine and chlorpromazine: a double-blind controlled study. Psychopharmacology (Berl) 66:211–217, 1979

Pande AC, Crockatt JG, Janney CA, et al: Gabapentin in bipolar disorder: a placebo-controlled trial of adjunctive therapy. Bipolar Disord 2:249–255, 2000

Peet M, Peters S: Drug-induced mania. Drug Saf 12:146–153, 1995

Perlis RH, Sachs GS, Lafer B: Effect of abrupt change from standard to low serum levels of lithium: a re-analysis of double-blind lithium maintenance data. Am J Psychiatry 159:1155–1159, 2002

Perlis RH, Baker RW, Zarate CA Jr, et al: Olanzapine versus risperidone in the treatment of manic or mixed states in bipolar I disorder: a randomized, double-blind trial. J Clin Psychiatry 67:1747–1753, 2006a

Perlis RH, Ostacher MJ, Patel JK, et al: Predictors of recurrence in bipolar disorder: primary outcomes from the Systematic Treatment Enhancement Program for Bipolar Disorder (STEP-BD). Am J Psychiatry 163:217–224, 2006b

Perlis RH, Welge JA, Vornik LA, et al: Atypical antipsychotics in the treatment of mania: a meta-analysis of randomized, placebo-controlled trials. J Clin Psychiatry 67:509–516, 2006c

Platman SR: A comparison of lithium carbonate and chlorpromazine in mania. Am J Psychiatry 127:351–353, 1970

Pope HG Jr, McElroy SL, Keck PE Jr, et al: Valproate in the treatment of acute mania: a placebo-controlled study. Arch Gen Psychiatry 48:62–68, 1991

Post RM, Uhde TW, Roy-Byrne PP: Antidepressant effects of carbamazepine. Am J Psychiatry 43:29–34, 1986

Post RM, Altshuler LL, Frye MA, et al: Rate of switch in bipolar patients prospectively treated with second-generation antidepressants as augmentation to mood stabilizers. Bipolar Disord 3:259–265, 2001

Post RM, Altshuler LL, Leverich GS, et al: Mood switch in bipolar depression: comparison of adjunctive venlafaxine, bupropion and sertraline. Br J Psychiatry 189:124–131, 2006

Potkin S, Keck PE Jr, Segal S, et al: Ziprasidone in acute bipolar mania: a 21-day randomized, double-blind, placebo-controlled replication trial. J Clin Psychopharmacol 25:301–310, 2005

Prien RF, Caffey EM Jr, Klett CJ: Comparison of lithium carbonate and chlorpromazine in the treatment of mania: report of the Veterans Administration and National Institute of Mental Health Collaborative Study Group. Arch Gen Psychiatry 26:146–153, 1972

Ramey TS, Giller EL, English EP: Ziprasidone efficacy and safety in acute bipolar mania: a 12-week study. Abstracts of the 6th International Conference on Bipolar Disorders, Pittsburgh, PA, June 16, 2003

Rea MM, Tompson M, Miklowitz DJ, et al: Family focused treatment vs. individual treatment for bipolar disorder: results from a randomized controlled trial. J Consult Clin Psychol 71:482–492, 2003

Rizvi S, Zaretsky AE: Psychotherapy through the phases of bipolar disorder: evidence for general efficacy and differential effects. J Clin Psychol 63:491–506, 2007

Rush AJ: Strategies and tactics in the management of maintenance treatment for depressed patients. J Clin Psychiatry 60 (suppl 14): 21–26, 1999

Sachs GS, Collins MC: A placebo-controlled trial of divalproex sodium in acute bipolar depression. Presented at the American College of Neuropsychopharmacology Annual Meeting, San Juan, PR, December 2001

Sachs GS, Lafer B, Stoll AL, et al: A double-blind trial of bupropion versus desipramine for bipolar depression. J Clin Psychiatry 55:391–393, 1994

Sachs GS, Koslow CL, Ghaemi SN: The treatment of bipolar depression. Bipolar Disord 2:256–260, 2000

Sachs GS, Grossman F, Ghaemi SN, et al: Combination mood stabilizer with risperidone or haloperidol for treatment of acute mania: a double-blind, placebo-controlled comparison of efficacy and safety. Am J Psychiatry 159:1146–1154, 2002

Sachs GS, Chengappa KN, Suppes T: Quetiapine with lithium or divalproex for the treatment of bipolar mania: a randomized, double-blind, placebo-controlled study. Bipolar Disord 6:213–223, 2004

Sachs GS, Sanchez R, Marcus R, et al: Aripiprazole in the treatment of acute manic or mixed episodes in patients with bipolar I disorder: a 3-week placebo controlled study. J Clin Psychopharmacol 20:536–546, 2006

Sachs GS, Nierenberg AA, Calabrese JR, et al: Effectiveness of adjunctive antidepressant treatment for bipolar depression. N Engl J Med 356:1711–1722, 2007

Salloum IM, Cornelius JR, Daley DC, et al: Efficacy of valproate maintenance in patients with bipolar disorder and alcoholism: a double-blind placebo-controlled study. Arch Gen Psychiatry 62:37–45, 2005

Scherk H, Pajonk FG, Leucht S: Second-generation antipsychotic agents in the treatment of acute mania: a systematic review and meta-analysis of randomized controlled trials. Arch Gen Psychiatry 64:442–455, 2007

Schwartz T, Loewenstein J, Isenberg KE: Maintenance ECT: indications and outcome. Convulsive Ther 11:14–23, 1995

Schou M, Juel-Nielson, Stomgren E, et al: The treatment of manic psychoses by administration of lithium salts. J Neurol Neurosurg Psychiatry 17:250–260, 1954

Scott J, Paykel E, Morriss R, et al: Cognitive behaviour therapy for severe and recurrent bipolar disorders: a randomized controlled trial. Br J Psychiatry 188:313–320, 2006

Segal J, Berk M, Brook S: Risperidone compared with both lithium and haloperidol in mania: a double-blind randomized controlled trial. Clin Neuropharmacol 21:176–180, 1998

Shelton RC, Stahl SM: Risperidone and paroxetine given singly and in combination for bipolar depression. J Clin Psychiatry 65:1715–1719, 2004

Shopsin B, Gershon S, Thompson H, et al: Psychoactive drugs in mania: a controlled comparison of lithium carbonate, chlorpromazine, and haloperidol. Arch Gen Psychiatry 32:34–42, 1975

Sikdar S, Kulhara P, Avasthi A: Combined chlorpromazine and electroconvulsive therapy in mania. Br J Psychiatry 164:806–810, 1994

Small JG: Anticonvulsants in affective disorders. Psychopharmacol Bull 26:25–36, 1990

Small JG, Klapper MH, Kellams JJ, et al: Electroconvulsive treatment compared with lithium in the management of manic states. Arch Gen Psychiatry 45:727–732, 1988

Small JG, Klapper MH, Milstein V, et al: Carbamazepine compared with lithium in the treatment of mania. Arch Gen Psychiatry 48:915–921, 1991

Smulevich AB, Khanna S, Eerdekens M, et al: Acute and continuation risperidone monotherapy in bipolar mania: a 3-week placebo-controlled trial followed by a 9-week double-blind trial of risperidone and haloperidol. Eur Neuropsychopharmacol 15:75–84, 2005

Solomon DA, Ryan CE, Keitner GI: A pilot study of lithium carbonate plus divalproex sodium for the continuation and maintenance treatment of patients with bipolar I disorder. J Clin Psychiatry 58:95–99, 1997

Spring G, Schweid D, Gray C, et al: A double-blind comparison of lithium and chlorpromazine in the treatment of manic states. Am J Psychiatry 126:1306–1310, 1970

Stokes PE, Shamoian CA, Stoll PM, et al: Efficacy of lithium as acute treatment of manic-depressive illness. Lancet 1(7713): 1319–1325, 1971

Stokes PE, Kocsis JH, Orestes JA: Relationship of lithium chloride dose to treatment response in acute mania. Arch Gen Psychiatry 33:1080–1084, 1976

Stoll AL, Severus WE, Freeman MP, et al: Omega 3 fatty acids in bipolar disorder. A preliminary double-blind, placebo-controlled trial. Arch Gen Psychiatry 56:407–412, 1999

Suppes T, Webb A, Paul B, et al: Clinical outcome in a randomized 1-year trial of clozapine versus treatment as usual for patients with treatment-resistant illness and a history of mania. Am J Psychiatry 156:1164–1169, 1999

Suppes T, Dennehy EB, Hirschfeld RMA, et al: The Texas Implementation of Medication Algorithms: update to the algorithms for the treatment of bipolar I disorder. J Clin Psychiatry 66:870–886, 2005

Swann AC, Bowden CL, Calabrese JR, et al: Differential effect of number of previous episodes of affective disorder on response to lithium or divalproex in mania. Am J Psychiatry 156:1264–1266, 1999

Takahashi R, Sakuma A, Itoh K, et al: Comparison of efficacy of lithium carbonate and chlorpromazine in mania: report of collaborative study group on treatment of mania in Japan. Arch Gen Psychiatry 32:1310–1318, 1975

Thase ME, Sachs GS: Bipolar depression: pharmacotherapy and related therapeutic strategies. Biol Psychiatry 48:558–572, 2000

Thase ME, Macfadden W, Weisler RH, et al: Efficacy of quetiapine monotherapy in bipolar I and II depression: a double-blind, placebo-controlled study. J Clin Psychopharmacol 26:600–609, 2006

Thase ME, Jonas A, Khan A, et al: Aripiprazole monotherapy in nonpsychotic bipolar I depression: results of 2 randomized, placebo-controlled studies. J Clin Psychopharmacol 28:13–20, 2008

Thomas J, Reddy B: The treatment of mania: a retrospective evaluation of the effects of ECT, chlorpromazine, and lithium. J Affective Disorder 4:85–92, 1982

Tohen M, Sanger TM, McElroy SL, et al: Olanzapine versus placebo in the treatment of acute mania. Am J Psychiatry 156:702–790, 1999

Tohen M, Jacobs TG, Grundy SL, et al: Efficacy of olanzapine in acute bipolar mania: a double-blind, placebo-controlled study. Arch Gen Psychiatry 57:841–849, 2000

Tohen M, Baker RW, Altshuler LL, et al: Olanzapine versus divalproex in the treatment of acute mania. Am J Psychiatry 159:1011–1017, 2002a

Tohen M, Chengappa KNR, Suppes T, et al: Efficacy of olanzapine in combination with valproate or lithium in the treatment of mania in patients partially nonresponsive to valproate or lithium monotherapy. Arch Gen Psychiatry 59:62–69, 2002b

Tohen M, Goldberg JF, Gonzalez-Pinto A, et al: A 12-week, double-blind comparison of olanzapine vs haloperidol in the treatment of acute mania. Arch Gen Psychiatry 60:1218–1226, 2003a

Tohen M, Ketter TA, Zarate CA Jr, et al: Olanzapine versus divalproex sodium for the treatment of acute mania and maintenance of remission: a 47-week study. Am J Psychiatry 160:1263–1271, 2003b

Tohen M, Vieta E, Calabrese J, et al: Efficacy of olanzapine and olanzapine-fluoxetine combination in the treatment of bipolar I depression. Arch Gen Psychiatry 60:1079–1088, 2003c

Tohen M, Chengappa KNR, Suppes T, et al: Relapse prevention in bipolar I disorder: 18-month comparison of olanzapine plus mood stabilizer vs mood stabilizer alone. Br J Psychiatry 184:337–345, 2004

Tohen M, Greil W, Calabrese JR, et al: Olanzapine versus lithium in the maintenance treatment of bipolar disorder: a 12-month, randomized, double-blind, controlled trial. Am J Psychiatry 162:1281–1290, 2005

Tohen M, Calabrese JR, Sachs GS, et al: Randomized, placebo-controlled trial of olanzapine as maintenance therapy in patients with bipolar I disorder. Am J Psychiatry 163:247–256, 2006

Vanelle JM, Loo H, Galinowski A, et al: Maintenance ECT in intractable manic-depressive disorders. Convuls Ther 10:195–205, 1994

Vasudev K, Goswami U, Kohli K: Carbamazepine and valproate monotherapy: feasibility, relative safety and efficacy, and therapeutic drug monitoring in manic disorders. Psychopharmacology 150:15–23, 2000

Van der Loos M, Nolen WA: Lamotrigine as add-on to lithium in bipolar depression, in Abstracts of the 160th Annual Meeting of the American Psychiatric Association Annual Meeting #286, San Diego, CA, May 21, 2007

Vieta E, Martinez-Aran A, Goikolea JM: A randomized trial comparing paroxetine and venlafaxine in the treatment of bipolar depressed patients taking mood stabilizers. J Clin Psychiatry 63:508–512, 2002

Vieta E, Bourin M, Sanchez R, et al: Effectiveness of aripiprazole vs haloperidol in acute bipolar mania: a double-blind, randomized, comparative 12-week trial. Br J Psychiatry 187:235–242, 2005a

Vieta E, Mullen J, Brecher M, et al: Quetiapine monotherapy for mania associated with bipolar disorder: combined analysis of two international, double-blind, randomized, placebo-controlled studies. Curr Med Res Opin 21:923–934, 2005b

Wagner KD, Kowatch RA, Emslie GJ: A double-blind, randomized, placebo-controlled trial of oxcarbazepine in the treatment of bipolar disorder in children and adolescents. Am J Psychiatry 163:1179–1186, 2006

Walton SA, Berk M, Brook S: Superiority of lithium over verapamil in mania: a randomized, controlled, single-blind trial. J Clin Psychiatry 57:543–546, 1996

Weisler RH, Dunn J, English P: Ziprasidone adjunctive treatment of acute bipolar mania: a randomized, double-blind placebo-controlled trial. Abstracts of the 16th Annual Meeting of the European College of Neuropsychopharmacol, Prague, Czech Republic, September 24, 2004a

Weisler RH, Kalali AH, Ketter TA: A multicenter, randomized, double-blind, placebo-controlled trial of extended release carbamazepine capsules as monotherapy for bipolar patients with manic or mixed episodes. J Clin Psychiatry 65:478–484, 2004b

Weisler RH, Keck PE Jr, Swann AC: Extended release carbamazepine capsules as monotherapy for acute mania in bipolar disorder: a multicenter, randomized, double-blind, placebo-controlled trial. J Clin Psychiatry 66:323–330, 2005

Weiss RD, Griffin ML, Kolodziej ME, et al: A randomized trial of integrated group therapy versus group drug counseling for patients with bipolar disorder and substance dependence. Am J Psychiatry 164:100–107, 2007

Yatham LN, Grossman F, Augustyns I, et al: Mood stabilizers plus risperidone or placebo in the treatment of acute mania. International, double-blind, randomized controlled trial. Br J Psychiatry 182:141–147, 2003

Yatham LN, Paulsson B, Mullen J, et al: Quetiapine versus placebo in combination with lithium or divalproex for the treatment of bipolar mania. J Clin Psychopharmacol 24:599–606, 2004

Yildiz-Yesiloglu A: Targeted treatment strategies in mania: antimanic effects of a PKC inhibitor—tamoxifen (abstract). Biol Psychiatry 61:23S, 2007

Young LT, Joffe RT, Robb JC, et al: Double-blind comparison of addition of a second mood stabilizer versus an antidepressant to an initial mood stabilizer for treatment of patients with bipolar depression. Am J Psychiatry 157:124–127, 2000

Young RC, Biggs JT, Ziegler VE, et al: A rating scale for mania: reliability, validity and sensitivity. Br J Psychiatry 133:429–435, 1978

Zajecka JM, Weisler R, Swann AC, et al: A comparison of the efficacy, safety, and tolerability of divalproex sodium and olanzapine in the treatment of bipolar disorder. J Clin Psychiatry 63:1148–1155, 2002

Zarate CA Jr, Payne LL, Quiroz J: Pramipexole for bipolar II depression: a placebo-controlled proof of concept study. Biol Psychiatry 56:54–60, 2004

Zarate CA Jr, Manji HK: Efficacy of a protein kinase C inhibitor (tamoxifen) in the treatment of acute mania: a double-blind, placebo-controlled study (abstract). Biol Psychiatry 61:7S, 2007

Zaretsky AE, Segal ZV, Gemar M: Cognitive therapy for bipolar depression: a pilot study. Can J Psychiatry 44:491–494, 1999

Zornberg GL, Pope HG Jr: Treatment of depression in bipolar disorder: new directions for research. J Clin Psychopharmacol 13:397–408, 1993

CHAPTER 55

Treatment of Schizophrenia

Tsung-Ung W. Woo, M.D., Ph.D.

Carla M. Canuso, M.D.

Joanne D. Wojcik, P.M.H.C.N.S.–B.C.

Mary F. Brunette, M.D.

Alan I. Green, M.D.

Schizophrenia is a debilitating brain disorder characterized by a chronic relapsing and remitting course of psychosis that is superimposed on persistent "deficit" features such as cognitive dysfunction and negative symptoms. It appears to be equally prevalent across geographical and cultural boundaries (see Jablensky et al. 1992), afflicting approximately 1% of the population (Perala et al. 2007).

The etiology and pathophysiology of schizophrenia remain poorly understood, but the importance of genetic factors is consistently supported by twin (Gottesman 1991; Kendler 1983), family (Gottesman 1991; Kendler 1983; Tsuang et al. 1980), and adoption (Kety et al. 1964, 1994) studies. In the past few years, a number of genes have been identified as being associated with schizophrenia. Furthermore, intensive research has focused on trying to understand how these candidate genes may play a role in the pathophysiology of schizophrenia (G. Harrison 2004; P.J. Harrison and Owen 2003; Porteous et al. 2006; Stefansson et al. 2004). Although the heritability of schizophrenia is high, it appears that environmental events, such as stress (Moghaddam and Jackson 2004), or epigenetic factors (E. Costa et al. 2003, 2006; Tsankova et al. 2007) also play an important role in modulating the expression of the dis-

ease genes and, therefore, in the development of particular schizophrenia phenotypes. This notion is highlighted by the observation that the concordance rate for schizophrenia in monozygotic twins is far less than 100%; it usually lies between 46% and 53% (Gottesman 1991). The environmental factors that have been suggested to contribute to the pathophysiology of schizophrenia include in utero virus (Browne et al. 2000; Buka et al. 2001; Mednick et al. 1988), toxoplasmosis (Dickerson et al. 2007; Hinze-Selch et al. 2007; Mortensen et al. 2007), malnutrition (A.S. Brown et al. 1996), cannabis use (Macleod et al. 2006), and obstetric or perinatal complications (Cannon 1997; Cannon et al. 2000; Geddes and Lawrie 1995). Although significant progress has been made in recent years toward understanding the neural basis of schizophrenia, the exact cascade of events—for example, how interactions between genes and environmental factors lead to the emergence of the illness—has yet to be elucidated (Ross et al. 2006; Tsankova et al. 2007; Weinberger 1996).

Considerable progress has been made in the pharmacological treatment of schizophrenia since the serendipitous discovery in the early 1950s of chlorpromazine as the first effective antipsychotic medication (Lehmann and

The authors would like to acknowledge the contribution of Holly L.L. Pierce in the preparation of this chapter.

Hanrahan 1954). Many other antipsychotic agents, all sharing chlorpromazine's dopamine D_2 receptor–blocking ability, were subsequently developed. These "conventional," or first-generation, antipsychotics are all effective in the treatment of positive symptoms of psychosis, but they all have limited beneficial effects on negative symptoms and cognitive deficits. Furthermore, these first-generation agents commonly produce extrapyramidal side effects (EPS), including parkinsonism, akathisia, and tardive dyskinesia.

Since 1990, a second generation of antipsychotic drugs has become available in the United States. These second-generation agents are also commonly referred to as "atypical" or "novel" antipsychotics, largely because of their reduced propensity, compared with the conventional agents, to cause EPS. It has been postulated that this unique property (i.e., the low risk of EPS) may reflect the potent serotonin$_{2A}$ (5-HT$_{2A}$) receptor antagonistic effects or, more specifically, the high ratio of 5-HT$_{2A}$ to D_2 receptor occupancy of these drugs (Meltzer 1989). More recently, it has been proposed that the rapid dissociation (high dissociation constant) of these drugs from D_2 receptors may be another very important pharmacological property that determines "atypicality" (Kapur and Remington 2001; Seeman 2002).

With the introduction and widespread use of the second-generation antipsychotics, the focus of treatment has been gradually expanding beyond targeting psychotic or positive symptoms of the illness alone. Second-generation agents have been reported to improve some aspects of negative symptoms and cognitive impairment—elements of the disorder not typically responsive to first-generation antipsychotics, at least the high-potency ones (see below). An ability to ameliorate cognitive deficits, in particular, would be important, because such deficits have been found to be strong predictors of long-term functional outcome of the illness (M.F. Green 1996; M.F. Green and Nuechterlein 1999). In fact, development of compounds that can improve cognition has rapidly become one of the main foci in schizophrenia research in just the past few years (Fenton et al. 2003; Hyman and Fenton 2003; Marder 2006).

It should be stressed, however, as will be elaborated in this chapter, that although some of the data on the efficacy of second-generation antipsychotics in the treatment of negative symptoms and cognitive impairment are encouraging, they are by no means conclusive. It may be that rational development of yet newer drugs with novel mechanisms may be necessary before negative symptoms and cognitive deficits can be treated in a clinically mean-

ingful manner (Carpenter and Gold 2002; M.F. Green 2002). This drug discovery and development process is likely to rely critically on an improved understanding of the neurobiological basis of both negative symptoms and cognitive deficits.

In recent years, the field has developed a focused interest in early diagnosis and early intervention in patients who are just becoming psychotic. Studies are under way to determine whether it is possible to delay or even prevent the emergence of psychosis. In the years to come, it is likely that this emphasis on early intervention will expand with further research on the treatment of prodromal states, in an attempt to improve the overall course or perhaps even prevent the actual onset of overt illness in individuals who appear likely to develop schizophrenia.

Clinical Manifestations of Schizophrenia

There is a growing consensus, following the seminal work of several investigators (e.g., Andreasen 1985; Crow 1985), that schizophrenia can be conceptualized as a disorder with at least two more or less orthogonal dimensions of symptomatology: positive and negative symptoms. Positive, or psychotic, symptoms usually are the symptoms that first trigger psychiatric attention, and traditionally, the onset of schizophrenia is clinically synonymous with the emergence of overt psychosis. This concept, however, is gradually changing, because accumulating evidence indicates that the schizophrenia disease process probably begins long before the onset of psychosis. For example, existing evidence from animal studies suggests that brain insults occurring during the first trimester of pregnancy and/or during the perinatal period could have late-occurring detrimental effects on the normal functioning of the brain (Bertolino et al. 2002; D.A. Lewis and Levitt 2002; O'Donnell et al. 2002; Waddington et al. 1998; Weinberger 1987). Interestingly, subtle neurological abnormalities, as well as intellectual and cognitive difficulties, have been observed in children who later show symptoms of schizophrenia (Walker et al. 1999). Finally, research suggests that patients begin to experience a gradual decline in their level of social and cognitive functioning for a period of up to 5 years before the onset of overt psychosis. During this time, they characteristically have symptoms that are similar to the negative symptoms of schizophrenia (Cannon et al. 2007; Hafner et al. 1994, 1999; Yung and McGorry 1996b). Furthermore, it appears that during this prodromal stage of the illness, several regions of the cerebral cortex undergo pronounced volumetric reduction (Borgwardt et al. 2007; Pantelis et al. 2003).

Positive Symptoms

Positive symptoms are perceptual or cognitive features that "normal" individuals usually do not experience. They include hallucinations, delusions, and disorganized thinking, although disorganization also can be conceptualized as an independent symptom dimension (Liddle et al. 1989). As a general rule, positive symptoms tend to respond to treatment with antipsychotic medications; traditionally, they have been the focus of treatment with these medications. Although positive symptoms are dramatic, and while in the midst of them, patients' ability to function is usually severely disrupted, studies have quite consistently shown that such symptoms do not appear to bear any significant association with or predict the long-term functional outcome of the illness (M.F. Green et al. 2000). It also should be emphasized that psychotic symptoms are not specific to schizophrenia; they can occur in a wide spectrum of other psychiatric, neurological, and medical disorders. Therefore, it is essential to rule out other possible causes of psychosis before a diagnosis of schizophrenia is made.

Negative Symptoms

Negative symptoms represent a "loss" of functions or abilities that people without schizophrenia normally possess. They include anhedonia, affective flattening, alogia, avolition, and asociality. Negative symptoms are somewhat associated with intellectual and neurocognitive impairment (Dickerson et al. 1996; Harvey et al. 1998), and they are better predictors of long-term functional outcome and psychosocial functioning of schizophrenia patients than are positive symptoms (Buchanan et al. 1994; Dickerson et al. 1996; Harvey and Keefe 1998). However, neurocognitive deficits, as discussed below, remain the strongest predictors of outcome (M.F. Green 1996). As mentioned above, negative symptoms may have developed long before the actual "onset" of the illness (Hafner et al. 1994, 1999; Yung and McGorry 1996b), which is traditionally defined as the beginning of psychosis. In fact, many prodromal symptoms of schizophrenia may be phenomenologically indistinguishable from negative symptoms. Importantly, EPS produced by antipsychotic medications can sometimes resemble negative symptoms of schizophrenia.

To clarify matters, the concepts of primary versus secondary negative symptoms have been introduced (Carpenter et al. 1988). Thus, *primary* negative symptoms represent the core negative symptoms reflecting the schizophrenia disease process. *Secondary* negative symptoms, on the other hand, may resemble primary negative symptoms, but they are caused by or are secondary to positive symptoms of psychosis or the antipsychotic medications themselves. This distinction has important treatment implications. For example, a reduction in medication dosage may alleviate some secondary negative symptoms, but this strategy is unlikely to have a beneficial effect on primary negative symptoms.

Diagnosis of Schizophrenia

According to DSM-IV-TR (American Psychiatric Association 2000), to make the diagnosis of schizophrenia, there must be evidence of continuous symptomatic disturbance for at least 6 months accompanied by a decline from the premorbid level of functioning. Thus, in line with the Kraepelinian concept (Kraepelin 1919/1971), DSM-IV-TR emphasizes the longitudinal course of deterioration of the illness. This 6-month period can include functional deterioration occurring during the prodromal phase before the onset of overt psychosis. Within the 6-month period, the patient must have two or more of the following symptoms for at least 1 month: delusions, hallucinations, disorganized speech, grossly disorganized or catatonic behavior, and negative symptoms. If the duration of psychotic symptoms is less than 1 month because of successful treatment with antipsychotic medication, a diagnosis of schizophrenia still may be made. Of course, before the diagnosis of schizophrenia is made, other medical or psychiatric conditions need to be considered and ruled out.

Neurocognitive Deficits in Schizophrenia

In the early Kraepelinian formulation of schizophrenia (or dementia praecox), cognitive impairments represented core deficits (Kraepelin 1919/1971). This Kraepelinian concept was somewhat displaced by an emphasis on psychotic symptoms in the diagnosis and treatment of schizophrenia until recently, when the field of schizophrenia research witnessed substantial resurgence of interest in neurocognitive dysfunction in schizophrenia. Research on cognition may facilitate the identification of endophenotypes (i.e., genetic traits) of schizophrenia and also may have significant treatment implications: cognitive deficits are strong predictors of long-term functional outcome of patients with schizophrenia, and unfortunately, they are also among the features that are most resistant to treatment (M.F. Green 1996; M.F. Green et al. 2000). Further research on cognitive deficits may result in the development of more effective pharmacological, cognitive, and psychosocial interventions in the management and perhaps treatment of these deficits.

Schizophrenia appears to be associated with a decline in general cognitive function at some point during the course of the illness. Various studies have shown that this decline may either predate the onset of psychosis (Aylward et al. 1984; David et al. 1997; Nelson et al. 1990; Russell et al. 1997; Simon et al. 2007) or occur concurrently with or subsequent to the first psychotic episode (Nelson et al. 1990). It appears that after this initial decline, the level of cognitive impairment follows a relatively stable course for several decades without evidence of further significant deterioration (Elvevag and Goldberg 2000; Goldberg et al. 1993). Several aspects of cognitive impairment that are well documented in schizophrenia are briefly discussed below.

Verbal Declarative Memory

Among the cognitive functions that are known to be disturbed in schizophrenia, verbal declarative memory impairment, which can be manifested as disturbances in the encoding, storage, and retrieval of mnemonic items, is one of the most consistent findings. It also represents one of the most severe deficits (Saykin et al. 1991, 1994) that is independent of other cognitive impairment, such as attentional deficits. Memory impairment may represent a core feature of the illness (Saykin et al. 1991), one that is stable over time and relatively independent of clinical course (Censits et al. 1997; Gur et al. 1998). It does not appear to be an artifact of antipsychotic medications because memory impairment occurs in drug-naive first-episode patients (Saykin et al. 1994). In addition, it also occurs in otherwise psychiatrically healthy close relatives of schizophrenia patients (Toomey et al. 1998), suggesting that verbal memory impairment may be an endophenotype of schizophrenia. Interestingly, an association between the degree of memory impairment and the severity of negative symptoms has been found (Harvey et al. 1998; Zakzanis 1998). Like memory deficits, negative symptoms also appear to be quite resistant to treatment and are relatively stable during the course of the illness. Thus, memory impairment and negative symptoms in schizophrenia may involve a shared neuroanatomical substrate. Because

memory function is largely mediated by medial temporal structures and negative symptoms are generally associated with prefrontal deficits, information-processing disturbances between the prefrontal and the temporal cortices may represent a prominent feature of schizophrenia (Gur et al. 1998; Heckers et al. 1998).

Working Memory

Working memory is the ability to hold information online when other perceptual, cognitive, or mnemonic information is not immediately present in order to guide future behavior and action (Baddeley 1986). This function is mediated by a neural system of which the prefrontal cortex is a key component (Goldman-Rakic 1996). There have been robust findings of impaired performance of schizophrenic patients on tasks that tap working memory (Park and Holzman 1992), impairments that do not appear to be caused by antipsychotic medications (Goldberg and Weinberger 1996). The fact that working memory impairment is also observed in many first-degree relatives of patients with schizophrenia (Park et al. 1995) suggests that this feature, like verbal declarative memory deficits, may conceivably represent an endophenotype of the illness. Finally, working memory has been extensively studied in nonhuman primates, and the neural elements that support working memory are relatively well understood (Fuster 2000; Goldman-Rakic 1996). Interestingly, postmortem studies have found that many of these neural elements appear to be disturbed in schizophrenia (D.A. Lewis and Lieberman 2000; D.A. Lewis et al. 2005).

Executive Function

Traditionally, the term *executive function* has been used to describe the specific role of the prefrontal cortex in the temporal organization, planning, and sequential execution of goal-directed behavior based on representational information that is constantly being generated and updated (Stuss and Benson 1986). Executive function deficits in schizophrenia, such as those tapped by the Wisconsin Card Sorting Test (WCST), have been frequently described. In a series of well-controlled experiments, Weinberger et al. (1986) showed that during the performance of the WCST, normal control subjects differed from schizophrenic subjects by the selective activation of the dorsolateral prefrontal cortex, as shown by a differential increase in the regional cerebral blood flow (rCBF) to this part of the prefrontal cortex. The lack of action of the prefrontal cortex has been referred to as "hypofrontality" (Ingvar and Franzen 1974). This observation was replicated in subsequent studies when the prefrontal cortex was functionally challenged with the performance of cognitive tasks (K.F. Berman and Weinberger 1999; Carter et al. 1998), although negative findings also have been reported (e.g., Frith et al. 1995; Manoach et al. 1999; Spence et al. 1998).

Attention

Attention plays a key role in mediating many cognitive processes. Attention deficits are well documented in schizophrenia and may in part contribute to the many cognitive disturbances seen in this illness (Braff 1993, 1999; Nuechterlein and Dawson 1984). For example, schizophrenic subjects tend to perform poorly on the Continuous Performance Test, a commonly used task to tap sustained attention. Attention deficit in schizophrenia may reflect an underlying "gating" deficit in which patients have difficulties "filtering out" information that is context-irrelevant or distracting (Braff 1993). One of the most consistent findings in patients with schizophrenia is a deficit in the phenomenon of *prepulse inhibition* (PPI). For example, a sound (prepulse) that occurs 30–500 msec before a sudden loud tone (i.e., a stimulus that normally triggers a startle response) will prevent or reduce the amplitude of the startle response (Braff et al. 1992). However, in patients with schizophrenia, this PPI of the response to the stimulus is diminished (Braff et al. 1992). Interestingly, PPI deficits are also observed in unaffected relatives of patients with schizophrenia (Cadenhead et al. 2000), a finding that is consistent with the notion that such deficits may serve as a trait marker or an endophenotype of schizophrenia.

Course of Schizophrenia

Schizophrenia is a chronic illness with the onset of psychotic symptoms usually occurring around late adolescence and early adulthood (D.A. Lewis and Lieberman 2000). The age at onset is approximately 5 years later in women than in men (Angermeyer et al. 1990; Faraone et al. 1994; Hambrecht et al. 1992; Szymanski et al. 1995). The onset of illness also tends to be more acute in women, as compared with the typically more insidious onset in men, and women tend to have had a higher level of premorbid functioning. Although there may be no clear sex differences in cross-sectional symptomatology of the illness (Hafner et al. 1993; Szymanski et al. 1995), the differences in the age at onset, tempo of onset, and level of premorbid functioning, all of which are prognostic fac-

tors, are consistent with the fact that women in general tend to have a more favorable outcome.

Accumulating evidence suggests that schizophrenia is a neurodevelopmental disorder (D.A. Lewis and Levitt 2002; Murray 1994; Pilowsky et al. 1993; Waddington 1993; Weinberger 1987, 1996). It has been postulated that disturbances in brain development during the first and second trimesters may contribute to the pathophysiology of the illness (Waddington 1993). Other factors such as obstetric complications may further alter the course of brain development (Cannon 1997; Cannon et al. 2000; Geddes and Lawrie 1995). Minor physical anomalies (Lane et al. 1997), neurological soft signs (Browne et al. 2000; Lawrie et al. 2001; Rosso et al. 2000), and neuromotor abnormalities (Walker et al. 1999) have been observed in children who later develop schizophrenia, consistent with the notion that the pathophysiological process leading to schizophrenia appears to have begun much earlier than the onset of psychosis.

For a period of 2–5 years before the onset of the first overt psychotic episode, up to three-quarters of the patients who eventually develop schizophrenia show a wide spectrum of "prodromal" symptoms (Docherty et al. 1978; Freedman and Chapman 1973; Hafner et al. 1992, 1993, 1994; G. Huber et al. 1980; Lieberman 2006; Simon et al. 2007; Varsamis and Adamson 1971; Yung and McGorry 1996a, 1996b). During the prodromal period, behavior changes, such as deterioration in school, work, social, and interpersonal functioning, are often noted. Prodromal symptoms are usually affective or cognitive in nature (e.g., depressed mood, social withdrawal, decreased concentration and attention, decreased motivation, agitation, anxiety, and sleep disturbances). Many of these symptoms are highly reminiscent of and, in fact, perhaps clinically indistinguishable from the negative symptoms and cognitive deficits seen in schizophrenia itself. Other symptoms occurring in the prodromal period, such as suspiciousness, magical thinking, and paranoia, may resemble positive or psychotic symptoms but tend to be transient and not particularly complex; these quasi-psychotic symptoms eventually coalesce into full-blown psychotic symptoms that characterize the onset of the illness.

After the onset of the first episode of psychosis, the course of the illness is often characterized by a gradual and at times continuous deterioration, especially in the first 2–5 years (McGlashan 1998). Some evidence suggests that functional deterioration may be accompanied by a gradual loss of gray matter volume of the cerebral cortex (DeLisi et al. 1997; Kasai et al. 2003a, 2003b; Salisbury et al. 2007; van Haren et al. 2007; Zipursky et al. 1992). In addition, there has been speculation that these observations of functional and structural brain changes after the onset of psychosis may reflect a neurodegenerative process (DeLisi 1999; DeLisi et al. 1997; Lieberman 1999). However, the available evidence in support of the neurodegeneration hypothesis of schizophrenia remains weak (Carpenter 1998; Weinberger and McClure 2002). Conventionally, the hallmark of neurodegeneration is neuronal death, which is generally not believed to be occurring, at least not in large scale, in schizophrenia (Selemon and Goldman-Rakic 1999). However, it is possible that, short of leading to cell death, neuronal injury can be manifested as loss of dendrites and synapses, which can contribute to the observation of progressive gray matter loss. Furthermore, gray matter volume reduction can alternatively be explained as reflecting an exaggerated synaptic pruning process that is normally occurring during the period of late adolescence and early adulthood (Huttenlocher 2002).

After an initial period of functional deterioration, symptoms tend to become more or less stabilized. Some degree of amelioration of positive symptoms (and, to a lesser extent, of disorganization symptoms) may not be uncommon in older patients (Davidson et al. 1995; Harding et al. 1987; Pfohl and Winokur 1982; Schultz et al. 1997). However, findings of amelioration of psychotic symptoms should be interpreted in light of the fact that these are also the symptoms most responsive to treatment with antipsychotic medication, making it difficult to distinguish between the natural course of the disorder and the accumulated response to treatment. Positive symptoms usually respond to treatment, whereas negative symptoms are believed to be relatively treatment resistant and may tend to become increasingly prominent during the course of the illness (Breier et al. 1991).

Many, but not all, studies (Ho et al. 2000) have implied that early intervention during the very first episode of psychosis could be associated with better overall prognosis, as measured by fewer relapses, shorter duration between initiation of antipsychotic treatment and response, and fewer residual symptoms (Birchwood 1992; Haas et al. 1998; Johnstone et al. 1986; Loebel et al. 1992). However, these same studies also have shown that the time between the onset of symptoms and the patient's first presentation to psychiatric care (i.e., the duration of untreated psychosis) is far from optimal: the average duration of untreated psychosis is about 1–2 years. Thus, a major goal in the treatment of schizophrenia is early recognition of illness and timely treatment.

Management of Schizophrenia

Acute Psychosis

The acute phase of schizophrenia is characterized by psychotic symptoms and often by agitation. Affective symptoms such as depression and mania also may occur. The severity of symptoms may vary widely, requiring careful evaluation to determine the most optimal treatment setting and management strategy. The decision to hospitalize a patient usually is based on whether the patient has the ability to care for him- or herself or whether he or she poses any risks of harm to self or others. Regardless of whether treatment is provided in a hospital or in an outpatient setting, acute psychosis requires use of antipsychotic medication.

Management of an acutely agitated and psychotic patient can pose a challenge. It may be necessary to physically restrain the patient for his or her own safety and also for the safety of others. Medications given orally or, in the event of severe agitation, parenterally may be indicated. Although the practice patterns for treatment of acute psychosis are changing following the introduction of atypical agents, for initial acute management of severe behavioral dyscontrol, many physicians still use a high-potency first-generation antipsychotic either alone or in conjunction with a benzodiazepine (such as lorazepam) and/or an anticholinergic drug (such as benztropine). Prior to medicating a patient, it is important to inquire about a history of allergic or severe adverse reactions to the medications to be prescribed. For example, the clinician should be particularly cautious when deciding to prescribe a high-potency first-generation antipsychotic agent to a patient with a history of acute dystonic reaction and should avoid such agents in a patient with a history of neuroleptic malignant syndrome.

If the patient has a history of treatment with antipsychotic medications, one needs to ascertain whether the current psychosis is the result of noncompliance or a "breakthrough" episode because of loss of therapeutic response to the medications. Noncompliance with antipsychotic medications is common and is one of the major causes of symptom exacerbation or full-blown relapse (Crow et al. 1986; Lieberman et al. 1993; Robinson et al. 1999). Causes of noncompliance vary, but the most common reasons are side effects, lack of insight into the illness, delusional interpretations about medication, substance abuse, and lack of a supportive environment (Kampman and Lehtinen 1999). If the psychotic episode appears to result from medication noncompliance, the clinician may decide to restart the same medications in the patient, but it is imperative to focus on improving adherence by providing psychoeducation to the patient (and family, if available) and discussing with the patient the reasons for nonadherence. Depot medications also should be considered if noncompliance is a persistent or recurring problem. Of course, in the case of apparent breakthrough psychosis, change in the patient's medication regimen may be indicated. Other causes of exacerbation of psychosis may include comorbid substance abuse or dependence and comorbid depression, as well as psychosocial stressors including difficulties with housing, employment, benefits, insurance, disability, family, and friends. Therefore, although medications are undoubtedly the mainstay for initial treatment of psychosis, other treatment such as psychotherapy, group therapy, family therapy, dual-diagnosis treatment, social skills training, and case management are important adjuncts to pharmacological management.

First-Episode Psychosis

Emphasis on the early diagnosis and treatment of the first psychotic episode of schizophrenia arises from the recent evidence from some, but not all (Ho et al. 2000), studies suggesting that the duration of untreated psychosis may be associated with poorer overall outcome (Birchwood 1992; Loebel et al. 1992; Wyatt 1991). One hypothesis to account for this observation is that shortening of duration of untreated psychosis by early treatment with antipsychotics may decrease the long-term morbidity of the illness. An alternative hypothesis is that prolonged duration of untreated psychosis represents a different, more severe form of schizophrenia that, by itself, is associated with poorer outcome (McGlashan 1999). For example, the delay in obtaining treatment may indicate a more insidious course of onset of psychosis, which is thought to be associated with increased long-term morbidity; alternatively, patients who seek treatment earlier may experience a more acute form of psychosis, which has been suggested to be a predictor of better prognosis (McGlashan 1999). This hypothesis, however, was not supported by a study in which the mode of onset of psychosis, whether insidious or acute, was not correlated with outcome (Loebel et al. 1992). In summary, although some studies have indicated that duration of untreated psychosis is correlated with outcome, whether a prolonged duration of untreated psychosis could be a marker or a determinant of poor outcome remains to be elucidated (McGlashan 1999).

Because of the more favorable neurological side-effect profile—mainly the reduced risks of adverse neurological events such as parkinsonism, akathisia, and tardive dyskinesia—the second-generation antipsychotics are often considered for the initial treatment of first-episode psychosis. However, as discussed below, many of these medications carry other medically important side effects, including weight gain. Because patients are likely to require long-term treatment, clinicians should pay close attention to antipsychotic side effects and to their potential morbidity. In general, a conservative titration schedule is appropriate for first-episode patients, in part to minimize side effects but also to take into account that these patients may require only low doses for the control and remission of symptoms (Remington et al. 1998; Robinson et al. 1999; Schooler et al. 2005; Wyatt 1995).

After remission of an initial episode of psychosis in a patient with a diagnosis of schizophrenia, potential discontinuation of medication, even if done very gradually, is controversial and often not attempted. Any decision about this should be made in light of studies showing that the relapse rate is very high after medication discontinuation in first-episode schizophrenia (Crow et al. 1986; Johnson 1985; Kane et al. 1982; Robinson et al. 1999). Gitlin et al. (2001), using a low threshold to define recurrence of symptoms, reported that the relapse rate in the first year after medication discontinuation was 78% and increased to 98% by the end of the second year. Moreover, Robinson et al. (1999) found that the relapse rate among self-selected first-episode patients who discontinued their medication was five times the rate among those who continued taking medication. Studies suggest that relapse rates may be lower if uninterrupted medication treatment occurs for at least 1 year after the resolution of psychosis (Kissling et al. 1991).

If a decision is made to initiate a trial of medication discontinuation, the discontinuation should be done very gradually, and the patient should continue to be monitored closely for an extended period. Fortunately, in one study of medication discontinuation in recent-onset patients (Gitlin et al. 2001), the combination of close clinical supervision after medication discontinuation and rapid reinstatement of treatment at the first signs of symptom exacerbation was able to prevent frank psychosis and rehospitalization in most patients.

Choice of Antipsychotics

Since the early 1990s, second-generation antipsychotics have been used widely with the belief that these agents were more effective, better tolerated, and ultimately more cost-effective than first-generation antipsychotics. However, little data comparing first- and second-generation antipsychotics existed. To address this knowledge gap, the National Institute of Mental Health (NIMH) sponsored the Clinical Antipsychotic Trials of Intervention Effectiveness (CATIE) study (Lieberman et al. 2005). The study was designed to compare the effectiveness of four second-generation antipsychotics (olanzapine, quetiapine, risperidone, ziprasidone) and a representative first-generation antipsychotic (perphenazine) in "real world" schizophrenia patients. The primary outcome parameter was discontinuation of treatment. Of the 1,432 subjects who received at least one dose, 74% discontinued study medication before 18 months: 64% of subjects on olanzapine discontinued, compared with 74%–82% on perphenazine, quetiapine, risperidone, and ziprasidone. More subjects receiving olanzapine discontinued due to weight gain and metabolic effects, whereas more subjects assigned to perphenazine discontinued due to EPS (Lieberman et al. 2005). Interestingly, individuals assigned to olanzapine and risperidone who were continuing with their baseline medication had significantly longer times until discontinuation than did those assigned to switch antipsychotics (Essock et al. 2006). Phase II of the CATIE study included two treatment pathways (efficacy and tolerability) with randomized follow-up medication based on the reason for discontinuation of the previous antipsychotic drug (McEvoy et al. 2006; Stroup et al. 2006). For subjects who failed to improve with an atypical antipsychotic, clozapine was more effective than switching to another atypical antipsychotic (McEvoy et al. 2006), and in patients who failed to respond to perphenazine, olanzapine and quetiapine were more effective than risperidone (Stroup et al. 2006). Moreover, in subjects who discontinued an atypical agent due to tolerability or efficacy but who were unwilling to be randomized to clozapine, risperidone and olanzapine were more effective than quetiapine or ziprasidone (Stroup et al. 2006). Finally, while the CATIE cost-effectiveness analysis found perphenazine to be less costly and similarly effective (based on quality adjusted life-years) than each of the atypical antipsychotics, the authors note that these results cannot be generalized to all patient populations, and they suggest that these findings do not warrant policies that would unconditionally restrict access to a particular medication (Rosenheck et al. 2006).

Similar to the NIMH-sponsored CATIE study, the United Kingdom's National Health Service funded the Cost Utility of the Latest Antipsychotic Drugs in Schizo-

phrenia Study (CUtLASS). This study of 227 schizophrenia-spectrum patients randomly assigned to first- and second-generation antipsychotics (other than clozapine) found no difference between the groups in quality of life, symptoms, or health care costs at 1 year (P.B. Jones et al. 2006). The applicability of these results to U.S. populations may be difficult as this study included several medications that are not available in the United States.

Neither the CATIE nor the CUtLASS study addressed the comparative effects of oral and long-acting injectable antipsychotics. Older mirror-image studies in which patients served as their own controls provide evidence of substantial benefit for first-generation long-acting injectable (LAI) antipsychotics over first-generation oral medications (Schooler 2003). Risperidone is the only second-generation antipsychotic currently available in an LAI formulation. Further research evaluating the comparative effects of risperidone LAI to oral atypical agents is needed.

Taken together, the CATIE and the CUtLASS studies indicate that antipsychotic medications are generally effective but have a variety of shortcomings. Moreover, the effectiveness of a given antipsychotic appears to vary according to clinical circumstances, suggesting the need for individualized therapy based on differences in efficacy and tolerability and, perhaps, reflecting why several medication trials may be necessary in the treatment of patients with schizophrenia (Stroup et al. 2007). Additionally, this variation in effectiveness may underlie the increasing use of antipsychotic polypharmacy, for which there is no empirical basis.

Physicians must thoroughly inquire about the patient's past experience with medications and side effects when selecting an antipsychotic, discuss risks and benefits of each treatment option, and consider the patient's preference. Attempts to optimize current medication regimens (e.g., dosage adjustments or psychosocial interventions) may be useful before deciding to switch medications (Essock et al. 2006). Clozapine should be considered for patients who have failed to respond to other second-generation medications. LAI antipsychotics may be considered for patients with poor adherence. Physicians need to be well informed about the differential tolerability of all antipsychotics. First-generation agents clearly have the highest risk of EPS and tardive dyskinesia (Glazer 2000b; Jeste et al. 1998; Tollefson et al. 1997). Risperidone and the newly available paliperidone tend to elevate serum prolactin levels and may cause EPS at higher doses. Although weight gain and metabolic disturbances are associated with all of the second-generation agents (with the possible exception of ziprasidone and aripiprazole), olanzapine and clozapine appear to have the highest likelihood of causing these side effects (Allison et al. 1999; American Diabetes Association et al. 2004). Sedation is commonly observed in patients receiving quetiapine, olanzapine, or clozapine. Both ziprasidone and paliperidone carry product labeling for QTc prolongation and should be used with caution in patients at risk for QTc prolongation. Finally, clozapine, because of its side effects of agranulocytosis, seizures, and myocarditis, is generally reserved for patients with treatment-resistant illness or suicidality.

Maintenance Treatment

The major goals of maintenance treatment are prevention of relapse and improvement in psychosocial and vocational function. The primary methods used to achieve these goals are, as at all phases, an integration of optimal psychopharmacological and psychosocial treatments. Treatment and prevention of other psychiatric comorbidities, such as substance abuse and dependence, are important aspects of maintenance treatment. Also, with the use of the second-generation antipsychotics in particular, treatment and prevention of medical comorbidities that may be associated with these drugs, as well as those that may result from the lifestyle of some patients with schizophrenia who are given these drugs, have become a very important part of long-term management.

Prevention of relapse improves long-term clinical outcomes (Wyatt et al. 1998) and reduces the associated economic burden of the illness (Bernardo et al. 2006). With each relapse, the time it takes to achieve clinical stability lengthens, with the possible consequence of ultimate unresponsiveness to treatment (Lieberman et al. 1993; Wyatt et al. 1998). Several studies have demonstrated that higher rates of relapse are associated with medication discontinuation (Beasley et al. 2003; Carpenter et al. 1990; Herz et al. 1991; Jolley et al. 1990; Kramer et al. 2007; Muller et al. 1992; Pietzcker et al. 1993; Schooler et al. 1997). All available atypical antipsychotics have been granted U.S. Food and Drug Administration (FDA) approval for the maintenance treatment of schizophrenia. Moreover, some evidence suggests that atypical antipsychotics may be more effective than conventional agents in forestalling relapse (Conley and Kelly 2002; Csernansky et al. 2002; Leucht et al. 2003a; Schooler 2006; Tran et al. 1998). While it is not clear whether this apparent advantage for atypicals over conventional antipsychotics is related to better tolerability and adherence (Leucht 2004),

nonadherence to medication is a significant predictor of relapse (Schooler 2006). LAI atypical antipsychotics have the potential to improve medication adherence and thus improve long-term outcomes, but this requires further research. New research on long-term clinical outcomes in patients with schizophrenia will be aided by the newly proposed and validated remission criteria for the disorder (Andreasen et al. 2005; van Os et al. 2006).

An ongoing treatment alliance among the patient, the family, and the treating clinicians is a crucial factor in maximizing medication and overall treatment adherence. Psychoeducation about illness, relapse, and side effects, as well as specific strategies to manage or avoid particular side effects in the context of an ongoing treatment partnership, helps to increase compliance. Medication adherence is the cornerstone of treatment throughout all phases of schizophrenia.

Treatment-Resistant Schizophrenia

Within this chapter, we have emphasized the pervasive nature of negative symptoms and neurocognitive deficits and their resistance to treatment. However, even if we focus only on psychotic symptoms, which tend to respond favorably to antipsychotic medications, at least 30% of patients still can be classified as having incomplete to poor response to antipsychotics, with persistent psychotic symptoms (Kane et al. 1988, 2007; Tamminga 1999). Furthermore, patients may show differential therapeutic response to medications; the fact that a patient fails to respond to one or two antipsychotic medications does not necessarily imply that he or she will not respond to a third agent. For research purposes, Kane et al. (1988) operationally defined *treatment resistance* as 1) lack of significant response to at least three adequate trials of neuroleptics from at least two different chemical classes in the past 5 years and 2) persistently poor social and occupational functioning.

Most of the available data suggest that clozapine is the most effective drug for treatment-resistant schizophrenia (Kane et al. 2001; S.W. Lewis et al. 2006; McEvoy et al. 2006). However, because of the serious side effects produced by clozapine and the requirement for frequent white blood cell count monitoring, some patients and some psychiatrists are reluctant to use it, and some patients are unable to tolerate it. However, whether the other second-generation agents even approach the effectiveness of clozapine for the treatment of these chronically ill patients is unclear. In studies that have compared the efficacy of risperidone and clozapine in treatment-resistant schizophrenia, risperidone has been shown to be either as effective as

(Bondolfi et al. 1998) or less effective than (Breier et al. 1999; Volavka et al. 2002) clozapine. Moreover, patients with treatment-resistant illness may require high doses of risperidone, increasing the likelihood of EPS. Some evidence has indicated that olanzapine at higher dosages (e.g., 30 mg/day) may be as effective as clozapine in improving both positive and negative symptoms (Tollefson et al. 2001; Volavka et al. 2002), although not all studies agree (Buchanan et al. 2005). Other preliminary data also suggest the possible utility of quetiapine, aripiprazole, and ziprasidone in treatment-resistant patients (Emsley et al. 2000; Kane et al. 2006, 2007).

In summary, clozapine remains the primary medication for treatment-resistant schizophrenia, although some studies suggest that other second-generation agents also may have a role in the management of this disorder. Clinically, judicious combinations of antipsychotics from different classes are sometimes used for patients who fail to respond to monotherapy (including those who fail to respond to clozapine), as may the addition of other agents, such as mood stabilizers. Unfortunately, however, no controlled data suggest that any specific combination is more effective than others. Some of the more commonly used regimens include the combination of an atypical agent with a high-potency conventional agent such as haloperidol and the combination of two atypical agents. Clearly, more research is needed to guide treatment in such patients.

Neurocognitive Deficits

Neurocognitive deficits, especially disturbances in executive functioning, memory, and attention (M.F. Green 1996; M.F. Green et al. 2000), are closely associated with the long-term functional outcome of patients with schizophrenia. It appears that second-generation antipsychotics may improve some aspects of cognition in schizophrenia, as found in a meta-analysis of 15 studies on the cognitive-enhancing effects of these drugs (Bilder et al. 2002). In contrast, conventional antipsychotics have usually been believed not to be efficacious in alleviating these deficits (Cassens et al. 1990; Spohn and Strauss 1989), although findings from the CATIE study suggest that at least some of them might be (Keefe et al. 2007). The therapeutic effects of the newer antipsychotics are most notable in measures of verbal fluency and executive functioning, whereas improvement in memory may be more limited. One recently published study suggested that clozapine, olanzapine, and risperidone all showed superiority over haloperidol in the improvement in global neurocognitive measures, including assessments of memory, attention, motor speed, and executive functions (Bilder et al. 2002). However, it must be noted that the available studies are limited, and many are methodologically compromised (Harvey and Keefe 2001). Thus, whether such improvement represents a genuine amelioration of cognitive deficits as a result of correction of the underlying neural system dysfunctions or rather simply epiphenomenal improvement resulting from the differential side-effect profiles between the first- and the second-generation drugs remains debatable (Carpenter and Gold 2002). Moreover, in contrast to the idea that second-generation drugs are superior to the older drugs in the treatment of neurocognitive deficits, data obtained from the CATIE trial (Keefe et al. 2007) show that at 18 months of treatment, perphenazine was actually more effective than any of the second-generation drugs in improving all domains of neurocognitive deficits (Keefe et al. 2007). The authors postulate that a number of factors could potentially explain this unexpected finding, including sample size, differences between mid-potency drugs such as perphenazine and high-potency drugs (e.g., haloperidol) that were commonly used in prior studies, the "real-world" features of the CATIE sample, and prior drug trials before entering the study (Keefe et al. 2007). Finally, regardless of the comparable efficacy of first- and second-generation compounds, a critical question that remains unanswered is whether any of the apparent statistically significant improvements in neurocognitive deficits measured in the laboratory can actually be translated into improved functional outcomes, for example, in terms of employment, school performance, or social role (for a discussion, see M.F. Green 2002).

Psychosocial Treatment of Schizophrenia

Despite the proven efficacy of antipsychotics in the treatment of schizophrenia, most patients continue to have some degree of residual positive symptoms, negative symptoms, and cognitive deficits, and many (even those who take their medications regularly) have difficulty attaining or regaining their desired level of social and occupational functioning. Thus, the optimal treatment of patients with schizophrenia requires the integration of pharmacotherapy with psychosocial interventions that target functional goals. Treatment is ideally offered by a multidisciplinary team that includes, at a minimum, a medication prescriber and a clinician who understands psychosocial rehabilitation but may also include employment and housing specialists. Programs that utilize clinical case managers to directly assist patients in accessing services and to provide the psychosocial interventions are ideal (Rapp and Goscha 2004). To date, several different types of psychosocial interventions have been empirically shown to reduce rates of relapse and rehospitalization, and a variety of treatments may assist patients in acquiring social and vocational skills and possibly in managing residual psychotic symptoms (Bustillo et al. 2001; Lauriello et al. 1999; Penn and Mueser 1996). Furthermore, the interaction between pharmacological and psychosocial treatments appears to be more than additive because each can enhance the effects of the other and affect different domains of outcome (Marder 2000).

Relapse Prevention

It has long been noted that patients with highly critical or overinvolved family members (so-called high-expressed-emotion [EE] families) have a higher risk of relapse (G.W. Brown and Rutter 1966). In a classic study, M.J. Goldstein et al. (1978) reported that a 6-week therapy focusing on teaching families more effective communication dispute-resolution skills reduced relapse rates for up to 6 months. Many other studies have since confirmed the efficacy of family psychoeducation interventions (involving education, training in problem-solving techniques, and/or in cognitive and behavioral management strategies) to prevent relapse and to improve other outcomes (Falloon et al. 1982; Pilling et al. 2002; Pitschel-Walz et al. 2001; Tarrier et al. 1988). In addition, the positive impact of family interventions seems to persist beyond the time of intervention (Sellwood et al. 2001). Finally, despite the fact that families and patients at different stages of the illness may have specific needs and preferences (e.g., first-episode patients may need more intensive and personalized intervention, whereas families of patients with long-term illness may need continuous long-term support [Montero et al. 2005]), the effectiveness of family psychoeducation in preventing relapse has been found to be independent of either the specific form or the intensity of the intervention (Bustillo et al. 2001).

Another psychosocial intervention that has been shown to be effective in preventing relapse or rehospitalization in schizophrenia is assertive community treatment (ACT). This intervention, which involves intensive multidisciplinary team management and service delivery in both community and inpatient settings, is designed for individuals who experience intractable symptoms and high levels of functional impairment. At least 30 studies of ACT have shown advantages over standard commu-

nity treatment in reducing symptoms, family burden, and hospitalization and in improving independent living, housing stability, and quality of life (Mueser et al. 1998; Phillips et al. 2001; Stein and Test 1980). However, it appears that the advantages of ACT do not persist after discontinuation of the program, even after prolonged delivery of services. Finally, ACT also does not have much effect on social adjustment or competitive employment.

Improvement of Psychosocial Functioning

Most patients with schizophrenia have personal goals that involve social and occupational functioning in the community. Hence, psychosocial treatment of patients with schizophrenia targets impairments in these areas. While past research (e.g., the Camarillo State Hospital Study [May et al. 1978]) showed that dynamic psychotherapy was unsuccessful in the treatment of patients with schizophrenia, other forms of individual and group psychotherapy may improve social adjustment and symptom management. In a 3-year study, Hogarty et al. (1997a) found that weekly individual personal therapy, in which an incremental psychoeducational approach based on the patient's phase of recovery was used, had a significant advantage over supportive therapy, family therapy, and combined treatment in improving social adjustment. Yet personal therapy did not appear to be more effective than the other treatments in preventing relapse (Hogarty et al. 1997b). Interestingly, cognitive-behavioral therapy (CBT) may have a role in the management of persistent psychotic symptoms, particularly delusions, in patients with schizophrenia (Chadwick et al. 1994; Granholm et al. 2005; Tarrier et al. 2000). CBT involves the use of techniques such as distraction, cognitive reframing of psychotic beliefs or experiences, and verbal challenge followed by reality testing (Penn and Mueser 1996). Review and meta-analyses of CBT for psychosis suggest a positive effect, although not for reducing relapse (Bellack 2004; C. Jones et al. 2004; Pilling et al. 2002). Further study is needed to demonstrate the efficacy of this treatment paradigm for the management of psychotic symptoms.

Social skills training (SST) is one treatment strategy to help individuals acquire interpersonal disease management and independent living skills that can be delivered in the context of a comprehensive treatment approach. Reviews of SST (Bellack and Mueser 1993; Kopelowicz et al. 2006) have described three models of SST: basic, social problem solving, and cognitive remediation. Within the *basic model,* complex social scenarios are broken down to simpler components, the therapist models correct behaviors, and the patient learns through repeated role-play. This model has been shown to be potentially effective in improving specific social skills for 1 year (Bellack and Mueser 1993). Additionally, the combination of this form of SST with antipsychotic medication appears to be more effective than medication alone in reducing relapse, provided weekly SST is maintained (Hogarty et al. 1986). However, despite skill acquisition, this learning does not appear to generalize to improved social competence within the community (Dilk and Bond 1996).

The *social problem-solving model* focuses on impaired information processing, which is thought to cause social skills deficits, in hopes of achieving a generalized improvement in social adjustment. This model targets symptom and medication management, recreation, basic conversation, and self-care in educational modules, and it has been shown to be effective in enhancing skills (Eckman et al. 1992), although improvements in adaptive functioning within the community are still modest (Liberman et al. 1998; Marder et al. 1996). To enhance generalization to community functioning, interventions that utilize cueing and support in everyday community interactions by "indigenous supporters" such as clinicians, friends, or family seem to improve transfer of newly learned social skills to everyday community interactions (e.g., Glynn et al. 2002).

Finally, the *cognitive remediation model* of SST targets more fundamental cognitive deficits, in areas such as attention, memory, and planning, with the aim of supporting more complex cognitive processes used in learning social skills. Although initial studies following this model have shown some benefit on basic cognitive processes (Brenner et al. 1992), small studies of more complex cognitive and social skills have been mixed (Hodel and Brenner 1994; Spencer et al. 1994; Wykes et al. 1999). One study of cognitive enhancement therapy, an integrated approach to the concomitant training of neurocognitive and social cognitive abilities as well as social skills, showed improvement in social adjustment (Hogarty et al. 2004) that persisted over 3 years (Hogarty et al. 2006).

Recent work to improve social functioning has focused on social cognition, the capacity to perceive the intentions and dispositions of others (Penn et al. 2006). Interventions targeting social cognition attempt to improve areas that are problematic in individuals with schizophrenia: 1) theory of mind (the ability to represent the mental states of others and make inferences about another's intentions); 2) attributional style; and 3) the ability to perceive facial affect in others. A preliminary study of social cognition and interaction training during 18 weekly sessions comprised of emotion training, figuring out situations, and integration of skills into real life suggests that this may be a promising approach for improving interpersonal functioning and for directly managing symptoms of psychosis (Combs et al. 2007).

Illness management and recovery (IMR) is a manualized package of empirically supported approaches (psychoeducation, cognitive-behavioral approaches for medication adherence, relapse prevention planning, SST, and coping skills training) delivered in weekly group or individual sessions that are utilized with a recovery focus that targets each individual's personal life goals (Mueser et al. 2006). Preliminary research shows that this combination of approaches results in improved symptoms and community functioning (Mueser et al. 2006).

Whereas family psychoeducation, CBT, SST, and IMR may improve symptoms and/or social functioning, they do not appear to affect employment status. In addition, traditional vocational rehabilitation programs have assisted with transitional and sheltered employment, but they have not been successful in helping patients with schizophrenia to obtain and maintain competitive employment (Lehman 1995). However, more than 14 studies suggest that supported employment programs, which use rapid job searches, on-the-job training, continuous job support, and integration with mental health treatment, are more effective than traditional methods in helping patients obtain competitive employment (Bond 2004). Research is currently under way to investigate modifications of supported employment, the role of cognitive remediation (McGurk et al. 2007), and other strategies to improve the ability of supported employment to help patients maintain employment.

In addition to employment, the ability to maintain a residence in the community is an important marker of community functioning and a frequently voiced personal goal of patients with schizophrenia. A variety of approaches have been studied to help these patients obtain and maintain stable community residential tenure. Simple provision of access to affordable housing by Section 8 certificates improves housing stability (Hurlburt et al. 1996b). Supported housing, broadly defined as access to independent housing of the patient's choice (often supported with housing subsidies) that is coupled with access to community mental health and support services, improves residential stability and reduces hospitalization (Rog 2004). ACT for homeless individuals has also been shown to reduce homelessness (Coldwell and Bender 2007).

As multiple effective psychosocial interventions exist and are still being developed, the choice of which inter-

vention to apply should depend not only on therapeutic efficacy but also on each individual's goals and preferences. Patients and their families need to be given information about treatment options and should be engaged in discussions with their treatment providers about how treatments can be useful in the context of an individual's symptoms, comorbidities, and needs and preferences.

Management of Medical Comorbidity

Obesity, Metabolic Syndrome, and Diabetes Mellitus

Medication side effects, as well as lifestyle and disease factors, place patients with schizophrenia at increased risk of developing obesity and metabolic side effects, including glucose intolerance, type 2 diabetes, diabetic ketoacidosis, and hyperlipidemia (Dixon et al. 2000; Meyer and Koro 2004; Wirshing et al. 2002, 2003). While clinically significant weight gain occurs in a substantial proportion of patients receiving an antipsychotic medication (Baptista 1999), a convincing body of evidence indicates that certain atypical antipsychotics cause more weight gain than other agents (Allison et al. 1999; Lieberman et al. 2005; Wirshing et al. 1999). A large meta-analytic study of atypical and typical antipsychotics (Wirshing et al. 1999) found a mean weight gain of 9.8 lbs with clozapine, 9.1 lbs with olanzapine, and 4.6 lbs with risperidone, compared with 2.4 lbs with haloperidol, while the atypical antipsychotic ziprasidone was associated with a less than 1-lb weight gain. Furthermore, the CATIE study demonstrated a greater than 7% weight gain from baseline in 30% of patients receiving olanzapine, 16% of those receiving quetiapine, 14% of those receiving risperidone, 12% of those receiving perphenazine, and 7% of those receiving ziprasidone (Lieberman et al. 2005).

Weight gain induced by antipsychotic medication is usually most rapid early in treatment and may plateau after 1–2 years (Allison et al. 1999; Stanton 1995). Young patients and those with a low baseline body mass index may be at increased risk for weight gain (Kinon 1998). This noticeable and often unacceptable side effect of antipsychotics may contribute to medication noncompliance and increase the risk of obesity-related comorbidities, such as diabetes and adverse serum lipid profile (Allison et al. 1999; A.I. Green et al. 2000).

Diabetes mellitus is estimated to occur two to four times more frequently in patients with schizophrenia compared to the general population (Dixon et al. 2000; Goff et

al. 2005; Henderson et al. 2000; Mukherjee et al. 1996; Wirshing et al. 1998). While the risk of diabetes in schizophrenia is likely multifactorial, accrued evidence indicates that atypical antipsychotics are associated with glucose dysregulation (Jin et al. 2004). Several case reports (Koller and Doraiswamy 2002; Koller et al. 2001, 2003), retrospective studies (Dixon et al. 2000; Wirshing et al. 2002), epidemiological investigations (Gianfrancesco et al. 2002), and limited prospective studies (Henderson et al. 2000) of hyperglycemia, new-onset diabetes mellitus, and diabetic ketoacidosis led to heightened attention to and concern over the metabolic effects of atypical antipsychotics, resulting in the issuance of warnings by regulatory authorities and class labeling (Jin et al. 2004). Moreover, in 2004 the American Psychiatric Association, together with the American Diabetes Association, published consensus guidelines on monitoring and described the differential risk of metabolic effects for the atypical antipsychotics (American Diabetes Association et al. 2004). Clozapine and olanzapine are described as having the greatest effect on weight (with increased risk for diabetes), whereas risperidone and quetiapine are described as having an effect on weight (but with unclear risk for diabetes). Aripiprazole and ziprasidone are described as having small or no effect on weight and without risk for diabetes.

Certain atypical antipsychotics (particularly clozapine, olanzapine, and quetiapine) and low-potency conventional agents have been shown to be associated with hyperlipidemia (Henderson et al. 2000; Meyer and Koro 2004; Osser et al. 1999), whereas ziprasidone and aripiprazole do not appear to carry this adverse effect (Kingsbury et al. 2001; Meyer and Koro 2004). The co-occurrence of atherogenic dyslipidemia with abdominal adiposity, insulin resistance, impaired fasting glucose or overt diabetes mellitus, and hypertension constitutes the cluster of clinical features known as the metabolic syndrome, or syndrome X. Given the well-established and close relationship between metabolic syndrome and coronary heart disease (Isomaa et al. 2001) and the growing awareness of a range of metabolic issues in patients with schizophrenia, researchers and clinicians are now focusing on identifying the metabolic syndrome in patients with schizophrenia. Baseline data from the CATIE study indicated that more than 40% of subjects had metabolic syndrome. Moreover, the CATIE males were 138% more likely to have metabolic syndrome than matched controls, and the CATIE females were 251% more likely to have metabolic syndrome than matched controls (McEvoy et al. 2005).

To minimize iatrogenic medical problems and to ensure optimal treatment outcome, prevention and man-

agement of weight gain and obesity-related conditions in patients with schizophrenia are essential. In addition to receiving ongoing education about the potential for weight gain, patients should be counseled about dietary choices, encouraged to exercise, and weighed frequently. In a recent review of behavioral interventions for weight management, the authors concluded that such interventions may prevent further weight gain and in some cases may result in weight loss (Loh et al. 2006).

Centrally acting weight-loss drugs that have the potential to increase biogenic amine activity could theoretically exacerbate symptoms of psychosis in this population. However, anecdotal reports suggesting the utility of nizatidine, citmetadine, metformin, topiramate, sibutramine, and amantadine in the prevention or treatment of antipsychotic-associated obesity exist (Werneke et al. 2002) but have not been substantiated with well-controlled trials. Orlistat, the non–centrally acting weight-control drug, may theoretically have a role in helping patients with schizophrenia lose weight, although no clinical trials have been reported to date (A.I. Green et al. 2000). One case series (Hamoui et al. 2004) suggested that bariatric surgery was as effective in promoting weight loss in patients with schizophrenia as it is in other obese patients.

The differential propensity of the various agents to cause weight gain, and glucose and lipid dysregulation, should be taken into consideration when treating individuals at increased risk. Clinicians should employ monitoring, such as that recommended by the American Diabetes Association–American Psychiatric Association consensus panel (American Diabetes Association et al. 2004). Patients who develop glucose intolerance or diabetes may require treatment with hypoglycemic agents, and those with hyperlipidemia may require lipid-lowering agents in collaboration with an internist. Although to the best of our knowledge no studies of the long-term effects of these simple interventions in minimizing the overall morbidity of this patient population have been done, such interventions may be important in the lowering of long-term morbidity.

Cigarette Smoking

Reports indicate that up to approximately 90% of patients with schizophrenia smoke cigarettes, over three times the rate seen in the general population (S. Brown et al. 2000; Dalack et al. 1998; Meyer and Nasrallah 2003). Heavy cigarette smoking contributes to the risk of coronary heart disease, which accounts for over 50% of the mortality in patients with schizophrenia (Hennekens et al. 2005). Beyond health, tobacco use results in financial consequences, with some schizophrenia patients spending nearly a third of their disability income on cigarettes (Steinberg et al. 2004). It has been proposed that the high rates of smoking may relate to abnormalities in brain reward circuitry (including presynaptic nicotinic acetylcholine receptors within mesolimbic and mesocortical dopamine pathways) and self-medication of clinical symptoms and cognitive deficits (George and Vessicchio 2001; Knott et al. 2006; Ripoll et al. 2004; Sacco et al. 2005). Indeed, such hypotheses and observations may provide insight into the neurobiology of schizophrenia and targets for treatment of both schizophrenia and nicotine addiction (Meyer and Nasrallah 2003).

Treatment of nicotine addiction in the schizophrenia population has been met with limited success and appears to be even more difficult for this patient population compared with both the general and other psychiatric populations (Covey et al. 1994). Nonetheless, evidence suggests that a multimodality approach, which integrates motivation-based treatment, addiction treatment, and tobacco dependence treatment into mental health settings, may be beneficial (Ziedonis et al. 2003). Group therapy, when combined with a nicotine patch, may help reduce smoking (George et al. 2000), and bupropion in combination with psychotherapy may reduce tobacco use in patients with schizophrenia (Evins et al. 2005; Weiner et al. 2001). Additionally, in a case series of patients previously unable to quit smoking despite tobacco dependence treatment, use of nicotine nasal spray was associated with substantial reduction in or abstinence from smoking in 9 of 12 patients (J.M. Williams et al. 2004). Interestingly, whereas typical antipsychotic medications may be associated with an increase in smoking (McEvoy et al. 1995a), treatment with clozapine may lead to a decrease (George et al. 1995; McEvoy et al. 1995b). Finally, some other atypical antipsychotic medications may facilitate the ability of the nicotine patch itself to decrease smoking (George et al. 2000).

HIV and Hepatitis Risks

Patients with schizophrenia, especially those with substance abuse, are at high risk for HIV and hepatitis B and C (Cournos and Bakalar 1996; Meyer and Nasrallah 2003; Rosenberg et al. 2001). A cross-sectional Medicaid claims analysis found that patients with schizophrenia spectrum illnesses were 1.5 times as likely to have a diagnosis of HIV compared to recipients without a diagnosis

of serious mental illness (Blank et al. 2002). Additionally, recent retrospective evaluations of both large Department of Veterans Affairs and civilian populations indicate that patients with schizophrenia or severe mental illness have rates of hepatitis C virus (HCV) seropositivity of approximately 20% (Huckans et al. 2006; Meyer and Nasrallah 2003) and that the rate of HCV infection in patients with schizophrenia is 11 times higher than found in the general population (Osher et al. 2003; Rosenberg et al. 2001). Risk factors such as unsafe sexual practices, combined with multiple partners, place patients with schizophrenia at heightened risk for sexually transmitted diseases (Sewell 1996). Patients should be asked about their sexual practices and, when indicated, tested for HIV and hepatitis. Discussions that provide education about safe sex are important. For those schizophrenic patients with HIV/AIDS or hepatitis, a close collaboration with a medical specialist is essential, as treatment may be complicated by poor adherence, neuropsychiatric consequences of antiviral therapies (e.g., interferon), and drug–drug and drug–disease interactions.

Extrapyramidal Side Effects

The term *extrapyramidal side effects* (EPS) describes a spectrum of adverse reactions, including akathisia, parkinsonism, and acute dystonia, induced in some patients by antipsychotic medications. Parkinsonism and acute dystonia are associated with the degree of dopamine D_2 receptor occupancy in the striatum (Kapur and Remington 1996). Thus, high-potency first-generation antipsychotics, such as haloperidol, have the greatest propensity (especially at high doses) to cause these side effects, but many second-generation agents, such as risperidone, olanzapine, and ziprasidone, also may cause EPS in a dose-dependent manner. The CATIE study found that the rate of drug discontinuation due to reported EPS was 8% in the patient group treated with the typical antipsychotic perphenazine, with rates of 4% for ziprasidone, 3% for risperidone and quetiapine, and 2% for olanzapine (Lieberman et al. 2005). Among the second-generation agents, quetiapine and clozapine do not appear to produce clinically significant parkinsonism or dystonia. In addition, aripiprazole has a low propensity to cause EPS (Ohlsen and Pilowsky 2005), although there are case reports of akathisia (Cohen et al. 2005) and parkinsonism (Cohen et al. 2005; Sharma and Sorrell 2006; Ziegenbein et al. 2006) occurring with this drug.

Akathisia, a disturbing sense of inner restlessness and the inability of the patient to stay still, is associated with

seemingly purposeless movements (such as tapping or pacing) that may be noticeable to the examiner. The restlessness of akathisia may be misdiagnosed as an increase in psychosis, one that worsens when treated by higher doses of antipsychotic medication. Like other EPS, akathisia appears less likely to occur with second-generation agents (Glazer 2000b). Although lowering the dose of the antipsychotic is an obvious treatment for akathisia, addition of a β-blocker (e.g., propranolol) is often effective. Anticholinergic drugs and benzodiazepines are generally not that effective but can be tried in patients who fail to respond to β-blockers, and anticholinergics also may be useful in patients with coexisting parkinsonism.

Parkinsonism (Osser 1999), characterized by tremor, rigidity, and bradykinesia, can occur early in treatment, usually within the initial weeks or months. Bradykinesia includes generalized slowing of movement and a mask-like face (with a loss of facial expression); it may be confused with depression or negative symptoms. One variant of parkinsonism, akinesia, can coexist with bradykinesia (but without tremor or rigidity) and may be associated with symptoms of apathy and fatigue. The "rabbit syndrome" (Casey 1999), occurring after months or years of antipsychotic drug treatment, is also a variant of parkinsonism and is characterized by a perioral and jaw tremor. As with other forms of EPS, the second-generation antipsychotics appear less likely to cause parkinsonism than the older agents (Glazer 2000b), although the rate of parkinsonism may be dose related with some of the newer agents. Anticholinergic medications are the treatment of choice and usually are effective. Lower doses of antipsychotics and a switch to an agent less likely to produce EPS also may be helpful.

Acute dystonia occurs most commonly during the week after initiation of antipsychotics or following an abrupt and rapid dose increase (Ayd 1961; Barnes and Spence 2000; Remington and Kapur 1996). Age is an important risk factor; dystonia occurs most commonly in children and young adults, especially in males. The dystonia may appear as torticollis, trismus, tongue protrusion, pharyngeal constriction, laryngospasm, blepharospasm, oculogyric crisis, or abnormal contractions of any part of the body. Clinically, in addition to the dystonic muscular contractions that may be immediately noticeable, the patient may complain of tongue thickening, throat tightening, and difficulty speaking or swallowing. Acute treatment with either an anticholinergic agent or an antihistamine is usually highly effective but may need to be repeated at intervals if acute dystonia recurs (before the dose of the anticholinergic is stabilized). Should res-

piratory difficulty develop, medications may need to be given parenterally.

Tardive Dyskinesia and Tardive Dystonia

Tardive dyskinesia, which is a syndrome of potentially irreversible involuntary movements, and tardive dystonia, which is characterized by sustained muscle contractions, can gradually emerge after a prolonged period of treatment with antipsychotic medications. Accumulating evidence suggests that the second-generation antipsychotics are less likely to cause these tardive syndromes than the first-generation drugs (Jeste et al. 1998; Kane et al. 1993; Marder et al. 2002; Margolese et al. 2005; Shirzadi and Ghaemi 2006; Tarsy and Baldessarini 2006; Tollefson et al. 1997). However, since many patients have had exposure to more than one second-generation agent, it is difficult to determine the risk associated with individual agents. It appears that compared with the first-generation agents, collectively the second-generation drugs carry one-fifth to one-twelfth the risk of causing tardive dyskinesia and tardive dystonia (Correll et al. 2004; Kane 2004; Leucht et al. 2003b; Margolese et al. 2005; Tarsy and Baldessarini 2006).

The most common form of tardive dyskinesia involves dyskinetic movements of the orofacial and buccolingual musculature, manifesting as grimacing, facial tics, lip smacking, chewing, and wormlike movements of the tongue. Involvement of the neck, axial, and extremity musculature also may occur in the form of choreoathetoid movements, which on rare occasions may involve laryngopharyngeal and respiratory muscles. Tardive dystonia may occur earlier in treatment than tardive dyskinesia and is characterized by slow, sustained twisting movements of the head, neck, trunk, and extremities; blepharospasm, torticollis, facial grimacing, back arching, and hyperextension and rotation of the limbs may also be seen (Simpson 2000).

Among the risk factors for tardive dyskinesia, age appears quite important; elderly individuals have an incidence five to six times higher than that in younger people (Kane 2004). Tardive dyskinesia occurs more frequently in older female patients (Jeste 2000; Saltz et al. 1991), whereas tardive dystonia is more common in younger patients and males. Other risk factors for tardive dyskinesia include mood disorders (Keck et al. 2000), race/ethnicity (African American) (Keck et al. 2000), high doses of medication (Glazer 2000a, 2000c), previous evidence of parkinsonian side effects from antipsychotics (Keck et al. 2000), early onset of extrapyramidal syndromes (Kane 2004), and substance abuse (Miller et al. 2005).

Although no treatment has been proven to be effective for tardive dyskinesia, several management strategies may be clinically useful. Clinicians should screen patients taking antipsychotic medications on a regular basis. If tardive dyskinesia develops, switching from a first-generation to a second-generation drug may be helpful. For those patients who are taking a second-generation agent, a switch to another second-generation drug may be considered. Among the second-generation drugs, evidence suggests that clozapine may reduce symptoms of tardive dyskinesia (Glazer 2000a; Lieberman et al. 1991). Symptoms may also be suppressed, at least temporarily, by increasing the dosage of the antipsychotic medications that produce tardive dyskinesia; however, this strategy runs the risk of causing or worsening EPS and possibly increasing tardive dyskinesia over time. Patients with tardive dyskinesia who are taking anticholinergic medications should have these medications discontinued, because they can worsen tardive dyskinesia. Finally, the symptoms of tardive dystonia may be alleviated by reducing the dosages of the antipsychotics, by switching from first-generation to second-generation agents (including clozapine), by using anticholinergics, and/or by administering dopamine-depleting agents, such as reserpine or tetrabenazine (Simpson 2000).

Neuroleptic Malignant Syndrome

Neuroleptic malignant syndrome (NMS), which occurs in about 1%–2% of patients receiving typical antipsychotic medication and is potentially fatal in up to 20% of the cases (without treatment), has been reported to occur during treatment with both the typical (Caroff and Mann 1993) and the atypical (Ananth et al. 2004; Hasan and Buckley 1998; Wirshing et al. 2000) antipsychotics. Several factors may increase risk, including intramuscular injections, rapid escalation of high doses of antipsychotic medication, dehydration, restraint use, and high temperatures. Catatonia and severe disorganization are clinical symptoms that may be associated with a high risk for NMS (Berardi et al. 2002). Symptoms of NMS include hyperpyrexia, altered consciousness, muscle rigidity and dystonia, autonomic nervous system dysfunction, and laboratory tests indicating elevated creatine phosphokinase, liver enzymes, and white blood cell count. Early detection and rapid treatment of this medical emergency are crucial and include discontinuation of the antipsychotic, treatment in a medical setting that can support vital functioning, and in some cases the use of a dopamine agonist such as bromocriptine or dantrolene, a muscle relaxant (Koppel 1998; Susman 2001).

Hyperprolactinemia

Antipsychotic medications—particularly typical agents, risperidone, and paliperidone—can produce an increase in serum prolactin levels (Dickson and Glazer 1999; Marder et al. 2004). Although early studies reported few negative consequences of long-term prolactin elevation (Meltzer 1985), this topic has received increased attention in recent years. It is well known that hyperprolactinemia secondary to medical disorders (e.g., pituitary tumor) can produce galactorrhea, hypogonadism (evidenced by sexual and menstrual dysfunction and diminished gonadal hormone levels), and osteoporosis, all of which have also been reported in patients with schizophrenia (Abraham et al. 1996; Ghadirian et al. 1982; Riecher-Rossler et al. 1994; Windgassen et al. 1996; Yazigi et al. 1997). Yet the relationships between antipsychotic-induced hyperprolactinemia and these conditions, perhaps with the exception of galactorrhea (Windgassen et al. 1996), remain unclear, with conflicting reports in the literature (Canuso et al. 2002; A.M. Costa et al. 2007; Hummer et al. 2005; Kinon et al. 2006; Kleinberg et al. 1999; O'Keane and Meaney 2005). Interestingly, several reports suggest that hypoestrogenism in schizophrenia occurs in women with and without hyperprolactinemia (Bergemann et al. 2005; Canuso et al. 2002; T.J. Huber et al. 2004). Thus, while prolactin-related hypogonadism may contribute to the increased risk of these conditions, it appears that patients with schizophrenia may be at inherent risk for hypogonadism. The important question of whether drug-induced hyperprolactinemia increases long-term breast cancer risk has also been raised. Although a large claims database analysis found a 16% increase in the risk of breast cancer in women exposed to dopamine antagonists, the authors concluded that these results are preliminary and potentially confounded and should not necessarily lead to changes in treatment strategies (Wang et al. 2002). Finally, a recent retrospective review of pharmacovigilance data suggested that treatment with potent D_2 receptor antagonists, such as risperidone, may be associated with increased risk for pituitary tumors (Szarfman et al. 2006). Prospective studies are needed to confirm this association.

Clinicians should inquire about possible adverse effects of hyperprolactinemia and aim to diminish them. If a patient is symptomatic, prolactin levels should be obtained and medical causes of hyperprolactinemia ruled out. Prolactin elevation associated with galactorrhea, or sexual and menstrual dysfunction, may be minimized by dosage reduction or by a medication change to an atypical antipsychotic with less prolactin-elevating potential (Canuso et al. 1998; Dickson and Glazer 1999). Because patients with schizophrenia generally require chronic treatment with antipsychotics, those who have had prolonged hyperprolactinemia may be at an increased risk for osteoporosis (Abraham et al. 1996) and may be appropriate candidates for screening with bone densitometry. Female patients should have routine mammography in accordance with the screening guidelines set forth for all women.

Psychiatric Conditions Comorbid With Schizophrenia and Their Treatment

Substance-Related Disorders

Nearly one-half of the patients with schizophrenia are reported to have a lifetime history of an alcohol or a substance use disorder, compared with 16% of the general population (Regier et al. 1990). Alcohol is the most commonly abused substance in chronically ill patients, followed by cannabis and cocaine (Selzer and Lieberman 1993; Sevy et al. 1990); first-episode patients appear more likely to abuse cannabis over other substances (Rolfe et al. 1999). As in the general population, men with schizophrenia are more likely to abuse substances than are women (Mueser et al. 1995).

The use of alcohol, marijuana, cocaine, and other substances can cause serious problems for patients with schizophrenia. Comorbid substance use has a deleterious effect on both physical health and the long-term course of schizophrenia itself (Grech et al. 1999); use of even small amounts can produce negative effects (D'Souza et al. 2005; Drake et al. 2001). Patients with schizophrenia and substance abuse are at increased risk for infectious diseases such as HIV, hepatitis B, and hepatitis C (Rosenberg et al. 2001); in addition, alcohol and substance use is associated with clinical worsening, poor functioning, and an increased rate of hospitalizations and homelessness (Dixon et al. 1990; Drake and Mueser 1996; Hurlburt et al. 1996a; Negrete et al. 1986; Soni and Brownlee 1991). In some studies, more than 50% of the first-episode patients have been reported to have cannabis use disorder (Rolfe et al. 1999), often complicating the diagnosis of a psychotic disorder (Addington 1999). Comorbid alcohol and substance use often has an overwhelmingly negative effect on the ability of patients to function at their highest possible level (Dickey and Azeni 1996).

Given the negative consequences of substance abuse in these patients, investigators have tried to understand

the basis of such use. One theory, the "self-medication" hypothesis, suggests that alcohol and substances of abuse help to decrease negative symptoms of schizophrenia and the EPS produced by antipsychotic medications (Glynn and Sussman 1990; Khantzian 1985; Siris 1990). However, although alcohol and substances of abuse may in fact transiently alleviate negative symptoms and EPS, our group has suggested that the existence of negative symptoms or EPS of antipsychotics may not be causally related to the substance use (A.I. Green et al. 1999). Some studies indicate that patients with few negative symptoms may actually use substances more than do those with more negative symptoms (Buchanan et al. 1997; Lysaker et al. 1994). Also, first-episode patients, who have not yet been exposed to antipsychotic medication and who therefore could not have EPS, are quite likely to use alcohol or substances (A.I. Green et al. 2004).

We (A.I. Green et al. 1999; Roth et al. 2005) have introduced a neurobiological formulation, based on animal studies (Svensson et al. 1995), suggesting that a deficiency in the dopamine-mediated mesocorticolimbic brain reward circuit of patients with schizophrenia may underlie the use of alcohol and substances in these patients. This formulation posits that alcohol and substances of abuse may ameliorate this deficiency by improving the "signal detection" capability of dopamine-rich systems, by which they reduce negative symptoms and EPS while enhancing the reward system (Fadda et al. 1989; Goeders and Smith 1986; A.I. Green et al. 1999). A related neurobiological formulation also has been proposed by Chambers et al. (2001).

Although obtaining information from patients about the use of substances of abuse should be a standard part of a medical history, alcohol or substance abuse is often underrecognized and undertreated in mental health settings (Ananth et al. 1989). Because patients often deny the use of alcohol and drugs, clinicians also should pursue collateral reports from family members, case managers, and others involved in the delivery of services to patients. Unfortunately, the traditional separation of mental health and substance abuse services compounds the problems of detection. Patients with schizophrenia and a comorbid alcohol or substance use disorder require specialized treatment for both disorders (Bellack and DiClemente 1999), optimally in programs that provide integrated mental health and substance abuse treatment, as well as medication management (Drake and Mueser 2001; Minkoff 1989; Osher and Kofoed 1989). Drake and Mueser (2001) reported that the treatment of comorbid substance abuse requires long-term comprehensive services (Osher and Kofoed 1989), including individual treatment planning

tailored to the patient's ability to engage in treatment and assertive outreach (Drake and Mueser 2000; Ziedonis et al. 2000), with interventions within the social support system. The specific integrated interventions for substance abuse in patients with schizophrenia with the most evidence are group counseling with cognitive-behavioral and motivational components (Bellack et al. 2006; Weiss et al. 2007), contingency management (Drebing et al. 2005; Ries et al. 2004), and, for patients who do not respond to less intensive interventions, long-term residential programs (Brunette et al. 2004).

Although there is no agreed-upon pharmacological treatment approach for patients with schizophrenia and comorbid alcohol or substance use disorders (A.I. Green et al. 2007, 2008; Wilkins 1997), some investigators have been interested in the potential role of atypical antipsychotics in these patients. The atypical antipsychotic that has been studied most in this population is clozapine. Three preliminary studies—a naturalistic study (Drake et al. 2000) and two retrospective studies (A.I. Green et al. 2003; Zimmet et al. 2000)—reported a large reduction in alcohol use in patients taking clozapine; evidence also was found for a reduction in cannabis and cocaine use. Two other studies (Buckley et al. 1999; Lee et al. 1998) also have reported this beneficial effect of clozapine in patients with schizophrenia and comorbid substance use disorder. Clozapine was also associated with reduced rates of relapse to substance abuse in patients who had been in remission (Brunette et al. 2006). Randomized trials of clozapine needed to confirm these preliminary studies are currently under way.

The data concerning the potential effect of the other atypical antipsychotics are even more preliminary. Reports on risperidone appear to be conflicted (Albanese 2000; A.I. Green et al. 2003), although a report by Smelson et al. (2000) found that cocaine-abusing schizophrenic patients treated with risperidone experienced less craving, had fewer relapses, and remained in treatment longer than did those treated with typical antipsychotics. Recently, Rubio et al. (2006) reported that the new LAI form of risperidone was more effective in improving substance abuse than a depot form of the typical agent zuclopenthixol (which is not available in the United States), but the difference was small and probably not clinically significant. However, a report of data from a large Veterans Administration treatment group showed no advantage for either risperidone or olanzapine compared with typical antipsychotics on clinical substance abuse measures (Petrakis et al. 2006). Two other open prospective studies of olanzapine treatment noted improvements in substance use, but one of them (Noordsy et al. 2001), which might have been limited by

statistical power, did not find significant advantages of olanzapine over typical antipsychotic treatment (Littrell et al. 2001; Noordsy et al. 2001). Two randomized trials of olanzapine's impact on cocaine craving and use compared to typical antipsychotics also reported conflicting results (Sayers et al. 2005; Smelson et al. 2006). Preliminary research on quetiapine and aripiprazole is promising. Two open studies of quetiapine (E.S. Brown et al. 2003; Potvin et al. 2006) and of aripiprazole (Beresford et al. 2005; E.S. Brown et al. 2005) suggest that these medications may be helpful for alcohol and/or cocaine use disorders in patients with schizophrenia. No research has assessed the impact of ziprasidone.

Other possible pharmacological options for treatment of alcohol or substance use disorder in schizophrenia include the following: 1) disulfiram (Kofoed et al. 1986), which one randomized, placebo-controlled trial (Petrakis et al. 2005) and one open trial (Mueser et al. 2003) suggest is effective for alcohol dependence in patients with schizophrenia but requires monitoring (Kofoed et al. 1986); 2) naltrexone, which was found to decrease alcohol use among patients with schizophrenia in two randomized, placebo-controlled trials (Petrakis et al. 2004, 2005); 3) the tricyclic antidepressants desipramine or imipramine for the treatment of comorbid cocaine disorders (Siris et al. 1993; Ziedonis et al. 1992); and 4) bupropion for the treatment of nicotine dependence in these patients (George et al. 2002). Acamprosate, although shown to be effective for alcohol dependence in placebo-controlled trials, has yet to be studied in patients with schizophrenia. Clearly, more studies need to be undertaken to develop optimal pharmacological strategies for the treatment of these comorbid disorders.

Depression

Schizophrenia is often associated with depressive states, from dysphoria to major depression. The Epidemiologic Catchment Area study suggests that those with schizophrenia have a 14-fold greater risk of depression than the general population (Fenton 2001). At various times, depression has been viewed as an aspect of schizophrenia (McGlashan and Carpenter 1976; Sax et al. 1996), as a response to psychosis (McGlashan and Carpenter 1976; Sax et al. 1996), or as a state occurring after the cessation of frank psychotic symptoms (Birchwood et al. 2000). Depressive symptoms can occur throughout the course of schizophrenia, including in first-episode patients (Hafner et al. 2005; Koreen et al. 1993), but in chronically ill patients in particular, these symptoms appear to be associ-

ated with risk of relapse (Mandel et al. 1982) and suicide (Drake et al. 1986).

Assessing patients with schizophrenia for the presence of depression requires knowledge of the types of depressive states in patients with schizophrenia and the conditions, such as negative symptoms and EPS, that can be confused with depression. In detecting depression, the presence of a core depressed mood and related neurovegetative symptoms should be distinguished from flatness of affect and anhedonia (McGlashan and Carpenter 1976). Depression occurring during an exacerbation of psychosis may remit with treatment of the psychosis (Birchwood et al. 2000; Koreen et al. 1993; Tollefson et al. 1999). However, postpsychotic depression classically develops after the resolution or improvement of psychotic symptoms, particularly in first-episode patients (Birchwood et al. 2000; Koreen et al. 1993). Moreover, dysphoria and demoralization frequently occur in patients with schizophrenia (Iqbal et al. 2000; Siris 2000a), as patients struggle with illness-related disability, but these symptoms may not be associated with the classical neurovegetative symptoms of depression (Bartels and Drake 1988).

Treatment of depression in patients with schizophrenia may include both psychopharmacological and psychosocial components (Siris 2000b). Because depression may presage an increase in psychosis, the adequacy of pharmacological treatment of psychotic symptoms should be assessed. Treatment of depression in acute psychosis may be accomplished through the use of antipsychotic medication alone, especially the atypical antipsychotics (Banov et al. 1994; Levinson et al. 1999; Marder et al. 1997; Tollefson et al. 1998). However, major depression developing after the remission of psychosis often requires more specific intervention, such as treatment with combinations of antipsychotics and antidepressants or mood stabilizers (Levinson et al. 1999). Postpsychotic depression may benefit from the addition of tricyclic antidepressants or serotonin reuptake inhibitors to the antipsychotic medication (Hogarty et al. 1995; Kirli and Caliskan 1998; Siris et al. 1987). However, demoralization and dysphoria do not appear to be responsive to antidepressants (Iqbal et al. 2000; Levinson et al. 1999); rather, appropriate psychosocial interventions (e.g., stress management, job training, cognitive therapy, support) may be most helpful (Siris 2000b).

Suicide

Suicide is the leading cause of premature death in patients with schizophrenia, who have a 10% lifetime risk of suicide. Nearly 50% of the patients with schizophrenia attempt suicide during their lifetime (Black et al. 1985; Tsuang et al. 1999a). The risk of suicide is as high in patients with schizophrenia as in patients with mood disorder and is 10-fold higher than in the general population (Baxter and Appleby 1999). Several factors are associated with an increased risk of suicide in patients with schizophrenia: depression and the diagnosis of schizoaffective disorder (Harkavy-Friedman et al. 2004; Radomsky et al. 1999), social isolation (Drake et al. 1986; G. Goldstein et al. 2006; Potkin et al. 2003), and feelings of hopelessness and disappointment over failure to meet high self-expectations (Kim et al. 2003; Westermeyer et al. 1991). Patients with a higher level of insight and awareness of their illness may be at increased risk (Amador et al. 1996; Bourgeois et al. 2004; Crumlish et al. 2005), as may patients with a poor level of functioning (Kaplan and Harrow 1996).

A history of suicide attempts is one of the strongest predictors of suicide in patients with schizophrenia (Rossau and Mortensen 1997; Roy 1982a). In a large 2-year prospective study of 980 schizophrenia and schizoaffective disorder patients at high risk for suicide, multivariate analysis found the number of lifetime suicide attempts, number of hospitalizations to prevent suicide in the previous 3 years, history of alcohol or substance abuse, baseline anxiety scale score, and severity of parkinsonism to be the strongest predictors of suicide (Potkin et al. 2003). Moreover, a recent meta-analysis of 29 case–control and cohort studies indicated that suicide risk factors included previous depressive disorders, drug abuse, agitation or motor restlessness, fear of mental disintegration, poor adherence to treatment, and recent loss (Hawton et al. 2005).

Gender also appears to be a risk factor (Rossau and Mortensen 1997); men with schizophrenia commit suicide at an earlier age than do women with schizophrenia (Roy 1982a). An increased risk of suicide is present in the early phase of the illness (Drake et al. 1985; Kuo et al. 2005; Ran et al. 2005), especially in those patients with an earlier age at onset of schizophrenia (Gupta et al. 1998). The risk of suicide appears to peak immediately after admission and shortly after discharge (Qin and Nordentoft 2005; Rossau and Mortensen 1997), especially in patients who are hospitalized for short periods (Qin and Nordentoft 2005) and in those who return to a socially isolated environment (Drake et al. 1986). Patients in an active phase of the illness (Heila et al. 1997) or with positive symptoms (Kelly et al. 2004) may be at risk, especially if they have prominent symptoms of suspiciousness and delusions (Fenton et al. 1997).

A national clinical survey conducted in Great Britain, based on a 4-year (1996–2000) sample of people who died

by suicide, found that the deaths of schizophrenia patients were characterized by more violent methods: they were more likely than others to be young, male, unmarried, and from an ethnic minority, with high rates of unemployment (Hunt et al. 2006). Moreover, rates of previous violence and drug abuse were high, and suicide victims were proportionally more likely to be inpatients at the time of death and to have been noncompliant with medication (Hunt et al. 2006). In another study (Roy 1982b), half of all patients who committed suicide had been seen in the week prior, and in another study (Heila et al. 1997), between 49% and 96% of the patients had been seen within 3 months of the suicide.

The treating clinician should regularly evaluate the patient's condition, assess for suicide risk factors, and aim to enhance protective factors such as social support and positive coping skills (Montross et al. 2005). Patients who present with suicidal thoughts or behavior require close follow-up and intensive outreach. For the isolated or newly diagnosed patient, a clear aftercare plan (often in a day treatment center) should be in place before discharge from the hospital (Drake et al. 1986; Harkavy-Friedman and Nelson 1997). Improved ward safety, effective substance abuse treatment, affective symptom control, and ensured medication adherence are all measures that may prevent suicide (Hawton et al. 2005; Hunt et al. 2006). Additionally, evidence suggests that community programs for early detection of schizophrenia may reduce suicidality risk (Melle et al. 2006).

Psychopharmacological treatment plays a crucial role in the prevention of suicide. In one study, more than half of the patients who committed suicide were either medication noncompliant or prescribed inadequate doses of antipsychotics, and 23% of the sample were thought to be nonresponsive to treatment (Heila et al. 1999). Moreover, a landmark study of nearly 1,000 patients with schizophrenia and schizoaffective disorder who were at risk for suicide (but who were not necessarily classically treatment resistant) indicated that treatment with clozapine was more likely to decrease suicidality than was treatment with olanzapine (Meltzer et al. 2003).

Obsessive-Compulsive Symptoms

Obsessive-compulsive symptoms are seen in 8.8%–30% of patients with schizophrenia (I. Berman et al. 1995a; Byerly et al. 2005; Cassano et al. 1998; Ongur and Goff 2005). Although obsessive-compulsive symptoms may be difficult to distinguish from delusions (Eisen et al. 1997), they are important to identify because they may indicate a poor prognosis, yet they may be responsive to specialized treatment regimens. Most studies have indicated that obsessive-compulsive symptoms are associated with unfavorable outcomes—with increased social isolation, longer hospitalizations, greater psychopathology, and poor treatment response (Fenton and McGlashan 1986; Hwang et al. 2000; Ongur and Goff 2005). By contrast, a more recent study (*N* = 58) suggested that the presence of obsessive-compulsive symptoms does not impact clinical outcomes (Byerly et al. 2005). The obsessive-compulsive symptoms in schizophrenia are similar to those found in obsessive-compulsive disorder (Tibbo et al. 2000), although they may not be ego-dystonic in patients with schizophrenia.

Treatment of obsessive-compulsive schizophrenia may require the use of a tricyclic antidepressant or a serotonin reuptake inhibitor with a typical antipsychotic (I. Berman et al. 1995b; Chang and Berman 1999; Poyurovsky et al. 2000). The data regarding the role of atypical agents in these patients are mixed (Fenton 2001). Some reports suggest that atypical antipsychotics may exacerbate obsessive-compulsive symptoms, whereas others suggest that they may be helpful (Baker et al. 1992, 1996; Kopala and Honer 1994; Morrison et al. 1998; Ongur and Goff 2005; Strous et al. 1999). Although the addition of a serotonin reuptake inhibitor to an atypical antipsychotic may decrease obsessive-compulsive symptoms in these patients (as the addition of a serotonin reuptake inhibitor to some typical agents does), the combined use of serotonin reuptake inhibitors with clozapine, especially, may require care because of the possible increase in blood levels of clozapine.

Future Directions

Novel Pharmacotherapeutic Treatment

Although all existing antipsychotic medications have effects on the dopamine system, other neurotransmitter systems are increasingly being recognized as possible therapeutic targets. For instance, the glutamate hypothesis of schizophrenia (Coyle 1996; Goff and Coyle 2001; Javitt and Zukin 1991; Olney and Farber 1995) suggests that modulation of glutamatergic activity could be a potential target for pharmacological treatment of schizophrenia. The glutamate hypothesis is, to a large extent, derived from the observation that treatment of healthy subjects with *N*-methyl-D-aspartate (NMDA) antagonists, such as ketamine and phencyclidine (PCP), produces symptoms reminiscent of schizophrenia (Adler et al. 1998; Newcomer et al. 1999). Most important, in addition to the psy-

chotic symptoms, which can be induced by a variety of central nervous system stimulants or hallucinogens, NMDA antagonists uniquely produce many of the cognitive deficits associated with schizophrenia (Krystal et al. 1994) and symptoms that resemble the negative symptoms of the illness (Abi-Saab et al. 2001). Thus, it would follow that drugs that enhance NMDA receptor function might be beneficial in the treatment of negative symptoms of schizophrenia (Javitt 2006; Javitt and Coyle 2004).

Because of the possible risks of neurotoxicity as a result of direct stimulation of NMDA receptors, drugs that indirectly enhance NMDA neurotransmission by modulating other binding sites on the NMDA receptor complex have been studied. For example, D-cycloserine (a partial agonist) (Goff et al. 1999), D-serine (Tsai et al. 1998), D-alanine (Tsai et al. 2006), glycine (Heresco-Levy et al. 1996a, 1996b; Javitt et al. 2001), agonists of the glycine binding site (located adjacent to the NMDA ion channel), and sarcosine (a glycine transporter-1 inhibitor) (Tsai et al. 2004) have been shown to have therapeutic potential. Preliminary data are quite promising, in that all of these agents appear to be effective in improving negative symptoms of schizophrenia, although their effects on positive symptoms, if any, tend to be very modest (Goff and Coyle 2001; Tsai et al. 1998), and it appears that they may not be effective in patients treated with clozapine (Goff et al. 1996; Potkin et al. 1999; but see Javitt et al. 2001).

Non-NMDA glutamate receptors may also be potential targets for treatment. For example, a recent preliminary study demonstrated that a selective agonist of metabotropic glutamate 2/3 (mGlu2/3) receptors, used as monotherapy, was efficacious in reducing both positive and negative symptoms in 196 patients with schizophrenia (Patil et al. 2007). MGlu2/3 agonists, which blunt the effects of PCP in animals, are thought to work in part by modulating glutamate release (Patil et al. 2007). This study suggests that agents that do not directly block dopamine receptors may have therapeutic potential in schizophrenia.

Another novel approach to the treatment of schizophrenia is the development of drugs that act as partial dopamine agonists. These drugs bind to dopamine receptors, including the presynaptic autoreceptors, with high affinity but with variable intrinsic activity, depending on the activity level of the target system (Tamminga 2002). Because of this, they exert a wide range of modulatory effects on the dopaminergic system. The first FDA-approved drug with this mechanism is aripiprazole.

Given the increasing evidence suggesting that neurocognitive deficits are pervasive in patients with schizophrenia and that they are important determinants of long-term functional outcome, there has been considerable interest in developing compounds that target these deficits. Drugs that may be effective, at least in theory, in the treatment of neurocognitive deficits include muscarinic agonists, alpha 7 nicotinic receptor agonists (Martin et al. 2007), ampakines (agonists of the AMPA [amino-3-hydroxy-5-methyl-4-isoxazole propionic acid] class of glutamate receptors) (Goff and Coyle 2001), class I metabotropic glutamate receptor agonists (Moghaddam 2004), dopamine D_1 receptor agonists (G.V. Williams and Castner 2006), and alpha 2 γ-aminobutyric acid (GABA) type A ($GABA_A$) receptor agonists (D.A. Lewis and Gonzalez-Burgos 2006). Although clinical experience with these drugs is quite limited, there are ongoing clinical trials to test the possible efficacy of at least some of these compounds.

Early Intervention and Prevention of Schizophrenia

As emphasized earlier in this chapter, some investigators have suggested that early detection and treatment of first-episode psychosis may improve the long-term prognosis of schizophrenia. In recent years, there have even been attempts to identify individuals who are in the prodromal phase of schizophrenia but have not yet developed psychosis (Yung and McGorry 1996b), with the notion that intervention, including psychopharmacological treatment, during this period of the illness may be able to prevent the onset of full-blown psychosis (McGorry et al. 2002). However, as has been discussed in this chapter, many of the prodromal symptoms, among which depression and anxiety are common manifestations, are not specific to schizophrenia and are not uncommonly observed in otherwise healthy adolescents (McGorry et al. 1995). The issue of misidentification of individuals who are not at risk for psychosis must be considered. The current challenge is to establish the predictive validity of specific traits or prodromal symptoms of the diagnosis or recognition of the prodrome as a syndrome. However, even if these individuals can be reliably identified, the modes of treatment, including the specific classes of medications, that may be most effective in preventing the onset of psychosis are at present virtually unknown (Cannon et al. 2007; McGlashan et al. 2007).

Another concept that may help clarify prodrome is the notion of schizotaxia, which was originally put forward by Meehl (1962, 1989) and reformulated by Faraone et al. (2001) to describe a constellation of negative symp-

toms and neuropsychological deficits present in 20%–50% of the first-degree relatives of patients with schizophrenia. Preliminary findings from treatment of six such relatives meeting criteria for schizotaxia with low-dose risperidone (up to 2 mg) for 6 weeks suggested that this treatment may improve the deficits associated with this condition (Tsuang et al. 1999b). If the validity of schizotaxia as a "preschizophrenic" trait could be established (Tsuang et al. 2000), it would be important to determine whether treatment of schizotaxia in individuals with prodromal symptoms could actually be associated with a decrease in the incidence of schizophrenia.

References

Abi-Saab WM, D'Souza C, Madonick S, et al: Targeting the glutamate system, in Current Issues in the Psychopharmacology of Schizophrenia. Edited by Breier A, Tran PV, Herrea JM, et al. Philadelphia, PA, Lippincott Williams & Wilkins, 2001, pp 304–332

Abraham G, Friedman RH, Verghese C: Osteoporosis demonstrated by dual energy x-ray absorptiometry in chronic schizophrenic patients. Biol Psychiatry 40:430–431, 1996

Addington J: Early intervention strategies for co-morbid cannabis use and psychosis. Presented at the Inaugural International Cannabis and Psychosis Conference, Melbourne, Australia, February 16–19, 1999

Adler CM, Goldberg TE, Malhotra AK, et al: Effects of ketamine on thought disorder, working memory, and semantic memory in healthy volunteers. Biol Psychiatry 43:811–816, 1998

Albanese MJ: Risperidone in substance abusers with bipolar disorder. Presented at the 39th Annual Meeting of the American College of Neuropsychopharmacology, San Juan, Puerto Rico, 2000

Allison DB, Mentore JL, Heo M, et al: Antipsychotic-induced weight gain: a comprehensive research synthesis. Am J Psychiatry 156:1686–1696, 1999

Amador XF, Friedman JH, Kasapis C, et al: Suicidal behavior in schizophrenia and its relationship to awareness of illness. Am J Psychiatry 153:1185–1188, 1996

American Diabetes Association, American Psychiatric Association, American Association of Clinical Endocrinologists, et al: Consensus development conference on antipsychotic drugs and obesity and diabetes. J Clin Psychiatry 65:267–272, 2004

American Psychiatric Association: Diagnostic and Statistical Manual of Mental Disorders, 4th Edition, Text Revision. Washington, DC, American Psychiatric Association, 2000

Ananth J, Vandewater S, Kamal M, et al: Missed diagnosis of substance abuse in psychiatric patients. Hosp Community Psychiatry 40:297–299, 1989

Ananth J, Parameswaran S, Gunatilake S, et al: Neuroleptic malignant syndrome and atypical antipsychotic drugs. J Clin Psychiatry 65:464–470, 2004

Andreasen NC: Positive vs. negative schizophrenia: a critical evaluation. Schizophr Bull 11:380–389, 1985

Andreasen NC, Carpenter WT Jr, Kane JM, et al: Remission in schizophrenia: proposed criteria and rationale for consensus. Am J Psychiatry 162:441–449, 2005

Angermeyer MC, Kuhn L, Goldstein JM: Gender and the course of schizophrenia: differences in treated outcomes. Schizophr Bull 16:293–307, 1990

Ayd FJ Jr: A survey of drug-induced extrapyramidal reactions. JAMA 175:1054–1060, 1961

Aylward E, Walker E, Bettes B: Intelligence in schizophrenia: meta-analysis of the research. Schizophr Bull 10:430–459, 1984

Baddeley AD: Working Memory. Oxford, UK, Oxford University Press, 1986

Baker RW, Chengappa KN, Baird JW, et al: Emergence of obsessive compulsive symptoms during treatment with clozapine. J Clin Psychiatry 53:439–442, 1992

Baker RW, Ames D, Umbricht DS, et al: Obsessive-compulsive symptoms in schizophrenia: a comparison of olanzapine and placebo. Psychopharmacol Bull 32:89–93, 1996

Banov MD, Zarate CA Jr, Tohen M, et al: Clozapine therapy in refractory affective disorders: polarity predicts response in long-term follow-up. J Clin Psychiatry 55:295–300, 1994

Baptista T: Body weight gain induced by antipsychotic drugs: mechanisms and management. Acta Psychiatr Scand 100:3–16, 1999

Barnes TRE, Spence SA: Movement disorders associated with antipsychotic drugs: clinical and biological implications, in Psychopharmacology of Schizophrenia. Edited by Reverly MA, Deakin JFW. New York, Oxford University Press, 2000, pp 178–210

Bartels SJ, Drake RE: Depressive symptoms in schizophrenia: comprehensive differential diagnosis. Compr Psychiatry 29:467–483, 1988

Baxter D, Appleby L: Case register study of suicide risk in mental disorders. Br J Psychiatry 175:322–326, 1999

Beasley CM Jr, Sutton VK, Hamilton SH, et al: A double-blind, randomized, placebo-controlled trial of olanzapine in the prevention of psychotic relapse. J Clin Psychopharmacol 23:582–594, 2003

Bellack AS: Skills training for people with severe mental illness. Psychiatr Rehabil J 27:375–391, 2004

Bellack AS, DiClemente CC: Treating substance abuse among patients with schizophrenia. Psychiatr Serv 50:75–80, 1999

Bellack AS, Mueser KT: Psychosocial treatment for schizophrenia. Schizophr Bull 19:317–336, 1993

Bellack AS, Bennett ME, Gearon JS, et al: A randomized clinical trial of a new behavioral treatment for drug abuse in people with severe and persistent mental illness. Arch Gen Psychiatry 63:426–432, 2006

Berardi D, Dell'Atti M, Amore M, et al: Clinical risk factors for neuroleptic malignant syndrome. Hum Psychopharmacol 17:99–102, 2002

Beresford TP, Clapp L, Martin B, et al: Aripiprazole in schizophrenia with cocaine dependence: a pilot study. J Clin Psychopharmacol 25:363–366, 2005

Bergemann N, Mundt C, Parzer P, et al: Plasma concentrations of estradiol in women suffering from schizophrenia treated with conventional versus atypical antipsychotics. Schizophr Res 73:357–366, 2005

Berman I, Kalinowski A, Berman SM, et al: Obsessive and compulsive symptoms in chronic schizophrenia. Compr Psychiatry 36:6–10, 1995a

Berman I, Sapers BL, Chang HH, et al: Treatment of obsessive-compulsive symptoms in schizophrenic patients with clomipramine. J Clin Psychopharmacol 15:206–210, 1995b

Berman KF, Weinberger DR: Neuroimaging studies of schizophrenia, in Neurobiology of Mental Illness. Edited by Charney DS, Nestler EJ, Bunney BS. New York, Oxford University Press, 1999, pp 246–257

Bernardo M, Ramon Azanza J, Rubio-Terres C, et al: Cost-effectiveness analysis of schizophrenia relapse prevention: an economic evaluation of the ZEUS (Ziprasidone-Extended-Use-In-Schizophrenia) study in Spain. Clin Drug Investig 26:447–457, 2006

Bertolino A, Roffman JL, Lipska BK, et al: Reduced N-acetylaspartate in prefrontal cortex of adult rats with neonatal hippocampal damage. Cereb Cortex 12:983–990, 2002

Bilder RM, Goldman RS, Volavka J, et al: Neurocognitive effects of clozapine, olanzapine, risperidone, and haloperidol in patients with chronic schizophrenia or schizoaffective disorder. Am J Psychiatry 159:1018–1028, 2002

Birchwood M: Early intervention in schizophrenia: theoretical background and clinical strategies. Br J Clin Psychol 31(pt 3):257–278, 1992

Birchwood M, Iqbal Z, Chadwick P, et al: Cognitive approach to depression and suicidal thinking in psychosis, I: ontogeny of post-psychotic depression. Br J Psychiatry 177:516–521, 2000

Black DW, Warrack G, Winokur G: The Iowa record-linkage study, I: suicides and accidental deaths among psychiatric patients. Arch Gen Psychiatry 42:71–75, 1985

Blank MB, Mandell DS, Aiken L, et al: Co-occurrence of HIV and serious mental illness among Medicaid recipients. Psychiatr Serv 53:868–873, 2002

Bond GR: Supported employment: evidence for an evidence-based practice. Psychiatr Rehabil J 27:345–359, 2004

Bondolfi G, Dufour H, Patris M, et al: Risperidone versus clozapine in treatment-resistant chronic schizophrenia: a randomized double-blind study. The Risperidone Study Group. Am J Psychiatry 155:499–504, 1998

Borgwardt SJ, McGuire PK, Aston J, et al: Structural brain abnormalities in individuals with an at-risk mental state who later develop psychosis. Br J Psychiatry Suppl 51:s69–s75, 2007

Bourgeois M, Swendsen J, Young F, et al: Awareness of disorder and suicide risk in the treatment of schizophrenia: results of the international suicide prevention trial. Am J Psychiatry 161:1494–1496, 2004

Braff DL: Information processing and attention dysfunctions in schizophrenia. Schizophr Bull 19:233–259, 1993

Braff DL: Psychophysiological and information processing approaches to schizophrenia, in Neurobiology of Mental Illness. Edited by Charney DS, Nestler EJ, Bunney BS. New York, Oxford University Press, 1999, pp 258–271

Braff DL, Grillon C, Geyer MA: Gating and habituation of the startle reflex in schizophrenic patients. Arch Gen Psychiatry 49:206–215, 1992

Breier A, Schreiber JL, Dyer J, et al: National Institute of Mental Health longitudinal study of chronic schizophrenia. Prognosis and predictors of outcome. Arch Gen Psychiatry 48:239–246, 1991

Breier AF, Malhotra AK, Su TP, et al: Clozapine and risperidone in chronic schizophrenia: effects on symptoms, parkinsonian side effects, and neuroendocrine response. Am J Psychiatry 156:294–298, 1999

Brenner HD, Hodel B, Roder V, et al: Treatment of cognitive dysfunctions and behavioral deficits in schizophrenia. Schizophr Bull 18:21–26, 1992

Brown AS, Susser ES, Butler PD, et al: Neurobiological plausibility of prenatal nutritional deprivation as a risk factor for schizophrenia. J Nerv Ment Dis 184:71–85, 1996

Brown ES, Nejtek VA, Perantie DC, et al: Cocaine and amphetamine use in patients with psychiatric illness: a randomized trial of typical antipsychotic continuation or discontinuation. J Clin Psychopharmacol 23:384–388, 2003

Brown ES, Jeffress J, Liggin JD, et al: Switching outpatients with bipolar or schizoaffective disorders and substance abuse from their current antipsychotic to aripiprazole. J Clin Psychiatry 66:756–760, 2005

Brown GW, Rutter M: The measurement of family activities and relationships: a methodological study. Human Relations 19:241–263, 1966

Brown S, Inskip H, Barraclough B: Causes of the excess mortality of schizophrenia. Br J Psychiatry 177:212–217, 2000

Browne S, Clarke M, Gervin M, et al: Determinants of neurological dysfunction in first episode schizophrenia. Psychol Med 30:1433–1441, 2000

Brunette MF, Mueser KT, Drake RE: A review of research on residential programs for people with severe mental illness and co-occurring substance use disorders. Drug Alcohol Rev 23:471–481, 2004

Brunette MF, Drake RE, Xie H, et al: Clozapine use and relapses of substance use disorder among patients with co-occurring schizophrenia and substance use disorders. Schizophr Bull 32:637–643, 2006

Buchanan RW, Strauss ME, Kirkpatrick B, et al: Neuropsychological impairments in deficit vs nondeficit forms of schizophrenia. Arch Gen Psychiatry 51:804–811, 1994

Buchanan RW, Strauss ME, Breier A, et al: Attentional impairments in deficit and nondeficit forms of schizophrenia. Am J Psychiatry 154:363–370, 1997

Buchanan RW, Ball MP, Weiner E, et al: Olanzapine treatment of residual positive and negative symptoms. Am J Psychiatry 162:124–129, 2005

Buckley P, McCarthy M, Chapman P, et al: Clozapine treatment of comorbid substance abuse in patients with schizophrenia. Schizophr Res 36:272, 1999

Buka SL, Tsuang MT, Torrey EF, et al: Maternal infections and subsequent psychosis among offspring. Arch Gen Psychiatry 58:1032–1037, 2001

Bustillo J, Lauriello J, Horan W, et al: The psychosocial treatment of schizophrenia: an update. Am J Psychiatry 158:163–175, 2001

Byerly M, Goodman W, Acholonu W, et al: Obsessive compulsive symptoms in schizophrenia: frequency and clinical features. Schizophr Res 76:309–316, 2005

Cadenhead KS, Swerdlow NR, Shafer KM, et al: Modulation of the startle response and startle laterality in relatives of schizophrenic patients and in subjects with schizotypal personality disorder: evidence of inhibitory deficits. Am J Psychiatry 157:1660–1668, 2000

Cannon TD: On the nature and mechanisms of obstetric influences in schizophrenia: a review and synthesis of epidemiologic studies. Int Rev Psychiatry 9:387–397, 1997

Cannon TD, Rosso IM, Hollister JM, et al: A prospective cohort study of genetic and perinatal influences in the etiology of schizophrenia. Schizophr Bull 26:351–366, 2000

Cannon TD, Cornblatt B, McGorry P: The empirical status of the ultra high-risk (prodromal) research paradigm. Schizophr Bull 33:661–664, 2007

Canuso CM, Hanau M, Jhamb KK, et al: Olanzapine use in women with antipsychotic-induced hyperprolactinemia. Am J Psychiatry 155:1458, 1998

Canuso CM, Goldstein JM, Wojcik J, et al: Antipsychotic medication, prolactin elevation, and ovarian function in women with schizophrenia and schizoaffective disorder. Psychiatry Res 111:11–20, 2002

Caroff SN, Mann SC: Neuroleptic malignant syndrome. Med Clin North Am 77:185–202, 1993

Carpenter WT Jr, Heinrichs DW, Wagman AM: Deficit and nondeficit forms of schizophrenia: the concept. Am J Psychiatry 145:578–583, 1988

Carpenter WT Jr, Hanlon TE, Heinrichs DW, et al: Continuous versus targeted medication in schizophrenic outpatients: outcome results. Am J Psychiatry 147:1138–1148, 1990

Carpenter WT Jr: New views on the course and treatment of schizophrenia. J Psychiatr Res 32:191–195, 1998

Carpenter WT Jr, Gold JM: Another view of therapy for cognition in schizophrenia. Biol Psychiatry 51:969–971, 2002

Carter CS, Perlstein W, Ganguli R, et al: Functional hypofrontality and working memory dysfunction in schizophrenia. Am J Psychiatry 155:1285–1287, 1998

Casey DE: Rabbit syndrome, in Movement Disorders in Neurology and Neuropsychiatry. Edited by Joseph AB, Young RR. Malden, MA, Blackwell Science, 1999, pp 119–122

Cassano GB, Pini S, Saettoni M, et al: Occurrence and clinical correlates of psychiatric comorbidity in patients with psychotic disorders. J Clin Psychiatry 59:60–68, 1998

Cassens G, Inglis AK, Appelbaum PS, et al: Neuroleptics: effects on neuropsychological function in chronic schizophrenic patients. Schizophr Bull 16:477–499, 1990

Censits DM, Ragland JD, Gur RC, et al: Neuropsychological evidence supporting a neurodevelopmental model of schizophrenia: a longitudinal study. Schizophr Res 24:289–298, 1997

Chadwick PDJ, Lowe CF, Horne PJ, et al: Modifying delusions: the role of empirical testing: innovations in cognitive-behavioral approaches to schizophrenia. Behav Ther 25:35–49, 1994

Chambers RA, Krystal JH, Self DW: A neurobiological basis for substance abuse comorbidity in schizophrenia. Biol Psychiatry 50:71–83, 2001

Chang HH, Berman I: Treatment issues for patients with schizophrenia who have obsessive-compulsive symptoms. Psychiatric Annals 29:529–532, 1999

Cohen ST, Rulf D, Pies R: Extrapyramidal side effects associated with aripiprazole coprescription in 2 patients. J Clin Psychiatry 66:135–136, 2005

Coldwell CM, Bender WS: The effectiveness of assertive community treatment for homeless populations with severe mental illness: a meta-analysis. Am J Psychiatry 164:393–399, 2007

Combs DR, Adams SD, Penn DL, et al: Social Cognition and Interaction Training (SCIT) for inpatients with schizophrenia spectrum disorders: preliminary findings. Schizophr Res 91:112–116, 2007

Conley RR, Kelly DL: Current status of antipsychotic treatment. Curr Drug Targets CNS Neurol Disord 1:123–128, 2002

Correll CU, Leucht S, Kane JM: Lower risk for tardive dyskinesia associated with second-generation antipsychotics: a systematic review of 1-year studies. Am J Psychiatry 161:414–425, 2004

Costa AM, de Lima MS, Faria M, et al: A naturalistic, 9-month follow-up, comparing olanzapine and conventional antipsychotics on sexual function and hormonal profile for males with schizophrenia. J Psychopharmacol 21:165–170, 2007

Costa E, Grayson DR, Guidotti A: Epigenetic downregulation of GABAergic function in schizophrenia: potential for pharmacological intervention? Mol Interv 3:220–229, 2003

Costa E, Dong E, Grayson DR, et al: Epigenetic targets in GABAergic neurons to treat schizophrenia. Adv Pharmacol 54:95–117, 2006

Cournos F, Bakalar N: AIDS and People With Severe Mental Illness: A Handbook for Mental Health Professionals. New Haven, CT, Yale University Press, 1996

Covey L, Hughes DC, Glassman AH, et al: Ever-smoking, quitting, and psychiatric disorders: evidence from the Durham, North Carolina, Epidemiologic Catchment Area. Tobacco Control 3:222–227, 1994

Coyle JT: The glutamatergic dysfunction hypothesis for schizophrenia. Harv Rev Psychiatry 3:241–253, 1996

Crow TJ: The two-syndrome concept: origins and current status. Schizophr Bull 11:471–486, 1985

Crow TJ, MacMillan JF, Johnson AL, et al: A randomised controlled trial of prophylactic neuroleptic treatment. Br J Psychiatry 148:120–127, 1986

Crumlish N, Whitty P, Kamali M, et al: Early insight predicts depression and attempted suicide after 4 years in first-episode schizophrenia and schizophreniform disorder. Acta Psychiatr Scand 112:449–455, 2005

Csernansky JG, Mahmoud R, Brenner R: A comparison of risperidone and haloperidol for the prevention of relapse in patients with schizophrenia. N Engl J Med 346:16–22, 2002

D'Souza DC, Abi-Saab WM, Madonick S, et al: Delta-9-tetrahydrocannabinol effects in schizophrenia: implications for cognition, psychosis, and addiction. Biol Psychiatry 57:594–608, 2005

Dalack GW, Healy DJ, Meador-Woodruff JH: Nicotine dependence in schizophrenia: clinical phenomena and laboratory findings. Am J Psychiatry 155:1490–1501, 1998

David AS, Malmberg A, Brandt L, et al: IQ and risk for schizophrenia: a population-based cohort study. Psychol Med 27:1311–1323, 1997

Davidson M, Harvey PD, Powchik P, et al: Severity of symptoms in chronically institutionalized geriatric schizophrenic patients. Am J Psychiatry 152:197–207, 1995

DeLisi LE: Defining the course of brain structural change and plasticity in schizophrenia. Psychiatry Res 92:1–9, 1999

DeLisi LE, Sakuma M, Tew W, et al: Schizophrenia as a chronic active brain process: a study of progressive brain structural change subsequent to the onset of schizophrenia. Psychiatry Res 74:129–140, 1997

Dickerson F, Boronow JJ, Ringel N, et al: Neurocognitive deficits and social functioning in outpatients with schizophrenia. Schizophr Res 21:75–83, 1996

Dickerson F, Boronow J, Stallings C, et al: Toxoplasma gondii in individuals with schizophrenia: association with clinical and demographic factors and with mortality. Schizophr Bull 33:737–740, 2007

Dickey B, Azeni H: Persons with dual diagnoses of substance abuse and major mental illness: their excess costs of psychiatric care. Am J Public Health 86:973–977, 1996

Dickson RA, Glazer WM: Neuroleptic-induced hyperprolactinemia. Schizophr Res 35 (suppl):S75–S86, 1999

Dilk MN, Bond GR: Meta-analytic evaluation of skills training research for individuals with severe mental illness. J Consult Clin Psychol 64:1337–1346, 1996

Dixon L, Haas G, Weiden P, et al: Acute effects of drug abuse in schizophrenic patients: clinical observations and patients' self-reports. Schizophr Bull 16:69–79, 1990

Dixon L, Weiden P, Delahanty J, et al: Prevalence and correlates of diabetes in national schizophrenia samples. Schizophr Bull 26:903–912, 2000

Docherty JP, Van Kammen DP, Siris SG, et al: Stages of onset of schizophrenic psychosis. Am J Psychiatry 135:420–426, 1978

Drake RE, Mueser KT: Alcohol-use disorder and severe mental illness. Alcohol Health Res World 20:87–93, 1996

Drake RE, Mueser KT: Psychosocial approaches to dual diagnosis. Schizophr Bull 26:105–118, 2000

Drake RE, Mueser KT: Substance abuse comorbidity, in Comprehensive Care of Schizophrenia. Edited by Lieberman JA, Murray RM. London, Martin Dunitz, 2001, pp 243–254

Drake RE, Gates C, Whitaker A, et al: Suicide among schizophrenics: a review. Compr Psychiatry 26:90–100, 1985

Drake RE, Gates C, Cotton PG: Suicide among schizophrenics: a comparison of attempters and completed suicides. Br J Psychiatry 149:784–787, 1986

Drake RE, Xie H, McHugo GJ, et al: The effects of clozapine on alcohol and drug use disorders among patients with schizophrenia. Schizophr Bull 26:441–449, 2000

Drake RE, Essock SM, Shaner A, et al: Implementing dual diagnosis services for clients with severe mental illness. Psychiatr Serv 52:469–476, 2001

Drebing CE, Van Ormer EA, Krebs C, et al: The impact of enhanced incentives on vocational rehabilitation outcomes for dually diagnosed veterans. J Appl Behav Anal 38:359–372, 2005

Eckman TA, Wirshing WC, Marder SR, et al: Technique for training schizophrenic patients in illness self-management: a controlled trial. Am J Psychiatry 149:1549–1555, 1992

Eisen JL, Beer DA, Pato MT, et al: Obsessive-compulsive disorder in patients with schizophrenia or schizoaffective disorder. Am J Psychiatry 154:271–273, 1997

Elvevag B, Goldberg TE: Cognitive impairment in schizophrenia is the core of the disorder. Crit Rev Neurobiol 14:1–21, 2000

Emsley RA, Raniwalla J, Bailey PJ, et al: A comparison of the effects of quetiapine ("Seroquel") and haloperidol in schizophrenic patients with a history of and a demonstrated, partial response to conventional antipsychotic treatment. PRIZE Study Group. Int Clin Psychopharmacol 15:121–131, 2000

Essock SM, Covell NH, Davis SM, et al: Effectiveness of switching antipsychotic medications. Am J Psychiatry 163:2090–2095, 2006

Evins AE, Cather C, Deckersbach T, et al: A double-blind placebo-controlled trial of bupropion sustained-release for smoking cessation in schizophrenia. J Clin Psychopharmacol 25:218–225, 2005

Fadda F, Mosca E, Colombo G, et al: Effect of spontaneous ingestion of ethanol on brain dopamine metabolism. Life Sci 44:281–287, 1989

Falloon IR, Boyd JL, McGill CW, et al: Family management in the prevention of exacerbations of schizophrenia: a controlled study. N Engl J Med 306:1437–1440, 1982

Faraone SV, Chen WJ, Goldstein JM, et al: Gender differences in age at onset of schizophrenia. Br J Psychiatry 164:625–629, 1994

Faraone SV, Green AI, Seidman LJ, et al: "Schizotaxia": clinical implications and new directions for research. Schizophr Bull 27:1–18, 2001

Fenton WS: Comorbid conditions in schizophrenia. Curr Opin Psychiatry 14:17–23, 2001

Fenton WS, McGlashan TH: The prognostic significance of obsessive-compulsive symptoms in schizophrenia. Am J Psychiatry 143:437–441, 1986

Fenton WS, McGlashan TH, Victor BJ, et al: Symptoms, subtype, and suicidality in patients with schizophrenia spectrum disorders. Am J Psychiatry 154:199–204, 1997

Fenton WS, Stover EL, Insel TR: Breaking the log-jam in treatment development for cognition in schizophrenia: NIMH perspective. Psychopharmacology (Berl) 169:365–366, 2003

Freedman B, Chapman LJ: Early subjective experience in schizophrenic episodes. J Abnorm Psychol 82:46–54, 1973

Frith CD, Friston KJ, Herold S, et al: Regional brain activity in chronic schizophrenic patients during the performance of a verbal fluency task. Br J Psychiatry 167:343–349, 1995

Fuster JM: Prefrontal neurons in networks of executive memory. Brain Res Bull 52:331–336, 2000

Geddes JR, Lawrie SM: Obstetric complications and schizophrenia: a meta-analysis. Br J Psychiatry 167:786–793, 1995

George T, Vessicchio J: Nicotine addiction and schizophrenia. Psychiatr Times 18:39–42, 2001

George TP, Sernyak MJ, Ziedonis DM, et al: Effects of clozapine on smoking in chronic schizophrenic outpatients. J Clin Psychiatry 56:344–346, 1995

George TP, Ziedonis DM, Feingold A, et al: Nicotine transdermal patch and atypical antipsychotic medications for smoking cessation in schizophrenia. Am J Psychiatry 157:1835–1842, 2000

George TP, Vessicchio JC, Termine A, et al: A placebo controlled trial of bupropion for smoking cessation in schizophrenia. Biol Psychiatry 52:53–61, 2002

Ghadirian AM, Chouinard G, Annable L: Sexual dysfunction and plasma prolactin levels in neuroleptic-treated schizophrenic outpatients. J Nerv Ment Dis 170:463–467, 1982

Gianfrancesco FD, Grogg AL, Mahmoud RA, et al: Differential effects of risperidone, olanzapine, clozapine, and conventional antipsychotics on type 2 diabetes: findings from a large health plan database. J Clin Psychiatry 63:920–930, 2002

Gitlin M, Nuechterlein K, Subotnik KL, et al: Clinical outcome following neuroleptic discontinuation in patients with remitted recent-onset schizophrenia. Am J Psychiatry 158:1835–1842, 2001

Glazer WM: Expected incidence of tardive dyskinesia associated with atypical antipsychotics. J Clin Psychiatry 61 (suppl 4): 21–26, 2000a

Glazer WM: Extrapyramidal side effects, tardive dyskinesia, and the concept of atypicality. J Clin Psychiatry 61 (suppl 3):16–21, 2000b

Glazer WM: Review of incidence studies of tardive dyskinesia associated with typical antipsychotics. J Clin Psychiatry 61 (suppl 4): 15–20, 2000c

Glynn SM, Sussman S: Why patients smoke. Hosp Community Psychiatry 41:1027–1028, 1990

Glynn SM, Marder SR, Liberman RP, et al: Supplementing clinic-based skills training with manual-based community support sessions: effects on social adjustment of patients with schizophrenia. Am J Psychiatry 159:829–837, 2002

Goeders NE, Smith JE: Reinforcing properties of cocaine in the medial prefrontal cortex: primary action on presynaptic dopaminergic terminals. Pharmacol Biochem Behav 25:191–199, 1986

Goff DC, Tsai G, Manoach DS, et al: D-cycloserine added to clozapine for patients with schizophrenia. Am J Psychiatry 153:1628–1630, 1996

Goff DC, Henderson DC, Evins AE, et al: A placebo-controlled crossover trial of D-cycloserine added to clozapine in patients with schizophrenia. Biol Psychiatry 45:512–514, 1999

Goff DC, Coyle JT: The emerging role of glutamate in the pathophysiology and treatment of schizophrenia. Am J Psychiatry 158:1367–1377, 2001

Goff DC, Sullivan LM, McEvoy JP, et al: A comparison of ten-year cardiac risk estimates in schizophrenia patients from the CATIE study and matched controls. Schizophr Res 80:45–53, 2005

Goldberg TE, Hyde TM, Kleinman JE, et al: Course of schizophrenia: neuropsychological evidence for a static encephalopathy. Schizophr Bull 19:797–804, 1993

Goldberg TE, Weinberger DR: Effects of neuroleptic medications on the cognition of patients with schizophrenia: a review of recent studies. J Clin Psychiatry 57 (suppl 9):62–65, 1996

Goldman-Rakic PS: Regional and cellular fractionation of working memory. Proc Natl Acad Sci U S A 93:13473–13480, 1996

Goldstein G, Haas GL, Pakrashi M, et al: The cycle of schizoaffective disorder, cognitive ability, alcoholism, and suicidality. Suicide Life Threat Behav 36:35–43, 2006

Goldstein MJ, Rodnick EH, Evans JR, et al: Drug and family therapy in the aftercare of acute schizophrenics. Arch Gen Psychiatry 35:1169–1177, 1978

Gottesman II: Schizophrenia Genesis: The Origins of Madness. New York, WH Freeman, 1991

Granholm E, McQuaid JR, McClure FS, et al: A randomized, controlled trial of cognitive behavioral social skills training for middle-aged and older outpatients with chronic schizophrenia. Am J Psychiatry 162:520–529, 2005

Grech A, Van Os J, Murray RM: Influence of cannabis on the outcome of psychosis. Schizophr Res 36:41, 1999

Green AI, Zimmet SV, Strous RD, et al: Clozapine for comorbid substance use disorder and schizophrenia: do patients with schizophrenia have a reward-deficiency syndrome that can be ameliorated by clozapine? Harv Rev Psychiatry 6:287–296, 1999

Green AI, Patel JK, Goisman RM, et al: Weight gain from novel antipsychotic drugs: need for action. Gen Hosp Psychiatry 22:224–235, 2000

Green AI, Burgess ES, Dawson R, et al: Alcohol and cannabis use in schizophrenia: effects of clozapine vs risperidone. Schizophr Res 60:81–85, 2003

Green AI, Tohen MF, Hamer RM, et al: First episode schizophrenia-related psychosis and substance use disorders: acute response to olanzapine and haloperidol. Schizophr Res 66:125–135, 2004

Green AI, Drake RE, Brunette MF, et al: Schizophrenia and co-occurring substance use disorder. Am J Psychiatry 164:402–408, 2007

Green AI, Noordsy DL, Brunette MF, et al: Substance abuse and schizophrenia: pharmacotherapeutic intervention. J Subst Abuse Treat 34:61–71, 2008

Green MF: What are the functional consequences of neurocognitive deficits in schizophrenia? Am J Psychiatry 153:321–330, 1996

Green MF: Recent studies on the neurocognitive effects of second-generation antipsychotic medications. Curr Opin Psychiatry 15:25–29, 2002

Green MF, Nuechterlein KH: Should schizophrenia be treated as a neurocognitive disorder? Schizophr Bull 25:309–319, 1999

Green MF, Kern RS, Braff DL, et al: Neurocognitive deficits and functional outcome in schizophrenia: are we measuring the "right stuff"? Schizophr Bull 26:119–136, 2000

Gupta S, Black DW, Arndt S, et al: Factors associated with suicide attempts among patients with schizophrenia. Psychiatr Serv 49:1353–1355, 1998

Gur RE, Cowell P, Turetsky BI, et al: A follow-up magnetic resonance imaging study of schizophrenia. Relationship of neuroanatomical changes to clinical and neurobehavioral measures. Arch Gen Psychiatry 55:145–152, 1998

Haas GL, Garratt LS, Sweeney JA: Delay to first antipsychotic medication in schizophrenia: impact on symptomatology and clinical course of illness. J Psychiatr Res 32:151–159, 1998

Hafner H, Riecher-Rossler A, Maurer K, et al: First onset and early symptomatology of schizophrenia. A chapter of epidemiological and neurobiological research into age and sex differences. Eur Arch Psychiatry Clin Neurosci 242:109–118, 1992

Hafner H, Maurer K, Loffler W, et al: The influence of age and sex on the onset and early course of schizophrenia. Br J Psychiatry 162:80–86, 1993

Hafner H, Maurer K, Loffler W, et al: The epidemiology of early schizophrenia. Influence of age and gender on onset and early course. Br J Psychiatry Suppl (23):29–38, 1994

Hafner H, Loffler W, Maurer K, et al: Depression, negative symptoms, social stagnation and social decline in the early course of schizophrenia. Acta Psychiatr Scand 100:105–118, 1999

Hafner H, Maurer K, Trendler G, et al: The early course of schizophrenia and depression. Eur Arch Psychiatry Clin Neurosci 255:167–173, 2005

Hambrecht M, Maurer K, Hafner H, et al: Transnational stability of gender differences in schizophrenia? An analysis based on the WHO study on determinants of outcome of severe mental disorders. Eur Arch Psychiatry Clin Neurosci 242:6–12, 1992

Hamoui N, Kingsbury S, Anthone GJ, et al: Surgical treatment of morbid obesity in schizophrenic patients. Obes Surg 14:349–352, 2004

Harding CM, Brooks GW, Ashikaga T, et al: The Vermont longitudinal study of persons with severe mental illness, II: long-term outcome of subjects who retrospectively met DSM-III criteria for schizophrenia. Am J Psychiatry 144:727–735, 1987

Harkavy-Friedman JM, Nelson E: Management of the suicidal patient with schizophrenia. Psychiatr Clin North Am 20:625–640, 1997

Harkavy-Friedman JM, Nelson EA, Venarde DF, et al: Suicidal behavior in schizophrenia and schizoaffective disorder: examining the role of depression. Suicide Life Threat Behav 34:66–76, 2004

Harrison G: Trajectories of psychosis: towards a new social biology of schizophrenia. Epidemiol Psichiatr Soc 13:152–157, 2004

Harrison PJ, Owen MJ: Genes for schizophrenia? Recent findings and their pathophysiological implications. Lancet 361:417–419, 2003

Harvey PD, Keefe RE: Cognition and the new antipsychotics. Journal of Advanced Schizophrenia Brain Research 1:2–8, 1998

Harvey PD, Keefe RS: Studies of cognitive change in patients with schizophrenia following novel antipsychotic treatment. Am J Psychiatry 158:176–184, 2001

Harvey PD, Howanitz E, Parrella M, et al: Symptoms, cognitive functioning, and adaptive skills in geriatric patients with lifelong schizophrenia: a comparison across treatment sites. Am J Psychiatry 155:1080–1086, 1998

Hasan S, Buckley P: Novel antipsychotics and the neuroleptic malignant syndrome: a review and critique. Am J Psychiatry 155:1113–1116, 1998

Hawton K, Sutton L, Haw C, et al: Schizophrenia and suicide: systematic review of risk factors. Br J Psychiatry 187:9–20, 2005

Heckers S, Rauch SL, Goff D, et al: Impaired recruitment of the hippocampus during conscious recollection in schizophrenia. Nat Neurosci 1:318–323, 1998

Heila H, Isometsa ET, Henriksson MM, et al: Suicide and schizophrenia: a nationwide psychological autopsy study on age- and sex-specific clinical characteristics of 92 suicide victims with schizophrenia. Am J Psychiatry 154:1235–1242, 1997

Heila H, Isometsa ET, Henriksson MM, et al: Suicide victims with schizophrenia in different treatment phases and adequacy of antipsychotic medication. J Clin Psychiatry 60:200–208, 1999

Henderson DC, Cagliero E, Gray C, et al: Clozapine, diabetes mellitus, weight gain, and lipid abnormalities: a five-year naturalistic study. Am J Psychiatry 157:975–981, 2000

Hennekens CH, Hennekens AR, Hollar D, et al: Schizophrenia and increased risks of cardiovascular disease. Am Heart J 150:1115–1121, 2005

Heresco-Levy U, Javitt DC, Ermilov M, et al: Double-blind, placebo-controlled, crossover trial of glycine adjuvant therapy for treatment-resistant schizophrenia. Br J Psychiatry 169:610–617, 1996a

Heresco-Levy U, Silipo G, Javitt DC: Glycinergic augmentation of NMDA receptor-mediated neurotransmission in the treatment of schizophrenia. Psychopharmacol Bull 32:731–740, 1996b

Herz MI, Glazer WM, Mostert MA, et al: Intermittent vs maintenance medication in schizophrenia. Two-year results. Arch Gen Psychiatry 48:333–339, 1991

Hinze-Selch D, Daubener W, Eggert L, et al: A controlled prospective study of Toxoplasma gondii infection in individuals with schizophrenia: beyond seroprevalence. Schizophr Bull 33:782–788, 2007

Ho BC, Andreasen NC, Flaum M, et al: Untreated initial psychosis: its relation to quality of life and symptom remission in first-episode schizophrenia. Am J Psychiatry 157:808–815, 2000

Hodel B, Brenner HD: Cognitive therapy with schizophrenic patients: conceptual basis, present state, future directions. Acta Psychiatr Scand Suppl 384:108–115, 1994

Hogarty GE, Anderson CM, Reiss DJ, et al: Family psychoeducation, social skills training, and maintenance chemotherapy in the aftercare treatment of schizophrenia, I: one-year effects of a controlled study on relapse and expressed emotion. Arch Gen Psychiatry 43:633–642, 1986

Hogarty GE, McEvoy JP, Ulrich RF, et al: Pharmacotherapy of impaired affect in recovering schizophrenic patients. Arch Gen Psychiatry 52:29, 1995

Hogarty GE, Greenwald D, Ulrich RF, et al: Three-year trials of personal therapy among schizophrenic patients living with or independent of family, II: effects on adjustment of patients. Am J Psychiatry 154:1514–1524, 1997a

Hogarty GE, Kornblith SJ, Greenwald D, et al: Three-year trials of personal therapy among schizophrenic patients living with or independent of family, I: description of study and effects on relapse rates. Am J Psychiatry 154:1504–1513, 1997b

Hogarty GE, Flesher S, Ulrich R, et al: Cognitive enhancement therapy for schizophrenia: effects of a 2-year randomized trial on cognition and behavior. Arch Gen Psychiatry 61:866–876, 2004

Hogarty GE, Greenwald DP, Eack SM: Durability and mechanism of effects of cognitive enhancement therapy. Psychiatr Serv 57:1751–1757, 2006

Huber G, Gross G, Schuttler R, et al: Longitudinal studies of schizophrenic patients. Schizophr Bull 6:592–605, 1980

Huber TJ, Borsutzky M, Schneider U, et al: Psychotic disorders and gonadal function: evidence supporting the oestrogen hypothesis. Acta Psychiatr Scand 109:269–274, 2004

Huckans MS, Blackwell AD, Harms TA, et al: Management of hepatitis C disease among VA patients with schizophrenia and substance use disorders. Psychiatr Serv 57:403–406, 2006

Hummer M, Malik P, Gasser RW, et al: Osteoporosis in patients with schizophrenia. Am J Psychiatry 162:162–167, 2005

Hunt IM, Kapur N, Windfuhr K, et al: Suicide in schizophrenia: findings from a national clinical survey. J Psychiatr Pract 12:139–147, 2006

Hurlburt MS, Hough RL, Wood PA: Effects of substance abuse on housing stability of homeless mentally ill persons in supported housing. Psychiatr Serv 47:731–736, 1996a

Hurlburt MS, Wood PA, Hough RL: Providing independent housing for the homeless mentally ill: a novel approach to evaluating long-term longitudinal housing patterns. Journal of Community Psychology 24:291–310, 1996b

Huttenlocher PR: Neural Plasticity: The Effects of Environment on the Development of the Cerebral Cortex. Cambridge, MA, Harvard University Press, 2002

Hwang MY, Morgan JE, Losconzcy MF: Clinical and neuropsychological profiles of obsessive-compulsive schizophrenia: a pilot study. J Neuropsychiatry Clin Neurosci 12:91–94, 2000

Hyman SE, Fenton WS: Medicine. What are the right targets for psychopharmacology? Science 299:350–351, 2003

Ingvar DH, Franzen G: Abnormalities of cerebral blood flow distribution in patients with chronic schizophrenia. Acta Psychiatr Scand 50:425–462, 1974

Iqbal Z, Birchwood M, Chadwick P, et al: Cognitive approach to depression and suicidal thinking in psychosis, II: testing the validity of a social ranking model. Br J Psychiatry 177:522–528, 2000

Isomaa B, Almgren P, Tuomi T, et al: Cardiovascular morbidity and mortality associated with the metabolic syndrome. Diabetes Care 24:683–689, 2001

Jablensky A, Sartorius N, Ernberg G, et al: Schizophrenia: manifestations, incidence and course in different cultures. A World Health Organization ten-country study. Psychol Med Monogr Suppl 20:1–97, 1992

Javitt DC: Is the glycine site half saturated or half unsaturated? Effects of glutamatergic drugs in schizophrenia patients. Curr Opin Psychiatry 19:151–157, 2006

Javitt DC, Coyle JT: Decoding schizophrenia. Sci Am 290:48–55, 2004

Javitt DC, Zukin SR: Recent advances in the phencyclidine model of schizophrenia. Am J Psychiatry 148:1301–1308, 1991

Javitt DC, Silipo G, Cienfuegos A, et al: Adjunctive high-dose glycine in the treatment of schizophrenia. Int J Neuropsychopharmacol 4:385–391, 2001

Jeste DV: Tardive dyskinesia in older patients. J Clin Psychiatry 61 (suppl 4):27–32, 2000

Jeste DV, Lacro JP, Bailey A: Lower incidence of tardive dyskinesia with risperidone compared with haloperidol in older patients. Presented at the 21st Congress of the Collegium Internationale Neuro-Psychopharmacologicum, Glasgow, Scotland, July 12–16, 1998

Jin H, Meyer JM, Jeste DV: Atypical antipsychotics and glucose dysregulation: a systematic review. Schizophr Res 71:195–212, 2004

Johnson DA: Antipsychotic medication: clinical guidelines for maintenance therapy. J Clin Psychiatry 46:6–15, 1985

Johnstone EC, Crow TJ, Johnson AL, et al: The Northwick Park Study of first episodes of schizophrenia, I: presentation of the illness and problems relating to admission. Br J Psychiatry 148:115–120, 1986

Jolley AG, Hirsch SR, Morrison E, et al: Trial of brief intermittent neuroleptic prophylaxis for selected schizophrenic outpatients: clinical and social outcome at two years. BMJ 301:837–842, 1990

Jones C, Cormac I, Silveira da Mota Neto JI, et al: Cognitive behaviour therapy for schizophrenia. Cochrane Database Syst Rev (4):CD000524, 2004

Jones PB, Barnes TR, Davies L, et al: Randomized controlled trial of the effect on Quality of Life of second- vs first-generation antipsychotic drugs in schizophrenia: Cost Utility of the Latest Antipsychotic Drugs in Schizophrenia Study (CUtLASS 1). Arch Gen Psychiatry 63:1079–1087, 2006

Kampman O, Lehtinen K: Compliance in psychoses. Acta Psychiatr Scand 100:167–175, 1999

Kane JM: Tardive dyskinesia rates with atypical antipsychotics in adults: prevalence and incidence. J Clin Psychiatry 65 (suppl 9): 16–20, 2004

Kane JM, Rifkin A, Quitkin F, et al: Fluphenazine vs placebo in patients with remitted, acute first-episode schizophrenia. Arch Gen Psychiatry 39:70–73, 1982

Kane JM, Honigfeld G, Singer J, et al: Clozapine for the treatment-resistant schizophrenic. A double-blind comparison with chlorpromazine. Arch Gen Psychiatry 45:789–796, 1988

Kane JM, Woerner MG, Pollack S, et al: Does clozapine cause tardive dyskinesia? J Clin Psychiatry 54:327–330, 1993

Kane JM, Handan G, Malhotra AK: Clozapine, in Current Issues in the Psychopharmacology of Schizophrenia. Edited by Breier A, Tran PV, Herrea JM, et al. Philadelphia, PA, Lippincott Williams & Wilkins, 2001, pp 209–223

Kane JM, Khanna S, Rajadhyaksha S, et al: Efficacy and tolerability of ziprasidone in patients with treatment-resistant schizophrenia. Int Clin Psychopharmacol 21:21–28, 2006

Kane JM, Meltzer HY, Carson WH Jr, et al: Aripiprazole for treatment-resistant schizophrenia: results of a multicenter, randomized, double-blind, comparison study versus perphenazine. J Clin Psychiatry 68:213–223, 2007

Kaplan KJ, Harrow M: Positive and negative symptoms as risk factors for later suicidal activity in schizophrenics versus depressives. Suicide Life Threat Behav 26:105–121, 1996

Kapur S, Remington G: Serotonin-dopamine interaction and its relevance to schizophrenia. Am J Psychiatry 153:466–476, 1996

Kapur S, Remington G: Dopamine D(2) receptors and their role in atypical antipsychotic action: still necessary and may even be sufficient. Biol Psychiatry 50:873–883, 2001

Kasai K, Shenton ME, Salisbury DF, et al: Progressive decrease of left Heschl gyrus and planum temporale gray matter volume in first-episode schizophrenia: a longitudinal magnetic resonance imaging study. Arch Gen Psychiatry 60:766–775, 2003a

Kasai K, Shenton ME, Salisbury DF, et al: Progressive decrease of left superior temporal gyrus gray matter volume in patients with first-episode schizophrenia. Am J Psychiatry 160:156–164, 2003b

Keck PE Jr, McElroy SL, Strakowski SM, et al: Antipsychotics in the treatment of mood disorders and risk of tardive dyskinesia. J Clin Psychiatry 61 (suppl 4):33–38, 2000

Keefe RS, Bilder RM, Davis SM, et al: Neurocognitive effects of antipsychotic medications in patients with chronic schizophrenia in the CATIE Trial. Arch Gen Psychiatry 64:633–647, 2007

Kelly DL, Shim JC, Feldman SM, et al: Lifetime psychiatric symptoms in persons with schizophrenia who died by suicide compared to other means of death. J Psychiatr Res 38:531–536, 2004

Kendler KS: Overview: a current perspective on twin studies of schizophrenia. Am J Psychiatry 140:1413–1425, 1983

Kety SS, Rosenthal D, Wender PH: The types and prevalence of mental illness in the biological and adoptive families of adopted schizophrenics. J Psychiatr Res 1:345–362, 1964

Kety SS, Wender PH, Jacobsen B, et al: Mental illness in the biological and adoptive relatives of schizophrenic adoptees. Replication of the Copenhagen Study in the rest of Denmark. Arch Gen Psychiatry 51:442–455, 1994

Khantzian EJ: The self-medication hypothesis of addictive disorders: focus on heroin and cocaine dependence. Am J Psychiatry 142:1259–1264, 1985

Kim CH, Jayathilake K, Meltzer HY: Hopelessness, neurocognitive function, and insight in schizophrenia: relationship to suicidal behavior. Schizophr Res 60:71–80, 2003

Kingsbury SJ, Fayek M, Trufasiu D, et al: The apparent effects of ziprasidone on plasma lipids and glucose. J Clin Psychiatry 62:347–349, 2001

Kinon BJ: The routine use of atypical antipsychotic agents: maintenance treatment. J Clin Psychiatry 59 (suppl 19):18–22, 1998

Kinon BJ, Ahl J, Liu-Seifert H, et al: Improvement in hyperprolactinemia and reproductive comorbidities in patients with schizophrenia switched from conventional antipsychotics or risperidone to olanzapine. Psychoneuroendocrinology 31:577–588, 2006

Kirli S, Caliskan M: A comparative study of sertraline versus imipramine in postpsychotic depressive disorder of schizophrenia. Schizophr Res 33:103–111, 1998

Kissling WJ, Kane JM, Barnes TRE, et al: Guidelines for neuroleptic relapse prevention in schizophrenia: towards a consensus view, in Guidelines for Neuroleptic Relapse Prevention in Schizophrenia. Edited by Kissling WJ. Berlin, Germany, Springer-Verlag, 1991, pp 155–163

Kleinberg DL, Davis JM, de Coster R, et al: Prolactin levels and adverse events in patients treated with risperidone. J Clin Psychopharmacol 19:57–61, 1999

Knott V, McIntosh J, Millar A, et al: Nicotine and smoker status moderate brain electric and mood activation induced by ketamine, an N-methyl-D-aspartate (NMDA) receptor antagonist. Pharmacol Biochem Behav 85:228–242, 2006

Kofoed L, Kania J, Walsh T, et al: Outpatient treatment of patients with substance abuse and coexisting psychiatric disorders. Am J Psychiatry 143:867–872, 1986

Koller EA, Doraiswamy PM: Olanzapine-associated diabetes mellitus. Pharmacotherapy 22:841–852, 2002

Koller E, Schneider B, Bennett K, et al: Clozapine-associated diabetes. Am J Med 111:716–723, 2001

Koller EA, Cross JT, Doraiswamy PM, et al: Risperidone-associated diabetes mellitus: a pharmacovigilance study. Pharmacotherapy 23:735–744, 2003

Kopala L, Honer WG: Risperidone, serotonergic mechanisms, and obsessive-compulsive symptoms in schizophrenia. Am J Psychiatry 151:1714–1715, 1994

Kopelowicz A, Liberman RP, Zarate R: Recent advances in social skills training for schizophrenia. Schizophr Bull 32 (suppl 1): S12–S23, 2006

Koppel BS: Neuroleptic malignant syndrome, in Principles and Practices of Emergency Medicine, 4th Edition. Edited by Schwartz GR, Hanke BK, Mayer TA. Baltimore, MD, Williams & Wilkins, 1998, pp 1155–1605

Koreen AR, Siris SG, Chakos M, et al: Depression in first-episode schizophrenia. Am J Psychiatry 150:1643–1648, 1993

Kraepelin E: Dementia Praecox and Paraphrenia (1919). New York, Robert E Krieger, 1971

Kramer M, Simpson G, Maciulis V, et al: Paliperidone extended-release tablets for prevention of symptom recurrence in patients with schizophrenia: a randomized, double-blind, placebo-controlled study. J Clin Psychopharmacol 27:6–14, 2007

Krystal JH, Karper LP, Seibyl JP, et al: Subanesthetic effects of the noncompetitive NMDA antagonist, ketamine, in humans. Psychotomimetic, perceptual, cognitive, and neuroendocrine responses. Arch Gen Psychiatry 51:199–214, 1994

Kuo CJ, Tsai SY, Lo CH, et al: Risk factors for completed suicide in schizophrenia. J Clin Psychiatry 66:579–585, 2005

Lane A, Kinsella A, Murphy P, et al: The anthropometric assessment of dysmorphic features in schizophrenia as an index of its developmental origins. Psychol Med 27:1155–1164, 1997

Lauriello J, Bustillo J, Keith SJ: A critical review of research on psychosocial treatment of schizophrenia. Biol Psychiatry 46:1409–1417, 1999

Lawrie SM, Byrne M, Miller P, et al: Neurodevelopmental indices and the development of psychotic symptoms in subjects at high risk of schizophrenia. Br J Psychiatry 178:524–530, 2001

Lee ML, Dickson RA, Campbell M, et al: Clozapine and substance abuse in patients with schizophrenia. Can J Psychiatry 43:855–856, 1998

Lehman AF: Vocational rehabilitation in schizophrenia. Schizophr Bull 21:645–656, 1995

Lehmann HE, Hanrahan GE: Chlorpromazine: new inhibiting agent for psychomotor excitement and manic states. AMA Arch Neurol Psychiatry 71:227–237, 1954

Leucht S, Barnes TR, Kissling W, et al: Relapse prevention in schizophrenia with new-generation antipsychotics: a systematic review and exploratory meta-analysis of randomized, controlled trials. Am J Psychiatry 160:1209–1222, 2003a

Leucht S, Wahlbeck K, Hamann J, et al: New generation antipsychotics versus low-potency conventional antipsychotics: a systematic review and meta-analysis. Lancet 361:1581–1589, 2003b

Leucht S: Amisulpride: a selective dopamine antagonist and atypical antipsychotic: results of a meta-analysis of randomized controlled trials. Int J Neuropsychopharmacol 7 (suppl 1): S15–S20, 2004

Levinson DF, Umapathy C, Musthaq M: Treatment of schizoaffective disorder and schizophrenia with mood symptoms. Am J Psychiatry 156:1138–1148, 1999

Lewis DA, Gonzalez-Burgos G: Pathophysiologically based treatment interventions in schizophrenia. Nat Med 12:1016–1022, 2006

Lewis DA, Levitt P: Schizophrenia as a disorder of neurodevelopment. Annu Rev Neurosci 25:409–432, 2002

Lewis DA, Lieberman JA: Catching up on schizophrenia: natural history and neurobiology. Neuron 28:325–334, 2000

Lewis DA, Hashimoto T, Volk DW: Cortical inhibitory neurons and schizophrenia. Nat Rev Neurosci 6:312–324, 2005

Lewis SW, Davies L, Jones PB, et al: Randomised controlled trials of conventional antipsychotic versus new atypical drugs, and new atypical drugs versus clozapine, in people with schizophrenia responding poorly to, or intolerant of, current drug treatment. Health Technol Assess 10:iii–iv, ix–xi, 1–165, 2006

Liberman RP, Wallace CJ, Blackwell G, et al: Skills training versus psychosocial occupational therapy for persons with persistent schizophrenia. Am J Psychiatry 155:1087–1091, 1998

Liddle PF, Barnes TR, Morris D, et al: Three syndromes in chronic schizophrenia. Br J Psychiatry Suppl (7):119–122, 1989

Lieberman JA: Is schizophrenia a neurodegenerative disorder? A clinical and neurobiological perspective. Biol Psychiatry 46:729–739, 1999

Lieberman JA: Neurobiology and the natural history of schizophrenia. J Clin Psychiatry 67:e14, 2006

Lieberman JA, Saltz BL, Johns CA, et al: The effects of clozapine on tardive dyskinesia. Br J Psychiatry 158:503–510, 1991

Lieberman JA, Jody D, Geisler S, et al: Time course and biologic correlates of treatment response in first-episode schizophrenia. Arch Gen Psychiatry 50:369–376, 1993

Lieberman JA, Stroup TS, McEvoy JP, et al: Effectiveness of antipsychotic drugs in patients with chronic schizophrenia. N Engl J Med 353:1209–1223, 2005

Littrell KH, Petty RG, Hilligoss NM, et al: Olanzapine treatment for patients with schizophrenia and substance abuse. J Subst Abuse Treat 21:217–221, 2001

Loebel AD, Lieberman JA, Alvir JM, et al: Duration of psychosis and outcome in first-episode schizophrenia. Am J Psychiatry 149:1183–1188, 1992

Loh C, Meyer JM, Leckband SG: A comprehensive review of behavioral interventions for weight management in schizophrenia. Ann Clin Psychiatry 18:23–31, 2006

Lysaker P, Bell M, Beam-Goulet J, et al: Relationship of positive and negative symptoms to cocaine abuse in schizophrenia. J Nerv Ment Dis 182:109–112, 1994

Macleod J, Davey Smith G, Hickman M: Does cannabis use cause schizophrenia? Lancet 367:1055, 2006

Mandel MR, Severe JB, Schooler NR, et al: Development and prediction of postpsychotic depression in neuroleptic-treated schizophrenics. Arch Gen Psychiatry 39:197–203, 1982

Manoach DS, Press DZ, Thangaraj V, et al: Schizophrenic subjects activate dorsolateral prefrontal cortex during a working memory task, as measured by fMRI. Biol Psychiatry 45:1128–1137, 1999

Marder SR: Integrating pharmacological and psychosocial treatments for schizophrenia. Acta Psychiatr Scand Suppl (407): 87–90, 2000

Marder SR: Drug initiatives to improve cognitive function. J Clin Psychiatry 67 (suppl 9):31–35; discussion 36–42, 2006

Marder SR, Wirshing WC, Mintz J, et al: Two-year outcome of social skills training and group psychotherapy for outpatients with schizophrenia. Am J Psychiatry 153:1585–1592, 1996

Marder SR, Davis JM, Chouinard G: The effects of risperidone on the five dimensions of schizophrenia derived by factor analysis: combined results of the North American trials. J Clin Psychiatry 58:538–546, 1997

Marder SR, Essock SM, Miller AL, et al: The Mount Sinai conference on the pharmacotherapy of schizophrenia. Schizophr Bull 28:5–16, 2002

Marder SR, Essock SM, Miller AL, et al: Physical health monitoring of patients with schizophrenia. Am J Psychiatry 161:1334–1349, 2004

Margolese HC, Chouinard G, Kolivakis TT, et al: Tardive dyskinesia in the era of typical and atypical antipsychotics, part 2: incidence and management strategies in patients with schizophrenia. Can J Psychiatry 50:703–714, 2005

Martin LF, Leonard S, Hall MH, et al: Sensory gating and alpha-7 nicotinic receptor gene allelic variants in schizoaffective disorder, bipolar type. Am J Med Genet B Neuropsychiatr Genet 144:611–614, 2007

May PR, Tuma AH, Dixon WJ: For better or worse? Outcome variance with psychotherapy and other treatments for schizophrenia. J Nerv Ment Dis 165:231–239, 1978

McEvoy JP, Freudenreich O, Levin ED, et al: Haloperidol increases smoking in patients with schizophrenia. Psychopharmacology (Berl) 119:124–126, 1995a

McEvoy J, Freudenreich O, McGee M, et al: Clozapine decreases smoking in patients with chronic schizophrenia. Biol Psychiatry 37:550–552, 1995b

McEvoy JP, Meyer JM, Goff DC, et al: Prevalence of the metabolic syndrome in patients with schizophrenia: baseline results from the Clinical Antipsychotic Trials of Intervention Effectiveness (CATIE) schizophrenia trial and comparison with national estimates from NHANES III. Schizophr Res 80:19–32, 2005

McEvoy JP, Lieberman JA, Stroup TS, et al: Effectiveness of clozapine versus olanzapine, quetiapine, and risperidone in patients with chronic schizophrenia who did not respond to prior atypical antipsychotic treatment. Am J Psychiatry 163:600–610, 2006

McGlashan TH: The profiles of clinical deterioration in schizophrenia. J Psychiatr Res 32:133–141, 1998

McGlashan TH: Duration of untreated psychosis in first-episode schizophrenia: marker or determinant of course? Biol Psychiatry 46:899–907, 1999

McGlashan TH, Carpenter WT Jr: Postpsychotic depression in schizophrenia. Arch Gen Psychiatry 33:231–239, 1976

McGlashan TH, Addington J, Cannon T, et al: Recruitment and treatment practices for help-seeking "prodromal" patients. Schizophr Bull 33:715–726, 2007

McGorry PD, McFarlane C, Patton GC, et al: The prevalence of prodromal features of schizophrenia in adolescence: a preliminary survey. Acta Psychiatr Scand 92:241–249, 1995

McGorry PD, Yung AR, Phillips LJ, et al: Randomized controlled trial of interventions designed to reduce the risk of progression to first-episode psychosis in a clinical sample with subthreshold symptoms. Arch Gen Psychiatry 59:921–928, 2002

McGurk SR, Mueser KT, Feldman K, et al: Cognitive training for supported employment: 2–3 year outcomes of a randomized controlled trial. Am J Psychiatry 164:437–441, 2007

Mednick SA, Machon RA, Huttunen MO, et al: Adult schizophrenia following prenatal exposure to an influenza epidemic. Arch Gen Psychiatry 45:189–192, 1988

Meehl PE: Schizotaxia, schizotypy, schizophrenia. Am Psychol 17:827–838, 1962

Meehl PE: Schizotaxia revisited. Arch Gen Psychiatry 46:935–944, 1989

Melle I, Johannesen JO, Friis S, et al: Early detection of the first episode of schizophrenia and suicidal behavior. Am J Psychiatry 163:800–804, 2006

Meltzer HY: Long-term effects of neuroleptic drugs on the neuroendocrine system. Adv Biochem Psychopharmacol 40:59–68, 1985

Meltzer HY: Clinical studies on the mechanism of action of clozapine: the dopamine-serotonin hypothesis of schizophrenia. Psychopharmacology (Berl) 99 (suppl):S18–S27, 1989

Meltzer HY, Alphs L, Green AI, et al: Clozapine treatment for suicidality in schizophrenia: International Suicide Prevention Trial (InterSePT). Arch Gen Psychiatry 60:82–91, 2003

Meyer JM, Koro CE: The effects of antipsychotic therapy on serum lipids: a comprehensive review. Schizophr Res 70:1–17, 2004

Meyer J, Nasrallah H: Medical Illness and Schizophrenia. American Psychiatric Publishing, 2003

Miller DD, McEvoy JP, Davis SM, et al: Clinical correlates of tardive dyskinesia in schizophrenia: baseline data from the CATIE schizophrenia trial. Schizophr Res 80:33–43, 2005

Minkoff K: An integrated treatment model for dual diagnosis of psychosis and addiction. Hosp Community Psychiatry 40:1031–1036, 1989

Moghaddam B: Targeting metabotropic glutamate receptors for treatment of the cognitive symptoms of schizophrenia. Psychopharmacology (Berl) 174:39–44, 2004

Moghaddam B, Jackson M: Effect of stress on prefrontal cortex function. Neurotox Res 6:73–78, 2004

Montero I, Hernandez I, Asencio A, et al: Do all people with schizophrenia receive the same benefit from different family intervention programs? Psychiatry Res 133:187–195, 2005

Montross LP, Zisook S, Kasckow J: Suicide among patients with schizophrenia: a consideration of risk and protective factors. Ann Clin Psychiatry 17:173–182, 2005

Morrison D, Clark D, Goldfarb E, et al: Worsening of obsessive-compulsive symptoms following treatment with olanzapine. Am J Psychiatry 155:855, 1998

Mortensen PB, Norgaard-Pedersen B, Waltoft BL, et al: Early infections of Toxoplasma gondii and the later development of schizophrenia. Schizophr Bull 33:741–744, 2007

Mueser KT, Bennett M, Kushner MG: Epidemiology of substance use disorders among persons with chronic mental illnesses, in Double Jeopardy: Chronic Mental Illness and Substance Abuse. Edited by Lehman AF, Dixon L. New York, Harwood Academic Publishers, 1995, pp 9–25

Mueser KT, Bond GR, Drake RE, et al: Models of community care for severe mental illness: a review of research on case management. Schizophr Bull 24:37–74, 1998

Mueser KT, Noordsy DL, Fox L, et al: Disulfiram treatment for alcoholism in severe mental illness. Am J Addict 12:242–252, 2003

Mueser KT, Meyer PS, Penn DL, et al: The Illness Management and Recovery program: rationale, development, and preliminary findings. Schizophr Bull 32 (suppl 1):S32–S43, 2006

Mukherjee S, Decina P, Bocola V, et al: Diabetes mellitus in schizophrenic patients. Compr Psychiatry 37:68–73, 1996

Muller P, Bandelow B, Gaebel W, et al: Intermittent medication, coping and psychotherapy. Interactions in relapse prevention and course modification. Br J Psychiatry Suppl (18):140–144, 1992

Murray RM: Neurodevelopmental schizophrenia: the rediscovery of dementia praecox. Br J Psychiatry Suppl (25):6–12, 1994

Negrete JC, Knapp WP, Douglas DE, et al: Cannabis affects the severity of schizophrenic symptoms: results of a clinical survey. Psychol Med 16:515–520, 1986

Nelson HE, Pantelis C, Carruthers K, et al: Cognitive functioning and symptomatology in chronic schizophrenia. Psychol Med 20:357–365, 1990

Newcomer JW, Farber NB, Jevtovic-Todorovic V, et al: Ketamine-induced NMDA receptor hypofunction as a model of memory impairment and psychosis. Neuropsychopharmacology 20:106–118, 1999

Noordsy DL, O'Keefe C, Mueser KT, et al: Six-month outcomes for patients who switched to olanzapine treatment. Psychiatr Serv 52:501–507, 2001

Nuechterlein KH, Dawson ME: Information processing and attentional functioning in the developmental course of schizophrenic disorders. Schizophr Bull 10:160–203, 1984

O'Donnell P, Lewis BL, Weinberger DR, et al: Neonatal hippocampal damage alters electrophysiological properties of prefrontal cortical neurons in adult rats. Cereb Cortex 12:975–982, 2002

O'Keane V, Meaney AM: Antipsychotic drugs: a new risk factor for osteoporosis in young women with schizophrenia? J Clin Psychopharmacol 25:26–31, 2005

Ohlsen RI, Pilowsky LS: The place of partial agonism in psychiatry: recent developments. J Psychopharmacol 19:408–413, 2005

Olney JW, Farber NB: Glutamate receptor dysfunction and schizophrenia. Arch Gen Psychiatry 52:998–1007, 1995

Ongur D, Goff DC: Obsessive-compulsive symptoms in schizophrenia: associated clinical features, cognitive function and medication status. Schizophr Res 75:349–362, 2005

Osher FC, Kofoed LL: Treatment of patients with psychiatric and psychoactive substance abuse disorders. Hosp Community Psychiatry 40:1025–1030, 1989

Osher FC, Goldberg RW, McNary SW, et al: Substance abuse and the transmission of hepatitis C among persons with severe mental illness. Psychiatr Serv 54:842–847, 2003

Osser DN: Neuroleptic-induced pseudoparkinsonism, in Movement Disorders in Neurology and Neuropsychiatry. Edited by Joseph AB, Young RR. Malden, MA, Blackwell Science, 1999, pp 61–68

Osser DN, Najarian DM, Dufresne RL: Olanzapine increases weight and serum triglyceride levels. J Clin Psychiatry 60:767–770, 1999

Pantelis C, Velakoulis D, McGorry PD, et al: Neuroanatomical abnormalities before and after onset of psychosis: a cross-sectional and longitudinal MRI comparison. Lancet 361:281–288, 2003

Park S, Holzman PS: Schizophrenics show spatial working memory deficits. Arch Gen Psychiatry 49:975–982, 1992

Park S, Holzman PS, Goldman-Rakic PS: Spatial working memory deficits in the relatives of schizophrenic patients. Arch Gen Psychiatry 52:821–828, 1995

Patil ST, Zhang L, Martenyi F, et al: Activation of mGlu2/3 receptors as a new approach to treat schizophrenia: a randomized phase 2 clinical trial. Nat Med 13:1102–1107, 2007

Penn DL, Mueser KT: Research update on the psychosocial treatment of schizophrenia. Am J Psychiatry 153:607–617, 1996

Penn DL, Addington J, Pinkham A: Social cognitive impairments, in Textbook of Schizophrenia. Edited by Lieberman JA, Stroup TS, Perkins DO. Washington, DC, American Psychiatric Publishing, 2006, pp 261–274

Perala J, Suvisaari J, Saarni SI, et al: Lifetime prevalence of psychotic and bipolar I disorders in a general population. Arch Gen Psychiatry 64:19–28, 2007

Petrakis IL, O'Malley S, Rounsaville B, et al: Naltrexone augmentation of neuroleptic treatment in alcohol abusing patients with schizophrenia. Psychopharmacology (Berl) 172:291–297, 2004

Petrakis IL, Poling J, Levinson C, et al: Naltrexone and disulfiram in patients with alcohol dependence and comorbid psychiatric disorders. Biol Psychiatry 57:1128–1137, 2005

Petrakis IL, Leslie D, Finney JW, et al: Atypical antipsychotic medication and substance use-related outcomes in the treatment of schizophrenia. Am J Addict 15:44–49, 2006

Pfohl B, Winokur G: The evolution of symptoms in institutionalized hebephrenic/catatonic schizophrenics. Br J Psychiatry 141:567–572, 1982

Phillips SD, Burns BJ, Edgar ER, et al: Moving assertive community treatment into standard practice. Psychiatr Serv 52:771–779, 2001

Pietzcker A, Gaebel W, Kopcke W: Intermittent versus maintenance neuroleptic long-term treatment in schizophrenia: 2 year results of German multicenter study. J Psychiatr Res 27:321–339, 1993

Pilling S, Bebbington P, Kuipers E, et al: Psychological treatments in schizophrenia, II: meta-analyses of randomized controlled trials of social skills training and cognitive remediation. Psychol Med 32:783–791, 2002

Pilowsky LS, Kerwin RW, Murray RM: Schizophrenia: a neurodevelopmental perspective. Neuropsychopharmacology 9:83–91, 1993

Pitschel-Walz G, Leucht S, Bauml J, et al: The effect of family interventions on relapse and rehospitalization in schizophrenia—a meta-analysis. Schizophr Bull 27:73–92, 2001

Porteous DJ, Thomson P, Brandon NJ, et al: The genetics and biology of DISC1—an emerging role in psychosis and cognition. Biol Psychiatry 60:123–131, 2006

Potkin SG, Jin Y, Bunney BG, et al: Effect of clozapine and adjunctive high-dose glycine in treatment-resistant schizophrenia. Am J Psychiatry 156:145–147, 1999

Potkin SG, Alphs L, Hsu C, et al: Predicting suicidal risk in schizophrenic and schizoaffective patients in a prospective two-year trial. Biol Psychiatry 54:444–452, 2003

Potvin S, Stip E, Lipp O, et al: Quetiapine in patients with comorbid schizophrenia-spectrum and substance use disorders: an open-label trial. Curr Med Res Opin 22:1277–1285, 2006

Poyurovsky M, Dorfman-Etrog P, Hermesh H, et al: Beneficial effect of olanzapine in schizophrenic patients with obsessive-compulsive symptoms. Int Clin Psychopharmacol 15:169–173, 2000

Qin P, Nordentoft M: Suicide risk in relation to psychiatric hospitalization: evidence based on longitudinal registers. Arch Gen Psychiatry 62:427–432, 2005

Radomsky ED, Haas GL, Mann JJ, et al: Suicidal behavior in patients with schizophrenia and other psychotic disorders. Am J Psychiatry 156:1590–1595, 1999

Ran MS, Xiang MZ, Mao WJ, et al: Characteristics of suicide attempters and nonattempters with schizophrenia in a rural community. Suicide Life Threat Behav 35:694–701, 2005

Rapp CA, Goscha RJ: The principles of effective case management of mental health services. Psychiatr Rehabil J 27:319–333, 2004

Regier DA, Farmer ME, Rae DS, et al: Comorbidity of mental disorders with alcohol and other drug abuse. Results from the Epidemiologic Catchment Area (ECA) Study. JAMA 264:2511–2518, 1990

Remington G, Kapur S: Neuroleptic-induced extrapyramidal symptoms and the role of combined serotonin/dopamine antagonist. J Clin Psychiatry 14:14–24, 1996

Remington G, Kapur S, Zipursky R: APA Practice guideline for schizophrenia: risperidone equivalents. American Psychiatric Association. Am J Psychiatry 155:1301–1302, 1998

Riecher-Rossler A, Hafner H, Stumbaum M, et al: Can estradiol modulate schizophrenic symptomatology? Schizophr Bull 20:203–214, 1994

Ries RK, Dyck DG, Short R, et al: Outcomes of managing disability benefits among patients with substance dependence and severe mental illness. Psychiatr Serv 55:445–447, 2004

Ripoll N, Bronnec M, Bourin M: Nicotinic receptors and schizophrenia. Curr Med Res Opin 20:1057–1074, 2004

Robinson DG, Woerner MG, Alvir JM, et al: Predictors of treatment response from a first episode of schizophrenia or schizoaffective disorder. Am J Psychiatry 156:544–549, 1999

Rog DJ: The evidence on supported housing. Psychiatr Rehabil J 27:334–344, 2004

Rolfe TJ, McGory P, Cooks J, et al: Cannabis use in first episode psychosis: incidence and short-term outcome. Schizophr Res 36:313, 1999

Rosenberg SD, Goodman LA, Osher FC, et al: Prevalence of HIV, hepatitis B, and hepatitis C in people with severe mental illness. Am J Public Health 91:31–37, 2001

Rosenheck RA, Leslie DL, Sindelar J, et al: Cost-effectiveness of second-generation antipsychotics and perphenazine in a randomized trial of treatment for chronic schizophrenia. Am J Psychiatry 163:2080–2089, 2006

Ross CA, Margolis RL, Reading SA, et al: Neurobiology of schizophrenia. Neuron 52:139–153, 2006

Rossau CD, Mortensen PB: Risk factors for suicide in patients with schizophrenia: nested case-control study. Br J Psychiatry 171:355–359, 1997

Rosso IM, Bearden CE, Hollister JM, et al: Childhood neuromotor dysfunction in schizophrenia patients and their unaffected siblings: a prospective cohort study. Schizophr Bull 26:367–378, 2000

Roth RM, Brunette MF, Green AI: Treatment of substance use disorders in schizophrenia: a unifying neurobiological mechanism? Curr Psychiatry Rep 7:283–291, 2005

Roy A: Risk factors for suicide in psychiatric patients. Arch Gen Psychiatry 39:1089–1095, 1982a

Roy A: Suicide in chronic schizophrenia. Br J Psychiatry 141:171–177, 1982b

Rubio G, Martinez I, Ponce G, et al: Long-acting injectable risperidone compared with zuclopenthixol in the treatment of schizophrenia with substance abuse comorbidity. Can J Psychiatry 51:531–539, 2006

Russell AJ, Munro JC, Jones PB, et al: Schizophrenia and the myth of intellectual decline. Am J Psychiatry 154:635–639, 1997

Sacco KA, Termine A, Seyal A, et al: Effects of cigarette smoking on spatial working memory and attentional deficits in schizophrenia: involvement of nicotinic receptor mechanisms. Arch Gen Psychiatry 62:649–659, 2005

Salisbury DF, Kuroki N, Kasai K, et al: Progressive and interrelated functional and structural evidence of post-onset brain reduction in schizophrenia. Arch Gen Psychiatry 64:521–529, 2007

Saltz BL, Woerner MG, Kane JM, et al: Prospective study of tardive dyskinesia incidence in the elderly. JAMA 266:2402–2406, 1991

Sax KW, Strakowski SM, Keck PE Jr, et al: Relationships among negative, positive, and depressive symptoms in schizophrenia and psychotic depression. Br J Psychiatry 168:68–71, 1996

Sayers SL, Campbell EC, Kondrich J, et al: Cocaine abuse in schizophrenic patients treated with olanzapine versus haloperidol. J Nerv Ment Dis 193:379–386, 2005

Saykin AJ, Gur RC, Gur RE, et al: Neuropsychological function in schizophrenia. Selective impairment in memory and learning. Arch Gen Psychiatry 48:618–624, 1991

Saykin AJ, Shtasel DL, Gur RE, et al: Neuropsychological deficits in neuroleptic naive patients with first-episode schizophrenia. Arch Gen Psychiatry 51:124–131, 1994

Schooler NR: Relapse and rehospitalization: comparing oral and depot antipsychotics. J Clin Psychiatry 64 (suppl 16):14–17, 2003

Schooler NR: Relapse prevention and recovery in the treatment of schizophrenia. J Clin Psychiatry 67 (suppl 5):19–23, 2006

Schooler NR, Keith SJ, Severe JB, et al: Relapse and rehospitalization during maintenance treatment of schizophrenia. The effects of dose reduction and family treatment. Arch Gen Psychiatry 54:453–463, 1997

Schooler NR, Rabinowitz J, Davidson M, et al: Risperidone and haloperidol in first-episode psychosis: a long-term randomized trial. Am J Psychiatry 162:947–953, 2005

Schultz SK, Miller DD, Oliver SE, et al: The life course of schizophrenia: age and symptom dimensions. Schizophr Res 23:15–23, 1997

Seeman P: Atypical antipsychotics: mechanism of action. Can J Psychiatry 47:27–38, 2002

Selemon LD, Goldman-Rakic PS: The reduced neuropil hypothesis: a circuit based model of schizophrenia. Biol Psychiatry 45:17–25, 1999

Sellwood W, Barrowclough C, Tarrier N, et al: Needs-based cognitive-behavioural family intervention for carers of patients suffering from schizophrenia: 12-month follow-up. Acta Psychiatr Scand 104:346–355, 2001

Selzer JA, Lieberman JA: Schizophrenia and substance abuse. Psychiatr Clin North Am 16:401–412, 1993

Sevy S, Kay SR, Opler LA, et al: Significance of cocaine history in schizophrenia. J Nerv Ment Dis 178:642–648, 1990

Sewell DD: Schizophrenia and HIV. Schizophr Bull 22:465–473, 1996

Sharma A, Sorrell JH: Aripiprazole-induced parkinsonism. Int Clin Psychopharmacol 21:127–129, 2006

Shirzadi AA, Ghaemi SN: Side effects of atypical antipsychotics: extrapyramidal symptoms and the metabolic syndrome. Harv Rev Psychiatry 14:152–164, 2006

Simon AE, Cattapan-Ludewig K, Zmilacher S, et al: Cognitive functioning in the schizophrenia prodrome. Schizophr Bull 33:761–771, 2007

Simpson GM: The treatment of tardive dyskinesia and tardive dystonia. J Clin Psychiatry 61 (suppl 4):39–44, 2000

Siris SG: Pharmacological treatment of substance-abusing schizophrenic patients. Schizophr Bull 16:111–122, 1990

Siris SG: Depression in schizophrenia: perspective in the era of "atypical" antipsychotic agents. Am J Psychiatry 157:1379–1389, 2000a

Siris SG: Management of depression in schizophrenia. Psychiatric Annals 30:13–19, 2000b

Siris SG, Morgan V, Fagerstrom R, et al: Adjunctive imipramine in the treatment of postpsychotic depression. A controlled trial. Arch Gen Psychiatry 44:533–539, 1987

Siris SG, Mason SE, Bermanzohn PC, et al: Adjunctive imipramine in substance-abusing dysphoric schizophrenic patients. Psychopharmacol Bull 29:127–133, 1993

Smelson DA, Williams J, Kaune M, et al: Reduced cue-elicited cocaine craving and relapses following treatment with risperidone. Presented at the 153rd Annual Meeting of the American Psychiatric Association, Chicago, IL, May 13–18, 2000

Smelson DA, Ziedonis D, Williams J, et al: The efficacy of olanzapine for decreasing cue-elicited craving in individuals with schizophrenia and cocaine dependence: a preliminary report. J Clin Psychopharmacol 26:9–12, 2006

Soni SD, Brownlee M: Alcohol abuse in chronic schizophrenics: implications for management in the community. Acta Psychiatr Scand 84:272–276, 1991

Spence SA, Hirsch SR, Brooks DJ, et al: Prefrontal cortex activity in people with schizophrenia and control subjects. Evidence from positron emission tomography for remission of "hypofrontality" with recovery from acute schizophrenia. Br J Psychiatry 172:316–323, 1998

Spencer T, Biederman J, Wilens T, et al: Is attention-deficit hyperactivity disorder in adults a valid disorder? Harv Rev Psychiatry 1:326–335, 1994

Spohn HE, Strauss ME: Relation of neuroleptic and anticholinergic medication to cognitive functions in schizophrenia. J Abnorm Psychol 98:367–380, 1989

Stanton JM: Weight gain associated with neuroleptic medication: a review. Schizophr Bull 21:463–472, 1995

Stefansson H, Steinthorsdottir V, Thorgeirsson TE, et al: Neuregulin 1 and schizophrenia. Ann Med 36:62–71, 2004

Stein LI, Test MA: Alternative to mental hospital treatment, I: conceptual model, treatment program, and clinical evaluation. Arch Gen Psychiatry 37:392–397, 1980

Steinberg ML, Williams JM, Ziedonis DM: Financial implications of cigarette smoking among individuals with schizophrenia. Tob Control 13:206, 2004

Stroup TS, Lieberman JA, McEvoy JP, et al: Effectiveness of olanzapine, quetiapine, risperidone, and ziprasidone in patients with chronic schizophrenia following discontinuation of a previous atypical antipsychotic. Am J Psychiatry 163:611–622, 2006

Stroup TS, Lieberman JA, McEvoy JP, et al: Effectiveness of olanzapine, quetiapine, and risperidone in patients with chronic schizophrenia after discontinuing perphenazine: a CATIE study. Am J Psychiatry 164:415–427, 2007

Strous RD, Patel JK, Zimmet S, et al: Clozapine and paroxetine in the treatment of schizophrenia with obsessive-compulsive features. Am J Psychiatry 156:973–974, 1999

Stuss DT, Benson DF: The Frontal Lobes. New York, Raven Press, 1986

Susman VL: Clinical management of neuroleptic malignant syndrome. Psychiatr Q 72:325–336, 2001

Svensson TH, Mathe JM, Andersson JL, et al: Mode of action of atypical neuroleptics in relation to the phencyclidine model of schizophrenia: role of 5-HT2 receptor and alpha 1-adrenoceptor antagonism [corrected]. J Clin Psychopharmacol 15:11S–18S, 1995

Szarfman A, Tonning JM, Levine JG, et al: Atypical antipsychotics and pituitary tumors: a pharmacovigilance study. Pharmacotherapy 26:748–758, 2006

Szymanski S, Lieberman JA, Alvir JM, et al: Gender differences in onset of illness, treatment response, course, and biologic indexes in first-episode schizophrenic patients. Am J Psychiatry 152:698–703, 1995

Tamminga CA: Principles of the pharmacotherapy of schizophrenia, in Neurobiology of Mental Illness. Edited by Charney DS, Nestler EJ, Bunney BS. New York, Oxford University Press, 1999, pp 272–290

Tamminga CA: Partial dopamine agonists in the treatment of psychosis. J Neural Transm 109:411–420, 2002

Tarrier N, Barrowclough C, Vaughn C, et al: The community management of schizophrenia. A controlled trial of a behavioural intervention with families to reduce relapse. Br J Psychiatry 153:532–542, 1988

Tarrier N, Kinney C, McCarthy E, et al: Two-year follow-up of cognitive—behavioral therapy and supportive counseling in the treatment of persistent symptoms in chronic schizophrenia. J Consult Clin Psychol 68:917–922, 2000

Tarsy D, Baldessarini RJ: Epidemiology of tardive dyskinesia: is risk declining with modern antipsychotics? Mov Disord 21:589–598, 2006

Tibbo P, Kroetsch M, Chue P, et al: Obsessive-compulsive disorder in schizophrenia. J Psychiatr Res 34:139–146, 2000

Tollefson GD, Beasley CM Jr, Tamura RN, et al: Blind, controlled, long-term study of the comparative incidence of treatment-emergent tardive dyskinesia with olanzapine or haloperidol. Am J Psychiatry 154:1248–1254, 1997

Tollefson GD, Sanger TM, Lu Y, et al: Depressive signs and symptoms in schizophrenia: a prospective blinded trial of olanzapine and haloperidol. Arch Gen Psychiatry 55:250–258, 1998

Tollefson GD, Andersen SW, Tran PV: The course of depressive symptoms in predicting relapse in schizophrenia: a double-blind, randomized comparison of olanzapine and risperidone. Biol Psychiatry 46:365–373, 1999

Tollefson GD, Birkett MA, Kiesler GM, et al: Double-blind comparison of olanzapine versus clozapine in schizophrenic patients clinically eligible for treatment with clozapine. Biol Psychiatry 49:52–63, 2001

Toomey R, Faraone SV, Seidman LJ, et al: Association of neuropsychological vulnerability markers in relatives of schizophrenic patients. Schizophr Res 31:89–98, 1998

Tran PV, Dellva MA, Tollefson GD, et al: Oral olanzapine versus oral haloperidol in the maintenance treatment of schizophrenia and related psychoses. Br J Psychiatry 172:499–505, 1998

Tsai G, Yang P, Chung LC, et al: D-serine added to antipsychotics for the treatment of schizophrenia. Biol Psychiatry 44:1081–1089, 1998

Tsai G, Lane HY, Yang P, et al: Glycine transporter I inhibitor, N-methylglycine (sarcosine), added to antipsychotics for the treatment of schizophrenia. Biol Psychiatry 55:452–456, 2004

Tsai GE, Yang P, Chang YC, et al: D-alanine added to antipsychotics for the treatment of schizophrenia. Biol Psychiatry 59:230–234, 2006

Tsankova N, Renthal W, Kumar A, et al: Epigenetic regulation in psychiatric disorders. Nat Rev Neurosci 8:355–367, 2007

Tsuang MT, Winokur G, Crowe RR: Morbidity risks of schizophrenia and affective disorders among first degree relatives of patients with schizophrenia, mania, depression and surgical conditions. Br J Psychiatry 137:497–504, 1980

Tsuang MT, Fleming JA, Simpson JC: Suicide and schizophrenia, in The Harvard Medical School Guide to Suicide Assessment and Intervention. Edited by Jacobs DG. San Francisco, CA, Jossey-Bass, 1999a, pp 287–299

Tsuang MT, Stone WS, Seidman LJ, et al: Treatment of nonpsychotic relatives of patients with schizophrenia: four case studies. Biol Psychiatry 45:1412–1418, 1999b

Tsuang MT, Stone WS, Faraone SV: Towards the prevention of schizophrenia. Biol Psychiatry 48:349–356, 2000

van Haren NE, Pol HE, Schnack HG, et al: Progressive brain volume loss in schizophrenia over the course of the illness: evidence of maturational abnormalities in early adulthood. Biol Psychiatry 63:106–113, 2007

van Os J, Drukker M, a Campo J, et al: Validation of remission criteria for schizophrenia. Am J Psychiatry 163:2000–2002, 2006

Varsamis J, Adamson JD: Early schizophrenia. Can Psychiatr Assoc J 16:487–497, 1971

Volavka J, Czobor P, Sheitman B, et al: Clozapine, olanzapine, risperidone, and haloperidol in the treatment of patients with chronic schizophrenia and schizoaffective disorder. Am J Psychiatry 159:255–262, 2002

Waddington JL: Schizophrenia: developmental neuroscience and pathobiology. Lancet 341:531–536, 1993

Waddington JL, Buckley PF, Scully PJ, et al: Course of psychopathology, cognition and neurobiological abnormality in schizophrenia: developmental origins and amelioration by antipsychotics? J Psychiatr Res 32:179–189, 1998

Walker E, Lewis N, Loewy R, et al: Motor dysfunction and risk for schizophrenia. Dev Psychopathol 11:509–523, 1999

Wang PS, Walker AM, Tsuang MT, et al: Dopamine antagonists and the development of breast cancer. Arch Gen Psychiatry 59:1147–1154, 2002

Weinberger DR: Implications of normal brain development for the pathogenesis of schizophrenia. Arch Gen Psychiatry 44:660–669, 1987

Weinberger DR: On the plausibility of "the neurodevelopmental hypothesis" of schizophrenia. Neuropsychopharmacology 14:1S–11S, 1996

Weinberger DR, Berman KF, Zec RF: Physiologic dysfunction of dorsolateral prefrontal cortex in schizophrenia, I: regional cerebral blood flow evidence. Arch Gen Psychiatry 43:114–124, 1986

Weinberger DR, McClure RK: Neurotoxicity, neuroplasticity, and magnetic resonance imaging morphometry: what is happening in the schizophrenic brain? Arch Gen Psychiatry 59:553–558, 2002

Weiner E, Ball MP, Summerfelt A, et al: Effects of sustained-release bupropion and supportive group therapy on cigarette consumption in patients with schizophrenia. Am J Psychiatry 158:635–637, 2001

Weiss RD, Griffin ML, Kolodziej ME, et al: A randomized trial of integrated group therapy versus group drug counseling for patients with bipolar disorder and substance dependence. Am J Psychiatry 164:100–107, 2007

Werneke U, Taylor D, Sanders TA: Options for pharmacological management of obesity in patients treated with atypical antipsychotics. Int Clin Psychopharmacol 17:145–160, 2002

Westermeyer JF, Harrow M, Marengo JT: Risk for suicide in schizophrenia and other psychotic and nonpsychotic disorders. J Nerv Ment Dis 179:259–266, 1991

Wilkins JN: Pharmacotherapy of schizophrenia patients with comorbid substance abuse. Schizophr Bull 23:215–228, 1997

Williams GV, Castner SA: Under the curve: critical issues for elucidating D1 receptor function in working memory. Neuroscience 139:263–276, 2006

Williams JM, Ziedonis DM, Foulds J: A case series of nicotine nasal spray in the treatment of tobacco dependence among patients with schizophrenia. Psychiatr Serv 55:1064–1066, 2004

Windgassen K, Wesselmann U, Schulze Monking H: Galactorrhea and hyperprolactinemia in schizophrenic patients on neuroleptics: frequency and etiology. Neuropsychobiology 33:142–146, 1996

Wirshing DA, Spellberg BJ, Erhart SM, et al: Novel antipsychotics and new onset diabetes. Biol Psychiatry 44:778–783, 1998

Wirshing DA, Wirshing WC, Kysar L, et al: Novel antipsychotics: comparison of weight gain liabilities. J Clin Psychiatry 60:358–363, 1999

Wirshing DA, Erhart SM, Pierre JM: Nonextrapyramidal side effects of novel antipsychotics. Curr Opin Psychiatry 13:45–50, 2000

Wirshing DA, Boyd JA, Meng LR, et al: The effects of novel antipsychotics on glucose and lipid levels. J Clin Psychiatry 63:856–865, 2002

Wirshing DA, Pierre JM, Erhart SM, et al: Understanding the new and evolving profile of adverse drug effects in schizophrenia. Psychiatr Clin North Am 26:165–190, 2003

Wyatt RJ: Neuroleptics and the natural course of schizophrenia. Schizophr Bull 17:325–351, 1991

Wyatt RJ: Early intervention for schizophrenia: can the course of the illness be altered? Biol Psychiatry 38:1–3, 1995

Wyatt RJ, Damiani LM, Henter ID: First-episode schizophrenia. Early intervention and medication discontinuation in the context of course and treatment. Br J Psychiatry Suppl 172:77–83, 1998

Wykes T, Reeder C, Corner J, et al: The effects of neurocognitive remediation on executive processing in patients with schizophrenia. Schizophr Bull 25:291–307, 1999

Yazigi RA, Quintero CH, Salameh WA: Prolactin disorders. Fertil Steril 67:215–225, 1997

Yung AR, McGorry PD: The initial prodrome in psychosis: descriptive and qualitative aspects. Aust N Z J Psychiatry 30:587–599, 1996a

Yung AR, McGorry PD: The prodromal phase of first-episode psychosis: past and current conceptualizations. Schizophr Bull 22:353–370, 1996b

Zakzanis KK: Neuropsychological correlates of positive vs. negative schizophrenic symptomatology. Schizophr Res 29:227–233, 1998

Ziedonis D, Richardson T, Lee E, et al: Adjunctive desipramine in the treatment of cocaine abusing schizophrenics. Psychopharmacol Bull 28:309–314, 1992

Ziedonis D, Williams J, Corrigan P, et al: Management of substance abuse in schizophrenia. Psychiatr Ann 30:67–75, 2000

Ziedonis D, Williams JM, Smelson D: Serious mental illness and tobacco addiction: a model program to address this common but neglected issue. Am J Med Sci 326:223–230, 2003

Ziegenbein M, Sieberer M, Calliess IT, et al: Aripiprazole-induced extrapyramidal side effects in a patient with schizoaffective disorder. Aust N Z J Psychiatry 40:194–195, 2006

Zimmet SV, Strous RD, Burgess ES, et al: Effects of clozapine on substance use in patients with schizophrenia and schizoaffective disorder: a retrospective survey. J Clin Psychopharmacol 20:94–98, 2000

Zipursky RB, Lim KO, Sullivan EV, et al: Widespread cerebral gray matter volume deficits in schizophrenia. Arch Gen Psychiatry 49:195–205, 1992

CHAPTER 56

Treatment of Anxiety Disorders

Jonathan R. T. Davidson, M.D.

Kathryn M. Connor, M.D., M.H.S.

Wei Zhang, M.D., Ph.D.

Over the past decade and a half, there has been substantial progress in our understanding of the anxiety disorders. Particularly fruitful has been the search to develop new treatments for the six major anxiety disorders: obsessive-compulsive disorder (OCD), panic disorder, social phobia (social anxiety disorder), specific phobia, generalized anxiety disorder (GAD), and posttraumatic stress disorder (PTSD). In this chapter, we review the main findings from double-blind, and some open-label, trials in each disorder. Both short-term and continuation/maintenance treatment studies are included.

Obsessive-Compulsive Disorder

When Kierkegaard wrote that "no grand inquisitor has in readiness such terrible tortures as has anxiety, which never lets him escape," he may well have been thinking of OCD, one of the few conditions that has the capacity to produce a lifetime of psychological torture. Before the existence of serotonin reuptake–inhibiting drugs, especially clomipramine, and selective serotonin reuptake inhibitors (SSRIs), biological treatments generally had little effect, producing mild palliation at best.

According to the Epidemiologic Catchment Area study (Myers et al. 1984; Robins et al. 1984), OCD carries a lifetime prevalence of 2.5% in the United States and 6-month and 1-month prevalence rates of 1.5% and 1.3%, respectively, although a more recent analysis from the National Comorbidity Survey Replication (NCS-R) suggested slightly lower rates of 1.6% and 1.0% for the lifetime and 12-month prevalence of OCD, respectively (Kessler et al. 2005a, 2005b). Its economic toll is also substantial (Hollander et al. 1997). OCD has been recognized as the tenth leading cause of disability worldwide (Murray and Lopez 1996). Treatment can be grouped broadly into psychosocial and psychopharmacological approaches, the latter being our focus here. First, we present information on monotherapy with serotonin reuptake–inhibiting drugs, followed by management of partial responders or nonresponders, and we conclude with comments on less frequently used treatments.

The chief rating scale for treatment studies of OCD remains the Yale-Brown Obsessive Compulsive Scale (Y-BOCS; Goodman et al. 1989), a 10-item observer-rated measure. Self-ratings are of less importance in the OCD literature and have traditionally received little weight.

Monotherapy

In 1967, Fernandez-Cordoba and Lopez-Ibor reported beneficial effects of the nonselective serotonin reuptake inhibitor (SRI) tricyclic antidepressant (TCA) clomipramine in treating OCD. Following this important insight, a series of placebo-controlled studies were completed in the late 1980s and the early 1990s, leading eventually to the first approved treatment of OCD in the United States and other countries (Clomipramine Collaborative Study Group 1991). Clomipramine differs from other tricyclic drugs in that it has a particularly potent serotonin reuptake–inhibiting effect. The drug is not selective for serotonin, however, in that its demethylated metabolite is a norepinephrine reuptake inhibitor. The anti-OCD effect of clomipramine correlates with the plasma level of the parent drug, which is an SRI, suggesting that reuptake inhibition of serotonin is the critical factor underlying the drug's benefit. Moreover, some studies have shown lack of effect for selective norepinephrine reuptake–inhibiting drugs, such as nortriptyline and desipramine, in OCD (Leonard et al. 1988; Thoren et al. 1980). An interesting aspect of the pharmacokinetics of clomipramine is the ability of fluvoxamine to inhibit its demethylation, thereby increasing the amount of clomipramine relative to desmethylclomipramine, which can produce a potentiating effect in partial responders.

In the influential Clomipramine Collaborative Study Group (1991) trial, the Y-BOCS score was reduced by about 40% in patients taking the drug as compared with 5% in patients receiving placebo, bearing out findings by Mavissakalian et al. (1990) that OCD has a remarkably low placebo response rate. At one point, it was thought that clomipramine may have a larger effect size than SSRIs in the treatment of OCD (Greist et al. 1995b), but subsequently this finding has been interpreted as more likely to have been due to sampling differences between studies. In general, it is held that clomipramine and SSRI drugs are equivalent in the treatment of OCD (Koran et al. 1996). Nonetheless, clomipramine still may be a drug to consider in SSRI nonresponders. For the most part, in view of its greater side effects and risks, as well as dose-related risks of seizures, clomipramine would be regarded as a second-line treatment.

Today, SSRIs are considered first-line treatments for OCD, particularly the SSRIs fluvoxamine, fluoxetine, sertraline, and paroxetine, all of which have a U.S. Food and Drug Administration (FDA) indication for the treatment of OCD (Greist et al. 1995a, 1995b; Tollefson et al. 1994). Clomipramine, fluvoxamine, fluoxetine, and sertraline also have been shown to be effective in treating OCD in children, with an indication for treatment in such patients (Flament et al. 1985; Liebowitz et al. 2002; March et al. 1998; Riddle et al. 2001). Escitalopram is also efficacious in OCD at a daily dose of 20 mg on all main measures of efficacy, while 10 mg of escitalopram and 40 mg of paroxetine were superior to placebo on some measures but took longer to work (D.J. Stein et al. 2007).

Paroxetine and fluoxetine appear to be more effective at higher doses, whereas no clear relation between dose and effect was seen with sertraline, although a paradoxical finding of lesser efficacy at 100 mg/day was most likely an artifact. The results for escitalopram suggest that possibly a higher does of 20 mg is preferred, although 10 mg is somewhat effective. Recent results (Ninan et al. 2006) suggest additional benefit for increasing the dosage of sertraline up to 400 mg/day in nonresponders. Thus, when an SSRI drug is to be used in the treatment of OCD, not only may it need to be given in higher doses, but also it may take a longer time to work effectively. Most people believe that treatment should be long term to reduce the chance of relapse (Pato et al. 1990), although the dosage might be lowered without loss of benefit (Ravizza et al. 1996).

Long-Term Treatment and Relapse Prevention

Long-term pharmacological treatments of OCD have suggested sustained response of an effective medication beyond the acute treatment phase. In addition, clomipramine, paroxetine, sertraline, and most recently, escitalopram all have been shown to be more effective than placebo in preventing relapse in OCD (Fineberg et al. 2005, 2007). SSRIs appear to be well tolerated in these studies.

Augmentation, Combination, and Other Strategies

Up to 60% of individuals with OCD show a response to SSRIs according to a conventional and conservative criterion, full remission is rare, and response is often no more than partial. Relapse can occur even while patients continue taking an SSRI, and comorbidity is often a complicating factor in managing the disorder. The following augmentation, combination, and other novel strategies have been reported as offering benefit:

- Combining fluvoxamine with clomipramine (Szegedi et al. 1996) and the intravenous use of clomipramine as monotherapy (Fallon et al. 1992; Koran et al. 1997) are both approaches to consider in individuals who have shown a partial response to clomipramine. The rationale for combining fluvoxamine with clomipramine was explained in the previous section, but some caution is in order given the possibility of increased side effects and risk of seizure. Monitoring of plasma levels and electrocardiograms is important with this combination. The use of intravenous clomipramine derives from the fact that first-pass metabolism is avoided, and there is some suggestion that side effects are less severe.
- The benzodiazepine clonazepam has been added to clomipramine with mixed benefits (Pigott et al. 1992) and to sertraline with no added benefit (Crockett et al.

1999). Each of these findings was based on a double-blind, placebo-controlled trial.

- Patients with OCD refractory to SRI treatments may benefit from additional antipsychotic augmentation. A meta-analysis of double-blind, randomized trials demonstrated significant benefits of haloperidol and risperidone over placebo augmentation for OCD patients who failed to show treatment response after an adequate trial of SRI, whereas evidence for the efficacy of olanzapine and quetiapine is less conclusive (Bloch et al. 2006). Despite the fact that this approach appeared to benefit only a limited number of subjects (although it was more beneficial among subjects who suffered from comorbid tic disorders), any increased chance of improvement is worth striving for.
- Greist and Jefferson (1998) have reported four studies in which SSRI and behavior therapy approaches were compared and/or combined. Three of these studies gave some modest support to the idea that combined treatment produces an enhanced effect. Also, rates of relapse after discontinuing behavior therapy are considerably lower than those after discontinuing drug therapy. Other studies of SRI and cognitive-behavioral therapy (CBT) using exposure and ritual prevention techniques have yielded inconsistent results as to the benefits of combining drug and CBT over CBT alone (Cottraux et al. 1993; Foa et al. 2005).
- The addition of lithium, buspirone, desipramine, or gabapentin has produced very limited benefits in studies to date, although there may be occasional patients for whom such combinations are helpful.

Other Approaches

One report suggested that St. John's wort (*Hypericum perforatum*) produced some improvement after 12 weeks of treatment in 12 patients with OCD (Taylor and Kobak 2000). The promise of this early finding has been dampened by failure of the same group to establish efficacy for St. John's wort in a subsequent and adequately powered placebo-controlled study (Kobak et al. 2005).

A double-blind trial of intravenous clomipramine suggested greater benefit than oral loading (Koran et al. 1997). Inositol, a naturally occurring second-messenger precursor, led to greater improvement than placebo at a dosage of 18 g/day for 6 weeks (Fux et al. 1996).

Neurosurgical approaches, wherein either cingulotomy or anterior capsulotomy are carried out, can be helpful for refractory OCD. Between 25% and 30% of the subjects show marked improvement, and the side-effect burden of this procedure is small (Baer et al. 1995; Jenike et al. 1991). Limited but promising studies also suggested other potential approaches such as deep brain stimulation for severely treatment-refractory OCD patients (B.D. Greenberg et al. 2006; Nuttin et al. 1999).

CBT is well established for treating OCD, and evidence for efficacy is strong (e.g., Eddy et al. 2004; Foa et al. 2005). In most types of CBT for this disorder, exposure with response prevention is used. CBT is a first-choice option for OCD.

Panic Disorder

Panic disorder is a chronic and costly (P.E. Greenberg et al. 1999) condition that affects approximately 1%–3% of the population (Alonso et al. 2004; Kessler et al. 2005b). It often presents as a medical emergency and is associated with substantial comorbidity and increased suicidal risks (Roy-Byrne et al. 2000). Effective treatment results in reduced emergency department and laboratory resource utilization (Roy-Byrne et al. 2001).

Five core areas of the disorder require treatment: 1) full and limited symptom panic attacks, 2) anticipatory anxiety, 3) phobias related to panic, 4) general well-being, and 5) disability (Ballenger et al. 1998a). Treatment outcome can be comprehensively and succinctly measured with the Panic Disorder Severity Scale (PDSS), which can be administered both as a clinician-rated and as a self-rated scale (Shear et al. 1997). The PDSS contains seven domains relevant to panic disorder and agoraphobia. Other widely used measures include the Sheehan Panic and Anticipatory Anxiety Scale (PAAS; Sheehan 1986) and the self-rated Marks-Matthews Fear Questionnaire (FQ; Marks and Matthews 1979). Ideally, as with all of the anxiety disorders, the desired endpoint is full remission. However, this is not always attainable.

The earliest groups of drugs to show robust efficacy relative to placebo were the TCAs and the monoamine oxidase inhibitors (MAOIs) (Mavissakalian and Perel 1989; Sheehan et al. 1980). However, even before any randomized clinical trials had been published to support the use of SSRI drugs, the experts who were convened for the International Psychopharmacology Algorithm Project (Jobson et al. 1995) indicated that their preferred first-line approach was to use an SSRI. The other main approach would be to use benzodiazepine drugs, such as alprazolam or clonazepam (Lydiard et al. 1992; Rosenbaum et al. 1997; Tesar et al. 1991). Initial drug selection, to be based on discussion between the patient and the physician, would take into account issues of prior response, proneness to abuse of medication, tolerability, safety, comorbidity, and presenting clinical picture (e.g., degree of agitation).

First-Line Drug Treatments

Selective Serotonin Reuptake Inhibitors

In 1995, Boyer reported that SSRI drugs were more effective than imipramine and alprazolam in treating panic disorder, although a recent meta-analysis by Otto et al. (2001) failed to confirm these findings. Evidence is now available in support of citalopram (Wade et al. 1997), escitalopram (Stahl et al. 2003), fluoxetine (Michelson et al. 1998, 2001), fluvoxamine (Asnis et al. 2001; Black et al. 1993), paroxetine (Ballenger et al. 1998b; Oehrberg et al. 1995; Sheehan et al. 2005), and sertraline (Londborg et al. 1998). In addition, clomipramine has been shown to have efficacy in panic disorder (Lecrubier et al. 1997). Fluoxetine, paroxetine, and sertraline have been approved by the FDA for treatment of panic disorder.

Although SSRI drugs are favored as first-line treatment, the following points need to be kept in mind. Patients with panic disorder are often extremely sensitive to activating effects of antidepressants and have poor tolerance of symptoms such as palpitations, sweating, and tremor. It is therefore not uncommon for them to quickly lose faith and discontinue treatment or even drop out without a full discussion having taken place. This problem can almost always be obviated, either by coprescribing a benzodiazepine or by starting with extremely low doses of an SSRI and gradually building up as tolerated. Also, perhaps of most importance is the availability of the physician and thorough and reassuring preparation of patients ahead of time. Other problems of SSRIs to be concerned about in panic disorder are those common to all other conditions for which SSRIs are used (e.g., problems associated with weight gain, sexual dysfunction, impairment of sleep, and potential drug–drug interactions). Discontinuation of treatment can be a significant concern in panic disorder. Besides the obvious issue of relapse, SSRIs, with the exception of fluoxetine, may sometimes produce troublesome discontinuation symptoms. Many of these symptoms mimic panic disorder itself and can be quite distressing. Gradual dosage reduction is usually recommended, along with adequate patient education and physician availability. Coping strategies, including behavior therapy (Otto et al. 1993), are an option. Switching to an SSRI such as fluoxetine also may be considered because this drug has a slow built-in taper. One also might consider using serotonin$_2$ (5-HT$_2$) or serotonin$_3$ (5-HT$_3$) re-

ceptor antagonists, such as mirtazapine, nefazodone, and ondansetron, to limit some of the symptoms that are mediated through these pathways (e.g., insomnia, agitation, gastrointestinal distress).

Benzodiazepines

In the late 1980s, alprazolam received an FDA indication for treatment of panic disorder, making it the first product so licensed. An important byproduct of this indication was raising general awareness of the condition as well as helping to differentiate panic disorder with agoraphobia from other kinds of anxiety. Several trials showed that alprazolam was more effective than placebo. These included the Cross-National Collaborative Panic Study (1992), wherein imipramine and alprazolam were both more effective than placebo. Lydiard et al. (1992) reported that alprazolam 2 mg/day was more effective than placebo, and benefit for alprazolam was shown in other trials. Efficacy for clonazepam was also demonstrated in panic disorder (Davidson and Moroz 1998; Rosenbaum et al. 1997; Tesar et al. 1991).

Although alprazolam has been widely used for panic disorder, it is now regarded more as a second-line treatment. Problems include the need for frequent administration, tendency to produce sedation at higher doses, abuse liability, and discontinuation-related distress. Lesser et al. (1992) showed that higher plasma levels (i.e., >70 ng/mL) were associated with greater likelihood of response as compared with lower levels (in the 20–40 ng/mL range). Thus, higher doses may have an advantage, particularly in managing phobic avoidance, but often at the price of more side effects or discontinuation difficulty. Comparable efficacy and tolerability have been demonstrated for the sustained-release formulation of alprazolam (Pecknold et al. 1994; Schweizer et al. 1993). Clonazepam, which is also FDA approved for panic disorder, has an advantage over alprazolam in that its half-life is considerably longer and the drug can be dosed once or twice a day. However, it shares the usual class effects of benzodiazepines and can produce sedation, depression, and discontinuation syndrome. A particular concern with benzodiazepines is their use in the elderly. The elderly are not only more prone to developing side effects, including sedation and falls that result in fractures and potential head injury, but also more likely to experience problems upon discontinuation of the drug. In a fixed-dose study, clonazepam 1 mg/day was more effective than placebo on nearly all major measures; however, clonazepam 0.5 mg/day was ineffective except on the Hamilton Anxiety Scale (Ham-

A; Hamilton 1959). In general, escalating the dosage up to 4 mg/day did not provide greater benefit, suggesting that such higher dosages should be reserved for patients who are refractory to treatment at lower dosages. In the clonazepam studies, ratings of actual panic attacks tended to be the least likely to detect drug and placebo differences. As pointed out by Bandelow et al. (1995), overreliance on reduction of panic attacks as the principal outcome measure is an unsatisfactory marker of overall treatment benefit. Despite the almost universal unhappiness with this measure, it continues to be chosen as a primary outcome for regulatory studies.

One interesting and important finding to emerge from the studies of clonazepam in panic disorder is its substantial benefits on quality of life and work productivity. A broad-spectrum effect was noted on all five measures of mental health–related quality of life. During a 6-week clinical trial, patients moved from the seventh percentile for all adult Americans with regard to mental health component score (MCS) of the Short Form–36 (SF-36) to the seventeenth percentile. By contrast, the placebo group moved only from the eighth to the twelfth percentile during this time. With respect to work productivity, the difference between the effects of clonazepam and placebo during a 6-week treatment period amounted to an additional 6 hours of full productivity during a 40-hour workweek (Jacobs et al. 1997).

Other Pharmacological Approaches

Tricyclic Antidepressants

Several studies have reported benefit for clomipramine and imipramine in the treatment of panic disorder (Andersch et al. 1991; Cross-National Collaborative Panic Study 1992; Fahy et al. 1992; Lecrubier et al. 1997; Mavissakalian and Perel 1989; Modigh et al. 1992). The norepinephrine reuptake inhibitor desipramine also was more effective than placebo (Lydiard et al. 1993).

TCAs are second-line treatments for panic disorder at best. They are certainly effective, but the associated autonomic side effects, cardiovascular problems, weight gain, and potential lethality in overdose are all matters of concern. Dosing with TCAs may be critical. Mavissakalian and Perel (1995), for example, found that phobic symptoms responded best if the plasma level of imipramine and desmethylimipramine was in the range of 110–140 ng/mL, whereas control of panic attacks tended to occur at lower plasma levels. As with SSRIs, low starting dosages in the range of 10–25 mg/day are in order, with gradual titration thereafter in accordance with patient tolerance.

Monoamine Oxidase Inhibitors

Sheehan et al. (1980) found that phenelzine, along with imipramine, was more effective than placebo in the treatment of panic disorder with agoraphobia, which they referred to as "endogenous anxiety." Lydiard and Ballenger (1987) expressed the opinion that MAOIs may be superior to TCAs. Although these debates were fruitful in the 1980s, MAOIs have been swept aside by the remorseless tide of history, as have TCAs to some degree. These drugs now have been relegated to a lower echelon. Although for some patients MAOIs may still be the best treatment, their overall role in managing anxiety disorders is now fairly small. The role of the safer reversible inhibitor of monoamine oxidase A (RIMA) in panic disorder is unclear. Brofaromine and moclobemide have shown comparable efficacy and tolerability to clomipramine (Bakish et al. 1993; Kruger and Dahl 1999) and moclobemide also to fluoxetine for up to 1 year (Tiller et al. 1999); however, the significance of these findings is questionable in the absence of a placebo control. When compared with CBT and placebo, the effect of moclobemide was no different from placebo and failed to enhance the effect of CBT (Loerch et al. 1999).

Other Drugs

The extended-release (XR) formulation of venlafaxine, a serotonin–norepinephrine reuptake inhibitor (SNRI), has demonstrated greater efficacy than placebo in patients with panic disorder (Bradwejn et al. 2005) and has received FDA approval for the treatment of panic disorder. Following 10 weeks of treatment, patients receiving venlafaxine XR (mean dosage = 163 mg/day) experienced fewer panic attacks, greater freedom from limited symptom attacks (but not full symptom attacks), improvement in anticipatory anxiety and avoidance, and higher rates of response and remission compared with placebo. The drug was well tolerated, with an adverse-effect profile comparable with that of the drug in depression and other anxiety disorders.

Mirtazapine, a noradrenergic and specific serotonergic antidepressant, has also demonstrated anxiolytic activity. Possible benefit in panic disorder has been reported for the drug (Boshuisen et al. 2001; Ribeiro et al. 2001; Sarchiapone et al. 2003); however, double-blind, placebo-controlled trials have yet to be conducted. It is noteworthy that mirtazapine has been associated with the induction of panic attacks in depressed patients undergoing dose escalation and discontinuation (Berigan 2003; Klesmer et al. 2000).

Reboxetine, a selective reuptake inhibitor of norepinephrine, has been found to produce greater benefit than placebo in patients with panic disorder (Versiani et al. 2002). At dosages of 6–8 mg/day, the drug produced greater improvement in the number of panic attacks and phobic symptoms, as well as reduction in score on the Hamilton Rating Scale for Depression (Ham-D; Hamilton 1960), the Hopkins Symptom Checklist–90, and the Sheehan Disability Scale. It also produced significantly higher levels of dry mouth than placebo but in general was well tolerated. In a more recent randomized, single-blind study comparing reboxetine with paroxetine, paroxetine was more effective on panic attacks, but no differences were noted between the treatments on anticipatory anxiety and avoidance (Bertani et al. 2004). These findings suggest perhaps different roles of norepinephrine and serotonin in the treatment of panic disorder. In those countries where reboxetine has been approved for depression and is therefore available, it might be a useful backup drug for use in SSRI and benzodiazepine nonresponders. Given its antidepressant properties, it might be advantageous over benzodiazepines. However, the selective noradrenergic reuptake inhibitor maprotiline appears to be ineffective in panic disorder (Den Boer and Westenberg 1988), while the data for bupropion are inconclusive (Sheehan et al. 1983; Simon et al. 2003).

Trazodone was less effective than imipramine and alprazolam in the treatment of panic disorder (Charney et al. 1986). Buspirone, a 5-HT$_{1A}$ partial agonist, was ineffective in panic disorder (Sheehan et al. 1990). The anticonvulsant gabapentin was also generally ineffective in panic disorder, though post hoc analyses suggest an anxiolytic effect in more severely ill patients (Pande et al. 2000). Possible benefit has been reported for other anticonvulsant drugs, including levetiracetam, tiagabine, and valproic acid (Keck et al. 1993; Papp 2006; Zwanzger et al. 2001), but double-blind trials have not been undertaken. Preliminary data suggest improvement in refractory panic disorder when atypical antipsychotics are prescribed to augment an SSRI (risperidone: Simon et al. 2006; olanzapine: Sepede et al. 2006) or at higher doses as monotherapy (olanzapine: Hollifield et al. 2005); however, double-blind, placebo-controlled trials are needed. Metabotropic glutamate type 2 receptor agonists have shown promise in preclinical models of anxiety but have yet to demonstrate clinical efficacy in panic disorder (Bergink and Westenberg 2005). Similarly, the effect of a cholecystokinin-B receptor antagonist was no different from placebo in patients with panic disorder (Pande et al. 1999a).

Combination Pharmacotherapy

The activating side effects of SSRIs can be quite troublesome for anxiety patients, particularly when beginning pharmacotherapy in patients with panic disorder. Coadministration of a long-acting benzodiazepine for the first several weeks of treatment may help improve SSRI tolerability and provide more rapid stabilization of panic symptoms than SSRI treatment alone (Goddard et al. 2001; Pollack et al. 2003).

Long-Term Management

Maintenance treatment is recommended for at least 12–24 months, if not longer. The long-term treatment of panic disorder has been reviewed elsewhere (Davidson 1998). In a controlled trial of paroxetine, clomipramine, and placebo, 84% of the paroxetine-treated patients eventually became panic free over the 9-month period (Lecrubier and Judge 1997). In a 4-year naturalistic follow-up study of 367 patients with panic disorder, greater improvements in panic attacks, phobic avoidance, and daily functioning were observed in those who received continuation treatment for 4 years, compared with 1 year (Katschnig et al. 1995), suggesting that recovery continues over several years.

Long-term randomized, controlled trials have reported efficacy for citalopram (Lepola et al. 1998), clomipramine (Fahy et al. 1992), fluoxetine (Michelson et al. 1999), paroxetine (Lecrubier and Judge 1997; Lydiard et al. 1998), and sertraline (Rapaport et al. 2001). In a relapse prevention trial following 3 months of successful open-label treatment with the drug, Ferguson et al. (2007) showed that over the course of 7 months, relapse on placebo was 50%, whereas relapse among those remaining on venlafaxine XR was 22%.

From an early long-term study of imipramine (Mavissakalian and Perel 1992), it appeared that relapse may diminish with the passage of time, provided effective psychopharmacological cover has been provided, but a later trial by the same group failed to confirm this (Mavissakalian and Perel 2002).

Discontinuation

Even though there is some similarity between symptoms of relapse and symptoms of drug withdrawal, the existence of discontinuation symptoms from stopping medication is unarguable. If poorly managed, discontinuation can be fraught with problems. Some strategies are likely to make withdrawal of medication more tolerable. The first strategy is a slow taper. Indeed, for some benzodiazepines, it may be necessary to taper the drug over many weeks or even months. Second, timing of the taper may be important. This is best accomplished when other variables in a patient's life are as stable as possible. Switching to a longer-acting benzodiazepine, such as clonazepam, also may be helpful. Some authors (Pages and Ries 1998) have advocated consideration of anticonvulsants, such as carbamazepine and valproate. Otto et al. (1993) also found behavior therapy to be helpful in this regard.

Various elaborations of CBT, including self-help books, and telephone- and Internet-delivered therapy, have demonstrated efficacy on a consistent basis for panic disorder, with the common elements being education, cognitive strategies, and exposure to feared sensations and situations (Clum and Surls 1993; Royal Australian and New Zealand College of Psychiatrists Clinical Practice Guidelines Team for Panic Disorder and Agoraphobia 2003). CBT is a first-line choice, and even when pharmacotherapy is given as main treatment, principles of CBT should be incorporated into the management plan. As noted, it can be of benefit during the process of drug discontinuation, and perhaps in lessening the chance of relapse afterwards.

Social Phobia

Social phobia, also referred to as social anxiety disorder, can be grouped into generalized and nongeneralized types. Generalized social phobia is more commonly seen in clinical settings, is usually more disabling, and is associated with greater levels of comorbidity and genetic loading than nongeneralized social phobia. Most of our knowledge about pharmacotherapy for social phobia derives from generalized social phobia, and the literature suggests that different medication approaches may be called for in treating the two subtypes.

Comprehensive treatment of social phobia requires that the symptoms of fear, avoidance, and physiological distress are brought under control, comorbidity is treated, disability and impairment are improved, and quality of life is enhanced. Furthermore, evidence from maintenance and relapse prevention studies has confirmed the value of long-term therapy in treatment responders.

Instruments commonly used to measure treatment change in social phobia include the clinician- and self-rated Liebowitz Social Anxiety Scale (LSAS; Liebowitz 1987), which assesses 24 performance or interpersonal situations for fear and avoidance. A score of 30 or less is con-

sidered to equate with remission. The Social Phobia Inventory (SPIN) is a useful 17-item self-rating instrument that assesses fear, avoidance, and physiological distress (Connor et al. 2000) and, like the LSAS, is able to detect treatment differences on all its subscales.

Pharmacotherapy

Most clinicians consider SSRI drugs as the first choice for generalized social phobia, with either β-blockers or benzodiazepines being the first choice for nongeneralized social phobia. Second-line drugs for generalized social phobia comprise the benzodiazepines, perhaps venlafaxine (an SNRI), and maybe other antidepressants, including nefazodone and mirtazapine. MAOIs also have a role. Bupropion and TCAs have been generally disappointing.

Serotonergic Drugs

Fluvoxamine has been widely studied and has the longest track record of success in the treatment of social phobia. In 1994, van Vliet et al. showed superiority for fluvoxamine over placebo, with response rates of 46% and 7%, respectively. M.B. Stein et al. (1999) later confirmed the efficacy of fluvoxamine relative to placebo on all symptom domains of social phobia (i.e., fear, avoidance, and physiological arousal). Studies have also looked at the controlled-released (CR) form of fluvoxamine and found it to be superior to placebo (Davidson et al. 2004c; Westenberg et al. 2004). In the study by Davidson et al. (2004c), baseline symptom severity was higher than in most other clinical trials, yet drug therapy was still effective. In addition to these studies conducted in the United States or Europe, a more recent study in Japan also found fluvoxamine to be effective compared to placebo in reducing symptoms and associated psychosocial disability among Japanese patients with generalized social anxiety disorder (Asakura et al. 2007).

Sertraline also has been studied (Blomhoff et al. 2001; Katzelnick et al. 1995; Liebowitz et al. 2003; Van Ameringen et al. 2001; Walker et al. 2000). In the study by Van Ameringen et al. (2001), 53% responded to sertraline as compared with 29% to placebo. As with the fluvoxamine study of M.B. Stein et al. (1999), the Brief Social Phobia Scale was a primary outcome measure, and in both instances, the drug was shown to produce benefit on all three symptom domains. In a primary care setting, Haug et al. (2000) showed that cognitive therapy and sertraline could be effectively delivered, although the combination did not really show any superiority over treatment with drug alone.

Effectiveness for paroxetine was shown relative to placebo in both short-term efficacy and relapse prevention. In the short-term studies by M.B. Stein et al. (1998), Allgulander (1999), and Baldwin et al. (1999), rates of response to paroxetine were 55%, 70%, and 66%, respectively, as compared with placebo response rates of 24%, 8%, and 32%. These differences are substantial and suggest a marked effect for paroxetine in social phobia. All subjects in the paroxetine trials fulfilled criteria for generalized social phobia and showed benefit on the primary measure, the LSAS. Between 2 and 4 weeks was required for paroxetine to show significant superiority.

Fluoxetine, while superior to placebo on primary outcomes in one study (Davidson et al. 2004c), failed to separate from placebo in another (Kobak et al. 2002). In the latter study, placebo seemed to yield a greater response (30%) than most other studies of SSRIs in social phobia. Another study comparing cognitive therapy, fluoxetine plus self-exposure, and placebo plus self-exposure in social phobia found cognitive therapy to be superior to fluoxetine plus self-exposure and placebo plus self-exposure on measures of social phobia, with no difference between the latter two groups (D.M. Clark et al. 2003). Interestingly, another serotonergic agent, nefazodone, also failed to separate from placebo on most outcome measures in a recent report of Canadian outpatients with social phobia (Van Ameringen et al. 2007).

Placebo-controlled data with citalopram have not been presented for social phobia. However, trials with escitalopram have shown superiority over placebo in short-term, long-term, and relapse prevention studies of generalized social phobia (Kasper et al. 2005; Lader et al. 2004; Montgomery et al. 2005). Venlafaxine XR has also shown superiority over placebo in two double-blind trials of generalized social phobia (Allgulander et al. 2004; Liebowitz et al. 2005). A double-blind, placebo-controlled trial of mirtazapine in women showed statistically significant superiority for drug over placebo (Muehlbacher et al. 2005).

Paroxetine, sertraline, and venlafaxine XR are currently the only FDA-approved drugs for the treatment of social phobia, although the controlled-release form of fluvoxamine is likely to be approved for social anxiety disorder in the near future.

Benzodiazepines

Three major placebo-controlled trials have shown efficacy for benzodiazepines in social phobia. First, Gelernter et al. (1991) showed a very modest effect for alprazolam over placebo and a generally inferior picture for alprazolam relative to phenelzine. The response rate with alprazolam, at a mean daily dose of 4.2 mg, was 38%, a rate significantly better than the 20% response rate to placebo. Davidson et al. (1993) conducted a moderately large trial in 75 patients taking clonazepam or placebo and found a substantial 70% response rate to clonazepam compared with a 20% response rate to placebo. Clonazepam worked rapidly and effectively and had a broad-spectrum effect in the disorder. Bromazepam also has been found to work more effectively than placebo (Versiani et al. 1997). A magnetic resonance spectroscopy study of clonazepam in social phobia has shown that even when clonazepam is effective, there are no changes in the extent of N-acetylaspartate, choline, and myo-inositol, suggesting that these particular changes within the central nervous system are not state dependent.

Some benzodiazepines (clonazepam and bromazepam) provide a marked response yet do not find favor as first-line drugs because of their more limited spectrum of action, as well as potential withdrawal difficulties. However, they work rapidly, are well tolerated, and may be particularly useful for individuals with periodic performance-related social anxiety.

Anticonvulsants

Gabapentin and pregabalin produce significant effects in social phobia. Pande et al. (1999b) found a superior effect for gabapentin over placebo, with response rates of 39% and 17%, respectively. Baseline symptom scores were comparatively high and overall response rates relatively low, suggesting a degree of treatment resistance in the population. A flexible dosage of gabapentin was used, ranging from 900 to 3,600 mg, with 2,100 mg/day being the most commonly chosen final dosage. The newer anticonvulsant drug pregabalin has shown benefit in generalized social phobia. Although 150 mg/day of pregabalin was no different from placebo, 600 mg/day produced greater effects than placebo, with response rates of 43% and 22%, respectively. At 600 mg/day, pregabalin produces a relatively high rate of side effects, and it is probably necessary to explore lower dosages for social phobia. Further work with anticonvulsants is called for because they are generally well tolerated, safe, and less likely to produce difficulties during discontinuation than many SSRIs and benzodiazepines.

Reversible Inhibitors of Monoamine Oxidase

Moclobemide initially appeared to be a safer and very promising alternative to older MAOIs. A study by Versiani et al. (1992) showed that moclobemide worked almost as effectively as phenelzine and significantly better than placebo but that it was slower to take effect compared with phenelzine. Response rates to moclobemide and placebo in the study were 65% and 15%, respectively, with a fairly high dosage of moclobemide being attained (581 mg/day). However, these exciting early findings have not been borne out by subsequent studies. For instance, Noyes et al. (1997) reported no significant advantage for moclobemide at several dosages as compared with placebo. Schneier et al. (1998) showed a poor effect for the drug in a single-center trial, and the International Multicenter Clinical Trial Group on Moclobemide in Social Phobia (1997) found a modestly greater response rate (47%) for moclobemide at 600 mg/day than for placebo (34%). Based on the two positive trials, moclobemide has received a license in some countries but is not available in the United States. Another RIMA, brofaromine, has shown promise in three trials, with response rates of 78%, 50%, and 73%, respectively, compared with placebo response rates of 23%, 19%, and 0% (Fahlen et al. 1995; Lott et al. 1997; van Vliet et al. 1992).

Irreversible Inhibitors of Monoamine Oxidase

Phenelzine has been studied in four double-blind, placebo-controlled trials and showed positive benefit in all cases (Gelernter et al. 1991; Heimberg et al. 1998; Liebowitz et al. 1992; Versiani et al. 1992). Response rates to phenelzine were 69%, 85%, 64%, and 65%, respectively, as compared with 20%, 15%, 23%, and 33%, respectively, to placebo. Even though phenelzine is so consistently effective, perhaps as a result of its combined noradrenergic, dopaminergic, and serotonergic effects, its poor tolerance, as well as greater risks, makes it an unsuitable choice for most patients. However, it should not be completely ignored and may make a major difference in the lives of some patients whose symptoms do not respond to other drugs.

Other Drugs

Olanzapine yielded greater improvement than placebo in a preliminary double-blind, placebo-controlled monotherapy trial of social anxiety disorder (Barnett et al. 2002), suggesting atypical antipsychotics may deserve further investigation in this area of research. Ondansetron, while producing a statistically significant effect relative to placebo, seems to be of very limited benefit (Bell and De-Veaugh-Geiss 1994; Davidson et al. 1997b), but it might be a useful backup or adjunct in some cases. Its cost is a major problem. Buspirone was ineffective in a double-

blind trial, producing only a 7% response rate (van Vliet et al. 1997).

Despite their intuitive appeal, β-blockers have shown poor effect in treating generalized social phobia. For example, atenolol failed to separate from placebo in two trials (Liebowitz et al. 1992; Turner et al. 1994). β-Blockers do show some value in performance social anxiety, perhaps by virtue of their ability to reduce peripheral autonomic arousal and block negative feedback. Nefazodone, bupropion, and selegiline have not shown impressive results in open-label reports (Emmanuel et al. 1991; Simpson et al. 1998; Van Ameringen et al. 1999).

A novel therapeutic approach is suggested by the findings of Hofmann et al. (2006), who administered a single dose of D-cycloserine or placebo to patients with social anxiety disorder treated with CBT. The drug was given prior to each CBT session and enhanced the benefit of CBT to a greater extent than did placebo. The postulated mechanism of action relates to drug-facilitated extinction of learned fear via glutamatergic pathways.

Treatment in Children and Adolescents

One interesting placebo-controlled trial of fluvoxamine in children ages 6–17 years showed that it was superior to placebo in social phobia, GAD, or the combination: 76% of the fluvoxamine group responded, as compared with 19% of the placebo group (Research Unit on Pediatric Psychopharmacology Anxiety Study Group 2001). Double-blind trials of paroxetine immediate-release (IR) (Wagner et al. 2004) and venlafaxine XR (March et al. 2007) have produced positive results in children and adolescents with generalized social anxiety disorder. Response rates for paroxetine and placebo were 78% and 38%, respectively; in the venlafaxine study, they were 56% and 37%. An open-label trial by Compton et al. (2001) suggested some value for sertraline in children and adolescents with social phobia, but we are unaware of any published placebo-controlled trials.

Duration of Treatment

Because social phobia is a chronic illness, treatment is generally recommended for years. Sutherland et al. (1996) reported that at 2-year follow-up, subjects who had received an active drug rather than placebo in a double-blind trial were doing better. Relatively few relapse prevention studies have been done. In a 12-month trial with clonazepam, Connor et al. (1998) showed a 20% relapse rate in those switched to placebo compared with 0% in those who continued taking clonazepam. On other measures, there was an upward drift in fear and phobia scores in subjects who were withdrawn from clonazepam. However, in the study with its very slow taper, it was encouraging that withdrawal symptoms were rare and not problematic. M.B. Stein et al. (1996) reported that 62% of the subjects relapsed when switched double-blind from paroxetine to placebo after 12 weeks, compared with only 12% who relapsed during maintenance treatment with paroxetine.

Other Issues

CBT is efficacious in social anxiety disorder, being comparable to pharmacotherapy (Davidson et al. 2004b; Fedoroff and Taylor 2001), but little is known as to whether adding CBT to medication lowers the relapse rate, and so far the limited evidence does not suggest any potentiating effects when the treatments are combined (Davidson et al. 2004b). It does appear as if exposure consistently produces gain, but adding cognitive elements does not confer further benefit (Haug et al. 2003; Hofmann 2004). In a comparative study of drug and psychotherapy, Heimberg et al. (1998) showed that phenelzine and CBT were approximately similar, although phenelzine had an edge in more severely symptomatic patients. On the other hand, when subjects who had discontinued treatment were followed up, rates of relapse tended to be lower in those who had received CBT than in those who had taken phenelzine. Turner et al. (1994) found that atenolol was not as good as social skills training, and D.B. Clark and Agras (1991) showed a relatively poor response with buspirone over exposure therapy in performance social phobia.

Despite the obvious benefits of drug therapy in social phobia, medication often falls short of producing remission, and a pressing need remains to find better drugs, better combinations, and the ways in which drug therapy and psychosocial treatments might be most productively used, whether in sequence, simultaneously, or according to some other formula. Nevertheless, compared with the situation 15 years ago, prospects for recovery from social phobia are perhaps better than they have ever been.

Specific Phobia

Specific phobia is among the most common psychiatric disorders, with a lifetime prevalence of 8%–12.5% (Alonso et al. 2004; Kessler et al. 2005b) and 12-month prevalence of 3.5%–9% (Alonso et al. 2004; Kessler et al. 2005a). While the disorder is characterized by an early age of onset (median age at onset is 7 years) (Kessler et al.

2005b), most of those with the disorder are unimpaired by their symptoms; hence, few individuals actually seek treatment for their specific phobia (Magee et al. 1996; Stinson et al. 2007; Zimmerman and Mattia 2000). However, for a minority of individuals, specific phobia causes significant disability and requires treatment. The generally accepted treatment of choice is exposure therapy, which is uniformly and rapidly effective, with techniques including virtual reality or in vivo exposure, and muscle tension exercises (for blood–injury phobia) (Swinson et al. 2006). Few studies have evaluated the efficacy of pharmacological approaches, and no drug has yet been approved by the FDA for treating specific phobia. No standard ratings exist for this disorder, although the Marks-Matthews FQ is quite suitable for blood–injury phobia and some other fears. A modification of this scale, the Marks-Sheehan Main Phobia Severity Scale (MSMPSS; Sheehan 1986) can be recommended.

Serotonergic drugs have shown efficacy in treating symptoms of fear and avoidance in a variety of anxiety disorders and thus would seem logical choices in treating specific phobias. It is therefore not surprising that studies of pharmacological treatments for specific phobia have focused on serotonergic agents. In a double-blind, controlled trial, 11 subjects were treated for 4 weeks with either paroxetine (up to 20 mg/day) or placebo (Benjamin et al. 2000). As measured by the Marks-Matthews FQ and the Ham-A, 60% of the subjects (3 of 5), compared with 17% taking placebo (1 of 6), responded to treatment with paroxetine. A more recent randomized, double-blind pilot trial compared the effects of escitalopram versus placebo over 12 weeks in 12 adults with specific phobia (Alamy et al. 2008). While no difference was observed on the primary outcome, response based on a Clinical Global Impression Scale (CGI) Improvement score of 1 or 2 was noted in 60% of subjects who received escitalopram, compared with 29% on placebo (effect size = 1.13). The findings from these two small trials suggest promise for the SSRIs in specific phobia; however, larger controlled trials are needed. In contrast, in a controlled trial of the serotonergic and noradrenergic drug imipramine in 218 phobic subjects (agoraphobic, mixed phobic, or simple phobic) receiving 26 weeks of behavior therapy, no difference was observed between imipramine and placebo (Zitrin et al. 1983). Intermittent use of benzodiazepines also may be helpful in the acute treatment of the somatic anxiety that accompanies specific phobia, although this usage has not been an area of active investigation.

In a long-term controlled study of clonazepam in social phobia, Davidson et al. (1994) observed that clonazepam was superior in reducing symptoms of anxiety related to blood–injury phobia as measured by changes in the blood–injury phobia subscale of the Marks-Matthews FQ. Some caution should be used with these drugs, however, because there is risk of physiological dependence.

Using a novel approach, Ressler et al. (2004) investigated the effect of a cognitive enhancer, D-cycloserine, as an adjunct to psychotherapy, hypothesizing that the drug would accelerate the associative learning processes that contribute to ameliorating psychopathology. D-Cycloserine is a *N*-methyl-D-aspartate (NMDA) receptor partial agonist that has demonstrated improvement in extinction in rodents. Subjects with acrophobia ($n=28$) were randomized to receive a single dose of D-cycloserine or placebo prior to each of two virtual reality exposure therapy sessions. The combination of D-cycloserine and exposure therapy was associated with greater improvement in the virtual-reality setting, as well as on a variety of anxiety domains. These changes were noted early in treatment and were maintained at 3-month follow-up.

Specific phobia tends to be a chronic condition. Although psychotherapeutic approaches can be beneficial in the short term, evidence suggests that the initial gains noted with treatment may not be sustained over the long term (Lipsitz et al. 1999). Pharmacological augmentation may help to extend the benefits of exposure therapy over time. It also has been hypothesized that specific phobia may represent a phenomenological marker for a vulnerability to developing other anxiety disorders that are characterized by more general avoidance (Goisman et al. 1998). As such, perhaps early recognition and treatment in individuals at risk could reduce the occurrence of more severe anxiety disorders in this population. Further study of these hypotheses is needed.

Generalized Anxiety Disorder

GAD is a common anxiety disorder, with a lifetime prevalence of 5%–6% (Wittchen and Hoyer 2001) and is the most prevalent anxiety disorder in primary care, with rates that exceed 8% (Goldberg and Lecrubier 1995). GAD tends to be a chronic and disabling condition with lifetime rates of comorbidity as high as 90% (Wittchen et al. 1994), particularly depression (prevalence rate greater than 60%) (Wittchen et al. 1994), which can increase the severity and burden of the disorder.

GAD is characterized by persistent and excessive worry that is difficult to control and is accompanied by symptoms of anxiety, tension, and autonomic arousal. Effective treatments include anxiolytic drugs, such as benzodiazepines and azapirones. These drugs can be helpful for symptoms of anxiety, but they are not generally considered satisfactory in the treatment of depression. In addition, the side-effect profile of benzodiazepines and potential for physiological dependence limit their use in many patients and have resulted in growing interest in the search for alternative treatments. In recent years, growing evidence supports the role for antidepressants in treating GAD, especially in patients with comorbid depression.

The goals of pharmacotherapy for GAD include treatment of the symptoms of worry, anxiety, tension, somatic distress, and autonomic arousal. Ideally, treatments will have a rapid onset of action in reducing these core symptoms; will be effective in treating the associated disability, psychosocial impairment, and comorbidity; and will be safe for longer-term use in chronic GAD.

Assessment of response in almost all pharmacotherapy trials of GAD has involved use of the clinician-administered Ham-A (Hamilton 1959), which measures psychic (i.e., psychological) and somatic symptoms of anxiety and broadly maps onto the clinical features of GAD. Remission is usually defined as a Ham-A score of 7 or less. The Hospital Anxiety and Depression Scale (HADS; Zigmond and Snaith 1983) is also widely used and is capable of detecting differences in treatment efficacy. An advantage of the HADS lies in the fact that its items are independent from the confounding influence of psychotropic drug side effects. It also has widely established population norms.

Anxiolytics

Benzodiazepines

Benzodiazepines have been widely used to treat acute and chronic anxiety since their introduction in the 1960s. Their activity is mediated through potentiation of the inhibitory neurotransmitter γ-aminobutyric acid (GABA) at the $GABA_A$ receptor. The efficacy and relative safety of benzodiazepines in short-term use, over several weeks or months, are well established (Rickels et al. 1983; Shader and Greenblatt 1993). However, the use of these drugs over longer periods is more controversial, and long-term use can be associated with the development of tolerance, physiological dependence, and withdrawal (if abruptly discontinued), as well as troublesome side effects, including ataxia, sedation, motor dysfunction, and cognitive impairment. Furthermore, these drugs should be avoided in patients with a history of substance disorders, and long-term use may infrequently lead to the development of major depression (Lydiard et al. 1987).

Benzodiazepines have been shown to be effective in GAD, as reported by Rickels et al. (1993) in an 8-week study of diazepam in patients with DSM-III (American Psychiatric Association 1980)–diagnosed GAD. The appeal of these drugs lies in their rapid onset of action, ease of use, tolerability, and relative safety. However, few controlled data support their use over the long term in GAD. Findings from several 6- to 8-month trials of maintenance treatment for chronic anxiety have indicated continued efficacy of benzodiazepines over time (Rickels et al. 1983, 1988a, 1988b; Schweizer et al. 1993). Because GAD tends to be a chronic disorder, many patients may need to continue pharmacotherapy with benzodiazepines or other drugs for many years.

Estimates suggest that approximately 70% of patients with GAD will respond to an adequate trial of a benzodiazepine (Greenblatt et al. 1983). An adequate treatment trial corresponds to the equivalent of a 3- to 4-week treatment course of up to 40 mg/day of diazepam or 4 mg/day of alprazolam (Schweizer and Rickels 1996). If a decision is made to discontinue treatment, the drug should be tapered slowly to minimize the effects of withdrawal, the development of rebound anxiety, and the potential for relapse. Some evidence suggests that benzodiazepines may be more effective in treating particular GAD symptoms, such as autonomic arousal and somatic symptoms, but less effective for the psychic symptoms of worry and irritability (Rickels et al. 1982; Rosenbaum et al. 1984).

As our understanding of the phenomenology of GAD has grown and as the diagnostic criteria have evolved from DSM-III to DSM-IV (American Psychiatric Association 1994), there has been a greater emphasis on the psychic component of the disorder, with de-emphasis of the autonomic and somatic components. Given these changes, along with the high rates of comorbid depression in GAD and the anxiolytic activity of many of the newer classes of antidepressants, the utility of benzodiazepines as a primary treatment for GAD is uncertain. However, even though somatic symptoms are no longer featured as diagnostic criteria, they are frequently seen as presenting clinical symptoms in practice. A degree of uncertainty still hangs over the most appropriate way to classify GAD. Even as DSM-IV was being crafted, debate centered around the extent to which GAD could be separated from mood disorders, such as dysthymia and major depression (Moras et al. 1996). This question has never been well resolved, and it is possible that with so much in common

between GAD and depressive disorders, its classification primarily as an anxiety disorder may change in DSM-V.

Azapirones

The azapirones are structurally distinct from the benzodiazepines and are believed to exert their anxiolytic effect through partial agonism of 5-HT_{1A} receptors. Several trials have indicated that buspirone is superior to placebo and comparable to benzodiazepines in treating GAD, with fewer side effects and without concerns for abuse, dependence, and withdrawal (Cohn et al. 1986; Enkelmann 1991; Petracca et al. 1990; Rickels et al. 1988b; Strand et al. 1990), although other studies have reported conflicting results (Fontaine et al. 1987; Olajide and Lader 1987; Ross and Matas 1987). Buspirone appears more effective in treating the psychic component of anxiety (Rickels et al. 1982) and possibly anxiety with mixed depressive symptoms (Rickels et al. 1991) than the somatic and autonomic symptoms of anxiety (Schweizer and Rickels 1988; Sheehan et al. 1990). An adequate trial of buspirone in GAD would be 3–4 weeks of treatment at a dosage of up to 60 mg/day, in divided doses. Treatment-limiting effects of the drug include greater potential for side effects at higher dosages, slower onset of action, more variable antidepressant effect, and possibly reduced effectiveness in patients with a prior favorable response to benzodiazepines (Schweizer et al. 1986).

Tricyclic Antidepressants

Retrospective studies of subjects with "anxiety neurosis" suggested that TCAs may be effective in treating anxiety states similar to GAD (Cohn et al. 1986; Johnstone et al. 1980). Data in support of these findings come from controlled studies of imipramine and trazodone in GAD (Hoehn-Saric et al. 1988; Rickels et al. 1993). In a 6-week trial comparing imipramine and alprazolam, similar improvement was observed with both treatments by week 2; however, imipramine appeared to be more effective in treating the psychic anxiety associated with GAD, whereas alprazolam was more effective in attenuating somatic symptoms (Hoehn-Saric et al. 1988). In an 8-week double-blind, placebo-controlled trial of imipramine, trazodone, and diazepam (Rickels et al. 1993), early onset of effect was noted with diazepam by week 2, with effect primarily on somatic symptoms. Over the next 6 weeks, however, symptoms of psychic anxiety were more responsive to treatment with the antidepressants. Overall, imipramine was more efficacious than diazepam, whereas the effect of trazodone was comparable to that of diazepam, and all treatments were superior to placebo. In a controlled trial comparing imipramine, paroxetine, and 2'-chlordesmethyldiazepam, early onset of action was again noted with the benzodiazepine by week 2, but overall greater improvement was noted with the antidepressants by week 4, with particular benefit noted in psychic symptoms (Rocca et al. 1997).

Potential advantages of the TCAs over the benzodiazepines include their ability to treat symptoms of both anxiety and depression, the absence of potential for abuse and physiological dependence, and their effectiveness in the management of discontinuation of long-term benzodiazepine therapy (Rickels et al. 2000a). TCAs, however, can be accompanied by a variety of troublesome side effects related to pharmacological blockade of histamine$_1$ (H$_1$), α_1-adrenergic, and muscarinic receptors, and these effects can limit their use. Frequently reported adverse effects include weight gain, orthostatic hypotension, edema, urinary retention, blurred vision, dry mouth, and constipation. Sedation is also commonly noted; for some patients this is an adverse event, whereas for others it is of therapeutic benefit. The utility of the TCAs is also limited by their cardiotoxic potential and lethality in overdose.

Selective Serotonin Reuptake Inhibitors and Serotonin–Norepinephrine Reuptake Inhibitors

A number of SSRIs are effective in GAD. Paroxetine IR at 20–50 mg per day has been shown to be as effective as imipramine and more effective than 2'-chlordesmethyldiazepam, with the antidepressants again demonstrating greatest effect on symptoms of psychic anxiety (Rocca et al. 1997). Compared with placebo, a similar dosage range of paroxetine IR was associated with significant reduction in anxiety after 8 weeks of treatment (Bellew et al. 2000; Pollack et al. 2001), with an improvement in psychic anxiety as measured by reduction in the anxious mood item of the Ham-A scale, observed as early as 1 week after initiating treatment (Pollack et al. 2001). Paroxetine IR also improves social functioning in patients with GAD (Bellew et al. 2000). Rickels et al. (2003) have reported superior benefit of paroxetine IR in GAD, relative to placebo.

Three 8-week placebo-controlled trials have found efficacy for escitalopram in a 10- to 20-mg dose range on a variety of measures, of both anxiety symptoms and disability or quality of life (Davidson et al. 2004a; Goodman et al. 2005). In a 6-month trial, Bielski et al. (2005) found equivalent benefit for paroxetine IR and escitalopram. In a larger placebo-controlled trial of three doses of escitalo-

pram and 20 mg paroxetine IR, 10 mg escitalopram demonstrated superiority over 20 mg paroxetine, 10 and 20 mg escitalopram were superior to placebo, while 5 mg escitalopram and 20 mg paroxetine IR were superior on some secondary outcomes (Baldwin et al. 2006). A relapse prevention study found that sustained treatment with escitalopram 20 mg/day up to 74 weeks reduced the rate of relapse relative to placebo substitution (Allgulander et al. 2006). Relapse rates were for 19% for escitalopram versus 56% for placebo.

Two studies have shown benefit for sertraline over placebo in GAD (Allgulander et al. 2004; Brawman-Mintzer et al. 2006).

Several placebo-controlled trials have confirmed the short-term efficacy of venlafaxine XR in GAD over 8 weeks, with improvement noted in both the psychic and the somatic symptoms of the disorder. In one trial, 365 adult outpatients received treatment with venlafaxine XR (75 mg/day or 150 mg/day), buspirone (30 mg/day), or placebo (Davidson et al. 1999). The adjusted mean scores on the Ham-A anxious mood and tension items were significantly improved at both dosages of venlafaxine XR compared with placebo; however, the adjusted mean Ham-A total score failed to distinguish between the groups. Venlafaxine XR was superior to buspirone on the Anxiety subscale of the HADS. In a second trial, 541 outpatients were given either venlafaxine XR (37.5 mg/day, 75 mg/day, or 150 mg/day) or placebo (Allgulander et al. 2001). By the end of the study, the 75-mg and 150-mg doses of venlafaxine showed superior efficacy to placebo on all primary outcome measures, whereas the 37.5-mg dose was superior on only one measure (the Anxiety subscale of the HADS). Significant improvement was noted in symptoms of psychic anxiety by week 2 of treatment with venlafaxine, with reduction of somatic symptoms noted a bit later, following 4–8 weeks of treatment. A third trial evaluated fixed dosages of venlafaxine XR at 75 mg/day, 150 mg/day, and 225 mg/day (Rickels et al. 2000b). Venlafaxine XR was superior to placebo on all outcome measures, although the most robust effects were observed with 225 mg/day. In addition, venlafaxine XR significantly reduced psychic anxiety but was no different from placebo in treating somatic symptoms of anxiety.

Venlafaxine XR also has shown long-term efficacy in GAD. In two 6-month controlled trials of fixed (37.5 mg, 75 mg, 150 mg/day) (Allgulander et al. 2001) and flexible (75–225 mg/day) (Gelenberg et al. 2000) doses of venlafaxine XR, significant improvement in anxiety was observed as early as 1 week, and efficacy was sustained over the 28-week treatment period. In the fixed-dose study, the greatest effect was observed with the 150-mg/day dose. In addition, significant improvement in social functioning was noted at the two higher doses by week 8 and sustained over the 6 months of the trial.

Venlafaxine XR is also effective in treating GAD with comorbid depression (Silverstone and Salinas 2001). After 12 weeks of treatment with venlafaxine XR (75–225 mg/day), fluoxetine, or placebo, significant reduction was observed in both anxiety and depression, as measured by the Ham-A and the Ham-D, respectively, only in subjects receiving venlafaxine XR. The response was delayed somewhat in subjects with comorbid GAD and depression, as compared with those with depression alone, suggesting that those with comorbidity may benefit from a longer course of treatment.

The traditional treatment goal for GAD and many other psychiatric disorders has been attainment of response, defined as 50% improvement relative to baseline. There is a growing consensus in the field, however, that this goal is not sufficient for many patients and that the goal of treatment should instead be remission, defined as 70% or greater improvement from baseline and/or minimal or absent symptoms (i.e., Ham-A score ≤7). Pooled analysis of data from the two long-term studies noted above has determined that remission is attainable in GAD (Meoni and Hackett 2000). By 2 months, approximately 40% of those receiving venlafaxine responded to treatment (response defined as ≥50% reduction in Ham-A score from baseline), and 42% attained remission (defined as a Ham-A score ≤7). By 6 months, the proportion of those in remission increased to almost 60%, whereas responders declined to 20%, in contrast to a remission rate of less than 40% with placebo.

Venlafaxine XR has some advantages over the benzodiazepines—notably, antidepressant activity, lack of potential for abuse and dependence, and efficacy in treating symptoms of psychic anxiety. Nonetheless, venlafaxine can be associated with some adverse effects, even though the incidence of these effects diminishes markedly with long-term treatment. Adverse events may be noted with long-term therapy, however, and include sexual dysfunction and blood pressure elevation in some patients. In addition, abrupt discontinuation of treatment can be associated with unpleasant side effects, most commonly dizziness, light-headedness, tinnitus, nausea, vomiting, and loss of appetite, and the discontinuation syndrome is worse if one abruptly stops from higher dosage levels (Allgulander et al. 2001).

Duloxetine, also an SNRI antidepressant, has shown superior efficacy to placebo in GAD (Allgulander et al.

2007; Rynn et al. 2008) in the range of 60–120 mg per day, as well as lessening the chance of relapse during maintenance therapy.

Noradrenergic and Specific Serotonergic Antidepressants (Mirtazapine, Bupropion)

The antidepressant mirtazapine also has demonstrated anxiolytic properties (Ribeiro et al. 2001). However, published reports of its effect in GAD are limited to a small open-label study in major depression and comorbid GAD (Goodnick et al. 1999). Although the results were encouraging, data from controlled trials are needed to adequately assess a possible role for mirtazapine in GAD.

One double-blind trial, published in abstract form, found that bupropion XL produced a higher remission rate than escitalopram, as well as better coping skills (Bystritsky et al. 2005). Notwithstanding these intriguing findings, the body of clinical evidence for now supports the use of serotonergic drugs, or dual serotonergic/noradrenergic reuptake inhibitors, before agents that are primarily noradrenergic in action. However, the Bystritsky et al. findings suggest the potential importance of noradrenergic mechanisms in GAD and its therapeutics.

Hydroxyzine

Hydroxyzine, a drug that blocks both H_1 and muscarinic receptors, has been studied in GAD. In one controlled study, hydroxyzine was superior to placebo following 1 week of treatment, and this difference was maintained over a 4-week trial (Ferreri and Hantouche 1998). In a larger controlled multicenter trial, hydroxyzine was compared with buspirone over 4 weeks (Lader and Scotto 1998). Changes in the Ham-A from baseline to day 28 indicated that hydroxyzine was superior to placebo, with no difference observed between buspirone and placebo. Of note, both hydroxyzine and buspirone were more efficacious than placebo on the secondary outcomes. Llorca et al. (2002) found that hydroxyzine 50 mg/day was superior to placebo and comparable to bromazepam in a 12-week trial.

Other Drugs

The $\alpha_2\delta$ calcium channel antagonist pregabalin was superior to placebo in four studies of GAD (Feltner et al. 2003; Pande et al. 2003; Pohl et al. 2005; Rickels et al. 2005). Efficacy was noted early in treatment, but the ability of this drug to successfully treat some of the comorbid disorders found with GAD is unknown. The GABA reuptake inhibitor tiagabine failed to separate from placebo on key measures in one multicenter trial (Pollack et al. 2005).

Evidence for antipsychotic monotherapy in GAD is limited. An open-label trial suggested benefit for ziprasidone (Snyderman et al. 2005). Flupenthixol is approved for the use of depression in some countries but is also widely used to treat GAD-like states. One controlled study showed that flupenthixol was superior to amitriptyline, clotiazepam, and placebo among subjects with refractory GAD (Wurthmann et al. 1995). Sulpiride is also used in similar situations (Bruscky et al. 1974; Chen et al. 1994). Use of antipsychotic drugs carries some concern about their tolerability and safety profile.

Riluzole, a presynaptic glutamate release inhibitor, has shown promise in a small open-label study at a daily dose of 100 mg (Mathew et al. 2005).

Complementary treatments, such as homeopathy and the herbal remedy kava kava, are ineffective in GAD (Bonne et al. 2003; Connor and Davidson 2002).

A meta-analysis of GAD studies by Hidalgo et al. (2007) showed that the effect sizes (in diminishing order from strongest to weakest) for each drug or drug group versus placebo were as follows: pregabalin, 0.50; hydroxyzine, 0.45; venlafaxine XR, 0.42; benzodiazepines, 0.38; SSRIs, 0.36; buspirone, 0.17; and homeopathy and herbal treatment, −0.31.

Drugs that have been approved in the United States for treating GAD or historical forerunners of the disorder include a large number of benzodiazepines, buspirone, paroxetine IR, escitalopram, venlafaxine XR, and duloxetine.

There is also convincing evidence in favor of efficacy for CBT in GAD, with sustained benefit over 2 years of follow-up. These findings have been well reviewed by Swinson et al. (2006). There are no clinically informative studies to compare, or combine, CBT and pharmacotherapy in GAD, but on pragmatic grounds, one may consider their combination in patients who have shown only a partial response to a thorough course of either CBT or medication alone.

Posttraumatic Stress Disorder

PTSD is a chronic and disabling disorder, with a lifetime prevalence of about 7% (Kessler et al. 2005a). The direct and indirect consequences of the disorder inflict an enormous burden on society, leading PTSD to be the primary cost driver in the annual $42 billion cost of anxiety disorders in the late 1990s (P.E. Greenberg et al. 1999).

Treatment of PTSD should target a range of presenting features. Clearly, effective therapy needs to reduce the core symptoms of the disorder. Treatment also should focus on improving resilience and coping with daily stress, improving quality of life, and reducing comorbidity and disability. For some, medication may serve to help seal over the distress and pain of the event and allow a return to normal daily activities. For others, medication may help them to engage in a treatment plan that involves uncovering the distress and allows for resolution of the traumatic experience.

Instruments that have been widely used in trials of pharmacotherapy comprise the DSM-IV criteria–linked Clinician-Administered PTSD Scale (CAPS; Weathers et al. 2001) and the more globally oriented Short PTSD Rating Instrument (SPRINT; Connor and Davidson 2001). Self-rating scales include the Davidson Trauma Scale (DTS; Davidson et al. 1997a), a 17-item, two-part assessment of the major DSM-IV symptoms of PTSD, and the SPRINT, which also has been validated as a self-rating. Most studies to date have evaluated monotherapy, but a growing number are examining augmentation approaches.

Antidepressants

The TCAs and MAOIs were among the first pharmacological agents studied in controlled trials of PTSD. More recently, findings from several controlled multicenter trials have shown efficacy for the SSRI and SNRI drugs. With the documented antidepressant and anxiolytic effects of these noradrenergic and serotonergic agents, and the high rates of comorbid depression in PTSD (Kessler et al. 1995), antidepressants would seem like a logical choice for treatment of PTSD.

Tricyclic Antidepressants

Positive evidence for the efficacy of TCAs has been found in two controlled trials involving male combat veterans with PTSD defined by DSM-III criteria. In one study, 46 World War II and Vietnam War veterans were given amitriptyline (50–300 mg/day) or placebo for 8 weeks. Greater improvement was noted with amitriptyline than with placebo; 50% of those receiving amitriptyline showed much or very much global improvement, compared with 17% of those receiving placebo (Davidson et al. 1990). A second study examined imipramine (50–300 mg/day) and placebo in 60 veterans of the Vietnam era. Greater reduction in symptoms was noted in subjects receiving imipramine, with a 25% reduction in Impact of Event Scale (IES; Horowitz et al. 1979) score from baseline for imipramine compared with 5% for placebo. Global improvement also was superior with imipramine (65%) compared with placebo (28%) (Kosten et al. 1991). Together, these studies showed that TCAs are more effective than placebo in the short-term treatment of PTSD in male combat veterans.

Monoamine Oxidase Inhibitors

In a study of male combat veterans, Kosten et al. (1991) compared phenelzine (15–75 mg/day) with placebo and found a 45% decrease in IES score from baseline for phenelzine, compared with a 5% decrease for placebo, but no improvement was noted in depressive symptoms with either treatment. The RIMA brofaromine has been assessed in two controlled trials of PTSD: a U.S. sample composed predominantly of combat veterans (n = 114) (Baker et al. 1995) and a civilian European sample with few veterans (n = 68) (Katz et al. 1994). The U.S. study failed to show a difference between the treatments. Findings from the European study also were mixed, depending on the measure used to assess change. Finally, the RIMA moclobemide was assessed in 20 subjects with PTSD meeting DSM-III-R (American Psychiatric Association 1987) criteria (Neal et al. 1997). Following 12 weeks of treatment, 11 subjects no longer met the full PTSD criteria, providing a signal that the drug might be effective in PTSD.

Selective Serotonin Reuptake Inhibitors

Three controlled trials support the efficacy of fluoxetine in PTSD. In these studies, fluoxetine was administered at dosages of 20–80 mg/day for 5–12 weeks in samples including both civilians and combat veterans with PTSD meeting DSM-III-R (Connor et al. 1999; van der Kolk et al. 1994) or DSM-IV (Martenyi et al. 2002a) criteria. Significant differences were observed in favor of fluoxetine, as measured by changes in clinician-rated structured interviews from baseline to the end of treatment. In the study by Connor et al. (1999), fluoxetine also was associated with a significant improvement in resilience, as measured by a reduction in stress vulnerability, and in disability. Martenyi et al. (2002a) showed that at a mean dosage of 57 mg/day, fluoxetine was associated with significant reduction in PTSD symptoms from baseline as early as week 6 and at week 12, in a sample predominantly made up of male combat veterans.

Two studies of maintenance therapy with fluoxetine over a period of 1 year have shown reductions in the rate of relapse, as compared with placebo substitution (Davidson et al. 2005; Martenyi et al. 2002b).

Two studies have shown efficacy for sertraline in PTSD (Brady et al. 2000; Davidson et al. 2001). At a mean dosage of approximately 150 mg/day, sertraline was more effective than placebo in reducing overall PTSD symptoms and avoidance; symptoms of arousal improved with sertraline in one study (Brady et al. 2000; Davidson et al. 2001), but no differences were noted in intrusive symptoms. Based on a response definition of a greater than 30% reduction in CAPS (Blake et al. 1995) score from baseline and a CGI score of 1 or 2 (much or very much improvement), response rates for sertraline ranged from 53% to 60%, compared with 32%–38% for placebo. A pooled analysis of these data showed the broad-spectrum effect of the drug, particularly on psychological symptoms of the disorder, with an early modulation of anger at 1 week preceding improvement in other symptoms (Davidson et al. 2002). This finding is of particular interest, given that angry temperament can be associated with impulsivity and violence and a greater risk for cardiac events (Williams et al. 2001), as well as increased heart rate and blood pressure, in PTSD (Beckham et al. 2002). Other short-term studies of sertraline in PTSD have been negative (Brady et al. 2005; Davidson et al. 2006b; Friedman et al. 2007) or inconclusive (Zohar et al. 2002).

Continued treatment with sertraline over 9 months was associated with sustained improvement in more than 90% of the subjects (Londborg et al. 2001). In those with more severe PTSD who did not improve with acute treatment over 12 weeks, more than 50% were likely to respond with continued treatment (Londborg et al. 2001). Over 15 months of treatment, improvement was sustained, with relapse rates of 5% with sertraline and 26% with placebo, thereby suggesting that the drug provides prophylactic protection against relapse (Davidson et al. 2001). Sertraline is also effective in improving quality of life and reducing functional impairment, with rapid improvement noted with acute treatment and more than 55% of patients functioning at levels within 10% of the general population. These gains are maintained with long-term treatment, and continued improvement can be noted, whereas treatment discontinuation is more likely to lead to deteriorating function, although not to levels observed prior to treatment (Rapaport et al. 2002).

The efficacy of paroxetine in PTSD has been shown in two 12-week controlled multicenter trials, including flexible-dose (n = 307; paroxetine 20–50 mg) (Tucker et al. 2001) and fixed-dose (n = 451; paroxetine 20 or 40 mg) (Marshall et al. 2001) regimens. Compared with placebo, paroxetine produced significant improvement in overall PTSD symptomatology, individual symptom clusters, and functional impairment. Response rates ranged from 54% to 62% for paroxetine compared with 37% to 40% for placebo.

Findings from two open-label studies of fluvoxamine, at dosages of 100–250 mg/day, have been reported, including those from an 8-week study in civilians (*n* = 15) and a 10-week study in combat veterans (*n* = 10) (Davidson et al. 1998; Marmar et al. 1996), in which the drug was effective in treating symptoms of PTSD. Treatment with fluvoxamine (mean = 194 mg/day) also has been associated with significant improvement in autonomic reactivity, with reductions in heart rate and blood pressure on exposure to trauma cues to levels that are indistinguishable from those of control subjects without PTSD (Tucker et al. 2000). These findings are encouraging, but larger controlled trials are needed to determine the efficacy of the drug in PTSD.

Two large multicenter studies have established efficacy for venlafaxine XR up to 300 mg per day, in one case for as long as 6 months. Rates of remission exceeded 50% in the longer-term trial, and resilience was significantly improved in one of the two studies (Davidson et al. 2006a, 2006b).

In summary, the SSRIs are efficacious in the treatment of PTSD, with two drugs, paroxetine IR and sertraline, approved for treatment of PTSD. SSRIs and SNRIs show a broad spectrum of activity, with significant reduction in some symptoms as early as 1–2 weeks after treatment initiation. SSRI and SNRI drugs not only improve symptoms with acute treatment but also result in sustained and continued improvement, and in some cases remission, with long-term treatment up to 15 months. These drugs are generally well tolerated, although some adverse effects (e.g., sexual dysfunction, sleep disturbances, and weight gain) may lead to treatment discontinuation.

Other Antidepressants

Results of one 8-week controlled trial of mirtazapine in 29 outpatients with PTSD have been reported. A clinician-rated global assessment found response rates to mirtazapine of 65% compared with response rates to placebo of 20%, with significant improvement on several measures of PTSD as well as general anxiety (Davidson et al. 2003).

Six open-label studies of nefazodone in civilians and combat veterans with PTSD have been reported (Hidalgo et al. 1999). Treatment with nefazodone (50–600 mg/day) over 6–12 weeks was associated with significant reduction in severity of overall PTSD, as well as in each of

the symptom clusters. Of particular note was improvement in sleep, which is often disrupted in PTSD, and these problems are frequently exacerbated by treatment with SSRIs. Davis et al. (2004) have demonstrated superior efficacy for the drug, relative to placebo, in combat veterans.

Anxiolytics

Benzodiazepines are often prescribed to treat acute anxiety in the aftermath of a trauma. However, findings have been disappointing. An open-label study of alprazolam and clonazepam in 13 outpatients with PTSD found reduced hyperarousal symptoms but no change in intrusion or avoidance/numbing (Gelpin et al. 1996). In a crossover design, subjects received 5 weeks of treatment with either alprazolam or placebo followed by 5 weeks of the alternative therapy (Braun et al. 1990). Minimal improvement was observed in anxiety symptoms overall, with no improvement in the core symptoms of PTSD. Clonazepam 2 mg was not different from placebo in controlling nightmares in a 2-week single-blind crossover study, where the test drug was added to preexisting treatment (Cates et al. 2004). Thus, the evidence does not yet support the use of benzodiazepines in PTSD, even though they appear to be widely used (Mellman et al. 2003). Their position in managing PTSD thus remains unclear.

Anticonvulsants

In the 1980s, Lipper et al. (1986) proposed that the pathophysiology of PTSD may involve sensitization and kindling processes and, to this end, that anticonvulsants might be of therapeutic benefit. In testing this hypothesis, these investigators found that 7 of 10 (70%) Vietnam War veterans who received open-label carbamazepine (600–1,000 mg/day) for 5 weeks had "moderate" or "very much" improvement with treatment, particularly in symptoms of intrusion and hyperarousal. Three subsequent open-label studies have been performed, including two with sodium valproate in combat veterans (R.D. Clark et al. 1999; Fesler 1991) and a study of adjunctive topiramate in a civilian PTSD sample (Berlant and van Kammen 2002). The treatments showed somewhat different effects, with sodium valproate (250–2,000 mg/day) improving symptoms of arousal and intrusion in one study (Fesler 1991) and arousal and avoidance in the other (R.D. Clark et al. 1999), whereas topiramate (15.5–500 mg/day) was most effective in reducing symptoms of intrusion, particularly nightmares and flashbacks (Berlant and van Kammen

2002). The largest placebo-controlled trial of an anticonvulsant to date found no difference between tiagabine, dosed up to 16 mg per day, and placebo in 232 patients in a 12-week multicenter trial (Davidson et al. 2007). In a small placebo-controlled trial of lamotrigine (200–500 mg per day) in 15 outpatients (Hertzberg et al. 1999), a response rate of 50% was noted with lamotrigine, compared with a placebo response rate of 25%.

Other Treatments

Antipsychotics

One placebo-controlled monotherapy trial of olanzapine has been published (Butterfield et al. 2001), in which 15 subjects were randomized 2:1 to treatment with olanzapine (up to 20 mg/day) or placebo. No differences were observed between the treatments, although olanzapine was associated with greater weight gain. It is difficult to interpret these findings in this small sample, especially given the high placebo response rate (60%). Other reports of antipsychotics are based on augmentation therapy in SSRI partial responders. Four placebo-controlled studies, mainly as augmentation, have found superior efficacy for low-dose risperidone (Bartzokis et al. 2005; Hamner et al. 2003; Monnelly et al. 2003; Reich et al. 2004) and olanzapine (M.B. Stein et al. 2002). In the Monnelly study, particular benefit was noted for irritability and in the Hamner study, psychotic symptoms were relieved. These antipsychotic studies in aggregate comprised 155 patients.

Prazosin and Guanfacine

Raskind et al. (2003) reported encouraging results for intractable PTSD-related nightmares in a placebo-controlled crossover study of prazosin, an α_1-adrenergic antagonist, at doses of up to 10 mg/day. The investigators have confirmed their initial findings in a second and larger placebo-controlled, double-blind augmentation trial conducted in combat veterans, using doses of up to 15 mg daily; benefits were most apparent on nightmares and sleep quality, but the drug also produced greater global improvement (Raskind et al. 2007). One possible mechanism of action may lie in the ability of prazosin to reduce the output of corticotropin-releasing hormone. Suppression of nightmare-generating non–rapid eye movement stage 1 sleep may be another explanation for this intriguing finding. Standing in contrast is a negative placebo-controlled study of the α_2-adrenergic agonist guanfacine in patients who, unlike those in the prazosin

studies, were not preselected for having troublesome nightmares (Neylan et al. 2006).

Other Drugs

Given the prevalence of comorbid depression with PTSD and the effectiveness of triiodothyronine (T_3) augmentation in some individuals with treatment-refractory depression, it is possible that T_3 augmentation also may be of benefit in PTSD. Five subjects with PTSD currently taking an SSRI were treated with open-label T_3 (25 μg/day) for 8 weeks (Agid et al. 2001). Improvement was noted as early as 2 weeks, and by the end of treatment, four of the five subjects showed at least partial improvement in depressive symptoms and hyperarousal. The mechanism for these effects is unknown, and further controlled studies of this augmentation strategy are therefore needed. Cyproheptadine, an antihistaminic drug, was no more effective than placebo for nightmares over 2 weeks in a series of 69 combat veterans with PTSD (Jacobs-Rebhun et al. 2000). The naturally occurring compound inositol was ineffective in a small placebo-controlled trial (Kaplan et al. 1996).

Acute Stress Disorder and the Immediate Aftermath of Trauma

Acute stress disorder (ASD) is characterized by the development of a constellation of symptoms shortly after a traumatic event and includes symptoms of dissociation and intrusive recollections, avoidance, and hyperarousal. These symptoms persist for 2–28 days following the trauma and cause significant distress and/or impairment. If the condition persists beyond 1 month, the individual usually qualifies for a diagnosis of PTSD. ASD was first included in the diagnostic nosology in DSM-IV, and little is known about the pharmacotherapy of this disorder. As noted earlier, it has been suggested that early intervention for trauma survivors might help to alter the course of PTSD, and this would imply early identification and treatment of those with or at risk for ASD.

The effects of open-label treatment with risperidone have been reported in four inpatient survivors of physical trauma with ASD; this drug showed possible benefit in flashback symptoms (Eidelman et al. 2000). A controlled pilot study assessed the effects of low-dose imipramine compared with choral hydrate in 25 pediatric burn patients with ASD (Robert et al. 1999a). After 1 week of treatment, 38% of the subjects responded to treatment with placebo, compared with 83% to imipramine, with an earlier report noting reduction in intrusion and hyperarousal symptoms (Robert et al. 1999b). Another study evaluated the effects of β-adrenergic blockade in reducing subsequent PTSD following acute trauma (Pitman et al. 2002). Within 6 hours of the trauma, subjects were treated with either propranolol (n=18; 40 mg qid) or placebo (n=23) for 10 days, followed by a 9-day taper period. One month after the trauma, PTSD was noted in 30% of the placebo group compared with 10% of the propranolol group. At 3-month follow-up, physiological arousal was assessed using personal script-driven imagery of the event, and 43% of the placebo group were physiological responders compared with 0% of the propranolol group. Although the dropout rate was higher with propranolol (7 of 18; 39%) than with placebo (3 of 23; 13%), these findings suggest that acute treatment with β-adrenergic-blocking agents may be effective in preventing the later development of PTSD, but further studies are needed. In one study of temazepam versus placebo for ASD or subthreshold PTSD, coupled with at least moderate sleep disturbance, there was no advantage for the drug, either during treatment or at follow-up 6 weeks posttrauma (Mellman et al. 2002). Two promising studies have found greater long-term benefit for short-term hydrocortisone versus placebo in high-risk subjects recovering from septic shock and from cardiac surgery (Schelling et al. 2006). In subpopulations with critical illness–related corticosteroid insufficiency, this might be an attractive treatment approach for preventing PTSD. One limitation of the authors' work, however, has been the absence of baseline PTSD ratings before administration of hydrocortisone.

CBT has been extensively studied in PTSD and shows efficacy in most cases (Bisson and Andrew 2005). Exposure is regarded as the key therapeutic principle in the numerous variants of CBT. Modest preservation of gains is found at long-term follow-up (Bradley et al. 2005), but much pathology remains. For this reason, it is unfortunate that there are almost no trials, either long or short term, combining CBT with drugs. Shortened forms of CBT appear to be effective for acute PTSD-like states, with persistence of gain at 4-year follow-up (Bryant et al. 1998, 2003).

Conclusion

Twenty years ago, few would have thought that one class of drugs, the SSRIs, which were all introduced initially for depression, would have established primacy in five of the six major anxiety disorder categories. Their position is based on solid category 1 randomized, controlled trial evidence, and they are now first-line drugs for treatment of these disorders. To the extent that studies have been conducted, SSRIs also offer some protection against relapse. However, they are not 100% successful, they carry some limiting side effects, and they may require supplementation with, or substitution by, drugs from other categories. We have reviewed what is known about these other drugs and expect further progress in the pharmacotherapy of anxiety, with both established drugs and novel categories (e.g., corticotropin-releasing hormone antagonist). Among many unexplored areas, we need to know more about the treatment of resistant anxiety disorders and comorbid anxiety disorder and the comparative efficacy, or contribution, of pharmacotherapy and psychosocial treatment in anxiety.

The rationale for using drugs rests, in part, on the broad-based evidence that vulnerability to each of the anxiety disorders includes shared and/or unique genetic risk factors, which usually coexist with environmental factors in respect of explaining variance. High trait neuroticism is a genetic risk factor for internalizing disorders as a whole and for comorbidity among the anxiety disorders and depression (Hettema et al. 2006). A diagnostically nonspecific genetic vulnerability may underlie fear proneness and amygdalar hyperreactivity (Hariri et al. 2005). Family and twin studies, as well as other types of studies, support genetic risk factors for generalized anxiety, panic disorder, phobias, and OCD (Hettema et al. 2001; Westenberg et al. 2007) and social anxiety disorder (Mathew and Ho 2007), for which some candidate genes are beginning to emerge. For PTSD, the evidence suggests a role for unique and shared genetic effects (Chantarujikapong et al. 2001; True et al. 1993), including common genetic liability for PTSD and major depression (Koenen et al. 2008). While detailed consideration of genetics goes beyond the scope of this chapter, it is of considerable interest to note the findings of M. B. Stein et al. (2006) and Denys et al. (2007), for example, that drug response in social anxiety disorder and OCD, respectively, may be related to genetic polymorphisms. These exciting findings may herald a time when we can more effectively individualize pharmacotherapy for anxiety.

References

Agid O, Shalev AY, Lerer B, et al: Triiodothyronine augmentation of selective serotonin reuptake inhibitors in posttraumatic stress disorder. J Clin Psychiatry 62:169–173, 2001

Alamy S, Zhang W, Varia I, et al: Escitalopram in specific phobia: results of a placebo-controlled pilot trial. J Psychopharmacol 22:157–161, 2008

Allgulander C: Paroxetine in social anxiety disorder: a randomized placebo-controlled study. Acta Psychiatr Scand 100:193–198, 1999

Allgulander C, Hackett D, Salinas E: Venlafaxine extended release (ER) in the treatment of generalised anxiety disorder: twenty-four-week placebo-controlled dose-ranging study. Br J Psychiatry 179:15–22, 2001

Allgulander C, Dahl AA, Austin C, et al: Efficacy of sertraline in a 12-week trial for generalized anxiety disorder. Am J Psychiatry 161:1642–1649, 2004

Allgulander C, Florea I, Huusom AK: Prevention of relapse in generalized anxiety disorder by escitalopram treatment. Int J Neuropsychopharmacol 9:495–505, 2006

Allgulander C, Hartford J, Russell J, et al: Pharmacotherapy of generalized anxiety disorder: results of duloxetine treatment from a pooled analysis of three clinical trials. Curr Med Res Opin 23:1245–1252, 2007

Alonso J, Angermeyer MC, Bernert S, et al: Sampling and methods of the European Study of the Epidemiology of Mental Disorders (ESEMeD) project. Acta Psychiatr Scand Suppl (420):8–20, 2004

American Psychiatric Association: Diagnostic and Statistical Manual of Mental Disorders, 3rd Edition. Washington, DC, American Psychiatric Association, 1980

American Psychiatric Association: Diagnostic and Statistical Manual of Mental Disorders, 3rd Edition, Revised. Washington, DC, American Psychiatric Association, 1987

American Psychiatric Association: Diagnostic and Statistical Manual of Mental Disorders, 4th Edition. Washington, DC, American Psychiatric Association, 1994

Andersch S, Rosenberg NK, Kullingsjo H, et al: Efficacy and safety of alprazolam, imipramine and placebo in treating panic disorder. A Scandinavian multicenter study. Acta Psychiatr Scand Suppl 365:18–27, 1991

Asakura S, Tajima O, Koyama T: Fluvoxamine treatment of generalized social anxiety disorder in Japan: a randomized double-blind, placebo-controlled study. Int J Neuropsychopharmacol 10:263–274, 2007

Asnis GM, Hameedi FA, Goddard AW, et al: Fluvoxamine in the treatment of panic disorder: a multi-center, double-blind, placebo-controlled study in outpatients. Psychiatry Res 103:1–14, 2001

Baer L, Rauch SL, Ballantine HT Jr, et al: Cingulotomy for intractable obsessive-compulsive disorder. Prospective long-term follow-up of 18 patients. Arch Gen Psychiatry 52:384–392, 1995

Baker DG, Diamond BI, Gillette G, et al: A double-blind, randomized, placebo-controlled, multi-center study of brofaromine in the treatment of post-traumatic stress disorder. Psychopharmacology (Berl) 122:386–389, 1995

Bakish D, Saxena BM, Bowen R, et al: Reversible monoamine oxidase-A inhibitors in panic disorder. Clin Neuropharmacol 16 (suppl 2):S77–S82, 1993

Baldwin D, Bobes J, Stein DJ, et al: Paroxetine in social phobia/social anxiety disorder. Randomised, double-blind, placebo-controlled study. Paroxetine Study Group. Br J Psychiatry 175:120–126, 1999

Baldwin DS, Huusom AK, Maehlum E: Escitalopram and paroxetine in the treatment of generalised anxiety disorder: ran-domised, placebo-controlled, double-blind study. Br J Psychiatry 189:264–272, 2006

Ballenger JC, Davidson JR, Lecrubier Y, et al: Consensus statement on panic disorder from the International Consensus Group on Depression and Anxiety. J Clin Psychiatry 59 (suppl 8):47–54, 1998a

Ballenger JC, Wheadon DE, Steiner M, et al: Double-blind, fixed-dose, placebo-controlled study of paroxetine in the treatment of panic disorder. Am J Psychiatry 155:36–42, 1998b

Bandelow B, Hajak G, Holzrichter S, et al: Assessing the efficacy of treatments for panic disorder and agoraphobia, I: methodological problems. Int Clin Psychopharmacol 10:83–93, 1995

Barnett SD, Kramer ML, Casat CD, et al: Efficacy of olanzapine in social anxiety disorder: a pilot study. J Psychopharmacol (Oxf) 16:365–368, 2002

Bartzokis G, Lu PH, Turner J, et al: Adjunctive risperidone in the treatment of chronic combat-related posttraumatic stress disorder. Biol Psychiatry 57:474–479, 2005

Beckham JC, Vrana SR, Barefoot JC, et al: Magnitude and duration of cardiovascular responses to anger in Vietnam veterans with and without posttraumatic stress disorder. J Consult Clin Psychol 70:228–234, 2002

Bell J, DeVeaugh-Geiss J: Multicenter trial of a 5-HT antagonist, ondansetron, in social phobia. Paper presented at the 33rd Annual Meeting of the American College of Neuropsychopharmacology, San Juan, Puerto Rico, December 12–16, 1994

Bellew KM, McCafferty JP, Iyengar M: Short-term efficacy of paroxetine in generalized anxiety disorder: a double-blind placebo-controlled trial (NR253). Paper presented at the 153rd Annual Meeting of the American Psychiatric Association, Chicago, IL, May 13–18, 2000

Benjamin J, Ben-Zion IZ, Karbofsky E, et al: Double-blind placebo-controlled pilot study of paroxetine for specific phobia. Psychopharmacology 149:194–196, 2000

Bergink V, Westenberg HG: Metabotropic glutamate II receptor agonists in panic disorder: a double blind clinical trial with LY354740. Int Clin Psychopharmacol 20:291–293, 2005

Berigan TR: Panic attacks during escalation of mirtazapine. Primary Care Companion to the Journal of Clinical Psychiatry 5:93, 2003

Berlant J, van Kammen DP: Open-label topiramate as primary or adjunctive therapy in chronic civilian posttraumatic stress disorder: a preliminary report. J Clin Psychiatry 63:15–20, 2002

Bertani A, Perna G, Migliarese G, et al: Comparison of the treatment with paroxetine and reboxetine in panic disorder: a randomized, single-blind study. Pharmacopsychiatry 37:206–210, 2004

Bielski RJ, Bose A, Chang CC: A double-blind comparison of escitalopram and paroxetine in the long-term treatment of generalized anxiety disorder. Ann Clin Psychiatry 17:65–69, 2005

Bisson J, Andrew M: Psychological treatment of post-traumatic stress disorder (PTSD). Cochrane Database Syst Rev (2):CD003388, 2005

Black DW, Wesner R, Bowers W, et al: A comparison of fluvoxamine, cognitive therapy, and placebo in the treatment of panic disorder. Arch Gen Psychiatry 50:44–50, 1993

Blake DD, Weathers FW, Nagy LM, et al: The development of a clinician-administered PTSD scale. J Trauma Stress 8:75–90, 1995

Bloch MH, Landeros-Weisenberger A, Kelmendi B, et al: A systematic review: antipsychotic augmentation with treatment refractory obsessive-compulsive disorder. Mol Psychiatry 11:622–632, 2006

Blomhoff S, Haug TT, Hellstrom K, et al: Randomised controlled general practice trial of sertraline, exposure therapy and combined treatment in generalised social phobia. Br J Psychiatry 179:23–30, 2001

Bonne O, Shemer Y, Gorali Y, et al: A randomized, double-blind, placebo-controlled study of classical homeopathy in generalized anxiety disorder. J Clin Psychiatry 64:282–287, 2003

Boshuisen ML, Slaap BR, Vester-Blokland ED, et al: The effect of mirtazapine in panic disorder: an open label pilot study with a single-blind placebo run-in period. Int Clin Psychopharmacol 16:363–368, 2001

Boyer W: Serotonin uptake inhibitors are superior to imipramine and alprazolam in alleviating panic attacks: a meta-analysis. Int Clin Psychopharmacol 10:45–49, 1995

Bradley R, Greene J, Russ E, et al: A multidimensional meta-analysis of psychotherapy for PTSD. Am J Psychiatry 162:214–227, 2005

Bradwejn J, Ahokas A, Stein DJ, et al: Venlafaxine extended-release capsules in panic disorder: flexible-dose, double-blind, placebo-controlled study. Br J Psychiatry 187:352–359, 2005

Brady K, Pearlstein T, Asnis GM, et al: Efficacy and safety of sertraline treatment of posttraumatic stress disorder: a randomized controlled trial. JAMA 283:1837–1844, 2000

Brady KT, Sonne S, Anton RF, et al: Sertraline in the treatment of co-occurring alcohol dependence and posttraumatic stress disorder. Alcohol Clin Exp Res 29:395–401, 2005

Braun P, Greenberg D, Dasberg H, et al: Core symptoms of posttraumatic stress disorder unimproved by alprazolam treatment. J Clin Psychiatry 51:236–238, 1990

Brawman-Mintzer O, Knapp RG, Rynn M, et al: Sertraline treatment for generalized anxiety disorder: a randomized, double-blind, placebo-controlled study. J Clin Psychiatry 67:874–881, 2006

Bruscky SB, Caldeira MV, Bueno JR: Clinical trials of sulpiride. Arq Neuropsiquiatr 32:234–239, 1974

Bryant RA, Harvey AG, Dang ST, et al: Treatment of acute stress disorder: a comparison of cognitive-behavioral therapy and supportive counseling. J Consult Clin Psychol 66:862–866, 1998

Bryant RA, Moulds ML, Nixon RV, et al: Cognitive behaviour therapy of acute stress disorder: a four-year follow-up. Behav Res Ther 41:489–494, 2003

Butterfield MI, Becker ME, Connor KM, et al: Olanzapine in the treatment of post-traumatic stress disorder: a pilot study. Int Clin Psychopharmacol 16:197–203, 2001

Bystritsky A, Kerwin L, Eiduson S, et al: A pilot controlled trial of bupropion vs. escitalopram in generalized anxiety disorder (GAD) [abstract]. Neuropsychopharmacology 30 (suppl 1): S101, 2005

Cates ME, Bishop MH, Davis LL, et al: Clonazepam for treatment of sleep disturbances associated with combat-related posttraumatic stress disorder. Ann Pharmacother 38:1395–1399, 2004

Chantarujikapong SI, Scherrer JF, Xian H, et al: A twin study of generalized anxiety disorder symptoms, panic disorder symptoms and post-traumatic stress disorder in men. J Nerv Ment Dis 103:133–145, 2001

Charney DS, Woods SW, Goodman WK, et al: Drug treatment of panic disorder: the comparative efficacy of imipramine, alprazolam, and trazodone. J Clin Psychiatry 47:580–586, 1986

Chen A, Zhao Y, Yu X: The clinical study of antianxiety and antidepressive effect of sulpiride. Chin J Neurol Psychiatry 27:220–222, 1994

Clark DB, Agras WS: The assessment and treatment of performance anxiety in musicians. Am J Psychiatry 148:598–605, 1991

Clark DM, Ehlers A, McManus F, et al: Cognitive therapy versus fluoxetine in generalized social phobia: a randomized placebo-controlled trial. J Consult Clin Psychol 71:1058–1067, 2003

Clark RD, Canive JM, Calais LA, et al: Divalproex in posttraumatic stress disorder: an open-label clinical trial. J Trauma Stress 12:395–401, 1999

Clomipramine Collaborative Study Group: Clomipramine in the treatment of patients with obsessive-compulsive disorder. Arch Gen Psychiatry 48:730–738, 1991

Clum GA, Surls R: A meta-analysis of treatments for panic disorder. J Consult Clin Psychol 61:317–326, 1993

Cohn JB, Bowden CL, Fisher JG, et al: Double-blind comparison of buspirone and clorazepate in anxious outpatients. Am J Med 80:10–16, 1986

Compton SN, Grant PJ, Chrisman AK, et al: Sertraline in children and adolescents with social anxiety disorder: an open trial. J Am Acad Child Adolesc Psychiatry 40:564–571, 2001

Connor KM, Davidson JRT: SPRINT: a brief global assessment of post-traumatic stress disorder. Int Clin Psychopharmacol 16:279–284, 2001

Connor KM, Davidson JRT: A placebo-controlled study of kava kava in generalized anxiety disorder. Int Clin Psychopharmacol 17:185–188, 2002

Connor KM, Davidson JR, Potts NL, et al: Discontinuation of clonazepam in the treatment of social phobia. J Clin Psychopharmacol 18:373–378, 1998

Connor KM, Sutherland SM, Tupler LA, et al: Fluoxetine in posttraumatic stress disorder. Randomised, double-blind study. Br J Psychiatry 175:17–22, 1999

Connor KM, Davidson JRT, Churchill EL, et al: Psychometric properties of the Social Phobia Inventory (SPIN). A new self-rating scale. Br J Psychiatry 176:379–386, 2000

Cottraux J, Mollard E, Bouvard M, et al: Exposure therapy, fluvoxamine, or combination treatment in obsessive-compulsive disorder: one-year follow-up. Psychiatry Res 49:63–75, 1993

Crockett BA, Davidson JRT, Churchill LE: Treatment of obsessive-compulsive disorder with clonazepam and sertraline versus placebo and sertraline. Paper presented at the 39th Annual Meeting of the New Clinical Drug Evaluation Unit, Boca Raton, FL, June 1, 1999

Cross-National Collaborative Panic Study: Drug treatment of panic disorder. Comparative efficacy of alprazolam, imipramine, and placebo. Br J Psychiatry 160:191–202, 1992

Davidson JRT: The long-term treatment of panic disorder. J Clin Psychiatry 59 (suppl 8):17–21, 1998

Davidson JRT, Moroz G: Pivotal studies of clonazepam in panic disorder. Psychopharmacol Bull 34:169–174, 1998

Davidson JRT, Kudler H, Smith R, et al: Treatment of posttraumatic stress disorder with amitriptyline and placebo. Arch Gen Psychiatry 47:259–266, 1990

Davidson JRT, Hughes DL, George LK, et al: The epidemiology of social phobia: findings from the Duke Epidemiological Catchment Area Study. Psychol Med 23:709–718, 1993

Davidson JRT, Tupler LA, Potts NL: Treatment of social phobia with benzodiazepines. J Clin Psychiatry 55 (suppl):28–32, 1994

Davidson JRT, Book SW, Colket JT, et al: Assessment of a new self-rating scale for post-traumatic stress disorder. Psychol Med 27:153–160, 1997a

Davidson JRT, Miner CM, DeVeaugh-Geiss J, et al: The Brief Social Phobia Scale: a psychometric evaluation. Psychol Med 27:161–166, 1997b

Davidson JRT, Weisler RH, Malik M, et al: Fluvoxamine in civilians with posttraumatic stress disorder. J Clin Psychopharmacol 18:93–95, 1998

Davidson JRT, DuPont RL, Hedges D, et al: Efficacy, safety, and tolerability of venlafaxine extended release and buspirone in outpatients with generalized anxiety disorder. J Clin Psychiatry 60:528–535, 1999

Davidson JRT, Pearlstein T, Londborg P, et al: Efficacy of sertraline in preventing relapse of posttraumatic stress disorder: results of a 28-week double-blind, placebo-controlled study. Am J Psychiatry 158:1974–1981, 2001

Davidson JRT, Landerman LR, Farfel GM, et al: Characterizing the effects of sertraline in post-traumatic stress disorder. Psychol Med 32:661–670, 2002

Davidson JRT, Weisler RH, Butterfield MI, et al: Mirtazapine vs. placebo in posttraumatic stress disorder: a pilot trial. Biol Psychiatry 53:188–191, 2003

Davidson JRT, Bose A, Korotzer A, et al: Escitalopram in the treatment of generalized anxiety disorder: double-blind, placebo controlled, flexible-dose study. Depress Anxiety 19:234–240, 2004a

Davidson JRT, Foa EB, Huppert JD, et al: Fluoxetine, comprehensive cognitive behavioral therapy (CCBT) and placebo in generalized social phobia. Arch Gen Psychiatry 61:1005–1013, 2004b

Davidson JRT, Yaryura-Tobias J, DuPont R, et al: Fluvoxamine-controlled release formulation for the treatment of generalized social anxiety disorder. J Clin Psychopharmacol 24:118–225, 2004c

Davidson JRT, Connor KM, Hertzberg MA, et al: Maintenance therapy with fluoxetine in posttraumatic stress disorder: a placebo-controlled discontinuation study. J Clin Psychopharmacol 25:166–169, 2005

Davidson JRT, Baldwin D, Stein DJ, et al: Treatment of posttraumatic stress disorder with venlafaxine extended release: a 6-month randomized controlled trial. Arch Gen Psychiatry 63:1158–1165, 2006a

Davidson JRT, Rothbaum BO, Tucker P, et al: Venlafaxine extended release in posttraumatic stress disorder: a sertraline- and placebo-controlled study. J Clin Psychopharmacol 26:259–267, 2006b

Davidson JRT, Brady K, Mellman TA, et al: The efficacy and tolerability of tiagabine in adult patients with post-traumatic stress disorder. J Clin Psychopharmacol 27:85–88, 2007

Davis LL, Jewell ME, Ambrose S, et al: A placebo-controlled study of nefazodone for the treatment of chronic posttraumatic stress disorder: a preliminary study. J Clin Psychopharmacol 24:291–297, 2004

Den Boer JA, Westenberg HG: Effect of a serotonin and noradrenaline uptake inhibitor in panic disorder; a double-blind comparative study with fluvoxamine and maprotiline. Int Clin Psychopharmacol 3:59–74, 1988

Denys D, van Nieuwerburgh F, Deforce D, et al: Prediction of response to paroxetine and venlafaxine by serotonin-related genes in obsessive-compulsive disorder in a randomized, double-blind trial. J Clin Psychiatry 68:747–753, 2007

Eddy K, Dutra L, Bradley R, et al: A multidimensional meta-analysis of psychotherapy and pharmacotherapy for obsessive-compulsive disorder. Clin Psychol Rev 24:1–30, 2004

Eidelman I, Seedat S, Stein DJ: Risperidone in the treatment of acute stress disorder in physically traumatized in-patients. Depress Anxiety 11:187–188, 2000

Emmanuel NP, Lydiard RB, Ballenger JC: Treatment of social phobia with bupropion. J Clin Psychopharmacol 11:276–277, 1991

Enkelmann R: Alprazolam versus buspirone in the treatment of outpatients with generalized anxiety disorder. Psychopharmacology (Berl) 105:428–432, 1991

Fahlen T, Nilsson HL, Borg K, et al: Social phobia: the clinical efficacy and tolerability of the monoamine oxidase-A and serotonin uptake inhibitor brofaromine. A double-blind placebo-controlled study. Acta Psychiatr Scand 92:351–358, 1995

Fahy TJ, O'Rourke D, Brophy J, et al: The Galway Study of Panic Disorder, I: clomipramine and lofepramine in DSM-III-R panic disorder. A placebo controlled trial. J Affect Disord 25:63–75, 1992

Fallon BA, Campeas R, Schneier FR, et al: Open trial of intravenous clomipramine in five treatment-refractory patients with obsessive-compulsive disorder. J Neuropsychiatry Clin Neurosci 4:70–75, 1992

Fedoroff I, Taylor S: Psychological and pharmacological treatments of social phobia: a meta-analysis. J Clin Psychopharmacol 21:311–324, 2001

Feltner DE, Crockatt JG, Dubovsky SJ, et al: A randomized, double-blind, placebo-controlled, fixed-dose, multicenter study of pregabalin in patients with generalized anxiety disorder. J Clin Psychopharmacol 23:240–249, 2003

Ferguson JM, Khan A, Mangano R, et al: Relapse prevention of panic disorder in adult outpatient responders to treatment with venlafaxine extended release. J Clin Psychiatry 68:58–68, 2007

Fernandez-Cordoba E, Lopez-Ibor JA: La monoclorimipramina en enfermos psiquitricos resistentes a otrostratiamentos. Actas Luso-Espanolas de Neurologia, y Psiquiatria Ciencias Afines 26:119–147, 1967

Ferreri M, Hantouche EG: Recent clinical trials of hydroxyzine in generalized anxiety disorder. Acta Psychiatr Scand Suppl 393:102–108, 1998

Fesler FA: Valproate in combat-related posttraumatic stress disorder. J Clin Psychiatry 52:361–364, 1991

Fineberg NA, Sivakumaran T, Roberts A, et al: Adding quetiapine to SRI in treatment-resistant obsessive-compulsive disorder: a randomized controlled treatment study. Int Clin Psychopharmacol 20:223–226, 2005

Fineberg NA, Tonnoir B, Lemming O, et al: Escitalopram prevents relapse of obsessive-compulsive disorder. Eur Neuropsychopharmacol 17:430–439, 2007

Flament MF, Rapoport JL, Berg CJ, et al: Clomipramine treatment of childhood obsessive-compulsive disorder. A double-blind controlled study. Arch Gen Psychiatry 42:977–983, 1985

Foa EB, Liebowitz MR, Kozak MJ, et al: Randomized, placebo-controlled trial of exposure and ritual prevention, clomipramine, and their combination in the treatment of obsessive-compulsive disorder. Am J Psychiatry 162:151–161, 2005

Fontaine R, Beaudry P, Beauclair L, et al: Comparison of withdrawal of buspirone and diazepam: a placebo controlled study. Prog Neuropsychopharmacol Biol Psychiatry 11:189–197, 1987

Friedman MJ, Marmar CR, Baker DG, et al: Randomized double-blind comparison of sertraline and placebo for posttraumatic stress disorder in a Department of Veterans Affairs setting. J Clin Psychiatry 68:711–720, 2007

Fux M, Levine J, Aviv A, et al: Inositol treatment of obsessive-compulsive disorder. Am J Psychiatry 153:1219–1221, 1996

Gelenberg AJ, Lydiard RB, Rudolph RL, et al: Efficacy of venlafaxine extended-release capsules in nondepressed outpatients with generalized anxiety disorder: a 6-month randomized controlled trial. JAMA 283:3082–3088, 2000

Gelernter CS, Uhde TW, Cimbolic P, et al: Cognitive-behavioral and pharmacological treatments of social phobia. A controlled study. Arch Gen Psychiatry 48:938–945, 1991

Gelpin E, Bonne O, Peri T, et al: Treatment of recent trauma survivors with benzodiazepines: a prospective study. J Clin Psychiatry 57:390–394, 1996

Goddard AW, Brouette T, Almai A, et al: Early coadministration of clonazepam with sertraline for panic disorder. Arch Gen Psychiatry 58:681–686, 2001

Goisman RM, Allsworth J, Rogers MP, et al: Simple phobia as a comorbid anxiety disorder. Depress Anxiety 7:105–112, 1998

Goldberg DP, Lecrubier Y: Form and frequency of mental disorders across centers, in Mental Illness in General Health Care: An International Study. Edited by Üstürn TB, Sartorius N. New York, Wiley, 1995, pp 323–334

Goodman WK, Price LH, Rasmussen SA, et al: The Yale-Brown Obsessive Compulsive Scale, II: validity. Arch Gen Psychiatry 46:1012–1016, 1989

Goodman WK, Bose A, Wang Q: Treatment of generalized anxiety disorder with escitalopram: pooled results from double-blind, placebo-controlled trials. J Affect Disord 87:161–167, 2005

Goodnick PJ, Puig A, DeVane CL, et al: Mirtazapine in major depression with comorbid generalized anxiety disorder. J Clin Psychiatry 60:446–448, 1999

Greenberg BD, Malone DA, Friehs GM, et al: Three-year outcomes in deep brain stimulation for highly resistant obsessive-compulsive disorder. Neuropsychopharmacology 31:2384–2393, 2006

Greenberg PE, Sisitsky T, Kessler RC, et al: The economic burden of anxiety disorders in the 1990s. J Clin Psychiatry 60:427–435, 1999

Greenblatt DJ, Shader RI, Abernethy DR: Drug therapy. Current status of benzodiazepines. N Engl J Med 309:410–416, 1983

Greist JH, Jefferson JW: Pharmacotherapy for obsessive-compulsive disorder. Br J Psychiatry Suppl (35):64–70, 1998

Greist JH, Chouinard G, DuBoff E, et al: Double-blind parallel comparison of three dosages of sertraline and placebo in outpatients with obsessive-compulsive disorder. Arch Gen Psychiatry 52:289–295, 1995a

Greist JH, Jefferson JW, Kobak KA, et al: Efficacy and tolerability of serotonin transport inhibitors in obsessive-compulsive disorder. A meta-analysis. Arch Gen Psychiatry 52:53–60, 1995b

Hamilton M: The assessment of anxiety states by rating. Br J Med Psychol 32:50–55, 1959

Hamilton M: A rating scale for depression. J Neurol Neurosurg Psychiatry 23:56–62, 1960

Hamner MB, Faldowski RA, Ulmer HG, et al: Adjunctive risperidone treatment in post-traumatic stress disorder: a preliminary controlled trial of effects on comorbid psychotic symptoms. Int Clin Psychopharmacol 18:1–8, 2003

Hariri AR, Drabant EM, Munoz KE, et al: A susceptibility gene for affective disorders and the response of the human amygdala. Arch Gen Psychiatry 62:145–152, 2005

Haug TT, Hellstrom K, Blomhoff S, et al: The treatment of social phobia in general practice: is exposure therapy feasible? Fam Pract 17:114–118, 2000

Haug TT, Blomoff S, Hellstrom K, et al: Exposure therapy and sertraline in social phobia: 1-year follow-up of a randomized controlled trial. Br J Psychiatry 182:312–318, 2003

Heimberg RG, Liebowitz MR, Hope DA, et al: Cognitive behavioral group therapy vs phenelzine therapy for social phobia: 12-week outcome. Arch Gen Psychiatry 55:1133–1141, 1998

Hertzberg MA, Butterfield MI, Feldman ME, et al: A preliminary study of lamotrigine for the treatment of posttraumatic stress disorder. Biol Psychiatry 45:1226–1229, 1999

Hettema JM, Neale MC, Kendler KS: A review and meta-analysis of the genetic epidemiology of anxiety disorders. Am J Psychiatry 158:1568–1578, 2001

Hettema JM, Neale MC, Myers JM, et al: A population-based twin study of the relationship between neuroticism and internalizing disorders. Am J Psychiatry 163:857–864, 2006

Hidalgo R, Hertzberg MA, Mellman T, et al: Nefazodone in posttraumatic stress disorder: results from six open-label trials. Int Clin Psychopharmacol 14:61–68, 1999

Hidalgo RB, Tupler LA, Davidson JRT: An effect-size analysis of pharmacological treatments for generalized anxiety disorder. J Psychopharmacol 21:864–872, 2007

Hoehn-Saric R, McLeod DR, Zimmerli WD: Differential effects of alprazolam and imipramine in generalized anxiety disorder: somatic versus psychic symptoms. J Clin Psychiatry 49:293–301, 1988

Hofmann SG: Cognitive mediation of change in social phobia. J Consult Clin Psychol 72:393–399, 2004

Hofmann SG, Meuret AE, Smits JA, et al: Augmentation of exposure therapy with D-cycloserine for social anxiety disorder. Arch Gen Psychiatry 63:298–304, 2006

Hollander E, Stein DJ, Kwon JH, et al: Psychosocial and economic costs of obsessive-compulsive disorder. CNS Spectr 2:16–25, 1997

Hollifield M, Thompson PM, Ruiz JE, et al: Potential effectiveness and safety of olanzapine in refractory panic disorder. Depress Anxiety 21:33–40, 2005

Horowitz M, Wilner N, Alvarez W: Impact of Event Scale: a measure of subjective stress. Psychosom Med 41:209–218, 1979

International Multicenter Clinical Trial Group on Moclobemide in Social Phobia: Moclobemide in social phobia. A double-blind, placebo-controlled clinical study. Eur Arch Psychiatry Clin Neurosci 247:71–80, 1997

Jacobs RJ, Davidson JR, Gupta S, et al: The effects of clonazepam on quality of life and work productivity in panic disorder. Am J Manag Care 3:1187–1196, 1997

Jacobs-Rebhun S, Schnurr PP, Friedman MJ, et al: Posttraumatic stress disorder and sleep difficulty. Am J Psychiatry 157:1525–1526, 2000

Jenike MA, Baer L, Ballantine T, et al: Cingulotomy for refractory obsessive-compulsive disorder. A long-term follow-up of 33 patients. Arch Gen Psychiatry 48:548–555, 1991

Jobson KO, Davidson JR, Lydiard RB, et al: Algorithm for the treatment of panic disorder with agoraphobia. Psychopharmacol Bull 31:483–485, 1995

Johnstone EC, Owens DG, Frith CD, et al: Neurotic illness and its response to anxiolytic and antidepressant treatment. Psychol Med 10:321–328, 1980

Kaplan Z, Amir M, Swartz M, et al: Inositol treatment of post-traumatic stress disorder. Anxiety 2:51–52, 1996

Kasper S, Stein DJ, Loft H, et al: Escitalopram in the treatment of social anxiety disorder: randomised, placebo-controlled, flexible-dosage study. Br J Psychiatry 186:222–226, 2005

Katschnig H, Amering M, Stolk JM, et al: Long-term follow-up after a drug trial for panic disorder. Br J Psychiatry 167:487–494, 1995

Katz RJ, Lott MH, Arbus P, et al: Pharmacotherapy of post-traumatic stress disorder with a novel psychotropic. Anxiety 1:169–174, 1994

Katzelnick DJ, Kobak KA, Greist JH, et al: Sertraline for social phobia: a double-blind, placebo-controlled crossover study. Am J Psychiatry 152:1368–1371, 1995

Keck PE Jr, McElroy SL, Tugrul KC, et al: Antiepileptic drugs for the treatment of panic disorder. Neuropsychobiology 27:150–153, 1993

Kessler RC, Sonnega A, Bromet E, et al: Posttraumatic stress disorder in the National Comorbidity Survey. Arch Gen Psychiatry 52:1048–1060, 1995

Kessler RC, Berglund P, Demler O, et al: Lifetime prevalence and age-of-onset distributions of DSM-IV disorders in the National Comorbidity Survey Replication. Arch Gen Psychiatry 62:593–602, 2005a

Kessler RC, Chiu WT, Demler O, et al: Prevalence, severity, and comorbidity of 12-month DSM-IV disorders in the National Comorbidity Survey Replication.[see comment]. Arch Gen Psychiatry 62:617–627, 2005b

Klesmer J, Sarcevic A, Fomari V: Panic attacks during discontinuation of mirtazapine. Can J Psychiatry 45:570–571, 2000

Kobak KA, Greist JH, Jefferson JW, et al: Fluoxetine in social phobia: a double-blind, placebo-controlled pilot study. J Clin Psychopharmacol 22:257–262, 2002

Kobak KA, Taylor LV, Bystritsky A, et al: St. John's wort versus placebo in obsessive-compulsive disorder: results from a double-blind study. Int Clin Psychopharmacol 20:299–304, 2005

Koenen KC, Fu QJ, Ertel K, et al: Common genetic liability to major depression and posttraumatic stress disorder in men. J Affect Disord 105:109–115, 2008

Koran LM, McElroy SL, Davidson JR, et al: Fluvoxamine versus clomipramine for obsessive-compulsive disorder: a double-blind comparison. J Clin Psychopharmacol 16:121–129, 1996

Koran LM, Sallee FR, Pallanti S: Rapid benefit of intravenous pulse loading of clomipramine in obsessive-compulsive disorder. Am J Psychiatry 154:396–401, 1997

Kosten TR, Frank JB, Dan E, et al: Pharmacotherapy for posttraumatic stress disorder using phenelzine or imipramine. J Nerv Ment Dis 179:366–370, 1991

Kruger MB, Dahl AA: The efficacy and safety of moclobemide compared to clomipramine in the treatment of panic disorder. Eur Arch Psychiatry Clin Neurosci 249 (suppl 1):S19–S24, 1999

Lader M, Scotto JC: A multicentre double-blind comparison of hydroxyzine, buspirone and placebo in patients with generalized anxiety disorder. Psychopharmacology (Berl) 139:402–406, 1998

Lader M, Stender K, Burger V, et al: Efficacy and tolerability of escitalopram in 12- and 24-week treatment of social anxiety disorder: randomised, double-blind, placebo-controlled, fixed-dose study. Depress Anxiety 19:241–248, 2004

Lecrubier Y, Judge R: Long-term evaluation of paroxetine, clomipramine and placebo in panic disorder. Collaborative Paroxetine Panic Study Investigators. Acta Psychiatr Scand 95:153–160, 1997

Lecrubier Y, Bakker A, Dunbar G, et al: A comparison of paroxetine, clomipramine and placebo in the treatment of panic disorder. Collaborative Paroxetine Panic Study Investigators. Acta Psychiatr Scand 95:145–152, 1997

Leonard H, Swedo S, Rapoport JL, et al: Treatment of childhood obsessive compulsive disorder with clomipramine and desmethylimipramine: a double-blind crossover comparison. Psychopharmacol Bull 24:93–95, 1988

Lepola UM, Wade AG, Leinonen EV, et al: A controlled, prospective, 1-year trial of citalopram in the treatment of panic disorder. J Clin Psychiatry 59:528–534, 1998

Lesser IM, Lydiard RB, Antal E, et al: Alprazolam plasma concentrations and treatment response in panic disorder and agoraphobia. Am J Psychiatry 149:1556–1562, 1992

Liebowitz MR: Social phobia. Mod Probl Pharmacopsychiatry 22:141–173, 1987

Liebowitz MR, Schneier F, Campeas R, et al: Phenelzine vs atenolol in social phobia. A placebo-controlled comparison. Arch Gen Psychiatry 49:290–300, 1992

Liebowitz MR, Turner SM, Piacentini J, et al: Fluoxetine in children and adolescents with OCD: a placebo-controlled trial. J Am Acad Child Adolesc Psychiatry 41:1431–1438, 2002

Liebowitz MR, DeMartinis NA, Weihs K, et al: Efficacy of sertraline in severe generalized social anxiety disorder: results of a double-blind, placebo-controlled study. J Clin Psychiatry 64:785–792, 2003

Liebowitz MR, Mangano RM, Bradwejn J, et al: A randomized controlled trial of venlafaxine extended release in generalized social anxiety disorder. J Clin Psychiatry 66:238–247, 2005

Lipper S, Davidson JR, Grady TA, et al: Preliminary study of carbamazepine in post-traumatic stress disorder. Psychosomatics 27:849–854, 1986

Lipsitz JD, Mannuzza S, Klein DF, et al: Specific phobia 10–16 years after treatment. Depress Anxiety 10:105–111, 1999

Llorca PM, Spadone C, Sol O, et al: Efficacy and safety of hydroxyzine in the treatment of generalized anxiety disorder: a 3-month double-blind study [see comment]. J Clin Psychiatry 63:1020–1027, 2002

Loerch B, Graf-Morgenstern M, Hautzinger M, et al: Randomised placebo-controlled trial of moclobemide, cognitive-behavioural therapy and their combination in panic disorder with agoraphobia. Br J Psychiatry 174:205–212, 1999

Londborg PD, Wolkow R, Smith WT, et al: Sertraline in the treatment of panic disorder. A multi-site, double-blind, placebo-controlled, fixed-dose investigation. Br J Psychiatry 173:54–60, 1998

Londborg PD, Hegel MT, Goldstein S, et al: Sertraline treatment of posttraumatic stress disorder: results of 24 weeks of open-label continuation treatment. J Clin Psychiatry 62:325–331, 2001

Lott M, Greist JH, Jefferson JW, et al: Brofaromine for social phobia: a multicenter, placebo-controlled, double-blind study. J Clin Psychopharmacol 17:255–260, 1997

Lydiard RB, Ballenger JC: Antidepressants in panic disorder and agoraphobia. J Affect Disord 13:153–168, 1987

Lydiard RB, Laraia MT, Ballenger JC, et al: Emergence of depressive symptoms in patients receiving alprazolam for panic disorder. Am J Psychiatry 144:664–665, 1987

Lydiard RB, Lesser IM, Ballenger JC, et al: A fixed-dose study of alprazolam 2 mg, alprazolam 6 mg, and placebo in panic disorder. J Clin Psychopharmacol 12:96–103, 1992

Lydiard RB, Morton WA, Emmanuel NP, et al: Preliminary report: placebo-controlled, double-blind study of the clinical and metabolic effects of desipramine in panic disorder. Psychopharmacol Bull 29:183–188, 1993

Lydiard RB, Steiner M, Burnham D, et al: Efficacy studies of paroxetine in panic disorder. Psychopharmacol Bull 34:175–182, 1998

Magee WJ, Eaton WW, Wittchen HU, et al: Agoraphobia, simple phobia, and social phobia in the National Comorbidity Survey. Arch Gen Psychiatry 53:159–168, 1996

March JS, Biederman J, Wolkow R, et al: Sertraline in children and adolescents with obsessive-compulsive disorder: a multicenter randomized controlled trial. JAMA 280:1752–1756, 1998

March JS, Entsuah AR, Rynn M, et al: A randomized controlled trial of venlafaxine ER versus placebo in pediatric social anxiety disorder. Biol Psychiatry 62:1149–1154, 2007

Marks IM, Mathews AM: Brief standard self-rating for phobic patients. Behav Res Ther 17:263–267, 1979

Marmar CR, Schoenfeld F, Weiss DS, et al: Open trial of fluvoxamine treatment for combat-related posttraumatic stress disorder. J Clin Psychiatry 57 (suppl 8):66–70, 1996

Marshall RD, Beebe KL, Oldham M, et al: Efficacy and safety of paroxetine treatment for chronic PTSD: a fixed-dose, placebo-controlled study. Am J Psychiatry 158:1982–1988, 2001

Martenyi F, Brown EB, Zhang H, et al: Fluoxetine versus placebo in posttraumatic stress disorder. J Clin Psychiatry 63:199–206, 2002a

Martenyi F, Brown EB, Zhang H, et al: Fluoxetine vs placebo in prevention of relapse in post-traumatic stress disorder. Br J Psychiatry 181:315–320, 2002b

Mathew SJ, Ho S: Etiology and neurobiology of social anxiety disorder. J Clin Psychiatry 67 (suppl 12):9–13, 2007

Mathew SJ, Amiel JM, Coplan JD, et al: Open-label trial of riluzole in generalized anxiety disorder. Am J Psychiatry 162:2379–2381, 2005

Mavissakalian MR, Perel JM: Imipramine dose-response relationship in panic disorder with agoraphobia. Preliminary findings. Arch Gen Psychiatry 46:127–131, 1989

Mavissakalian M, Perel JM: Protective effects of imipramine maintenance treatment in panic disorder with agoraphobia. Am J Psychiatry 149:1053–1057, 1992

Mavissakalian MR, Perel JM: Imipramine treatment of panic disorder with agoraphobia: dose ranging and plasma level-response relationships. Am J Psychiatry 152:673–682, 1995

Mavissakalian MR, Perel JM: Duration of imipramine therapy and relapse in panic disorder with agoraphobia. J Clin Psychopharmacol 22:294–299, 2002

Mavissakalian MR, Jones B, Olson S: Absence of placebo response in obsessive-compulsive disorder. J Nerv Ment Dis 178:268–270, 1990

Mellman TA, Bustamante V, David D, et al: Hypnotic medication in the aftermath of trauma. J Clin Psychiatry 63:1183–1184, 2002

Mellman TA, Clark RE, Peacock WJ: Prescribing patterns for patients with posttraumatic stress disorder. Psychiatr Serv 54:1618–1621, 2003

Meoni P, Hackett D: Characterization of the longitudinal course of long-term venlafaxine-ER treatment of GAD. Paper presented at the 13th Annual Meeting of the European College of Neuropsychopharmacology, Munich, Germany, September 11, 2000

Michelson D, Lydiard RB, Pollack MH, et al: Outcome assessment and clinical improvement in panic disorder: evidence from a randomized controlled trial of fluoxetine and placebo. The Fluoxetine Panic Disorder Study Group. Am J Psychiatry 155:1570–1577, 1998

Michelson D, Pollack M, Lydiard RB, et al: Continuing treatment of panic disorder after acute response: randomised, placebo-controlled trial with fluoxetine. The Fluoxetine Panic Disorder Study Group. Br J Psychiatry 174:213–218, 1999

Michelson D, Allgulander C, Dantendorfer K, et al: Efficacy of usual antidepressant dosing regimens of fluoxetine in panic disorder: randomised, placebo-controlled trial. Br J Psychiatry 179:514–518, 2001

Modigh K, Westberg P, Eriksson E: Superiority of clomipramine over imipramine in the treatment of panic disorder: a placebo-controlled trial. J Clin Psychopharmacol 12:251–261, 1992

Monnelly EP, Ciraulo DA, Knapp C, et al: Low-dose risperidone as adjunctive therapy for irritable aggression in posttraumatic stress disorder. J Clin Psychopharmacol 23:193–196, 2003

Montgomery SA, Nil R, Durr-Pal N, et al: A 24-week randomized, double-blind, placebo-controlled study of escitalopram for the prevention of generalized social anxiety disorder. J Clin Psychiatry 66:1270–1278, 2005

Moras K, Borkovec TD, DiNardo PA, et al: Generalized anxiety disorder, in DSM-IV Sourcebook. Edited by Widiger TA, Frances AJ, Pincus HA, et al. Washington, DC, American Psychiatric Association, 1996, pp 607–621

Muehlbacher M, Nickel MK, Nickel C, et al: Mirtazapine treatment of social phobia in women: a randomized, double-blind, placebo controlled trial. J Clin Psychopharmacol 25:580–583, 2005

Murray CJL, Lopez AD: The Global Burden of Disease. Cambridge, MA, Harvard School of Public Health, 1996

Myers JK, Weissman MM, Tischler GL, et al: Six-month prevalence of psychiatric disorders in three communities 1980 to 1982. Arch Gen Psychiatry 41:959–967, 1984

Neal LA, Shapland W, Fox C: An open trial of moclobemide in the treatment of post-traumatic stress disorder. Int Clin Psychopharmacol 12:231–237, 1997

Neylan TC, Lenoci M, Samuelson KW, et al: No improvement of posttraumatic stress disorder symptoms with guanfacine treatment. Am J Psychiatry 163:2186–2188, 2006

Ninan PT, Koran LM, Kiev A, et al: High-dose sertraline strategy for nonresponders to acute treatment for obsessive-compulsive disorder: a multicenter double-blind trial. J Clin Psychiatry 67:15–22, 2006

Noyes R Jr, Moroz G, Davidson JR, et al: Moclobemide in social phobia: a controlled dose-response trial. J Clin Psychopharmacol 17:247–254, 1997

Nuttin B, Cosyns P, Demeulemeester H, et al: Electrical stimulation in anterior limbs of internal capsules in patients with obsessive-compulsive disorder. Lancet 354:1526, 1999

Oehrberg S, Christiansen PE, Behnke K, et al: Paroxetine in the treatment of panic disorder. A randomised, double-blind, placebo-controlled study. Br J Psychiatry 167:374–379, 1995

Olajide D, Lader M: A comparison of buspirone, diazepam, and placebo in patients with chronic anxiety states. J Clin Psychopharmacol 7:148–152, 1987

Otto MW, Pollack MH, Sachs GS, et al: Discontinuation of benzodiazepine treatment: efficacy of cognitive-behavioral therapy for patients with panic disorder. Am J Psychiatry 150:1485–1490, 1993

Otto MW, Tuby KS, Gould RA, et al: An effect-size analysis of the relative efficacy and tolerability of serotonin selective reuptake inhibitors for panic disorder. Am J Psychiatry 158:1989–1992, 2001

Pages KP, Ries RK: Use of anticonvulsants in benzodiazepine withdrawal. Am J Addict 7:198–204, 1998

Pande AC, Davidson JR, Jefferson JW, et al: Treatment of social phobia with gabapentin: a placebo-controlled study. J Clin Psychopharmacol 19:341–348, 1999a

Pande AC, Greiner M, Adams JB, et al: Placebo-controlled trial of the CCK-B antagonist, CI-988, in panic disorder. Biol Psychiatry 46:860–862, 1999b

Pande AC, Pollack MH, Crockatt J, et al: Placebo-controlled study of gabapentin treatment of panic disorder. J Clin Psychopharmacol 20:467–471, 2000

Pande AC, Crockatt JG, Feltner DE, et al: Pregabalin in generalized anxiety disorder: a placebo-controlled trial. Am J Psychiatry 160:533–540, 2003

Papp LA: Safety and efficacy of levetiracetam for patients with panic disorder: results of an open-label, fixed-flexible dose study. J Clin Psychiatry 67:1573–1576, 2006

Pato MT, Hill JL, Murphy DL: A clomipramine dosage reduction study in the course of long-term treatment of obsessive-compulsive disorder patients. Psychopharmacol Bull 26:211–214, 1990

Pecknold J, Luthe L, Munjack D, et al: A double-blind, placebo-controlled, multicenter study with alprazolam and extended-release alprazolam in the treatment of panic disorder. J Clin Psychopharmacol 14:314–321, 1994

Petracca A, Nisita C, McNair D, et al: Treatment of generalized anxiety disorder: preliminary clinical experience with buspirone. J Clin Psychiatry 51 (suppl):31–39, 1990

Pigott T, L'Hereux F, Rubinstein CS: A controlled trial of clonazepam augmentation in OCD patients with clomipramine or fluoxetine (NR82). Paper presented at the 145th Annual Meeting of the American Psychiatric Association, May 2–7, 1992

Pitman RK, Sanders KM, Zusman RM, et al: Pilot study of secondary prevention of posttraumatic stress disorder with propranolol. Biol Psychiatry 51:189–192, 2002

Pohl RB, Feltner DE, Fieve RR, et al: Efficacy of pregabalin in the treatment of generalized anxiety disorder: double-blind, placebo-controlled comparison of BID versus TID dosing. J Clin Psychopharmacol 25:151–158, 2005

Pollack MH, Zaninelli R, Goddard A, et al: Paroxetine in the treatment of generalized anxiety disorder: results of a placebo-controlled, flexible-dosage trial. J Clin Psychiatry 62:350–357, 2001

Pollack MH, Simon NM, Worthington JJ, et al: Combined paroxetine and clonazepam treatment strategies compared to paroxetine monotherapy for panic disorder. J Psychopharmacol (Oxf) 17:276–282, 2003

Pollack MH, Roy-Byrne PP, Van Ameringen M, et al: The selective GABA reuptake inhibitor tiagabine for the treatment of generalized anxiety disorder: results of a placebo-controlled study. J Clin Psychiatry 66:1401–1408, 2005

Rapaport MH, Wolkow R, Rubin A, et al: Sertraline treatment of panic disorder: results of a long-term study. Acta Psychiatr Scand 104:289–298, 2001

Rapaport MH, Endicott J, Clary CM: Posttraumatic stress disorder and quality of life: results across 64 weeks of sertraline treatment. J Clin Psychiatry 63:59–65, 2002

Raskind MA, Peskind ER, Kanter ED, et al: Reduction of nightmares and other PTSD symptoms in combat veterans by prazosin: a placebo-controlled study. Am J Psychiatry 160:371–373, 2003

Raskind MA, Peskind ER, Hoff DJ, et al: A parallel group placebo controlled study of prazosin for trauma nightmares and sleep disturbance in combat veterans with post-traumatic stress disorder. Biol Psychiatry 61:928–934, 2007

Ravizza L, Barzega G, Bellino S, et al: Drug treatment of obsessive-compulsive disorder (OCD): long-term trial with clomipramine and selective serotonin reuptake inhibitors (SSRIs). Psychopharmacol Bull 32:167–173, 1996

Reich DB, Winternitz S, Hennen J, et al: A preliminary study of risperidone in the treatment of posttraumatic stress disorder related to childhood abuse in women. J Clin Psychiatry 65:1601–1606, 2004

Research Unit on Pediatric Psychopharmacology Anxiety Study Group: Fluvoxamine for the treatment of anxiety disorders in children and adolescents. N Engl J Med 344:1279–1285, 2001

Ressler KJ, Rothbaum BO, Tannenbaum L, et al: Cognitive enhancers as adjuncts to psychotherapy: use of D-cycloserine in phobic individuals to facilitate extinction of fear. Arch Gen Psychiatry 61:1136–1144, 2004

Ribeiro L, Busnello JV, Kauer-Sant'Anna M, et al: Mirtazapine versus fluoxetine in the treatment of panic disorder. Braz J Med Biol Res 34:1303–1307, 2001

Rickels K, Weisman K, Norstad N, et al: Buspirone and diazepam in anxiety: a controlled study. J Clin Psychiatry 43:81–86, 1982

Rickels K, Case WG, Downing RW, et al: Long-term diazepam therapy and clinical outcome. JAMA 250:767–771, 1983

Rickels K, Fox IL, Greenblatt DJ, et al: Clorazepate and lorazepam: clinical improvement and rebound anxiety. Am J Psychiatry 145:312–317, 1988a

Rickels K, Schweizer E, Csanalosi I, et al: Long-term treatment of anxiety and risk of withdrawal. Prospective comparison of clorazepate and buspirone. Arch Gen Psychiatry 45:444–450, 1988b

Rickels K, Amsterdam JD, Clary C, et al: Buspirone in major depression: a controlled study. J Clin Psychiatry 52:34–38, 1991

Rickels K, Downing R, Schweizer E, et al: Antidepressants for the treatment of generalized anxiety disorder. A placebo-controlled comparison of imipramine, trazodone, and diazepam. Arch Gen Psychiatry 50:884–895, 1993

Rickels K, DeMartinis N, Garcia-Espana F, et al: Imipramine and buspirone in treatment of patients with generalized anxiety disorder who are discontinuing long-term benzodiazepine therapy. Am J Psychiatry 157:1973–1979, 2000a

Rickels K, Pollack MH, Sheehan DV, et al: Efficacy of extended-release venlafaxine in nondepressed outpatients with generalized anxiety disorder. Am J Psychiatry 157:968–974, 2000b

Rickels K, Zaninelli R, McCafferty J, et al: Paroxetine treatment of generalized anxiety disorder: a double-blind, placebo-controlled study. Am J Psychiatry 160:749–756, 2003

Rickels K, Pollack MH, Feltner DE, et al: Pregabalin for treatment of generalized anxiety disorder: a 4-week, multicenter, double-blind, placebo-controlled trial of pregabalin and alprazolam. Arch Gen Psychiatry 62:1022–1030, 2005

Riddle MA, Reeve EA, Yaryura-Tobias JA, et al: Fluvoxamine for children and adolescents with obsessive-compulsive disorder: a randomized, controlled, multicenter trial. J Am Acad Child Adolesc Psychiatry 40:222–229, 2001

Robert R, Blakeney PE, Villarreal C, et al: Imipramine treatment in pediatric burn patients with symptoms of acute stress disorder: a pilot study. J Am Acad Child Adolesc Psychiatry 38:873–882, 1999a

Robert R, Meyer WJ 3rd, Villarreal C, et al: An approach to the timely treatment of acute stress disorder. J Burn Care Rehabil 20:250–258, 1999b

Robins LN, Helzer JE, Weissman MM, et al: Lifetime prevalence of specific psychiatric disorders in three sites. Arch Gen Psychiatry 41:949–958, 1984

Rocca P, Fonzo V, Scotta M, et al: Paroxetine efficacy in the treatment of generalized anxiety disorder. Acta Psychiatr Scand 95:444–450, 1997

Rosenbaum JF, Woods SW, Groves JE, et al: Emergence of hostility during alprazolam treatment. Am J Psychiatry 141:792–793, 1984

Rosenbaum JF, Moroz G, Bowden CL: Clonazepam in the treatment of panic disorder with or without agoraphobia: a dose-response study of efficacy, safety, and discontinuance. Clonazepam Panic Disorder Dose-Response Study Group. J Clin Psychopharmacol 17:390–400, 1997

Ross CA, Matas M: A clinical trial of buspirone and diazepam in the treatment of generalized anxiety disorder. Can J Psychiatry 32:351–355, 1987

Royal Australian and New Zealand College of Psychiatrists Clinical Practice Guidelines Team for Panic Disorder and Agoraphobia: Australian and New Zealand clinical practice guidelines for the treatment of panic disorder and agoraphobia. Aust N Z J Psychiatry 37:641–656, 2003

Roy-Byrne PP, Stang P, Wittchen HU, et al: Lifetime panic-depression comorbidity in the National Comorbidity Survey. Association with symptoms, impairment, course and help-seeking. Br J Psychiatry 176:229–235, 2000

Roy-Byrne PP, Clary CM, Miceli RJ, et al: The effect of selective serotonin reuptake inhibitor treatment of panic disorder on emergency room and laboratory resource utilization. J Clin Psychiatry 62:678–682, 2001

Rynn M, Russell JM, Erickson J, et al: Efficacy and safety of duloxetine in the treatment of generalized anxiety disorder: a flexible-dose, progressive-titration, placebo-controlled trial. Depress Anxiety 25:182–189, 2008

Sarchiapone M, Amore M, De Risio S, et al: Mirtazapine in the treatment of panic disorder: an open-label trial. Int Clin Psychopharmacol 18:35–38, 2003

Schelling G, Roozendaal B, Krauseneck T, et al: Efficacy of hydrocortisone in preventing posttraumatic stress disorder following critical illness and major surgery. Ann N Y Acad Sci 1071:46–53, 2006

Schneier FR, Goetz D, Campeas R, et al: Placebo-controlled trial of moclobemide in social phobia. Br J Psychiatry 172:70–77, 1998

Schweizer E, Rickels K: Buspirone in the treatment of panic disorder: a controlled pilot comparison with clorazepate. J Clin Psychopharmacol 8:303, 1988

Schweizer E, Rickels K: Pharmacological treatment for generalized anxiety disorder, in Long-term Treatments of Anxiety Disorders. Edited by Mavissakalian M, Prien RF. Washington, DC, American Psychiatric Press, 1996, pp 201–220

Schweizer E, Rickels K, Lucki I: Resistance to the anti-anxiety effect of buspirone in patients with a history of benzodiazepine use. N Engl J Med 314:719–720, 1986

Schweizer E, Patterson W, Rickels K, et al: Double-blind, placebo-controlled study of a once-a-day, sustained-release preparation of alprazolam for the treatment of panic disorder. Am J Psychiatry 150:1210–1215, 1993

Sepede G, De Berardis D, Gambi F, et al: Olanzapine augmentation in treatment-resistant panic disorder: a 12-week, fixed-dose, open-label trial. J Clin Psychopharmacol 26:45–49, 2006

Shader RI, Greenblatt DJ: Use of benzodiazepines in anxiety disorders. N Engl J Med 328:1398–1405, 1993

Shear MK, Brown TA, Barlow DH, et al: Multicenter collaborative panic disorder severity scale. Am J Psychiatry 154:1571–1575, 1997

Sheehan DV: The Anxiety Disease. Bantam Books, New York, 1986

Sheehan DV, Ballenger J, Jacobsen G: Treatment of endogenous anxiety with phobic, hysterical, and hypochondriacal symptoms. Arch Gen Psychiatry 37:51–59, 1980

Sheehan DV, Davidson J, Manschreck T, et al: Lack of efficacy of a new antidepressant (bupropion) in the treatment of panic disorder with phobias. J Clin Psychopharmacol 3:28–31, 1983

Sheehan DV, Raj AB, Sheehan KH, et al: Is buspirone effective for panic disorder? J Clin Psychopharmacol 10:3–11, 1990

Sheehan DV, Burnham DB, Iyengar MK, et al: Efficacy and tolerability of controlled-release paroxetine in the treatment of panic disorder. J Clin Psychiatry 66:34–40, 2005

Silverstone PH, Salinas E: Efficacy of venlafaxine extended release in patients with major depressive disorder and comorbid generalized anxiety disorder. J Clin Psychiatry 62:523–529, 2001

Simon NM, Emmanuel N, Ballenger J, et al: Bupropion sustained release for panic disorder. Psychopharmacol Bull 37:66–72, 2003

Simon NM, Hoge EA, Fischmann D, et al: An open-label trial of risperidone augmentation for refractory anxiety disorders. J Clin Psychiatry 67:381–385, 2006

Simpson HB, Schneier FR, Marshall RD, et al: Low dose selegiline (L-deprenyl) in social phobia. Depress Anxiety 7:126–129, 1998

Snyderman SH, Rynn MA, Rickels K: Open-label pilot study of ziprasidone for refractory generalized anxiety disorder. J Clin Psychopharmacol 25:497–499, 2005

Stahl SM, Gergel I, Li D: Escitalopram in the treatment of panic disorder: a randomized, double-blind, placebo-controlled trial. J Clin Psychiatry 64:1322–1327, 2003

Stein DJ, Andersen EW, Tonnoir B, et al: Escitalopram in obsessive-compulsive disorder: a randomized, placebo-controlled, paroxetine-referenced, fixed-dose, 24-week study. Curr Med Res Opin 23:701–711, 2007

Stein MB, Chartier MJ, Hazen AL, et al: Paroxetine in the treatment of generalized social phobia: open-label treatment and double-blind placebo-controlled discontinuation. J Clin Psychopharmacol 16:218–222, 1996

Stein MB, Liebowitz MR, Lydiard RB, et al: Paroxetine treatment of generalized social phobia (social anxiety disorder): a randomized controlled trial. JAMA 280:708–713, 1998

Stein MB, Fyer AJ, Davidson JR, et al: Fluvoxamine treatment of social phobia (social anxiety disorder): a double-blind, placebo-controlled study. Am J Psychiatry 156:756–760, 1999

Stein MB, Kline NA, Matloff JL: Adjunctive olanzapine for SSRI-resistant combat-related PTSD: a double-blind, placebo-controlled study. Am J Psychiatry 159:1777–1779, 2002

Stein MB, Seedat S, Gelernter J: Serotonin transporter gene promoter polymorphism predicts SSRI response in generalized social anxiety disorder. Psychopharmacology (Berl) 187:168–172, 2006

Stinson FS, Dawson DA, Patricia Chou S, et al: The epidemiology of DSM-IV specific phobia in the USA: results from the National Epidemiologic Survey on Alcohol and Related Conditions. Psychol Med 37:1047–1059, 2007

Strand M, Hetta J, Rosen A, et al: A double-blind, controlled trial in primary care patients with generalized anxiety: a comparison between buspirone and oxazepam. J Clin Psychiatry 51 (suppl):40–45, 1990

Sutherland SM, Tupler LA, Colket JT, et al: A 2-year follow-up of social phobia. Status after a brief medication trial. J Nerv Ment Dis 184:731–738, 1996

Swinson RP, Antony MM, Bleau P, et al: Clinical practice guidelines. Management of anxiety disorders. Can J Psychiatry 51 (suppl 2):1–92, 2006

Szegedi A, Wetzel H, Leal M, et al: Combination treatment with clomipramine and fluvoxamine: drug monitoring, safety, and tolerability data. J Clin Psychiatry 57:257–264, 1996

Taylor LH, Kobak KA: An open-label trial of St John's wort (Hypericum perforatum) in obsessive-compulsive disorder. J Clin Psychiatry 61:575–578, 2000

Tesar GE, Rosenbaum JF, Pollack MH, et al: Double-blind, placebo-controlled comparison of clonazepam and alprazolam for panic disorder. J Clin Psychiatry 52:69–76, 1991

Thoren P, Asberg M, Cronholm B, et al: Clomipramine treatment of obsessive-compulsive disorder, I: a controlled clinical trial. Arch Gen Psychiatry 37:1281–1285, 1980

Tiller JW, Bouwer C, Behnke K: Moclobemide and fluoxetine for panic disorder. International Panic Disorder Study Group. Eur Arch Psychiatry Clin Neurosci 249 (suppl 1):S7–S10, 1999

Tollefson GD, Rampey AH Jr, Potvin JH, et al: A multicenter investigation of fixed-dose fluoxetine in the treatment of obsessive-compulsive disorder. Arch Gen Psychiatry 51:559–567, 1994

True WR, Rice J, Eisen SA, et al: A twin study of genetic and environmental contributions to liability for posttraumatic stress symptoms. Arch Gen Psychiatry 50:257–264, 1993

Tucker P, Smith KL, Marx B, et al: Fluvoxamine reduces physiologic reactivity to trauma scripts in posttraumatic stress disorder. J Clin Psychopharmacol 20:367–372, 2000

Tucker P, Zaninelli R, Yehuda R, et al: Paroxetine in the treatment of chronic posttraumatic stress disorder: results of a placebo-controlled, flexible-dosage trial. J Clin Psychiatry 62:860–868, 2001

Turner SM, Beidel DC, Jacob RG: Social phobia: a comparison of behavior therapy and atenolol. J Consult Clin Psychol 62:350–358, 1994

Van Ameringen M, Mancini C, Oakman JM: Nefazodone in social phobia. J Clin Psychiatry 60:96–100, 1999

Van Ameringen MA, Lane RM, Walker JR, et al: Sertraline treatment of generalized social phobia: a 20-week, double-blind, placebo-controlled study. Am J Psychiatry 158:275–281, 2001

Van Ameringen M, Mancini C, Oakman J, et al: Nefazodone in the treatment of generalized social phobia: a randomized, placebo-controlled trial. J Clin Psychiatry 68:288–295, 2007

van der Kolk BA, Dreyfuss D, Michaels M, et al: Fluoxetine in posttraumatic stress disorder [see comment]. J Clin Psychiatry 55:517–522, 1994

van Vliet IM, den Boer JA, Westenberg HG: Psychopharmacological treatment of social phobia: clinical and biochemical effects of brofaromine, a selective MAO-A inhibitor. Eur Neuropsychopharmacol 2:21–29, 1992

van Vliet IM, den Boer JA, Westenberg HG: Psychopharmacological treatment of social phobia: a double blind placebo controlled study with fluvoxamine. Psychopharmacology (Berl) 115:128–134, 1994

van Vliet IM, den Boer JA, Westenberg HG, et al: Clinical effects of buspirone in social phobia: a double-blind placebo-controlled study. J Clin Psychiatry 58:164–168, 1997

Versiani M, Nardi AE, Mundim FD, et al: Pharmacotherapy of social phobia. A controlled study with moclobemide and phenelzine. Br J Psychiatry 161:353–360, 1992

Versiani M, Nardi AE, Figueria J: Double-blind placebo-controlled trial with bromazepam in social phobia. J Bras Psiquiatr 46:167–171, 1997

Versiani M, Cassano G, Perugi G, et al: Reboxetine, a selective norepinephrine reuptake inhibitor, is an effective and well-tolerated treatment for panic disorder. J Clin Psychiatry 63:31–37, 2002

Wade AG, Lepola U, Koponen HJ, et al: The effect of citalopram in panic disorder. Br J Psychiatry 170:549–553, 1997

Wagner KD, Berard R, Stein MB, et al: A multicenter, randomized, double-blind, placebo-controlled trial of paroxetine in children and adolescents with social anxiety disorder. Arch Gen Psychiatry 61:1153–1162, 2004

Walker JR, Van Ameringen MA, Swinson R, et al: Prevention of relapse in generalized social phobia: results of a 24-week study in responders to 20 weeks of sertraline treatment. J Clin Psychopharmacol 20:636–644, 2000

Weathers FW, Keane TM, Davidson JRT: Clinician-administered PTSD scale: a review of the first ten years of research. Depress Anxiety 13:132–156, 2001

Westenberg HG, Stein DJ, Yang H, et al: A double-blind placebo-controlled study of controlled release fluvoxamine for the treatment of generalized social anxiety disorder. J Clin Psychopharmacol 24:49–55, 2004

Westenberg HG, Fineberg N, Denys D: Neurobiology of obsessive-compulsive disorder: serotonin and beyond. CNS Spectr 12 (suppl 3):14–27, 2007

Williams JE, Nieto FJ, Sanford CP, et al: Effects of an angry temperament on coronary heart disease risk: the Atherosclerosis Risk in Communities Study. Am J Epidemiol 154:230–235, 2001

Wittchen HU, Hoyer J: Generalized anxiety disorder: nature and course. J Clin Psychiatry 62 (suppl 11):15–19, 2001

Wittchen HU, Zhao S, Kessler RC, et al: DSM-III-R generalized anxiety disorder in the National Comorbidity Survey. Arch Gen Psychiatry 51:355–364, 1994

Wurthmann C, Klieser E, Lehmann E: [Differential pharmacologic therapy of generalized anxiety disorders—results of a study with 30 individual case experiments]. Fortschritte der Neurologie-Psychiatrie 63:303–309, 1995

Zigmond AS, Snaith RP: The Hospital Anxiety and Depression Scale. Acta Psychiatr Scand 67:361–370, 1983

Zimmerman M, Mattia JI: Principal and additional DSM-IV disorders for which outpatients seek treatment. Psychiatr Serv 51:1299–1304, 2000

Zitrin CM, Klein DF, Woerner MG, et al: Treatment of phobias, I: comparison of imipramine hydrochloride and placebo. Arch Gen Psychiatry 40:125–138, 1983

Zohar J, Amital D, Miodownik C, et al: Double-blind placebo-controlled pilot study of sertraline in military veterans with post-traumatic stress disorder. J Clin Psychopharmacol 22:190–195, 2002

Zwanzger P, Baghai TC, Schule C, et al: Tiagabine improves panic and agoraphobia in panic disorder patients. J Clin Psychiatry 62:656–657, 2001

CHAPTER 57

Treatment of Agitation and Aggression in the Elderly

Carl Salzman, M.D.

Pierre N. Tariot, M.D.

Severe agitation—restlessness, wandering, or screaming—may accompany late-life psychosis or dementia, with particularly high prevalence rates in nursing homes. Aggression and assaultiveness may also occur as a consequence of the delusions or hallucinations of late-life psychosis from dementia, depression, or a combination of these factors. Behavioral and psychiatric symptoms develop in as many as 60% of community-dwelling dementia patients (Lyketsos et al. 2000; Ryu et al. 2005; Tractenberg et al. 2003; Wragg and Jeste 1988). The lifetime risk of behavioral complications of dementia approaches 100% (Lyketsos et al. 2000). Rates of physical aggression range from 11% to 46% among community-dwelling dementia patients and from 31% to 42% among patients in institutional settings (Billig et al. 1991; Brodaty et al. 2003; Cohen-Mansfield et al. 1995; Peabody et al. 1987; Wragg and Jeste 1988; Zimmer et al. 1984). The etiology of agitation and aggression in late-life psychosis or dementia is unknown, although environmental and biological factors, such as drug toxicity, medical illness, pain, frustration, loneliness, reduced sensory input, new surroundings, diminished nutritional status, and altered central nervous system (CNS) function, alone or in combination, may play important roles (Mintzer and Brawman-Mintzer 1996).

In recent years, researchers and clinicians have begun to categorize disruptive behavioral syndromes according to associated etiology, as agitation and aggression of 1) psychosis, 2) dementia with psychosis, and 3) nonpsychotic dementia (Jeste et al. 2006). At present, there are no specific diagnostic categories of "psychosis with dementia" or "dementia-related agitation," so that all treatments are "off label." Psychotic and nonpsychotic patients have been mixed together in clinical trials, a practice that may have confused the outcomes and clinical recommendations. A distinct category of "psychosis of Alzheimer's disease and related dementia" may improve research examining late-life agitation and aggression (Jeste and Finkel 2000).

No drugs have been approved by the U.S. Food and Drug Administration (FDA) for the treatment of persisting psychosis, agitation, or aggression associated with dementia. Nevertheless, despite only modest benefits and frequent warnings about adverse effects and inappropriate use, antipsychotic drugs continue to be used as first-line agents. An increasing number of other medication classes, including anticonvulsants, antidepressants, and cognitive enhancers, are also being used as second-line choices for management of agitation and aggression in dementia that cannot be managed without medication (Docherty et al. 1998; Jeste et al. 2008; Kindermann et al. 2002; Raivio et al. 2007; Salzman 2000; Salzman and Tune 2001; Salzman et al. 2008; Small et al. 1997).

Antipsychotic Treatment

First-Generation (Conventional, Typical) Antipsychotics

Before the second-generation (atypical) antipsychotics, with their superior side-effect profiles, became available, first-generation antipsychotics (FGAs; sometimes called conventional or typical antipsychotics), especially haloperidol, were the mainstay of treatment of late-life agitation. Extrapyramidal side effects (EPS), however, are common with haloperidol, especially in the elderly, limiting its usefulness. Tardive dyskinesia, a late-appearing EPS, develops more rapidly and at lower antipsychotic doses in elderly patients than in younger ones (Caligiuri et al. 1999; Jeste et al. 1999; Karson et al. 1990; Lieberman et al. 1984; Saltz et al. 1989). Tardive dyskinesia is also more common in patients with evidence of cortical atrophy and in dementia patients (Sweet and Pollock 1992). When antipsychotics are discontinued, tardive dyskinesia symptoms are less likely to disappear in older patients than in younger adults (Smith and Baldessarini 1980; Yassa et al. 1984), although the symptoms may not increase in severity (Yassa et al. 1992). These concerns regarding tardive dyskinesia and other EPS have contributed to the switch in clinical preference for the newer antipsychotic drugs.

Second-Generation Antipsychotics

Second-generation antipsychotics (SGAs; sometimes called atypical antipsychotics) have replaced conventional antipsychotics as the first-choice treatment for agitation and aggression in the elderly. As a class, these newer antipsychotics carry a lower risk of EPS and tardive dyskinesia. Although pharmacokinetic data are not available for all of the newer SGAs, studies of risperidone indicate that clearance of risperidone and its 9-hydroxy metabolite does not decline with age, whereas clearance of quetiapine is reduced with increasing age (Jaskiw et al. 2004; Maxwell et al. 2002).

SGAs are as effective as FGAs for treating agitation and aggression, with or without associated psychosis (Ballard and Waite 2006; Sink et al. 2005). Ballard and Waite (2006), for example, found a significant improvement in aggression with risperidone and olanzapine compared with placebo and a significant improvement in dementia-associated psychosis among risperidone-treated patients. These observations have been supported by numerous other studies. Katz et al. (1999) reported the superiority of risperidone compared with placebo for the treatment of

agitation in Alzheimer's disease. Street et al. (2000) reported that olanzapine was superior to placebo for agitation associated with Alzheimer's disease. Meehan et al. (2002) studied acute treatment of agitation with intramuscular olanzapine in 272 inpatients or nursing home residents with Alzheimer's disease and/or vascular dementia. Patients were given up to three injections of olanzapine (2.5 mg or 5.0 mg), lorazepam (1.0 mg or 0.5 mg), or placebo and assessed within a 24-hour period. Olanzapine was found to be superior to placebo in treating agitation at 2 hours and 24 hours. Adverse events were not significantly different between groups. Aripiprazole was also reported to be superior to placebo for treatment of psychosis of Alzheimer's disease in outpatients (Laks et al. 2006).

Not all studies of SGAs have reported positive results, however. In a placebo-controlled multicenter trial comparing quetiapine and haloperidol versus placebo for psychosis associated with dementia, Tariot et al. (2006) reported no benefit of either active treatment, with one secondary measure of agitation suggesting benefit. This led to a subsequent placebo-controlled multicenter trial of quetiapine at fixed dosages (100 mg/day and 200 mg/day), which found overall superiority for quetiapine compared with placebo in the management of agitation (Zhong et al. 2006, 2007). Ballard and Waite (2006) conducted a placebo-controlled trial of quetiapine versus rivastigmine in which no benefit of either treatment was observed on behavioral outcomes; cognition worsened in the quetiapine group, a worrisome result that has not been seen in any other study of quetiapine.

The Clinical Antipsychotic Trials of Intervention Effectiveness—Alzheimer's Disease (CATIE-AD) addressed the relative effectiveness of commonly used atypical antipsychotics (Schneider et al. 2006). Outpatients with Alzheimer's disease and psychosis, aggression, or agitation were randomly assigned to treatment with olanzapine (mean dosage = 5 mg/day), quetiapine (mean dosage ≅ 50 mg/day), risperidone (mean dosage ≅ 1 mg/day), or placebo. No conventional antipsychotic was included in the study because of concerns about tardive dyskinesia. The primary measure of effectiveness was time to all-cause discontinuation; secondary measures addressed time to discontinuation due to lack of efficacy, significant safety concerns, or death, as well as improvement in Clinical Global Impression Scale Change scores. There was no significant difference among the drugs in the primary outcomes, although time to discontinuation due to lack of efficacy was longer with olanzapine and risperidone versus quetiapine or placebo. Conversely, time to discontinuation due to adverse events or drug intolerability was longer for all active treatments than for placebo. The CATIE-AD trial, therefore, confirmed the modest efficacy of atypical antipsychotic drugs as a class.

Meta-analytic reviews also suggest that the overall efficacy of SGAs for treatment of agitation and aggression is modest, as is the difference between active drug and placebo. Overall response rates in CATIE-AD ranged from 48% to 65% with active treatment versus 30%–48% with placebo, showing an incremental treatment benefit of about 18% for active drug over placebo (Schneider et al. 2006).

Studies comparing SGAs with FGAs have reported significantly greater efficacy for second-generation agents than for first-generation ones (Suh et al. 2004), and in all studies, the FGAs were associated with more EPS than the SGAs (Chan et al. 2001; De Deyn et al. 1999; Suh et al. 2004). The CATIE-AD study, lacking an FGA arm, could not add to these observations.

Side Effects of Antipsychotic Drugs

In addition to modest efficacy, reports of serious side effects other than EPS and tardive dyskinesia have raised concerns regarding the use of antipsychotics as first-line treatments for agitation or aggression, with or without psychosis, in elderly populations. An initial report indicating an increased risk of cerebrovascular adverse events (CVAEs; e.g., stroke, transient ischemic attack [TIA], death) in male nursing home residents older than 85 years who were treated with risperidone (Wooltorton 2002) led to further investigation. Similar suggestive evidence was reported for olanzapine and ultimately for other SGAs (Kryzhanovskaya et al. 2006; Percudani et al. 2005; Wooltorton 2004). Taken together, these observations of increased CVAEs in elderly individuals receiving SGAs stimulated an examination of all studies, which supported concerns regarding a possible increased risk of CVAEs when either of these drugs is given to elderly patients with dementia. Data from 11 olanzapine or risperidone studies collectively suggested that 2.2% of drug-treated subjects experienced CVAEs, compared with 0.8% of placebo-treated subjects. The combined relative risk was 2.7. Ballard and Waite (2006) concluded that despite the modest efficacy of these drugs, the significance of the adverse events dictates that "neither risperidone nor olanzapine should be used routinely to treat dementia patients with aggression or psychosis unless there is marked risk or severe distress."

In 2003, the FDA issued a black box warning regarding a possible increased risk of CVAEs associated with use of atypical antipsychotics in older adults with dementia. The warning was eventually extended to include aripiprazole, olanzapine, and risperidone. The death rate in clinical trials was 3.5% with SGAs versus 2.3% with placebo, leading the FDA to impose a black box warning for all SGAs. Studies examining large public databases (Ballard and Waite 2006; Schneider et al. 2006) have found similar rates of death among elderly people receiving FGAs (Schneeweiss et al. 2007; Wang et al. 2005).

The FDA warning has generated considerable controversy. Some researchers, examining the data on which the FDA's warning was based, have become concerned that methodological faults in many of the studies may have compromised the meta-analyses and led to an overly harsh interpretation of the data and an unwarranted concern for safety. Some studies failed to find an increase in death rate or incidence of CVAEs. For example, Herrmann et al. (2004), as well as Haupt et al. (2006) and Gill et al. (2005), found no significant increase in the risk of ischemic stroke with either FGAs or SGAs or among those receiving SGAs compared with FGAs. The American College of Neuropsychopharmacology has issued a White Paper (Jeste et al. 2008) concluding that further research data are needed to clarify the ongoing significance, if any, of increased development of CVAEs. An expert consensus conference held in 2006 (Salzman et al. 2008) essentially made the same point.

Most recently, a retrospective study of 254 very frail patients with dementia (mean age = 86 years) from seven nursing homes and two hospitals in Finland found that neither SGAs nor FGAs increased mortality (the use of SGAs actually should lower the risk of mortality) (Raivio et al. 2007).

Clinicians currently struggle with a difficult treatment dilemma when confronted with an elderly patient with dementia who is possibly psychotic and whose behavior is characterized by extreme agitation and/or aggression that cannot be controlled without medications. The essential conclusion of the CATIE-AD study, and a sensible statement about the role of antipsychotics (Jeste et al. 2008; Salzman et al. 2008; Sink et al. 2005), was that on average, patients receive modest benefit without being harmed: these are the patients for whom continued therapy is rational. The following clinical conclusions appear to be warranted at this time:

1. Recognizing that the use of antipsychotic drugs to treat agitation or aggression is "off label," clinicians must be certain that the behavior cannot be managed nonpharmacologically and that the severity of the

disruptive behavior warrants the selection of this class of drugs. If an FGA such as haloperidol is selected, doses should be kept low to minimize the likelihood of developing EPS.

2. SGAs are still preferred to FGAs because of the lower likelihood of EPS and tardive dyskinesia.

3. Clinicians should confer with the patient's family or significant others regarding the use of these drugs and should attempt to obtain some form of informed consent, balancing the possible risk of using these medications against the likelihood of worsening behavior and clinical status without such treatment.

4. Clinicians should follow these patients closely for early warning signs of a CVAE.

Non-Antipsychotic Treatment

A growing body of clinical experience, research, and anecdotal reports suggests that agents such as trazodone, anticonvulsants (mood stabilizers), buspirone, serotonergic antidepressants, and cognitive enhancers may help manage a variety of agitated behaviors refractory to more conventional treatment. These drugs, however, are ineffective in treating symptoms of psychosis.

Benzodiazepines

Although benzodiazepines are quite widely used in this population, there have been no studies of benzodiazepine treatment of agitation or aggression in nearly a decade. Most of the older studies were not placebo controlled, but they nonetheless suggested that on average, agitation could be reduced with short-term benzodiazepine therapy (Loy et al. 1999). For example, Coccaro et al. (1990) compared oxazepam (10–60 mg/day) with low-dose haloperidol in patients with mixed dementia diagnoses. Five percent of patients in the benzodiazepine group improved, compared with 24% of those in the haloperidol group, a difference that was not statistically significant, perhaps because of the small sample size. Christensen and Benfield (1998) compared alprazolam (0.5 mg twice daily) with haloperidol (0.6 mg/day) in a crossover study. Adverse events were not significantly different between groups. The dosages of both agents used in this study were probably too low to expect an effect, and none was seen. Meehan et al. (2002) noted that intramuscular lorazepam 1.0 mg or 0.5 mg was superior to placebo at 2 hours but not at 24 hours.

Possible side effects of benzodiazepines given to elderly individuals include ataxia, falls, confusion, antero-

grade amnesia, sedation, light-headedness, and tolerance and withdrawal syndromes (Patel and Tariot 1995). This profile, along with the scant evidence of efficacy, suggests that use of benzodiazepines for agitation should be time limited or on an as-needed basis, with chronic use only for those patients in whom other agents have proven ineffective. Drugs with simpler metabolisms and relatively short half-lives, such as lorazepam, are always preferred.

Anticonvulsants (Mood Stabilizers)

Although Chambers et al. (1982) reported no benefit of carbamazepine in a crossover study in 19 patients with agitation, most subsequent studies suggest that anticonvulsants are modestly helpful for controlling agitation and aggression in elderly individuals with dementia. In a placebo-controlled crossover study in 25 agitated dementia patients, Tariot et al. (1994) reported improvement with carbamazepine. This was supported by a confirmatory parallel-group study of 51 patients in which the mean daily dosage was 300 mg (Tariot et al. 1998). Carbamazepine was well tolerated in both studies; sedation and ataxia were the most common side effects (Tariot et al. 1998, 2002). Another small ($n = 21$) placebo-controlled study of carbamazepine (400 mg/day) reported modest benefit. Adverse events were reported as mild (Olin et al. 2001). Despite these preliminary findings, there is a relative dearth of evidence of efficacy from controlled clinical trials. Given the high risk of drug–drug interactions with carbamazepine and the frequent side effects seen in other populations (including rashes, sedation, hematological abnormalities, hepatic dysfunction, and altered electrolytes), carbamazepine should not be considered a first-choice treatment in this population.

Valproic acid, and its enteric-coated derivative divalproex sodium, has been the subject of a number of case reports or case series in patients with dementia and agitation, in which about two-thirds of patients with dementia and agitation have been described as clinically improved. The first randomized, placebo-controlled, parallel-group study of valproate was conducted as a precursor to a larger multicenter trial (Porsteinsson et al. 2001); a secondary measure of agitation showed improvement that was also seen in an open-label extension (Porsteinsson et al. 2003). Side effects seen with valproate included sedation, gastrointestinal distress, and ataxia, as well as the expected decrease in average platelet count (about 20,000/mm^3). A small placebo-controlled crossover study of valproate used for aggressive behavior found no benefit on primary measures of aggression (Sival et al. 2002). There were no drug–placebo differences in rates or types of adverse events. A 6-week randomized, placebo-controlled multicenter study of divalproex sodium in 172 nursing home residents with dementia and agitation who also met criteria for secondary mania used a target dosage of 10 mg/kg/day for 10 days (Tariot et al. 2001b). There was a high dropout rate (n = 100 completers), with 19 divalproex sodium–treated patients (22%) and 3 placebo-treated patients (4%) withdrawing from the study because of adverse events, primarily somnolence (typically occurring at daily dosages ≥15 mg/kg).There were no significant drug–placebo differences in change in manic features, although a significant drug effect on agitation was seen. Sedation occurred in 36% of the drug group versus 20% of the placebo group, and mild thrombocytopenia occurred in 7% of the drug group versus none of the placebo-treated patients. There were no other significant drug–placebo differences in adverse effects. The results from this trial were used to amend prescribing information by cautioning against the use of similar high doses and/or titration rates in the elderly. The largest (n = 153) placebo-controlled trial prospectively addressing agitation, conducted by the Alzheimer's Disease Cooperative Study, found no benefit from divalproex (Tariot et al. 2005). In a comprehensive review, Sink et al. (2005) likewise failed to find benefit for divalproex, and they noted mixed results regarding the efficacy of carbamazepine in patients with dementia. A Cochrane review of valproate for agitation in dementia (Lonergan et al. 2004) concluded that low-dose valproate was ineffective and that high-dose valproate was associated with an unacceptable rate of adverse effects.

There are no placebo-controlled studies of lamotrigine, gabapentin, or topiramate in the treatment of behavioral symptoms in dementia. Despite the absence of controlled studies, however, anticonvulsants are used in clinical practice when other drug treatments fail or are poorly tolerated. The greatest amount of clinical data are available for gabapentin, with almost all reports noting improvement in a majority (but not all) of the subjects. Dosages used ranged from 200 to 1,200 mg/day (Alkhalil et al. 2004; Goldenberg et al. 1998; Herrmann et al. 2000; Moretti et al. 2003; Roane et al. 2000). A review of case reports described worsening of behavior in Lewy body dementia patients who received gabapentin (Rossi et al. 2002). A small retrospective review of topiramate found that agent modestly helpful for aggressive behavior in dementia (Fhager et al. 2003). A single letter to the editor reported the usefulness of lamotrigine for the treatment of aggression in dementia (Devarajan and Dursun 2000).

In an effort to develop more innovative clinical trial designs, as well as to address the public health significance of psychopathology in Alzheimer's disease, the Alzheimer's Disease Cooperative Study organized the first multicenter trial addressing secondary prevention of psychopathology in Alzheimer's disease (Tariot et al. 2002). This multicenter study is examining whether valproate therapy can delay, attenuate, or prevent the emergence of agitation or psychosis in patients lacking these features at baseline. The design incorporates traditional measures of illness progression as secondary outcomes, based on the potential for neuroprotective effects of chronic administration, and may contribute to improved understanding of mechanisms of action of valproate therapy via use of biological markers selected for their relevance to mechanism of action as well as pathobiology of Alzheimer's disease. The study has completed enrollment and will end in early 2009.

Serotonergic Drugs

Sink et al. (2005) found little overall evidence of efficacy for antidepressants in the treatment of neuropsychiatric symptoms other than depression. However, because depression, including irritability, is commonly seen in people with dementia, serotonergic antidepressants are often used in their treatment.

The antidepressant drug trazodone has been reported to be effective in treating agitation and severely disruptive behavior (Greenwald et al. 1986; Nair et al. 1973; Pinner and Rich 1988; Simpson and Foster 1986; Tingle 1986), although these studies did not distinguish between psychotic and nonpsychotic patients. Extensive clinical experience suggests that trazodone is effective at dosages of 50–200 mg/day, with few side effects other than sedation. The mechanism of trazodone's effect is unknown. There have been two double-blind, controlled studies of trazodone in the treatment of dementia-associated agitation. The first was a brief crossover study in only 28 patients, comparing trazodone at a mean dosage of 220 mg/day with haloperidol at a mean dosage of 2.5 mg/day (Sultzer et al. 1997). Agitation improved equally in both drug groups, with better tolerability seen in the trazodone group. The Alzheimer's Disease Cooperative Study reported negative results for all active treatments in a multicenter outpatient study contrasting trazodone, haloperidol, placebo, and caregiver training (Teri et al. 2000). Although there is negative as well as positive evidence of trazodone's efficacy, clinical experience suggests that trazodone is often extremely helpful as an add-on medication when antipsychotics or other drugs alone cannot control disruptive behavior. Priapism is a rare side effect of trazodone in elderly men.

Selective serotonin reuptake inhibitor (SSRI) antidepressants may also have modest antiagitation properties in elderly patients with dementia (Burke et al. 1997; Swartz et al. 1997). Citalopram (Kim et al. 2000; Pollock et al. 2002) and sertraline (Kaplan 1998), in particular, have demonstrated efficacy. In a double-blind study, citalopram was found to be effective, and superior to perphenzine, in treating behavioral disturbances in hospitalized elderly patients with dementia (Pollock et al. 2002). Sertraline in combination with a cognitive-enhancing medication (donepezil) was reported to decrease agitation, although a fulminant chemical hepatitis developed in one patient, necessitating discontinuation (Verrico et al. 2000). In contrast to these positive reports, Olafsson et al. (1992) failed to show the effectiveness of fluvoxamine in the treatment of behavioral disruption in elderly patients with dementia. One review suggested that when antipsychotics cannot be used, SSRIs should be considered first-line treatment (Burke et al. 1997), especially for verbal aggression (Ramadan et al. 2000). Further research of the antiagitation properties of the SSRIs is essential, however, because these antidepressants also tend to be activating and may actually increase agitation, especially in the late stages of a dementing illness.

Buspirone, a nonbenzodiazepine antianxiety agent with effects at serotonin receptors, was reported to be effective in controlling disruptive behavior in older patients in one study (Colenda 1988) but not in another (Strauss 1988). No randomized, placebo-controlled, double-blind studies of buspirone have been conducted, and available studies were small in size. There is insufficient evidence to inform about dosing, titration, safety, tolerability, and efficacy. A small (n = 20) single-blind, placebo-controlled trial reported improvement on measures of aggression, but only 60% of the 20 subjects completed that study (Levy et al. 1994). In a crossover study (n = 10) comparing buspirone with trazodone, Lawlor (1994) found no relative benefit of buspirone. Cantillon et al. (1996) compared buspirone 15 mg/day versus haloperidol 1.3 mg/day in a nursing home population with Alzheimer's disease (n = 26); they reported no significant benefit of either drug. Even when buspirone is effective, disruptive behavior may not decrease for 1 or 2 weeks at full therapeutic doses. Side effects are modest, although one elderly patient with dementia experienced oral dyskinesia that persisted for at least 4 months after symptom onset (Strauss 1988). An occasional patient may become more agitated. Research studies have not yet compared buspirone's effect

with that of placebo or other drugs for treating agitation. The average total daily dosage range is 20–80 mg in divided doses.

Beta-Blockers

β-Blockers, given at low dosages (10–100 mg/day), have been used to reduce agitated and assaultive behavior in elderly patients (Greendyke et al. 1984; Petrie and Ban 1981; Sky and Grossberg 1994). Not all studies of β-blockers have yielded positive findings, however (Risse and Barnes 1986; Weiler et al. 1988). Most evidence is derived from older reports in patients with nonspecific diagnoses (Tariot et al. 1995). Shankle et al. (1995) reported decreased aggression in 8 of 12 patients treated with low doses of propranolol (30–80 mg/day). Side effects of note include bradycardia, hypotension, worsening of congestive heart failure, and asthma. β-Blockers should be used only sparingly for this purpose. Furthermore, these drugs can be given only to those elderly patients without cardiovascular disease and chronic obstructive pulmonary disease (particularly asthma). Typical side effects include sedation, orthostatic hypotension, and decreased cardiac output.

Hormones

There are no rigorous studies of either estrogenic or antiandrogenic approaches, although roughly a dozen published anecdotes exist (Rosenquist et al. 2000). The available evidence suggests occasional benefit for hormonal agents, but this is unproven. A single case report (Kyomen et al. 1991) noted that estrogen (diethylstilbestrol 1 mg/day or conjugated estrogen 0.625 mg/day) reduced the number of incidents of physical aggression, but not of verbal aggression or physical or verbal repetitive behaviors, in elderly male patients with dementia. Medroxyprogesterone has been reported to rapidly and safely treat sexual acting-out behavior in elderly men with dementia (Cooper 1987).

Cognitive-Enhancing Drugs

Cholinergic Agents

As summarized by Cummings (2000), there is increasing evidence that cholinergic agents, especially cholinesterase inhibitors, may have modest behavioral benefits in some patients with dementia. However, most data come from multicenter studies primarily addressing cognitive or global outcomes, using behavioral measures as secondary outcomes.

A prospective clinical trial of metrifonate versus placebo found modest average reductions in neuropsychiatric symptoms, as assessed with the Neuropsychiatric Inventory (NPI), in the drug group versus the placebo group (Morris et al. 1998). A retrospective analysis of two 26-week double-blind, placebo-controlled multicenter trials of metrifonate found a behavioral effect size of 15%, with significant improvement observed on measures of agitation/aggression and aberrant motor behavior as well as hallucinations, dysphoria, and apathy (Cummings et al. 2001; Raskind and Risse 1986).

In a 5-month study of galantamine, Tariot et al. (2000) showed reduced symptoms of cognitive and attentional dysfunction on drug versus placebo in outpatients who generally lacked psychopathology at baseline. In a placebo-controlled trial of donepezil in nursing home residents with probable Alzheimer's disease complicated by behavioral symptoms, there was no evidence of improved behavior on a global measure, although a secondary analysis showed some evidence of reduced agitation (Tariot et al. 2001a). Another study of donepezil in mild to moderate Alzheimer's disease found overall improvement, with modest improvement in behavioral symptoms (Holmes et al. 2004). A subsequent study, however, failed to find improvement in behavioral symptoms with rivastigmine (Ballard and Waite 2006). There appears to be no reliable evidence for the therapeutic effect of this drug on psychosis or behavioral symptoms of dementia and related behavioral disruption. The cholinesterase inhibitors donepezil, rivastigmine, and galantamine have each been reported to reduce restlessness in a small number of elderly individuals with Lewy body dementia (Herrmann et al. 2004; Maclean et al. 2001; Skjerve and Nygaard 2000).

Memantine

Memantine, a noncompetitive inhibitor of N-methyl-D-aspartate (NMDA) receptors approved by the FDA for treatment of moderate to severe Alzheimer's disease, has been examined in several multicenter trials, none addressing behavior as a primary objective. A placebo-controlled study of memantine 10 mg/day in patients with severe dementia showed no benefit on the single behavior item that was used (Winblad and Poritis 1999). A subsequent placebo-controlled study of memantine 20 mg/day also did not find significant behavioral benefit (Reisberg et al. 2003). However, a study in which memantine or placebo was administered to patients already receiving donepezil found significant benefit from memantine on behavior (Cummings et al. 2006a, 2006b; Tariot et al.

2004). In a meta-analysis, Sink et al. (2005) found that cholinesterase inhibitors had a small but statistically significant benefit for behavioral symptoms, whereas memantine had no significant benefit. Trinh et al. (2003) also reported slight overall benefit from cholinesterase inhibitors in patients with mild to moderate Alzheimer's disease. More recently, modest behavioral benefits of memantine have been reported (Swanberg 2007; Winblad and Poritis 1999; Winblad et al. 2007), including data from unpublished trials. Memantine added to donepezil also has been shown to have modest benefit for behavioral disruption in Alzheimer's disease (Tariot et al. 2004). More research is needed on the use of these drugs for treatment of dementia-associated agitation.

Conclusion

Good clinical care of the agitated and/or aggressive elderly patient with dementia requires careful appraisal of factors that may be contributing to the disruptive behavior. Special attention should be paid to recent changes in medical status, treatment with nonpsychiatric medications, and alterations in the environment (Jeste et al. 2008; Salzman et al. 2008). When psychiatric medications become necessary, clinicians now may choose among several classes of psychotropic agents: antipsychotic drugs, mood stabilizers, and serotonergic antidepressants. Available data would suggest that antipsychotic agents are still the first-choice class of drugs, especially for the most severely agitated and aggressive elderly person. This class of drugs, however, carries a potential increased risk of side effects, including extrapyramidal symptoms, cerebrovascular events (including stroke), and possibly premature death. Clinicians must endeavor to use these medications carefully, therefore, monitoring patients closely and informing family members (or significant responsible individuals) of these risks. Initial doses should be modest, with careful dose increments, following the geriatric maxim "Start low and go slow." Other recommended classes of psychotropic drug treatment, in order of preference, are mood stabilizers, serotonergic antidepressants, and cognitive enhancers. These medications are less reliably effective but lack the side effects of antipsychotic drugs. Clinical choice depends on the physical health, prior drug response, and vulnerability to side effects of the elderly individual.

Future research will continue to elucidate the risks versus benefits of different classes of psychotropic drugs while also developing nonpharmacological approaches for the treatment of the common yet serious disruptive behavioral problems associated with dementia.

References

Alkhalil C, Tanvir F, Alkhalil B, et al: Treatment of sexual disinhibition in dementia: case reports and review of the literature. Am J Ther 11:231–235, 2004

Ballard C, Waite J: The effectiveness of atypical antipsychotics for the treatment of aggression and psychosis in Alzheimer's disease. Cochrane Database Syst Rev (1):CD003476, 2006

Billig N, Cohen-Mansfield J, Lipson S: Pharmacological treatment of agitation in a nursing home. J Am Geriatr Soc 39:1002–1005, 1991

Brodaty H, Ames D, Snowdon J, et al: A randomized placebo-controlled trial of risperidone for the treatment of aggression, agitation, and psychosis of dementia. J Clin Psychiatry 64:134–143, 2003

Burke WJ, Dewan V, Wengel SP, et al: The use of selective serotonin reuptake inhibitors for depression and psychosis complicating dementia. Int J Geriatr Psychiatry 12:519–525, 1997

Caligiuri MP, Laero JP, Jeste DV: Incidence and predictors of drug-induced parkinsonism in older psychiatric patients treated with very low doses of neuroleptics. J Clin Psychopharmacol 19:322–328, 1999

Cantillon M, Brunswick R, Molina D, et al: Buspirone vs haloperidol: a double-blind trial for agitation in a nursing home population with Alzheimer's disease. Am J Geriatr Psychiatry 4:263–267, 1996

Chambers CA, Bain J, Rosbottom R, et al: Carbamazepine in senile dementia and overactivity—a placebo controlled double blind trial. IRCS Medical Science 10:505–506, 1982

Chan WC, Lam LC, Choy CN, et al: A double-blind randomized comparison of risperidone and haloperidol in the treatment of behavioral and psychological symptoms in Chinese dementia patients. Int J Geriatr Psychiatry 16:1156–1162, 2001

Christensen DB, Benfield WR: Alprazolam as an alternative to low-dose haloperidol in older, cognitively impaired nursing facility patients. J Am Geriatr Soc 46:620–625, 1998

Cohen-Mansfield J, Werner P, Watson V, et al: Agitation among elderly persons at adult day-care center: the experiences of relatives and staff members. Int Psychogeriatr 7:447–458, 1995

Colenda CC: Buspirone in treatment of agitated demented patient. Lancet 1(8595):1169, 1988

Cooper AJ: Medroxyprogesterone acetate (MPA) treatment of sexual acting out in med suffering from dementia. J Clin Psychiatry 48:368–370, 1987

Coccaro EF, Kramer E, Zemishlany Z, et al: Pharmacology treatment of noncognitive behavioral disturbances in elderly demented patients. Am J Psychiatry 147:1640–1645, 1990

Cummings JL: Cholinesterase inhibitors: a new class of psychotropic compounds. Am J Psychiatry 157:4–16, 2000

Cummings JL, Nadel A, Masterman D, et al: Efficacy of metrifonate in improving the psychiatric and behavioral disturbances of patients with Alzheimer's disease. J Geriatr Psychiatry Neurol 14:101–108, 2001

Cummings JL, McRae T, Zhang R, et al: Effects of donepezil on neuropsychiatric symptoms in patients with dementia and severe behavioral disorders. Donepezil-Sertraline Study Group. Am J Geriatr Psychiatry 14:605–612, 2006a

Cummings JL, Schneider E, Tariot PN, et al: Behavioral effects of memantine in Alzheimer disease patients receiving donepezil treatment. Neurology 67:57–63, 2006b

De Deyn P, Rabheru K, Rasmissen A, et al: A randomized trial of risperidone, placebo, and haloperidol for behavioral symptoms of dementia. Neurology 53:946–955, 1999

Devarajan S, Dursun SM: Aggression in dementia with lamotrigine treatment (letter). Am J Psychiatry 157:1178, 2000

Docherty JP, Frances A, Kahn DA: Treatment of agitation in older persons with dementia: The Expert Consensus Guideline Series. A Postgraduate Medicine Special Report, 1998

Fhager B, Meiri IM, Sjögren M, et al: Treatment of aggressive behavior in dementia with the anticonvulsant topiramate: a retrospective pilot study. Int Psychogeriatr 15:307–309, 2003

Gill SS, Rochon PA, Hermann N, et al: Atypical antipsychotic drugs and risk of ischemic stroke: population based retrospective cohort study. BMJ 330:445, 2005

Goldenberg G, Kahner, Basavarju N, et al: Gabapentin for disruptive behavior in an elderly demented patients (letter). Drugs Aging 13:183–184, 1998

Greendyke RM, Schuster DB, Wooton JA: Propranolol in the treatment of assaultive patients with organic brain disease. J Clin Psychopharmacol 4:282–285, 1984

Greenwald BS, Marin DB, Silverman SM: Serotonergic treatment of screaming and banging dementia (letter). Lancet 2(8521–22):1464–1465, 1986

Haupt M, Cruz-Jentoft A, Jeste D: Mortality in elderly dementia patients treated with risperidone. J Clin Psychopharmacol 26:566–570, 2006

Herrmann N, Lanctot K, Myszak M: Effectiveness of gabapentin for the treatment of behavioral disorders in dementia. J Clin Psychopharmacol 20:90–93, 2000

Herrmann N, Mamdani M, Lanctot KL: Atypical antipsychotics and risk of cerebrovascular accidents. Am J Psychiatry 161:1113–1115, 2004

Holmes C, Wilkinson D, Dean C, et al: The efficacy of donepezil in the treatment of neuropsychiatric symptoms in Alzheimer disease. Neurology 63:214–219, 2004

Jaskiw GE, Thyrum PT, Fuller MA, et al: Pharmacokinetics of quetiapine in elderly patients with selected psychotic disorders. Clin Pharmacokinet 43:1025–1035, 2004

Jeste DV, Finkel SI: Psychosis of Alzheimer's disease and related dementias. Am J Geriatr Psychiatry 8:29–32, 2000

Jeste DV, Lacro JP, Palmer B, et al: Incidence of tardive dyskinesia in early stages of low-dose treatment with typical neuroleptics in older patients. Am J Psychiatry 156:309–311, 1999

Jeste DV, Meeks TW, Kim DS, et al: Research agenda for DSM-V: diagnostic categories and criteria for neuropsychiatry syndromes in dementia. J Geriatr Psychiatry Neurol 19:160–171, 2006

Jeste DV, Blazer D, Casey D, et al: ACNP white paper on the use of antipsychotic drugs in elderly persons with dementia. Neuropsychopharmacology 33:957–970, 2008

Kaplan EW: Retrospective review of the effects of sertraline on 32 outpatients with dementia (letter). Am J Geriatr Psychiatry 6:184, 1998

Karson CG, Bracha HS, Powell A, et al: Dyskinetic movements, cognitive impairment, and negative symptoms in elderly neuropsychiatric patients. Am J Psychiatry 147:1646–1649, 1990

Katz IR, Jeste DV, Mintzer JE, et al: Comparison of risperidone and placebo for psychosis and behavioral disturbances associated with dementia: a randomized, double-blind trial. J Clin Psychiatry 60:107–115, 1999

Kim KY, Bader GM, Jones E: Citalopram for verbal agitation in patients with dementia. J Geriatr Psychiatry Neurol 13:53–55, 2000

Kindermann SS, Dolder CR, Bailey A, et al: Pharmacologic treatment of psychosis and agitation in elderly patients with dementia: four decades of experience. Drugs Aging 19:257–276, 2002

Kryzhanovskaya LA, Jeste DV, Young CA, et al: A review of treatment-emergent adverse events during olanzapine clinical trials in elderly patients with dementia. J Clin Psychiatry 67:933–945, 2006

Kyomen HH, Nobel KW, Wei JY: The use of estrogen to decrease aggressive physical behavior in elderly men with dementia. J Am Geriatr Soc 39:1110–1112, 1991

Laks J, Miotto R, Marinho V, et al: Use of aripiprazole for psychosis and agitation in dementia. Int Psychogeriatr 18:335–340, 2006

Lawlor BA: A pilot placebo-controlled study of trazodone and buspirone in Alzheimer's disease. Int J Geriatr Psychiatry 9:55–59, 1994

Levy MA, Burgio LD, Sweet R, et al: A trial of buspirone for the control of disruptive behaviors in community-dwelling patients with dementia. Int J Geriatr Psychiatry 9:841–848, 1994

Lieberman J, Kane JM, Woerner M, et al: Prevalence of tardive dyskinesia in elderly samples. Psychopharmacol Bull 20:22–26, 1984

Lonergan ET, Cameron M, Luxenberg J: Valproic acid for agitation in dementia. Cochrane Database Syst Rev (2):CD003945, 2004

Loy R, Tariot PN, Rosenquist K: Alzheimer's disease: behavioral management, in Annual Review of Gerontology and Geriatrics: Focus on Psychopharmacologic Interventions in Late Life. Edited by Katz IR, Oslin D, Lawton MP. New York, Springer, 1999, pp 136–194

Lyketsos CG, Steinberg M, Tschanz JT, et al: Mental and behavioral disturbances in dementia: findings from the Cache County Study on memory in aging. Am J Psychiatry 157:708–714, 2000

Maclean LE, Collins CC, Byrne EJ: Dementia with Lewy bodies treated with rivastigmine: effects on cognition, neuropsychiatric systems, and sleep. Int Psychogeriatr 13:277–288, 2001

Maxwell RA, Sweet RA, Mulsant BH, et al: Risperidone and 9-hydroxyrisperidone concentrations are not dependent on age or creatinine clearance among elderly subjects. J Geriatr Psychiatry Neurol 15:77–81, 2002

Meehan KM, Wang H, David SR, et al: Comparison of rapidly acting intramuscular olanzapine, lorazepam, and placebo: a double-blind, randomized study in acutely agitated patients with dementia. Neuropsychopharmacology 26:494–504, 2002

Mintzer JE, Brawman-Mintzer O: Agitation as a possible expression of generalized anxiety disorder in demented elderly patients: toward a treatment approach. J Clin Psychiatry 57:55–63, 1996

Moretti R, Torre O, Antonello RM, et al: Gabapentin for the treatment of behavioral alterations in dementia: preliminary 15-month investigation. Drugs Aging 20:1035–1040, 2003

Morris JC, Cyrus PA, Orazem J, et al: Metrifonate benefits cognitive, behavioral, and global function in patients with Alzheimer's disease. Neurology 50:1222–1230, 1998

Nair NPV, Ban TA, Hontela S, et al: Trazodone in the treatment of organic brain syndrome, with special reference to psychogeriatrics. Curr Ther Res 15:769–775, 1973

Olafsson K, Jorgensen S, Jensen HV, et al: Fluvoxamine in the treatment of demented elderly patients: a double-blind, placebo-controlled study. Acta Psychiatr Scand 85:453–456, 1992

Olin JT, Fox LS, Pawluczyk S, et al: A pilot randomized trial of carbamazepine for behavioral symptoms in treatment-resistant outpatients with Alzheimer disease. Am J Geriatr Psychiatry 9:400–405, 2001

Patel S, Tariot PN: Use of benzodiazepines in behaviorally disturbed patients: risk–benefit ratio, in Behavioral Complications of Alzheimer's Disease. Edited by Lawler BA. Washington, DC, American Psychiatric Press, 1995, pp 153–170

Peabody CA, Warner MD, Whiteford HA, et al: Neuroleptics and the elderly. J Am Geriatr Soc 35:233–238, 1987

Percudani M, Barbui C, Fortino I, et al: Second-generation antipsychotics and risk of cerebrovascular accidents in the elderly. J Clin Psychopharmacol 25:468–470, 2005

Petrie WM, Ban TA: Propranolol in organic agitation. Lancet 1(8215):324, 1981

Pinner E, Rich CL: Effects of trazodone on aggressive behavior in seven patients with organic mental disorders. Am J Psychiatry 145:1295–1296, 1988

Pollock BG, Mulsant BH, Rosen J, et al: Comparison of citalopram, perphenazine, and placebo for the acute treatment of psychosis and behavioral disturbances in hospitalized, demented patients. Am J Psychiatry 159:460–465, 2002

Porsteinsson AP, Tariot PN, Erb R, et al: Placebo-controlled study of divalproex sodium for agitation in dementia. Am J Geriatr Psychiatry 9:58–66, 2001

Porsteinsson AP, Tariot PN, Jakimovich LJ, et al: Valproate therapy for agitation in dementia: open-label extension of a double-blind trial. Am J Geriatr Psychiatry 11:434–440, 2003

Ramadan FH, Naughton BJ, Bassanelli AG: Treatment of verbal agitation with a selective serotonin reuptake inhibitor. J Geriatr Psychiatry Neurol 13:56–59, 2000

Raivio MM, Laurila JV, Strandberg TE, et al: Neither atypical nor conventional antipsychotics increase mortality or hospital admissions among elderly patients with dementia: a two-year prospective study. Am J Geriatr Psychiatry 15:416–424, 2007

Raskind MA, Risse SC: Antipsychotic drugs and the elderly. J Clin Psychiatry 5 (suppl):17–22, 1986

Reisberg B, Doody R, Stamer A, et al: Memantine in moderate-to-severe Alzheimer's disease. The Memantine Study Group. N Engl J Med 348:1333–1341, 2003

Risse SC, Barnes R: Pharmacologic treatment of agitation associated with dementia. J Am Geriatr Soc 34:368–376, 1986

Roane DM, Feinberg TE, Meckler L, et al: Treatment of dementia-associated agitation with gabapentin. J Neuropsychiatry Clin Neurosci 12:40–43, 2000

Rosenquist K, Tariot PN, Loy R: Treatments for behavioral and psychological symptoms in Alzheimer's disease and other dementias, in Dementia, 2nd Edition. Edited by Ames D, Burns A, O'Brien J. London, Chapman & Hall, 2000, pp 571–601

Rossi P, Serrao M, Pozzessere G: Gabapentin-induced worsening of neuropsychiatric symptoms in dementia with Lewy bodies: case reports. Eur Neurol 47:56–57, 2002

Ryu SH, Katona C, Rive B, et al: Persistence of and changes in neuropsychiatric symptoms in Alzheimer disease over 6 months: the LASER-AD study. Am J Geriatr Psychiatry 13:976–983, 2005

Saltz BL, Kane JM, Woerner MG, et al: Prospective study of tardive dyskinesia in the elderly. Psychopharmacol Bull 25:52–56, 1989

Salzman C: Treatment of the agitation of late-life psychosis and Alzheimer's disease. Eur Psychiatry 15:1–4, 2000

Salzman C, Tune L: Neuroleptic treatment of late-life schizophrenia. Harv Rev Psychiatry 77:77–83, 2001

Salzman C, Jeste D, Meyer RE, et al: Elderly patients with dementia-related symptoms of severe agitation and aggression: consensus statement on treatment options, clinical trials methodology, and policy. J Clin Psychiatry 69:889–898, 2008

Schneeweiss S, Setoguchi S, Brookhart A, et al: Risk of death associated with the use of conventional versus atypical antipsychotic drugs among elderly patients. CMAJ 176:627–632, 2007

Schneider LS, Tariot PN, Dagerman KS, et al: Effectiveness of atypical antipsychotic drugs in patients with Alzheimer's disease. N Engl J Med 355:1525–1538, 2006

Shankle WR, Nielson KA, Cotman CW: Low-dose propranolol reduces aggression and agitation resembling that associated with orbitofrontal dysfunction in elderly demented patients. Alzheimer Dis Assoc Disord 9:233–237, 1995

Simpson DM, Foster D: Improvement in organically disturbed behavior with trazodone treatment. J Clin Psychiatry 47:191–193, 1986

Sink KM, Holden KF, Yaffe K: Pharmacological treatment of neuropsychiatric symptoms of dementia: a review of the evidence. JAMA 293:596–608, 2005

Sival RC, Haffmans PM, Jansen PA, et al: Sodium valproate in the treatment of aggressive behavior in patients with dementia—a randomized placebo controlled clinical trial. Int J Geriatr Psychiatry 17:579–585, 2002

Skjerve A, Nygaard HA: Improvement in sundowning in dementia with Lewy bodies after treatment with donepezil. Int J Geriatr Psychiatry 15:1147–1151, 2000

Sky AJ, Grossberg GT: The use of psychotropic medication in the management of problem behaviors in the patient with Alzheimer's disease. Med Clin North Am 78:811–823, 1994

Small GW, Rabins PV, Barry PP, et al: Diagnosis and treatment of Alzheimer disease and related disorders: consensus statement of the American Association for Geriatric Psychiatry, the Alzheimer's Association, and the American Geriatrics Society. JAMA 278:1363–1371, 1997

Smith JM, Baldessarini RJ: Changes in prevalence, severity and recovery in tardive dyskinesia with age. Arch Gen Psychiatry 37:1368–1373, 1980

Strauss A: Oral dyskinesia associated with buspirone use in an elderly woman. J Clin Psychiatry 49:322–323, 1988

Street JS, Clark WS, Gannon KS, et al: Olanzapine treatment of psychotic and behavioral symptoms in patients with Alzheimer disease in nursing care facilities: a double-blind, randomized, placebo-controlled trial. The HGEU Study Group. Arch Gen Psychiatry 57:968–976, 2000

Suh GH, Son HG, Ju YS, et al: A randomized, double-blind crossover comparison of risperidone and haloperidol in Korean dementia patients with behavioral disturbances. Am J Geriatr Psychiatry 12:509–516, 2004

Sultzer DL, Gray KF, Gunay I, et al: A double-blind comparison of trazodone and haloperidol for treatment of agitation in patients with dementia. Am J Geriatr Psychiatry 5:60–69, 1997

Swanberg MM: Memantine for behavioral disturbances in front temporal dementia: a case series. Alzheimer Dis Assoc Disord 21:164–166, 2007

Swartz JR, Miller BL, Lesser IM, et al: Front-temporal dementia: treatment response to serotonin selective reuptake inhibitors. J Clin Psychiatry 58:212–216, 1997

Sweet RA, Pollock G: Neuroleptics in the elderly: guidelines for monitoring. Harv Rev Psychiatry Neurol 5:156–161, 1992

Tariot PN, Erb R, Leibovici A, et al: Carbamazepine treatment of agitation in nursing home patients with dementia: a preliminary study. J Am Geriatr Soc 42:1160–1166, 1994

Tariot PN, Schneider LS, Katz IR: Anticonvulsant and other non-neuroleptic treatment of agitation in dementia. J Geriatr Psychiatry Neural 8:S28–S39, 1995

Tariot PN, Erb R, Podgorski CA, et al: Efficacy and tolerability of carbamazepine for agitation and aggression in dementia. Am J Psychiatry 155:54–61, 1998

Tariot PN, Solomon PR, Morris JC, et al: Galantamine USA-10 Study Group: a 5-month, randomized placebo-controlled trial of galantamine in AD. Neurology 54:2269–2276, 2000

Tariot PN, Cummings JL, Katz IR, et al: A randomized, double-blind, placebo-controlled study of the efficacy and safety of donepezil in patients with Alzheimer's disease in the nursing home setting. J Am Geriatr Soc 49:1590–1599, 2001a

Tariot PN, Schneider L, Mintzer J, et al: Safety and tolerability of divalproex sodium for the treatment of signs and symptoms of mania in elderly patients with dementia: results of a double-blind, placebo-controlled trial. Curr Ther Res 62:51–67, 2001b

Tariot PN, Loy R, Ryan JM, et al: Mood stabilizers in Alzheimer's disease: symptomatic and neuroprotective rationales. Adv Drug Deliv Rev 54:1567–77, 2002

Tariot PN, Farlow PR, Grossberg GT, et al: Memantine treatment in patients with moderate to severe Alzheimer disease already receiving donepezil. JAMA 291:317–324, 2004

Tariot PN, Raman R, Jakimovich L, et al: Divalproex sodium in nursing home residents with possible or probable Alzheimer disease complicated by agitation: a randomized, controlled trial. Am J Geriatr Psychiatry 13:942–949, 2005

Tariot PN, Schneider L, Katz IR, et al: Quetiapine treatment of psychosis associated with dementia: a double-blind, randomized, placebo-controlled clinical trial. Am J Geriatr Psychiatry 14:767–776, 2006

Teri L, Logsdon RG, Peskind E, et al: Treatment of agitation in AD: a randomized, placebo-controlled clinical trial. Neurology 55:1271–1278, 2000

Tingle D: Trazodone in dementia (letter). J Clin Psychiatry 47:482, 1986

Tractenberg RE, Weiner MF, Patterson MB, et al: Comorbidity of psychopathological domains in community-dwelling persons with Alzheimer's disease. J Geriatr Psychiatry 16:94–99, 2003

Trinh NH, Hoblyn J, Mohanty S, et al: Efficacy of cholinesterase inhibitors in the treatment of neuropsychiatric symptoms and functional impairment in Alzheimer's disease: a meta-analysis. JAMA 289:210–216, 2003

Verrico MM, Nace DA, Towers AL: Fulminant chemical hepatitis possibly associated with donepezil and sertraline therapy. J Am Geriatr Soc 48:1659–1663, 2000

Wang PS, Schneeweiss S, Avorn J, et al: Risk of death in elderly users of conventional vs atypical antipsychotic medications. N Engl J Med 353:2335–2341, 2005

Weiler PG, Mungas D, Bernick C: Propranolol for the control of disruptive behavior in senile dementia. J Geriatr Psychiatry Neurol 1:226–230, 1988

Winblad B, Poritis N: Memantine in severe dementia: results of the 9M-Best Study (Benefit and Efficacy in Severely Demented patients during treatment with Memantine). Int J Geriatr Psychiatry 14:135–146, 1999

Winblad B, Jones RW, Wirth Y, et al: Memantine in moderate to severe Alzheimer's disease: a meta-analysis of randomized clinical trials. Dement Geriatr Cogn Disord 24:20–27, 2007

Wooltorton E: Risperidone: increased rate of cerebrovascular events in dementia trials. CMAJ 26:1269–1270, 2002

Wooltorton E: Olanzapine: increased incidence of cerebrovascular events in dementia trials. CMAJ 170:1395, 2004

Wragg RE, Jeste DV: Neuroleptics and alternative treatments: management of behavioral symptoms and psychosis in Alzheimer's disease and related conditions. Psychiatr Clin North Am 11:195–214, 1988

Yassa R, Nair V, Schwartz G: Tardive dyskinesia: a two year follow-up study. Psychosomatics 25:852–855, 1984

Yassa R, Nastase C, Dupont D, et al: Tardive dyskinesia in elderly psychiatric patients: a 5-year study. Am J Psychiatry 149:1206–1211, 1992

Zhong KX, Sweitzer DE, Hamer RM, et al: Comparison of quetiapine and risperidone in the treatment of schizophrenia: a randomized, double-blind, flexible-dose, 8-week study. J Clin Psychiatry 67:1093–1103, 2006

Zhong KX, Tariot PN, Mintzer J, et al: Quetiapine to treat agitation in dementia: a randomized, double-blind, placebo-controlled study. Curr Alzheimer Res 4:81–93, 2007

Zimmer JG, Watson N, Trent A: Behavior problems among patients in skilled nursing facilities. Am J Public Health 74:1118–1121, 1984

Treatment of Substance-Related Disorders

Charles P. O'Brien, M.D., Ph.D.

Charles A. Dackis, M.D.

Drugs that produce substance use disorders all activate the brain reward system, but each class of drugs activates the system by a different pharmacological mechanism. Thus, this chapter is organized according to pharmacological class. The emphasis is on pharmacotherapy, but all treatment using medications should be accompanied by counseling or psychotherapy according to the patient's needs. Medication combines very well with psychotherapy, including self-help groups such as Alcoholics Anonymous (AA). The majority of patients also have an additional mental disorder (besides the addictive disorder) such as depression, anxiety, or bipolar disorder. These comorbidities require specific treatment including medication and psychotherapy. The best treatments for addiction complicated by additional psychiatric disorders are delivered in an integrated fashion, preferably from the same therapist. All psychiatrists should be able to manage substance use disorders, especially those that co-occur with other psychiatric diagnoses.

Alcohol

The 12-month prevalence of alcohol use disorders in the United States in the most recent epidemiological survey was 7.35%, and combined with other drug use disorders the total was more than 8.4% (Compton et al. 2007). Alcohol is the number one substance chosen by both adults and teenagers. The annual loss of life for all causes, but often through accidents, is over $185 billion per year. In a

2005 survey among twelfth-grade students, 53% had used alcohol in the past 30 days and 34% had been drunk during the same period (Johnston 2006). As with all substance use disorders, the best treatments involve a combination of psychotherapy and pharmacotherapy. A variety of medications have been used at the important stages of alcohol use disorder treatment. The first stage is detoxification, which means clearing of the alcohol from the body. After detoxification, the relapse prevention stage should be continued for months or even years.

Alcohol Detoxification

Detoxification involves the clearing of alcohol from the body and the readjustment of all systems to functioning in the absence of alcohol. The alcohol withdrawal syndrome at the mild end may include only headache and irritability, but about 5% of alcoholic patients have severe withdrawal symptoms manifested by tremulousness, tachycardia, rapid respiration, and even seizures. The presence of malnutrition, electrolyte imbalance, or infection increases the possibility of cardiovascular collapse.

Significant progress has been made in establishing safe and effective medications for alcohol withdrawal. Pharmacotherapy with a benzodiazepine is the treatment of choice for the prevention and treatment of the signs and symptoms of alcohol withdrawal. Many patients, however, detoxify from alcohol dependence without specific treatment or medications. It is difficult to determine accurately which persons require medication for alcohol withdrawal. Clinicians should learn to use a formal alcohol withdrawal scale such as the Clinical Institute Withdrawal Assessment (CIWA AD; Sellers et al. 2000) in order to rate the severity of withdrawal and the response to medication. Patients in good physical condition with uncomplicated mild to moderate alcohol withdrawal symptoms usually can be treated as outpatients.

A typical outpatient regimen requires the patient to attend the clinic daily for 5–10 days to receive clinical evaluations, multiple vitamins, and gradually decreasing benzodiazepine pharmacotherapy. A typical medication dosing regimen involves giving enough benzodiazepine on the first day of treatment to relieve withdrawal symptoms. The dose should be adjusted if withdrawal symptoms increase or if the patient complains of excessive sedation. Over the next 5–7 days, the dose of benzodiazepine is tapered to zero. Most clinicians use longer-acting benzodiazepines such as clonazepam, chlordiazepoxide, or diazepam. The usual starting dose of medication on the first day is 25–50 mg of chlordiazepoxide or 10 mg of diazepam given every 6 hours. In an outpatient setting, oxazepam may be particularly useful because it is associated with less abuse and does not require hepatic biotransformation, an important consideration for alcoholics with liver disease.

The diagnosis of delirium tremens is given to patients who have marked confusion and severe agitation in addition to the usual alcohol withdrawal symptoms. It is important to remember that there is a risk of mortality approaching 5% in patients with severe alcohol withdrawal symptoms. Patients who have medically complicated or severe alcohol withdrawal must be treated in a hospital. Benzodiazepines usually will be sufficient to calm agitated patients; however, some patients may require intravenous medication to control extreme agitation.

Relapse Prevention

All patients should be engaged in long-term outpatient care after detoxification. Referral to an AA group is often very useful, but this should not be expected to replace a case manager or therapist. A multipronged approach involving AA, counseling, and medication has the best chance of being successful. Three different kinds of medication have received U.S. Food and Drug Administration (FDA) approval.

Disulfiram

In 1951, disulfiram (Antabuse) became the first medication to be approved by the FDA for the treatment of alcohol dependence other than detoxification. Disulfiram inhibits a key enzyme, aldehyde dehydrogenase, involved in breakdown of ethyl alcohol. After drinking, the alcohol–disulfiram reaction produces excess blood levels of acetaldehyde, which is toxic in that it produces facial flushing, tachycardia, hypotension, nausea and vomiting, and physical discomfort. The usual maintenance dosage of disulfiram is 250 mg/day.

There have been only a few randomized, controlled trials of disulfiram, and these trials have had mixed results for drug efficacy (Peachy and Naranjo 1984). The most comprehensive trial was the Veterans Administration (VA) Cooperative Study of disulfiram treatment of alcoholism. This study was conducted with male veterans and found no differences between disulfiram, 250 mg/day and 1 mg/day (an ineffective dose), and placebo groups in total abstinence, time to first drink, employment, or social stability. Among patients who drank, those in the 250-mg disulfiram group reported significantly fewer drinking days (Fuller et al. 1986).

The main problem with disulfiram is that frequently patients stop taking it and relapse to drinking (Goodwin 1992). Disulfiram is most effective when it is used in a clinical setting that emphasizes abstinence and offers a mechanism to ensure that the medication is taken. Drug compliance may be successfully ensured either by giving the medication at 3- to 4-day intervals in the physician's office or at the treatment center or by having a spouse or family member administer it.

Naltrexone

Naltrexone is a specific opiate receptor antagonist developed for the treatment of heroin addiction. In animal models of alcohol drinking, it was found to reduce the self-administration of alcohol. Beginning in 1983, it was tested as an adjunctive therapy for alcoholism and was found to prevent relapse in some, but not all, patients (Volpicelli et al. 1990, 1992).

After replication of these findings by other researchers (O'Malley et al. 1992), naltrexone was approved by the FDA for use in alcoholism. The first use of naltrexone was to test the hypothesis that at least a part of the reward from alcohol is mediated by the endogenous opioid system. Studies in animal models and in humans have supported that hypothesis (Volpicelli et al. 1995). There have also been reports of reduction in alcohol craving (O'Malley et al. 2002). Alcoholics in treatment get no adverse effects if they drink alcohol while on naltrexone, but they frequently report that it is no longer rewarding. In 2006, the FDA approved an extended-release depot version of naltrexone that is effective with only one injection per month. This is a major treatment advance because the requirement of daily dosing of the oral form led to poor adherence and more relapse. Of course, opioid peptides may not be the only brain system involved in alcohol reinforcement. Norepinephrine, dopamine, serotonin, and γ-aminobutyric acid (GABA) may also be involved in alcohol craving and consumption. Medications aimed at these neurotransmitters are currently in development.

Acamprosate

Another FDA-approved pharmacotherapy for alcohol dependence is acamprosate, whose chemical name is calcium acetyl homotaurinate. Structurally, acamprosate is similar to the amino acid taurine and has been shown to have several actions on the GABA–N-methyl-D-aspartate (NMDA) complex. Acamprosate has been reported to be a safe and effective treatment for alcoholism in several controlled studies. In 1985, Lhuintre et al. published the results of a double-blind study in which 85 subjects, described as severely alcoholic, were randomly assigned to 3 months of treatment with either acamprosate or placebo. Seventy subjects completed the trial, and of these, 20 of 33 (61%) acamprosate-treated subjects and 12 of 37 (32%) placebo-treated subjects were abstinent during the study. Positive results were reported for two subsequent placebo-controlled trials (Lhuintre et al. 1990; Paille et al. 1995) in which the total number of abstinent days was higher for acamprosate-treated subjects compared with placebo-treated subjects. In 1996, the reports of two German double-blind, placebo-controlled studies were published. In the first trial, Sass et al. (1996) studied 272 subjects randomly assigned to a year of treatment with either acamprosate or placebo and evaluated for an additional 12 months following the discontinuation of study medication. Compared with placebo-treated subjects, the subjects who received acamprosate had a significantly lower dropout rate, a greater number of days before their first drink, and a greater number of days of total abstinence during the study.

The second study, which had a similar design, involved 455 subjects and was conducted by Whitworth et al. (1996). The results of this trial were that acamprosate was superior to placebo with respect to the number of dropouts, relapse rate, and total days of abstinence. Interestingly, 18% of the acamprosate-treated subjects, compared with 7% of the placebo-treated subjects, remained continuously abstinent a year after discontinuation of study medication. Subsequently, acamprosate was studied

in a multiclinic trial in the United States (Mason and Ownby 2000) and in a large National Institutes of Health–sponsored trial comparing acamprosate, naltrexone, and placebo (Anton et al. 2006). Although acamprosate trials in the United States have not been positive, the clear results of the European trials were sufficient to merit FDA approval in 2004.

Alcoholism With Other Coexisting Mental Disorders

Depression commonly occurs in alcoholic individuals. The above anticraving medications can be used in combination with all antidepressants, including monoamine oxidase inhibitors (MAOIs), if they are otherwise indicated. Antidepressants alone have not been found to be consistently useful in reducing drinking, but in depressed persons with alcoholism, they are effective in improving mood and overall well-being.

Nicotine

According to the 2000 National Household Survey, an estimated 65.5 million Americans, or 29% of the population, reported current use of tobacco. Most tobacco users, 55.7 million, smoked cigarettes, whereas the remainder smoked cigars and pipes or used smokeless tobacco (Substance Abuse and Mental Health Services Administration 2001). Tobacco accounts for approximately 400,000 deaths per year. Since the mid-1960s, the incidence of smoking in the United States has progressively decreased by about 1% per year (Substance Abuse and Mental Health Services Administration 2001). This remarkable change in tobacco use is a consequence of the realization by society that tobacco-related mortality and morbidity are entirely preventable. Most of these smokers have symptoms that meet the DSM-IV-TR (American Psychiatric Association 2000) criteria for the substance use disorder nicotine dependence. The behavioral aspects of nicotine dependence are similar to those for alcohol and opiate dependence, as well as the production of tolerance and physical dependence. In about 80% of smokers (Gross and Stitzer 1989), nicotine abstinence leads to well-described withdrawal signs and symptoms (Hughes and Hatsukami 1986).

Pharmacotherapy in the form of nicotine replacement has been a key element in reducing withdrawal symptoms and initiating smoking cessation. More recently, nonnicotine medications that can be used in combination with nicotine replacement have become available.

Nicotine Replacement

Nicotine replacement can be obtained over the counter in the form of gum, patch, or nasal spray. Nicotine replacement reduces irritability and withdrawal symptoms such as sleep disturbance, difficulty concentrating, and restlessness. Transdermal nicotine is initially administered in 15- to 21-mg patches for 4–12 weeks, followed by lower-dose patches for up to another 8 weeks. Transdermal nicotine also has excellent documentation for its ability to decrease the severity of withdrawal symptoms and also to decrease craving for tobacco (Daughton et al. 1991; Tonnesen et al. 1991).

Neither gum nor transdermal nicotine has any long-term effect in preventing weight gain after cessation of smoking. Both nicotine preparations provide a significant advantage over placebo in smoking cessation. Stitzer (1991) reviewed seven double-blind, placebo-controlled smoking cessation trials in which nicotine gum was used. Abstinence rates at 4–6 weeks were 73% for nicotine gum compared with 49% for placebo gum. Most of the transdermal nicotine double-blind studies were reviewed by Palmer et al. (1992), who found that quit rates at 4–6 weeks were 39%–71% for transdermal nicotine compared with 13%–41% for the placebo patches. The FDA approved nicotine gum in 1981 and transdermal nicotine in 1991 as prescription medications, and in 1996 both were approved for over-the-counter (nonprescription) use. Beyond the initiation of abstinence, nicotine preparations are associated with a progressive relapse to smoking. After 1 year, abstinence rates are about 25% for the nicotine gum and patch compared with 12% for placebo (Benowitz 1993).

The nasal spray and the inhaler are preparations that provide rapid-release forms of nicotine. The potential advantage of these rapid-release preparations is that they closely simulate smoking by providing a rapid plasma concentration and oral and sensory stimulation. The results from the initial trials for the nasal spray (Schneider et al. 1995; Sutherland et al. 1992) and the inhaler (Tonnesen et al. 1993) are similar to those for the gum and patch.

Nonnicotine Pharmacotherapies

Bupropion, a monocyclic antidepressant that has noradrenergic and dopaminergic effects, was approved by the FDA as a pharmacotherapeutic agent for smoking cessation. Bupropion reduces craving for nicotine, but the mechanism by which this occurs is not well understood. The results from several studies indicate that the bupropion anticraving effect is related to its action on central nervous system dopamine (Covey et al. 2000). In an initial double-blind trial (Ferry et al. 1992) in which 42 men were randomly assigned to 12 weeks of treatment with bupropion 300 mg/day or placebo, the results showed significantly longer continuous abstinence for bupropion-treated subjects at the end of treatment, as well as 6 and 12 months after treatment. Hurt et al. (1997) conducted a study that clearly established the efficacy of bupropion as pharmacotherapy for nicotine dependence. The trial involved 615 nondepressed subjects (50% female) who were randomly assigned to either bupropion 300 mg/day or placebo for an 8-week medication phase. At 1 year, the smoking cessation rate was 23% for the bupropion group compared with 12% for the placebo group. Jorenby et al. (1999) reported on a multisite smoking study with 893 subjects in which placebo, bupropion, nicotine patch, and bupropion plus nicotine patch were compared for efficacy as pharmacotherapy for nicotine dependence. The 12-month abstinence rates were 15.5% for placebo, 16.4% for nicotine patch, 30.3% for bupropion, and 35.5% for bupropion plus nicotine patch. Bupropion, alone or in combination with the nicotine patch, was superior to the nicotine patch or placebo. Bupropion has also been found to be useful in adolescent smokers, a time of great vulnerability to addiction (Killen et al. 2006).

Varenicline is the newest medication that was approved in 2006 by the FDA as an aid to smoking cessation. It is an $\alpha4$, $\beta2$ nicotinic acetylcholine receptor partial agonist. Laboratory data suggest that this receptor is involved in the reinforcing effects of nicotine through activation of the brain reward system. Varenicline was tested against bupropion and placebo in two identical multisite studies. In one study (Gonzales and Weiss 1998) of 1,025 smokers, those randomized to varenicline had significantly greater abstinence rates (44%) at 12 weeks than placebo- or bupropion-treated patients. Continuous abstinence to 52 weeks was 29.1% for varenicline, 16.1% for bupropion, and 8.4% for placebo. In the second study (Jorenby et al. 2006), the varenicline group also had significantly greater abstinence rates than the placebo or bupropion groups by week 12, and the rates of continuous abstinence to 52 weeks were 23% for varenicline, 14.6% for bupropion, and 10.3% for placebo. Thus, the clinician has three pharmacotherapy options to aid in smoking cessation, along with a behavioral treatment program.

Smoking and Psychiatric Disorders

The incidence of smoking in persons who abuse alcohol, stimulants, and opiates is about 90%; however, compared with the other two groups, alcoholic patients smoke the most cigarettes (Burling and Ziff 1988). Many of those who work with psychiatric patients have observed that cigarette smoking is extremely common among patients with schizophrenia. Research not only supports this observation but also clearly shows the extraordinarily high rate of smoking in schizophrenic inpatients and outpatients. Goff et al. (1992) studied schizophrenic outpatients and found that 74% smoked, compared with a national average of less than 30%. Between 80% and 90% of a group of institutionalized schizophrenic patients were found to smoke (Matherson and O'Shea 1984). There is no known reason for the high rate of nicotine use by schizophrenic patients. Some have speculated that the dopamine-augmenting effect of nicotine may counterbalance a relative dopamine deficiency that exists in schizophrenic patients (Glassman 1993). However, nicotine-induced changes in other neurotransmitters (e.g., serotonin) (Benwell and Balfour 1982) may help to explain why so many schizophrenic patients smoke. Also, there is speculation that nicotine ameliorates the cognitive deficits in schizophrenia (Sacco et al. 2005). Further research is needed to understand nicotine's involvement in the pathophysiology of schizophrenia. It is not unreasonable to expect that future antipsychotics not only will ameliorate psychiatric symptoms but also may decrease nicotine dependence in schizophrenic patients.

Glassman et al. (1988) conducted pioneering research establishing the link between major depression and cigarette smoking. Based on data from the Epidemiologic Catchment Area (ECA) survey (Regier et al. 1984), they found that 76% of persons with a lifetime history of major depression "had ever smoked" compared with 52% of persons without a depression history. Similarly, the incidence of depression was 6.6% in smokers compared with 2.9% in nonsmokers, and smokers with a history of depression had a low rate of cessation. These findings have been replicated by several investigators, and the association between depression and smoking is well supported. Another observation is that depressive symptoms appear during smoking cessation in persons with a history of depression (Covey et al. 1990). These researchers also found that alcoholism had the highest association with smoking. Smoking rates among persons with anxiety disorders are at least twice those of persons without a psychiatric diagnosis.

It is unclear what role smoking plays in psychopathology of these disorders. There is some information supporting smoking in these populations as a maladaptive coping strategy (Revell et al. 1985). Future research on smoking in these targeted psychiatric populations may indicate the most efficient treatment approaches for patients who suf-

fer from a combination of nicotine dependence and another psychiatric disorder. Ignoring the nicotine addiction in psychiatric patients, however, is no longer considered acceptable practice.

Benzodiazepines and Other Sedatives

The benzodiazepines have largely replaced older sedative-hypnotic agents, such as barbiturates and meprobamate, in clinical use. To a great extent, the benzodiazepines are popular because they are safe in overdose situations and because, when first marketed, they were thought to have no (or almost no) abuse potential. Clinical experience and scientific study have since shown that although the benzodiazepines, as a class of drugs, are certainly safer in isolated overdose situations than the older agents, physiological dependence is possible and occurs with long-term use, even at therapeutic doses.

These findings have touched off a controversy that has yet to be settled. Most patients who are, in fact, physiologically dependent on benzodiazepines do not increase the dose of medication above the physician's prescription or in any other way abuse the prescribed medication. However, if the benzodiazepine were to be abruptly discontinued, the patient would, in all probability, experience a withdrawal abstinence syndrome that could be extremely severe (O'Brien 2005). For instance, abrupt discontinuation of high therapeutic doses of alprazolam has frequently been reported to cause seizures. Thus, any patient receiving a benzodiazepine for a significant length of time, that is, longer than 3–6 months, should be slowly tapered off his or her medication; this does not preclude the possibility of reemergence of the patient's anxiety symptoms, which may necessitate continued use of the medication.

The fact that patients become physiologically dependent on therapeutic doses of benzodiazepines has led some people in the field to equate any use of benzodiazepines in any patient for long-term treatment with abuse of the drug. This is undoubtedly an overstatement of the abuse of these agents. Significant abuse of benzodiazepines does, in fact, occur but is usually seen in patients abusing other drugs also, not in patients who are carefully monitored and are stable taking therapeutically indicated benzodiazepines.

In general, patients who abuse only benzodiazepines are rare; benzodiazepine abuse in combination with abuse of other drugs is much more common. Alcoholic patients will not infrequently abuse benzodiazepines if the opportunity presents, and patients who abuse cocaine and opioids are also likely to use benzodiazepines concomitantly. Studies in alcoholic patients admitted for detoxification have shown that the rate of benzodiazepine use among these patients is between 28% and 41%, as determined by urinalysis (Crane et al. 1988; Ogborne and Kapur 1987; Soyka et al. 1989); generally only about one-third of the patients with a positive urine test result for benzodiazepines admitted to using the drugs. A variety of studies from Europe have examined benzodiazepine use in patients who use illicit opioids and have found that up to 90% of patients use benzodiazepines to some extent, although most patients deny that they use benzodiazepines or state that they use them to mitigate insomnia or anxiety or to reduce withdrawal symptoms.

Methadone-maintained patients often use benzodiazepines, but generally on a sporadic basis. Magura et al. (1987) showed that 40% of patients in four methadone programs in New York had urine test results that were positive for benzodiazepines, whereas studies in England showed rates of benzodiazepine-positive urine test results of 54% (Lipsedge and Cook 1987) and 59% (Beary et al. 1987) in methadone-maintained patients. In patients who use benzodiazepines in conjunction with other drugs, the issues of abuse and physiological dependence take on a much different meaning than in stable patients taking long-term prescribed benzodiazepines. If these patients use or abuse more than one substance, the use or abuse of benzodiazepines can seriously interfere with drug abuse treatment for other substances; for example, the patient may be discharged from his or her methadone maintenance program for having urine test results that are consistently positive for illicit benzodiazepines. These patients require detoxification from benzodiazepines, with either a benzodiazepine or a phenobarbital taper; evaluation for underlying psychiatric disorders such as generalized anxiety or panic disorder; and relapse prevention techniques for benzodiazepine abuse.

Cocaine

Cocaine abuse in the United States reached epidemic status in the early 1980s. Over the next decade, cocaine use initially decreased and then stabilized. In 2000, an estimated 1.2 million Americans age 12 years and older were current cocaine users. The estimated number of current crack users in 2000 was 265,000 (Substance Abuse and Mental Health Services Administration 2001). According to data from the 2000 Drug Abuse Warning Network (DAWN) Report, cocaine was the illicit substance most

frequently associated with hospital emergencies (Substance Abuse and Mental Health Services Administration 2001). In 2000, the rate of cocaine mentions was 71 per 100,000 population. This rate has remained essentially the same since 1994.

The selection of potential pharmacotherapies has been based on the current understanding of the neurochemical changes that result from chronic stimulant use (see Chapter 49, "Neurobiology of Substance Abuse and Addiction"). Cocaine administration results in increased levels of dopamine in the region of the nucleus accumbens in rats, which is an important part of the brain reward pathways. Cocaine and other abused substances that increase nucleus accumbens dopamine also *decrease* the threshold for brain stimulation reward (Kornetsky and Porrino 1992) and increase the threshold during cocaine withdrawal after chronic cocaine (Koob et al. 2004). A large number of human imaging and animal model studies demonstrate that chronic cocaine exposure dysregulates dopamine function in reward-related brain regions (Dackis and O'Brien 2003).

Pharmacotherapy for cocaine dependence must be considered separately from pharmacotherapy used to treat complications involved in cocaine abuse such as depression and psychotic reactions. Gawin and Kleber (1986) initially described a three-phase cocaine withdrawal syndrome consisting of crash, withdrawal, and extinction. Although this description of cocaine withdrawal found quick acceptance by many clinicians, it was not observed to be valid in several inpatient trials (Miller et al. 1993; Satel et al. 1991; Weddington et al. 1990). In these trials, only mild abstinence symptoms, including depression, anxiety, fatigue, and impaired concentration, were found; the symptoms declined in a linear fashion over the course of 1–2 weeks (Satel et al. 1991; Weddington et al. 1990). However, despite the fact that cocaine withdrawal is not considered to be medically significant, cocaine withdrawal symptom severity is important because of its predictive value. Kampman et al. (2004b) used an instrument called the Cocaine Selective Severity Assessment to measure cocaine withdrawal symptom severity. They found that cocaine withdrawal symptom severity at the start of treatment predicted outcome in several trials. Severe cocaine withdrawal may result from cocaine-induced neuroadaptations and may identify patients with more persistent hedonic dysregulation (Dackis 2005).

Over the past three decades, many agents have been tested and demonstrated to be ineffective as treatments for cocaine dependence. It is noteworthy that dopamine antagonists actually destabilize cocaine-addicted individuals (Grabowski et al. 2000; Kampman et al. 2003), perhaps by exacerbating cocaine-induced dopamine dysregulation. Conversely, the dopamine-enhancing agents disulfiram and modafinil promoted abstinence in controlled trials (Carroll et al. 2004; Dackis et al. 2005). Modafinil also blunted cocaine-induced euphoria in three controlled human laboratory studies (Dackis et al. 2003; Myrick et al. 2004; Hart et al. 2006) and is under current investigation in three large clinical trials.

Advances in the neurobiology of cocaine dependence have guided medication development by identifying neuronal mechanisms associated with specific aspects of cocaine dependence, such as euphoria, withdrawal, and cue-induced craving (Dackis 2005). While dopamine-enhancing agents may reverse neuroadaptations that interfere with the attainment of abstinence, GABA-enhancing agents may prevent relapse in abstinent patients by dampening cue-induced craving, which is a persistent clinical phenomenon that leads directly to recidivism. Topiramate, a GABA-enhancing agent, may promote abstinence by dampening cue-induced craving (Kampman et al. 2004a). Similarly, modafinil and vaccines that reduce cocaine's entry into the brain may promote abstinence by blocking cocaine-induced euphoria (Sofuoglu and Kosten 2005).

The lack of success in identifying an effective medication for treating cocaine dependence has not dampened scientific enthusiasm or impeded further research. On the contrary, there is renewed interest in studying various methods of altering the physiological effects of cocaine. One promising type of relapse prevention pharmacotherapy is not a medicine but a vaccine capable of stimulating the production of cocaine-specific antibodies. Several cocaine vaccines are under development. One of these vaccines, called TACD, works by stimulating the production of cocaine-specific antibodies that bind to cocaine molecules and prevent them from crossing the blood–brain barrier. Because cocaine is inhibited from entering the brain, its euphoric and reinforcing effects are reduced. Cocaine itself is too small a molecule to provoke an immune response, so the vaccine attaches a large protein molecule to a cocaine molecule, thus allowing the immune system to recognize cocaine and produce antibodies against it. TACD can stimulate the production of cocaine-specific antibodies in rats and mice, and the vaccine is effective in reducing cocaine self-administration in rodent models (Fox et al. 1996; Kantak et al. 2000). TACD was administered to 34 former cocaine users in a Phase I trial. The vaccine was well tolerated, and dose-related levels of anticocaine antibodies were detected (Kosten et al. 2002; Martell et al. 2005).

Methamphetamine

In recent years, methamphetamine abuse has become a severe problem, especially in Hawaii and western continental United States. Methamphetamine is a stimulant that possesses stronger dopamine augmentation than cocaine and for a longer duration. While cocaine temporarily blocks dopamine reuptake at synapses, amphetamines also reverse the transporter, thus releasing even more of the neurotransmitter into synapses. Amphetamine, dextroamphetamine, methamphetamine, phenmetrazine, methylphenidate, and diethylpropion all produce behavioral activation similar to that of cocaine. Intravenous or smoked methamphetamine produces an abuse/dependence syndrome similar to that of cocaine, but paranoid psychosis appears to be more common with amphetamine abuse. A different picture arises when oral stimulants are prescribed in a weight reduction program. These drugs do reduce appetite, with accompanying weight loss, on a short-term basis, but the effects diminish over time as tolerance develops. In rodents, there is a rebound of appetite and weight gain when amphetamine use is stopped. In obese humans, weight loss after amphetamine treatment is usually temporary. Anorectic medications, therefore, are not considered to be a treatment for obesity by themselves but rather a short-term adjunct to behavioral treatment programs. Drug abuse manifested by drug-seeking behavior occurs in only a small proportion of patients given stimulants to facilitate weight reduction.

No medication has yet achieved FDA approval for the treatment of methamphetamine addiction, but several that have received positive reports in cocaine addiction treatment such as modafinil are currently in clinical trials for methamphetamine (Ling et al. 2006).

Opioids

Pharmacotherapy for opioid dependence has a long history, in part because "heroinism" was one of the first recognized drug problems in the United States and because therapeutically used congeners of the drug of abuse, heroin, were readily available. Later studies have shown only limited success with nonpharmacological treatment.

Detoxification From Opioid Dependence

The classical method of opioid detoxification was, and remains, short-term substitution therapy. The medication traditionally used has been methadone, at a sufficient dose to suppress signs and symptoms of heroin withdrawal; the methadone is then tapered over a period ranging from 1 week to 6 months. The idea behind a rapid (i.e., 1- to 2-week) detoxification regimen is to achieve total opioid abstinence quickly so that treatment can be continued in a drug-free setting. Detoxification usually can be accomplished in 4–7 days in an inpatient setting, whereas more time is often required in the outpatient setting to minimize patient discomfort. Most practitioners consider 21 days sufficient for short-term outpatient detoxification. However, many patients have very chaotic lives when presenting for treatment and require a period of stabilization before they can hope to maintain a drug-free lifestyle. There is no evidence that more rapid detoxification leads to better long-term outcomes. As discussed below, the regulations for opioid treatment facilities require that patients be dependent on opioids for at least 1 year before they may be admitted to methadone maintenance. The 6-month stabilization/detoxification regimen allows these patients to work on the most acute personal and employment problems while they are stabilized at a relatively low dosage (30–40 mg/day) of methadone and then are detoxified from methadone to continue treatment in a drug-free setting. Unfortunately, the relapse rate after detoxification and drug-free counseling is very high, and long-term maintenance on medication is usually necessary.

The partial opiate agonist buprenorphine received FDA approval in 2002 for the treatment of opioid withdrawal and for maintenance. A major change in the U.S. approach to addiction treatment occurred with passage of a law in 2000 that allows physicians who have a special federal certification to prescribe buprenorphine in their office rather than limiting access, as is the case with methadone.

Buprenorphine has been studied for efficacy in suppressing withdrawal signs and symptoms. In outpatient trials, Bickel et al. (1988) showed that buprenorphine was as effective as methadone in a 10-week double-blind trial (4 weeks on medication taper followed by 6 weeks of placebo). In an open trial, Kosten and Kleber (1988) compared three doses of buprenorphine and found that 4 mg, administered sublingually, was superior to 2 or 8 mg in suppressing signs and symptoms of withdrawal, although illicit opiates were present in the urine of approximately equal numbers of patients in both the 2-mg and the 4-mg dose groups.

There has always been concern about substitution detoxification on the basis that the physician is prolonging the problem by prescribing an addictive medication, even with a tapering regimen. Many of the symptoms of opioid withdrawal (e.g., diaphoresis, hyperactivity, and irritability) appear to be mediated by overactivity in the sympathetic nervous system. This led Gold et al. (1978, 1980) to attempt to depress this overactivity and thereby ameliorate the withdrawal abstinence syndrome by using adrenergic agents that have no abuse potential. Clonidine, an α-adrenergic agonist with inhibitory action primarily at an autoreceptor in the locus coeruleus, was effective in inpatient populations in decreasing the signs and symptoms of opioid withdrawal. Outpatient detoxification with clonidine has not been as successful as inpatient treatment. Inpatient studies reported an 80%–90% success rate, whereas outpatient studies reported success rates as low as 31% in detoxifying patients from methadone and 36% in detoxifying patients from heroin. The problems identified in outpatient clonidine detoxification include 1) access to heroin and other opioids, 2) lethargy, 3) insomnia, 4) dizziness, and 5) oversedation. The last four adverse effects were noted in inpatient populations during detoxification with clonidine but were easily managed in the hospital setting.

Because the side effects of clonidine were unacceptable to many patients, other α-adrenergic agonists have been investigated for use in detoxifying opioid-dependent patients. Lofexidine is widely used for this purpose in the United Kingdom and is in clinical trials in the United States (Gerra et al. 2001).

Ultrarapid detoxification under general anesthesia has been used in some settings with claims of a painless and rapid method to attain the opiate-free state. A randomized comparison of this procedure with a standard buprenorphine detoxification was conducted, and the results showed no advantage for the ultrarapid procedure (Collins et al. 2005). The major hurdle for the treatment of opiate addiction is prevention of relapse, and the method or duration of the detoxification makes no difference.

Maintenance Treatment of Opioid Dependence

Methadone maintenance has been the mainstay of the pharmacotherapy for opioid dependence since its introduction by Dole and Nyswander (1965). Since the 1970s, levo-α-acetylmethadol (LAAM), a long-acting congener of methadone, has been used experimentally for maintenance treatment. It was approved by the FDA for this purpose in 1993 but was later withdrawn from the U.S. market by the pharmaceutical company because of concerns about possible cardiac arrhythmias. With the availability of buprenorphine in 2002, there are again two options for agonist maintenance treatment: methadone and buprenorphine.

Methadone

As discussed earlier in this chapter, methadone has been used for both short- and long-term detoxification from opioids. Methadone maintenance, however, is designed to support patients with opioid dependence for months or years while the patient engages in counseling and other therapy to change his or her lifestyle. Experience with methadone encompassing approximately 1.5 million person-years strongly showed methadone to be safe and effective (Gerstein 1992). Furthermore, this experience has shown that although patients on methadone maintenance show physiological signs of opioid tolerance, there are minimal side effects, and patients' general health and nutritional status improve.

This approach to the treatment of opioid dependence has been controversial since its beginning. Physicians and other treatment professionals who consider addiction to be a brain disease have little or no problem treating patients with an active drug for long periods of time, especially in light of repeated treatment failures in the absence of active medication therapy. However, many people view methadone maintenance as simply substituting a legal drug for an illegal one and refuse to accept any outcome other than total abstinence from all drugs. These people point to long-term follow-up studies of methadone maintenance patients (see Maddux and Desmond 1992) that show that only 10%–20% of the patients are completely abstinent (defined as not being enrolled in methadone maintenance and not using illicit opioids) 5 years after discharge from the maintenance program. However, long-term follow-up studies of patients discharged from drug-free treatment programs show that only 10%–19% of opioid-dependent patients are abstinent at 3- or 5-year time points (see Maddux and Desmond 1992) when the same definition is used. The DSM course specifier "on agonist therapy" applies to those patients who do well on methadone or buprenorphine while continuing the medication and do not use illegal drugs.

Outcome studies conducted with patients in maintenance treatment consistently show that these patients have marked improvement in various measures. Investigators have shown up to an 85% decrease in criminal behavior, measured by self-report or arrest records. Employment among maintenance patients ranges from 40% to 80%. Gerstein (1992) quoted a Swedish study published in 1984 showing the results over 5 years in 34 patients who applied for treatment to the only methadone clinic in Sweden at the time. The 34 patients were randomly assigned to either methadone maintenance or outpatient drug-free therapy; the patients in drug-free treatment could not apply for methadone for a minimum of 24 months after being accepted into the study. After 2 years, 71% of the methadone patients were doing well, compared with 6% of the patients admitted to drug-free treatment. After 5 years, 13 of 17 (76%) patients remained on methadone and were free of illicit drugs, whereas 4 of 17 (24%) patients had been discharged from treatment for continued drug use. Of the 17 drug-free treatment patients, 9 (53%) had subsequently been switched to methadone treatment, were free of illicit drug use, and were "socially productive." Of the remaining 8 patients, 5 (63%) were dead (allegedly from overdose), 2 (25%) were in prison, and 1 (13%) was drug free.

Furthermore, although previous generations of drug abusers had hepatitis B, endocarditis, and other infections, in this age when injection drug use and concomitant sharing of needles and syringes place a patient at risk for HIV infection, the medical consequences of heroin dependence must be taken into account when determining appropriate therapy for a patient. These issues are currently being studied by a variety of methods, but the overall clinical impression of increased general health in methadone maintenance patients is very strong. Additionally, Metzger et al. (1993) undertook a study of HIV seroconversion rates in opioid-dependent subjects. In this study, 152 subjects were in methadone maintenance treatment and 103 subjects were out of treatment. At baseline, 12% of the subjects were HIV positive (10% of in-treatment and 16% of out-of-treatment subjects); follow-up of HIV-negative subjects over 18 months showed conversion rates of 3.5% for in-treatment subjects and 22% for those remaining out of treatment. These data suggest that although transmission of HIV still occurs, opioid-abusing injection drug users in methadone maintenance programs have a significantly lower likelihood of becoming infected than do patients who are not in treatment.

Methadone maintenance programs in the United States are accredited by agencies such as Joint Commission on Accreditation of Healthcare Organizations, approved under regulations by the Center for Substance Abuse Treatment (CSAT) in the Substance Abuse and Mental Health Services Administration (SAMHSA) of the Department of Health and Human Services and the Drug Enforcement Agency (DEA). A program must be accredited and its physicians licensed for a methadone maintenance program in order to prescribe or dispense more than a 2-week supply of any opioid to a patient known or suspected to be dependent on opioids. Most clinics treat ambulatory outpatients and are open 6–7 days per week, requiring patients to come into the clinic daily to receive medication unless and until a patient has "earned" privileges (take-home medication) by compliance with the clinic rules and abstinence from illicit substances. For a person to be eligible for methadone maintenance, he or she must be at least 18 years old (or have consent of the legal guardian) and must be physiologically dependent on heroin or other opioids for at least 1 year. The treatment regulations define a 1-year history of addiction to mean that the patient was addicted to an opioid narcotic at some time at least 1 year before admission and was addicted, either continuously or episodically, for most of the year immediately before admission to the methadone maintenance program. A physician must document evidence of current physiological dependence on opioids before a patient can be admitted to the program; such evidence may be a precipitated abstinence syndrome in response to a naloxone challenge or, more commonly, signs and symptoms of opioid withdrawal, evidence of intravenous injections, or evidence of medical complications of intravenous injections. Exceptions to these requirements are patients who have recently been in penal or chronic care, previously treated patients, or pregnant patients; in these cases, patients need not show evidence of current physiological dependence, but the physician must justify their enrollment in methadone maintenance. A person younger than 18 years must have documented evidence of at least two attempts at short-term detoxification or drug-free treatment (the episodes must be separated by at least 1 week) and have the consent of his or her parent or legal guardian.

Dosage of methadone is an important variable and should be adjusted according to the level of physical dependence. A careful study of performance of methadone programs showed continued heroin use among low-dose patients. Among patients receiving at least 71 mg/day of methadone, no heroin use was detected, whereas patients receiving 46 mg/day of methadone or lower were five times more likely to use heroin than those receiving higher doses (Ball and Ross 1991). Furthermore, McLellan et al. (1993) showed, in a comparison of three levels of treatment services in which all patients received at least 60 mg/day of methadone, that "enhanced methadone services" patients (methadone plus counseling and on-site medical/psychiatric, employment, and family therapy) had fewer positive urine test results for illicit substances than did patients in the "standard services"

(methadone plus counseling) group or the "minimum services" (methadone alone) group. The standard services group did significantly better in treatment than did the minimum services group, and in fact, 69% of the minimum services group required transfer to a standard program 12 weeks into the study because of unremitting use of opioids or other illicit drugs.

Yet another issue that has engendered a great deal of controversy is the treatment of opioid dependence in pregnant women. Those who are philosophically opposed to methadone treatment would advocate that any woman using illicit opioids (heroin) or enrolled in methadone maintenance who became pregnant should be detoxified. It is currently estimated that up to 3% of infants born each year have had intrauterine exposure to opioids. Because many women with substance abuse problems fear all organizations, including medical ones, they frequently have little or no prenatal care, exposing themselves and their babies to the complications of unsupervised pregnancy in addition to the severe stressor of maternal addiction. The complications and treatment of maternal opioid addiction and the effects on the fetus and neonate have been discussed by Finnegan (1991) and Finnegan and Kandall (1992). For the purposes of this chapter, it should be noted that current evidence shows that pregnant women who wish to be detoxified from opioids (either heroin or methadone) should not be detoxified before gestational week 14 because of the potential risk of inducing abortion or after gestational week 32 because of possible withdrawal-induced fetal stress (see Finnegan 1991). Most clinicians dealing with pregnant opioid-dependent patients advocate methadone maintenance at a dose of methadone that maintains homeostasis and eliminates opioid craving; this dose must be individualized for each patient and managed in concert with the obstetrician.

Buprenorphine

Buprenorphine is a partial agonist of μ opioid–type receptor and is a clinically effective analgesic agent with an estimated potency of 25–40 times that of morphine (Cowan et al. 1977). Buprenorphine was approved by the FDA for the treatment of opiate addiction in 2002 in addition to its use as an analgesic agent. Human pharmacology studies have shown buprenorphine to be 25–30 times as potent as morphine in producing pupillary constriction, but buprenorphine was less effective in producing morphine-like subjective effects (Jasinski et al. 1978). Furthermore, these studies showed that the physiological and subjective effects of morphine (15–120 mg) were significantly attenuated when morphine was administered 3 hours after buprenorphine in patients maintained on 8 mg/day of buprenorphine; the physiological and subjective effects of 30 mg of morphine also were tested at 29.5 hours after the last dose of chronically administered buprenorphine and were again significantly attenuated.

Studies in opiate-abusing patients have shown that buprenorphine can be administered sublingually rather than subcutaneously, the route most commonly used for analgesic effect, with only a moderate decrease in potency, 1.0 mg subcutaneously being equal to 1.5 mg sublingually (Jasinski et al. 1989). Early clinical trials with opioid-dependent patients found that patients would tolerate the sublingual route, that the dose of buprenorphine could be rapidly escalated to effective doses without significant side effects or toxicity (Johnson et al. 1989), and that detoxification from heroin dependence using buprenorphine was as effective as using methadone (Bickel et al. 1988) or clonidine (Kosten and Kleber 1988). Johnson et al. (1992) compared buprenorphine (8 mg/day sublingually) and methadone (20 mg/day or 60 mg/day) in a 25-week maintenance study and found that buprenorphine was as effective as 60 mg/day of methadone in reducing illicit opioid use and keeping patients in treatment. Both buprenorphine and methadone 60 mg/day were superior to methadone 20 mg/day in this study. A multicenter study compared sublingual doses of 1 mg of buprenorphine with 8 mg of buprenorphine in more than 700 patients. The 8-mg dose was significantly better than the 1-mg dose on outcome measures of opiate-free urine tests and retention in treatment (Ling et al. 1998).

Results from a review of the controlled studies suggest that buprenorphine is as effective as moderate dosages of methadone (e.g., 60 mg/day), although it is not clear whether it can be as effective as higher methadone dosages (80–100 mg/day) in patients requiring higher dosages for maintenance therapy. A Swedish randomized trial of buprenorphine/naloxone combination versus standard methadone treatment reported equal results as measured by opiate-free urines and improvement on the Addiction Severity Index (Kakko et al. 2007).

Both detoxification and maintenance studies have shown that the abrupt discontinuation of buprenorphine in a blind fashion causes only very minor elevations in withdrawal scores on any withdrawal scale (Bickel et al. 1988; Fudala et al. 1990; Jasinski et al. 1978; Johnson et al. 1989; Kosten and Kleber 1988). Because the issue of take-home medication is likely to arise in any opiate

maintenance program and because methadone take-home medication has the potential for being diverted to illegal channels, the option of every-other-day buprenorphine dosing has been explored. After 19 heroin-dependent patients were stabilized on buprenorphine, 8 mg/day, for 2 weeks, 9 patients continued to receive buprenorphine daily while the other 10 patients, in a blind fashion, received alternate-day buprenorphine doses, 8 mg/dose, for 4 weeks. Patients reported some dysphoria on days on which they received placebos, and it was also noted that pupils were less constricted on placebo days in the patients on alternate-day therapy, but patients tolerated the 48-hour dosing interval without significant signs or symptoms of opiate withdrawal abstinence (Fudala et al. 1990). This leaves open the possibility of alternate-day medication in the treatment setting, eliminating the need for take-home medication.

Buprenorphine is currently marketed in 4:1 combinations with naloxone (buprenorphine/naloxone sublingual tablets of 2 mg/0.5 mg and 8 mg/2 mg). The goal is to reduce abuse of prescribed buprenorphine by injection instead of sublingual dosage. Mendelson et al. (1999) showed that buprenorphine-to-naloxone combination ratios of 2:1 and 4:1 might be useful in treating opiate dependence by causing significant opiate withdrawal symptoms when the combination is taken intravenously. A multicenter clinical trial compared the efficacy of a sublingual tablet of buprenorphine/naloxone, in a 4:1 ratio, with that of placebo and a buprenorphine mono sublingual tablet. The results showed that both the buprenorphine/naloxone combination and the buprenorphine mono tablets were significantly more effective than placebo in reducing illicit opioid use, reducing opioid craving, and improving global functioning. No difference was noted between the efficacy of the combination and the mono products, and the combination product was as acceptable to the subjects as was the mono product (Fudala et al. 1999). Because the buprenorphine/naloxone combination is now widely prescribed throughout the United States, a monitoring program has been in place since 2002 to detect signs of street use of the medication. Thus far, nonprescribed use is minimal, and careful interviews have found that it is most often used to self-treat withdrawal symptoms but not to get high (C.R. Schuster, C.E. Johanson, T. Cicero, C. O'Brien, S. Schnoll, J. Anthony, C. Boyd, R. Schottenfeld, and M. Ensminger, "Surveillance Report—Subutex/Suboxone (July 1–September 30, 2007)," personal communication, December 24, 2007).

Drug Addiction Treatment Act of 2000

The Drug Addiction Treatment Act of 2000 (DATA) allows for the use of opioid medications in the office-based treatment of opioid dependence, provided that both the medication and the physician meet the criteria set forth by the act. The medication must be approved by the FDA for the treatment of opioid dependence and be scheduled in C-III, C-IV, or C-V; medications in Schedule C-II, such as methadone, are not included in the act. The physician must be a "qualified" physician and have an addendum to his or her DEA license to prescribe medications under DATA 2000. Qualifying physicians under this law, however, will be able to more effectively treat opioid dependence in their offices, without referring patients to opioid treatment clinics. The only medications currently available that meet the requirements of DATA are buprenorphine and buprenorphine/naloxone combinations.

Relapse Prevention

As has been noted earlier in this chapter, various methods of detoxifying patients from opioids have been developed, from substitution and rapidly tapering the dose of opioid to long-term methadone maintenance and a very gradual methadone taper. These methodologies are, by and large, unsuccessful in achieving permanent opioid abstinence in patients. It has long been thought that both conditioned reactivity to drug-associated cues (O'Brien et al. 1977; Wikler 1973) and protracted withdrawal symptoms (Martin and Jasinski 1969) contribute to the high rate of opioid relapse. The use of a blocking dose of a pure opioid antagonist would allow the patient to extinguish the conditioned responses to opioids by blocking the positive reinforcing effects of the illicit drugs. Naltrexone was shown to be orally effective in blocking the subjective effects of morphine for up to 24 hours (Martin et al. 1973). Patients using naltrexone maintenance for relapse prevention need to be carefully screened because they must be opioid free at the start of naltrexone administration. Many practitioners administer a naloxone challenge, which must be negative, before starting naltrexone. Naltrexone is usually administered either daily (50 mg) or three times weekly (100 mg, 100 mg, and 150 mg). Although naltrexone is pharmacologically able to block the reinforcing effects of opioids, the patient must take the medication in order for it to be effective. Many opioid-addicted patients have very little motivation to remain abstinent. Fram et al. (1989) reported that of 300 inner-city patients offered naltrexone, only 15 (5%) agreed to take the medication, and 2 months later, only 3 patients were still taking naltrexone. However, patients with better-identified motivation, among them groups of recovering professionals (e.g., physicians, attorneys) and federal probationers who face loss of license to practice a profession or legal consequences, have significantly better success with naltrexone.

A group of federal probationers with a history of opiate addiction were randomly assigned to either naltrexone or treatment as usual. The group receiving naltrexone had significantly fewer opiate-positive urines, and most importantly, the reincarceration rate of the naltrexone group was half that of the control group at 6 months. In 2006, a depot formulation was approved by the FDA for the treatment of alcoholism (Garbutt et al. 2005). Approval for opiate addiction was not requested, but laboratory studies showed the medication to be effective for 30–40 days in blocking usual doses of injected opiates (Bigelow et al. 2006). A clinical trial of another formulation of depot naltrexone, not yet FDA approved, was found to be effective in a placebo-controlled clinical trial (Comer et al. 2006). Thus, the marketed depot version of naltrexone is yet another option for long-term relapse prevention in patients detoxified from opiate addiction.

Hallucinogens

The use and abuse of hallucinogens wax and wane much more than the use of some other drugs, such as alcohol and opioids. The major drugs of abuse that fall into this classification are cannabis and related compounds, lysergic acid diethylamide (LSD) and other indolealkylamines (psilocybin), phencyclidine (PCP) and its congeners, and hallucinogenic amphetamine congeners such as methylenedioxymethamphetamine (MDMA, "ecstasy"). Cannabis has a relatively constant rate of use, but its use alone usually does not cause the user to seek medical attention. That has changed somewhat in recent years, as will be described below. LSD (and related compounds) use has changed from the pattern set in the 1960s, when users lived together communally and the lifestyle of the group frequently revolved around the psychedelic experience. Today, LSD use occurs in isolated groups, polysubstance abusers, and adolescents and young adults who frequent "rave" clubs. Most users of LSD and related compounds are not seen in emergency departments, but occasionally patients experiencing acute adverse reactions to these drugs are brought to medical attention. The most frequent adverse effects of LSD and related compounds are acute panic reactions. Most acute panic reactions, the "bad trips," do not require any intervention other than a calm atmosphere and reassurance, but occasionally a patient will be seen who benefits from a low dose of a benzodiazepine to decrease the anxiety associated with the experience. Likewise, intoxication with MDMA rarely requires more than reassurance or, occasionally, acute benzodiazepine administration, again to enable the patient to deal with the anxiety associated with an adverse experience. However, more recently, as MDMA use has become more popular, particularly in dance or "rave" club situations, more serious effects have been noted. These effects include things such as grinding of the teeth, causing dental problems, as well as more significant medical complications, most notably severe dehydration. It is not known whether the combination of alcohol and MDMA increases the risk of dehydration, but the combination is a frequent occurrence.

PCP intoxication, however, can have serious psychiatric and medical complications. An acute psychotic state can be produced by very low doses of PCP, but behavioral disinhibition, frequently accompanied by anxiety, rage, aggression, and panic rather than by the core psychotic effects, necessitates treatment in most cases in which treatment is mandated. There is no convincing evidence of the superiority of either benzodiazepines or neuroleptics in treating the acute reaction to PCP. Benzodiazepines are frequently used because they have a rapid onset of action and because they can be titrated intravenously. If a neuroleptic is to be used, haloperidol is the most commonly used agent because many other neuroleptics have significant interaction with the anticholinergic properties of PCP itself. There is a paucity of information on chronic use of PCP and on treatment, if indicated, of the chronic user.

Marijuana

Marijuana is mentioned as an hallucinogen, but its use is so common that it deserves special consideration. The cannabis plant has been cultivated for centuries both for the production of hemp fiber and for its presumed medicinal and psychoactive properties. The smoke from burning cannabis contains many chemicals, including 61 different cannabinoids that have been identified. One of these, delta-9-tetrahydrocannabinol (Δ-9-THC), produces almost all of the characteristic pharmacological effects of smoked marijuana (Iversen 2000). The pharmacological effects of Δ-9-THC vary according to the dose, route of administration, experience of the user, vulnerability to psychoactive effects, and setting of use. Intoxication with marijuana produces changes in mood, perception, and motivation, but the effect sought after by most users is the "high" and "mellowing out." This is described as different from the stimulant high and the opiate high. The effects vary with dose, but the typical marijuana smoker experiences a high that lasts about 2 hours. Some users progress to daily use, which is associated with true dependence (addiction) as well as low motivation and possibly increased risk for schizophrenia (Ferdinand et al. 2005).

Rates of marijuana consumption in adults 18 years and older held relatively steady at 4% of respondents in 2002. However, rates of marijuana-related disorders—discrete conditions defined according to criteria established by the American Psychiatric Association—increased from 1.2% to 1.5% of respondents, or from 30.2% overall to 35.6% among marijuana smokers (Compton et al. 2007). In 2007, the National Survey Results on Drug Use estimated that 31.7% of twelfth grade students used marijuana during 2007 (Figure 58–1).

Marijuana is one of the four major substances of abuse; the others are alcohol, cocaine, and heroin. According to the 2000 DAWN report, marijuana had one of the highest emergency department drug mentions, at 39 per 100,000. From 1994 to 2000, marijuana mentions increased from 17 to 39, or by 141% (Substance Abuse and Mental Health Services Administration 2002). After alcohol use disorders, marijuana abuse had the second highest rate of treatment, with 700,000 persons (Substance Abuse and Mental Health Services Administration 2001).

The usual treatment interventions for marijuana abuse include drug monitoring, individual and group psychotherapy, and education (Hubbard et al. 1999). No pharmacotherapy is available for marijuana abuse. This may soon change, given the recent remarkable discoveries concerning cannabinoids.

There has been an explosive growth of marijuana research. Key to this have been the discoveries of cannabinoid receptors and endocannabinoids (naturally occurring cannabis substances) in humans. The neurobehavioral and genetic aspects of cannabinoids are the focus of numerous ongoing studies (see review by Onaivi 2006). The recent scientific discoveries are significant first steps in understanding the mechanisms by which cannabinoids cause physiological effects.

Marijuana has been proposed for several medical indications, including nausea associated with cancer chemotherapy, glaucoma, and wasting disorders. Also, the dis-

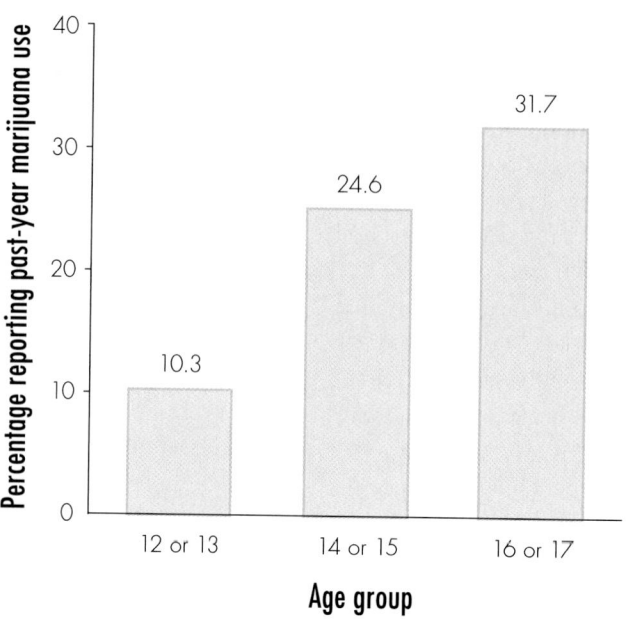

FIGURE 58–1.   Percentages of youths ages 12–17 years reporting past-year marijuana use, by age group: 2000.

Source.   Reprinted from Substance Abuse and Mental Health Services Administration: 2000 National Household Survey on Drug Abuse Report: Marijuana Use Among Youth. Substance Abuse and Mental Health Services Administration, July 2002. Used with permission.

covery of cannabinoid receptors opens the opportunity for the development of specific agonists and antagonists at these receptors that may have important medical value.

Self-Help Groups

Self-help groups—such as Alcoholics Anonymous, Narcotics Anonymous, and Cocaine Anonymous—that are based on a 12-Step method of recovery can be a valuable source of support for the recovering patient. These groups are a fellowship of recovering people interested in helping themselves and others lead drug-free lives. The groups are very good for reminding people of the adverse consequences of relapse and of the benefits of abstinence. Many recovering people feel that it is easier and more relevant to hear about some aspects of recovery from another recovering person. Patients can attend meetings as frequently as necessary and can learn more effective management of leisure time. A sponsor, a person in the group with a prolonged time in a drug-free lifestyle, can provide a good role model for a person in recovery, in addition to providing support and encouragement. Self-help groups are also available to non-drug-abusing family members to help them understand the addictive process and how family member dynamics can affect the drug-abusing or recovering family member.

Conclusion

Addictive disorders can be caused by a variety of drugs that activate the reward system. The common clinical feature of all addictions is loss of control over drug use so that recurrent compulsive drug taking occurs. Treatment, as with other chronic disorders, is generally effective for at least the short term, but relapses are always possible and even likely. Randomized, controlled clinical trials have demonstrated that the combination of antiaddiction medications and psychotherapy provides the best treatment for addictive disorders.

References

American Psychiatric Association: Diagnostic and Statistical Manual of Mental Disorders, 4th Edition, Text Revision. Washington, DC, American Psychiatric Association, 2000

Anton RF, O'Malley SS, Ciraulo DA, et al: Combined pharmacotherapies and behavioral interventions for alcohol dependence: the COMBINE study: a randomized controlled trial. JAMA 295:2003–2017, 2006

Ball JC, Ross A: The Effectiveness of Methadone Maintenance Treatment. New York, Springer-Verlag, 1991

Beary MD, Christofides J, Fry D, et al: The benzodiazepines as substances of abuse. Practitioner 231:19–20, 1987

Benowitz NL: Nicotine replacement therapy: what has been accomplished—can we do better? Drugs 45:157–170, 1993

Benwell ME, Balfour DJ: The effects of nicotine administration on 5-HT uptake and biosynthesis in rat brain. Eur J Pharmacol 84:71–77, 1982

Bickel WE, Stitzer ML, Bigelow GE, et al: A clinical trial of buprenorphine: comparison with methadone in the detoxification of heroin addicts. Clin Pharmacol Ther 43:72–78, 1988

Bigelow G, Preston K, Schmittner J, et al: A randomized, single-dose, opioid challenge study of extended-release naltrexone in opioid-using adults. Neuropsychopharmacology 31:S199, 2006

Burling TA, Ziff DC: Tobacco smoking: a comparison between alcohol and drug abuse in patients. Addict Behav 13:185–190, 1988

Carroll KM, Fenton LR, Ball SA, et al: Efficacy of disulfiram and cognitive behavior therapy in cocaine-dependent outpatients: a randomized placebo-controlled trial. Arch Gen Psychiatry 61:264–272, 2004

Collins ED, Kleber HD, Whittington RA, et al: Anesthesia-assisted vs buprenorphine- or clonidine-assisted heroin detoxification and naltrexone induction: a randomized trial. JAMA 294:903–913, 2005

Comer SD, Sullivan MA, Yu E, et al: Injectable, sustained-release naltrexone for the treatment of opioid dependence: a randomized, placebo-controlled trial. Arch Gen Psychiatry 63:210–218, 2006

Compton W, Thomas Y, Stinson F, et al: Prevalence, correlates, disability, and comorbidity of DSM-IV drug abuse and dependence in the United States. Arch Gen Psychiatry 64:566–576, 2007

Covey LS, Glassman AH, Stetner F: Depression and depressive symptoms in smoking cessation. Compr Psychiatry 31:350–354, 1990

Covey LS, Sullivan MA, Johnston J, et al: Advances in non-nicotine pharmacotherapy for smoking cessation. Drugs 59:17–31, 2000

Cowan A, Lewis JW, Macfarlane IR: Agonist and antagonist properties of buprenorphine, a new antinociceptive agent. Br J Pharmacol 60:537–545, 1977

Crane M, Sereny G, Gordis E: Drug use among alcoholism detoxification patients: prevalence and impact on alcoholism treatment. Drug Alcohol Depend 22:33–36, 1988

Dackis CA: New treatments for cocaine abuse. Drug Discovery Today 2:79–86, 2005

Dackis C, O'Brien C: Glutamatergic agents for cocaine dependence. Ann N Y Acad Sci 1003:328–345, 2003

Dackis CA, Lynch KG, Yu E, et al: Modafinil and cocaine: a double-blind, placebo-controlled drug interaction study. Drug Alcohol Depend 70:29–37, 2003

Dackis CA, Kampman KM, Lynch K, et al: A double-blind, placebo-controlled trial of modafinil for cocaine dependence. Neuropsychopharmacology 30:205–211, 2005

Daughton DM, Heatley SA, Pendergast JJ, et al: Effect of transdermal nicotine delivery as an adjunct to low-intervention smoking cessation therapy. Arch Intern Med 151:749–752, 1991

Dole VP, Nyswander M: A medical treatment for diacetylmorphine (heroin) addiction: a clinical trial with methadone hydrochloride. JAMA 193:646–650, 1965

Ferdinand RF, van der Ende J, Bongers I, et al: Cannabis-psychosis pathway independent of other types of psychopathology. Schizophr Res 79:289–295, 2005

Ferry LH, Robbins AS, Scariati PD, et al: Enhancement of smoking cessation using the antidepressant bupropion hydrochloride: abstract from the 65th Scientific Sessions of the American Heart Association, New Orleans, LA. Circulation 86 (suppl 1): 671, 1992

Finnegan LP: Treatment issues for opioid-dependent women during the perinatal period. J Psychoactive Drugs 23:191–201, 1991

Finnegan LP, Kandall SR: Maternal and neonatal effects of alcohol and drugs, in Substance Abuse: A Comprehensive Textbook. Edited by Lowinson JH, Ruiz P, Millman RB, et al. Baltimore, MD, Williams & Wilkins, 1992, pp 628–656

Fox BS, Kantak KM, Edwards MA, et al: Efficacy of a therapeutic cocaine vaccine in rodent models. Nat Med 2:1129–1132, 1996

Fram DH, Marmo J, Holden R: Naltrexone treatment—the problem of patient acceptance. J Subst Abuse Treat 6:119–122, 1989

Fudala PJ, Jaffe JH, Dax EM, et al: Use of buprenorphine in the treatment of opiate addiction, II: physiologic and behavioral effects of daily and alternate-day administration and abrupt withdrawal. Clin Pharmacol Ther 47:525–534, 1990

Fudala PJ, Bridge TP, Herbert S, et al: A multi-site efficacy evaluation of a buprenorphine/naloxone product for opiate dependence treatment. NIDA Res Monogr 179:105, 1999

Fuller RK, Branchey L, Brightwell DR, et al: Disulfiram treatment of alcoholism: a Veterans Administration cooperative study. JAMA 256:1449–1455, 1986

Garbutt JC, Kranzler HR, O'Malley SS, et al: Efficacy and tolerability of long-acting injectable naltrexone for alcohol dependence: a randomized controlled trial. JAMA 293:1617–1625, 2005

Gawin FH, Kleber HD: Abstinence symptomatology and psychiatric diagnosis in cocaine abusers. Arch Gen Psychiatry 43:107–113, 1986

Gerra G, Zaimovic A, Giusti F, et al: Lofexidine versus clonidine in rapid opiate detoxification. J Subst Abuse Treat 21:11–17, 2001

Gerstein DR: The effectiveness of drug treatment, in Addictive States, Vol 70. Edited by O'Brien CP, Jaffe JH. New York, Raven, 1992, pp 253–282

Glassman AH: Cigarette smoking: implications for psychiatric illness. Am J Psychiatry 150:546–553, 1993

Glassman AH, Stetner F, Walsh Raizman PS, et al: Heavy smokers, smoking cessation, and clonidine: results of a double-blind, randomized trial. JAMA 259:2863–2866, 1988

Goff DC, Henderson DC, Amico E: Cigarette smoking in schizophrenia: relationship to psychopathology and medication side effects. Am J Psychiatry 149:1189–1194, 1992

Gold MS, Redmond DE, Kleber HD: Clonidine blocks acute opiate withdrawal symptoms. Lancet 2(8090):599–602, 1978

Gold MS, Pottach AC, Sweeney DR, et al: Opiate withdrawal using clonidine. JAMA 243:343–346, 1980

Gonzales RA, Weiss F: Suppression of ethanol-reinforced behavior by naltrexone is associated with attenuation of the ethanol-induced increase in dialysate dopamine levels in the nucleus accumbens. J Neurosci 18:10663–10671, 1998

Goodwin DW: Alcohol: clinical aspects, in Substance Abuse—A Comprehensive Textbook. Edited by Lowinson JH, Ruiz P, Millman RB. Baltimore, MD, Williams & Wilkins, 1992, pp 144–151

Grabowski J, Rhoades H, Siverman P, et al: Risperidone for the treatment of cocaine dependence: randomized double-blind trial. J Clin Psychopharmacol 20:305–310, 2000

Gross J, Stitzer ML: Nicotine replacement: ten-week effects on tobacco withdrawal symptoms. Psychopharmacology 93:334–341, 1989

Hart CL, Haney M, Ruben E, et al: Smoked cocaine self-administration decreased by modafinil maintenance: preliminary findings. Presented at International Study Group for the Investigation of Drug as Reinforcers Annual Meeting, Scottsdale, AZ, June 2006

Hubbard JR, Franco SE, Onaivi ES: Marijuana: medical implications. Am Fam Physician 60:2583–2588, 1999

Hughes JR, Hatsukami D: Signs and symptoms of tobacco withdrawal. Arch Gen Psychiatry 43:289–294, 1986

Hurt RD, Sachs DP, Glover ED, et al: A comparison of sustained-release bupropion and placebo for smoking cessation [see comments]. N Engl J Med 337:1195–1202, 1997

Iversen LL: The Science of Marijuana. New York, Oxford University Press, 2000

Jasinski DR, Pevnick JS, Griffith JD: Human pharmacology and abuse potential of the analgesic buprenorphine. Arch Gen Psychiatry 35:501–516, 1978

Jasinski DR, Fudala PJ, Johnson RE: Sublingual versus subcutaneous buprenorphine in opiate abusers. Clin Pharmacol Ther 45:513–519, 1989

Johnson RE, Cone EJ, Henningfield JE, et al: Use of buprenorphine in the treatment of opiate addiction, I: physiologic and behavioral effects during a rapid dose induction. Clin Pharmacol Ther 46:335–343, 1989

Johnson RE, Jaffe JH, Fudala PJ: A controlled trial of buprenorphine treatment for opioid dependence. JAMA 267:2750–2755, 1992

Johnston L: Monitoring the Future 2005, in Monitoring the Future: National Survey Results on Drug Use, 1975–2005. Edited by Johnston L, O'Malley P, Bachman J, et al. Bethesda, MD, National Institute on Drug Abuse, 2006, pp 139–262

Jorenby DE, Leischow SJ, Nides MA, et al: A controlled trial of sustained-release bupropion, a nicotine patch, or both for smoking cessation [see comments]. N Engl J Med 340:685–691, 1999

Jorenby DE, Hays JT, Rigotti NA, et al: Efficacy of varenicline, an alpha4beta2 nicotinic acetylcholine receptor partial agonist, vs placebo or sustained-release bupropion for smoking cessation: a randomized controlled trial. JAMA 296:56–63, 2006

Kakko J, Gronbladh L, Svanborg KD, et al: A stepped care strategy using buprenorphine and methadone versus conventional methadone maintenance in heroin dependence: a randomized controlled trial. Am J Psychiatry 164:797–803, 2007

Kampman KM, Pettinati H, Lynch KG, et al: A pilot trial of olanzapine for the treatment of cocaine dependence. Drug Alcohol Depend 70:265–273, 2003

Kampman KM, Pettinati H, Lynch KG, et al: A pilot trial of topiramate for the treatment of cocaine dependence. Drug Alcohol Depend 75:233–240, 2004a

Kampman KM, Pettinati HM, Volpicelli JR, et al: Cocaine dependence severity predicts outcome in outpatient detoxification from cocaine and alcohol. Am J Addict 13:74–82, 2004b

Kantak KM, Collins SL, Lipman EG, et al: Evaluation of anti-cocaine antibodies and a cocaine vaccine in a rat self-administration model. Psychopharmacology 148:251–262, 2000

Killen JD, Fortmann SP, Murphy GM, et al: Extended treatment with bupropion SR for cigarette smoking cessation. J Consult Clin Psychol 74:286–294, 2006

Koob GF, Ahmed SH, Boutrel B, et al: Neurobiological mechanisms in the transition from drug use to drug dependence. Neurosci Biobehav Rev 27:739–749, 2004

Kornetsky C, Porrino LJ: Brain mechanisms of drug-induced reinforcement, in Addictive States, Vol 70. Edited by O'Brien CP, Jaffe JH. New York, Raven, 1992, pp 59–78

Kosten TR, Kleber HD: Buprenorphine detoxification from opioid dependence: a pilot study. Life Sci 42:635–641, 1988

Kosten TR, Rosen M, Bond J, et al: Human therapeutic cocaine vaccine: safety and immunogenicity. Vaccine 20:1196–1204, 2002

Lhuintre JP, Daoust M, Moore ND, et al: Ability of calcium bis acetyl homotaurine, a GABA agonist, to prevent relapse in weaned alcoholics. Lancet 1(8436):1014–1016, 1985

Lhuintre JP, Moore N, Tran G, et al: Acamprosate appears to decrease alcohol intake in weaned alcoholics. Alcohol Alcohol 25:613–622, 1990

Ling W, Charuvastra C, Collins JF, et al: Buprenorphine maintenance treatment of opiate dependence: a multicenter, randomized clinical trial. Addiction 93:475–486, 1998

Ling W, Rawson R, Shoptaw S, et al: Management of methamphetamine abuse and dependence. Curr Psychiatry Rep 8:345–354, 2006

Lipsedge MS, Cook CCH: Prescribing for drug addicts. Lancet 2(8556):451–452, 1987

Maddux JF, Desmond DP: Methadone maintenance and recovery from opioid dependence. Am J Drug Alcohol Abuse 18:63–74, 1992

Magura S, Goldsmith D, Casriel C, et al: The validity of methadone clients' self-reported drug use. Int J Addict 22:727–750, 1987

Martell BA, Mitchell E, Poling J, et al: Vaccine pharmacotherapy for the treatment of cocaine dependence. Biol Psychiatry 58:158–164, 2005

Martin WR, Jasinski DR: Physical parameters of morphine dependence in man: tolerance, early abstinence, protracted abstinence. J Psychiatry Res 7:9–17, 1969

Martin WR, Jasinski D, Mansky P: Naltrexone, an antagonist for the treatment of heroin dependence. Arch Gen Psychiatry 28:784–791, 1973

Mason BJ, Ownby RL: Acamprosate for the treatment of alcohol dependence: a review of double-blind, placebo-controlled trials. CNS Spectr 5:58–69, 2000

Matherson E, O'Shea B: Smoking and malignancy in schizophrenia. Br J Psychiatry 145:429–432, 1984

McLellan AT, Arndt IO, Metzger DS, et al: The effects of psychosocial services on substance abuse treatment. JAMA 269:1953–1959, 1993

Mendelson J, Jones RT, Welm S, et al: Buprenorphine and naloxone combinations: the effects of three dose ratios in morphine-stabilized, opiate-dependent volunteers. Psychopharmacology 141:37–46, 1999

Metzger DS, Woody GE, McLellan AT, et al: Human immunodeficiency virus seroconversion among in- and out-of-treatment intravenous drug users: an 18-month prospective follow-up. J Acquir Immune Defic Syndr Hum Retrovirol 6:1049–1056, 1993

Miller N, Summers G, Gold M: Cocaine dependence: alcohol and other drug dependence and withdrawal characteristics. J Addict Dis 12:1712–1716, 1993

Myrick H, Malcolm R, Taylor B, et al: Modafinil: preclinical, clinical, and post-marketing surveillance—a review of abuse liability issues. Ann Clin Psychiatry 16:101–109, 2004

O'Brien CP: Benzodiazepine use, abuse, and dependence. J Clin Psychiatry 66 (suppl 2):28–33, 2005

O'Brien CP, Testa T, O'Brien TJ, et al: Conditioned narcotic withdrawal in humans. Science 195:1000–1002, 1977

Ogborne AC, Kapur BM: Drug use among a sample of males admitted to an alcohol detoxification center. Alcohol Clin Exp Res 11:183–185, 1987

O'Malley SS, Jaffe AJ, Chang G, et al: Naltrexone and coping skills therapy for alcohol dependence. Arch Gen Psychiatry 49:881–887, 1992

O'Malley SS, Krishnan-Sarin S, Farren C, et al: Naltrexone decreases craving and alcohol self-administration in alcohol-dependent subjects and activates the hypothalamo-pituitary-adrenocortical axis. Psychopharmacology (Berl) 160:19–29, 2002

Onaivi ES: Neuropsychobiological evidence for the functional presence and expression of cannabinoid CB2 receptors in the brain. Neuropsychobiology 54:231–246, 2006

Paille FM, Guelfi JD, Perkins AC, et al: Double-blind randomized multicentre trial of acamprosate in maintaining abstinence from alcohol. Alcohol Alcohol 30:239–247, 1995

Palmer KJ, Buckley MM, Faulds D: Transdermal nicotine: a review of its pharmacodynamic and pharmacokinetic properties and therapeutic efficacy as an aid to smoking cessation. Drugs 44:498–529, 1992

Peachy JE, Naranjo CA: The role of drugs in the treatment of alcoholism. Drugs 27:171–182, 1984

Regier DA, Myers JK, Kramer M, et al: The NIMH Epidemiologic Catchment Area Program: historical context, major objectives, and study population characteristics. Arch Gen Psychiatry 41:934–941, 1984

Revell AD, Warburton DM, Wesnes K: Smoking as a coping strategy. Addict Behav 10:209–224, 1985

Sacco KA, Termine A, Seyal A, et al: Effects of cigarette smoking on spatial working memory and attentional deficits in schizophrenia: involvement of nicotinic receptor mechanisms. Arch Gen Psychiatry 62:649–659, 2005

Sass H, Soyka M, Mann K, et al: Relapse prevention by acamprosate: results from a placebo-controlled study on alcohol dependence. Arch Gen Psychiatry 53:673–680, 1996

Satel SL, Price LH, Palumbo JM, et al: Clinical phenomenology and neurobiology of cocaine abstinence: a prospective inpatient study. Am J Psychiatry 148:1712–1716, 1991

Schneider NG, Olmstead R, Mody FV, et al: Efficacy of a nicotine nasal spray in smoking cessation: a placebo-controlled trial. Addiction 90:1671–1682, 1995

Sellers EM, Sullivan JT, Somer G, et al: Clinical Institute Withdrawal Assessment for Alcohol (CIWA-AD), in Task Force for the Handbook of Psychiatric Measures, Washington, DC, American Psychiatric Association, 2000, pp 479–481

Sofuoglu M, Kosten TR: Novel approaches to the treatment of cocaine addiction. CNS Drugs 19:13–25, 2005

Soyka M, Lutz W, Kauert G, et al: Epileptic seizures and alcohol withdrawal: significance of additional use (and misuse) of drugs and electroencephalographic findings. Epilepsy 2:109–113, 1989

Stitzer ML: Nicotine-delivery products: demonstrated and desirable effects, in New Developments in Nicotine-Delivery Systems. Edited by Henningfield JE, Stitzer ML. Ossining, NY, Cortland Communications, 1991, pp 35–45

Substance Abuse and Mental Health Services Administration: Summary of Findings From the 2000 National Household Survey on Drug Abuse. Rockville, MD, U.S. Government Printing Office, 2001

Substance Abuse and Mental Health Services Administration: Emergency Department Trends From the Drug Abuse Warning Network, Preliminary Estimates January–June 2001 With Revised Estimates 1994 to 2000. Rockville, MD, U.S. Government Printing Office, 2002

Sutherland G, Stapleton JA, Russell MAH, et al: Randomised controlled trial of nasal nicotine spray in smoking cessation. Lancet 340:324–329, 1992

Tonnesen P, Norregaard J, Simonsen K, et al: A double-blind trial of a 16-hour transdermal nicotine patch in smoking cessation. N Engl J Med 325:311–315, 1991

Tonnesen P, Norregaard J, Mikkelson K, et al: A double-blind trial of a nicotine inhaler for smoking cessation. JAMA 269:1268–1271, 1993

Volpicelli JR, O'Brien CP, Alterman AI, et al: Naltrexone and the treatment of alcohol dependence: initial observations, in Opioids, Bulimia, Alcohol Abuse, and Alcoholism. Edited by Reid LB. New York, Springer-Verlag, 1990, pp 195–214

Volpicelli JR, Alterman AI, Hayashida M, et al: Naltrexone in the treatment of alcohol dependence. Arch Gen Psychiatry 49:876–880, 1992

Volpicelli JR, Watson NT, King AC, et al: Effect of naltrexone on alcohol "high" in alcoholics. Am J Psychiatry 152:613–615, 1995

Weddington WW, Brown BS, Haertzen CA, et al: Changes in mood, craving, and sleep during short-term abstinence reported by male cocaine addicts: a controlled, residential study. Arch Gen Psychiatry 47:861–868, 1990

Whitworth AB, Fischer F, Lesch OM, et al: Comparison of acamprosate and placebo in long-term treatment of alcohol dependence [see comments]. Lancet 347:1438–1442, 1996

Wikler A: Dynamics of drug dependence. Arch Gen Psychiatry 28:611–616, 1973

Treatment of Eating Disorders

W. Stewart Agras, M.D.

Eating disorders are seen frequently in the clinic, reflecting a combined prevalence in women for anorexia nervosa (AN), bulimia nervosa (BN), and binge-eating disorder (BED) of about 3.5% for the full disorder and 6% if subthreshold disorders are included (Hudson et al. 2007). Males are affected less frequently; about 10% of all cases of AN and BN are in males, with the proportion rising to about 30% for BED in clinical samples. Because much comorbid psychopathology is associated with each of these disorders, including current major depression in about 25% of cases, the treatment plan must take any such disorders into account. Two forms of treatment, psychopharmacological and psychotherapeutic, are effective in the treatment of BN and BED, and possibly in AN. Hence, determining how to sequence or combine treatment modalities is an important issue.

Historical Background

Case histories of starvation, binge eating, and purging have been documented, mostly as rare curiosities, for centuries. The histories of saintly women in the thirteenth to fifteenth centuries who had all the symptoms of AN, including self-induced vomiting, are particularly well documented both in their own writings and in the accounts of others. For these women, starvation was in the service of their religious beliefs (Bynum 1987). Cases of BN were rarely seen in the clinic until their relatively sudden increase throughout the Western world in the late 1970s (Garner et al. 1985). This apparent increase in the prevalence of BN has been attributed to increasing societal pressures on women to maintain a thin body shape.

Hence, the motivation for excessive dieting may vary according to the cultural pressures of the times.

Research into the psychopathology and treatment of the eating disorders was relatively slow to develop as compared with such research in depression and the anxiety disorders. This was probably because of the low prevalence of AN and the relatively recent increase in the number of cases of BN. Moreover, BED was only recently recognized as a syndrome, although there is now a large body of literature on the condition. Despite this slow start, sufficient controlled treatment trials are now available to provide guidance to the clinician. This is particularly true for BN, for which psychopharmacological and psychotherapeutic studies began at the same time. Because of the similarity between BN and BED, treatments successful for BN were then applied to BED with some success.

Bulimia Nervosa

BN has its onset in late adolescence or early adult life, with a prodromal period characterized by dissatisfaction with body shape and a fear of becoming overweight, followed by dietary restriction and weight loss. Sooner or later, periods of dietary restriction are followed by episodes of binge eating experienced as a loss of control over dietary intake. This, in turn, further aggravates dissatisfaction with body shape and fears of weight gain. Ultimately, the bulimic patient discovers purging, usually in the form of self-induced vomiting, with or without laxative or diuretic use, excessive exercise, or (less commonly) fasting; and in rare cases in the form of chewing food and spitting it out.

DSM-IV-TR (American Psychiatric Association 2000) distinguishes two forms of BN: purging and non-purging types, the latter characterized by the use of exercise or fasting rather than other compensatory behaviors. The implications of this classification for treatment are unknown. Medical complications of BN are relatively rare; the most serious are potassium depletion and dental caries. Other complications include salivary gland enlargement and exercise injuries. Comorbid psychopathology includes major depression; anxiety disorders, including obsessive-compulsive disorder, social phobia, and panic disorder; alcoholism; and personality disorders, particularly those in the Cluster B spectrum.

Assessment

Assessment should begin with a history of the development of disordered eating, including the psychosocial factors involved in its development. Areas that should be explored include binge eating, purging methods, exercise, and concerns about weight and shape. Eating binges comprise two features: a feeling of loss of control over eating and the eating of a large amount of food. Loss of control appears to be facilitated by the experience of negative affect often deriving from faulty interpersonal interactions (Agras and Apple 2007; Agras and Telch 1998). An objective binge involves eating an amount of food equivalent to an intake of two or more meals. Such binges are required to meet criteria for the diagnosis. Subjective binges consist of a feeling of loss of control but eating less than the required amount for an objective binge. These binges are often quite small and may involve eating a "forbidden" food. The most common method of purging is self-initiated vomiting. It is important to inquire about the use of ipecac to facilitate vomiting because of its toxic cardiovascular effects. The next most frequent method of purging is the use of laxatives. Diuretics also may be used, but less frequently than laxatives. Chewing food and spitting it out and the use of enemas as purgative methods are occasionally seen. Exercise is also used frequently in an attempt to control weight and shape. It is important to distinguish such exercise from normal exercise patterns. The most common distinguishing feature is an exercise regimen that results in exhaustion or that is compulsively adhered to and that would cause anxiety if it were omitted from the daily routine.

In addition to the history, an electrolyte panel is needed, particularly to check potassium levels, which are low and require correcting in about 5% of individuals with BN. A hematocrit is also useful because anemia may

be present. Serum amylase levels also may be elevated. If the patient is not receiving regular dental care, then a referral for such care should be considered because of the erosion of dental enamel and periodontal disease that frequently accompany bulimia. Finally, the assessment should document both past and present comorbid psychiatric disorders because these conditions may have to be taken into account in planning treatment. For example, current major depression may interfere with the patient's ability to adhere to treatment and should be treated together with the eating disorder.

Pharmacological Treatment

Antidepressants

The use of antidepressants in the treatment of BN was sparked by the observation that depression is often a comorbid feature of the disorder (Pope and Hudson 1982). In 1982, two groups of researchers conducted small-scale uncontrolled studies indicating that both tricyclic antidepressants and monoamine oxidase inhibitors reduced binge eating and purging (Pope and Hudson 1982; Walsh et al. 1982). These observations were followed by a series of double-blind, placebo-controlled studies confirming the utility of antidepressants in treating BN, at least in the short term.

A wide range of antidepressant drugs have been found effective, including imipramine (Agras et al. 1987; Mitchell et al. 1990; Pope et al. 1983), desipramine (Agras et al. 1991; Barlow et al. 1988; Blouin et al. 1989; Hughes et al. 1986), phenelzine (Walsh et al. 1988), brofaromine (Kennedy et al. 1993), trazodone (Pope et al. 1989), fluoxetine (Fluoxetine Bulimia Nervosa Collaborative Study Group 1992), fluvoxamine (Milano et al. 2005), and citalopram (Leombruni et al. 2006). Fluoxetine is the only medication approved by the U.S. Food and Drug Administration for the treatment of BN. In these studies, the median rate of decrease in binge eating and purging was 69%, the median recovery rate was 32%, and the mean dropout rate was 23%. In one study involving 77 BN patients (Walsh et al. 2006b) that examined the rate of decline in bulimic symptoms with desipramine, the authors found that those unlikely to respond to the antidepressant could be reliably identified after 2 weeks of treatment.

Antidepressants are prescribed for BN at the same dosages used for treating depression, with the exception of fluoxetine, for which a dosage of 60 mg/day was found to be more effective than 20 mg/day in reducing binge eating and purging in a placebo-controlled trial involving 387 bulimic women (Fluoxetine Bulimia Nervosa Collaborative Study Group 1992). One problem with medication given at times other than bedtime is that a significant amount may be purged through subsequent vomiting. Side effects and reasons for discontinuation of the various medications are similar to those observed in the treatment of depression. However, a study of bupropion found that a higher-than-expected proportion of patients developed grand mal seizures (Horne et al. 1988). The authors concluded that bupropion should not be used for the treatment of BN.

Overall, most antidepressants appear effective for the short-term treatment of BN, with little difference between them (Bacaltchuk and Hay 2003). An interesting recent study involving 47 patients with BN (Monteleone et al. 2005) examined the association of the 5-HTTLPR serotonin transporter genotype with antidepressant response, finding that those with the long form had a tenfold higher likelihood of attaining remission with a selective serotonin reuptake inhibitor (SSRI). As the authors pointed out, these results, if replicated, could allow therapists to prescribe SSRIs to those patients with BN who would be most likely to respond to these agents.

Less is known about the long-term effectiveness of medication. Three small-scale uncontrolled studies found that about one-third of the patients continuing antidepressant medication over periods of 6 months to 2 years relapsed (Pope et al. 1985; Pyle et al. 1990; Walsh et al. 1991). In a larger-scale examination of this issue, 147 women with BN who had decreased their vomiting by at least 50% while taking 60 mg of fluoxetine over an 8-week period were randomly allocated to continue medication or to be switched to placebo (Romano et al. 2002). A survival analysis found that the group receiving active medication experienced a longer time to relapse (or dropout) than did the placebo group. However, it should be noted that at the 3-month assessment, 55% of the fluoxetine group and 78% of the placebo group had either relapsed or dropped out of the study. At the 12-month follow-up, 83% of the fluoxetine group and 92% of the placebo group had experienced a relapse. The authors suggest that given these results, a multimodal approach to the treatment of BN, including cognitive-behavioral therapy (CBT), should be considered.

To date, only one study has compared different lengths of antidepressant treatment, in this case with desipramine. Patients with BN treated for 16 weeks relapsed to pretreatment levels of binge eating when medication was withdrawn. On the other hand, those treated for 24 weeks maintained remission after withdrawal and at 1-year follow-up (Agras et al. 1991, 1994a). This study suggests that patients who respond to antidepressant treatment should be given a minimum trial of 6 months on medication. For the most part, however, controlled studies of antidepressants are of relatively short duration, as is the assessment of bulimic symptoms. Both of these factors may somewhat exaggerate the clinical efficacy of these medications.

Other Medications

Although considerable evidence from controlled trials indicates that most antidepressants are useful in the treatment of BN, few controlled studies of other pharmacological agents have appeared in the literature. However, topiramate (an anticonvulsant drug) has been evaluated in two controlled trials. In the first of these studies, patients meeting criteria for DSM-IV-TR bulimia nervosa were allocated at random to treatment with either topiramate ($n=35$) or placebo ($n=34$) over a 10-week period (Hoopes et al. 2003). Twenty-two (63%) of those in the topiramate group completed the trial, and topiramate was statistically superior in reducing binge eating and purging, and 22% of completers were recovered at the end of treatment. In the second study (Nickel et al. 2005), 30 patients with BN were randomly allocated to either topiramate or placebo. Topiramate was statistically superior to placebo in reducing binge eating and purging; however, no data on remission or recovery were reported. Although no direct comparison between topiramate and an antidepressant has been made, the data so far suggest that topiramate is about as effective as the antidepressants in the treatment of BN.

Combined Treatment

CBT for BN was developed in parallel with the use of antidepressants. CBT in either individual or group format has been shown to be more effective in reducing binge eating and/or purging than placebo (Mitchell et al. 1990), supportive psychotherapy plus self-monitoring of eating behavior (Agras et al. 1989), stress management (Laessle et al. 1991), behavior therapy (Fairburn et al. 1993), and psychodynamic forms of psychotherapy (Garner et al. 1993; Walsh et al. 1997). The existence of two different and effective treatments, antidepressant medications and CBT, naturally led to the question of whether the combined treatments would be more effective than either treatment alone.

The first study of this question used a randomized 2×2 design with four experimental groups: 1) imipramine combined with group psychosocial treatment, 2) imipramine with no psychosocial treatment, 3) placebo combined with group psychosocial treatment, and 4) placebo with no psychosocial treatment (Mitchell et al. 1990). Treatment was preceded by a single-blind placebo washout phase. One hundred and seventy-one women with BN entered treatment, which lasted for 10 weeks. The psychosocial treatment was an intensive group variant of CBT, with 5 daily sessions in the first week and 22 treatment sessions overall. The mean daily dosage of imipramine was 217 mg for the psychosocial treatment group and 266 mg for the group receiving medication alone. As might be expected, the dropout rate was significantly higher for those receiving medication (34%) compared with those taking placebo (15%). Imipramine was superior to placebo; however, CBT, with a remission rate of 51%, was superior to imipramine, with a remission rate of 16%, and combining the two treatments did not result in any additional advantage in reducing binge eating and purging. The combined treatment was, however, significantly superior to CBT in reducing depression.

In the second study (Agras et al. 1991, 1994a), 71 participants were randomly allocated to one of three groups: 1) desipramine (mean daily dosage = 168 mg), 2) CBT, and 3) combined treatment. Half of the desipramine participants were withdrawn from medication at 16 weeks and the remainder at 24 weeks. CBT lasted for 24 weeks. Eighteen percent of the participants stopped taking desipramine before the end of treatment, compared with a treatment dropout of 4.3% of those participants receiving CBT. CBT, with a 48% remission rate, was significantly superior to desipramine, with a 33% remission rate, in reducing the frequency of binge eating and purging, and the combined treatment was no more effective than CBT alone. At 1-year follow-up of 61 of the original 71 patients, 77% of the combined treatment group were abstinent, compared with 54% of those receiving CBT alone (Agras et al. 1994a). This difference was not statistically significant. However, receiving desipramine alone for 24 weeks was the most cost-effective approach in terms of the cost of treatment per recovered patient at 1-year follow-up (Koran et al. 1995).

Another study involving 120 women with BN used a more sophisticated medication regimen consisting of desipramine followed by fluoxetine if the first medication was either ineffective or poorly tolerated (Walsh et al. 1997). It is important to note that the two-medication combination was used by two-thirds of the patients assigned to active medication, suggesting that a two-medication combination is closer to clinical reality than the use of a single medication. This study used a five-cell design: CBT combined with placebo or active medication, psychodynamically oriented therapy combined with placebo or active medication, and medication alone. CBT (plus placebo) was more effective than psychodynamic therapy (plus placebo) in reducing both binge eating and purging. The average dosage of desipramine was 188 mg/day and of fluoxetine was 55 mg/day. Forty-three percent of the patients receiving medication dropped out of the study, compared with 32% of those receiving psychotherapy. Patients receiving active medication (in combination with psychological treatments) reduced binge eating significantly more than did those receiving placebo. Finally, antidepressant medication combined with CBT was superior to medication alone in reducing purging frequency. Of those receiving CBT plus medication, 50% were in remission, compared with 25% of those receiving medication alone. These findings suggest that the combination of CBT plus antidepressant medication may be the most effective approach to the treatment of BN. A meta-analysis confirmed this impression (Bacaltchuk et al. 2000).

Treatment After Psychotherapy Failure

In a small-scale double-blind, randomized, controlled trial, participants who had failed to respond to either CBT or interpersonal therapy in a multisite trial were randomly allocated to either fluoxetine 60 mg/day or placebo (Walsh et al. 2000). Twenty-three participants entered the study with a median of 22 binges and 30 purges over a 4-week period. Of those receiving fluoxetine, 38% were abstinent (over a 4-week period) at the end of treatment compared with none in the placebo group. This finding suggests that fluoxetine may be useful for those who do not respond to psychological treatments.

Comprehensive Treatment

Patients with BN are best treated as outpatients, unless there are either medical or psychiatric reasons for hospitalization (e.g., an intercurrent physical illness or a comorbid psychiatric disorder requiring hospitalization, such as major depression with suicidality). One reason that outpatient treatment is useful for the BN patient is that gains made in the hospital may not carry over to the patient's natural environment, where more complex food stimuli and greater stress are present than in the hospital.

The research evidence to date suggests that the combination of antidepressant medication and CBT is likely to be somewhat more effective than either therapy alone. Because CBT is more effective than antidepressant med-

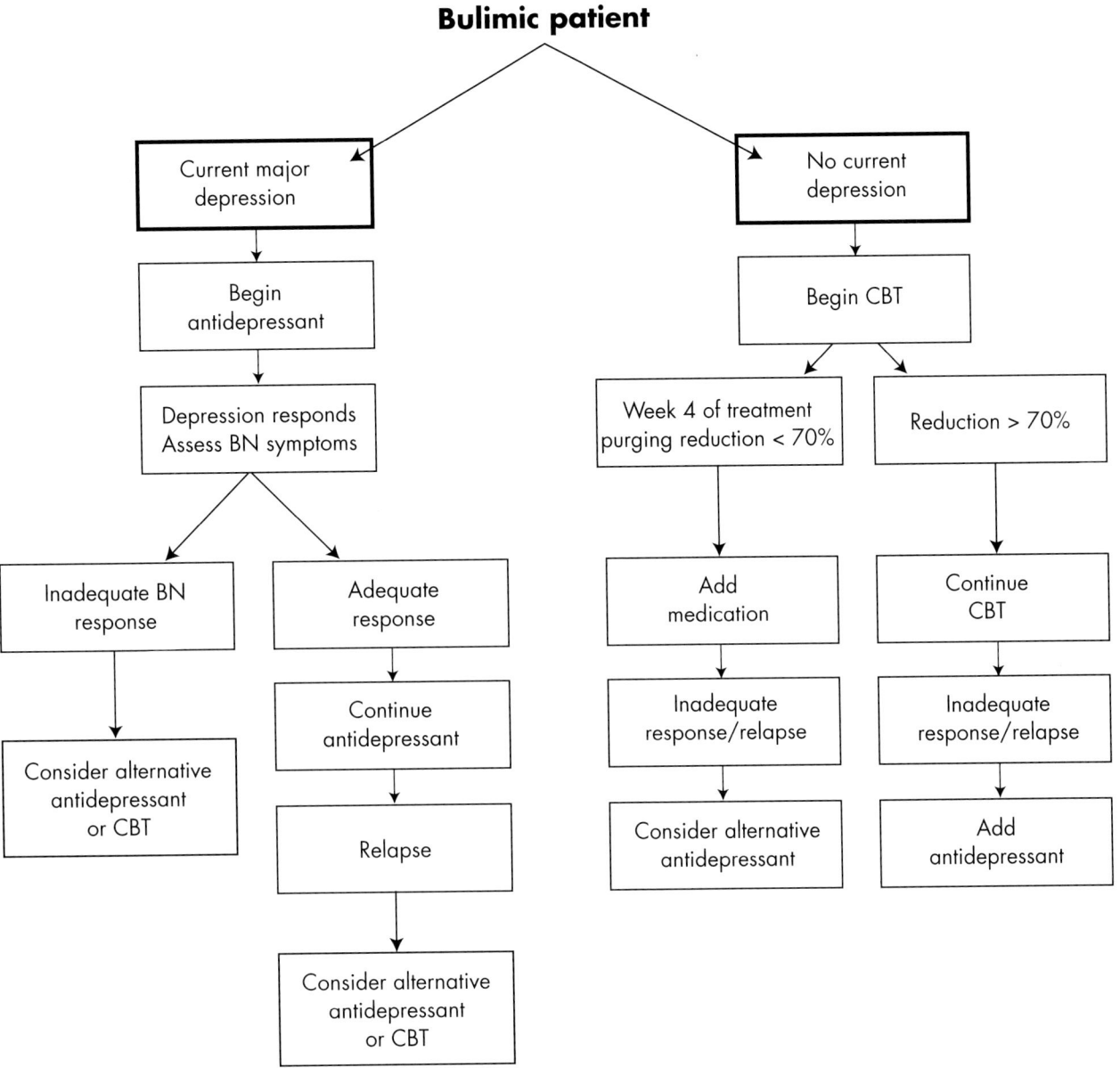

Bulimic patient

FIGURE 59-1. Flow chart depicting different treatment sequences for bulimia nervosa (BN).

CBT = cognitive-behavioral therapy.

ication, having fewer dropouts than medication, in the ideal case, this should be the first therapy offered to the patient. However, CBT is not always available, and in such circumstances, medication will be the only choice. In addition, patient preferences for one or another treatment should be taken into account.

The flow chart in Figure 59–1 presents an algorithm as guidance to the overall treatment of BN. The first decision to make is whether the patient has current major depression, which is seen in approximately 25% of bulimic patients presenting for treatment. Because depressive symptoms can interfere with the conduct of CBT for BN,

antidepressant medication should precede CBT in such patients. When the patient has sufficiently recovered from depression, the eating disorder should be reevaluated. If the patient has not recovered from the eating disorder, then CBT should be added.

As shown in Figure 59–1, after 4 weeks (six sessions) of therapy, if the reduction in purging with CBT is less than 70%, an antidepressant should be added. This algorithm is based on the findings of a multisite study involving 194 women with BN, which found that the initial treatment response to CBT predicted outcome reasonably well (Agras et al. 2000). Those reducing purging less than 70%

after 4 weeks of treatment were more likely to be nonresponders. If there is an inadequate response to antidepressant treatment or a relapse, an alternative antidepressant should be used. For those who complete CBT with insufficient improvement, despite having reduced their purging at session 6, then an antidepressant should be advised.

Binge-Eating Disorder

Although the association between binge eating and obesity has been noted from time to time in case reports in the literature, it was not until the upsurge of research into the psychopathology and treatment of BN that systematic attention was paid to BED. The principal features of BED are episodes of binge eating at a frequency of at least 2 days a week for 6 months, marked distress caused by binge eating, and binge eating that does not occur during the course of BN or AN. Purging does not occur in this condition, although about 10% of the patients with BED have a history of BN.

Between 1% and 2% of women in the general population meet criteria for BED (Bruce and Agras 1992). In clinical populations, the ratio of women to men with BED is approximately 3:2, the highest rate for men for any eating disorder. Although obesity is not a requirement for the diagnosis of BED, there is a substantial overlap between BED and obesity. Studies have shown that about one-quarter of obese subjects have symptoms that meet criteria for BED and that the prevalence of binge eating increases as body mass index increases (Marcus et al. 1985; Spitzer et al. 1993; Telch et al. 1988). Because binge eating often precedes the onset of becoming overweight, binge eating may be a risk factor for obesity and the multiple health problems associated with being overweight. Moreover, the syndrome is associated with comorbid psychopathology similar to that of BN and causes much distress; hence, it is an entity deserving of treatment in its own right. One study that compared individuals with BED with weight-matched non-binge-eating obese individuals found that subjects with BED were significantly more likely to receive diagnoses of major depression (51%), panic disorder (9%), and borderline personality disorder (9%) than were those without BED (Yanovski et al. 1992).

Pharmacological Treatment

Antidepressants

Double-blind, placebo-controlled studies suggest that antidepressants are at least as useful in the treatment of BED as in BN. Early placebo-controlled studies found desipramine to be effective in reducing binge eating, with an abstinence rate of 60% (McCann and Agras 1990). Studies of SSRIs suggest moderate efficacy for fluoxetine, sertraline, and citalopram (Appolinario and McElroy 2004; McElroy et al. 2000). Other studies have found no effect for fluoxetine on binge eating (Devlin et al. 2005; Grilo et al. 2005b). These conflicting results may be due to the relatively high placebo response observed in some studies. There has also been considerable variability in weight losses experienced by patients with BED treated with antidepressants, from essentially no weight loss to several pounds. Although the McCann and Agras (1990) study found that antidepressants reduced binge eating, patients who stopped binge eating did not lose weight. In another controlled study, 108 overweight women with BED received 3 months of CBT, followed by 6 months of weight-loss treatment combined with desipramine. No additive effect of desipramine on binge eating was found; however, women in the medication group lost significantly more weight (4.8 kg) than those in the comparison group (Agras et al. 1994b).

The serotonin–norepinephrine reuptake inhibitor sibutramine (15 mg/day) and the selective norepinephrine reuptake inhibitor reboxetine (8 mg/day) also appeared to be useful in the treatment of BED in open-label studies (Shapira et al. 2000; Silveira et al. 2005). Weight losses were relatively large with both of these medications. A placebo-controlled study of sibutramine in 60 obese women with BED confirmed these early studies (Appolinario et al. 2003), with 52% achieving abstinence from binge eating compared with 32% in the placebo group. Weight losses were 7.4 kg for the sibutramine group compared with a small increase in weight for the placebo group.

Other Medications

Anticonvulsants such as topiramate and zonisamide also appear useful in the treatment of BED (McElroy et al 2006). A multisite study in which more than 400 participants with BED were allocated at random to either topiramate or placebo provided further evidence of the efficacy of topiramate (McElroy et al. 2007). The median dosage of topiramate was 300 mg/day. Dropouts were equivalent between groups (29% topiramate; 30% placebo). Fifty-eight percent of those in the topiramate group and 29% in the placebo group were in remission at the end of the study period. The mean weight loss was 4.5 kg in the topiramate group versus a small gain in the placebo group. The most common side effects specific to topiramate were paresthesia and difficulty concentrating. Hence, topiramate leads to a reasonable rate of remission combined with substantial weight loss.

Finally, a placebo-controlled study comprising 50 overweight participants with BED compared orlistat (120 mg three times daily) with placebo, both groups receiving an abbreviated form of CBT (Grilo et al. 2005a). At the end of treatment, 64% of those in the orlistat group and 36% of those in the placebo group were in remission. The proportions achieving at least a 5% weight loss were 36% for orlistat and 8% for placebo. However, after discontinuation of both treatments, there was no difference in abstinence rates between groups (52% in both groups).

Comprehensive Treatment

BED presents three problems to the clinician: binge eating, overweight, and comorbid psychopathology, particularly depression. Hence, a comprehensive treatment should address all of these problems. There are few direct comparisons of psychotherapy and medication, and the situation is further complicated by the larger placebo responses found in BED as compared with BN, probably accounting for the lack of efficacy of pharmacological agents in some studies. For patients who prefer to try medication, it appears on present evidence that sertraline and topiramate are the most effective in terms of reducing both binge eating and weight. Less is known about medications that may add to the effects of psychotherapies such as CBT and interpersonal therapy, both of which are associated with substantial reductions in binge eating that appear to be well maintained, although weight losses are small. Hence, it appears reasonable to augment psychotherapy with either sertraline or another SSRI, topiramate, or orlistat.

Anorexia Nervosa

AN is a relatively rare disorder characterized by marked weight loss (at least 15% below ideal body weight), intense fear of gaining weight, disturbance in the experience of body shape (i.e., feeling fat in the face of marked weight loss), and (in females) amenorrhea. It is the most lethal psychiatric disorder. Follow-up studies document an aggregate mortality rate of about 5.6% per decade; about half of these deaths are a result of suicide, and the remainder are largely due to cardiovascular instability (Casiero and Fishman 2006). Because of the chronicity of the condition, it has become apparent that identification

and treatment of the disorder early in its course are essential. A specific family therapy for adolescents that aims to help parents take charge of their child's eating appears to be successful in both the short and the long term, with about 70% of adolescent patients with anorexia recovered both at the end of treatment and at follow-up (Lock et al. 2005, 2006).

Most patients with anorexia can be treated as outpatients. However, treatment can be difficult because of the patient's reluctance to gain weight. Weight should be monitored at every outpatient visit, and it is important that weight be measured in a hospital gown to prevent the use of lead weights to which some patients with anorexia resort. Other methods of inflating weight are less easy to detect, such as drinking large quantities of water before being weighed. Indications for hospitalization include weight less than 75% of ideal body weight for age and height, heart rate below 40 beats/minute, blood pressure below 90/60 mm Hg, potassium levels below 3 mEq/L, temperature below 97°F, and very rapid weight loss. In addition, because of the associated psychopathology in this disorder, the usual indications for hospitalization for severe psychopathology should be followed.

Because the disorder is rare, it is difficult in any one center to acquire an adequate sample size for a study in a reasonable time; thus, satisfactory randomized, double-blind medication trials are difficult to accomplish. Moreover, medication trials should be long enough and use optimal medication dosages to adequately show effects in this chronic relapsing disorder. Unfortunately, few trials meet these criteria; many are of short duration, use inadequate dosages of medication, or have been carried out in inpatients.

Pharmacological Treatment

Most studies of antipsychotic agents in the treatment of AN, including chlorpromazine, pimozide, and sulpiride, showed no evidence of efficacy (Dally and Sargant 1960; Vandereycken 1984; Vandereycken and Pierloot 1982). Recent case reports, however, suggest that risperidone may lead to weight gains (Newman-Toker 2000). The effects of olanzapine were studied in 34 patients with anorexia nervosa receiving day care treatment who were allocated to active drug or placebo. The mean dosage of olanzapine was 6.61 mg/day. Those allocated to olanzapine recovered more quickly than those on placebo and gained about 0.6 kg more than those on placebo. Obsessive thinking was also decreased in those receiving olanzapine, but there were no other differences in psychopathology between groups (Bissada et al. 2008). Further studies with larger sample sizes are needed. Moreover, the clinical impression is that olanzapine is not well accepted by patients with AN.

An important study found that fluoxetine was not effective in hospitalized patients with AN (Attia et al. 1998). In this study, 31 women hospitalized with AN participated in a 7-week randomized, double-blind trial of fluoxetine at a mean dosage of 56 mg/day. Four patients in each group terminated the trial early. Although all patients in the study showed improvement, no significant differences were seen between active medication and placebo. In addition, there was no apparent effect of medication on depression or obsessional symptoms. This study suggested that fluoxetine had no effect over and above that of an inpatient program and adds to the consistent failure to show a beneficial effect of antidepressant medication during the period of weight regain.

Despite the findings of an earlier small-scale outpatient study (Kaye et al. 2001), a more recent study of 93 adult outpatients found no benefit of fluoxetine in either promoting weight maintenance or prolonging time to relapse in a double-blind, placebo-controlled trial (Walsh et al. 2006a). As is usual in this population, there was a large proportion of dropouts or early terminations from treatment (51% of fluoxetine-treated and 63% of placebo-treated patients). A fairly high proportion of patients were dissatisfied with treatment. The very high dropout rates make a statistical comparison between groups difficult because of the large amount of data being carried forward in an intent-to-treat analysis. Nonetheless, the only difference between groups was a statistical advantage for fluoxetine in reducing anxiety levels.

Given the findings that fluoxetine confers no benefit for adult patients with AN either during the weight gain period in hospital or during outpatient treatment, one must conclude that the use of fluoxetine is not indicated in the treatment of AN except for the treatment of comorbid psychopathology. At this point, however, there have been no satisfactory studies of SSRIs in adolescents with AN, and such studies would appear warranted given the high priority for treatment early in the course of AN.

Conclusion

The place of psychopharmacological agents in the treatment of BN has been well worked out. Treatment with sequential trials of different antidepressants should result in abstinence rates of about 40%. The addition of CBT en-

hances the effectiveness of antidepressants. It is becoming clear that agents such as topiramate and similar anticonvulsants are useful in the treatment of BED, with the added advantage of facilitating substantial weight loss in the overweight patient. In the case of AN, there is little evidence that pharmacological agents are helpful in either inpatient or outpatient treatment of the adult patient, except to treat comorbid psychiatric disorders. There is insufficient information regarding adolescent anorexia to provide guidance regarding the use of medication at this point.

References

Agras WS, Apple RF: Overcoming Eating Disorders: Therapist Guide. New York, Oxford University Press, 2007

Agras WS, Telch CF: The effects of caloric deprivation and negative affect on binge eating in obese binge-eating disordered women. Behav Ther 29:491–503, 1998

Agras WS, Dorian B, Kirkley BG, et al: Imipramine in the treatment of bulimia: a double-blind controlled study. Int J Eat Disord 6:29–38, 1987

Agras WS, Schneider JA, Arnow B, et al: Cognitive-behavioral and response prevention treatment for bulimia nervosa. J Consult Clin Psychol 57:215–221, 1989

Agras WS, Rossiter EM, Arnow B, et al: Pharmacologic and cognitive-behavioral treatment for bulimia nervosa: a controlled comparison. Am J Psychiatry 159:325–333, 1991

Agras WS, Rossiter EM, Arnow B, et al: One-year follow-up of psychosocial and pharmacologic treatments for bulimia nervosa. J Clin Psychiatry 55:179–183, 1994a

Agras WS, Telch CF, Arnow B, et al: Weight loss, cognitive-behavioral, and desipramine treatments in binge-eating disorder: an additive design. Behav Ther 25:225–238, 1994b

Agras WS, Crow SJ, Halmi KA, et al: Outcome predictors for the cognitive-behavioral treatment of bulimia nervosa: data from a multisite study. Am J Psychiatry 157:1302–1308, 2000

American Psychiatric Association: Diagnostic and Statistical Manual of Mental Disorders, 4th Edition, Text Revision. Washington, DC, American Psychiatric Association, 2000

Appolinario JC, McElroy SL: Pharmacologic approaches to the treatment of binge eating disorder. Curr Drug Targets 5:301–307, 2004

Appolinario JC, Bacaltchuk J, Sichieri R, et al: A randomized double-blind, placebo-controlled study of sibutramine in the treatment of binge eating disorder. Arch Gen Psychiatry 60:1109–1116, 2003

Attia E, Haiman C, Walsh BT, et al: Does fluoxetine augment the inpatient treatment of anorexia nervosa? Am J Psychiatry 155:548–551, 1998

Bacaltchuk J, Hay P: Antidepressants versus placebo for people with bulimia nervosa. Cochrane Database Syst Rev (4): CD003391, 2003

Bacaltchuk J, Trefiglio IR, Oliveria P, et al: Combination of antidepressants and psychological treatments for bulimia nervosa: a systematic review. Acta Psychiatr Scand 101:256–267, 2000

Barlow J, Blouin J, Blouin A, et al: Treatment of bulimia with desipramine: a double-blind crossover study. Can J Psychiatry 33:129–133, 1988

Bissada H, Tasca GA, Barber AM, et al: Olanzapine in the treatment of low body weight and obsessive thinking in women with anorexia nervosa: a randomized, double-blind, placebo-controlled trial. Am J Psychiatry 165:1281–1288, 2008

Blouin J, Blouin A, Perez E: Bulimia: independence of antibulimic and antidepressant properties of desipramine. Can J Psychiatry 34:24–29, 1989

Bruce B, Agras WS: Binge-eating in females: a population-based investigation. Int J Eat Disord 12:365–373, 1992

Bynum CW: Holy Feast and Holy Fast: The Religious Significance of Food to Medieval Women. Berkeley and Los Angeles, University of California Press, 1987

Casiero D, Fishman WH: Cardiovascular complications of eating disorders. Cardiol Rev 14:227–231, 2006

Dally PJ, Sargant W: A new treatment of anorexia nervosa. BMJ 1:1770–1773, 1960

Devlin MJ, Golfein, JA, Petkova E, et al: Cognitive-behavioral therapy and fluoxetine as adjuncts to group behavioral therapy for binge eating disorder. Obes Res 13:1077–1088, 2005.

Fairburn CG, Jones R, Peveler RC, et al: Psychotherapy and bulimia nervosa: longer-term effects of interpersonal psychotherapy, behavior therapy, and cognitive behavior therapy. Arch Gen Psychiatry 50:419–428, 1993

Fluoxetine Bulimia Nervosa Collaborative Study Group: Fluoxetine in the treatment of bulimia nervosa. Multicenter, placebo-controlled, double-blind trial. Arch Gen Psychiatry 49:139–147, 1992

Garner DM, Olmsted MP, Garfinkel PE: Similarities among bulimic groups selected by weight and weight history. J Psychiatr Res 19:129–134, 1985

Garner DM, Rockert I, Davis R, et al: Comparison between cognitive-behavioral and supportive-expressive therapy for bulimia nervosa. Am J Psychiatry 150:37–46, 1993

Grilo CM, Masheb RM, Salant SL: Cognitive behavioral therapy, guided self-help and orlistat for the treatment of binge eating disorder: a randomized double-blind placebo-controlled trial. Biol Psychiatry 57:1193–1201, 2005a

Grilo CM, Masheb RM, Wilson GT: Efficacy of cognitive behavioral therapy and fluoxetine for the treatment of binge eating disorder: a randomized double-blind placebo-controlled comparison. Biol Psychiatry 57:301–309, 2005b

Hoopes SP, Reimherr FW, Hedges DW, et al: Treatment of bulimia nervosa with topiramate in a randomized, double-blind, placebo-controlled trial, part 1: improvement in binge and purge measures. J Clin Psychiatry 64:1335–1341, 2003

Horne RL, Ferguson JM, Pope HG, et al: Treatment of bulimia with bupropion: a multicenter controlled trial. J Clin Psychiatry 49:262–266, 1988

Hudson JI, Hiripi E, Pope HG, et al: The prevalence and correlates of eating disorders in the national comorbidity survey replication. Biol Psychiatry 61:348–358, 2007

Hughes PL, Wells LA, Cunningham CI, et al: Treating bulimia with desipramine. A double-blind, placebo-controlled study. Arch Gen Psychiatry 43:182–187, 1986

Kaye WH, Nagata T, Weltzin TE, et al: Double-blind placebo-controlled administration of fluoxetine in restricting- and restricting-purging-type anorexia nervosa. Biol Psychiatry 49:644–652, 2001

Kennedy SH, Goldbloom DS, Ralevski E, et al: Is there a role for selective monoamine oxidase inhibitor therapy in bulimia nervosa? A placebo-controlled trial. J Clin Psychopharmacol 13:415–422, 1993

Koran LM, Agras WS, Rossiter E, et al: Comparing the cost-effectiveness of psychiatric treatments: bulimia nervosa. Psychiatry Res 58:13–21, 1995

Laessle PJ, Beumont PJV, Butow P, et al: A comparison of nutritional management with stress management in the treatment of bulimia nervosa. Br J Psychiatry 159:250–261, 1991

Leombruni P, Amianto F, Delsedime N, et al: Citalopram versus fluoxetine for the treatment of patients with bulimia nervosa: a single-blind randomized controlled trial. Adv Ther 23:481–494, 2006

Lock J, Agras WS, Bryson S, et al: A comparison of short- and long-term family therapy for adolescent anorexia nervosa. J Am Acad Child Adolesc Psychiatry 44:632–639, 2005

Lock J, Couturier J, Agras WS: Comparison of long term outcomes in adolescents with anorexia nervosa treated with family therapy. J Am Acad Child Adolesc Psychiatry, 45:666–672, 2006

Marcus MD, Wing RR, Lamparski DM: Binge-eating and dietary restraint in obese patients. Addict Behav 10:163–168, 1985

McCann UD, Agras WS: Successful treatment of compulsive binge-eating with desipramine: a double-blind placebo-controlled study. Am J Psychiatry 147:1509–1513, 1990

McElroy SL, Casuto LS, Nelson EB, et al: Placebo-controlled trial of sertraline in the treatment of binge eating disorder. Am J Psychiatry 157:1004–1006, 2000

McElroy SL, Kotwal R, Guerdjikova A, et al: Zonisamide in the treatment of binge eating disorder with obesity: a randomized controlled trial. J Clin Psychiatry 67:1897–1906, 2006

McElroy SL, Hudson JI, Capece JA, et al: Topiramate for the treatment of binge eating disorder associated with obesity: a placebo-controlled study. Biol Psychiatry 61:1039–1048, 2007

Milano W, Siano C, Putrella C, et al: Treatment of bulimia nervosa with fluvoxamine: a randomized controlled trial. Adv Ther 22:278–283, 2005

Mitchell JE, Pyle RL, Eckert ED, et al: A comparison study of antidepressants and structured intensive group psychotherapy in the treatment of bulimia nervosa. Arch Gen Psychiatry 47:149–160, 1990

Monteleone P, Santonastaso P, Tortorella A, et al: Serotonin transporter polymorphism and potential response to SSRIs in bulimia. Mol Psychiatry 10:716–718, 2005

Newman-Toker J: Risperidone in anorexia nervosa. J Am Acad Child Adolesc Psychiatry 39:941–942, 2000

Nickel C, Tritt K, Muehlbacher M, et al: Topiramate treatment in bulimia nervosa patients: a randomized, double-blind, placebo-controlled trial. Int J Eat Disord 38:295–300, 2005

Pope HG, Hudson JI: Treatment of bulimia with antidepressants. Psychopharmacology (Berl) 78:176–179, 1982

Pope HG, Hudson JI, Jonas JM, et al: Bulimia treated with imipramine: a placebo-controlled double-blind study. Am J Psychiatry 140:554–558, 1983

Pope HG, Hudson JI, Jonas JM, et al: Antidepressant treatment of bulimia: a two-year follow-up study. J Clin Psychopharmacol 5:320–327, 1985

Pope HG, Keck PE, McElroy SL, et al: A placebo-controlled study of trazodone in bulimia nervosa. J Clin Psychopharmacol 9:254–259, 1989

Pyle RL, Mitchell JE, Eckert ED, et al: Maintenance treatment and 6-month outcome for bulimic patients who respond to initial treatment. Am J Psychiatry 147:871–875, 1990

Romano SJ, Halmi KA, Sarka NP, et al: A placebo-controlled study of fluoxetine in continued treatment of bulimia nervosa after successful acute fluoxetine treatment. Am J Psychiatry 159:96–102, 2002

Shapira NA, Goldsmith TD, McElroy SL: Treatment of binge-eating disorder with topiramate: a clinical case series. J Clin Psychiatry 61:368–372, 2000

Silveira RO, Zanatto V, Appolinario JC, et al: An open trial of reboxetine in obese patients with binge eating disorder. Eat Weight Disord 10:e93–e96, 2005

Spitzer RL, Yanovski S, Wadden T, et al: Binge eating disorder: its further validation in a multisite study. Int J Eat Disord 13:137–153, 1993

Telch CF, Agras WS, Rossiter EM: Binge-eating increases with increasing adiposity. Int J Eat Disord 7:115–119, 1988

Vandereycken W: Neuroleptics in the short-term treatment of anorexia nervosa: a double-blind placebo-controlled study with sulpiride. Br J Psychiatry 144:288–292, 1984

Vandereycken W, Pierloot R: Pimozide combined with behavior therapy in the short-term treatment of anorexia nervosa: a double-blind placebo-controlled cross over study. Acta Psychiatr Scand 66:445–450, 1982

Walsh BT, Stewart JW, Wright L, et al: Treatment of bulimia with monoamine oxidase inhibitors. Am J Psychiatry 139:1629–1630, 1982

Walsh BT, Gladis M, Roose SP, et al: Phenelzine vs placebo in 50 patients with bulimia. Arch Gen Psychiatry 45:471–475, 1988

Walsh BT, Hadigan CM, Devlin MJ, et al: Long-term outcome of antidepressant treatment for bulimia nervosa. Am J Psychiatry 148:1206–1212, 1991

Walsh BT, Wilson GT, Loeb KL, et al: Medication and psychotherapy in the treatment of bulimia nervosa. Am J Psychiatry 154:523–531, 1997

Walsh BT, Agras WS, Devlin MJ, et al: Fluoxetine for bulimia nervosa following poor response to psychotherapy. Am J Psychiatry 157:1332–1334, 2000

Walsh BT, Kaplan AS, Attia E, et al: Fluoxetine after weight restoration in anorexia nervosa: a randomized controlled trial. JAMA 295:2605–2612, 2006a

Walsh BT, Sysko R, Parides MK: Early response to desipramine among women with bulimia nervosa. Int J Eat Disord 39:72–75, 2006b

Yanovski SZ, Nelson JE, Dubbert BK, et al: Association of binge-eating disorder and psychiatric comorbidity in the obese. Am J Psychiatry 150:1472–1479, 1992

CHAPTER 60

Treatment of Insomnia

Martin Reite, M.D.

Our conceptualization of insomnia has undergone a dramatic shift during the past few years, from an annoying but not particularly serious symptom to the recognition that 1) sleep loss from any cause has serious consequences, 2) chronic insomnia and the impaired sleep it represents are highly comorbid with (or indeed may cause) many other medical and psychiatric disorders, and 3) chronic insomnia in some cases may represent a separate medical disorder in itself, with an independent neurobiological basis. It has been suggested that certain chronic insomnias be considered on a par with depression as a serious disorder with a tendency toward chronicity whose treatment needs independent assessment and possibly long-term management (Jindal et al. 2004). This increase in complexity is in part offset by improved treatment options, both pharmacological and nonpharmacological. This chapter will review these areas in what we hope is a clinically useful manner.

Morbidity of Insomnia and Consequences of Sleep Loss

The 2005 National Institutes of Health (NIH) Consensus Conference on Chronic Insomnia in Adults estimated that 30% of the general population has symptoms or complaints consistent with insomnia (http://consensus.nih.gov/2005/2005InsomniaSOS026html.htm). The symptoms of insomnia may include complaints of not being able to get to sleep, not being able to stay asleep, waking too early, or sleep that is not refreshing—and often a combination of the foregoing. Individuals with insomnia report diminished quality of life, including impaired con-

centration and memory, decreased ability to accomplish daily tasks, decreased ability to accomplish daily tasks, and decreased ability to enjoy interpersonal relationships (Ancoli-Israel and Roth 1999). Untreated insomnia is associated with increases in new-onset anxiety and depression, increased daytime sleepiness, and increased health-related concerns (Richardson 2000), as well as increased use of health-related services (Novak et al. 2004). Patients with primary insomnia demonstrate impaired memory consolidation during sleep (Backhaus et al. 2006), and recent evidence suggests they may have diminished hippocampal volumes (Riemann et al. 2007).

New data on the effects of sleep loss in otherwise healthy adults affirm the importance of adequate sleep. Going without sleep for 17–21 hours, not uncommon in many occupations and life situations, may lead to psychomotor performance decrements similar to those seen with legal alcohol intoxication (Dawson and Reid 1997), which may not be apparent to the individual concerned. Going without sleep for a single night following a hepatitis A immunization may lead to a 50% reduction in hepatitis A antibody formation a month later (Lange et al. 2003). Relatively mild sleep loss may result in significant decline in cognitive performance, and sleep restriction to 4 hours per night for 2 nights in healthy males has been shown to decrease leptin and increase ghrelin production, with potentially adverse effects on the potential to develop obesity (Spiegel et al. 2004). Both short-term total and partial sleep deprivation have been shown to increase C reactive protein levels in otherwise healthy adults (Meier-Ewert et al. 2004). Although an insomnia complaint is not isomorphic with sleep deprivation, individuals with insomnia have been shown to get less sleep and therefore are at greater risk for the adverse events accompanying sleep deprivation. Data are emerging suggesting a relationship between sleep loss and the development of both insulin resistance and the individual components of the metabolic syndrome (Wolk and Somers 2007), an issue of special concern in an American population thought to be generally mildly sleep deprived and in which obesity and type 2 diabetes are serious public health issues.

We now recognize that the insomnia complaint may reflect dysfunction of several underlying neurobiological systems supporting sleep, including the homeostatic Process S and circadian Process C systems, as well as influences from comorbid medical and/or psychiatric conditions and the effects of environmental stress and poor sleep habits. Quite often, several of these factors interact to produce the insomnia-based symptom complex that patients present with, a circumstance that serves to highlight the importance of accurate and comprehensive differential diagnosis of an insomnia complaint before embarking on treatment.

This chapter advances the position that most patients with insomnia complaints can be helped if sufficient attention is paid to accurate differential diagnosis, with recognition and appropriate treatment of their underlying pathologies contributing to their complaints.

Sleep Architecture

Sleep architecture refers to the characteristic scalp electroencephalogram (EEG) patterns that characterize the different waking and sleep states (wakefulness, rapid eye movement [REM] sleep) and non-REM sleep stages (1 through 4). EEG rhythms are defined primarily by their frequency in cycles per second (termed Hertz [Hz]), with the major frequency bands being delta (<4 Hz), theta (>4 to <8 Hz), alpha (~8 to ~12 Hz), beta (~13 to ~20 Hz), and gamma (>20 Hz). Sometimes 12- to 14-Hz "sleep spindle" activity is termed *sigma* activity.

Wakefulness is normally accompanied by what is termed a "low-voltage, fast" scalp-recorded EEG, with frequencies usually greater than 8 Hz and amplitudes in the vicinity of 50 μV or less. The most prominent EEG rhythm of quiet, relaxed wakefulness is the so-called alpha rhythm, seen over the top and back of the head (visual receptive regions) when the eyes are closed. Alpha rhythm consists of rhythmical 8- to 12-Hz activity, usually about 50 μV in amplitude.

The transition from wakefulness to sleep—normally stage 1 non-REM sleep—is indicated by the appearance in the EEG of slower 5- to 7-Hz theta activity of generally low voltage. The subject is not responsive at this point but can be easily aroused. stage 1 sleep usually constitutes only about 5%–7% of total sleep time.

After a few minutes, the typical subject transitions into stage 2 sleep, characterized by further slowing of the EEG and the appearance of sleep spindles and K complexes. Spindles are short (usually <1 second) bursts of 12- to 14-Hz activity dominant over high central regions that wax and wane in amplitude—hence the term *spindle*.

Stage 3 and stage 4 sleep usually follow stage 2 and are characterized by increased slowing and increased amplitude of the EEG. Stage 3 sleep contains between 20% and 50% of high-voltage (>75 mV) slow (<2 Hz) delta activity, and stage 4 sleep contains >50% slow delta activity. Stage 3 and stage 4 sleep are often grouped together and termed *delta sleep* or slow-wave sleep (SWS). Stage 3 and 4 sleep constitute about 20%–25% of sleep time in adults, but that percentage is higher in adolescents and lower in healthy elderly individuals as well as in many pathological conditions, including depression, schizophrenia, and many insomnia disorders. Older individuals may have slow-wave delta activity, but it is not of sufficient amplitude (75 μV) to be formally scored as stage 3 or 4.

After the typical adult has been asleep (in non-REM sleep) for about 90 minutes, the EEG transitions to a lower-voltage, faster pattern. The subject remains asleep, but the eyes can now be seen rapidly moving beneath the closed lids. Consequently, this stage of sleep is called rapid eye movement or REM sleep. If awakened during this stage, the subject will often report dreaming. The time from sleep onset (i.e., stage 1) to the onset of the first REM period is termed *REM latency*, which has diagnostic implications. In some psychiatric disorders (e.g., major affective disorders, schizophrenia, and eating disorders), and occasionally in narcolepsy, REM latency is shorter than normal. REM latency tends to decrease with advancing age, but, as a rule of thumb, nocturnal REM latency of less than 60 minutes in an adult should be considered unusually short and might suggest a major affective disorder. REM sleep usually constitutes about 20% of total sleep time in adults.

Until very recently, conventional EEG sleep scoring was still largely based on the sleep atlas of Rechtschaffen and Kales (1968), which dates from the time that sleep records were recorded on paper EEG machines, usually run at a speed of 10–30 mm/second, and included only those EEG frequencies easily visible to the naked eye (very low [<0.5 Hz] and very high [>50 Hz] frequencies were usually not recorded). We can probably expect some significant revisions in scoring techniques in the near future based on availability of computerized EEG recording and analytical techniques. Altered sleep morphology not captured by conventional scoring includes the presence of "cyclic alternating patterns" that appear during sleep and may be associated with daytime fatigue (Guilleminault et al. 2006), computer quantification of slow-wave activity indexing sleep drive and/or quality (Armitage et al. 2007), and the presence of very-high-frequency (gamma-band) EEG activity (Perlis et al. 2001a, 2001b). Such issues have begun to be addressed in "The AASM Manual for the Scoring of Sleep and Associated Events: Rules, Terminology and Technical Specification," recently published by the American Academy of Sleep Medicine (2007).

Sleep Physiology as It Relates to Insomnia

It is necessary to have a basic understanding of the neurobiological mechanisms underlying sleep if we are to understand insomnia.

Perhaps the most basic issue is that there are fundamentally two quite different types of sleep, non-REM and REM, each with its own neuroanatomy, physiology, function, developmental course across the life span, and pathologies. These differences are summarized in Table 60–1.

At any single point in time, the brain will usually be in only a single "state"—that is, either awake, in non-REM sleep, or in REM sleep. Admixtures of state, however, are possible and usually present as unusual sleep pathologies. For example, "sleep paralysis" and cataplexy are admixtures of REM sleep and awake. Sleepwalking is an admixture of partial (motor—not conscious) arousal and non-REM sleep. The major indicator of what state we are in is the type of EEG patterns and related physiological and behavioral activity present at the moment.

A second basic issue is that we usually conceptualize sleep as reflecting the balance of two fundamental processes—Process S, a homeostatic process in which the tendency to go into non-REM sleep is increased by previous time awake, and Process C, a circadian arousal process that tends to offset Process S so that we don't go to sleep until we are ready to—that is, when 1) Process S has built up and 2) the Process C arousal tendency begins to decrease.

These different types of sleep and control processes should become clearer as we outline them in the following sections.

Wakefulness, Non-REM Sleep, and the Biology of Process S

The neuronal systems that regulate our daily cycle of sleep and wakefulness, while quite complex, are becoming better defined. Discovery of the ascending reticular activating system (ARAS), a wakefulness-promoting neurophysiological circuit that originates in the lower and more central parts of the brain, was based in part on von Economo's observations of brain pathology in individuals who died of the epidemic of sleeping sickness or encephalitis lethargica that was seen in Europe and the United States in the early twentieth century. Mediated through two major pathways, one to the thalamus and a second more direct one to the hypothalamus and cortex, these cell groups when active promote wakefulness. The ARAS depends significantly on acetylcholine and monoamines, as well as other neuropeptide neurotransmitter systems.

TABLE 60–1. Characteristics of non-REM and REM sleep

	NON-REM SLEEP	REM SLEEP
Neuroanatomy	Basal forebrain, VLPO neurons	Pontine tegmentum
Physiology	↓HR, ↓RR, ↓BP, ↓BT, ↓EMG	↕HR, ↕RR, ↕BP, poikilothermic, ↓↓↓EMG
Control mechanism	Process S and Process C	Independent pontine oscillator
Developmental course across life span	Appears during first year, ↑ in early adolescence, then stabilizes in adulthood	High at birth, decreases by age 6 years to adult levels
Function	Neurometabolic restoration, synaptic pruning	Early mammalian brain development
Pathologies	Insomnia, parasomnias, hypersomnias	Nightmares, RBD, narcolepsy

Note. ↑=increased; ↓=decreased; ↓↓↓=very greatly decreased; ↕ =highly variable.
BP=blood pressure; BT=body temperature; EMG=electromyograph; HR=heart rate; REM=rapid eye movement; RBD=REM sleep behavior disorder; RR=respiratory rate; VLPO=ventrolateral preoptic area.

A second set of competing systems located primarily in hypothalamic and contiguous regions, and emphasizing neuronal activity in the ventrolateral preoptic (VLPO) region of the hypothalamus, promotes non-REM or slow-wave sleep and inhibits wakefulness. These neuronal systems depend significantly on the inhibitory neurotransmitters galanin and γ-aminobutyric acid (GABA) (which most hypnotics are thought to modulate). Cells in the VLPO system appear to be activated by a buildup of adenosine secondary to duration of preceding wakefulness (Basheer et al. 2004). The longer a person has been awake, the more likely it is that sleep will be triggered, and the adenosine antagonist caffeine tends to prolong wakefulness.

Although the ARAS and the VLPO system are competing (increased activity in one decreases activity in the other), normally only one system at a time is predominant, for as a rule we are either awake or asleep and spend relatively little time in intermediate (and biologically less useful states) states. This suggests from an engineering view a type of biological flip-flop switch. Recent research indicates that such a switch may indeed exist, mediated by the lateral hypothalamic neuropeptides orexin and hypocretin, serving the function of a stabilizing system to keep the brain in either a wakeful or sleep state and preventing rapid oscillation from one state to the other (Saper et al. 2005). The role of orexin in modulating the sleep–wake system is not yet well understood, although preliminary animal studies suggest orexin antagonists induce sleep in animals and humans (Brisbare-Roch et al. 2007).

The REM State

REM sleep constitutes the third major physiological state (wakefulness and slow-wave sleep being the others), with neuronal generating and control systems essentially independent of wakefulness and non-REM or slow-wave sleep. The REM state is uniquely different from either wakefulness or slow-wave sleep, may include elements of both, yet may be independent of both.

Brain stem neuronal systems that have independent oscillation frequencies appear to account for the periodic generation of the REM state in all mammals, including humans. These systems largely reside in the pontine tegmentum and may constitute a separate component of the ARAS. The periods of these independent oscillations appear to be a function of body size, being approximately 2 hours in elephants, 90 minutes in humans, 60 minutes in Old World monkeys, 30 minutes in cats, 12 minutes in rats, and 6 minutes in mice. Cholinergic systems appear

involved in activating REM states, and monoamines in suppressing them. Agents that increase acetylcholine (ACh) activity, such as the acetylcholinesterase inhibitor physostigmine, increase REM sleep, and agents that increase monoamine activity, such as monoamine oxidase–inhibiting antidepressants, decrease REM sleep. It has recently been suggested that a type of neurophysiological toggle switch also exists for controlling transitions into and out of the REM state, consisting of mutually inhibitory neuronal populations that are GABA-ergic in nature, with independent pathways mediating EEG and atonia effects (Lu et al. 2006). This switch is thought to be subsidiary to the putative wake–sleep toggle switch, preventing transitions into REM during wakefulness, absent pathologies such as narcolepsy, which is thought to involve a weakened wake side of the wake–sleep switch due to loss of orexin neurons. Such a model would help explain a number of disorders in which impaired REM regulation is seen.

Process C: Circadian Physiology and Sleep

A second major neurobiological system controlling the timing of sleep is termed Process C (for circadian).

Like most living organisms, humans have prominent daily, or circadian, biological rhythms, which have important implications for normal sleep regulation and sleep disorders. The body's major circadian oscillator is located in the suprachiasmatic nucleus (SCN) of the hypothalamus. The SCN can oscillate independently, and animal studies suggest that separate genes control the phase, period, and amplitude of its oscillations. Recent studies have linked specific human circadian clock genes to circadian-based sleep disorders (Hamet and Tremblay 2006). The SCN controls many biological rhythms, including those of body temperature, various hormones, and the sleep–wake cycle, or perhaps more precisely the circadian alerting tendency, which is here termed Process C. This rhythm appears coupled to the temperature rhythm, with higher body temperatures being associated with an increased tendency to wakefulness, and vice versa.

The normal sleep–wake rhythm is a 24-hour rhythm that is usually synchronized to the circadian temperature and cortisol rhythm. The sleep–wake rhythm may become desynchronized when the sleep–wake schedule is abruptly changed (as occurs with a rapid time zone shift), during which the circadian oscillator initially remains on its original schedule. This desynchrony between the attempted sleep–wake schedule in the new time zone and the underlying circadian rhythm is one cause of "jet lag."

Human subjects who live in caves or other dimly lit, time cue–free environments will typically adopt a sleep–wake rhythm of approximately 24.2 hours (Czeisler et al. 1999). This suggests that the normal free-running circadian period is slightly longer than 24 hours and must be "phase advanced" about 12 minutes each day to stay in synchrony with the 24-hour rhythm of the sun. Overall, it appears easier to phase-delay than to phase-advance the body's rhythms, since a phase delay is going in the "direction" of a free-running rhythm. This has practical implications in the adaptation to a new time zone. A phase delay, as in East-to-West travel (with a later bedtime), is generally easier and more quickly adjusted to than a phase advance, such as when going West to East (with an earlier bedtime).

Light is a major synchronizer of circadian rhythms, and it has become apparent that, as in most other organisms, circadian rhythms in humans can be reset by appropriately timed exposure to bright light (Czeisler et al. 1986). Recent evidence suggests that short-wavelength light (shifted toward the blue end of the spectrum; wavelength ~460 nm) is more effective at modulating the activity of the SCN compared to longer-wavelength light (Lockley et al. 2006). The phase–response curve (PRC) plots how the timing of light exposure affects circadian rhythm timing. The human PRC suggests that exposure to bright light immediately before or shortly after onset of the sleep period (i.e., typically in the late evening) will tend to delay the circadian system, whereas exposure late in the sleep period, shortly before or after awakening (i.e., early morning), will tend to advance the circadian system. Light sensitivity may be related to the time of the lowest body temperature (the "nadir" of the body temperature circadian rhythm), with light exposure just prior to the body temperature nadir phase delaying the circadian rhythms and light exposure just after the nadir phase advancing the circadian rhythms. The human PRC provides useful information for timing the use of bright-light exposure as a therapeutic modality for treatment of jet lag or circadian rhythm disorders resulting from shift work.

The hormone melatonin, secreted by the pineal gland at night, appears to influence circadian rhythms. Its secretion is regulated by light information relayed to the pineal gland from the SCN. Melatonin secretion can be blocked by exposure to bright light during normally dark times. There is emerging evidence that melatonin can be used to reset the circadian system, to treat circadian rhythm disorders, and possibly to treat jet lag and work shift change (Brzezinski 1997), although it generally does not work well as a hypnotic agent. Although the therapeutic use of melatonin is receiving considerable media attention, it has been classified as a food supplement and is available over the counter.

The take-away point here is that both Process S and Process C have specific biological underpinnings, and pathologies in either or both can result in disturbed sleep and complaints of insomnia. Part of the differential diagnosis of insomnia is attempting to separate the two systems in terms of their independent contribution to the complaint, as this impacts treatment.

Functions of Sleep

Sleep is a function of the brain and is thought to support proper brain function. Emerging data clearly suggest sleep has a major role in both memory consolidation and brain (synaptic) plasticity (Walker and Stickgold 2006). Sleep spindle activity has been related specifically to improved memory recall performance (Clemens et al. 2005; Schabus et al. 2004), and very localized increases in very slow delta activity during sleep has been related to performance improvement in sleep-dependent learning of motor tasks, supporting its role in synaptic "pruning and tuning" (Huber et al. 2004).

Sleep is likely intimately related to regulation of overall energy metabolism as well, as suggested by the effect of mild sleep restriction on changes in leptin (decreases) and ghrelin (increases) production (Spiegel et al. 2004). Both sleep restriction and excessive sleep have been reported as risk factors in the development of insulin resistance and type 2 diabetes (Yaggi et al. 2006), and it has been postulated that chronic sleep loss may be a risk factor for obesity and insulin resistance, as well as type 2 diabetes (Chaput et al. 2008; Gangwisch et al. 2007; Spiegel et al. 2005).

The role of REM sleep in adult animals remains to be clearly defined, but its role in the development of the immature mammalian brain seems apparent, specific mechanisms notwithstanding. Human newborns have about 50% REM sleep, and human premature infants 80%. Newborn infants of altricial mammals like rats and cats have greater percentages of REM sleep than adult animals, while newborn infants of precocial animals like guinea pigs have lower adultlike levels of REM sleep at birth. It has been suggested that the periodic ascending brain activation associated with REM sleep may be important in developing species-appropriate neuronal pathways in the developing brain. Its role in adult animals has been postulated as involving learning and memory functions, but studies to date are inconclusive in this regard.

The Insomnia Complaint

The duration of an insomnia complaint has a major impact on its differential diagnosis and treatment. Transient and short-term insomnias are usually stress- or environmentally related, and the cause is obvious. Although they rarely come to the attention of health care providers, their treatment is also generally straightforward, and they should, as a rule, be treated when found to prevent them from becoming more chronic. The chronic insomnia complaint requires a more systematic differential diagnosis procedure, also fortunately usually fairly straightforward. We first consider the transient and short-term complaint and then move on to a discussion of the chronic insomnia complaint.

Transient and Short-Term Insomnias

Transient (several days) and short-term (several weeks) insomnias are quite common. Most individuals experience short-term trouble with sleep latency or sleep maintenance at times of stress, excitement, or anticipation; during an illness; after going to high altitudes; or accompanying sleep time changes (e.g., shift work, jet lag). Such problems rarely come to the attention of the clinician in the early stages, although, of course, clinicians will experience these problems themselves. Symptoms of insomnias can nonetheless be decreased, and daytime functioning improved, if certain guidelines are followed. Stress-related insomnia, or temporary trouble sleeping in response to excitement or worry (e.g., anticipating a trip or a forthcoming interview or examination), may appropriately be treated with a night or two of a short-half-life hypnotic agent (e.g., zolpidem 5 or 10 mg at bedtime). This medication need not necessarily be taken in anticipation of trouble sleeping; it can be placed at the bedside and taken only after the patient has been unable to fall asleep for 30–60 minutes, because it has a rapid onset and relatively short duration of action. Awakening in the middle of the night with inability to fall asleep again can be treated with zaleplon 10 mg (half-life approximately 1 hour), as long as at least 4 hours are still available for sleep.

Short-term insomnias are due to more serious and prolonged stressful situations and may last up to several weeks. The concern is that, if not treated, a conditioned or learned insomnia may develop in response to concerns about not being able to go to sleep that can result in a more chronic insomnia.

The appropriate treatment of transient and short-term insomnia not only improves daytime performance but also may prevent the insomnia from developing into a chronic problem. There is no reason that responsible patients who know they are susceptible to transient insomnia in relation to predictable stressful events cannot have a hypnotic agent available to use prophylactically. Bereavement is often associated with a short-term insomnia, which has been reported to respond favorably to sedative tricyclic agents (Pasternak et al. 1991).

Altitude-Related Insomnia

Altitude-related insomnia may occur when individuals rapidly travel to higher altitudes, such as skiing and mountain climbing trips. High-altitude insomnia results primarily from periodic breathing with increases in sleep-related central apneas and hypopneas, which can be diminished by several days' administration of acetazolamide (125 mg once or twice a day). Acetazolamide also appears to decrease risk of developing altitude sickness. A short-acting hypnotic may also be useful for several nights. It has been demonstrated that both zaleplon (10 g) and zolpidem (10 mg) improve sleep quality at altitude without adverse effects on respiration, attention, alertness, or mood (Beaumont et al. 2007). Altitude-related insomnia normally improves spontaneously after several days, at least at altitudes below 15,000 feet. Altitude-related sleep problems can also be seen in infants but normally resolve spontaneously without specific treatment after the first night (Yaron et al. 2004).

Shift Work– and Jet Lag–Related Insomnia

Attempts to sleep at times substantially different from what one is accustomed to, commonly associated with long-distance travel (jet lag) or shift work, often result in disrupted sleep and insomnia complaints. In both cases sleep is being attempted when the Process C system may be in the high arousal state, and wakefulness may be necessary when the Process C is in the low arousal state. In both shift work– and jet lag–related insomnia, there can be significant problems with both sleep and wakefulness.

Shift work is the more serious of the two since it is often prolonged and is known to be associated with health and performance impairments. More than 6 million Americans work night shifts on a regular or rotating basis, and shift work sleep disorder is common in this group, with increased incidence of gastrointestinal and cardiovascular disorders and impaired family and social functioning, as well as an increased risk of accidents (Schwartz and Roth 2006). When working shifts is necessary, efforts must be made to preserve sleep as much as possible as well as to maintain wakefulness during the work period. Such efforts can be both pharmacological and behavioral. Modafinil (200 mg) has been shown to help maintain wakefulness during work hours, but because it has a relatively long half-life (~12–15 hours), it should be taken early so as not to interfere with later sleep. The use of hypnotics to improve sleep during the sleep period must be considered in terms of the risk–benefit ratio. Bright light early during the work period, with protection from bright light late in the work period and on the way home in the morning, can help with subsequent sleep (Schwartz and Roth 2006).

Jet lag also involves travel-related rapid time zone changes such that waking activities are required during the circadian sleep time and sleep is required during the circadian wake time. Symptoms are due both to this circadian desynchrony and sleep loss. Paying proper attention to light exposure following transoceanic travel and remembering that initially the circadian system responds to light as though it is still on the time zone one departed from can facilitate rapid entrainment to the new light–dark schedule. Protection of sleep with short-acting hypnotic agents during the new sleep periods for the first few nights can be helpful, as is appropriate supplemental melatonin administration (Cardinali et al. 2006).

Chronic Insomnia

Chronic insomnia is of greater concern than short-term insomnia, as it is both common (the National Sleep Foundation estimates that 10%–15% of adults experience chronic insomnia) and results in substantial adverse effects on health, quality of life, and overall function, as reviewed by Krystal (2007). Chronic insomnia in adults is a risk factor for the development of anxiety and depression (Neckelmann et al. 2007; Richardson 2000). Chronic insomnia in adolescents is a risk factor for development of early adult depression and substance abuse (Roane and Taylor 2008). Chronic insomnia should be viewed not just as a sleep problem but also as a problem affecting the individual 24 hours a day.

Differential Diagnosis of the Chronic Insomnia Complaint: A Six-Step Decision Process

The differential diagnosis and effective treatment of chronic insomnia can challenge the most skilled clinician. With chronic insomnias, unlike transient and short-term insomnias, the primary cause is rarely immediately

apparent, and the likelihood of more than one cause is high. Accurate diagnosis is important because different causes of insomnia can present in a similar fashion, and the appropriate treatment for one may aggravate another. Failure to systematically pursue a complete differential diagnosis may yield misdiagnoses, treatment failures, and dissatisfied patients. Most patients with chronic insomnia present with a straightforward complaint of insomnia; however, it is important to realize that a substantial disturbance in nocturnal sleep can present as complaints of chronic fatigue, impaired daytime performance, and excessive daytime sleepiness (EDS), which raises the question of a possible excessive sleep disorder. A careful history should identify such patients so that a more appropriate inquiry into nocturnal sleep habits and patterns can be undertaken. Similarly, a large variety of medical and psychiatric disorders (and sometimes their treatments) are accompanied by insomnia complaints.

First in order in any patient is a *detailed sleep history*, which will include the type of insomnia problem (sleep onset, sleep maintenance, early awakening), when it began (childhood, recently, at time of major stress or life event), when it occurs (every night, weeknights only, at times of stress), what has been done when and by whom, previous response to treatment, how the insomnia affects daytime functioning, and similar issues. Family history is important since there are substantial genetic contributions both to basic sleep control mechanisms and to sleep pathologies (Hamet and Tremblay 2006). Development of atypical sleep-related habits counter to those of good sleep hygiene should be inquired about. A sleep diary kept for 1–2 weeks may be helpful in establishing the type, perceived severity, and periodicity of the insomnia.

For this group of insomnias, the clinician should first establish that the patient has a true insomnia and is not just a typical short sleeper. Short sleepers, although not common, do exist and may get along fine on 4–5 hours of sleep a night. They do not complain of EDS or fatigue, and usually they have no sleep complaints. Their families, however, see the patient up until midnight and then out of bed again at 4:00 A.M. and assume that he or she has a sleep problem and convince him or her to seek professional help. Such individuals need no specific treatment, although an explanation is helpful for family members.

It is also important to decide whether the insomnia reflects a problem with non-REM or slow-wave sleep (more often) or REM sleep (less often). REM sleep–related insomnia complaints can result from frequent awakenings from frightening dreams or nightmares or from REM sleep behavior disorder (RBD). RBD is most often seen in older males and results from failure of proper skeletal muscle inhibition during REM such that patients can act out their dreams, often resulting in very disturbed sleep. Memory of dream content during the episode suggests RBD, which can be confirmed by polysomnography (Schenck and Mahowald 2005).

With this information on hand, the differential diagnosis is facilitated by a systematic approach such as that outlined in the schematic decision tree in Figure 60–1.

Step 1—Medical Conditions Affecting Sleep

Medical conditions, as well as the pharmacological treatments of medical conditions, can result in insomnia complaints. The endocrinopathies are notorious for being associated with sleep-related complaints, as are conditions associated with chronic pain, breathing difficulties, cardiac arrhythmias, arthritis, renal failure, and central nervous system (CNS) disorders, especially the dementias. Evaluation may include a complete medical history and, if appropriate, a physical examination with relevant laboratory tests. Keep in mind the fact that the incidence of medical disorders accompanied by sleep complaints increases with age. Some of the more common medical disorders associated with impaired sleep are listed in Table 60–2.

Sleep-related breathing disorders are frequently associated with insomnia complaints. Obstructive and mixed apneas are usually accompanied by other symptoms, such as snoring, excessive daytime sleepiness, and possibly cognitive problems. Central apnea is an occasional, albeit uncommon, cause of chronic insomnia, especially in older patients and at higher altitudes. The clinician should inquire whether the patient has had any subjective sense of trouble getting his or her breath or feeling like his or her breathing is interfered with, especially during the transition from wakefulness to sleep. Also ask the bed partner whether the patient has irregular breathing or pauses in his or her breathing during sleep. Snoring may be another clue (although it is more likely related to an obstructive component). Frequent apneas cause sleep fragmentation, which results in insomnia complaints and often complaints of increased daytime sleepiness (Bonnet and Arand 1997). Central sleep apnea is frequently associated with medical and neurological disorders (Thalhofer and Dorow 1997), but it may also occur in otherwise healthy individuals. It is more frequently encountered in older individuals (Ancoli-Israel et al. 1997). Both oxygen and continuous positive airway pressure (CPAP) can be used in the treatment of central apnea in patients with medical disorders (Franklin et al. 1997; Granton et al. 1996). The pharmacological treatment of central sleep apnea is less than optimal. Therapeutic options might include protriptyline (5–20 mg at bedtime), fluoxetine (10–20 mg/day), or theophylline (300–600 mg/day) (Ancoli-Israel et al. 1997), although their efficacy has yet to be clearly established in well-controlled studies.

Step 1. Do history and physical suggest a medical disorder?	Yes ⇨	Evaluate medical condition as a possible cause of insomnia
Next ⇩		
Step 2. Is there evidence of significant anxiety, panic attacks, depression, or other psychiatric symptoms?	Yes ⇨	Evaluate possible insomnia related to psychiatric disorder
Next ⇩		
Step 3. Does patient use sedative-hypnotics, alcohol, or drugs of abuse regularly or to excess?	Yes ⇨	Evaluate possible substance-related insomnia
Next ⇩		
Step 4. Is sleep per se normal, but it occurs at the wrong time?	Yes ⇨	Evaluate possible circadian rhythm disorder
Next ⇩		
Step 5. Does patient have evidence of kicking during sleep or uncomfortable feelings in legs?	Yes ⇨	Evaluate possible periodic limb movements of sleep or restless legs syndrome
Next ⇩		
Step 6. Does patient respond to treatment for conditioned or primary insomnia?	Yes ⇨	Probable conditioned or primary insomnia or sleep state misperception syndrome
No ⇩		
Consider referral to sleep disorder center		

FIGURE 60–1. Differential diagnosis decision tree for chronic insomnia.

Note. SMSS = sleep state misperception syndrome.

Also, a number of prescription drugs may result in insomnia complaints (prescription drug use also tends to increase with age). Commonly used medications that can produce insomnia complaints in some patients are listed in Table 60–3.

TABLE 60–2. Medical conditions commonly associated with impaired sleep

Cardiovascular disorders

   Angina

   Congestive heart failure

   Ischemic heart disease

Pulmonary disorders

   Chronic obstructive pulmonary disease

   Cystic fibrosis

   Asthma

   Sleep apnea

   Dyspnea from any cause

Neurological disorders

   Dementias

   Parkinson's disease

   Central nervous system degenerative disorders

   Traumatic brain injury

   Central nervous system neoplasms

Endocrinological disorders

   Hyperthyroidism

   Hypothyroidism

   Cushing's syndrome

   Addison's disease

Gastrointestinal disorders

   Gastroesophageal reflux

   Peptic ulcer disease

Genitourinary disorders

   Nocturia

   Renal failure

Immunological and rheumatic disorders

   Rheumatoid arthritis

   Osteoarthritis

   Fibromyalgia

Pain and fever from any cause

Metabolic disorders such as diabetes

TABLE 60–3. Commonly used drugs with insomnia as a side effect

β-Blockers

Corticosteriods

Adrenocorticotropic hormone

Monoamine oxidase inhibitors

Phenytoin

Calcium channel blockers

α-Methyldopa

Bronchodilators

Stimulating tricyclics

Stimulants

Some selective serotonin reuptake inhibitors

Thyroid hormones

Oral contraceptives

Antimetabolites

Some decongestants

Thiazides

No specific sleep abnormalities are usually associated with most medical disorders other than usually a decrease in total sleep, an increase in awakenings, and perhaps decreases in REM sleep. Fibromyalgia and chronic fatigue syndrome are very frequently associated with sleep complaints. On occasion, fibromyalgia is associated with an alpha–delta type of sleep abnormality, in which alpha frequency activity is accentuated in the slow-wave-sleep background, with a complaint of nonrestorative sleep. This pattern suggests a state of CNS hyperarousal. Sleep complaints are very common in chronic fatigue syndrome and can include insomnia, hypersomnia, nonrestorative sleep, and sleeping at the wrong time of the 24-hour period (circadian rhythm abnormalities). Conventional polysomnographic findings are generally nonspecific and include decreased sleep efficiency, decreased slow-wave sleep, increased sleep latency, and alpha–delta sleep EEG patterns (VanHoof et al. 2007). Chronic fatigue–related disturbances in regulation of underlying sleep control mechanisms are supported by several studies. One recent study found an increase in the cyclic alternating pattern in polysomnograms of chronic fatigue patients complaining of nonrestorative sleep (Guilleminault et al. 2006), and there is also evidence of decreased sleep drive (Process S) in chronic fatigue syndrome (Armitage et al. 2007).

Treatment of insomnia associated with medical conditions involves first isolating and appropriately treating the medical condition and then, if the insomnia complaint persists, evaluating the possibility of a separate additional sleep disorder. Conditioned insomnia can complicate insomnia complaints in this population, and it must be separately addressed (as outlined below). Similarly, it is quite possible for a patient with primary insomnia also to have a medical condition that further disrupts sleep. A study by Rybarczyk et al. (2005) indicated that cognitive-behavioral therapy (CBT) may be effective in older patients with insomnia comorbid with other medical conditions, such as osteoarthritis, coronary artery disease, or pulmonary disease, suggesting that CBT should be considered in these conditions.

Insomnia associated with acute medical conditions is appropriately treated with short-half-life hypnotic agents (e.g., zolpidem 5–10 mg, triazolam 0.125–0.25 mg, or eszopiclone 2–3 mg at bedtime) if no other contraindication to their use exists. Insomnia complaints associated with fibromyalgia and chronic fatigue syndrome are frequently resistant to treatment, although small doses of amitriptyline (10–50 mg at bedtime) or cyclobenzaprine (10 mg three times a day) have been reported to be helpful, and occasionally zolpidem (5–10 mg) will help with the associated insomnia complaints.

Scharf et al. (2003) reported that treatment with sodium oxybate (Zyrem) improved both sleep abnormalities and symptoms of pain and fatigue in patients with fibromyalgia. Edinger et al. (2005) found that CBT was effective in treating sleep complaints in patients with fibromyalgia. Modafinil has been reported to decrease daytime fatigue and sleepiness in fibromyalgia patients, but its impact on sleep has not yet been reported (Schaller and Behar 2001). If a medical disorder is suspected of causing or contributing to the sleep complaint, a change of or alterations in treatment that might improve sleep should be considered. It is important, however, to remember that the differential diagnosis of a chronic insomnia complaint does not stop here—the remainder of the differential diagnosis should be completed.

Dementing illnesses such as Alzheimer's disease are often associated with severe insomnia complaints that are quite disruptive to patients and families and often are the factors precipitating institutional care. Disease-associated neuropathological changes in the sleep and circadian rhythm control centers in the hypothalamus and SCN may contribute to these symptoms. Patients with Alzheimer's disease demonstrate phase delayed body temperature and activity rhythms, with delayed sleep onset, increased nocturnal activity, and fragmented sleep, likely related to disease-associated SCN lesions. Some evidence suggests that a melatonin deficiency may be present in some patients with Alzheimer's disease (Liu et al. 1999). Sleep is also disturbed in dementia with Lewy bodies (DLB), which has been found in up to 20% of dementia cases referred to autopsy (McKeith 2000); this disturbance is often in the realm of increased motor activity suggestive of an REM behavior disorder (Boeve et al. 1998; Ferman et al. 1999). Clearly, then, sleep and activity abnormalities associated with dementia may result

from very different pathophysiologies and thus might respond to different treatments. Until such specific treatments can be based on specific pathophysiology, we should adhere to optimal environmental circadian principles (quiet, dark nocturnal environment; bright, socially stimulating daytime environment). Possible supplementation with evening melatonin and additional morning bright light may prove useful, in addition to the appropriate use of sedative-hypnotic agents, with the proviso that CNS lesions may significantly impact the response to hypnotic agents. There is evidence that behavioral treatment methods may benefit some Alzheimer's patients (McCurry et al. 2004).

Step 2—Psychiatric Disorders

The presence of significant anxiety, dysphoric or cyclic mood, or frank depression with sleep complaints should alert the clinician to a possible *psychiatric-related insomnia*. Nocturnal panic attacks can result in insomnia complaints, even in individuals who do not have typical panic episodes during the day. Accordingly, the clinician should pay special attention to evidence of nocturnal arousals accompanied by autonomic symptoms such as tachycardia, rapid breathing, and the sense of anxiety or fearfulness. Insomnias related to psychiatric causes usually covary with the degree of psychiatric symptoms. The fear of not being able to get to sleep seen in patients with conditioned insomnia ("I can't turn off my thoughts") sometimes can be difficult to distinguish from anxiety, but treatments may differ (e.g., CBT for conditioned insomnia, anxiolytics for anxiety).

Psychiatric disorders, especially disorders associated with anxiety or depression, frequently include insomnia as an associated symptom. Chronic anxiety is not infrequently associated with sleep-onset insomnia or sleep-maintenance insomnia, whereas depression is not infrequently associated with early-morning awakening. These associations are not specific enough to be diagnostic, however, and a systematic psychiatric evaluation is necessary. Many depressive disorders appear to be accompanied by shortened REM latency, increased REM density during the first REM period of the night, and deficient slow-wave sleep. To date, however, such findings are not sufficiently specific to merit the cost of a polysomnogram.

Antidepressant agents, although effective for the patient's depression, may have significantly different effects on sleep—a possibility that is useful to bear in mind. Table 60–4 shows sleep-related effects of the major antidepressant groups.

TABLE 60–4. Overview of the effects of antidepressants on sleep

DRUG	CONTINUITY	SWS	REM SLEEP	SEDATION
TCAs				
Amitriptyline (Elavil)	↑↑↑	↑	↓↓↓	++++
Doxepin (Sinequan)	↑↑↑	↑↑	↓↓	++++
Imipramine (Tofranil)	↔↑	↑	↓↓	++
Nortriptyline (Pamelor)	↑	↑	↓↓	++
Desipramine (Norpramin)	↔	↑	↓↓	+
Clomipramine (Anafranil)	↑↔	↑	↓↓↓↓	±
MAOIs				
Phenelzine (Nardil)	↓	↔	↓↓↓↓	↔
Tranylcypromine (Parnate)	↓↓	↔	↓↓↓↓	↔
SSRIs				
Fluoxetine (Prozac)	↓	↔↓	↔↓	±
Paroxetine* (Paxil)	↓	↔↓	↓↓	±
Sertraline (Zoloft)	↔	↔	↓↓	↔
Citalopram (Celexa)	↓	↔	↓	↔
Fluvoxamine (Luvox)	↓	↔	↓	+
Others				
Bupropion (Wellbutrin)	↓↔	↔	↑	↔
Venlafaxine (Effexor)	↓	↔	↓↓	++
Trazodone (Desyrel)	↑↑↑	↔↑	↓	++++
Mirtazapine (Remeron)	↑↑	↔↑	↔↓	++++
Duloxetine (Cymbalta)	↔	↔	↓	↔

Note. ↑=increased; ↓=decreased; ↔=no change; +=slight effect; ++=small effect; +++=moderate effect; ++++=great effect; ±=no significant effect. EEG=electroencephalogram; MAOIs=monoamine oxidase inhibitors; REM=rapid eye movement; SSRIs=selective serotonin reuptake inhibitors; SWS=slow-wave sleep; TCAs=tricyclic antidepressants.
*When taken at bedtime, paroxetine potentially decreases sleep continuity less than other SSRIs.
Source. Adapted from Winoker A, Reynolds C: "Overview of Effects of Antidepressant Therapies on Sleep." *Primary Psychiatry* 1:22–27, 1994. Used with permission.

The choice of an antidepressant agent for a specific patient, all other things being equal, might well take into account the type of accompanying sleep complaint and the therapeutic effect on sleep desired. Typically, resolution of the depression will be accompanied by reduction in the sleep complaints. If, for a patient already complaining of insomnia, an antidepressant with a known high incidence of insomnia side effects is chosen, it may be useful to augment it with a hypnotic agent early in the course of treatment.

Treatment of insomnia associated with anxiety can incorporate a benzodiazepine with sedative-hypnotic properties with a sufficient bedtime dose to augment sleep. Many antianxiety agents, such as sedative tricyclics, have

sedative-hypnotic properties as well, which facilitate the management of the insomnia component. Panic attacks can occasionally arise exclusively from sleep (Rosenfeld and Furman 1994); treatment in such cases should probably follow conventional panic attack treatment strategies. Mirtazapine, an antidepressant with antianxiety properties (Anttila and Leinonen 2001), may be helpful in the management of some cases of anxiety with insomnia.

Bipolar disorder may be accompanied by prominent sleep disruption. Manic and hypomanic episodes may be accompanied by marked decreases in sleep, although not necessarily insomnia complaints. Sedative antidepressants have been shown to increase the risk of a shift to mania in treating insomnia complaints in bipolar depressed patients (Saiz-Ruiz et al. 1994), and the use of other hypnotic agents would therefore be more advisable in these patients. Milder cyclic mood disorders also may have associated insomnia complaints, which can be mistaken for a primary insomnia or a conditioned arousal insofar as the patients find it difficult to turn off their thinking at sleep onset or after awakening during the night. If these patients are questioned carefully, evidence of a cyclic mood component will suggest that treatment with a mood stabilizer might be appropriate for the chronic insomnia complaint in these patients.

Posttraumatic stress disorder (PTSD) is a psychiatric disorder in which sleep disturbances are a hallmark. Patients with PTSD may exhibit increased sleep latency, decreased sleep efficiency, recurrent traumatic dreams, and evidence of increased REM density (Mellman et al. 1997), as well as evidence of impaired skeletal muscle inhibition during REM sleep (Ross et al. 1994). Chronic nightmares in PTSD have been successfully treated with CBT (Davis and Wright 2007). Recent reviews suggest that a variety of medications may be useful for insomnia problems associated with PTSD, including the atypical antipsychotic olanzapine and the α_1-adrenoreceptor antagonist prazosin, and possibly serotonin 2 (5-HT$_2$) receptor antagonists (van Liempt et al. 2006), and residual insomnia in PTSD patients has been treated with CBT (Deviva et al. 2005). Overall, however, satisfactory treatment of sleep problems in PTSD remains elusive.

Step 3—Substance Misuse

A careful drug history will help to identify those patients who have used sedatives or hypnotics, including alcohol, nightly for many months to years in order to fall asleep and who have developed a chronic *insomnia secondary to substance misuse*. Similarly, a history of stimulant use or other inappropriate drug use may result in a sleep disorder. A history of chronic or excessive drug or alcohol use recounted by the patient or, equally important, by a family member or friend suggests that further workup in this area is required. Psychotropic dependence—the perceived need to "take a pill" to diminish anxiety about potentially not being able to sleep—is not always easy to distinguish from physical dependence—the actual need for the physiological effects of medication in order to maintain sleep.

Alcohol remains a significant problem, as do stimulants and other drugs of abuse. Alcohol-dependent sleep disorder occurs in those who habitually "self-medicate" with alcohol to induce sleep. Alcohol does tend to decrease sleep latency and wakefulness during the first 3–4

hours of sleep. It also suppresses REM sleep and leads to REM rebound (with the possibility of vivid dreams or nightmares), with fragmented sleep during the latter part of the night. Treatment includes withdrawal of alcohol, with long-term abstinence as the goal. When necessary, sedation can be provided by judicious use of antihistamines (e.g., diphenhydramine [25–50 mg] or cyproheptadine [4–24 mg]).

Chronic use of stimulants leads to prolonged sleeplessness, and their withdrawal is followed by a period of hypersomnolence. A chronic insomnia complaint is often seen in long-term stimulant abusers even when they are not actively abusing the agents. Treatment is similar to that of alcohol-induced sleep disorder. Antikindling agents such as carbamazepine (100–600 mg/day) or divalproex (250–1,500 mg/day) may help when CNS hyperarousal/kindling is evident, as is sometimes seen in postcocaine panic disorder in polysubstance abusers.

Habituation to benzodiazepine agents does not usually result in insomnia unless they are too rapidly withdrawn, in which case the withdrawal syndrome may include insomnia. Doses should be tapered by one therapeutic dose per week.

In all cases of substance abuse sleep disorders, the insomnia complaint should emphasize behavioral treatment strategies to the fullest extent possible because psychoactive agents have already proved to be a problem.

Step 4—Circadian Rhythm Disorders

Circadian rhythm disorders often present as sleep complaints. The most common is the delayed sleep phase syndrome (DSPS), which presents as sleep-onset insomnia. Typically, individuals with DSPS cannot get to sleep until 3:00–4:00 A.M. If they can then sleep until 10:00 A.M. or noon the next day, they can do fine, indicating that they may have no trouble initiating or maintaining sleep, but if they are required to arise early to get to school or work, they complain of insomnia, and they are, of course, sleep deprived. Individuals with DSPS typically sleep in on weekends to recoup lost sleep. They often have already tried hypnotics, which are generally ineffective other than in inducing drowsiness, and their complaints are usually long-standing. DSPS typically appears in adolescence or early adulthood, and it is frequently familial. Often first-degree relatives have a history of similar sleep patterns.

In DSPS patients, evidence indicates that temperature rhythms and sleep rhythms are delayed and that possibly sleep persists for a longer time following the body temperature low point, suggesting that these patients may continue to sleep through the period when bright light would be most effective in phase-advancing their circadian system (Ozaki et al. 1988). Melatonin rhythms also may be phase-delayed in DSPS (Shibui et al. 1999).

Other forms of circadian rhythm disorders presenting as sleep complaints include advanced sleep phase syndrome (ASPS) and non-24-hour sleep–wake syndrome, also known as hypernychthemeral syndrome (Richardson and Malin 1996). ASPS is accompanied by retiring very early in the evening and correspondingly arising very early in the morning, a schedule that sometimes mimics that of terminal insomnia. Patients with the hypernychthemeral syndrome experience a failure of the circadian clock to entrain normally to the 24-hour day, and they sometimes experience a free-running 25-hour rhythm. This disorder is especially prevalent in blind persons, for whom light is unable to synchronize the circadian system. Some blind persons, however, are sensitive to light as an entrainer of the circadian system so long as the retina and retinohypothalamic tract are functioning normally.

Treatment of circadian rhythm–based sleep disorders now most often includes both bright light and melatonin. Early-morning bright-light exposure administered after the body temperature low point, with restriction of light exposure in the evening, has been found to be effective for phase-advancing the circadian system in DSPS (Regestein and Pavlova 1995; Rosenthal et al. 1990). Evening bright-light treatment has been found to be effective in phase-delaying the circadian system and in effectively treating ASPS (Chesson et al. 1999). Melatonin has also been used successfully in the treatment of DSPS (Dahlitz et al. 1991; Lamberg 1996; Szeinberg et al. 2006), and a case report indicated its successful use in entraining the circadian system in a blind, mentally retarded child who was unresponsive to bright light (Lapierre and Dumont 1995). Melatonin is also effective in synchronizing the free-running circadian rhythm in blind persons (Lewy et al. 2006).

Step 5—Movement Disorders: Restless Legs Syndrome and Periodic Leg Movements in Sleep

Restless legs syndrome (RLS) is not a true sleep disorder but rather a movement disorder that interferers with sleep. RLS is characterized by uncomfortable sensations in the calves at sleep onset that require that the patient get up and "walk them out." RLS symptoms are often maximal between the hours of 10 P.M. and 2 A.M., thus interfering with sleep. Severe untreated cases can be associated with significant sleep impairment and even skeletal

injury (Kuzniar and Silber 2007). RLS is increased in pregnancy, iron deficiency, renal disease, and diabetic neuropathy. There are genetic contributions to RLS, and several candidate gene loci have been identified (Winkelmann et al. 2007). While its pathophysiology remains unclear, some evidence suggests that RLS is associated with increased intracortical excitability that can be reversed by the dopamine D_2 receptor agonist cabergoline (Nardone et al. 2006).

Treatment for RLS should take into account severity, and division of patients into three groups has been suggested: 1) those with intermittent RLS symptoms, 2) those with daily RLS symptoms, and 3) those with symptoms refractory to common treatments. Both behavioral and pharmacological strategies should be employed, and treatment algorithms are available (Hening 2007). Dopamine agonists have been used for treatment of RLS. Carbidopa or levodopa was used initially but frequently led to augmentation, or worsening of symptoms, with time. Ropinirole 0.5–6 mg/day in divided doses, and pramipexole 0.125–0.75 mg have been shown to be effective in treating RLS. Gabapentin 300–1,200 mg has also been found helpful (Happe et al. 2003)

Because iron deficiency can be a cause of RLS, iron supplementation can often be helpful, especially if serum ferritin levels are below 45 μg/L (O'Keeffe 2005). Some evidence suggests a deficiency of iron transport into the CNS in RLS (Connor et al. 2003), and the use of intravenous iron has been reported to be helpful in severe cases but is not yet an approved treatment modality.

Periodic leg movements in sleep (PLMS; formerly termed nocturnal myoclonus) consist of periodic leg jerks occurring during sleep. Physiologically they appear to consist of extensions of the great toe and dorsiflexion of the ankle, knee, and hip, and they may represent the release of Babinski-type reflexes due to enhanced spinal cord excitability during light sleep. Associated muscle contractions are usually short (0.5–1.0 second) in duration and periodic (every 20–40 seconds), with recurrent episodes. They may be associated with EEG arousals or with cyclic-alternating-pattern discharges in the EEG. There is disagreement as to whether PLMS constitutes a form of sleep pathology that should be evaluated for treatment (Hogl 2007) or a normal variant with little clinical significance and not requiring treatment (except perhaps for the bed partner experiencing the kicking activity) (Mahowald 2007). In any case, dopaminergic agents as used for RLS are the treatments of choice, but the issue remains unresolved, and individual cases should be evaluated in the context of the latest medical literature.

Step 6—Conditioned Insomnia, Primary Insomnia, and Sleep State Misperception Syndrome Group

Finally, after the foregoing causes have been ruled out, a persistent chronic insomnia complaint likely falls into what we term the *conditioned insomnia/primary insomnia/sleep state misperception syndrome category*. This group has often been characterized as "psychophysiological insomnia" (American Academy of Sleep Medicine 2005), a term recently resurrected in the latest International Classification of Sleep Disorders (ICSD) that, while likely correct in that insomnia has both psychological and physiological components, is not of great help in separating independent causes that may respond to separate treatments. *Primary insomnia* is a DSM-IV-TR (American Psychiatric Association 2000) diagnostic with emerging information on the pathophysiology underlying its apparent chronic physiological hyperarousal. *Conditioned insomnia* is, as the name suggests, a "learned insomnia" in which a susceptible individual, after having trouble sleeping for a few nights, becomes fearful, with accompanying hyperarousal, about the very thought of going to bed or even going into the bedroom. The *sleep state misperception syndrome* is an interesting if still poorly understood condition that can be initially confusing, for these individuals appear unable to recognize that they have been asleep. These three types (as used here) of chronic insomnia tend to have a commonality of treatment approaches, which will likely continue to be the case until we have more data on their specific independent pathophysiologies. From a statistical and epidemiological standpoint, this category, in combination with the psychiatric causes of poor sleep, represents overall the largest group of the chronic insomnias. We believe it useful to attempt to separate the members of this category, even though they respond to the same treatment approaches. We will consider these three syndromes independently, first defining each as best we can and then discussing the common differential diagnosis and treatments options.

Conditioned Insomnia

The presenting symptoms for conditioned insomnia are as follows:

- Insomnia complaint, in a susceptible individual, beginning at a time of stress but persisting after the resolution of the stress
- Fear of going to bed because of the difficulty getting to sleep

- Racing thoughts when finally lying down and trying to sleep (must be differentiated from anxiety and mood dysregulation)
- May not be present in alternative sleep environment (couch, sleep lab, another home)

Conditioned insomnia is a learned arousal state. Typically beginning at a time of stress in susceptible individuals (those with a history of fragile or easily interrupted sleep), a few nights of trouble getting to sleep or staying asleep lead to development of a fear of going to bed because of concern that sleep again will be difficult to initiate or maintain. This fear is associated with increased cognitive and physiological arousal, and soon a vicious cycle is established in which merely going into the bedroom to prepare for sleep results in a conditioned arousal response sufficient to interfere with sleep. More specifically, these individuals develop a "conditioned arousal" to the normal sleep environment.

The conditioned arousal can continue long after resolution of the initial stress, and the resulting insomnia complaint can be quite chronic. Such individuals may be able to sleep on the living room couch, because they are conditioned to arouse only in their own bedroom. They may be able to nap during the day, and often sleep well on vacation or in a new environment. They may also sleep normally in the sleep lab, which is a new environment in which they may not experience conditioned arousal. Thus, a normal polysomnogram does not mean that the patient does not experience insomnia at home. Frequently, such individuals complain of not being able to turn off their thoughts at bedtime and recognize that they become fearful and aroused at the thought of going to bed. The differential diagnosis includes anxiety disorders and racing thoughts associated with a mildly hypomanic state, such as may accompany bipolar II disorder. Not surprisingly, conditioned arousal can co-occur with and complicate other causes (e.g., medical, psychiatric) of insomnia, having developed in response to the sleep difficulties associated with those disorders.

Primary Insomnia

The presenting symptoms for primary insomnia are as follows:

- Complaint of chronic insomnia 1 month or more in duration (sometimes years), that may wax and wane in intensity and appears independent of stressful or life events.

- Little evidence of fear about going to bed or complaints of racing thoughts.
- Other causes of chronic insomnia have been ruled out, or if present appropriately treated.

DSM-IV-TR criteria for primary insomnia are listed in Table 60–5.

Recent evidence suggests a state of hyperarousal may accompany and possibly be a cause of primary insomnia. These patients evidence increases in brain metabolism using positron emission tomography (PET) neuroimaging both while awake and during sleep compared with normally sleeping control subjects (Nofzinger et al. 2004), and evidence of increased metabolism during NREM sleep using single photon emission computed tomography (SPECT) imaging (Smith et al. 2002). They also evidence increased fast-EEG activity during sleep (Merica et al. 1998; Perlis et al 2001a, 2001b). There may be genetic contributions, although specifics remain to be determined (Heath et al. 1990). The important point is that this may be a bona fide medical disorder requiring long-term management, including possibly long-term medication for sleep.

Sleep State Misperception Syndrome

Sleep state misperception syndrome (SSMS), a somewhat confusing term and a still poorly understood condition, characterizes individuals who may go to sleep, spend time asleep, and awaken, and yet not be aware of having slept. If sleep lab studies are performed to investigate the chronic insomnia complaint, findings may appear normal. However, despite evidence of normal or near-normal sleep, SSMS patients may still have symptoms seen in other patients with chronic insomnia, such as disturbed daytime vigilance (Sugerman et al. 1985). Interestingly, a "reverse sleep state misperception syndrome" has also been reported, in which a patient reported having slept normally while objectively awake (Attarian et al. 2004).

Physiological studies are sparse. One study reported evidence of increased basal metabolic rate in patients with SSMS compared with control subjects, but not as high as in psychophysiological insomnia (Bonnet and Arand 1997), and there is evidence of possible sleep EEG differences (increased faster rhythms) in SSMS (Edinger and Krystal 2003).

The extent to which sleep misperception may constitute a clinically meaningful subtype of chronic insomnia remains to be determined. Because the syndrome has yet to be objectively defined and requires objective evidence of

TABLE 60–5. DSM-IV-TR diagnostic criteria for primary insomnia

A. The predominant complaint is difficulty initiating or maintaining sleep, or nonrestorative sleep, for at least 1 month.

B. The sleep disturbance (or associated daytime fatigue) causes clinically significant distress or impairment in social, occupational, or other important areas of functioning.

C. The sleep disturbance does not occur exclusively during the course of narcolepsy, breathing-related sleep disorder, circadian rhythm sleep disorder, or a parasomnia.

D. The disturbance does not occur exclusively during the course of another mental disorder (e.g., major depressive disorder, generalized anxiety disorder, a delirium).

E. The disturbance is not due to the direct physiological effects of a substance (e.g., a drug of abuse, a medication) or a general medical condition.

lack of awareness of being in a state of EEG-defined sleep, the issue of etiology remains moot, although the usual suspects (genetics, impaired arousal regulation (cause), conditioning or learning, stress responses) come to mind.

Differential Diagnosis for the Conditioned Arousal, Primary Insomnia, and Sleep State Misperception Syndrome Group

Since other causes having already been eliminated, the major differential in the case of conditioned insomnia, sleep state misperception, and primary insomnia rests upon history, symptoms, and perhaps a polysomnogram (may be helpful in SSMS). An important aspect of conditioned insomnia is that it frequently complicates insomnias resulting from other causes, and requires independent assessment and treatment.

In conditioned insomnia, the history will often disclose a stressful event as initiating the insomnia, which continues after the event resolves. In conditioned insomnia, sleep complaints tend to be fixed over time, but they may covary with the degree of daytime stress. These patients often tend to be tense or "wired" individuals; thus, some individuals may be more prone than others to the development of psychophysiological insomnia. Sleep-onset insomnia does not always characterize this disorder. Some patients may be able to fall asleep rather easily, but then they may have several hours of wakefulness later in the night, again unable to turn off their thoughts. Primary insomnia tends to be more chronic without clear-cut stressful initiating events. The separation of primary insomnia from chronic mild anxiety is sometimes difficult. SSMS patients may complain of getting absolutely no sleep at all—which of course is unlikely. The DSM-IV-TR criteria for primary insomnia need to be met. SSMS may not be suggested until a laboratory study (actigraphy or polysomnography) suggests a dissociation between subjective complaints and objective findings.

Sleep Laboratory Studies

Are sleep laboratory studies useful in any of the insomnias? In most cases—no. An all-night sleep study or polysomnogram may be indicated in chronic insomnia patients who are suspected of having either PLMS possibly causing insomnia or a SRBD, where identification and quantification is useful. Some conditioned insomnia patients may have less trouble sleeping in the laboratory environment than at home, which results in more normal-appearing polysomnographic findings. Thus, the presence of a relatively normal polysomnogram result in the laboratory does not exclude the possibility of real sleep difficulties in the patient's regular sleep environment. A polysomnogram can be helpful in the case of SSMS, where the findings may be within normal limits even though the patient believes he or she has obtained little or no sleep. It is questionable, however, whether the cost–benefit ratio merits a polysomnogram in the latter cases, unless there are other reasons for the study (e.g., treatment nonresponsiveness).

Conventional polysomnography is designed primarily to quantify respiratory and related physiology as well as muscle activity, but it does not typically sample brain activity with sufficient temporal and spatial resolution to provide useful information about other insomnia conditions. A polysomnogram in insomnia typically shows evidence of increased sleep latency, more frequent awakenings, and lower-than-normal total sleep and sleep efficiency, but the patient has already told you that. Functional neuroimaging studies (high-density EEG or magnetoencephalography, PET, SPECT) are research tools of potential value in better understanding disturbances in brain function underlying insomnia complaints, but they are not yet of routine diagnostic utility for most insomnia patients.

Actigraphy, providing an objective measure of minute-to-minute activity over several days or weeks, may be helpful in suggesting a circadian rhythm disorder and sometimes SSMS, but while activity measures often correlate well with polysomnogram-determined sleep measures, actigraphy alone has not yet been shown to be accurate for diagnosis (Littner et al. 2003).

Treatment of Chronic Insomnia

It is very important to realize that more than one cause of chronic insomnia may be present—in fact, it might be stated that *comorbidity is the rule, not the exception*. A patient may, for example, have a medical cause and a psychiatric cause in addition to PLMS or another movement disorder–related insomnia, and may then go on to develop a "conditioned" component. Patients who are depressed with comorbid insomnia may also have a primary insomnia disorder. Thus a complete differential diagnosis should be done for each patient, which should not stop when the first likely cause is identified. Similarly, treatments should be designed to cover all appropriate causes. The question of whether all appropriate treatments should be initiated together rather than waiting to see if the first treatment modality works alone before adding another is an important issue with no clear answer. Starting several at once risks overtreatment, whereas starting only one modality to see if it works before starting the others can mean delay in obtaining relief, furthering the belief that the insomnia is intractable and possibly even leading to the development or aggravation of a conditioned component. In the absence of firm rules, good clinical judgment and a good understanding of the patient are paramount.

Combined Treatment Approach for Chronic Insomnia

Recent years have seen major advances in both pharmacological and nonpharmacological (behavioral) treatments for insomnia (Erman 2005). These treatments will often be supplementary to the treatments designed specifically for medical, psychiatric, and other comorbidities, which may also be concurrent. As a general rule, a combined approach—utilizing both behavioral and pharmacological components—is preferable, recognizing that behavioral components may not always be available.

The mainstay of nonpharmacological behavioral treatments is CBT, which has been well documented as an effective strategy. Additional behavioral treatments include improved sleep hygiene, biofeedback, sleep restriction, progressive relaxation, and various meditation techniques. From the pharmacological standpoint, recent years have seen the development of a series of new non-benzodiazepine hypnotic agents that are both more effective and less troublesome than the older benzodiazepine agents.

Nonpharmacological Treatments for Chronic Insomnia

Cognitive-Behavioral Therapy

CBT for chronic insomnia has proved effective in a number of recent studies (Morin 2004; Smith and Perlis 2006). CBT has three components—education, behavioral modification, and cognitive therapy (Morin 2004). The literature on CBT as an effective treatment for insomnia is extensive and compelling and was nicely reviewed by Morin (2004). Smith and Perlis (2006) outline its use as a first-line treatment for chronic insomnia, including insomnia comorbid with medical and psychiatric disorders. One recent study using CBT in the treatment of insomnia associated with breast cancer suggested improvement in both sleep and immunological function resulting from CBT (Savard et al. 2003). Two issues of concern are which patients are optimally suited (or not well suited) for CBT (Smith and Perlis 2006) and whether therapists trained in CBT are available. Recent reports indicate that CBT need not be a long-term and complex treatment program; indeed, a very brief two-session form of CBT has recently been described that can be effective in primary care settings (Edinger and Sampson 2003). Perlis et al. (2005) has published a manualized step-by-step cognitive-behavioral treatment program for insomnia that clinicians should be able to implement effectively.

Sleep Hygiene

Sleep hygiene should be emphasized in the treatment of any chronic insomnia, including psychophysiological insomnia. Principles of good sleep hygiene are summarized in Table 60–6.

Biofeedback

Biofeedback treatment that directly teaches patients how to control autonomic functioning may be a useful therapeutic strategy (Hauri et al. 1982). Biofeedback may serve the dual function of enhancing a sense of self-control and reducing autonomic arousal. Although electromyography (EMG) and skin temperature biofeedback systems are perhaps the most commonly available forms, EEG biofeedback has been shown to be useful in some cases of chronic insomnia (Cortoos et al. 2006).

Sleep Restriction

Some patients with chronic insomnia (especially elderly patients) spend greater and greater amounts of time in bed

achieving less and less sleep, such that they may be in bed 10 hours or more and sleep only 6 hours. Sleep tends to spread out among the hours spent in bed, and this process further fragments nocturnal sleep. The principle of sleep restriction is to decrease substantially the time spent in bed so that sleep will consolidate to that time (Spielman et al. 1987). Restricting time available for sleep results in enhanced consolidation (which has important benefits in terms of improving actual and perceived sleep quality) and an improved subjective sense of self-control over sleep habits. The steps involved include the following:

1. Have the patient maintain a sleep diary for at least 5 nights. This diary should include a) time to bed at night, b) estimated time of sleep onset, c) number and estimated time of awakenings during the night, d) time of final awakening in the morning, and e) time out of bed. From this 5-night sleep diary data, calculate the mean value for estimated total sleep time (TST) and percentage sleep efficiency: TST divided by total time in bed.
2. Set the beginning total time in bed to equal the mean TST. For example, if the patient's estimate of his or her TST per night averaged over 5 nights is 5½ hours, set the time in bed to no more than 5½ hours, perhaps having the patient go to bed at 12:30 A.M. and get up again at 6:00 A.M. This restriction will result in increased daytime sleepiness the first several days, so the patient may need encouragement to continue with the program.
3. Instruct the patient to call in, usually to an answering machine, every morning while in the program and report his or her sleep data for the previous night, including time to bed, time of awakenings during sleep, time of final awakening, and time out of bed.
4. Calculate TST and sleep efficiency for each night. When mean sleep efficiency for 5 consecutive nights reaches 85% or better, increase time in bed by 15 minutes, by allowing the patient to go to bed 15 minutes earlier. If mean sleep efficiency declines to less than 85%, decrease time in bed by 15 minutes (but not within the first 10 days of treatment). Naps outside the prescribed time in bed are not allowed.
5. Repeat the above procedure until the patient is maintaining a sleep efficiency of 85% or better and obtaining what he or she considers to be a subjectively adequate amount of nocturnal sleep.

Sleep restriction results in some unavoidable sleepiness at the beginning of the regimen, and not all patients

TABLE 60–6.   Sleep hygiene

Regular sleep time	Establishing a regular sleep–wake schedule is very important, especially a regular time to awaken in the morning, with no more than 1-hour deviation from day to day, including weekends. Arousal time is perhaps the most important synchronizer of circadian rhythms. Awakening at 6:00 A.M. on weekdays to go to work and then sleeping until noon on weekends should be discouraged.
Proper sleep environment	Sleep interruptions should be minimized. The bedroom should be cool, dark, and quiet. The clinician needs to inquire specifically about noise, because patients may habituate to a noisy sleep environment and may not remember the noise, even though it continues to disrupt their sleep pattern. Patients who have convinced themselves that they can sleep only with the radio or television on should be discouraged from this practice. Attention to the radio or television may prevent their minds from wandering, or may keep them from beginning to worry about other matters, and thus assist with sleep latency, but the continuing noise will be a disruptive factor during the course of the night. Clock radios that automatically turn off may be useful.
Wind-down time	Time to wind down before sleep is important. The clinician should advise patients to stop work at least 30 minutes before sleep-onset time and to change their activities to something different and non-stressful, such as reading or listening to music.
Stimulus control	This procedure, an important component of sleep hygiene, involves removing from the bedroom all stimuli that are not associated with sleep. The bedroom should be used for sleep and, of course, sexual activity (which is often conducive to sleep). Activities such as eating, drinking, arguing, discussing the day's problems, and paying bills should be done elsewhere, because their associated arousal may interfere with sleep onset.
Avoidance of poorly timed alcohol and caffeine	Caffeine is quite disruptive of nocturnal sleep in many patients, and it has a long half-life. Thus, caffeine consumption should be limited to the forenoon and in some individuals not be continued after noon. A glass of wine or beer in the evening may help some individuals relax, but regularly having several drinks before bedtime for the express purpose of using the alcohol as a sedative should be discouraged. Alcohol in large doses can substantially disrupt and fragment sleep. Cigarette smoking may produce or aggravate insomnia in some patients.
Late-night high-tryptophan snack	A bedtime snack such as a glass of milk, a cookie, a banana, or a similar high-tryptophan food may help promote sleep onset in some patients.
Regular exercise	Periods of exercise for 20–30 minutes at least 3–4 days a week should be encouraged. Improved aerobic fitness has been shown experimentally to promote slow-wave sleep. Exercise should not occur within 3 hours of bedtime, however, because the autonomic arousal accompanying the exercise may serve to delay sleep onset.

can complete this treatment. However, those who can have a substantial chance of improving their sleep efficiency and achieving greater satisfaction with their sleep.

Pharmacological Treatment Options for Chronic Insomnia

The use of hypnotic agents in the treatment of insomnia has a long and checkered history. Early sedative-hypnotic agents such as the barbiturates, and then agents such as Noludar, Placidyl, Quaalude, and Doriden, with their potential lethality, disruption of sleep morphology, and addiction and/or habit-forming tendencies, gave the word "hypnotic" a bad reputation, to a considerable extent well deserved at the time. Such agents no longer have a place in the routine treatment of insomnia. Although chloral hydrate (500–1,000 mg) is still available for hypnotic use,

it is associated with increased addiction potential and has a relatively limited range between effective and lethal dose; thus, it might best be reserved for occasional use when indicated for other reasons.

Mendelson and Jain (1995) suggested that the ideal hypnotic would have a therapeutic profile characterized by rapid sleep induction and no residual effects (including memory effects). Its pharmacokinetic profile would include rapid absorption and optimal half-life, as well as specific receptor binding and lack of active metabolites. Its pharmacodynamic profile would include lack of tolerance or physical dependence and no CNS or respiratory depression. Although the ideal hypnotic agent has yet to be developed, hypnotic agents are being systematically improved with respect to most of the foregoing issues.

When the benzodiazepines came on the scene in the latter part of the twentieth century, with their prominent

TABLE 60–7. Benzodiazepine agents for treatment of insomnia

DRUG	HALF-LIFE (HOURS)	ABSORPTION	TYPICAL DOSE (MG)	ACTIVE METABOLITE
Triazolam (Halcion)	2–5	Fast	2.5–10	No
Temazepam (Restoril)	8–12	Moderate	7.5–30	No
Estazolam (ProSom)	12–20	Moderate	1–2	Minimal
Quazepam (Doral)	50–200	Fast	7.5–15	Yes
Flurazepam (Dalmane)	50–200	Fast	15–30	Yes

and useful sedative, hypnotic, anxiolytic, and anticonvulsant effects, safety was improved, but habituation, tolerance, and altered sleep morphology (decreased SWS) were side effects of concern. Because these agents activate the multiple benzodiazepine receptors in the brain and enhance CNS GABAergic inhibition, they have a role in insomnia related to anxiety, where their anxiolytic and GABAergic hypnotic effects are useful. Benzodiazepine agents approved by the U.S. Food and Drug Administration (FDA) for the treatment of insomnia are listed in Table 60–7.

The benzodiazepine compounds differ substantially in terms of half-life, and the clinician can choose the agent with a half-life most appropriate for the clinical situation. A long-half-life hypnotic such as flurazepam (15–30 mg) or quazepam (7.5–15.0 mg) might be appropriate for an anxious patient in whom daytime anxiolytic effects are helpful if the interference with psychomotor performance is acceptable and tolerable and if both patient and physician realize that considerable buildup in blood level can be expected. Patients with difficulty sleeping through the night might benefit from intermediate-half-life agents such as temazepam (15–30 mg) or estazolam (1–2 mg). Patients who must be alert in the morning without residual daytime sedation would best be managed with a short-half-life agent such as triazolam (0.125–0.25 mg). Many other benzodiazepines have been used for insomnia because of their sedative-hypnotic properties, but current thinking suggests that these agents might best be reserved for those patients who have significant anxiety or who have perhaps not responded to newer hypnotic agents.

Several new nonbenzodiazepine hypnotic agents have been developed that appear to act on the omega$_1$ benzodiazepine receptor but carry less potential for the problems that may accompany benzodiazepine use, such as habituation, tolerance, and altered sleep patterns. These newer nonbenzodiazepine agents generally have in common demonstrated efficacy in treating insomnia, differing primarily in half-life and effective duration of action (Table 60–8).

Zolpidem is an imidazopyridine agent active at the omega$_1$ benzodiazepine receptor but without the same degree of potential for tolerance or rebound seen with the benzodiazepines. Zolpidem has shown no evidence of rebound insomnia after being used at 10 mg/day for up to 35 days (Monti et al. 1994; Scharf et al. 1994; Ware et al. 2007). An extended-release (XR) form of zolpidem is available that extends duration of action about 1.5 hours. Its use over a 6-month period is associated with minimal residual and rebound effects (Owen 2006a).

Zaleplon is a nonbenzodiazepine pyrazolopyrimidine sedative-hypnotic agent that also acts as a benzodiazepine receptor agonist. With a short half-life of about 1.5 hours, this agent can be administered during middle-of-the-night awakenings as long as the patient has 4 hours of possible sleep time remaining (Zammit et al. 2006). Its short duration of action provides a somewhat more favorable safety profile for adult and elderly patients (Israel and Kramer 2002).

Eszopiclone is a nonbenzodiazepine cyclopyrrolone agent with rapid absorption and a half-life of about 6

TABLE 60–8. Nonbenzodiazepine agents for treatment of insomnia

DRUG	HALF-LIFE (HOURS)	ABSORPTION	TYPICAL DOSE (MG)	ACTIVE METABOLITE
Zaleplon (Sonata)	1–1.5	Fast	5–20	No
Ramelteon (Rozerem)	1–2.6	Fast	4–8	Yes
Zolpidem (Ambien)	1.5–2.6	Fast	2.5–10	No
Zolpidem ER (Ambien CR)	2.8	Fast	6.12–12.5	No
Eszopiclone (Lunesta)	6	Fast	7.5–15	Yes

hours. Eszopiclone is extensively metabolized by oxidation and demethylation, and the cytochrome P450 (CYP) isozymes CYP3A4 are involved, thus agents that induce or inhibit these enzymes may influence the metabolism of eszopiclone. Some individual report a bitter taste as a side effect (Najib 2006).

As a group, these agents appear to be relatively safe and effective for insomnia complaints, differing primarily in regard to half-life. With this increased safety and resulting increased worldwide use has come potentially significant problems associated with their inappropriate use or misuse, most often involving either 1) routine prescription without adequate preliminary differential diagnosis (the clinician's problem), and/or 2) taking the medication at an inappropriate time such as before having retired to bed (most often the patient's problem), resulting in inappropriate and potentially dangerous drug-induced waking behaviors. This is an issue related to proper differential diagnosis and proper treatment planning and monitoring, which needs to be addressed by improved education (still unfortunately often relatively sparse in medical school curricula). The 2005 NIH Consensus Conference on Chronic Insomnia in Adults recommended that these newer nonbenzodiazepine hypnotic agents be considered as the first-line treatment for insomnia rather than the traditional benzodiazepines. While not significantly altering sleep morphology, these agents do not specifically increase SWS, an attribute thought to be possibly desirable based on the role of SWS in memory function.

Additional recently developed agents include the melatonin MT_1 and MT_2 receptor agonist ramelteon, approved for use in insomnia with no long-term-use restrictions (Owen 2006b). Ramelteon is thought to promote sleep by influencing homeostatic sleep signaling mediated by the suprachiasmatic nucleus (Pandi-Perumal et al. 2007). It was shown to be effective for treatment of primary insomnia in elderly adults at a dose of 4 mg or 8 mg, with no evidence of adverse next-day effects (Roth et al. 2007b).

Several agents that are not yet formally approved for the treatment of insomnia have been found to selectively increase SWS. Sodium oxybate, a sedative-hypnotic agent that has been shown to increase SWS, is currently FDA approved only for use in treating narcolepsy. Its potential for abuse and limited availability are issues of concern. Tiagabine, a GABA reuptake inhibitor that increases synaptic GABA through selective inhibition of the GABA transporter type 1 (GAT-1), has been shown to increase SWS in a dose-dependent fashion in primary insomnia at doses up to 8 mg (Walsh et al. 2006). Gaboxadol, a selective extra-synaptic $GABA_A$ agonist, has been demonstrated to increase SWS at a dose of 15 mg (Deacon et al. 2007) and to improve sleep in a phase-advance model of insomnia (Walsh et al. 2007a). Lankford et al. (2008) reported results of two randomized, placebo-controlled studies of the use of gaboxidal over a 30-night period in both young adult and elderly patient with primary insomnia. Subjects treated with gaboxidal demonstrated enhancement of PSG-measured sleep maintenance and SWS as well as improvement in subjective sleep measures. The unique extra-synaptic mechanism of action of gaboxadol involves a $GABA_A$ receptor well represented in the thalamus, suggesting a mechanism of action quite different from that of most other GABA agents (Wafford and Ebert 2006).

The FDA has recommended limitations on quantities and duration of use for many hypnotic agents, although several recently approved agents (e.g., eszopiclone, zolpidem ER, ramelteon) have no such limitations.

There are a number of other sedative agents, many of them among the tricyclic antidepressant arsenal, that have been used for insomnia, including amitriptyline, nortriptyline, trimipramine, and doxepin (which are generally antihistaminic). Trazodone is also frequently prescribed. While clearly indicated when insomnia complicates depression, their general use for insomnia has neither FDA approval nor solid scientific backing. Special caution should be used in patients with increased risk factors such as cardiac conduction defects, glaucoma, or seizure disorders. Similar considerations exist for sedating atypical antipsychotic agents, which while often quite useful for insomnia complaints, should remain in the domain of patients experiencing cognitive symptoms suggestive of possible thought disorder. That being said, the author has had patients with chronic insomnia nonresponsive to usual hypnotic agents that does respond well to very low bedtime doses of sedative tricyclics such as nortriptyline. It should be noted that a recent placebo-controlled study has found doxepin doses of 1,3, and 6 mg to be effective for treatment of primary insomnia, demonstrating improvement of both PSG-determined and patient-reported sleep measures. Presumably at this dose the drug is acting primarily as an H_1 selective antagonist (Roth et al. 2007a). FDA approval for doxepin in this dose range for insomnia is pending.

Over-the-counter sleep agents and various herbal remedies found in health food stores have generally not been evaluated for hypnotic efficacy in well-controlled double-blind studies. Although some have modest sedative effects, consumers should be cautious, especially as concerns regular or excessive use of such agents.

The future may see the use of orexin-modulating agents in insomnia. Orexins are involved in sleep–wake stabilization and are deficient in narcolepsy, which is accompanied by excessive sleepiness. An orexin antagonist has been shown to induce sleep in both animals and humans, but is not yet available for clinical use (Brisbare-Roch et al. 2007).

Long-Term Use of Hypnotic Agents for Chronic Insomnia

The long-term use of hypnotic agents employed in the treatment of chronic insomnia is a topic of considerable concern. Short-term intermittent use is often recommended and remains a good overall principle. If a specific etiology, such as a medical or psychiatric disorder, can be identified and treated, the insomnia may resolve. Many, although not all, circadian rhythm disorders can be effectively managed with bright-light or melatonin treatment. Many patients with primary insomnia, however, may require long-term pharmacological management. In a recent study, long-term (6-month) treatment of chronic primary insomnia with eszopiclone 3 mg led to enhanced quality of life, reduced work limitations, and improved patient satisfaction with sleep without evidence of rebound insomnia following medication discontinuation (Walsh et al. 2007b). Several similar placebo-controlled studies reported that 12.5 mg zolpidem ER administered 3–7 nights per week over a 6-month period resulted in improved daytime concentration and work performance as well as improved satisfaction with nocturnal sleep (Erman et al. 2008; Krystal et al. 2008).

The use of the lowest dose of the most innocuous but most effective agent is a good rule. Unnecessary withholding of treatment should be avoided, however. Considering the known adverse effects of chronic sleep loss, in the context of the current availability of relatively safe and effective hypnotic agents, there would appear to be no reason to withhold or to limit treatment in those patients for whom a comprehensive and thorough diagnostic evaluation has established the presence of a primary insomnia disorder that would benefit from long-term treatment. The cost–benefit ratio of chronic pharmacological treatment must be carefully evaluated on an individual patient basis.

Given the demonstrated effectiveness of CBT, it seems any patients being considered for long-term hypnotic treatment should at least be given the option of trying CBT to see if it might decrease the need for hypnotic use. The following three general rules might be useful to keep in mind when considering the long-term use of hypnotics:

1. Use the lowest effective dose and the shortest clinically indicated duration of use.
2. Do not put a patient on long-term hypnotic use for a chronic insomnia condition without including at the very least a good trial of behavioral treatment for insomnia.
3. Do not hesitate to prescribe long-term use of one of the newer and safer hypnotic agents when clinically indicated for an appropriately evaluated chronic insomnia condition (including but not limited to primary insomnia).

Insomnia in the Elderly

Up to 50% of older Americans report chronic difficulties with their sleep (Foley et al. 1995), and similar numbers have been reported from other cultures. In addition to resulting dissatisfaction with sleep and aspects of daytime performance, those with sleep complaints use health services to a greater extent (Novak et al. 2004). While the differential diagnosis and treatment strategies are similar in elderly individuals, there are both physiological and behavioral aspects of aging that impact sleep that require emphasis.

Normal Aging and Sleep Control Mechanisms

CNS changes associated with aging may adversely impact both Process S and Process C sleep control systems. There is evidence that the number of non-REM-promoting VLPO neurons in the hypothalamus decreases with age, beginning about after age 50 years, with the decrease being more pronounced in women than men (Hofman and Swaab 1989). By age 85 years, there may be a loss of 50% of VLPO neurons. To the extent that these VLPO neurons support the integrity of non-REM sleep, or Process S, this cell loss could be related to the increase in insomnia complaints in the elderly, especially women (Ancoli-Israel and Ayalon 2006). Additionally, the nocturnal production of melatonin decreases with age, significantly so by age 60 years, which may lead to impairment in the Process C circadian arousal control system (Cardinali et al. 2006). The possible impact of such changes should be taken into account in evaluating sleep complaints in the elderly—the use of hypnotics and/or melatonin supplementation may be especially useful (Haimov et al. 1995).

Those medical and psychiatric conditions adversely impacting sleep and sometimes comorbid with insomnia increase in frequency in the elderly, and specific sleep disorders, such as RLS, sleep apnea, and REM sleep behavior disorder, also increase in incidence with age. The comorbidity of insomnia and sleep-related breathing disorders in the elderly is associated with significant impairment (Gooneratne et al. 2006). Elderly people frequently take a variety of medications that, for a variety of reasons, may either interact or act differently in the elderly person and result in altered sleep patterns or sleep behavior.

Adverse Sleep Habits and Environments in the Elderly

Even the healthy elderly may live a lifestyle of restricted interests and decreased mental and physical activities, which can contribute to poorer sleep. Process S appears to be stimulated by the amount and intensity of the preceding day's mental and physical activity, and reductions in such can be expected to adversely impact Process S. Maintenance of a sleep-healthy lifestyle with vigorous mental and physical as well as social activities can certainly help here. The impact of exercise on sleep is still somewhat unclear (Driver and Taylor 2000; Kubitz et al. 1996); however, the role of improved aerobic fitness in health and well-being generally is well established.

The less healthy elderly, who may reside in more restrictive environments or nursing homes, are at special risk, not only because of the foregoing but because of the adverse impact of factors such as irregular schedules, excessive nocturnal lighting, noise, and other issues adversely affecting sleep. Efforts should be made to modify and improve the living and sleeping environment before routinely moving to pharmacological interventions such as sedative-hypnotic agents.

Treatment of Insomnia in Elderly Patients

Strict attention to good sleep hygiene is important, including not spending excessive time in bed and improving aerobic fitness if possible. Excessive use of caffeine, including that contained in over-the-counter analgesics, should be curtailed.

Bright-light treatment has been useful in treating sleep disorders, including morning bright light for certain cases of sleep-onset insomnia (possibly caused by a mild circadian phase delay), in elderly patients. Evening bright light has been found to be effective in sleep-maintenance insomnia

in healthy elderly subjects (Campbell et al. 1995). It should be kept in mind that elderly individuals may be less responsive to bright light and therefore might require a greater duration or intensity of treatment (Duffy et al. 2007).

Use of pharmacological agents must be tempered by the awareness that half-lives may be extended, that risk of multiple drug interactions may be increased, and that lower-than-usual doses may be adequate. Zaleplon, because of its short half-life, may be a relatively safe agent in the elderly, and indiplon (15 mg), a nonbenzodiazepine hypnotic active at the benzodiazepine alpha$_1$ subunit, was shown to improve sleep in elderly patients with primary insomnia during a 2-week treatment period with no significant side effects (Lydiard et al. 2006). Indiplon could potentially be released as a hypnotic in the near future.

Some have suggested that use of hypnotics in elderly patients should be very conservative, with an emphasis on nonpharmacological strategies (Bain 2006; Sivertsen et al. 2007) and CBT, which has been shown to be effective in elderly patients with insomnia. While concerns have been expressed about a relationship between hypnotic use and falls in the elderly, a recent study found that insomnia, but not hypnotic use, was associated with a greater risk of subsequent falls (Avidan et al. 2005).

Considering the cognitive difficulties experienced by many elderly individuals possibly related to sleep impairment, a recent study demonstrating improved cognitive function in an animal model of genetically induced impaired sleep following treatment with a benzodiazepine to help improve sleep might be important (Pallier et al. 2007). It has yet to be determined whether nonpharmacological treatment of insomnia is as effective as pharmacological in reversing the adverse cognitive effects of insomnia.

Conclusion

It is gratifying that the available treatment strategies for insomnia have improved coincidentally with our recognition of the importance of protecting sleep and treating insomnia in recent years. We are still left with an unclear understanding of the basic pathophysiology of many insomnia-related syndromes, however, and until our knowledge base improves, we must depend on systematic differential diagnosis and treatment planning using the information available. Fortunately, with this approach, most patients with insomnia complaints can be significantly helped.

References

American Academy of Sleep Medicine: The International Classification of Sleep Disorders, 2nd Edition. Rochester, MN, Johnson Printing, 2005

American Academy of Sleep Medicine: The AASM Manual for the Scoring of Sleep and Associated Events: Rules, Terminology and Technical Specification. Westchester, IL, American Academy of Sleep Medicine, March 2007

American Psychiatric Association: Diagnostic and Statistical Manual of Mental Disorders, 4th Edition, Text Revision. Washington, DC, American Psychiatric Association, 2000

Ancoli-Israel S, Poceta JS, Stepnowsky C, et al: Identification and treatment of sleep problems in the elderly. Sleep Med Rev 1:3–17, 1997

Ancoli-Israel S, Roth T: Characteristics of insomnia in the United States: results of the 1991 National Sleep Foundation Survey, I. Sleep 22 (suppl 2):S347–S353, 1999

Ancoli-Israel S, Ayalon L: Diagnosis and treatment of sleep disorders in older adults. Am J Geriatr Psychiatry 14:95–103, 2006

Anttila SA, Leinonen EV: A review of the pharmacological and clinical profile of mirtazapine. CNS Drug Rev 7:249–264, 2001

Armitage R, Landis C, Hoffmann R, et al: The impact of a 4-hour sleep delay on slow wave activity in twins discordant for chronic fatigue syndrome. Sleep 30:657–662, 2007

Attarian HP, Duntley S, Brown KM: Reverse sleep state misperception. Sleep Med 5:269–272, 2004

Avidan AY, Fries BE, James ML: Insomnia and hypnotic use, recorded in the minimum data set, as predictors of falls and hip fractures in Michigan nursing homes. J Am Geriatr Soc 53:955–962, 2005

Backhaus J, Junghanns K, Born J, et al: Impaired declarative memory consolidation during sleep in patients with primary insomnia: influence of sleep architecture and nocturnal cortisol release. Biol Psychiatry 60:1324–1330, 2006

Bain KT: Management of chronic insomnia in elderly persons. Am J Geriatr Pharmacother 4:168–192, 2006

Basheer R, Strecker RE, Thakkar MM, et al: Adenosine and sleep-wake regulation. Prog Neurobiol 73:379–396, 2004

Beaumont M, Batejat D, Pierard C, et al: Zaleplon and zolpidem objectively alleviate sleep disturbances in mountaineers at a 3,613 meter altitude. Sleep 30:1527–1533, 2007

Boeve BF, Silber MH, Ferman TJ, et al: REM sleep behavior disorder and degenerative dementia: an association likely reflecting Lewy body disease. Neurology 51:363–370, 1998

Bonnet MH, Arand DL: Physiological activation in patients with sleep state misperception. Psychosom Med 59:533–540, 1997

Brisbare-Roch C, Dingemanse J, Koberstein R, et al: Promotion of sleep by targeting the orexin system in rats, dogs and humans. Nat Med 13:150–155, 2007

Brzezinski A: Melatonin in humans. N Engl J Med 336:186–195, 1997

Campbell SS, Terman M, Lewy AJ, et al: Light treatment for sleep disorders: consensus report, V: age-related disturbances. J Biol Rhythms 10:151–154, 1995

Cardinali DP, Furio AM, Reyes MP, et al: The use of chronobiotics in the resynchronization of the sleep-wake cycle. Cancer Causes Control 17:601–609, 2006

Chaput JP, Despres JP, Bouchard C, et al: The association between sleep duration and weight gain in adults: a 6-year prospective study from the Quebec Family Study. Sleep 31:517–523, 2008

Chesson AL Jr, Anderson WM, Littner M, et al: Practice parameters for the nonpharmacologic treatment of chronic insomnia. An American Academy of Sleep Medicine report. Standards of Practice Committee of the American Academy of Sleep Medicine. Sleep 22:1128–1133, 1999

Clemens Z, Fabo D, Halasz P: Overnight verbal memory retention correlates with the number of sleep spindles. Neuroscience 132:529–535, 2005

Connor JR, Boyer PJ, Menzies SL, et al: Neuropathological examination suggests impaired brain iron acquisition in restless legs syndrome. Neurology 61:304–309, 2003

Cortoos A, Verstraeten E, Cluydts R: Neurophysiological aspects of primary insomnia: implications for its treatment. Sleep Med Rev 10:255–266, 2006

Czeisler CA, Allan JS, Strogatz SH, et al: Bright light resets the human circadian pacemaker independent of the timing of the sleep-wake cycle. Science 233:667, 1986

Czeisler CA, Duffy JF, Shanahan TL, et al: Stability, precision, and near-24-hour period of the human circadian pacemaker. Science 284:2177–2181, 1999

Dahlitz M, Alvarez B, Vignau J, et al: Delayed sleep phase syndrome response to melatonin. Lancet 337:1121–1124, 1991

Davis JL, Wright DC: Randomized clinical trial for treatment of chronic nightmares in trauma-exposed adults. J Trauma Stress 20:123–133, 2007

Dawson D, Reid K: Fatigue, alcohol and performance impairment. Nature 388:235, 1997

Deacon S, Staner L, Staner C, et al: Effect of short-term treatment with gaboxadol on sleep maintenance and initiation in patients with primary insomnia. Sleep 30:281–287, 2007

Deviva JC, Zayfert C, Pigeon WR, et al: Treatment of residual insomnia after CBT for PTSD: case studies. J Trauma Stress 18:155–159, 2005

Driver HS, Taylor SR: Exercise and sleep. Sleep Med Rev 4:387–402, 2000

Duffy JF, Zeitzer JM, Czeisler CA: Decreased sensitivity to phase-delaying effects of moderate intensity light in older subjects. Neurobiol Aging 28:799–807, 2007

Edinger JD, Krystal AD: Subtyping primary insomnia: is sleep state misperception a distinct clinical entity? Sleep Med Rev 7:203–214, 2003

Edinger JD, Sampson WS: A primary care "friendly" cognitive behavioral insomnia therapy. Sleep 26:177–182, 2003

Edinger JD, Wohlgemuth WK, Krystal AD, et al: Behavioral insomnia therapy for fibromyalgia patients: a randomized clinical trial. Arch Intern Med 165:2527–2535, 2005

Erman MK: Therapeutic options in the treatment of insomnia. J Clin Psychiatry 66:18–23, 2005

Erman M, Guiraud A, Joish VN, et al: Zolpidem extended-release 12.5 mg associated with improvements in work performance in a 6-month randomized, placebo-controlled trial. Sleep 31:1371–1378, 2008

Ferman TJ, Boeve BF, Smith GE, et al: REM sleep behavior disorder and dementia: cognitive differences when compared with AD. Neurology 52:951–957, 1999

Foley DJ, Monjan AA, Brown SL, et al: Sleep complaints among elderly persons: an epidemiologic study of three communities. Sleep 18:425–432, 1995

Franklin KA, Eriksson P, Sahlin C, et al: Reversal of central sleep apnea with oxygen. Chest 111:163–169, 1997

Gangwisch JE, Heymsfield SB, Boden-Albala B, et al: Sleep duration as a risk factor for diabetes incidence in a large US sample. Sleep 30:1667–1673, 2007

Gooneratne NS, Gehrman PR, Nkwuo JE, et al: Consequences of comorbid insomnia symptoms and sleep-related breathing disorder in elderly subjects. Arch Intern Med 166:1732–1738, 2006

Granton JT, Naughton MT, Benard DC, et al: CPAP improves inspiratory muscle strength in patients with heart failure and central sleep apnea. Am J Respir Crit Care Med 153:277–282, 1996

Guilleminault C, Poyares D, Rosa A, et al: Chronic fatigue, unrefreshing sleep and nocturnal polysomnography. Sleep Med 7:513–520, 2006

Haimov I, Lavie P, Laudon M, et al: Melatonin replacement therapy of elderly insomniacs. Sleep 18:598–603, 1995

Hamet P, Tremblay J: Genetics of the sleep-wake cycle and its disorders. Metabolism 55:S7–S12, 2006

Happe S, Sauter C, Klosch G, et al: Gabapentin versus ropinirole in the treatment of idiopathic restless legs syndrome. Neuropsychobiology 48:82–86, 2003

Hauri PJ, Percy L, Hellekson C, et al: The treatment of psychophysiologic insomnia with biofeedback: a replication study. Biofeedback Self Regul 7:223–235, 1982

Heath AC, Kendler KS, Eaves LJ, et al: Evidence for genetic influences on sleep disturbance and sleep pattern in twins. Sleep 13:318–335, 1990

Hening WA: Current guidelines and standards of practice for restless legs syndrome. Am J Med 120:S22–S27, 2007

Hofman MA, Swaab DF: The sexually dimorphic nucleus of the preoptic area in the human brain: a comparative morphometric study. J Anat 164:55–72, 1989

Hogl B: Periodic limb movements are associated with disturbed sleep. J Clin Sleep Med 3:12–14, 2007

Huber R, Ghilardi MF, Massimini M, et al: Local sleep and learning. Nature 430:78–81, 2004

Israel AG, Kramer JA: Safety of zaleplon in the treatment of insomnia. Ann Pharmacother 36:852–859, 2002

Jindal RD, Buysse DJ, Thase ME: Maintenance treatment of insomnia: what can we learn from the depression literature? Am J Psychiatry 161:19–24, 2004

Krystal A: Treating the health, quality of life, and functional impairments in insomnia. J Clin Sleep Med 3:63–72, 2007

Krystal AD, Erman M, Zammit GK, et al: Long-term efficacy and safety of zolpidem extended-release 12.5 mg, administered 3 to 7 nights per week for 24 weeks, in patients with chronic primary insomnia: a 6-month, randomized, double-blind, placebo-controlled, parallel-group, multicenter study. Sleep 31:79–90, 2008

Kubitz KA, Landers DM, Petruzzello SJ, et al: The effects of acute and chronic exercise on sleep: a meta-analytic review. Sports Med 21:277–291, 1996

Kuzniar TJ, Silber MH: Multiple skeletal injuries resulting from uncontrolled restless legs syndrome. J Clin Sleep Med 3:60–61, 2007

Lamberg L: Melatonin potentially useful but safety, efficacy remain uncertain. JAMA 276:1011–1014, 1996

Lange T, Perras B, Fehm HL, et al: Sleep enhances the human antibody response to hepatitis A vaccination. Psychosom Med 65:831–835, 2003

Lankford DA, Corser BC, Zheng YP, et al: Effect of gaboxadol on sleep in adult and elderly patients with primary insomnia: results from two randomized, placebo-controlled, 30-night polysomnography studies. Sleep 31:1359–1370, 2008

Lapierre O, Dumont M: Melatonin treatment of a non-24-hour sleep-wake cycle in a blind retarded child. Biol Psychiatry 38:119–122, 1995

Lewy AJ, Emens J, Jackman A, et al: Circadian uses of melatonin in humans. Chronobiol Int 23:403–412, 2006

Littner M, Kushida CA, Anderson WM, et al: Practice parameters for the role of actigraphy in the study of sleep and circadian rhythms: an update for 2002. Sleep 26:337–341, 2003

Liu RY, Zhou JN, vanHeerikhuize J, et al: Decreased melatonin levels in postmortem cerebral spinal fluid in relation to aging, Alzheimer's disease, and apolipoprotein E-episilon4/4 genotype. J Clin Endocrinol Metab 84:323–327, 1999

Lockley SW, Evans EE, Scheer FA, et al: Short-wavelength sensitivity for the direct effects of light on alertness, vigilance, and the waking electroencephalogram in humans. Sleep 29:161–168, 2006

Lu J, Sherman D, Devor M, et al: A putative flip-flop switch for control of REM sleep. Nature 441:589–594, 2006

Lydiard RB, Lankford DA, Seiden DJ, et al: Efficacy and tolerability of modified-release indiplon in elderly patients with chronic insomnia: results of a 2-week double-blind, placebo-controlled trial. J Clin Sleep Med 2:309–315, 2006

Mahowald MW: Periodic limb movements are NOT associated with disturbed sleep: con. J Clin Sleep Med 3:15–17, 2007

McCurry SM, Logsdon RG, Vitiello MV, et al: Treatment of sleep and nighttime disturbances in Alzheimer's disease: a behavior management approach. Sleep Med 5:373–377, 2004

McKeith IG: Clinical Lewy body syndromes. Ann N Y Acad Sci 920:1–8, 2000

Meier-Ewert HK, Ridker PM, Rifai N, et al: Effect of sleep loss on C-reactive protein, an inflammatory marker of cardiovascular risk. J Am Coll Cardiol 43:678–683, 2004

Mellman TA, Nolan B, Hebding J, et al: A polysomnographic comparison of veterans with combat-related PTSD, depressed men, and non-ill controls. Sleep 20:46–51, 1997

Mendelson WB, Jain B: An assessment of short-acting hypnotics. Drug Saf 13:257–270, 1995

Merica H, Blois R, Gaillard JM: Spectral characteristics of sleep EEG in chronic insomnia. Eur J Neurosci 10:1826–1834, 1998

Monti JM, Attali P, Monti D, et al: Zolpidem and rebound insomnia—a double-blind, controlled polysomnographic study in chronic insomniac patients. Pharmacopsychiatry 27:166–175, 1994

Morin CM: Cognitive-behavioral approaches to the treatment of insomnia. J Clin Psychiatry 65:33–40, 2004

Najib J: Eszopiclone, a nonbenzodiazepine sedative-hypnotic agent for the treatment of transient and chronic insomnia. Clin Ther 28:491–516, 2006

Nardone R, Ausserer H, Bratti A, et al: Cabergoline reverses cortical hyperexcitability in patients with restless legs syndrome. Acta Neurol Scand 114:244–249, 2006

Neckelmann D, Mykletun A, Dahl AA: Chronic insomnia as a risk factor for developing anxiety and depression. Sleep 30:873–880, 2007

Nofzinger EA, Buysse DJ, Germain A, et al: Functional neuroimaging evidence for hyperarousal in insomnia. Am J Psychiatry 161:2126–2128, 2004

Novak M, Mucsi I, Shapiro CM, et al: Increased utilization of health services by insomniacs—an epidemiological perspective. J Psychosom Res 56:527–536, 2004

O'Keeffe ST: Iron deficiency with normal ferritin levels in restless legs syndrome. Sleep Med 6:281–282, 2005

Owen RT: Extended-release zolpidem: efficacy and tolerability profile. Drugs Today (Barc) 42:721–727, 2006a

Owen RT: Ramelteon: profile of a new sleep-promoting medication. Drugs Today (Barc) 42:255–263, 2006b

Ozaki N, Iwata T, Itoh A, et al: Body temperature monitoring in subjects with delayed sleep phase syndrome. Neuropsychobiology 20:174–177, 1988

Pallier PN, Maywood ES, Zheng Z, et al: Pharmacological imposition of sleep slows cognitive decline and reverses dysregulation of circadian gene expression in a transgenic mouse model of Huntington's disease. J Neurosci 27:7869–7878, 2007

Pandi-Perumal SR, Srinivasan V, Poeggeler B, et al: Drug Insight: the use of melatonergic agonists for the treatment of insomnia-focus on ramelteon. Nat Clin Pract Neurol 3:221–228, 2007

Pasternak RE, Reynolds CF III, Schlernitzauer M, et al: Acute open-trial nortriptyline therapy of bereavement-related depression in late life. J Clin Psychiatry 52:307–310, 1991

Perlis ML, Kehr EL, Smith MT, et al: Temporal and stagewise distribution of high frequency EEG activity in patients with primary and secondary insomnia and in good sleeper controls. J Sleep Res 10:93–104, 2001a

Perlis ML, Smith MT, Andrews PJ, et al: Beta/Gamma EEG activity in patients with primary and secondary insomnia and good sleeper controls. Sleep 24:110–117, 2001b

Perlis ML, Jungquist C, Smith MT, et al: Cognitive Behavioral Treatment o Insomnia: A Session by Session Guide. New York, Springer, 2005

Rechtschaffen A, Kales A: A Manual of Standardized Terminology, Techniques and Scoring System for Sleep Stages of Human Subjects (NIH publication no. 204). Washington, DC. U.S. Government Printing Office, 1968

Regestein QR, Pavlova M: Treatment of delayed sleep phase syndrome. Gen Hosp Psychiatry 17:335–345, 1995

Richardson GS: Managing insomnia in the primary care setting: raising the issues. Sleep 23 (suppl 1):S9–S12, 2000

Richardson GS, Malin HV: Circadian rhythm sleep disorders: pathophysiology and treatment. J Clin Neurophysiol 13:17–31, 1996

Riemann D, Voderholzer U, Spiegelhalder K, et al: Chronic insomnia and MRI-measured hippocampal volumes: a pilot study. Sleep 30:955–958, 2007

Roane BM, Taylor DJ: Adolescent insomnia as a risk factor for early adult depression and substance abuse. Sleep 31:1351–1356, 2008

Rosenfeld DS, Furman Y: Pure sleep panic: two case reports and a review of the literature. Sleep 17:462–465, 1994

Rosenthal NE, Joseph-Vanderpool JR, Levendosky AA, et al: Phase-shifting effects of bright morning light as treatment for delayed sleep phase syndrome. Sleep 13:354–361, 1990

Ross RJ, Ball WA, Dinges DF, et al: Motor dysfunction during sleep in posttraumatic stress disorder. Sleep 17:723–732, 1994

Roth T, Rogowski R, Hull S, et al: Efficacy and safety of doxepin 1 mg, 3 mg, and 6 mg in adults with primary insomnia. Sleep 30:1555–1561, 2007a

Roth T, Seiden D, Wang-Weigand S, et al: A 2-night, 3-period, crossover study of ramelteon's efficacy and safety in older adults with chronic insomnia. Curr Med Res Opin 23:1005–1014, 2007b

Rybarczyk B, Stepanski E, Fogg L, et al: A placebo-controlled test of cognitive-behavioral therapy for comorbid insomnia in older adults. J Consult Clin Psychol 73:1164–1174, 2005

Saiz-Ruiz J, Cebollada A, Ibanez A: Sleep disorders in bipolar depression: hypnotics vs sedative antidepressants. J Psychosom Res 38:55–60, 1994

Saper CB, Scammell TE, Lu J: Hypothalamic regulation of sleep and circadian rhythms. Nature 437:1257–1263, 2005

Savard J, Laroche L, Simard S, et al: Chronic insomnia and immune functioning. Psychosom Med 65:211–221, 2003

Schabus M, Gruber G, Parapatics S, et al: Sleep spindles and their significance for declarative memory consolidation. Sleep 27:1479–1485, 2004

Schaller JL, Behar D: Modafinil in fibromyalgia treatment. J Neuropsychiatry Clin Neurosci 13:530–531, 2001

Scharf MB, Roth T, Vogel GW, et al: A multicenter, placebo-controlled study evaluating zolpidem in the treatment of chronic insomnia. J Clin Psychiatry 55:192–199, 1994

Scharf MB, Baumann M, Berkowitz DV: The effects of sodium oxybate on clinical symptoms and sleep patterns in patients with fibromyalgia. J Rheumatol 30:1070–1074, 2003

Schenck CH, Mahowald MW: Rapid eye movement sleep parasomnias. Neurol Clin 23:1107–1126, 2005

Schwartz JR, Roth T: Shift work sleep disorder: burden of illness and approaches to management. Drugs 66:2357–2370, 2006

Shibui K, Uchiyama M, Okawa M: Melatonin rhythms in delayed sleep phase syndrome. J Biol Rhythms 14:72–76, 1999

Sivertsen B, Nordhus IH: Management of insomnia in older adults. Br J Psychiatry 190:285–286, 2007

Smith MT, Perlis ML, Park A, et al: Comparative meta-analysis of pharmacotherapy and behavior therapy for persistent insomnia. Am J Psychiatry 159:5–11, 2002

Smith MT, Perlis ML: Who is a candidate for cognitive-behavioral therapy for insomnia? Health Psychol 25:15–19, 2006

Spiegel K, Tasali E, Penev P, et al: Brief communication: sleep curtailment in healthy young men is associated with decreased leptin levels, elevated ghrelin levels, and increased hunger and appetite. Ann Intern Med 141:846–850, 2004

Spiegel K, Knutson K, Leproult R, et al: Sleep loss: a novel risk factor for insulin resistance and Type 2 diabetes. J Appl Physiol 99:2008–2019, 2005

Spielman AJ, Saskin P, Thorpy MJ: Treatment of chronic insomnia by restriction of time in bed. Sleep 10:45–56, 1987

Sugerman JL, Stern JA, Walsh JK: Daytime alertness in subjective and objective insomnia: some preliminary findings. Biol Psychiatry 20:741–750, 1985

Szeinberg A, Borodkin K, Dagan Y: Melatonin treatment in adolescents with delayed sleep phase syndrome. Clin Pediatr 45:809–818, 2006

Thalhofer S, Dorow P: Central sleep apnea. Respiration 64:2–9, 1997

VanHoof E, DeBecker P, Lapp C, et al: Defining the occurrence of alpha-delta sleep in chronic fatigue syndrome. Am J Med Sci 333:78–84, 2007

van Liempt S, Vermetten E, Geuze E, et al: Pharmacotherapy for disordered sleep in post-traumatic stress disorder: a systematic review. Int Clin Psychopharmacol 21:193–202, 2006

Wafford KA, Ebert B: Gaboxadol—a new awakening in sleep. Curr Opin Pharmacol 6:30–36, 2006

Walker MP, Stickgold R: Sleep, memory, and plasticity. Annu Rev Psychol 57:139–166, 2006

Walsh JK, Perlis M, Rosenthal M, et al: Tiagabine increases slow-wave sleep in a dose-dependent fashion without affecting traditional efficacy measures in adults with primary insomnia. J Clin Sleep Med 2:35–41, 2006

Walsh JK, Deacon S, Dijk DJ, et al: The selective extrasynaptic GABAA agonist, gaboxadol, improves traditional hypnotic efficacy measures and enhances slow wave activity in a model of transient insomnia. Sleep 30:593–602, 2007a

Walsh JK, Krystal AD, Amato DA, et al: Nightly treatment of primary insomnia with eszopiclone for six months: effect on sleep, quality of life, and work limitations. Sleep 30:959–968, 2007b

Ware JC, Walsh JK, Scharf MB, et al: Minimal rebound insomnia after treatment with 10-mg zolpidem. Clin Neuropharmacol 20:116–125, 2007

Winkelmann J, Polo O, Provini F, et al: Genetics of restless legs syndrome (RLS): state-of-the-art and future directions. Mov Disord 22 (suppl 18):S449–S458, 2007

Wolk R, Somers VK: Sleep and the metabolic syndrome. Exp Physiol 92:67–78, 2007

Yaggi HK, Araujo AB, McKinlay JB: Sleep duration as a risk factor for the development of type 2 diabetes. Diabetes Care 29:657–661, 2006

Yaron M, Lindgren K, Halbower AC, et al: Sleep disturbance after rapid ascent to moderate altitude among infants and preverbal young children. High Alt Med Biol 5:314–320, 2004

Zammit GK, Corser B, Doghramji K, et al: Sleep and residual sedation after administration of zaleplon, zolpidem, and placebo during experimental middle-of-the-night awakening. J Clin Sleep Med 2:417–423, 2006

CHAPTER 61

Treatment of Personality Disorders

Daphne Simeon, M.D.

Eric Hollander, M.D.

What Does Medication Change in Treating Personality?

Personality disorders are some of the more challenging psychiatric conditions and have traditionally been viewed by many clinicians as more difficult to treat than numerous Axis I conditions, often requiring investment in more lengthy treatments that involve a variety of modalities and approaches. It is also common to attain lesser and more modest degrees of success in treating personality disorders, with a recognition, however, that even partial modifications in people's dysfunctional interpersonal relationships, coping mechanisms, and symptomatology can bring about notably better adaptations. Psychotherapy continues to be the treatment foundation for all personality disorders, and psychotherapy studies of personality disorders on the whole find that patients with these disorders improve with treatment, with large treatment effects—two to four times greater than the improvement found in the control conditions (Perry and Bond 2000). In more recent years, the traditional psychodynamic therapy approaches have become enriched with more eclectic possibilities and structured therapies, such as dialectical-behavioral therapy for borderline personality disorder (BPD) (Linehan 1993) and various other cognitive psychotherapies (Tyrer and Davidson 2000). Although medications continue to be an adjunct to the treatment of personality disorders, and research medication treatment trials in personality disorders continue to be much fewer than those available in Axis I disorders, medications undoubtedly can play a useful role in the treatment of personality disorders, at least in some disorders and for some patients.

The main indications for using medications in treating personality disorders are periods of decompensation, crises, and hospitalizations; the longer-term management of symptom clusters that are maladaptive and may be responsive to medication; and the reappearance or worsening of comorbid Axis I conditions. Frameworks have been previously described conceptualizing the medication treatment of personality disorders (Coccaro 1993; Gabbard 2000; Kapfhammer and Hippius 1998). Such frameworks must address several interesting questions. Can medication treat the underlying personality disorder per se or simply some of its symptomatic manifestations? Is medication effective at targeting Axis II symptom clusters that lie on a dimensional continuum and are subclinical variants of Axis I conditions? Can medication, in addition, treat unique symptomatology that may be more temperament related and less Axis I bound? Reflecting on these questions necessitates a brief overview of the foundations of personality, as well as an overview of the kinds of changes over time that medication treatment studies of personality disorders examine and the methodological issues involved.

Overview of Personality

Personality can be broadly conceptualized as an admixture of *temperament*, which is strongly determined by genetics, and *character*, which is mainly environmentally shaped. Evidence from population twin studies indicates that personality disorders have a heritable component that presumably is attributable largely to temperament

(Coolidge et al. 2001; Torgersen et al. 2000), with heritability estimates ranging from approximately 0.30 to 0.80, depending on the personality disorder. Additionally, symptom clusters within a personality disorder may have distinct heritabilities. For example, there is evidence in BPD that affective and impulsive traits show independent familial transmission (Silverman et al. 1991).

One of the more widely used temperament models in the mainstream psychiatric literature is Cloninger's psychobiological model of personality, which delineates four basic and independent temperaments—novelty seeking, harm avoidance, reward dependence, and persistence—which contribute about 50% to the formation of personality (Cloninger et al. 1993). It was initially postulated that there was a single neurochemical axis underlying each temperament: dopamine for novelty seeking, serotonin for harm avoidance, and norepinephrine for reward dependence. However, recent genetic studies have not lent support to this simplistic conceptualization but have rather begun to suggest that each temperament dimension may be more complexly determined by several neurochemical systems and specific receptor types (Comings et al. 2000). In addition, we do not yet have behavioral genetic studies confirming the genetic nature of temperament and the nongenetic nature of character, and thus this traditional dichotomy must not be taken for granted (Cravchik and Goldman 2000).

Conversely, when character is being reflected on, other aspects of the personality are evoked, those presumed to be shaped by early parental influences, other environmental effects, trauma, and life stressors, leading to intrapsychic structure or organization characterized by particular self-representations, mechanisms for regulating self-cohesion and self-esteem, internalized object relations, defensive styles, and predominant cognitive schemata. The widely held assumption is that these constituents of character are not predominantly biologically driven and, therefore, are not highly amenable to medication treatment. Although the clinical wisdom of this outlook is largely taken for granted, some caution is called for. The degree to which aspects of character are biologically determined is a largely unexplored area, notable for the absence of studies rather than the presence of negative studies. This is due, at least in part, to the complexity of character concepts, which makes them more difficult to operationalize and study than simple symptoms, as well as the traditional divergence and absence of collaboration between psychodynamic and phenomenologically or biologically oriented scientists. On a second note of caution, the assumption that if something is strongly biologically driven, it will respond better to

pharmacotherapy, and if it is more environmentally determined, it will be more amenable to psychotherapy, is partially a fallacy. Genetically, high cholesterol can be partly treated with appropriate diet. In strongly biologically driven disorders such as obsessive-compulsive disorder (OCD), pharmacotherapy and cognitive-behavioral therapy can have comparable therapeutic efficacy and are accompanied by similar brain activity changes (for details, see Baxter et al. 1992; Schwartz et al. 1996).

Medication and Personality Disorders

Unfortunately, aspects of character organization, and measures of these, traditionally have been excluded from pharmacological trials in treating personality disorders; thus, again we are faced with an absence of studies rather than negative studies. In one small study that partially addressed this question (Mullen et al. 1999), defense mechanisms as measured by the Defense Style Questionnaire and personality organization as measured by the Inventory of Personality Organization were assessed before and after treatment of major depression. Compared with the nonresponders, the responders showed a significant reduction in the use of primitive defenses. Personality organization did not change, but this was assessed in only a small subgroup of patients.

It does make sense that treating symptoms such as affective and impulse dysregulation could have a notable effect on self-perception, self-esteem, and relationships with others and thus could positively affect character, even if not modifying its core. Indeed, several treatment studies of Axis I disorders found a decrease in comorbid Axis II disorders after treatment of the target disorder, and this finding may in part reflect some shift in character structure when gross symptomatology is stabilized (Baer et al. 1992; Noyes et al. 1991). Furthermore, some evidence indicates that patterns of relationships between the more "biologically driven" temperament traits and the more "experience driven" character traits may exist within a given personality disorder. For example, in BPD, the trait of affective instability has been found to be associated with the defenses of splitting, projection, acting out, passive aggression, undoing, and autistic fantasy, whereas the trait of impulsive aggression was positively associated with the defense of acting out and negatively associated with the defenses of suppression and reaction formation (Koenigsberg et al. 2001).

Another caveat in the biological versus nonbiological conceptualization of personality disorders is that some are typically viewed, with some supporting evidence, as more biologically driven than others, possibly lying on a continuum with biologically well-characterized Axis I disorders (Siever et al. 1991). The main biologically driven personality disorders are schizotypal personality disorder, which can be conceptualized as a schizophrenia spectrum disorder with supporting familial and biological data; BPD, which can be viewed as a mood spectrum disorder; and avoidant personality disorder, which may lie on a continuum with social phobia.

Gitlin (1993) described three conceptual frameworks for the pharmacotherapy of personality. The first is categorical, proposing that the medications treat the disorder itself as a whole. This model may be more plausible when one is considering the aforementioned more strongly biologically driven personality disorders. Although it is compelling to speculate that medications may treat more than the manifest symptoms of personality, as we just described, evidence for this is lacking, and we hope that it will be addressed by future study designs.

The second framework is dimensional, most supported by the literature to date, and the one adopted in this chapter. It proposes that pharmacotherapy targets core trait vulnerabilities, manifested as symptom clusters, that may cut across the various personality disorders or may even represent Axis I subclinical variants. The major four such dimensions that are consistently cited in the literature are cognitive–perceptual, impulsivity–aggression, mood instability–lability, and anxiety–behavioral inhibition (see Siever and Davis 1991; Soloff 1990). The various personality disorders thus present with various admixtures of these trait symptom clusters (these are described further in the sections detailing the pharmacological treatment of each disorder).

The third conceptual model speculates that in treating Axis II personality disorders with medication, efficacy results from the treatment of Axis I disorders that may be masked or distorted by the prominent personality features. For example, individuals with avoidant personality disorder may in fact have a very chronic and pervasive generalized type of social phobia that is being interpreted as personality pathology. This model, in our view, has become less useful in recent times as both clinicians and researchers have become more educated and adept in diagnosing on both axes and reflecting on their interactions.

Another important area in critically assessing the medication treatment trials of personality disorders is an awareness of the significant methodological challenges that face this field (Coccaro 1993; Gitlin 1993). A historical issue relates to the fact that the classification of personality disorders changed dramatically with the advent of DSM-III-R in 1987 (American Psychiatric Association 1987); therefore, treatment trials prior to that time can be extrapolated to only currently defined disorders. Fortunately, at least from a research point of view, DSM-IV (American Psychiatric Association 1994) did not introduce much change in classifying Axis II disorders.

Pharmacological treatment studies of personality disorders have assessed to varying degrees the comorbid Axis I or Axis II disorders that may be affecting treatment outcome. Also, personality disorders, particularly those of Cluster B, can notoriously differ in how they manifest at differing points in time. For example, BPD patients can be much more or less symptomatic, depending on a variety of environmental factors. Therefore, the traditional 8- to 12-week trial design that establishes a very-short-term baseline and then measures short-term change to an arbitrary endpoint may not be as ideally suited for studying Axis II as it is for Axis I disorders. Trials that use a more broadly defined baseline, or examine more long-term change across multiple time points, might be more suited to studying Axis II disorders.

Finally, the choice of instruments used to measure Axis II change is critical. Traditionally, these are directly borrowed from Axis I studies, such as the Hamilton Rating Scale for Depression and the Hamilton Anxiety Scale. However, other types of scales measuring less tightly Axis I bound symptoms and concepts such as mood intensity, mood lability, parasuicidal tendencies, aggressive outbursts, and subtle cognitive distortions may be better suited to accurately track Axis II symptomatology. A good example is the Overt Aggression Scale (Coccaro et al. 1991; Yudofsky et al. 1986), which measures and quantifies various types of verbally and physically aggressive behaviors against the self, objects, and others. It is currently widely used in Axis II treatment trials and had no good analog prior to its conception, exemplifying the dimensional approach to personality disorder pathology. Just as important, symptom scales are typically used in Axis II treatment studies rather than measures of character such as defenses, self-concept, personality organization, and interpersonal relationships. Character measures have been pervasively absent from trials to date, and we hope that they will become more prevalent in future studies.

Overview of the Chapter

In this chapter, we review the existing medication trials for the treatment of personality disorders. The chapter is organized by personality disorder clusters, beginning with Cluster B, which has by far the largest number of studies, and followed by Clusters A and C, in which the much fewer existing studies partly overlap with those in Cluster B. We take this pragmatic approach in presenting the treatment studies because the large majority of them selected subjects by personality disorder diagnosis as the major inclusion criterion, although in reviewing these studies, it is always useful to keep in mind the target symptom dimensional approach. Following these sections, the chapter ends with a section on Axis I comorbidity, in which three pertinent questions are addressed: 1) How does the presence of Axis II comorbidity affect the likelihood of medication treatment for Axis I conditions? 2) What is the compliance rate with such treatment? and 3) What is the likelihood of this treatment being efficacious?

Pharmacotherapy for Cluster B Personality Disorders

By far the most extensive literature on pharmacological treatment of Cluster B, or any Axis II disorders for that matter, refers to BPD. The symptom clusters typically targeted in this condition, although varying from trial to trial and in instruments used, are dysregulated impulsivity and aggression, affective lability and hyperreactivity, cognitive-perceptual disorganization, anxiety, and dissociation. Dysregulation of impulses and affective instability are widely viewed as the hallmark symptoms of BPD. The remaining symptom clusters are examined less systematically in BPD studies—for example, when there is a focus on psychotic spectrum or trauma spectrum pathology.

Summary of Medication Trials

Conventional Antipsychotics

Cognitive-perceptual symptoms, such as paranoia, perceptual aberrations, and subtle thought disorder, although not figuring as prominently in the diagnosis of Cluster B as in Cluster A personality disorders, are definitely present in at least a subgroup of BPD patients, especially under periods of stress and decompensation. The presence of such target symptoms, more prominent in the older BPD trials that included schizotypal subgroups of patients, was the impetus for the early neuroleptic trials. Studies from the late 1970s and early 1980s began to report some efficacy of low-dose neuroleptics in treating BPD, although these studies were not placebo controlled (Brinkley et al. 1979; Leone 1982).

Serban and Siegel (1984) reported on a large trial of 52 outpatients with personality disorders (46 completers:

16 with BPD, 14 with schizotypal personality disorder, 16 with both) treated for 12 weeks in a randomized, double-blind design with thiothixene 9.4 mg/day or haloperidol 3 mg/day (mean dosages). Of the total subjects, 84% showed moderate to marked improvement. The main symptoms that improved were cognitive disturbance, derealization, ideas of reference, anxiety, depression, self-esteem, and social functioning, suggesting that medicating target symptoms may have a wide-reaching effect. Outcome did not vary by borderline or schizotypal diagnosis. In another study (Montgomery and Montgomery 1982), patients with personality disorders, mostly borderline, presenting acutely with a suicide attempt and with histories of at least two prior attempts were treated with a low-dose depot neuroleptic (flupenthixol 20 mg every 4 weeks) or placebo. The neuroleptic was highly effective in reducing suicide attempts at 4–6 months of treatment. Shortly after and for the next decade, several placebo-controlled, randomized trials were published examining conventional antipsychotics in the treatment of BPD and comparing these agents with other classes of medications such as antidepressants, mood stabilizers, and benzodiazepines.

Goldberg et al. (1986) studied 50 outpatients (17 with BPD, 13 with schizotypal personality disorder, 20 with both) with a bias toward psychotic presentation: at least one psychotic symptom was required for inclusion. Subjects were treated for 12 weeks with thiothixene (average dosage = 9 mg/day) or placebo. Thiothixene was significantly better than placebo in treating psychosis (especially for greater symptom severity at baseline), obsessive-compulsive symptoms, and phobic anxiety, but not depression. The results suggested narrow efficacy, because total scores for borderline pathology, schizotypal pathology, and global assessment did not change. When the results were analyzed by diagnosis, the pure BPD subgroup showed the smallest medication effect, implying that neuroleptics may have target specificity for psychotic spectrum symptoms.

Another study, however, suggested that low-dose neuroleptics have a more global effect in treating BPD (Soloff et al. 1986, 1989). Ninety acutely hospitalized inpatients (35 with BPD, 4 with schizotypal personality disorder, and 51 with both) were treated for 5 weeks with haloperidol (average dosage = 5 mg/day), amitriptyline (average dosage = 150 mg/day), or placebo. Haloperidol was found to have a broad-spectrum effect in symptom domains, including schizotypal, affective, and impulsive-behavioral, and was superior to amitriptyline in all areas with the exception of a comparable weak antidepressant effect. As in the Goldberg et al. (1986) study, more severe psychotic spectrum symptoms predicted a better response to halo-peridol, although overall improvement was still modest.

However, these results were not replicated by the same investigator group in a subsequent large study with a very similar design, consisting of 108 consecutively admitted inpatients (42 with BPD, 66 with BPD and schizotypal personality disorder) treated for 5 weeks with haloperidol, the monoamine oxidase inhibitor (MAOI) phenelzine, or placebo (Soloff et al. 1993). This study failed to replicate efficacy for haloperidol (average dosage = 4 mg/day), with the exception of some measures of overt hostile or aggressive behavior. The investigators attributed this discrepancy to the presence of more severely ill psychotic spectrum patients in the earlier studies and suggested that in less impaired BPD populations, low-dose neuroleptics had little to contribute and were poorly tolerated in terms of side effects. The above acute treatment study was extended into a 16-week outpatient continuation trial with 54 continuing participants (Cornelius et al. 1993), which again yielded essentially negative results. Haloperidol was effective only in treating irritability, and two-thirds of the subjects dropped out.

Another frequently cited medication trial in BPD is a double-blind, placebo-controlled comparison of the typical antipsychotic trifluoperazine (average dosage = 8 mg/day), the benzodiazepine anxiolytic alprazolam (average dosage = 5 mg/day), the anticonvulsant and mood stabilizer carbamazepine (average dosage = 820 mg/day), and the MAOI tranylcypromine (average dosage = 40 mg/day) (Cowdry and Gardner 1988). This study found very modest effects for neuroleptic treatment. Trifluoperazine was only associated with a trend toward lessened behavioral dyscontrol, whereas alprazolam led to paradoxical disinhibition and worsening of severe behavioral dyscontrol. Psychotic-like symptoms were not assessed. Conventional antipsychotic studies in BPD are summarized in Table 61–1.

Atypical Antipsychotics

The question of efficacy of atypical antipsychotics in BPD has received growing attention (see Table 61–1), and earlier smaller trials have now been followed by larger studies. An open trial of clozapine in 15 severely disturbed patients with refractory BPD and pronounced psychotic symptoms reported an overall 33% improvement during a 2- to 9-month treatment (Frankenburg and Zanarini 1993). Given the weekly monitoring and the common compliance difficulties of BPD patients, this antipsychotic is clearly not the optimal choice for the average patient. A case report noted partial to good response to ari-

piprazole treatment in 2 out of 3 patients (Mobascher et al. 2006). A small 8-week placebo-controlled risperidone trial in BPD reported similar modest symptomatic improvement in the two treatment groups (Schulz et al. 1998). An open-label trial of risperidone in 15 BPD outpatients with prominent histories of aggressive behavior and no current major Axis I disorders, using a final mean dosage of 3.3 mg/day, reported a marked reduction in aggression, along with a reduction in depressive symptoms and improved global functioning (Rocca et al. 2002).

To date, there are three published quetiapine treatment trials in BPD, all open-label. In one 12-week trial in 23 outpatients, at a mean dosage of 250 mg/day, impulsivity significantly improved, as did most other outcome measures and global functioning (Villeneuve and Lemelin 2005). Another 12-week trial in 14 outpatients employed an average dosage of about 300 mg/day and reported significant improvement in various symptom domains, particularly impulsiveness/aggressiveness (Bellino et al. 2006). The third open trial followed 29 outpatients for 12 weeks, at a higher average dosage of 540 mg/day, and reported a highly significant improvement in a number of BPD features, including aggression and low mood; transient thrombocytopenia occurred in 2 patients (Perrella et al. 2007). Finally, a case report described a marked improvement in severe self-mutilation in two BPD patients treated with quetiapine (Hilger et al. 2003).

An 8-week open trial examined the efficacy of olanzapine (average dosage = 8 mg/day) in 11 BPD outpatients with comorbid dysthymia, 7 of whom also had schizotypal personality disorder, and reported moderate significant improvement in all symptom domains (Schulz et al. 1999). In a small controlled olanzapine trial of 28 women with BPD (Zanarini and Frankenburg 2001), longer duration of treatment was undertaken for 6 months, a time frame more reflective of clinical reality, at a mean end dose of 5.3 mg/day. Olanzapine was found to be significantly better than placebo in decreasing anxiety, paranoia, anger/hostility, and interpersonal sensitivity, but not depression.

More recently, two much larger randomized, controlled multicenter trials have yielded mixed findings on the efficacy of olanzapine in treating BPD. One 12-week study used flexibly dosed olanzapine (range 2.5–20 mg/day) versus placebo in 314 outpatient participants with moderate disorder severity, and although both treatment groups significantly improved during treatment, there was no difference in overall change between the two groups (P = 0.66), with response rates of 65% for olanzapine and 54% for placebo group (Schulz et al. 2007). The second 12-week study of 451 BPD participants was overall similar

TABLE 61–1. Summary of medication treatment trials with antipsychotics in borderline personality disorder (BPD)

Study	Subjects	Antipsychotic(s)	Other agent(s)	Duration	Outcome
Typical antipsychotics					
Montgomery and Montgomery 1982	30 BPD	Depot flupenthixol	Placebo	4–6 months	Decreased suicide attempts
Serban and Siegel 1984	16 BPD, 14 SPD, 16 both	Thiothixene, haloperidol	—	12 weeks	Improvement on multiple domains
Goldberg et al. 1986	17 BPD, 13 SPD, 20 both	Thiothixene	Placebo	12 weeks	Decreased psychosis, anxiety
Soloff et al. 1986, 1989	35 BPD, 4 SPD, 51 both	Haloperidol	Amitriptyline, placebo	5 weeks	General improvement
Cowdry and Gardner 1988	16 BPD	Trifluoperazine	Alprazolam, carbamazepine, tranylcypromine, placebo	6-week crossover	Minimal decrease in behavioral dyscontrol; psychoticism not measured
Soloff et al. 1993	42 BPD, 66 BPD and SPD	Haloperidol	Phenelzine, placebo	5 weeks	Largely ineffective
Cornelius et al. 1993	Continuation of above study			16-week extension	
Atypical antipsychotics					
Frankenburg and Zanarini 1993	15 refractory BPD	Clozapine	—	2–9 months	33% overall improvement
Schulz et al. 1998	BPD	Risperidone	Placebo	8 weeks	Modest improvement, no better than placebo
Schulz et al. 1999	11 BPD (7 also SPD)	Olanzapine	—	8 weeks	General modest to moderate improvement
Zanarini and Frankenburg 2001	28 BPD	Olanzapine	Placebo	6 months	Decreased anger, paranoia, anxiety, interpersonal sensitivity
Rocca et al. 2002	15 BPD with marked aggression	Risperidone	—	8 weeks	Decreased aggression, improved global functioning
Villeneuve and Lemelin 2005	23 BPD	Quetiapine	—	12 weeks	Improved impulsivity, other measures, and global function
Bellino et al. 2006	14 BPD	Quetiapine	—	12 weeks	Improvement especially for impulsiveness/aggressiveness
Perrella et al. 2007	29 BPD	Quetiapine	—	12 weeks	Improvement especially in aggression and low mood
Schulz et al. 2007	314 BPD	Olanzapine 2.5–20 mg/day	Placebo	12 weeks	No difference in overall symptom improvement between groups
Zanarini et al. 2007	451 BPD	Low-dose olanzapine (2.5 mg/day), moderate-dose olanzapine (5–10 mg/day)	Placebo	12 weeks	Greater overall improvement on moderate-dose olanzapine compared with two other groups

Note.   SPD=schizotypal personality disorder.

in design and illness severity but differed in using two fixed dosages of olanzapine, low (2.5 mg/day) and moderate (5–10 mg/day), versus placebo (Zanarini et al. 2007). Treatment with the higher olanzapine dose resulted in significantly greater overall improvement than the lower dose (P=0.018) and the placebo (P=0.006), with response rates of 74%, 60%, and 58%, respectively. Furthermore, both olanzapine-treated groups showed significantly greater improvement on irritability, suicidality, and family life functioning relative to placebo. Adverse events more common on olanzapine included somnolence and weight gain (3.2 kilograms for the higher dose).

Antidepressants

Tricyclic antidepressants (TCAs) have a limited role in treating BPD (Soloff et al. 1986, 1989). The few MAOI trials that have been conducted have yielded mixed results. Soloff et al. (1993) and Cornelius et al. (1993) found that phenelzine had only modest efficacy in BPD and was superior to placebo only against anger and hostility, but not in measures of depression, atypical depression, psychoticism, impulsivity, or global borderline severity. The investigators speculated that the short duration of treatment, the use of suboptimal phenelzine dosing (average dosage=60 mg/day), and the fact that the atypical depression characteristics known to be responsive to MAOIs were not highly prominent in the patient samples may have contributed to these studies' failure to show efficacy for phenelzine. In contrast, a crossover placebo-controlled study of four classes of medications in BPD (Cowdry and Gardner 1988) found that the MAOI tranylcypromine was significantly superior to placebo, according to both clinicians and patients, in global ratings and in most domains that were measured, including depression, anxiety, anger, rejection sensitivity, impulsivity, and suicidality. This finding was more in accordance with an earlier report of phenelzine efficacy in BPD patients, all of whom had concurrent atypical depression (Parsons et al. 1989).

Regardless of efficacy, both TCAs and MAOIs pose serious overdose and dangerous adverse effect risks that are of particular concern in this unstable, impulsive population. Investigations of newer antidepressants in treating BPD appear more promising. Preliminary reports in small open trials first suggested that the selective serotonin reuptake inhibitor (SSRI) fluoxetine at dosages ranging from 20 to 60 mg/day might be beneficial in treating depression and impulsive aggression in BPD (Coccaro et al. 1990; Cornelius et al. 1991; Norden 1989). A larger open trial (Markovitz et al. 1991) involved 22 patients

with BPD or schizotypal personality disorder treated for 12 weeks with high-dose fluoxetine (80 mg/day). There was a 74% decline in self-mutilation, as well as an overall improvement in depressive symptoms, obsessive-compulsive symptoms, anxiety, interpersonal sensitivity, psychoticism, and paranoia. In a comparable open trial by the same group (Markovitz 1995), 23 BPD patients were treated openly for an initial 12-week period with sertraline 200 mg/day, and about half showed improvement in self-injurious behavior, anxiety, depression, and suicidality. Of note, half of the responders had previously failed to respond to fluoxetine, underlining the usefulness of trying more than one SSRI in this population, given the variability of responses across SSRIs. The trial was continued to a 1-year duration, and dosages in nonresponders were increased to more than 300 mg/day. By the completion of the study, on average, depression had decreased by 56% and self-injurious episodes had decreased by 93%. In another small open trial of sertraline in nine patients with personality disorders, dosages of 100–200 mg/day resulted in a decrease of impulsive aggression over 8 weeks (Kavoussi et al. 1994).

Subsequently, three controlled trials of SSRIs in borderline spectrum patients have been described. In a small double-blind trial, 17 BPD patients were randomly assigned to high-dose fluoxetine (80 mg/day) or placebo for 14 weeks. A statistically significant improvement was seen in the fluoxetine group, compared with placebo, on all measures used, including global symptomatology, anxiety, and depression (Markovitz 1995). A larger study randomly assigned 27 patients with borderline disorder or traits, at the milder end of the severity spectrum and without current major depression, to fluoxetine (average dosage=40 mg/day) or placebo (Salzman et al. 1995). The main finding after 12 weeks of treatment was a significantly greater decrease in anger and depression with fluoxetine, despite a pronounced placebo response. Finally, in the largest trial reported (Coccaro and Kavoussi 1997), the effects of fluoxetine were investigated over a 12-week period in 40 subjects with personality disorder with marked impulsive aggression as the major entry criterion and without current major depression. About half of the subjects met Cluster B criteria (one-third of the total had BPD), 40% met Cluster C criteria, and 28% met Cluster A criteria. Compared with placebo, fluoxetine at dosages of 20–60 mg/day led to a consistent and significant decrease in aggression and irritability and in global improvement apparent by the second month of treatment, and this effect was irrespective of changes in depression or anxiety.

In addition to SSRIs, newer antidepressants have been tried in BPD. In an open trial of the serotonin–norepinephrine reuptake inhibitor (SNRI) venlafaxine, 45 subjects were entered and 39 completed a 12-week treatment with an average dosage of 315 mg/day (Markovitz and Wagner 1995). A highly significant overall reduction of 41% occurred on a scale of global symptomatology. Of the 7 patients who were self-injurious at baseline, only 2 remained self-injurious at the end of treatment. Although the study was not placebo controlled, this was a fairly large trial, and the results appear promising. Studies of antidepressant treatment in BPD are summarized in Table 61–2.

Mood Stabilizers

Mood stabilizers also have emerged as highly promising in treating BPD. The literature on lithium is unfortunately limited to older studies but looks promising. Most studies examined the effects of lithium on aggression in mentally retarded or violent inmate populations and reported some efficacy (reviewed by Wickham and Reed 1987). More directly relevant to BPD, an older study had first documented the efficacy of lithium in treating mood lability (other symptoms were not measured) in a 6-week placebo-controlled trial of 21 subjects with "emotionally unstable character disorder" (Rifkin et al. 1972). Description of the characteristics of this disorder, such as mood swings, overreactivity, impulsivity, and chronic maladaptive behaviors, clearly overlaps with current BPD criteria, although these patients may have had a bipolar variant. Finally, a single small controlled study examined lithium in subjects meeting clear BPD criteria (Links et al. 1990). Seventeen subjects received 6 weeks each of lithium, the TCA desipramine, and placebo in a randomized crossover design, and 10 completed at least two medication trials. Neither medication was better than placebo for depressive symptoms, but lithium resulted in a significant decrease in anger and suicidality according to clinician, but not patient, perception. A larger study is clearly warranted but has not been done.

Anticonvulsants are used more widely than lithium in treating BPD. Cowdry and Gardner (1988) found that carbamazepine led to a dramatic and highly significant decrease in behavioral dyscontrol but had much more modest effects on mood, and patients subjectively did not feel better while taking it. This was a 6-week double-blind, placebo-controlled crossover design, comparing alprazolam (average dosage = 5 mg/day), carbamazepine (average dosage = 820 mg/day), trifluoperazine (average dosage = 8 mg/day), and tranylcypromine (average dosage = 40 mg/

day) (Cowdry and Gardner 1988). Subjects were 16 female outpatients with BPD, with additional inclusion criteria of presence of prominent behavioral dyscontrol and absence of current major depression. However, another carbamazepine study, involving 20 inpatients with BPD without concurrent depression or concomitant medications, yielded negative results (De La Fuenta and Lotstra 1994). After 4 weeks of treatment at standard therapeutic drug levels, carbamazepine was no better than placebo in treating depression, behavioral dyscontrol, or global symptomatology.

More recently, anticonvulsant trials have focused on valproate and, to a lesser extent, on the newer anticonvulsants. In one open trial, 11 patients with BPD were treated openly with valproate for 8 weeks, attaining blood levels of 50–100 µg/mL, and 8 patients completed the trial (Stein et al. 1995). Half of the completers were rated as overall responders, with significant decreases in depression, anxiety, anger, impulsivity, rejection sensitivity, and irritability. The trial was summarized as modestly helpful, and larger controlled studies were called for to establish valproate efficacy in BPD. In another open-label trial, 20 BPD patients were treated for 12 weeks with extended-release valproate, leading to significant overall improvement and decline in irritability and aggression (Simeon et al. 2007). In another small but placebo-controlled trial, 16 outpatients with BPD were treated for 10 weeks with valproate or placebo (Hollander et al. 2001). Global improvement was significant by two measures in patients treated with valproate, but the small sample size and dropout rate precluded statistically significant findings. In another controlled valproate study, efficacy was examined in 30 women with comorbid BPD and bipolar II disorder over 6 months of treatment (Frankenburg and Zanarini 2002). Valproate at an average dosage of 850 mg/day (with blood levels ranging between 50 and 100 µg/mL) was well tolerated and resulted in significant improvement in interpersonal sensitivity, hostility/anger, and aggression compared with placebo.

More importantly, there is now a large placebo-controlled multicenter trial of valproate focusing on the treatment of impulsive aggression in Cluster B personality disorders (Hollander et al. 2003). Ninety-one outpatients selected for the presence of prominent impulsive aggression and absence of bipolar I disorder or current major depression were randomly assigned to 12 weeks of treatment with placebo or valproate, at an average end dosage of 1,400 mg/day with an end mean blood level of 66 µg/mL. About 10% were taking concomitant stable doses of antidepressants, and there was an approximately equal drop-

TABLE 61–2. Summary of medication treatment trials with antidepressants in borderline personality disorder (BPD)

STUDY	SUBJECTS	ANTIDEPRESSANT(S)	OTHER AGENT(S)	DURATION	OUTCOME
Soloff et al. 1986, 1989	35 BPD, 4 SPD, 51 both	Amitriptyline	Haloperidol, placebo	5 weeks	Minimally effective and only for depression
Soloff et al. 1993	42 BPD, 66 BPD and SPD	Phenelzine	Haloperidol, placebo	5 weeks	Modest efficacy, better than placebo
Cornelius et al. 1993	Continuation of above study			16-week extension	Only for hostility/anger
Cowdry and Gardner 1988	16 BPD	Tranylcypromine	Alprazolam, carbamazepine, trifluoperazine, placebo	6-week crossover	Decreased depression, anxiety, anger, rejection sensitivity, impulsivity, suicidality
Markovitz et al. 1991	22 BPD or SPD	Fluoxetine	—	12 weeks	Marked decline in self-mutilation, depression, anxiety, interpersonal sensitivity, paranoia
Markovitz 1995	23 BPD	Sertraline	—	12 weeks	Half of subjects showed improvement in self-injury, anxiety, depression, suicidality
	Continuation of above study			1 year	Decline in depression 56%, self-injury 93%
Kavoussi et al. 1994	9 personality disorder with impulsive aggression	Sertraline	—	8 weeks	Decreased impulsive aggression
Markovitz 1995	17 BPD	Fluoxetine	Placebo	14 weeks	Global improvement on all measures
Salzman et al. 1995	27 BPD or BPD traits	Fluoxetine	Placebo	12 weeks	Decreased anger, depression
Coccaro and Kavoussi 1997	40 impulsive-aggressive personality disorder (one-third BPD), no major depression	Fluoxetine	Placebo	12 weeks	Marked decrease in aggression and irritability irrespective of changes in anxiety/depression
Markovitz and Wagner 1995	45 BPD	Venlafaxine	—	12 weeks	40% global improvement, less self-injury

Note. SPD = schizotypal personality disorder.

out rate of almost half of the subjects in each group. Valproate was well tolerated overall, with 17% of the subjects discontinuing for valproate-related adverse events. The main finding of the study was a significant decrease in impulsive aggression in the last month of treatment, reflected in significantly greater than placebo declines in overall aggression, including verbal assault, assault against objects, and assault against others, and in overall irritability. When the BPD subgroup of the above study was examined separately (Hollander et al. 2005), it was found that divalproex was indeed superior to placebo in reducing impulsive aggression in this subgroup. Divalproex-treated patients responded better as a function of higher baseline trait impulsivity symptoms and state aggression symptoms. These two effects appeared to be independent of one another, while baseline affective instability did not influence differential treatment response.

With respect to the newer anticonvulsants, there is a report of a small open trial of lamotrigine, 75–300 mg/day, while concomitant psychotropic medications were tapered off, in eight patients with BPD without concurrent major depression (Pinto and Akiskal 1998). Two subjects were discontinued secondary to adverse events or noncompliance, and three did not respond. The remaining three were described as robust responders, with a marked increase in their overall level of functioning; a cessation of impulsive behaviors such as promiscuity, substance abuse, and suicidality; and maintenance of response at 1-year follow-up. We can probably expect further trials of new anticonvulsants in BPD. Medication trials of mood stabilizers in BPD are summarized in Table 61–3.

Other Medications

Another class of medications for which very limited data exist on treating BPD is the opioid antagonists. A more extensive literature supports the efficacy of naltrexone in treating impulsive addictive behaviors such as alcoholism and gambling, and therefore naltrexone would be a consideration in borderline patients with these types of problems. An open trial of naltrexone at daily dosages of 100–400 mg in 15 women with BPD found that it led to a significant decrease in dissociative symptoms and flashbacks over a course of treatment of at least 2 weeks (Bohus et al. 1999).

Conclusions and Treatment Guidelines

In conclusion, several open and controlled pharmacological treatment trials of BPD have been conducted. Interpretation of the findings is somewhat complicated by the diversity of patient presentations at treatment entry, including inpatient or outpatient status; overall severity of baseline pathology; presence of comorbid personality disorders; presence or absence of major depression, including atypical symptoms; emphasis on varying symptomatology, such as psychoticism or impulsive aggression; and use of a wide range of change measures. In addition, some of the core features of the disorder, such as identity diffusion, interpersonal vicissitudes, and primitive defensive structure, were never examined, and thus the assumption that these features are less medication responsive has not been empirically proven. As mentioned earlier, it is not unreasonable to assume that stabilization and alleviation of dysregulated affect, cognition, and impulses could have a beneficial effect on "deeper" aspects of character structure. Furthermore, concomitant psychotherapy is rarely mentioned as an exclusion criterion in the BPD medication trials, and clinical knowledge of these populations makes it reasonable to assume that it must have commonly co-occurred, even if of a general exploratory and supportive nature and not specifically geared to the structured treatment of the condition. We therefore cannot underestimate the potential influence of general placebo effects and concomitant therapies in many of these studies, and medications continue to be viewed as adjuvant features of treating patients with Cluster B disorders.

Notwithstanding, it is reasonable to conclude that three classes of medications emerge as the most useful in treating BPD: serotonin reuptake inhibitors, mood stabilizers, and atypical antipsychotics. Fluoxetine, valproate, and olanzapine are the three best-studied medications to date regarding efficacy. Comparison trials of these three classes of medications, including combination strategies, have not been reported and would be of great interest in the future.

Dosing guidelines are also not entirely clear because most trials aim to minimize possible undertreatment and tend to use relatively high dosages. Therefore, SSRIs may be efficacious at lower dosages than the 60 or 80 mg/day fluoxetine target dosages that have been studied. There are also no guidelines for targeted blood levels of valproate in treating BPD, although a recent large trial reported efficacy at a mean endpoint blood level of 66 μg/mL (Hollander et al. 2003). For olanzapine, it appears that moderate doses are more effective than low doses (Zanarini et al. 2007). In clinical settings, it makes sense to start with lower doses because these are generally better tolerated and gradually increase the dosage while carefully monitoring response to increasing dose. Symptoms of the disorder are often chronic and by their nature con-

TABLE 61–3. Summary of medication treatment trials with mood stabilizers in borderline personality disorder (BPD)

STUDY	SUBJECTS	MOOD STABILIZER(S)	OTHER AGENT(S)	DURATION	OUTCOME
Rifkin et al. 1972	21 emotionally unstable character disorder	Lithium	Placebo	6 weeks	Decreased mood lability
Cowdry and Gardner 1988	16 BPD	Carbamazepine	Trifluoperazine, tranyl-cypromine, alprazolam, placebo	6-week crossover	Marked decrease in behavioral dyscontrol
Links et al. 1990	17 BPD	Lithium	Desipramine, placebo	6-week crossover	Decreased anger and suicidality
De La Fuenta and Lotstra 1994	20 BPD without depression	Carbamazepine	Placebo	4 weeks	No effect for depression, behavioral dyscontrol, global symptoms
Stein et al. 1995	11 BPD	Valproate	—	8 weeks	Modest benefit, half responders, less depression, anxiety, anger, impulsivity, rejection sensitivity
Pinto and Akiskal 1998	8 BPD without depression	Lamotrigine	—	1 year	Two discontinued; three robust global responders with decreased impulsivity and suicidality
Frankenburg and Zanarini 2002	30 BPD	Valproate	Placebo	6 months	Significant improvement in hostility, anger, aggression, interpersonal sensitivity
Hollander et al. 2003	91 impulsive-aggressive Cluster B	Valproate	Placebo	12 weeks	Significant decrease in impulsive aggression
Simeon et al. 2007	20 BPD	Valproate extended release	—	12 weeks	Overall improvement, decreased irritability and aggression

siderably fluctuating; thus, the effect of each medication and dose can be more reliably assessed over longer rather than shorter durations.

With respect to specific target symptoms, certain algorithms can be extrapolated from the existent trials and have been proposed on the basis of the types of symptoms that are most prevalent in each patient and the degree of response to the various medication pathways (American Psychiatric Association 2001; Soloff 1998). These algorithms give useful practical guidance, although they tend to become quickly outdated with findings of new trials. On the basis of the existent algorithms in the literature and modifying them according to the results of the latest medication trials, we propose a medication treatment approach outline for BPD as summarized in Table 61–4.

Almost all Cluster B personality disorder trials have focused primarily on BPD. Although some of these trials, as individually mentioned in the overview above, included mixed samples of Cluster B participants, they did not present separate analyses for non-BPD diagnoses. Therefore, the general principle to follow in treating these other disorders would be to target symptom clusters with medications as per the guidelines developed above for BPD. In general, narcissistic and histrionic personality disorders are not characterized by the severe degree of either mood lability or impulse dyscontrol encountered in BPD, but in individuals in whom such features are more prominent or problematic, medication trials can be attempted. With regard to antisocial personality disorder, the general treatment guideline is that individuals who meet full criteria for the disorder are generally treatment noncompliant and nonresponsive. Very few pharmacological studies have been done in patients with antisocial personality disorder (Coccaro 1993), and those closest to showing at least temporary benefits are some of the earlier lithium studies that reported decreased impulsive-aggressive behavior in prison inmates (Wickham and Reed 1987). More recently, a report on four antisocial personality disorder inpatients in a maximum-security facility found decreases in impulsivity, hostility, aggressiveness, irritability, and rage reactions with quetiapine treatment at dosages of 600–800 mg/day (Walker et al. 2003). Generally, borderline patients who have some antisocial traits are more responsive to medication treatment than purely antisocial patients. Recent studies with the mood stabilizer valproate suggest that subjects with antisocial personality disorder are less responsive to the pharmacotherapy than are subjects with other Cluster B personality disorders (Hollander et al. 2003). It also has been found that borderline patients are significantly more likely than

TABLE 61–4. Psychopharmacological treatment guidelines for borderline personality disorder

If most prominent symptoms are depression, interpersonal sensitivity, and impulsivity and aggression

1. Start with selective serotonin reuptake inhibitor (SSRI) (or related antidepressant).
2. *If good response*, maintain.
   If partial response, add mood stabilizer.
   If no response, switch to mood stabilizer.
3. *If significant residual anger, anxiety, dyscontrol*, add atypical antipsychotic.

If most prominent symptoms are mood lability, impulsivity and aggression, and family history of bipolar spectrum

1. Start with mood stabilizer (valproate; carbamazepine or lithium as alternatives).
2. *If good response*, maintain.
   If partial response, add mood stabilizer.
   If no response, switch to mood stabilizer.
3. *If significant residual anger, anxiety, dyscontrol*, add atypical antipsychotic.

If most prominent symptoms are paranoia, psychoticism, hostility, and overwhelming anxiety

1. Start with atypical antipsychotic (olanzapine and risperidone most studied).
2. *If good response*, maintain.
   If partial response, add SSRI or mood stabilizer.
   If no response and minimal mood symptoms, switch to typical antipsychotic.

antisocial personality disorder patients to have received adequate medication trials, including anxiolytics and antidepressants (Zanarini et al. 1988).

Pharmacotherapy for Cluster A Personality Disorders

Cluster A personality disorders are characterized by cognitive distortions, perceptual distortions, mild thought disorder, constricted affectivity, and interpersonal mistrust and distance. Schizotypal personality disorder is the prime example of all these symptom clusters, whereas in paranoid and schizoid personality disorders, the cognitive-perceptual and thought disorder disturbances are not prominent. Cluster A symptoms are reminiscent of both the positive and the negative symptoms of schizophrenia,

and dopaminergic dysregulation has been postulated to underlie them (Siever and Davis 1991). Schizotypal personality disorder is by far the most extensively investigated disorder of the cluster in terms of biological underpinnings (Siever 1985; Siever et al. 1990), relation to Axis I as a schizophrenia spectrum disorder (Asarnow et al. 2001; Kendler et al. 1994), and pharmacological treatment trials. All the treatment trials to date, however, have included subjects typically with BPD or with mixed personality disorders. They have been presented already in the Cluster B section, and we summarize them again here with respect to schizotypy findings. We are not aware of any medication trials examining specifically paranoid or schizoid personality disorder.

Serban and Siegel (1984) treated a sample of patients, one-third of whom had schizotypal personality disorder and one-third of whom had schizotypal personality disorder and BPD, with either thiothixene or haloperidol, without placebo, and found marked improvement in psychotic spectrum symptoms. Goldberg et al. (1986) treated a similar sample with thiothixene or placebo and found a significant improvement in psychotic symptoms with thiothixene that was more pronounced in the patients with the schizotypal rather than the borderline diagnosis. Soloff et al. (1986, 1989), in a sample containing a sizable proportion of combined schizotypal personality disorder and BPD patients, found significantly better efficacy for haloperidol compared with placebo for schizotypal symptoms but were not able to replicate this finding in a subsequent haloperidol trial with similar diagnoses (Soloff et al. 1993). They speculated that their failure to replicate might have been because the later trial included a less disturbed group of subjects with less prominent psychotic symptoms.

With regard to the treatment of schizotypy with atypical antipsychotics, Schulz et al. (1999) reported improvement in psychotic symptoms in a small group of patients who received olanzapine, most of whom had schizotypal personality disorder that was comorbid with BPD. There is one published randomized, placebo-controlled trial of an atypical antipsychotic focusing exclusively on schizotypal personality disorder, which found risperidone to be significantly more efficacious than placebo (Koenigsberg et al. 2002). In this 9-week study in 25 schizotypal personality disorder patients, with low incidence of comorbid depression or BPD, low-dose risperidone was used, titrated up from 0.25 to 2 mg/day. Active medication resulted in a significantly greater decrease in negative and positive symptoms compared to placebo, and side effects were generally well tolerated.

With regard to the effect of antidepressants on schizotypal personality disorder, Markovitz et al. (1991) conducted an open trial of fluoxetine in patients with BPD and schizotypal personality disorder (proportions of each unspecified) and reported improvement in psychoticism and paranoia, among numerous other symptoms. Although the results were not analyzed with respect to diagnosis, it is notable that no worsening of psychotic spectrum symptoms was found. This finding is difficult to interpret in that improved paranoia could be consequent to better affective regulation in subjects with prominent borderline traits. Of note, an older trial reported increased hostility and paranoia in a subgroup of patients treated with the TCA amitriptyline (Soloff et al. 1986, 1989). Finally, a large trial of fluoxetine that found significant benefits for impulsive aggression across Axis II disorders (Coccaro and Kavoussi 1997) included 28% Cluster A subjects, but results did not focus on psychotic spectrum symptoms and were not presented separately by cluster.

In summary, the limited trials of Cluster A disorders suggest, not surprisingly, that the medications of choice are conventional antipsychotics. Given the probable need for long-term treatment of the chronic, stable psychotic spectrum symptoms in these populations, the better safety profile of atypical antipsychotics with regard to tardive dyskinesia suggests that they should be tried first, although more data exist in the literature to date examining conventional neuroleptics. Finally, in subjects with mixed traits and prominent additional affective or impulsive symptoms, SSRIs appear to cause no worsening of psychosis and may be of some adjuvant benefit.

Pharmacotherapy for Cluster C Personality Disorders

Anxiety and behavioral inhibition are the main symptoms that characterize individuals with Cluster C personality disorders, although the focus of the anxiety varies across disorders. It centers on social interaction in avoidant personality disorder, need for control of uncertainty in obsessive-compulsive personality disorder, and conflicts surrounding autonomy in dependent personality disorder. The medication trials in these disorders are very limited to date and are summarized below. In addition, limited indirect information and insights can be gauged from studies either of related Axis I disorders or of personality traits or dimensions that are characteristic of the Cluster C personality disorders.

Avoidant personality disorder has received the most attention in terms of pharmacological treatment of the Cluster C disorders because it is often viewed as lying on a continuum with Axis I social phobia. Clinically, it can be difficult to distinguish pervasive, generalized social phobia of long-standing duration from avoidant personality disorder. The latter tends to be characterized by deeper interpersonal difficulties, impairments in interpersonal skills, and a very small number of close relationships, which is often not the case even in very socially phobic individuals (Turner et al. 1986). Numerous studies have convincingly shown the efficacy of MAOIs and SSRIs in social phobia, including its generalized subtype. Although, unfortunately, these studies did not report on the presence or change in avoidant personality, they do suggest that these medications may be worth trying in treating the Axis II variant. Indeed, a few open trials and case reports have reported promising findings.

Deltito and Perugi (1986) reported the case of a man with pervasive social phobia and avoidant personality disorder who responded well to phenelzine 45 mg/day, with an overall improvement in his social adjustment. Subsequently, another four cases were described of individuals with avoidant personality disorder who responded to MAOIs or fluoxetine, showing increased social confidence and well-being (Deltito and Stam 1989). Liebowitz et al. (1988) also described a sizable proportion of generalized social phobia patients who also met avoidant personality disorder criteria and showed substantial overall gain in social and occupational functioning when they were given phenelzine. However, in all these reports, most, if not all, avoidant subjects had comorbid social phobia, and the criteria used to differentiate the two conditions and their medication response were not clearly defined. In a more systematic approach, Reich et al. (1989) openly treated 14 patients with DSM-III-R social phobia with alprazolam for 8 weeks at a mean daily dosage of 3 mg and specifically measured treatment response in nine avoidant personality traits based on the DSM-III-R diagnostic criteria for avoidant personality disorder. Six of the nine avoidant traits showed significant improvement during treatment, correlating with a change in subjective anxiety and disability. Further pharmacological studies with precise dissection of social phobia from avoidant personality would be of great interest.

There is hardly any literature on the pharmacological treatment of obsessive-compulsive personality disorder. Although Axis I OCD is well known to respond to serotonin reuptake inhibitors, and the older psychodynamic literature merged the two conditions as obsessional neu-

rosis, recent studies dispute the notion that the Axis I and II variants are related. The older literature suggested the presence of definite obsessional traits in as many as two-thirds of patients with OCD, but structured personality assessments were not used. In more recent standardized evaluations, only a minority of patients with OCD had DSM-III-R obsessive-compulsive personality disorder, but other personality disorders such as avoidant or dependent were more common (Thomsen and Mikkelsen 1993). In addition, personality disorders may be more common in the presence of longer OCD duration, suggesting that they could be secondary to the Axis I disorder, and criteria for personality disorders may no longer be met after successful treatment of the OCD (Baer et al. 1990, 1992). However, a recent study presented evidence in favor of a familial spectrum of OCD and obsessive-compulsive personality disorder (Samuels et al. 2000). Regardless, no medication trials have examined this personality disorder per se, and SSRI trials in severe obsessive-compulsive personality disorder would be of some interest.

One report from the early 1990s claimed that major depression in the presence of comorbid compulsive personality disorder showed better response to serotonin reuptake inhibitors than that in the absence of comorbid compulsive personality (Ansseau et al. 1991). However, this finding has not been replicated, and methodological issues have been raised, including the validity of the distinction between preexisting obsessional personality and depression-related obsessional states (Pollitt and Tyrer 1992).

We are also not aware of studies examining the pharmacological treatment of dependent personality disorder. It has been reported in the presence of comorbid Axis I panic disorder, in particular, that the initial rate of dependent personality traits was to a large extent state related and waned with the treatment of panic over a 3-year period (Noyes et al. 1991).

Finally, one study examined change in core symptoms of Cluster C disorders, as measured by personality inventories in the absence of categorical Axis II assessment, in patients treated pharmacologically for Axis I disorders (Brody et al. 2000). In 37 patients treated with SSRIs for major depression or OCD, an increase in social dominance and a decrease in social hostility were found, irrespective of treatment response for Axis I, supporting the notion that serotonin reuptake inhibitors may be useful to treat avoidant personality traits. Similarly, a decrease in harm avoidance was found with treatment, which was greater in the Axis I treatment responders, again supporting the notion that serotonin reuptake inhibitors may be useful in treating obsessive-compulsive and dependent

personality traits. More pharmacological studies using this dimensional approach to symptom change would be of interest in Cluster C personality disorders.

Treatment Issues in the Presence of Axis I Comorbidity

This section focuses not on the direct treatment of Axis II disorders but rather on the widely asked question of whether the presence of Axis II disorders affects the likelihood of, compliance in, or success of treating major Axis I disorders, primarily depression and anxiety. The literature in this area often shows contradictory results, and lore blends with evidence-based reality. Here we summarize the major empirical findings against the background of a widely espoused belief, not necessarily substantiated by fact, that the presence of personality disorders generally impedes the recognition and successful treatment of Axis I disorders.

A community survey, conducted as part of a 1981 epidemiological study that used DSM-III (American Psychiatric Association 1980) diagnostic criteria, examined the association between Axis I and II disorders and the need for and likelihood of treatment (Samuels et al. 1994). Among subjects with any Axis I disorder, 87% of those with personality disorders were in need of treatment compared with 46% of those without, a highly significant difference. Furthermore, 18% of the subjects with personality disorders were actually receiving treatment compared with 6% of the subjects without. In essence, then, although those with comorbid personality disorders were proportionately more likely to be receiving some type of psychiatric treatment if in need of it, about 80% of the total individuals with personality disorders who were deemed as needing treatment were not receiving it.

The literature is most extensive for depressive disorders. Earlier studies from the 1980s reported that depressed patients with personality disorders were less likely to receive medication treatment (Black et al. 1988; Charney et al. 1981) or received it for shorter periods (Pfohl et al. 1987) than did those without personality disorders. However, Downs et al. (1992) found that patients with Axis II comorbidity were not less likely to receive medications. Based on chart review, they were actually likely to receive greater numbers of medications, especially if they had BPD, than patients without personality disorder. In regard to the question of compliance, patients with major depression who dropped out of controlled medication trials were characterized by a significantly higher

prevalence of "image distorting" defense mechanisms, such as projective identification, splitting, omnipotence, and idealization/devaluation (Mullen et al. 1999).

Two review studies have examined the impact of Axis II disorders on the efficacy of pharmacotherapy in depressed patients. A descriptive review study (Mulder 2002) examined more than 50 relevant trials and concluded that better-designed treatment trials were least supportive of an adverse effect of personality pathology on depression outcome. A negative impact of personality on depression treatment was most consistently found for high neuroticism scores, whereas Cloninger's personality dimensions bore no consistent relation to depression outcome. Similarly, when personality disorders were measured by categorical diagnostic instruments, results among the various studies were quite inconsistent, and the best-designed studies that used structured diagnostic interviews and randomized, controlled designs showed the least effect. A more recent meta-analytic review study (Kool et al. 2005) reported similar findings. When all randomized, controlled trials in adult ambulatory patients with major depression and comorbid personality disorders were examined according to strict methodological criteria, the difference in depression remission rates between the groups with and without Axis II disorders was a mere 3%, a difference neither statistically significant nor clinically pertinent. However, another study reported that acute response of major depressive disorder to electroconvulsive therapy (ECT) was poorer in patients with comorbid BPD than in patients with other or no personality disorders, a finding not accounted for by age, gender, or medication-resistance status (Feske et al. 2004).

Addressing a somewhat different question, a recent 11-year prospective study examined whether the presence of Axis II comorbidity increases the likelihood of major depression recurrence or relapse and found that it did (Khan et al. 2007). In a sample of 168 outpatients receiving long-term treatment with an SSRI, Cluster A, B, and C dimensional personality traits were highly inversely correlated with duration of stability without mood disorder. Similar findings were reported when Axis II pathology was examined categorically; patients without personality disorders remained in remission from depression almost twice as long as did patients with at least one personality disorder.

Less literature exists examining the relation between the treatment of Axis I bipolar disorder and the presence of Axis II personality disorder. A study of 200 bipolar I and II disorder patients examining various factors affecting medication compliance found that personality disor-

der comorbidity was the factor most strongly associated with poor compliance (Colom et al. 2000). About one-quarter of the subjects had at least one comorbid Axis II disorder, and of these, 17% were assessed as having good compliance, 37% medium compliance, and 44% poor compliance.

Fewer studies have examined the relation between Axis II comorbidity and treatment of Axis I anxiety disorders. A recent report claims to be the first one to examine the amount of psychiatric treatment received in anxiety disorder patients as a function of comorbid personality disorder (Phillips et al. 2001). This large study examined several hundred anxious patients with a variety of Axis I diagnoses: panic disorder, generalized anxiety disorder, social phobia, OCD, posttraumatic stress disorder, and agoraphobia. Despite minor discrepancies between the two time-point assessments (1991 and 1996), the findings were fairly consistent: similar percentages of anxious subjects with and without personality disorders received medication treatment. If medicated, those with personality disorders, and especially those with BPD, were likely to be receiving a greater number of medications, specifically heterocyclic antidepressants. Thus, these investigators found no evidence for medication undertreatment of patients with Axis II comorbidity. They proposed, in reviewing trends in the pertinent literature, that influential biological studies and medication trials of Axis II disorders from the late 1980s and the early 1990s may have led toward a more favorable shift in medicating patients with personality disorders who previously may have been more likely to be assessed as needing only psychotherapy.

Conclusion

In this chapter, we reviewed the pharmacological treatment of personality disorders, providing a conceptual framework, highlighting methodological limitations, and summarizing treatment trials to date. Almost all of these trials focused on symptom clusters, such as psychoticism, impulsivity, hostility/aggression, mood instability, and anxiety/inhibition. Trials were largely limited to BPD, although from some trials, additional conclusions can be drawn about other personality disorders in mixed-group study designs or by extrapolation of comparable symptom clusters. It is becoming increasingly established that medication treatment can play a very important role, albeit adjunctive to psychotherapy, in the treatment of personality disorders. Even if benefits are more modest than those encountered with medication treatment of some

Axis I conditions, they can still make a significant contribution to symptom reduction, functional improvement, and overall adaptation. Continued medication trials of Axis II disorders that also focus on broader dimensions of personality, including aspects of character, are eagerly awaited.

References

American Psychiatric Association: Diagnostic and Statistical Manual of Mental Disorders, 3rd Edition. Washington, DC, American Psychiatric Association, 1980

American Psychiatric Association: Diagnostic and Statistical Manual of Mental Disorders, 3rd Edition, Revised. Washington, DC, American Psychiatric Association, 1987

American Psychiatric Association: Diagnostic and Statistical Manual of Mental Disorders, 4th Edition. Washington, DC, American Psychiatric Association, 1994

American Psychiatric Association: Practice guideline for the treatment of patients with borderline personality disorder. Am J Psychiatry 158 (suppl):44–46, 2001

Ansseau M, Troisfontaines B, Papart P, et al: Compulsive personality as predictor of response to serotonergic antidepressants. BMJ 303:760–761, 1991

Asarnow RF, Nuechterlein KH, Fogelson D, et al: Schizophrenia and schizophrenia-spectrum personality disorders in the first-degree relatives of children with schizophrenia: the UCLA family study. Arch Gen Psychiatry 58:581–588, 2001

Baer L, Jenike MA, Ricciardi JN, et al: Standardized assessment of personality disorders in obsessive-compulsive disorder. Arch Gen Psychiatry 47:826–830, 1990

Baer L, Jenike MA, Black DW, et al: Effect of Axis II diagnoses on treatment outcome with clomipramine in 55 patients with obsessive-compulsive disorder. Arch Gen Psychiatry 49:862–866, 1992

Baxter LR, Schwartz JM, Bergman KS, et al: Caudate glucose metabolic rate changes with both drug and behavior therapy for obsessive-compulsive disorder. Arch Gen Psychiatry 49:681–689, 1992

Bellino S, Paradiso E, Bogetto F: Efficacy and tolerability of quetiapine in the treatment of borderline personality disorder: a pilot study. J Clin Psychiatry 67:1042–1046, 2006

Black DW, Bell S, Hulbert J, et al: The importance of Axis II in patients with major depression: a controlled study. J Affect Disord 14:115–122, 1988

Bohus MJ, Landwehrmeyer B, Stiglmayr CE, et al: Naltrexone in the treatment of dissociative symptoms in patients with borderline personality disorder: an open-label trial. J Clin Psychiatry 60:598–603, 1999

Brinkley JR, Beitman BD, Friedel RO: Low-dose neuroleptic regimens in the treatment of borderline patients. Arch Gen Psychiatry 36:319–326, 1979

Brody AL, Saxena S, Fairbanks LA, et al: Personality changes in adult subjects with major depressive disorder or obsessive-compulsive disorder treated with paroxetine. J Clin Psychiatry 61:349–355, 2000

Charney DS, Nelson JC, Quinlan D: Personality traits and disorders in depression. Am J Psychiatry 138:1601–1604, 1981

Cloninger CR, Svrakic DM, Prybeck TR: A psychobiological model of temperament and character. Arch Gen Psychiatry 50:975–990, 1993

Coccaro EF: Psychopharmacological studies in patients with personality disorders: review and perspective. J Personal Disord 7 (suppl):181–192, 1993

Coccaro EF, Kavoussi RJ: Fluoxetine and impulsive aggressive behavior in personality-disordered subjects. Arch Gen Psychiatry 54:1081–1088, 1997

Coccaro EF, Astill JL, Herbert JL, et al: Fluoxetine treatment of impulsive aggression in DSM-III-R personality disorder patients. J Clin Psychopharmacol 10:373–375, 1990

Coccaro EF, Harvey PD, Kupsaw-Lawrence E, et al: Development of neuropharmacologically based behavioral assessment of impulsive aggressive behavior. J Neuropsychiatry Clin Neurosci 3:S44–S51, 1991

Colom F, Vieta E, Martinez-Aran A, et al: Clinical factors associated with treatment noncompliance in euthymic bipolar patients. J Clin Psychiatry 61:549–555, 2000

Comings DE, Gade-Andavolu R, Gonzalez N, et al: A multivariate analysis of 59 candidate genes in personality traits: the temperament and character inventory. Clin Genet 58:375–385, 2000

Coolidge FL, Thede LL, Jang KL: Heritability of personality disorders in childhood: a preliminary investigation. J Personal Disord 15:33–40, 2001

Cornelius JR, Soloff PH, Perel JM, et al: A preliminary trial of fluoxetine in refractory borderline patients. J Clin Psychopharmacol 11:116–120, 1991

Cornelius JR, Soloff PH, Perel JM, et al: Continuation pharmacotherapy of borderline personality disorder with haloperidol and phenelzine. Am J Psychiatry 150:1843–1848, 1993

Cowdry RW, Gardner DL: Pharmacotherapy of borderline personality disorder: alprazolam, carbamazepine, trifluoperazine, and tranylcypromine. Arch Gen Psychiatry 45:111–119, 1988

Cravchik A, Goldman D: Neurochemical individuality: genetic diversity among human dopamine and serotonin receptors and transporters. Arch Gen Psychiatry 57:1105–1114, 2000

De La Fuenta JM, Lotstra F: A trial of carbamazepine in borderline personality disorder. Eur Neuropsychopharmacol 4: 479–486, 1994

Deltito JA, Perugi G: A case of social phobia with avoidant personality disorder treated with MAOI. Compr Psychiatry 27:255–258, 1986

Deltito JA, Stam M: Psychopharmacological treatment of avoidant personality disorder. Compr Psychiatry 30:498–504, 1989

Downs NS, Swerdlow NR, Zisook S: The relationship of affective illness and personality disorders in psychiatric outpatients. Ann Clin Psychiatry 4:87–94, 1992

Feske U, Mulsant BH, Pilkonis PA, et al: Clinical outcome of ECT in patients with major depression and comorbid borderline personality disorder. Am J Psychiatry 161:2073–2080, 2004

Frankenburg FR, Zanarini MC: Clozapine treatment of borderline patients: a preliminary study. Compr Psychiatry 34:402–405, 1993

Frankenburg FR, Zanarini MC: Divalproex sodium treatment of women with borderline personality disorder and bipolar II disorder: a double-blind placebo-controlled pilot study. J Clin Psychiatry 63:442–446, 2002

Gabbard GO: Combining medication with psychotherapy in the treatment of personality disorders, in Psychotherapy for Personality Disorders (Review of Psychiatry Series, Vol 19; Oldham JM and Riba MB, series eds). Edited by Gunderson JG, Gabbard GO. Washington, DC, American Psychiatric Press, 2000, pp 65–94

Gitlin MJ: Pharmacotherapy of personality disorders: conceptual framework and clinical strategies. J Clin Psychopharmacol 13:343–353, 1993

Goldberg SC, Schulz C, Schulz PM, et al: Borderline and schizotypal personality disorders treated with low-dose thiothixene vs placebo. Arch Gen Psychiatry 43:680–686, 1986

Hilger E, Barnas C, Kasper S: Quetiapine in the treatment of borderline personality disorder. World J Biol Psychiatry 4:42–44, 2003

Hollander E, Allen A, Lopez RP, et al: A preliminary double-blind, placebo-controlled trial of divalproex sodium in borderline personality disorder. J Clin Psychiatry 62:199–203, 2001

Hollander E, Tracy KA, Swann A, et al: Divalproex in the treatment of impulsive aggression: efficacy in Cluster B personality disorders. Neuropsychopharmacology 28:1186–1197, 2003

Hollander E, Swann AC, Coccaro EF, et al: Impact of trait impulsivity and state aggression on divalproex versus placebo response in borderline personality disorder. Am J Psychiatry 162:621–624, 2005

Kapfhammer HP, Hippius J: Special feature: pharmacotherapy in personality disorders. J Personal Disord 12:277–288, 1998

Kavoussi RJ, Liu J, Coccaro EF: An open trial of sertraline in personality disordered patients with impulsive aggression. J Clin Psychiatry 55:137–141, 1994

Kendler KS, Gruenberg AM, Kinney DK: Independent diagnoses of adoptees and relatives as defined by DSM-III in the provincial and national samples of the Danish Adoption Study of Schizophrenia. Arch Gen Psychiatry 51:456–468, 1994

Khan SJ, Peselow ED, Orlowski B: Personality traits and prophylactic treatment with selective serotonin reuptake inhibitors. Presented at the 160th Annual Meeting of the American Psychiatric Association, San Diego, CA, May 19–24, 2007 (No. 82)

Koenigsberg HW, Harvey PD, Mitropoulou V, et al: Are the interpersonal and identity disturbances in the borderline personality disorder criteria linked to the traits of affective instability and impulsivity? J Personal Disord 15:358–370, 2001

Koenigsberg HW, Reynolds D, Goodman M, et al: Risperidone in the treatment of schizotypal personality disorder. J Clin Psychiatry 64:628–634, 2002

Kool S, Schoevers R, de Maat S, et al: Efficacy of pharmacotherapy in depressed patients with and without personality disorders: a systematic review and meta-analysis. J Affect Disord 88:269–278, 2005

Leone NF: Response of borderline patients to loxapine and chlorpromazine. J Clin Psychiatry 43:148–150, 1982

Liebowitz MR, Gorman JM, Fyer AJ, et al: Pharmacotherapy of social phobia: an interim report of a placebo-controlled comparison of phenelzine and atenolol. J Clin Psychiatry 49:252–257, 1988

Linehan MM: Cognitive-Behavioral Treatment for Borderline Personality Disorder. New York, Guilford, 1993

Links PS, Steiner M, Boiage I, et al: Lithium therapy for borderline patients: preliminary findings. J Personal Disord 4:173–181, 1990

Markovitz PJ: Pharmacotherapy of impulsivity, aggression, and related disorders, in Impulsivity and Aggression. Edited by Hollander E, Stein DJ. New York, Wiley, 1995, pp 263–288

Markovitz PJ, Wagner SC: Venlafaxine in the treatment of borderline personality disorder. Psychopharmacol Bull 31:773–777, 1995

Markovitz PJ, Calabrese JR, Schultz SC, et al: Fluoxetine in the treatment of borderline and schizotypal personality disorders. Am J Psychiatry 148:1064–1067, 1991

Mobascher A, Mobascher J, Schlemper V, et al: Aripiprazole pharmacotherapy of borderline personality disorder. Pharmacopsychiatry 39:111–112, 2006

Montgomery SA, Montgomery D: Pharmacological prevention of suicidal behaviour. J Affect Disord 4:291–298, 1982

Mulder RT: Personality pathology and treatment outcome in major depression: a review. Am J Psychiatry 159:359–371, 2002

Mullen LS, Blanco C, Vaughan SC, et al: Defense mechanisms and personality in depression. Depress Anxiety 10:168–174, 1999

Norden MJ: Fluoxetine in borderline personality disorder. Prog Neuropsychopharmacol Biol Psychiatry 13:885–893, 1989

Noyes R Jr, Reich JH, Suelzer M, et al: Personality traits associated with panic disorder: change associated with treatment. Compr Psychiatry 32:283–294, 1991

Parsons B, Quitkin FM, McGrath PJ, et al: Phenelzine, imipramine, and placebo in borderline patients meeting criteria for atypical depression. Psychopharmacol Bull 25:524–534, 1989

Perrella C, Carrus D, Costa E, et al: Quetiapine for the treatment of borderline personality disorder: an open-label study. Prog Neuropsychopharmacol Biol Psychiatry 31:158–163, 2007

Perry JC, Bond M: Empirical studies of psychotherapy for personality disorders, in Psychotherapy for Personality Disorders (Review of Psychiatry Series, Vol 19; Oldham JM and Riba MB, series eds). Edited by Gunderson JG, Gabbard GO. Washington, DC, American Psychiatric Press, 2000, pp 1–31

Pfohl B, Coryell W, Zimmerman M, et al: Prognostic validity of self-report and interview measures of personality disorder in depressed inpatients. J Clin Psychiatry 48:468–472, 1987

Phillips KA, Shea MT, Warshaw M, et al: The relationship between comorbid personality disorders and treatment received in patients with anxiety disorders. J Personal Disord 15:157–167, 2001

Pinto OC, Akiskal HS: Lamotrigine as a promising approach to borderline personality: an open case series without concurrent DSM-IV major mood disorder. J Affect Disord 51:333–343, 1998

Pollitt J, Tyrer P: Compulsive personality as predictor of response to serotonergic antidepressants. Br J Psychiatry 161:836–838, 1992

Reich J, Noyes R, Yates W: Alprazolam treatment of avoidant personality traits in social phobic patients. J Clin Psychiatry 50:91–95, 1989

Rifkin A, Quitkin F, Carrillo C, et al: Lithium carbonate in emotionally unstable character disorder. Arch Gen Psychiatry 27:519–523, 1972

Rocca P, Marchiaro L, Cocuzza E, et al: Treatment of borderline personality disorder with risperidone. J Clin Psychiatry 63:241–244, 2002

Salzman C, Wolfson AN, Schatzberg A, et al: Effect of fluoxetine on anger in symptomatic volunteers with borderline personality disorder. J Clin Psychopharmacol 15:23–29, 1995

Samuels JF, Nestadt G, Romanoski AJ, et al: DSM-III personality disorders in the community. Am J Psychiatry 151:1055–1062, 1994

Samuels J, Nestadt G, Bienvenu OJ, et al: Personality disorders and normal personality dimensions in obsessive-compulsive disorder. Br J Psychiatry 177:457–462, 2000

Schulz SC, Camlin KL, Berry SA, et al: A double-blind study of risperidone for BPD (NR270). Poster presented at the 151st annual meeting of the American Psychiatric Association, Toronto, Ontario, Canada, May 30–June 4, 1998

Schulz SC, Camlin KL, Berry SA, et al: Olanzapine safety and efficacy in patients with borderline personality disorder and comorbid dysthymia. Biol Psychiatry 46:1429–1435, 1999

Schulz SC, Zanarini MC, Detke HC, et al: Olanzapine for the treatment of borderline personality disorder: a flexible-dose 12-week randomized double-blind placebo-controlled study. Presented at the 160th Annual Meeting of the American Psychiatric Association, San Diego, CA, May 19–24, 2007 (No. 83)

Schwartz JM, Stoessel PW, Baxter LR, et al: Systematic changes in cerebral glucose metabolic rate after successful behavior modification treatment of obsessive-compulsive disorder. Arch Gen Psychiatry 53:109–113, 1996

Serban G, Siegel S: Response of borderline and schizotypal patients to small doses of thiothixene and haloperidol. Am J Psychiatry 141:1455–1458, 1984

Siever LJ: Biological markers in schizotypal personality disorder. Schizophr Bull 11:564–575, 1985

Siever LJ, Davis KL: A psychobiological perspective on the personality disorders. Am J Psychiatry 148:1647–1658, 1991

Siever LJ, Keefe R, Bernstein DP, et al: Eye tracking impairment in clinically identified patients with schizotypal personality disorder. Am J Psychiatry 147:740–745, 1990

Siever LJ, Bernstein DP, Silverman JM: Schizotypal personality disorder: a review of its current status. J Personal Disord 5:178–193, 1991

Silverman JM, Pinkham L, Horvath TB, et al: Affective and impulsive personality disorder traits in the relatives of patients with borderline personality disorder. Am J Psychiatry 148:1378–1385, 1991

Simeon D, Baker B, Chaplin W, et al: An open-label trial of extended release valproate in the treatment of borderline personality disorder. CNS Spectr 12:439–443, 2007

Soloff PH: What's new in personality disorders? An update on pharmacological treatment. J Personal Disord 4:233–243, 1990

Soloff PH: Algorithms for pharmacological treatment of personality dimensions: symptom-specific treatments for cognitive-perceptual, affective, and impulsive-behavioral dysregulation. Bull Menninger Clin 62:195–214, 1998

Soloff PH, George A, Nathan S, et al: Progress in pharmacotherapy of borderline disorders: a double-blind study of amitriptyline, haloperidol, and placebo. Arch Gen Psychiatry 43:691–697, 1986

Soloff PH, George A, Nathan RS, et al: Amitriptyline versus haloperidol in borderlines: final outcomes and predictors of response. J Clin Psychopharmacol 9:238–246, 1989

Soloff PH, Cornelius J, George A, et al: Efficacy of phenelzine and haloperidol in borderline personality disorder. Arch Gen Psychiatry 50:377–385, 1993

Stein DJ, Simeon D, Frenkel M, et al: An open trial of valproate in borderline personality disorder. J Clin Psychiatry 56:506–510, 1995

Thomsen PH, Mikkelsen HU: Development of personality disorders in children and adolescents with obsessive-compulsive disorder: a 6- to 22-year follow-up study. Acta Psychiatr Scand 87:456–462, 1993

Torgersen S, Lygren S, Anders Oien P, et al: A twin study of personality disorders. Compr Psychiatry 41:416–425, 2000

Turner SM, Beidel DC, Dancu CV: Psychopathology of social phobia and comparison to avoidant personality disorder. J Abnorm Psychol 95:389–394, 1986

Tyrer P, Davidson K: Cognitive therapy for personality disorders, in Psychotherapy for Personality Disorders (Review of Psychiatry Series, Vol 19; Oldham JM and Riba MB, series eds). Edited by Gunderson JG, Gabbard GO. Washington, DC, American Psychiatric Press, 2000, pp 131–149

Villeneuve E, Lemelin S: Open-label study of atypical neuroleptic quetiapine for treatment of borderline personality disorder: impulsivity as main target. J Clin Psychiatry 66:1298–1303, 2005

Walker C, Thomas J, Allen TS: Treating impulsivity, irritability, and aggression of antisocial personality disorder with quetiapine. Int J Offender Ther Comp Criminol 47:556–567, 2003

Wickham EA, Reed JV: Lithium for the control of aggressive and self-mutilating behavior. Int Clin Psychopharmacol 2:181–190, 1987

Yudofsky SC, Silver JM, Jackson W, et al: The Overt Aggression Scale for the objective rating of verbal and physical aggression. Am J Psychiatry 143:335–339, 1986

Zanarini MC, Frankenburg FR: Olanzapine treatment of female borderline personality disorder patients: a double-blind, placebo-controlled pilot study. J Clin Psychiatry 62:849–854, 2001

Zanarini MC, Frankenburg FR, Gunderson JG: Pharmacotherapy of borderline outpatients. Compr Psychiatry 29:372–378, 1988

Zanarini MC, Schulz SC, Detke HC, et al: A dose comparison of olanzapine for the treatment of borderline personality disorder: a 12-week randomized double-blind placebo-controlled study. Presented at the 160th Annual Meeting of the American Psychiatric Association, San Diego, CA, May 19–24, 2007 (No. 84)

CHAPTER 62

Treatment of Psychiatric Emergencies

Margaret B. Weigel, M.D.

David C. Purselle, M.D., M.S.

Barbara D'Orio, M.D., M.P.A

Steven J. Garlow, M.D., Ph.D.

Psychiatric emergencies occur in many different situations in both clinical and nonclinical settings. While often managed in specialized psychiatric emergency and crisis stabilization units, psychiatric emergencies may also surface in other settings, such as general medical/surgical units and outpatient clinics, general emergency departments, and other nonclinical settings. The resources and personnel available in a facility will significantly affect the thoroughness of the evaluation, options for short-term stabilization, and ultimate disposition of the patient. A fully staffed, freestanding psychiatric emergency room will provide more options for patient care than will an ambulatory clinic or a general emergency medicine department.

The effective practice of emergency psychiatry requires a broad range of clinical skills, including elements of psychosomatic psychiatry, behavioral neurology, psychopharmacology, individual and family psychotherapy, and addiction psychiatry. In addition, a basic knowledge of forensic and legal issues is essential. With recent large-scale changes in mental health care delivery, including the deinstitutionalization of the mentally ill and the elimination and downsizing of inpatient mental health facilities with an emphasis on cost containment, the role of an emergency psychiatrist in the mental health field has expanded dramatically. These changes impact not only specialized psychiatric facilities but also general emergency room departments. According to one study that used the National Hospital Ambulatory Medical Care Survey (NHAMCS), from 1992 until 2001 there were 53 million mental health–related general emergency room visits. This represented an increase from 4.9% to 6.3% of all emergency room visits across the decade (Larkin et al. 2005).

Decision making in psychiatric emergencies involves gathering objective data from the medical history and mental status examination, the same process as in other fields of medicine. But in emergent situations, this assessment may occur without the luxury of time to develop a comprehensive differential diagnosis. Patients with emergent behavioral and psychiatric syndromes are often unable or unwilling to provide accurate historical details; therefore, the clinician must rely on collateral sources of information, including friends, family, and previous treatment providers. One consequence of this process of data collection is that absolute patient confidentiality, the standard of care in other clinical settings, is more tenuous. In the context of a psychiatric emergency, the need to acquire critical information supersedes the individual's right to privacy. In emergent situations, resources such as medical records, friends, and relatives may provide critical data for diagnosis and treatment. And depending on the patient's condition, it may not be possible to obtain his or her consent to acquire this information. This is one situation in which it is appropriate to stretch the boundaries of confidentiality in order to provide the best clinical care. The focus is on obtaining components of history while not disclosing protected information. There are other circumstances in which there is a mandated breach of confidentiality, which includes a patient's risk of harm to self or others, and the knowledge of child and elder abuse. Requirements vary by jurisdiction.

Another consequence of the need to make diagnostic and treatment decisions with limited information is that these decisions should be conservative. For example, care must be taken not to rashly make a diagnosis such as schizophrenia in response to the presence of psychotic symptoms when the data do not justify this conclusion. A 1-year study of diagnostic stability suggested that 38.7% of psychiatric emergency room patients were given a different discharge diagnosis from the inpatient service (Woo et al. 2006). Use of "rule out," "provisional," and "not otherwise specified (NOS)" qualifiers helps ensure that a patient does not receive an incorrect diagnosis that may cause additional problems in the future (American Psychiatric Association 2000). The setting in which the patient is evaluated will have a significant effect on the diagnostic formulation. A patient evaluated in a crisis stabilization facility with a 24- to 48-hour secure observation unit should receive a more definitive diagnosis than one evaluated in an emergency medicine department in a general hospital that is not equipped or staffed for long-term psychiatric observation.

Following the principles of Hippocrates, the emphasis is to make treatment decisions in the best interests of the patient while balancing the need to prevent further harm. The ultimate goals are to provide adequate treatment of the underlying pathology based on a careful but succinct evaluation of the patient and to provide this treatment in the least restrictive environment while maintaining the safety of patient, clinician, and staff.

Psychiatric emergencies can be divided into those that do not call for pharmacological intervention, those that may require adjunctive pharmacological intervention, and those that usually demand pharmacological intervention. The remainder of this chapter is divided along these lines.

Nonpharmacological Psychiatric Emergencies

Situations that require emergent psychiatric intervention but not psychopharmacological treatment include evalu-

TABLE 62–1. Psychiatric emergencies that do not require pharmacological intervention

EMERGENCY	INTERVENTION
Suicidal state	Risk assessment Decision to admit
Homicidal state	Establish or rule out presence of psychiatric disorder Risk assessment Decision to admit *Tarasoff* notification
Grave disability, unable to care for self	Patient identification (if wandered from caregivers) Medical evaluation Decision to admit
Child, elder, spouse abuse	Notify/report to law enforcement and other agencies Referral to safe shelters

ation of need for hospitalization, assessment of suicide or homicide risk, determination of ability to care for self, and requirements to notify third parties to ensure safety of the patient or others (Table 62–1). Emergency psychiatrists are in a unique position of having to make predictions about patients' future behavior (e.g., suicide, homicide) and (to the best of their abilities) take appropriate preemptive action to prevent these outcomes. The focus is on the welfare of the patient and the safety of others with whom the psychiatrist has no therapeutic relationship. All states have civil commitment laws that allow for the involuntary hospitalization of persons who by virtue of a mental illness may be considered an imminent risk to themselves or others. Typically, these laws allow for commitments of 48–72 hours in secure receiving facilities for assessment and stabilization. Involuntary hospitalization beyond this holding period for observation and treatment generally involves some form of judicial review.

Need for Hospitalization

The decision to hospitalize a psychiatric patient is dependent on several factors, but the welfare of the patient is of the greatest importance. There should be clear, definable treatment objectives for hospitalization, and the facility in which the patient is hospitalized should be able to meet these needs. Beyond consideration of the patient's welfare, other factors can contribute to the decision of whether to hospitalize a patient (R.I. Simon 1998). These include availability of psychiatric hospital beds and admission authorization by third-party payers. A decrease in funding of mental health services has resulted in a decrease in available inpatient resources. Thus, the clinician must balance the availability of resources with the needs of individual patients. And while third-party payers may limit the ability to admit a patient to a hospital, the onus of providing appropriate care ultimately falls on the clinician.

Once the decision is made to hospitalize a patient, every effort should be made to have this occur on a voluntary basis. This is the first step in establishing therapeutic rapport with patients. The indiscriminate use of involuntary commitments can set up the perception of an adversarial relationship between patients and treatment providers (Olofsson and Jacobson 2001). Patients with chronic, persisting mental illnesses will most likely require multiple hospitalizations in the course of their illness. Avoiding experiences that elicit the perception of being "locked up" against one's will is one way of facilitating the long-term care of the mentally ill patient.

Suicidal State

Suicide is the eleventh leading cause of death in the United States across all age groups. As a public health issue, suicide continues to be a major problem, with a population rate around 11 deaths per 100,000, which has remained invariant over the past four decades. But there are several recent studies that suggest a slight decrease in U.S. suicide rates since selective serotonin reuptake inhibitors (SSRIs) have been introduced. Historically, one of the truly vexing problems in psychiatry is the lack of effect of specific psychiatric treatments on the suicide rate. Several studies have failed to find any association between the availability of psychiatric treatment resources and the suicide rate (Garlow et al. 2002; Lewis et al. 1994).

Predicting imminent suicide in any individual patient is difficult and can provoke significant anxiety in the clinician (Pokorny 1983, 1993). Completed suicide is a rare event, but it has profound effects on both the surviving family members and friends of the victim and the physician and treatment staff (Gitlin 1999; Hendin et al. 2000). There are also potential legal ramifications of a patient's committing suicide if he or she has been in recent contact with psychiatrists and other mental health providers (R.I. Simon 2000).

Recently, a relationship between antidepressant use and suicidal behaviors has been reported in the media and psychiatric literature. The impetus for this focus was the addition of a black box warning by the U.S. Food and Drug Administration (FDA) on the potential increased risk of suicidal ideation in children, adolescents, and young adults treated with SSRIs. Of note, within the study population from which the original warning was issued, there were no completed suicides. This warning stirred a debate on the risk versus the potential beneficial effects of treatment with this class of medications. Subsequent analysis of the FDA database using a standardized algorithm for assessing suicidal events, termed the Columbia Classification Algorithm of Suicide Assessment (C-CASA), suggests that misclassification of suicidal events may have led to an overestimation of true risk (Posner et al. 2007). Observational studies have shown that treatment, specifically the use of SSRIs, has a protective effect on emergent suicidal behavior (Gibbons et al. 2005, 2007; G.E. Simon and Savarino 2007). Additional research has shown the highest number of suicide attempts in the month before treatment, suggesting that suicidal behavior is often a precipitant for seeking treatment rather than a consequence of antidepressant use (G.E. Simon and Savarino 2007). This particular study compared patients entering psychotherapy to those receiving antidepressant medication, and there was no difference in the rates of suicide-related behaviors in either treatment group, strongly suggesting that suicidality is a reflection of the underlying disease and not of the treatment. One way of solving this conundrum is to use toxicological analysis to determine the presence of antidepressants in suicide victims. One study of more than 5,000 adult suicides found most had not taken antidepressants immediately prior to death, despite being diagnosed as being depressed (Isacsson et al. 1997). Similar results were found in adolescent populations (Isacsson et al. 2005). With the addition of the black box warning and the subsequent publicity, utilization of antidepressants in the pediatric and adolescent populations has fallen, with a coincident increase in suicide-related behaviors (Nemeroff et al. 2007). In summary, despite claims to the contrary, the evidence suggests that antidepressant medications exert a protective effect on suicide risk.

The relationship between suicidal ideation, attempted suicide, and completed suicide is complex (Moscicki 1997). No direct relation exists between any one of these states and the others. In one population-based study of completed suicides, 56% of the individuals were successful on the first attempt (Isometsa and Lonnqvist 1998). In another comprehensive study of completed suicides, 75% of the cohort had no contact with mental health providers in the year prior to death (Appleby et al. 1999). One ominous finding in this study was that 16% of the suicides occurred while the victims were inpatients in psychiatric wards, and 24% occurred within 3 months after discharge from psychiatric facilities. In a 10-year follow-up study of patients admitted to the hospital for a medically serious suicide attempt, 25% of the cohort made a second attempt, and 12% eventually died by suicide, with the highest rate of completed suicides occurring in the 2 years following the index admission (Isometsa and Lonnqvist 1998). The expression of suicidal ideation and a history of previous suicide attempts appear to identify a large group of at-risk patients, but only a small percentage of these patients go on to complete suicide. Understanding which patients will go on to complete suicide involves a comprehensive assessment of suicide risk factors.

Suicide risk is estimated by assessing both acute and chronic risk factors (Table 62–2), which include patient characteristics, nature of suicidal behavior, availability of a high-lethality means, and level of and access to psychosocial support systems (e.g., family, friends, community) (R.C. Hall et al. 1999; R.I. Simon and Gutheil 2002). This is an example of a psychiatric emergency in which acquiring reliable and accurate past and collateral history is essential, which may lead to some breach of patient confidentiality. Acute risk factors are most predictive of emergent suicidality and should carry the most weight in the decision to hospitalize a patient (Fawcett et al. 1991).

Acute Risk Factors

Acute risk factors are much more predictive of emergent suicidality than chronic risk factors. Acute risk factors include increasing anxiety and frank panic attacks, psychic turmoil, global insomnia, mood-congruent nihilistic delusions, profound hopelessness, and recent discharge from a psychiatric hospital (Busch et al. 2003; Fawcett 1992; Fawcett et al. 1991). Patients who are experiencing the first three of these symptoms should be viewed as being at particularly high risk regardless of whether they verbalize suicidal ideation. In terms of recent psychiatric hospitalization, the 3-month period following discharge poses a significant period of vulnerability, with one population study indicating 7.8% of the suicide victims completed suicide within 1 month of discharge (Deisenhammer et al. 2007).

Active substance intoxication is another acute risk factor. Recent alcohol consumption plays a role in 25%–50% of all suicides, and the consumption of both alcohol and cocaine may be particularly dangerous (Cornelius et al. 1998). Alcohol intoxication is related to higher rates of completed suicide, while cocaine intoxication is related to higher rates of suicidal ideation (Garlow 2002; Garlow et al. 2003). In this comprehensive series of sui-

cide victims, 40% had alcohol or cocaine detected at the time of autopsy, indicating that the substance was consumed within 48 hours of death (Garlow 2002). Fully 21% of these suicide victims had blood alcohol levels above the legal limit for intoxication (0.08 µg/mL). Cocaine intoxication doubles the risk of suicide in white teenagers compared with African American teenagers (Garlow et al. 2007).

Previous suicide attempts are known precursors for completed suicide; thus, nonlethal suicide attempts are acute risk factors (Deisenhammer et al. 2007; Isometsa and Lonnqvist 1998; Tejedor et al. 1999). The risk for completion is notably higher in the time period following a suicide attempt (Conwell et al. 1996). Consideration should be given to the actual lethality of the attempt; the patient's perception of that lethality; efforts made by the patient to ensure detection or nondetection; calls for help by the patient to medical or law enforcement agencies; contacts to friends or family during the attempt; and use of a firearm. All of these factors illuminate the actual suicidal intent of a patient. A person who took a lethal overdose in a secluded location with no contact to others and who was discovered by accident represents a much higher risk than a person who took a sublethal overdose in a witnessed situation or who immediately called someone to report the overdose or ask for help. Access to firearms must always be determined in a suicide attempt and in someone who appears to be at high risk (Conwell et al. 2002; Miller et al. 2002; Romero and Wintemute 2002).

Other behaviors that should be noted include giving away possessions, placing financial and legal affairs in order, and showing extreme social withdrawal or severing previous interpersonal relationships. Reliable assessment of these behaviors requires collateral history from individuals close to the patient.

Chronic Risk Factors

Chronic risk factors for suicide set the background on which acute risk factors are evaluated. They are derived from population-based analyses of suicides and often are not amenable to any therapeutic intervention, since they are primarily demographic characteristics of people who have died by suicide (Kessler et al. 1999; Moscicki 1997). Males complete suicide four times more often than females do, but females attempt suicide three times more often than males. Males tend to choose more lethal and violent means of suicide than do females. Among males, firearms are the most commonly used (57.6%) method of suicide (National Center for Injury and Prevention and

TABLE 62–2. Acute and chronic risk factors for suicide

ACUTE	CHRONIC
Increasing anxiety/frank panic attacks	Gender (male:female = 4:1)
Psychic turmoil	Age (18–24 years; >65 years)
Global insomnia	Chronic illness
Mood-congruent nihilistic delusions	Race (white:nonwhite = 2:1)
Profound hopelessness	Presence of a mental illness
Recent discharge from a psychiatric hospital	Substance abuse/dependence
Substance intoxication	Access to high-lethality means
Access to high-lethality means	Previous suicide attempts
Previous suicide attempts	Family history of suicide

Control 2005). Individuals age 65 years and older constitute 13% of the population but account for 19% of the suicides, making older age a significant chronic risk factor. The suicide rate for white men older than 85 years is 65 deaths per 100,000 population. A coincident risk factor is chronic illness, especially if it was diagnosed in the previous year. Another at-risk group is teenagers and young adults between the ages of 18 and 24 years, in whom suicide is the third leading cause of death.

Whites complete suicide two times more often than nonwhites, with white males accounting for 73% of the suicides in 1998 (National Center for Injury Prevention and Control 2002). The suicide rates for Native Americans are 1.5 times the national average. Suicide rates for specific ethnic groups change with the age and gender of the individual, so blanket statements of risk are not necessarily accurate. In one study, African American males constituted the largest group, numerically and statistically, of teenage suicide victims but accounted for only 26% of victims from all age groups. In this same data set, African American females accounted for only 3% of all suicides, with only one occurring in an individual older than 45 years (Garlow et al. 2005).

Approximately 90%–95% of suicide victims have a major psychiatric illness, of which approximately half have a mood disorder (Angst et al. 2002; Fawcett 1992; Harris and Barraclough 1997). Male bipolar patients are at higher risk, especially those at an earlier phase of the illness, those who are currently in a depressed state, and those with comorbid substance abuse (Simpson and Jamison 1999). Patients with alcohol and other substance use disorders have higher rates of completed suicide than the national average, with alcoholic patients having a suicide rate twice the national average (Fowler et al. 1986). For alcoholic patients, comorbid depression and recent inter-

personal loss increase risk (Murphy and Wetzel 1990; Murphy et al. 1992). A family history of suicide increases suicide risk independent of a family history of mental illness (Qin et al. 2002, 2003).

Patients with personality disorders often express ongoing suicidal ideation; as a result, suicidality becomes embedded in their sense of self (Soloff et al. 1994). This can manifest as repeated acts of parasuicidal or gestural self-injurious behavior, such as cutting and sublethal overdoses. These patients can be very difficult to manage and can put a great deal of strain on the mental health services delivery system. A consistently applied treatment plan, restrained responses on the part of clinicians and staff (minimizing countertransference behaviors), and use of secure 24-hour patient observation areas can be particularly useful in managing these patients. The goal is to allow patients to deescalate and calm down so that they can ultimately be discharged back into their ongoing outpatient treatment regimens (Maltsberger and Buie 1974).

Protective Factors

In formulating a suicide risk assessment, it is important to note protective factors in addition to the presence or absence of acute and chronic risk factors. One study of depressed patients without a history of suicide attempts found that the following served as protective factors: an expression of more responsibility toward family, more fear of social disapproval, more moral objections to suicide, greater coping skills, and greater fear of suicide (Malone et al. 2000). Social connectivity also serves a protective role for depressed patients, as first described by Emile Durkheim (1951). Having close familial relationships, living with another person (family or friend), and having dependent children are all protective factors. Being involved in cultural groups such as organized religion and having moral objections to suicide are associated with lower rates of suicide (Dervic et al. 2004, 2006).

Generating a comprehensive suicide risk assessment involves organizing and balancing risk with protective factors. Clear documentation of these risk/protective factors, steps taken toward intervention, and associated clinical reasoning are essential. A basic statement indicating competency should also be included. In the case of a chronically suicidal patient, clearly documenting this pattern and obtaining a second opinion to corroborate the treatment plan and objectives may be beneficial.

Management of Suicidal Patients

Ensuring safety is the first and most important step in managing a potentially suicidal patient. This can best be accomplished through admission to a secure patient holding area. If no such facility is available, close observation of the patient by a staff member is another option. In this circumstance, moving the patient to a more secure location is the first treatment goal. Patients who are considered to be particularly high risk may require close observation even after they have been admitted to a secure unit. It is important to note that in one study of inpatient suicides on whom information on precaution status was available, 42% were on 15-minute checks or were observed within 15 minutes of the suicide. Furthermore, 9% of this group was on one-to-one observation at the time of suicide (Busch et al. 2003). Staff assigned to monitor patients should be given specific instructions regarding their role and responsibilities. Furthermore, there should be guidelines for how to manage attempts toward self-injurious behaviors.

Use of extended observation areas can be useful in clarifying the clinical picture while the patient is maintained in safe surroundings. Patients who are intoxicated and expressing suicidal ideation can be allowed to sober up prior to a more definitive assessment. In one psychiatric emergency setting, cocaine use, but not ethanol use, was associated with suicidal ideation, although the mood state was usually transient, resolving in 48–72 hours (Garlow et al. 2003).

The decision to hospitalize a potentially suicidal patient should take into account both acute and chronic risk factors; specific treatment needs of the patient; availability of other treatment options, including partial hospitalization, day treatment, and crisis group home settings; and social support network for the patient. No-harm contracts between patients and clinicians are not useful in making

treatment decisions with suicidal patients (Kroll 2000; R.I. Simon 1999). Of psychiatric inpatients who committed suicide, 50% had made such no-harm contracts, and 67% had denied suicidal ideation on the day of the suicide (R.I. Simon 1999). Focusing on the acute behavioral state of the patient (anxiety, agitation, and insomnia), the presence of chronic risk factors, and access to high-lethality means (firearms) is much more relevant to making the decision to hospitalize the patient.

Patients who are not hospitalized require close follow-up, including a detailed treatment plan, an identified treatment provider, and instructions for the patient and family members on what to do in case of symptom worsening. For individuals not hospitalized and for those recently discharged from the hospital, interventions should be made to improve the safety of the patient's living environment. Individuals with access to high-lethality means should be advised to remove these items from the home. Firearms and medications lethal in overdose should be neither in the home nor readily accessible. Family members and friends may be consulted to assist with the removal of these items from the patients' possession (Mann et al. 2005).

Homicidal State

Establishment of a psychiatric diagnosis is the first step in developing a management plan for a patient expressing homicidal ideation. Whereas suicide most often occurs in the context of a mental illness, homicide and homicidal behaviors often do not. There is a relation between sadness and other negative affective states and suicide, but there is no correlation between these mood states and homicidal or violent acts (Apter et al. 1991). Nonetheless, a patient may develop homicidal ideation in the context of a psychotic disorder, particularly disorders that include firmly held paranoid, persecutory, or erotomanic delusions. If such delusional beliefs are driving the expression of homicidal ideation, involuntary hospitalization would be the appropriate course of action.

Expressions of anger, hostility, rage, and violent intent occur in many interpersonal situations and conflicts in which the perpetrator is not afflicted with a psychiatric disorder. In these cases, once a determination has been made that the individual is not psychotic or delusional or expressing homicidal ideation on the basis of some other psychiatric disorder, appropriate interventions are in the domain of law enforcement agencies and not psychiatrists. Such an individual would not benefit from a psychiatric hospitalization but would instead divert scarce resources away from patients who truly would benefit from such an intervention.

If a patient who is expressing homicidal ideation is not admitted to a psychiatric facility, the clinician must give very careful consideration to the need to notify the intended victim and law enforcement agencies based on the principles set forth in *Tarasoff v. Regents of the University of California* (1976; R.I. Simon 1998; Walcott et al. 2001). This case established a precedent for mental health workers to breach confidentiality to notify an intended victim and law enforcement agencies if they are aware of a patient's plan to harm that victim. Clinicians should consider making a *Tarasoff* notification to the intended victim any time a patient who has expressed homicidal ideation is discharged, regardless of whether that patient has a psychiatric diagnosis. Adoption of the principles set forth in the *Tarasoff* ruling varies by state; therefore, awareness of and adherence to the particular laws within one's own jurisdiction are essential.

Predicting which individuals may act on homicidal ideation is very difficult (Resnick and Scott 2000). Factors that contribute to this assessment are the specificity of the plan, identity of the victim, access to high-lethality means (firearms), capacity of the patient to persist in the plan, and proximity of the perpetrator to the intended victim (Borum and Reddy 2001). Even with a careful history, assessment, and appropriate intervention, preventing an adverse outcome may not be possible. In the *Tarasoff* case, the police determined that the perpetrator was not a threat when they interviewed him, but he eventually carried out the lethal act 3 months later.

Grave Disability and Inability to Care for Self

Another condition for which involuntary commitment laws exist is for patients who by virtue of a mental illness are unable to care for themselves; some states also include "as a result of substance abuse disorders" under this heading (K.T. Hall and Appelbaum 2002). The consideration is whether the patient cannot provide adequately for basic needs, shelter, food, and medical attention because of a mental illness. Common manifestations of this situation include when the patient with a psychotic disorder is living on the streets, without regular or adequate nutrition, and is possibly neglecting ongoing medical conditions. This situation is not the same as that in which a person is homeless because of some other occurrence or circumstance, because homelessness does not in itself constitute grave disability. Another common situation that falls under this heading is when a patient with dementia or other

profound cognitive impairments has wandered away from his or her caregivers. In this case, effort should be focused on establishing the identity of the individual and returning him or her to the appropriate facility. If this is a new-onset cognitive impairment, the patient should be hospitalized for definitive evaluation and diagnosis.

Notification of Third Parties

As noted earlier, the principles set forth by the *Tarasoff* ruling in California encourage clinicians to act in the best interests of the intended victim, with notification of the intended victim and law enforcement agencies in the case of expressed homicidal ideation. As in the case of assessment of suicidal and homicidal risk, this may result in a breach of patient confidentiality. This places a unique burden on psychiatrists—to predict future behavior of a patient and to assume responsibility for the welfare of another person with whom the psychiatrist does not have a therapeutic relationship.

Another circumstance that requires breach of patient confidentiality is notification of authorities in cases of suspected child abuse and neglect. All states have statutes that require clinicians of all disciplines to notify the appropriate agency in the case of suspected child abuse. Many states also have laws for reporting elder abuse and abuse of other vulnerable individuals. Specifics of these laws vary with each jurisdiction.

Psychiatric Emergencies Requiring Minimal or Adjunctive Pharmacological Intervention

Psychiatric emergencies requiring minimal or adjunctive pharmacological intervention occur in many different situations, although many share a common thread of developing in response to some discrete, identifiable stressor (Table 62–3). The practice of crisis intervention psychiatry involves identifying the root cause or stressor of the presenting syndrome and developing a focused treatment plan. The principal therapeutic goals are to alleviate short-term distress, rapidly return the patient to his or her previous level of functioning, and prevent the development of a more serious long-term syndrome. The judicious use of psychopharmacological agents, in concert with psychotherapeutic, psychosocial, and family system interventions, can be particularly effective in these emergencies.

Some conditions in this category require a more thorough diagnostic evaluation and long-term pharmacologi-

TABLE 62–3. Psychiatric emergencies requiring minimal or adjunctive pharmacological intervention

EMERGENCY	INTERVENTION
Adjustment disorder or acute grief	Diagnostic/psychosocial assessment
	Psychotherapy
	Social and family system intervention
	Short course of sedative-hypnotic
	Short course of benzodiazepine
	Selective serotonin reuptake inhibitor
Rape, assault, or trauma	Medical evaluation and treatment
	Law enforcement
	Psychotherapy
	Short course of sedative-hypnotic
	Short course of benzodiazepine
	Insult-specific psychotherapy
	Rape counseling
	Spousal abuse counseling
	Violence victim counseling
Borderline personality disorder	Controlled environment/deescalation
	Structured psychotherapies
	Low-dose neuroleptics
Panic disorder	Medical evaluation
	Short course of benzodiazepine
	Treatment referral

cal management, but in the short term, these agents may or may not be required. Examples of this situation are new-onset panic disorder, dissociative states, catatonia, mania, and conversion disorders. Any of these conditions occurring in a previously well individual, with no history of mental illness, require comprehensive medical evaluation and diagnosis. The long-term management of patients with panic disorder, mania, or psychotic disorders will undoubtedly involve psychopharmacological agents, but these agents may not be required in the immediate setting, depending on the severity of the presenting behavioral syndrome.

Adjustment Disorder

Adjustment disorders are defined as the maladaptive response to an identifiable psychosocial stressor within 3 months of onset of the stressor, with the symptoms having persisted for no more than 6 months (American Psychiatric Association 2000).

The common clinical manifestations of adjustment disorders encountered in psychiatric emergency settings are patients experiencing a mixture of anxiety, depressive,

and neurovegetative symptoms in response to some external stressor or crisis. DSM-IV-TR (American Psychiatric Association 2000) nosology provides subtype designations for characterization of the predominant symptoms of the adjustment disorder: with depressed mood, with anxiety, with mixed anxiety and depressed mood, with disturbance of conduct, and with mixed disturbance of emotions and conduct. The potential stressors are myriad, including death of a family member or friend, job loss, diagnosis of a serious medical condition, divorce and other disturbances of family function, financial hardship, and many other circumstances.

The principal interventions for adjustment disorders are psychotherapeutic, educational, and psychosocial. Most crises have a natural time course and resolution. Feelings of distress in response to many of these insults are innate and expected. Psychoeducational interventions are aimed at helping the patient realize that the syndrome is self-limited and expectable in response to the stressor. Often, these patients have a sleep disturbance, so the short-term use of a soporific (diphenhydramine 25–50 mg, hydroxyzine 25 mg, trazodone 50–100 mg, mirtazapine 7.5–15.0 mg), a sedative-hypnotic (zolpidem 5–10 mg, zaleplon 5–10 mg, eszopiclone 2–3 mg, ramelteon 8 mg), or a benzodiazepine (lorazepam 1–2 mg, diazepam 5 mg) could be considered to assist in reestablishing a normal sleep–wake cycle. If daytime anxiety symptoms are particularly severe and debilitating, daytime use of a benzodiazepine may be considered, but this must be done cautiously, because there is no evidence indicating that the early use of such agents prevents the eventual development of more serious disorders such as posttraumatic stress disorder (PTSD) (Gelpin et al. 1996). The goal of any of these interventions is to assist the patient to return to his or her previous functional level as rapidly as possible.

Bereavement falls into this category and can be on the severe end of the spectrum, especially with the loss of a spouse or child. Because many reactions to such losses are culture-bound, a patient's response to a loss must be evaluated against the background of culturally normative behavior. In normal grief reactions, additional therapeutic focus should be on the involvement of family, friends, religious and spiritual figures, and other members of the patient's community.

Bereavement can be distinguished from a major depressive episode on the basis of several criteria. The presence of suicidal ideation, excessive guilt, prominent psychomotor retardation, hallucinations, preoccupation with worthlessness, or symptoms that last for longer than 2 months are not consistent with a diagnosis of uncomplicated bereavement. Further evaluation and more intensive interventions are necessary in these cases.

Acute Trauma

Patients who have been exposed to an acute psychological trauma are at risk for developing acute stress disorder (ASD) or PTSD. The DSM-IV-TR definition of traumatic events includes direct personal experience of an event that involves actual or threatened death, injury, or threat to one's physical integrity or witnessing such an event or learning about such an event happening to a family member or close associate. Most people who experience such traumas do not go on to develop any psychiatric disorder, but a significant minority, up to 30%, will develop PTSD. One theoretical formulation of PTSD is the failure of the normal recovery process after experiencing a trauma (Foa et al. 1989).

Psychological debriefing has become one of the standard interventions after traumatic events (Mitchell 1983). A trained moderator conducts the debriefing with the goal of encouraging the expression of thoughts and feelings about an event shortly after it has occurred. This type of intervention is commonly offered to both the victims of a trauma and the care providers (e.g., police officers, firefighters, emergency medical technicians) that were involved. Evidence shows that the timing of the debriefing is critical and that this might not be the ideal posttraumatic intervention in all situations (Campfield and Hills 2001; Greenberg 2001). An evolving approach to immediate trauma intervention is to assess the risk of a patient developing PTSD and educate the patient about normal reactions to trauma and potential symptoms of PTSD. Theoretical frameworks suggest that adrenergic activation during times of stress contribute to the solidification of memories in the hippocampus. Attempts have been made to test this theory by administering a β-adrenergic antagonist within 6 hours of the traumatic event to assess whether blocking this receptor may lead to a decreased intensity and imprinting of the stored memory. Results of such investigations are promising but warrant the need for further investigation (Pitman et al. 2002; Vaiva et al. 2003).

Treatment referrals should be made to appropriate providers in the event that a patient develops symptoms of ASD or PTSD over time. Behavioral indicators of risk of developing PTSD include heightened levels of arousal and coping via disengagement after a traumatic event (Mellman et al. 2001). Personalization of the traumatic event, especially thoughts that one might die, is another risk factor. The typical time course for posttraumatic re-

actions to resolve is on the order of 4 weeks. During this time, it is extremely common for all trauma victims to experience some of the symptoms of PTSD. One of the main early therapeutic goals should be to educate patients about this time course and to encourage them to return to treatment if these symptoms persist past 4 weeks or become particularly debilitating. Referral to trauma-specific psychotherapies (rape crisis, violent crime, survivor groups) can be helpful to victims of these specific insults.

The role of the emergency psychiatrist in the face of a national disaster was assessed following the attacks on the United States on September 11, 2001. In the wake of the terrorist attacks on 9/11, studies have assessed access to mental health care. Some early reports suggested that 44% of Americans reported "substantial symptoms" of psychological distress following the attacks (Schuster et al. 2001). Another study suggests that the residents of the communities that were directly affected by the attacks were significantly distressed by the events, while U.S. communities as a whole did not experience an increase in emergent mental health–related complaints (Catalano et al. 2004). In the wake of a national disaster, the emergency psychiatrist should be prepared to deal with trauma-related symptoms of stress.

Medication recommendations are the same as for adjustment disorders. Two SSRIs, sertraline and paroxetine, have a U.S. Food and Drug Administration (FDA)–approved indication for treatment of PTSD symptoms once the full-blown syndrome has developed. Other SSRIs may share a similar pharmacological profile and subsequent clinical utility. Whether the early use of SSRIs after a trauma prevents the development of PTSD is an open question. One study using animal models suggested that immediate postexposure administration of an SSRI (in this case, sertraline) reduced anxiety-like and avoidant behavior, decreased hyperarousal responses, and diminished the overall incidence of extreme (PTSD-like) behavioral responses, compared with a delayed treatment (7 days posttrauma) regimen and with saline controls (Matar et al. 2006). Other studies have evaluated the use of brief cognitive-behavioral therapy for patients with acute PTSD. One such study indicated accelerated rates of recovery in patients who received this intervention, although it did not influence the long-term outcome (Sijbrandij et al. 2007).

The use of benzodiazepines is controversial in the context of acute trauma. While these medications may be useful in decreasing overall levels of anxiety, there is no clinical evidence supporting their use as prophylaxis against the development of PTSD. The Consensus Statement on

PTSD from the International Consensus Group on Depression and Anxiety discouraged the use of benzodiazepines secondary to limited efficacy, concern for tolerance and withdrawal, and the possibility of "impairment of learning" (Ballenger et al. 2000, 2004). In general, these agents should be considered to have a secondary or augmentation role in the treatment of PTSD. If the decision is made to use these medications, long-half-life agents, such as clonazepam and diazepam, minimize the risk of withdrawal or rebound anxiety (Davidson 2004).

If PTSD symptoms persist after 4 weeks or become increasingly debilitating 2–3 weeks after a traumatic event, consideration should be given to use of an SSRI. In addition to SSRIs, recent studies suggest a role for a novel psychotherapeutic treatment, eye movement desensitization and reprocessing (EMDR), in the treatment of adult trauma survivors. In one study, 75.0% of adult-onset versus 33.3% of child-onset PTSD subjects receiving EMDR achieved asymptomatic end-state functioning, compared with none in the SSRI group (van der Kolk et al. 2007).

Conditions That Require Medical Evaluation

With any acute change in mental status or sudden-onset change in behavior in a previously well individual, organic causes must be considered first, before it is assumed that the symptoms are a manifestation of a previously undiagnosed psychiatric disorder (Frame and Kercher 1991; R.C. Hall et al. 1978, 1981). This is especially true when the syndrome occurs outside of the usual age-based window of vulnerability. For example, new-onset psychotic symptoms in a patient older than 40 years or mania in a patient older than 50 years should be considered to be due to a medical condition until proven otherwise. Other psychiatric disorders do not have as clearly defined windows of vulnerability as schizophrenia and bipolar disorder, but should on initial presentation be suspected as due to a medical condition.

Panic Disorder

A patient presenting for the very first time with dyspnea, tachycardia, diaphoresis, chest pain, and light-headedness should receive a thorough medical evaluation before being assigned a diagnosis of panic disorder. Many different conditions can present with some or all of these symptoms, including unstable angina and myocardial infarction, hypoglycemia, anemia, pulmonary embolism, asthma, obstructive pulmonary disease, gastroesophageal reflux disease, irritable bowel disease, hyperparathyroid-

ism, hyperthyroidism, pheochromocytoma, Huntington's disease, Parkinson's disease, seizure disorder, and autoimmune disorders, such as systemic lupus erythematosus (Roy-Byrne et al. 2006). Only after these medical conditions have been ruled out should a diagnosis of panic disorder be entertained. During the initial attack, use of a benzodiazepine may be helpful to make the patient more comfortable, but care should be taken not to mask symptoms of a more serious underlying condition. Current FDA-approved medications for panic disorder include alprazolam (a benzodiazepine), sertraline and paroxetine (SSRIs), and venlafaxine (serotonin–norepinephrine reuptake inhibitor). SSRIs tend to be utilized first line because of their general tolerability, lack of potential for dependence/misuse, and safety profile (Katon 2006). Currently, the gold standard of clinical practice in the definitive long-term management of panic disorder is the use of SSRIs in concert with cognitive-behavioral therapy.

Dissociative Episodes

Amnestic and acute confusional states should always be considered to be due to a medical or neurological condition until proven otherwise. Amnestic symptoms are common after head injury, during cerebrovascular accidents and transient ischemic accidents, in postictal states, with brain tumors, in intentional and unintentional intoxications, and in many other medical conditions. Another important diagnostic consideration is of a delirium, which could have any number of medical or metabolic causes. Establishing the correct diagnosis in this type of patient is facilitated by extended observation, with repeated assessments. This allows for detection of the fluctuating levels of consciousness and awareness common in delirium and of the temporal evolution of the amnestic symptoms. Unobtrusive observation of these patients also allows for assessment of purposeful, deliberate, and organized behaviors, which usually are observed in patients with psychogenic or factitious amnestic conditions but often are not seen in those with an organic condition.

Catatonia

Catatonia is a syndrome of motor dysregulation characterized by the presence of at least two of the following symptoms for more than 24 hours: mutism, immobility, negativism, posturing, staring, rigidity, stereotypy, mannerisms, echophenomena, perseveration, and automatic obedience (Fink and Taylor 2006; Taylor and Fink 2003). Catatonia can be diagnosed in 7%–15% of psychiatric patients in acute inpatient services and emergency room settings

(Fink and Taylor 2006). Although commonly classified as a psychotic spectrum disorder, catatonia is more frequently associated with mania, melancholia, and psychotic depression than it is with schizophrenia. If a patient has not had documented previous episodes of catatonia in conjunction with one of these psychiatric disorders, a medical cause should be sought vigorously. Episodes of catatonic behavior can occur in a variety of neurological and medical conditions, including metabolic encephalopathies, viral encephalitis, cerebrovascular accidents, epileptic episodes, hypercalcemia, and adverse medication (neuroleptic) and drug (phencyclidine [PCP]) side effects. These conditions should be ruled out before a psychiatric diagnosis is made. Although no established standard of care exists for the treatment of catatonia, acceptable treatment options include high-dose intravenous barbiturates (e.g., amobarbital) and benzodiazepines (e.g., lorazepam), as well as electroconvulsive therapy (ECT) (Fink 2001; Rosebush et al. 1990). However, definitive treatment is based on the underlying diagnosis.

Mania and Psychosis

New-onset mania and psychosis should always be approached as potentially due to a medical condition. The clinical context will guide the urgency of the medical evaluation. New-onset psychotic symptoms in a 40-year-old and new-onset mania in a 50-year-old should prompt an urgent medical evaluation. Such symptoms appearing in an adolescent or a young adult should still be evaluated medically, although not with the same urgency as in the older adult. These symptoms can be caused by brain tumors, cerebrovascular accidents, autoimmune disorders, multiple sclerosis, and hyperthyroidism. Many medications, including exogenously administered steroids and stimulants, as well as illicit drugs can provoke manic and psychotic symptoms. Therefore, a thorough physical examination and a urine drug screen are essential components of the diagnostic workup.

Conversion Disorder

Conversion disorder is a diagnosis of exclusion. Accordingly, new-onset neurological symptoms, including nonepileptic seizures, nonanatomical movement disorders, paresthesias, paresis, and amnestic syndromes, should be thoroughly evaluated before being attributed to a psychogenic cause. Management of conversion symptoms includes a complete medical assessment and reassurance that the symptoms will resolve with time. In one case report describing treatment of a patient with acute conver-

sion disorder, use of intravenous lorazepam in combination with hypnosis led to a full recovery (Stevens 1990). Long-term management involves both physical rehabilitation and treatment of the underlying psychological conflict or distress. Family therapy can be a useful tool, given that family dynamics are often an essential part of the psychosomatic response to stress (Hurwitz 2004). Similar treatment strategies can be used for the treatment of somatization disorder.

Psychiatric Emergencies That Usually Require Pharmacological Intervention

Management of severe behavioral emergencies usually requires psychopharmacological intervention prior to definitive diagnosis (Table 62–4). Many psychiatric patients will have episodes of disorganized, disinhibited, agitated, aggressive, or violent behavior. These behavioral states can occur in patients who are psychotic, manic, or intoxicated as well as in those who have organic syndromes such as dementia or delirium. Patients who are experiencing severe medication side effects or adverse events also require pharmacological intervention, as do patients with substance use disorders in withdrawal states.

Assaultive, Aggressive, or Violent Behavior

Assaultive, aggressive, and violent behaviors can have many different etiologies, including psychotic or delusional ideation secondary to a primary psychotic or mood disorder, substance intoxication, acute confusional states associated with dementia and delirium, rage attacks in patients with personality disorders, and deliberate, volitional acts by antisocial individuals. The most important chronic risk factor for predicting violent behavior is a history of such behavior. Acute risk factors include over- or undercontrolled behavior. The former refers to a patient with decreased psychomotor activity, tension, anger, and paranoia, whereas the latter refers to a patient who is agitated, intrusive, and verbally provocative. Intoxication is an independent acute risk factor that can potentiate violent behaviors in patients with many different diagnoses.

The initial diagnostic effort should be to globally assess the behavioral state causing the aggressive behaviors, because this will affect subsequent treatment decisions. Concurrently, the focus should be to maintain a safe environment for the patient, other patients, and the staff. A well-

TABLE 62–4. Psychiatric emergencies that usually require pharmacological intervention

EMERGENCY	INTERVENTION
Assaultive, aggressive, or violent behavior	Calm, controlled staff Adequate staff/"show of force" Seclusion/stimulus minimization Physical restraint

Primary psychotic or mood disorder	Medication:
	  Lorazepam
	  Haloperidol
	  Atypical antipsychotics
	Definitive diagnosis and treatment plan

Delirium	Diagnose delirium vs. other disorder Definitive medical diagnosis Treat underlying cause Intravenous (iv) or intramuscular (im) haloperidol
Ethanol or sedative-hypnotic withdrawal	Benzodiazepine to stabilize withdrawal symptoms Controlled taper under supervision Refer to chemical dependency treatment
Alcohol withdrawal delirium	Medical intensive care Supportive measures Benzodiazepine taper
Medication side effects	

Neuroleptic-induced dystonia	Acute:
	  Diphenhydramine 25–50 mg iv
	Maintenance:
	  Diphenhydramine 25–100 mg qd, or
	  Benztropine 0.5–4.0 mg qd, or
	  Trihexyphenidyl 2–10 mg qd

Neuroleptic-induced akathisia	Lower antipsychotic dose Propranolol 10 mg two to three times daily Benzodiazepine

Neuroleptic malignant syndrome	Discontinue offending agent
	Medical intensive care/support:
	  Cooling
	  Hydration
	  Anticoagulation
	Medical intensive care/support:
	  Cooling
	  Hydration
	  Anticoagulation
	Dantrolene
	Benzodiazepine
	Electroconvulsive therapy

Anticholinergic delirium	Discontinue offending agent(s) Supportive measures

TABLE 62–4. Psychiatric emergencies that usually require pharmacological intervention (continued)

EMERGENCY	INTERVENTION
Medication side effects (continued)	
Hypertensive crisis	Management of blood pressure Supportive measures
Serotonin syndrome	Discontinue offending agent Medical supportive measures/intensive care Benzodiazepine
Priapism	Discontinue offending agent Medical supportive measures Urology evaluation if condition does not resolve
Selective serotonin reuptake inhibitor discontinuation syndrome	Reassurance; restart medications

trained staff of an adequate number in an appropriately designed facility is the best preventive strategy for minimizing violent episodes. Staff members who are trained to respond in a calm, deliberate, and nonthreatening manner help to establish an atmosphere of order and control. Preventing a violent act from occurring is preferable to responding to a violent act after it has occurred; thus, ongoing assessment of patients is essential, as is the proactive use of sedating medications. It is better to have a patient take a medication voluntarily and orally before his or her behavior has escalated than to be required to involuntarily medicate the patient after a crisis has occurred. This cooperation of care is the first step in establishing a therapeutic alliance, which in turn can further mitigate the risk of escalation.

There are several options in the acute management of the agitated patient. Orally available agents include several benzodiazepines and atypical antipsychotics. Lorazepam in 2-mg doses given every 45–60 minutes usually will sedate most patients by the second dose. Other alternatives are 15–20 mg of olanzapine, 4–6 mg of risperidone, or 5 mg of haloperidol in a single oral dose. The decision of which agent to use is based on the underlying diagnosis. If a patient with a known diagnosis of schizophrenia or bipolar disorder appears to be experiencing a psychotic or manic decompensation, then an atypical antipsychotic should be used. If the diagnosis is not known or is unclear, then lorazepam is a better choice. This is especially true given that acute intoxication with some agents—for example, anticholinergics like diphenhydramine—may be worsened by the addition of atypical antipsychotics. Lorazepam is also most appropriate for patients who are violent as a result of intoxication with drugs or alcohol.

The administration of oral medications is preferred over the use of parenteral medications when the agitated patient is willing to accept such an intervention. Research has suggested that clinicians may overutilize intramuscular injections out of ease of treatment. One study in a Geneva, Switzerland, psychiatric emergency service evaluated the rates of involuntary injections in patients being observed for psychomotor agitation. The results supported the theory of overutilization, as there was a 27% reduction in involuntary injections during a 3-month observation of treatment (Damsa et al. 2006). Given these findings, efforts should be made to encourage voluntary administration of medications if possible.

New alternatives to the established pill or tablet formulation of second-generation antipsychotics exist and demonstrate positive results in comparative trials. Risperidone M-Tab, Zyprexa Zydis, and Abilify disc melt are currently available rapidly dissolving forms of their parent agents. Risperidone is also available in an oral concentrate solution. These formulations exhibit benefit over the traditional pill formulation in patients who may "cheek," or store the administered medication in their cheek, and dispose of it prior to consumption (Allen et al. 2001, 2005). These formulations display similar pharmacokinetics compared with the traditional pill formulation.

When staff attempts to redirect an actively or imminently violent patient fail, quick and decisive action must be taken. The most direct means to ensure safety of the patient and all others in the immediate area is seclusion and restraint. Adequate numbers of well-trained staff are required to accomplish this rapidly and with minimal chance of injury to the patient and staff. Staff should be trained to manage the situation assertively while maintaining professionalism—that is, not acting in a manner that is punitive or reactive to the patient's behavior. Patients who are restrained also should receive medication, usually via the intramuscular or intravenous route. However, because establishment of intravenous access in a combative patient is often very difficult and is potentially dangerous to the patient and staff, intramuscular is usually the preferred route.

Involuntary administration of psychotropic medications is allowed in emergencies that are considered life-threatening, although rather wide variation exists in the legal definition of life-threatening emergencies and in the practice of administering involuntary medication. Clinicians should be well informed on the local definitions and regulations regarding involuntary administration of psychotropic medication. Accurate and timely documentation of the need for restraint and involuntary medication administration is essential.

Currently, six medications are suitable for intravenous or intramuscular administration in behavioral emergencies. These are lorazepam, diazepam, haloperidol, and injectable preparations of three atypical antipsychotics—olanzapine, ziprasidone, and aripiprazole. Lorazepam is the most useful and should be the mainstay for controlling behavioral emergencies (Battaglia et al. 1997; Foster et al. 1997; Salzman et al. 1991). Lorazepam is rapidly absorbed from intramuscular injections, has a rapid onset of action, has a short half-life, and is anxiolytic as well as sedating. Patients who are being combative generally are experiencing high levels of fear or anxiety, so the anxiolytic properties of lorazepam are an additional advantage. Intramuscular diazepam can be absorbed erratically and thus is not particularly useful. Haloperidol should be reserved for patients who are clearly psychotic, with the expectation that they will receive long-term treatment with an antipsychotic agent.

A sufficiently large dose should be given with the first injection in a behavioral emergency to ensure rapid onset of sedation and to minimize the need for a second or third injection. Lorazepam should be administered in 2-mg doses that can be repeated at 45 minutes if the initial dose is not sufficient. Very rarely will any additional injections be required after a second 2-mg dose of lorazepam. The initial haloperidol injection should be 2.5–5.0 mg and should not be repeated for at least 2 hours. Sufficient time must be given for the medication to be absorbed and for maximal sedation to occur. Under no circumstances should a patient receive more than 5 mg of haloperidol in a single injection or more than two injections (10 mg) in 24 hours, which can provoke a severe dystonic reaction. To prevent dystonia, 1 mg of benztropine should be included with intramuscular haloperidol. Alternatively, 25 mg of diphenhydramine may be added to prevent dystonia while providing additional sedation via its antihistaminergic mechanism of action. The combination of lorazepam and haloperidol in a ratio of 2 mg of lorazepam to 5 mg of haloperidol is often used to provide adequate sedation and anxiolysis while treating the underlying psychosis. However, unless the patient is obviously psychotic and the plan is for long-term antipsychotic treatment, this combination should be avoided. On the other hand, benztropine is not needed if lorazepam has been given with haloperidol.

The injectable atypical antipsychotics should be reserved for patients who will be given an oral atypical agent after the immediate emergency has resolved. Intramuscular ziprasidone was approved in 2002, and it has been studied in patients with schizophrenia who were psychotic and agitated and is currently indicated for the treatment of these conditions (Daniel et al. 2001; Lesem et al. 2001). In these clinical trials, patients received an initial injection of 10 mg, followed by injections of 5–20 mg every 4–6 hours, for a maximum dose of 80 mg in 24 hours. At the end of 3 days of intramuscular treatment, these patients were converted to the oral preparation of ziprasidone. The intramuscular ziprasidone package insert (Geodon 2008) recommends doses of 10–20 mg, with 10-mg doses repeatable at 2-hour intervals and 20-mg doses at 4-hour intervals. The maximum recommended intramuscular dose in 24 hours is 40 mg. Studies of intramuscular ziprasidone in the treatment of acute agitation note overall efficacy in reducing agitation while relieving anxiety. Intramuscular ziprasidone appears to have a low incidence of extrapyramidal side effects compared with intramuscular haloperidol (Brook et al. 2000). Results from one naturalistic study suggest that the use of intramuscular ziprasidone may reduce time in restraints for agitated patients compared with treatment with a conventional agent (Preval et al. 2005). One drawback of the intramuscular ziprasidone preparation is that it has to be reconstituted with sterile water immediately prior to administration.

Injectable olanzapine has been studied for use in agitated patients with schizophrenia, bipolar mania, and dementia (Breier et al. 2002; Meehan et al. 2001, 2002; Wright et al. 2001). In the schizophrenia trials, patients received up to three individual injections of 2.5–10.0 mg in 24 hours, with the higher doses producing more significant and sustained reduction of agitation. In the bipolar trials, patients received up to three injections of 5 or 10 mg of olanzapine in 24 hours, with significant reduction in agitated behaviors. In the dementia trial, agitated patients received up to three olanzapine injections of 2.5 or 5 mg in 24 hours, with significant reduction in agitation. A recent review of the literature by Tulloch and Zed (2004) concluded that injectable olanzapine was superior to placebo in all study populations and to intramuscular lorazepam in patients with bipolar affective disorder. However, this review further concluded that injectable olanzapine did not differ significantly from intramuscular haloperidol or lorazepam in the management of agitation associated with schizophrenia/schizoaffective disorder or dementia. It is relevant to note that olanzapine is FDA approved for the treatment of schizophrenia and bipolar mania, but not agitation associated with dementia.

Injectable aripiprazole was FDA approved for the treatment of agitation in patients with schizophrenia and bipolar mania in 2006. With a unique mechanism of action as a dopamine partial agonist, aripiprazole presents a new treatment approach in the management of acute agitation. Efficacy studies demonstrate injectable aripiprazole at a dose of 9.75 mg is superior to placebo and comparable to injectable olanzapine. Injectable aripiprazole demonstrated tolerability and symptom reduction without oversedation (Trans-Johnson et al. 2007). One benefit of this formulation is that it is packaged in a 9.75 mg/1.3 mL ready-to-use single vial.

Schizophrenia

Atypical antipsychotics represent the current standard of care for the treatment of acute agitation in patients with schizophrenia (American Psychiatric Association 2004). With proven efficacy in comparison with haloperidol and improved tolerability, these agents represent the first-line treatment in the agitated psychotic patient (Aleman and Kahn 2001; Currier and Trenton 2002; Yildiz et al. 2003). The only patients in whom this is not the case are those who have been stable long term (5 or more years) while taking a typical antipsychotic. The optimal intervention in a patient with schizophrenia who is experiencing an acute exacerbation is to rapidly initiate treatment with an atypical antipsychotic. In this regard, risperidone and olanzapine are the most useful agents, because both can be initiated at a high therapeutic dose (15–20 mg for olanzapine; 4–6 mg for risperidone) and can be given in multiple oral doses (two or three doses) over a period of 24 hours. Both of these medications, as well as aripiprazole, are available in an orally disintegrating formulation if compliance is in question. However, if compliance is a concern, then one must assess the utility of oral medications in general, and consider an intramuscular medication.

In a patient who is too disorganized or combative to take medication orally, intramuscular administration is the only viable route. Currently, haloperidol, ziprasidone, olanzapine, and aripiprazole are available as injectable preparations. In a patient who is psychotic and agitated, the coadministration of a benzodiazepine during the first few days of treatment can be particularly effective in controlling behavior while the antipsychotic response develops. Studies suggest that this combination may reduce the total antipsychotic dose and potentially result in fewer adverse antipsychotic effects (Salzman et al. 1991; Yildiz et al. 2003). One caveat to this choice of treatment is the recent attention surrounding an increased risk of sedation and cardiorespiratory depression in patients treated with intramuscular olanzapine and intramuscular lorazepam, leading to a warning in the prescribing information provided by Eli Lilly, the manufacturer of olanzapine (Zyprexa 2005).

Bipolar Disorder

Although behavioral emergencies can occur during both manic and depressive mood states, they tend to occur more often during mania. The goal of managing these patients is the establishment of a long-term definitive treatment regimen, which means initiating treatment with a mood-stabilizing agent such as lithium (10–20 mg/kg) or valproic acid (20–30 mg/kg) as soon as possible. Prior to initiating either of these two agents, a serum pregnancy test should be obtained and documented as negative, since both agents are teratogenic. Patients should be monitored for signs and symptoms of adverse side effects and toxicity. Both lithium and valproic acid require time to reach a therapeutic blood level and may take up to 14 days to become fully effective. Until steady state is established, behavioral control can be achieved with oral or intramuscular lorazepam or another benzodiazepine on an as-needed basis or with an atypical antipsychotic such as olanzapine, risperidone, ziprasidone, quetiapine, or aripiprazole, all of which are FDA approved for the treatment of acute bipolar mania. Olanzapine, risperidone, and quetiapine have the advantage of being sedating, which can be useful in an emergency room–type setting. In fact, atypical agents may be preferable to benzodiazepines in the management of acute bipolar mania according to recent studies. A recent review of the literature indicated that intramuscular olanzapine was superior to lorazepam monotherapy in the treatment of agitated manic patients (Tulloch and Zed 2004). Focusing on the long-term treatment goals is of the essence. If the long-term plans do not include an antipsychotic, then lorazepam or another benzodiazepine should be used for short-term behavioral control. If, however, it is known that the patient will require both a mood stabilizer and an antipsychotic for long-term management, then the antipsychotic should be substituted for the benzodiazepine.

Another treatment option in both manic and depressed bipolar patients is ECT. With a rapid onset of action and known efficacy, especially in terms of short-term stabilization, this is a viable treatment option. This could be considered a treatment of choice in patients who are pregnant. Unfortunately, many facilities are not equipped to provide this treatment, and there are legal issues around obtaining informed consent to administer ECT emergently.

Substance Intoxication

Violent and combative behavior by intoxicated patients is a very common occurrence in psychiatric and medical emergency departments. Alcohol, cocaine, and PCP are the main culprits, but methamphetamines, γ-hydroxybutyrate, and hallucinogens also can lead to violent behavior.

Ethanol intoxication is a very common cause of violent behavior in many settings. The appropriate interventions are physical restraint and sedation with a benzodiazepine, in conjunction with haloperidol if the agitation is significant, to allow the patient to become sober while serving as a seizure prophylaxis. Once a patient's blood alcohol level is below the legal limit for intoxication, a more definitive evaluation can be carried out, focusing on presence of an underlying psychiatric diagnosis or other treatment needs. Follow-up options include referral to substance abuse treatment, involuntary commitment if allowed in that jurisdiction, admission to a dual-diagnosis unit or program, or discharge.

Prolonged cocaine use can lead to development of both mood and psychotic syndromes. Transient paranoid states are very common in cocaine users, as are frank delusions and hallucinations. Agitated, paranoid states accompanying cocaine intoxication can lead to significant violent behavior. Interventions are as described previously, including seclusion and restraint, use of intramuscular lorazepam, and possibly use of an antipsychotic if the patient is frankly psychotic. When the patient is no longer intoxicated, the presence of underlying psychopathology can be assessed. Disposition is as described for alcohol: admission to a dual-diagnosis program if the patient has another psychiatric disorder, referral to chemical dependency treatment, or discharge.

PCP intoxication can be particularly provocative of agitated, combative, and violent behavior. Fortunately (or unfortunately), PCP use tends to occur in localized geographical regions and not in others. In areas where PCP use is common, intoxicated persons are common in emergency facilities. PCP intoxication can present with frank psychotic symptoms, agitation, disorientation, and disorganized behavior. Violent outbursts can be sudden, unprovoked, and unexpected. Patients in the throes of PCP intoxication can be very insensitive to pain, so they are prone to continue to fight even if seriously injured. Adequate numbers of well-trained staff are essential when dealing with patients who have been using PCP. The expectation should be that these patients will require seclusion and restraint. Restraint rooms should be dark and quiet so as to minimize stimulation. Intramuscular lorazepam should be used to sedate the patient, and he or she should be allowed to become fully sober before definitive assessment. The half-life of PCP is 20 hours, so these behavioral states can persist for several days before fully resolving.

Methamphetamine, hallucinogens, γ-hydroxybutyrate, and cannabis can cause agitated, disorganized, and even violent behavior. Methamphetamine in particular can have behavioral consequences very similar to those of cocaine. Because of the long half-life of methamphetamine compared with cocaine, this drug can be particularly provocative of frank paranoid and psychotic symptoms. Like PCP use, methamphetamine use tends to be limited to certain geographical regions and not others.

From 1991 to 1994, methamphetamine-related emergency cases tripled nationwide, making it a growing clinical phenomenon (Centers for Disease Control and Prevention 1995). Presenting symptoms often include agitation, hallucinations, suicidal ideation, and chest pain (Derlet et al. 1989). Distinguishing stimulant intoxication from other clinical diagnoses can be challenging given the symptom overlap. Generally, stimulant-induced psychosis tends to be distinguishable from primary psychotic disorders by the absence of a thought disorder and a prominence of visual hallucinations (Harris and Batki 2000). However, given the potential for comorbidity, a positive drug screen does not completely discount the diagnosis of a mood or psychotic disorder. Treatment should focus on maintaining the patient's safety while awaiting the drug's metabolism and dissipation from the patient's system. A more complete diagnostic workup can be completed once the patient is no longer intoxicated.

Delirium

Patients with delirium can become disorganized, agitated, and combative. Delirium is defined as a state of a disturbed level of consciousness with a change in cognition or with perceptual disturbances, during which the symptoms occurs rapidly and tend to fluctuate with time. Delirium may be due to a general medical condition, substance intoxication or withdrawal, or secondary to multiple etiologies (American Psychiatric Association 2000). Delirium is a medical emergency and carries a very high burden of morbidity and mortality. The definitive treatment of delirium requires diagnosing the underlying

cause and taking corrective action toward that particular pathology. Interventions aimed at controlling behavior include soft or leather restraints, environmental modification including frequent reorientation of the patient, and use of intravenous haloperidol. Behavioral control is essential so that the patient does not further injure him- or herself or interfere with treatment and to protect staff and other patients. The first intravenous dose of haloperidol should be 2.5 mg. If the patient is still agitated after 2 hours, the dose should be increased to 5 mg. This dose can be repeated in another 2 hours if the patient continues to be agitated. Once the patient is stabilized, a routine neuroleptic regimen should be initiated, dividing the total dose into two or four regular doses. The neuroleptic can be decreased and discontinued as the delirium clears. Benzodiazepines are generally contraindicated in cases of delirium, because they can exacerbate behavioral dysregulation and potentiate the altered level of consciousness.

Dementia

Patients with dementia can become agitated, combative, or psychotic for many different reasons. The most common cause for this is a delirium overlying the dementia. Delirium in these patients can be caused by side effects from medications; infectious processes, which can appear quite minimal or clinically insignificant; and metabolic disturbances from many medical causes. Definitive diagnosis and treatment of the underlying disorder are essential to achieving adequate long-term resolution. Patients with dementia who are not delirious can become agitated as a result of confusion or psychosis inherent in the dementing pathology. In these cases, the best interventions are nonpharmacological, including environmental modification, behavior modification, and supportive measures. Aggressive behavior in patients with dementia can be treated pharmacologically, in the short term with lorazepam or low-dose neuroleptics and in the long term with low-dose neuroleptics, the anticonvulsants carbamazepine or valproic acid, propranolol, serotonin reuptake inhibitors, or buspirone. As is the case in all geriatric medicine, low doses and slow titration schedules are the appropriate course. Recent data suggest an increased mortality risk associated with the administration of neuroleptics in the management of dementia-related psychosis (Schneider et al. 2005). It is important to note that second-generation antipsychotics are not approved for the treatment of dementia-related psychosis and that a black box warning has been placed on the prescribing information of these agents in this population regarding an increased risk of cerebrovascular events and adverse events that are infectious in nature.

Substance Withdrawal States

Alcohol and Sedative-Hypnotics

Alcohol and sedative-hypnotic withdrawal can result in a frank delirium that is life-threatening (Marco and Kelen 1990; Olmedo and Hoffman 2000). The acute signs of early alcohol, sedative-hypnotic, and benzodiazepine withdrawal are similar and include autonomic instability, tremulousness, diaphoresis, and gastrointestinal disturbances. Autonomic signs include tachycardia, hypertension, and hyperthermia. Treatment of this withdrawal state is best accomplished with a long-half-life benzodiazepine. Use of long-half-life agents such as diazepam or chlordiazepoxide prevents peaks and troughs in blood levels, thereby leading to a smoother taper. During the first 24 hours, vital signs should be taken at 2- to 4-hour intervals and additional benzodiazepine given if vital signs are still elevated. After 24 hours, the total dose should be added up and given as four divided doses, which are then decreased 10%–20% per day. In patients with significant liver disease, lorazepam or oxazepam should be used in preference to other benzodiazepines because their metabolism is not as dependent on hepatic function. It is important to consider concomitant medications, since β-blockers prescribed for a general medical condition may mask the autonomic signs of withdrawal.

Alcohol withdrawal delirium (delirium tremens) is a life-threatening medical condition (Erwin et al. 1998). This syndrome has a very high mortality rate—up to 35% of untreated patients and as high as 5%–15% in optimally treated patients. The delirium usually develops 48–72 hours after discontinuation of alcohol or sedative-hypnotics, peaks around day 4, and can persist for 2 weeks. The symptoms include autonomic instability, fever, disorientation, perceptual disturbances and hallucinations, agitation, and confusion. Patients with delirium tremens should be treated in a medical intensive care unit. These patients typically require physical restraint and vigorous supportive measures. Intravenous haloperidol can be used to control agitation and psychosis, but by the time a patient develops delirium tremens, benzodiazepines are not particularly useful.

Wernicke-Korsakoff syndrome is another consequence of long-term alcohol use. Wernicke encephalopathy is the symptom complex of ophthalmoplegia, ataxia, and an acute confusional state. Wernicke-Korsakoff syndrome is diagnosed if persistent learning and memory deficits are additionally present. Alcoholic patients should receive three daily 100-mg doses of thiamine via the intramuscular route from the day of presentation, followed by three daily oral doses to prevent development of this syndrome. Patients should receive the first intramuscular dose before oral or intravenous administration of a carbohydrate load in order to prevent rapid thiamine depletion and emergent development of Wernicke-Korsakoff syndrome. Patients should also be given folic acid and magnesium replacement supplementation, because nutritional deficiencies are common in alcohol-dependent patients.

Another potentially emergent situation is a patient presenting with an alcohol–disulfiram reaction. Disulfiram (Antabuse) blocks alcohol dehydrogenase, leading to a buildup of acetaldehyde. Subsequent consumption of alcohol produces unpleasant symptoms, including headache, flushing, nausea, and vomiting, creating an aversive reaction to alcohol consumption. No treatment for these mild symptoms is necessary. Serious symptoms such as arrhythmias and respiratory depression can occur and should be treated immediately with supportive measures.

Opiates

Opiate withdrawal can be exceedingly uncomfortable for the patient but, unlike alcohol and sedative-hypnotic withdrawal, is generally not life-threatening. Accordingly, the goal of opiate withdrawal treatment is relief of pain and suffering. Symptoms of opiate withdrawal include dysphoria, anxiety, irritability, craving, mydriasis, piloerection, diaphoresis, nausea, vomiting, diarrhea, rhinorrhea, lacrimation, insomnia, fever, and hypertension. Onset of this syndrome depends on the half-life of the drug used and with heroin is usually 6–8 hours after the last use. The syndrome can last 2–5 days, depending on the individual patient. Most of the symptoms are attributable to upregulation of α_2-adrenergic receptors; as a result, α_2 agonists such as clonidine are very useful. Clonidine in doses of 0.1–0.3 mg every 3 hours, up to 0.8 mg/day, can be given to suppress signs of opiate withdrawal (Ahmadi-Abhari et al. 2001; Akhondzadeh et al. 2000; Charney et al. 1981; Gossop 1988). A major side effect of this regimen is hypotension, so the regimen must be carried out in a medically supervised setting. Clonidine should be avoided in patients who are dependent on both opiates and alcohol or a sedative-hypnotic; clonidine may mask the autonomic signs of ethanol withdrawal without actually preventing the emergence of delirium tremens.

Another approach to opiate withdrawal is to substitute a long-half-life agent such as methadone at a dose of

30–80 mg and then taper off this agent at a rate of 10%–20% per day. This is best accomplished in a "cocktail" that keeps the patient "blind" to the daily dose. This type of detoxification regimen is recommended in patients who are dually addicted to opiates and ethanol or sedative-hypnotics. A long-half-life opiate and long-half-life benzodiazepine are used to detoxify both dependencies.

Psychotropic Medication Side Effects

Antipsychotics

Several adverse events can occur in patients taking typical antipsychotics and to a lesser degree in patients taking atypical antipsychotics. Dystonic reactions are characterized by extreme muscle contraction and rigidity in a patient with stable vital signs and a clear sensorium. These occur most frequently with high-potency, first-generation antipsychotics (Moleman et al. 1982; Schillevoort et al. 2001). Young males are particularly susceptible to dystonic reactions. Most dystonic reactions are extremely uncomfortable and frightening to the patient. Treatment of these reactions is typically 1–2 mg of benztropine via the oral or intramuscular route. An alternative is diphenhydramine in doses of 25–50 mg via the oral or intramuscular route. Dystonias that include the eyes, the so-called oculogyric crises, are particularly frightening, as are dystonias that cause laryngeal spasms, which can compromise the airway. These reactions should be treated with 50 mg of intravenous diphenhydramine, which provides rapid relief. Maintenance treatment of 1–2 mg of benztropine twice a day or 25–50 mg of diphenhydramine twice a day should be initiated after the acute reaction has resolved (Keepers et al. 1983).

Akathisia is a syndrome characterized by internal restlessness, often perceived as the need to be in motion. This leads to increased psychomotor activity, including pacing, rocking, leg tapping and bouncing, and moving frequently between sitting and standing. The patient may complain of feeling anxious, irritable, or that his or her "skin is crawling." Treatment providers may interpret the anxiety, irritability, and increased motor activity common to patients with akathisia as worsening of psychotic symptoms, resulting in increased administration of antipsychotics. This further provokes the akathisia and consequently worsens the behavioral state. Lowering the dose of the antipsychotic or switching to an atypical antipsychotic are treatment options; the atypical drugs cause akathisia at lower rates compared with typical agents. Propranolol in doses of 10 mg two or three times a day is an effective treatment for akathisia.

Neuroleptic malignant syndrome (NMS) is a potentially fatal delirium that develops in some patients in response to antipsychotic agents (Susman 2001). The diagnosis is made on the triad of symptoms of altered level of consciousness, muscular rigidity (often described as lead-pipe rigidity), and autonomic instability. The autonomic instability includes hyperthermia, tachycardia, labile blood pressure, diaphoresis, incontinence, and occasional dysphagia and bowel obstruction. Associated findings include elevated creatine phosphokinase (CPK), elevated white blood cell count, and metabolic acidosis. Later complications include rhabdomyolysis and renal failure. The main interventions in NMS are discontinuation of the offending agent and provision of general supportive measures, including cooling, rehydration, intensive nursing care, and anticoagulation. A few drugs have been used to treat NMS, including benzodiazepines, bromocriptine (15 mg/day), dantrolene (100–300 mg/day), and amantadine (200 mg/day). ECT also has been used to treat NMS.

The atypical antipsychotic clozapine can cause catastrophic agranulocytosis in up to 1% of patients treated. This usually occurs within 6 weeks to 6 months of initiating therapy with clozapine. As a result, a surveillance program has been put in place so that all patients taking clozapine have weekly blood counts for the first 6 months of therapy, then every other week for 6 months, followed by monthly counts for the duration of treatment. A white blood cell count of less than $3,500/mm^3$ or a granulocyte count of less than $1,500/mm^3$ warrants discontinuation of the medication. Other signs of impending marrow failure are fever, flulike symptoms, and sore throat. Discontinuation of the clozapine, supportive measures, and treatment of specific infections if identified are the main interventions for agranulocytosis, and in life-threatening cases, growth factors (filgrastim [Neupogen]) can be used.

Antidepressants

Older-generation antidepressants can cause severe adverse events, whereas the newer agents, especially the SSRIs, are remarkably safe.

Adverse events associated with tricyclic antidepressants include anticholinergic delirium, cardiac conduction delays, and seizures. Anticholinergic delirium is more common in elderly and impaired individuals and may be potentiated by concomitant anticholinergic medications. The principal intervention is to decrease or discontinue the offending agent. Furthermore, the coadministration of an SSRI or other drug known to inhibit the cytochrome P450 2D6 enzyme with a tricyclic antidepressant can cause dramatic increases in tricyclic antidepressant blood levels and resultant delirium. This can occur in a patient taking a low dose of the tricyclic antidepressant, and pharmacokinetic interactions must be considered in an emerging delirium in a patient taking what would otherwise be a safe dose of a tricyclic antidepressant. These drugs also can affect cardiac conduction, can lower seizure thresholds, and are lethal in overdose.

A hypertensive crisis can occur in a patient who is taking monoamine oxidase inhibitors. This usually happens after ingestion of a large dose of tyramine, which can be found in certain food products or after an interaction with another drug, such as meperidine, other antidepressants, and sympathomimetic agents. Discontinuation of the monoamine oxidase inhibitor and management of the hypertension are the appropriate treatments. Blood pressure control can be achieved with intravenous phentolamine or intramuscular or oral chlorpromazine.

Serotonin syndrome is a delirium characterized by altered level of consciousness, autonomic instability, and neuromuscular abnormalities including myoclonus, hyperreflexia, nystagmus, akathisia, and muscle rigidity (Martin 1996; Mason et al. 2000). Several different drugs, usually administered in combination, can cause this adverse event. Drugs reported to provoke serotonin syndrome include SSRIs, tricyclic antidepressants, monoamine oxidase inhibitors, venlafaxine, trazodone, nefazodone, lithium, tryptophan, meperidine, sumatriptan, buspirone, duloxetine, milnacipran, and amphetamines. Discontinuation of the offending agent and general supportive measures are the principal interventions. Unlike in NMS, bromocriptine can worsen the serotonin syndrome. Other drugs useful in treating this condition are benzodiazepines, cyproheptadine, chlorpromazine, methysergide, and propranolol.

Although not a life-threatening emergency, SSRI discontinuation syndrome can be very frightening and distressing to patients. This syndrome develops after abrupt discontinuation of a short-half-life SSRI, with paroxetine and venlafaxine the two most common agents. Symptoms include dizziness, malaise, nausea, paresthesias, tremor, ataxia, confusion, myoclonus, anxiety, and vivid dreaming. Symptoms usually develop 48 hours after the last dose, peak around day 4–5, and can last as long as 2 weeks. Interventions include reassuring the patient and restarting the medicine, followed by a very gradual taper. Another approach is to switch to a long-half-life agent such as fluoxetine during the final days of SSRI treatment, which will then result in a more gradual clearing of the drug and a much lower chance of provoking the discontinuation syndrome.

Priapism is a rare but potentially serious adverse event that has been associated with psychotropic medications including trazodone. This physiological condition is usually self-limiting. However, a patient with an erection lasting for more than 4 hours warrants an evaluation and treatment by appropriate medical personnel (Montague et al. 2003). Patients should be warned of this rare but serious potential side effect.

Conclusion

In the modern era, with changes in the mental health care delivery systems and the resultant limitations placed on the utilization of inpatient treatment resources, the emergency psychiatrist will increasingly be called upon to diagnose and initiate definitive treatment of patients with a wide range of psychiatric disorders. Emergency psychiatrists must balance the needs of individual patients with those of the larger community, the health care system, and the third-party payer system with a focus on delivering care that is both efficacious and cost-effective. This will require a broad knowledge base, incorporating elements of all branches of psychiatry, and consideration toward thorough yet expeditious evaluation, diagnosis, and treatment of patients with mental illnesses.

References

Ahmadi-Abhari SA, Akhondzadeh S, Assadi SM, et al: Baclofen versus clonidine in the treatment of opiates withdrawal, side-effects aspect: a double-blind randomized controlled trial. J Clin Pharm Ther 26:67–71, 2001

Akhondzadeh S, Ahmadi-Abhari SA, Assadi SM, et al: Double-blind randomized controlled trial of baclofen vs clonidine in the treatment of opiates withdrawal. J Clin Pharm Ther 25:347–353, 2000

Aleman A, Kahn RS: Effects of the atypical antipsychotic risperidone on hostility and aggression in schizophrenia: a meta-analysis of controlled trials. Eur Neuropsychopharmacol 11:289–293, 2001

Allen MH, Currier GW, Hughes DH, et al: Expert Consensus Panel for Behavioral Emergencies. The Expert Consensus Guideline Series. Treatment of behavioral emergencies. Postgraduate Medicine (Spec No):1–88; quiz 89–90, 2001

Allen MH, Currier GW, Carpenter D, et al: Expert Consensus Panel for Behavioral Emergencies 2005. The expert consensus guideline series. Treatment of behavioral emergencies 2005. J Psychiatr Pract 11 (suppl 1):5–108; quiz 110–112, 2005

American Psychiatric Association: Diagnostic and Statistical Manual of Mental Disorders, 4th Edition, Text Revision. Washington, DC, American Psychiatric Association, 2000

American Psychiatric Association: Practice guidelines for the treatment of schizophrenia, 2nd edition. Am J Psychiatry 61 (suppl 2):1–56, 2004

Angst F, Stassen HH, Clayton PJ, et al: Mortality of patients with mood disorders: follow-up over 34–38 years. J Affect Disord 68:167–181, 2002

Appleby L, Shaw J, Amos T, et al: Suicide within 12 months of contact with mental health services: national clinical survey. BMJ 318:1235–1239, 1999

Apter A, Kotler M, Sevy S, et al: Correlates of risk of suicide in violent and nonviolent psychiatric patients. Am J Psychiatry 148:833–877, 1991

Ballenger JC, Davidson J, Lecrubier Y, et al: Consensus statement on posttraumatic stress disorder from the International Consensus Group on Depression and Anxiety. J Clin Psychiatry 61:60–66, 2000

Ballenger JC, Davidson JRT, Lecrubier Y, et al: Consensus statement update on posttraumatic stress disorder from the International Consensus Group on depression and anxiety. J Clin Psychiatry 65:55–62, 2004

Battaglia J, Moss S, Rush J, et al: Haloperidol, lorazepam, or both for psychotic agitation? A multicenter, prospective, double-blind, emergency department study. Am J Emerg Med 15:335–340, 1997

Borum R, Reddy M: Assessing violence risk in Tarasoff situations: a fact based model of inquiry. Behav Sci Law 19:375–385, 2001

Breier A, Meehan K, Birkett M, et al: A double-blind, placebo-controlled dose-response comparison of intramuscular olanzapine and haloperidol in the treatment of acute agitation in schizophrenia. Arch Gen Psychiatry 59:441–448, 2002

Brook S, Lucey JV, Gunn KP: Intramuscular ziprasidone compared with intramuscular haloperidol in the treatment of acute psychosis. J Clin Psychiatry 61:933–941, 2000

Busch KA, Fawcett J, Jacobs DG: Clinical correlates of inpatient suicide. J Clin Psychiatry 64:14–19, 2003

Campfield KM, Hills AM: Effect of timing of critical incident stress debriefing (CISD) on posttraumatic symptoms. J Trauma Stress 15:327–340, 2001

Catalano RA, Kessell ER, McConnell W, et al: Psychiatric emergencies after the terrorist attacks of September 11, 2001. Psychiatr Serv 55:163–166, 2004

Centers for Disease Control and Prevention: Increasing morbidity and mortality associated with abuse of methamphetamine—United States, 1991–1994. MMWR Morb Mortal Wkly Rep 44:882–886, 1995

Charney DS, Sternberg DE, Kleber HD, et al: The clinical use of clonidine in abrupt withdrawal from methadone: effects on blood pressure and specific signs and symptoms. Arch Gen Psychiatry 38:1273–1277, 1981

Conwell Y, Duberstein PR, Cox C, et al: Relationships of age and Axis I diagnoses in victims of completed suicide: a psychological autopsy study. Am J Psychiatry 153:1001–1008, 1996

Conwell Y, Duberstein PR, Connor K, et al: Access to firearms and risk for suicide in middle-aged and older adults. Am J Geriatr Psychiatry 10:407–416, 2002

Cornelius JR, Thase ME, Salloum IM, et al: Cocaine use associated with increased suicidal behavior in depressed alcoholics. Addict Behav 23:119–121, 1998

Currier GW, Trenton A: Pharmacological treatment of psychotic agitation. CNS Drugs 16:219–228, 2002

Damsa C, Ikelheimer D, Adam E, et al: Heisenberg in the ER: observation appears to reduce involuntary intramuscular injections in a psychiatric emergency service. Gen Hosp Psychiatry 28:431–433, 2006

Daniel DG, Potkin SG, Reeves KR, et al: Intramuscular (IM) ziprasidone 20 mg is effective in reducing acute agitation associated with psychosis: a double-blind, randomized trial. Psychopharmacology (Berl) 155:128–134, 2001

Davidson JR: Use of benzodiazepines in social anxiety disorder, generalized anxiety disorder, and posttraumatic stress disorder. J Clin Psychiatry 65:29–33, 2004

Deisenhammer EA, Huber M, Kemmler G, et al: Psychiatric hospitalizations during the last 12 months before suicide. Gen Hosp Psychiatry 29:63–65, 2007

Derlet RW, Rice P, Horowitz BZ, et al: Amphetamine toxicity: experience with 127 cases. J Emerg Med 7:157–161, 1989

Dervic K, Oquendo MA, Grunebaum MF, et al: Religious affiliation and suicide attempt. Am J Psychiatry 161:2303–2308, 2004

Dervic K, Oquendo MA, Currier D, et al: Moral objections to suicide: can they counteract suicidality in patients with cluster B psychopathology. J Clin Psychiatry 67:620–625, 2006

Durkheim E: Suicide. Translated by Spaulding JA, Simpson G. New York, Free Press, 1951

Erwin WE, Williams DB, Speir WA: Delirium tremens. South Med J 91:425–432, 1998

Fawcett J: Suicide risk factors in depressive disorders and panic disorder. J Clin Psychiatry 53 (suppl):9–13, 1992

Fawcett J, Scheftner WA, Fogg L, et al: Time-related predictors of suicide in major affective disorders. Am J Psychiatry 147:1189–1194, 1991

Fink M: Catatonia: syndrome or schizophrenia subtype? Recognition and treatment. J Neural Transm 108:637–644, 2001

Fink M, Taylor MA: Catatonia: subtype or syndrome in DSM? Am J Psychiatry 163:1875–1876, 2006

Foa EB, Steketee G, Rothbaum BO: Behavioral/cognitive conceptualizations of post-traumatic stress disorder. Behav Ther 20:155–176, 1989

Foster S, Kessel J, Berman ME, et al: Efficacy of lorazepam and haloperidol for rapid tranquilization in a psychiatric emergency room setting. Int Clin Psychopharmacol 12:175–179, 1997

Fowler RC, Rich CL, Young D: San Diego Suicide Study, II: substance abuse in young cases. Arch Gen Psychiatry 43:962–965, 1986

Frame DS, Kercher EE: Acute psychosis: functional versus organic. Emerg Med Clin North Am 9:123–136, 1991

Garlow SJ: Age, gender, and ethnicity differences in patterns of cocaine and ethanol use preceding suicide. Am J Psychiatry 159:615–619, 2002

Garlow SJ, D'Orio B, Purselle DC: The relationship of restrictions on state hospitalization and suicides among emergency psychiatric patients. Psychiatr Serv 53:1297–1300, 2002

Garlow SJ, Purselle DC, D'Orio B: Cocaine use disorders and suicidal ideation. Drug Alcohol Depend 70:101–104, 2003

Garlow SJ, Purselle D, Heninger M: Ethnic differences in patterns of suicide across the life cycle. Am J Psychiatry 162:319–323, 2005

Garlow SJ, Purselle D, Heninger M: Cocaine and alcohol use preceding suicide in African American and white adolescents. J Psychiatr Res 41:530–536, 2007

Gelpin E, Bonne O, Peri T, et al: Treatment of recent trauma survivors with benzodiazepines: a prospective study. J Clin Psychiatry 57:390–394, 1996

Geodon (ziprasidone mesylate) for injection: U.S. package insert, revised June 2008. Available at: http://www.geodon.com/b_ppi.asp. Accessed September 2008.

Gibbons RD, Hur K, Bhaumik DK, et al: The relationship between antidepressant medication use and rate of suicide. Arch Gen Psychiatry 62:165–172, 2005

Gibbons RD, Brown CH, Hur K, et al: Relationship between antidepressants and suicide attempts: an analysis of the Veterans Health Administration data sets. Am J Psychiatry 164:1044–1049, 2007

Gitlin MJ: A psychiatrist's reaction to a patient's suicide. Am J Psychiatry 156:1630–1634, 1999

Gossop M: Clonidine and the treatment of the opiate withdrawal syndrome. Drug Alcohol Depend 21:253–259, 1988

Greenberg N: A critical review of psychological debriefing: the management of psychological health after traumatic experiences. J R Nav Med Serv 87:158–161, 2001

Hall KT, Appelbaum PS: The origins of commitment for substance abuse in the United States. J Am Acad Psychiatry Law 30:33–45, 2002

Hall RC, Popkin MK, Devaul RA, et al: Physical illness presenting as psychiatric disease. Arch Gen Psychiatry 35:1315–1320, 1978

Hall RC, Gardner ER, Popkin MK, et al: Unrecognized physical illness prompting psychiatric admission: a prospective study. Am J Psychiatry 138:629–635, 1981

Hall RC, Platt DE, Hall RC: Suicide risk assessment: a review of risk factors for suicide in 100 patients who made severe suicide attempts: evaluation of suicide risk in a time of managed care. Psychosomatics 40:18–27, 1999

Harris D, Batki SL: Stimulant psychosis: symptom profile and acute clinical course. Am J Addict 9:28–37, 2000

Harris EC, Barraclough B: Suicide as an outcome of mental disorders: a meta-analysis. Br J Psychiatry 170:205–228, 1997

Hendin H, Lipschitz A, Maltsberger JT: Therapists' reactions to patients' suicides. Am J Psychiatry 157:2022–2027, 2000

Hurwitz TA: Somatization and conversion disorder. Can J Psychiatry 49:172–178, 2004

Isacsson G, Holmgren P, Druid H, et al: The utilization of antidepressants—a key issue in the prevention of suicide: an analysis of 5,281 suicides in Sweden during the period 1992–1994. Acta Psychiatr Scand 96:94–100, 1997

Isacsson G, Holmgren P, Ahlner J: Selective serotonin reuptake inhibitor antidepressants and the risk of suicide: a controlled forensic database study of 14,857 suicides. Acta Psychiatr Scand 111:286–290, 2005

Isometsa ET, Lonnqvist JK: Suicide attempts preceding completed suicide. Br J Psychiatry 173:531–535, 1998

Katon WJ: Clinical practice. Panic disorder. N Engl J Med 354:2360–2367, 2006

Keepers GA, Clappison VJ, Casey DE: Initial anticholinergic prophylaxis for neuroleptic-induced extrapyramidal syndromes. Arch Gen Psychiatry 40:1113–1117, 1983

Kessler RC, Borges G, Walters EE: Prevalence of and risk factors for lifetime suicide attempts in the National Comorbidity Survey. Arch Gen Psychiatry 56:617–626, 1999

Kroll J: Use of no-harm contracts by psychiatrists in Minnesota. Am J Psychiatry 157:1684–1686, 2000

Larkin GL, Claassen CA, Emond JA, et al: Trends in US emergency department visits for mental health conditions, 1992–2001. Psychiatr Serv 56:671–677, 2005

Lesem MD, Zajecka JM, Swift RH, et al: Intramuscular ziprasidone, 2 mg versus 10 mg, in the short-term management of agitated psychotic patients [erratum appears in J Clin Psychiatry 62:209, 2001]. J Clin Psychiatry 62:12–18, 2001

Lewis G, Appleby L, Jarman B: Suicide and psychiatric services. Lancet 344:822, 1994

Malone KM, Oquendo MA, Haas GL, et al: Protective factors against suicidal acts in major depression: reasons for living. Am J Psychiatry 157:1084–1088, 2000

Maltsberger JT, Buie DH: Countertransference hate in the treatment of suicidal patients. Arch Gen Psychiatry 30:625–633, 1974

Mann JJ, Apter A, Bertolote J, et al: Suicide prevention strategies: a systematic review. JAMA 294:2064–2074, 2005

Marco CA, Kelen GD: Acute intoxication. Emerg Med Clin North Am 8:731–748, 1990

Martin T: Serotonin syndrome. Ann Emerg Med 28:520–526, 1996

Mason PJ, Morris VA, Balcezak TJ: Serotonin syndrome: presentation of 2 cases and review of the literature. Medicine (Baltimore) 79:201–209, 2000

Matar MA, Cohen H, Kaplan Z, et al: The effect of early poststressor intervention with sertraline on behavioral responses in an animal model of post-traumatic stress disorder. Neuropsychopharmacology 31:2610–2618, 2006

Meehan K, Zhang F, David S, et al: A double-blind, randomized comparison of the efficacy and safety of intramuscular injections of olanzapine, lorazepam, or placebo in treating acutely agitated patients diagnosed with bipolar mania. J Clin Psychopharmacol 21:389–397, 2001

Meehan KM, Wang H, David SR, et al: Comparison of rapidly acting intramuscular olanzapine, lorazepam, and placebo: a double-blind, randomized study in acutely agitated patients with dementia. Neuropsychopharmacology 26:494–504, 2002

Mellman TA, David D, Bustamante V, et al: Predictors of post-traumatic stress disorder following severe injury. Depress Anxiety 14:226–231, 2001

Miller M, Azael D, Hemenway D: Household firearm ownership and suicide rates in the United States. Epidemiology 13:517–524, 2002

Mitchell J: When disaster strikes: the critical incident stress debriefing process. JEMS 8:36–39, 1983

Moleman P, Schmitz PJ, Ladee GA: Extrapyramidal side effects and oral haloperidol: an analysis of explanatory patient and treatment characteristics. J Clin Psychiatry 43:492–496, 1982

Montague DK, Jarow J, Broderick GA, et al: American Urological Association guideline on the management of priapism. J Urol 170(4 pt 1):1318–1324, 2003

Moscicki EK: Identification of suicide risk factors using epidemiologic studies. Psychiatr Clin North Am 20:499–517, 1997

Murphy GE, Wetzel RD: The lifetime risk of suicide in alcoholism. Arch Gen Psychiatry 47:383–392, 1990

Murphy GE, Wetzel RD, Robins E, et al: Multiple risk factors predict suicide in alcoholism. Arch Gen Psychiatry 49:459–463, 1992

National Center for Injury Prevention and Control: Web-Based Injury Statistics Query and Reporting System (WISQARS). Atlanta, GA, National Center for Injury Prevention and Control, 2002

National Center for Injury Prevention and Control: Web-Based Injury and Statistics Query and Reporting System (WIS-

CARS). Atlanta, GA, National Center for Injury Prevention and Control, 2005

Nemeroff CB, Kalali A, Keller MB, et al: Impact of publicity concerning pediatric suicidality data on physician practice patterns in the United States. Arch Gen Psychiatry 64:466–472, 2007

Olmedo R, Hoffman RS: Withdrawal syndromes. Emerg Med Clin North Am 18:273–288, 2000

Olofsson B, Jacobsson L: A plea for respect: involuntarily hospitalized psychiatric patients' narratives about being subjected to coercion. J Psychiatr Ment Health Nurs 8:357–366, 2001

Pitman RK, Sanders KM, Zusman RM, et al: Pilot study of secondary prevention of posttraumatic stress disorder with propranolol. Biol Psychiatry 51:189–192, 2002

Pokorny AD: Prediction of suicide in psychiatric patients: report of a prospective study. Arch Gen Psychiatry 40:249–257, 1983

Pokorny AD: Suicide prevention revisited. Suicide Life Threat Behav 23:1–10, 1993

Posner K, Oquendo MA, Gould M, et al: Columbia Classification Algorithm of Suicide Assessment (C-CASA): classification of suicidal events in the FDA's pediatric suicidal risk analysis of antidepressants. Am J Psychiatry 164:1035–1043, 2007

Preval H, Klotz SG, Southard R, et al: Rapid-acting ziprasidone in a psychiatric emergency service: a naturalistic study. Gen Hosp Psychiatry 27:140–144, 2005

Qin P, Agerbo E, Mortensen PB: Suicide risk in relation to family history of completed suicide and psychiatric disorders: a nested case-control study based on longitudinal registers. Lancet 360:1126–1130, 2002

Qin P, Agerbo E, Mortensen PB: Suicide risk in relation to socioeconomic, demographic, psychiatric, and familial factors: a national register-based study of all suicides in Denmark, 1981–1997. Am J Psychiatry 160:765–772, 2003

Resnick PJ, Scott CL: The prediction of violence, in Aggression and Physical Violence: An Introductory Text. Edited by Hersen M, VanHassett V. Needham Heights, MA, Allyn & Bacon, 2000, pp 284–302

Romero MP, Wintemute GJ: The epidemiology of firearm suicide in the United States. J Urban Health 79:39–48, 2002

Rosebush PI, Hildebrand AM, Fulong BG, et al: Catatonic syndrome in a general psychiatric inpatient population: frequency, clinical presentation, and response to lorazepam. J Clin Psychiatry 51:357–362, 1990

Roy-Byrne PP, Craske MG, Stein MB: Panic disorder. Lancet 368:1023–1032, 2006

Salzman C, Solomon D, Miyawaki E, et al: Parenteral lorazepam versus parenteral haloperidol for the control of psychotic disruptive behavior. J Clin Psychiatry 52:177–180, 1991

Schillevoort I, de Boer A, Herings RM, et al: Risk of extrapyramidal syndromes with haloperidol, risperidone, or olanzapine. Ann Pharmacother 35:1517–1522, 2001

Schneider LS, Dagerman KS, Insel P: Risk of death with atypical antipsychotic drug treatment for dementia: Meta-analysis of randomized placebo-controlled trials. JAMA 294:1934–1943, 2005

Schuster MA, Stein BD, Jaycox L, et al: A national survey of stress reactions after the September 11, 2001, terrorist attacks. N Engl J Med 345:1507–1512, 2001

Sijbrandij M, Olff M, Reitsma JB, et al: Treatment of acute posttraumatic stress disorder with brief cognitive behavioral therapy: a randomized controlled trial. Am J Psychiatry 164:82–90, 2007

Simon GE, Savarino J: Suicide attempts among patients starting depression treatment with medications or psychotherapy. Am J Psychiatry 164:1029–1034, 2007

Simon RI: Psychiatrists' duties in discharging sicker and potentially violent inpatients in the managed care era. Psychiatr Serv 49:62–67, 1998

Simon RI: The suicide prevention contract: clinical, legal, and risk management issues. J Am Acad Psychiatry Law 27:445–450, 1999

Simon RI: Taking the "Sue" out of suicide: a forensic psychiatrist's perspective. Psychiatr Ann 30:399–407, 2000

Simon RI, Gutheil TG: A recurrent pattern of suicide risk factors observed in litigated cases: lessons in risk management. Psychiatr Ann 32:384–387, 2002

Simpson SG, Jamison KR: The risk of suicide in patients with bipolar disorders. J Clin Psychiatry 60 (suppl 2):53–56; discussion 75–76, 113–116, 1999

Soloff PH, Lis JA, Kelly TM, et al: Risk factors for suicidal behavior in borderline personality disorder. Am J Psychiatry 151:1316–1326, 1994

Stevens CB: Lorazepam in the treatment of acute conversion disorder. Hosp Community Psychiatry 41:1255–1257, 1990

Susman VL: Clinical management of neuroleptic malignant syndrome. Psychiatr Q 72:325–336, 2001

Tarasoff v Regents of the University of California, 551 P2d 334 (Cal. 1976)

Taylor M, Fink M: Catatonia in psychiatric classification: a home of its own. Am J Psychiatry 160:1–9, 2003

Tejedor MC, Diaz A, Castillon JJ, et al: Attempted suicide: repetition and survival—findings of a follow-up study. Acta Psychiatr Scand 100:205–211, 1999

Trans-Johnson TK, Sack, DA, Marcus RN, et al: Efficacy and safety of intramuscular aripiprazole in patients with acute agitation: a randomized, double-blind, placebo-controlled trial. J Clin Psychiatry 68:111–119, 2007

Tulloch KJ, Zed PJ: Intramuscular olanzapine in the management of acute agitation. Ann Pharmacother 38:2128–2135, 2004

van der Kolk BA, Spinazzola J, Blaustein ME, et al: A randomized clinical trial of eye movement desensitization and reprocessing (EMDR), fluoxetine, and pill placebo in the treatment of posttraumatic stress disorder: treatment effects and long-term maintenance. J Clin Psychiatry 68:37–46, 2007

Vaiva G, Ducrocq F, Jezequel K, et al: Immediate treatment with propranolol decreases posttraumatic stress disorder two months after trauma. Biol Psychiatry 54:947–949, 2003

Walcott DM, Cerundolo P, Beck JC: Current analysis of the Tarasoff duty: an evolution towards the limitations of the duty to protect. Behav Sci Law 19:325–343, 2001

Woo BK, Sevilla CC, Obrocea GV: Factors influencing the stability of psychiatric diagnoses in the emergency setting: review of 934 consecutively inpatient admissions. Gen Hosp Psychiatry 28:434–436, 2006

Wright P, Birkett M, David SR, et al: Double-blind, placebo-controlled comparison of intramuscular olanzapine and intramuscular haloperidol in the treatment of acute agitation in schizophrenia. Am J Psychiatry 158:1149–1151, 2001

Yildiz A, Sachs GS, Turgay A: Pharmacological management of agitation in emergency settings. Emerg Med J 20:339–346, 2003

Zyprexa: US prescribing information, updated May 26, 2005. Available at: http://pi.lilly.com/us/zyprexa-pi.pdf. Accessed October 2005.

CHAPTER 63

Treatment of Child and Adolescent Disorders

Karen Dineen Wagner, M.D., Ph.D.

Steven R. Pliszka, M.D.

This chapter focuses on the psychopharmacology of psychiatric disorders in children and adolescents. However, nonpharmacological treatment interventions are also an important component of a child's psychiatric care. Individual psychotherapy, group therapy, and family therapy may improve clinical outcome. Working closely with school personnel is another ingredient in the treatment of a child with a psychiatric disorder. Case management for the child and support for the family are other facets of treatment for children.

It is important for clinicians to be aware of the evidence base for the use of psychotropic medications for children and adolescents. In this chapter, data from the literature, with a focus on controlled studies, are presented. On the basis of these findings, clinical recommendations regarding pharmacotherapy for childhood psychiatric disorders are offered. The appendix and tables contain specific information about dosages, monitoring, and adverse effects of psychotropics in children.

Psychotropic Medication for Children and Adolescents

Attention has been focused on the need for controlled studies to assess the safety and efficacy of psychotropic medication for children and adolescents. Although there has been a substantial increase in the use of psychotropic medications for children (Safer et al. 1996) and for preschoolers (Zito et al. 2000), there is a significant gap between empirical treatment research and clinical practice with these agents (Jensen et al. 1999). The pressing need to expand the empirical basis for the treatment of children has resulted in a substantial increase in National Institute of Mental Health (NIMH)–funded research for clinical trials in children and adolescents with psychiatric disorders (Vitiello 2001). The U.S. Food and Drug Administration Modernization Act (FDAMA) of 1997, which provides a 6-month extension of market exclusivity for selected medications for children, has resulted in a significant increase in the number of industry-sponsored studies of psychotropic medications in youths. Following this act, the U.S. Food and Drug Administration (FDA) issued "Regulations Requiring Manufacturers to Assess

---

Portions of the Attention-Deficit/Hyperactivity Disorder section of this chapter were adapted from Wagner KD: "Management of Treatment Refractory Attention-Deficit/Hyperactivity Disorder in Children and Adolescents." *Psychopharmacology Bulletin* 36:130–142, 2002. Used with permission.

the Safety and Effectiveness of New Drugs and Biological Products in Pediatric Patients" (U.S. Food and Drug Administration 1998), which became effective in April 1999. This rule allows the FDA to require pediatric studies of certain new and marketed drugs, especially those that are likely to be commonly used for children. The information obtained from these studies will allow product labeling to include directions for the safe and effective use of these medications in children. To date, however, there are relatively few FDA-approved psychotropic medications for children and adolescents.

Evaluation

Prior to the initiation of psychotropic medication for children and adolescents, it is essential to conduct a comprehensive evaluation to ensure the accuracy of the diagnosis. A thorough history and careful attention to the clinical presentation are central components of the evaluation. The clinician should interview the child and parents separately so that both may have the opportunity to freely express their concerns. Extended family members, school personnel, and school records are other potential sources of information.

Clinicians must be skilled at differential diagnosis of childhood disorders, given that there is a significant overlap of symptoms among these disorders (e.g., bipolar disorder and attention-deficit/hyperactivity disorder [ADHD]). Knowledge of commonly occurring comorbid disorders is also necessary. Medical conditions, such as seizure disorders and hypothyroidism, should be considered within the differential diagnosis and adequately assessed.

Disorder-specific rating scales at baseline and during the course of treatment may be useful in assisting with the measurement of clinical outcome.

Clinical Issues Affecting Response to Pharmacotherapy

Whenever a child fails to respond to initial pharmacotherapy, several clinical issues should be addressed before initiating alternative or adjunctive medication, as discussed below.

Diagnostic Accuracy

The diagnosis should be reassessed. Often there is symptomatic overlap among disorders that may lead to misdiagnosis. For example, symptoms of excessive energy and distractibility are common features of both ADHD and bipolar disorder. Similarly, irritability and sleep distur-

bance often occur in children with major depression, bipolar disorder, and posttraumatic stress disorder (PTSD).

Comorbid Disorders

Unrecognized comorbid disorders may adversely affect treatment outcome. As an illustration, children with comorbid internalizing disorders have been reported to have lower response rates to methylphenidate than children without comorbidity (Tannock et al. 1995).

Psychosocial Factors

Child abuse, domestic violence, family conflict, parental psychopathology, and bullying by peers may lead to symptoms that mimic or exacerbate a preexisting psychiatric disorder. As examples, ostracism by peers may lead to depression in a child, or a parent with depression who has a negative cognitive style may heighten the pessimistic views of a child with depression.

Medication Compliance

Some children and adolescents are reluctant to take medication because of such reasons as denial of illness, perceived stigma, and side effects. To increase medication compliance, it is essential that the child or adolescent, as well as the parent, understand the youth's disorder, course of illness, and goals of treatment. It is important for parents to participate in monitoring their child's medication compliance.

Nonpharmacological Treatment

Psychotherapy may be a component of treatment, either alone or in conjunction with medication. Specific psychotherapies have been found to be effective in the treatment of some childhood disorders. As examples, cognitive-behavioral therapy (CBT) (Brent et al. 1997) and interpersonal therapy (Mufson and Sills 2006) have demonstrated efficacy in the treatment of adolescents with depression. Similarly, CBT is commonly used for the treatment of childhood anxiety disorders (Roblek and Piacentini 2005). Behavior therapy has led to improvement in symptoms of ADHD for children (Pelham et al. 1998), although stimulants have demonstrated superiority to behavioral treatment (MTA [Multimodal Treatment of ADHD] Cooperative Group 1999). Adjunctive psychoeducation to medication treatment has shown benefit in the treatment of children with bipolar disorder (Fristad et al. 2003). Social skills training can be a useful component of treatment in autism spectrum disorders (Krasny et al. 2003).

Informed Consent

Informed consent is necessary prior to prescribing psychotropic medication to any patient, but it is particularly important in pediatric psychopharmacology because there are few FDA-approved medications and few controlled studies to address safety and efficacy in children. There are five recommended components of informed consent for prescribing psychotropic medications to children and adolescents (Popper 1987). The child's parent(s) and the child/adolescent should be provided with the following information:

1. The purpose (benefits) of the treatment
2. A description of the treatment process
3. An explanation of the risks of the treatment, including risks that would ordinarily be described by the psychiatrist and risks that would be relevant to making the decision
4. A statement of the alternative treatments, including nontreatment
5. A statement that there may be unknown risks of these medications (This is particularly essential for children, because there is a paucity of information on the potential long-term effects of psychotropic medications.)

Evidence Base

It is important for clinicians to be aware of the evidence base for medication treatment of each childhood psychiatric disorder. Clinical treatment guidelines generally rely on the strength of the available data in determining first-line agents (Hughes et al. 2007; Kowatch et al. 2005). In most cases, clinicians should select a medication within the group of first-line agents when initiating medication treatment with a child. Additional factors that will dictate medication choice are prior medication history, medical history, side-effect profile of the drug, and adolescent and parent preferences.

Major Depressive Disorder

The prevalence of major depression in children and adolescents is estimated to range from 1.8% to 4.6% (Kashani and Sherman 1988; Kroes et al. 2001). DSM-IV-TR (American Psychiatric Association 2000) criteria are used to establish a diagnosis of major depression in children and adolescents. The mean length of an episode of major depression in youth ranges from 8 to 13 months,

and relapse rates range from 30% to 70% (Birmaher et al. 2002). There is increasing evidence for the continuity of depression from youth into adulthood (Dunn and Goodyer 2006).

Recently, a number of double-blind, placebo-controlled multicenter medication studies for treating major depression in children and adolescents have been reported. In the following subsections, medication groups are discussed in order of largest to smallest evidence base.

Selective Serotonin Reuptake Inhibitors

Fluoxetine

Fluoxetine is the only selective serotonin reuptake inhibitor (SSRI) medication to have FDA approval for the treatment of major depression in children and adolescents. There have been three positive medication trials.

In the first study of fluoxetine, 96 child and adolescent outpatients (ages 8–17 years) with major depression were randomly assigned to fluoxetine (20 mg/day) or placebo for an 8-week trial (Emslie et al. 1997). The fluoxetine group, with 27 youths (56%) much or very much improved, showed statistically significant greater improvement in Clinical Global Impressions (CGI) scores than did the placebo group, with 16 youths (33%) much or very much improved. Remission, which was defined as a Children's Depression Rating Scale—Revised (CDRS-R; Poznanski et al. 1985) score ≤28, occurred in 31% of the fluoxetine group and 23% of the placebo group. Medication side effects leading to discontinuation in the study were manic symptoms in 3 patients and severe rash in 1 patient.

In a double-blind, placebo-controlled multicenter study of fluoxetine, 219 child and adolescent outpatients (ages 8–17 years) with major depression were randomly assigned to fluoxetine (20 mg/day) or placebo for an 8-week trial (Emslie et al. 2002). The fluoxetine group showed statistically significant greater improvement in depression, as assessed by CDRS-R scores, than did the placebo group. Fifty-two percent of patients treated with fluoxetine were rated as much or very much improved, compared with 37% of patients treated with placebo. Remission rates were 39% in the fluoxetine group and 20% in the placebo group. Headache was the only side effect that was reported more frequently in the group treated with fluoxetine than in the group treated with placebo.

Fluoxetine alone, fluoxetine with CBT, CBT alone, and placebo were compared in a multicenter trial of 439 adolescent outpatients with a diagnosis of major depression (Treatment for Adolescents with Depression Study

[TADS] Team 2004). Patients were randomly assigned to 12 weeks of fluoxetine (10–40 mg/day), fluoxetine (10–40 mg/day) with CBT, CBT alone, or placebo. Compared with placebo, the combination of fluoxetine with CBT was significantly superior on CDRS-R scores. Combination treatment with fluoxetine and CBT was significantly superior to fluoxetine alone and CBT alone. Fluoxetine monotherapy was superior to CBT. Based on CGI scores of much or very much improved, the response rates were 71% for fluoxetine–CBT combination therapy, 61% for fluoxetine, 43% for CBT, and 35% for placebo. At the end of 12 weeks, only 23% of youths achieved remission (CDRS-R≤28). Remission rates were significantly higher in the combination group (37%) than in the fluoxetine (23%), CBT (16%), and placebo (17%) groups (Kennard et al. 2006).

Citalopram

There have been two controlled trials of citalopram, one with positive and one with negative results in the treatment of depression in youth.

The efficacy of citalopram was demonstrated in a double-blind, placebo-controlled multicenter trial of 174 outpatient children and adolescents (ages 7–17 years) with major depression (Wagner et al. 2004b). Patients were randomly assigned to citalopram (dosage range = 20–40 mg/day; mean daily dose = 23 mg for children, 24 mg for adolescents) or placebo for an 8-week trial. The group treated with citalopram showed statistically significant greater improvement in depression (CDRS-R scores) than did the placebo group. The response rates (CDRS-R score <28) were 36% for patients receiving citalopram and 24% for patients receiving placebo. The most frequent adverse events were headache, nausea, rhinitis, abdominal pain, and influenza-like symptoms. The discontinuation rate for adverse events was 5% in both the group being treated with citalopram and the group receiving placebo.

A European double-blind, placebo-controlled multicenter study (Knorring et al. 2006) of citalopram in 224 adolescents with major depression failed to show superiority of citalopram to placebo on the primary efficacy measures of Schedule for Affective Disorders and Schizophrenia for School-Age Children, Present Episode version (Kiddie-SADS-P; Chambers et al. 1985) and the Montgomery-Åsberg Depression Rating Scale (MADRS; Montgomery et al. 1979). Interpretation of these findings is confounded by the allowed use of psychotherapy and other psychotropic medications during the course of the trial. The most commonly reported adverse events were headache, nausea, and vomiting.

Paroxetine

There have been three double-blind, placebo-controlled trials of paroxetine for treatment of depression in children and adolescents, all of which have negative findings on the primary outcome measure.

In a study of 275 adolescent outpatients (ages 12–18 years) with major depression, patients were randomly assigned to paroxetine (dosage range = 20–40 mg/day; mean daily dose = 28 mg), imipramine (dosage range = 200–300 mg; mean daily dose = 205 mg/day), or placebo for an 8-week trial (Keller et al. 2001). Although there was no statistically significant difference among the treatment groups on the primary efficacy measure of reduction in the Hamilton Rating Scale for Depression (Ham-D; Hamilton 1960) total score, there was statistically significant greater global improvement for the group receiving paroxetine. Sixty-six percent of the group receiving paroxetine was much or very much improved, compared with 52% of the group receiving imipramine and 48% of the group receiving placebo. The most common side effects reported for paroxetine were headache, nausea, dizziness, dry mouth, and somnolence, which (with the exception of somnolence) occurred at rates similar to those in the placebo group. The most common side effects reported for imipramine were dizziness, dry mouth, headache, nausea, and tachycardia.

Two hundred six children and adolescents (ages 7–17 years) with major depression were included in an 8-week double-blind, placebo-controlled, randomized multicenter study of paroxetine treatment (Emslie et al. 2006). Patients were randomly assigned to paroxetine (10–50 mg/day) or placebo. There was no statistically significant difference between paroxetine-treated patients and placebo-treated patients on change from baseline in CDRS-R total score at endpoint. Adverse events reported for paroxetine with an incidence of >5% and at least twice that of placebo were dizziness, cough, dyspepsia, and vomiting.

A 12-week international placebo-controlled multicenter trial of paroxetine in 286 adolescents with major depression failed to show superiority of paroxetine compared with placebo on change from baseline in MADRS or Schedule for Affective Disorders and Schizophrenia for School-Aged Children—Lifetime version (Kiddie-SADS-L; Kaufman et al. 1997) total scores (Berard et al. 2006).

Sertraline

The efficacy of sertraline was assessed in two identical double-blind, placebo-controlled multicenter studies of 376 outpatient children and adolescents with major depression (Wagner et al. 2003a). Patients were randomly assigned to sertraline (dosage range = 50–200 mg per day; mean daily dose = 131 mg) or placebo for a 10-week trial. The group receiving sertraline showed a statistically significant greater improvement in depression (CDRS-R scores) than did the placebo group. Response rates (decrease >40% in baseline CDRS-R scores) were 69% in the group treated with sertraline and 59% in the group treated with placebo. The most common side effects in the group treated with sertraline were headache, nausea, insomnia, upper respiratory tract infection, abdominal pain, and diarrhea. In a 24-week open follow-up of 226 of these patients, continued improvement in depressive symptoms was shown with sertraline treatment. At endpoint, 86% of youths met response criteria (Rynn et al. 2006).

Sertraline, CBT, and combined CBT plus medication were compared for the treatment of 73 adolescents with depressive disorders (Melvin et al. 2006). All treatments showed statistically significant improvement on all outcome measures; there were no significant advantages of combined treatment.

Escitalopram

There has been one controlled study of escitalopram that failed to demonstrate significant improvement on CDRS-R scores at endpoint between escitalopram and placebo (Wagner et al. 2006a). In this study, 264 children and adolescents were randomly assigned to escitalopram (10–20 mg/day) or placebo for 8 weeks. In a post hoc analysis of adolescent completers, escitalopram showed significantly improved CDRS-R scores compared with placebo. Headache and abdominal pain were the only adverse events reported in more than 10% of the patients in the escitalopram group.

Other Antidepressants

Venlafaxine

Two double-blind, placebo-controlled multicenter studies have evaluated the efficacy of venlafaxine extended-release (XR) for the treatment of major depression in 165 and 169 child and adolescent outpatients, ages 7–17 years, respectively (Emslie et al. 2007a, 2007b). Patients were randomly assigned to venlafaxine XR (37.5–225 mg/day) for 8-week trials. Both studies were negative on the primary outcome measure of change from baseline to endpoint in the CDRS-R scores. A post hoc analysis of the pooled data showed greater improvement on CDRS-R scores with venlafaxine XR for adolescents than for children. The most common adverse events were anorexia

and abdominal pain (Emslie et al. 2007a). In a 6-month open-label follow-up study, it was found that most improvement with venlafaxine XR occurred in the first 6 weeks of treatment. At the end of week 6, mean CDRS-R scores decreased from 60 to 36.3, and to 33.8 at 6 months (Emslie et al. 2007b).

Nefazodone

The efficacy of nefazodone was assessed in a double-blind, placebo-controlled multicenter trial of 195 adolescents (ages 12–17 years) with major depression (Rynn et al. 2002). Adolescents were randomly assigned to nefazodone (dosage range = 300–600 mg/day; mean daily dose = 444 mg) for an 8-week trial. The nefazodone group showed greater improvement than the placebo group; however, this difference missed statistical significance (P<0.055), based on the comparison of mean CDRS-R score from baseline to endpoint between the group being treated with nefazodone and the group receiving placebo. The most common side effects with nefazodone were headache, abdominal pain, nausea, vomiting, somnolence, and dizziness, all of which were reported with greater frequency in the nefazodone group than in the group receiving placebo.

In a second double-blind, placebo-controlled multicenter trial of nefazodone in both children and adolescents (ages 7–17 years) with major depression, nefazodone did not differentiate from placebo (U.S. Food and Drug Administration 2004b).

Bupropion

There are no controlled trials of bupropion for the treatment of pediatric depression.

In an 8-week study of bupropion sustained release (SR) (dosage range = 100–400 mg/day; mean daily dose = 362 mg) for treating 11 adolescents (ages 12–17 years) with major depression, 8 adolescents (79%) showed a 50% reduction in depression score from baseline (Glod et al. 2000).

Bupropion SR was assessed in an 8-week open study for the treatment of comorbid depression and ADHD in 24 adolescents (Daviss et al. 2001). Bupropion SR dosages were flexibly titrated up to 4 mg/kg taken twice daily (mean dose = 2.2 mg/kg in A.M. and 1–7 mg/kg in P.M.). Global improvement was reported for 14 subjects (58%) for both depression and ADHD, 7 subjects (29%) for depression only, and 1 subject (4%) for ADHD only. Common side effects were headache, nausea, rash, and irritability.

Mirtazapine

There have been two double-blind, placebo-controlled multicenter trials of mirtazapine for the treatment of child and adolescent outpatients (ages 7–17 years) with major depression. These studies, which included 126 and 133 patients, respectively, who were randomly assigned to mirtazapine (15–45 mg/day) or placebo for an 8-week trial, failed to distinguish mirtazapine from placebo on the primary efficacy measure of change from baseline to endpoint in CDRS-R scores (U.S. Food and Drug Administration 2004b).

Duloxetine

There are no published reports of the use of duloxetine for the treatment of major depression in children and adolescents. There are two case reports of duloxetine treatment for pediatric chronic pain and comorbid major depressive disorder (Meighen 2007) and one case report of duloxetine treatment for pediatric depression with pain and dissociative symptoms (Desarkar et al. 2006) that described improvement in depressive symptoms.

Tricyclic Antidepressants

There have been eight double-blind, placebo-controlled studies of tricyclic antidepressants (TCAs) in children and adolescents. No significant differences between TCA and placebo were found in any of these studies (Birmaher et al. 1998; B. Geller et al. 1990, 1992; Keller et al. 2001; Kutcher et al. 1994; Kye et al. 1996; Puig-Antich et al. 1987; Tancer et al. 1992). Response rates for TCA-treated patients ranged from 8% to 92% (B. Geller et al. 1990; Kye et al. 1996) and from 17% to 92% for patients treated with placebo (B. Geller et al. 1992; Kye et al. 1996). Several open trials with TCAs have reported a response rate of 60%–80% (Ambrosini et al. 1994; B. Geller et al. 1986; Preskorn et al. 1982; Puig-Antich et al. 1979).

Monoamine Oxidase Inhibitors

One chart review found a response rate of 74% in 23 adolescents treated with monoamine oxidase inhibitors (MAOIs) who had been unresponsive to TCAs. Dietary noncompliance was noted for 6 of these adolescents; 1 developed headache and hypertension, and 1 developed myoclonic jerks (Ryan et al. 1988).

Suicidality and FDA Warning

In a combined analysis of 24 short-term placebo-controlled trials of antidepressant medications in child and adolescent major depressive disorder, obsessive-compulsive disorder (OCD), or other psychiatric disorders, the risk of suicidality (suicidal thinking and behavior) was 4%, twice the placebo rate (2%). There were no suicides in any of the clinical trials. The FDA directed manufacturers to add a black box warning to the health professional label of antidepressant medications to describe the increased risk of suicidal thoughts and behavior in children and adolescents being treated with antidepressant medications and to emphasize the need for close monitoring of patients on the medications (U.S. Food and Drug Administration 2004a). Parents and patients should be advised of the black box warning for antidepressant medication.

In a subsequent meta-analysis of 27 trials of pediatric major depression, the rates of suicidal ideation and attempts were 3% in the youths treated with antidepressants and 2% in the youth who received placebo (Bridge et al. 2007). These investigators reported that the number needed to treat was 10, whereas the number needed to harm was 112, and therefore the benefits of antidepressants outweigh the potential risk from suicidal ideation or attempt.

A number of recent studies, in both the United States and Europe, have failed to demonstrate an association between antidepressant use and youth suicide (Gibbons et al. 2006; Markowitz and Cuellar 2007; Simon et al. 2006; Søndergård et al. 2006). Noteworthy, there was an increase in the suicide rate in youth following the black box warning on antidepressants (Hamilton et al. 2007). The FDA advisory has been associated with significant decreases in the rates of diagnosis and treatment in pediatric depression (Libby et al. 2007).

Clinical Recommendations for Major Depressive Disorder

An evidence-based consensus medication algorithm for the treatment of childhood major depression has been recently updated (Texas Children's Medication Algorithm Project [TMAP]; Hughes et al. 2007). Based on research evidence and panel discussion, four stages of medication treatment were identified:

- Stage 1: SSRI (fluoxetine, citalopram, sertraline)
- Stage 2: Alternate SSRI (fluoxetine, sertraline, citalopram, escitalopram, paroxetine [adolescents only if paroxetine])
- Stage 2A (if partial response to SSRI): SSRI + lithium, bupropion, or mirtazapine

- Stage 3: Different class of antidepressant medication (venlafaxine, bupropion, mirtazapine, duloxetine)
- Stage 4: Reassess, treatment guidance

If a child fails to respond to treatment in one stage, the clinician should move to the next stage of treatment. It was recommended by the consensus panel that dosage titration should occur in youths who do not have significant improvement in symptoms by 4–6 weeks of treatment. Additional dose adjustments should be made at 8–10 weeks of treatment before moving to another stage of treatment.

It was further recommended that antidepressants be continued for 6–12 months after symptom remission. At the time of discontinuation of an antidepressant, the dose should be tapered slowly (i.e., no more than 25% per week). The typical tapering and discontinuation period is 2–3 months.

Bipolar Disorder

The prevalence of bipolar disorder in a community sample of adolescents was found to be 1% (Lewinsohn et al. 1995). Although DSM-IV-TR criteria are used to diagnose bipolar disorder in youths, the clinical features in children may differ from those in adolescents and adults. Children with bipolar disorder frequently exhibit mixed mania and rapid cycling (B. Geller et al. 2000). One-year recovery rates of 87% and relapse rates of 64% have been reported in children with bipolar disorder (B. Geller et al. 2004). Despite the severity of bipolar disorder and its significant adverse effects on a child's social, emotional, and academic functioning, it has yet to be determined whether pharmacotherapy alters the course of the illness (Birmaher et al. 2006).

Lithium

Lithium is the only medication with FDA approval for the treatment of mania in adolescents.

There is only one small double-blind, placebo-controlled study of lithium treatment for adolescent bipolar disorder and substance dependence (B. Geller et al. 1998). Twenty-five adolescent outpatients were randomly assigned to either lithium (mean serum level = 0.97 mEq/L) or placebo for a 6-week trial. There was significantly greater improvement in global functioning with lithium than with placebo. It was found that onset of bipolar disorder preceded substance dependence by approximately 6 years. Side effects in the group treated with lithium were polyuria, thirst, nausea, vomiting, and dizziness.

There have been six controlled studies of lithium in the treatment of bipolar disorder in youths. In four of these double-blind crossover studies, significant improvement was found with lithium, compared with placebo (DeLong and Nieman 1983; Gram and Rafaelsen 1972; Lena 1979; McKnew et al. 1981). However, small sample size, diagnostic issues, and short treatment duration limit these findings.

In a 4-week open trial, 100 adolescents with mania received lithium (mean serum level 0.93 mEq/L) (Kafantaris et al. 2003). Forty-six of these youths also received concomitant antipsychotic medication. The lithium response rate was 55%, based on a ≥50% reduction in Young Mania Rating Scale (YMRS; Young et al. 1978) scores. The most common side effects were polydipsia, polyuria, weight gain, gastrointestinal symptoms, headache, and tremor.

Kafantaris et al. (2004) conducted a controlled discontinuation study with 40 adolescents who had responded to lithium in the open trial. Responders were randomly assigned to continue or discontinue lithium during a 2-week double-blind, placebo-controlled phase. There was no statistically significant difference on symptom exacerbation rate between the lithium (52.6%) and placebo (61.9%) groups. The investigators concluded that 4 weeks of lithium monotherapy may be insufficient for symptom remission in adolescents.

The efficacy of lithium, divalproex, and carbamazepine was compared in a 6-week randomized, open-label trial of 42 children and adolescents (ages 8–18 years) with bipolar disorder (Kowatch et al. 2000b). There were no significant differences in response rates (defined as ≥50% reduction in YMRS from baseline to endpoint) among lithium, divalproex, and carbamazepine. The lithium response rate was 38%, and the effect size was 1.06.

Lithium treatment for adolescents with bipolar depression was investigated in a 6-week open study of 27 adolescents. The response rate (≥50% reduction in baseline CDRS-R score) was 48% (Patel et al. 2006).

Anticonvulsants
Divalproex

A 4-week double-blind, placebo-controlled multicenter trial of 150 youths (ages 10–17 years) with bipolar I disorder (mixed or manic) failed to show a significant difference in scores on the YMRS from baseline to endpoint between divalproex extended release (ER) and placebo (Abbott Laboratories, accessed 2007). The mean modal dose of divalproex ER was 1,286 mg. There were no statistically significant differences in adverse-event incidents between the divalproex ER and placebo groups. Gastrointestinal symptoms were more commonly reported in divalproex ER than in placebo groups.

In a multisite open study of divalproex treatment for youths, 40 children and adolescents (ages 7–19 years) with bipolar disorder received divalproex for a period of 2–8 weeks (Wagner et al. 2002). Sixty-one percent of the subjects showed >50% improvement on the YMRS from baseline to endpoint. Twenty-three patients (58%) discontinued the study; of those, 16 patients had a comorbid diagnosis, including ADHD, conduct disorder, or oppositional defiant disorder (ODD). Headache, nausea, vomiting, diarrhea, and somnolence were the most common side effects.

In the previously mentioned active-comparator study of lithium, divalproex, and carbamazepine, the response rate (≥50% reduction in baseline YMRS scores) was 53% for divalproex. The effect size for divalproex was 1.63. The most common side effects of divalproex were nausea and sedation (Kowatch et al. 2000b).

The efficacy of divalproex was compared with that of quetiapine in 50 hospitalized adolescents with bipolar I disorder, manic or mixed (DelBello et al. 2006). Twenty-five adolescents were randomly assigned to divalproex (serum level 80–120 μg/mL) or quetiapine (400–600 mg/day). There were no significant differences between divalproex and quetiapine across the 28 days of the study. The CGI-BP-I overall response rate (CGI-BP-I overall score ≤2 at endpoint) was 40%, and the CGI-BP-I mania response rate was 56% for divalproex, which were significantly lower than the rates for quetiapine. The rate of remission (YMRS ≥12) for divalproex was 28%.

Carbamazepine

In a 6-week active-comparator study of lithium, divalproex, and carbamazepine (Kowatch et al. 2000b), carbamazepine had a response rate (defined as ≥50% reduction in YMRS from baseline to endpoint) of 38% (vs. 38% for lithium and 53% for divalproex) and an effect size of 1.00 (vs. 1.6 for lithium and 1.63 for divalproex). The most common side effects of carbamazepine were sedation, nausea, dizziness, and rash.

Oxcarbazepine

There is one double-blind, placebo-controlled multicenter trial of oxcarbazepine for the treatment of youths with bipolar I disorder, manic or mixed, that failed to show superiority of oxcarbazepine to placebo. One hundred sixteen youths (ages 7–18 years) were randomly as-

signed to oxcarbazepine (mean dosage = 1,515 mg/day) or placebo for a 7-week trial (Wagner et al. 2006b). There was no significant difference in YMRS scores at endpoint between the oxcarbazepine and placebo groups. The most common side effects in the oxcarbazepine-treated patients were dizziness, nausea, somnolence, diplopia, fatigue, and rash.

Topiramate

A double-blind, randomized, placebo-controlled multicenter study assessing the efficacy of topiramate treatment in children and adolescents with acute mania was designed as a 200-patient study but was terminated after randomizing 56 patients (ages 6–17 years) when adult mania trials failed to show efficacy (DelBello et al. 2005). Patients were titrated to 400 mg/day (mean dosage = 278 mg/day). Over a 4-week period, no significant difference was found between the topiramate and placebo groups. The most common adverse events in the topiramate group included decreased appetite, nausea, diarrhea, paresthesias, and somnolence.

Lamotrigine

In a 12-week open-label single-center outpatient study in adolescents diagnosed with bipolar disorder I, depressed or mixed, 23 patients entered, and 13 completed the trial (Swope et al. 2004). The mean dosage of lamotrigine was 241 mg/day. There was improvement on depression and mania ratings at study endpoint. No subjects discontinued for adverse events related to the study drug.

Lamotrigine as monotherapy or adjunctive treatment for 20 adolescents with bipolar depression was assessed in an 8-week open-label trial (Chang et al. 2006). The mean dosage of lamotrigine was 132 mg/day. Seven adolescents were also taking other psychotropic medications. The response rate (CGI-I≤2) was 84%, and the remission rate (CDRS-R≤28 and CGI-S≤2) was 58%. The most common side effects were headache, fatigue, nausea, sweating, and difficulty sleeping. There were no significant rashes during the trial.

The use of lamotrigine as adjunctive therapy for treatment-refractory bipolar depression in adolescents was assessed in an open-label study (Kusumakar and Yatham 1997). Twenty-two adolescents whose bipolar depression was refractory to treatment with a combination of divalproex plus another mood stabilizer and antidepressant were treated with lamotrigine added to divalproex for 6 weeks. Sixteen of the adolescents (72%) had a positive response by week 6.

Atypical Antipsychotics

Olanzapine

There is one reported double-blind, placebo-controlled multicenter study of olanzapine (2.5–20 mg/day) for the treatment of adolescent outpatients with bipolar I disorder, mixed or manic (Tohen et al. 2007). Adolescents were randomly assigned to olanzapine (n=107) or placebo (n=54) for 3 weeks. Response rates (defined as ≥50% decrease in YMRS and a CGI-BP mania score≤3) were significantly greater for the olanzapine group (44.8%) than for the placebo group (18.5%). Remission rates (defined as YMRS<12 and CGI-BP mania score≤3) were significantly greater for the olanzapine (35.2%) than for the placebo (11.1%) group. Adverse effects in the olanzapine group were hyperprolactinemia, weight gain (mean=3.7 kg), somnolence, and sedation.

In an open study, 23 children (ages 5–14 years) with bipolar disorder received olanzapine (2.5 mg/day) for 8 weeks (Frazier et al. 2001). Using a response definition of 30% or greater improvement on the YMRS, the response rate was 61%. No significant side effects except weight gain (mean=5 kg) were reported.

The use of olanzapine in preschoolers is an area of recent interest. An 8-week open-label study of olanzapine and risperidone in children (ages 4–6 years) with bipolar disorder (manic, mixed, or hypomanic) was conducted by Biederman et al. (2005b). Fifteen children were treated with olanzapine (mean dosage=6.3 mg/day). The response rate (CGI-I≤2 or YMRS reduction≥30%) was 53% for olanzapine. Mean weight increase was 3.2 kg for olanzapine-treated children. The most common side effects of olanzapine were increased appetite, cold symptoms, headache, and sedation.

Risperidone

There are no data available from controlled trials of risperidone for the treatment of bipolar disorder in youth.

An 8-week open-label study of risperidone (mean dosage=1.25 mg/day) for 30 youths (ages 6–17 years) with bipolar disorder (manic, mixed, or hypomanic) was conducted by Biederman et al. (2005c). Twenty-two of 30 youths completed the study. The response rate (CGI-I in mania score≤2 at endpoint) was 70%. Significant side effects included weight increase (mean 2.1 kg) and a four-fold increase in prolactin levels from baseline.

In the previously mentioned open-label study of preschoolers with bipolar disorder (Biederman et al. 2005b), 16 children received risperidone (mean dosage=1.4 mg/

day). The response rate (CGI-I≤2 or YMRS reduction of ≥30%) was 69% in the risperidone group. Weight increase was a mean of 2.2 kg in the risperidone-treated children. The most common side effects were increased appetite, cold symptoms, headaches, and sedation.

Quetiapine

The efficacy of quetiapine was compared with divalproex in 50 hospitalized adolescents with bipolar I disorder, manic or mixed (DelBello et al. 2006). Twenty-five adolescents were randomly assigned to quetiapine (400–600 mg/day). There was no statistically significant difference in YMRS scores across the 28 days of the study between quetiapine and divalproex. Response rates of 72% (CGI-BP-I overall score≤2) and of 84% (CGI-BP-I mania score≤2) for quetiapine were significantly higher than those for divalproex. The rate of remission (YMRS≤12) was 60% in the quetiapine group. Improvement occurred more rapidly in the quetiapine group than in the divalproex group.

Aripiprazole

There are no published controlled studies of aripiprazole treatment for bipolar disorder in children and adolescents.

Three chart reviews reported clinical global improvement in symptoms for youth with bipolar disorder who were treated with aripiprazole (Barzman et al. 2004; Biederman et al. 2005a; Gibson et al. 2007).

Ziprasidone

There are no data available from controlled trials of ziprasidone for the treatment of bipolar disorder in youth.

In a study of 30 children and adolescents with bipolar disorder given open-label ziprasidone (mean dosage=56 mg/day) for a mean treatment duration of 359 days, 70% of patients responded to ziprasidone (CGI-I score of much or very much improved) (Barnett and Cohen 2004).

The comparative efficacy of atypical antipsychotics was assessed in youths with mania (Biederman 2005). In this study, 21 youths received ziprasidone (mean dosage=56 mg/day) in an 8-week open-label trial. There were significant reductions in YMRS scores for all atypical antipsychotics, with no significant difference among them. The CGI≤2 response rate was 57% for ziprasidone. Mean weight gain was 0.6 kg for ziprasidone.

Combination Treatment

Some children may not respond to initial monotherapy treatment or may need combination treatment over the course of the illness. For example, following acute 6-week treatment with one mood stabilizer, Kowatch et al. (2000a) reported that 20 of 35 youths (58%) required additional psychotropic medication over the next 16 weeks. The response rate to combination treatment with two mood stabilizers was high (80%) for those youths who did not respond to monotherapy.

The effectiveness of combination lithium and divalproex sodium was assessed in an open trial (Findling et al. 2003a). Ninety youths (ages 5–17 years) with bipolar I or II disorder were treated for up to 20 weeks with divalproex sodium (mean blood level=79.8 μg/mL) and lithium (mean blood level=0.9 mmol/L). The clinical remission rate (defined as contiguous weekly ratings of YMRS ≤12.5, CDRS-R ≤40, Children's Global Assessment Scale [CGAS] ≥51, clinical stability, and no mood cycling) was 42%.

Lithium and adjunctive haloperidol were used to treat five adolescents with psychotic mania (Kafantaris et al. 2001b). In this trial, haloperidol was discontinued within 1 week of therapeutic lithium levels. All of these adolescents had a rapid return to symptoms, which responded to restarting haloperidol.

In a larger open trial (Kafantaris et al. 2001a), 28 acutely manic adolescents with psychotic features received combination lithium and antipsychotic medication for 4 weeks. At the end of 4 weeks, only 14 (50%) were clinically stable enough to have the antipsychotic medication discontinued. On lithium monotherapy, 8 adolescents remained stable over a 4-week period, and 6 adolescents had an exacerbation of symptoms. These investigators concluded that adjunctive antipsychotic medication needs to be continued for more than 4 weeks for most adolescents with psychotic mania.

The efficacy of combination risperidone and lithium or divalproex sodium was assessed in a 6-month open-label trial (Pavuluri et al. 2004). Thirty-seven youths (ages 5–18 years) with bipolar I disorder (manic or mixed) received risperidone (mean dosage=0.75 mg) plus divalproex sodium (mean serum level=106 μg/mL) or risperidone (mean dosage=0.70 mg) plus lithium (mean serum level=0.9 mEq/L). Response rates (≥50% reduction in baseline YMRS scores) were similar for both combinations: 80% for divalproex sodium plus risperidone, and 82.4% for lithium plus risperidone. There were no significant differences between the groups in safety and tolerability.

Risperidone augmentation of lithium nonresponders was assessed in a 1-year open-label study (Pavuluri et al. 2006). Twenty-one of 38 youths (ages 4–17 years) who failed to respond to lithium monotherapy or relapsed after

initial response were given risperidone (mean dosage=0.99 mg) for 11 months. Response rates in the lithium plus risperidone group were 85.7%.

In a double-blind, placebo-controlled study of quetiapine, 30 adolescents with bipolar disorder received divalproex (20 mg/kg) and were randomly assigned to adjunctive quetiapine (mean daily dose=432 mg) or placebo for 6 weeks (DelBello et al. 2002). Response rates (YMRS reduction from baseline ≥50%) were significantly higher in the group receiving divalproex and quetiapine (87%) than in the group receiving divalproex and placebo (53%).

Maintenance Treatment

There is only one reported maintenance study for children and adolescents with bipolar disorder. Sixty youths who had responded to a combination of lithium and divalproex in a 20-week trial were randomly assigned in a double-blind trial to either lithium or divalproex for 18 months (Findling et al. 2005). There was no significant difference in the time to relapse between the groups (median days: divalproex 112, lithium 114).

Clinical Recommendations for Bipolar Disorder

Treatment guidelines were developed by expert consensus and review of the available treatment literature for children and adolescents (ages 6–17 years) with bipolar I disorder, manic or mixed (Kowatch et al. 2005). Six stages were identified:

- Stage 1: Monotherapy with mood stabilizer or atypical antipsychotic (lithium, valproate, carbamazepine, olanzapine, quetiapine, risperidone)
- Stage 2: Switch monotherapy agent (drug class not tried in stage 1)
- Stage 3: Switch monotherapy agent (drug class not tried in stage 1 or 2) OR combination treatment (2 agents)
- Stage 4: Combination treatment (2 agents) OR combination treatment (3 agents)
- Stage 5: Alternative monotherapy (drugs not tried in stages 1, 2, 3)
- Stage 6: Electroconvulsive therapy (adolescents) or clozapine

If a child fails to respond to treatment in one stage, the clinician should move to the next stage of treatment. For treatment of bipolar I disorder, manic or mixed with psychosis, it was recommended that initial treatment be a mood stabilizer plus an atypical antipsychotic. A minimum of 4–6 weeks at therapeutic blood levels and/or adequate doses for each medication was recommended. Following sustained remission of at least 12–24 months, medication taper should be considered.

Anxiety Disorders

Obsessive-Compulsive Disorder

OCD has a prevalence rate of 2%–4% in youths (Douglass et al. 1995; Zohar 1999). The DSM-IV-TR criteria for OCD are the same in children and adults, with the exception that children may not recognize that their obsessions or compulsions are unreasonable (American Psychiatric Association 2000). The course of OCD in youths is chronic. In a 2- to 7-year follow-up of 54 children and adolescents with OCD, 23 subjects (43%) continued to meet diagnostic criteria for OCD, and only 3 subjects (6%) achieved complete remission (Leonard et al. 1993).

Serotonin Reuptake Inhibitors

Four medications have received FDA approval for the treatment of OCD in children and adolescents: clomipramine (≥10 years old), fluvoxamine (≥7 years old), sertraline (≥6 years old), and fluoxetine (≥7 years old).

Fluvoxamine. The safety and efficacy of fluvoxamine were evaluated in a double-blind, placebo-controlled multicenter study (Riddle et al. 2001). One hundred twenty outpatient children and adolescents (ages 8–17 years) with OCD were randomly assigned to fluvoxamine (dosage range=50–200 mg/day; mean daily dose=165 mg) or placebo for a 10-week trial. Patients who did not respond after 6 weeks could discontinue the double-blind phase and enter an open-label trial of fluvoxamine. Mean CY-BOCS scores were significantly different between the group treated with fluvoxamine and the group treated with placebo at weeks 1, 2, 3, 4, 6, and 10. Response rates (>25% reduction in CY-BOCS scores) were 42% in the group being treated with placebo. Adverse events occurring at a placebo-adjusted frequency of >10% were insomnia and asthenia.

To assess the safety and effectiveness of fluvoxamine in the long-term treatment of pediatric OCD, 99 patients who completed the acute double-blind, placebo-controlled fluvoxamine study (Riddle et al. 2001) participated in a 1-year open-label extension study (Walkup et

al. 1998). Fluvoxamine dosages were titrated to 200 mg/day over the first 4 weeks. Patients experienced a 42% reduction in CY-BOCS scores by the end of long-term treatment. Clinical improvement plateaued at about 6 months of treatment. The most common side effects were insomnia, asthenia, nausea, hyperkinesias, and nervousness. There were no clinically significant laboratory or vital sign abnormalities.

Sertraline. In a double-blind, placebo-controlled multicenter study, 187 children and adolescents (ages 6–17 years) with OCD were randomly assigned to sertraline or placebo (March et al. 1998). Sertraline dosages were titrated to a maximum of 200 mg/day during the first 4 weeks of the trial, and these dosages were maintained for an additional 8 weeks. The mean dosage of sertraline was 167 mg/day at endpoint. Compared with patients receiving placebo, patients receiving sertraline showed significantly greater improvement on the CY-BOCS, the NIMH Global Obsessive Compulsive Rating Scale (NIMH GOCS), and the Clinical Global Impression Severity of Illness (CGI-S) and Improvement (CGI-I) rating scales. Forty-two percent of patients in the sertraline group and 26% of patients in the placebo group were rated as very much or much improved. Side effects of insomnia, nausea, agitation, and tremor occurred significantly more often in the group receiving sertraline than in the group receiving placebo.

To assess the long-term safety and effectiveness of sertraline for pediatric OCD, 137 patients who completed the 12-week double-blind, placebo-controlled sertraline study (March et al. 1998) were given open-label sertraline (mean dosage=120 mg/day) in a 52-week extension study. Significant improvement was found on CY-BOCS, NIMH GOCS, and CGI scores. Rates of response (defined as >25% decrease in CY-BOCS and a CGI-I score of 1 or 2) were 72% for children and 61% for adolescents (Cook et al. 2001). Full remission (defined as a CY-BOCS score >8) was achieved in 47% of patients, and an additional 25% achieved partial remission (CY-BOCS score <15 but >8) (Wagner et al. 2003b). The most common side effects were headache, nausea, diarrhea, somnolence, abdominal pain, hyperkinesias, nervousness, dyspepsia, and vomiting. There were no clinically significant electrocardiogram (ECG), vital sign, or laboratory abnormalities.

The relative and combined efficacy of sertraline and CBT was assessed in a 12-week trial for 112 children and adolescents (ages 7–17 years) with OCD (Pediatric OCD Treatment Study [POTS] Team 2004). Patients were randomly assigned to sertraline, CBT, combined sertraline and CBT, or placebo. Combined treatment was significantly superior to CBT alone and sertraline alone, which did not differ from each other.

Group cognitive-behavioral therapy (GCBT) was compared with sertraline treatment for OCD in a randomized trial with 40 youths (ages 9–17 years) (Asbahr et al. 2005). Both GCBT and sertraline yielded significant improvement in CY-BOCS scores after 12 weeks of treatment. After a 9-month follow-up period, GCBT-treated patients had a significantly lower rate of relapse compared with the sertraline-treated group (5.3% vs. 50%, respectively).

Paroxetine.   The efficacy and safety of paroxetine were assessed in a double-blind, placebo-controlled multicenter study of 203 outpatient children and adolescents (ages 7–17 years) with OCD (D.A. Geller et al. 2004). Patients were randomly assigned to paroxetine (dosage range = 10–50 mg/day; mean daily dose = 23 mg) or placebo for a 10-week trial. There was a statistically significant greater reduction in CY-BOCS scores from baseline to endpoint in patients treated with paroxetine than in patients treated with placebo. Response rates (>25% reduction in CY-BOCS scores) were 64.9% in the paroxetine-treated patients and 41.2% in the placebo-treated patients. The most common adverse effects in the paroxetine group were headache, abdominal pain, nausea, respiratory disorder, somnolence, hyperkinesias, and trauma.

The efficacy of paroxetine in 335 outpatients (ages 7–17 years) with OCD was assessed in a 16-week open-label multicenter study of paroxetine (10–60 mg/day), followed by double-blind randomization of responders to paroxetine or placebo for an additional 16 weeks (Emslie et al. 2000). The rate of response (defined as >25% reduction in CY-BOCS scores) was 68.7% in the open-label phase. No significant differences in response rates were found between the group receiving paroxetine and the group receiving placebo in the randomization phase. However, fewer patients receiving paroxetine relapsed than did patients receiving placebo (34.7% and 43.9%, respectively).

A post hoc analysis of the study by Emslie et al. (2000) found that the response rates in patients with comorbid ADHD, tic disorder, or ODD (56%, 53%, and 39%, respectively) were significantly lower than those in patients without comorbid disorders (75%). Behavioral adverse events, such as insomnia, nervousness, and hyperkinesia, were also significantly more frequent in patients with psychiatric comorbidity (D.A. Geller et al. 2001a).

Fluoxetine.   The safety and efficacy of fluoxetine were assessed in a 13-week double-blind, placebo-controlled

multicenter trial (D.A. Geller et al. 2001b). One hundred three children and adolescents (ages 7–17 years) with OCD were randomly assigned in a 2:1 ratio to either fluoxetine (dosage range = 10–60 mg/day; mean daily dose = 24.6 mg) or placebo. The group treated with fluoxetine showed a statistically significant reduction in OCD severity compared with the group treated with placebo, as assessed by CY-BOCS scores. Rates of response (defined as >40% reduction in CY-BOCS score) were 49% in the fluoxetine group and 25% in the placebo group. There were no significant differences in treatment-emergent adverse events between the fluoxetine and placebo groups. There were significant differences for change in weight and blood pressure between the groups, in the direction of mild weight loss and slight decrease in blood pressure for the fluoxetine group.

In post hoc subgroup analyses of the study by D.A. Geller et al. (2001b), no predictive factors in response to fluoxetine treatment for pediatric OCD were found (D.A. Geller et al. 2001c). There were no statistically significant differences in treatment effect between children versus adolescents, females versus males, patients with versus without a family history of depression or OCD, or patients with age at onset <7 years versus ≥7 years.

Fluoxetine was compared with placebo in a controlled trial in 43 youths with OCD (Liebowitz et al. 2002). It was found that after 16 (but not 8) weeks of treatment, the fluoxetine group had significantly lower CY-BOCS scores than the placebo group. These investigators concluded that fluoxetine's full effect took longer than 8 weeks to develop.

In a smaller double-blind crossover trial of fixed-dosage fluoxetine (20 mg/day) and placebo, 14 children and adolescents (ages 8–15 years) with OCD participated in a 20-week trial with crossover at 8 weeks (Riddle et al. 1992). CY-BOCS scores decreased significantly more after 8 weeks of treatment with fluoxetine than after treatment with placebo (44% and 27%, respectively). The most frequently reported side effects were insomnia, fatigue, motoric activation, and nausea.

Citalopram.   Twenty-three child and adolescent outpatients (ages 9–18 years) with OCD were administered open-label citalopram (dosage range = 10–40 mg/day; mean daily dose = 37 mg) in a 10-week trial (Thomsen 1997). There was a statistically significant improvement in CY-BOCS scores from baseline to endpoint. Over 75% of youths showed a moderate to marked improvement in OCD symptoms. Adverse effects were minimal and transient.

In an 8-week open-label citalopram study of 15 youths (ages 6–17 years) with OCD, 14 patients showed significant improvement in CY-BOCS scores from baseline to end-point. Sedation ($n = 1$) and insomnia ($n = 1$) were reported in the first week of treatment (Mukaddes and Abali 2003).

In a long-term, open study of 30 adolescents with OCD, citalopram (dosage range = 20–70 mg/day; mean daily dose = 46.5 mg) was administered for 1–2 years (Thomsen et al. 2001). There was a significant reduction in CY-BOCS scores from baseline to assessment at 2 years. No serious adverse events were reported, and the most common side effects were sedation, sexual dysfunction, and weight gain.

Clomipramine

Clomipramine has been shown to be efficacious in the treatment of pediatric OCD in two double-blind, placebo-controlled trials. In the first study (Flament et al. 1985), 19 children (ages 10–18 years) with OCD were randomly assigned to clomipramine (dosage range = 100–200 mg/day; mean daily dose = 141 mg) or placebo for 5 weeks. Significant improvement in observed and self-reported obsessions and compulsions was found for patients who received clomipramine. The most common side effects were tremor, dry mouth, dizziness, and constipation. One patient had a grand mal seizure.

In an 8-week double-blind, placebo-controlled multicenter study of 60 children and adolescents (ages 10–17 years) with OCD, it was found that patients who received clomipramine (up to 200 mg/day) had significantly greater reductions in scores on the Children's Yale-Brown Obsessive Compulsive Scale (CY-BOCS; Goodman et al. 1991) compared with the placebo group (37% and 8%, respectively). Forty-seven patients continued in a 1-year open-label extension trial, and effectiveness was maintained with long-term treatment. The most frequent side effects were dry mouth, somnolence, dizziness, fatigue, tremor, headache, constipation, and anorexia (DeVeaugh-Geiss et al. 1992).

In a 10-week double-blind crossover trial of clomipramine and desipramine for 48 children and adolescents (ages 7–19 years) with OCD, clomipramine was shown to be significantly superior to desipramine in reducing obsessive-compulsive symptoms (Leonard et al. 1989). Sixty-four percent of patients who received clomipramine as their first active treatment showed some signs of relapse during treatment with desipramine.

Leonard et al. (1991) further assessed whether patients who were maintained on long-term clomipramine would relapse following double-blind desipramine substitution. Twenty-six children and adolescents with OCD who received maintenance treatment (mean duration = 17.1 months; range = 4–32 months) entered an 8-month double-blind desipramine substitution trial. Eight of 9 patients (89%) in the desipramine group and 2 of 11 patient (18%) in the clomipramine group relapsed during the comparison period.

Anxiolytics

Buspirone. In a case report of an 11-year-old girl with treatment-refractory OCD, buspirone (up to 300 mg/day) over a 3-week period was noted to produce a substantial reduction in obsessive-compulsive symptoms (Alessi and Bos 1991).

Benzodiazepines. A case report of a 14-year-old boy with OCD who received clonazepam (up to 2 mg/day) found a marked decrease in obsessive-compulsive symptoms over an 11-week period (Ross and Pigott 1993). A 16-year-old boy with OCD who had failed to respond to prior trials of clomipramine, fluoxetine, fluvoxamine, and buspirone augmentation showed a 75% improvement in obsessive-compulsive symptoms when his fluoxetine dosage (60 mg/day) was augmented with clonazepam (4 mg/day) (Leonard et al. 1994).

Atypical Antipsychotic Augmentation

Adjunctive risperidone (≤2 mg daily) was investigated in an open trial for 17 adolescents with OCD who failed to respond to two serotonin reuptake inhibitor monotherapy trials. A significant reduction in CY-BOCS scores was reported (Thomsen 2004).

Aripiprazole augmentation of CBT was found to be effective in the case of an adolescent who had a partial response to combined CBT and sertraline (Storch et al. 2008).

Generalized Anxiety Disorder

The prevalence of generalized anxiety disorder (GAD) in children and adolescents is estimated to range from 2.9% to 7.3% (J.C. Anderson et al. 1987; Kashani and Orvaschel 1988). Children with GAD have excessive anxiety and worry about several events or activities (e.g., school performance), have difficulty controlling the worry, and have at least one associated symptom, such as restlessness, fatigue, concentration difficulties, irritability, muscle tension, and sleep disturbance (American Psychiatric Association 2000). Most symptoms of childhood overanxious disorder were subsumed within GAD. Therefore, overanxious disorder was eliminated from DSM-IV (American Psychiatric Association 1994). The course of GAD in youths tends to be chronic (Keller et al. 1992).

Venlafaxine

The efficacy and safety of venlafaxine XR were evaluated in an 8-week double-blind, placebo-controlled multicenter trial (Kunz et al. 2002). One hundred fifty-eight children and adolescents (ages 6–17 years) with GAD were randomly assigned to venlafaxine XR (dosage range = 37.5–225 mg/day) or placebo. There was a statistically significant greater reduction in anxiety scores in the venlafaxine XR group compared with the placebo group. Forty-nine patients (64%) receiving venlafaxine were much or very much improved, compared with five patients (6%) receiving placebo. The most common treatment-related adverse events were hyperkinesia, somnolence, and epistaxis.

Sertraline

Twenty-two children and adolescents (ages 5–17 years) with GAD were randomly assigned to sertraline or placebo in a 9-week double-blind trial (Rynn et al. 2001). The maximum dosage of sertraline was 50 mg/day. Significant differences in favor of sertraline over placebo were observed on Hamilton Anxiety Scale (Ham-A; Hamilton 1959) scores and on CGI-S and CGI-I ratings. Side effects found to be more common (but not statistically significant so) with sertraline than with placebo were dry mouth, drowsiness, leg spasm, and restlessness.

Buspirone

There have been two open studies of buspirone for the treatment of GAD in youths. In an open study of adolescents with GAD, a significant decrease in anxiety clinical ratings after 6 weeks of treatment with buspirone (mean dosage range = 15–30 mg/day) was reported (Kutcher et al. 1992). Simeon (1993) reported the results of an open trial of buspirone for 13 children with anxiety disorders; 9 of these patients had DSM-III-R (American Psychiatric Association 1987) overanxious disorder as a primary or secondary diagnosis. Patients received buspirone (maximum dosage = 30 mg/day) over 4 weeks. Significant improvement in anxiety was found on clinical ratings and parent, teacher, and patient reports. Mild and transient side effects were reported, including sleep difficulties, tiredness, nausea, stomachaches, and headaches.

Benzodiazepines

A few studies have demonstrated some effectiveness of high-potency benzodiazepines in treating children and adolescents with GAD. Twelve patients (ages 8–16 years) with a DSM-III-R diagnosis of overanxious disorder or avoidant disorder received alprazolam (maximum dosage = 0.5–1.5 mg/day) in a 4-week open trial (Simeon and Ferguson 1987). Significant improvement in anxiety was found on clinical ratings and parent questionnaires. Parental reports indicated a decrease in the frequency and severity of sleep problems. The most commonly reported adverse effects were initial daytime sleepiness, agitation, headaches, and nausea. No significant changes in blood pressure, pulse, or respiration were observed.

This open study was followed by a double-blind, placebo-controlled study of alprazolam in the treatment of 30 children (ages 8–16 years) with a DSM-III-R diagnosis of overanxious disorder (n = 21) or avoidant disorder (n = 9) (Simeon et al. 1992). Patients were randomly assigned to alprazolam (dosage range = 0.5–3.5 mg/day; mean daily dose = 1.57 mg) or placebo for a 4-week trial. On the basis of global ratings of improvement, alprazolam was superior to placebo, but this difference was not statistically significant. Side effects were mild and included dry mouth and fatigue. No rebound or withdrawal symptoms occurred, and no adverse cognitive effects were noted.

Social Anxiety Disorder

The prevalence of social anxiety disorder (social phobia) is estimated to range from 0.9% to 7% of children and adolescents (J.C. Anderson et al. 1987; Stein et al. 2001). The diagnostic criteria for social anxiety disorder in children and adolescents are the same as the diagnostic criteria used in adults (American Psychiatric Association 2000). Social anxiety disorder in youths is a chronic condition, and it increases the risk of depression (Stein et al. 2001). Social anxiety disorder during adolescence has been shown to persist into adulthood (Pine et al. 1998).

Selective Serotonin Reuptake Inhibitors

Paroxetine.   The efficacy and safety of paroxetine were evaluated in a 16-week double-blind, placebo-controlled multicenter trial in 322 outpatient children and adolescents (ages 8–17 years) with social anxiety disorder (Wagner et al. 2004a). Paroxetine was significantly superior to placebo, with rates of response (defined as CGI-I score = 1 or 2) of 77.6% and 38.3%, respectively. Side effects more common with paroxetine than with placebo were insomnia, decreased appetite, and vomiting.

Sertraline.   Fourteen outpatient children and adolescents (ages 10–17 years) with a diagnosis of social anxiety disorder received sertraline (dosage range = 100–200 mg/day; mean daily dose = 123 mg) in an 8-week open trial (Compton et al. 2001). Five of the patients (36%) were much or very much improved, and four of the patients (29%) had a partial response by the end of the 8-week trial. A significant clinical response was noted by week 6. Sertraline was well tolerated, and no patient developed significant behavioral disinhibition or mania (Compton et al. 2001).

Citalopram.   Chavira and Stein (2002) investigated the effectiveness of a combined psychoeducational and pharmacological treatment program for youths with social anxiety disorder. Twelve children and adolescents (ages 8–17 years) with social anxiety disorder received citalopram (mean daily dose = 35 mg) and eight 15-minute counseling sessions over a 12-week period. On the basis of clinical global ratings of change, 41.7% of youths ($n = 5$) were very much improved, and 41.7% of youths ($n = 5$) were much improved.

Nefazodone

A 15-year-old boy with social anxiety who was treated with nefazodone (up to 350 mg/day) over a 5-month period had resolution of social anxiety symptoms (Mancini et al. 1999).

Buspirone

A 16-year-old boy with social anxiety disorder and a mixed personality disorder with predominantly schizotypal features was treated with buspirone (up to 20 mg/day). At the end of 12 days of buspirone treatment, he was noted to have a significant reduction in anxiety, which persisted over a 1-year follow-up period (Zwier and Rao 1994).

Selective Mutism

The prevalence of selective mutism in children is estimated to be less than 1% (Dow et al. 1995). Selective mutism is characterized by an absence of speech in at least one specific social situation, usually school, despite the child's ability to speak in other situations (American Psychiatric Association 2000). Selective mutism has been viewed as a variant of social anxiety disorder (Black and Uhde 1992).

Selective Serotonin Reuptake Inhibitors

Fluoxetine.   Fifteen children and adolescents (ages 6–11 years) with selective mutism were randomly assigned to fluoxetine (dosage range = 12–27 mg/day; mean daily dose = 21.4 mg) or placebo for a 12-week trial (Black and Uhde 1994). Significant improvements on ratings of selective mutism were observed in both fluoxetine-treated and placebo-treated subjects. The group treated with fluoxetine showed significantly more improvement on parent ratings of mutism change and global change than did the group receiving placebo. However, most patients in the study continued to be very symptomatic at study end. Side effects were minimal and not significantly different between the groups.

In a 9-week open trial of fluoxetine (dosage range = 10–60 mg/day; mean daily dose = 28.1 mg) in 21 children (ages 5–14 years) with selective mutism, 76% of patients showed improvement, with decreased anxiety and increased speech in public settings (Dummit et al. 1996).

In case reports of a 4-year-old girl (Wright et al. 1995) and a 12-year-old girl (Black and Uhde 1992) with selective mutism, fluoxetine treatment resulted in clinically significant improvement of symptoms.

Fluvoxamine.   A 6-year-old girl was reported to have resolution of symptoms of selective mutism when treated with fluvoxamine (100 mg/day) (Lafferty and Constantino 1998).

Monoamine Oxidase Inhibitors

Phenelzine.   Case studies of five children treated with phenelzine (30–60 mg/day) reported positive response (Golwyn and Sevlie 1999; Golwyn and Weinstock 1990). Weight gain was the most common side effect.

Separation Anxiety Disorder

The prevalence of separation anxiety in children is estimated to be 3.5% (J.C. Anderson et al. 1987). Children with separation anxiety disorder have excessive anxiety and worry about separation from home or from a person to whom they are attached (American Psychiatric Association 2000). School refusal or school phobia may be a symptom of separation anxiety disorder. A long-term follow-up of children with school phobia found that in adulthood, these individuals lived with their parents more often, had fewer children, and more psychiatric consultation than did a general population comparison group (Flakierska-Praquin et al. 1997).

Tricyclic Antidepressants

Imipramine. Imipramine has been the most studied medication for the treatment of separation anxiety disorder, and the treatment results have been mixed. In a 6-week double-blind, placebo-controlled trial, 35 children with school phobia were randomly assigned to imipramine (dosage range = 100–200 mg/day; mean daily dose = 152 mg) or placebo (Gittelman-Klein and Klein 1971). All children received concurrent behavioral treatment. Imipramine treatment was significantly superior to placebo in rates of school return (81% and 47%, respectively). However, in another controlled study of imipramine for separation anxiety disorder (Klein et al. 1992), no significant superiority was found for imipramine (dosage range = 75–275 mg/day; mean daily dose = 153 mg), compared with placebo, in reduction of anxiety symptoms. The most frequent imipramine side effect was irritability or angry outbursts.

Imipramine was compared with alprazolam in an 8-week controlled study in which 24 children and adolescents (ages 7–17 years) with school refusal were randomly assigned to imipramine (dosage range = 150–200 mg/day; mean daily dose = 164.3 mg), alprazolam (dosage range = 1–3 mg/day; mean daily dose = 1.8 mg), or placebo (Bernstein et al. 1990). There was a significant reduction in anxiety ratings from baseline to endpoint in both groups treated with medication, compared with the group receiving placebo. Side effects were mild, with abdominal pain, headaches, and drowsiness the most commonly reported.

The efficacy of imipramine versus placebo in combination with CBT was assessed in the treatment of school refusal in adolescents (Bernstein et al. 2000). Sixty-three adolescents with school refusal were randomly assigned to either imipramine (mean daily dose = 182 mg) plus CBT or placebo plus CBT for an 8-week trial. The group treated with imipramine plus CBT showed a significantly higher rate of school attendance than did the group treated with placebo plus CBT (70% vs. 28%, respectively). In a 1-year follow-up of 41 of the 63 subjects, no significant differences between the two groups were found in prevalence of anxiety diagnoses (Bernstein et al. 2001).

Clomipramine. A 12-week double-blind, placebo-controlled trial of clomipramine (dosage range = 40–75 mg/day) in 46 children and adolescents with school refusal failed to show a significant positive effect (Berney et al. 1981).

Benzodiazepines

Graae et al. (1994) conducted a double-blind crossover trial of 4 weeks of clonazepam therapy (dosage range = 0.5– 2.0 mg/day) and 4 weeks of placebo in 15 children (ages 7–13 years) with anxiety disorders, predominantly separation anxiety disorder. No significant improvement was found relative to baseline for clonazepam or placebo. Two boys discontinued the study because of significant disinhibition and marked irritability, aggression, and tantrums, and 1 boy was noncompliant with the protocol. The most common clonazepam side effects were drowsiness, irritability, and oppositional behavior.

In an open-label study, 9 children (ages 8–11 years) with school refusal received chlordiazepoxide (10–30 mg daily) for 5–30 days (D'Amato 1962). Eight of the children (89%) regularly attended school after 2 weeks of treatment. Drowsiness was the only reported side effect.

Gabapentin

Two adolescents with school refusal who received gabapentin (dosage range = 1,200–2,000 mg/day) were reported to have a positive response to treatment (Durkin 2002).

Posttraumatic Stress Disorder

The prevalence of PTSD in adolescents is reported to be 6.3% (Giaconia et al. 1995). The criteria for diagnosing PTSD in youths are the same as those used for adults (American Psychiatric Association 2000). PTSD symptoms in children tend to vary over time, and although the disorder is chronic, the course is prolonged with greater severity of the stressor (Clarke et al. 1993).

Citalopram

Eight adolescents with PTSD received citalopram in a fixed daily dose of 20 mg in a 12-week open-label study (Seedat et al. 2001). Core PTSD symptoms of reexperiencing, avoidance, and hyperarousal showed statistically significant improvement at week 12, with a 38% reduction in total score on the Clinician-Administered PTSD Scale—Child and Adolescent Version (CAPS-CA; Nader et al. 1996). Citalopram was well tolerated, and the most common side effects were increased sweating, nausea, headache, and tiredness.

In a larger 8-week open trial, Seedat et al. (2002) treated 24 children and adolescents with citalopram (dosage range = 20–40 mg/day; mean daily dose 20 mg). Both the children and adolescents had a significant reduction in CAPS-CA scores at endpoint. Common side effects of citalopram were drowsiness, headache, nausea, and increased sweating.

Clonidine

Seven preschool children (ages 3–6 years) with a diagnosis of PTSD received open treatment with clonidine at a dosage range of 0.05–0.15 mg/day (Harmon and Riggs 1996). To decrease sedation, oral clonidine was subsequently converted to a clonidine patch. The majority of children showed at least moderate improvements in hyperarousal, hypervigilance, insomnia, nightmares, and mood lability.

Guanfacine

A 7-year-old girl with PTSD received guanfacine 0.5 mg daily, which suppressed PTSD nightmares for the 7-week period of administration (Horrigan 1996).

Carbamazepine

Twenty-eight children and adolescents (ages 8–17 years) with a diagnosis of PTSD received carbamazepine (dosage range = 300–1,200 mg/day) for an average of 35 days. Twenty-two patients (78%) became asymptomatic, and the remaining six patients were significantly improved during the course of treatment (Looff et al. 1995).

Propranolol

Eleven children (ages 6–12 years) with a diagnosis of PTSD participated in an off–on–off medication design of 4 weeks of propranolol treatment (Famularo et al. 1988). Propranolol was initiated at 0.8 mg/kg/day and titrated to a maximum of 2.5 mg/kg/day. A significant improvement in PTSD symptoms was found during the treatment period. Side effects included sedation and mildly lowered blood pressure and pulse.

Panic Disorder

The prevalence of panic disorder in children and adolescents ranges from 0.6% to 5.0% in the community and from 0.2% to 9.6% in clinical settings (Masi et al. 2001). The diagnostic criteria for panic disorder in children and adolescents are the same as those for adults (American Psychiatric Association 2000). Panic disorder in youths is a chronic condition, and there is continuity between pediatric and adult panic disorder (Biederman et al. 1997).

Selective Serotonin Reuptake Inhibitors

In an open-label trial, 12 children and adolescents (ages 7–17 years) with panic disorder were treated with an SSRI for 6–8 weeks (Renaud et al. 1999). Mean daily doses of SSRIs were fluoxetine 34 mg, paroxetine 20 mg, and sertraline 125 mg. Adjunctive benzodiazepines were used for 8 patients. Seventy-five percent of patients showed much to very much clinical improvement while receiving treatment with SSRIs. At the end of the trial, 8 patients (67%) no longer fulfilled panic disorder criteria. No significant side effects were found.

Paroxetine. A chart review was conducted of 18 child and adolescent outpatients (ages 7–16 years) with a diagnosis of panic disorder who received monotherapy with paroxetine (dosage range = 10–40 mg/day; mean daily dose = 23 mg) (Masi et al. 2001). The mean paroxetine treatment duration was 11.7 months. Fifteen patients (83%) had a CGI score of much or very much improved. The most common side effects were nausea, tension–agitation, sedation, insomnia, palpitations, and headache.

Citalopram. Three youths (ages 9, 13, and 16 years) with panic disorder and school phobia were treated with citalopram (up to 20 mg/day) over an 8- to 15-month period. All patients experienced resolution of panic attacks during the course of citalopram treatment (Lepola et al. 1996).

Tricyclic Antidepressants

An 11-year-old girl with panic disorder and agoraphobia was treated with imipramine (75 mg/day), which resulted in cessation of panic attacks (Ballenger et al. 1989). A 9-year-old boy with panic disorder and Tourette's syndrome was treated with imipramine (25 mg daily). Within 1 week of treatment onset, the boy's panic episodes ceased, and the cessation was maintained over a 2-year period (Sverd 1988).

Two cases of children (ages 8 and 13 years) with panic disorder and agoraphobia were reported in which the combination of imipramine and alprazolam resulted in complete remission of symptoms (see Ballenger et al. 1989).

Benzodiazepines

In a 2-week open trial, four adolescents with panic disorder were treated with clonazepam (0.5 mg twice daily). A significant reduction in panic attacks (from 3 attacks per week to 0.25 per week) was reported (Kutcher and MacKenzie 1988).

Mixed Anxiety Disorders

Selective Serotonin Reuptake Inhibitors

Fluvoxamine.   One hundred twenty-eight outpatient children and adolescents (ages 6–17 years) with GAD, social anxiety disorder, or separation anxiety disorder (who had received 3 weeks of open treatment with supportive psychoeducational therapy without improvement) were randomly assigned to fluvoxamine (up to 300 mg) or placebo for an 8-week trial (Research Units on Pediatric Psychopharmacology Anxiety Study Group 2001). The group treated with fluvoxamine had a significantly greater reduction in scores on the Pediatric Anxiety Rating Scale (Research Units on Pediatric Psychopharmacology Anxiety Study Group 2002a) than did the group treated with placebo. On the CGI-I scale, the response rate was 76% in the group treated with fluvoxamine and 29% in the group receiving placebo. Adverse effects of abdominal discomfort and increased motor activity were more common in the group treated with fluvoxamine than in the group treated with placebo. Following completion of the 8-week placebo-controlled study, the 128 patients entered a 6-month open-label treatment phase (Research Units on Pediatric Psychopharmacology Anxiety Study Group 2002b). Anxiety symptoms remained low in 33 of 35 (94%) subjects who initially responded to fluvoxamine. Of 14 fluvoxamine nonresponders switched to fluoxetine, anxiety symptoms significantly improved in 10 (71%) patients. Among 48 placebo nonresponders, 27 (56%) showed significant improvement in anxiety on fluvoxamine.

Fluoxetine.   Seventy-four youths (ages 7–17 years) with GAD, separation anxiety disorder, and/or social phobia were randomly assigned to fluoxetine (20 mg/day) or to placebo for 12 weeks (Birmaher et al. 2003). Sixty-one percent of fluoxetine-treated patients and 35% of placebo-treated patients were much or very much improved. Fluoxetine was well tolerated, with mild headache and gastrointestinal symptoms reported as adverse events.

Fluoxetine's efficacy in long-term treatment of children with GAD, separation anxiety disorder, and/or social phobia was assessed in a 1-year open treatment (Clark et al. 2005) following the acute-phase study (Birmaher et al. 2003). Compared with youths taking no medication, those taking fluoxetine ($n=42$) showed significantly superior outcome in anxiety measures. These investigators concluded that fluoxetine is effective in maintenance treatment of anxiety disorders in youth.

Clinical Recommendations for Anxiety Disorders

SSRIs are the medication treatment of choice for OCD in children and adolescents (Riddle 1998). Clomipramine is also effective in the treatment of this disorder; however, anticholinergic side effects often make this a less tolerable agent than SSRIs. A 10- to 12-week trial at adequate dosages is required to determine whether a child with OCD will respond to an SSRI (Greist et al. 1995). If a child fails to respond to one SSRI, switching to another SSRI is a reasonable strategy. Clomipramine may be a third treatment option, either as monotherapy or as augmentation of an SSRI. Other possible SSRI augmentation strategies are clonazepam, antipsychotics, lithium, and buspirone; however, these agents have not received systematic study in children (American Academy of Child and Adolescent Psychiatry 1998). Some children may require long-term medication maintenance; however, it is reasonable to attempt medication discontinuation 1 year after symptom resolution. Medication should be tapered gradually to assess for relapse and to avoid discontinuation symptoms (Grados et al. 1999).

In regard to other childhood anxiety disorders, SSRIs are first-line treatment (Reinblatt and Walkup 2005). Venlafaxine has also demonstrated efficacy for the treatment of childhood GAD. Other treatment options include buspirone, TCAs, and benzodiazepines (Bernstein et al. 1996). However, benzodiazepines should be used only on a short-term basis (i.e., weeks) because of the potential for abuse and dependence in youths (Riddle et al. 1999).

Attention-Deficit/Hyperactivity Disorder

The prevalence of ADHD in children and adolescents is estimated to range from 5% to 12% (Barbaresi et al. 2002; Centers for Disease Control and Prevention 2005; Rowland et al. 2002), although only about half of children diagnosed with ADHD receive treatment (Centers for Disease Control and Prevention 2005). In addition to the core behavioral features of inattention, hyperactivity, and impulsivity, children with ADHD often have significant impairment in social and academic functioning (Barkley 2005). About 4% of adults in the general population meet criteria for ADHD (Kessler et al. 2006). Of all of the childhood psychiatric disorders, ADHD has the greatest number of pharmacological treatment studies.

Psychostimulants

The classes of psychostimulants include methylphenidate, dexmethylphenidate, dextroamphetamine, mixed amphetamine salts, and L-lysine-D-amphetamine (lisdexamfetamine). By the 1980s, there were already hundreds of randomized, controlled trials showing the efficacy of stimulants for the treatment of ADHD in school-age children (Greenhill et al. 1999). Beginning in the late 1980s and 1990s, the intensive study of the pharmacokinetics and pharmacodynamics of stimulant medications was undertaken, pioneered by the group at the University of California at Irvine. Analog classroom settings were used to examine the hour-by-hour effects of stimulant medications on behavior and cognition and its relationship to serum stimulant medications. Such studies led to the development of methylphenidate (Swanson et al. 1998, 1999, 2000, 2002, 2003), mixed salts of amphetamine–dextroamphetamine (Greenhill et al. 2003; McCracken et al. 2003), extended-release methylphenidate (Swanson et al. 2004; Wigal et al. 2003), dexmethylphenidate hydrochloride (Quinn et al. 2004), and lisdexamfetamine dimesylate (Findling et al. 2006a).

Subsequently, numerous large-scale clinical trials proved the efficacy of these new agents (Biederman et al. 2002; Greenhill et al. 2002, 2005; McCracken et al. 2003; Pelham et al. 1999; Wigal et al. 2005a; Wolraich 2000; Wolraich et al. 2001). A methylphenidate transdermal patch (Findling and Lopez 2005; Pelham et al. 2005) has been recently approved for use in the treatment of ADHD. In the study of the transdermal patch, 270 children with ADHD were randomly assigned to receive either a placebo patch or varying dosages of the methylphenidate patch in a double-blind design. At the end of the 5-week study, 72% of those on the active patch were classified as responders compared to 24% on placebo; side effects were similar to oral methylphenidate (decreased appetite, insomnia, weight loss, tics).

Lisdexamfetamine dimesylate is a "prodrug" in which D-amphetamine is covalently bound to L-lysine (Findling et al. 2006a). In the bloodstream, the lysine is hydrolyzed to yield the active stimulant. The prodrug appears to have lower potential than amphetamine for oral or intravenous abuse (Jasinski and Krishman 2006a, 2006b). In the pivotal trials, 290 children (ages 6–12 years) with ADHD were randomly assigned to either placebo ($n=72$) or different dosages of lisdexamfetamine dimesylate (30, 50, 70 mg/day). All doses of lisdexamfetamine dimesylate were superior to placebo ($P<0.0001$) throughout the 4-week trial at three different time points during the day (10 A.M.,

2 P.M., and 6 P.M.). Common side effects of lisdexamfetamine dimesylate were decreased appetite (39%), irritability (10%), insomnia (19%), nausea/vomiting (6%–9%), and weight loss (9%). No serious adverse events were reported. The medication was well tolerated in long-term follow-up, with no significant laboratory or ECG abnormalities reported (Childress et al. 2006).

Initial research with long-acting stimulants was carried out in school-age children, but recent controlled trials of stimulants have focused on adolescents (T.J. Spencer et al. 2006b; Wilens et al. 2006b) and adults (Biederman et al. 2006a; Weisler et al. 2006). These studies in older individuals show response rates to stimulants similar to those of children; with adequate response for most subjects being obtained with 70–100 mg of methylphenidate or 40–60 mg of amphetamine a day.

Preschoolers with ADHD have also been the focus of recent work. In the NIMH Preschool ADHD Treatment Study (PATS), 183 children (ages 3–5 years) underwent an open-label trial of methylphenidate; subsequently 165 of these subjects were randomized into a double-blind, placebo-controlled crossover trial of methylphenidate lasting 6 weeks (Greenhill et al. 2006b). One hundred forty subjects who completed this second phase went on to enter a long-term maintenance study of methylphenidate. Parents of subjects in this study were required to complete a 10-week course of parent training before their child was treated with medication. Of note, only 37 of 279 enrolled parents felt that the behavior training resulted in significant or satisfactory improvement (Greenhill et al. 2004).

Results from the short-term, open-label run-in and double-blind crossover studies do show that methylphenidate is effective in preschoolers with ADHD (Wigal et al. 2006). The mean optimal dose of methylphenidate was found to be 0.7+0.4 mg/kg/day, which is lower than the mean of 1.0 mg/kg/day found to be optimal in the Multimodal Treatment of ADHD (MTA) study with school-age children. Eleven percent of subjects discontinued methylphenidate because of adverse events (Wigal et al. 2006). Also relative to the MTA study, the preschool group showed a higher rate of emotional adverse events, including crabbiness, irritability, and proneness to crying. The conclusion was that the dose of methylphenidate (or any stimulant) should be titrated more conservatively in preschoolers than in school-age patients, and lower mean doses may be effective. A pharmacokinetic study done as part of the PATS protocol showed that preschoolers metabolized methylphenidate more slowly than did school-age children, perhaps explaining these results (McGough et al. 2006).

Longer-term open-label studies of these agents, often lasting up to 2 years (McGough et al. 2005; Wilens et al. 2003b, 2005), have also been performed, giving the field more data about efficacy and safety after prolonged use. These studies do not show the presence of any major medical adverse events, with no abnormalities of hematological or chemical measures (Biederman et al. 2002; Greenhill et al. 2002; McCracken et al. 2003; Wolraich 2000; Wolraich et al. 2001).

Atomoxetine

Atomoxetine is a noradrenergic reuptake inhibitor that has indirect effects on dopamine reuptake in cortex but not in the striatum (Bymaster et al. 2002). Numerous double-blind, placebo-controlled trials have demonstrated its efficacy in the treatment of ADHD in children, adolescents, and adults (Michelson et al. 2001, 2002, 2003). Given its pharmacokinetic half-life of 5 hours, it is generally dosed twice a day. While open trials comparing methylphenidate with atomoxetine showed the two agents to have similar efficacy (Kratochvil et al. 2002), double-blind, placebo-controlled trials comparing atomoxetine with amphetamine (Biederman et al. 2006b; Wigal et al. 2005b) and methylphenidate (Michelson 2004) have shown the stimulants to be more efficacious.

Atomoxetine is effective in treating ADHD in those with comorbid tics and may also reduce tics (Allen et al. 2005). It is also useful in children with ADHD who have comorbid anxiety, showing effectiveness in treating anxiety and inattention (Sumner et al. 2005). Atomoxetine is well tolerated in long-term use. In a global multicenter study, 416 children and adolescents who responded to an initial 12-week open-label period of treatment with atomoxetine were randomly assigned to continued atomoxetine treatment or placebo for 9 months under double-blind conditions. Atomoxetine was significantly superior to placebo in preventing relapse (defined as a return to 90% of baseline symptom severity), 22.3% and 37.9%, respectively (Michelson 2004). Data from 13 atomoxetine studies (6 double-blind, 7 open-label) were pooled for subjects ages 12–18 years with ADHD (Wilens et al. 2006b). Of the 601 atomoxetine-treated subjects in this meta-analysis, 537 (89.4%) completed 3 months of acute treatment. At the time of publication, a total of 259 subjects (48.4%) were continuing atomoxetine treatment; 219 of these subjects had completed at least 2 years of treatment. Symptoms remained improved up to 24 months without dosage escalation. During the 2-year treatment period, 99 (16.5%) subjects discontinued treat-

ment due to lack of effectiveness, and 31 (5.2%) subjects discontinued treatment due to adverse events. No clinically significant abnormalities in height, weight, blood pressure, pulse, mean laboratory values, or ECG parameters were found.

Tricyclic Antidepressants

Before the advent of atomoxetine, TCAs were the primary alternative to stimulant treatment of ADHD. There have been 15 double-blind, placebo-controlled studies of TCAs demonstrating the efficacy of desipramine, imipramine, amitriptyline, nortriptyline, and clomipramine in the treatment of children with ADHD (Daly and Wilens 1998; Popper 2000; Prince et al. 2000). Desipramine is rarely used today because of isolated reports in the 1990s of sudden death at therapeutic dosages (Popper and Ziminitzky 1995). In general, there has been a decline in the use of TCAs for the treatment of ADHD due to the need to monitor ECG (see Appendix) and the risk of death in the event of overdose.

Bupropion

Bupropion is an antidepressant with noradrenergic and dopaminergic actions. Simeon et al. (1986) conducted a 14-week single-blind study consisting of placebo baseline for 4 weeks, bupropion (dosage range = 50–150 mg; mean daily dose = 135 mg) for 8 weeks, and placebo posttreatment for 2 weeks. Seventeen boys with ADHD and conduct disorder (ages 7–13 years) participated in the study. Significant improvement in hyperactivity, conduct problems, and global functioning was found.

A double-blind, placebo-controlled four-center study was conducted to assess the efficacy of bupropion in the treatment of childhood ADHD (Conners et al. 1996). One hundred nine children (ages 6–12 years) with ADHD were randomly assigned to bupropion ($n = 72$) or placebo ($n = 37$) for a 6-week trial. Dosages of bupropion ranged from 3 to 6 mg/kg/day. Significant treatment effects were found for hyperactivity, impulsivity, conduct problems, and attention. Moderate effect sizes of bupropion that were somewhat less than those for stimulant treatment of ADHD were found. The most frequent adverse effects with bupropion were rash, urticaria, nausea, and vomiting. Although no patients experienced a seizure, 6 of 72 children who received bupropion had electroencephalograms (EEGs) that changed from normal at baseline to abnormal on the final day of treatment (approximately 4 weeks later) (Conners et al. 1996).

Bupropion was compared with methylphenidate in a small double-blind crossover study (Barrickman et al. 1995). Fifteen children and adolescents (ages 7–17 years) were randomly assigned to bupropion or methylphenidate for 6 weeks, underwent washout for 2 weeks, and were crossed over to the other medication. The dosage range of bupropion was 1.4–5.7 mg/kg/day (mean daily dose = 3.3 mg/kg) and the dosage range of methylphenidate was 0.4–1.3 mg/kg/day (mean daily dose = 0.7 mg/kg). Bupropion and methylphenidate produced significant and similar improvement in ADHD symptoms. Despite this finding, however, the two medications have never been compared in more rigorous parallel-group designs, and clinical experience strongly suggests that the effect size for bupropion is not as great as that for stimulants.

Clonidine

A review of the literature from 1980 to 1999 found 39 studies regarding the use of clonidine for symptoms of childhood ADHD, and 11 of the studies ($n = 150$) had sufficient data to be included in a meta-analysis (Connor et al. 1999). Of these 150 subjects, 42 received clonidine for ADHD, and the others received clonidine for ADHD comorbid with tic disorders ($n = 67$), developmental disorders ($n = 15$), or conduct disorders ($n = 26$). The mean daily dose of clonidine was 0.18 mg, and the average length of treatment was 10.9 weeks. Clonidine showed a moderate effect size of 0.58 on symptoms of ADHD, which is smaller than the effect size (0.82) reported for stimulant treatment of ADHD (Swanson et al. 1995).

Guanfacine

Two open trials and one controlled trial provide some support for the use of guanfacine in the treatment of youths with ADHD. In a study by Hunt et al. (1995), 13 children and adolescents with ADHD received guanfacine (mean daily dose = 3.2 mg) for 1 month. Significant improvements in hyperactivity and inattention were found. In another study by Chappell et al. (1995b), 10 children and adolescents with comorbid ADHD and Tourette's syndrome received guanfacine (mean daily dose = 1.5 mg) over a 4- to 20-week period. Four of the 10 children (40%) had moderate to marked improvement in ADHD symptoms.

In an 8-week double-blind, placebo-controlled trial, 34 children and adolescents (ages 7–14 years) with ADHD and tic disorder were randomly assigned to guanfacine (dosage range = 1.5–3.0 mg/day) or placebo (Scahill et al. 2001). There was a 37% improvement in ADHD

symptoms for children treated with guanfacine, compared with an 8% improvement in ADHD symptoms for children receiving placebo. The most common side effects of guanfacine were sedation and dry mouth. There were no significant changes in pulse or blood pressure with guanfacine.

An extended-release formulation of guanfacine has been recently studied in a double-blind, placebo-controlled Phase III multicenter trial (Melmed et al. 2006). Children and adolescents ages 6–17 years were randomly assigned to placebo or 2, 3, or 4 mg/day of guanfacine. All three doses of guanfacine were superior to placebo in reducing symptoms of ADHD. The most commonly reported side effects were headache, somnolence, and fatigue. No serious adverse events were reported. In healthy young adults (ages 19–24 years), abrupt discontinuation of 4 mg of extended-release guanfacine did not lead to increases in blood pressure or ECG abnormalities (Kisicki et al. 2006).

Modafinil

Modafinil, a nonstimulant activator of the cortex approved for the treatment of narcolepsy, was studied to determine its efficacy in the treatment of ADHD. A 9-week double-blind, placebo-controlled trial randomly assigned 248 subjects to either placebo or modafinil (dosage range = 170–425 mg once per day) (Biederman et al. 2005d). At study termination, 48% of subjects on modafinil were rated as much or very much improved compared to 17% of those on placebo (effect size vs. placebo = 0.69). The most common adverse events reported were insomnia (29%), headache (20%), and decreased appetite (16%). In a second controlled trial, 200 subjects were randomly assigned to placebo or modafinil (Greenhill et al. 2006a); 52% of those on modafinil were classified as responders versus 18% of subjects on placebo ($P < 0.001$). A double-blind, placebo-controlled discontinuation study involving 189 patients with ADHD also demonstrated efficacy of modafinil in ADHD (Swanson et al. 2006b). While the medication was well tolerated by most subjects in open-label follow-up studies, one case of suspected Stevens-Johnson syndrome was reported, and the FDA declined to approve the medication for clinical use (U.S. Food and Drug Administration 2006c). Given the low response rate (~50%) relative to that seen with stimulants (65%–85%), it is not likely that modafinil would have emerged as a first-line treatment for ADHD. Clinicians face a dilemma if they choose to use modafinil (Provigil) off label for the treatment of ADHD; this should be attempted only if all other agents have failed and the patient and family are informed of the reason for the FDA's failure to approve the medication.

Other Antidepressants

Fenfluramine, a potent serotonergic agonist, was found to be ineffective in the treatment of ADHD (Donnelly et al. 1989). Thus, findings from open trials suggesting improvement in ADHD symptoms with SSRI treatment (Barrickman et al. 1991; Gammon and Brown 1993) must be greeted with skepticism. In the Gammon and Brown (1993) study, improvement in mood and attention was seen when fluoxetine was added to methylphenidate when the clinical response after monotherapy with the stimulant was deemed insufficient in a sample of 32 children and adolescents with ADHD. However, in a later open-label study of sertraline or fluoxetine in the treatment of seven children and adolescents with ADHD and major depression, Findling (1996) found no improvement in ADHD symptoms for any patient treated with SSRIs. More recently, the addition of fluvoxamine to methylphenidate was not demonstrated to be effective relative to addition of placebo in a sample of children with ADHD and comorbid anxiety (Abikoff et al. 2005).

In an open trial of venlafaxine, 7 of 16 children and adolescents (44%) showed some improvement in ADHD symptoms of hyperactivity and impulsivity; however, no improvement was seen in cognitive symptoms (Olvera et al. 1996). The mean daily dose of venlafaxine was 60 mg. Four patients (25%) were unable to tolerate the medication, with 3 of the patients discontinuing medication because of worsening hyperactivity. Other side effects included drowsiness, irritability, and nausea. No effects on blood pressure or heart rate were found. No double-blind, placebo-controlled trials have ever proven the efficacy of venlafaxine in the treatment of ADHD. Given concerns about antidepressants increasing the risk of suicidal ideation, anti-depressants without proven efficacy in the treatment of ADHD should not be used in its treatment. They may be used in conjunction with an established medication treatment for ADHD to treat a comorbid anxiety or depressive disorder.

Clinical Recommendations for Attention-Deficit/Hyperactivity Disorder

Recently, the Texas Children's Medication Algorithm Project (CMAP) has revised the algorithm for the treatment of ADHD (Pliszka et al. 2006a). Based on current research and panel discussion, the stages of medication treatment were established as follows:

- Stage 1: Psychostimulant
- Stage 2: Alternative psychostimulant
- Stage 3: Atomoxetine
- Stage 3a: Combination of stimulant and low-dose atomoxetine
- Stage 4: Bupropion or TCA
- Stage 5: Alternative antidepressant from stage 5
- Stage 6: Alpha agonist (guanfacine or clonidine)

Arnold (2000) reviewed studies in which subjects underwent a trial of both amphetamine and methylphenidate. This review suggested that approximately 41% of subjects with ADHD responded equally to both methylphenidate and amphetamine, while 44% responded preferentially to one of the classes of stimulants. This suggests the initial response rate to stimulants may be as high as 85% if both stimulants are tried (in contrast to the finding of 65%–75% response when only one stimulant is tried). There is at present, however, no method to predict which stimulant will produce the best response in a given patient. The recent practice parameters of the American Academy of Child and Adolescent Psychiatry (2007) characterize all FDA-approved agents (stimulants and atomoxetine) as appropriate for initial treatment of ADHD, with antidepressants and alpha agonists as second line.

Disruptive Behavior Disorders and Aggression

Oppositional Defiant Disorder and Conduct Disorder

Oppositional defiant disorder (ODD) is a pattern of negativistic, defiant, angry behavior that is persistent and causes impairment in the child's social functioning. Conduct disorder (CD) consists of antisocial and aggressive behavior (lying, stealing, fighting, fire setting, destruction of property, truancy, running away) (American Psychiatric Association 2000). ODD and CD are highly comorbid with ADHD, particularly in younger children (Maughan et al. 2004; Pliszka et al. 1999).

Psychostimulants

The efficacy of methylphenidate in treating 84 youths (ages 6–15 years) with CD, with and without ADHD, was assessed in a 5-week double-blind, placebo-controlled trial. Ratings of antisocial behaviors specific to CD were significantly reduced by methylphenidate treatment (up to 60 mg/day) (Klein et al. 1997). The severity of the ADHD did not affect the response of CD symptoms to the stimulant studies. Since this study, multiple double-blind, placebo-controlled trials have shown that ODD responds to stimulant medication, yielding an effect size similar to that for the ADHD symptoms (American Psychiatric Association 2000; Pelham et al. 2001; T.J. Spencer et al. 2006a).

Atomoxetine

Children and adolescents (ages 8–18 years) with ADHD were treated for approximately 8 weeks with placebo or atomoxetine under randomized, double-blind conditions. Of the 293 subjects, 39% were diagnosed with comorbid ODD and 61% were not (Newcorn et al. 2005). Treatment group differences and differences between patients with and without comorbid ODD were examined post hoc for changes on numerous clinical measures. Youths with ADHD and comorbid ODD showed statistically significant improvement in ADHD and ODD symptoms as well as in quality-of-life measures on atomoxetine relative to placebo. Treatment response was similar in youths with and without ODD, although the comorbid group may require higher doses to achieve response than those with ADHD alone.

In general, a child with ODD or CD should be treated with a stimulant or atomoxetine before proceeding to the use of other psychotropic agents. The use of more potent agents (mood stabilizers, antipsychotics) is generally reserved for those with severe aggression, and then only after a behavioral treatment has failed (Pappadopulos et al. 2003; Pliszka et al. 2006a).

Aggressive Behavior

While ODD and CD are *syndromes*, aggression is a *symptom*. Although many children and adolescents with CD are aggressive, a child can meet criteria for CD without being aggressive; aggression may present as a problematic symptom in children with depression, psychosis or bipolar disorder without the child meeting criteria for CD. Thus, the clinician must be clear whether ODD/CD or aggression is the target of treatment, as studies have addressed the problems separately. Treatments for ADHD have been used to target ODD/CD, whereas mood stabilizers and antipsychotics have been used in patients with severe aggressive outbursts, regardless of diagnosis (Pappadopulos et al. 2006).

Psychostimulants

In a meta-analysis of the literature from 1970 to 2001 that utilized 28 studies to determine the effect size for stimu-

lants on overt and covert aggression-related behaviors in children with ADHD, it was found that the mean effect size for aggressive behaviors was similar to that for core behaviors of ADHD (Connor et al. 2002; Pappadopulos et al. 2006).

Risperidone

A significant body of research has accumulated showing the effectiveness of risperidone in the treatment of aggression, although most of these studies involve patients with subaverage intelligence (Pappadopulos et al. 2006). One hundred ten children (ages 5–12 years) with an IQ of 36–84 with a disruptive behavior disorder were enrolled in a clinical trial of risperidone consisting of a 1-week single-blind, placebo run-in period followed by a 6-week double-blind, placebo-controlled period (Snyder et al. 2002). Eighty percent of subjects had comorbid ADHD. Risperidone dosages ranged from 0.02 to 0.06 mg/kg/day. The risperidone-treated subjects showed a significant ($P<0.001$) reduction (47.3%) in mean scores versus placebo-treated subjects (20.9%) on the Conduct Problem subscale of the Nisonger Child Behavior Rating Form (NCBRF) ($P<0.001$). The effect of risperidone was unaffected by diagnosis, presence/absence of ADHD, psychostimulant use, and IQ status. Risperidone produced no changes on the cognitive variables, and the most common side effects were somnolence, headache, appetite increase, and dyspepsia. Somnolence did not predict response of aggressive symptoms. Side effects related to extrapyramidal symptoms were reported in 7 (13.2%) and 3 (5.3%) of the subjects in the risperidone and placebo groups, respectively ($P=0.245$).

Other double-blind, placebo-controlled trials of risperidone in children and adolescents with disruptive behavior disorders (and subaverage IQ) have yielded similar results, with no negative trials reported (Aman et al. 2002; Buitelaar et al. 2001; LeBlanc et al. 2005). Weight gain was a significant side effect in these studies, but there has not been evidence of adverse neuropsychological effects (Gunther et al. 2006). Addition of stimulant does not appear to increase rates of side effects and enhances treatment of hyperactivity (Aman et al. 2004). Indeed adding risperidone to a stimulant to control aggression has become a common practice, although a recent controlled study showed that aggression was equally reduced when either placebo or risperidone was added to psychostimulant medication (Armenteros et al. 2007). The sample in this study was small ($N=25$), but the study should caution clinicians that aggression can respond to psychosocial events, like the expectations of a study.

Because of weight gain and increased prolactin associated with risperidone, concern exists regarding its long-term use (Correll and Carlson 2006). The long-term safety and efficacy of risperidone in disruptive behavior disorders in children with subaverage IQ were studied in a 48-week open-label extension study of risperidone in 77 children (Turgay et al. 2002). Subjects received risperidone at daily doses of between 0.02 and 0.06 mg/kg. Adverse events were reported for 76 participants; none were serious, and most were mild/moderate in severity. Somnolence (52%), headache (38%), and weight gain (36%) were the most common adverse events. The degree of sedation was mild and not associated with cognitive deterioration. Mean weight gain was 8.5 kg, half of this attributable to normal growth. Asymptomatic peak prolactin levels were observed within 4 weeks of beginning risperidone treatment and declined over time to within normal range. At study endpoint, mean prolactin levels were statistically significantly greater than baseline only in male participants but within the normal range. Twenty participants experienced mild or moderate extrapyramidal symptoms, but these did not cause withdrawal from the study.

The pooled database of five studies of the long-term use of risperidone (n=700) included 700 children ages 5–15 years who had received risperidone for 11 or 12 months (Dunbar et al. 2004). Subjects also had baseline and 11- or 12-month height measurements (n=350); girls ≥9 years and boys ≥10 years also had baseline and 11- or 12-month Tanner staging (n=222). Risperidone-treated children had a mean increase in height 1.2 cm greater than the reference population, and they experienced no delay in progression through Tanner staging. Transient increases in prolactin did not correlate with growth or sexual maturation. The authors concluded that there was no evidence of statistically or clinically significant growth failure or delay in pubertal onset or progression in children treated for up to 1 year with risperidone.

A full review of all studies of risperidone in the treatment of childhood aggression was recently published (Pandina et al. 2006). This review pooled adverse-event data from these studies (n=688), showing the most common side effects of risperidone to be somnolence (33%), weight gain (20%), hyperprolactinemia (10.2%), and fatigue (10%). In the pooled studies, there was an excess mean weight gain (over normal growth) of 6.0+7 kg after 35–43 weeks of treatment. Of the 688 patients, 651 were free of dyskinetic movements at baseline, and only 1 patient developed new dyskinetic movements during the follow-up period (these symptoms resolved even though risperidone was continued). There was no worsening of dyskinetic movements in those with such preexisting symptoms. Rates of extrapyramidal side effects were low throughout the long-term follow-up period. It should be noted that the dosages of risperidone used in these studies were quite low (1–2 mg/day); thus, these results may not apply to dosages in the 6 mg/day range.

Quetiapine

Quetiapine has been studied in an open trial with aggressive children with CD (Findling et al. 2006b) The 8-week trial enrolled 17 children ages 6–12 years. Outcome measures included the Rating of Aggression Against People and/or Property Scale (RAAPPS), the NCBRF, and the Conners Parent Rating Scale (CPRS-48). Blood sampling for pharmacokinetic analyses occurred at the end of weeks 2 and 8: the mean dose of quetiapine at week 8 was 4.4±1.1 mg/kg. Significant decreases in baseline scores of the RAAPPS, and in several subscales of the NCBRF and the CPRS, were found by the end of the study (P<0.05). No patients discontinued because of an adverse event or experienced extrapyramidal side effects. These preliminary data suggest that aggressive children with CD may benefit from quetiapine. The pharmacokinetics of quetiapine supports twice-daily dosing in children. Nine of the subjects in this study were subsequently enrolled in a 26-week open-label trial; they were treated with dosages of quetiapine ranging from 75 to 300 mg/day. Aggression remained well controlled, no subject developed extrapyramidal side effects, and 1 subject had a significant weight gain but remained in the study.

The efficacy and tolerability of quetiapine and divalproex for the treatment of impulsivity and reactive aggression were studied in 33 subjects with bipolar disorder and disruptive behavior disorders (Barzman et al. 2006). The subjects were randomly assigned to quetiapine (400–600 mg/day) or divalproex (serum level 80–120 microgram/mL) for 28 days in this double-blinded study. Repeated-measures analysis of variance (ANOVA) demonstrated statistically significant within-treatment-group effects for divalproex (baseline=20.6, endpoint=13.3, P<0.0001) and quetiapine (baseline=18.8, endpoint=10.8, P<0.0001) for the Positive and Negative Syndrome Scale (PANSS) Excited Component (EC), but there was no significant difference in the rate of improvement in the PANSS EC scores between the two treatment groups; thus, the two agents showed similar efficacy for the treatment of impulsivity and reactive aggression in this study. No double-blind, placebo-controlled trials of quetiapine in the treatment of aggression have been performed.

Other Atypical Antipsychotics

There have only been small open trials and case reports of the use of aripiprazole, olanzapine, and ziprasidone in the treatment of aggression (Hazaray et al. 2004; Khan et al. 2006; Rugino and Janvier 2005; Staller and Staller 2004; Stephens et al. 2004; Valicenti-McDermott and Demb 2006). In most of these studies, children had primary psychiatry diagnoses other than ODD or CD, such as mood disorders or developmental disorders.

Rugino and Janvier (2005) reported on the use of aripiprazole in a mixed sample (n = 17) of children with bipolar disorder and developmental disorders. Only 4 of the subjects responded, but coadministration of alpha$_2$ agonists in a large proportion of the sample may have confounded the results. A retrospective chart review of 32 children (ages 5–19 years) with developmental disabilities treated with aripiprazole was conducted (Valicenti-McDermott and Demb 2006). Twenty-four had diagnoses within the autistic spectrum, and 18 had mental retardation. Other disorders included ADHD/disruptive behavior disorders (n = 13), mood disorders (n = 7), reactive attachment disorder (n = 2), and sleep disorders (n = 2). Target symptoms included aggression, hyperactivity, impulsivity, and self-injurious behaviors. The mean daily aripiprazole starting dose was 7.1±0.32 mg (0.17 mg/kg/day), and the mean daily maintenance dose was 10.55±6.9 mg (0.27 mg/kg/day). While improvement in target symptoms was found in 56% of the sample, side effects were reported in 16 (50%), with the most frequent being sleepiness (n = 6). Mean body mass index (BMI) rose significantly, and weight gain was more pronounced in children younger than 12 years.

Inpatient children who received intramuscular ziprasidone or olanzapine for emergency treatment of aggression were found to have similar lengths of stay and number of restraints, but those administered ziprasidone required many more injections and were more likely to require coadministration of lorazepam (Khan et al. 2006).

The effects of olanzapine on aggressive behavior and tic severity was examined in 10 subjects (ages 7–13 years) with a primary diagnosis of Tourette's syndrome and a history of aggressive behavior (Stephens et al. 2004). They were treated in a 2-week single-blind placebo run-in followed by an 8-week treatment-phase trial. The starting dose of olanzapine was 1.25–2.5 mg/day and was titrated at biweekly intervals, as tolerated. The mean dosage at the end of the trial was 14.5 mg/day. Olanzapine produced clinically and statistically significant reductions of aggression and tic severity from baseline to trial completion, as measured by the Achenbach Child Behavior Checklist (CBCL) and Yale Global Tic Severity Scale (YGTSS). Weight gain during the treatment period was the most common adverse effect (range = 2–20 lbs; group mean = 12.0 lbs±5.71). No other significant adverse effects were observed during the 10-week trial.

Lithium

The efficacy of lithium in the treatment of CD in youths has been demonstrated in three of the four double-blind, placebo-controlled studies reported to date. Haloperidol, lithium, and placebo were compared in a double-blind, randomized trial for 61 hospitalized children with aggression (ages 5–12 years) and CD. The optimal dosages of haloperidol ranged from 1 to 6 mg/day; the optimal dosages of lithium ranged from 500 to 2,000 mg/day. Both haloperidol and lithium were found to be significantly superior to placebo in reducing aggression. However, there were more adverse effects associated with haloperidol than with lithium, including excessive sedation, acute dystonic reaction, and drooling. Stomachache, headache, and tremor were more common with lithium than with haloperidol (Campbell et al. 1984).

In a subsequent study, Campbell et al. (1995) conducted a 6-week double-blind, placebo-controlled trial of lithium treatment for 50 hospitalized children (ages 5–12 years) with aggression and CD. The mean optimal daily dose of lithium was 1,248 mg, and the mean serum level was 1.12 mEq/L. Lithium was significantly superior to placebo in reducing aggression. The most common lithium side effects were stomachache, nausea, vomiting, headache, tremor, and urinary frequency.

Eighty-six inpatients (ages 10–17 years) with CD were randomly assigned to treatment with lithium (mean daily dose = 1,425 mg; mean serum level = 1.07 mmol/L) or placebo in a 4-week double-blind trial. Aggression ratings decreased significantly for the group treated with lithium, compared with the group treated with placebo. More than 50% of patients in the lithium group experienced nausea, vomiting, and urinary frequency (Malone et al. 2000).

Rifkin et al. (1997) found no significant differences between lithium and placebo in aggression ratings in a 2-week double-blind study of 33 inpatients with CD. The short duration of treatment may have accounted for the lack of efficacy, suggesting that a 4- to 6-week trial is necessary to show response. In a clinical series of 17 hospitalized children, approximately 75% showed reduction of aggression when treated with lithium (Vetro et al. 1985).

Divalproex

Twenty outpatient children and adolescents (ages 10–18 years) with CD or ODD were randomly assigned to divalproex (dosage range = 750–1,500 mg/day; mean blood level = 82 µg/mL) or placebo in a 6-week double-blind, placebo-controlled crossover study. Of the 15 patients who completed both phases, 12 patients (80%) had a statistically significant superior response to divalproex. Increased appetite was the only significant side effect (Donovan et al. 2000).

Steiner et al. (2003) randomly assigned 71 adolescents with CD in a residential facility for juvenile offenders to either therapeutic or low doses of divalproex for 7 weeks; both subjects and outcome raters were blind to treatment status. Reduction in aggression severity ($P = 0.02$), improvement in impulse control ($P < 0.05$), and global improvement ($P = 0.0008$) were greater in the group with therapeutic divalproex levels than in the low-dose condition. Serum level and "Immature defenses" (as assessed by the Weinberger Adjustment Inventory) predicted response to divalproex, but psychiatric comorbidity did not (Saxena et al. 2005).

Saxena et al. (2006) conducted a 12-week open trial of divalproex in 24 children of bipolar parents who had mixed (but nonbipolar) diagnoses (major depression, cyclothymia, ADHD, and ODD). At the end of the study, 71% of the subjects were determined to be divalproex responders based on reductions in aggression as assessed by the Overt Aggression Scale.

Clonidine

Seventeen outpatients (ages 5–15 years) with CD or ODD received open treatment with clonidine for 1–18 months. Aggression decreased significantly in 15 children (88%). The major side effect of clonidine was drowsiness (Kemph et al. 1993).

Despite controversy over its safety (Swanson et al. 1995; see Appendix), clonidine has often been combined with stimulants to treat comorbid aggression in children with ADHD. In a 2-month randomized comparison of clonidine, methylphenidate, and clonidine combined with methylphenidate in the treatment of 24 children and adolescents (ages 6–16 years) with ADHD and CD or ODD, it was found that all three treatment groups showed significant improvement in oppositional and CD symptoms (Connor et al. 2000). No significant ECG changes were noted.

Children ages 6–14 years with ADHD currently taking methylphenidate were randomly assigned to receive clonidine syrup 0.10–0.20 mg/day ($n = 37$) or placebo ($n = 29$) for 6 weeks (Hazell and Stuart 2003). Analysis showed that significantly more clonidine-treated children than controls were responders on the Conduct subscale (21 of 37 vs. 6 of 29; $P < 0.01$) of the parent-report Conners Behavior Checklist but not the Hyperactive Index subscale (13 of 37 vs. 5 of 29). Compared with placebo, clonidine was associated with a greater reduction in systolic blood pressure measured standing and with transient sedation and dizziness. Clonidine-treated individuals had a greater reduction in a number of unwanted effects associated with psychostimulant treatment compared with placebo. The findings supported the use of clonidine in combination with psychostimulant medication to reduce conduct symptoms associated with ADHD.

Beta-Blockers

Propranolol. In an open study of 16 patients (ages 4–24 years) with aggressive outbursts treated with propranolol (mean daily dose = 164 mg), 19 patients (63%) showed a significant reduction in aggressive outbursts. Fatigue was the most common side effect (Kuperman and Stewart 1987). In a retrospective study of propranolol (dosage range = 50–1,600 mg/day; median optimal daily dose = 160 mg) for uncontrolled rage outbursts in 30 patients (ages 7–35 years [4 adults]) with organic brain dysfunction, approximately 75% of patients showed moderate to marked improvement in rage outbursts. The most common side effects were somnolence, lethargy, and hypotension (Williams et al. 1982). There was a lack of standardized outcome measures, however, and the wide dosage range is puzzling. Results of this study have never been confirmed by a controlled trial in children or adolescents.

Nadolol. Nadolol is a beta-blocker that does not cross the blood–brain barrier; thus, any clinical effect would be due to its action on the peripheral sympathetic nervous system. Its use as an adjunctive pharmacological treatment for aggression and/or inattention/overactivity was studied in a developmentally delayed child, adolescent, and young adult population (Connor et al. 1997). Twelve subjects (mean age = 13.8 years, range = 9–24 years) completed a 5-month trial of nadolol (mean dosage = 109 mg/day, range = 30–220 mg/day) with baseline, weekly, and end-of-study assessments of aggression and inattention/overactivity. Ten subjects (83%) showed clinical improvement while receiving nadolol. Significant improvements were noted on observer-rated overt categorical aggression, severity of illness, and global impressions of improvement. No significant effects were found for inattention/overactivity, although blood pressure and pulse were significantly reduced. Nadolol was well tolerated, with few side effects. While the study suggests usefulness of this agent in treating aggression, the sample size was small and no controlled trials have been performed. The effectiveness of beta-blockers in the treatment of aggression must be viewed as unproven; beta-blockers can induce asthma attacks and significant bradycardia so should be used only as a last resort.

Clinical Recommendations for Disruptive Behavior Disorders and Aggression

The Center for the Advancement of Children's Mental Health at Columbia University joined with the New York State Office of Mental Health to develop guidelines for treatment of aggression, which led to the Treatment Recommendations for the Use of Antipsychotics for Aggressive Youth (TRAAY) (Pappadopulos et al. 2003; Schur et al. 2003). These recommendations call first for a thorough psychiatric evaluation of the child with severe aggression. Next, a psychosocial intervention should be used first when the aggression is the primary problem (such as in ODD/CD or intermittent explosive disorder). The clinician should then treat any primary condition, such as ADHD, psychosis, or mood disorder, that may be causing or contributing to the aggression. If the aggression does not respond to these steps, then an atypical antipsychotic should be used. Different atypical antipsychotics should be tried as monotherapy before moving to polypharmacy (e.g., adding a classic mood stabilizer such as lithium or divalproex to the antipsychotic). Monitoring of weight and laboratory measures of glucose, cholesterol, and triglycerides is mandatory (Correll and Carlson 2006).

Alpha agonists may be used in more mild aggression or temper outbursts since their effect size on aggression is more modest (Hazell and Stuart 2003). Beta-blockers should be used only as a last resort. Recently, the Intercontinental Schizophrenia Outpatient Health Outcomes study compared the response of aggressiveness to clozapine, olanzapine, quetiapine, risperidone, or haloperidol in a very large sample of adult schizophrenia patients (*n* = 3,135) who had 6 months of monotherapy (Bitter et al. 2005). Olanzapine and risperidone were significantly superior to haloperidol and clozapine for reducing aggression. Given that typical antipsychotics have higher rates of tardive dyskinesia than atypical antipsychotics (Correll et al. 2004) and now have been shown to be less ef-

fective for the treatment of aggression, the use of typical antipsychotics to treat children with aggression is contraindicated.

Tourette's Syndrome

The prevalence of Tourette's syndrome is estimated to be 0.7% in children (Comings et al. 1990). Tourette's syndrome is characterized by multiple motor tics and by one or more vocal tics that occur frequently for longer than 1 year (American Psychiatric Association 2000). The average age at onset of tics is at about age 5 years. Tics tend to increase in severity in the prepubertal years, but they diminish significantly by age 18 years (Leckman 2002).

α-Adrenergic Receptor Agonists

Clonidine

Two of three controlled studies support the efficacy of clonidine treatment for Tourette's syndrome. In a 12-week double-blind, placebo-controlled trial, 39 children and adolescents with Tourette's syndrome were randomly assigned to clonidine (dosage range = 3.2–5.7 µg/kg/day; mean daily dose = 4.4 µg/kg) or placebo. The group treated with clonidine had a statistically significant greater improvement on Tourette's Syndrome Global Scale (TSGS) scores than did the group receiving placebo. Clonidine was most effective for motor tics and tics that were noticeable to others. The most common side effects were sedation, fatigue, dry mouth, dizziness, and irritability (Leckman et al. 1991).

Thirteen children and adolescents (ages 9–16 years) with Tourette's syndrome were randomly assigned to a 20-week single-blind, placebo-controlled trial of clonidine (mean daily dose = 5.5 µg/kg). Six patients (46%) had a positive response to clonidine, as determined by TSGS scores. The most common side effects of clonidine were sedation, headache, and early-morning awakening (Leckman et al. 1985).

Twenty-four children and adolescents with Tourette's syndrome completed a double-blind crossover study that included two 12-week treatment phases—one phase with clonidine (either 0.0075 mg/kg/day or 0.015 mg/kg/day) and the other phase with placebo. However, in this study, clonidine did not significantly reduce motor tics, vocalizations, or behaviors. The most common side effects were sedation, dry mouth, and restlessness. There were no clinically significant changes in blood pressure or pulse (Goetz et al. 1987).

A retrospective study of 53 children and adolescents (ages 5–18 years) with Tourette's syndrome was conducted to determine predictors of response to clonidine treatment. Patients who had a longer duration of vocal tics had a good behavioral response to clonidine. Of 47 patients who received clonidine for tic control, 57% had a good tic response. The authors concluded that clonidine is a useful medication for 40%–60% of patients with mild to moderate tics (Lichter and Jackson 1996).

Clonidine was compared with risperidone in the treatment of children and adolescents with Tourette's syndrome (Gaffney et al. 2002). Following a single-blind placebo lead-in, 21 subjects (ages 7–17 years) were randomly assigned to 8 weeks of double-blind treatment with clonidine or risperidone. Research scales evaluated tics and comorbid obsessive-compulsive and attention-deficit/hyperactivity symptoms. Risperidone (mean dosage = 1.5±0.9 mg/day) and clonidine (mean dosage = 0.175±0.075 mg/day) appeared equally effective in the treatment of tics in an intent-to-treat analysis, as rated by the YGTSS. Risperidone produced a mean reduction in the YGTSS of 21%; clonidine produced a 26% reduction. There was a nonsignificant trend for subjects with comorbid obsessive-compulsive symptoms to respond better to risperidone (63%) than to clonidine (33%). Both treatments caused mild sedation that resolved with time; no clinically significant extrapyramidal symptoms were observed.

Guanfacine

Scahill et al. (2001) randomly assigned 34 children (mean age 10.4 years) with comorbid ADHD and tic disorders to receive either placebo or guanfacine for 8 weeks in a double-blind fashion. Tic severity declined by an average of 31% in the guanfacine group versus 0% in the placebo group. Globally, 9 of 17 subjects were rated as much or very much improved on the CGI compared with none so rated in the placebo group. One subject withdrew due to sedation; guanfacine was associated with insignificant decreases in blood pressure. In contrast, in a 4-week double-blind, placebo-controlled study of guanfacine in 24 children (ages 6–16 years) with Tourette's syndrome, there was no significant improvement in tic severity for guanfacine-treated patients compared with placebo-treated patients (Cummings et al. 2002).

Lofexidine

Lofexidine is an α_2 agonist used for the treatment of opiate withdrawal in the United Kingdom, similar to the use of clonidine in the United States. Forty-four medication-free subjects (41 boys and 3 girls; mean age = 10.4 years) with ADHD, combined type, and a tic disorder participated in an 8-week trial of lofexidine (Niederhofer et al. 2003). Lofexidine was associated with a mean improvement of 41% in the total score on the teacher-rated ADHD Rating Scale, compared with 7% improvement for placebo. Eleven of 22 subjects who received lofexidine were blindly rated on the CGI-I as either much improved or very much improved, compared with none of 22 subjects who received placebo. Tic severity decreased by 27% in the lofexidine group, compared with 0% in the placebo group. One lofexidine subject withdrew because of sedation at week 4. Lofexidine was associated with insignificant decreases in blood pressure and pulse. Lofexidine appears to be a safe and effective treatment for children with tic disorders and ADHD, although it is not clear if it has any advantage over clonidine or guanfacine.

Atypical Antipsychotics

Risperidone

Risperidone is the atypical antipsychotic most studied for the treatment of Tourette's syndrome and tic disorders. Risperidone was compared with pimozide in a 12-week double-blind, placebo-controlled multicenter study of 50 patients (ages 10–65 years) with Tourette's syndrome. Patients treated with both risperidone (mean daily dose = 3.8 mg) and pimozide (mean daily dose = 2.9 mg) showed significant improvement on the Tourette's Syndrome Severity Scale (TSSS; Shapiro et al. 1988). Fourteen of 26 patients (54%) treated with risperidone and 9 of 24 patients (38%) treated with pimozide had very mild or no symptoms on the TSSS at endpoint. Fewer patients treated with risperidone than with pimozide reported extrapyramidal side effects. Side effects common to both treatment groups were depression, fatigue, and somnolence (Bruggeman et al. 2001).

In a double-blind, placebo-controlled trial in 48 adolescent and adult outpatients (ages 14–49 years) with Tourette's syndrome, patients were randomly assigned to risperidone (dosage range = 1–6 mg/day; median daily dose = 2.5 mg) or placebo for an 8-week trial. Risperidone was significantly superior to placebo on the global severity rating of the TSSS. Adverse effects more common in the group treated with risperidone than in the group treated with placebo were hypokinesia, tremor, fatigue, and somnolence (Dion et al. 2002).

The efficacy of risperidone was further assessed in an 8-week randomized, double-blind, placebo-controlled trial using the Total Tic score of the YGTSS as the primary outcome variable (Scahill et al. 2003). Thirty-four medication-free subjects (26 children and 8 adults) ranging in age from 6 to 62 years (mean = 19.7±17.0 years) participated. After 8 weeks of treatment, the 16 subjects receiving risperidone (mean daily dose = 2.5±0.85) showed a 32% reduction in tic severity from baseline, compared with a 7% reduction for the 18 subjects receiving placebo (*P* = 0.004). The 12 children randomly assigned to risperidone showed a 36% reduction in tic symptoms, compared with an 11% decrease in the 14 children on placebo (*P* = 0.004). Two children on risperidone showed acute social phobia, which resolved with dose reduction in 1 subject but resulted in medication discontinuation in the other. A mean increase in body weight of 2.8 kg was observed in the risperidone group compared with no change in placebo (*P* = 0.0001). No extrapyramidal symptoms and no clinically significant alterations in cardiac conduction times or laboratory measures were observed.

Risperidone was compared to pimozide in the treatment of children and adolescents with tic disorders in a randomized, double-blind crossover study (Gilbert et al. 2004). Nineteen children (ages 7–17 years) with Tourette's syndrome or chronic motor tic disorder were randomly assigned to 4 weeks of treatment with pimozide or risperidone, followed by the alternate treatment after a 2-week placebo washout. The primary efficacy outcome measure was change in tic severity assessed by the YGTSS. Compared to pimozide treatment, risperidone treatment was associated with significantly lower tic severity scores (YGTSS: baseline 43.3±17.5, pimozide 34.2±14.2, risperidone 25.2±13.6; *P* = 0.05). Weight gain during the 4-week treatment periods was greater for risperidone (mean 1.9 kg) than pimozide (1.0 kg). No patient suffered a serious adverse event, but 6 of 19 subjects failed to complete the protocol. Neither medication was associated with ECG changes. While risperidone appeared superior to pimozide for tic suppression, it was associated with greater weight gain.

Most recently, a 6-week open-label study examined the effects of risperidone in the treatment of chronic tic disorder or Tourette's disorder in children and adolescents (Kim et al. 2005). The subjects were 15 young children and adolescents (mean age 10±2.4 years). Seven subjects were diagnosed with Tourette's disorder and 8 subjects with chronic tic disorder. Ten of the 15 subjects were administered risperidone for the first time, and 5 of the 15 subjects had been previously treated with traditional drugs (haloperidol or pimozide). Clinical responses were measured at baseline and after 1, 3, and 6 weeks of drug

treatment by using the Korean version of the YGTSS and the Global Assessment of Functioning Scale. The mean dosage of risperidone was 0.53±0.13 mg for the first week, 0.90±0.28 mg for the third week, and 1.23±0.37 mg for the sixth week. Comparison between periods according to the Korean version of the YGTSS showed significant differences (*P* < 0.01) between the first week and the third week. After 6 weeks of administration, tic severity scale scores revealed a 36% reduction in overall tic symptoms; 13 of the 15 subjects showed significant improvement, 1 subject showed no difference in symptoms, and 1 subject showed worsening of symptoms.

Olanzapine

An open-label trial was performed to explore efficacy and safety of olanzapine for treatment of Tourette's disorder (Budman et al. 2001). Ten adult patients (ages 20–44 years) with Tourette's disorder were treated using an open-label, flexible-dosing schedule for 8 weeks. Three patients who continued olanzapine were reevaluated after 6 months. Three subjects were psychotropic medication naive, 5 patients experienced intolerable side effects with conventional antipsychotics, and 2 patients had a past history of successful response to conventional antipsychotics. Tic severity was rated by the YGTSS; weight, vital signs, and adverse effects were assessed weekly. Two of 10 patients prematurely discontinued olanzapine owing to excessive sedation. Of 8 patients who completed the 8-week trial, 4 (50%) demonstrated reduction of global tic severity scores by ≥20 points, and 6 (75%) demonstrated reductions by ≥10 points. Sedation, weight gain, increased appetite, dry mouth, and transient asymptomatic hypoglycemia were the most common side effects. Tic improvements were maintained in 3 patients reassessed 6 months later. Final olanzapine dosages ranged from 2.5 mg to 20 mg daily (mean = 10.9 mg/day).

The effects of olanzapine on aggressive behavior and tic severity were further examined in children with Tourette's syndrome, as described above in the aggression section of this chapter (Stephens et al. 2004). Olanzapine significantly reduced tics in the 10-week trial.

Ziprasidone

In an 8-week double-blind, placebo-controlled trial, 28 children and adolescents (ages 7–17 years) with Tourette's syndrome were randomly assigned to ziprasidone (dosage range = 10–40 mg/day; mean daily dose = 28 mg) or placebo. The group treated with ziprasidone had a statistically significant reduction in scores on the YGTSS, compared with the group treated with placebo. The most common adverse event was somnolence. No clinically significant changes in vital signs or ECG parameters were reported (Sallee et al. 2000).

Nonetheless, concerns continue to be raised about possible cardiovascular effects of ziprasidone. A sudden death occurred in a child who participated in a clinical trial of ziprasidone for Tourette's (Scahill et al. 2005). Despite the fact that a single dose of ziprasidone did not produce abnormal ECG changes (Sallee et al. 2006), ECG changes were found in the children treated with ziprasidone for Tourette's syndrome in a long-term open-label safety study (Blair et al. 2005). In 20 children treated with ziprasidone, there were statistically significant changes from baseline to peak values in heart rate, pulse rate, and QTc intervals, but not in QRS complex width. The mean QTc prolongation was 28 ± 26 milliseconds and not related to dose ($r = 0.16$, $P = .07$). The peak QTc of three subjects reached or exceeded 450 milliseconds; one subject experienced a 114-millisecond prolongation. These findings, occurring at doses low by current treatment standards, suggest that electrocardiographic monitoring is warranted when prescribing ziprasidone to children.

Quetiapine

The short-term safety and effectiveness of quetiapine in the treatment of children and adolescents with Tourette's disorder were studied in an 8-week open-label trial that included 12 subjects with a mean age of 11.4 ± 2.4 years (Mukaddes and Abali 2003). Clinical responses, as measured by the Turkish version of the YGTSS, revealed a statistically significant reduction in tic scores ranging from 30% to 100%. The mean dosage of quetiapine at the end of the study was 72.9 ± 22.5 mg/day. Three subjects complained of sedation in the first week of treatment.

In a retrospective study of clinic patients, 12 patients (ages 8–18 years) with Tourette's syndrome received quetiapine therapy at a starting dose of 25 mg/day, which was increased to a mean dosage of 175.0 ± 116.6 mg/day by the eighth week of the study (Copur et al. 2007). The YGTSS score, which was 21.6 ± 4.0 at baseline, showed significant decreases at 4 and 8 weeks (reducing to 7.5 ± 7.4 and 5.6 ± 8.1, respectively; $P < 0.003$). Routine laboratory parameters and serum prolactin levels were all normal and did not change throughout treatment. Mild but significant increases in both body weight and BMI at 4 and 8 weeks compared with baseline were observed. No controlled trials of quetiapine in the treatment of tic disorders have been performed.

Aripiprazole

Murphy et al. (2005) reported six cases of children and adolescents (age range = 8–19 years, mean age = 12.1 years) who had comorbid tic disorder and OCD and were treated with aripiprazole (mean dosage = 11.7 mg/day; range = 5–20 mg/day) for 12 weeks. The subjects experienced a mean reduction of 56% in the severity of their tics as assessed by YGTSS. Similarly, Yoo et al. (2006) treated 15 children and adolescents with tic disorder with aripiprazole (mean dosage = 10.89 mg/day; range = 12.5–15 mg/day) and reported a mean reduction of 40% in YGTSS scores; side effects were minimal. Two subjects experienced nausea, 1 had weight gain, and 1 suffered sedation that responded to dosage reduction.

A case series of 11 consecutive patients with Tourette's syndrome (age range = 7–50 years; mean age = 7 years) were treated with aripiprazole; the majority of these had been refractory to other treatments with other antipsychotics (Davies et al. 2006). Ten of the 11 patients who were treated with aripiprazole improved, although to variable degrees. In the majority of patients, response was sustained with aripiprazole doses ranging from 10 to 20 mg daily. Side effects were mild and transient.

Typical Antipsychotics: Pimozide and Haloperidol

In a controlled trial comparing pimozide, haloperidol, and placebo in 57 patients (ages 8–65 years) with Tourette's syndrome, both active treatments were significantly more effective than placebo, and haloperidol was slightly more effective than pimozide. No significant differences in side effects were found between haloperidol and pimozide (Shapiro et al. 1989).

Sallee et al. (1997) conducted a 24-week double-blind, placebo-controlled crossover study of haloperidol (mean daily dose = 3.5 mg) and pimozide (mean daily dose = 3.4 mg) in 22 children and adolescents (ages 7–16 years) with Tourette's syndrome. Only pimozide was significantly superior to placebo on TSGS scores. There was a threefold higher frequency of serious side effects (depression, anxiety, and severe dyskinesias) with haloperidol (41%) than with pimozide (14%) in these youths. Extrapyramidal side effects were reported significantly more often with haloperidol than with pimozide.

In an open clinical trial in 31 patients (ages 10–50 years) with Tourette's syndrome treated for, on average, 1–2 years, 23 patients (74.2%) receiving pimozide, compared with 14 patients (45.2%) receiving haloperidol, had significant clinical improvement (Shapiro et al. 1983).

Long-term (6–84 months) treatment with pimozide (0.5–9 mg/day) was reported to produce a good clinical response in 81% of 65 patients (ages 6–54 years) (Regeur et al. 1986). A 1- to 15-year follow-up of 33 patients (ages 9–50 years) with Tourette's syndrome treated with pimozide (2–18 mg/day), haloperidol (2–15 mg/day), or no medications found that significantly more patients discontinued haloperidol than pimozide because of adverse side effects, especially dyskinesias and dystonias (Sandor et al. 1990). Thus, pimozide appears superior to haloperidol for treatment of tics.

Other Agents

Metoclopramide

Metoclopramide is a dopamine antagonist used for the treatment of gastroesophageal reflux; it blocks dopamine$_2$ receptors in the striatum but not in the cerebral cortex. Acosta and Castellanos (2004) reported that metoclopramide improved tics in 10 patients with tic disorders, with negligible adverse events. Nicolson et al. (2005) randomly assigned 27 children and adolescents with tic disorders to receive either placebo or metoclopramide in an 8-week double-blind, placebo-controlled trial. Metoclopramide was started at 5 mg/day and titrated to a maximum dose of 40 mg/day. In the active-drug group, there was a 39% reduction in tics versus a 13% reduction on placebo ($P = 0.001$). No extrapyramidal side effects were reported, and side effects were not different between metoclopramide and placebo. Further large-scale double-blind, placebo-controlled trials of this agent are needed.

Nicotine

In a double-blind, placebo-controlled trial, 74 patients (mean age = 11 years) with Tourette's syndrome who received haloperidol were randomly assigned to adjunctive transdermal nicotine (7 mg/24 hours) or placebo. Transdermal nicotine was significantly superior to placebo in reducing symptoms of Tourette's syndrome (Silver et al. 2001b). A transdermal nicotine patch (7 mg/24 hours) as adjunctive treatment to antipsychotics was shown to produce significant improvement in tic severity for 16 children and adolescents with Tourette's syndrome (Silver et al. 1996).

In a trial of nicotine gum (2 mg) added to haloperidol treatment, 10 youths with Tourette's syndrome had marked reduction in tics (Sanberg et al. 1989). In a fol-low-up study with 10 additional patients, nicotine gum added to haloperidol was shown to reduce tic frequency during and after 1 hour of gum chewing (McConville et al. 1991). In a controlled study comparing nicotine gum plus haloperidol, nicotine gum only, and placebo gum in 19 patients with Tourette's syndrome, the combined treatment of nicotine gum plus haloperidol showed the greatest reduction in tic frequency and severity (McConville et al. 1992).

Mecamylamine

Mecamylamine is a nicotine receptor antagonist that has been used as an antihypertensive agent and for smoking cessation. In an 8-week double-blind, placebo-controlled multicenter trial, 61 children and adolescents (ages 8–17 years) with Tourette's syndrome were randomly assigned to mecamylamine (dosage range = 2.5–7.5 mg/day) or placebo (Silver et al. 2001a). No significant difference was found on ratings of Tourette's symptoms between the group treated with mecamylamine and the group treated with placebo. The most common side effects were weakness, vomiting, muscle twitching, hypersomnia, and dysphoria.

In one retrospective open-label study of 19 children and adolescents and 5 adults with Tourette's syndrome treated with mecamylamine (2.5–6.25 mg/day) for 8–550 days, a significant improvement in severity of illness from baseline was reported (Macaluso et al. 2000). In another retrospective study that included 9 children with Tourette's syndrome, concomitant use of mecamylamine was found to improve symptoms of Tourette's syndrome (Sanberg et al. 1998). Given that this agent is rarely used in adults for its indicated purposes, further controlled studies are needed before it is used widely for tic disorders.

Common Comorbid Conditions

Obsessive-Compulsive Disorder

Tourette's syndrome is frequently comorbid with OCD (Leckman 2002), necessitating treatment of both conditions. The Pediatric OCD Treatment Study (POTS) (March et al. 2007) randomly assigned 112 children with OCD (17 of whom had comorbid tics) to CBT, sertraline, a combination of sertraline and CBT, or placebo. In patients without tics, combination therapy was superior to CBT alone which in turn was superior to sertraline; all treatments were superior to placebo. In the small subset of patients with tics, sertraline was not superior to placebo for the treatment of OCD, but combined treatment was. An earlier study randomly assigned children with OCD and tics to either sulpiride (a typical antipsychotic) or fluvoxamine for a double-blind treatment period, followed by a single-blind period of combined treatment (George et al. 1993). Fluvoxamine, whether alone or with sulpiride, did not ameliorate tics but was effective for OCD. In contrast, sulpiride did reduce tics when used as monotherapy.

Attention-Deficit/Hyperactivity Disorder

ADHD is a common comorbid disorder with Tourette's syndrome. Treatment of both disorders is often necessary in children. Although prior literature has cautioned against the use of psychostimulants to treat ADHD in Tourette's syndrome because of potential exacerbation of tics, recent studies do not support this view. Methylphenidate in low to moderate doses did not produce a clinically significant increase in motor tics for youths with tic disorders or Tourette's disorder and ADHD (Castellanos et al. 1997; Gadow et al. 1995). In a 2-year longitudinal follow-up of 29 children with ADHD and tic disorders (predominantly Tourette's syndrome) treated with methylphenidate, there was no evidence that methylphenidate increased motor or vocal tics (Gadow et al. 1999).

In a 16-week double-blind, placebo-controlled multicenter study, 136 youths with tic disorder and ADHD were randomly assigned to clonidine (mean daily dose = 0.25 mg), methylphenidate (mean daily dose = 26 mg), combination methylphenidate plus clonidine (mean daily dose = 0.28 mg), or placebo. Compared with placebo, active treatment groups showed a significant reduction in tic severity, with combination treatment showing the greatest improvement in tics (Tourette's Syndrome Study Group 2002). This is in contrast to an earlier smaller ($N = 37$) double-blind, placebo-controlled trial which found that clonidine did not reduce tic severity in children with Tourette's syndrome and ADHD (Singer et al. 1995).

Atomoxetine was studied in children and adolescents (ages 7–17 years) who met criteria for ADHD and Tourette's syndrome or chronic motor tic disorder (Allen et al. 2005). Patients were randomly assigned to double-blind treatment with placebo ($n = 72$) or atomoxetine (0.5–1.5 mg/kg/day, $n = 76$) for up to 18 weeks. Atomoxetine treatment was associated with greater reduction of tic severity at endpoint relative to placebo, approaching significance on the YGTSS total score ($P = 0.063$) and Tic Symptom Self-Report total score ($P = 0.095$) and achieving significance on the Clinical Global Impressions (CGI) tic/neurological severity scale score ($P = 0.002$). Atomoxetine was effective for ADHD symptoms and clearly did not exacerbate tic symptoms.

In a double-blind, placebo-controlled trial with 37 children with Tourette's syndrome and ADHD, desipramine, compared with clonidine, was reported to be more effective for both disorders (Singer et al. 1995). Compared with placebo, desipramine was found to be significantly more effective for the reduction of both tics and ADHD symptoms in 41 children and adolescents (T. Spencer et al. 2002). The earlier noted reports of sudden death limit its use. Nortriptyline has also been reported in retrospective studies to be effective in treating the symptoms of both ADHD and Tourette's syndrome in children and adolescents (T. Spencer et al. 1993).

Clinical Recommendations for Tourette's Syndrome

If a tic is not severe or socially impairing, observation may be in order, as the natural history of tics is to wax and wane; in general, tics improve over time (Leckman 2002). Often, psychosocial treatment such as habit reversal training is highly effective at reducing tics (Piacentini and Chang 2006). If conservative treatment fails, use of an alpha agonist would be desirable, owing to the risk of weight gain and dyslipidemia with atypical antipsychotics. Due to lower efficacy and higher risk of tardive dyskinesia with typical antipsychotics, the atypical antipsychotics are preferred. Haloperidol and pimozide should be used only as a last resort when several atypical agents have failed.

In children with comorbid ADHD, a stimulant can be used, but a nonstimulant is indicated if the stimulant exacerbates tics (Pliszka et al. 2006a). Often stimulants must be combined with alpha agonists or antipsychotics to control both the ADHD and the tics (Pliszka et al. 2006a; Tourette's Syndrome Study Group 2002). In children with OCD and comorbid tics, CBT or CBT combined with a serotonin reuptake inhibitor should be tried first before proceeding with treatment of the tics with alpha agonists or antipsychotics (March et al. 2007).

Schizophrenia

The prevalence of schizophrenia in children younger than 13 years is very rare; however, the prevalence rises in adolescence, with peak onset from 15 to 30 years (McClellan and Werry 2001). The clinical features of the disorder are similar in youths and adults, and the same DSM-IV-TR criteria are used to establish a diagnosis (American Psychiatric Association 2000). The outcome of childhood-onset schizophrenia is reported to be poor (Eggers and Bunk 1997). Typical antipsychotics have been studied in small randomized, controlled trials of youths with schizophrenia. Recently, the results of large controlled multicenter trials of atypical antipsychotics in adolescents with schizophrenia have been reported.

Atypical Antipsychotics

Clozapine

There has been one 6-week double-blind, placebo-controlled comparison of clozapine and haloperidol for 21 children and adolescents (ages 6–18 years) with schizophrenia (Kumra et al. 1996). Clozapine (mean dosage = 176 mg/day; range = 25–525 mg/day) was significantly superior to haloperidol (mean dosage = 16 mg/day; range = 7–27 mg/day) in reducing positive and negative symptoms of schizophrenia. Clozapine improved interpersonal functioning and enabled patients to live in a less restrictive setting. Side effects, however, were significant with clozapine. One patient had a seizure, and 3 patients were given anticonvulsants after they became more irritable and aggressive and experienced epileptiform changes on EEG. Mild to moderate neutropenia, weight gain, and sinus tachycardia were the other major side effects. One-third of the clozapine group discontinued use of the medication. One patient was discontinued from the haloperidol treatment group because of early signs of neuroleptic malignant syndrome.

Clozapine was found to be effective for the treatment of aggressive behavior in children and adolescents with treatment-refractory schizophrenia (Kranzler et al. 2005). Twenty youths received clozapine (mean daily dose = 476 mg at week 24) in an open-label study. A significant reduction in the frequency of receiving emergency oral medications and emergency injectable medications, as well as a decreased use of seclusion, was found on clozapine compared with before clozapine treatment.

Olanzapine

A positive double-blind, placebo-controlled multicenter study of olanzapine (mean dosage = 11.1 mg/day) for the treatment of adolescents with schizophrenia was recently reported (Kryzhanovskaya et al. 2006). One hundred adolescents were randomly assigned to olanzapine (n = 72) or placebo (n = 35) for a 6-week trial. Olanzapine-treated adolescents had significant improvements on the Brief Psychiatric Rating Scale for Children (BPRS-C; Overall and Pfefferbaum 1984) and CGI-S compared with the placebo group. There was no significant difference in response rate (≥30% decrease in BPRS-C and CGI severity ≤3) between olanzapine (37.5%) and placebo (25.7%) groups. Significantly more olanzapine-treated adolescents had treatment-emergent high AST/SGOT, ALT/SGPT, and prolactin and low bilirubin and hematocrit during treatment. There was a significant increase in fasting triglycerides at endpoint in the olanzapine-treated adolescents.

In an 8-week open-label trial of olanzapine (mean dosage = 17.5 mg/day) in the treatment of eight children and adolescents with schizophrenia, there was a 17% improvement on the BPRS, a 27% improvement on the Scale for the Assessment of Negative Symptoms, and a 1% improvement on the Scale for the Assessment of Positive Symptoms (Kumra et al. 1998). The magnitude of the effect size for olanzapine was reported to be greater than that for clozapine. The most common side effects reported for olanzapine were increased appetite, constipation, nausea, vomiting, headache, somnolence, insomnia, sustained tachycardia, transient elevation of liver transaminase levels, increased agitation, and difficulty concentrating. Average weight gain during a 6-week period of olanzapine was 3.4 kg.

In an 8-week open-label prospective trial of olanzapine (mean total daily dose = 12.4 mg/day) in 16 adolescents (age range = 12–17 years), statistically significant reductions in total PANSS scores and improvement in global functioning were found (Findling et al. 2003b).

Risperidone

The first positive double-blind, placebo-controlled multicenter trial of risperidone in the treatment of adolescents with schizophrenia was recently reported (Haas et al. 2007). One hundred sixty patients were randomly assigned to risperidone 1–3 mg/day (n = 55), risperidone 4–6 mg/day (n = 51), or placebo (n = 54) for a 6-week trial. Both dosage ranges of risperidone were significantly superior to placebo on the primary efficacy measure, PANSS total change score at endpoint. The most common adverse events were somnolence (24%), agitation (15%), and headache (13%) in the risperidone 1–3 mg/day group. Extrapyramidal disorder (16%), dizziness (14%), and hypertonia (14%) were the most common adverse events in the risperidone 4–6 mg/day group. The investigators concluded that the overall risk–benefit ratio favored the lower dosage range of risperidone.

Aripiprazole

The results of a large double-blind, placebo-controlled multicenter trial of aripiprazole for the treatment of schizophrenia in adolescents were recently reported (Findling et al. 2007). Three hundred and two patients were randomly assigned to aripiprazole 10 mg, aripiprazole 30 mg (after 5- or 11-day titration), or placebo over a 6-week period. Both the 10-mg and 30-mg doses of aripiprazole showed statistically significant differences from placebo on the PANSS total score at week 6 (Robb et al. 2007). The most common adverse events associated with aripiprazole were extrapyramidal disorder, somnolence, and headache.

Quetiapine

No data are available from double-blind, placebo-controlled trials of quetiapine for the treatment of schizophrenia in youth. There have been two open trials assessing the effectiveness of quetiapine in adolescents with psychotic disorders. J.A. Shaw et al. (2001) conducted an 8-week open trial of quetiapine (467 mg/day; range 300–800 mg/day) in 15 adolescents with a diagnosis of psychotic disorder (including 5 with a diagnosis of schizophrenia). Quetiapine significantly reduced psychotic symptoms in these adolescents. Mean weight gain over the 8-week period was 3.4 kg. There were no changes in prolactin and cholesterol levels or in ECG or ophthalmic examination findings. The most common adverse effects were somnolence, agitation, drowsiness, and headache. McConville et al. (2000) assessed the effectiveness of quetiapine in 10 adolescents with psychotic disorders (7 with schizoaffective disorder, 3 with bipolar disorder). Improvement in both positive and negative symptoms was observed during the course of the 25-day inpatient trial.

In a long-term study of an adolescent treated with quetiapine, it was reported that continued improvement in positive symptoms was evident up to 8 months after initiation of treatment, and negative symptoms were still improving at 18 months. After 28 months of treatment, there were no apparent adverse effects (Hayden 2001).

Comparison of Atypical Antipsychotics

In an open-label 12-week trial, risperidone (mean dosage = 1.6 mg/day) was compared with olanzapine (mean dosage = 8.2 mg/day) in the treatment of 25 children with schizophrenia (Mozes et al. 2006). Both groups showed similar significant improvement in the PANSS total and subscale scores. Eleven (91.7%) of the olanzapine-treated children and 9 (69.2%) of the risperidone-

treated children completed the 12-week study. Both groups showed significant weight increase from baseline to endpoint (mean 5.8 kg for olanzapine group and mean 4.5 kg for risperidone group).

In an 8-week double-blind study, 50 youths (ages 8–19 years) with psychotic disorders were randomly assigned to risperidone (mean dosage = 4 mg/day), olanzapine (mean dosage = 12.3 mg/day), or haloperidol (mean dosage = 5 mg/day) (Sikich et al. 2004). Eighty-eight percent of patients treated with olanzapine, 74% treated with risperidone, and 53% treated with haloperidol met response criteria (CGI-I scores of much or very much improved and at least a 20% reduction in BPRS-C total score). Sedation, extrapyramidal symptoms, and weight gain were the most common side effects.

Clozapine was compared with olanzapine in an 8-week double-blind, randomized trial (P. Shaw et al. 2006). Twenty-five youths (ages 7–16 years) with schizophrenia who were resistant to treatment with at least two antipsychotics participated in the trial. Clozapine (mean dosage = 327 mg/day) showed significant improvement in all outcome measures, compared with olanzapine (mean dosage = 19.1 mg/day), which showed improvement on some outcome measures. Improvement in negative symptoms was significantly greater for the clozapine group. Clozapine produced more adverse events, including nocturnal enuresis, tachycardia, and hypertension. Prolactin levels showed significantly greater increases in the olanzapine group. At 2-year follow-up, 15 patients who were receiving clozapine had continued clinical improvement, although lipid abnormalities (n = 6) and seizures (n = 1) had occurred.

Typical Antipsychotics

Haloperidol

Haloperidol has been compared with placebo and other typical antipsychotics in controlled trials in youths. In a 10-week double-blind, placebo-controlled crossover study, the safety and efficacy of haloperidol were assessed in 12 hospitalized children (ages 5–12 years) with schizophrenia. Haloperidol (optimal dosage range = 0.5–3.5 mg/day) was significantly superior to placebo in improving overall clinical functioning and reducing ideas of reference, delusions, and hallucinations. Common side effects were acute dystonic reaction, drowsiness, and dizziness (E.K. Spencer et al. 1992).

Haloperidol was compared with fluphenazine in a 12-week double-blind study of 30 outpatients (ages 6–12 years) with schizophrenia. Both haloperidol and fluphenazine were very effective in improving symptoms. There was no significant difference between their overall efficacy; 87% of haloperidol patients and 93% of fluphenazine patients were much or very much improved. The most common side effects were extrapyramidal symptoms, which occurred more frequently with fluphenazine than with haloperidol (Engelhardt et al. 1973). In an 8-week double-blind comparison trial of haloperidol and fluphenazine in 60 children (ages 5–12 years) with schizophrenia, both medications were effective in improving symptoms; however, haloperidol was more effective than fluphenazine in reducing provocativeness and autism (Faretra et al. 1970).

Haloperidol and loxapine were compared in a 4-week double-blind, placebo-controlled study of 75 adolescent inpatients with schizophrenia. Both haloperidol and loxapine were significantly superior to placebo, and there was no significant difference in efficacy between the two medications. Response rates (based on CGI improvement) were 87.5% for loxapine, 70% for haloperidol, and 36.4% for placebo. Common side effects were sedation, extrapyramidal symptoms, and somnolence (Pool et al. 1976).

Thiothixene

Thiothixene was compared with thioridazine in a 6-week single-blind study of 21 adolescent inpatients with schizophrenia. Thiothixene (optimal mean dosage = 16.2 mg/day) and thioridazine (optimal mean dosage = 178 mg/day) were equally effective in controlling symptoms, although most of the adolescents continued to be quite impaired. Thiothixene was less sedating than thioridazine (Realmuto et al. 1984). Thiothixene was also compared with trifluoperazine in an 8-week double-blind study of 16 children (ages 8–15 years) with schizophrenia (Wolpert et al. 1967). The effects of both medications were similar in terms of decreasing avoidance behavior, reducing stereotypic behavior, and increasing peer socialization. Side effects were minimal in both groups.

In a single-blind study, thiothixene (10–24 mg/day) was administered to 18 children (ages 5–13 years) with schizophrenia. All patients experienced global clinical improvement, with significant improvement noted in motor activity, stereotyped behavior, coordination, sleeping, affect, exploratory behavior, concentration, eating habits, and range of communication. Common side ef-

fects were extrapyramidal symptoms and increased salivation (Waizer et al. 1972).

Trifluoperazine

A study of four children with schizophrenia who received trifluoperazine (4 mg/day) reported that the medication had little influence in improving classroom behavior for three of the four children (Simpson 1977).

Pimozide

Pimozide (dosage range = 1–2 mg/day) produced improvement in affective contact and social behavior in youths with schizophrenia in a small open study followed by placebo discontinuation (Pangalila-Ratulangi 1973).

Clinical Recommendations for Schizophrenia

Both typical and atypical antipsychotics have demonstrated some effectiveness in the treatment of schizophrenia in youths, although the sample sizes have been small in the trials of typical antipsychotics. Given fewer reported extrapyramidal side effects and tardive dyskinesia with atypical antipsychotics, it would be reasonable to initiate treatment with an atypical antipsychotic for a child with schizophrenia. Clozapine, however, should not be initiated unless at least two other antipsychotics have been tried without success. It is important to monitor weight and metabolic parameters for children who receive atypical antipsychotics.

Antipsychotics should be administered for a period of no less than 4–6 weeks at adequate dosages in order to determine efficacy. If there is no response or intolerable side effects, then a trial of a different antipsychotic should be initiated (American Academy of Child and Adolescent Psychiatry 2001).

There are no data to guide maintenance treatment. Because the majority of youths will have a second psychotic episode within 5–7 years of stabilization, there is a significant risk of relapse with medication withdrawal (Kumra 2000). It is recommended that first-episode patients receive maintenance pharmacological treatment for 1–2 years after the initial episode, given the risk of relapse (American Academy of Child and Adolescent Psychiatry 2001). If medication discontinuation is attempted, the dosage should be gradually reduced over several months.

Autistic Disorder and Other Pervasive Developmental Disorders

The prevalence of autistic disorder and other pervasive developmental disorders is estimated to be up to 18.7 per 10,000 population (Howlin 2000). Core features of these disorders are impairments in communication and social skills and the restriction of interests and activities (American Psychiatric Association 2000). Associated behavioral features include hyperactivity, stereotypies, attentional problems, self-injurious behavior, aggression, mood lability, anxiety, obsessions, and compulsions. The majority of children with autistic disorder will continue to have significant social and communication impairments throughout adulthood, although some individuals will be able to live independently (Buitelaar and Willemsen-Swinkels 2000).

Pharmacotherapy is one component of a treatment plan for children with autism. Although there are controlled studies, open trials, and case reports of a variety of pharmacological agents, no medication has been identified that effectively treats the core symptoms of autism and other pervasive developmental disorders (Tanguay 2000). Pharmacotherapy is aimed at target symptoms in order to increase the ability of these children to participate in educational and other psychosocial interventions (Volkmar et al. 1999).

Atypical Antipsychotics

Risperidone

Risperidone has received FDA approval for the treatment of irritability associated with autistic disorder in children and adolescents, including symptoms of aggression toward others, deliberate self-injuriousness, temper tantrums, and quickly changing moods.

Risperidone was chosen as the first drug to be studied by the Research Units on Pediatric Psychopharmacology (RUPP) network funded by NIMH, which was designed to investigate the safety and efficacy of medications for treating maladaptive symptoms and behaviors associated with autistic disorders (McDougle et al. 2000b). One hundred one children ranging in age from 5 to 17 years with autistic disorder participated in an 8-week double-blind, placebo-controlled trial of risperidone (dosage range=0.5–3.5 mg/day; mean=1.8 mg/day). A significantly greater positive response—defined as a 25% decrease in the irritability subscale of the Aberrant Behavior Checklist and a rating of much or very much improved

on the CGI-I scale—was found for the risperidone group (69%) compared with the placebo group (12%). Adverse events of increased appetite, fatigue, drowsiness, dizziness, and drooling were more common in the risperidone group than in the placebo group. Mean weight gain was 2.7 kg in the risperidone group and 0.8 kg in the placebo group. An 18-month follow-up showed that the majority of subjects who responded to risperidone during intermediate-length treatment continued to show improvement (McDougle et al. 2004).

In an 8-week double-blind, placebo-controlled trial, 79 children (ages 5–12 years) with autism and other pervasive developmental disorders were randomly assigned to either placebo or risperidone (mean dosage=1.5 mg/day). Risperidone-treated patients exhibited a 64% improvement over baseline irritability, compared with a 30.7% improvement in placebo-treated subjects (Shea et al. 2004).

In a 6-month placebo-controlled study of 40 children (ages 2–9 years) with autism, risperidone (1 mg/day) decreased aggressiveness, hyperactivity, and irritability and improved social responsiveness and nonverbal communication. Appetite increase, weight gain, sedation, and transient dyskinesias in the risperidone-treated children were reported (Nagaraj et al. 2006).

The long-term effects of risperidone were assessed in youths (ages 5–17 years) with autism spectrum disorders (Troost et al. 2005). Twenty-four youths received risperidone for 6 months, followed by a double-blind discontinuation to placebo or continued risperidone. Risperidone was superior to placebo in preventing relapse, with relapse rates of 25% and 75%, respectively. Weight gain, increased appetite, fatigue, and anxiety were the most common side effects.

Similar rates of relapse were reported after placebo substitution following 4 months of risperidone treatment in 32 children with autism. The relapse rates were 62.5% in the placebo substitution group and 12.5% in those who continued risperidone treatment (Research Units on Pediatric Psychopharmacology Autism Network et al. 2005).

Olanzapine

In a 12-week open-label study of olanzapine (mean dosage=7.8 mg/day) in eight patients (ages 5–42 years) with autistic disorder or pervasive developmental disorder not otherwise specified, the six patients who completed the trial showed much or very much global improvement (Potenza et al. 1999). Significant improvements were found in hyperactivity, social relatedness, affectual responses, sensory responses, language usage, self-injurious behavior, aggression, irritability, anxiety, and depression. The most significant adverse effects were increased appetite and weight gain in six patients and sedation in three patients.

In a 3-month open study of olanzapine (dosage range = 1.25–20 mg/day) in 25 subjects (ages 6–16 years) with pervasive developmental disorder, significant global improvement was reported. The most common side effect was weight gain (mean = 4.8 kg) (Kemner et al. 2002).

Olanzapine was compared with haloperidol in a 6-week open trial in 12 children (ages 4–11 years) with autistic disorder (Malone et al. 2001). Both the olanzapine treatment (mean dosage = 7.9 mg/day) and the haloperidol treatment (mean dosage = 1.4 mg/day) reduced symptoms of social withdrawal and stereotypies and improved speech and object relations.

Quetiapine

The effectiveness of quetiapine (dosage range = 100–350 mg/day) was assessed in a 16-week open-label trial in six children with autistic disorder (Martin et al. 1999). No significant behavioral improvements were found from baseline to endpoint. Only two subjects completed the full 16 weeks of treatment; subjects terminated early because of nonresponse and sedation. One patient had a possible seizure during the fourth week of treatment; other side effects included behavioral activation, increased appetite, and weight gain.

In a 12-week open-label study of quetiapine of nine adolescents (mean age = 14.6 years) with autistic disorder, only two patients were much or very much improved at study endpoint (Findling et al. 2004). The most common side effects reported were sedation and weight gain.

Ziprasidone

The use of ziprasidone (mean daily dose = 59.23) for the treatment of autistic children, adolescents, and young adults was evaluated in an open-label study of 12 patients (ages 8–20 years) for at least 6 weeks (McDougle et al. 2002). Fifty percent of patients were responders based on a CGI scale rating of much improved or very much improved. Transient sedation was the most common side effect.

Clozapine

A case series of three children with autistic disorder treated with clozapine (up to 100 mg/day) for 3 months reported a 40% improvement in measures of abnormal object relationships, negativism, fidgetiness, and hyperactivity. After 8 months of clozapine treatment (mean daily dose = 200 mg), two of the children showed a substantial improvement in language and communication skills (Zuddas et al. 1996).

Typical Antipsychotics

Haloperidol

Haloperidol has been the most widely studied typical antipsychotic for the treatment of autism in children and adolescents. In double-blind, placebo-controlled studies, haloperidol has been shown to be significantly superior to placebo in reducing maladaptive behaviors and facilitating learning on discrimination tasks (Campbell et al. 1982); in increasing retention of discrimination learning and decreasing maladaptive behaviors in the classroom (L. T. Anderson et al. 1984); in decreasing occurrence of stereotypies and increasing orienting reactions of children (Cohen et al. 1980); and in decreasing hyperactivity, temper tantrums, withdrawal, and stereotypies and increasing relatedness (L. T. Anderson et al. 1989). Optimal dosages of haloperidol in these studies ranged from 0.25 to 4 mg/day. The most common side effects were sedation, increased irritability, and acute dystonic reactions. Weight gain was modest (0.2 kg) in autistic children who received haloperidol 0.25–3.5 mg/day for a 6-month period (Silva et al. 1993).

Haloperidol was compared with behavioral therapy in a double-blind, placebo-controlled trial in 40 children (ages 2–7 years) with autistic disorder (Campbell et al. 1978). For children older than 4.5 years, haloperidol was found to be significantly superior to placebo in reducing the severity of withdrawal behaviors and stereotypies. The combination of behavior therapy and haloperidol was the most effective in facilitating the acquisition of imitative speech.

The long-term efficacy of haloperidol was assessed in 48 children (ages 2–8 years) with autism who received haloperidol for 6 months (Perry et al. 1989). Haloperidol remained effective throughout the 6-month treatment period, and it was equally effective whether it was given continuously or on a discontinuous schedule consisting of 5 days on haloperidol and 2 days on placebo. Children who had symptoms of irritability, angry and labile affect, and uncooperativeness were the best responders to haloperidol.

Reversible haloperidol-related dyskinesias have been reported in 29% of autistic children (Campbell et al. 1988a). Factors related to the development of haloperidol-induced dyskinesias in acute studies of autistic children include female gender (Campbell et al. 1988a) and prenatal and perinatal complications (Armenteros et al. 1995). In a long-term prospective study of haloperidol treatment for 118 children with autism, withdrawal dyskinesias developed in 40 children (33.9%), with 20 children having more than one dyskinetic episode (Campbell et al. 1997). Female gender, prenatal and perinatal complications, greater cumulative haloperidol dose, and/or longer exposure to haloperidol increased the risk of withdrawal dyskinesias.

Pimozide

Pimozide was compared with haloperidol and placebo in a controlled crossover trial that included 34 children with autistic disorder (Naruse et al. 1982). Pimozide and haloperidol were significantly more effective than placebo in reducing maladaptive behavior, such as lack of interest, self-centeredness, and aggressiveness. There was no significant difference between pimozide and haloperidol. An open study of 8 children treated with pimozide (mean dosage = 4.9 mg/day) reported improved behavioral functioning (Ernst et al. 1992).

Serotonin Reuptake Inhibitors

The only placebo-controlled studies of serotonin reuptake inhibitors are with fluoxetine and fluvoxamine treatment of autistic disorders.

Fluoxetine

The efficacy of liquid fluoxetine was assessed to treat repetitive behaviors in children and adolescents with autism spectrum disorders. Forty-five youths were randomly assigned to two 8-week acute phases in a double-blind crossover study. Low-dose liquid fluoxetine (mean dosage = 9.9 mg/day) was superior to placebo in reducing repetitive behaviors (Hollander et al. 2005).

In an open study of fluoxetine (dosage range = 20 mg every other day to 80 mg/day) in 23 patients (ages 7–28 years) with autistic disorder, 15 patients (65%) experienced significant clinical global improvement (Cook et al. 1992). The most common side effects were restlessness, hyperactivity, agitation, decreased appetite, and insomnia. Case reports and a retrospective chart review of fluoxetine treatment for youths with autistic disorder reported improvements in irritability, stereotypies, and inappropriate speech (Fatemi et al. 1998; Ghaziuddin et al. 1991; Todd 1991).

Fluvoxamine

A double-blind, placebo-controlled study of fluvoxamine treatment (mean dosage = 106.9 mg/day) in 34 children

and adolescents with autistic disorder did not find significant clinical improvement with fluvoxamine (McDougle et al. 2000a).

Sertraline

Open-label sertraline (dosage range = 25–50 mg/day) was administered to nine children with autistic disorder (Steingard et al. 1997). Eight of the nine patients showed clinically significant improvement in ability to tolerate changes in their routine or environment without displaying symptoms of anxiety, irritability, or agitation. Clinical response tended to occur in 2–8 weeks. In two cases, behavioral worsening was observed when the dosage was raised to 75 mg/day.

Citalopram

Seventeen children with autistic spectrum disorders were treated with citalopram for at least 2 months (Couturier and Nicolson 2002). Ten children (59%) were judged to be much or very much improved on measures of aggression, anxiety, and stereotypies. Common adverse side effects were insomnia and agitation.

Paroxetine

A child with autistic disorder who received paroxetine (up to 10 mg/day) showed a significant reduction in preoccupations and temper tantrums within 6 weeks of treatment initiation (Posey et al. 1999). Snead et al. (1994) described a case of an adolescent with autistic disorder whose symptom of self-injurious behavior resolved within 2 weeks of treatment initiation with paroxetine (20 mg/day).

Escitalopram

In a 10-week open-label study, 28 youths (ages 6–17 years) with pervasive developmental disorder received escitalopram. There was significant improvement in irritability and clinical global functioning. Twenty-five percent of youths responded at escitalopram daily doses less than 10 mg, and 36% of youths responded at doses greater than or equal to 10 mg (Owley et al. 2005).

Other Antidepressants

Clomipramine

The results of controlled trials with clomipramine in the treatment of autistic disorder have yielded mixed results. Clomipramine and haloperidol were compared in a placebo-controlled crossover study for 7 weeks with active treatment (Remington et al. 2001). Thirty-six patients (ages 10–36 years) with autistic disorder were randomly assigned to clomipramine (mean dosage = 128.4 mg/day; range = 100–150 mg/day), haloperidol (mean dosage = 1.3 mg/day; range = 1–1.5 mg), or placebo. A significant advantage for haloperidol was found on global measures of autistic symptom severity and on specific measures of irritability and hyperactivity. Clomipramine was comparable to haloperidol only in patients who were able to complete a full therapeutic trial. However, significantly fewer patients receiving clomipramine versus haloperidol were able to complete the trial (37.5% vs. 69.7%, respectively) for reasons related to inefficacy, side effects, or behavioral problems.

Clomipramine was compared with desipramine for the treatment of autistic disorder in a double-blind crossover study with a sample of 30 patients ranging from 6 to 23 years of age (Gordon et al. 1993). Clomipramine was significantly superior to both desipramine and placebo on ratings of autistic symptoms, including stereotypies, anger, and compulsive ritualized behaviors. No differences were found between desipramine and placebo. One patient had a grand mal seizure during the second week of clomipramine therapy. Clomipramine dosage reduction was necessary in two patients because of QT interval prolongation in one case and severe tachycardia in the other. Increased irritability, temper outbursts, and aggression occurred in 8 of the 12 subjects receiving desipramine.

Mirtazapine

In an open-label study of mirtazapine (dosage range = 7.5–45 mg/day; mean = 30.3 mg/day) in 26 patients (ages 3–23 years) with pervasive developmental disorders, 9 patients (34.6%) were judged much or very much improved in symptoms of aggression, self-injury, irritability, hyperactivity, anxiety, depression, and insomnia (Posey et al. 2001). Mirtazapine did not improve symptoms of social or communication impairment. Common side effects included increased appetite, irritability, and transient sedation.

Venlafaxine

The effectiveness of venlafaxine was assessed in an open retrospective study of 10 patients (ages 3–21 years) with pervasive developmental disorders (Hollander et al. 2000). Six of 10 patients who received venlafaxine (mean dosage = 24.4 mg/day; range = 6.25–50 mg/day) over an average of 5 months were much or very much improved. Improvements were shown in repetitive behaviors, restricted interests, social deficits, communication and language function, inattention, and hyperactivity. Side effects of venlafaxine included behavioral activation, nausea, inattention, and polyuria.

Mood Stabilizers

Lamotrigine

Twenty-eight children (ages 3–11 years) with autistic disorder participated in a double-blind, placebo-controlled study of lamotrigine (mean maintenance dosage = 5 mg/kg/day) for a 12-week study period (Belsito et al. 2001). There were no significant differences between the lamotrigine and placebo groups on severity of behavioral symptoms. Insomnia and hyperactivity were the most frequently reported side effects. No children in the study were withdrawn because of rash.

Lithium

Case studies have reported the effectiveness of lithium in improving manic-like symptoms in children with autism (Kerbeshian et al. 1987; Shafey 1986; Steingard and Biederman 1987).

Anxiolytics

Buspirone

In a 6- to 8-week open trial, 22 children and adolescents with pervasive developmental disorders or autistic disorder were treated with buspirone (dosage range = 15–45 mg/day) (Buitelaar et al. 1998). Sixteen patients (73%) showed moderate to marked improvement in anxiety and irritability symptoms. In a 4-week open trial comparing buspirone with fenfluramine or methylphenidate in children with autistic disorder, two of three children who received buspirone showed improvement in hyperactivity (Realmuto et al. 1989). One patient who received fenfluramine had a slight decrease in hyperactivity. Behavioral deterioration was found in one of two patients treated with methylphenidate.

Other Agents

Flumazenil

One of two children who received flumazenil (a benzodiazepine antagonist) showed a mild increase in interpersonal engagement (Wray et al. 2000). No adverse effects were seen in either child.

Naltrexone

Double-blind, placebo-controlled trials of naltrexone in the treatment of children with autistic disorder have reported modest improvement of symptoms, including reductions in autistic symptomatology (Scifo et al. 1996); decreased self-injurious behavior, improved socialization, and increased attentiveness and communication (Leboyer et al. 1992); improved socialization, decreased withdrawal, increased proximity seeking, increased eye contact, increased attentiveness, and decreased restlessness and affective lability (Leboyer et al. 1990); decreased irritability (Willemsen-Swinkels et al. 1995); decreased hyperactivity and irritability (Willemsen-Swinkels et al. 1996); decreased restlessness and hyperactivity (Kolmen et al. 1995); decreased self-injury (Barrett et al. 1989); decreased hyperactivity (Campbell et al. 1993); and global improvement as assessed by teacher ratings (Kolmen et al. 1997). Dosage ranges of naltrexone were 0.5–1.5 mg/kg in these studies. There were no significant changes in cardiovascular parameters of heart rate or systolic blood pressure for children with autism treated with naltrexone (Herman et al. 1993).

In other controlled trials, naltrexone demonstrated no superiority over placebo in producing beneficial changes in social behavior (Willemsen-Swinkels et al. 1995), social and stereotypic behavior (Willemsen-Swinkels et al. 1996), social behavior and activity level (Bouvard et al. 1995), discrimination learning (Campbell et al. 1993), and communication (Feldman et al. 1999).

During 6-month continuation treatment for naltrexone-responsive children with autism, the hyperactivity-reducing effect of naltrexone was maintained (Willemsen-Swinkels et al. 1999). However, no additional gains in social interaction, communication, or stereotypic behaviors were observed after the 4-week acute phase. Moreover, parents did not request to continue treatment with naltrexone for their autistic children. These researchers therefore did not advocate the routine use of naltrexone for children with autism.

Clonidine

A double-blind, placebo-controlled crossover study with transdermal clonidine (0.005 mg/kg/day or placebo by a weekly transdermal patch) in nine patients (ages 5–33 years) with autistic disorder was conducted for a total 8-week active period (Fankhauser et al. 1992). Significant improvement with clonidine, compared with placebo, was found on measures of social relationship, affectual responses, and sensory responses. In a double-blind, pla-

cebo-controlled crossover trial of clonidine in eight children with autistic disorder, clonidine was found to be modestly effective in reducing irritability and hyperactivity (Jaselskis et al. 1992).

Methylphenidate

There have been two small double-blind, placebo-controlled crossover studies of methylphenidate for the treatment of autistic disorder in children ranging in age from 5 to 11 years. In a study that included 10 children, a modest but statistically significant improvement in hyperactivity was found with methylphenidate treatment, compared with placebo (Quintana et al. 1995). No significant side effects, such as worsening of behavior or of stereotypic movements, were observed. In a study that included 13 children, 6 patients had a significant decrease in hyperactivity, stereotypies, and inappropriate speech (Handen et al. 2000). However, there were no changes found on the Child Autism Rating Scale. Significant adverse side effects occurred in some children and included social withdrawal and irritability, particularly at a methylphenidate dosage of 0.6 mg/kg/day.

Fenfluramine

Fenfluramine, a serotonin agonist, has been studied in autism. It was marketed as an anti-obesity agent but was withdrawn from the market because of pulmonary hypertension when used in combination with phentermine.

Following the report of significant clinical improvement and an increase in the IQs of three boys who received fenfluramine (E. Geller et al. 1982), a number of double-blind, placebo-controlled studies were conducted to assess the efficacy and safety of fenfluramine in the treatment of children with autism. The results of these studies have been mixed, with modest improvements in autistic symptoms found in a few studies.

Children who received fenfluramine, compared with placebo, were reported to have decreased hyperactivity, decreased stereotypies, increased eye contact, increased socialization, and increased use of appropriate language (Ritvo et al. 1983); decreased motor activity, decreased distractibility, and improved mood (August et al. 1984); increased social awareness, eye contact, and attention to schoolwork (Ritvo et al. 1984); increased IQ, increased communication, and increased socialization (Ritvo et al. 1986); decreased respiratory stereotypies (Gastaut et al. 1987); reduction in motor activity, anxiety, mood disturbance, and distractibility (Barthelemy et al. 1989); improved attention span and activity level (Groden et al.

1987); increased language and awareness of environment in children with IQs above 40 (Stubbs et al. 1986); and decreased activity level, increased attention, and decreased hyperactivity (August et al. 1985). Open studies with fenfluramine reported improvement in relatedness, hyperactivity, irritability, and aggressiveness (Campbell et al. 1986) and improved communication and social awareness (Klykylo et al. 1985).

However, numerous reports of controlled trials failed to show significant superiority of fenfluramine relative to placebo in the treatment of children with autistic disorder (Beeghly et al. 1987; Beisler et al. 1986; Campbell et al. 1988b; Coggins et al. 1988; Ekman et al. 1989; Ho et al. 1986; Kohler et al. 1987; Leventhal et al. 1993; Ross et al. 1987; Sherman et al. 1989; Stern et al. 1990; Yarbrough et al. 1987). The average dose of fenfluramine was 1.5 mg/day in these studies.

In a review of the literature, Aman and Kern (1989) concluded that there was no evidence that IQ was increased by fenfluramine. Fenfluramine may enhance social relatedness, reduce stereotypic behavior, lessen overactivity, and improve attention span in some children, although the results are inconsistent. In another review, du Verglas et al. (1988) concluded that fenfluramine may have positive effects in reducing hyperactivity and stereotypic behaviors in 33% of children and noted that the best responders were children with the highest baseline IQs.

There had been concern about the untoward effects of fenfluramine in children with autism. Realmuto et al. (1986) described listlessness, food refusal, and stomach upset in the initial phase of treatment, followed by irritability, agitation, and crying with continued medication use. Decreased appetite, lethargy, irritability, and behavioral regression were also reported with fenfluramine use (Piggott et al. 1986). In a 2-year follow-up of autistic children treated with fenfluramine, reasons for discontinuing the medication included development of tolerance, appetite and weight changes, and the need for other interventions, particularly other psychotropic medications (Varley and Holm 1990). Significant concern had also been raised about possible neurotoxicity with the use of fenfluramine in children, based on studies of the neurotoxic effects of fenfluramine in animals (Schuster et al. 1986).

Famotidine

The efficacy of famotidine, a histamine$_2$ receptor antagonist, was assessed in a randomized, double-blind, placebo-controlled crossover study in nine children (ages 3–8 years) with a diagnosis of pervasive developmental disor-

der (Linday et al. 2001). The maximum daily dose of famotidine was 100 mg (2 mg/kg/day). Four of nine children (44%) randomly assigned to famotidine showed increased social interaction and affection. Children with marked stereotypy did not respond.

Amantadine

Thirty-nine children and adolescents (ages 5–19 years) with autistic disorder were randomly assigned in a 9-week double-blind, placebo-controlled trial to amantadine (5 mg/kg/day) or placebo (King et al. 2001). Parent ratings did not demonstrate a statistically significant change in irritability and hyperactivity, with a mean placebo response rate of 37% versus 47% for amantadine. However, clinician ratings of improvement in behavioral changes of hyperactivity and inappropriate speech were significantly higher in the amantadine group than in the placebo group. Overall clinical functioning was rated higher in the amantadine group than in the placebo group (53% improved vs. 25% improved, respectively). The most common side effects were insomnia and somnolence.

Amisulpride

Nine children (ages 4–13 years) with autistic disorder participated in a randomized, double-blind crossover trial of amisulpride (1.5 mg/kg/day) and bromocriptine (0.15–0.20 mg/kg/day) for two consecutive 8-week treatment periods (Dollfus et al. 1992). Neither amisulpride nor bromocriptine showed a statistically significant effect on global autism scores. However, the two agents differed in their effects on specific autistic symptoms, with amisulpride having a more positive effect on behavioral inhibition and withdrawal symptomatology and bromocriptine having a more positive effect on motor hyperactivity and attention symptoms. The most common side effects were insomnia and anorexia for amisulpride and bromocriptine, respectively. Amisulpride is not available in the United States or Canada.

Sulpiride

Sulpiride (up to 400 mg/day) was reported to significantly reduce abnormal speech and withdrawal in a teenager with autistic disorder (Scott and Eames 1988). Sulpiride is not available in the United States or Canada.

Secretin

Following the report of marked improvement in socialization and communication skills in three children with autism who had received secretin during an upper endoscopy (Horvath et al. 1998), there was a flurry of media reports about the success of this neuropeptide hormone. It is estimated that approximately 2,500 children have received secretin injections for the treatment of autism (Kastner 1998). However, randomized, double-blind, placebo-controlled trials of single-dose intravenous secretin for the treatment of children with autism have produced no evidence that secretin is effective for the treatment of autism or pervasive developmental disorder in 174 children and adolescents who participated in the studies. There have been no significant changes in parents' perceptions of autistic behaviors or language skills (Coniglio et al. 2001), no improvement in either primary or secondary features of autism (Sandler et al. 1999), and no change in social and communication skills (Owley et al. 2001).

The efficacy of repeated doses of secretin in the treatment of autism was assessed in a double-blind, placebo-controlled trial in 64 children (ages 2–7 years) who received two doses of secretin 6 weeks apart (Roberts et al. 2001). No differences between the secretin and placebo groups were found on measures of language, cognition, or autistic symptomatology. Similarly, in a controlled study of 12 children with autism, there were no significant differences between secretin and placebo groups on language or social assessments (Corbett et al. 2001).

Clinical Recommendations for Autistic Disorder and Other Pervasive Developmental Disorders

There is no evidence that pharmacotherapy is effective in treating the core social and communication deficits in autistic disorder. However, medications have been shown to be useful in treating associated symptoms, such as hyperactivity, inattention, stereotypies, self-injurious behavior, tantrums, aggression, mood lability, and anxiety. Antipsychotics may decrease withdrawal, stereotypies, and aggression and may facilitate learning. To date, the most data available support the use of risperidone for treating irritability, aggression, self-injurious behavior, temper tantrums, and mood lability associated with autistic disorder in children and adolescents. Serotonin reuptake inhibitors and other antidepressants have been shown to reduce compulsions, anxiety, and depression in children with autism. In some cases, naltrexone may reduce hyperactivity, irritability, and self-injurious behavior. Stimulants may increase attention span and reduce hyperactivity. Given concerns about the potential neurotoxicity and limited effectiveness of fenfluramine, this agent should be used with ex-

treme caution in children with autism. Secretin is not recommended for use because it has no established efficacy.

There are limited data on the long-term use of pharmacotherapy in children with autism. After receiving an intermediate-length (4–6 months) course of treatment with risperidone, children withdrawn from the medication through placebo substitution had high relapse rates (Research Units on Pediatric Psychopharmacology Autism Network et al. 2005; Troost et al. 2005). Therefore, clinicians must weigh the risk–benefit ratio of maintenance medication treatment in this population and carefully monitor children for side effects.

References

Abbott Laboratories: Multicenter Controlled Trial of Divalproex ER for Pediatric Bipolar I Disorder. Abbott Park, IL, Abbott Labs, 2007. Available at: http://www.clinicalstudyresults.org. Accessed May 24, 2007.

Abikoff H, McGough J, Vitiello B et al: Sequential pharmacotherapy for children with comorbid attention-deficit/hyperactivity and anxiety disorders. J Am Acad Child Adolesc Psychiatry 44:418–427, 2005

Acosta MT, Castellanos FX: Use of the "inverse neuroleptic" metoclopramide in Tourette syndrome: an open case series. J Child Adolesc Psychopharmacol 14:123–128, 2004

Alessi N, Bos T: Buspirone augmentation of fluoxetine in a depressed child with obsessive-compulsive disorder. Am J Psychiatry 148:1605–1606, 1991

Allen AJ, Kurlan RM, Gilbert DL, et al: Atomoxetine treatment in children and adolescents with ADHD and comorbid tic disorders. Neurology 65:1941–1949, 2005

Aman MG, Kern RA: Review of fenfluramine in the treatment of the developmental disabilities. J Am Acad Child Adolesc Psychiatry 28:549–565, 1989

Aman MG, De Smedt G, Derivan A, et al: Double-blind, placebo-controlled study of risperidone for the treatment of disruptive behaviors in children with subaverage intelligence. Am J Psychiatry 159:1337–1346, 2002

Aman MG, Binder C, Turgay A: Risperidone effects in the presence/absence of psychostimulant medicine in children with ADHD, other disruptive behavior disorders, and subaverage IQ. J Child Adolesc Psychopharmacol 14:243–254, 2004

Ambrosini PJ, Bianchi MD, Metz C, et al: Evaluating clinical response of open nortriptyline pharmacotherapy in adolescent major depression. J Child Adolesc Psychopharmacol 4:233–244, 1994

American Academy of Child and Adolescent Psychiatry: Practice parameters for the assessment and treatment of children and adolescents with obsessive-compulsive disorder. J Am Acad Child Adolesc Psychiatry 37 (10 suppl):27S–45S, 1998

American Academy of Child and Adolescent Psychiatry: Practice parameters for the assessment and treatment of children and adolescents with schizophrenia. J Am Acad Child Adolesc Psychiatry 40 (7 suppl):4S–23S, 2001

American Academy of Child and Adolescent Psychiatry: Practice parameter for the assessment and treatment of children and adolescents with attention-deficit/hyperactivity disorder. J Am Acad Child Adolesc Psychiatry 46:894–921, 2007

American Diabetes Association, American Psychiatric Association, American Association of Clinical Endocrinologists, et al: Consensus development conference on antipsychotic drugs and obesity and diabetes. Diabetes Care 27:596–601, 2004

American Psychiatric Association: Diagnostic and Statistical Manual of Mental Disorders, 3rd Edition, Revised. Washington, DC, American Psychiatric Association, 1987

American Psychiatric Association: Diagnostic and Statistical Manual for Mental Disorders, 4th Edition. Washington, DC, American Psychiatric Association, 1994

American Psychiatric Association: Diagnostic and Statistical Manual of Mental Disorders, 4th Edition, Text Revision. Washington, DC, American Psychiatric Association, 2000

Anderson JC, Williams S, McGee R, et al: DSM-III disorders in preadolescent children. Prevalence in a large sample from the general population. Arch Gen Psychiatry 44:69–76, 1987

Anderson LT, Campbell M, Grega DM, et al: Haloperidol in the treatment of infantile autism: effects on learning and behavioral symptoms. Am J Psychiatry 141:1195–1202, 1984

Anderson LT, Campbell M, Adams P, et al: The effects of haloperidol on discrimination learning and behavioral symptoms in autistic children. J Autism Dev Disord 19:227–239, 1989

Armenteros JL, Adams PB, Campbell M, et al: Haloperidol-related dyskinesias and pre- and perinatal complications in autistic children. Psychopharmacol Bull 31:363–369, 1995

Armenteros JL, Lewis JE, Davalos M: Risperidone augmentation for treatment-resistant aggression in attention-deficit/hyperactivity disorder: a placebo-controlled pilot study. J Am Acad Child Adolesc Psychiatry 46:558–565, 2007

Arnold LE: Methylphenidate vs amphetamine: comparative review. J Attention Disord 3:200–211, 2000

Asbahr FR, Castillo AR, Montenegro L, et al: Group cognitive-behavioral therapy versus sertraline for the treatment of children and adolescents with obsessive-compulsive disorder. J Am Acad Child Adolesc Psychiatry 44:1128–1136, 2005

August GJ, Raz N, Papanicolaou AC, et al: Fenfluramine treatment in infantile autism. Neurochemical, electrophysiological, and behavioral effects. J Nerv Ment Dis 172:604–612, 1984

August GJ, Raz N, Baird TD: Effects of fenfluramine on behavioral, cognitive, and affective disturbances in autistic children. J Autism Dev Disord 15:97–107, 1985

Ballenger JC, Carek DJ, Steele JJ, et al: Three cases of panic disorder with agoraphobia in children. Am J Psychiatry 146:922–924, 1989

Barbaresi WJ, Katusic SK, Colligan RC, et al: How common is attention-deficit/hyperactivity disorder? Incidence in a population-based birth cohort in Rochester, Minn. Arch Pediatr Adolesc Med 156:217–224, 2002

Barbey JT, Roose SP: SSRI safety in overdose. J Clin Psychiatry 59 (suppl 15):42–48, 1998

Barkley RA: Attention Deficit Hyperactivity Disorder: A Clinical Handbook, 3rd Edition. New York, Guilford, 2005

Barnett M, Cohen S: Ziprasidone's metabolic effects in pediatric bipolar disorder. Presented at the 51st annual meeting of American Academy of Child and Adolescent Psychiatry, Washington, DC, October 19–24, 2004

Barrett RP, Feinstein C, Hole WT: Effects of naloxone and naltrexone on self-injury: a double-blind, placebo controlled analysis. Am J Ment Retard 93:644–651, 1989

Barrickman L, Noyes R, Kuperman S, et al: Treatment of ADHD with fluoxetine: a preliminary trial. J Am Acad Child Adolesc Psychiatry 30:762–767, 1991

Barrickman LL, Perry PJ, Allen AJ, et al: Bupropion versus methylphenidate in the treatment of attention-deficit hyperactivity disorder. J Am Acad Child Adolesc Psychiatry 34:649–657, 1995

Barthelemy C, Bruneau N, Jouve J, et al: Urinary dopamine metabolites as indicators of the responsiveness to fenfluramine treatment in children with autistic behavior. J Autism Dev Disord 19:241–254, 1989

Barzman DH, DelBello MP, Kowatch RA, et al: The effectiveness and tolerability of aripiprazole for pediatric bipolar disorders: a retrospective chart review. J Child Adolescent Psychopharmacol 14:593–600, 2004

Barzman DH, DelBello MP, Adler CM, et al: The efficacy and tolerability of quetiapine versus divalproex for the treatment of impulsivity and reactive aggression in adolescents with co-occurring bipolar disorder and disruptive behavior disorder(s). J Child Adolesc Psychopharmacol 16:665–670, 2006

Beeghly JH, Kuperman S, Perry PJ, et al: Fenfluramine treatment of autism: relationship of treatment response to blood levels of fenfluramine and norfenfluramine. J Autism Dev Disord 17:541–548, 1987

Beisler JM, Tsai LY, Stiefel B: The effects of fenfluramine on communication skills in autistic children. J Autism Dev Disord 16:227–233, 1986

Belsito KM, Law PA, Kirk KS, et al: Lamotrigine therapy for autistic disorder: a randomized, double-blind, placebo-controlled trial. J Autism Dev Disord 31:175–181, 2001

Berard R, Fond R, Carpenter DJ, et al: An international, multicenter, placebo-controlled trial of paroxetine in adolescents with major depressive disorder. J Child Adolesc Psychopharmacol 16:59–75, 2006

Berney T, Kolvin I, Bhate SR, et al: School phobia: a therapeutic trial with clomipramine and short-term outcome. Br J Psychiatry 138:110–118, 1981

Bernstein GA, Garfinkel BD, Borchardt CM: Comparative studies of pharmacotherapy for school refusal. J Am Acad Child Adolesc Psychiatry 29:773–781, 1990

Bernstein GA, Borchardt CM, Perwien AR: Anxiety disorders in children and adolescents: a review of the past 10 years. J Am Acad Child Adolesc Psychiatry 35:1110–1119, 1996

Bernstein GA, Borchardt CM, Perwien AR, et al: Imipramine plus cognitive-behavioral therapy in the treatment of school refusal. J Am Acad Child Adolesc Psychiatry 39:276–283, 2000

Bernstein GA, Hektner JM, Borchardt CM, et al: Treatment of school refusal: one-year follow-up. J Am Acad Child Adolesc Psychiatry 40:206–213, 2001

Biederman J: Comparative efficacy of atypical antipsychotics for pediatric bipolar disorder. Poster presented at the 158th annual meeting of the American Psychiatric Association, Atlanta, GA, May 21–26, 2005

Biederman J, Faraone SV, Marrs A, et al: Panic disorder and agoraphobia in consecutively referred children and adolescents. J Am Acad Child Adolesc Psychiatry 36:214–223, 1997

Biederman J, Lopez FA, Boellner SW, et al: A randomized, double-blind, placebo-controlled, parallel-group study of SLI381 (Adderall XR) in children with attention-deficit/hyperactivity disorder. Pediatrics 110:258–266, 2002

Biederman J, McDonnell MA, Wozniak J, et al: Aripiprazole in the treatment of pediatric bipolar disorder: a systematic chart review. CNS Spectr 10:141–148, 2005a

Biederman J, Mick E, Hammerness P, et al: Open-label, 8-week trial of olanzapine and risperidone for the treatment of bipolar disorder in preschool-age children. Biol Psychiatry 58:589–594, 2005b

Biederman J, Mick E, Wozniak J, et al: An Open-label trial of risperidone in children and adolescents with bipolar disorder. J Child Adolesc Psychopharmacol 15:311–317, 2005c

Biederman J, Swanson JM, Wigal SB, et al: Efficacy and safety of modafinil film-coated tablets in children and adolescents with attention-deficit/hyperactivity disorder: results of a randomized, double-blind, placebo-controlled, flexible-dose study. Pediatrics 116:e777–e784, 2005d

Biederman J, Mick E, Surman C, et al: A randomized, placebo-controlled trial of OROS methylphenidate in adults with attention-deficit/hyperactivity disorder. Biol Psychiatry 59:829–835, 2006a

Biederman J, Wigal SB, Spencer TJ, et al: A post hoc subgroup analysis of an 18-day randomized controlled trial comparing the tolerability and efficacy of mixed amphetamine salts extended release and atomoxetine in school-age girls with attention-deficit/hyperactivity disorder. Clin Ther 28:280–293, 2006b

Birmaher B, Waterman GS, Ryan ND, et al: Randomized, controlled trial of amitriptyline versus placebo for adolescents with "treatment resistant" major depression. J Am Acad Child Adolesc Psychiatry 37:527–535, 1998

Birmaher B, Arbelaez C, Brent D: Course and outcome of child and adolescent major depressive disorder. Child Adolesc Psychiatry Clin North Am 11:619–637, 2002

Birmaher B, Axelson DA, Monk K, et al. Fluoxetine for the treatment of childhood anxiety disorders. J Am Acad Child Adolesc Psychiatry 42:415–423, 2003

Birmaher B, Axelson D, Strober M, et al: Clinical course of children and adolescents with bipolar spectrum disorders. Arch Gen Psychiatry 63:175–183, 2006

Bitter I, Czobor P, Dossenbach M, et al: Effectiveness of clozapine, olanzapine, quetiapine, risperidone, and haloperidol monotherapy in reducing hostile and aggressive behavior in outpatients treated for schizophrenia: a prospective naturalistic study (IC-SOHO). Eur Psychiatry 20:403–408, 2005

Black B, Uhde TW: Elective mutism as a variant of social phobia. J Am Acad Child Adolesc Psychiatry 31:1090–1094, 1992

Black B, Uhde TW: Treatment of elective mutism with fluoxetine: a double-blind, placebo-controlled study. J Am Acad Child Adolesc Psychiatry 33:1000–1006, 1994

Blair J, Scahill L, State M, et al: Electrocardiographic changes in children and adolescents treated with ziprasidone: a prospective study. J Am Acad Child Adolesc Psychiatry 44:73–79, 2005

Bouvard MP, Leboyer M, Launay JM, et al: Low-dose naltrexone effects on plasma chemistries and clinical symptoms in autism: a double-blind, placebo-controlled study. Psychiatry Res 58:191–201, 1995

Brent DA, Holder D, Kolko D, et al: A clinical psychotherapy trial for adolescent depression comparing cognitive, family, and supportive therapy. Arch Gen Psychiatry 54:877–885, 1997

Bridge JA, Iyengar S, Salary CB, et al: Clinical response and risk for reported suicidal ideation and suicide attempts in pediatric antidepressant treatment: a meta-analysis of randomized controlled trials. JAMA 297:1683–1696, 2007

Bruggeman R, van der Linden C, Buitelaar JK, et al: Risperidone versus pimozide in Tourette's disorder: a comparative double-blind parallel-group study. J Clin Psychiatry 62:50–56, 2001

Budman CL, Gayer A, Lesser M, et al: An open-label study of the treatment efficacy of olanzapine for Tourette's disorder. J Clin Psychiatry 62:290–294, 2001

Buitelaar JK, van der Gaag RJ, van der Hoeven J: Buspirone in the management of anxiety and irritability in children with pervasive developmental disorders: results of an open-label study. J Clin Psychiatry 59:56–59, 1998

Buitelaar JK, Willemsen-Swinkels SH: Medication treatment in subjects with autistic spectrum disorders. Eur Child Adolesc Psychiatry 9 (suppl 1):I85–I97, 2000

Buitelaar JK, Van der Gaag RJ, Cohen-Kettenis P, et al: A randomized controlled trial of risperidone in the treatment of aggression in hospitalized adolescents with subaverage cognitive abilities [comment]. J Clin Psychiatry 62:239–248, 2001

Bymaster FP, Katner JS, Nelson DL, et al: Atomoxetine increases extracellular levels of norepinephrine and dopamine in prefrontal cortex of rat: a potential mechanism for efficacy in attention deficit/hyperactivity disorder. Neuropsychopharmacology 27:699–711, 2002

Campbell M, Anderson LT, Meier M, et al: A comparison of haloperidol and behavior therapy and their interaction in autistic children. J Am Acad Child Psychiatry 17:640–655, 1978

Campbell M, Anderson LT, Small AM, et al: The effects of haloperidol on learning and behavior in autistic children. J Autism Dev Disord 12:167–175, 1982

Campbell M, Small AM, Green WH, et al: Behavioral efficacy of haloperidol and lithium carbonate: a comparison in hospitalized aggressive children with conduct disorder. Arch Gen Psychiatry 41:650–656, 1984

Campbell M, Perry R, Polonsky BB, et al: An open study of fenfluramine in hospitalized young autistic children. J Autism Dev Disord 16:495–506, 1986

Campbell M, Adams P, Perry R, et al: Tardive and withdrawal dyskinesia in autistic children: a prospective study. Psychopharmacol Bull 24:251–255, 1988a

Campbell M, Adams P, Small AM, et al: Efficacy and safety of fenfluramine in autistic children. J Am Acad Child Adolesc Psychiatry 27:434–439, 1988b

Campbell M, Anderson LT, Small AM, et al: Naltrexone in autistic children: behavioral symptoms and attentional learning. J Am Acad Child Adolesc Psychiatry 32:1283–1291, 1993

Campbell M, Adams PB, Small AM, et al: Lithium in hospitalized aggressive children with conduct disorder: a double blind and placebo controlled study. J Am Acad Child Adolesc Psychiatry 34:445–453, 1995

Campbell M, Armenteros JL, Malone RP, et al: Neuroleptic-related dyskinesias in autistic children: a prospective, longitudinal study. J Am Acad Child Adolesc Psychiatry 36:835–843, 1997

Cantwell DP, Swanson J, Connor DF: Case study: adverse response to clonidine. J Am Acad Child Adolesc Psychiatry 36:539–544, 1997

Castellanos FX, Giedd JN, Elia J, et al: Controlled stimulant treatment of ADHD and comorbid Tourette's syndrome: effects of stimulant and dose. J Am Acad Child Adolesc Psychiatry 36:589–596, 1997

Centers for Disease Control and Prevention: Mental health in the United States. Prevalence of diagnosis and medication treatment for attention deficit/hyperactivity disorder—United States 2003. MMWR Morb Mortal Wkly Rep 54:842–847, 2005

Chambers WJ, Puig-Antich J, Hirsch M, et al: The assessment of affective disorders in children and adolescents by semistructured interview. Test-retest reliability of the schedule for affective disorders and schizophrenia for school-age children, present episode version. Arch Gen Psychiatry 42:696–702, 1985

Chang K, Saxena K, Howe M, et al: An open-label study of lamotrigine adjunct or monotherapy for the treatment of adolescents with bipolar depression. J Am Acad Child Adolesc Psychiatry 45:298–304, 2006

Chappell PB, Riddle MA, Scahill L, et al: Guanfacine treatment of comorbid attention-deficit hyperactivity disorder and Tourette's syndrome: preliminary clinical experience. J Am Acad Child Adolesc Psychiatry 34:1140–1146, 1995b

Chavira DA, Stein MB: Combined psychoeducation and treatment with selective serotonin reuptake inhibitors for youth with generalized social anxiety disorder. J Child Adolesc Psychopharmacol 12:47–54, 2002

Charach A, Figueroa M, Chen S, et al: Stimulant treatment over 5 years: effects on growth. J Am Acad Child Adolesc Psychiatry 45:415–421, 2006

Childress AC, Krishman S, McGough JJ, et al: Interim analysis of a long-term, open-label, single-arm study of lisdexamfetamine (LDX), an amphetamine prodrug, in children with ADHD. Presented at the 53rd Annual Meeting of the American Academy of Child and Adolescent Psychiatry, San Diego, CA, October 27, 2006

Clark DB, Birmaher B, Axelson D, et al: Fluoxetine for the treatment of childhood anxiety disorder: open-label, long-term extension to a controlled trial. J Am Acad Child Adolesc Psychiatry 44:1263–1270, 2005

Clarke GN, Sack WH, Ben R, et al: English language skills in a group of previously traumatized Khmer adolescent refugees. J Nerv Ment Dis 181:454–456, 1993

Coggins TE, Morisset C, Krasney L, et al: Brief report: does fenfluramine treatment enhance the cognitive and communicative functioning of autistic children? J Autism Dev Disord 18:425–434, 1988

Cohen IL, Campbell M, Posner D, et al: Behavioral effects of haloperidol in young autistic children. An objective analysis using a within-subjects reversal design. J Am Acad Child Psychiatry 19:665–677, 1980

Comings DE, Himes JA, Comings BG: An epidemiologic study of Tourette's syndrome in a single school district. J Clin Psychiatry 51:463–469, 1990

Compton SN, Grant PJ, Chrisman AK, et al: Sertraline in children and adolescents with social anxiety disorder. J Am Acad Adolesc Psychiatry 40:564–571, 2001

Coniglio SJ, Lewis JD, Lang C, et al: A randomized, double-blind, placebo-controlled trial of single-dose intravenous secretin as treatment for children with autism. J Pediatr 138:649–655, 2001

Conners CK, Casat CD, Gualtieri CT, et al: Bupropion hydrochloride in attention deficit disorder with hyperactivity. J Am Acad Child Adolesc Psychiatry 35:1314–1321, 1996

Connor DF, Ozbayrak KR, Benjamin S, et al: A pilot study of nadolol for overt aggression in developmentally delayed individuals. J Am Acad Child Adolesc Psychiatry 36:826–834, 1997

Connor DF, Fletcher KE, Swanson JM: A meta-analysis of clonidine for symptoms of attention-deficit hyperactivity disorder. J Am Acad Child Adolesc Psychiatry 38:1551–1559, 1999

Connor DF, Barkley RA, Davis HT: A pilot study of methylphenidate, clonidine, or the combination in ADHD comorbid with aggressive oppositional defiant disorder or conduct disorder. Clin Pediatr 39:15–25, 2000

Connor DF, Glatt SJ, Lopez ID, et al: Psychopharmacology and aggression, I: a meta-analysis of stimulant effects on overt/covert aggression-related behaviors in ADHD. J Am Acad Child Adolesc Psychiatry 41:253–261, 2002

Cook EH, Rowlett R, Jaselskis C, et al: Fluoxetine treatment of children and adults with autistic disorder and mental retardation. J Am Acad Child Adolesc Psychiatry 31:739–745, 1992

Cook EH, Wagner KD, March JS, et al: Long-term sertraline treatment of children and adolescents with obsessive-compulsive disorder. J Am Acad Child Adolesc Psychiatry 40:1175–1181, 2001

Copur M, Arpaci B, Demir T, et al: Clinical effectiveness of quetiapine in children and adolescents with Tourette's syndrome: a retrospective case-note survey. Clin Drug Investig 27:123–130, 2007

Corbett B, Khan K, Czapansky-Beilman D, et al: A double-blind, placebo-controlled crossover study investigating the effect of porcine secretin in children with autism. Clin Pediatr 40:327–331, 2001

Correll CU, Carlson HE: Endocrine and metabolic adverse effects of psychotropic medications in children and adolescents. J Am Acad Child Adolesc Psychiatry 45:771–791, 2006

Correll CU, Leucht S, Kane JM: Lower risk for tardive dyskinesia associated with second-generation antipsychotics: a systematic review of 1-year studies. Am J Psychiatry 161:414–425, 2004

Correll CU, Penzer JB, Parikh UH, et al: Recognising and monitoring adverse events of second-generation antipsychotics in children and adolescents. Child Adolesc Psychiatric Clin N Am 15:177–206, 2006

Couturier JL, Nicolson R: A retrospective assessment of citalopram in children and adolescents with pervasive developmental disorders. J Child Adolesc Psychopharmacol 12:243–248, 2002

Cummings DD, Singer HS, Krieger M, et al: Neuropsychiatric effects of guanfacine in children with mild Tourette syndrome: a pilot study. Clin Neuropharmacol 25:325–332, 2002

Daly JM, Wilens T: The use of tricyclic antidepressants in children and adolescents. Pediatr Clin North Am 45:1123–1135, 1998

D'Amato G: Chlordiazepoxide in management of school phobia. Dis Nerv Syst 23:292–295, 1962

Davanzo PA, McCracken JT: Mood stabilizers in the treatment of juvenile bipolar disorder: advances and controversies. Child Adolesc Psychiatr Clin N Am 9:159–182, 2000

Davies L, Stern JS, Agrawal N, et al: A case series of patients with Tourette's syndrome in the United Kingdom treated with aripiprazole. Hum Psychopharmacol. 21:447–453, 2006

Daviss WB, Bentivoglio P, Racusin R, et al: Bupropion sustained release in adolescents with co morbid attention-deficit/hyperactivity disorder and depression. J Am Acad Child Adolesc Psychiatry 40:307–314, 2001

DelBello MP, Kowatch RA: Pharmacological interventions for bipolar youth: developmental considerations. Dev Psychopathol 18:1231–1246, 2006

DelBello M, Schwiers ML, Rosenberg HL: A double-blind, randomized, placebo-controlled study of quetiapine as adjunctive treatment for adolescent mania. J Am Acad Child Adolesc Psychiatry 41:1216–1223, 2002

DelBello MP, Findling RL, Kushner S, et al: A pilot controlled trial of topiramate for mania in children and adolescents with bipolar disorder. J Am Acad Child Adolesc Psychiatry 44:539–547, 2005

DelBello MP, Kowatch RA, Adler CM, et al: A double-blind randomized pilot study comparing quetiapine and divalproex for adolescent mania. J Am Acad Child Adolesc Psychiatry, 45:305–313, 2006

DeLong GR, Nieman GW: Lithium-induced behavior changes in children with symptoms suggesting manic-depressive illness. Psychopharmacol Bull 19:258–265, 1983

DeVeaugh-Geiss J, Moroz G, Biederman J, et al: Clomipramine hydrochloride in childhood and adolescent obsessive-compulsive disorder—a multicenter trial. J Am Acad Child Adolesc Psychiatry 31:45–49, 1992

Desarkar P, Das A, Sinha VK: Duloxetine for childhood depression with pain and dissociative symptoms. Eur Child Adolesc Psychiatry 15:496–499, 2006

Dion Y, Annable L, Sandor P, et al: Risperidone in the treatment of Tourette syndrome: a double blind, placebo controlled trial. J Clin Psychopharmacol 22:31–39, 2002

Dollfus S, Petit M, Menard JF, et al: Amisulpride versus bromocriptine in infantile autism: a controlled crossover comparative study of two drugs with opposite effects on dopaminergic function. J Autism Dev Disord 22:47–60, 1992

Donnelly M, Rapoport JL, Potter WZ, et al: Fenfluramine and dextroamphetamine treatment of childhood hyperactivity. Clinical and biochemical findings. Arch Gen Psychiatry 46:205–212, 1989

Donovan SJ, Stewart JW, Nunes EV, et al: Divalproex treatment for youth with explosive temper and mood lability: a double-blind, placebo-controlled crossover design. Am J Psychiatry 157:818–820, 2000

Douglass HM, Moffitt TE, Dar R, et al: Obsessive-compulsive disorder in a birth cohort of 18-year-olds: prevalence and predictors. J Am Acad Child Adolesc Psychiatry 34:1424–1431, 1995

Dow SP, Sonies BC, Scheib D, et al: Practical guidelines for the assessment and treatment of selective mutism. J Am Acad Child Adolesc Psychiatry 34:836–846, 1995

du Verglas G, Banks SR, Guyer KE: Clinical effects of fenfluramine on children with autism: a review of the research. J Autism Dev Disord 18:297–308, 1988

Dummit ES III, Klein RG, Tancer NK, et al: Fluoxetine treatment of children with selective mutism: an open trial. J Am Acad Child Adolesc Psychiatry 35:615–621, 1996

Dunbar F, Kusumakar V, Daneman D, et al: Growth and sexual maturation during long-term treatment with risperidone. Am J Psychiatry 161:918–920, 2004

Dunn V, Goodyer IM: Longitudinal investigation into childhood- and adolescence-onset depression: psychiatric outcome in early adulthood. Br J Psychiatry 188:216–222, 2006

Durkin JP 2nd: Gabapentin in complicated school refusal. J Am Acad Child Adolesc Psychiatry 41:632–633, 2002

Eggers C, Bunk D: The long-term course of childhood-onset schizophrenia: a 42-year follow-up. Schizophr Bull 23:105–117, 1997

Ekman G, Miranda-Linne F, Gillberg C, et al: Fenfluramine treatment of twenty children with autism. J Autism Dev Disord 19:511–532, 1989

Emslie GJ, Rush AJ, Weinberg WA, et al: A double-blind, randomized, placebo-controlled trial of fluoxetine in children and adolescents with depression. Arch Gen Psychiatry 54:1031–1037, 1997

Emslie GJ, Wagner KD, Riddle M, et al: Efficacy and safety of paroxetine in juvenile OCD. Poster presented at the 153rd annual meeting of the American Psychiatric Association, Chicago, IL, May 13–18, 2000

Emslie GJ, Heiligenstein JH, Wagner KD, et al: Fluoxetine for acute treatment of depression in children and adolescents: a placebo-controlled, randomized clinical trial. J Am Acad Child Adolesc Psychiatry 41:1205–1215, 2002

Emslie GJ, Wagner KD, Kutcher S, et al: Paroxetine treatment in children and adolescents with major depressive disorder: a randomized, multicenter, double-blind, placebo-controlled trial. J Am Acad Child Adolesc Psychiatry 45:709–719, 2006

Emslie GJ, Findling RL, Yeung PP, et al: Venlafaxine ER for the treatment of pediatric subjects with depression: results of two placebo-controlled trials. J Am Acad Child Adolesc Psychiatry 46:479–488, 2007a

Emslie GJ, Yeung PP, Kunz NR: Long-term, open-label venlafaxine extended-release treatment in children and adolescents with major depressive disorder. CNS Spectr 12:223–233, 2007b

Engelhardt DM, Polizos P, Waizer J, et al: A double-blind comparison of fluphenazine and haloperidol in outpatient schizophrenic children. J Autism Child Schizophr 3:128–137, 1973

Ernst M, Magee HJ, Gonzalez NM, et al: Pimozide in autistic children. Psychopharmacol Bull 28:187–191, 1992

Famularo R, Kinscherff R, Fenton T: Propranolol treatment for childhood posttraumatic stress disorder, acute type: a pilot study. Am J Dis Child 142:1244–1247, 1988

Fankhauser MP, Karumanchi VC, German ML et al: A double blind, placebo-controlled study of the efficacy of transdermal clonidine in autism. J Clin Psychiatry 53:77–82, 1992

Faretra G, Dooher L, Dowling J: Comparison of haloperidol and fluphenazine in disturbed children. Am J Psychiatry 126:1670–1673, 1970

Fatemi SH, Realmuto GM, Khan L, et al: Fluoxetine in treatment of adolescent patients with autism: a longitudinal open trial. J Autism Dev Disord 28:303–307, 1998

Feldman HM, Kolmen BK, Gonzaga AM, et al: Naltrexone and communication skills in young children with autism. J Am Acad Child Adolesc Psychiatry 38:587–593, 1999

Fenichel R: Combining methylphenidate and clonidine: the role of post-marketing surveillance. J Child Adolesc Psychopharmacol 5:155–156, 1995

Findling RL: Open-label treatment of comorbid depression and attentional disorders with co-administration of serotonin reuptake inhibitors and psychostimulants in children, adolescents, and adults: a case series. J Child Adolesc Psychopharmacol 6:165–175, 1996

Findling RL, Lopez FA: Efficacy of transdermal methylphenidate with reference to Concerta in ADHD. Presented at the 25th annual meeting of the American Academy of Child and Adolescent Psychiatry, Toronto, CA, October 18–23, 2005

Findling RL, McNamara NK, Gracious BL, et al: Combination lithium and divalproex sodium in pediatric bipolarity. J Am Acad Child Adolesc Psychiatry 42:895–901, 2003a

Findling RL, McNamara NK, Youngstrom EA, et al. A prospective, open-label trial of olanzapine in adolescents with schizophrenia. J Am Acad Child Adolesc Psychiatry 42:170–175, 2003b

Findling RL, McNamara NK, Gracious BL: Quetiapine in nine youths with autistic disorder. J Child Adolesc Psychopharmacol 14:287–294, 2004

Findling RL, McNamara NK, Youngstrom EA, et al. Double-blind 18-month trial of lithium versus divalproex maintenance treatment in pediatric bipolar disorder. J Am Acad Child Adolesc Psychiatry 44:409–417, 2005

Findling RL, Krishman S, Biederman J: Efficacy and safety of lisdexamfetamine (LDX) in children aged 6 to 12 years with attention-deficit/hyperactivity disorder (ADHD). Presented at the 53rd Annual Meeting of the American Academy of Child and Adolescent Psychiatry, San Diego, CA, October 28, 2006a

Findling RL, Reed MD, O'Riordan MA, et al: Effectiveness, safety, and pharmacokinetics of quetiapine in aggressive children with conduct disorder. J Am Acad Child Adolesc Psychiatry 45:792–800, 2006b

Findling RL, Nyilas M, Auby P, et al: Tolerability of aripiprazole in the treatment of adolescents with schizophrenia. New research poster presented at the 160th annual meeting of the American Psychiatric Association, San Diego, CA, May 19–24, 2007

Flakierska-Praquin N, Lindstrom M, Gillberg C: School phobia with separation anxiety disorder: a comparative 20- to 29-year follow-up study of 35 school refusers. Compr Psychiatry 38:17–22, 1997

Flament MF, Rapoport JL, Berg CJ, et al: Clomipramine treatment of childhood obsessive-compulsive disorder. A double-blind controlled study. Arch Gen Psychiatry 42:977–983, 1985

Frazier JA, Biederman J, Tohen M, et al: A prospective open-label treatment trial of olanzapine monotherapy in children and adolescents with bipolar disorder. J Child Adolesc Psychopharmacol 11:239–250, 2001

Fristad MA, Goldberg-Arnold JS, Gavazzi SM, et al: Multifamily psychoeducation groups in the treatment of children with mood disorders. J Marital Fam Ther 29:491–504, 2003

Gadow KD, Sverd J, Sprafkin J, et al: Efficacy of methylphenidate for attention-deficit hyperactivity disorder in children with tic disorder. Arch Gen Psychiatry 52:444–455, 1995

Gadow KD, Sverd J, Sprafkin J, et al: Long-term methylphenidate therapy in children with comorbid attention-deficit hyperactivity disorder and chronic multiple tic disorder [see comments]. Arch Gen Psychiatry 56:330–336, 1999

Gaffney GR, Perry PJ, Lund BC, et al: Risperidone versus clonidine in the treatment of children and adolescents with Tourette's syndrome. J Am Acad Child Adolesc Psychiatry 41:330–336, 2002

Gammon GD, Brown TE: Fluoxetine and methylphenidate in combination for treatment of attention deficit and comorbid depressive disorder. J Child Adolesc Psychopharmacol 3:1–10, 1993

Gastaut H, Zifkin B, Rufo M: Compulsive respiratory stereotypies in children with autistic features: polygraphic recording and treatment with fenfluramine. J Autism Dev Disord 17:391–406, 1987

Geller B, Cooper TB, Chestnut EC, et al: Preliminary data on the relationship between nortriptyline plasma level and response in depressed children. Am J Psychiatry 143:1283–1286, 1986

Geller B, Cooper TB, Graham DL, et al: Double-blind placebo-controlled study of nortriptyline in depressed adolescents using a "fixed plasma level" design. Psychopharmacol Bull 26:85–90, 1990

Geller B, Cooper TB, Graham DL, et al: Pharmacokinetically designed double-blind placebo-controlled study of nortriptyline in 6- to 12-year-olds with major depressive disorder. J Am Acad Child Adolesc Psychiatry 31:34–44, 1992

Geller B, Cooper TB, Sun K, et al: Double blind and placebo controlled study of lithium for adolescent bipolar disorders with secondary substance dependency. J Am Acad Child Adolesc Psychiatry 37:171–178, 1998

Geller B, Zimerman B, Williams M, et al: Diagnostic characteristics of 93 cases of prepubertal and early adolescent bipolar disorder phenotype by gender, puberty and comorbid attention deficit hyperactivity disorder. J Child Adolesc Psychopharmacol 10:157–164, 2000

Geller B, Tillman MS, Craney JL, et al: Four-year prospective outcome and natural history of mania in children with a prepubertal and early adolescent bipolar disorder phenotype. Arch Gen Psychiatry 61:459–467, 2004

Geller DA, Biederman J, Wagner KD, et al: Comorbid psychiatric illness and response to treatment, relapse rates, and behavioral adverse event incidence in pediatric OCD. Poster presented at the 41st annual meeting of the New Clinical Drug Evaluation Unit, Phoenix, AZ, May 28–31, 2001a

Geller DA, Hoog SL, Heiligenstein JH, et al: Fluoxetine treatment for obsessive-compulsive disorder in children and adolescents: a placebo-controlled clinical trial. J Am Acad Child Adolesc Psychiatry 40:773–779, 2001b

Geller DA, Hoog SL, Heiligenstein JH, et al: Predictive factors in response to fluoxetine treatment for pediatric OCD. Poster presented at the 48th annual meeting of the American Academy of Child and Adolescent Psychiatry, Honolulu, HI, October 23–28, 2001c

Geller DA, Wagner KD, Emslie G, et al: Paroxetine treatment in children and adolescents with obsessive-compulsive disorder: a randomized, multicenter, double-blind, placebo-controlled trial. J Am Acad Child Adolesc Psychiatry 43:1387–1396, 2004

Geller E, Ritvo ER, Freeman BJ, et al: Preliminary observations on the effect of fenfluramine on blood serotonin and symptoms in three autistic boys. N Engl J Med 307:165–169, 1982

Gelperin K: Psychiatric adverse events associated with drug treatment of ADHD: review of postmarketing safety data. U.S. Food and Drug Administration Pediatric Advisory Committee, March 22, 2006. Available at: http://www.fda.gov/ohrms/dockets/ac/06/slides/2006-4210s_15_Gelperin_Review%20of%20Postmarking%20Safety.ppt. Accessed December 2008.

George MS, Trimble MR, Robertson MM: Fluvoxamine and sulpiride in comorbid obsessive compulsive disorder and Gilles de la Tourette's syndrome. Hum Psychopharmacol 8:327–334, 1993

Ghaziuddin M, Tsai L, Ghaziuddin N, et al: Fluoxetine in autism with depression. J Am Acad Child Adolesc Psychiatry 30:508–509, 1991

Giacona RM, Reinherz HZ, Silverman AB, et al: Traumas and posttraumatic stress disorder in a community population of older adolescents. J Am Acad Child Adolesc Psychiatry 34:1369–1380, 1995

Gibbons RD, Hur K, Bhaumik DK, et al: The relationship between antidepressant prescription rates and rate of early adolescent suicide. Am J Psychiatry 163:1898–1904, 2006

Gibson AP, Crismon ML, Mican LM, et al: Effectiveness and tolerability of aripiprazole in child and adolescent inpatients: a retrospective evaluation. Int Clin Psychopharmacol 22:101–105, 2007

Gilbert DL, Batterson JR, Sethuraman G, et al: Tic reduction with risperidone versus pimozide in a randomized, double-blind, crossover trial. J Am Acad Child Adolesc Psychiatry 43:206–214, 2004

Gittelman-Klein R, Klein DF: Controlled imipramine treatment of school phobia. Arch Gen Psychiatry 25:204–207, 1971

Gittelman-Klein R, Mannuzza S: Hyperactive boys almost grown up, III: methylphenidate effects on ultimate height. Arch Gen Psychiatry 45:1131–1134, 1988

Glod CA, Lynch A, Flynn E, et al: Bupropion SR in the treatment of adolescent depression. Poster presented at the 40th Annual Meeting of the New Clinical Drug Evaluation Unit, Boca Raton, FL, 2000

Goetz CG, Tanner CM, Wilson RS, et al: Clonidine and Gilles de la Tourette's syndrome: double-blind study using objective rating methods. Ann Neurol 21:307–310, 1987

Golwyn DH, Sevlie CP: Phenelzine treatment of selective mutism in four prepubertal children. J Child Adolesc Psychopharmacol 9:109–113, 1999

Golwyn DH, Weinstock RC: Phenelzine treatment of elective mutism: a case report. J Clin Psychiatry 51:384–385, 1990

Goodman WK, Price LH, Rasmusen SA et al: Children's Yale-Brown Obsessive Compulsive Scale (CY-BOCS). New Haven, CT, Department of Psychiatry, Yale University School of Medicine, 1991

Gordon CT, State RC, Nelson JE, et al: A double-blind comparison of clomipramine, desipramine, and of autistic disorder. Arch Gen Psychiatry 50:441–447, 1993

Graae F, Milner J, Rizzotto L, et al: Clonazepam in childhood anxiety disorders. J Am Acad Child Adolesc Psychiatry 33:372–376, 1994

Grados M, Scahill L, Riddle MA: Pharmacotherapy in children and adolescents with obsessive-compulsive disorder. Child Adolesc Clin N Am 8:617–634, 1999

Gram LF, Rafaelsen OJ: Lithium treatment of psychotic children and adolescents. A controlled clinical trial. Acta Psychiatr Scand 48:253–260, 1972

Green WH: Child and Adolescent Clinical Psychopharmacology, 3rd Edition. Philadelphia, PA, Lippincott Williams & Wilkins, 2001

Greenhill LL, Halperin JM, Abikoff H: Stimulant medications. J Am Acad Child Adolesc Psychiatry 38:503–512, 1999

Greenhill LL, Findling RL, Swanson JM: A double-blind, placebo-controlled study of modified-release methylphenidate in children with attention-deficit/hyperactivity disorder. Pediatrics 109:e39, 2002

Greenhill LL, Swanson JM, Steinhoff K, et al: A pharmacokinetic/pharmacodynamic study comparing a single morning dose of Adderall to twice-daily dosing in children with ADHD. J Am Acad Child Adolesc Psychiatry 42:1234–1241, 2003

Greenhill LL, Vitiello B, Abikoff HB, et al: Outcome results from the NIMH, multi-site, preschool ADHD treatment study (PATS). Presented at the 51st Annual Meeting of the American Academy of Child and Adolescent Psychiatry, Washington, DC, October 19–24, 2004

Greenhill LL, Ball R, Levine AJ, et al: Extended release dexmethylphenidate in children and adolescents with ADHD. Presented at the 158th Annual Meeting of the American Psychiatric Association, Atlanta, GA, May 21–25, 2005

Greenhill LL, Biederman J, Boellner SW, et al: A randomized, double-blind, placebo-controlled study of modafinil film-coated tablets in children and adolescents with attention-deficit/hyperactivity disorder. J Am Acad Child Adolesc Psychiatry 45:503–511, 2006a

Greenhill LL, Kollins S, Abikoff H, et al: Efficacy and safety of immediate-release methylphenidate treatment for preschoolers with ADHD. J Am Acad Child Adolesc Psychiatry 45:1284–1293, 2006b

Gunther T, Herpertz-Dahlmann B, Jolles J, et al: The influence of risperidone on attentional functions in children and adolescents with attention-deficit/hyperactivity disorder and comorbid disruptive behavior disorder. J Child Adolesc Psychopharmacol 16:725–735, 2006

Greist JH, Jefferson JW, Kobak KA, et al: Efficacy and tolerability of serotonin transport inhibitors in obsessive-compulsive disorder. Arch Gen Psychiatry 52:53–60, 1995

Groden G, Groden J, Dondey M, et al: Effects of fenfluramine on the behavior of autistic individuals. Res Dev Disabil 8:203–211, 1987

Haas M, Unis AS, Copenhaver M, et al: Efficacy and safety of risperidone in adolescents with schizophrenia. Presented at the 160th Annual Meeting of the American Psychiatric Association, San Diego, CA, May 19–24, 2007

Hamilton BE, Minino AM, Martin JA, et al: Annual summary of vital statistics: 2005. Pediatrics 119:345–360, 2007

Hamilton M: The assessment of anxiety states by rating. Br J Med Psychol 32:50–55, 1959

Hamilton M: A rating scale for depression. J Neurol Neurosurg Psychiatry 23:56–62, 1960

Hammerness PG, Vivas FM, Geller DA: Selective serotonin reuptake inhibitors in pediatric psychopharmacology: a review of the evidence. J Pediatr 148:158–165, 2006

Handen BL, Johnson CR, Lubetsky M: Efficacy of methylphenidate among children with autism and symptoms of attention-deficit hyperactivity disorder. J Autism Dev Disord 30:245–255, 2000

Harmon RJ, Riggs PD: Clonidine for posttraumatic stress disorder in preschool children. J Am Acad Child Adolesc Psychiatry 35:1247–1249, 1996

Hayden F: Long-term remission of schizophrenia in an adolescent treated with quetiapine. J Child Adolesc Psychopharmacol 11:289–293, 2001

Hazaray E, Ehret J, Posey DJ, et al: Intramuscular ziprasidone for acute agitation in adolescents. J Child Adolesc Psychopharmacol 14:464–470, 2004

Hazell PL, Stuart JE: A randomized controlled trial of clonidine added to psychostimulant medication for hyperactive and aggressive children. J Am Acad Child Adolesc Psychiatry 42:886–894, 2003

Herman BH, Asleson GS, Powell A, et al: Cardiovascular and other physical effects of acute administration of naltrexone in autistic children. J Child Adolesc Psychopharmacol 3:157–168, 1993

Ho HH, Lockitch G, Eaves L, et al: Blood serotonin concentrations and fenfluramine therapy in autistic children. J Pediatr 108:465–469, 1986

Hollander E, Kaplan A, Cartwright C, et al: Venlafaxine in children, adolescents, and young adults with autism spectrum disorders: an open retrospective clinical report. J Child Neurol 15:132–135, 2000

Hollander E, Phillips A, Chaplin W, et al: A placebo controlled crossover trial of liquid fluoxetine on repetitive behaviors in childhood and adolescent autism. Neuropsychopharmacology 30:582–589, 2005

Horrigan JP: Guanfacine for PTSD nightmares. J Am Acad Child Adolesc Psychiatry 35:975–976, 1996

Horvath K, Stafanatos G, Sokolski KN, et al: Improved social and language skills after secretin administration in patients with autistic spectrum disorders. J Assoc Acad Minor Phys 9:9–15, 1998

Howlin P: Autism and intellectual disability: diagnostic and treatment issues. J R Soc Med 93:351–355, 2000

Hughes CW, Emslie GJ, Crismon MJ, et al: The Texas Children's Medication Algorithm Project: Update from Texas Consensus Conference Panel on Medication Treatment of Childhood Major Depressive Disorder. J Am Acad Child Adolesc Psychiatry 46:667–686, 2007

Hunt RD, Capper L, O'Connell P: Clonidine in child and adolescent psychiatry. J Child Adolesc Psychopharmacol 1:87–102, 1990

Hunt RD, Amsten AF, Asbell MD: An open trial of guanfacine in the treatment of attention-deficit hyperactivity disorder. J Am Acad Child Adolesc Psychiatry 34:50–54, 1995

Jaselskis CA, Cook EH, Fletcher KE, et al: Clonidine treatment of hyperactive and impulsive children with autistic disorder. J Clin Psychopharmacol 12:322–327, 1992

Jasinski D, Krishman S: Abuse liability of intravenous lisdexamfetamine (LDX; NRP104). Presented at the 58th Institute on Psychiatric Services, New York, NY, October 6, 2006a

Jasinski D, Krishman S: A double-blind, randomized, placebo- and active-controlled, 6-period crossover study to evaluate the likeability, safety, and abuse potential of lisdexamfetamine dimesylate (LDX) in adult stimulant abusers. Presented at the 2006 US Psychiatric and Mental Health Congress, New Orleans, LA, November 17, 2006b

Jensen PS, Bhatara VS, Vitiello B, et al: Psychoactive medication prescribing practices for US children: gaps between research and clinical practice. J Am Acad Child Adolesc Psychiatry 38:557–565, 1999

Kaufman J, Birmaher B, Brent D, et al: Schedule for Affective Disorders and Schizophrenia for School Age Children, Present and Lifetime Versions (K-SADS-PL): initial reliability and validity data. J Am Acad Child Adolesc Psychiatry 36:980–988, 1997

Kafantaris V, Coletti DJ, Dicker R, et al: Adjunctive antipsychotic treatment of adolescents with bipolar psychosis. J Am Acad Child Adolesc Psychiatry 40:1448–1456, 2001a

Kafantaris V, Dicker R, Coletti DJ, et al: Adjunctive antipsychotic treatment is necessary for adolescents with psychotic mania. J Am Acad Child Adolesc Psychopharmacol 11:409–413, 2001b

Kafantaris V, Coletti DJ, Dicker R, et al: Lithium treatment of acute mania in adolescents: a large open trial. J Am Acad Child Adolesc Psychiatry 42:1038–1045, 2003

Kafantaris V, Coletti DJ, Dicker R, et al: Lithium treatment of acute mania in adolescents: a placebo-controlled discontinuation study. J Am Acad Child Adolesc Psychiatry 43:984–993, 2004

Kappagoda C, Schell DN, Hanson RM, et al: Clonidine overdose in childhood: implications of increased prescribing. J Paediatr Child Health 34:508–512, 1998

Kashani JH, Orvaschel H: Anxiety disorders in mid-adolescence: a community sample. Am J Psychiatry 145:960–964, 1988

Kashani JH, Sherman DD: Childhood depression: epidemiology, etiological models, and treatment implications. Integr Psychiatry 6:1–8, 1988

Kastner T: Secretin and autism. Except Health Care 9:45–46, 1998

Keller MB, Lavori PW, Wunder J, et al: Chronic course of anxiety disorder in children and adolescents. J Am Acad Child Adolesc Psychiatry 31:595–599, 1992

Keller MB, Ryan ND, Strober M, et al: Efficacy of paroxetine in the treatment of adolescent major depression: a randomized, controlled trial. J Am Acad Child Adolesc Psychiatry 40:762–772, 2001

Kemner C, Willemsen-Swinkels SHN, DeJonge M, et al: Open-label study of olanzapine in children with pervasive developmental disorder. J Clin Psychopharmacol 22:455–460, 2002

Kemph JP, DeVane CL, Levin GM, et al: Treatment of aggressive children with clonidine: results of an open pilot study. J Am Acad Child Adolesc Psychiatry 32:577–581, 1993

Kennard B, Silva S, Vitiello B, et al: Remission and residual symptoms after short-term treatment in the treatment of adolescents with depression study (TADS). J Am Acad Child Adolesc Psychiatry 45:1404–1411, 2006

Kerbeshian J, Burd L, Fisher W: Lithium carbonate in the treatment of two patients with infantile autism and atypical bipolar symptomatology. J Clin Psychopharmacol 7:401–405, 1987

Kessler RC, Adler L, Barkley R, et al: The prevalence and correlates of adult ADHD in the United States: results from the National Comorbidity Survey Replication. Am J Psychiatry 163:716–723, 2006

Khan SS, Mican LM, Khan SS, et al: A naturalistic evaluation of intramuscular ziprasidone versus intramuscular olanzapine for the management of acute agitation and aggression in children and adolescents. J Child Adolesc Psychopharmacol 16:671–677, 2006

Kim BN, Lee CB, Hwang JW, et al: Effectiveness and safety of risperidone for children and adolescents with chronic tic or Tourette disorders in Korea. J Child Adolesc Psychopharmacol 15:318–324, 2005

King BH, Wright DM, Handen BL, et al: Double-blind, placebo-controlled study of amantadine hydrochloride in the treatment of children with autistic disorder. J Am Acad Child Adolesc Psychiatry 40:658–665, 2001

Kisicki J, Fiske K, Scheckner B, et al: Abrupt cessation of guanfacine extended release in healthy young adults. Presented at the 53rd Annual Meeting of the American Academy of Child and Adolescent Psychiatry, San Diego, CA, October 24–29, 2006

Klein RG, Koplewicz HS, Kanner A: Imipramine treatment of children with separation anxiety disorder. J Am Acad Child Adolesc Psychiatry 31:21–28, 1992

Klein RG, Abikoff H, Klass E, et al: Clinical efficacy of methylphenidate in conduct disorder with and without attention deficit hyperactivity disorder. Arch Gen Psychiatry 54:1073–1080, 1997

Klykylo WM, Feldis D, O'Grady D, et al: Clinical effects of fenfluramine in ten autistic subjects. J Autism Dev Disord 15:417–423, 1985

Knorring A, Olsson GI, Thomsen PH, et al: A randomized, double-blind, placebo-controlled study of citalopram in adolescents with major depressive disorder. J Clin Psychopharmacol 26:311–315, 2006

Kofoed L, Tadepalli G, Oesterheld JR, et al: Case series: clonidine has no systematic effects on PR or QTc intervals in children. J Am Acad Child Adolesc Psychiatry 38:1193–1196, 1999

Kohler JA, Shortland G, Rolles CJ: Effect of fenfluramine on autistic symptoms. Br Med J (Clin Res Ed) 295:885, 1987

Kolmen BK, Feldman HM, Handen BL, et al: Naltrexone in young autistic children: a double-blind, placebo-controlled crossover study. J Am Acad Child Adolesc Psychiatry 34:223–231, 1995

Kolmen BK, Felman HM, Handen BL, et al: Naltrexone in young autistic children: replication study and learning measures. J Am Acad Child Adolesc Psychiatry 36:1570–1578, 1997

Kowatch RA, Carmody TJ, Suppes T, et al: Acute and continuation pharmacological treatment of children and adolescents with bipolar disorders: a summary of two previous studies. Acta Neuropsychiatrica 12:145–149, 2000a

Kowatch RA, Suppes T, Carmody TJ, et al: Effect size of lithium, divalproex sodium, and carbamazepine in children and adolescents with bipolar disorder. J Am Acad Child Adolesc Psychiatry 39:713–720, 2000b

Kowatch RA, Fristad M, Birmaher B, et al: Treatment guidelines for children and adolescents with bipolar disorder. J Am Acad Child Adolesc Psychiatry 44:213–235, 2005

Kramer JR, Loney J, Ponto LB, et al: Predictors of adult height and weight in boys treated with methylphenidate for childhood behavior problems. J Am Acad Child Adolesc Psychiatry 39:517–524, 2000

Kranzler H, Roofeh D, Gerbino-Rosen G, et al: Clozapine: its impact on aggressive behavior among children and adolescents with schizophrenia. J Am Acad Child Adolesc Psychiatry 44:55–63, 2005

Krasny L, Williams BJ, Provencal S, et al: Social skills interventions for the autism spectrum: essential ingredients and a model curriculum. Child Adolesc Psychiatric Clin N Am 12:107–122, 2003

Kratochvil CJ, Heiligenstein JH, Dittmann R, et al: Atomoxetine and methylphenidate treatment in children with ADHD: a prospective, randomized, open-label trial. J Am Acad Child Adolesc Psychiatry 41:776–784, 2002

Kratochvil CJ, Vaughan BS, Harrington MJ, et al: Atomoxetine: a selective noradrenaline reuptake inhibitor for the treatment of attention-deficit/hyperactivity disorder. Expert Opin Pharmacother 4:1165–1174, 2003

Kroes M, Kalfe AC, Kessels AG, et al: Child psychiatric diagnoses in a population of Dutch schoolchildren aged 6 to 8 years. J Am Acad Child Adolesc Psychiatry 40:1401–1409, 2001

Kryzhanovskaya L, Schultz C, McDougle J, et al: A double-blind, placebo-controlled study of olanzapine in adolescents with schizophrenia. Presented at the 159th annual meeting of the American Psychiatric Association, Toronto, Canada, May 20–25, 2006

Kumra S: The diagnosis and treatment of children and adolescents with schizophrenia: "My mind is playing tricks on me." Child Adolesc Psychiatr Clin N Am 9:183–199, 2000

Kumra S, Frazier JA, Jacobsen LK, et al: Childhood-onset schizophrenia. A double-blind clozapine-haloperidol comparison. Arch Gen Psychiatry 53:1090–1097, 1996

Kumra S, Jacobsen LK, Lenane M, et al: Childhood-onset schizophrenia: an open-label study of olanzapine in adolescents. J Am Acad Child Adolesc Psychiatry 37:377–385, 1998

Kunz NR, Khan A, Nicoloacopoulos E, et al: Venlafaxine extended-release for GAD treatment in children and adolescents. Poster presented at the 155th annual meeting of the American Psychiatric Association, Philadelphia, PA, May 18–23, 2002

Kuperman S, Stewart MA: Use of propranolol to decrease aggressive outbursts in younger patients. Psychosomatics 28:315–319, 1987

Kusumakar V, Yatham LN: An open study of lamotrigine in refractory bipolar depression. Psychiatry Res 72:145–148, 1997

Kutcher SP, MacKenzie S: Successful clonazepam treatment of adolescents with panic disorder. J Clin Psychopharmacol 8:299–301, 1988

Kutcher SP, Reiter S, Gardner DM, et al: The pharmacotherapy of anxiety disorders in children and adolescents. Psychiatr Clin North Am 15:41–67, 1992

Kutcher SP, Boulos C, Ward B, et al: Response to desipramine treatment in adolescent depression: a fixed-dose, placebo-controlled trial. J Am Acad Child Adolesc Psychiatry 33:686–694, 1994

Kye CH, Waterman GS, Ryan ND, et al: A randomized, controlled trial of amitriptyline in the acute treatment of adolescent major depression. J Am Acad Child Adolesc Psychiatry 35:1139–1144, 1996

Lafferty JE, Constantino JN: Fluvoxamine in selective mutism. J Am Acad Child Adolesc Psychiatry 37:12–13, 1998

Law SF, Schachar RJ: Do typical clinical doses of methylphenidate cause tics in children treated for attention-deficit hyperactivity disorder? J Am Acad Child Adolesc Psychiatry 38:944–951, 1999

LeBlanc JC, Binder CE, Armenteros JL, et al: Risperidone reduces aggression in boys with a disruptive behaviour disorder and below average intelligence quotient: analysis of two placebo-controlled randomized trials. Int Clin Psychopharmacol 20:275–283, 2005

Leboyer M, Bouvard MP, Lensing P, et al: Opioid excess hypothesis of autism: a double-blind study of naltrexone. Brain Dysfunction 3:285–298, 1990

Leboyer M, Bouvard MP, Launay JM, et al: Brief report: a double-blind study of naltrexone in infantile autism. J Autism Dev Disord 22:309–319, 1992

Leckman JF: Tourette's syndrome. Lancet 360:1577–1586, 2002

Leckman JF, Detlor J, Harcherik DF, et al: Short- and long-term treatment of Tourette's syndrome with clonidine: a clinical perspective. Neurology 35:343–351, 1985

Leckman JF, Hardin MT, Riddle MA, et al: Clonidine treatment of Gilles De La Tourette's syndrome. Arch Gen Psychiatry 48:324–328, 1991

Lena B: Lithium in child and adolescent psychiatry. Arch Gen Psychiatry 36:854–855, 1979

Leonard HL, Swedo SE, Rapoport JL, et al: Treatment of obsessive-compulsive disorder with clomipramine and desipramine in children and adolescents. A double-blind crossover comparison. Arch Gen Psychiatry 46:1088–1092, 1989

Leonard HL, Swedo SE, Lenane MC, et al: A double-blind desipramine substitution during long-term clomipramine treatment in children and adolescents with obsessive-compulsive disorder. Arch Gen Psychiatry 48:922–927, 1991

Leonard HL, Swedo SE, Lanane MC, et al: A 2- to 7-year follow-up study of 54 obsessive-compulsive children and adolescents. Arch Gen Psychiatry 50:429–439, 1993

Leonard HL, Topol D, Bukstein O, et al: Clonazepam as an augmenting agent in the treatment of childhood-onset obsessive-compulsive disorder. J Am Acad Child Adolesc Psychiatry 33:792–794, 1994

Lepola U, Leinonen E, Koponen H: Citalopram in the treatment of early onset panic disorder and school phobia. Pharmacopsychiatry 29:30–32, 1996

Leventhal BL, Cook EH Jr, Morford M, et al: Clinical and neurochemical effects of fenfluramine in children with autism. J Neuropsychiatry Clin Neurosci 5:307–315, 1993

Lewinsohn PM, Klein DN, Seeley JR: Bipolar disorders in a community sample of older adolescents: prevalence, phenomenology, comorbidity, and course. J Am Acad Child Adolesc Psychiatry 34:454–463, 1995

Libby AM, Brent DA, Morrato EH, et al: Decline in treatment of pediatric depression after FDA advisory on risk suicidality with SSRIs. Am J Psychiatry 164:884–891, 2007

Liberthson RR: Sudden death from cardiac causes in children and young adults. N Engl J Med 334:1039–1044, 1996

Lichter DG, Jackson LA: Predictors of clonidine response in Tourette's syndrome: implications and inferences. J Child Neurol 11:93–97, 1996

Liebowitz MR, Turner SM, Piacentini J, et al: Fluoxetine in children and adolescents with OCD: a placebo-controlled trial. J Am Acad Child Adolesc Psychiatry 41:1431–1438, 2002

Linday LA, Tsiouris JA, Cohen IL, et al: Famotidine treatment of children with autistic spectrum disorders: pilot research using single subject research design. J Neural Transm 108:593–611, 2001

Looff D, Grimley P, Kuller F, et al: Carbamazepine for PTSD. J Am Acad Child Adolesc Psychiatry 34:703–704, 1995

Macaluso E, Frith CD, Driver J: Modulation of human visual cortex by cross-modal spatial attention. Science 289:1206–1208, 2000

Malone RP, Delaney MA, Luebbert JF, et al: A double-blind placebo-controlled study of lithium in hospitalized aggressive children and adolescents with conduct disorder. Arch Gen Psychiatry 57:649–654, 2000

Malone RP, Cater J, Sheikh RM, et al: Olanzapine versus haloperidol in children with autistic disorder: an open pilot study. J Am Acad Child Adolesc Psychiatry 40:887–894, 2001

Mancini C, Van Amerigen M, Oakman JM, et al: Serotonergic agents in the treatment of social phobia in children and adolescents: a case series. Depress Anxiety 10:33–39, 1999

March JS, Biederman J, Wolkow R, et al: Sertraline in children and adolescents with obsessive-compulsive disorder: a multicenter randomized controlled trial. JAMA 280:1752–1756, 1998

March JS, Franklin ME, Leonard H, et al: Tics moderate treatment outcome with sertraline but not cognitive-behavior therapy in pediatric obsessive-compulsive disorder. Biol Psychiatry 61:344–347, 2007

Markowitz S, Cuellar A: Antidepressants and youth: healing or harmful? Soc Sci Med 64:2138–2151, 2007

Martin A, Koenig K, Scahill L, et al: Open-label quetiapine in the treatment of children and adolescents with autistic disorder. J Child Adolesc Psychopharmacol 9:99–107, 1999

Masi G, Toni C, Mucci M, et al: Paroxetine in child and adolescent outpatients with panic disorder. J Child Adolesc Psychopharmacol 11:151–157, 2001

Maughan B, Rowe R, Messer J, et al: Conduct disorder and oppositional defiant disorder in a national sample: developmental epidemiology. J Child Psychol Psychiatry 45:609–621, 2004

McClellan J, Werry J: Practice parameter for the assessment and treatment of children and adolescents with schizophrenia. American Academy of Child and Adolescent Psychiatry. J Am Acad Child Adolesc Psychiatry 40 (7 suppl):4S–23S, 2001

McClellan J, Kowatch R, Findling RL: Practice parameter for the assessment and treatment of children and adolescents with bipolar disorder. J Am Acad Child Adolesc Psychiatry 46:107–125, 2007

McConville BJ, Fogelson MH, Norman AB, et al: Nicotine potentiation of haloperidol in reducing tic frequency in Tourette's disorder. Am J Psychiatry 148:793–794, 1991

McConville BJ, Sanberg PR, Fogelson MH, et al: The effects of nicotine plus haloperidol compared to nicotine only and placebo nicotine only in reducing tic severity and frequency in Tourette's disorder. Biol Psychiatry 31:832–840, 1992

McConville BJ, Arvanitis L, Thyrum P, et al: Pharmacokinetics, tolerability, and clinical effectiveness of quetiapine in adolescents with selected psychotic disorders. Eur Neuropsychopharmacol 9 (suppl 5):S267, 1999

McCracken JT, Biederman J, Greenhill LL, et al: Analog classroom assessment of a once-daily mixed amphetamine formulation, SLI381 (Adderall XR), in children with ADHD. J Am Acad Child Adolesc Psychiatry 42:673–683, 2003

McDougle CJ, Kresch LE, Posey DJ: Repetitive thoughts and behavior in pervasive developmental disorders: treatment with serotonin reuptake inhibitors. J Autism Dev Disord 30:427–435, 2000a

McDougle CJ, Scahill L, McCracken JT, et al: Research Units on Pediatric Psychopharmacology (RUPP) Autism Network. Background and rationale for an initial controlled study of risperidone. Child Adolesc Psychiatr Clin N Am 9:201–224, 2000b

McDougle CJ, Kem DL, Posey DJ: Case series: use of ziprasidone for maladaptive symptoms in youths with autism. J Am Acad Child Adolesc Psychiatry 41:921–927, 2002

McDougle CJ, Martin A, Aman M, et al: New findings from the RUPP autism network study of risperidone. Presented at the 51st annual meeting of the American Academy of Child and Adolescent Psychiatry, Washington, DC, October 19–24, 2004

McGough JJ, Biederman J, Wigal SB, et al: Long-term tolerability and effectiveness of once-daily mixed amphetamine salts (Adderall XR) in children with ADHD. J Am Acad Child Adolesc Psychiatry 44:530–538, 2005

McGough J, McCracken J, Swanson J, et al: Pharmacogenetics of methylphenidate response in preschoolers with ADHD. J Am Acad Child Adolesc Psychiatry 45:1314–1322, 2006

McKnew DH, Cytryn L, Buchsbaum MS, et al: Lithium in children of lithium-responding parents. Psychiatry Res 4:171–180, 1981

Mei Z, Grummer-Strawn LM, Thompson D, et al: Shifts in percentiles of growth during early childhood: analysis of longitudinal data from the California Child Health and Development Study. Pediatrics 113:e617–e627, 2004

Meighen KG: Duloxetine treatment of pediatric chronic pain and comorbid major depressive disorder. J Child Adolesc Psychopharmacol 17:121–127, 2007

Melmed RD, Patel A, Konow J, et al: Efficacy and safety of guanfacine extended release for ADHD treatment. Presented at the 53rd annual meeting of the American Academy of Child and Adolescent Psychiatry, San Diego, CA, October 24–29, 2006

Melvin GA, Tonge BJ, King NJ, et al: A comparison of cognitive-behavioral therapy, sertraline, and their combination for adolescent depression. J Am Acad Child Adolescent Psychiatry 45:1151–1161, 2006

Messenheimer JA: Rash in adult and pediatric patients treated with lamotrigine. Can J Neurol Sci 25:S14–S18, 1998

Michelson D: Active comparator studies in the atomoxetine clinical development program. Presented at the 51st Annual Meeting of the American Academy of Child and Adolescent Psychiatry, San Francisco, CA, October 19–24, 2004

Michelson D, Faries D, Wernicke J, et al: Atomoxetine in the treatment of children and adolescents with attention-deficit/hyperactivity disorder: a randomized, placebo-controlled, dose-response study. Pediatrics 108:1–9, 2001

Michelson D, Allen AJ, Busner J, et al: Once-daily atomoxetine treatment for children and adolescents with attention deficit hyperactivity disorder: a randomized, placebo-controlled study. Am J Psychiatry 159:1896–1901, 2002

Michelson D, Adler L, Spencer T, et al: Atomoxetine in adults with ADHD: two randomized, placebo-controlled studies. Biol Psychiatry 53:112–120, 2003

Montgomery SA, Asberg M: A new depression scale designed to be sensitive to change. Br J Psychiatry 134:382–389, 1979

Mosholder A: Psychiatric adverse events in clinical trials of drugs for attention deficit hyperactivity disorder (ADHD). Available at: Food and Drug Administration Website, 2006

Mozes T, Ebert T, Michal SE, et al: An open-label randomized comparison of olanzapine versus risperidone in the treatment of childhood-onset schizophrenia. J Child Adolesc Psychopharmacol 16:393–403, 2006

Mufson L, Sills R: Interpersonal Psychotherapy for depressed adolescents (IPT-A): an overview. Nord J Psychiatry 60:431–437, 2006

Mukaddes NM, Abali O: Quetiapine treatment of children and adolescents with Tourette's Disorder. J Child Adolesc Psychopharmacol 13:295–299, 2003

Murphy TK, Bengtson MA, Soto O, et al: Case series on the use of aripiprazole for Tourette syndrome. Int J Neuropsychopharmacol 8:489–490, 2005

MTA Cooperative Group: 14 Month randomized clinical trial of treatment strategies for children and attention deficit hyperactivity disorder. Arch Gen Psychiatry 56:1073–1086, 1999

MTA Cooperative Group: National Institute of Mental Health Multimodal Treatment Study of ADHD follow-up: changes in effectiveness and growth after the end of treatment. Pediatrics 113:762–769, 2004

MTA Cooperative Group: Effects of stimulant medication on growth rates across 3 years in the MTA follow-up. J Am Acad Child Adolesc Psychiatry 46:1015–1027, 2007

Nader KO, Kriegler JA, Blake DD, et al: Clinician administered PTSD Scale for Children and Adolescents for (DSM-IV) (CAPS-CA). Current and Lifetime Diagnostic Version, and Instruction Manual. A National Center for PTSD/UCLA Trauma Psychiatry Program. Los Angeles, CA, National Center for PTSD and UCLA Trauma Psychiatry Program, 1996

Nagaraj R, Singhi P, Malhi P: Risperidone in children with autism: randomized, place-controlled, double-blind study. J Child Neurol 21:450–455, 2006

Naruse H, Nagahata M, Nakane Y, et al: A multi-center double-blind trial of pimozide (Orap), haloperidol and placebo in children with behavioral disorders, using crossover design. Acta Paedopsychiatr 48:173–184, 1982

Newcorn JH, Spencer TJ, Biederman J, et al: Atomoxetine treatment in children and adolescents with attention-deficit/hyperactivity disorder and comorbid oppositional defiant disorder. J Am Acad Child Adolesc Psychiatry 44:240–248, 2005

Nicolson R, Craven-Thuss B, Smith J, et al: A randomized, double-blind, placebo-controlled trial of metoclopramide for the treatment of Tourette's disorder. J Am Acad Child Adolesc Psychiatry 44:640–646, 2005

Niederhofer H, Staffen W, Mair A: A placebo-controlled study of lofexidine in the treatment of children with tic disorders and attention deficit hyperactivity disorder. J Psychopharmacol 17:113–119, 2003

Olvera RL, Pliszka SR, Luh J, et al: An open trial of venlafaxine in children and adolescents with ADHD. J Child Adolesc Psychopharmacol 6:241–250, 1996

Overall J, Pfefferbaum B: A Brief Psychiatric Rating Scale for Children. Innovations 3:264, 1984

Owley T, McMahon W, Cook EH, et al: Multisite, double-blind, placebo-controlled trial of porcine secretin in autism. J Am Acad Child Adolesc Psychiatry 40:1293–1299, 2001

Owley T, Walton L, Salt J, et al: An open-label trial of escitalopram in pervasive developmental disorders. J Am Acad Child Adolesc Psychiatry 44:343–348, 2005

Pandina GJ, Aman MG, Findling RL, et al: Risperidone in the management of disruptive behavior disorders. J Child Adolesc Psychopharmacol 16:379–392, 2006

Pangalila-Ratulangi EA: Pilot evaluation of Orap (pimozide, R 6238) in child psychiatry. Psychiatr Neurol Neurochir 76:17–27, 1973

Pappadopulos E, Macintyre Ii JC, Crismon ML, et al: Treatment recommendations for the use of antipsychotics for aggressive youth (TRAAY), Part II. J Am Acad Child Adolesc Psychiatry 42:145–161, 2003

Pappadopulos E, Woolston BA, Chait A, et al: Pharmacotherapy of aggression in children and adolescents: efficacy and effect size. J Am Acad Child Adolesc Psychiatry 15:27–39, 2006

Patel NC, DelBello MP, Bryan HS, et al: Open-label lithium for the treatment of adolescents with bipolar depression. J Am Acad Child Adolesc Psychiatry 45:289–297, 2006

Pavuluri MN, Henry DB, Carbray JA, et al: Open-label prospective trial of risperidone in combination with lithium or divalproex sodium in pediatric mania. J Affect Disord 82 (suppl 1):S103–S111, 2004

Pavuluri MN, Henry DB, Carbray JA, et al: A one-year open-label trial of risperidone augmentation in lithium nonresponder youth with preschool-onset bipolar disorder. J Child Adolesc Psychopharmacol 16:336–350, 2006

Pediatric OCD Treatment Study (POTS) Team: Cognitive-behavior therapy, sertraline, and their combination for children and adolescents with obsessive-compulsive disorder. JAMA 292:1969–1976, 2004

Pelham WE, Wheeler T, Chronis A: Empirically supported psychosocial treatments for attention deficit hyperactivity disorder. J Clin Child Psychol 27:190–205, 1998

Pelham WE, Burrows-MacLean L, Gnagy E, et al: Once-a-day OROS methylphenidate versus tid methylphenidate in natural settings. Presented at the 46th Annual Meeting of the American Academy of Child and Adolescent Psychiatry, Chicago, IL, October 19–24, 1999

Pelham WE, Gnagy EM, Burrows-MacLean L, et al: Once-a-day Concerta methylphenidate versus three-times-daily methylphenidate in laboratory and natural settings. Pediatrics 107:e105, 2001

Pelham WE, Burrows-MacLean L, Gnagy EM, et al: Transdermal methylphenidate, behavioral, and combined treatment for children with ADHD. Exp Clin Psychopharmacol 13:111–126, 2005

Perry R, Campbell M, Adams P, et al: Long-term efficacy of haloperidol in autistic children: continuous versus discontinuous drug administration. J Am Acad Child Adolesc Psychiatry 28:87–92, 1989

Piacentini JC, Chang SW: Behavioral treatments for tic suppression: habit reversal training. Adv Neurol 99:227–233, 2006

Piggott LR, Gdowski CL, Villanueva D, et al: Side effects of fenfluramine in autistic children. J Am Acad Child Psychiatry 25:287–289, 1986

Pine DS, Cohen P, Gurley D, et al: The risk for early adulthood anxiety and depressive disorders in adolescent with anxiety and depressive disorders. Arch Gen Psychiatry 55:56–64, 1998

Pliszka SR, Carlson CL, Swanson JM: ADHD With Comorbid Disorders: Clinical Assessment and Management. New York, Guilford, 1999

Pliszka SR, Crismon ML, Hughes CW, et al: The Texas Children's Medication Algorithm Project: revision of the algorithm for pharmacotherapy of attention-deficit/hyperactivity disorder. J Am Acad Child Adolesc Psychiatry 45:642–657, 2006a

Pliszka SR, Matthews TL, Braslow KJ, et al: Comparative effects of methylphenidate and mixed salts amphetamine on height and weight in children with attention-deficit/hyperactivity disorder (ADHD). J Am Acad Child Adolesc Psychiatry 45:520–526, 2006b

Pool D, Bloom W, Mielke DH, et al: A controlled evaluation of loxitane in seventy-five adolescent schizophrenic patients. Curr Ther Res Clin Exp 19:99–104, 1976

Popper CW: Medical unknowns and ethical consent: prescribing psychotropic medications for children in the face of uncertainty, in Psychiatric Pharmacosciences of Children and Adolescents. Edited by Popper CW. Washington, DC, American Psychiatric Press, 1987, pp 127–161

Popper CW: Pharmacologic alternatives to psychostimulants for the treatment of attention-deficit/hyperactivity disorder. Child Adolesc Psychiatr Clin N Am 9:605–646, 2000

Popper CW, Ziminitzky B: Sudden death putatively related to desipramine treatment in youth: a fifth case and a review of speculative mechanisms. J Child Adolesc Psychopharmacol 5:283–300, 1995

Posey DJ, Walsh KH, Wilson GA, et al: Risperidone in the treatment of two very young children with autism. J Child Adolesc Psychopharmacol 9:273–276, 1999

Posey DJ, Guenin KD, Kohn AE, et al: A naturalistic open-label study of mirtazapine in autistic and other pervasive developmental disorders. J Child Adolesc Psychiatry 11:267–277, 2001

Potenza MN, Holmes JP, Kanes SJ, et al: Olanzapine treatment of children, adolescents, and adults with pervasive developmental disorders: an open-label pilot study. J Clin Psychopharmacol 19:37–44, 1999

Poulton A: Growth on stimulant medication: clarifying the confusion: a review. Arch Dis Child 90:801–806, 2005

Poznanski EO, Freman LN, Mokros HB: Children's Depression Rating Scale–Revised. Psychopharmacol Bull 21:979–989, 1985

Preskorn SH, Weller EB, Weller RA: Depression in children: relationship between plasma imipramine levels and response. J Clin Psychiatry 43:450–453, 1982

Prince JB, Wilens TE, Biederman J, et al: A controlled study of nortriptyline in children and adolescents with attention deficit hyperactivity disorder. J Child Adolesc Psychopharmacol 10:193–204, 2000

Puig-Antich J, Perel JM, Lupatkin W, et al: Plasma levels of imipramine (IMI) and desmethylimipramine (DMI) and clinical response in prepubertal major depressive disorder: a preliminary report. J Am Acad Child Psychiatry 18:616–627, 1979

Puig-Antich J, Perel JM, Lupatkin W, et al: Imipramine in prepubertal major depressive disorders. Arch Gen Psychiatry 44:81–89, 1987

Quinn D, Wigal S, Swanson J, et al: Comparative pharmacodynamics and plasma concentrations of d-threo-methylphenidate hydrochloride after single doses of d-threo-methylphenidate hydrochloride and d,l-threo-methylphenidate hydrochloride in a double-blind, placebo-controlled, crossover laboratory school study in children with attention-deficit/hyperactivity disorder. J Am Acad Child Adolesc Psychiatry 43:1422–1429, 2004

Quintana H, Birmaher B, Stedge D, et al: Use of methylphenidate in the treatment of children with autistic disorder. J Autism Dev Disord 25:283–294, 1995

Rasgon NL: The relationship between polycystic ovary syndrome and antiepileptic drugs: a review of the evidence. J Clin Psychopharmacol 24:322–334, 2004

Realmuto GM, Erickson WD, Yellin AM, et al: Clinical comparison of thiothixene and thioridazine in schizophrenic adolescents. Am J Psychiatry 141:440–442, 1984

Realmuto GM, Jensen J, Klykylo W, et al: Untoward effects of fenfluramine in autistic children. J Clin Psychopharmacol 6:350–355, 1986

Realmuto GM, August GJ, Garfinkel BD: Clinical effect of buspirone in autistic children. J Clin Psychopharmacol 9:122–125, 1989

Regeur L, Pakkenberg B, Fog R, et al: Clinical features and long-term treatment with pimozide in 65 patients with Gilles de la Tourette's syndrome. J Neurol Neurosurg Psychiatry 49:791–795, 1986

Reinblatt SP, Walkup JT: Psychopharmacologic treatment of pediatric anxiety disorders. Child Adolesc Psychiatric Clin N Am 14:877–908, 2005

Remington G, Sloman L, Konstantareas M, et al: Clomipramine versus haloperidol in the treatment of autistic disorder: a double-blind, placebo-controlled, crossover study. J Clin Psychopharmacol 21:440–444, 2001

Renaud J, Birmaher B, Wassick SC, et al: Use of selective serotonin reuptake inhibitors for the treatment of childhood panic disorder: a pilot study. J Child Adolescent Psychopharmacology 9:73–83, 1999

Research Units on Pediatric Psychopharmacology Anxiety Study Group: Fluvoxamine for the treatment of anxiety disorders in children and adolescents. N Engl J Med 344:1279–1285, 2001

Research Units on Pediatric Psychopharmacology Anxiety Study Group: The pediatric anxiety rating scale (PARS): development and psychometric properties. J Am Acad Child Adolesc Psychiatry 41:1061–1069, 2002a

Research Units on Pediatric Psychopharmacology Anxiety Study Group: Treatment of pediatric anxiety disorders: an open-label extension of the Research Units on Pediatric Psychopharmacology anxiety study. J Am Acad Child Adolesc Psychiatry 12:175–188, 2002b

Research Units on Pediatric Psychopharmacology Autism Network: Risperidone treatment of autistic disorder: longer-term benefits and blinded discontinuation after 6 months. Am J Psychiatry 162:1361–1369, 2005

Riddle M: Obsessive-compulsive disorder in children and adolescents. Br J Psychiatry 173 (35 suppl):91–96, 1998

Riddle MA, Scahill L, King RA, et al: Double-blind, crossover trial of fluoxetine and placebo in children and adolescents with obsessive-compulsive disorder. J Am Acad Child Adolesc Psychiatry 31:1062–1069, 1992

Riddle MA, Bernstein GA, Cook EH, et al: Anxiolytics, adrenergic agents, and naltrexone. J Am Acad Child Adolesc Psychiatry 38:546–556, 1999

Riddle MA, Reeve EA, Yaryura-Tobias JA, et al: Fluvoxamine for children and adolescents with obsessive-compulsive disorder: a randomized, controlled, multicenter trial. J Am Acad Child Adolesc Psychiatry 40:222–229, 2001

Rifkin A, Karajgi B, Dicker R, et al: Lithium treatment of conduct disorders in adolescents. Am J Psychiatry 154:554–555, 1997

Ritvo ER, Freeman BJ, Geller E, et al: Effects of fenfluramine on 14 outpatients with the syndrome of autism. J Am Acad Child Psychiatry 22:549–558, 1983

Ritvo ER, Freeman BJ, Yuwiler A, et al: Study of fenfluramine in outpatients with the syndrome of autism. J Pediatr 105:823–828, 1984

Ritvo ER, Freeman BJ, Yuwiler A, et al: Fenfluramine treatment of autism: UCLA collaborative study of 81 patients at nine medical centers. Psychopharmacol Bull 22:133–140, 1986

Robb AS, Auby P, Nyilas M, et al: Efficacy of aripiprazole in the treatment of adolescents with schizophrenia. New research poster presented at the 160th Annual Meeting of the American Psychiatric Association, San Diego, CA, May 19–24, 2007

Roberts W, Weaver L, Brian J, et al: Repeated doses of porcine secretin in the treatment of autism: a randomized, placebo-controlled trial. Pediatrics 107:e71, 2001

Roblek T, Piacentini J: Cognitive-behavior therapy for childhood anxiety disorders. Child Adolesc Psychiatric Clin N Am 14:863–876, 2005

Ross DC, Piggott LR: Clonazepam for OCD. J Am Acad Child Adolesc Psychiatry 32:470–471, 1993

Ross DL, Klykylo WM, Hitzemann R: Reduction of elevated CSF beta-endorphin by fenfluramine in infantile autism. Pediatr Neurol 3:83–86, 1987

Rowland AS, Umbach DM, Stallone L, et al: Prevalence of medication treatment for attention deficit-hyperactivity disorder among elementary school children in Johnston County, North Carolina. Am J Public Health 92:231–234, 2002

Rugino TA, Janvier YM: Aripiprazole in children and adolescents: clinical experience. J Child Neurol 20:603–610, 2005

Ryan ND, Puig-Antich J, Rabinovich H, et al: MAOIs in adolescent major depression unresponsive to tricyclic antidepressants. J Am Acad Child Adolesc Psychiatry 27:755–758, 1988

Rynn MA, Siqueland L, Rickels K: Placebo-controlled trial of sertraline in the treatment of children with generalized anxiety disorder. Am J Psychiatry 158:2008–2014, 2001

Rynn MA, Findling RL, Emslie GJ, et al: Efficacy and safety of nefazodone in adolescents with MDD. Poster presented at the

155th annual meeting of the American Psychiatric Association, Philadelphia, PA, May 18–23, 2002

Rynn M, Wagner KD, Donnelly C, et al: Long-term sertraline treatment of children and adolescents with major depressive disorder. J Child Adolescent Psychopharmacol 16:103–113, 2006

Safer D, Zito JM, Fine EM: Increased methylphenidate usage for attention deficit disorder in the 1990s. Pediatrics 98:1084–1088, 1996

Sallee FR, Nesbitt L, Jackson C, et al: Relative efficacy of haloperidol and pimozide in children and adolescents with Tourette's disorder. Am J Psychiatry 154:1057–1062, 1997

Sallee FR, Kurlan R, Goetz CG, et al: Ziprasidone treatment of children and adolescents with Tourette's syndrome: a pilot study. J Am Acad Child Adolesc Psychiatry 39:292–299, 2000

Sallee FR, Miceli JJ, Tensfeldt T, et al: Single-dose pharmacokinetics and safety of ziprasidone in children and adolescents. J Am Acad Child Adolesc Psychiatry 45:720–728, 2006

Sanberg PR, McConville BJ, Fogelson HM, et al: Nicotine potentiates the effects of haloperidol in animals and in patients with Tourette syndrome. Biomed Pharmacother 43:19–23, 1989

Sanberg PR, Shytle RD, Silver AA: Treatment of Tourette's syndrome with mecamylamine. Lancet 352:705–706, 1998

Sandler AD, Sutton KA, DeWeese J, et al: Lack of benefit of a single dose of synthetic human secretin in the treatment of autism and pervasive developmental disorder. N Engl J Med 341:1801–1806, 1999

Sandor P, Musisi S, Moldofsky H, et al: Tourette syndrome: a follow-up study. J Clin Psychopharmacol 10:197–199, 1990

Saxena K, Silverman MA, Chang K, et al: Baseline predictors of response to divalproex in conduct disorder. J Clin Psychiatry 66:1541–1548, 2005

Saxena K, Howe M, Simeonova D, et al: Divalproex sodium reduces overall aggression in youth at high risk for bipolar disorder. J Child Adolesc Psychopharmacol 16:252–259, 2006

Scahill L, Chappell PB, Kim YS, et al: A placebo-controlled study of guanfacine in the treatment of children with tic disorders and attention deficit hyperactivity disorder. Am J Psychiatry 158:1067–1074, 2001

Scahill L, Leckman JF, Schultz RT, et al: A placebo-controlled trial of risperidone in Tourette syndrome. Neurology 60:1130–1135, 2003

Scahill L, Blair J, Leckman JF, et al: Sudden death in a patient with Tourette syndrome during a clinical trial of ziprasidone. J Psychopharmacol 19:205–206, 2005

Schur SB, Sikich L, Findling RL, et al: Treatment recommendations for the use of antipsychotics for aggressive youth (TRAAY). Part I: a review. J Am Acad Child Adolesc Psychiatry 42:132–144, 2003

Schuster CR, Lewis M, Seiden LS: Fenfluramine: neurotoxicity. Psychopharmacol Bull 22:148–151, 1986

Scifo R, Cioni M, Nicolosi A, et al: Opioid-immune interactions in autism: behavioural and immunological assessment during a double-blind treatment with naltrexone. Ann Ist Super Sanita 32:351–359, 1996

Scott DW, Eames P: Use of sulpiride in a case of atypical autism. J Autism Dev Disord 18:144–146, 1988

Seedat S, Lockhat R, Kaminer D, et al: An open trial of citalopram in adolescents with post-traumatic stress disorder. Int Clin Psychopharmacol 16:21–25, 2001

Seedat S, Stein DJ, Ziervogel C, et al: Comparison of response to a selective serotonin reuptake inhibitor in children, adolescents, and adults with posttraumatic stress disorder. J Child Adolesc Psychopharmacology 12:37–46, 2002

Shafey H: Use of lithium and flupenthixol in a patient with pervasive developmental disorder. Am J Psychiatry 143:681, 1986

Shapiro AK, Shapiro E, Eisenkraft GJ: Treatment of Gilles de la Tourette's syndrome with clonidine and neuroleptics. Arch Gen Psychiatry 40:1235–1240, 1983

Shapiro A, Shapiro E, Young J, et al: Gilles de la Tourette Syndrome, 2nd Edition. New York, Raven, 1988

Shapiro E, Shapiro AK, Fulop G, et al: Controlled study of haloperidol, pimozide, and placebo for the treatment of Gilles de la Tourette's syndrome. Arch Gen Psychiatry 46:722–730, 1989

Shaw JA, Lewis JE, Pascal S, et al: A study of quetiapine: efficacy and tolerability in psychotic adolescents. J Child Adolesc Psychopharmacol 11:415–424, 2001

Shaw P, Sporn A, Gogtay N, et al: Childhood-onset schizophrenia: a double-blind, randomized clozapine-olanzapine comparison. Arch Gen Psychiatry 63:721–730, 2006

Shea S, Turgay A, Carroll A, et al: Risperidone in the treatment of disruptive behavioral symptoms in children with autistic and other pervasive developmental disorders. Pediatrics 114:634–641, 2004

Sherman J, Factor DC, Swinson R, et al: The effects of fenfluramine (hydrochloride) on the behaviors of fifteen autistic children. J Autism Dev Disord 19:533–543, 1989

Sikich L, Hamer RM, Bashford RA, et al: A pilot study of risperidone, olanzapine, and haloperidol in psychotic youth: a double-blind, randomized, 8-week trial. Neuropsychopharmacology 29:133–145, 2004

Silva RR, Malone RP, Anderson LT, et al: Haloperidol withdrawal and weight changes in autistic children. Psychopharmacol Bull 29:287–291, 1993

Silver AA, Shytle RD, Philipp MK, et al: Case study: long-term potentiation of neuroleptics with transdermal nicotine in Tourette's syndrome. J Am Acad Child Adolesc Psychiatry 35:1631–1636, 1996

Silver AA, Shytle RD, Philipp MK, et al: Transdermal nicotine and haloperidol in Tourette's disorder: a double-blind placebo-controlled study. J Clin Psychiatry 62:707–714, 2001a

Silver AA, Shytle RD, Sheehan KH, et al: Multicenter, double-blind, placebo-controlled study of mecamylamine monotherapy for Tourette's disorder. J Am Acad Child Adolesc Psychiatry 40:1103–1110, 2001b

Simeon JG: Use of anxiolytics in children. Encephale 19:71–74, 1993

Simeon JG, Ferguson HB: Alprazolam effects in children with anxiety disorders. Can J Psychiatry 32:570–574, 1987

Simeon JG, Ferguson HB, Van-Wyck-Fleet J: Bupropion effects in attention deficit and conduct disorders. Can J Psychiatry 31:581–585, 1986

Simeon JG, Ferguson HB, Knott V, et al: Clinical, cognitive, and neurophysiological effects of alprazolam in children and adolescents with overanxious and avoidant disorders. J Am Acad Child Adolesc Psychiatry 31:29–33, 1992

Simon GE, Savarino J, Operskalski B, et al: Suicide risk during antidepressant treatment. Am J Psychiatry 163:41–47, 2006

Simpson RL: The effects of an antipsychotic medication on the classroom behavior of four schizophrenic male children. J Autism Child Schizophr 7:349–358, 1977

Singer HS, Brown J, Quaskey S, et al: The treatment of attention-deficit hyperactivity disorder in Tourette's syndrome: a double

blind placebo controlled study with clonidine and desipramine. Pediatrics 95:74–81, 1995

Snead RW, Boon F, Presberg J: Paroxetine for self-injurious behavior. J Am Acad Child Adolesc Psychiatry 33:909–910, 1994

Snyder R, Turgay A, Aman M, et al: Effects of risperidone on conduct and disruptive behavior disorders in children with subaverage IQs. J Am Acad Child Adolesc Psychiatry 41:1026–1036, 2002

Søndergård L, Kvist K, Andersen PK, et al: Do antidepressants precipitate youth suicide? A nationwide pharmacoepidemiological study. Eur Child Adolesc Psychiatry 15:232–240, 2006

Spencer EK, Kafantaris V, Padron-Gayol MV, et al: Haloperidol in schizophrenic children: early findings from a study in progress. Psychopharmacol Bull 28:183–186, 1992

Spencer T, Biederman J, Steingard R, et al: Nortriptyline treatment of children with attention deficit hyperactivity disorder and tic disorder or Tourette's syndrome. J Am Acad Child Adolesc Psychiatry 32:205–210, 1993

Spencer T, Biederman J, Coffey B, et al: A double-blind comparison of desipramine and placebo in children and adolescents with chronic tic disorder and comorbid attention-deficit/hyperactivity disorder. Arch Gen Psychiatry 59:649–656, 2002

Spencer TJ, Abikoff HB, Connor DF, et al: Efficacy and safety of mixed amphetamine salts extended release (Adderall XR) in the management of oppositional defiant disorder with or without comorbid attention-deficit/hyperactivity disorder in school-aged children and adolescents: a 4-week, multicenter, randomized, double-blind, parallel-group, placebo-controlled, forced-dose-escalation study. Clin Ther 28:402–418, 2006a

Spencer TJ, Wilens TE, Biederman J, et al: Efficacy and safety of mixed amphetamine salts extended release (Adderall XR) in the management of attention-deficit/hyperactivity disorder in adolescent patients: a 4-week, randomized, double-blind, placebo-controlled, parallel-group study. Clin Ther 28:266–279, 2006b

Staller JA, Staller JA: Intramuscular ziprasidone in youth: a retrospective chart review. J Child Adolesc Psychopharmacol 14:590–592, 2004

Stein MB, Fuetsch M, Muller N, et al: Social anxiety disorder and the risk of depression: a prospective community study of adolescents and young adults. Arch Gen Psychiatry 58:251–256, 2001

Steiner H, Petersen ML, Saxena K, et al: Divalproex sodium for the treatment of conduct disorder: a randomized controlled clinical trial. J Clin Psychiatry 64:1183–1191, 2003

Steingard R, Biederman J: Lithium responsive manic-like symptoms in two individuals with autism and mental retardation. J Am Acad Child Adolesc Psychiatry 26:932–935, 1987

Steingard RJ, Zimnitzky B, DeMaso RD, et al: Sertraline treatment of transition-associated anxiety and agitation in children with autistic disorder. J Child Adolesc Psychopharmacol 7:9–15, 1997

Stephens RJ, Bassel C, Sandor P, et al: Olanzapine in the treatment of aggression and tics in children with Tourette's syndrome—a pilot study. J Child Adolesc Psychopharmacol 14:255–266, 2004

Stern LM, Walker MK, Sawyer MG, et al: A controlled crossover trial of fenfluramine in autism. J Child Psychol Psychiatry 31:569–585, 1990

Storch EA, Lehmkuhl H, Geffken GR, et al: Aripiprazole augmentation of incomplete treatment response in an adolescent male with obsessive-compulsive disorder. Depress Anxiety 25:172–174, 2008

Stubbs EG, Budden SS, Jackson RH, et al: Effects of fenfluramine on eight outpatients with the syndrome of autism. Dev Med Child Neurol 28:229–235, 1986

Sumner CS, Donnelly C, Lopez FA, et al: Atomoxetine treatment for pediatric patients with ADHD and comorbid anxiety. Presented at the annual meeting of the American Psychiatric Association, Atlanta, GA, May 2005

Sverd J: Imipramine treatment of panic disorder in a boy with Tourette's syndrome. J Clin Psychiatry 49:31–32, 1988

Swanson JM, Flockhart D, Udrea D, et al: Clonidine in the treatment of ADHD: questions about safety and efficacy. J Child Adolesc Psychopharmacol 5:301–304, 1995

Swanson JM, Wigal SB, Udrea D, et al: Evaluation of individual subjects in the analog classroom setting, I: examples of graphical and statistical procedures for within-subject ranking of responses to different delivery patterns of methylphenidate. Psychopharmacol Bull 34:825–832, 1998

Swanson J, Gupta S, Guinta D, et al: Acute tolerance to methylphenidate in the treatment of attention deficit hyperactivity disorder in children. Clin Pharmacol Ther 66:295–305, 1999

Swanson J, Greenhill L, Pelham W, et al: Initiating Concerta (OROS methylphenidate HCl) qd in children with attention-deficit hyperactivity disorder. J Clin Res 3:59–76, 2000

Swanson JM, Gupta S, Williams L, et al: Efficacy of a new pattern of delivery of methylphenidate for the treatment of ADHD: effects on activity level in the classroom and on the playground. J Am Acad Child Adolesc Psychiatry 41:1306–1314, 2002

Swanson J, Gupta S, Lam A, et al: Development of a new once-a-day formulation of methylphenidate for the treatment of attention-deficit/hyperactivity disorder: proof-of-concept and proof-of-product studies. Arch Gen Psychiatry 60:204–211, 2003

Swanson JM, Wigal SB, Wigal T, et al: A comparison of once-daily extended-release methylphenidate formulations in children with attention-deficit/hyperactivity disorder in the laboratory school (the Comacs Study). Pediatrics 113:e206–e216, 2004

Swanson JM, Greenhill LL, Lopez FA, et al: Modafinil film-coated tablets in children and adolescents with attention-deficit/hyperactivity disorder: results of a randomized, double-blind, placebo-controlled, fixed-dose study followed by abrupt discontinuation. J Clin Psychiatry 67:137–147, 2006a

Swanson JM, Greenhill LL, Wigal T, et al: Stimulant-related reduction of growth rates in the preschool ADHD treatment study (PATS). J Am Acad Child Adolesc Psychiatry 45:1304–1313, 2006b

Swope GS, Hoopes SP, Amy LS, et al: An open-label study of lamotrigine in adolescents with bipolar mood disorder. New research poster presented at the 157th annual meeting of the American Psychiatric Association, New York, May 1–6, 2004

Tancer NK, Klein RG, Koplewicz HS, et al: Rate of atypical depression and tricyclic drug response in adolescents. J Am Acad Child Adolesc Psychiatry 31:576, 1992

Tanguay PE: Pervasive developmental disorders: a 10-year review. J Am Acad Child Adolesc Psychiatry 39:1079–1095, 2000

Tannock R, Ickowicz A, Schachar R: Differential effects of methylphenidate on working memory in ADHD children with and without comorbid anxiety. J Am Acad Child Adolesc Psychiatry 34:886–896, 1995

Thomsen PH: Child and adolescent obsessive-compulsive disorder treated with citalopram: findings from an open trial of 23 cases. J Child Adolesc Psychopharmacol 7:157–166, 1997

Thomsen PH: Risperidone augmentation in the treatment of severe adolescent OCD in SSRI-refractory cases: a case-series. Ann Clin Psychiatry 16:201–207, 2004

Thomsen PH, Ebbesen C, Persson C: Long-term experience with citalopram in the treatment of adolescent OCD. J Am Acad Child Adolesc Psychiatry 40:895–902, 2001

Todd RD: Fluoxetine in autism. Am J Psychiatry 148:1089, 1991

Tohen M, Kryzhanovskaya L, Carlson G, et al: Olanzapine versus placebo in the treatment of adolescents with bipolar mania. Am J Psychiatry 164:1547–1556, 2007

Tourette's Syndrome Study Group: Treatment of ADHD in children with tics: a randomized controlled trial. Neurology 58:527–536, 2002

Treatment for Adolescents with Depression Study (TADS) Team: Fluoxetine, cognitive-behavioral therapy, and their combination for adolescents with depression. TADS randomized controlled trial. JAMA 292:807–820, 2004

Troost PW, Lahuis BE, Steenhuis MP, et al: Long-term effects of risperidone in children with autism spectrum disorders: a placebo discontinuation study. J Am Acad Child Adolesc Psychiatry 44:1137–1144, 2005

Turgay A, Binder C, Snyder R, et al: Long-term safety and efficacy of risperidone for the treatment of disruptive behavior disorders in children with subaverage IQs. Pediatrics 110:e34, 2002

U.S. Food and Drug Administration: FDA, Final Rule, Regulations Requiring Manufacturers to Assess the Safety and Effectiveness of New Drugs and Biological Products in Pediatric Patients, 63 Fed. Reg. 66,631 (1998); see also 21 CFR §201.23 (1999); 21 CFR §314.55 (1999); 21 CFR §601.27 (1999)

U.S. Food and Drug Administration: FDA News: FDA launches a multi-pronged strategy to strengthen safeguards for children treated with antidepressant medication. October 15, 2004a. Available at: http://www.fda.gov/bbs/topics/news/2004/NEW01124.html. Accessed December 2008.

U.S. Food and Drug Administration: Joint Meeting of the Psychopharmacologic Drugs Advisory Committee and Pediatric Advisory Committee. September 13–14, 2004b. Available at: http://www.fda.gov/ohrms/dockets/ac/04/briefing/2004–4065b1.htm. Accessed December 2008.

U.S. Food and Drug Administration: FDA Alert [09/05]: Suicidal thinking in children and adolescents. Available at: Food and Drug Administration Website, 2005

U.S. Food and Drug Administration: New warning for Strattera. Available at: Food and Drug Administration Website, 2006a

U.S. Food and Drug Administration: Pediatric advisory committee briefing information (March 22, 2006). Available at: Food and Drug Administration Website, 2006b

U.S. Food and Drug Administration: Psychopharmacological drugs advisory committee briefing information (March 23, 2006). Available at: Food and Drug Administration Website, 2006c

U.S. Food and Drug Administration: FDA News: FDA Proposes New Warnings About Suicidal Thinking, Behavior in Young Adults Who Take Antidepressant Medications,.May 2, 2007. Available at: http://www.fda.gov/bbs/topics/NEWS/2007/NEW01624.html. Accessed December 2008.

Valicenti-McDermott MR, Demb H: Clinical effects and adverse reactions of off-label use of aripiprazole in children and adolescents with developmental disabilities. J Child Adolesc Psychopharmacol 16:549–560, 2006

Varley CK, Holm VA: A two-year follow-up of autistic children treated with fenfluramine. J Am Acad Child Adolesc Psychiatry 29:137–140, 1990

Vetro A, Szentistvanyi I, Pallag L, et al: Therapeutic experience with lithium in childhood aggressivity. Neuropsychobiology 14:121–127, 1985

Villalaba L: Follow-up review of AERS search identifying cases of sudden death occurring with drugs used for the treatment of attention deficit hyperactivity disorder (ADHD). Available at: Food and Drug Administration Website, 2006

Vitiello B: Psychopharmacology for young children: clinical needs and research opportunities. Pediatrics 108:983–989, 2001

Volkmar F, Cook EH Jr, Pomeroy J, et al: Practice parameters for the assessment and treatment of children, adolescents, and adults with autism and other pervasive developmental disorders. American Academy of Child and Adolescent Psychiatry Working Group on Quality Issues. J Am Acad Child Adolesc Psychiatry 38 (12 suppl):32S–54S, 1999

Wagner KD, Weller E, Carlson G, et al: An open-label trial of divalproex in children and adolescents with bipolar disorder. J Am Acad Child Adolesc Psychiatry 41:1224–1230, 2002

Wagner KD, Ambrosini P, Rynn M, et al: Efficacy of sertraline in the treatment of children and adolescents with major depressive disorder: two randomized controlled trials. JAMA 290:1033–1041, 2003a

Wagner KD, Cook Eh, Chung H, et al: Remission status after long-term sertraline treatment of pediatric obsessive-compulsive disorder. J Child Adolesc Psychopharmacol 13 (suppl 1):S53–S60, 2003b

Wagner KD, Berard R, Stein MB, et al. A multicenter, randomized, double-blind, placebo-controlled trial of paroxetine in children and adolescents with social anxiety disorder. Arch Gen Psychiatry 61:1153–1162, 2004a

Wagner, KD, Robb AS, Findling RL, et al: A randomized, placebo-controlled trial of citalopram for the treatment of major depression in children and adolescents: Am J Psychiatry 161:1079–1083, 2004b

Wagner KD, Jonas J, Findling RL, et al: A double-blind, randomized, placebo-controlled trial of escitalopram in the treatment of pediatric depression. J Am Acad Child Adolesc Psychiatry 45:280–288, 2006a

Wagner KD, Kowatch RA, Emslie GJ, et al: A double-blind, randomized, placebo-controlled trial of oxcarbazepine in the treatment of bipolar disorder in children and adolescents. Am J Psychiatry 163:1179–1186, 2006b

Waizer J, Polizos P, Hoffman SP, et al: A single-blind evaluation of thiothixene with outpatient schizophrenic children. J Autism Child Schizophr 2:378–386, 1972

Walkup JT, Reeve E, Yaryura-Tobias J, et al: Fluvoxamine for childhood OCD: long-term treatment. Poster presented at the 45th Annual Meeting of the American Academy of Child and Adolescent Psychiatry, Anaheim, CA, October 27–November 1, 1998

Weisler RH, Biederman J, Spencer TJ, et al: Mixed amphetamine salts extended-release in the treatment of adult ADHD: a randomized, controlled trial. CNS Spectr 11:625–639, 2006

Weiss G, Hechtman L: Hyperactive Children Grown Up, 2nd Edition. New York, Guilford, 2003

Wigal SB, Sanchez DY, Decroy DY, et al: Selection of the optimal dose ratio for a controlled-delivery formulation of methylphenidate. J Appl Res 3:46–63, 2003

Wigal S, McGough J, Abikoff HB, et al: Behavioral effects of methylphenidate transdermal system in children with ADHD. Presented at the 52nd Annual Meeting of the American Academy of Child and Adolescent Psychiatry, Toronto, CA, October 18–23, 2005a

Wigal SB, McGough JJ, McCracken JT, et al: A laboratory school comparison of mixed amphetamine salts extended release (Adderall XR) and atomoxetine (Strattera) in school-aged children with attention deficit/hyperactivity disorder. J Atten Disord 9:275–289, 2005b

Wigal T, Greenhill LL, Chuang S, et al: Safety and tolerability of methylphenidate in preschool children with ADHD. J Am Acad Child Adolesc Psychiatry 45:1294–1303, 2006

Wilens TE, Faraone SV, Biederman J, et al: Does stimulant therapy of attention-deficit/hyperactivity disorder beget later substance abuse? A meta-analytic review of the literature. Pediatrics 111:179–185, 2003a

Wilens T, Pelham W, Stein M, et al: ADHD treatment with once-daily OROS methylphenidate: interim 12-month results from a long-term open-label study. J Am Acad Child Adolesc Psychiatry 42:424–433, 2003b

Wilens T, McBurnett K, Stein M, et al: ADHD treatment with once daily OROS methylphenidate treatment: final results from a long term open-label study. J Am Acad Child Adolesc Psychiatry 44:1015–1023, 2005

Wilens TE, McBurnett K, Bukstein O, et al: Multisite controlled study of OROS methylphenidate in the treatment of adolescents with attention-deficit/hyperactivity disorder. Arch Pediatr Adolesc Med 160:82–90, 2006a

Wilens TE, Newcorn JH, Kratochvil CJ, et al: Long-term atomoxetine treatment in adolescents with attention-deficit/hyperactivity disorder. J Pediatr 149:112–119, 2006b

Willemsen-Swinkels SH, Buitelaar JK, Weijen FG, et al: Placebo-controlled acute dosage naltrexone study in young autistic children. Psychiatry Res 58:203–215, 1995

Willemsen-Swinkels SH, Buitelaar JK, van Engeland H: The effects of chronic naltrexone treatment in young autistic children: a double-blind placebo controlled crossover study. Biol Psychiatry 39:1023–1031, 1996

Willemsen-Swinkels SH, Buitelaar JK, van Berckelaer-Onnes IA, et al: Brief report: six months continuation treatment in naltrexone-responsive children with autism: an open-label case-control design. J Autism Dev Disord 29:167–169, 1999

Williams DT, Mehl R, Yudofsky S, et al: The effect of propranolol on uncontrolled rage outbursts in children and adolescents with organic brain dysfunction. J Am Acad Child Psychiatry 21:129–135, 1982

Wolpert A, Hagamen MB, Merlis S: A comparative study of thiothixene and trifluoperazine in childhood schizophrenia. Curr Ther Res Clin Exp 9:482–485, 1967

Wolraich ML: Evaluation of efficacy and safety or OROS methylphenidate HCI (MPH) extended release tablets, methylphenidate tid, and placebo in children with ADHD. Pediatr Res 47:36A, 2000

Wolraich ML, Greenhill LL, Pelham W, et al: Randomized, controlled trial of OROS methylphenidate once a day in children with attention-deficit/hyperactivity disorder. Pediatrics 108:883–892, 2001

Wray JA, Yoon JH, Vollmer T, et al: Pilot study of the behavioral effects of flumazenil in two children with autism. J Autism Dev Disord 30:619–620, 2000

Wright HH, Cuccaro ML, Leonhardt TV, et al: Case study: fluoxetine in the multimodal treatment of a preschool child with selective mutism. J Am Acad Child Adolesc Psychiatry 34:857–862, 1995

Yarbrough E, Santat U, Perel I, et al: Effects of fenfluramine on autistic individuals residing in a state developmental center. J Autism Dev Disord 17:303–314, 1987

Yoo HK, Kim JY, Kim CY: A pilot study of aripiprazole in children and adolescents with Tourette's disorder. J Child Adolesc Psychopharmacol 16:505–506, 2006

Young RC, Biggs JT, Ziegler VE, et al: A rating scale for mania: reliability, validity and sensitivity. Br J Psychiatry 133:429–435, 1978

Zito JM, Safer DJ, dosReis S, et al: Trends in the prescribing of psychotropic medications in preschoolers. JAMA 283:1025–1030, 2000

Zohar AH: The epidemiology of obsessive-compulsive disorder in children and adolescents. Child Adolesc Psychiatr Clin N Am 8:445–460, 1999

Zuddas A, Ledda MG, Fratta A, et al: Clinical effects of clozapine on autistic disorder. Am J Psychiatry 153:738, 1996

Zwier KJ, Rao U: Buspirone use in an adolescent with social phobia and mixed personality. J Am Acad Child Adolesc Psychiatry 33:1007–1011, 1994

Appendix

Psychotropic Medications Commonly Prescribed for Children and Adolescents

This Appendix describes common classes of psychotropic medications used to treat children and adolescents. Dosages, common side effects, and monitoring schedules are presented for each medication class.

Antidepressants

Dosage and monitoring. The starting and target doses of antidepressants for children and adolescents are listed in Table 63–1.

Premedication laboratories include complete blood count, blood chemistries, and liver function tests. Blood pressure should be monitored during dose titration with venlafaxine.

The FDA has issued the following black box warning, which applies to all antidepressants (U.S. Food and Drug Administration 2007):

> Antidepressants increased the risk compared to placebo of suicidal thinking and behavior (suicidality) in children, adolescents, and young adults in short-term studies of major depressive disorder (MDD) and other psychiatric disorders. Anyone considering the use of [*Name of Antidepressant*] or any other antidepressant in a child, adolescent, or young adult must balance this risk with the clinical need. Short-term studies did not show an increase in the risk of suicidality with antidepressants compared with placebo in adults beyond age 24 years; there was a reduction in risk with antidepressants compared with placebo in adults ages 65 years and older. Depression and certain other psychiatric disorders are themselves associated with increases in the risk of suicide. Patients of all ages who are started on antidepressant therapy should be monitored appropriately and observed closely for clinical worsening, suicidality, or unusual changes in behavior. Families and caregivers should be advised of the need for close observation and communication with the prescriber.

Side effects. Common side effects of selective serotonin reuptake inhibitors (SSRIs) are headache, nausea, abdominal pain, dry mouth, insomnia, and somnolence (Emslie et al. 2002; Keller et al. 2001; Wagner et al. 2003a, 2004b, 2006a). Potential serious adverse events include serotonin syndrome, extrapyramidal symptoms (tics, myoclonus), amotivational syndrome, and increased bleeding (Hammerness et al. 2006). A major advantage of SSRIs is their safety in overdose (Barbey and Roose 1998).

TABLE 63–1. Clinical use of antidepressants in children and adolescents

MEDICATION	TYPICAL STARTING DOSE (MG)		TARGET DOSE (MG/DAY)
	CHILD	ADOLESCENT	
Citalopram	5–10	10	20–40
Escitalopram	5	10	10–20
Fluoxetine	5–10	10	20–40
Paroxetine	5–10	10	20–40
Sertraline	25	50	100–200
Mirtazapine	15	15	30–45
Venlafaxine	37.5	37.5	150–225
Bupropion	50 bid	50 bid	100–200

Common side effects of mirtazapine are somnolence, increased appetite, weight gain, dizziness, dry mouth, and constipation (Green 2001).

Common side effects of venlafaxine include anorexia, abdominal pain, insomnia, somnolence, dizziness, dry mouth, increased sweating and nervousness, and elevated blood pressure with dose increase (Emslie et al. 2007a; Green 2001).

Common side effects of bupropion are headache, nausea, rash, irritability, drowsiness, fatigue, and anorexia (Barrickman et al. 1995; Conners et al. 1996; Daviss et al. 2001). Bupropion is contraindicated in children with seizure disorders, since it may lower the seizure threshold.

Atomoxetine

Dosage and monitoring. Atomoxetine can be given in the late afternoon or evening, whereas stimulants generally cannot; atomoxetine may have less pronounced effects on appetite and sleep than stimulants, though it may produce relatively more nausea or sedation. Gastrointestinal distress can be minimized by taking the medication after a meal. In children and young adolescents, atomoxetine is initiated at a dosage of 0.3 mg/kg/day and titrated over 1–3 weeks to a maximum dosage of 1.2–1.8 mg/kg/day (Kratochvil et al. 2003). Adults or adult-sized adolescents should be started on atomoxetine 40 mg daily and titrated to atomoxetine 80–100 mg/day over 1–3 weeks, if needed (Kratochvil et al. 2003). Atomoxetine's labeling recommends both once-daily and twice-daily dosing, although its elimination half-life of 5 hours (as well as clinical experience) suggests that twice-daily dosing (early A.M. and early P.M) is more effective and less prone to cause side effects. Michelson et al. (2002) showed that while atomoxetine was superior to placebo at week 1 of the trial, its greatest effects were observed at week 6, suggesting that patients should be maintained at the full therapeutic dose for at least several weeks in order to observe the drug's full effects.

Side effects.   Side effects of atomoxetine that occurred more often than placebo in clinical trials included gastrointestinal distress, sedation, and decreased appetite. These can generally be managed by dosage adjustment and often attenuate with time. On December 17, 2004, the FDA required that a warning be added to atomoxetine due to reports of two patients (an adult and child) who developed severe liver disease (U.S. Food and Drug Administration 2006a). Both patients recovered. The FDA has also issued an alert regarding suicidal thinking with atomoxetine in children and adolescents (U.S. Food and Drug Administration 2005). A black box warning is included in the package insert. In 12 controlled trials involving 1,357 patients on atomoxetine and 851 on placebo, the average risk of suicidal thinking was 4 per 1,000 in the atomoxetine-treated group versus none in the placebo group.

Atypical Antipsychotics

Dosage and monitoring.   Typical starting and target dosages of atypical antipsychotics are listed in Table 63–2.

Premedication laboratories include complete blood count, blood chemistries, and liver function tests. In addition, the American Diabetes Association et al. (2004) recommendations should be followed. These include baseline body mass index (BMI), waist circumference, blood pressure, and fasting glucose and lipid panels. BMI should be followed monthly for 3 months, and then measured quarterly. Blood pressure, fasting glucose, and lipid panels should be followed up at 3 months and then yearly. Monitoring should also be done for extrapyramidal side effects.

Side effects.   Side effects of atypical antipsychotics include weight gain, dyslipidemia, insulin resistance and diabetes, hyperprolactinemia, extrapyramidal side effects and akathisia, QTc prolongation, sedation, liver toxicity, neutropenia, and neuroleptic malignant syndrome. Clozapine has also been associated with seizures, agranulocytosis, and myocarditis (Correll et al. 2006).

Clonidine

Dosage and monitoring.   Clonidine is initiated at 0.05 mg/day, with dose increases of 0.05 mg every 3 days.

TABLE 63–2.   Clinical use of atypical antipsychotics in children and adolescents

MEDICATION	TYPICAL STARTING DOSE (MG)	TARGET DOSE (MG/DAY)
Clozapine	25 twice daily	200–400
Olanzapine	2.5 twice daily	10–20
Quetiapine	50 twice daily	400–600
Risperidone	0.25 twice daily	1–2
Ziprasidone	20 twice daily	80–120
Aripiprazole	2.5–5.0 at bedtime	10–25

Source.   DelBello and Kowatch 2006.

Typical dosages for ADHD are in the range of total 0.15–0.3 mg/day (on a three-times-per-day schedule). Transdermal clonidine delivers doses of 0.1, 0.2, or 0.3 mg/day. During initial treatment, a temporary worsening of motor and phonic tics in Tourette's syndrome may occur, which usually resolves within 2–4 weeks. Clonidine should be tapered by 0.05 mg/day upon discontinuation (Hunt et al. 1990).

Given the reports of adverse cardiovascular side effects in children taking clonidine, recommendations have been made regarding cardiovascular monitoring (Cantwell et al. 1997). Pulse and blood pressure should be measured at baseline, weekly during titration of dose, and every 4–6 weeks during maintenance treatment. ECGs should be obtained at baseline and after the maximal dose of clonidine is achieved. Abrupt discontinuation of clonidine is not recommended, because it increases the risk of adverse cardiovascular side effects, particularly hypertension.

Side effects.   Common side effects of clonidine in children are sedation, depression, irritability, hypotension, sleep disturbance, dry mouth, and dizziness. Skin irritation and erythema are common with the clonidine patch (Connor et al. 1999; Hunt et al. 1990). Rebound tachycardia and hypertension may occur if clonidine is abruptly discontinued, particularly after chronic use (Popper 2000).

Safety concerns have been raised about the combination of clonidine and methylphenidate, following the report of four cases of sudden death in children on this medication combination (Cantwell et al. 1997; Fenichel 1995). Swanson et al. (1995) described two types of clonidine-related cardiovascular side effects. In one type, fatigue and sedation were associated with a decrease in pulse and blood pressure and changes in ECG. In the other, tachycardia and tachypnea occurred, which led to anxiety, fever, and changes in mental status. Adverse cardiovascular side effects, including bradycardia and depressed level of consciousness, have been reported with clonidine overdose in children (Kappagoda et al. 1998). However, in a retrospective study of 42 children treated with clonidine alone or clonidine plus stimulants, no systematic effects were found on ECG parameters of pulse rate or QTc intervals (Kofoed et al. 1999).

Guanfacine

Dosage and monitoring.   Guanfacine is initiated at a daily dose of 0.5 mg, with an upward titration of 0.5 mg every 3 days, based on clinical response and tolerability, to a maximum daily dose of 4 mg (Hunt et al. 1995).

Pulse and blood pressure should be monitored during guanfacine treatment. Guanfacine should be tapered over a 4-day period upon discontinuation.

Side effects.   Common side effects of guanfacine in children are sedation, fatigue, headache, dizziness, stomachache, and decreased appetite (Chappell et al. 1995b; Hunt et al. 1995; Melmed et al. 2006; Scahill et al. 2001). Rebound hypertension, nervousness, and anxiety may occur if guanfacine is abruptly discontinued (Green 2001).

Mood Stabilizers

Dosage and monitoring.   The starting dose and target doses and therapeutic serum levels of mood stabilizers are listed in Table 63–3.

Premedication laboratories in general include complete blood count, liver function tests, and pregnancy test (for females).

For lithium, baseline thyroid function tests, electrolytes, urinalysis, blood urea nitrogen, creatinine, and serum calcium should also be obtained. Lithium levels, renal function, thyroid function, and urinalysis should be monitored every 3–6 months.

For divalproex, drug serum levels, complete blood count, and liver function tests should be monitored every 3–6 months. Given concerns about a possible relationship between divalproex and polycystic ovarian syndrome (PCOS) (Rasgon 2004), female adolescents taking divalproex should be monitored for signs of PCOS, including menstrual abnormalities, weight gain, acne, and hirsutism (DelBello and Kowatch 2006; McClellan et al. 2007). Parents and their female adolescents should be apprised about this possible association prior to initiating medication.

For oxcarbazepine, children should be monitored for hyponatremia.

Side effects.   Common side effects of lithium in children and adolescents include hypothyroidism, nausea, polyuria, polydypsia, acne, tremor, and weight gain (DelBello and Kowatch 2006).

Common side effects of divalproex in children and adolescents include weight gain, nausea, sedation, and tremor (DelBello and Kowatch 2006). Concern has been raised about a possible association between divalproex and PCOS (Rasgon 2004). Other potential side effects of concern are hepatic failure, pancreatitis, thrombocytopenia, behavioral deterioration, and hair loss (Davanzo and McCracken 2000; Green 2001).

Side effects of topiramate include decreased appetite, weight loss, nausea, diarrhea, paresthesias, somnolence, and word-finding difficulties (DelBello and Kowatch 2006; DelBello et al. 2005).

TABLE 63–3.   Clinical use of mood stabilizers in children and adolescents

MEDICATION	TYPICAL STARTING DOSE (MG)	TARGET DOSE	THERAPEUTIC SERUM LEVEL
Carbamazepine	7 mg/kg/day	Based on response and serum level	8–11 µg/L
Lamotrigine	12.5 mg once daily	Based on response	NA
Lithium	25 mg/kg/g (2–3 daily doses)	30 mg/kg/day (2–3 daily doses)	0.8–1.2 mEq/L
Oxcarbazepine	150 mg twice daily	20–29 kg (900 mg/day) 30–39 kg (1,200 mg/day) >39 kg (1,800 mg/day)	NA
Topiramate	25 mg once daily	100–400 mg/day	NA
Valproic acid, divalproex sodium	20 mg/kg/day (2 daily doses)	20 mg/kg/day (2–3 daily doses)	90–120 µg/mL

Source.   DelBello and Kowatch 2006.

TABLE 63–4.   Clinical use of psychostimulants in children and adolescents

MEDICATION	DOSAGE FORM	TYPICAL STARTING DOSE	FDA MAX/DAY	OFF-LABEL MAX/DAY
Amphetamine preparations				
Adderall	5, 7.5, 10, 12.5, 15, 20, 30 mg	3–5 yr: 2.5 mg qd ≥6 yr: 5 mg qd–bid	40 mg	>50 kg: 60 mg
Dexedrine	5 mg	3–5 yr: 2.5 mg qd ≥6 yr: 5 mg qd-bid	40 mg	>50 kg: 60 mg
DextroStat	5, 10 mg	3–5 yr: 2.5 mg qd ≥6 yr: 5 mg qd–bid	40 mg	>50 kg: 60 mg
Dexedrine Spansule	5, 10, 15 mg	≥6 yr: 5–10 mg qd–bid	40 mg	>50 kg: 60 mg
Adderall XR	5, 10, 15, 20, 25, 30 mg	≥6 yr: 10 mg qd	30 mg	>50 kg: 60 mg
Vyvanse	30, 50, 70 mg	30 mg qd	70 mg	Not determined
Methylphenidate preparations				
Focalin	2.5, 5, 10 mg	2.5 mg bid	20 mg	50 mg
Focalin XR	5, 10, 15, 20 mg	5 mg q A.M.	30 mg	50 mg
Methylin	5, 10, 20 mg	5 mg bid	60 mg	>50 kg: 100 mg
Metadate ER	10, 20 mg	10 mg q A.M.	60 mg	>50 kg: 100 mg
Methylin ER	10, 20 mg	10 mg q A.M.	60 mg	>50 kg: 100 mg
Ritalin SR	20 mg	10 mg q A.M.	60 mg	>50 kg: 100 mg
Metadate CD	10, 20, 30, 40, 50, 60 mg	20 mg q A.M.	60 mg	>50 kg: 100 mg
Ritalin LA	20, 30, 40 mg	20 mg q A.M.	60 mg	Not yet known
Concerta	18, 27, 36, 54 mg	18 mg q A.M.	72 mg	108 mg
Daytrana patch	10-, 15-, 20-, 30-mg patches	Begin with 10-mg patch qd, then titrate up by patch strength	30 mg	Not yet known

Note.   qd = once daily; bid = twice daily; q A.M. = every morning.

Side effects of oxcarbazepine in children include dizziness, nausea, somnolence, diplopia, fatigue, and rash (Wagner et al. 2006b). Hyponatremia is also a side effect of oxcarbazepine.

Common side effects of lamotrigine in children include ataxia, nausea, vomiting, and constipation. Of concern is the incidence of serious rash, including Stevens-Johnson syndrome, in pediatric patients reported to be 1%. This high incidence of serious rash may be attributable to the prior use of high doses of lamotrigine with concomitant divalproex (Messenheimer et al. 1998). The current dosing guidelines may reduce this rash incidence in pediatric patients.

Psychostimulants

Dosage and monitoring.   The American Academy of Child and Adolescent Psychiatry (2007) recently revised its parameters for the diagnosis and treatment of attention-deficit/hyperactivity disorder ADHD). A wide variety of stimulant preparations are available; Table 63–4 describes their use in clinical practice. Each stimulant has a maximum dose suggested by the U.S. Food and Drug Administration (FDA)–approved package insert, but higher off-label doses are commonly used with careful monitoring. In terms of safety monitoring, pulse, blood pressure, weight, and height should be obtained at baseline and at least annually. No laboratory measures or electrocardiogram (ECG) monitoring is required.

Side effects.   Common side effects of psychostimulants are insomnia, diminished appetite, weight loss, irritability, abdominal pain, and headaches (American Academy of Child and Adolescent Psychiatry 2007). Rebound symptoms of worsening behavior may occur when the effects of the short-acting psychostimulants dissipate. Switching to sustained-release or longer-acting psychostimulants may ameliorate rebound symptoms.

There is no evidence that psychostimulants increase substance abuse in youths with ADHD. On the contrary, youths with ADHD who were treated with psychostimulants were at less risk for developing substance abuse than those youths with ADHD who did not receive stimulants (Wilens et al. 2003a). Motor tics may develop during treatment with stimulants, but one study reported no increase in tics for children with or without preexisting tics who received typical clinical doses of methylphenidate compared with placebo (Law and Schachar 1999).

The FDA and its Pediatric Advisory Committee have reviewed data regarding psychiatric adverse events to stimulant medication (U.S. Food and Drug Administration 2006b). Data from both controlled trials and postmarketing safety data from sponsors and the FDA Adverse Events Reporting System (AERS), also referred to as MedWatch, were reviewed. For most of the agents, these events were slightly more common in the active-drug group relative to placebo in the controlled trials, but these differences did not reach statistical significance (Mosholder 2006). Postmarketing safety data were also reviewed for reports of mania/psychotic symptoms, aggression, and suicidality (Gelperin 2006). Rare events of suicidal thoughts, manic-like activation, or psychosis were reported. At the time, the Pediatric Advisory Committee did not recommend a black box warning regarding psychiatric adverse events but did suggest clarifying labeling regarding these phenomena. No changes to the stimulant medication labeling were suggested regarding suicide or suicidal ideation.

There have been rare reports of sudden death in patients taking stimulant medication The FDA has record of 20 cases of sudden death with amphetamine or dextroamphetamine (14 children, 6 adults), while there were 14 pediatric and 4 adult cases of sudden death with methylphenidate (Villalaba 2006). It is important to note that the rate of sudden death in the general pediatric population has been estimated at 1.3–8.5 per 100,000 patient-years (Liberthson 1996). The rate of sudden death among those with a history of congenital heart disease can be as high as 6% by age 20 years (Liberthson 1996). Villalaba (2006) estimated the rate of sudden death in treated ADHD children for the exposure period January 1, 1992, to December 31, 2004, to be 0.2 per 100,000 patient-years for methylphenidate, 0.3 per 100,000 patient-years for amphetamine, and 0.5 per 100,000 patient-years for atomoxetine (the differences between the agents are not clinically meaningful). Thus, the rate of sudden death of children on ADHD medications does not appear to exceed the base rate of sudden death in the general popula-

tion; therefore, cardiac monitoring of healthy children during treatment with stimulants is not required. Children with preexisting heart disease (or significant symptoms suggesting the condition) should obtain a cardiology consultation prior to starting a stimulant.

Poulton (2005) reviewed growth data and concluded that stimulant treatment may be associated with a reduction in expected height gain, at least in the first 1–3 years of treatment. The National Institute of Mental Health (NIMH) Multimodal Treatment of ADHD (MTA) study showed reduced growth rates in ADHD patients after 2 years of stimulant treatment compared with patients who received no medication (MTA Cooperative Group 2004), and these deficits persisted at 36 months (MTA Cooperative Group 2007). The PATS study followed a group of 140 preschoolers who received methylphenidate for up to a year for ADHD (Swanson et al. 2006b). The subjects had less than expected mean gains in height (−1.38 cm) and weight (−1.3 kg). Charach et al. (2006) found that higher doses of stimulant correlated with reduced gains in height and weight and that the effect did not become significant until the dose in methylphenidate equivalents was >2.5 mg/kg/day for 4 years. Pliszka et al. (2006b) did not find that children with ADHD treated with monotherapy with either amphetamine or methylphenidate showed any failure to achieve expected height; furthermore the two stimulant classes did not have any differential effect on height, but amphetamine had somewhat greater effects on weight than methylphenidate. The subjects in this study had drug holidays averaging 31% of time during their treatment course, which may have contributed to the lack of effect of the stimulant on height.

In assessing for clinically significant growth reduction, it is recommended to use serial plotting of height and weight on growth charts labeled with lines showing the major percentiles (5th, 10th, 25th, 50th, 75th, 90th, and 95th) (Mei et al. 2004). This should occur one to two times per year, and more frequently if practical. If the patient has a change in height or weight that crosses 2 percentile lines, this suggests an aberrant growth trajectory. In these cases, a drug holiday should be considered, if return of symptoms during weekends or summers does not lead to marked impairment of functioning. The clinician should also consider switching the patient to another ADHD medication. It is important for the clinician to carefully balance the benefits of medication treatment with the risks of small reductions in height gain, which as of yet have not been shown to be related to reductions in adult height (Gittelman-Klein and Mannuzza 1988; Kramer et al. 2000; Weiss and Hechtman 2003).

CHAPTER 64

Psychopharmacology During Pregnancy and Lactation

D. Jeffrey Newport, M.D.

Susana V. Fernandez, B.A.

Sandra Juric, B.A.

Zachary N. Stowe, M.D.

The management of mental illness during pregnancy and lactation represents a unique and complex clinical situation involving a minimum of two concomitant medical conditions (i.e., pregnancy and a psychiatric disorder) and also demanding consideration of the welfare of at least two patients (i.e., mother and child), not to mention the potential impact of maternal illness on the family at large. The American College of Obstetricians and Gynecologists Practice Bulletin on the use of psychotropic medications during pregnancy and lactation acknowledges the potential adverse impact of untreated or inadequately treated maternal mental illness (American College of Obstetricians and Gynecologists 2007).

Given the high incidence of psychiatric disorders among women during the childbearing years, the increasing proportion of women who plan to nurse, and the introduction of new psychotropic medications that are less likely to interfere with female reproductive physiology (e.g., second-generation antipsychotics [SGAs]), clinicians will be more frequently confronted with this complex dilemma. The most common scenarios in which physicians provide care for a patient with a mental disorder while she is pregnant or nursing include the following:

- Preconception consultation with a patient who wishes to have a baby but who has a history of a chronic or re-

current psychiatric illness and/or who currently takes one or more psychotropic medications
- Urgent consultation in early pregnancy with a patient who has inadvertently conceived during treatment with one or more psychotropic medications
- Provision of treatment to a patient who is experiencing an exacerbation of a preexisting mental illness during pregnancy or the postpartum, often after having discontinued pharmacological treatment proximate to conception
- Provision of treatment to a patient who is experiencing the onset of a new mental illness during pregnancy or the postpartum
- Formulation of plans during pregnancy to provide prophylactic treatment at some juncture to a patient who is at high risk for postpartum mental illness

Despite rapid advances, the extant literature regarding psychotropic therapy during pregnancy and lactation remains hampered by a cadre of confounds that preclude definitive treatment guidelines. Existing studies lack methodological consistency and are often without the requisite sample size or study design necessary to establish a significant causal relation for deleterious effects of psychotropic medications. Specific methodological concerns include 1) limited effort to control for the concomitant effect of maternal illness on obstetrical and infant outcome; 2) limited effort to control for the potentially confounding effects of other nonpsychotropic exposures that might accompany maternal mental illness; 3) failure to provide objective confirmation of purported exposures, with a tacit assumption of full maternal psychotropic compliance and disclosure of other concomitant exposures (e.g., tobacco, alcohol); and 4) widespread reliance on retrospective recall to document exposures and/or outcomes (even in many so-called prospective studies) months or even years after delivery, with a potential for systematic recall bias. As early as 6 months after delivery, maternal retrospective reports demonstrate systematically biased underreporting of depression and use of nonpsychotropic agents during pregnancy, whereas use of psychotropic agents is accurately reported (Newport et al. 2008b).

The proper assessment of the risk to offspring attributable to psychotropic exposure must consider the baseline frequencies of obstetrical complications and developmental anomalies, the timeline of embryonic and fetal development, the potential risks of exposure to nonpsychotropic medications, and the potential risks associated with untreated maternal psychiatric illness. In the United States, 84.5% of pregnancies result in a live delivery (Kiely 1991; McBride 1972). Recent birth registry data collectively comprising nearly 2.5 million deliveries in New York State and Sweden indicate that 3%–4% of these infants will suffer from major malformations (New York State Department of Health 2005; Swedish Centre for Epidemiology 2004). Most major malformations occur during the embryonic period (i.e., the third through the eighth week of gestation), and most organ systems (with the notable exception of the central nervous system [CNS]) are developed by the conclusion of week 11 (Sadler 1985). Finally, it must be noted that medications are prescribed to up to 80% of pregnant women (Cohen et al. 1989), and more than one-third take a psychotropic medication at some point during pregnancy (Doering and Stewart 1978).

Because clinical experience indicates that the principal goal of both patient and clinician is to minimize potentially harmful offspring exposure, we propose in this chapter a rational model for developing perinatal treatment guidelines that is founded on the shared conviction that minimizing infant exposure to the effects of both maternal illness and maternal treatment is the preeminent objective. We subsequently review the available data regarding pharmacokinetic and pharmacodynamic alterations during pregnancy and lactation and describe the clinical relevance of these data for psychotropic dose

management and forecasting of offspring exposure. We then review the available data regarding the potential risks of pharmacotherapy during pregnancy or lactation with specific psychotropic agents from various medication classes, including antidepressants, mood stabilizers, antipsychotics, and anxiolytics. We conclude the chapter with a review of the future directions for perinatal psychiatric research and a discussion of potential modifications of previously suggested treatment guidelines, emphasizing the need for an individualized risk–benefit assessment.

A Model for Treatment Guidelines During Pregnancy and Lactation: Minimizing Offspring Exposure

The clinical management of any medical condition during pregnancy and lactation is one of "relative safety" that must consider the reproductive safety of available therapies, the likelihood of illness relapse or exacerbation in the absence of continued treatment, and the potential impact of untreated maternal illness. Minor ailments, including headaches, nausea, insomnia, and localized infections, are routinely treated during pregnancy with medications that often have limited reproductive safety data. Conversely, women with mental illness are often encouraged to discontinue psychotropic medication during pregnancy and lactation. The underlying desire to avoid offspring psychotropic exposure is laudable; however, such recommendations are often made with limited knowledge of the potential adverse obstetrical effects of maternal mental illness and an assumption that psychotropic medications are poorly represented in the reproductive safety database. Comprehensive treatment guidelines for perinatal psychiatric illness must therefore incorporate an appraisal of the clinical consequences of offspring exposure to both maternal illness and available therapies.

When the clinician conducts a risk–benefit assessment for new or expectant mothers with mental illness, it must first be acknowledged that the possibility of offspring exposure, to either treatment or illness, is always present. Advising a pregnant or breast-feeding patient to discontinue psychotropic medication does not eliminate offspring exposure; it simply exchanges the risks of psychotropic exposure for the risks of untreated maternal illness. A thorough risk–benefit assessment also requires an understanding of the pathways of offspring exposure. In the context of perinatal psychiatric illness, fetal/neonatal exposure may occur either directly or indirectly (Stowe et al. 2001). *Direct exposure* is imparted by any biological or pharmacological substrate that comes into direct contact with the child. *Indirect exposure* is conferred by the influence of such a substrate on the child's environment.

Direct exposure to psychotropic agents is a given. All psychotropics studied to date cross the placenta (Hendrick et al. 2003b; Newport et al. 2005, 2007; Stowe et al. 1997), are present in amniotic fluid (Hostetter et al. 2000), and are excreted into breast milk (Newport et al. 2002a). Clinicians often assume that liability exists only for those direct exposures to medications that are under their immediate control, but other exposures should engender concern. The fetus and breast-feeding infant are also directly exposed to maternal illness via changes in the hormonal and immunological constituents within the fetomaternal circulation (Wadhwa et al. 1998) and breast milk (Cox et al. 2000). The magnitude and clinical significance of these direct exposures to the substrates of maternal illness remain obscure.

Indirect exposures to illness or treatment are also possible, although less readily apparent. Indirect effects of maternal psychiatric illness on offspring may be mediated by poor maternal compliance with prenatal care, inadequate maternal nutrition, exposure to other prescription or over-the-counter medications or herbal remedies, increased use of alcohol and tobacco, deficits in mother–infant bonding, and disruptions within the family environment. Indirect exposure to psychotropic therapy may be conferred by treatment-emergent side effects (e.g., somnolence, alterations in appetite).

Assessing the risks of offspring exposure to maternal psychiatric illness must consider both the likelihood that an episode of illness will occur and the evidence that the illness may be harmful to the child. The clinician can estimate a patient's likelihood of peripartum recurrence or exacerbation by carefully synthesizing prevalence data from epidemiological studies with evidence from the patient's own history. Gathering comprehensive personal and family psychiatric histories is critical to treatment planning. Patients with frequent episodes of psychiatric illness, a declining course, or a history of prior perinatal illness are more likely to become ill in the current puerperium. Because many psychiatric disorders are more prevalent in women than in men, and most begin early in life, typically during or even before the reproductive years, clinicians routinely provide treatment to women for mental illnesses during the childbearing years. Efforts to determine the precise incidence of perinatal psychiatric illness are hindered by several factors: 1) the overlap of symptoms between certain mental illnesses and the normal sequelae of pregnancy, 2) the reliance on retrospec-

tive reports in many studies, and 3) the limited assessment of comorbid medical disorders that could contribute to psychiatric symptoms (e.g., anemia, thyroid dysfunction) (Pedersen et al. 1993).

Prevalence of Psychiatric Disorders During Pregnancy and the Postpartum Period

Despite the clinical lore that pregnancy is a time of emotional well-being, rates of depression during pregnancy are comparable to those of nonpuerperal depression (Buesching et al. 1988; Cutrona 1986; Kumar and Robson 1984; Manly et al. 1982; O'Hara et al. 1982; Watson et al. 1984). Two large investigations, collectively comprising 122,400 women, found a 14%–20% incidence of major depressive disorder during pregnancy (Marcus et al. 2003; Oberlander et al. 2006). In fact, more than 11% of women presenting for evaluation of postpartum depression report symptom onset during pregnancy (Stowe et al. 2005). Treatment discontinuation can be especially problematic. In a recent study by our group, pregnant women with a history of depression who discontinued antidepressant therapy proximate to conception were 2.6 times more likely to experience a relapse before delivery in comparison with those who continued antidepressant treatment (68% vs. 26%) (Cohen et al. 2006).

The perinatal course and management of bipolar disorder have come under increased scrutiny in the past decade. In an initial retrospective study, Grof et al. (2000) described a benign course for women with lithium-responsive bipolar disorder during pregnancy; however, most evidence indicates that pregnant women with bipolar disorder are highly vulnerable to recurrence without continued pharmacotherapy. For example, three retrospective studies have reported 45%–52% bipolar disorder recurrence rates during pregnancy (Blehar et al. 1998; Freeman et al. 2000; Viguera et al. 2000). More recently, we have reported, in two separate prospective samples, relapse rates of 84%–100% among pregnant women with bipolar disorder who discontinue mood stabilizer therapy versus 30%–38% among those who continue mood stabilizer therapy (Newport et al. 2008b; Viguera et al. 2007).

Psychotic disorders have also been observed to worsen during pregnancy (Glaze et al. 1991; McNeil et al. 1984a, 1984b). Furthermore, women with schizophrenia have been reported to have high rates of unplanned and unwanted pregnancies (Miller 1997; Miller and Finnerty 1996) that may further escalate as SGAs with little impact on prolactin physiology (Dickson and Edwards 1997; Kaplan et al. 1996) become mainstays of therapy.

Although perinatal data regarding obsessive-compulsive disorder (OCD) are limited, it is noteworthy that 15%–39% of women with OCD report symptom onset during pregnancy (Neziroglu et al. 1992; K.E. Williams and Koran 1997). The course of OCD during pregnancy appears to be variable, with 73% of women reporting no symptom change, 14% reporting symptom exacerbation, and 14% reporting symptom improvement (Jenike et al. 1990; K.E. Williams and Koran 1997). The course of panic disorder during gestation is also highly variable, with 19% of patients experiencing more frequent panic attacks, 30% having reduced attacks, and 51% showing no change (Hertzberg and Wahlbeck 1999; Wisner et al. 1996a). Finally, a traumatic labor and delivery experience can precipitate posttraumatic stress disorder (Allen 1998; Fones 1996).

Postpartum psychiatric illness has been documented for millennia and has been substantiated by recent research. For example, a widely cited study by Kendler et al. (1993) reported a dramatic rise in psychiatric hospitalizations during the first postpartum month. In fact, up to 13% of all psychiatric admissions for women occur during the first postpartum year (Duffy 1983). Postpartum depression affects between 10% and 22% of adult women and up to 26% of adolescent mothers (Stowe and Nemeroff 1995; Troutman and Cutrona 1990). The postpartum is also a time of heightened risk for women with bipolar disorder (Kendell et al. 1987; Targum et al. 1979). Postpartum psychosis is thankfully a rare condition, occurring in only 1–2 of every 1,000 live births. Most postpartum psychoses appear to be psychotic episodes of a mood disorder (McGorry and Conell 1990).

Effect of Maternal Psychiatric Disorders

Not only the likelihood but also the potential impact of maternal psychiatric illness on child well-being must be considered in the risk–benefit assessment. A salient feature of most mental disorders is impairment of function (American Psychiatric Association 2000), and intervention is clearly warranted if the impairment precludes a woman's participation in prenatal care or in some other manner jeopardizes the pregnancy or infant.

Obstetrical and developmental outcomes have been best studied in women experiencing depressive symptoms. For example, prenatal maternal depression may

slow fetal growth (Hedegaard et al. 1996; Schell 1981), result in smaller infant head circumferences (Lou et al. 1994), increase the risk of preterm delivery and other obstetrical complications (Korebrits et al. 1998; Oberlander et al. 2006; Orr and Miller 1995; Perkin et al. 1993; Steer et al. 1992), and even precipitate long-standing behavioral changes in the offspring (Luoma et al. 2001, 2004; Meijer 1985; T.G. O'Connor et al. 2003; Stott 1973). Depressed gravidas are also more likely to abuse alcohol, engage in suicidal behavior, neglect prenatal care, and receive inadequate nutrition (Zuckerman et al. 1989), causing significant risk to the fetus (Perkin et al. 1993).

Maternal depression during pregnancy is also associated with neurobiological alterations in the offspring. For example, elevated serum concentrations of cortisol and catecholamines in depressed third-trimester gravidas are correlated with urinary concentrations of these substrates in their infants 24 hours after delivery (Lundy et al. 1999).

Postnatal maternal depression also carries deleterious consequences for infant development. As early as 3 months, infants of depressed mothers exhibit less facial expression, less head orientation, less crying, and more fussiness than do infants of nondepressed mothers (Martinez et al. 1996). As they age, the children of depressed mothers display ineffective emotional regulation (Downey and Coyne 1990), slowed motor development evident as early as 6 months (Galler et al. 2000), and poorly integrated interactions even when the children of depressed mothers are interacting with nondepressed mothers (Jameson et al. 1997), and these children also show lower self-esteem beginning in preschool (Downey and Coyne 1990), more fear and anxiety (Lyons-Ruth et al. 2000), more aggression (Jameson et al. 1997), and more insecure and disorganized attachment behaviors (Martins and Gaffan 2000) than do children of nondepressed mothers. Children of depressed mothers are ultimately more likely to experience emotional instability, to have behavioral problems and suicidal behavior, and to require psychiatric treatment (Lyons-Ruth et al. 2000; Weissman et al. 1984).

The effect of other maternal psychiatric disorders on infant and neonatal development is less well investigated. Although formal studies are lacking, the poor judgment and reckless behavior that characterize manic episodes of bipolar disorder inarguably convey a host of risks to the developing child. The risks, if any, associated with maternal hypomania are less clear.

Perinatal exacerbation of schizophrenia and other psychotic illnesses also warrants concern. Women with schizophrenia have a higher prevalence of substance abuse during pregnancy (Miller and Finnerty 1996) and often exhibit bizarre ideas regarding contraception, pregnancy, and child rearing that complicate their perinatal course (McEvoy et al. 1983). Left untreated, schizophrenia during the peripartum can have devastating consequences for both mother and child. Cases exist of maternal self-mutilation (Coons et al. 1986; Yoldas et al. 1996), infanticide (Bucove 1968), and denial of pregnancy with consequent refusal of prenatal care (Slayton and Soloff 1981). In addition, children born to mothers with schizophrenia are more likely to suffer from obstetrical complications (Miller and Finnerty 1996), although a recent investigation did not confirm this finding (Bennedsen et al. 2001). Maternal schizophrenia is also associated with a higher rate of perinatal death (Rieder et al. 1975). Furthermore, mothers with schizophrenia often exhibit aberrant parenting styles that may contribute to the development of avoidant behaviors in their children (Riordan et al. 1999).

The impact of anxiety disorders on obstetrical outcomes remains obscure. A case series of eight women with OCD during pregnancy reported that two developed preeclampsia, three delivered prematurely, and five underwent cesarean section (Maina et al. 1999).

The clinical data regarding the obstetrical and developmental consequences of maternal mental illness are complemented by an extensive line of laboratory animal research bearing homology to depression and other stress-related psychiatric disorders (for a review, see Newport et al. 2002b). Consistent with the limited human database, animal research indicates that prenatal stress adversely affects offspring growth (Herrenkohl and Gala 1979; Schneider et al. 1999), learning ability (Jaiswal and Bhattacharya 1993; Smith et al. 1981; Weller et al. 1988), and postnatal development (Fride and Weinstock 1984).

Furthermore, preclinical research indicates that certain biobehavioral aberrations induced by prenatal stress may persist into adulthood. For example, prenatally stressed adult rats continue to demonstrate depression-like behaviors (Secoli and Teixeira 1998), anxiety-like behaviors in novel situations (Fride and Weinstock 1988; Poltyrev et al. 1996; Szuran et al. 1991; Vallee et al. 1997; Weinstock et al. 1988), and exaggerated "emotional" responses to stress (Fride et al. 1986; Pfister and Muir 1992; Wakshlak and Weinstock 1990). Prenatally stressed primates also exhibit diminished exploratory behavior (Clarke and Schneider 1993; Schneider 1992).

These behavioral alterations are accompanied by lasting neurobiological alterations. In particular, prenatally stressed animals demonstrate multiple alterations in hypothalamic-pituitary-adrenal (HPA) axis function, including the following: 1) increased basal concentrations of plasma corticosterone and adrenocorticotropic hormone (ACTH) (McCormick et al. 1995; Takahashi 1998; Takahashi and Kalin 1991), 2) heightened production of corticotropin-releasing factor (CRF) in the fetal hypothalamus (Fujioka et al. 1999), and 3) exaggerated corticosterone responses to subsequent mild stressors (Fride and Weinstock 1984; Henry et al. 1994; Peters 1982; Weinstock et al. 1992). The activity of catecholamine (Alonso et al. 1994, 1997; Fride et al. 1985; Henry et al. 1995; Peters 1982, 1984) and serotonin (Hayashi et al. 1998; Peters 1982, 1986, 1988, 1990) systems is also altered in prenatally stressed laboratory animals.

Laboratory paradigms that interfere with maternal care (e.g., maternal separation, variable foraging) precipitate similar adverse biobehavioral outcomes in the offspring. Offspring from these neonatal maternal stress protocols exhibit insecure attachment behaviors (Andrews and Rosenblum 1988, 1991, 1994; Rosenblum and Paully 1984), depression-like and anxiety-like behaviors (Levine 1967), and alterations in stress-respondent neurobiological systems (Coplan et al. 1996, 1998; Pauk et al. 1986; Pihoker et al. 1993; Walker et al. 1991). Although direct correlations between laboratory animal stress models and human psychiatric illness are difficult to sustain, these preclinical data underscore the potential long-term effects of maternal stress during the peripartum.

Treatment Issues During Pregnancy and Lactation

An appraisal of the risks and benefits afforded by psychotropic treatment is the other major facet of the perinatal risk–benefit assessment. The theoretical risks of fetal and neonatal medication exposure may be classified as either acute or developmental adverse effects (Table 64–1). *Acute effects* are typically immediately evident and are not

TABLE 64–1.   Risks of perinatal medication exposure

	ACUTE	DEVELOPMENTAL
Pregnancy	Neonatal toxicity Neonatal withdrawal Drug–drug interactions	Somatic teratogenesis Neurobehavioral teratogenesis
Lactation	Infant toxicity Drug–drug interactions	Neurobehavioral teratogenesis

dependent on the developmental window of exposure. Examples of acute effects include drug toxicity, drug withdrawal, and drug–drug interactions. *Developmental effects* are, by definition, dependent on the developmental window of exposure and are often not evident until later. These effects include somatic teratogenesis (i.e., major and minor malformations) and so-called neurobehavioral teratogenesis (i.e., alterations in brain development that affect the child's subsequent behavior, cognitive abilities, and emotional regulation). The window of vulnerability to somatic teratogenesis is limited to the embryonic phase of development, but because CNS development continues long after delivery, the fetus and breast-feeding infant are vulnerable to the theoretical risk of neurobehavioral teratogenesis.

The risks of psychopharmacological exposure can be averted by using nonpharmacological treatment alternatives. Some of these therapies, including interpersonal psychotherapy (O'Hara et al. 2000; Spinelli 1997), cognitive-behavioral therapy (Appleby et al. 1997), sleep deprivation (B.L. Parry et al. 2000), and electroconvulsive therapy (Miller 1994), have been used in the peripartum and warrant consideration (Cohen et al. 1989; Miller 1991). These alternatives are not without shortcomings. They are often costly or unavailable in the rapidly evolving managed care environment, and they may take longer to work than psychotropic medications. Any delay in therapeutic benefit thus extends the child's exposure to the risks associated with maternal mental illness. A recent meta-analysis that the treatment effect of perinatal psychotherapy is less than that of antidepressant pharmacotherapy, although synergistic effects can be achieved with concomitant administration of antidepressants and psychotherapy (Bledsoe et al. 2006). Consequently, psychotropic medications remain the principal treatment offering for many, if not most, women with perinatal mental illness.

Deciding whether to use psychotropic medication during pregnancy and/or lactation carries complicated clinical, ethical, and potentially legal ramifications. A rapidly expanding data set regarding the reproductive safety of psychotropic medications has in part addressed many of these concerns, but these data span a broad literature in psychiatry, obstetrics, pediatrics, and basic science journals, limiting the ease of availability. In addition, the current literature regarding psychotropic medications during pregnancy and lactation reveals numerous methodological problems. The most glaring deficiency is the absence of an appropriate control group for comparison; therefore, psychotropic outcome studies are subject to the confounding effects of maternal psychiatric

illness that may be misinterpreted as medication effects. Despite these limitations, ethical considerations preclude the possibility that well-controlled clinical trials will ever be conducted for psychotropic medication among pregnant or lactating women.

The use of psychotropic medications during pregnancy and lactation continues to generate considerable debate, and a final consensus is unlikely to be forthcoming. Adequately controlled studies to resolve these issues are equally unlikely. The pregnancy and lactation reproductive safety database for psychotropic medications is therefore composed of a diverse conglomeration of isolated case reports, case series by pharmaceutical companies and academic centers, birth registries, retrospective surveys, reports from teratology or poison control centers, more extensive clinical and preclinical pharmacokinetic investigations, an increasing array of review articles summarizing data from these primary sources, the American Academy of Pediatrics (2001) breast-feeding rating system, and the U.S. Food and Drug Administration (FDA) pregnancy rating system (Table 64–2). In the absence of controlled trials, it is not surprising that the FDA has not to date approved any psychotropic medication for use during pregnancy or lactation. The FDA pregnancy rating system is not without shortcomings. One potential confounder of this system is that medications that have been available longer are more likely to have accrued a greater number of adverse case reports than newer, less studied medications. Similarly, it is often difficult to track the process that actually contributes to the individual category ratings.

Reviewing the reproductive safety database is only one aspect of assessing the relative utility of psychopharmacological treatment. A meticulous review of the patient's clinical history is also important. Obtaining comprehensive medical and obstetrical histories, particularly screening for a history of placental insufficiency, preeclampsia, and urinary or gastrointestinal disorders, is imperative. Early identification of probable perinatal comorbidities may guide the selection of psychotropic agents. For example, psychotropics with potent antihistaminic properties may complicate the course of overt or gestational diabetes during pregnancy, whereas other psychotropic agents (e.g., selective serotonin reuptake inhibitors [SSRIs]) may actually improve glycemic control. Potential drug interactions with medications used to manage medical comorbidities or with analgesic and anesthetic medications used at delivery should also be considered. Obtaining the patient's psychiatric history and family psychiatric history is also important, not only for

TABLE 64–2. U.S. Food and Drug Administration (FDA) use-in-pregnancy ratings

CATEGORY	INTERPRETATION
A	**Controlled studies show no risk:** Adequate, well-controlled studies in pregnant women have failed to demonstrate risk to the fetus.
B	**No evidence of risk in humans:** Either animal findings show risk, but human findings do not; or, if no adequate human studies have been done, animal findings are negative.
C	**Risk cannot be ruled out:** Human studies are lacking, and animal studies are either positive for fetal risk or lacking as well. However, potential benefits may justify the potential risk.
D	**Positive evidence of risk:** Investigational or postmarketing data show risk to the fetus. Nevertheless, potential benefits may outweigh risks.
X	**Contraindicated in pregnancy:** Studies in animals or humans, or investigational or postmarketing reports, have shown fetal risk that clearly outweighs any possible benefit to the patient.

Source. Physicians' Desk Reference 2007.

clarifying the psychiatric diagnosis but also for providing documentation of responses to previous therapeutic trials of psychotropic medications. Regardless of the volume of reproductive safety data, a medication that has been poorly tolerated or ineffective for a particular patient is of little value.

Pharmacokinetics and Pharmacodynamics of Pregnancy and Lactation: Implications for Dose Management

When the decision is made to use a psychotropic medication during pregnancy or lactation, it is important to administer the *minimum effective dose*. Clinicians commonly reduce the dose of psychotropic medication upon learning that a patient is pregnant, in a well-meaning effort to reduce fetal medication exposure. However, indiscriminate dosage reduction also increases the patient's vulnerability to relapse. Inadequate dosing therefore unduly exposes the child to the risks of both medication and maternal illness, yet administering doses higher than those necessary to achieve and sustain remission is equally inadvisable. Inordinately high doses expose the child to unnecessarily high medication concentrations. The therapeutic goals of psychopharmacological treatment during pregnancy and lactation are 1) to eliminate the child's exposure to maternal illness by achieving clinical remission while 2) minimizing the child's exposure to psychotropic medication. To accomplish these concomitant goals, dose management during pregnancy and lactation must be informed by an understanding of the factors governing the placental passage and breast milk excretion

of psychotropic medications as well as of the impact of the physiological changes of pregnancy on the pharmacological effects of these medicines.

It is well recognized that dosage adjustments are often required to maintain the therapeutic efficacy of medications during pregnancy. For example, it may be necessary to increase the dose of tricyclic antidepressants (TCAs) to approximately 1.6 times the preconception dose to maintain therapeutic concentrations in late pregnancy (Altshuler et al. 1996; Wisner et al. 1993). Similar increases may be required with SSRIs during the early third trimester to sustain euthymia (Hostetter et al. 2000). However, the pattern of dose adjustment during gestation is not uniform for all medications. For example, among anticonvulsant/mood-stabilizing medications, serum concentrations of lamotrigine (I. Ohman et al. 2000; Pennell et al. 2000; Tran et al. 2002) and valproic acid (Otani 1985; Philbert et al. 1985) decline steadily across gestation, whereas carbamazepine concentrations (Bardy et al. 1982b; Battino et al. 1982; Bologa et al. 1991; Dam et al. 1979; Lander et al. 1980; Omtzigt et al. 1993; Otani 1985; Tomson et al. 1994; Yerby et al. 1985) exhibit smaller changes that are primarily evident only in late pregnancy. Increasing evidence indicates that these alterations in drug concentrations and dosing requirements are a consequence of the impact of the physiological changes of pregnancy on the pharmacokinetics (Boobis and Lewis 1983; Frederiksen 2001; Little 1999; Wyska and Jusko 2001), and possibly the pharmacodynamics (Wyska and Jusko 2001), of psychotropic medications.

Each of the four generally recognized phases of the pharmacokinetic sequence—absorption, distribution, metabolism, and excretion—is affected by pregnancy. Several factors serve to increase the *absorption* of orally administered medications during gestation. Decreases in the rate of gastric emptying (Hunt and Murray 1958) and intestinal motility (E. Parry et al. 1970) lengthen the transit time of oral medications and thus increase the time for absorption across the intestinal mucosa. In addition, heightened blood flow to the digestive tissues (Mattison 1986) increases the rate of absorption.

Drug *distribution* is also altered during gestation. Both plasma volume (Lund and Donovan 1967; Mattison et al. 1991) and extracellular fluid volume (Mattison et al. 1991; Petersen 1957; Plentl and Gray 1959) increase dramatically. In addition, increases in body fat during pregnancy (Mattison et al. 1991) further expand the volume of distribution for psychotropic medications, which are almost uniformly highly lipophilic compounds. The dilutional effect of the increased volume of distribution is offset somewhat by decreased concentrations of circulating plasma proteins such as albumin (Frederiksen et al. 1986; Mendenhall 1970; Perucca and Crema 1982), serving to increase the distribution of many compounds into the bioavailable free fraction. However, plasma concentrations of some plasma proteins are relatively unchanged (e.g., α_1-acid glycoprotein [Wood and Wood 1981]) or even increased (e.g., sex hormone–binding globulin [Perucca and Crema 1982]) during pregnancy. Alterations in the unbound fraction arising from gestational changes in plasma protein concentrations impact the availability of medications not only for bioactivity but also for metabolic degradation.

Rates of drug *metabolism* during pregnancy are also affected by other mechanisms. First, tissue delivery of medication is increased during pregnancy by the increase (up to 50%) in cardiac output (Lees et al. 1967), but a smaller percentage of this heightened cardiac output is delivered to the liver as more blood is diverted to the uterus and other organs (Robson et al. 1990). Second, pregnancy is associated with numerous changes in the activity of various hepatic and extrahepatic enzymes. The activity of the hepatic cytochrome P450 (CYP) 3A4 (Bologa et al. 1991; Homma et al. 2000) isoenzyme is increased during gestation but that of CYP1A2 (Bologa et al. 1991; Tsutsumi et al. 2001) is decreased. CYP2D6 activity is increased during pregnancy in all women except those who are pharmacogenetically poor CYP2D6 metabolizers (Wadelius et al. 1997). Many CYP isoenzymes are also present in placental tissue, although the activity of the placental enzymes appears to be considerably lower than that of their hepatic counterparts (Hakkola et al. 1996).

Finally, drug *elimination* during pregnancy is affected by increases in renal blood flow (Metcalfe et al. 1955) and glomerular filtration rate (Davison and Hytten 1974; Dunlop 1981). In summary, the pharmacokinetic alterations of pregnancy are governed by a complex set of interdependent variables that remain obscure but may ultimately provide a basis from which to construct rational models for dosing guidelines during gestation.

Dose management during the peripartum may also be affected by alterations in the pharmacodynamics of psychotropic agents. Even less is known regarding the impact of the physiology of pregnancy on pharmacodynamics, but indications that postpartum depression is associated with alterations in the binding affinity of platelet serotonin transporters for radiolabeled imipramine and paroxetine (Hannah et al. 1992; Newport et al. 2004) lend credence to the existence of puerperal pharmacodynamic alterations. Pharmacodynamic indirect response models and signal transduction models (Wyska and Jusko 2001) offer plausible mechanisms whereby drug activity is altered during gestation. Additional candidate models of pharmacodynamic alterations during pregnancy remain to be explored.

The extent of fetal psychotropic exposure is the other principal consideration when administering medication during gestation. Fetal psychotropic exposure is largely dictated by placental passage of the medication, and all psychotropic medications are presumed to cross the placenta. Rates of placental transfer can be grouped into three categories (Pacifici and Nottoli 1995):

- *Type I: complete transfer*—Medication concentrations rapidly equilibrate between the maternal and fetal compartments.
- *Type II: excessive transfer*—Fetal concentrations are greater than maternal concentrations.
- *Type III: incomplete transfer*—Fetal concentrations are less than maternal concentrations.

Although there is no immediate evidence of placental filtering of psychotropic medications, there are significant differences in the rates of placental passage among antidepressants (Hendrick et al. 2003b) and antipsychotics (Newport et al. 2007). The primary mechanism of placental transport is simple diffusion, and its rate largely depends on the physicochemical properties of the particular medication. The major determinants of a medication's rate of diffusion across the placenta are molecular weight, lipid solubility, degree of ionization, and protein binding (Audus 1999; W.M. Moore et al. 1966; Pacifici and Nottoli 1995); however, the relative importance and critical thresholds for the respective physicochemical properties are yet to be delineated. At least one transplacental active transport mechanism has been identified. Placental glycoprotein (PGP) actively transports substrates from the fetal circulation back to the maternal circulation. Consequently, medications with greater affinity for PGP should be associated with relatively lower fetal-to-maternal medication ratios, as we recently demonstrated in an investigation of antipsychotic placental passage (Newport et al. 2007). Further clarification of the pharmacological attributes governing placental passage may ultimately contribute to the identification and development of efficacious psychotropic agents with minimal rates of placental transfer (Wang et al. 2007).

Fetal plasma concentrations are not, however, the ultimate measure of functional psychotropic exposure and may even underestimate the more critical measure, fetal brain concentration. Certain physiological attributes of the human fetus, including high cardiac output, increased blood–brain barrier permeability, low plasma protein concentrations and plasma protein binding affinity, and low hepatic enzyme activity (Bertossi et al. 1999; Morgan 1997; Oesterheld 1998), may result in higher fetal CNS concentrations of psychotropic medications than might be anticipated from circulating levels. Preclinical investigations from our group have demonstrated that transplacental passage results in high levels in fetal brain tissues and significant binding at neurotransmitter uptake sites (A.D. Fisher et al. 2001; Graybeal et al. 2002; Owens et al. 1997).

Similar considerations apply when endeavoring to minimize the psychotropic exposure of infants whose mothers are receiving psychiatric medication during lactation. After delivery, the neonate continues to exhibit unique physiological characteristics, including relatively low activity of hepatic enzymes. Hepatic maturation in the infant appears to occur at a highly variable rate (Warner 1986) and is more delayed in premature infants. Both glucuronidation and oxidation systems are initially immature at birth (as low as 20% of adult levels). The latter system typically matures by age 3 months (Atkinson et al. 1988). In addition, rates of glomerular filtration and tubular secretion are relatively low in neonates—30%–40% and 20%–30% lower than adult levels, respectively (Welch and Findlay 1981). Hence, the potential that psychotropic exposure may be higher than anticipated remains a consideration for breast-fed infants.

Because medications predominantly enter breast milk by passive diffusion of the nonionized, unbound fraction (J.T. Wilson et al. 1980), the pH gradient between maternal serum and breast milk plays a significant role in the amount of medication that is excreted into breast milk. Medications may in certain instances become iontrapped in milk. The lower pH of human milk may alter the molecular structure of a medication, preventing its reperfusion into the maternal circulation (Agatonovic-Kustrin et al. 2002). In addition, active secretory mechanisms also exist that can further concentrate drugs in breast milk (Kari et al. 1997; Oo et al. 1995; Toddywalla et al. 1997). A model to predict rates of breast milk excretion from descriptive characteristics of the molecular structure of candidate medications has recently been proposed (Agatonovic-Kustrin et al. 2002).

One purpose of such models is to provide a means to forecast infant exposure without performing invasive procedures on the child. Most familiar approaches utilize maternal serum concentrations and/or breast milk concentrations to calculate a milk-to-plasma ratio that is in turn used to calculate the infant's "daily dose" acquired through breast-feeding. Unfortunately, many existing studies calculate the milk-to-plasma ratio from a single random breast milk sample. This simplistic approach ignores the pharmacokinetics of medication excretion in breast milk and may thus provide an inaccurate prediction of infant exposure.

Accurately forecasting the level of infant exposure via lactation necessitates consideration of two well-described excretion gradients: distribution gradient and time gradient (Stowe et al. 1997, 2000). First, a distribution gradient of medication concentration in human milk exists during the course of a single feeding. As a rule, psychotropic medications are highly lipophilic and therefore present in higher concentrations in the fatty hindmilk. Consequently, a milk–plasma ratio calculated from an isolated random milk sample can vary widely between foremilk and hindmilk collections. In addition, a dose-to-dose time gradient for psychotropic excretion into breast milk also exists. The time course of psychotropic excretion into breast milk is largely consistent with the gastrointestinal absorptive phase of these medications and thus can largely be predicted by their known pharmacokinetics. For example, peak breast milk concentrations of sertraline occur at about 8 hours after the last dose, whereas the nadir occurs just prior to the next dose. Accurate prediction of daily infant dose via breast-feeding requires a model that acknowledges these excretion gradients. Utilizing this type of model, our group completed a detailed study of both the pharmacokinetics of excretion and infant serum measures for sertraline demonstrating that the maximum calculated infant dose is typically less than 1/500 of the maternal dose (Stowe et al. 1997).

Antidepressants

Antidepressant medications are used to treat a variety of neuropsychiatric illnesses. Commonly prescribed antidepressants are listed in Table 64–3. According to recent reports, 6.6% of pregnant women receive a prescription for an antidepressant at some point during pregnancy (Andrade et al. 2008).

Selective Serotonin Reuptake Inhibitors

SSRI antidepressants, among the best-studied medications in pregnancy and the single best-studied class of medications in lactation, have emerged as first-line agents for treating depression during pregnancy and lactation.

Prospective reports of first-trimester SSRI use currently consist of 4,679 fluoxetine exposures resulting in 126 (2.7%) children with major malformations (Briggs et al. 2005; Chambers et al. 1996; GlaxoSmithKline 2005; Goldstein et al. 1997; Hallberg and Sjöblom 2005; McElhatton et al. 1996; Pastuszak et al. 1993; Wilton et al. 1998), 3,393 sertraline exposures with 66 (1.9%) major malformations (GlaxoSmithKline 2005; Hallberg and Sjöblom 2005; Kulin et al. 1998; Wilton et al. 1998), 2,688 citalopram exposures with 73 (2.7%) major malformations (Ericson et al. 1999; GlaxoSmithKline 2005; Hallberg and Sjöblom 2005; Heikkinen et al. 2002; Sivojelezova et al. 2005), 2,687 paroxetine exposures with 94 (3.5%) major malformations (GlaxoSmithKline 2005; Hallberg and Sjöblom 2005; Kulin et al. 1998; McElhatton et al. 1996; Wilton et al. 1998), 235 escitalopram exposures with 8 (3.4%) major malformations (GlaxoSmithKline 2005), 147 fluvoxamine exposures with 1 (0.7%) major malformation (GlaxoSmithKline 2005; Kulin et al. 1998; McElhatton et al. 1996; Wilton et al. 1998), and 395 exposures to unspecified SSRIs with 6 (1.5%) major malformations (Einarson et al. 2001; Ericson et al. 1999; Hendrick et al. 2003a; Simon et al. 2002; Sivojelezova et al. 2005). The 2.6% (n=374) overall SSRI malformation rate among these 14,224 pregnancies is consistent with rates reported in the general population (New York State Department of Health 2005; Rimm et al. 2004; Swedish Centre for Epidemiology 2004).

Despite these reassuring and voluminous data, some concerns have been raised. For example, a preliminary analysis of a managed care database demonstrated a statistically higher odds ratio for major malformations, particularly cardiovascular malformations, after first-trimester paroxetine exposure in comparison to exposure to other antidepressants (GlaxoSmithKline 2005), leading the FDA to reclassify paroxetine's pregnancy category

(U.S. Food and Drug Administration 2005). Although the FDA deemed the data sufficiently compelling to alter the pregnancy classification, definitive conclusions are precluded by numerous limitations in this data set (e.g., there is no nonexposed control group, the paroxetine malformation rates reported in this study approximate population norms, and the significant finding in one arm of the study is eliminated when those with exposure to other known teratogens are excluded).

Three recent large-scale case–control studies of first-trimester SSRI exposure have likewise produced generally reassuring results, although some concerns have emerged. One of these studies comparing 9,622 cases (infants with malformations) and 4,092 controls (infants without malformations) found no evidence to suggest that SSRI exposure was associated with higher rates of cardiovascular defects but did report small increases in the risk for three uncommon malformations—anencephaly (odds ratio [OR] = 2.4), craniosynostosis (OR = 2.5), and omphalocele (OR = 2.8) (Alwan et al. 2007). Conversely, a study comparing 9,489 cases and 5,860 controls found no evidence of increased risk for heart defects of these other three malformations with first-trimester SSRI exposure (Louik et al. 2007). Analysis of individual antidepressants in the second study did demonstrate an increased risk for omphalocele (OR = 5.7) and septal defects (OR = 2.0) with sertraline exposure, and for right ventricular outflow tract obstruction defects (OR = 3.3) with paroxetine exposure. Finally, a nested case–control study of 1,403 infants, including 101 with major malformations, found no evidence that SSRI or paroxetine use was associated with an increased risk for cardiovascular or other major malformations, unless women were administered ≥25 mg of paroxetine per day, in which case their infants were at higher risk for cardiovascular malformations (OR = 3.1) and overall malformations (OR = 2.2).

The first investigation of the neurobehavioral impact of prenatal SSRI exposure was a landmark study by Nulman et al. (1997a) of children exposed in utero to antidepressant medications (55 fluoxetine-exposed children, 80 TCA-exposed children, 84 children with no antidepressant exposure). Children between 16 months and 7 years of age were evaluated with an extensive battery of neurodevelopmental tools measuring global intelligence quotient (IQ), language development, temperament, mood, activity level, and behavior. No significant differences on any of the neurodevelopmental measures were detected among the three groups of children in the study. Furthermore, global IQ and language development were nearly identical among all the groups. In conclusion, there was

TABLE 64–3.   Antidepressant medications

GENERIC NAME	TRADE NAME	DAILY DOSE (MG/DAY)[a]	RISK CATEGORY[b]	AMERICAN ACADEMY OF PEDIATRICS RATING[c]
Selective serotonin uptake inhibitors				
Citalopram	Celexa	20–60	C	Unknown, but of concern
Escitalopram	Lexapro	5–20	C	N/A
Fluoxetine	Prozac	20–60	C	Unknown, but of concern
Fluvoxamine	Luvox	50–300	C	Unknown, but of concern
Paroxetine	Paxil	20–50	D	Unknown, but of concern
Sertraline	Zoloft	50–200	C	Unknown, but of concern
Tricyclic antidepressants				
Amitriptyline	Elavil, Endep	150–300	D	Unknown, but of concern
Amoxapine	Asendin	150–400	C_m	Unknown, but of concern
Clomipramine	Anafranil	150–250	C_m	Unknown, but of concern[d]
Desipramine	Norpramin	150–300	C	Unknown, but of concern
Doxepin	Sinequan, Adapin	150–300	C	Unknown, but of concern
Imipramine	Tofranil	150–300	D	Unknown, but of concern
Maprotiline	Ludiomil	140–225	B_m	N/A
Nortriptyline	Pamelor, Aventyl	75–150	D	N/A
Protriptyline	Vivactil	15–60	C	N/A
Monoamine oxidase inhibitors				
Isocarboxazid	Marplan	30–60	C	N/A
Phenelzine	Nardil	45–90	C	N/A
Tranylcypromine	Parnate	30–60	C	N/A
Other antidepressants				
Bupropion	Wellbutrin	150–450	C	Unknown, but of concern
Duloxetine	Cymbalta	30–90	C	N/A
Mirtazapine	Remeron	15–45	C	N/A
Nefazodone	Serzone	300–600	C	N/A
Trazodone	Desyrel	200–300	C	Unknown, but of concern
Venlafaxine[e]	Effexor	150–375	C	N/A

Note.   N/A=not available.

[a]Dosing strategies adapted from Schatzberg and Cole 1991; Kaplan and Sadock 1993; and, for newer medications, the manufacturers' package inserts.

[b]Risk category adapted from Briggs et al. 2005 and/or *Physicians' Desk Reference* 2007; "m" subscript indicates data taken from the manufacturer's package insert.

[c]American Academy of Pediatrics 2001.

[d]Original committee report 1994 listed as "compatible," and a correction was later published.

[e]Not listed in Briggs et al. 1994. Risk category taken from *Physicians' Desk Reference* (1992, 1993, 1994, and 1996 editions).

no apparent neurobehavioral impact of prenatal exposure to fluoxetine or TCAs on children of preschool or early elementary school age.

To date, few studies have systematically assessed child development after prenatal antidepressant exposure. The first two reports, from the same group, assessed children between 15 and 86 months of age, collectively comparing 126 children exposed prenatally to a TCA and 90 children exposed to fluoxetine with 120 children of women with no history of depression. Using age-adjusted rating instruments, they found no differences with respect to global cognition, psychomotor development, or language development (Nulman et al. 1997a, 2002). The third study, assessing children between 6 and 40 months of age, compared 13 children whose mothers were depressed but did not take antidepressant medication during pregnancy with 31 children who were prenatally exposed to an SSRI (Casper et al. 2003). Like the Nulman et al. studies, this group also found no differences in global cognition; however, lower psychomotor scores were reported for the SSRI-exposed children.

Unfortunately, limitations of these three studies render their implications speculative at best. First, children were not age-matched in any of these studies. Although the authors reported age-adjusted index scores, the predictive validity of these indices across child developmental stages has not been established (Black and Matula 2000). Consequently, groupwise differences in the ages of the children might confound the results. Second, the Casper et al. (2003) study is further confounded by the fact that 29% of the participants were enrolled after delivery. This inclusion of a retrospective (postnatally enrolled) sampling could result in an overrepresentation of children with developmental abnormalities.

Another recent investigation (Oberlander et al. 2004) evaluated children at fixed time points (2 months and 8 months of age), thereby eliminating the age adjustment confound. This study reported no difference between 46 SSRI-exposed infants and 23 children of healthy volunteers with respect to either cognitive or motor development. Finally, a recent assessment of externalizing and attentional behaviors in 4-year-old children found no evidence that prenatal SSRI exposure affected these outcomes (Oberlander et al. 2007).

Although evidence regarding the developmental effects of SSRI exposure has been reassuring, data on the impact of prenatal antidepressant exposure on vulnerability to miscarriage, preterm delivery, and/or low birth weight are decidedly mixed. Some investigators have reported an association with such outcomes (Chambers et al. 1996; Chun-Fai-Chan et al. 2005; Oberlander et al. 2006; Pastuszak et al. 1993; Simon et al. 2002), whereas others have not (Einarson et al. 2001, 2003; Kulin et al. 1998; Sivojelezova et al. 2005). This is further complicated by yet other studies reporting an association of prenatal maternal stress and/or depression with prematurity and low birth weight (Orr et al. 2002; Steer et al. 1992). As such, no definitive conclusions can be drawn as to whether antidepressant use during gestation conveys an adverse impact on fetal growth or the timing of parturition.

Finally, a transient self-limited syndrome of neonatal symptoms, most commonly respiratory difficulty and tremulousness/jitteriness, associated with fetal exposure to serotonergic antidepressants proximate to delivery has drawn increasing attention (Moses-Kolko et al. 2005). Most controlled prospective studies suggest that there may be an association between SSRI exposure and poor neonatal adaptation (Chambers et al. 1996; Costei et al. 2002; Källén 2004; Laine et al. 2003; Oberlander et al. 2004, 2006; Sivojelezova et al. 2005; Zeskind and Stephens 2004), although one recent study found no such association (Maschi et al. 2008) and closer scrutiny of these reports reveals a cadre of methodological shortcomings. Little effort has been made to mask those evaluating the neonates as to fetal antidepressant exposure, only one study (Oberlander et al. 2006) has endeavored to control for the impact of maternal mental illness, and key confounding exposures such as gestational age at delivery, maternal smoking, and/or maternal use of other medications have been either ignored altogether or controlled in the crudest fashion (as dichotomous variables derived from unconfirmed maternal self-report). The most recent and arguably best designed of these studies (Oberlander et al. 2006) reported a significant association of SSRI exposure with neonatal respiratory difficulty and small-for-gestational-age birth weight; however, the authors failed to highlight the significant associations in their data of maternal depression during pregnancy with cesarean section delivery, preterm delivery, longer duration of neonatal hospital stay, and neonatal feeding problems.

A putative mechanism for SSRI-associated neonatal respiratory difficulty has been suggested by a recent retrospective case–control study (Chambers et al. 2006) reporting an overrepresentation of SSRI exposure after gestational week 20 among neonates with persistent pulmonary hypertension (PPHN) (OR=6.1). However, the fact that only 3.7% of the neonates with PPHN were exposed to an SSRI in late pregnancy, coupled with the recognition that PPHN is itself a relatively rare condition affecting approximately 0.19% of newborns (Greenough et al. 2005), raises questions as to whether this statistically significant finding is as clinically meaningful as the authors contend.

Another recent case–control study, comparing the exposures of neonates who "required observation" with those of "healthy" neonates (Misri et al. 2004), further highlights the importance of controlling for confounding factors. In this study, in which all neonates (n=46) were exposed to antidepressants and born to mothers who fulfilled diagnostic criteria for major depressive disorder, the mothers of infants who required observation had significantly higher scores on the Hamilton Rating Scale for Depression (21.7 vs. 16.2) and the Hamilton Anxiety Scale (21.1 vs. 13.6), were significantly more likely to have a comorbid anxiety disorder (92.8% vs. 53.1%), and were on average exposed to higher doses of clonazepam (0.43 mg/day vs. 0.14 mg/day).

Pharmacokinetic data regarding the placental passage of SSRI antidepressants remain limited. A recent study by Hendrick et al. (2003b) demonstrated that mean fetal–maternal ratios of the plasma concentrations of several SSRIs (i.e., fluoxetine, fluvoxamine, paroxetine, and sertraline) and their active metabolites are uniformly less than 1, although considerable differences exist between medications. Data on in vivo placental passage of citalopram are not yet available. Investigations that will enable the elaboration of comprehensive pharmacodynamic models to guide SSRI dose management throughout gestation are currently under way.

Published reports pertaining to SSRIs and lactation now exceed the published literature for any other class of medications, encompassing numerous exposures to sertraline (Altshuler et al. 1995; Birnbaum et al. 1999; Dodd et al. 2000; C. Epperson et al. 1997; N. Epperson et al. 2001; Hendrick et al. 2001; Kristensen et al. 1998; Mammen et al. 1997; Stowe et al. 1997, 2000; Wisner et al. 1998), fluoxetine (Birnbaum et al. 1999; Burch and Wells 1992; Nonacs and Cohen 2002; Kristensen et al. 1999; Lester et al. 1993; Taddio et al. 1996; Yoshida et al. 1998a), paroxetine (Birnbaum et al. 1999; Hendrick et al. 2001; R. Ohman et al. 1999; Spigset et al. 1996; Stowe et al. 2000), escitalopram (Rampono et al. 2006), fluvoxamine (Hendrick et al. 2001; Piontek et al. 2001; Wright et al. 1991), and citalopram (Jensen et al. 1997; Schmidt et al. 2000; Spigset et al. 1997). Although infant follow-up data are limited, only a few isolated cases of adverse effects have been reported. Long-term neurobehavioral studies of infants exposed to SSRI antidepressants during lactation have not been conducted, although a study of 12 infants exposed to sertraline during nursing detected no adverse effects on growth or achievement of developmental milestones (Llewellyn et al. 1997).

Pharmacokinetic studies of SSRIs in lactation constitute a confusing array of investigations employing varying assay sensitivities and inconsistent collection methods that complicate efforts to compare rates of breast milk excretion between compounds. The pharmacokinetic profiles of breast milk excretion, including delineation of distribution gradients and time gradients, are best defined for sertraline (Hendrick et al. 2002b; Stowe et al. 1997), paroxetine (Stowe et al. 2000), and fluoxetine (Suri et al.

2002). Collectively, findings from these studies indicate that quantitative infant SSRI exposure during lactation is considerably lower than transplacental exposure to these same medications during gestation.

Tricyclic Antidepressants

TCAs have been available in the United States since 1963 and were widely used during pregnancy and lactation before the proliferation of reproductive safety data regarding the SSRIs. No clear association has been demonstrated between TCA exposure and congenital malformations. Early studies suggested that TCA exposure might be associated with limb anomalies (Barson 1972; Elia et al. 1987; McBride 1972), but a meta-analysis by Altshuler et al. (1996) of 14 studies representing more than 300,000 live births identified a congenital malformation incidence of only 3.14% ($n = 13$) among 414 infants exposed to a TCA during the first trimester. A review of data from the European Network of Teratology Information Services revealed similar rates of malformation after TCA exposure (McElhatton et al. 1996). These rates are well within the normal baseline incidence of 2%–4%. Furthermore, the landmark study by Nulman et al. (1997a) involving 80 children exposed to a TCA during gestation found no evidence that prenatal exposure to these medications is associated with adverse neurobehavioral effects.

Few data exist regarding the acute effects of TCA exposure on fetal and neonatal well-being. There are case reports of fetal tachycardia (Prentice and Brown 1989) and numerous neonatal symptoms, including tachypnea, tachycardia, cyanosis, irritability, hypertonia, clonus, and spasm (Eggermont 1973; Miller 1991; Webster 1973). A small ($n = 18$) prospective study identified no evidence of increased complications during labor and delivery but did report transient withdrawal symptoms among TCA-exposed neonates (Misri and Sivertz 1991).

In a pharmacokinetic investigation addressing nortriptyline dose management during gestation, Wisner et al. (1993) reported that dose increases approximately 1.6 times higher than the preconception dose might be required in late pregnancy to maintain therapeutic serum concentrations and thereby sustain clinical benefit.

TCAs also have been widely used during lactation. The only adverse event reported to date is respiratory depression in a nursing infant exposed to doxepin, leading the authors to conclude that doxepin should be avoided but that most TCAs are safe for use during breast-feeding (Matheson et al. 1985). This clinical finding is paralleled by the pharmacokinetic data regarding TCAs in which all

TCAs are evident in breast milk, but infant plasma concentrations are considerably higher for doxepin than for other TCAs (for a review, see Wisner et al. 1996b). The time gradient for excretion also has been reported, with peak breast milk concentrations occurring 4–6 hours after an oral dose of both amitriptyline (Pittard and O'Neal 1986) and desipramine (Stancer and Reed 1986).

Monoamine Oxidase Inhibitors

Although the monoamine oxidase inhibitors (MAOIs) were introduced more than 40 years ago, clinical data regarding their use during pregnancy and lactation are limited. The currently available MAOIs (i.e., isocarboxazid, phenelzine, and tranylcypromine) are all FDA Category C medications; however, a small prospective study (Heinonen et al. 1977) suggested that prenatal tranylcypromine exposure is associated with increased risk for fetal malformations. Laboratory animal studies also have reported teratogenic potential from embryonic exposure to MAOIs (Poulson and Robson 1964). The utility of MAOIs during pregnancy and lactation is severely limited by the potential for hypertensive crisis, which necessitates dietary constraints and avoidance of numerous medications that are commonly used during pregnancy (e.g., pseudoephedrine) or labor and delivery (e.g., meperidine). These restrictions can be avoided, at least in part, with the so-called reversible MAOIs (i.e., brofaromine and moclobemide). The reversible MAOIs are not currently available in the United States. The single published case report regarding moclobemide exposure during gestation reported no perinatal complications and indicated that the child demonstrated normal somatic and motoric development up to 14 months of age (Rybakowski 2001).

Other Antidepressants

Reproductive safety data are considerably more limited for most of the agents comprising the heterogeneous assortment of other antidepressants, including bupropion, duloxetine, mirtazapine, nefazodone, trazodone, and venlafaxine.

Prospective reports of first-trimester use of these agents consist of 2,550 bupropion exposures producing 56 (2.2%) children with major malformations (Boshier et al. 2003; Briggs et al. 2005; Chun-Fai-Chan et al. 2005; Cole et al. 2007; GlaxoSmithKline 2005), 771 venlafaxine exposures with 14 (1.4%) major malformations (Einarson et al. 2001; GlaxoSmithKline 2005), 404 trazodone exposures with 10 (2.5%) major malformations (Briggs et al. 2005;

GlaxoSmithKline 2005; McElhatton et al. 1996), 140 nefazodone exposures with 2 (1.4%) major malformations (GlaxoSmithKline 2005), 125 mirtazapine exposures with 2 (1.6%) major malformations (Djulus et al. 2006; GlaxoSmithKline 2005), and an additional combined report of 121 nefazodone or trazodone exposures with 2 (1.7%) major malformations (Einarson et al. 2003). There are no published data on first-trimester duloxetine exposure.

Pharmacokinetic data during pregnancy are available only for venlafaxine. The pharmacokinetic study by Hendrick et al. (2002b) reported that fetal–maternal plasma ratios for both venlafaxine and its active metabolite, O-desmethylvenlafaxine, are greater than 1. This higher rate of placental passage may be a consequence of certain physicochemical properties of venlafaxine, including its relatively low molecular weight and low binding to plasma proteins.

Data regarding the use of atypical antidepressants during lactation are likewise extremely limited. The existing literature includes reports of one infant exposed to bupropion (Briggs et al. 1993) and three infants exposed to venlafaxine (Ilett et al. 1998). No adverse effects were reported for any of these four children. Bupropion was undetectable in the plasma of the infant whose mother was taking that antidepressant (Briggs et al. 1993), but the plasma concentration of O-desmethylvenlafaxine was higher in one of the venlafaxine-exposed infants than in her mother (Ilett et al. 1998).

Mood-Stabilizing Medications

The perinatal management of bipolar disorder has received considerable attention and continues to be one of the most difficult challenges of modern psychiatric practice. The current mainstays of treatment for bipolar disorder are lithium, valproate, carbamazepine, and lamotrigine (Table 64–4).

Lithium

Used routinely since the 1950s, lithium remains the cornerstone of the available pharmacotherapies for bipolar disorder. Early reports of congenital malformations following in utero lithium exposure led to the establishment of the Danish Registry of Lithium Babies in 1969. Additional registries were later established in Canada and the United States, culminating in the International Register of Lithium Babies.

Early retrospective data suggested that lithium exposure was associated with a 400-fold increase in the vulner-

TABLE 64–4. Mood-stabilizing and antiepileptic medications

GENERIC NAME	TRADE NAME	DAILY DOSAGE (MG/DAY)[a]	RISK CATEGORY[b]	AMERICAN ACADEMY OF PEDIATRICS RATING[c]
Carbamazepine	Tegretol	400–1,600	C_m	Compatible
Clonazepam	Klonopin	0.5–10	C	N/A
Gabapentin	Neurontin	900–1,800	C	N/A
Lamotrigine	Lamictal	300–500	C	Unknown, but of concern
Levetiracetam	Keppra	500–3,000	C	N/A
Lithium carbonate	Eskalith, Lithobid, Lithonate	900–2,100	D	Contraindicated
Oxcarbazepine	Trileptal	600–1,200	C	Unknown, but of concern
Tiagabine	Gabatril	160–320	C	N/A
Topiramate	Topamax	200–800	C	Unknown, but of concern
Valproic acid	Depakote (divalproex sodium)	750–1,500	D	Compatible

Note. N/A=not available.
[a]Dosing strategies adapted from Schatzberg and Cole 1991; Kaplan and Sadock 1993; and for newer medications, the manufacturers' package inserts.
[b]Risk category adapted from Briggs et al. 2005 and/or *Physicians' Desk Reference* 2007; "m" subscript indicates data taken from the manufacturer's package insert.
[c]American Academy of Pediatrics 2001.

ability to congenital heart disease, with particular susceptibility to a malformation of the tricuspid valve known as Ebstein's anomaly (Nora et al. 1974; Weinstein and Goldfield 1975), but a subsequent meta-analysis of the available data calculated the risk ratio for cardiac malformations to be 1.2–7.7 and the risk ratio for overall congenital malformations to be 1.5–3.0 (Cohen et al. 1994). Altshuler et al. (1996) estimated that the risk for Ebstein's anomaly after prenatal lithium exposure rises from 1 in 20,000 to 1 in 1,000. A series of more recent yet small studies also failed to confirm the early estimates regarding the teratogenic potential of lithium (Friedman and Polifka 2000; Jacobsen et al. 1992; Källén and Tandberg 1983), although these studies had limited statistical power. Laboratory animal studies had indicated that neurobehavioral alterations also might be a concern for prenatal lithium exposure, but a 5-year follow-up of 60 school-age children exposed to lithium during gestation found no overt evidence of adverse neurobehavioral sequelae (Schou 1976).

Preconception counseling with a psychiatrist, obstetrician, and perhaps a genetic counselor should be the standard of care for women with bipolar disorder. Cohen et al. (1994) suggested the following treatment guidelines for women who are maintained on lithium and plan to conceive: 1) lithium should be gradually (>2 weeks) tapered prior to conception in women who experience mild and infrequent episodes of illness; 2) lithium should be tapered prior to conception but reinstituted after organogenesis in women who have more severe episodes but are only at moderate risk for relapse in the short term; 3) lithium should be continued throughout gestation for women who have especially severe and frequent episodes of illness in conjunction with counseling regarding reproductive risks. Prenatal assessment for fetal anomalies, including a fetal echocardiogram between weeks 16–18 of gestation, should be performed for women treated with lithium during the first trimester. In the event of unplanned conception during lithium therapy, the decision to continue or discontinue lithium should also be informed by the severity and course of the patient's illness as well as the time point in gestation when the exposure comes to attention. Discontinuing lithium therapy after cardiogenesis is complete at approximately 9–11 weeks gestation may be ill advised.

In addition to the developmental consequences of exposure, lithium's low therapeutic index also raises concerns regarding acute perinatal toxicities. Lithium exposure later in gestation can produce fetal and neonatal cardiac arrhythmias (N. Wilson et al. 1983), hypoglycemia and nephrogenic diabetes insipidus (Mizrahi et al. 1979), reversible changes in thyroid function (Karlsson et al. 1975), polyhydramnios, premature delivery, and a "floppy infant syndrome" similar to that witnessed with benzodiazepine exposure (Llewellyn et al. 1998). The neonate may exhibit signs of lithium toxicity at serum concentrations lower than maternal concentrations. Neonatal symptoms of lithium toxicity, including flaccidity, lethargy, and poor suck reflexes, may persist for more than 7 days (Woody et al. 1971).

In a pooled analysis of lithium placental passage and neonatal outcomes (Newport et al. 2005), we determined that 1) higher neonatal lithium concentrations were associated with significantly lower Apgar scores, longer hospital stays, and higher rates of CNS and neuromuscular complications; 2) umbilical cord (i.e., fetal) plasma concentrations were uniformly equivalent to maternal concentrations, suggesting that lithium rapidly equilibrates across the placenta; and 3) withholding lithium therapy for 24–48 hours prior to delivery resulted in a 0.28 mEq/L reduction in maternal (and presumably fetal) lithium concentrations, thereby likely improving neonatal outcomes. Consequently, scheduled deliveries, which afford opportunity for temporary suspension of lithium therapy for 24–48 hours, are advised for women taking lithium during late gestation.

The physiological alterations of pregnancy are of particular importance in the perinatal management of lithium. Changes in renal clearance across pregnancy and the potential for abrupt volume changes during delivery due to copious diaphoresis and the loss of blood and amniotic fluid mandate careful monitoring of lithium levels during pregnancy and especially at delivery. Furthermore, nonsteroidal anti-inflammatory drugs, which inhibit renal clearance of lithium, should be avoided in mother and infant alike during the early postpartum period.

The existing database regarding lithium and lactation encompasses 21 maternal–infant nursing dyads (Fries 1970; Schou and Amdisen 1973; Skausig and Schou 1977; Sykes et al. 1976; Tunnessen and Hertz 1972; Viguera et al. 2007; Weinstein and Goldfield 1969; Woody et al. 1971). Adverse events, including lethargy, hypotonia, hypothermia, cyanosis, electrocardiogram changes, and elevated thyroid-stimulating hormone level, were reported in 4 (19%) of these children (Skausig and Schou 1977; Tunnessen and Hertz 1972; Viguera et al. 2007; Woody et al. 1971), including 1 infant who developed frank lithium toxicity with a serum concentration of 1.4 mEq/L, which was double the maternal level (Skausig and Schou 1977). The American Academy of Pediatrics (2001) discourages the use of lithium during lactation. The largest pharmacokinetic study of lithium in lactation demonstrated a milk-to-plasma ratio of 0.53 and an infant-to-maternal plasma ratio of 0.24 (Viguera et al. 2007). In other studies, nursing infants have exhibited lithium concentrations generally ranging from 5% to 65% of maternal levels (Fries 1970; Kirksey and Groziak 1984; Schou and Amdisen 1973; Sykes et al. 1976; Tunnessen

and Hertz 1972; Weinstein and Goldfield 1969), excluding the lone infant whose serum concentration was 200% of the maternal concentration (Skausig and Schou 1977). Because dehydration can increase the vulnerability to lithium toxicity, the hydration status of nursing infants of mothers taking lithium should be carefully monitored (Llewellyn et al. 1998). There are no available reports regarding the long-term neurobehavioral sequelae of lithium exposure during lactation.

Valproate (Valproic Acid)

Several anticonvulsants, including valproate, lamotrigine, and carbamazepine, are now used in the treatment of bipolar disorder. The widespread use of valproate raises serious concerns for the reproductive safety of women with bipolar disorder. Prenatal exposure to valproate has been associated with numerous congenital malformations, including neural tube defects (Bjerkedal et al. 1982; Centers for Disease Control 1992; Jager-Roman et al. 1986; Lindhout and Schmidt 1986); craniofacial anomalies, including craniosynostosis (Assencio-Ferreira et al. 2001; Lajeunie et al. 1998, 2001; Paulson and Paulson 1981); limb abnormalities (Rodriguez-Pinilla et al. 2000); and cardiovascular anomalies (Dalens et al. 1980; Koch et al. 1983; Sodhi et al. 2001).

Valproate exposure prior to neural tube closure, during the fourth week of gestation, confers a 1%–2% risk for spina bifida, which is 10–20 times greater than the prevalence in the general population (Bjerkedal et al. 1982; Centers for Disease Control 1992; Rosa 1991). One meta-analysis placed the risk for neural tube defects even higher, at 3.8%, with particular vulnerability for the infants of women whose daily dose exceeds 1,000 mg (Samrén et al. 1997). Other studies support this dose–response relationship (Canger et al. 1999; Kaneko et al. 1999; Omtzigt et al. 1992; Samrén et al. 1999), leading one group to recommend that daily dosages not exceed a maximum of 1,000 mg and that maternal serum concentrations not exceed a maximum of 70 µg/mL to reduce the risk for malformations (Kaneko et al. 1999). In a case–control study examining the incidence of limb malformations in a cohort of more than 44,000 children, 67 of whom were exposed to valproate in the first trimester, Rodriguez-Pinilla et al. (2000) reported an odds ratio of 6.17 for limb abnormalities among children exposed to valproate and estimated the risk of limb abnormalities from valproate exposure at 0.42%.

A *fetal valproate syndrome* was initially reported by Di Liberti et al. (1984) and subsequently confirmed by other investigators (Ardinger et al. 1988; Martinez-Frias 1990; Winter et al. 1987). The phenotypic attributes of fetal valproate syndrome include stereotypical facial features such as bifrontal narrowing, midface hypoplasia, a broad nasal bridge, a short nose with anteverted nares, epicanthal folds, micrognathia, a shallow philtrum, a thin upper lip, and a thick lower lip (McMahon and Braddock 2001; S.J. Moore et al. 2000). Many of the congenital malformations previously associated with valproate exposure, including neural tube defects, congenital heart defects, cleft lip, cleft palate, limb abnormalities, urogenital defects, and abdominal wall defects, have been recognized as components of the fetal valproate syndrome (McMahon and Braddock 2001). Whereas the association between neural tube defects and folate deficiency is well established, valproate's antagonistic effect on folate may also underlie the full spectrum of fetal valproate syndrome. A case–control study comparing 57 children with fetal anticonvulsant syndromes, 46 of whose mothers were treated with valproate, with 152 control children found a significantly higher rate of a homozygosity for a mutation in the gene for methylenetetrahydrofolate reductase (MTHFR), a key enzyme in folate metabolism (Dean et al. 1999).

Neurodevelopmental outcomes associated with prenatal valproate exposure are equally concerning. A review indicated that developmental delay is evident in 20% and mental retardation in 10% of children exposed to valproate monotherapy prenatally (Kozma 2001). An interim report from a prospective multicenter investigation of the neurodevelopmental effects of prenatal antiepileptic drug exposure indicated that 24% of 2-year-olds with prenatal valproate exposure had mental developmental indexes of less than 70, more than doubling the rate of other antiepileptic drugs (Meador et al. 2006). Retrospective reports indicate that varying degrees of cognitive impairment may be present in children manifesting the physical sequelae of fetal valproate syndrome (Adab et al. 2001; Gaily et al. 1990; S.J. Moore et al. 2000). Fetal valproate syndrome has also been associated with pervasive developmental disorders, including autism (Bescoby-Chambers et al. 2001; S.J. Moore et al. 2000; G. Williams et al. 2001; P.G. Williams and Hersh 1997) and Asperger's syndrome (S.J. Moore et al. 2000).

Valproate exposure during gestation is also associated with risks for numerous fetal and neonatal toxicities, including hepatotoxicity (Kennedy and Koren 1998), coagulopathies (Mountain et al. 1970), and neonatal hypoglycemia (Ebbesen et al. 2000; Thisted and Ebbesen 1993). Ten of 13 infants who demonstrated neonatal hypoglyce-

mia after prenatal valproate exposure developed withdrawal symptoms—including irritability, jitteriness, hypertonia, seizures, and vomiting—that began 12–24 hours after delivery and lasted up to 1 week (Ebbesen et al. 2000).

Pharmacokinetic studies in women with epilepsy indicate that maternal valproate concentrations steadily decline across pregnancy, reaching levels up to 50% lower than preconception concentrations (Yerby et al. 1990, 1992). Consistent findings from other studies demonstrate that valproate is more rapidly cleared during gestation, and especially during the final month of pregnancy (Nau et al. 1982b; Otani 1985; Philbert et al. 1985). Dosage increases during pregnancy may therefore be required to maintain therapeutic concentrations. Valproate readily crosses the human placenta, with fetal concentrations at delivery equal to or slightly higher than maternal concentrations (Froescher et al. 1984b; Philbert et al. 1985; Yerby et al. 1990, 1992).

The published literature regarding valproate and lactation includes 41 mother–infant nursing dyads (Alexander 1979; Bardy et al. 1982a; Dickinson et al. 1979; Froescher et al. 1981; Nau et al. 1981; Piontek et al. 2000; Stahl et al. 1997; Tsuru et al. 1988; von Unruh et al. 1984; Wisner and Perel 1998). From these cases, only one adverse event, thrombocytopenia and anemia in an infant, has been reported (Stahl et al. 1997). The pharmacokinetic data indicate that valproate milk-to-plasma ratios are uniformly low and that serum concentrations of nursing infants are 2%–40% of maternal concentrations (Alexander 1979; Bardy et al. 1982a; Piontek et al. 2000; Stahl et al. 1997; von Unruh et al. 1984; Wisner et al. 1996b). Studies of the neurobehavioral effects of valproate exposure during lactation have not been conducted.

In summary, among all psychotropic agents, valproate bears the greatest burden for fetal risk, leading the principal investigator of the multicenter Neurodevelopmental Effects of Antiepileptic Drugs study, Kimford Meador, M.D., to conclude that it "should never be used as a first-line choice in women of childbearing age" (Cassels 2006). If valproate must be used during pregnancy, its risk may be reduced by being careful not to exceed 1,000 mg per day or a serum concentration of 70 μg/ml. Folate supplementation (4–5 mg per day) is also recommended, although there is no evidence that this reduces the risk of valproate-associated anomalies. Because nearly half of pregnancies in the United States are unplanned, and women with unplanned pregnancies typically first recognize that they are pregnant during the sixth week of gestation or even later (2 full weeks after neural tube closure), all women of childbearing potential who are treated with valproate should receive concomitant folate supplementation, regardless of whether they plan to conceive. The preliminary evidence that aspects of fetal valproate syndrome other than neural tube defects may be associated with valproate's antagonism of folate metabolism suggests that folate supplementation should be administered not only in the first trimester but also throughout gestation. Because of the potential for valproate-associated neonatal coagulopathies, oral vitamin K supplementation (10–20 mg per day) may be considered during the final month of gestation. Prenatal surveillance for congenital abnormalities should include maternal serum α-fetoprotein, fetal echocardiography, and a level 2 ultrasound at approximately 16–18 weeks' gestation. Finally, genetic screening of women taking valproate for mutations in the MTHFR gene warrants future consideration but cannot yet be recommended for routine clinical practice.

In contrast to the marked risks of its use during pregnancy, valproate therapy during lactation appears to be well tolerated by nursing infants. Nevertheless, periodic assays of platelet count and serum liver enzymes of nursing infants are recommended because of the risks for thrombocytopenia and hepatotoxicity associated with valproate therapy.

Carbamazepine

Carbamazepine is associated with many of the same risks as valproate during gestation, although in many cases with less frequency or severity. For example, first-trimester carbamazepine exposure is associated with a risk for neural tube defects, although the 0.5%–1.0% risk in carbamazepine-exposed infants (Rosa 1991) is approximately half that seen with valproate exposure (Lindhout and Schmidt 1986; Rosa 1991). A meta-analysis of five prospective studies encompassing 1,255 prenatal exposures indicated that carbamazepine exposure in utero is associated with an increased risk of neural tube defects, cleft palate, cardiovascular abnormalities, and urinary tract anomalies (Matalon et al. 2002). An epidemiological study indicated that periconceptional folate supplementation was associated with a lower rate of neural tube defects among the children of women taking carbamazepine during pregnancy (Hernandez-Diaz et al. 2001).

A *fetal carbamazepine syndrome* manifested by a short nose, long philtrum, epicanthal folds, hypertelorism, upslanting palpebral fissures, and fingernail hypoplasia has also been described (Jones et al. 1989) but has received considerably less attention than fetal valproate syndrome.

A subsequent study found the phenotypic characteristics of fetal carbamazepine syndrome evident in 6 of 47 children exposed to carbamazepine monotherapy during gestation (Ornoy and Cohen 1996). Other investigations have confirmed this association with facial anomalies (S.J. Moore et al. 2000; Nulman et al. 1997b; Scolnick et al. 1994; Wide et al. 2000), but one of these studies demonstrated similar facial abnormalities among children born to women with epilepsy who were untreated during pregnancy (Nulman et al. 1997b). This fetal carbamazepine syndrome has also been associated with developmental delay in up to 20% of exposed children (Jones et al. 1989; S.J. Moore et al. 2000; Ornoy and Cohen 1996), although other investigators have failed to demonstrate evidence of cognitive dysfunction in carbamazepine-exposed children (Gaily et al. 1990, 2004; Meador et al. 2006; Scolnick et al. 1994; van der Pol 1991; Wide et al. 2000).

Potential fetal/neonatal toxicities associated with carbamazepine exposure include blood dyscrasias, coagulopathies, skin reactions, and hepatotoxicity. Most of these risks remain theoretical, although neonatal hepatotoxicity has been reported in a carbamazepine-exposed infant (Frey et al. 2002).

Pharmacokinetic studies of carbamazepine clearance during gestation have yielded mixed results. Some investigators have reported statistically significant increases in carbamazepine clearance during the third trimester (Battino et al. 1982; Dam et al. 1979; Lander et al. 1980), but others have found no changes in carbamazepine clearance (Bardy et al. 1982b; Otani 1985; Yerby et al. 1985). Placental pharmacokinetic studies indicate that the placental transfer of carbamazepine is lower than that of other anticonvulsants (Nau et al. 1982a; Yerby et al. 1990, 1992), with fetal-to-maternal plasma ratios equaling 0.5–0.8 (Nau et al. 1982a).

The literature on carbamazepine and lactation includes 12 published reports and 144 mother–infant nursing pairs (Brent and Wisner 1998; Frey et al. 1990, 2002; Froescher et al. 1984a; Kaneko et al. 1982; Kok et al. 1982; Kuhnz et al. 1983; Merlob et al. 1992; Niebyl et al. 1979; Pynnonen and Sillanpaa 1975; Pynnonen et al. 1977; Wisner and Perel 1998), representing the most extensive data set for any mood stabilizer in lactation. This includes 8 reports of adverse events: 1 drowsy, irritable infant with an undetectable serum concentration of carbamazepine (Kok et al. 1982); 2 "hyperexcitable" infants in whom carbamazepine levels were not reported (Kuhnz et al. 1983); 2 infants with cholestatic hepatitis in whom carbamazepine levels were not reported (Frey et al. 1990, 2002); 1 infant with poor nursing effort (Froescher et al. 1984a); 1 infant with an increased serum concentration of γ-glutamyl transpeptidase (GGT) but no overt clinical sequelae whose serum concentration was 33% of the maternal concentration (Merlob et al. 1992); and 1 infant with a "seizurelike" phenomenon whose carbamazepine level was 8% of the maternal level (Brent and Wisner 1998). Serum carbamazepine concentrations in the 8 nursing infants in whom these levels were assessed ranged from undetectable to 65% of the maternal level (Brent and Wisner 1998; Kok et al. 1982; Merlob et al. 1992; Pynnonen and Sillanpaa 1975; Pynnonen et al. 1977; Wisner and Perel 1998).

Although the risks associated with in utero carbamazepine exposure are marginally better than those for valproate exposure, the clinical recommendations are quite similar. Carbamazepine should be avoided in pregnancy, especially during the first trimester. Folate supplementation (4–5 mg/day) is also recommended not only during gestation but also throughout the reproductive years because of the high prevalence of inadvertent conception in the United States. Women taking carbamazepine during gestation should receive prenatal surveillance for congenital abnormalities, including maternal serum α-fetoprotein, fetal echocardiography, and a level 2 ultrasound at approximately 16–18 weeks' gestation. Carbamazepine has by far the most extensive database for mood stabilizers in lactation, but reports of hepatic dysfunction in nursing infants certainly raise concern. Periodic assays of blood counts and serum liver enzymes of nursing infants are recommended in light of the risks for blood dyscrasias and hepatotoxicity associated with carbamazepine therapy.

Lamotrigine

Reproductive safety data regarding lamotrigine have rapidly accrued during the past decade and compare favorably with safety data for other agents available in the treatment of bipolar disorder. The overall risk of major fetal malformations following first-trimester prenatal exposure to lamotrigine is 2.6% (83 per 3,176 exposures, including 0.32% [8 per 2,537 exposures] for midline cleft formations) (Dominguez-Salgado et al. 2004; GlaxoSmithKline 2007; Holmes et al. 2006; Meador et al. 2006; Morrow et al. 2006; Sabers et al. 2004; Vajda et al. 2003), rates that are within the range of births not involving drug exposures. A recent report by the North American Pregnancy Registry (Holmes et al. 2006) noted a relatively high rate of midline facial clefts (0.89% of 564 exposures); however, the collective rate of orofacial clefts in the other registries was only 0.15% (2 per 1,937 exposures) (Dominguez-Salgado et al. 2004; GlaxoSmithKline 2007;

Meador et al. 2006; Morrow et al. 2006; Sabers et al. 2004; Vajda et al. 2003). Furthermore, a forthcoming case–control study by the European Surveillance of Congenital Anomalies (EUROCAT), encompassing 5,511 children with orofacial clefts and 80,052 children without clefts, reports an adjusted odds ratio of 0.67 for clefts with lamotrigine exposure (Dolk et al. 2008). The United Kingdom Epilepsy and Pregnancy Register reported a higher risk of malformations at maternal daily doses exceeding 200 mg (Morrow et al. 2006), although this was not confirmed in a subsequent analysis of the manufacturer's registry (GlaxoSmithKline 2007). Despite these reassuring findings, folate supplementation is recommended for all women of childbearing age taking any antiepileptic drug, including lamotrigine. Prospective neurodevelopmental data have also been favorable among children with prenatal lamotrigine exposure (Meador et al. 2006).

The pharmacokinetics of lamotrigine during pregnancy are well studied, with numerous studies consistently reporting that lamotrigine clearance steadily increases across gestation (De Haan et al. 2004; Pennell et al. 2004; Petrenaite et al. 2005; Tran et al. 2002). Indeed, seizure control in pregnant women with epilepsy can be maximized by regular monitoring of plasma concentrations and periodic dose changes as necessary (Pennell et al. 2008). These studies are limited by the cotherapy of lamotrigine with other anticonvulsants, which are known to alter the metabolism of lamotrigine. It is unclear whether similar dose changes would be necessary to maintain mood stability in patients with bipolar disorder and whether the common adjunctive agents used to treat bipolar disorder would have similar effects on lamotrigine metabolism. Studies in epilepsy patients taking lamotrigine also reveal that its rate of clearance abruptly declines after delivery (I. Ohman et al. 2000; Pennell et al. 2004; Tran et al. 2002). Therefore, dosage reductions may be necessary after delivery to avoid maternal symptoms of lamotrigine toxicity, such as dizziness, nausea and vomiting, and diplopia (Tran et al. 2002).

Published reports are also available regarding the placental passage of lamotrigine with a series of small studies to indicate that lamotrigine concentrations in fetal circulation at delivery are equal to maternal concentrations (Myllynen et al. 2003; I. Ohman et al. 2000; Sathanandar et al. 2000; Tomson et al. 1997). There have been no reports of acute adverse events observed in neonates exposed to lamotrigine.

Reports regarding lamotrigine and lactation (GlaxoSmithKline 2007; Liporace et al. 2004; Newport et al. 2008b; I. Ohman et al. 2000; Page-Sharp et al. 2006; Rambeck et al. 1997; Tomson et al. 1997) collectively encompass 55 maternal–infant nursing dyads. There have been no adverse events observed in these breast-fed infants, although 7 infants were observed to have a benign thrombocytosis (Newport et al. 2008a). In the largest (n=30) of these studies (Newport et al. 2008a), the mean milk-to-plasma ratio was 41.3%, the relative infant dose equaled 9.2%, and the infant-to-maternal plasma ratio equaled 18.3%. Long-term neurobehavioral outcomes have not been studied in nursing infants exposed to lamotrigine.

Other Anticonvulsants

Other antiepileptic drugs (gabapentin, levetiracetam, zonisamide) may be utilized in the treatment of mental illnesses, although efficacy trials for these agents have not been impressive.

Clinicians should be aware that more pharmaceutical companies are initiating postmarketing surveillance registries for antiepileptic drugs.

Second-Generation Antipsychotics

The older first-generation antipsychotics (FGAs) such as haloperidol and chlorpromazine have historically been used to manage the agitated behavior that often accompanies a manic episode; however, these agents are not effective mood stabilizers. Recent interest has focused on the mood-stabilizing utility of the SGAs (i.e., aripiprazole, clozapine, olanzapine, paliperidone, quetiapine, risperidone, and ziprasidone). With the exception of the newest of these agents, paliperidone, all SGAs now carry an FDA indication for one or more phases of bipolar disorder management.

The reproductive safety database for the SGAs, which is reviewed in the following section, contains scant data. Given this paucity of information, the SGAs cannot yet be recommended as first-line agents for the management of bipolar disorder during the peripartum. However, a risk–benefit assessment after inadvertent conception by a patient who is taking an SGA to manage bipolar disorder may indicate that continuing the SGA is preferable to switching to another mood stabilizer.

Antipsychotics

Second-Generation Antipsychotics

The advent of SSRIs in the 1980s revolutionized the treatment of depression, and a similar revolution has now taken place in the treatment of psychosis. The psycho-

pharmacological armamentarium available to treat psychotic disorders has expanded beyond the traditional FGAs (e.g., haloperidol, chlorpromazine) to include a growing array of SGAs.

Commonly prescribed antipsychotic medications, as well as agents used to treat the side effects of FGAs, are listed in Table 64–5. The SGAs currently available in the United States are aripiprazole, clozapine, olanzapine, paliperidone, quetiapine, risperidone, and ziprasidone. Compared with the older FGAs, these new agents are less likely to produce tardive dyskinesia and extrapyramidal side effects (EPS) and arguably more effective in managing the negative symptoms of schizophrenia. The SGAs have consequently supplanted the FGAs as first-line medications for psychotic disorders and are being increasingly used for other psychiatric indications, including bipolar disorder, OCD, and treatment-resistant depression. Despite these agents' rapidly expanding use, the reproductive safety database regarding SGAs remains extremely limited.

Clozapine

The extant literature regarding the reproductive safety of clozapine, the oldest of the SGAs, is limited to case reports (Barnas et al. 1994; Di Michele et al. 1996; Kornhuber and Weller 1991; Waldman and Safferman 1993), case series (McKenna et al. 2005; Stoner et al. 1997; Tenyi and Tixler 1998), and a retrospective review (Dev and Krupp 1995), collectively encompassing 79 children exposed to clozapine during pregnancy and/or lactation. Adverse sequelae associated with perinatal clozapine therapy include maternal gestational diabetes (Dickson and Hogg 1998); several minor anomalies, including cephalohematoma, hyperpigmentation folds, and a coccygeal dimple, in an infant (Stoner et al. 1997); transient low-grade fever at delivery in an infant whose was mother receiving lithium cotherapy (Stoner et al. 1997); and floppy infant syndrome in a newborn whose mother was taking clozapine and lorazepam during gestation (Di Michele et al. 1996). In a review of 61 children exposed to clozapine perinatally, Dev and Krupp (1995) reported 5 cases of congenital malformations and 5 cases of neonatal syndromes, although many of these mothers were taking other psychotropic medications during pregnancy. The lone case report of clozapine use during lactation reported no adverse impact on the nursing infant (Kornhuber and Weller 1991).

The only investigation of the perinatal pharmacokinetics of clozapine demonstrated similar medication concentrations in maternal serum and amniotic fluid but markedly higher concentrations in fetal serum and breast

TABLE 64–5. Antipsychotic medications

GENERIC NAME	TRADE NAME	DAILY DOSAGE (MG/DAY)[a]	RISK CATEGORY[b]	AMERICAN ACADEMY OF PEDIATRICS RATING[c]
First-generation antipsychotics				
Chlorpromazine	Thorazine	200–800	C	Unknown, but of concern
Fluphenazine	Prolixin	5–10	C	N/A
Haloperidol	Haldol	5–10	C_m	Unknown, but of concern
Loxapine	Loxitane	20–80	C	N/A
Mesoridazine	Serentil	100–400	C	Unknown, but of concern
Molindone	Moban	20–80	C	N/A
Perphenazine	Trilafon	8–32	C	Unknown, but of concern
Pimozide[d]	Orap	1–10	C	N/A
Thioridazine	Mellaril	200–600	C	N/A
Thiothixene	Navane	10–40	C	N/A
Trifluoperazine	Stelazine	10–40	C	Unknown, but of concern
Second-generation antipsychotics				
Aripiprazole	Abilify	10–30	C_m	N/A
Clozapine	Clozaril	100–800	B_m	Unknown, but of concern
Olanzapine	Zyprexa	5–20	C_m	N/A
Paliperidone	Invega	3–12	C_m	N/A
Quetiapine	Seroquel	25–800	C	Unknown, but of concern
Risperidone[d]	Risperdal	1–16	C	N/A
Ziprasidone	Geodon	40–160	C	Unknown, but of concern
Medications for side effects				
Amantadine	Symmetrel	100–400	C_m	N/A
Benztropine	Cogentin	0.5–6.0	C	N/A
Diphenhydramine	Benadryl	25–150	B_m	N/A
Propranolol	Inderal	20–120	C_m	Compatible
Trihexyphenidyl	Artane	2–15	C	N/A

Note. N/A = not available.
[a]Dosing strategies adapted from Schatzberg and Cole 1991; Kaplan and Sadock 1993; and for newer medications, the manufacturers' package inserts.
[b]Risk category adapted from Briggs et al. 2005 and/or Physicians' Desk Reference 2007; "m" subscript indicates data taken from the manufacturer's package insert.
[c]American Academy of Pediatrics 2001.
[d]Not listed in Briggs et al. 1994. Risk category taken from *Physicians' Desk Reference* (1992, 1993, 1994, and 1996 editions).

milk (Barnas et al. 1994), leading the authors to conclude that clozapine accumulates in the fetal circulation and breast milk. Although no cases of agranulocytosis have been reported in infants of women taking clozapine during pregnancy or lactation, this theoretical risk and the consequent requirement for monitoring of leukocyte counts in newborns and nursing infants limit the utility of clozapine during the peripartum.

Olanzapine

Of the remaining SGAs, the earliest reproductive safety data were reported for olanzapine. A published birth registry of 23 prospectively ascertained olanzapine-exposed pregnancies and 2 retrospectively ascertained cases of olanzapine lactation exposure from the Lilly Worldwide Pharmacovigilance Safety Database reported no major congenital malformations, 13% spontaneous abortions, 5% preterm deliveries, and 5% rate of fetal demise (Goldstein et al. 2000). A prospective study comparing outcomes among 151 pregnant women with SGA exposure (olanzapine, $n=60$; risperidone, $n=49$; quetiapine, $n=36$; clozapine, $n=6$) to 151 pregnant control subjects reported no differences in rates of spontaneous abortion, stillbirth, major malformations, prematurity, or low birth weight (McKenna et al. 2005). In this study, only one SGA-exposed child (olanzapine) was observed to have any major malformations (a series of midline defects including an oral cleft, encephalocele, and aqueductal stenosis).

In a recent study of antipsychotic placental passage rates and neonatal outcomes (Newport et al. 2007), umbilical cord concentrations in olanzapine-exposed neonates ($n=14$) were 72.1% of maternal concentrations (higher than rates for haloperidol, risperidone, and quetiapine). In this study, there were trends toward higher rates of low birth weight (30.8%; $P<0.06$) and neonatal intensive care unit admission (30.8%; $P<0.09$) among neonates exposed to olanzapine than those exposed to the other agents.

Case reports of 16 infants exposed to olanzapine during lactation with no evidence of infant toxicity currently appear in the literature (Croke et al. 2002; Friedman et al. 2003; Gardiner et al. 2003; Goldstein et al. 2000; Kirchheiner et al. 2000). Pharmacokinetic studies of olanzapine exposure during lactation have reported that plasma concentrations were undetectable in infants during nursing (Gardiner et al. 2003; Kirchheiner et al. 2000) and that the median infant daily dose via breast-feeding was approximately 1.0%–1.6% of the maternal dose (Ambresin et al. 2004; Croke et al. 2002; Gardiner et al. 2003).

There are no available data regarding the neurodevelopmental effects of olanzapine exposure during pregnancy or lactation.

Risperidone

There are two prospective reports of pregnancy outcome for women with first-trimester risperidone exposure. In the first, an assessment of the collective outcomes for several SGAs (McKenna et al. 2005) included 49 women with risperidone exposure. There were no children born with major malformations in this sample. The second study, including 68 women with first-trimester exposure and known outcomes, reported 9 (13.2%) spontaneous abortions, 1 (1.5%) stillbirth, and 2 (2.9%) children with major malformations (Coppola et al. 2007). The reproductive safety literature for risperidone encompasses 49 women and is limited to a single case report.

In our recent analysis of antipsychotic placental passage, risperidone concentrations in neonates ($n=6$) were 49.2% of maternal levels (Newport et al. 2007). Pharmacokinetic studies of risperidone excretion into breast milk have reported milk-to-plasma ratios of less than 0.5 for both risperidone and 9-hydroxyrisperidone (R.C. Hill et al. 2000; Ilett et al. 2004) and infant doses ranging from 2.3% to 4.7% of the maternal dose (Ilett et al. 2004).

There are no available data regarding the neurodevelopmental effects of risperidone exposure during pregnancy or lactation.

Quetiapine

The reproductive safety literature for first-trimester quetiapine exposure is limited to the McKenna et al. (2005) study, which reported no major malformations among 36 infants exposed to quetiapine. In the Newport et al. (2007) study of antipsychotic placental passage, quetiapine concentrations among neonates ($n=21$) were 23% of maternal concentrations. To our knowledge, this is the lowest placental passage rate ever reported for a psychotropic agent.

A single case of quetiapine use during lactation following use during pregnancy estimated the nursing infant dose at 0.09% of the maternal daily dose (Lee et al. 2004).

There are no available data regarding the neurodevelopmental effects of quetiapine exposure during pregnancy or lactation.

Aripiprazole

There are currently no reports regarding the use of aripiprazole during pregnancy or lactation.

Paliperidone

There are currently no reports regarding the use of paliperidone during pregnancy or lactation.

Ziprasidone

There are currently no reports regarding the use of ziprasidone during pregnancy or lactation.

First-Generation Antipsychotics

In contrast to the SGAs and most other classes of psychotropic medications, the FGAs have a large reproductive safety database that addresses concerns of both somatic and neurobehavioral teratogenicity. Furthermore, the widespread use of phenothiazines to treat pregnancy-associated emesis (typically at low doses) aids in separating the effects of psychiatric illness and antipsychotic drugs on pregnancy outcome. Chlorpromazine, haloperidol, and perphenazine have received the greatest scrutiny, with no significant associations between these compounds and major congenital malformations forthcoming (Goldberg and DiMascio 1978; R.M. Hill and Stern 1979; Nurnberg and Prudic 1984).

In a study of 100 women treated with haloperidol (mean dosage = 1.2 mg/day) for hyperemesis gravidarum, no differences in gestational duration, fetal viability, or birth weight were noted (Van Waes and Van de Velde 1969). In a large prospective study encompassing nearly 20,000 women treated primarily with phenothiazines for emesis, Milkovich and Van den Berg (1976) found no significant association with neonatal survival rates or severe anomalies after controlling for maternal age, medication, and gestational age at exposure. Similar results have been obtained in several retrospective studies of women treated with trifluoperazine for repeated abortions and emesis (Moriarty and Nance 1963; Rawlings et al. 1963). In contrast, Rumeau-Rouquette et al. (1977) reported a significant association of major anomalies with prenatal exposure to aliphatic side-chain phenothiazines but not with piperazine- or piperidine-class agents. Reanalysis of the data obtained by Milkovich and Van den Berg (1976) did find a significant risk of malformations associated with phenothiazine exposure in weeks 4 through 10 of gestation (Edlund and Craig 1976).

Clinical neurobehavioral outcome studies encompassing 203 children exposed to FGAs during gestation detected no significant differences in IQ scores at 4 years of age (Kris 1965; Slone et al. 1977), although relatively low antipsychotic doses were used by many women in these studies. Conversely, several laboratory animal studies (Hoffeld et al. 1968; Ordy et al. 1966; Robertson et al. 1980), although not all (Dallemagne and Weiss 1982), have demonstrated persistent deficits in learning and memory among offspring prenatally exposed to FGA medications.

Beyond the teratogenic potential of the FGAs lies the possibility of fetal and infant toxicities such as neuroleptic malignant syndrome (James 1988) and EPS manifested by heightened muscle tone and increased rooting and tendon reflexes persisting for several months (Cleary 1977; R.M. Hill et al. 1966; M.O. O'Connor et al. 1981). Furthermore, prenatal exposure to SGAs has been reported to produce neonatal jaundice (Scokel and Jones 1962) and postnatal intestinal obstruction (Falterman and Richardson 1980).

In our recent study of antipsychotic placental passage, neonatal haloperidol (n = 13) concentrations were 66% of maternal concentrations (Newport et al. 2005).

In lactation, chlorpromazine is the most widely studied typical antipsychotic, with 7 infants exposed to chlorpromazine during nursing exhibiting no developmental deficits at 16-month and 5-year follow-up evaluations (Kris and Carmichael 1957). However, 3 infants in another study whose mothers were prescribed both chlorpromazine and haloperidol exhibited evidence of developmental delay at 12–18 months (Yoshida et al. 1998b). Pharmacokinetic investigations of FGAs during lactation, including haloperidol (Stewart et al. 1980; Whalley et al. 1981; Yoshida et al. 1998b), trifluoperazine (J.T. Wilson et al. 1980; Yoshida et al. 1998b), perphenazine (J.T. Wilson et al. 1980), thioxanthenes (Matheson and Skjaeraasen 1988), and chlorpromazine (Yoshida et al. 1998b), have uniformly reported milk-to-plasma ratios of less than 1, although adequate control for distribution and time gradients is lacking in these studies. One group postulated that the physicochemical properties of perphenazine could lead it to become "trapped" in breast milk (J.T. Wilson et al. 1980).

Fetal and infant exposure to any of the various agents available for the management of EPS (e.g., diphenhydramine, benztropine, amantadine) also raises concern. Results of the Collaborative Perinatal Project indicate that first-trimester exposure to diphenhydramine, the best studied of these medications, is associated with major and minor congenital anomalies (Miller 1991; Wisner and Perel 1988). A case–control study demonstrated a significantly higher rate of prenatal diphenhydramine exposure among 599 infants with oral clefts than among 590 control infants (Saxén 1974). Clinical studies of the teratogenic potential of benztropine and amantadine are lacking, although laboratory animal studies indicate that amantadine is associated with an elevated risk of congenital malformations (Hirsch and Swartz 1980). Perinatal toxicities, including neonatal intestinal obstruction after gestational exposure to benztropine (Falterman and Richardson 1980) and a possible neonatal diphenhydramine withdrawal syndrome manifested by tremulousness and diarrhea (Parkin 1974), also warrant concern.

In summary, FGAs have been widely used for almost 50 years, and the paucity of data linking these agents to either teratogenic or toxic effects suggests that the risk associated with these medications is minimal. In particular, piperazine phenothiazines (e.g., trifluoperazine, perphenazine) may have especially limited teratogenic potential (Rumeau-Rouquette et al. 1977). Given the greater perinatal risks associated with anticholinergic medications, their use should be avoided if possible. Consequently, FGAs used during the peripartum should be kept at the lowest effective dose to minimize the need for adjunctive medications to manage EPS.

Early data regarding the teratogenic potential of the SGAs have been reassuring; however, the limited volume of SGA data to date precludes definitive conclusions regarding their reproductive safety. Therefore, the routine use of SGAs during pregnancy and lactation cannot yet be recommended. Nonetheless, if a woman who is taking an SGA inadvertently conceives, a comprehensive risk–benefit assessment may indicate that continuing the SGA (to which the fetus has already been exposed) during gestation is preferable to switching to an FGA (to which the fetus has not yet been exposed). Monitoring of blood glucose and weight gain should be an integral aspect of clinical management during pregnancy.

Anxiolytics

Benzodiazepines and antidepressants are the most commonly used medications for the treatment of anxiety disorders. Benzodiazepines have a wide spectrum of clinical indications, including the full array of anxiety disorders, insomnia, alcohol detoxification, muscle relaxation, adjunctive treatment of seizure disorders, and conscious sedation during invasive medical procedures. A retrospective survey of Medicaid prescription records for more than 100,000 pregnant women between 1980 and 1983 found that at least 2% were prescribed a benzodiazepine during gestation (Bergman et al. 1992). Table 64–6 lists the benzodiazepine and nonbenzodiazepine anxiolytics and sedative-hypnotics used in the treatment of anxiety disorders and insomnia.

The earliest studies of benzodiazepine-associated teratogenic effects reported an increased risk of oral clefts after in utero exposure to diazepam (Aarskog 1975; Saxén 1975; Saxén and Saxén 1974), but later studies failed to confirm this association (Entman and Vaughn 1984; Rosenberg et al. 1984; Shiono and Mills 1984). Prospective studies of first-trimester alprazolam exposure encompassing approximately 1,300 pregnancies demonstrated no excess of oral clefts or other congenital anomalies (Barry and St. Clair 1987; Schick-Boschetto and Zuber 1992; St. Clair and Schirmer 1992). A subsequent meta-analysis by Altshuler et al. (1996), which pooled data from several studies, demonstrated that prenatal benzodiazepine exposure does confer an increased risk of oral

cleft, although the absolute risk increased by only 0.01%, from 6 in 10,000 to 7 in 10,000. This conclusion is consistent with the findings of a recent case–control study that reported no difference in the rate of prenatal benzodiazepine exposure between more than 38,000 infants with congenital anomalies and nearly 23,000 control children without congenital defects (Eros et al. 2002).

Longitudinal follow-up studies to evaluate the neurobehavioral effects of prenatal benzodiazepine exposure are urgently needed. A "benzodiazepine exposure syndrome," including growth retardation, dysmorphism, and both mental and psychomotor retardation in infants exposed prenatally to benzodiazepines (Laegreid et al. 1987), has been reported, although other investigators have disputed this finding (Gerhardsson and Alfredsson 1987; Winter 1987). A second group found no differences in the incidence of behavioral abnormalities at age 8 months or in IQ scores at age 4 years among children exposed to chlordiazepoxide during gestation (Hartz et al. 1975). Nevertheless, a series of laboratory animal studies continues to raise concerns that prenatal benzodiazepine exposure may be associated with long-term deficits in memory and learning ability (Frieder et al. 1984; Hassmannova and Myslivecek 1994; Myslivecek et al. 1991).

Although the data regarding the teratogenic effects of benzodiazepine exposure remain somewhat controversial, the occurrence of neonatal toxicity and withdrawal syndromes is well documented. Numerous groups have described a floppy infant syndrome characterized by hypothermia, lethargy, poor respiratory effort, and feeding difficulties after maternal use of benzodiazepines shortly before delivery (Erkkola et al. 1983; J.N. Fisher et al. 1985; Haram 1977; Kriel and Cloyd 1982; McAuley et al. 1982; Sanchis et al. 1991; Speight 1977; Woods and Malan 1978). In a study of 53 infants born to women who were administered lorazepam prior to delivery, term infants whose mothers had taken oral lorazepam (up to 2.5 mg three times daily) showed no evidence of toxicity other than a minimal delay in establishing feeding, but preterm infants and term infants whose mothers had received larger intravenous doses of lorazepam exhibited a constellation of symptoms consistent with floppy infant syndrome (Whitelaw et al. 1981). Neonatal withdrawal syndromes characterized by restlessness, hypertonia, hyperreflexia, tremulousness, apnea, diarrhea, and vomiting have been described in infants whose mothers were taking alprazolam (Barry and St. Clair 1987), chlordiazepoxide (Athinarayanan et al. 1976; Bitnum 1969; Stirrat et al. 1974), or diazepam (Backes and Cordero 1980; Mazzi 1977). Symptoms of these neonatal syndromes

TABLE 64–6. Anxiolytic and hypnotic medications

GENERIC NAME	TRADE NAME	DAILY DOSAGE (MG/ DAY)[a]	RISK CATEGORY[b]	AMERICAN ACADEMY OF PEDIATRICS RATING[c]
Benzodiazepines				
Alprazolam	Xanax	0.5–6.0	D_m	Unknown, but of concern
Chlordiazepoxide	Librium	15–100	D	N/A
Clonazepam	Klonopin	0.5–10	C	N/A
Clorazepate	Tranxene	7.5–60	D	N/A
Diazepam	Valium	2–60	D	Unknown, but of concern
Estazolam[d]	ProSom	1–2	X	N/A
Flurazepam	Dalmane	15–30	X_m	N/A
Halazepam[d]	Paxipam	60–160	N/A	N/A
Lorazepam	Ativan	2–6	D_m	Unknown, but of concern
Oxazepam	Serax	30–120	D	N/A
Prazepam[d]	Centrax	20–60	D	Unknown, but of concern
Quazepam[d]	Doral	7.5–30	X_m	Unknown, but of concern
Temazepam	Restoril	15–30	X_m	Unknown, but of concern
Triazolam	Halcion	0.125–0.25	X_m	N/A
Nonbenzodiazepines				
Buspirone[d]	BuSpar	20–30	B_m	N/A
Chloral hydrate	Noctec	500–1,500	C_m	Compatible
Eszopiclone	Lunesta	2–6	C	N/A
Ramelteon	Rozerem	8	C	N/A
Zaleplon	Sonata	5–20	C	Unknown, but of concern
Zolpidem tartrate[d]	Ambien	5–10	C	N/A

Note.   N/A = not available.

[a]Dosing strategies adapted from Schatzberg and Cole 1991; Kaplan and Sadock 1993; and for newer medications, the manufacturers' package inserts.

[b]Risk category adapted from Briggs et al. 2005 and/or *Physicians' Desk Reference* 2007; "m" subscript indicates data taken from the manufacturer's package insert.

[c]American Academy of Pediatrics 2001.

[d]Not listed in Briggs et al. 1994. Risk category taken from *Physicians' Desk Reference* (1992, 1993, 1994, and 1996 editions).

have been reported to persist for as long as 3 months after delivery (for a review, see Miller 1991).

Pharmacokinetic studies during pregnancy indicate that benzodiazepines as a class readily traverse the placenta and that some of these drugs may accumulate in the fetus after prolonged administration (Mandelli et al. 1975; Shannon et al. 1972). For example, the fetal–maternal ratio of plasma diazepam concentrations at delivery is generally greater than 1 (Erkkola et al. 1974), likely a result, at least in part, of the fact that the fetal rate of metabolizing diazepam is considerably slower than the adult rate (Mandelli et al. 1975). In addition, particularly high concentrations of diazepam are sequestered in lipophilic

fetal tissues, including the fetal brain, lungs, and heart (Mandelli et al. 1975). A study reporting that fetal–maternal ratios of lorazepam are typically less than 1 (Whitelaw et al. 1981) suggests that placental transfer of lorazepam is lower than that of other benzodiazepines. Neonatal clearance of lorazepam is slow, with detectable levels evident 8 days after delivery (Whitelaw et al. 1981), and the clearance of chlordiazepoxide appears to be even slower (Athinarayanan et al. 1976).

Buist et al. (1990) concluded that benzodiazepines at relatively low doses present no contraindication to nursing. However, infants with an impaired capacity to metabolize benzodiazepines may exhibit sedation and poor feeding even with low maternal doses (Wesson et al. 1985). Overall, benzodiazepines exhibit lower milk-to-plasma ratios than other classes of psychotropics. For example, Wreitland (1987) found a milk-to-plasma ratio of 0.1–0.3 for oxazepam and calculated that the infant daily dose via lactation is 1/1,000 of the maternal dose. The percentage of the maternal dose of lorazepam to which a nursing infant is exposed has been estimated to be 2.2% (Summerfield and Nielsen 1985).

In summary, benzodiazepines do not appear to carry a significant risk of somatic teratogenesis, but neurobehavioral sequelae remain obscure. Because benzodiazepines are associated with a risk for neonatal toxicity and withdrawal syndromes, these drugs should be tapered prior to delivery when possible. Benzodiazepines should not, however, be abruptly withdrawn during pregnancy. Clonazepam (FDA Category C) appears to have minimal teratogenic risks (Sullivan and McElhatton 1977). Because lorazepam and oxazepam are less dependent on hepatic metabolism, they theoretically have less potential for fetal accumulation during pregnancy. Finally, when judicious doses are utilized, benzodiazepines can be safely administered during lactation. However, breast-feeding should be discontinued if an infant exhibits sedation or other signs of benzodiazepine toxicity, regardless of maternal dose.

Recently, newer agents, including buspirone, a nonbenzodiazepine anxiolytic, and zolpidem and zaleplon, nonbenzodiazepine hypnotics, have been added to the psychotropic armamentarium. There are no published reports of the use of these agents in pregnancy or lactation.

Future Directions and General Recommendations

The development of treatment guidelines for mental illness during pregnancy and lactation continues to be hampered by the haphazard accrual of research data with inconsistent methodologies. Whereas there are limited clinical data to support the contention that most psychotropic medications are teratogenic, laboratory animal studies, which typically attain maternal concentrations markedly higher than those achieved in clinical care, demonstrate clear somatic and neurobehavioral teratogenic effects (Elia et al. 1987). Such discrepancies between the clinical and preclinical data hinder efforts to construct reliable treatment recommendations. Because pregnant and nursing women are generally excluded from clinical trials of pharmacological agents, definitive clarification is unlikely to be forthcoming in the near future.

This raises questions about the future of clinical research in pregnancy and lactation. Some investigators have argued that conducting clinical trials in pregnant and nursing women is on its face unethical (Kerns 1986). Although such a view is understandable, the failure to conduct such studies may deprive some women of available treatment and may over time increase the overall risk to women and their infants. Alternative ethical positions regarding perinatal clinical research have been raised. In an investigation of alternative interventions following evidence of in utero failure to thrive, obstetrical researchers have advocated application of the *uncertainty principle* (Peto and Baigent 1998) to the ethical question of clinical research during gestation (Vail et al. 2001). The uncertainty principle mandates that a patient, even a pregnant patient, should be ethically eligible to participate in a randomized clinical trial if the preferred clinical course of action is uncertain. Because the relative risks to fetus and infant of exposure to maternal psychiatric illness compared with exposure to maternal psychotropic medication are often unclear, the uncertainty principle may be equally applicable to the study of psychiatric treatment during pregnancy and lactation. These questions must be deliberated so that perinatal psychiatric research can be advanced in an ethically responsible, yet expeditious, manner.

Meanwhile, given the current state of our knowledge, a thorough risk–benefit analysis should be completed for each woman presenting with concerns of psychiatric illness during pregnancy and lactation. This risk–benefit analysis should consider factors such as maternal psychiatric history, the potential deleterious effects of untreated illness on both the mother and her infant, and the potential adverse effects of offspring exposure to different classes of psychotropic medications within particular developmental windows. Table 64–7 and Table 64–8 summarize the basic risk–benefit assessments for pregnancy and lactation, which should be individualized according to the patient's history and treatment goals.

Initial Treatment Approach for Women of Reproductive Age

When treating women of reproductive age, it is advisable to assume at all times that pregnancy is imminent. More than 50% of pregnancies in the United States are unplanned; however, it is not cost effective to screen for pregnancy at all routine outpatient psychiatric visits.

By factoring reproductive safety considerations into all treatment decisions for women of child-bearing age, whether or not the patient is pregnant or actively trying

TABLE 64–7. Risk–benefit assessment for pregnancy: summary of facts

Known

85% of all pregnancies produce live births.

7%–14% of deliveries are preterm.

2%–4% of live births result in infants with significant malformations, and up to 12% have minor anomalies.

>60% of all women take at least one prescription medication during pregnancy.

In the ideal pregnancy, as defined by the Centers for Disease Control and Prevention, maternal weight is ±15% of ideal body weight, and the mother was taking prenatal vitamins with folic acid for 6 weeks before conception.

Most women learn of pregnancy at 5–8 weeks' gestation and therefore may be past the window of risk for fetal anomalies associated with psychotropic medications.

Pregnancy is not protective against psychiatric illness.

Increasing data

Major depressive episodes occur with similar incidence during pregnancy as during nongravid periods.

Obsessive-compulsive disorder may have its onset or may worsen during pregnancy.

The incidence of psychotic disorders varies throughout pregnancy; there are limited data suggesting a need to decrease dosage of antipsychotic medications.

The teratogenic risk of psychotropic medications has been historically overestimated.

Increasing data on obstetrical outcome and follow-up of infants of mothers taking psychotropic medications are comparable in study sample sizes to data on most other prescription drugs.

Untreated maternal mental illness may adversely affect obstetrical outcome and infant development.

Unknown

The long-term neurobehavioral effects of in utero exposure to psychotropic medications are unknown, although initial studies have not reported adverse effects for several medications.

TABLE 64–8. Risk–benefit assessment for lactation: summary of facts

Known: postpartum

>60% of women plan to breast-feed.

5%–17% of all nursing women take a prescription medication during breast-feeding.

12%–20% of nursing women smoke cigarettes.

Breast-feeding is supported by numerous professional organizations as the ideal form of nutrition for the infant.

The postnatal period is a high-risk time for onset or relapse of psychiatric illness.

All psychotropic medications studied to date are excreted in breast milk.

Increasing data

Untreated maternal mental illness has an adverse effect on mother–infant attachment and later infant development.

The adverse effects of psychotropic agents on infants are limited to case reports.

The nursing infant's daily dose of psychotropic agents is less than the maternal daily dose.

The nursing infant's exposure to psychotropic medications is less than the fetal exposure.

Psychotropic medications are excreted in breast milk with a specific individual time course, allowing the minimization of infant exposure with continuation of breast-feeding.

Unknown

The long-term neurobehavioral effects of infant exposure to psychotropic medications through breast-feeding are unknown.

---

to conceive, clinicians can maximize reproductive safety when inadvertent conception occurs.

Assuming that the clinician has already exhausted reasonable nonpharmacological interventions, we offer the following general treatment recommendations for the care of a patient with a mental disorder during pregnancy and lactation.

Informed Consent

It is impossible to provide an exhaustive list of all the risks for any given psychotropic medication, but the evidence (or lack thereof) for adverse activational effects (e.g., toxicity, withdrawal) and organizational effects (e.g., somatic teratogenesis, neurobehavioral teratogenesis) of each medication should be reviewed. It is equally important to discuss with the patient the risks of the untreated illness to both the mother and the infant. Finally, it is important to document that other treatment modalities have been attempted or considered.

Choice of Medication

When the decision is made to use a psychotropic medication, the goal is to maximize efficacy so that offspring exposure to maternal mental illness can most reliably be eliminated while avoiding offspring exposure to multiple medications. The most important factor in choosing a medication is therefore treatment history. If a patient has a history of a positive response to a particular medication, a novel agent should not be started during pregnancy or lactation. Such an approach only increases the risk of off-spring exposure to multiple medications and continued maternal illness. Prior offspring exposures also warrant consideration. If a patient was taking a particular medication earlier in gestation (and it was efficacious), continuing or restarting that medication is usually preferable to switching to a new medication. Switching medications in this manner automatically increases the child's number of medication exposures and may extend the duration of maternal illness. In addition to data from the treatment history, medications with the following characteristics should be sought:

- *Greatest reproductive safety database*—Medications with some published pregnancy and/or lactation safety data are preferred. Being the first to use a particular medication in pregnancy or nursing is not advisable. Medications that have been available for a longer time usually have a larger database.
- *Lower FDA risk category (B > C > D)*—The FDA is empirically conservative and has access to the greatest amount of pre- and postmarketing data. Although this rating may be controversial for some medications, medicolegal considerations support this approach.
- *Few or no metabolites*—Data from both pregnancy and lactation suggest that drug metabolites, which typically have longer elimination half-lives relative to the parent drug, may achieve higher steady-state levels in both fetal circulation and nursing infant serum. The issue of active versus inactive metabolites is unresolved with respect to teratogenic effects.
- *Fewer side effects and drug interactions*—Medications with fewer hypotensive and anticholinergic side effects are preferable. Additionally, the effect on seizure threshold and potential interaction with commonly used obstetrical anesthetic and analgesic agents should be minimized.
- *Concordant data*—Medications with conflicting data should be avoided; a clinically comparable alternative should be used, if available. Adherence to this recommendation also should reduce any potential legal liability.

Dosage

The goal of treatment during pregnancy and lactation is adequate treatment for syndrome remission. Partial treatment only enhances risk by continuing to expose mother and infant to both illness and medications. The minimum effective dose should be maintained throughout treat-

ment, and the clinician should remain mindful that dosage requirements might change during pregnancy. To minimize the potential for neonatal withdrawal and maternal toxicity after delivery, careful monitoring of side effects and serum concentrations may be indicated. Adjusting the feeding and dose schedule and discarding the peak breast milk concentrations for several agents can minimize exposure of nursing infants.

Communication With Other Physicians

It is highly recommended that the psychiatrist discuss the medication and potential interactions with both the patient's obstetrician and, if the patient chooses to nurse, her infant's pediatrician.

Monitoring Exposure of Nursing Infants

Most clinical laboratory assays lack the sensitivity necessary to detect the typical serum concentrations of nursing infants, and even detectable infant serum concentrations are uninterpretable; therefore, infant serum monitoring is not routinely indicated for most psychotropic medications. One noteworthy exception is the child who is exhibiting potential medication side effects. A small proportion of breast-feeding children may be metabolic outliers for a particular medication and thus may accumulate especially high serum concentrations. If there is a reasonable index of suspicion that the child's symptoms represent a medication effect, then breast-feeding should be discontinued, regardless of infant serum concentration. Consequently, we recommend checking an infant's serum concentration when the child is suspected to be experiencing a medication side effect. Furthermore, infant serum concentrations and other laboratory studies (e.g., blood counts, electrolytes, hepatic profiles) should be monitored when nursing mothers are taking medications (e.g., certain anticonvulsants) with low therapeutic indices or known systemic toxicities.

Conclusion

The use of pharmacological therapies during pregnancy and lactation will continue to be a complex clinical endeavor that will certainly generate anxiety among patients and clinicians. There is a propensity in the medical literature and the news media to emphasize adverse outcomes, whereas negative study results seldom garner much attention. This is true for both medication and illness exposures. Consequently, clinicians must practice with access to incomplete information.

Thoughtful consideration of "pregnancy potential" in the treatment planning for women of reproductive capacity serves to reduce the consternation precipitated by a positive pregnancy test. By inquiring routinely about birth control during all visits when treating women during the reproductive years, clinicians can provide a conduit for discussion and treatment planning that aims to reduce risk for mother and child.

References

Aarskog D: Letter: Association between maternal intake of diazepam and oral clefts. Lancet 2(7941):921, 1975

Adab N, Jacoby A, Smith D, et al: Additional educational needs in children born to mothers with epilepsy. J Neurol Neurosurg Psychiatry 70:15–21, 2001

Agatonovic-Kustrin S, Ling LH, Tham SY, et al: Molecular descriptors that influence the amount of drugs transfer into human breast milk. J Pharm Biomed Anal 29:103–119, 2002

Alexander FW: Sodium valproate and pregnancy. Arch Dis Child 54:240, 1979

Allen S: A quantitative analysis of the process, mediating variables, and impact of traumatic childbirth. J Reprod Infant Psychol 16:107–131, 1998

Alonso SJ, Navarro E, Rodriguez M: Permanent dopaminergic alterations in the nucleus accumbens after prenatal stress. Pharmacol Biochem Behav 49:353–358, 1994

Alonso SJ, Navarro E, Santana C, et al: Motor lateralization, behavioral despair and dopaminergic brain asymmetry after prenatal stress. Pharmacol Biochem Behav 58:443–448, 1997

Altshuler LL, Burt VK, McMullen M, et al: Breastfeeding and sertraline: a 24-hour analysis. J Clin Psychiatry 56:243–245, 1995

Altshuler LL, Cohen LS, Szuba MP, et al: Pharmacologic management of psychiatric illness in pregnancy: dilemmas and guidelines. Am J Psychiatry 153:592–606, 1996

Alwan S, Reefhuis J, Rasmussen SA, et al: Use of selective serotonin-reuptake inhibitors in pregnancy and the risk of birth defects. N Engl J Med 356:2684–2692, 2007

Ambresin G, Berney P, Schulz P, et al: Olanzapine excretion into breast milk: a case report. J Clin Psychopharmacol 24:93–95, 2004

American Academy of Pediatrics, Committee on Drugs: The transfer of drugs and other chemicals into human milk. Pediatrics 108:776–789, 2001

American College of Obstetricians and Gynecologists: ACOG Practice Bulletin No. 87, November 2007: Use of psychiatric medications during pregnancy and lactation. Obstet Gynecol 110:1179–1198, 2007

American Psychiatric Association: Diagnostic and Statistical Manual of Mental Disorders, 4th Edition, Text Revision. Washington, DC, American Psychiatric Association, 2000

Andrade SE, Raebel MA, Brown J, et al: Use of antidepressant medications during pregnancy: a multisite study. Am J Obstet Gynecol 198(2):194.e1–194.e5, 2008

Andrews M, Rosenblum L: Relationship between foraging and affiliative social referencing in primates, in Ecology and Behavior of Food-Enhanced Primate Groups. Edited by Fa J, Southwick C. New York, Alan R Liss, 1988, pp 247–268

Andrews M, Rosenblum L: Attachment in monkey infants raised in variable and low-demand environments. Child Dev 62:686–693, 1991

Andrews M, Rosenblum L: Developmental consequences of altered dyadic coping patterns in bonnet macaques, in Current Primatology: Social Development, Learning and Behavior. Edited by Roeder J, Thierry B, Anderson J, et al. Strasbourg, France, Universitie Louis Pasteur, 1994, pp 265–271

Appleby L, Warner R, Whitton A, et al: A controlled study of fluoxetine and cognitive-behavioral counseling in the treatment of postnatal depression. BMJ 314:932–936, 1997

Ardinger H, Atkin J, Blackston RD, et al: Verification of the fetal valproate syndrome phenotype. Am J Med Genet 29:171–185, 1988

Assencio-Ferreira VJ, Abraham R, Veiga JC, et al: Metopic suture craniosynostosis: sodium valproate teratogenic effect: case report [Portuguese]. Arquivos de Neuro-Psiquiatria 59(2-B):417–420, 2001

Athinarayanan P, Peirog SH, Nigam SK, et al: Chlordiazepoxide withdrawal in the neonate. Am J Obstet Gynecol 124:212–213, 1976

Atkinson HC, Begg EJ, Darlow BA: Drugs in human milk: clinical pharmacokinetic considerations. Clin Pharmacokinet 14:217–240, 1988

Audus KL: Controlling drug delivery across the placenta. Eur J Pharmacol Sci 8:161–165, 1999

Backes CR, Cordero L: Withdrawal symptoms in the neonate from presumptive intrauterine exposure to diazepam: report of case. J Am Osteopath Assoc 79:584–585, 1980

Bardy AH, Granström ML, Hiilesmaa VK: Valproic acid and breast feeding, in Epilepsy, Pregnancy, and the Child. Edited by Janz D, Dam M, Richens A. New York, Raven Press 1982a, pp 359–360

Bardy AH, Teramo K, Hiilesmaa VK: Apparent plasma clearances of phenytoin, phenobarbitone, primidone, and carbamazepine during pregnancy: results of the prospective Helsinki study, in Epilepsy, Pregnancy, and the Child. Edited by Janz D, Dam M, Richens A, et al. New York, Raven Press, 1982b, pp 141–145

Barnas C, Bergant A, Hummer A, et al: Clozapine concentrations in maternal and fetal plasma, amniotic fluid, and breast milk. Am J Psychiatry 151:945, 1994

Barry WS, St. Clair SM: Exposure to benzodiazepines in utero. Lancet 1(8547):1436–1437, 1987

Barson AJ: Malformed infants. BMJ 2:45, 1972

Battino D, Avanzini G, Bossi L, et al: Monitoring of antiepileptic drug plasma levels during pregnancy and puerperium, in Epilepsy, Pregnancy, and the Child. Edited by Janz D, Dam M, Richens A, et al. New York, Raven Press, 1982, pp 147–154

Bennedsen BE, Mortensen PB, Olesen AV, et al: Obstetric complications in women with schizophrenia. Schizophr Res 47:167–175, 2001

Bergman U, Rosa FW, Baum C, et al: Effects of exposure to benzodiazepine during fetal life. Lancet 340:694–696, 1992

Bertossi M, Virgintino D, Errede M, et al: Immunohistochemical and ultrastructural characterization of cortical plate microvasculature in the human fetus telencephalon. Microvasc Res 58:49–61, 1999

Bescoby-Chambers N, Forster P, Bates G: Foetal valproate syndrome and autism: additional evidence of an association. Dev Med Child Neurol 43:847, 2001

Birnbaum C, Cohen LS, Bailey JW, et al: Serum concentrations of antidepressants and benzodiazepines in nursing infants: a case series. Pediatrics 104:1–6, 1999

Bitnum S: Possible effects of chlordiazepoxide on the foetus. Can Med Assoc J 100:351, 1969

Bjerkedal T, Czeizel A, Goujard J, et al: Valproic acid and spina bifida. Lancet 2(8307):109, 1982

Black MM, Matula K: Essentials of Bayley Scales of Infant Development—II Assessment. New York, Wiley, 2000

Bledsoe SE, Grote NK: Treating depression during pregnancy and the postpartum: a preliminary meta-analysis. Res Soc Work Pract 16:109–120, 2006

Blehar MC, DePaulo JR, Gershon ES, et al: Women with bipolar disorder: findings from the NIMH Genetics Initiative sample. Psychopharmacol Bull 34:239–243, 1998

Bologa M, Tang B, Klein J, et al: Pregnancy-induced changes in drug metabolism in epileptic women. J Pharmacol Exp Ther 267:735–740, 1991

Boobis AR, Lewis PJ: Pharmacokinetics in pregnancy, in Clinical Pharmacology in Obstetrics. Edited by Lewis P. Boston, MA, Wright-PSG, 1983, pp 6–54

Boshier A, Wilton LV, Shakir SA: Evaluation of the safety of bupropion (Zyban) for smoking cessation from experience gained in general practice use in England in 2000. Eur J Clin Pharmacol 59:767–773, 2003

Brent NB, Wisner KL: Fluoxetine and carbamazepine concentrations in a nursing mother/infant pair. Clin Pediatr 37:41–44, 1998

Briggs GG, Samson JH, Ambrose PJ, et al: Excretion of bupropion in breast milk. Ann Pharmacother 27:431–433, 1993

Briggs GG, Freeman RK, Yaffe SJ: Drugs in Pregnancy and Lactation, 4th Edition. Philadelphia, PA, Lippincott Williams & Wilkins, 1994

Briggs GG, Freeman RK, Yaffe SJ: Drugs in Pregnancy and Lactation, 7th Edition. Philadelphia, PA, Lippincott Williams & Wilkins, 2005

Bucove AD: A case of prepartum psychosis and infanticide. Psychiatr Q 42:263–270, 1968

Buesching DP, Glasser ML, Frate DA: Progression of depression in the prenatal and postpartum periods. Women Health 11:61–78, 1988

Buist A, Norman TR, Dennerstein L: Breastfeeding and the use of psychotropic medication: a review. J Affect Disord 19:197–206, 1990

Burch K, Wells B: Fluoxetine/norfluoxetine concentrations in human milk. Pediatrics 89:676–677, 1992

Canger R, Battino D, Canevini MP, et al: Malformations in offspring of women with epilepsy: a prospective study. Epilepsia 40:1231–1236, 1999

Casper RC, Fleisher BE, Lee-Ancajas JC, et al: Follow-up of children of depressed mothers exposed or not exposed to antidepressant drugs during pregnancy. J Pediatr 142:402–408, 2003

Cassels C: Valproate should not be used as first-line therapy in women of childbearing age. Medscape Today. Medscape Medical News. August 7, 2006. Available at: http://www.medscape.com/viewarticle/542424. Accessed March 2008.

Centers for Disease Control: Spina bifida incidence at birth—United States, 1983–1990. MMWR Morb Mortal Wkly Rep 41:497–500, 1992

Chambers CD, Johnson KA, Dick LM, et al: Birth outcomes in pregnant women taking fluoxetine. N Engl J Med 335:1010–1015, 1996

Chambers CD, Hernandez-Diaz S, Van Marter LJ, et al: Selective serotonin-reuptake inhibitors and risk of persistent pulmonary hypertension of the newborn. N Engl J Med 354:579–587, 2006

Chun-Fai-Chan B, Koren G, Fayez I, et al: Pregnancy outcome of women exposed to bupropion during pregnancy: a prospective comparative study. Am J Obstet Gynecol 192:932–936, 2005

Clarke AS, Schneider ML: Prenatal stress has long-term effects on behavioral responses to stress in juvenile rhesus monkeys. Dev Psychobiol 26:293–304, 1993

Cleary MF: Fluphenazine decanoate during pregnancy. Am J Psychiatry 134:815–816, 1977

Cohen LS, Heller VL, Rosenbaum JF: Treatment guidelines for psychotropic drug use in pregnancy. Psychosomatics 30:25–33, 1989

Cohen LS, Friedman JM, Jefferson JW, et al: A reevaluation of risk of in utero exposures to lithium. JAMA 271:146–150, 1994

Cohen LS, Altshuler LL, Harlow BL, et al: Relapse of major depression during pregnancy in women who maintain or discontinue antidepressant treatment. JAMA 295:499–507, 2006 [Erratum in JAMA 296:170, 2006]

Cole JA, Ephross SA, Cosmatos IS, et al: Paroxetine in the first trimester and the prevalence of congenital malformations. Pharmacoepidemiol Drug Saf 16:1075–1085, 2007

Coons PM, Ascher-Svanum H, Bellis K: Self-amputation of the female breast. Psychosomatics 27:667–668, 1986

Coplan J, Andrews M, Rosenblum LA, et al: Persistent elevations of cerebrospinal fluid concentrations of corticotropin-releasing factor in adult nonhuman primates exposed to early life stressors: implications for the pathophysiology of mood and anxiety disorders. Proc Natl Acad Sci U S A 93:1619–1623, 1996

Coplan J, Trost R, Owens M, et al: Cerebrospinal fluid concentrations of somatostatin and biogenic amines in grown primates reared by mothers exposed to manipulated foraging conditions. Arch Gen Psychiatry 55:473–477, 1998

Coppola D, Russo LJ, Kwarta RF, et al: Evaluating the postmarketing experience of risperidone use during pregnancy: pregnancy and neonatal outcomes. Drug Saf 30:247–264, 2007

Costei AM, Kozer E, Ho T, et al: Perinatal outcome following third trimester exposure to paroxetine. Arch Pediatr Adolesc Med 156:1129–1132, 2002

Cox MT, Stowe ZN, Hostetter A, et al: Cortisol concentrations in the breast milk of women with major depression. Paper presented at the American Psychiatric Association 153rd Annual Meeting, Chicago, IL, May 13–18, 2000

Croke S, Buist A, Hackett LP, et al: Olanzapine excretion in human breast milk: estimation of infant exposure. Int J Neuropsychopharmacol 5:243–247, 2002

Cutrona CE: Causal attributions and perinatal depression. J Abnorm Psychol 92:161–172, 1986

Dalens B, Raynaud EJ, Gaulme J: Teratogenicity of valproic acid. J Pediatr 97:332–333, 1980

Dallemagne G, Weiss B: Altered behavior of mice following postnatal treatment with haloperidol. Pharmacol Biochem Behav 16:761–767, 1982

Dam J, Christiansen J, Munck O, et al: Antiepileptic drugs: metabolism in pregnancy. Clin Pharmacokinet 4:53–62, 1979

Davison JM, Hytten FE: Glomerular filtration during and after pregnancy. Br J Obstet Gynaecol 81:588–595, 1974

Dean JC, Moore SJ, Osborne A, et al: Fetal anticonvulsant syndrome and mutation in the maternal MTHFR gene. Clin Genet 56:216–220, 1999 de Haan GJ, Edelbroek P, Segers J, et al: Gestation-induced changes in lamotrigine pharmacokinetics: a monotherapy study. Neurology 63:571–573, 2004

Dev V, Krupp P: The side-effects and safety of clozapine. Rev Contemp Pharmacother 6:197–208, 1995

Di Liberti JH, Farndon PA, Dennis NR, et al: The fetal valproate syndrome. Am J Med Genet 19:473–481, 1984

Di Michele V, Ramenghi LA, Sabatino G: Clozapine and lorazepam administration in pregnancy. Eur Psychiatry 11:214, 1996

Dickinson RG, Harland RC, Lynn RK, et al: Transmission of valproic acid (Depakene) across the placenta: half-life of the drug in mother and baby. J Pediatr 94 832–835, 1979

Dickson RA, Edwards A: Clozapine and fertility. Am J Psychiatry 154:582–583, 1997

Dickson RA, Hogg L: Pregnancy of a patient treated with clozapine. Psychiatr Serv 49:1081–1083, 1998

Djulus J, Koren G, Einarson TR, et al: Exposure to mirtazapine during pregnancy: a prospective, comparative study of birth outcomes. J Clin Psychiatry 67:1280–1284, 2006

Dodd S, Stocky A, Buist A, et al: Sertraline in paired blood plasma and breast-milk samples from nursing mothers. Hum Psychopharmacol 15:261–264, 2000

Doering JC, Stewart RB: The extent and character of drug consumption during pregnancy. JAMA 239:843–846, 1978

Dolk H, Jentink J, Loane M, et al: Does Lamotrigine use in pregnancy increase orofacial cleft risk relative to other malformations? Neurology 71:714–722, 2008

Dominguez-Salgado M, Morales A, Santiago Gomez R, et al: Gestational lamotrigine monotherapy: congenital malformations and psychomotor development (abstract). Epilepsia 45 (suppl 7):229–230, 2004

Downey G, Coyne JC: Children of depressed parents: an integrative review. Psychol Bull 108:50–76, 1990

Duffy CL: Postpartum depression: identifying women at risk. Genesis 11:21, 1983

Dunlop W: Serial changes in renal haemodynamics during pregnancy. Br J Obstet Gynaecol 8:1–9, 1981

Ebbesen F, Joergensen AM, Hoseth E, et al: Neonatal hypoglycaemia and withdrawal symptoms after exposure in utero to valproate. Arch Dis Child Fetal Neonatal Ed 83:F124–F129, 2000

Edlund MJ, Craig TJ: Antipsychotic drug use and birth defects: an epidemiologic reassessment. Compr Psychiatry 25:244–248, 1976

Eggermont E: Withdrawal symptoms in neonates associated with maternal imipramine therapy. Lancet 2(7830):680, 1973

Einarson A, Fatoye B, Sarkar M, et al: Pregnancy outcome following gestational exposure to venlafaxine: a multicenter prospective controlled study. Am J Psychiatry 158:1728–1730, 2001

Einarson A, Bonari L, Voyer-Lavigne S, et al: A multicentre prospective controlled study to determine the safety of trazodone and nefazodone use during pregnancy. Can J Psychiatry 48:106–110, 2003

Elia J, Katz IR, Simpson GM: Teratogenicity of psychotherapeutic medications. Psychopharmacol Bull 23:531–586, 1987

Entman SS, Vaughn WK: Lack of relation of oral clefts to diazepam use in pregnancy. N Engl J Med 310:1121–1122, 1984

Epperson C, Anderson G, McDougle C: Sertraline and breast-feeding. N Engl J Med 336:1189–1190, 1997

Epperson N, Czarkowski KA, Ward-O'Brien D, et al: Maternal sertraline treatment and serotonin transport in breast-feeding mother-infant pairs. Am J Psychiatry 158:1631–1637, 2001

Ericson A, Kallen B, Wiholm BE: Delivery outcome after the use of antidepressants in early pregnancy. Eur J Clin Pharmacol 55:503–508, 1999

Erkkola R, Kanto J, Sellman R: Diazepam in early human pregnancy. Acta Obstet Gynecol Scand 53:135–138, 1974

Erkkola R, Kero P, Kanto J, et al: Severe abuse of psychotropic drugs during pregnancy with good perinatal outcome. Ann Clin Res 15:88–91, 1983

Eros E, Czeizel AE, Rockenbauer M, et al: A population-based case-control teratologic study of nitrazepam, medazepam, tofisopam, alprazolam, and clonazepam treatment during pregnancy. Eur J Obstet Gynecol Reprod Biol 101:147–154, 2002

Falterman CG, Richardson CJ: Small left colon syndrome associated with maternal ingestion of psychotropic drugs. J Pediatr 97:308–310, 1980

Fisher AD, Brown JS, Newport DJ, et al: Fetal CNS exposure after maternal SSRI: a rodent model (NR137), in 2001 New Research Program and Abstracts, American Psychiatric Association 154th Annual Meeting, New Orleans, LA, May 5–10, 2001. Washington, DC, American Psychiatric Association, 2001, p 12

Fisher JN, Edgren BE, Mammel MC, et al: Neonatal apnea associated with clonazepam therapy: a case report. Obstet Gynecol 66:348–358, 1985

Fones C: Posttraumatic stress disorder occurring after painful childbirth. J Nerv Ment Dis 184:195–196, 1996

Frederiksen MC: Physiologic changes in pregnancy and their effect on drug disposition. Semin Perinatol 25:120–123, 2001

Frederiksen MC, Ruo TI, Chow MJ, et al: Theophylline pharmacokinetics in pregnancy. Clin Pharmacol Ther 40:321–328, 1986

Freeman MP, Smith KW, Freeman SA, et al: The impact of reproductive events on the course of bipolar disorder in women. J Clin Psychiatry 63:284–287, 2000

Frey B, Schubiger G, Musy JP: Transient cholestatic hepatitis in a neonate associated with carbamazepine exposure during pregnancy and breast-feeding. Eur J Pediatr 150:136–138, 1990

Frey B, Braegger CP, Ghelfi D: Neonatal cholestatic hepatitis from carbamazepine exposure during pregnancy and breast feeding. Ann Pharmacother 36:644–647, 2002

Fride E, Weinstock M: The effects of prenatal exposure to predictable or unpredictable stress on early development in the rat. Dev Psychobiol 17:651–660, 1984

Fride E, Weinstock M: Prenatal stress increases anxiety related behavior and alters cerebral lateralization of dopamine activity. Life Sci 36:1059–1065, 1988

Fride E, Dan Y, Gavish M, et al: Prenatal stress impairs maternal behavior in a conflict situation and reduces hippocampal benzodiazepine receptors. Life Sci 36:2103, 1985

Fride E, Dan Y, Feldon J, et al: Effects of prenatal stress on vulnerability to stress in prepubertal and adult rats. Physiol Behav 37:681–687, 1986

Frieder B, Epstein S, Grimm VE: The effects of exposure to diazepam during various stages of gestation or during lactation on the development and behavior of rat pups. Psychopharmacology 83:51–55, 1984

Friedman JM, Polifka JE: Teratogenic Effects of Drugs: A Resource for Clinicians (TERIS), 2nd Edition. Baltimore, MD, Johns Hopkins University Press, 2000, pp ix–x

Friedman SH, Rosenthal MB: Treatment of perinatal delusional disorder: a case report. Int J Psychiatry Med 33:391–394, 2003

Fries H: Lithium in pregnancy. Lancet 1(7658):1233, 1970

Froescher W, Eichelbaum M, Nieson M, et al: Antiepileptic therapy with carbamazepine and valproic acid during pregnancy and the lactation period, in Advances in Epileptology: The 12th Epilepsy International Symposium. Edited by Dam M, Gram L, Penry JK. New York, Raven Press, 1981, pp 581–588

Froescher W, Eichelbaum M, Niesen M, et al: Carbamazepine levels in breast milk. Ther Drug Monit 6:266–271, 1984a

Froescher W, Gugler R, Niesen M, et al: Protein binding of valproic acid in maternal and umbilical cord serum. Epilepsia 25:244–249, 1984b

Fujioka T, Sakata Y, Yamaguchi K, et al: The effects of prenatal stress on the development of hypothalamic paraventricular neurons in fetal rats. Neuroscience 92:1079–1088, 1999

Gaily E, Kantola-Sorsa E, Granstrom ML: Specific cognitive dysfunction in children with epileptic mothers. Dev Med Child Neurol 32:403–414, 1990

Gaily E, Kantola-Sorsa E, Hiilasmaa V et al: Normal intelligence in children with prenatal exposure to carbamazepine. Neurology 62:8–9, 2004

Galler JR, Harrison RH, Ramsey F, et al: Maternal depressive symptoms affect infant cognitive development in Barbados. J Child Psychol Psychiatry 41:747–757, 2000

Gardiner SJ, Kristensen JH, Begg EJ, et al: Transfer of olanzapine into breast milk, calculation of infant drug dose, and effect on breast-fed infants. Am J Psychiatry 160:1428–1431, 2003

Gerhardsson M, Alfredsson L: In-utero exposure to benzodiazepines. Lancet 1(8533):628, 1987

GlaxoSmithKline: Epidemiology study: Updated preliminary report on bupropion and other antidepressants, including paroxetine in pregnancy and the occurrence of cardiovascular and major congenital malformations (study EPIP083). 2005. Available at: http://ctr.gsk.co.uk/summary/paroxetine/epip083part2.pdf. Accessed January 2008.

GlaxoSmithKline Corp: International Pregnancy Registry: interim report (1 September 1992 through 31 March 2007). Wilmington, NC, Inveresk, 2007

Glaze R, Chapman G, Murray D: Recurrence of puerperal psychosis during late pregnancy. Br J Psychiatry 159:567–569, 1991

Goldberg HL, DiMascio A: Psychotropic drugs in pregnancy, in Psychopharmacology: A Generation of Progress. Edited by Lipton HL, DiMascio A, Killam KF. New York, Raven, 1978, pp 1047–1055

Goldstein DJ, Sundell KL, Corbin LA: Birth outcomes in pregnant women taking fluoxetine. N Engl J Med 336:872–873, 1997

Goldstein DJ, Corbin LA, Fung MC: Olanzapine-exposed pregnancies and lactation: early experience. J Clin Psychopharmacol 20:399–403, 2000

Graybeal S, Newport DJ, Fisher A, et al: Antidepressants in pregnancy, minimizing fetal exposure: clinical and preclinical data (NR280), in 2002 New Research Program and Abstracts, American Psychiatric Association 155th Annual Meeting, Philadelphia, PA, May 18–23, 2002. Washington, DC, American Psychiatric Association, 2002, p 25

Greenough A, Khetriwal B: Pulmonary hypertension in the newborn. Paediatr Respir Rev 6:111–116, 2005

Grof PR, Robbins W, Alda M, et al: Protective effect of pregnancy in women with lithium-responsive bipolar disorder. J Affect Disord 61:31–39, 2000

Hakkola J, Pasanen M, Hukkanen J, et al: Expression of xenobiotic-metabolizing cytochrome P450 forms in human full-term placenta. Biochem Pharmacol 51:403–411, 1996

Hallberg P, Sjöblom V: The use of selective serotonin reuptake inhibitors during pregnancy and breast-feeding: a review and clinical aspects. J Clin Psychopharmacol 25:59–73, 2005

Hannah P, Adams D, Glover V, et al: Abnormal platelet 5-hydroxytryptamine uptake and imipramine binding in postnatal dysphoria. J Psychiatr Res 26:69–75, 1992

Haram K: "Floppy infant syndrome" and maternal diazepam. Lancet 2(8038):612–613, 1977

Hartz SC, Heinonen OP, Shapiro S, et al: Antenatal exposure to meprobamate and chlordiazepoxide in relation to malformations, mental development, and childhood mortality. N Engl J Med 292:726–728, 1975

Hassmannova J, Myslivecek J: Inhibitory and excitatory adult learning after prenatal diazepam application. Studia Psychologica 36:323–326, 1994

Hayashi A, Nagaoka M, Yamada K, et al: Maternal stress induces synaptic loss and developmental disabilities of offspring. Int J Dev Neurosci 16:209–216, 1998

Hedegaard M, Henriksen T, Sabroe S, et al: The relationship between psychological distress during pregnancy and birth weight for gestational age. Acta Obstet Gynecol Scand 75:32–39, 1996

Heikkinen T, Ekblad U, Kero P, et al: Citalopram in pregnancy and lactation. Clin Pharmacol Ther 72:184–191, 2002

Heinonen OP, Stone D, Shapiro S: Birth Defects and Drugs in Pregnancy. Littleton, MA, Publishing Sciences Group, 1977

Hendrick V, Fukuchi A, Altshuler LL, et al: Use of sertraline, paroxetine, and fluvoxamine by nursing women. Br J Psychiatry 179:163–166, 2001

Hendrick V, Smith LM, Suri R, et al: Birth outcomes after prenatal exposure to antidepressant medication. Am J Obstet Gynecol 188:812–815, 2003a

Hendrick V, Stowe ZN, Altshuler LL, et al: Placental passage of antidepressant medication. Am J Psychiatry 160:993–996, 2003b

Henry C, Kabbaj M, Simon H, et al: Prenatal stress increases the hypothalamo-pituitary-adrenal axis response in young and adult rats. J Neuroendocrinol 6:341–345, 1994

Henry C, Guegant G, Cador M, et al: Prenatal stress in rats facilitates amphetamine-induced sensitization and induces long-lasting changes in dopamine receptors in the nucleus accumbens. Brain Res 685:179–186, 1995

Hernandez-Diaz S, Werler MM, Walker AM, et al: Neural tube defects in relation to use of folic acid antagonists during pregnancy. Am J Epidemiol 153:961–968, 2001

Herrenkohl LR, Gala RR: Serum prolactin levels and maintenance of progeny by prenatally stressed female offspring. Experientia 35:702–704, 1979

Hertzberg T, Wahlbeck K: The impact of pregnancy and puerperium on panic disorder: a review. J Psychosom Obstet Gynecol 20:59–64, 1999

Hill RC, McIvor RJ, Wojnar-Horton RE, et al: Risperidone distribution and excretion into human milk: case report and estimated infant exposure during breast-feeding. J Clin Psychopharmacol 20:285–286, 2000

Hill RM, Stern L: Drugs in pregnancy: effects on the fetus and newborn. Curr Ther 20:131–150, 1979

Hill RM, Desmond MM, Kay JL: Extrapyramidal dysfunction in an infant of a schizophrenic mother. J Pediatr 69:589–595, 1966

Hirsch MS, Swartz MN: Antiviral agents. N Engl J Med 302:903–907, 1980

Hoffeld DR, McNew J, Webster RL: Effect of tranquilizing drugs during pregnancy on activity of offspring. Nature 218:357–358, 1968

Holmes LB, Wyszynski DF, Baldwin EJ, et al: Increased risk for nonsyndromic cleft palate among infants exposed to lamotrigine during pregnancy (abstract). Birth Defects Res Part A Clin Mol Teratol 76:318, 2006

Homma M, Beckerman K, Hayashi S, et al: Liquid chromatographic determination of urinary 6-hydroxycortisol to assess cytochrome P450 3A activity in HIV positive pregnant women. J Pharm Biomed Anal 23:629–635, 2000

Hostetter A, Ritchie JC, Stowe ZN: Amniotic fluid and umbilical cord blood concentrations of antidepressants in three women. Biol Psychiatry 48:1032–1034, 2000

Hunt JN, Murray FA: Gastric function in pregnancy. Br J Obstet Gynaecol 65:78–83, 1958

Ilett K, Hackett L, Dusci L, et al: Distribution and excretion of venlafaxine and O-desmethylvenlafaxine in human milk. Br J Clin Pharmacol 45:459–462, 1998

Ilett KF, Hackett LP, Kristensen JH, et al: Transfer of risperidone and 9-hydroxyrisperidone into human milk. Ann Pharmacother 38:273–276, 2004

Jacobsen SJ, Jones K, Johnson K, et al: Prospective multicentre study of pregnancy outcome after lithium exposure during first trimester. Lancet 339:530–533, 1992

Jager-Roman E, Deichl A, Jakob S, et al: Fetal growth, major malformations, and minor anomalies in infants born to women receiving valproic acid. J Pediatr 108:997–1004, 1986

Jaiswal A, Bhattacharya S: Effects of gestational undernutrition, stress and diazepam treatment on spatial discrimination learning and retention in young rats. Indian J Exp Biol 31:353–359, 1993

James ME: Neuroleptic malignant syndrome in pregnancy. Psychosomatics 29:112–119, 1988

Jameson PB, Gelfand DM, Kulcsar E, et al: Mother-toddler interaction patterns associated with maternal depression. Dev Psychopathol 9:537–550, 1997

Jenike MA, Hyman S, Baer L, et al: A controlled trial of fluvoxamine in obsessive-compulsive disorder: implications for a serotonergic theory. Am J Psychiatry 147:1209–1215, 1990

Jensen P, Olesen O, Bertelsen A, et al: Citalopram and desmethylcitalopram concentrations in breast milk and in serum of mother and infant. Ther Drug Monit 19:236–239, 1997

Jones KL, Lacro RV, Johnson KA, et al: Pattern of malformations in the children of women treated with carbamazepine during pregnancy. N Engl J Med 320:1661–1666, 1989

Källén B: Neonate characteristics after maternal use of antidepressants in late pregnancy. Arch Pediatr Adolesc Med 158:312–316, 2004

Källén B, Tandberg A: Lithium and pregnancy: a cohort of manic-depressive women. Acta Psychiatr Scand 68:134–139, 1983

Kaneko S, Suzuki K, Sato T, et al: The problems of antiepileptic medication in the neonatal period: is breast-feeding advisable? in Epilepsy, Pregnancy and the Child. Edited by Janz D, Dam M, Richens A. New York, Raven Press, 1982, pp 343–348

Kaneko S, Battino D, Andermann E, et al: Congenital malformations due to antiepileptic drugs. Epilepsy Res 33:145–158, 1999

Kaplan B, Modai I, Stoler M, et al: Clozapine treatment and risk of unplanned pregnancy. J Am Board Fam Pract 8:239–241, 1996

Kaplan HI, Sadock BJ: Pocket Handbook of Psychiatric Drug Treatment. Baltimore, MD, Williams & Wilkins, 1993

Kari FW, Weaver R, Neville MC: Active transport of nitrofurantoin across the mammillary epithelium in vivo. J Pharmacol Exp Ther 280:664–668, 1997

Karlsson K, Lindstedt G, Lundberg PA, et al: Letter: Transplacental lithium poisoning: reversible inhibition of fetal thyroid. Lancet 1(7919):1295, 1975

Kendell R, Chalmers J, Platz C: Epidemiology of puerperal psychosis. Br J Psychiatry 150:662–673, 1987

Kendler KS, Kessler RC, Neale MC, et al: The prediction of major depression in women: toward an integrated etiologic model. Am J Psychiatry 150:1139–1148, 1993

Kennedy D, Koren G: Valproic acid use in psychiatry: issues in treating women of reproductive age. J Psychiatry Neurosci 23:223–228, 1998

Kerns LL: Treatment of mental disorders in pregnancy: a review of psychotropic drug risks and benefits. J Nerv Ment Dis 174:652–659, 1986

Kiely M: Reproductive and Perinatal Epidemiology. Boca Raton, FL, CRC Press, 1991

Kirchheiner J, Berghofer A, Bolk-Weischedel D: Healthy outcome under olanzapine treatment in a pregnant woman. Pharmacopsychiatry 33:78–80, 2000

Kirksey A, Groziak SM: Maternal drug use: evaluation of risks to breast-fed infants. World Rev Nutr Diet 43:60–79, 1984

Koch S, Jager-Roman E, Rating D, et al: Possible teratogenic effect of valproate during pregnancy. J Pediatr 103:1007–1008, 1983

Kok TH, Taitz LS, Bennett MJ, et al: Drowsiness due to clemastine transmitted in breast milk. Lancet 1(8277):914–915, 1982

Korebrits C, Ramirez M, Watson L, et al: Maternal corticotropin-releasing hormone is increased with impending preterm birth. J Clin Endocrinol Metab 83:1585–1591, 1998

Kornhuber J, Weller M: Postpartum psychosis and mastitis: a new indication for clozapine? Am J Psychiatry 148:1751–1752, 1991

Kozma C: Valproic acid embryopathy: report of two siblings with further expansion of the phenotypic abnormalities and a review of the literature. Am J Med Genet 98:168–175, 2001

Kriel RL, Cloyd J: Clonazepam and pregnancy. Ann Neurol 11:544, 1982

Kris EB: Children of mothers maintained on pharmacotherapy during pregnancy and postpartum. Curr Ther Res 7:785–789, 1965

Kris EB, Carmichael D: Chlorpromazine maintenance therapy during pregnancy and confinement. Psychiatr Q 31:690–695, 1957

Kristensen J, Ilett K, Dusci L, et al: Distribution and excretion of sertraline and N-desmethylsertraline in human milk. Br J Clin Pharmacol 45:453–457, 1998

Kristensen J, Ilett K, Hackett L, et al: Distribution and excretion of fluoxetine and norfluoxetine in human milk. Br J Clin Pharmacol 48:521–527, 1999

Kuhnz W, Jager-Roman E, Rating D, et al: Carbamazepine and carbamazepine-10,11-epoxide during pregnancy and postnatal period in epileptic mothers and their nursed infants: pharmacokinetics and clinical effects. Pediatr Pharmacol 3:199–208, 1983

Kulin N, Pastuszak A, Sage S, et al: Pregnancy outcome following maternal use of the new selective serotonin reuptake inhibitors: a prospective controlled multicenter study. JAMA 279:609–610, 1998

Kumar R, Robson KM: A prospective study of emotional disorders in childbearing women. Br J Psychiatry 144:35–47, 1984

Laegreid L, Olegard R, Wahlstrom J, et al: Abnormalities in children exposed to benzodiazepines in utero. Lancet 1(8524):108–109, 1987

Laine K, Heikkinen T, Ekblad U, et al: Effects of exposure to selective serotonin reuptake inhibitors during pregnancy on serotonergic symptoms in newborns and cord blood monoamine and prolactin concentrations. Arch Gen Psychiatry 60:720–726, 2003

Lajeunie E, Le Merrer M, Marchac D, et al: Syndromal and nonsyndromal primary trigonocephaly: analysis of 237 patients. Am J Med Genet 75:211–215, 1998

Lajeunie E, Barcik U, Thorne JA, et al: Craniosynostosis and fetal exposure to sodium valproate. J Neurosurg 95:778–782, 2001

Lander CM, Livingstone I, Tyrer JH, et al: The clearance of anticonvulsant drugs in pregnancy. Clin Exp Neurol 17:71–78, 1980

Lee A, Giesbrecht E, Dunn E, et al: Excretion of quetiapine in breast milk. Am J Psychiatry 161:1715–1716, 2004

Lees MM, Taylor SH, Scott DM, et al: A study of cardiac output at rest throughout pregnancy. Br J Obstet Gynaecol 74:319–328, 1967

Lester B, Cucca J, Andreozzi L, et al: Possible association between fluoxetine hydrochloride and colic in an infant. J Am Acad Child Adolesc Psychiatry 32:1253–1255, 1993

Levine S: Maternal and environmental influences on the adrenocortical response to stress in weanling rats. Science 156:258–260, 1967

Lindhout D, Schmidt D: In-utero exposure to valproate and neural tube defects. Lancet 1(8494):329–333, 1986

Liporace J, Kao A, D'Abreu A: Concerns regarding lamotrigine and breast-feeding. Epilepsy Behav 5:102–105, 2004

Little BB: Pharmacokinetics during pregnancy: evidence-based maternal dose formulation. Obstet Gynecol 93:858–868, 1999

Llewellyn AM, Stowe ZN, Nemeroff CB: Infant outcome after sertraline exposure, in 1997 New Research Program and Abstracts, American Psychiatric Association 150th Annual Meeting, San Diego, CA, May 17–22, 1997. Washington, DC, American Psychiatric Association, 1997, p 176

Llewellyn AM, Stowe ZN, Strader JR: The use of lithium and management of women with bipolar disorder during pregnancy and lactation. J Clin Psychiatry 59 (suppl 6):57–64, 1998

Lou HC, Hansen D, Nordentoft M, et al: Prenatal stressors of human life affect fetal brain development. Dev Med Child Neurol 36:826–832, 1994

Louik C, Lin AE, Werler MM, et al: First-trimester use of selective serotonin-reuptake inhibitors and the risk of birth defects. N Engl J Med 356:2675–2683, 2007

Lund CV, Donovan JC: Blood volume during pregnancy: significance of plasma and red cell volumes. Am J Obstet Gynecol 98:394–403, 1967

Lundy BL, Jones NA, Field T, et al: Prenatal depression effects on neonates. Infant Behav Dev 22:119–129, 1999

Luoma I, Tamminen T, Kaukonen P, et al: Longitudinal study of maternal depressive symptoms and child well-being. J Am Acad Child Adolesc Psychiatry 40:1367–1374, 2001

Luoma I, Kaukonen P, Mäntymaa M, et al: A longitudinal study of maternal depressive symptoms, negative expectations and perceptions of child problems. Child Psychiatry Hum Dev 35:37–53, 2004

Lyons-Ruth K, Wolfe R, Lyubchik A: Depression and the parenting of young children: making the case for early preventive mental health services. Harv Rev Psychiatry 8:148–153, 2000

Maina G, Albert U, Bogetto F, et al: Recent life events and obsessive-compulsive disorder (OCD): the role of pregnancy/delivery. Psychiatry Res 89(1):49–58, 1999

Mammen O, Perel JM, Rudolph G, et al: Sertraline and norsertraline levels in three breastfed infants. J Clin Psychiatry 58:100–103, 1997

Mandelli M, Morselli PL, Nordio S, et al: Placental transfer of diazepam and its disposition in the newborn. Clin Pharmacol Ther 17:564–572, 1975

Manly PC, McMahon RJ, Bradley CF, et al: Depressive attributional style and depression following childbirth. J Abnorm Psychol 91:245–254, 1982

Marcus SM, Flynn HA, Blow FC, et al: Depressive symptoms among pregnant women screened in obstetrics settings. J Womens Health (Larchmt) 12:373–380, 2003

Martinez A, Malphurs J, Field T, et al: Depressed mothers' and their infants' interactions with nondepressed partners. Infant Ment Health J 17:74–80, 1996

Martinez-Frias ML: Clinical manifestation of prenatal exposure to valproic acid using case reports and epidemiologic information. Am J Med Genet 37:277–282, 1990

Martins C, Gaffan EA: Effects of early maternal depression on patterns of infant-mother attachment: a meta-analytic investigation. J Child Psychol Psychiatry 41:737–746, 2000

Maschi S, Clavenna A, Campi R, et al: Neonatal outcome following pregnancy exposure to antidepressants: a prospective controlled cohort study. BJOG 115:283–289, 2008

Matalon S, Schechtman S, Goldzweig G, et al: The teratogenic effect of carbamazepine: a meta-analysis of 1255 exposures. Reprod Toxicol 16:9–17, 2002

Matheson I, Pande H, Alertson AR: Respiratory depression caused by N-desmethyldoxepine in breast milk. Lancet 2(8464):1124, 1985

Matheson I, Skjaeraasen J: Milk concentrations of flupenthixol, nortriptyline and zuclopenthixol and between breast differences in two patients. Eur J Clin Pharmacol 35:217–220, 1988

Mattison DR: Physiologic variations in pharmacokinetics during pregnancy, in Drug and Chemical Action in Pregnancy: Pharmacologic and Toxicologic Principles. Edited by Fabro S, Scialli A. New York, Marcel Dekker, 1986, pp 37–102

Mattison DR, Blann E, Malek A: Physiological alterations during pregnancy: impact on toxicokinetics. Fundam Appl Toxicol 16:215–218, 1991

Mazzi E: Possible neonatal diazepam withdrawal: a case report. Am J Obstet Gynecol 129:586–587, 1977

McAuley DM, O'Neill MP, Moore J, et al: Lorazepam premedication for labour. Br J Obstet Gynecol 89:149–154, 1982

McBride WG: Limb deformities associated with iminodibenzyl hydrochloride. Med J Aust 1:175–178, 1972

McCormick CM, Smythe JW, Sharma S, et al: Sex-specific effects of prenatal stress on hypothalamic-pituitary-adrenal responses to stress and brain glucocorticoid receptor density in adult rats. Brain Res 84:55–61, 1995

McElhatton PR, Garbis HM, Elefant E, et al: The outcome of pregnancy in 689 women exposed to therapeutic doses of antidepressants. A collaborative study of the European Network of Teratology Information Services (ENTIS). Reprod Toxicol 10:285–294, 1996

McEvoy JP, Hatcher A, Appelbaum PS, et al: Chronic schizophrenic women's attitudes toward sex, pregnancy, birth control, and childrearing. Hosp Community Psychiatry 34:536–539, 1983

McGorry P, Conell S: The nosology and prognosis of puerperal psychosis: a review. Compr Psychiatry 31:519–534, 1990

McKenna K, Koren G, Tetelbaum M, et al: Pregnancy outcome of women using atypical antipsychotic drugs: a prospective comparison study. J Clin Psychiatry 66:444–449, 2005

McMahon CL, Braddock SR: Septo-optic dysplasia as a manifestation of valproic acid embryopathy. Teratology 64:83–86, 2001

McNeil TF, Kaij L, Malmquist-Larson A: Women with nonorganic psychosis: mental disturbance during pregnancy. Acta Psychiatr Scand 70:127–139, 1984a

McNeil TF, Kaij L, Malmquist-Larson A: Women with nonorganic psychosis: pregnancy's effect on mental health during pregnancy. Acta Psychiatr Scand 70:140–148, 1984b

Meador KJ, Baker GA, Finnell RH, et al: In utero antiepileptic drug exposure: fetal death and malformations. Neurology 67:407–412, 2006

Meijer A: Child psychiatric sequelae of maternal war stress. Acta Psychiatr Scand 72:505–511, 1985

Mendenhall HW: Serum protein concentrations in pregnancy, I: concentrations in maternal serum. Am J Obstet Gynecol 106:388–399, 1970

Merlob P, Mor N, Litwin A: Transient hepatic dysfunction in an infant of an epileptic mother treated with carbamazepine during pregnancy and breastfeeding. Ann Pharmacother 26:1563–1565, 1992

Metcalfe J, Romney SL, Ramsey LH, et al: Estimation of uterine blood flow in women at term. J Clin Invest 34:1632–1638, 1955

Milkovich L, Van den Berg BJ: An evaluation of the teratogenicity of certain antinauseant drugs. Am J Obstet Gynecol 125:244–248, 1976

Miller LJ: Clinical strategies for the use of psychotropic drugs during pregnancy. Psychiatr Med 9:275–298, 1991

Miller LJ: Use of electroconvulsive therapy during pregnancy. Hosp Community Psychiatry 45:444–450, 1994

Miller LJ: Sexuality, reproduction, and family planning in women with schizophrenia. Schizophr Bull 23:623–635, 1997

Miller LJ, Finnerty M: Sexuality, pregnancy, and childrearing among women with schizophrenia-spectrum disorders. Psychiatr Serv 47:502–506, 1996

Misri S, Sivertz K: Tricyclic drugs in pregnancy and lactation: a preliminary report. Int J Psychiatry Med 21:157–171, 1991

Misri S, Oberlander TF, Fairbrother N, et al: Relation between prenatal maternal mood and anxiety and neonatal health. Can J Psychiatry 49:684–689, 2004

Mizrahi EM, Hobbs JF, Goldsmith DI: Nephrogenic diabetes insipidus in transplacental lithium intoxication. J Pediatr 94:493–495, 1979

Moore SJ, Turnpenny P, Quinn A, et al: A clinical study of 57 children with fetal anticonvulsant syndromes. J Med Genet 37:489–497, 2000

Moore WM, Hellegers AE, Battaglia FC: In vitro permeability of different layers of human placenta to carbohydrates and urea. Am J Obstet Gynecol 96:951–955, 1966

Morgan DJ: Drug disposition in mother and foetus. Clin Exp Pharmacol Physiol 24:869–873, 1997

Moriarty AJ, Nance NR: Trifluoperazine and pregnancy. Can Med Assoc J 88:375–376, 1963

Morrow J, Russell A, Guthrie E, et al: Malformation risks of antiepileptic drugs in pregnancy: a prospective study from the UK Epilepsy and Pregnancy Register. J Neurol Neurosurg Psychiatry 77:193–198, 2006

Moses-Kolko EL, Bogen D, Perel J, et al: Neonatal signs after late in utero exposure to serotonin reuptake inhibitors: literature review and implications for clinical applications. JAMA 293:2372–2383, 2005

Mountain KR, Hirsh J, Gallus AS: Neonatal coagulation defect due to anticonvulsant drug treatment in pregnancy. Lancet 1(7641):265–268, 1970

Myllynen PK, Pienimaki PK, Vahakangas KH: Transplacental passage of lamotrigine in a human placental perfusion system in vitro and in maternal and cord blood in vivo. Eur J Clin Pharmacol 58:677–682, 2003

Myslivecek J, Hassmannova J, Josifko M: Impact of prenatal low-dose diazepam or chlorpromazine on reflex and motor development and inhibitory-learning. Homeost Health Dis 33:77–88, 1991

Nau H, Rating D, Koch S, et al: Valproic acid and its metabolites: placental transfer, neonatal pharmacokinetics, transfer via mother's milk and clinical status in neonates of epileptic mothers. J Pharmacol Exp Ther 219:768–777, 1981

Nau H, Kuhnz W, Egger HJ, et al: Anticonvulsants during pregnancy and lactation: transplacental, maternal and neonatal pharmacokinetics. Clin Pharmacokinet 7:508–543, 1982a

Nau H, Wittfoht W, Rating D, et al: Pharmacokinetics of valproic acid and its metabolites in a pregnant patient: stable isotope methodology, in Epilepsy, Pregnancy, and the Child. Edited by Janz D, Bossi L, Dam M, et al: New York, Raven Press, 1982b, pp 131–139

New York State Department of Health: Congenital Malformations Registry Summary Report: Statistical Summary of Children Born in 1998–2001 and Diagnosed Through 2003. Troy, NY, Congenital Malformations Registry, New York State Department of Health, 2005. Available at: http://www.health.state.ny.us/nysdoh/cmr/docs/98report.pdf. Accessed November 2007.

Newport DJ, Wilcox M, Stowe ZN: Antidepressants during pregnancy and lactation: defining exposure. Semin Perinatol 25:177–190, 2001

Newport DJ, Hostetter A, Arnold A, et al: The treatment of postpartum depression: minimizing infant exposures. J Clin Psychiatry 63 (suppl 7):31–44, 2002a

Newport DJ, Stowe ZN, Nemeroff CB: Parental depression: animal models of an adverse life event. Am J Psychiatry 159:1265–1283, 2002b

Newport DJ, Owens MJ, Knight DL, et al: Alterations in platelet serotonin transporter binding in women with postpartum onset major depression. J Psychiatr Res 38:467–473, 2004

Newport DJ, Viguera AC, Beach AJ, et al: Lithium placental passage and obstetrical outcome: implications for clinical management during late pregnancy. Am J Psychiatry 162:2162–2170, 2005

Newport DJ, Calamaras MR, DeVane CL, et al: Atypical antipsychotic administration during late pregnancy: placental passage and obstetrical outcomes. Am J Psychiatry 164:1214–1220, 2007

Newport DJ, Pennell PB, Calamaras MR, et al: Lamotrigine in breast milk and nursing infants: determination of exposure. Pediatrics 122:e223–e231, 2008a

Newport DJ, Stowe ZN, Viguera AC, et al: Lamotrigine in bipolar disorder: efficacy during pregnancy. Bipolar Disord 10:432–436, 2008b

Neziroglu FN, Anemone MA, Yaryura-Tobias JA: Onset of obsessive-compulsive disorder in pregnancy. Am J Psychiatry 149:947–950, 1992

Niebyl JR, Blake DA, Freeman JM, et al: Carbamazepine levels in pregnancy and lactation. Obstet Gynecol 53:139–140, 1979

Nonacs R, Cohen LS: Depression during pregnancy: diagnosis and treatment options. J Clin Psychiatry 63 (suppl 7):24–30, 2002

Nora JJ, Nora AH, Toews WH: Letter: Lithium, Ebstein's anomaly, and other congenital heart defects. Lancet 2(7880):594–595, 1974

Nulman I, Rovet J, Stewart DE, et al: Neurodevelopment of children exposed in utero to antidepressant drugs. N Engl J Med 336:258–262, 1997a

Nulman I, Scolnick D, Chitayat D, et al: Findings in children exposed in utero to phenytoin and carbamazepine monotherapy: independent effects of epilepsy and medications. Am J Med Genet 68:18–24, 1997b

Nulman I, Rovet J, Stewart DE, et al: Child development following exposure to tricyclic antidepressants or fluoxetine throughout fetal life: a prospective, controlled study. Am J Psychiatry 159:1889–1895, 2002

Nurnberg HG, Prudic J: Guidelines for treatment of psychosis during pregnancy. Hosp Community Psychiatry 35:67–71, 1984

Oberlander TF, Misri S, Fitzgerald CE, et al: Pharmacologic factors associated with transient neonatal symptoms following prenatal psychotropic medication exposure. J Clin Psychiatry 65:230–237, 2004

Oberlander TF, Warburton W, Misri S, et al: Neonatal outcomes after prenatal exposure to selective serotonin reuptake inhibitor antidepressants and maternal depression using population-based linked health data. Arch Gen Psychiatry 63:898–906, 2006

Oberlander TF, Reebye P, Misri S, et al: Externalizing and attentional behaviors in children of depressed mothers treated with a selective serotonin reuptake inhibitor antidepressant during pregnancy. Arch Pediatr Adolesc Med 161:22–29, 2007

O'Connor MO, Johnson GH, James DI: Intrauterine effect of phenothiazines. Med J Aust 1:416–417, 1981

O'Connor TG, Heron J, Golding J, et al: Maternal antenatal anxiety and behavioural/emotional problems in children: a test of a programming hypothesis. J Child Psychol Psychiatry 44:1025–1036, 2003

Oesterheld JR: A review of developmental aspects of cytochrome P450. J Child Adolesc Psychopharmacol 8:161–174, 1998

O'Hara MW, Rehm LP, Campbell SB: Predicting depressive symptomatology: cognitive-behavioural models and postpartum depression. J Abnorm Psychol 91:457–461, 1982

O'Hara MW, Stuart S, Gorman LL, et al: Efficacy of interpersonal psychotherapy for postpartum depression. Arch Gen Psychiatry 57:1039–1045, 2000

Ohman I, Vitols S, Tomson T: Lamotrigine in pregnancy: pharmacokinetics during delivery, in the neonate, and during lactation. Epilepsia 41:709–713, 2000

Ohman R, Hagg S, Carleborg L, et al: Excretion of paroxetine into breast milk. J Clin Psychiatry 60:519–523, 1999

Omtzigt JG, Nau H, Los FJ, et al: The disposition of valproate and its metabolites in the late first trimester and early second trimester of pregnancy in maternal serum, urine, and amniotic fluid: effect of dose, co-medication, and the presence of spina bifida. Eur J Clin Pharmacol 43:381–388, 1992

Omtzigt JG, Los FJ, Meijer JW, et al: The 10,11-epoxide-10, 11-diol pathway of carbamazepine in early pregnancy in maternal serum, urine, and amniotic fluid: effect of dose, comedication, and relation to outcome of pregnancy. Ther Drug Monit 15:1–10, 1993

Oo CY, Kuhn RJ, Desai N, et al: Active transport of cimetidine into human milk. Clin Pharmacol Ther 58:548–555, 1995

Ordy JM, Samorajski T, Collins RL: Prenatal chlorpromazine effects on liver survival and behavior of mice offspring. J Pharmacol Exp Ther 151:110–125, 1966

Ornoy A, Cohen E: Outcome of children born to epileptic mothers treated with carbamazepine during pregnancy. Arch Dis Child 75:517–520, 1996

Orr S, Miller C: Maternal depressive symptoms and the risk of poor pregnancy outcome. Epidemiol Rev 17:165–170, 1995

Orr ST, James SA, Blackmore Prince C: Maternal prenatal depressive symptoms and spontaneous preterm births among African-American women in Baltimore, Maryland. Am J Epidemiol 156:797–802, 2002

Otani K: Risk factors for the increased seizure frequency during pregnancy and puerperium. Folia Psychiatr Neurol Jpn 39:33–41, 1985

Owens M, Hostetter AL, Knight DL, et al: Fetal exposure to SERT antagonist antidepressants in rats. Presented at the annual meeting of the Society for Neuroscience, New Orleans, LA, October 25–30, 1997

Pacifici GM, Nottoli R: Placental transfer of drugs administered to the mother. Clin Pharmacokinet 28:235–269, 1995

Page-Sharp M, Kristensen JH, Hackett LP, et al: Transfer of lamotrigine into breast milk. Ann Pharmacother 40:1470–1471, 2006

Parkin DE: Probable Benadryl withdrawal manifestations in a newborn infant. J Pediatr 85:580, 1974

Parry BL, Javeed S, Laughlin GA, et al: Cortisol circadian rhythms during the menstrual cycle and with sleep deprivation in premenstrual dysphoric disorder and normal control subjects. Biol Psychiatry 48:920–931, 2000

Parry E, Shields R, Turnbull AC: Transit time in the small intestine in pregnancy. Br J Obstet Gynaecol 77:900–901, 1970

Pastuszak A, Schick-Boschetto B, Zuber C, et al: Pregnancy outcome following first trimester exposure to fluoxetine (Prozac). JAMA 269:2246–2248, 1993

Pauk J, Kuhn C, Field T, et al: Positive effects of tactile versus kinesthetic or vestibular stimulation on neuroendocrine and ODC activity in maternally deprived rat pups. Life Sci 39:2081–2087, 1986

Paulson GW, Paulson RB: Teratogenic effects of anticonvulsants. Arch Neurol 38:140–143, 1981

Pedersen CA, Stern RA, Pate J, et al: Thyroid and adrenal measures during late pregnancy and the puerperium in women who have been major depressed or who become dysphoric postpartum. J Affect Disord 29:201–211, 1993

Pennell P, Gleba J, Clements S: Antiepileptic drug monitoring during pregnancy in women with epilepsy. Epilepsia 41:200, 2000

Pennell PB, Newport DJ, Stowe ZN, et al: The impact of pregnancy and childbirth on the metabolism of lamotrigine. Neurology 62:292–295, 2004

Pennell PB, Peng L, Newport DJ, et al: Lamotrigine in pregnancy: clearance, therapeutic drug monitoring, and seizure frequency. Neurology 70(22 pt 2):2130–2136, 2008

Perkin R, Bland J, Peacock J, et al: The effect of anxiety and depression during pregnancy on obstetric complications. Br J Obstet Gynaecol 100:629–634, 1993

Perucca E, Crema A: Plasma protein binding of drugs in pregnancy. Clin Pharmacokinet 7:336–352, 1982

Peters D: Prenatal stress: effects on brain biogenic amine and plasma corticosterone levels. Pharmacol Biochem Behav 17:721–725, 1982

Peters D: Prenatal stress: Effect on development of rat brain adrenergic receptors. Pharmacol Biochem Behav 21:417–422, 1984

Peters D: Prenatal stress increases the behavioral response to serotonin agonists and alters open field behavior in the rat. Pharmacol Biochem Behav 25:873–877, 1986

Peters D: Effects of maternal stress during different gestational periods on the serotonergic system in adult rat offspring. Pharmacol Biochem Behav 31:839–843, 1988

Peters D: Maternal stress increases fetal brain and neonatal cerebral cortex 5-hydroxytryptamine synthesis in rats: a possible mechanism by which stress influences brain development. Pharmacol Biochem Behav 35:943–947, 1990

Petersen VP: Body composition and fluid compartments in normal, obese and underweight human subjects. Acta Med Scand 108:103–111, 1957

Peto R, Baigent C: Trials: the next 50 years. BMJ 317:1170–1171, 1998

Petrenaite V, Sabers A, Hansen-Schwartz J. Individual changes in lamotrigine plasma concentrations during pregnancy. Epilepsy Research 65:185–188, 2005

Pfister H, Muir J: Prenatal exposure to predictable and unpredictable novelty stress and oxytocin treatment affects offspring development and behavior in rats. Int J Neurosci 62:227–241, 1992

Philbert A, Pederson B, Dam M: Concentration of valproate during pregnancy in the newborn and in breast milk. Acta Neurol Scand 72:460–463, 1985

Physicians' Desk Reference (PDR), 61st Edition. Montvale, NJ, Thomson Healthcare, 2007

Pihoker C, Owens M, Kuhn C, et al: Maternal separation in neonatal rats elicits activation of the hypothalamic-pituitary-adrenocortical axis: a putative role for corticotropin-releasing factor. Psychoneuroendocrinology 7:485–493, 1993

Piontek CM, Baab S, Peindl KS, et al: Serum valproate levels in 6 breast-feeding mother-infant pairs. J Clin Psychiatry 61:170–172, 2000

Piontek CM, Wisner KL, Perel JM, et al: Serum fluvoxamine levels in breastfed infants. J Clin Psychiatry 52:111–113, 2001

Pittard WB, O'Neal W: Amitriptyline excretion in human milk. J Clin Psychopharmacol 6:383–384, 1986

Plentl AA, Gray MJ: Total body water, sodium space and total exchangeable sodium in normal and toxemic pregnant women. Am J Obstet Gynecol 78:472–478, 1959

Poltyrev T, Keshet G, Kay G, et al: Role of experimental conditions in determining differences in exploratory behavior of prenatally stressed rats. Dev Psychobiol 29:453–462, 1996

Poulson E, Robson JM: Effect of phenelzine and some related compounds in pregnancy. J Endocrinol 30:205–215, 1964

Prentice A, Brown R: Fetal tachyarrhythmia and maternal antidepressant treatment. BMJ 298:190, 1989

Pynnonen S, Sillanpaa M: Letter: carbamazepine and mother's milk. Lancet 2(7934):563, 1975

Pynnonen S, Kanto J, Sillanpaa M, et al: Carbamazepine: placental transport, tissue concentrations in foetus and newborn, and level in milk. Acta Pharmacol Toxicol 41:244–253, 1977

Rambeck B, Kurlemann G, Stodieck SR, et al: Concentrations of lamotrigine in a mother on lamotrigine treatment and her newborn child. Eur J Clin Pharmacol 51:481–484, 1997

Rampono J, Hackett LP, Kristensen JH, et al: Transfer of escitalopram and its metabolite desmethylescitalopram into breast-milk. Br J Clin Pharmacol 62:316–322, 2006

Rawlings WJ, Ferguson R, Maddison TG: Phenmetrazine and trifluoperazine. Med J Aust 1:370, 1963

Rieder RO, Rosenthal D, Wender P, et al: The offspring of schizophrenics: fetal and neonatal deaths. Arch Gen Psychiatry 32:200–211, 1975

Rimm AA, Katayama AC, Diaz M, et al: A meta-analysis of controlled studies comparing major malformation rates in IVF and ICSI infants with naturally conceived children. J Assist Reprod Genet 21:437–443, 2004

Riordan D, Appleby L, Faragher B: Mother-infant interaction in post-partum women with schizophrenia and affective disorders. Psychol Med 29:991–995, 1999

Robertson RT, Majka JA, Peter CP, et al: Effects of prenatal exposure to chlorpromazine on postnatal development and behavior of rats. Toxicol Appl Pharmacol 53:541–549, 1980

Robson SC, Mutch E, Boy RJ, et al: Apparent liver blood flow during pregnancy: a serial study using indicyanine green clearance. Br J Obstet Gynaecol 97:720–724, 1990

Rodriguez-Pinilla E, Arroyo I, Fondevilla J, et al: Prenatal exposure to valproic acid during pregnancy and limb deficiencies: a case-control study. Am J Med Genet 90:376–381, 2000

Rosa FW: Spina bifida in infants of women treated with carbamazepine during pregnancy. N Engl J Med 324:674–677, 1991

Rosenberg L, Mitchell AA, Parsells JL, et al: Lack of relation of oral clefts to diazepam use during pregnancy. N Engl J Med 309:1281–1285, 1984

Rosenblum L, Paully G: The effects of varying environmental demands on maternal and infant behavior. Child Dev 55:305–314, 1984

Rumeau-Rouquette C, Goujard J, Huel G: Possible teratogenic effect of phenothiazines in human beings. Teratology 15:57–64, 1977

Rybakowski JK: Moclobemide in pregnancy. Pharmacopsychiatry 34:82–83, 2001

Sabers A, Dam M, A-Rogvi-Hansen B, et al: Epilepsy and pregnancy: lamotrigine as main drug used. Acta Neurol Scand 109:9–13, 2004

Sadler TW (ed): Langman's Medical Embryology, 5th Edition. Baltimore, MD, Williams & Wilkins, 1985, pp 58–88

Samrén E, van Duijn C, Koch S, et al: Maternal use of antiepileptic drugs and the risk of major congenital malformations: a joint European prospective study of human teratogenesis associated with maternal epilepsy. Epilepsia 38:981–990, 1997

Samrén E, van Duijn C, Christiaens G, et al: Antiepileptic drug regimens and major congenital abnormalities in the offspring. Ann Neurol 46:739–746, 1999

Sanchis A, Rosique D, Catala J: Adverse effects of maternal lorazepam on neonates. Ann Pharmacother 25:1137–1138, 1991

Sathanandar S, Blesi K, Tran T, et al: Lamotrigine clearance increases markedly during pregnancy. Epilepsia 41:246, 2000

Saxén I: Cleft palate and maternal diphenhydramine intake. Lancet 1(7854):407–408, 1974

Saxén I: Association between oral clefts and drugs taken during pregnancy. Int J Epidemiol 4:37–44, 1975

Saxén I, Saxén L: Association between maternal intake of diazepam and oral clefts. Lancet 2(7933):498, 1974

Schatzberg AF, Cole JO: Manual of Clinical Psychopharmacology, 2nd Edition. Washington, DC, American Psychiatric Press, 1991

Schell L: Environmental noise and human prenatal growth. Am J Physiol Anthropol 56:63–70, 1981

Schick-Boschetto B, Zuber C: Alprazolam exposure during early human pregnancy. Teratology 45:460, 1992

Schmidt K, Olesen O, Jensen P: Citalopram and breast-feeding: serum concentration and side effects in the infant. Biol Psychiatry 47:164–165, 2000

Schneider M: Prenatal stress exposure alters postnatal behavioral expression under conditions of novelty challenge in rhesus monkey infants. Dev Psychobiol 25:529–540, 1992

Schneider M, Roughton E, Koehler A, et al: Growth and development following prenatal stress exposure in primates: an examination of ontogenetic vulnerability. Child Dev 70:263–274, 1999

Schou M: What happened later to the lithium babies?: follow-up study of children born without malformations. Acta Psychiatr Scand 54:193–197, 1976

Schou M, Amdisen A: Lithium and pregnancy, III: lithium ingestion by children breast-fed by women on lithium treatment. BMJ 2:138, 1973

Scokel PW, Jones WD: Infant jaundice after phenothiazine drugs for labor: an enigma. Obstet Gynecol 20:124–127, 1962

Scolnick D, Nulman I, Rovet J, et al: Neurodevelopment of children exposed in utero to phenytoin and carbamazepine monotherapy. JAMA 271:767–770, 1994

Secoli S, Teixeira N: Chronic prenatal stress affects development and behavioral depression in rats. Stress 2:273–280, 1998

Shannon RW, Fraser GP, Aitken RG, et al: Diazepam in preeclamptic toxaemia with special reference to its effect on the newborn infant. Br J Clin Pract 26:271–275, 1972

Shiono PH, Mills JL: Oral clefts and diazepam use during pregnancy. N Engl J Med 311:919–920, 1984

Simon GE, Cunningham ML, Davis RL: Outcomes of prenatal antidepressant exposure. Am J Psychiatry 159:2055–2061, 2002

Sivojelezova A, Shuhaiber S, Sarkissian L, et al: Citalopram use in pregnancy: prospective comparative evaluation of pregnancy and fetal outcome. Am J Obstet Gynecol 193:2004–2009, 2005

Skausig OB, Schou M: Breast feeding during lithium therapy [Danish]. Ugeskrift for Laeger 139:400–401, 1977

Slayton RI, Soloff PH: Psychotic denial of third-trimester pregnancy. J Clin Psychiatry 42:471–473, 1981

Slone D, Siskind V, Heinonen OP, et al: Antenatal exposure to the phenothiazines in relation to congenital malformations, perinatal mortality rate, birth weight, and intelligence quotient score. Am J Obstet Gynecol 128:468–486, 1977

Smith B, Wills G, Naylor D: The effects of prenatal stress on rat offsprings' learning ability. J Psychol 107:45–51, 1981

Sodhi P, Poddar B, Parmar V: Fatal cardiac malformation in fetal valproate syndrome. Indian J Pediatr 68:989–990, 2001

Speight AN: Floppy-infant syndrome and maternal diazepam and/or nitrazepam. Lancet 2(8043):878, 1977

Spigset O, Carleborg L, Norstrom A, et al: Paroxetine level in breast milk. J Clin Psychiatry 57:39, 1996

Spigset O, Carleborg L, Ohman R, et al: Excretion of citalopram in breast milk. Br J Clin Pharmacol 44:295–298, 1997

Spinelli MG: Interpersonal psychotherapy for depressed antepartum women: a pilot study. Am J Psychiatry 154:1028–1030, 1997

St. Clair SM, Schirmer RG: First trimester exposure to alprazolam. Obstet Gynecol 80:843–846, 1992

Stahl MM, Neiderud J, Vinge E: Thrombocytopenic purpura and anemia in a breast-fed infant whose mother was treated with valproic acid. J Pediatr 130:1001–1003, 1997

Stancer HC, Reed KL: Desipramine and 2-hydroxydesipramine in human breast milk and the nursing infant's serum. Am J Psychiatry 143:1597–1600, 1986

Steer R, Scholl T, Hediger M, et al: Self-reported depression and negative pregnancy outcomes. Epidemiology 45:1093–1099, 1992

Stewart R, Karas B, Springer P: Haloperidol excretion in human milk. Am J Psychiatry 137:849–850, 1980

Stirrat GM, Edington P, Berry DJ: Transplacental passage of chlordiazepoxide. BMJ 2:729, 1974

Stoner SC, Sommi RW, Marken PA, et al: Clozapine use in two full-term pregnancies. J Clin Psychiatry 58:364–365, 1997

Stott D: Follow-up study from birth of the effects of prenatal stresses. Dev Med Child Neurol 15:770–787, 1973

Stowe ZN, Nemeroff CB: Women at risk for postpartum-onset major depression. Am J Obstet Gynecol 173:639–645, 1995

Stowe ZN, Owens MJ, Landry JC, et al: Sertraline and desmethylsertraline in human breast milk and nursing infants. Am J Psychiatry 154:1255–1260, 1997

Stowe ZN, Cohen LS, Hostetter A, et al: Paroxetine in breast milk and nursing infants. Am J Psychiatry 157:185–189, 2000

Stowe ZN, Calhoun K, Ramsey C, et al: Mood disorders during pregnancy and lactation: defining exposure and treatment issues. CNS Spectr 6:150–166, 2001

Stowe Z, Hostetter A, Newport D: The onset of postpartum depression: implications for clinical screening in obstetrical and primary care. Am J Obstet Gynecol 192:522–526, 2005

Sullivan FM, McElhatton PR: A comparison of the teratogenic activity of the antiepileptic drugs carbamazepine, clonazepam, ethosuximide, phenobarbital, phenytoin, and pyrimidone in mice. Toxicol Appl Pharmacol 40:365–378, 1977

Summerfield RJ, Nielsen MS: Excretion of lorazepam into breast milk. Br J Anaesth 57:1042–1043, 1985

Suri R, Stowe ZN, Hendrick V, et al: Estimates of nursing infant daily dose of fluoxetine through breast milk. Biol Psychiatry 52:446–451, 2002

Swedish Centre for Epidemiology: Registration of congenital malformations in the Swedish Health Registers. Stockholm, Sweden, National Board of Health and Welfare, Centre for Epidemiology, June 18, 2004. Available at: http://www.socialstyrelsen.se/Publicerat/2004/5120/2004-112-1.htm. Accessed December 2007

Sykes PA, Quarrie J, Alexander FW: Lithium carbonate and breast-feeding. BMJ 2:1299, 1976

Szuran T, Zimmerman E, Pliska V, et al: Prenatal stress effects on exploratory activity and stress-induced analgesia in rats. Dev Psychobiol 24:361–372, 1991

Taddio A, Ito S, Koren G: Excretion of fluoxetine and its metabolite norfluoxetine in human breast milk. J Clin Pharmacol 36:42–47, 1996

Takahashi LK: Prenatal stress: consequences of glucocorticoids on hippocampal development and function. Int J Dev Neurosci 16:199–207, 1998

Takahashi L, Kalin N: Early developmental and temporal characteristics of stress-induced secretion of pituitary-adrenal hormones in prenatally stress rat pups. Brain Res 558:75–78, 1991

Targum S, Davenport Y, Webster M: Postpartum mania in bipolar manic-depressive patients withdrawn from lithium carbonate. J Nerv Ment Dis 167:572–574, 1979

Tenyi T, Tixler M: Clozapine in the treatment of pregnant schizophrenic women. Psychiatria Danubina 10:15–18, 1998

Thisted E, Ebbesen F: Malformations, withdrawal manifestations, and hypoglycaemia after exposure to valproate in utero. Arch Dis Child 69:288–291, 1993

Toddywalla VS, Kari FW, Neville MC: Active transport of nitrofurantoin across a mouse mammillary epithelial monolayer. J Pharmacol Exp Ther 280:669–676, 1997

Tomson T, Lindborn U, Ekqvist B, et al: Disposition of carbamazepine and phenytoin in pregnancy. Epilepsia 35:131–135, 1994

Tomson T, Ohman I, Vitols S: Lamotrigine in pregnancy and lactation: a case report. Epilepsia 38:1039–1041, 1997

Tran TA, Leppik IE, Blesi K, et al: Lamotrigine clearance during pregnancy. Neurology 59:251–255, 2002

Troutman B, Cutrona C: Nonpsychotic postpartum depression among adolescent mothers. J Abnorm Psychol 99:69, 1990

Tsuru N, Maeda T, Tsuruoka M: Three cases of delivery under sodium valproate—placental transfer, milk transfer and probable teratogenicity of sodium valproate. Jpn J Psychiatry Neurol 42:89–96, 1988

Tsutsumi K, Kotegawa T, Matsuki S, et al: The effect of pregnancy on cytochrome P450 1A2, xanthine oxidase, and N-acetyltransferase activities in humans. Clin Pharmacol Ther 70:121–125, 2001

Tunnessen WW, Hertz CG: Toxic effects of lithium in newborn infants: a commentary. J Pediatr 81:804–807, 1972

U.S. Food and Drug Administration: FDA advising of risk of birth defects with Paxil: agency requiring updated product labeling. FDA News P05–P97, 2005

Vail A, Hornbuckle J, Spiegelhalter DJ, et al: Prospective application of Bayesian monitoring and analysis in an open randomized clinical trial. Stat Med 20:3777–3787, 2001

Vajda FJ, O'Brien TJ, Hitchcock A, et al: The Australian registry of anti-epileptic drugs in pregnancy: experience after 30 months. J Clin Neurosci 10:543–549, 2003

Vallee M, Mayo W, Dellu F, et al: Prenatal stress induces high anxiety and postnatal handling induces low anxiety in adult offspring: correlation with stress-induced corticosterone secretion. J Neuroscience 17:2626–2636, 1997

Van der Pol MC, Hadders-Algra M, Huisjes MJ, et al: Antiepileptic medication in pregnancy: late effects on the children's nervous system development. Am J Obstet Gynecol 164:121–128, 1991

Van Waes A, Van de Velde EJ: Safety evaluation of haloperidol in the treatment of hyperemesis gravidarum. J Clin Pharmacol 9:224–227, 1969

Viguera AC, Nonacs R, Cohen LS, et al: Risk of recurrence of bipolar disorder in pregnant and nonpregnant women after discontinuing lithium maintenance. Am J Psychiatry 157:179–184, 2000

Viguera AC, Whitfield T, Baldessarini RJ, et al: Risk of recurrence in women with bipolar disorder during pregnancy: prospective study of mood stabilizer discontinuation. Am J Psychiatry 164:1817–1824, 2007

von Unruh GE, Froescher W, Hoffmann F, et al: Valproic acid in breast milk: how much is really there? Ther Drug Monit 6:272–276, 1984

Wadelius M, Darj E, Frenne G, et al: Induction of CYP2D6 in pregnancy. Clin Pharmacol Ther 62:400–407, 1997

Wadhwa PD, Porto M, Garite TJ, et al: Maternal corticotropin-releasing hormone levels in the early third trimester predict length of gestation in human pregnancy. Am J Obstet Gynecol 179:1079–1085, 1998

Wakshlak A, Weinstock M: Neonatal handling reverses behavioral abnormalities induced in rats by prenatal stress. Physiol Behav 48:289–292, 1990

Waldman MD, Safferman AZ: Pregnancy and clozapine. Am J Psychiatry 150:168–169, 1993

Walker C, Scribner K, Cascio C, et al: The pituitary-adrenocortical system of neonatal rats is responsive to stress throughout development in a time-dependent and stressor-specific fashion. Endocrinology 128:1385–1395, 1991

Wang JS, Newport DJ, Stowe ZN, et al: The emerging importance of transporter proteins in the psychopharmacological treatment of the pregnant patient. Drug Metabolism Reviews 39:723–746, 2007

Warner A: Drug use in the neonate: inter-relationships of pharmacokinetics, toxicity and biochemical maturity. Clin Chem 32:721–727, 1986

Watson JP, Elliott SA, Rugg AJ, et al: Psychiatric disorder in pregnancy and the first postnatal year. Br J Psychiatry 144:453–462, 1984

Webster PA: Withdrawal symptoms in neonates associated with maternal antidepressant therapy. Lancet 2(7824):318–319, 1973

Weinstein MR, Goldfield M: Lithium carbonate treatment during pregnancy; report of a case. Dis Nerv System 30:828–832, 1969

Weinstein MR, Goldfield MD: Cardiovascular malformations with lithium use during pregnancy. Am J Psychiatry 132:529–531, 1975

Weinstock M, Fride E, Hertzberg R: Prenatal stress effects on functional development of the offspring. Prog Brain Res 73:319–331, 1988

Weinstock M, Matlina E, Maor G, et al: Prenatal stress selectively alters the reactivity of the hypothalamic-pituitary-adrenal system in female rats. Brain Res 595:195–198, 1992

Weissman MM, Prusoff BA, Gammon GD, et al: Psychopathology in the children (ages 6–18) of depressed and normal parents. J Am Acad Child Adolesc Psychiatry 23:78–84, 1984

Welch R, Findlay J: Excretion of drugs in human breast milk. Drug Metab Rev 12:261–277, 1981

Weller A, Glaubman H, Yehuda S, et al: Acute and repeated gestational stress affect offspring learning and activity in rats. Physiol Behavior 43:139–143, 1988

Wesson DR, Camber S, Harkey M, et al: Diazepam and desmethyldiazepam in breast milk. J Psychoactive Drugs 17:55–56, 1985

Whalley LJ, Blain PG, Prime JK: Haloperidol secreted in breast milk. BMJ 282:1746–1747, 1981

Whitelaw AGL, Cummings AJ, McFadyen IR: Effect of maternal lorazepam on the neonate. BMJ 282:1106–1108, 1981

Wide K, Winbladh B, Tomson BWT, et al: Psychomotor development and minor anomalies in children exposed to antiepileptic drugs in utero: a prospective population based study. Dev Med Child Neurol 42:87–92, 2000

Williams G, King J, Cunningham M, et al: Fetal valproate syndrome and autism: additional evidence of an association. Dev Med Child Neurol 43:202–206, 2001

Williams KE, Koran L: Obsessive-compulsive disorder in pregnancy, the puerperium, and the premenstruum. J Clin Psychiatry 58:330–334, 1997

Williams PG, Hersh JH: A male with fetal valproate syndrome and autism. Dev Med Child Neurol 39:632–634, 1997

Wilson JT, Brown RD, Cherek DR, et al: Drug excretion in human breast milk: principles, pharmacokinetics and projected consequences. Clin Pharmacokinet 5:1–66, 1980

Wilson N, Forfar JC, Godman MJ: Atrial flutter in the newborn resulting from maternal lithium ingestion. Arch Dis Child 58:538–549, 1983

Wilton LV, Pearce GL, Martin RM, et al: The outcomes of pregnancy in women exposed to newly marketed drugs in general practice in England. Br J Obstet Gynaecol 105:882–889, 1998

Winter RM: In utero exposure to benzodiazepines. Lancet 1(8533):627, 1987

Winter RM, Donnai D, Burn J, et al: Fetal valproate syndrome: is there a recognizable phenotype? J Med Genet 24:692–695, 1987

Wisner KL, Perel JM: Psychopharmacologic agents and electroconvulsive therapy during pregnancy and the puerperium, in Psychiatric Consultation in Childbirth Settings: Parent- and Child-Oriented Approaches. Edited by Cohen RL. New York, Plenum, 1988, pp 165–206

Wisner KL, Perel JM: Serum levels of valproate and carbamazepine in breastfeeding mother-infant pairs. J Clin Psychopharmacol 18:167–169, 1998

Wisner KL, Perel JM, Wheeler SB: Tricyclic dose requirements across pregnancy. Am J Psychiatry 150:1541–1542, 1993

Wisner KL, Peindl KS, Hanusa BH: Effect of childbearing on the natural history of panic disorder with comorbid mood disorder. J Affect Disord 41:173–180, 1996a

Wisner KL, Perel JM, Findling RL: Antidepressant treatment during breast-feeding. Am J Psychiatry 153:1132–1137, 1996b

Wisner K, Perel J, Blumer J: Serum sertraline and N-desmethylsertraline levels in breast-feeding mother-infant pairs. Am J Psychiatry 155:690–692, 1998

Wood M, Wood AJJ: Changes in plasma drug binding and alpha-1-acid glycoprotein in mother and newborn infant. Clin Pharmacol Ther 29:522–526, 1981

Woods DL, Malan AF: Side effects of maternal diazepam on the newborn infant. S Afr Med J 54:636, 1978

Woody JN, London WL, Wilbanks GD: Lithium toxicity in a newborn. Pediatrics 47:94–96, 1971

Wreitland MA: Excretion of oxazepam in breast milk. Eur J Clin Pharmacol 33:209–210, 1987

Wright S, Dawling S, Ashford J: Excretion of fluvoxamine in breast milk. Br J Clin Pharmacol 31:209, 1991

Wyska E, Jusko WJ: Approaches to pharmacokinetic/pharmacodynamic modeling during pregnancy. Semin Perinatol 25:124–132, 2001

Yerby MS, Friel PN, Miller DQ: Carbamazepine protein binding and disposition in pregnancy. Ther Drug Monit 7:269–273, 1985

Yerby MS, Friel PN, McCormick K, et al: Pharmacokinetics of anticonvulsants in pregnancy: alterations in plasma protein binding. Epilepsy Res 5:223–228, 1990

Yerby MS, Friel PN, McCormick K: Antiepileptic drug disposition during pregnancy. Neurology 42:12–16, 1992

Yoldas Z, Iscan A, Yoldas T, et al: A woman who did her own cesarean section. Lancet 348:135, 1996

Yoshida K, Smith B, Craggs M, et al: Fluoxetine in breast-milk and developmental outcome of breast-fed infants. Br J Psychiatry 172:175–178, 1998a

Yoshida K, Smith B, Craggs M, et al: Neuroleptic drugs in breast-milk: a study of pharmacokinetics and of possible adverse effects in breast-fed infants. Psychol Med 28:81–91, 1998b

Zeskind PS, Stephens LE: Maternal selective serotonin reuptake inhibitor use during pregnancy and newborn neurobehavior. Pediatrics 113:368–375, 2004

Zuckerman B, Amaro H, Bauchner H, et al: Depressive symptoms during pregnancy: relationship to poor health behaviors. Am J Obstet Gynecol 160:1107–1111, 1989

CHAPTER 65

Treatment During Late Life

Steven P. Roose, M.D.

Bruce G. Pollock, M.D., Ph.D.

D. P. Devanand, M.D.

Adverse events caused by medication have been estimated to be between the fourth and sixth leading cause of death in the United States (Lazarou et al. 1998). The elderly bear the greatest burden of medical illness and are subject to extensive medication regimens; in consequence, they experience more adverse drug events than do other segments of the population. In a large study of ambulatory Medicare enrollees, 38% of adverse drug events were serious, life-threatening, or fatal and 28% were considered preventable (Gurwitz et al. 2005). Moreover, psychotropics are among the most common medications associated with preventable adverse drug events in elderly patients in long-term care settings (Gurwitz et al. 2000).

Pharmacokinetics of Psychotropic Medications in the Elderly

In general, age-associated pharmacokinetic changes result in higher and more variable drug concentrations. Nonetheless, specific information on the pharmacokinetics of most psychoactive medications is inadequate, particularly with regard to medical subgroups and potential drug interactions. The limited information that does exist for older subjects is largely derived from classical pharmacokinetic modeling (Pollock 2005). For example, with fluoxetine, the only published data on disposition in older subjects are limited to a study of single doses in 11 healthy volunteers (Bergstrom et al. 1988). Traditional pharmacokinetic studies require a large number of plasma drug samples ob-

tained from a small number (i.e., 6–12) of volunteers. Single-dose pharmacokinetic studies usually are not adequate to rule out the possibility of nonlinear kinetics. Moreover, it is difficult to generalize from these studies because of the small numbers, the virtual absence of elderly subjects and those with illness, and the concurrent medication use typical at this age (DeVane and Pollock 1999). It should also be appreciated that age or illness-associated differences in pharmacodynamics are not interpretable in the absence of drug concentration data. Population pharmacokinetics provides a means for addressing heterogeneous drug exposure for elders using minimal sampling methods (Bigos et al. 2006). For example, using this approach, our laboratory analyzed 199 citalopram concentration samples obtained on clinic visits from 109 patients across a wide age range. After correcting for weight effects, a significant relationship between age and clearance was observed, with the clearance of citalopram decreasing from approximately 30 L/hour at 18 years of age to as low as 5 L/hour at 93 years of age (Bies et al. 2004). Similarly, among 171 elders treated with paroxetine, we found that weight, sex, and cytochrome P450 (CYP) 2D6 genotype had significant pharmacokinetic effects (Feng et al. 2006).

Although individuals older than 65 years now account for more than one-third of prescription drug expenditures in the United States, they are often excluded from clinical and regulatory trials (Atkin et al. 1999). While regulatory authorities have developed guidelines for pharmaceutical companies regarding new medications that are likely to have significant use in the elderly, the full impact of these guidelines has yet to be realized. In addition, the trials that do include elders rarely include the "oldest old" (i.e., 85+ years), those having multiple comorbidities, or those taking multiple medications. These exclusions raise questions about the generalizability of psychotropic data to the frail elderly. The lack of information on new pharmaceuticals has resulted in an escalating pattern of recommended dosage decreases for neuropharmacological drugs after there has been clinical experience in older patients (Cross et al. 2002).

Age-associated pharmacokinetic differences may be due to changes in absorption, distribution, metabolism, or elimination of a drug (Table 65–1). The multidimensional changes associated with aging are heterogeneous, and only the most superficial generalizations can be made (Lotrich and Pollock 2005; Pollock 1998).

Absorption

Absorption of nutrients, such as iron, thiamine, and calcium, is often impaired in the elderly. Nonetheless, the rate and extent of passive drug absorption do not appear to be affected by normal aging. Antacids, high-fiber supplements, and cholestyramine may significantly diminish the absorption of medications.

Distribution

For most psychotropics that are lipid soluble, the loss of lean body mass with aging will lead to increases in their volumes of distribution, resulting in longer half-lives and drug accumulation. This is because a drug's half-life is directly proportional to its apparent volume of distribution. Conversely, for water-soluble drugs such as lithium and digoxin, volumes of distribution will be diminished in older patients, reducing the margin of safety after acute increases in plasma drug concentration.

Reductions in serum albumin with age and possible increases in α_1-acid glycoprotein with illness may affect the extent of drug bound to plasma proteins. However, it is now recognized that changes in plasma protein binding are of clinical significance only when therapeutic drug monitoring is used to adjust dosing, because total drug concentrations (free+protein bound) are usually reported (Benet and Hoener 2002). Total drug levels may be interpreted as too low if a drug's free fraction is increased by diminished plasma proteins or drug displacement. The use of free drug levels in older patients has been found to be useful for lidocaine, theophylline, phenytoin, and digitoxin. More data regarding the use of therapeutic plasma levels are needed for elders treated with valproate, given its greater risks for thrombocytopenia and hepatotoxicity in the aged (Conley et al. 2001).

Metabolism

Available evidence suggests that there is no uniform age-associated decline in liver metabolism by CYP enzymes (Pollock et al. 1992b; Schmucker 2001). Nonetheless, reductions in hepatic mass and blood flow with aging place greater emphasis on interindividual differences in drug metabolic capacity. These metabolic differences may be either genetic or the result of interactions from multiple medications. Enzyme specificity suggests that inhibition or induction of a given CYP enzyme will affect all drugs metabolized by that specific enzyme (Pollock 1998).

CYP2D6 is the enzyme responsible for metabolizing tricyclic antidepressants (TCAs) and venlafaxine as well as several older neuroleptics and risperidone. Among the white population, 5%–10% are genetically poor CYP2D6 metabolizers, which has been shown in older patients to affect nortriptyline doses (Murphy et al. 2001) and the severity of perphenazine-associated adverse effects (Pollock

TABLE 65–1.   Physiological changes in the elderly associated with altered pharmacokinetics

ORGAN SYSTEM	CHANGE	PHARMACOKINETIC CONSEQUENCE
Gastrointestinal tract	Decreased intestinal and splanchnic blood flow	Decreased rate of drug absorption
Circulatory	Decreased concentration of plasma albumin and increased α_1-acid glycoprotein	Increased or decreased free concentration of drugs in plasma
Kidney	Decreased glomerular filtration rate	Decreased renal clearance of active metabolites
Muscle	Decreased lean body mass and increased adipose tissue	Altered volume of distribution of lipid-soluble drugs, leading to increased elimination half-life
Liver	Decreased liver size; decreased hepatic blood flow; minimal effects on cytochrome P450 enzyme activity	Decreased hepatic clearance

et al. 1995). Concern also has been raised about poor CYP2D6 metabolizers treated with venlafaxine or extensive metabolizers given venlafaxine and concomitant 2D6 inhibitors (Johnson et al. 2006; Lessard et al. 1999, 2001; Whyte et al. 2006).

Drugs metabolized by CYP3A4, such as alprazolam, triazolam, sertraline, mirtazapine, and nefazodone, appear to be cleared less well in elderly patients (Barbhaiya et al. 1996; Greenblatt et al. 1991; Ronfeld et al. 1997; Timmer et al. 1996). However, this may be because metabolism of CYP3A4 drugs is typically perfusion limited (i.e., dependent on hepatic blood flow, which is known to decline substantially with age) (Wynne et al. 1990). CYP3A4 makes up 30% of total hepatic CYP and nearly all of drug-metabolizing enzyme in the small bowel, and therefore is substantially responsible for "first-pass" or presystemic drug disposition (Shimada et al. 1994). Minimally, 50% of clinically used medications are at least partly dependent on CYP3A4 for their clearance. Serious toxicity has occurred when the 3A4-mediated clearance of terfenadine, astemizole, cisapride, cerivastatin, midazolam, and triazolam was inhibited (Dresser et al. 2000). CYP3A4 activity may be inhibited by grapefruit juice, protease inhibitors, macrolide antibiotics, and triazole antifungals. Among antidepressants, nefazodone and fluvoxamine are the most potent inhibitors of CYP3A4, followed by fluoxetine, through its demethylated metabolite. The very long half-life of norfluoxetine may result in interactions occurring many weeks after the initiation of fluoxetine treatment. The 3A4 enzyme is also potently induced by other drugs, such as carbamazepine, phenytoin, topiramate, modafinil, barbiturates, steroids, and St. John's wort. CYP3A4 induction will increase the likelihood of therapeutic failure for concurrently prescribed 3A4 substrate drugs. Many CYP3A4 inhibitors (e.g., diltiazem) and inducers (e.g., St. John's wort) also have been found to inhibit or induce the P-glycoprotein drug transporter, amplifying their effects on 3A4 (Yu 1999).

CYP1A2 metabolizes clozapine, olanzapine, fluvoxamine, and theophylline and contributes to the demethylation of some tertiary TCAs. This enzyme is induced by cigarette smoking, cruciferous vegetables, and charcoaled meats as well as by medications such as omeprazole and phenobarbital. Estrogen replacement therapy in postmenopausal women has been found to inhibit CYP1A2 metabolism (Pollock et al. 1999). CYP2C9 metabolizes several drugs with a narrow therapeutic index (i.e., phenytoin, tolbutamide, ibuprofen, and warfarin). It is therefore important to recognize that this enzyme may be inhibited by fluvoxamine and fluoxetine. CYP2B6 has been found

to metabolize bupropion, and in vitro evidence indicates that fluoxetine, paroxetine, and sertraline may cause inhibition (Hesse et al. 2000).

Excretion

The well-established age-associated decline in renal clearance may affect excretion of psychotropic drug metabolites and lithium in older patients. The magnitude of this decline varies greatly among the aged (Pollock et al. 1992b), being exacerbated by concomitant conditions (e.g., diabetes and hypertension) and medications (e.g., nonsteroidal anti-inflammatory drugs). Accumulation of active TCA metabolites in the elderly was previously a subject of concern (Pollock et al. 1992a). Higher concentrations of bupropion and venlafaxine metabolites also have been observed in older patients and those with renal impairment, with uncertain clinical consequences (Sweet et al. 1995; Whyte et al. 2006).

Pharmacodynamics of Psychotropic Medications in the Elderly

Interindividual differences in pharmacodynamics become evident when those with similar plasma drug concentrations experience different effects. In general, older patients are more sensitive to adverse effects of psychotropics at lower concentrations (Pollock 1999). Homeostatic mechanisms, such as postural control, water balance, orthostatic circulatory responses, and thermoregulation, are frequently less robust in the aged. This factor may interfere with the ability to physiologically adapt to medication. For example, all psychotropics, including selective serotonin reuptake inhibitors (SSRIs), may increase the risk of falls and hip fractures (Liu et al. 1998). Similarly, the syndrome of inappropriate antidiuretic hormone secretion has been reported as an age-associated adverse effect of all SSRIs and of venlafaxine (see Kirby and Ames 2001).

Reductions in dopamine or acetylcholine function with age may increase sensitivity to antipsychotics and SSRIs (which indirectly reduce dopamine outflow) as well as medications with antimuscarinic effects. Even low serum anticholinergic levels may be associated with cognitive impairment in depressed and nondepressed elderly persons (Mulsant et al. 2002; Nebes et al. 2005). Unfortunately, anticholinergic drugs continue to be widely prescribed in older patients, including those with cognitive impairment (Roe et al. 2002).

Anticoagulant–antidepressant interactions may be both pharmacokinetic and pharmacodynamic. Fluvoxamine and fluoxetine pose the greatest risk of pharmacokinetic interactions through CYP2C9 inhibition, reducing the clearance of warfarin's active S-enantiomer. However, increased bleeding times with SSRIs alone or in combination with anticoagulants also may be possible as a result of depleting platelets of serotonin and attenuating their aggregation (Pollock et al. 2000b).

At present, evidence is limited that genetic differences may influence pharmacodynamics in older patients. Depressed elderly patients with the long–long (LL) serotonin transporter promoter genotype were found to have a more rapid initial response to paroxetine (Pollock et al. 2000a). This is consistent with results obtained with other SSRIs in younger patients (Serretti et al. 2006). Another study in geriatric major depression found that carriers of the short (S) allele experienced more severe adverse events during paroxetine treatment (Murphy et al. 2004). Interestingly, findings in Koreans with late-life depression were in the opposite direction—that is, better responses among carriers of the S allele (Kim et al. 2006).

Serotonin transporter polymorphisms also may influence the probability that those with dementia will manifest aggressive or psychotic disturbances (Sweet et al. 2001). Similarly, the serotonin 5-HT$_{2A}$ receptor C102/C102 genotype was found significantly more frequently in Alzheimer's disease patients with psychosis (Nacmias et al. 2001). These intriguing reports reinforce the possibility that serotonergic dysfunction plays a prominent role in the psychiatric symptoms of dementia (Pollock et al. 2002, 2007). Given the extensive use of risperidone in the treatment of late-life psychoses and its potent affinity for the 5-HT$_{2A}$ receptor, it is also of interest that the C102/C102 genotype was found to be associated with a more robust risperidone response in younger patients with acutely exacerbated schizophrenia than in younger patients without this genotype (Lane et al. 2002). This same variation in the 5-HT$_{2A}$ receptor was associated with more side effects and more study discontinuations in geriatric patients treated with paroxetine but not mirtazapine (Murphy et al. 2003). Although findings from these early association studies are tenuous, it is encouraging that attempts are now being made to parse medication response by genotype in older subjects.

Antidepressants in the Elderly

Treatment of Late-Life Depression

The combined prevalence of major depressive disorder and dysthymia in late life is 5%–12% in epidemiological studies; this rate is similar to the rate in the younger adult population. However, the symptom pattern and frequency of specific depressive subtypes appear to be different; older patients have more somatic symptoms, and both the melancholic and the delusional subtypes of depression increase in frequency in older populations. In addition, some degree of cognitive impairment, whether manifest only concurrently with the depressive episode or as a function of age, is common.

As in younger patients, untreated depression in late life causes significant social, vocational, and interpersonal morbidity, and depression in late life is associated with a significant risk of mortality. Comorbid depression adversely affects the course of several disease processes; this has been best documented for ischemic heart disease. Patients with unstable angina, post–myocardial infarction, or congestive heart failure who are depressed have a higher cardiac mortality rate than do medically comparable patients who are not depressed (Musselman et al. 1998). Furthermore, the suicide rate in men (in the United States, specifically white men) increases dramatically after age 60 years and continues to rise significantly as a function of age.

Depression in late life probably represents a heterogeneous group of disorders with distinct etiologies; for example, late-onset depression, defined as having a first episode after age 60 years, is associated with brain imaging findings consistent with significant vascular disease (Figiel et al. 1991), and late-life dysthymia in men is associated with low testosterone levels (Seidman and Roose 2000). Thus, late-life depression is not simply an episode of major depression in a patient 70 years old rather than a patient 40 years old.

Studies of Antidepressant Treatment in Older Patients

The pharmacological treatment of late-life depression has long been influenced by three widely held clinical beliefs about older patients: 1) they do not respond at the same rate or as robustly as younger patients; 2) they take longer to respond to antidepressant medication, and therefore a 12-week trial is mandatory; and 3) they experience a higher rate of side effects and adverse events. Until recently, there has been a relative paucity of rigorous randomized, controlled trials of antidepressant treatment in late-life depression; consequently, these clinical beliefs have gone untested. However, perhaps stimulated by the prevalence and clinical significance of late-life depression and the need to establish safe and effective treatments, there has been a recent increase in the number of studies of antidepressant treatment for late-life depression (although most are sponsored by the pharmaceutical industry). In addition, analyses of extant data address the issue of optimal duration of treatment.

Considering the physiological changes associated with aging and the differences in the phenomenology and possible etiology of depression in late life compared with earlier in life, it is expected that clinical trials of antidepressants in late life will have a unique set of patient moderators and study design mediators that may significantly affect results. Variability in results of randomized, controlled trials of antidepressants in late-life depression may result from heterogeneity in the patient population. Treatment moderators that have been identified as significant for late-life depression include

- Subtype (e.g., melancholic or atypical)
- Severity
- Medical burden
- Social support
- Abnormalities on magnetic resonance scans indicating vascular disease
- Pattern of neurocognitive abnormalities labeled "executive dysfunction"

With respect to mediators of treatment response, the standard considerations in study design—namely, randomization, placebo versus comparator control, dosage, duration, and criteria for response and remission—are all important, but specifically the value of placebo-controlled trials versus comparator trials and optimal duration of treatment have been systematically reexamined. Sneed et al. (2008) conducted a meta-analysis of all studies published in peer-reviewed journals from 1985 to 2006 that were randomized, placebo-controlled or comparator (a comparison of two active conditions) trials of antidepressants for the treatment of late-life depression. The intent of the meta-analysis was to determine whether rates of response to medications in comparator trials are significantly higher than rates of response to comparable medications in placebo-controlled trials—that is, whether study design significantly affects treatment outcome. Sixteen studies (9 comparator trials and 7 placebo-controlled trials) met the rigorous inclusion criteria for the meta-analysis. As hypothesized, antidepressant response rates were significantly higher in the comparator trials compared to placebo-controlled trials; the estimated probability of antidepressant response in a placebo-controlled trial was 46% as compared with 60% in a comparator trial. One possible explanation for the higher response rate to

the same medication in a comparator trial is that patient, doctor, and even research rater expectations of response are higher when it is known that the subject is receiving an active medication. Irrespective of the reason that response rates are higher in comparator trials, the results of the study suggest that when clinicians want to make evidence-based treatment decisions and communicate likelihood of response to patients, data from comparator trials may be more appropriate than results of placebo-controlled trials, since comparator trials more closely approximate the clinical situation in that both patient and doctor know that an active medication is being prescribed.

Although it would be optimal if the numerous randomized, controlled trials of antidepressant treatment in late-life depression all had comparable patients, the same rigorous study design, and similar data analysis, few (if any) studies are without problems. Thus, the review of specific antidepressants that follows does not attempt to be inclusive of all studies but rather aims to illustrate the effect of medication by reviewing data from the best studies available.

Tricyclic Antidepressants

There are scores of randomized, placebo-controlled or comparator (usually an SSRI) trials of TCA treatment for late-life depression. The problem is that most of the placebo-controlled trials involving TCAs were done before the use of plasma-level measurements to ensure optimal TCA treatment. Later randomized, controlled trials that compared TCAs with SSRIs were invariably supported by the pharmaceutical industry, which had no desire to compare their new compound against optimal TCA treatment. Consequently, the preponderance of studies of TCA treatment in late-life depression reported on inadequate doses of the tertiary-amine tricyclics amitriptyline and imipramine. Nonetheless, the results of these studies established that TCAs are an effective treatment for depression in geriatric patients.

Nortriptyline. Of the tricyclics, nortriptyline has been found to induce the least orthostatic hypotension and has a documented "therapeutic window" that permits optimal dosing (Roose et al. 1981). Consequently, nortriptyline has emerged as the choice of this class of medications issued to treat late-life depression. However, there are no rigorous placebo-controlled trials of nortriptyline in late-life depression; thus, the relative effectiveness of this medication is inferred from two open trials and three randomized comparator trials.

In a study reported by Flint and Rifat (1996), 101 patients meeting DSM-III-R (American Psychiatric Association 1987) criteria for major depressive disorder were treated openly with nortriptyline. The dosing schedule was as follows: all patients achieved a dose of 75 mg by the end of week 1, and then the dose was adjusted if necessary to achieve a plasma level within the therapeutic window of 50–150 ng/mL. The treatment duration was 6 weeks, and the remission criterion was a final Hamilton Rating Scale for Depression (Ham-D; 17-item) score of 10 or less; 60% of the intent-to-treat sample and 75% of the completers met the remission criteria. To establish speed of response, the authors determined the week of treatment that the 61 patients who met criteria for remission at the end of the study first achieved sustained remission. Not surprisingly, at the end of week 1, no patient met the criteria for remission, and thus the cumulative response rate was 0%. At week 2, 11% of the sample met the remission criteria, and at week 3, 33% met the remission criteria (thus, the cumulative rate at the end of week 3 was 11%+33%, or 44%). At weeks 4 and 5, 25% and 20%, respectively, met the remission criteria. Thus, the accumulated remission rate at the end of week 5 was 89%. Although it is widely believed that late-life depression patients should have longer treatment trials, specifically 12 weeks, this study found that 89% of the patients who eventually recovered did so by the end of week 5. With respect to tricyclics, it may be that the slower dose escalation often used for older patients, rather than an intrinsic difference in the rapidity of response between young and old, is the critical factor accounting for delayed response.

A second open study of a therapeutic plasma level of nortriptyline reported on 42 inpatients (mean age=70 years) with cardiac disease and melancholic depression who also were treated for 6 weeks (Roose et al. 1994). The remission criterion was a final Ham-D (21-item) score of 8 or less; the intent-to-treat remission rate was 67%, the completer remission rate was 82%, and the dropout rate was 19%.

Three randomized, controlled trials compared nortriptyline with an SSRI; two studies compared a therapeutic plasma level of nortriptyline with paroxetine, and one study compared flexible-dose nortriptyline with sertraline. Mulsant et al. (2001a) compared nortriptyline with paroxetine in 116 inpatients and outpatients (mean age=72 years) in a 12-week trial. Patients were considered to be in remission if the final Ham-D (17-item) score was 10 or less; the intent-to-treat remission rate was 57% for the nortriptyline group and 55% for the paroxetine group. The rate of dropout due to side effects in the

nortriptyline group was significantly higher than that in the paroxetine group (33% vs. 16%; P=0.04).

A second randomized, controlled trial comparing nortriptyline (targeted to a therapeutic plasma level) with paroxetine is included in this chapter, although technically it should not be considered a geriatric study because the mean age of the patients was 58 years (Nelson et al. 1999). However, it is the only other study comparing a therapeutic plasma level of a tricyclic with an SSRI, and the results are consistent with those of the Mulsant et al. (2001a) study. In this trial, 81 outpatients with ischemic heart disease were treated with medication for 6 weeks. The remission criterion was a final Ham-D (17-item) score of 8 or less; in the intent-to-treat analysis, 63% of the nortriptyline group and 61% of the paroxetine group were remitters. The dropout rate for nortriptyline (35%) was significantly higher than the dropout rate for paroxetine (10%) (P<0.05). The rate of remission in study completers was 85% for nortriptyline and 68% for paroxetine, which was not a statistically significant difference, although the power of this comparison was limited by the small size of the completer group.

The randomized, controlled trial comparing sertraline with nortriptyline included 210 patients (mean age=68 years) randomly assigned to 12 weeks of medication treatment (Bondareff et al. 2000). This study did not report remission rates but only response rates, defined as a 50% reduction in Ham-D (24-item) score from baseline. The response rates for nortriptyline and sertraline were 41% and 52%, respectively.

Tricyclic side effects and safety.   Unfortunately, despite their robust effectiveness, the clinical utility of TCAs in the late-life population is limited by their side-effect and safety profiles. Tricyclics have significant anticholinergic effects, and although the total anticholinergic load is lower for desipramine and nortriptyline compared with the tertiary tricyclics, even in these medications, it is still considerable. The anticholinergic effects of tricyclics result in dry mouth, constipation, and blurred vision, and more important, the geriatric population is particularly susceptible to anticholinergic-induced urinary retention and confusional states.

The major safety problem with respect to the tricyclics is cardiovascular effects (Glassman et al. 1993). Tricyclics are lethal in overdose, and as little as three times the daily dose can result in death from heart block or arrhythmias. The TCAs have type 1A antiarrhythmic activity similar to that of moricizine and quinidine and consequently are presumed to confer an increased risk of sudden cardiovascular death if given to patients with ischemic heart disease. Given the prevalence of occult and manifest ischemic heart disease in both men and women older than 60 years, the use of tricyclics in this population must reflect a careful consideration of the risk–benefit ratio.

Selective Serotonin Reuptake Inhibitors

As in younger depressed patients, the SSRIs are the most prescribed class of antidepressants for late-life depression. However, strikingly few rigorous placebo or comparator randomized, controlled trials have reported response and remission data. Within this class, the various SSRIs appear to have equivalent efficacy and side-effect profiles. There are differences in pharmacokinetics and potential for drug–drug interactions, which are of importance in the geriatric population and have been discussed earlier in this chapter.

Fluoxetine.   Four large studies of fluoxetine in late-life depression have been done: 1) placebo-controlled study; 2) three-cell study comparing venlafaxine, placebo, and fluoxetine; 3) randomized, controlled trial with a comparator drug; and 4) open treatment. In the first study, fluoxetine was compared with placebo in 671 patients (Tollefson et al. 1995). The dosing schedule was fluoxetine 20 mg/day for 6 weeks, and the remission criterion was a Ham-D (17-item) score of 7 or less after 4 weeks. The intent-to-treat analysis remission rate was 23% for fluoxetine and 13% for placebo; in the completer analysis, the remission rate was 27% for fluoxetine and 16% for placebo. Although fluoxetine was significantly more effective than placebo in both the intent-to-treat and the completer analyses, this was the first large SSRI trial in a geriatric population, and in comparison to the clinical experience with therapeutic plasma levels of tricyclics, the remission rates in this study were disappointingly low.

In the comparator randomized clinical trial, patients were randomly assigned to either fluoxetine 20–40 mg or sertraline 50–100 mg for 12 weeks (Newhouse et al. 2000). The sample of 225 patients (mean age = 68 years) was somewhat unusual because the mean duration of the current episode of major depression was 9 years. The intent-to-treat remission rate was 46% for fluoxetine and 45% for sertraline, the completer remission rate was 60% for fluoxetine and 59% for sertraline, and the dropout rate was 33% for fluoxetine and 32% for sertraline. This study also reported an intriguing analysis of the response pattern of a subsample of 75 patients (42 treated with sertraline, 33 treated with fluoxetine) with a mean age of 75

years. For both sertraline and fluoxetine, 95% of the patients who achieved a 50% reduction in baseline Ham-D score did so by the end of week 8. As with the Flint and Rifat (1996) study of a therapeutic plasma level of nortriptyline, these data challenge the clinical wisdom that antidepressant trials in late-life depression must be extended to 12 weeks.

Finally, 308 patients meeting DSM-III (American Psychiatric Association 1980) criteria for major depressive disorder (mean age = 66 years) were treated openly with 20 mg of fluoxetine for 8 weeks (Mesters et al. 1992). The remission criterion was a final Ham-D (24-item) score of 10 or less; the intent-to-treat remission rate was 35%, the completer remission rate was 50%, and the dropout rate was 29%.

Sertraline.   In addition to the two randomized, controlled comparator trials previously described, nortriptyline versus sertraline and fluoxetine versus sertraline, a large rigorous placebo-controlled trial of sertraline in late-life depression was recently completed (Schneider et al. 2003). In this study, 716 patients (mean age = 70 years) were randomly assigned to flexible-dose sertraline 50–100 mg or placebo in an 8-week clinical trial. The criterion for remission was a final Ham-D (17-item) score of 10 or less; the intent-to-treat remission rate was 29% in the sertraline group, compared with 23% in the placebo group (P<0.05).

Paroxetine.   In addition to the two previously described trials that compared nortriptyline at a therapeutic plasma level with paroxetine and in which the intent-to-treat remission rates (final 17-item Ham-D score≤10) were 55% and 61%, respectively, a third recently completed trial compared mirtazapine with paroxetine (Schatzberg et al. 2002). In this study, 255 patients (mean age = 72 years) were randomly assigned to mirtazapine 30–45 mg or paroxetine 30–40 mg in an 8-week clinical trial. The criterion for remission was a final Ham-D (17-item) score of 7 or less; the intent-to-treat remission rates were 38% for mirtazapine and 28% for paroxetine and were not statistically different.

Citalopram and escitalopram.   Many of the studies of citalopram in a geriatric population included patients with depression and dementia or significant cognitive impairment; therefore, the results of these studies are not comparable to those of other antidepressant trials in late-life depression (Gottfries 1996). However, two studies do provide information on citalopram in this population; the first is a single-blind comparison between citalopram and a therapeutic plasma level of nortriptyline, and the second is a recently completed comparison of citalopram with placebo in depressed patients older than 75 years.

In the first study, 58 patients (mean age = 71 years) were randomly assigned to treatment with 30–40 mg of citalopram or a therapeutic plasma level of nortriptyline in a 12-week clinical trial (Navarro et al. 2001). The criterion for remission was a final Ham-D (17-item) score of 7 or less; the intent-to-treat remission rates were 69% for citalopram and 93% for nortriptyline. The remission rates for both medications were strikingly high in comparison to those in other trials; whether this results from differences in patient population or study design is not obviously apparent.

The second trial is unique in the literature because it is the only study to focus on treatment of depression in the "old-old." In this study, 174 patients were randomly assigned to treatment with either citalopram 20–40 mg or placebo in an 8-week clinical trial (Roose et al. 2002). The population was 58% female, with a mean age of 80 years and a mean baseline Ham-D (24-item) score of 24. The intent-to-treat response rate (50% reduction from baseline Ham-D score) was 41% in the citalopram group and 39% in the placebo group. The sample was divided for secondary analyses into patients with "severe" and "not severe" depression, which were defined as being either above or below the mean Ham-D score, respectively. The "not severe" group had a baseline Ham-D score of 22 and included 47 patients randomly assigned to citalopram and 59 patients randomly assigned to placebo. The criterion for remission was a final Ham-D score of 10 or less. In this group, the intent-to-treat remission rate was 34% for citalopram and 41% for placebo. The "severe" patient group had a mean baseline Ham-D score of 28 and included 37 patients randomly assigned to citalopram and 31 patients randomly assigned to placebo. In this group, the intent-to-treat remission rate was 36% for citalopram and 19% for placebo ($P<0.05$). Thus, citalopram is significantly more effective than placebo in the "severe" patient population, but this difference resulted not from an increased efficacy of citalopram compared with "not severe" patients but from a decreased efficacy of placebo.

A third recent study—an 8-week randomized, controlled trial—compared citalopram (flexible dose 10–20 mg/day) and venlafaxine (flexible dose 75–150 mg/day) in the treatment of late-life depression (Allard 2004). The study included 151 patients (mean age = 73 years; 73% female) with a baseline Montgomery-Åsberg Depression Rating Scale (MADRS) score of 27±4. The response rates for venlafaxine versus citalopram were 75%

and 73%, respectively, and the remission rates were 19% and 23%, respectively. The differences between the response rates and the remission rates are quite striking; it is unusual to see such a differential.

There is one randomized, controlled trial of escitalopram in the treatment of late-life depression (Kasper 2005). In this study, 517 patients (mean age = 75 years; 75% female; mean baseline MADRS score = 28±4) were randomly assigned to escitalopram (10 mg/day), fluoxetine (20 mg/day), or placebo. There was no significant difference in response rates across the three treatment conditions (response rates: escitalopram 46%, fluoxetine 37%, and placebo 47%).

SSRI side effects and safety.   As a group of medications, the SSRIs have the same side-effect profile in older patients as in younger patients: specifically, gastrointestinal distress, agitation, insomnia, and sexual dysfunction. Discontinuation rates for SSRIs are not statistically different from the discontinuation rates reported for a therapeutic plasma level of nortriptyline in the geriatric samples.

With respect to safety, the SSRIs offer a significant advantage over the tricyclics. SSRIs are relatively benign in overdose (Barbey and Roose 1998) and have been extensively tested in patients with ischemic heart disease, in patients with congestive heart failure, and immediately post–myocardial infarction (Glassman et al. 2002; Roose et al. 1998). In contrast to the tricyclics, the SSRIs have a relatively benign cardiovascular profile and specifically do not have an effect on blood pressure, heart rate, cardiac conduction, or cardiac arrhythmias and have no indication that they carry significant cardiac risk. In a randomized, controlled trial of depressed patients post–myocardial infarction who received sertraline or placebo, the patients treated with sertraline had significantly fewer major cardiovascular events than did the patients receiving placebo. The beneficial effect of medication in this study may not exclusively or even in part result from the effective treatment of depression. SSRIs have been established to have significant "antiplatelet" effects and therefore have anticoagulant benefit above and beyond that of aspirin in patients with significant vascular disease (Musselman et al. 1998).

Other Antidepressants

Venlafaxine.   One study reported meaningful information about venlafaxine in a geriatric population (Schatzberg and Cantillon 2000). In this 8-week randomized, controlled clinical trial, 204 patients (mean age = 71 years) were randomly assigned to treatment with venlafaxine 75–225 mg/day, fluoxetine 20–60 mg/day, or placebo. Remission was defined as a Ham-D (24-item) score less than 8; the intent-to-treat remission rate was 42% for venlafaxine, 29% for fluoxetine, and 38% for placebo (no statistically significant differences). Significantly more patients treated with venlafaxine (27%) and fluoxetine (19%) discontinued study participation because of side effects than did those given placebo (9%) (*P*<0.05). Cardiovascular measures, including heart rate and measures of cardiac conduction (including pulse rate, QRS, and QTc intervals), were assessed, and neither medication induced a significant change compared with placebo in any of these measures.

Duloxetine. There is one randomized, controlled trial of duloxetine for the treatment of late-life depression. In this study 311 patients (mean baseline Ham-D score = 22±4) were randomly assigned in a 2-to-1 allocation favoring duloxetine (Raskin et al. 2007). The response and remission (final Ham-D score = ≤7) rates were significantly greater for duloxetine than for placebo (response rates: duloxetine 37%, placebo 27% [*P*<0.001]; remission rates: duloxetine 19%, placebo 15% [*P*=0.002]). However, as with many other trials of antidepressant medication for the treatment of late-life depression, the remission rates are distressingly low.

Mirtazapine. As previously discussed, in one randomized, controlled comparator trial of mirtazapine versus paroxetine in a geriatric population, the intent-to-treat remission rates were 38% for the mirtazapine group and 28% for the paroxetine-treated patients (Schatzberg et al. 2002). In this study, the rate of discontinuation due to adverse events was similar in both groups: 33% for mirtazapine and 29% for paroxetine.

Bupropion. One randomized, controlled comparator trial of bupropion versus paroxetine in late-life depression has been published, and this represents the only data available on bupropion in this population (Weihs et al. 2000). In this 6-week clinical trial, 100 patients (mean age = 70 years), with a baseline Ham-D (24-item) score of 27, were randomly assigned to treatment with either bupropion 100–300 mg/day or paroxetine 10–40 mg/day. Rates of response (defined as a 50% reduction from baseline Ham-D score) in the intent-to-treat analysis were 71% in the bupropion group and 77% in the paroxetine group. Remission data were not reported. Discontinuation rates were 17% in the bupropion group and 15% in the paroxetine group.

Duration of Antidepressant Treatment

A long-standing adage is that older patients take longer to respond to antidepressant treatment than do younger patients as a result of either the physiological effects of aging or the more treatment-resistant nature of mood disorders over time. Also, a longer time to response in the elderly may result from slower dose escalation. It is commonly believed that a lower starting dose and slower dose escalation of antidepressant medication will improve tolerability among geriatric patients. However, the "start low and go slow" paradigm evolved in the era when TCAs were the primary treatment for depression and the tertiary tricyclics amitriptyline and imipramine were more widely used than nortriptyline. In fact, the evidence does not support the view that side effects such as orthostatic hypotension or anticholinergic phenomena are minimized by slow dose escalation of the TCAs. Furthermore, the utility of the "start low and go slow" strategy for treatment with SSRIs or other antidepressants is essentially untested.

The belief that patients with late-life depression take longer to respond than younger patients has led to the dictum that for the elderly the minimum duration necessary for an adequate antidepressant trial is 12 weeks. Do all patients require a 12-week trial before they can be considered nonresponders? An affirmative answer implies that patients who are still quite ill at week 11 may improve dramatically and meet remission criteria by week 12.

Data on this issue are sparse and somewhat contradictory. Georgotas et al. (1989) reported that extending a nortriptyline trial from 7 to 9 weeks resulted in a significantly higher response rate. In this study, at the end of 7 weeks, 54% (26 of 48) of the nortriptyline-treated patients had responded, and 4 additional patients responded during the 2-week extension, bringing the total response rate to 63%. The number of slow responders to nortriptyline was small, and the slow responders had low plasma levels of nortriptyline in the early weeks of the trial and required a dosage increment. Despite these caveats, this study is frequently cited as yielding findings supporting the need for longer treatment trials in late-life depression.

Other studies suggest that speed of response to TCAs is not slowed in older patients. Studies of depressed patients older than 60 years receiving a therapeutic plasma level of TCA (either imipramine, nortriptyline, or desipramine) reached by week 2 of treatment reported that 90% of the patients who met response criteria did so by the end of week 4 (Roose 1990).

In contrast to the studies of tricyclic treatment, two 12-week randomized, controlled trials of SSRIs in late-life depression comparing sertraline with fluoxetine and sertraline with nortriptyline both reported an increase in response rates at week 12 compared with week 8 (Bondareff et al. 2000; Newhouse et al. 2000). Hypothetically, the increased number of patients meeting the response criteria at 12 weeks represents two different groups: 1) patients who were close to meeting the response criteria by week 8 and crossed the threshold by week 12, and 2) patients who had no significant symptom reduction by week 8 but then improved dramatically over the next 4 weeks to meet the response criteria at week 12 (so-called late responders). If the significantly higher response rate at week 12 is due to patients who experienced most of their improvement between weeks 8 and 12, this would imply that all patients deserve a 12-week trial, even those who have no significant improvement by week 8. However, if the responders at week 12 already had shown significant improvement by week 8, this would imply that the additional weeks of treatment benefit only those who are well on their way to remission.

Recently, new data analyses of 12-week antidepressant treatment trials in late-life depression focused on time to response and the early identification of nonresponders (Sackeim and Roose 2002). Data for these analyses came from two industry-sponsored trials, one comparing sertraline with fluoxetine and the other, fluoxetine with nortriptyline.

In the first study, 236 patients were randomly assigned to treatment with either fluoxetine (20–40 mg/day) or sertraline (50–100 mg/day) for 12 weeks. In the second study, 210 patients were randomly assigned to treatment with either sertraline (50–150 mg/day) or nortriptyline (50–100 mg/day), also for 12 weeks. The patients who completed the 12-week trials did not differ in demographic or clinical features, nor did the groups differ in rates of response or remission. Therefore, those who completed the trial in the four groups were combined for the purpose of enhancing sample size with respect to other analyses.

For the total sample of completers (N=304), the response rate was 69%. When the criterion for remission was a final Ham-D (24-item) score of 10 or less, the remission rate was 59%; for a final Ham-D score of 6 or less, the remission rate was 34%. The median time to onset of sustained remission was 4 weeks if remission was defined as a final Ham-D score of 10 or less, but 36% of the patients required 8 or more weeks to reach this point. If the remission criterion was a final Ham-D score of 6 or less, then the time to sustained remission was 8 weeks, with 29% reaching the criterion only in week 12. Thus, not surprisingly, time to remission is dependent on the remission criteria. However,

given a remission criterion of a final Ham-D score of 10 or less, which is often used in late-life depression trials, the median time to onset of remission (4 weeks) is not prolonged compared with reports on younger depressed patients. Neither the overall response or remission rates nor the time to achieve sustained remission supports the belief that patients with late-life depression are less responsive to antidepressant medication or take longer to respond.

With respect to the early identification of nonresponders, when a remission criterion of a final Ham-D score of 6 or less is used, if a patient does not have at least a 30% improvement in the Ham-D score by week 2, he or she has only a 22% probability of being in remission at week 12, and this probability progressively decreases, so that by week 6, if a patient does not have a 30% reduction in baseline Ham-D score, the probability of remission at the end of week 12 is only 7%. As would be expected, if the remission criterion is a final Ham-D score of 10 or less, there was still strong predictive power, but it was somewhat delayed (i.e., by week 6, if a patient did not achieve a 30% reduction from baseline Ham-D score, then there was a 22% chance of being in remission at the end of the study, and this decreased to 19% by week 8). The results suggest that if there is not a moderate degree of symptomatic improvement early in treatment, clinicians can have a high level of accuracy in predicting that the patient will not adequately respond to this treatment within 12 weeks.

The most important clinical implication of these data is that clinicians no longer have to mandate a 12-week trial of antidepressant medication to all depressed patients older than 60 years. Rather, they can make informed decisions about changing or continuing treatment at the 4- and 6-week time points based on the probability that given the patient's improvement to date, he or she will or will not meet remission criteria by week 12.

Antipsychotics in the Elderly

Antipsychotic medications are increasingly being used in geriatric patients, particularly in dementia (Colenda et al. 2002). In the elderly, antipsychotic use in neurodegenerative disorders exceeds antipsychotic use in schizophrenia because of the difference in disease prevalence rates. In the elderly, the population prevalence of schizophrenia remains below 1%, whereas the prevalence of dementia is approximately 2%–5% for people older than 60 years, and the prevalence increases to 15%–40% for people older than 85 years of age (Thomas et al. 2001). Psychosis and behavioral dyscontrol occur in the majority of patients with dementia during their course of illness (Devanand et al. 1997; Lyketsos et al. 2000). Consequently, use of antipsychotics is greater in elderly patients with dementia than in those with schizophrenia, even though antipsychotic medications are not U.S. Food and Drug Administration (FDA) approved for the treatment of psychosis or behavioral dyscontrol in dementia (i.e., their use represents an off-label indication).

Antipsychotics: Special Issues in the Elderly

Side Effects of Antipsychotics

Older patients are more sensitive to the side effects of antipsychotics, which can include sedation, cardiac effects (e.g., tachycardia, orthostatic hypotension), anticholinergic side effects (e.g., dry mouth, blurred vision, constipation, urinary retention), neuroleptic malignant syndrome with hyperpyrexia, autonomic instability and tachycardia, pigmentary retinopathy, weight gain and associated metabolic changes, allergic reactions, and seizures (Arana 2000). In the elderly, the risk of orthostatic hypotension leading to falls and fractures, anticholinergic side effects, and the neurological syndromes of extrapyramidal side effects (EPS) and tardive dyskinesia (TD) are particularly important.

The antipsychotics most likely to cause orthostatic hypotension are low-potency conventional (or typical) antipsychotics such as chlorpromazine and thioridazine and the atypical antipsychotics clozapine, risperidone, olanzapine, and quetiapine (Tandon 1998). Low-potency conventional antipsychotics and clozapine have the most anticholinergic effects. At comparable doses, low-potency conventional antipsychotics are less likely to cause EPS than are than high-potency conventional antipsychotics such as haloperidol, but up to 50% of patients 60–80 years of age receiving conventional antipsychotics develop either EPS or TD (Jeste et al. 1999). Saltz et al. (1991) reported an incidence of TD of 31% after 43 weeks of conventional antipsychotic treatment in a sample of elderly patients, and antipsychotic-induced TD is five to six times more prevalent in elderly than in younger patients (Jeste 2000). Besides age, other risk factors for TD include early development of EPS, cumulative use of antipsychotics, duration of antipsychotic treatment, and history of alcohol abuse and/or dependence (Lohr et al. 2002). The susceptibility of older patients to the side effects of typical antipsychotics, particularly the neurological side effects of EPS and TD, requires the use of doses lower than those commonly used in young adults. Atypical antipsychotics have a lower potential for TD compared with typical antipsychotics (Jeste 2000). Although neurological side effects are less of a concern with most atypical antipsychotics, lower doses are still needed because of the older patient's susceptibility to the other side effects of antipsychotics, including anticholinergic and cardiovascular side effects.

Mortality Risks of Antipsychotics

The use of antipsychotics is associated with an increased risk of sudden cardiac death (Ray et al. 2001). Among the antipsychotics, thioridazine appears to carry the highest risk of sudden unexplained death that is believed to be due to cardiac causes (Reilly et al. 2002). Risperidone prolongs the QTc interval but has no effect on QT dispersion (Yerrabolu et al. 2000). Prolongation of the QTc interval, which is associated with the development of torsades de pointes and sudden death, is known to occur with several antipsychotics including the atypical antipsychotic ziprasidone, but aripiprazole, a new atypical antipsychotic, may reduce the QTc interval (Goodnick et al. 2002).

Based on a review of double-blind, placebo-controlled trials of atypical antipsychotics in patients with dementia, the FDA concluded that there was a significantly greater mortality risk (1.6–1.7 times) for patients treated with these medications compared with those treated with placebo and that all antipsychotic medications must carry a black box warning to this effect (Jeste et al. 2007). Most deaths were due to cardiac or infectious causes, which generally are the most common causes of death in patients with dementia. At this time, there is no clear explanation as to why use of atypical antipsychotics is associated with an increased mortality risk in patients with dementia. There appears to be a small increase in the risk of stroke (Brodaty et al. 2003), for which the mechanism has not been identified (Jeste et al. 2007). However, the increase in stroke risk does not by itself account for the increased mortality risk (Jeste et al. 2007).

The metabolic syndrome with glucose dysregulation is a potential side effect of all antipsychotic medications, to varying degrees. New-onset type 2 diabetes mellitus or diabetic ketoacidosis may be more common with clozapine and olanzapine compared with other antipsychotics, and blood glucose levels need to be monitored in elderly patients (Jin et al. 2004). Fasting lipid levels may rise more with olanzapine than with risperidone (Meyer 2002). Weight gain is a problematic side effect of several antipsychotics, particularly olanzapine and clozapine. There is evidence that treatment with clozapine or typical antipsychotics leads to increased leptin concentrations (Hagg et al. 2001).

Sedation is one of the most common side effects of antipsychotic medications, with low-potency antipsychotics being potent sleep inducers. In addition, low-potency antipsychotics have a greater propensity to cause anticholinergic side effects, and daytime confusion and disorientation are potential complications of antipsychotic use in the elderly.

Elderly patients are often taking a large number of medications, and drug interactions need to be considered when prescribing antipsychotics. Specifically, adding fluoxetine to risperidone raises risperidone levels (Bondolfi et al. 2002), and similar effects have been reported when fluoxetine is combined with typical antipsychotics (Solai et al. 2001).

Pharmacokinetics and Pharmacodynamics of Antipsychotics in the Elderly

Age-related decreases in gut motility and the anticholinergic effects of antipsychotics may decrease absorption rates. Antipsychotic drugs undergo biotransformation primarily in the liver, with the gastrointestinal tract, lungs, and kidneys being secondary sites. Antipsychotics have slightly longer half-lives in the elderly than in the rest of the adult population (Hicks and Davis 1980). Therefore, drugs take longer to reach therapeutic blood levels and also take longer to leave the system, thereby prolonging side effects. The concomitant use of antacids may lower antipsychotic blood levels (Fann et al. 1973).

Dopamine neurons degenerate with aging, particularly after age 70 years, and decreases in the number of cholinergic receptors occur in Alzheimer's disease (AD) (Davies and Maloney 1976; Perry et al. 1977). The decrease in the number of available dopaminergic receptors reduces the tolerance of elderly patients to antipsychotics, thereby increasing the likelihood of neurological side effects, including EPS and TD.

Blockade of dopamine$_2$ (D$_2$) receptors is believed to be the primary mechanism of action of antipsychotics. Atypical antipsychotics are more potent antagonists at the serotonin 5-HT$_{2A}$ receptor compared to the D$_2$ receptor, resulting in fewer EPS and less TD compared with typical antipsychotics (Jeste et al. 1999).

Treatment of Behavioral Complications of Dementia

Patients with dementia often develop behavioral disturbances (e.g., agitation and aggression) or psychotic features (e.g., delusions and hallucinations). As used here,

the term *behavioral complications* denotes both behavioral disturbances and psychotic features. Behavioral complications occur in most forms of dementia, lead to considerable burden for caregivers, and are common precipitants of institutionalization.

Personality changes occur early in dementia and include apathy, anhedonia, irritability, inability to pay attention, depression, and loss of emotional connection (Rubin and Kinscherf 1989). In later stages, varying degrees of agitation may occur in more than half of AD patients in outpatient clinics (Devanand et al. 1997) and nursing homes (Cohen-Mansfield et al. 1989), with aggressive behavior also becoming common (Devanand et al. 1997; Swearer et al. 1988). Other disinhibited behaviors include pacing, wandering, verbal and physical aggression, repetitive calling out and screaming, and (rarely) self-mutilating behaviors. Catastrophic reactions, including bursts of anger and even violent behavior, can occur when patients are required to perform tasks beyond their cognitive capacities (Devanand et al. 1992a). Stubbornness, or refusal to complete essential activities of daily life, can be particularly frustrating for caregivers.

Psychotic symptoms are common in dementia, with the prevalence ranging from 10% to 70% across studies. The prevalence of delusions ranges from 0% to 50% in different samples of AD patients (Devanand et al. 1997; Lyketsos et al. 2000; Reisberg et al. 1989). Isolated delusional thoughts are more common than diagnosable psychotic disorders, and paranoid delusions of theft and suspicion are the most frequent types of delusions. Systematized complex delusions and grandiose delusions are relatively rare in AD and other dementias. Delusional processes in dementia can be chronic or intermittent, a feature that distinguishes them from delusions in schizophrenia. Hallucinations, which can be visual or auditory, occur in 5%–15% of patients with dementia. In AD, a typical hallucination is the conviction that someone else is in the house (i.e., phantom boarder syndrome). Diagnostic criteria for psychosis in AD have been developed on the basis of these clinical features (Jeste and Finkel 2000).

In a series of 235 patients with mild to moderate AD who were followed prospectively for up to 5 years, approximately half of the patients who manifested paranoid delusions or hallucinations at baseline were likely to manifest the same symptom 6 months later (Devanand et al. 1997), a finding consistent with other reports (Ballard et al. 1997; Paulsen et al. 2000). However, paranoid delusions or hallucinations were evident at three out of four consecutive visits (over a period of 2 years) in only 10%–15% of patients, which raises the question, still unanswered, of how long patients need to continue taking psychotropic medications after treatment response. Psychosis and behavioral dyscontrol often coexist in AD, and treatment with antipsychotics is often prescribed for one or both sets of symptoms.

Assessment of Psychopathology in Alzheimer's Disease

In elderly patients, assessment and treatment of psychopathology should occur after reversible medical conditions (e.g., occult urinary tract infection, metabolic imbalance, iatrogenic or medication-induced symptoms) have been ruled out. Because of the intrinsic nature of AD and other dementias, most rating scales have been developed as informant-based interviews. Commonly used rating scales for measurement of neuropsychiatric symptoms of AD include the Neuropsychiatric Inventory (NPI; Cummings et al. 1994), the Neuropsychiatric Inventory—Nursing Home Version (Wood et al. 2000), the Behavioral Pathology in Alzheimer's Disease Rating Scale (BEHAVE-AD; Reisberg et al. 1987), the Consortium to Establish a Registry for Alzheimer's Disease (CERAD) Behavior Rating Scale (Tariot et al. 1995), the Cohen-Mansfield Agitation Inventory (Cohen-Mansfield et al. 1989), and the Columbia University Scale for Psychopathology in Alzheimer's Disease (CUSPAD; Devanand et al. 1992b). Currently, the NPI, which uses a quantitative time-efficient, decision-tree approach, is the most widely used scale for evaluating the effects of antipsychotic treatment in patients with dementia.

Neurobiological Mechanisms of Psychosis in Dementia

AD patients with psychosis have been found to have significantly more plaques and tangles in the medial temporal–prosubicular area and the middle frontal cortex (Zubenko et al. 1991) and four to five times higher levels of abnormal paired helical filament (PHF)–tau protein in the entorhinal and temporal cortices (Mukaetova-Ladinska et al. 1993). A decrease in serotonin in the prosubiculum of the cerebral cortex has been reported in patients with psychotic compared with nonpsychotic dementia (Lawlor et al. 1995; Zubenko et al. 1991). Decreases in acetylcholine have been correlated with increases in thought disorder (Sunderland et al. 1997). Cholinergic agents, including the acetylcholinesterase inhibitors (donepezil, rivastigmine, galantamine) that are used to treat cognitive impairment in AD, may also reduce behavioral symptoms (Bodick et al. 1997; Kaufer et al. 1996; Raskind

1999). Higher levels of norepinephrine in the substantia nigra (Zubenko et al. 1991) and higher levels of β-adrenergic receptors (Russo-Neustadt and Cotman 1997) in multiple brain regions have been reported in psychotic compared with nonpsychotic patients with AD. These data suggest an enhanced responsiveness of catecholamines that may be associated with increased psychosis in AD (Peskind et al. 1995). Homozygosity of the 1 and 2 alleles of the dopamine receptor *DR3* gene (Holmes et al. 2001; Sweet et al. 1998) and homozygosity for the C102 allele of the 5-HT$_{2A}$ receptor gene (Nacmias et al. 2001) may be associated with psychosis in AD. However, the precise pathophysiology underlying psychosis in AD is still unknown.

Psychotropic Medication Use in Dementia

Earlier studies indicated that nearly half of inpatients with dementia in Veterans Administration hospitals (Prien et al. 1975) and in other settings (Michel and Kolakowska 1981) received psychotropic medications, primarily antipsychotics and benzodiazepines (Ray et al. 1980). The neurological side effects of typical antipsychotics, particularly in dementia patients in nursing homes, led to the promulgation of the Omnibus Budget Reconciliation Act (OBRA) of 1987 (Elon and Pawlson 1992), which became effective in 1990. OBRA required identification of target symptoms, justification for the use of antipsychotics, and mandatory attempts to decrease or stop the antipsychotic medication every 3 months. Nonetheless, antipsychotic medications remain the treatment of choice for behavioral complications in dementia (Devanand et al. 1998; Katz et al. 1999; Schneider et al. 1990; Street et al. 2000), and drug utilization studies show that antipsychotics are used in 30%–50% of elderly institutionalized patients (Giron et al. 2001; Lantz et al. 1990).

Studies of Antipsychotics in Dementia

The results of an earlier meta-analysis of placebo-controlled treatment trials indicated that typical antipsychotic treatment in dementia was significantly more efficacious than placebo, with the magnitude of the advantage over placebo averaging 18% (Schneider et al. 1990). In placebo-controlled clinical trials with typical or atypical antipsychotics, response rates varied between 45% and 60% for active medication and between 20% and 45% for placebo (De Deyn et al. 1999; Devanand et al. 1998; Katz et al. 1999; Street et al. 2000), with an overall advantage for antipsychotic over placebo in the range of 18%–26% (Kindermann et al. 2002; Lanctot et al. 1998). Differences in response have been moderate on average, and clinically, a complete "cure" of the target psychotic and behavioral symptoms is uncommon.

In schizophrenia, antipsychotics are often assumed to be specific for the treatment of psychosis, and improvement in behavioral dyscontrol is believed to be secondary to improvement in psychosis. However, in patients with dementia, placebo-controlled studies consistently show comparable advantages for antipsychotics over placebo for symptoms of both psychosis and behavioral dyscontrol (Brodaty et al. 2003; De Deyn et al. 1999; Devanand et al. 1998; Katz et al. 1999; Street et al. 2000).

Typical antipsychotics. Early placebo-controlled studies of typical antipsychotics used in the management of behavioral complications of dementia showed moderate efficacy with a high placebo response rate, and considerable EPS occurred even at moderate doses (Barnes et al. 1982; Finkel et al. 1995; Petrie et al. 1982; Rada and Kellner 1976). In a double-blind, placebo-controlled, randomized comparison of standard-dose (2–3 mg/day) and low-dose (0.50–0.75 mg/day) haloperidol in 71 outpatients with AD (Devanand et al. 1998), standard-dose haloperidol was efficacious and superior to both low-dose haloperidol and placebo, as measured by scores on the Brief Psychiatric Rating Scale (BPRS) psychosis factor ($P<0.03$ and $P<0.05$, respectively) and psychomotor agitation ($P<0.03$ and $P<0.04$, respectively). EPS tended to be greater for haloperidol 2–3 mg/day than for the other two conditions, primarily because of a subgroup (20%) that developed moderate to severe EPS. Other somatic side effects, cognitive performance, and daily functioning did not differ among the three treatment conditions. Low-dose haloperidol did not differ from placebo on any measure of efficacy or side effects. The results indicated a favorable therapeutic profile for haloperidol at a dosage of 2–3 mg/day, although a subgroup did develop moderate to severe EPS (Devanand et al. 1998). In another study that compared the SSRI citalopram, the typical antipsychotic perphenazine, and placebo, citalopram was comparable to perphenazine in efficacy and significantly superior to placebo, with an advantageous side-effect profile (Pollock et al. 2002). While intriguing, replication of these findings with an SSRI antidepressant is needed before citalopram can be recommended for treatment of behavioral complications in dementia.

A multicenter study yielded findings that contradicted the earlier literature on typical antipsychotics, reporting no significant advantage for haloperidol over either trazodone or placebo in 149 patients with AD (Teri et al. 2000). However, that study had several methodological flaws, including the assignment of a subset of patients at only some of the sites to receive behavioral treatment that was not administered in a double-blind manner (Teri et al. 2000).

Atypical antipsychotics. Because of their more favorable safety profile, the atypical antipsychotics have gradually replaced typical antipsychotics in the treatment of behavioral complications in dementia. Atypical antipsychotics can be safely administered with cholinesterase inhibitors (e.g., donepezil, rivastigmine, galantamine), which are used to treat the cognitive impairment of dementia (Weiser et al. 2002). The choice of atypical antipsychotic depends on the patient's clinical profile and the medication's side-effect profile (e.g., a patient prone to falls should receive a medication that is not likely to cause orthostatic hypotension). Clozapine, risperidone, paliperidone (risperidone metabolite), olanzapine, quetiapine, aripiprazole, and ziprasidone are the atypical antipsychotics that are currently available.

Clozapine. Clozapine was the first atypical antipsychotic available in the United States. Clozapine causes substantial serotonergic blockade and has antiadrenergic and antimuscarinic properties (Lieberman 1998). Clozapine may be more efficacious than other antipsychotics in schizophrenia, and it carries essentially no risk of TD (Kane et al. 1988). Circulating levels of clozapine rise with dose and age and may be slightly higher in women than in men; sedation is common, and seizure potential is elevated (Centorrino et al. 1994; Kurz et al. 1998). Clozapine's anticholinergic properties can lead to dry mouth and constipation and can adversely affect cognition in the elderly. Also, intensive monitoring is required for blood dyscrasias, particularly agranulocytosis, which is reported to occur in 0.38% of patients (Kane et al. 1988). These factors, as well as the increased risk of falls and fractures related to the side effect of orthostatic hypotension, limit the use of clozapine in the elderly. Partly because of these safety concerns, there have been no double-blind, placebo-controlled trials using clozapine to treat behavioral complications in dementia. The few retrospective reviews and case reports available indicate moderate efficacy but with significant adverse events, suggesting very low tolerability (Chengappa et al. 1995; Oberholzer et al. 1992; Pitner et al. 1995). Therefore, clozapine is rarely used in patients with dementia. Its use should be considered only when other antipsychotic medication treatment has failed to yield improvement.

Risperidone. Risperidone has serotonin 5-HT$_2$ and dopamine D$_2$ blocking properties, α_1- and α_2-adrenergic blocking properties, minimal histaminergic H$_1$ blocking properties, and little affinity for cholinergic receptors (Janssen et al. 1988). Its elimination half-life is between 20 and 22 hours, allowing for once-a-day dosing (Byerly and DeVane 1996).

In a multicenter study of young adults with schizophrenia that compared risperidone 2, 6, 12, and 16 mg/day with haloperidol 20 mg/day, risperidone 6 mg/day was efficacious and had the best therapeutic profile, with a low propensity for EPS (Chouinard et al. 1993). However, the optimal risperidone dosage range is much lower in elderly patients (Katz et al. 1999). Compared with the other atypical antipsychotics, risperidone may be more likely to lead to EPS and TD, although this risk is considerably lower than with typical antipsychotics such as haloperidol (Jeste 2000). In 255 elderly institutionalized patients with dementia and without baseline TD who were treated with risperidone at an average daily dose of 0.96 (SD=0.53) mg, the 1-year cumulative incidence of persistent emergent TD was a relatively low 2.6% (Jeste et al. 2000). Risperidone is mildly sedating and has the potential to cause orthostatic hypotension, although the latter effect is uncommon when low doses are used in the elderly (Katz et al. 1999).

In a multicenter study, 625 nursing home patients (mean age=83 years) with dementia (73% AD, 15% vascular, 12% mixed dementia; mean 30-item Mini-Mental State Examination [MMSE] score=6.6) who had behavioral complications were randomly assigned to receive risperidone—at 0.5 mg/day, 1.0 mg/day, or 2.0 mg/day—or placebo for 12 weeks (Katz et al. 1999). The clinical trial was completed by 435 (70%) patients, with discontinuations primarily due to adverse events (12% of patients receiving placebo; 8%, 16%, and 24% of patients receiving 0.5, 1.0, and 2.0 mg/day of risperidone, respectively). At study endpoint, response rates for risperidone 1 mg/day (45%) and 2 mg/day (50%) were significantly superior to rates for placebo and risperidone 0.5 mg/day, which showed similar response rates (33%). Patients receiving risperidone 2 mg/day were more likely than those receiving risperidone 0.5 mg/day or 1 mg/day to develop EPS and sedation, suggesting a relatively narrow therapeutic window. Orthostatic hypotension was a relatively infrequent side effect in this study (Katz et al. 1999). Therefore, a risperidone starting dosage of 0.5 mg/day, with gradual upward dosage titration to 1–2 mg/day, is recommended. This dosage range is far lower than the optimal risperidone dosage of 6 mg/day in adults with schizophre-

nia (Chouinard et al. 1993). A meta-analysis of four placebo-controlled trials with risperidone found that it was superior to placebo in treating psychosis and agitation, particularly in severely disturbed patients (Katz et al. 2007). Although a long-acting injectable risperidone preparation is available, that formulation has not been studied in the treatment of behavioral complications of dementia. This issue is particularly relevant for patients who may not take oral medications on a regular basis.

Paliperidone. Paliperidone, or 9-OH risperidone, is a metabolite of risperidone that has been recently approved for the treatment of schizophrenia. Paliperidone extended-release (ER) tablets need to be taken once daily. There is a lack of information on use of paliperidone ER in patients with dementia. In a 6-week randomized, placebo-controlled, double-blind trial of paliperidone in adults diagnosed with schizophrenia, paliperidone ER 6 mg/day and 12 mg/day led to comparable improvement in positive and negative symptoms, but only the 6-mg/day dosage was associated with improvement in personal and social functioning (Marder et al. 2007). The medication showed comparable efficacy to a treatment arm with olanzapine 10 mg/day in the same study. Another study showed that paliperidone at dosages of 3–9 mg/day was superior to placebo in the treatment of schizophrenia (Davidson et al. 2007). Paliperidone ER provides a useful treatment alternative in patients whose compliance may be suboptimal. However, further studies are needed to evaluate its side-effect profile in the elderly, particularly in patients with dementia.

Olanzapine. Olanzapine blocks multiple receptor sites, including serotonin 5-HT$_{2A/2C}$ and dopamine D$_{4/3/2/1}$ (serotonin-to-dopamine receptor binding ratio of 8:1), histaminergic H$_1$ receptors, muscarinic acetylcholine receptors, and noradrenergic α_1 receptors (Bymaster et al. 1996). Olanzapine is well absorbed, is unaffected by food, and with a mean half-life of 30 hours, it can be used once a day (Fulton and Goa 1997).

Sedation and weight gain are prominent side effects of olanzapine, and its use has been associated with the development of metabolic syndrome. Orthostatic hypotension is also of concern because it can lead to falls and fractures, but this side effect is uncommon when low doses are used in elderly patients (Street et al. 2000). Intramuscular olanzapine is a useful alternative to intramuscular haloperidol in the treatment of acutely psychotic, agitated patients with schizophrenia (Breier et al. 2002a) and may be a useful alternative to intramuscular lorazepam in patients with dementia (Meehan et al. 2002).

In an 8-week double-blind, randomized treatment trial of 238 elderly AD outpatients with behavioral complications (mean age = 78.6 years), olanzapine at an average daily dose of 2.4 mg was not superior to placebo. The lack of efficacy, however, may have been attributable to use of suboptimal dosages (Satterlee and Sussman 1998). In a second double-blind, placebo-controlled multicenter clinical trial, 206 nursing home patients (mean age = 83 years) with AD (mean MMSE score = 6.9) and behavioral complications were randomly assigned to placebo or fixed-dose olanzapine 5 mg/day, 10 mg/day, or 15 mg/day for 6 weeks. Olanzapine 5 mg/day was significantly more efficacious than placebo, but the 10-mg/day and 15-mg/day dosages were not superior to placebo. The prominent side effects of sedation and weight gain were limiting factors at the higher dosages (Street et al. 2000). Clinically, a starting dose of 2.5 mg/day with gradual upward titration is recommended.

Quetiapine. Quetiapine acts as an antagonist at multiple neurotransmitter receptors in the brain, including dopamine D_1, D_2, serotonin 5-HT_{1A} and 5-HT_2, histamine H_1, and α_1- and α_2-adrenergic receptors. D_2 receptor affinity is less than 5-HT_2 receptor affinity. Quetiapine has no appreciable binding affinity to cholinergic muscarinic or benzodiazepine receptors (Casey 1996). Although it has a short half-life (approximately 3–6 hours; Fulton and Goa 1997), efficacy has been documented with twice-daily administration (McManus et al. 1999).

The incidence of EPS is very low. The risk of a rare lenticular and corneal opacity was reported in pre-drug-release studies (Shahzad et al. 2002). However, it remains unclear whether this potential side effect occurs in elderly patients, because the high prevalence of lenticular opacities in the normal elderly population makes it difficult to evaluate this possible side effect (Tariot et al. 2006).

In a study of 284 elderly patients with dementia, quetiapine (average dose 96.9 mg) and haloperidol (average dose 1.9 mg) were indistinguishable from placebo on most measures of efficacy, although haloperidol led to more EPS (Tariot et al. 2006). The optimal dose for quetiapine is undetermined because dose comparison studies have not been conducted in patients with dementia. Wide dose ranges from 25 to 800 mg/day are used in clinical practice. In the absence of double-blind, placebo-controlled data clearly demonstrating its superiority over placebo, quetiapine cannot be recommended as a first-line antipsychotic medication to treat behavioral complications in patients with dementia. However, physicians often do prescribe quetiapine because of its relatively benign side-effect profile. Sedation is the most common side effect with this medication.

Ziprasidone. Ziprasidone is used at dosages of 80–160 mg/day in adults (Arato et al. 2002). Unlike the other atypical antipsychotics, it causes little weight gain, produces minimal to no EPS, and has no anticholinergic side effects. However, ziprasidone can cause prolongation of the QTc interval on the electrocardiogram, and this side effect may limit its use in elderly patients with cardiovascular disease. There is a lack of published data on the use of ziprasidone in elderly patients and no controlled trials in dementia. Ziprasidone's potential to prolong the QTc interval on the electrocardiogram requires monitoring, but it causes less weight gain than most other antipsychotics (Arato et al. 2002).

Aripiprazole. A placebo-controlled study of aripiprazole in 208 outpatients with AD who had behavioral complications showed no advantage for aripiprazole on the main outcome measure (NPI score), but there was superiority on secondary outcome measures (BPRS psychosis and Core scores). The average dosage used was 10 mg/day, and it was generally well tolerated (De Deyn et al. 2005). These limited data suggest that aripiprazole can play a role as a second-line atypical antipsychotic treatment in AD patients with behavioral complications.

Comparisons among antipsychotics. Head-to-head comparison studies show few differences between typical antipsychotics in the treatment of behavioral complications in dementia (Barnes et al. 1982; Carlyle et al. 1993; Petrie et al. 1982; Smith et al. 1974; Tsuang et al. 1971). In the first comparison of a typical and an atypical antipsychotic, patients with dementia and behavioral complications were randomly assigned to receive flexible-dose risperidone, haloperidol, or placebo (De Deyn et al. 1999). In 344 patients, risperidone (average dosage = 1.1 mg/day), haloperidol (average dosage = 1.2 mg/day), and placebo showed improvement rates of 54%, 63%, and 47%, respectively, at week 12 ($P = 0.25$). Likewise, no significant differences in improvement were seen between the groups on psychosis scores. In post hoc analyses, both haloperidol and risperidone were significantly better than placebo at reducing the total BEHAVE-AD and aggression cluster scores ($P = 0.01$), and risperidone was superior to haloperidol on the aggression cluster score ($P = 0.05$). Patients taking haloperidol had significantly higher EPS scores at endpoint than did patients taking either risperidone or placebo, with no significant difference in EPS scores between patients receiving risperidone and placebo (De Deyn et al. 1999). Overall, risperidone's efficacy was comparable to that of haloperidol, with a superior side-effect profile.

Early studies reported conflicting data on whether atypical antipsychotics show superior efficacy when compared with typical antipsychotics in mixed-age samples of schizophrenic patients (Arvanitis and Miller 1997; Geddes et al. 2000; Kane et al. 1988). The Clinical Antipsychotic Trials of Intervention Effectiveness (CATIE) in adults with schizophrenia showed only marginal superiority in antipsychotic effectiveness for olanzapine compared with typical and other atypical antipsychotics (Lieberman et al. 2005). In England, the Cost Utility of the Latest Antipsychotic Drugs in Schizophrenia Study (CUtLASS) of 227 patients with schizophrenia did not show any differences in treatment response for atypical versus typical antipsychotics (Jones et al. 2006).

In dementia, comparisons of haloperidol and risperidone led to equivocal results (Chan et al. 2001; De Deyn et al. 1999; Suh et al. 2004). In the 421 elderly patients who participated in the AD component of CATIE that compared risperidone, olanzapine, quetiapine, and placebo (first randomized phase), there were no significant differences in time to discontinuation because the superior efficacy of risperidone and olanzapine was compromised by their increased propensity to side effects; quetiapine was indistinguishable from placebo (Schneider et al. 2006). These findings indicate that efficacy must be weighed against side effects when prescribing risperidone or olanzapine in a patient with dementia and that quetiapine may not be effective.

Studies of antipsychotics versus benzodiazepines in dementia. The few studies that compared antipsychotics with benzodiazepines suffered from methodological flaws, particularly in sample selection and study design (Burgio et al. 1992; Covington 1975; Kirven and Montero 1973; Stotsky 1984; Tewfik et al. 1970). The data available from these studies do not indicate superiority for benzodiazepines over antipsychotics in the treatment of behavioral complications in patients with dementia.

Benzodiazepines are known to have deleterious effects on learning and memory in healthy subjects (Ghoneim et al. 1981; Jones et al. 1978; Liljequist et al. 1978), particularly in the elderly (Pomara et al. 1991). Benzodiazepines can lead to tolerance and dependence, and worsening of cognition is a concern. Therefore, benzodiazepines should be used in low doses and restricted to short-term crisis management of agitated and anxious behaviors if antipsychotics or other medications are ineffective.

Studies of anticonvulsants and other agents in dementia. A small-sample study suggested that carbamazepine was effective in the treatment of behavioral complications of AD (Tariot et al. 1998), and there were suggestions that valproate was efficacious in a single-site study by the same research group (Porsteinsson et al. 2001). However, valproate at an average dosage of 800 mg/day did not show superiority over placebo in a larger study of 153 nursing home patients who participated in a double-blind, placebo-controlled trial (Tariot et al. 2005). Nonetheless, anticonvulsants such as valproate are prescribed commonly in nursing homes, presumably because of their relatively benign side-effect profile. To date, no published studies have compared an antipsychotic with an anticonvulsant in the treatment of behavioral complications in patients with dementia.

Studies with other medications, such as buspirone (Lawlor et al. 1994), trazodone (Sultzer et al. 1997; Teri et al. 2000), lithium (Holton and George 1985), and propranolol (Shankle et al. 1995; Weiler et al. 1988), have involved case series or small samples, usually without placebo control. These medications can be considered as therapeutic options only after antipsychotic treatment has failed.

Choice of Antipsychotic for Treatment of Behavioral Complications of Dementia

Given the relative lack of differences in efficacy among antipsychotics (except the possible lower efficacy for quetiapine) for treating behavioral complications in dementia, the potential side-effect profile should determine the choice for individual patients (Ellingrod et al. 2002). Because of its problematic side-effect profile and its requirement for extensive blood-level monitoring, clozapine should be reserved for those patients who do not respond to the other available antipsychotics. Patients prone to orthostatic hypotension (e.g., patients receiving β-blockers) may develop this side effect while taking risperidone or olanzapine, although postural hypotension is uncommon at low doses (Katz et al. 1999; Street et al. 2000). Olanzapine causes weight gain and is strongly sedating, but the latter side effect may be advantageous in patients with prominent insomnia. The metabolic syndrome can occur with all antipsychotics but is most likely to occur with olanzapine. Quetiapine is generally well tolerated, but it can be sedating. Among the atypical antipsychotics, risperidone is the most likely to cause EPS, so olanzapine or quetiapine should be preferred in elderly patients who have parkinsonian features. The incidence of TD is much lower with atypical antipsychotics than with the typical antipsychotic haloperidol (Jeste et al. 2000). In a study of 35 agitated patients with dementia who were switched from haloperidol to risperidone, the crossover was generally safe and effective (Lane et al. 2002). Overall, the decreased likelihood of neurological side effects, both short-term and long-term, makes atypical antipsychotics the treatment of choice in these patients.

Optimal Antipsychotic Dosing Strategy

It is important to avoid using excessive antipsychotic doses in elderly patients with dementia, who are particularly prone to side effects (e.g., EPS). On the other hand, using too low a dose may reduce efficacy. As already described, several placebo-controlled studies have compared different doses of antipsychotic medications: haloperidol (Devanand et al. 1998), risperidone (Katz et al. 1999), and olanzapine (Street et al. 2000). The studies with haloperidol and risperidone produced similar results: very low doses were ineffective, whereas high doses led to side effects, suggesting a relatively narrow therapeutic window for these medications in dementia patients who develop behavioral complications. The optimal dosage for olanzapine appears to be 5 mg/day, based on the study comparing 5, 10, and 15 mg/day, although the lack of superior efficacy for the higher dosages (10–15 mg/day) is a little puzzling (Street et al. 2000). As discussed earlier, the optimal quetiapine dosage remains uncertain. To date, there is no published information available on the optimal dose of ziprasidone in this patient population.

These dose-finding and related studies have helped refine the dosing strategy for treating behavioral complications in dementia. In patients with AD, risperidone should be started at 0.25–0.50 mg/day at bedtime (or twice-daily dosing), with a 0.5-mg/day increase per week to a maximum of 2 mg/day (or possibly 3 mg/day). Olanzapine should be started at 2.5 mg/day or 5.0 mg/day at bedtime and slowly increased to a target daily dose of 5–10 mg. Quetiapine should be started at 25 mg twice daily, with dose increases as tolerated up to 300 mg twice daily, based solely on clinical response and side effects, because the optimal dosage range for quetiapine has not been identified. If a typical antipsychotic is used, a starting dose equivalent to haloperidol 0.5 mg/day is suggested, with subsequent individualized titration to achieve an optimal tradeoff between efficacy and side effects.

Use of Concomitant Psychotropics

Anticholinergic agents to treat EPS should be avoided, particularly in AD, in which the cholinergic deficit is be-

lieved to underlie much of the cognitive impairment. In some patients, the concomitant use of a hypnotic (e.g., zolpidem 5–10 mg or zaleplon 5–10 mg) may be required. Trazodone at dosages of 25–200 mg/day can also be used as a hypnotic in these patients. As noted earlier, benzodiazepine use should be limited to short-term crisis management of anxiety or agitation.

Optimal Duration of Antipsychotic Treatment in Dementia

A trial of 6–12 weeks usually is sufficient to determine the outcome of an antipsychotic treatment trial. If the optimal antipsychotic dose is reached quickly, clinical response may occur within the first 1 or 2 weeks. On the other hand, the need to adjust the dosage because of side effects may require a relatively prolonged trial period.

The expected natural course of target symptoms during the course of dementia should be considered in determining the duration of antipsychotic treatment. Delusions and hallucinations are moderately persistent, whereas agitation usually persists for several months to years during the course of AD (Devanand et al. 1997). Currently, there is conflicting evidence on how long these patients need to be continued on antipsychotic medications. One report suggested that antipsychotics and other psychotropics can be discontinued in nursing home patients with dementia without increased risk of relapse (Cohen-Mansfield et al. 1999), but other reports indicate a moderate to high rate of relapse after discontinuation (Avorn et al. 1992; Fitz and Mallya 1992; Horwitz et al. 1995). Until large-scale systematic, controlled discontinuation trials are conducted to clarify the optimal duration of treatment, a reasonable approach is to attempt gradual tapering of the antipsychotic medication after 1 year of continuous treatment.

Antipsychotic Effects on Cognition and Activities of Daily Living

One concern associated with use of antipsychotic medications in dementia is that the anticholinergic activity of antipsychotics may further compromise the already damaged central cholinergic projections in AD. The level of cognitive impairment may be increased by the use of antipsychotics with strong anticholinergic properties or by the addition of anticholinergic agents to treat drug-induced EPS. Therefore, if EPS develops following antipsychotic treatment in a patient with dementia, switching to an antipsychotic that is less likely to cause EPS is preferable to adding an anticholinergic medication to treat the EPS. At another level, the sedation produced by antipsychotics may worsen the degree of disorientation and cognitive impairment in AD.

Antipsychotic Blood-Level Monitoring

Little work has examined the utility of monitoring antipsychotic blood levels in patients with dementia. In a study that compared haloperidol 2–3 mg/day, haloperidol 0.5–0.75 mg/day, and placebo, plasma haloperidol levels were detectable in all patients at the 2–3 mg daily dosage, and blood levels showed stronger correlations with efficacy and EPS than did oral dosages (Pelton et al. 2003). Few of the patients had ever received antipsychotics prior to entering the study, and this lack of previous exposure to antipsychotics may have precluded the alterations in drug absorption and metabolism that occur with chronic antipsychotic treatment in schizophrenia, with resultant distortion of the relationship between oral dosage and blood level. Interestingly, in this series of AD patients, therapeutic effects occurred at haloperidol blood levels that were invariably below the postulated therapeutic window of 5–15 ng/mL in schizophrenia (Van Putten et al. 1992; Volavka et al. 1992). Also, EPS developed in some patients at these low blood levels, suggesting that the increased sensitivity to antipsychotics seen in dementia is not likely to be attributable to pharmacokinetic changes. A pharmacodynamic explanation (e.g., loss of dopamine receptors leading to greater sensitivity to even low oral dosages of antipsychotic medication) is more likely. In contrast to the associations observed with the typical antipsychotic haloperidol, clinically relevant associations between blood levels of atypical antipsychotics and either efficacy or side effects have not been demonstrated (Jeste 2000).

Monitoring Treatment of Behavioral Complications in Dementia

The heterogeneous nature of behavioral complications suggests that specific target symptoms should be identified before initiating antipsychotic treatment, and these target symptoms should be monitored serially during the course of treatment. A scale like the NPI can also be used. In addition to neurological and other common antipsychotic side effects, cognition and activities of daily living need to be monitored, preferably with brief instruments such as the MMSE. In patients who are being maintained for extended periods on antipsychotics, assessment for TD using the Abnormal Involuntary Movement Scale should be conducted at regular intervals. Periodic attempts should be made to taper or discontinue the anti-

psychotic, although the optimal duration of continuation antipsychotic treatment remains to be established.

Antipsychotics in Other Neurodegenerative Disorders in the Elderly

The relative efficacy of antipsychotics in different subtypes of dementia (e.g., AD and vascular dementia) has not been studied extensively. The antipsychotic treatment trials that included patients with vascular, mixed, and other forms of dementia did not reveal any differences in treatment response among the diagnostic subtypes of dementia (De Deyn et al. 1999; Katz et al. 1999). With the exceptions of diffuse Lewy body disease and Parkinson's disease, the recommendations for the use of antipsychotics in AD generally apply to their use in other types of dementia.

Diffuse Lewy body disease (DLBD) is a subtype of dementia characterized by prominent EPS, fluctuating clinical course, hallucinations, and extreme sensitivity to the neurological side effects of antipsychotics (McKeith 2006). DLBD has features that overlap with those of AD and Parkinson's disease, and the boundaries of DLBD as a diagnostic entity remain controversial. Sensitivity to typical antipsychotics is one of the defining criteria for DLBD (McKeith 2006), and atypical antipsychotics may be safer to use in these patients. A post hoc analysis of the olanzapine dose comparison study in AD suggested that olanzapine was safe and effective for the subgroup of patients who met diagnostic criteria for DLBD (Cummings et al. 2002).

Patients with Parkinson's disease can develop iatrogenic psychosis caused by the levodopa–carbidopa combination (Sinemet) or dopamine agonists. Lowering the dose of the dopaminergic agent will often lead to remission of psychotic symptoms, but the price paid may be an unacceptable increase in parkinsonian symptoms (Breier et al. 2002b). In such cases, antipsychotics with a very low propensity to cause EPS can be considered. However, in a series of five Parkinson's disease patients who developed psychosis, olanzapine was not effective in treating psychosis and was associated with worsening motor function and sedation (Marsh et al. 2001), and two double-blind, placebo-controlled trials did not find an advantage for olanzapine over placebo in these patients (Breier et al. 2002b). Clozapine may be of some value in patients with Parkinson's disease (J. H. Friedman and Fernandez 2002), but quetiapine may be the preferred antipsychotic in this disorder. Long-term quetiapine use is generally well tolerated in patients with Parkinson's disease or DLBD (Fernandez et al. 2002).

In patients with delirium, short-term antipsychotic administration is a standard treatment strategy, particularly antipsychotic medications with low anticholinergic properties, such as haloperidol (Tune 2002). Atypical antipsychotics are useful in the management of delirium, and olanzapine has been reported to be safe and efficacious for the treatment of symptoms of delirium in hospitalized patients (Breitbart et al. 2002).

Antipsychotics in Late-Life Schizophrenia

The majority of elderly schizophrenic patients were first diagnosed as young adults, but a minority of patients are first diagnosed with schizophrenia later in life. The International Late-Onset Schizophrenia Group reached a consensus that the diagnoses of late-onset schizophrenia (onset after age 40 years) and very-late-onset schizophrenia (onset after age 60 years) have face validity and clinical utility (Howard et al. 2000). Although age at onset affects the clinical presentation to some extent (Sable and Jeste 2002), it does not appreciably influence the likelihood of response to antipsychotics or the occurrence of side effects (Sable and Jeste 2002).

Studies of Antipsychotics in Elderly Patients With Schizophrenia

Most elderly schizophrenic patients with disease onset in young adulthood have been maintained on antipsychotic medications for many years, often decades, as they enter old age. Tapering and stopping antipsychotic medications in schizophrenia is associated with a high risk of relapse (Csernansky and Schuchart 2002). This risk has made it difficult to conduct placebo-controlled trials in samples of elderly schizophrenic patients (Sable and Jeste 2002). However, because many of these patients have taken typical antipsychotics for many years and have developed EPS and/or TD over time, there is often a need to switch from a typical to an atypical antipsychotic to reduce the neurological toxicity profile. In elderly schizophrenic patients, switching from typical antipsychotics to risperidone has been reported to be effective and well-tolerated (Barak et al. 2002). Atypical antipsychotics appear to be at least as efficacious as and better tolerated than typical antipsychotics in the elderly, and a study of veterans suggested that adherence to atypical antipsychotics is slightly higher than adherence to typical antipsychotics (Dolder et al. 2002).

In a 4-month comparison trial of flexible-dose risperidone (n=175) and quetiapine (n=553) in 728 mixed-age patients with a variety of psychotic disorders, quetiapine was as effective as risperidone and less likely to require adjustment of concomitant antiparkinsonian medication. However, quetiapine was associated with more sedation, dry mouth, and dizziness (Mullen et al. 2001). In another study of patients with treatment-refractory schizophrenia in a long-stay state hospital, olanzapine and risperidone showed comparable efficacy (Dinakar et al. 2002). Quetiapine was evaluated in a sample of 151 elderly psychotic patients (mean age=77 years), among whom 40% had schizophrenia, bipolar disorder, or psychotic depression; 50% had psychosis associated with AD; and 10% had psychosis associated with Parkinson's disease. The median quetiapine dosage was 100 mg/day (range=100–400 mg/day). Significant improvement was seen in the primary outcome measure of psychosis as measured by the Brief Psychiatric Rating Scale (P<0.0001) and Clinical Global Impressions (P<0.01). The prominent side effects included somnolence in 32%, dizziness or postural hypotension in 13%, and EPS in 6% (McManus et al. 1999).

In 184 elderly patients (mean age=76.1 years), 72% with AD and 28% with other psychoses (mainly schizophrenia), open-label quetiapine was administered over 52 weeks. A total of 89 patients remained on quetiapine for the entire year, with the main reasons for withdrawal being lack of efficacy (19%), adverse events or intercurrent illness (15%), and failure to return for follow-up (13%). In this sample, quetiapine at a median dosage of 137.5 mg/day was effective, with 49% of the patients showing a 20% or greater decline in BPRS scores. The main side effects were sedation (31%), dizziness (17%), and postural hypotension (15%) (Tariot et al. 2000). EPS-related adverse events occurred in 13% of the patients, but overall ratings on an EPS scale showed a small improvement from baseline, and new-onset TD did not develop in any patient over the 1-year period. Although limited by the lack of placebo control or comparison with another antipsychotic to establish efficacy, the relatively benign side-effect profile of quetiapine is noteworthy. The CATIE studies suggested that quetiapine's lack of efficacy compared with olanzapine and risperidone (quetiapine did not separate from placebo) should be an equally important consideration (Lieberman et al. 2005; Schneider et al. 2006).

Few data on the use of ziprasidone in elderly schizophrenic patients have been published, perhaps because of its increased propensity to prolong the QT interval on the electrocardiogram, which may be problematic in elderly patients.

In all age groups, it has been difficult to demonstrate that the atypical antipsychotics approved for use in the United States improve negative symptoms (e.g., anhedonia, apathy), even though this putative effect was one of the factors driving the development of these compounds. However, medications approved in Europe (e.g., amisulpride) have been shown to be efficacious in improving the negative symptoms of schizophrenia in controlled studies (Moller 2001).

Treatment and Dosing

In elderly patients with schizophrenia, a thorough evaluation followed by treatment with low doses of atypical antipsychotics is the optimal strategy. When appropriate, antipsychotic treatment may need to be combined with psychosocial intervention (Sable and Jeste 2002).

The doses of typical antipsychotics used in elderly patients with schizophrenia need to be lower than the doses used in young adults (Jeste 2000), but published dose-comparison studies of individual antipsychotics in these patients are lacking. Abrupt withdrawal of atypical antipsychotics, particularly quetiapine, has not been shown to cause major adverse effects, but nonetheless, gradual withdrawal over a few days is advisable for all antipsychotics (Cutler et al. 2002). Although atypical antipsychotics can be safely combined with cholinesterase inhibitors in schizophrenia, a study in patients receiving risperidone found no cognitive benefit from adding donepezil compared with adding placebo (J.I. Friedman et al. 2002).

Antipsychotics in Other Psychotic Disorders in the Elderly

Late-onset delusional disorder is uncommon. As is the case in young adults, this disorder is difficult to treat, and the delusions often do not remit even with adequate antipsychotic treatment. The diagnosis of paraphrenia overlaps considerably with current nomenclature for late-onset schizophrenia, and atypical antipsychotics are the treatment of choice for this disorder (Howard et al. 2000).

Psychotic depression is an uncommon but clinically important diagnosis in the elderly. Based on studies in mixed-age samples, antipsychotics combined with antidepressants are the pharmacological treatment of choice in psychotic depression, but electroconvulsive therapy (ECT) is still considered the most effective treatment for this disorder (Mulsant et al. 2001b; Sackeim et al. 1995; Spiker et al. 1985). Expert consensus guidelines suggest that antipsychotic medication should be continued for 6 months following treatment response in psychotic depression (Alexopoulos et al. 2001), although sparse informa-

tion from controlled trials is available on this issue. In a sample of 29 elderly patients with psychotic depression who responded to combination antipsychotic–antidepressant or ECT, 25% relapsed during continuation treatment (Meyers et al. 2001). No significant difference in relapse rates was found between patients receiving nortriptyline plus perphenazine and patients receiving nortriptyline alone. However, combination therapy was associated with more EPS, increased risk of TD, and falls. Although these data suggest that continuation treatment with antidepressant alone may be sufficient and perhaps optimal in geriatric psychotic depression, more data from controlled studies with typical or atypical antipsychotics are needed before this approach can be recommended for standard clinical practice.

Antipsychotics are used widely in the treatment of the manic phase of bipolar disorder across the life span (Levine et al. 2000). In bipolar disorder, there is ample evidence for the efficacy of typical and atypical antipsychotics, both individually and in combination with mood stabilizers (Sachs et al. 2002; Tohen et al. 2002). However, there is a surprising lack of data on the use of antipsychotics in geriatric patients with bipolar disorder. Lithium's toxicity, particularly in the neurological domain, is problematic in the elderly (McDonald 2000). Hence, anticonvulsants and atypical antipsychotics are used frequently to treat mania in elderly patients. However, in the absence of controlled data, the optimal choice of antipsychotic and the optimal dose to use in these patients are open questions that need to be answered in future research.

Although obsessive-compulsive disorder is not considered a psychotic illness, there is evidence that atypical antipsychotics are useful adjunctive medications in adults with this disorder (Denys et al. 2002). However, comparable data are lacking in geriatric patients.

Conclusion

Clearly, antipsychotic medications, particularly atypical antipsychotics, have an important role to play in the treatment of psychosis and behavioral dyscontrol in AD, other types of dementia, and other neurodegenerative conditions. Antipsychotics remain the first-line treatment for schizophrenia and other psychotic disorders across the life span. When antipsychotic medications are used in elderly patients, monitoring of target symptoms, somatic side effects, potential drug interactions, cognition, and activities of daily living is necessary.

References

Alexopoulos GS, Katz IR, Reynolds CF III, et al: Pharmacotherapy of depressive disorders in older patients. Postgrad Med (Special Report) October 2001, pp 35–39

Allard P, Gram L, Timdahl K, et al: Efficacy and tolerability of venlafaxine in geriatric outpatients with major depression: a double-blind, randomized 6-month comparative trial with citalopram. Int J Geriatr Psychiatry 19:1123–1130, 2004

American Psychiatric Association: Diagnostic and Statistical Manual of Mental Disorders, 3rd Edition. Washington, DC, American Psychiatric Association, 1980

American Psychiatric Association: Diagnostic and Statistical Manual of Mental Disorders, 3rd Edition, Revised. Washington, DC, American Psychiatric Association, 1987

Arana GW: An overview of side effects caused by typical antipsychotics. J Clin Psychiatry 61 (suppl 8):5–11; discussion 12–13, 2000

Arato M, O'Connor R, Meltzer HY: A 1-year, double-blind, placebo-controlled trial of ziprasidone 40, 80 and 160 mg/day in chronic schizophrenia: the Ziprasidone Extended Use in Schizophrenia (ZEUS) study. Int Clin Psychopharmacol 17:207–215, 2002

Arvanitis LA, Miller BG: Multiple fixed doses of "Seroquel" (quetiapine) in patients with acute exacerbation of schizophrenia: a comparison with haloperidol and placebo. The Seroquel Trial 13 Study Group. Biol Psychiatry 42:233–246, 1997

Atkin PA, Veitch PC, Veitch EM, et al: The epidemiology of serious adverse drug reactions among the elderly. Drugs Aging 14:141–152, 1999

Avorn J, Soumerai SB, Everitt DE, et al: A randomized trial of a program to reduce the use of psychoactive drugs in nursing homes. N Engl J Med 327:168–173, 1992

Ballard C, O'Brien J, Coope B, et al: A prospective study of psychotic symptoms in dementia sufferers: psychosis in dementia. Int Psychogeriatr 9:57–64, 1997

Barak Y, Shamir E, Weizman R: Would a switch from typical antipsychotics to risperidone be beneficial for elderly schizophrenic patients? A naturalistic, long-term, retrospective, comparative study. J Clin Psychopharmacol 22:115–120, 2002

Barbey JT, Roose SP: SSRI safety in overdose. J Clin Psychiatry 59 (suppl 15):42–48, 1998

Barbhaiya RH, Buch AB, Greene DS: A study of the effect of age and gender on the pharmacokinetics of nefazodone after single and multiple doses. J Clin Psychopharmacol 16:19–25, 1996

Barnes R, Veith R, Okimoto J, et al: Efficacy of antipsychotic medications in behaviorally disturbed dementia patients. Am J Psychiatry 139:1170–1174, 1982

Benet LZ, Hoener B: Changes in plasma protein binding have little clinical relevance. Clin Pharmacol Ther 71:115–121, 2002

Bergstrom RF, Lemberger L, Farid NA, et al: Clinical pharmacology and pharmacokinetics of fluoxetine: a review. Br J Psychiatry 153 (suppl 3):47–50, 1988

Bies RR, Feng Y, Lotrich FE, et al: Utility of sparse concentration sampling for citalopram in elderly clinical trial subjects. J Clin Pharmacol 44:1352–1359, 2004

Bigos KL, Bies RR, Pollock BG: Population pharmacokinetics in geriatric psychiatry. Am J Geriatric Psychiatry 14:993–1003, 2006

Bodick NC, Offen WW, Shannon HE, et al: The selective muscarinic agonist xanomeline improves both the cognitive deficits and behavioral symptoms of Alzheimer disease. Alzheimer Dis Assoc Disord 11 (suppl 4):S16–S22, 1997

Bondareff W, Alpert M, Friedhoff AJ, et al: Comparison of sertraline and nortriptyline in the treatment of major depressive disorder in late-life. Am J Psychiatry 157:729–736, 2000

Bondolfi G, Eap CB, Bertschy G, et al: The effect of fluoxetine on the pharmacokinetics and safety of risperidone in psychiatric patients. Pharmacopsychiatry 35:50–56, 2002

Breier A, Meehan K, Birkett M, et al: A double-blind, placebo-controlled dose-response comparison of intramuscular olanzapine and haloperidol in the treatment of acute agitation in schizophrenia. Arch Gen Psychiatry 59:441–448, 2002a

Breier A, Sutton V, Feldman P, et al: Olanzapine in the treatment of dopamimetic-induced psychosis in patients with Parkinson's disease. Biol Psychiatry 52:438–447, 2002b

Breitbart W, Tremblay A, Gibson C: An open trial of olanzapine for the treatment of delirium in hospitalized cancer patients. Psychosomatics 43:175–182, 2002

Brodaty H, Ames D, Snowdon J, et al: A randomized placebo-controlled trial of risperidone for the treatment of aggression, agitation, and psychosis of dementia. J Clin Psychiatry 64:134–143, 2003

Burgio LD, Reynolds CFI, Janosky JE, et al: A behavioral microanalysis of the effects of haloperidol and oxazepam in demented psychogeriatric inpatients. Int J Geriatr Psychiatry 7:253–262, 1992

Byerly MJ, DeVane CL: Pharmacokinetics of clozapine and risperidone: a review of recent literature. J Clin Psychopharmacol 16:177–187, 1996

Bymaster FP, Calligaro DO, Falcone JF, et al: Radioreceptor binding profile of the atypical antipsychotic olanzapine. Neuropsychopharmacology 14:87–96, 1996

Carlyle W, Ancill RJ, Sheldon L: Aggression in the demented patient: a double-blind study of loxapine versus haloperidol. Int Clin Psychopharmacol 8:103–108, 1993

Casey DE: Extrapyramidal syndromes and new antipsychotic drugs: findings in patients and non-human primate models. Br J Psychiatry 29 (suppl):32–39, 1996

Centorrino F, Baldessarini RJ, Kando JC, et al: Clozapine and metabolites: concentrations in serum and clinical findings during treatment of chronically psychotic patients. J Clin Psychopharmacol 14:119–125, 1994

Chan WC, Lam LC, Choy CN, et al: A double-blind randomized comparison of risperidone and haloperidol in the treatment of behavioral and psychological symptoms in Chinese dementia patients. Int J Geriatr Psychiatry 16:1156–1162, 2001

Chengappa KNR, Baker RW, Kreinbrook SB, et al: Clozapine use in female geriatric patients with psychoses. J Geriatr Psychiatry Neurol 8:12–15, 1995

Chouinard G, Jones B, Remington G, et al: A Canadian multicenter placebo-controlled study of fixed doses of risperidone and haloperidol in the treatment of chronic schizophrenic patients. J Clin Psychopharmacol 13:25–40, 1993

Cohen-Mansfield J, Marx MS, Rosenthal AS: A description of agitation in a nursing home. Gerontology 44:M77–M84, 1989

Cohen-Mansfield J, Lipson S, Werner P, et al: Withdrawal of haloperidol, thioridazine, and lorazepam in the nursing home: a controlled, double-blind study. Arch Intern Med 159:1733–1740, 1999

Colenda CC, Mickus MA, Marcus SC, et al: Comparison of adult and geriatric psychiatric practice patterns: findings from the American Psychiatric Association's practice research network. Am J Geriatr Psychiatry 10:609–617, 2002

Conley EL, Coley K, Pollock BP, et al: Prevalence and risk of thrombocytopenia with valproic acid: experience at a psychiatric teaching hospital. Pharmacotherapy 21:1325–1330, 2001

Covington JS: Alleviating agitation, apprehension, and related symptoms in geriatric patients. South Med J 58:719–724, 1975

Cross J, Lee H, Westelinck A, et al: Postmarketing drug dosage changes of 499 FDA-approved new molecular entities, 1980–1999. Pharmacoepidemiol Drug Saf 11:439–446, 2002

Csernansky JG, Schuchart EK: Relapse and rehospitalisation rates in patients with schizophrenia: effects of second generation antipsychotics. CNS Drugs 16:473–484, 2002

Cummings JL, Miller B, Hill MA, et al: Neuropsychiatric aspects of multi-infarct dementia and dementia of the Alzheimer type. Arch Neurol 44:389–393, 1987

Cummings JL, Mega M, Gray K, et al: The Neuropsychiatric Inventory: comprehensive assessment of psychopathology in dementia. Neurology 44:2308–2314, 1994

Cummings JL, Street J, Masterman D, et al: Efficacy of olanzapine in the treatment of psychosis in dementia with Lewy bodies. Dement Geriatr Cogn Disord 13:67–73, 2002

Cutler AJ, Goldstein JM, Tumas JA: Dosing and switching strategies for quetiapine fumarate. Clin Ther 24:209–222, 2002

Davidson M, Emsley R, Kramer M, et al: Efficacy, safety, and early response of paliperidone extended release tablets (paliperidone ER): results of a 6-week, randomized, placebo-controlled study. Schizophr Res 93:117–130, 2007

Davies P, Maloney AJF: Letter: Selective loss of central cholinergic neurons in Alzheimer's disease. Lancet 2(8000):1403, 1976

De Deyn PP, Rabheru K, Rasmussen A, et al: A randomized trial of risperidone, placebo, and haloperidol for behavioral symptoms of dementia. Neurology 53:946–955, 1999

De Deyn P, Jeste DV, Swanink R, et al: Aripiprazole for the treatment of psychosis in patients with Alzheimer's disease: a randomized, placebo-controlled study. J Clin Psychopharmacol 25:463–467, 2005

Denys D, van Megen H, Westenberg H: Quetiapine addition to serotonin reuptake inhibitor treatment in patients with treatment-refractory obsessive-compulsive disorder: an open-label study. J Clin Psychiatry 63:700–703, 2002

Devanand DP, Brockington CD, Moody BJ, et al: Behavioral syndromes in Alzheimer's disease. Int Psychogeriatr 4:161–184, 1992a

Devanand DP, Miller L, Richards M, et al: The Columbia University Scale for Psychopathology in Alzheimer's disease. Arch Neurol 49:371–376, 1992b

Devanand DP, Jacobs DM, Tang M-X, et al: The course of psychopathology in mild to moderate Alzheimer's disease. Arch Gen Psychiatry 54:257–263, 1997

Devanand DP, Marder K, Michaels KS, et al: A randomized, placebo-controlled, dose-comparison trial of haloperidol for psychosis and disruptive behaviors in Alzheimer's disease. Am J Psychiatry 155:1512–1520, 1998

DeVane CL, Pollock BG: Pharmacokinetic considerations of antidepressant use in the elderly. J Clin Psychiatry 60 (suppl 20): 38–44, 1999

Dinakar HS, Sobel RN, Bopp JH, et al: Efficacy of olanzapine and risperidone for treatment-refractory schizophrenia among long-stay state hospital patients. Psychiatr Serv 53:755–757, 2002

Dolder CR, Lacro JP, Dunn LB, et al: Antipsychotic medication adherence: is there a difference between typical and atypical agents? Am J Psychiatry 159:103–108, 2002

Dresser GK, Spence JD, Bailey DG: Pharmacokinetic-pharmacodynamic consequences and clinical relevance of cytochrome P450 3A4 inhibition. Clin Pharmacokinet 38:41–57, 2000

Ellingrod VL, Schultz SK, Ekstam-Smith K, et al: Comparison of risperidone with olanzapine in elderly patients with dementia and psychosis. Pharmacotherapy 22:1–5, 2002

Elon R, Pawlson LG: The impact of OBRA on medical practice within nursing facilities. J Am Geriatr Soc 40:958–963, 1992

Fann WE, Davis J, Janowsky D, et al: Chlorpromazine: effects of antacids on its gastrointestinal absorption. J Clin Pharmacol 13:388–390, 1973

Feng Y, Pollock BG, Ferrell RE, et al: Paroxetine: population pharmacokinetics analysis in late-life depression using sparse concentration sampling. Br J Clin Pharmacol 61:558–569, 2006

Fernandez HH, Trieschmann ME, Burke MA, et al: Quetiapine for psychosis in Parkinson's disease versus dementia with Lewy bodies. J Clin Psychiatry 63:513–515, 2002

Figiel GS, Krishnan KRR, Doraiswamy PM, et al: Subcortical hyperintensities on brain magnetic resonance imaging: a comparison between late age onset and early onset elderly depressed subjects. Neurobiol Aging 26:245–247, 1991

Finkel SI, Lyons JS, Anderson RL, et al: A randomized, placebo-controlled trial of thiothixene in agitated, demented nursing home patients. Int J Geriatr Psychiatry 10:129–136, 1995

Fitz D, Mallya A: Discontinuation of a psychogeriatric program for nursing home residents: psychotropic medication changes and behavioral reactions. J Appl Gerontol 11:50–63, 1992

Flint A, Rifat S: The effect of sequential antidepressant treatment on geriatric depression. J Affect Disord 36:95–105, 1996

Friedman JH, Fernandez HH: Atypical antipsychotics in Parkinson-sensitive populations. J Geriatr Psychiatry Neurol 15:156–170, 2002

Friedman JI, Adler DN, Howanitz E, et al: A double blind placebo controlled trial of donepezil adjunctive treatment to risperidone for the cognitive impairment of schizophrenia. Biol Psychiatry 51:349–357, 2002

Fulton B, Goa K: Olanzapine: a review of its pharmacological properties and therapeutic efficacy in the management of schizophrenia and related psychoses. Drugs 53:281–298, 1997

Geddes J, Freemantle N, Harrison P, et al: Atypical antipsychotics in the treatment of schizophrenia: systematic overview and meta-regression analysis. BMJ 321:1371–1376, 2000

Georgotas A, McCue RE, Cooper TBN, et al: Factors affecting the delay of antidepressant effect in responders to nortriptyline and phenelzine. Psychiatry Res 28:1–9, 1989

Ghoneim NM, Mewaldt SP, Berie JL, et al: Memory and performance effects of single and 3-week administration of diazepam. Psychopharmacology (Berl) 73:147–151, 1981

Giron MS, Forsell Y, Bernsten C, et al: Psychotropic drug use in elderly people with and without dementia. Int J Geriatr Psychiatry 16:900–906, 2001

Glassman AH, Roose SP, Bigger JT Jr: The safety of tricyclic antidepressants in cardiac patients—risk/benefit reconsidered. JAMA 269:2673–2675, 1993

Glassman AH, O'Connor CM, Califf RM, et al: Sertraline treatment of major depression in patients with acute MI or unstable angina. JAMA 288:701–709, 2002

Goodnick PJ, Jerry J, Parra F: Psychotropic drugs and the ECG: focus on the QTc interval. Expert Opin Pharmacother 3:479–498, 2002

Gottfries CG: Scandinavian experience with citalopram in the elderly. Int Clin Psychopharmacol 11 (suppl 1):41–44, 1996

Greenblatt DJ, Harmatz JS, Shader RI: Clinical pharmacokinetics of anxiolytics and hypnotics in the elderly: therapeutic considerations. Clin Pharmacokinet 21:165–177, 1991

Gurwitz JH, Field TS, Avorn J, et al: Incidence and preventability of adverse drug events in nursing homes. Am J Med 109:87–94, 2000

Gurwitz JH, Field TS, Harrold LR, et al: Incidence and preventability of adverse drug events among older persons in the ambulatory setting. JAMA 289:1107–1116, 2005

Hagg S, Soderberg S, Ahren B, et al: Leptin concentrations are increased in subjects treated with clozapine or conventional antipsychotics. J Clin Psychiatry 62:843–848, 2001

Hesse LM, Venkatakrishnan K, Court MH, et al: CYP2B6 mediates the in vitro hydroxylation of bupropion: potential drug interactions with other antidepressants. Drug Metab Dispos 28:1176–1183, 2000

Hicks R, Davis J: Pharmacokinetics in geriatric psychopharmacology, in Psychopharmacology of Aging. Edited by Eisdorfer C, Fann W. New York, Spectrum Publications, 1980, pp 169–212

Holmes C, Smith H, Ganderton R, et al: Psychosis and aggression in Alzheimer's disease: the effect of dopamine receptor gene variation. J Neurol Neurosurg Psychiatry 71:777–779, 2001

Holton A, George K: The use of lithium carbonate in severely demented patients with behavioral disturbance. Br J Psychiatry 146:99–100, 1985

Horwitz GJ, Tariot PN, Mead K, et al: Discontinuation of antipsychotics in nursing home patients with dementia. Am J Geriatr Psychiatry 3:290–299, 1995

Howard R, Rabins PV, Seeman MV, et al: Late-onset schizophrenia and very-late-onset schizophrenia-like psychosis: an international consensus. The International Late-Onset Schizophrenia Group. Am J Psychiatry 157:172–178, 2000

Janssen PA, Niemegeers CJ, Awouters F, et al: Pharmacology of risperidone (R 64 766), a new antipsychotic with serotonin-S2 and dopamine-D2 antagonistic properties. J Pharmacol Exp Ther 244:685–693, 1988

Jeste DV: Tardive dyskinesia in older patients. J Clin Psychiatry 61 (suppl 4):27–32, 2000

Jeste DV, Finkel SI: Psychosis of Alzheimer's disease and related dementias: diagnostic criteria for a distinct syndrome. Am J Geriatr Psychiatry 8:29–34, 2000

Jeste DV, Lacro JP, Palmer B, et al: Incidence of tardive dyskinesia in early stages of low-dose treatment with typical antipsychotics in older patients. Am J Psychiatry 156:309–311, 1999

Jeste DV, Okamoto A, Napolitano J, et al: Low incidence of persistent tardive dyskinesia in elderly patients with dementia treated with risperidone. Am J Psychiatry 157:1150–1155, 2000

Jeste DV, Blazer D, Casey D, et al: ACNP white paper: update on use of antipsychotic drugs in elderly persons with dementia. Neuropsychopharmacology 33:1–14, 2007

Jin H, Meyer JM, Jeste DV: Atypical antipsychotics and glucose dysregulation: a systematic review. Schizophr Res 71:195–212, 2004

Johnson E, Whyte EM, Mulsant BH, et al: Cardiovascular changes associated with venlafaxine in the treatment of late-life depression. Am J Geriatr Psychiatry 14:796–802, 2006

Jones DM, Lewis MJ, Spriggs TLB: The effects of low doses of diazepam on human performance in group administered tasks. Br J Clin Pharmacol 6:333–337, 1978

Jones PB, Barnes TR, Davies L, et al: Randomized controlled trial of the effect on Quality of Life of second- vs first-generation antipsychotic drugs in schizophrenia: Cost Utility of the Latest Antipsychotic Drugs in Schizophrenia Study (CUtLASS 1). Arch Gen Psychiatry 63:1079–1087, 2006

Kane J, Honigfeld G, Singer J, et al: Clozapine for the treatment-resistant schizophrenic: a double-blind comparison with chlorpromazine. Arch Gen Psychiatry 45:789–796, 1988

Kasper S, deSwart H, Anderson HF: Escitalopram in the treatment of depressed elderly patients. Am J Geriatr Psychiatry 13:884–891, 2005

Katz IR, Jeste DV, Mintzer JE, et al: Comparison of risperidone and placebo for psychosis and behavioral disturbances associated with dementia: a randomized, double-blind trial. Risperidone Study Group. J Clin Psychiatry 60:107–115, 1999

Katz I, de Deyn PP, Mintzer J, et al: The efficacy and safety of risperidone in the treatment of psychosis of Alzheimer's disease and mixed dementia: a meta-analysis of 4 placebo-controlled clinical trials. Int J Geriatr Psychiatry 22:475–484, 2007

Kaufer DI, Cummings JL, Christine D: Effect of tacrine on behavioral symptoms in Alzheimer's disease: an open-label study. J Geriatr Psychiatry Neurol 9:1–6, 1996

Kim H, Lim SW, Kim S, et al: Monoamine transporter gene polymorphisms and antidepressant response in Koreans with late-life depression. JAMA 296:1609–1618, 2006

Kindermann SS, Dolder CR, Bailey A, et al: Pharmacological treatment of psychosis and agitation in elderly patients with dementia: four decades of experience. Drugs Aging 19:257–276, 2002

Kirby D, Ames D: Hyponatraemia and selective serotonin reuptake inhibitors in elderly patients. Int J Geriatr Psychiatry 16:484–493, 2001

Kirven LG, Montero EF: Comparison of thioridazine and diazepam in the control of nonpsychotic symptoms associated with senility: double-blind study. J Am Geriatr Soc 21:546–551, 1973

Kurz M, Hummer M, Kemmler G, et al: Long-term pharmacokinetics of clozapine. Br J Psychiatry 173:341–344, 1998

Lanctot KL, Best TS, Mitmann N, et al: Efficacy and safety of neuroleptics in behavioral disorders associated with dementia. J Clin Psychiatry 59:550–561; quiz 562–563, 1998

Lane H-Y, Chang Y-C, Chiu C-C, et al: Association of risperidone treatment response with a polymorphism in the 5-HT2A receptor gene. Am J Psychiatry 159:1593–1595, 2002

Lantz MS, Louis A, Lowenstein G, et al: A longitudinal study of psychotropic prescriptions in a teaching nursing home. Am J Psychiatry 147:1637–1639, 1990

Lawlor BA, Radcliffe J, Molchan SE, et al: A pilot placebo-controlled study of trazodone and buspirone in Alzheimer's disease. Int J Geriatr Psychiatry 9:55–59, 1994

Lawlor BA, Ryan TM, Bierer LM, et al: Lack of association between clinical symptoms and postmortem indices of brain serotonin function in Alzheimer's disease. Biol Psychiatry 37:895–896, 1995

Lazarou J, Pomeranz BH, Corey PN: Incidence of adverse drug reactions in hospitalized patients: a meta-analysis of prospective studies. JAMA 279:1200–1205, 1998

Lessard E, Yessine MA, Hamelin BA, et al: Influence of CYP-2D6 activity on the disposition and cardiovascular toxicity of the antidepressant agent venlafaxine in humans. Pharmacogenetics 9:435–443, 1999

Lessard E, Yessine MA, Hamelin BA, et al: Diphenhydramine alters the disposition of venlafaxine through inhibition of CYP2D6 activity in humans. J Clin Psychopharmacol 21:175–184, 2001

Levine J, Chengappa KN, Brar JS, et al: Psychotropic drug prescription patterns among patients with bipolar I disorder. Bipolar Disorder 2:120–130, 2000

Lieberman JA: Maximizing clozapine therapy: managing side effects. J Clin Psychiatry 59 (suppl 3):38A–43A, 1998

Lieberman JA, Stroup TS, McEvoy JP, et al: Effectiveness of antipsychotic drugs in patients with chronic schizophrenia. Clinical Antipsychotic Trials of Intervention Effectiveness (CATIE) Investigators. N Engl J Med 353:1209–1223, 2005

Liljequist R, Linnoila M, Mattila MJ: Effect of diazepam and chlorpromazine on memory functions in man. Eur J Clin Pharmacol 13:339–343, 1978

Liu B, Anderson G, Mittmann N, et al: Use of selective serotonin-reuptake inhibitors or tricyclic antidepressants and risk of hip fractures in elderly people. Lancet 351:1303–1307, 1998

Lohr JB, Caligiuri MP, Edson R, et al: Treatment predictors of extrapyramidal side effects in patients with tardive dyskinesia: results from Veterans Affairs Cooperative Study 394. J Clin Psychopharmacol 22:196–200, 2002

Lotrich FE, Pollock BG: Aging and clinical pharmacology: implications for antidepressants. J Clin Pharmacol 45:1106–1122, 2005

Lyketsos CG, Steinberg M, Tschanz JT, et al: Mental and behavioral disturbances in dementia: findings from the Cache County Study on Memory in Aging. Am J Psychiatry 157:708–714, 2000

Marder SR, Kramer M, Ford L, et al: Efficacy and safety of paliperidone extended-release tablets: results of a 6-week, randomized, placebo-controlled study. Biol Psychiatry 62:1363–1370, 2007

Marsh L, Lyketsos C, Reich SG: Olanzapine for the treatment of psychosis in patients with Parkinson's disease and dementia. Psychosomatics 42:477–481, 2001

McDonald WM: Epidemiology, etiology, and treatment of geriatric mania. J Clin Psychiatry 61 (suppl 13):3–11, 2000

McKeith IG: Consensus guidelines for the clinical and pathologic diagnosis of dementia with Lewy bodies (DLB): report of the Consortium on DLB International Workshop. J Alzheimers Dis 9 (3 suppl):417–423, 2006

McManus DQ, Arvanitis LA, Kowalcyk BB, et al: Quetiapine, a novel antipsychotic: experience in elderly patients with psychotic disorders. Seroquel Trial 48 Study Group. J Clin Psychiatry 60:292–298, 1999

Meehan KM, Wang H, David S, et al: Comparison of rapidly acting intramuscular olanzapine, lorazepam, and placebo: a double-blind, randomized study in acutely agitated patients with dementia. Neuropsychopharmacology 26:494–504, 2002

Mesters P, Ansseau M, Brasseur R, et al: An open multicentre study to evaluate the efficacy and tolerance of fluoxetine 20 mg in depressed ambulatory patients. Acta Psychiatr Belg 92:232–245, 1992

Meyer JM: A retrospective comparison of weight, lipid, and glucose changes between risperidone- and olanzapine-treated inpatients: metabolic outcomes after 1 year. J Clin Psychiatry. 63:425–433, 2002

Meyers BS, Klimstra SA, Gabriele M, et al: Continuation treatment of delusional depression in older adults. Am J Geriatr Psychiatry 9:415–422, 2001

Michel K, Kolakowska T: A survey of prescribing psychotropic drugs in two psychiatric hospitals. Br J Psychiatry 138:217–221, 1981

Moller HJ: Amisulpride: efficacy in the management of chronic patients with predominant negative symptoms of schizophrenia. Eur Arch Psychiatry Clin Neurosci 251:217–224, 2001

Mukaetova-Ladinska EB, Harrington CR, Roth M, et al: Biochemical and anatomical redistribution of tau protein in Alzheimer's disease. Am J Pathol 143:565–578, 1993

Mullen J, Jibson MD, Sweitzer D: A comparison of the relative safety, efficacy, and tolerability of quetiapine and risperidone in outpatients with schizophrenia and other psychotic disorders: the Quetiapine Experience With Safety and Tolerability (QUEST) study. Clin Ther 23:1839–1854, 2001

Mulsant BH, Pollock BG, Nebes R, et al: A twelve-week, double-blind randomized comparison of nortriptyline and paroxetine in older depressed patients and outpatients. Am J Geriatr Psychiatry 9:406–414, 2001a

Mulsant BH, Sweet RA, Rosen J, et al: A double-blind randomized comparison of nortriptyline plus perphenazine versus nortriptyline plus placebo in the treatment of psychotic depression in late life. J Clin Psychiatry 62:597–604, 2001b

Mulsant BH, Pollock BG, Kirshner M, et al: Serum anticholinergic activity in a community-based geriatric sample: relationship with cognitive performance. Am J Geriatr Psychiatry 10 (suppl 1):58, 2002

Murphy GM, Pollock BG, Kirshner M, et al: CYP 2D6 genotyping with oligonucleotide microarrays predicts nortriptyline levels in geriatric depression. Neuropsychopharmacology 25:737–743, 2001

Murphy GM Jr, Kremer C, Rodrigues HE, et al: Pharmacogenetics of antidepressant medication intolerance. Am J Psychiatry 160:1830–1835, 2003

Murphy GM Jr, Hollander SB, Rodrigues HE, et al: Effects of the serotonin transporter gene promoter polymorphism on mirtazapine and paroxetine efficacy and adverse events in geriatric major depression. Arch Gen Psychiatry 61:1163–1169, 2004

Musselman DL, Evans DL, Nemeroff CB: The relationship of depression to cardiovascular disease. Arch Gen Psychiatry 55:580–592, 1998

Nacmias B, Tedde A, Forleo P, et al: Association between 5-HT2A receptor polymorphism and psychotic symptoms in Alzheimer's disease. Biol Psychiatry 50:472–475, 2001

Navarro V, Gasto C, Torres X, et al: Citalopram versus nortriptyline in late-life depression: a 12-week randomized single-blind study. Acta Psychiatr Scand 103:435–440, 2001

Nebes RD, Pollock BG, Meltzer CC, et al: Cognitive effects of serum anticholinergic activity and white matter hyperintensities. Neurology 65:1487–1489, 2005

Nelson JC, Kennedy JS, Pollock BG, et al: Treatment of major depression with nortriptyline and paroxetine in patients with ischemic heart disease. Am J Psychiatry 156:1024–1028, 1999

Newhouse PA, Krishnan KRR, Doraiswami PM, et al: A double blind comparison of sertraline and fluoxetine in depressed elderly outpatients. J Clin Psychiatry 61:559–568, 2000

Oberholzer AF, Hendriksen C, Monsch AU, et al: Safety and effectiveness of low-dose clozapine in psychogeriatric patients: a preliminary study. Int Psychogeriatr 4:187–195, 1992

Paulsen JS, Salmon DP, Thal LJ, et al: Incidence of and risk factors for hallucinations and delusions in patients with probable AD. Neurology 54:1965–1971, 2000

Pelton GH, Devanand DP, Bell K, et al: Usefulness of plasma haloperidol levels for monitoring clinical efficacy and side effects in Alzheimer patients with psychosis and behavioral dyscontrol. Am J Geriatr Psychiatry 11:186–193, 2003

Perry EK, Gibson PH, Blessed G, et al: Neurotransmitter enzyme abnormalities in senile dementia. J Neurol Sci 34:247–265, 1977

Peskind ER, Raskind MA, Wingerson D, et al: Enhanced hypothalamic-pituitary-adrenocortical axis responses to physostigmine in normal aging. J Gerontol A Biol Sci Med Sci 50:M114–M120, 1995

Petrie WM, Ban TA, Berney S, et al: Loxapine in psychogeriatrics: a placebo- and standard-controlled investigation. J Clin Psychopharmacol 2:122–126, 1982

Pitner JK, Mintzer JE, Pennypacker LC, et al: Efficacy and adverse effects of clozapine in four elderly psychotic patients. J Clin Psychiatry 56:180–185, 1995

Pollock BG: Drug interactions, in Geriatric Psychopharmacology. Edited by Nelson JC. New York, Marcel Dekker, 1998, pp 43–60

Pollock BG: Adverse reactions of antidepressants in elderly patients. J Clin Psychiatry 60 (suppl 20):4–8, 1999

Pollock BG: The pharmacokinetic imperative in late-life depression. J Clin Psychopharmacology 25 (suppl 1):S19–S23, 2005

Pollock BG, Everett G, Perel JM: Comparative cardiotoxicity of nortriptyline and its isomeric 10-hydroxymetabolites. Neuropsychopharmacology 6:1–10, 1992a

Pollock BG, Perel J, Altieri L, et al: Debrisoquine hydroxylation phenotyping in geriatric psychopharmacology. Psychopharmacol Bull 28:163–168, 1992b

Pollock BG, Mulsant BH, Sweet RA, et al: Prospective cytochrome P450 2D6 phenotyping for neuroleptic treatment in dementia. Psychopharmacol Bull 31:327–331, 1995

Pollock BG, Wylie M, Stack JA, et al: Inhibition of CYP1A2 mediated metabolism by estrogen replacement therapy in postmenopausal women. J Clin Pharmacol 39:936–940, 1999

Pollock BG, Ferrell RE, Mulsant BH: Allelic variation in the serotonin transporter promoter affects onset of paroxetine treatment response in late-life depression. Neuropsychopharmacology 23:587–590, 2000a

Pollock BG, Laghrissi-Thode F, Wagner WR: Evaluation of platelet activation in depressed patients with ischemic heart disease after paroxetine or nortriptyline treatment. J Clin Psychopharmacol 20:137–140, 2000b

Pollock BG, Mulsant BH, Rosen J, et al: Comparison of citalopram, perphenazine and placebo for the acute treatment of psychosis and behavioral disturbances in hospitalized, demented patients. Am J Psychiatry 159:460–465, 2002

Pollock BG, Mulsant BH, Rosen J, et al: A double-blind comparison of citalopram and risperidone for the treatment of behavioral and psychotic symptoms associated with dementia. Am J Geriatr Psychiatry 15:942–952, 2007

Pomara N, Deptula D, Singh R, et al: Cognitive toxicity of benzodiazepines in the elderly, in Anxiety in the Elderly: Treatment and Research. Edited by Salzman C, Lebowitz BD. New York, Springer, 1991, pp 175–196

Porsteinsson AP, Tariot PN, Erb R, et al: Placebo-controlled study of divalproex sodium for agitation in dementia. Am J Geriatr Psychiatry 9:58–66, 2001

Prien Y, Haber PA, Caffey EMJ: The use of psychoactive drugs in elderly patients with psychiatric disorders: survey conducted in twelve Veterans Administration hospitals. J Am Geriatr Soc 23:104–112, 1975

Rada RT, Kellner R: Thiothixene in the treatment of geriatric patients with chronic organic brain syndrome. J Am Geriatr Soc 24:105–107, 1976

Raskin J, Wiltse CG, Siegal A, et al: Efficacy of duloxetine on cognition, depression, and pain in elderly patients with major depressive disorder: an 8-week, double-blind, placebo-controlled trial. Am J Psychiatry 164:900–909, 2007

Raskind MA: Evaluation and management of aggressive behavior in the elderly demented patient. J Clin Psychiatry 60 (suppl 15):45–49, 1999

Ray WA, Federspiel CF, Schaffner W: A study of antipsychotic drug use in nursing homes: epidemiologic evidence suggesting misuse. Am J Public Health 70:485–491, 1980

Ray WA, Meredith S, Thapa PB, et al: Antipsychotics and the risk of sudden cardiac death. Arch Gen Psychiatry 58:1161–1167, 2001

Reilly JG, Ayis SA, Ferrier IN, et al: Thioridazine and sudden unexplained death in psychiatric in-patients. Br J Psychiatry 180:515–522, 2002

Reisberg B, Borenstein J, Salob SP, et al: Behavioral symptoms in Alzheimer's disease: phenomenology and treatment. J Clin Psychiatry 48:9–15, 1987

Reisberg B, Franssen E, Sclan S, et al: Stage specific incidence of potentially remediable behavioral symptoms in aging and Alzheimer's disease: a study of 120 patients using the BEHAVE-AD. Bull Clin Neurosci 54:95–112, 1989

Roe CM, Anderson MJ, Spivack B: Use of anticholinergic medications by older adults with dementia. J Am Geriatr Soc 50:836–842, 2002

Ronfeld RA, Tremaine LM, Wilner KD: Pharmacokinetics of sertraline and its N-demethyl metabolite in elderly and young male and female volunteers. Clin Pharmacokinet 32 (suppl 1):22–30, 1997

Roose SP: Methodological issues in the diagnosis, treatment and study of refractory depression, in Treatment Strategies for Refractory Depression. Edited by Roose SP, Glassman AH. Washington, DC, American Psychiatric Press, 1990, pp 3–9

Roose SP, Glassman AH, Siris SG, et al: Comparison of imipramine and nortriptyline induced orthostatic hypotension: a meaningful difference. J Clin Psychopharmacol 1:316–319, 1981

Roose SP, Glassman AH, Attia E, et al: Comparative efficacy of the selective serotonin reuptake inhibitors and the tricyclics in the treatment of melancholia. Am J Psychiatry 151:1735–1739, 1994

Roose SP, Laghrissi-Thode F, Kennedy JS, et al: Comparison of paroxetine and nortriptyline in depressed patients with ischemic heart disease. JAMA 279:287–291, 1998

Roose S, Alexopoulos G, Burke W, et al: Treatment of depression in the "old-old": a randomized, double-blind, placebo-controlled trial of citalopram in patients at least 75 years of age, in New Research, American Association of Geriatric Psychiatry, Orlando, FL, March 2002

Rubin EH, Kinscherf DA: Psychopathology of very mild dementia of the Alzheimer type. Am J Psychiatry 146:1017–1021, 1989

Russo-Neustadt A, Cotman CW: Adrenergic receptors in Alzheimer's disease brain: selective increases in the cerebella of aggressive patients. J Neurosci 17:5573–5580, 1997

Sable JA, Jeste DV: Antipsychotic treatment for late-life schizophrenia. Curr Psychiatry Rep 4:299–306, 2002

Sachs GS, Grossman F, Ghaemi SN, et al: Combination of a mood stabilizer with risperidone or haloperidol for treatment of acute mania: a double-blind, placebo-controlled comparison of efficacy and safety. Am J Psychiatry 159:1146–1154, 2002

Sackeim H, Roose S: How long should antidepressant trials be in geriatric depression? Paper presented at the 155th annual meeting of the American Psychiatric Association, Philadelphia, PA, May 18–23, 2002

Sackeim HA, Devanand DP, Nobler MS: Electroconvulsive therapy, in Psychopharmacology: The Fourth Generation of Progress. Edited by Bloom F, Kupfer D. New York, Raven, 1995, pp 1123–1141

Saltz BL, Woerner MG, Kane JM, et al: Prospective study of tardive dyskinesia incidence in the elderly. JAMA 266:2402–2406, 1991

Satterlee JS, Sussman MR: Unusual membrane-associated protein kinases in higher plants. J Membr Biol 164:205–213, 1998

Schatzberg AF, Cantillon M: Antidepressant early response and remission with venlafaxine or fluoxetine in depressed geriatric outpatients. Poster presented at the European College of Neuropsychopharmacology, 2000

Schatzberg AF, Kremer C, Rodrigues HE, et al: Double-blind randomized comparison of mirtazapine and paroxetine in elderly depressed patients. Am J Geriatr Psychiatry 10:541–550, 2002

Schmucker DL: Liver function and phase 1 drug metabolism in the elderly. Drugs Aging 18:837–851, 2001

Schneider LS, Pollock VE, Lyness SA: A meta-analysis of controlled trials of neuroleptic treatment in dementia. J Am Geriatr Soc 38:553–563, 1990

Schneider LS, Nelson JC, Clary CM, et al: An 8-week multicenter, parallel-group, double-blind, placebo-controlled study of sertraline in elderly outpatients with major depression. Am J Psychiatry 160:1277–1285, 2003

Schneider LS, Tariot PN, Dagerman KS, et al: Effectiveness of atypical antipsychotic drugs in patients with Alzheimer's disease. N Engl J Med 355:1525–1538, 2006

Seidman SN, Roose SP: The relationship between depression and erectile dysfunction. Curr Psychiatry Rep 2:201–205, 2000

Serretti A, Cusin C, Rausch JL, et al: Pooling pharmacogenetic studies on the serotonin transporter: a mega-analysis. Psychiatry Res 145:61–65, 2006

Shahzad S, Suleman MI, Shahab H, et al: Cataract occurrence with antipsychotic drugs. Psychosomatics 43:354–359, 2002

Shankle WR, Nielson KA, Cotman CW: Low-dose propranolol reduces aggression and agitation resembling that associated with orbitofrontal dysfunction in elderly demented patients. Alzheimer Dis Assoc Disord 9:233–237, 1995

Shimada T, Yamazaki H, Mimura M, et al: Interindividual variations in human liver cytochrome P-450 enzymes involved in the oxidation of drugs, carcinogens and toxic chemicals: studies with liver microsomes of 30 Japanese and 30 Caucasians. J Pharmacol Exp Ther 270:414–423, 1994

Smith GR, Taylor CW, Linkous P: Haloperidol versus thioridazine for the treatment of psychogeriatric patients: a double-blind clinical trial. Psychosomatics 15:134–138, 1974

Sneed JR, Rutherford BR, Rindskopf D, et al: Design makes a difference: a meta-analysis of antidepressant response rates in placebo-controlled versus comparator trials of late-life depression. Am J Geriatr Psychiatry 16:65–73, 2008

Solai LK, Mulsant BH, Pollock BG: Selective serotonin reuptake inhibitors for late-life depression: a comparative review. Drugs Aging 18:355–368, 2001

Spiker DG, Weiss JC, Dealy RS, et al: The pharmacological treatment of delusional depression. Am J Psychiatry 142:430–436, 1985

Stotsky B: Multicenter studying thioridazine with diazepam and placebo in elderly, nonpsychotic patients with emotional and behavioral disorders. Clin Ther 6:546–559, 1984

Street JS, Clark WS, Gannon KS, et al: Olanzapine treatment of psychotic and behavioral symptoms in patients with Alzheimer disease in nursing care facilities: a double-blind, randomized, placebo-controlled trial. The HGEU Study Group. Arch Gen Psychiatry 57:968–976, 2000

Suh GH, Son HG, Ju YS, et al: A randomized, double-blind, crossover comparison of risperidone and haloperidol in Korean dementia patients with behavioral disturbances. Am J Geriatr Psychiatry 12:509–516, 2004

Sultzer DL, Gray KF, Gunay I, et al: A double-blind comparison of trazodone and haloperidol for treatment of agitation in patients with dementia. Am J Geriatr Psychiatry 5:60–69, 1997

Sunderland T, Molchan SE, Little JT, et al: Pharmacologic challenges in Alzheimer disease and normal controls: cognitive modeling in humans. Alzheimer Dis Assoc Disord 11 (suppl 4): S23–S26, 1997

Swearer J, Drachman D, O'Donnell B: Troublesome and disruptive behaviors in dementia. J Am Geriatr Soc 36:784–790, 1988

Sweet RA, Pollock BG, Wright B, et al: Single and multiple dose bupropion pharmacokinetics in elderly patients with depression. J Clin Pharmacol 35:876–884, 1995

Sweet R, Nimgaonkar VL, Kamboh MI, et al: Dopamine receptor genetic variation, psychosis, and aggression in Alzheimer's disease. Arch Neurol 55:1335–1340, 1998

Sweet RA, Pollock BG, Sukonick DL, et al: The 5HTTLPR-polymorphism confers liability to a combined phenotype of psychotic and aggressive behavior in Alzheimer's disease. Int Psychogeriatr 13:401–409, 2001

Tandon R: Impact of antipsychotic treatment on long-term course of schizophrenic illness: an introduction. J Psychiatr Res 32:119–120, 1998

Tariot PN, Mack JL, Patterson MB, et al: The CERAD Behavior Rating Scale for Dementia (BRSD). Am J Psychiatry 152:1349–1357, 1995

Tariot PN, Erb R, Podgorski CA, et al: Efficacy and tolerability of carbamazepine for agitation and aggression in dementia. Am J Psychiatry 155:54–61, 1998

Tariot PN, Salzman C, Yeung PP, et al: Long-term use of quetiapine in elderly patients with psychotic disorders. Clin Ther 22:1068–1084, 2000

Tariot PN, Raman R, Jakimovich L, et al: Divalproex sodium in nursing home residents with possible or probable Alzheimer disease complicated by agitation: a randomized, controlled trial.

Alzheimer's Disease Cooperative Study; Valproate Nursing Home Study Group. Am J Geriatr Psychiatry 13:942–949, 2005

Tariot PN, Schneider L, Katz IR, et al: Quetiapine treatment of psychosis associated with dementia: a double-blind, randomized, placebo-controlled clinical trial. Am J Geriatr Psychiatry 14:767–776, 2006

Teri L, Logsdon RG, Peskind E, et al: Treatment of agitation in AD: a randomized, placebo-controlled clinical trial. Neurology 55:1271–1278, 2000

Tewfik GI, Jain VK, Harcup M, et al: Effectiveness of various tranquilizers in the management of senile restlessness. Gerontologia Clinica 12:351–359, 1970

Thomas VS, Darvesh S, MacKnight C, et al: Estimating the prevalence of dementia in elderly people: a comparison of the Canadian Study of Health and Aging and National Population Health Survey approaches. Int Psychogeriatr 13 (suppl 1):169–175, 2001

Timmer CJ, Paanakker JE, Van Hal HJM: Pharmacokinetics of mirtazapine from orally administered tablets: influence of gender, age and treatment regimen. Hum Psychopharmacol 11:497–509, 1996

Tohen M, Baker RW, Altshuler LL, et al: Olanzapine versus divalproex in the treatment of acute mania. Am J Psychiatry 159:1011–1017, 2002

Tollefson GD, Bosomworth JC, Heiligenstein JH, et al: A double-blind, placebo-controlled clinical trial of fluoxetine in geriatric patients with major depression. Int Psychogeriatr 7:89–104, 1995

Tsuang M, Lu LM, Stotsky BA, et al: Haloperidol versus thioridazine for hospitalized psychogeriatric patients: double-blind study. J Am Geriatr Soc 19:593–600, 1971

Tune L: The role of antipsychotics in treating delirium. Curr Psychiatry Rep 4:209–212, 2002

Van Putten T, Marder SR, Mintz J, et al: Haloperidol plasma levels and clinical response: a therapeutic window relationship. Am J Psychiatry 149:500–505, 1992

Volavka J, Cooper T, Czobor P, et al: Haloperidol blood levels and clinical effects. Arch Gen Psychiatry 49:354–361, 1992

Weihs KL, Settle EC Jr, Batey SR, et al: Bupropion sustained release versus paroxetine for the treatment of depression in the elderly. J Clin Psychiatry 61:196–202, 2000

Weiler P, Mungas D, Bernick C: Propranolol for the control of disruptive behavior in senile dementia. J Geriatr Psychiatry Neurol 4:226–230, 1988

Weiser M, Rotmensch HH, Korczyn AD, et al: A pilot, randomized, open-label trial assessing safety and pharmacokinetic parameters of co-administration of rivastigmine with risperidone in dementia patients with behavioral disturbances. Int J Geriatr Psychiatry 17:343–346, 2002

Whyte E, Mulsant BH, Kirshner M, et al: CYP2D6 genotype and venlafaxine-XR concentrations in the depressed elderly. Int J Geriatr Psychiatry 21:542 549, 2006

Wood S, Cummings JL, Hsu MA, et al: The use of the Neuropsychiatric Inventory in nursing home residents: characterization and measurement. Am J Geriatr Psychiatry 8:75–83, 2000

Wynne HA, Goudevenos J, Rawlins MD, et al: Hepatic drug clearance: the effect of age using indocyanine green as a model compound. Br J Clin Pharmacol 30:634–637, 1990

Yerrabolu M, Prabhudesai S, Tawam M, et al: Effect of risperidone on QT interval and QT dispersion in the elderly. Heart Dis 2:10–12, 2000

Yu DK: The contribution of P-glycoprotein to pharmacokinetic drug-drug interactions. J Clin Pharmacol 39:1203–1211, 1999

Zubenko GS, Moossy J, Martinez AJ, et al: Neuropathologic and neurochemical correlates of psychosis in primary dementia. Arch Neurol 48:619–624, 1991

Treatment of Chronic Pain Syndromes

Kurt Kroenke, M.D.

Erin E. Krebs, M.D., M.P.H.

Matthew J. Bair, M.D., M.S.

Pain is the most common symptom reported in both the general population and the general medical setting (Kroenke 2003b; Sternbach 1986; Verhaak et al. 1998). Pain complaints account for more than 40% of all symptom-related outpatient visits, or over 100 million ambulatory encounters in the United States alone each year (Schappert 1992). Pain costs the United States more than $100 billion each year in health care and lost productivity (Stewart et al. 2003). Pain medications are the second most commonly prescribed class of drugs (after cardiac–renal drugs), accounting for 12% of all medications prescribed during ambulatory office visits in the United States (Turk 2002). Yet nonopioid analgesics fail to provide adequate relief in many patients (Curatolo and Bogduk 2001), and physicians' concerns about regulatory restrictions as well as risks of tolerance or addiction constrain the prescribing of opioid analgesics for noncancer pain (Joranson et al. 2002). Moreover, opioids themselves may produce only moderate reductions in chronic pain (Furlan et al. 2006; Martell et al. 2007; Turk 2002) and may fail to improve (or may even worsen) psychological outcomes (e.g., depression) or functional status even when they do alleviate the pain (Moulin et al. 1996). At the same time, clinicians are being pressured to respond to pain as the "fifth vital sign" (Joint Commission on Accreditation of Healthcare Organizations 2000). In House Resolution 1863, the National Pain Care Policy Act of 2003, Congress declared this the "Decade of

Pain Control and Research." Indeed, persistent pain is a major international health problem (Gureje et al. 1998), prompting the World Health Organization to endorse a global campaign against pain (Breivik 2002). Persistent pain may lead to excessive surgery or other expensive or invasive procedures and is the leading reason for use of complementary and alternative medicine (CAM) (Astin 1998). Pain is also among the most common reasons for temporary as well as permanent work disability (B.H. Smith et al. 2001). Many pain treatment recommendations are based principally on expert consensus rather than on clinical trial results (Bair et al. 2005) and have yet to influence primary care practice (Chodosh et al. 2001).

Psychiatric Comorbidity

Pain is even more prevalent in patients with psychiatric comorbidity, particularly mood disorders. The overlap between pain and depression ranges from 30% to 60% (Ang et al. 2006; Bair et al. 2003; Magni et al. 1993). Pain is a strong predictor of both the onset and persistence of depression (Ohayon and Schatzberg 2003), and depression is likewise a powerful predictor of pain, particularly persistent pain (Bair et al. 2003; Gureje et al. 1998). Concurrent pain and depression have a much greater impact than either disorder alone on multiple domains of functional status as well as health care utilization (Bair et al. 2003).

Comorbid depression worsens disability and decreases active coping in patients suffering from pain (Arnow et al. 2006; Demyttenaere et al. 2006). Comorbidity decreases the likelihood of a favorable response of either condition to treatment and also diminishes patient satisfaction with treatment (Bair et al. 2004; Karp et al. 2005; Kroenke et al. 2008; Mavandadi et al. 2007; Thielke et al. 2007). Thus, reliable methods for assessing the presence and severity of pain in patients with depression (particularly those not responding to initial treatment) and strategies for effectively and efficiently integrating evidence-based depression care into the management of patients with chronic pain are sorely needed (Kroenke 2003a).

Although not as extensively studied, the comorbidity of pain with anxiety appears to be nearly as strong as its comorbidity with depression (Kroenke 2003b; Kroenke and Price 1993; Kroenke et al. 1994, 1997; McWilliams et al. 2003). Indeed, a global study conducted by the World Health Organization in 17 countries involving more than 85,000 community-dwelling adults showed that pain is associated with mood and anxiety disorders, but not with alcohol abuse or dependence (Gureje et al. 2008). The prevalence of specific mood and anxiety disorders was lowest among persons with no pain, intermediate among those with one pain site, and highest among those with multiple pain sites. Relative to persons not reporting pain, the age–sex adjusted odds ratios were 1.8 (95% confidence interval [CI] = 1.7–2.0) for mood disorders and 1.9 (95% CI = 1.8–2.1) for anxiety disorders for persons with single-site pain, and 3.7 (95% CI = 3.3–4.1) for mood disorders and 3.6 (95% CI = 3.3–4.0) for anxiety disorders among those with multisite pain.

Definition and Classification of Pain

The International Association for the Study of Pain (IASP) defines pain as "an unpleasant sensory and emotional experience associated with actual or potential tissue damage, or described in terms of such damage." Although there are more complex approaches to classifying pain, a pragmatic and frequently used system broadly classifies pain as either *nociceptive* or *neuropathic* (Basbaum et al. 2005). Nociceptive pain includes most cases of acute pain in which a strong, noxious stimulus impacts the skin or deep tissue. Acute pain resolves after the noxious stimulus has been removed, but inflammatory and other mechanisms may lead to persistence of nociceptive pain for weeks, months, or years (i.e., chronic pain). Many pain conditions, including arthritis and other musculoskeletal disorders, migraine and tension headache, and chronic widespread pain conditions such as fibromyalgia, would be classified under the broad rubric of nociceptive pain.

A second type of chronic pain, neuropathic pain, arises from injury to the peripheral or central nervous system. Examples include postherpetic neuralgia, painful diabetic neuropathy, phantom limb pain, and sciatica. Neuropathic pain is often characterized as burning, paroxysmal, stabbing, buzzing, or electric shock–like. Some conditions, such as low back pain, may include both nociceptive components (arising from the muscles or contiguous tissues) and neuropathic components (radicular pain or sciatica).

Persons with chronic pain often suffer from spontaneous ongoing pain. Also, stimuli that are normally not painful (movement, light touch) become painful, a phenomenon known as *allodynia*. Examples include pain produced by touching sunburned skin or moving an arthritic joint. *Hyperalgesia* is exacerbated pain produced by a stimulus that is expected to be only mildly painful (e.g., slapping sunburned skin). These phenomena may be related to central sensitization, which has been proposed as a common mechanism underlying unexplained pain syndromes such as fibromyalgia.

Sometimes the broader category of nociceptive pain is subclassified into *somatic* pain (triggered in the skin, muscles, joints, or fascia) and *visceral* pain (heart, lungs, gastrointestinal or genitourinary system, or other deeper organs). The latter is diffuse and poorly localized, reflecting differences in innervation between somatic and visceral tissue. Somatosensory fibers are precisely located in the spinal cord and brain, whereas afferent viscerosensory fibers overlap each other and converge at several levels within the nervous system. Although some of the principles of pain management are relevant to visceral pain, in this chapter we concentrate on the management of chronic pain due to nociceptive pain of the somatic variety and neuropathic pain conditions. Together, these account for the majority of chronic pain conditions seen in clinical practice. Moreover, visceral pain is more commonly a harbinger of a serious underlying disorder with specific treatments targeting the disease itself rather than mere analgesia. In contrast, pain itself becomes the primary "disease" or target of therapy in a large proportion of chronic somatic and neuropathic pain disorders.

Treatment of Pain

Overview

The focus of this chapter is twofold. First, we discuss major classes of medications as they relate to pain management. Because a number of drugs are effective across multiple types of pain disorders, it is useful to consider them in a cross-cutting as well as a disease-specific fashion. Nonpharmacological treatments are also reviewed. In the following main section ("Selected Pain Disorders"), we briefly address several specific categories of disorders chosen because they 1) account for the most common types of chronic pain, 2) are conditions for which pain management is the principal focus, and 3) have been studied in numerous clinical trials. In short, prevalence, pain management as a priority rather than disease modification, and evidence-based therapy are the three selection criteria for the discussion of specific disorders. Even within these two broad foci (disorders and treatments), there will perforce be some intermingling. For example, certain drug classes have been heavily studied within certain pain disorders, and conversely, certain pain disorders have been a common target of several classes of medications or other treatments.

The prototypical diseases discussed are musculoskeletal disorders (principally fibromyalgia, low back pain, and osteoarthritis) and neuropathic pain. Musculoskeletal disorders account for more than two-thirds of pain-related outpatient visits, and neuropathic pain not only is common but also is a popular target for clinical trials in pain management and therefore a common reason for seeking U.S. Food and Drug Administration (FDA) approval of pain as a drug indication. Although pharmacotherapy receives the greatest attention in this chapter, we briefly review nonpharmacological treatments due to their important role in the management of chronic pain. Acute pain (e.g., injuries, postoperative pain), cancer pain, headache, and visceral pain are not addressed. Although a moderate amount of the information presented in this chapter is relevant to the treatment of pain in these and other conditions (especially the discussion of specific analgesics), a detailed discussion of these specialized topics is beyond the scope of this chapter.

Strength of Evidence

The majority of the information in this chapter was derived from meta-analyses and systematic reviews published since 2005. Individual randomized, controlled trials (RCTs) are not presented unless they reported on a promising treatment for which multiple trials had not yet been performed. Certainly, evidence is strongest for those treatments that have shown efficacy in multiple trials rather than a single RCT, particularly because individual trials sometimes yield contradictory findings. Uncontrolled or open-label studies provide still weaker evidence and are cited only in a few instances.

In meta-analyses and systematic reviews, the magnitude of a treatment's effect on particular domains such as pain and physical function is often reported as an *effect size*. The effect size is a standard way to determine the degree of improvement (or change) related to a particular therapy compared with a placebo or other type of control group. The effect size is calculated as the mean change in the treatment group minus the mean change in the control group, divided by the pooled standard deviation. By convention, an effect size of less than 0.2 is considered trivial; 0.2–0.5, small; 0.5–0.8, moderate; 0.8–1.2, important; and 1.2 or greater, very important (Cohen 1998).

Effect size can be useful when comparing continuous variables such as mean differences (e.g., in pain scores). When comparing response rates on a categorical variable (e.g., "improved" or "≥50% reduction in pain"), the *number needed to treat* (NNT) is another common metric. The NNT is calculated as the reciprocal of the absolute difference between treatment groups. For example, if a clinical trial demonstrates that 60% of subjects improve while taking a new analgesic versus 35% of subjects receiving a placebo, that is an absolute difference of 25%. The NNT is the reciprocal of that: 1/0.25=4. This means that for every four patients who receive the analgesic, one additional patient would achieve a therapeutic response over and above placebo (i.e., the other three patients may have done just as well taking the placebo). Actually, an NNT of ≤5 typically represents a reasonably good analgesic.

When studying the same pain condition, the NNT may also be useful in comparing different drugs. For example, in one study of acute pain after certain operative procedures, 10 mg of morphine, 30 mg of ketorolac, and 100 mg of meperidine (all administered by intramuscular injection) and 1,000 mg of acetaminophen (administered orally) all had NNTs between 3 and 4; furthermore, their 95% confidence intervals overlapped, implying no significant difference in the analgesic efficacy between intramuscular opioids, intramuscular nonsteroidal anti-inflammatory drugs (NSAIDs), and oral acetaminophen (Barden et al. 2004). However, analgesic effect may depend on the type of pain condition being treated or clinical context as well. For example, one study found that the NNT for acetaminophen after dental extraction was 3.8, compared with 1.9 after orthopedic surgery (Barden et al. 2004). Also, small sample sizes may affect the precision of NNT estimates; some feel that NNT calculations based on trial data involving fewer than 500 subjects should be interpreted cautiously. Second, it is more problematic to compare the NNTs of different drugs estimated from separate studies than when NNTs are estimated for different drugs tested in the same clinical trial. Third, NNTs derived from studying analgesics in acute pain conditions may not be readily generalizable to their efficacy in the treatment of chronic pain.

Pharmacotherapy

Nonopioid Analgesics

The anti-inflammatory properties of the extract of willow bark have been known for centuries. Salicylic acid was discovered as the extract's active ingredient in the nineteenth century and was subsequently acetylated to improve its gastrointestinal tolerability; acetylsalicylic acid became the prototypical analgesic aspirin. Aspirin and other related compounds constitute a class of drugs known as NSAIDs. All NSAIDs have three desirable pharmacological effects—anti-inflammatory, analgesic, and antipyretic. NSAIDs and acetaminophen are among the most commonly prescribed medications for acute and chronic pain and can also be obtained without a prescription.

Acetaminophen has analgesic and antipyretic effects similar to those of the NSAIDs but lacks a specific anti-inflammatory effect. Despite its widespread use, the analgesic mechanism of acetaminophen is poorly understood. Acetaminophen is a slightly weaker analgesic than NSAIDs (<10 point difference on a 100-point visual analog pain scale) (Lee et al. 2004; Towheed et al. 2006; Wegman et al. 2004) but is a reasonable first-line option because of its more favorable safety profile and low cost. However, acetaminophen is associated with asymptomatic elevations of aminotransferase levels at dosages of 4 g/day even in healthy adults, although the clinical significance of these findings is uncertain (Watkins et al. 2006).

NSAIDs block the enzymatic activity of cyclo-oxygenase (COX), which uses arachidonic acid to generate prostanoids. Prostanoids influence immune, cardiovascular, gastrointestinal, renovascular, pulmonary, central nervous system, and reproductive function. Although gastrointestinal adverse effects have traditionally been considered the most common and worrisome complication, cardiovascular risk has gained increasing attention (Antman et al. 2007). Aspirin was the first and at one time the most commonly used NSAID.

There are two major COX isoenzymes: COX-1 is expressed constantly in most tissues, whereas COX-2 is induced by inflammation. NSAIDs vary in their chemical structure and relative ability to block the COX-1 versus the COX-2 isoenzymes. Several prostaglandins are both hyperalgesic and gastroprotective. Thus, nonselective COX inhibition with NSAIDs like aspirin, ibuprofen, in-

domethacin, and naproxen, which inhibit both COX-1 and COX-2 enzymes, provides effective pain relief for inflammatory conditions but carries a risk for erosive gastritis and gastrointestinal bleeding. Selective COX-2 inhibitors (valdecoxib, rofecoxib, celecoxib) have less gastrointestinal toxicity because of the relative paucity of COX-2 expression in the gastrointestinal tract relative to inflammatory tissue. However, data from meta-analyses and registries have shown an increased risk of cardiovascular events and mortality from COX-2 use, particularly in patients with known cardiovascular disease who receive prolonged treatment. Rofecoxib (Vioxx) has been withdrawn from the market, and all COX-2 inhibitors should be used cautiously, if at all, in patients with cardiovascular disease or risk factors for cardiovascular disease. All NSAIDs, including nonselective COX inhibitors and COX-2 agents, appear equally effective in the treatment of pain disorders (Chou et al. 2006). The NSAID that appears to be the safest in terms of cardiovascular risk is naproxen.

Opioid Analgesics

> The analgesic effects of opium have been known to mankind for more than 5,000 years. However, their inherent risk of abuse soon became evident. Ever since, society has attempted to find a balance between licit and illicit use, therapeutic versus adverse effects, and medical needs and legal issues. Despite all the legal, administrative, and social interference, no other class of drugs has remained in use for as long as opioids. (Schug 2005)

Opioids have a leading place in the treatment of acute pain and advanced cancer pain of moderate to severe intensity, because in both instances treatment is expected to be of short to medium duration. In contrast, opioid treatment for chronic noncancer pain is frequently delayed until first- or second-line treatments have failed because of less clarity about the benefits of chronic use and greater concerns about addiction, long-term effects (e.g., immunological, reproductive), opioid-induced hyperalgesia, and regulatory difficulties.

The Controlled Substances Act of 1970 divided substances to be regulated into five schedules, as determined by the U.S. Drug Enforcement Administration. These schedules govern the legal distribution and use of most substances with a significant abuse liability. Schedule I drugs have the highest abuse potential; they are available for research only and have no approved medical uses. Schedule II–IV substances have decreasing abuse liabilities (II is the highest) and approved medical uses. Physicians are licensed to prescribe these compounds, and pharmacies can dispense them, although pharmacies do not stock all of these substances. Schedule II compounds have more stringent record-keeping and storage requirements than do Schedule III and Schedule IV substances. Schedule V substances have a recognized abuse liability (and approved medical uses) but are generally not as highly regulated vis-à-vis record keeping. Many of these substances are used in common over-the-counter medicines. Including compounds on this schedule facilitates state and local regulations deemed appropriate in some jurisdictions (e.g., an individual state may impose restrictions on some substance considered to have an unexpectedly high abuse liability).

Propoxyphene and tramadol. Two drugs are "on the border" of what are traditionally considered opioids. Propoxyphene is a lower-scheduled drug than other opioids, and tramadol has been an unscheduled drug. Still, the efficacy and toxicity of both drugs are related, at least in part, to opioid effects, and thus they are discussed within this category.

Propoxyphene (Darvon) had, until recently, been one of the most widely prescribed analgesics for mild to moderate pain. It is often used in combination with acetaminophen (as Darvocet) or aspirin (Darvon Compound). Experts increasingly advise against its use for several reasons (Pasero et al. 1999). First, its therapeutic–toxicity ratio is not particularly favorable. Propoxyphene is only one-half to one-third as potent as codeine. Its recommended dose of 100 mg is equal in analgesic effect to 60 mg of codeine, which is known to be equal to 600 mg (less than two 325-mg tablets) of aspirin. Yet at equianalgesic doses, propoxyphene has the same incidence of minor side effects as codeine. More importantly, propoxyphene and its active metabolite, norpropoxyphene, can accumulate in the body and produce severe toxicity with repeated doses. Respiratory depression, sedation, and cognitive impairment can occur with excessive accumulation or when propoxyphene is used in combination with alcohol or sedating medications, and elderly patients may be particularly sensitive due to poorer renal clearance.

Tramadol (Ultram) is unique in that it has both opioid and nonopioid effects. Although its mode of action is not completely understood, it exerts an analgesic effect through binding to the μ opioid receptor as an agonist (opioid effect) and weakly inhibiting the reuptake of serotonin and norepinephrine (nonopioid effect), similar to the effect of tricyclic antidepressants (TCAs). Tramadol is available in both short- and long-acting formulations. The starting dosage for the short-acting formulation is 50 mg

once or twice daily, with gradual titration to a maximum of 400 mg/day. Dosage reduction is necessary in those with renal or hepatic disease. The risk of respiratory depression and, presumably, addiction is lower than with other opiates. Because tramadol is an unscheduled drug, clinicians may not be aware of its opioid effect. However, it still should be used with some caution in persons recovering from substance use disorders. Dose reduction is recommended in older adult patients (>75 years) and in those with renal impairment (creatinine clearance <30 mL/minute) or cirrhosis of the liver. Multiple trials have demonstrated the efficacy of tramadol in pain disorders, particularly osteoarthritis, fibromyalgia, and neuropathic pain.

Hollingshead et al. (2006) conducted a systematic review of six trials evaluating tramadol in neuropathic pain. All four trials comparing tramadol with placebo showed benefit with tramadol: the NNT with tramadol versus placebo to reach at least 50% pain relief was 3.8. Single trials comparing tramadol with clomipramine or morphine were inconclusive.

In summary, the clinical trial evidence across a number of pain disorders is much stronger for tramadol, which has led to its recommendation as at least a second-line treatment for conditions such as osteoarthritis, fibromyalgia, and neuropathic pain. In contrast, the benefits of propoxyphene have not been clearly shown to exceed its potential risks.

Efficacy of opioids. Furlan et al. (2006) conducted a meta-analysis of opioid use for chronic noncancer pain. Included were 41 trials involving 6,019 patients: 80% of the patients had nociceptive pain (osteoarthritis, rheumatoid arthritis, or back pain); 12%, neuropathic pain (postherpetic neuralgia, diabetic neuropathy, or phantom limb pain); 7%, fibromyalgia; and 1%, mixed pain. For certain analyses, the authors classified opioids as weak (propoxyphene, tramadol, codeine) and strong (all other opioids). Tramadol was the agent studied in 17 trials (3,433 patients), propoxyphene or dextropropoxyphene in 3 trials (1,074 patients), codeine in 7 trials (444 patients), oxycodone in 6 trials (517 patients), and morphine in 8 trials (551 patients). Average duration of treatment was 5 weeks (range, 1–16 weeks). On average, 33% of patients in the opioid groups dropped out (15% because of inadequate pain relief and 21% because of side effects; some patients reported both reasons), as did 38% in the placebo groups (30% because of inadequate pain relief and 10% because of side effects).

Opioids were more effective than placebo for both pain and functional outcomes in patients with nociceptive or neuropathic pain. The only opioid studied for fibromyalgia was tramadol (2 trials, 228 patients), where it proved effective. The effect size for opioids compared with placebo was moderate for pain (–0.60) and small for functional outcomes (–0.31). Only 8 trials compared opioids with other analgesics; in these trials, opioids did not differ significantly from nonopioids in terms of pain relief (effect size, –0.05) and were significantly worse than nonopioids in terms of functional outcomes, although only slightly so (effect size, 0.16). The authors concluded that the strong opioids (oxycodone, morphine) were significantly more effective than other drugs (effect size, –0.34), but this was based on only 2 trials, one of which was an open-label study (Furlan et al. 2006).

A systematic review reported on 11 studies (2,877 patients) that assessed quality of life in patients with chronic nonmalignant pain receiving long-term opioid treatment (Devulder et al. 2005). Six studies were randomized trials and five were observational studies. Of the 4 trials in which baseline values were reported, 3 showed an improvement in quality of life. Similarly, it improved in 4 of the 5 observational studies. While this suggests potential quality-of-life benefits, the authors concluded that further methodologically rigorous studies are needed to confirm these findings and to elucidate the potential adverse effects of physical tolerance, withdrawal, and addiction on functional status.

Adverse effects.   Moore and McQuay (2005) conducted a systematic review of 34 trials with 4,212 patients that provided information on adverse events related to opioid use in treating noncancer pain. Most opioids used (accounting for 90% of patients) were for treating moderate rather than severe pain. Dry mouth (affecting 25% of patients), nausea (21%), and constipation (15%) were the most common adverse events. A substantial proportion of patients taking opioids (22%) withdrew because of adverse events. Because most trials were short (<4 weeks) and did not use titrated doses, the implications for long-term use in clinical practice are less certain. Eisenberg et al. (2006) also reported on adverse events in their systematic review of opioids for neuropathic pain. Compared with placebo recipients, opioid recipients had higher rates of nausea (33% vs. 9%), constipation (33% vs. 10%), drowsiness (29% vs. 12%), dizziness (21% vs. 6%), and vomiting (15% vs. 3%). Among studies reporting causes of withdrawal, more patients receiving opioids withdrew because of adverse effects (11% vs. 4%). Finally, in the review by Furlan et al. (2006), only three side effects occurred significantly more frequently with opioids than

with placebo: nausea, constipation, and somnolence. These rates were 14%, 9%, and 6% higher in opioid recipients, respectively.

A large population-based study from Denmark found that opioid usage was significantly associated with more severe pain, poorer self-rated health, lower quality of life, less physical activity, lower employment, higher levels of health care utilization, and more subjects living alone (Højsted and Sjøgren 2007). The cross-sectional nature of the study does not prove causation, and it is certainly possible that the opioid users would have fared worse without opioid treatment. However, it does raise questions of whether opioid treatment of chronic pain is achieving the key goals of pain relief, improved functional status, and better quality of life.

Studies have indicated that endocrinological abnormalities such as hypogonadism and erectile dysfunction may be associated with opioid therapy (Ballantyne and Mao 2003; Daniell 2002). In women, opioid use has been associated with amenorrhea and decreased sex hormone levels (Daniell 2008). Two small trials evaluating opioid use in chronic pain reported analyzable data regarding sexual activity, and both found that patients taking opioids had better self-reported sexual function than those taking placebo (Furlan et al. 2006). Improvement of well-being secondary to better pain control may account for this. Clearly, the incidence and clinical significance of opioid-related hypogonadism need to be better defined.

A feared consequence of long-term opioid use is cognitive dysfunction. Studies have suggested that opioid treatment for chronic pain may be associated with impaired neuropsychological performance regarding reaction times, psychomotor speed, and working memory (Højsted and Sjøgren 2007). However, many other factors may be playing a role, including pain itself, concomitant medications, and psychiatric comorbidity. A systematic review concluded that stable doses of opioids do not impair driving performance (Fishbain et al. 2003).

Tolerance and addiction.   The risks of prescription opioid addiction, abuse, and diversion among chronic pain patients are not well understood. In part, this is due to inconsistent use of terminology and the difficulty of defining addiction and abuse in patients receiving opioids for chronic pain (Heit 2003; Savage et al. 2003). The term *dependence* is particularly problematic because confusion can occur between physical dependence, psychological dependence, and substance dependence (as defined in DSM-IV-TR [American Psychiatric Association 2000]). Some experts believe that the term *addiction* should be reserved for the specific condition defined as substance dependence in DSM-IV-TR. *Misuse* describes other problematic opioid use, including DSM-IV-TR substance abuse and other nontherapeutic uses that do not meet DSM-IV-TR criteria. *Diversion* includes selling, sharing, and trading of prescription opioids.

A systematic review of the literature on the risk of iatrogenic addiction in patients treated with opioids for acute and subacute pain yielded 41 eligible articles (Wasan et al. 2006). However, there were no randomized trials or comparative longitudinal studies, and the results of nine studies of low methodological quality yielded conflicting findings. The authors concluded that it is not known whether the risk for iatrogenic addiction among patients treated for acute or subacute pain is relatively high (>10%) or low (<0.1%).

In a 10-year follow-up study of patients treated with opioids for chronic pain, tolerance was not a problem in the majority of patients (Jensen et al. 2006). In contrast, a retrospective study of 104 chronic pain patients younger than 50 years and 102 patients older than 60 years showed that younger patients and those with nociceptive pain (as compared with neuropathic pain) had much higher escalation of opioid doses over a 15-month follow-up period (Buntin-Mushock et al. 2005). Another worrying finding of this study was that although the younger patients had a dosage increase of 640% (from 49 to 365 mg/day of morphine equivalent) during the observation period, the pain visual analog scale scores did not change at all. Although this does not mean that addiction is playing an important role, it does suggest that decisions about dose escalation may need to vary depending on the type of pain, patient age, treatment response, and other factors. Failure of pain to improve with moderate dosage increases in an individual patient may indicate that opioids are not the optimal treatment rather than that continuing dose escalations are needed. Some experts have classified patients or pain syndromes as opioid responsive versus opioid resistant (H.S. Smith 2005). Indeed, some patients may develop opioid-induced hyperalgesia where the balance between antinociceptive and pro-nociceptive systems is upregulated after opioid exposure, leading to an enhanced vulnerability to pain (Angst and Clark 2006; Højsted and Sjøgren 2007).

Højsted and Sjøgren (2007) reviewed some important predictors of opioid use. The "rush" the patient experiences after administration of an opioid is caused by a rapid and large increase in dopamine in the brain reward system. Important factors for abuse liability associated with the drug include the speed of access and the concentration at the target sites. On a scale of opioid attractiveness,

sustained-release oxycodone had the highest rating and the fentanyl patch had the lowest score; oral transmucosal fentanyl, methadone, and sustained-release morphine had intermediate scores. However, research demonstrating higher abuse potential of one opioid versus another is limited. Risk factors for opioid abuse in patients with chronic pain are young age, male gender, past alcohol or cocaine abuse, previous drug conviction, mental health disorders, pain in multiple regions, and pain after motor vehicle accidents.

A randomized trial of 11,352 participants with chronic noncancer pain compared the abuse potential of tramadol, NSAIDs, and hydrocodone (Adams et al. 2006). Abuse was defined by an algorithm including increasing doses without physician approval, use for purposes other than the ones intended, inability to stop using the drug, and withdrawal. The percentage of subjects who scored positive for abuse at least once during the 12-month follow-up period was 2.5% with NSAIDs, 2.7% with tramadol, and 4.9% with hydrocodone. When more than one algorithm criterion was required, abuse rates were 0.5% with NSAIDs, 0.7% with tramadol, and 1.2% with hydrocodone. Although the authors concluded that the prevalence of abuse/dependence was significantly less with NSAIDs and tramadol than with hydrocodone, the rates are overall quite low and the between-group differences are rather small.

General principles of opioid use. Useful suggestions for management of chronic opioid therapy have been published (Ballantyne 2006; Kahan et al. 2006; Pasero et al. 1999). The use of very high doses of opioids is rarely helpful. Purely on the basis that the highest daily dosage of opioids used in existing trials is 180 mg of morphine or its equivalent, opioid reduction or rotation should be considered at this point. Because of incomplete cross-tolerance (i.e., patients may be tolerant to high doses of the first opioid yet have a lower tolerance to the new opioid), the initial dosage of a new opioid should be equivalent to 50% or less of the dosage of the original opioid. Equianalgesic doses of oral and transdermal opioids are summarized in Table 66–1. When trials of several opioids are ineffective in chronic pain, it is appropriate to consider weaning patients off the drug and discontinuing its use. Weaning can usually be accomplished over 10 days, but the exact weaning schedule depends on dose, drug, and duration of treatment. In cases of addiction, referral to an addiction specialist may be preferable to drug discontinuation. Opioids are often best used as an adjunctive treatment rather than as the sole therapy for chronic

TABLE 66–1.   Oral and transdermal opioid analgesic equivalence

DRUG	DOSE (MG)	DURATION (HOURS)[a]
Morphine	20–30	2–4
Codeine	200[b]	3–4
Hydrocodone	30[c]	4–6
Oxycodone	20	3–4
Hydromorphone	7.5	3–4
Meperidine	300[b]	2–4
Methadone	20[d]	4–8
Fentanyl (transdermal)	0.001/hour (1 μg/hour)[e]	48–72

[a]Duration of analgesia is dose-dependent; the higher the dose, usually the longer the duration.

[b]These high doses of codeine and meperidine are not recommended clinically.

[c]Equianalgesic data not available for hydrocodone.

[d]For opioid-tolerant patients converted to methadone, starting doses should be 10%–25% of the equianalgesic dose. Also, the half-life of methadone can vary widely, from 12 to 190 hours.

[e]1 μg/hour transdermally is approximately equal to morphine 2 mg/24 hours orally.

pain. Before starting opioid therapy, patients should understand that the goal of treatment is not the complete elimination of pain but a 25%–50% reduction in its intensity and improvement in mood and functioning.

Whether patients at risk for addiction should be excluded from opioid therapy is controversial. Current evidence suggests that such patients do well in controlled programs and should not be denied opioid treatment of pain solely on the basis of existing addiction comorbidities. A written agreement may be helpful for obtaining informed consent about the risks and benefits of opioid therapy and setting out terms of use, including the following:

• Obtaining opioids only from a single provider
• Reporting lost or stolen drugs promptly
• Not using more than is prescribed or requesting early refills on a regular basis
• Testing urine periodically to determine that opioids are being taken by the patient (and not diverted for economic gain) and that illicit drugs are not being taken

Some experts recommend a universal precautions approach for all patients receiving opioids because clinical factors are not sufficiently predictive of who will have problems with abuse or addiction. At each visit, the clinician should document the "4 As" (McCarberg and Passik 2005):

• Analgesic (pain relief)
• Activities of daily living (physical and psychosocial functioning)

• Adverse effects (side effects)
• Aberrant drug taking (taking more than prescribed, diversion, etc.)

Long-acting opioids.   Chou (2008) conducted an evidence-based review of 25 randomized trials ($N = 2,752$) that evaluated long-acting opioids in patients with chronic noncancer pain. The review included 2 or more clinical trials of transdermal fentanyl and long-acting oral oxycodone, morphine, codeine, and dihydrocodeine. Methadone and levorphanol were each studied in only a single trial, and no trials evaluated long-acting hydromorphone. Only 5 trials compared one long-acting opioid with another; 7 compared a long-acting opioid with a short-acting opioid, and 13 compared a long-acting opioid with a nonopioid agent or placebo. Ten trials used a crossover design. The number of subjects in the trials averaged 110 (range, 12–680). The pain disorder was osteoarthritis in 5 trials, back pain in 7, neuropathic pain in 7, heterogeneous pain conditions in 4, phantom limb pain in 1, and chronic pancreatitis in 1. Nearly all of the trials were of relatively short duration, ranging from 5 days to 16 weeks. All trials excluded persons with past or current substance abuse. The majority of trials recruited patients from specialty clinics, most commonly from rheumatology or pain practices.

The authors concluded that there is insufficient evidence from either the 20 trials comparing long-acting opioids with other types of drugs or with placebo or the 5 head-to-head trials to suggest that one long-acting opioid is superior to another. The largest (680 subjects) and longest (13 months) randomized trial found that transdermal fentanyl and twice-daily morphine were similar in efficacy for patients with chronic low back pain who had not previously received strong opioids on a regular basis (Allan et al. 2005). Also, the 7 trials comparing long- versus short-acting opioids were unable to demonstrate superior efficacy or lesser side-effect rates with long-acting opioids. The single fair-quality trial comparing differences in adverse events among long-acting opioids found less constipation with fentanyl than with morphine (31% vs. 48%) but also a trend toward a higher rate of withdrawals due to any adverse event with fentanyl (37% vs. 31%).

Methadone. Until recently, methadone has been used primarily as maintenance drug to prevent withdrawal in opioid-addicted adults. The stigma as a "drug for addicts" has been one factor limiting its use as an analgesic in clinical practice. It has gained increased use in the treatment of intractable pain in end-of-life care and other palliative care settings. Concerns regarding use of methadone for pain relate to its long and unpredictable half-life and the associated risk of a delayed overdose. Furthermore, there are large individual variations in presumed equianalgesic doses of methadone relative to other opioids. This prevents the use of simple equianalgesic tables to calculate the required dose of methadone during rotation from other opioids.

Although methadone has increasingly been used for the treatment of chronic noncancer pain, published data are rather modest. In a literature review of 21 studies, only 1 small randomized trial ($N=19$) was found; the remainder were either cases series ($N=7$) or case reports ($N=13$) (Sandoval et al. 2005). Methadone was administered primarily when previous opioid treatment was ineffective or poorly tolerated. Thus, the evidence base is currently inadequate and does not support a first-line role for methadone in chronic pain therapy.

Antidepressants

Tricyclic antidepressants and selective serotonin reuptake inhibitors. TCAs have the longest track record in the treatment of multiple pain conditions. Typically, lower doses of TCAs have been used in clinical trials of pain (e.g., 25–100 mg of amitriptyline or equivalent) than the doses usually necessary for treating depression. Advantages of TCAs include good evidence from multiple clinical trials, decades of clinical experience with TCAs in pain management, and the low cost of these generic agents. Disadvantages include the side effects asso-

ciated with TCAs (which may be less, however, when prescribing the lower doses used for analgesia), including worrisome cardiovascular side effects (e.g., hypertension, postural hypotension, arrhythmias) and a risk of falling in elderly patients, and potential lethality in overdoses.

A meta-analysis of 96 RCTs evaluating antidepressants for the treatment of conditions manifested by somatic symptoms (the majority involving painful symptoms) included 55 TCA trials, of which 76% showed benefits; 28 trials using anti-serotonin agents (principally headache trials using mianserin, a drug approved in Europe but not in the United States), of which 57% showed benefits; and 17 trials using selective serotonin reuptake inhibitor (SSRI) antidepressants, of which 47% showed positive results (O'Malley et al. 1999). Only a few trials were head-to-head comparisons of two antidepressants. Indirect comparisons did not show a significant difference by type of antidepressant using meta-regression, but TCAs were superior to SSRIs ($P<0.02$) using a bivariate tally procedure. Admittedly, such statistical comparisons are not as conclusive as direct comparisons of antidepressants within the same trial. Another review concluded that SSRIs appeared to have a relatively weak effect in ameliorating chronic pain (Jung et al. 1997).

Serotonin–norepinephrine reuptake inhibitors. Duloxetine has proven superior to placebo in three 12-week randomized, placebo-controlled trials that enrolled patients with pain due to diabetic peripheral neuropathy (Goldstein et al. 2005; Raskin et al. 2005; Wernicke et al. 2006). Both 60-mg and 120-mg daily dosages of duloxetine separated from placebo, but not from one another. Duloxetine showed no adverse effects on diabetes control. Duloxetine showed rapid onset of action, with separation from placebo beginning at week 1. Both patients with depression and those without depression were enrolled in the trials, although path analysis estimated that more than 90% of the analgesic effect in duloxetine-treated patients with diabetic neuropathy was attributable to a direct analgesic effect, with less than 10% possibly explained by an antidepressant effect (Perahia et al. 2006).

Some have questioned the strength of the evidence regarding the analgesic effect of serotonin–norepinephrine reuptake inhibitors (SNRIs). A recent meta-analysis of five trials in depressed patients reported a very small and statistically nonsignificant ($P=0.057$) analgesic effect for duloxetine (Spielmans 2008). Another meta-analysis that examined the evidence comparing duloxetine with SSRIs in treating the painful physical symptoms of depression likewise concluded that there was insufficient evidence of a superior analgesic effect with duloxetine (Krebs et al. 2008b). On the other hand, placebo-controlled trials of duloxetine have shown a significant analgesic effect of duloxetine not only for neuropathic pain but for the chronic widespread pain of fibromyalgia as well (Arnold et al. 2004, 2005, 2007b).

Several factors related to these trials should be considered. Pain was typically examined as a secondary outcome in major depression trials, and an important proportion of patients had no pain. Thus, the depression studies were not optimally designed to test analgesic effects. In contrast, the neuropathic pain and fibromyalgia studies were designed primarily to examine treatment effects on pain. Of note, major depression trials in which the sample was enriched with patients reporting at least moderate pain showed that duloxetine had an analgesic effect that was independent of its effect on depression (Brannan et al. 2005; Brecht et al. 2007). The analgesic effect of duloxetine in the pain trials was compared with placebo rather than with another antidepressant. Head-to-head comparisons of a particular antidepressant with an active comparator are few, so it is harder to draw conclusions about the superiority of duloxetine or other SNRIs compared with other antidepressants or pain treatments. In summary, there is reasonably good evidence that duloxetine is more effective than placebo in treating neuropathic pain and fibromyalgia. Evidence regarding its separation from placebo in treating the secondary painful symptoms of major depression is inconclusive, and its relative effectiveness for pain compared with other antidepressants or analgesic therapies requires head-to-head clinical trials.

Other antidepressants.   Mirtazapine was studied in a 6-week open-label trial of 594 patients with a primary diagnosis of at least one chronic pain syndrome (≥3 months) and a clinical diagnosis of depression (Freynhagen et al. 2006). The mean daily dose was 35±10 mg at study endpoint, and a statistically significant reduction in pain ($P<0.0001$) was found. Pain improvement was not related to age or type of pain syndrome.

Anticonvulsants

Anticonvulsant drugs have been used in the management of pain since the 1960s. The clinical impression is that they are useful for chronic neuropathic pain, especially when the pain is lancinating or burning. Three of the most extensively studied anticonvulsants are gabapentin, pregabalin, and carbamazepine. Gabapentin and pregabalin have the strongest evidence for the treatment of pain.

These two *gabapentinoids* act as neuromodulators by selectively binding to the $\alpha_2\delta$-subunit protein of calcium channels in various regions of the brain and the superficial dorsal horn of the spinal cord. This results in inhibition of the release of excitatory neurotransmitters that are important in the production of pain. Gabapentin and pregabalin are analogs of γ-aminobutyric acid (GABA), but they have no activity at GABA receptors and do not alter GABA uptake or degradation.

Gabapentin.   A systematic review of 15 trials (1,468 participants) evaluating gabapentin included 1 acute pain trial and 14 trials involving neuropathic pain (7 studies of diabetic neuropathy, 2 of postherpetic neuralgia, and 1 each of cancer-related neuropathy, phantom limb pain, spinal cord injury, Guillain-Barré syndrome, and miscellaneous neuropathies) (Wiffen et al. 2005b). In the 14 chronic neuropathic pain trials, 42% of participants improved taking gabapentin versus 19% taking placebo, and the NNT for improvement in all trials with evaluable data was 4.3 (95% CI = 3.5–5.7). Withdrawal rates were 14% for gabapentin versus 10% for placebo. The study of acute postoperative pain (70 patients) showed no benefit for gabapentin. Thus, there is good evidence that gabapentin is more effective than placebo in the treatment of chronic neuropathic pain.

Pregabalin.   Pregabalin is a novel compound that has analgesic, anticonvulsant, and anxiolytic effects (Shneker and McAuley 2005). The FDA approved pregabalin for treatment of neuropathic pain associated with diabetic peripheral neuropathy and postherpetic neuralgia and for treatment of fibromyalgia; evidence from the supporting trials is discussed in the "Neuropathic Pain" and "Fibromyalgia" sections of this chapter. Pregabalin is also approved as an adjunctive therapy for adults with partial-onset seizures. The U.S. Drug Enforcement Administration has placed pregabalin in Schedule V of the Controlled Substance Act (indicating a low potential for abuse), possibly because of withdrawal symptoms that were found during clinical trials. The most common adverse events are related to the central nervous system and include somnolence, dizziness, and peripheral edema. Dose-related weight gain can occur, highest at a dosage of 600 mg/day. For pain disorders, the usual dosage is 300–450 mg/day, administered in twice-daily doses.

Carbamazepine.   A systematic review of 12 trials (404 participants) included 4 placebo-controlled trials of trigeminal neuralgia, of which 2 with evaluable data yielded an NNT of 1.8 (95% CI = 1.4–2.8) (Wiffen et al. 2005c). For diabetic neuropathy the data were insufficient to calculate an NNT. There was no evidence that carbamazepine was effective for acute pain. In summary, carbamazepine appears effective for trigeminal neuralgia, but the amount and quality of evidence for gabapentin are stronger for other types of neuropathic pain.

Other anticonvulsants. A systematic review that included other anticonvulsants found an NNT of 2.1 (95% CI = 1.5–3.6) for phenytoin in a single trial of diabetic neuropathic pain (Wiffen et al. 2005a). Sodium valproate was ineffective in a single trial of acute pain.

Other Pharmacological Agents

Skeletal muscle relaxants. Most skeletal muscle relaxants are approved by the FDA for treating either spasticity (baclofen, dantrolene, and tizanidine) or musculoskeletal pain (carisoprodol, chlorzoxazone, cyclobenzaprine, metaxalone, methocarbamol, and orphenadrine) (Chou and Peterson 2005). There is insufficient evidence to prove that skeletal muscle relaxants differ in their efficacy, adverse events, or safety. Most trials have focused on acute rather than chronic pain. Cyclobenzaprine has been studied in several fibromyalgia trials and is discussed further in the "Fibromyalgia" section (under "Pharmacotherapy"). Indeed, cyclobenzaprine is the best-studied muscle relaxant in musculoskeletal disorders overall; in 21 fair-quality trials, it has consistently proven superior to placebo for relieving pain, reducing muscle spasms, and improving functional status. Cyclobenzaprine 5-mg doses are equally effective as 10-mg doses (each given three times a day) but cause fewer side effects. Also, 20-mg doses (thrice daily) are not more effective than 10-mg doses and cause more side effects.

Topical analgesics. A potential advantage of topical agents is avoidance of the systemic side effects often associated with oral medications. Disadvantages are that only localized areas of pain can be effectively treated and that irritating skin reactions occur in a minority of patients. Several topical analgesics—lidocaine, capsaicin, and salicylate—have been studied in multiple trials. Postherpetic neuralgia is an FDA-approved indication for the lidocaine 5% patch, which is discussed in more detail in the "Neuropathic Pain" section. In a meta-analysis of systemic administration of local anesthetics for neuropathic pain, Tremont-Lukats et al. (2005) reviewed 19 studies (706 patients total; 10 trials of lidocaine and 9 trials of mexiletine, an antiarrhythmic agent that is also used off-label for

pain). Lidocaine (most commonly 5 mg/kg administered intravenously over 30–60 minutes) and mexiletine (median dosage = 600 mg/day administered orally) were similar in efficacy and tolerance to morphine, amitriptyline, and gabapentin. However, the effects of parenteral lidocaine are short lived, and mexiletine is not yet widely used or recommended as first- or second-line therapy.

Capsaicin is an alkaloid derived from chili peppers that acts on vanilloid type 1 receptors; repeated application of capsaicin is thought to desensitize cation channel receptors, leading to depletion of substance P from primary afferent neurons (Chong and Hester 2007). The main disadvantage of capsaicin is the initial burning sensation, which may persist for days. Capsaicin must be applied three to four times per day over the entire painful area for up to 8 weeks before optimal pain relief can be achieved. Mason et al. (2004a) reviewed the clinical trial evidence for using capsaicin to treat chronic pain. Six double-blind, placebo-controlled trials (656 patients) were pooled for analysis of neuropathic conditions, and three double-blind, placebo-controlled trials (368 patients) were pooled for analysis of musculoskeletal conditions. In patients with neuropathic pain, 57% of patients achieved at least 50% pain relief with capsaicin versus 42% of patients taking placebo. In patients with musculoskeletal conditions, the response rates were 38% versus 25%. Approximately one-third of patients experienced local adverse events with capsaicin. The authors concluded that capsaicin has moderate to poor efficacy in the treatment of chronic musculoskeletal or neuropathic pain but may be useful as an adjunctive therapy or sole therapy for a small number of patients who are unresponsive to, or intolerant of, other treatments.

The same authors also reviewed the evidence for topical salicylate (Mason et al. 2004b). In three trials evaluating 182 patients with acute conditions, topical salicylate was significantly more efficacious in relieving pain than placebo (NNT = 2.1; 95% CI = 1.7–2.8). In six trials evaluating 429 patients with chronic conditions, topical salicylate was also better than placebo (NNT = 5.3; 95% CI = 3.6–10.2). However, larger, more rigorous trials tended to have negative results. Based on limited information, the authors concluded that topical salicylates may be efficacious in the treatment of acute pain, although trials of its use in treating musculoskeletal and arthritic pain suggested moderate to poor efficacy. Finally, systematic reviews (J. Lin et al. 2004; Mason et al. 2004c) as well as a recent RCT suggest that topical NSAIDs may be beneficial (ibuprofen for osteoarthritis of the knee has been studied the most) (Underwood et al. 2008).

Cannabinoids. The presence of specific high-affinity cannabinoid type 1 (CB_1) receptor binding sites has been demonstrated in the central nervous system and in certain peripheral tissues, whereas CB_2 receptors are expressed in high quantities in immune tissues and cells. Two main endogenous cannabinoids have been described, and their role in modulating pain has been increasingly recognized. The social stigma associated with cannabinoids and the politicolegal issues related to cannabis use for medical purposes have been barriers to research.

Nonetheless, six RCTs published since 2005 have shown promising results (Beaulieu and Ware 2007). The largest study enrolled 502 patients with multiple sclerosis; the primary outcome was objective spasticity rather than pain. Five smaller trials involving a total of 217 patients measured short-term outcomes (trial duration, 1–5 weeks) of five different pain conditions, including multiple sclerosis, rheumatoid arthritis, upper motor neuron syndrome, human immunodeficiency virus (HIV) neuropathy, and heterogeneous chronic pain. The agents studied included oral tetrahydrocannabinol in three trials, nabilone in two trials, and smoked marijuana in one trial. Five of the six trials (including the large trial) showed benefits.

In a recent review, Lever and Rice (2007) were more circumspect about the role of cannabinoids in chronic pain:

> Preclinical studies demonstrate that cannabinoids can reduce pain response in a range of inflammatory and neuropathic pain models. In contrast, the clinical effectiveness of cannabinoids as analgesics is less clear. Progress in this area requires the development of cannabinoids with a more favourable therapeutic index than those currently available for human use, and the testing of their efficacy and side effects in high-quality clinical trials. (p. 265)

In summary, cannabinoids can be considered promising at this point but still experimental for the treatment of chronic pain. Despite this, cannabinoids now appear as adjunctive agents in treatment guidelines for neuropathic pain in Europe (Attal et al. 2006) and Canada (Moulin et al. 2007).

Nonpharmacological Treatments

Nonpharmacological treatments will not be discussed in detail but need to be mentioned because of their important role in the management of chronic pain. Medications are typically targeted to the symptoms, but dysfunctional beliefs, attitudes, coping styles, and behaviors frequently develop in patients with chronic pain and con-

tribute to its perpetuation and their disability. Moreover, just as in other chronic medical disorders, pharmacotherapy is necessary but not sufficient for optimizing outcomes. For example, the patient with diabetes not only needs insulin or other hypoglycemic drugs but also requires dietary changes, exercise, and other lifestyle modifications to achieve target blood glucose levels.

Psychotherapy and Behavioral Interventions

Cognitive-behavioral therapy. Cognitive-behavioral therapy (CBT) has by far the largest body of evidence supporting its effectiveness in the treatment of various types of chronic pain disorders. Kroenke and Swindle (2000) reviewed 31 trials of CBT for the treatment of somatic syndromes, of which more than half involved pain conditions, including 5 trials of back pain, 3 of irritable bowel syndrome, 3 of noncardiac chest pain, 2 of fibromyalgia, and 4 of other pain disorders. Most of those trials (14 of 17) involving pain disorders found CBT to be beneficial. A recent update of this review found additional more recent studies confirming the effectiveness of CBT (Jackson et al. 2006). Also, a recent systematic review of treatment for somatoform disorders (in which multiple pain symptoms are often present) found CBT was effective in 11 of 13 RCTs (Kroenke 2007). Both group CBT and individual CBT appeared effective, as did briefer courses of CBT (e.g., 3–6 sessions). When administered for pain and other somatic disorders, it is important that CBT be *somatically focused*, having a somewhat different orientation than CBT provided for depressive and anxiety disorders. Patients with chronic pain and other somatic syndromes present with physical rather than psychological symptoms and often attribute their symptoms to physical disorders (i.e., medical factors). Thus, the mental health professional accustomed to providing CBT for psychiatric disorders may require some additional training in CBT appropriate for treating chronic pain and other somatic syndromes.

Pain self-management programs. Pain self-management (PSM) programs that emphasize self-efficacy have consistently demonstrated effectiveness in improving health outcomes and reducing health care utilization among patients with various rheumatic conditions (Heuts 2005; Lorig 2003; Lorig and Holman 1993); benefits included cost-effectiveness (Lorig et al. 1993) and improved psychological functioning (Barlow et al. 1998). Self-management for both acute (Damush et al. 2003) and chronic (Von Korff and Moore 2001) low back pain has also proven effective. Indeed, CBT and PSM are the two best-established psychobehavioral approaches to treating chronic musculoskeletal pain (Bradley and Alberts 1999). In fact, PSM incorporates important components of CBT with additional educational and behavioral strategies. Another important component of PSM programs is emotional coping and management (Lorig and Holman 2003). One advantage of PSM compared with CBT in the medical setting is that it may be effectively administered by varying levels of trained individuals, including lay personnel (Cohen et al. 1986).

Hypnosis.   A systematic review of hypnosis found that its effects on chronic pain tend to be similar, on average, to the effects of progressive muscle relaxation, biofeedback, and other types of relaxation training, all of which often include hypnosis-like suggestions (Jensen and Patterson 2006). None of the published studies have compared hypnosis with an equally credible placebo or minimally effective pain treatment. Therefore, conclusions cannot yet be made about whether hypnotic analgesia treatment is specifically effective over and above patients' expectancies.

Other psychological interventions.   Other reviews of psychological interventions for pain have shown a similar predominance of CBT trials. A meta-analysis of 27 RCTs of psychological interventions for treating arthritis found that CBT was used in 23 trials, stress management in 5, and biofeedback, emotional disclosure, and hypnosis in 1 trial each (several trials used more than one intervention) (Dixon et al. 2007). The reduction in pain was statistically significant but clinically rather small (pooled effect size, 0.18). Three systematic reviews of psychological treatments for somatic syndromes (many of which are manifested predominantly by pain) have also been heavily weighted with CBT studies (Allen et al. 2002; Henningsen et al. 2007; Raine et al. 2002). A large trial ($N=1,337$ patients) of telephone-based, nurse-administered problem-solving therapy (which is one of the evidence-based psychotherapies for depression) proved the therapy beneficial in primary care patients with chronic pain (Ahles et al. 2006), although further research is needed before one could recommend this over CBT or PSM programs.

Exercise

Exercise has been extensively studied in chronic pain patients and has been demonstrated to be an effective adjunctive treatment for several types of chronic pain disorders. Evidence regarding its effectiveness is discussed in more detail in the "Fibromyalgia" and "Osteoarthritis" sections. Six general issues relevant to initiating and maintaining an exercise program for chronic pain are summarized in Table 66–2.

Complementary and Alternative Medicine

A comprehensive review of CAM therapies for chronic pain was recently published (Tan et al. 2007). Although it is beyond the scope of this chapter to discuss this subject in detail, the authors concluded there was reasonable evidence for the effectiveness of the following therapies:

- Acupuncture for chronic low back pain and probably premenstrual syndrome–related pain
- Massage therapy for low back and shoulder pain
- Chiropractic therapy for several types of musculoskeletal pain
- Yoga for low back pain
- Meditation (as well as hypnosis) for several types of chronic pain

Two CAM treatments in particular—acupuncture and the use of magnets—have been the topic of several recent systematic reviews (Table 66–3). Acupuncture has proven effective in treating back pain and possibly osteoarthritis of the knee, although osteoarthritis trials have been fewer and the results less conclusive (Manheimer et al. 2005, 2007; A. White et al. 2007). Although headache pain is not the focus of this chapter, it should be noted that a systematic review of 13 trials of acupuncture for migraine headaches found inconclusive evidence supporting its efficacy, although most studies had serious design limitations (Griggs and Jensen 2006). Acupuncture's effects on experimental pain appear to be mediated through the release of neurohormonal factors, some of which can be inhibited by the opioid antagonist naloxone (Staud 2007). Compared with the pain relief associated with placebo use, acupuncture-related pain relief takes considerable time to develop and to wear off.

Static magnets represent a multibillion-dollar industry (Pittler et al. 2007). As many as one-quarter of patients with rheumatoid arthritis, osteoarthritis, or fibromyalgia use magnets or copper bracelets for pain relief. The mechanisms for magnets' putative efficacy are not established. One theory is that magnetic fields attenuate nociceptive C-fiber depolarization by shifting the membrane resting potential. Another theory suggests that magnetic fields promote an increase in blood flow through the skin and subcutaneous and muscular tissues, which reduces pain. However, the empirical data for effi-

TABLE 66–2.   Key principles for initiating and maintaining exercise for chronic pain

PRINCIPLE	COMMENTS
Type of exercise	Aerobic exercise is particularly important for some types of chronic pain (e.g., fibromyalgia), whereas strengthening and flexibility exercises may be helpful in others (back pain, osteoarthritis).
Catastrophizing as a barrier	Fear that movement or activity will worsen pain is common. Emphasizing that gradual activity will not cause further harm but instead can be beneficial is essential to activation and rehabilitation.
Stage of change	For patients in precontemplation phase, motivating them to initiate exercise is the challenge. For many others who begin an exercise program, getting them to maintain regular exercise more than a few months is the critical issue. This is analogous to weight loss, smoking cessation, and other lifestyle or behavioral changes.
Graduated program	Patients should not try to do too much initially. Instead, they should begin slowly and increase the amount of exercise gradually over a matter of weeks to months.
Structured vs. home based	The benefits of structured exercise programs demonstrated in some research studies may have a "voltage drop" when patients are instructed to begin an exercise program on their own. Exercise conducted in clinical settings (e.g., physical therapy, rehabilitation programs) or community settings (e.g., YMCA, fitness centers) may be reinforced by motivation, group participation, expert leadership, guidance, and/or an externally imposed regular schedule.
Monotherapy vs. bundled	Many studies of exercise have included other components, such as education about the particular pain disorder, self-management techniques, relaxation, and other cognitive-behavioral strategies. Certainly, exercise coupled with one or more of these is ideal.

cacy are inconclusive. A qualitative review found that static magnets were effective across a variety of pain conditions (Eccles 2005). However, a quantitative meta-analysis found no significant effects of static magnets, except possibly (though not conclusively) in treating osteoarthritis (Pittler et al. 2007). Pulsed electromagnetic energy has been much less studied and in a review of five trials was found ineffective (McCarthy et al. 2006).

Combination Therapy

Over time, the treatment of chronic pain often includes stepwise addition to a patient's regimen (and deletion if a therapy shows no benefit) of medications from several classes (Black and Sang 2005; Gallagher 2005). In addition to medications given to produce analgesia, pain management may include medications to treat the side effects of the analgesics, such as laxatives or stool softeners for patients receiving opioids, gastroprotective medications for those receiving NSAIDs, and psychostimulants to combat excessive somnolence.

Very few studies have tested combinations of treatments to determine their additive value, if any, compared with monotherapy. Only limited data suggest that the combination of acetaminophen with NSAIDs has additive pain-relieving effects (Schug 2005). More data show a beneficial effect in combining acetaminophen with opi-

oids, including codeine, tramadol, and morphine. Indeed, one of the more common fixed combinations in a single pill has been the coupling of an opioid, such as codeine, tramadol, oxycodone, or hydrocodone, with a nonopioid analgesic such as acetaminophen or aspirin. One important consideration in using fixed-dose combinations is that the maximum daily dosages of one component may restrict flexibility in optimizing the dosage of the other component. For example, when oxycodone 5 mg is combined with acetaminophen 500 mg, the maximum number of tablets that can be administered is eight in a 24-hour period (i.e., 4,000 mg of acetaminophen). If this is insufficient to manage the patient's pain, the opioid and nonopioid should be given as separate medications to allow further upward titration of the opioid.

Head-to-head clinical trials comparing different analgesics, separately or in combination, are rare. One example is a small (57 subjects enrolled; 41 trial completers) randomized, double-blind crossover trial in patients with neuropathic pain, which showed that gabapentin and morphine combined achieved better analgesia at lower doses of each drug than either as a single agent (Gilron et al. 2005). On the other hand, the gabapentin–morphine combination resulted in a higher frequency of constipation than gabapentin alone and a higher frequency of dry mouth than morphine alone.

TABLE 66–3. Acupuncture and magnets for painful disorders: summary of systematic reviews

TREATMENT	STUDY	CONDITION	REVIEW TYPE (*N*)	BENEFITS	STRENGTH OF EVIDENCE	COMMENTS
Acupuncture						
Acupuncture	Manheimer et al. 2005	Back pain	Meta-analysis (33 trials)	Yes	Good	Acupuncture was more effective than sham acupuncture (ES=0.54) or no treatment (ES=0.69) in chronic low back pain.
Acupuncture	Manheimer et al. 2007	Knee OA	Meta-analysis (11 trials)	Mixed	Moderate	Acupuncture was more effective than wait-list (ES=0.96) or usual-care controls but only slightly more effective than sham acupuncture for short-term (ES=0.35) and long-term (ES=0.13) pain improvement.
Acupuncture	A. White et al. 2007	Knee OA or pain	Meta-analysis (13 trials)	Yes	Moderate	In 5 studies that could be combined (*N*=1,334), acupuncture was superior to sham acupuncture for pain and function and was also superior to no-intervention controls.
Magnetism						
Static magnets	Eccles 2005	Various	Systematic (21 trials)	Yes	Moderate	Eleven of 18 better-quality trials were positive. Multiple types of pain conditions were studied.
Static magnets	Pittler et al. 2007	Various	Meta-analysis (25 trials)	No	Moderate	Meta-analysis showed no significant effects. Evidence was encouraging only for one condition—osteoarthritis.
PEMF stimulation	McCarthy et al. 2006	Knee OA	Systematic (five trials)	No	Moderate	PEMF therapy yielded insignificant improvement in pain and function.

Note. ES = effect size (mean difference between groups divided by pooled standard deviation); OA = osteoarthritis; PEMF = pulsed electromagnetic field.

The common decision in clinical practice when optimal pain relief has not been achieved is whether to switch to a new treatment or to add it to what is currently being provided. Given the paucity of combination drug trials, this decision is currently guided by practical considerations. Switching to another monotherapy is often less costly than combining two or more treatments and often is done when a patient has had only a minimal response to and/or poor tolerance of the initial treatment. On the other hand, adding a second treatment may be favored when there has been at least a partial response to the first therapy or when the second treatment has a different mechanism of action that may complement the original treatment. Factors influencing combination therapy decisions include not only added efficacy but also costs, side effects, adherence, and patient preferences. Sometimes, the secondary effects of a drug may influence the decision to use it in a particular patient. For example, the side effect of sedation that occurs with certain medications (e.g., gabapentin or pregabalin) may be troublesome in one patient whereas in another it may be useful to treat comorbid insomnia, particularly if taken at bedtime. Likewise, the antidepressant effects of a particular adjunctive pain medication (e.g., SNRIs like duloxetine or venlafaxine) may reduce both pain and mood disturbances in the patient with diabetic neuropathic pain and comorbid major depression. TCAs could serve the same purpose, although higher doses of TCAs are typically required for antidepressant action than for analgesic action, in which case the side effects of higher-dose TCAs, especially their cardiovascular effects, must be considered as well.

Selected Pain Disorders

Neuropathic Pain

Chou et al. (2007a) summarized several key points regarding the prevalence, etiology, and classification of neuropathic pain:

> Neuropathic pain (NP) is often classified by etiology or by the presumed site of neurologic involvement (central or peripheral). More complex classification systems based on symptoms, signs, anatomical distribution, or hypotheses regarding etiologies have been proposed, but it is not clear if such classifications are accurate or reproducible. NP is characterized by continuous or intermittent spontaneous pain, typically characterized by patients as burning, aching, or shooting. Up to 3% of the general population reports NP at some time. NP is most commonly associated with painful diabetic neu-

ropathy, post-herpetic neuralgia (PHN), or lumbar nerve root compression. Diabetic neuropathy occurs in approximately 10% of persons with diabetes. The most common form of diabetic peripheral neuropathy is a distal symmetric polyneuropathy, typically manifested by symptoms beginning in the feet. PHN is defined as pain persisting or recurring at the site of acute herpes zoster 3 or more months after the acute episode. It occurs in up to 25% of patients following an episode of shingles. Symptomatic spinal stenosis and lumbar disc herniation with nerve root compression occur in approximately 3% and 4% of patients with low back pain, respectively. Other causes of NP include cancer-related pain, spinal cord injury, post-stroke pain, HIV-associated neuropathy, and phantom limb pain. Uncommon but potentially debilitating NP conditions include trigeminal neuralgia (incidence 4/100,000 population). In the U.S., health care and disability-related costs associated with NP are estimated at almost $40 billion annually. (Chou et al. 2007a, p. 6)

Four drugs are FDA approved for the treatment of diabetic neuropathy or postherpetic neuralgia: gabapentin, pregabalin, duloxetine, and lidocaine (the lidocaine patch) (Chou et al. 2007a). Recommendations regarding the dosing of these drugs for neuropathic pain are summarized in Table 66–4. Venlafaxine and lidocaine gel also have some evidence for efficacy in treatment of neuropathic pain but do not have an FDA indication for this use. Other drugs have been used for neuropathic pain—particularly TCAs and anticonvulsants—besides those listed above, but have not been approved by the FDA for this indication. The one exception is carbamazepine, which was approved to treat trigeminal neuralgia based on three trials that included a total of 150 patients, published in the 1960s.

In their evidence-based review commissioned by the Agency for Healthcare Research and Quality, Chou et al. (2007a) highlighted several key findings:

1. Gabapentin (12 trials), pregabalin (8 trials), and duloxetine (3 trials) have proven superiority to placebo.
2. Trials of topical lidocaine patch or gel and venlafaxine are inconclusive.
3. Although indirect comparisons suggest the potential superiority of TCAs compared to gabapentin, direct analyses of 3 head-to-head trials found no difference between gabapentin and TCAs for pain relief, though the estimates are relatively imprecise. Additionally, 1 small trial found no difference between venlafaxine and imipramine.
4. Indirect analyses of trials found gabapentin and pregabalin moderately superior to both other anticon-

TABLE 66–4.   First-line drugs for neuropathic pain

DRUG	TRADE NAME	LABELED INDICATION	RECOMMENDED DAILY DOSAGE FOR NEUROPATHIC PAIN	DAILY DOSAGE RANGE IN RCTs (MEDIAN)
Anticonvulsants				
Gabapentin	Neurontin	Postherpetic neuralgia	Start at 300 mg, titrate to 900 mg, increase up to 1,800 mg (in three doses)	900–3,600 mg (1,800 mg)
Pregabalin	Lyrica	Diabetic neuropathy Postherpetic neuralgia	Start at 150 mg, increase up to 300 mg (in two to three doses)	75–600 mg (300 mg)
SNRI antidepressants				
Duloxetine	Cymbalta	Diabetic neuropathy	60 mg once daily	20–120 mg (90 mg)
Topical analgesic				
Lidocaine 5% patch	Lidoderm	Postherpetic neuralgia	Up to three patches for up to 12 hours within a 24-hour period	1–3 patches

Note.   NA = not applicable; RCTs = randomized, controlled trials; SNRI = serotonin–norepinephrine reuptake inhibitor.

vulsants (carbamazepine, lamotrigine, topiramate, and valproic acid) and SSRIs. However, such indirect analyses must be interpreted cautiously.

Chou et al. (2007a) also summarized the results of 6 systematic reviews that evaluated the benefits of gabapentin, pregabalin, SNRIs, or topical lidocaine for neuropathic pain. All of the newer medications for neuropathic pain were superior to placebo in at least one systematic review. The systematic reviews included a total of 17 unique placebo-controlled trials of gabapentin, 5 trials of pregabalin, 3 trials of venlafaxine, 6 trials of topical lidocaine, and 2 trials of duloxetine. None of the systematic reviews found any published reports of a head-to-head trial of one of these drugs versus another. Several of the reviews also concluded that TCAs were effective (the best evidence was for amitriptyline), and there were limited data for the effectiveness of SSRIs. It should also be noted that many of the TCA studies performed several decades ago had smaller samples than trials of currently approved drugs. For example, the sum total of patients with diabetic neuropathy studied in all TCA trials was less than 120 (Chong and Hester 2007). Also, a number of the TCA studies used a crossover design rather than a parallel-group design.

Eisenberg et al. (2006) conducted a systematic review of trials evaluating the use of opioids for neuropathic pain. Of 23 trials, 14 were classified as short-term (<24 hours), and 9 as intermediate-term (median, 28 days; range, 8–70 days). The short-term trials had contradictory results. In contrast, all 9 intermediate-term trials

demonstrated opioid efficacy: 13 points lower (95% CI = –16 to –9) than placebo on a scale of 1–100.

The European Federation of Neurological Sciences published guidelines on pharmacological treatment of neuropathic pain in 2006 (Attal et al. 2006), which are generally concordant with the Agency for Healthcare Research and Quality evidence-based report. The European Federation of Neurological Sciences concluded that there was level A evidence for the efficacy of TCAs, gabapentin, pregabalin, and opioids in neuropathic pain, followed by topical lidocaine in postherpetic neuralgia and SNRIs in diabetic neuropathy. They also concluded that diabetic and nondiabetic painful polyneuropathies are similar in symptomatology and response to treatment. The only exceptions noted were that HIV- and chemotherapy-induced neuropathy may be more refractory to treatment. The principal opioids studied have been oxycodone and tramadol, both of which have proven superior to placebo. Trials of topical capsaicin have provided discrepant results. The antiarrhythmic drug mexiletine, the N-methyl-D-aspartate antagonist memantine, and topical capsaicin have not shown convincing efficacy.

A consensus panel from the IASP likewise concluded that first-line treatments for neuropathic pain include certain antidepressants (i.e., TCAs and SNRIs), calcium channel $\alpha_2\delta$-ligands (i.e., gabapentin and pregabalin), and topical lidocaine (Dworkin et al. 2007). Opioid analgesics and tramadol were recommended as second-line treatments. The IASP also noted: "Although few clinical trials have been conducted, no medications have demonstrated efficacy in patients with lumbosacral radiculopathy, which is probably the most common type of neuropathic pain" (Dworkin et al. 2007, p. 237). Indeed, an RCT evaluating nortriptyline, morphine, and their combination in patients with chronic lumbar root pain found no greater efficacy with the combination than with either medication alone or placebo (Khoromi et al. 2007). The IASP also noted that little is known regarding the treatment response of those with mild to moderate neuropathic pain because most trials have enrolled patients with more severe neuropathic pain, and long-term effectiveness is unknown because most RCTs have been of less than 3 months' duration. The IASP also favored secondary-amine TCAs (nortriptyline and desipramine) over tertiary-amine TCAs (amitriptyline and imipramine) because of their comparable analgesia (Max et al. 1992; Rowbotham et al. 2005; Watson et al. 1998) and fewer side effects. Finally, the IASP concluded that the magnitude of pain reduction associated with opioid analgesics is at least as great as that obtained with other treatments for neuropathic pain.

No clear first choice emerges among FDA-approved drugs for neuropathic pain. The most common adverse events for gabapentin and pregabalin include dizziness, somnolence, and weight gain, and nausea can be a perplexing side effect of SNRIs. Sometimes, a drug may be preferentially chosen because of comorbid conditions (e.g., gabapentin or pregabalin for the patient with neuropathic pain and insomnia, or duloxetine when neuropathic pain is accompanied by major depression). Also, lower doses of two drugs may produce better analgesia with fewer side effects in selected patients (Gilron et al. 2005). Finally, switching or adding medications will frequently be necessary because no more than 40%–60% of patients obtain partial relief from a single agent (Dworkin et al. 2007).

Fibromyalgia

Mechanisms and Evaluation

Fibromyalgia is one of the most common musculoskeletal disorders seen in rheumatology practice as well as primary care. It is often classified among the functional somatic syndromes (FSSs), which include irritable bowel syndrome, chronic fatigue syndrome, temporomandibular joint disorder, interstitial cystitis, and other symptom-based conditions manifested by a cluster of symptoms for which the pathophysiological mechanism is not well understood (Aaron and Buchwald 2001). Patients with one FSS often suffer from one or more other FSSs as well as psychological comorbidity, including depression, anxiety,

and histories of abuse during childhood or as adults. The distinction between FSS and somatoform disorders is also being revisited (Kroenke et al. 2007). However, it does not appear that FSSs are entirely explained by psychological factors (Henningsen et al. 2003), and emerging research also shows biological factors that may be causative or contributory.

The American College of Rheumatology core diagnostic criteria for fibromyalgia are quite simple and do not require any laboratory or radiological testing. They are twofold:

1. Generalized pain that is both widespread (i.e., on both the right and left sides of the body, upper and lower halves, and axial as well as proximal arms and legs) and chronic (lasting ≥3 months)
2. Multiple tender points on physical examination (located in the front and back of the neck, upper chest and back areas, iliosacral and posterior gluteal areas, elbows and knees)

Although the American College of Rheumatology criteria technically require a tender point threshold (≥11 of 18), many clinicians do not actually count tender points but rather establish that the patient is tender at multiple areas, which can be done in 5–10 seconds. Besides multiple tender points, the other diagnostically useful finding is that, unlike patients with arthritic conditions (e.g., osteoarthritis, rheumatoid arthritis, systemic lupus) who mainly suffer from arthralgias (pain and tenderness over the joints or periarticular regions), fibromyalgia patients experience myalgias (pain and tender points in nonarticular regions). In fact, recent research shows that fibromyalgia patients feel tenderness wherever you apply pressure, including areas previously considered to be "control points" (Clauw 2007). The tenderness simply reflects the fibromyalgia patient's tendency toward allodynia (experiencing pain from stimuli that would normally be nonpainful) or hyperalgesia (experiencing more severe pain from stimuli that would normally be only mildly painful). Given that the symptoms seem to arise from disturbances in the central processing of pain and that tender points are a relatively nonspecific finding, some have recently advocated calling the condition *chronic widespread pain*.

The primary problem in fibromyalgia appears to be not that there is too much input coming from the pressure nociceptors peripherally but rather that there is inadequate filtering of that activity, perhaps because of decreased activity of descending anti-nociceptive pathways. In fact, multiple mechanisms seem to be operative in fibromyalgia (Abeles et al. 2007). Two key mechanisms are as follows:

1. Functional imaging studies in fibromyalgia patients have shown increased blood flow to pain-relevant areas of the brain at lower thresholds of nociceptive input.
2. There appears to be dysregulation of descending inhibitory pain pathways. Thus, the pain "amplifier" is turned up, and the "mute" button is turned down in fibromyalgia patients. Collectively, this is known as *central sensitization*.

Not only is fibromyalgia accompanied by psychiatric comorbidity, it also can coexist with other rheumatological disorders. For example, as many as one-quarter of patients with rheumatoid arthritis and other systemic arthritides may also have fibromyalgia. Thus, if an individual with arthritis or another musculoskeletal disorder also has chronic widespread pain, therapies effective for fibromyalgia should be added to the treatment regimen. Also, communication with the patient, including explanations about central sensitization and abnormal pain processing, may be helpful. Despite assumptions that being "labeled" with fibromyalgia may adversely affect patients, it has been shown that patients have had significant improvement in health satisfaction and symptoms after having received this diagnosis (K.P. White et al. 2002).

Pharmacotherapy

Five types of medications are effective in fibromyalgia: 1) TCAs, 2) cyclobenzaprine, 3) tramadol, 4) SNRIs (duloxetine, milnacipran), and 5) $\alpha_2\delta$-ligand anticonvulsants (pregabalin, gabapentin). Although classified as a muscle relaxant, cyclobenzaprine has a chemical structure closely related to that of the TCAs, which may partly account for its effectiveness in fibromyalgia. Although multiple trials have shown the effectiveness of tramadol in fibromyalgia, the few studies of stronger opioids have not established their efficacy. Also, the few studies of NSAIDs in fibromyalgia have also had negative results, suggesting that a class of drugs considered first-line treatment for arthritis and other musculoskeletal disorders may not be effective in treating fibromyalgia.

Perhaps because clinicians are more familiar with traditional analgesics than with medications proven effective in treating fibromyalgia, there is a disconnect between current practice and evidence. This was highlighted by Clauw (2007):

Market surveys suggest that the no. 1 class of drugs currently used to treat fibromyalgia in the United States is NSAIDs, whereas opioids are no. 3 or 4, even although there is no evidence that either of these classes of drugs works in fibromyalgia. Moreover, most fibromyalgia patients are not being given adequate education about their disease, nor are they given access to exercise and cognitive-behavioral therapy programs. So it should not be surprising that these patients are frustrated and trying to prove that they really have something wrong with them when they come in to see us. (Clauw 2007, p. 107)

A meta-analysis of antidepressants published in 2000 found 13 trials with evaluable data involving three classes of antidepressants: TCAs (9 trials), SSRIs (3 trials), and S-adenosyl-L-methionine (2 trials) (O'Malley et al. 2000). Overall, antidepressants were superior to placebo, with an NNT of 4. The effect sizes for pain, fatigue, sleep, and overall well-being were all moderate (range = 0.39–0.52). In the 5 studies where there was adequate assessment for treatment response independent of depression, only 1 study found a correlation between symptom improvement and depression scores. Antidepressant class did not make a difference, although only 3 trials tested SSRIs. Since this meta-analysis, 2 more trials of SSRIs in fibromyalgia have been published: a flexible-dose trial showing that fluoxetine (mean dosage = 45 mg/day) was superior to placebo in 60 women (Arnold et al. 2002), and an inconclusive trial of citalopram in 40 patients (Anderberg et al. 2000). There is more conclusive evidence for TCAs in treating fibromyalgia than for SSRIs; however, evidence for the superiority of TCAs compared with SSRIs in treating this condition is not as convincing as the evidence for their superiority in treating neuropathic pain.

A meta-analysis of 4 trials found that cyclobenzaprine (10–40 mg/day) was also superior to placebo (Arnold et al. 2000). Again, this is not surprising, given that its structure and pharmacological properties are quite similar to those of the TCAs. Finally, 2 trials—with 100 patients (Russell et al. 2000) and 313 patients (Bennett et al. 2003), respectively—showed that tramadol was superior to placebo in treating fibromyalgia, although the largest trial combined tramadol with acetaminophen.

The most research in terms of pharmacotherapy for fibromyalgia over the past 5 years has involved the SNRI antidepressants and the $\alpha_2\delta$-ligand anticonvulsants (Table 66–5). Pregabalin, duloxetine, and milnacipran have each proven effective in several positive Phase III RCTs (Arnold et al. 2004, 2005, 2007b; Clauw et al. 2007a, 2007b; Crofford et al. 2005; Gendreau et al. 2005; Russell

TABLE 66–5.   Efficacy of SNRI antidepressants and anticonvulsants in fibromyalgia: summary of randomized, placebo-controlled clinical trials

Drug	Study	N	Study duration (weeks)	Primary endpoint	Beneficial?
Pregabalin[a]	Crofford et al. 2005	529	8	Mean pain score	Yes
Pregabalin[a]	Arnold et al. 2007c[b]	750	14	Mean pain score	Yes
Duloxetine[a]	Arnold et al. 2004	207	12	Fibromyalgia Impact Questionnaire (total and pain scores)	Yes
Duloxetine[a]	Arnold et al. 2005	354	12	Brief Pain Inventory (average pain severity)	Yes
Duloxetine[a]	Russell et al. 2008	520	26	Brief Pain Inventory (average pain severity) Patient Global-Rated Improvement	Yes
Milnacipran	Gendreau et al. 2005	125	12	Pain intensity (pain diary) Average daily pain score	Yes
Milnacipran	Clauw et al. 2007b[b]	888	24	Composite (pain severity plus global improvement plus physical function)	Yes
Milnacipran	Clauw et al. 2007a[b]	1,196	24	Composite (pain severity plus global improvement)	Yes
Gabapentin	Arnold et al. 2007a	150	12	Brief Pain Inventory (average pain severity)	Yes

Note.   SNRI = serotonin–norepinephrine reuptake inhibitor.
[a]Pregabalin and duloxetine are U.S. Food and Drug Administration (FDA)–approved for the treatment of fibromyalgia. It is expected that applications for FDA approval of milnacipran will be submitted in 2009.
[b]Presented in abstract form but not yet published.

et al. 2008). Pregabalin and duloxetine are the first FDA-approved drugs for the treatment of fibromyalgia, and the makers of milnacipran will be seeking approval. Gabapentin, another $\alpha_2\delta$-ligand, has been evaluated in a single trial, the results of which were positive (Arnold et al. 2007a). Another SNRI, venlafaxine, was tested in a low-dose trial (75 mg/day) and did not differ in efficacy from placebo (Zijlstra et al. 2002). Certainly, the strongest evidence exists for pregabalin, duloxetine, and milnacipran. Pregabalin and duloxetine (as well as milnacipran if FDA approval is obtained) could be considered first-line pharmacotherapies for fibromyalgia, along with TCAs, cyclobenzaprine, and tramadol. Given their longer track record, evidence of efficacy, and low cost, TCAs or cyclobenzaprine might be tried initially, assuming that the patient does not have any contraindications. Tramadol could be a second-line choice, although the fact that it is a weak opioid should be taken into consideration. Generic gabapentin and venlafaxine would be less expensive than the other drugs shown in Table 66–5, although there is only a single trial supporting the use of gabapentin and no positive RCT results for venlafaxine.

In the Phase III trials summarized in Table 66–5, pregabalin dosages were 300–450 mg/day (divided into twice-daily doses), duloxetine dosages were 60–120 mg once a day, and milnacipran dosages were 100–200 mg once a day. In all trials, the difference in efficacy between the highest and lowest dosages of each drug was small to minimal, whereas side-effect rates increased somewhat at higher dosages. Thus, the majority of fibromyalgia patients who respond to these drugs will do so with 300 mg of pregabalin, 60 mg of duloxetine, or 100 mg of milnacipran per day. The most bothersome side effect of duloxetine and of milnacipran (as well as venlafaxine) is nausea, which may be lessened by starting therapy at lower dosages (e.g., duloxetine 30 mg/day or venlafaxine 37.5 mg/day) for the first 1–2 weeks and by taking the drug with food. The most bothersome side effects with pregabalin and gabapentin are somnolence (which often improves with treatment and may be reduced by using low initial doses and having the patient take the only dose or the highest dose at bedtime), dizziness, and weight gain.

Nonpharmacological Treatment

More than with most other pain disorders, nonpharmacological treatment for fibromyalgia is especially important, and few patients should be treated with medication only. Several systematic reviews have shown that the three treatments with the most evidence of efficacy are exercise (particularly aerobic exercise), education about fibromyalgia (either individually or in groups), and CBT (Goldenberg et al. 2004; Henningsen et al. 2007; Sim and Adams 2002; van Koulil et al. 2007). A systematic review of 34 RCTs (involving 2,276 subjects) evaluated exercise in fibromyalgia and found that aerobic-only exercise had moderate positive effects on global well-being (effect size, 0.49), physical function (effect size, 0.66), and pain (effect size, 0.65) (Busch et al. 2007). Strength and flexibility exercises were underevaluated. A review of 8 RCTs of balneotherapy (pool exercise) also showed beneficial results in fibromyalgia (Gowans and deHueck 2007), and this may be an alternative as an initial form of exercise for individuals with arthritis, to reduce weight bearing on arthritic joints, or for patients who fear exercise will exacerbate their pain. Seven RCTs of CBT (2 of which also included exercise) involving a total of 595 patients showed benefits for CBT in 5 of the 7 trials (van Koulil et al. 2007). Education about fibromyalgia has been studied in numerous trials, both individually and coupled with one or more other interventions, and appears to have a positive effect (Goldenberg et al. 2004; Sim and Adams 2002). Education coupled with exercise seems a particularly valuable bundled intervention (Burckhardt 2006; Karjalainen et al. 2000; Rooks et al. 2007). Educational and self-management resources are readily available online from organizations like the National Fibromyalgia Association, the American College of Rheumatology, and the Arthritis Foundation. Finally, there are insufficient data to recommend acupuncture, chiropractic therapy, massage therapy, trigger point injections, or other nonpharmacological or CAM treatments for fibromyalgia

(Goldenberg et al. 2004; Henningsen et al. 2007; Mayhew and Ernst 2007; Sim and Adams 2002; Tan et al. 2007).

Low Back Pain

A series of systematic reviews by Chou and colleagues (Chou and Huffman 2007a, 2007b; Chou et al. 2007b) provides a comprehensive update on the evaluation and management of low back pain. The authors describe the burden of back pain:

> Low back pain is the fifth most common reason for all physician office visits in the U.S. and the second most common symptomatic reason. Approximately one quarter of U.S. adults reported having low back pain lasting at least 1 whole day in the past 3 months, and 7.6% reported at least 1 episode of severe acute low back pain within a 1-year period. Low back pain is also very costly: Total incremental direct health care costs attributable to low back pain in the U.S. were estimated at $26.3 billion in 1998. In addition, indirect costs related to days lost from work are substantial, with approximately 2% of the U.S. work force compensated for back injuries each year. (Chou et al. 2007b, p. 478)

The authors go on to describe several other key points relevant to the clinical epidemiology of low back pain. Most low back pain (85%) is nonspecific—that is, it cannot be attributed to a specific disease or spinal abnormality. Classification schemes frequently conflict with one another, and there is little evidence that labeling patients by using specific anatomical diagnoses improves outcomes. In a primary care setting, low back pain is only occasionally caused by a specific serious disorder, such as cancer (0.7% of cases), compression fracture (4%), or spinal infection (0.01%). The estimated prevalence of ankylosing spondylitis in primary care patients ranges from 0.3% to 5%. Spinal stenosis and symptomatic herniated disc are present in about 3% and 4% of patients, respectively. The cauda equina syndrome, due to massive midline disc herniation, is very rare (occurring in 0.04% of patients with low back pain). Urinary retention is 90% sensitive, and the probability of the cauda equina syndrome in back pain patients without urinary retention is approximately 1 in 10,000. The probability of cancer in patients presenting with back pain increases from approximately 0.7% to 9% in patients with a history of cancer (not including nonmelanoma skin cancer). In patients with any one of three other risk factors (unexplained weight loss, failure to improve after 1 month, and age >50 years), the likelihood of cancer only increases to approximately 1.2%.

TABLE 66–6.   Key aspects of evaluation and management of low back pain

Most back pain (>70%–80%) improves in the first 2–6 weeks. Thus, a 4-week wait (i.e., a conservative approach) is warranted (even with sciatica) in the absence of red flags.

Red flags that may prompt earlier diagnostic testing or referral include the following:
  Cancer: history of cancer (strong predictor) or unexplained weight loss, failure to improve after 4 weeks, and age greater than 50 years (all weaker predictors)
  Infection (vertebral): fever, intravenous drug use, recent infection (none well studied)
  Compression fracture: older age, osteoporosis, steroid use
  Cauda equina syndrome rare (0.04%); urinary retention 90% sensitive.

Physical examination focuses on a few cardinal neurological parts of the lower-body exam:
  Straight-leg raising (SLR) in which the hip is flexed while the knee remains extended. Ipsilateral-positive SLR is 91% sensitive but only 26% specific for radiculopathy, whereas a crossed-positive SLR (i.e., sciatica in the other leg) is only 29% sensitive but 88% specific.
  Lower-extremity motor and sensory exam:
    Knee strength and reflexes (L4 nerve root); screen with squat and rise
    Great toe and foot dorsiflexion strength (L5 nerve root); screen with heel walking
    Foot plantar-flexion and ankle reflexes (S1 nerve root); screen with walking on toes

Diagnostic tests are needed in only a minority of cases (with red flags or persistent neurological signs).
  MRI is the preferred imaging study (less radiation and better visualization of soft tissue, vertebral marrow, and the spinal canal).
  With some weaker red flags (e.g., age >50 years), plain films and ESR may be obtained first and MRI obtained only if these tests are abnormal or symptoms persist.

Psychological factors are a stronger predictor of chronicity and functional outcomes such as disability than physical exam findings or the severity or duration of pain.

Treatment: No treatment for back pain has good-quality (grade A) evidence of substantial benefit. The following have fair-quality (grade B) evidence of moderate benefit or small benefits but no significant harm, costs, or burdens:
  Pharmacotherapy: acetaminophen, NSAIDs, TCAs, tramadol/opiates, benzodiazepines
  Nonpharmacological: chiropractic, acupuncture, massage, yoga, exercise, progressive relaxation, cognitive-behavioral therapy, intensive interdisciplinary rehabilitation

Note.   ESR = erythrocyte sedimentation rate; MRI = magnetic resonance imaging; NSAIDs = nonsteroidal anti-inflammatory drugs; TCAs = tricyclic antidepressants.

Table 66–6 outlines some key recommendations with respect to the evaluation and management of low back pain. In the absence of red flags, a conservative approach for at least 4 weeks is usually warranted, even if sciatica is present. Magnetic resonance imaging is the preferred imaging procedure but can be reserved for the minority of patients with red flags or persistent symptoms, especially neurological findings. The two most common indications for surgery are herniated disc with persistent symptoms (especially radiculopathy) and spinal stenosis, which together account for less than 10% of cases of chronic back pain. Recent trial data suggest that surgery may be only marginally beneficial for pain due to a herniated disc but more helpful for spinal stenosis (Weinstein et al. 2006, 2008). Psychological factors are stronger predictors of low back pain treatment outcomes than either physical examination findings or the severity or duration of pain. Psychosocial factors that may predict poorer low back pain outcomes include presence of depression, passive coping strategies, job dissatisfaction, higher disability levels, disputed compensation claims, and somatization.

Medications are the most frequently recommended intervention for low back pain. The most commonly prescribed medications for low back pain are NSAIDs, skeletal muscle relaxants, and opioid analgesics (Chou and Huffman 2007a). Benzodiazepines, systemic corticosteroids, antidepressant medications, and antiepileptic drugs are also prescribed. Frequently used over-the-counter medications include acetaminophen, aspirin, and certain NSAIDs. No treatments for back pain have grade A evidence supporting their use—that is, good-quality evidence of substantial benefits. Table 66–6 summarizes treatments with grade B evidence. For pharmacotherapy, this includes acetaminophen, NSAIDs, tramadol, and TCAs. For all medications, the evidence of beneficial effects on functional outcomes is limited. Skeletal muscle relaxants, which may be beneficial for acute back pain, do not have established efficacy for chronic pain. Although systematic reviews of opioids for various chronic pain conditions have shown moderate benefits, the evidence for opioids specifically for low back pain is sparse and inconclusive (Martell et al. 2007). A recent prospective study found that early prescription of opioids for acute occupational low back injury was associated with an increased risk of work disability at 1 year, even after adjustment for severity of pain, function, and initial injury (Franklin et al. 2008). A systematic review of 25 trials involving 2,206 patients found no benefits for either continuous or intermittent traction in the treatment of low back pain (Clarke et al. 2007). There is also good evidence that systemic corticosteroids are ineffective for low back pain with or without sciatica. One systematic review identified only 7 trials evaluating medications for sciatica (Vroomen et al. 2000). Two small trials suggest that gabapentin may be useful in the subset of patients with radiculopathy.

Ten trials were included in two systematic reviews of antidepressants (Salerno et al. 2002; Staiger et al. 2003). In all of the trials, the duration of therapy ranged from 4 to 8 weeks. Antidepressants were consistently superior to placebo for pain relief, whereas the benefits in terms of functional outcomes were uncertain. The pooled effect size for pain relief was moderate (0.41). Indirect comparisons suggested modest benefits with TCAs but not with paroxetine or trazodone. A recent review did not identify any relevant trials in back pain for SNRI antidepressants such as duloxetine or venlafaxine (Chou and Huffman 2007a).

Osteoarthritis

Osteoarthritis is one of the most common musculoskeletal pain disorders (along with low back pain and fibromyalgia) in both primary care and specialty settings. It typically increases with age (particularly after age 50), with the majority of individuals older than 65 years having at least one joint affected by osteoarthritis. Common joints involve the distal and proximal interphalangeal (but not metacarpal) joints of the fingers, the base of the thumb, the knees, the hips, and the cervical and lumbar regions of the spine. The shoulder and elbow are rarely involved. The most common finding on physical examination is an increase in joint size secondary to osteophyte formation. Plain radiographs are typically the only diagnostic test required to confirm the diagnosis of osteoarthritis, which is manifested by loss of joint space and/or osteophyte formation.

Unlike in rheumatoid arthritis and other inflammatory types of arthritis, the structural changes in osteoarthritis are not amenable to specific disease-modifying treatments. Thus, the focus of treatment in osteoarthritis is reduction of pain and preservation of function. Acetaminophen and NSAIDs, which are inexpensive and available without a prescription, are the mainstays of pharmacotherapy. A systematic review of 13 trials in patients with osteoarthritis of the knee found that both aerobic exercise and home-based quadriceps-strengthening exercise reduced pain (effect size, 0.52 and 0.39, respectively) and disability (effect size, 0.46 and 0.32) (Roddy et al. 2005). Benefits of aerobic and strengthening exercises in osteoarthritis patients were confirmed in a second systematic review (Brosseau et al. 2003). For advanced disease with progressive pain and functional impairment, total hip arthroplasty and knee arthroplasty are effective. In contrast, a systematic review of 23 studies found inconclusive evidence for the benefits of arthroscopic lavage and/or debridement in knee osteoarthritis (Samson et al. 2007). Glucosamine, chondroitin, and intra-articular hyaluronic acid have been the most popular CAM treatments for osteoarthritis, but 4 systematic reviews as well as an overall review (Table 66–7) found that the evidence regarding the efficacy of each of these three treatments is still inconclusive (Arrich et al. 2005; Distler and Anguelouch 2006; Reichenbach et al. 2007; Samson et al. 2007; Vlad et al. 2007).

Avouac et al. (2007) conducted a meta-analysis of trials evaluating opioid therapy in osteoarthritis patients. Of the 18 placebo-controlled trials, 13 assessed pain intensity for 2,438 participants receiving opioids and 1,295 receiving placebo. Six studies evaluated stronger opioids (oxycodone in 4 studies, fentanyl and morphine in 1 study each) and 7 studies examined weaker opioids (tramadol in 4 studies, tramadol–acetaminophen combination in 2 studies, and codeine in 1 study). The median trial duration was 12 weeks. The pooled effect size for pain intensity was moderate, at −0.79 (95% CI = −0.98 to −0.59). Sensitivity analysis showed no changes in the conclusions by type of opioid studied, type of scale used to assess pain, or methodological quality of the study. Physical function was assessed in 5 trials, with 1,429 participants receiving opioids (tramadol–acetaminophen in 2 studies; morphine, tramadol, and codeine in 1 study each) and 595 receiving placebo. The median trial duration was 4 weeks. The pooled effect size for physical function was small, at −0.31 (95% CI = −0.39 to −0.24). Again, sensitivity analyses did not change the conclusions. The average treatment discontinuation rate for toxicity was 25% in the opioid group (31% for strong opioids and 19% for weak opioids) versus 7% in the placebo group.

Unlike the many trials of antidepressants for neuropathic pain, fibromyalgia, and chronic low back pain, antidepressants have not been well studied as a treatment

TABLE 66–7.   Glucosamine, chondroitin, and hyaluronic acid for osteoarthritis (OA): summary of systematic reviews

TREATMENT	STUDY	CONDITION	REVIEW TYPE	BENEFITS	STRENGTH OF EVIDENCE	COMMENTS
Glucosamine	Vlad et al. 2007	Knee or hip OA	Meta-analysis (15 trials, 2,825 patients)	Not known	Moderate	Glucosamine hydrochloride (three trials) did not have a significant effect size (0.06), but glucosamine sulfate (12 trials) did (0.44). However, large heterogeneity among trials made conclusions about efficacy uncertain.
Chondroitin	Reichenbach et al. 2007	Knee or hip OA	Meta-analysis (20 trials, 3,846 patients)	No	Moderate	Minimal to no effect on symptoms. Only three large high-quality trials, which accounted for 40% of patients.
Glucosamine and/ or chondroitin	Distler and Anguelouch 2006	Knee or hip OA	Review of prior reviews	No	Moderate	Review of four prior meta-analyses and large GAIT trial concluded that neither glucosamine nor chondroitin is effective in OA.
Glucosamine and/ or chondroitin	Samson et al. 2007	Knee OA	Systematic (21 trials)	Not known	Moderate	Evidence from small trials inconclusive. The GAIT study in 1,583 patients showed no difference from placebo.
Hyaluronic acid (intra-articular)	Arrich et al. 2005	Knee OA	Meta-analysis (22 trials)	No	Moderate	Small but clinically insignificant effect on pain. Only four high-quality trials.
Hyaluronic acid (intra-articular)	Samson et al. 2007	Knee OA	Systematic (42 trials)	Not known	Moderate	Generally some modest benefits compared with placebo but unclear clinical significance.

Note.   GAIT = Glucosamine–Chondroitin Arthritis Intervention Trial.

for the pain of osteoarthritis. However, recent studies have shown that when depression co-occurs with arthritis, it can explain as much of the variance in pain intensity as objective severity of the arthritis (Katon et al. 2007). Also, RCTs have shown that treatment of depression in arthritis patients may reduce pain as well as depression (Bair et al. 2008; E.H. Lin et al. 2003). Thus, while antidepressants cannot currently be recommended in osteoarthritis patients without depression, screening for and comanaging depression may benefit patients in their pain outcomes.

Algorithmic Approach to Treatment of Chronic Pain

This chapter focuses on the main classes of treatments for chronic pain, with a particular emphasis on pharmacotherapy but also briefer synopses of nonpharmacological treatments. Four of the most common disorders in which pain is a predominant treatment target are discussed: neuropathic pain, fibromyalgia, low back pain, and osteoarthritis. Acute pain and cancer pain are not specifically addressed, nor are two other common sources of chronic pain—headache and regional pain syndromes—reviewed. Based on our reviews within these parameters, an evidence-based algorithm for treating pain is summarized in Figure 66–1.

Other Issues

Treatment of Pain Comorbid With Depression or Anxiety

As mentioned earlier, there is substantial evidence for a pain-depression dyad and probably a pain–depression–anxiety triad (see "Psychiatric Comorbidity"). The comorbidity among these disorders ranges from 30% to 60%, and they have reciprocal adverse effects on quality of life, disability, health care use, and treatment response. In particular, the presence of pain negatively affects depression outcomes, while depression in turn makes pain treatments less effective. Anxiety may have a similar effect, although the research in this area is less substantial than for depression.

Several trials have shown that depression treatment also benefits patients in pain outcomes, although the effect size for pain is only about half that for depression (Bair et al. 2008; Greco et al. 2004; E.H. Lin et al. 2003).

Until more trials are conducted in those with depression and comorbid pain, several suggestions may be considered. First, pain should be asked about when treating depressed or anxious patients, particularly in those who are not achieving remission or optimal responses. Likewise, psychiatric screening should be considered in patients with persistent pain, possibly with brief measures that screen for both depression and anxiety (Kroenke et al., in press). Second, it may be that antidepressant selection is important when pain is a major problem. For some types of pain conditions, TCAs and SNRI antidepressants appear to be more effective than SSRI or other antidepressants, although head-to-head trials are still few. Third, adding CBT, PSM (pain self-management) programs, or other nonpharmacological treatments proven effective for pain could be considered. Fourth, optimizing analgesic management in patients with depression and pain, rather than simply focusing on depression medications, may be important. Increasingly, we may need to consider pain and depression as dual diagnoses, where attention to both is necessary to optimize patients' outcomes.

Placebo Effect

As with other symptom-based conditions (e.g., depression, anxiety, somatoform disorders), pain has a placebo response in the 30%–40% range or higher. This can make it challenging to separate the specific effects of a pain treatment—medication or nonpharmacological—from placebo or other nonspecific effects. Furthermore, it means that the more successful a trial is in masking the patient to active versus control treatment (typically greatest in a placebo-controlled drug trial), the lower the estimated differences from placebo are likely to be. In contrast, less effective masking (e.g., attention–placebo control groups for psychotherapy or behavioral interventions, sham procedures for acupuncture or chiropractic manipulation) or nonexistent masking (e.g., wait-list or treatment-as-usual control groups) are more likely to overestimate the effect of a pain treatment.

At the same time, the role of placebo effects on pain outcomes can be useful in clinical practice, including patient expectancy for an analgesic outcome and the clinical benefits of a positive therapeutic relationship. Pain is the most frequent reason for seeking CAM care (Astin 1998). Although evidence for several CAM treatments may still be lacking, their placebo effects coupled with frustration among many allopathic physicians and patients in the context of chronic pain may account for the popularity of CAM treatments for pain.

Step 1: Does the patient have: (1) neuropathic pain, (2) fibromyalgia/chronic widespread pain, or (3) back pain?
- <u>Yes:</u> Start TCA and simple analgesics
- <u>No:</u> Go to simple analgesic algorithm

TCAs: try at least two before considering a failure
1. Amitriptyline, start at 10–25, titrate to 100 mg (max 50 mg if taking an SSRI/SNRI)
2. Nortriptyline, start at 10–25, titrate to 100 mg (max 50 mg if taking an SSRI/SNRI)

Simple analgesics
1. Acetaminophen 1,000 mg q6h (max 2,000 mg if cirrhosis or ≥ 3 alcoholic drinks/day)
2. NSAIDs: try at least 2;
   a. First line: naproxen 500 mg q12h or 500 q am plus 250 bid (max 1,000)(114; 117; 126)
   b. Second line: 1) salsalate 1,000 mg q8h or 1,500 mg q12h (max 3,000 mg/day); 2) etodolac 300 mg q8h or 500 mg q12h (max 1,000 mg/day); 3 ibuprofen 600 mg q6h (max 2,400 mg/day); 4) diclofenac 50 mg q8h (max 150 mg/day)
3. Adjunct: Consider topical analgesic if neuropathic pain or localized musculoskeletal pain (e.g., knee osteoarthritis). For example, capsaicin cream applied 4 times a day for at least 3–4 weeks

Step 2: Tramadol
1. Start 25 mg BID or TID and titrate to 100 mg QID (max 300 mg if age > 75; max 100 mg BID if CrCl < 30, 50 mg BID if CrCl < 10; max 50 mg BID if cirrhosis)
2. Use concurrent acetaminophen, 500–1,000 mg dosed with tramadol TID-QID (or an NSAID)

Step 3

- **Neuropathic pain**
  1. Gabapentin, titrate up to 900–1,200 tid
  2. Duloxetine (60 mg qd) or Pregabalin (300–450 mg qd, divided into bid doses)
  3. If neuropathic pain involves focal area: Lidocaine 5% patch (maximum, 3 patches)
  4. Go to opioid algorithm

- **Fibromyalgia/chronic widespread pain**
  1. Cyclobenzaprine, titrate to 10 mg TID
  2. Pregabalin (300–450 mg qd, divided into bid doses) or Duloxetine (60 mg qd)
  3. If FDA approval is obtained: Milnacipran 100 mg qd)

- **Musculoskeletal pain:** Go to opioid algorithm in step 4

Step 4: Opioids
1. Acetaminophen/codeine
2. Acetaminophen/hydrocodone
3. Acetaminophen/oxycodone
4. Morphine SR
5. Fentanyl patch
6. Methadone

Nonpharmacological treatments can be considered at any step. Ones that have proven effective in several types of pain conditions include: exercise, cognitive-behavioral therapy, pain self-management, and acupuncture.

FIGURE 66–1.   Analgesic algorithm for chronic pain.

Algorithm for an evidence-based approach to treatment selection in the management of chronic pain. Nonpharmacological treatments can be considered at any step; ones that have proven effective in several types of pain conditions include exercise, cognitive-behavioral therapy, pain self-management, and acupuncture. CrCl = creatinine clearance; FDA = U.S. Food and Drug Administration; max = maximum; NSAID = nonsteroidal anti-inflammatory drug; SNRI = serotonin–norepinephrine reuptake inhibitor; SR = sustained release; SSRI = selective serotonin reuptake inhibitor; TCAs = tricyclic antidepressants.

Experimental work has also revealed some interesting physiological effects of placebo. A meta-analysis of 12 studies (1,183 participants) was conducted to examine the effects of placebo and an opioid antagonist, naloxone, on pain (Sauro and Greenberg 2005). Placebo adminis- tration was associated with a decrease in self-reported pain, and a hidden or blind injection of naloxone re- versed placebo-induced analgesia. A recent experimental study in 20 healthy subjects found that the placebo and nocebo effects (i.e., the therapeutic and adverse effects, respectively, of inert substances or sham procedures) are associated with opposite responses of dopaminergic and endogenous opioid neurotransmission in a distributed network of regions throughout the brain (Scott et al. 2008). The results support other literature showing that the belief in and expectation of analgesia induce discrete physiological changes, leading to relief from pain, and this response may be mediated by endogenous opioids.

Assessment and Monitoring of Pain

Clinical trials have often used a wide variety of pain measures in assessing outcomes, and until recently, consensus has been lacking on a standard or optimal approach. This is not unlike other psychiatric disorders or symptom-based conditions where patient-reported measures are necessary to assess clinical outcomes, in contrast to disorders where a universally agreed-on physical measure (e.g., blood pressure) or laboratory test (e.g., for serum cholesterol levels) is the criterion standard. In a review of pain clinical trials published in seven top-tier medical journals in 2003, a total of 50 studies used 28 types of pain assessments (Litcher-Kelly et al. 2007). The most frequently used assessments were a single-item visual analog scale and a single-item 0–10 numeric rating scale (NRS); multidimensional inventories were used infrequently.

Inadequate pain assessment has been identified as a key barrier to appropriate pain management. Important initiatives have aimed to increase awareness of pain as a clinical problem by promoting better pain assessment. The U.S. Department of Veterans Affairs (VA) campaign promoting "pain as the fifth vital sign" requires all VA facilities to assess patients using an NRS of 0–10 for current pain. Even more far-reaching, the Joint Commission on Accreditation of Healthcare Organizations (2000) pain assessment and management standards, implemented in 2001, require accredited health care facilities to assess all patients for pain in both inpatient and ambulatory care settings. Although Joint Commission standards do not mandate a specific method of pain assessment, many organizations have responded by adopting use of an NRS of pain as the "fifth vital sign" (Dahl 2002). A verbal (interviewer-administered) and visual (self-rated) version of this single-item NRS for pain assessment is shown in Figure 66–2. As a result, assessment of current pain intensity with a single-item rating scale has become nearly ubiquitous in many U.S. health care settings. However, this movement has not led to clear improvements in the quality or outcomes of chronic pain management, and studies have shown that the NRS may not be the optimal mea-

Verbal

"On a scale of zero to ten, where zero means no pain and ten equals the worst possible pain, what is your current pain level?"

Visual

0	1	2	3	4	5	6	7	8	9	10
No pain		Mild			Moderate			Severe		Worst possible pain

FIGURE 66–2. Pain numeric rating scale (NRS). Interviewer-administered (verbal) and self-administered (visual) versions of the single-item NRS for pain, also referred to "the fifth vital sign."

sure for assessing and monitoring chronic pain in clinical practice (Krebs et al. 2007; Mularski et al. 2006). An important limitation of single-item pain measurement is that it provides an overly simplified picture of a complex subjective experience.

Recent consensus recommendations from the Initiative on Methods, Measurement, and Pain Assessment in Clinical Trials (IMMPACT) recommend four core chronic pain outcome domains for monitoring treatment response: pain intensity (i.e., severity), physical functioning (i.e., pain-specific disability), emotional functioning (largely depression), and patient-rated overall improvement (Dworkin et al. 2008). The first two domains are captured in the recently validated PEG pain scale based on three items from the Brief Pain Inventory (average pain severity, interference with enjoyment of life, and interference with general activities), shown in Figure 66–3 (Krebs et al. 2008a). For emotional functioning, a clinical or patient-rated assessment of depression is recommended. For overall improvement, the single-item Patient Global Impression of Change scale uses a seven-point rating scale with the options "very much improved," "much improved," "minimally improved," "no change," "minimally worse," "much worse," and "very much worse."

The competing demands of clinical practice in which visits are short and pain is often a secondary focus make efficiency as well as validity of assessment a paramount concern. At the same time, there must be a balance between number of items and key operating characteristics such as reliability, validity, and responsiveness to therapy. For example, "ultrabrief" depression measures containing two or three items perform better than single-item depression measures (Mitchell and Coyne 2007). In this sense, the three-item PEG may be preferable to the single item NRS, which is currently promulgated by various accrediting bodies but which has substantial limitations, as dem-

1. What number best describes your pain on average in the past week?

     0   1   2   3   4   5   6   7   8   9   10
     No | | | | | | | | | Pain as bad
     pain   as you can
                                             imagine

2. What number best describes how, during the past week, pain has interfered with your general activity?

     0   1   2   3   4   5   6   7   8   9   10
     Does not | | | | | | | | | Completely
     interfere   interferes

3. What number best describes how, during the past week, pain has interfered with your enjoyment of life?

     0   1   2   3   4   5   6   7   8   9   10
     Does not | | | | | | | | | Completely
     interfere   interferes

FIGURE 66–3. PEG three-item pain scale.

The PEG three-item pain scale—an ultrabrief measure for assessing and monitoring pain—is based on three items from the Brief Pain Inventory: average **P**ain severity, interference with **E**njoyment of life, and interference with **G**eneral activities.

Source. Krebs EE, Bair MJ, Damush TM, Sutherland JM. Used with the authors' permission.}

onstrated in two recent studies (Krebs et al. 2007; Mularski et al. 2006). Moreover, the PEG captures both the severity and the functional interference dimensions of pain, whereas the NRS captures only pain severity. This is essential in pain management because pain interference has been shown to have an even greater impact than simple severity on quality of life and other patient-centered outcomes (Von Korff et al. 1992).

Economic Issues

As mentioned in the introduction to this chapter, pain costs the United States more than $100 billion each year in health care and lost productivity (Stewart et al. 2003), and pain medications are the second most prescribed class of drugs (Turk 2002). Despite the importance of considering drug costs, a recent review of 142 chronic pain–related economic evaluations published between 1988 and 2006 found important methodological shortcomings (Vetter 2007). Only a few studies combined the economic analysis along with an RCT, the economic endpoints had limited time horizons, and there was a failure to address the protracted costs versus benefits of treating long-term and often recurrent chronic pain conditions. Unlike many cardiology and oncology trial–based economic evaluations with societal perspectives and protracted time horizons (e.g., longer-term survival or death), many of the economic analyses related to chronic

pain treatment have been restricted to a third-party insurer perspective and have used a limited time horizon of less than 1 year. For example, it is possible that a more expensive medication may be more cost-effective than a lower-cost medication if it were shown that time lost from work was less or enhancements in quality in life were greater. In an economic evaluation of controlled-release oxycodone compared with oxycodone–acetaminophen for osteoarthritis, the more costly controlled-release medication proved more effective and less costly from a societal perspective, including greater gains in quality-adjusted life years and lower costs associated with time lost from work or other activities (Marshall et al. 2006). In a similar evaluation of pregabalin versus gabapentin for neuropathic pain, the authors concluded that pregabalin was more cost-effective, costing about $15 for each additional day with no pain or only mild pain and about $600 for each additional patient with no pain or mild pain (Rodríguez et al. 2007). Both studies used simulated analyses from existing trial data rather than head-to-head comparisons in an RCT, so the conclusions must be interpreted with caution. Nonetheless, pharmacoeconomic decision making needs to incorporate not only drug costs but also differential efficacy and side effects, impacts on work and quality of life, and the adjudication of patient, insurer, employer, and societal perspectives.

Gaps in Knowledge Base Regarding Treatment of Chronic Pain

There are several important gaps in our knowledge regarding treatment that in fact are probably not unique to chronic pain. First, there is a paucity of head-to-head trials, meaning that although we can draw conclusions about the effectiveness of a particular monotherapy compared with a placebo or minimal treatment, we have much less information about the comparative effectiveness of different treatments. Second, few trials have evaluated different strategies for choosing initial treatment, so that deciding between first-line and subsequent treatments is more a matter of expert consensus, clinician experience, and patient preferences. Third, evidence is sparse on the effectiveness of dual-medication or other combination therapy versus monotherapy or sequential treatment, even though patients are frequently prescribed more than one medication or treatment. Fourth, most treatment trials have been short-term, so evidence of benefits sustained beyond 4–12 weeks is often lacking; this is a critical gap given the fact that our focus is on the management of chronic pain.

Despite these gaps, substantial evidence has accumulated over the past several decades about what works and what does not work for treating chronic pain. Avoiding ineffective treatments and maximizing the use of treatments proven beneficial in clinical trials are likely to produce better outcomes than have often been experienced by clinicians and patients in the management of chronic pain.

References

Aaron LA, Buchwald D: A review of the evidence for overlap among unexplained clinical conditions. Ann Intern Med 134:868–881, 2001

Abeles AM, Pillinger MH, Solitar BM, et al: Narrative review: the pathophysiology of fibromyalgia. Ann Intern Med 146:726–734, 2007

Adams EH, Breiner S, Cicero TJ, et al: A comparison of the abuse liability of tramadol, NSAIDs, and hydrocodone in patients with chronic pain. J Pain Symptom Manage 31:465–476, 2006

Ahles TA, Wasson JH, Seville JL, et al: A controlled trial of methods for managing pain in primary care patients with or without co-occurring psychosocial problems. Ann Fam Med 4:341–350, 2006

Allan L, Richarz U, Simpson K, et al: Transdermal fentanyl versus sustained release oral morphine in strong-opioid naive patients with chronic low back pain. Spine 30:2484–2490, 2005

Allen LA, Escobar JI, Lehrer PM, et al: Psychosocial treatments for multiple unexplained physical symptoms: a review of the literature. Psychosom Med 64:939–950, 2002

American Psychiatric Association: Diagnostic and Statistical Manual of Mental Disorders, 4th Edition, Text Revision. Washington, DC, American Psychiatric Association, 2000

Anderberg UM, Marteinsdottir I, von Knorring L: Citalopram in patients with fibromyalgia: a randomized, double-blind, placebo-controlled study. Eur J Pain 4:27–35, 2000

Ang DC, Kroenke K, McHorney CA: Impact of pain severity and location on health-related quality of life. Rheumatol Int 26:567–572, 2006

Angst MS, Clark JD: Opioid-induced hyperalgesia: a qualitative systematic review. Anesthesiology 104:570–587, 2006

Antman EM, Bennett JS, Daugherty A, et al: Use of nonsteroidal antiinflammatory drugs: an update for clinicians: a scientific statement from the American Heart Association. Circulation 115:1634–1642, 2007

Arnold LM, Keck PE Jr, Welge JA: Antidepressant treatment of fibromyalgia: a meta-analysis and review. Psychosomatics 41:104–113, 2000

Arnold LM, Hess EV, Hudson JI, et al: A randomized, placebo-controlled, double-blind, flexible-dose study of fluoxetine in the treatment of women with fibromyalgia. Am J Med 112:191–197, 2002

Arnold LM, Lu Y, Crofford LJ, et al: A double-blind, multicenter trial comparing duloxetine with placebo in the treatment of fibromyalgia patients with or without major depressive disorder. Arthritis Rheum 50:2974–2984, 2004

Arnold LM, Rosen A, Pritchett YL, et al: A randomized, double-blind, placebo-controlled trial of duloxetine in the treatment of women with fibromyalgia with or without major depressive disorder. Pain 119:5–15, 2005

Arnold LM, Goldenberg DL, Stanford SB, et al: Gabapentin in the treatment of fibromyalgia: a randomized, double-blind, placebo-controlled, multicenter trial. Arthritis Rheum 56:1336–1344, 2007a

Arnold LM, Pritchett YL, D'Souza DN, et al: Duloxetine for the treatment of fibromyalgia in women: pooled results from two randomized, placebo-controlled clinical trials. J Womens Health (Larchmt) 16:1145–1156, 2007b

Arnold L, Russell J, Duan W, et al: A 14-week, randomized, double-blind placebo-controlled, monotherapy trial of pregabalin (bid) in patients with fibromyalgia syndrome (FMS). J Pain 8:S24, 2007c

Arnow BA, Hunkeler EM, Blasey CM, et al: Comorbid depression, chronic pain, and disability in primary care. Psychosom Med 68:262–268, 2006

Arrich J, Piribauer F, Mad P, et al: Intra-articular hyaluronic acid for the treatment of osteoarthritis of the knee: systematic review and meta-analysis. CMAJ 172:1039–1043, 2005

Astin JA: Why patients use alternative medicine: results of a national study. JAMA 279:1548–1553, 1998

Attal N, Cruccu G, Haanpaa M, et al: EFNS guidelines on pharmacological treatment of neuropathic pain. Eur J Neurol 13:1153–1169, 2006

Avouac J, Gossec L, Dougados M: Efficacy and safety of opioids for osteoarthritis: a meta-analysis of randomized controlled trials. Osteoarthr Cartil 15:957–965, 2007

Bair MJ, Robinson RL, Katon W, et al: Depression and pain comorbidity: a literature review. Arch Intern Med 163:2433–2445, 2003

Bair MJ, Robinson RL, Eckert GJ, et al: Impact of pain on depression treatment response in primary care. Psychosom Med 66:17–22, 2004

Bair MJ, Richardson KM, Dobscha SK, et al: Chronic pain management guidelines: a systematic review of content and strength of evidence (abstract). J Gen Intern Med 20 (suppl 1):62, 2005

Bair MJ, Damush TM, Wu J, et al: Optimizing antidepressant therapy in primary care patients with musculoskeletal pain and depression: a randomized controlled trial. J Gen Intern Med 23:353–354, 2008

Ballantyne JC: Opioids for chronic nonterminal pain. South Med J 99:1245–1255, 2006

Ballantyne JC, Mao J: Opioid therapy for chronic pain. N Engl J Med 349:1943–1953, 2003

Barden J, Edwards JE, McQuay HJ, et al: Pain and analgesic response after third molar extraction and other postsurgical pain. Pain 107:86–90, 2004

Barlow JH, Turner AP, Wright CC: Long-term outcomes of an arthritis self-management programme. Br J Rheumatol 37:1315–1319, 1998

Basbaum A, Bushnell C, Devor M: Pain: basic mechanisms, in Pain 2005—An Updated Review: Refresher Course Syllabus. Edited by Justins DM. Seattle, WA, IASP Press, 2005, pp 3–18

Beaulieu P, Ware M: Reassessment of the role of cannabinoids in the management of pain. Curr Opin Anaesthesiol 20:473–477, 2007

Bennett RM, Kamin M, Karim R, et al: Tramadol and acetaminophen combination tablets in the treatment of fibromyalgia pain: a double-blind, randomized, placebo-controlled study. Am J Med 114:537–545, 2003

Black DR, Sang CN: Advances and limitations in the evaluation of analgesic combination therapy. Neurology 65 (suppl):S3–S6, 2005

Bradley LA, Alberts KR: Psychological and behavioral approaches to pain management for patients with rheumatic disease. Rheum Dis Clin North Am 25:215–232, viii, 1999

Brannan SK, Mallinckrodt CH, Brown EB, et al: Duloxetine 60 mg once-daily in the treatment of painful physical symptoms in patients with major depressive disorder. J Psychiatr Res 39:43–53, 2005

Brecht S, Courtecuisse C, Debieuvre C, et al: Efficacy and safety of duloxetine 60 mg once daily in the treatment of pain in patients with major depressive disorder and at least moderate pain of unknown etiology: a randomized controlled trial. J Clin Psychiatry 68:1707–1716, 2007

Breivik H: International Association for the Study of Pain: update on WHO-IASP activities. J Pain Symptom Manage 24:97–101, 2002

Brosseau L, MacLeay L, Robinson V, et al: Intensity of exercise for the treatment of osteoarthritis. Cochrane Database Syst Rev (2):CD004259, 2003

Buntin-Mushock C, Phillip L, Moriyama K, et al: Age-dependent opioid escalation in chronic pain patients. Anesth Analg 100:1740–1745, 2005

Burckhardt CS: Multidisciplinary approaches for management of fibromyalgia. Curr Pharm Des 12:59–66, 2006

Busch AJ, Barber KA, Overend TJ, et al: Exercise for treating fibromyalgia syndrome. Cochrane Database Syst Rev (3):CD003786, 2007

Chodosh J, Ferrell BA, Shekelle PG, et al: Quality indicators for pain management in vulnerable elders. Ann Intern Med 135:731–735, 2001

Chong MS, Hester J: Diabetic painful neuropathy: current and future treatment options. Drugs 67:569–585, 2007

Chou R: Drug class review on long-acting opioid analgesics. Final report. Portland, OR, Oregon Health and Science University, 2008. Available at: http://www.ohsu.edu/ohsuedu/research/policycenter/DERP/about/final-products.cfm. Accessed December 16, 2008.

Chou R, Huffman LH: Medications for acute and chronic low back pain: a review of the evidence for an American Pain Society/American College of Physicians clinical practice guideline. Ann Intern Med 147:505–514, 2007a

Chou R, Huffman LH: Nonpharmacologic therapies for acute and chronic low back pain: a review of the evidence for an American Pain Society/American College of Physicians clinical practice guideline. Ann Intern Med 147:492–504, 2007b

Chou R, Peterson K: Drug class review on skeletal muscle relaxants. Portland, OR, Oregon Health and Science University, 2005. Final report. Available at: http://www.ohsu.edu/ohsuedu/research/policycenter/customcf/derp/product/SMR_Final_Report_Update%2022.pdf. Accessed December 16, 2008.

Chou R, Helfand M, Peterson K, et al: Drug class review on cyclooxygenase (COX)–2 inhibitors and nonsteroidal anti-inflammatory drugs (NSAIDs). Final report update 3. Portland, OR, Oregon Health and Science University, 2006. Available at: http://www.ohsu.edu/ohsuedu/research/policycenter/custom

cf/derp/product/NSAIDS_Final_Report_Update%203.pdf. Accessed December 16, 2008.

Chou R, Norris SL, Carson S, et al: Drug class review on drugs for neuropathic pain. Final report. Portland, OR: Oregon Health and Science University, 2007a. Available at: http://www.ohsu.edu/ohsuedu/research/policycenter/customcf/derp/product/NP_Final_Report_Original.pdf. Accessed December 16, 2008.

Chou R, Qaseem A, Snow V, et al: Diagnosis and treatment of low back pain: a joint clinical practice guideline from the American College of Physicians and the American Pain Society. Ann Intern Med 147:478–491, 2007b

Clarke JA, van Tulder MW, Blomberg SE, et al: Traction for low-back pain with or without sciatica. Cochrane Database Syst Rev (2):CD003010, 2007

Clauw DJ: Fibromyalgia: update on mechanisms and management. J Clin Rheumatol 13:102–109, 2007

Clauw DJ, Palmer RH, Thacker K, et al: Milnacipran efficacy in the treatment of fibromyalgia syndrome: a 15-week, randomized, double-blind, placebo-controlled trial (abstract). Arthritis Rheum 56:4231, 2007a

Clauw DJ, Palmer RH, Vitton O, et al: The efficacy and safety of milnacipran in the treatment of fibromyalgia (abstract). Arthritis Rheum 56:4231, 2007b

Cohen J: Statistical Power Analysis for the Behavioral Sciences. Hillsdale, NJ, Lawrence Erlbaum, 1998

Cohen JL, Sauter SV, deVellis RF, et al: Evaluation of arthritis self-management courses led by laypersons and by professionals. Arthritis Rheum 29:388–393, 1986

Crofford LJ, Rowbotham MC, Mease PJ, et al: Pregabalin for the treatment of fibromyalgia syndrome: results of a randomized, double-blind, placebo-controlled trial. Arthritis Rheum 52:1264–1273, 2005

Curatolo M, Bogduk N: Pharmacologic pain treatment of musculoskeletal disorders: current perspectives and future prospects. Clin J Pain 17:25–32, 2001

Dahl JL: Working with regulators to improve the standard of care in pain management: the U.S. experience. J Pain Symptom Manage 24:136–146, 2002

Damush TM, Weinberger M, Perkins SM, et al: Randomized trial of a self-management program for primary care patients with acute low back pain: short-term effects. Arthritis Rheum 49:179–186, 2003

Daniell HW: Hypogonadism in men consuming sustained-action oral opioids. J Pain 3:377–384, 2002

Daniell HW: Opioid endocrinopathy in women consuming prescribed sustained-action opioids for control of nonmalignant pain. J Pain 9:28–36, 2008

Demyttenaere K, Bonnewyn A, Bruffaerts R, et al: Comorbid painful physical symptoms and depression: prevalence, work loss, and help seeking. J Affect Disord 92:185–193, 2006

Devulder J, Richarz U, Nataraja SH: Impact of long-term use of opioids on quality of life in patients with chronic, non-malignant pain. Curr Med Res Opin 21:1555–1568, 2005

Distler J, Anguelouch A: Evidence-based practice: review of clinical evidence on the efficacy of glucosamine and chondroitin in the treatment of osteoarthritis. J Am Acad Nurse Pract 18:487–493, 2006

Dixon KE, Keefe FJ, Scipio CD, et al: Psychological interventions for arthritis pain management in adults: a meta-analysis. Health Psychol 26:241–250, 2007

Dworkin RH, O'Connor AB, Backonja M, et al: Pharmacologic management of neuropathic pain: evidence-based recommendations. Pain 132:237–251, 2007

Dworkin RH, Turk DC, Wyrwich KW, et al: Interpreting the clinical importance of treatment outcomes in chronic pain clinical trials: IMMPACT recommendations. J Pain 9:105–121, 2008

Eccles NK: A critical review of randomized controlled trials of static magnets for pain relief. J Altern Complement Med 11:495–509, 2005

Eisenberg E, McNicol E, Carr DB: Opioids for neuropathic pain. Cochrane Database Syst Rev (3):CD006146, 2006

Fishbain DA, Cutler RB, Rosomoff HL, et al: Are opioid-dependent/tolerant patients impaired in driving-related skills? A structured evidence-based review. J Pain Symptom Manage 25:559–577, 2003

Franklin GM, Stover BD, Turner JA, et al: Early opioid prescription and subsequent disability among workers with back injuries: the Disability Risk Identification Study Cohort. Spine 33:199–204, 2008

Freynhagen R, Muth-Selbach U, Lipfert P, et al: The effect of mirtazapine in patients with chronic pain and concomitant depression. Curr Med Res Opin 22:257–264, 2006

Furlan AD, Sandoval JA, Mailis-Gagnon A, et al: Opioids for chronic noncancer pain: a meta-analysis of effectiveness and side effects. CMAJ 174:1589–1594, 2006

Gallagher RM: Pain science and rational polypharmacy: an historical perspective. Am J Phys Med Rehabil 84 (suppl):S1–S3, 2005

Gendreau RM, Thorn MD, Gendreau JF, et al: Efficacy of milnacipran in patients with fibromyalgia. J Rheumatol 32:1975–1985, 2005

Gilron I, Bailey JM, Tu D, et al: Morphine, gabapentin, or their combination for neuropathic pain. N Engl J Med 352:1324–1334, 2005

Goldenberg DL, Burckhardt C, Crofford L: Management of fibromyalgia syndrome. JAMA 292:2388–2395, 2004

Goldstein DJ, Lu Y, Detke MJ, et al: Duloxetine vs. placebo in patients with painful diabetic neuropathy. Pain 116:109–118, 2005

Gowans SE, deHueck A: Pool exercise for individuals with fibromyalgia. Curr Opin Rheumatol 19:168–173, 2007

Greco T, Eckert G, Kroenke K: The outcome of physical symptoms with treatment of depression. J Gen Intern Med 19:813–818, 2004

Griggs C, Jensen J: Effectiveness of acupuncture for migraine: critical literature review. J Adv Nurs 54:491–501, 2006

Gureje O, Von Korff M, Simon GE, et al: Persistent pain and well-being: a World Health Organization Study in Primary Care. JAMA 280:147–151, 1998

Gureje O, Von KM, Kola L, et al: The relation between multiple pains and mental disorders: results from the World Mental Health Surveys. Pain 135:82–91, 2008

Heit HA: Addiction, physical dependence, and tolerance: precise definitions to help clinicians evaluate and treat chronic pain patients. J Pain Palliat Care Pharmacother 17:15–29, 2003

Henningsen P, Zimmermann T, Sattel H: Medically unexplained physical symptoms, anxiety, and depression: a meta-analytic review. Psychosom Med 65:528–533, 2003

Henningsen P, Zipfel S, Herzog W: Management of functional somatic syndromes. Lancet 369:946–955, 2007

Heuts PH, de Bie RA, Drietelaar M, et al: Self-management in osteoarthritis of hip or knee: a randomized clinical trial in a primary healthcare setting. J Rheumatol 32:543–549, 2005

Højsted J, Sjøgren P: An update on the role of opioids in the management of chronic pain of nonmalignant origin. Curr Opin Anaesthesiol 20:451–455, 2007

Hollingshead J, Duhmke RM, Cornblath DR: Tramadol for neuropathic pain. Cochrane Database Syst Rev (3):CD003726, 2006

Jackson JL, O'Malley PG, Kroenke K: Antidepressants and cognitive-behavioral therapy for symptom syndromes. CNS Spectr 11:212–222, 2006

Jensen M, Patterson DR: Hypnotic treatment of chronic pain. J Behav Med 29:95–124, 2006

Jensen MK, Thomsen AB, Højsted J: 10-year follow-up of chronic non-malignant pain patients: opioid use, health related quality of life and health care utilization. Eur J Pain 10:423–433, 2006

Joint Commission on Accreditation of Healthcare Organizations: Pain Assessment and Management: An Organizational Approach. Oakbrook Terrace, IL, JCAHO, 2000

Joranson DE, Carrow GM, Ryan KM, et al: Pain management and prescription monitoring. J Pain Symptom Manage 23:231–238, 2002

Jung AC, Staiger T, Sullivan M: The efficacy of selective serotonin reuptake inhibitors for the management of chronic pain. J Gen Intern Med 12:384–389, 1997

Kahan M, Srivastava A, Wilson L, et al: Opioids for managing chronic non-malignant pain: safe and effective prescribing. Can Fam Physician 52:1091–1096, 2006

Karjalainen K, Malmivaara A, van Tulder M, et al: Multidisciplinary rehabilitation for fibromyalgia and musculoskeletal pain in working age adults. Cochrane Database Syst Rev (2):CD001984, 2000

Karp JF, Scott J, Houck P, et al: Pain predicts longer time to remission during treatment of recurrent depression. J Clin Psychiatry 66:591–597, 2005

Katon W, Lin EH, Kroenke K: The association of depression and anxiety with medical symptom burden in patients with chronic medical illness. Gen Hosp Psychiatry 29:147–155, 2007

Khoromi S, Cui L, Nackers L, et al: Morphine, nortriptyline and their combination vs. placebo in patients with chronic lumbar root pain. Pain 130:66–75, 2007

Krebs EE, Carey TS, Weinberger M: Accuracy of the pain numeric rating scale as a screening test in primary care. J Gen Intern Med 22:1453–1458, 2007

Krebs EE, Bair MJ, Damush TM, et al: Development and initial validation of a 3-item brief pain inventory. J Gen Intern Med 23:278–279, 2008a

Krebs EE, Gaynes BN, Gartlehner G, et al: Treating the physical symptoms of depression with second-generation antidepressants: a systematic review and meta-analysis. Psychosomatics 49:191–198, 2008b

Kroenke K: The interface between physical and psychological symptoms. Prim Care Companion J Clin Psychiatry 5 (suppl 7):11–18, 2003a

Kroenke K: Patients presenting with somatic complaints: epidemiology, psychiatric comorbidity and management. Int J Methods Psychiatr Res 12:34–43, 2003b

Kroenke K: Efficacy of treatment for somatoform disorders: a review of randomized controlled trials. Psychosom Med 69:881–888, 2007

Kroenke K, Price RK: Symptoms in the community: prevalence, classification, and psychiatric comorbidity. Arch Intern Med 153:2474–2480, 1993

Kroenke K, Swindle R: Cognitive-behavioral therapy for somatization and symptom syndromes: a critical review of controlled clinical trials. Psychother Psychosom 69:205–215, 2000

Kroenke K, Spitzer RL, Williams JBW, et al: Physical symptoms in primary care: predictors of psychiatric disorders and functional impairment. Arch Fam Med 3:774–779, 1994

Kroenke K, Jackson JL, Chamberlin J: Depressive and anxiety disorders in patients presenting with physical complaints: clinical predictors and outcome. Am J Med 103:339–347, 1997

Kroenke K, Sharpe M, Sykes R: Revising the classification of somatoform disorders: key questions and preliminary recommendations. Psychosomatics 48:277–285, 2007

Kroenke K, Shen J, Oxman TE, et al: Impact of pain on the outcomes of depression treatment: results from the RESPECT trial. Pain 134:209–215, 2008

Kroenke K, Spitzer RL, Williams JBW, et al: An ultra-brief screening scale for anxiety and depression: the PHQ-4. Psychosomatics (in press)

Lee C, Straus WL, Balshaw R, et al: A comparison of the efficacy and safety of nonsteroidal antiinflammatory agents versus acetaminophen in the treatment of osteoarthritis: a meta-analysis. Arthritis Rheum 51:746–754, 2004

Lever IJ, Rice AS: Cannabinoids and pain. Handb Exp Pharmacol (177):265–306, 2007

Lin EH, Katon W, Von Korff M, et al: Effect of improving depression care on pain and functional outcomes among older adults with arthritis: a randomized controlled trial. JAMA 290:2428–2429, 2003

Lin J, Zhang W, Jones A, Doherty M: Efficacy of topical non-steroidal anti-inflammatory drugs in the treatment of osteoarthritis: meta-analysis of randomized controlled trials. BMJ 329:324–329, 2004

Litcher-Kelly L, Martino SA, Broderick JE, et al: A systematic review of measures used to assess chronic musculoskeletal pain in clinical and randomized controlled clinical trials. J Pain 8:906–913, 2007

Lorig K: Self-management education: more than a nice extra. Medical Care 41:699–701, 2003

Lorig K, Holman H: Arthritis self-management studies: a twelve-year review. Health Educ Q 20:17–28, 1993

Lorig KR, Holman H: Self-management education: history, definition, outcomes, and mechanisms. Ann Behav Med 26:1–7, 2003

Lorig KR, Mazonson PD, Holman HR: Evidence suggesting that health education for self-management in patients with chronic arthritis has sustained health benefits while reducing health care costs. Arthritis Rheum 36:439–446, 1993

Magni G, Marchetti M, Moreschi C, et al: Chronic musculoskeletal pain and depressive symptoms in the National Health and Nutrition Examination, I: epidemiologic follow-up study. Pain 53:163–168, 1993

Manheimer E, White A, Berman B, et al: Meta-analysis: acupuncture for low back pain. Ann Intern Med 142:651–663, 2005

Manheimer E, Linde K, Lao L, et al: Meta-analysis: acupuncture for osteoarthritis of the knee. Ann Intern Med 146:868–877, 2007

Marshall DA, Strauss ME, Pericak D, et al: Economic evaluation of controlled-release oxycodone vs oxycodone-acetaminophen for osteoarthritis pain of the hip or knee. Am J Manag Care 12:205–214, 2006

Martell BA, O'Connor PG, Kerns RD, et al: Systematic review: opioid treatment for chronic back pain: prevalence, efficacy, and association with addiction. Ann Intern Med 146:116–127, 2007

Mason L, Moore RA, Derry S, et al: Systematic review of topical capsaicin for the treatment of chronic pain. BMJ 328:991–994, 2004a

Mason L, Moore RA, Edwards JE, et al: Systematic review of efficacy of topical rubefacients containing salicylates for the treatment of acute and chronic pain. BMJ 328:995–997, 2004b

Mason L, Moore RA, Edwards JE, et al: Topical NSAIDs for chronic musculoskeletal pain: systematic review and meta-analysis. BMC Musculoskelet Disord 5:28, 2004c

Mavandadi S, Ten Have TR, Katz IR, et al: Effect of depression treatment on depressive symptoms in older adulthood: the moderating role of pain. J Am Geriatr Soc 55:202–211, 2007

Max MB, Lynch SA, Muir J, et al: Effects of desipramine, amitriptyline, and fluoxetine on pain in diabetic neuropathy. N Engl J Med 326:1250–1256, 1992

Mayhew E, Ernst E: Acupuncture for fibromyalgia—a systematic review of randomized clinical trials. Rheumatology (Oxford) 46:801–804, 2007

McCarberg B, Passik SD (eds): Expert Guide to Pain Management. Philadelphia, PA, American College of Physicians, 2005

McCarthy CJ, Callaghan MJ, Oldham JA: Pulsed electromagnetic energy treatment offers no clinical benefit in reducing the pain of knee osteoarthritis: a systematic review. BMC Musculoskelet Disord 7:51, 2006

McWilliams LA, Cox BJ, Enns MW: Mood and anxiety disorders associated with chronic pain: an examination in a nationally representative sample. Pain 106:127–133, 2003

Mitchell AJ, Coyne JC: Do ultra-short screening instruments accurately detect depression in primary care? A pooled analysis and meta-analysis of 22 studies. Br J Gen Pract 57:144–151, 2007

Moore RA, McQuay HJ: Prevalence of opioid adverse events in chronic non-malignant pain: systematic review of randomised trials of oral opioids. Arthritis Res Ther 7:R1046–R1051, 2005

Moulin DE, Iezzi A, Amireh R, et al: Randomised trial of oral morphine for chronic non-cancer pain. Lancet 347:143–147, 1996

Moulin DE, Clark AJ, Gilron I, et al: Pharmacological management of chronic neuropathic pain—consensus statement and guidelines from the Canadian Pain Society. Pain Res Manag 12:13–21, 2007

Mularski RA, White-Chu F, Overbay D, et al: Measuring pain as the 5th vital sign does not improve quality of pain management. J Gen Intern Med 21:607–612, 2006

Ohayon MM, Schatzberg AF: Using chronic pain to predict depressive morbidity in the general population. Arch Gen Psychiatry 60:39–47, 2003

O'Malley PG, Jackson JL, Santoro J, et al: Antidepressant therapy for unexplained symptoms and symptom syndromes. J Fam Pract 48:980–990, 1999

O'Malley PG, Balden E, Tomkins G, et al: Treatment of fibromyalgia with antidepressants: a meta-analysis. J Gen Intern Med 15:659–666, 2000

Pasero C, Portenoy RK, McCaffery M: Opioid analgesics, in Pain Clinical Manual. Edited by McCaffery M, Pasero C. St. Louis, MO, CV Mosby, 1999, pp 161–299

Perahia DG, Pritchett YL, Desaiah D, et al: Efficacy of duloxetine in painful symptoms: an analgesic or antidepressant effect? Int Clin Psychopharmacol 21:311–317, 2006

Pittler MH, Brown EM, Ernst E: Static magnets for reducing pain: systematic review and meta-analysis of randomized trials. CMAJ 177:736–742, 2007

Raine R, Haines A, Sensky T, et al: Systematic review of mental health interventions for patients with common somatic symptoms: can research evidence from secondary care be extrapolated to primary care? BMJ 325:1082–1085, 2002

Raskin J, Pritchett YL, Wang F, et al: A double-blind, randomized multicenter trial comparing duloxetine with placebo in the management of diabetic peripheral neuropathic pain. Pain Med 6:346–356, 2005

Reichenbach S, Sterchi R, Scherer M, et al: Meta-analysis: chondroitin for osteoarthritis of the knee or hip. Ann Intern Med 146:580–590, 2007

Roddy E, Zhang W, Doherty M: Aerobic walking or strengthening exercise for osteoarthritis of the knee? A systematic review. Ann Rheum Dis 64:544–548, 2005

Rodríguez MJ, Díaz S, Vera-Llonch M, et al: Cost-effectiveness analysis of pregabalin versus gabapentin in the management of neuropathic pain due to diabetic polyneuropathy or postherpetic neuralgia. Curr Med Res Opin 23:2585–2596, 2007

Rooks DS, Gautam S, Romeling M, et al: Group exercise, education, and combination self-management in women with fibromyalgia: a randomized trial. Arch Intern Med 167:2192–2200, 2007

Rowbotham MC, Reisner LA, Davies PS, et al: Treatment response in antidepressant-naive postherpetic neuralgia patients: double-blind, randomized trial. J Pain 6:741–746, 2005

Russell IJ, Kamin M, Bennett RM, et al: Efficacy of tramadol in treatment of pain in fibromyalgia. J Clin Rheumatol 6:250–257, 2000

Russell IJ, Mease PJ, Smith TR, et al: Efficacy and safety of duloxetine for treatment of fibromyalgia in patients with or without major depressive disorder: results from a 6-month, randomized, double-blind, placebo-controlled, fixed-dose trial. Pain 136:432–444, 2008

Salerno SM, Browning R, Jackson JL: The effect of antidepressant treatment on chronic back pain: a meta-analysis. Arch Intern Med 162:19–24, 2002

Samson DJ, Grant MD, Ratko TA, et al: Treatment of primary and secondary osteoarthritis of the knee. Evid Rep Technol Assess (Full Rep) 157:1–157, 2007

Sandoval JA, Furlan AD, Mailis-Gagnon A: Oral methadone for chronic noncancer pain: a systematic literature review of reasons for administration, prescription patterns, effectiveness, and side effects. Clin J Pain 21:503–512, 2005

Sauro MD, Greenberg RP: Endogenous opiates and the placebo effect: a meta-analytic review. J Psychosom Res 58:115–120, 2005

Savage SR, Joranson DE, Covington EC, et al: Definitions related to the medical use of opioids: evolution towards universal agreement. J Pain Symptom Manage 26:655–667, 2003

Schappert SM: National Ambulatory Medical Care Survey: 1989 summary. National Center for Health Statistics. Vital Health Stat 13(110):1–80, 1992

Schug SA: Clinical pharmacology of non-opioid and opioid analgesics, in Pain 2005—An Updated Review: Refresher Course Syllabus. Edited by Justins DM. Seattle, WA, IASP Press, 2005, pp 31–40

Scott DJ, Stohler CS, Egnatuk CM, et al: Placebo and nocebo effects are defined by opposite opioid and dopaminergic responses. Arch Gen Psychiatry 65:220–231, 2008

Shneker BF, McAuley JW: Pregabalin: a new neuromodulator with broad therapeutic indications. Ann Pharmacother 39:2029–2037, 2005

Sim J, Adams N: Systematic review of randomized controlled trials of nonpharmacological interventions for fibromyalgia. Clin J Pain 18:324–336, 2002

Smith BH, Elliott AM, Chambers WA, et al: The impact of chronic pain in the community. Fam Pract 18:292–299, 2001

Smith HS: Taxonomy of pain syndromes, in The Neurological Basis of Pain. Edited by Pappagallo M. New York, McGraw-Hill, 2005, pp 289–300

Spielmans GI: Duloxetine does not relieve painful physical symptoms in depression: a meta-analysis. Psychother Psychosom 77:12–16, 2008

Staiger TO, Gaster B, Sullivan MD, et al: Systematic review of antidepressants in the treatment of chronic low back pain. Spine 28:2540–2545, 2003

Staud R: Mechanisms of acupuncture analgesia: effective therapy for musculoskeletal pain? Curr Rheumatol Rep 9:473–481, 2007

Sternbach RA: Survey of pain in the United States: the Nuprin Pain Report. Clin J Pain 2:49–53, 1986

Stewart WF, Ricci JA, Chee E, et al: Lost productive time and cost due to common pain conditions in the US workforce. JAMA 290:2443–2454, 2003

Tan G, Craine MH, Bair MJ, et al: Efficacy of selected complementary and alternative medicine interventions for chronic pain. J Rehabil Res Dev 44:195–222, 2007

Thielke SM, Fan MY, Sullivan M, et al: Pain limits the effectiveness of collaborative care for depression. Am J Geriatr Psychiatry 15:699–707, 2007

Towheed TE, Maxwell L, Judd MG, et al: Acetaminophen for osteoarthritis. Cochrane Database Syst Rev (1):CD004257, 2006

Tremont-Lukats IW, Challapalli V, McNicol ED, et al: Systemic administration of local anesthetics to relieve neuropathic pain: a systematic review and meta-analysis. Anesth Analg 101:1738–1749, 2005

Turk DC: Clinical effectiveness and cost-effectiveness of treatments for patients with chronic pain. Clin J Pain 18:355–365, 2002

Underwood M, Ashby D, Cross P, et al: Advice to use topical or oral ibuprofen for chronic knee pain in older people: randomised controlled trial and patient preference study. BMJ 336:138–142, 2008

van Koulil S, Effting M, Kraaimaat FW, et al: Cognitive-behavioural therapies and exercise programmes for patients with fibromyalgia: state of the art and future directions. Ann Rheum Dis 66:571–581, 2007

Verhaak PF, Kerssens JJ, Dekker J, et al: Prevalence of chronic benign pain disorder among adults: a review of the literature. Pain 77:231–239, 1998

Vetter TR: The application of economic evaluation methods in the chronic pain medicine literature. Anesth Analg 105:114–118, 2007

Vlad SC, LaValley MP, McAlindon TE, et al: Glucosamine for pain in osteoarthritis: why do trial results differ? Arthritis Rheum 56:2267–2277, 2007

Von Korff M, Moore JC: Stepped care for back pain: activating approaches for primary care. Ann Intern Med 134:911–917, 2001

Von Korff M, Ormel J, Keefe FJ, et al: Grading the severity of chronic pain. Pain 50:133–149, 1992

Vroomen PC, de Krom MC, Slofstra PD, et al: Conservative treatment of sciatica: a systematic review. J Spinal Disord 13:463–469, 2000

Wasan AD, Correll DJ, Kissin I, et al: Iatrogenic addiction in patients treated for acute or subacute pain: a systematic review. J Opioid Manag 2:16–22, 2006

Watkins PB, Kaplowitz N, Slattery JT, et al: Aminotransferase elevations in healthy adults receiving 4 grams of acetaminophen daily: a randomized controlled trial. JAMA 296:87–93, 2006

Watson CP, Vernich L, Chipman M, et al: Nortriptyline versus amitriptyline in postherpetic neuralgia: a randomized trial. Neurology 51:1166–1171, 1998

Wegman A, van der Weindt, D, van Tulder M, et al: Nonsteroidal antiinflammatory drugs or acetaminophen for osteoarthritis of the hip or knee? A systematic review of evidence and guidelines. J Rheumatol 31:344–354, 2004

Weinstein JN, Tosteson TD, Lurie JD, et al: Surgical vs nonoperative treatment for lumbar disk herniation: the Spine Patient Outcomes Research Trial (SPORT): a randomized trial. JAMA 296:2441–2450, 2006

Weinstein JN, Tosteson TD, Lurie JD, et al: Surgical versus nonsurgical therapy for lumbar spinal stenosis. N Engl J Med 358:794–810, 2008

Wernicke JF, Pritchett YL, D'Souza DN, et al: A randomized controlled trial of duloxetine in diabetic peripheral neuropathic pain. Neurology 67:1411–1420, 2006

White A, Foster NE, Cummings M, et al: Acupuncture treatment for chronic knee pain: a systematic review. Rheumatology (Oxford) 46:384–390, 2007

White KP, Nielson WR, Harth M, et al: Does the label "fibromyalgia" alter health status, function, and health service utilization? A prospective, within-group comparison in a community cohort of adults with chronic widespread pain. Arthritis Rheum 47:260–265, 2002

Wiffen P, Collins S, McQuay H, et al: Anticonvulsant drugs for acute and chronic pain. Cochrane Database Syst Rev (3):CD001133, 2005a

Wiffen PJ, McQuay HJ, Edwards JE, et al: Gabapentin for acute and chronic pain. Cochrane Database Syst Rev (3):CD005452, 2005b

Wiffen PJ, McQuay HJ, Moore RA: Carbamazepine for acute and chronic pain. Cochrane Database Syst Rev (3):CD005451, 2005c

Zijlstra TR, Barendregt PJ, van de Laar MAF: Venlafaxine in fibromyalgia: results of a randomized, placebo-controlled, double-blind trial (abstract). Arthritis Rheum 46 (suppl 9):S105, 2002

PART V

Ethical Issues

Ethical Considerations in Psychopharmacological Treatment and Research

Jinger G. Hoop, M.D., M.F.A.

Joseph B. Layde, M.D., J.D.

Laura Weiss Roberts, M.D., M.A.

The discovery of chlorpromazine's effectiveness in treating symptoms of schizophrenia in 1952 (Delay and Deniker 1952) launched the modern era of pharmacological treatment of psychiatric disease and was a critical development in the compassionate care of people living with mental illness and in the reduction of the societal burden of mental disease. Chlorpromazine's introduction was followed in 1958 by the introduction of imipramine as a treatment for depression (Kuhn 1958) and in 1960 by that of chlordiazepoxide for anxiety (Shorter 1997). Within years, these medications eased the symptoms of hundreds of thousands of the most severely and persistently ill individuals—many of whom otherwise would have endured a lifetime of suffering, disability, and institutionalization, as had millions before them.

As the ensuing decades have shown, the use of psychotropic medications has deep ethical as well as clinical and social implications. This is because psychopharmacological agents have the power not only to relieve severe mental illness symptoms but also to profoundly influence an individual's most fundamental personal attributes—for example, the abilities to experience emotions fully, to relate to others in an empathic and loving way, to engage in focused and sustained thought, to understand oneself more completely, and to extinguish maladaptive or hurtful impulsive behaviors. Taking a selective serotonin reuptake inhibitor may cause a chronically depressed person to experience herself for the first time as relaxed and outgoing. A highly distractible child who is prescribed a psychostimulant may suddenly perceive himself to be smart and likeable. The ability of psychotropic agents to influence personality, mood, cognitions, and psyche raises a number of questions about their ethical use. For example, under what circumstances is it acceptable to use sedating or antipsychotic medications coercively to prevent severely mentally ill individuals from harming themselves or others? When, if ever, is it acceptable to use psychotropic medications for enhancement of personality or intellectual performance—that is, to help psychiatrically healthy persons to become "better than well" (Kramer 1993)?

As psychopharmacology becomes more innovative, extending further into relatively uncharted territory such as the treatment of cognitive dysfunction and substance abuse, we will be challenged by an expanding number of ethical questions regarding treatment selection, the process of informed consent, and related issues (Roberts 2002c; Roberts and Dyer 2004). Furthermore, the acceleration in pharmacological research involving mentally ill adults and children provokes its own set of ethical concerns (Hoop et al. 2008; Roberts and Krystal 2003). The nature of psychiatric illness itself can pose barriers to informed consent for research participation, and protocol features such as placebo control groups and symptom provocation may expose individual research participants to risks that are difficult to understand prospectively and may be significant (Roberts and Roberts 1999). Investigators must continue to address these issues in an explicit, thoughtful manner to maintain the public's trust.

For all these reasons, excellence in psychopharmacology requires sensitivity to a growing range of ethical considerations. The aim of this chapter is to introduce the reader to these issues and to provide a framework for analyzing them. We begin with a discussion of why ethical psychopharmacology is vital to maintaining public trust in psychiatry, and we describe essential ethics skills for psychopharmacologists. We then discuss a number of ethical concerns and controversies in psychopharmacology. The topics covered are not exhaustive but were selected to give the reader a sense of the scope of issues in this important field. We finish by addressing one of psychiatry's most pressing concerns: the need to anticipate and manage the ethical issues that arise in relation to overlapping roles and potential conflicts of interest in interactions with industry.

Ethics, Psychopharmacology, and the Public Trust

Clear standards of ethics and professional behavior help preserve public trust in psychiatry (Roberts and Dyer 2004). Consequently, as the practice of psychiatry has become increasingly devoted to delivering biologically based treatments, creating ethical standards for psychopharmacological interventions has become a matter of growing importance (Ghaemi 2006). The ethics of psychopharmacology is relatively uncharted territory, however, compared with our detailed understanding of other ethical aspects of clinical psychiatry, including boundary issues in psychotherapy and psychoanalysis, the appropriate use of power in involuntary treatment, and the duty to warn third parties about treatments' potential harm (Dyer 1988; Gabbard 1999; Levine 1972; Roberts and Dyer 2004). The ethical issues involved in clinical psychopharmacology have received relatively little attention in the psychiatric literature, with a handful of important exceptions (Brown and Pantelis 1999; Tasman et al. 2000). A major current goal of our profession is to clearly articulate whether, and if so, precisely how, the psychophar-

macologist's ethical obligations differ from those of the psychoanalyst, the forensic specialist, or the emergency psychiatrist.

Clarity about the ethical duties of the psychopharmacologist is needed in part because psychiatrists practice in the context of an enduring public debate about the medical model of mental illness and its biological treatments (Szasz 1960). Some of this controversy can be attributed to a Calvinistic view of psychological suffering as an integral aspect of the human condition rather than as a symptom of disease (Kramer 1993; Sperry and Prosen 1998). Individuals and groups who reject the medical view of mental illness may perceive psychopharmacology as inappropriate attempt to avoid suffering rather than enduring or learning from it. Even those who are generally supportive of psychiatric care may feel that Americans have become too reliant on psychotropic medications as "quick fixes" for their problems. Within the psychiatric community, the increased prescribing of these drugs over the past several decades (Wong et al. 2004) is generally attributed to better recognition of psychopathology and the introduction of safer and more efficacious medications (Arehart-Treichel 2004). Among psychiatry's critics, however, increased prescribing may be interpreted as the overuse of drugs to treat social or moral problems or to perform "cosmetic pharmacology"—that is, to use medication to enhance normal functioning rather than to treat illness (Bjorklund 2005; Elliott 2003; Kramer 1993).

Public trust in psychiatry may also be affected by negative or inaccurate perceptions of psychopharmacology. On the one hand, a psychotropic medication may be viewed, for instance, as more harmful than the underlying condition or than other treatment approaches, such as psychotherapy. Medications may indeed be more likely to cause side effects, more stigmatizing (i.e., apparently indicating more severe pathology), and more easily misused (Bjorklund 2005; Elliott 2003; McHenry 2005; Sperry and Prosen 1998). On the other hand, the marketing of over-the-counter medications with psychotropic properties may suggest that these medications are relatively mild or benign when they may in fact have very potent but poorly understood effects (Beaubrun and Gray 2000; Werneke 2006). Medications for mental disorders may also be perceived as less "scientific" than treatments for other diseases (McHenry 2005), because relatively little is known about the mechanism of action of many psychiatric medications.

Public trust is also affected by the activities of the pharmaceutical industry (McHenry 2006). Direct-to-consumer advertising to encourage individuals to seek treatment for depression, social anxiety disorder, attention-deficit/hyperactivity disorder, and other conditions can be justified ethically by its ability to increase public awareness and perhaps decrease social stigma. Still, this form of advertising may also leave some observers with the impression that psychiatric diagnosis and treatment are linked to the sale of pharmaceuticals (Bjorklund 2005; Elliott 2003; Halasz 2004).

Conflicts of interest or the appearance of conflicts of interest among psychiatrists with ties to pharmaceutical companies have therefore become a major concern (Carlat 2007; Harris and Roberts 2007; Moncrieff et al. 2005). Many educational activities in psychiatry have been funded by the pharmaceutical industry, from large symposia at meetings of professional societies to one-on-one "detailing" by pharmaceutical representatives who meet with psychiatrists and residents in clinic offices (Carlat 2007; Hill 2006; Lurie et al. 2005; Wazana 2000). Although many physicians do not believe that such encounters affect their prescribing practices, empirical evidence suggests that these interactions are more influential than has been realized or acknowledged (Orlowski and Wateska 1992; Wazana 2000). The pharmaceutical industry also funds a significant proportion of treatment research in psychiatry, a phenomenon that has been criticized by some for resulting in a biased evidence base regarding pharmaceuticals (Melander et al. 2003). Finally, industry provides direct payments to many psychiatrists for educational, clinical, or research activities—for example, via fees for giving presentations, attending industry-sponsored activities, referring patients to research studies, or conducting clinical trials.

Arrangements such as these create potential conflicts of interest (Roberts and Dyer 2004). While such conflicts occur naturally throughout all of medicine, they may lead to ethical lapses and/or create an appearance of unethical behavior that endangers the public trust. Clinicians and clinical scientists are experts, patient care advocates, and organizational resources to society, and it is logical that they would be the individuals who would be approached by industry to assume overlapping roles related to their knowledge and various professional efforts. The roles themselves are not inherently or necessarily unethical. However, certain activities may be fundamentally incompatible with the professional obligations of being a physician—for example, appearing in advertisements for unproven treatments (American Medical Association Council on Ethical and Judicial Affairs 2002). Furthermore, the multiplicity of roles and competing obligations of the various roles, taken together, may in fact adversely affect a clinician's or clinician-scientist's decisions in

small and large ways. Finally, the perception of conflict of interest may raise public concerns that undermine the integrity of the profession (Harris 2007; Harris and Roberts 2007). Managing potential conflicts and overlapping roles requires careful attention to issues such as disclosing potential conflicts of interest and establishing safeguards for patients and research participants, approaches that are discussed in detail at the end of this chapter (see "Management of Overlapping Roles and Conflicts of Interest in Psychopharmacology").

All of these factors highlight the importance of establishing clear and consistent standards for ethical psychopharmacology to maintain the trust in the profession's ability to diagnose and treat mental disorders in an unbiased and scientifically sound manner. This is especially important today, while the evidence base for psychiatric treatments is modest and potentially controversial practices such as off-label prescribing are unavoidable if we are to provide treatment for certain understudied disorders and populations (Gazarian et al. 2006; Miskimen et al. 2003). Without the confidence of the public, funding for much-needed research may suffer and the stigma of mental illness may deepen, making it even more difficult for individuals in need to seek, obtain, and adhere to psychopharmacological treatments.

Essential Ethics Skills of Psychopharmacologists

In contrast to the view that ethics and professionalism cannot be taught and learned, we believe that ethical behavior, like clinical acumen, is based on a set of skills that are learned and honed over time (Roberts and Dyer 2004; Roberts et al. 1996). Six key ethics skills are crucial to psychiatric practice, as discussed below, and all are directly relevant to clinical psychopharmacology and psychopharmacological research (Table 67–1).

1. The first essential ethics skill is ethical sensitivity, the ability to detect ethical issues when they arise. To recognize ethical issues requires an awareness of the meaning of bioethics concepts such as autonomy, beneficence, and justice (Table 67–2) and an understanding of the dilemmas that occur when these principles are in conflict (Table 67–3). As a simple example, the psychiatrist who evaluates a pregnant woman with bipolar disorder should recognize that the selection of treatment has an ethical dimension, because of the possibility of teratogenicity, which re-

TABLE 67–1.   Essential ethics abilities in psychopharmacology

The ability to identify the ethical features in caring for patients or conducting research

The ability to anticipate ethically risky or problematic situations

The ability to see how the physician's own life experience, attitudes, and knowledge may influence the care of the patient

The ability to identify one's areas of expertise (i.e., scope of clinical or research competence) and to work within these boundaries

The ability to gather additional information and to seek consultation and additional expertise in order to clarify and, ideally, to resolve ethical conflicts

The ability to build additional ethical safeguards into one's work

Source.   Reprinted from Roberts LW, Dyer AR: "Clinical Decision-Making and Ethics Skills," in *Concise Guide to Ethics in Mental Health Care.* Washington, DC, American Psychiatric Publishing, 2004, p. 20. Used with permission.

quires careful consideration along with the clinical indications.

2. A second related skill is the ability to anticipate that ethical conflicts are likely to arise in certain situations. In the clinical sphere, such situations include involuntary treatment, which may pit a clinicians' duty to respect autonomy against the duty to act with beneficence. In research, ethically higher-risk situations include protocols that involve medication washout periods or placebo groups, which in the absence of adequate safeguards may pose harm for some research participants.

3. The third essential ethics skill is the psychopharmacologist's ability to monitor how his or her own moral beliefs and values may affect ethically important thinking and decision making. For instance, a psychiatrist who has been personally devastated by the suicide of a patient may recognize that this experience has made him or her more driven to "do good" for patients via aggressive pharmacotherapy and less capable of respecting the decisionally capable patient's right to refuse treatment. Similarly, a researcher whose spiritual beliefs include a high value on social justice may realize that this influences his or her thinking about subject recruitment and that it is helpful to discuss this aspect of protocol design with collaborators who do not share the same values.

4. A fourth key ethics skill is the ability to recognize and respect one's professional limits. Our appropriate sphere of professional activity is properly bounded by the extent of our education, training, and experience

and by the relative availability of more qualified colleagues. Some psychopharmacologists may not have the training or experience to conduct combined medication management/psychodynamic psychotherapy, whereas others may lack qualifications to treat psychiatrically ill patients during childhood, pregnancy, or old age or those with concomitant medical illness. Physicians who practice in remote or isolated communities may ethically provide a broader range of services than those who practice in large urban centers with many subspecialists. No one person is able to provide every kind of medical or psychiatric evaluation and treatment; referring patients demonstrates humility and self-awareness as well as dedication to the principles of nonmaleficence and beneficence.

5. A fifth skill is the willingness to seek and use ethics consultations or guidelines in appropriate situations. Clinicians who are faced with ethical challenges have many resources to guide them, including written ethics standards, codes, and guidelines. All psychopharmacologists should be familiar with ethics resource documents of the American Psychiatric Association, such as *The Principles of Medical Ethics With Annotations Especially Applicable to Psychiatry* (American Psychiatric Association 2001; available online at http://www.psych.org/psych_pract/ethics/ethics.cfm), and of the American Medical Association Council on Ethical and Judicial Affairs (2002). In addition, many hospitals and academic centers have ethics committee members or ethics consultants who can be contacted for help in defining an ethical problem and identifying a range of acceptable solutions. Researchers can seek guidance from the relevant institutional review board, through a formal protocol review and/or informal consultation.

6. The final essential skill for psychiatrists is the ability to create ethical safeguards to anticipate, prevent, and/or ameliorate future ethical problems. For example, a clinician may establish specific informed consent procedures to follow when prescribing off label or when prescribing agents with high addiction potential. Similarly, researchers can build safeguards into their protocols, such as clearly defined benchmarks for ongoing consent for participation in trials and appropriate disenrollment and referral procedures for participants who experience relapse during medication-free intervals (Roberts 1999). As a final example, the potential harms associated with conflicts of interest may be anticipated and prevented by identifying and appropriately managing overlapping roles and conflicting interests.

TABLE 67–2.   Glossary of ethics terms

Altruism.   The virtue of acting for the good of another rather than for oneself, at times entailing self-sacrifice.

Autonomy.   Literally "self-rule." In medical ethics, autonomy is the ability to make deliberated or reasoned decisions for oneself and to act on the basis of such decisions.

Beneficence.   An action done to benefit others. The principle of beneficence in medicine signifies an obligation to benefit patients and to seek what will do them good.

Coercion.   The use of some form of pressure to persuade or compel an individual to agree to a belief or action.

Compassion.   Literally, "suffering with" another person, with kindness and an active regard for his or her welfare. Compassion is more closely related to empathy than to sympathy, as sympathy connotes the more distanced experience of "feeling sorry for" the individual.

Confidentiality.   The obligation of physicians not to disclose information obtained from patients or observed about them without their permission. In clinical care, it entails taking precautions to protect the personal information about patients. Confidentiality is a privilege linked to the legal right of privacy and may at times be overridden by exceptions stipulated in law.

Conflict of interest.   In medicine, a situation in which a physician has competing roles, relationships, or interests that could potentially interfere with the ability to care for patients. Such situations may naturally occur in clinical care and research, and they are not inherently unethical. They must be recognized and managed appropriately to safeguard the well-being of vulnerable individuals (e.g., patients, research participants) and to prevent exploitative practices.

Empathy.   Entering into someone else's frame of reference in terms of thoughts, feelings, and experiences, to have an authentic understanding of the other person's experiences imaginatively as one's own.

Fidelity.   The virtue of promise keeping, truthfulness, and honor. In clinical care, it refers to the faithfulness with which a clinician commits to the duty of helping patients and acting in a manner that is in keeping with the ideals of the profession.

Fiduciary.   An entity in a position of trust with a duty to act on behalf of another, for the other's good. Physicians are fiduciaries with respect to their patients.

Honesty.   A virtue in which one conveys the truth fully, without misrepresentation through deceit, bias, or omission.

Human dignity.   The principle that every person, intrinsically, is valued and worthy of respect. In medical ethics, every patient is believed to have innate and inalienable worth as a human being that requires he or she be treated with respect and compassion and full interpersonal regard as expressed in attitudes, behaviors, and nondiscriminatory practices.

Informed consent.   In the clinical setting, a legal and ethical obligation for clinicians to inform patients about their illness and alternatives for care and to assist them in making reasoned, authentic decisions about treatment. In the research setting, a similar obligation of a researcher to inform participants about the research protocol and help them make reasoned, authentic decisions about research participation.

Integrity.   A virtue literally defined as wholeness or coherence. It connotes professional soundness and reliability of intention and action.

Justice.   The ethical principle of fairness. Distributive justice refers to the fair and equitable distribution of resources and burden through society.

Medical decision making.   The intentional process associated with making a choice in clinical care. It pertains to a patient's capacity to make decisions related to his or her health or health care and to the clinician's process of deliberation, consultation, and data gathering that results in the development of a diagnosis and of therapeutic alternatives for a patient.

Medical negligence.   The legal concept of a breach of duty of medical care. It rests on the existence of a duty of care, failure to fulfill that duty, and resultant harm.

Nonmaleficence.   The duty to avoid doing harm.

Personhood.   Having full moral status as a human being.

Quality of life.   The expression of a value judgment by an individual regarding the experience of life as a whole or some aspect of it.

Respect.   The virtue of fully regarding and according intrinsic value to someone or something. In clinical care, it is reflected in treating another individual with genuine consideration and attentiveness to that person's life history, values, and goals.

Self-understanding.   Awareness of one's own values and motivations. Self-understanding based on insight and careful self-scrutiny is a key ethics skill of special importance to mental health care ethics.

Therapeutic boundaries.   The set of concepts, rules, and duties that structures the clinician–patient relationship to ensure psychological safety, to optimize therapeutic benefit, and to prevent potentially exploitative practices.

TABLE 67–2. Glossary of ethics terms *(continued)*

Trustworthiness.   A virtue that pertains to a disposition that inspires confident belief in and reliance on the physician's character and ability to act beneficently and honestly.

Voluntariness.   The attribute in which a belief or act derives from one's own free will and is not coerced or unduly influenced by others.

Vulnerability.   The capacity to be wounded or hurt physically, emotionally, spiritually, or socially and being without the means to defend or advocate for oneself fully.

Source.   Adapted from Roberts LW, Dyer AR: Appendix A, in *Concise Guide to Ethics in Mental Health Care*. Washington, DC, American Psychiatric Publishing, 2004, pp. 319–320. Used with permission.

Selected Ethical Issues in Psychopharmacology

The Doctor–Patient Relationship

The therapeutic relationship in medicine and psychiatry is rooted in the principles of beneficence and respect for autonomy. Historically, an emphasis on beneficence over autonomy has been the hallmark of paternalism, in which the physician acts benevolently and at times unilaterally, like a parent, in dealings with patients. By contrast, an emphasis on respect for autonomy over beneficence in the therapeutic relationship highlights the importance of patients' rights. Patients' rights in pharmacotherapy have been described as including the following: "access to treatment; provision of necessary information [about treatment]; the freedom to accept or refuse treatment; and a voice in the selection of specific drugs and the conditions under which to take them" (Brown and Pantelis 1999, p. 257). At its most extreme, a strictly beneficence-based practice may diminish the ill individual, violating the cardinal ethical principle that governs all actions in medicine and human science: respect for persons. On the other hand, a strictly autonomy-based practice at its most extreme appears to be akin to a mere business transaction—a trade of goods and services between two "equal" individuals, one with a product or service and the other with an identified interest or need, with no specific moral obligation between the two parties (Dyer 1988; Wise 2007).

To avoid these two extremes, Dyer suggests that the therapeutic relationship be viewed as a fiduciary partnership (Dyer and Bloch 1987). A *fiduciary* in health care is one whose actions are worthy of trust. A *fiduciary partnership* has been described as being characterized by "sincerity without reserve" and "loving care" (Guttentag 1968). Through such a trusting partnership and through the process of informed consent, physicians and patients may achieve a relationship in which optimal healing can oc-

cur (Brown and Pantelis 1999; Dyer 1988; Roberts and Dyer 2004). The physician provides information and compassionate care while respecting the patient's privacy, values, and preferences in a manner that helps the patient identify and adhere to optimal treatments.

Although the psychodynamics of the doctor–patient relationship have been most exhaustively studied in the psychoanalytical literature, many features pertain across a wide range of clinician–patient encounters (Roberts and Dyer 2004). In all types of health care settings, patients have needs and clinicians have the knowledge and ability to attempt to meet those needs, establishing a power differential between clinician and patient. Transference and countertransference arise and can complicate treatment if not recognized and addressed (Gabbard 2000; Tasman et al. 2000). For example, patients may act out feelings of negative transference through treatment nonadherence, and a prescriber may act out countertransference anger toward such a patient by becoming overly authoritative (Gabbard 2000; Tasman et al. 2000). Furthermore, a therapeutic frame exists in the practice of psychopharmacology as in the practice of psychotherapy. This frame may differ in some ways—frequency of appointments is the most obvious—but like any therapeutic frame, it has boundaries that must be maintained by the clinician.

Maintenance of Therapeutic Boundaries in Psychopharmacological Treatment

Gabbard (1999) has defined professional boundaries as the "'edge' or limit of appropriate behavior by the psychiatrist in the clinical setting" (p. 142). Boundaries include the circumstances under which patients are seen—such as for a set fee, in the physician's office, during office hours—and the professional conduct of the psychiatrist during the encounter. Maintaining appropriate boundaries demonstrates respect for the individual patient, who is in an unequal relationship with the clinician and therefore vulnerable to possible exploitation.

TABLE 67–3. Ethical tensions in clinical psychopharmacology

CLINICAL SITUATION	RELEVANT ETHICAL PRINCIPLE(S)	CONFLICTS AND TENSIONS
A patient refuses a medically indicated medication.	Autonomy and beneficence	The patient's right to make his or her own decisions is in tension with the physician's duty to do good by providing medically indicated treatment.
A colleague asks a psychiatrist to write a prescription for a sleep medicine.	Nonmaleficence	The desire to oblige a colleague may conflict with the psychiatrist's duty to avoid harming a patient by prescribing without conducting a thorough medical evaluation and establishing a treatment relationship.
A rural psychiatrist's patient needs a treatment that the psychiatrist is not competent to provide; no other practitioner is available.	Nonmaleficence	The psychiatrist's duty to avoid harming the patient by practicing outside his or her scope of competency is in conflict with the obligation to avoid harming the patient by leaving him or her without a treatment provider.
A pharmaceutical company offers a psychiatrist an unusually large fee for referring patients to a research trial.	Fidelity	Financial self-interest threatens the psychiatrist's duty to remain faithful to the goals of treatment and to the role of a healer.
A patient's severe psychiatric illness responds only to a medication that is contraindicated because of a concomitant medical condition.	Nonmaleficence and beneficence	The psychiatrist's duty to do good by treating the psychiatric illness is in tension with the risk of worsening the medical condition.
A pregnant woman has a severe mental illness that responds best to psychotropic medication that may pose a risk to her fetus; the patient is ambivalent about the pregnancy and her treatment options.	Nonmaleficence, beneficence, and respect for autonomy	The psychiatrist's duty to do good by treating the psychiatric illness is in tension with the possibility of harming the fetus. Respecting the patient's autonomous right to select a treatment is complicated by her ambivalence.

Source. Adapted from Roberts LW, Hoop JG, Dunn LB: "Ethical Tensions in Common Clinical Situations," in *The American Psychiatric Publishing Textbook of Psychiatry*, 5th Edition. Edited by Hales RE, Yudofsky SC, Gabbard GO. Washington, DC, American Psychiatric Publishing, 2008, pp. 1770–1771. Used with permission.

Boundary violations occur when clinicians act in a way that transgresses the normal professional limits and may harm the patient. Sexual contact between psychiatrist and patient is a severe boundary violation that has been shown to cause lasting damage to patients (R.S. Epstein 1994b), is prohibited by the American Psychiatric Association (2001), and is illegal in many jurisdictions (Milne 2002). Characteristics of psychiatrists who commit sexual boundary violations include narcissistic pathology, poor training, and isolation from colleagues (R.S. Epstein 1994a). Insights drawn from therapeutic work with physicians and therapists who have had sexual contact with patients and from analysis of cases where ethics complaints have been brought forward related to sexual boundary violations indicate that these clinicians may not appreciate the exploitative nature of their actions. The "lovesick" caregiver, as Gabbard (1999) suggests, may in fact be "well-intended" but has confused his or her own need for fulfillment and gratification with the needs of the patient and has failed to adhere to the primary ethical imperatives of clinical care: respect for persons, beneficence, and nonmaleficence. Nonsexual boundary violations include engaging in other forms of physical contact, seeing patients outside the office or hospital setting, accepting large gifts from patients, or exploiting patients for social or business purposes (R.S. Epstein 1994a; Frick 1994; Gabbard 1999). The defining characteristic of these violations is the subordination or eclipse of the patient's needs by the self-interested objectives, whether intentional or not, of the professional.

As opposed to boundary violations, boundary *crossings* are subtle transgressions that serve to advance the treatment—for example, accepting a token gift to help a patient feel more comfortable in the therapeutic relationship (Gabbard 1999; Gutheil and Gabbard 1993, 1998). Boundary crossings are therefore not inherently unethical. Still, they should be undertaken in a deliberate fashion (e.g., after being discussed with a peer, supervisor, or consultant; occurring only in certain contexts or with certain kinds of issues or with healthier patients) and always be oriented toward the goals of treatment.

Most psychiatrists have been trained in the importance of respect for boundaries in the therapeutic relationship in psychotherapy; in psychopharmacological practice, such respect is no less crucial, although the less intense nature of the therapeutic relationship may make it more difficult for clinicians to notice a tendency toward making subtle boundary violations. Seeking supervision or consultation can help ensure that what the clinician perceives is a useful boundary crossing is not potentially detrimental to the patient—for example, making a house call to visit a favorite patient when that is not one's usual practice.

Informed Consent for Psychopharmacotherapy

In clinical care, the process of informed consent is a fundamental and ethically important activity of the physician. Informed consent represents an ongoing exchange between physician and patient in which the clinician fulfills the role of teacher as well as diagnostician and healer. Through this process, physicians demonstrate respect for patients, enhance patients' ability to act in concert with their authentic wishes, and strengthen the therapeutic alliance. Informed consent is an example of shared decision making (R.M. Epstein et al. 2004), as opposed to the paternalistic view of medical decision making as solely the domain of the physician (Faden and Beauchamp 1980). Shared decision making appears to increase treatment adherence and improve doctor–patient communication (R.M. Epstein et al. 2004).

Informed consent is a legal as well as an ethical concept. The 1914 landmark opinion of the New York Court of Appeals in *Schloendorff v. Society of New York Hospital*, written by Justice Benjamin Cardozo, set forth the basic principle of American law regarding consent to medical procedures: "Every human being of adult years and sound mind has a right to determine what shall be done with his own body; and a surgeon who performs an operation without the patient's consent commits an assault, for which he is liable in damages." Subsequent court cases have enshrined in law the ethical principle that a patient's consent must be truly informed (Morris et al. 2005).

Informed consent has been described as consisting of three elements, each of which is vital to the process: information provision, decision-making capacity, and voluntariness (Figure 67–1) (Faden et al. 1986; Roberts and Dyer 2004). These elements are described below:

1. Information provision is the domain of the provider, who must give patients all relevant information about the potential advantages and disadvantages of contemplated treatment, as well as any viable alternatives to the treatment, including no treatment at all. Information provision is a process that requires dialogue between the patient and the provider. From a legal standpoint, the amount and type of information that must be disclosed vary across jurisdictions. Some adhere to a *professional standard*—that is, the amount and type of information that most physicians would disclose to patients. Other states use the *reasonable person standard*—that is, the amount of information a reasonable person would want to know. It is not possible to create a one-size-fits-all information-sharing session that can be used for any patient with a given diagnosis. The clinician should be attuned to the intellectual, emotional, and relational needs of the patient in deciding how to provide information about treatment options.

2. The second feature of informed consent is the decision-making capacity of the patient, which is itself defined as consisting of four abilities (Appelbaum and Grisso 1995). First, the patient must be capable of communicating a preference. This is demonstrated by patients who have the physical ability to speak, write, or gesture in such a way that others can understand. Second is the ability to comprehend the information necessary for making the medical decision, a primarily cognitive task that is affected by factors such as patients' educational background. Because patients vary in the ability to comprehend complex medical data, providers should use language, examples, and illustrations tailored to the needs of individual patients. Third is the ability to appreciate the significance of the medical decision that is to be made. Although a patient may comprehend the facts about the medical situation (e.g., "I understand that lithium is an effective treatment for mania"), lack of insight may impair the ability to appreciate how that information is relevant to the current situation (e.g., "I am not manic and therefore have no need to take lithium"). The ability to appreciate the significance of medical information is influenced by one's beliefs and values, and it can be difficult to thoroughly assess whether someone is truly capable of appreciating clinical material (Roberts et al. 2008a). The final element of decisional capacity is the ability to reason—to weigh options and consequences in order to come to a considered judgment. The outcome of this reasoning process does not

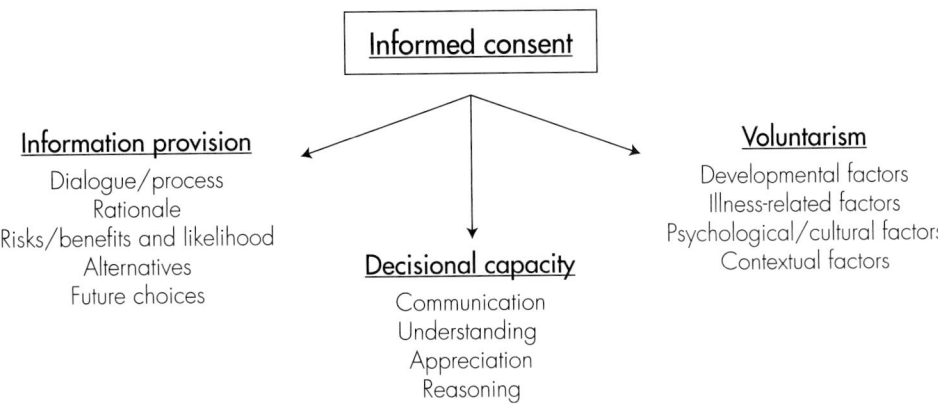

FIGURE 67–1. Elements of informed consent.

Source. Reprinted from Roberts LW, Dyer AR: "Informed Consent and Decisional Capacity," in *Concise Guide to Ethics in Mental Health Care*. Washington, DC, American Psychiatric Publishing, 2004, p. 52. Used with permission.

necessarily have to be considered a rational decision by others.

Predictable variations in decisional capacity occur with various illness states. Patients with delirium are likely to have waxing and waning capacity. Patients with dementias generally become less capable of making treatment decisions as their disease progresses. Individuals with psychotic disorders may be decisional at some times in the course of their disorder and non-decisional at other times. Those who are depressed may become more pessimistic about the possibility of successful treatment if the depression worsens. Clinicians who are aware of these likely variations in cognitive capacity may properly take advantage of moments when patients are decisionally capable to clarify patient preferences regarding their treatment and persons who may act as alternative decision makers for them.

3. The third element of informed consent is the patient's level of voluntariness, or *voluntarism*: the ability to make choices that are free from coercive pressure and are in concert with the individual's authentic wishes. Voluntarism has been described as depending on four types of factors: 1) developmental factors; 2) illness-related factors; 3) psychological and cultural factors; and 4) contextual factors and pressures (Roberts 2002c).

As an example, a 19-year-old male patient with new-onset psychosis may have numerous factors bearing on his ability to voluntarily consent to the use of antipsychotic medication. These could include the patient's developmental level and amount of relevant life experience; the nature of the psychotic process;

whether he has received involuntary treatment in the past (e.g., medication, hospitalization); his personal and cultural beliefs about suffering, mental illness, and the use of medications that affect the brain; and pressures from family, the treating physician, and perhaps the courts. Clinicians who are aware of the presence of these issues can anticipate and address them when informing the patient about treatment options. Understanding the array of influences on voluntarism, moreover, can help clinicians to target ways to enhance the voluntary nature of their patients' decision-making process—for example, by providing emotional support for someone who has symptoms or experiences that have felt disempowering in the past, by allowing the patient ample time for making decisions that are not urgent, and by providing an opportunity to share information with valued family members who might help advocate for the patient's preferences—or, alternatively, by helping to shield the patient from inappropriate pressure by someone who does not have the patient's wishes and best interests at heart.

When are decisional capacity, voluntarism, and information sharing considered sufficient to enable a patient to consent to or refuse medication treatment? There is no single answer to this question, and many experts adhere to the notion of a *sliding scale for consent* (Drane 1984), in which the standards for consent are dependent on the likely seriousness of risks accompanying the decision. Standards for consent for a low-risk treatment, such as the one-time use of diphenhydramine for insomnia, are generally considered lower than standards for consent to a treatment with a greater potential for adverse effects, such as clozapine or a monoamine oxidase inhibitor. Of course, individuals who are clearly incapable of comprehending the information necessary to make a decision regarding their medical care, of appreciating the implications of their consent to or refusal of contemplated care, of reasoning rationally in arriving at a treatment choice, or of communicating their decision are not able to negotiate the process of giving or withholding informed consent for even low-risk pharmacotherapy.

The sliding scale paradigm suggests that, in general, there is a higher standard for refusing recommended treatment than for consenting to it, because treatment refusal typically involves higher risk. This is an important concept, ethically and clinically. The naïve individual may initially reject the notion that, under some circumstances, there appear to be different standards for accepting or refusing treatments. In fact, the standards are not different—it is just that the standard for decision making is determined by the level of risk and benefit hinging upon the decision. In other words, use of a very dangerous medication for a mild illness will entail an extremely high standard for decision making, as it should. Alternatively, the decision to decline a relatively benign medication for a severe and life-threatening illness will also entail an extremely high standard for decision making. This approach to assessing an individual's capacity for clinical decision making is governed by the principle of beneficence—seeking to do good—and, even more, by the principle of nonmaleficence—seeking to avoid harm.

Exceptions to Informed Consent and Involuntary Intervention

There are a few exceptions to the ethical and legal requirement to obtain the informed consent of patients before providing treatment. Necessary medical treatment may be given in emergencies to those who are unconscious or otherwise unable to give informed consent. Treatment may also be provided to individuals who lack decisional capacity if consent is obtained from the appropriate alternative decision maker, such as the parent of a child or the health care proxy of a decisionally incapable adult. This is discussed in more detail below. Traditionally, it was also acceptable to provide treatment without consent to patients who were considered likely to become too emotionally distraught from the disclosure of relevant medical information to be able to rationally choose to accept or refuse proposed treatment (Morris et al. 2005). This practice, known as the *therapeutic privilege*, has fallen substantially out of favor with ethicists, courts, and phy-

sicians in recent years as paternalistic approaches to patient care have given way to the contemporary ideal of shared or participatory decision making.

The pharmacotherapy of children requires special attention to the issues of informed consent. Parents and legal guardians of children and unemancipated minors have the legal right to make decisions about medical treatment for minor patients. The age of majority differs in some jurisdictions for obtaining mental health, substance abuse, or reproductive health treatment, so clinicians who treat children and adolescents should be familiar with local laws regarding the age of majority. Even if a guardian must provide consent, minor children should also be educated about the medications they are being prescribed, in a manner that is appropriate to their cognitive level. According to the "rule of sevens" guideline (Hoop et al. 2008), cognitively normal children younger than about 7 years are presumed not to have the capacity to give informed consent; those between about ages 7 and 14 years are capable of some level of decision making; and adolescents 14 years and older have many of the abilities required to make an informed treatment decision.

In the case of pharmacotherapy for patients who are decisionally compromised due to cognitive impairment, the judicial appointment of a legal guardian to make health care decisions is often required. During the informed consent process, the guardian must take into consideration any previously expressed wishes of the patient regarding treatments. For example, a spouse who is the guardian of a patient with dementia should endeavor to make medical decisions that align with the previously expressed wishes of the ill spouse—a standard known as *substituted judgment*. When a guardian has no idea of a patient's wishes, as is the case with patients with severe developmental disorders who have never been able to formulate or express treatment preferences, the guardian may make treatment decisions based on what is believed to be in the best interest of the patient.

In some jurisdictions, patients with mental disorders whose ability to make decisions fluctuates during the course of illness may create an advanced directive for psychiatric care, to give health care providers guidance regarding treatment preferences should the patient become incapacitated at a later time. In the absence of such a document, legal interventions allow for treatment permission to be granted by a substitute decision maker (sometimes a judge or a medical professional not involved in the care of the patient). The decision maker may rely on substituted judgment if the wishes of the patient (expressed while the patient was decisional) are known, but often the decision maker must make a determination of what he or she believes to be in the best interest of the patient.

Involuntary treatment may be necessary for patients whose mental illness makes them a danger to themselves or others, and it has been ethically justified on the grounds of beneficence—to do good both for the patient and for any person who may be endangered by the patient's actions. Involuntary treatment represents a rare occurrence in contemporary medicine, in which the clinician's duty of beneficence is allowed to trump the duty to respect patient autonomy. The ethics of involuntary treatment has long been a matter of discussion (Bartlett 2003; Levenson 1986–1987; Rosenman 1998), with a few experts and advocates arguing that any such treatment should be impermissible as a violation of human rights (Szasz 1976) and a larger contingent seeing it as necessary and beneficial, if implemented with appropriate checks and balances. Especially in the extreme situations that lead to involuntary treatment, clinicians should endeavor to respond to patients therapeutically, compassionately, and respectfully (Roberts and Dyer 2004). Strategies for doing so are presented in Table 67–4.

Working With "Difficult" Patients

A wide range of clinical issues leads physicians to perceive patients as "difficult": they may have severe or treatment-resistant illness, or they may have a personality disorder or be self-destructive, needy, angry, help rejecting, nonadherent, narcissistic, rich, famous, or simply too much like the clinician in some crucial way (McCarty and Roberts 1996; Robbins et al. 1988). Treating such patients can be deeply challenging, because their maladaptive behaviors may push clinicians toward reactions that lack compassion or are even unethical (Gabbard 2000; Roberts et al. 2008b).

Consider, for example, the reactions of the prescribing physician treating a patient whose major depressive disorder has continued unabated for several months despite adequate trials of several antidepressant medications. The clinician's frustration at the situation may cause him or her to emotionally detach from the treatment relationship, blame the patient for the treatment failure, or become overzealous and suggest unnecessarily risky treatments. Another example is the clinician whose patient with schizophrenia does well while taking an antipsychotic medication but because of lack of insight is unable to adhere to the medication for any extended period. Repeated cycles of clinical improvement, stabilization, nonadherence, and then decompensation may exhaust the clinician's ability to work compassionately with the pa-

TABLE 67–4. Working therapeutically with patients receiving involuntary medication treatment

Understand treatment refusal as a possible expression of distress

Ascertain the reasons for refusal

Allow the patient to discuss his or her preferences and fears

Explain the reason for the intervention in simple language

Offer options for the disposition of treatment

Appropriately enlist the assistance of family and friends

Request support from nursing and support staff

Assess the patient's decisional capacity and, if necessary, have recourse to the courts

Attend to side effects—both long- and short-term, serious and bothersome

Work to preserve the therapeutic alliance

Consult with the patient's legal guardian, or utilize his or her advance directive where appropriate

Source. Reprinted from Roberts LW, Dyer AR: "Working Therapeutically in the Ethical Use of Power," in *Concise Guide to Ethics in Mental Health Care.* Washington, DC, American Psychiatric Publishing, 2004, p. 93. Used with permission.

tient. A third example is the patient who is perceived as medication seeking. Clinicians feel varying levels of comfort with and tolerance for working with patients who seek care because of a desire for benzodiazepines, psychostimulants, or cosmetic pharmacology via selective serotonin reuptake inhibitors as personality enhancers.

A three-step approach to working therapeutically with difficult patients has been described (McCarty and Roberts 1996). As a first step, the clinician analyzes the situation to understand precisely what makes it difficult. Next, the clinician adjusts his or her perspective to view the problematic behavior as a *clinical sign*, an observable indication or form of communication that is key to better understanding the patient and the treatment relationship. Finally, the clinician pauses and reflects before reacting to the patient's behavior. Consultation or supervision may also be invaluable in helping the clinician develop a therapeutic and respectful response.

This framework suggests that a useful response to the medication-seeking patient is to compassionately and nonjudgmentally explore with the patient the reasons for the request for the medication—rather than responding reflexively with an adversarial, withholding stance. This approach may allow the patient to discuss feelings and/or symptoms that had not previously been fully disclosed. This strategy should also strengthen the therapeutic alliance and help ensure that the patient remains in treatment even if the request for medication cannot be fulfilled. When talking with a medication-seeking patient about such a request, it is useful to maintain one's focus on the actual risks and benefits of the requested treatment for the patient, including a forthright discussion of the risks of addiction or abuse. It is also important to give genuine and careful consideration to the merits of the request, which may in fact be justified by the patient's symptoms. In rare cases, the psychiatrist may have evidence that the request for unnecessary prescriptions truly represents antisocial acting out by the patient. The clinician is of course obligated to demur in such situations.

A similar strategy can be employed when working with chronically nonadherent patients. The treating psychiatrist should work compassionately with the patient to learn why the patient has not adhered to the treatment plan. One possibility is lack of decisional capacity; another is an inadequate understanding of the benefits of taking the prescribed medication on a regular basis. Other issues that may underlie nonadherence include lack of insight into the illness, forgetting doses or forgetting to refill prescriptions, inability to pay for the medication, homelessness or other chaotic living situations that make routine medication use difficult or impossible, bothersome side effects such as weight gain and sedation, or personal/cultural/religious beliefs about mental illness and medications (Cooper et al. 2007). Once the underlying reasons for nonadherence are identified, the psychiatrist can work with the patient to develop a therapeutic strategy that is more congruent with the patient's needs and preferences. This may involve providing psychoeducation, prescribing a less costly medication, enrolling the patient in a financial assistance program, changing medications or doses to ameliorate side effects, prescribing injectable depot preparations, or enrolling the patient in case management services.

Ethical Use of High-Risk Pharmacotherapy

Prescribing psychopharmacological treatments with a high potential for adverse consequences requires keen attention to ethical issues and to the informed consent process. For example, consider the case of a formerly suicidal patient whose severe bipolar disorder responds only to divalproex sodium but who has just been diagnosed with a low-grade chronic infection with hepatitis C. Further treatment with divalproex carries with it an increased risk for severe liver damage in such a patient, while discontinuing the medication carries the risk of relapse and perhaps suicide. The clinician is faced with the possibility of causing serious harm with either action.

To handle this type of situation in a clinically and ethically appropriate manner, the clinician would be wise to do the following:

- Consider all clinical options.
- Look for ways to safeguard the patient (for example, through ordering laboratory tests more frequently, involving the family, or hospitalizing the patient).
- Consult with more experienced colleagues or obtain a second opinion.
- Engage the patient in a thorough discussion of the options and their risks.

Most likely, there will be a range of ethically appropriate responses, and patient preferences should guide the decision. If the patient is unable or unwilling to participate in the decision, it may be possible to bring family members or other loved ones into the process. Such situations are likely to provoke anxiety or other strong emotional responses among clinicians; self-awareness may prevent clinicians from allowing those responses to subtly or overtly influence the patient's decision.

Ethical Use of Long-Acting Medications

Injectable depot antipsychotic medications (long-acting preparations) are an important treatment option for many patients, particularly those who have the most severe and persistent psychotic disorders and those for whom medication adherence presents a major challenge. The scientific literature suggests that these agents may offer some benefits over oral preparations, in terms of pharmacokinetics and bioavailability, convenience, cost, treatment adherence, and outcomes such as hospitalization (Barnes and Curson 1994; Gerlach 1995; Kane et al. 2003; Knapp et al. 2002; Marder et al. 2002; Swartz et al. 2001). The risks appear similar to those of oral preparations of the same agent, but there may be additional difficulty in managing side effects or adverse events should they occur (Adams et al. 2001; Glazer and Kane 1992).

From an ethical perspective, the use of depot medications has traditionally raised concerns about coercion and impaired voluntarism (Patel et al. 2005; Roberts and Geppert 2004). As mentioned above, voluntarism is the ability to make authentic decisions freely about one's life and body. For example, a patient who decides to discontinue an oral antipsychotic can rid his or her body of the drug within a relatively short period of time simply by not taking the next dose. A patient who is prescribed a depot preparation of the same medication does not have this level of control. If the patient wishes to discontinue the drug, the ability to act on this desire may be thwarted by the medication's extended half-life, and the patient may be forced to live with the drug's effects for days to weeks (Wiles et al. 1990). In effect, the drug's pharmacokinetics coerces the patient to remain on the medication for an extended period. The flip side of this is that the drug's pharmacokinetics may save patients from the suffering that could occur if doses are accidentally missed or a prescription refill is forgotten. Moreover, the patient may have improved decision-making abilities for longer periods of time and therefore have paradoxically greater ability to give informed consent (or refusal) for treatment while on depot treatments (Roberts and Geppert 2004). Nevertheless, the persistence of these drugs in the body raises deep concerns about their use in decisionally incapable patients, because the long-acting medication may persist in the patient's body long after the patient's decision-making capacity is restored (Eastwood and Pugh 1997; Roberts and Geppert 2004).

Concerns about coercion and impaired voluntarism must be balanced by psychiatrists' ethical duty of beneficence, which may be exemplified by prescribing depot preparations when they have demonstrated advantages over oral agents. The number of clinical situations in which these preparations are indicated may grow now that a long-acting form of an atypical antipsychotic has been introduced (Möller 2007). Bolstering this view are empirical data regarding patients' feelings about being prescribed depot preparations. Although these data are limited, a 2001 review of the literature found that most patients expressed positive attitudes toward depot forms of typical antipsychotics (Walburn et al. 2001). Much more empirical work in this area is needed to further clarify patients' attitudes, including opinions about depot preparations of atypical antipsychotics. Meanwhile, prescribing long-acting medications can be ethically justified on beneficent grounds, especially for decisionally capable patients with severe and persistent illness who have difficulty adhering to treatment (Roberts and Geppert 2004). In fact, the underuse of depot preparations among populations of patients who could benefit from them may be perceived as an ethical failing of the health care system to provide fair and equitable access to innovative forms of treatment (Heres et al. 2006; Roberts and Geppert 2004).

Ethics of Off-Label Prescribing and Clinical Innovation

Every day, many patients seek psychiatric care for severe symptoms for which there are few or no treatments approved by the U.S. Food and Drug Administration (FDA). The psychiatric treatment of special populations, especially children and adolescents, is profoundly hindered by the scarcity of clinical evidence regarding the efficacy and safety of psychotropics in these patients. In response, many psychiatrists prescribe medications *off label*—that is, for conditions or populations for which the FDA has not, or not yet, given approval. This practice has at times been characterized in the popular media and on the Internet as an unprofessional deviation from medical norms (Harris 2007), although it is common practice for nonpsychiatric drugs such as chemotherapeutic agents, and some indications (such as lithium for suicide prevention) are believed to lack FDA approval primarily because no pharmaceutical company has sought the indication (Daly 2007).

Off-label prescribing falls under the rubric of *clinical innovation* if its intention is to help individual patients, and it is considered *medical research* if it is done in a systematic attempt to gather generalizable data (U.S. Department of Health and Human Services 2001). Clinical innovation can be considered ethically justified if it occurs under specific circumstances, as shown in Figure 67–2 and described below:

1. There must be a substantial clinical need. For example, off-label prescribing is not justified if a patient presents with a previously untreated condition for which a safe, effective, and FDA-approved medication exists.
2. Standard treatment efforts must have been exhausted without success. All medications that have been approved for the condition and would be appropriate for the individual must have been given reasonable trials.
3. Scientific evidence must exist in support of the innovation providing a benefit. The amount of evidence required depends on the severity of the condition, the known risks and benefits of the treatment, and the patient's preferences. For example, relatively modest evidence of efficacy may be required to justify the use of an innovative agent that has excellent safety data if the patient prefers to try the new treatment and has severe treatment-resistant symptoms.
4. The anticipated likely risks of the intervention *and* the relatively rare but entirely possible risks must not be significantly greater than the risks associated with

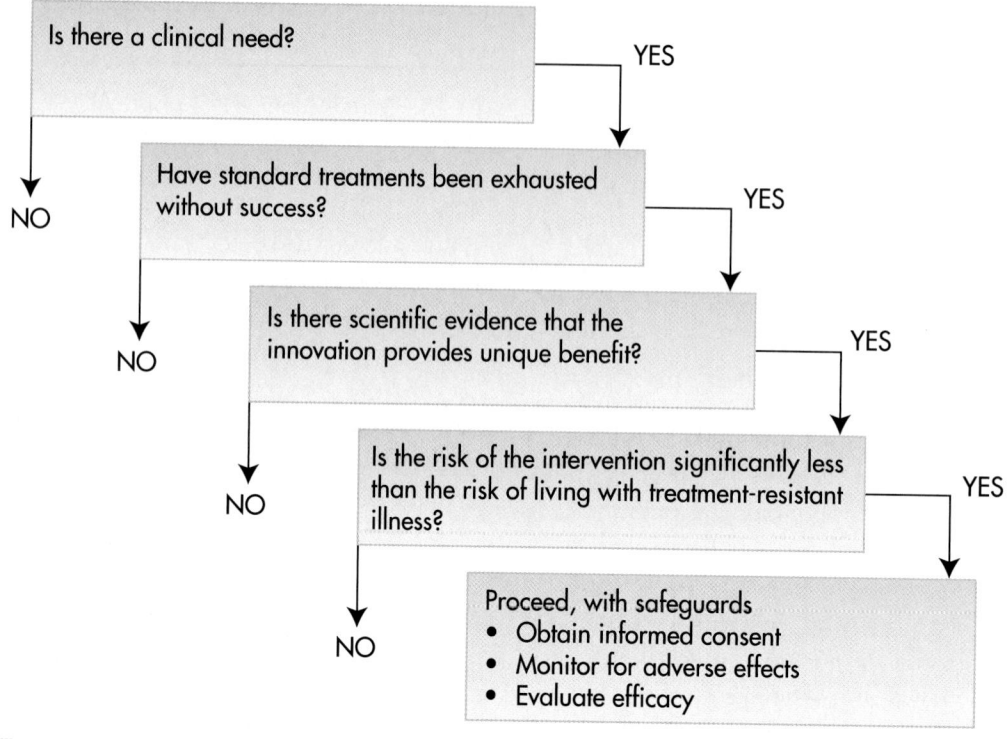

FIGURE 67–2.   Decision tree for ethical use of clinical innovation.

the underlying illness or condition. For example, the use of clozapine as an innovative treatment for transient mild anxiety would be inappropriate given the risks of significant side effects associated with this drug. In addition, appropriate safeguards to identify risks and side effects must be feasible and put in place.

When off-label prescribing or another clinical innovation is indicated by the reasons listed above, treatment may proceed with appropriate safeguards. The foremost safeguard is the process of obtaining informed consent, as described above (see "Informed Consent for Psychopharmacotherapy"). Information provision is an important part of this process, and the psychiatrist should make clear to the patient that the FDA has not approved this use of the medication. The psychiatrist should clarify the status of the science supporting the off-label use of the medication and should describe how widespread the off-label use is in psychiatric practice. Only by clearly informing the patient of the status of the medication can the psychiatrist ensure that the patient has the opportunity to give genuinely informed consent to the treatment. When treating decisionally incapable patients, clinicians should provide all information to the appropriate alternative or substitute decision makers. Other safeguards include clinical monitoring for adverse effects, evaluating the medi-

cation's efficacy, and reevaluating both the patient's need for the medication and the scientific evidence supporting its use on an ongoing basis.

Management of the Split-Treatment Relationship

The relationship of a prescribing psychiatrist to affiliated psychologists or other therapists who care for the same patients can present numerous issues that affect patients' care, including interpersonal conflicts, confidentiality concerns, splitting, and scope-of-practice issues (Lazarus 2001). Asking patients to provide a continuing *release of information* agreement that allows the prescriber and other therapists to talk about the case over time is an important step in ensuring that communication is adequate to keep the goals of psychotherapy and psychopharmacology aligned. It is also important that psychiatrists and therapists who treat patients with pharmacotherapy and psychotherapy in a split-therapy model do so in a manner that respects and supports the contribution of the other professional. Different mental health disciplines have different theoretical orientations and practices, which can lead to disagreements among professionals regarding the appropriate care of the patient. Frequent, open, and respectful communication is necessary to ensure that patient care is optimal (Roberts et al. 2008b).

Ethical Issues in Psychopharmacological Research

To be ethical, clinical research must meet several criteria, as summarized below (Emanuel et al. 2000; Roberts 1999, 2001a):

- The research question must be important.
- The study design and methodology must be adequate to answer the question and must minimize risks and maximize benefits.
- By training and experience, research personnel must be capable of performing the research in a scientific and ethical manner.
- Participants must be selected and recruited fairly and then be adequately informed about the study.
- Study data must be kept confidential.
- The entire process must be overseen by peer reviewers such as members of institutional review boards.
- Results must be reported in an appropriate manner.

All of these ethical considerations pertain to medication trials in psychiatry; perhaps the most controversy has surrounded issues related to informed consent (Roberts 2002b; Rosenstein and Miller 2003) and specific study design features such as the use of placebo control subjects and medication-free intervals (Carpenter et al. 1997; Roberts et al. 2003; Weijer and Appelbaum 1996).

Because psychiatric disorders may interfere with or disrupt a person's ability to receive and understand information, decision making, and sense of voluntarism, ethical concerns have long been raised about informed consent for psychopharmacological trials, especially for drugs to treat disorders associated with cognitive impairment or psychosis. However, efforts to protect psychiatric patients from exploitation in the research setting may, if applied too broadly, cause unintended harm and injustice by unfairly preventing entire diagnostic categories from receiving needed research attention (Roberts et al. 2008a; Rosenstein and Miller 2003). Empirical data on this issue have helped to establish that a broad-based approach may not be necessary or just. For example, survey data gathered by one of us (L.W.R.) suggest that schizophrenia patients are capable of making nuanced judgments about research participation (Roberts et al. 2000, 2003). Ethically rigorous methods for including decisionally impaired individuals in research include educational interventions to enhance their decision-making capacity (Carpenter et al. 2000; Dunn and Roberts 2005; Dunn et al. 2006; Moser et al. 2006), the use of alternative decision makers (Roberts et al. 2000), and the use of advance directives for research participation (Muthappan et al. 2005; Roberts and Dyer 2004).

Specific design elements in psychopharmacological research studies have also sparked controversy and debate (Carpenter et al. 1997, 2003; Charney et al. 2002; Frank et al. 2003; Kong and Whitaker 1998; Miller 2000; National Bioethics Advisory Commission 1998; Roberts 2002a; Roberts et al. 2001b; Rosenstein and Miller 2003). Among the most controversial procedures are the use of placebo control subjects and the use of medication-free intervals. In both cases, the investigator's ethical duty to provide meaningful data on research questions of high import is in tension with the duty to minimize risks to participants. Strategies for resolving this dilemma involve using the least risky protocol necessary to answer the research question and implementing safeguards to protect individual research participants (Emanuel et al. 2000; Roberts 1999; Roberts and Heinrich 2005). Appropriate safeguards might include close monitoring for symptom emergence, coupled with procedures to disenroll individuals for whom the risks of continued study participation become too great (Roberts and Heinrich 2005). An additional level of safeguarding is provided by having a data safety and monitoring board oversee the study (Carandang et al. 2007; National Institutes of Health 1998; Roberts 1999). Data safety and monitoring boards are independent groups of experts who are charged with monitoring study data and adverse events and are invested with the authority to halt or suspend studies if necessary to protect participants.

Management of Overlapping Roles and Conflicts of Interest in Psychopharmacology

Psychiatrists are called upon to fulfill multiple roles in contemporary society because of their combined expertise in mental illness, psychology, and medicine. Psychiatrists are intellectual resources not just for patients but also for students and trainees, agencies and institutions, and private industry. The result is that many psychiatrists, especially in academia, have ethical obligations related to multiple professional roles. The ethical demands of these overlapping roles may not fully align, however, and when this occurs, the physician may be placed in an ethical bind. For example, a physician-educator may feel caught between the pragmatic need to allow students to learn by practicing and the doctor's ethical duty to provide the best possible care to each patient. Similarly, the researcher with professional ties to both academia and industry may be caught between the obligation for truth telling inherent in the academic role and the requirement to protect trade secrets.

Managing such conflicts is an important task, the rules of which are still being written. The recent attention focused by media worldwide on the interaction of the pharmaceutical industry with physicians, and with psychiatrists in particular, makes this issue one of the most urgent unresolved ethical issues in our field (Harris 2007; Lewis et al. 2006). Conflicts of interest have traditionally been managed primarily through disclosure—that is, overlapping relationships are described explicitly so that others can make informed decisions about whether a role has been compromised. For example, many psychiatric journals have dealt with concerns about bias toward pharmaceuticals in research by creating policies requiring authors to disclose any relationships with pharmaceutical companies (Fava 2004; Perlis et al. 2005).

In the clinical sphere, there are no uniform standards for disclosing to patients that the clinician has a relationship with a pharmaceutical company, be it as a highly paid consultant, an occasional speaker, or a one-time attendee at a sponsored conference or dinner. One approach is to consider what information a patient might reasonably want to know about the psychiatrist's relationship with the pharmaceutical industry; if a patient could reasonably think that knowing about the details of that relationship would help him or her to understand why the psychiatrist is recommending a particular medication, the psychiatrist should make the disclosure. Following this logic, physician-scientists whose work is funded by the pharmaceutical industry should disclose this fact to their patients, particularly when recommending medications manufactured by that company.

Recently, methods of handling conflicts of interest that go beyond mere disclosure have begun to gain support (Fava 2007; Roberts and Dyer 2004; Roberts et al. 2008a, 2008b; Warner and Roberts 2004), such as the following:

1. *Role separation:* One strategy is deliberate role separation so that specific conflicts do not arise. This may require individuals to withdraw from certain activities. For example, clinician-researchers may design study protocols in which research participants receive clin-

ical care from nonresearch personnel rather than from investigators affiliated with the study.
2. *Role restrictions:* Similarly, certain public institutions, such as state medical colleges, may not allow employed physicians to engage in roles that entail paid involvement with industry.
3. *Oversight:* A third strategy is institutional oversight and management. Policies in some academic departments, for example, may place limits on the amount of money that a faculty member can earn through involvement with industry.

The increased attention given in recent years to the problems associated with physicians' conflicts of interest is likely to continue. Professional societies in particular will need to continue to strive to minimize the damage such problems can cause both to clinicians' relationships with their patients and to the reputation of the field of psychiatry. Psychiatrists should closely follow developments in this area, keeping in mind the obligation of the medical profession and its organizations to deal with the conflicts responsibly.

Conclusion

Psychopharmacology can be viewed as an intrinsically ethical activity, because it is designed to meet the moral imperative to relieve human suffering—and the suffering caused by mental disorders is indisputably widespread and devastating to individuals, families, and society. The clinical psychopharmacologist embodies the ethical principles of beneficence, nonmaleficence, and respect for persons whenever he or she thoroughly and empathically evaluates an individual with mental illness, carefully considers therapeutic alternatives, and engages the patient in a partnership for selecting and implementing a treatment.

As psychopharmacology has become increasingly relevant to psychiatric practice, it has also become important to identify and work through the unique ethical concerns that arise from this form of psychiatric treatment. One of our greatest needs is to establish procedures and safeguards appropriate to the current limited evidence base for psychopharmacological treatment. More research is needed, for example, to learn how well individuals with a variety of mental illnesses understand informed consent for treatment, particularly when it involves off-label prescribing, and how clinicians can best inform and safeguard patients when prescribing agents about which we have limited safety and efficacy data. Such research should provide evidence that helps us work ethically during this time of expanding growth in our understanding of the etiology and treatment of mental illness.

References

Adams CE, Fenton MK, Quraishi S, et al: Systematic meta-review of depot antipsychotic drugs for people with schizophrenia. Br J Psychiatry 179:290–299, 2001

American Medical Association Council on Ethical and Judicial Affairs: Code of Medical Ethics: Current Opinions With Annotations. Chicago, IL, American Medical Association, 2002

American Psychiatric Association: The Principles of Medical Ethics With Annotations Especially Applicable to Psychiatry, 2001 Edition. Washington, DC, American Psychiatric Association, 2001

Appelbaum PS, Grisso T: The MacArthur competence study I, II, III. Law Hum Behav 19:105–174, 1995

Arehart-Treichel J: Rapid rise in psychotropic use becomes global phenomenon. Psychiatr News 39(24):1–33, 2004

Barnes TR, Curson DA: Long-term depot antipsychotics: a risk-benefit assessment. Drug Saf 10:464–479, 1994

Bartlett P: The test of compulsion in mental health law: capacity, therapeutic benefit and dangerousness as possible criteria. Med Law Rev 11:326–352, 2003

Beaubrun G, Gray GG: A review of herbal medicines for psychiatric disorders. Psychiatr Serv 51:1130–1134, 2000

Bjorklund P: Can there be a "cosmetic" psychopharmacology? Prozac unplugged: the search for an ontologically distinct cosmetic psychopharmacology. Nurs Philos 6:131–143, 2005

Brown P, Pantelis C: Ethical aspects of drug treatment, in Psychiatric Ethics, 3rd Edition. Edited by Bloch S, Chodoff P, Green SA. New York, Oxford University Press, 1999, pp 245–274

Carandang C, Santor D, Gardner D, et al: Data safety monitoring boards and other study methodologies that address subject safety in "high-risk" therapeutic trials in youths. J Am Acad Child Adolesc Psychiatry 46:489–490, 2007

Carlat D: Diagnosis: conflict of interest. The New York Times, June 13, 2007, p A23

Carpenter WT, Schooler NR, Kane JM: The rationale and ethics of medication-free research in schizophrenia. Arch Gen Psychiatry 54:401–407, 1997

Carpenter WT, Gold JM, Lahti AC, et al: Decisional capacity for informed consent in schizophrenia research. Arch Gen Psychiatry 57:533–538, 2000

Carpenter WT, Appelbaum PS, Levine RJ: The Declaration of Helsinki and clinical trials: a focus on placebo-controlled trials in schizophrenia. Am J Psychiatry 160:356–362, 2003

Charney DS, Nemeroff CB, Lewis L, et al: National Depressive and Manic-Depressive Association consensus statement on the use of placebo in clinical trials of mood disorders. Arch Gen Psychiatry 59:262–270, 2002

Cooper C, Bebbington P, King M, et al: Why people do not take their psychotropic drugs as prescribed: results of the 2000 National Psychiatric Morbidity Survey. Acta Psychiatr Scand 116:47–53, 2007

Daly R: APA urges change in FDA-monitored medication guides. Psychiatr News 42:1, 2007

Delay J, Deniker P: Le traitement des psychoses par une methode neurolytique derivee de l'hibernotherapie. Congres des Medecins Alienistes et Neurologistes de France 50:497–502, 1952

Drane J: Competency and giving informed consent. JAMA 252:925–927, 1984

Dunn LB, Roberts LW: Emerging findings in ethics of schizophrenia research. Curr Opin Psychiatry 18:111–119, 2005

Dunn LB, Candilis PJ, Roberts LW: Emerging empirical evidence on the ethics of schizophrenia research. Schizophr Bull 32:47–68, 2006

Dyer AR: Ethics and Psychiatry: Toward Professional Definition. Washington, DC, American Psychiatric Press, 1988,

Dyer AR, Bloch S: Informed consent and the psychiatric patient. J Med Ethics 13:12–16, 1987

Eastwood N, Pugh R: Long-term medication in depot clinics and patients' rights: an issue for assertive outreach. Psychiatr Bull R Coll Psychiatr 21:273–275, 1997

Elliott C: Better Than Well: American Medicine Meets the American Dream. New York, WW Norton, 2003

Emanuel EJ, Wendler D, Grady C: What makes clinical research ethical? JAMA 283:2701–2711, 2000

Epstein RS: The nature and function of therapeutic boundaries, in Keeping Boundaries: Maintaining Safety and Integrity in the Psychotherapeutic Process. Washington, DC, American Psychiatric Press, 1994a, pp 15–34

Epstein RS: Psychological characteristics of therapists who commit serious boundary violations, in Keeping Boundaries: Maintaining Safety and Integrity in the Psychotherapeutic Process. Washington, DC, American Psychiatric Press, 1994b, pp 239–254

Epstein RM, Alper BS, Quill TE: Communicating evidence for participatory decision making. JAMA 291:2359–2366, 2004

Faden RR, Beauchamp TL: Decision-making and informed consent: a study of the impact of disclosed information. Soc Indic Res 7:313–336, 1980

Faden RR, Beauchamp TL, King N: A History and Theory of Informed Consent. New York, Oxford University Press, 1986

Fava GA: Conflict of interest in psychopharmacology: can Dr. Jekyll still control Mr. Hyde? Psychother Psychosom 73:1–4, 2004

Fava GA: Financial conflicts of interest in psychiatry. World Psychiatry 6:19–24, 2007

Frank E, Novick DM, Kupfer DJ: Beyond the question of placebo controls: ethical issues in psychopharmacological drug studies. Psychopharmacology (Berl) 171:19–26, 2003

Frick DE: Nonsexual boundary violations in psychiatric treatment, in American Psychiatric Press Review of Psychiatry, Vol 13. Edited by Oldham JM, Riba MB. Washington, DC, American Psychiatric Press, 1994, pp 415–432

Gabbard GO: Boundary violations, in Psychiatric Ethics, 3rd Edition. Edited by Bloch S, Chodoff P, Green SA. New York, Oxford University Press, 1999, pp 141–160

Gabbard GO: Psychodynamic Psychiatry in Clinical Practice, 3rd Edition. Washington, DC, American Psychiatric Press, 2000, pp 134–143

Gazarian M, Kelly M, McPhee JR, et al: Off-label use of medicines: consensus recommendations for evaluating appropriateness. Med J Aust 185:544–548, 2006

Gerlach J: Depot neuroleptics in relapse prevention: advantages and disadvantages. Int Clin Psychopharmacol 9 (suppl 5):17–20, 1995

Ghaemi SN: Paradigms of psychiatry: eclecticism and its discontents. Curr Opin Psychiatry 19:619–624, 2006

Glazer WM, Kane JM: Depot neuroleptic therapy: an underutilized treatment option. J Clin Psychiatry 53:426–433, 1992

Gutheil TH, Gabbard GO: The concept of boundaries in clinical practice: theoretical and risk-management dimensions. Am J Psychiatry 150:188–196, 1993

Gutheil TH, Gabbard GO: Misuses and misunderstandings of boundary theory in clinical and regulatory settings. Am J Psychiatry 155:409–414, 1998

Guttentag OE: The role of the physician in today's society, in Ethical Issues in Medicine: The Role of the Physician in Today's Society. Edited by Torrey EF. Boston, MA, Little, Brown, 1968, pp 195–226

Halasz G: Hidden truths: the politics of brain, mind and soul in Australian psychiatry. Australas Psychiatry 12:3–10, 2004

Harris G: Psychiatrists top list in drug maker gifts. The New York Times, June 27, 2007, p A1

Harris G, Roberts J: After sanctions, doctors get drug company pay. The New York Times, June 3, 2007, p A1

Heres S, Hamann J, Kissling W, et al: Attitudes of psychiatrists toward antipsychotic depot medication. J Clin Psychiatry 67:1948–1953, 2006

Hill KP: Free lunch? Am J Psychiatry 163:569–570, 2006

Hoop JG, Smyth AC, Roberts LW: Ethical issues in psychiatric research on children and adolescents. Child Adolesc Psychiatr Clin N Am 17:127–148, 2008

Kane JM, Eerdekens M, Lindenmayer JP, et al: Long-acting injectable risperidone: efficacy and safety of the first long-acting atypical antipsychotic. Am J Psychiatry 160:1125–1132, 2003

Knapp M, Ilson S, David A: Depot antipsychotic preparations in schizophrenia: the state of the economic evidence. Int Clin Psychopharmacol 17:135–140, 2002

Kong D, Whitaker R: Doing harm: research on the mentally ill. The Boston Globe, November 15–18, 1998:A1

Kramer PD: Listening to Prozac. New York, Penguin Books, 1993

Kuhn R: The treatment of depressive states with G22355 (imipramine hydrochloride). Am J Psychiatry 115:459–464, 1958

Lazarus JA: Ethics in split treatment. Psychiatr Ann 31:611–614, 2001

Levenson JL: Psychiatric commitment and involuntary hospitalization: an ethical perspective. Psychiatr Q 58:106–112, 1986–1987

Levine M: Psychiatry and Ethics. New York, G Braziller, 1972

Lewis DA, Michels R, Pine DS, et al: Conflict of interest. Am J Psychiatry 163:571–573, 2006

Lurie P, Tran T, Wolfe SM, et al: Violations of exhibiting and FDA rules at an American Psychiatric Association annual meeting. J Public Health Policy 26:389–399, 2005

Marder SR, Davis JM, Erehefsky L, et al: Partial compliance: the need for long-acting atypical antipsychotics, in The Journal of Clinical Psychiatry Audiograph Series., Vol 5 Memphis, TN, Physicians Postgraduate Press, 2002

McCarty T, Roberts LW: The difficult patient, in Medicine: A Primary Care Approach. Edited by Rubin RH, Voss C, Derksen DJ, et al. Philadelphia, PA, WB Saunders, 1996, pp 395–399

McHenry L: On the origin of great ideas: science in the age of big pharma. Hastings Cent Rep 35:17–19, 2005

McHenry L: Ethical issues in psychopharmacology. J Med Ethics 32:405–410, 2006

Melander H, Ahlqvist-Rastad J, Meijer G, et al: Evidence b(i)ased medicine—selective reporting from studies sponsored by pharmaceutical industry: review of studies in new drug applications. BMJ 326:1171–1173, 2003

Miller FG: Placebo-controlled trials in psychiatric research: an ethical perspective. Biol Psychiatry 47:707–716, 2000

Milne D: Psychologists' disciplinary failure leads to new law in Ohio. Psychiatr News 37:18, 2002

Miskimen T, Marin H, Escobar J: Psychopharmacological research ethics: special issues affecting US ethnic minorities. Psychopharmacology (Berl.) 171:98–104, 2003

Möller HJ: Long-acting injectable risperidone for the treatment of schizophrenia: clinical perspectives. Drugs 67:1541–1566, 2007

Moncrieff J, Hopker S, Thomas P: Psychiatry and the pharmaceutical industry: who pays the piper? Psychiatr Bull R Coll Psychiatr 29:84–85, 2005

Morris GH, Neumark D, Haroun AM: Informed consent in psychopharmacology [guest editorial]. J Clin Psychopharmacol 25:403–406, 2005

Moser DJ, Reese RL, Hey CT, et al: Using a brief intervention to improve decisional capacity in schizophrenia research. Schizophr Bull 32:116–120, 2006

Muthappan P, Forster H, Wendler D: Research advance directives: protection or obstacle? Am J Psychiatry 162:2389–2391, 2005

National Bioethics Advisory Commission: Research Involving Persons With Mental Disorders That May Affect Decision-making Capacity. Rockville, MD, National Bioethics Advisory Commission, 1998

National Institutes of Health: NIH policy for data and safety monitoring, 1998. Available at: http://grants.nih.gov/grants/guide/notice-files/not98-084.html. Accessed September 14, 2007.

Orlowski JP, Wateska L: The effects of pharmaceutical firm enticements on physician prescribing patterns. Chest 102:270–273, 1992

Patel MX, DeZoysa N, Baker D, et al: Antipsychotic depot medication and attitudes of community psychiatric nurses. J Psychiatr Ment Health Nurs 12:237–244, 2005

Perlis RH, Perlis CS, Wu Y, et al: Industry sponsorship and financial conflict of interest in the reporting of clinical trials in psychiatry. Am J Psychiatry 162:1957–1960, 2005

Robbins JM, Beck PR, Mueller DP, et al: Therapists' perceptions of difficult psychiatric patients. J Nerv Ment Dis 176:490–497, 1988

Roberts LW: Ethical dimensions of psychiatric research: a constructive criterion-based approach to protocol preparation: the Research Protocol Ethics Assessment Tool (RePEAT). Biol Psychiatry 46:1106–1119, 1999

Roberts LW: Ethics and mental illness research. Psychiatr Clin North Am 25:525–545, 2002a

Roberts LW: Ethics in psychiatry: principles, skills, and evidence. Psychiatric Times 19:34–36, 2002b

Roberts LW: Informed consent and the capacity for voluntarism. Am J Psychiatry 159:705–712, 2002c

Roberts LW, Dyer A: Concise Guide to Ethics in Mental Health Care. Washington, DC, American Psychiatric Publishing, 2004

Roberts LW, Geppert CM: Ethical use of long-acting medications in the treatment of severe and persistent mental illnesses. Compr Psychiatry 45:161–167, 2004

Roberts LW, Heinrich T: Walking a tightrope: ethics and neuropsychiatric research. Psychiatric Times, October 2005:25–26

Roberts LW, Krystal J: A time of promise, a time of promises: ethical issues in advancing psychopharmacological research. Psychopharmacology (Berl) 171:1–5, 2003

Roberts LW, Roberts B: Psychiatric research ethics: an overview of evolving guidelines and current ethical dilemmas in the study of mental illness. Biol Psychiatry 46:1025–1038, 1999

Roberts LW, Hardee JT, Franchini G, et al: Medical students as patients: a pilot study of their health care needs, practices, and concerns. Acad Med 71:1225–1232, 1996

Roberts LW, Warner TD, Brody JL: Perspectives of patients with schizophrenia and psychiatrists regarding ethically important aspects of research participation. Am J Psychiatry 157:67–74, 2000

Roberts LW, Geppert CM, Brody JL: A framework for considering the ethical aspects of psychiatric research protocols. Compr Psychiatry 42:351–363, 2001a

Roberts LW, Lauriello J, Geppert CM, et al: Paradoxes and placebos in psychiatric research: an ethics perspective. Biol Psychiatry 49:887–893, 2001b

Roberts LW, Warner TD, Nguyen KP, et al: Schizophrenia patients' and psychiatrists' perspectives on ethical aspects of symptom re-emergence during psychopharmacological research participation. Psychopharmacology (Berl) 171:58–67, 2003

Roberts LW, Hoop JG, Dunn LB: Ethical aspects of psychiatry, in The American Psychiatric Publishing Textbook of Psychiatry, 5th Edition. Edited by Hales RE, Yudofsky SC, Gabbard GO. Washington, DC, American Psychiatric Publishing, 2008a, pp 1767–1803

Roberts LW, Hoop JG, Dunn LB, et al: Ethics and professionalism: an overview for mental health clinicians, researchers, and learners, in Professionalism and Ethics: A Question-and-Answer Self-Study Guide for Mental Health Professionals. Edited by Roberts LW, Hoop JG, Anderson TT, et al. Washington, DC, American Psychiatric Publishing, 2008b, pp 27–111

Rosenman S: Psychiatrists and compulsion: a map of ethics. Aust N Z J Psychiatry 32:785–793, 1998

Rosenstein DL, Miller FG: Ethical considerations in psychopharmacological research involving decisionally impaired subjects. Psychopharmacology (Berl) 171:92–97, 2003

Schloendorff v Society of New York Hospital, 211 N.Y. 125, 105 N.E. 92, 1914

Shorter E: A History of Psychiatry. New York, Wiley, 1997

Sperry L, Prosen H: Contemporary ethical dilemmas in psychotherapy: cosmetic psychopharmacology and managed care. Am J Psychother 52:54–63, 1998

Swartz MS, Swanson JW, Wagner HR, et al: Effects of involuntary outpatient commitment and depot antipsychotics on treatment adherence in persons with severe mental illness. J Nerv Ment Dis 189:583–592, 2001

Szasz TS: The myth of mental illness. Am Psychol 15:113–118, 1960

Szasz TS: Involuntary psychiatry. Univ Cincinnati Law Rev 45:347–365, 1976

Tasman A, Riba MB, Silk KR: The Doctor–Patient Relationship in Pharmacotherapy: Improving Treatment Effectiveness. New York, Guilford, 2000

U.S. Department of Health and Human Services: Mental Health: Culture, Race, and Ethnicity—Supplement to Mental Health: Report of the Surgeon General. Rockville, MD, U.S. Department of Health and Human Services, Substance Abuse and Mental Health Service Administration, Center for Mental Health Services, 2001

Walburn J, Gray R, Gournay K, et al: Systematic review of patient and nurse attitudes to depot antipsychotic medication. Br J Psychiatry 179:300–307, 2001

Warner TD, Roberts LW: Scientific integrity, fidelity and conflicts of interest in research. Curr Opin Psychiatry 17:381–385, 2004

Wazana A: Physicians and the pharmaceutical industry: is a gift ever just a gift? JAMA 283:373–380, 2000

Weijer C, Appelbaum P: Placebo controls are not good science. IRB 18(5):8–10, 1996

Werneke U: Complementary medicines in psychiatry: review of effectiveness and safety. Br J Psychiatry 188:109–121, 2006

Wiles DH, McCreadie RG, Whitehead A: Pharmacokinetics of haloperidol and fluphenazine decanoates in chronic schizophrenia. Psychopharmacology (Berl) 101:274–281, 1990

Wise TN: Commentary, in Professionalism and Ethics: A Question-and-Answer Self-Study Guide for Mental Health Professionals. Edited by Roberts LW, Hoop JG, Anderson TT, et al. Washington, DC, American Psychiatric Publishing, 2007, pp 19–23

Wong IC, Murray ML, Camilleri-Novak D, et al: Increased prescribing trends of paediatric psychotropic medications. Arch Dis Child 89:1131–1132, 2004

Index

*Page numbers printed in **boldface** type refer to tables or figures.*

Autoimmune disorders, 201
  depression and, 210
  thyroiditis, in depression, 910
  tumor necrosis factor-α antagonists
    for, 210–211, 214
Automatic thoughts, 1099
Autonomic nervous system (ANS)
  in alcohol or sedative-hypnotic
    withdrawal, 1303
  in childhood mental disorders, 1070
  in depression, 204, 213
  immune system and, 206–207
  in Lewy body dementia, 585
  in neuroleptic malignant syndrome,
    547, 1150, 1304, 1423
Autonomy, 1479, **1481**, 1482, **1483**
Autoreceptors, 5–6
Autosomes, 60, 85, 87
Aventyl. *See* Nortriptyline
Avoidant personality disorder,
  1279–1280
  metarepresentational abnormalities
    in, 1048
  pharmacotherapy for, 1280
  relationship with social anxiety
    disorder, 1269, 1280
Avolition, in schizophrenia, 1137
AVP (arginine vasopressin).
  See Vasopressin
Awareness, disturbances of, 1049–1050
Azapirones, 488–489, 1182
  buspirone, 491–493, 1181, 1182
  gepirone, 496

B cells, 202–203, **203**
  corticotropin-releasing hormone
    effects on, 208
  in depression, 204
BACE (beta-site APP cleaving enzyme),
  996
Back pain, 1442, 1443, 1461–1463
  burden of, 1461
  causes of, 1461
  evaluation and management of,
    1462, **1462**
  pharmacotherapy for, 1462–1463
    duloxetine, 458
    tricyclic antidepressants, 275
  sertraline-induced, 315
  surgical treatment of, 1462
Baclofen, 1451
Bacteriophages, 67
BAD (Bcl-x/Bcl-2–associated death
  promoter), 47, **48**, 49

"Bad trips," 1225
Balanced translocations, 85, 90
Barbital, 831
Barbitone, 832
Barbiturates, 465, 477, 831–834
  contraindications to, 833
  dependence on, 833
  drug interactions with, 833–834,
    1415
    paroxetine, 344
    tricyclic antidepressants, 281
  effects on sleep stages, **828**, 833
  for electroconvulsive therapy, 877
  history and discovery of, 831
  indications for, 833
    catatonia, 1297
    insomnia, 833, 1258
  intravenous, 833
  mechanism of action of, 831–832
  overdose of, 833
  pharmacokinetics and disposition of,
    832
  pharmacological profile of,
    831–832
    control of chloride ion channels,
      832
    GABA$_A$ receptor affinity, 29,
      823, 831–832, 838
  side effects and toxicology of, 833
  structure–activity relations for, 831,
    832
  suicide and, 833
  tolerance to effects of, 832, 833
  withdrawal from, 833
Barbituric acid, 831, **832**
Bariatric surgery, 1148
Barnes Akathisia Rating Scale (BAS),
  622, 672
Basal ganglia
  GABAergic neurons in, 123, **123**
  in mood disorders, **921**, 921–922
  nigrostriatal projection to, 124, **124**
  in obsessive-compulsive disorder,
    1075
  in schizophrenia, 948
Basal (core) promoters, 60
BCAA-T (branched-chain amino acid
  aminotransferase), gabapentin
  effects on, 767
BChE (butyrylcholinesterase), 811, 990
Bcl-2, 39, 47, **48**, 49
  lithium effects on, 720
  valproate effects on, 720

Bcl-x/Bcl-2–associated death promoter
  (BAD), 47, **48**, 49
BDI (Beck Depression Inventory), 310,
  927, **1092**, 1093
BDNF. *See* Brain-derived neurotrophic
  factor
Beck, Aaron, 1099
Beck Depression Inventory (BDI), 310,
  927, **1092**, 1093
BED. *See* Binge-eating disorder
BEHAVE-AD (Behavioral Pathology in
  Alzheimer's Disease Rating Scale),
  1425, 1428
Behavior. *See also* Eating/feeding
    behavior; Self-injurious behavior;
    Violent behavior
  in autism, 633, 655
  cytokine-induced sickness behavior,
    210–211, 924
  drug-seeking, 1007, 1008, 1010, 1012
    relapse to, 1014–1020
  management of behavioral
    disturbances in dementia,
    1201–1208, 1424–1431
  neurobiology of disruptive behavior
    disorders in children,
    1061–1076
  in schizophrenia, 946
Behavior therapy. *See also* Cognitive-
    behavioral therapy
  in attention-deficit/hyperactivity
    disorder, 1310
  in borderline personality disorder,
    587
  for insomnia, 837
  in obsessive-compulsive disorder,
    356, 1173
Behavioral activation therapy, for
  depression, 1099, 1100
Behavioral genetics, 1065, 1268
Behavioral Pathology in Alzheimer's
  Disease Rating Scale (BEHAVE-
  AD), 1425, 1428
Benadryl. *See* Diphenhydramine
Beneficence, 1479, **1481**, 1482, **1483**
Benperidol, **534**
Benzamides, **534**, 538.
  See also Antipsychotics
Benzhexol hydrochloride, 673.
  See also Trihexyphenidyl
Benzodiazepine agonists, 826, **827**
Benzodiazepine antagonists, 826, **827**
Benzodiazepine inverse agonists, 826,
  827

passage across blood–brain barrier, 504

regulation of release of, 491, 971, 1089

in specific disorders
  anxiety and fear, 971
  bipolar disorder, 908, **909**
  childhood anxiety disorders, 163
  depression, 155, 156, 162–163, 204, 212, 504, 511, 904, 905, 906, 907, **907**, 1089
    with psychotic features, 908
  panic disorder, 163, 969, 971
  posttraumatic stress disorder, 163–165, 971
  schizoaffective disorder, 908
  schizophrenia, 908
  social anxiety disorder, 163
in stress response, 503, 971
"Cosmetic pharmacology," 1478
Cost containment, 1287
Cost Utility of the Latest Antipsychotic Drugs in Schizophrenia Study (CUtLASS), 535, 538, **542,** 542–543, 553, 558–559, 1142, 1429
Cough, drug-induced
  haloperidol, **635**
  paroxetine, 1312
  risperidone, **635**
Cough syrups, interaction with monoamine oxidase inhibitors, 394
Counterclockwise hysteresis curves, 190, **191**
Countertransference, 1482
COX (cyclo-oxygenase) inhibitors
  Alzheimer's disease and, 992, 999
  for pain, 1444
CP-88059. See Ziprasidone
CPAP. See Continuous positive airway pressure
CpG islands, 62
CPK (creatine phosphokinase), 847, 1304
m-CPP (m-chlorophenylpiperazine), 296, 404, 407–408, 411, 1036
CPRS (Conners Parent Rating Scale), 1332
CR (conditioned response), 966
Crack cocaine, 1218.
  See also Cocaine abuse
Creatine phosphokinase (CPK), 847, 1304
Creativity, lithium effects on, 706

CREB (cAMP response element–binding protein), **39,** 42, 47, **48,** 63, **64,** 353, 368, 381
  antidepressant effects on, 517–518, 519, 918
CREB-binding protein (CBP), 63
CREs (cAMP response elements), 63
CRF (corticotropin-releasing factor). See Corticotropin-releasing hormone
CRH. See Corticotropin-releasing hormone
Cross-National Collaborative Panic Study, 1174
CS (conditioned stimulus), 966, 967
CSAQT (Center for Substance Abuse Treatment), 1221
CSF2RA gene, in schizophrenia, 97
CSFQ (Changes in Sexual Functioning Questionnaire), 379
Cue-induced drug craving, 1014, 1015–1018, **1016**
Current clamp, 143
Cushing's disease, 167
  depression in, 504, 905
  dexamethasone suppression test for, 907
  mifepristone for, 908
CUSPAD (Columbia University Scale for Psychopathology in Alzheimer's Disease), 1425
Cutaneous effects of drugs
  antipsychotics, **549,** 551
  barbiturates, 833
  benzodiazepines, 830
  bupropion, 421, 423
  carbamazepine, 746, 747, 1117, 1316
  lamotrigine, 787–789, **789,** 1121–1122, 1124
  modafinil and, 851
  oxcarbazepine, 748, 1316
  topiramate, 802
  tricyclic antidepressants, 279
CUtLASS (Cost Utility of the Latest Antipsychotic Drugs in Schizophrenia Study), 535, 538, **542,** 542–543, 553, 558–559, 1142, 1429
Cyamemazine, **534**
CY-BOCS (Children's Yale-Brown Obsessive Compulsive Scale), 311, 356, 374, 1319–1321

Cyclic adenosine monophosphate (cAMP) signaling cascade, 5, 12, **12,** 13, 14, **16, 19, 22,** 30, 34, **41,** 266, 326, 517–518
  carbamazepine effects on, 740
  G protein mediation of, 41–42
  phosphodiesterase inactivation of, 518
Cyclic guanosine monophosphate (cGMP), 37
  carbamazepine effects on, 740
Cyclobenzaprine
  for chronic fatigue syndrome, 1250
  for fibromyalgia, 1250, 1451, 1459, 1460
  interaction with monoamine oxidase inhibitors, **395**
Cyclo-oxygenase (COX) inhibitors
  Alzheimer's disease and, 992, 999
  for pain, 1444
Cycloplegia, drug-induced
  antipsychotics, 551
  trihexyphenidyl, 673
D-Cycloserine (DCS)
  in anxiety disorders, 916, 967
    social anxiety disorder, 1179
    specific phobias, 1181
  in depression, 514, 916
  in schizophrenia, 26, 579, 1155
Cyclosporine–drug interactions
  buspirone, 494
  carbamazepine and oxcarbazepine, **751**
  nefazodone, 410
Cymbalta. See Duloxetine
Cyproheptadine, 911
  for alcohol-related insomnia, 1252
  for drug-induced sexual dysfunction, 338, 393
  for myoclonic jerks, 393
  for posttraumatic stress disorder, 1188
  for serotonin syndrome, 1305
Cytidine 5'-diphosphocholine (CDP-choline), for vascular dementia, 815
Cytochrome P450 (CYP) enzymes, 184–185
  age-related changes in, 269
  amphetamines and, 846, 848
  antidepressants and, 196, **197**
    bupropion, 281, 417, 423–424
    cyclic antidepressants, 263, 268–269, 280–281

Duloxetine, drug interactions with
  (*continued*)
    diphenhydramine, 461
    monoamine oxidase inhibitors,
      461
    tricyclic antidepressants, 280
  efficacy of
    vs. escitalopram, 371, 456, **457**
    vs. fluoxetine, 456, **457**
    vs. paroxetine, 329, 456, **457**
    vs. venlafaxine, **457**
  for elderly persons, 1421
  history and discovery of, 453
  indications for, 456–460
    depression, 453, 456–458, **457**
      in pediatric patients, 1314
    fibromyalgia, 453, 456, 458, 1450,
      1459–1461, **1460**
    generalized anxiety disorder, 335,
      453, 456, 458, 1184
    neuropathic pain, 297, 456, 458,
      1449–1450, 1456–1458,
      1457
    stress urinary incontinence, 460
  mechanism of action of, 455–456,
    1096
  metabolites of, 456
  overdose of, 461
  pharmacokinetics and disposition of,
    456
  pharmacological profile of, 453–455,
    455
  in pregnancy and lactation, **1383,**
    1386
  side effects and toxicology of, 460,
    1096
  sleep effects of, **1251**
  structure–activity relations for, 453,
    454
  switching to/from monoamine
    oxidase inhibitor, 461
Duty to warn, 1293
Dynorphins, 32, **33,** 975
Dysarthria, amantadine-induced, 678
Dysbindin gene, in schizophrenia, 951,
  955–956
Dyskinesia Identification System
  Condensed User Scale (DISCUS),
  672
Dyslipidemia, drug-induced
  antipsychotics, 550, **607,** 1147
    clozapine, 564–566, 1147
    olanzapine, 565, 590, **607,** 623,
      659, 1147

    quetiapine, **607,** 659, 1147
    risperidone, 565, 634
    ziprasidone, 658–659
  carbamazepine, 748
  oxcarbazepine, 749
  valproate, 728
Dyspepsia, drug-induced
  aripiprazole, 622
  bupropion, **422**
  haloperidol, **635**
  quetiapine, **606**
  risperidone, **606,** 634, **635,** 1118
  sertraline, 1319
  valproate, 727
Dysphoria, premenstrual.
  See Premenstrual dysphoric disorder
Dysthymic disorder, 1081, 1087–1088
  depression and, 866, 1087–1088
  diagnostic criteria for, 1087,
    1087
  in elderly persons, 1416
  gender and, 1082
  prevalence of, 905
  treatment of
    mirtazapine, 431
    sertraline for children and
      adolescents, 314
    tricyclic antidepressants, 274
Dystonic reactions, acute (ADRs), 670,
  1149–1150.
  See also Extrapyramidal side effects
  antipsychotic-induced, 535, 539,
    545–546, **548, 606,** 635, 670,
    1304
  clinical features of, 670
  etiology of, 671, 672
  laryngeal, 547, 670, 681
  prevalence of, 670–671
  prophylaxis for, 686
  risk factors for, 686, **686,** 1149
  sertraline-induced, 315
  tardive, 547, 670, 671
  timing of, 670, 686
  treatment of, 547, 682–683,
    1149–1150
    anticholinergics, 673–676, **674,**
      682–683
    botulinum toxin, 681
    clonazepam, 680
    emergency interventions, **1298,**
      1304

EAATs (excitatory amino acid
  transporters), 23, 514

Early life stress
  adult substance abuse and,
    1013–1014
  animal studies of, 156–157
  behavioral effects of, 1377
  effect on hypothalamic-pituitary-
    adrenal axis development, 1083
  hippocampal volume in adult
    survivors of, 156
  as risk factor for depression, 1083,
    1089
Eating Disorder Inventory Drive for
  Thinness, 1031
Eating disorders, 1027–1038,
  1231–1238.
  See also Anorexia nervosa; Binge-
    eating disorder; Bulimia nervosa
  appetite regulation in, 1027, 1032
  body image distortion in, 1027, 1028,
    1031
  clinical phenomenology of, 1027,
    1028
  course of, 1028
  depression and, 1027, 1231
  distinction between anorexia nervosa
    and bulimia nervosa, 1027
  etiology of, 1028
  family studies of, 1027
  genetics of, **83,** 1029–1030
    associations with other behavioral
      phenotypes, 1030
    candidate gene studies,
      1029–1030
    family and twin studies, 1029
  historical background of, 1231
  neurobiology of, 1030–1038
  neuroendocrinology of, 167–168,
    1033
  neuroimaging in, 1031, 1032, 1035,
    1036–1038
  neurotransmitters in, 1032–1038
    monoamine systems, 1035–1038
      dopamine, 1035
      serotonin, 295–296,
        1035–1038
    neuropeptides, 1032–1035
      cholecystokinin, 1033, 1034
      corticotropin-releasing
        hormone, 1033
      ghrelin, 1035
      leptin, 1034–1035
      neuropeptide Y, 1033–1034
      opioid peptides, 1033
      peptide YY, 1033–1034

Statins
Alzheimer's disease risk and, 992, 993
for vascular dementia, 815
Statistical analysis and power, 254–256
Statistical significance, 246, 247
STATs (signal transducers and activators
of transcription), 29, 36, 207, 213
Status epilepticus, 863, 864
electroconvulsive therapy for, 869
Steady-state drug concentration, 182,
188, 188–189, **189**, 192.
See also Plasma drug concentration
drug interactions affecting, 195–196,
196
Stelazine. *See* Trifluoperazine
STEP-BD (Systematic Treatment
Enhancement Program for Bipolar
Disorder), 729
Stereochemistry, 192
Stereotypies, amphetamine-induced,
848
Steroid hormones, 36–37
Stevens-Johnson syndrome.
See also Rash
carbamazepine and, 746, 1117
lamotrigine and, 788, 1370
modafinil and, 852
Stimulants. *See* Psychostimulants
Stimulus control therapy, for insomnia,
837
Stool softeners, 277
Stress response
animal models of, 154–155
effects of early life stress, 156–157
learned helplessness, 154
cytokines in, 923
in depression, 155, **204**, 204–206,
503–512, 1089
inflammation and, 205, 923–924,
924
dopamine in, 155
growth hormone in, 170
hippocampal effects of, 519, 920,
921
hypothalamic-pituitary-adrenal axis
in, 125, 156–157, 161, 204,
503–504, 906, 923–924,
969–970
immune system and, 203–205, 206
new-generation antidepressants
targeting, 503–513, **505**
corticotropin-releasing hormone
antagonists, 504–510,
508–510, 970

glucocorticoid receptor
antagonists, 511–512
inhibitors of glucocorticoid
synthesis, 512–513
vasopressin receptor antagonists,
510–511, 970
in persons exposed to early trauma,
1083
in substance abuse relapses, 1014,
1016, 1018–1019
substance P in, 125
vasopressin in, 503–504
Stress urinary incontinence, duloxetine
for, 456, 460
Stresscopin, 504
Stresscopin-related peptide, 504
Stress–diathesis model of depression,
905, **906**
Stressful life events. *See also* Early life
stress; Traumatic events
adjustment disorder due to,
1294–1295
behavioral effects of perinatal stress,
1377
depression and, 1083, 1089
genetic risk factors and, 82, 84
insomnia due to, 836, 1246
substance abuse and, 1013–1014
Stroke
antipsychotic-associated risk in
elderly dementia patients, 585,
620, 634, 655–656, 1203–1204,
1302–1303, 1423
depression after, 378, 853
drug use in patients with
citalopram, 378
escitalopram, 378
monoamine oxidase inhibitors,
395, 396
psychostimulants, 853
STRs (short tandem repeats), 88
Structured association method, 94
Structured Interview Guide for the
Ham-D, 1092
STS. *See* Selegiline transdermal system
Stupor, idiopathic recurring, 826
Stuttering, sertraline-induced, 315
Subgenual cingulate, in mood disorders,
920, **920**
Substance Abuse and Mental Health
Services Administration
(SAMHSA), 1221
Substance K, **33**
Substance P, **33**, 125, 207

in anxiety and stress response, 125
brain distribution of, 125
carbamazepine effects on, 740
in depression, 125, 515
Substance use disorders, 1007–1022,
1213–1226.
See also specific substances of abuse
in adolescence, 1014
animal models of, 1010–1011, 1012,
1018–1019
anticholinergic abuse, 675
benzodiazepine abuse, 474–477, 480,
1217–1218
comorbidity with
anorexia nervosa, 1028
depression, nefazodone for, 409
impulsive aggression, neural
correlates of, 1020–1021
schizophrenia, 559, 1151–1153
definitions related to, 474, **475**, 1007
drug addiction, 474, 1007–1010
(*See also* Addiction)
gender differences in, 1009
racial/ethnic differences in,
1009–1010
stage model of, 1007, **1008**,
1008–1009
transition from drug use to,
1011–1012
drug dependence, 474, **475**, 1007
environmental factors and, **1008**,
1013–1014
genetics of, **1008**, 1012–1013
γ-hydroxybutyrate abuse, 834
insomnia and, **837**
neurobiology of, 1007–1022
neurodevelopmental factors and,
1014
neuroimaging in, 1011, 1014, 1015,
1019, 1022
personality and, 1013
polydrug abuse, 476
relapse of, 1007, 1014–1020
conditioned drug cues for, 1014,
1015–1018, **1016**
drug-primed reinstatement,
1014–1015, **1016**,
1019–1020
models of neurobiological
mechanisms of, 1014–1015,
1016
stress-related, 1014, **1016**,
1018–1019
socioeconomic costs of, 1007